A Complete NEXT-Centric Approach

FMGE SOLUTIONS

For **Foreign Medical Graduates** Appearing for *Indian Medical Registration*

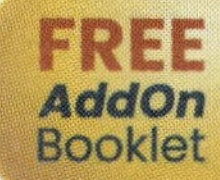

Includes **Important Key Points** *of all 19 subjects for* **Last-minute revision**

Eighth Edition

Deepak Marwah
Director
Medicine Buster Classes

Siraj Ahmad
Faculty (Pharmacology)
AllenNEXT

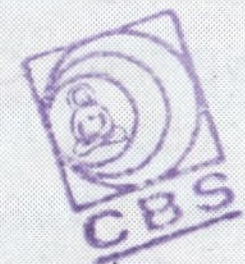

CBS Publishers and Distributors Pvt Ltd

• New Delhi • Bengaluru • Chennai • Kochi • Kolkata • Lucknow
• Mumbai • Hyderabad • Nagpur • Patna • Pune • Vijayawada

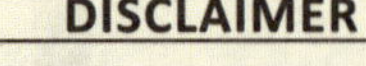

DISCLAIMER

This book contains questions based on topics asked in previous years' MCI Screening Exams. Often repeated topics and sub-topics have been included for students' benefit. We do not claim that these questions are exact or similar to the questions asked in MCI Exams. If any such similarity is found, it is purely coinicidental and by chance.

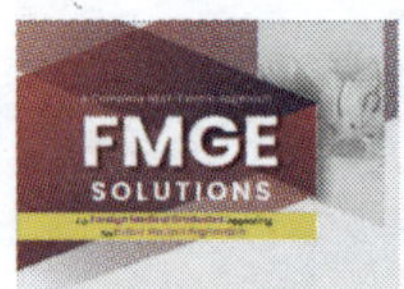

Set ISBN: 978-93-94525-45-0

Eight Edition: 2024

Seventh Edition: 2023

Published by **Satish Kumar Jain** and produced by **Varun Jain** for

CBS Publishers and Distributors Pvt Ltd

4819/XI Prahlad Street, 24 Ansari Road, Daryaganj, New Delhi 110 002, India.
Ph: +91-11-23289259, 23266861, 23266867 Website: www.cbspd.com Fax: 011-23243014
e-mail: delhi@cbspd.com; cbspubs@airtelmail.in.

Corporate Office: 204 FIE, Industrial Area, Patparganj, Delhi 110 092
Ph: +91-11-4934 4934 Fax: 4934 4935
e-mail: feedback@cbspd.com; bhupesharora@cbspd.com

Branches

- **Bengaluru:** Seema House 2975, 17th Cross, K.R. Road, Banasankari 2nd Stage, Bengaluru 560 070, Karnataka
  Ph: +91-80-26771678/79 Fax: +91-80-26771680 e-mail: bangalore@cbspd.com
- **Chennai:** 7, Subbaraya Street, Shenoy Nagar, Chennai-600 030, Tamil Nadu
  Ph: +91-44-26680620, 26681266 Fax: +91-44-42032115 e-mail: chennai@cbspd.com
- **Kochi:** 68/1534, 35, 36-Power House Road, Opp. KSEB, Cochin-682018, Kochi, Kerala
  Ph: +91-484-4059061-65 Fax: +91-484-4059065 e-mail: kochi@cbspd.com
- **Kolkata:** Hind Ceramics Compound, 1st floor, 147, Nilganj Road, Belghoria, Kolkata-700056, West Bengal
  Ph: +033-2563-3055/56 e-mail: kolkata@cbspd.com
- **Lucknow:** Basement, Khushnuma Complex, 7-Meerabai Marg (Behind Jawahar Bhawan), Lucknow-226001, Uttar Pradesh
  Ph: +0522-4000032 e-mail: tiwari.lucknow@cbspd.com
- **Mumbai:** PWD Shed, Gala No. 25/26, Ramchandra Bhatt Marg, Next to J.J. Hospital Gate No. 2, Opp. Union Bank of India, Noor Baug, Mumbai-400009, Maharashtra
  Ph: +91-22-66661880/89 Fax: +91-22-24902342 e-mail: mumbai@cbspd.com

Representatives

- **Hyderabad** +91-9885175004
- **Pune** +91-9623451994
- **Patna** +91-9334159340
- **Vijayawada** +91-9000660880

Printed at: Goyal Offset Works Pvt. Ltd.

Dedicated to

My Loving wife **Renuka**

Dr Deepak Marwah

My adorable daughter **Sarah S. Ahmad**
and
My Loving wife **Dr Sadia H. Ahmad**

Dr Siraj Ahmad

Preface to the Eighth Edition

Dear Students,

We are happy to announce the release of the much-awaited 8th edition of FMGE SOLUTIONS for all of you after going through all the mind-boggling recalls collection.

This book has been divided into four sections:

1. Recall-based questions of all 19 subjects up to July 2023
2. Clinical Case-Based Scenarios
3. Image-Based Questions
4. Key Points Covering Important Points of All the Subjects for Last Minute Revision.

The latest pattern of examination typically has turned out more toward clinical scenarios, but at the same time, many short MCQs are also asked as per the feedback we have received. We have adapted to the new pattern and introduced many new features to the book including the clinical-based scenarios. In order to maintain the balance, we have kept some short questions as well in the book. Since, it has been a trend that exact MCQs are barely repeated, the topics are repeated frequently. So, our readers are advised to focus on explanations given for each MCQs, be it short or long. The recent edition of book not only includes clinical vignettes but also additional image-based questions to enhance students' skills and increase the strike rate in the actual exam.

This examination has always been challenging for the students and they describe it as a barrier in their career. In order to overcome this barrier, you will have to be ready in the format it is anticipated. For this, your preparation level should be from the very basics and it should be continued with persistence, and remember, persistence is a great substitute for talent.

"A river cuts through the rock, NOT because of its power but because of its persistence."

As we always mention in our classes that ***Hard work beats talent, when talent doesn't work hard.*** This examination tests not only your talent, but also your dedication, your hard work, your capacity to sit for 12–14 hours per day. We have seen all of you studying the same matter with similar dedication, but only a handful of people taste the success of crossing the boundary line. Many a time, the most talented ones are also left behind. Ever wondered what is the thing that separates the winners from the rest of the population? The reasons can be many. But we could recite a few:

First and foremost is the **faith and belief that you can do it**. It is said, "***if you have acquired this belief that you can do it, half of the battle is already won.***" Now the question arises, is it just enough to believe that you can do it? The answer is NO. In addition to this belief, you also need to show the **consistency** and **will** to challenge what comes next. You will have to work accordingly.

Secondly, ***"the extra mile they ran"***. After your full day exhaustive classes, it is practically impossible to sit with the notes once again for the next few hours. But dear students, this is what that makes the difference between a topper and an average performer. A top ranked student shows this toughness, aggressiveness and will to run that extra mile on the same evening. It is this very attitude that brings him or her one step closer to victory every day. Therefore, it is very much advisable to all of you, to revive yourself after all the tiredness and do the revision of that day, the same evening itself. ***"This is your battle, push yourself for one more step, no one else is going to do it for you, the success lies right there."***

Thirdly, the **willingness to explore the new and to accept the challenge**. Remember "***if it doesn't challenge you, it won't change you***" and ***"old ways won't open new doors."***

As the level of examination has been in most unpredictable way, you will have to accept the challenge and be ready to learn the new things that comes along. Remember, the percentage of repeat questions in the examination is very less but **"the topics are often repeated"**. Hence, your analytical and reading skills will determine your score. In the book, the explanation section covers information over and above those asked in the questions in each topic. Therefore, we would suggest you to read all the explanations in detail with at least 3–4 revisions including the **"Extra Mile"** boxes which are add-ons and golden points for your examination.

In order to keep it up to the exam, this time we have segregated the book in separate segments including *Clinical Questions, Image-Based Questions and "Key Points"*, which will be your most important revision tool in last few days of revision.

Last but not least, it is the proper strategy and time management that make all the difference. Remember, you all get only 5–6 months for your preparation and in the same time, you have to finish the classes of all 19 subjects, revise them, give tests, which certainly is a lot of work in a very short span of time. Hence, you are advised to finish the first reading in first 3–4 months. In the 4th to 5th month your revisions should start. Whenever you start revision, remember to do 2 to 3 subjects per day (for example—One clinical/major subject + One paraclinical/Pre clinical + One Minor subject). Dry subjects, like Anatomy, Biochemistry, Microbiology should be in continuous touch. Give at least 90 minutes every day on your subjects alternatively and follow them religiously on priority basis.

"The key is NOT to prioritize what's on your schedule, but to schedule your priorities."

One more point which we would like to highlight is, keep yourself away from negative thoughts and negative people. It somehow degrades your confidence level from within. With positive mindset, you acquire the power to take tasks and be optimistic at all times.

"Your mind is a powerful thing, when you fill it with positive thoughts, your life will start to change."

Every possible effort has been made to bring this book in the best shape possible. However, in case of any typographical errors, queries or suggestions, please write to us on: **marwahmedicine@gmail.com/sirajahmad9@gmail.com**

With these words we would like to extend our best wishes to all our readers across the globe.

Best Wishes!

Deepak Marwah

Siraj Ahmad

Preface to the Previous Edition

Dear Students,

We convey our sincere regards and thanks to all our readers for the huge response to the previous edition of FMGE Solutions and making it as the best book for FMGE aspirants. In order to improvise further we are coming up with the 4th edition of this book.

The first edition of this book was launched in 2014 and since then it has been among the favourite books, not only for the FMGE students, but also among other NBE preparing students. The basic purpose and concept behind this book was to orient students with true concepts of exam pattern question and also to provide them genuine information and data from standard references all at one place. We continued to follow the same protocol in the further editions with more number of recent pattern questions, tabulated data and additional images.

The first edition was quite successful, and since then the students named it as "Bible for FMGEs" because of its easy tabulated contents and most recent hands-on information in the most simplified way. The huge belief of Readers and our continuous effort, dedication and persistency for this book, have made it as the most sought-after book among aspirants and the previous edition was labelled as the best-seller. The multi-coloured edition has given an edge to all the image pattern questions and the important mnemonics and tabulated data which are highlighted. At the end of the book, a separate section has been given entitled "Key Points" which includes the recent pattern question in one-liner forms, additional important tables and data all at one place for the last-minute revision.

The students are advised to go through all the explanations as there are a huge number of questions which have been asked on the topics being explained in the recent examinations. As we have mentioned earlier also that percentage of repeat question in this examination is very less, however the topics are often being repeated. Therefore, readers are advised to go through the book from cover to cover at least 3–4 times (as also recommended by toppers). The "extra mile/also know" boxes at the end of explanations have always been a saviour according to previous toppers. So for keeping yourself in continuous touch with the explanations, going through these important boxes is always advised.

Remember, there are hardly any obstacles that cannot be overcome by repeated practice; therefore, it is very important to practice the test and do multiple revisions. By continuously practicing the test, you are exposing yourself to the real-time exam experience, which will increase your mental training for exam and decrease the exam-day anxiety, so constant practice plays a crucial role in your performance.

Best Wishes!

Deepak Marwah

Siraj Ahmad

Acknowledgments

We would like to thank all our readers across the globe and the people who helped and motivated us in bringing and shaping this book.

- Our parents whose prayers and blessings have given us the strength to keep working.
- All our students in India and abroad for their continuous feedback, appraisal and criticism, which helped in shaping this book.
- Our teachers whose valuable lessons and teachings are always with us at each and every step.
- This book would be lacking its charisma without the contributions of subject matter specialists who have given their valuable time in rectifying the errors and providing constructive suggestions in shaping this book.
  - Microbiology: Dr Sadia Hassaan, Resident, Microbiology at JNMC, AMU. It was next to impossible to complete this book on time without her dedicated contributions. Dr Sonu Panwar, MD Microbiology for his continual guidance for shaping Microbiology as per the latest standards.
  - Preventive and Social Medicine: Dr Ashwini Ranjan MD, PSM from AIIMS, New Delhi
  - Pathology: Dr Preeti Sharma, MD Pathology from VMMC and Safdarjung Hospital
  - Biochemistry: Dr Amit Jain, MD Biochemistry, MAMC, New Delhi
  - Ophthalmology: Dr Sashwat Ray, MS Ophthalmology from MAMC, New Delhi
  - Psychiatry: Dr Ankur Jain, MD Psychiatry from PGI, Rohtak
  - Forensic Medicine: Dr Magendran, for his continuous support and doing proofreading of entire forensic medicine.
  - Orthopedics: Dr Yusuf Ali Tyagi his priceless suggestions and round the clock availability for all the ortho-related queries.
  - Dr Maddineni Srinivas (Dr MSD), Consultant Dermatologist, Hyderabad, for his wonderful suggestions and feedback to improvise the content.
  - Dr Sravan, MD (Pediatrics), for his impressive support in pediatrics section and for all his continuous support.
  - Dr Azam, Faculty of Anatomy, for his constant backing in completion of this book.
  - Dr Manoj Kumar Bhoomigari, MS (Anatomy) for his worthy support and advises.
  - Dr Abirami MD (Physiology) for her valuable suggestions and contribution in the completion of this book.
- Not to forget the constant feedback and support of our colleagues: Dr Ankit Goel, MD Psychiatry, Dr Naveen Porwal MD (Physiology), KGMU, Lucknow, Dr Sushant Soni, MD Pathology, Dr Sandeep, MS Surgery, Dr Arshad Ansari, MD, Dr Shanthan V, MD Medicine, Dr Saleem, MD (Preventive Medicine), for being a cool and supportive friend, Mohd Raza, for being the most effective and best friend one can ever pray for.
- We sincerely thank and appreciate the continuous support and words of wisdom from Mr David Pillai, Mr Kadwin Pillai and Dr Herlad Miller from King's International Medical Academy and Transworld Educare.
- All others who showed interest and provided feedback on the previous edition which helped us in improvising the latest edition of this book. To mention some: Dr Megrath Donold, Dr Omkar, Dr Angad Rai, Dr Mansoori, Dr R Chaudhary, Dr Ali, Dr Amresh, Dr Khalid Ziaullah. There are many names we couldn't recall but our heartfelt gratitude and blessings are due to every single person who contributed to completion of this journey.
- We thank our office staff members, Mr Naveen and Mr Mukesh for their true efforts in completion of this book.
- No words can describe the role of all Medical Graduate Students in India and abroad, with whom we have ever interacted through online or offline mode. We sincerely extend our thanks and appreciation to these students for helping us while giving this book its final shape.

We would like to thank **Mr Satish Kumar Jain** (Chairman) and **Mr Varun Jain** (Managing Director), M/s CBS Publishers and Distributors Pvt Ltd for providing us the platform in bringing out the book. We have no words to describe the role, efforts, inputs and initiatives undertaken by **Mr Bhupesh Aarora** [Sr Vice President – Publishing and Marketing (Health Sciences Division)] for helping and motivating us.

FMGE SOLUTIONS

We sincerely thank the entire CBS team for bringing this colorful edition with utmost care and amazing presentation. We would like to thank Ms Nitasha Arora (Publishing Head & Content Strategist – PGMEE & Nursing Division), Ms Daljeet Kaur (Assistant Publishing Manager), Dr Anju Dhir (Product Manager cum Commissioning Editor – Medical), Mr Shivendu Bhushan Pandey (Senior Manager and Team Leader), Mr Ashutosh Pathak (Senior Proofreader cum Team Coordinator) for putting their hard work and efforts to bring out this book on time and all the production team members for devoting laborious hours in designing and typesetting of the book.

From the Publisher's Desk

We request all the readers to provide us their valuable suggestions/errors (*if any*) at:

feedback@cbspd.com

so as to help us in further improvement of this book in the subsequent editions.

Contents

CONTENTS

ANATOMY

1

MOST RECENT QUESTIONS 2023

1. A patient underwent extraction of 3rd molar tooth and after this the patient was observed to have a loss of sensation from the anterior 2/3rd of the tongue and floor of the mouth. Which nerve is most likely to be damaged? ***(Most Recent Question July 2023)***

a. Hypoglossal nerve
b. Lingual nerve
c. Accessory nerve
d. Inferior alveolar nerve

2. A person had a road traffic accident and suffered from injury to the membranous urethra. Which will be the location of collection of urine due to this injury? ***(Most Recent Question July 2023)***

a. Superficial perineal pouch
b. Peritoneal cavity
c. Anterior abdominal wall
d. Ischiorectal fossa

3. A needle has to be inserted by an intern for thoracentesis. Which is the most preferred site for this clinical procedure? ***(Most Recent Question July 2023)***

a. Lower border of the upper rib
b. Upper border of the lower rib
c. Middle of the intercostal space
d. Lower border of the lower rib

4. What is the vertebral level for the red colored line shown in the image? ***(Most Recent Question July 2023)***

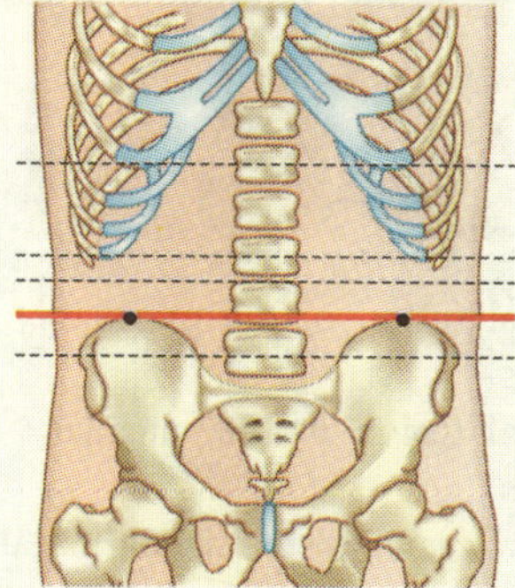

a. L2–L3
b. L3–L4
c. L4–L5
d. L5–S1

5. A maid in the house complained of pain and swelling at the knee. Which bursa can be involved in this condition? ***(Most Recent Question July 2023)***

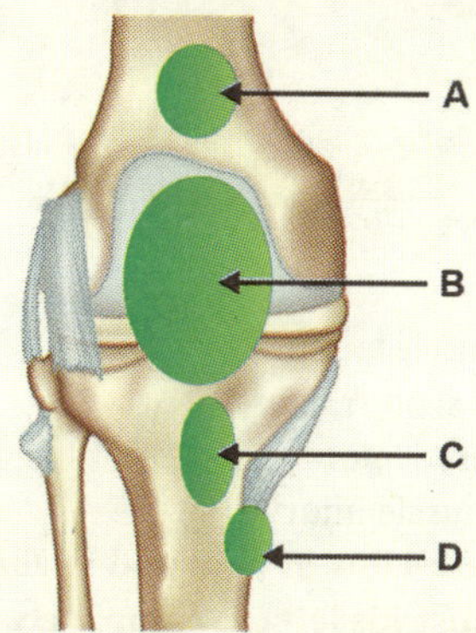

a. A
b. B
c. C
d. D

6. Which congenital deformity is shown in the image? ***(Most Recent Question July 2023)***

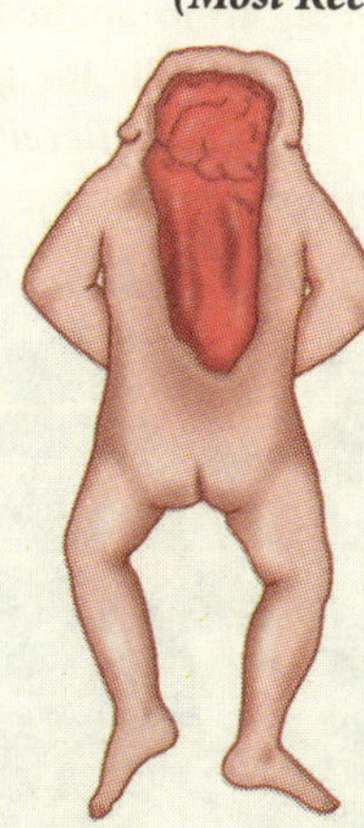

a. Anencephaly
b. Craniorachischisis
c. Meningomyelocele
d. Spina bifida occulta

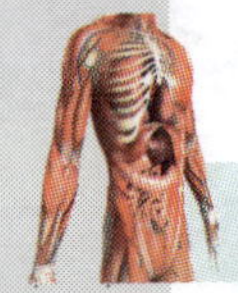

7. Post-delivery a female is complaining of pain in the anterolateral aspect of the thigh. Which nerve is most likely to be damaged? *(Most Recent Question July 2023)*

a. Femoral nerve
b. Lateral femoral cutaneous nerve
c. Obturator nerve
d. Tibial nerve

8. Which of the following conditions is shown in the image? *(Most Recent Question July 2023)*

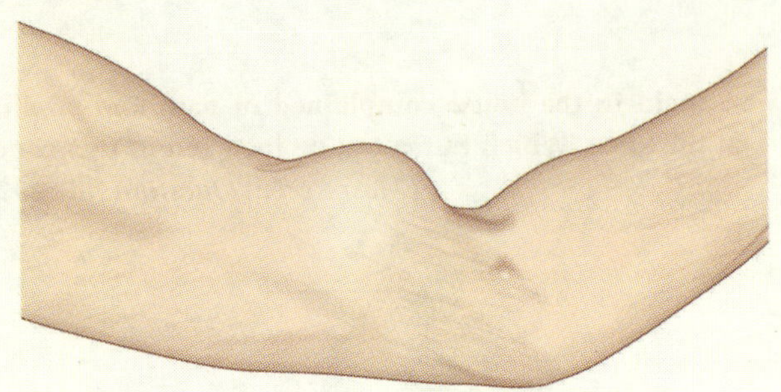

a. Biceps muscle rupture
b. Humerus shaft fracture
c. Radial nerve injury
d. Triceps muscle injury

9. A patient complains of pain and swelling below the ear. He cannot close his left eye completely and is having difficulty in eating food. Which nerve is most likely to be damaged? *(Most Recent Question July 2023)*

a. Greater auricular nerve
b. Auriculotemporal nerve
c. Facial nerve
d. Inferior alveolar nerve

10. A patient is suffering from aortic dissection. Injury to which marked structure in the image will cause hiccups? *(Most Recent Question July 2023)*

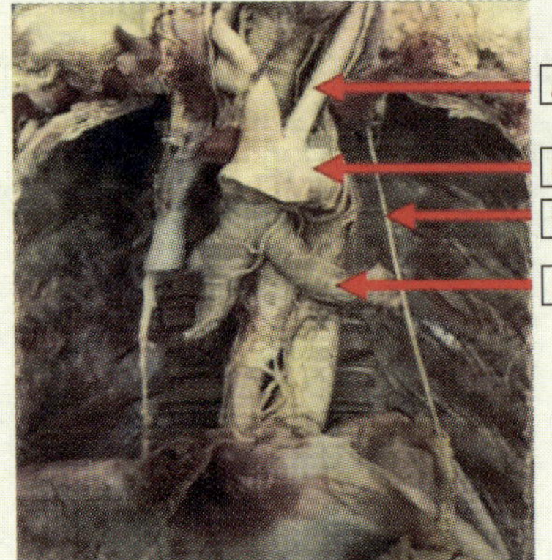

a. A
b. B
c. C
d. D

11. Which underlying cause is responsible for the congenital deformity shown in the image? *(Most Recent Question July 2023)*

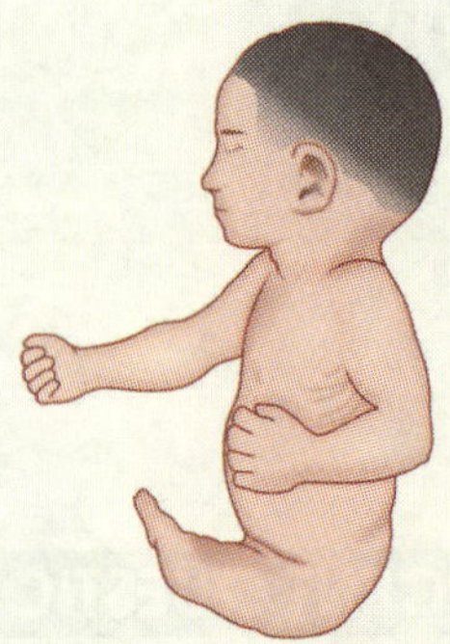

a. Morulation
b. Neurulation
c. Lateral rotation
d. Gastrulation

12. At which time does the talus bone gets ossified in the intrauterine life? *(Most Recent Question July 2023)*

a. 3 months
b. 6 months
c. 7 months
d. 9 months

13. Identify the arrow-marked structure in the given image. *(Most Recent Question Jan 2023)*

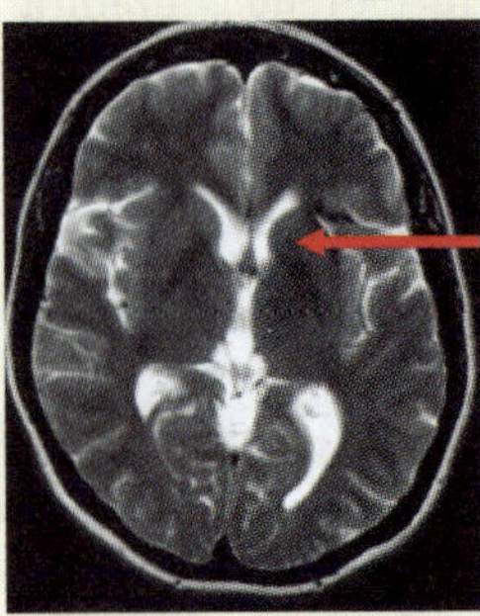

a. External capsule
b. Internal capsule
c. Claustrum
d. Globus pallidus

14. Which embryological basis is correct about the malformation shown in the image? *(Most Recent Question Jan 2023)*

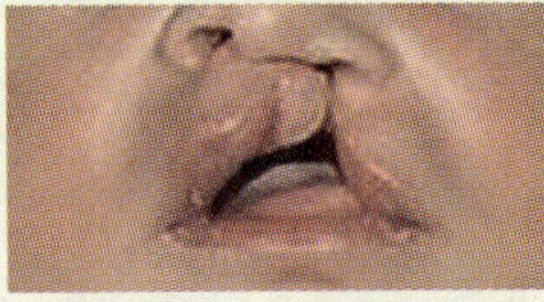

a. Abnormal fusion of the maxillary and medial nasal processes
b. Abnormal fusion of the maxillary and lateral nasal processes
c. Abnormal fusion of the medial nasal and lateral nasal processes
d. Abnormal fusion of the mandibular and medial nasal processes

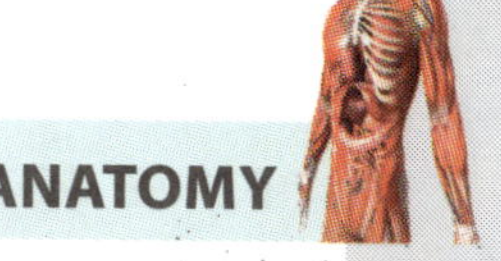

15. In the given image which landmark carries splenic vessels? ***(Most Recent Question Jan 2023)***

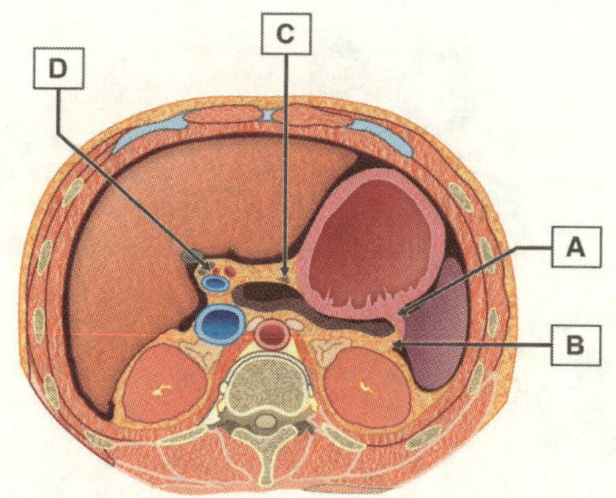

a. A
b. B
c. C
d. D

16. If the fracture occurs at an arrow marked location, then which nerve is most likely to be involved? ***(Most Recent Question Jan 2023)***

a. Ulnar nerve
b. Median nerve
c. Radial nerve
d. Musculocutaneous nerve

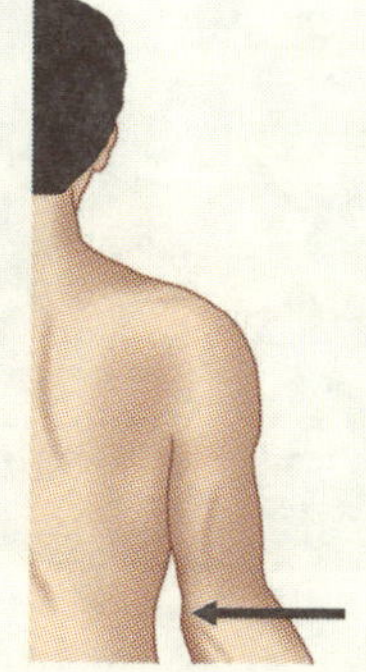

17. Which structure passes through arrow-marked area? ***(Most Recent Question Jan 2023)***

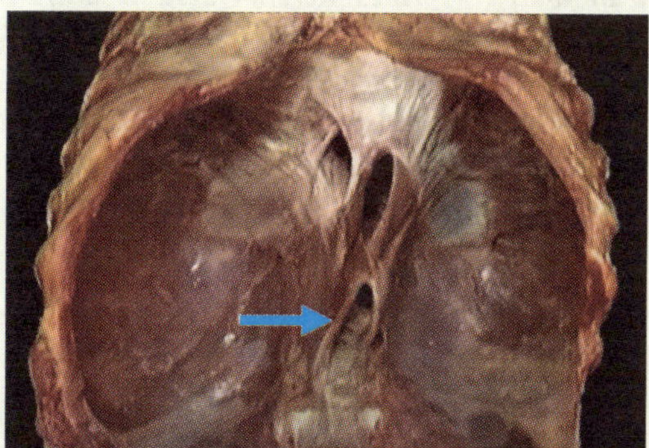

a. Inferior vena cava
b. Thoracic duct
c. Sympathetic trunk
d. Esophagus

18. If the paracentral lobule of the brain is involved, then which region of the body will be affected? ***(Most Recent Question Jan 2023)***

a. Brain and neck
b. Trunk and leg
c. Trunk and arm
d. Perineum and leg

19. During the examination, when a patient was asked to stand on the left foot, a drop of right hip/side was observed. Which muscles are paralyzed in this case? ***(Most Recent Question Jan 2023)***

a. Right gluteus medius and gluteus minimus
b. Left gluteus medius and gluteus minimus
c. Right gluteus maximus
d. Left gluteus maximus

20. At the level of elbow, fracture is observed as seen in the image. Due to this the forearm is pulseless. Which of the following structure is most likely injured? ***(Most Recent Question Jan 2023)***

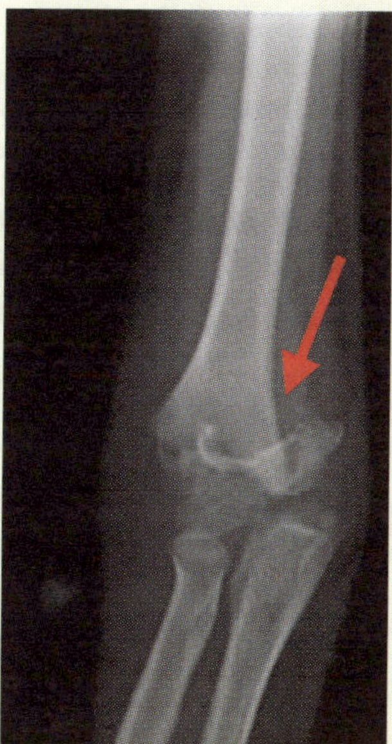

a. Brachial artery
b. Radial artery
c. Ulnar artery
d. Anterior interosseous artery

21. A cyst is observed at the anterior border of the sternocleidomastoid in a 25-year-old man. This cyst is due to persistence of which of the following cleft? ***(Most Recent Question Jan 2023)***

a. 1st
b. 2nd
c. 3rd
d. 4th

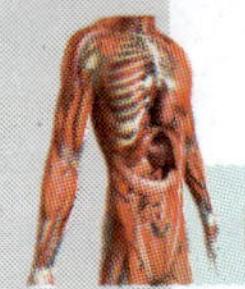

22. Identify the type of epithelium shown in the image. *(Most Recent Question Jan 2023)*

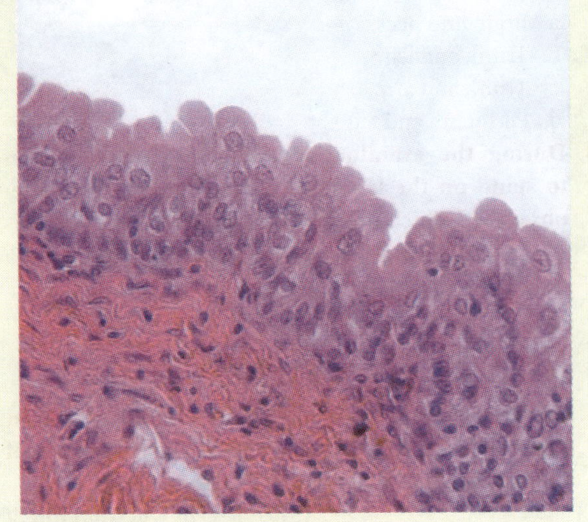

a. Transitional epithelium
b. Keratinized stratified squamous epithelium
c. Nonkeratinized stratified squamous epithelium
d. Ciliated pseudostratified columnar epithelium

EMBRYOLOGY, HISTOLOGY AND OSTEOLOGY

23. The section along the frontal plane (as shown in diagram) is called: *(Most Recent Question Dec 2021)*

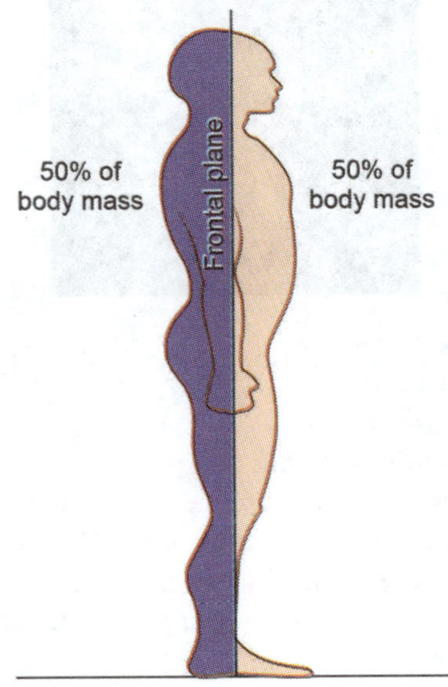

a. Sagittal
b. Coronal
c. Transverse
d. Median

24. Identify the arrow marked follicle: *(Most Recent Question Dec 2021)*

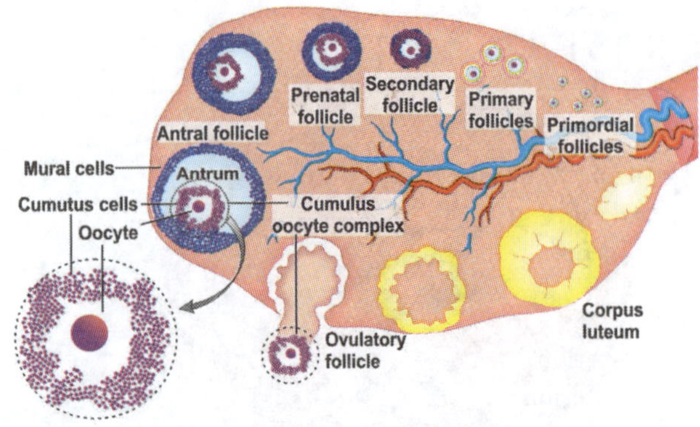

a. Primordial
b. Primary
c. Preantral
d. Antral

25. Fallopian tube epithelium is: *(Most Recent Question Dec 2021)*

a. Simple squamous
b. Ciliated cuboidal
c. Ciliated columnar
d. Pseudostratified columnar

26. The marked cell in the HPE image of thyroid follicles secrete which hormone? *(Most Recent Question Dec 2021)*

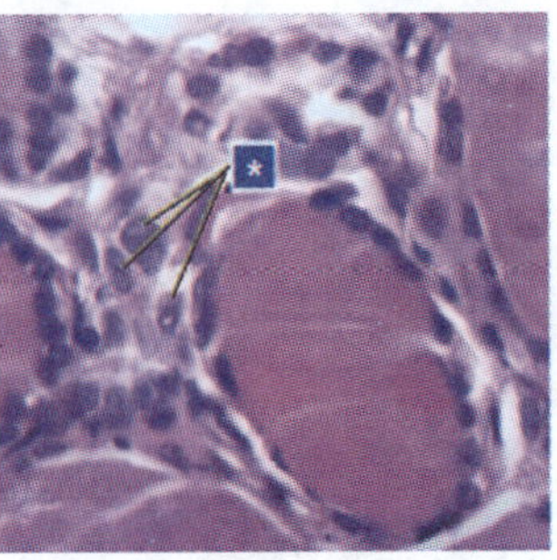

a. Thyroxine
b. Calcitonin
c. Adrenaline
d. Prolactin

27. What is the embryological basis of the following congenital anomaly? *(Most Recent Question June/Dec 2021)*

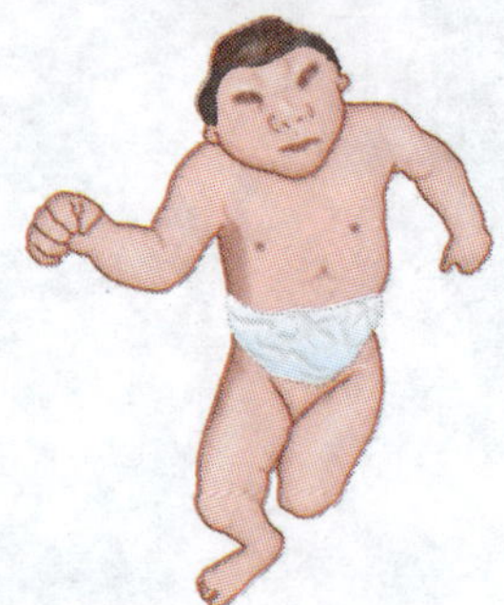

a. Nonclosure of anterior neuropore
b. Nonclosure of posterior neuropore
c. Nonclosure of entire neural tube
d. Nonclosure of skull bones

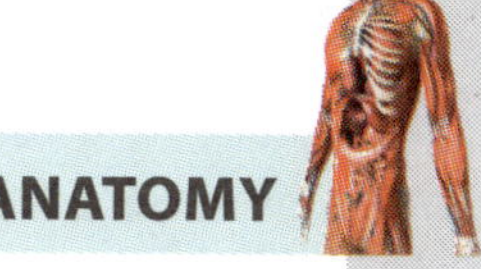

28. Identify the encircled structure:
(Most Recent Question Dec 2020)

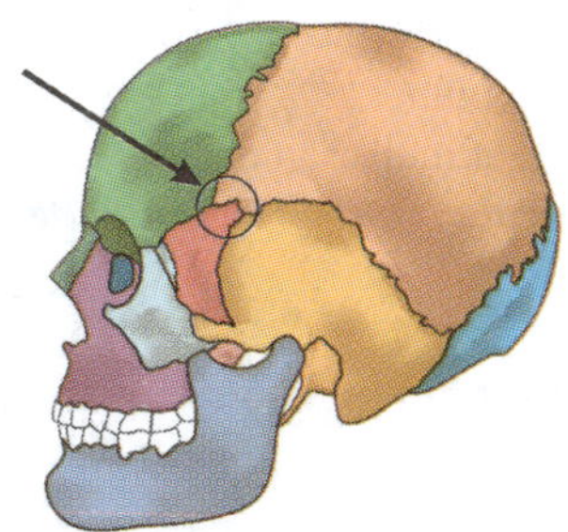

a. Pterion
b. Glabella
c. Asterion
d. Nasion

29. Ductus arteriosus develops from which pharyngeal arch artery? *(Most Recent Question Aug 2020)*
a. 3
b. 4
c. 5
d. 6

30. Structure developing in dorsal mesogastrium:
(Most Recent Question Aug 2020)
a. Lesser omentum
b. Falciform ligament
c. Spleen
d. Liver

31. Skin receptor responsible for detecting rapid vibration sense. *(Most Recent Question Aug 2020)*
a. Meissner corpuscle
b. Pacinian corpuscle
c. Merkel cell
d. Ruffini's corpuscle

32. Failure of closure of rostral neuropore at 25th day leads to: *(Most Recent Question 2019)*
a. Craniorachischisis
b. Spina bifida
c. Anencephaly
d. Hydranencephaly

33. Fetal midgut rotates in intrauterine life by:
(Recent Pattern Question 2018-19)
a. 270 degree clockwise
b. 360 degree clockwise
c. 270 degree anticlockwise
d. 360 degree anticlockwise

34. Rotation of mid gut loop occurs around:
(Recent Pattern Question 2018-19)
a. Superior mesenteric artery
b. Inferior mesenteric artery
c. Middle-colic artery
d. Superior rectal artery

35. Neural crest cell migration is due to:
(Recent Pattern Question 2018)
a. Heparin
b. Heparan sulfate
c. Hyaluronic acid
d. Dermal sulfate

36. Which of the following is the derivative of ultimo-branchial body? *(Recent Pattern Question 2018)*
a. Thyroid
b. Parafollicular 'C' cells
c. Capsule of thyroid
d. 2nd branchial pouch

37. Which of the following is the derivative of tumor from Rathke's pouch? *(Recent Pattern Question 2018)*
a. Meningioma
b. Craniopharyngioma
c. Ependymoma
d. Low grade glioma

38. Hardest bone of the body is:
(Recent Pattern Question 2017)
a. Head of humerus
b. Calcaneum
c. Tibial condyle
d. Osseus labyrinth

39. Which of the following structure is derived from umbilical artery? *(Recent Pattern Question 2017)*
a. Ligamentum arteriosum
b. Medial umbilical ligament
c. Ligamentum venosum
d. Ligamentum teres

40. Labia majora is homologous to ________ in a male.
(Recent Pattern Question 2017)
a. Glans penis
b. Scrotum
c. Corpus cavernosa
d. Shaft of penis

41. Morula cell stage has how many cells?
(Recent Pattern Question 2017)
a. 8
b. 16
c. 32
d. >64

42. Umbilical cord has: *(Recent Pattern Question 2017)*
a. One artery, two veins and umbilical artery going to fetus
b. One artery, two veins and umbilical artery going to placenta
c. Two arteries and one vein, umbilical artery supplying towards fetus
d. Two arteries and one vein, umbilical vein supplying towards fetus

43. In the Umbilical cord which of the following structure does not get obliterated during fetal life?
(Recent Pattern Question 2017)
a. Vitelline duct
b. Vitelline vessels
c. Allantois
d. Umbilical vessels

44. What is correct about embryogenesis?
(Recent Pattern Question 2017)
a. Branchial cleft: Mesoderm
b. Branchial arch: Ectoderm
c. Branchial pouch: Endoderm
d. All are correct

45. Superior vena cava is derived from:
(Recent Pattern Question 2017)
a. Aortic arch
b. Pharyngeal arch
c. Cardinal vein
d. Vitelline vein

46. Arch of aorta is derived from:
(Recent Pattern Question 2017)
a. 2nd aortic arch
b. 3rd aortic arch
c. 3rd pharyngeal arch
d. 4th pharyngeal arch

47. Common carotid artery is derived from:
(Recent Pattern Question 2017)
a. 2nd aortic arch
b. 3rd pharyngeal arch
c. 4th pharyngeal arch
d. 6th pharyngeal arch

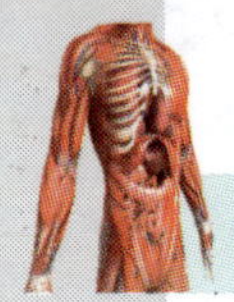

48. Stylohyoid ligament is derived from: ***(Recent Pattern Question 2017)***

a. 1st branchial arch
b. 2nd branchial arch
c. 1st branchial pouch
d. 2nd branchial pouch

49. Sphenomandibular ligament is derived from which branchial arch? ***(Recent Pattern Question 2017)***

a. 1
b. 2
c. 3
d. 4

50. Which of the following is a derivative of 2nd branchial arch? ***(Recent Pattern Question 2017)***

a. Stylohyoid ligament
b. Sphenomandibular ligament
c. Spine of sphenoid
d. Greater cornu of hyoid

51. Lesser cornu of hyoid bone is derived from which arch?

a. 1st mandibular arch
b. 2nd branchial arch
c. 3rd branchial arch
d. 4th branchial arch

52. Superior portion of hyoid bone is derived from which branchial arch?

a. I
b. II
c. III
d. IV

53. All of the following muscles are derived from 6th branchial arch; EXCEPT:

a. Lateral cricoarytenoid
b. Posterior cricoarytenoid
c. Interarytenoid
d. Cricothyroid

54. Which of the following does not develop from branchial pouch?

a. Superior parathyroid
b. Inferior parathyroid
c. Thymus
d. Thyroid

55. The auricle develops from:

a. 1st branchial cleft
b. 1st branchial arch
c. 1st, 2nd and 3rd branchial arch
d. 1st and 2nd branchial arch

56. Inferior parathyroid gland develops from: ***(Recent Pattern Question 2017)***

a. Branchial arch 3rd
b. Branchial arch 4th
c. Branchial pouch 3rd
d. Branchial pouch 4th

57. Tonsil is derived from: ***(Recent Pattern Question 2017)***

a. 1st pouch
b. 2nd pouch
c. 3rd pouch
d. 4th pouch

58. Which of the following is not derived from 1st pharyngeal pouch?

a. Middle ear
b. Eustachian tube
c. Tympanic membrane
d. Palatine tonsils

59. External auditory canal is formed from: ***(Recent Pattern Question 2017)***

a. Ventral part of 1st cleft
b. Dorsal part of 1st cleft
c. Ventral part of 2nd cleft
d. Dorsal part of 2nd cleft

60. Lower 1/3 of vagina is formed by: ***(Recent Pattern Question 2017)***

a. Mesonephric duct
b. Paramesonephric duct
c. Sinovaginal bulb
d. Mesoderm of mullerian duct

61. Hypoblast forms: ***(Recent Pattern Question 2017)***

a. Notochord
b. Apical ligament of atlas
c. Endoderm
d. Prochordal plate

62. First organ to attain functional maturity is: ***(Recent Pattern Question 2017)***

a. CVS
b. CNS
c. GIT
d. Lungs

63. Gastrulation occurs in which week of embryonic development? ***(Recent Pattern Question 2017)***

a. Week 1
b. Week 2
c. Week 3
d. Week 4

64. First germ layer to be formed is: ***(Recent Pattern Question 2017)***

a. Ectoderm
b. Endoderm
c. Mesoderm
d. All of them develop simultaneously

65. Notochord is formed by: ***(Recent Pattern Question 2017)***

a. Nucleus pulposus
b. Epiblast
c. Hypoblast
d. Myeloblast

66. Homeobox gene is responsible for: ***(Recent Pattern Question 2017)***

a. Segmental organization of embryo in craniocaudal direction
b. Proper organization along dorsal ventral axis
c. Stimulation for lengthening of limbs
d. All of the above

67. Chromaffin cells are derived from: ***(Recent Pattern Question 2017)***

a. Neural crest
b. Surface ectoderm
c. Neuroectoderm
d. Endoderm

68. Proximal umbilical artery forms: ***(Recent Pattern Question 2017)***

a. Superior vesical artery
b. Median umbilical fold
c. Lateral umbilical fold
d. Ligamentum teres

69. Ligamentum teres is a remnant of:

a. Ductus venosus
b. Ductus arteriosus
c. Hypogastric artery
d. Umbilical vein

70. Remnant of ductus venosus will be:

a. Ligamentum teres
b. Ligamentum venosum
c. Ligamentum arteriosum
d. Falciform ligament

71. Left horn of sinus venosus forms: ***(Recent Pattern Question 2017)***

a. Coronary sinus
b. Smooth part of right atrium
c. Superior vena cava
d. Inferior vena cava

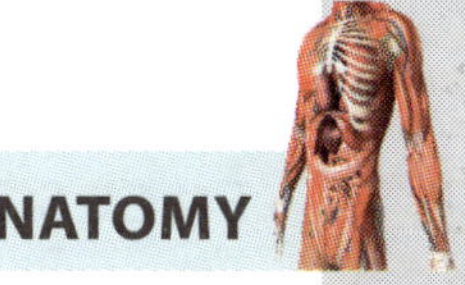

72. Stapedial artery is derived from which aortic arch:
(Recent Pattern Question 2017)
a. 1
b. 2
c. 3
d. 4

73. Fossa ovalis is a remnant of:
(Recent Pattern Question 2017)
a. Septum primum
b. Septum secondum
c. Bulbus cordis
d. Conus

74. In a fetus, testis lies at superficial inguinal ring at:
(Recent Pattern Question 2017)
a. 6th month
b. 7th month
c. 8th month
d. 9th month

75. Pons is derived from: *(Recent Pattern Question 2017)*
a. Metencephalon
b. Mylencephalon
c. Mesencephalon
d. Prosencephalon

76. Glomerulus is derived from:
(Recent Pattern Question 2017)
a. Metanephros
b. Mesonephros
c. Ureteric bud
d. Urogenital sinus

77. Prostate gland is derived from:
(Recent Pattern Question 2017)
a. Urogenital sinus
b. Urogenital folds
c. Labioscrotal swelling
d. Gubernaculum

78. Collecting duct is derived from:
a. Ureteric bud
b. Mesonephros
c. Metanephros
d. Allantois

79. Synovial fluid is produced by:
(Recent Pattern Question 2017)
a. Type A synoviocytes
b. Type B synoviocytes
c. Type C synoviocytes
d. Type D synoviocytes

80. Blue color cartilage is: *(Recent Pattern Question 2017)*
a. Hyaline
b. Elastic
c. Fibrocartilage
d. Synchondrosis

81. Tyson's glands are: *(Recent Pattern Question 2017)*
a. Apocrine glands
b. Holocrine gland
c. Eccrine gland
d. Endocrine gland

82. Fecal fistula at the umbilicus is due to:
(Recent Pattern Question 2017)
a. Persistent urachus
b. Persistent vitellointestinal duct
c. Raspberry tumor
d. Sister Joseph nodules

83. Ribs develop from: *(Recent Pattern Question 2017)*
a. Endothoracic fascia
b. Para-axial mesenchyme
c. Deep intercostal fascia
d. Superficial intercostal fascia

84. Pituitary develops from: *(Recent Pattern Question 2017)*
a. Posterior neural ridge
b. Rathke pouch
c. Neural crest
d. Neural plate

85. What is true about spermatogenesis?
a. It takes 74 days
b. Takes place in spermatic cord
c. Meiosis occurs only after secondary spermatocyte
d. Spermatid is formed from spermatozoa

86. Which of the following has the largest size?
a. Spermatogonium
b. Primary spermatocyte
c. Secondary spermatocyte
d. Spermatozoa

87. Spermatogonium to spermatozoon transformation takes place in:
a. 64 days
b. 74 days
c. 84 days
d. 94 days

88. Sperm acquires motility in:
a. Seminiferous tubule
b. Fallopian tube
c. Epididymis
d. Spermatic cord

89. All the following statements about seminal vesicles are true; EXCEPT:
a. Stores the spermatozoa
b. Actively depends on the level of testosterone
c. Secretion has abundant fructose
d. Lined by pseudostratified columnar epithelium

90. At what stage of embryonic development does an embryo normally begin to implant in the endometrium?
a. Blastocyst
b. Four-cell stage
c. Morula
d. Trilaminar embryo

91. Embryo term is used till:
a. 12 weeks after LMP
b. 10 weeks after fertilization
c. 10 weeks after LMP
d. 8 weeks of fertilization

92. Fetal stage is termed:
a. From the day of implantation
b. From 6th week of gestation
c. From 8th week of gestation
d. From 10th week of gestation

93. Which is not a derivative of midgut?
a. Appendix
b. Jejunum
c. Ascending colon
d. Descending colon

94. Which of the following artery mainly supplies hind gut?
a. Celiac trunk
b. Superior mesenteric artery
c. Inferior mesenteric artery
d. Rectal artery

95. Adrenal medulla is derived from:
a. Ectoderm
b. Endoderm
c. Mesoderm
d. Neural crest

96. Germ cells develop from:
a. Yolk sac
b. Surface ectoderm
c. Coelomic endoderm
d. Trophoblastic layer

97. How many ossification centers are there for the hyoid bone?
a. 5
b. 4
c. 6
d. 3

98. Trigone of urinary bladder develops from:
a. Endoderm
b. Ectoderm
c. Mesoderm
d. None

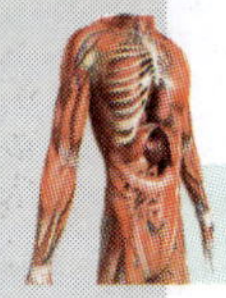

99. What are the vessels in umbilical cord?
a. 1 artery, 2 veins
b. 2 arteries, 1 vein
c. 1 artery, 1 vein
d. 2 arteries, 2 veins

100. Testosterone in male is secreted from:
a. Leydig cell
b. Sertoli cell
c. Seminal vesicle
d. Epididymis

101. Gallbladder is lined by:
a. Ciliated columnar cells
b. Brush bordered columnar epithelium
c. Striated columnar epithelium
d. Pseudostratified columnar cells

102. Hassall's corpuscles are found in:
a. Liver
b. Spleen
c. Kidney
d. Thymus

103. Malphigian corpuscles are seen in:
a. Thyroid
b. Kidney
c. Neurons
d. Liver

104. Cord of billroth is seen in:
a. Liver
b. Spleen
c. Kidney
d. Thymus

105. T cells are derived from:
a. Tonsils
b. Thymus
c. Thalamus
d. Thyroid

UPPER LIMB

106. Name the type of joint present at the arrow marked region: ***(Most Recent Question June 2022)***

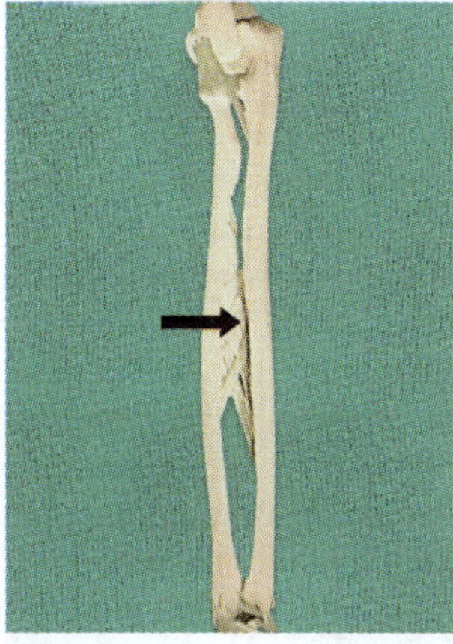

a. Synchondrosis
b. Syndesmosis
c. Symphysis
d. Synostosis

107. A patient presents to emergency room with pain and swelling in the right shoulder. A fracture clavicle is suspected. The most common site of fracture is; ***(Most Recent Question June 2022)***
a. Junction of medial 1/3 and lateral 2/3
b. Junction of medial 2/3 and lateral 1/3
c. Medial 1/3
d. Lateral 1/3

108. In case of frozen shoulder, the marked muscle is involved. Identify which movement has been compromised at the joint. ***(Most Recent Question June 2022)***

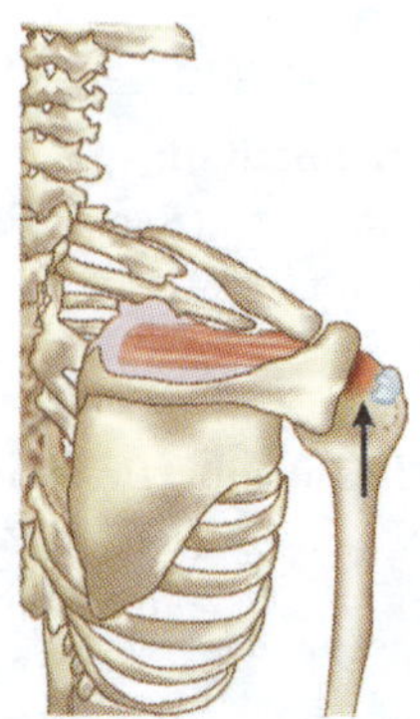

a. Abduction
b. Adduction
c. Flexion
d. Extension

109. Identify the arrow marked tendon: ***(Most Recent Question June 2022)***

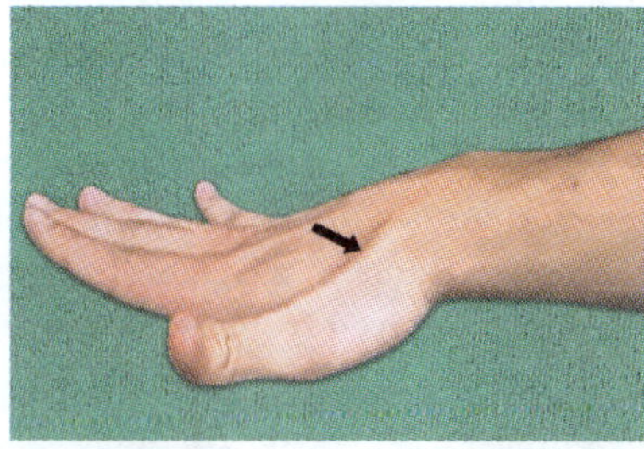

a. Abductor policis longus
b. Abductor policis brevis
c. Extensor policis longus
d. Extensor policis brevis

110. Biceps brachii functions as which types of muscle for lifting forearm: ***(Most Recent Question June/Dec 2021)***
a. Prime mover
b. Fixator
c. Antagonist
d. Synergist

111. A known case of leprosy has presented with the following deformity. The nerve compromised is: ***(Most Recent Question June/Dec 2021)***

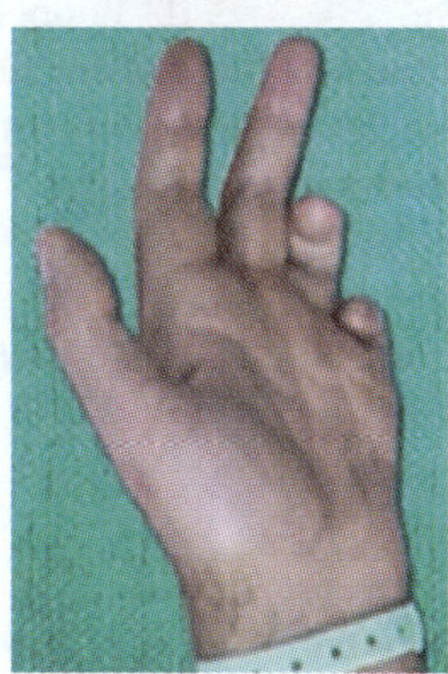

a. Ulnar
b. Median
c. Ulnar and median
d. Radial

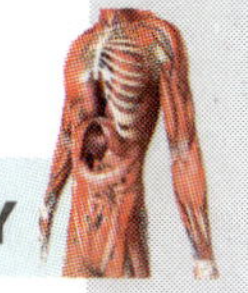

112. Tendon marked 'X' in the given image is:
(Most Recent Question Dec 2020)

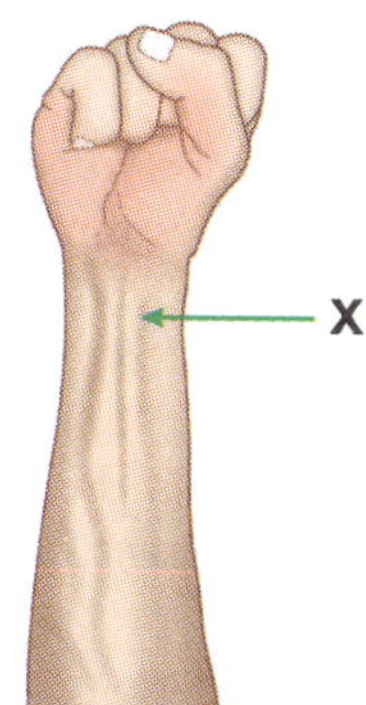

a. Flexor digitorum superficialis
b. Flexor digitorum profundus
c. Flexor carpi radialis
d. Flexor carpi ulnaris

113. A young computer operator presents with tingling sensation and paresthesia on medial side of hand. Which structure is most likely affected?
(Most Recent Question Dec 2020)

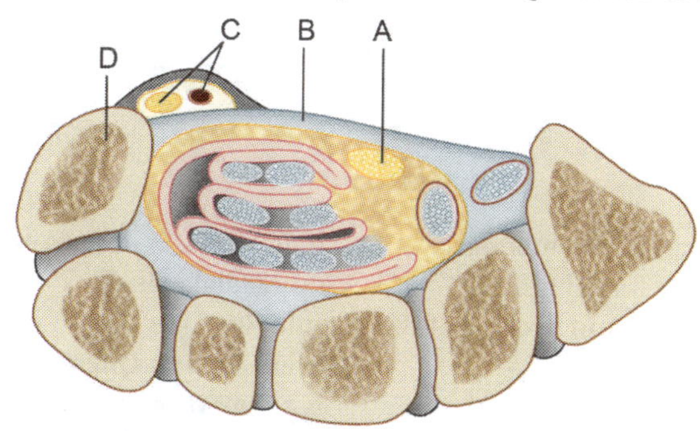

a. A
b. B
c. C
d. D

114. The highlighted muscle is supplied by which nerve?
(Most Recent Question Dec 2020)

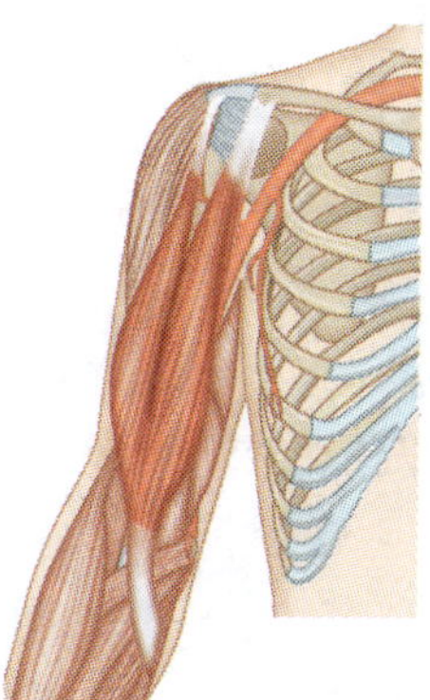

a. Radial nerve
b. Ulnar nerve
c. Median nerve
d. Musculocutaneous nerve

115. Nerve involved in injury to the marked structure:
(Most Recent Question Dec 2020)

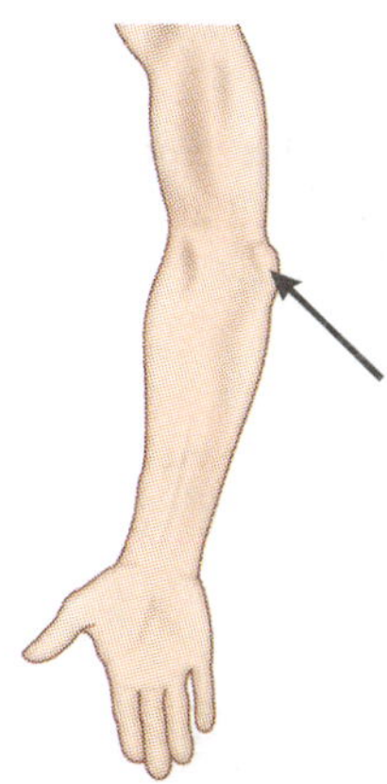

a. Axillary nerve
b. Ulnar nerve
c. Median nerve
d. Radial nerve

116. Which of the following nerves get compromised in a lesion at the arrow marked area?
(Most Recent Question Aug 2020)

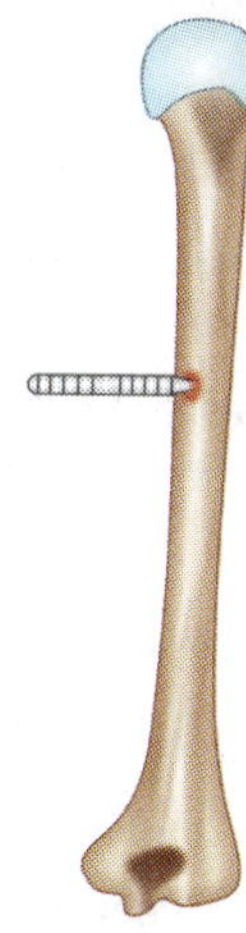

a. Axillary nerve
b. Radial nerve
c. Medial nerve
d. Ulnar nerve

117. An injury to the shown area can lead to fracture of which bone?
(Most Recent Question 2019)

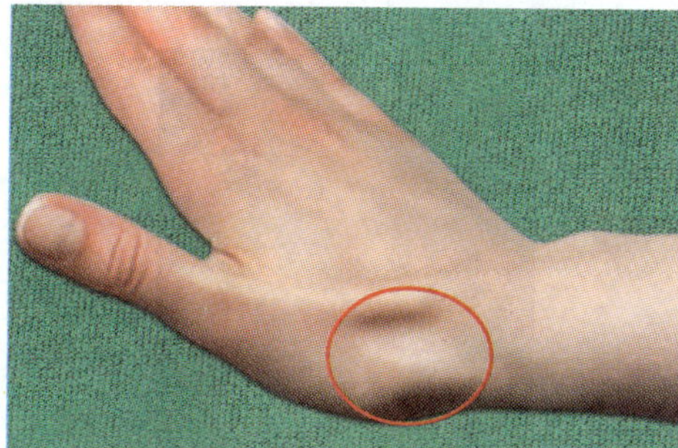

a. Scaphoid
b. Lunate
c. Trapezium
d. Hamate

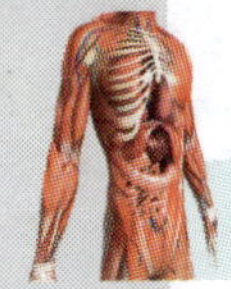

118. Which muscle originates from medial epicondyle of humerus? *(Most Recent Question 2019)*

a. Supinator
b. Pronator teres
c. Pronator quadratus
d. Brachioradialis

119. A patient presents with hypothenar muscle wasting and loss of sensation of medial one and a half digits. Which nerve is involved? *(Most Recent Question 2019)*

a. Ulnar nerve
b. Median nerve
c. Radial nerve
d. Musculocutaneous nerve

120. Identify the muscle marked in the diagram. *(Most Recent Question 2019)*

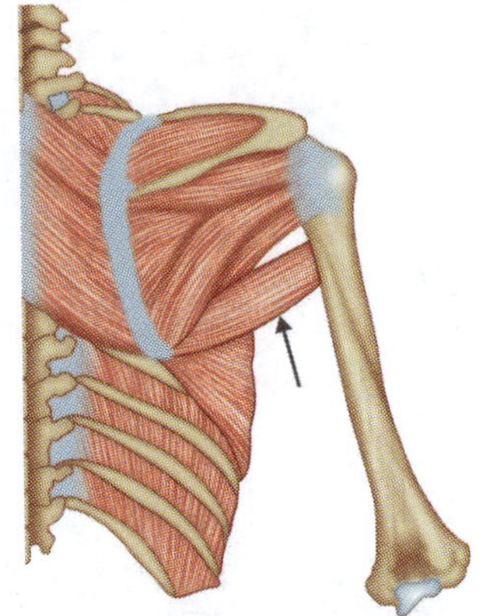

a. Teres major
b. Teres minor
c. Infraspinatus
d. Supraspinatus

121. Inferior scapular angle is at which level? *(Most Recent Question 2019)*

a. T4
b. T6
c. T8
d. T2

122. Flexion, adduction and medial rotation of arm is done by which muscle? *(Most Recent Question 2019)*

a. Pectoralis minor
b. Pectoralis major
c. Subclavius
d. Serratus Anterior

123. Upper lateral cutaneous nerve of arm is a branch of: *(Most Recent Question 2019)*

a. Radial nerve
b. Ulnar nerve
c. Axillary nerve
d. Musculocutaneous nerve

124. Identify the marked bone: *(Recent Pattern Question 2018-19)*

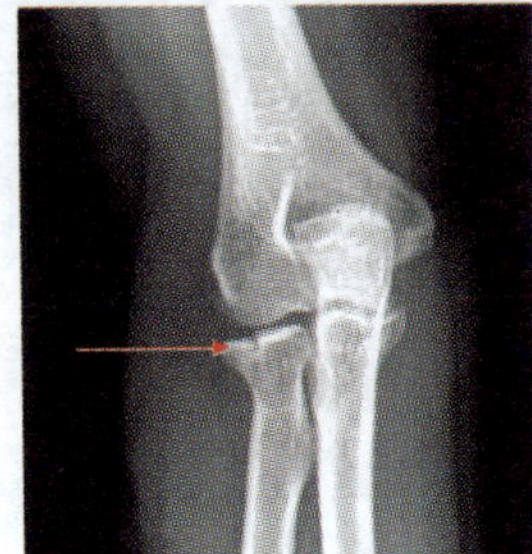

a. Capitulum
b. Olecranon
c. Trochlea
d. Radial head

125. Retraction of scapula is by: *(Recent Pattern Question 2018-19)*

a. Serratus anterior
b. Trapezius
c. Suprascapularis
d. Deltoid muscle

126. In a patient with Fracture of upper radius and ulna at the insertion of pronator teres muscle, which movement is restricted: *(Recent Pattern Question 2018-19)*

a. Pronation
b. Supination
c. Hyperpronation
d. Hyperabduction

127. Which of the following is the insertion of the shown muscle? *(Recent Pattern Question 2018-19)*

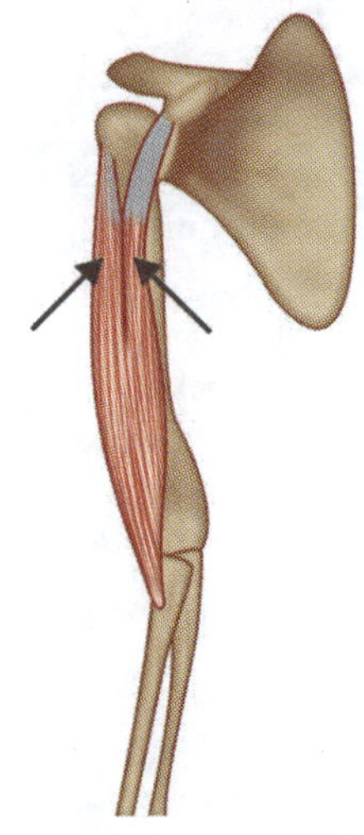

a. Radial tuberosity
b. Olecranon process
c. Radial head
d. Medial malleolus

128. Coracoid process of the scapula is: *(Recent Pattern Question 2018)*

a. Pressure epiphysis
b. Traction epiphysis
c. Atavistic epiphysis
d. Aberrant epiphysis

129. Which of the following is *not* a component of carpal tunnel? *(Recent Pattern Question 2018)*

a. Ulnar nerve
b. Median nerve
c. Flexor digitorum superficialis
d. Flexor digitorum profundus

130. Which structure passes through Guyon's canal? *(Recent Pattern Question 2018)*

a. Ulnar nerve
b. Median nerve
c. Radial nerve
d. Flexor carpi radialis

131. Which is the nerve root of biceps jerk? *(Recent Pattern Question 2017)*

a. C5-C6
b. C6-C8
c. C7-C8
d. C8-T1

132. Angle of humeral torsion is_____ degrees: *(Recent Pattern Question 2017)*

a. 15
b. 35
c. 135
d. 164

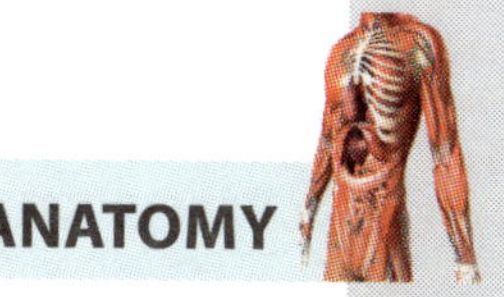

133. Which carpal bone has a hook?
(Recent Pattern Question 2017)
a. Capitate b. Lunate
c. Hamate d. Pisiformis

134. Which is the 1st carpal bone to ossify?
(Recent Pattern Question 2017)
a. Capitate b. Lunate
c. Hamate d. Pisiformis

135. Which is not a part of proximal row of carpal bones?
(Recent Pattern Question 2017)
a. Scaphoid b. Lunate
c. Triquetral d. Hamate

136. Which is the most commonly fractured carpal bone?
a. Hamate b. Lunate
c. Scaphoid d. Capitates

137. Articulation of pisiform bone is with:
a. Triquetral b. Lunate
c. Scaphoid d. Trapezoid

138. Middle trunk of branchial plexus is formed of:
(Recent Pattern Question 2017)
a. C6, C7 b. C7, C8
c. C8, T1 d. C7

139. Regimental band anesthesia is due to lesion of:
(Recent Pattern Question 2017)
a. Musculocutaneous nerve
b. Axillary nerve
c. Long thoracic nerve
d. Spinal accessory nerve

140. Screwing movement in upper limb is possible with:
(Recent Pattern Question 2017)
a. Brachioradialis b. Anconeus
c. Supinator d. Pronator teres

141. Radial artery ends as: *(Recent Pattern Question 2017)*
a. Superficial palmar arch b. Deep palmar arch
c. Both of above d. Profunda brachii artery

142. The largest bursa in the body is:
(Recent Pattern Question 2017)
a. Prepatellar bursa b. Infrapatellar bursa
c. Subacromial bursa d. Trochanteric bursa

143. Which is the nerve passing through medial epicondyle?
a. Ulnar b. Radial
c. Median d. Posterior interosseus

144. Anastomosis of subscapular artery are formed by all EXCEPT:
a. Transverse cervical artery
b. Suprascapular artery
c. 1st part of subclavian artery
d. 2nd part of axillary artery

145. Which structure is present in the anatomical snuff box?
a. Ulnar artery b. Radial artery
c. Median nerve d. Radial nerve

146. Anatomical snuff box contains:
a. Axillary nerve b. Radial artery
c. Brachial artery d. Ulnar artery

147. The medial boundary of the anatomical snuffbox is formed by the:
a. Ext. pollicis brevi b. Ext Carpi radialis longus
c. Extensor pollicis longus d. Ext Carpi radialis brevis

148. Surgical neck fracture leads to all; EXCEPT:
a. Teres major palsy b. Teres minor palsy
c. Weakness of abduction d. Deltoid muscle palsy

149. Which of the following artery is affected in anterior shoulder dislocation?
a. Radial b. Axillary
c. Median d. Ulnar

150. Which among the following muscles receives Dual Nerve supply?
a. Flexor digitorum profundus
b. Flexor digitorum superficialis
c. Palmaris longus
d. Extensor carpi radialis

151. All of the following structures are passing deep to flexor retinaculum; EXCEPT:
a. Flexor pollicis longus
b. Flexor digitorum superficialis
c. Palmaris longus
d. Flexor digitorum profundus

152. Which structure passes superficial to flexor retinaculum?
a. Ulnar nerve
b. Median nerve
c. Flexor digitorum superficialis
d. Flexor digitorum profundus

153. Root value to axillary nerve:
a. C5, C6 b. C6, C7, C8
c. C5, C6, C7 d. C5-T1

154. Musculocutaneous nerve arises from which cord:
a. Medial cord b. Lateral cord
c. Anterior cord d. Posterior cord

155. Root of radial nerve:
a. C6, C7, T1 b. C5, C6, C7, T1
c. C5, C6, C7, C8, T1 d. C4, C5, C6, C7, C8, T1

156. Winging of scapula is due to damage of:
a. Axillary nerve b. Long thoracic nerve
c. Median nerve d. Ulnar nerve

157. Winging of scapula is due to paralysis of:
a. Serratus anterior muscle
b. Latissimus dorsi muscle
c. Rhomboidus major muscle
d. Pectoralis major muscle

158. Winging of scapula is due to paralysis of:
a. Serratus anterior muscle b. Latissimus dorsi muscle
c. Rhomboid major muscle d. Pectoralis major muscle

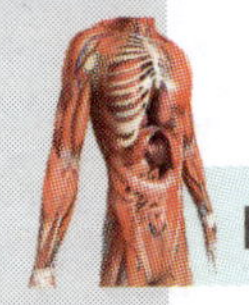

159. 'Dropped shoulder' occurs due to paralysis of:
a. Teres minor b. Deltoid
c. Teres major d. Trapezius

160. Trapezius muscle is attached to all structures; EXCEPT:
a. First rib b. Clavicle
c. Scapula d. Occiput

161. All of the following show ulnar nerve injury; EXCEPT:
a. Clawing of medial 2 digits
b. Abductor pollicis palsy
c. Adductor pollicis palsy
d. Weak grip

162. Pointing finger injury is due to injury of which nerve?
a. Radial nerve b. Ulnar nerve
c. Median nerve d. Axillary nerve

163. Claw hand is due to:
a. Median nerve b. Ulnar nerve
c. Median and ulnar both d. Radial nerve

164. Ape thumb deformity is due to injury of which nerve?
a. Radial nerve b. Ulnar nerve
c. Median nerve d. Axillary nerve

165. Compression of which of the following nerves lead to carpal tunnel syndrome:
a. Ulnar nerve b. Median nerve
c. Radial nerve d. Both a and b

166. Median nerve supplies all; EXCEPT:
a. Abductor pollicis longus
b. Pronator quadratus
c. Flexor pollicis longus
d. Flexor carpi radialis

167. All are muscles of rotator cuff; EXCEPT:
a. Teres major b. Teres minor
c. Infraspinatous d. Supraspinatous

168. Most common injured muscle in rotator cuff is:
a. Supraspinatous muscle b. Infraspinatous muscle
c. Teres minor d. Subscapularis

169. In a man lifting up a suitcase, downward dislocation of glenohumeral joint is prevented by:
a. Deltoid b. Latissimus dorsi
c. Coracobrachialis d. Supra spinatous

170. Short head of biceps is innervated by:
a. Musculo cutaneous nerve
b. Radial nerve
c. Axillary nerve
d. Median nerve

171. Muscle which covers both elbow and shoulder joint:
a. Biceps
b. Biceps brachialis
c. Coracobrachialis
d. Long head of triceps brachii

172. Which one of the following is a multipennate muscle?
a. Tibialis anterior b. Deltoid
c. Tibialis posterior d. Latissimus dorsi

173. Fracture of shaft of humerus leads to:
a. Radial nerve injury
b. Ulnar nerve injury
c. Median nerve injury
d. Musculocutaneous nerve injury

174. Posterior wall of axilla is formed by all; EXCEPT:
a. Teres major
b. Subscapularis
c. Supraspinatus
d. Latissimus dorsi

175. Location of level III axillary lymph node in relation to pectoralis minor is:
a. Anterior
b. Posterior
c. Superior
d. Inferior

176. Supination and pronation of upper limb is due to:
a. Wrist joint b. Radioulnar joint
c. Elbow joint d. Carpometacarpal joint

177. Medial border of cubital fossa is formed by:
a. Pronator teres b. Brachioradialis
c. Supinator d. Brachialis

178. All are contents of the cubital fossa; EXCEPT:
a. Ulnar artery b. Median nerve
c. Brachial artery d. Ulnar nerve

179. All are contents of cubital fossa; EXCEPT:
a. Median nerve b. Ulnar nerve
c. Biceps tendon d. Brachial artery

180. Boundary of triangle of auscultation is formed by all; EXCEPT:
a. Scapula b. Trapezius
c. Serratus anterior d. Latissimus dorsi

LOWER LIMB

181. Which arterial pulse is being taken?
(Most Recent Question June 2022)

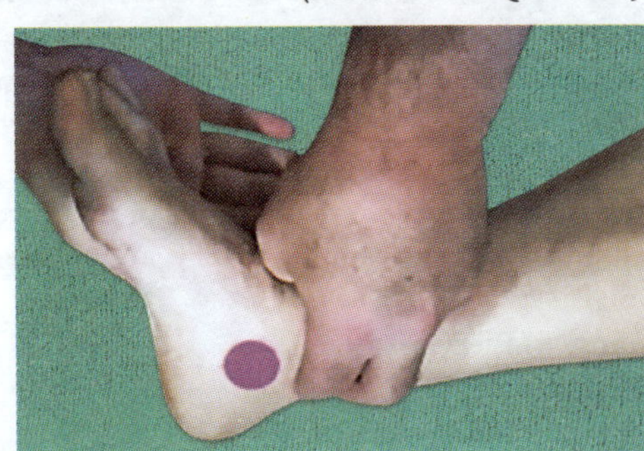

a. Anterior tibial artery
b. Posterior tibial artery
c. Dorsalis pedis artery
d. Medial plantar artery

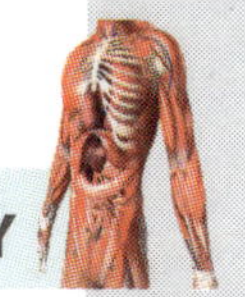

182. The examiner is palpating which artery in the following diagram: *(Most Recent Question June/Dec 2021)*

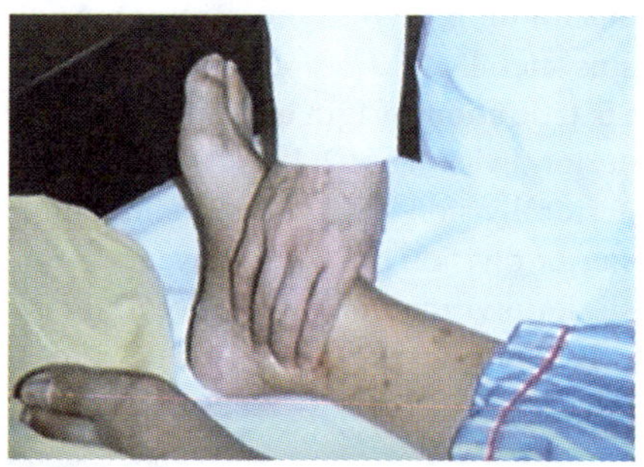

a. Anterior tibial b. Posterior tibial
c. Dorsalis pedis d. Medial plantar

183. The dermatome of the area marked with arrow is: *(Most Recent Question June/Dec 2021)*

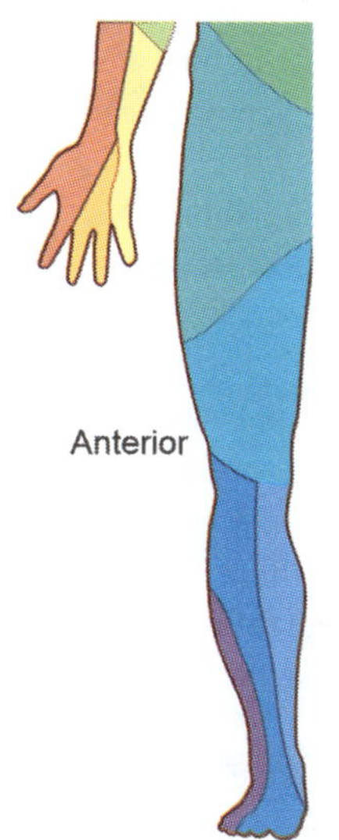

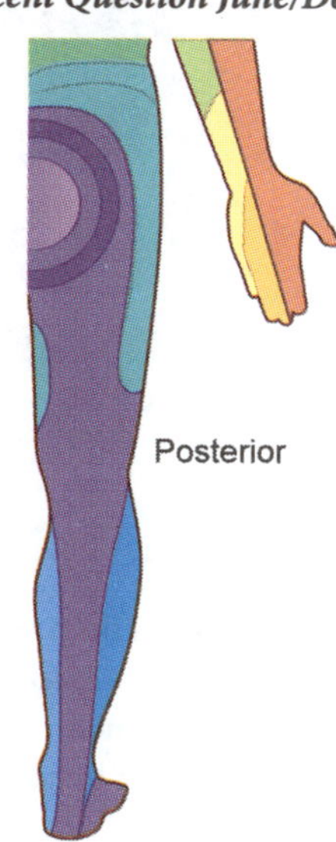

a. L2 b. L3
c. L4 d. L5

184. Nerve involved in the difficulty in eversion of foot and loss of sensation in dorsal aspect of foot is: *(Most Recent Question Dec 2020)*

a. Deep peroneal nerve b. Superficial peroneal nerve
c. Sural nerve d. Saphenous nerve

185. Which muscle tendon is stretched in patellar tendon reflex? *(Most Recent Question Dec 2020)*

a. Biceps femoris b. Quadriceps femoris
c. Addactur magnus d. Quadratus

186. A 45-year-old policeman comes from duty with complain of pain in right leg and starts from right buttock. On examination pulse in right popliteal fossa was absent where as in left side it was normal. The block is at which level? *(Most Recent Question Dec 2020)*

a. Femoral b. External iliac
c. Aortoiliac d. Popliteal

187. What is the name of marked artery? *(Most Recent Question Dec 2020)*

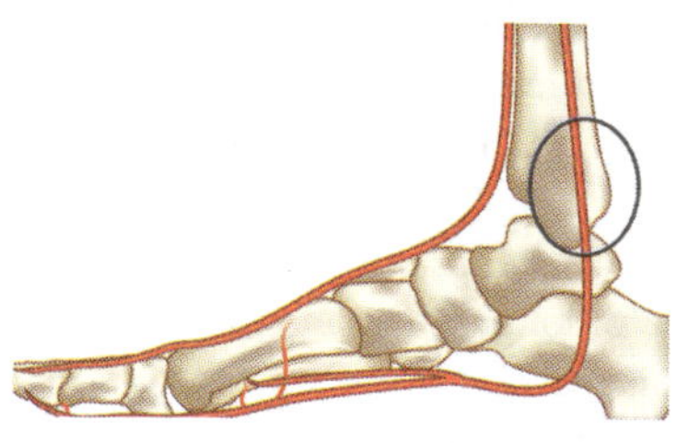

a. Posterior tibial artery b. Deep phalangeal artery
c. Lateral planter d. Medial plantar

188. Identify the arrow marked tarsal bone in the given image: *(Most Recent Question Dec 2020)*

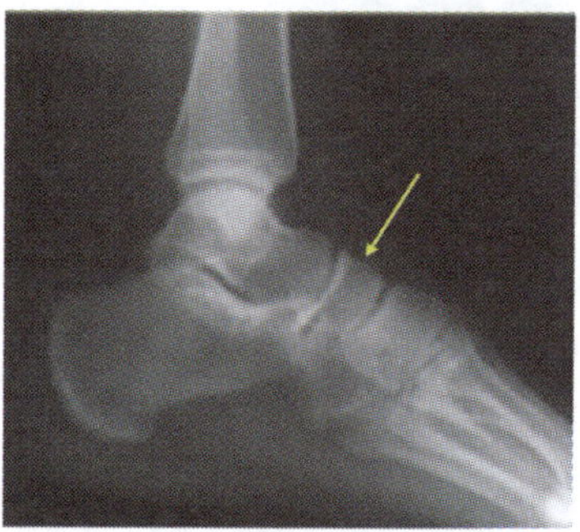

a. Cuboid b. Talus
c. Navicular d. Cuneiform

189. Posterior tibial artery pulse is felt: *(Most Recent Question Aug 2020)*

a. Between medial malleolus & medial border of tendon calcaneus in inversion
b. Between medial malleolus & medial border of tendon calcaneus in eversion
c. Between medial malleolus & lateral border of tendon calcaneus in inversion
d. Between medial malleolus & lateral border of tendon calcaneus in eversion

190. Identify the marked muscle tendon in the diagram: *(Most Recent Question 2019)*

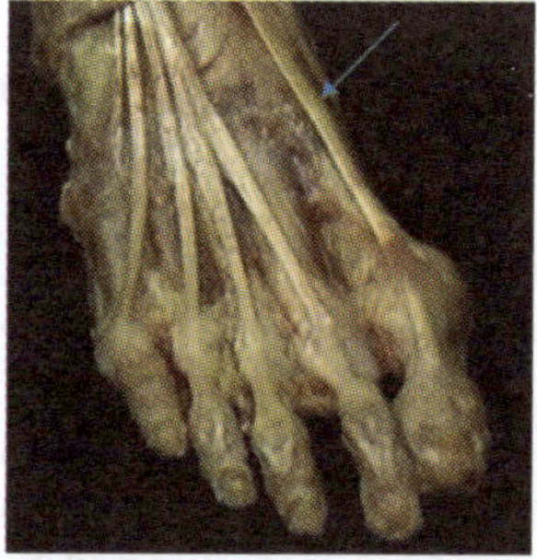

a. Flexor hallucis longus b. Extensor hallucis longus
c. Extensor digitorum longus
d. Tibialis anterior

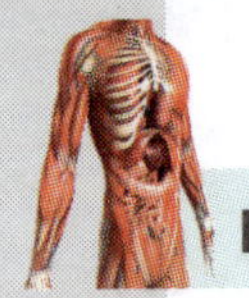

191. Abduction at the hip joint is done by: *(Most Recent Question 2019)*
a. Gluteus maximus b. Obturator internus
c. Quadratus femoris d. Gluteus medius

192. Tibial and common peroneal nerve supplies: *(Recent Pattern Question 2018-19)*
a. Adductor magnus muscle
b. Adductor longus muscle
c. Gracilis muscle
d. Biceps Femoris muscle

193. Which of the following muscle is supplied by obturator nerve? *(Recent Pattern Question 2018-19)*
a. Gluteus medius b. Obturator internus
c. Sartorius d. Adductor brevis

194. Which of the following muscle is evertor of foot? *(Recent Pattern Question 2018-19)*
a. Tibialis anterior muscle
b. Tibialis posterior
c. Peroneus longus muscle
d. Extensor digitorum longus

195. Most common nerve damaged in leg: *(Recent Pattern Question 2018)*
a. Common peroneal nerve b. Femoral nerve
c. Sciatic nerve d. Tibial nerve

196. Femoral triangle base is formed by: *(Recent Pattern Question 2018)*
a. Medial border of sartorius
b. Inguinal ligament
c. Medial border of adductor longus
d. Iliacus

197. Medial compartment of thigh is supplied by which nerve? *(Recent Pattern Question 2018)*
a. Tibial nerve b. Obturator nerve
c. Femoral nerve d. Common peroneal

198. First web space of foot is supplied by: *(Recent Pattern Question 2018)*
a. Common peroneal nerve
b. Superficial peroneal nerve
c. Deep peroneal nerve
d. Sural nerve

199. Which bone in foot is not attached by any muscle? *(Recent Pattern Question 2017)*
a. Talus b. Calcaneum
c. Metatarsals d. Fibula

200. Which muscle originates from anterior superior iliac spine? *(Recent Pattern Question 2017)*
a. Iliofemoral ligament b. Sartorius
c. Vastus lateralis d. Vastus medialis

201. Tibialis posterior muscle is supplied by which nerve? *(Recent Pattern Question 2017)*
a. Posterior tibial nerve b. Deep peroneal nerve
c. Femoral nerve d. Sural nerve

202. Adductor canal lateral boundary is formed by: *(Recent Pattern Question 2017)*
a. Adductor longus b. Rectus medialis
c. Vastus lateralis d. Vastus medialis

203. Which is true about origin of Femoral nerve root value?
a. Anterior division of L2, L3, L4 ventral rami
b. Anterior division of L1, L2, L3 ventral rami
c. Posterior division of L2, L3, L4 ventral rami
d. Posterior division of L1, L2, L3 ventral rami

204. Which is the muscle marked as A in the femoral triangle? *(Recent Pattern Question 2017)*

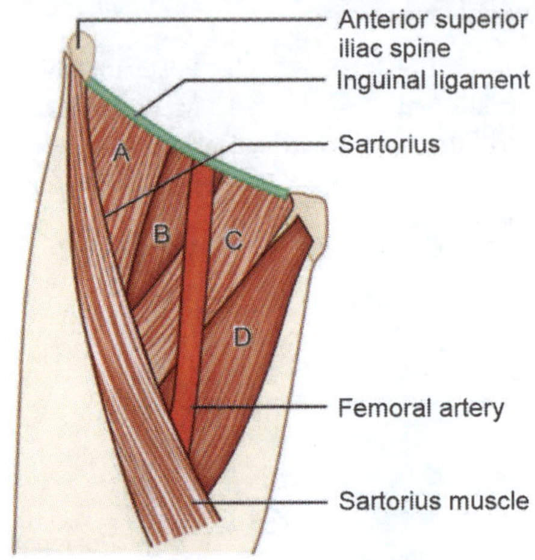

a. Iliacus b. Psoas major
c. Pectineus d. Adductor longus

205. Biceps femoris does which of the following function? *(Recent Pattern Question 2017)*
a. Adduction of knee
b. Flexion of knee
c. Extension of knee
d. Abduction of knee

206. Chief extensor of thigh at hip joint is supplied by: *(Recent Pattern Question 2017)*
a. Inferior gluteal nerve
b. Superior gluteal nerve
c. Sciatic nerve
d. Peroneal nerve

207. Which of the following muscles is an evertor of foot? *(Recent Pattern Question 2017)*
a. Peroneus tertius b. Tibialis anterior
c. Extensor hallicus longus d. Extensor digitorum longus

208. What is the nerve supply of popliteus muscle? *(Recent Pattern Question 2017)*
a. Tibial nerve b. Popliteal nerve
c. Common peroneal nerve d. Deep peroneal nerve

209. Which is not a cause of positive trendelenburg sign? *(Recent Pattern Question 2017)*
a. Paralysis of gluteus maximus
b. Congenital dislocation of hip
c. Ununited fracture of neck
d. Coxa vara

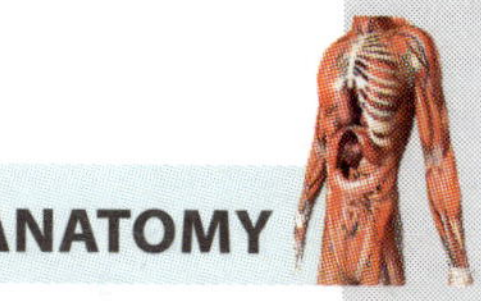

210. Which of the following nerve injury leads to positive trendelenberg test?
a. Inferior gluteal b. Obturator
c. Tibial d. Superior gluteal nerve

211. Trendelenburg test is done for:
a. Gluteus medius, minimus
b. Gluteus maximus, minimus
c. Gluteus maximus, medius
d. Gluteus maximus, medius, minimus

212. Capsule of knee joint is supplied by: *(Recent Pattern Question 2017)*
a. Genital branch of genitofemoral nerve
b. Femoral branch of genitofemoral nerve
c. Genicular branch of obturator nerve
d. Femoral branch of obturator nerve

213. Fabella is present in: *(Recent Pattern Question 2017)*
a. Medial head of gastrocnemius
b. Lateral head of gastrocnemius
c. Adductor magnus
d. Adductor longus

214. Which is the nerve supply of soleus muscle? *(Recent Pattern Question 2016)*
a. Tibial nerve
b. Common peroneal nerve
c. Superficial peroneal nerve
d. Deep peroneal nerve

215. What is true about iliotibial tract? *(Recent Pattern Question 2016)*
a. Thickening of fascia lata
b. Gluteus medius is inserted into it
c. Insertion at medial aspect of tibia
d. Runs along the medial aspect of thigh

216. Which muscle is responsible for sitting to standing position? *(Recent Pattern Question 2016)*
a. Gluteus medius
b. Gluteus maximus
c. Gluteus minimus
d. Tensor fascia lata

217. All are branches of femoral artery; EXCEPT:
a. Superficial epigastric artery
b. Superficial circumflex artery
c. Inferior epigastric artery
d. Descending genicular artery

218. Gluteus maximus is inserted on:
a. Lesser trochanter b. Gluteal tuberosity
c. Iliotibial tract d. Iliac crest

219. Iliotibial band has insertion of all of the following muscles; EXCEPT:
a. Tensor fasciae latae b. Gluteus maximus
c. Gluteus minimus d. Vastus lateralis

220. Which is the longest muscle of the body:
a. Sartorius b. Extraocular muscle
c. External oblique d. Popliteal muscle

221. Which of the following muscles has attachment on the capsule of hip joint?
a. Sartorius b. Rectus femoris
c. Vastus lateralis d. Vastus medialis

222. This muscle is part of hamstrings muscle:
a. Semimembranous
b. Gracilis
c. Short head of biceps femoris
d. Sartorius

223. Gluteus medius is supplied by:
a. Superior gluteal nerve
b. Inferior gluteal nerve
c. Nerve to obturator internus
d. Nerve to quadratus femoris

224. Which of the following nerve supplies gluteus maximus?
a. Superior gluteal nerve b. Inferior gluteal nerve
c. Anterior gluteal nerve d. Posterior gluteal nerve

225. Which is the nerve supplying gamellus inferior muscle?
a. Nerve to obturator internus
b. Nerve to obturator externus
c. Nerve to quadratus femoris
d. Ventral rami to S1 and S2

226. All of the following structures pass through lesser sciatic foramen; EXCEPT:
a. Pudendal nerve
b. Internal pudendal vessels
c. Nerve to obturator internus
d. Nerve to obturator externus

227. Which is the main extensor of knee?
a. Biceps femoris b. Quadriceps femoris
c. Semitendinosus d. Semimembranosus

228. Which muscle is responsible for unlocking of knee?
a. Popliteus b. Quadriceps femoris
c. Semitendinosus d. Semimembranosus

229. Which of the following bone has no muscle attachment?
a. Navicular b. Calcaneum
c. Talus d. Cuboid

230. In injury to the neck of fibula, which of the following nerve is usually injured?
a. Superficial peroneal nerve
b. Deep peroneal nerve
c. Common peroneal nerve
d. Tibial nerve

231. Medial border of Hesselbach's triangle is formed by:
a. Linea alba
b. Linea semilunaris
c. Inferior epigastric artery
d. Conjoint tendon

232. Poupart's ligament forms which border of hesselbach's triangle:
a. Anterior b. Posterior
c. Superior d. Inferior

233. All of the following are true about lateral cutaneous nerve of thigh; EXCEPT:

a. Supplies skin over the lateral skin of thigh
b. Supplies skin over the medial aspect of thigh
c. Arises from L2 and L3
d. It is a purely sensory nerve

234. What is the nerve Root value of superior gluteal nerve:

a. $L_{4,5,}$ S_1
b. $L_{4,5}$, S_1, S_2
c. $L_{4,5}$, S_1,S_2, S_3
d. L_5, S_1, S_2

235. Root value of the posterior cutaneous nerve of the thigh:

a. S_1, S_2
b. S_1, S_2, S_3
c. S_2, S_3
d. S_2, S_3, S_4

236. Root value of sciatic nerve is:

a. $S_1S_2S_3$
b. $L_4L_5S_1S_2S_3$
c. $L_1L_2L_3$
d. $L_2L_3L_4$

237. Nerve root of pudendal nerve is:

a. $S_1S_2S_3$
b. $S_2S_3S_4$
c. S_3-S_4
d. S_2-S_3

THORAX AND ABDOMEN

238. Identify the arrow marked structure in the dissected specimen: *(Most Recent Question June 2022)*

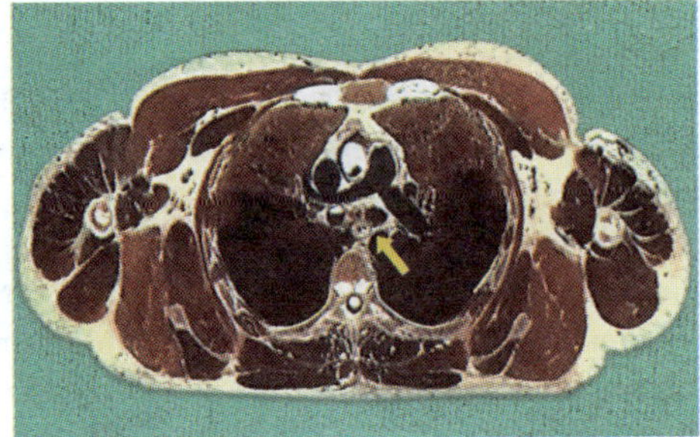

a. Oesophagus
b. Superior vena cava
c. Inferior vena cava
d. Descending aorta

239. The marked line corresponds to vertebral level *(Most Recent Question June 2022)*

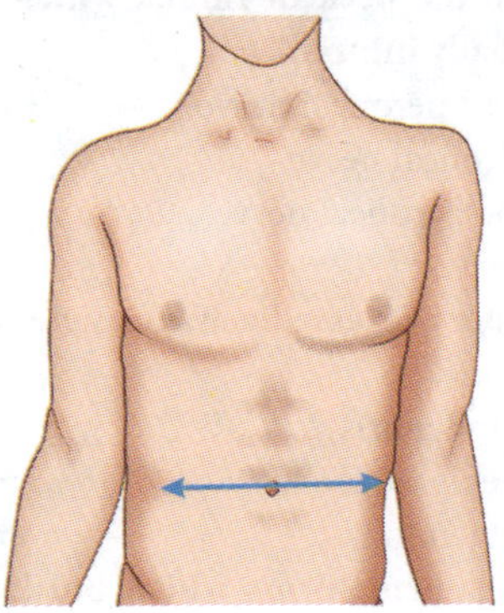

a. T – 12
b. L – 1
c. L – 2
d. L – 3

240. Identify the chamber marked with arrow: *(Most Recent Question June/Dec 2021)*

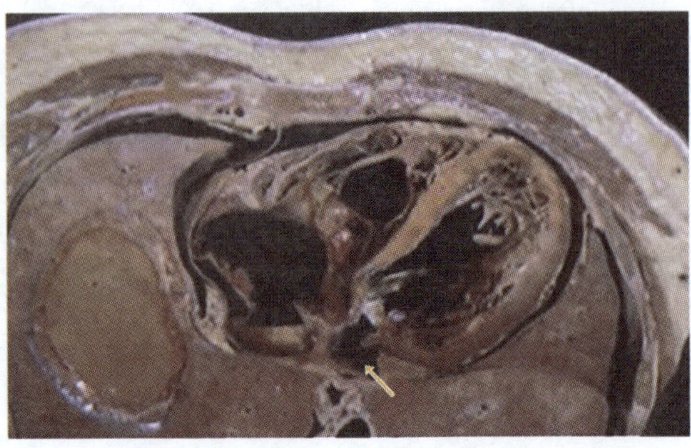

a. Right atrium
b. Left atrium
c. Right ventricle
d. Left ventricle

241. The neurovascular bundle in anterior wall of abdomen lies between: *(Most Recent Question June/Dec 2021)*

a. External and internal oblique muscle
b. Internal oblique and transverse abdominis muscle
c. External oblique and transversus abdominis muscle
d. Transversus abdominis and transversalis fascia

242. Structure marked in the image will terminate at: *(Most Recent Question Dec 2020)*

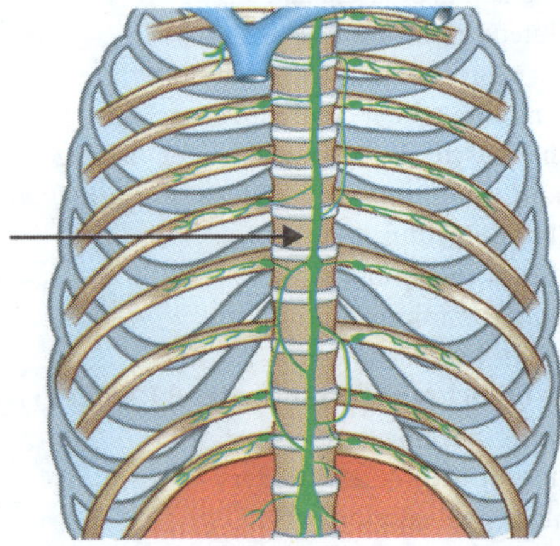

a. Junction of Left jugular vein and subclavian vein
b. Brachiocephalic vein
c. Superior vena cava
d. Right subclavian vein

243. A baby at 9 to 10 month develops which curvature in vertebral spine: *(Most Recent Question Aug 2020)*

a. Secondary curvature at cervical spine
b. Secondary curvature at thoracic spine
c. Secondary curvature at lumbar spine
d. Secondary curvature at sacral spine

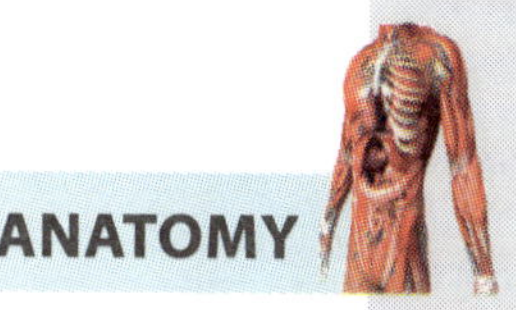

244. Identify the structure marked with pointer:

(Most Recent Question Aug 2020)

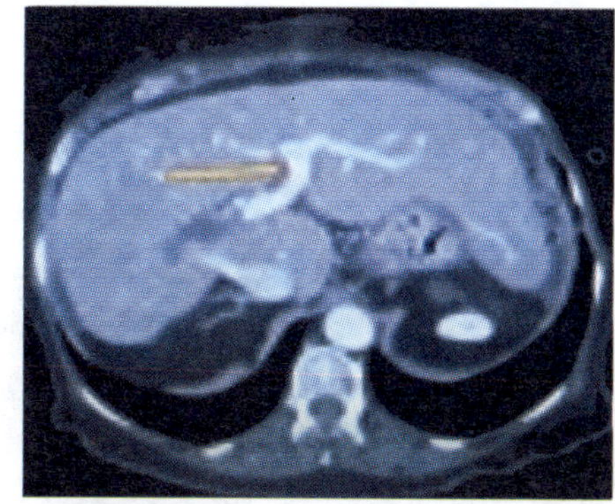

a. Hepatic artery
b. Hepatic vein
c. Inferior vena cava
d. Portal vein

245. Testicular artery is a branch of:

(Most Recent Question 2019)

a. Common iliac artery
b. Abdominal aorta
c. Internal iliac artery
d. External iliac artery

246. Which of the following structure is present over the mediastinal surface of right lung?

(Recent Pattern Question 2018-19)

a. Azygos vein
b. Right thoracic duct
c. Aorta
d. Trachea

247. Which of the following structures is not found in superior mediastinum?

a. Pulmonary trunk
b. Thymus
c. Left intercostal artery
d. Arch of aorta

248. Which of these is true about bronchopulmonary segment? *(Recent Pattern Question 2018)*

a. Nonresectable
b. Spherical in shape
c. Artery is intersegmental
d. Pulmonary veins are intersegmental

249. Left anterior descending artery is a branch of:

(Recent Pattern Question 2018)

a. Right coronary artery
b. Left coronary artery
c. Ascending aorta
d. Coronary sinus

250. VAN (vein, artery, nerve) sequence is present in intercostal space at: *(Recent Pattern Question 2017)*

a. Upper border of rib
b. Middle border of rib
c. Lower border of rib
d. Middle portion of intercostal space

251. Which of the following rib is known as floating rib?

(Recent Pattern Question 2017)

a. 8
b. 9
c. 10
d. 11

252. Which is not a true rib:

a. 5th
b. 6th
c. 7th
d. 8th

253. Xiphoid process unites with the body at age of _______ years? *(Recent Pattern Question 2017)*

a. 10
b. 20
c. 30
d. 40

254. Which structure passes though foramen of langer?

(Recent Pattern Question 2017)

a. Inguinal canal
b. Tail of spence
c. CN V3
d. CN VII

255. Sappey's plexus drains? *(Recent Pattern Question 2017)*

a. Breast
b. Thyroid
c. Adrenal
d. Porta hepatis

256. Lingula is which part of lung?

(Recent Pattern Question 2017)

a. Left lower lobe
b. Left upper lobe
c. Right lower lobe
d. Right upper lobe

257. Which muscle is involved in violent expiratory efforts?

(Recent Pattern Question 2017)

a. Diaphragm
b. Latissimus dorsi
c. External oblique
d. Internal intercostal

258. Right coronary artery supplies all; EXCEPT:

a. Right atrium
b. Posterior part of interventricular septum
c. Anterior interventricular groove
d. SA node

259. Base of the heart is formed by:

a. RA
b. RV
c. LA
d. LV

260. All of these form right heart border; EXCEPT?

a. SVC
b. IVC
c. Right atrium
d. Right ventricle

261. What is the length of trachea?

a. 5 cm
b. 10 cm
c. 20 cm
d. 25 cm

262. What is the diameter of trachea?

a. 0.5 cm
b. 2 cm
c. 3 cm
d. 5 cm

263. Most commonly foreign body lodges in which part of esophagus?

a. Where it crosses the aortic arch
b. Cricopharyngeus
c. Where it is crossed by left bronchus
d. Where it pierces the diaphragm

264. Which is not an accessory muscle of respiration?

a. Sternocleidomastoid
b. Scalaneus
c. Erector spinae
d. None of these

265. 75% respiration is due to:

a. Diaphragm
b. Internal intercostals
c. Intercostals
d. Serratus anterior

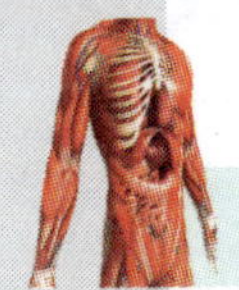

266. Which is the motor supply of diaphragm?
a. Phrenic nerve
b. Thoracodorsal nerve
c. Intercostals
d. Sympathetic nerves

267. Intercostal veins drain into:
a. Left subclavian vein
b. Internal jugular vein
c. Azygous vein
d. Inferior vena cava

ABDOMEN

268. Celiac artery is seen at which vertebral level?
(Most Recent Question Dec 2020)
a. T9
b. T10
c. T12
d. L2

269. Identify the branch originating from Celiac trunk:
(Recent Pattern Question 2018-19)
a. Splenic artery
b. Left gastric artery
c. Left gastroepiploic artery
d. Left renal artery

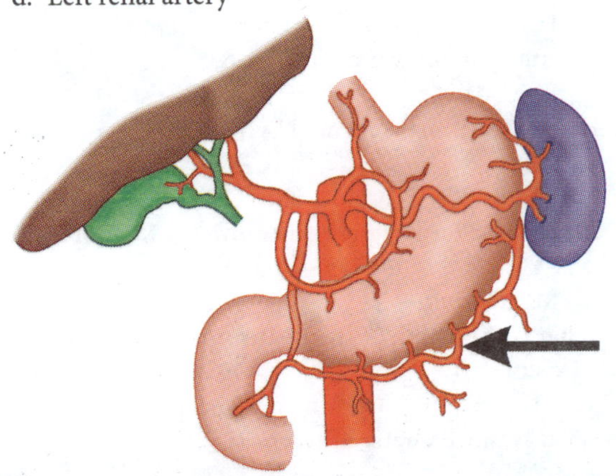

270. Tail of pancreas is present in:
(Recent Pattern Question 2018-19)
a. Gastrosplenic ligament
b. Splenorenal ligament
c. Hepatogastric ligament
d. Gastroduodenal ligament

271. Sternum attached to scapula via:
(Recent Pattern Question 2018-19)
a. Manubrium
b. First rib
c. Second rib
d. Clavicle

272. Vasa Brevia is the name of:
(Recent Pattern Question 2018-19)
a. Long gastric arteries
b. Short gastric arteries
c. Duodenal arteries
d. Renal arteries

273. Identify the part of duodenum marked below:
(Recent Pattern Question 2018)
a. 1st part
b. 2nd part
c. 3rd part
d. 4th part

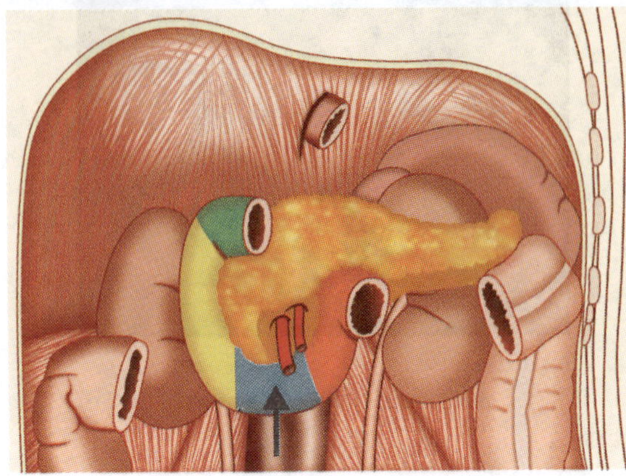

274. Cords of billroth in spleen are found in:
(Recent Pattern Question 2018)
a. White pulp
b. Trabecular zone
c. Red pulp
d. Mantle zone

275. Which is the water shed area of inferior mesenteric artery and internal iliac artery? *(Recent Pattern Question 2017)*
a. Griffith's point
b. Sigmoid colon
c. Ano rectal junction
d. Sudeck's point

276. Portal vein starts at level of____?
(Recent Pattern Question 2017)
a. L2
b. L3
c. L4
d. L5

277. Which is not a derivative of dorsal mesogastrium?
(Recent Pattern Question 2017)
a. Greater omentum
b. Gastrosplenic ligament
c. Gastro-phrenic ligament
d. Coronary ligament

278. Which of the following is not a part of pancreatic bed?
(Recent Pattern Question 2017)
a. Splenic vein
b. Right suprarenal gland
c. Aorta
d. Left crus of diaphragm

279. Smallest branch of celiac artery is:
(Recent Pattern Question 2017)
a. Right gastric artery
b. Splenic artery
c. Left gastric artery
d. Cystic artery

280. Constriction of diaphragm will not cause constriction of which opening: *(Recent Pattern Question 2016)*
a. Aortic opening
b. Esophageal opening
c. IVC opening
d. Thoracic duct aperture

281. Identify the intestinal segment:

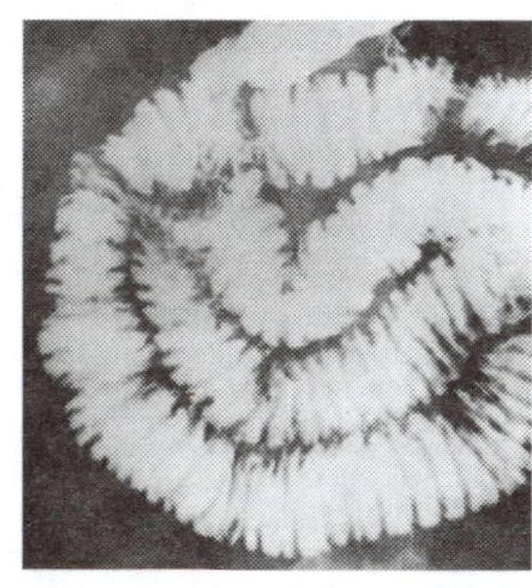

a. Ileum b. Jejunum
c. Caecum d. Large intestine

282. Shape of left adrenal gland:

a. Oval b. Semilunar
c. Triangular d. Trapezoid

283. All of the following form boundary of Left supra renal gland; EXCEPT:

a. Greater sac of stomach forms anterior border
b. Psoas major forms posterior border
c. Spleen forms anterolateral border
d. Left kidney forms inferior border

284. What is the weight of adrenal gland?

a. 4 grams b. 8 grams
c. 10 grams d. 15 grams

285. Aortic hiatus pierces diaphragm at what level?

a. T 8 b. T10
c. T11 d. T12

286. Structures passing through aortic opening in diaphragm are all; EXCEPT:

a. Aorta b. Azygous vein
c. Thoracic duct d. Vagus nerve

287. Right phrenic nerve passes through this diaphragmatic opening:

a. Aortic opening b. Caval opening
c. Esophageal opening d. Phrenic nerve opening

288. Structures passing through esophageal opening are all; EXCEPT:

a. Esophagus b. Phrenic nerve
c. Vagus nerve d. Gastric artery branches

289. Which of the following structure does not pass through diaphragm?

a. Aorta b. IVC
c. Esophagus d. Cisterna chyli

290. All of the following vessels are valveless; EXCEPT:

a. Inferior vena cava b. Superior vena cana
c. Pulmonary vein d. Internal jugular vein

291. Which of the follwing vessel has value to prevent bach-flow of blood.:

a. Internal jugular vein b. Portal vein
c. Superior vena cava d. Inferior vena cava

292. All are muscular arteries; EXCEPT?

a. Aorta b. Femoral artery
c. Popliteal artery d. Splenic artery

293. Inferior vena cava is formed at which level:

a. L2 b. L3
c. L4 d. L5

294. Portal vein forms at which vertebral level?

a. L1 b. L5
c. S1 d. S5

295. Brunner glands are seen in:

a. Duodenum b. Esophagus
c. Cardia of stomach d. Small intestine

296. Brunner's gland in the duodenum secretes:

a. Mucinus alkaline b. Acid
c. Pepsin d. Gastrin

297. All of the following form visceral relation of spleen; EXCEPT:

a. Fundus of stomach b. Left kidney
c. Splenic flexure of colon d. Duodenum

298. Which of the following forms the posterior wall of kidney?

a. Latissimus dorsi b. Quadratus lumborum
c. Transverse abdominis d. External oblique

299. Which of the following is not in anterior relationship with left kidney?

a. Jejunal flexure b. Splenic flexure
c. Head of pancreas d. Left suprarenal gland

300. Which of these is present anterior to right kidney:

a. Suprarenal gland b. Right colic flexure
c. Intestinal looping d. Duodenum 2nd part

301. Which of the following structure will affect or stop the ascent of kidney in fetal development?

a. Superior mesenteric artery
b. Inferior mesenteric artery
c. Left splenic vein
d. Celiac trunk

302. Kidney cortex contains:

a. Loop of henle
b. Pyramids
c. Collecting tubule and duct
d. Calyces

303. Which is the longest part of duodenum?

a. First part b. Second part
c. Third part d. Fourth part

304. Which of the following is dermatome of umbilicus:

a. T8 b. T10
c. T12 d. L1

305. Commonest position of the appendix is:

a. Paracecal b. Retrocecal
c. Pelvic d. Subcecal

306. Which is the least common position of appendix?

a. Retroceacal b. Preileal
c. Postileal d. Pelvic

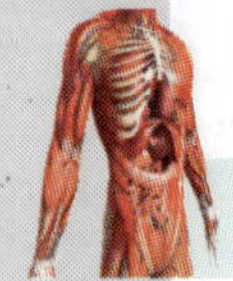

307. All are tributaries of portal vein; EXCEPT:
- a. Left gastric vein
- b. Right gastric vein
- c. Inferior pancreatoduodenal vein
- d. Superior mesenteric vein

308. Which are the correct boundaries of Calot triangle?
- a. Cystic artery, liver, right hepatic duct
- b. Cystic duct, liver, common hepatic duct
- c. Cystic duct, liver, cystic artery
- d. Common bile duct, cystic duct, liver

309. Superior boundary of calot's triangle is formed by:
- a. Hepatic duct
- b. Superior surface of liver
- c. Inferior surface of liver
- d. Cystic duct

310. All of the structures pass through Calot's triangle; EXCEPT:
- a. Portal vein
- b. Cystic artery
- c. Right hepatic artery
- d. Lymph node of Lund

311. Structures at the transpyloric plane include all; EXCEPT:
- a. Fundus of gallbladder
- b. Termination of portal vein
- c. Hilum of kidneys
- d. Pylorus of stomach

312. Which is true regarding portal venous system?
- a. Whole system is valve less
- b. Valves are present at the junction of superior mesenteric artery and splenic artery
- c. Valves are present in the intrahepatic system
- d. There are about 10–12 valves along the entire course

313. Chief cells are found in which area of stomach?
- a. Fundus
- b. Pit
- c. Neck
- d. Body

314. Average weight of spleen in adult:
- a. 5 ounce
- b. 7 ounce
- c. 14 ounce
- d. 21 ounce

315. Which is the most mobile part of rectum?
- a. Upper 1/3rd
- b. Middle 1/3rd
- c. Lower 1/3rd
- d. Lower 2/3rd

316. What is the length of rectum?
- a. 5 cm
- b. 12 cm
- c. 15 cm
- d. 20 cm

317. Which of the following is not in posterior relationship to rectum?
- a. Sacral vertebra
- b. Superior rectal artery
- c. Seminal vesicles
- d. Middle rectal artery

318. Opening of anal epithelium is made up of:
- a. Squamous cell
- b. Columnar
- c. Transitional
- d. Cuboidal

319. The puborectalis covers anorectal angle:
- a. Completely
- b. Anteriorly
- c. Posteriorly
- d. Laterally

320. All of the following arteries supply pancreas; EXCEPT:
- a. Gastroduodenal artery
- b. Superior mesenteric artery
- c. Inferior mesenteric artery
- d. Pancreatic branch of splenic artery

321. Which of the following is *not* a ventral branch of abdominal aorta?
- a. Gonadal artery
- b. Celiac trunk
- c. Superior mesenteric artery
- d. Inferior mesenteric artery

322. All of the following are branches of external iliac artery; EXCEPT:
- a. Femoral artery
- b. Deep circumflex artery
- c. Inferior epigastric artery
- d. Gonadal artery

NEUROANATOMY, HEAD AND NECK

323. Name the dural venous sinus arrow marked in the radiograph: ***(Most Recent Question June 2022)***

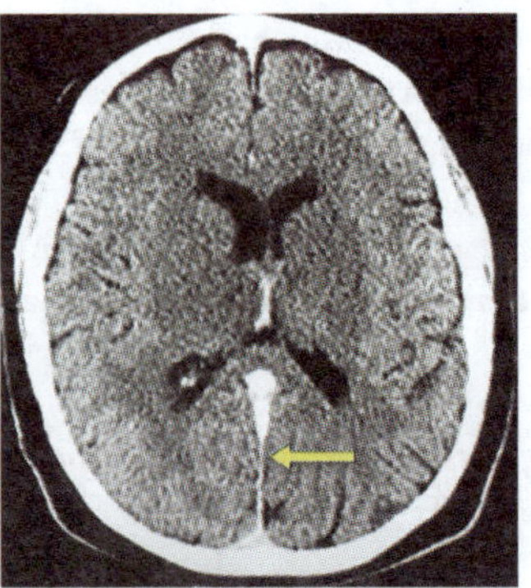

- a. Straight sinus
- b. Superior sagittal sinus
- c. Inferior sagittal sinus
- d. Confluence of sinuses

324. Identify the arrow marked structure in the radiograph: ***(Most Recent Question June 2022)***

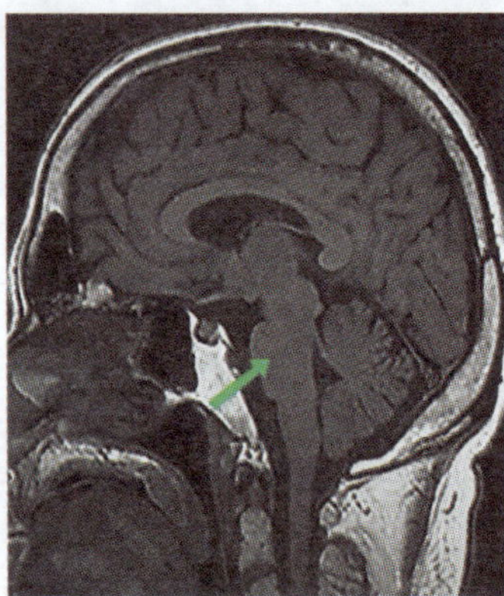

- a. Midbrain
- b. Pons
- c. Medulla oblongata
- d. Spinal cord

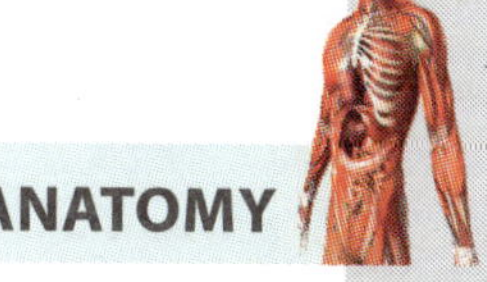

325. In unilateral hypoglossal nerve lesion, position of tongue on protrusion is: *(Most Recent Question June 2022)*

a. Midline
b. Deviates to ipsilateral side
c. Deviates to contralateral side
d. No protrusion possible

326. Identify the muscle shown in the figure below: *(Most Recent Question June/Dec 2021)*

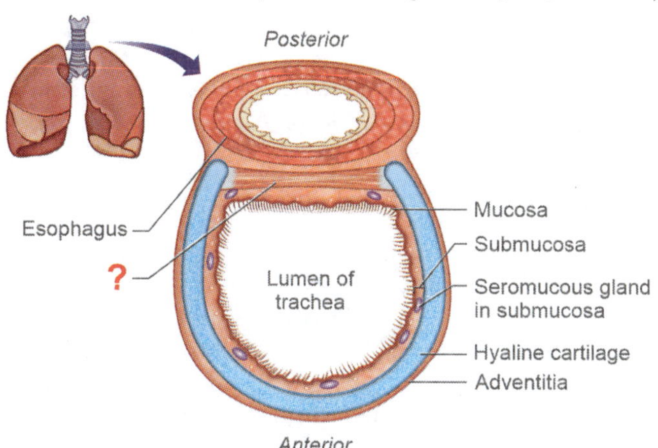

a. Interarytenoid
b. Longitudinal muscle of oesophagus
c. Circular muscle of oesophagus
d. Trachealis

327. A patient presented where physician noted that all extraocular muscles have been paralyzed. The most probable level of lesion is: *(Most Recent Question June/Dec 2021)*

a. Midbrain
b. Pons
c. Upper medulla
d. Lower medulla

328. The marked structure is: *(Most Recent Question June/Dec 2021)*

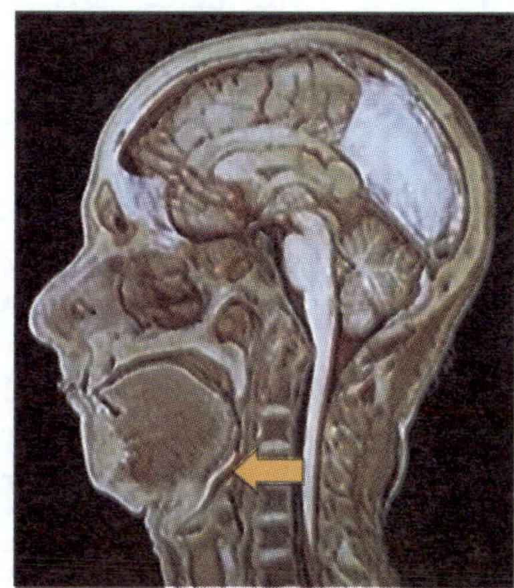

a. Epiglottis b. Uvula
c. Glottis d. Tongue

329. Termination of spinal cord in a newborn lies at which vertebral level: *(Most Recent Question June/Dec 2021)*

a. Lower borer of L1 b. Lower border of L2
c. Lower border of L3 d. Lower border of S2

330. Identify the muscle marked 'X' in the given image: *(Most Recent Question June/Dec 2021)*

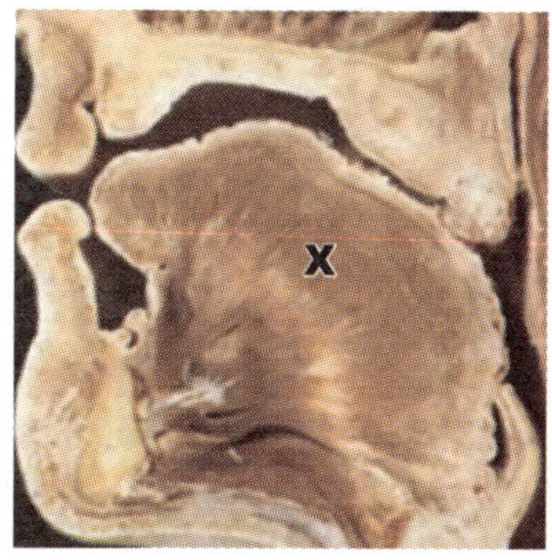

a. Styloglossus b. Genioglossus
c. Hyoglossus d. Palatoglossus

331. All are paired cartilages; EXCEPT: *(Most Recent Question June/Dec 2021)*

a. Arytenoid b. Corniculate
c. Thyroid d. Cuneiform

332. Which of the following is an abductor of vocal cords? *(Most Recent Question June/Dec 2021)*

a. Posterior cricoarytenoid b. Lateral cricoarytenoid
c. Cricothyroid d. Thyroarytenoid

333. All of the following are true; EXCEPT: *(Most Recent Question June/Dec 2021)*

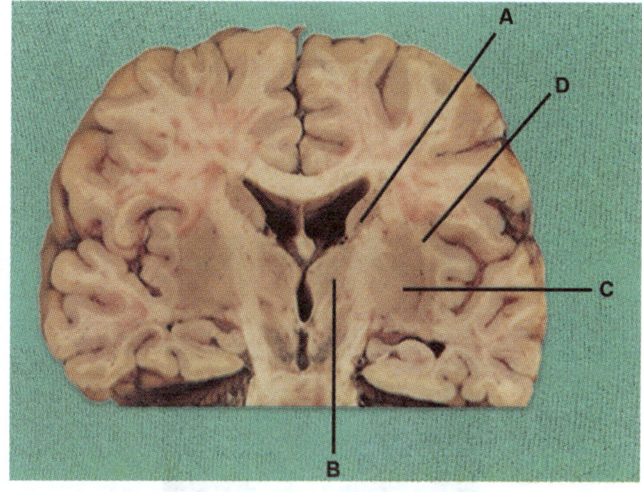

a. A – Caudate nucleus b. B – Thalamus
c. C- Lentiform nucleus d. D- Internal capsule

334. Corticospinal tract crosses at the level of: *(Most Recent Question June/Dec 2021)*

a. Midbrain b. Pons
c. Upper medulla d. Lower medulla

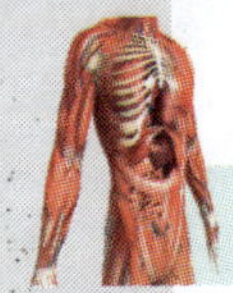

335. Killian's dehiscence is seen between: *(Most Recent Question June/Dec 2021)*
a. Coricopharyngeus and thyropharyngeus
b. Stylopharyngeus and palatopharyngeus
c. Palatopharyngeus and salpingopharyngeus
d. Stylopharyngeus and salpingopharyngeus

336. Which of the following is the safety muscle of tongue? *(Most Recent Question Dec 2020)*
a. Genioglossus b. Hyoglossus
c. Palatoglossus d. Styloglossus

337. Lacrimal gland is supplied through parasympathetic system. It is supplied by which ganglion? *(Most Recent Question Dec 2020)*
a. Ciliary ganglia b. Otic ganglia
c. Pterygopalatine d. Submandibular

338. The structure which doesn't pass through the parotid gland? *(Most Recent Question Dec 2020)*
a. Facial nerve
b. Internal carotid artery
c. Branch of external carotid artery
d. Retromandibular vein

339. Protraction of jaw is due to which of the following muscle? *(Most Recent Question Dec 2020)*
a. Serratus anterior b. Pectoralis major
c. Pectoralis minor d. Lateral pterygoid

340. Middle meningeal artery is branch of: *(Most Recent Question Dec 2020)*
a. Maxillary artery b. Mandibular
c. Facial artery d. Ophthalmic artery

341. The muscle which is required to open eustachian tube: *(Most Recent Question Dec 2020)*
a. Tensor veli palatini muscle
b. Salpingo pharengeous
c. Tensor veli tympani
d. Levator veli palatini

342. Identify the structure marked with arrow: *(Most Recent Question Aug 2020)*

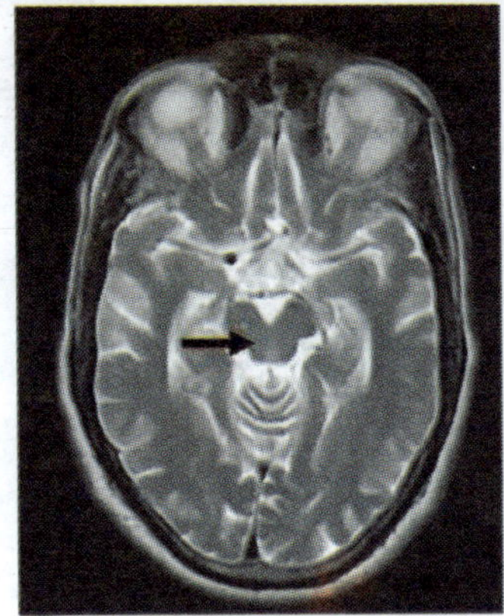

a. Midbrain b. Pons
c. Medulla oblongata d. Spinal cord

343. Killian dehiscence is formed due to: *(Most Recent Question 2019)*
a. Superior constrictor muscle
b. Inferior constrictor muscle
c. Middle pharyngeal constrictor muscle
d. Esophageal fibers

344. Glossopharyngeal nerve supplies which of the following gland? *(Most Recent Question 2019)*
a. Parotid gland b. Submandibular gland
c. Sublingual gland d. Lacrimal gland

345. Which branch of facial nerve supplies muscles of lower lip? *(Recent Pattern Question 2018-19)*
a. Temporal branch
b. Cervical branch
c. Buccal branch
d. Mandibular branch

346. Lower lip blood supply: *(Recent Pattern Question 2018-19)*
a. Angular artery b. Lateral nasal artery
c. Labial artery d. Greater palatine artery

347. Landmark of facial nerve in parotid gland: *(Recent Pattern Question 2018-19)*
a. Tragal pointer
b. Anterior belly of digastric muscle
c. Helical point
d. Suprameatal triangle

348. Trismus is due to spasm of which muscle? *(Recent Pattern Question 2018-19)*
a. Orbiculis
b. Lateral pterygoid
c. Mentalis
d. Medial pterygoid

349. Accessory muscle of mastication: *(Recent Pattern Question 2018-19)*
a. Risorius b. Orbicularis oris
c. Buccinator d. Platysma

350. Parotid duct opens into: *(Recent Pattern Question 2018-19)*
a. First mandibular molar
b. First maxillary pre-molar
c. Second mandibular molar
d. Second maxillary molar

351. Mammillary body projects via: *(Recent Pattern Question 2018-19)*
a. Thalamus b. Corpus callosum
c. Pituitary gland d. Fornix

352. Which structure connects the Broca's area and Wernicke area? *(Recent Pattern Question 2018-19)*
a. Arcuate fasciculus b. Anterior commissure
c. Corpus callosum d. Fornix

353. The nerve passing through cavernous sinus: *(Recent Pattern Question 2018)*
a. Optic nerve b. Olfactory
c. Abducens d. Facial

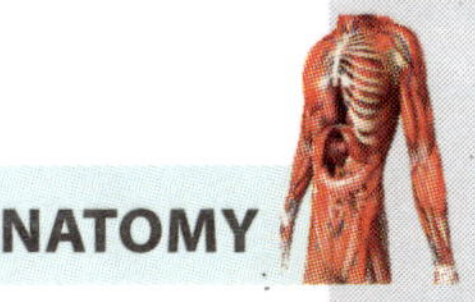

354. The blood supply of abdominal part of esophagus: *(Recent Pattern Question 2018)*
a. Bronchial vein and arch of aorta
b. Right gastric artery
c. Left gastric artery
d. Pulmonary trunk

355. Most medially located nuclei of cerebellum is: *(Recent Pattern Question 2018)*
a. Putamen b. Lentiform
c. Caudate d. Fastigii

356. Which cranial nerve supplies lateral rectus muscle? *(Recent Pattern Question 2017)*
a. Trochlear b. Trigeminal
c. Abducens d. Glossopharyngeal

357. Blood supply of spinal cord is _______ spinal arteries? *(Recent Pattern Question 2017)*
a. 1 anterior and 2 posterior
b. 2 anterior and 1 posterior
c. 2 anterior and 2 posterior
d. 1 anterior and 1 posterior

358. Anterior 2/3rd of spinal cord is supplied by: *(Recent Pattern Question 2017)*
a. Anterior choroidal artery
b. Anterior communicating artery
c. Anterior cerebral artery
d. Anterior spinal artery

359. Which muscle is attached to the temporal bone? *(Recent Pattern Question 2017)*
a. Stapedius muscle b. Postauricular muscle
c. Tensor tympani muscle d. Digastric muscle

360. Ipsilateral deviation of tongue occurs due to which intact tongue muscle? *(Recent Pattern Question 2017)*
a. Palatoglossus b. Styloglossus
c. Genioglossus d. Pharyngoglossus

361. Arteria thyroidea ima originates from: *(Recent Pattern Question 2017)*
a. External carotid artery b. Thyrocervical trunk
c. Vertebral artery d. Arch of aorta

362. Thyroid gland is situated at the level of: *(Recent Pattern Question 2017)*
a. C4-C8 b. C4-T1
c. C5-T1 d. C6-T2

363. How many lobes are present in cerebellum? *(Recent Pattern Question 2017)*
a. 2 b. 4
c. 6 d. 8

364. Which is the smallest lobe of cerebellum? *(Recent Pattern Question 2017)*
a. Flocculonodular lobe
b. Lingular lobe
c. Pyramidal lobe
d. Archicerebellum

365. Vertebral artery is derived from: *(Recent Pattern Question 2017)*
a. First part of subclavian artery
b. Second part of subclavian artery
c. Third part of subclavian artery
d. Fourth part of subclavian artery

366. Which of the following is a branch of 3rd part of subclavian artery? *(Recent Pattern Question 2017)*
a. Thyrocervical trunk b. Dorsal scapular artery
c. Vertebral artery d. Internal thoracic artery

367. Cavernous sinus is a collection of venous sinuses on either side of pituitary. Which of the following does not pass through the lateral wall of the cavernous sinus? *(Recent Pattern Question 2017)*
a. CN III
b. CN V2
c. Post ganglionic sympathetic fibers
d. Internal carotid artery

368. Anterior inferior cerebellar artery is a branch of: *(Recent Pattern Question 2017)*
a. Subclavian artery b. Vertebral artery
c. Basilar artery d. Middle cerebral artery

369. Smallest branch of external carotid artery is: *(Recent Pattern Question 2017)*
a. Superior thyroid artery
b. Ascending pharyngeal artery
c. Facial artery
d. Maxillary artery

370. Subarachnoid space extends up to: *(Recent Pattern Question 2017)*
a. Lower border L1
b. Upper border L1
c. Upper border of S2
d. Lower border of S2

371. Which of the following cranial nerve carries parasympathetic fibers? *(Recent Pattern Question 2017)*
a. CN 1 b. CN 2
c. CN 3 d. CN 4

372. Which of the following cranial nerve is a pure sensory nerve? *(Recent Pattern Question 2017)*
a. CN 3 b. CN 5
c. CN 8 d. CN 9

373. Leptomeninges is formed by: *(Recent Pattern Question 2017)*
a. Dura mater and Arachnoid
b. Arachnoid and pia mater
c. Dura and pia mater
d. Dura, arachnoid and pia matter

374. Sylvian fissure separates: *(Recent Pattern Question 2017)*
a. Temporal lobe from occipital lobe
b. Temporal lobe from frontoparietal areas
c. Temporal lobe from opposite frontal lobe
d. Temporal lobe from cerebellum

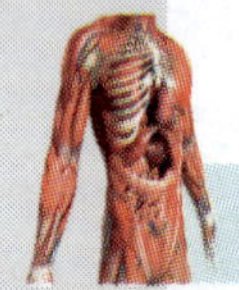

375. Superior vena cava is formed by fusion of__________: *(Recent Pattern Question 2017)*
a. Internal and external jugular veins
b. Subclavian and internal jugular veins
c. Left and right brachiocephalic veins
d. Left and right common iliac veins

376. Which is these is a Bi-condylar joint? *(Recent Pattern Question 2017)*
a. TM joint
b. Atlanto-occipital
c. Interphalangeal
d. Intermetatarsal joint

377. Which structure is not transmitted by foramen ovale? *(Recent Pattern Question 2017)*
a. Middle meningeal artery
b. Accessory meningeal artery
c. Lesser petrosal nerve
d. Emissary vein

378. Maxillary nerve is transmitted via: *(Recent Pattern Question 2017)*
a. Foramen ovale
b. Foramen rotundum
c. Foramen lacerum
d. Foramen spinosum

379. Foramen transversarium is found at: *(Recent Pattern Question 2017)*
a. Anterior cranial fossa
b. Middle cranial fossa
c. Posterior cranial fossa
d. Cervical vertebra

380. Nerve carrying taste sensation from anterior 2/3rd of tongue is called: *(Recent Pattern Question 2017)*
a. Arnold nerve
b. Jacobson nerve
c. Criminal nerve of grassi
d. Nerve of wrisberg

381. Which of the following areas of the brain is not a primary sensory cortex? *(Recent Pattern Question 2017)*
a. 1
b. 2
c. 3
d. 4

382. Which is a part of limbic system: *(Recent Pattern Question 2017)*
a. Corpus callosum
b. Pineal gland
c. Cingulate gyrus
d. Tegmentum

383. Nucleus ambiguus is composed of: *(Recent Pattern Question 2017)*
a. Sensory to 9, 10, 11 cranial nerve nucleus
b. Motor to 9, 10, 11 cranial nerve nucleus
c. Sensory to 7, 9, 10 cranial nerve nucleus
d. Motor to 7, 9, 10 cranial nerve nucleus

384. IInd cranial nerve is: *(Recent Pattern Question 2017)*
a. Optic nerve
b. Abducens nerve
c. Trigeminal nerve
d. Occulomotor nerve

385. Lower one-third of auricle is supplied by:
a. Auriculotemporal nerve
b. Vagus nerve
c. Greater auricular nerve
d. Greater retrasal nerve

386. All are related to facial nerve; EXCEPT:
a. Maxillary process
b. Stylomastoid foramen
c. Posterior belly of diagstric muscle
d. Parotid gland

387. Parotid duct opens:
a. Opposite to lower 1st molar tooth
b. Opposite to lower 2nd molar tooth
c. In floor of mouth
d. In relation with upper 2nd molar tooth

388. Which of the following is not a test for integrity of 7th and 9th nerve:
a. Position of uvula
b. Palate symmetry
c. Deviation of tongue
d. Taste sensation of anterior 2/3rd of tongue

389. Opening of mouth is caused by:
a. Lateral pterygoid
b. Medial pterygoid
c. Temporalis
d. Masseter

390. Sensory supply to anterior 2/3rd of tongue given by:
a. Facial nerve
b. Trigeminal nerve
c. Hypoglossal nerve
d. Glossopharyngeal nerve

391. Taste sensation is not carried by:
a. CN V
b. CN VII
c. CN IX
d. CN XI

392. Taste sensation from mucosal membranes of oral side of tongue is carried by:
a. Lingual nerve
b. Vagus nerve
c. Hypoglossal nerve
d. Glossopharyngeal nerve

393. What is the site of lesion affecting cranial nerve VI, VII and VIII?
a. Pons
b. Midbrain
c. Medulla
d. Junction between pons and medulla

394. Which of the following cranial nerve decussate within the brain?
a. Optic
b. Occulomator
c. Trochlear
d. Trigeminal

395. Which cranial nerve has the largest intracranial course?
a. Vagus nerve
b. Oculomotor nerve
c. Trochlear nerve
d. Abducens nerve

396. Which of the following nerve is known as criminal nerve of grassi?
a. Hypoglossal nerve
b. Trigeminal nerve
c. Thyroglossal nerve
d. Vagus nerve

397. Which nerve pierces the thyroid gland?
a. Superior laryngeal nerve
b. Inferior laryngeal nerve
c. Recurrent laryngeal nerve
d. Posterior laryngeal nerve

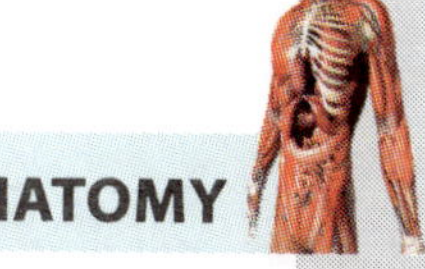

398. All of the following structures pass through superior orbital fissure; EXCEPT:
a. Inferial ophthalmic vein b. Lacrimal nerve
c. Trigeminal nerve d. Nasociliary nerve

399. Which cranial nerve is not transmitted by superior orbital fissure? ***(Recent Pattern Question 2017)***
a. 2 b. 3
c. 4 d. 5

400. Which is the following structure passes through the lateral part of superior orbital fissure?
a. Superior ophthalmic vein
b. Inferior ophthalmic vein
c. Abducent nerve
d. Nasociliary nerve

401. All these nerves pass through superior orbital fissure; EXCEPT?
a. Mandibular nerve b. Abducens nerve
c. Trochlear nerve d. Oculomotor nerve

402. Which of the following structure passes through inferior orbital fissure?
a. Infraorbital nerve b. Infraorbital artery
c. Both d. None

403. Which of the following causes injury to cranial nerve 3rd, 4th and 1st branch of CN 5?
a. Sphenoid bone tumor b. Parotid gland tumor
c. Petrous bone tumor d. Acoustic neuroma

404. What is the root value of phrenic nerve?
a. C2, C3, C4 b. C4, C5, T1
c. C3, C4, C5 d. C5, T1, T2

405. Which of the following is the most common congenital anomaly?
a. Cleft lip
b. Cleft palate
c. Cleft lip and cleft palate both
d. None

406. Which is the dangerous layer of scalp?
a. Subcutaneous layer
b. Musculoapneurotic layer
c. Loose subaponeurotic layer
d. Periosteum layer

407. Which of the following layer of scalp is made up of a tough layer of dense fibrous tissue:
a. Subcutaneous layer
b. Musculoaponeurotic layer
c. Loose subaponeurotic layer
d. Galea aponeurotica

408. Medial wall of orbit is formed by which bone:
a. Lesser wing of sphenoid
b. Frontal process of maxilla
c. Greater wing of sphenoid
d. Arterial and posterior ethmoidal canals

409. Which of the following nerve supplies the muscles of palate?
a. Hypoglossal nerve b. Greater palatine nerve
c. Glossopharyngeal nerve d. Trigeminal nerve

410. Safety muscle of tongue is?
a. Genioglossus b. Palatoglossus
c. Styloglossus d. Hyoglossus

411. Safety muscle of larynx is:
a. Aryepiglotticus b. Cricoarytenoid
c. Thyroarytenoid d. Posterior cricoarytenoid

412. At the end of C6 which is not true:
a. Trachea bifurcates b. Pharynx ends
c. Esophagus begins d. Larynx ends

413. Adult larynx extends between cervical spine:
a. C_7 to T_1 b. C_2 to C_3
c. C_3 to C_4 d. C_3 to C_6

414. Anterior fontannel corresponds to all; EXCEPT:
a. Frontal bones b. Coronal suture
c. Lambdoid suture d. Saggital suture

415. Which is not a T.M. joint ligament?
a. Temporomandibular
b. Sphenomandibular
c. Stylomandibular ligament
d. Tympanomandibular

416. What is the location of Hyoid bone in terms of cervical vertebral level:
a. C2 b. C3
c. C4 d. C5

417. What is the level of Isthmus of the thyroid gland across tracheal ring?
a. 3rd to 5th b. 2nd to 4th
c. 5th to 6th d. 2nd to 3rd

418. Which of the following artery supplies parathyroid glands?
a. Superior thyroid artery b. Inferior thyroid artery
c. Common carotid artery d. Middle thyroid artery

419. Which of the following is not a part of lower motor neuron?
a. Anterior nerve root b. Peripheral ganglia
c. Peripheral nerve d. Anterior horn cells

420. All of the following are pneumatic bones; EXCEPT:
a. Maxilla b. Frontal
c. Mandible d. Ethmoid

421. Which of the following is a pneumatic bone?
a. Tibia b. Frontal bone
c. Clavicle d. Femur

422. Gustatory cortex is situated in:
a. Superior temporal gyrus b. Inferior frontal gyrus
c. Superior frontal gyrus d. Inferior parietal gyrus

423. Maximum contribution to the floor of orbit is by which bone?
a. Maxillary b. Zygomatic
c. Sphenoid d. Palatine

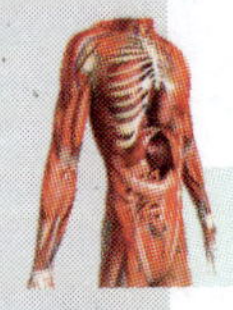

424. Angular vein infection causes thrombosis in:
a. Cavernous sinus
b. Suprasaggital sinus
c. Transverse sinus
d. Inferior petrosal sinus

425. Left spinal leminiscus contains which fibers?
a. Left sided pain, touch, temperature
b. Left sided position, vibration sense
c. Right sided pain, touch, temperature
d. Right sided position, vibration sense

426. All of the following muscles are attached to the apex of orbit; EXCEPT:
a. Superior oblique
b. Superior rectus
c. Medial rectus
d. Inferior oblique

427. Which nerve helps in looking laterally and downward:
a. Abducent
b. Trochlear
c. Trigeminal
d. Occulomotor

428. All of the following are parts of nasal septum; EXCEPT:
a. Septal cartilage
b. Lateral cartilage
c. Crest of maxilla
d. Peripendicular plate of ethmoid

429. Which is not a part of basal ganglia?
a. Caudate nucleus
b. Thalamus
c. Lenticular nucleus
d. Globus pallidus

430. Cerebellar cortex contains:
a. Pyramidal cells
b. Purkinje cells
c. Stromal cells
d. Kupffer cells

431. Cerebellar connection to other parts of the brain is projected through which cell?
a. Golgi cells
b. Basket cells
c. Purkinje cells
d. Oligodendrocytes

432. In adults, the spinal cord normally ends at:
a. Lower border of L1
b. Lower border of L3
c. Lower border of L5
d. Lower border of S1

433. The spinal cord in infants ends at the level of:
a. L1
b. L2
c. L3
d. L4

434. Which nerve passes from paraphyrangeal space?
a. VI
b. VII
c. VIII
d. X

435. Which of the following tracts is seen in the posterior column of spinal cord?
a. Lateral spinothalamic tract
b. Fasciculus gracilis
c. Rubrospinal tract
d. Posterior spinocerebellar

436. Which is the most prominent spinous process?
a. T1
b. C7
c. C6
d. L5

437. The movement at the following joint permits a person to say NO by head movement:
a. Atlanto-occipital joint
b. Atlantoaxial joint
c. C2-C3 joint
d. C3-C4 joint

438. 'Chassaignac's tubercle' is:
a. Erb's point
b. Carotid tubercle on C6 vertebra
c. Found on first rib
d. Medial condyle of humerus

PELVIS AND PERINEUM

439. Injury to bulbar urethra leads to extravasation of urine in all; EXCEPT: ***(Most Recent Question June/Dec 2021)***
a. Deep perineal pouch
b. Superficial perineal pouch
c. Scrotum
d. Thigh

440. Which of the following muscle is attached to the arrow marked structure? ***(Most Recent Question Dec 2020)***

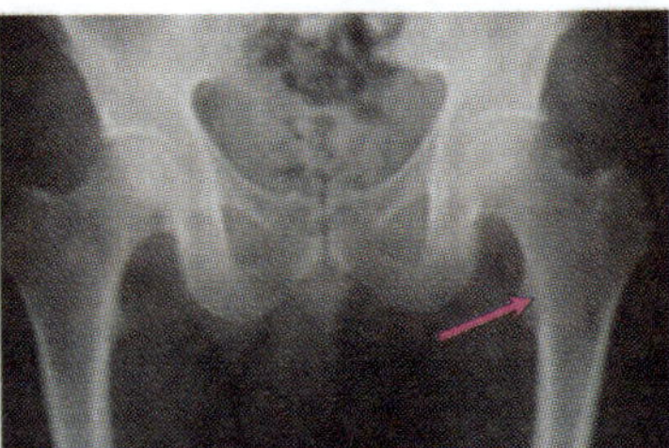

a. Gluteus maximus
b. Gluteus medius
c. Gluteus minimus
d. Iliopsoas

441. Identify the arrow marked joint in the given image: ***(Most Recent Question Dec 2020)***

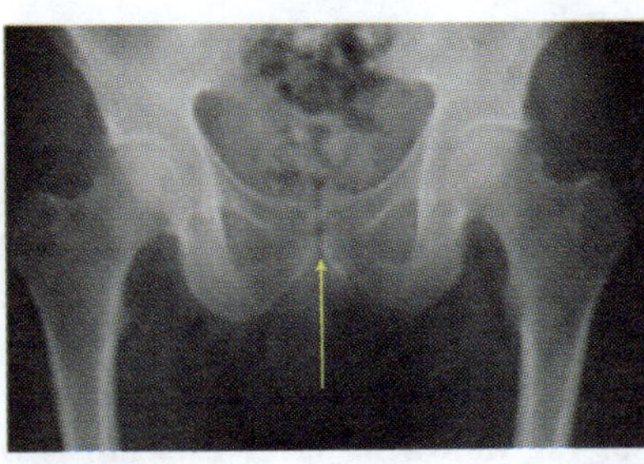

a. Syndesmosis
b. Primary cartilaginous joint
c. Secondary cartilaginous joint
d. Synchondrosis

442. Trigone of bladder is derived from: ***(Most Recent Question Dec 2020)***
a. Distal part of paramesonephric duct
b. Distal part of mesonephric duct
c. Ventral part of mesonephric duct
d. Ventral part of urogenital sinus

443. Identify the marked structure:
(Most Recent Question Dec 2020)

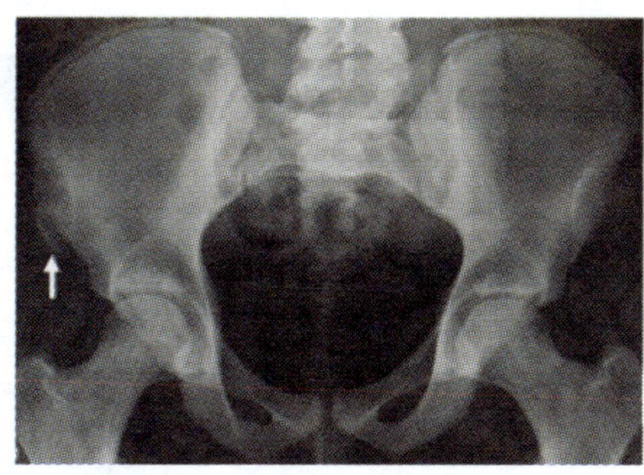

a. Anterior superior iliac spine
b. Anterior inferior iliac spine
c. Ischial tuberosity
d. Pubic symphysis

444. Highest point of iliac crest is seen at:
(Most Recent Question Dec 2020)

a. L3 b. L4
c. S1 d. S2

445. Which type of joint is present at the arrow mark shown in the diagram (encircled):
(Most Recent Question Aug 2020)

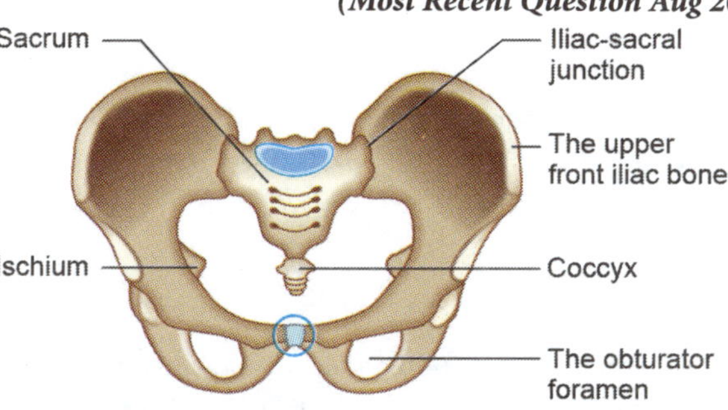

a. Primary cartilaginous b. Secondary cartilaginous
c. Fibrous d. Synovial

446. Deep inguinal ring is a defect in:
(Most Recent Question Aug 2020)

a. External oblique muscle aponeurosis
b. Internal oblique muscle aponeurosis
c. Transversus abdominal muscle aponeurosis
d. Transversalis fascia

447. Deep inguinal ring is formed in:
(Most Recent Question 2019)

a. Transversus abdominis
b. Transversalis fascia
c. External oblique aponeurosis
d. Internal oblique aponeurosis

448. Inguinal ligament is formed due to:
(Most Recent Question 2019)

a. External oblique aponeurosis
b. Transversus abdominis
c. Internal oblique aponeurosis
d. Inguinal muscle

449. The patient is having bleeding from hemorrhoids. Which of the following artery is the source of bleeding?
(Recent Pattern Question 2018-19)

a. Superior rectal vein b. Superior rectal artery
c. Middle rectal artery d. Middle rectal vein

450. Blood supply of bulb of the penis:
(Recent Pattern Question 2018)

a. Scrotal artery
b. Superficial pudendal artery
c. Bulbourethral artery
d. Bulbocavernosus artery

451. Cremasteric muscle nerve supply:
(Recent Pattern Question 2018)

a. Ilioinguinal nerve
b. Iliohypogastric nerve
c. Genital branch of genitofemoral nerve
d. Femoral nerve

452. Which of the following is the artery for endometrial blood supply?
(Recent Pattern Question 2018)

a. Endometrial artery b. Myometrial artery
c. Spiral artery d. Cervical artery

453. Alcock's canal transmits:
(Recent Pattern Question 2017)

a. Pudendal nerve b. Epididymis
c. CN VIII d. Fallopian tube

454. Posterior superior iliac spine is at which level?
(Recent Pattern Question 2016)

a. S1 b. S2
c. L1 d. L2

455. Coccyx has how many vertebra:
(Recent Pattern Question 2016)

a. 1 b. 2
c. 3 d. 4

456. Muscles of the perineal body include all of the following; EXCEPT:

a. External anal sphincter
b. Iliococcygeus
c. Superficial transverse perinei
d. Bulbocavernosus

457. Structures forming perineal body are all; EXCEPT:

a. Levator ani muscle
b. Bulbospongiosus
c. Deep transverse perinei
d. Ischiococcygeus

458. Pelvic diaphragm is made of all; EXCEPT:

a. Iliococcygeus b. Ischiococcygeus
c. Pubococcygeus d. Puborectalis

459. Which is true regarding prostate gland?

a. Only glandular tissue
b. Glandular tissue covered with transitional epithelium
c. Glandular tissue and fibromuscular stroma
d. Entire gland is composed of collagen

460. What is the normal weight of uterus?

a. 20 g b. 40 g
c. 60 g d. 100 g

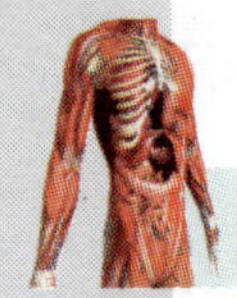

ANSWERS WITH EXPLANATIONS

MOST RECENT QUESTIONS 2023

1. Ans. (b) Lingual nerve

- The lingual nerve is a branch of the trigeminal nerve that supplies sensation to the anterior 2/3rd of the tongue and the floor of the mouth.
- Damage to the lingual nerve during tooth extraction can lead to sensory loss.
- This nerve runs alongside the lingual side of the mandible.
- Its injury can result in numbness in the tongue and floor of the mouth.

Extra Mile

- Hypoglossal nerve: Supplies the tongue with motor innervation.
- Accessory nerve: Supplies the sternocleidomastoid muscle and the trapezius muscle.
- Inferior alveolar nerve: Supplies sensation to the lower teeth and the lower lip.

2. Ans. (c) Anterior abdominal wall

Urethral Injury

Type	Deep extravasation	Superficial extravasation
Cause	Instrumentation - least dilatable part of the urethra Pelvic Fractures – RTA	Straddle-type injuries from falls or kicks
Area of spread	Upwards into the extraperitoneal space of the pelvis around bladder and prostate into the anterior abdominal wall	Between **perineal membrane** and the membranous layer of the superficial fascia **(Colles Fascia)** • Superficial perineal space • Scrotum • Penis • Lower part of the ant abdominal wall
Not spread to	Peritoneum	Ischioanal fossa or the thigh by the firm attachment of the membranous layer of superficial fascia
	Urinary bladder; Rupture of membranous part of urethra **FIGURE:** Extravasation of urine due to rupture of membranous urethra	Urinary bladder; Perineal body; Rupture of penile part of urethra; Scrotal sac; Penis **FIGURE:** Extravasation of urine due to rupture of penile urethra

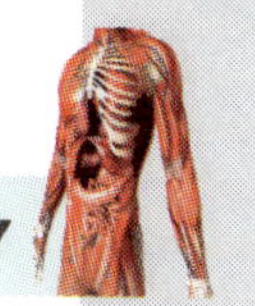

3. Ans. (b) Upper border of the lower rib

- Thoracentesis is done to remove pleural effusion fluid for diagnostic or therapeutic purposes. It is ultrasound guided procedure.
- The upper border of the lower rib is the safest site for needle insertion because it is the farthest away from the neurovascular bundle that travels below each rib.

4. Ans. (c) L4–L5

- The red-colored line in the image represents the location of the iliac crest, a prominent bony structure in the pelvic region. In most individuals, the iliac crest corresponds to the vertebral level of L4–L5.
- The lumbar vertebrae are numbered L1–L5. The line is located between the L4 and L5 vertebrae.
- Clinically, the iliac crest serves as an important anatomical landmark for various procedures, including lumbar punctures and the identification of lumbar vertebral levels.
- The L2–L3, L3–L4 vertebrae are located in the thoracic region of the spine.
- The L5–S1 vertebrae are located in the sacral region of the spine.

5. Ans. (b) B

- **Housemaid's knee, also known as prepatellar bursitis,** is an inflammation of the prepatellar bursa, which is a fluid-filled sac that lies in front of the kneecap.
- It is caused by repetitive kneeling, such as when scrubbing floors or doing housework.
- Option C infrapatellar bursa is located between the patella and the kneecap. It is a fluid-filled sac that helps to cushion the knee joint, and its inflammation is called clergyman knee.

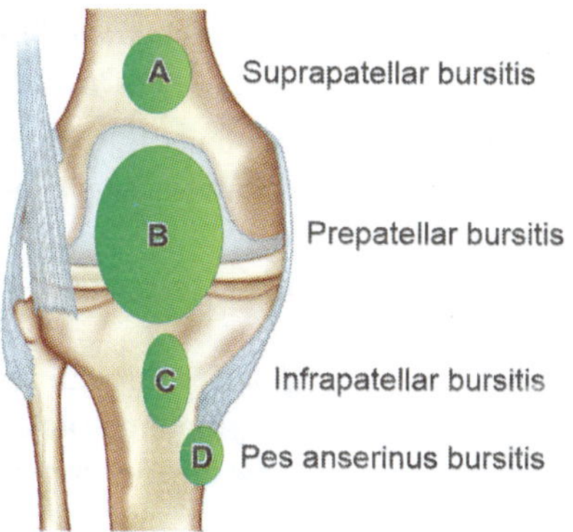

6. Ans. (b) Craniorachischisis

- The image shows both brain and spinal cord of body being malformed. This disease is a combination of anencephaly and myelomeningocele, and is called craniorachischisis.
- Meningomyelocele is a congenital defect in which the meninges and spinal cord protrude through a defect in the spine.
- Spina bifida occulta is can only be detected on X-ray of lumbosacral spine.

7. Ans. (b) Lateral femoral cutaneous nerve

- The lateral femoral cutaneous nerve is a sensory nerve supplying the skin of the anterolateral thigh.
- Post pregnancy, the nerve can be compressed due to stretching or pressure from the gravid uterus, leading to meralgia paresthetica, causing pain and sensory disturbances in this area.
- The femoral nerve primarily innervates the anterior thigh and lower leg, the obturator nerve supplies the medial thigh, and the tibial nerve covers the posterior thigh and leg.

Extra Mile

- **Femoral nerve:** Primarily supplies the anterior thigh and hip region.
- **Obturator nerve:** Innervates the medial thigh.
- **Tibial nerve:** Responsible for sensory and motor functions in the posterior thigh and leg.

8. Ans. (a) Biceps muscle rupture

- A biceps muscle rupture occurs when the tendon connecting the biceps muscle to the bone tears, leading to a bulging appearance in the upper arm known as the **"Popeye deformity."**
- This condition can result from excessive force, sudden contraction, or repeated strain on the biceps muscle and tendon.
- It is different from humerus shaft fractures, which involve break in the bone, radial nerve injuries, which can cause wrist drop, and tennis elbow, characterized by lateral epicondylitis.

9. Ans. (c) Facial nerve

- This constellation of symptoms is suggestive of facial nerve (cranial nerve VII) dysfunction.
- Facial nerve palsy can cause difficulty in closing the eye (eye closure muscles affected) and difficulty in eating (mouth muscles affected).
- Swelling below the ear could indicate involvement of the parotid gland, which innervates the facial nerve

10. Ans. (c) C

- Structure C corresponds to the phrenic nerve, which innervates the diaphragm.
- Irritation or compression of the phrenic nerve can lead to hiccups.

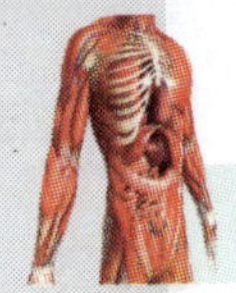

- The phrenic nerve originates from cervical spinal nerves and passes through the thoracic cavity, so aortic dissection involving the region could irritate it.

11. Ans. (d) Gastrulation

- Limbs are fused in the shown image, which is also called caudal dysgenesis (sirenomelia).
- Gastrulation is a critical early developmental process where the three primary germ layers (ectoderm, mesoderm, and endoderm) are formed.
- Disruptions in this process can lead to a variety of congenital anomalies like sirenomelia/caudal dysgenesis.

12. Ans. (b) 6 months

- The ossification of the talus bone typically begins around the 6th month of intrauterine life during fetal development.
- The talus bone is one of the early bones to start ossifying in the fetal skeleton.

13. Ans. (b) Internal capsule

Ref: Gray's Anatomy: The Anatomical Basis of Clinical Practice, 41st ed. pg. 365

- The arrow in the image points to the internal capsule, which is a prominent white matter structure in the brain that carries motor and sensory fibers to and from the cerebral cortex.
- The internal capsule separates the thalamus and the caudate nucleus from the lentiform nucleus.

Extra Mile

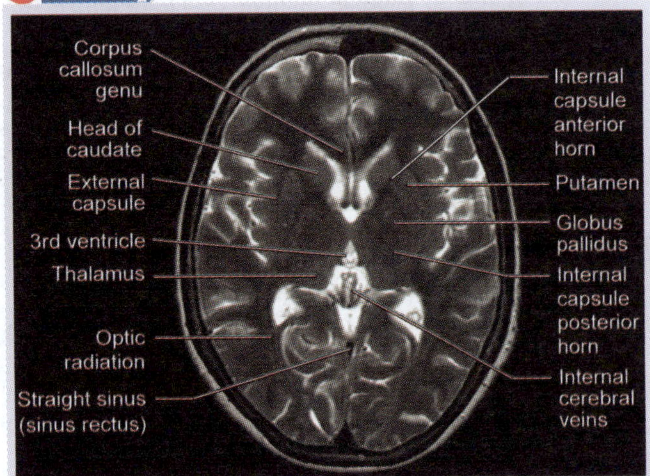

14. Ans. (a) Abnormal fusion of the maxillary and medial nasal processes

Ref: Gray's Anatomy: The Anatomical Basis of Clinical Practice, 41st ed. pg. 617

- The image likely shows a cleft lip.
- The embryological basis for the cleft lip is described as the abnormal fusion of the maxillary and medial nasal processes.

15. Ans. (b) B

- The lienorenal ligament, also known as the splenorenal ligament, is a structure that connects the hilum of the spleen to the anterior surface of the left kidney. It is marked as B in the provided image.
- This ligament plays an important role in supporting and stabilizing the spleen in its anatomical position.
- One of the significant structures contained within the lienorenal ligament is the splenic artery. The splenic artery is a large blood vessel that arises from the celiac trunk and supplies oxygenated blood to the spleen.

Extra Mile

Splenic Ligament	Attachments
• Phrenicocolic ligament	Diaphragm to the splenic flexure of the colon.
• Phrenicosplenic ligament	Posterior abdominal wall to the upper pole of the spleen.
• Splenorenal (lienorenal) ligament	Hilum of the spleen to the anterior surface of the left kidney Tail of the pancreas Splenic artery and vein
• Gastrosplenic ligament	Greater curvature of the stomach to the upper pole of the spleen Left gastroepiploic artery

16. Ans. (a) Ulnar nerve

Ref: Gray's Anatomy: The Anatomical Basis of Clinical Practice, 41st ed. pg. 783

- The arrow in the image points to the region near the medial epicondyle of the humerus, which is a common site of injury.
- Fractures in this area can lead to ulnar nerve compression or damage.
- The ulnar nerve, which passes through this region, can be affected, resulting in symptoms such as numbness, tingling, or weakness in the ulnar nerve distribution.

17. Ans. (b) Thoracic duct

Ref: Gray's Anatomy: The Anatomical Basis of Clinical Practice, 41st ed. pg. 1038

- The arrow in the image points to aortic opening. Among the given choices, thoracic duct passes through this opening

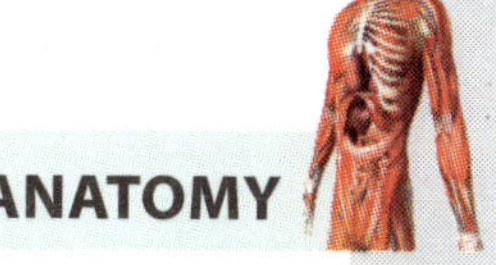

Structures passing through the aortic opening are as follows:

1. Aorta
2. Thoracic duct
3. Azygos vein
4. Hemiazygos vein

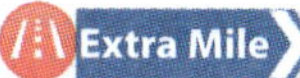

Extra Mile

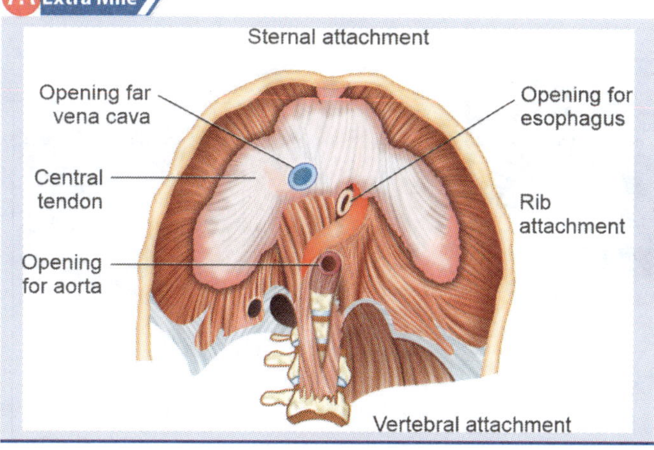

18. Ans. (d) Perineum and leg

Ref: Gray's Anatomy: The Anatomical Basis of Clinical Practice, 41st ed. pg. 898

- The paracentral lobule is a region of the cerebral cortex, located in the medial aspect of the precentral gyrus.
- It plays a crucial role in motor control, particularly for the lower limbs.
- Lesions in the paracentral lobule lead to:
  - Weakness and loss of sensation in the **contralateral lower limb** (paraplegia).
  - Urinary incontinence
  - Fecal incontinence

19. Ans. (b) Left gluteus medius and gluteus minimus

Ref: Gray's Anatomy: The Anatomical Basis of Clinical Practice, 41st ed. pg. 1358

- The gluteus medius and minimus muscles stabilize the pelvis and help maintain an upright position. When these muscles are paralyzed, the pelvis sinks on the unsupported side when standing on the affected limb. This is known as a positive Trendelenburg sign.
- The Trendelenburg sign is a clinical test used to assess the strength of the hip abductor muscles, specifically the gluteus medius and gluteus minimus.
- In this case, the left gluteus medius and gluteus minimus are affected, causing the drop of the right hip/side.

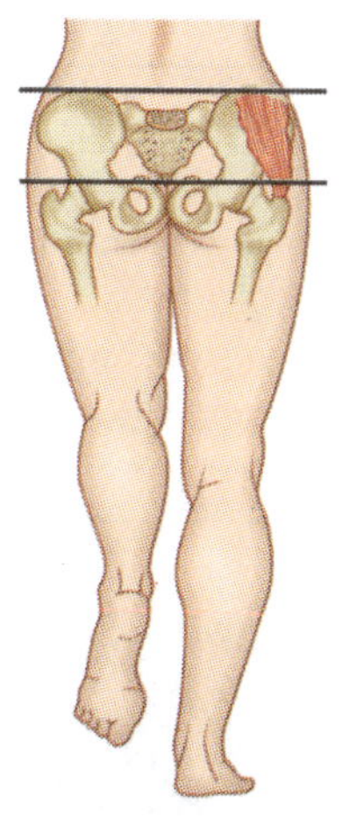

Normal

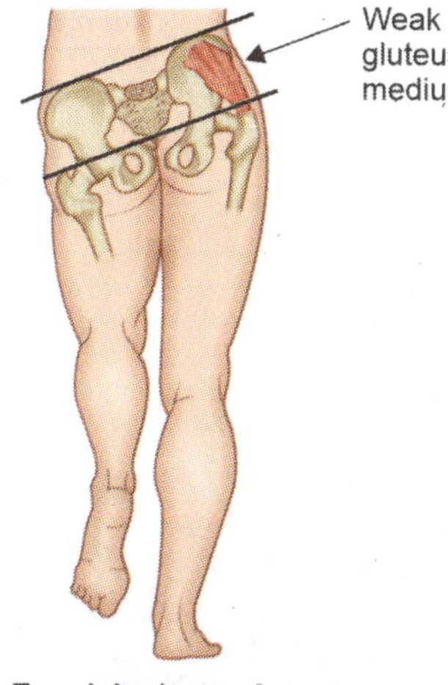

Trendelenburg sing
Drop of pelvis when lifting leg opposite to weak gluteus medius

20. Ans. (a) Brachial artery

Ref: Gray's Anatomy: The Anatomical Basis of Clinical Practice, 41st ed. pg. 873

- In the given scenario, where a fracture is observed at the level of the elbow and the forearm is pulseless, the most likely injured structure is the brachial artery.
- The brachial artery is a major blood vessel located in the upper arm, and its injury can lead to the absence of a pulse distal to the site of injury.

21. Ans. (b) 2nd

Ref: Gray's Anatomy: The Anatomical Basis of Clinical Practice, 41st ed. pg. 898

- The cyst observed at the anterior border of the sternocleidomastoid is due to the persistence of the 2nd branchial cleft.
- During embryonic development, the branchial arches and clefts form, and the 2nd branchial cleft normally disappears.
- However, if it fails to close properly, a cyst can develop in the region of the anterior border of the sternocleidomastoid muscle.

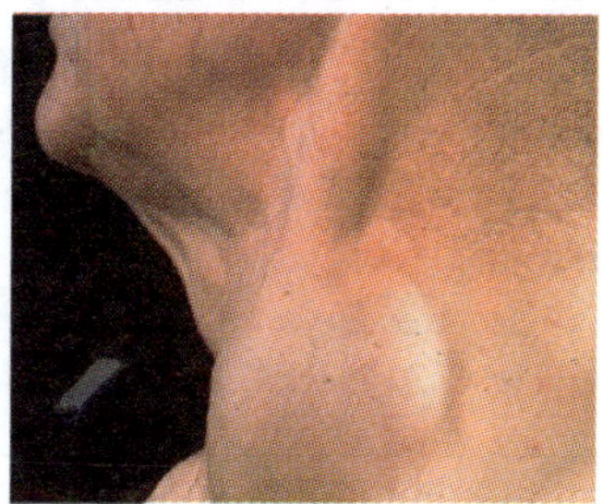

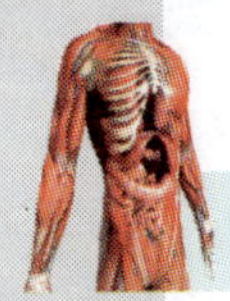

22. **Ans. (a) Transitional epithelium**

Ref: Inderbir Singh's Textbook of Human Histology, 8th ed. pg. 21

- The image depicts transitional epithelium. Notice the spherical cells on top that can flatten when stretched.
- Transitional epithelium is a specialized type of stratified epithelium found in organs such as the urinary bladder, ureters, and part of the urethra.
- It is characterized by its ability to undergo stretching and recoil, allowing the organs to accommodate changes in volume.

Extra Mile

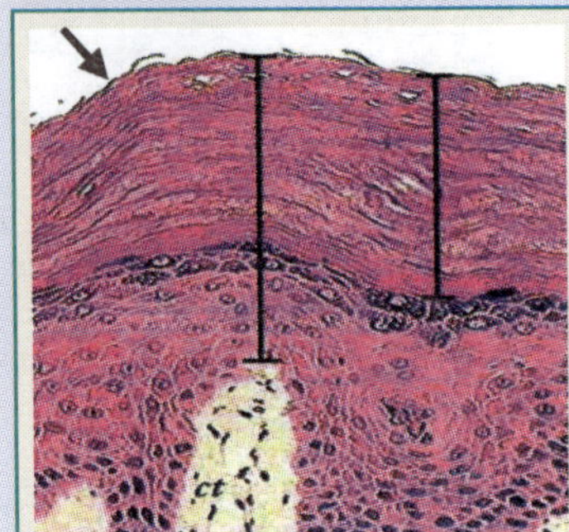

Keratinized stratified squamous epithelium: found in the epidermis of the skin

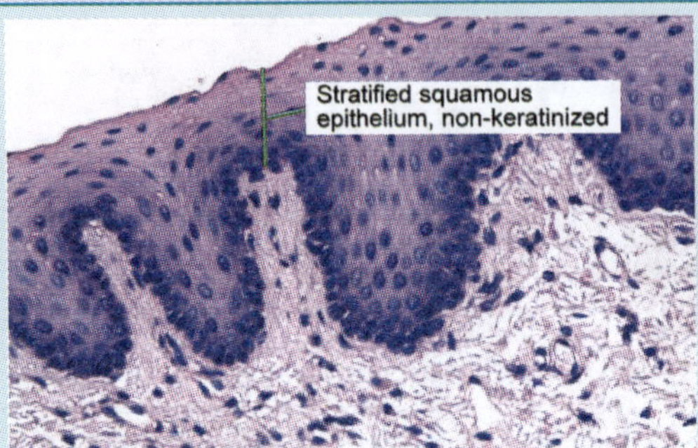

Nonkeratinized stratified squamous epithelium: Found in oral cavity, esophagus, vagina

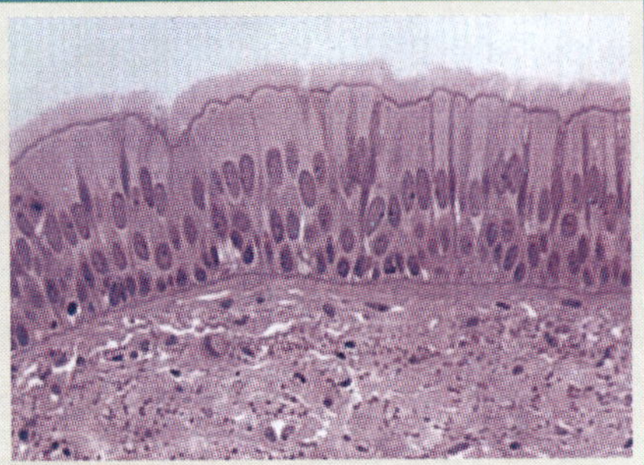

Ciliated pseudostratified columnar epithelium: Found in respiratory tract

EMBRYOLOGY, HISTOLOGY AND OSTEOLOGY

23. **Ans. (a) Coronal**

Ref: Gray's Anatomy, 42nd ed, pg. 16

There are three planes commonly used; sagittal, coronal and transverse.

1. Sagittal plane — a vertical line which divides the body into a left section and a right section.
2. Coronal plane — a vertical line which divides the body into a front (anterior) section and back (posterior) section.
3. Transverse plane — a horizontal line which divides the body into an upper (superior) section and a lower (inferior) section.

24. **Ans. (d) Antral**

Ref: Gray's Anatomy, 42nd ed, pg. 1323

- Antral follicles are small follicles (about 2–9 mm in diameter) that we can see — and measure and count — with ultrasound.
- Antral follicles are also referred to as resting follicles or also known as Graafian follicle.

25. **Ans. (c) Ciliated columnar**

Ref: Gray's Anatomy, 42nd ed, pg. 30

- The wall of the fallopian tube includes an elaborately folded mucosa (endosalpinx) surrounded by a muscularis (myosalpinx).
- The mucosa is lined by a ciliated columnar epithelium with secretory cells, and is folded out into the lumen so that an ovum in the lumen will always be close to the cilia for transport to the uterus.

26. **Ans. (b) Calcitonin**

Ref: Gray's Anatomy, 42nd ed, pg. 92

- The marked cell in the image is large polyhedral cells with oval and eccentric nuclei and is called C cell. It secretes calcitonin. They lie between adjoining follicular cells but donot reach the lumen.
- Calcitonin is a hormone that plays a role in regulating the level of calcium in your blood.
- It reduces calcium level by inhibiting osteoclastic activity.

27. **Ans. (a) Nonclosure of anterior neuropore**

Ref: Gray's Anatomy, 42nd ed, pg. 233

- Anterior neuropore closes around day 25 and posterior neuropore closes around day 28
- Failure of closure of the anterior neuropore during embryogenesis will lead to anencephaly, the failure of the brain and skull to develop.
- **Note:** Failure of closure of posterior neuropore may leads to spina bifida, meningocele, myelomeningocele, etc.

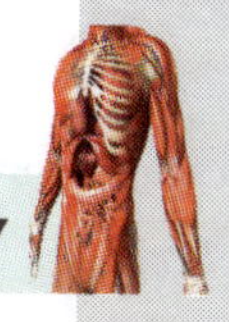

28. Ans. (a) Pterion

- The marked structure in the image is pterion. *(Most repeated question in FMGE).*
- Pterion is the area where frontal, parietal, temporal and greater wing of sphenoid bone join together.

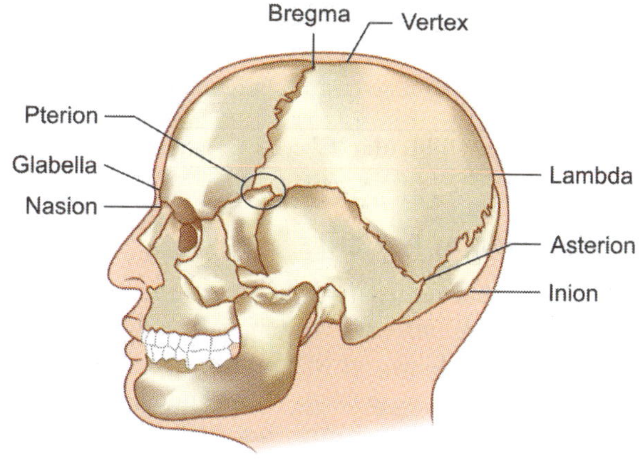

29. Ans. (d) 6

Ref: BD Chaurasia, 7th ed. Vol. I, pg. 87

Blood vessels derived from different arches

Arch	Derived blood vessel
First arch (Mandibular arch)	Maxillary artery
Second arch (Hyoid arch)	Stapedial artery
Third arch	Internal and common carotid artery
Fourth arch	Aortic arch on left side Part of subclavian artery on right side
Sixth arch	• Pulmonary arteries (on each side) • Ductus arteriosus on left side

Contd...

30. Ans. (c) Spleen

Ref: BD Chaurasia, 7th ed. Vol. II, pg. 326

- Spleen develops in the mesoderm in the cephalic part of left layer of dorsal mesogastrium.
- The development occurs in sixth week of intrauterine life.
- Number of nodules develop which soon fuse to form a lobulated spleen.

31. Ans. (b) Pacinian corpuscle

Ref: Gray's Anatomy, 41st ed. pg. 61

There are 4 types of mechanoreceptors in skin:

Receptor	Function
• Meissner corpuscles	Fine touch Slow vibration
• Merkel cell	Sensitive to edges and corners
• Pacinian corpuscles	Rapid vibration
• Ruffini's endings	Pressure sensation

32. Ans. (c) Anencephaly

- Cranial (rostral) neuropore closes by day 25
- Caudal neuropore closes by day 28
- Failure of cranial neuropore to close at day 25 results in anencephaly
- Failure of caudal neuropore to close results in spina bifida.

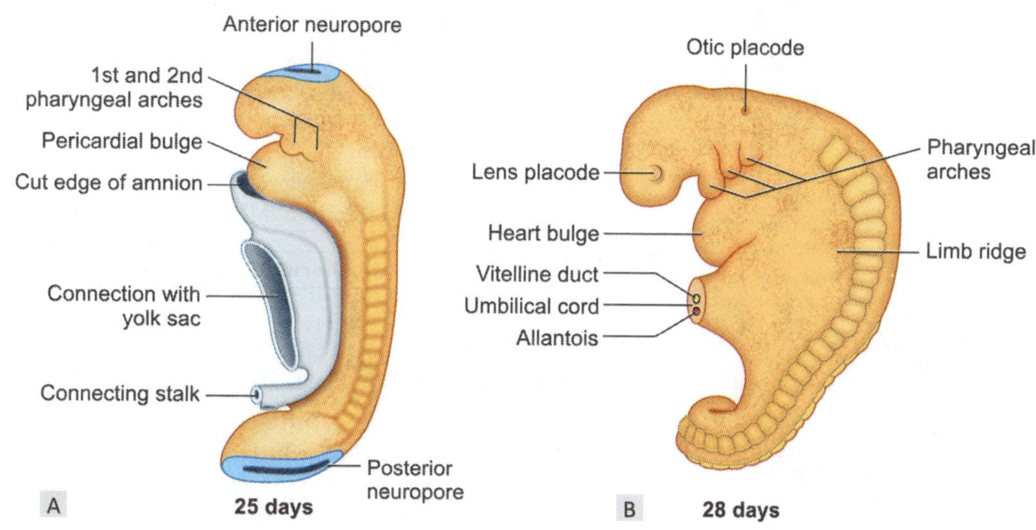

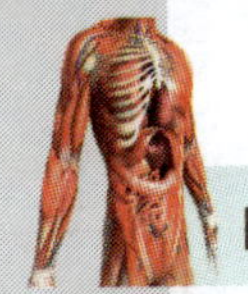

33. Ans. (c) 270 degree anticlockwise

Ref: Textbook of Clinical Embryology by Vishram Singh, pg. 148

- The rotation of midgut occurs when herniated intestinal loop returns back to the abdominal cavity.
- It begins at the end of third month of intrauterine life
- The primary intestinal loop rotates around an axis formed by the superior mesenteric artery, which divides the midgut loop into 2 segments:
  1. **Proximal (prearterial) segment**- present cranially
     - Give rise to: Distal half of duodenum, Jejenum, Ileum; EXCEPT its terminal part
  2. **Distal (postarterial) segment**- present caudally
     - Give rise to terminal part of ileum, Cecum, appendix, ascending colon, proximal 2/3rd of transverse colon.
- In order to return to abdominal cavity, the midgut loop undergoes anticlockwise rotation of 90° thrice → total rotation of 270°.
  - The first 90° rotation occurs outside abdominal cavity (within umbilicus), remaining 2 rotations in abdominal cavity

34. Ans. (a) Superior mesenteric artery

Ref: Gray's Anatomy, 41st ed. pg. 1054

Rotation of Midgut Loop

- Midgut loop has 2 ends: Cranial end and caudal end.
- The primary intestinal loop rotates around an axis formed by the superior mesenteric artery

Refer to above explanation for more detailed explanation

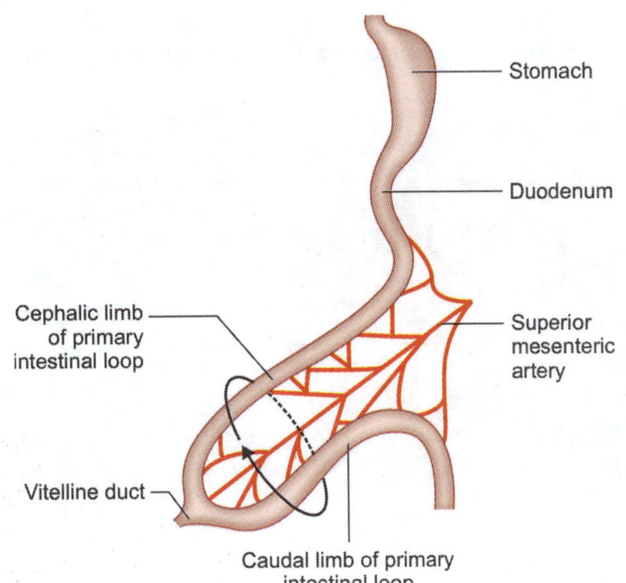

35. Ans. (c) Hyaluronic acid

Ref: Gray's Anatomy, E-book, 41st ed. pg. 188

- Hyaluronic acid and chondroitin sulfate are present in the migration pathways of neural crest cells.
- Hyaluronic acid is synthesized by the neural crest cells, ectoderm, somites and neural tube cells.
- The role of hyaluronic acid is to expand the extracellular spaces and facilitate migration of neural crest cells.

36. Ans. (b) Parafollicular 'C' cells

Ref: Gray's Anatomy, E-book. pg. 61

ENDODERMAL POUCHES

- **1st pouch:** Dorsal part forms tubotympanic recess which forms the middle ear cavity and eustachian tube.
- **2nd pouch:** Joins with ventral part of 1st pouch to form palatine tonsil. Also forms parts of middle ear.
- **3rd pouch:** Dorsal part forms the inferior parathyroid gland and ventral forms thymus.
- **4th pouch:** Dorsal part forms the superior parathyroid gland.
  - Ventral part forms the ultimobranchial body which forms the parafollicular C-cells of thyroid.

37. Ans. (b) Craniopharyngioma

Ref: Gray's Anatomy, E-Book 2015 ed. pg. 431

- In embryogenesis Rathke's pouch is an evagination at the roof of the developing mouth in front of buccopharyngeal membrane. It gives rise to anterior pituitary (adenohypophysis).
- Craniopharyngioma are benign cystic lesions derived from Rathke's pouch, most frequently in children. It is associated with hypopituitarism, growth retardation and diabetes insipidus.
- **Clinical features:**
  1. Raised ICT
  2. Presents before 20 years of age
  3. Visual field abnormalities
  4. Weight gain
  5. Cranial nerve damage
- **Investigation:** MRI is superior to CT.

38. Ans. (d) Osseus labyrinth

Ref: Gray's Anatomy, 41st ed. pg. 644

- Osseous labyrinth is considered as hardest bone of the body. It is embedded in petrous part of temporal bone, which is also known as "rock bone".
- **American edition of British encyclopedia states:** *"The labyrinth of the ear is formed of cochlea, 3 semicircular canals and a small cavity known as vestibulum into*

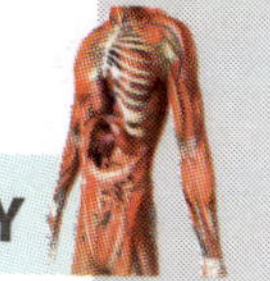

which cochlea and semicircular canal opens. These parts are formed of the hardest bone in body, almost equal in solidity to ivory and petrous portion of temporal bone.

39. Ans. (b) Medial umbilical ligament

Ref: Langman Embryology, pg. 148

Fetal structure	Adult structure
Foramen Ovale	Fossa Ovalis
Umbilical vein (intra-abdominal part)	Ligamentum teres
Ductus venosus	Ligamentum venosum
Umbilical arteries and Proximal part of umbilical artery	Medial umbilical ligaments Superior vesicular artery (supplies bladder)
Ductus arteriosus	Ligamentum arteriosum

40. Ans. (b) Scrotum

Ref: D.C. Dutta, 8th ed. pg. 1

- Labia majora is homologous to scrotum in male.
- Round ligament terminates at upper border of labia majora

41. Ans. (b) 16

Ref: D.C. Dutta, 8th ed. pg. 22

MORULA FORMATION

- Morula is a 16 cell stage where embryo is enclosed in zona pellucida.
- After the zygote formation, typical mitotic division of the nucleus occurs producing two blastomeres.
- The two cell stage is reached *approximately 30 hours* after fertilization. Each contains equal cytoplasmic volume and chromosome numbers.
- The blastomeres continue to divide by binary division through 4, 8, 16 cell stage until a cluster of cell is formed which is called *morula*, resembling a mulberry. As the total volume of the cell mass is not increased and the zona pellucida remains intact, the morula after spending about 3 days in the uterine tube *enters the uterine cavity through the narrow uterine ostium (1 mm) on the 4th day in the 16–64 cell stage.*

42. Ans. (d) Two arteries and one vein, umbilical vein supplying toward fetus

"Remember 2AV"

- Umbilical cord is the structure which connects mother to fetus and acts as a bridge for transfer of blood and other nutrients from mother to baby.
- It contains *2 arteries and one vein.* Arteries carry deoxygenated blood from fetus to mother while *vein carries oxygenated blood from mother towards fetus.*
- Cord contains Wharton's jelly and the structures embedded in this are:
  - 2 arteries and 1 vein
  - Allantois and
  - Remains of vitellointestinal duct

43. Ans. (d) Umbilical vessels

Ref: Textbook of Human Embroyology, pg. 56

- *The structures of the umbilical cord, i.e., vitelline duct, vitelline vessels and allantois also get obliterated and are converted into* ***Wharton's jelly.*** *The only structures which remain functional in Wharton's jelly are the umbilical vessels.*

Extra Mile

- Obliterated umbilical artery gives rise to medial umbilical ligament
- Obliterated umbilical veins give rise to ligamentum teres

44. Ans. (c) Branchial pouch: Endoderm

Ref: Netter's Essential Histology, 2nd ed. pg. 355

The branchial apparatus is composed up of branchial clefts, arches and pouch

Branchial **C**lefts	**E**ctoderm
Branchial **A**rches	**M**esoderm
Branchial **P**ouches	**E**ndoderm

45. Ans. (c) Cardinal vein

Ref: Langman's Essesntial Medical Embroyology, pg. 57

- During early embryonic development (through 4th week), paired cardinal veins drain the body. *Anterior cardinal* veins drain the head and upper limb buds, while *posterior cardinal veins* drain the body. Both the anterior and posterior veins on each side unite at the common cardinal veins that flow into the sinus venosus and ultimately into the common atrium.
- Most of the posterior segment on the left disappears; EXCEPT for that forming the left superior intercostal vein, whereas the right anterior segment forms the superior vena cava.

46. Ans. (d) 4th pharyngeal arch

Ref: Gray's Anatomy, 41st ed. pg. 607

Derivatives of the Pharyngeal Arches

Arch number	Arch name	Embryonic cartilage	Cartilage derivative	Muscle	Nerve	Artery
1	Mandibular	Quadrate Meckel's	Incus Malleus Anterior ligament of malleus Spine of sphenoid Sphenomandibular ligament Genial tubercle of mandible	Tensor tympani Muscles of mastication Mylohyoid Anterior belly of digastric Tensor veli palatine	Trigeminal (V) Mandibular division	First aortic arch artery (transitory)
2	Hyoid	Reichert's	• Stapes • Styloid process of temporal bone • Styloid process of temporal bone • Stylohyoid ligament • Lesser horn and upper part of body of hyoid bone	• Stapedius • Stylohyoid muscle • Facial muscles, include. ▪ Buccinator ▪ Platysma ▪ Posterior belly digastric	Facial (VII)	Stapedial artery (transitory)
3	Third		Greater horn and lower part of body of hyoid bone	Stylopharyngeus	Glossopharyngeal (IX)	**Common carotid artery**
4	Fourth		Thyroid cartilage Corniculate cartilage Cuneiform cartilage	Pharyngeal and extrinsic laryngeal muscles, levator veli palatini	Vagus (X) Pharyngeal branch	• Proximal part of subclavian artery on the right • **Arch of aorta** between origins of left common carotid and left subclavian arteries
6	Sixth		Arytenoid cartilages	Intrinsic laryngeal muscles	Vagus (X) Recurrent laryngeal branch	Part between the pulmonary trunk and dorsal aorta becomes ductus arteriosus on left, disappears on right

47. Ans. (b) 3rd pharyngeal arch

Ref: Gray's Anatomy, 41st ed. pg. 607

- The common carotid and first part of internal carotid artery is derived from 3rd **pharyngeal arch**
- The common carotid arteries differ on the right and left sides with respect to their origins. **On the right**, the common carotid arises from the brachiocephalic artery as it passes behind the sternoclavicular joint.
- **On the left**, the common carotid artery comes directly from the arch of the aorta in the superior mediastinum. The right common carotid, therefore, has only a cervical part whereas the left common carotid has cervical and thoracic parts.

48. Ans. (b) 2nd branchial arch

Ref: Gray's Anatomy, 41st ed. pg. 449

- The stylohyoid ligament is a fibrous cord extending from the tip of the styloid process to the lesser cornu of the hyoid bone. It gives attachment to the highest fibers of the middle pharyngeal constrictor and is intimately related to the lateral wall of the oropharynx. Below, it is overlapped by hyoglossus.
- The ligament is derived from the cartilage of the **second branchial arch,** and may be partially calcified.

49. Ans. (a) 1

Ref: Gray's Anatomy, 41st ed. pg. 607

50. Ans. (a) Stylohyoid ligament

Ref: Gray's Anatomy, 41st ed. pg. 607

51. Ans. (b) 2nd branchial arch

Ref: Inderbir Singh's Embroyology, 9th ed. pg. 116-117, 7th ed. pg. 119-120

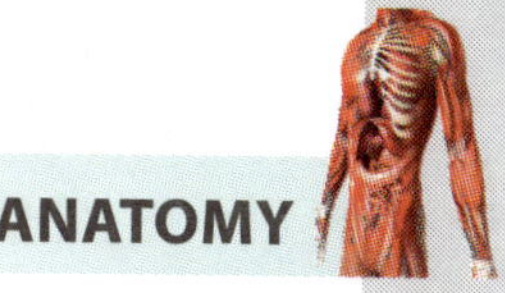

- At first there are 6 arches. The 5th arch disappears.
- ***Upper half and lesser cornu of hyoid bone is derived from 2nd arch.***
- *Lower half and greater of hyoid bone is derived from 3rd arch.*
- Palatine tonsil derived from 2nd branchial pouch.

52. Ans. (b) II

Ref: I.B. Singh, 9th ed. pg. 116

53. Ans. (d) Cricothyroid

Ref: I.B. Singh, 9th ed. pg. 116

- Cricothyroid muscle is derived from fourth branchial arch. It is the only intrinsic laryngeal muscle not derived from 6th branchial arch
- **Nerve supply:** Superior laryngeal nerve

54. Ans. (d) Thyroid

Ref: I.B. Singh, 9th ed. pg. 116–17

- Superior parathyroid is derived from 4th branchial pouch
- Inferior parathyroid and thymus develop from 3rd branchial pouch
- ***Most of the thyroid gland develops from thyroglossal duct (endodemal duct at foramen cecum).***

55. Ans. (d) 1st and 2nd branchial arch

Ref: P.L. Dhingra, 6th ed. pg. 11

- The auricle develops from fusion of mesenchyme of **1st and 2nd branchial arch**.
- External ear canal develops from the ectoderm of 1st branchial cleft.
- Tympanic membrane is derived from all three germ layers contributed by 1st pharyngeal/ branchial arch.

56. Ans. (c) Branchial pouch 3rd

Ref: Netter's Essential Histology, 2nd ed. pg. 227

- **Third** branchial pouch forms the **thymus** and **Inferior** parathyroid glands.
- Fourth branchial pouch forms superior parathyroid glands and ultimobranchial body.
- Aberrant development of third and fourth branchial pouches results in *Di-george syndrome.* It leads to thymic and inferior parathyroid gland hypoplasia. The infant develops recurrent pneumonia episodes and hypocalcemia.
- 2nd branchial pouch forms tonsils.
- 1st branchial pouch *ventral* part forms tongue
- 1st branchial pouch *dorsal* part forms tubotympanic recess, Eustachian tube, middle ear cavity and inner part of Eustachian tube.

57. Ans. (b) 2nd pouch

Ref: Netter's Essential Histology, 2nd ed. pg. 227

Tonsil is derived from 2nd branchial pouch.

58. Ans. (d) Palatine tonsils

Ref: I.B. Singh, 9th ed. pg. 1118

- First pharyngeal pouch is located between 1st and 2nd pharyngeal arch
- **Palatine tonsil is a derivative of 2nd pharyngeal pouch**
- Eustachean tube, Middle ear, mastoid antrum and tympanic membrane is derived from 1st pharyngeal pouch.

59. Ans. (b) Dorsal part of 1st cleft

Ref: Netter's Essentials of Human Embryology, 3rd ed. pg. 235

- The dorsal part of 1st cleft forms the *external auditory canal* while the *ventral part of first cleft obliterates.*
- The 2nd to 4th clefts form temporary cervical sinuses and failure to obliterate leads to branchial cleft cyst.

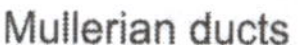

60. Ans. (c) Sinovaginal bulb

Ref: Human Embroyology: The Ultimate USMLE step 1, pg. 45

- In females, the paired embryonic paramesonephric duct forms the uterine tubes, uterus, cervix and superior part of vagina.
- The **lower 3rd of vagina** develops from **sinovaginal bulbs**, which are paired evaginations of the wall of the urogenital sinus.
- At around 15 weeks of embroyologic development, the **mullerian system** which forms the **upper 2/3rd of vagina**, fuses with the invaginating cloaca or **urogenital sinus to form the lower 1/3rd of vagina.**
- These two parts of vagina, i.e. paramesonephric duct part and sinovaginal bulb part canalize to form a single, complete vaginal canal.

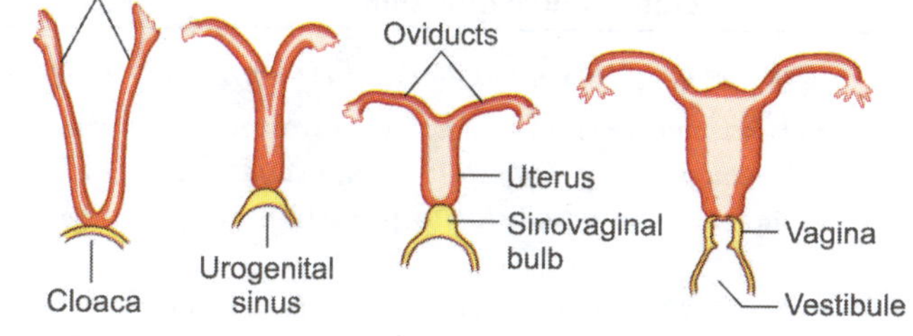

61. Ans. (d) Prochordal plate

Ref: Netter's Clinical Anatomy, 3rd ed. pg. 39

- Hypoblast and epiblast are 2 germ layers in the second week of embryonic development.

- The *hypoblast* gives rise to prochordal plate which is the future site of mouth and forms the cranio-caudal axis.
- Notochord is formed by *epiblast* cells.
- Epiblast is also the source of all three germ layers.
- *First germ layer* to be formed is the *endoderm.*[Q]
- *Remnants of notochord* are nucleus pulposus and apical ligament of atlas.

62. Ans. (a) CVS

Ref: Netter's Clinical Anatomy, 3rd ed. pg. 35

- CVS is the first fully functional organ system in fetus and first to attain maturity from functional perspective.

63. Ans. (c) Week 3

Ref: Netter's Clinical Anatomy, 3rd ed. pg. 39

- Gastrulation is defined as formation of 3 germ layers in 3rd week of embryonic development.
- The 3rd week of development is also called stage of trilaminar germ disk.
- *Gastrulation begins* with formation of primitive streak by proliferation of epiblast cells near the caudal end of embryonic disk. Primitive disc regresses by fourth week.

64. Ans. (b) Endoderm

Ref: Netter's Atlas of Embryology, 2012 ed. pg. 47

- Epiblast is the source of all three germ layers and *endoderm* is the *first germ layer* to be formed.

65. Ans. (b) Epiblast

Ref: Netter's Atlas of Neurosciences, 3rd ed. pg. 126

- Notochord is formed by epiblast cells and it provides central axis to the embryronic disc. It induces the overlying ectodermal cells to become neuro-ectodermal cells and form the neural tube.

66. Ans. (a) Segmental organization of embryo is craniocaudal direction

Ref: Netter's Atlas of Human Embryology, 2012 ed. pg. 10

- *Homeobox (HOX)* gene is involved in *segmental organization of embryo in cranio-caudal* direction. The mutation in gene leads to formation of appendages in wrong locations.
- *Sonic hedge-hog gene* is involved in patterning in *A-P axis.* The mutation in this gene leads to holoprosencephaly.

67. Ans. (a) Neural crest

Ref: Netter's Atlas of Neurosciences, 3rd ed. pg. 133

Derivatives of neural crest (mnemonic: **N.O.P.E**)

- MelaNocytes
- SchwaNn cells
- Adrenal medulla (ChromaffiN cells)
- **O**dontoblasts
- **P**arasympathetic ganglia of gut
- **P**arafollicular cells of thyroid
- **P**ia and arachnoid matters
- **E**ndocardial cushions and aortopulmonary septum in heart

Extra Mile

Derivatives of neuroectoderm:
- All CNS neurons astrocytes, oligodendrocytes, ependymocytes, neurohypophysis and pineal gland.

68. Ans. (a) Superior vesical artery

Ref: Netter's Atlas of Human Embryology, 2012 ed. pg. 86

Structure name	Derivative
Obliterated umbilical artery	Medial umbilical ligament
Proximal part of umbilical artery	*Superior vesical artery*
Inferior epigastric artery	Lateral umbilical fold
Left umbilical vein	Ligamentum teres
Right umbilical vein	Disappears
Ductus venosus	Ligamentum venosum
Urachus	Median umbilical ligament
Vitello-intestinal duct	Meckel's diverticulum

69. Ans. (d) Umbilical vein

Ref: Langeman's, 8th pg. 264, 259

70. Ans. (b) Ligamentum venosum

Ref: Langeman's, 8th pg. 264, 259

71. Ans. (a) Coronary sinus

Ref: Netter's Atlas of Human Embryology: 2012 ed. pg. 96

Heart tube embryonic derivatives

Embryonic structure	Gives rise to
• Proximal 1/3rd of bulbus cordis	Primitive trabeculated left ventricle
• Middle 1/3rd of bulbus cordis	Right and left ventricular outflow tract
• Distal 1/3rd of bulbus cordis (truncus arteriosus)	Ascending aorta and pulmonary trunk
• Left horn of sinus venosus	Coronary sinus
• Right horn of sinus venosus	Smooth part of right atrium
Right common cardinal nerve and right anterior cardinal nerve	SVC (superior vena cava)

72. Ans. (b) 2

Ref: Netter's Atlas of Human Embryology: 2012 ed. pg. 88

- There are six pairs of aortic arches which develop in cephalo-caudal direction.
- The 5th aortic arch completely disappears whereas 1st and 2nd disappear partially.
- *The stapedial artery is derived from the 2nd aortic arch.*
- Inferior alveolar artery is derived from the 1st aortic arch.

73. Ans. (a) Septum primum

Ref: Netter's Clinical Anatomy, 3rd ed. pg. 113

- *Fossa ovalis* is the remnant of **septum primum.**
- *Foramen ovale* is opening between the upper and lower limbs of **septum secundum.**
- This is a very closely worded question, so get the perspectives right.

74. Ans. (c) 8th month

Ref: Netter's Clinical Anatomy, 3rd ed. pg. 325

Descent of testis

3rd month	Iliac fossa
7th month	*Deep inguinal ring*
7th month	Transits through inguinal canal
8th month	*Superficial inguinal ring*
9th month	Enters the scrotum

75. Ans. (a) Metencephalon

Ref: Netter's Atlas of Neurosciences, 3rd ed. pg. 136

Parts of Developing Brain

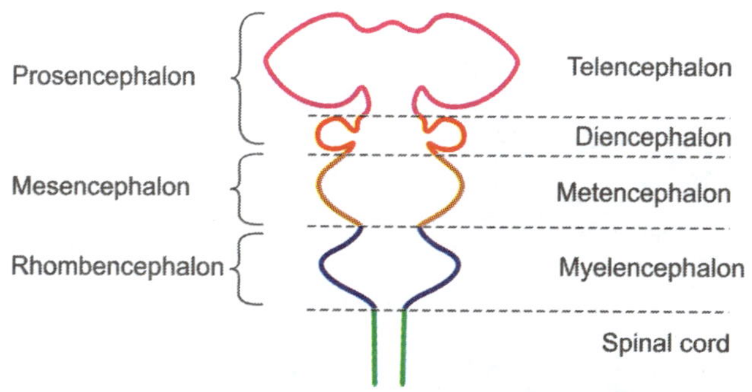

Myelencephalon	Medulla oblongata
Metencephalon	*Pons, cerebellum and 4th ventricle*
Mesencephalon	Midbrain and aqueduct of slyvius
Diencephalon	Thalamus, hypothalamus and 3rd *ventricle*
Telencephalon	Cerebral hemispheres and lateral ventricles

76. Ans. (a) Metanephros

Ref: Netter's Atlas of Human Embryology: 2012 ed. pg. 162

- Metanephros forms the definitive adult kidney. *It gives rise to renal parenchyma.* The nephrons form PCT, DCT, Henle's Loop and glomerulus.
- *Ureteric bud* gives rise to *collecting parts of the kidney* which is pelvis of kidney, major and minor calcyces with collecting tubules.
- *Urogenital sinus* develops into bladder, urethra and allantois.

77. Ans. (a) Urogenital sinus

Ref: Netter's Atlas of Human Embryology: 2012 ed. pg. 159

Genital Homologues in Male and Female

Choice number	Male	Female
A: Urogenital Sinus	• Corpus spongiosum • Bulbourethral glands of Cowper • Prostate gland	• Vestibular bulbs • Vestibular glands of bartholin • Urethral and paraurethral glands of skene
B: Urogenital Folds	Ventral shaft of penis (penile urethra)	Labia minora
C: Labio-scrotal Swelling	Scrotum	Labia majora
D: Gubernaculum	Gubernaculum testis	Ovarian and round ligaments

78. Ans. (a) Ureteric bud

Ref: I.B. Singh, 9th ed. pg. 252

- During the fifth week of gestation, the mesonephric duct develops an outpouching, the ureteric bud, near its attachment to the cloaca. This bud, also called the metanephrogenic diverticulum, grows posteriorly and towards the head of the embryo.
- *The elongated stalk of the ureteric bud, called the metanephric duct, later forms the ureter. As the cranial end of the bud extends into the intermediate mesoderm, it undergoes a series of branchings to form the collecting duct system of the kidney. It also forms the major and minor calyces and the renal pelvis.*

79. Ans. (b) Type B synoviocytes

Ref: Netter's Essential Histology, 2nd ed. pg. 156

Type A synoviocytes	Type B synoviocytes
• Resemble *macrophages* and contain extensive golgi apparatus	• Specialised *fibroblasts producing synovial fluid* and contain abundant Rough endoplasmic reticulum

80. Ans. (a) Hyaline

Ref: Netter's Essential Histology, 2nd ed. pg. 133

Hyaline cartilage is blue colored while *elastic cartilage is yellow* and *fibrocartilage is white.*

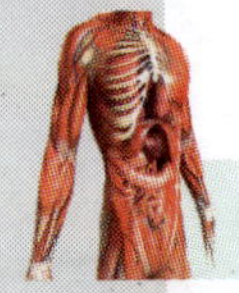

Extra edge

Hyaline cartilage
The most abundant and common cartilage
All long bones are pre-formed in hyaline cartilage; EXCEPT clavicle.
Types (**Mnemonic** L.A.N.C.E.T- T.B)
1. **L**arynx (Arytenoid lower end, cricoid)
2. **A**rticular cartilage
3. **N**asal cartilage
4. **C**ostal cartilage
5. **E**mbryonic cartilage
6. **T**racheal cartilage
7. **T**hyroid cartilage
8. **B**ronchial cartilage

81. Ans. (b) Holocrine gland

***Ref:** Netter's Essential Histology, 2nd ed. pg. 259*

- Tyson glands are located on external surface of prepuce and are holocrine glands.
- Holocrine glands are characterised by *disentigration of entire cell which discharges its secretions.*
- The holocrine glands are found everywhere; EXCEPT palms and soles.
- Sebaceous glands are usually associated with hair follicles; EXCEPT in following locations
  - **Eyelids:** Glands of zeis and meibomian glands
  - **Nipple and areola:** Montgomery tubercle
  - **Tyson glands:** Prepuce

82. Ans. (b) Persistent vitellointestinal duct

***Ref:** Kulkarni Clinical Anatomy, 2nd ed. pg. 590*

Urinary fistula at umbilicus	Persistent urachus
Faecal fistula at umbilicus	Persistent vitellointestinal duct
Raspberry tumor	Umbilical adenoma
Sister joseph nodule	Metastatic adenocarcinoma at umbilicus

83. Ans. (b) Para-axial mesenchyme

***Ref:** Gray's Anatomy, 41st ed. pg. 212*

- The axial skeleton, vertebrae and ribs are derived from paraxial mesenchyme
- The skull is derived from paraxial mesenchyme and neural crest mesenchyme
- The skeletal elements in the limbs are derived from somatopleuric mesenchyme, which forms the limb buds.

84. Ans. (b) Rathke pouch

***Ref:** Hypothalamic-pituitary Development: Genetic and Clinical Aspect, pg. 2-3*

- The anterior pituitary and intermediate lobe of pituitary develops from Rathke's pouch, which is initially derived from the anterior neural ridge, adjacent to cells in the neural plate.
- Neural plate contributes to ventral diencephalon.
- **Posterior lobe** of pituitary develops from the **infundibulum,** an evagination of the ventral diencephalon.

85. Ans. (a) It takes 74 days

***Ref:** Textbook of Human Embroyology, pg. 24*

- **Spermatogenesis** - Process of formation of spermatozoa from primitive germ cell (spermatogonia)
- **Spermiogenesis** - Formation of spermatozoa from spermatid.
- Spermatogenesis begins at-puberty (oogenesis begins intrauterine life)
- Spermatogenesis continues-throughout life (oogenesis-stops at menopause)
- **Average time**-74 days
- **Site**- seminiferous tubule
- **Sperm size**- 55–65 μm
- **Parts**- head, neck, middle piece, principal piece, end piece.
- **Acquire motility in**- epididymis.

86. Ans. (b) Primary spermatocyte

***Ref:** I.B. Singh, 9th ed. pg. 14-15*

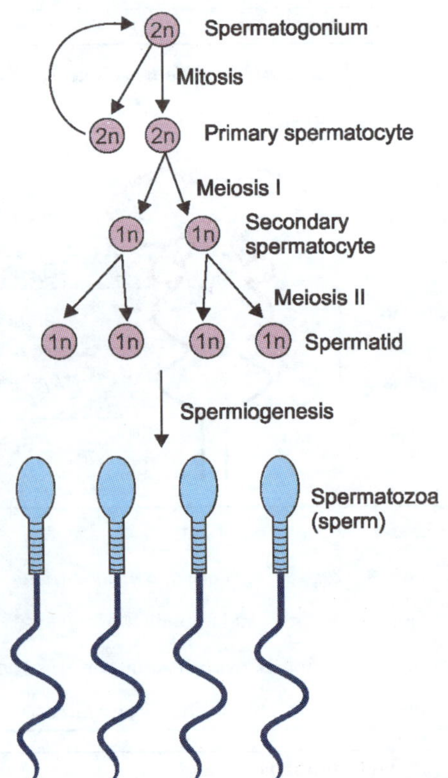

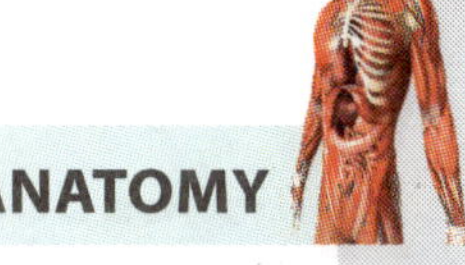

- Spermatogonium undergoes mitotic division and forms primary spermatocyte, which further forms secondary spermatocyte and spermatid after first and 2nd meiotic division respectively.
- Microscopically primary spermatocyte is largest in size among all.
- **The formation of spermatogonium to spermatozoa takes around 74 days.**

87. Ans. (b) 74 days

Ref: I.B. Singh, 9th ed. pg. 14-15

88. Ans. (c) Epididymis

Ref: I.B. Singh, 9th ed. pg. 15

89. Ans. (a) Stores the spermatozoa

Ref: I.B. Singh, 9th ed. pg. 15

- Seminal vesicles are two lobulated sacs, situated between the bladder and rectum.
- Each vesicles is about **5 cm long**, and is directed upwards and laterally and is lined by pseudostratified columnar epithelium.
- The lower narrow end forms the duct of the seminal vesicle which joins the ductus deferens to form the ejaculatory duct.
- **The seminal vesicles do not form a reservoir for spermatozoa.**
- Their secretion is slightly alkaline and contains fructose and a coagulating enzyme called the vesiculase.
- The secretion depends on level of testosterone.

90. Ans. (a) Blastocyst

Ref: I.B. Singh, 9th ed. pg. 43-44

- After fertilization, the fertilized ovum begins to divide as it migrates through the uterine tube.

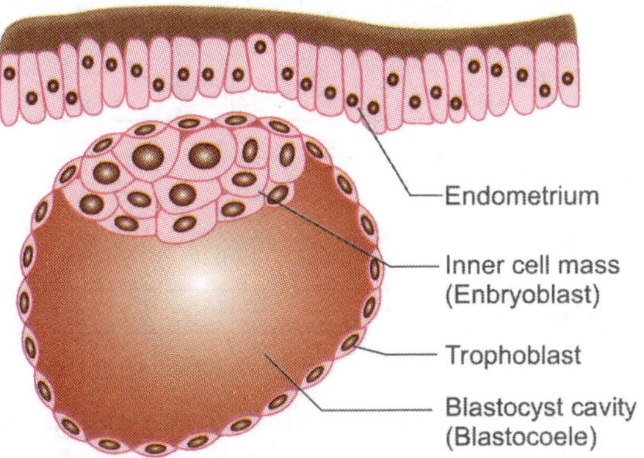

- It undergoes cleavage till a 16 cell stage and is called morula.
- Cells of morula differentiate into an inner cell mass which is completely surrounded by an outer layer of cells, which further gives rise to a structure called trophoblast.
- It reaches the blastocyst stage (approximately 110 cells) on about day 5 and it enters the uterus on about day 6.
- Implantation normally begins on day 6 with the syncytiotrophoblast of the embryonic pole of the blastocyst eroding into the endometrium.

91. Ans. (d) 8 weeks of fertilization

Ref: Dutta's Obstetrics, 7th ed. pg. 41

The prenatal period can be divided into:

Period	Product (known as)	Extends
• Ovular/ Germinal	Ovum	1st 2 weeks after ovulation
• Embryonic	Embryo	From fertilization (2nd week of gestation) to 8th week of development after fertilization (10th week AOG)
• Fetal	Fetus	From 8th week of fertilization (10th week AOG) till delivery

92. Ans. (d) From 10th week of gestation

Ref: Dutta's Obstetrics, 7th ed. pg. 41

Refer to above explanation.

93. Ans. (d) Descending colon

Ref: Langman's Medical Embryology, 9th ed. pg. 298

- *"Descending colon is a derivative of Hindgut"*

Part	Part in adult	Gives rise to	Arterial supply
Foregut	Esophagus to first 2 sections of the duodenum	Esophagus, stomach, duodenum (1st and 2nd parts), liver, gallbladder, pancreas, spleen, superior portion of pancreas	Celiac trunk
Midgut	Lower duodenum, to the first two-thirds of the transverse colon	Lower duodenum, ***jejunum***, ileum, cecum, ***appendix***, ***ascending colon***, and first 2/3rd of the transverse colon	Branches of the superior mesenteric artery
Hindgut	Last third of the transverse colon, to the upper part of the anal canal	Last third of the transverse colon, ***descending colon***, rectum, and upper part of the anal canal	Branches of the inferior mesenteric artery

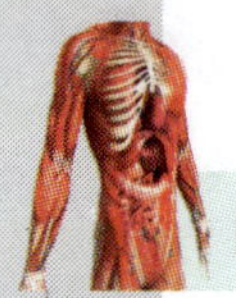

94. Ans. (c) Inferior mesenteric artery

Ref: Langman's Medical Embryology, 9th ed. pg. 298

95. Ans. (d) Neural crest

Ref: Keith L. Moore, 5th ed. pg. 318

- The adrenal cortex derives from mesoderm and secretes corticosteroids and androgens
- The adrenal medulla derives from **neural crest cells** and secretes catecholamines (mostly epinephrine).

96. Ans. (a) Yolk sac

Ref: I.B. Singh, 9th ed. pg. 252

- Umbilical vesicle (Yolk sac) attains full development and is large at *32 days (4–5 weeks).* It can be observed sonographically early in 5th week.
- By 10 weeks, it shrinks to pear shaped 5 mm in diameter and after 20 weeks it is not visible.
- Although umbilical vesicle contains no yolk, it's essential because:
  - Site of origin of primordial germ cells is *endodermal lining of wall of umbilical vesicle.*
  - In 3rd week blood first develops in vascularized extraembryonic mesoderm covering the wall of umbilical vesicle, and continues to form there until hemopoietic activity begins in liver during 6th week
  - Endoderm which is derived from epiblast, gives rise *to epithelium of trachea, bronchi, lungs and digestive tract (form primordial gut in 4th week).*

97. Ans. (c) 6

Ref: Internet Source

- Hyoid bone has a body, two greater and two lesser cornua or horns.
- The hyoid bone develops from 2nd & 3rd pharyngeal arches, the lesser cornu from 2nd the greater cornu from 3rd and body from fused ventral, ends of both.
- Ossification proceeds from 6 centers i.e. a pair for body and one for each conu. Ossification begins in the greater cornu towards the end of intrauterine life, in body shortly after birth and in lesser cornu around puberty.

98. Ans. (c) Mesoderm

Ref: BDC, Vol-2 pg. 382

- *Trigone of bladder is formed by the absorption of mesonephric ducts and is mesodermal in origin.*

99. Ans. (b) 2 arteries, 1 vein

Ref: I.B. Singh, 9th ed. pg. 59

Refer to Explanation of Question 68

100. Ans. (a) Leydig cell

Ref: I.B. Singh, 9th ed. pg. 14-16

- **Leydig cell** secretes testosterone
- **Sertoli cells** help in maturation of spermatozoa
- **Epididymis:** Store sperm
- **Seminal vesicle:** Secretes thick alkaline fluid.

101. Ans. (b) Brush bordered columnar epithelium

Ref: BDC, 6th ed. Vol. II, pg. 288-89

MICROVILLI

- When microvilli are of same height & arranged regularly, they are termed as **striated** border, as observed in small intestine.
- *If they are of irregular height, they will constitute the **brush border** as seen in **gallbladder** and proximal convoluted tubules of kidney - (Gray's anatomy).*

102. Ans. (d) Thymus

Ref: Gray's, 41st ed. pg. 619

- **Corpuscle** means any small body.
- **Hassall's corpuscles** are spherical or ovoid bodies *found in the medulla of the thymus,* composed of concentric arrays of epithelial cells which contain keratohyaline and bundles of cytoplasmic filaments.

Extra Mile

Some Other Known Corpuscles

- **Lamellated corpuscle** a type of large encapsulated nerve ending found throughout the body, concerned with perception of sensations.
- **Malpighian corpuscles:** Found in Nephrons (kidney) and in spleen (white pulp)
- **Meissner's corpuscle:** A type of medium sized encapsulated nerve ending in the skin, chiefly in the palms and soles.
- **Paciniform corpuscles** a type of rapidly adapting lamellated corpuscles responding to muscle stretch and light pressure.
- **Red corpuscle:** Red Blood Cells
- **White corpuscle:** White Blood Cells

103. Ans. (b) Kidney

Please refer to above explanation

104. Ans. (b) Spleen

Ref: BDC, 6th ed. Vol. II, pg. 297

The **Cords of Billroth** are also known as **splenic cords** or **red pulp cords**. They are found in the red pulp of the spleen between the sinusoids consisting of fibrils and connective tissue cells with a large population of monocytes and macrophages. *These cords contain half of the human body's monocytes.*

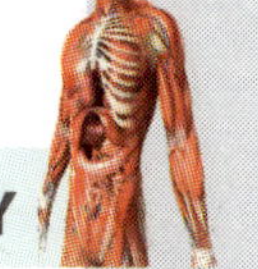

105. Ans. (b) Thymus

Ref: BDC, 6th ed. Vol. II, pg. 147

T cells originate in the bone marrow but mature in the thymus. So, T stands for 'Thymus'.

- Thymus and bone marrow are primary lymphoid organs.
- Lymph node and spleen are secondary lymphoid organs.

UPPER LIMB

106. Ans. (b) Syndesmosis

Ref: BD Chaurasia's Handbook of General Anatomy, 6th ed, pg. 93

- The type of joint represented in the above picture is Syndesmosis. It is a fibrous union between bones.
- It may be represented as interosseous ligament as in inferior tibiofibular joint or a tense membrane.

107. Ans. (b) Junction of medial 2/3 and lateral 1/3

Ref: BD Chauraisia's Human Anatomy, Volume 1, 8th ed, pg. 8

- The most common site of clavicle fracture is the junction between the two curvatures of the bone, i.e. the Junction of Medial 2/3rd and lateral 1/3, which is the weakest point.
- The lateral fragment is displaced downwards by the weight of limbs as trapezius muscle alone is unable to support the weight of upper limb.

108. Ans. (a) Abduction

Ref: BD Chauraisia's Human Anatomy, Volume 1, 8th ed, pg. 163

- Frozen shoulder is a common occurrence due to injury to rotator cuff muscles.
- The two layers of the synovial membrane become adherent to each other. The patient complains of progressively increasing pain in the shoulder, stiffness and restriction of Movements particularly **abduction**.
- As the contribution of the glenohumeral joint is reduced, the patient shows altered scapulohumeral rhythm due to excessive use of scapular motion while performing abduction.

109. Ans. (c) Extensor policis longus

Ref: BD Chauraisia's Human Anatomy, Volume 1, 8th ed, pg. 144

- The arrow marked tendon is of Extensor Policis Longus. The anatomical snuffbox is a triangular depression on the posterolateral side of the wrist. It is seen best when the thumb is extended.
- The tendon of Extensor policis longus form the medial/posterior boundary of anatomical snuffbox.

110. Ans. (a) Prime mover

Ref: Gray's Anatomy, 42nd ed, pg. 908

- The biceps brachii is on the anterior side of the humerus and is the prime mover (agonist) responsible for flexing the forearm.

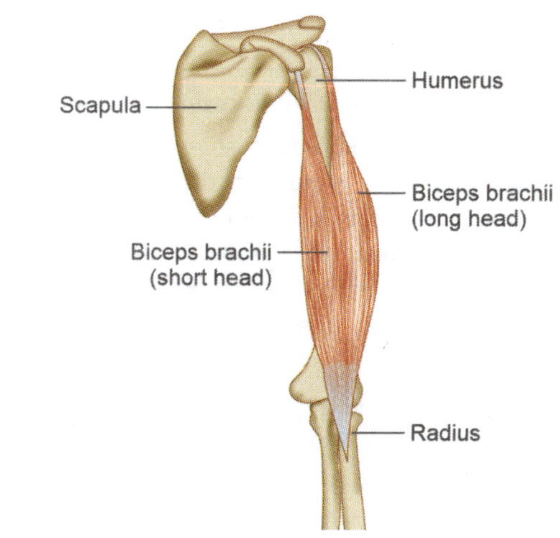

111. Ans. (a) Ulnar

Ref: Gray's Anatomy, 42nd ed, pg. 882

- An ulnar claw, also known as partial claw hand or 'spinster's claw', is a deformity or an abnormal attitude of the hand that develops due to ulnar nerve damage causing paralysis of the lumbricals.
- Deficit is primarily in 4th and 5th fingers.
- Complete claw hand involves ulnar nerve and median nerve.

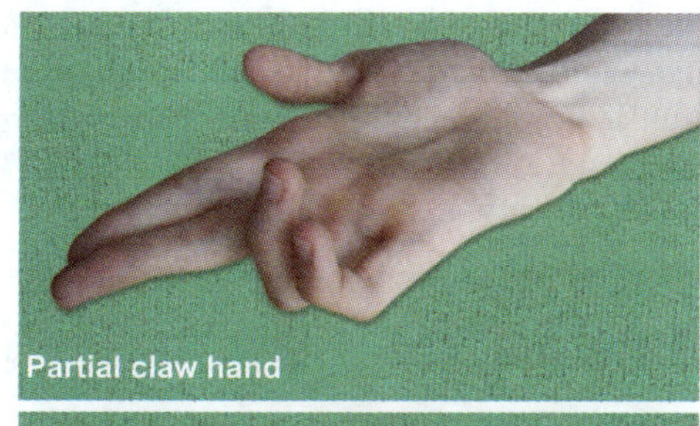

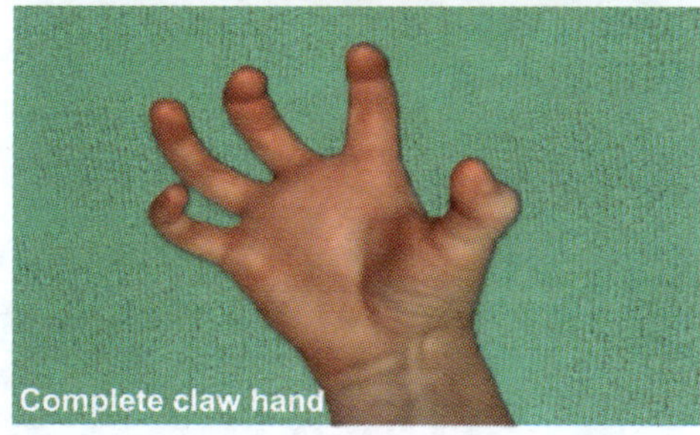

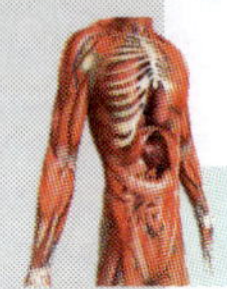

112. Ans. (c) Flexor carpi radialis

Ref: BD Chaurasia 7th ed. Vol. I, pg. 108

- The flexor carpi radialis is one of four muscles in the superficial layer of the anterior compartment of the forearm.
- The tendon of the flexor carpi radialis is visible on the anterior surface of the forearm, just proximal to the wrist, when the wrist is flexed. It is the tendon seen most lateral, closest to the thumb.

113. Ans. (a) A

Ref: BD Chaurasia 7th ed. Vol. I, pg. 130

- Carpal tunnel syndrome, also called median nerve compression, is a condition that causes numbness, tingling, or weakness in the hand.
- It happens because of pressure on the median nerve, which runs the length of the arm, goes through a passage in the wrist called the carpal tunnel, and ends in the hand.

A: Median nerve
B: Transverse carpal ligament
C: Ulnar nerve and artery
D: Pisiform bone

114. Ans. (d) Musculocutaneous nerve

Ref: BD Chaurasia 7th ed. Vol. I, pg. 93

- The highlighted muscle in the diagram is biceps brachii.
- It receives its innervation from the C5 and C6 fibers of the musculocutaneous nerve.
- The brachialis muscle originates on the distal portion of the anterior humerus, and inserts on both the coronoid process and tuberosity of the ulna.

115. Ans. (b) Ulnar nerve

Ref: BD Chaurasia 7th ed. Vol. I, pg. 17

- The arrow marked area in the image is medial epicondyle.
- In injury to medial epicondyle, the nerve that is damaged is ulnar nerve, since that nerve is passing through the ulnar groove.

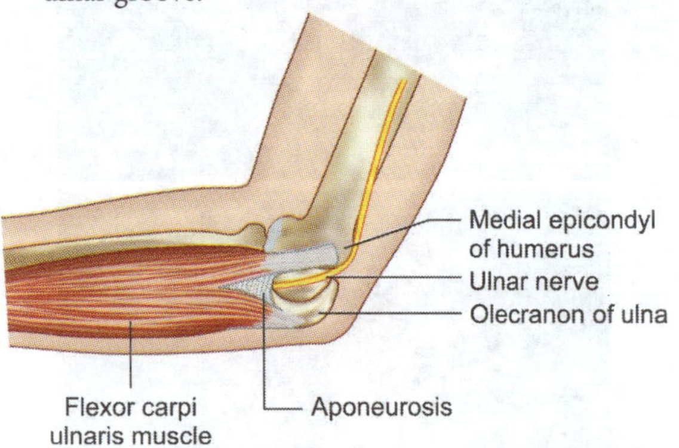

116. Ans. (b) Radial nerve

Ref: BD Chaurasia, 7th ed. Vol. I, pg. 17

- The marking shows fracture of shaft of humerus which causes lesion of radial nerve
- Surgical neck injury causes lesion of axillary nerve.
- Lesion to the ulnar nerve is caused by the fracture at supracondylar region.

117. Ans. (a) Scaphoid

- The floor of the anatomical snuff box is formed by the scaphoid bone. An injury to this area increases the suspicion of scaphoid fracture

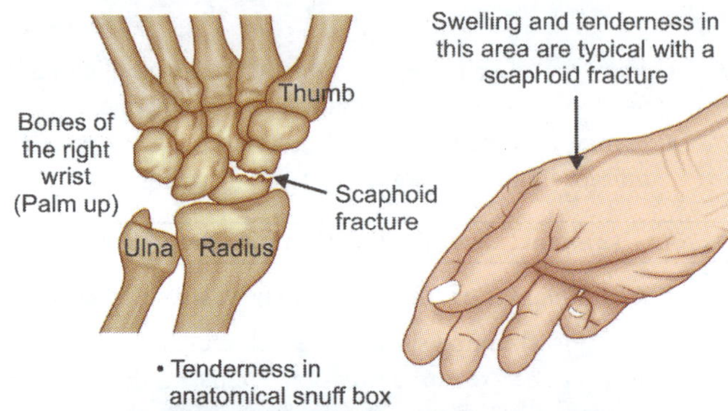

- Tenderness in anatomical snuff box
- X-ray fracture line

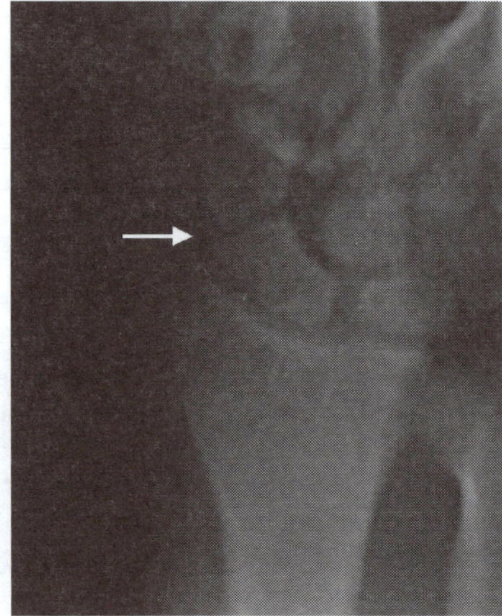

118. Ans. (b) Pronator teres

- Among given options pronator teres originates from medial epicondyle.
- Pronator teres muscle (from anterior arm, superior group of muscle):
  - **Action:** Pronates and flexes forearm

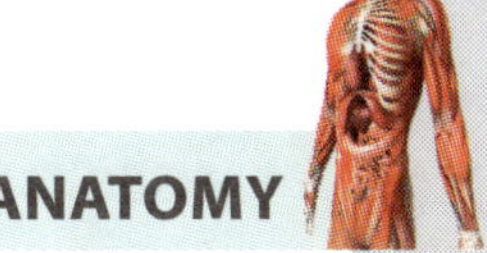

- **Origin:** Medial epicondyle of humerus, coronoid process of ulna
- **Insertion:** Lateral surface of radius

- **Muscles originating from medial epicondyle of humerus:**
  - Pronator teres
  - Flexor carpi radialis
  - Palmaris longus
  - Flexor carpi ulnaris

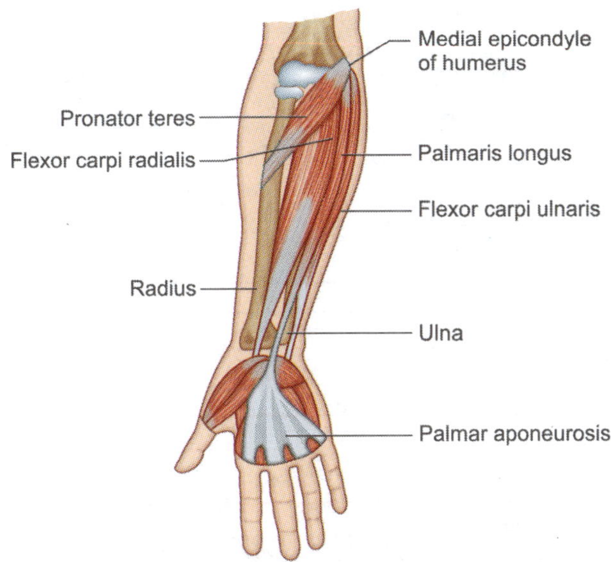

119. Ans. (a) Ulnar nerve

- The shown course of nerve is of ulnar nerve
- Please refer the image as follows:

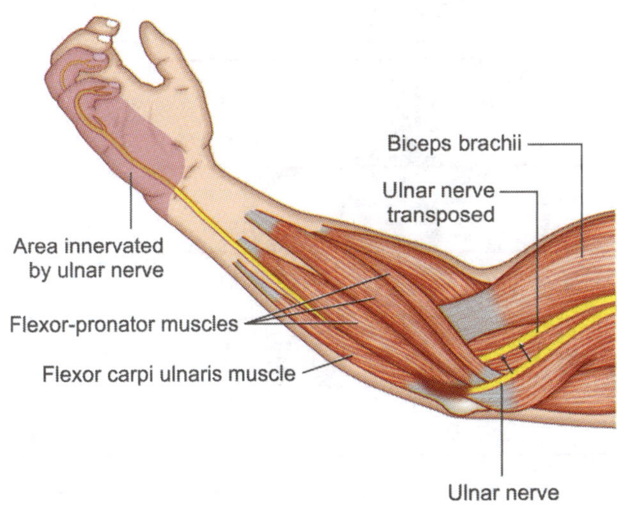

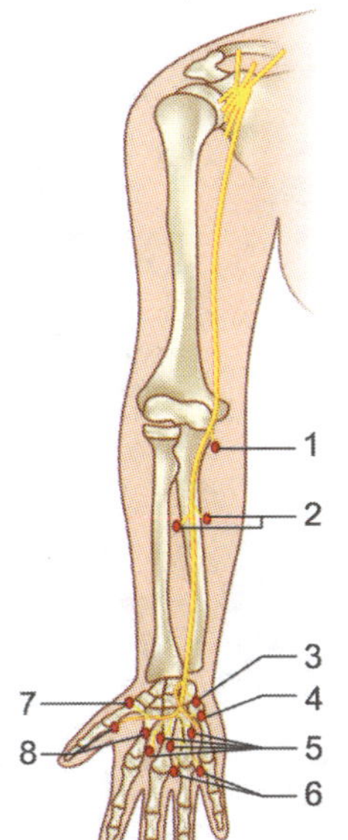

Ulnar nerve

Distribution of the motor branches

1. Flexor carpi ulnaris
2. Flexor digitorum profundus ulnar portion
3. Hypothenar muscles: abductor, short flexor, opponens of little finger
4. Palmaris brevis
5. All dorsal and palmar interossei
6. Ulnar lumbricals
7. Deep head of flexor pollicus brevis
8. Adductor pollicus

120. Ans. (a) Teres major

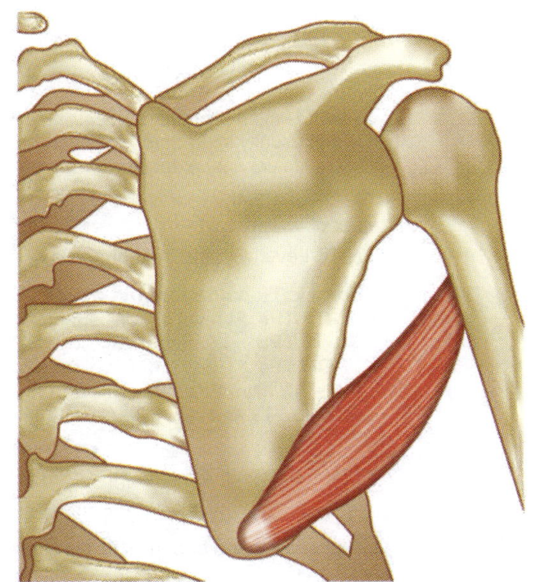

- The shown muscle in the image is teres major.
- Origin-Inferior angle of scapula
- Insertion-Intertubecular sulcus of humerus
- Action
  - Extends arm at shoulder joint
  - Assist in adduction and medial rotation of arm at shoulder joint
- Nerve supply
  - Lower subscapular nerve

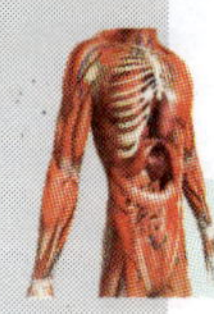

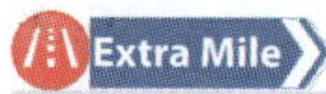

Identify the deep muscles of shoulder in image

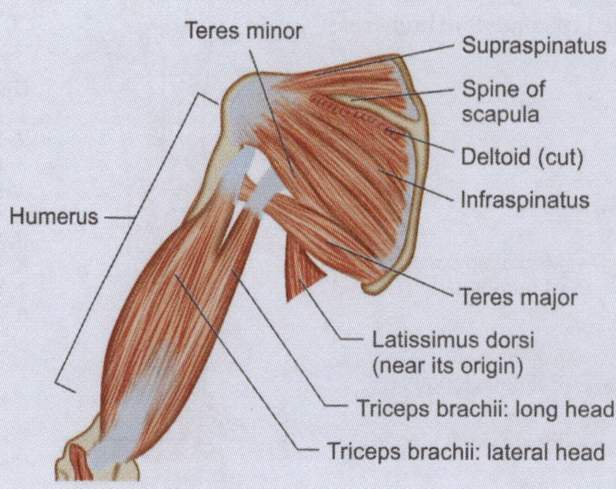

121. Ans. (c) T8

- Inferior scapular angle lies at the anatomical level of T8

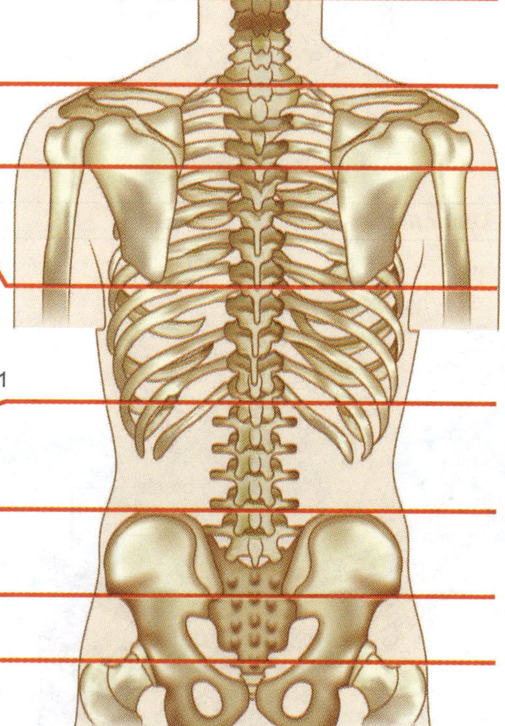

SP: Spinous process, TP: Thoracic process

122. Ans. (b) Pectoralis major

Anatomy of pectoralis major muscle:

- **Origin:** Clavicle, sternum and costal cartilage 2nd–6th ribs
- **Insertion:** Lateral lip of intertubercular groove of humerus
- **Function:** Flexion, adduction and medial rotation of arm

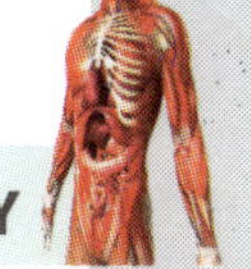

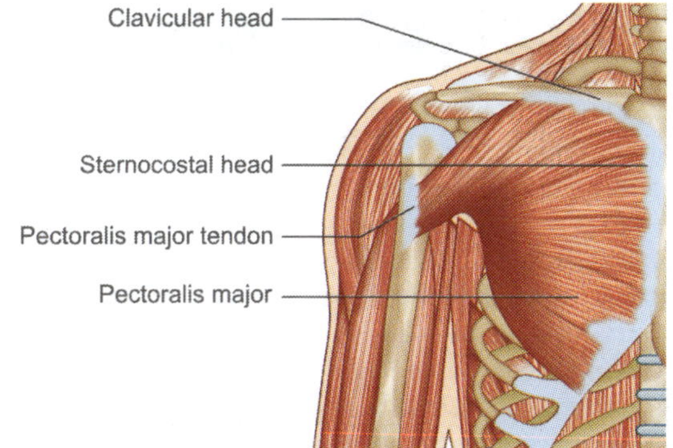

123. Ans. (c) Axillary nerve

- Upper lateral cutaneous nerve of the arm is a branch of axillary nerve.
- Supplies skin over lower half of deltoid.

124. Ans. (d) Radial head

Ref: Gray's Anatomy, 41st ed. pg. 839

- The arrow here points towards radial head.
- The radial head articulates with humeral capitulum

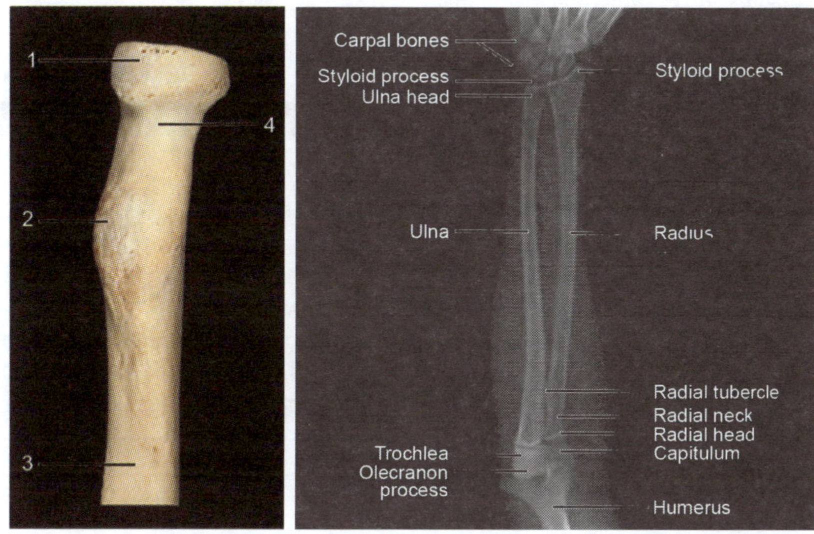

FIGURE: The proximal end of the left radius, anterior view. Key 1. head; 2. radial tuberosity; 3. shaft; 4. neck

125. Ans. (b) Trapezius

Ref: Gray's Anatomy, 41st ed. pg. 810, 786.e1

- **Protraction:** Involves moving the scapula away from midline (abduction)
- **Retraction:** Involves moving the scapula towards the midline (adduction) and is done by middle part of trapezius and Rhomboids muscle

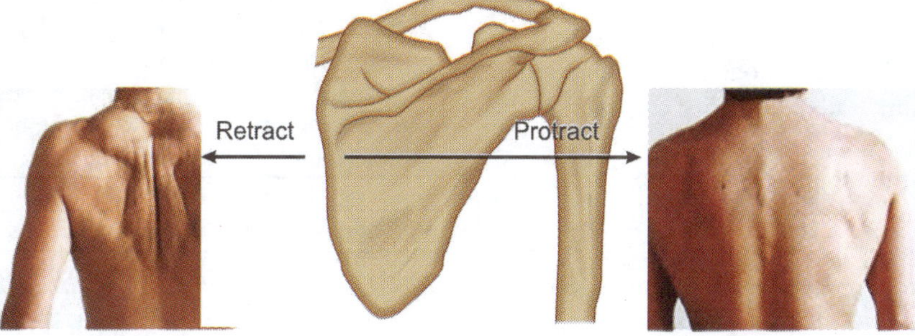

Muscles of Scapular Stabilization:

- **Trapezius:**
  - Retraction (middle part)
  - Elevation (superior part)

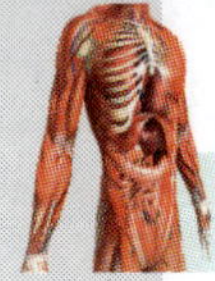

  - Depression (Inferior part)
  - Upward rotation (superior + middle)
- **Rhomboid:** Retraction
- **Levator scapulae:** Elevation
- **Serratus anterior and Pectoralis major:** Protraction

126. Ans. (a) Pronation

Ref: Gray's Anatomy, 41st ed. pg. 846-48

- Pronator teres muscle is involved in pronation of forearm, by rotating the radius medially on the ulna.
- Proximally movements at the humeroradial joint and distally at radioulnar joints pronate and supinate the hand.
- In pronation, the radius turns anteromedially and obliquely across the ulna.
  - Proximal end remains lateral to the ulna while its distal end lies medially and the interosseous membrane becomes spiralled.
- If there is fracture at this pronator muscle insertion area → it may be detached → Forearm acquired supination.
- The movement pronation is restricted.

127. Ans. (a) Radial tuberosity

Ref: Gray's Anatomy, 41st ed. pg. 824

- The shown muscle in the image is biceps brachii.
- It has two proximal heads (hence the name). Their attachments are:
  - **Short head:** Tip of coracoid process
  - **Long head:** Supraglenoid tubercle of scapula
- **Insertion:**
  - Radial tuberosity and fascia of forearm via bicipital aponeurosis
- **Innervation:** Musculocutaneous nerve (C5, C6)
- **Action:** Supination of forearm and flexion of shoulder joint

128. Ans. (c) Atavistic epiphysis

Ref: Clinical Anatomy, Kulkarni 2nd ed. pg. 73

TYPES OF EPIPHYSIS

- **Pressure:** Seen at the end of long bones subjected to pressure. E.g. Femur, head of humerus, condyles of tibia and femur.
- **Traction:** Formed due to pull of muscles. E.g. Mastoid process, tibial tuberosity, tubercles, trochanters.
- **Atavistic:** Functional in lower animals. Degenerated in humans e.g. Coracoid process of scapula, os trigonum of talus
- **Abberant:** It is an extra epiphysis. E.g. Proximal end of 1st metacarpal bone.

129. Ans. (a) Ulnar nerve

Ref: Gray's Basic Anatomy E-book, pg. 399

Carpal Tunnel Anatomy

- Posterior border
  - Carpal bones
- Anterior border
  - Transverse carpal ligament
- Boundaries
  - Proximally—pisiform and tubercle of navicular
  - Distally—hook of hamate and tubercle of trapezium
- Contents
  - Flexor digitorum superficialis
  - Flexor digitorum profundus
  - Flexor pollicis longus
  - Median nerve

130. Ans. (a) Ulnar nerve

Ref: Gray's Anatomy, review E-book, pg. 336

Clinical Correlates: Guyon's Canal Syndrome

- Guyon's canal (ulnar tunnel) is formed by the pisiform, hook of the hamate, and pisohamate ligament, deep to the palmaris brevis and palmar carpal ligament and transmits the ulnar nerve and artery.
- Guyon's canal syndrome is an entrapment of the ulnar nerve in the Guyon's canal.
- **Symptoms:** Pain, numbness, and tingling in the ring and little fingers, followed by loss of sensation and motor weakness.
- **Rx:** Surgical decompression of the nerve.

131. Ans. (a) C5-C6

Ref: Gray's Anatomy, 41st ed. pg. 792

- **Biceps jerk (C5, 6)** The elbow is flexed to a right angle and slightly pronated. A finger is placed on the biceps tendon and struck with a percussion hammer; this should elicit flexion and slight supination of the forearm.

Extra Mile

- **Triceps jerk (C6–8)** The arm is supported at the wrist and flexed to a right angle. Triceps tendon is struck with a percussion hammer just proximal to the olecranon; this should elicit extension of the elbow.
- **Radial jerk (C7, 8)** The radial jerk is a periosteal, not a tendon reflex. The elbow is flexed to a right angle and the forearm placed in the mid pronation/supination position. The radial styloid is struck with the percussion hammer. This elicits contraction of brachioradialis, which causes flexion of the elbow.

132. Ans. (d) 164

Ref: Vishram Singh, Vol. I: 2nd ed. pg. 22

- Angle of humeral torsion is 164 degrees in contrast to femoral torsion of 15 degrees.
- The angle of humeral torsion is due to *angulation* between the *long axis of articular surface of the upper and lower ends of humerus*. This is because the upper end appears to have rotated laterally

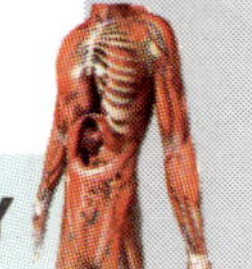

133. Ans. (c) Hamate

Ref: Kulkarni Clinical Anatomy, 2nd ed. pg. 80

The largest carpal bone is capitate and the carpal bone with **H**ook is **H**amate.

Extra Mile

- Proximal row of carpals (Lateral to Medial): **S**caphid, **L**unate, **T**riquetral and **P**isiform
- Distal row of carpals: **T**rapezium, **T**rapezoid, **C**apitate and **H**amate Pisiform bone is a *sesamoid* bone lying in the tendon of *flexor carpi ulnaris.*
- Mnemonic to remember carpal bones *"She Looks Too Petite, Try To Catch Her"*

134. Ans. (a) Capitate

Ref: Kulkarni Clinical Anatomy, 2nd ed. pg. 80

- The carpal bones are cartilaginous at birth. Capitate is the first bone to ossify at 1 year and pisiform the last one to ossify at 12 years.

Extra Mile

- Scaphoid is boat-shaped. Its neck or waist subdivides the scaphoid into proximal and distal segments. A tubercele projects from its lateral side. It lies in the floor of anatomical snuff-box, where it can be palpated.
- Lunate is shaped like lunar crescent (shape of half moon).
- Triquetral is pyramidal in shape.
- Pisiform is pea-shaped. It is a sesamoid bone in the tendon of flexor carpi ulnaris.
- Trapezium is quadrilateral and bears a crest and groove (for lodging tendon of flexor carpi radialis). It takes part in the first carpometacarpal joint, which imparts unique mobility to human thumb.
- Trapezoid is irregular like a baby's shoe.
- Capitate bears a big head. It is largest carpal bone.
- Hamate has a hook-shaped process.

135. Ans. (d) Hamate

Ref: Kulkarni Clinical Anatomy, 2nd ed. pg. 80

Proximal row of carpals (Lateral to Medial): Scaphoid, Lunate, **T**riquetral and **P**isiform.

136. Ans. (c) Scaphoid

Ref: BDC, 6th ed. Vol. I, pg. 26

- The scaphoid is a BOAT SHAPED carpal bone and has a tubercle in its lateral side.
- Scaphoid bone is the most commonly fractured carpal bone.
- Lunate (crescent shaped) is the 2nd most commonly fractured carpal bone.
- Scaphoid fracture is usually caused by a fall on an outstretched hand with the weight landing on the palm.
- Scaphoid bone forms the floor of the anatomical snuff box.
- It articulates with the following bones: radius, lunate, capitate, trapezium, and trapezoid.

137. Ans. (a) Triquetral

Ref: BDC, 6th ed. Vol. I, pg. 25; Snell's 8th ed. pg. 402

PISIFORM

- It is a sesamoid bone in the tendon of flexor carpi ulnaris.
- ***Its dorsal surface presents a smooth, oval facet, for articulation with the triquetral***
- The palmar surface is rounded and rough, and gives attachment to the transverse carpal ligament, and to the Flexor carpi ulnaris and Abductor digiti quinti.

138. Ans. (d) C7

Ref: Kulkarni Clinical Anatomy, 2nd ed. pg. 18

- Brachial plexus is composed of anterior rami of spinal nerves C5 to T1.
- *C5 and C6* join to form the *upper* trunk
- Root *C7* forms the *middle* trunk
- Root *C8* and *T1* join to form the *lower* trunk

139. Ans. (b) Axillary nerve

Ref: Kulkarni Clinical Anatomy, 2nd ed. pg. 30

The damage to axillary nerve leads to regimental badge anesthesia.

Axillary nerve injury leads to *deltoid* and *teres minor* paralysis. The manifestations are:

- *Loss of rounded contour of shoulder*
- Sensory loss in skin covering lower part of deltoid.
- Loss of abduction from 15° to 90° is due to deltoid paralysis.

140. Ans. (b) Anconeus

Ref: Kulkarni Clinical Anatomy, 2nd ed. pg. 73

- The screwing movement is due to action of muscle aconeus.
- The anconeus muscle is a small triangular muscle located at the elbow. It *originates* at the *dorsal side of the lateral epicondyle* of the humerus and *inserts* at the *olecranon of ulna.*
- It is *supplied by* motor branch of *radial nerve (C6-C8)* which arises at the radial sulcus of the humerus.

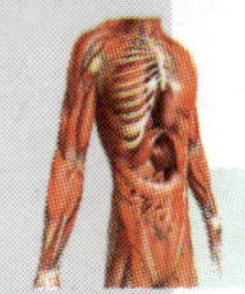

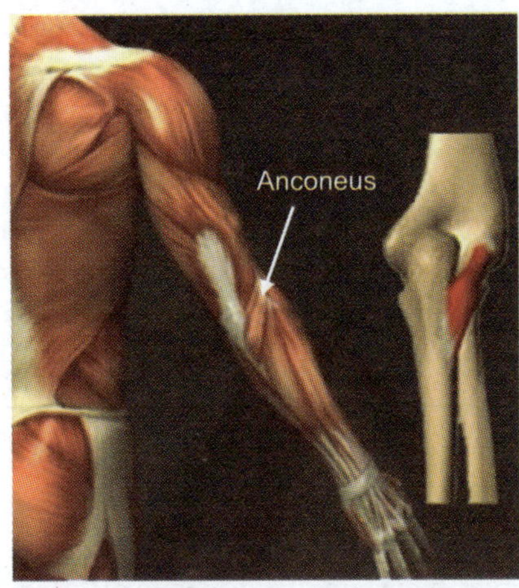

141. Ans. (b) Deep palmar arch

Ref: Kulkarni Clinical Anatomy, 2nd ed. pg. 20

- *Radial* artery ends as **deep palmar arch** while the *ulnar* artery ends as **superficial palmar arch**.
- Branches of branchial artery which *terminates* as *radial and ulnar* artery:
  - Muscular artery
  - Profunda brachii artery (accompanies the radial nerve in spiral groove)
  - Superior and inferior ulnar collateral artery

142. Ans. (c) Subacromial bursa

Ref: Kulkarni Clinical Anatomy, 2nd ed. pg. 48

The subacromial bursa is the *largest bursa* of the body

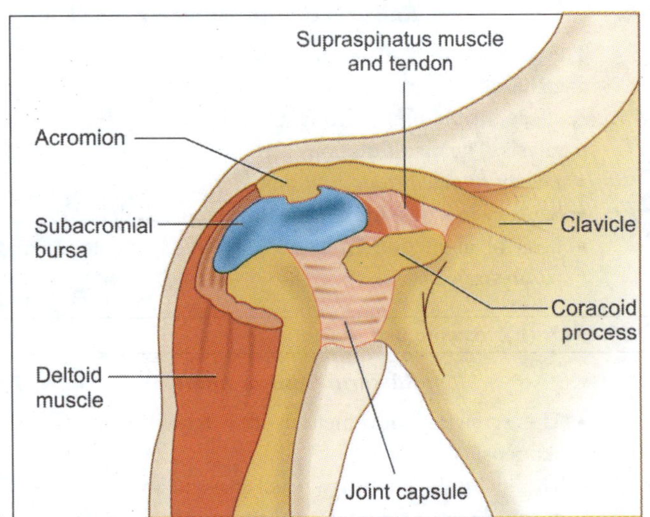

143. Ans. (a) Ulnar

Ref: BDC, 6th ed. Vol. I, pg. 93; Gray, 822,29,37

- Nerve passing through medial epicondyle is ulnar nerve. Very often when we hit our elbow on any surface, the current like feeling in arm, is due to ulnar nerve injury.
- **Medial epicondyle fracture causes injury to ulnar nerve.**
  - Ulnar nerve palsy causes partial claw hand.
  - **Claw hand**-sensory loss of medial 1 ½ digits.
  - Weakness of grip (paralysis of intrinsic muscle)
  - Loss of flexion of MCP (lumbricals and interossei)
  - Loss of adduction of thumb

144. Ans. (d) 2nd part of axillary artery

Ref: BDC, 6th ed. Vol. I, pg. 73

- The extreme mobility of shoulder may result in kinking of axillary artery.
- To compensate this, an arterial anastomosis exists between branches of 1st part of subclavian artery and *3rd part of axillary artery (NOT 2nd part axillary artery).*
- It also provides collateral circulation when the subclavian artery is obstructed *(Eg: by a cervical rib or fibrous band)*
- **This anastomosis involves:**
  - *Suprascapular artery and deep branch of transverse (superficial) cervical arteries-* ***both arising from thyrocervical trunk of 1st part of subclavian artery***
  - *Subscapular artery & its circumflexscapular branch (arising from 3rd part of axillary artery).*

145. Ans. (b) Radial artery

Ref: BDC, 6th ed. Vol. I, pg. 122; Gray's 41st ed. pg. 790

- The anatomical snuffbox is formed by the tendons of extensor polloicis longus and brevis, and abductor pollicis longus.
- It has the radial artery running in the floor of the snuffbox, and the radial nerve passing to the dorsum of the hand.
- **Boundaries of snuff box:**
  - **Postero-medial border** is the tendon of the extensor pollicis longus.
  - **Anterolateral border** is a pair of parallel and intimate tendons of the **extensor pollicis brevis** and the **abductor pollicis longus.**
  - The **proximal border** is formed by the styloid process of the radius.
  - The **distal border** is formed by the approximate apex of the schematic snuffbox isosceles.

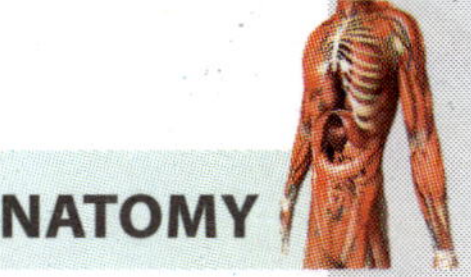

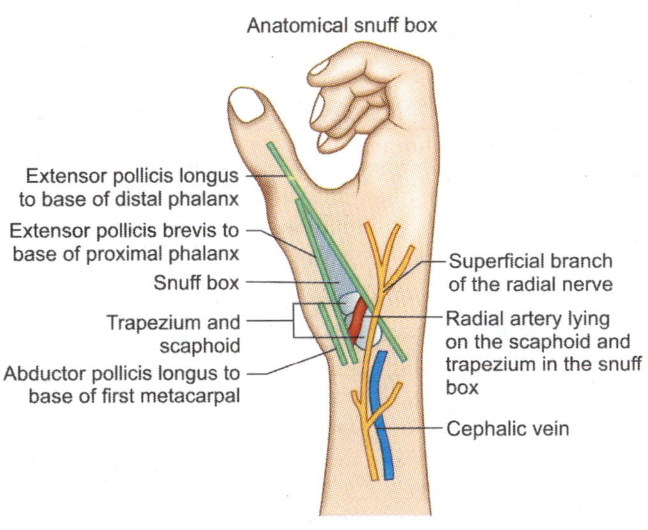

146. Ans. (b) Radial artery

Ref: BDC, 6th ed. Vol. I, pg. 22, 5th ed. pg. 102

Please refer to above explanation.

147. Ans. (c) Extensor pollicus longus

Ref: Gray's 41st ed. pg. 790

148. Ans. (a) Teres major palsy

Ref: BDC, 4th ed. Vol. I / 62, 171; Gray's 41st ed. /831-33

- Axillary nerve (C5, C6) is injured due to surgical neck fracture or due to shoulder dislocation.

Motor injury	Sensory injury
• **Deltoid muscle palsy:** Loss of rounded contour of shoulder • Weakness of abduction • Teres minor palsy	• Lateral cutaneous nerve of arm • Sensory loss over lower half of deltoid *(regimental batch area)*

Note: Teres Major is supplied by lower subscapular nerve.

149. Ans. (b) Axillary

Ref: Gray's 41st ed. pg. 831e-2; Keith L. Moore 5th ed. pg. 760

- Anterior shoulder dislocation can cause injury to axillary nerve
- Axillary nerve passes inferior to the humeral head and winds around the surgical neck of the humerus. The axillary nerve is usually injured during fracture of this part of the humerus.
- It may also be damaged during dislocation of the gleno-humeral joint and by compression from the incorrect use of crutches.

150. Ans. (a) Flexor digitorum profundus

Ref: Gray's, 41st ed. pg. 851

- **Composite** or **hybrid muscles** are those muscles which have more than one set of fibers but perform the same function and are usually supplied by different nerves for different set of fibers
- The muscles of the anterior compartment are innervated mostly by the median nerve, but one and a half muscles are innervated by the ulnar nerve which are FLEXOR CARPI ULNARIS and HALF OF FLEXOR DIGITORUM PROFUNDUS.

OTHER HYBRID/COMPOSITE MUSCLES

- **Adductor magnus:** Adductor part is innervated by **OBTURATOR NERVE** whereas the Hamstring part is innervated by **SCIATIC NERVE**
- **Biceps femoris:** Its long head is supplied by the **TIBIAL BRANCH OF SCIATIC NERVE** whereas the short head is supplied by the **COMMON PERONEAL NERVE.** This reflects the composite derivation from the flexor and extensor musculature.
- **Pectineus:** Its anterior set of fibers are supplied by the femoral nerve, whereas posterior set of fibers are supplied by the obturator nerve.
- **Iliopsoas:** It is a composite muscle performing flexion at the hip.

151. Ans. (c) Palmaris longus

Ref: BDC, 6th ed. Vol. I, pg. 113

- **Palmaris longus** passes **superficial** to flexor retinaculum.
- **Structures Deep to flexors retinaculum:**
  - Flexor digitorum superficialis (FDS)
  - Flexor digitorum profundus (FDP)
  - Flexor pollicis longus (FPL)
  - Flexor carpi radialis
  - *Median nerve*
- **Structures Superficial to flexor retinaculum:**
  - **Palmaris longus**
  - *Ulnar nerve and artery*
  - Palmar cutaneous branches of median and ulnar nerves

152. Ans. (a) Ulnar nerve

Ref: BDC, 6th ed. Vol. I, pg. 113

- Ulnar nerve passes above (superficial) to flexor retinaculum especially the palmar cutaneous branch of ulnar nerve.

153. Ans. (a) C5, C6

Ref: BDC, 6th ed. Vol. I, pg. 55-56; Clinical Anatomy by Harold Ellis, 11th ed. pg. 189-190

Brachial Plexus in a Nutshell

- **Five *roots*** derived from the anterior primary rami of C5, 6, 7, 8 and T1; link up into:

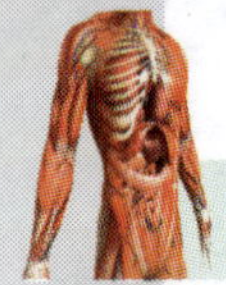

- **Three *trunks*** formed by the union of
  - C5 and 6 (upper);
  - C7 alone (middle);
  - C8 and T1 (lower)

Which split into:

- **Six *divisions*** formed by each trunk dividing into an anterior and posterior division; which link up again into:
- **Three *cords***
  - A lateral, from the fused anterior divisions of the upper and middle trunks;
  - A medial, from the anterior division of the lower trunk;
  - A posterior, from the union of all three posterior divisions.

Division is remembered as "RTDC"

*"The **roots** lie between the anterior and middle scalene muscles. **The trunks** traverse the posterior triangle of the neck. The **divisions** lie behind the clavicle. **The cords** lie in the axilla"*

The cords continue distally to form the main nerve trunks of the upper limb thus:

- The lateral cord continues as the *musculocutaneous nerve*;
- The medial cord, as the *ulnar nerve*;
- The posterior cord, as the *radial nerve* and the *axillary nerve*;
- A cross-communication between the lateral and medial cords forms the *median nerve*.

Note

- 5 BRANCHES of Posterior cord and their root nerve:
  - Upper subscapular Nerve **(C5, C6)**
  - Lower subscapular Nerve **(C5, C6)**
  - Nerve to latissimus dorsi **(C6, 7, 8)**
  - **AXILLARY NERVE (C5, C6)** → *SUPPLIES DELTOID AND TERES MINOR*
  - Radial nerve **(C5 to T1)**

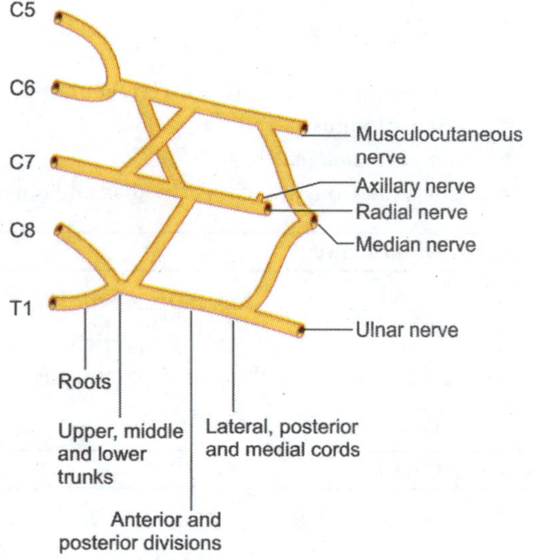

154. Ans. (b) Lateral cord

Ref: BDC, 6th ed. Vol. I, pg. 55-56

155. Ans. (c) C5, C6, C7, C8, T1

Ref: BDC, 6th ed. Vol. I, pg. 55-56

156. Ans. (b) Long thoracic nerve

Ref: BDC, 6th ed. Vol. I, pg. 55-56; 3rd ed. Vol. I, pg. 45-50; 180,181

- Winging of scapula is due to damage of long thoracic nerve due to paralysis of serratus anterior muscle.
- **Serratus anterior** helps in *vertical overhead abduction* (assisted by trapezius), *forward punch* (assisted by pectoralis minor) & *forced inspiration.*
- *Its paralysis leads to winging of scapula.*
- Nerve Supply of Serratus anterior: **Long Thoracic Nerve** *(Nerve of Bell) (C5, C6, C7)*
- ***Action of Serratus anterior muscle***
  - Rotates the scapula so that glenoid cavity is raised upward & forward- Helps in *Vertical over head abduction* (in this action *assisted by Trapezius muscle).*
  - Draws the scapula forward around the thoracic wall so *paralysis leads to winging of scapula.*
  - Also used when arm is pushed forward in horizontal position as in *forward punch (helped by Pectoralis minor in this action).*
  - Steadies the scapula during weight carrying.
  - Helps in *forced inspiration* (Accessory muscle of inspiration).
  - Because of greater pull exerted on the inferior angle, inferior angle passes laterally and forward and the glenoid cavity is raised upward & forward; in this action the muscle is assisted by trapezius.

157. Ans. (a) Serratus anterior muscle

Ref: Gray's Anatomy, 41st ed. pg. 819

- Winging of scapula is due to paralysis of **serratus anterior muscle.**
- **Nerve supplying serratus anterior muscle: Long thoracic nerve** (C5, 6, 7). Therefore long thoracic nerve palsy can also lead to winging of scapula.
- **Vascular supply:** Serratus anterior is supplied by **superior** and **lateral thoracic arteries,** and by branches from the thoracodorsal artery after it divides in latissimus dorsi.

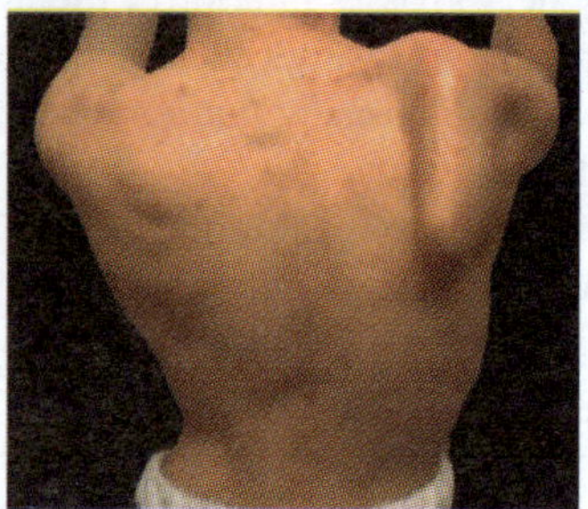

WINGING OF SCAPULA

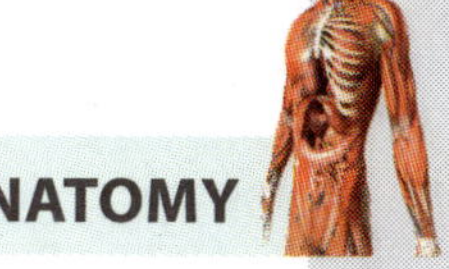

158. Ans. (a) Serratus anterior muscle

Ref: BDC, 6th ed. Vol. I, pg. 55-56

159. Ans. (d) Trapezius

Ref: Gray's, 41st ed. pg. 817

Dropped Shoulder Versus Winged Scapula

- The position of the scapula on the posterior wall of thorax is maintained by the tone and balance of the muscles attached to it.
- If one of these muscles is paralyzed, the balance is upset, as in dropped shoulder, which occurs with paralysis of the trapezius or winged scapula caused by paralysis of serratus anterior.

160. Ans. (a) First rib

Ref: Gray's, 41st ed. pg. 816-817

- **Origin of trapezius muscle is from:**
  - External occipital protuberance
  - Superior nuchal line
  - Ligament nuchae,
  - C_1 spine and
  - Spines of T_1 to T_{12} vertebrae.
- Insertion of trapezius muscle is on lateral third of clavicle (upper fibers), medial border of acromion process (middle fibers), and upper margin of spine of scapula (lower fibers).

161. Ans. (b) Abductor pollicis palsy

Ref: BDC, 6th ed. Vol. I, pg. 109-110, 120

- In ulnar nerve palsy grip is weak due to paralysis of intrinsic muscles *(all interossei, lateral 3rd & 4th lumbricals, hypothenar and adductor pollicis muscles).*
- Sensory supply of ulnar nerve is medial 1½ fingers.
- *Abductor pollicis is supplied by median nerve.*
- **Finger drop** i.e. loss of extension of metacarpophalangeal joint is seen in Radial & Posterior interosseous nerve palsy

Signs of Ulnar Nerve palsy *(remembered as BCDEF)*

- **Book test/Fromet sign:** While holding the book between thumb and rest of hand, there is overaction of flexor pollicis longus due to adductor pollicis nerve palsy.
- **Claw hand:** Clawing of medial 2 digits
- **Card test:** for testing palmar interossei, i.e. adduction of fingers. *(PAD)*
- **aDDuctor pollicis paralysis:** Adduction of thumb lost
- **Egawa's test:** To test dorsal interossei i.e. abduction of fingers *(DAB).*
- **Froment sign**

Extra Mile

- In low ulnar nerve palsy forearm muscles are spared but the clawing is more (as compared to high ulnar n. palsy) this phenomenon is known as ***ulnar paradox.***
- Lower the lesion, more the clawing.

162. Ans. (c) Median nerve

Ref: BDC, 6th ed. Vol. I, pg. 126-127, Vol. I, pg. 109,159; Clinical Anatomy, Vishram Singh/58

- Median nerve is the main nerve of the front of the forearm. It also supplies the muscles of thenar eminence.
- Median nerve aka *labourer's nerve* as it supplies most of the long muscles of the front of forearm.

Extra Mile

- ***Deformities that may occur due to median nerve paralysis:***
  - Carpal tunnel syndrome
  - Pointing index finger
  - Ape thumb deformity aka ape hand deformity
  - Claw hand (median + ulnar)
- ***Deformities that may occur due to radial nerve paralysis***
  - Wrist drop
  - Saturday night palsy
- ***Deformities that may occur due to ulnar nerve paralysis***
  - Ulnar claw hand
  - Cubital tunnel syndrome

163. Ans. (c) Median and ulnar both

Ref: BDC Vol. I, pg. 109,159; Clinical Anatomy, Vishram Singh/58

164. Ans. (c) Median nerve

Ref: BDC Vol. I, pg. 109,159; Clinical anatomy, Vishram Singh/58

- Median nerve is the main nerve of the front of the forearm. It also supplies the muscles of thenar eminence.
- The ape hand deformity or ape thumb deformity of hand is due to paralysis of thenar muscles which is supplied by median nerve.

Presenting Feature of Ape Thumb Deformity

- Thumb is laterally rotated and adducted
- Loss of thenar eminence
- Loss of opposition of thumb

165. Ans. (b) Median nerve

Ref: BDC, 6th ed. Vol. I, pg. 126

- Median nerve is the main nerve of the front of the forearm. It also supplies the muscles of thenar eminence.

- Carpal tunnel syndrome occurs as a result of compression of the median nerve. The median nerve runs from your forearm through a passageway in the wrist (carpal tunnel) to the hand. It provides sensation to the palm, side of the thumb and fingers, with the; exception of the little finger. It also provides nerve signals to move the muscles around the base of the thumb.

166. Ans. (a) Abductor pollicis longus

Ref: BDC, 6th ed. Vol. I, pg. 126-128

- Median nerve is formed by combination of lateral cord (C5, 6, 7) and medial cord (C8, T1)
- Median nerve is the main nerve of the front of the forearm. It also supplies the muscles of thenar eminence. All the muscles of anterior compartment of forearm is innervated by Median Nerve; EXCEPT: FLEXOR CARPI ULNARIS, HALF OF FLEXOR DIGITORUM PROFUNDUS.
- Muscles of the extensor compartment are innervated by Radial Nerve. **Abductor Pollicis Longus belongs to this group of muscles.**

167. Ans. (a) Teres major

Ref: BDC, 6th ed. Vol. I, pg. 68-69, 73

- The rotator cuff is a group of tendons and muscles in the shoulder, connecting the upper arm (humerus) to the shoulder blade (scapula). The rotator cuff tendons provide stability to the shoulder; the muscles allow the shoulder to rotate.

The Muscles in the Rotator Cuff Include

- Teres minor
- Infraspinatus
- Supraspinatus
- Subscapularis

- Each muscle of the rotator cuff inserts at the scapula, and has a tendon that attaches to the humerus. Together, the tendons and other tissues form a cuff around the humerus.

Mnemonic: SITS [Supraspinatous, Infraspinatous, Teres minor, Subscapularis].

Teres major is not a part of rotator cuff muscles.

168. Ans. (a) Supraspinatous muscle

Ref: BDC, 6th ed. Vol. I, pg. 68-69

- Four of the Intrinsic shoulder muscles collectively forms the Rotator cuff muscles.
- Injury or disease may damage the musculotendinous rotator cuff, producing instability of the glenohumeral joint. Trauma may tear or rupture one or more of the tendons of the SITS muscles; and ***supraspinatus** is most commonly involved.*

169. Ans. (c) Coracobrachialis

Ref: Gray's, 41st ed. pg. 819-821

- The coracobrachialis is an elongated muscle in the superomedial part of the arm. The coracobrachialis helps flex and adduct the arm and stabilize the glenohumeral joint.
- With the deltoid and long head of the triceps, it serves as a shunt muscle, resisting downward dislocation of the head of the humerus, as when carrying a heavy suitcase.
- The median nerve and/or the brachial artery may run deep to the coracobrachialis and be compressed by it.
- Nerve supply 2 Musculocutaneous nerve.

170. Ans. (a) Musculo cutaneous nerve

Ref: BDC, 6th ed. Vol. I, pg. 88

- Short head of biceps comes under anterior compartment of arm. All the muscles of the anterior compartment of arm are innervated by musculocutaneous nerve.
- Posterior compartment muscles are innervated by radial nerve.

171. Ans. (d) Long head of triceps brachii

Ref: BDC, 6th ed. Vol. I, pg. 96-97

- The **triceps brachii muscle** is the large muscle on the avoid back of the upper limb.
- It originates from the infraglenoid tubercle of scapula and inserts at the elbow joint in olecranon process of ulna.
- It is the muscle principally responsible for extension of the elbow joint (straightening of the arm).

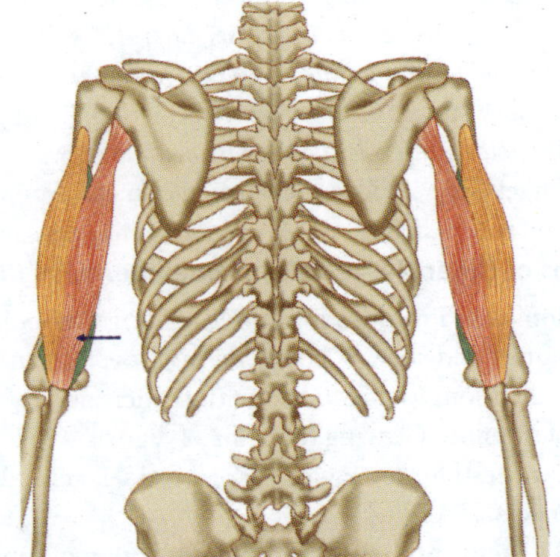

Since it has three heads, all of them have different origin:

1. **Long head:** Infraglenoid tubercle of scapula
2. **Lateral head:** Above the radial sulcus
3. **Medial head:** Below the radial sulcus

Insertion: Olecranon process of ulna

172. Ans. (b) Deltoid

Ref: Gray's Anatomy, 41st ed. pg. 113

Unipennate	• Extensor digitorum longus • Flexor pollicis longus • Soleus
Bipennate	• Rectus femoris • Dorsal interossei • Gastrocnemius
Multipennate	• Deltoid
Circumpennate	• Tibialis anterior

173. Ans. (a) Radial nerve injury

Ref: BDC, 6th ed. Vol. I, pg. 98

- Radial nerve gets injured in cases of humerus shaft fracture.
- Ulnar nerve injury may take place when there is damage to medial epicondyle of humerus and in cases of tardive ulnar palsy.
- Median nerve damage can be secondary to compression (for ex-carpal tunnel syndrome), which may lead to gun stock deformity, ape thumb deformity.

Extra Mile

- **Median nerve aka labourer's nerve** as it supplies most of the long muscles of the front of forearm.
- **Ulnar nerve aka musician's nerve** as it controls the fine movements of hand.

174. Ans. (c) Supraspinatus

Ref: BDC, 6th ed. Vol. I /47; Gray's Anatomy, 39th ed/ 841

Boundaries of Axilla

- Anterior wall: Pectoralis major, Pectoralis minor, Clavipectoral fascia
- ***Posterior wall: Subscapularis, Teres major, Latissimus dorsi***
- Medial wall: First 4 ribs & their associated intercostal muscles, Serratus anterior
- Lateral wall: Intertubercular (bicipital groove), Biceps tendon.

175. Ans. (c) Superior

Ref: Clinical Anatomy, 11th ed. pg. 160-161

The axillary lymph nodes (some 20–30|in number) drain not only the lymphatics of the breast, but also those of the pectoral region, upper abdominal wall and the upper limb, and are arranged in five groups:

- **Anterior**—lying deep to pectoralis major along the lower border of pectoralis minor;
- **Posterior**—along the subscapular vessels;
- **Lateral**—along the axillary vein;
- **Central**—in the axillary fat;
- **Apical** *(through which all the other axillary nodes drain)*—immediately behind the clavicle at the apex of the axilla above pectoralis minor and along the medial side of the axillary vein.

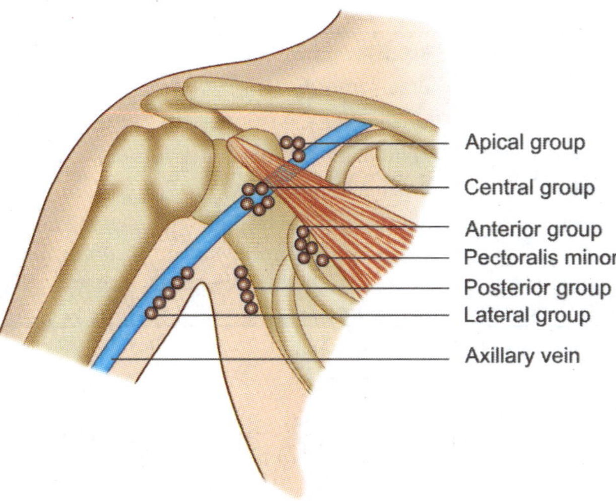

Clinicians and pathologists often define metastatic axillary node spread simply into three levels:

- Level I—nodes inferior to pectoralis minor
- Level II—nodes behind pectoralis minor
- **Level III—nodes above pectoralis minor.**

176. Ans. (b) Radioulnar joint

Ref: BDC, 6th ed. Vol. I, pg. 153-154; Clinically Oriented Anatomy by Keith, Moore, 5th ed. pg. 865

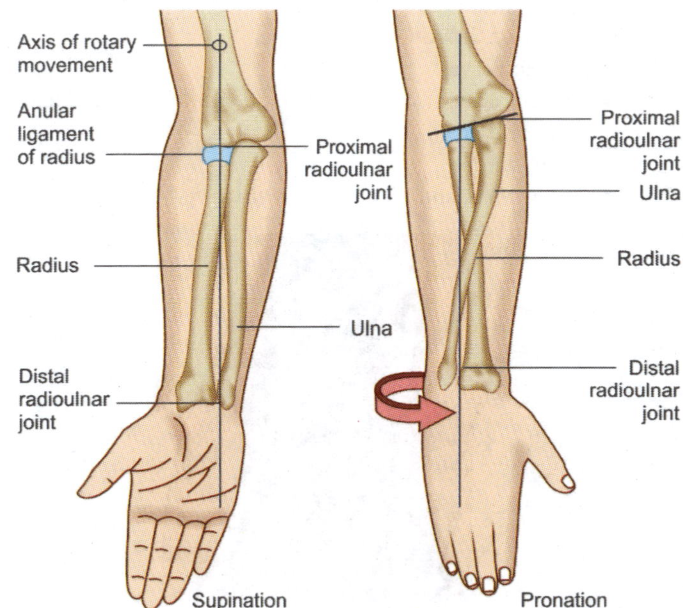

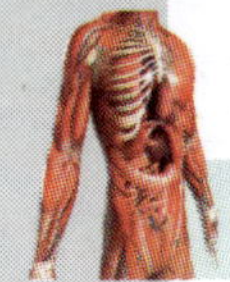

- During supination radius rotates laterally and palm faces anteriorly
- During pronation, radius rotates medially and palm faces posteriorly
- This movement takes place around distal radioulnar joint.

177. Ans. (a) Pronator teres

TABLE: Cubital fossa boundaries

Medial boundary	Pronator teres
Lateral boundary	Brachioradialis
Base	Line joining the two epicondyles of humerus
Apex	Point joining lateral and medial boundaries
Floor	Brachialis, supinator
Roof	Skin, superficial fascia *(containing medial cubital vein, lateral and medial cutaneous nerve of forearm)*, deep facia, bicipital aponeurosis

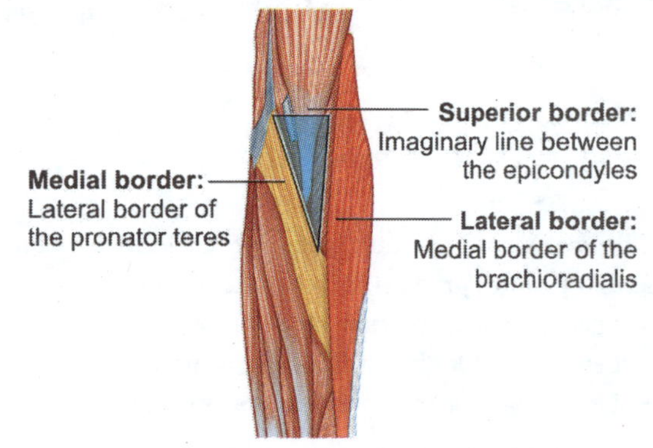

Cubital fossa (Left hand)

178. Ans. (d) Ulnar nerve

Ref: BDC, 6th ed. Vol. I, pg. 94

Contents of Cubital Fossa

- Median nerve
- Brachial artery *(termination and beginning of radial and ulnar arteries)*
- Biceps tendon
- Radial nerve and Radial collateral artery

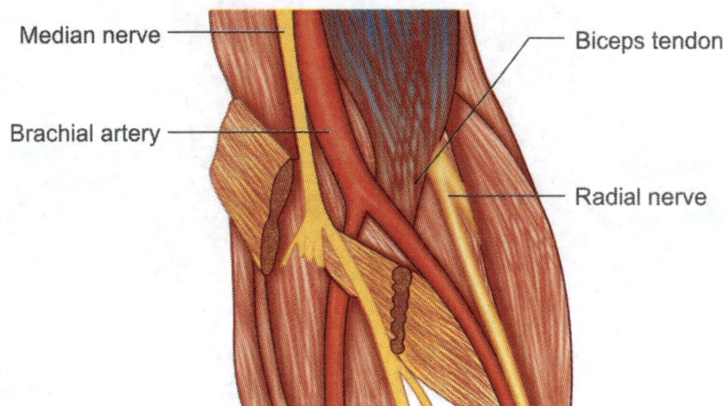

179. Ans. (b) Ulnar nerve

Ref: BDC, 6th ed. Vol. I, pg. 94

180. Ans. (c) Serratus anterior

Ref: Gray's, 41st pg. 749

- **Triangle of auscultation is bounded by:**
  - **Medially:** Trapezius
  - **Laterally:** Scapula
  - **Inferiorly:** Latissimus dorsi

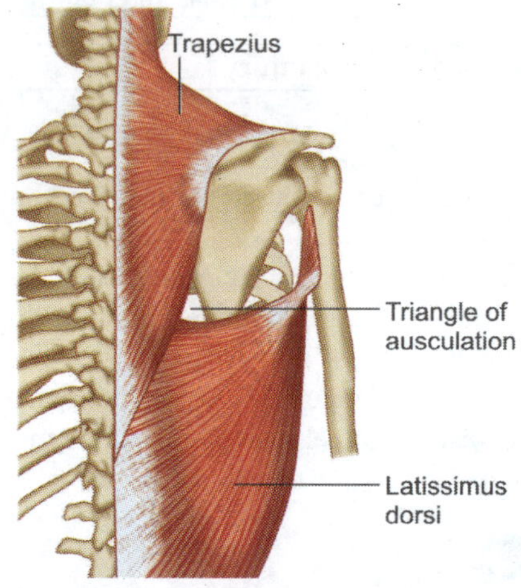

LOWER LIMB

181. Ans. (b) Posterior tibial artery

Ref: BD Chauraisia's Human Anatomy, Volume 2, 8th ed, pg. 132

- The arterial pulse being taken in above picture is of Posterior tibial artery. The posterior tibial pulse can be felt against the calcaneum about 2 cm below and behind the medial malleolus.
- It is palpated in doubtful cases of intermittent claudication where a person gets cramps and severe pain in calf muscles due to lack of blood supply.

182. Ans. (b) Posterior tibial

Ref: Gray's Anatomy, 42nd ed, pg. 1335

- The arterial pulse being taken in above picture is of Posterior tibial artery
- The posterior tibial artery of the lower limb is an artery that carries blood to the posterior compartment of the leg and plantar surface of the foot.
- The posterior tibial pulse can be felt against the calcaneum about 2 cm below and behind the medial malleolus.
- It is palpated in doubtful cases of intermittent claudication where a person gets cramps and severe pain in calf muscles due to lack of blood supply.

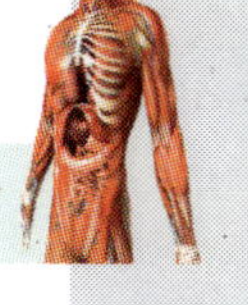

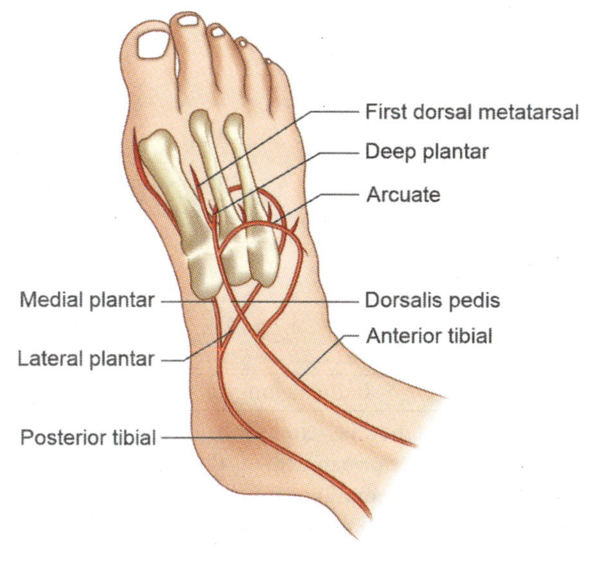

183. Ans. (c) L4

Ref: Gray's Anatomy, 42nd ed, pg. 1341

The dermatome L4 corresponds with the medial lower leg

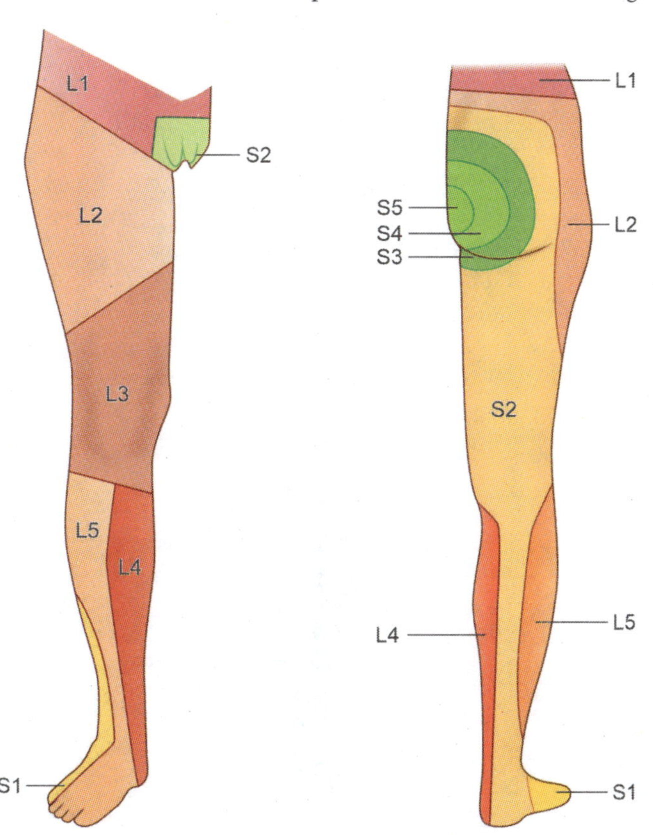

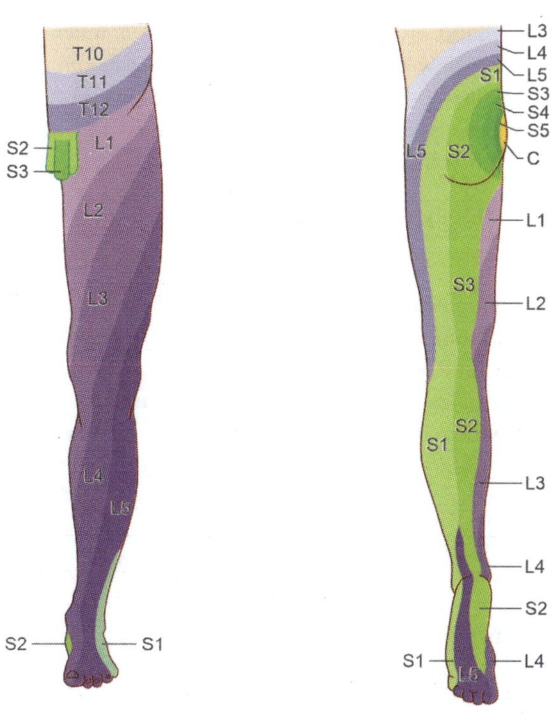

184. Ans. (b) Superficial peroneal nerve

Ref: BD Chaurasia 7th ed, Vol. II, pg. 190

- Injury to the superficial peroneal nerve can result in an inability to evert the foot and loss of sensation over the dorsum of the foot (with the; exception of the first web space between the great toe and the second toe, where the deep peroneal nerve innervates).
- **Note:** Deep peroneal nerve is involved in foot dorsiflexion and toe extension

185. Ans. (b) Quadriceps femoris

Ref: BD Chaurasia 7th ed. Vol. II, pg. 23

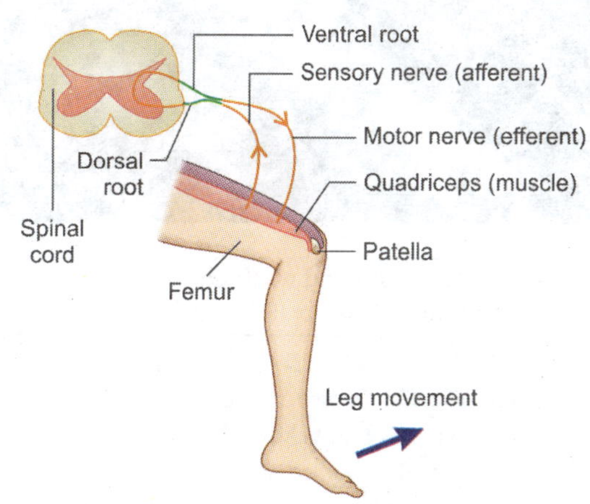

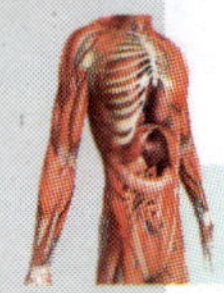

- Striking of the patellar tendon with a reflex hammer just below the patella stretches the muscle spindle in the quadriceps muscle. From there, an alpha motor neuron conducts an efferent impulse back to the quadriceps femoris muscle, triggering contraction.

186. Ans. (b) External iliac

Ref: BD Chaurasia 7th ed. Vol. II, pg. 85

- Sudden blockage of the lower aorta where it divides into the common iliac arteries causes both legs to suddenly become painful, pale, and cold.
- No pulse can be felt in the legs, which may become numb. Sudden blockage of an iliac artery causes symptoms in only one leg. These symptoms indicate a medical emergency.

187. Ans. (a) Posterior tibial artery

Ref: BD Chaurasia 7th ed. Vol. II, pg. 120

- The posterior tibial artery is a branch of the popliteal artery that supplies the posterior compartment of the leg and the sole of the foot.
- It is located in the posterior compartment of the leg, coursing from the inferior margin of the popliteus muscle up to behind the medial malleolus.

188. Ans. (c) Navicular

Ref: BD Chaurasia 7th ed. Vol. II, pg. 36

- The marked bone in the image is navicular bone.
- Identify and learn the radiological anatomy of other tarsal bone through the given image:

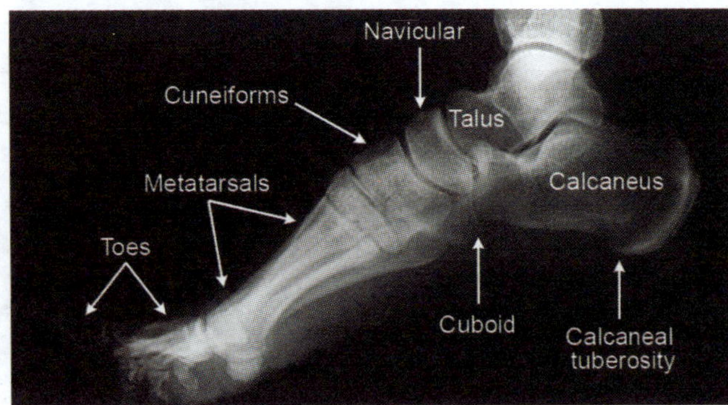

189. Ans. (a) Between medial malleolus & medial border of tendon calcaneus in inversion

Ref: BD Chaurasia, 7th Vol. II, pg. 121

- The posterior tibial pulse can be felt against the calcaneum about 2 cm below and behind the medial malleolus.
- The posterior tibial pulse is palpated in doubtful cases of intermittent claudication where a person gets cramps and severe pain in calf muscles due to lack of blood supply.

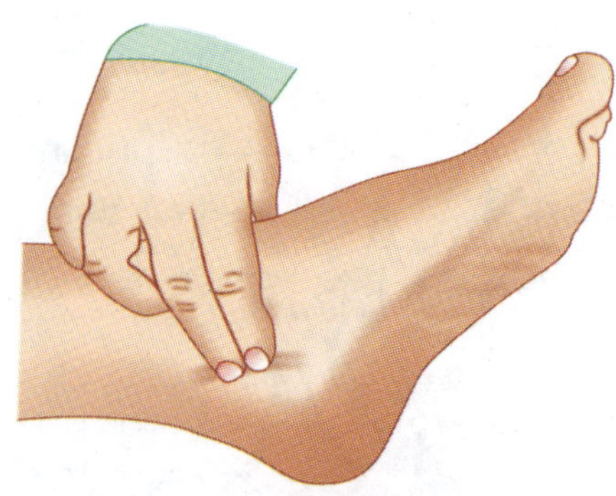

190. Ans. (b) Extensor hallucis longus

- The shown tendon is extensor hallucis longus.
- **Origin:** Anterior surface of fibula and the adjacent interosseous membrane
- **Insertion**: Base of dorsal center of distal phalanx of great toe
- **Function:** Dorsal flexion and eversion of foot and extension of toes.
- **Innervation:** Deep peroneal nerve (L4, L5, S1)

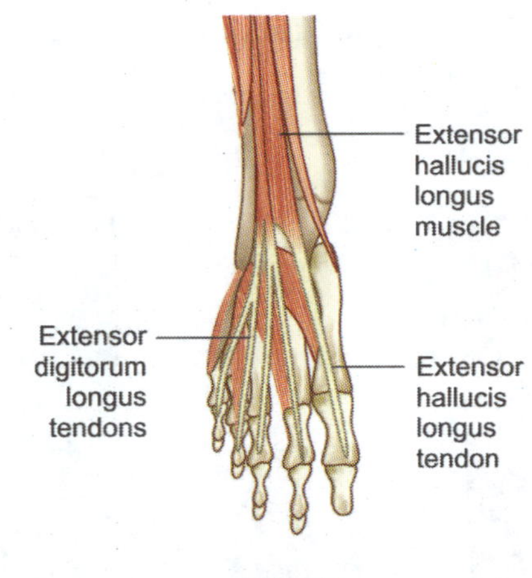

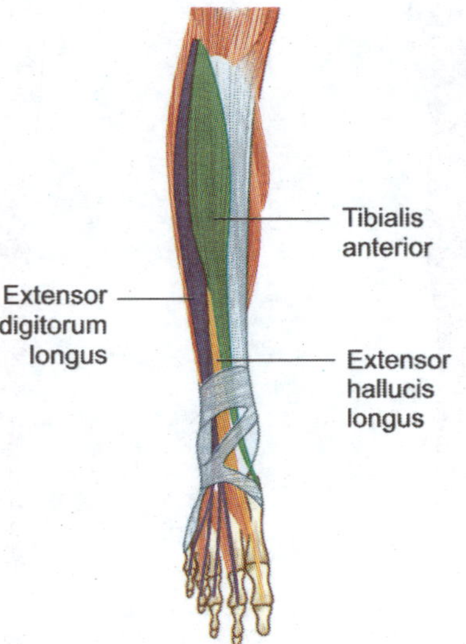

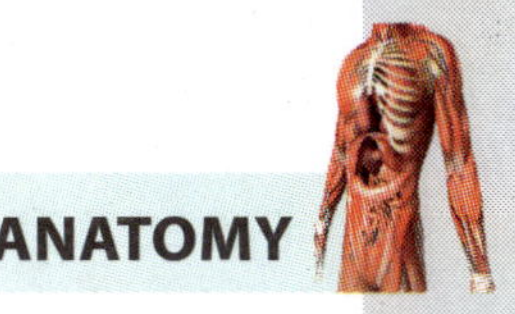

191. Ans. (d) Gluteus medius

Gluteus medius
- Posterior part covered by gluteus maximus

Origin
- Outer surface of ilium b/w iliac crest above and posterior gluteal line behind and middle gluteal line below.

Insertion
- Lateral surface of greater trochanter
- **Nerve**-superior gluteal nerve

Action
- With Gluteus minimus and tensor fascia lata-powerful abductor at hip
- Anterior fibers medially rotate the thigh
- Walking and running
- Holds opposite side of pelvis horizontally when foot is off the ground

192. Ans. (d) Biceps Femoris muscle

Ref: Gray's Anatomy, 41st ed. pg. 1324. e2

- The posterior compartment includes semitendinosus, semimembranosus and biceps femoris
  - *Note: Biceps femoris is the only muscle of the thigh that is attached distally to the fibula, and has no tibial attachment*
- Biceps femoris muscle is supplied by tibial and common peroneal nerve.
- While in posterior descent, sciatic nerve is crossed by the long head of biceps femoris and divides it into the tibial and common fibular (peroneal) nerves proximal to the knee.
- The short head of biceps femoris is supplied by the lateral (common fibular/peroneal) component.
- Long head of biceps femoris is supplied by tibial component.

193. Ans. (d) Adductor brevis

Ref: Gray's Anatomy, 41st ed. pg. 1364

- Adductor brevis is muscle of medial compartment of thigh. Muscles of this compartment are:
- **Muscles:**
  - Adductor longus
  - Adductor brevis
  - Adductor magnus (Adductor portion)
  - Gracilis
- **Action**

Adduction of HIP joint
- **Nerve supply:**

Obturator nerve

194. Ans. (c) Peroneus longus muscle

Ref: Gray's Anatomy, 41st ed. pg. 1324.e2

- Eversion of foot is the movement of foot when side of the sole is turned out laterally.

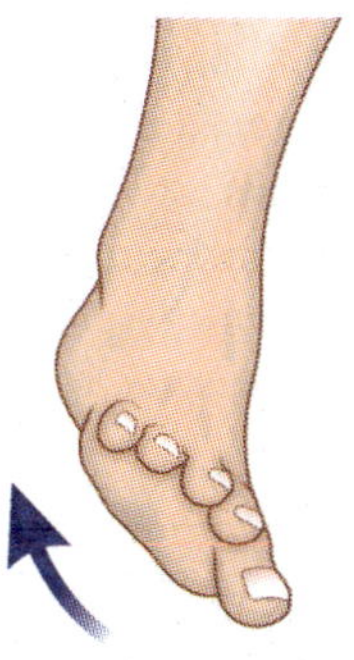

Foot eversion

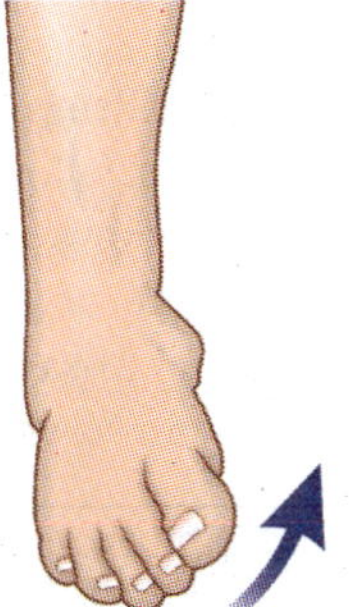

Foot inversion

- Muscles causing eversion:
  - Peroneus/Fibularis longus
  - Peroneus/Fibularis brevis
  - Peroneus/Fibularis tertius

TABLE: Ankle muscles, its actions and nerve supply

Ankle	Dorsiflexion	Tibialis anterior	Deep fibular n.
		Extensor digitorum longus	Deep fibular n.
		Extensor hallucis longus	Deep fibular n.
		Fibularis tertius	Deep fibular n.
	Plantar flexion	Gastrocnemius	Tibial n.
		Soleus	Tibial n.
		Flexor digitorum longus	Tibial n.
		Flexor hallucis longus	Tibial n.
		Fibularis longus	Superficial fibular n.
		Tibialis posterior	Tibial n.
	Inversion	Tibialis anterior	Deep fibular n.
		Tibialis posterior	Tibial n.
	Eversion	Fibularis longus	Superficial fibular n.
		Fibularis tertius	Deep fibular n.
		Fibularis brevis	Superficial fibular n.

195. Ans. (a) Common peroneal nerve

Ref: Neuromuscular Diseases: A Practical Approach to Diagnosis and Management By Schwartz, pg. 134

- **Book states:** *"In leg the common peroneal nerve is most often affected nerve"*. Nerves may be damaged at the time

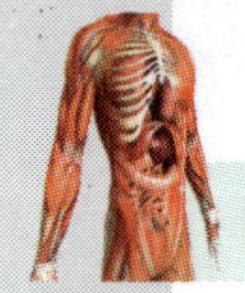

of fracture or afterwards from the effects of movement or of reduction of a dislocation.

- Iatrogenic injuries occur from penetrating injury to nerves. These usually occur during intramuscular injection of drugs, for example, a sciatic nerve injury may occasionally follow drug injections into the buttock. The femoral nerve is also vulnerable in the thigh. Attempted cannulation of veins or arteries, especially in the antecubital fossa where the median nerve is vulnerable, may cause a severe nerve injury.

196. Ans. (b) Inguinal ligament

Ref: Gray's Basic Anatomy E-book, P 280

FEMORAL TRIANGLE

A triangular depressed area situated in the upper part of the medial aspect of the thigh just below the inguinal ligament.

BOUNDARIES

Superiorly (base): The inguinal ligament
Laterally: Medial border of sartorius
Medially: Medial border of adductor longus
Apex: Continuous with adductor canal
Anterior wall: Fascia lata
Posterior wall: Consists of iliopsoas, pectineus and adductor longus from lateral to medial side.

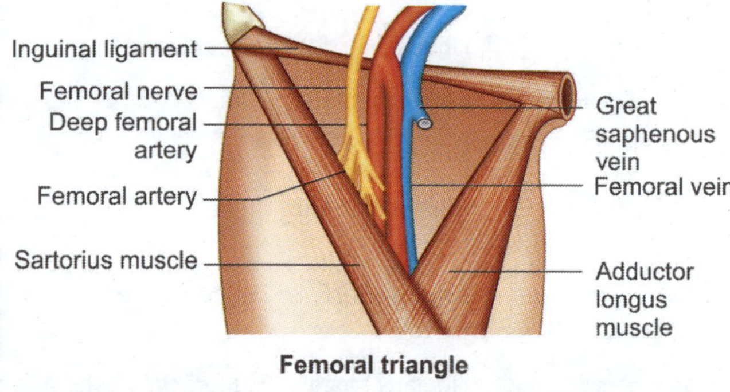

Femoral triangle

197. Ans. (b) Obturator nerve

Ref: Gray's Basic Anatomy E-book, pg. 205

Obturator nerve is a branch of lumbar plexus.
Related to ala of sacrum.
Forms the lateral boundary of ovarian fossa.
Emerges out of the obturator foramen and divides into anterior and posterior.

Branches of Obturator Nerve
A. Anterior division: Gives off:
▪ **Muscular branches to 3 muscles:** Adductor longus, adductor brevis and gracilis
▪ **Articular branch** to the hip joint
▪ **Cutaneous branch** to the skin of the medial side of the thigh.
B. Posterior division: Gives off:
▪ **Muscular branches** to 2 muscles
▪ Obturator externus and adductor magnus (pubic part)
▪ **Articular branch** to the knee joint.

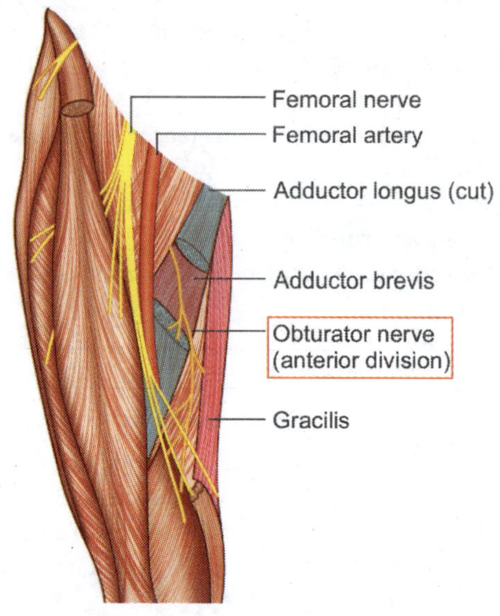

198. Ans. (c) Deep peroneal nerve

Ref: Anatomy of Foot and Ankle, pg. 12

Nerve	Motor innervation	Sensory distribution
Common peroneal (L4, L5, S1, S2)	Deep and superficial peroneal	Articular branches to knee; anterolateral aspect proximal leg (via lateral sural nerve)
Deep peroneal	Tibialis anterior, EDL, EHL, peroneus tertius Lateral branch: EDB	**Medial branch:** Dorsal first web space lateral hallux, medial second toe. **Lateral branch:** Tarsal and metatarsal joints
Superficial peroneal	Peroneus longus and brevis	Anterolateral distal two thirds of leg; dorsum of foot and toes

199. (a) Talus

Ref: Snell's Clinical Anatomy, pg. 354

Ref states: "*Numerous important ligaments are attached to talus, but no muscles are attached to this bone*"

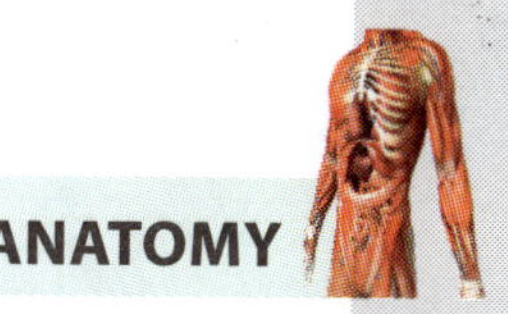

Extra Mile

Superficial group of muscles in the posterior compartment of leg (spinal segments in bold are the major segments innervating the muscle)

Muscle	Innervation	Function
Gastrocnemius	Tibial nerve [S1, S2]	Plantar flexes the foot and the knee
Plantaris	Tibial nerve [S1, S2]	Plantar flexes the foot and the knee
Soleus	Tibial nerve [S1, S2]	Plantar flexes the foot

200. Ans. (b) Sartorius

Ref: Gray's Anatomy, pg. 630

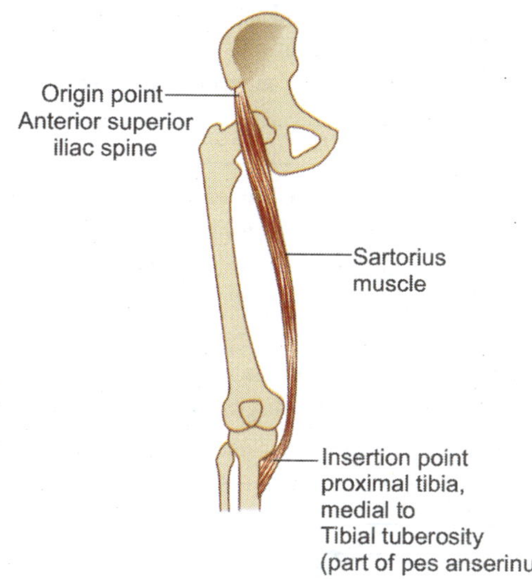

- The **anterior superior iliac spine** is a bony projection of the iliac bone and an important landmark of surface anatomy.
- It provides attachment for the inguinal ligament, and sartorius muscle.

201. (a) Posterior tibial nerve

Ref: Mac Glamry's Textbook of Foot and Ankle Surgery, pg. 196

- Posterior tibial muscle is supplied by L5, S1 (posterior tibial nerve)
  - *Action*: Inversion of the foot at the ankle.
  - *Test*: The patient holds his foot in the inverted position while the examiner pushes outward toward eversion.
- Anterior tibial muscle is supplied by L4, 5 (deep peroneal nerve)
  - *Action:* Dorsiflexion of the foot at the ankle.
  - *Test:* The patient dorsiflexes the foot and the examiner try to push the foot downward towards plantar extension.

202. (d) Vastus medialis

Ref: Gray's Anatomy, 41st ed. pg. 1319, 1339

- Adductor canal is also known as subsartorial canal or *hunter's canal.*
- It is an intramuscular space situated below the Sartorius muscle in anteromedial aspect of the distal 2/3rd of the thigh.

Boundary

- **Anterolaterally** by vastus medialis
- **Posteromedially** by adductor longus and adductor magnus.
- Its anteromedial boundary *(often referred to as the roof)* is a strong and dense fascia that extends from the medial surface of vastus medialis to the medial edge of the adductors longus and magnus, overlapping in its stride the femoral vessels in the adductor canal.

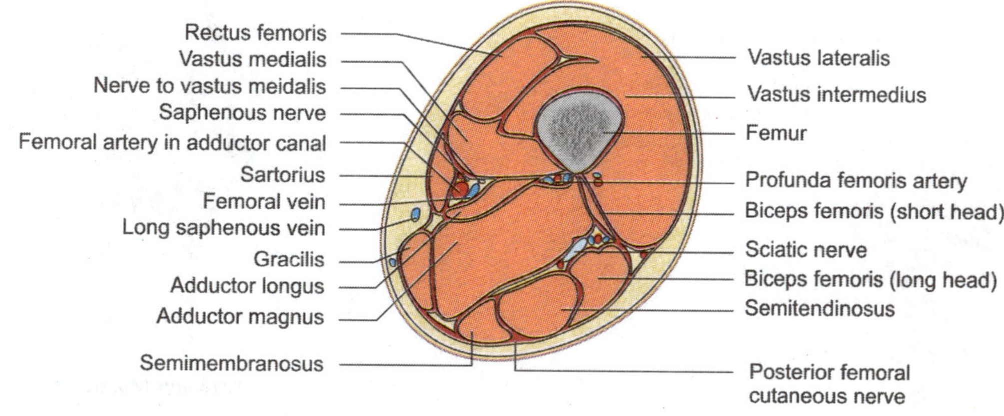

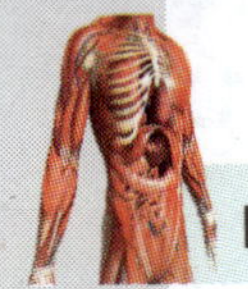

Contents of adductor canal:
- Femoral artery and its branch, descending genicular artery
- Femoral vein
- Saphenous nerve
- Nerve to vastus medialis

203. Ans. (c) Posterior division of L2, L3, L4 ventral rami

Ref: Gray's Anatomy, 41st ed. pg. 1322

- The femoral nerve is the nerve of the anterior compartment of the thigh.
- It arises from the **posterior divisions of the second to fourth lumbar ventral rami**, descends through psoas major and emerges on its lateral border to pass between it and iliacus.

Table: Root values

- Femoral nerve (L2–4)
- Obturator nerve (L2–4)
- Sciatic nerve (L4, L5, S1–3)
- Tibial nerve (L4, L5, S1–3)
- Common fibular nerve (L4, L5, S1, S2)
- Gluteal nerves (L4, L5, S1, S2)

204. Ans. (a) Iliacus

Ref: Netter's Clinical Anatomy, 3rd ed. pg. 191

Boundaries of femoral triangle
Upper border formed by: Inguinal ligament
Lateral border formed by: Sartorius
Medial border formed by: Lateral border of adductor longus
Contents of femoral triangle
A = Iliacus
B = Psoas major
C = Pectineus
D = Adductor longus

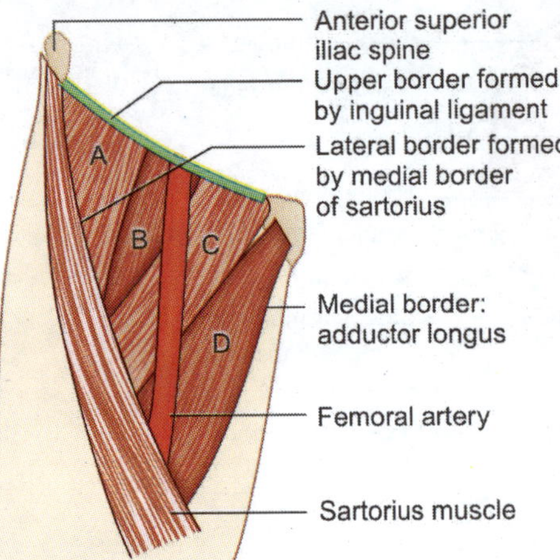

205. Ans. (b) Flexion of knee

Ref: Netter's Clinical Anatomy, 3rd ed. pg. 288

- Biceps femoris is present in posterior compartment of thigh and forms hamstrings. It is responsible for flexion of knee.
- The other hamstrings are semitendinosus and semimembranosus. All these muscles originate from the ischial tuberosity and are innervated by tibial part of sciatic nerve (L5, S1 and S2).

206. Ans. (a) Inferior gluteal nerve

Ref: Netter's Clinical Anatomy, 3rd ed. pg. 279-280

- The chief extensor of thigh at hip joint is gluteus maximus and helps in rising from sitting position.
- It is supplied by inferior gluteal nerve (L5, S1, S2). *(mnemonic: M.I.G- 512)*
- Gluteus medius are minimus are powerful abductor of thigh and are supplied by superior gluteal nerve (L4, 5, S1).

207. Ans. (a) Peroneus tertius

Ref: Kulkarni Clinical Anatomy, 2nd ed. pg. 864

- Peroneus tertius in an evertor of foot.
- Tibialis anterior muscle is an invertor of foot.
- Dorsiflexors of foot are:
  - Tibialis anterior
  - Extensor halluces longus
  - Extensor digitorum longus
  - Peroneus tertius

208. Ans. (a) Tibial nerve

Ref: Kulkarni Clinical Anatomy, 2nd ed. pg. 832

- **Origin:** Anterior part of the popliteal groove on lateral surface of lateral femoral condyle

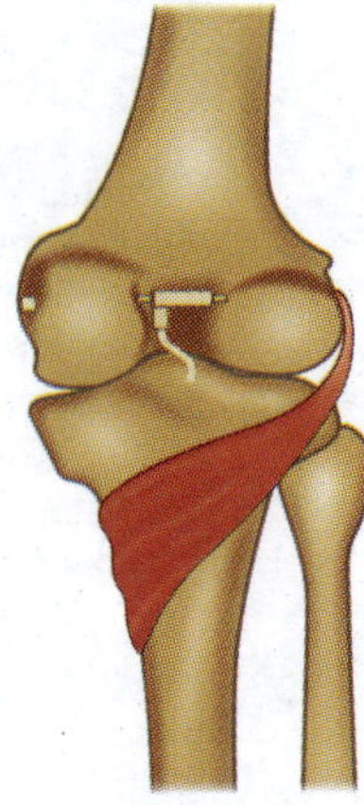

Popliteus Muscle

- **Insertion:** Posterior surface of tibia in a fan-like fashion, just superior to the popliteal line

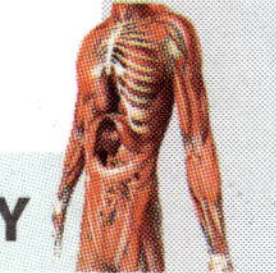

- **Action:** Rotates knee medially and flexes the leg on the thigh
- **Innervation:** Tibial nerve (L4, L5, S1)
- **Arterial supply:** Medial inferior genicular branch of popliteal artery and muscular branch of posterior tibial artery

209. Ans. (a) Paralysis of gluteus maximus

Ref: Maheswari Orthopaedics, 5th ed. pg. 135

- When a person stands on one leg, the tendency of unsupported side to sag down is *counteracted* by *gluteus medius and minimus*. These two muscles form the abductor mechanism of hip.

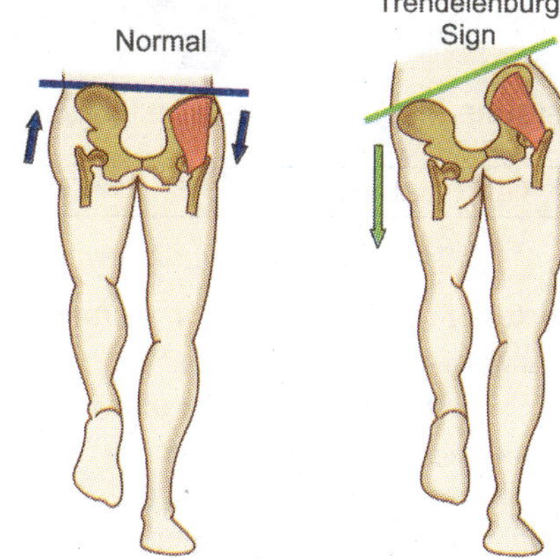

- In case the *abductor mechanism is defective*, unsupported side of the pelvis drops and is called *Positive Trendelenburg sign*. It is seen in:
  - Paralysis of gluteus medius and minimus
  - Congenital dislocation of Hip
  - Ununited fracture
  - Coxa vara

210. Ans. (d) Superior gluteal nerve

Ref: BDC 6th ed. Vol. II / 68-69, 70; Keith L. Moore 5th ed./619-621

- **Trendelenburg's sign** is found in people with weak or paralyzed abductor muscles of the hip, namely gluteus medius and gluteus minimus.
- **Superior gluteal** nerve, if injured, paralyses the 3 muscles: **gluteus medius, gluteus minimus** and tensor fascia latae and hence leads to positive **Trendelenberg test**.
- These 3 muscles, especially the gluteus medius raises the unsupported hip during walking, which otherwise will be pulled down by the gravity.
- In Trendelenberg test this action of gluteus medius (superior pelvic tilt of contralateral hip) is absent and we actually observe that there is a downward drop of the unsupported hip- due to unopposed action of gravity.
- This leads to Lurching gait in the patient.

Extra Mile

- Trendelenburg test becomes positive in congenital dislocation of hip/ long standing fracture of neck of femur.
- Inferior gluteal nerve supplies gluteus maximus.

211. Ans. (a) Gluteus medius, minimus

Ref: BDC 6th ed. Vol. II / 69-70; Keith L. Moore 5th ed. / 619-621

Please refer to above explanation.

212. Ans. (c) Genicular branch of obturator nerve

Ref: Netter's Atlas of Neurosciences, 3rd ed. pg. 194

- The capsule of knee joint is supplied by genicular branch of *obturator nerve* which pierces the oblique popliteal ligament.
- The *genitofemoral nerve* mediates the *cremasteric reflex*.

213. Ans. (b) Lateral head of gastrocnemius

Ref: Kulkarni Clinical Anatomy, 2nd ed. pg. 580

- Fabella is a small sesamoid bone present in tendon of origin of lateral *head of gastrocnemius*.

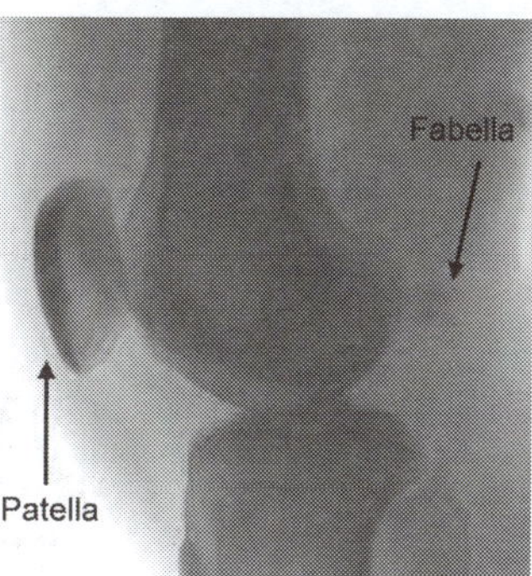

214. Ans. (a) Tibial nerve

Ref: Gray's Anatomy, 41st ed. pg. 1324e1-e2

Points to know about soleus:

- Soleus muscle is located immediately deep (anterior) to gastrocnemius.
- **Origin:** Upper third of fibula and soleal line of tibia.
- **Insertion:** Inserted with gastrocnemius into calcaneal tendon.
- **Action:** Flexes foot.
- **Nerve supply:** Soleus is innervated by two branches from the tibial nerve, S1 and S2.
- **Vascular supply:**
  - The superior arises from the popliteal artery at about the level of the soleal arch, and
  - The inferior arises from the proximal part of the fibular artery or sometimes from the posterior tibial artery.

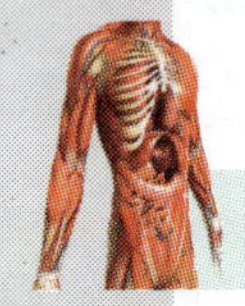

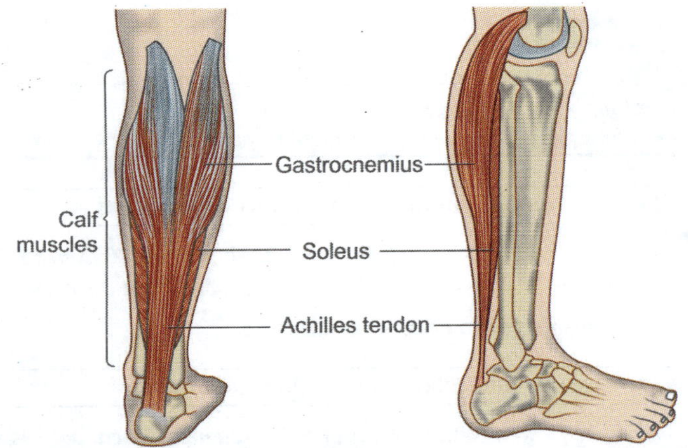

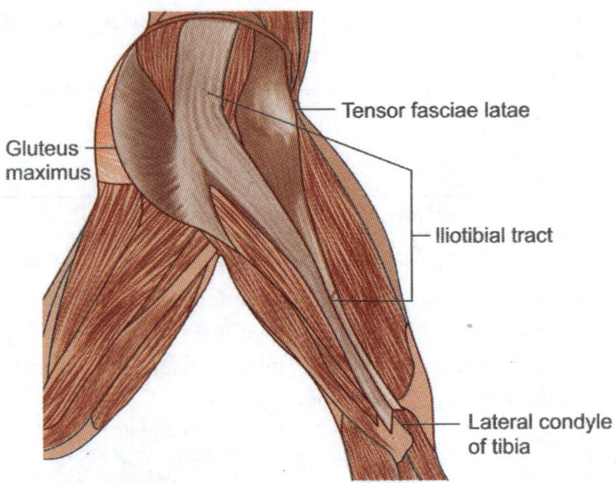

FIGURE: Important muscles of the limb

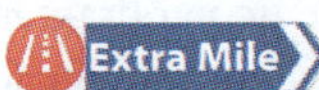

Extra Mile

TABLE: The movements and muscles tested to determine with details of innervation

Movement	Muscle	Spinal nerve level	Nerve
Hip flexion	Iliopsoas	L1, 2	Femoral
Hip adduction	Adductors	L2, 3	Obturator
Hip extension	Gluteus maximus	L5, S1	Inferior gluteal
Knee flexion	Hamstrings	S1	Sciatic
Knee extension	Quadriceps femoris	L3, 4	Femoral
Ankle dorsiflexion	Tibialis anterior	L4	Deep fibular
Ankle eversion	Fibularis longus and fibularis brevis	L5, S1	Superficial fibular
Ankle inversion	Tibialis posterior	L4, 5	Tibial
Ankle plantar flexion	**Gastrocnemius/ soleus**	S1, 2	**Tibial**
Great toe extension	Extensor hallucis longus	L5	Deep fibular

215. Ans. (a) Thickening of fascia lata

Ref: Gray's Anatomy, 41st ed. pg. 1337-38

- The iliotibial tract is a **thickened portion of the deep fascia of the thigh (fascia lata)**. This tract runs from the lateral aspect of the iliac crest to Gerdy's tubercle and produces the flattened appearance of the lateral thigh.
- The attachment on Gerdy's tubercle is on the **anterior aspect of the lateral condyle** that is usually approximately **1 cm inferior to the joint** line and about 2 cm superolateral to the tibial tuberosity.
- The upper end of the tract splits into two layers, where it encloses and anchors tensor fasciae latae and receives, posteriorly, most of the tendon of **gluteus maximus.**

216. Ans. (b) Gluteus maximus

Ref: Grays Anatomy, 41st ed. pg. 1318

The muscles of the gluteal region include:

- Three named gluteal muscles and
- The deeper short lateral rotators of the hip joint

Gluteus maximus lies most superficially

- **Origin:** Iliac, sacrum and coccyx
- **Insertion:** Gluteal tuberosity, iliotibial band
- **Function:** It is a powerful extensor of the hip joint, acting more often to extend the trunk on the femur than to extend the limb on the trunk.
- Therefore **used for changing position from sitting to standing.**

Gluteus medius and minimus

- **Attachment:** Proximally to the outer surface of the ilium and distally to the greater trochanter of the femur
- **Function:**
  - They are **abductors of the hip**;
  - Their most important action is to stabilize the pelvis on the femur during locomotion, and they are helped in this function by tensor fasciae latae.

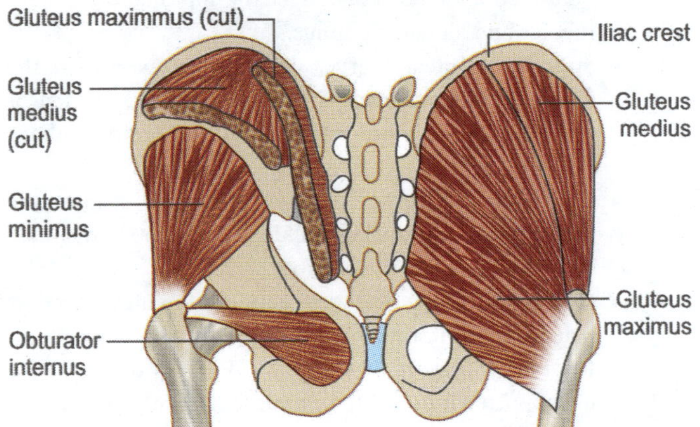

FIGURE: Gluteal and lateral rotators, posterior view

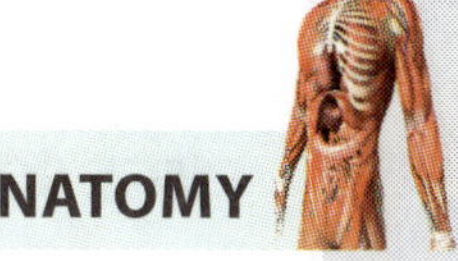

217. Ans. (c) Inferior epigastric artery

Ref: BDC, 6th ed. Vol. II, pg. 49-50

- Inferior epigastric artery is a branch of external iliac artery.
- The branches of the femoral artery are: **3 superficial** branches and **5 deep branches**

SUPERFICIAL BRANCHES (*Mn: triple S*)

- **Superficial epigastric artery**—For skin and fascia of lower part of anterior abdominal wall.
- **Superficial iliac circumflex artery**—For skin along iliac crest.
- **Superficial external pudendal artery**—For skin of external genital organ.

DEEP BRANCHES

Mnemonic: *Deep branches: Put My Dog Down Please!*

- *P*rofunda Femoris
- *M*uscular Branches
- *D*eep external pudendal branches
- *D*escending genicular arteries
- *P*erforating Branches

218. Ans. (c) Iliotibial tract

Ref: BDC, 6th ed. Vol. II, pg. 68

- **Gluteus maximus:**
  - **Origin: Iliac crest**, posterior gluteal line of ilium and area above and behind it, sacrum, coccyx, sacrotuberous ligament.
  - **Insertion:** Gluteal tuberosity and iliotibial tract.
  - Major 3/4th part inserted into iliotibial tract.
  - 1/4th part inserted into Gluteal tuberosity.

219. Ans. (c) Gluteus minimus

Ref: BDC, 6th ed. Vol. II, pg. 67-68

- **Iliotibial band is the thickened band of fascia lata. It receives insertion of three muscles:**
  - Tensor fasciae latae
  - Gluteus maximus
  - Few fibers of vastus lateralis

220. Ans. (a) Sartorius

Ref: BDC, 6th ed. Vol. II, pg. 53

- Sartorius muscle is the longest muscle of the body.
- It is also known as tailor's muscle (Sartor = tailor)

221. Ans. (b) Rectus femoris

Ref: BDC, 6th ed. Vol. II, pg. 54

- **Rectus femoris arises by two tendons**: One, the anterior or straight head, from the anterior inferior iliac spine; the other, the posterior or reflected head, from a groove above the brim of the acetabulum and the capsule of hip joint.
- The two unite at an acute angle, and are inserted into the base of the patella.

222. Ans. (a) Semimembranous

Ref: BDC, 6th ed. Vol. II, pg. 83

Hamstring muscles are

1. Semimembranosus
2. Semitendinosus
3. Long head of biceps femoris and
4. Ischial head of adductor magnus.

223. Ans. (a) Superior gluteal nerve

- Gluteus medius and minimus are supplied by superior gluteal nerve whereas gluteus maximus is supplied by inferior gluteal nerve.

Extra Mile

TABLE: Important muscles and their nerve supply

Nerve supply	Muscle
Superior gluteal nerve	• Gluteus medius • Gluteus minimus • Tensor fascia lata
Inferior gluteal nerve	• Gluteus maximus
Nerve to obturator internus	• Obturator internus • Gamellus superior
Nerve to quadratus femoris	• Gamellus inferior • Quadratus femoris

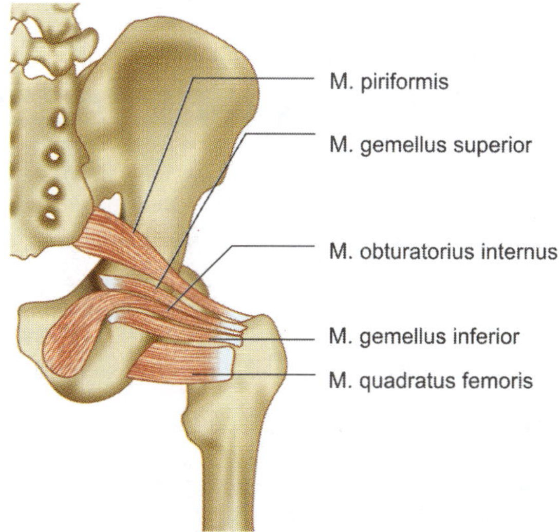

224. Ans. (b) Inferior gluteal nerve

Ref: BDC, 6th ed. Vol. II, pg. 69; Gray's Anatomy 40th ed. pg. 1384

225. Ans. (c) Nerve to quadratus femoris

Ref: BDC, 6th ed. Vol. II, pg. 69; Grays Anatomy 40th ed. pg. 1384

- **Quadratus femoris and gamellus inferior muscle are arranged together. Nerve which is bifurcating to supply quadratus femoris muscle, supplies gamellus inferior muscle as well**

Extra Mile

- Nerve supply of piriformis: Ventral rami to S1 and S2
- Nerve supply of obturator externus muscle: Posterior division of obturator nerve

226. Ans. (d) Nerve to obturator externus

Ref: BDC, 6th ed. Vol. II, pg. 74

Mnemonic to Remember this Often Asked Question

N. to obturatour internus	**Not**
Tendon of obturatour internus.	**Tonight**
Pudendal vessels and nerve.	**Please**

227. Ans. (b) Quadriceps femoris

Ref: BDC, vol II, pg. 155

- **Quadriceps femoris is the main and only extensor of knee.**
- It produces locking action as a result of medial rotation of the femur during the last stage of extension.
- To reverse this lock popliteus muscle comes into action and does so by the lateral rotation of femur

Remember: **Lock is: Quadriceps femoris muscle and, Key is popliteus muscle.**

TABLE: Muscles producing movements at the knee joint

Movement	Principal muscles
A. Flexion	• Biceps femoris • Semitendinosus • Semimembranosus
B. Extension	Quadriceps femoris
C. Medial rotation of flexed leg	• Popliteus • Semimembranosus • Semitendinosus
D. Lateral rotation of flexed leg	• Biceps femoris

Extra Mile

- **Quadriceps femoris incudes:** Rectus femoris, Vastus Lateralis, Vastis Medialis, Vastus Intermedius.
- Rectus femoris is also known as "**kicking muscle**"

228. Ans. (a) Popliteus

Ref: BDC, Vol. II, pg. 155

Please refer to above explanation

229. Ans. (c) Talus

Ref: BDC, 6th ed. Vol. II, pg. 30

- *Talus has no muscle attachment.*
- Talus also has a precarious blood supply because blood enters it distally ie. Retrograde blood supply.
- ***Remember incus in ear also has no muscle attachment.***

230. Ans. (c) Common peroneal nerve

Ref: BDC 6th ed. Vol. II, pg. 29; Snell's Anatomy, pg. 273

Common peroneal nerve is palpated against the neck of the fibula. It is a superficial nerve hence; it is unprotected as compared to tibial nerve. It may be injured in the fracture of neck of the fibula or due to a pressure of a tightly applied plaster cast. It is also affected in leprosy where it gets thickened and tender.

Clinical significance

Common peroneal nerve injury causes paralysis of dorsiflexors of the ankle joint and the evertors of the foot supplied through its superficial and deep perosneal nerve branches respectively. The paralysis of the muscles may result in **'foot drop',** where the patient walks on his toes.

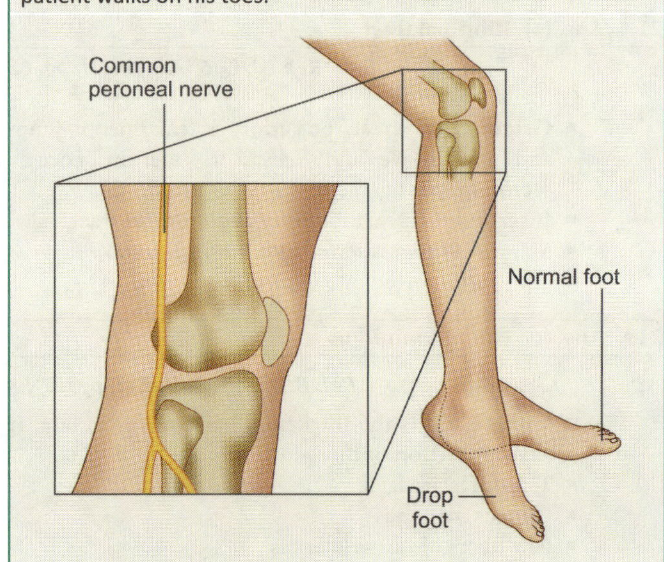

231. Ans. (b) Linea semilunaris

Ref: Gray's, 41st ed. pg. 1080-81; Keith L Moore Clinical Anatomy, 4th ed. pg.193-4

HESSELBACH'S TRIANGLE

- **Medial border:** Lateral margin the rectus sheath, also called linea semilunaris
- **Superolateral border:** Inferior epigastric vessels
- **Inferior border:** Inguinal ligament, sometimes referred to as Poupart's ligament.

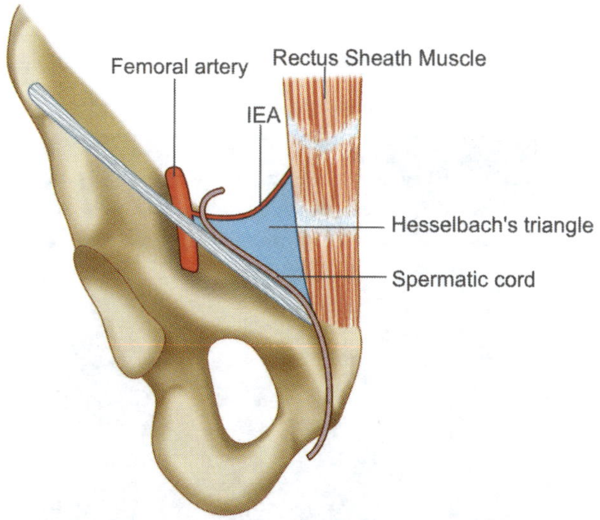

232. Ans. (d) Inferior

Ref: Gray's, 41st pg. 1080-81

233. Ans. (b) Supplies skin over the medial aspect of thigh

Ref: Clinical Anatomy, 11th ed. pg. 251

- ***The femoral nerve supplies the skin of the medial and anterior aspects of the thigh via its medial and intermediate cutaneous branches.***
- The lateral aspect is supplied by the *lateral cutaneous nerve of the thigh* (L2–3).
- As its name suggests, it is purely sensory.
- It arises from L2 and L3, travels downward lateral to the psoas muscle, crosses the iliacus muscle (deep to fascia), passes either through or underneath the lateral aspect of the inguinal ligament, and finally travels onto innervate the lateral thigh.

234. Ans. (a) $L_{4,5,}$ S_1

Ref: BDC, 6th ed. Vol. II, pg. 173

Nerve	Root valve
• **Sciatic nerve** • Tibial nerve • Common peroneal nerve	$L_{4,5}$ $S_{1,2,3}$ $L_{4,5}$, $S_{1,2,3}$ $L_{4,5,}$ $S_{1,2}$
• Superior gluteal nerve	$L_{4,5}$, S_1
• Inferior gluteal nerve	L_5, $S_{1,2}$
• Nerve to quadratus femoris	$L_{4,5}$, S_1
• Nerve to obturatus internus	L_5, $S_{1,2}$
• Superior gemellus	$L_{4,5,}$ S_1
• Inferior gemellus	$L_{4,5}$, $S_{1,2}$
• **Posterior cutaneous nerve of thigh**	$S_{1,2,3}$
• Pudendal nerve	S_2 S_3 S_4
• Perforating cutaneous nerve	$S_{2,3}$

Contd...

235. Ans. (b) S_1, S_2, S_3

Ref: BDC, 6th ed. Vol. II, pg. 173

236. Ans. (b) $L_4L_5S_1S_2S_3$

Ref: BDC, 6th ed. Vol. II, pg. 173-74

237. Ans. (b) $S_2S_3S_4$

Ref: BDC, 6th ed. Vol. II, pg. 173-174

THORAX AND ABDOMEN

238. Ans. (d) Descending aorta

Ref: BD Chauraisia's Human Anatomy, Volume 1, 8th ed, pg. 314

The arrow marked structure in the figure is Descending aorta. It is the continuation of Arch of aorta. It lies in the posterior mediastinum. It continues as abdominal aorta which ends by dividing into right and left common iliac arteries.

239. Ans. (b) L–3

Ref: BD Chauraisia's Human Anatomy, Volume 2, 8th ed, pg. 220

- The marked line in the above image corresponds to **L-3 vertebral** level.
- Umbilicus lies between L3 and L4
- The skin around umbilicus is innervated by T10

Mnemonic: T10 for Belly ButTEN

240. Ans. (b) Left atrium

Ref: Gray's Anatomy, 42nd ed, pg. 1000

- The marked structure in the image is left atrium. It is located below left ventricle.
- Left atria forms mainly the base of the heart.
- Blood enters via to left atria via pulmonary veins and exits through the mitral valve to left ventricle.

241. Ans. (b) Internal oblique and transverse abdominis muscle

Ref: Gray's Anatomy, 42nd ed, pg. 1005

The neurovascular bundle, consisting of the intercostal nerve and vessels, lies in between the internal oblique and the transverse abdominis muscle.

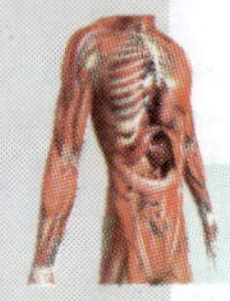

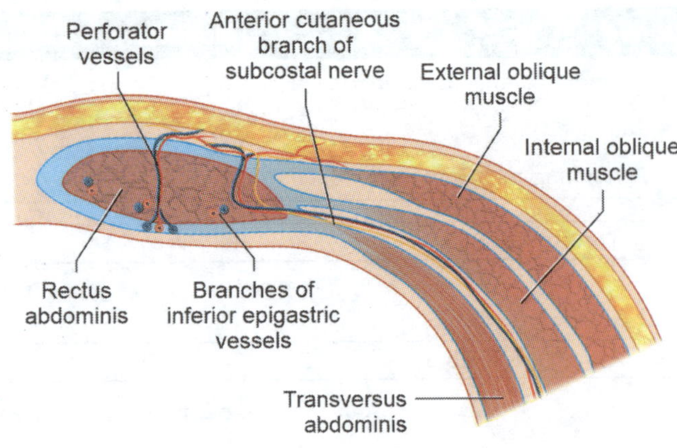

242. Ans. (a) Junction of Left jugular vein and subclavian vein

Ref: BD Chaurasia 7th ed. Vol. I, pg. 302

- Structure marked is thoracic duct.
- The thoracic duct terminates at the junction of the left subclavian vein and internal jugular vein.

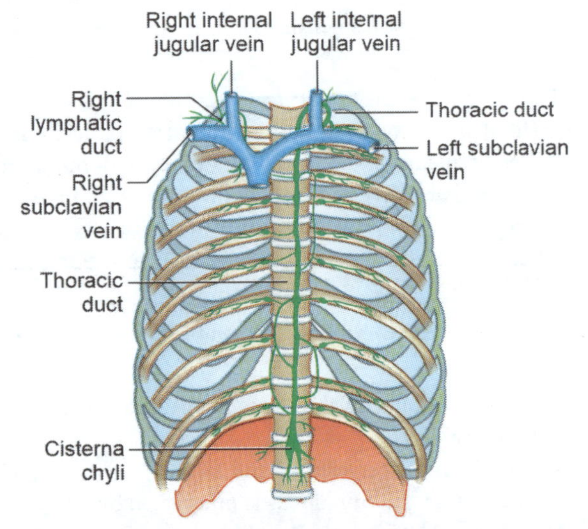

243. (c) Secondary curvature at lumbar spine

Ref: Gray Anatomy for Students, pg. 53, 115

- During fetal period and at birth the vertebral column shows a continuous curvature with the concavity direct forwards. In fully developed spine, thoracic and sacral curvature are concave forwards, and are called primary curvature.
- Cervical and lumbar curves are convex forwards, and are termed as secondary curvature, because they develop after birth.
- Cervical curvature develop 3-4 month after birth and lumbar curvature develops 12-15 months after birth.

244. Ans. (d) Portal vein

Ref: BD Chaurasia, 7th Vol. II, pg. 475

- The marked structure in image is portal vein

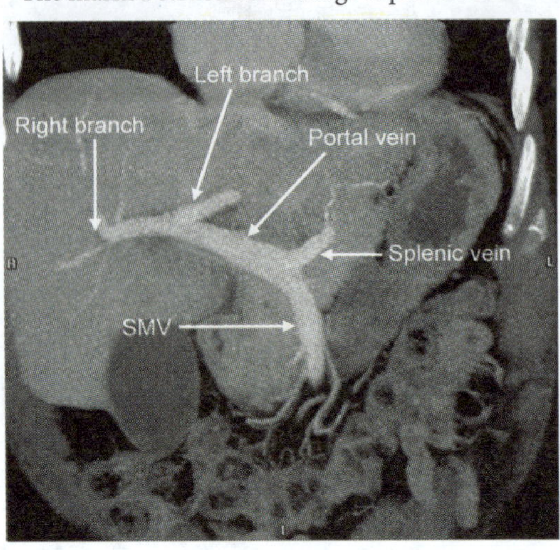

245. Ans. (b) Abdominal aorta

- Testicular artery is a branch of abdominal aorta.
- *Please refer the image given as follows:*

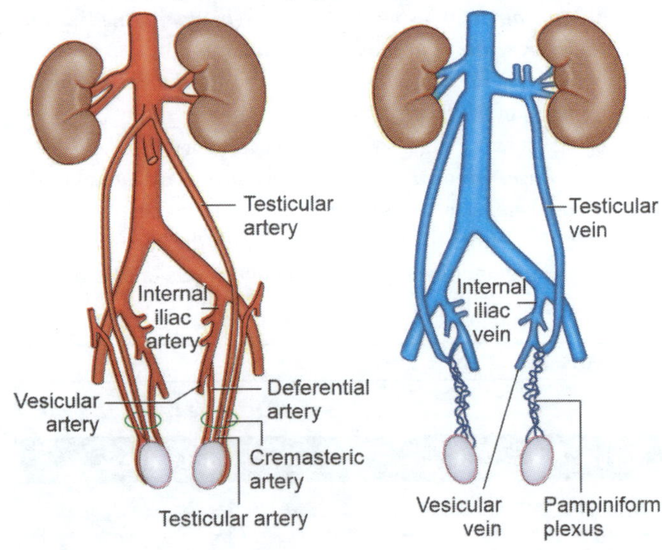

246. Ans. (a) Azygos vein

Ref: Gray's Anatomy, 41st ed. P 955

Mediastinal Surface of Right Lung

On the mediastinal surface of the right lung, you find these structures:

- **Azygos vein** and **its arch** (posterior and over the root of the lung).
- **Vagus nerve** posterior to the root of the lung.

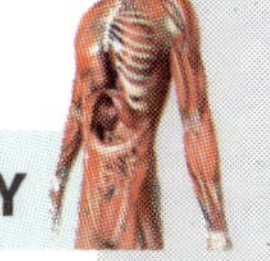

- **Esophagus** posterior to the root.
- **Phrenic nerve** anterior to the root of the lung.
- **Cardiac impression:** Related to right atrium.
- **Below hilum and in front of pulmonary ligament:** Groove for IVC.

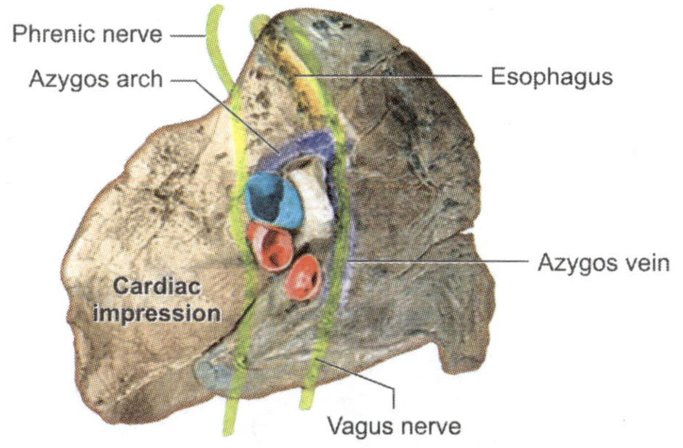

247. Ans. (c) Left intercostal artery

Ref: Gray's Anatomy, 41st ed. pg. 976

- The superior mediastinum lies between the manubrium sternum anteriorly and the upper four thoracic vertebrae posteriorly, and is bounded laterally by the mediastinal pleura.
- It accommodates the thymus, trachea, esophagus, aortic arch, pulmonary trunk, brachiocephalic trunk, left common carotid and subclavian arteries (the vertebral artery sometimes arises from the aortic arch between them), the internal thoracic arteries, the left superior intercostal, hemiazygos, internal thoracic and inferior thyroid veins, and numerous lymph nodes, including those from the tracheobronchial, paratracheal and brachiocephalic groups.

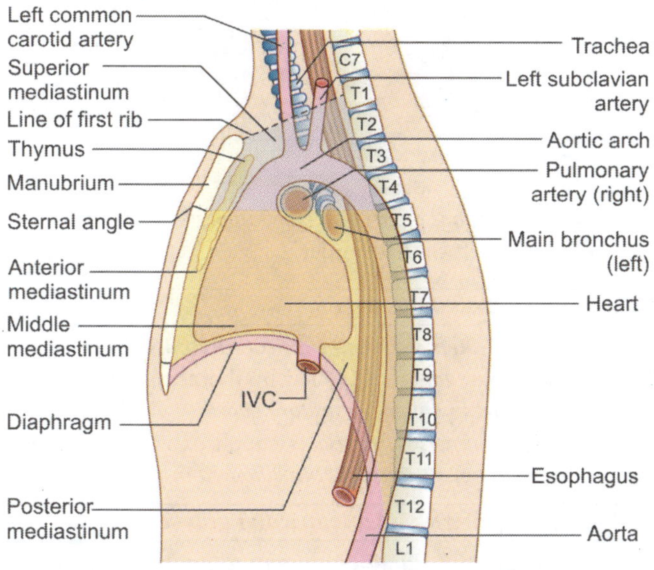

248. Ans. (d) Pulmonary veins are intersegmental

Ref: Gray's Basic Anatomy E-book, pg. 87

Characteristics of Bronchopulmonary Segments

Pulmonary artery
Segmental branches
Pulmonary vein
Terminal bronchiole
Alveolus

- It is a subdivision of a lung lobe.
- It is pyramidal in shape, its apex lies toward the root, while its base lies on the lung surface.
- It is surrounded by connective tissue septa.
- It has a segmental. bronchus, a segmental artery, lymph vessels, and autonomic nerves.
- The segmental vein lies in the intersegmental CT septa between the segments.
- A diseased segment can be removed surgically, because it is a structural unit.

249. Ans. (b) Left coronary artery

Ref: Gray's Anatomy, Review E-book, pg. 80

Left anterior descending artery is a branch of left coronary artery.

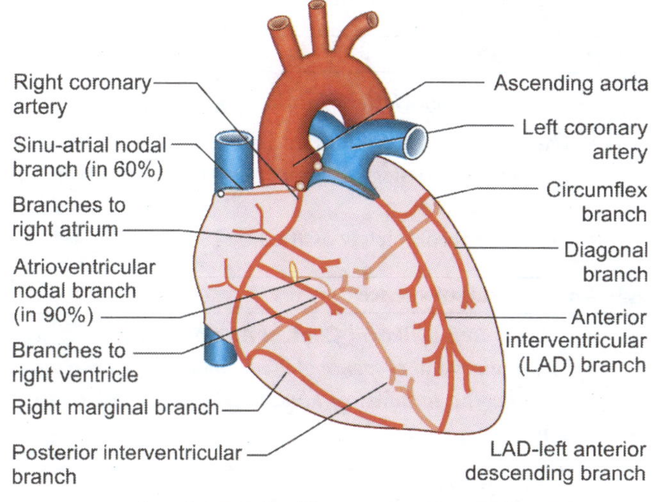

Arterial supply of heart coronary arteries

250. Ans. (c) Lower border of rib

Ref: Snell's Clinical Anatomy, pg. 41

- There are 11 **intercostal spaces** within the thoracic wall. The spaces are filled in by 3 layers of intercostal muscles and their related fasciae and are bounded superiorly and inferiorly by the adjacent ribs.
- The ***costal groove*** *is located along the inferior border of each rib* (upper aspect of the intercostal space) and provides protection for the vein which is most superior and the nerve which is inferior in the groove (VAN).

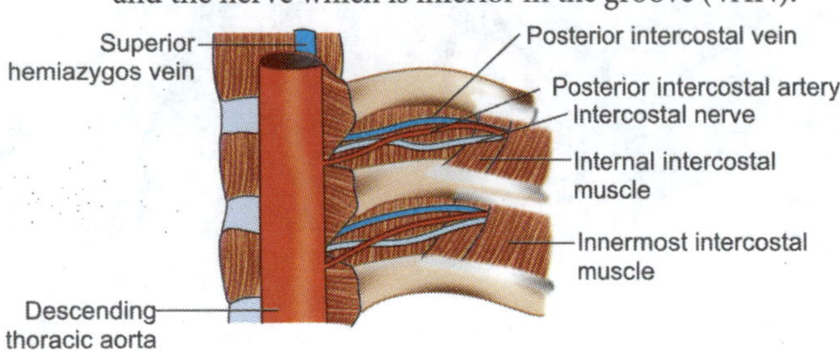

251. Ans. (d) 11

Ref: Netter's Clinical Anatomy, 3rd ed. pg. 89

- The 11th and 12th ribs are *floating ribs* as they are free at their ends.
- The 8th, 9th and 10th ribs are *false ribs* as they are joined to form cartilage of rib immediately above.
- The first 7 pair of ribs are *true ribs.*

252. Ans. (d) 8th

Ref: BDC, 6th Vol. I, pg. 196-97

- **True ribs:** Ribs directly articulating with sternum through costal cartilage. **They are ribs 1 to 7**
- **False ribs:** Ribs that do NOT articulate directly with sternum. **Ribs 8 to 12th.**

253. Ans. (d) 40

Ref: Netter's Clinical Anatomy, 3rd ed. pg. 90

- The xiphoid process unites with the body at about 40 years.
- The manubrio-sternal joint persists as cartilaginous throughout life.
- The body is completely ossified by 25 years.

254. Ans. (b) Tail of spence

Ref: Kulkarni Clinical Anatomy, 2nd ed. pg. 182

- The *axillary tail of spence of breast* pierces the *deep fascia* through the *foramen of langer* and comes to lie in the axilla.

255. Ans. (a) Breast

Ref: Kulkarni Clinical Anatomy, 2nd ed. pg. 11

- The lymphatic plexus below the areola is the *Sub-areolar plexus of sappey.*
- 75% of breast lymphatics drain to axillary lymph nodes.

Extra Mile

Quadrant wise breast lymphatic drainage

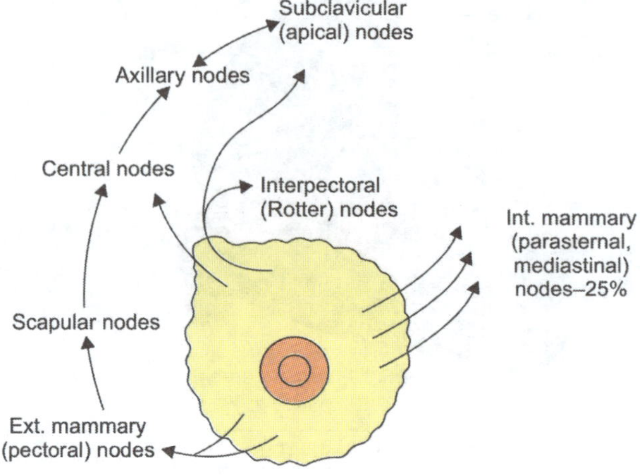

There is a quadrant-wise drainage:

- **Lateral quadrant:** Axillary nodes and supraclavicular through the pectoral, interpectoral and deltopectoral.
- **Medial quadrant:** Parasternal nodes.
- **Lower quadrant:** Inferior phrenic (abdominal) nodes.

256. Ans. (b) Left upper lobe

Ref: Kulkarni Clinical Anatomy, 2nd ed. pg. 943

- Left upper lobe is divided into apical lobe and lingular lobe.

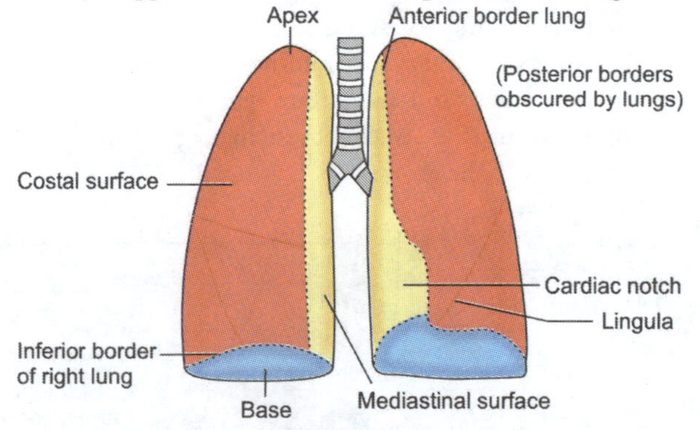

- *The Lingula is a part of the Left upper lobe of lung*
- It forms left cardiac border.

257. Ans. (b) Latissimus dorsi

Ref: Kulkarni Clinical Anatomy, 2nd ed. pg. 38

- *Latissimus dorsi* is supplied by thoracodorsal nerve. It *takes part in violent expiratory efforts.*
- *Serratus anterior muscle* is supplied by long thoracic nerve of bell. It *takes part in laboured inspiration.*

258. Ans. (c) Anterior interventricular groove

Ref: BDC's Human Anatomy, 6th ed. Vol: 1 pg. 264-65

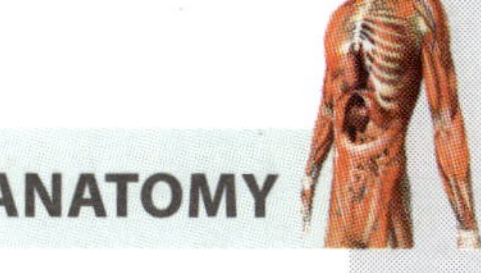

- The entire heart is supplied by two coronary arteries, arising from the ascending aorta. They run in coronary sulcus.
- Anterior interventricular groove is supplied by left coronary artery.

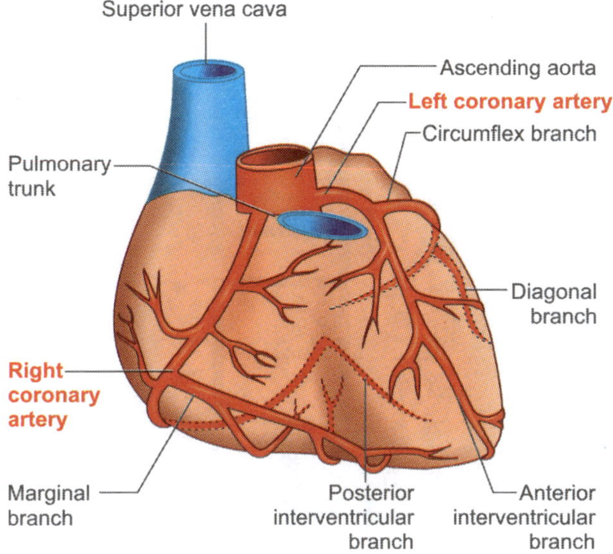

Right Coronary Artery Supplies

- Right atrium
- A large part of right ventricle; EXCEPT the area surrounding the anterior interventricular groove
- Posterior part of interventricular septum, and
- Whole of the conducting system of the heart; EXCEPT a branch of the AV bundle.

Left Coronary Artery Supplies

- Left atrium
- A large part of left ventricle; EXCEPT the area surrounding the posterior interventricular groove and a small part of the right ventricle surrounding the anterior interventricular groove.
- Anterior part of the Interventricular septum
- A part of the left branch of the AV bundle.

259. Ans. (c) LA

Ref: BDC, 6th ed. Vol. I, pg. 253; Snell's Anatomy, pg. 137

- **Right ventricle** is located between RA and LV. It doesn't form any boundary of heart
- **Right atrium** forms the right border
- **Left atrium** is located posteriorly. Forms the base of heart
- **Left ventricle** forms the left border. Apex is formed by LV.

260. Ans. (d) Right ventricle

Ref: BDC, 6th ed. Vol. I, pg. 253; Keith L. Moore 5th ed. pg. 147

BORDERS OF HEART

- **Right border** (slightly convex): Formed by the right atrium, SVC and the IVC.
- **Left border (nearly horizontal):** Formed by the left ventricle and slightly by the left auricle.
- **Inferior border** (oblique, nearly vertical), formed mainly by the right ventricle and slightly by the left ventricle.
- **Superior border:** Formed by the right and left atria and auricles in an anterior view.

261. Ans. (b) 10 cm

Ref: BDC's Human Anatomy, 6th ed. Vol: 1 pg. 280

TRACHEA

- The trachea is **10 to 15 cm** in length
- Diameter varies: About **2 cm in males** and about **1.5 cm in females.**

Some Important Lengths to Remember

- Length of esophagus 25 cm
- Length of ureters- 25 cm
- Length of male urethra- 20 cm
- Length of female urethra- 4 cm
- C- shaped rings in trachea- 16–20

262. Ans. (b) 2 cm

Ref: BDC, 6th ed. Vol. I, pg. 280

Please refer to above explanation

263. Ans. (b) Cricopharyngeus

Ref: BDC, 6th ed. Vol. I, pg. 282

- The first constriction present at the root of the neck is bounded by Cricopharyngeus muscle. Foreign body most commonly lodges here because of its strong constriction.

The Esophagus Shows 4 Constrictions at the Following Levels

1. At its beginning, **15 cm** from the **incisor teeth**
2. Where it is crossed by the aortic arch, **22.5 cm** from the **incisor teeth**
3. Where it is crossed by the left bronchus, **27.5 cm** from the **incisor teeth**
4. Where it pierces the diaphragm **37.5 cm** from the **incisor teeth.**

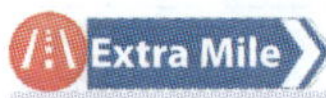

- *Most common foreign body which lodges in esophagus is food particle.*

264. Ans. (d) None

Ref: Snell Anatomy 7th ed. pg. 499; BDC, 6th ed. Vol. I /180

- All the given options are accessory muscles of respiration.
- Muscles used for forceful breathing are accessory muscles of respiration.

Accessory muscle for inspiration	Accessory muscle for expiration
• SCM • Serratus anterior • Serratus posterior • Pectoralis major • Pectoralis minor • Erector spinae • Scalene	• Internal intercostals • Innermost intercostals • Transverse thoracis • Lattissimus dorsi • Abdominal muscle

265. Ans. (a) Diaphragm

Ref: Snell Anatomy, 7th ed. pg. 499; BDC 6th ed. Vol. I, pg. 212-13

- Diaphragm is major respiratory muscle
- Inspiration is an active process and requires contraction of inspiratory muscles.
- During quiet breathing expiration is a passive process.
- During inspiration all the 3 dimensions of the thoracic cavity expand
  - **Vertical-75% (by diaphragm)**
  - AP 25% (external intercostals and internal intercostals)
  - Transverse
  - Increase in vertical diameter is brought about by downward movement of diaphragm—which account for 70% of the thoracic expansion.

266. Ans. (a) Phrenic nerve

Ref: BDC, 6th Vol. I, pg. 192

NERVE SUPPLY OF DIAPHRAGM

- **Motor supply:** Phrenic nerve
- **Sensory supply:**
  - Peripheral part: Lower 6 intercostal nerves
  - Central part: Phrenic nerve

267. Ans. (c) Azygous vein

Ref: BDC 6th ed. Vol. I / 221-222; Keith L. Moore 5th ed. / 105

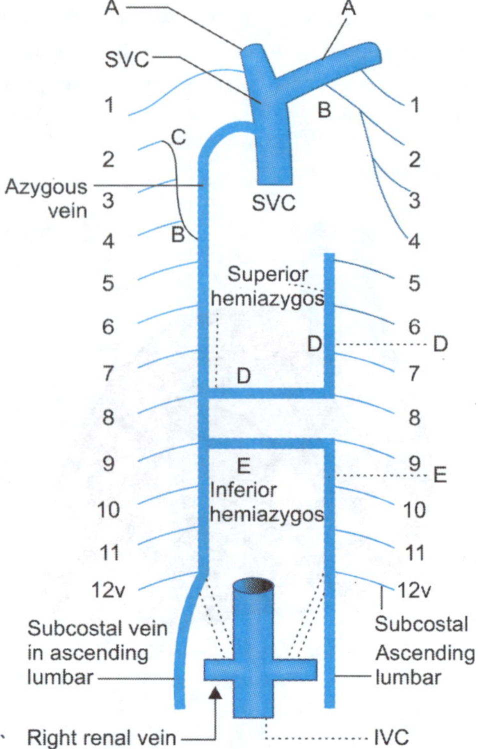

POSTERIOR INTERCOSTAL VEINS

- One in each of the 11 spaces
- **On the right:**
  - 1st drains into Rt. innominate vein (A)
  - 2nd, 3rd & sometimes the 4th unite to form Rt. Superior Intercostal vein (B) which drains into azygos vein.
  - From 5th to 11th & subcostal veins drain into azygos vein (C).
- **On the left:**
  - 1st drains into Lt. innominate vein (A)
  - 2nd, 3rd & sometimes the 4th join to form Lt. Superior intercostal vein which drains into Lt innominate vein vein (B)
  - 5th, 6th, 7th & 8th form *superior hemiazygos vein* to azygos vein (D)
  - 9th, 10th, 11th & subcostal form *inferior hemiazygos veins drain* to azygos vein (E).

ABDOMEN

268. Ans. (c) T12

Ref: BD Chourasia 7th ed. Vol. II, pg. 302

- The celiac trunk, also known as the celiac artery, is a short vessel that arises from the aorta and passes below

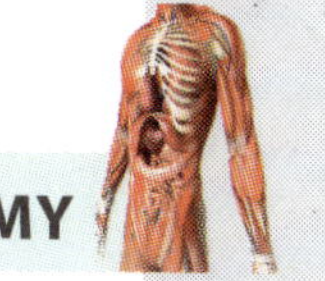

the median arcuate ligament, just as the aorta enters the abdomen at the level of the T12 vertebra.

- The celiac trunk measures about 1.5 cm to 2 cm in length.

269. Ans. (c) Left gastroepiploic artery

Ref: Gray's Anatomy, 41st ed. pg. 1116

- The shown artery in the image is left gastroepiploic artery, the largest branch of splenic artery.
- **Origin and course:** Arises near splenic hilum and runs anteroinferiorly between the layers of the gastrosplenic ligament into the upper gastrocolic omentum → descends and anastomose with right gastroepiploic artery.
- **Size:** Up to 8 cm long (longer than right gastroepiploic artery)
- Supplies gastric fundus and body.

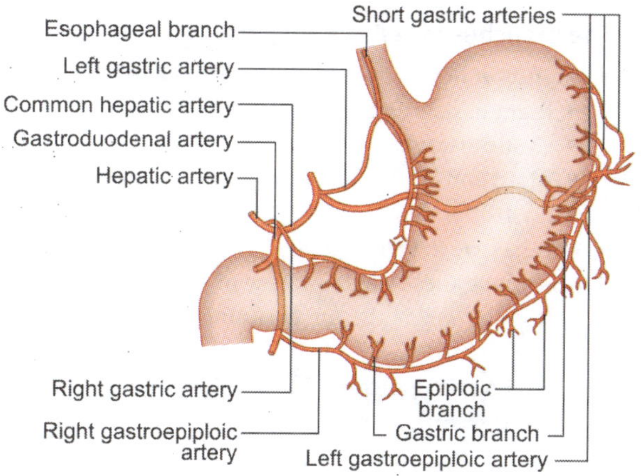

FIGURE: Arteries around stomach

270. Ans. (b) Splenorenal ligament

Ref: Gray's Anatomy, 41st ed. pg. 1181

- Most lateral and narrowest portion of pancreas is pancreatic tail
- **Length:** 1.5–3.5 cm
- Lies between layers of splenorenal ligament

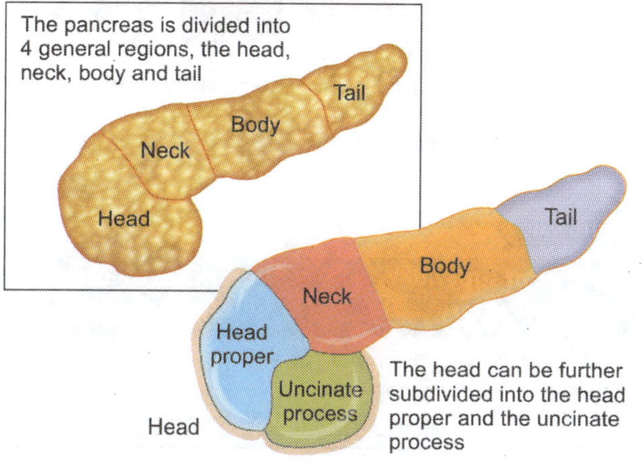

271. Ans. (d) Clavicle

Ref: Gray's Anatomy, 41st ed. pg. 799-800

- Clavicle/collar bone is the connection between sternum and scapula
- **Sternal/Medial end:** Attaches to manubrium of sternum and first coastal cartilage
- **Acromial end/Lateral end:** Attaches to acromion on scapula → supports shoulder

	Sternoclavicular joint	Acromioclavicular joint
Type	Saddle type of synovial joint	Plane type of synovial joint
Bone forming	Sternal end of clavicle and manubrium of sternum	Lateral end of clavicle with acromion process of scapula
Ligaments	Costoclavicular ligament between 1st rib and clavicle	Coracoclavicular ligament–very strong–between coracoid process of scapula and clavicle. Two parts–Conoid and Trapezoid ligaments

272. Ans. (b) Short gastric arteries

Ref: Grey Henry, Anatomy of Human Body, pg. 606

- The **short gastric arteries** also known as *vasa brevia* consist of five to seven small branches, which *arise* from the end of the splenic artery (aka lienal artery), and from its terminal divisions.
- They pass from left to right, between the layers of the gastrolienal ligament, and are distributed to the greater curvature of the stomach, anastomosing with branches of the left gastric and left gastroepiploic arteries

273. Ans. (c) 3rd part

Ref: Gray's Anatomy, Review E-book, pg. 183

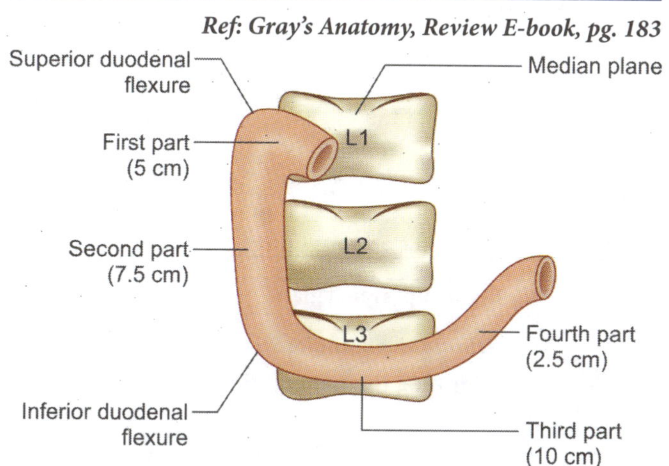

274. Ans. (c) Red pulp

Ref: General Anatomy E-book, pg. 170

The **Cords of Billroth *also*** known as **red pulp cords or splenic cord** are found in the red pulp of the spleen between the sinusoids, consisting of fibrils and connective tissue cells with a large population of monocytes and macrophages.

The white pulp consists of thick layer of lymphocytes surrounding the arteries that have left the trabeculae. They form a periarterial sheath which contains mainly T cells. The sheaths expand to form well developed lymphoid nodules called malphigian nodules.

275. Ans. (d) Sudeck's point

Ref: Yamada's Textbook of Gastroenterology, Vol I, pg. 104

- **Watershed area:** It is the medical term referring to regions of the body that receive dual blood supply from the most distal branches of two large arteries.
- **Griffith's critical point:** A potential watershed area present between superior and inferior mesenteric arterial system. It is located at the splenic flexure.
- **Sudeck's point:** Located at the watershed area between inferior mesenteric artery and internal iliac artery. This point is located near the rectosigmoid junction.

276. Ans. (a) L2

Ref: Netter's Clinical Anatomy, 3rd ed. pg. 202

- Portal vein starts at level of *L2 vertebra* and is formed by *junction of superior mesenteric vein and splenic vein.* It is *8 cm* long and lies behind the neck of pancreas.
- Normal portal vein pressure is *5–10 mm Hg.*

277. Ans. (d) Coronary ligament

Ref: Netter's Clinical Anatomy, 3rd ed. pg. 205

Derivatives of Dorsal Mesogastrium
Greater omentum
Gastrosplenic ligament
Gastrophrenic ligament
Lienorenal ligament
Derivatives of Ventral Mesogastrium
Lesser omentum
Falciform ligament
Coronary ligament
Right and left triangular ligament

278. Ans. (b) Right suprarenal gland

Ref: Vishram singh Anatomy: Volume 2: 2nd ed. pg. 97

Structures forming the pancreatic bed

- Splenic vein
- Aorta and superior mesenteric artery
- Left renal vessels and left kidney
- Left supra-renal gland
- Left crus of diaphragm

Extra Mile

Structures forming the tonsillar bed	
1.	Buccopharyngeal fascia
2.	Superior constrictor muscles
3.	Palatopharyngeus
4.	Glossopharyngeus Nerve
5.	Pharyngo-basiliar fascia

279. Ans. (c) Left gastric artery

Ref: Netter's Clinical Anatomy, 3rd ed. pg. 181

The branches of celiac artery are:

- **Common hepatic artery** which gives rise to
  - Right gastric artery
  - Cystic artery
  - Right and left hepatic artery
  - Gastroduodenal artery
- **Left gastric artery:** *Smallest branch* of celiac artery and runs along the lesser curvature of stomach
- **Splenic artery** is the *largest branch* of celiac artery and gives rise to:
  - Pancreatic branches
  - Short gastric branches
  - Left gastroepiploic artery

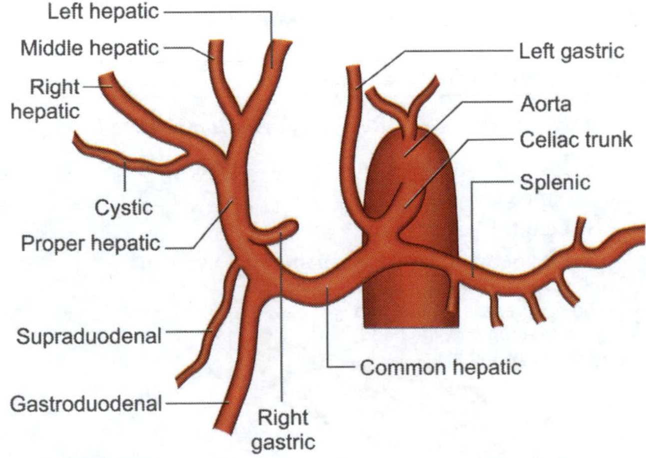

Extra Mile

Branches of superior mesenteric artery	Branches of inferior mesenteric artery
Supplies all derivatives of mid gut from major duodenal papilla to right 2/3rd of transverse colon	Superior rectal artery Sigmoid artery Left colic artery

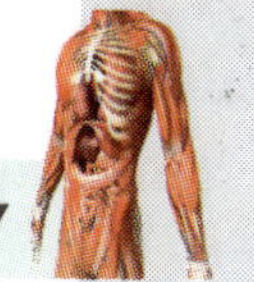

280. Ans. (c) IVC opening

- IVC passes through **tendon opening** and tendon is noncontracting part of muscle. Therefore constriction of diaphragm will not cause constriction of IVC.

281. Ans. (b) Jejunum

Ref: BDC, 6th ed. Vol. II, pg. 264

- Jejunum has valvulae conniventes, which are spaced regularly, concentrically giving a ladder effect.
- **Ileum:** Featureless or very thin valvulae coniventes
- **Caecum:** Rounded gas shadow in right iliac fossa
- **Large bowel:** Haustral folds, spaced regularly.

282. Ans. (b) Semilunar

Ref: BDC, 6th ed. Vol. II, pg. 326

- Left adrenal gland is **crescenteric/semilunar**
- Right adrenal gland is **pyramidal in shape**
- The average weight of adrenal **gland: 4-6 g**

283. Ans. (a) Greater sac of stomach forms anterior border

Ref: Clinical Anatomy, 11th ed. pg. 151

- The suprarenal glands cap the upper poles of the kidneys and lie against the crura of the diaphragm.
- ***The left is related anteriorly to the stomach across the lesser sac,*** the right lies behind the right lobe of the liver and tucks medially behind the inferior vena cava.
- Posteriorly both kidney and adrenals are guarded by psoas major muscle.
- Spleen is anterolateral to left adrenal gland.

Extra Mile

- Each gland, although weighing only **4 to 6 gm,** has three arteries supplying it:
  - **SUPERIOR:** A branch from the phrenic artery;
  - **MIDDLE:** A direct branch from the aorta;
  - **INFERIOR:** A branch from the renal artery.
- **VENOUS DRAINAGE:**
  - IVC on RIGHT
  - RENAL VEIN on the LEFT.
  - *The stubby right suprarenal vein, coming directly from the inferior vena cava, presents the most dangerous feature in performing an adrenalectomy.*

284. Ans. (a) 4 grams

Ref: BDC, 6th ed. Vol. II, pg. 326

285. Ans. (d) T12

Ref: BDC, 6th ed. Vol. II, pg. 333

- Diaphragm has several openings for the passage of structures from thorax to abdomen.

TABLE: Main openings in the diaphragm and their levels

Opening	Level	Structure passing
AORTIC OPENING- osseoaponeurotic opening (not a true opening) *Str passing: "Remember ATA"*	T12	• Aorta • Thoracic duct • Azygous vein
ESOPHAGEAL OPENING- lies in muscular part of diaphragm	T10	• Esophagus • Gastric or vagus nerve • Esophagheal branch of left gastric artery
VENA CAVAL OPENING- lies in central tendon of diaphragm	T8	• Inferior vena cava • Right phrenic nerve branches

Extra Mile

- Only motor nerve to diaphragm- PHRENIC NERVE (C3, C4, C5)
- It is the principle muscle of inspiration

Extra Mile

Structures and level of piercing in diaphragm: ***(Mn: I ate, 10 Eggs, At 12)***
- IVC: T8
- Esophagus: T10
- Aorta: T12

286. Ans. (d) Vagus nerve

Ref: BDC, 6th ed. Vol. II, pg. 333

287. Ans. (b) Caval opening

Ref: BDC, 6th ed. Vol. II, pg. 333

288. Ans. (b) Phrenic nerve

Ref: BDC, 6th ed. Vol. II, pg. 333, 5th ed. pg. 336

289. Ans. (d) Cisterna chyli

Ref: Clinically Oriented Anatomy by Keith, Moore, 5th ed. pg. 387; Gray's Anatomy 40th ed. pg. 180

- The **cisterna chyli** is a normal anatomical structure seen as saccular area of dilatation in the lymphatic channels that is located in the **retrocrural space,** usually to the immediate right of the abdominal aorta. It originates at the level of L1/2 vertebral body and extends 5–7 cm in the caudocephalad axis.
- **Thoracic duct originates from the chyle cistern in the abdomen and ascends through the aortic hiatus in the diaphragm.** Thoracic duct ascends in the posterior mediastinum among the thoracic aorta on its left, the azygos vein on its right, the esophagus anteriorly, and

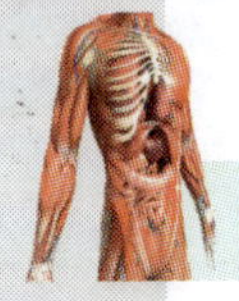

the vertebral bodies posteriorly. At the level of the T4, T5, or T6 vertebra, the thoracic duct crosses to the left, posterior to the esophagus, and ascends into the superior mediastinum.

- **Note:** *Although thoracic duct derives from cisterna chyli, it is the thoracic duct that passes through diaphragm and not the cisterna chyli.*

290. Ans. (a) Inferior vena cava

Ref: Gray's 41st ed. pg. 1021, 1027, 1167

- *Most of the venous system has valves to prevent backflow of blood in order to maintain venous return.*
- IVC has only one valve present at the junction where it drains into right atrium. This valve is named ***Eustachean valve***
- *Thebesian the besian valve is present in coronary sinus.*
- Veins contain valves to help keep blood flowing toward the heart at all times.
- Veins which are valveless can be remembered as: **IPSS**
  - Internal jugular vein
  - Pulmonary vein, Portal vein
  - Superior vena cava
  - Sinuses of brain

291. Ans. (d) Inferior vena cava

Ref: Gray's, 41st ed. pg. 127-128; Repeat question

Please refer to above explanation

292. Ans. (a) Aorta

- Aorta is an elastic artery with diameter ~ 25 mm.
- Systemic arteries can be subdivided into two types- muscular and elastic-according to the relative compositions of elastic and muscle tissue in their tunica media as well as their size and the makeup of the internal and external elastic lamina.
- The larger arteries (>10 mm diameter) are generally elastic and the smaller ones (0.1-10 mm) tend to be muscular.

293. Ans. (d) L5

Clinically Oriented Anatomy by Keith, Moore, 5th ed. pg. 340

- The IVC begins anterior to **the L5 vertebra** by the union of the common iliac veins.
- This union occurs approximately 2.5 cm to the right of the median plane, inferior to the bifurcation of the aorta and posterior to the proximal part of the right common iliac artery.
- Renal vein at the level of **L1**
- **Portal veins form at L1**
- Hepatic veins form at **T8**

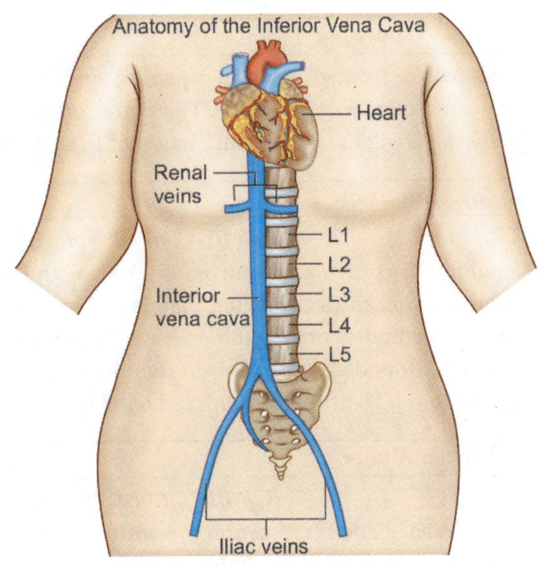

294. Ans. (a) L1

Ref: Clinically Oriented Anatomy by Keith, Moore, 5th ed. pg. 340

295. Ans. (a) Duodenum

Ref: BDC, 5th ed. Vol. II, pg. 268

- Brunner's gland is found in duodenum above sphincter of oddi.
- Main function of these glands is to produce mucus rich alkaline secretion which protects duodenum from gastric acidic contents.
- It also facilitates activation of intestinal enzymes which helps in absorption.

296. Ans. (a) Mucinus alkaline

Ref: BDC, 5th ed. Vol. II, pg. 268

- Brunner's glands are also known as duodenal glands.
- These are small compound tubuloacinar glands which secrete mucus that protects duodenum from gastric acidic contents.
- They also facilitate activation of intestinal enzymes which helps in absorption.

Extra Mile

- The gastric glands situated in the fundus and body of stomach contain parietal/oxyntic cells which secrete acid, mucus, pepsin and other digestive enzymes.

297. Ans. (d) Duodenum

Ref: BDC, 6th ed. Vol. II, pg. 303

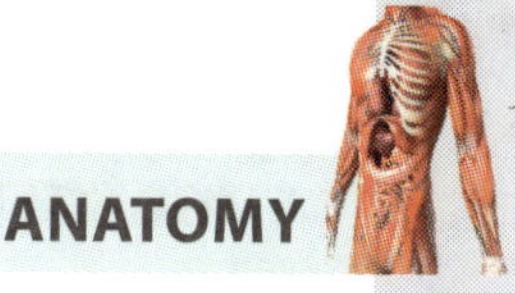

VISCERAL RELATIONS OF SPLEEN

- Spleen forms visceral relation with the following nearby organs:
  - Fundus of the stomach
  - The anterior surface of the left kidney
  - Splenic flexure of the colon and
  - The tail of the pancreas

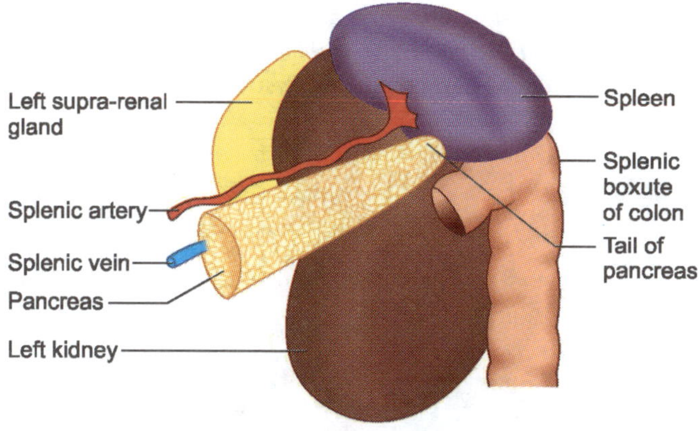

298. Ans. (b) Quadratus lumborum

Ref: BDC, 6th ed. Vol. II, pg. 313-314

- The kidneys are reddish brown and measure approximately 10 cm in length, 5 cm in width, and 2.5 cm in thickness.
- **Superiorly:** The kidneys are associated with the diaphragm, which separates them from the pleural cavities and the 12th pair of ribs.
- **Posterior surfaces** of the kidney are related to **the *quadratus lumborum muscle.*** The subcostal nerve and vessels and the iliohypogastric and ilioinguinal nerves descend diagonally across the posterior surfaces of the kidneys.
- **Anterior surface** The kidneys are associated with liver, duodenum, ascending colon and supra renal glands.
- *The right kidney is separated from the liver by the hepatorenal recess.* ***The left kidney is related to the stomach, spleen, pancreas, jejunum, and descending colon***

299. Ans. (c) Head of pancreas

Refer to above explanation.

300. Ans. (c) Intestinal looping

Ref: BDC, 6th ed. Vol. II, pg. 313-314

THE RELATIONS OF THE RIGHT KIDNEY

- **Anteriorly**—suprarenal gland, liver, second part of duodenum, right colic flexure
- **Posteriorly**—diaphragm, 12th rib, costodiaphragmatic recess of the pleura, psoas muscle, quadratus lumborum muscle, transversus abdominis muscle

THE RELATIONS OF THE LEFT KIDNEY

- **Anteriorly**—suprarenal gland, spleen, stomach, pancreas, left colic flexure, coils of jejunum.
- **Posteriorly**—diaphragm, costodiaphragmatic recess of the pleura, 11th and 12th rib, psoas muscle, quadratus lumborum muscle, transversus abdominis muscle.

301. Ans. (b) Inferior mesenteric artery

Ref: Gray's, 41st ed. pg. 1206

The embryonic kidneys are close together in the pelvis. In approximately 1 in 600 fetuses, the inferior poles (rarely, the superior poles) of the kidneys fuse to form a horseshoe kidney. This U-shaped kidney usually lies at the level of **L3-L5 vertebrae** because the root of the **inferior mesenteric artery** prevents normal ascent of the abnormal kidney. Horseshoe kidney usually produces no symptoms; however, associated abnormalities of the kidney and renal pelvis may be present, obstructing the ureter.

302. Ans. (c) Collecting tubule and duct

Ref: BDC, 6th ed. Vol. II, pg. 315-16

- **The kidney consists of an outer renal cortex and an inner renal medulla that contains the renal pyramids which drain into → Calyx → Pelvis.**
- Cortex forms a continuous smooth outer zone with a number of projections (cortical columns) that extend down between the pyramids.
- It contains the renal corpuscles and the renal *tubules; EXCEPT for parts of the loop of Henle* which descend into the renal medulla. ***It also contains blood vessels and cortical collecting ducts.***
- The renal cortex is the part of the kidney where ultrafiltration occurs.

303. Ans. (c) Third part

Ref: BDC, 6th ed. Vol. II, pg. 261

304. Ans. (b) T10

Ref: BDC, 6th ed. Vol. II, pg. 198

- Dermatome of umbilicus is at T10.
- **T10 segment also supplies to:**
  - Appendix: T9 - T10
  - Stomach: T6 – T10
  - Testis/Ovary: T10
  - Intestine: T9 –T11

305. Ans. (b) Retrocecal

Ref: BDC, 6th ed. Vol. II, pg. 269-70

- ***Most common position of vermiform appendix is retrocaecal,*** (12 o'clock- 65%) followed by pelvic (4 O'clock position).

TABLE: Types of appendix and their relative position

Appendix	Position	Prevalence/comment
Retrocecal	12 o'clock	***65%; most common***
Pelvic	4 o'clock	30%; 2nd most common
Subcecal	6 o'clock	2.5%; points towards midinguinal point
Preileal	2 o'clock or splenic	1%; points towards spleen & lie infront of ileum
Postileal	2 o'clock or splenic	**0.5%;** point towards spleen & lie behind ileum
Paracolic	11 o'clock	

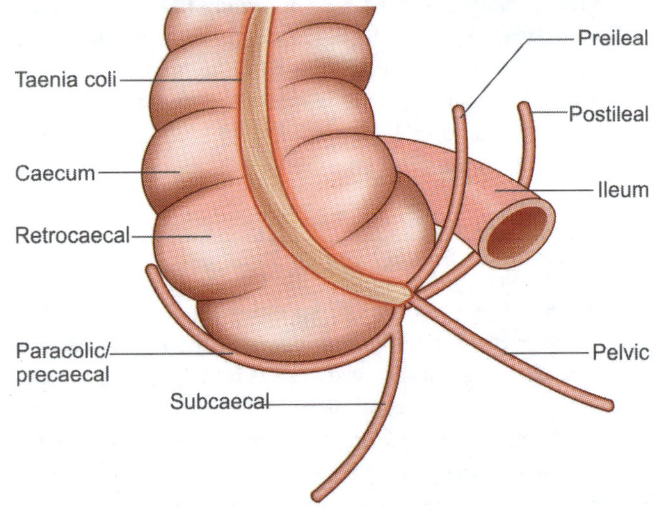

306. Ans. (c) Postileal

Ref: BDC, 6th ed. Vol. II, pg. 269-70

307. Ans. (c) Inferior pancreatoduodenal vein

Tributaries of Portal Vein

1. Left Gastric vein
2. Right Gastric vein
3. Superior Pancreatoduodenal vein
4. Splenic vein
5. Superior mesenteric vein
6. Inferior mesenteric vein
7. Cystic vein

Extra Mile

- Hepatic portal vein is a blood vessel that conducts blood from GIT and spleen to the liver.
- ***Liver receives 75% of its blood through hepatic portal vein, and the remainder from hepatic artery proper.***
- Note: blood leaves the liver to the heart in the hepatic vein.

308. Ans. (b) Cystic duct, liver, common hepatic duct

Ref: Gray's Anatomy, 41st ed. pg. 1175

The Calot's Triangle Aka Hepatobiliary Triangle or Cystohepatic Triangle.

- **Boundaries** (Cystic duct, Liver, Common hepatic duct):
  - **Medial:** Common hepatic duct
  - **Infero-lateral:** Cystic duct
  - ***Superior:*** *Inferior surface of liver*
- **Content of Calot triangle –Cystic artery.**

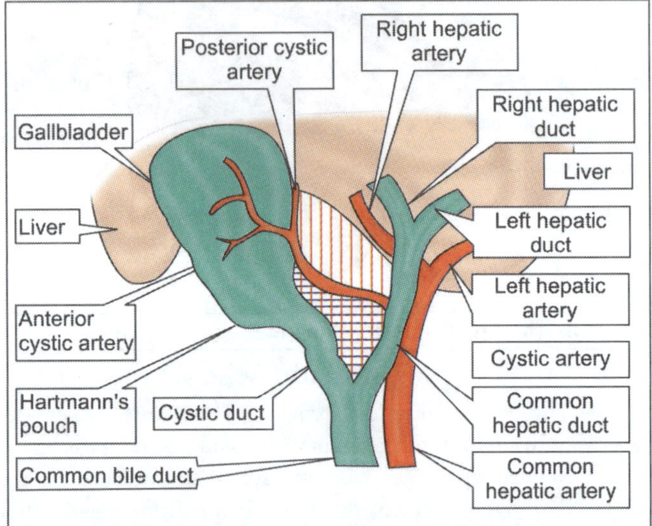

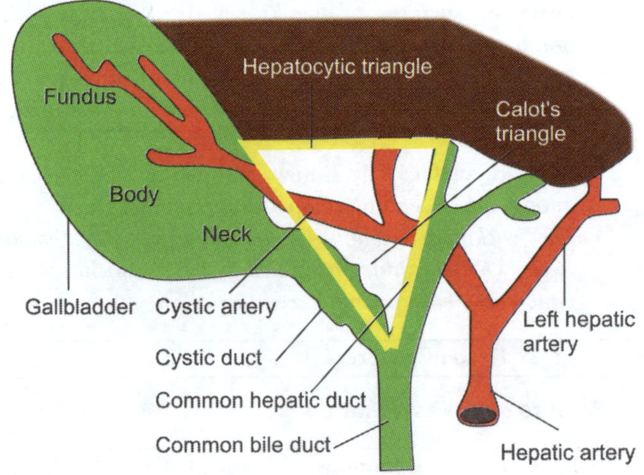

309. Ans. (c) Inferior surface of liver

Ref: Gray's Anatomy, 39th ed. pg. 1229

Please refer to above explanation

310. Ans. (a) Portal vein

Ref: Gray's Anatomy, 41st ed. pg. 1175

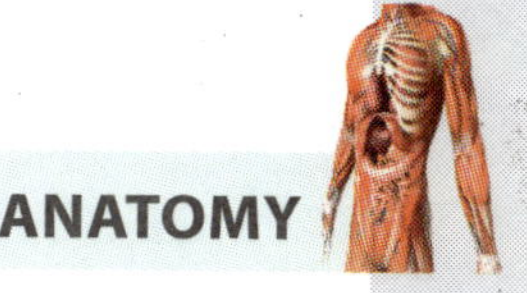

Contents of Calot's Triangle

- Cystic artery (Main)
- Right hepatic artery
- Lymph node of Lund

311. Ans. (b) Termination of portal vein

- The kidneys occupy the epigastric, hypochondriac lumbar and umbilical regions
- Vertically they extend from the upper border of twelfth thoracic vertebra to the center of the body of third lumbar vertebra.
- The right kidney is slightly lower than the left and the left kidney is a little nearer to the median plane than the right.
- The transpyloric plane passes through the upper part of the hilus of the right kidney; and through the lower part of the hilus of the left kidney.

Structures at the Level of Transpyloric Plane

- Origin of superior mesenteric artery.
- Origin of portal vein.
- Hilum of left kidney.
- Origin of renal artery.
- Termination of spinal cord.
- Level of duodenojejunal flexure.

312. Ans. (a) Whole system is valve less

Ref: BDC, 4th ed. Vol. II/268-71, Gray's 39th ed. pg. 1218-19

- In adults, the portal vein and its tributaries have no valves.
- In fetal life and for a short postnatal period valves are demonstrable in its tributaries, but they usually get atrophied.
- Rarely some persist in an atrophic form into adulthood.

313. Ans. (a) Fundus

Ref: Gray's, 41st ed. pg. 1120

- Chief cells are usually **fundal** in position.
- Chief (Peptic) cells are the source of digestive enzymes like pepsin and lipase.
- These cells are cuboidal with round nucleus and contain lots of zymogen granules.
- **Parietal/Oxyntic cells** produce HCl and the intrinsic factor.
- These cells are oval with centrally placed nucleus.
- They are mainly located in the apical half of the **body** of gland, reaching as far as the **neck**.
- Surface mucus cells are distributed in the **gastric pit**-region of the gastric mucosa.
- Mucus neck cells are abundant in the neck region as the name is also suggesting.
- Neuroendocrine cells are situated mainly in the deeper/basal parts of the glands, along with the chief cells.

Extra Mile

Goblet cell: Mucus (protect stomach lining)
Parietal cell: Gastric acid (HCl), intrinsic factor
Chief cell: Pepsinogen
D cell: Somatostatin
G cell: Gastrin
ECL cell: Histamine

314. Ans. (b) 7 ounce

Ref: BDC, 6th ed. Vol. II, pg. 294

- On an average the spleen is 1 inch or 2.5 cm thick, 3 inches or 7.5 cm broad, 5 inches or 12.5 cm long *and 7 ounces in weight.*

Some Must Know Weights

- Weight of liver: 1.5 kg.
- Weight of thyroid gland: 25 g
- Weight of prostate: **8 g.**

315. Ans. (c) Lower 1/3rd

Ref: BDC, 6th ed. Vol. II, pg. 407-408

ANATOMY OF RECTUM

- This is continuous with the sigmoid colon at the midpiece of the sacrum.
- It has a length of about **12 cm**.
- It descends along the **sacro-coccygeal concavity** as the **sacral flexure**.
- It eventually joins the **anal canal** at the **anorectal junction**, **2–3 cm** in front of the **coccygeal tip**.
- The bend at this point is known as the **perineal flexure of the rectum**.
- The rectum is covered by **peritoneum:**
  - **UPPER 1/3rd: on anterior surface and sides,**
  - **MIDDLE 1/3rd: anterior surface**
  - **LOWER 1/3rd: not covered by peritoneum** → ***thus making it more mobile.***
- The lower part of the rectum is dilated as the **rectal ampulla**.
- The upper part has **3 transverse rectal folds** (upper and lower on the left, the middle on the right).
- The upper part of the rectum above the middle fold may contain faeces, but the lower part only contains faeces in **chronic constipation** or **during the call to defecate**.
- *The rectum ends antero-inferior to the tip of the coccyx, immediately before a sharp posteroinferior angle **(the anorectal flexure of the anal canal)** that occurs as the gut perforates the pelvic diaphragm (levator ani). The roughly **80°degree anorectal flexure** is an important mechanism for fecal continence, being maintained during the resting state by the tonus of the puborectalis muscle and by its active contraction during peristaltic contractions if defecation is not to occur.*

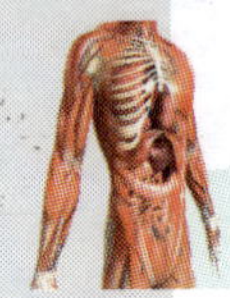

- *With the flexures of the* ***rectosigmoid junction superiorly and the anorectal junction inferiorly, the rectum has an S shape when viewed laterally.***

316. Ans. (b) 12 cm

Ref: BDC, 6th ed. Vol. II, pg. 407-408

317. Ans. (c) Seminal vesicles

Ref: BDC, 6th ed. Vol. II, pg. 408

- Rectum is a 12 cm structure which is in conitunation of sigmoid colon and terminates at anal canal.

TABLE: Relationship of rectum

	Anterior	Posterior	Laterally
Males	• Base of bladder • **Seminal vesicles** • Rectovesical pouch • Ileum • Ductus deferens • Terminal ureter • Prostate gland	• S3-S5 vertebrae • Coccyx • Median sacral artery and vein • Middle rectal artery • Superior rectal artery and vein	• Sigmoid colon • Ileum • Pelvic plexuses • Coccygeus muscle • Levator ani muscle
Fe-males	• Uterus • Vagina • Rectouterine pouch • Ileum • Sigmoid colon	Same as for male	Same as for male

318. Ans. (a) Squamous cell

Ref: Keith L. Moore, 5th ed. pg. 447-48

- The anal canal is divided into three parts. The zona columnaris is the upper half of the canal and is lined by simple columnar epithelium. The lower half of the anal canal, below the pectinate line, is divided into two zones separated by **Hilton's white line.**
- The two parts are the zona hemorrhagica and zona cutanea, *lined by stratified squamous non-keratinized and stratified squamous keratinized*, respectively.

319. Ans. (c) Posteriorly

Ref: Gray's, 41st ed. pg. 1148, 1153

Refer to above explanation.

320. Ans. (c) Inferior mesenteric artery

Ref: BDC, Vol. II, pg. 286-287

- **Superior pancreatoduodenal artery** from gastroduodenal artery and the **inferior pancreatoduodenal from superior mesenteric artery** supplies the head of the pancreas.
- Pancreatic branch of splenic artery also supplies the neck, body and tail.
- Inferior mesenteric artery supplies the left one third of transverse colon, the descending colon, sigmoid colon, rectum and upper part of anal canal.

321. Ans. (a) Gonadal artery

Ref: Gray's, 41st ed. pg. 1047

Ventral Branches of Abdominal Aorta and Level

- Celiac trunk - T_{12}
- Superior mesenteric artery - L1
- Inferior mesenteric artery - L3

Paired/Lateral Branches of Abdominal Aorta

- Inferior phrenic artery
- Middle suprarenal artery
- Renal arteries

Testicular or Ovarian Artery

- Four paired lumbar arteries

Branches of External Iliac Artery

- Inferior epigastric artery
- Deep circumflex iliac artery
- Femoral artery

322. Ans. (d) Gonadal artery

Ref: Clinically Oriented Anatomy by Keith, Moore, 5th ed. pg. 252-253

- Gonadal artery arises from abdominal aorta (Lateral Branch)

NEUROANATOMY, HEAD AND NECK

323. Ans. (a) Straight sinus

Ref: BD Chauraisia's Human Anatomy, Volume 3, 8th ed, pg. 220

- The arrow in the above figure represents Straight Sinus. It lies in the median plane within the junction of Falx cerebri and tentorium cerebelli.
- It is formed anteriorly by the union of the inferior sagittal sinus with the great cerebral vein, and ends at the internal occipital protuberance by continuing as transverse sinus.

324. Ans. (b) Pons

Ref: BD Chauraisia's Human Anatomy, Volume 4, 8th ed, pg. 107

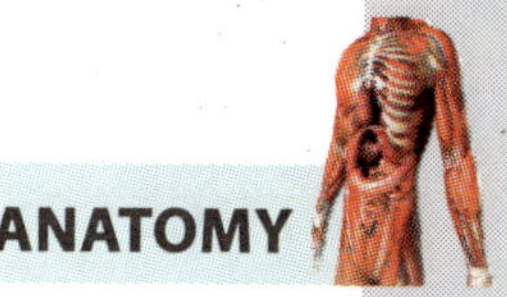

- The arrow marked structure in the above radiograph is Pons, a part of the Brainstem.
- It is also called metencephalon. It is 2.5 cm long and extends from cranial end of medulla oblongata to the cerebral peduncles of Midbrain.
- Cranial Nerves 5, 6, 7, and 8 are attached here.
- Anteriorly it is related to clivus, laterally middle cerebral peduncle and posteriorly to fourth ventricle.

325. Ans. (b) Deviates to ipsilateral side

Ref: BD Chauraisia's Human Anatomy, Volume 4, 8th ed, pg. 95

- The hypoglossal nerve 12th cranial nerve, is tested clinically by asking the patient to protrude his/her tongue. Normally, the tongue is protruded straight forwards.
- If the nerve is paralyzed, the tongue deviates to the paralyzed site.
- An infranuclear unilateral lesion of the hypoglossal nerve produces paralysis of the tongue on that side.
- On protrusion, its tip deviates to paralyzed side as normal genioglossus muscle pulls the base toward normal side.

326. Ans. (d) Trachealis

Ref: Gray's Anatomy, 42nd ed, pg. 1025

- The trachealis muscle is a thick band of smooth muscle that bridges the ends of each of the horseshoe-shaped cartilage rings that help to stabilize the entire length of the windpipe.

327. Ans. (a) Midbrain

Ref: Gray's Anatomy, 42nd ed, pg. 391

- The third and fourth cranial nerves originate from the midbrain: oculomotor nerve (CN III) trochlear nerve (CN IV).
- The extraocular muscles are supplied by oculomotor nerve (CN III) trochlear nerve (CN IV).
- A lesion at the midbrain can cause paralysis of these cranial nerves.

328. Ans. (a) Epiglottis

Ref: Gray's Anatomy, 42nd ed, pg. 574

- The marked structure in the image is epiglottis
- The epiglottis is a leaf-shaped flap in the throat that prevents food and water from entering the windpipe and the lungs.

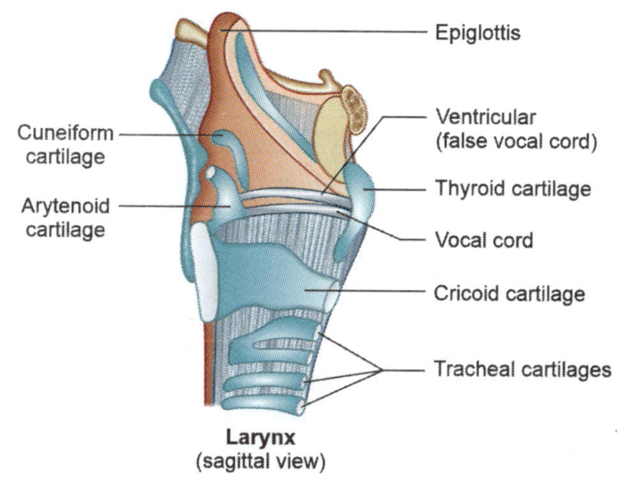

Larynx
(sagittal view)

329. Ans. (c) Lower border of L3

Ref: Gray's Anatomy, 42nd ed, pg. 818

- The spinal cord ends at approx.
  - Lower border of L3 in infants, and
  - Approx. L1–L2 in adults

330. Ans. (b) Genioglossus

Ref: Gray's Anatomy, 42nd ed, pg. 586

- The genioglossus muscle is a fan-shaped muscle that is involved in forming most of the tongue mass.
- It emerges from the superior mental spines and inserts on the hyoid bone as well as the inferior portion of the tongue.

331. Ans. (c) Thyroid

Ref: Gray's Anatomy, 42nd ed, pg. 719

- **There are a total of 9 cartilages in larynx.**
- **Three paired cartilages (6) and three unpaired cartilages (3):**
  - Arytenoid
  - Cuneiform
  - Corniculate
- **Unpaired cartilages are:**
  - Epiglottis
  - Cricoid
  - Thyroid

332. Ans. (a) Posterior cricoarytenoid

Ref: Gray's Anatomy, 42nd ed, pg. 727

- The sole abductor of the vocal cord is posterior cricoarytenoid muscle.

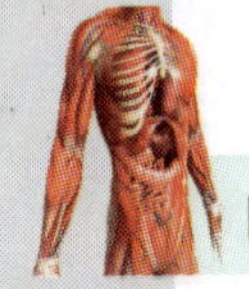

- The muscles lateral cricoarytenoid, thyroarytenoid, interarytenoid, and cricothyroid, all act together to adduct the vocal folds.

333. Ans. (d) D- Internal capsule

Ref: Gray's Anatomy, 42nd ed, pg. 389

The structure marked 'D' is Putamen.

Basal Ganglia

These structures are **involved in** the control of posture and movement. They are sometimes referred to anatomically as the corpus striatum but **clinically**, as basal ganglia.

The putamen and globus pallidus are called the **lentiform or lenticular** nucleus. The corpus striatum are **connected with** thalamus; subthalamus of diencephalon and substantia nigra of midbrain.

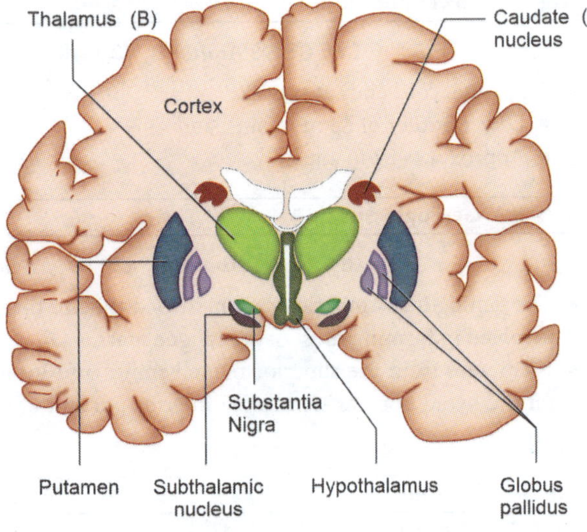

334. Ans. (d) Lower medulla

Ref: Gray's Anatomy, 42nd ed, pg. 390

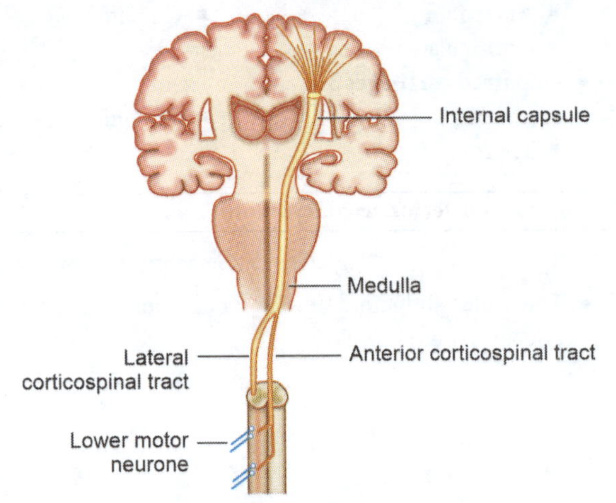

- Decussation of the corticospinal tract occurs at the junction of the medulla oblongata and spinal cord while the corticonuclear tracts decussate above each relevant cranial nerve nuclei.

335. Ans. (a) Coricopharyngeus and thyropharyngeus

Ref: Gray's Anatomy, 42nd ed, pg. 713

- Killian's dehiscence (also known as Killian's triangle) is a triangular area in the wall of the pharynx between the cricopharyngeus and thyropharyngeus which are the two parts of the inferior constrictors.

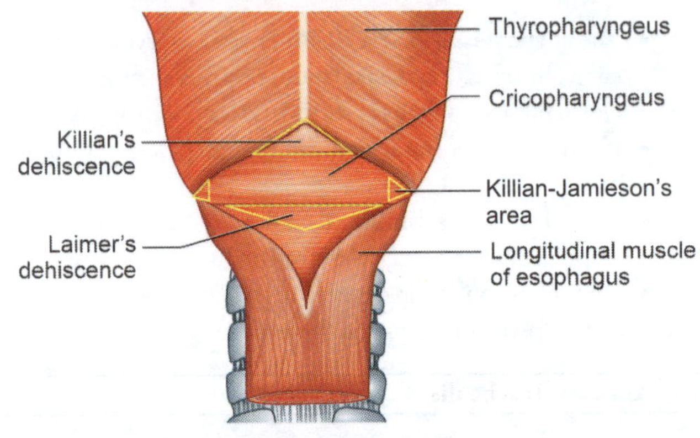

336. Ans. (a) Genioglossus

- The genioglossus muscle plays an important role in maintaining upper airway patency. The GG is responsible for tongue protrusion and stiffens the tongue and prevents posterior tongue displacement and upper airway closure.
- The genioglossus is a phasic respiratory muscle.

337. Ans. (c) Pterygopalatine

Ref: BD Chaurasia 7th ed. Vol. III, pg. 260

- The pterygopalatine ganglion supplies the lacrimal gland, paranasal sinuses, glands of the mucosa of the nasal cavity and pharynx, the gingiva, and the mucous membrane and glands of the hard palate.
- It communicates anteriorly with the nasopalatine nerve.

338. Ans. (b) Internal carotid artery

Ref: BD Chaurasia 7th ed. Vol. III, pg. 110

- Internal carotid artery doesn't pass through parotid gland
- The facial nerve and its branches pass through the parotid gland, as does the external carotid artery and retromandibular vein.
- The external carotid artery forms its two terminal branches within the parotid gland: maxillary and superficial temporal artery.

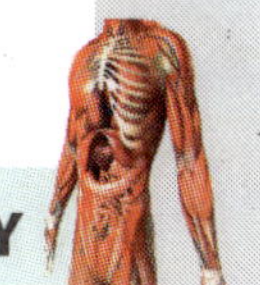

- The gland usually contains several intraparotid lymph nodes.

339. Ans. (d) Lateral pterygoid

Ref: BD Chaurasia 7th ed. Vol. III, pg. 33

- Acting bilaterally, the lateral pterygoids protract the mandible, pushing the jaw forwards.
- Unilateral action produces the 'side to side' movement of the jaw.
- **Note:** Contraction of the lateral pterygoid will produce lateral movement on the contralateral side.

340. Ans. (a) Maxillary artery

Ref: BD Chaurasia 7th ed. Vol. III, pg. 122

- Maxillary artery (a branch of external carotid artery) has 5 branches from the first group (before lateral pterygoid):
  - Middle meningeal artery
  - Accessory meningeal artery
  - Anterior tympanic branch
  - Deep auricular branch
  - Inferior alveolar artery

Image: Branches of maxillary artery

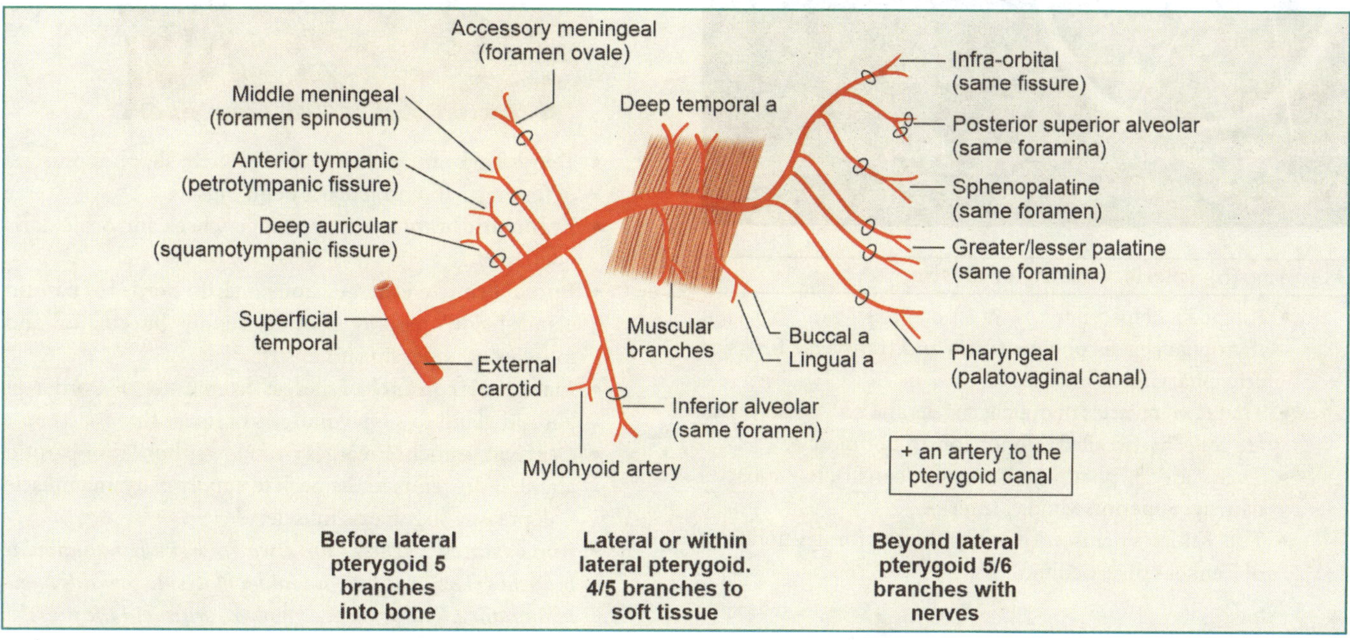

341. Ans. (a) Tensor veli palatini muscle

Ref: BD Chaurasia 7th ed. Vol. III, pg. 17; Image: Dhingra's ENT

- The muscle is at the base of the skull, in the shape of an inverse triangle. The motion of the muscle is activated when a patient swallows or yawns. This motion opens the Eustachian tube because normally, this tube remains closed.

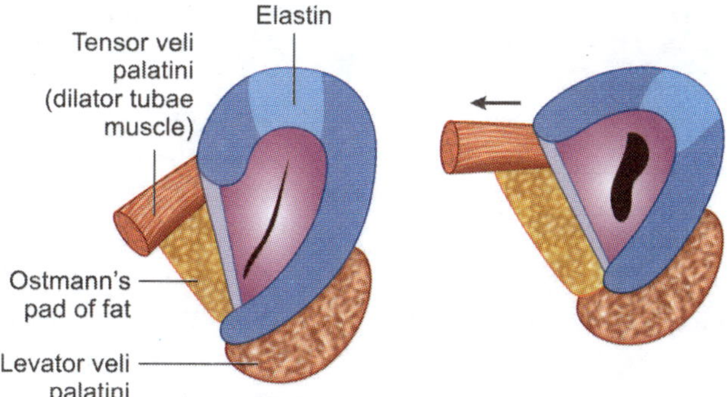

342. Ans. (a) Midbrain

Ref: BD Chaurasia, seventh ed. Vol. IV, pg. 180

- The marked structure in brain MRI is midbrain.

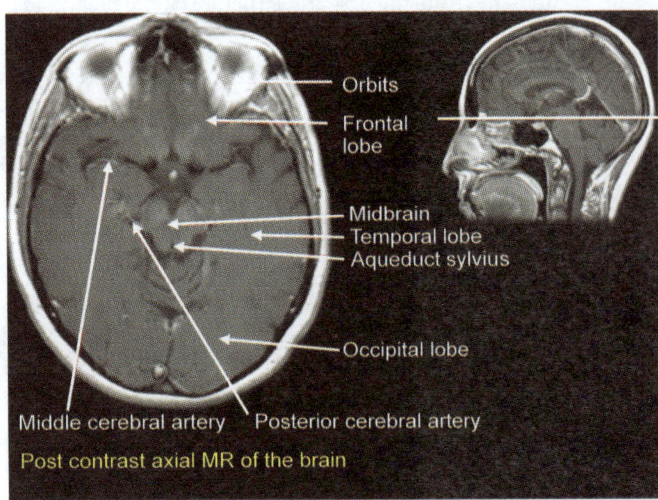

Post contrast axial MR of the brain

343. Ans. (b) Inferior constrictor muscle

- Killian's dehiscence is a potential gap between thyropharyngeus oblique fibers and transverse fibers of cricopharyngeus muscle.
- These two muscles thyropharyngeus and cricopharyngeus are collectively called inferior constrictor muscle.
- There are 3 pharyngeal circular/constrictor muscles namely: Superior, Middle, Inferior.
- This Killian's dehiscence is also the site for development of Zenker's diverticulum.

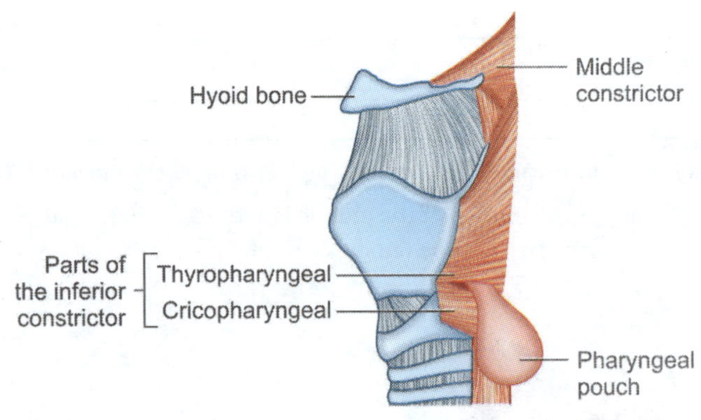

344. Ans. (a) Parotid gland

- All the glands in the face (like submandibular, sublingual, lacrimal gland) are supplied by facial nerve; EXCEPT parotid gland, which is supplied by glossopharyngeal nerve.

345. Ans. (d) Mandibular branch

Ref: Gray's Anatomy, 41st ed. pg. 502

Branches of facial nerve on face:

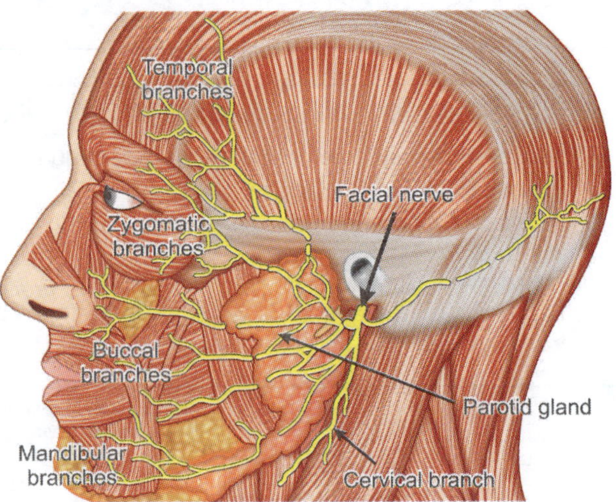

- **Temporal branch:** Aka frontal branch; supplies muscles of forehead and orbicularis oculi muscle
- **Zygomatic branch:** Supplies upper cheek and orbicularis oculi muscle
- **Buccal branch:** Emerges from anterior border of parotid gland below parotid duct to supply buccinator and muscles of upper lip and nostril.
- **Mandibular branch:** Emerges from anterior border of parotid gland to supply muscles of **lower lip**.
- **Cervical branch:** Emerges from lower border of parotid gland, it descends in the neck to supply platysma muscle + depressor anguli oris muscle.
- **Book states:** *"There are two marginal mandibular branches. They run forward under platysma towards angle of mandible. The branches supply risorius and the muscles of the lower lip and chin, and filaments communicate with the mental nerve"*

Extra Mile

- Orbicularis oris muscle is also supplied by mandibular branch of facial nerve

346. Ans. (c) Labial artery

Ref: Gray's Anatomy, 41st ed. pg. 498

- External carotid artery gives rise to facial artery branch, which has several branches over face.
- *Superior labial*–supplies to upper lip and antero-inferior part of nasal septum.
- *Inferior labial*–supplies to lower lip.
- *Lateral nasal*–to the ala and dorsum of nose.
- Angular–supplies the lacrimal sac and orbicularis oculi.

347. Ans. (a) Tragal pointer

Ref: Gray's Anatomy, 41st ed. pg. 412

Surgical Landmark of Parotid Gland

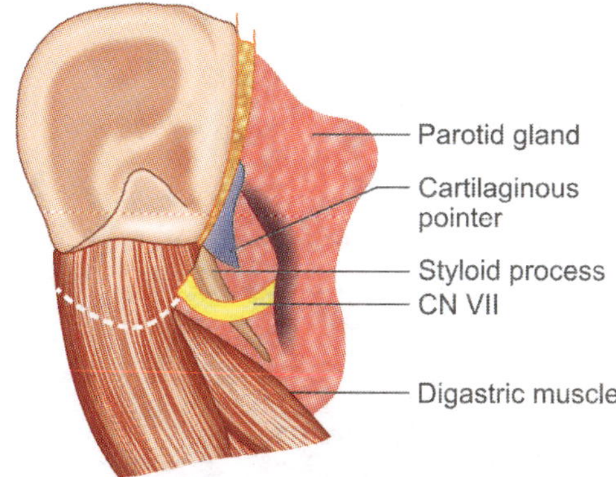

- **Tympano-mastoid suture in posterior canal wall:** 5–8 mm medial mastoid segment of facial nerve
- **Digastric ridge in mastoid tip:** Leads antero-medially to mastoid segment of facial nerve
- **Groove between mastoid and bony EAC meatus:** Bisected by facial nerve
- **Tragal pointer:** 1 cm antero-infero-medial is facial nerve
- **Root of styloid process:** Lateral to it lies facial nerve
- **Superior border of posterior belly of digastric:** Superior and parallel to it lies facial nerve

348. Ans. (d) Medial pterygoid

Ref: Gray's Anatomy, 41st ed. pg. 552

- **Trismus/Lock jaw** is painful reflex muscle spasm. It occurs due to spasm of muscle of mastication and leads to inability to open the oral cavity
- Trismus occurs due to involvement of masseter or medial pterygoid muscle or due to sub mucosal fibrosis.
- **Note:** Infection of pterygomandibular region can cause trismus, which usually affects medial pterygoid muscle.

349. Ans. (c) Buccinator

Ref: Gray's Anatomy, 41st ed. pg. 495

- It is a thin quadrilateral muscle of cheek, occupies the interval between maxilla and mandible.
- It compresses the cheek against the teeth and gums during mastication and assists the tongue in directing the food between teeth.

Classically the muscles of mastication are:

- *Masseter*
- *Lateral Pterygoid*
- *Medial Pterygoid*
- *Temporalis*

Accessory muscles of mastication

- *Anterior belly of digastric*
- *Mylohyoid muscle*
- *Geniohyiod muscle*
- *Buccinator*

350. Ans. (d) Second maxillary molar

Ref: Gray's Anatomy, 41st ed. pg. 411, 505

Parotid Duct/Stensen Duct

- It is a 5 cm long duct of parotid gland that originates from anterior border of upper part of parotid gland by the confluence of two main tributaries.
- **Course:** It then passes horizontally across masseter, midway between angle of mouth and zygomatic arch. Down the course it also crosses through buccal fat and buccinators muscle opposite the crown of upper third molar tooth.
- It then opens on a small papilla opposite the second upper molar crown.

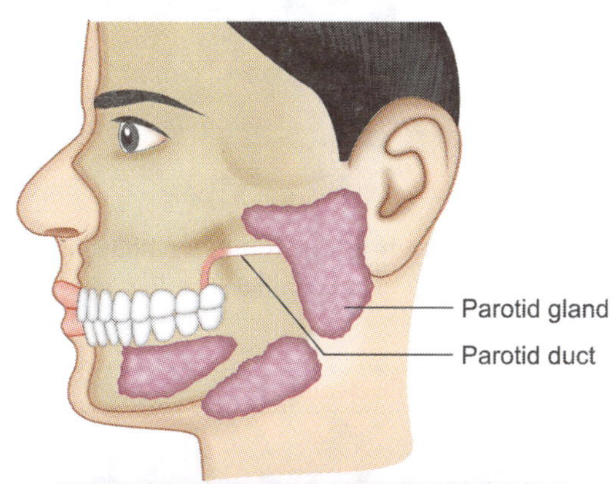

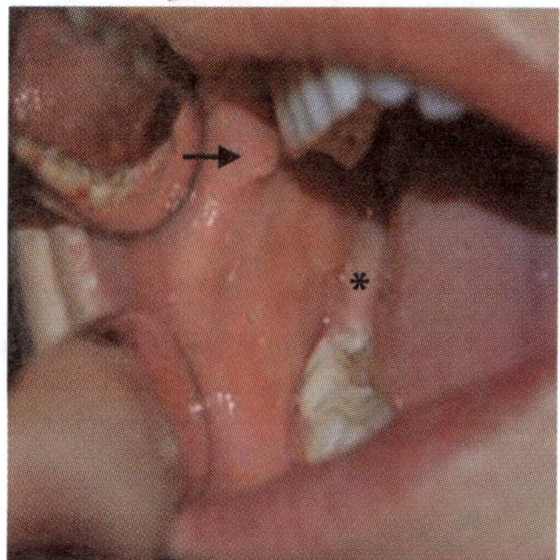

351. Ans. (d) Fornix

Ref: Gray's Anatomy, 41st ed. pg. 356

- The mammillary bodies are hemispherical, pea-sized eminences, lying side by side, anterior to the posterior perforated substance, each with nuclei enclosed in fascicles of fibers derived largely from the fornix.

The ***fornix*** is a white matter structure leaving the ***hippocampus*** that projects mainly to the ***mammillary bodies*** (hypothalamus) which, in turn, mainly projects to the ***thalamus*** via mammillothalamic tracts.

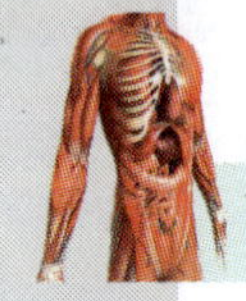

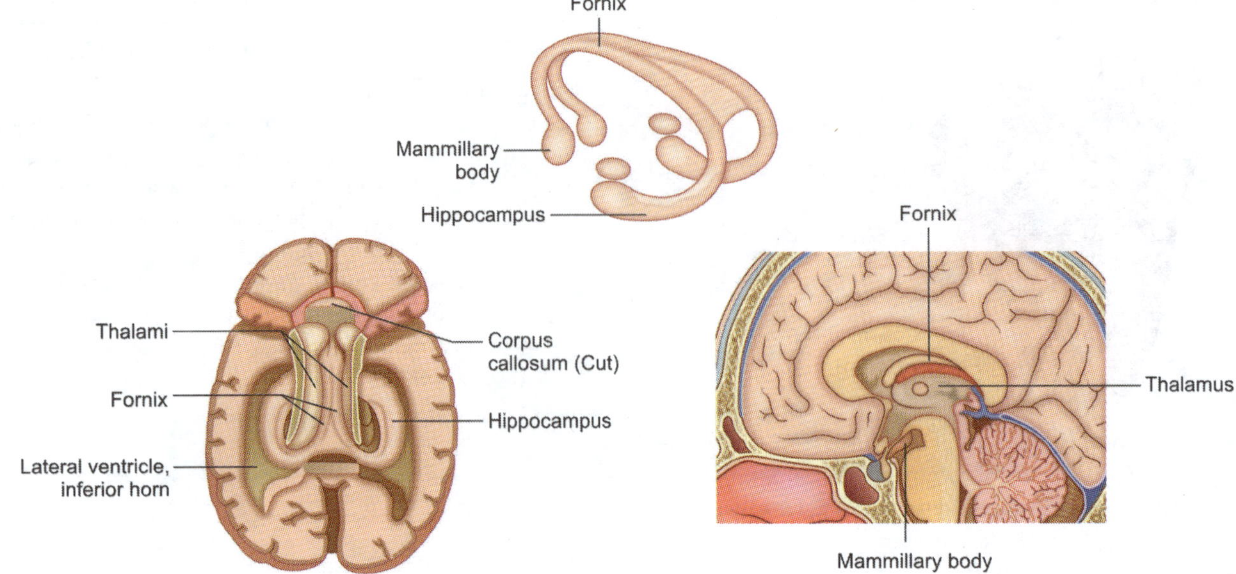

- Mammillary body is important for recollective memory.
- **Note:** Damage to mammillary bodies due to thiamine deficiency, is important in pathogenesis of Wernicke-Korsakoff syndrome.

352. Ans. (a) Arcuate fasciculus

Ref: Gray's Anatomy, 41st ed. pg. 391, 393

- Arcuate fasciculus is a white matter tract which connects broca's area and wernicke's area through the temporal, parietal and frontal lobes.
- It allows coordinated, comprehensive speech.
- **Note:** If damaged → Conduction Aphasia (auditory comprehension and speech articulation is present, but patient finds it difficult to repeat the heard speeches)

Extra Mile

1. **Uncinate fasciculus** connects frontal to temporal lobe
2. **Superior longitudinal fasciculus:** Connects the frontal, occipital, parietal, and temporal lobes
3. **Arcuate fasciculus:** Connect gyri in frontal to temporal lobes
4. **Inferior longitudinal fasciculus:** Connects occipital to temporal pole
5. **Cingulum:** Connects frontal and parietal lobes to the parahippocampal gyrus and adjacent temporal gyri

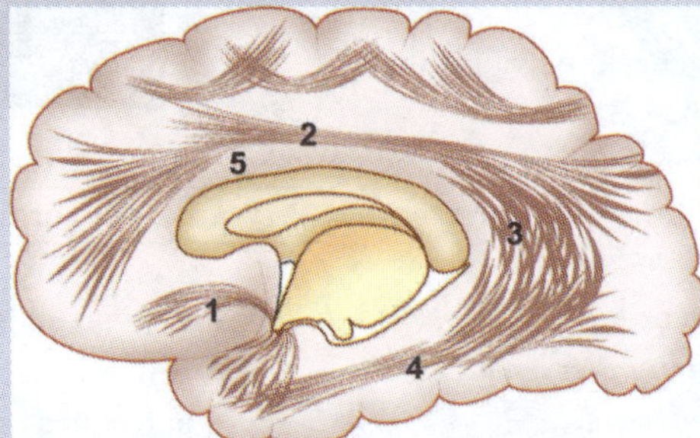

353. Ans. (c) Abducens

Ref: Textbook of Clinical Neuroanatomy 2015 ed. pg. 191

Abducens nerve passes through cavernous sinus. Other nerves like CN III, IV, V1 and V2 run in the wall of cavernous sinus.

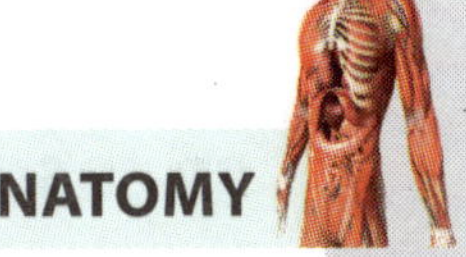

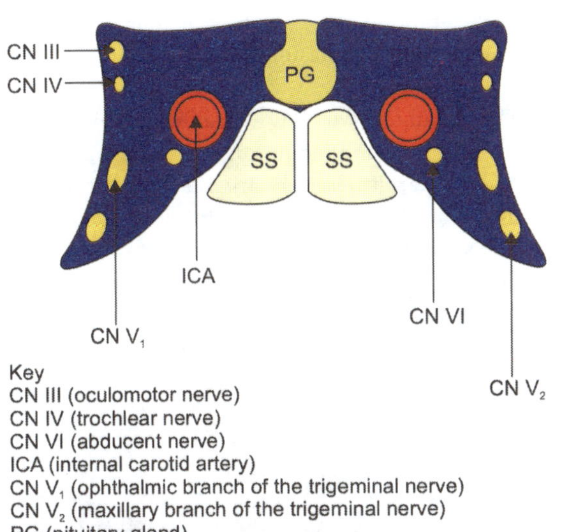

Cavernous sinus

354. Ans. (c) Left gastric artery

Ref: Gray's Anatomy, for Students E-book. pg. 222

Blood Supply of the Esophagus

- The upper third of the esophagus is supplied by the interior thyroid artery
- The middle third by branches from the descending thoracic aorta

Contd...

- The lower third by branches from the left gastric artery
- The veins from the upper third drain into the inferior thyroid veins, from the middle third into the azygos veins, and from the lower third into the left gastric vein, a tributary of the portal vein.

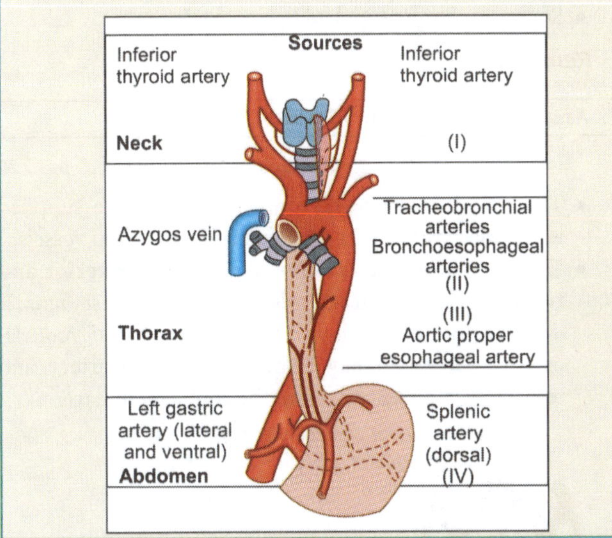

355. Ans. (d) Fastigii

Ref: Gray's Anatomy, E-book, pg. 337

- Cerebellar nuclei are arranged with dentate nucleus being most laterally located and nucleus fastigii being most medially located.

Cerebellar Nuclei (Nuclei = Deep Cluster of Neurons)

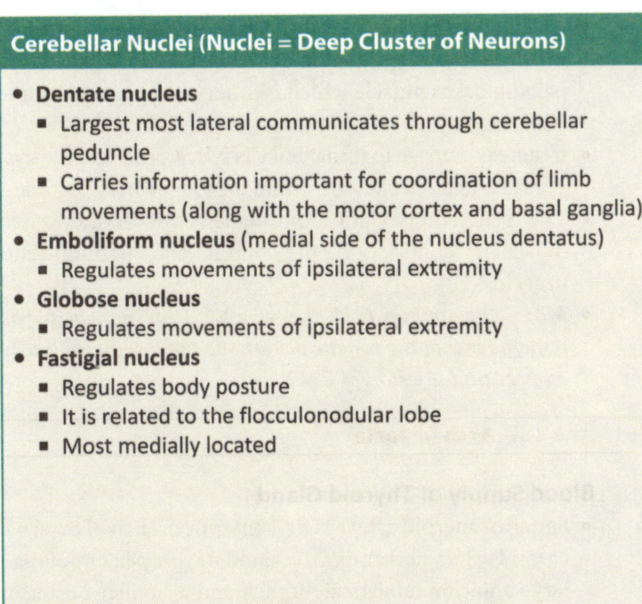

- **Dentate nucleus**
  - Largest most lateral communicates through cerebellar peduncle
  - Carries information important for coordination of limb movements (along with the motor cortex and basal ganglia)
- **Emboliform nucleus** (medial side of the nucleus dentatus)
  - Regulates movements of ipsilateral extremity
- **Globose nucleus**
  - Regulates movements of ipsilateral extremity
- **Fastigial nucleus**
  - Regulates body posture
  - It is related to the flocculonodular lobe
  - Most medially located

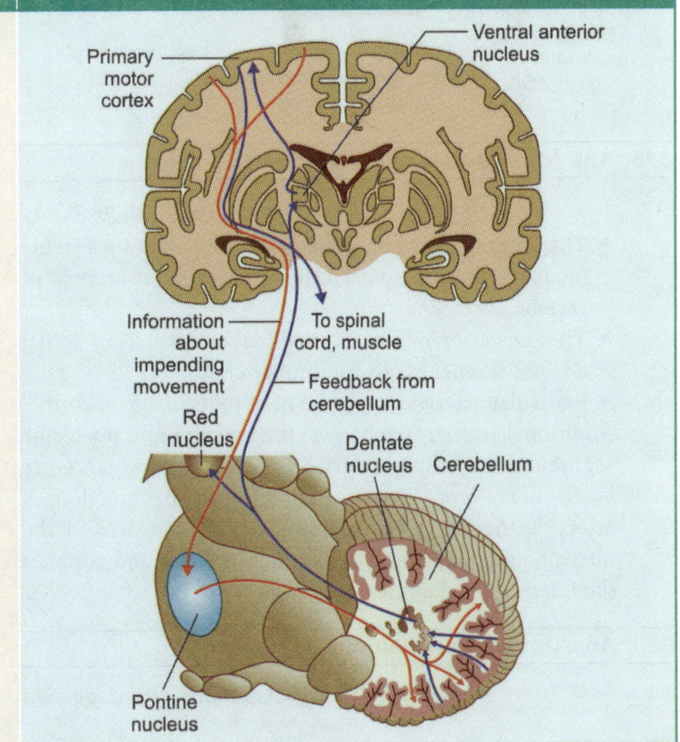

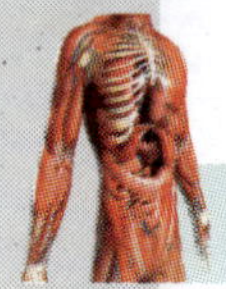

356. Ans. (c) Abducens

- All the extraocular muscles are supplied by CN III; EXCEPT lateral rectus and superior oblique.
- Lateral rectus supplied by—CN VI
- Superior oblique supplied by—CN IV

Remember- LR6; SO_4

357. Ans. (a) 1 anterior and 2 posterior

Ref: Gray's Anatomy, 41st ed. pg. 770

- The spinal cord and its roots and nerves are supplied with blood by both longitudinal and segmental vessels.
- Three major longitudinal vessels, **a single anterior and two posterior spinal arteries** *(each of which is sometimes doubled to pass on either side of the dorsal rootlets)* originate intracranially from the vertebral artery and terminate in a plexus around the conus medullaris.

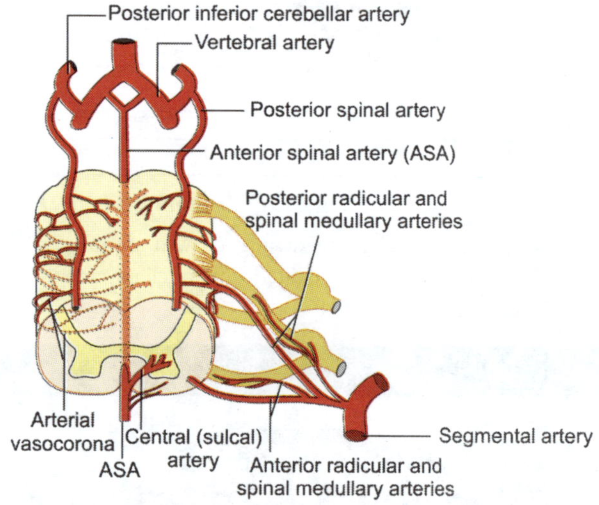

358. Ans. (d) Anterior spinal artery

Ref: Netter's Clinical Anatomy, 3rd ed. pg. 83-84

- The anterior 2/3rd of spinal cord is supplied by a single median anterior spinal artery which is a branch of vertebral artery.
- The posterior 1/3rd is supplied by posterior spinal arteries (branches of verterbral artery).
- Radicular arteries supply the neve roots of spinal cord.

Additional arterial supply is via the **anterior and posterior segmental medullary arteries**—small vessels which enter via the nerve roots. The largest anterior segment medullary artery is the artery of **Adamkiewicz**. It arises from the interior intercostal or upper lumbar arteries and supplies the inferior 2/3rd of the spinal cord.

359. Ans. (b) Postauricular muscle

Ref: Gray's Anatomy, 41st ed. pg. 628

- Each temporal bone consists of four components: the squamous, petromastoid and tympanic parts and the styloid process.
- The squamous part has a shallow mandibular fossa associated with the temporomandibular joint. The petromastoid part is relatively large; its petrous portion houses the auditory apparatus and is formed of compact bone.
- The **auricularis posterior** consists of two or three fleshy fasciculi that arise by short aponeurotic fibers from the mastoid part of the temporal bone and insert into the ponticulus on the eminentia conchae.

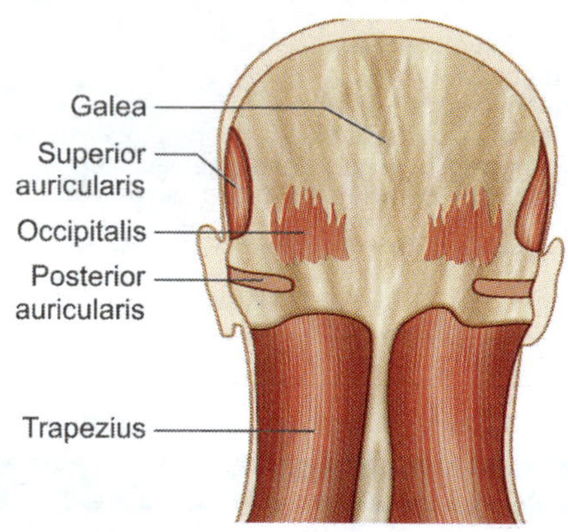

360. Ans. (c) Genioglossus

Ref: Lippincott's Illustrated, Review of Anatomy and Embryology, pg. 214

- All the intrinsic and extrinsic muscles of the tongue are innervated by hypoglossal nerve (CN XII); EXCEPT the palatoglossus muscle which is innervated by vagus nerve (CN X).
- If there is damage to ipsilateral CN XII, it produces the dysarthria and fasciculations within the tongue musculature.
- The ipsilateral deviation of tongue is due to unopposed muscular contraction of contralateral **genioglossus muscle.**
- ***Mn:*** *"The tongue licks the wound" (this will help you remember that the tongue deviates to the ipsilateral side in a lower motor lesion of CN XII)*

361. Ans. (d) Arch of aorta

Blood Supply of Thyroid Gland

- Superior thyroid artery is first anterior branch of external carotid artery and enters the gland near superior pole as a large anterior superficial branch and a smaller posterior branch.
- Inferior thyroid artery, a branch of thyrocervical trunk of subclavian artery passes behind the carotid sheath running medially reaching the posterolateral aspect of the gland.

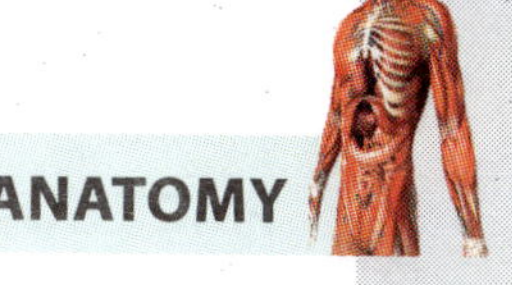

- Thyroidea ima artery, a branch of aorta or brachiocephalic artery enters the isthmus or lower pole of one of the lateral lobes (3%).
- Tracheal and esophageal branches serve blood supply to retained thyroid gland after thyroidectomy.

362. Ans. (c) C5-T1

- Thyroid gland is located in anterior triangle of the neck and weighs 20 grams. Gland lies against C5 to T1 vertebra.
- Isthmus extends from 2–4th tracheal rings

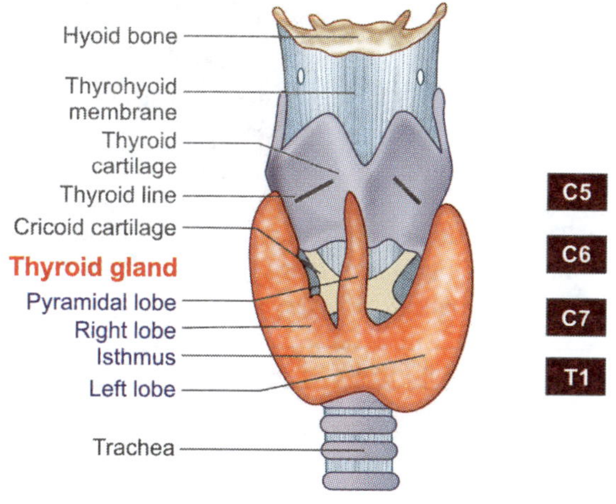

363. Ans. (c) 6

Ref: Netter's Atlas of Neurosciences, 3rd ed. pg. 247

- There are *2 cerebellar hemispheres* with each divided into *3 lobes*, thus making 6 lobes in all.
- The anterior is separated from middle lobe by *fissure primura.*
- There are 4 pairs of cerebellar nuclei.

D: Nucleus Dentatus
E: Nucleus emboliformis
F: Nucleus fastigii
G: Nucleus globosus

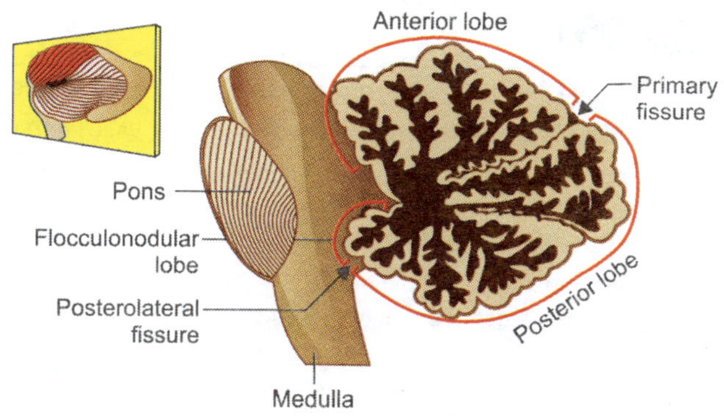

364. Ans. (a) Flocculonodular lobe

Ref: Netter's atlas of Neurosciences, 3rd ed. pg. 409

- The flocconodular lobe is the *smallest lobe.*

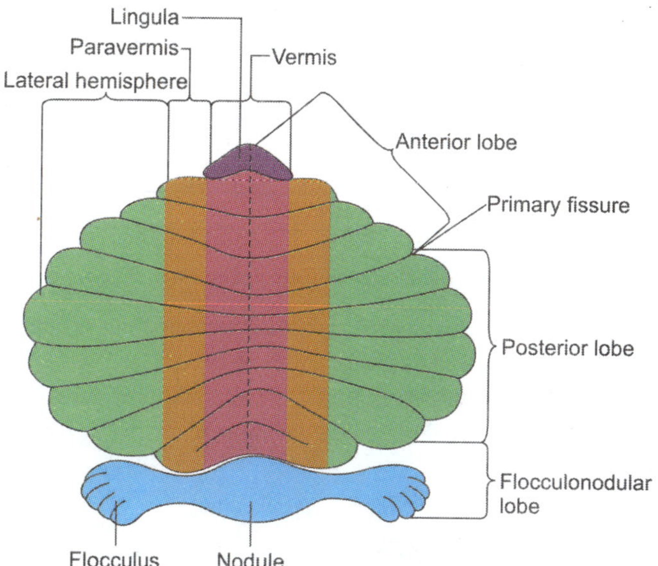

- Most *primitive part* of cerebellum is archi-cerebellum and most *recent part* is neo-cerebellum.

365. Ans. (a) First part of subclavian artery

Ref: Netter's atlas of neurosciences, 3rd ed. pg. 110

- Subclavian artery is divided into three parts by **scalaneus anticus muscle *(Mn: VIT CD)***

Branches from 1st part	Branches from 2nd part	Branches from 3rd part
• Vertebral artery	• No branch on left side	• Dorsal scapular branch
• Internal thoracic artery	• Gives costocervical trunk on right side	
• Thyrocervical trunk		
• Costocervical branch on left side		

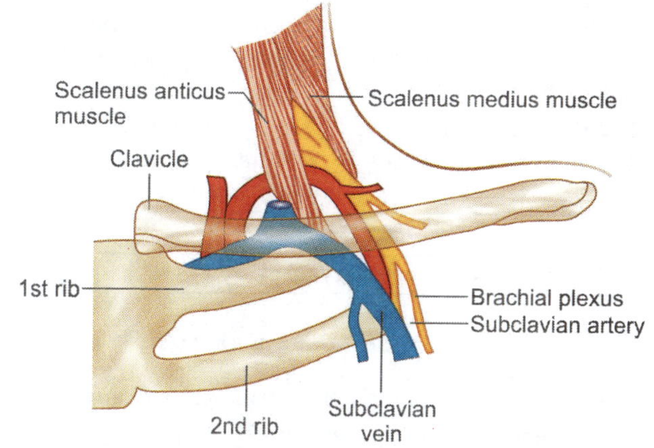

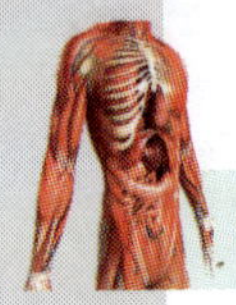

366. Ans. (b) Dorsal scapular artery

Ref: Netter's Clinical Anatomy, 3rd ed. pg. 504

- Dorsal scapular artery is a branch of 3rd part of subclavian artery.

367. Ans. (d) Internal carotid artery

Ref: Netter's Clinical Anatomy, 3rd ed. pg. 420

- The free floating structure in cavernous sinus is cranial nerve VI and internal carotid artery.
- The cranial nerves III, IV, V1, V2 and post ganglionic fibers pass through the lateral wall of the cavernous sinus.

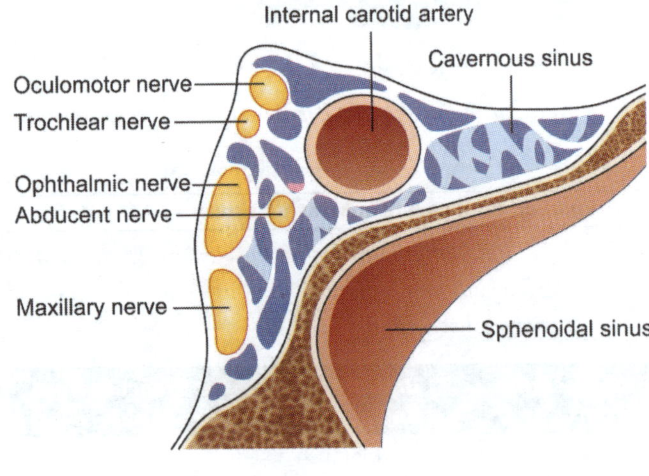

368. Ans. (c) Basilar artery

Ref: Netter's Clinical Anatomy, 3rd ed. pg. 426

Branches of Basilar artery (mnemonic: P.A.L.S)	Branches of Vertebral artery
• Posterior cerebral artery • Pontine artery • Anterior inferior cerebellar artery • Labyrinthine artery • Superior cerebellar artery	• Post inferior cerebellar artery *(largest branch)* • Anterior spinal artery *(single artery and runs in anterior median fissure)* • *Posterior Spinal Artery* • *Basilar Artery*

369. Ans. (b) Ascending pharyngeal artery

Ref: Netter's Clinical Anatomy, 3rd ed. pg. 487

- The smallest branch of external carotid artery is the ascending pharyngeal artery.

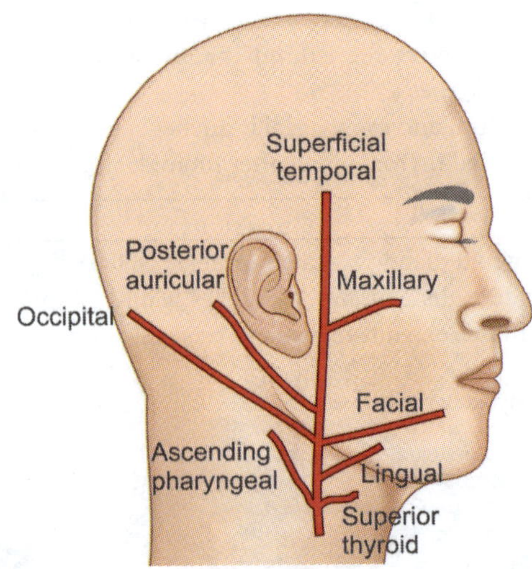

- The common carotid artery divides at the level of upper border of thyroid cartilage (C4 Level) into the internal and external carotid artery.

370. Ans. (d) Lower border of S2

Ref: Netter's Clinical Anatomy, 3rd ed. pg. 420

- The subarachnoid space extends up to *lower border of S2* where the dura fuses with filum terminale and obliterates the subarachnoid space.
- The *spinal cord* extends from *upper border of atlas* to *lower border of L1* or upper border of L2. The spinal cord ends in a sharp tip called conus medullaris.
- The *conus* is continuous with *filum terminale*, which is a fine connective tissue element which descends up to the dorsum of the *first coccygeal ligament*.

371. Ans. (c) CN 3

Ref: Netter's Atlas of Neurosciences, pg. 265

The cranial nerves carrying parasympathetic fibers are 3, 7, 9, 10.

Extra Mile

• *CN having longest intraosseous course*	Facial nerve
• *CN having longest extracranial coursel*	Vagus nerve
• *Thinnest* and most slender cranial nerve • Only one to *originate from the dorsal surface* • *Longest intracranial course*	Trochlear
• *Thickest* and largest cranial nerve • *Largest branch* of trigeminal is mandibular nerve.	Trigeminal
False localising sign in raised ICP	Abducens
Longest intra-osseus course	Facial
Cranial nerve with both motor and sensory components	5, 7, 9, 10

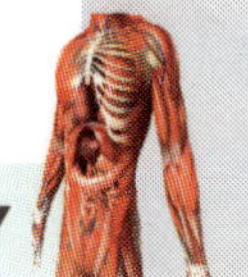

372. Ans. (c) CN 8

Ref: Netter's Atlas of Neurosciences, pg. 265

- Cranial nerve 3 is pure motor nerve and performs ocular movement.
- Cranial nerve 5 performs mastication and is sensory to face.
- Cranial nerve 9 is a mixed nerve and carries taste from posterior 1/3rd of tongue and performs swallowing with help of stylopharyngeus.
- CN 8th is pure sensory. Associated with hearing and balancing.

373. Ans. (b) Arachnoid and pia mater

Ref: Netter's Clinical Anatomy, 3rd ed. pg. 25

- *Meninx* implies all three layers—dura, arachnoid and inner pia matter.
- The dura mater is called *pachymeninx*.
- The middle arachnoid and inner pia matter is called as *leptomeninges*.
- The arachnoid does not follow the convolutions of brain and looks like a loose fitting sac. Multiple arachnoid granulations pass through subarachnoid space and blends with pia matter.

374. Ans. (b) Temporal lobe from fronto-parietal areas

Ref: Netter's Atlas of Neurosciences, 3rd ed. pg. 52

The Slyvian fissure separates the temporal lobes inferiorly from the fronto-parietal lobes.

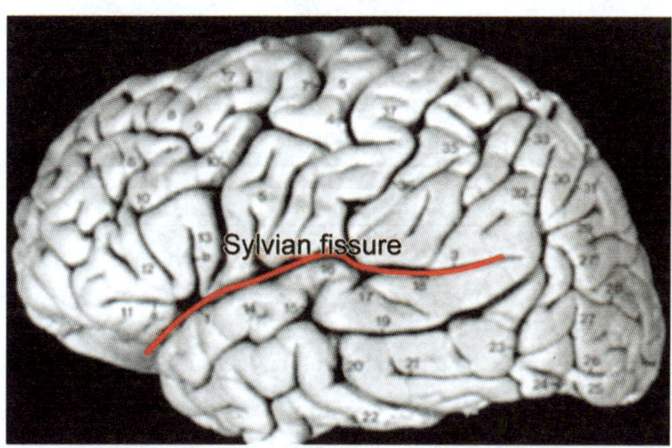

375. Ans. (c) Left and right brachiocephalic veins

Ref: Atlas of Human Anatomy, 6th ed. pg. 59

- *Superior vena cava is formed* by junction of *2 brachiocephalic veins* and has No valves.
- *Inferior vena cava* is formed by union of *2 common iliac veins*.
- *Portal vein* is formed by union of superior mesenteric vein and splenic vein.
- *External jugular vein* is formed by union of *posterior division of retromandibular vein and posterior* auricular vein.

376. Ans. (a) TM joint

Ref: Kulkarni Clinical Anatomy, 2nd ed. pg. 24

TM joint	Bi-condylar joint
Atlanto-occipital joint	Ellipsoid joint/bi-axial joint
Interphalangeal joint	Hinge joint/uniaxial joint
Inter-metatarsal joint	Plane joint

Extra Mile

- **Bi-condylar joints:** Knee joint and temporomandibular joint
- **Pivot joint/Trochoid joint:** Superior and inferior radioulnar joint, median atlanto-axial joint

377. Ans. (a) Middle meningeal artery

Ref: Netter's Clinical Anatomy, 3rd ed. pg. 460

Structures transmitted via foramen ovale (M.A.L.E.)

- **M**andibular nerve-V3
- **A**ccessory meningeal artery
- **L**esser petrosal nerve
- **E**missary vein

Extra Mile

Foramen rotundum	Maxillary nerve V2
Foramen Lacerum	Internal carotid artery Lesser petrosal nerve Greater petrosal nerve Deep petrosal nerve
Foramen spinosum	Middle meningeal artery Nervus spinosus (Meningeal Branch of mandibular nerve) Posterior trunk of middle meningeal vein
Carotid canal	Internal carotid artery Venous and sympathetic plexus around the artery

Since lots of questions are asked on the topic of base of skull, students are expected to memorise this diagram by drawing it yourself.

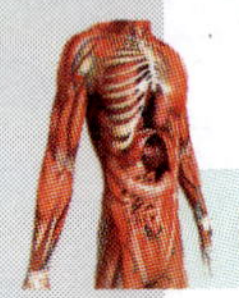

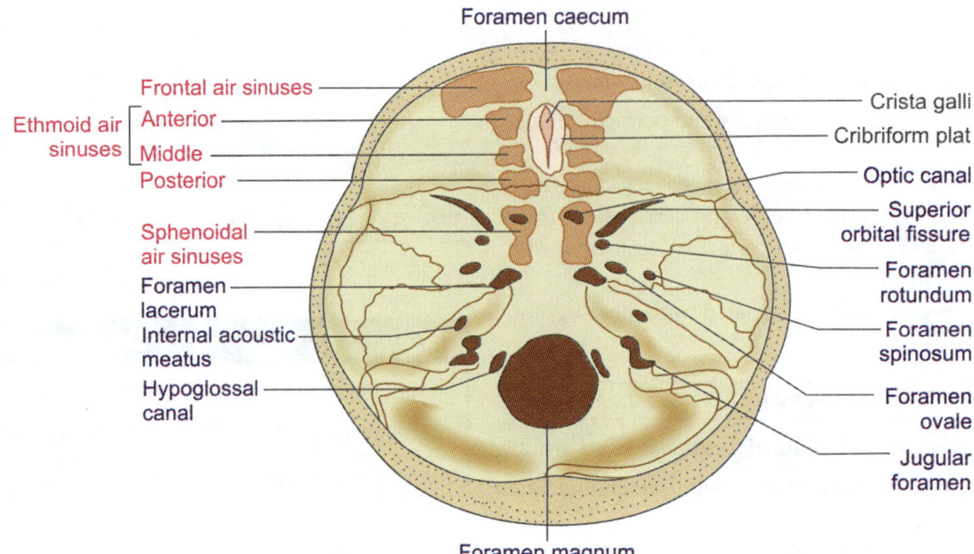

378. Ans. (b) Foramen rotundum

Ref: Netter's Clinical Anatomy, 3rd ed. pg. 352

Trigeminal nerve branches transmitted via—

V1 (Ophthalmic nerve)	Superior orbital Fissure
V2 (Maxillary nerve)	Foramen Rotundum
V3 (Mandibular nerve)	Foramen Ovale

379. Ans. (d) Cervical vertebra

Ref: Kulkarni Clinical Anatomy, 2nd ed. pg. 330

- Foramen transversarium is found only in cervical vertebra and transmits the vertebral artery.
- Another feature peculiar to cervical vertebra is bifid spinous process which is absent in C7 and has a small body.

Extra Mile

Flexion and extension of neck	Atlanto-occipital joint
Rotational movement of neck	Atlanto-axial joint

380. Ans. (d) Nerve of wrisberg

Ref: Netter's Atlas of Human Anatomy, 5th ed. pg. 62

Nerve and its Details

Arnold nerve (choice A)	Auricular branch of vagus (alderman nerve)
Jacobson nerve (choice B)	Tympanic branch of glossopharyngeal nerve
Criminal nerve of grassi (choice C)	Branch of right posterior vagus that passes to left behind oesophagus ending in gastric cardia It is cut in highly selective vagotomy to avoid recurrent peptic ulceration
Nerve of wrisberg (choice D)	Sensory component of facial nerve which carries taste sensation from anterior 2/3 of tongue

Extra Mile

Vidian nerve	Nerve of pterygoid canal
Nerve of latarjet	Branch of anterior gastric nerve and supplies the pylorus. It is left intact in highly selective vagotomy so that the function of gastric emptying remains intact.

381. Ans. (d) 4

Ref: Netter's Atlas of Neurosciences, 3rd ed. pg. 53

- The primary sensory cortex lies in the post central gyrus and is area 1, 2, 3
- Area 4 is the primary voluntary cortex.

Brodmann Areas of Cerebral Cortex

1, 2, 3	Primary sensory cortex lies in Post central gyrus
4	Primary voluntary cortex lies in precentral gyrus
17	Primary visual cortex and lies in calcarine cortex
18, 19	Visual association cortex
22	*Wernicke's* area (*Superior Temporal lobe*)
41	Primary auditory area
44, 45	*Broca* area (*inferior frontal gyrus*)

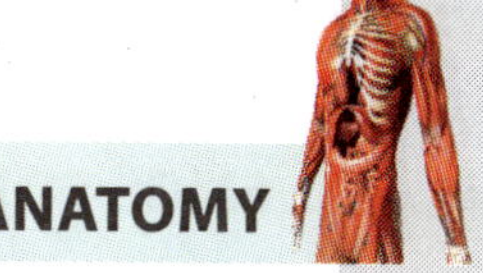

382. Ans. (c) Cingulate gyrus

Ref: Netter's Correlative Imaging of Neuroanatomy, pg. 147

The limbic system is composed of following contents:
1. Cingulate gyrus
2. Hippocampus
3. Fornix
4. Mammillary bodies

The limbic system manages the emotional behaviour, sexual behaviour and food habits.

383. Ans. (b) Motor to 9, 10, 11 cranial nerve nucleus

Ref: Netter's Atlas of Neurosciences, 3rd ed. pg. 251

The cells in nucleus ambiguus contain *motor neurons* concerned with three cranial nerves
1. Rostral pole = *Glossopharyngeal*
2. Middle part = *Vagus*
3. Caudal pole = *Spino-accessory*
   - Axons arising from nucleus ambiguus pass laterally and slightly ventrally to exit the medulla just dorsal to the inferior olive.
   - These axons then course with the three cranial nerves: IX (glossopharyngeal), X (vagus) and XI (spinoaccessory) to innervate the striated muscles of the soft palate, pharynx, larynx, and upper part of the esophagus.

384. Ans. (a) Optic nerve

Ref: Gray's Anatomy, 41st ed. pg. 310

- The cranial nerves are individually named and numbered, using Roman numerals, in a rostro-caudal sequence, reflecting their order of attachment to the brain. They are named as follows:

TABLE: Cranial nerves

CN number	CN name	Attachment/Comments
I	Olfactory nerve	Arises from the olfactory epithelium in the nasal cavity and terminates directly in cortical and subcortical areas of the frontal and temporal lobes
II	Optic nerve	The axons of the optic nerve (II) pass into the optic chiasma, where medially positioned axons decussate; all of the axons emerge as the optic tract, which terminates in the lateral geniculate nucleus of the thalamus

Contd...

CN number	CN name	Attachment/Comments
III	Occulomotor nerve	Arise in, and are attached to, the midbrain.
IV	Trochlear nerve	
V	Trigeminal nerve	Attaches to the pons, medial to the middle cerebellar peduncle.
VI	Abducens nerve	Attaches to the brainstem at, or close to, the pontomedullary junction.
VII	Facial nerve	
VIII	Vestibulocochlear N.	
IX	Glossopharyngeal N.	Attached to the medulla
X	Vagus nerve	
XI	Spinal accessory nerve	Arises from cervical levels C1–C5/C6, enters the cranium through the foramen magnum and then exits via the jugular foramen, together with the glossopharyngeal and vagus nerves.
XII	Hypoglossal nerve	Attached to the medulla

385. Ans. (c) Greater auricular nerve

Ref: Dhingra, 6th ed. pg. 4

Nerve supply of Auricle/Pinna

- **Lateral Surface**
  - Greater auricular nerve (most part)
  - Auriculotemporal nerve (supplies anteriorly, Tragus, some part of helix)
  - CN- X and CN- VII (Concha)
- **Medial Surface**
  - Upper 1/3 by Lesser occipital N.
  - ***Lower 2/3 by Greater Auricular N.***
  - Concha/Root of auricle by Auricular br. Of vagus N. + Facial nerve

386. Ans. (a) Maxillary process

Ref: BDC, Vol-3 pg. 355-356

- The facial nerve leaves the skull by passing through the **stylomastoid foramen.**
- Branches and Distribution:
  - Within the facial canal:
    - **Greater petrosal nerve**- *to the eye (lacrimal gland)*
    - **The nerve to the stapedius**- *to the stapedius muscle in middle ear*
    - **The chorda tympani**- *to the tongue*

- At its exit from the stylomastoid foramen it gives out branches to Posterior auricular, **Digastrics** and stylohyoid.
- It has terminal branches within the **parotid gland** also like, temporal, Zygomatic, Buccal, Marginal mandibular and Cervical.

387. Ans. (d) In relation with upper 2nd molar tooth

Ref: Clinical Anatomy by Systems by Richard S. Snell/55

Gland	Type of gland	Duct	Duct opening
Parotid	Serous	Stensons duct	Vestibule of mouth opposite second upper molar
Sub-mandibular	Mixed but predominantly serous	Whartons duct	On the floor of mouth on summit of sublingual papilla at the side of frenulum of tongue
Sublingual	Mixed but predominantly mucus	Bartholins duct	On the floor of mouth on summit of sublingual papilla

388. Ans. (c) Deviation of tongue

- Facial nerve gives sensory supply to tongue.
- Chorda tympani nerve is a sensory branch of facial nerve (CN VII) which gives taste sensation of anterior 2/3rd of tongue.
- Glossopharyngeal nerve (CN IX) gives the taste sensation from posterior 2/3rd of tongue.
- Motor supply to tongue is by hypoglossal nerve (CN XII). Injury to hypoglossal nerve paralyzes ipsilateral half of tongue.
- If CN XII is functioning normally, tongue protrudes evenly in midline.
- If CN XII is paralyzed: When tongue is protruded, its tip deviates towards the paralyzed side because of unopposed action of genioglossus muscle on the normal side of tongue.(TDS)

389. *Ans. (a)* Lateral pterygoid

Ref: Gray's, 41st ed. pg. 507-508

- The primary function of the lateral pterygoid muscle is to pull the head of the condyle out of the mandibular fossa along the articular eminence to protrude the mandible.
- **The effort of the lateral pterygoid muscles acts in helping lower the mandible and open the jaw** whereas unilteral action of a lateral pterygoid produces contralateral excursion (a form of mastication), usually performed in concert with the medial pterygoids.
- Unlike the other three muscles of mastication, the lateral pterygoid is the only muscle of mastication that assists in depressing the mandible i.e. opening the jaw. At the beginning of this action it is assisted by the digastric, mylohyoid and geniohyoid muscles.

390. Ans. (a) Facial nerve

Ref: BDC, 5th ed. Vol. III, pg. 252-253

- Basically, facial nerve supplies the taste sensation of anterior 2/3rd of the tongue, but since this option is given with this question, the best suited option is facial nerve.

According to BDC

- Sensory supply of anterior 2/3rd of the tongue is by facial nerve (CN VII).
- ***Its lingual branch is for general sensation.***
- *Corda tympani branch is for taste*
- **Sensory supply for posterior 1/3rd** - glossopharyngeal nerve/ CN IX (general and taste sensation both).
- **Posterior most or valeculla** is supplied by vagus nerve (internal laryngeal branch).

391. Ans. (d) CN XI

Ref: BDC, 5th ed. Vol. III, pg. 252-253

- Sensory supply of anterior 2/3rd of the tongue is by facial nerve (CN VII).
  - Its lingual branch is for general sensation.
  - Corda tympani branch is for taste
- Sensory supply for posterior 1/3rd - glossopharyngeal nerve/ CN IX (general and taste sensation both).
- Posterior most or valeculla is supplied by vagus nerve *(internal laryngeal branch).*

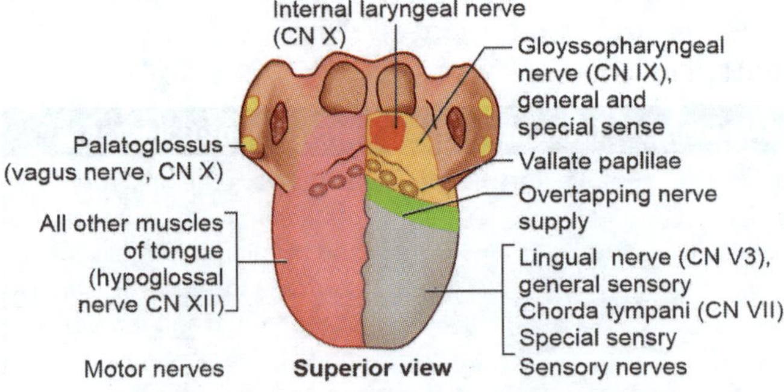

392. Ans. (a) Lingual nerve

Please refer to above explanation

393. Ans. (a) Pons

Ref: BDC, 6th ed. Vol. III, pg. 364, 70, 71

- CN 3rd and 4th cranial nerve attach to midbrain

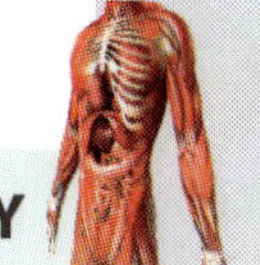

- CN 5th, 6th, 7th, and 8th attach to Pons
- CN 9th, 10th, 11th and 12th from medulla
- Vestibular component of vestibulocochlear nerve (CN 8th) arises from junction of pons and medulla.

Extra Mile

- Acoustic neuroma is most common cerebellopontine angle tumor.
- Earliest CN involved is CN 5th, which is followed by 8th, 9th, 10th, 7th and 6th.

394. Ans. (c) Trochlear

Ref: BDC, 6th ed. Vol. II, pg. 364

TROCHLEAR (IV) NERVE

- **Smallest cranial nerve**
- **Most slender cranial**
- Only nerve to emerge from dorsal (posterior) surface of brain stem (mid brain)
- Passes anteriorly around the brain stem, running the longest intracranial (subarachnoid) course
- Nerve crosses the midline within the midbrain, emerges from its dorsal aspect and immediately decussates with the nerve of opposite side
- It supplies superior oblique, the only extra ocular muscle that uses pulley/trochlea to redirect its line of action

395. Ans. (c) Trochlear nerve

Ref: BDC 6th ed. Vol. III, pg. 362

- **Trochlear nerve** is the only cranial nerve to emerge dorsally from the brain stem.
  - *It has the longest intracranial course* and it is the most slender cranial nerve in terms of axon contents.
- Largest cranial nerve: Trigeminal N. (CN 5th)
- CN which has most extensive distribution beyond head and neck: Vagus Nerve (CN 10th).
- Most frequently paralyzed CN: Facial Nerve (CN 7th)-due to wide intraosseous course.
- Pure sensory CN: CN 1, 2, 8
- Pure motor CN: CN 3, 4, 6, 11, 12
- Mixed CN: CN 5, 7, 9, 10

396. Ans. (d) Vagus nerve

Ref: BDC, 6th ed. Vol. III, pg. 379-81

- The "criminal nerve" of Grassi is the first gastric branch of the posterior vagus nerve. This nerve may branch proximal or distal to the celiac division of the posterior vagus nerve.
- The importance of this nerve is during Truncal vagotomy, since failure to transect the nerve of Grassi proximal to its origin will result in an incomplete vagotomy.

397. Ans. (c) Recurrent laryngeal nerve

Ref: BDC, Vol. 3 pg. 171, 172,173, 176.

- It is recurrent laryngeal nerve that pierces the thyroid gland.

Must know about Thyroid

- The gland consists of 2 lobes that are joined to each other by the isthmus
- The gland extends against vertebrae C5, C6, C7 and T1
- It weighs about 25 g.
- The thyroid gland is supplied by the superior and inferior thyroid arteries.
  - The superior thyroid artery is the first anterior branch of the external carotid artery.
  - The inferior thyroid artery is a branch of thyro cervical trunk
- Nerve supply
  - Nerves are derived mainly from the middle cervical ganglion and partly also from the superior and inferior cervical ganglia. Follicular
- It is made of following two types of Secretory cells
  - Follicular cells lining the follicles of the gland secrete T3 and T4.
  - Parafollicular cells (C cells) are fewer and lie in between the follicles. They secrete thyrocalcitonin.

Extra Mile

What is the function of thyrocalcitonin?
- It promotes deposition of calcium salts in skeletal and other tissues, and tends to produce hypocalcaemia.

398. Ans. (c) Trigeminal nerve

Ref: Gray's 41st ed. pg. 667, BDC, 6th ed. Vol. III, pg. 206-7

TABLE: Structures passing through superior orbital fissure

Superior orbital fissure		
Upper part/ Lateral	**Middle part (through tendinous ring)**	**Lower/Medial part**
• Superior ophthalmic vein • Lacrimal nerve • Frontal nerve • Trochlear nerve ***Mn – "Superior LFT"***	• Nasociliary nerve • Occulomotor nerve • Abducent nerve ***Mnemonic –"NOA"***	• Inferior ophthalmic vein • Sympathetic nerves around internal carotid artery ***Mn: Inferior sympathy***

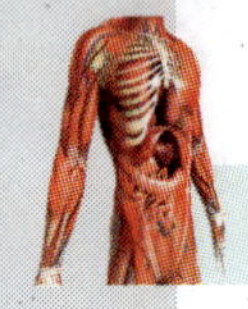

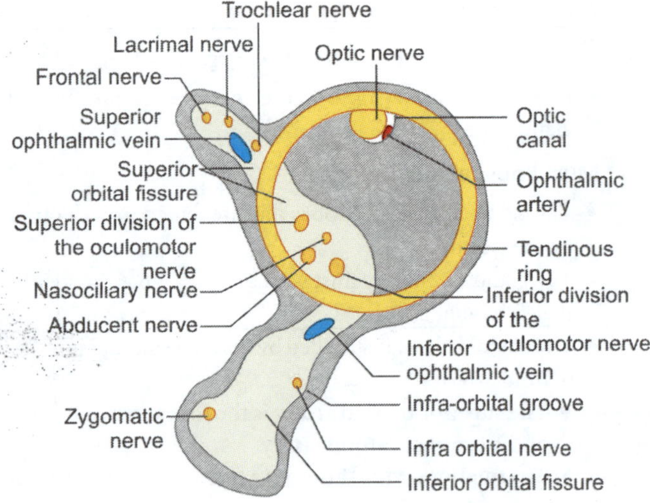

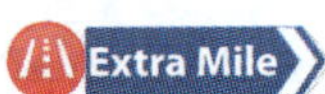
Extra Mile

Structures passing through Inferior orbital fissure
- Zygomatic branch of maxillary nerve
- Infraorbital nerve & vessels
- Rami of Pterygoid ganglion
- Communicating vein b/w inferior ophthalmic & pterygoid plexus of veins.

Mn-"ZIPC"

399. Ans. (a) 2

Ref: Netter's Clinical Anatomy, 3rd ed. pg. 442

Structures transmitted via the superior orbital fissure
- Cranial nerve III, IV, V1 (ophthalmic nerve) and VI
- Inferior ophthalmic vein

The optic nerve is transmitted via the optic canal. The optic canal transmits optic nerve, ophthalmic artery and central retinal vein.

400. Ans. (a) Superior ophthalmic vein

Ref: Gray's, 41st ed. pg. 667

401. Ans. (a) Mandibular nerve

Ref: Keith L. Moore, 5th ed. pg. 899

402. Ans. (c) Both

Ref: Gray's, 41st ed. pg. 667

403. Ans. (a) Sphenoid bone tumor

Ref: Gray's Anatomy, pg. 801-805

TABLE: CN injury and their cause

Cranial Nerve	Usual cause
CN III, IV, first division of V	***Invasive sphenoid bone tumor***
CN VII, VIII	Petrous bone tumor
CN V, VII, VIII	Acoustic neuroma, Meningioma
CN IX, X, XI, XII	Parotid gland and carotid body tumor and Metastasis

404. Ans. (c) C3, C4, C5

Ref: Gray's, 38th ed. pg. 1265

TABLE: Phrenic nerve

Root value	Anterior primary rami of C3, C4, C5 (chiefly C4) Mnemonic. "C3,4,5 keeps the diaphragm alive
Relations	Front of scalenus anterior and behind prevertebral fascia in neck Behind brachiocephalic vein and front of subclavian artery in thorax entry Passes in front of hilum of lung **Rt. Phrenic:** Pass through vena caval opening (T8) **Lt. phrenic:** Muscular part of diaphragm
Supply	Motor: Diaphragm Sensory: Pleura diaphragmatic, pericardium (fibrous & parietal), coronary and falciform ligament of liver, IVC, adrenals and gallbladder.

405. Ans. (c) Cleft lip and cleft palate both

Ref: Clinical Anatomy, Vishram Singh, pg. 306

- The cleft lip and palate are the most common congenital anomalies of the head and neck, occurring in 1 per 750 live births.

406. Ans. (c) Loose subaponeurotic layer

Ref: BDC, 6th ed. Vol. III, pg. 61-63

The 5 layers of scalp can be remembered as **SCALP:**
- **Skin:** Consist of hair follicles, sebaceous gland and sweat glands.
- Sub Cutaneous layer: Contains blood vessels, nerves of the scalp
- Aponeurotic layer aka **galea aponeurotica.** It is a tough layer of dense fibrous tissue which runs from the frontalis muscle anteriorly to the occipitalis posteriorly
- **Loose subaponeurotic tissue** containing the emissary veins and allowing free movement of layers 1 to 3 as a unit. *Layer 4 is a **"dangerous area"*** because it allows spread of infection even, by way of the emissary veins, to intracranial structures.

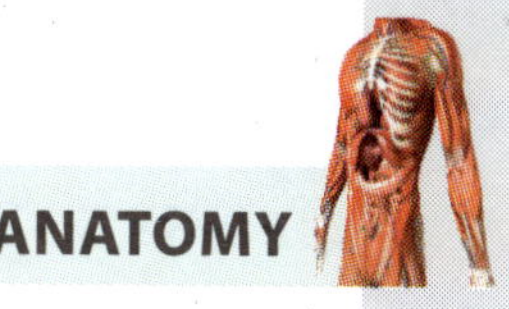

- Pericranium, is the periosteum of the skull bones providing nutrition.

407. Ans. (d) Galea aponeurotica

Ref: BDC, 6th ed. Vol. III, pg. 61-63

408. Ans. (b) Frontal process of maxilla

Ref: BDC, 6th ed. Vol. III, pg. 28

Orbit wall	Formed by
• Medial wall *Mn – "uSMLE*	Sphenoid (body) , Maxilla (frontal process), Lacrimal bone, Ethmoid (orbital plate)
• **Lateral wall** Mn – "ZyGS"	Zygomatic (frontal process) Greater wing of Sphenoid
• **Roof**	Frontal bone and Lesser wing of sphenoid
• Floor	Palatine (orbital process), Maxilla, Zygomatic

409. Ans. (d) Trigeminal nerve

Ref: Gray's, 41st ed. pg. 315-16, 20-21

- ***Muscles of soft palate are supplied by pharyngeal plexus (of cranial accessory & vagus nerves) and mandibular division (V2) of trigeminal nerve.***
- General sensation by lesser palatine branch of maxillary division (V2) of trigeminal nerve & glossopharyngeal nerve.
- Secretomotor parasympathic post ganglionic fibers through lesser palatine nerves (pterygopalatine ganglion) & otic ganglion.
- *Taste by facial nerve (through lesser palatine nerve)*
- Hard palate is supplied by greater palatine & nasopalatine branches of maxillary nerve in place of lesser palatine nerve. All 3 (greater, lesser & naso) palatine nerves pass through pterygopalatine ganglion.
- Palate is supplied by trigeminal (maxillary, mandibular), facial, glossopharyngeal, cranial accessory & vagus nerves.

410. Ans. (a) Genioglossus

Ref: BDC, 5th ed. pg. 252

- Genioglossus is a fan shaped, *bulkiest muscle of tongue.*
- It is originated from upper genial tubercle of mandible and inserted into tip of tongue and into hyoid bone.
- **Function:** It retracts and depresses the tongue. It is also known as life saving muscle because it pulls the posterior part of tongue forwards and protrudes the tongue forwards.

Extra Mile

- **MOTOR:** All the extrinsic and intrinsic muscles of tongue are supplied by hypoglossal nerve; EXCEPT palatoglossus, which is supplied by the cranial root of accessory nerve through the pharyngeal plexus.
- **SENSORY:** Anterior 2/3rd by facial nerve (lingual branch); posterior 1/3rd glossopharyngeal.

Posterior most or valeculla is supplied by vagus nerve.

411. Ans. (d) Posterior cricoarytenoid

Ref: Dhingra, 5th pg. 300

- Posterior cricoarytenoid is the most important muscle of the larynx as it is the only abductor of vocal cord.
- Paralysis of posterior cricoarytenoid will lead to adduction of vocal cord, which may lead to dyspnea resulting in death.

412. Ans. (a) Trachea bifurcates

Ref: BDC, 6th ed. Vol. II, pg. 280-81

- Trachea *begins* at lower border of cricoid cartilage opposite to the *lower border of C6 vertebra.*
- Trachea extends up to upper border of T5
- Tracheal bifurcation (carina) is at T4–T5 level.
- Length of trachea is 10–12 cm
- Thyroid cartilage is over 3, 4 & 5 tracheal rings

At C6 vertebral level: *Landmark is Cricoid cartilage*

- Larynx ends; Trachea begins
- Pharynx ends; Esophagus begins
- Inferior thyroid artery crosses posterior to carotid sheath.
- Middle cervical sympathetic ganglion behind inferior thyroid artery
- Inferior laryngeal nerve enters the larynx.
- Vertebral artery enters the transverse foramen of C6.

413. Ans. (d) C_3 to C_6

Ref: Gray, 41st ed. pg. 586

- In adult male at rest, larynx lies at the level of the bodies of C_3 to C_6 vertebra. Although it is somewhat higher in adult females and children.
- In infants between 6-12 months, the tip of epiglottis (the highest part of the larynx) is a little above the junction of the dens and body of axis (C_2) vertebrae.

414. Ans. (c) Lambdoid suture

Ref: Gray, 41st ed. pg. 418-419

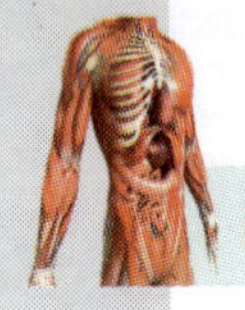

- Anterior fontanel is formed by frontal bone and parietal bone. It is diamond shaped and closes at 18 months.
- Posterior fontanel is formed by parietal bone and occipital bone. It is triangular shaped and closes immediately after birth or within 2–3 months.

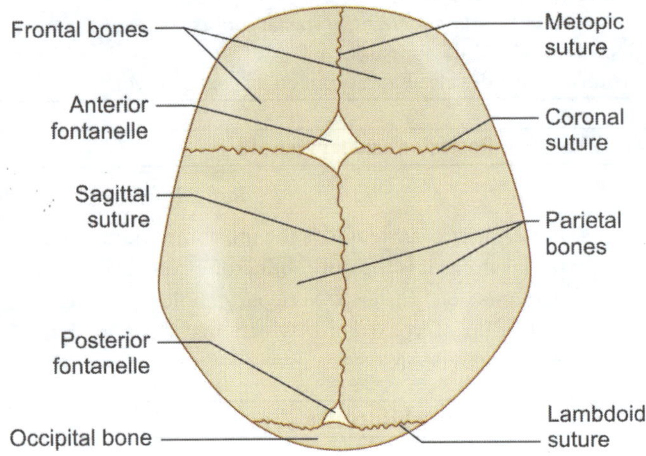

415. Ans. (d) Tympanomandibular

Ref: Gray's, 41st ed. pg. 541

TABLE: Ligaments of TM Joint

Main	Accessory
Fibrous capsule Lateral or Temporomandibular	Sphenomandibular Stylomandibular

416. Ans. (b) C3

Ref: Gray's Anatomy, 39th ed. pg. 444, 634

- The hyoid bone may be felt a few centimeters below and behind the chin, especially if the neck is extended. It may be palpated between finger and thumb and moved from side to side.
- ***The hyoid bone lies approximately at the level of the third cervical vertebra.***

417. Ans. (b) 2nd to 4th

Ref: Gray's, 41st ed. pg. 470

- Thyroid gland lies against C_5, C_6, C_7& T_1 vertebra
- Isthmus extends from 2nd to 4th tracheal ring
- Each lobe extends from middle of thyroid cartilage to $4^{th}/5^{th}$ tracheal ring.

418. Ans. (b) Inferior thyroid artery

Ref: Gray's, 41st ed. pg. 472

- Both upper & lower parathyroid glands are supplied by the inferior thyroid artery

Extra Mile

- The superior parathyroid glands usually lie at the level of inferior border of cricoids cartilage.
- The inferior glands are usually within thyroid fascia 1 cm below the inferior thyroid arteries behind the lower poles.
- **Color of thyroid gland:** Deep red color
- **Color of parathyroid gland:** Brownish yellow color

419. Ans. (b) Peripheral ganglia

Ref: Gray's, 41st ed. pg. 231, 303

Lower motor neuron (LMN): It consists of:

- Anterior horn cells or homologous cells in brainstem
- Anterior spinal nerve root
- Peripheral nerve

420. Ans. (c) Mandible

Ref: Gray's, 38th ed. pg. 431

- **Pneumatic Bone:** Some cranial bones have air filled cavities for making skull light weight, resonance of voice & air conditioning.
- Maxilla, Mastoid, Ethmoid, Sphenoid & Frontal bones are pneumatic bones.

TABLE: Types of bone

Sesamoid bones	Pneumatic bone *(Mn: It has Maximum Spherical Front Mass)*	Membranous (Dermal) bone
• Patella • Pisiform • Fabella	• Ethmoid • Maxilla • Sphenoid • Frontal • Mastoid (temporal)	• Skull vault bones • Facial bones

421. Ans. (b) Frontal bone

Ref: Gray, 38th ed. pg. 436

- Pneumatic bones are bones which contain air filled cavities for making the skull light weight, and aid resonance of voice and air conditioning. These include: Frontal, Ethmoid, Maxilla, Sphenoid and mastoid.

Extra Mile

- **Sesamoid bones** are patella, pisiform and fabella.
- **Membranous (dermal) bones** are skull vault bones and facial bones.

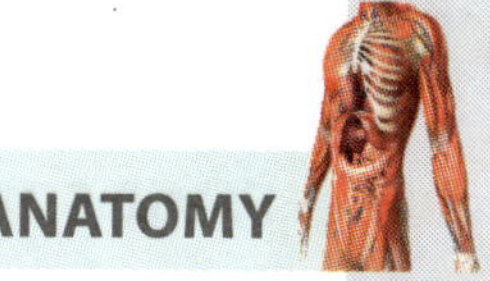

422. Ans. (d) Inferior parietal gyrus

Ref: Gray's, 41st ed. pg. 313

- The sense of taste (SVA-special visceral efferent) is transduced by gustatory hair (**neuroepithelium**), taste buds and is conveyed via **three** of the twelve cranial nerves.
  - The facial nerve carries taste sensations from the anterior two thirds of the tongue (**excluding** the circumvallate papillae) and **soft palate**.
  - The glossopharyngeal nerve carries the taste sensations from the posterior one third of the tongue (**including** the circumvallate papillae) and,
  - A branch of the vagus nerve carries some taste sensations from the back of the oral cavity (i.e. posterior-most tongue, pharynx and epiglottis).
- Impulses generated by the gustatory taste hairs on the superior surface of the tongue, travel from the tongue to medulla oblongata, to the thalamus, ***ending up in the gustatorial area of the cortex of the parietal lobe (inferior gyrus) of the cerebrum.***
- The axons from these cranial nerves ascend in the spinal cord without crossing over. These fibers terminate in the medulla, ventral posterior medial (VPM) nucleus of the thalamus, and then project to the somatosensory cortex within the brain.
- Thus, a lesion of the nucleus tractus solitarius (NTS) or **solitario-thalamic tract** results in loss of taste from the ipsi-lesional, the same side as the lesion, half of the tongue.

423. Ans. (a) Maxillary

Ref: Gray's Anatomy, 39th ed. pg. 477, 479

- The maxillae are the largest of the facial bones, other than the mandible, and jointly form the whole of the upper jaw. Each bone forms the greater part of the floor and lateral wall of the nasal cavity, and of the floor of the orbit
- *"Orbital surface of maxilla is smooth and triangular, and forms most of the floor of the orbit"*
- **The seven bones that articulate with orbit are:**
  - Frontal bone (Roof)
  - Lacrimal bone (Medial wall of orbit)
  - Ethmoid bone (Medial wall of orbit)
  - Maxillary bone (Floor of orbit)
  - Palatine bone (Floor of orbit)
  - Sphenoid bone (Lateral wall of orbit)
  - Zygomatic (Lateral wall of orbit)

Extra Mile

- ***Maxilla is also the most common fracture of orbital floor.***
- The floor (inferior wall) is formed by the orbital surface of maxilla, the orbital surface of Zygomatic bone and the orbital process of palatine bone.

Note: The nasal bone does not form part of the orbit.

424. Ans. (a) Cavernous sinus

Ref: Gray's Anatomy, 40th ed. Ch. 29

- The upper most segment of the facial vein, above its junction with the superior labial vein, is also called the angular vein.
- Any infection of the mouth or face can spread via the angular veins to the cavernous sinuses resulting in thrombosis.

425. Ans. (c) Right sided pain, touch, temperature

Ref: Gray's, 41st ed. pg. 299, 309

- First order neuron carrying pain, touch, temperature enter the spinal cord, relay in same side.
- Second order neurons cross over to other side and travel up in anterior and lateral spino-thalamic tract and enter the medulla.
- Same fibers are now known as spinal lemniscus and they relay at thalamus. ***So spinal lemniscus on the left contain pain touch temperature from right side of the body.***

426. Ans. (d) Inferior oblique

Ref: Gray's, 41st ed. pg. 671, Gray's, 39th ed. pg. 693

- All the rectus muscles are attached to the orbital apex.
- Aside from rectus muscles, superior oblique also attaches to orbital apex, while inferior oblique has no attachment with orbital apex.

427. Ans. (b) Trochlear

Ref: Gray's, 41st ed. pg. 671

- Superior oblique muscle is supplied by trochlear nerve.
- Its actions are: aBBduct, Intort & Depress ("BID") eye in primary position.

428. Ans. (b) Lateral cartilage

Ref: Gray's, 41st ed. pg. 560

Nasal septum is an osseocartilagenous structure contributed by

Part of septum	Main structure	Contributory structures
Bony septum	• Vomer • *Ethmoid (perpendicular plate)*	• Nasal spine of frontal bone • *Nasal crests of maxillary, nasal & palatine bones* • Rostrum & crest of sphenoid
Cartilaginous septum	• Septal cartilage	• Inferior nasal cartilage (Septal process)

429. Ans. (b) Thalamus

Ref: Textbook of Neuroanatomy, pg. 82, 83

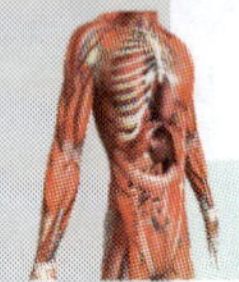

Basal ganglia include following nuclei:
- Caudate nucleus
- Putamen
- *Globus pallidus*
- Subthalamic nucleus
- Substantia nigra

Lenticulate nucleus = putamen + globus pallidus

Function of basal ganglia—Planning and programming of movements.

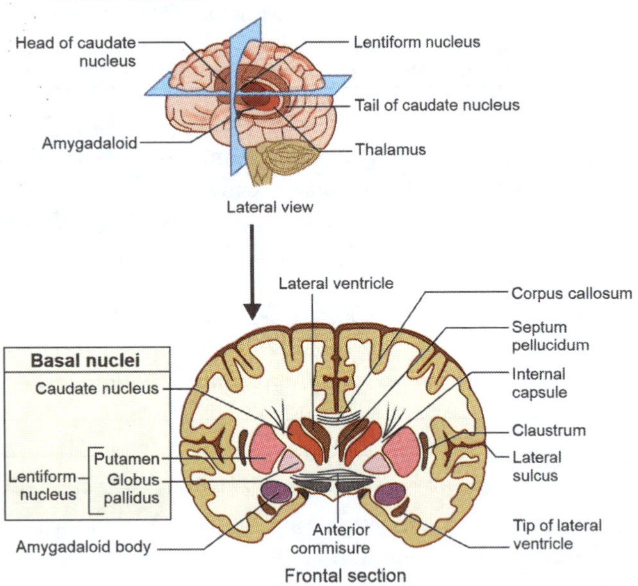

430. Ans. (b) Purkinje cells

Ref: Gray's, 41st ed. pg. 335-336

- The cerebellar cortex contains five types of neurons: Purkinje, Granule, Basket, Stellate and Golgi Cells.

431. Ans. (c) Purkinje cells

Ref: Gray's, 41st ed. pg. 335-336

- The axons of purkinje cells are the only output through cerebellar cortex.
- However, it should be kept in mind that the output from the cerebellum is through deep nuclei, and purkinje cells axons generally pass to deep nuclei.

432. Ans. (a) Lower border of L1

Ref: IB Singh, 8th ed. pg. 31

- Spinal cord begins at foramen magnum and, in adults, ends at lower border of L1.
- In newborn, spinal cord ends at L3 vertebrae.

433. Ans. (c) L3

Ref: IB Singh, 8th ed. pg. 31

434. Ans. (d) X

Ref: BDC, 5th ed. Vol. III, pg. 78

Parapharyngeal space contains
- Carotid vessel
- Jugular vein
- Last 4 cranial nerves (9,10,11,12)
- Sympathetic chain

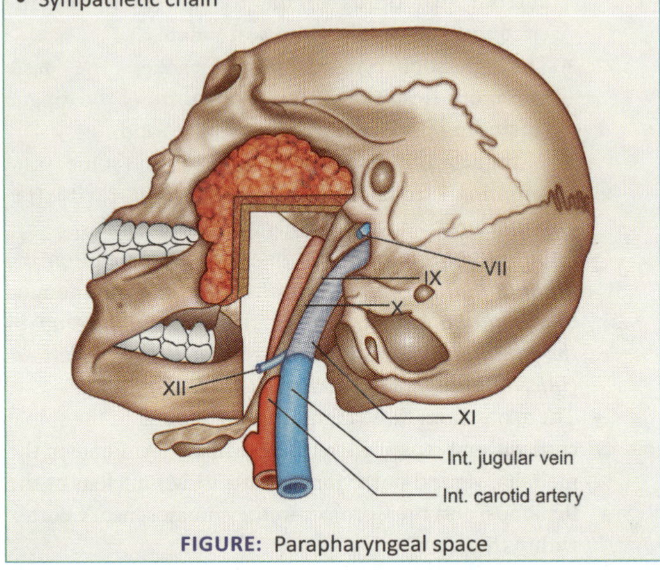

FIGURE: Parapharyngeal space

435. Ans. (b) Fasciculus gracilis

Ref: Gray's, 41st ed. pg. 296-97, 311

NERVE PATHWAYS
- **Posterior**-Fasciculus gracilis, fasciculus cuneatus
- **Lateral**-Lateral spinothalamic, anterior and posterior spinocerebellar, spino-olivary, spinotectal
- **Anterior**-Anterior spinothalamic

436. Ans. (b) C7

Ref: BDC, 5th ed. Vol. III, pg. 43

- The C7 vertebra is also known as the vertebra prominence because of its long spinous process.
- Atypical cervical vertebra are: 1, 2, and 7 (atlas, axis and vertebra prominens respectively)

437. Ans. (b) Atlantoaxial joint

Ref: Gray's, 38th ed. pg. 521

- **Atlanto-occipital (between skull and C1)** joint permits *nodding of head* (as when indicating approval or yes)
- **Atlantoaxial joint** permits the head to be **turned from side to side** i.e. rotation (as indicating disapproval, the NO movement).

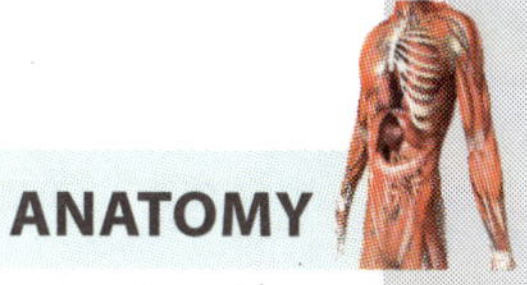

438. Ans. (b) Carotid tubercle on C6 vertebra

Ref: Gray's, 41st ed. pg. 414, Color Atlas of Human Anatomy, pg. 446

- Chassaignac's tubercle (carotid tubercle) is the other name of anterior tubercle of transverse process of C6 vertebra.
- It is the longest tubercle of Cervical (C6) Vertebra.

PELVIS AND PERINEUM

439. Ans. (a) Deep perineal pouch

Ref: Gray's Anatomy, 42nd ed, pg. 1283

- The most accurate answer here is deep perineal pouch as straddle Injury leads to rupture of bulbar urethra, below the perineal membrane.
- As a result extravasation of urine can take place at four places: Superficial perineal pouch, scrotum, penis and anterior abdominal wall. However, urine cannot extravasate in three places:
  1. Deep perineal pouch because it is prevented by intact perineal membrane.
  2. Ischiorectal fossa because it is prevented by Colle's fascia.
  3. It cannot enter thigh because it is prevented by Fascia Lata.

440. Ans. (d) Iliopsoas

Ref: BD Chaurasia 7th ed. Vol. II, pg. 184

- The marked structure in the image is lesser trochanter. The muscle attached is iliopsoas muscle.
- The iliopsoas muscles are the flexors of the hip. An abdominal X-ray often demonstrates the lateral edge of the psoas muscles as a near straight line.
- The iliacus muscles are not visible, as they lie over the iliac bones of the pelvis.

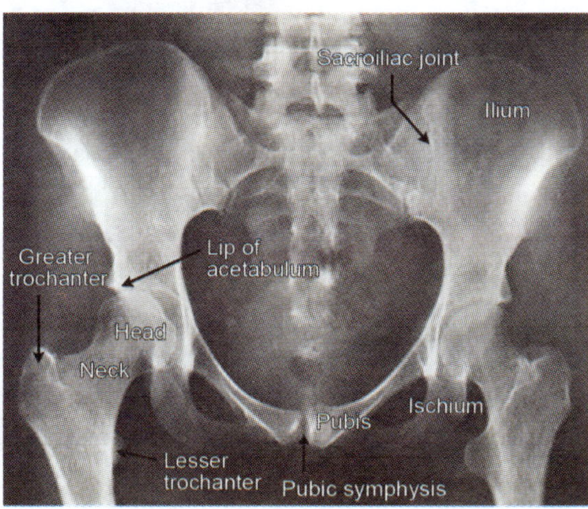

441. Ans. (c) Secondary cartilaginous joint

Ref: BD Chaurasia 7th ed, Vol. II, pg. 147

- The shown structure in the image is symphysis pubis, which is a secondary cartilaginous joint.

Secondary Cartilaginous Joint

- These are permanent joints called symphyses and are composed of fibrocartilage. They are considered amphiarthroses, meaning that they allow only slight movement and are all found at the skeletal midline.
- Example—manubriosternal joint (between the manubrium and the sternum), intervertebral discs, and the pubic symphysis.

442. Ans. (b) Distal part of mesonephric duct

Ref: BD Chaurasia 7th ed. Vol. III, pg. 276

- As the bladder grows and expands, the distal ends of the mesonephric ducts are absorbed into the wall of the bladder as the TRIGONE.

443. Ans. (a) Anterior superior iliac spine

Ref: BD Chaurasia 7th ed. Vol. II, pg. 184

- The marked structure in the image is anterior superior iliac spine (ASIS)
- The ASIS is the site of attachment for sartorius muscle and inguinal ligament and is most commonly avulsed in adolescent athletes.

Image: Some important pelvic bone structure and muscle attachment over it

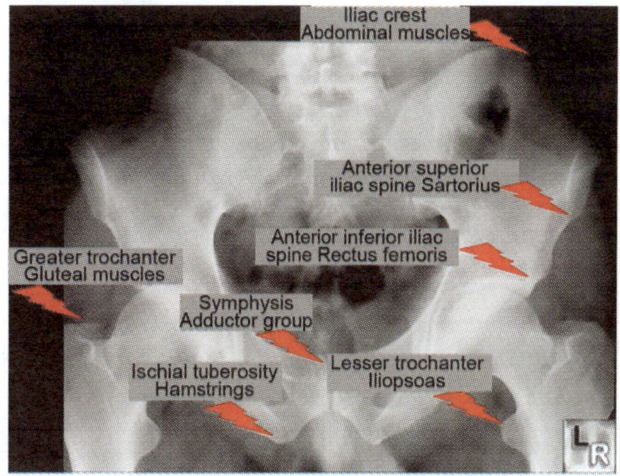

444. Ans. (b) L4

Ref: BD Chaurasia 7th ed. Vol. II, pg. 7

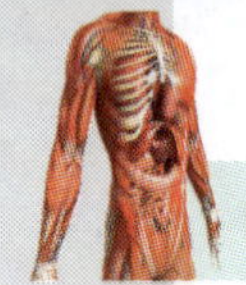

- The top of the iliac crests also marks the level of the fourth lumbar vertebral body (L4), above or below which lumbar puncture may be performed.

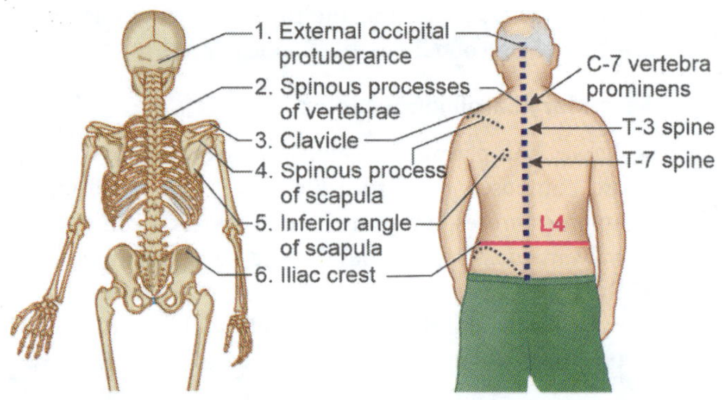

Extra Mile

TABLE: Facetal anatomy of the greater trochanter

Facet	Related structure
Superolateral	Gluteus medius tendon
Anterior	Gluteus minimus tendon
Lateral	Gluteus medius tendon
Posterior	Submaximus/trochanteric bursa

445. Ans. (b) Secondary cartilaginous

Ref: BD Chaurasia, 7th ed. Vol. II, pg. 464

- The marked structure in image is pubic symphysis
- The pubic symphysis is a secondary cartilaginous joint, which means there is a wedge-shaped fibrocartilaginous interpubic disc situated between two layers of hyaline cartilage, which line the oval-shaped medial articular surfaces of the pubic bones.
- These are permanent joints called symphyses and are composed of fibrocartilage. They are considered amphiarthroses, meaning that they allow only slight movement and are all found at the skeletal midline.

446. Ans. (d) Transversalis fascia

Ref: BD Chaurasia, 7th Vol. II, pg. 229

- The initial opening of the inguinal canal is located at the midpoint of the inguinal ligament, and is referred to as the deep (lateral) inguinal ring.
- It is an oval defect in the transversalis fascia, which is widest along the vertical axis of the opening.

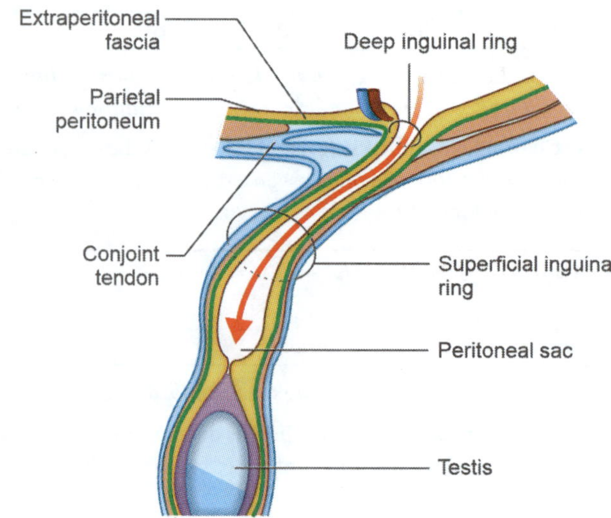

447. Ans. (b) Transversalis fascia

- **Deep inguinal ring** is an oval opening formed in transversalis fascia.
- It lies about 0.5 inch (1.3 cm) above inguinal ligament midway between anterior superior iliac supine and symphysis pubis.
- Medial to deep inguinal ring is inferior epigastric vessels.

Extra Mile

- Superficial inguinal ring: A triangular shaped opening in the aponeurosis of external oblique muscle and lies immediately above and medial to pubic tubercle.

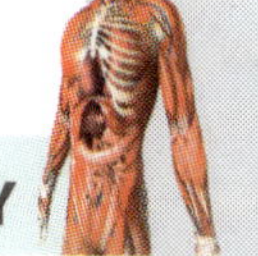

448. Ans. (a) External oblique aponeurosis

- Inguinal ligament is a fibrous, thickened, folded margin of the external oblique aponeurosis.
- It extends from anterior superior iliac spine to pubic tubercle.

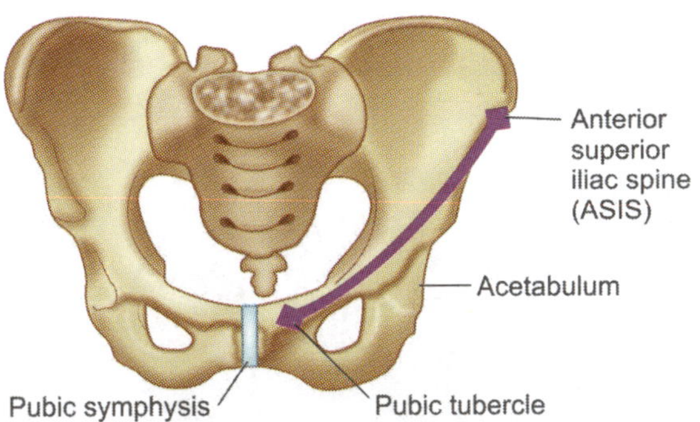

449. Ans. (a) Superior rectal vein

Ref: Gray's Anatomy, 41st ed. pg. 1153, 1158

- Source of bleeding in haemorrhoids are usually the internal haemorrhoids which are symptomatic anal cushions and lie in 3, 7 and 11 o'clock position *(left-lateral, right-posterior and right-anterior quadrants of the wall of the canal).*
- **Book states:** *"The cushions help to seal the anal canal and contribute to the maintenance of continence to flatus and fluid. The anal cushions are important in the pathogenesis of haemorrhoids."*
  - Haemorrhoids develop due to degeneration of the supporting connective tissue of anal cushion.
  - This degeneration causes downward displacement of cushions and abnormal venous dilatation.
- The superior haemorrhoidal veins draining the upper half of the anal canal above the dentate line, pass upwards to become the rectal veins: These unite to form the **superior rectal vein**, which later becomes the **inferior mesenteric vein**.
- In the middle anal canal, there are 6–10 vertical mucosal folds and the anal columns. These columns mainly contain the superior rectal vein, artery and some middle and inferior rectal vessels.

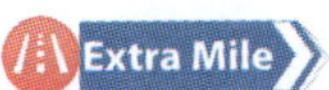

- Dilated veins in the subepithelial tissue below the dentate line contribute to an external haemorrhoidal venous plexus

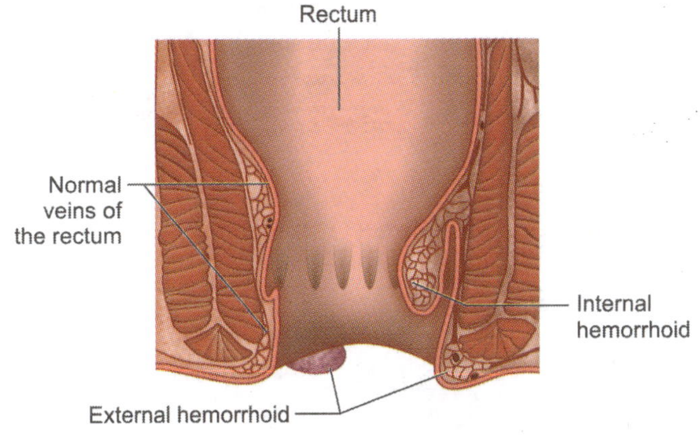

450. Ans. (c) Bulbourethral artery

Ref: Gray's Anatomy, for Students E-book, pg. 516

- Blood supply to the skin of the penis is from the left and right superficial external pudendal arteries, which arise from the femoral artery.
  - The superficial external pudendal arteries branch into dorsolateral and ventrolateral branches, which collateralize across the midline.
  - In addition, branches in the skin form an extensive subdermal vascular plexus.
- The blood supply to the ventral penile skin is based on the posterior scrotal artery, a superficial branch of the deep internal pudendal artery.
- The blood supply to deep structures of the penis is derived from a continuation of the internal pudendal artery, after it gives off the perineal branch. Three branches of the internal pudendal artery flow to the penis, as follows:
- **Bulbourethral artery:** Artery of the bulb passes through the deep penile (Buck) fascia to enter and supply the bulb of the penis and penile (spongy) urethra.
- The dorsal artery travels along the dorsum of the penis between the dorsal nerve and deep dorsal vein and gives off circumflex branches that accompany the circumflex veins; the terminal branches are in the glans penis.
- **Cavernosal artery:** Deep penile artery is usually a single artery that arises on each side and enters the corpus cavernosum at the crus and runs the length of the penile shaft, giving off the helicine arteries, which are an integral component of the erectile process.

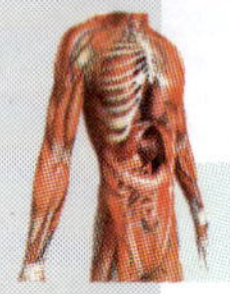

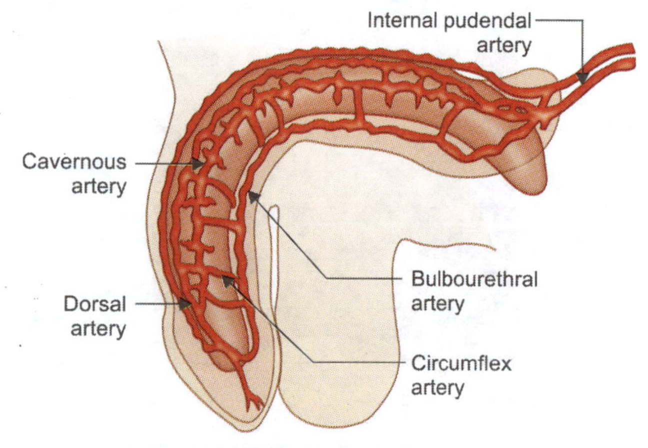

451. Ans. (c) Genital branch of genitofemoral nerve

Ref: Gray's Anatomy, Review E-book, pg. 221

- The **cremaster muscle** is a muscle that covers the testis and the spermatic cord.
- The cremaster muscle is supplied by the cremasteric artery which is a branch of inferior epigastric artery.
- The cremaster muscle is innervated from the genital branch of the genitofemoral nerve. It receives distinctly different innervation and vascular supply in comparison to the internal oblique.

452. Ans. (c) Spiral artery

Ref: Gray's Anatomy, E-book, pg. 172

- Spiral artery, a branch of radial artery, chiefly supplies endometrium.
- Endometrium and myometrium are supplied mainly by ovarian and uterine artery.

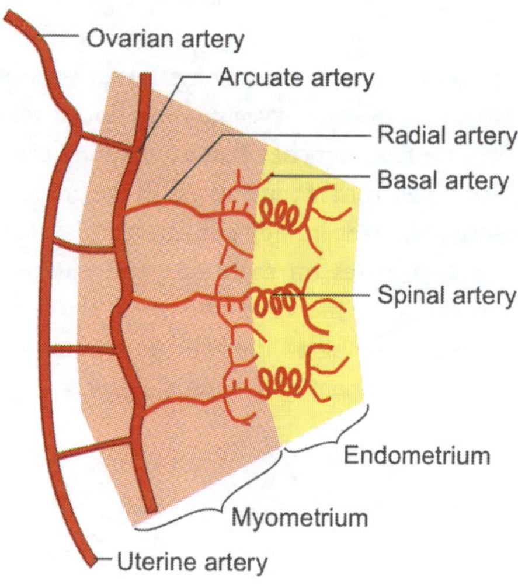

453. Ans. (a) Pudendal nerve

Ref: Netter's Clinical Anatomy, 3rd ed. pg. 252

Alcock's canal/pudendal canal is a fascial tunnel in the lateral wall *of ischiorectal fossa* and *contains* the *pudendal nerve and internal pudendal vessels.*

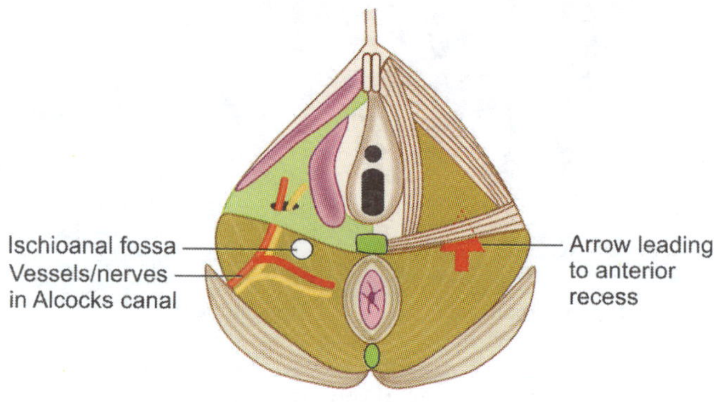

454. Ans. (b) S2

Anatomic level of some important structures:

- **Posterior Superior Iliac Spine (PSIS):** S2
- **Anterior Superior Iliac Spine (ASIS):** S1
- **Pylorus and Celiac trunk:** L1
- **Inferior mesenteric artery:** L3
- **Umbilicus:** Between L3 and L4

Extra Mile

TABLE: Vertebral body level as landmark for the viscera *(Table extracted from Gray's Anatomy 41st ed.)*

Vertebral body level	Viscera
C6	Cricoid cartilage, start of oesophagus
C7-T1	Lung apex
Upper T4	Aorta reaches vertebral column; medial part of scapular spine
T4-5 disk	Sternal plane/angle of Louis
Upper T5	• Tracheal bifurcation • Concavity of aortic arch • Azygos vein—superior venacava junction • Bifurcation of pulmonary trunk • Upper border of heart
Upper T8	• Inferior angle of scapula • Lower border of heart • Inferior vena cava crosses diaphragm • Central tendon of diaphragm

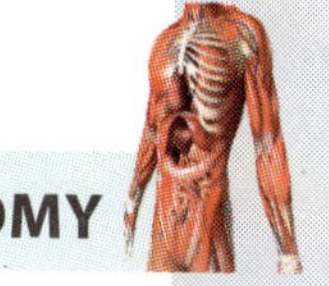

Extra Mile

Vertebral body level	Viscera
Upper T11	• Lower border of lung • Cardia of stomach • Upper border of kidney
Mid L1	• Lowest level of pleura • Pylorus; transpyloric plane • Hilum of left kidney • Origin of renal arteries and superior mesenteric artery • Pancreas **(neck)** • Spinal cord termination
Mid L2	Pancreas **(head)**; duodenojejunal flexure
Mid L3	Lower border of kidney
Mid L4	Bifurcation of aorta
Mid L5	Formation of inferior vena cava

455. Ans. (d) 4

Ref: Gray's Anatomy, 41st ed. pg. 729

- The coccyx is a small, **asymmetrical**, triangular bone of the spine, the distal most.
- It usually **consists of four fused rudimentary vertebrae**, although the **number varies from three to five**, and the first is sometimes separate.
- The bone is directed downwards and ventrally from the sacral apex.

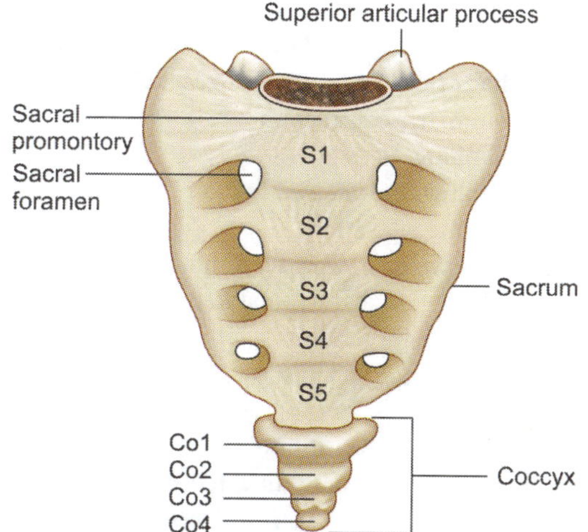

FIGURE: Coccyx, anterior view

456. Ans. (d) Bulbocavernosus

Ref: BDC Vol. II, pg. 429-32; Keith Moore, 7th ed. 493-32

STRUCTURES FORMING PERINEAL BODY

- Levator Ani (Pubo and Iliococcygeus)
- Bulbo- Spongiosus
- Superficial and Deep Transverse perinei
- Sphincters i.e. External anal sphincter and sphincter urethrae

Clinical Significance

In episiotomy all muscles of perineal body; EXCEPT two sphincter (i.e. sphincter urethrae and external anal sphincter) are cut

UROGENITAL DIAPHRAGM

- Sphincter urethrae
- Deep Transverse Perinei
- Perineal membrane (Inferior fascia of urogenital diaphragm)
- Superior fascia of urogenital diaphragm

PELVIC DIAPHRAGM: TRUE PELVIC FLOOR

- Levator anii
  - Muscles (Iliococcygeus and Pubococcygeus)
- **Ischiococcygeus**

457. Ans. (d) Ischiococcygeus

Refer to above explanation

458. Ans. (d) Puborectalis

Refer to above explanation

459. Ans. (c) Glandular tissue and fibromuscular stroma

Ref: Gray's Anatomy, 39th ed. pg. 1302

- The anterior part of the prostate is composed mainly of fibromuscular stroma, which is continuous with detrusor fibers.
- Toward the apex of the gland, this fibromuscular tissue blends with striated muscle from the levator.
- Pubosprostatic ligaments also blend with this area.

460. Ans. (c) 60 g

Ref: William's OB, 23rd ed. Ch 1

- ***William's states*** *"In nonparous women, the uterus averages **50 to 70 g**, whereas in parous women it averages **80 g** or more"*
- Since this question is asking just the normal weight of uterus, 60 gm is most appropriate given the option.

UTERUS

- **Shape**- pyriform
- **Size**- 7.5 cm long × 5 cm broad × 2.5 cm thick
- **Weight**- 60 g
- **Position**- 90 degree with the long axis of vagina
- ***Angulation****- anteverted, anteflexed*

PHYSIOLOGY

2

MOST RECENT QUESTIONS 2023

1. **Two medical students are planning a trip to Leh. They want to study the effects of acclimatization in high altitude. Which of the following changes will not be seen in high altitude during the process of acclimatization?** ***(Most Recent Question July 2023)***
   a. Increase in RBC count b. Increase in capillary density
   c. Increase in myoglobin d. Hypoventilation
2. **The transporter GLUT2 transports glucose at which of the following sites?** ***(Most Recent Question July 2023)***
   a. Large intestine b. Kidney
   c. Liver d. Brain
3. **Which of the following glucose transporter is present on the basolateral membrane of the intestinal epithelial cell?** ***(Most Recent Question July 2023)***
   a. GLUT1 b. GLUT2
   c. GLUT3 d. GLUT4
4. **In the given graph of intravesical muscle contraction, Phase Ib represents which one of the following properties?** ***(Most Recent Question July 2023)***

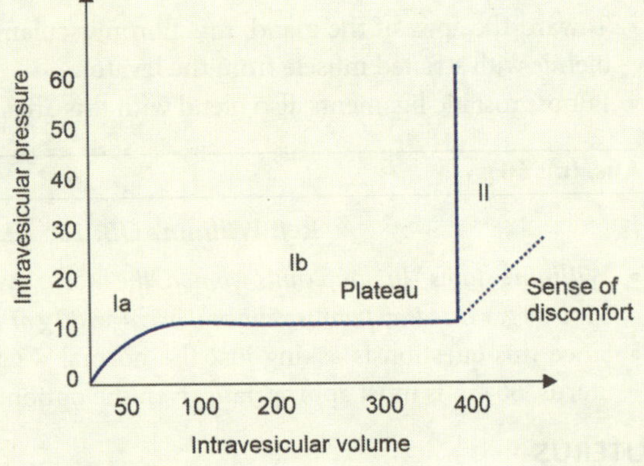

   a. Elasticity
   b. Plasticity
   c. Contractility
   d. Relaxation
5. **Serosa is not present in which of the following?** ***(Most Recent Question July 2023)***
   a. Stomach b. Esophagus
   c. Small intestine d. Large intestine
6. **Upon IV injection of an irritant substance, bradycardia, hypotension and apnea developed in the subject. This represents which of the following reflex?** ***(Most Recent Question July 2023)***
   a. Bezold-Jarisch reflex b. Brainbridge reflex
   c. Cushing's reflex d. Physiological reflex
7. **A 5-year-old boy is brought by his mother as he is having significant difficulty walking. At the age of 11 months, he began to walk. Four months ago, his mother realized he was having trouble rising from the floor. His calves are bilaterally hypertrophied upon inspection. He carefully gets up from the floor, supporting himself with his hands on his thighs. Which of the following defect is the cause of the patient's condition?** ***(Most Recent Question Jan 2023)***
   a. Titin b. Dystrophin
   c. Desmin d. Actinin
8. **The first heart sound (S1) coincides with which phase of the cardiac cycle?** ***(Most Recent Question Jan 2023)***
   a. Isovolumetric contraction
   b. Rapid filling
   c. Early filling
   d. Isovolumic relaxation
9. **Large "v" wave on JVP is seen in which of the following conditions?** ***(Most Recent Question Jan 2023)***
   a. Tricuspid regurgitation
   b. DCM
   c. PDA
   d. Constrictive pericarditis
10. **Which of the following is an extrinsic clotting factor?** ***(Most Recent Question Jan 2023)***
    a. VI
    b. VII
    c. VIII
    d. IX

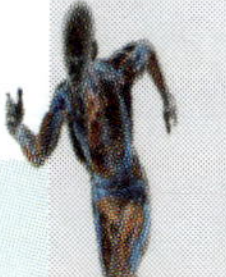

11. Which of the following is true regarding creatinine clearance? *(Most Recent Question Jan 2023)*
a. Creatinine clearance is lesser than inulin clearance
b. Creatinine clearance is greater than inulin clearance
c. Creatinine clearance is equal to inulin clearance
d. None of the above

12. What is the cause of death in diabetic ketoacidosis? *(Most Recent Question Jan 2023)*
a. Sepsis b. Dehydration
c. Hypokalemia d. Cerebral edema

CELL AND NERVE-MUSCLE PHYSIOLOGY

13. Insulin stimulates glucose uptake by cells via GLUT 4. This is an example of: *(Most Recent Question June 2022)*
a. Primary active transport b. Secondary active transport
c. Simple diffusion d. Facilitated diffusion

14. ABG of patient shows pH = 7.23, pCO_2 = 60 mm Hg, pO_2 = 82 mm Hg and HCO_3 = 26 mEq. Diagnosis is: *(Most Recent Question June 2022)*
a. Respiratory acidosis b. Respiratory alkalosis
c. Metabolic acidosis d. Metabolic alkalosis

15. The gut flora is symbiotic with human body. These bacteria produce ammonia that can cross the cell membrane. The transport is an example of: *(Most Recent Question June 2022)*
a. Osmosis
b. Facilitated diffusion
c. Carrier mediated transport
d. Non-ionic diffusion

16. Which of the following is not an attachment protein? *(Most Recent Question June 2022)*
a. Titin b. Desmin
c. Nebulin d. Tropomyosin

17. Which of the following is correct about ROMK channel? *(Most Recent Question June 2022)*
a. Uniport b. Symport
c. Antiport d. All of these

18. Gower sign has been demonstrated in a child in your OPD. Work up shows decreased/altered dystrophin protein. Diagnosis is: *(Most Recent Question Dec 2021)*
a. Duchenne muscular dystrophy
b. Becker's muscular dystrophy
c. Congenital myopathy
d. All of the above

19. When ORS is given to the patient, Glucose is absorbed by: *(Most Recent Question Dec 2021)*
a. Simple diffusion b. Osmosis
c. Facilitative diffusion d. Secondary active transport

20. Identify the antibody based on the structure given below. *(Most Recent Question June 2021)*

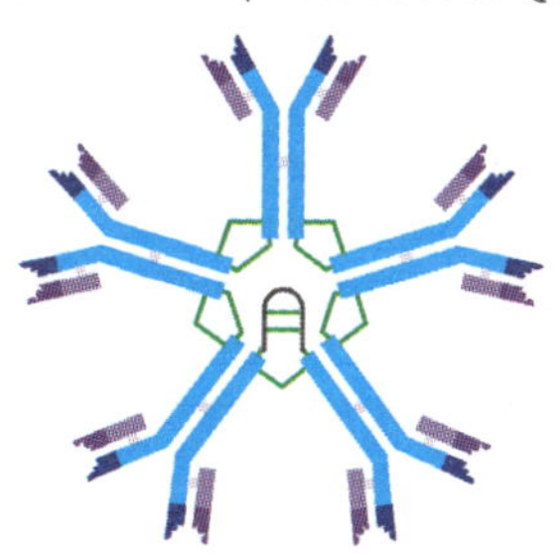

a. IgA b. IgG
c. IgM d. IgE

21. A child was defecating in open air in village when was attacked by pack of dogs. One of the attacking dogs was found dead the next day. Considering the high risk of rabies in the child he has admitted to District hospital and was given antirabies serum (ARS) and Rabipur vaccine. Which of the following is responsible for transport of rabies virus to brain? *(Most Recent Question Aug 2020)*
a. Dynein b. Kinesin
c. Actin d. Vimentin

22. In which of the following imbalances increased nerve excitability is seen? *(Most Recent Question Aug 2020)*
a. Hyponatremia b. Hypokalemia
c. Hypocalcemia d. Hypochloremia

23. A patient with HbA1c of 11.4% has come to your clinic with severe pain in feet at night. Which nerve fibers are involved in this patient? *(Most Recent Question Aug 2020)*
a. Aα b. Aβ
c. Aγ d. C

24. Serotonin is found in highest concentration in: *(Most Recent Question Dec 2019)*
a. Limbic system b. Chromaffin cells
c. Sympathetic ganglia d. Platelets

25. Which of the following is not seen in Intracellular Fluid? *(Recent Pattern Question 2018-19)*
a. Calcium b. Magnesium
c. Potassium d. Protein

26. Which of the following is not a calcium binding protein? *(Recent Pattern Question 2018-19)*
a. Calbindin b. Calmodulin
c. Troponin d. Clathrin

27. Inverse stretch reflex is mediated *via*: *(Recent Pattern Question 2018-19)*
a. Golgi tendon b. Muscle spindle
c. Unmyelinated C fibers d. Dorsal Column

28. Organelle having DNA is____. *(Recent Pattern Question 2018-19)*
a. Mitochondria b. Golgi complex
c. SER d. RER

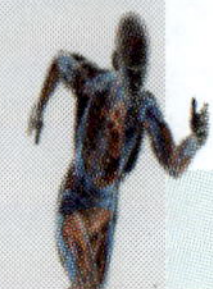

29. Delivery of stimulus above threshold intensity leads to a constant amplitude of AP and is known as:

a. All or none law *(Recent Pattern Question 2018-19)*
b. Electrotonic potential
c. Absolute refractory period
d. Relative refractory period

30. Which is correct about malignant Hyperthermia in adults? *(Recent Pattern Question 2018)*

a. Increase calcium transport *via* L type calcium channels in T-tubule
b. Increase calcium Transport *via* T type calcium channels in T-tubule
c. Decrease calcium transport *via* L type calcium channels in T-tubule
d. Decrease calcium transport *via* T type calcium channels in T-tubule

31. Which of the following ion plays a role in exocytosis? *(Recent Pattern Question 2018)*

a. Sodium b. Potassium
c. Calcium d. Magnesium

32. Dense bodies are found in smooth muscle at which of the following sites? *(Recent Pattern Question 2018)*

a. A band b. Z line
c. M line d. H band

33. Which of the following is not a molecular motor? *(Recent Pattern Question 2018)*

a. Dynein b. Kinesin
c. Myosin d. Actin

34. Which is correct about function of antiporter?

a. Both molecules go in *(Recent Pattern Question 2018)*
b. One molecule goes in and other molecule goes out
c. Both molecules go out
d. One molecule goes in and two exit out

35. Which of these is true about SGLT1? *(Recent Pattern Question 2018)*

a. Secondary active transport of glucose in brain
b. Secondary active transport of glucose in intestine
c. Secondary active transport of in prostate
d. Secondary active transport of glucose in rods and cones

36. Which of the following has maximum smooth muscle as compared to wall thickness? *(Recent Pattern Question 2018)*

a. Respiratory bronchiole b. Alveoli
c. Terminal bronchiole d. Alveolar ducts

37. During a 100 m sprint which of the following is used by the muscle for meeting energy demands? *(Recent Pattern Question 2018)*

a. Phosphofructokinase
b. Phosphocreatine
c. Glucose 1-phosphate
d. Creatine phosphokinase

38. Golgi tendon is innervated by which nerve fiber? *(Recent Pattern Question 2017)*

a. Ia b. Ib
c. II d. III

39. Pain and temperature is carried by: *(Recent Pattern Question 2017)*

a. Anterior spinothalamic tract
b. Lateral spinothalamic tract
c. Dorsal column pathway
d. Ventral column pathway

40. SGLT1 is located on: *(Recent Pattern Question 2017)*

a. Brain b. Liver
c. Intestine d. RBC

41. Steroid synthesis occurs in which organelle?

a. Lysosome *(Recent Pattern Question 2017)*
b. Smooth endoplasmic reticulum
c. Rough endoplasmic reticulum
d. Lysozyme

42. Fiber mainly affected by local anesthesia: *(Recent Pattern Question 2017)*

a. A beta b. A delta
c. B fibers d. C fibers

43. Which is true about rheobase? *(Recent Pattern Question 2017)*

a. Minimum time required to produce action potential
b. Maximum time required to produce action potential
c. Minimum strength of stimulus to produce action potential
d. Maximum strength of stimulus to produce action potential

44. Which of these sends K^+ inside cells: *(Recent Pattern Question 2016)*

a. Insulin b. Glucagon
c. TSH d. FSH

45. Placenta to fetus glucose is transported by: *(Recent Pattern Question 2016)*

a. Endocytosis
b. Active transport
c. Facilitated diffusion
d. Simple diffusion

46. During excitatory synaptic transmission all are true; EXCEPT: *(Recent Pattern Question 2016)*

a. Release Ach
b. Calcium influx increase
c. Decrease K efflux
d. Increase chloride influx

47. Maximum excitation of cell occurs in which phase? *(Recent Pattern Question 2016)*

a. Depolarization
b. Hyperpolarization
c. After hyperpolarization
d. Repolarization

48. Which is true about paracrine communication?

a. Action across synaptic cleft
b. Directly from cell to cell
c. By diffusion in interstitial fluid
d. By circulating body fluids

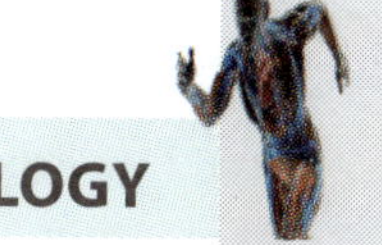

49. The electrogenic Na/K ATPase plays a critical role in cellular physiology by?
   a. Using energy in ATP to extrude 3 Na^+ out of cells in exchange for taking two K^+ into the cell
   b. Using energy in ATP to extrude $3K^+$ out of cells in exchange for taking Na^+ into the cell
   c. Using the energy in moving Na^+ into the cell or K^+ outside the cell to make ATP
   d. Using energy in moving Na^+ outside of cell or K^+ inside the cell to make ATP

50. All of the following are calcium binding proteins in muscles; EXCEPT?
   a. Troponin I
   b. Calmodulin
   c. Dystrophin
   d. Calcineurin

51. Which of the following is a *correct* statement?
   a. Desmosomes help to attach the cells to basal lamina
   b. Hemi-desmosomes help to attach cells to each other
   c. Tight junctions permit passage of some solutes between cells
   d. Gap junctions prevent the movement of proteins in the plane of cell membrane

52. All are true about body fluids and electrolytes; EXCEPT?
   a. Intracellular fluid constitutes 40% of body weight
   b. Interstitial fluid constitutes 15% of body weight
   c. Insensible losses are 400–800 ml per day
   d. Chloride inside cells is more than outside cells

53. Motor neuron of spinal cord is?
   a. Unipolar cell
   b. Bipolar cell
   c. Pseudo-unipolar cells
   d. Multipolar cells

54. A person after Saturday night partying falls asleep with one arm under the head. When he awakens the arm is weak and it tingles and hurts. True reason for this is?
   a. A fibers are more susceptible to hypoxia than B fibers
   b. A fibers are more sensitive to pressure than C fibers
   c. C fibers are more sensitive to pressure than A fibers
   d. Motor fibers are more affected by sleep than sensory fibers

55. All are true about cardiac muscle; EXCEPT:
   a. Phase 1 of depolarization is due to opening of voltage gated sodium channels
   b. Phase 2 of depolarization is due to slow opening of voltage gated calcium channels
   c. Phase 3 of repolarization is due to K^+ efflux
   d. Tetany of cardiac muscle is never seen

56. Which of the following is responsible for skeletal muscle relaxation?
   a. Dystrophin b. Tropomyosin
   c. Myosin d. Actin

57. Which of the following is a unique feature of smooth muscle?
   a. Tetany
   b. Plasticity
   c. Excitation contraction coupling
   d. Not recalled

58. All are second messengers; EXCEPT:
   a. cAMP b. DAG
   c. IP3 d. Guanylyl cyclase

59. Transport of Na^+ with sugar from enterocytes is example of?
   a. Diffusion b. Active transport
   c. Facilitated diffusion d. Secondary active transport

60. Permeability of which of the following ion leads to resting membrane potential?
   a. Chloride b. Potassium
   c. Sodium d. Calcium

61. Decrease extracellular calcium leads to?
   a. Decrease excitability of nerves
   b. Decrease membrane stability of nerves
   c. Increase amount of depolarization needed
   d. Increase amount of repolarization

62. Which of the following is a neurotransmitter at preganglionic area?
   a. ATP b. Epinephrine
   c. Norepinephrine d. Acetylcholine

63. Resting membrane potential of RODS?
   a. –70 mV b. –50 mV
   c. –40 mV d. –30 mV

64. RMP of RBC?
   a. –90 mV b. –70 mV
   c. –60 mV d. –12 mV

65. Nerve fibers first affected in case of hypoxia?
   a. A fibers b. B fibers
   c. C fibers d. D fibers

66. Fastest conducting nerve fiber is?
   a. Alpha b. Beta
   c. Gamma d. Epsilon

67. Which of the following fiber is preganglionic:
   a. Myelinated A alpha and A delta
   b. Unmyelinated A beta and A gamma
   c. Myelinated B fibers
   d. Unmyelinated C fiber

68. True about neuropraxia:
   a. Neuronal degeneration
   b. Disruption of conduction
   c. Disrupted axon and sheath
   d. Structural change of nerve

69. Exchange between lung capillaries and alveoli is?
   a. Facilitated diffusion b. Passive diffusion
   c. Filtration d. Active transport

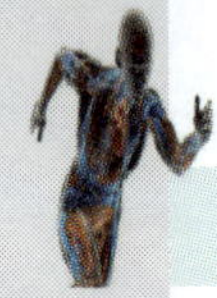

70. Which of the nerve fiber carry pain:
a. A-Alpha
b. A-Beta
c. A-Gamma
d. C-fibers

71. Tickling and itching is carried by which pathway?
a. Lateral spinothalamic tract
b. Anterior spinothalamic tract
c. Posterior spinothalamic tract
d. Dorsal column

72. All of the following muscle bands are covered by actin filament; EXCEPT:
a. A band
b. H band
c. I band
d. Z band

RENAL PHYSIOLOGY

73. The following graph represents handling of ____ by Glomerulus. *(Most Recent Question June 2021)*

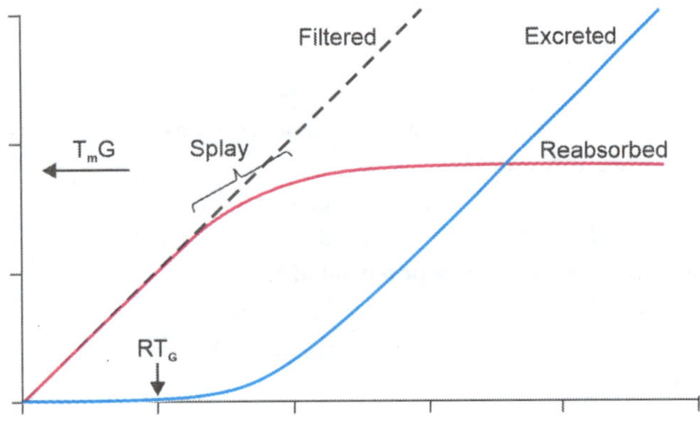

a. Urea
b. Glucose
c. Chloride
d. Inulin

74. Maximum water absorption occurs from which part of nephron? *(Most Recent Question Dec 2020)*

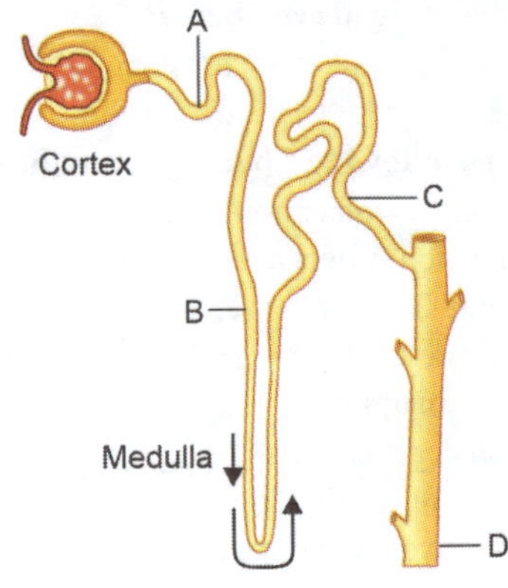

a. A
b. B
c. C
d. D

75. Sodium potassium and Chloride cotransporter for ultrafiltrate in tubules is located in: *(Most Recent Question Dec 2020)*
a. PCT
b. DCT
c. Thick ascending limb of loop of henle
d. Collecting duct

76. Sodium chloride cotransporter is present in which part of nephron? *(Most Recent Question Aug 2020)*
a. PCT
b. DCT
c. Loop of henle
d. Collecting duct

77. A 60-year-old known case of Diabetes mellitus has been noticed on laboratory work up to have microalbuminuria. What is the site of reabsorption of proteins in the ultrafiltrate? *(Most Recent Question Aug 2020)*
a. Podocytes
b. Proximal convoluted tubule
c. Distal convoluted tubule
d. Collecting duct

78. Normal anion gap value is___ mmol/L. *(Recent Pattern Question 2019)*
a. 4–6
b. 6–12
c. 12–24
d. 24–50

79. Glucose is absorbed from: *(Recent Pattern Question 2018-19)*
a. Upper part of PCT
b. Ascending limb of LOH
c. Cortical Collecting duct
d. Medullary collecting duct

80. Correct about solute excretion in water diuresis: *(Recent Pattern Question 2018-19)*
a. First increases then decreases
b. First decreases and then increases
c. Increased all through
d. Remains unchanged

81. Pressure diuresis lowers arterial pressure because it? *(Recent Pattern Question 2017)*
a. Lowers blood volume
b. Lowers renal release of renin
c. Lowers systemic vascular resistance
d. Causes renal vasodilation

82. Thiazide diuretics act on: *(Recent Pattern Question 2017)*
a. PCT mainly
b. DCT mainly
c. Loop of henle
d. All part of tubule

83. Maximum vitamin C concentration is seen in: *(Recent Pattern Question 2017)*
a. Adrenal
b. Liver
c. Kidney
d. Lung

84. Which cells in the kidney are involved in acid secretion?
a. Lacis cells
b. Principal cells
c. Intercalated cells
d. Granular cells

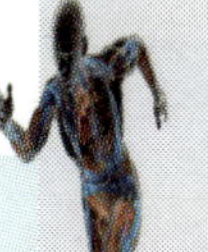

85. Macula densa is responsible for?
a. Tubulo-glomerular feedback
b. Glomerulo-tubular feedback
c. Reno-renal reflex
d. Maintaining filtration fraction

86. All of the following increase vasopressin secretion; EXCEPT:
a. Vomiting b. ECF volume shrinkage
c. Alcohol d. Tumor

87. Which of the following is the principal buffer in plasma?
a. Haemoglobin
b. Carbonic acid
c. Compounds containing histidine
d. H_2PO_4

88. Which cells in the kidney produce 1,25 dihydroxy-cholecalciferol?
a. Granular cells
b. Proximal convoluted tubular cells
c. Mesangial cells
d. Peritubular cells

89. Percentage of GFR to renal plasma flow:
a. 20% b. 38%
c. 50% d. 60%

90. Which of the following combination is true about hormone and its site of action in renal tubules?
a. Aldosterone in collecting ducts
b. Angiotensin in distal tubule
c. ANP in loop of Henle
d. ADH in proximal tubule

91. Aldosterone acts at:
a. Collecting duct
b. Glomerulus
c. Proximal convoluted tubule
d. Loop of Henle

92. CO_2 is mainly transported in blood in which form:
a. Dissolved form
b. HCO_3
c. Carbamino compound
d. Gas form

93. The tubuloglomerular feedback is mediated by:
a. Sensing of water concentration in the macula densa
b. Sensing of Na^+ concentration in macula densa
c. Sensing of sugar concentration in macula densa
d. Sensing of NaCl concentration in macula densa

94. In proximal convoluted tubule H^+ is exchanged for:
a. HCO_3^- b. K^+
c. Cl^- d. Na^+

95. Osmotic diuretics act on?
a. PCT mainly
b. DCT mainly
c. Ascending limb of loop of henle
d. Collecting duct

96. HCO_3 is absorbed through:
a. PCT b. DCT
c. Loop of Henle d. Collecting duct

97. RAAS mechanism is mainly regulated by:
a. Beta stimulation b. Alpha blocker
c. Aldosterone antagonism d. $Na^+ K^+$ ATPase

98. Osmotic difference in renal calyx is maintained by:
a. Water b. Sodium
c. HCO_3 d. Ammonia

99. 25(OH) cholecalciferol is converted to 1,25-dihydroxy-cholecalciferol in:
a. Skin b. Lung
c. Liver d. Kidney

100. Water is maximally reabsorbed in:
a. Collecting duct
b. Loop of Henle
c. Distal convoluted tubule
d. Proximal convoluted tubule

GASTROINTESTINAL PHYSIOLOGY

101. Pancreatic cell tumor leading to secretory diarrhea is:
(Most Recent Question June 2022)
a. VIPoma
b. Glucagonoma
c. Insulinoma
d. Zollinger Ellison syndrome

102. Identify the event taking place in the intestine.
(Most Recent Question Dec 2020)

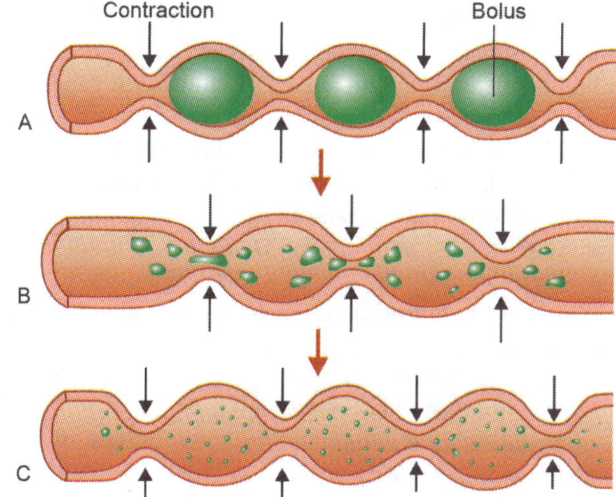

a. Peristalsis b. Segmentation
c. Passive diffusion d. Basal electrical rhythm

103. Why is sugar added to ORS?
(Recent Pattern Question 2019)
a. Enhance acceptability b. Enhance salt absorption
c. Enhance shelf life d. Enhance taste

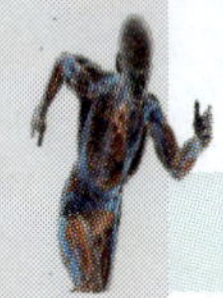

104. Esters of fat-soluble vitamins are digested by: *(Recent Pattern Question 2018-19)*
a. Pancreatic lipase b. Cholesterol esterase
c. Colipase d. Carboxypeptidase

105. Enterokinase is an activator of: *(Recent Pattern Question 2018-19)*
a. Trypsinogen b. Trypsin
c. Chymotrypsin d. Antitrypsin

106. Histamine is secreted by: *(Recent Pattern Question 2018-19)*
a. Enterochromaffin cell b. Parietal cell
c. Oxyntic cell d. Chief cell

107. Colipase is an enzyme found in ________. *(Recent Pattern Question 2018)*
a. Saliva b. Bile
c. Pancreatic juice d. Succus entericus

108. Parietal cell secretes *(Recent Pattern Question 2016)*
a. Pepsin b. Mucin
c. Acid d. Gastrin

109. Function of secretin is: *(Recent Pattern Question 2016)*
a. Relax pyloric sphincter
b. Increase gastric acid secretion
c. Increase gastric motility
d. Bicarbonate secretion from pancreas

110. D xylose absorption test is used to assess which of the following conditions: *(Recent Pattern Question 2016)*
a. Colon cancer b. PUD
c. Celiac disease d. Ulcerative colitis

111. A 41-year-old patient presented with chronic diarrhea from last 3 months. AD xylose absorption test will reveal which of the following: *(Recent Pattern Question 2016)*
a. Carbohydrate malabsorption due to mucosal disorder
b. Carbohydrate malabsorption due to chronic pancreatitis
c. Fat malabsorption due to mucosal disorder
d. Fat malabsorption due to chronic pancreatitis

112. Hydrochloric acid is produced by?
a. G-cell b. D-cell
c. Oxyntic cells d. Chief cells

113. Which of the following statements is true about gastric emptying?
a. Increased by Secretin
b. Decreased by Cholecystokinin
c. Decreased by Gastrin
d. Increased by GIP

114. Gastric emptying is maximum affected by:
a. Lipids b. Amino acid
c. Carbohydrates d. Fiber

115. All are correct about stomach; EXCEPT:
a. Parietal cells secrete intrinsic factor
b. Pylorus has more acid secreting cells
c. Lots of goblet cells are present in mucous lining
d. Chief cells secrete pepsinogen

116. Starch is hydrolyzed in the mouth by:
a. Mucin b. Ptyalin
c. Pancreatic amylase d. Lipase

117. Fecal mass is mainly derived from:
a. Undigested food b. Digested food
c. Intestinal secretion d. Intestinal absorption

118. Most sensitive taste sensation is:
a. Salt b. Bitter
c. Sweet d. Acid

119. D cells of Islet of Langerhans of pancreas secrete?
a. Insulin b. Glucagon
c. Gastrin d. Somatostatin

120. The rate of absorption of sugars by the small intestine is highest for?
a. Pentose b. Disaccharides
c. Hexoses d. Polysaccharides

121. Chymotrypsinogen is activated into chymotrypsin by?
a. Trypsin b. Pepsin
c. Enterokinase d. Bile salts

122. Enterogastric reflex is stimulated by all; EXCEPT:
a. Alkaline content of small intestine
b. Hyper-osmolality of chime
c. Distension of duodenum
d. Intense pain

123. Transporter of iron into enterocytes is?
a. Ferroportin b. Transferrin
c. Hepcidin d. Divalent metal transporter

124. All are functions of CCK; EXCEPT:
a. Gallbladder contraction
b. Contraction of sphincter of oddi
c. Stimulation of pancreatic secretion
d. Inhibits gastric emptying

125. CCK is produced by:
a. Neuro-endocrine cells in the gut
b. Entero-endocrine cells in the gut
c. Interstitial cells of Cajal
d. Hepatocytes

126. All are principal digestive enzymes produced by exocrine pancreas; EXCEPT:
a. Trypsinogen b. Lipase
c. Lactase d. Amylase

127. All are correct about somatostatin hormone; EXCEPT:
a. Paracrine action in GIT
b. Produced by D cells
c. Growth hormone inhibiting hormone
d. Gastro-ileal reflex

128. Incorrect about bilirubin:
a. Conjugation by UDPq Glucorornyl transferase in liver
b. Breakdown by glucoronidase in gut to increase free pool of unconjugated bilirubin
c. Normally excreted in urine
d. Can cross blood brain barrier

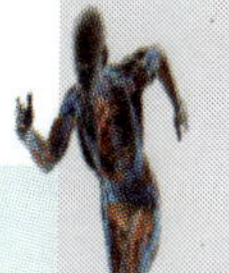

129. Initiation of basic electrical Rhythm of intestine is by:
 a. Interstitial cells of Cajal b. Entero-chromaffin cells
 c. Auerbach plexus d. Meissner plexus

ENDOCRINE AND REPRODUCTIVE PHYSIOLOGY

130. Comment on the hormone produced by marked cells. *(Most Recent Question Dec 2021)*

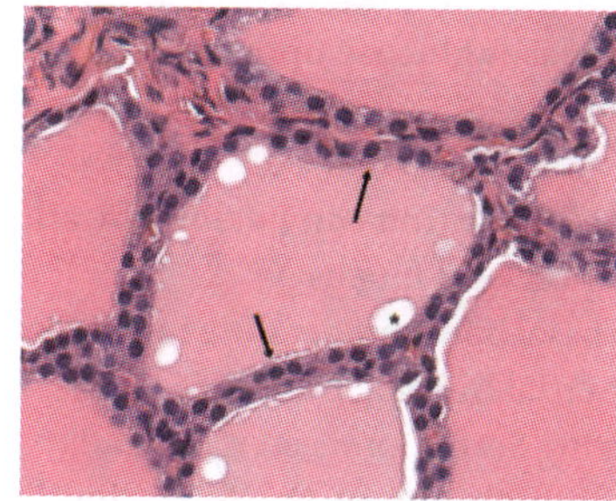

 a. Parathyroid hormone b. Calcitonin
 c. Thyroid hormone d. TSH

131. A female complains of cramps in the breast while breast feeding which hormone is responsible: *(Most Recent Question June 2021)*
 a. Prolactin b. Oxytocin
 c. Prostaglandin d. Somatostatin

132. Hormone that regulates serum calcium levels. *(Most Recent Question June 2021)*
 a. Calcitonin b. Vitamin D
 c. Parathyroid hormone d. All of these

133. A monkey is having increased sexual activity, increased appetite, anger and no fear, injury to which structure is suspected? *(Most Recent Question June 2021)*
 a. Amygdala b. Thalamus
 c. Cingulate gyrus d. Hypothalamus

134. Dopamine in low dose acts as: *(Most Recent Question June 2021)*
 a. Vasodilator b. Increase GFR
 c. Has ionotropic affect d. Increase in pressure

135. Which of the following hormone will regulate release of Prolactin from the anterior pituitary? *(Most Recent Question Dec 2020)*
 a. Corticotropin-releasing hormone
 b. Gonadotropin-releasing hormone
 c. Follicle stimulating hormone
 d. Thyrotropin-releasing hormone

136. Which of the following hormone is involved in milk ejection reflex? *(Most Recent Question Aug 2020)*
 a. Prolactin b. Progesterone
 c. Estrogen d. Oxytocin

137. Thyroxine has maximum affinity for which of the following? *(Most Recent Question Aug 2020)*
 a. Thyroxine binding pre-albumin
 b. Thyroxine binding globulin
 c. Albumin
 d. Prothrombin

138. All are Glucogenic hormones; EXCEPT? *(Recent Pattern Question 2018-19)*
 a. ADH
 b. Glucagon
 c. Thyroxine
 d. Glucocorticoids

139. Active form of Vitamin D3 is: *(Recent Pattern Question 2018-19)*
 a. Calcitriol
 b. Calciferol
 c. Calcidiol
 d. Ergocalciferol

140. Inhibin-A is produced by: *(Recent Pattern Question 2018-19)*
 a. Sertoli cell
 b. Leydig cell
 c. Hilus cell
 d. Placenta

141. Which hormone receptor has 4 subunits and 2 units for tyrosine kinase receptor binding? *(Recent Pattern Question 2018-19)*
 a. Insulin b. Glucagon
 c. T3 d. ADH

142. Name the hormone marked on the picture: *(Recent Pattern Question 2018-19)*

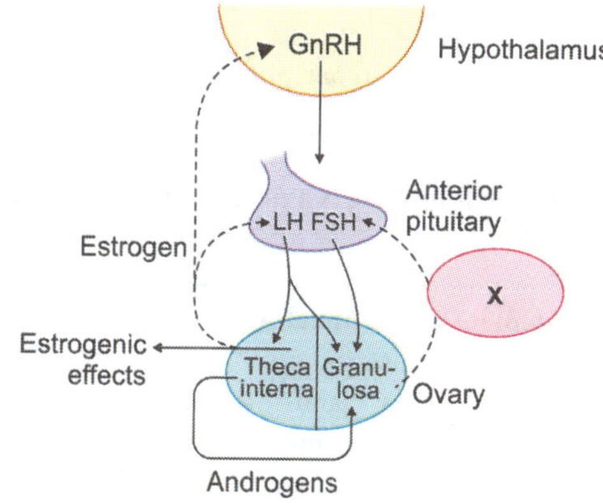

 a. Inhibin A b. Inhibin B
 c. Progesterone d. DHEAS

143. The blood levels of 1,25 dihydroxycholecalciferol is positively regulated by: *(Recent Pattern Question 2018)*
 a. PTH b. Calcium
 c. Magnesium d. 25 OH cholecalciferol

144. Which acts on intracellular receptor: *(Recent Pattern Question 2016)*
 a. TSH b. FSH
 c. Glucagon d. Epinephrine

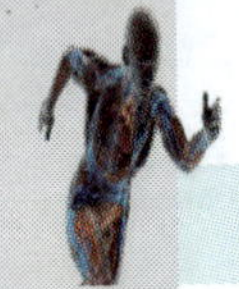

145. During spermatogenesis Sertoli cells secrete ***(Recent Pattern Question 2016)***
a. FSH b. LH
c. Inhibin d. Testosterone

146. Somatostatin is secreted by:
a. Alpha cells b. Beta cells
c. Gamma cells d. Delta cells

147. Adrenal medulla secretes all; EXCEPT?
a. Cortisol b. Epinephrine
c. Nor epinephrine d. Dopamine

148. Adrenal medulla secretes:
a. Neurohormones b. Cortisol
c. Aldosterone d. Vasopressin

149. All of the following are actions of cortisol; EXCEPT:
a. Increase blood amino acid
b. Decrease liver amino acid
c. Decrease blood amino acid
d. Increase liver amino acid

150. Milk ejection is facilitated by:
a. Prolactin b. Oxytocin
c. Growth hormone d. ACTH

151. Which of the following promotes formation of growth hormone?
a. Cortisol b. REM sleep
c. Glucose d. Glucagon

152. Prolactin secretion is *not* stimulated by:
a. Levodopa b. Sleep
c. Estrogen d. Pregnancy

153. TSH is produced by:
a. Anterior pituitary b. Post pituitary
c. Hypothalamus d. Thyroid gland

154. T4 to T3 conversion in peripheral tissues done by?
a. Thyroxine peroxidase b. D1 Deiodinase
c. D2 Deiodinase d. D3 Deiodinase

155. Which of the following is a negative feedback hormone?
a. ACTH b. Growth hormone
c. TSH d. GnRH

156. True statement about Melatonin are all; EXCEPT:
a. Secreted by pituitary gland
b. Secreted by pineal gland
c. Associated with sleep mechanism
d. Can be used to treat jet lag

157. Separation of first polar body occurs at the time of:
a. Menstruation b. Ovulation
c. Fertilization d. Implantation

158. Sperm head contains:
a. Axoneme b. Mitochondria
c. Nucleus d. None of these

159. Sertoli cell secretes which hormone:
a. Testosterone b. Inhibin
c. LH d. FSH

160. All are true about capacitation; EXCEPT:
a. Changes that occur in sperm to penetrate ova
b. Occurs in female genital tract
c. Occurs in male genital tract
d. Sperm loses its cholesterol content in the process

161. Defect in leptin leads to:
a. Obesity b. Anorectic
c. Both d. None of these

162. GLUT receptor on pancreas is?
a. GLUT 1 b. GLUT 2
c. GLUT 4 d. GLUT 5

163. Insulin increases glucose uptake in?
a. Small intestine b. Skeletal muscle
c. RBC d. Kidney

164. Diagnosis of ovulation can be done by all; EXCEPT:
a. Study of cervical mucus
b. Rise in basal body temperature in the second half of cycle
c. Endometrial histology
d. Measuring Serum progesterone on day 14 of the cycle

165. Release of which one of the following hormones is an example of neuroendocrine secretion?
a. Growth hormone
b. Cortisol
c. Oxytocin
d. Thyroxine

166. All are true about testosterone; EXCEPT:
a. Produced by Leydig cells
b. Produced from Androstenedione secreted by adrenal cortex
c. Carbon 17 steroid
d. Secretion under control of LH

167. Correct about menstrual cycle:
a. Proliferative phase by progesterone
b. Secretory phase by Estrogen
c. Superficial 1/3rd of endometrium is shed
d. Menstrual blood is predominantly arterial

168. Inhibin regulates:
a. FSH
b. LH
c. GnRH
d. Testosterone

169. All hormones peak at term; EXCEPT:
a. Estriol
b. Progesterone
c. Prolactin
d. hCG

170. Spinnbarkeit refers to:
a. Cervical mucus
b. Uterine gland thickness
c. Cervical os appearance
d. Proliferation of breast alveoli

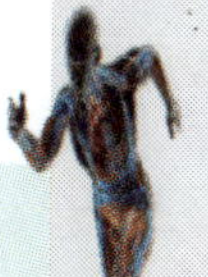

RESPIRATORY PHYSIOLOGY

171. Left shift of Oxygen dissociation curve is seen in: *(Most Recent Question Dec 2021)*

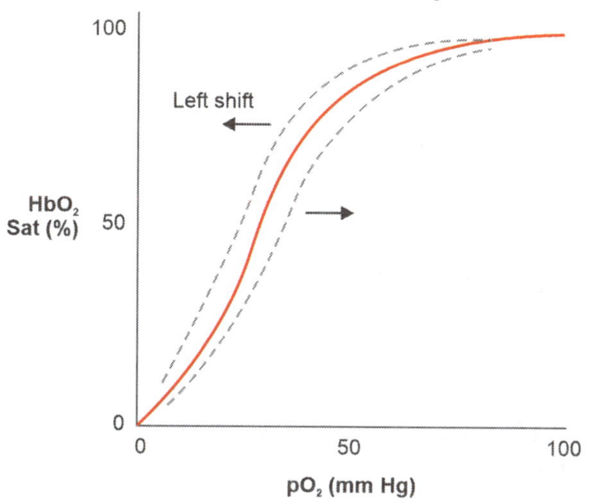

a. Increased in temperature
b. Increased 2, 3 BPG
c. Increased pH
d. Increased pCO_2

172. In gestational life surfactant are produced by which cells? *(Most Recent Question June 2021)*

a. Type 1 pneumocytes
b. Type 2 pneumocytes
c. Basal cells
d. Clara cells

173. Pressure volume graph of cardiac hemodynamics is shown below. What does point B indicate?

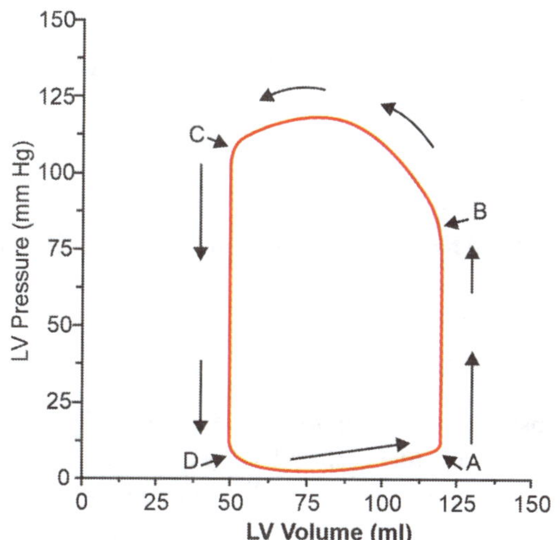

a. Opening of aortic valve
b. Opening of mitral valve
c. Closing of aortic valve
d. Closing of mitral valve

174. A 60-year-old patient has complaints of breathlessness on climbing stairs. On auscultation Heart sounds are normal and normal breath sounds are heard in bilateral lung fields. Flow volume loop is shown/marked in color blue. Comment on diagnosis? *(Most Recent Question Aug 2020)*

Flow volume loops

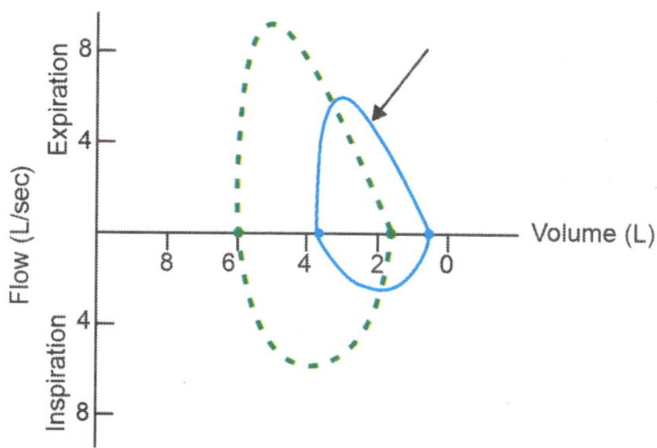

a. Obstructive airway disease
b. Parenchymal restrictive airway disease
c. Extra-parenchymal Restrictive airway disease
d. Normal report

175. Which of the following is correct about CO_2 dissociation curve shown below? *(Most Recent Question Aug 2020)*

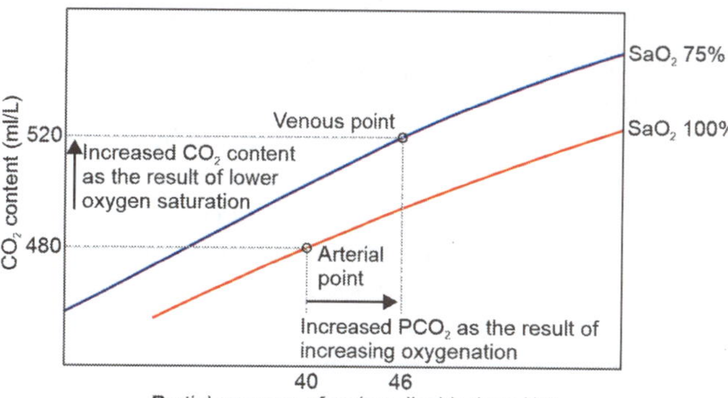

a. Bohr effect
b. Hamburger phenomenon
c. Chloride shift
d. Haldane effect

176. The human lung never empties in spite of forceful expiration. This is due to lining of alveoli by surfactant. This surfactant is cleared by: *(Most Recent Question Aug 2020)*

a. G-CSF
b. GM-CSF
c. Surfactant protein A
d. Surfactant protein B

177. Adequate oxygen delivery at cellular level is present in which type of hypoxia? *(Recent Pattern Question 2019)*

a. Histotoxic
b. Hypoxic
c. Stagnant
d. Anaemic

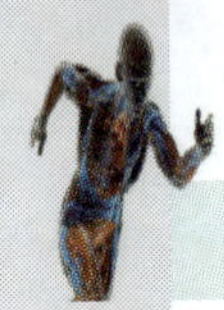

178. Comment on the breathing pattern of a patient with prolonged inspiratory spasms that resemble breath holding? ***(Recent Pattern Question 2019)***
a. Biot breathing b. Apneustic breathing
c. Cheyne stokes breathing d. Kussmaul breathing

179. Transpulmonary pressure is the difference between? ***(Recent Pattern Question 2017)***
a. The bronchus and atmospheric pressure
b. Pressure in alveoli and intrapleural pressure
c. Atmosphere and intrapleural pressure
d. Atmosphere and intraalveolar pressure

180. Respiratory quotient of the brain is? ***(Recent Pattern Question 2017)***
a. 0.6–0.7 b. 0.7–0.8
c. 0.8–0.9 d. 0.9–1.0

181. Mean pulmonary artery pressure:
a. 25 mm Hg b. 8 mm Hg
c. 16 mm Hg d. 20 mm Hg

182. pO_2 pressure at sea level:
a. 140 b. 150
c. 160 d. 180

183. Which is correct regarding lungs in an upright posture?
a. V/Q ratio is high at the apex of the lung
b. V/Q ratio is low at the apex of the lung
c. V/Q ratio is equal at apex and base
d. None of the above

184. Which of the following statement is true about functional residual capacity?
a. Tidal volume + Volume Expired forcefully
b. Volume remaining after forced expiration
c. Tidal volume + Volume inspired forcefully
d. Volume remaining after normal expiration

185. Production of Surfactant is by:
a. Alveolar macrophages b. Type I Pneumocytes
c. Type II Pneumocytes d. Clara cells

186. Bronchial secretions contain?
a. Immunoglobulin G b. Immunoglobulin M
c. Immunoglobulin A d. Immunoglobulin E

187. Peripheral chemoreceptors are stimulated by?
a. CO_2 b. Hydrogen ions
c. pH d. Oxygen

188. The main danger during deep sea diving is due to?
a. Oxygen and nitrogen
b. Oxygen only
c. Nitrogen only
d. CO_2 and nitrogen

189. At high altitude acclimatization happens due to?
a. Increased hemoglobin content and RBC
b. Increased reticulocyte index
c. Decreased pulmonary ventilation
d. Decreased ability of tissues to use oxygen

190. Which of the following is true about hypoxic hypoxia?
a. Due to inadequate carrying capacity
b. Due to inability to utilize oxygen
c. Due to inadequate gas exchange
d. Due to slow circulation

191. Over-inflation of lung is prevented by?
a. Chemo-receptor b. Hering-Breuer reflex
c. Surfactant d. Clara cells

192. Oxygen hemoglobin dissociation curve shifts to right in all of the following conditions; EXCEPT:
a. Hyperthermia b. Decreased pH
c. Decreased H^+ d. Increase CO_2

193. PCO_2 increase leads to:
a. Shift of Oxy-Hb dissociation curve to left
b. Shift of Oxy-Hb dissociation curve to right
c. Shift of Oxy-Hb dissociation curve upwards
d. Shift of Oxy-Hb dissociation curve downwards

194. S shaped curve of oxygen hemoglobin dissociation curve is due to?
a. Atmospheric pressure decreases affinity of O_2 binding with Hemoglobin
b. Binding of oxygen to hemoglobin decreases affinity of Hb for CO_2
c. Falling of pH decreases oxygen affinity for Hemoglobin
d. Binding of oxygen molecule increases affinity of binding other oxygen molecule

195. Which of the following is not responsible for causing a right shift of the oxygen dissociation curve:
a. Increased carbon dioxide
b. Temperature
c. Exercise
d. Alkalosis

196. Pulmonary Chemo-reflex is characterized by?
a. Reflex bradycardia
b. Rise in blood pressure
c. Reflex tachycardia
d. Pulmonary oligaemia

197. What will happen to respiration if both vagi are cut?
a. Becomes slow and deep
b. Becomes fast and shallow
c. Increase in depth of respiration
d. Increase in rate of breathing

198. "Obstructive sleep apnea" is defined as temporary pause in breathing during sleep lasting at least?
a. 40 seconds b. 30 seconds
c. 20 seconds d. 10 seconds

199. Damage to pneumotaxic center will cause?
a. Apneusis
b. Apnea
c. Slower breathing with greater tidal volume
d. Faster breathing with lesser tidal volume

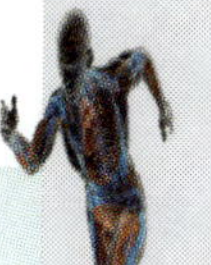

200. Damage to J receptors in lungs will result in?

a. Apnea followed by Rapid shallow breathing
b. Hyperpnea followed by rapid shallow breathing
c. Cardiac arrest
d. Hering Breur reflex

201. Myoglobin binds to ________ molecules of oxygen?

a. 1 b. 2
c. 3 d. 4

202. Normal ventilation/perfusion ratio is?

a. 0.8 b. 1.2
c. 1.6 d. 2.0

203. Normal respiratory minute volume is?

a. Tidal volume × Respiratory rate
b. Tidal volume/Respiratory rate
c. TLC/Respiratory rate
d. FRC/Respiratory rate

204. Which of the following statement is true about inspiratory capacity:

a. Tidal volume + volume expired forcefully
b. Volume remaining after forced expiration
c. Tidal volume + volume inspired forcefully
d. Volume remaining after normal expiration

205. Which of the following is seen in placenta?

a. Bohr effect b. Double Bohr effect
c. Hamburger phenomenon d. Haldane effect

206. Cut off limit for deoxygenated hemoglobin for appearance of cyanosis is?

a. >4 gm% b. >5 gm%
c. < 2 gm% d. <4 gm%

207. Which is the site of generation of respiratory rhythm?

a. Botzinger complex
b. Pre-Botzinger complex
c. Dorsal respiratory group of neurons in medulla
d. Ventral respiratory group of neurons in medulla

CARDIOVASCULAR AND CIRCULATORY PHYSIOLOGY

208. Which of the following is correct about jugular venous pressure? ***(Most Recent Question Dec 2020)***

a. Measured from xiphisternum
b. V wave occurs in Isovolumetric contraction
c. Rises with deep inspiration in normal person
d. Y descent occurs in rapid ventricular filling phase

209. A 55-year-old man has chest pain on rest for last 6 hours. ECG was performed on admission and showed findings of myocardial ischemia. His biomarkers report was sent to the lab for diagnostic workup. Which of the following will help in diagnosis? ***(Most Recent Question Aug 2020)***

a. LDH1 b. LDH2
c. LDH3 d. LDH4

210. What is the cause of dicrotic notch? ***(Recent Pattern Question 2019)***

a. Passive filling of blood in ventricles
b. Rapid ejection phase
c. Peripheral resistance
d. Isovolumic contraction

211. Which of the following is correct about Isovolumeteric relaxation? ***(Recent Pattern Question 2019)***

a. AV valves are closed
b. Corresponds to QT interval
c. C wave of JVP
d. Semilunar valves open

212. If radius of a vessel is doubled then the blood flow is increased by? ***(Recent Pattern Question 2019)***

a. 8 times
b. 16 times
c. 32 times
d. 256 times

213. Which is true about heart sound? ***(Recent Pattern Question 2017)***

a. First heart sound has maximum frequency
b. First heart sound has maximum duration
c. First heart sound is due to semilunar valve closure
d. Second heart sound is due to AV valve closure

214. Purkinje fibers are: ***(Recent Pattern Question 2016)***

a. Nerve fibers
b. Modified muscle fibers
c. Modified connective tissue fibers
d. Retinal fibers

215. Forward blood flow in the fetal venous system is in this phase ***(Recent Pattern Question 2016)***

a. Preload b. After load
c. Systolic volume d. All of these

216. What is the reason for increased interstitial fluid? ***(Recent Pattern Question 2016)***

a. Increase hydrostatic pressure, increase oncotic pressure
b. Decrease hydrostatic pressure, decrease oncotic pressure
c. Increase hydrostatic pressure, decrease oncotic pressure
d. Decrease hydrostatic pressure, increase oncotic pressure

217. All of the following statements are false; EXCEPT:

a. Right ventricle work more than left ventricle
b. Left ventricle works more than right ventricle
c. Both ventricle work equal
d. Maximum ventricular filing occurs in isovolumetric contraction

218. All are true; EXCEPT:

a. SA is dominant pacemaker
b. AV node shows fast conduction
c. Purkinje fibers have fastest conduction
d. AV nodal delay is 0.1 sec.

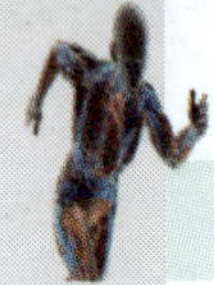

219. All of the following statements are false about stroke volume; EXCEPT:
   a. Determined by after load
   b. Determined by pre-diastolic volume
   c. Decreases by increase in heart rate
   d. Increased by increase in heart rate

220. Severe HTN cut off is
   a. >140 mm Hg
   b. >150 mm Hg
   c. >160 mm Hg
   d. >170 mm Hg

221. In JVP, "a- wave" is due to:
   a. Atrial relaxation
   b. Atrial filling
   c. Atrial contraction
   d. Ventricular relaxation

222. Which of the following is true about Coronary blood flow?
   a. Stable throughout the cardiac cycle
   b. Maximum during diastole
   c. Maximum during systole
   d. Regulated by sympathetic vasodilatory activity

223. Repolarization in isolated muscle piece fiber proceeds from?
   a. Epicardium to endocardium
   b. Endocardium to epicardium
   c. Left to right
   d. Right to left

224. Sympathetic Stimulation causes all of the following; EXCEPT
   a. Increase in heart rate
   b. Increase in blood pressure
   c. Increase in total peripheral resistance
   d. Increase in venous capacitance

225. Incorrect about ECG?
   a. Normal axis of heart is –30 to +110 degrees
   b. ST segment is 0.40 seconds
   c. Holter is ambulatory recording
   d. AV nodal delay is 0.1 seconds

226. Dicrotic notch corresponds to?
   a. Closure of AV valves
   b. Closure of aortic and pulmonic valves
   c. Opening of AV valves
   d. Opening of aortic and pulmonic valves

227. Which of the following is correct about Frank starling law?
   a. Explains the increase in heart rate produced by exercise
   b. Explains the increase in cardiac output when venous return is increased
   c. Explains the decrease in heart rate in spinal shock
   d. Explains the decrease in heart rate by Valsava manoeuvre

228. Cardiac output is measured by all; EXCEPT:
   a. Doppler
   b. Oscillometry
   c. Thermo-dilution method
   d. Fick's principle

229. All are true about circulating changes in exercising muscle; EXCEPT:
   a. Complete flow stops on maximal tension reaching 70%
   b. Blood supply increases by 30 times between contractions
   c. Dilation of arterioles and pre-capillaries
   d. Peripheral resistance increases

230. Which represent ventricular systole?
   a. Start of P to end of T wave
   b. End of P to end of T wave
   c. Middle of R to end of T wave
   d. Start of q to end of S wave

231. Dromotropy is:
   a. Increase in Rate of transmission
   b. Increase in Force of contraction
   c. Increase in RMP potential
   d. Increase in action potential duration

232. Not a component of JVP?
   a. A wave bigger than V wave
   b. C wave is called as Dicrotic notch
   c. X wave is seen ventricular systole
   d. Y descent in ventricular diastole

233. Traube Hering waves are due to?
   a. Fluctuation in BP with respiration
   b. Fluctuations in JVP with respiration
   c. Fluctuation in CVP with respiration
   d. Fluctuation in ICP with respiration

234. Which of the following has maximum cross sectional area?
   a. Aorta
   b. Artery
   c. Venule
   d. Arteriole

235. Normal arm to tongue circulation time is
   a. 5 seconds b. 10 seconds
   c. 15 seconds d. 30 seconds

CNS AND PNS PHYSIOLOGY

236. A person with head injury is admitted to ER with GCS of 8/15. NCCT Head is scheduled. Which is not correct about Cushing reflex? ***(Most Recent Question June 2022)***
   a. Trigger is Fall in Cerebral perfusion
   b. Activation of cardioinhibitory center
   c. Widening of pulse pressure
   d. Abolished by blockade of chemoreceptors

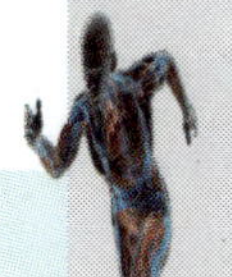

237. Arrange the following in right order:
(Most Recent Question Dec 2021)

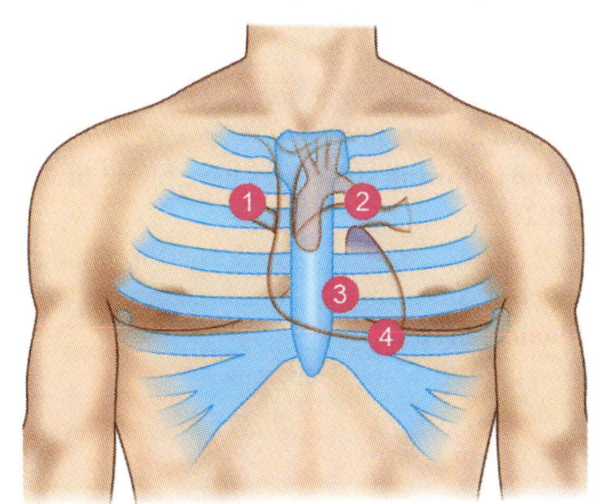

a. 1 = Aortic area, 2 = pulmonic area, 3 = tricuspid area, 4 = mitral area
b. 1 = pulmonic area, 2=aortic area, mitral area, 4 tricuspid area
c. 1 = Aortic area, 2 = mitral area, 3 = pulmonic area 4 = tricuspid area
d. 1 = aortic area, 2 = pulmonic area, 3 mitral area, 4 = tricuspid area

238. Brown-Séquard syndrome leads to damage to:
(Most Recent Question Dec 2020)
a. Ascending sensory and descending motor pathways in spinal cord
b. Descending motor and ascending sensory pathways in spinal cord
c. Ascending motor and ascending sensory pathways in spinal cord
d. Descending motor and descending sensory pathways in spinal cord

239. A 25-year-old patient after head trauma presented to the Emergency room. On neurological examination, he was found to have normal handwriting and could copy shapes of objects but could not speak. Localize the CNS lesion of this patient: *(Most Recent Question Dec 2020)*
a. Wernicke's area b. Broca's area
c. Arcus fasciculus d. Internal capsule

240. Resistance against passive stretch is called:
(Recent Pattern Question 2018-19)
a. Tone b. Spasticity
c. Rigidity d. Paratonia

241. Which structure connects the Broca's area and Wernicke area? *(Recent Pattern Question 2018-19)*
a. Arcuate fasciculus
b. Anterior commissure
c. Corpus callosum
d. Fornix

242. Reward center in the brain is?
(Recent Pattern Question 2018-19)
a. Amygdala b. Thalamus
c. Hippocampus d. Ventral tegmental area

243. Which part of thalamus is related to motor control?
(Recent Pattern Question 2018-19)
a. Ventrolateral thalamus
b. Ventral posteromedial
c. Ventral posterolateral
d. Superior and inferior colliculi

244. In case a small stimulus causes more pain, it is called:
(Recent Pattern Question 2018-19)
a. Hypersensitivity b. Causalgia
c. Hyperalgesia d. Allodynia

245. Stretch stimulus is mediated by which of the following receptors? *(Recent Pattern Question 2018)*
a. Merkel's disc b. Meissner
c. Pacinian d. Muscle spindle

246. During sleep which hormone is increased?
(Recent Pattern Question 2017)
a. Serotonin b. Dopamine
c. GABA d. Ach

247. Which is true about sleep cycle?
(Recent Pattern Question 2017)
a. REM is half of sleep cycle
b. Muscle tone is absent in REM sleep
c. NREM is 25% of sleep cycle
d. Muscle tone is absent in NREM sleep

248. mGluR 4 is associated with which taste?
(Recent Pattern Question 2016)
a. Sweet b. Sour
c. Bitter d. Umami

249. Which cells secrete glutamate in cerebellum?
(Recent Pattern Question 2016)
a. Stellate cell b. Basket cells
c. Granular cell d. Golgi cell

250. Excitatory neurotransmitter of brain is?
(Recent Pattern Question 2016)
a. GABA b. Aspartate
c. Glutamate d. Glycine

251. Not a part of basal ganglia is?
a. Caudate nucleus b. Corpus striatum
c. Lenticular nucleus d. Sub-Fornical organ

252. True about GABA:
a. Excitatory neurotransmitter
b. Inhibitory to neuron
c. Facilitatory neurotransmitter
d. Stimulatory to neuron

253. Brain contains which neurotransmitter:
a. Tyrosine b. Glutamate
c. Serine d. Tryptophan

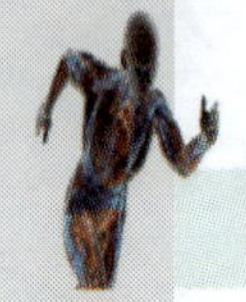

254. All of the following cells are present in cerebellar cortex; EXCEPT:
a. Granular cell b. Purkinje cell
c. Golgi cell d. Bipolar cell

255. Posterior pre-frontal cortex contains which of the following areas?
a. Wernicke's area b. Broca's area
c. Brodmann's area d. Limbic association area

256. Broca's area is located at:
a. Inferior frontal gyrus
b. Superior temporal gyrus
c. Inferior temporal gyrus
d. Superior frontal gyrus

257. Which of the following vascular occlusion is the most common cause of hemiplegia?
a. Basilar artery b. Vertebral artery
c. Anterior cerebral artery d. Middle cerebral artery

258. Auditory receptor is present in:
a. Broca's area
b. Cingulate gyrus
c. Superior temporal gyrus
d. Inferior temporal gyrus

259. Damage to preoptic nuclei of brain leads to?
a. Decrease heart rate, decrease arterial pressure
b. Increase heart rate, increase arterial pressure
c. Increase heart rate, decrease arterial pressure
d. Decrease heart rate, increase arterial pressure

260. Which is the Longest duration NREM Stage?
a. Stage 1 b. Stage 2
c. Stage 3 d. Spread throughout

261. Teeth grinding is seen in which stage of sleep:
a. NREM 1 b. NREM 2
c. NREM 3 d. NREM 4

262. The alpha rhythm appearing in EEG has the following characteristic feature?
a. Produces 20–30 waves per second
b. Disappear when a patient opens eyes
c. Associated with deep sleep
d. Replaced by slower, larger waves during REM sleep

263. Hippocampal formation includes all; EXCEPT?
a. Dentate gyrus b. Subiculum
c. Amygdaloid nucleus d. Entorhinal cortex

264. The inability to perceive the texture & shape an object occurs in lesion of?
a. Lateral Spinothalamic tract
b. Nucleus gracilis
c. Spino-reticular tract
d. Nucleus cuneatus

265. EEG rhythm recorded from the surface of the scalp during REM sleep?
a. Alpha b. Beta
c. Delta d. Theta

266. Which of the following phrase adequately describes Pacinian corpuscles?
a. A type of pain receptors
b. Slowly adapting touch receptors
c. Rapidly adapting touch receptors
d. Located in the joints

267. All of the following structures have blood brain barrier; EXCEPT:
a. Optic tract b. Posterior pituitary
c. Superior colliculus d. Basal ganglia

268. Paradoxical sleep is?
a. Seen in obstructive sleep apnea
b. REM sleep
c. NRM sleep
d. Narcolepsy

269. All are hyperkinetic movements; EXCEPT:
a. Chorea b. Atheotosis
c. Akinesia d. Ballism

270. Glycinergic inhibitory interneuron in spinal cord is?
a. Renhaw cell b. Purkinje cell
c. Basket cell d. Golgi cell

271. Clonus is due to?
a. Upper motor neuron damage
b. Lower motor neuron damage
c. Extrapyramidal damage
d. Cerebellar damage

272. Clasp knife effect is seen in?
a. Flaccidity b. Rigidity
c. Spasticity d. All of these

273. Rebound phenomenon is seen due to:
a. Damage to cerebrum
b. Damage to cerebellum
c. Damage to extrapyramidal pathway
d. Damage to rubrospinal pathway

274. First reflex to reappear after spinal shock?
a. Myotactic reflex b. Withdrawal reflex
c. Stretch reflex d. Inverse stretch reflex

275. Corpus striatum is formed by?
a. Caudate and putamen
b. Caudate and subthalamic nucleus
c. Caudate and lenticular nucleus
d. Caudate and amygdaloid nucleus

276. Inverse stretch reflex is__________?
a. Monosynaptic reflex
b. Bi-Synaptic reflex
c. Polysynaptic reflex
d. Occurs when Ia spindle fibers are inhibited

277. Inverse stretch reflex is mediated by:
a. Muscle spindle b. Golgi tendon organ
c. Unmyelinated C fibers d. B fibers

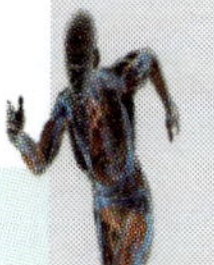

278. Lowest level of Integration of Stretch reflex is at:
a. Cerebral cortex b. Medulla
c. Lower medulla d. Spinal Cord

279. Twitch of a single motor unit is called:
a. Myoclonic-jerk b. Fasciculation
c. Tremor d. Chorea

280. Not a component of light reflex:
a. Lateral geniculate body
b. Edinger westphal nucleus
c. Occipital radiation
d. Optic nerve

281. Globus pallidus and putamen are present in:
a. Pons b. Thalamus
c. Cerebellum d. Basal ganglia

282. Phantom limb phenomenon is due to:
a. Weber Fechner Law
b. Law of Projection
c. Doctrine of specific nerve energies
d. Bell Magendie Law

PHYSIOLOGY OF BLOOD

283. Most common macrocytic anemia is:
(Most Recent Question June 2022)
a. Megaloblastic anemia b. Alcoholic hepatitis
c. Bone marrow disorders d. Hemolytic Anemia

284. Which is correct about action of Vitamin K?
(Recent Pattern Question 2018)
a. γ-carboxylation of glutamic acid residues to clotting factor 2, 7, 9 and 10
b. β-carboxylation of glutamic acid residues to clotting factor 2, 7, 9 and 10
c. α-carboxylation of asparatic acid residues to clotting factor 2, 7, 9 and 10
d. γ-carboxylation of aspartic acid residues clotting factor 2, 7, 9 and 10

285. One hemoglobin molecule can carry how many oxygen molecules? ***(Recent Pattern Question 2017)***
a. 1 b. 2
c. 3 d. 4

286. Bilirubin is synthesised from
(Recent Pattern Question 2016)
a. Amino acid b. Hemoglobin
c. Myoglobin d. WBCs

287. During intrauterine life, *hepatic stage* of erythropoiesis starts at?
a. 2nd week b. 5th week
c. 12th week d. 18th week

288. The biochemical role of vitamin K in the post-translational modification of clotting factors is by?
a. Glycosylation b. Carboxylation
c. Acetylation d. Phosphorylation

289. All are true about serum; EXCEPT:
a. Lacks clotting factors
b. Higher serotonin content
c. Does not clot
d. Constitutes 5% of body weight

290. All of the following proteins are synthesized by the liver; EXCEPT:
a. Haptoglobin b. Antithrombin-III
c. Von Willebrand factor d. Hemopexin

291. During second trimester of pregnancy, erythropoiesis occurs in the fetus primarily in:
a. Liver b. Spleen
c. Red bone marrow d. Lymph nodes

292. Which one of the following is NOT a function of albumin?
a. Osmoregulation b. Solubilization of glucose
c. Transport of hormones d. Transport of bilirubin

293. Which of the following is major mechanisms causing heat loss from a normal person when the environmental temperature is 21°C?
a. Conduction b. Convection
c. Radiation d. Evaporation

294. Shivering is caused by?
a. Stimulation of fibers coming from anterior hypothalamus
b. Stimulation of fibers coming from posterior hypothalamus
c. Stimulation of fibers coming from intermediate lobe of hypothalamus
d. Stimulation of median eminence

295. Which of the following plasma proteins is not synthesized primarily in liver?
a. Angiotensinogen
b. C-reactive protein
c. Angiotensin converting enzyme
d. Fibrinogen

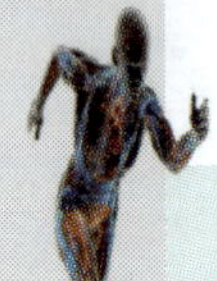

ANSWERS WITH EXPLANATIONS

MOST RECENT QUESTIONS 2023

1. Ans. (d) Hypoventilation

Ref: Guyton and Hall Textbook of Medical Physiology, 13th ed. pg. 554, 555

- In an environment with decreased oxygen levels, the body attempts to compensate by increasing respiratory rate and depth to maximize oxygen intake. This response is known as hyperventilation.
- Hypoventilation, on the other hand, refers to reduced ventilation, resulting in inadequate oxygen uptake. This would undermine the acclimatization process, as it would limit the body's ability to cope with the reduced oxygen tension at high altitudes. Adequate oxygen uptake is crucial for sustaining bodily functions and preventing hypoxia-related issues.
- **Note:** At high altitude, there will be increase in RBC count and myoglobin. Increased RBC count will increase the oxygen-carrying capacity and myoglobin which is a muscle protein, facilitating oxygen storage and release in muscle cells. Increased capillary density allows more effective diffusion of oxygen from capillaries to muscle cells.

2. Ans. (c) Liver

Ref: Ganong's Review of Medical Physiology, 26th ed. pg. 48, 52, 53, 426

- GLUT2 is primarily found in the liver, intestinal epithelial cells and pancreatic β-cells.
- In the liver, GLUT2 is involved in glucose uptake, storage as glycogen, and release as needed to maintain blood glucose levels within a normal range.
- In pancreatic β-cells, GLUT2 plays a role in glucose sensing and insulin release, contributing to the regulation of blood glucose levels.

3. Ans. (b) GLUT2

Ref: Ganong's Review of Medical Physiology, 26th ed. pg. 48, 52, 53, 426

- Glucose transporters, known as GLUTs, play a crucial role in facilitating the movement of glucose across cell membranes. Different GLUT isoforms are found in various tissues, each specialized for specific functions.
- GLUT2 isoform of the glucose transporter is primarily present on the basolateral membrane of intestinal epithelial cells.
- After absorption in the small intestine, glucose needs to enter the bloodstream to be transported to different tissues for energy utilization.
- GLUT2 assists in transporting glucose from the intestinal cells into the bloodstream, ensuring its distribution to various parts of the body.
- **Note:** GLUT5 is present in the mucosal surface of small intestine, sperm and also on kidneys.

4. Ans. (b) Plasticity

Ref: Ganong's Review of Medical Physiology, 25th ed. pg. 118, 207, 238

- The terms "elasticity" and "plasticity" are used to describe the mechanical properties of tissues. The graph shows pressure changes in urinary bladder as it progressively fills up with urine.
- Phase Ib on the graph represents plasticity. Ia represent elasticity.
- Plasticity refers to the ability of certain tissues to undergo deformation that is not fully reversible upon removal of the deforming force.

5. Ans. (b) Esophagus

Ref: Guyton and Hall Textbook of Medical Physiology, 14th ed. pg. 789, 790

- The serosa is a thin, protective layer of connective tissue that covers the external surfaces of some organs within body cavities.
- Serosa is not present in the esophagus.
- The esophagus is part of the gastrointestinal tract and lacks the serosa layer, which is typically found in abdominal organs.

6. Ans. (a) Bezold-Jarisch reflex

Ref: Guyton and Hall Textbook of Medical Physiology, 14th ed. pg. 224, 225

- The **Bezold-Jarisch reflex** is a cardiovascular reflex characterized by bradycardia, hypotension, and apnea in response to certain stimuli, particularly the infusion of irritant substances into the coronary arteries.
- This reflex is a protective response that can occur when the heart senses irritation or ischemia, leading to a decrease in heart rate and blood pressure.
- **Brainbridge reflex** is caused by stimulation of the brainstem and results in a decrease in heart rate and blood pressure. It is thought to be involved in the regulation of blood flow to the brain.

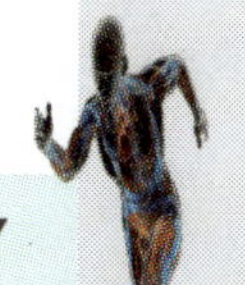

- **Cushing's reflex** is thought to be involved in the body's response to stress. There is an increase in heart rate, blood pressure, and respiratory rate.

7. Ans. (b) Dystrophin

Ref: Nelson Textbook of Pediatrics, 21st ed. pg. 3281

- This patient is suffering from Duchenne muscular dystrophy. Dystrophin protein (sarcolemma protein) is absent in patients with DMD due to a mutation in the dystrophin gene.

8. Ans. (a) Isovolumetric contraction

Ref: Ganong's Review of Medical Physiology, 26th ed. pg. 529

- First heart sound corresponds to the isovolumetric contraction phase in the cardiac cycle where ventricles contract against closed mitral valves.

Heart sound	Phase in cardiac cycle
S1	Isovolumetric contraction
S2	Isovolumetric relaxation
S3	Early diastole
S4	Atrial contraction
Systolic clicks	Mid systole
Opening snap	Early diastole

9. Ans. (a) Tricuspid regurgitation

Ref: Harrison's Principles of Internal Medicine, 20th ed. pg. 1768

- Large "v" wave on JVP examination is seen in **tricuspid regurgitation**.
- **In tricuspid regurgitation**, an S3 gallop, and a palpable RV heave along the left sternal border can be noted.
- Other features of tricuspid regurgitation include hepatomegaly, pulsatile liver, tenderness in the right upper quadrant, and pitting pedal edema.

Important conditions and JVP findings:

• Constrictive pericarditis	Elevated and prominent JVP with steep "y" descent
• Cardiac tamponade	Elevated JVP with absent or jugular venous pulsation
• Superior vena cava obstruction	Elevated JVP with distended neck veins
• Pulmonary hypertension	Elevated JVP with prominent "a" wave
• Tricuspid regurgitation	Elevated JVP with prominent "v" wave and regurgitant waves

10. Ans. (b) VII

- Extrinsic clotting factors are proteins involved in the coagulation cascade that are activated outside of the blood vessels.
- Factor VII is an extrinsic clotting factor.
- Factor VII, also known as proconvertin, is activated by tissue factor (also called factor III), which is released from damaged tissues in response to tissue injury.
- Once activated, factor VII initiates the extrinsic pathway of coagulation, leading to the formation of a fibrin clot.
- Intrinsic factor starts from factor XII → XI → IX which activate factor X.

11. Ans. (b) Creatinine clearance is greater than inulin clearance

Ref: Ganong's Review of Medical Physiology, 26th ed. pg. 667

- Creatinine clearance is a measure of kidney function and is used to estimate the glomerular filtration rate.
- Creatinine is a waste product produced by the breakdown of creatine in muscle tissue. It is filtered by the glomerulus and excreted in the urine.
- Inulin is a substance that is freely filtered by the glomerulus and is used as a marker to measure the GFR accurately.
- Creatinine clearance is a commonly used approximation of GFR because creatinine is easily measured in the blood and urine.
- In general, creatinine clearance overestimates GFR because a small amount of creatinine is secreted by the renal tubules, leading to an overestimation of the amount of creatinine cleared by the kidneys.
- However, inulin clearance provides a more accurate measurement of GFR as it is not subject to tubular secretion.
- Therefore, creatinine clearance is greater than inulin clearance.

12. Ans. (d) Cerebral edema

Ref: Harrison's Principles of Internal Medicine, 21st ed. pg. 3117

- Cerebral edema is a severe complication that can occur in DKA, especially in children.
- Acidosis induced damage to blood barrier explains cerebral edema. Next important cause of death will be dehydration.

CELL AND NERVE-MUSCLE PHYSIOLOGY

13. Ans. (d) Facilitated diffusion

Ref: Ganong 26th ed. pg. 426

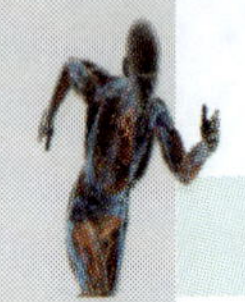

- Insulin regulates peripheral glucose uptake and glucose production within the liver — a family of five transmembrane proteins, known as GLUT which transport glucose *via* facilitated diffusion across the cell plasma membrane.
- The primary regulatory mechanism by which glucose uptake takes place is *via* insulin-stimulated transport of glucose into skeletal muscle and adipose tissue, primarily mediated by glucose transporter protein type-4 called GLUT 4.

14. Ans. (a) Respiratory acidosis

Ref: Ganong 25th ed. pg. 635

pH shows Acidosis. The elevated levels of Carbon dioxide and low pO_2 values indicate respiratory acidosis. HCO_3 values are on higher side of normal.

15. Ans. (d) Non-ionic diffusion

Ref: Ganong 26th ed. pg. 48

Ammonia is a weak base that can cross the membrane of cells in non-ionized form but not in ionized form. Option a, osmosis occurs across solute gradient. Option b occurs *via* carrier protein specific.

16. Ans. (d) Tropomyosin

Ref: Ganong 26th ed. pg. 101-102

- Option d is answer as tropomyosin is an contractile protein along with actin, myosin-II and Troponin.
- Structural proteins that are important in skeletal muscle function include actinin, titin and desmin.
- Actinin binds to actin to Z lines. Titin is the largest known protein that connects Z line to M lines and provides scaffolding for sarcomere. Desmin adds structure to Z lines.

17. Ans. (a) Uniport

Ref: Ganong 26th ed. pg. 48

ROMK is a carrier protein that transports potassium and is called uniport. Option b transports two or more substances from one side of membrane to other in same direction. Option c transports substances in opposite direction like Na-H exchanger or Na-K pump.

18. Ans. (b) Becker's muscular dystrophy

Ref: Ganong 26th ed. pg. 102

The key word is decreased dystrophin protein indicating Becker's muscular dystrophy. In contrast, if the report says absent dystrophin protein it indicates Duchenne's muscular dystrophy.

19. Ans. (d) Secondary active transport

Ref: Berne and Levy Physiology, 6th ed. pg. 19

- In the intestine and renal proximal tubule, glucose is transported against a concentration gradient by a secondary active transport mechanism.
- In secondary active transport mechanism, glucose is co-transported with sodium ions.

20. Ans. (c) IgM

Ref: Ananth-Narayana and Panicker's Textbook of Microbiology, 10th ed. pg. 98-99

- The image shows a pentameric structure of Immunoglobulin M which are each comprised two heavy-chains (mu-chains) and two light chains, bound together by disulfide bonds and a so-called J-chain.

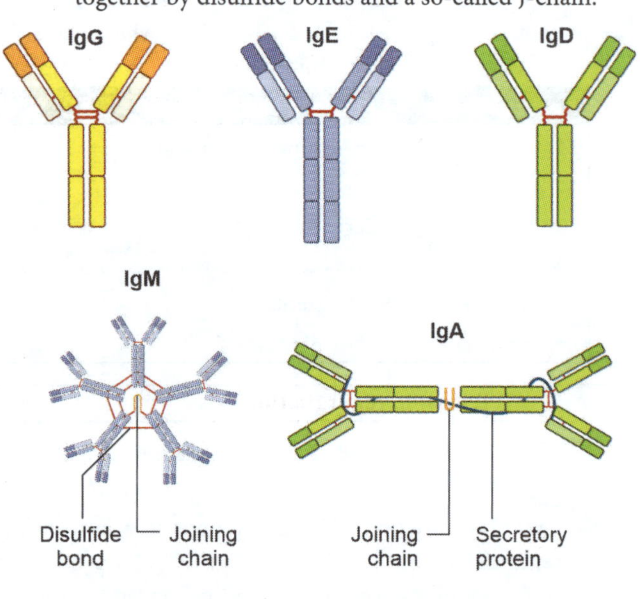

21. Ans. (a) Dynein

Ref: Ganong 26th ed. pg. 40

- The Rabies virus travels via the axons of nerve retrogradely towards the brain. The molecular motor responsible for this retrograde transport is Dynein.
- Kinesin is responsible for anterograde movement.
- Neuroinvasive viruses, such as alpha herpesviruses (αHV) and rabies virus (RABV), initially infect peripheral tissues, followed by invasion of the innervating axon termini. Virus particles now undergo long distance retrograde axonal transport to reach the neuron cell bodies in the peripheral or central nervous system.

22. Ans. (c) Hypocalcemia

Ref: Ganong 26th ed. pg. 370

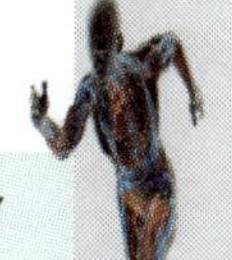

- Low serum calcium lowers the threshold potential of nerves. It means less inward current is required to depolarize the nerve. In other words, it increases neuromuscular excitability of median nerve and can lead to carpopedal spasm.
- Option a leads to seizures
- Option b can lead to muscle weakness and paralysis.

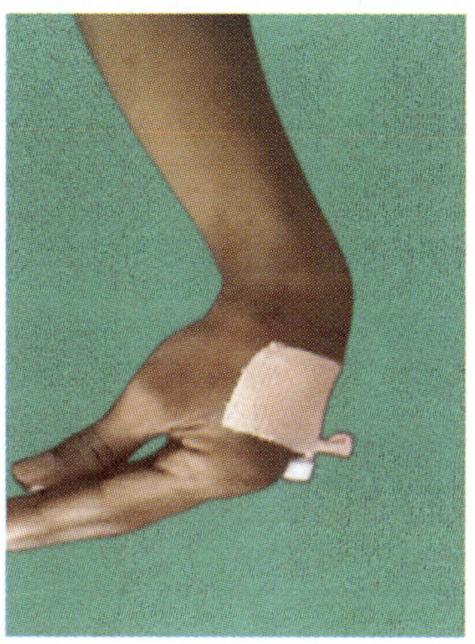

23. Ans. (d) C

Ref: Ganong 26th ed. pg. 92

Diabetic neuropathy is a microvascular complication that affects unmyelinated C fibers that mediate pain sensation.

Fiber Type	Function
Aα	Proprioception; somatic motor
Aβ	Touch, pressure
Aγ	Motor to muscle spindles
Aδ	Pain, temperature
B	Preganglionic autonomic
C, Dorsal root	Pain, temperature
C, sympathetic	Postganglionic sympathetic

24. Ans. (d) Platelets

Ref: Ganong 26th ed. pg. 148

Serotonin/5 hydroxytryptamine is present in highest concentration in blood platelets and gastrointestinal tract where it is found in enterochromaffin cells and myenteric plexus. It is also found within the brainstem in midline raphe nuclei which project to CNS including hypothalamus, limbic system and neocortex.

25. Ans. (a) Calcium

Ref: Ganong 25th ed. pg. 5

- Potassium, magnesium, and phosphate are the three most common electrolytes in the ICF.

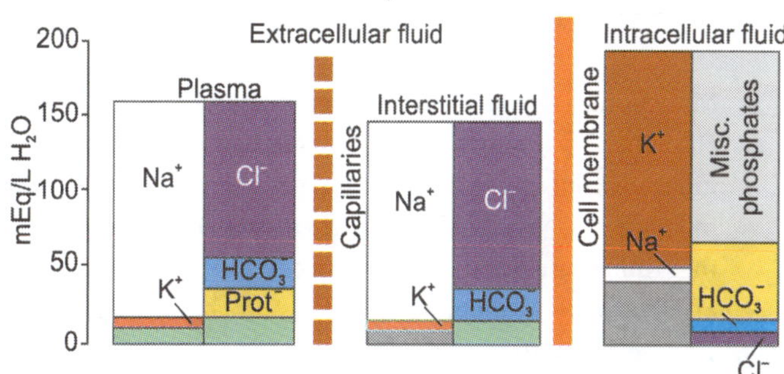

- Intracellular fluid is the place where most of the fluid in the body is contained (40% body weight).
- Magnesium is the second most important intracellular cation after potassium. Less than 1% of total body magnesium is found in red blood cells. It is distributed principally between the bone, muscle, and soft tissues.

26. Ans. (d) Clathrin

Ref: Ganong 25th ed. pg. 56

- Clathrin plays a role in endocytosis.
- Calcium binding proteins are troponin, Calmodulin, at Calbindin.
- The major role of *calbindin* is to facilitate the vitamin D dependent movement of calcium through the cytosolic compartment of the intestinal or renal cell. It also plays a role in different cell types in protecting against apoptotic cell death
- *Troponin* is a calcium binding protein involved in contraction of skeletal muscle.
- *Calmodulin* plays a role in smooth muscle contraction.

Extra Mile

Calcineurin is a phosphatase that inactivates calcium channels by dephosphorylating them. It also plays a role in activating T cells and is inhibited by immunosuppressants.

27. Ans. (a) Golgi tendon

Ref: Ganong 25th ed. pg. 232

- Up to a certain point, harder a muscle is stretched the stronger it will contract. However when the tension becomes great enough, contraction ceases and muscle relaxes. This relaxation in response to strong stretch is called inverse stretch reflex.
- The receptor for the same is called Golgi tendon organ. It is a net like connection of knobby nerve findings amongst the fascicles of a tendon.

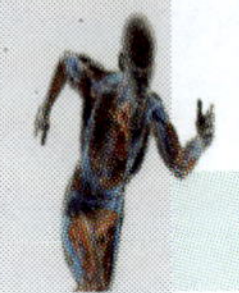

- There are 3–25 muscle fibers per Golgi tendon organ.
- The fibers from Golgi tendon organ make up I_b group of myelinated rapidly conducting sensory nerve fibers.

28. Ans. (a) Mitochondria

Ref: Ganong 25th ed. pg. 36

Mitochondria have their own genome and contain DNA. Human mitochondrial DNA has a circular double stranded molecule containing 16,500 base pairs compared to a billion in nuclear DNA. Mitochondria are derived from ovum, their inheritance is maternal. Since, the repair mechanism of DNA is poor, mutation rate for mitochondrial DNA is 10 times more than nuclear DNA.

29. Ans. (a) All or none law

Ref: Ganong 25th ed. pg. 92

- The action potential fails to occur if stimulus is subthreshold. It occurs with constant amplitude regardless of strength of stimulus if the stimulus provided is above the threshold intensity. This is called "All or none law".
- Anodal current producing hyperpolarization is called electrotonic potential. The magnitude of response decreases as the distance between the stimulating and recording electrodes is increased.
- During Absolute refractory period no stimulus irrespective of strength will excite the nerve. However, during relative refractory period, the stronger stimuli can cause excitation.

30. Ans. (a) Increase Calcium Transport *via* L type calcium channels in T-tubule

Ref: Harrison 19th ed. pg. 40-41

- The pathophysiology of malignant hyperthermia involves dysregulation of calcium transport primarily caused by abnormal functioning of Excitation contraction coupling.
- *The EC complex is localized to the T-tubules/Sarcoplasmic reticulum of skeletal muscle.*
- The T-tubule *consists of pentameric L-type Calcium channel* (DHPR) which is a voltage gated calcium channel.
- It is triggered by inhalation of volatile inhalational agents and NM blocking agent succinylcholine.
- Clinical manifestation is intraoperative hyperthermia, respiratory acidosis, hyperkalemia and DIC.
- DOC for management is Dantrolene sodium.

Extra Mile

Basic difference between T & L type Ca^{++} channels

L-type Ca^{++} Channels	T-type Ca^{++} Channels
• Long lasting	• Short acting
• Also known as DHP receptors	• T for "transient"
• HVA (High voltage activated receptors)	• LVG (Low voltage Gated)
• Found in ▪ Skeletal muscle ▪ Smooth muscle ▪ Bone (osteoblasts) ▪ Ventricular myocytes (responsible for prolonged action potential in cardiac cell; also termed DHP receptors) ▪ Dendrites and dendritic spines of cortical neurons	• Found in ▪ Neurons ▪ Cells that have pacemaker activity ▪ Bone (osteocytes)

31. Ans. (c) Calcium

Ref: Ganong 25th ed. pg. 46

- *Exocytosis is a calcium dependent process* where vesicles containing material for export are targeted to the cell membrane.
- This area of fusion then breaks down leaving the contents of vesicle outside the cell membrane intact.
- The reverse of exocytosis is called *endocytosis* and is mediated by the protein *Clathrin.*

32. Ans. (b) Z line

Ref: Ganong 25th ed. pg. 115

- Choices a and d are ruled out as bands are not present in smooth muscles.
- Smooth muscles lack visible cross striations. Actin and myosin are present and they slide on each other to produce contractions.
- *Instead of Z lines, smooth muscles contain dense bodies in the cytoplasm* and are attached to cell membrane. They act by binding alpha actinin to actin filaments.

Smooth muscles are different from cardiac fibers due to the following reasons:

1. Absence of striations
2. Presence of dense bodies at site of Z lines
3. Absent troponins
4. Less extensive sarcoplasmic reticulum
5. Energy generation via glycolysis and few mitochondria

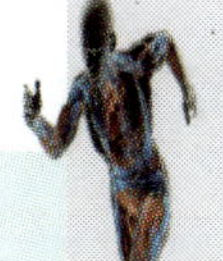

Actin and myosin contractile proteins are not organized into sarcomeres; instead the fibers attach to the dense bodies under the cell membrane	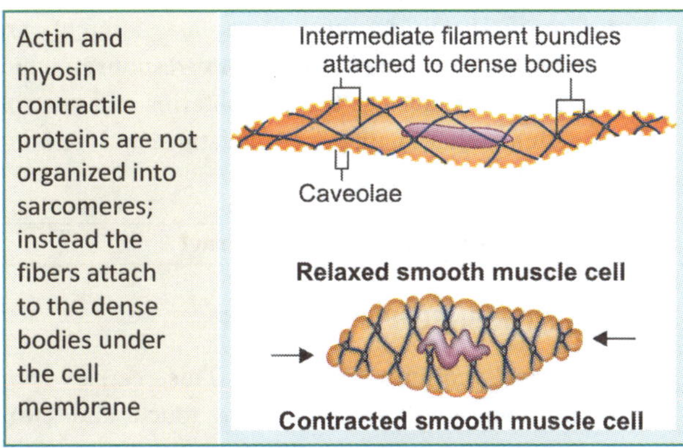

33. Ans. (d) Actin

Ref: Ganong 25th ed. pg. 39

Molecular motors are involved in movement of proteins, organelles and cell parts to all parts of the cell. There are three super families of molecular motors.

1.	Kinesin
2.	Dynein
3.	Myosin

These molecular motors connect to cargo at one end and actin filaments forming microtubules at the other end.

Extra Mile

Functions of actin
1. Cellular contraction
2. Cell migration
3. Cell signaling
4. Backbone for muscle contraction

34. Ans. (b) One molecule goes in and other molecule goes out

Ref: Ganong 25th ed. pg. 48

Uniport	Transport only one substance
Symport	More than one substance
Antiport	Exchange substance one for the other

Extra Mile

- *Na-H antiporter in distal convoluted tubule*
- The malfunction of this antiporter leads to inability to absorb salt leading to salt wasting. The inability to excrete Hydrogen ions leads to metabolic acidosis called Renal tubular acidosis type 1.

35. Ans. (b) Secondary active transport of glucose in intestine

Ref: Ganong Physiology: 25th ed. pg. 432

SGLT 1 is located in GIT and SGLT 2 in proximal convoluted tubules of kidney.

Extra Mile

Type of SGLT	Major sites	Functions: transport of
SGLT 1	Small intestine, heart, trachea, kidney (S3)	Na, glucose galactose
SGLT 2	Kidney (S1, S2)	Na, glucose
SGLT 3	Small intestine, uterus, lung, thyroid, testis	Na
SGLT 4	Small intestine, kidney, liver, stomach, lung	Glucose, mannose
SGLT 5	Kidney	Unknown
SGLT 6	Spinal cord, kidney, brain, small intestine	Myoinositol, glucose

36. Ans. (c) Terminal bronchiole

Ref: Ganong 25th ed. pg. 623

The cellular transition from conducting airways to alveoli (shown below in the image) and the amount smooth muscle decreases progressively.

Between two close options the answer is terminal bronchiole as respiratory bronchiole is more distal and has less cartilage.

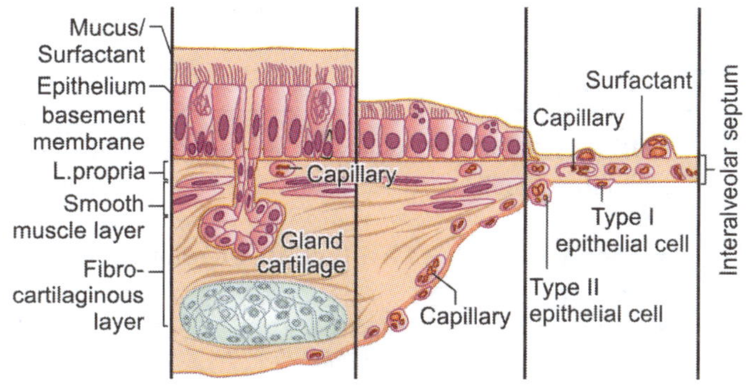

37. Ans. (b) Phosphocreatinine

Ref: Ganong 25th ed. pg. 108–109

During a 100 meter sprint that takes about 10 seconds anaerobic synthesis of ATP occurs. This supply comes from Phosphocreatine.

Distance covered	Contribution from anaerobic pathways
100 meter dash	85%
2 mile race	20%
Long distance race 60 minutes	5%

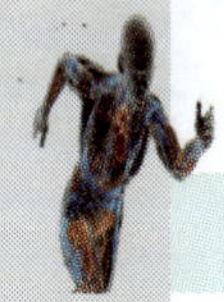

ENERGY SOURCES IN WORKING MUSCLES

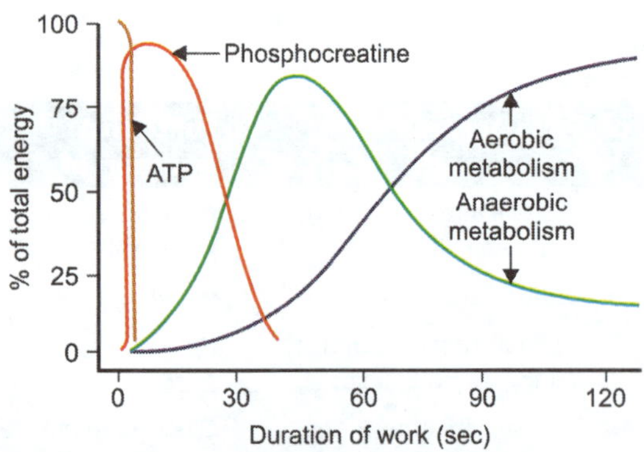

COMPARISON BETWEEN SYSTEMS

Characteristic	ATP-PC*	Lactic acid	Aerobic
Fuel/s	ATP stores and Phosphocreatine	Glycogen	CHO, Fats Then Protein
ATP production per molecule of energy source	Less than 1	Approx. 2	Glucose = 38 Fats = 460
Speed/rate of ATP production	Small amounts instantly	Limited amounts rapidly	Unlimited amount slowly
Intensity	Maximal effort	Near maximal (85–95%)	Sub-maximal (<85%)
Duration	0–10 secs	30 secs–2 minutes	5 minutes +
Oxygen requirements	Nil	Nil	O_2 required

* *ATP-Phosphocreatine*

38. Ans. (b) Ib

GOLGI TENDON ORGAN is embedded within the musculotendinous junction (90%) and in the tendon itself (10%).

- **They are stimulated by: Increased tension at muscle tendon**
- **Afferent:** Ib fiber (myelinated).
- Mediates inverse stretch reflex

Extra Mile

Reflex	Afferent fiber	Stimulus	Response
Golgi tendon reflex	Ib	Muscle contraction	Relaxation of the muscle
Stretch reflex	Ia	Muscle is stretched	Contraction of the muscle
Flexor – withdrawal reflex	II, III, and IV	Pain, touch	Ipsilateral flexion, contralateral extension

- Group III/IV afferent fibers are afferent arm of cardiovascular ventilatory reflex responses which are mediated in nucleus tractus solitarius and ventrolateral medulla. They facilitate central fatigue and are important in endurance sports.

39. Ans. (b) Lateral spinothalamic tract

SOMATOSENSORY PATHWAYS

- **Dorasal column pathway:** This carries pressure, vibration, proprioception, fine touch and two-point discrimination.
- **Anterior spinothalamic tract:** This carries crude touch and pressure (less role).
- **Lateral spinothalamic tract:** This carries pain and temperature.

40. Ans. (c) Intestine

***Ref:** Ganong, 25th ed. pg. 478; Harper 30th ed. pg. 518*

	Major site of expression	Proposed functions
SGLT1	Intestine and kidney	Glucose reabsorption in intestine and kidney
SGLT2	Kidney (PCT)	Low affinity and high selectivity for glucose
SGLT3	Small intestine, skeletal muscle	Glucose activated Na^+ channel

Extra Mile

- SGLT2 inhibitors, also called *gliflozins*, are used in the treatment of type 2 diabetes.
- Examples include dapagliflozin, canagliflozin and empagliflozin.

41. Ans. (b) Smooth endoplasmic reticulum

- The smooth endoplasmic reticulum is continuous with the rough endoplasmic reticulum and does not contain any ribosomes. Although it has several functions, the sER is specialized for the production of steroid hormones in cells of the adrenal cortex.
- Remember that cholesterol is the main precursor for steroid hormones produced in the adrenal cortex and the gonads.

42. Ans. (b) A delta

***Ref:** Miller's Anaesthesia, 7th ed. pg. 921-922*

Susceptibility order of nerve fibers are as follows:

- **Pressure:** Aα > Aβ > Ag > Aδ > B > C

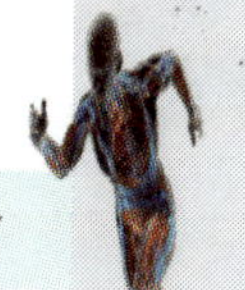

- **Local anesthetic:** Susceptibility order Aγ & Aδ>> Aα & Aβ>> B>> C (Some people with zero patient experience are quoting this as wrong answer and create controversy).
- **Hypoxia:** Susceptibility order B > A > C
- **Paresthesias** (inappropriate sensations such as burning or prickling) usually seen when A-delta is involved.

43. Ans. (c) Minimum strength of stimulus to produce action potential

- **Rheobase:** The ***minimum strength*** of a stimulus, which is able to produce AP in an excitable tissue (e.g. Nerve, muscle), regardless of the duration it takes.
- **Utilization time:** Minimum ***time (duration)*** for which ***the rheobase*** has to be applied for excitation of tissue.
- **Chronaxie:** Minimum ***time (duration)*** for which a stimulus ***double the rheobase*** has to be applied for excitation of tissue.

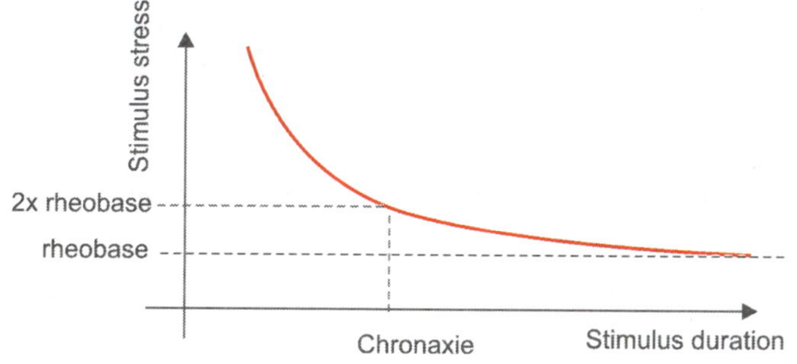

44. (a) Insulin

Ref: Quantitative Human Physiology; An Introduction. pg. 191-92

Insulin has two major roles: Sends glucose and potassium both intracellular, thereby decreasing their level (i.e. hypoglycaemia and hypokalemia).

45. Ans. (c) Facilitated diffusion

Ref: Quantitative Human Physiology; An Introduction. pg. 126-27

Since the transport of glucose to placenta is via GLUT, it is called a facilitated transfer of glucose.

	Simple diffusion	Facilitated diffusion
Energy	Not required	Not required
Carrier molecule	Not involved	Involved
Saturation	Not saturable (No Tm)	Saturable (has a Tm)
Follows	Fick's law of diffusion	Enzyme-substrate kinetics of Michaelis menten
Example:	O_2 and CO_2 exchange in alveoli	Glucose transport by glucose transporters (GLUT)

46. Ans. (d) Increase chloride influx

Ref: Quantitative Human Physiology; An Introduction. pg. 259-60

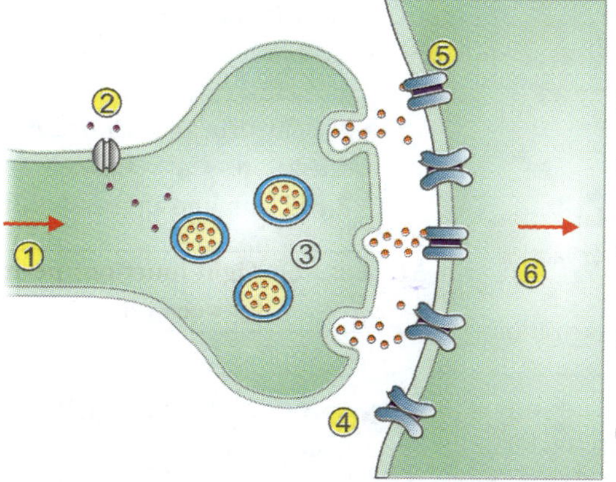

FIGURE: Summary of neurotransmission

- Most essential step in neurotransmission: Depolarization of neurons at pre-synapse

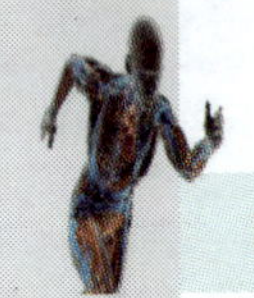

TABLE: Concept of EPSP and IPSP

EPSP (Excitatory post-synaptic potential)	IPSP (Inhibitory post-synaptic potential)
Excitatory Neurotransmitter: Glutamate and Aspartate	**Inhibitory Neurotransmitter: GABA and Glycine**
Due to influx of Calcium, Na^+ and closure of K^+ channel	Due to influx of Chloride (Cl^-) and efflux of K^+
• Fast EPSP: Na^+ and Ca^+ Influx ▪ Latency: 0.5 ms • Slow EPSP: K^+ channel closure ▪ Latency: 100 - 500 ms • Late slow EPSP: K^+ channel closure ▪ Latency: 1–5 sec	• **FAST IPSP:** Cl^- entry ▪ Latency: 0.5 ms • **Slow IPSP:** K^+ efflux/ closure of channel ▪ Latency: 100–500 ms

47. Ans. (c) After hyperpolarization

Ref: Quantitative Human Physiology; An Introduction, pg. 215-16

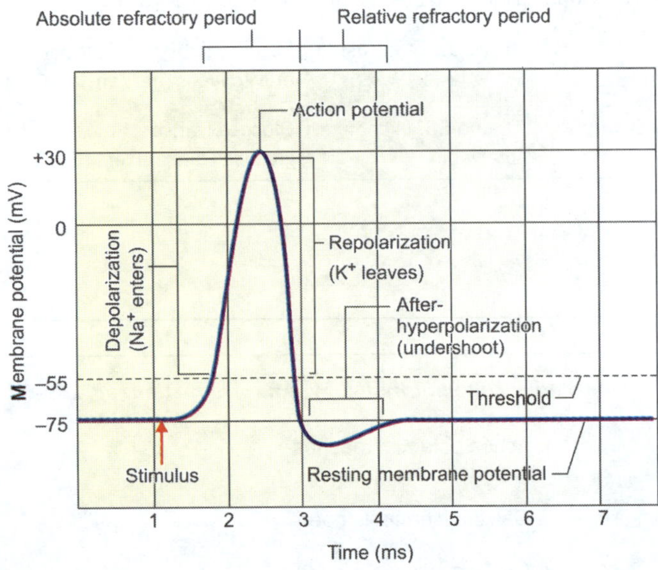

- Maximum excitation is seen after hyperpolarization state. In this phase cell is ready for another action potential, **given just the threshold stimulus.**
- Cell is in absolute refractory phase in depolarization phase. In this phase no matter how much stimulus is given, there will be no further AP.
- During repolarization phase, cell is in relative refractory phase. Action potential may ensue, if a **higher strength** of stimulus is provided.

48. Ans. (c) By diffusion in interstitial fluid

Ref: Ganong, 25th ed. pg. 752

Modalities of Communication Between Cells

Action across synaptic cleft	Synaptic transmission
Directly from cell to cell	Gap junctions
By diffusion in interstitial fluid	Paracrine and autocrine
Endocrine	By circulating body fluids

49. Ans. (a) Using energy in ATP to extrude 3 Na^+ out of cells in exchange of taking two K^+ into the cell

- Na^+ K^+ ATPase catalyse the hydrolysis of ATP to adenosine diphosphate and uses energy to extrude three Na^+ from the cell and take two K^+ into the cell for each molecule of ATP hydrolyzed.
- It is therefore said to have a coupling ratio of 3:2
- Its activity is inhibited by Ouabain and related digitalis glycosides which are used for CHF.
- Active transport of sodium and potassium is a major energy consuming process in the body. In body it accounts for 24% of energy utilized by cells and 70% of energy utilized by neurons.

Hormones increasing Na-K ATPase activity are

- Thyroid hormones
- Aldosterone
- Insulin

50. Ans. (c) Dystrophin

Ref: Ganong, 25th ed. pg. 56

Calcium binding proteins are:

- Troponin = Involved in contraction of skeletal muscle and cardiac muscle.
- Calmodulin = Helps in phosphorylation of myosin and muscle contraction
- Calbindin = Vitamin D dependant Calcium binding proteins
- Calcineurin = Calmodulin activated protein which inactivates Ca^{++} channels and *plays role in activating T Cells.* Immunosuppressive drugs can inhibit it.

51. Ans. (c) Tight junctions permit passage of some solutes between cells

Ref: Ganong, 25th ed. pg. 41

- Desmosomes help to hold the cells together. Hence, choice a is wrong
- Hemi-desmosomes and focal adhesions attach cells to basal lamina. Hence, choice b is wrong
- Gap junction is a cytoplasmic tunnel for diffusion of small molecules <1000 Da between two neighbouring cells. Hence, choice d is wrong.

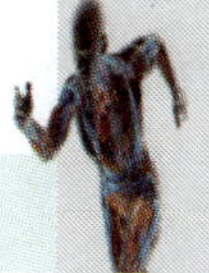

- *The function of tight junctions is:*
  1. Passage of some ions and solutes in between adjacent cells called para-cellular pathway.
  2. Prevent movement of proteins in the plane of membrane.

52. Ans. (d) Chloride inside cells is more than outside cells

Ref: Ganong, 25th ed. pg. 5 & 9

Composition of Body Fluids and Electrolytes into Compartments

Intracellular fluid	40%
Interstitial fluid	15%
Blood, plasma	5%

Concentration of ions inside/outside mammalian spinal motor neurons in mEq/dl

Ions	Inside cell	Outside cell
Chloride	9	125
Potassium	150	5.5
Sodium	15	150

53. Ans. (d) Multipolar cells

Ref: Ganong, 25th ed. pg. 87

Unipolar cells	Invertebrate cells
Bipolar cells	Bipolar cells of retina
Pseudo-unipolar cells	Ganglion cell of dorsal root
Multi-polar cells	*Motor neuron of spinal cord* *Pyramidal cell of hippocampus* *Purkinje cell of cerebellum*

54. Ans. (b) A fibers are more sensitive to pressure than C fibers

Ref: Miller's Anesthesia, pg. 77, 922

Susceptibility to	Most susceptible	Intermediate	Least susceptible
Pressure	*A*	*B*	*C*
Local anesthesia	$A\gamma > A\delta > A\alpha$	*B*	*C*
Hypoxia	*B*	*A*	*C*

55. Ans. (a) Phase 1 of depolarization is due to opening of voltage gated sodium channels

Phase 0	Rapid depolarization due to opening of voltage sensitive sodium channels
Phase 1	*Rapid repolarization* due to *closure of sodium channels* and opening of one type of K channels
Phase 2	Plateau phase due to slow and prolonged opening of voltage gated calcium channels
Phase 3 and 4	Final repolarization to RMP is due to closure of Ca^{++} channels and a slow delayed increase of K^+ efflux

Since, cardiac muscle remains in refractory period until phase 4, tetanic contractions which can occur in skeletal muscle cannot occur in cardiac muscle.

56. Ans. (b) Tropomyosin

Ref: Ganong, 25th ed. pg. 101

- Tropomyosin acts as a relaxing protein at rest by covering the sites where myosin binds to action
- Dystrophin is a sarcolemmal protein providing calcium input to sarcoplasmic reticulum. This Ca^{++} is useful in coupling of actin-myosin complex.

57. Ans. (b) Plasticity

Ref: Ganong, 25th ed. pg. 118

- Smooth muscle has 20% of myosin content and 100 fold difference in ATP use when compared to skeletal muscle, yet it can generate similar force per cross sectional area. *This special feature of smooth muscle is called as plasticity where it behaves like a viscous mass rather than rigid structured tissue.*
- An example of plasticity is that urinary bladder tension rises very slowly when urine amount is minimal. But when the amount of urine approximates about 150 ml, the bladder can contract forcefully.

58. Ans. (d) Guanylyl cyclase

Ref: Ganong, 25th ed. pg. 59

- Guanylyl cyclase is an enzyme that catalyses the formation of cGMP.
- cGMP is important for vision in both rods and cones.
- Second messengers bring about short term changes by altering enzyme function, triggering exocytosis and can also lead to alteration of transcription of various genes
- *Examples of secondary messengers*
  - cAMP: Produced by action of adenyl cyclase enzyme and stimulates protein kinase A which catalyses

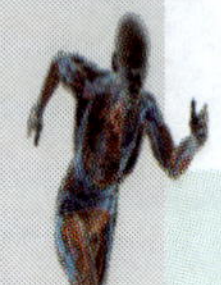

phosphorylation of proteins and altering there activity. For example *cholera toxin increases cAMP levels whereas pertussis toxin inhibits it.*

- IP3: Inositol phosphate diffuses into endoplasmic reticulum and triggers calcium release.
- DAG: Diacyglycerol works with IP3.

59. Ans. (d) Secondary active transport

Ref: Ganong, 25th ed. pg. 48–51

Secondary active transport	Luminal membrane of mucosal cells in small intestine contain a symport that transports glucose into the cell only if sodium binds to protein and transported into cell at the same time
Active transport	Glucose movement from ECF into cytoplasm of the cell *requires carriers and utilises energy* and is called as active transport.
Facilitated diffusion	When *carrier proteins move substances* in the *direction of their chemical or electrical gradients, no energy input is required* and the process is called as facilitated diffusion

60. Ans. (b) Potassium

Ref: Ganong, 22nd ed. BRS Physiology, 4th ed. pg. 11

Ionic Basis of Nerve Resting Membrane Potential

- **RMP:** Resting membrane potential is potential difference across the cell membrane in millivolts, ***which is by convention –70 mV.***
- RMP is established by diffusion potential that results from concentration differences of permeable ions.
- Resting membrane potential (–70 mV) is close to equilibrium potential of K^+ and Cl^- (both-85 mV) and far from the equilibrium potential of Na^+ (+65 mV). ***That means at rest the nerve membrane is more permeable to K^+ than Na^+***
- Na+ is actively transported out of neurons and other cells and K^+ is actively transported into cells, ***but because K^+ permeability at rest is greater than Na^+ permeability, K^+ channels maintain the resting membrane potential.***

61. Ans. (b) Decrease membrane stability of nerves

Ref: Ganong's, 22nd ed. chapter 2.

- A *decrease in extracellular Ca^{++}* concentration *increases the excitability of nerve* and muscle cells by decreasing the amount of depolarization necessary to initiate the action potential.
- Conversely, an increase in extracellular Ca^{++} concentration "stabilizes the membrane" by decreasing excitability.

62. Ans. (d) Acetylcholine

Ref: Ganong's, 25th ed. pg. 259, 266

- Acetylcholine is released at the nerve terminal of all preganglionic neuron, postganglionic parasympathetic ganglion and a few postganglionic sympathetic ganglion(e.g.: Sweat gland and sympathetic vasodilator fibers). The remaining sympathetic postganglionic neuron release norepinephrine.

63. Ans. (c) –40 mV

- *In the dark, the resting membrane potential (RMP) of photoreceptors is –40 mV unlike other* neural receptors where the RMP is about –70 to –80 mV. This is due to dark current'.
- In the dark, the Na^+ channels in the outer segment of photoreceptors are open as they bind with cGMP. So, Na^+ enters into the cell decreasing the RMP.

64. Ans. (d) –12 mV

• Skeletal muscle cells: –95 mV
• Smooth muscle cells: –50 mV
• Astrocytes: –80/–90 mV
• Neurons: –70 mV
• Erythrocytes: –10 to –12 mV

65. Ans. (b) B fibers

Ref: Miller's Anesthesia pg. 77

- In case of hypoxia, first nerve fiber affected is B fibers.
- Nerve fibers in decreasing order of susceptibility in different situations:
  - **Pressure:** A-B-C *(fiber A is most susceptible followed by B and then C in case of Pressure)*
  - **Local anesthetics:** A-B-C *(fiber A is most susceptible followed by B and C in case of LA)*
  - ***Hypoxia: B-A-C*** *(fiber B is most susceptible followed by A and then C in case of Hypoxia)*
- ***Remember:*** *A and B fibers are Myelinated and C fibers are unmyelinated.*

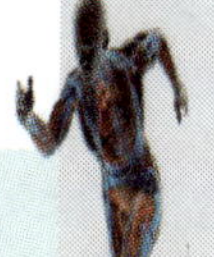

66. Ans. (a) Alpha

Ref: Ganong, 25th ed. pg. 95, Miller's Anesthesia pg. 77

Group		Myelination	Conduction velocity (m/s)	Function
Erlanger and Gasser	Lloyd & Hunt			
A α	I	Heavily myelinated	70–120 maximum	Proprioception Motor supply to skeletal muscle (extrafusal to muscle spindle)
A β	II	Myelinated	25–70	Touch, kinesthetic sense, pressure
A γ	-	Slightly myelinated	15–30	Motor supply to intrafusal muscle fibers (muscle spindle)
A δ	III	Partially myelinated	5–30	Pain, temperature, pressure, touch (cold/font sharp pain)
B	–	Partially myelinated	3–14	Preganglionic autonomic fibers
C	IV	Un-myelinated	0.2–2	Pain, temperature pressure, post-ganglionic autonomic fibers (Hot temp/slow, visceral pain)

67. Ans. (c) Myelinated B fibers

Ref: Ganong, 25th ed. pg. 94

- *Myelinated B fibers are preganglionic, autonomic.*
- Unmyelinated C fibers are postganglionic.
- Refer to the table in above explanation.

68. Ans. (b) Disruption of conduction

Ref: Maheswari Orthopedics, 3rd ed. pg. 51

Neuropraxia *refers to physiological disruption of conduction only*. No anatomical disruption is seen.

- *Both axon and sheath are intact.*
- **No structural change** *or* **degeneration** *occurs in case of neuropraxia.*
- Neuronal degeneration is seen in:
  - Crush nerve injury
  - Fetal development
  - Senescence

Extra Mile

Axontemesis

- Axon and myelin sheath disrupted but endoneural perineurium and epineurium sheath is intact.
- Neural degeneration present

Neurontemesis

- Complete division of nerve
- Axon & neural tube (i.e. perineurium, epineurium, and endoneural sheath) are divided.
- Neural degeneration present.

69. Ans. (b) Passive diffusion

Ref: Ganong's 25th ed. pg. 634-635

- Exchange of oxygen and CO_2 across the lung capillary and alveoli is passive diffusion.
- Diffusion of O_2 occur from alveoli to capillary (towards the pressure gradient), and diffusion of CO_2 is in opposite direction *(from capillary to alveoli).*
- *Facilitated diffusion requires special carrier proteins.*

Extra Mile

- Rate of diffusion is directly proportional to:
  - Pressure gradient
  - Surface area of respiratory membrane
  - Solubility of gas
- Rate of diffusion is inversely proportional to:
  - Thickness of respiratory membrane
  - Molecular weight of gas

70. Ans. (d) C-fibers

Ref: Ganong, 25th ed. pg. 94; Guyton Physiology, 11th ed. pg. 576-577

- **Pain** is carried by A δ and C-fibers
- **General classification of Nerve Fibers**
  - In the general classification, the fibers are divided into types A, B and C.
    - Type A fibers are further subdivided into α, β, γ, and δ fibers.
  - Type A fibers are the typical large and medium-sized myelinated fibers of spinal nerves.
  - Type B fibers are Myelinated, Pre-ganglionc autonomic.
  - Type C fibers are the small unmyelinated nerve fibers that conduct impulses at low velocities.

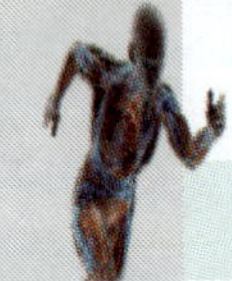

Nerve Fiber Type and Function

Fiber type	Function
A fiber	
α	Proprioception; Somatic motor
β	Touch, pressure, motor
γ	Motor to muscle spindle
δ	Pain, cold, touch
B fiber	Preganglionic Autonomic
C fiber	
Dorsal root	Pain, temperature, reflex responses
Sympathetic root	Postganglionic sympathetic

71. Ans. (b) Anterior spinothalamic tract

Ref: Guyton, 12th ed. pg. 573-74

- *Fibers* for crude touch (itch and tickle): C- Fiber
- *Pathway* for crude touch: Anterior spinothalamic tract
- Pathway for pain and temperature: Lateral spinothalamic tract
- Pathway for proprioception, fine touch, vibration, joint position is be: Posterior column/Dorsal column.

72. Ans. (b) H band

Ref: Ganong's, 25th ed. pg. 101

- ***The area between two adjacent Z lines is called a sarcomere***
- The thick filaments, which are about twice the diameter of the thin filaments, are made up of myosin; the thin filaments are made up of actin, tropomyosin and troponin
- *The lighter H bands in the center of the A bands are the regions where, when the muscle is relaxed, the thin filaments do not overlap the thick filaments.*
- The Z lines transect the fibrils and connect to the thin filaments. If a transverse section through the A band is examined under the electron microscope, each thick filament is seen to be surrounded by six thin filaments in a regular hexagonal pattern.
- Here is a quick reminder of all the structures involved in muscle contraction:
  - **Myofibril:** A cylindrical organelle running the length of the muscle fiber, containing actin and myosin filaments.
  - **Sarcomere:** The functional unit of the myofibril, divided into I, A and H bands.
  - **Actin**: A thin, contractile protein filament, containing 'active' or 'binding' sites.
  - **Myosin**: A thick, contractile protein filament, with protrusions known as myosin heads.
  - **Tropomyosin:** An actin-binding protein which regulates *muscle relaxation.*
  - **Troponin:** A complex of three proteins, regulating muscle contraction.

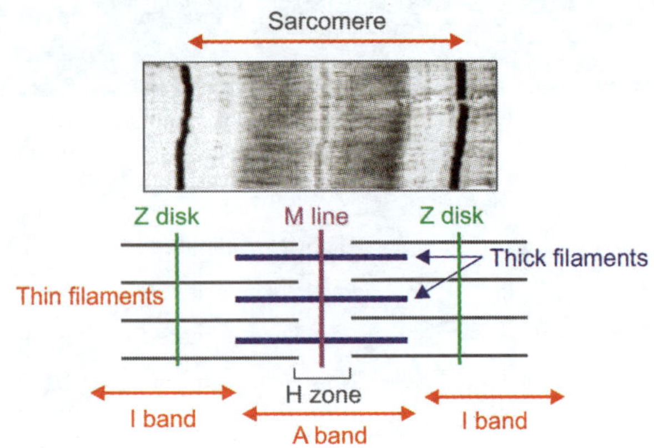

RENAL PHYSIOLOGY

73. Ans. (b) Glucose

Ref: Berne and Levy Physiology, 6th ed. pg. 1000

- The image shows T_mG which is a transport maximum for glucose tubular transport. In adult human, value is about 375 mg/min.
- Normally, filtered glucose is about 125 mg/min.
- The PCT is responsible for reabsorbing most of the glucose, amino acids, and small peptides that enter the ultrafiltrate.
- The PCT contains numerous secondary active, sodium-coupled transporters for glucose (SGLT2) and amino acids.

74. Ans. (a) A

Ref: Ganong 26th ed. pg. 673

- Proximal tubules reabsorb about 65% of water, sodium, potassium and chloride, 100% of glucose, 100% amino acids, and 85–90% of bicarbonate.
- This reabsorption occurs due to the presence of channels on the basolateral and apical membranes.
- There are two routes through which reabsorption can take place: Paracellular and transcellular.
- The transcellular route is transporting solutes through a cell. The paracellular route is transporting solutes through the intercellular space.
- The driving force for the reabsorption in the PCT is sodium.

75. Ans. (c) Thick ascending limb of loop of Henle

Ref: Ganong 26th ed. pg. 670

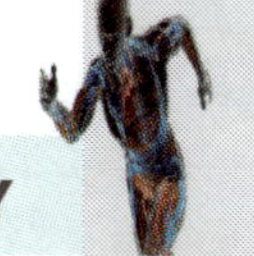

Sodium potassium chloride cotransporter is present in Thick ascending limb of loop of Henle. Disease that occurs due to malfunction of this transporter is Bartter syndrome.

TABLE: Transport proteins involved in the movement of Na^+ and Cl^- across the apical membranes of renal tubular cells

Site	Apical transporter	Function
Proximal tubule	Na/glucose CT	Na^+ uptake, glucose uptake
	Na^+/P_1 CT	Na^+ uptake, P_1 uptake
	Na^+ amino acid CT	Na^+ uptake, amino acid uptake
	Na/lactate CT	Na^+ uptake, lactate uptake
	Na/H exchanger	Na^+ uptake, H^+ extrusion
	Cl/base exchanger	Cl^- uptake
Thick ascending limb	Na–K–2Cl CT	Na^+ uptake, Cl^- uptake, K^+ uptake
	Na/H exchanger	Na^+ uptake, H^+ extrusion
	K^+ channels	K^+ extrusion (recycling)
Distal convoluted tubule	NaCl CT	Na^+ uptake, Cl^- uptake
Collecting duct	Na^+ channel (ENaC)	Na^+ uptake

76. Ans. (b) DCT

Ref: Ganong 26th ed. pg. 670

The sodium chloride co transporter is present in Distal convoluted tubule. The disease that occurs due to malfunction of this cotransporter is Gitelman syndrome.

77. Ans. (b) Proximal convoluted tubule

Ref: pg. 293, Harrison 20th edition

Proximal tubular reabsorption of albumin by endocytosis includes both nonspecific fluid-phase endocytosis as well as receptor-mediated endocytosis. Two important proteins involved are megalin and cubilin.

78. Ans. (b) 6–12

Ref: Harrison 20th ed. pg. 316

Normal anion gap is Sodium minus sum of chloride and bicarbonate.

$$\text{Anion gap} = Na^+ - (Cl^- + HCO_3^-)$$

It is approximately 6-12 mmol/L with average of 10 mmol/L

79. Ans. (a) Upper part of PCT

Ref: Ganong 25th ed. pg. 680

Glucose, amino acids and bicarbonate are absorbed along with sodium in early portion of proximal tubule. Essentially all of the glucose is reabsorbed and no more than few mg will reappear in urine. The renal threshold for glucose is the plasma level at which glucose appears in the urine. For venous blood is blood level of 180 mg/dL.

80. Ans. (d) Remains unchanged

Ref: Ganong 25th ed. pg. 686-687

Water diuresis is increased urine flow rate after drinking water. The increased water intake leads to development of reduced secretion of ADH from the neurohypophysis. This decreases the water permeability of collecting duct and distal tubule leading to increased water loss initially followed by constant water load being excreted. *However, there is no change in urinary excretion of solutes in water diuresis unlike osmotic diuresis which leads to increase of urine flow as well as excretion of solutes.*

Comparison of water and osmotic diuresis

Water diuresis	Osmotic diuresis
Increased urine flow rate (No change in urine excretion of solutes)	Increases urine flow rate as well as the excretion of solutes
Causes: • Excess ingestion of water • Lack of ADH • Defect in ADH receptors in Distal segment of nephron (nephrogenic diabetes insipidus)	Causes: • Increase plasma glucose level (DM) • Increase level of poorly reabsorbed solutes/anions • Diuretic drugs (Lasix)
Diuresis is mainly due to decrease in water reabsorption in distal segment of nephron. No change to the water reabsorbed proximally	Diuresis is mainly due to decrease in reabsorption of solute in PCT or LOH. Decrease solute reabsorption results in decrease in water reabsorption proximally as well as distally

81. Ans. (a) Lowers blood volume

- Pressure diuresis lowers arterial pressure by lowering blood volume and, thereby, lowering cardiac output.
- All of the other choices do lower arterial pressure, but are not caused by pressure diuresis.

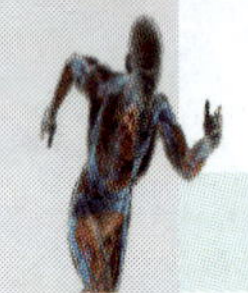

82. Ans. (b) DCT mainly

Diuretic class	Drugs	MOA	Site of action
Osmotic diuretic	Mannitol	Inhibit water and solute reabsorption	All part of tubule, ***but mainly proximal tubule***
Loop diuretics	Furosemide Torsemide	Inhibit Na^+-K^+-$2Cl^-$ co-transport	Thick ascending loop of henle
Thiazide diuretic	Hydrochlorothiazide Benzthiazide Chlorthalidone Indapamide	Inhibit Na^+- Cl^- co-transport	Distal tubule
K^+ sparing diuretic	Spironolactone Triamterene Amiloride	Decrease Na^+ reabsorption Decrease K^+ secretion	Collecting tubule
Carbonic anhydrase inhibitor	Acetazolamide	Inhibit H^+ secretion and HCO_3 reabsorption, which reduces Na^+ reabsorption	Proximal tubule

83. Ans. (a) Adrenal

Ref: Modern Nutrition in Health and Disease, pg. 913

Vitamin C content of human Tissues

Organ/tissue	Vitamin C concentration	Organ/tissue	Vitamin C concentration
Pituitary gland	40–50	Lungs	7
Adrenal gland	30–40	Skeletal muscle	3–4
Eye lens	25–31	Testes	3
Liver	10–16	Thyroid	2
Brain	13–15	Cerebrospinal fluid	3.8
Pancreas	10–15	Plasma	0.4–1
Spleen	10–15	Saliva	9.07–0.09
Kidneys	5–15		

84. Ans. (c) Intercalated cells

Ref: Ganong, 25th ed. pg. 672

Lacis cells	Are cells that lie between macula densa (Sensor for distal tubule) and renin secreting granular cells
Principal cells	Seen in epithelium of collecting ducts and are involved in sodium absorption and vasopressin mediated water re-absorbtion
Intercalated cells	*Seen in collecting ducts and distal tubules and are concerned with acid secretion and HCO_3 transport.*
Granular cells	Seen in JG apparatus and secrete renin

85. Ans. (a) Tubulo-glomerular feedback

Ref: Ganong, 25th ed. pg. 682

Tubulo-glomerular feedback	Mantains the constancy of load delivered to distal tubule and the sensor for this response is macula densa
Glomerulo-tubular feedback	Decrease in GFR promotes solute reabsorption in proximal tubule and thick ascending limb of Henle
Reno-renal Reflex	Increase in ureteral pressure in one kidney leads to decrease in efferent nerve activity to contralateral kidney. This permits an increase in excretion of sodium and water
Filtration fraction	Ratio of GFR to renal plasma flow with normal fraction of 0.16–0.20 In hypotension GFR is lesser than renal plasma flow because of efferent arteriolar constriction

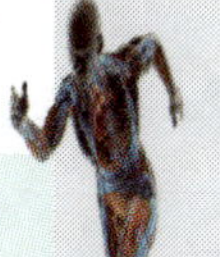

86. Ans. (c) Alcohol

Ref: Ganong, 25th ed./Table 38-1 pg. 696

Factors Affecting Vasopressin Secretion

Increased vasopressin secretion	Decreased vasopressin secretion
• Increased effective osmotic pressure of plasma • Decreased ECF volume • Pain, emotion, stress Nausea vomiting • Tumours leading to SIADH- oat cell cancer of lung, • Carcinoid tumours	• Decreased effective osmotic pressure of plasma • Increased ECF volume • Alcohol

87. Ans. (b) Carbonic acid

Ref: Ganong, 25th ed. pg. 717; Indu Khurana

Buffers in whole blood

Buffer Type	Buffering capacity (%)
Haemoglobin	35%
Bicarbonate	53% (plasma 35% + RBC 18%)
Organic phosphates	3%
Plasma protein	7%
Inorganic	2%

Most abundant buffer in the body is proteins.

Most important buffer in the body is bicarbonate.

88. Ans. (b) Proximal convoluted tubular cells

Ref: Contemporary Nephrology, 1st ed. pg. 164 and Indu Khurana

Granular cells	Produce renin
Proximal convoluted cells	Contain 1 alpha hydroxylase that is essential to produce vitamin D_3
Mesangial cells	Regulate RBC leakage
Peritubular cells	Produce erythropoietin

89. Ans. (a) 20%

Ref: Guyton's Physiology, 11th ed. pg. 316

- *GFR Is About 20 Per Cent of the Renal Plasma Flow.*
- In an average adult GFR is about 125 ml/min, or 180 L/day.
- Renal plasma flow is 650 ml/min
- The *filtration fraction* is calculated as follows: GFR/Renal plasma flow
- Therefore, $\frac{125 \text{ ml/min}}{650 \text{ ml/min}} = 0.2$
- The fraction of the renal plasma flow that is filtered (the filtration fraction) averages about 0.2; this means that about 20 per cent of the plasma flowing through the kidney is filtered through the glomerular capillaries.

Extra Mile

- The entire plasma volume is only about 3 liters, whereas the GFR is about 180 L/day, the entire plasma can be filtered and processed about 60 times each day.

90. Ans. (a) Aldosterone in collecting ducts

Ref: Guyton, 10th ed. pg. 290, 304

Hormones and their site of Action

Hormones	Site of action in kidney
Angiotensin II	Constricts afferent arterioles, helps to reduce GFR
Aldosterone	Cortical collecting duct & distal tubules
ADH	Medullary collecting duct
ANP	Collecting duct

91. Ans. (a) Collecting duct

Ref: Ganong, 23rd ed. pg. 648

- Aldosterone is secreted from adrenal cortex.
- Action of aldosterone is localized to distal tubule and collecting duct.
- Mechanism: Stimulates Na^+K^+ ATPase at basolateral end, which generate gradient for movement of sodium ion from apical membrane causing an increase in sodium reabsorption.

92. Ans. (b) HCO_3

Ref: Ganong, 25th ed. pg. 641-44

- CO_2 is transported in blood in 3 forms:
  1. **As HCO_3**- CO_2 is **mainly transported** in bicarbonate form ~ 70%. When CO_2 diffuses into RBC, it reacts chemically with water and with help of enzyme carbonic anhydrase it is converted into $HCO_3^- + H^+$
  $CO_2 + H_2O \rightarrow HCO_3 + H^+$
  2. **As dissolved CO_2:** 6–7% of CO_2 transport
  3. **As carbamino compound of Hb and other plasma proteins**: 20% of CO_2 transport.

93. Ans. (d) Sensing of NaCl concentration in macula densa

Ref: Guyton, 11th ed. pg. 323-324

- To perform the function of auto regulation, the kidneys have a feedback mechanism known as tubulo-glomerular feedback which links changes in sodium chloride concentration at the macula densa (tubular component) with the control of renal arteriolar resistance.

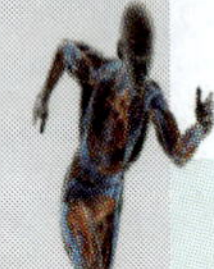

- **Macula densa**
  - It is the short segment of renal tubule *at the end of thick ascending limb* & continues into distal tubule.
  - It contains *specialized group of epithelial cells* in the distal tubule *that comes in contact with the efferent and particularly afferent arteriole.*
  - Juxta glomerular apparatus consists of macula densa (in DCT) and JG cells in afferent and efferent arterioles.
  - The macula densa senses the changes in sodium chloride concentration
  - The Na^+ and Cl^- enter the macula densa cells via the Na^+ –K^+ –$2Cl^-$ cotransporter.

94. Ans. (d) Na^+

Ref: Guyton Physiology, 11th ed. pg. 55

- Sodium-hydrogen counter-transport occurs in several tissues.
- An important example is in the proximal tubules of the kidneys, where sodium ions move from the lumen of the tubule to the interior of the tubular cell, while hydrogen ions are counter transported into the tubule lumen.

95. Ans. (a) PCT mainly

Ref: Renal Physiology, 5th ed. pg. 168

Diuretic class	Drugs	MOA	Site of action
Osmotic diuretic	Mannitol	Inhibit water and solute reabsorption	All part of tubule, ***but mainly proximal tubule***
Loop diuretics	Furosemide Torsemide	Inhibit Na^+-K^+-$2Cl^-$ co-transport	Thick ascending loop of henle
Thiazide diuretic	Hydrochlorthiazide Benzthiazide Chlorthalidone Indapamide	Inhibit Na^+- Cl^- co-transport	Distal tubule
K+ sparing diuretic	Spironolactone Triamterene Amiloride	Decrease Na^+ reabsorption Decrease K^+ secretion	Collecting tubule
Carbonic anhydrase inhibitor	Acetazolamide	Inhibit H^+ secretion and HCO_3 reabsorption, which reduces Na^+ reabsorption	Proximal tubule

96. Ans. (a) PCT

Ref: Ganong, 25th ed. pg. 713

- 80-90% of bicarbonate is reabsorbed in PCT.
- Absorption of HCO_3 is indirect (due to secretion of H^+ by PCT)
- $H^+ + HCO_3 \rightarrow H_2CO_3 \rightarrow H_2O + CO_2 \rightarrow CO_2$ diffuses into epithelial cell and generate HCO_3 ion which is then reabsorbed.

Extra Mile

- **PCT reabsorbs:** Na^+, Cl, HCO_3, PO_4, K^+, Glucose and amino acid
- **PCT secretes:** H^+ ion, organic acid and bases (oxalate, urate)
- PCT is highly permeable to water.

97. Ans. (a) Beta stimulation

Ref: Harrison, 19th ed. pg. 1613

- The Renin-Angiotensin-Aldosterone System (RAAS) contributes to the regulation of arterial pressure primarily *via* the vasoconstrictor properties of angiotensin II and the sodium-retaining properties of aldosterone.

There are Three Primary Stimuli for Renin Secretion

1. Decreased NaCl transport in the distal portion of the thick ascending limb of the loop of Henle.
2. Decreased pressure or stretch within the renal afferent arteriole (baroreceptor mechanism)
3. **Sympathetic nervous system stimulation of renin-secreting cells via β1 adrenoreceptors.**

Conversely, RAAS can be Inhibited by

- Increased NaCl transport in the thick ascending limb of the loop of Henle
- Increased stretch within the renal afferent arteriole
- β1 receptor blockade.

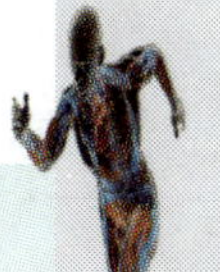

98. Ans. (b) Sodium

Ref: Ganong, 22nd ed. pg. 717

- Hyperosmolarity at renal medulla is due to counter current mechanism acting at loop of henle.
- Maximum osmotic gradient is 1200–1400 mOsm/L found in the inner part of medulla at pelvic tip.
- Prime driving force (initiating event) for the counter-current multiplier system is active reabsorption of Na^+ from thick ascending limb.
- **Renal medullary hyperosmolarity is due to:**
  1. **NaCl** (most important factor causing hyperosmolarity)
  2. Urea
  3. Potassium

99. Ans. (d) Kidney

Ref: Ganong, 23rd ed. pg. 674

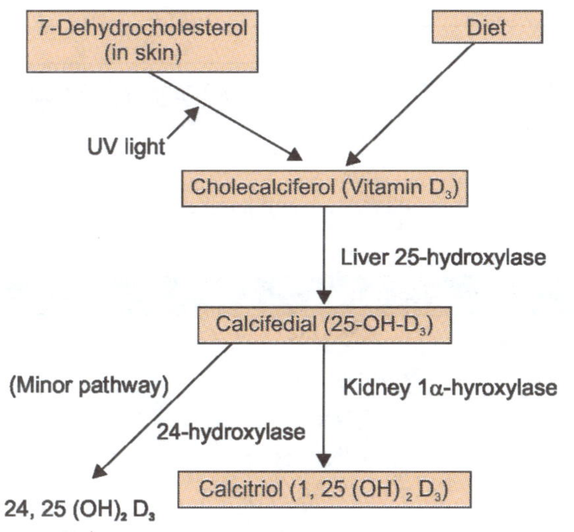

100. Ans. (d) Proximal convoluted tubule

Ref: Ganong, 25th ed. pg. 680, 683

About 2/3rd of filtered water is reabsorbed in the proximal convoluted tubule along with salt absorption. Other molecules absorbed here are bicarbonate, glucose, amino-acids and phosphate.

GASTROINTESTINAL PHYSIOLOGY

101. Ans. (a) VIPoma

Ref: Ganong 26th ed. pg. 459

- Vasoactive intestinal peptide leads to activation of water channels in gut and leads to secretory diarrhea.
- Option B leads to impaired glucose tolerance. Option C leads to recurrent episodes of hypoglycemia.
- Option d leads to hypergastrinemia and hyperchlorhydria. The increased acid can damage mucosa of duodenum and can cause osmotic diarrhea.

102. Ans. (b) Segmentation

Ref: Ganong 26th ed. pg. 486

- The image shows food getting broken down in the gut with *contractions occurring at both sides of the gut.* The objective is to mix the intestinal contents. This is called segmentation. Notice that in image marked B, contractions are starting in center of segment of gut to force the contents backwards and forwards and help in mixing.
- Peristalsis will show a sequential contraction and relaxation of a forward moving wave.
- Option D is ruled as BER does not itself cause muscle contraction but spike potentials. It leads to spontaneous rhythmic fluctuations in membrane potential between –65 and –45 mV.

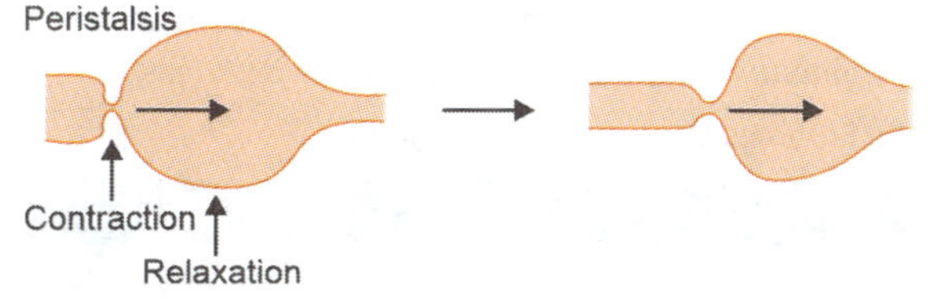

103. Ans. (b) Enhance salt absorption

Ref: Ganong 25th ed. pg. 478

In diarrhea, only salt is lost but sugar is added as it helps to absorb salt and sugar by process of symport. The transporter in the gut is SGLT-1.

104. Ans. (b) Cholesterol Esterase

Ref: Ganong, 25th ed. pg. 482

Cholesterol esterase is a pancreatic lipase activated by bile acids. It causes the following actions:

- Hydrolysis of cholesterol esters
- Hydrolysis of esters of fat-soluble vitamins
- Hydrolysis of phospholipids

Most of the fat digestion begins in the duodenum and pancreatic lipase is the most important enzyme. Colipase is activated by trypsin and allows lipase to remain associated with droplets of dietary lipid even in the presence of bile acids.

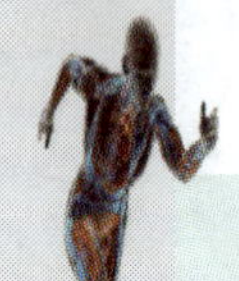

105. Ans. (a) Trypsinogen

Ref: Ganong, 25th ed. pg. 479

- Trypsinogen is converted to active enzyme trypsin by enterokinase when the pancreatic juice enters into the duodenum. Enterokinase contains 41% polysaccharide and this high polysaccharide content prevents the enterokinase from getting digested.
- The trypsin, chymotrypsin and elastase act at interior peptide bonds in the peptide molecules and are called endopeptidases.

106. Ans. (a) Enterochromaffin cell

Ref: Ganong, 25th ed. pg. 457

Enterochromaffin cell is responsible for histamine and serotonin secretion. Chief cells produce pepsinogen.

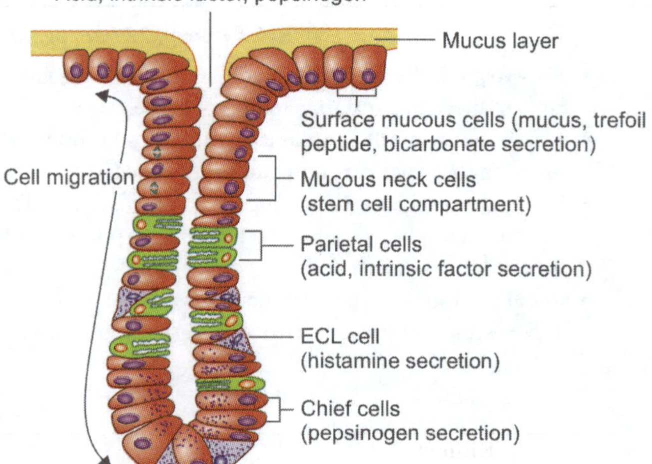

107. Ans. (c) Pancreatic juice

Ref: Ganong, 25th ed. pg. 461

- *Colipase* is secreted in pancreatic juice in inactive form. It is activated in intestinal lumen by trypsin.
- *Lingual lipase* is secreted by Von Ebner's glands.
- *Intestinal lipase* is secreted in succus entericus. Succus entericus is secreted by small intestine and has a pH of 8.3.

TABLE: Enzymes involved in fat digestion

Area	Juice	Enzyme	Substrate
Mouth	Saliva	Lingual lipase	Triglycerides
Stomach	Gastric juice	• Gastric lipase (weak lipase) • Pancreatic lipase • Cholesterol ester hydrolase • Phospholipase A	• Triglycerides • Triglycerides • Cholesterol ester • Phospholipids
Small intestine	Pancreatic juice	• Phospholipase B • Colipase • Bile-salt-activated lipase	• Lysophospholipids • Facilitates action of pancreatic lipase • Phospholipids • Cholesterol esters
Small intestine	Succus entericus	Intestinal lipase	Triglycerides

108. Ans. (c) Acid

Ref: Quantitative Human Physiology; An Introduction. pg. 705

Gastric Cells and their Secretion

Cells	Location in stomach	Their secretion
Parietal cell/Oxyntic cell	Body	HCl and intrinsic factor
Chief cells/Peptic cell	Body	Pepsinogen
G cells	Antrum	Gastrin
Mucus neck cells	Oxyntic glands	Mucus

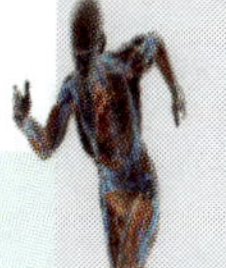

109. Ans. (d) Bicarbonate secretion from pancreas

Ref: Quantitative Human Physiology; An Introduction, pg. 711-712

TABLE: Important differences between GIT hormones (Gastrin, CCK, Secretin, GIP)

	Gastrin	CCK	Secretin	GIP
Site	Main site: G cells (antrum)	I-cells of the proximal two-thirds of small intestine	S-cells: Upper small intestine	K-cells: Proximal intestinal crypts
Actions	**Major:** • Stimulate acid and pepsin secretion • Stimulate gastric motility • Act as growth factor to stimulate mucosal proliferation	**Major:** • Stimulate pancreatic acinar cell enzyme secretion • Stimulate GB contraction • Relaxes sphincter of oddi • Inhibits gastric acid secretion and gastric emptying • Pyloric sphincter contraction	• **Major:** Secretion of HCO_3 from biliary and pancreatic ductular cell and Brunner gland. • Inhibit gastric acid secretion • Stimulate pyloric sphincter • Increases bile flow • Augments the action of CCK	**Major:** Stimulate insulin release from pancreas
Major stimulus	Peptides **(most potent)** Distension of stomach Calcium GRP (gastrin releasing peptides)	Peptides **(most potent)** Fatty acid (BUT NOT TG)	Acid **(most potent)** Digestive protein	Glucose, fat and amino acid

110. Ans. (c) Celiac disease

Ref: Methods in Disease: Investigating the Gastrointestinal Tract by Victor R Preddy pg. 43

- **D-xylose absorption test** is a medical test performed to diagnose conditions that present with malabsorption of the proximal small intestine *due to defects in the integrity of the gastrointestinal mucosa.*
- D-xylose is a monosaccharide, or simple sugar, that **does not require enzymes** for digestion prior to absorption. Its absorption requires an intact mucosa only.
- In this test, the patient ingests D-xylose *(a nondigestible but absorbable carbohydrate)* by mouth, and then the urinary D-xylose is measured.
- Urine excretion below certain levels *(depending on the amount of D-xylose ingested)* implies poor absorption of D-xylose and, therefore, disease of the small intestine.
- Alternatively, a blood level of xylose is measured 2 hours after the D-xylose is taken by mouth. Low levels in the blood imply poor absorption. Abnormal D-xylose tests are most frequently associated with disorders of the small intestine **such as celiac sprue.**
- Malabsorbtion can also occur in pancreatic insufficiency, **but D-xylose test should be normal.**

111. Ans. (a) Carbohydrate malabsorption due to mucosal disorder

Ref: Methods in Disease: Investigating the Gastrointestinal Tract by Victor R Preddy pg. 43

- *Xylose is a pentose sugar and is absorbed directly from intestinal nucosa.*
- D xylose will reveal carbohydrate malabsorption due to mucosal disorder, **but in malabsorption due to pancreatic disease, the D-xylose test should be normal.**
- Due to high false positives and ease of obtaining small intestinal biopsy after endoscopy, intestinal biopsy is the preferred method.

112. Ans. (c) Oxyntic cells

Ref: Ganong, 23rd ed. pg. 431-32

Secretion in Stomach

- **Oxyntic cell (parietal cell)** secretes: HCl and intrinsic factor of castle
- Chief cell (zymogen or peptic cell) secrete: pepsinogen
- G cell secrete: Gastrin
- D cell secrete: Somatostatin
- ECL cells secrete: Histamine

113. Ans. (b) Decreased by cholecystokinin

Ref: Ganong Review of Medical Physiology, 22nd ed. pg. 484-86

Factors Affecting Gastric Emptying

Decrease emptying	Increase emptying
Cholecystokinin Secretin GIP (Gastric inhibitory peptide) Somatostatin Hyperosmolality of duodenal contents	Carbohydrate rich food leaves stomach in few hours. Protein rich food leaves more slowly & *emptying is slowest after fat rich meal.*

114. Ans. (a) Lipids

Ref: Ganong Review of Medical Physiology, 23rd ed. Chapter 28

- *The presence of fat in the small intestine is the most potent inhibitor of gastric emptying, resulting in relaxation of the proximal stomach and diminished contractions of the distal, "gastric grinder" - when the fat has been absorbed, the inhibitory stimulus is removed and productive gastric motility resumes.*
- If the fluid is hypertonic or acidic or rich in nutrients such as fat or certain amino acids, the rate of gastric emptying will be considerably slower and non-exponential.
- Indeed, the rate of gastric emptying of any meal can be predicted rather accurately by knowing its nutrient density.
- Nutrient density is sensed predominantly in the small intestine by osmoreceptors and chemoreceptors, and relayed to the stomach as inhibitory neural and hormonal messages that delay emptying by altering the patterns of gastric motility.

115. Ans. (b) Pylorus has more acid secreting cells

Ref: Ganong, 25th ed. pg. 457

- Pylorus is mostly populated with mucus-secreting cells.

GASTRIC GLANDS

- They can be divided into three groups—the pyloric, principal (in the body and fundus) and cardiac glands.

A. Pyloric Glands

- Pyloric glands are mostly *populated with mucus-secreting cells*, parietal cells are few and chief cells scarce. In contrast, neuroendocrine cells are numerous, especially G cells, which secrete gastrin when activated by appropriate mechanical stimulation (causing increased gastric motility and secretion of gastric juices).

B. Principal Glands

- Located in body and fundus
- *Contain distinct cell types: Chief, parietal, mucous neck, stem and neuroendocrine*
    1. **Chief cells:** Source of pepsinogen, rennin and lipase. Contain zymogens, contain abundant RNA and hence, intensely basophilic
    2. **Parietal (oxyntic) cells:** Are the source of gastric acid and intrinsic factor.
    3. **Neuroendocrine cells:** Synthesize a number of biogenic amines and polypeptides important for the control of motility and glandular secretion. In the stomach they include cells designated as G cells secreting gastrin, D cells (somatostatin), and ECL (enterochromaffin-like) cells (histamine).

C. Cardiac Glands

- *Mucus-secreting cells predominate* and parietal and chief cells are few.

116. Ans. (b) Ptyalin

Ref: Guyton's Physiology, 11th ed. pg. 793

- Saliva contains two major types of protein secretion:
    - ***Serous secretion***- contains ptyalin, an enzyme for digesting starches.
    - ***Mucus secretion***

Gland	Secretion	Content	Function
Parotid gland	Serous type	Ptyalin	Digest starches
Submandibular gland	Serous and mucous type	Mucin	Lubricating and for surface protective purposes
Buccal gland	Only mucus	Mucin	Lubricating

- Saliva has a pH between 6.0 and 7.0, a favorable range for the digestive action of ptyalin.
- But before food and its accompanying saliva become completely mixed with the gastric secretions, as much as 30 to 40% of the starches will have been hydrolyzed mainly to form *maltose.*
- *In small intestine the remaining starch Digestion takes place by Pancreatic Amylase.* Pancreatic secretion is almost identical in its function with the α-amylase of saliva but is several times more powerful.

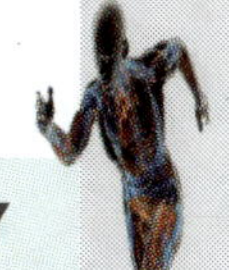

- Hence, within 15–30 minutes after the chyme empties from the stomach into the duodenum and mixes with pancreatic juice, nearly all the carbohydrates will have become digested.

117. Ans. (a) Undigested food

Ref: Ganong, 25th ed. pg. 502

- Fecal mass is derived from undigested food.
- Feces are the particles of waste matter that is left over after the body has processed and absorbed nourishment from the foods we eat.
- It contains water, dietary fiber, inorganic salts, dead cells, bacteria, and anything the body cannot or will not absorb.

118. Ans. (b) Bitter

Ref: Ganong, 25th ed. pg. 224

- There are 5 types of taste sensations commonly recognized by humans. Sweet, umami, salty, sour, and bitter.
- None of these tastes are elicited by single chemical. Also, there are different thresholds for detection of taste that differ among chemicals. **The taste having lowest threshold will be most sensitive** *(please refer to table)*

Taste	Substance	Threshold for tasting
Salty	Sodium chloride	0.01 M
Sweet	Sucrose	0.01 M
Umami	Glutamate	0.0007 M
Sour	Hydrochloric acid	0.09 M
Bitter	Quinine	0.000008 M

119. Ans. (d) Somatostatin

Ref: Ganong, 25th ed. pg. 154

Somatostatin is found in the D cells of pancreatic islets. It inhibits the secretion of insulin, glucagon, and pancreatic polypeptide and may act locally within the pancreatic islets in a paracrine fashion.

120. Ans. (c) Hexoses

Ref: Harrison, 19th ed./Table 26.1 pg. 477

- Hexoses are absorbed most rapidly; Amongst hexoses, glucose and galactose are absorbed more rapidly than others.
- Mannose and pentose are absorbed more slowly.

121. Ans. (a) Trypsin

Ref: Ganong's Physiology, 23rd ed. ch. 27

- *Trypsin converts chymotrypsinogens into chymotrypsins and other proenzymes into active enzymes.* Trypsin can also activate trypsinogen; therefore, once some trypsin is formed, there is an auto-catalytic chain reaction.
- Trypsin, the chymotrypsins, and elastase act at interior peptide bonds in the peptide molecules and are called **endopeptidases**.
- The powerful protein-splitting enzymes of the pancreatic juice are *secreted as inactive proenzymes.*
- *Trypsinogen is converted to the active enzyme trypsin by enterokinase when the pancreatic juice enters the duodenum.*
- Enterokinase *contains 41% polysaccharide,* and this high polysaccharide content apparently *prevents it from being digested itself* before it can exert its effect.

122. Ans. (a) Alkaline content of small intestine

Ref: Guyton's, 11th ed. pg. 776, 784-90

Enterogastric reflex inhibits stomach secretions and motility based on the signals from small intestine and colon.

Enterogastric reflex is stimulated by
Duodenal acidic pH
Duodenal distension
Duodenal hypertonicity
Sympathetic stimulation
Intense pain
Increased osmolality of gastric chime
Inhibited by
Parasympathetic stimulation
Increased volume and fluidity of gastric content

123. Ans. (d) Divalent metal transporter

Ref: Ganong, 25th ed. pg. 484

- All iron absorption occurs in the duodenum.
- *Transport of iron into the enterocytes occurs via divalent metal transporter 1 (DMT1)*
- Some is stored in form of ferritin and the rest is transported out of enterocytes by basolateral transporter called ferroportin 1
- In plasma Fe^{2+} is converted to Fe^{3+} and bound to transport protein transferrin

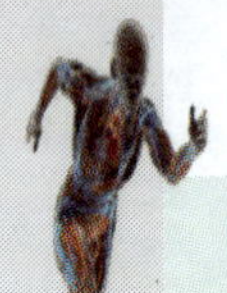

Transferrin saturation	35%
Plasma iron	110-130 mg/dl

124. Ans. (b) Contraction of Sphincter of oddi

Ref: Ganong, 25th ed. pg. 479

Functions of CCK

- CCK mediates digestion in the small intestine by *inhibiting gastric emptying* and decreasing gastric acid secretion.
- It *stimulates the acinar cells of the pancreas* to release digestive enzymes which catalyze the digestion of fat, protein, and carbohydrates.
- CCK also causes the increased production of hepatic bile
- Stimulates the *contraction of the gall bladder*
- *Relaxation of the Sphincter of Oddi* (Glisson's sphincter), resulting in the delivery of bile into the duodenum.
- Site of CCK release is epithelial cells in the mucosal lining of the small intestine (mostly in the duodenum and jejunum)
- The presence of fatty acids and/or certain amino acids in the chyme entering the duodenum is the greatest stimulator of CCK release.

125. Ans. (b) Entero-endocrine cells in the gut

Ref: Ganong, 25th ed. pg. 470, 500

- Site of CCK release is epithelial cells called I *cells* in the mucosal lining of the small intestine (mostly in the duodenum and jejunum)

126. Ans. (c) Lactase

Ref: Ganong, 25th ed. pg. 461

The enzymes produced by exocrine pancreas are:

1. Trypsinogen
2. Chymotrypsinogens
3. Elastase
4. Carboxypeptidase A and B
5. Colipase
6. Pancreatic lipase
7. Pancreatic alpha amylase
8. Phospholipase A2

Lactase is produced by *cells of intestinal mucosa* to breakdown lactose.

127. Ans. (d) Gastro-ileal reflex

Ref: Ganong, 25th ed. pg. 502

- When the food leaves the stomach, caecum relaxes and the passage of chyme through ileocaecal valve increases. This is called as gastro-ileal reflex and is mediated via vagal action.
- Somatostatin is a *growth hormone inhibiting hormone* isolated from hypothalamus and is secreted as paracrine by D cells in pancreatic islets.

Actions of Somatostatin

1. Inhibits VIP, GIP, secretin and motilin
2. Inhibits GH release
3. Inhibits gastric acid secretion and motility
4. Inhibits gall bladder contraction

128. Ans. (c) Normally excreted in urine

Ref: Ganong, 25th ed. pg. 511

- Bilirubin excretion in the urine is seen in obstructive jaundice when conjugated bilirubin regurgitates back into the blood stream since it cannot be excreted secondary to obstruction. This bilirubinuria seen in obstructive jaundice leads to mustard yellow discoloration of the urine. Hence, bilirubin in urine indicates a pathology.
- The conjugated bilirubin in normal people is broken down by an enzyme by name of beta-glucoronidase to form unconjugated bilirubin. This is called enterohepatic cycle. Choice b is correct
- *Conjugation of bilirubin occurs in liver and in case of defective conjugation (Criggler najar syndrome) the levels of unconjugated bilirubin increases to level that it crosses the blood brain barrier and leads to kernicterus. Choice a and d are correct.*

129. Ans. (a) Interstitial cells of Cajal

Ref: Ganong, 25th ed. pg. 496

The basal electrical rhythm is initiated by *interstitial cells of Cajal* which are *stellate mesenchymal parenchymal cells* that send long multiple branched processes into the intestinal smooth muscle.

ENDOCRINE AND REPRODUCTIVE PHYSIOLOGY

130. Ans. (c) Thyroid hormone

Ref: Berne and Levy Physiology, 6th ed. pg. 1240

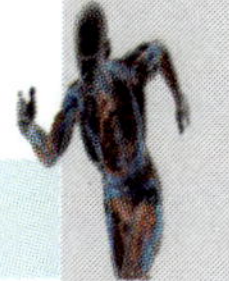

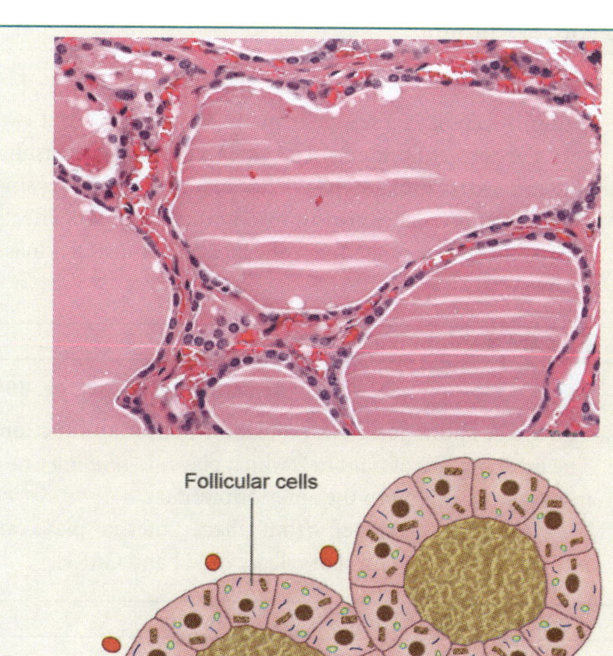

- The image shows colloid filled follicles. The arrow is marked at the Follicular cells.
- These follicular cells are the derivates of the endoderm and secrete thyroid hormone.
- If the arrow was present in the septa separating the follicles, then para follicular cells would have been the answer.
- The circulating form of this hormone is thyroxine, which is tetraiodothyronine (T4) along with a small quantity of triiodothyronine (T3).

131. Ans. (b) Oxytocin

Ref: Berne and Levy Physiology, 6th ed. pg. 1216

- Breastfeeding can bring on postpartum cramping or make it more intense.
- That's because baby's sucking triggers the release of the hormone oxytocin.
- This is as oxytocin acts on myoepithelial cells

132. Ans. (d) All of these

Ref: Berne and Levy Physiology, 6th ed. pg. 170

- Three major hormones (vitamin D, PTH and calcitonin) interact to maintain a constant concentration of calcium, despite variations in intake and excretion.
- PTH and Calcitonin regulate serum calcium by bone remodeling. Vitamin D3 helps in maintaining values of calcium by increasing intestinal absorption of calcium.

133. Ans. (a) Amygdala

Ref: Berne and Levy Physiology, 6th ed. pg. 195,196

- Amygdala is located deep in the brain's medial temporal lobe and it has a key role in the processing of emotions and encoding memories.
- Damage to the temporal lobe results in profound changes in fear reactivity, feeding, and sexual behavior.

134. Ans. (a) Vasodilator

Ref: Berne and Levy Physiology, 6th ed. pg. 994

- Dopamine is an endogenous catecholamine which at low doses (≤3 μg/kg/min), may selectively activate dopamine receptors and promote renal vasodilatation

135. Ans. (d) Thyrotropin-releasing hormone

Ref: Ganong 26th ed. pg. 309

- TRH and VIP are polypeptides that are found in hypothalamus and can stimulate prolactin secretion.
- TRH stimulates the release of both TSH and Prolactin.
- Prolactin releasing Hormone/PRH is postulated to exist but has not been isolated.

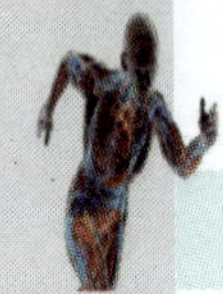

136. Ans. (d) Oxytocin

Milk production in breast acini is due to action of prolactin. The sight, smell, sound of cry of baby and suckling will cause release of oxytocin. It is released from posterior pituitary and causes contraction of myoepithelial cells lining the breast ducts that causes milk let down into mouth of the baby.

137. Ans. (b) Thyroxine binding globulin

Ref: Ganong 26th ed. pg. 359

The plasma proteins that bind thyroid hormones are:
- Albumin: It has the largest capacity but affinity for T4 and T3 is lesser than that for TBG
- Transthyretin (formerly called Thyroxine binding pre-albumin
- Thyroxine binding globulin: Highest affinity to bind to T4 and T3.

TABLE: Binding of thyroid hormones to plasma proteins in normal adult humans.

Protein	Plasma concentration (mg/dL)	Amounts of circulating hormone bound (%)	
		T_4	T_3
Thyroxine-binding globulin (TBG)	2	67	46
Transthyretin (thyroxine-binding (prealbumin, TBPA)	15	20	1
Albumin	3500	13	53

138. Ans. (a) ADH

Ref: Ganong, 25th ed. pg. 442

Glucagon, thyroxine, cortisol and growth hormone increase blood sugar levels and are glucogenic. ADH regulates water re-absorption *via* the collecting duct.

139. Ans. (a) Calcitriol

Ref: Ganong, 25th ed. pg. 378

The active metabolite of vitamin D3 is produced in kidney and is called calcitriol or 1,25 dihyroxycholecalciferol. The cells of proximal convoluted tubule produce an enzyme by name of 1 alpha hydroxylase that converts 25 hydroxycholecalcifero! into 1,25 dihyroxycholecalciferol.

140. Ans. (d) Placenta

Ref: Ganong, 25th ed. pg. 409, 425

- *Inhibin A is produced by placenta and corpus luteum.* It is used in quadruple screening for prenatal detection of down Syndrome.
- *Inhibin B* inhibits FSH in both males and females. It is *produced by Sertoli cells* in male and *granulosa cells* in female.

141. Ans. (a) Insulin

Ref: Ganong, 25th ed. pg. 434

Insulin receptor is a tetramer made of two alpha and two beta glycoprotein proteins. The alpha subunits bind insulin and are extracellular while beta subunits have tyrosine kinase activity. The growth promoting anabolic effects of insulin are mediated by phosphatidyl inositol kinase pathway.

142. Ans. (b) Inhibin B

Ref: Ganong, 25th ed. pg. 409

The image shows feedback regulation of ovarian function. The marking X is of inhibin B which plays an *inhibitory* role in release of FSH from the anterior pituitary.

In contrast oestrogen from theca interna plays an inhibitory role in control of release of LH and GnRH.

143. Ans. (a) PTH

Ref: Harrison 19th ed. pg. 2464

- For formation of active form of vitamin D3, proximal convoluted tubule of kidney is the main site.
- *The major inducers of activity of 1-α-hydroxylase are PTH and phosphate.*
- The repressors of activity of 1-α-hydroxylase are FGF23, calcium and 1,25 (OH)2D.
- The main concept is that 25 hydroxy D regulates its own enzyme 25 hydroxylase activity and 1,25(OH)2 D regulates its own enzyme 1 α Hydroxylase. The two *do not* regulate each others activity.

144. Ans. (a) TSH

Receptors for Hormones
- **Membrane receptor:** They mainly bind peptide hormones and catecholamines
- **Nuclear receptor:** Bind small molecules that can diffuse across the cell membrane, such as steroids and vitamin D.

Note:
- **Guyton states:** *"Amino acid derivatives and peptide hormones interact with cell surface membrane receptors."*
- *Steroids,* **thyroid hormones,** *vitamin D and retinoids are lipid soluble and interact with intracellular nuclear receptors.*

TABLE: Receptors and their respective hormones

Nuclear receptors *(Mn: TOAD)*	Thyroxine Estrogen Vitamin A Vitamin D
Cytoplasmic receptors	All steroids except Estrogen
Cell membrane via G protein stimulation	All others like ACTH, LH, FSH, GH

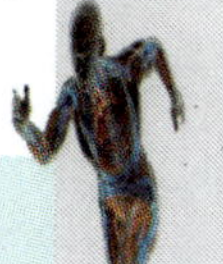

145. Ans. (c) Inhibin

Ref: Ganong Physiology, 24th ed. pg. 419 and 420; Guyton's Physiology, 11th ed. pg. 1007

- The walls of the seminiferous tubules are **lined by primitive germ cells and Sertoli cells.**
- **Maturation** of spermatozoa takes place in deep folds of the cytoplasm of the sertoli cells.
- Mature spermatozoa are released from the Sertoli cells and become free in the lumens of the tubules. ***The sertoli cells secrete androgen binding protein (ABP), inhibin, and MIS.***
- Inhibin inhibits follicle-stimulating hormone (FSH) secretion.
- Inhibin has a strong direct effect on the anterior pituitary gland to inhibit the secretion of FSH and possibly a slight effect on the hypothalamus to inhibit secretion of GnRH.

Extra Mile

- **Testosterone,** secreted by the *Leydig cells*
- **Luteinizing hormone**—by anterior pituitary gland, stimulates the Leydig cells to secrete testosterone.
- **FSH**—also by the anterior pituitary gland, stimulates the *Sertoli cells*; essential for spermatogenesis.

146. Ans. (d) Delta cells

Ref: Guyton's Physiology, 11th ed. pg. 961

- The human pancreas has 1–2 million islets of Langerhans cells
- These islets contain three major types of cells: *alpha*, *beta*, and *delta* cells
- **Beta cells**—60% of all the cells of the islets, lie mainly in the middle of each islet and secrete *insulin* and *amylin*.
- **Alpha cells**—about 25% of the total islets- secrete *glucagon*.
- **Delta cells**—about 10% of the total islets-secrete *somatostatin*.

Extra Mile

The hormones secreted act as control of secretion of some hormones by other hormones:

- Insulin inhibits glucagon secretion
- Amylin inhibits insulin secretion
- Somatostatin inhibits both insulin and glucagon secretion.

In addition to these, somatostatin has other functions:

- It decreases the motility of the stomach, duodenum, and gallbladder.
- It decreases both secretion and absorption in the gastrointestinal tract.

Doing so, somatostatin has following effects:

- It extends the time period over which the food nutrients are absorbed into the blood.
- By inhibiting insulin and glucagon secretion, it prevents rapid utilization of nutrients by the tissues.

Remember: Somatostatin is also known as *growth hormone inhibitory hormone,* which is also secreted in the hypothalamus and suppresses anterior pituitary gland growth hormone secretion.

147. Ans. (a) Cortisol

Ref: Ganong, 22nd ed. ch. 20

- ***Cortisol is secreted by adrenal cortex not medulla.***
- Norepinephrine, epinephrine, and dopamine are secreted by the adrenal medulla.

148. Ans. (a) Neurohormones

Ref: Lange Medical Physiology by Ganong, ch. 20

Adreno-medullary hormones are *catecholamines* secreted from the adrenal medulla by chromaffin cells, neurosecretory cells connected to the central nervous system.

The synthesis, storage (in chromaffin cells) and release of *catecholamines is co-regulated by synaptic input from their respective pre-synaptic sympathetic neurons, as well as hormonal and local inputs.* The adreno-medullary hormones are:

1. Epinephrine
2. Norepinephrine
3. Dopamine

149. Ans. (c) Decrease blood amino acid

Ref: Berne & Levy's Physiology, 5th ed. pg. 909 and chapter 20: Lange medical physiology by Ganong 23rd ed.

- *Cortisol raises the free amino acids in the serum. It does this by inhibiting collagen formation, decreasing amino acid uptake by muscle, and inhibiting protein synthesis.*
- Glucocorticoids promote protein degradation and inhibit entry of amino acids in tissues (Primarily Branch chain amino acids).
- Glucocorticoids also lead to utilization of amino acids by promoting gluconeogenesis directly and by permissive effect on Growth hormone.

150. Ans. (b) Oxytocin

TABLE: Hormones from Anterior Pituitary

Hormones	Major functions
Growth hormone	Stimulates protein synthesis and overall growth of most cells and tissues
TSH	Stimulates synthesis and secretion of thyroid hormones (T3 & T4)
Adrenocorticotropic hormone (ACTH)	Stimulates synthesis and secretion of adrenocortical hormones (cortisol, androgens, and aldosterone)

Contd...

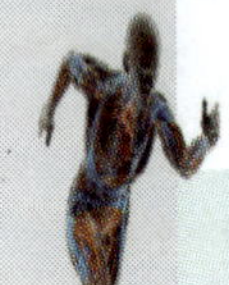

Hormones	Major functions
Prolactin	Promotes development of the female breast and *secretion of milk*
Follicle-stimulating hormone (FSH)	Causes growth of follicles in the ovaries and sperm maturation in sertoli cells of testes
Luteinizing hormones (LH)	Stimulates testosterone synthesis in Leydig cells of testes; stimulates ovulation, formation of corpus luteum, and estrogen and progesterone synthesis in ovaries

TABLE: Hormones from Posterior Pituitary

Antidiuretic hormone (ADH)/ Vasopressin	Increase water reabsorption by the kidneys and cause vasoconstriction and increased blood pressure
Oxytocin	***Stimulates milk ejection*** from breasts and uterine contractions

151. Ans. (d) Glucagon

- GH secretion is regulated by GHRH released from hypothalamus in a pulsatile fashion.
- Large burst of secretion occurs at night during the onset of deep sleep (NREM sleep).

Stimuli that increase secretion of GH	Stimuli that decreases secretion of GH
• Hypoglycemia • Exercise • Fasting • Protein meals • Stress • **Glucagon** • Estrogens, androgens, L-dopa and alpha adrenergics	• Sleep • Glucose • Cortisol • FFA • GH

152. Ans. (a) Levodopa

Ref: Ganong's, 23rd ed. pg. 333

TABLE: Factors affecting Prolactin secretion

Increase prolactin	Decrease prolactin
• Sleep • Pregnancy; Estrogen • Opioids • TRH • Phenothiazines	• L-Dopa • Apomorphine • Bromocriptine related ergot derivative

153. Ans. (a) Anterior pituitary

Ref: Guyton Physiology 11th ed. pg. 907

- Thyroid stimulating hormone is secreted by anterior pituitary after getting stimulus by TRH (thyrotropin releasing hormone) from hypothalamus.

154. Ans. (b) D1 Deiodinase

Ref: Harrison, 18th ed./Figure 341-1

- Deiodination is the foremost pathway of thyroid hormone metabolism.
- Three iodothyronine deiodinases (D1-D3) are identified as *seleno cysteino-containing membrane proteins with their active enzymatic sites located in the cytoplasm.*
- *D1 and D2 convert T4 to T3.*
- D3 has only inner ring deiodination activity and inactivates T4 and T3 to rT3 and T2, respectively

155. Ans. (c) TSH

Ref: Guyton & Hall Textbook of Physiology, 11th ed. pg. 939 and chapter 18: Lange Medical Physiology by Ganong

Increased thyroid hormone in the body fluids decreases secretion of TSH by the anterior pituitary. When the level of thyroid hormone secretion rises to about 1.75 times the normal, the rate of TSH secretion falls essentially to zero. *Almost all this feedback depressant effect occurs even when the anterior pituitary has been separated from the hypothalamus.*

156. Ans. (a) Secreted by pituitary gland

Ref: Ganong's 24th ed. pg. 278; Guyton pg. 1009-1010

- Melatonin is *secreted by pineal*[Q] *gland*. Its synthesis and *secretion is increased remarkably in the dark period of the day* and maintained at low levels in the daylight.
- It is associated with sleep mechanism.
- *Melatonin based drugs can be used to treat jet lag and insomnia in elderly.*
- It also acts as inhibitor of gonadotropic hormone secretion and the gonads become inhibited and even partly involuted.

157. Ans. (b) Ovulation

Ref: Guyton Physiology, 11th ed. pg. 1027

- While still in the ovary, the ovum is in the primary oocyte stage.
- *Right before it is released from the ovarian follicle*, its nucleus divides by meiosis and a *first polar body* is *expelled from the nucleus of the oocyte.*

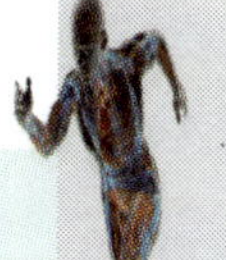

- The primary oocyte then becomes the secondary oocyte.
- In this process, each of the 23 pairs of chromosomes loses one of its partners, which becomes *incorporated in a polar body that is expelled.*
- This leaves 23 unpaired chromosomes in the secondary occyte. It is at this time that the ovum, still in the secondary oocyte stage, is ovulated into the abdominal cavity.

158. Ans. (c) Nucleus

Ref: Guyton Physiology, 11th ed. pg. 997-998

- Each spermatozoon is composed of a head and a tail
- *The head comprises the condensed nucleus* of the cell with only a thin cytoplasmic and cell membrane layer around its surface.
- Golgi apparatus form a thick cap called the acrosome which is on the outside of the anterior two thirds of the head.
- The tail of the sperm, called the flagellum, has three major components:
  - A central skeleton constructed of 11 microtubules, collectively called the axoneme
  - A thin cell membrane covering the axoneme
  - A collection of mitochondria surrounding the axoneme in the proximal portion of the tail (called the body of the tail)

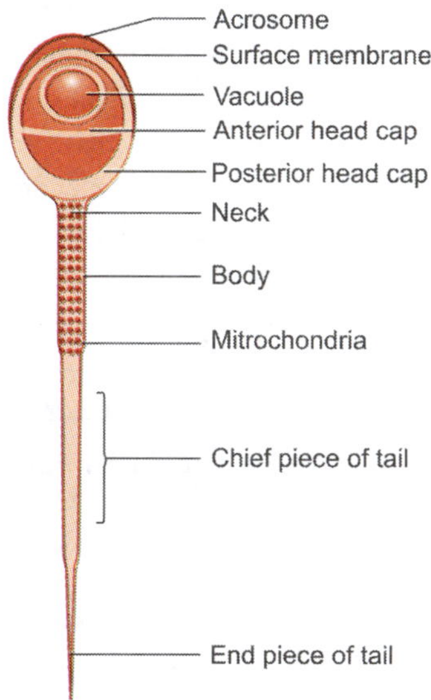

159. Ans. (b) Inhibin

Ref: Ganong Physiology, 24th ed. pg. 419 and 420; Guyton's Physiology, 11th ed. pg. 1007

- The walls of the seminiferous tubules are lined by primitive germ cells and sertoli cells.
- Maturation of spermatozoa takes place in deep folds of the cytoplasm of the sertoli cells.
- Mature spermatozoa are released from the Sertoli cells and become free in the lumens of the tubules. *The sertoli cells secrete* **androgen binding protein** (ABP), **inhibin**, and **MIS**.
- *Inhibin inhibits follicle-stimulating hormone (FSH) secretion.*
- Inhibin also has a strong direct effect on the anterior pituitary gland to inhibit the secretion of FSH and possibly a slight effect on the hypothalamus to inhibit secretion of GnRH.

Extra Mile

- *Testosterone*, secreted by the *Leydig cells*
- *Luteinizing hormone*- Secreted by anterior pituitary gland, stimulates the Leydig cells to secrete testosterone.
- *FSH*- also secreted by the anterior pituitary gland, stimulates the *Sertoli cells*; essential for spermatogenesis.

160. Ans. (c) Occurs in male genital tract

- Capacitation is a process which makes spermatozoa to undergo the physical changes necessary to fertilize an egg in female genital tract.
- Spermatozoa in male genital tract are exposed to floating vesicles from seminiferous tubules which contain large amount of cholesterol that cover up the sperm acrosome, which make the membrane tough.
- *After ejaculation,* the sperm deposited in vagina swim away from cholesterol vesicle upward into the uterine cavity and hence, lose excess cholesterol and *membrane of the head of sperm becomes weaker, which makes the penetration in ova easy.*

161. Ans. (a) Obesity

Ref: Guyton Physiology, 11th ed. pg. 871

- Leptin gives a sensation of satiety.
- In case it is defective, person develops irresistible eating tendency, which may lead to obesity.
- *Hypothalamus senses energy storage* through the actions of *leptin*, a peptide hormone *released from adipocytes*, which once released in the circulation occupies its receptors in hypothalamus especially POMC neurons of arcuate nuclei.
- Mutations that render Fat cells unable to produce leptin or mutations that cause defective leptin receptors in the hypothalamus leads to marked hyperphagia and ultimately morbid obesity occurs.

162. Ans. (b) GLUT 2

Transporter	Function	Site of action
SGLT1	Absorption of glucose	Small intestine, renal tubules
SGLT2	Absorption of glucose	Renal tubules

Contd...

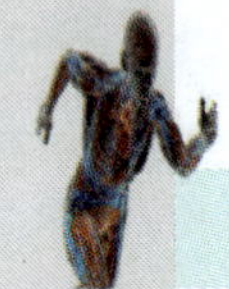

Facilitated diffusion		
GLUT1	Basal glucose uptake	Placenta, blood-brain barrier, brain, red cells, kidneys, colon
GLUT2	B-cell glucose sensor; transport out of intestinal and renal epithelial cells	B cells islets, liver, epithelial cells of small intestine, kidneys
GLUT3	Basal glucose uptake	Brain, placenta, kidneys
GLUT4	Insulin – stimulated glucose uptake	Skeletal and cardiac muscle, adipose tissue, other tissues
GLUT5	Fructose transport	Jejunum, sperm
GLUT6	Unknown	Brain, spleen and leukocytes
GLUT7	Glucose 6-phosphate transporter in endoplasmic reticulum	Liver

163. Ans. (b) Skeletal muscle

- Insulin increases glucose uptake in skeletal muscle.
- Insulin dependent glucose transportation is mediated by GLUT4 which is expressed in skeletal muscles, cardiac muscles and adipose tissue.
- Both GLUT1 and GLUT4 are expressed in skeletal muscle but GLUT4 is main glucose transporter in the tissue.
- GLUT 1 mediates *basal* glucose uptake, whereas GLUT 4 mediates *insulin stimulated* glucose uptake.

164. Ans. (d) Measuring serum progesterone on day 14 of the cycle

Study of cervical mucus	• Estrogen makes the mucus thinner and more alkaline, a change that promotes the survival and transport of sperms. • Progesterone makes it thick, tenacious, and cellular. • The mucus is thinnest at the time of ovulation, and its elasticity, or spinnbarkeit, increases such that by mid-cycle, a drop can be stretched into a long, thin thread that may be 8-23 cm or more in length. • In addition, it *dries in an arborizing, fern-like pattern* when a thin layer is spread on a slide. • After ovulation and during pregnancy, it becomes thick and fails to form pattern.
Basal body temperature	• A convenient and reasonably reliable indicator of the time of ovulation is a change, usually a rise in the basal body temperature. The rise starts 1-2 days after ovulation.

Contd...

	• A surge in LH secretion triggers ovulation and ovulation normally occurs about 9 hours after the peak of the LH surge at mid-cycle. The ovum lives for approximately 72 hours after it is extruded from the follicle, but it is fertilizable for a much shorter time than this.
Endometrial histology	• At the end of menstruation, new endometrium regrows under the influence of estrogens. • The endometrium increases rapidly in thickness from the fifth to 14th day of the menstrual cycle. • As the thickness increases, the uterine glands are drawn out so that they length but they do not become convoluted or secrete to any degree. • These endometrial changes are called proliferative, and this part of the menstrual cycle is sometimes called the *proliferative phase*. It is also called the pre-ovulatory or follicular phase of the cycle. • After ovulation, the endometrium becomes highly vascularized and slightly edematous under the influence of estrogen and progesterone from the corpus luteum. The glands become coiled and tortuous and they begin to secrete a clear fluid, consequently, this phase of the cycle is called the *secretory or luteal phase*.

165. Ans. (c) Oxytocin

Ref: Ganong, 25th ed. pg. 313

- Oxytocin and vasopressin are typical neural hormones, ie, hormones secreted into the circulation by nerve cells.
- They are secreted from the nerve endings of the supra-optic and paraventricular nuclei of the hypothalamus. These endings are located in the posterior pituitary.

166. Ans. (c) Carbon 17 steroid

Ref: Ganong, 25th ed. pg. 421

- *Testosterone is a C19 steroid with hydroxyl group at 17 position*
- The synthesis occurs from cholesterol in the leydig cells and is formed from androstenedione secreted by adrenal cortex.
- The secretion of testosterone is under the control of LH and the mechanism by which LH stimulates leydig cells involves increased formation of cAMP. This cyclic AMP promotes conversion of cholesterol to pregnenolone and testosterone eventually.

167. Ans. (d) Menstrual blood is predominantly arterial

Ref: Ganong, 25th ed. pg. 401

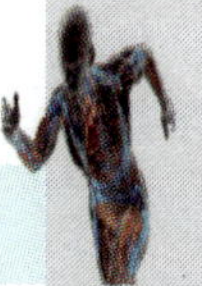

Proliferative phase by progesterone (Choice a)	Incorrect	It is due to estrogen and endometrial thickness increases from 5th to 14th days of menstrual cycle.
Secretory phase by estrogen (Choice b)	Incorrect	It is due to progesterone and when corpus luteum regresses, there is coiling of spiral arteries.
Superifical 1/3rd of endometrium is shed (Choice c)	Incorrect	Whole of the endometrium except basal layer is shed
Menstrual blood is predominantly arterial (Choice d)	Correct	The menstrual blood is predominantly arterial with only 25% being venous and contains prostaglandins and fibrinolysin.

168. Ans. (a) FSH

Ref: Ganong, 25th ed. pg. 425

Inhibin is a factor of testicular origin that inhibits FSH secretion.

Testosterone from the testis regulates LH secretion.

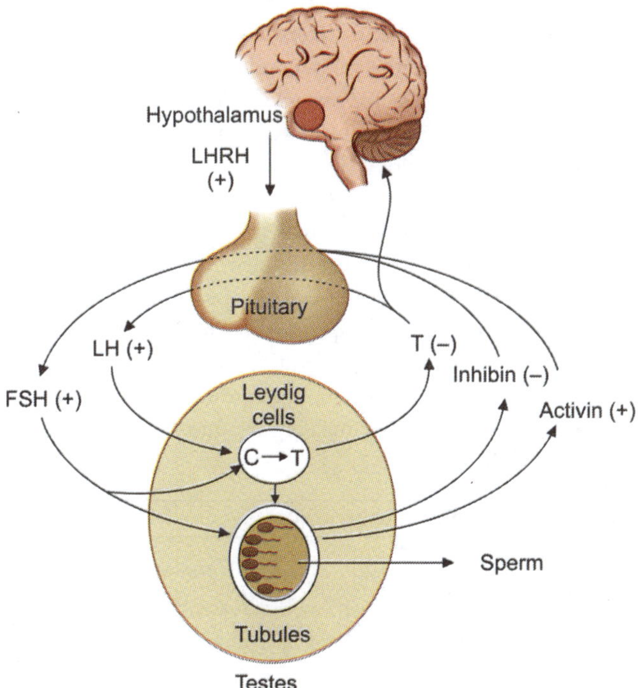

169. Ans. (d) hCG

Ref: Ganong, 25th ed./Table 22.5 pg. 412

Hormone	Time of peak secretion
hCG	First trimester
Relaxin	First trimester
hCS (human chorionic Somatotropin)	Term
Estradiol	Term
Estriol	Term
Progesterone	Term
Prolactin	Term

170. Ans. (a) Cervical mucus

Ref: Ganong 25th ed. pg. 402

- The cervical mucus is thinnest at time of ovulation and its elasticity or spinnbarkeit increases such that by mid-cycle one drop can be stretched into a long, thin thread that may be 8–12 cm or more in length.
- *It dries on a slide in an arborizing fern like pattern.*
- After ovulation, it becomes thick and fails to form the fern pattern.

RESPIRATORY PHYSIOLOGY

171. Ans. (c) Increased pH

Ref: Berne and Levy Physiology, 6th ed. pg. 773, 774

- A shift to the left indicates increased hemoglobin affinity for oxygen and an increased reluctance to release oxygen.
- It is due to the following reasons: decreased temperature, decreased hydrogen ion concentration.
- The right shift in the oxygen dissociation curve is due to an increase in pCO_2 or a decrease in pH. High pCO_2, H^+ concentration and temperature favor dissociation of oxygen from oxyhaemoglobin and show the reduced affinity of haemoglobin for oxygen.

172. Ans. (b) Type 2 pneumocytes

Ref: Berne and Levy Physiology, 6th ed. pg. 706

- Type II pneumocytes are identified as the synthesizing cells of the alveolar surfactant, which has important properties in maintaining alveolar and airway stability.
- Lung surfactant can reduce the surface tension and prevent alveolar collapse and the airway walls collapse.

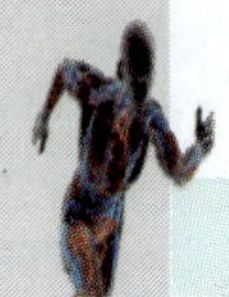

173. Ans. (a) Opening of aortic valve

Ref: Ganong 26th ed. pg. 529

A = Start of LV contraction as pressure begins to rise
B = Opening of Aortic valve as blood ejects into the aorta
C = End of ejection as Aortic valve closes
D = Relaxation of LV as pressure in chamber drops to initiate filling

174. Ans. (b) Parenchymal Restrictive airway disease

Ref: Harrison 20th ed. pg. 1947

The image shows a flow volume curve marked in color blue that is shifted to left and has lesser surface area covered as compared to baseline which is marked in color dotted green. Since the Residual volume and Total lung capacity in curve is reduced it implies patient is having parenchymal restrictive lung disease.

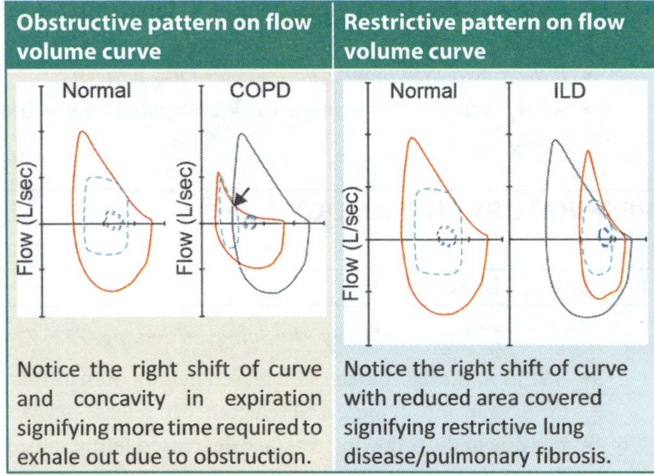

175. Ans. (d) Haldane effect

Ref: Ganong 26th ed. pg. 632

- The image shows carbon dioxide dissociation curve. The total concentration of CO_2 in all forms (ml/L) is plotted as function of Carbon dioxide partial pressure in blood. You will notice that at any given pCO_2 the total CO_2 content is greater in blood with a reduced oxygen content as compared to fully oxygenated blood. This is called as Haldane effect.
- Simply put it ensures more CO_2 in venous blood as compared to arterial blood because of this effect in body tissues. This CO_2 is then sent to lungs for expiration.
- Option A describes hemoglobin's lower affinity for oxygen secondary to increases in the partial pressure of carbon dioxide and/or decreased blood pH. This lower affinity, in turn, enhances the unloading of oxygen into tissues to meet the oxygen demand of the tissue.
- Option B and C are same and deal with exit of HCO_3 out of RBC and entry of chloride inside RBC via anion exchanger.

Extra Mile

Salient features of CO_2 dissociation curve
- Curve is more linear and steep than oxyhemoglobin dissociation curve
- Has no plateau
- Arterial point corresponds to pCP_2 = 40 mm Hg and content of CO_2 is 480 ml/L
- Mixed venous point pCP_2 = 46 mm Hg. CO_2 content is 520 ml/L

176. Ans. (b) GM-CSF

Ref: Ganong 26th ed. pg. 620

The surfactant is produced by type 2 cells of alveoli and is degraded by GM-CSF. Defective degradation of GM-CSF leads to accumulation of surfactant in alveoli and development of Pulmonary alveolar proteinosis.

177. Ans. (a) Histotoxic

Ref: Ganong, 25th ed. pg. 651

- Histotoxic hypoxia refers to a reduction in ATP production by the mitochondria *due to a defect in the cellular usage of oxygen while the delivery to tissues is normal*. The problem lies with extraction.
- Choice b, Hypoxic hypoxia occurs when the PO_2 of arterial blood falls. This could occur because inspired PO_2 is lower than normal (high altitude) or it could be due to a respiratory problem (e.g., hypoventilation, diffusion impairment caused by pulmonary oedema)
- Choice c, Stagnant hypoxia in terms of oxygen transport there is a decreased blood flow/hypoperfusion and thus the problem resides with the cardiovascular system.
- Choice d will have low delivery due to shortage of oxy-Hb values

178. Ans. (b) Apneustic breathing

Ref: Ganong: 25th ed. pg. 656

Prolonged inspiratory spasm that resemble breath holding is called apneusis. It occurs in case of damage to pneumotaxic center with cut vagi.

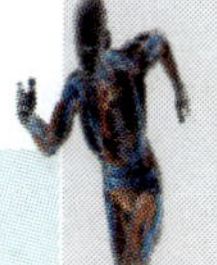

Pattern	Description	Causes	Pattern	Description	Causes
Bradypnea 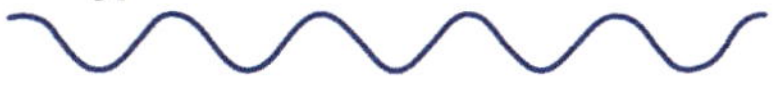	Slow respirations <10 breaths/min	CVA diabetic coma, head injury, increased ICP, metabolic disorder, opioid overdose, sleep	**Cheyne–stokes** 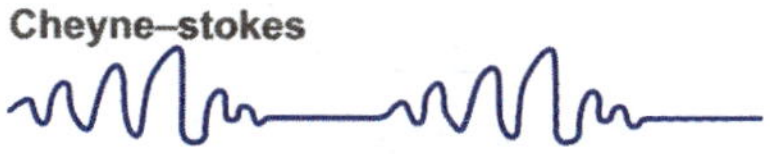	Increasing depth followed by apnea	Altitude sickness, brain stem injury, CO poisoning, CHF, CVA, increasing ICP, metabolic encephalopathy, uremia
Tachypnea 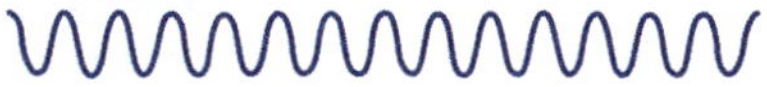	Fast, shallow respirations >24 breaths/min	Anxiety, exercise, fever, shock	**Air trapping** 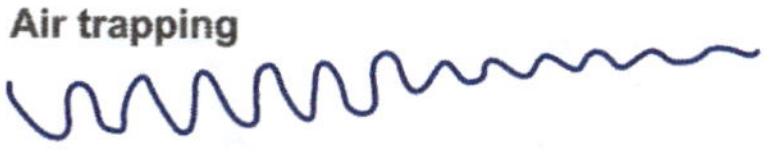	Increasing expiratory difficulty	Asthma, bronchiolitis obliterans syndrome, chronic bronchitis, emphysema
Hyperpnea 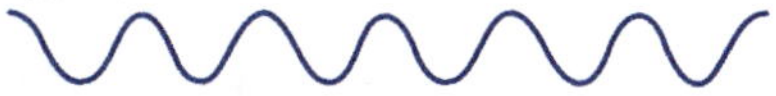	Deep, regular, respirations at normal rate	Diabetic ketoacidosis, emotional stress	**Obstructive** 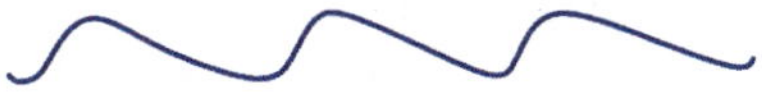	Prolonged expirations	Asthma, COPD
Kussmaul 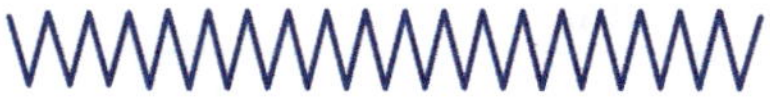	Regular, rapid, deep respirations	Diabetic ketoacidosis, exercise, metabolic acidosis, renal failure	**Sighing** 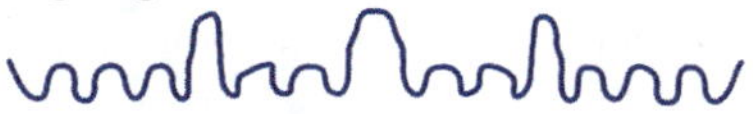	Regular breathing with frequent deep breaths	Anxiety, asthma, fatigue, hyperventilation syndrome
Hypopnea 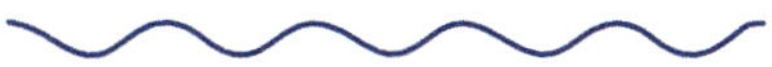	Shallow, regular, respirations at normal rate	Anxiety, asthma, hyperventilation, obesity, pneumonia, pulmonary edema, sedatives, shock, tonsilitis	**Apneustic** 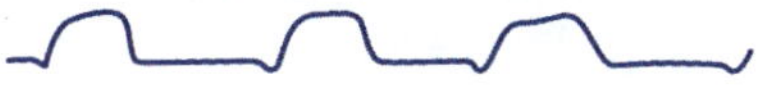	Prolonged inspiration and expiration	Brain stem lesion, CVA, brain stem injury
Ataxic 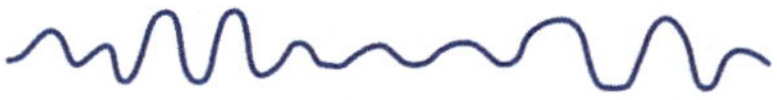	Irregular, disorganized, varying depth	CVA, medullary brain trauma	**Agonal** 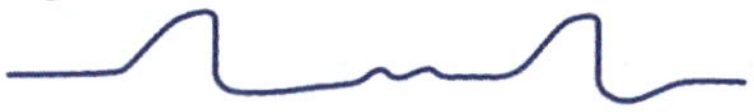	Occasional reflex driven gasps	Anoxia, cardiac arrest, cerebral ischemia, hypoxia
Biot 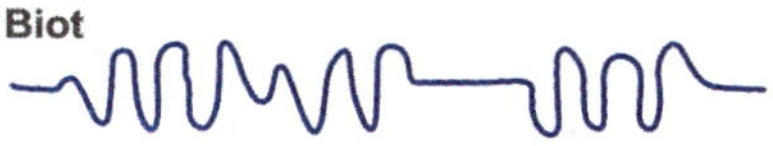	Irregular, disorganized with periods of apnea	Brain trauma, CNS disorder, CVA, opioid overdose, spinal meningitis	**Apnea**	Absence of breathing	CVA, brain trauma, deceased

179. Ans. (b) Pressure in alveoli and intrapleural pressure

- Transpulmonary pressure is the difference between *intrapulmonary* (also known as intraalveolar or airway) pressure and *intrapleural pressure*

180. Ans. (d) 0.9–1.0

- Respiratory quotient (RQ) is the ratio in the steady state of the volume of carbon dioxide produced to the volume of oxygen consumed per unit time.
- RQ of the brain is 0.97–0.99; this is *because the principal fuel for the brain is carbohydrates.*

181. Ans. (c) 16 mm Hg

Ref: Guyton's Physiology, 11th ed. pg. 162

- Pulmonary artery systolic pressure averages about 24 mm Hg and diastolic pressure 8 mm Hg, with *a mean pulmonary arterial pressure of only 16 mm Hg.*
- The mean pulmonary capillary pressure averages only 7 mm Hg.
- Mean pressure in the aorta is high, averaging about 100 mm Hg.

182. Ans. (c) 160

- At sea level the atmosphere exerts a total pressure of 760 mm Hg. Since the atmosphere is 21% O_2 (by volume), the partial pressure of oxygen (pO_2) = 0.21 × 760 = 160 mm Hg.
- The partial pressure of CO_2 (pCO_2) at sea level is 0.23 mm Hg.

183. Ans. (a) V/Q ratio is high at the apex of the lung

Ref: Ganong, 24th ed. pg. 636-37

- The ratio of pulmonary ventilation to pulmonary blood flow for the whole lung at rest is about 0.8.
- There is marked difference in this ventilation/perfusion ratio in various parts of the normal lung as a result of the effect of gravity.
- The ventilation/perfusion ratios are high in the upper portions of the lungs.
- In an upright posture ventilation (V) is high and perfusion (Q) is low at the apex of lung.
- While on the other hand ventilation is low and perfusion is high at the base of lung.

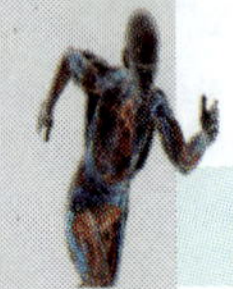

184. Ans. (d) **Volume remaining after normal expiration**

Ref: Ganong, 25th ed. pg. 629

LUNG VOLUME

Tidal volume (TV) **N = 500 ml**	Air that moves in or out of the lung with each normal inspiration or expiration t
Inspiratory reserve volume (IRV) **N = 3300 ml**	The air inspired with a maximal inspiratory effort in excess of tidal volume
Expiratory reserve volume (ERV) **N = 1000 ml**	The air expelled with a maximal expiratory effort in excess of tidal volume
Residual volume (RV) **N = 1200 ml**	The amount of air remaining in the lungs even after forced expiration

LUNG CAPACITIES

Inspiratory capacity (I.C) = (TV + IRV) **N = 3800 ml**	Total amount of air that can be breathed in.
Vital capacity; ***VC = TV + IRV + ERV*** **N = 4800 ml**	Maximum amount of air that can be expelled out force fully after a maximal (deep) inspiration
Functional residual capacity ***FRC = ERV + RV*** **N = 2200 ml**	It is the volume of air remaining in the lung after normal expiration (after normal tidal expiration)
Total lung capacity TLC = TV + IRV + ERV + RV *N = 6000 ml. (4.2-6 lit)*	The amount of air present in the lung after a maximal inspiration. This is the maximum volume to which the lungs can be expanded.

185. Ans. (c) **Type II Pneumocytes**

Ref: Guyton, 11th ed. pg. 474

- The smaller type II pneumocytes are often more numerous than type I pneumocytes, but they contribute less than 10% of the surface area.
- They are rounded cells which protrude from the alveolar surface, particularly at the angles between alveolar profiles.
- In the human lung they are often associated with interalveolar pores of Kohn. Their cytoplasm contains numerous characteristic secretory lamellar bodies, which they can recycle.
- Ultrastructurally, the lamellar bodies are comprised of concentric whorls of phospholipid-rich membrane, the precursors of alveolar surfactant.
- ***"Surfactant is stored in lamellar bodies and secreted in the form of tubular myelin (unrelated to myelin of the nervous system) by type II pneumocytes.*** It is recycled by type II pneumocytes, or cleared (phagocytosed) by alveolar macrophages.
- Clara cells of the bronchiolar epithelium serve as progenitor cells. They are nonciliated cuboidal epithelial cells in terminal bronchioles.

186. Ans. (c) **Immunoglobulin A**

Ref: Ganong, 24th ed. pg. 77-78

- The activated B cells proliferate and transform into memory B cells and plasma cells.
- The plasma cells secrete large quantities of antibodies into the general circulation known as immunoglobulins.

Immunoglobulins	Function
IgG	Complement activation
IgA	Localized protection in external secretions (tears, intestinal secretions, etc)
IgM	Complement activation[Q]
IgD	Antigen recognition by B cells
IgE	Reagin activity; releases histamine from basophils and mast cells

187. Ans. (d) **Oxygen**

Ref: Ganong 25th ed. Table 36. 1 pg. 657 & 659 and Guyton's, 11th ed. pg. 516

- The ultimate goal of respiration is to maintain proper concentration of oxygen, carbon dioxide and hydrogen ions in the tissues.
- Excess carbon dioxide or excess hydrogen ions in the blood mainly act directly on the respiratory center.
- Oxygen, in contrast, does not have a significant direct effect on the respiratory center of the brain in controlling respiration.
- Instead oxygen acts almost entirely on peripheral chemoreceptors located in the carotid and aortic bodies, and these in turn transmit appropriate nervous signals to the respiratory center for control of respiration by detecting O_2 level in blood.

Extra Mile

Central Chemoreceptors
- More powerful, less rapid than peripheral chemoreceptor
- Highly sensitive to changes in $PaCO_2$ or H^+
- *$PaCO_2$: Most important stimulus for central chemoreceptor.*
- High $PaCO_2$ stimulates respiratory center which then increases alveolar ventilation and vice versa.

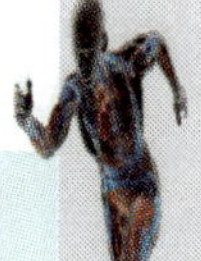

188. Ans. (a) Oxygen and nitrogen

Ref: Ganong's, 22nd ed. Chapter 37

Potential problems associated with exposure to increased barometric pressure under water:

- **Oxygen toxicity:** Lung damage, Convulsions
- **Nitrogen narcosis:** Euphoria, Impaired performance
- **High-pressure nervous syndrome:** Tremors, somnolence
- **Decompression sickness:** Pain, Paralysis
- **Air embolism:** Sudden death

189. Ans. (a) Increased hemoglobin content and RBC

Ref: Guyton's Physiology, 11th ed. pg. 539-541

- **Acclimatization:** Adaptation to new temperature or altitude so that hypoxia causes lesser effect to body.
- At high altitude there is low oxygen. When a person remains exposed to low oxygen, the hematocrit rises slowly from a normal value of 40–45 to an average of about 60.

Extra Mile

- A person remaining at high altitudes for days, weeks, or years becomes more and more *acclimatized* to the low pO_2.
- The principle means by which acclimatization comes about are:
  - **Increased** pulmonary ventilation
  - **Increased** numbers of RBC.
  - Increased diffusing capacity of the lungs.
  - increased vascularity of the peripheral tissues, and
  - **Increased** ability of the tissue cells to use oxygen despite low PO_2

- And an increase in hemoglobin concentration from normal of 15 g/dL to about 20 g/dL.
- In addition, the blood volume also increases, often by 20 to 30 per cent.

190. Ans. (c) Due to inadequate gas exchange

Ref: Ganong, 25th ed. pg. 651

- Hypoxic hypoxia is due to *inadequate gas exchange*, in which the oxygen content of arterial blood and PO_2 are reduced. Example: COPD, High altitude.

Types of Hypoxia and causes

Type of hypoxia	Pathophysiology	Example
Anemic Hypoxia	Due to reduced oxygen carrying capacity	Anemia (Reduced RBC, Reduced Hb); CO poisoning
Hypoxic Hypoxia	Due to Inadequate gas exchange	High altitude Respiratory disease (COPD)
Histotoxic Hypoxia	Inability of cells to utilize available O_2	Cyanide poisoning
Stagnant Hypoxia	Due to slow circulation	Circulatory Shock Congestive heart failure

191. Ans. (b) Hering Breur Reflex

Ref: Ganong, 25th ed. pg. 662

- Hering- Breuer reflex is reflex *triggered to prevent over inflation of lung*.
- Smooth muscles of lung have pulmonary stretch receptors which respond to excessive stretching of lung during large inspirations.
- The reflex limits the tidal volume while increasing the respiratory frequency
- Hering Breur inflation reflex is increase in duration of expiration produced by steady lung inflation.
- Hering breur deflation reflex is a decrease in duration of expiration produced by steady lung deflation.
- Surfactant prevents collapse of the lung.

192. Ans. (c) Decreased H+

Ref: Ganong, 25th ed. pg. 640-641

OXYGEN HEMOGLOBIN DISSOCIATION CURVE

- Oxygen- hemoglobin dissociation curve is sigmoid 'S' shaped because *binding of one oxygen molecule to heme increases the affinity of second heme molecule for oxygen* and so on.

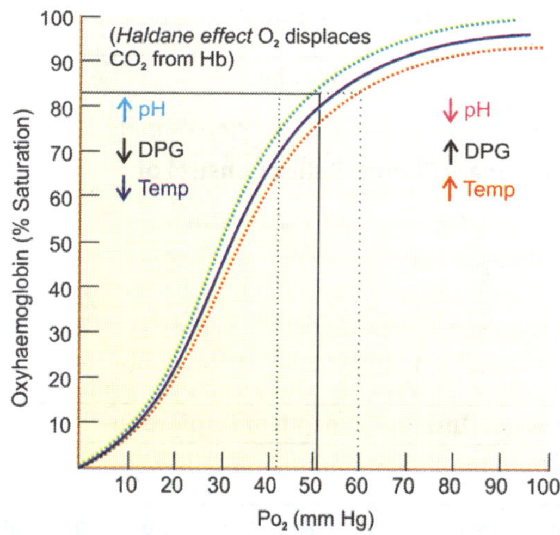

Factors affecting affinity of Hb for oxygen and causing the shift of curve are:

Left shift	Right shift
• This means the *affinity of oxygen to Hb is increased and oxygen is bound more tightly to hemoglobin* • Factors leading to left shift are ▪ *Alkalosis or ↑pH* ▪ *↓ pCO_2* (CO_2 content of blood) ▪ *↓ Temperature* (Hypothermia) ▪ ↓ 2,3 DPG	• This means the affinity of O_2 to Hb is decreased which *favors release of oxygen to tissue.* • Factors leading to right shift are: ▪ *Acidosis or ↓ pH* ▪ *↑ pCO_2* (CO_2 content of blood) ▪ *↑ Temperature* (Hypothermia) ▪ ↑ 2,3 DPG

193. Ans. (b) Shift of Oxy-Hb dissociation curve to right

Ref: Ganong's Physiology, 23rd ed. pg. 611 and Ganong, 25th ed. pg. 640-41

Refer to the above question. Increased carbon dioxide in blood will lead to respiratory acidosis, and shift curve to right.

194. Ans. (d) Binding of oxygen molecule increases affinity of binding other oxygen molecule

Ref: Ganong's, 23rd ed. pg. 610

- S-shape of O_2-Hb dissociation curve is formed when one oxygen molecule (among the 4 that is supposed to bind with Hb) binds with a hemoglobin molecule with greatest affinity and this binding increases affinity of other heme molecule to bind oxygen.
- Fall in pH due to increase pCO_2, decreases oxygen affinity of Hb. This phenomenon is known as ***Bohr's effect.***
- Binding of O_2 to Hb reduces affinity of Hb to CO_2. This phenomenon is known as ***Haldane effect.***

195. Ans. (d) Alkalosis

Ref: Ganong, 25th ed. pg. 640-41

Refer to above explanation

196. Ans. (a) Reflex bradycardia

Ref: Ganong, 25th ed. pg. 662

Pulmonary Chemo-Reflex Consists of:[Q]

1. Apnea followed by Rapid breathing
2. Bradycardia
3. Hypotension

It is caused by Stimulation of J receptors by intravenous or intra-cardiac administration of chemicals like capsaicin.

197. Ans. (c) Increase in depth of respiration

Ref: Ganong, 25th ed. pg. 656

Manifestation after both vagi are cut	Stretching of the lungs during inspiration initiates impulses in afferent pulmonary vagal discharges These impulses inhibit inspiratory discharge. Hence after Vagotomy the impulses inhibiting inspiratory discharge are absent and this will result in *increase of depth of respiration.*
Manifestation after Pneumotaxic center is damaged	Pneumotaxic center is dorsal pons which contains neurons active in active inspiration and expiration When this area is damaged *respiration will become slower and tidal volume greater.*
Manifestation after both vagi are cut along with damage to Pneumotaxic center	If vagi are cut after damage to pneumotaxic center, *apneusis[Q] (Prolonged inspiratory spasms that resemble breath holding) will develop*

Contd...

198. Ans. (d) 10 seconds

Ref: Harrison, 18th ed. pg. 2186

- Apneas are defined in adults as breathing pauses lasting >10 secs. and hypopneas as events >10 secs in which there is continued breathing but ventilation is reduced by at least 50% from the previous baseline during sleep.
- Obstructive sleep apnea/hypopnea syndrome is defined as the coexistence of unexplained excessive daytime sleepiness with at least five obstructed breathing events per hour of sleep.
- **Epworth sleepiness score** is used to assess the severity of the problem.

199. Ans. (c) Slower Breathing with greater tidal volume

Ref: Ganong, 25th ed. pg. 656

- Pneumotaxic center is dorsal pons which contains neurons active in active inspiration and expiration.
- When this area is damaged respiration will become slower and tidal volume greater.

200. Ans. (a) Apnea followed by rapid shallow breathing

Ref: Ganong, 25th ed. pg. 592

- Since the C fiber endings are close to pulmonary vessels, they are called J (Juxta-capillary) receptors.
- They are stimulated by hyperinflation of the lung.
- Activation of chemo-sensitive vagal C fibers in the cardio-pulmonary region causes profound bradycardia, hypotension and apnea followed by rapid shallow breathing. This is called pulmonary chemo-reflex.

Hering breuer reflexes are mediated by vagal afferent activity is mediated by slowly adapting receptors and causes shortening of inspiration.

- *Hering Breur inflation reflex is an* increase in duration of expiration produced by steady lung inflation
- *Hering Breur deflation reflex* is a decrease in duration of expiration produced by marked deflation of lung.

201. Ans. (a) 1

Ref: Ganong, 25th ed. pg. 641

Myoglobin is an iron containing pigment found in skeletal muscle and binds to 1 rather than 4 mol of O_2.

- The lack of cooperative binding is reflected in myoglobin dissociation curve which is rectangular hyperbola.
- The steepness of the curve shows that oxygen is released at low pO_2 values like at exercise.

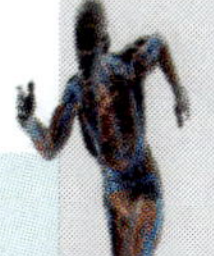

202. Ans. (a) 0.8

Ref: Ganong, 25th ed. pg. 636

Ventilation = 4.2 L/min
Perfusion = 5.5 L/min blood flow
Ventilation/perfusion ratio = 0.8

203. Ans. (a) Tidal volume × Respiratory rate

Ref: Ganong, 25th ed. pg. 629

RMV: Respiratory minute volume: 500 mL × 12 breaths/min = 6 L

204. Ans. (c) Tidal volume + Volume inspired forcefully

Functional residual Capacity	It represents the volume of air remaining in the lungs after expiration of a normal breath.
Inspiratory capacity	*It is the maximum amount of air inspired from end expiratory level.*
Vital lung capacity	Maximum amount of air expired from fully inflated lung.
Total lung capacity	Inspiratory reserve volume + Tidal volume + Expiratory reserve volume + Residual volume

205. Ans. (b) Double Bohr Effect

Ref: Fetal Medicine 1st ed. pg. 403 and Ganong, 25th ed. pg. 641-2

Double[Q] Bohr Effect is seen in placenta as CO_2 liberated by fetus enters the maternal circulation and shifts the maternal O_2 Hemoglobin dissociation curve to the right but shifts fetal curve to the left.

Haldane effect	Increased capacity of deoxygenated hemoglobin to bind and carry carbon dioxide leading to venous blood carrying CO_2.
Bohr effect	Decrease in oxygen affinity of hemoglobin when there is a fall in pH of blood.
Hamburger phenomenon	It is also called chloride shift. • When RBC's take up carbon dioxide, it is converted into bicarbonate inside the RBC • This bicarbonate is negatively charged and leaves the RBC *via anion exchanger[Q] 1 /Band 3 protein.* • *In return chloride enters the RBC.* • *Hence there is gain of osmotic molecule inside the RBC leading to entry of water into the cell leading the RBC to swell up.*

206. Ans. (b) >5 gm%

Ref: Ganong, 25th ed. pg. 642

Cyanosis appears whenever the magnitude of reduced hemoglobin level of blood in capillaries is >5 gm%.

207. Ans. (b) Pre-botzinger complex

Ref: Ganong, 25th ed. pg. 656

Prebotzinger complex-located between nucleus ambiguous and lateral reticular nucleus on either side of medulla is the site of generation of respiratory rhythm.

CARDIOVASCULAR AND CIRCULATORY PHYSIOLOGY

208. Ans. (d) Y descent occurs in rapid ventricular filling phase

Ref: Ganong, 26th ed. pg. 530

- Option a is incorrect as JVP is calculated from Manubrium of sternum and not xiphisternum.
- Option b is seen with iso-ventricular relaxation.
- Option c is incorrect as JVP falls with deep inspiration
- Option d is correct as Y descent occurs when AV valves open and free flow of blood occurs into ventricles.

209. Ans. (a) LDH1

Ref: Mosby manual of diagnostic methods E-book, pg. 339

Myocyte necrosis causes release of LDH_1 isoenzyme.

- **In normal serum**, LDH_2 is predominant isoenzyme.
- In myocardial infarction, LDH_1 levels is are greater than LDH_2, called flipped pattern
- Muscular dystrophy, LDH_5 is increased

210. Ans. (c) Peripheral resistance

Ref: Ganong 26th ed. pg. 530

Dicrotic notch is seen in pulse tracing after closing of aortic valve. The peripheral resistance generates an aberration in tracing while the aortic valves are closing. In simple words it is the pressure exerted by the vascular tree back upon the aortic valve.

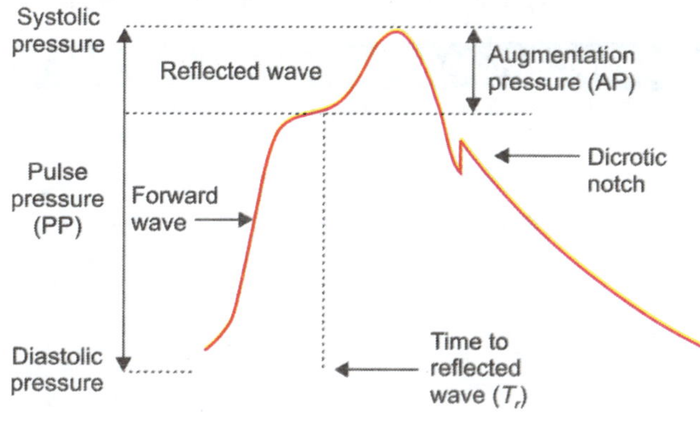

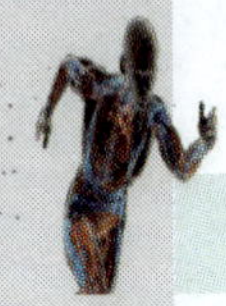

211. Ans. (a) AV valves are closed

Ref: Ganong 25th ed. pg. 539

Isovolumetric relaxation is characterised by initiation of relaxation of heart and venous return is initiated. The blood will however not enter into ventricles since *Atrio-ventricular valves are closed.*

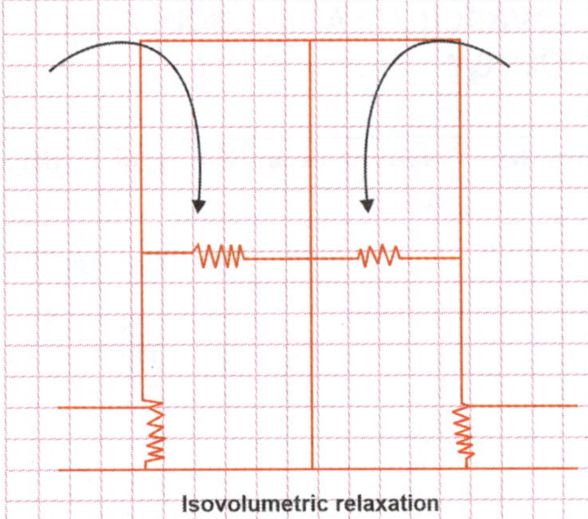

Choice b, QT interval corresponds to ventricular contraction and relaxation.

Choice c, c wave of JVP occurs in Isovolumetric contraction

Choice d, Semilunar valves opening occurs in ejection phase of cardiac cycle.

212. Ans. (b) 16 times

Ref: Ganong: 26th ed. pg. 563

- The influence of lumen diameter on resistance is dramatic. This is because resistance is inversely proportional to the radius of the blood vessel (one-half of the vessel's diameter) raised to the fourth power ($R = 1/r^4$).
- This means, that if an artery or arteriole constricts to one-half of its original radius, the resistance to flow will increase 16 times. And if an artery or arteriole dilates to twice its initial radius, then resistance in the vessel will decrease to 1/16 of its original value and flow will increase 16 times.

213. Ans. (b) First heart sound has maximum duration

Heart sound	Frequency	Duration	Associated event
First heart	25–45 Hz	0.15 sec	Closure of A-V valves—onset of ventricular systole
Second heart sound	50 Hz	0.12 sec	Closure of semilunar valves—onset of ventricular diastole
Third heart sound	Low	0.1 sec	First rapid filling phase of ventricular diastole
Fourth heart sound	Below 20 Hz	0.1 sec	Last rapid filling phase of ventricular diastole due to atrial contraction

214. Ans. (b) Modified muscle fibers

- Purkinje fibers are **modified myocardial muscle fibers** (NOT nerve fibers) that lead from the A-V node through the A-V bundle into the ventricles.
- These fibers have functional characteristics that are quite **the opposite of those of the A-V nodal fibers** *(except for the initial portion of these fibers where they penetrate the A-V fibrous barrier)*
- **Purkinje fibers are very large fibers**, larger than AV nodal fibers and even larger than the normal ventricular muscle fibers.
- Hence they transmit **action potentials at a velocity of 1.5 to 4.0 m/sec**, *which is about **6 times** that in the usual ventricular muscle and **150 times that in some of the A-V nodal fibers.***
- This allows almost instantaneous transmission of the cardiac impulse throughout the entire remainder of the ventricular muscle.

215. Ans. (b) After load

Ref: Current Obstetric and Gynecology by Mukherjee pg. 52

- In the normal fetuses, blood flow in the ductus venosus is always antegrade throughout the cardiac cycle. **Forward flow in the venous system is a function of cardiac compliance, contractility and afterload.**
- The typical waveform of fetal blood flow in the venous vessels consists of 3 phases related to the cardiac cycle *(on Doppler):*
  - **Peak S wave:** Corresponds to ventricular systole
  - **Peak D wave:** Corresponds to early diastole
  - **Peak A wave:** Corresponds to atrial contraction.

216. Ans. (c) Increase hydrostatic pressure, decrease oncotic pressure

- Starling's hypothesis states that the fluid movement due to filtration across the wall of a capillary is dependent on the balance between the hydrostatic pressure gradient and the oncotic pressure gradient across the capillary.

The four Starling's forces are:

1. Hydrostatic pressure in the capillary (Pc)
2. Hydrostatic pressure in the interstitium (Pi)
3. Oncotic pressure in the capillary (pc)
4. Oncotic pressure in the interstitium (pi)

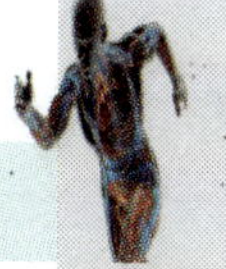

The balance of these forces allows calculation of the net driving pressure for filtration.

Net Driving Pressure = [(Pc - Pi) - (pc - pi)]

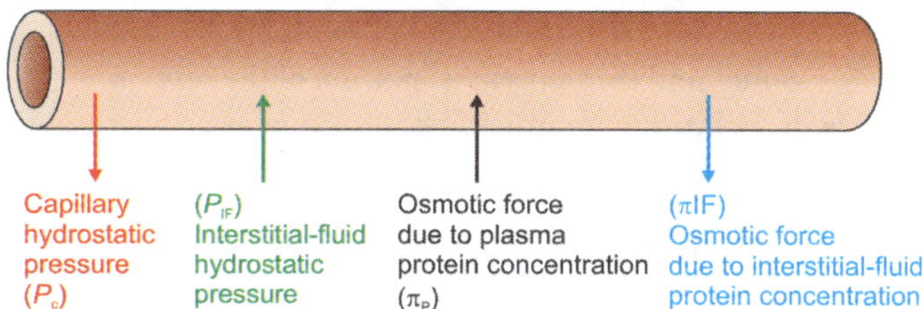

217. Ans. (b) Left ventricle works more than right ventricle

Ref: Guyton Physiology, 11th ed. pg. 110

- Right ventricular external work output is normally about *one sixth the work output of the left ventricle* because of the six-fold difference in systolic pressures that the two ventricles pump.

218. Ans. (b) AV node shows fast conduction

219. Ans. (c) Decreases by increase in heart rate

Ref: Ganong, 25th ed. pg. 570-71

- *Basically it is asking here about the TRUE statement among the given choices.*
- Stroke volume is indirectly proportional to heart rate
- Stroke volume = cardiac output/heart rate
- *As the heart rate increases, stroke volume decreases.*
- After load is determined by peripheral resistance. Therefore, it has nothing to do with stroke volume determination.
- Stroke volume depends upon end diastolic volume *(NOT pre-diastolic volume)*

220. Ans. (d) >170 mm Hg

Ref: Harrison's, 19th ed. pg. 1616

TABLE: Guidelines for threshold values between normal and high blood pressure

	Clinic measurement (mm Hg)	Home measurement (mm Hg)
Optimal control	<140/85	<130/80
Mild hypertension	140–150/90–100	135–145/85–95
Moderate hypertension	150–170/100–110	145–165/95–105
Severe hypertension	>170/110	>165/105

The question mentioned was severe hypertension, however if the grading of hypertension is asked, then answer must be according to this table:

BP classification	Systolic mm Hg	Diastolic, mm Hg
Normal	<120	and <80
Pre-hypertension	120–129	<80
Stage I HTN	130–139	80–89
Stage II HTN	>140	>90
Isolated systolic HTN	>140	and <90

221. Ans. (c) Atrial contraction

Ref: Harrison's Internal Medicine, 17th ed. Chapter 220, PE of CVS.

NORMAL JVP WAVEFORM

- Classically three upward deflections and two downward deflections have been described.
- ***The 'a' wave corresponds to right Atrial contraction*** and ends synchronously with the carotid artery pulse. The peak of the 'a' wave demarcates the end of atrial systole.
- ***The 'c' wave corresponds to right ventricular contraction*** causing the tricuspid valve to bulge towards the right atrium.
- ***The 'x' descent*** follows the 'a' wave and corresponds to atrial relaxation and rapid atrial filling due to low pressure.
- The 'x' (x prime) descent follows the 'c' wave and occurs as a result of the right ventricle pulling the tricuspid valve downward during ventricular systole.
- ***The 'v' wave*** corresponds to venous filling when the tricuspid valve is closed and venous pressure increases from venous return – this occurs during and following the carotid pulse.
- ***The 'y' descent*** corresponds to the rapid emptying of the atrium into the ventricle following the opening of the tricuspid valve.

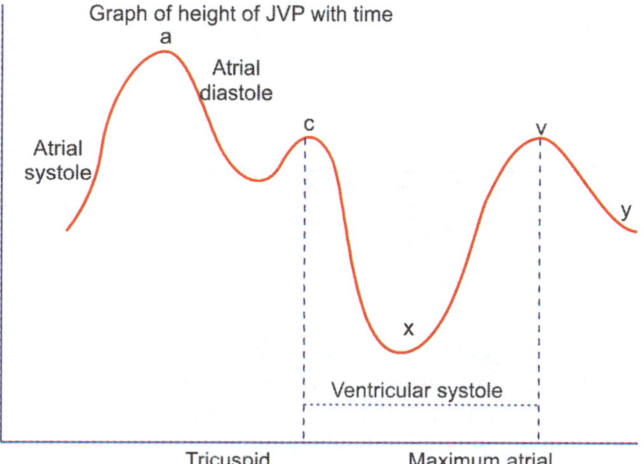

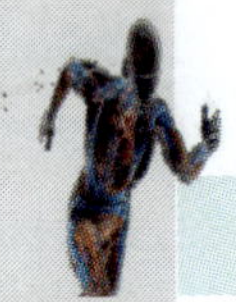

Extra Mile

About JVP

Raised JVP, Normal waveform	**Raised JVP, absent pulsation:**	**Large 'a' wave (increased atrial contraction pressure)**
Bradycardia Fluid overload Heart Failure	Superior vena cava syndrome **Cardiac Tamponade**	Tricuspid stenosis Right heart failure Pulmonary hypertension
Cannon 'a' wave (atria contracting against closed tricuspid valve)	**Absent 'a' wave (no unifocal atrial depolarization)**	**Paradoxical JVP (Kussmaul's sign: JVP rises with inspiration, drops with expiration)**
Atrial flutter Premature atrial rhythm (or tachycardia) Third degree heart block Ventricular ectopics Ventricular tachycardia	Atrial fibrillation	Pericardial effusion Constrictive pericarditis Pericardial tamponade

- **Large 'v' wave (c-v wave):** Tricuspid regurgitation
- Slow 'y' descent: Tricuspid stenosis

222. Ans. (b) Maximum during diastole

Ref: Ganong 25th ed. pg. 611

- The Flow in coronary arteries occurs in the sub-endocardial portion of the left ventricle only during diastole, although the force is sufficiently dissipated in the more superficial portions of the left ventricular myocardium to permit some flow in this region throughout the cardiac cycle.
- Because *no blood flow occurs during systole in the sub-endocardial portion of the left ventricle, this region is prone to ischemic damage* and is the most common site of myocardial infarction.

223. Ans. (b) Endocardium to epicardium

Ref: Ganong's Physiology, 23rd ed. chapter 30

- Depolarization: From endocardium to epicardium
- Repolarization always proceeds from epicardium to endocardium leading to positive T wave in all leads.
- Depolarization of the ventricular muscle starts at the left side of the interventricular septum and moves first to the right across the mid portion of the septum.
- The wave of depolarization then spreads down the septum to the apex of the heart.
- It returns along the ventricular walls to the AV groove, proceeding from the endocardial to the epicardial surface.
- The last parts of the heart to be depolarized are the postero-basal portion of the left ventricle, the pulmonary conus, and the uppermost portion of the septum.
- In isolated myocardial fiber direction of depolarization and repolarization is same

224. Ans. (d) Increase in venous capacitance

Ref: Ganong's Physiology, 23rd ed. chapter 17

SYMPATHETIC STIMULATION

Beta 1 Receptor–

- **SA node:** Increase in heart rate
- **AV node:** Increase in conduction velocity
- **HIS Purkinje system:** Increase in conduction velocity
- **Atria:** Increase in contractility and conduction velocity
- **Ventricle:** Increase in contractility

Alpha 1 Receptor–

- Increase in total peripheral resistance leads to increase in BP.

225. Ans. (b) ST segment is 0.40 seconds

Ref: Ganong, 25th ed. pg. 524

ECG INTERVALS

PR interval	0.12-0.2 sec	Atrioventricular conduction
QRS	0.08 sec-0.1 sec	Ventricular depolarization
QT interval	0.40-0.43 sec	Ventricular action potential
ST segment		*Plateau portion of the ventricular action potential*

Normal AV nodal delay is due to slow propogation via the AV node and is 0.1 seconds.

226. Ans. (b) Closure of aortic and pulmonic valves

Ref: Ganong, 25th ed. pg. 540

The Dicrotic notch is small oscillations on the falling phase of the pulse wave caused by vibrations set up when the aortic valve snaps shut.

227. Ans. (b) Explains the increase in cardiac output when venous return is increased

Ref: Ganong, 25th ed. pg. 546

- Frank starling law states that energy of contraction is directly proportional to initial length of cardiac muscle fiber.
- *Hence in case of more blood coming on to the right side of the heart, the length of muscle fiber will increase and this will result in increase in force of contraction of heart.*

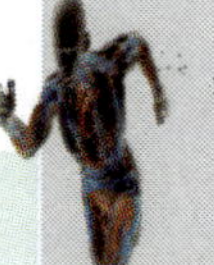

228. Ans. (b) Oscillometry

Ref: Ganong, 25th ed. pg. 543

Doppler	Based on acoustics of sound waves
Thermodilution method	Cold Saline is injected into right atrium and temperature change in blood is recorded in pulmonary artery. The temperature change in pulmonary artery shall be inversely related to blood flow.
Fick's principle	Amount of substance taken up by an organ is equal to arterial level of substance minus the venous level of substance times the blood flow.

229. Ans. (d) Peripheral resistance increases

Ref: Ganong, 25th ed. pg. 549

- Blood flow of resting skeletal muscle is low (2-4 ml/100 gm/min)
- When the muscle contracts, it compresses the vessels and when it develops 70% of its maximal tension, blood is completely interrupted.
- Between contractions the flow is increased by 30 times
- This is due to dilatation of arterioles and precapillary sphincters cause of 10-100 times increase in open capillaries
- *During exercise there is a net fall in peripheral resistance*, due to vasodilation in exercising muscles. Hence the SBP increases moderately and diastolic pressure remains unchanged or falls.

230. Ans. (c) Middle of R to end of T wave

Ref: Ganong, 25th ed. pg. 541

Atrial systole	Beginning of P wave and peak of R wave
Ventricular systolet	Middle of R wave and end of T wave
Ventricular diastole	End of T wave and beginning of next P wave

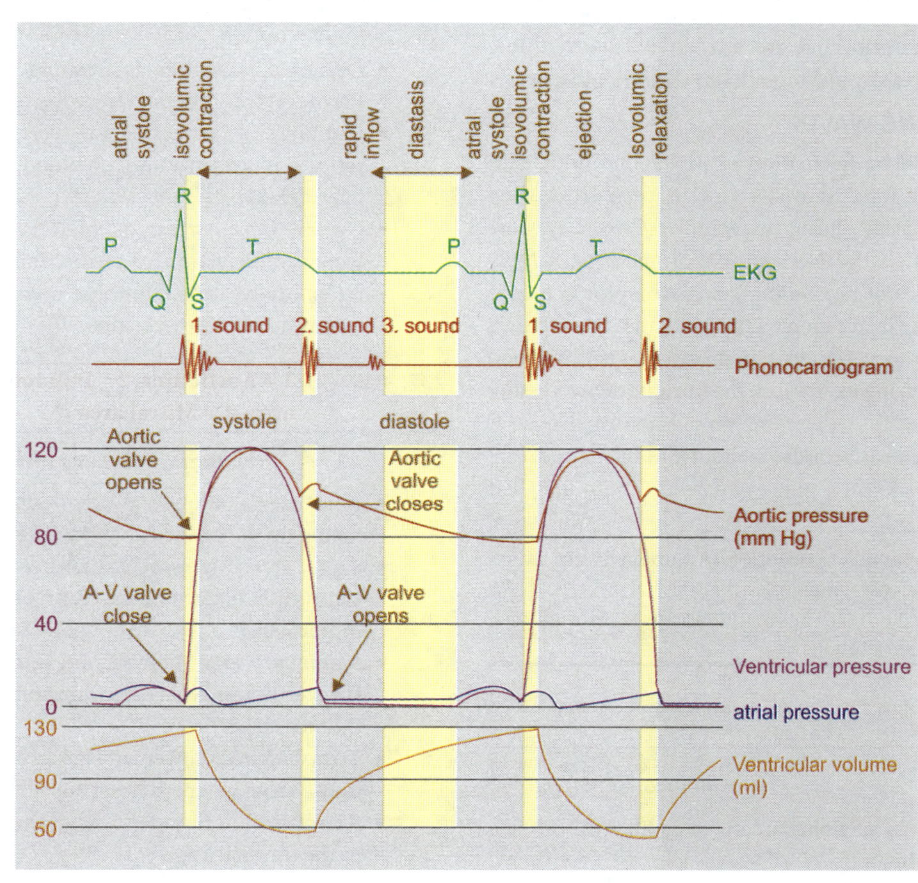

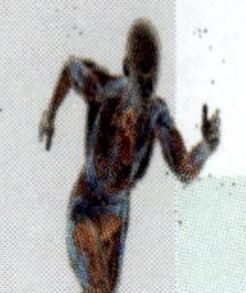

231. Ans. (a) Increase in rate of transmission

Ref: Ganong, 25th ed. pg. 545

Effect on heart rate = Chronotropic action
Effect on force of contraction = Inotropic action
Effect on rate of transmission = Dromotropic action

232. Ans. (b) C wave is called as dicrotic notch

Ref: Ganong, 25th ed. pg. 542

A wave	Atrial systole
C wave	Bulge of tricuspid valve into right atrium during isovolumetric contraction
X descent	Atrial relaxation
V wave	Beginning of isovolumetric relaxation
Y descent	Ventricular relaxation

Dicrotic Notch is seen in Pulse recording.

233. Ans. (a) Fluctuation in BP with respiration

Ref: Textbook of Medical Physiology, 2nd ed. pg. 435

Traube Hering Waves are oscillations in BP that occur with a frequency of 4/min, and are attributable to rhythmic oscillations in intensity of sympathetic vasomotor discharge.

TRAUBE–HERING WAVES

These are formed by fluctuation in BP synchronous with respiration. The wave shows a rise in pressure during inspiration and a fall during expiration. *These waves are produced due to change in vagal and sympathetic activity in different phases of respiration.* The vasomotor center is stimulated during inspiration by the irradiation of impulses from the inspiratory centers which causes rise in blood pressure. Also during expiration, the intrathoracic pressure becomes less negative, therefore venous return decreases which in turn decreases cardiac output and BP.

Extra Mile

- **Traube semilunar space:** A crescentic space about 12 cm wide, just above the costal margin.
- **Traube sign:** A murmur heard in auscultation over arteries in significant aortic regurgitation.

234. Ans. (c) Venule

Ref: Ganong, 25th ed. pg. 568

- Maximum cross sectional area is of capillaries. But it is *not* given in choices.
- The second most extensive cross sectional area is of venules.
- *However the maximum of percentage of blood volume is in venules + veins and vena cava and constitutes 54% of total blood volume contained.*

Vessel	Cross sectional area	% of blood volume contained
Capillary	4500 cm^2	5%
Venule	4000 cm^2	54%
Arteriole	400 cm^2	1%
Artery	20 cm^2	8%
Aorta	4.5 cm^2	2%

235. Ans. (c) 15 seconds

Ref: Ganong, 25th ed. pg. 573

The normal arm to tongue circulation time is 15 seconds and is measured by injecting a bile salt preparation into the arm vein and timing when the bitter taste will appear in the tongue of the patient.

CNS AND PNS PHYSIOLOGY

236. Ans. (d) Abolished by blockade of chemoreceptors

Ref: Ganong 26th ed. pg. 582

- Option d is answer as Cushing reflex is mediated by Baroreceptors and not chemoreceptors.
- Option a is correct as low cerebral perfusion causes reflex vasoconstriction of blood vessels and resultant hypertension.
- Option b is correct as high BP will cause negative feedback/activation of cardioinhibitory center to cause reflex bradycardia. Option c is correct high BP leads to widening of pulse pressure.

237. Ans. (a) 1 = Aortic area, 2 = Pulmonic area, 3 = Tricuspid area, 4 = Mitral area

Ref: Berne and Levy Physiology, 6th ed. pg. 490

- Heart auscultation is usually performed with the patient sitting up or reclined at about 45 degrees.
- *Aortic area:* Right second intercostal space close to the sternum is where the ascending aorta is nearest to the thoracic cage.
- *Pulmonary area:* Left second intercostal space close to the sternum is where the infundibulum is closest to the thoracic cage.
- *Tricuspid area:* Lower left sternal edge is the point closest to the valve in which heart auscultation is possible.
- *Mitral area:* At the apex beat, as the left ventricle is closest to the thoracic cage.

238. Ans. (a) Ascending sensory and descending motor pathways in spinal cord

Ref: Ganong 26th ed. pg. 168

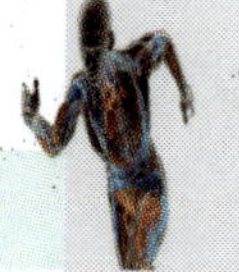

Brown-Séquard Syndrome

A functional hemisection of the spinal cord causes a characteristic and easily recognized clinical picture that reflects damage to *ascending sensory* (dorsal column pathway, ventrolateral spinothalamic tract) and *descending motor* (corticospinal tract) pathways, which is called the **Brown-Séquard syndrome**. The lesion to fasciculus gracilis and/or fasciculus cuneatus leads to ipsilateral loss of discriminative touch, vibration, and proprioception below the level of the lesion. The loss of the spinothalamic tract leads to contralateral loss of pain and temperature sensation beginning one or two segments below the lesion. Damage to the corticospinal tract produces weakness and spasticity in certain muscle groups on the same side of the body. The syndrome is common because it can be caused by a spinal cord tumor, spinal cord trauma, degenerative disk disease, and ischemia.

239. Ans. (b) Broca's area

Ref: Ganong 26th ed. pg. 206

- Speaking with logic, syntax (grammar) and fluency are functions of Broca's area. Wernicke's area is for understanding/Comprehension.
- Since patient can understand written words and write them Wernicke's area is working fine.
- However, the expression part is compromised in this patient post head injury and implies damage to Broca's area
- Option C is ruled out as repetition only is impaired. Understanding and producing speech output is normal.
- Option D presents as dense hemiplegia/hemianesthesia due to damage to corticospinal pathways.

240. Ans. (a) Tone

Ref: Ganong, 25th ed. pg. 232-33

- The resistance of muscle to stretch is called tone or tonus
- *Spasticity* is found with upper motor neuron injuries and manifests as a marked resistance to the initiation of rapid passive movement. This initial resistance gives way and then there is less resistance over the remaining range of motion (clasp-knife phenomenon).
- *Rigidity* is an increase in tone that persists throughout the passive range of motion. This has been termed "lead pipe" rigidity and is common with extrapyramidal disease, especially Parkinson's disease.
- *Paratonia* is a phenomenon in which the patient is essentially unable to relax during passive movements. You will note that the resistance is irregular and generally greatest when you change the pattern of movement. Extreme paratonia is common in patients with dementia.

241. (a) Arcuate fasciculus

Ref: Ganong, 25th ed. pg. 292

Arcus Fasiciculus connects the Broca's area to Wernicke's area. It is a white matter tract and damage to this area will result in conduction aphasia where repetition will be affected.

Extra Mile

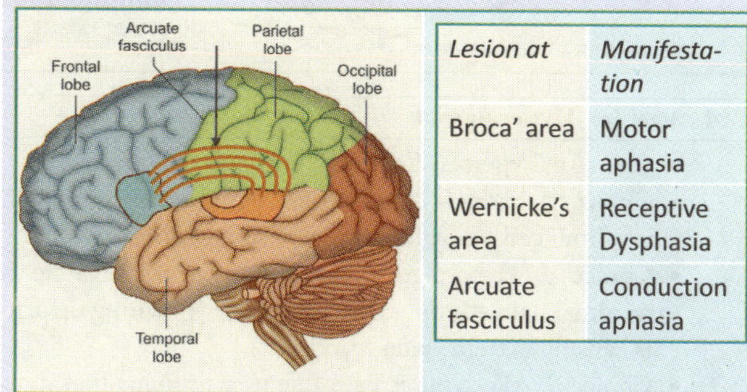

Lesion at	*Manifestation*
Broca' area	Motor aphasia
Wernicke's area	Receptive Dysphasia
Arcuate fasciculus	Conduction aphasia

242. Ans. (d) Ventral tegmental area

Ref: Harrison, 20th ed. pg. 174

Neurons in forebrain ventral tegmental area and nucleus accumbens are involved in motivated behaviours like laughter, pleasure, addiction and fear. These areas are called reward center. The mesocortical dopaminergic neurons that project from midbrain to nucleus accumbens and frontal cortex are also involved.

Extra Mile

Highly addictive drugs like morphine, heroin, cocaine increase the Dopamine which acts on D3 receptors in nucleus accumbens and is responsible for addictive behaviour.

243. Ans. (a) Ventrolateral thalamus

Ref: Ganong, 25th ed. pg. 270

Part of thalamus	Function
Ventrolateral and Ventro-anterior nuclei	Motor function. They receive input from basal ganglia and cerebellum and project to motor nucleus.
Medial geniculate body Lateral geniculate body	Specific sensory relay nuclei Medial geniculate relays auditory and lateral geniculate body relays motor information.
Ventral posteromedial Ventral posterolateral	Relay somatosensory information to post central gyrus

Contd...

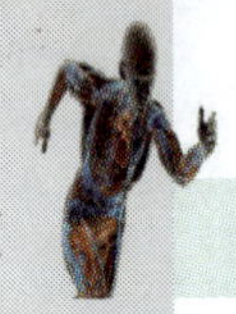

Part of thalamus	Function

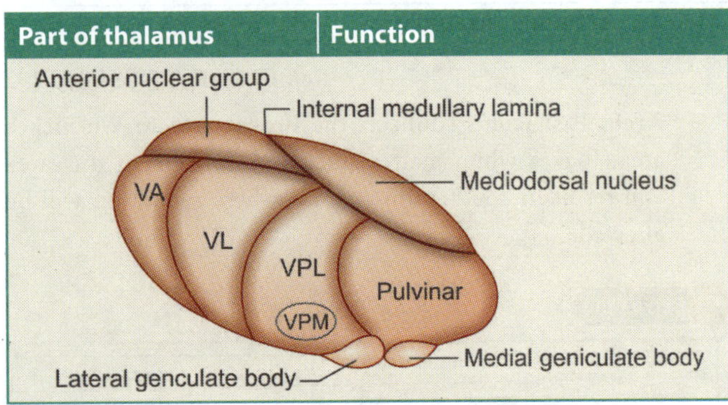

244. Ans. (c) Hyperalgesia

- Choice a, hypersensitivity is a non-specific term.
- Choice b, causalgia characterized by severe burning pain in a limb caused by injury to a peripheral nerve.
- Choice c, Hyperalgesia is heightened response to a minimal pain stimulus. Example gently pinching on arm is causing extreme pain reaction.
- Choice d, Allodynia is pain due to a stimulus that does not usually provoke pain example cold air from AC duct is causing sensation of pain

245. Ans. (d) Muscle spindle

Ref: Ganong 25th ed. Table 8.1: pg. 160

- The stretch stimulus is mediated by muscle spindle and tension by golgi tendon organ.
- Choice a Merkel's disc perceives touch and pressure.
- Choice b Meissner corpuscle perceives tap and flutter at 5–40 Hz.
- Choice c Pacinian corpuscle mediates deep pressure and vibration at 60–300 Hz.

Stimulus	Receptor cell types
Tap, flutter 5–40 Hz	Meissner corpuscles
Motion	Hair follicle receptors
Deep pressure, vibration 60–300 Hz	Pacinian corpuscles
Touch, pressure	Merkel cells
Sustained pressure	Ruffinil corpuscles
Stretch	Muscle spindles
Tension	Golgi tendon organ
Thermal	Cold and warm receptors
Chemical, thermal, and mechanical	Polymodal receptors or chemical, thermal, and ical nociceptors
Chemical	Chemical nociceptor
Light	Rods, cones
Sound	Hair cells (cochlea)
Angular acceleration	Hair cells (semicircular canals)
Linear acceleration, gravity	Hair cell (otolith organs)
Chemical	Olfactory sensory neuron
Chemical	Taste buds

246. Ans. (d) Ach

- **Awake state:** Increase activity of norepinephrine- and serotonin-containing neurons (locus coeruleus and raphe nuclei) and reduced level of activity in acetylcholine-containing neurons (pontine reticular formation). Reduced GABA release and increase histamine release is also there.
- **REM state:** Decrease activity of norepinephrine- and serotonin-containing neurons and increased level of acetylcholine containing neurons.
- **NREM sleep:** Increased release of GABA and reduced release of histamine.

Extra Mile

- **Serotonin: Old concept**—necessary to obtain and maintain behavioral sleep (permissive role on sleep).
- **Serotonin; recent concept**—suggests that during waking, serotonin may complement the action of noradrenaline and acetylcholine in promoting cortical responsiveness and participate to the inhibition of REM-sleep effector neurons of the brainstem **(inhibitory** role on REM sleep).
- Cortical Ach: Greatest during REM sleep > waking and reduced during non-REM (NREM) sleep.

247. Ans. (b) Muscle tone is absent in REM sleep

Physiological process	NREM (slow wave sleep)	REM (paradoxical sleep)
Time spent	75 % of total sleep duration	25% of total sleep duration
Brain activity	Decreases from wakefulness	Increases in motor and sensory areas are similar to NREM
Heart rate BP Blood flow to brain respiration	Decreases from wakefulness	Increases and varies compared to NREM
Sympathetic nerve activity	Decreases from wakefulness	Increases significantly from wakefulness
Muscle tone	**Similar to wakefulness**	**Absent in all muscle except facial and extraocular muscles**
Sexual arousal	Occurs infrequently	Greater than NREM
Dreams	Nonrecallable dream	Recallable dream (so called dream)

248. Ans. (d) Umami

Ref: Ganong, 25th ed. pg. 222

- Most taste buds on the tongue and other regions of the mouth **can detect umami taste,** irrespective of their location.
- Biochemical studies have identified the **taste receptors responsible for the sense of umami** as modified forms of **mGluR4, mGluR1** and **taste receptor type 1** (T1R1 + T1R3), all of which have been found in all regions of the tongue bearing taste buds.

249. Ans. (c) Granular cell

Ref: Barr's Human Nervous System, 9th ed. pg. 161

- The granular cells also make excitatory synapses with Purkinje cells.
- The excitatory transmitter is glutamate.
- *All other cerebellar neurons make inhibitory synapses with GABA as the transmitter.*
- The excitatory input to the cortex is modified by intra-cortical circuits that inhibit the Purkinje cells.
- The granular cells are the most numerous cerebellar interneurons with others being the golgi cells and basket cells.
- The axons afferent to the cerebellum make excitatory connections. Before reaching the cortex all the afferent axons give off collateral branches that contact the neurons in cerebellar nucleus.

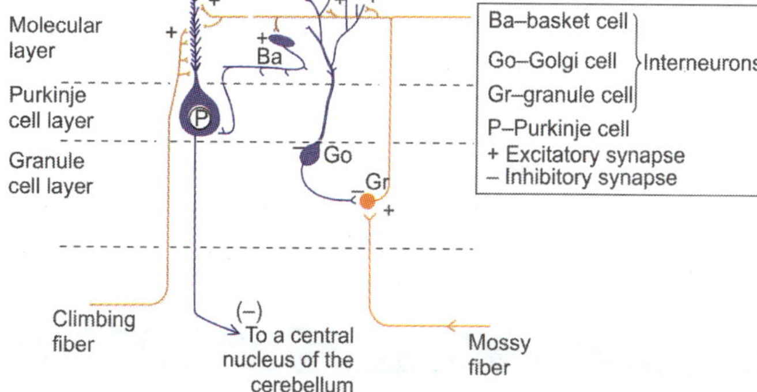

FIGURE: Neurons in the cerebellar cortex showing excitatory and inhibitory synapses. The diagram represents a longitudinally sectioned folium, with an edge on view of the dendritic tree of the Purkinje cell. Glutamatergic (excitatory) neurons are red: GABA-ergic (inhibitory) neurons are blue

250. Ans. (c) Glutamate

- The most prevalent transmitter is glutamate, which is excitatory at well over 90% of the synapses in the human brain.
- The next most prevalent is Gamma-Aminobutyric Acid, or GABA, which is inhibitory at synapses in the human brain.

251. Ans. (d) Sub-fornical Organ

- The **subfornical organ (SFO)**, situated on the ventral surface of the fornix (the reasoning behind the organ's name), at the interventricular foramina (foramina of Monroe), is one of the circumventricular organs of the brain, meaning that it is highly vascularized and does not have a blood-brain barrier, unlike the vast majority of regions in the brain.
- The SFO is a sensory circumventricular organ responsive to a wide variety of hormones and neurotransmitters, as opposed to a secretory circumventricular organ.

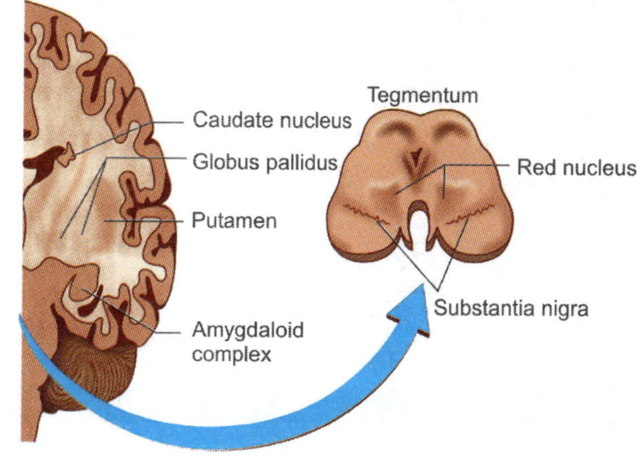

252. Ans. (b) Inhibitory to neuron

Ref: Guyton's Physiology, 11th ed. pg. 563

- GABA (gamma-aminobutyric acid) is secreted by nerve terminals in the spinal cord, cerebellum and basal ganglia. It always causes inhibition.

Extra Mile

Hormone	Source	Function
Dopamine	Neurons in substantia nigra	Inhibition
GABA	*Nerve terminals in spinal cord, baralgaylia and cerebeluar*	***Inhibition***
Glutamate	Presynaptic terminal in CNS and cerebral cortex	Excitation
Serotonin	Nuclei that originate in the median Raphe of Braine stern	Inhibition of pain pathology
Glycine	Synapses in spinal cord	Inhibition

253. Ans. (b) Glutamate

Ref: Lange Medical Physiology by Ganong, 23rd ed. ch. 15

- *Glutamate is the most abundant excitatory neurotransmitter in the vertebrate nervous system.*
- At chemical synapses, glutamate is stored in vesicles. Nerve impulses trigger release of glutamate from the presynaptic cell. Glutamate acts on ionotropic and metabotropic (G-protein coupled) receptors.

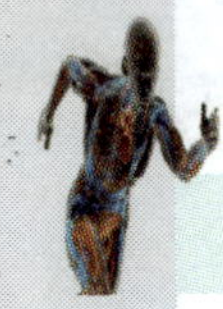

- Because of its role in synaptic plasticity, glutamate is involved in cognitive functions such as learning and memory in the brain.
- *Excitotoxicity due to excessive glutamate* release and impaired uptake occurs as part of the ischemic cascade and is associated with *stroke, autism*, some forms of intellectual disability, and diseases such as amyotrophic lateral sclerosis, lathyrism, and Alzheimer's disease.
- In contrast, *decreased glutamate release* is observed in *classical phenylketonuria*

254. Ans. (d) Bipolar cell

- Cerebellar cortex contain 5 types of neuron cells. They are:

1. Golgi cells
2. Purkinje cells
3. Basket cells
4. Granule cells
5. Stellate cells

255. Ans. (b) Broca's area

Ref: Guyton Physiology, 11th ed. pg. 717

	Location	Function
Broca's area	*Posterior* part of inferior frontal gyrus	Word formation
Limbic Association area	• Anterior pole of temporal lobe • Ventral portion of frontal lobe • Cingulate gyrus	Behavior Emotion motivation
Wernicke's area	Posterior superior temporal lobe	Language comprehension

256. Ans. (a) Inferior frontal gyrus

- Broca's area is now typically defined in terms of the pars opercularis and pars triangularis of the *inferior frontal gyrus*, represented in Brodmann's cytoarchitectonic map as areas 44 and 45 of the dominant hemisphere.
- Damage to Broca's area leads to Motor Aphasia

257. Ans. (d) Middle cerebral artery

Ref: Harrison's, 17th ed. Chapter 23

- The Middle cerebral artery is by far the largest cerebral artery and is the vessel most commonly affected by cerebrovascular accident (CVA) as it is the direct continuation of the internal carotid artery.
- The MCA supplies most of the outer convex brain surface, nearly all the basal ganglia, and the posterior and anterior internal capsules. *Hence it is most commonly affected and its occlusion most commonly leads to hemiplegia.*

258. Ans. (c) Superior temporal gyrus

Ref: Guyton's Physiology, 9th ed. pg. 658

- Auditory cortex lies principally on the supratemporal plane of the superior temporal gyrus but also extends onto the lateral side of the temporal lobe.

259. Ans. (b) Increase heart rate, increase arterial pressure

Ref: Guyton's Physiology 26th ed. pg. 733

- ***Pre-optic nucleus in hypothalamus plays a role in cardiovascular regulation and it decreases heart rate and arterial pressure.***
- ***But once this area is damaged there is no control over heart rate and arterial pressure. Hence it rises.***

Extra Mile

- **Other functions of preoptic area:**
  - It acts as temperature sensor
  - Serve as a thermostatic body temperature control center.
  - Increase thirst
  - Sweating

260. Ans. (b) Stage 2

NREM 1

- NREM Stage 1 (N1 – light sleep, somnolence, drowsy sleep – *5–10% of total sleep in adults and lasts 1–7 minutes)*
- This is a stage of sleep that usually occurs between sleep and wakefulness, and sometimes occurs between periods of deeper sleep and periods of REM.
- The muscles are active, and the eyes roll slowly, opening and closing moderately.
- The brain transitions from alpha waves having a frequency of 8–13 Hz (common in the awake state) to *theta waves* having a frequency of 4–7 Hz.
- Sudden twitches and hypnic jerks, also known as positive myoclonus, may be associated with the onset of sleep during N1. Some people may also experience hypnagogic hallucinations during this stage.

NREM 2

- NREM Stage 2 *(N2 – 45–55% of total sleep in adults and constitutes 10–25 minutes of initial sleep activity and progressively lengthens).*
- In this stage, theta activity is observed and sleepers become gradually harder to awaken; the alpha waves of the previous stage are interrupted by abrupt activity called *sleep spindles* (or thalamocortical spindles) and *K-complexes*. Sleep spindles range from 11 Hz to 16 Hz (most commonly 12–14 Hz).
- During this stage, muscular activity as measured by EMG decreases, and *conscious awareness of the external environment disappears.*

NREM 3

- NREM Stage 3 *(N3 – deep sleep, slow-wave sleep – 15–25% of total sleep in adults):*
- Formerly divided into stages 3 and 4, this stage is called slow-wave sleep (SWS) or deep sleep.

Contd...

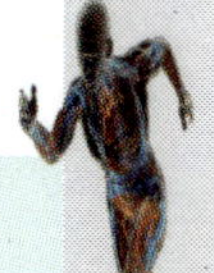

- The sleeper is less responsive to the environment; *many environmental stimuli no longer produce any reactions.*
- Slow-wave sleep is thought to be the *most restful form of sleep*, the phase which most relieves subjective feelings of sleepiness and restores the body.
- This stage is characterized by the presence of a minimum of 20% *delta waves* ranging from 0.5 Hz to 2 Hz and having a peak-to-peak amplitude >75 µV. (EEG standards define delta waves to be from 0 to 4 Hz, but sleep standards in both the original R&K, as well as the new 2007 AASM guidelines have a range of 0.5–2 Hz.)
- *This is the stage in which parasomnias such as* **night terrors, nocturnal enuresis, sleepwalking**, and **somniloquy occur**.

Extra Mile

NREM Stage 4 is currently merged into stage 3 by some authors

- NREM stage 4 has similar attributes to stage 3, except there are a greater proportion of EEG delta waves.
- These high voltage, slow EEG waves make up 50% or more of the record.
- This is the deepest stage of sleep; a more intense stimulus is needed to wake someone from stage 4 sleep than any other stage of NREM sleep.
- Children typically spend 20-25% of sleep in stages 3 and 4 slow wave sleep; this decreases to less than 10% by age 60. **Sleepwalking**, **sleep terrors**, and **sleep-related enuresis** episodes generally occur in stages 3 or 4, or during arousals from this stage.

261. Ans. (b) NREM 2

Ref: Ganong, 25th pg. 273-74

Bruxism: tooth grinding occurring during stage 2 of NREM period.

Nightmare
- Vivid, anxiety producing dreams during sleep.
- Patient wakes up and is able to recall the nightmare vividly.
- *Occurs in REM.*
- Treatment: REM suppressants such as tricyclic antidepressants, SSRIs, benzodiazepines.

Sleep terror (night terror)
- Arousal in the first one-third of the night.
- Invariably start with piercing scream or cry with intense panic.
- No recall on waking up the next day.
- *Occurs in NREM period (stages 3 and 4)*
- Seen especially in children, more common in boys.
- EEG is advised to rule out seizure (temporal lobe epilepsy).
- No specific treatment required

Sleep walking (somnambulism)
- Rising from bed with walking about in the first-third of the night.
- No recall on waking up the next day.
- *Occurs in* **NREM period** *(stages 3 and 4).*
- Occurs between 4 and 8 years, spontaneous recovery in adolescence.

Sleep talking (Somniloquy) occurs in all stages of sleep

Sleep-related head banging (Jactatio Capitis Nocturna): Rhythmic to-and-fro head rocking occurring just before or during sleep.

262. Ans. (b) Disappear when a patient opens eyes

Ref: Ganong 25th ed. pg. 273

- **Alpha activity** refers to activity in the range of 8–13 Hz.
- **Alpha rhythm** is 8–13 Hz activity occurring during wakefulness over the posterior head regions which is present when the eyes are closed and the patient relaxed and which is attenuated by eye opening or alerting of the patient.

EEG Waves and their Significance

Band	Frequency (Hz)	Location	Normally seen in	Pathologically seen in
Delta	<4	Frontally in adults, posteriorly in children; high-amplitude waves	Adult slow-wave sleep	• Subcortical lesions • Diffuse lesions • Metabolic encephalopathy Hydrocephalus
Theta	4–7	Found in locations not related to task at hand	Drowsiness in adults (It has been found to spike in situations where as persons is actively trying to repress a response or action).	• Subcortical lesions • Metabolic encephalopathy
Alpha	8–13	Posterior regions of head, both sides, higher in amplitude on dominant side.	Relaxed/reflecting Closing the eyes	• Coma
Beta	13–30	Both sides, symmetrical distribution, most evident frontally; low-amplitude waves	**Active thinking, focus, high alert, anxious**	• Benzodiazepines
Gamma	>30	Somatosensory cortex	Displays during cross-modal sensory processing (perception that combines two different senses, such as sound and sight)	• May be associated with cognitive decline

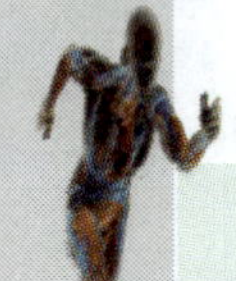

263. Ans. (c) Amygdaloid nucleus

Ref: Ganong, 25th ed. pg. 288, Atlas of Neuroanatomy, 2nd ed. pg. 203

- The **hippocampal formation** is a compound structure in the medial temporal lobe of brain containing
  - Dentate gyrus
  - Hippocampus proper
  - Subiculum
  - Entorhinal cortex.
- Amygadala primary role in the processing of memory, decision-making, and emotional reactions, the amygdalae are considered part of the limbic system.

264. Ans. (d) Nucleus Cuneatus

Ref: Harrison, 19th ed. pg. 160 and Diagnostic Clinical Neuropsychology, 3rd ed. pg. 32

- Astereognosis is impaired or lost ability to discriminate between various forms, as well as deficits in finger localization and in graphesthesia (ability to recognize palm writing). If a lesion occurs at or above the level of the thalamus, it commonly results in astereognosis.
- *Now Since Nucleus cuneatus gets information from T5 upwards including the upper limb, its lesion results in astereognosis.*
- The fasciculus gracilis (graceful, like a ballerina's legs) conveys information from the lower part of the body T6 and below.
- Together the fasciculus gracilis and cuneatus are referred to as the posterior columns, because they occupy a position at the posterior of the spinal cord.
- The posterior columns travel up the ipsilateral side of the spinal cord and synapse in the nucleus gracilis and nucleus cuneatus at the level of the medulla. From there, the fibers decussate (cross over) and continue on toward the thalamus in a pathway synapses in the thalamus, and from there the information is relayed to the postcentral gyrus, known as the somatosensory cortex.

265. Ans. (b) Beta

Ref: Ganong's Physiology, 23rd ed. chapter 15

There are two kinds of sleep: Rapid eye movement (REM) sleep and non-REM (NREM) sleep.

NREM Sleep is Divided into Four Stage

A person falling asleep enters

Stage 1	The EEG begins to show a low-voltage, mixed frequency pattern. A theta rhythm (4–7 Hz) can be seen at this early stage of slow-wave sleep. Throughout NREM sleep, there is some activity of skeletal muscle but no eye movements occur
Stage 2	It is marked by the appearance of sinusoidal waves called sleep spindles (12–14 Hz) and occasional high -voltage biphasic waves called K complexes.
Stage 3	A high-amplitude delta rhythm (0.5–4 Hz) dominates the EEG waves
Stage 4	Maximum slowing with large waves is seen in stage 4

REM sleep is so named because of the characteristic eye movements that occur during this stage of sleep.

The high-amplitude slow waves seen in the EEG during sleep are periodically replaced by rapid, low-voltage EEG activity, which resembles that seen in the awake, aroused state (beta wave). For this reason, ***REM sleep is also called paradoxical sleep.***

266. Ans. (c) Rapidly adapting touch receptors

Ref: Ganong, 25th ed. pg. 161; Basic Clinical Neurosciences 2nd ed. pg. 131

- When a maintained stimulus of constant strength is applied to a receptor, the frequency of the action potentials in its sensory nerve declines over time. This phenomenon is known as **adaptation or desensitization.**
- Receptors can be classified into **rapidly adapting** (phasic) receptors and **slowly adapting** (tonic) receptors.
- *Meissner and Pacinian corpuscles are examples of rapidly adapting receptors,* and Merkel cells and Ruffini endings are examples of slowly adapting receptors. Other examples of slowly adapting receptors are muscle spindles and nociceptors.

Meissner corpuscles	Tactile shapes and surfaces
Merkel disc	Tactile indentation
Hair follicle receptors	Tactile (hairy skin)
Ruffini nerve endings	Stretching
Pacinian corpuscles	Vibration
Muscle spindle	Proprioception
AS mechanical encapsulated	Pinprick
Free nerve endings	Cold/warmth

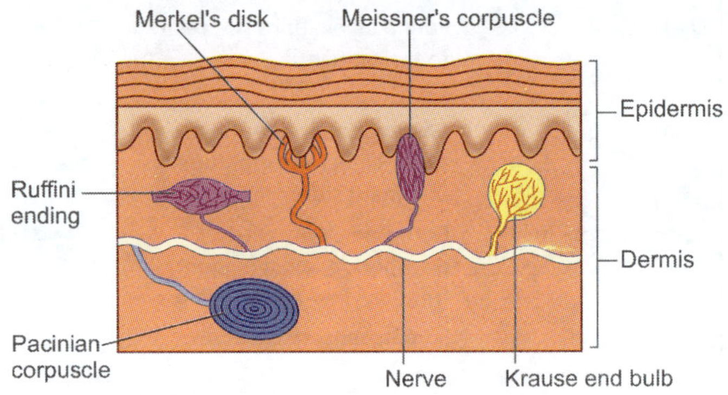

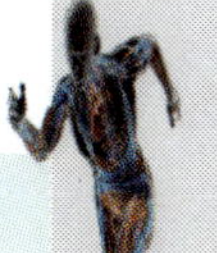

267. Ans. (b) Posterior pituitary

Ref: Ganong, 25th ed. pg. 606

List of brain structures outside the blood brain barrier called circumventricular organs:

1. Posterior pituitary and median eminence of hypothalamus
2. Area postrema (Chemoreceptor trigger zone)
3. Organum vasculosum of lamina terminalis (Osmoreceptor for vasopressin release)
4. Sub-fornical organ

All these structures have fenestrated capillaries and because of permeability are said to be outside the blood brain barrier.

268. Ans. (b) REM sleep

Ref: Ganong, 25th ed. pg. 274

- In REM sleep, the high amplitude slow waves in EEG during sleep are periodically replaced by rapid low voltage EEG activity which is identical to awake aroused state.
- Now the point is that the person is sleeping while EEG record is like that of an awake patient. Hence REM sleep is called as paradoxical sleep.

269. Ans. (c) Akinesia

Ref: Ganong, 25th ed. pg. 246

Hyperkinetic Movements and Sites of Lesion

Chorea	Lesion in Caudate nucleus
Atheotosis	Lesion in Globus pallidus
Ballism	Lesion in Sub-thalamic nucleus

270. Ans. (a) Renshaw cell

Ref: Ganong, 25th ed. pg. 233, 249

Neurons in Cerebellar Cortex

Purkinje cells	Biggest neurons in CNS
Granule cells	Innervate purkinje cells and give rise to parallel fibers
Basket cells	Located in molecular layer and receive excitatory input from parallel fibers.
Stellate cells	Same as basket cells but located more superficially
Golgi cells	Located in granular layer of cerebellum

Renshaw cell is an interneuron in spinal cord which has an inhibitory function and operates via a neurotransmitter called glycine.

271. Ans. (a) Upper motor neuron damage

Ref: Ganong, 25th ed. pg. 233

Clonus is characterised by repeated rhythmic contractions of muscle subjected to sudden maintained stretch.

It is Caused by

- Increased Gamma motor neuron discharge
- Spinal cord injury causing damage to Renshaw cell which is an inhibitory inter-neuron.

Conditions in Which Clonus is seen:

1. Amyotrophic lateral sclerosis
2. Stroke
3. Multiple sclerosis
4. Spinal cord damage
5. Hepatic encephalopathy

Clonazepam and botulinum toxin is useful in management of clonus.

272. Ans. (c) Spasticity

Ref: Ganong, 25th ed. pg. 232-33

- A muscle is said to be spastic in case the resistance to stretch is high. A sequence of resistance followed by sudden decrease in resistance is when the limb is moved passively and is known as clasp knife effect since it shows similarity to closing of a pocket knife.
- Ganong also calls it the lengthening reaction since it is the response of the spastic muscle to lengthening.

273. Ans. (b) Damage to cerebellum

Ref: Ganong, 25th ed. pg. 252

- The cerebellum acts as a brake to stop a particular movement.
- In case of cerebellar lesion, the movement of the arm can be stopped and it moves in a wide arc called rebound phenomenon.

Features of Cerebellar Lesion

- Gait ataxia
- Scanning speech
- Dysmetria
- Intention tremor
- Rebound phenomenon
- Dysaidokinesia
- Nystagmus
- Pendular knee jerks

274. Ans. (b) Withdrawal reflex

Ref: Ganong, 25th ed. pg. 235

- In days following development of spinal shock patient will have low threshold for elicitation of withdrawal reflex
- Minimal noxious stimulus to arm will lead to withdrawal of one extremity and marked flexion-extension pattern of other 3 limbs.

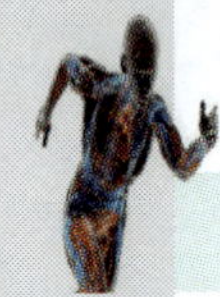

- Later the Deep tendon reflexes become brisk
- Application of minor noxious stimulus will lead to evacuation of bladder and rectum called mass reflex.

275. Ans. (a) Caudate and Putamen

Ref: Ganong 25th ed. pg. 244

Corpus Striatum	Caudate nucleus and putamen
Lenticular nucleus	Putamen and globus pallidus

276. Ans. (b) Bi-synaptic reflex

Ref: Ganong, 25th ed. pg. 232

A Golgi Tendon Reflex/Inverse Stretch Reflex Operates as follows:

- As the tension applied to a tendon increases, the Golgi tendon organ (sensor) is stimulated.
- Nerve impulses (action potentials) arise and propagate along the 1b sensory nerve fibers into the spinal cord.
- *Within the spinal cord, the 1b sensory nerve fibers synapse and generate an IPSP (inhibitory postsynaptic potential) on the motor neurons that supply the muscles form which the fibers arise*
- The muscle relaxes and excess tension is relieved.

277. Ans. (b) Golgi Tendon organ

Ref: Ganong, 25th ed. pg. 232

Refer to the explanation of above question.

278. Ans. (d) Spinal Cord

Ref:. Ganong's Physiology, 23rd ed. chapter 9

- When a skeletal muscle with an intact nerve supply is stretched, it contracts. This response is called the **stretch reflex.**
- The stimulus that initiates the reflex is stretch of the muscle, and the response is contraction of the muscle being stretched.
- The sense organ is a small encapsulated spindle like or fusiform shaped structure called the muscle spindle, located within the fleshy part of the muscle.
- The impulses originating from the spindle are transmitted to the CNS by fast sensory fibers that pass directly to the motor neurons which supply the same muscle.
- The neurotransmitter at the central synapse is glutamate. The stretch reflex is the best known and studied monosynaptic reflex and is typified by the **knee jerk reflex.**

279. Ans. (b) Fasciculation

Ref: Harrison, 18th ed. pg. 182

Fasciculation: Visible or palpable twitch within a muscle due to the spontaneous discharge of a motor unit.

Tremor: Involuntary, repetitive, oscillatory movements of a part of the body around a fixed point due to alternate contraction and relaxation of groups of muscles with their antagonists.

Chorea: Brief, rapid, jerky, explosive, Non-Repetitive, quasi-purposive involuntary movements chiefly involving face, tongue and limbs.

Myoclonic Jerk: Sudden, rapid, irregular, jerky involuntary movements of a limb due to contraction of a single muscle or a group of muscles.

280. Ans. (c) Occipital radiation

Ref: Ganong, 25th ed. pg. 190

281. Ans. (d) Basal ganglia

Ref: Ganong, 25th ed. pg. 244

282. Ans. (b) Law of Projection

Ref: Ganong, 25th ed. pg. 171

Law of projection states that irrespective of the site of application of the stimulus in the sensory pathway, the conscious perception of sensation evoked is felt at the site where receptor is present. This forms the basis of the Phantom Limb.

PHYSIOLOGY OF BLOOD

283. Ans. (a) Megaloblastic anemia

Ref: Harrison 20th ed. pg. 766

Most common cause of Macrocytic anemia is megaloblastic anemia. This is due to impaired DNA synthesis. Although DNA synthesis is impaired, RNA synthesis is unaffected, leading to a buildup of cytoplasmic components in a slowly dividing cell. This results in a larger-than-normal cell. The nuclear chromatin of these cells also has an altered appearance.

Major cause of non-megaloblastic macrocytic anemia is:

- Bone marrow disorders
- Liver disease
- Hemolytic anemia

284. Ans. (a) γ-carboxylation of glutamic acid residues to clotting factor 2, 7, 9 and 10

Ref: Ganong 25th ed. pg. 566-67

- Vitamin K is a necessary cofactor for the enzyme that catalyses the conversion of glutamic acid residues to ϒ-carboxyglutamic acid residues.

- A total of 6 proteins involved in clotting require conversion before being released into circulation. These are factor 2, 7, 9, 10 and protein C and S.

285. Ans. (d) 4

O_2 TRANSPORT

Transport occurs via two processes:

- Hemoglobin bound O_2 (99%)
- Dissolved O_2 (1%)

Note:

- 1 Hb can carry 4 oxygen molecules.
- Molecule of oxygen bound to hemoglobin depends on saturation of Hb (SaO_2/SpO_2) with oxygen. SaO_2 depends on PaO_2

CALCULATION OF HB-BOUND O_2

In arterial blood	In venous blood
• 97% hemoglobin is saturated with oxygen, at PaO_2 of 95 mm Hg. • With this saturation, 1 g of Hb, contains 1.34 mL of O_2. • Therefore 100 mL of blood contains 20.1 mL of oxygen (when normal Hb = 15 gm%) • When hemoglobin is 100% saturated with O_2, hemoglobin binds 1.39 mL O_2 per gm of Hb [This is known as oxygen capacity (O_2cap) of Hemoglobin]	• At PvO_2 of 40 mm Hg, Hb is only 75% saturated (SO_2= 75%). • Therefore, 100 mL of venous blood would carry 14.4 mL of O_2

286. Ans. (b) Hemoglobin

Ref: Quantitative Human Physiology; An Introduction. pg. 432-33

- An average weighing adult turns over approx 6 gm of Hb daily
- 1 g of Hb yield ~35 mg of Bilirubin
- Therefore daily bilirubin formation in an adult is approx 250–350 mg

287. Ans. (c) 12th week

Ref: Diagnostic Pediatric Hematopathology By Maria A. Proytcheva 2011 ed. pg. 6

Fetal liver is the major site for erythropoeisis between 11 and 24 weeks of gestation.

	Primitive hematopoiesis	Definitive hematopoiesis
Hematopoietic site	Yolk sac and vascular endothelium	Fetal liver and fetal bone narrow Hematopoietic niches
Type of Hematopoiesis	Mostly erythoid	Multileneage Hematopoiesis
RBC Characteristics	Remain Nucleated during their entire lifespan	Enucleated RBCs
Cell Size	Macrocytic	MCV decreases with gestational age
Sensitivity to EPO	Increased	Lower sensitivity
Lifespan	Short	Increases with gestation
Hemoglobin type	Embryonic: Gower 1, Gower 2 and Portland	Fetal Hb (a_2y_2) and adult Hb ($\alpha 2\ \beta 2$)

288. Ans. (b) Carboxylation

Vitamin	Action	Deficiency symptoms	Sources
K group	Catalyze γ, carboxylation of glutamic acid residues on various proteins concerned with blood clotting	Hemorrhage	Leafy green vegetables

289. Ans. (d) Constitutes 5% of body weight

Ref: Ganong, 25th ed. pg. 561

Serum is different from plasma in the following ways:

- Fibrinogen is not present
- Factor II, V, and VIII are not present
- Higher serotonin content

Plasma constitutes 5% of body weight and choice D is wrong.

290. Ans. (c) Von Willebrand factor

Ref: Ganong, 25th ed. pg. 563

Von Wilebrand factor is synthesized by endothelial cells.

Haptoglobin	Binds and transports free hemoglobin in blood released after intravascular hemolysis
Anti-thrombin III	Protease inhibitor of intrinsic coagulation system
Hemopexin	Binds to porphyrins particularly for heme recycling.

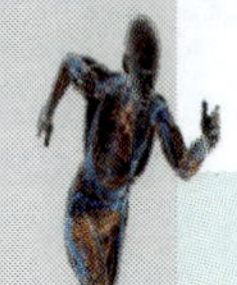

291. Ans. (a) Liver

Sites of Haematopoiesis

Yolk sac at 2 weeks	Earliest Hemoglobin to be formed is Gower 1. This is followed by Gower 2 and finally Portland.
In fetus in liver and partly spleen.	HbF appears at 14 weeks
At birth it shifts to the bone marrow	HbA appears at 38 weeks

292. Ans. (b) Solubilization of glucose

Ref: Harper, 26th pg. 584

- Bilirubin formed in peripheral tissues is transported to the liver by plasma albumin
- Smaller amounts of cortisol and other hormones are bound to albumin.
- Half-life of albumin is 21 days.

293. Ans. (c) Radiation

Ref: Ganong, 25th ed. pg. 317

From the skin, heat is lost to the environment mainly through radiation

Body heat lost in % (at 21°C) by various means:

Radiation and conduction	70%
Vaporization of heat	27%
Respiration	2%
Urination and defecation	1%

294. Ans. (b) Stimulation of fibers coming from posterior hypothalamus

Ref: Essentials of Medical Physiology, 6th ed. pg. 362

- The hypothalamus is said to integrate body temperature information from sensory receptors (primarily cold receptors) in the skin, deep tissues spinal cord, extra-hypothalamic portions of the brain, and the hypothalamus itself.
- *The reflex responses activated by cold are controlled from the posterior hypothalamus.*
- Those activated by warmth are controlled primarily from the anterior hypothalamus.

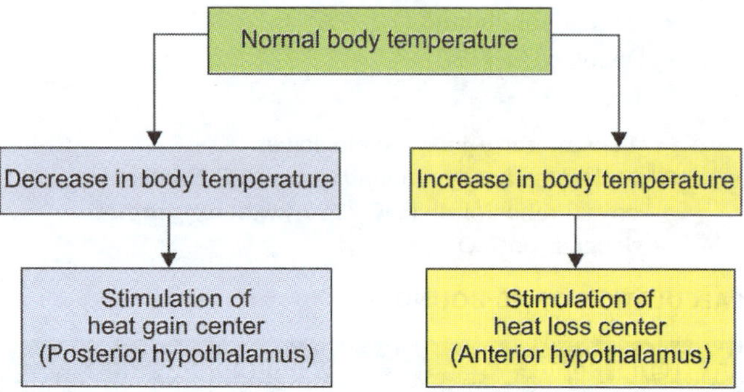

- Stimulation of the anterior hypothalamus causes cutaneous vasodilation and sweating, and lesion in this region cause hyperthermia, with rectal temperatures sometimes reaching 43°C (109.4°F).
- The threshold is >37°C for sweating and vasodilation, 36.8°C vasoconstrictions 36°C for non-shivering thermogenesis, and 35.5°C for shivering.

295. Ans. (c) Angiotensin converting enzyme

- The lungs activate the physiologically inactive decapeptide angiotensin I to the pressor, aldosterone-stimulating octapeptide angiotensin II in the pulmonary circulation. The reaction occurs in other tissues as well, but it is particularly prominent in the lungs.
- Large amounts of the angiotensin-converting enzyme responsible for this activation are *located on the surface of the endothelial cells of the pulmonary capillaries.*

BIOCHEMISTRY

3

MOST RECENT QUESTIONS 2023

1. Which of the following mineral is best known for stabilization of insulin secretion?

(Most Recent Question July 2023)

a. Copper
b. Cadmium
c. Iron
d. Zinc

2. A 65-year-old man with coronary artery disease comes to the physician for a follow-up examination. He is 183 cm (5 ft) tall and weighs 84 kg, BMI is 25 kg/m^2. His blood pressure is 130/80 mm Hg. Serum studies show a glucose concentration of 95 mg/dL and homocysteine concentration of 19.3 μmol/L (N = 5–15). Serum lipid concentrations are within the reference range. Which of the following enzyme deficiency is most likely to be found in this patient? *(Most Recent Question July 2023)*

a. Homogentisate oxidase
b. HGPRTase
c. Cystathionine β-synthase
d. Cystathionine γ-synthase

3. Which of the following is best known location for cardiolipin within the cells? *(Most Recent Question July 2023)*

a. Cytosol
b. Inner mitochondrial membrane
c. Outer mitochondrial membrane
d. Mitochondrial matrix

4. A child who has accompanied his father to a fish farming area in his hometown accidentally ingests a white odorless compound. Later he developed toxicity of the drug. Which of the following toxin is most likely to cause this condition? *(Most Recent Question July 2023)*

a. Alkyl guanidines
b. Cyanide
c. Antimycin A
d. BAL

5. A 40-year-old lady presented to OPD with a bleeding disorder and she was also found to have dental caries. Which of the following vitamin supplementation would be most appropriate in treating this condition?

(Most Recent Question July 2023)

a. Vitamin B_{12}
b. Vitamin B_9
c. Vitamin D
d. Vitamin K

6. A chronic alcoholic patient presents with loss of coordination, confusion and unsteady gait. Which vitamin deficiency is most likely seen in this patient?

(Most Recent Question July 2023)

a. Vitamin B_1
b. Vitamin C
c. Vitamin D
d. Vitamin A

7. Which of the following is the rate-limiting enzyme of heme synthesis pathway?

(Most Recent Question July 2023)

a. δ-aminolevulinic acid dehydratase
b. δ-aminolevulinic acid synthase
c. Ferrochelatase
d. HMB synthase

8. A full-term neonate who is born normally and is on breastfed, presents with hypoglycemia, hypophosphatemia, lactic acidosis, mild icterus. Urine shows positive Benedict's test. The most probable enzyme defect is:

(Most Recent Question July 2023)

a. Lactase
b. Fructokinase
c. Galactokinase
d. Galactose-1-phosphate uridyltransferase

9. Which of the following is best known to facilitate entry of cholera toxin through the intestinal mucosa?

(Most Recent Question July 2023)

a. GM1 ganglioside
b. GM2 ganglioside
c. GM3 ganglioside
d. Gi receptor

10. Which of the following intermediates of TCA cycle is formed from aspartate? *(Most Recent Question July 2023)*

a. Fumarate
b. Alpha-ketoglutarate
c. Oxaloacetate
d. Succinyl CoA

11. Which of the following pathways only takes place in a cell's cytoplasm? *(Most Recent Question Jan 2023)*

a. Glycolysis
b. Beta-oxidation
c. TCA
d. Urea cycle

12. Which of the following is not a microelement?

(Most Recent Question Jan 2023)

a. Copper
b. Calcium
c. Zinc
d. Selenium

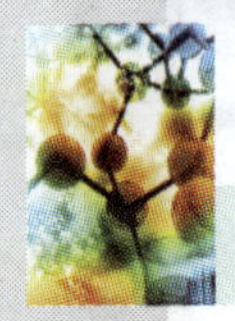

13. Melanin is synthesized from which of the following amino acid? *(Most Recent Question Jan 2023)*
a. Tyrosine
b. Tryptophan
c. Leucine
d. Phenylalanine

14. Which of the following enzyme is found to be deficient in Von Gierke's disease? *(Most Recent Question Jan 2023)*
a. Glucose-6-phosphatase
b. Debranching enzyme
c. Branching enzyme
d. Myophosphorylase

15. Which of the following options plays a role in collagen maturation? *(Most Recent Question Jan 2023)*
a. Copper and zinc
b. Ascorbic acid
c. Proline
d. Phenylalanine

16. Nitric oxide is formed from which amino acid? *(Most Recent Question Jan 2023)*
a. Tryptophan
b. Leucine
c. Arginine
d. Lysine

17. Breastfeeding is contraindicated in which of the following conditions? *(Most Recent Question Jan 2023)*
a. Galactosemia
b. CMV
c. Hepatitis B
d. West Nile virus

18. A patient who was in excruciating pain all over his body was taken to the hospital. In recent years, he has experienced these incidents frequently. When exercising vigorously, the ache begins. Anemia was detected by blood examination, along with elongated red blood cells as opposed to concave ones. It was determined that he had sickle cell anemia. The substitution that takes place in sickle cell anemia is: *(Most Recent Question Jan 2023)*
a. Substitution of valine (Val) by glutamic acid (Glu) at the 6th position
b. Substitution of glutamic acid (Glu) by valine (Val) at the 6th position
c. Substitution of glutamic acid (Glu) by valine (Val) at the 5th position
d. Substitution of valine (Val) by glutamic acid (Glu) at the 5th position

19. A patient presented to the OPD with complaint of diarrhea. The patient was later diagnosed with dementia and photosensitive dermatitis in sun-exposed areas. Which vitamin deficiency is responsible for this condition? *(Most Recent Question Jan 2023)*
a. Vitamin B_6
b. Niacin
c. Ascorbic acid
d. Biotin

20. Vitamin A deficiency leads to: *(Most Recent Question Jan 2023)*
a. Xerophthalmia
b. Beriberi
c. Pellagra
d. Neuropathy

21. In liver, apoB gene is completely translated to apoB100 and in intestine it is translated to apoB48. Which of the following mechanisms explains this? *(Most Recent Question Jan 2023)*
a. RNA editing
b. Gene splicing
c. Alternative polyadenylation
d. Gene rearrangements

CARBOHYDRATE

22. Complex IV inhibitors: *(Most Recent Question June 2022)*
a. Cyanide
b. Carbon dioxide
c. Oligomycin
d. Qubain

23. Which of the following condition is true about fed state? *(Most Recent Question June/Dec 2021)*
a. Increase in insulin level and decrease in glucagon level
b. Increase in glucagon level and decrease in insulin level
c. Both insulin and glucagon levels decrease
d. Only insulin levels increase

24. Glucagon activates all; EXCEPT: *(Most Recent Question June/Dec 2021)*
a. Gluconeogenesis
b. Lipolysis
c. Ketone body synthesis
d. Glycolysis

25. Thermogenin is present in: *(Most Recent Question June/Dec 2021)*
a. Mitochondria
b. Cytoplasm
c. Lysosomes
d. Peroxisomes

26. Enzyme deficient in Gaucher's disease: *(Most Recent Question June/Dec 2021)*
a. Beta galacto cerebrosidase
b. Glucose 6 phosphate
c. Glucose 6 phosphatase
d. Gluco cerebrosidase

27. Fat sugar baby is seen in: *(Most Recent Question June/Dec 2021)*
a. Diabetes
b. Kwashiorkor
c. Marasmus
d. Hypothyroidism

28. A vegetarian patient presents with anemia and hyper segmented neutrophil. The most probable diagnosis is: *(Most Recent Question June/Dec 2021)*
a. Anemia of chronic disease
b. Iron deficiency anemia
c. Megaloblastic anemia
d. Sideroblastic anemia

29. Which of the following enzyme deficiency is most likely to cause classical galactosemia in infants:
(Most Recent Question June/Dec 2021)
a. GALT – (galactose 1 phosphate uridyl transferase)
b. Galactokinase
c. UDP galactose 4 epimerase
d. Glucose 6 phosphatase

30. The subcellular organelle which is associated with killing viruses and bacteria is:
(Most Recent Question June/Dec 2021)
a. Peroxisome b. Mitochondria
c. Lysosome d. Golgi apparatus

31. Enzyme deficient in Tay-Sachs disease is:
(Most Recent Question Aug 2020)
a. Hexosaminidase A b. Glucocerebrosidase
c. G-6-PD d. Hexosaminidase A & B

32. Enzyme deficiency in Von Gierke disease:
(Most Recent Question Dec 2019-20)
a. Glucose-6-phosphatase
b. Branching enzyme
c. Acid maltase
d. Glycogen phosphorylase

33. Gluconeogenesis is inhibited by:
(Most Recent Question Dec 2019-20)
a. Glucagon b. Insulin
c. Cholecystokinin d. 5 alpha reductase

34. Which of the following is one of the uses of dietary fibres? *(Most Recent Question Dec 2019-20)*
a. Increased blood glucose level
b. Reduces intestinal transit time
c. No role in metabolism
d. Causes constipation

35. Which of the following is present in skeletal muscle?
(Most Recent Question Dec 2019-20)
a. GLUT 2 b. GLUT 4
c. GLUT 5 d. GLUT 7

36. Each of the following is a physiological uncoupler; EXCEPT:
(Most Recent Question 2019)
a. 2,4 dinitrophenol b. Thyroid hormone
c. Unconjugated bilirubin d. Long chain fatty acid

37. In glycolysis which of the following is not involved?
(Most Recent Question 2019)
a. Pyruvate dehydrogenase
b. Phosphofructokinase
c. Glucokinase
d. Pyruvate kinase

38. Urea cycle takes place in:
(Recent Pattern Question 2018-19)
a. Nucleus and endoplasmic reticulum
b. Mitochondria and Golgi apparatus
c. Mitochondria and cytoplasm
d. Only mitochondria

39. Which of the following is a physiological uncoupler?
(Recent Pattern Question 2018-19)
a. 2,4-Dinitrophenol b. Dinitrocresol
c. Aspirin d. Unconjugated bilirubin

40. Gluconeogenesis is mainly seen in:
(Recent Pattern Question 2018)
a. Kidney b. Liver
c. Spleen d. Heart

41. Glucose-6-phosphate dehydrogenase deficiency causes:
(Recent Pattern Question 2018)
a. Megaloblastic anemia
b. Hemolytic anemia
c. Sickle cell anemia
d. Microcytic anemia

42. Essential fructosuria is due to the deficiency of which enzyme? *(Recent Pattern Question 2017)*
a. Aldolase A b. Aldolase B
c. Fructokinase d. Glucokinase

43. Identify the glycogen storage disease with exercise induced myoglobinuria: *(Recent Pattern Question 2017)*
a. McArdle's disease
b. Pompe's disease
c. Von gierke disease
d. Anderson disease

44. All of the following enzymes catalyze irreversible steps in glycolysis; EXCEPT:
a. Hexokinase b. PFK-I
c. Enolase d. Pyruvate kinase

45. The net ATP yield when one molecule of pyruvate is completely oxidized to CO_2 and H_2O is:
a. 10 b. 15
c. 18 d. 30

46. Which of the following enzymes causes Substrate level phosphorylation in Glycolysis:
a. Glyceraldehyde 3 Phosphate dehydrogenase
b. Pyruvate kinase
c. Phosphofructokinase
d. Enolase

47. Glucose-6-phosphatase enzyme is absent in:
a. Liver b. Kidney
c. Brain d. Muscles

48. Which of the following doesn't occur in the mitochondria?
a. Cori cycle b. Urea cycle
c. FA oxidation d. Kreb's cycle

49. In which cells or tissue, Lactate will convert to pyruvate:
a. Muscles b. Liver
c. Erythrocytes d. Brain

50. Source of ATP in RBC cells:
a. Fatty acid oxidation
b. Oxidative phosphorylation
c. NADPH paroxidase
d. EMP pathway

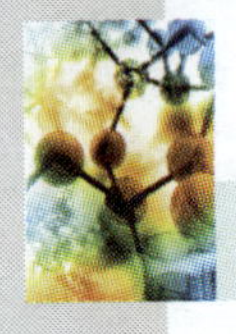

51. In glycolysis, insulin affects all of the following enzymes; EXCEPT:
a. Phosphofructokinase
b. Pyruvate kinase
c. Glucokinase
d. Hexokinase

52. Insulin is essential for entry of glucose in which of the following tissue:
a. Most neurons in cerebral cortex
b. Renal tubular cells
c. Skeletal muscles
d. Mucosa of small intestine

53. All of the following metabolic pathways occur in both Cytoplasm and Mitochondria; EXCEPT:
a. Glycolysis
b. Gluconeogenesis
c. Heme synthesis
d. Urea cycle

54. Which of the following occurs in both cytoplasm and mitochondria?
a. Glycolysis
b. Gluconeogenesis
c. Glycogenolysis
d. Glycogenesis

55. Gluconeogenesis is inhibited by:
a. Insulin
b. Glucagon
c. Glucocorticoids
d. GnRH

56. Cytoplasm to Mitochondria substrate shuttle is:
a. Glycerophosphate shuttle
b. Malate shuttle
c. Phosphoenol pyruvate
d. Oxaloacetate

57. What is not given in fructose intolerance patient:
a. Glucose
b. Galactose
c. Fructose
d. Maltose

58. Aldolase is an enzyme whose substrate is
a. Glucose -6-phosphate
b. Fructose-6-phosphate
c. Fructose
d. Fructose-1 biphosphate

59. On weaning off from milk and addition of fruit juices, an infant had frequent attacks of vomiting and tremors. Urine reducing sugar was positive but glucose was negative. The infant is likely to have:
a. Fructokinase deficiency
b. Galactokinase deficiency
c. Glucose-6-phosphatase deficiency
d. Aldolase - B deficiency

60. An enzyme involved in the catabolism of fructose to pyruvate in the liver is:
a. Glyceraldehydes-3-phosphate dehydrogenase
b. Phosphoglucomutase
c. Lactate-dehydrogenase
d. Glucokinase

61. Which is true for glucoronidation?
a. Water solubility is decreased
b. Phase II reaction
c. Phase I reaction
d. Done by CYP enzyme

62. Glucagon receptors are NOT found in which organ:
a. Cornea
b. Kidney
c. Stomach
d. Adrenal gland

63. Sodium fluoride is a good in-vitro preservative of glucose in blood samples because it inhibits:
a. Enolase
b. Hexokinase
c. Phosphofructokinase
d. Pyruvate dehydrogenase

64. Muscle is NOT involved in which type of glycogen storage disease:
a. Type 1
b. Type 2
c. Type 5
d. Type 7

65. Enzyme deficiency in Glycogen storage disease type V is?
a. Glucose-6-phosphatase
b. Acid maltase
c. Debranching enzyme
d. Myophosphorylase deficiency

66. Regarding HMP shunt, all of the following are true; EXCEPT:
a. Occurs in the cytosol
b. No ATP is produced in the cycle
c. It is active in Adipose tissue, Liver and Gonads
d. The oxidative phase generates NADH and the Non oxidative phase generates pyruvate.

67. Pentose phosphate pathway produces:
a. NADPH
b. ATP
c. Acetyl CoA
d. ADP

68. What is the composition of lugols solution?
a. 4% iodine 10% potassium iodide
b. 5% iodine and 10% potassium iodide
c. 2.5% iodine and 5% potassium iodide
d. 10% iodine and 6% potassium iodide

69. NADPH is used for:
a. Glycolysis
b. Lipid synthesis and glutathione reaction
c. Krebs cycle
d. All of the above

LIPIDS

70. Cholesterol is synthesized from: ***(Most Recent Question June/Dec 2021)***
a. Acetyl CoA
b. Malonyl CoA
c. Oxaloacetate
d. Bile acid

71. Dash DIET includes the following food; EXCEPT: ***(Most Recent Question June/Dec 2021)***
a. Rich in potassium
b. Rich in calcium
c. Rich in sodium
d. Rich in magnesium

72. Fats are stored in which of the following forms in tissues: ***(Most Recent Question June/Dec 2021)***
a. Fatty acid
b. Cholesterol
c. TGs
d. Cholesterol esters

73. In fatty liver, which is not given:
(Most Recent Question Aug 2020)
a. Choline b. Ethanol
c. Folic acid d. Methionine

74. Which of the following is cardioprotective?
(Most Recent Question Dec 2019-20)
a. HDL b. LDL
c. VLDL d. Chylomicron

75. First fatty acid to form in fatty acid synthesis:
(Most Recent Question 2019)
a. Palmitic acid b. Stearic acid
c. Oleic acid d. Pantothenic acid

76. Principle building block in fatty acid synthesis:
(Recent Pattern Question 2018-19)
a. Acetyl CoA b. Palmitoyl CoA
c. Malonyl CoA d. Oleate

77. Ideal total cholesterol to HDL cholesterol ratio is:
a. 1.5 b. 2.5
c. 3.5 d. 4.5

78. Niemann's pick disease is due to deficiency of which enzyme:
a. Sphingomyelinase b. Hexosaminidase-A
c. Aryl suplhatase d. Galactosidase-A

79. Which organelle is involved in the case of sphinghomyelin deficiency:
a. Lysosome b. Nucleus
c. Mitochondria d. Cell membrane

80. The most common lysosomal storage disorder is:
a. Gaucher's disease b. Taysach's disease
c. Wolman disease d. Niemann pick's disease

81. Enzyme replacement is mostly done for:
a. Niemann pick's b. Gangliosidosis
c. Gaucher's disease d. Phenylketonuria

82. Enzyme deficient in Tay-sach's disease:
a. α galactosidase b. Hexosaminidase A
c. β galactosidase d. β glucosidase

83. The enzyme is the rate limiting enzyme in cholesterol synthesis is:
a. HMG CoA synthetase b. HMG CoA reductase
c. HMG CoA lyase d. Catalase

84. Main LDL receptors is:
a. Apo-A b. Apo-B-100
c. Apoc-100 d. Apo-100 & Apo-E

85. Receptor present in liver for uptake of LDL:
a. Apo C b. Apo A and Apo E
c. Apo E and Apo B 48 d. Apo B 100

86. In primary familial hypercholesterolemia, there is defect in:
a. LDL-receptors b. Apoprotein
c. Apoprotein B d. VLDL

87. Which of the following has maximum cholesterol content:
a. HDL b. LDL
c. VLDL d. Chylomicrons

88. Which of the following lipoprotein transport triglyceride from liver to plasma:
a. LDL b. VLDL
c. Chylomicrons d. HDL

89. What is true regarding medium chain fatty acids:
a. Don't require pancreatic lipase
b. Diffuse directly into portal circulation
c. Not deposited in adipose tissue
d. All of the above

90. Auto oxidation is seen in:
a. Cholesterol b. Arachidonic acid
c. Stearic acid d. Palmitic acid

91. Which of the following is an Omega-3 fatty acid?
a. Linoleic acid b. α-Linolenic acid
c. Oleic acid d. Arachidonic acid

92. Which one of the following is an example of omega-3 fatty acids:
a. Gamma linolenic acid
b. Oleic acid
c. Docosahexaenoic acid
d. Palmitoleic acid

93. All of the following are derivative of omega-6; EXCEPT:
a. Alpha linolenic acid
b. Gamma linolenic acid
c. Arachidonic acid
d. Linoleic acid

94. Ketones body production occurs in:
a. Cytoplasm b. Mitochondria
c. Golgi Body d. Nucleus

95. Which enzyme activity is increased in starvation:
a. Pyruvate decarboxylase
b. Pyruvate kinase
c. Pyruvate carboxylase
d. Pyruvate dehydrogenase

96. In 3rd day to 2nd week starvation the body depends on:
a. Amino acid b. Ketone bodies
c. FA d. Glucose

97. Which of the following is a Monounsaturated Fatty acid (MUFA):
a. Linolenic acid b. Oleic acid
c. Lauric acid d. Stearic acid

98. The product of oxidation of odd chain fatty acids is:
a. Aceto-acetyl CoA
b. Malonyl CoA
c. Propionyl CoA
d. Fumaryl COA

99. Beta oxidation of odd chain fatty acid produces acetyl CoA and_____?
a. Malonyl CoA
b. Succinyl CoA
c. Propionyl CoA
d. Methylmanoyl CoA

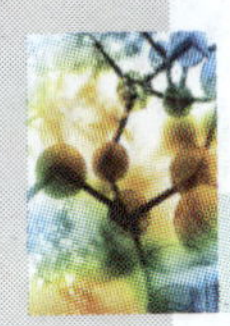

NUCLEIC ACID

100. A patient has swelling in metacarpophalangeal joints. Serum uric acid levels was raised. Doctor prescribed medicine for same. The medicine act by inhibiting which enzyme. ***(Most Recent Question June 2022)***

a. Thymidylate synthase
b. Xanthine oxidase
c. ADA (Adenosine deaminasae)
d. HGPRT

101. Severe combined immune deficiency is seen in: ***(Most Recent Question June/Dec 2021)***

a. HGPRTase deficiency
b. ADA deficiency
c. MCAD deficiency
d. Purine nucleoside phosphorylase deficiency

102. A patient with intellectual disability was found to have hyperuricemia. Self-mutation behaviour was also noticed. Which of the following enzyme is deficient? ***(Most Recent Question June/Dec 2021)***

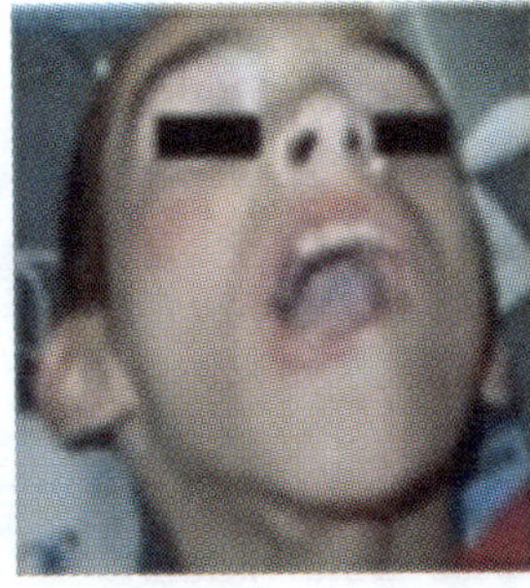

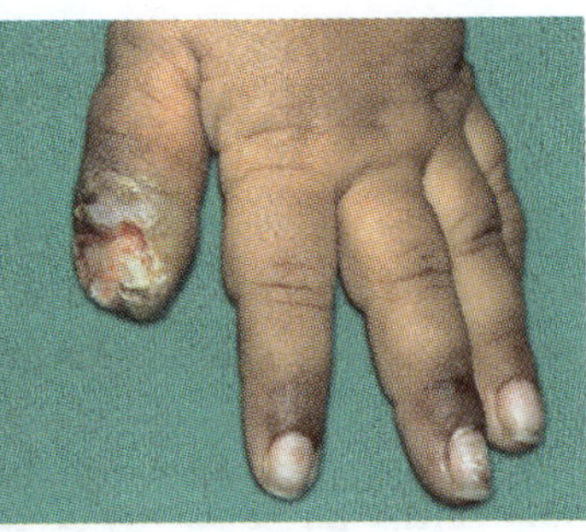

a. Alpha galactosidase A
b. Glucocerebrosidase
c. HGPRT
d. Sphingomyelinase

103. Which of the following is underlying cause of xeroderma pigmentosa development? ***(Most Recent Question June/Dec 2021)***

a. Base excision repair
b. Nucleotide excision repair
c. Mismatch repair
d. Homologous recombination

104. In a disease inheritance, Mother side uncle has a disease, her son also has same disease. Identify the type of inheritance. ***(Most Recent Question Aug 2020)***

a. X-linked recessive
b. X-linked dominant
c. Autosomal dominant
d. Autosomal recessive

105. Reverse transcriptase is used in: ***(Most Recent Question Dec 2019-20)***

a. RNA amplification
b. DNA amplification
c. DNA dependent DNA polymerase
d. RNA polymerase

106. The bases which are present in human DNA: ***(Most Recent Question Dec 2019-20)***

a. Adenine – Guanine and Thiamine – Uracil
b. Adenine – Guanine and Cytosine – Uracil
c. Adenine – Guanine and Cytosine – Thiamine
d. Adenosine – Guanosine and Cytosine – Tyrosine

107. Which of the following X-linked condition presents as urolithiasis with gouty arthritis? ***(Recent Pattern Question 2018-19)***

a. Holt oram syndrome
b. Lesch nyhan syndrome
c. SCID
d. Cystic fibrosis

108. Initiator codon in prokaryotes: ***(Recent Pattern Question 2018-19)***

a. UAA
b. UGA
c. AUG
d. UAG

109. Correct PCR staging sequence: ***(Recent Pattern Question 2018-19)***

a. Denature of DNA → Extension of primer → Annealing of Primer
b. Annealing of primer → Extension of primer → DNA denature
c. Denature of DNA → Annealing of primers → Extension of primer
d. Annealing of primer → DNA denature → Extension of primer

110. Which of the following is NOT seen in DNA? ***(Recent Pattern Question 2018-19)***

a. Cytosine
b. Adenine
c. Guanine
d. Uracil

111. Lac operon is: ***(Recent Pattern Question 2018)***

a. Repressor
b. Inducer
c. Operator
d. Activator

112. True about DNA polymerase 1: ***(Recent Pattern Question 2018)***

a. DNA polymerase III activity
b. 3′ – 5′ exonuclease activity
c. 5′ – 3′ exonuclease activity
d. All of the above

113. Reverse transcriptase PCR analyzes? ***(Recent Pattern Question 2017)***

a. DNA
b. RNA
c. Amino acid
d. Protein particle

114. Ionizing radiation damages DNA by which mechanism: ***(Recent Pattern Question 2017)***

a. Free radical damage
b. DNA helicase damage
c. Mismatch of bases
d. Bulky adducts formation

115. X chromosome belongs to which group: ***(Recent Pattern Question 2017)***

a. A
b. B
c. C
d. D

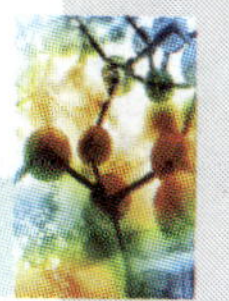

116. Which is Not true about Cockayne syndrome? *(Recent Pattern Question 2017)*
a. Autosomal recessive b. DNA mismatch repair
c. Related to XP d. Usually recurs

117. How many stop codons are seen? *(Recent Pattern Question 2017)*
a. 1 b. 2
c. 3 d. 4

118. Which is true about stop codon? *(Recent Pattern Question 2017)*
a. 3 codon coding for one amino acid
b. 3 codon coding for whole DNA
c. 3 codon coding for whole RNA
d. 3 codon act as terminator codon

119. Anti-codon arm is seen in *(Recent Pattern Question 2016)*
a. m-RNA b. r-RNA
c. t-RNA d. sn-RNA

120. Alpha helix is which structure *(Recent Pattern Question 2016)*
a. Primary b. Secondary
c. Tertiary d. Quaternary

121. Bend of DNA is made of which amino acid *(Recent Pattern Question 2016)*
a. Glycine b. Alanine
c. Cysteine d. Lysine

122. Enzyme involved in post-transcriptional capping at 5' end *(Recent Pattern Question 2016)*
a. 5 methyl transferase b. 7 methyl transferase
c. 5 methyl reductase d. 7 methyl reductase

123. Which of the following nitrogen base is not seen in RNA? *(Recent Pattern Question 2016)*
a. Adenine b. Thymine
c. Guanine d. Cytosine

124. Which of the following amino acid is common in Purine and pyridimines?
a. Alanine b. Glutamine
c. Guanine d. Uracil

125. In Pyrimidine synthesis rate limiting enzyme is:
a. Aspartate transcarbomylase
b. Carbamoyl phosphate synthetase II
c. Dihydroorotase dehydrogenase
d. OMP. Decarboxylase

126. The Watson's Crick double helix model of DNA is:
a. Right handed anti parallel
b. Left handed anti parallel
c. Right handed parallel
d. Left handed parallel

127. Equal number of nucleotide bases are seen between which pair of nucleotides:
a. A≡G b. G=T
c. G≡C d. A=C

128. Frame shift mutation:
a. Substitution of amino acid
b. Changed mRNA base at 3rd nucleotide of codon
c. Due to stop codon
d. Deletion of 2 bases

129. Frameshift mutation leads to cellular changes to which of the following processes:
a. Translation b. Transcription
c. Replication d. Spontaneous

130. Frame shift mutation DOESN'T occur in multiples of:
a. 2 b. 3
c. 4 d. 5

131. Sickle cell disease is present with which mutation:
a. Cross-linked defect b. Base pair defect
c. Mismatch defect d. Base pair substitution

132. Which of the following is not a part of DNA correction mechanism:
a. Nucleoside correction b. Pre replication
c. Post replication d. Base pair correction

133. 5' to 3' exonuclease activity is seen in:
a. Proof reading b. Repair of damaged DNA
c. DNA synthesis d. DNA polymerase

134. Radiation affects:
a. RNA b. DNA
c. Mitochondria d. Cytoskeleton protein

135. True about Chaperones:
a. For misfolding of protein
b. HSP 70 family of chaperones bind with hydrophobic amino acid
c. HSP 60 and 70 are similar in structure
d. Has no role in unfolding

136. DNA repair defect is seen in:
a. Xeroderma pigmentosum b. Li-fraumani syndrome
c. Retinoblastoma d. None

137. DNA enzyme for aging:
a. Telosomerase b. Topoisomerase
c. Telomerase d. DNA polymerase

138. Protein synthesis occurs in which part of the cell:
a. Smooth endoplasmic reticulum
b. Rough endoplasmic reticulum
c. Golgi body
d. All of the above

139. Protein synthesis occurs in:
a. Golgi bodies b. Endoplasmic reticulum
c. Mitochondria d. Peroxisomes

140. Protein synthesized in rough Endoplasmic reticulum will first go to:
a. Mitochondria b. Cytosol
c. Golgi body d. Lysosome

141. Which of the following structure is *not affected* in protein denaturation?
a. Primary structure b. Secondary structure
c. Tertiary structure d. Quaternary structure

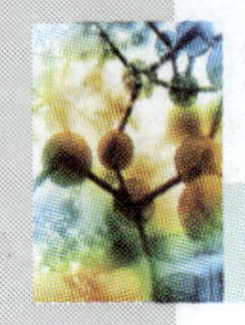

142. True about Lesch-Nyhan syndrome:
a. Patient have normal intellectual capacity
b. Pyrimidine overproduction is the cause
c. Uric acid stones are frequently formed
d. X- Linked dominant

143. All of the following are features of Lesch-Nyhan syndrome; EXCEPT:
a. Hyperuricaemia
b. Self-mutilation
c. Mental retardation
d. Immunodeficiency

144. The main catabolic product/products of purine nuleotides in humans is which one of the following:
a. Ammonia + CO_2 b. Ammonia
c. Uric acid d. CO_2 and water

145. Hyperuricemia occur due to all; EXCEPT:
a. Xanthine oxidase
b. Phosphoribosyl pyrophosphate synthetase
c. Glucose 6 phosphatase
d. Hypoxanthine-guanine phosphoribosyl-transferase

146. Hypouricaemia is associated with deficiency of which of the following:
a. Xanthine oxidase
b. Von Gierke's disease
c. Hypoxanthine guanine phosphoribosyl transferase
d. Adenine phosphoribosyl transferase

147. The technique used for separation and detection of RNA is which one of the following?
a. Northern blot b. Southern blot
c. Eastern blot d. Western blot

148. Carrier of genetic material:
a. DNA cistrons b. Codons of m RNA
c. Anti-codons of t RNA d. None

149. All of the following are true regarding cytosolic eukaryotic gene expression; EXCEPT:
a. Capping helps in attachment of mRNA to 40 S Ribosome
b. N formyl methionine t-RNA will be the first t-RNA to come into action
c. EF2 shifts between GDP & GTP
d. Releasing factor releases the polypeptide chain from the P site

150. Most common RNA is
a. t-RNA b. m-RNA
c. r-RNA d. sn-RNA

151. RNA silencing is seen with:
a. t-RNA b. m-RNA
c. Sn-RNA d. mi-RNA

152. SNURPS are:
a. Single nucleotide units for recycling of proteins
b. Small Nuclear Ribo-nucleoproteins
c. Small nuclear units for misfolded proteins
d. Single nuclear unit for recycling of misfolded proteins

153. Lac operon is classically activated by:
a. Increased glucose concentration, increased cAMP
b. Decreased glucose concentration, decreased cAMP
c. Decreased glucose concentration, increased cAMP
d. Increased glucose concentration, decreased cAMP

AMINO ACID

154. A child presents with complaints of urine turning black on standing. What is the diagnosis?
(Most Recent Question June 2022)
a. Homocystinuria b. Tyrosinemia
c. Alkaptonuria d. Maple syrup urine disease

155. Which of the following is considered as universal methyl donor in biochemical reactions?
(Most Recent Question June/Dec 2021)
a. SAM b. PAPS
c. Methyl cobalamin d. Methionine

156. Which of the following amino acid is excreted in urine in maple syrup urine disease?
(Most Recent Question June/Dec 2021)
a. Tryptophan b. Phenylalanine
c. Leucine d. Arginine

157. A patient has swelling in metacarpophalangeal joints. Serum uric acid levels were raised. Doctor prescribed a medicine for same. The medicine act by inhibiting which enzyme: ***(Most Recent Question Aug 2020)***
a. Thymidylate synthase b. Xanthine oxidase
c. ADA (adenosine deaminase)
d. HGPRT

158. Nitric oxide is synthesized from:
(Most Recent Question Aug 2020)
a. L -Hydroxy proline b. Arginine
c. D-histidine d. Cysteine

159. Which is involved in protein folding?
(Most Recent Question Aug 2020)
a. Chaperone b. Ubiquitin
c. Proline d. Arginine

160. A 40-year-old man presented with black pigmentation of pinna and sclera of eyes. The color of urine changes to black on long standing. What is the diagnosis?
a. Alkaptonuria ***(Most Recent Question Dec 2019-20)***
b. Phenylketonuria
c. Maple syrup urine disease
d. Hartnup disease

161. Nitrogenous waste are excreted from the body in the form of: ***(Most Recent Question Dec 2019-20)***
a. Glutamine b. Urea
c. Uric acid d. Nitric oxide

162. Which structure of protein is not denatured after heating up to 100 degree? ***(Most Recent Question Dec 2019-20)***
a. Primary b. Secondary
c. Tertiary d. Quaternary

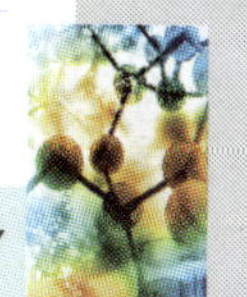

163. Synovial fluid contains:
(Most Recent Question Dec 2019-20)
a. Chondroitin sulphate b. Keratan sulphate
c. Hyaluronic acid d. Dermatan sulphate

164. Melanin is derived from which amino acid?
(Most Recent Question Dec 2019-20)
a. Tyrosine b. Tryptophan
c. Phenylalanine d. Alanine

165. 1 g of protein yields how much energy?
(Most Recent Question Dec 2019-20)
a. 9 cal b. 40 cal
c. 4 cal d. 1 cal

166. Ammonia formed in brain is converted into:
(Most Recent Question Dec 2019-20)
a. Glutamine b. Glycine
c. Cysteine d. Urea

167. Most abundant amino acids found in collagen:
(Most Recent Question Dec 2019-20)
a. Glycine b. Proline
c. Hydroxyproline d. Lysine

168. Which is a specific test for uric acid for gout?
(Most Recent Question Dec 2019-20)
a. Plasma uric acid b. Uric acid in urine
c. Synovial uric acid d. Serum uric acid

169. A child presents with complaints of urine turning black on standing. What is the diagnosis?
(Most Recent Question Dec 2019-20)
a. Homocystinuria b. Tyrosinemia
c. Alkaptonuria d. Maple syrup urine disease

170. Nitric oxide is synthesized from this amino acid:
(Most Recent Question 2019)
a. Arginine b. Lysine
c. Leucine d. Isoleucine

171. Enzyme deficient in maple syrup urine disease:
(Most Recent Question 2019)
a. Branched chain alpha keto acid decarboxylase
b. Methionine adenosyltransferase
c. Fumarylacetoacetate hydrolase
d. Tyrosine aminotransferase

172. Amino acid abundant in collagen:
(Most Recent Question 2019)
a. Glycine b. Lysine
c. Leucine d. Isoleucine

173. Strenuous exercise is not done in this glycogen storage disease: *(Most Recent Question 2019)*
a. McArdle disease b. Anderson disease
c. Pompe disease d. Von Gierke disease

174. Hartnup disease can present with:
(Recent Pattern Question 2018-19)
a. Pellagra like symptoms b. Nephrolithiasis
c. Protein intolerance d. Microcephaly

175. All of the following are derivatives of tryptophan; EXCEPT: *(Recent Pattern Question 2018-19)*
a. Melatonin b. Serotonin
c. Niacin d. Creatinine

176. Prostaglandins are derived from:
(Recent Pattern Question 2018-19)
a. Stearic acid b. Arachidonic acid
c. Glutamic acid d. Aspartic acid

177. Mental retardation is a clinical feature of:
(Recent Pattern Question 2018-19)
a. Alkaptonuria b. Albinism
c. Hawkinsinuria d. Phenylketonuria

178. Precursor of melanin synthesis:
(Recent Pattern Question 2018-19)
a. Tyrosine b. Glycine
c. Phenylalanine d. Lysine

179. Collagen contains amino acids Proline, Lysine and:
(Recent Pattern Question 2018-19)
a. Glycine b. Isoleucine
c. Cysteine d. Methionine

180. Disulfide bonds are formed in which amino acid:
(Recent Pattern Question 2018-19)
a. Glycine b. Cysteine
c. Proline d. Isoleucine

181. Which is not a biological derivative of tyrosine?
(Recent Pattern Question 2018)
a. Melanin b. Melatonin
c. Epinephrine d. Dopamine

182. The composition of creatine is:
(Recent Pattern Question 2018)
a. Glycine, arginine, methionine
b. Glycine and histidine
c. Glycine, glutamate, aspartate
d. Histidine and methionine

183. All of the following are branched chain amino acids; EXCEPT: *(Recent Pattern Question 2018)*
a. Leucine b. Lysine
c. Isoleucine d. Valine

184. Protein folding is done by: *(Recent Pattern Question 2017)*
a. Chaperone b. Endoplasmic reticulum
c. Peroxisome d. Lysosome

185. Which is the common amino acid between urea cycle and TCA? *(Recent Pattern Question 2017)*
a. Asparate b. Alanine
c. Asparagine d. Glutamate

186. Which amino acid is acidic? *(Recent Pattern Question 2017)*
a. Aspartic acid b. Valine
c. Leucine d. Aspartate

187. Guanidine combines with which amino acid?
(Recent Pattern Question 2017)
a. Tyrosine b. Arginine
c. Methionine d. Proline

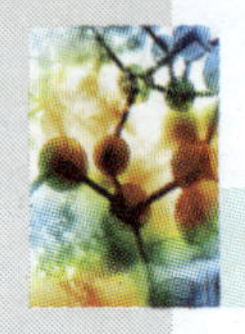

188. Dihydrobiopterin is used in management of which amino acid defect? ***(Recent Pattern Question 2017)***
a. Alanine b. Tyrosine
c. Phenylalanine d. Tryptophan

189. HbA1c does glycosylation with which amino acid? ***(Recent Pattern Question 2017)***
a. Arginine b. Glutamate
c. Valine d. Leucine

190. Test done to check protein purity? ***(Recent Pattern Question 2017)***
a. Mass Spectrophotometry b. SDS –PAGE
c. Western blot d. Sanger's technique

191. LDH1 is seen in: ***(Recent Pattern Question 2017)***
a. Liver b. Skeletal muscle
c. Heart d. Kidney

192. Non-essential amino acid ***(Recent Pattern Question 2016)***
a. Tryptophan b. Tyrosine
c. Arginine d. Histidine

193. True about lysine ***(Recent Pattern Question 2016)***
a. Deficient in pulses b. Deficient in cereals
c. Nonessential amino acid d. Acidic amino acid

194. Homocysteine is ***(Recent Pattern Question 2016)***
a. Protein D alpha amino acid
b. Protein L amino acid
c. Non-protein alpha amino acid
d. Seen in protein

195. Which of the following releases ammonia ***(Recent Pattern Question 2016)***
a. Aspartate dehydrogenase b. Glutaminase
c. Adenosine deaminase d. Aspartate synthetase

196. Carnitine is useful in transport of ***(Recent Pattern Question 2016)***
a. Aromatic amino acid b. Aliphatic amino acid
c. Fatty acid d. Glucose

197. PKU is due to deficiency of which enzyme: ***(Recent Pattern Question 2016)***
a. Phenylalanine reductase b. Phenylalanine hydroxylase
c. Tyrosine hydroxylase d. Tyrosine reductase

198. Which protein is abundant in our body: ***(Recent Pattern Question 2016)***
a. Collagen b. Albumin
c. Myoglobin d. Hemoglobin

199. Which is a niacin sparing amino acid:
a. Tryptophan b. Methionine
c. Cysteine d. Tyrosine

200. Which vitamin can be synthesized from tryptophan:
a. Niacin b. Riboflavin
c. Cobalamin d. Folic acid

201. Disease entity due to deficiency of alpha keto-decarboxylase enzyme:
a. Hartnup's disease b. Maple syrup disease
c. Alkaptonuria d. Alport syndrome

202. Limiting amino acid in maize:
a. Niacin b. Tyrosine
c. Tryptophan d. Methionine

203. In Alkaptonuria deficiency is:
a. Phosphofructo kinase
b. HMG CoA reductase
c. Homogentisate oxidase
d. Xanthine oxidase

204. First product of tryptophan catabolism is:
a. Kynerunine b. Bradykinin
c. PAF d. Xantheurenate

205. Urea is formed from which substrate:
a. Arginine b. Orginine
c. Citrulline d. Aspartate

206. Hydrolysis occurs at which step of urea cycle:
a. Cleavage of Arginine
b. Formation of Argininosuccinate
c. Formation of citrulline
d. Formation of ornithine

207. Polyamine like putrescine is derived from:
a. Arginine b. Ornithine
c. Yohimibine d. Arginosuccine

208. All are true about selenocystiene; EXCEPT:
a. Considered 21st Amino acid
b. Coded by UGA
c. Occurs in glutathione peroxidase
d. Made of cystiene and methionine

209. Cystinuria is due to the accumulation of:
a. Cysteine b. Lysine
c. Ornithine d. Cysteine

210. Nitric oxide is synthesized from:
a. L-arginine b. L- citrulline
c. Lysine d. Tryptophan

211. Smooth muscle relaxant nitric oxide is synthesized from:
a. Methionine b. Cyseine
c. Arginine d. Ornithine

212. Carnitine is made-up of:
a. Leusine b. Lysine
c. Lysine & methionine d. Arginine

213. β alanine is a product of:
a. Dihydrouracil b. Carnitine
c. Kynurenine d. Cyano-cobalamin

214. The structural polysaccharide chitin is a polymer of which of the following:
a. Galactosamine
b. Glucosamine
c. N. Acetyl Galactosamine
d. N-Acetyl Glucosamine

215. The initiation of hemoglobin synthesis requires:
a. Histidine b. Glycine
c. Folate d. Iron

216. In Hartnup's disease which of the following is excreted in the urine:
a. Ornithine b. Glycine
c. Tryptophan d. Cystine

217. Intestinal flora (bacteria) digests all; EXCEPT:
a. Cellulose b. Lignin
c. Pectin d. Starch

218. Amino acid which contributes to biosynthesis of purine ribonucleotide are all; EXCEPT:
a. Aspartate b. Histidine
c. Glutamate d. Glycine

219. Which of the following amino acid is used in biosynthesis of purines?
a. Alanine b. Glycine
c. Threonine d. Ornithine

220. Glutathione is composed of:
a. Glycine b. Cycteine
c. Glutamate d. All of these

221. Vitamin C is necessary in the formation of collagen. It is required for the conversion of:
a. Proline to hydroxyproline
b. Beta-carotene to vitamin A
c. Glutamate to gamma-carboxyglutamate
d. Pyridoxine to pyridoxal phosphate

222. What changes the conformation of alpha helix in collagen
a. Methionine b. Proline
c. Alanine d. Tyrosine

223. Used in Transamination:
a. Pyridoxal phosphate b. NADPH
c. NADP d. FAD

VITAMINS, MINERALS AND ENZYMES

224. Identify the image and its vitamin deficiency.
(Most Recent Question June 2022)

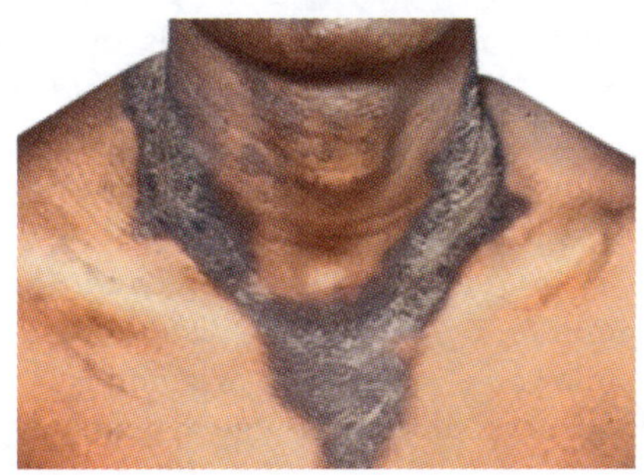

a. Niacin b. Copper
c. Iron d. Selenium

225. Vitamin deficiency causes tingling sensation:
(Most Recent Question June 2022)
a. Vitamin A b. Vitamin B_1
c. Folic acid d. Vitamin B_6

226. Menke's kink hair disease is due to:
(Most Recent Question June/Dec 2021)
a. P53 defect b. Copper excess
c. Copper deficiency d. Zinc deficiency

227. A patient came to OPD with complaints of diarrhea, dermatitis and dementia. It was also found that he was a maize eater. Which of the following could be most probably deficient? ***(Most Recent Question June/Dec 2021)***
a. Thiamin b. Riboflavin
c. Niacin d. Biotin

228. A 40-year-old female patient came to OPD with features of anemia. She had undergone subtotal gastrectomy few months back. General examination showed the following changes in the tongue as shown in the image. Which of the following vitamin is responsible for this?
(Most Recent Question June/Dec 2021)

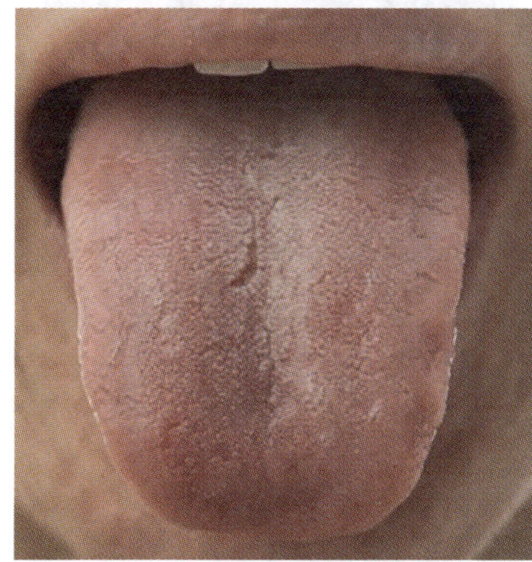

a. Vitamin A b. Vitamin B12
c. Vitamin C d. Vitamin B2

229. Patient who is a chronic alcoholic has signs of B1 deficiency. Which of the following is the marker for vitamin B1 deficiency? ***(Most Recent Question June/Dec 2021)***
a. RBC transketolase activity
b. RBC glyceraldehyde reductase activity
c. Homocysteine activity
d. Pyridoxal 5'-phosphate

230. A 70-year-old male has bruising under the eyes. Which of the following vitamin deficiency leads to easy bruising and bleeding gums?
(Most Recent Question June/Dec 2021)
a. Vitamin B12 b. Vitamin B_2
c. Vitamin B6 d. Vitamin C

231. The micronutrient that is deficients after ileal resection:
(Most Recent Question June/Dec 2021)
a. Folate b. B_{12}
c. Iron d. Copper

232. Which of the following explains the role of sunlight in vitamin D metabolism?
(Most Recent Question June/Dec 2021)
a. Conversion of cholecalciferol to 25 OH cholecalciferol
b. Conversion of 25 OH cholecalciferol to calcitoriol
c. Conversion of 25 OH cholecalciferol to 24,25 di OH cholecalciferol
d. Conversion of 7 dehydro cholesterol to cholecalciferol

233. Which vitamin deficiency will lead to the following?
(Most Recent Question June/Dec 2021)

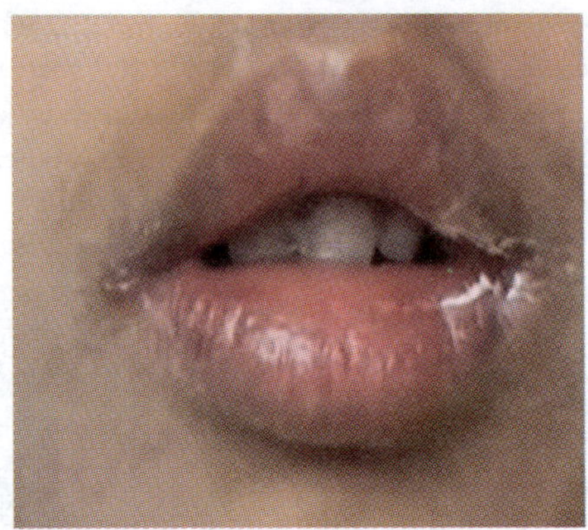

a. Vitamin A b. Vitamin B_2
c. Vitamin B_3 d. Vitamin C

234. A patient has macrocytic anemia and high homocysteine levels. His methyl malonyl CoA levels are normal. What is the diagnosis? ***(Most Recent Question June/Dec 2021)***
a. Vitamin B_6 deficiency
b. Vitamin B_9 deficiency
c. Vitamin B_{12} deficiency
d. Anemia of chronic disease

235. Glutathione peroxidase contains which metal?
(Most Recent Question June/Dec 2021)
a. Selenium b. Copper
c. Zinc d. Manganese

236. A patient having fatigue and weakness. On examination, his Hb was low, iron levels were low. Patient noted that his wound healing is delayed since last 1 year. Which vitamin deficiency is possible in this patient?
(Most Recent Question June/Dec 2021)
a. Vitamin C b. Vitamin A
c. Vitamin B12 d. Vitamin B2

237. Enzyme deficiency in Von gierke disease
(Most Recent Question June/Dec 2021)
a. Branching enzyme b. Muscle phosphorylase
c. Debranching enzyme d. Glucose 6-phosphatase

238. Alcoholic patient presents with neurological symptoms. There is deficiency of which vitamin:
(Most Recent Question Aug 2020)
a. B_1 b. A
c. B_9 d. B_{12}

239. A female patient with macrocytic anemia, homocystinuria & normal methylmalonate levels. Which vitamin therapy can help in this?
(Most Recent Question Aug 2020)
a. Folate plus vitamin B_{12}
b. Folate
c. Vitamin A
d. Vitamin C

240. A heart patient suddenly has chest pain. Which isoenzyme of LDH enzyme is elevated?
(Most Recent Question Aug 2020)
a. LDH-1 b. LDH-5
c. LDH-2 d. LDH-4

241. Cofactor for mitochondrial superoxide dismutase:
(Most Recent Question Aug 2020)
a. Mn b. Cu
c. Zn d. Mb

242. Which of the following is not a micronutrient?
(Most Recent Question Dec 2019-20)
a. Zinc b. Copper
c. Calcium d. Iodine

243. Most sensitive screening test for vitamin A deficiency?
(Most Recent Question Dec 2019-20)
a. Retinol < 10 b. Beta carotene <10
c. Bitot spot d. Night blindness

244. Which enzyme level is tested in thiamine deficiency?
(Most Recent Question Dec 2019-20)
a. PDH b. Pyruvate kinase
c. Transketolase d. Kinase

245. Keshan disease is due to deficiency of:
(Most Recent Question Dec 2019-20)
a. Selenium b. Zinc
c. Copper d. Iron

246. Zinc is cofactor of which enzyme?
(Most Recent Question Dec 2019-20)
a. Carbonic anhydrase b. Lysyl oxidase
c. Carboxylase d. Deiodinase

247. Which of the following vitamin is most potent antioxidant? ***(Most Recent Question 2019)***
a. Vitamin D b. Vitamin E
c. Vitamin K d. Vitamin B

248. Vitamin which helps in iron absorption:
(Most Recent Question 2019)
a. Vitamin A b. Vitamin B
c. Vitamin C d. Vitamin E

249. Wernicke encephalopathy is due to deficiency of:
(Most Recent Question 2019)
a. Thiamine b. Biotin
c. Niacin d. Hydroxycobalamin

250. Menkes disease is due to deficiency of:
(Recent Pattern Question 2018-19)
a. Selenium b. Copper
c. Chromium d. Manganese

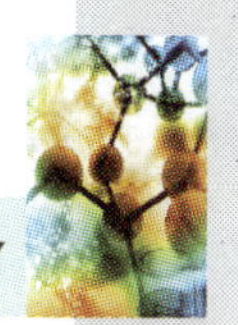

251. G6PD is enzyme of: ***(Recent Pattern Question 2018-19)***
a. Mitochondria b. Cell membrane
c. Golgi organ d. Endoplasmic reticulum

252. Inheritance pattern of G6PD: ***(Recent Pattern Question 2018-19)***
a. AR b. AD
c. X-linked d. Familial

253. Activator of trypsinogen is mainly by:
a. Chymotrypsinogen b. Enteropeptidase
c. Trypsin d. Hexokinase

254. Which of the following is a function of chaperone protein? ***(Recent Pattern Question 2018-19)***
a. It degrades proteins that have folded improperly
b. It provides a template for how the proteins should fold
c. It rescues proteins that have folded improperly and allows them to refold properly
d. It degrades proteins that have folded properly

255. In case of cyanide poisoning, antidote of amyl nitrate is given. This is an example of: ***(Recent Pattern Question 2018)***
a. Receptor antagonism
b. Chemical antagonism
c. Physical antagonism
d. Physiological antagonism

256. Synthesis of type I collagen requires which vitamin? ***(Recent Pattern Question 2018)***
a. Vitamin A b. Vitamin C
c. Vitamin D d. Vitamin K

257. cAMP is formed from: ***(Recent Pattern Question 2018)***
a. AMP b. GMP
c. ATP d. MTP

258. Among the following, which is the most effective antioxidant: ***(Recent Pattern Question 2018)***
a. Vitamin A b. Vitamin C
c. Vitamin E d. Vitamin K

259. Selenium deficiency causes: ***(Recent Pattern Question 2017)***
a. Menke's disease b. Wilson's disease
c. Keshan disease d. Kashinbeck disease

260. Which is correct about vitamin K? ***(Recent Pattern Question 2017)***
a. Shortest half life b. Exist in three forms
c. All are fat soluble d. All are water soluble

261. Peroxidases belong to which enzyme group? ***(Recent Pattern Question 2017)***
a. Oxidase-Reductase b. Lipase
c. Hydrolase d. Transferase

262. Impaired Glucose intolerance is caused by deficiency of ***(Recent Pattern Question 2016)***
a. Chromium b. Selenium
c. Copper d. Cobalt

263. Lactate dehydrogenase enzyme requires which metal ***(Recent Pattern Question 2016)***
a. Selenium b. Copper
c. Magnesium d. Zinc

264. True about competitive inhibition with first order kinetics ***(Recent Pattern Question 2016)***
a. K_m increased, V_{max} same
b. V_{max} increased, K_m same
c. K_m same, V_{max} decrease
d. K_m same, V_{max} increase

265. Methylcobalamin is required for which of the following enzymes:
a. Homocysteine deaminase
b. Homocysteine methyl transferase
c. Methionine synthase
d. Methionine reductase

266. True about Riboflavin is:
a. Deficiency causes Beri Beri
b. Consist of flavin group which is required in oxidation-reduction reaction
c. Pyridoxal phosphate act as a cofactor
d. Green leafy vegetables are major sources

267. Which vitamin is associated with carboxylation reactions:
a. Thiamine b. Riboflavin V
c. Biotin d. Folic acid

268. In pregnancy, neural tube defect arises in the fetus due to deficiency of which of the following in the mother?
a. Vitamin b. Folic acid
c. Vitamin A d. Vitamin C

269. Pellagra is due to:
a. Utilization of tryptophan b. Deficiency of tryptophan
c. Deficiency of thiamine d. Utilization of niacin

270. Menadione is analog of:
a. Vitamin K b. Vitamin A
c. Vitamin D d. Vitamin C

271. Which of the following is water soluble form of vitamin K:
a. Menaquinone b. Phylloqumone
c. Menadione d. Primidone

272. Water soluble form of Vitamin K
a. Phylloquinone b. Menaquinone
c. Menadione d. None

273. All of the following vitamins are anti-oxidants; EXCEPT:
a. Beta- carotene b. Ascorbic acid
c. Vitamin E d. Vitamin K

274. Which of the following vitamin deficiency is seen with biliary obstruction:
a. Vitamin K b. Vitamin C
c. Vitamin B_{12} d. Vitamin B_2

275. Of the following which is absent in eggs:
a. Vitamin B_{12} b. Vitamin C
c. Vitamin A d. Vitamin B_2

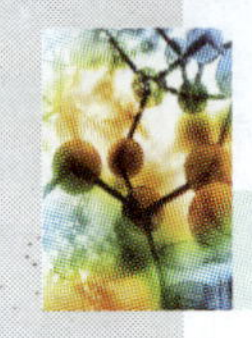

276. A child with alopecia, hyperpigmentation, hypogonadism and rash of genital area and mouth is likely to suffer from:
a. Iron deficiency
b. Zinc deficiency
c. Calcium deficiency
d. Copper deficiency

277. Toxicity of cholera toxin in due to which one of the following:
a. Decrease in activity of Gi protein
b. Decrease in activity of Gs protein
c. ADP-ribosylation of Gs alpha sub-unit
d. ADP-ribosylation of G1 alpha sub-unit

278. The normal pH of the human blood is which one of the following:
a. 70-72
b. 7.25-7.35
c. 7.36-7.44
d. 7.50-7.55

279. The best index for calculation of the nutritional value of protein is which one of the following:
a. Biological Value
b. Net protein utilization
c. Protein digestibility
d. Protein efficiency rates

280. Malonyl aciduria is seen in deficiency of:
a. Vitamin B_{12}
b. Vitamin B_2
c. Pyridoxine
d. Folic acid

281. Sunflower cataract is caused due to:
a. Iron deposit
b. Sorbitol deposit
c. Glucose deposit
d. Copper deposit

282. Marfan's syndrome is due to the defect in:
a. Collagen
b. Fibrillin
c. Elastin
d. Laminin

283. Which enzyme is used to convert phenylalanine to tyrosine:
a. Tyrosine synthase
b. Tyrosine hydroxylase
c. Phenylalanine hydroxylase
d. Phenylethanolamine methyltransferase

284. Which one of the following is a precursor of tyrosine?
a. Epinephrine
b. Phenylalanine
c. DOPA
d. Norepinephrine

285. Copper containing enzyme is:
a. Dopamine hydroxylase
b. Dopamine decarboxylase
c. Dopamine carboxylase
d. Tyrosine hydroxylase

286. Enzyme involved with copper as coenzyme
a. Lysyl oxidase
b. Phenylalanine Hydroxyalse
c. Alcohol dehydrogenase
d. None of these

287. Which of the following enzyme requires molybdenum for its activity?
a. Cytochrome oxidase
b. Xanthine oxidase
c. Carbonic anhydrase
d. Phosphogluco mutase

288. Which of the following elements is required for conversion of pro-collagen to collagen?
a. Zinc
b. Iron
c. Selenium
d. Copper

289. Which of the following ion is used in PCR?
a. Mn^{2+}
b. Mg^{2+}
c. Ca^{2+}
d. Mo

290. In Non competitive inhibition of enzyme:
a. Decreased K_m, increase V_{max}
b. Increase K_m, Increase V_{max}
c. Normal K_m, decrease V_{max}
d. Normal K_m, increase V_{max}

291. All enzymes are oxidoreductases; EXCEPT:
a. Glucokinase
b. Peroxidase
c. Oxidase
d. Oxygenase

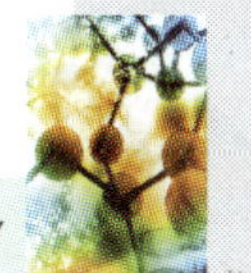

ANSWERS WITH EXPLANATIONS

MOST RECENT QUESTIONS 2023

1. Ans. (d) Zinc

Ref: Lehninger Principles of Biochemistry, 4th ed. pg. 126

Zinc is known to play a major role in the stabilization of insulin hexamers and in the pancreatic storage of insulin because it can enhance insulin binding to hepatocyte membranes.

2. Ans. (c) Cystathionine β-synthase

Ref: Lehninger Principles of Biochemistry, 4th ed. pg. 653

- High level of homocysteine in the patient directs toward homocystinuria.
- It is caused by cystathionine β-synthase (CBS) deficiency and is characterized by involvement of the eye (ectopia lentis and/or severe myopia), skeletal system (excessive height, long limbs, scoliosis, and pectus excavatum), vascular system (thromboembolism), and CNS (developmental delay/intellectual disability).

3. Ans. (b) Inner mitochondrial membrane

Ref: Lehninger Principles of Biochemistry, 4th ed. pg. 342

- Cardiolipin (CL) is a unique phospholipid which is localized and synthesized in the inner mitochondrial membrane (IMM).
- It is now widely accepted that CL plays a central role in many reactions and processes involved in mitochondrial function and dynamics.

4. Ans. (c) Antimycin A

Ref: Lehninger Principles of Biochemistry, 4th ed. pg. 698, 326

- Antimycin A is a known insecticide used in fisheries and an inhibitor of ETC complex III.
- Antimycin binds to the complex III and inhibits electron transfer. Inhibition of complex III stops the electron transport chain. Thus, ATP synthesis by oxidative phosphorylation is also stopped.
- **Symptoms of antimycin A toxin includes:**
  - Incoordination, impaired reflexes, respiratory distress, and central nervous system depression.
  - **Inhibitors of oxidative phosphorylation:**

Complex I	Rotenone (it is also a pesticide used in fisheries)
Complex II	Carboxin
Complex III	Antimycin A
Complex IV	Cyanide, azide, carbon monoxide
ATP synthase	Oligomycin
ATP-ADP translocase	Atractyloside

Contd...

5. Ans. (d) Vitamin K

Ref: Lehninger Principles of Biochemistry, 4th ed. pg. 532

Vitamin K deficiency in the clinical setting is characterized by a bleeding tendency as a consequence of low concentrations of the coagulation factors II, VII, IX, and X.

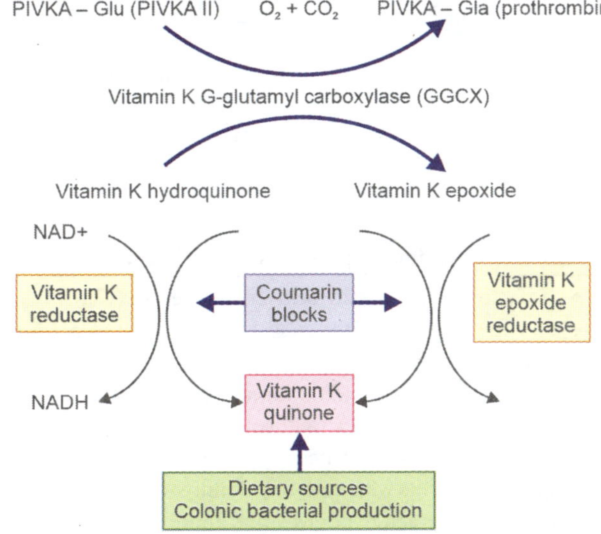

6. Ans. (a) Vitamin B_1

Ref: Park's Textbook of Preventive and Social Medicine, 25th ed. pg. 675

- Wernicke-Korsakoff syndrome mainly causes vision changes, loss of coordination, confusion and unsteady gait, ataxia and impaired memory.
- This occurs due to thiamine (vitamin B_1) deficiency. This can occur due to Wernicke encephalopathy, eating disorders, malnutrition, and alcohol abuse. It is usually secondary to prolonged alcohol abuse.

Extra Mile

- **Vitamin C deficiency** can cause fatigue, easy bruising, and bumpy skin.
- **Vitamin D deficiency** can cause rickets, osteomalacia, impaired calcium metabolism, osteoporosis, increased risk of fracture.
- **Vitamin A deficiency** can cause vision trouble, difficulty conceiving, dry or inflamed skin, chest infections.

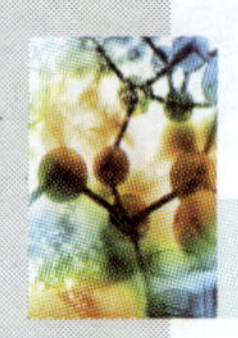

7. Ans. (b) δ-aminolevulinic acid synthase

Ref: Lehninger Principles of Biochemistry, 4th ed. pg. 313

- Current models for regulation of heme synthesis during erythropoiesis propose that the first enzyme of the pathway, **5-aminolevulinate synthase** (ALAS), is the rate-limiting enzyme.

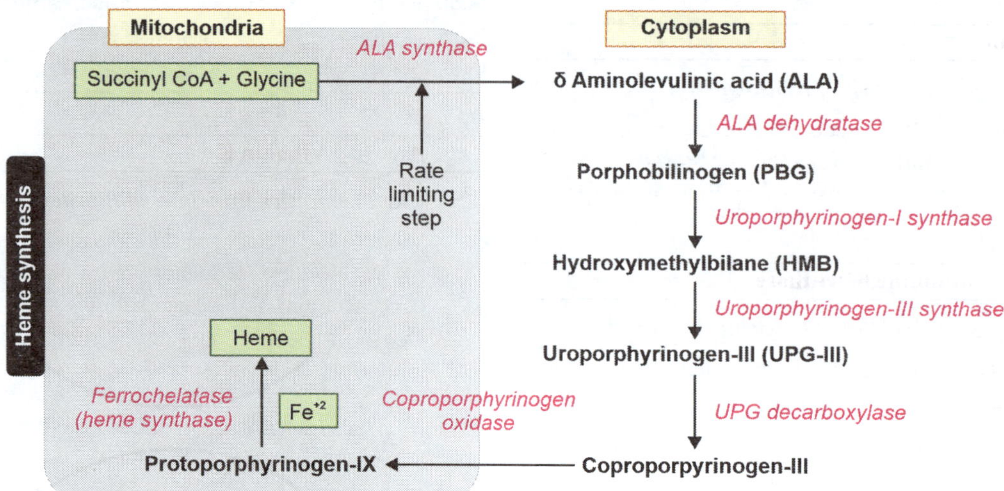

8. Ans. (d) Galactose-1-phosphate uridylyltransferase

- Galactose-1-phosphate uridylyltransferase (GALT) is an enzyme responsible for converting ingested galactose to glucose.
- Deficiency of GALT causes **classic galactosemia**. Galactosemia is an autosomal recessive inherited disorder detectable in newborns and childhood.
- Patient presents with vomiting, failure to thrive, jaundice, oil-drop cataract, hypoglycemia, anorexia, etc.

Other options:

- **Lactase deficiency** causes lactose intolerance. Patient presents with bloating, diarrhea, nausea, abdominal pain after lactose-rich food intake.
- **Fructokinase deficiency** leads to high levels of fructose in the blood and urine.
- **Galactokinase deficiency** (Type II Galactosemia) is caused by an inborn error of metabolism that affects the body's ability to metabolize galactose.

9. Ans. (a) GM1 ganglioside

Ref: Lehninger Principles of Biochemistry, 4th ed. pg. 262

Cholera is caused by cholera toxin produced by *Vibrio cholerae*, when taken up by cells in the intestine, the toxin causes diarrhea, and the ganglioside GM1 (a glycolipid) has long been considered the main receptor for cholera toxin.

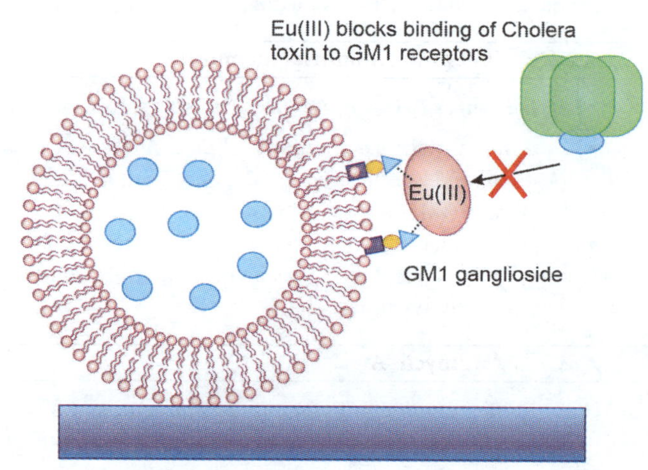

10. Ans. (c) Oxaloacetate

Ref: Lehninger Principles of Biochemistry, 4th ed. pg. 518

Aspartate transaminase catalyzes the **interconversion of aspartate and α-ketoglutarate to oxaloacetate and glutamate**. As a prototypical transaminase, AST relies on PLP (vitamin B_6) as a cofactor to transfer the amino group from aspartate or glutamate to the corresponding ketoacid.

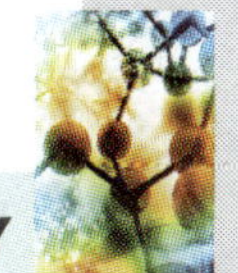

TCA cycle:

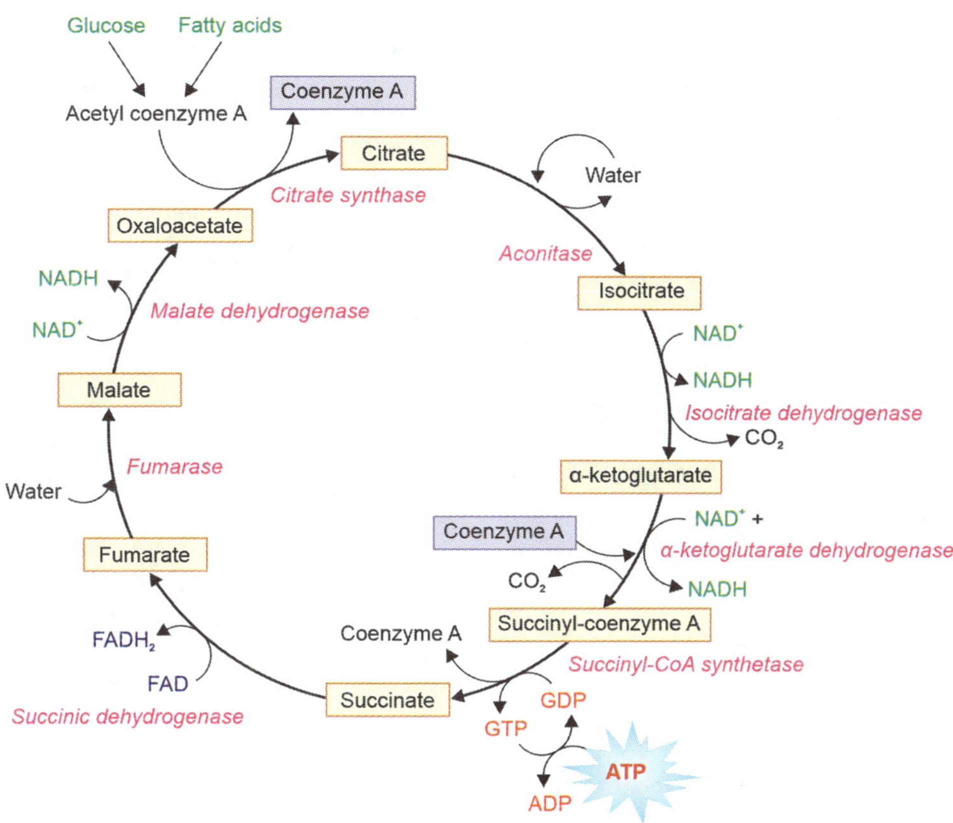

11. Ans. (a) Glycolysis

Ref: Harper's Illustrated Biochemistry, 31st ed. pg. 157

- Glycolysis is a metabolic pathway that occurs in the cytoplasm of cells.
- It is the initial step in the breakdown of glucose and involves a series of enzymatic reactions.
- During glycolysis, glucose is converted into pyruvate, and in the process, ATP and NADH are generated.
- Glycolysis is an ancient and highly conserved pathway that occurs in all living organisms. It is the main source of energy production in anaerobic conditions and serves as a precursor for other metabolic pathways.
- The other options, b. Beta-oxidation, c. TCA, and d. Urea cycle, occur in the mitochondria and are involved in the metabolism of fatty acids, citric acid cycle, and urea synthesis, respectively.

12. Ans. (b) Calcium

Ref: DM Vasudevan's Textbook of Biochemistry for Medical Students, 7th ed. pg. 502

- Calcium is not considered a microelement because it is required in larger amounts and is classified as a macromineral.
- Calcium plays a vital role in various physiological processes, including bone formation, muscle contraction, nerve transmission, and blood clotting.

13. Ans. (a) Tyrosine

Ref: Harper's Illustrated Biochemistry, 31st ed. pg. 300

- Melanin, the pigment responsible for skin, hair, and eye color, is synthesized from the amino acid tyrosine.
- Tyrosine undergoes enzymatic reactions, including the action of tyrosinase, to form melanin.

Extra Mile

- **Tryptophan** is an essential amino acid involved in the synthesis of various molecules, including neurotransmitters like serotonin and melatonin. However, it is not directly involved in melanin synthesis.
- **Leucine** is an essential amino acid involved in protein synthesis and regulation of muscle metabolism.
- **Phenylalanine** is an essential amino acid and a precursor for the synthesis of tyrosine. While it is indirectly linked to melanin synthesis through the conversion to tyrosine, it is not directly involved in melanin synthesis.

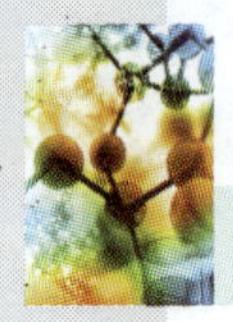

14. Ans. (a) Glucose-6-phosphatase

Ref: Harper's Illustrated Biochemistry, 31st ed. pg. 186

- Von Gierke's disease, also known as Glycogen storage disease type Ia, is caused by a deficiency of the enzyme glucose-6-phosphatase.
- This enzyme plays a critical role in glucose metabolism by catalyzing the conversion of glucose-6-phosphate to glucose, allowing glucose to be released from the liver and maintain blood glucose levels.

Note: *Other glycogen storage diseases are discussed later in this subject.*

Other options:

- **Debranching enzyme** is deficient in Glycogen storage disease type III—Cori disease.
- **Branching enzyme** is deficient in Glycogen storage disease type IV—Andersen disease.
- **Myophosphorylase** is deficient in Glycogen storage disease type V—McArdle disease.

15. Ans. (b) Ascorbic acid

Ref: Harper's Illustrated Biochemistry, 31st ed. 595

- Ascorbic acid, also known as vitamin C, plays a crucial role in collagen maturation.
- It is involved in the hydroxylation of proline and lysine residues in the collagen molecule, which is essential for the formation of stable collagen triple helices.
- Deficiency of ascorbic acid leads to impaired collagen synthesis and results in a condition known as scurvy.

16. Ans. (c) Arginine

Ref: Harper's Illustrated Biochemistry, 31st ed. pg. 297

- Nitric oxide (NO) is synthesized from the amino acid arginine by the enzyme nitric oxide synthase (NOS).
- Arginine is converted into citrulline and NO in a process known as the arginine-NO pathway.
- Nitric oxide plays a crucial role in regulating blood vessel dilation, neurotransmission, and immune response.

Extra Mile

- **Tryptophan** is an essential amino acid involved in the synthesis of various molecules, including neurotransmitters like serotonin and melatonin.
- **Leucine** is an essential amino acid involved in protein synthesis and regulation of muscle metabolism.
- **Lysine** is an essential amino acid involved in protein synthesis and plays a role in collagen formation.

17. Ans. (a) Galactosemia

Ref: Harper's Illustrated Biochemistry, 31st ed. pg. 189

- Galactosemia is a metabolic disorder characterized by the inability to metabolize galactose, a sugar found in milk.
- Infants with galactosemia lack the enzyme galactose-1-phosphate uridylyltransferase (GALT) needed to convert galactose into glucose.
- Therefore, breastfeeding is contraindicated in infants with galactosemia because their bodies cannot process the galactose present in breast milk.

18. Ans. (b) Substitution of glutamic acid (Glu) by valine (Val) at the 6th position

Ref: Harper's Illustrated Biochemistry, 31st ed. pg. 536

- Sickle cell anemia is caused by a point mutation in the gene encoding the beta-globin chain of hemoglobin.
- In this mutation, the nucleotide sequence is altered, leading to the substitution of glutamic acid (Glu) with valine (Val) at the 6th position of the beta-globin chain.
- This amino acid substitution results in the production of abnormal hemoglobin (HbS), which causes red blood cells to become sickle-shaped and less flexible.

19. Ans. (b) Niacin

Ref: Harper's Illustrated Biochemistry, 31st ed. pg. 534

- The patient's symptoms of diarrhea, dementia, and photosensitive dermatitis are indicative of pellagra, which is caused by niacin (vitamin B_3) deficiency.
- Niacin plays a crucial role in energy metabolism and the maintenance of healthy skin, digestive system, and nervous system.
- Deficiency of niacin can lead to various symptoms, including the ones observed in the patient.

Extra Mile

- **Vitamin B_6 deficiency** primarily manifests as neurological symptoms such as peripheral neuropathy and dermatitis is not commonly associated with B_6 deficiency.
- **Vitamin C deficiency** leads to scurvy, which is characterized by symptoms such as bleeding gums, joint pain, and fatigue.
- **Biotin deficiency** can lead to symptoms such as hair loss, dermatitis, and neurological manifestations. However, the specific symptoms of diarrhea, dementia, and photosensitive dermatitis are more consistent with niacin deficiency.

20. Ans. (a) Xerophthalmia

Ref: Harper's Illustrated Biochemistry, 31st ed. pg. 534

- Vitamin A deficiency can lead to a condition called xerophthalmia, which is characterized by dryness, inflammation, and night blindness of the eyes.
- Vitamin A plays a crucial role in maintaining healthy vision, and its deficiency can cause various eye-related problems.

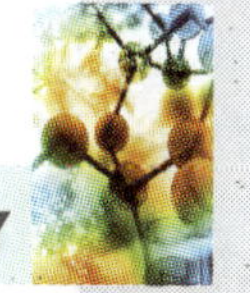

Extra Mile

- **Beri Beri** is caused by thiamine (vitamin B_1) deficiency and is associated with symptoms such as neurological issues, muscle weakness, and heart problems.
- **Pellagra** is caused by niacin (vitamin B_3) deficiency and is characterized by symptoms such as dermatitis, diarrhea, and dementia.
- **Neuropathy** refers to nerve damage and dysfunction, and it can be caused by various factors, including deficiencies of certain vitamins like B_{12}.

21. Ans. (a) RNA editing

Ref: Harper's Illustrated Biochemistry, 31st ed. pg. 238

- The differential translation of the apoB gene in the liver and intestine is achieved through a process called RNA editing.
- RNA editing involves the post-transcriptional modification of mRNA by inserting or deleting nucleotides, which alters the coding sequence.
- In the case of apoB mRNA, a Cytidine (C) to Uridine (U) deamination reaction occurs, converting a specific cytidine residue to uridine, leading to the creation of a premature stop codon in the intestine.
- This results in the synthesis of a shorter form of apoB, known as apoB48.

Extra Mile

- **Gene splicing** refers to the process of removing introns and joining exons together during mRNA processing.
- **Alternative polyadenylation** is a mechanism where different polyadenylation sites are used to generate distinct mRNA isoforms.
- **Gene rearrangements** involve the rearrangement of genetic material, such as gene segments, during processes like DNA recombination.

CARBOHYDRATE

22. Ans. (a) Cyanide

Ref: Lippincott's Illustrated Reviews, 6th ed. pg. 166

- Cyanide has been long recognized as an inhibitor of mitochondrial electron transport due to its binding to the heme prosthetic group in Complex IV.
- The shutdown of aerobic ATP generation is recognized as the primary mode of cyanide's cytotoxic action in eukaryotes.
- Cyanide binds to Fe^{3+} in heme-containing proteins. This inhibits the terminal cytochrome complex IV of the electron transport chain. The block of complex IV by cyanide depletes ATP culminating in cell death.

23. Ans. (a) Increase in insulin level and decrease in glucagon level

Ref: Lippincott's Illustrated Reviews, 6th ed. pg. 453

High insulin to low glucagon ratio occurs in the fed state activating anabolic pathways, such as storage of glucose and fatty acids as triglycerides.

24. Ans. (d) Glycolysis

Ref: Lippincott's Illustrated Reviews, 6th ed. pg. 441

- Glucagon turns off glycolysis in the liver, causing glycolytic intermediates to be shuttled to gluconeogenesis.
- Glucagon also regulates the rate of glucose production through lipolysis. Glucagon induces lipolysis in humans under conditions of insulin suppression (such as diabetes mellitus type 1).

25. Ans. (a) Mitochondria

Ref: Lippincott's Illustrated Reviews, 6th ed. pg. 170

Thermogenin or uncoupling protein (UCP) is a 33kDa dimeric protein found in the inner mitochondrial membrane of brown adipose tissue which supplies heat by allowing the dissipation of the proton gradient without ATP synthesis.

26. Ans. (d) Gluco cerebrosidase

Ref: Lippincott's Illustrated Reviews, 6th ed. pg. 332

Gaucher's disease is one of the most common lysosomal storage diseases, in which deficiency of the enzyme **glucocerebrosidase (Beta-glucosidase)** results in the accumulation of harmful quantities of certain fats (lipids), specifically the glycolipid glucocerebroside, throughout the body especially within the bone marrow, spleen and liver.

27. Ans. (b) Kwashiorkor

Ref: Lippincott's Illustrated Reviews, 6th ed. pg. 510

- Kwashiorkor, also known as "edematous malnutrition" because of its association with edema (fluid retention), is a nutritional disorder most often seen in regions experiencing famine.
- It is a form of protein energy malnutrition caused by a lack of protein in the diet or excessive dietary intake of carbohydrates "sugar babies."
- In these children edema results from lack of adequate blood proteins, primarily albumin. Hence, they have a general, **fat sugar baby** appearance.

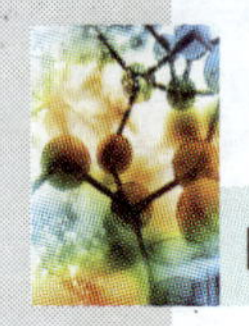

28. Ans. (c) Megaloblastic anemia

Ref: Lippincott's Illustrated Reviews, 6th ed. pg. 526

- Megaloblastic anemia is **a condition in which the bone marrow produces unusually large, structurally abnormal, immature red blood cells** (megaloblasts). The most common causes of megaloblastic anemia are deficiency of either **cobalamin (vitamin B_{12}) or folate (vitamin B_9).**
- Vitamin B_{12} is synthesized only by microorganism, and it is not present in plants/plant sources. It is present in appreciable amounts in liver, red meat, fish, eggs, dairy products.
- Nutritional deficiency of vitamin B_{12} is common in vegetarians who do not take milk or milk products, non-vegetarian foods or consume only vegetarian sources of this vitamin. Hence, megaloblastic anemia is commonly seen in vegetarians.

29. Ans. (a) GALT - (galactose 1 phosphate uridyl transferase)

Ref: Lippincott's Illustrated Reviews, 6th ed. pg. 244

- Galactosemia is a disorder that affects how the body processes a simple sugar called galactose.
- Classical galactosemia occurs due to GALT - (galactose 1 phosphate uridyl transferase enzyme deficiency. It is an autosomal recessive disorder.
- There is accumulation of galactose 1-phosphate and galacititol in the liver, brain, and eyes causing liver damage, brain damage and cataracts.

30. Ans. (c) Lysosome

Ref: Lippincott's Illustrated Reviews, 6th ed. pg. 12

- Lysosomes are spherical vesicles that contain hydrolytic enzymes that are involved in breakdown of biomolecules-carbohydrates, lipids, proteins and nucleic acids.
- Lysosomes are abundantly present in macrophages. They can breakdown bacteria and other microorganisms following the phagocytosis of these particles.

31. Ans. (a) Hexosaminidase A

Ref: Lippincott's Biochemistry, 6th ed. pg. 875

- Tay-Sachs disease is a genetic disorder (autosomal recessive) characterized by destruction of nerve cells in brain and spinal cord.
- It is caused by mutation in the HEXA gene on chromosome 15, which codes for a subunit of the hexosaminidase enzyme known as hexosaminidase A.

32. Ans. (a) Glucose-6-phosphatase

Ref: Lippincott's Illustrated Reviews, Biochemistry 7th ed. pg. 134-35

- Von Gierke disease is an inherited disease that results in the liver being unable to properly break down stored glycogen. This impairment disrupts the liver's ability to break down stored glycogen that is necessary to maintain adequate blood sugar levels.
- **It is caused by a deficiency in the enzyme glucose-6-phosphatase.**
- Since glycogenolysis is the principal metabolic mechanism by which the liver supplies glucose to the body during periods of fasting, deficiencies cause severe low blood sugar and, over time, excess glycogen storage in the liver and (in some cases) the kidneys.
- The principal metabolic effects of deficiency of glucose-6-phosphatase are hypoglycemia, lactic acidosis, hypertriglyceridemia, and hyperuricemia.

33. Ans. (b) Insulin

Ref: Lippincott's Illustrated Reviews, Biochemistry 7th ed. pg. 311

- Insulin promotes glucose storage mostly in three tissues-liver, muscle and adipose tissues.
- Decreased gluconeogenesis and glycogenolysis, decreases production of glucose from non-carbohydrate substrates, primarily in the liver (the vast majority of endogenous insulin arriving at the liver never leaves the liver); decrease of insulin causes glucose production by the liver from assorted substrates.

TABLE: Inducer and inhibitor of gluconeogenesis

Activators/inducers	Inhibitors/repressors
Glucagon	Insulin
Acetyl CoA	AMP
Citrate	Fasting state/hypoglycemia
ATP	Diabetes
Glycogenic amino acids	Carbohydrate feeding
Cortisol	

34. Ans. (b) Reduces intestinal transit time

Ref: Lippincott's Illustrated Reviews, Biochemistry 7th ed. pg. 365

- Dietary fiber increases food volume without increasing caloric content to the same extent as digestible carbohydrates, providing satiety appetite.
- It also:
  - Lowers total and LDL cholesterol, which may reduce the risk of cardiovascular diseases.

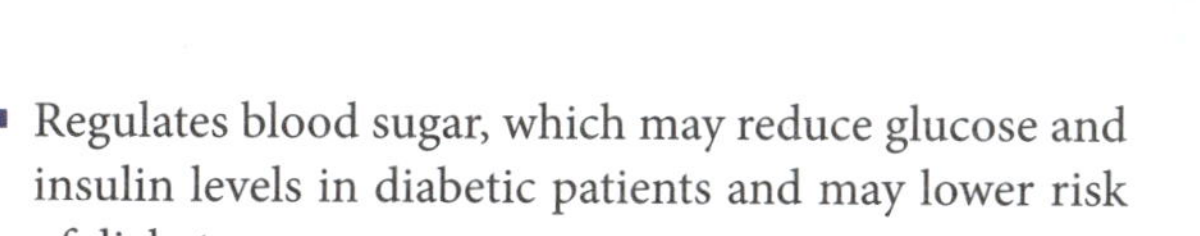

- Regulates blood sugar, which may reduce glucose and insulin levels in diabetic patients and may lower risk of diabetes.
- Speeds the passage of foods through the digestive system, which facilitates regular defecation.
- Adds bulk to the stool, which alleviates constipation and Balances intestinal pH and stimulates intestinal fermentation production of short-chain fatty acids

35. Ans. (b) GLUT 4

TABLE: GLUT receptors, their location and function

Receptor	Location on tissue	Function
GLUT 1	Brain, kidney, colon, placenta, RBC	Glucose uptake
GLUT 2	Liver, pancreatic beta cell, small intestine, Kidney	Rapid uptake or release of glucose
GLUT 3	Brain, kidney and placenta	Glucose uptake
GLUT 4	Heart, skeletal muscles, adipose tissue	Insulin-stimulated glucose uptake
GLUT 5	Small intestine	Absorption of fructose
GLUT 6	Spleen	—
GLUT 7	Liver, Endoplasmic reticulum	Glucose transport in endoplasmic reticulum

36. Ans. (a) 2,4 dinitrophenol

- Compounds that can uncouple or delink the ETC from oxidative phosphorylation, such compounds are known as uncouplers
- As a result ATP synthesis doesn't occur.
- 2,4 Dinitrophenol is an example of chemical uncoupler.

Chemical uncouplers	Physiological uncouplers
• 2, 4 dinitrophenol (has been extensively studied)	• Thyroid hormones • UCP-1
• Dinitrocresol	• Long chain fatty acids
• Pentachlorophenol	• Unconjugated bilirubin
• Tri fluoro carbonyl cyanide phenyl hydra zone (FCCP)	• These act as uncouplers only at high concentration
• Aspirin (high doses)	

37. Ans. (a) Pyruvate dehydrogenase

- The enzyme Pyruvate dehydrogenase irreversibly converts pyruvate, the end product of glycolysis, into acetyl CoA, a major fuel for the TCA cycle and the building block for fatty acid synthesis
- Thus, this enzyme pyruvate dehydrogenase is utilized in citric acid cycle and fatty acid synthesis.
- The reaction of pyruvate dehydrogenase, forming acetyl-CoA, is irreversible, and for every two carbon unit from acetyl-CoA that enters the citric acid cycle, there is a loss of two carbon atoms as carbon dioxide before oxaloacetate is reformed.
- This means that acetyl-CoA (and hence, any substrates that yield acetyl-CoA) can never be used for gluconeogenesis.

38. Ans. (c) Mitochondria and cytoplasm

Ref: Harper's Biochemistry, 30th ed. pg. 294-95

Urea Cycle

- Urea is the end product of nitrogen catabolism in humans
- It takes place in both mitochondria and cytoplasm
- Some reactions of urea synthesis occur in the matrix of the mitochondrion, other reactions in the cytosol
- Synthesis of 1 mol of urea requires 3 mol of ATP plus 1 mol each of ammonium ion and of the amino nitrogen of aspartate.
- **Undergoes 5 steps in urea synthesis:**
  - Steps 1 and 2 take place in mitochondria
  - Steps 3, 4 , 5 take place in cytosol

For more details please refer to mother book explanation 121

39. Ans. (d) Unconjugated bilirubin

- Uncouplers inhibit oxidative phosphorylation. They are hydrophobic molecules with a dissociable protein.
- They uncouple the ETC form oxidative phosphorylation
- Physiological uncouplers acts only at high dose.

Chemical Uncouplers	Physiological Uncouplers
• y 2,4-dinitrophenol (has been extensively studied). • Dinitrocresol • Pentachlorophenol • Tri fluoro carbonyl cyanide phenylhydrazone (FCCP). • Aspirin (high doses)	• Thyroid hormones. • UCP-1/thermogenin • Long chain fatty acids. • Unconjugated Bilirubin. These act as Uncouplers only at high concentration

Extra Mile

Inhibitors of Electron Transport Chain

Inhibitors of Oxidative Phosphorylation

- **Complex I:** **Rotenone**
- **Complex II:** Carboxin
- **Complex III:** Antimycin A
- **Complex IV:** H_2S, Cyanide, Azide, Carbon monoxide
- **ATP synthase:** Oligomycin
- **ATP-ADP translocase:** Atractyloside (a plant glycoside)

40. Ans. (b) Liver

Ref: Vasudevan Biochemistry 8th ed. pg. 136

SITE OF GLUCONEOGENESIS

- **Major site of gluconeogenesis:** Liver (90%)
- **Secondary site:** Kidney cortex and in small intestine under some conditions (10%).
- It takes place in the mitochondria and cytoplasm.
- The production of glucose is necessary for use as a fuel source by the brain, testes, erythrocytes, kidney medulla, lens and cornea of the eye and exercising muscles.

41. Ans. (b) Hemolytic anemia

Ref: Vasudevan Biochemistry, 8th ed. pg. 426

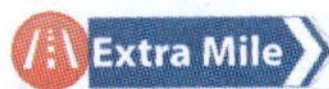

- G6PD deficiency causes hemolytic anemia, since RBCs become susceptible to oxidative stress

Other causes of hemolytic anemias are:

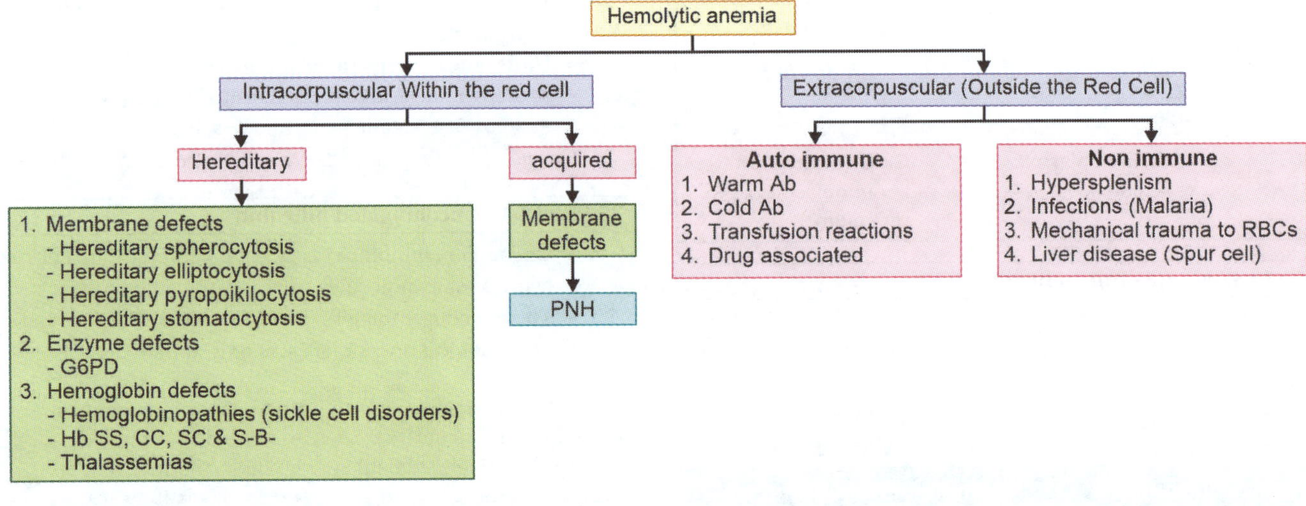

42. Ans. (c) Fructokinase

Ref: Harper, pg. 169

*"Deficiencies in the enzymes of fructose and galactose metabolism lead to **essential fructosuria** and **galactosemias.**"*

*"Lack of hepatic fructokinase causes **essential fructosuria,** and absence of hepatic aldolase B, which cleaves fructose 1-phosphate, leads to **hereditary fructose intolerance.**"*

Metabolism of fructose. Aldolase A is found in all tissues, whereas aldolase B is the predominant form in liver. (*, not found in liver)

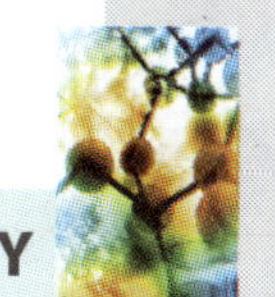

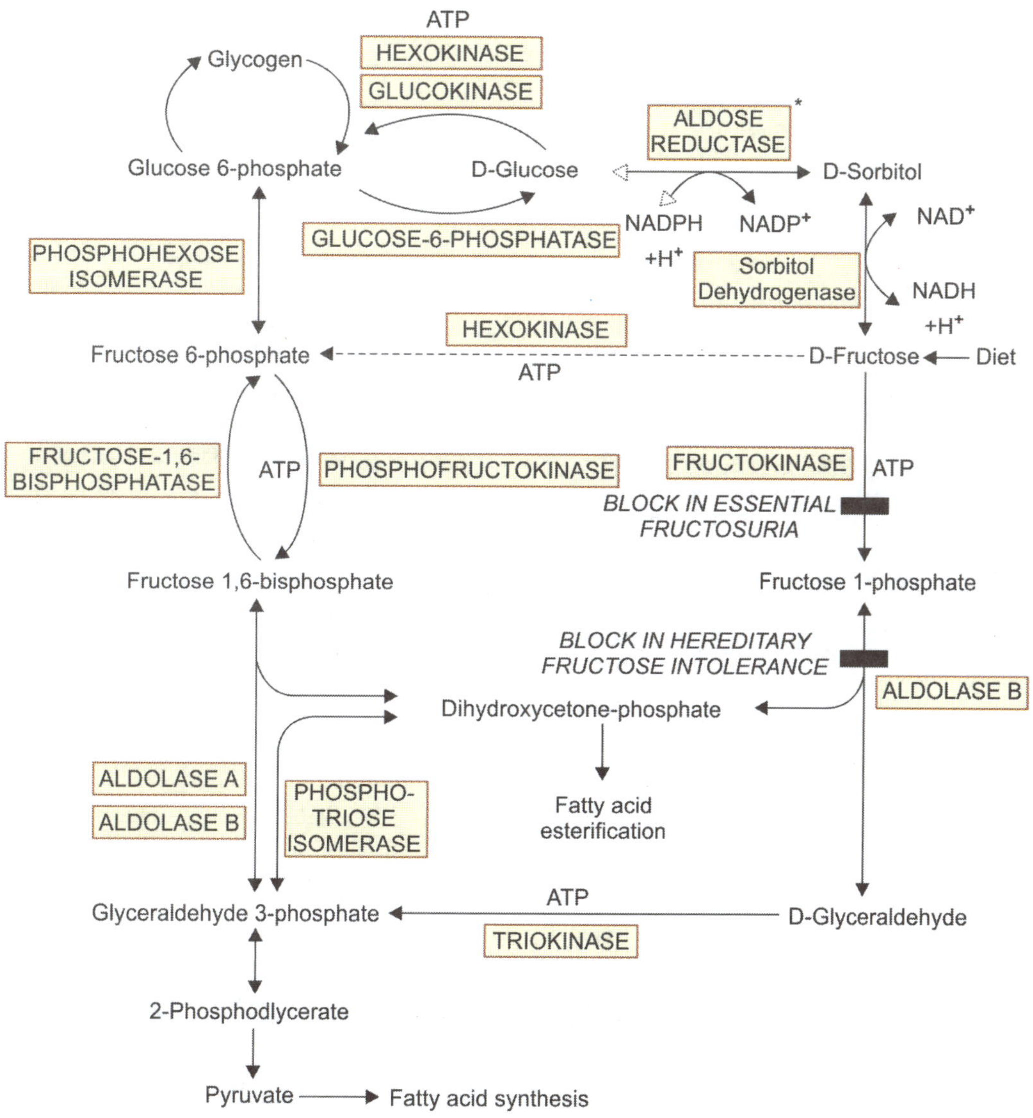

ATP
HEXOKINASE
GLUCOKINASE
Glycogen
ALDOSE REDUCTASE *
Glucose 6-phosphate
D-Glucose
D-Sorbitol
NADPH +H^+
$NADP^+$
NAD^+
GLUCOSE-6-PHOSPHATASE
Sorbitol Dehydrogenase
NADH +H^+
PHOSPHOHEXOSE ISOMERASE
HEXOKINASE
Fructose 6-phosphate
ATP
D-Fructose
Diet
FRUCTOSE-1,6-BISPHOSPHATASE
ATP
PHOSPHOFRUCTOKINASE
FRUCTOKINASE
ATP
BLOCK IN ESSENTIAL FRUCTOSURIA
Fructose 1,6-bisphosphate
Fructose 1-phosphate
BLOCK IN HEREDITARY FRUCTOSE INTOLERANCE
ALDOLASE B
Dihydroxycetone-phosphate
ALDOLASE A
ALDOLASE B
PHOSPHO-TRIOSE ISOMERASE
Fatty acid esterification
ATP
Glyceraldehyde 3-phosphate
D-Glyceraldehyde
TRIOKINASE
2-Phosphodlycerate
Pyruvate
Fatty acid synthesis

43. Ans. (a) McArdle's disease

Ref: Harper's Biochemistry, pg. 145

- **Glycogen storage diseases** are a group of inherited disorders characterized by deficient mobilization of glycogen or deposition of abnormal forms of glycogen, leading to muscular weakness or even death.
- **Nelson 20th ed states:** *"Approximately 50% patients with GSD type V, report burgundy colored urine after exercise, which is a consequence of exercise-induced myoglobinuria secondary to rhabdomyolysis"*

44. Ans. (c) Enolase

Ref: Harper's Biochemistry, 30th ed. pg. 170-171

Reversible steps of glycolysis are catalyzed by	Irreversible steps of glycolysis are catalyzed by
• Phosphohexose isomerase • Aldolase • Phosphotriose isomerase • Glyceraldehyde 3-phosphate dehydrogenase • Phosphoglycerate kinase • Phosphoglycerate mutase • **Enolase**	• Glucokinase/Hexokinase • Phosphofructokinase-I • Pyruvate kinase

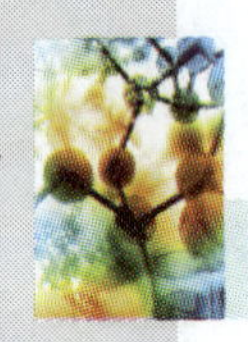

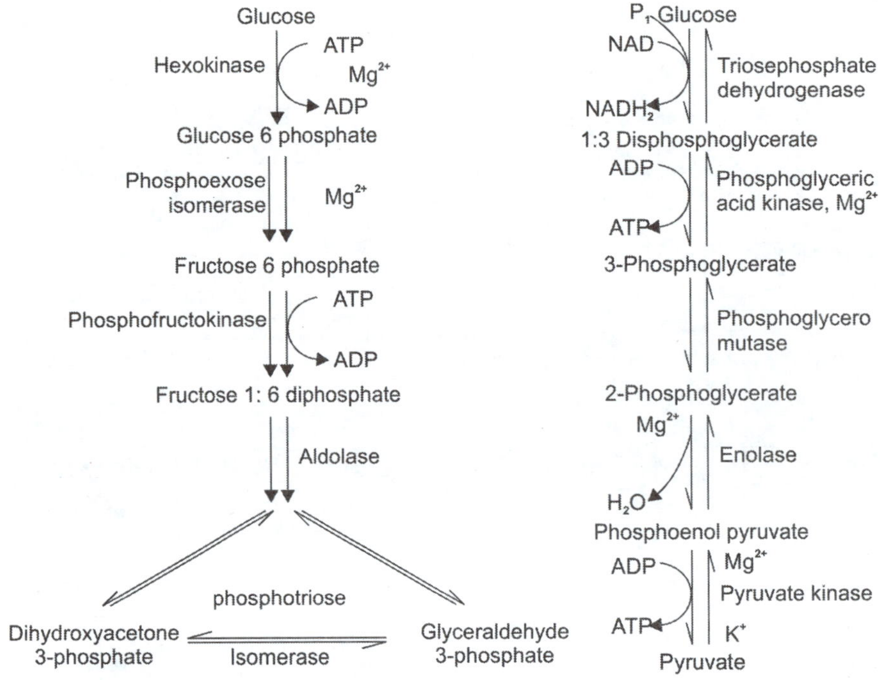

45. Ans. (a) 10

Ref: Harper's Biochemistry, 30th ed. pg. 169-170

- In glycolytic pathway, one molecule of glucose gives 2 pyruvate.
- The 2 molecules of pyruvate are further metabolized in citric acid cycle, giving out 20 ATP.
- Since, the question here is asking about one molecule of pyruvate, the answer will be the half of 20, i.e., 10.
- **In simple words:** 2 molecules of pyruvate give 20 ATP. Hence, one molecule will give 10 ATP.

Step	Coenzyme yield	ATP	Source of ATP
Glycolysis preparatory phase		−2	Phosphorylation of glucose and fructose 6-phosphate uses two ATP from the cytoplasm
Glycolysis pay-off phase		4	Substrate-level phosphorylation
	2 NADH *(2 x 2.5)*	5	Oxidative phosphorylation-Each NADH produces net 2 ATP due to NADH transport over the mitochondrial membrane
Oxidative decarboxylation of pyruvate	2 NADH *(2 x 2.5)*	5	Oxidative phosphorylation
NET ATP TILL PHOSPHORYLATION OF PYRUVATE: 5 + 5 + 4 = 14 − 2 = **12**		= 12	
Krebs cycle		2	**Substrate-level phosphorylation**
	6 NADH *(6 x 2.5)*	15	Oxidative phosphorylation
	2 FADH2 *(2 x 1.5)*	3	Oxidative phosphorylation
Total yield		**32 ATP**	From the complete oxidation of one glucose molecule to carbon dioxide and oxidation of all the reduced coenzymes.

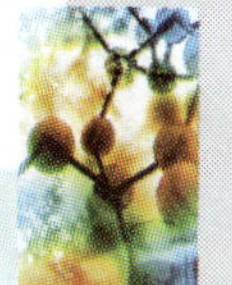

- Net generation of ATP in glycolytic pathway: 9–2 = **7**
  Oxidative phosphorylation of pyruvate: **5**
- Generation of ATP during Citric acid cycle: **20**
- Net generation of ATP from one glucose molecule = **32**

46. Ans. (b) Pyruvate kinase

Ref: Harper's Biochemistry, 30th ed. pg. 169, 171

- **Substrate-level phosphorylation** is *a type of metabolism that results in the formation and creation of adenosine triphosphate (ATP) or guanosine triphosphate (GTP) by the direct transfer and donation of a phosphoryl (PO_3) group to adenosine diphosphate (ADP) or guanosine diphosphate (GDP) from a phosphorylated reactive intermediate.*
- Note that the phosphate group does not have to directly come from the substrate. By convention, the phosphoryl group that is transferred is referred to as a phosphate group.
- We use the term substrate level phosphorylation because ATP formation in glycolysis is powered by the addition/removal of phosphate groups (phosphorylation) to molecules of glucose (the substrate). Hence the term substrate-level phosphorylation.

Extra Mile

Some Important Pathways and their Rate Limiting Enzyme

Pathway	Rate limiting enzyme
• Glycolysis	Phosphofructo kinase-1
• Glycogenesis	Glycogen synthase
• Glycogenolysis	Phosphorylase
• Cholesterol synthesis	*HMG - COA Reductase*
• Ketone body formation	*HMG - COA synthase*
• Bile acid synthesis	7α-hydroxylase
• Fatty acid synthesis	Acetyl COA carboxylase
• Uric acid synthesis	Xanthine oxidase

Examples of Substrate Level Phosphorylation that Occurs

- **The production of 1st ATP** when 1,3 bisphophoglycerate is converted into 3 phosphoglycerate by the enzyme **phosphoglycerate kinase**
- **Production of 2nd ATP** when phosphoenolpyruvate is converted to pyruvate by the enzyme **pyruvate kinase.**

47. Ans. (d) Muscles

Ref: Harper's Biochemistry, 30th ed. pg. 187

- *The conversion of glucose 6-phosphate to glucose is catalyzed by glucose 6-phosphatase is present in liver and kidney,* ***but absent from muscle and adipose tissue, which cannot export glucose into the bloodstream.*** Therefore in order to use muscle glycogen and lactate for gluconeogenesis two separate processes arepresent in body. They are:
  - **Cori's cycle:** Lactate, formed by glycolysis in skeletal muscle and transported to the liver and kidney where it reforms glucose, which again is available via the circulation for oxidation in the tissues.
    - **Glucose alanine cycle:** In the fasting state, there is a considerable output of all skeletal muscle, far in excess of its concentration in the muscle proteins that is catabolized. It is formed by transamination of pyruvate produced by glycolysis and glycogen, and is exported to the liver, where, after transamination back is a substrate for gluconeogenesis. This glucose-alanine cycle thus provides an indirect way of utilizing muscle glycogen to maintain blood glucose in the fasting state.

48. Ans. (a) Cori cycle

Ref: Harper's Biochemistry, 30th ed. pg. 190-191

The Cori cycle is the only one that is not dependent on the mitochondrial enzymes. This cycle is basically the transport of lactate from the muscle to the liver to be converted via gluconeogenesis to glucose to be transported back to the muscle.

Extra Mile

Mitochondria Mn: KEBOK in all cap	Cytoplasm	Both mitochondria and cytoplasm (Mn: Primary HUG for both)
• Kreb cycle • ETC • Bet oxidation of FA • Oxidative phosphorylation • Ketogenesis	• Glycolysis • Glycogenesis • Glycogenolysis • HMP Shunt • FA synthesis • Cholesterol synthesis • Bile acid/Salt synthesis	• Gluconeogenesis • Urea synthesis • Heme synthesis • Pyrimidine synthesis

49. Ans. (b) Liver

Ref: Harper's Biochemistry, 30th ed. pg. 190-191

- Each day the body has an excess production of about 1500 mmols of lactate (about 20 mmols/kg/day) *which enters the blood stream and is subsequently* ***metabolised mostly in the liver.***
- All tissues can produce lactate under anaerobic conditions but tissues with active glycolysis produce excess lactate from glucose under normal conditions

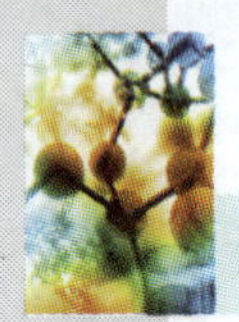

and this lactate tends to spill over into the blood. Lactate is produced from pyruvate in a reaction catalysed by lactate dehydrogenase:

Pyruvate + NADH + H^+<=> Lactate + NAD^+

50. Ans. (d) EMP pathway

51. Ans. (d) Hexokinase

- **These are the enzymes of glycolysis whose action is increased by insulin (regulates positively):**
  - Glucokinase
  - Phosphofructokinase
  - Pyruvate kinase
- **Note:** Insulin doesn't regulate Hexokinase

52. Ans. (c) Skeletal muscles

Ref: Harper's Biochemistry, 30th ed. pg. 191-192

- **Insulin** increases the number and activity of GLUT 4 receptor. Thereby facilitating the entry of glucose in tissues having GLUT4 receptor.
- **Tissues with abundant GLUT4 receptor are: *Skeletal muscles, Heart and Adipose tissue***
- Thus, among the given choices, skeletal muscle is the one which required for entry of glucose.

Extra Mile

TABLE: GLUT receptors, their location and function

Receptor	Location on tissue	Function
GLUT 1	Brain, kidney, colon, placenta, RBC, retina	Glucose uptake
GLUT 2	Liver, pancreatic beta cell, small intestine, Kidney	Rapid uptake or release of glucose
GLUT 3	Brain, kidney and placenta	Glucose uptake
GLUT 4	Heart, skeletal muscles, adipose tissue	Insulin-stimulated glucose uptake
GLUT 5	Small intestine	Absorption of fructose
GLUT 6	Spleen, leukocyte	—
GLUT 7	Liver, endoplasmic reticulum	Glucose transporter in endoplasmic reticulum

53. Ans. (a) Glycolysis

Ref: Harper's Biochemistry, 30th ed. pg. 142-144

- **Glycolysis occurs in cytoplasm.**
- ***There are two major sites for gluconeogenesis, the liver and the kidneys.***
- The liver accounts for 90% of gluconeogenesis in the body and the remaining 10% occur in the kidney and other tissues of the body.
- The liver and kidneys maintain the glucose level in the blood so that the brain, muscle and red blood cells have sufficient glucose to meet their metabolic demands.

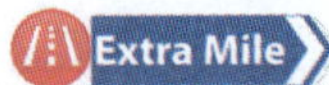

Extra Mile

Cycle occurs in both cytoplasm and mitochondria-
- Gluconeogenesis
- Urea cycle
- Heme synthesis

54. Ans. (b) Gluconeogenesis

Ref: Harper's Biochemistry, 30th ed. pg. 142-144

Please refer to above explanation

55. Ans. (a) Insulin

Ref: Harper's Biochemistry, 30th ed. pg. 191-192

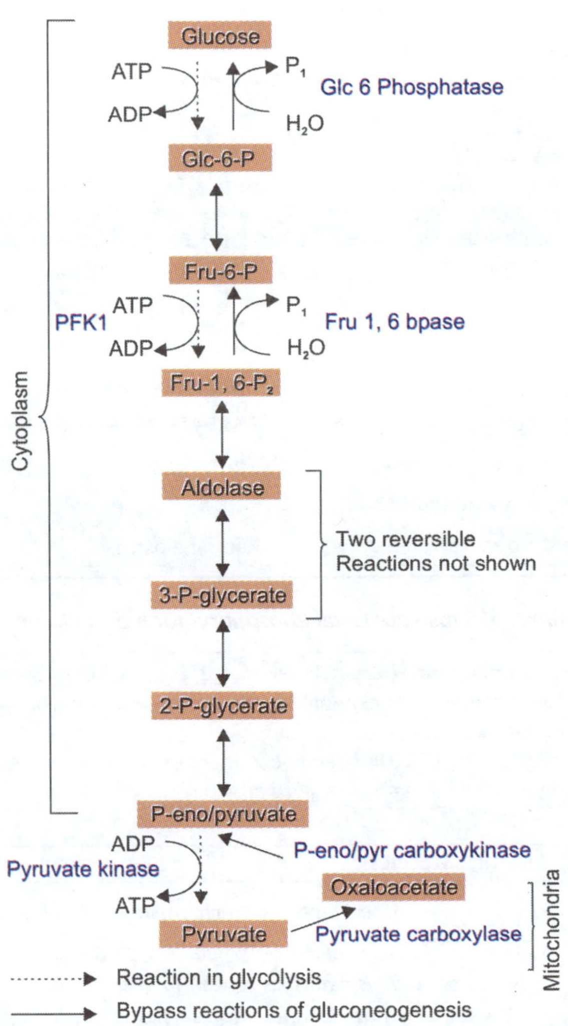

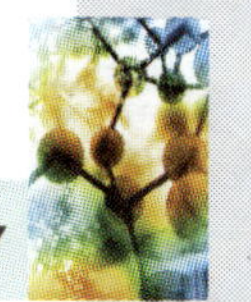

- Synthesis of glucose from non-carbohydrate source is called Gluconeogenesis.

Hormonal Regulation

↑ Glucagon, epinephrine, glucocorticoids.
↓ Insulin

- **Gluconeogenesis is regulated by 4 key enzymes:**
  - Pyruvate carboxylase
  - Phosphoenolpyruvate carboxylase
  - F16 bisphosphatase
  - G-6-phosphatase

56. Ans. (b) Malate shuttle

Ref: Harper's Biochemistry, 30th ed. pg. 134-135

- There are certain shuttle systems that operate for transport of reducing equivalents from cytosol into mitochondria. These shuttle systems operate because mitochondrial membrane is impermeable to cytosolic NADH produced during glycolysis. In order to gain entry of NADH into mitochondrial electron transport chain, these shuttle systems are helpful.
- **Malate shuttle (aka malate-aspartate shuttle):** It is most common and universal shuttle system. Mitochondrial NADH which gains entry from cytosol is oxidized by mitochondrial ETC, leading to formation of 2.5 molecules of ATP.
- **Glycerophosphate shuttle:** In this mechanism, cytosolic NADH is used to reduce dihydroxyacetone phosphate to glycerol-3 phosphate which diffuse through the outer mitochondrial membrane into the inter-membrane space of the mitochondria. In this space, glycerol 3-phosphate is reoxidized to dihydroxyacetone phosphate and the reducing equivalents are transferred to FAD to form $FADH_2$. $FADH_2$ is oxidized in ETC to form 1.5 molecules of ATP.

57. Ans. (c) Fructose

Ref: Harper's Biochemistry, 30th ed. pg. 205

Fructose —(Fructokinase; ATP → ADP)→ Fructose 1-phosphate —(Aldolase B)→ DHAP + Glyceraldehyde —(Triokinase; ATP → ADP)→ Glyceraldehyde 3-phosphate

- Hereditary fructose intolerance (HFI) is an inborn error of fructose metabolism caused by a deficiency of the enzyme aldolase-B.
- In the deficiency of Aldolase B enzyme, *if fructose is ingested, it will lead to an accumulation of fructose-1-phosphate.* This accumulation has downstream effects on gluconeogenesis and regeneration of ATP.
- **Symptoms of HFI include:** Vomiting, hypoglycemia, jaundice, hemorrhage, hepatomegaly, hyperuricemia and potentially kidney failure.
- **The key identifying feature of HFI:** *Appearance of symptoms with the introduction of fructose to the diet.*
- Sucrose, sorbitol should also be restricted in diet.

58. Ans. (d) Fructose-1, biphosphate

Ref: Harper's Biochemistry, 30th ed. pg. 202-203

- **Aldolase B** is preferentially expressed in the liver, while **aldolase A** is expressed in muscle and erythrocytes and **aldolase C** is expressed in the brain. Slight differences in isozyme structure result in different activities for the two substrate molecules: Fructose 1,6-Biphosphate and fructose 1-phosphate. *Aldolase B exhibits no preference and thus catalyzes both reactions, while aldolases A and C prefer FBP.*
- **Aldolase A** is an enzyme that catalyses a reversible aldol reaction: The substrate, fructose 1,6-bisphosphate (F-1,6-BP) is broken down into glyceraldehyde 3-phosphate and dihydroxyacetone phosphate (DHAP).
- Sucrose is composed of glucose and fructose and hence, cannot be tolerated by patients of HFI.

59. Ans. (d) Aldolase - B deficiency

Ref: Harper's Biochemistry, 30th ed. pg. 202-203

- **Hereditary fructose intolerance** is an in-born error of fructose metabolism caused by a deficiency of the enzyme aldolase B. Individuals affected with Hereditary fructose intolerance are asymptomatic until they ingest fructose. If fructose is ingested, the enzymatic block at aldolase B causes an accumulation of fructose-l-phosphate. This accumulation has downstream effect on gluconeogenesis and regeneration of adenosine triphosphate (ATP).
- **Symptoms:** Vomiting, hypoglycemia, jaundice, hemorrhage, hepatomegaly, hyperuricemia and potentially kidney failure.

60. Ans. (c) Lactate-dehydrogenase

Ref: Harper's Biochemistry 30th ed. pg. 171, 321

- Excess dietary fructose can be converted to pyruvate, this then enters the Krebs cycle and emerges as citrate directed toward free fatty acid synthesis in the cytosol of hepatocytes.

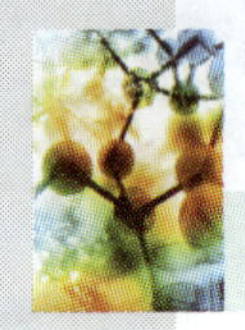

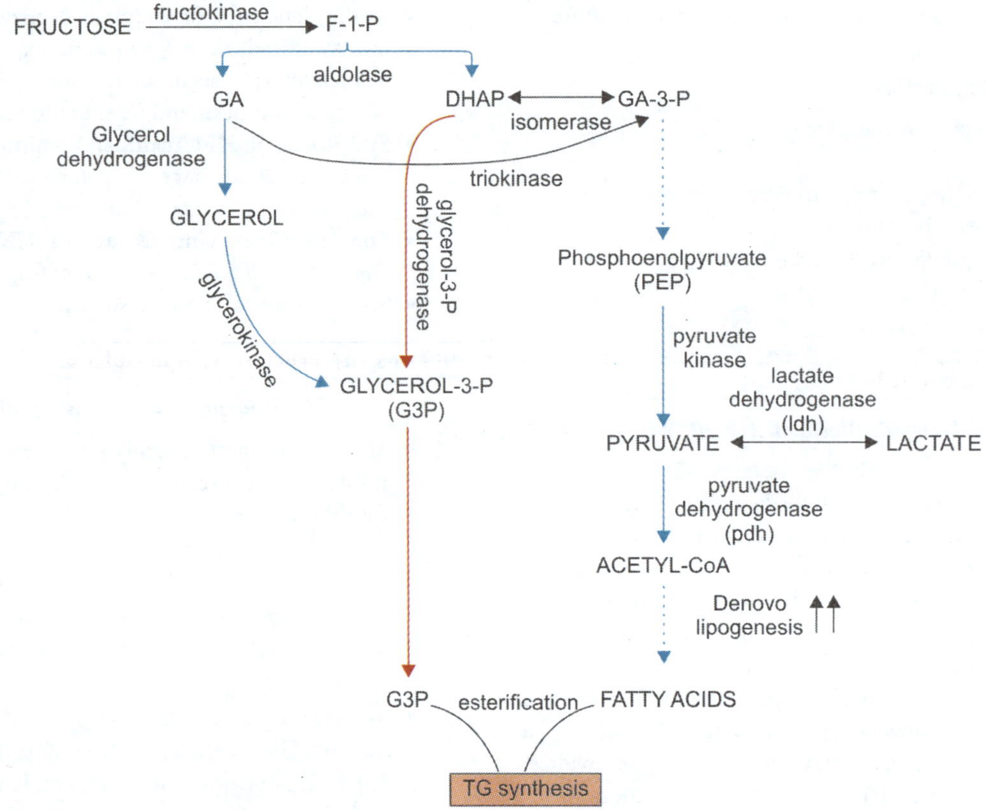

61. Ans. (b) Phase II reaction

Ref: Harper's Biochemistry, 30th ed. pg. 586

METABOLISM OF XENOBIOTICS

- **In phase 1,** the major reaction involved is hydroxylation, catalyzed by enzymes mono-oxygenases or cytochrome P450s. The reactions are:
  - **Hydroxylation**
  - Deamination
  - Dehalogenation
  - Desulfuration
  - Epoxidation
  - Peroxygenation
  - Reduction
- **In phase 2,** compounds produced in phase 1 are converted to various polar metabolites by conjugation with glucuronic acid, sulfate, acetate, glutathione, or certain amino acids, or by methylation.
- The overall purpose of the two phases of metabolism of xenobiotics is to increase their water solubility (polarity) and thus excretion from the body.
  Glucuronidation: UDP Glucuronic acid is the glucuronyl donor, and a variety of glucuronosyl transferases, present in both the endoplasmic reticulum and cytosol, are the catalysts.
- **Phase II reactions are:**
  - **Glucuronidation:** Is probably the most frequent conjugation reaction.
  - Sulfation
  - Conjugation with Glutathione
  - Acetylation
  - Methylation

62. Ans. (a) Cornea

Ref: Harper's Biochemistry, 30th ed. pg. 140

Glucagon receptors are mainly expressed in liver and in kidney with lesser amounts found in heart, adipose tissue, spleen, thymus, adrenal glands, pancreas, cerebral cortex, and gastrointestinal tract.

63. Ans. (a) Enolase

Ref: Harper's Biochemistry, 30th ed. pg. 170-171

- **Enolase**, also known as phosphopyruvate hydratase, is a metallo-enzyme responsible for the catalysis of the conversion of 2-phosphoglycerate to phosphoenol pyruvate, the ninth and penultimate step of glycolysis.

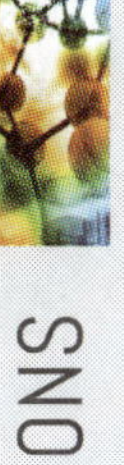

- If the sample for blood glucose is kept for some time, the Red blood cells will start consuming the sugar available and hence the final report shall be lower than actual.
- Sodium flouride shall inhibit enolase and ensure an accurate result.

64. Ans. (a) Type 1

Ref: Harper's Biochemistry, 30th ed. pg. 178-179

Number	Enzyme deficiency	Eponym	Hypoglycemia	Development/prognosis
GSD type I	Glucose 6-phosphate	Von Gierke's disease	Yes	Growth failure
GSD type II	Acid alpha-glucosidase	Pompe's disease	No	Death by age -2 years (infantile variant)
GSD type III	Glycogen debranching enzyme	Cori's disease of Forbes's disease	Yes	
GSD type IV	Glycogen Branching enzyme	Andersen disease	No	Failure to thrive, death at age -5 years
GSD type V	Muscle gklycogen phosphory-lase	McArdi disease	No	
GSD type VI	Liver glycogen phosphorylase	Her's disease	Yes	Growth retardation
GSD type VII	Muscle phosphofructokinase	Tarui's disease	No	Delayed motor development, Growth retardation
GSD type IX	Phosphorylase kinase PHKA2		Yes	

"Mn: Von Pump Cori and Make Her Tired"

65. Ans. (d) Myophosphorylase deficiency

Ref: Harper's Biochemistry, 30th ed. pg. 178-179

Please refer to above explanation.

66. Ans. (d) The oxidative phase generates NADH and the Non oxidative phase generates pyruvate

Ref: Harper's Biochemistry, 30th ed. pg. 198-199

- The **pentose phosphate pathway** (also called the **phosphogluconate pathway** and the **hexose monophosphate shunt**) is a process that generates NADPH and pentoses.
- There are two distinct phases in the pathway. The first is the oxidative phase, in which NADPH is generated, and the second is the non-oxidative synthesis of 5-carbon sugars. *This pathway is an alternative to glycolysis.*
- **The PPP occurs exclusively in the cytoplasm,** and is found to be most active in the liver, mammary gland and adrenal cortex in the human. The PPP is one of the three main ways the body creates molecules with reducing power, accounting for **approximately 60% of NADPH production in humans.**
- One of the uses of NADPH in the cell is to prevent oxidative stress.

67. Ans. (a) NADPH

Ref: Harper's Biochemistry, 30th ed. pg. 198-199

68. Ans. (b) 5% iodine and 10% potassium iodide

Solution	Iodine (w/v)	Potassium iodide (w/v)
Aqueous iodine (lugol's iodine)	5%	10%
Weak iodine solution (tincture of iodine)	2%	2.5%
Strong iodine solution	10%	6%

Uses of Lugol's Iodine

- During colposcopy, lugol's iodine is applied to the vagina and cervix.: Schiller's test
- Lugol's iodine may also be used to better visualize the muco-gingival junction in the mouth.
- Lugol's solution can also be used in various experiments to observe how a cell membrane uses osmosis and diffusion.
- Oxidizing germicide

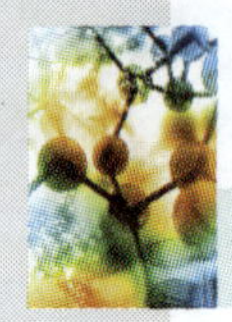

69. Ans. (b) Lipid synthesis and glutathione reaction

Ref: Harper's Biochemistry, 30th ed. pg. 234-35

NADPH is used for:

- Lipid synthesis
- Cholesterol synthesis
- Fatty acid chain elongation
- Regeneration of reduced glutathione (which protects against Reactive oxygen species)

LIPIDS

70. Ans. (a) Acetyl CoA

Ref: Lippincott's Illustrated Reviews, 6th ed. pg. 345

- Cholesterol Biosynthesis takes place in hepatic cytosol, beginning with acetyl-CoA. All carbon atoms are derived from acetyl CoA.
- Steps involved are:
  - **Condensation** of 3 acetate units to mevalonate
  - **Conversion** of mevalonate to activated isoprene
  - **Polymerization** of isoprene to form squalene
  - **Cyclization** of squalene to create the steroid nucleus

Steps in Cholesterol Synthesis

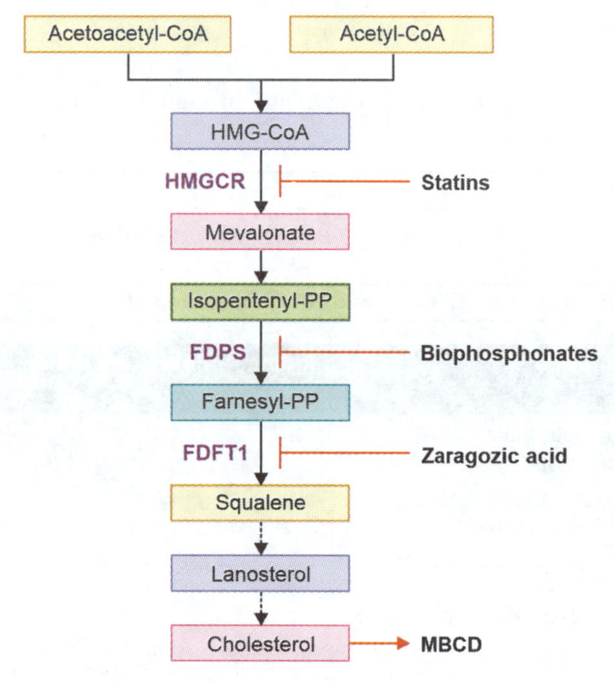

71. Ans. (c) Rich in sodium

Ref: Harrison's Medicine 20th ed. pg. 1901

- The DASH diet is **a healthy-eating plan designed to help, treat or prevent high blood pressure (hypertension).**
- The DASH diet includes foods that are rich in potassium, calcium and magnesium. These nutrients help to control blood pressure.
- The diet limits foods that are high in sodium, saturated fat and added sugars.

72. Ans. (c) TGs

Ref: Lippincott's Illustrated Reviews, 6th ed. pg. 293

- In adipose tissues, fats are stored in form of triglycerides upon excess intake of glucose/energy.
- In fasting stage, the triglyceride from adipocyte is broken down to release fatty acid to provide the ATP.

73. Ans. (b) Ethanol

Ref: Lippincott's Biochemistry, 6th ed. pg. 578

- Ethanol inhibits fatty acid oxidation in hepatocytes by competitive substrate oxidation, that results in an increased availability of long chain free fatty acids and enhances esterification leading to accumulation of triglycerides in liver.

74. Ans. (a) HDL

- HDL is the cardioprotective cholesterol
- Functions of HDL:
  - HDL causes reverse cholesterol transport (transports tissue cholesterol to liver)
  - Cholesterol is excreted through bile. This excretion need prior esterification with poly unsaturated fatty acid (PUFA).
  - PUFA reduces serum cholesterol level. It is also an anti-atherogenic fatty acid.

75. Ans. (a) Palmitic acid

- Palmitic acid is the most common fatty acid found in animals, plant and microbes.
- Excess carbohydrates and proteins are converted to palmitic acid.
- Palmitic acid is the first fatty acid synthesized during fatty acid synthesis.
- **Note:** First step in fatty acid synthesis is transfer of acetate units from mitochondrial acetyl CoA to the cytosol.

76. Ans. (a) Acetyl CoA

- **Principle building block in fatty acid synthesis: Acetyl CoA**
- **Cofactors required:** NADPH, ATP, Mn^{2+} and HCO_3
- **Source of Acetyl CoA:** From mitochondria (after aerobic glycolysis and Fatty acid oxidation)
- **Site of FA synthesis:** Liver, Kidney, Brain, Lungs, Adipose tissue, Lactating breast

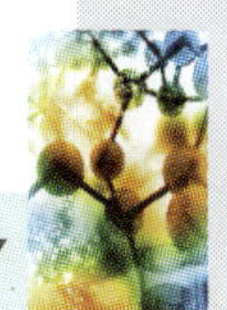

- **Organelle:** Extra-mitochondrial system in cytosol
- **Enzyme:**
  - Acetyl CoA carboxylase-*rate limiting enzyme*
  - Fatty acid synthase

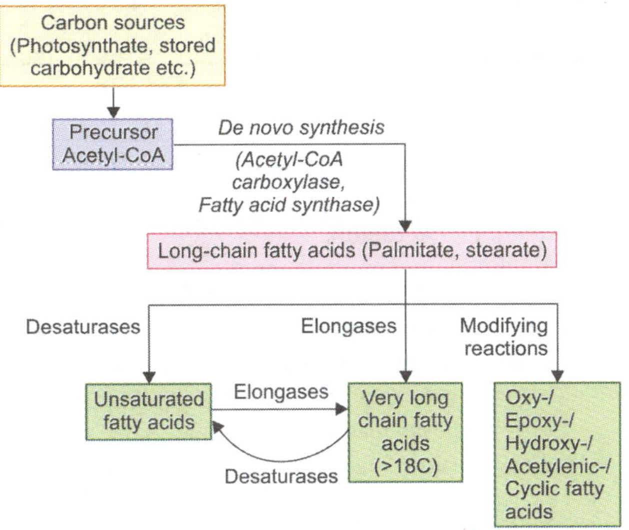

77. Ans. (c) 3.5

***Ref:* Harrison's, 18th ed. pg. ch 356**

- The total cholesterol to HDL cholesterol ratio is a number that is helpful in predicting an individual's risk of developing atherosclerosis.
- High ratios indicate higher risks of heart attacks, low ratios indicate lower risk.
- ***Ideally ratio should be kept below 4.***

78. Ans. (a) Sphingomyelinase

***Ref:* Harper's Biochemistry, 30th ed. pg. 250**

- Niemann's Pick diseases are genetic diseases which are classified in a subgroup of lipid storage disorders in which harmful quantities of fatty substances, or lipids, accumulate in the spleen, liver, lungs, bone marrow, and brain.
- In the classic infantile type-A variant, a mis-sense mutation causes complete deficiency of sphingomyelinase which leads to niemann pick disease.

Extra Mile

Other lysosomal storage disease and deficient enzymes

- **Hurler's syndrome:** Alpha-L-iduronidase deficiency
- **Hunter's syndrome:** Iduronate-2-sulfatase deficiency
- **Gaucher's:** β-Glucosidase deficiency
- **Farber's disease:** Ceramidase deficiency
- **Fabry disease:** Alpha Galactosidase-A
- **Tay-sach's:** Hexosaminidase A deficiency
- **Sandhoff's disease:** β-Hexosaminidase A and B
- **Metachromatic leukodystrophy:** *Arylsulfatase* A enzyme deficiency
- ***Krabbe disease:*** *β-Galactosidase*

79. Ans. (a) Lysosome

***Ref:* Harper's Biochemistry, 30th ed. pg. 251**

- Sphinghomyelin is a major neural tissue component, the core structure of which is formed by ceramide.
- ***It is the only sphingholipid without sugar.***
- The common sphinghomyelin deficiency is Neiman-Pick disease. The organelle which is involved is the lysosomes which allow accumulation of sphinghomyelin.
- **Signs & symptoms of Niemen pick's:** Hepatosplenomegaly, decreased appetite, unsteady gait, ataxia, slurring of speech (due to accumulation of sphingholipids in neural tissue).

80. Ans. (a) Gaucher's disease

***Ref:* Harper's Biochemistry, 30th ed. pg. 251**

LYSOSOMAL STORAGE DISEASE

- Lyzosomal storage disorders are a group of approximately 50 rare inherited metabolic disorders that result from defects in lysosomal function.
- Lysosomal storage disorders are caused by lysosomal dysfunction usually as a consequence of deficiency of a single enzyme required for the metabolism of lipids, glycoproteins (sugar containing proteins) or so-called mucopolysaccharides.
- **Gaucher's disease is the most common of the lysosomal storage diseases**. It is a form of sphingolipidosis (a subgroup of lysosomal storage diseases), as it involves dysfunctional metabolism of sphingolipids.
- *The disorder is characterized by bruising, fatigue, anemia, low blood platelets, and enlargement of the liver and spleen.*

81. Ans. (c) Gaucher's disease

***Ref:* Harper's Biochemistry, 30th ed. pg. 251**

Management of Gaucher's Disease

- *Regular, intravenous enzyme therapy is currently the treatment of choice in affected patients and is highly efficacious and safe in diminishing the hepatosis and improving bone marrow involvement and hematologic findings.*
- Symptomatic management of the blood cytopenias and joint replacement continue to have important roles in management
- The bone disease is decreased but not eliminated by enzyme therapy. Adults benefit from adjunctive treatment with bisphosphonates to improve bone mass.

82. Ans. (b) Hexosaminidase A

***Ref:* Harper's Biochemistry, 30th ed. pg. 251**

- **Tay–Sach's disease** (also known as **GM2 gangliosidosis** or **hexosaminidase A deficiency**) is a rare autosomal recessive genetic disorder.

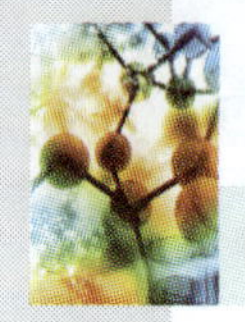

- In its most common variant (known as infantile Tay–Sachs disease), it causes a progressive deterioration of nerve cells and of mental and physical abilities that commences around six months of age and usually results in death by the age of four.

83. Ans. (b) HMG CoA reductase

Ref: Harper's Biochemistry, 30th ed. pg. 267

- ***HMG CoA reductase is the rate limiting ezyme in cholesterol synthesis.***
- HMG CoA Synthetase is involved in the formation of ketone bodies while HMG CoA lyase is involved also in the ketogenesis and also in the processing of leucine.
- Catalase on the other hand is an oxidoreductase which is involved in the connversion of hydrogen peroxide to water and oxygen.

84. Ans. (b) Apo B-100

Ref: Harper's Biochemistry, 30th ed. pg. 254

- The low-density-lipoprotein (LDL) receptor is a cell-surface protein that plays an important part in the metabolism of cholesterol by mediating the uptake of LDL from plasma into cells.
- Although LDL particles bind to the LDL receptor through their apolipoprotein B (apo B) and apolipoprotein E (apo E) moieties, other apo E-containing particles, like chylomicron remnants, are not dependent on the LDL receptor for uptake into cells.
- ApoB100 levels are associated with coronary heart disease, and are even a better predictor of it than is LDL level. A simple way of explaining this observation is to use the idea that ApoB-100 reflects lipoprotein particle number (independent of their cholesterol content). In this way, one can infer that the number of ApoB100-containing lipoprotein particles is a determinant of atherosclerosis and heart disease.

Extra Mile

- Most important apoprotein in HDL: **Apo A-I**
- Most important apoprotein in chylomicrons: **Apo B-48, E**
- Most important apoprotein in LDL, IDL, VLDL: **Apo B-100**
- Apo protein for IDL → **Apo B 100 and E**

85. Ans. (d) Apo-B 100

Ref: Harper's Biochemistry, 30th ed. pg. 253-254

86. Ans. (a) LDL-receptors

Ref: Harper's Biochemistry, 30th ed. pg. 275

- **Familial hypercholesterolemia** is a genetic disorder characterized by high cholesterol levels, specifically very high levels of low-density lipoprotein in the blood and early cardiovascular disease.
- *These patients have mutations in the LDLR gene that encodes the LDL receptor protein, which normally removes LDL from the circulation.*
- The high cholesterol levels in FH are less responsive to the kinds of cholesterol control methods that are usually more effective in people without FH (such as dietary modification and statin tablets), because the body's underlying biochemistry is slightly different. However, treatment (including higher statin doses) can often be successful.
- Heterozygous FH is normally treated with statins, bile acid sequestrants or other hypo-lipidemic agents that lower cholesterol levels.
- Homozygous FH often does not respond to medical therapy and may require other treatments, including LDL apheresis (removal of LDL in a method similar to dialysis) and occasionally liver transplantation.

87. Ans. (b) LDL

Ref: Harper's Biochemistry, 30th ed. pg. 254; Harper 26th ed. pg. 206

- **Max cholesterol**- LDL
- **Max TG**- chylomicrons *(in form of triacylglycerol)*
- **Max exogenous TG**- Chylomicron
- **Max endogenous TG**- VLDL

TABLE: Lipoprotein, its source, composition, main lipid component and its apolipoprotein

Lipoprotein	Source	Composition		Main lipid component	Apo-lipoprotein
		Protein (%)	Lipid (%)		
Chylomicrons	Intestine	1-2	98-99	Triacylglycerol	A-I, A-II, A-IV, B-48, C-I, C-II, C-III, E
VLDL	Liver (intestine)	7-10	90-93	Triacylglycerol	**B-100, C-I, C-II, C-III**
IDL	VLDL	11	89	Triacylglycerol, cholesterol	B-100, E

Contd...

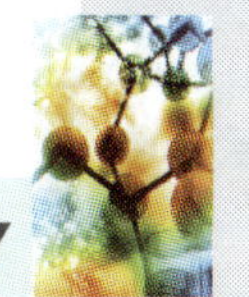

Lipoprotein	Source	Composition		Main lipid component	Apo-lipoprotein
		Protein (%)	Lipid (%)		
LDL	VLDL	21	79	Cholesterol	B-100
HDL	Liver, intestine, VLDL, chylomicrons	32	68	Phospholipids, Cholesterol	A-I, A-II, A-IV, C-I, C-II, C-III, D, E
Albumin	Adipose tissue	99	1	Free fatty acid	

88. Ans. (b) VLDL

Ref: Harper's Biochemistry, 30th ed. pg. 271-272

Lipoprotein	Transport
• HDL	Tissue → liver (good cholestrol)
• VLDL	Liver → plasma
• LDL	Liver → tissue (bad cholestrol)
• CHYLOMICRON	Intestine → plasma

89. Ans. (d) All of the above

Ref: Harper's Biochemistry, 30th ed. pg. 213-214

Medium chain fatty acid contain 8-14 carbon atoms

- Examples: caproic acid (10 C), lauric acid (12C), Myristic acid (14C), Palmitic acid (16C), Stearic Acid (18C).
- They do not require prolonged digestion
- Do not require Pancreatic lipase and bile salts
- Diffuse directly into portal circulation
- Preferentially oxidized by peripheral cells and therefore do not get deposited into adipose.

90. Ans. (b) Arachidonic acid

Ref: Harper's Biochemistry, 30th ed. pg. 238-40

- Auto oxidation is any oxidation that occurs in open air or in presence of oxygen and/or radiation and forms peroxides and hydro-peroxides.
- Unsaturated fatty acids undergo auto-oxidation in presence of oxygen due to presence of highly reactive double bonds. Unsaturated fatty acids have one or more double bonds between carbon atoms.
- The carbon atoms in the chain that are bound next to either side of the double bond can occur as *cis* or *trans* configuration.
  - A cis configuration means that adjacent hydrogen atoms are on the same side of 1 double bond.
  - A trans configuration, by contrast, means that the next two hydrogen atoms are box: To opposite sides of the double bond. As a result, they do not cause the chain to bound much, and their shape is similar to straight saturated fatty acids.

91. Ans. (b) α-Linolenic acid

Ref: Harper's Biochemistry, 30th ed. pg. 214

- PUFA are carboxylic acid with hydrocarbon tails of varying length containing two or more C=C double bonds.
- There are two families of PUFA: Omega-3 and Omega-6.
- In Omega-3 PUFA, the first C=C double bond is located at carbon 3 counting from terminal or omega methyl group tail.
- In Omega-6 PUFA, the first C=C double bond is located at carbon 3 counting-from terminal or omega methyl group tail.

Remember

TABLE: Different omega families and their respective members

ω3 family (DATE)	ω6 family	ω7 family	ω9 family
• Docosahexaenoic acid (DHA) • Alpha linolenic • Timnodonic • EPA (Enol Pyruvic Acid)	• Gamma linolenic • Arachidonic • Linoleic	Palmitoleic	Oleic Elaidic

92. Ans. (c) Docosahexaenoic acid

Ref: Harper's Biochemistry, 30th ed. pg. 214

Please refer to above table.

93. Ans. (a) Alpha linolenic acid

Ref: Harper's Biochemistry, 30th ed. pg. 214

Please refer to above explanation

94. Ans. (b) Mitochondria

- Enzymes responsible for ketone body formation are associated mainly with the mitochondria.
- Under conditions like starvation, Oxidation of fatty acids occurring in mitochondria, liver produces ketone bodies. Enzyme used is: **Pyruvate carboxylase**

- Acetoacetate, 3-hydroxybutyrate (Acetoacetate continually undergoes spontaneous decarboxylation to yield acetone) and Acetone are collectively known as the ketone bodies.

95. Ans. (c) Pyruvate carboxylase

Pyruvate carboxylase plays a crucial role in:
- Gluconeogenesis
- Lipogenesis
- In the biosynthesis of neurotransmitters
- Glucose-induced insulin secretion by pancreatic islets.

96. Ans. (b) Ketone bodies

Ref: Harper's Biochemistry, 30th ed. pg. 141, 149, 227-29

- ***Initially up to 24 hours glycogen stores are utilized.***
- Later it is fatty acid oxidation leading to ketone production which becomes the source of fuel.
- After 2 weeks proteins in muscles are catabolized to produce amino acids which act as substrate to produce energy.

TABLE: Source of Energy During Starvation

STAGE	I	II	III
DURATION	1st 2–3 days	Upto 2 weeks (longest)	**<1 week**
Energy source	Carbohydrate	Fats	**Proteins**
Metabolism	Initially Glycogenolysis then gluconeogenesis	Lipolysis and ***KETONE BODY formation***	**Breakdown of protein**

97. Ans. (b) Oleic acid

Ref: Harper's Biochemistry, 30th ed. pg. 213

- Oleic acid is a monounsaturated fatty acid.
- Polyunsaturated fatty acid are: Palmitate, stearate etc.

Extra Mile

- Essential fatty acid are:
  - ***Linoleic Acid: Most essential fatty acid***
  - Linolenic Acid
  - Arachidonic acid
- Richest source of ω6 essential fatty acid: Safflower oil
- Richest source of ω3 essential fatty acid: Flaxseed oil
- Richest source of saturated fatty acid: Coconut oil
- Richest source of medium chain fatty acid: Coconut oil
- Richest source of MUFA: Olive oil > Mustard oil.

98. Ans. (c) Propionyl CoA

Ref: Harper's Biochemistry, 30th ed. pg. 224-26

Propionyl-CoA is a coenzyme A derivative of propionic acid. There are several different ways in which it is formed:
- It is formed as a product of beta-oxidation of odd-chain fatty acids.
- It is also a product of metabolism of isoleucine and valine.
- It is a product of alpha-ketobutyric acid, which in turn is a product of digestion of threonine and methionine.

99. Ans. (c) Propionyl CoA

Ref: Harper's Biochemistry, 30th ed. pg. 224-26

- Fatty acids with an odd number of carbon atoms are oxidized by the pathway of **beta-oxidation**, producing **acetyl-CoA**, until a **three-carbon (propionyl-CoA)** residue remains.
- **Odd-chain fatty acid is the only part of a fatty acid that is glucogenic.**

NUCLEIC ACID

100. Ans. (b) Xanthine oxidase

Ref: Lippincott's Illustrated Reviews, 6th ed. pg. 581

The given case is of Gout, which is treated with Xanthine oxidase inhibitors like Allopurinol.

101. Ans. (b) ADA deficiency

Ref: Lippincott's Illustrated Reviews, 6th ed. pg. 712

- Severe combined immunodeficiency (SCID) is a group of rare disorders caused by mutations in different genes involved in the development and function of infection-fighting immune cells.
- The best-known form of autosomal recessive SCID is caused by adenosine deaminase (ADA) deficiency, in which infants lack the ADA enzyme necessary for T-cell survival.
- The function of the adenosine deaminase enzyme is **to eliminate a molecule called deoxyadenosine**, which is generated when DNA is broken down.
- Adenosine deaminase converts deoxyadenosine, which is toxic to lymphocytes, to another molecule called deoxyinosine, which is non harmful.
- Infants with SCID appear healthy at birth but are highly susceptible to severe infections.

102. Ans. (c) HGPRT

Ref: Lippincott's Illustrated Reviews, 6th ed. pg. 578

- Lesch-Nyhan syndrome is an **X-linked** inherited disorder of purine metabolism associated with virtually complete deficiency of enzyme HGPRT.

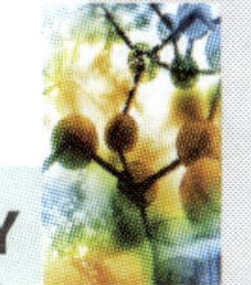

- Different types of mutations in HGPRTase gene have been identified in patients with Lesch-Nyhan syndrome.
- The disease is characterized by **self-mutilation**, (biting of lips and fingers), mental retardation, excessive uric acid production leading to hyperuricemia. The hyperuricemia frequently results in the formation of uric acid stones in the kidneys and deposition of urate crystals in the joints (gout)

103. Ans. (b) Nucleotide excision repair

Ref: Lippincott's Illustrated Reviews, 6th ed. pg. 606

Xeroderma Pigmentosum is an autosomal recessive genetic condition, commonly caused due to mutation in nucleotide excision repair enzymes.

104. Ans. (a) X-linked recessive

- X-linked recessive diseases most often occurs in males. Males have only one X chromosome. A single recessive gene on that X chromosome will cause the disease.
- Y chromosome doesn't contain most of the genes of the X chromosome, so it doesn't protect the male.
- Example: Hemophilia, Duchenne muscular dystrophy.

105. Ans. (a) RNA amplification

Ref: Lippincott's Illustrated Reviews, Biochemistry 7th ed. pg. 485

- Reverse transcriptase (RT) is an enzyme used to generate complementary DNA (cDNA) from an RNA template, a process termed reverse transcription.
- Reverse transcriptases are used by certain viruses such as HIV and the hepatitis B virus to replicate their genomes, by retrotransposon mobile genetic elements to proliferate within the host genome, and by eukaryotic cells to extend the telomeres at the ends of their linear chromosomes.
- In retroviruses and retrotransposons, cDNA can then integrate into the host genome, from which new RNA copies can be made via host-cell transcription.
- The same sequence of reactions is widely used in the laboratory to convert RNA to DNA for use in molecular cloning, RNA sequencing, polymerase chain reaction (PCR), or genome analysis.

106. Ans. (c) Adenine – Guanine and Cytosine – Thiamine

Ref: Lippincott's Illustrated Reviews, Biochemistry 7th ed. pg. 411-13

- Adenine, thymine, cytosine and guanine are the four nucleotides found in DNA.
- Traits as diverse as the color of a person's eyes and the scent of a rose are determined by the information contained in DNA.
- The Order of Nucleotides in a Gene Is Revealed by DNA Sequencing. Through the technique of DNA sequencing, first developed by Frederick Sanger, we can determine the exact order of nucleotides in an organism's genes.

107. Ans. (b) Lesch Nyhan syndrome

Ref: Harrison's 20th ed. pg. 3001

Lesch Nyhan Syndrome

- XLR condition
- Occurs due to complete deficiency of HGPRTase enzyme → accumulation of purine
- Degradation of purine → Increased uric acid
- The syndrome is characterized by hyperuricemia, nephrolithiasis, obstructive uropathy, self-mutilative behaviour, choreoathetosis, spasticity, and mental retardation.

Extra Mile

- Partial deficiency of HGPRTase enzyme → Kelley-Seegmiller syndrome.
    - Associated with hyperuricemia, nephrolithiasis, obstructive uropathy but low IQ central nervous system manifestations.

108. Ans. (c) AUG

Ref: Lippincott's Biochemistry, 6th ed. pg. 457 - 458

- Initiator codon in eukaryotes: **AUG** (codes for methionine)
- Initiator codon In prokaryotes: **AUG** (codes for N-Formyl methi-onine)
- **Stop codons:**
    - **UAG:** Amber
    - **UGA:** Opal
    - **UAA:** Ochre

109. Ans. (c) Denature of DNA → Annealing of primers → Extension of primer

Ref: Lippincott's Biochemistry 6th ed. pg. 480 – 81

Steps in PCR cycle:

- **DNA denaturation:** DNA to be amplified is heated → to separate dsDNA into single strands
- **Annealing of primers:** Separated ssDNA cooled → allowed to anneal to 2 primers
- **Extension of primer:** New chain synthesis which is complimentary to original DNA chains.

Steps	Temperature	Time (sec)
Denaturation	90°–96°C	20–60 sec
Annealing	50°–70°C	20–90 sec
Extension	68°–75°C	10–60 sec

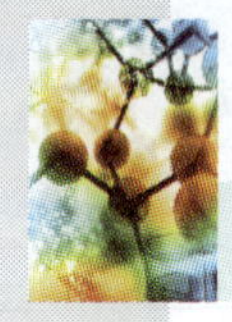

110. Ans. (d) Uracil

- Uracil is present in RNA.
- Nitrogen base pairs present in RNA: Adenine, Guanine, Uracil, Cytosine

Structure of DNA

- Double helix, right handed, anti-parallel to each other
- Two strands of DNA are held together with help of hydrogen bonds
  - 2 hydrogen bonds between A = T
  - 3 hydrogen bonds between G ≡ C
- 6 types of DNA have been described: A, B, C, D, E, Z
  - Z is left handed

Extra Mile

Important differences between DNA types:

Types of DNA	No. of base pairs per turns	Physical character	Orientation
A – DNA	11	Short and broad	Right handed
B – DNA *(MC form)*	10.5	Long and thin	Right handed
Z – DNA	12	Elongated and thin	Left handed

111. Ans. (b) Inducer

Ref: Instant Notes in Biochemistry, pg. 174

- Lac operon induces the production of structural genes in the absence of repressor.
- Repressor is inactivated by allolactose or simply lactose.
- In the *lac* operon, the structural genes are the *lacZ*, *lacY* and *lacA* genes encoding β-galactosidase, the permease and the transacetylase, respectively. They are transcribed to yield a single **polycistronic mRNA** that is then translated to produce all three enzymes. The existence of a polycistronic mRNA ensures that the amounts of all the gene products are regulated. Transcription occurs from a single promoter (P_{lac}) that lies upstream of these structural genes and binds RNA polymerase. Also present are an operator site (O_{lac}) between the promoter and the structural genes and a *lac*I gene that codes for the lac **repressor** protein.

112. Ans. (d) All of the above

Ref: Vasudevan Biochemistry, 7th ed. pg. 580

- Multiple DNA polymerase molecules engage in DNA replication. These share three important properties:
  - **Chain elongation:** Rate (in nucleotides per second) at which polymerization occurs.
  - **Processivity:** Number of nucleotides added to the nascent chain before the polymerase disengages from the template.
  - **Proofreading:** Identifies copying errors and corrects them.
- In *E. coli,* polymerase III (pol III) functions at the replication fork. Of all polymerases, it catalyzes the highest rate of chain elongation and is the **most processive**. It has 3′ to 5′ activity.
- Polymerase II (pol II) is mostly involved in proofreading and DNA repair. It has 3′ to 5′ activity.
- Polymerase I (pol I) completes chain synthesis between Okazaki fragments on the lagging strand. Eukaryotic cells have counterparts for each of these enzymes plus some additional ones.
  - **5′ to 3′ activity:** For repair and proofreading.
  - **3′ to 5′ activity:** For polymerization

Extra Mile

Classes of proteins involved in replication

Protein	Function
DNA polymerases	Deoxynucleotide polymerization
Helicases	Processive unwinding of DNA
Topoisomerases	Relieve torsional strain that results from helicase-induced unwinding
DNA primase	Initiates synthesis of RNA primers
Single-strand binding proteins	Prevent premature reannealing of dsDNA
DNA ligase	Seals the single strand nick between the nascent chain and Okazaki fragments on lagging strand

A COMPARISON OF PROKARYOTIC AND EUKARYOTIC DNA POLYMERASES

E. coli	Mammalian	Function
I	α	Primer synthesis Gap filling and synthesis of lagging strand
II	ε	DNA proofreading and repair
	β	Base excision repair (DNA repair)
	γ	Mitochondrial DNA synthesis
III	δ	Processive, leading strand synthesis

113. Ans. (b) RNA

- This technique is the PCR amplification of a reverse transcriptase product.
- It amplifies very small amount of any kind of RNA like mRNA, tRNA, rRNA and analyses the expressed mRNA sequence.
- Reverse transcriptase enzyme generates cDNA of mRNA.
- This method is used to obtain relative expression of gene in a cell.

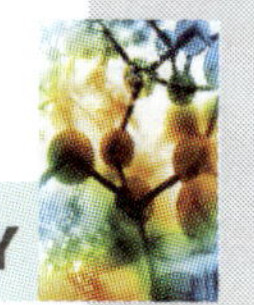

Extra Mile

- A **real-time polymerase chain reaction**, also known as quantitative polymerase chain reaction (qPCR), monitors the amplification of a targeted DNA molecule during the PCR, i.e. in real-time, and not at its end, as in conventional PCR.

114. Ans. (a) Free radical damage

- Ionizing radiation can be divided into X-rays, gamma rays, alpha and beta particles and neutrons.
- It is a type of high-energy radiation that is able to release electrons from atoms and molecules generating ions which can break covalent bonds.
- Ionizing radiation directly affects DNA structure by inducing **DNA breaks, particularly, double stranded breaks.** Secondary effects are the generation of **reactive oxygen species** that oxidize proteins and lipids, and also induce several damages to DNA, like generation of abasic sites and single strand breaks (SSB).
- Collectively, all these changes induce cell death and mitotic failure.

Damaging agent	Defect	Repair mechanism	Associated disorder
• Ionizing radiation	• Double strand break • Single strand break • Intrastrand crosslinking • Interstrand crosslinking	• Non homologous End joining repair • Homologous repair	• SCID • Ataxia Telangiectasia • Werner Syndrome • Breast CA susceptibility • Bloom Syndrome

Extra Mile

- UV light creates bulky adducts and pyrimidine dimers, which is repaired by nucleotide excision repair. A defect in nucleotide excision repair can cause disorders like **Xeroderma pigmentosa, Cockayne syndrome, Trichothiodystrophy.**

115. Ans. (c) C

X chromosome belongs to group C.

Different groups of chromosomes

Groups	Chromosome
A	1–3
B	4–5
C	6–12, X
D	13–15
E	16–18
F	19–20
G	21, 22, Y

Note:

- **X chromosome belongs to group C. They are submetacentric**
- **Y chromosome belongs to group G. They are small acrocentric**
- **The largest chromosome is chromosome 1**

116. Ans. (b) DNA mismatch repair

Ref: Harrisons, 19th ed. pg. 94e.4

- **Cockayne syndrome:** Includes a number of **autosomal recessive disorders** with features such as impaired neurologic growth, photosensitivity (xeroderma pigmentosa), and death during childhood years. These disorders are caused by mutations in the genes for **DNA excision repair proteins**, *ERCC-6* and *ERCC-8*.
- **Disorder associated with mismatch repair:** Hereditary non- polyposis colon cancer

117. Ans. (c) 3

- Stop codons are a normal part of protein synthesis—they are the reason that all proteins do not go on 'forever'. During translation, it is stop codon on mRNA sequence, that *terminates the process*. Therefore they are known to act as terminator codon.
- There are three stop codons namely:
  - UAG: Amber
  - UGA: Opal
  - UAA: Ochre

Extra Mile

Initiator codon:
- In eukaryotes: **AUG** (codes for methionine)
- In prokaryotes: **AUG** (codes for N-Formyl methionine)
- UGA codes for tryptophan in mitochondrial DNA.

118. Ans. (d) 3 codon act as terminator codon

Please refer to above explanation

119. Ans. (c) t-RNA

- **There are three main types of RNA:** tRNA, mRNA, and rRNA.
- The most abundant form of RNA is rRNA or ribosomal RNA because it is responsible for coding and producing all the proteins in cells.
- tRNA (transfer RNA): RNA which transfers amino acid from cytoplasm to ribosomal protein synthesizing machinery.
- **Secondary structure: Clover leaf shape**
- Tertiary structure: L shaped

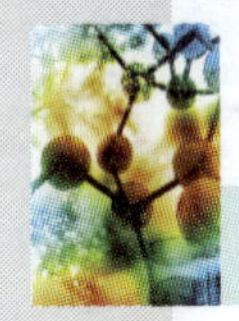

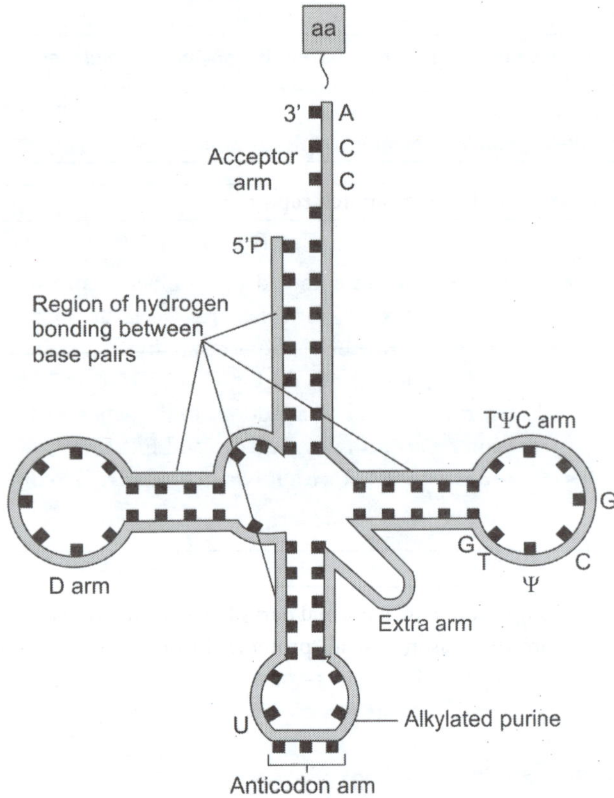

tRNA Arms

- **Acceptor arm:**
  - It is 3' end of tRNA, and has 3 unpaired nucleotide, CCA
  - It is the site of amino acid attachment
- **Anticodon arm:**
  - It has trinucleotide sequence complimentary to the codon of the amino acid, which mRNA carries.
  - Codon of mRNA and anti-codon of tRNA are anti-parallel in their complimentary.
- **DHU arm/D-arm:**
  - Recognizes the specific amino acyl tRNA synthetase enzyme
- **Pseudouridine arm:**
  - Binds the charged tRNA to the ribosome
- **Variable arm/Extra arm:**
  - Most variable feature of tRNA. It differentiates the different class of tRNA.

120. Ans. (b) Secondary

Structural organization of amino acid can be of following types:

- **Primary structure:**
  - Linear sequence of amino acid, held together by peptide bond (a type of covalent bond).
- **Secondary structure:**
  - Folding of short ~ 3–30 residue, contiguous segment of polypeptide.
  - Joined together **by non-covalent bond** primarily.
    - **Hydrogen bond:** Most important bond
    - Vander walls force
    - Hydrophobic bond
    - Electrostatic bond
- **Tertiary structure:** 3D conformation of polypeptide. Bonds are non-covalent *(similar to secondary structure)*
- **Quaternary structure:**
  - When more than one polypeptide aggregate to form one functional protein. The spatial relationship between these polypeptide subunit is called quaternary structure.
  - Bonds are non-covalent *(similar to secondary structure)*

Alpha Helix

- It is an example of **secondary structure.**
- It is the **most common** and **stable secondary structure**. Right handed spiral
- Each turn of alpha helix is formed by 3.6 amino acyl residues.
- Size of 1 turn of alpha helix: 0.54 nm
- Proteins whose major secondary structure is alpha-helix:
  - Haemoglobin and Myoglobin

121. Ans. (a) Glycine

- Most abundant amino acid in bend/turn is proline > Glycine.
- Since proline is NOT given in option, glycine is our next best choice.

122. Ans. (b) 7 methyl transferase

Ref: PubMed

Post-transcriptional modification of mRNA:

- **7 methyl guanosine capping** at 5' end is one of the post-transcriptional modification of mRNA.
- It takes place in two steps:

	Step I	Step II
Step	Guanosine triphosphate is attached to 5' end of hnRNA	Methylation of guanosine triphosphate
Enzyme	Guanylyl tranferase	**7 methyl transferase**
Site	Nucleus	Cytoplasm

123. Ans. (b) Thymine

Ref: Harper's Biochemistry, 30th pg. 341, 29th ed. pg. 344

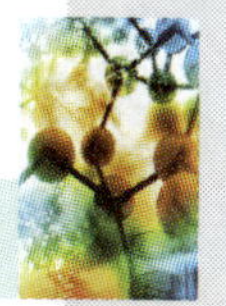

Nitrogen Bases present in RNA are:	Nitrogen Bases present in DNA are:
• Adenine	• Adenine
• Guanine	• Guanine
• Uracil	• Thymine
• Cytosine	• Cytosine

124. Ans. (b) Glutamine

Ref: Harper's Biochemistry, 29th ed. pg. 332

- AA for purine synthesis-glycine, aspartate, glutamine
- AA for pyrimidine synthesis-glutamine, aspartic acid (aspartate)
- Hence, 2 AA are common i.e., glutamine and aspartate

125. Ans. (b) Carbamoyl phosphate synthetase II

Ref: Harper's Biochemistry, 30th ed. pg. 340, 353

- ***Harper 27th ed pg. 305 says*** Aspartate transcarbomylase is the rate limiting enzyme of the pyrimidine synthesis in which case it does not make any differentiating remark between prokaryotic and eukaryotic pyrimidine synthesis.
- ***"Pyrimidine synthesis is regulated by ACTase in bacteria (prokaryotes) and CPS-II in animals (eukaryotes) as there rate limiting enzymes respectively"***
- Sources of a pyrimidine:
  - Asparatic acid (Nl, C4, C5, C6)
  - Amine N2 of glutamine (N3)
  - CO2 (C2)

Note: *UMP is the first pyrimidine to be synthesized.*

126. Ans. (a) Right handed anti parallel

Ref: Harper's Biochemistry, 30th ed. pg. 360-361

- Helical structure assumed by two strands of deoxyribonucleic acid, held together throughout their length by hydrogen bonds between bases on opposite strands, referred to as Watson-Crick base pairing. The structure is right handed anti-parallel structure.

127. Ans. (c) G≡C

Ref: Harper's Biochemistry, 30th ed. pg. 360-361

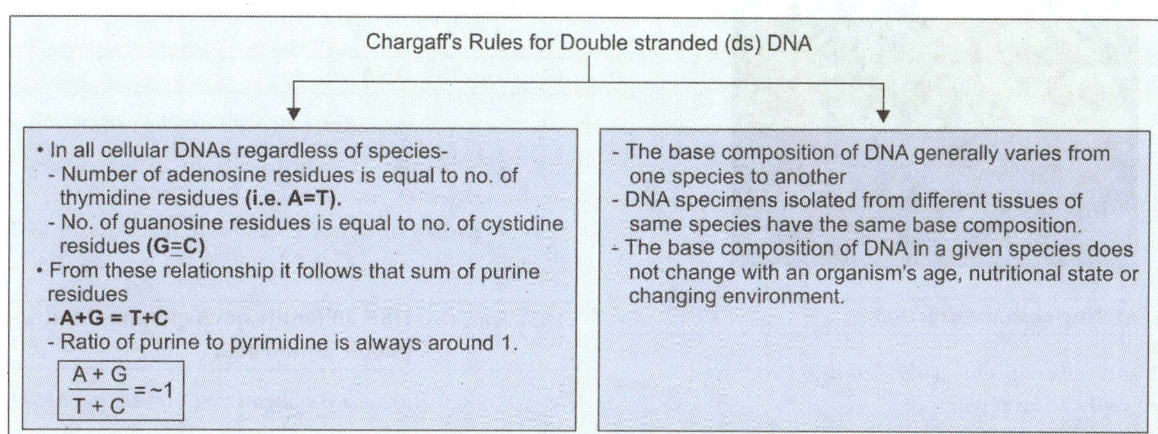

128. Ans. (d) Deletion of 2 bases

Ref: Harper's Biochemistry, 30th ed. pg. 417-18

Somatic Mutation Include

- **Point mutation**- (mutation of single nucleotide)
  - **Silent mutation:** If the changed base in the mRNA molecule at the third nucleotide of a codon, leads to no detectable effect.
  - **Mis-sense mutation:** Substitution of amino acid
  - **Non sense mutation:** Appearance of stop codon due to mutation
- **Frame shift mutation**-due to deletion/insertion, of one or two bases, which causes shift in reading frame. Whole reading frame is changed leading to entirely different protein molecule synthesis, called garbled protein.
- **Trinucleotide repeat mutation**-repeat more than 55 times.

129. Ans. (a) Translation

Ref: Harper's Biochemistry, 30th ed. pg. 417-418

- Frameshift mutations take place when there is an insertion or removal of 1 or 2 base pairs into the codon sequence. ***When the translation of the codon takes place, as it is read in triplets , the amino acid sequence of the protein synthesized is changed which leads to a "shift" in the frame that is being translated.*** But during the replicative or transcription processes there will be no problems as in the structure or stability of the DNA molecule.
- *Frameshift mutations also do not occur in multiples of 3* because in that case, only an amino acid is skipped in the translation process and the sequence is maintained.

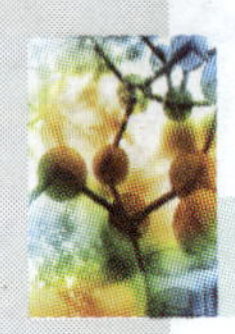

130. Ans: (b) 3

Ref: Harper's Biochemistry, 30th ed. pg. 417-18

- Frame-shift mutations
- *The genetic code is read in form of triplets of nucleotides which are known as codons.*
- If one or two base pairs from the code are removed or inserted, the genetic code will be misread from that change onwards, because the genetic code is not punctuated. Therefore the amino acid sequence translated from the change onwards will be completely changed. This is known as frame shift mutation.
- However *if the removal /insertion happens in multiples of three, rest of the reading frame doesn't change and hence the amino acid sequence will not change.*

131. Ans. (d) Base pair substitution

Ref: Harper's Biochemistry, 30th ed. pg. 416-17

A partial missense mutation (type of base pair substitution) glutamic acid, the normal amino acid in position 6 of the β chain, has been replaced by valine.

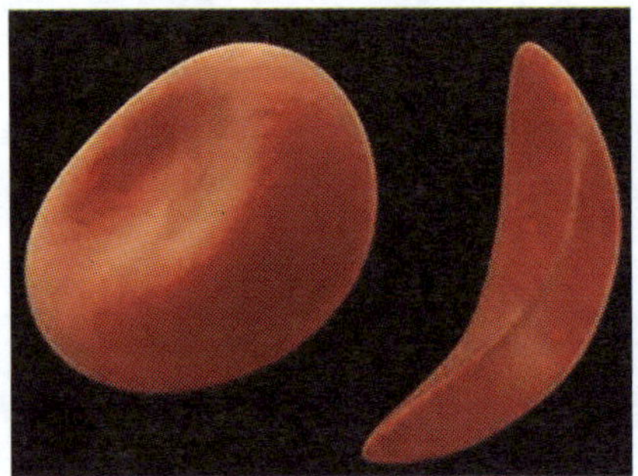

132. Ans. (a) Nucleoside correction

DNA correction has been divided into two types:

- **Pre replication repair:**
  - Most efficient form of repair
  - Done by: excision repair, photoreactivation, base replacement
- **Post replication repair:**
  - Done by: Daughter strand Gap repair, error prone induced repair.

TABLE: Mechanism of Dna Repair

Mechanism	Problem	Solution
Mismatch repair	Copying errors (single base or Two-to five-base unpaired loops)	Methyl-directed strand cutting, exonuclease digestion, and replacement
Double-strand break repair	Ionizing radiation, chemotherapy, oxidative free radicals	Synapsis, unwinding, alignment, ligation
Base excision-repair	Spontaneous, chemical, or radiation damage to a single base	Base removal by N-glycosylase, abasic sugar removal, replacement
Nucleotide excision-repair	Spontaneous, chemical, or radiation damage to a DNA segment	Removal of an approximately 30-nucleotide oligomer and replacement

Contd...

133. Ans. (b) Repair of damaged DNA

Ref: Harper's Biochemistry, 30th ed. pg. 389-90

Two types of exonuclease activity has been described:

- **5' to 3' exonuclease activity:** Responsible for cleavage of phosphodiester bond starting from 5' end of the strand. It is considered as the error correcting activity in damaged DNA.
- **3' to 5' exonuclease activity:** Responsible for cleavage of phosphodiester bond starting from 3' end of the strand. This activity provides a means for proofreading if in case any wrong base is mistakenly incorporated by DNA polymerase III during DNA synthesis.

134. Ans. (b) DNA

Ref: Harper's Biochemistry, 30th ed. pg. 724

- Radiation exposure leads to increased destruction of DNA.
- Radiation causes pyrimidine diamerisation– leading to DNA damage.

135. Ans. (b) HSP 70 family of chaperones bind with hydrophobic amino acid

Ref: Harper's Biochemistry, 30th ed. pg. 618-20, 26th ed. pg. 36-37

- ***Over half of mammalian protein folding is done by Chaperone proteins.***
- Chaperones prevent aggregation, thus providing an opportunity for the formation of appropriate secondary structural elements.
- **There are 2 families of HSP:** HSP 60 and HSP 70.
- The HSP 60 family of chaperones, sometimes called chaperonins, ***differ in sequence and structure from hsp70 and its homologs.***
- The HSP 70 (70-kDa heat shock protein) ***family of chaperones binds short sequences of hydrophobic amino acids in newly synthesized polypeptides, shielding them from solvent.***
- Hsp 60 acts later in the folding process, ***often together with an HSP 70 chaperone.***

- Hsp 60 chaperone is donut shaped, which provides a sheltered environment in which a polypeptide can fold until all hydrophobic regions are buried in its interior, eliminating aggregation.
- **Chaperone proteins can also "rescue" proteins** that have become thermodynamically trapped in a misfolded dead end. They rescue it ***by unfolding hydrophobic regions and providing a second chance to fold productively.***

136. Ans. (a) Xeroderma pigmentosum

Ref: Harper's Biochemistry, 30th ed. pg. 389-90, 28th ed. pg. 330-32

- **Xeroderma pigmentosum** is an **autosomal recessive** genetic disease which arises due to defect in DNA repair particularly of thymidine dimers.

Examples of Conditions Arising due to DNA Repair Defects:

- Xeroderma pigmentosa
- Ataxia telangiectasia
- Fanconi's syndrome
- Bloom syndrome
- HNPCC

137. Ans. (c) Telomerase

Ref: Harper's Biochemistry, 30th ed. pg. 374, 732, 26th ed. pg. 318

- The ends of each chromosome contain structures called telomeres.
- Telomeres consist of short, repeat TG-rich sequences. Human telomeres have a variable number of repeats of the sequence 5'-TTAGGG-3', which can extend for several kilobases.
- **Telomerase,** is related to viral RNA-dependent DNA polymerases (reverse transcriptases) and *is the enzyme responsible for telomere synthesis* and thus for maintaining the length of the telomere.
- Telomere shortening has been associated with both aging and malignant transformation. Because of this reason, telomerase has become an attractive target for cancer chemotherapy and drug development.

138. Ans. (b) Rough endoplasmic reticulum

Ref: Harper's Biochemistry, 30th ed. pg. 576-77

- The surface of the rough endoplasmic reticulum is studded with protein-manufacturing ribosomes giving it a "rough" appearance.
- The ribosomes bound to ER are not a stable part of this organelle's structure as they are constantly being bound and released from the membrane.
- A ribosome only binds to the RER once a specific protein-nucleic acid complex forms in the cytosol. This special complex forms when a free ribosome begins translating the mRNA of a protein destined for the secretory pathway.
- **Protein once produced from RER will go to golgi apparatus → secretory vesicles → which is further released.**

139. Ans. (b) Endoplasmic reticulum

Ref: Harper's Biochemistry 30th ed. pg. 576-77

Please refer to above explanation

140. Ans. (c) Golgi body

Ref: Ganong's Physiology, 25th ed. pg. 43-44

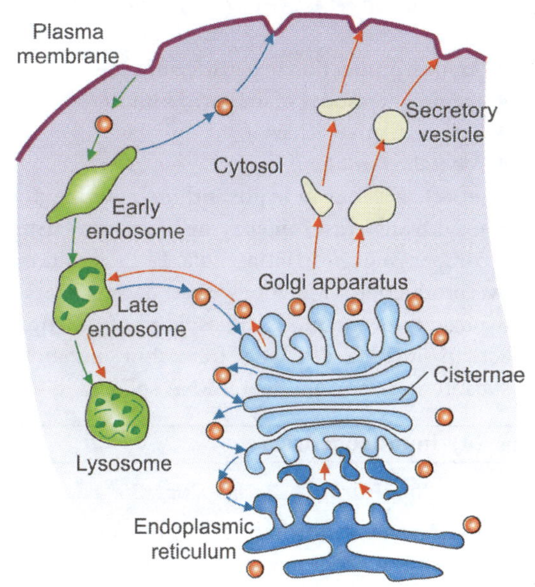

141. Ans. (a) Primary structure

Ref: Harper's Biochemistry, 30th ed. pg. 26-29, 618-19

PROTEIN DENATURATION

- In **quaternary structure** denaturation, protein sub-units are dissociated and/or the spatial arrangement of protein subunits is disrupted.
- **Primary structure**, such as the sequence of amino acids held together by covalent peptide bonds, is **not disrupted by denaturation.**
- In **secondary structure** denaturation proteins adopt a random coil as they lose all regular repeating patterns such as alpha-helices and beta-pleated sheets, and configuration.

- **Tertiary structure** denaturation involves the disruption of:
  1. **Covalent interactions** between amino acid side-chains (such as disulfide bridges between cysteine groups)
  2. **Non-covalent dipole-dipole interactions** between polar amino acid side-chains (and the surrounding solvent)
  3. **Van der Waals (induced dipole) interactions** between nonpolar amino acid side-chains.

142. Ans. (c) Uric acid stones are frequently formed

Ref: Harper's Biochemistry, 30th ed. pg. 354-55, 26th ed. pg. 300

LESCH-NYHAN SYNDROME

- It is a X-linked recessive disorder which is characterized by:
  - An overproduction hyperuricemia
  - Frequent episodes of ***uric acid lithiasis***
  - Self-mutilative behavior,
  - *Mental retardation.*
- It reflects a defect in **hypoxanthine-guanine phosphoribosyl transferase, an enzyme of purine salvage.** The accompanying rise in intracellular PRPP results in purine overproduction. Mutations that decrease or abolish hypoxanthine-guanine phosphoribosyl transferase activity include deletions, frameshift mutations, base substitutions, and aberrant mRNA splicing.

143. Ans. (d) Immunodeficiency

Ref: Harper's Biochemistry, 30th ed. pg. 354-355

- **Lesch–Nyhan syndrome** is a rare inherited disorder caused by a deficiency of the enzyme hypoxanthine-guanine phosphoribosyl transferase (HGPRT), produced by mutations in the HPRT gene located on X chromosome.

Clinical Features

- **One of the first symptoms of the disease is the presence of sand-like crystals** of uric acid in the diapers of the affected infant. *Overproduction of uric acid may lead to the development of uric acid crystals or stones in the kidneys, ureters, or bladder.* Such crystals deposited in joints later in the disease may produce gout-like arthritis, with swelling and tenderness
- **Irritability** is most often noticed along with the first signs of nervous system impairment. Within the first few years of life, extrapyramidal involvement causes abnormal involuntary muscle contractions such as dystonia, atheotosis and opisthotonus.
- **Cognitive impairment:** Affected persons have behavioral disturbances that emerge between 2–3 years of age. The self-injury begins with biting of the lips and tongue at the age of 3 years.

Remember

- A less severe related disease is **partial HGPRT deficiency** is known as Kelley-Seegmiller Syndrome *(Lesch-Nyhan Syndrome involves total HGPRT deficiency).* Symptoms generally involve less neurological involvement but the disease still causes gout and kidney stones.
- The prognosis for individuals with severe LNS is poor. *Death is usually due to renal failure or complications from hypotonia (PNEUMONIA), in the first or second decade of life.*

144. Ans. (c) Uric acid

Ref: Harper's Biochemistry, 30th ed. pg. 347-357

Purines are metabolized by several enzymes:

GUANINE

- A nuclease frees the nucleotide
- A nucleotidase creates guanosine
- Purine nucleoside phosphorylase converts guanosine to guanine
- Guanase converts guanine to xanthine
- *Xanthine oxidase (a form of xanthine oxidoreductase) catalyzes the oxidation of xanthine to uric acid*

ADENINE

- A nuclease frees the nucleotide
  - A nucleotidase creates adenosine, then adenosine deaminase creates inosine
  - Alternatively, AMP deaminase creates inosinic acid, then a nucleotidase creates inosine
- Purine nucleoside phosphorylase acts upon inosine to create hypoxanthine
- *Xanthine* oxidoreductase catalyzes the biotransformation of hypoxanthine to xanthine
- *Xanthine oxido-reductase acts upon xanthine to create uric acid*

145. Ans. (a) Xanthine oxidase

Ref: Harper's Biochemistry, 30th ed. pg. 355, 120, 26th ed. pg. 300

- **Xanthine oxidase** deficiency leads to hypouricemia.
- **Hypouricemia** and increased excretion of hypoxanthine and xanthine are associated with **xanthine oxidase deficiency due to a genetic defect or to severe liver damage.**
- **Patients with a severe enzyme deficiency may exhibit xanthinuria and xanthine lithiasis**

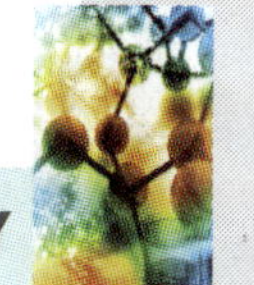

There are at least three different inherited defects that lead to early development of severe hyperuricemia and gout:

- Glucose-6-phosphatase (G6PT) deficiency **(as seen in Von gierke's disease)**
- Severe and partial hypoxanthine-guanine phosphoribosyl-transferase (HGPRT) deficiency: **(As seen in Lesch Nyhan syndrome)**
- **Elevated** 5'-phosphoribosyl-1'-pyrophosphate synthetase (PRPP synthetase) activity.

Extra Mile

DRUGS CAUSING HYPERURICEMIA:
(Mn: LEAD Poisoning Causes Stone and Nephropathy)

- Levodopa
- Ethcrynic acid
- Alcohol
- Diuretics
- Pyrazinamide
- Cyclosporine
- Salicylates
- Nicotinic acid

146. Ans. (a) Xanthine oxidase

Ref: Harper's Biochemistry, 30th ed. pg. 120, 355, 26th pg. 300

147. Ans. (a) Northern blot

Ref: Harper's Biochemistry, 30th ed. pg. 362-63

Northern blot	The **northern blot** is a technique used in molecular biology research to study gene expression by detection of **RNA** (or isolated mRNA) in a sample.
Southern blot	A **Southern blot** is a method routinely used in molecular biology for detection of a specific DNA sequence in **DNA** samples
Eastern blot	The **eastern blot** is a biochemical technique used to analyze **protein post translational modifications (PTM) such as lipids, phosphomoieties and glycoconjugates.** *It is most often used to detect carbohydrate epitopes. Thus, Eastern blotting can be considered an extension of the biochemical technique of Western blotting.*
Western blot	The **western blot** (sometimes called the protein immunoblot) is a widely accepted analytical technique used to detect specific **proteins** in a sample of tissue homogenate or extract

148. Ans. (a) DNA cistrons

Ref: Harper's Biochemistry, 30th ed. pg. 359-62

- DNA cistrons are a section of DNA that contain the genetic code for a single polypeptide and functions as a hereditary unit.

149. Ans. (b) N formyl methionine t-RNA will be the first t-RNA to come into action

Ref: Harper's Biochemistry, 30th ed. pg. 433-37

- *Methionine t-RNA is the first t-RNA involved in eukaryotic protein synthesis.*

150. Ans. (c) r-RNA

Ref: Harper's Biochemistry, 30th ed. pg. 366-67

- **There are three main types of RNA:** tRNA, mRNA, and rRNA.
- The most abundant form of RNA is rRNA or ribosomal RNA because it is responsible for coding and producing all of the proteins in cells.
- rRNA is found in the cytoplasm of cells and is associated with ribosomes. It takes the coded information delivered from the nucleus by mRNA and translates it so that proteins can be produced and modified.

151. Ans. (d) mi-RNA

Ref: Harper's Biochemistry, 30th ed. pg. 368, 28th ed. pg. 307-320, Lippincott 5th ed. pg. 402

TYPES OF RNA

Coding Vs Non-Coding

- **Coding RNA** – mRNA
- **Non-coding RNA** - RNA that do not encode protein. Rest all type of RNA are non coding i.e. t-RNA, r-RNA, sn RNA, sno RNA, sca RNA, mi RNA, siRNA, piRNA, etc.

miRNA

- Non-coding RNA, 21-25 nucleotide long
- Transcribed from RNA polymerase II
- All known mi RNA cause inhibition of gene expression by decreasing specific protein production via translational arrest or mRNA degradation. And thus the gene that it produces is silenced.
- Noble prize was awarded for the discovery of mi RNA in 2006.

152. Ans. (b) Small Nuclear Ribo-nucleoproteins

Ref: Harper's Biochemistry, 30th ed. pg. 365-67, 94-95, 26th ed. pg. 354

- *"SNURPS" are **small nuclear ribonucleic proteins***
- *They are RNA-protein complexes that combine with unmodified pre-mRNA and various other proteins to form a spliceosome, a large RNA-protein molecular complex with which splicing of pre-mRNA occurs.*

153. Ans. (c) Decreased glucose concentration, increased cAMP

Ref: Harper's Biochemistry, 30th ed. pg. 430-31

- The ***lac* operon** aka lactose operon is an operon required for the transport and metabolism of lactose in *Escherichia coli* and some other enteric bacteria.

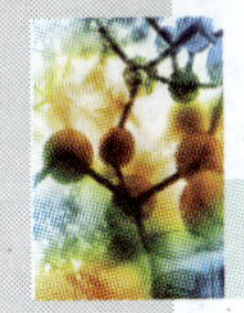

- **It has three adjacent structural genes,** which encodes:***(Mn: ZiYA ki GaLaThi)***
  - ***lacZ***: Encodes β-ga**lac**tosidase
  - ***lacY***: Encodes **lac**tose permease
  - ***lacA***: Encodes **thi**ogalactoside transacetylase (or galactoside O-acetyltransferase)
- The *lac* operon uses a two-part control mechanism to ensure that the cell spends energy only when necessary. In the absence of lactose, the *lac* repressor stops production of the enzymes encoded by the *lac* operon.
- In the presence of glucose, the catabolite activator protein (CAP), required for production of the enzymes, remains inactive, and EIIA shuts down lactose permease to prevent transport of lactose into the cell.
- In the absence of glucose, there is an **increase in the concentration of cAMP** and this leads to the activation of the lac operon which leads to the enzyme production in order to consume the lactose present in the cells.

AMINO ACID

154. Ans. (c) Alkaptonuria

Ref: Lippincott's Illustrated Reviews, 6th ed. pg. 409

- Alkaptonuria is an **autosomal recessive** condition
- The metabolic defect is the deficiency of enzyme **homogentisate oxidase.**
- This results in excretion of **homogentisic** acid in urine. It is compatible with fairly normal life. The only abnormality is the **blackening of urine** on standing.
- The homogentisic acid is oxidized by polyphenol oxidase to **benzoquinone acetate.** It is then polymerized to black colored **alkaptone bodies.**

155. Ans. (a) SAM

Ref: Lippincott's Illustrated Reviews, 6th ed. pg. 399

- The methyl group attached to sulfur in S-adenosylmethionine (SAM), is activated and can be transferred by methyltransferases to a variety of acceptors.
- Hence, SAM is considered universal methyl donor in biochemical reactions.

156. Ans. (c) Leucine

Ref: Lippincott's Illustrated Reviews, 6th ed. pg. 408

- Maple syrup urine disease is an **autosomal recessive** disorder in which there is Partial or complete deficiency of Branched chain alpha keto acid dehydrogenase.
- The mitochondrial enzyme that oxidatively decarboxylates leucine, isoleucine, and valine. These branched chain amino acids and their corresponding alpha keto acids accumulate in the blood.
- There is a characteristic maple syrup-like odor of the urine because of excretion of **leucine** in urine.

157. Ans. (b) Xanthine oxidase

Ref: Lippincott's Biochemistry, 6th ed. pg. 546

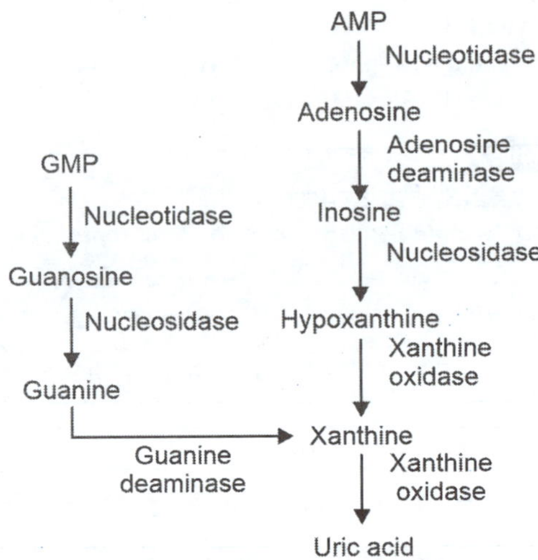

- In purine metabolism, Xanthine oxidase is responsible for conversion of Xanthine into uric acid, which gets accumulated in joints and cause swelling and pain (gout).
- Also, serum uric acid levels are also raised. To treat hyperuricemia, Xanthine oxidase inhibitors like Allopurinol is used.

158. Ans. (b) Arginine

Ref: Lippincott's Biochemistry, 6th ed. pg. 287

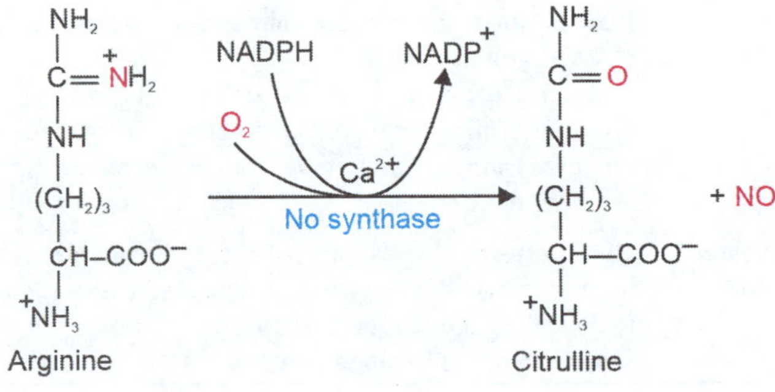

- Nitric oxide is synthesized as a byproduct in the conversation of arginine to citrulline with the help of nitric oxide synthase.

159. Ans. (a) Chaperone

Ref: Lippincott's Biochemistry, 6th ed. pg. 805

- Chaperones are proteins that assist the conformational folding or unfolding and the assembly or disassembly of other macromolecular structures.

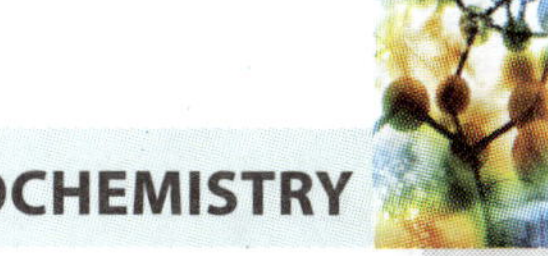

- Chaperones are present when the macromolecules perform their normal biological functions and have correctly completed the processes of folding and/or assembly.
- The chaperones are concerned primarily with protein folding.

160. Ans. (a) Alkaptonuria

Ref: Lippincott's Illustrated reviews, Biochemistry 7th ed. pg. 274

- Alkaptonuria involves deficiency of homogentisic acid oxidase.
- **The illness has three characteristic features:**
  - The urine has high levels of homogentisic acid—which is oxidised to a dark pigment on standing—hence the black color,
  - Large joint arthritis, and
  - Black ochronotic pigmentation of cartilage and connective tissue.
- Patients are usually asymptomatic until about 40 years of age.

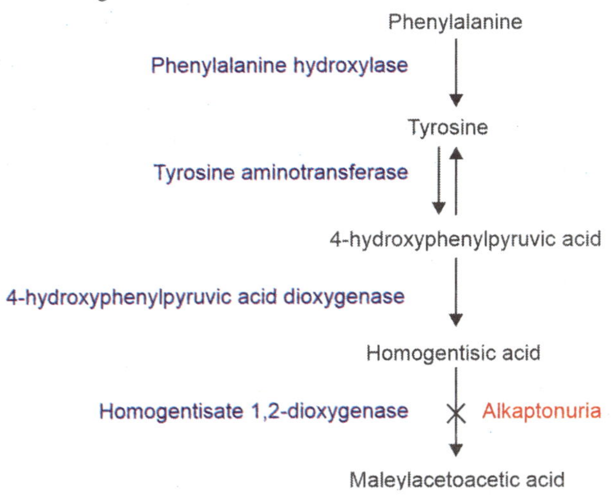

161. Ans. (b) Urea

Ref: Lippincott's Illustrated Reviews, Biochemistry 7th ed. pg. 253

- Urea is the major disposal form of amino groups derived from amino acids and accounts for about 90% of the nitrogen-containing components of urine.
- The carbon and oxygen of urea are derived from CO_2 (as HCO_3^-).
- Urea is produced by the liver and then is transported in the blood to the kidneys for excretion in the urine.
- Urea is a less toxic compound than ammonia; two nitrogen atoms are eliminated through it and less water is needed for its excretion.
- It requires 0.05 L of water to excrete 1 g of nitrogen, approximately only 10% of that required in ammonotelic organisms.
- Generally, a high blood urea nitrogen level means kidney is not working well. But elevated blood urea nitrogen can also be due to: Urinary tract obstruction. Congestive heart failure or recent heart attack.

162. Ans. (a) Primary

Ref: Lippincott's Illustrated Reviews, Biochemistry 7th ed. pg. 13

- In proteins, amino acids are joined covalently by peptide bonds, which are basically amide linkages.
- For example, glycine and alanine can form the dipeptide glycylalanine through the formation of a peptide bond.
- Peptide bonds are resistant to conditions that denature proteins, such as heating and high concentrations of urea. They can be destroyed by exposure to acids or bases.

Extra Mile

Causes of protein denaturation

Denaturing action	Mechanism of operation
Heat	Hydrogen bonds are broken by increased translational and vibrational energy (coagulation of egg white albumin on frying)
Ultraviolet radiation	Similar to heat (sunburn)
Strong acids or bases	Salt formation; disruption of hydrogen bonds (skin blisters and burns, protein precipitation)
Urea solution	Competition for hydrogen bonds. (precipitation of soluble proteins)
Some organic solvents (e.g. ethanol and acetone)	Change in dielectric constant and hydration of ionic groups (disinfectant action and precipitation of protein)
Agitation	Shearing of hydrogen bonds (beating egg white albumin into a meringue)

163. Ans. (c) Hyaluronic acid

Ref: Lippincott's Illustrated reviews, Biochemistry 7th ed. pg. 159

- Hyaluronic acid is a major component of the synovial fluid, and was found to increase the viscosity of the fluid. Along with lubricin, it is one of the fluid's main lubricating components.
- Hyaluronic acid is an important component of articular cartilage, where it is present as a coat around each cell (chondrocyte). When aggrecan monomers bind to hyaluronan in the presence of HAPLN1 (hyaluronic acid

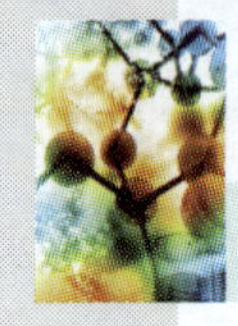

and proteoglycan link protein 1), large, highly negatively charged aggregates form. These aggregates imbibe water and are responsible for the resilience of cartilage (its resistance to compression).

- The molecular weight (size) of hyaluronan in cartilage decreases with age, but the amount increases.

164. Ans. (a) Tyrosine

Ref: Lippincott's Illustrated reviews, Biochemistry 7th ed. pg. 288

- Precursor of skin pigment melanin is tyrosine.
- The first step of the biosynthetic pathway for both eumelanin and pheomelanin is catalyzed by tyrosinase.

Tyrosine
↓ Tyrosin hydroxylase
DOPA
↓ Tyrosinase
Dopaquinone
→ Leucodopachrome → 5,6-Dihydroxyindole → (Tyrosinase) Indole 5-6-quinone → Melanochrome → **Melanin black polymers**
→ Cysteine → **Melanin red polymers**

165. Ans. (c) 4 cal

Ref: Lippincott's Illustrated reviews, Biochemistry 7th ed. Pg. 359

- Carbohydrates provide 4 calories per gram, protein provides 4 calories per gram, and fat provides 9 calories per gram. The energy content of food is calculated from the heat released by the total combustion of food in a calorie meter.
- It is expressed in kilo calories. The energy content of fat is more than twice that of carbohydrate or protein.

Nutrient	Calories per Gram
Carbohydrate	4
Protein	4
Fat	9
Alcohol	7

166. Ans. (a) Glutamine

Ref: Lippincott's Illustrated reviews, Biochemistry 7th ed. pg. 256-57

- Ammonia formed in the brain is converted to glutamine.
- In the kidneys, most of ammonia is excreted into the urine as NH_4^+, which provides an important mechanism for maintaining the body's acid–base balance through the excretion of protons.
- In the liver, the ammonia is detoxified to urea and excreted.
- Ammonia is also generated by intestinal glutaminase. The intestinal mucosal cells obtain glutamine either from the blood or from digestion of dietary protein. Glutamate Synthetase in the brain participates in the metabolic regulation of glutamate, the detoxification of brain ammonia, the assimilation of ammonia, recyclization of neurotransmitters, and termination of neurotransmitter signals.
- Glutamate synthetase, in the brain, is found primarily in astrocytes. Astrocytes protect neurons against excitotoxicity by taking up excess ammonia and glutamate.
- In hyperammonemic environments, astroglial swelling occurs.

167. Ans. (a) Glycine

Ref: Lippincott's Illustrated reviews, Biochemistry 7th ed. pg. 45

- The triple-helical structure of collagen arises from an abundance of three amino acids: glycine, proline, and hydroxyproline; glycine being the most common.
- These amino acids make up the characteristic repeating motif Gly-Pro-X, where X can be any amino acid. Each amino acid has a precise function.
- The side chain of glycine, an H atom, is the only one that can fit into the crowded center of a three-stranded helix. Hydrogen bonds linking the peptide bond NH of a glycine residue with a peptide carbonyl (C=O) group in an adjacent polypeptide help hold the three chains together.
- The fixed angle of the C – N peptidyl-proline or peptidyl-hydroxyproline bond enables each polypeptide chain to fold into a helix with a geometry such that three polypeptide chains can twist together to form a three-stranded helix. Although the rigid peptidyl-proline linkages disrupt the packing of amino acids in an α helix, they stabilize the rigid three-stranded collagen helix

168. Ans. (c) Synovial uric acid

Ref: Lippincott's Illustrated reviews, Biochemistry 7th ed. pg. 299

- Gout is a disorder initiated by high levels of uric acid which is the end product of purine catabolism in blood. It is a result of either the overproduction or under excretion of uric acid.

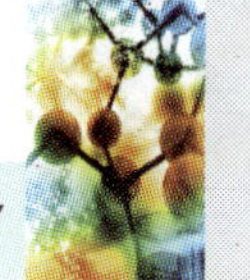

- Hyperuricemia can lead to deposition of monosodium urate crystals in the joints and inflammatory response to the crystals causing first acute and then progressing to chronic gouty arthritis.
- Formation of uric acid stones in the kidney and soft tissues may also be seen. Hyperuricemia is not sufficient to cause gout but gout is always preceded by hyperuricemia.
- The definite diagnosis of gout requires aspiration and examination of the synovial fluid to confirm the presence of monosodium urate crystals (needle shaped).

169. Ans. (c) Alkaptonuria

Ref: Nelson 20th ed. pg. 636

- This is a presentation of alkaptonuria. It occurs due to deficiency of the *hepatic* enzyme homogentisate 1,2-dioxygenase which forces the accumulation of homogentisic acid, which is rapidly cleared in the kidney and excreted.
- Upon contact with air, homogentisic acid is oxidized to form a pigmentlike polymeric material responsible for the black color of standing urine.

170. Ans. (a) Arginine

- Nitric oxide is synthesized from L-Arginine
- Reaction is catalysed from enzyme nitric oxide synthase.
- **Function:**
  - Similar in reactive oxygen species in their function
  - Potent microbial killer
  - Produced by endothelial cells and by activated macrophages

171. Ans. (a) Branched chain alpha keto acid decarboxylase

- Maple syrup urine disease is an inherited disorder characterized by the deficiency of branched-chain alpha-keto acid decarboxylase complex.
- This enzyme is required for breakdown of specific amino acid in body like valine, isoleucine and leucine.
- Due to the enzyme deficiency, these amino acid is not metabolized and hence there is accumulation in cells and body fluids → producing burnt sugar/maple syrup smelling urine.

172. Ans. (a) Glycine

- Collagen is rich in glycine and proline amino acid.
- Glycine is the smallest amino acid, present in every third position of chain, therefore it fits into the spaces where the three chains of helix comes together.
- This repeating structure, represented as (Gly-X-Y) n, is an absolute requirement for the formation of the triple helix. While X and Y can be any other amino acid, about 100 of the X positions are proline and about 100 of the Y positions are hydroxyproline. Proline and hydroxyproline confer rigidity on the collagen molecule.

173. Ans. (a) McArdle disease

- **McArdle disease** is an **AR condition**, one of **the type V glycogen storage disease**.
- Enzyme deficient: Myophosphorylase enzyme
- Due to enzyme deficiency there is inability to breakdown the muscle glycogen and prevents lactate production.
- Patients usually complain of exercise intolerance and muscle pain on exercise. Therefore strenuous exercise is contraindicated.

TABLE: Gycogen-storage diseases

Type	Defective enzyne	Organ affected	Glycogen in the affected organ	Clinical features
I. Von Gierke	Glucose 6-phosphatase or transport system	Liver and kidney	Increased amount; normal structure	Massive enlargement of the liver. Failure to thrive, Severe hypoglycemia, ketosis, hyperuricemia, heperlipemia
II. Pompe	α-1, 4–Glucosidase (lysosomal)	All organs	Massive increase in amount; normal structure	Cardiorespiratory failure causes death, usually before age 2
III. Cori	Amylo-1,6-glucosidase (debranching enzyme)	Muscle and liver	Increased amount; short outer branches	Like type I, but milder course
IV. Andersen	Branching enzyme (α-1,4 → α-1,6)	Liver and spleen	Normal amount; very long outer branches	Progressive cirrhosis of the liver. Liver failure causes death, usually before age 2

Contd...

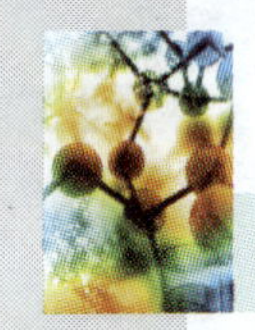

Type	Defective enzyne	Organ affected	Glycogen in the affected organ	Clinical features
V. McArdle	Phosphorylase	Muscle	Moderately increased amount; normal structure	Limited ability to perform strenuous exercise because of painful muscle cramps. Otherwise patient is normal and well developed
VI. Hers	Phosphorylase	Liver	Increased amount	Like type I, but milder course
VII.	Phosphofructokinase	Muscle	Increased amount; normal structure	Like type V
VIII.	Phosphorylase kinase	Liver	Increased amount; normal structure	Mild liver enlargement. Mild hypoglycemia

Note: Types I through VII are inherited as autosomal recessives. Type VIII is sex linked.

174. Ans. (a) Pellagra like symptoms

Ref: Harrison's 20th ed. pg. 3021

Hartnup Disease
- It is an AR condition, mainly seen due to defect in the transport of tryptophan and other neutral amino acids from the renal tubules and intestine
- **Molecular defect:** SLC6A19 gene (encode transporter protein of these amino acid)

Clinical Features:
- **MC:** Cutaneous photosensitivity
- Constant neutral aminoaciduria
- Intermittent pellagra like symptoms
- Intermittent ataxia (unsteady wide based gait)

Diagnosis: Obermeyer test (urinary test for indole compound)
Treatment: High protein diet and Nicotinic acid

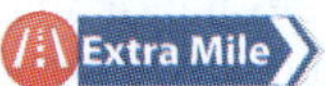

- **Drummond syndrome/Blue diaper syndrome:** Tryptophan transport defect lies only in intestine, NOT in kidney

Class of substance and disorder	Individual substrates	Tissues manifesting transport defect	Major clinical manifestations	Inheritance
Amino acids				
Cystinuria	Cystine, lysine, arginine, ornithine	Proximal renal tubule, jejunal mucosa	Cystine nephrolithiasis	AR
Lysinuric protein intolerance	Lysine arginine, ornithine	Proximal renal tubule, jejunal mucosa	Protein intolerance, hyperammonemia, intellectual disability	AR
Hartnup disease	Neutral amino acids	Proximal renal tubule, jejunal mucosa	Constant neutral aminoaciduria, intermittent symptoms of pellagra	AR
Brain branched-chain amino acid deficiency	Leucine, isoleucine, valine	Plasma membrane of blood brain barrier	Microcephaly, intellectual disability, seizures	AR
Citrullinemia type 2	Aspartate, glutamate, malate	Inner mitochondrial membrane	Sudden behavioral changes with stupor, coma, hyperammonemia	AR

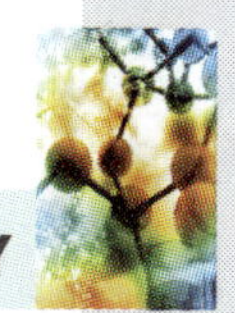

175. Ans. (d) Creatinine

- Tryptophan is one of the essential aromatic amino acid
- Metabolic fate of tryptophan: Metabolized by enzyme Tryptophan oxygenase (pyrrolase)
- **Derivatives of tryptophan:**
  - Niacin (Nicotinic acid)
  - Serotonin
  - Melatonin
- **Note:** Creatinine is synthesized from 3 amino acids namely: Glycine, Arginine, Methionine

176. Ans. (b) Arachidonic acid

Ref: Lippincott's Biochemistry, 6th ed. pg. 213

- Prostaglandin is derived from the metabolism of arachidonic acid with the help of cyclooxygenase (COX) enzyme.

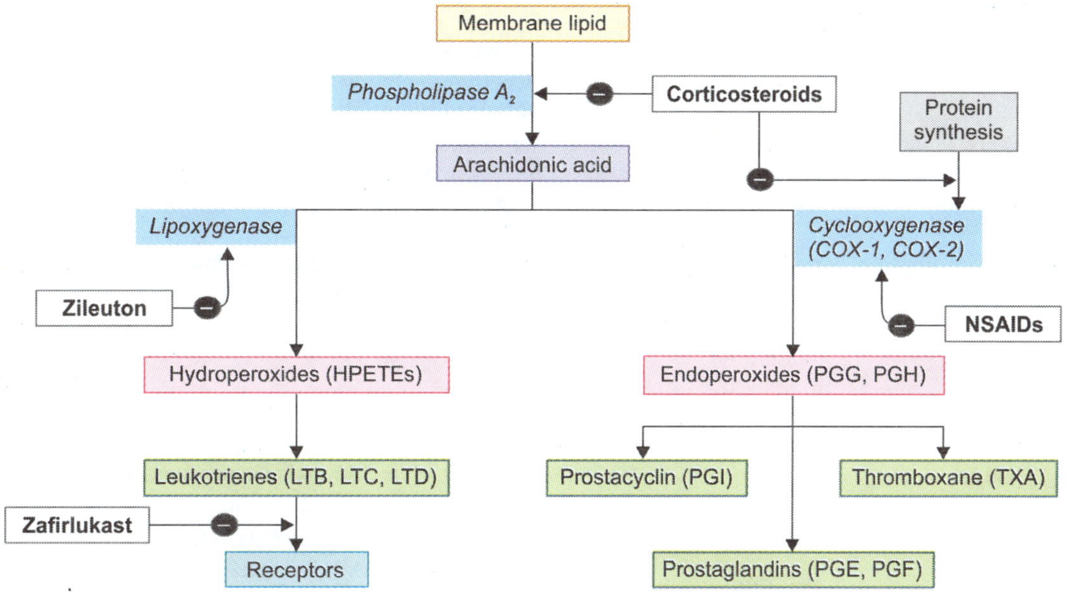

177. Ans. (d) Phenylketonuria

Ref: Harrison's 20th ed. pg. 3015–16

Phenylketonuria

- MC metabolic disorder of amino acid
- Seen due to deficiency of enzyme: Phenylalanine Hydroxylase
- Increased phenylalanine in blood → metabolized to phenylketones → excreted in urine → hence the name Phenylketonuria (PKU).
- MC organ damaged due to phenylalaninemia: Brain

Clinical Feature

- Gradual development of mental retardation (intellectual disability)
  - Infants normal at birth
- Excessive vomiting
- Autistic, choreiform movement
- Unpleasant, musty odor

Diagnosis

- Guthrie test-screening test in blood sample
- Ferric chloride test: Screening test in urine sample
- Tandem mass spectrometry: **IOC**

TABLE: Inherited disorders of Amin Acid Metabolism

Amino acid(s)	Condition	Enzyme defect	Clinical findings	Inheritance
Phenyla-la-nine	DNAJC12 Deficiency	Hydroxylase Co-chaperone	Dystonia, parkinsonism, intellectual disability	AR
	Phenylketonuria	Phenylalanine hydroxylase	Intellectual disability, microcephaly, hypopigmented skin and hairs, eczema, "mousy" odor	AR
	DHPR deficiency	Dihydroptendine reductase	Intellectual disability, hypotonia, spasticity, myoclonus	AR

Contd...

Amino acid(s)	Condition	Enzyme defect	Clinical findings	Inheritance
	PTPS deficiency	6-Pyruvoyl-tetrahydropterin synthase	Dystonia, neurologic deterioration, seizures, intellectual disability	AR
	GTP cyclohydrolase I deficiency	GTP cyclohydrolase I	Intellectual disability, seizures, dystonia, temperature instability	AR
	Carbinolamine dehydratase deficiency	Pterin-4α-carbinolamine dehydratase	Transient hyperphenylatanimenia (benign)	AR
Tyrosine	Tyrosinemia type I (hepatorenal)	Fumarylacetoacetate hydrolase	Liver failure, cirrhosis, rickets, failure to thrive, peripheral neuropathy, "boiled cabbage" odor	AR
	Tyrosinemia type II (oculocutaneous)	Tyrosine transaminase	Palmoplantar keratosis, painful corneal erosions with photophobia, learning disability	AR
	Tyrosinemia type III	4-Hydroxyphenyl pyruvate dioxygenase	Hypertyrosinemia with normal liver function, occasional mental delay	AR
	Hawkinsinuria type III	4-Hydroxyphenyl pyruvate dioxygenase	Transient failure to thrive, metabolic acidosis in infancy	AD
	Alkaptonuria	Homogentisic acid oxidase	Ochronosis. arthritis, cardiac valve involvement, coronary artery calcification	AR
	Albinism (oculocutaneous)	Tyrosinase	Hypopigmentation of hair, skin, and optic fundus; visual loss; photophobia	AR
	Albinism (ocular)	Different enzymes or transporters	Hypopigmentation of optic fundus, visual loss	AR, XL
	DOPA-responsive dystonia	Tyrosine hydroxylase	Rigidity, truncal hypotonia, tremor, intellectual disability	AR

178. Ans. (a) Tyrosine

Ref: Harper's Biochemistry, 30th ed. pg. 618-20, 26th ed. pg. 288

- **Melanin** is pigment of skin, hair and eyes, synthesized from tyrosine in the epidermis by the melanocytes.
- **Function:** Protect underlying cells from UV rays of sun.
- **Defect in melanin production:** Albinism
- **Generalized Albinism** aka Oculocutaneous albinism (OCA) is mainly classified into 3 types:
  - **OCA 1:** Tyrosinase deficient
  - **OCA 2:** Tyrosinase positive- MC type of albinism
  - **OCA 3:** Red OCA
- **Localized albinism:** Piebaldism, Waardenburg syndrome

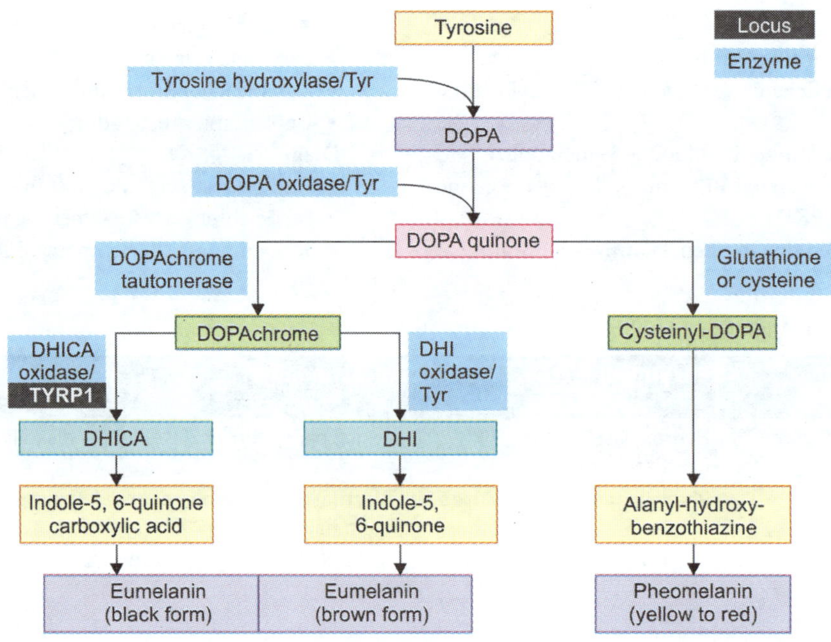

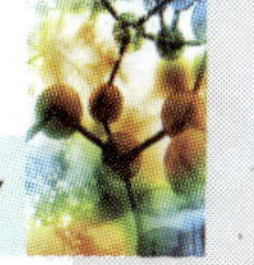

Extra Mile

- Specialized products from glycine: Creatinine, Heme, Purine nucleotide, Glutathione

179. Ans. (a) Glycine

Glycine
- In collagen every third amino acid is glycine
- Glycine is considered as the simplest amino acid
- Properties of glycine: Non-essential, Glucogenic and optically inactive amino acid
- **Acts as a conjugating agent:**
  - Conjugation of benzoic acid
  - Conjugation of bile acid
- As neurotransmitter, it has both properties excitatory and inhibitory.

Other amino acids present in collagen are: Proline, Hydroxyproline, Hydroxylysine

Lysine (K)
- An essential amino acid which is predominantly ketogenic
- It is an amino acid which is deficient in cereals
- **Functions:**
  - Important for covalent cross linkingin collagen
  - Precursor of carnitine = Lysine + Methionine

180. Ans. (b) Cysteine

- –SH group of 2 cysteine in proteins can be oxidized to form a covalent disulfide bond.
- It significantly stabilizes tertiary structures of protein
- This bond plays crucial role in structures of many proteins by forming covalent links.

Extra Mile

- Amino acid that decreases ageing process: **Cysteine and Taurine**
- Amino acid that accelerate ageing: **Homocysteine**

181. Ans. (b) Melatonin

Ref: Vasudevan Biochemistry, 8th ed. pg. 273

- Melatonin is released from pineal gland.

TYROSINE

- Neural cells convert tyrosine to epinephrine and norepinephrine. While dopa is also an intermediate in the formation of melanin, different enzymes hydroxylate tyrosine in melanocytes. Dopa decarboxylase, a pyridoxal phosphate-dependent enzyme, forms dopamine.
- β-oxidase then forms norepinephrine. In the adrenal medulla, phenylethanolamine-*N*-methyltransferase utilizes *S*-adenosylmethionine to methylate the primary amine of norepinephrine, forming epinephrine.
- Tyrosine is also a precursor of triiodothyronine and thyroxine.

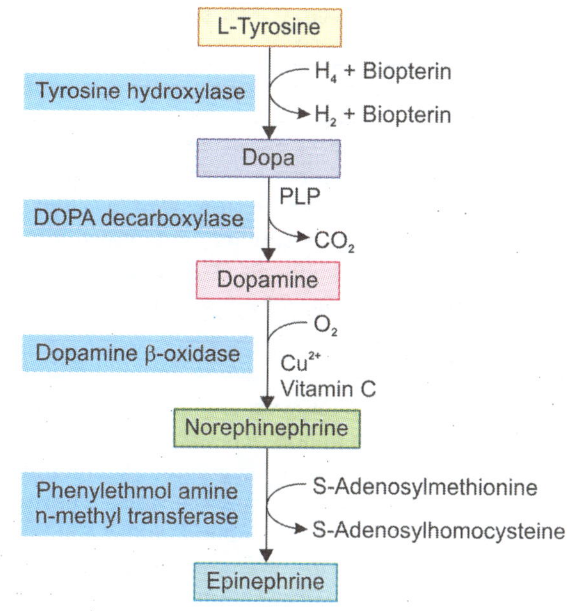

182. Ans. (a) Glycine, arginine, methionine

Ref: Vasudevan Biochemistry, 8th ed. pg. 269

- Creatinine is formed in muscle from creatine phosphate by irreversible, nonenzymatic dehydration and loss of phosphate.
- Glycine, arginine, and methionine all participate in creatine biosynthesis.
- Synthesis of creatine is completed by methylation of guanidinoacetate by *S*-adenosylmethionine.

183. Ans. (b) Lysine

Ref: Vasudevan Biochemistry, 8th ed, pg. 281-82

Based on variable side chain, amino acid can be classified into: Aliphatic amino acid and aromatic amino acid.

Aliphatic amino acid	Aromatic amino acid
It is further classified into several subtypes: • **Simple AA:** Glycine, alanine • **Branched chain AA:** Leucine, isoleucine, Valine • **Sulfur containing:** Cysteine, methionine • **With –OH group:** Serine, threonine • **With amide group:** Asparagine, glutamine • **Acidic AA:** Aspartic acid, glutamic acid • **Basic AA:** Arginine, lysine	• Histidine • Tyrosine • Tryptophan • Phenylalanine

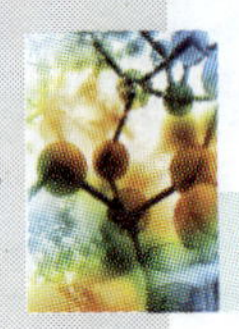

Extra Mile

- **Basic amino acid:** Histidine, arginine, lysine *(Histidine is also basic in nature, but it is aromatic)*
- **-OH containing AA:** Threonine, serine, tyrosine
- **Most basic amino acid:** Arginine

184. (a) Chaperone

Ref: Harper's Biochemistry, 26th ed. pg. 36-37

- Chaperone proteins participate in the ***folding of over half of mammalian proteins.*** The hsp70 (70-kDa heat shock protein) ***family of chaperones binds short sequences of hydrophobic amino acids in newly synthesized polypeptides, shielding them from solvent.***

185. Ans. (a) Asparate

Ref: Satyanarayan Biochemistry, pg. 339

Role of Aspartate in urea cycle:

- Aspartate participates in urea cycle for condensation with citrulline to form Argino succinic acid. The reaction is catalyzed by Argino succinic acid synthetase (Asparate provides one out of the two nitrogens of urea, the other nitrogen is contributed by Glutamate).
- In the subsequent reaction, Argino succinic acid undergoes a lytic reaction to form Arginine and fumarate. Fumarate forms a link between TCA cycle and urea. Fumarate can be recycled to form oxaloacetate, through intermediate formation of malate that can be transminated to form aspartate, to get reutilized in the urea cycle

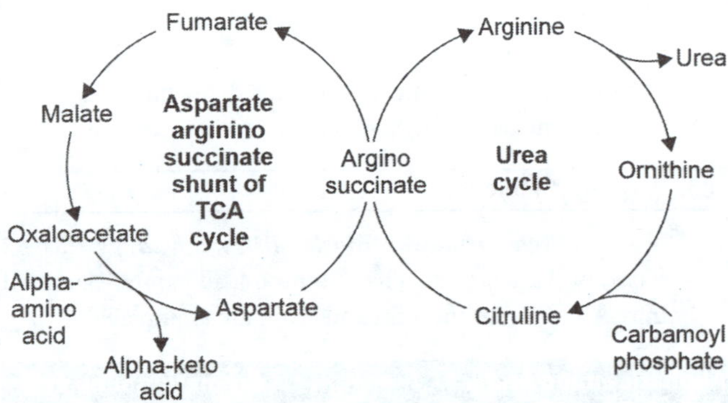

Link between TCA and urea cycle

Role of Aspartate in TCA cycle

- Oxaloacetate, the keto acid obtained from Aspartate by transamination is an intermediate of TCA cycle.
- Oxaloacetate can either be utilized in TCA cycle or be channeled to the pathway of gluconeogenesis.
- Hence asparatate is a common intermediate of TCA cycle (through oxaloacetate) and urea cycle (directly)

186. Ans. (a) Aspartic acid

Based in variable side chain, amino acid can be classified into: Aliphatic amino acid and Aromatic amino acid.

Aliphatic amino acid	Aromatic amino acid
It is further classified into several subtypes: • **Simple AA:** Glycine, Alanine • **Branched chain AA:** Leucine, Isoleucine, Valine • **Sulphur containing:** Cysteine, Methionine • **With –OH group:** Serine, Threonine • **With amide group:** Asparagine, Glutamine • **Acidic AA:** Aspartic acid, Glutamic acid • **Basic AA:** Arginine, Lysine	• Histidine • Tyrosine • Tryptophan • Phenylalanine

Extra Mile

- **Basic amino acid:** Histidine, Arginine, Lysine *(Histidine is also basic in nature, but it is aromatic)*
- **-OH containing AA:** Threonine, Serine, Tyrosine
- **Most basic amino acid:** Arginine

187. Ans. (b) Arginine

TABLE: Special groups present in amino acid

Special group	Amino acid
Guanidinium	Arginine
Phenol	Tyrosine
Thioether linkage	Methionine
Pyrrolidine	Proline
Benzene	Phenylalanine
Indole	Tryptophan
Thioalcohol	Cysteine
Imidazole	Histidine

188. Ans. (c) Phenylalanine

Ref: Lippincott's Biochemistry, pg. 268

Phenylketonuria (PKU), caused by a deficiency of *phenylalanine hydroxylase* and is the most common clinically encountered inborn error of amino acid metabolism (prevalence 1:11,000). **Hyperphenylalaninemia** may also be caused by deficiencies in the enzymes that synthesize or reduce the coenzyme **tetrahydrobiopterin (BH_4)**. It is important to distinguish among the various forms of hyperphenylalaninemia, because their clinical management is different. For example, a small fraction of PKU is a result of a deficiency in either *dihydropteridine (BH_2) reductase or BH_2 synthetase*. These mutations prevent synthesis of BH_4, and indirectly raise phenylalanine concentrations, because *phenylalanine hydroxylase* requires BH_4 as a coenzyme. BH_4 is also required for *tyrosine hydroxylase* and *tryptophan hydroxylase*, which catalyze reactions leading to the synthesis of neurotransmitters, such as serotonin and catecholamines.

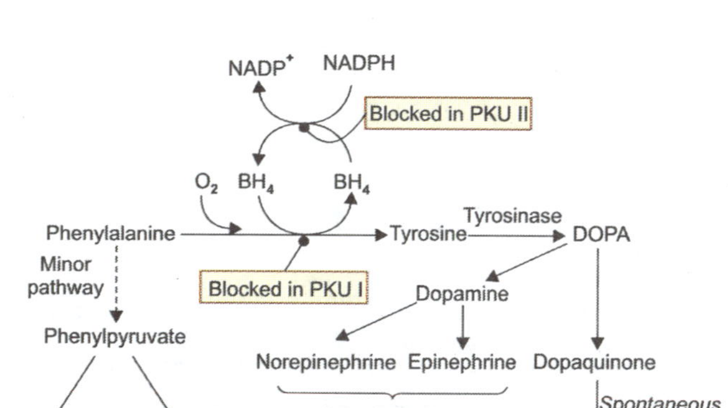

189. Ans. (c) Valine

Glycated hemoglobins arise from the non-enzymatic attachment of glucose to hemoglobin. They are formed and accumulate in the red cell in proportion to the blood glucose level. Their concentration reflects the long-term average glucose level and is thus *useful as an indicator of diabetic control.*

Types of glycated hemoglobin

- **HbA1a1:** Fructokinase 1,6 diphosphate N terminal valine
- **HbA1a2:** Glucose 6 phosphate N terminal valine
- **HbA1b:** Unknown carbohydrate N terminal valine
- **HbA1c:** Attachment of glucose to N terminal of amino acid valine

190. Ans. (b) SDS–PAGE

Ref: Harper's Biochemistry, pg. 24

- *The most widely used method for determining the purity of a protein is SDS-PAGE—polyacrylamide gel electrophoresis (PAGE) in the presence of the anionic detergent sodium dodecyl sulfate (SDS)*
- Electrophoresis separates charged biomolecules based on the rates at which they migrate in an applied electrical field. For SDS-PAGE, acrylamide is polymerized and crosslinked to form a porous matrix. SDS denatures and binds to proteins at a ratio of one molecule of SDS per two peptide bonds.

Extra Mile

- **Mass spectrometry** is considered as the method of choice for protein identification.
- **Sanger's technique** was the first technique to determine the sequence of protein.
- **Western blot detects** Protein by antigen-antibody interaction.
- **Southern blot** detects DNA by DNA-DNA hybridization.
- **Northern blot** detect RNA by RNA-cDNA hybridization.

191. Ans. (c) Heart

TABLE: Isoenzyme of LDH, its subunit, origin tissue and their respective electrophoretic activity

LDH isoenzyme	Subunit	Origin tissue	Electrophoretic activity
LDH 1	H4	Heart, RBC	Fastest
LDH 2	H3M1	Reticuloendothelial system	↓
LDH 3	H2M2	Lungs	
LDH 4	H1M3	Kidney, placenta pancreas	
LDH 5	M4	Liver and skeletal muscle	Slowest

192. Ans. (b) Tyrosine

- **TYROSINE:** nonessential AA, which is converted to Melanin, T3, T4 hormone by enzyme Tyrosinase.
  - Deficiency of Tyrosinase → Albinism
  - Deficiency of melanocyte →Vitiligo

AMINO ACIDS AT A GLANCE: Total AA = 20 in number

ESSENTIAL AA: *can't be synthesized. (Mn: TV TILL 8 PM)*	**Semi-essential AA:** *can be synthesized under normal condition as per demand.*	**Non-Essential AA:** *synthesized in body readily*
Threonine, Valine, Tryptophan, Isoleucine, Lysine, Leucine, Phenyalanine, Methionine	Histidine Arginine	The remaining 10 AA are Non-essential (including tyrosine).

193. Ans. (b) Deficient in cereals

- Lysine is an essential amino acid.
- It is **deficient in cereals and maize.**
- It is a basic amino acid. **Basic amino acids are:**
  - Arginine
  - Lysine
  - Histidine (Aromatic)
- **Acidic amino acids are:**
  - Aspartic acid
  - Glutamic acid

Food item	Limiting amino acids
• Pulses	Methionine & cysteine
• Cereals	Threonine & Lysine
• Maize	Tryptophan & Lysine

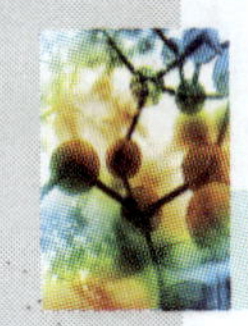

194. Ans. (c) Non-protein alpha amino acid

Ref: Harrisons, 19th ed. pg. 434e2

- Homocysteine is a non-protein alpha amino acid.
- It is a derived amino acid (from methionie) not seen in protein.
- Two fates of methionine
  - Derived as homocysteine
  - Derived as cysteine

TABLE: Diseases associated with homocysteine and it clinical features

Amino acid	Disease	Enzyme deficient	Clinical manifestation/ inheritance
Homo-cysteine	Homocyst-inuria—Classical	Cystathionine β-synthase	Lens dislocation, thrombotic vascular disease, intellectual disability, osteoporosis/AR
	Homocyst-inuria—Nonclas-sical	5, -1-10-Meth-ylene tet-rahydrofolate reductase	Intellectual disability, gait and psychiatric abnormalities, recurrent strokes/AR
	Homocyst-inuria	Methionine synthase	Intellectual disability, hyptonia, seizures, megaloblastic anemia/AR
	Homocyst-inuria and methyl-malonic acidemia	Vitamin B_{12} lysosomal efflux and metabolism	Intellectual disability, lethargy, failure to thrive, hypotonia, seizures megaloblastic anemia/AR

195. Ans. (b) Glutaminase

- In amino acid metabolism, there is detachment of NH_2. Since this amino group is toxic to body in free form, it is neutralized in form of glutamate by the process of transamination.
- This glutamate is converted to glutamine → which carries the ammonia to liver.
- In liver:

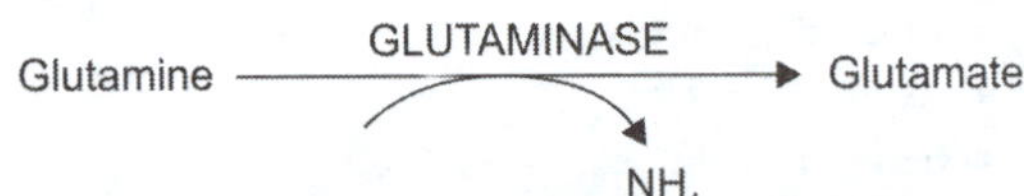

- It releases ammonia by hydrolytic cleavage and again gets converted to glutamate.
- Enzyme required here is: **Glutaminase.**

196. Ans. (c) Fatty acid

Ref: PubMed

- **Carnitine** is a quaternary ammonium compound biosynthesized from the amino acids lysine and methionine.
- It is required for the **transport of fatty acids** from the inter-membranous space in the mitochondria, into the mitochondrial matrix during the breakdown of lipids for the generation of metabolic energy.

Extra Mile

- Abnormalities in *carnitine* metabolism can cause dilated or restrictive cardiomyopathies, usually in children

197. Ans. (b) Phenylalanine hydroxylase

Ref: Harrisons, 19th ed. pg. 434e1

- PKU is an autosomal recessive disorder characterized by an increased concentration of phenylalanine and its by-products in body fluids and by severe mental retardation if untreated in infancy.
- It results from reduced activity of **phenylalanine hydroxylase.**
- The accumulation of phenylalanine:
  - Inhibits the transport of other amino acids required for protein or neurotransmitter synthesis
  - Reduces synthesis and increases degradation of myelin, and leads to inadequate formation of norepinephrine and serotonin.
- To prevent intellectual disability, diagnosis and initiation of dietary therapy must be started **before 2 weeks of age**

198. Ans. (a) Collagen

Ref: Harrisons, 19th ed. pg. 2504

- Collagen is the most abundant protein in the body.
- Harrisons states: "The first genes cloned for connective tissues were the two genes coding for **type I collagen, the most abundant protein** in bones, skin, tendons, and several other tissues.

199. Ans. (a) Tryptophan

Ref: Harper's Biochemistry 30th ed. pg. 316, 547, 5517; Food-facts and principles by N. Shakuntala, pg. 71

- Niacin can be synthesized by the bacteria of the intestinal flora and is formed in the tissues from amino acid tryptophan, which has *niacin sparing activity.* This explains why some food rich in tryptophan e.g. milk and egg, have a far greater niacin potency than would be expected from their actual content of niacin.
- In humans, deficiency of niacin results in weakness and indigestion followed by ulcerated mouth and tongue.

TRYPTOPHAN

- It is an essential amino acid, which is a precursor of melatonin, 5-HIAA and serotonin

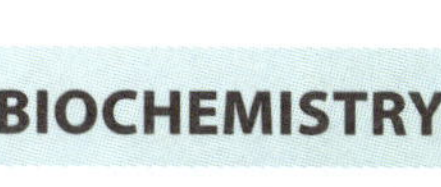

60 mg of tryptophan $\xrightarrow{\text{Vit B6}}$ 1 mg of Niacin.

- **In** deficiency of vitamin B6, the pathyway altered and leads to formation of xanthuric acid. **Thus XANTHURIC ACID IS THE INDEX OF VITAMIN B6 DEFICIENCY.**
- **Sulphur containing amino acid: CYSTEINE AND METHIONINE**
- **BASIC AMINO ACID:**
  - HISTIDINE
  - LYSINE
  - ARGININE (*most basic amino acid*)
- Most stable amino acid at physiologic pH: **HISTIDINE**
- **TYROSINE:** Non-essential AA, which is converted to Melanin, T3, T4 hormone by enzyme Tyrosinase.
  - Deficiency of Tyrosinase → Albinism
  - Deficiency of melanocyte → Vitiligo

200. Ans. (a) Niacin

Ref: Harper's Biochemistry, 30th ed. pg. 557

- Niacin is synthesized from tryptophan via kynurenine and quinolinic acids as key biosynthetic intermediates.
- *Refer to above explanation for more details.*

201. Ans. (b) Maple syrup disease

Ref: Harper's Biochemistry, 30th ed. 309, 27th ed. pg. 257

- Branched chain amino acids are remembered as VIL (Valine, Isoleucine, **Leucine**).
- These amino acids are converted to alpha-keto acid and then undergo oxidative decarboxylation by ***enzyme alpha keto-decarboxylase.*** *Deficiency of this enzyme leads to MSUD, which is characterized by burnt sugar or maple syrup smell in urine or sometimes in ear wax also.*
- In patients with deficiency of alpha keto-decarboxylase enzyme, there is **increased concentration of valine, Isoleucine and Leucine.**
- **Management** is done by restricted dietary intake of branched chain amino acid.

Extra Mile

Diseases and Deficiency
- **HARTNUP DISEASE:** TRYPTOPHAN
- **ALKAPTONURIA:** Homogentisate oxidase
- **ALPORT SYNDROME:** due to antibody against type IV collagen.

202. Ans. (c) Tryptophan

Ref: Harper's Biochemistry, 30th ed. pg. 281, 544

Food item	Limiting amino acids
• *Pulses*	Methionine & cysteine
• *Cereals*	Threonine & Lysine
• *Maize*	Tryptophan & lysine

203. Ans. (c) Homogentisate oxidase

Ref: Harper's Biochemistry, 30th ed. pg. 304

The defect in Alkaptonuria is lack of homogentisate oxidase. Most imp features are:
- The urine darkens on exposure to air due to oxidation of excreted homogentisate.
- Deposits called ochronosis occur in sclera, ear, nose, cheeks, intervertebral disc space. There may be calcification of inter vertebral discs.
- **Ochronosis arthritis**- affects shoulder, hip and knee.
- **Benedicts reaction is strongly positive and gives green brown precipitate.**
- **Fehling test** reagent gives blue green color.

204. Ans. (a) Kynerunine

Ref: Harper's Biochemistry, 30th ed. pg. 306-307

- Tryptophan is degraded to amphibolic intermediates via the kynurenine-anthranilate pathway. Tryptophan oxygenase (tryptophan pyrrolase) opens the indole ring, incorporates molecular oxygen, and forms N-formyl kynurenine.
- ***Hydrolytic removal of the formyl group of N-formylkynurenine, catalyzed by kynurenine formylase, produces kynurenine.***
- Since kynureninase requires pyridoxal phosphate, excretion of xanthurenate in response to a tryptophan load is diagnostic of vitamin B_6 deficiency.
- Hartnup disease reflects impaired intestinal and renal transport of tryptophan and other neutral amino acids.

205. Ans. (d) Aspartate

Ref: Harper's Biochemistry, 30th ed. pg. 294-95

NH_3 + HCO_3 + Aspartate + 3ATP → Urea + Fumarate + 2 ADP + AMP + 4 P.

UREA CYCLE

- Urea Is the Major End Product of Nitrogen Catabolism in Humans
- Some reactions of urea synthesis occur in the matrix of the mitochondrion, other reactions in the cytosol
- *Synthesis of 1 mol of urea requires 3 mol of ATP plus 1 mol each of ammonium ion and of the amino nitrogen of aspartate.*

STEPS OF UREA METABOLISM

Step -1: Site: Mitochondria

- Carbamoyl Phosphate Synthase I Initiates Urea Biosynthesis
- Condensation of CO_2, ammonia, and ATP to form carbamoyl phosphate is catalyzed by mitochondrial carbamoyl phosphate synthase I.
- Carbamoyl phosphate synthase I, the rate-limiting enzyme of the urea cycle, is active only in the presence of its allosteric activator N-acetylglutamate
- *The step requires 2 ATPs*

Step - 2: Site: Mitochondria

- Carbamoyl Phosphate Plus Ornithine Forms Citrulline
- L-Ornithine transcarbamoylase catalyzes the reaction Next 3 steps take place in cytosol

Step -3 : Site : Cytosol

- Citrulline plus Aspartate forms Argininosuccinate
- Argininosuccinate synthase links aspartate and Citrulline via the amino group of aspartate and provides the second nitrogen of urea. The reaction requires ATP.

Step: 4 : Site : Cytosol

- Cleavage of Argininosuccinate Forms Arginine & Fumarate catalyzed by argininosuccinase.

Step: 5 : Site : Cytosol

- Cleavage of Arginine Releases Urea & Re-Forms Ornithine
- Hydrolytic cleavage of the guanidino group of arginine, catalyzed by liver arginase, releases urea
- The other product, ornithine, reenters liver mitochondria for additional rounds of urea synthesis.

206. Ans. (a) Cleavage of Arginine

Ref: Harper's Biochemistry, 30th ed. pg. 299-300

Please refer to above explanation.

207. Ans. (b) Ornithine

- Polyamines like spermine, spermidine and putrescine metabolite are produced from L-ornithine by action of ODC (ornithine decarboxylase).
- S-Adenosylmethionine, the methyl group donor for many biosynthetic processes, also participates directly in spermine and spermidine biosynthesis.

208. Ans. (d) Made of cystiene and methionine

Ref: Harper's Biochemistry, 30th ed. pg. 299-300, 295

SELENOCYSTEINE

- Considered to be the 21st proteinogenic amino acid. It exists naturally in all kingdoms of life as a building block of selenoproteins.
- It is utilized only when required for protein functions.
- **Selenocysteine is present in several enzymes** for example:
  - **Gutathione peroxidases**
  - Tetraiodothyronine 5' deiodinases
  - Thioredoxin reductases and
  - Some hydrogenases
- Selenocysteine is not coded directly in the genetic code. Instead, **it is encoded in a special way by a UGA codon,** which is normally a stop codon. Such a mechanism is called translational receding and its efficiency depends on the seleno-protein being synthesized and on translation initiation factors.
  - The UGA codon is made to encode Selenocysteine by the presence of a SECI Selement (Seleno-Cysteine Insertion Sequence) in the mRNA.

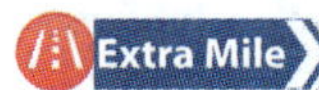

- ***Pyrrolysine is 22nd amino acid.***

209. Ans. (d) Cysteine

Ref: Harper's Biochemistry, 30th ed. pg. 301

- ***The clinical disease is due to the accumulation of cysteine which forms stones.***
- **MC inborn error of AA transport**

Causes of Cysteinuria:

- Due to the defective transport in the proximal and jejunal transport of dibasic amino acids such as cysteine, lysine, arginine and ornithine.
- **Cystinuria** (cystin-lysin-uria)- kidney is not able to reabsorb mainly 4 AA- cystine, ornithine, lysine, arginine (**COLA**)- excess amount excreted in urine.

Extra Mile

- **Cystinosis-** (cystine storage disorder)- cystine accumulates in the lysosome in many tissue and there is generalized **aminoaciduria.**

210. Ans. (a) L-arginine

Ref: Harper's Biochemistry, 30th ed. pg. 314, 660-61, 26th ed. pg. 269

- Nitric oxide, known as the *endothelium-derived relaxing* factor is biosynthesized endogenously from L-arginine, oxygen and NADPH by various nitric oxide synthase

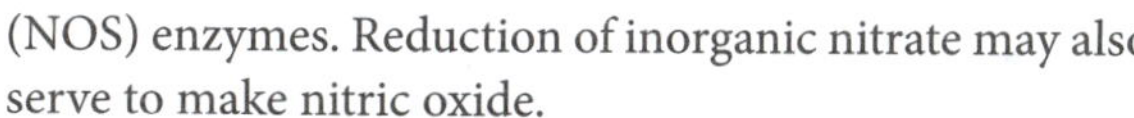

(NOS) enzymes. Reduction of inorganic nitrate may also serve to make nitric oxide.

- The endothelium of blood vessels uses nitric oxide to signal the surrounding smooth muscle to relax, thus resulting in vasodilation and increasing blood flow.

211. Ans. (c) Arginine

Ref: Harper's Biochemistry, 30th ed. pg. 314, 660-61

212. Ans. (c) Lysine & methionine

Ref: Harper's Biochemistry, 30th ed. pg. 223-24

- **Carnitine** is a quaternary ammonium compound biosynthesized from the amino acid lysine and methionine.
- It is required for the transport of fatty acids from the intermembraneous space in the mitochondria, into the mitochondrial matrix during the breakdown of lipids for the generation of metabolic energy.

213. Ans. (a) Dihydrouracil

Ref: Harper's Biochemistry, 30th ed. pg. 318

- βalanine *is formed in vivo by the* ***degradation of dihydrouracil and carnosine.***
- β-**Alanine** *is not used in the biosynthesis of any major proteins or enzymes. However,* It is a component of the naturally occurring peptidescarnosine and anserine and also of pantothenic acid (vitamin B_5), which itself is a component of coenzyme A. *Under normal conditions, β-alanine is metabolized into acetic acid.*
- β-Alanine is the rate-limiting precursor of carnosine, i.e. *carnosine levels are limited by the amount of available β-alanine.*

214. Ans. (d) N-Acetyl Glucosamine

Ref: Harper's Biochemistry, 30th ed. pg. 157-58

- Chitin is a long-chain polymer of *N*-acetyl-glucosamine, a derivative of glucose. Chitin's properties as a flexible and strong material make it favorable as a surgical thread. Its bio-degradibility means it wears away with time as the wound heals. Moreover, chitin has been reported to have some unusual properties that accelerate healing of wounds in humans.

215. Ans. (b) Glycine

Ref: Harper's Biochemistry, 30th ed. pg. 326-28

- Heme is synthesized in a complex series of steps involving enzymes in the mitochondrion and in the cytosol of the cell
- The first step in heme synthesis takes place in the mitochondrion. Steps in heme synthesis are:
    - **Condensation of succinyl CoA and glycine by ALA synthase to form 5-aminolevulic acid (ALA).**
    - 5 ALA is transported to the cytosol where a series of reactions produce a ring structure called coproporphyrinogen III. This molecule returns to the mitochondrion where an addition reaction produces protoporhyrin IX.
    - The enzyme ferrochelatase inserts iron into the ring structure of protoporphyrin IX to produce heme.

216. Ans. (c) Tryptophan

Ref: Harper's Biochemistry, 30th ed. pg. 308, 557; Harrison's, 19th ed. pg. 435e-2

- Hartnup disease is an **autosomal recessive** disorder caused by impaired neutral amino acid transport in the apical brush border membrane of the small intestine and the proximal tubule of the kidney.
- Patients of hartnup disease present with pellagra like skin eruptions, cerebellar ataxia, and gross aminoaciduria.
- Amino acids which are retained within the intestinal lumen due to impaired transport, are converted by bacteria to indolic compounds that can be toxic to the CNS. Amino acid like ***Tryptophan is converted to indole in the intestine.***
- Following absorption, indole is converted to 3-hydroxyindole (i.e, indoxyl, indican) in the liver, where it is conjugated with potassium sulfate or glucuronic acid. Subsequently, it is transported to the kidneys for excretion (i.e, indicanuria).
- Other tryptophan degradation products which are excreted in urine are: kynurenine and serotonin.
- In these patients Tubular renal transport is also defective, contributing to gross aminoaciduria.

217. Ans. (b) Lignin

- Gut flora's primary benefit to the host is the gleaning of energy from the fermentation of undigested carbohydrates and the subsequent absorption of short chain fatty acids. *They can even digest even products like cellulose, pectin and starch.*
- **The most important of these are:** Butyrates, metabolised by the colonic epithelium; propionates by the liver; and acetates by the muscle tissue.
- Intestinal bacteria also play a role in synthesizing vitamin B and vitamin K as well as metabolising bile acids, sterols and xenobiotics.
- *The human body carries about 100 trillion microorganisms in its intestines, a number ten times greater than the total number of human cells in the body*
- Lignin or lignen is a complex polymer of aromatic alcohols known as monolignols. It is most commonly

derived from wood, and is an integral part of the secondary cell walls of plants.

218. Ans. (b) Histidine

Ref: Harper's Biochemistry, 30th ed. pg. 340-42

- N1 of purine is derived from amino group of aspartate
- N3 & N9 are obtained from amide group of glutamine
- C4, C5, & N7 of the purine ring of nucleotides are contributed by glycine.

219. Ans. (b) Glycine

Ref: Harper's Biochemistry 30th ed. pg. 325-27; 26th/ 264

- **Glycine** is required for the biosynthesis of **heme, purines** and **creatine** and is conjugated to **bile acids.**
- **Serine** is required for the **phospholipid** and **sphingosine** synthesis apart from **purines** and **thymine.**
- **S-Adenosyl methionine** (the methyl group donor) for many biosynthetic processes, also participates directly in **spermine and spermidine** synthesis.

220. Ans. (d) All of these

Ref: Harper's Biochemistry 30th ed. pg. 22-23, 748

- *Glutathione (GSH) is a tripeptide with a gamma peptide linkage between the amine group of cysteine (which is attached by normal peptide linkage to a glycine) and the carboxyl group of the glutamateside-chain.*
- It is an antioxidant, preventing damage to important cellular components caused by reactive oxygen species such as free radicals and peroxides.

221. Ans. (a) Proline to hydroxyproline

Ref: Harper's Biochemistry, 30th ed. pg. 47, 562

- *Ascorbic acid is needed for a variety of biosynthetic pathways, by accelerating hydroxylation and amidation reactions.*
- In the synthesis of collagen, ascorbic acid is required as a cofactor for following enzymes:
  - Prolyl hydroxylase
  - Lysyl hydroxylase
- ***These two enzymes are responsible for the hydroxylation of the proline and lysine amino acids in collagen.***
- ***Remember,*** *Hydroxyproline and hydroxylysine are important for stabilizing collagen by cross-linking the propeptides in collagen.*
- Clinical effects if there is defective collagen fibrillogenesis:
  - Impaired wound healing.
  - Impaired bone bormation
  - Abnormal bleeding due to fragile capillaries.

222. Ans. (b) Proline

Ref: Harper's Biochemistry, 30th ed. pg. 141, 298-99

- Proline is the amino acid which changes the conformation of the alpha helix in collagen due to the nature of proline having a cyclical structure. It also forms the ends of the beta sheets in the secondary structures.

223. Ans. (a) Pyridoxal phosphate

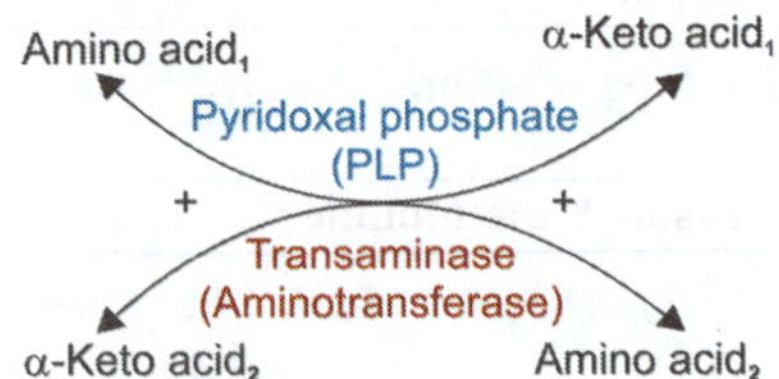

- Transamination involves reversible transfer of alpha amino group of alpha amino acid to an alpha-keto-acid to form a new amino acid and a new keto-acid.
- Enzyme catalyze this reaction is called transaminase (aminotransferase)
- All transaminase require **pyridoxal phosphate (Vit B6)** as a coenzyme
- **Example of transaminase are:**
  - Alanine transferase (ALT)
  - Aspartate transaminase (AST)
- Transamination reactions are **reversible**
- Transamination reactions occur **via ping pong mechanism** in which the 1st substrate bound and its product is realeased prior to binding of second substarte.
- Most amino acid undergo transamination **except lysine, theonine, proline, and hydroxyproline**

VITAMINS, MINERALS AND ENZYMES

224. Ans. (a) Niacin

Ref: Lippincott's Illustrated Reviews, 6th ed. pg. 532

- The image shows Casal's necklace pattern, which is seen in Pellagra.
- It is caused by deficiency of Vitamin B3 commonly known as **Niacin.**
- It involves skin, gastrointestinal tract, and CNS
- The symptoms of pellagra progress through the three Ds: dermatitis, diarrhea, and dementia. If untreated, death (a fourth D) occurs.

225. Ans. (d) Vitamin B_6

Ref: Lippincott's Illustrated Reviews, 6th ed. pg. 529

- Vitamin B_6 is the only water-soluble vitamin with significant toxicity.
- Neurologic symptoms (sensory neuropathy) occur at intakes above 500 mg/day.
- Symptoms include pain, tingling sensation, pins-and-needles sensation, numbness and weakness.

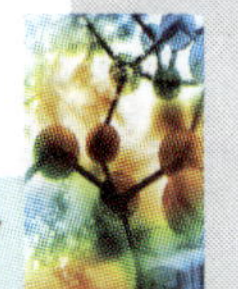

226. Ans. (c) Copper deficiency

Ref: Lippincott's Illustrated Reviews, 6th ed. pg. 556

- Menkes disease (MNK), also known as Menkes syndrome, is an X-linked recessive disorder caused by mutations in genes coding for the copper-transport protein **ATP7A**, leading to copper deficiency.
- Characteristic findings include kinky hair, growth failure, and nervous system deterioration.

227. Ans. (c) Niacin

Ref: Lippincott's Illustrated Reviews, 6th ed. pg. 532

- Pellagra can be common in people who obtain most of their food energy from corn, notably rural South America, where maize is a staple food.
- If maize is not nixtamalized, it is a poor source of tryptophan, as well as niacin, that can lead to pellagra.
- Nixtamalization is done to remove the toxins from the maize and other grains by soaking and cooking it in an alkaline solution (like lime water) followed by washing and removing its shell.

228. Ans. (b) Vitamin B12

Ref: Lippincott's Illustrated Reviews, 6th ed. pg. 525

- Vitamin B12 is one of important nutritional components that affect oral health.
- Individuals with decreased levels of vitamin B12 have been reported to exhibit various oral manifestations such as glossitis, glossodynia, recurrent ulcers, cheilitis, dysgeusia, lingual paresthesia, burning sensations, and pruritus.

229. Ans. (a) RBC transketolase activity

Ref: Lippincott's Illustrated Reviews, 6th ed. pg. 530

- Vitamin B1 (thiamine) is an essential nutrient that acts as a cofactor for a number of metabolic processes, particularly in energy metabolism.
- Symptoms of classic thiamine deficiency are recognized as beriberi, although clinical symptoms are nonspecific and recognition of subclinical deficiency is difficult. Therefore, reliable biomarkers of thiamine status are required.
- Thiamine diphosphate is a cofactor for transketolase, including erythrocyte transketolase (ETK). The ETK activity assay as an indirect, functional marker of thiamine status.

230. Ans. (d) Vitamin C

Ref: Lippincott's Illustrated Reviews, 6th ed. pg. 528

- Symptoms can manifest after 3 months of deficient intake of vitamin C-containing foods.
- Ascorbic acid is required for collagen synthesis. Its deficiency usually manifests with bleeding gums, ecchymoses, easy bruising, petechiae, coiled hairs and hyperkeratosis.

231. Ans. (b) B_{12}

Ref: Lippincott's Illustrated Reviews, 6th ed. pg. 527

- Vitamin B_{12} binds to the protein in the foods we eat. In the stomach, hydrochloric acid and enzymes unbind vitamin B_{12} into its free form. From there, vitamin B_{12} combines with a glycoprotein called intrinsic factor so that it can be absorbed further down in the small intestine.
- The cobalamin-IF complex travels through the intestine and binds to **cubulin** receptors on surface of mucosal cells of ileum, **which transports Vitamin B_{12} into general circulation.**
- Hence, ileal resection will lead to deficiency of Vitamin B_{12}.

232. Ans. (d) Conversion of 7 dehydro cholesterol to cholecalciferol

Ref: Lippincott's Illustrated Reviews, 6th ed. pg. 539

- 7-Dehydrocholestrol, an intermediate in cholesterol synthesis, is converted to cholecalciferol in the dermis and epidermis of humans exposed to ultraviolet light from sunlight and transported to liver bound to Vitamin-D binding protein.
- Vitamin-D is also known as '**Sunshine Vitamin**'

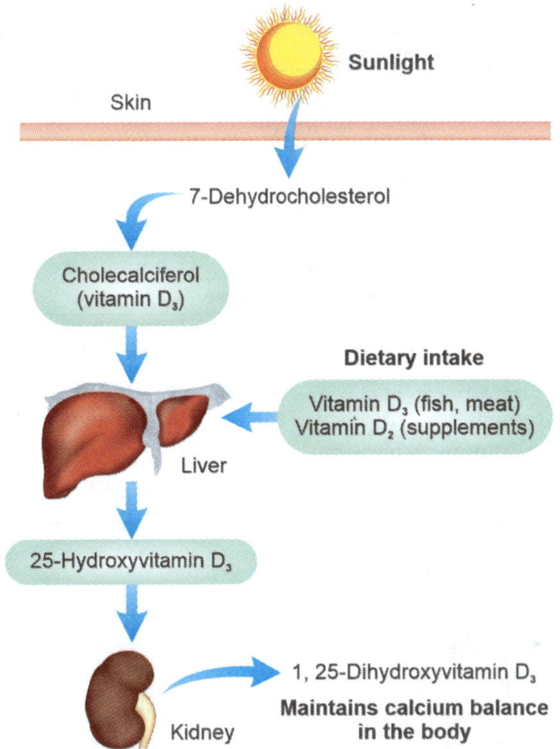

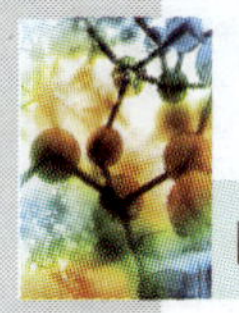

233. Ans. (b) Vitamin B_2

Ref: Lippincott's Illustrated Reviews, 6th ed. pg. 532

- The condition represents cheilosis (fissuring at the corners of the mouth) which is a common deficiency symptom seen in case of Vitamin B_2 or Riboflavin deficiency.
- Other symptoms of vitamin B_2 deficiency include dermatitis and glossitis (Tongue appearing smooth and dark).

234. Ans. (b) Vitamin B_9 deficiency

Ref: Lippincott's Illustrated Reviews, 6th ed. pg. 523

- Folate deficiency also results in elevated levels of homocysteine because of reduced activity of the methionine synthase–catalyzed reaction.
- Total homocysteine concentration, which comprises the sum of all homocysteine species in plasma/serum, including free and protein-bound forms, can be measured in plasma or serum.

235. Ans. (a) Selenium

Ref: Lippincott's Illustrated Reviews, 6th ed. pg. 561

- Selenocysteine is present at the catalytic site of glutathione peroxidase, and selenium availability regulates glutathione peroxidase enzyme activity.
- As a component of the glutathione cycle, it protects the liver from reactive oxygen metabolites.

236. Ans. (a) Vitamin C

Ref: Lippincott's Illustrated Reviews, 6th ed. pg. 528

- Vitamin C and iron deficiencies are both manifested by decreased collagen synthesis, which can result in delayed healing and capillary fragility.
- Wounds may fail to heal because scar tissue doesn't form.

237. Ans. (d) Glucose 6-phosphatase

Ref: Lippincott's Illustrated Reviews, 6th ed. pg. 235

Von Gierke disease is an **autosomal recessive** disorder caused by a deficiency of the enzyme glucose-6-phosphate translocase, which transports glucose-6-phosphate into the endoplasmic reticulum for further metabolism.

238. Ans. (a) B1

Ref: Lippincott's Biochemistry, 6th ed. pg. 693

- Thiamine deficiency is the established cause of an alcohol linked neurological disorder known as Wernicke-Korsakoff syndrome. It also contributes to other forms of alcohol induced brain injury.

239. Ans. (b) Folate

Ref: Lippincott's Biochemistry, 6th ed. pg. 684

- Folic acid deficiency causes macrocyclic Anemia and homocystinuria due to methyltetrahydrofolate deficiency that results from the poor metabolism of folate or lack of working of this enzyme. But the level of methyl malonate is normal, unlike vit B_{12} deficiency, where there is its high level.

240. Ans. (a) LDH-1

LDH (lactate dehydrogenase) has 5 isoenzymes:

• LDH 1	Heart and RBC
• LDH 2	WBC Very less amount in heart and RBC
• LDH 3	Lung tissue
• LDH 4	WBC, kidney, pancreatic cells and lymph nodes
• LDH 5	Liver and skeletal muscle

- Normally concentration of LDH 1 is lower than LDH 2, but after myocardial infarction, LDH 1 concentration becomes elevated and exceeds the concentration of LDH 2.

241. Ans. (a) Mn

Ref: Lippincott's Biochemistry, 6th ed. pg. 148

Superoxide dismutase is classified based on protein fold and metal cofactor:

- **Cu/Zn type**- cytosol of eukaryotes
- **Fe/Mn type**- prokaryotes, protista, mitochondria, chloroplast
  Mn SOD is found in human mitochondria
- **Ni type** – prokaryotes

242. Ans. (c) Calcium

Ref: Lippincott's Illustrated Reviews, Biochemistry 7th ed. pg. 399

- The macro minerals include: Calcium, Phosphorus (which is present as the inorganic phosphate), magnesium, sodium, chloride and potassium.
- Most other minerals are micronutrients for example: copper iron, manganese and zinc.
- Micro minerals can be further classified as trace micro minerals (for example iron and copper) and Ultra trace micro minerals like selenium and iodine.

243. Ans. (a) Retinol < 10

Ref: Lippincott's Illustrated reviews, Biochemistry 7th ed. pg. 386

- Retinol level estimation is a sensitive test.

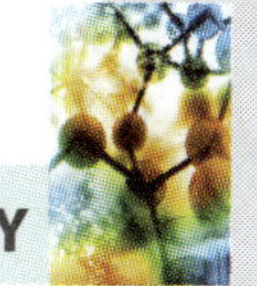

- Beta-carotene is obtained from plant foods and the conversion to vitamin A is inefficient and the vitamin activity of beta carotene is only about 1/12 that of retinol.
- Retinol is a primary alcohol which is the storage form of vitamin A.
- Night blindness and bitot spot are not a good test or the most sensitive test for vitamin A deficiency because they are not present in every person with vitamin A deficiency.

244. Ans. (c) Transketolase

Ref: Lippincott's Illustrated reviews, Biochemistry 7th ed. pg. 383

- Transketolase is a thiamine-dependent enzyme of the pentose phosphate pathway of glycolysis. This path forms a metabolic duct between the pentose/hexose phosphate shunt and the glycolytic pathway.
- The pentose phosphate shunt serves two major roles: to generate pentose sugars for nucleic acid and amino acid biosynthesis and to recover carbon that enters the pentose phosphate shunt via the oxidative route.
- Traditionally the erythrocyte transketolase saturation test, which is a measure of the stimulation of the transketolase reaction, has been used to assess thiamine status. A more sensitive test, however, is the measurement of thiamin-phosphorylated esters in plasma.

245. Ans. (a) Selenium

- Keshan disease is due to the deficiency of selenium.
- It can cause endemic cardiomyopathy.

Note:

- **Selenosis:** Chronic ingestion of large amount of selenium. Characterized by hair loss and nail brittleness, garlic breath odor, rash, myopathy etc.
- **Kashin-Beck disease:** A condition also due to selenium deficiency. It presents with osteochondropathy (long bone and skeletal deformity)

246. Ans. (a) Carbonic anhydrase

- **Zinc act as cofactor for important enzymes like:**
  - Carbonic anhydrase
  - Alcohol dehydrogenase
  - Lactate dehydrogenase
  - Carboxypeptidase

247. Ans. (b) Vitamin E

- Vitamins which act as anti-oxidants are: Vitamin A, C and E (tocopherol)
- Beta Carotene (Vit A) is an anti-oxidant at low PO_2.

These antioxidants are of two types:

1. **Preventive antioxidants:** Reduce the rate of chain initiation. Includes: Catalase, EDTA, DTPA
2. **Chain breaking antioxidant:** Interfere with chain propagation. Includes: SOD, Vitamin E.

248. Ans. (c) Vitamin C

- Vitamin C reduces ferric iron to ferrous form, thereby facilitating the absorption of dietary iron from the intestine.

249. Ans. (a) Thiamine

- The active form of thiamine (Vitamin B1) is thiamine pyrophosphate which is formed by the transfer of a pyrophosphate group from adenosine triphosphate (ATP) to thiamine.
- Thiamine deficiency is diagnosed by an increase in erythrocyte transketolase activity observed on addition of TPP

Deficiency of thiamine leads to:

- **Beri Beri:** A severe thiamine deficiency syndrome occurs due to intake of polished rice.
- **Wernicke-Korsakoff syndrome:** Associated with chronic alcoholism, which occurs due to dietary insufficiency or impaired dietary absorption of the vitamin. In some alcoholics there is development of Wernicke-Korsakoff syndrome, a thiamine deficiency syndrome characterized by confusion, ataxia and nystagmus with Wernicke's encephalopathy as well as memory problems, hallucination and dementia.

250. Ans. (b) Copper

Ref: Harrison's 20th ed. pg. 2318

Menkes Kinky Hair Syndrome

- X-Linked metabolic disturbance of copper metabolism
- Characterized by:
  - Mental retardation
  - Hypocupremia
  - Decreased circulating ceruloplasmin
- Due to mutation in **ATP7-A gene** (copper transporting gene)
- **Cause of death:** Dissecting aneurysm or cardiac rupture (usually <5 years of age)

Extra Mile

- **Wilson's disease:** Copper accumulation in liver, brain; due to mutation in ATP7-B gene.
- **Acrodermatitis enteropathica:** AR condition. Due to zinc deficiency
- **Chromium** potentiates the action of insulin and improves lipid profile
- **Keshan disease:** Endemic cardiomyopathy, due to dietary deficiency of selenium
- **Kashin-Beck disease:** Seen due to selenium deficiency and characterized by osteochondropathy

251. Ans. (b) Cell membrane

Ref: Lippincott's Biochemistry 6th ed. pg. 151-152

- G6PD enzyme is located at the cell membrane. RBC membrane is one such example, and is associated with severe pathology
- Location: X chromosome at q28 locus. (G6PD enzyme is X-linked gene)
- It protects the RBC from the deleterious effects of oxidizing agents by reducing themselves to NADPH.
- In deficiency of G6PD enzyme → impaired ability of RBC to form NADPH → Hemolysis

252. Ans. (c) X-Linked

Ref: Lippincott's Biochemistry 6th ed. pg. 151-152

- G6PD deficiency is most common disease producing enzyme abnormality in humans
- It is a X-linked disorder

253. Ans. (b) Enteropeptidase

- The pancreatic enzyme trypsinogen is activated to form trypsin with the help of enzyme enteropeptidase/ enterokinase.

Activation of some pancreatic zymogens

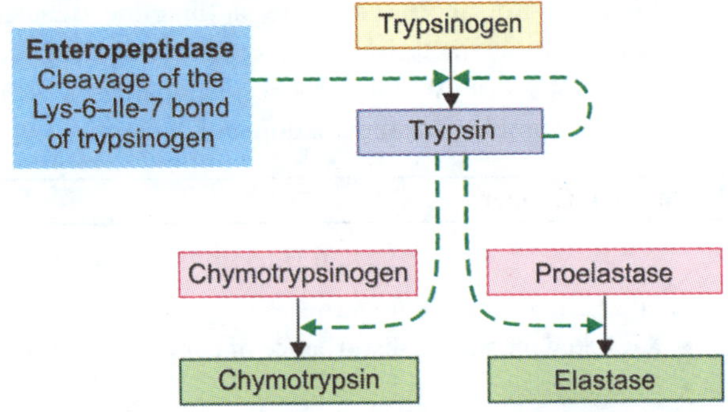

254. Ans. (c) It rescues proteins that have folded improperly and allows them to refold properly

Ref: Harper's Biochemistry, 30th ed. pg. 618-20, 26th ed. pg. 36-37

- **Over half of mammalian protein folding is done by Chaperone proteins.**
- Chaperones prevent aggregation, thus providing an opportunity for the formation of appropriate secondary structural elements.
- **There are 2 families of hsp:** hsp 60 and hsp 70.
- The hsp 60 family of chaperones, sometimes called chaperonins, differ in sequence and structure from hsp 70 and its homologs.
- The HSP 70 (70-kDa heat shock protein) **family of chaperones binds short sequences of hydrophobic amino acids in newly synthesized polypeptides, shielding them from solvent.**
- **Chaperone proteins can also "rescue" proteins** that have become thermodynamically trapped in a misfolded dead end. They rescue it **by unfolding hydrophobic regions and providing a second chance to fold productively.**

Extra Mile

- Chaperones for eukaryotes: Hsp 70
- Force favourable for protein folding: Hydrophobic interaction

255. Ans. (b) Chemical antagonism

Ref: Vasudevan Biochemistry, 8th ed. pg. 321

- **Chemical:** A type of antagonism where a drug counters the effect of another by simple chemical reaction/ neutralization (not binding to the receptor).
- **Physiological:** Two drugs act on two different types of receptor and antagonize action of each other.
- **Competitive:** Both drugs bind to same receptor.

256. Ans. (b) Vitamin C

Ref: Vasudevan Biochemistry, 8th ed. pg. 481

TABLE: The vitamins

Vitamin		Functions
A	Retinol, β-carotene	Visual pigments in the retina; regulation of gene expression and cell differentiation; β-carotene is an antioxidant
D	Calciferol	Maintenance of calcium balance; enhances intestinal absorption of Ca^{2+} and mobilizes bone mineral
E	Tocopherols, tocotrienols	Antioxidant, especially in cell membranes
K	Phylloquinone, menaquinones	Coenzyme in formation of γ-carboxyglutamate in enzymes of blood clotting and bone matrix
B_1	Thiamine	Coenzyme in pyruvate and α-ketoglutarate, dehydrogenases, and transketolase; poorly defined function in nerve conduction
B_2	Riboflavin	Coenzyme in oxidation and reduction reactions; prosthetic group of flavoproteins
Niacin	Nicotinic acid, nicotinamide	Coenzyme in oxidation and reduction reactions, functional part of NAD and NADP
B_6	Pyridoxine, pyridoxal, pyridoxamine	Coenzyme in transamination and decarboxylation of amino acids and glycogen phosphorylase; role in steroid hormone action
	Folic acid	Coenzyme in transfer of one-carbon fragments

Contd...

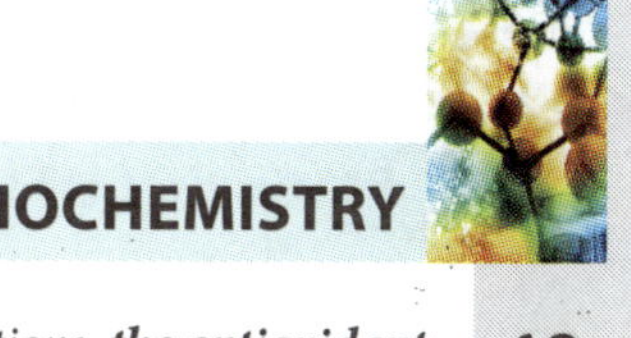

Vitamin		Functions
B_{12}	Cobalamin	Coenzyme in transfer of one-carbon fragments and metabolism of folic acid
	Pantothenic acid	Functional part of CoA and acyl carrier protein; fatty acid synthesis and metabolism
H	Biotin	Coenzyme in carboxylation reactions in gluconeogenesis and fatty acid synthesis
C	Ascorbic acid	Coenzyme in hydroxylation of proline and lysine in collagen synthesis; antioxidant; enhances absorption of iron

257. Ans. (c) ATP

Ref: Vasudevan Biochemistry, 8/e. P 531

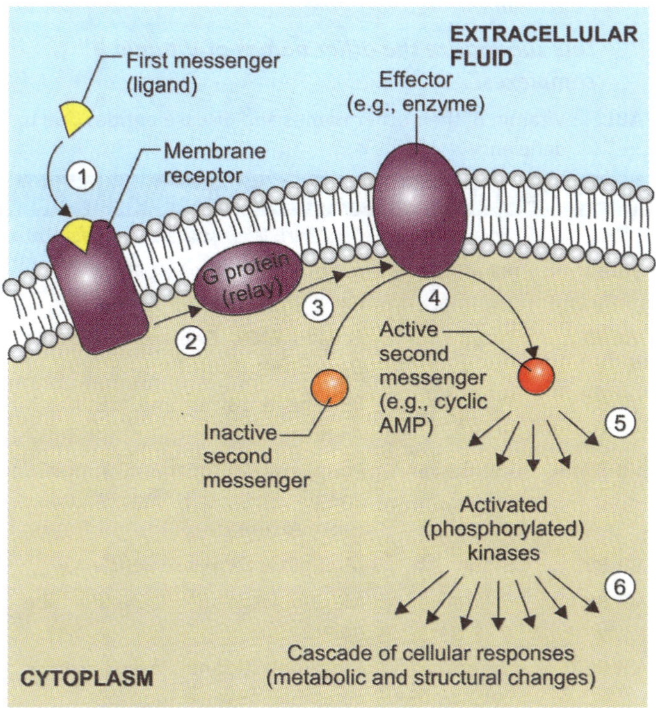

- **Cyclic AMP (cAMP)** is formed from cytosolic ATP by **adenylyl cyclase**, an enzyme that is anchored in the plasma membrane
- The enzyme is inactive until bound to activated Gs_{α}; (by receptor-ligand stimulated acquisition of GTP and release (from $Gs_{\beta\gamma}$)
- Gi_{α} inhibits adenylyl cyclase

258. Ans. (c) Vitamin E

Ref: Harper's Biochemistry, 30th ed. pg. 553, 564

- *Vitamin E has many biological functions,* ***the antioxidant function being the most important and/or best known.***
- **Other functions include:**
  - Enzymatic activities
  - Gene expression
  - Neurological function and
  - Cell signalling
- As an antioxidant, **vitamin E acts as a peroxyl radical scavenger,** preventing the propagation of free radicals in tissues.
- It does so by reacting with ROS to form a tocopheryl radical, which will then be reduced by a hydrogen donor (such as vitamin C) to its reduced state. As it is fat-soluble, it is incorporated into cell membranes, which protects them from oxidative damage.

259. Ans. (c) Keshan disease

- **Keshan disease** is an endemic cardiomyopathy found in children and young women of chinese regions due to dietary deficiency of selenium.
- **Kashin beck disease:** Occurs due to selenium deficiency. It is characterized by osteochondropathy.
- **Selenosis:** Due to selenium toxicity-characterized by hair loss, brittle nail, myopathy etc.

260. Ans. (b) Exist in three forms

TABLE: Forms of VITAMIN K

	Vitamin K1	Vitamin K2	Vitamin K3
Also known as	Phylloquinone	Menaquinone	Menadione
Source	Several green vegetables and prepared synthetically	Synthesized by GI bacteria, supplies 50% human requirement	Synthetic, Analog of 1,4-naphtho-quinone
Solubility	Fat soluble	Fat soluble	***Diphosphate salt is Water soluble***

261. Ans. (a) Oxidase-Reductase

Oxidoreductase enzyme groups can be remembered by mnemonic DOOP

- Dehydrogenases
- Oxidases
- Oxygenases
- Peroxidases

262. Ans. (a) Chromium

Ref: Harrisons, 19th ed. pg. 96e-9

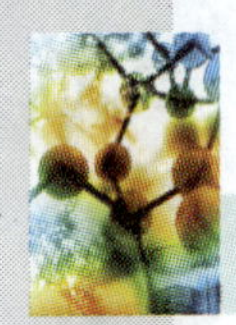

- A deficiency of chromium can cause impaired glucose tolerance.
- Physiologically, chromium potentiates the action of insulin in patients with impaired glucose tolerance, presumably by increasing insulin receptor-mediated signalling.
- Rich food sources of chromium include yeast, meat, and grain products.
- **Note:**
  - **Deficiency of Selenium:** Can cause cardiomyopathy **(Keshan disease)**
  - **Selenium toxicity:** Can cause selenosis **(Kashinbeck disease)**

263. Ans. (d) Zinc

TABLE: Important minerals and their respective action as cofactor

Minerals	Function
Selenium	• Cofactor for ▪ Glutathione peroxidase ▪ Deiodinase ▪ Thioredoxin reductase
Manganese	• Cofactor for: ▪ Arginase ▪ Kinase ▪ Carboxylase ▪ Glucosyl transferase ▪ Enolase
Zinc	• Cofactor for: ▪ Carbonic anhydrase ▪ Alcohol dehydrogenase ▪ **Lactate dehydrogenase** ▪ Carboxypeptidase

264. Ans. (a) K_m increased, V_{max} same

Type of Inhibition	Km	Vmax
Competitive inhibition	INCREASED	SAME
Non-competitive inhibition	Same	DECREASED

Competitive Inhibtion: Substrate and inhibitor, both compete for same site on enzyme.
Non-competitive Inhibition: Substrate and inhibitor both bind at different sites in the enzyme.

265. Ans. (c) Methionine synthase

Ref: Harper's Biochemistry, 30th ed. pg. 558

CONVERSION OF HOMOCYSTEINE TO METHIONINE

- Active form in this reaction is methycobalamin. This reaction requires both methylcobalamin and folic acid. The reaction is catalyzed by methionine synthase which is a methylcobalamin dependent reaction.

$$\text{Homocysteine} \xrightarrow[\textit{Methylcobalamin + folic acid}]{\text{Methionine synthase}} \text{Methionine}$$

266. Ans. (b) Consist of flavin group which is required in oxidation-reduction reaction

Ref: Harper's Biochemistry, 30th ed. pg. 556

RIBOFLAVIN is vitamin B_2 which contains isoelloxazine ring. It gives yellow color, therefore used to fortify some foods.

- ***It consists of flavin group which is required in oxidation-reduction reactions.***
- **Source:** Meat products, liver, egg, whole grain, vegetables
  - *Green leafy vegetables are major sources of folic acid (B9)*
- **Deficiency causes:** Angular stomatitis, cheilosis, dermatitis, Glossitis, geographic tongue Lesion on mouth and genitalia.

Lets summarize the other names of Vitamin B complexes:

TABLE: Vitamin B, their other names and disease entities due to deficiency

Vitamin	Other name	Deficiency causes
Vit B1	Thiamine	***Beri Beri,*** *Wernicke's encephalopathy*
Vit B2	Riboflavin	Angular stomatitis, cheilosis, dermatitis, Glossitis
Vit B3	Niacin	Pellagra ***(4D's- Dementia, Diarrhea, Dermatitis, Death)***
Vit B5	Pantothenic acid	Burning foot syndrome, Liener disease
Vit B6	Pyridoxine	Peripheral neuropathy, Sideroblastic anemia, Pellagra, Homocystinuria, Hartnup disease
Vit B7	Biotin	Multiple carboxylase deficiency
Vit B9	Folic acid	Megaloblastic anemia, Neural tube defect
Vit B12	Cyano-cobalamin	Megaloblastic anemia, subacute combined degeneration (SACD)

267. Ans. (c) Biotin

Ref: Harper's Biochemistry, 30th ed. pg. 560-61

- Acetyl-C0A carboxylase is a biotin-depenent enzyme that catalyzes the irreversible carboxylation of acetyl-CoA to produce malonyl-CoA through its two catalytic activities, biotin carboxylase and carboxyl transferase

268. Ans. (b) Folic acid

Ref: Harper's Biochemistry, 30th ed. pg. 299, 559-560, 26th ed. pg. 494

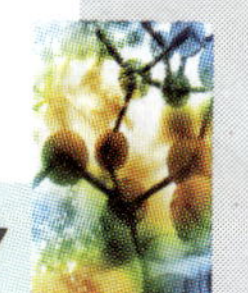

269. Ans. (b) Deficiency of tryptophan

Ref: Harper's Biochemistry 30th ed. pg. 546, 557, 29th ed. pg. 540

- Pellagra is seen due to deficiency of niacin (vitamin B3) aka nicotinic acid.
- **Nicotinic acid can be formed in the body from tryptophan**. 60 mg of tryptophan forms 1 mg of niacin. Henceforth, deficiency of tryptophan causes deficiency of niacin leading to pellagra.

Extra Mile

- **Deficiency of thiamine causes:** Beri-Beri, Wernicke's encephalopathy, Lactic acidosis
- **Deficiency of Vitamin B12 causes:** Pernicious anemia, Megaloblastic anemia, SCID, methymalonic acidura.
- **Deficiency of vitamin B9/Folic acid:** Megaloblastic anemia, NTD.

270. Ans. (a) Vitamin K

Ref: Harper's Biochemistry, 30th ed. pg. 554

- Menadione is the water soluble form of vitamin K.

TABLE: Forms of VITAMIN K

	Vitamin K1	Vitamin K2	Vitamin K3
Aka	Phylloquinone	Menaquinone	Menadione
Source	Several green vegetables and prepared synthetically	Synthesized by GI bacteria, supplies 50% human requirement	Synthetic, Analog of 1,4-naphthoquinone
Solubility	Fat soluble	Fat soluble	Diphosphate salt is Water soluble

- Vitamin K Is the Coenzyme for Carboxylation of Glutamate in Postsynthetic Modification of Calcium Binding Proteins. Vitamin K Is Also Important in Synthesis of Bone Calcium Binding Proteins.
- ***Dicumarol is an anticoagulant that functions as a vitamin K antagonist.***

271. Ans. (c) Menadione

Ref: Harper's Biochemistry, 30th ed. pg. 554

Please refer to above table

272. Ans. (c) Menadione

Ref: Harper's Biochemistry, 30th ed. pg. 554

273. Ans. (d) Vitamin K

Ref: Harper's Biochemistry, 30th ed. pg. 554-555

- Anti-oxidants are vitamin A, C and vitamin E (ACE). *Most important of all is vitamin E.*
- Free-radicals are formed from exposure to sunlight and pollution and also as a byproduct of cell metabolism.
- Alcohol, cigarette smoke, stress and even diet also affect the level of free-radical development in the body. Excellent antioxidants include Vitamin A, Vitamin E, Vitamin C, zinc, selenium, ginkgo biloba, grape seed extract, and green tea extract.

274. Ans. (a) Vitamin K

Ref: Harper's Biochemistry, 30th ed. pg. 5341-42, 554, 26th ed. pg. 481

Apart from **dietary inadequacy,** conditions affecting the digestion and absorption of the lipid-soluble vitamins (vitamins **A, D, E and K)** such as **steatorrhea and disorders of the biliary system,** all can lead to deficiency syndromes, including: night blindness and xerophthalmia (vitamin A); rickets in young children and osteomalacia in adults (vitamin D); neurologic disorders and anemia of the newborn (vitamin E); and hemorrhage of the newborn (vitamin K).

Vitamin K is also important in the synthesis of bone calcium-binding proteins like osteocalcin and bone matrix Gla protein. In fact, the release into the circulation of **osteocalcin provides an index of vitamin D status.**

275. Ans. (b) Vitamin C

Ref: K. Park, 23rd ed. pg. 630

- ***Eggs has all the nutrients except vitamin C and carbohydrate.***
- Eggs are also a source of folate , biotin pantothenic acid, choline, phosporous, iodine and selenium in terms of minerals and vitamins.
- ***Egg contains Avidin, which interferes with biotin absorption.***

276. Ans. (b) Zinc deficiency

Ref: Harrison's, 19th ed. pg. 96e-9

- Zinc is an essential trace nutrient required for the proper function of more than 100 enzymes and plays a crucial role in nucleic acid metabolism.
- Acrodermatitis enteropathica is an **autosomal recessive** disorder postulated to occur as a result of mutations in the ***SLC39A4* gene** located on band **8q24.3.**

- This protein is highly expressed in the **enterocytes in the duodenum and jejunum.** Therefore, affected individuals have a decreased ability to absorb zinc from dietary sources. Absence of a binding ligand needed to transport zinc may further contribute to zinc malabsorption.
- **Clinical manifestations include** diarrhea, alopecia, muscle wasting, depression, irritability, and a rash involving the extremities, face, and perineum. The rash is characterized by vesicular and pustular crusting with scaling and erythema.
- Features of acrodermatitis enteropathica **start appearing in the first few months of life,** if mother discontinues breast milk.

TABLE: Deficiency and toxicity of several metals

Element	Deficiency	Toxicity
Boron	No biologic function determined	Developmental defects, male sterility, testicular atrophy
Calcium	Reduced bone mass, osteoporosis	Renal insufficiency (milk-alkali syndrome)[Q] nephrolithiasis, impaired iron absorption, thiazide diuretics.
Copper	Anemia, growth retardation, defective keratinization and pigmentation of hair, hypothermia, degenerative changes in aortic elastin[Q], osteopenia, mental deterioration.	Nausea, vomiting, diarrhea, hepatic failure, tremor, mental deterioration, hemolytc anemia, renal dysfunction
Chromium	Impaired glucose tolerance[Q]	*Occupational*;Renal failure, dermatitis, pulmonary cancer
Fluoride	↑Dental caries[Q]	Dental and skeletal flurosis[Q], osteosclerosis
Iodine	Thyroid enlargement, ↓T_4 cretinism	Thyroid dysfunction, acne-like eruptions[Q].
Iron	Muscle abnormalities, koilonychia, pica anemia, ↓work performance, impaired cognitive development, premature labor, ↑perinatal maternal death	Gastrointestinal effects, (nausea, vomiting, diarrhea, constipation), iron overload with organ damage, acute and chronic systemic toxicity, increased susceptibility to malaria, increased risk association with certain chronic diseases (e.g. diabetes)
Manganese	Impaired growth and skeletal development reproduction, lipid and carbohydrate metabolism, upper body rash	*General:* Neurotoxicity, Parkinson-like symptoms[Q] *Occupational*: Encephalitis like syndrome, Parkinson like syndrome, psychosis, pneumoconiosis.
Molybdenum	Severe neurologic abnormalities	Reproductive and fetal abnormalities
Selenium	Cardiomyopathy, heart failure, striated muscle degeneration	*General:* Alopecia , nausea, vomiting, abnormal nails, emotional
Phosphorus	Rickets (osteomalacia) proximal muscle weakness, rhabdomyolysis, paresthesia, ataxia, seizure confusion, heart failure, hemolysis acidosis.	Hyperphosphatemia
Zinc	Growth retardation, ↓taste and smell alopecia, dermatitis, diarrhea, immune dysfunction, failure to thrive, gonasal atrophy, congenital malfomations.	General: Reduced copper, absorption, gastritis, sweating fever,nausea, vomiting *Occupational;* Respiratory distress, pulmonary fibrosis

277. Ans. (c) ADP-ribosylation of Gs alpha sub-unit

Ref: Harper's Biochemistry, 30th ed. pg. 250

Cholera Toxin Acts by the Following Mechanism

- The B subunit ring of the cholera toxin binds to GM1 gangliosides on the surface of target cells. Once bound, the entire toxin complex is endocytosed by the cell and the cholera toxin **A1 (CTA1) chain is released** and leads to ADP ribosylation of G_S subunit massive fluid efflux in GI lumen.
- *Cholera toxin ADP-ribosylates G proteins, causing* ↑cAMp and *massive fluid secretion from the lining of the small intestine, resulting in life-threatening diarrhea.*
- ADP-ribosylation is also responsible for the actions of some bacterial toxins, such as cholera toxin, diphtheria toxin, pertussis toxin, and heat-labile enterotoxin.

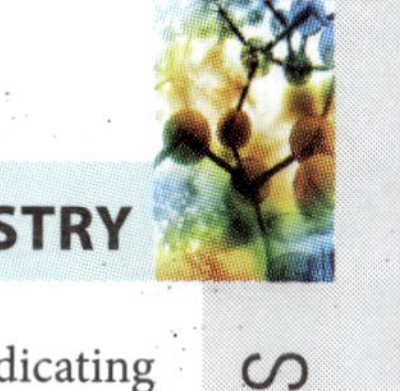

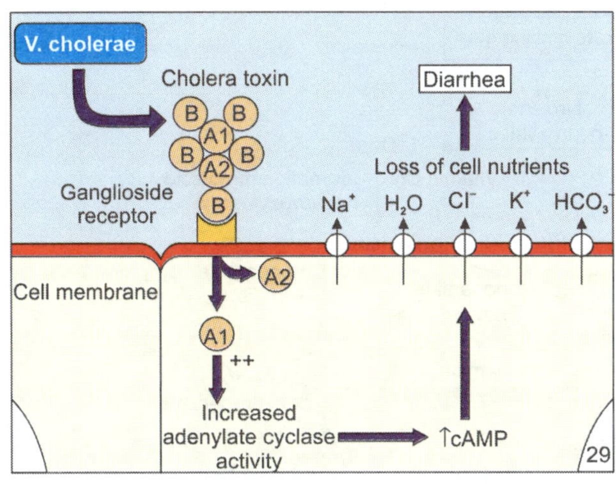

Extra Mile

- Active subunit of cholera toxin: A
- Binding subunit of cholera toxin: B

278. Ans. (c) 7.36-7.44

Ref: Harper's Biochemistry, 30th ed. pg. 10-13

Well I think this one is too simple for an explanation.
Also remember pH of urine = 4.6-8.0

Extra Mile

- Values of pH going above 7.4 is alkalosis and value of pH going below 7.4 is acidosis
- pH of Aqueous Humor - 7.2

TABLE: Conditions arising due to low and high pH

Low pH	High pH
• Metabolic acidosis • Respiratory acidosis	• Metabolic alkalosis • Repiratory alkalosis

279. Ans. (b) Net protein utilization

Ref: K.Park 23th ed.

- The **net protein utilization**, or NPU, is the ratio of amino acid converted to proteins to the ratio of amino acids supplied. This figure is somewhat affected by the salvage of essential amino acids within the body, but is profoundly affected by the level of limiting amino acids within a foodstuff.
- NPU can range from 1 to 0, with a value of 1 indicating 100% utilization of dietary nitrogen as protein and a value of 0 an indication that none of the nitrogen supplied was converted to protein. Certain foodstuffs, such as eggs or milk, rate as 1 on an NPU chart.

280. Ans. (a) Vitamin B_{12}

Ref: Harper's Biochemistry 30th ed. pg. 559

- Increased methyl malonic acid levels may indicate a vitamin B_{12} deficiency. However, it is sensitive but not specific. MMA is elevated in 90-98% of patients with B_{12} deficiency.
- The coenzyme A is linked form of methylmalonic acid. Methylmalonyl-CoA, is converted into succinyl-CoA by methylmalonyl-CoA mutase, in a reaction that requires vitamin B_{12} as a cofactor.

$$\text{Methylmalonyl - CoA} \xrightarrow[\text{Vitamin } B_{12}]{\text{Methylmalonyl-CoA mutase}} \text{Succinyl - CoA}$$

$$\text{Methylmalonyl - CoA} \xrightarrow{\text{Methylmalonyl-CoA mutase}} \text{Succinyl - CoA}$$

- In this way, it enters the Krebs cycle, and is thus part of one of the anaplerotic reactions.

281. Ans. (d) Copper deposit

Ref: Harper's Biochemistry, 30th ed. pg. 496

- Wilson's disease is also associated with sunflower cataracts exhibited by brown or green pigmentation of the anterior and posterior lens capsule.
- *For more details about the different types of cataract, please refer to ophthalmology section.*

282. Ans. (b) Fibrillin

Ref: Harrison's, 19th ed.

- Fibrillin-1 is a major component of the microfibrils that form a sheath surrounding the amorphous elastin. It is believed that the microfibrils are composed of end-to-end polymers of fibrillin. To date, 3 forms of fibrillin have been described and mutations in the FBN1 gene cause Marfan's syndrome. This protein and its genes are found on chromosome 15.
- **Mutation in Fibrillin 1 gene (FBN 1) primarily affects: Skeletal system, Cardiovascular system and Eye.**

283. Ans. (c) Phenylalanine hydroxylase

Ref: Harper's Biochemistry, 30th ed. pg. 509-510

Please refer to explanation fig.

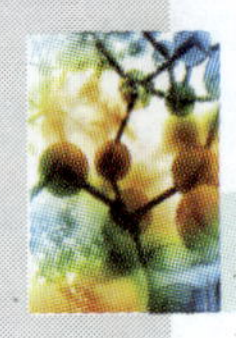

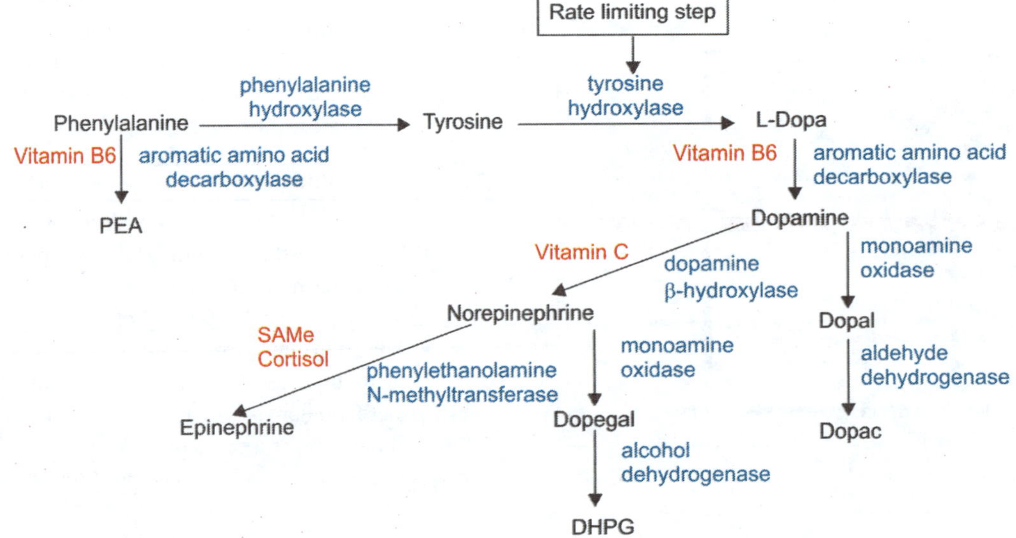

- **Phenylalanine hydroxylase**: for conversion of Phenylalanine to tyrosine conversion
- **Tyrosine hydroxylase**: for conversion of tyrosine to L-Dopa
- **Phenylethanolamine-*N*-methyltransferase:** for conversion of norepinephrine to epinephrine

284. Ans. (b) Phenylalanine

Ref: Harper's Biochemistry, 30th ed. pg. 509-10, 26th ed. pg. 255, 446

285. Ans. (a) Dopamine hydroxylase

Ref: Harper's Biochemistry, 30th ed. pg. 561

- Those enzymes that require inorganic metal ions as their cofactor are termed as metalloenzymes aka cofactors.
- ***Dopamine hydroxylase is a copper-containing enzyme involved in the synthesis of the catecholamines: Norepinephrine*** and Epinephrine from tyrosine in the adrenal medulla and central nervous system.
- Ascorbic acid is also linked with copper containing hydroxylases such as peptidoglycine hydroxylase and dopamine hydroxylase. Dopamine decarboxylase requires pyridoxal phosphate for the conversion of L-dopa to 3,4-dihydroxyphenylethylamine.

TABLE: Metals and their Metalloenzymes

Metal	Metalloenzymes
Copper	**Cytochrome oxidase, Lysyl oxidase, Dopamine Hydroxylase,** ascorbic acid oxidase, Tyrosinase, Ferroxidase (Ceruloplasmin), Superoxide Dismutase
Magnesium	**Hexokinase,** PFK, Glucose-6-phosphatase, Kinases, **Thermostable DNA polymerases, Enolase,** Creatinine kinase
Selenium	**Glutathione peroxidase**
Molybdenum	**Xanthine oxidase**
Calcium	**Lipase, Lecithinase**
Iron	**Cytochrome oxidase, Xanthine oxidase, Catalase, Peroxidase**
Nickel	**Urease**

Contd...

286. Ans. (a) Lysyl oxidase

Ref: Harper's Biochemistry, 30th ed. pg. 628

- Lysyl oxidase is an extracellular copper enzyme that catalyzes formation of aldehydes from lysine residues in collagen and elastin precursors.

Please refer to above table

287. Ans. (b) Xanthine oxidase

Ref: Harper's Biochemistry, 30th ed. pg. 120

288. Ans. (d) Copper

Ref: Harper's Biochemistry, 30th ed. pg. 629-30

- Copper plays a role in collagen cross linking and is catalyzed by lysyl oxidase.
- This enzyme utilizes copper as cupric ion.
- The genetic deficiency of lysyl oxidase is seen in Ehler danlos syndrome.

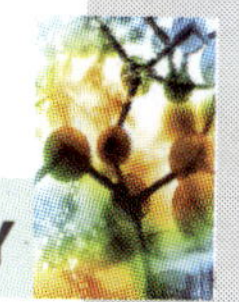

289. Ans. (b) Mg^{2+}

Ref: Harper's Biochemistry, 30th ed. pg. 458-59

- Magnesium is required as a co-factor for thermostable DNA polymerase, which is required for PCR.
- Taq polymerase is a magnesium-dependent enzyme and determining the optimum concentration to use is critical to the success of the PCR reaction.
- Some of the components of the reaction mixture such as template concentration, dNTPs and the presence of chelating agents (EDTA) or proteins can reduce the amount of free magnesium present thus reducing the activity of the enzyme.
- Primers which bind to incorrect template sites are stabilized in the presence of excessive magnesium concentrations and so result in decreased specificity of the reaction.
- Excessive magnesium concentrations also stabilize double stranded DNA and prevent complete denaturation of the DNA during PCR reducing the product yield.

290. Ans. (c) Normal K_m, decrease V_{max}

Ref: Harper's Biochemistry, 30th ed. pg. 81-82

Type of Inhibition	Km	Vmax
Competitive inhibition	INCREASED	SAME
Non-competitive inhibition	Same	DECREASED

Competitive Inhibition: Substrate and inhibitor Both compete for same site on enzyme.

Non-Competitive Inhibition: Substrate and Inhibitor both bind at different site in the enzyme.

291. Ans. (a) Glucokinase

Ref: Harper's Biochemistry, 30th ed. pg. 61-62

- Glucokinase is an enzyme which phosphorylates the glucose to glucose 6 phosphate in the cells. It is a phosphorylase enzyme and not an oxidoreductase. *Please see below Table.*

TABLE: Enzymes according to their family

I	II	III	IV	V	VI
Oxidoreductases	**Transferases**	**Hydrolases**	**Lyases**	**Isomerases**	**Ligases**
• Dehydrogenases • Oxidases • Oxygenases • Peroxidases • Catalase	Amino transferase Methyl-transferase Phosphorylases Kinases	• Phosphatases • Phosphodiesterases • Proteases • Peptidase Lipases Nuclease, Nucleotidase, Nucleosidase	Carbonic anhydrase Aldolase Decarboxylases	RECEMASES Epimerase Mutases	Carboxylases Synthetases Synthase
Mn: DOOP–Cat	*Mn: Amir Me & P-K*	*Mn: P4-LN*	*Mn: CAD*	Mn: REM	

PHARMACOLOGY

4

MOST RECENT QUESTIONS 2023

1. **An elderly male bought two bottles of alcohol from the local liquor shop. After consuming, he developed symptoms like ataxia, drowsiness and blurred vision. Which of the following is preferred for this patient?**
(Most Recent Question July 2023)
   a. Flumazenil b. Naloxone
   c. Ethyl alcohol d. Fomepizole
2. **Which of the following agent is preferred in treatment of benzodiazepine overdose?**
(Most Recent Question July 2023)
   a. Fomepizole b. Naloxone
   c. Flumazenil d. Folinic acid
3. **A thalassemia patient with history of multiple blood transfusion was brought with chronic iron overload. Which of the following will be preferred oral agent for managing his chronic iron overload symptoms?**
(Most Recent Question July 2023)
   a. Vitamin B_{12} supplementation
   b. EDTA
   c. D-penicillamine
   d. Deferiprone
4. **A female with history of HIV positive, not taking any antiretroviral therapy delivered a baby. What should be the initial treatment that should be started immediately to the newborn?** *(Most Recent Question July 2023)*
   a. Nevirapine for 6 weeks
   b. Nevirapine + Zidovudine for 6 weeks
   c. Nevirapine for 6 months
   d. Nevirapine + Zidovudine for 6 months
5. **A new drug Bedaquiline is approved for the treatment of MDR-TB. What is the mechanism of action of this drug?**
(Most Recent Question July 2023)
   a. Inhibits adenosine triphosphate synthase of mycobacteria
   b. Inhibits DNA-dependent RNA polymerase of mycobacteria
   c. Inhibits arabinosyltransferase of mycobacteria
   d. Inhibits catalase peroxidase of mycobacteria
6. **A 30-year-old female patient was brought by her husband in OPD with symptoms of depression. She was started in antidepressant therapy and now presented with insomnia, restlessness, agitation, anxiety, diarrhea and headache. Husband states that these symptoms were not there prior to starting the therapy. Which of the following drug could have caused these symptoms?**
(Most Recent Question July 2023)
   a. Lithium b. Fluoxetine
   c. Buspirone d. Haloperidol
7. **A 70-year-old patient was brought to the OPD with complaints of urinary hesitancy and incomplete urination. USG shows enlarged prostate gland and residual urine volume of 130 mL. Which of the following agent is used in the treatment of this patient?**
(Most Recent Question July 2023)
   a. 5-alpha-reductase inhibitor
   b. Calcium channel blocker
   c. ACE inhibitor
   d. Aldosterone receptor antagonist
8. **A 44-year-old patient with history of HIV positive, presents to OPD with complaints of blurred vision and floaters in the left eye. Fundoscopy reveals cotton wool spots and pizza pie appearance and the diagnosis of CMV retinitis is made. Which of the following is most appropriate treatment for this patient?**
(Most Recent Question July 2023)
   a. Aciclovir
   b. Cotrimoxazole
   c. Ganciclovir
   d. Tenofovir
9. **A patient with history of psychiatric condition and on some medication was brought to emergency with sudden hypertensive episode after consuming wine. Which of the following drug he might be consuming?**
(Most Recent Question July 2023)
   a. Phenelzine
   b. Amitriptyline
   c. Fluoxetine
   d. Trazodone

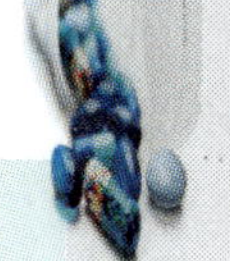

10. Which of the following adverse effect is not seen even after a year of lithium therapy? *(Most Recent Question July 2023)*

a. Hypothyroidism b. Diabetes insipidus
c. Tardive dyskinesia d. Tremors

11. A young person is planning for a trip to Ladakh. To prevent the motion sickness, which of the following should be preferred? *(Most Recent Question July 2023)*

a. Scopolamine b. Promethazine
c. Acetazolamide d. Sumatriptan

12. Thyroid hormone acts via which receptor? *(Most Recent Question July 2023)*

a. Tyrosine kinase receptor
b. Nuclear receptor
c. Ligand-gated receptor
d. G-protein-coupled receptor

13. Which of the following agent is preferred in patient with facial palsy? *(Most Recent Question July 2023)*

a. Prednisolone b. Aciclovir
c. Ceftriaxone d. Naproxen

14. Which of the following agent is not used in bacterial vaginosis? *(Most Recent Question July 2023)*

a. Metronidazole b. Tinidazole
c. Erythromycin d. Clindamycin

15. Which of the following is not acceptable as emergency contraceptive method? *(Most Recent Question July 2023)*

a. COCP two tablets immediately and two tablets after 12 hours within 2 days
b. Ulipristal 30 mg single dose within 5 days
c. Centchroman 50 mg two tablets 12 hours apart within 24 hours
d. Levonorgestrel 0.075 mg two tablets within 24 hours

16. A patient was given penicillin and within hours he developed swelling on face and lips. Which of the following hypersensitivity reaction is this? *(Most Recent Question July 2023)*

a. Type 1 b. Type 2
c. Type 3 d. Type 4

17. A patient treated for leprosy developed type 2 lepra reaction. Identify the type of hypersensitivity reaction: *(Most Recent Question July 2023)*

a. Type 1 b. Type 2
c. Type 3 d. Type 4

18. A patient of pheochromocytoma underwent surgery. Which of the following agent is given to prior to surgery control the intraoperative hypertension of the patient? *(Most Recent Question July 2023)*

a. Alpha-adrenergic blockers
b. Beta-blockers
c. 5-alpha-reductase blockers
d. Phosphodiesterase inhibitors

19. A patient consumed an antiemetic metoclopramide. Which of the following statement is incorrect about this drug? *(Most Recent Question July 2023)*

a. Can cause hyperprolactinemia
b. Can cause extrapyramidal symptoms like dystonia
c. Crosses BBB
d. Safer than domperidone in children

20. A 55 year patient diagnosed with cervical cancer. DOC for cervical cancer is: *(Most Recent Question July 2023)*

a. Cisplatin b. Tamoxifen
c. Paclitaxel d. Adriamycin

21. A 60-year-old female presented with cervical carcinoma. She was started on cisplatin therapy. Which of the following is most important toxicity of cisplatin? *(Most Recent Question July 2023)*

a. GI toxicity b. Neurotoxicity
c. Nephrotoxicity d. Pulmonary fibrosis

22. Which of the following causes thymidine-less death of cancer cells? *(Most Recent Question July 2023)*

a. 5-fluorouracil b. 6-mercaptopurine
c. Methotrexate d. Cyclophosphamide

23. A 5-year-old child was brought to OPD by parents with complaints of squint and decreased vision. For doing the refraction testing which of the following drug will be most suitable for this patient? *(Most Recent Question July 2023)*

a. Atropine ointment 1% b. Tropicamide 1%
c. Timolol 0.5% d. Loteprednol 0.5%

24. Which of the following is correct regarding STEP criteria of drugs? *(Most Recent Question July 2023)*

a. Related to drug metabolism
b. Related to clinical trials
c. Related to concept of P-drug
d. Related to volume of distribution of drug

25. Which of the following is correct protocol for treatment of pulmonary tuberculosis (PTB) in children? *(Most Recent Question July 2023)*

a. 4 HRZE + 2 HR
b. 2 HRZE + 4 HR + Steroids
c. 4 HRZE + 2 HRE
d. 2 HRZE + 4 HRE

26. A female patient was having pain in her great toe (metatarsal joint) with swelling and redness present over it. Her uric acid level is also high. She was treated with a proper drug therapy and her symptoms subsided. The drug that has reduced her uric acid level must have act by: *(Most Recent Question Jan 2023)*

a. Xanthine oxidase inhibition
b. HGPRTase inhibition
c. Thymidylate synthase inhibitor
d. Phosphoribosyltransferase inhibitor

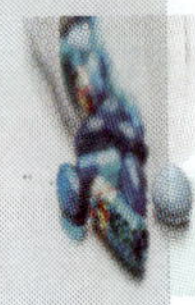

27. A patient had chronic pain related to gout for a month and it subsided after medication. What will be added for the excretion of uric acid in urine? ***(Most Recent Question Jan 2023)***

a. Allopurinol b. Febuxostat
c. Colchicine d. Probenecid

28. A patient had history of night sweats and cough for last 2 month and was brought to hospital. Work reveals pleural effusion and raised level of Adenosine deaminase. Which of the following antibiotic will be given in initial 2 months of therapy? ***(Most Recent Question Jan 2023)***

a. Linezolid b. Streptomycin
c. Ethambutol d. Levofloxacin

29. Which of the following diuretics act at the site marked with arrow? ***(Most Recent Question Jan 2023)***

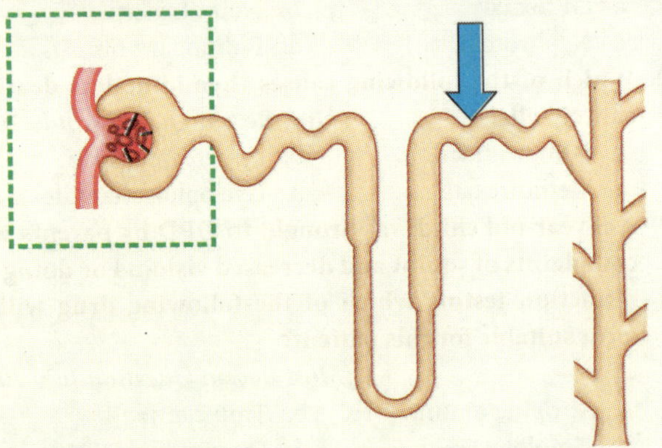

a. Furosemide b. Acetazolamide
c. Spironolactone d. Hydrochlorothiazide

30. Which of the following correctly describes Dale's reversal phenomenon? ***(Most Recent Question Jan 2023)***

a. Fall in BP upon giving epinephrine in a patient pretreated with phentolamine
b. Increased BP and HR upon isoprenaline administration
c. Decreased BP upon repeated ephedrine administration
d. Increased BP upon giving alpha-blocker in patient pretreated with beta-blocker

31. Which of the following statement correctly describes the mechanism of action of labetalol? ***(Most Recent Question Jan 2023)***

a. It decreases peripheral vascular resistance by directly acting at the vascular smooth muscles
b. Beta plus alpha-receptor blocker
c. Dilates arteries and results in reflex tachycardia
d. Mainly a venodilator

32. Which of the following agent decreases mortality in a patient with chronic congestive heart failure? ***(Most Recent Question Jan 2023)***

a. Metoprolol b. Torsemide
c. Prazosin d. Furosemide

33. Which of the following drug is represented by the shown image? ***(Most Recent Question Jan 2023)***

a. Epinephrine b. Norepinephrine
c. Isoprenaline d. Dopamine

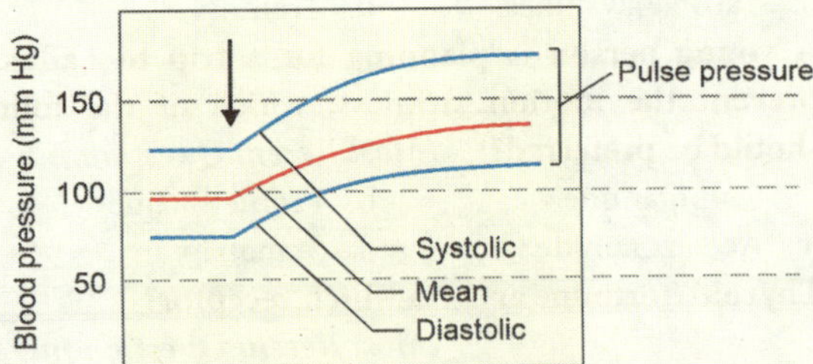

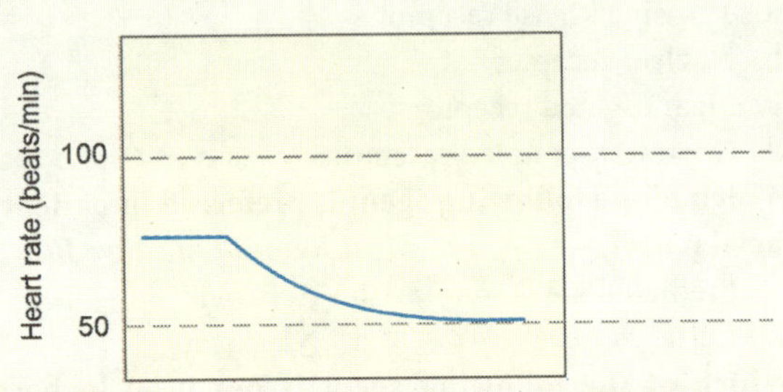

34. A child consumed multiple iron tablets and brought to emergency with vomiting and abdominal pain. Which of the following is antidote of choice? ***(Most Recent Question Jan 2023)***

a. D-penicillamine b. Deferoxamine
c. EDTA d. BAL

35. A patient comes to you with breathlessness, dry cough with reduced exercise capacity. On X-ray examination, diagnosis of pulmonary fibrosis is made. Which of the following drug is used to decrease the progression of fibrosis? ***(Most Recent Question Jan 2023)***

a. Roflumilast b. Pirfenidone
c. Busulfan d. Ipratropium

36. Which of the following agent acts at the marked site in the image? ***(Most Recent Question Jan 2023)***

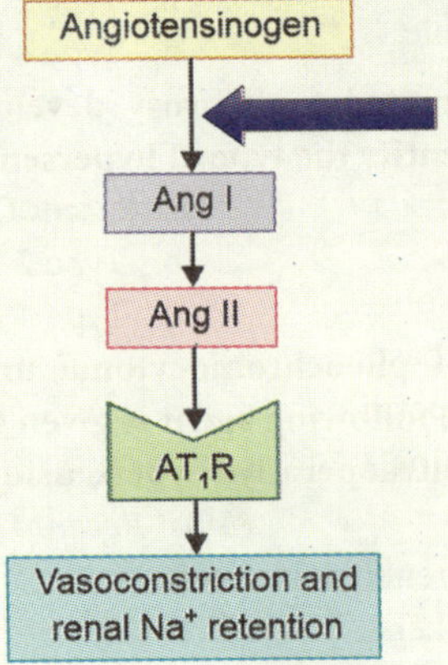

a. Aliskiren b. Ramipril
c. Losartan d. Spironolactone

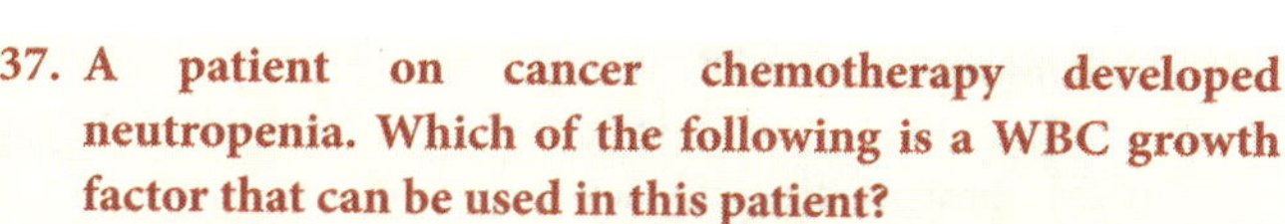

37. A patient on cancer chemotherapy developed neutropenia. Which of the following is a WBC growth factor that can be used in this patient?

(Most Recent Question Jan 2023)

a. Filgrastim b. Darbepoetin
c. Oprelvekin d. Romiplostim

38. Which of the following statements about drugs is false?

(Most Recent Question Jan 2023)

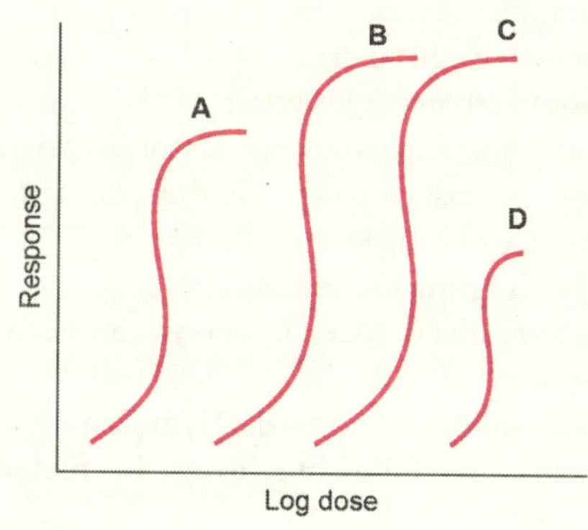

a. Drug B is more potent than C
b. Drug D is least potent
c. Drug B is more efficacious than A
d. Drug A is most efficacious

39. Which of the following antidyslipidemic drugs work by stimulating PPAR-alpha?

(Most Recent Question Jan 2023)

a. Simvastatin
b. Ezetimibe
c. Gemfibrozil
d. Colestipol

40. Which of the following agent will be used for treatment of diarrhea in a patient who was treated for colorectal carcinoma with 5-FU and irinotecan?

(Most Recent Question Jan 2023)

a. Ciprofloxacin
b. Ornidazole
c. Atropine
d. Loperamide

41. Which drugs are used for chemotherapy-induced nausea and vomiting? ***(Most Recent Question Jan 2023)***

a. Granisetron + Dexamethasone + Aprepitant
b. Dexamethasone + Metoclopramide + Domperidone
c. Prochlorperazine + Granisetron + Domperidone
d. Doxylamine + Granisetron + Aprepitant

42. A patient on antidepressant therapy complained of some sexual side effects. Which of the following antidepressant is least likely associated with sexual side effects?

(Most Recent Question Jan 2023)

a. Bupropion b. Fluoxetine
c. Escitalopram d. Venlafaxine

43. A female patient on lithium therapy developed symptoms of lithium overdose. Which of the following statement is false about lithium overdose?

a. Hemodialysis is not useful in this patient
b. Lithium causes hypothyroidism
c. Lithium toxicity is increased by thiazide diuretics
d. It is teratogenic

44. Which of the following is statement is correct about mechanism of action of Dicumarol?

(Most Recent Question Jan 2023)

a. It inhibits conversion of plasminogen to plasmin by inhibiting tissue plasminogen activator
b. It acts by inhibiting Vitamin K epoxide reductase which is involved in activation of clotting factor II, VII, IX, X
c. It chelates calcium and reduces calcium level in coagulation cascade
d. It acts by increasing AT3 level, which chelates factor IIa and Xa

45. An HIV patient presented with neck rigidity and seizure. CSF examination confirms diagnosis of cryptococcal meningitis. Which of the following antifungal is the preferred agent in this patient?

(Most Recent Question Jan 2023)

a. Voriconazole b. Liposomal amphotericin B
c. Fluconazole high dose d. 5-Flucytosine + Fluconazole

46. In a clinical trial, a drug is found to have therapeutic index of 25. Which of the following best describes therapeutic index of the drug?

(Most Recent Question Jan 2023)

a. Ratio between a dose producing lethality in 50% and effect in 50%
b. Ratio between therapeutic dose and maximum lethal dose
c. It represents first pass metabolism and is calculated by duration of action of drug by the half-life of drug
d. It represents extent of drug absorption and is calculated by AUC and time graph

GENERAL PHARMACOLOGY

47. LD_{50} stands for: ***(Most Recent Question June 2022)***

a. 50% of animal mortality in an experiment after exposure of drug
b. 50% effect of the drug in animal sample
c. Death of 50 animals in an experiment
d. 50% reduction of infection in the given population of animals

48. Histamine acts on H1 receptor causing bronchoconstriction, and adrenaline acting on Beta receptor causing bronchodilation. Type of antagonism:

(Most Recent Question Aug 2020)

a. Chemical b. Physiological
c. Physical d. Pharmacological

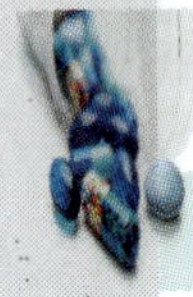

49. After which phase of drug trial, post marketing surveillance starts? *(Most Recent Question Dec 2019-20)*
- a. Phase 1
- b. Phase 2
- c. Phase 3
- d. Phase 4

50. Which of the following drugs follows zero order kinetics? *(Most Recent Question Dec 2019-20)*
- a. Phenytoin
- b. Clopidogrel
- c. Morphine
- d. Propranolol

51. Therapeutic drug monitoring is done for: *(Most Recent Question Dec 2019-20)*
- a. Phenytoin
- b. Heparin
- c. Aspirin
- d. Metformin

52. 100% Bioavailability is seen with this route: *(Repeated Frequently)*
- a. Oral
- b. Intravenous
- c. Intramuscular
- d. Subcutaneous

53. Healthy volunteers are recruited in which phase of clinical trials? *(Most Recent Question 2019)*
- a. Phase 1
- b. Phase 2
- c. Phase 3
- d. Phase 4

54. Good clinical practice is NOT needed in which phase of clinical trial: *(Recent Pattern Question 2018-19)*
- a. Preclinical stage
- b. Phase 2
- c. Phase 3
- d. Phase 4

55. Drug not given with ketoconazole: *(Recent Pattern Question 2018)*
- a. Aminoglycoside
- b. Cisapride
- c. Indinavir
- d. All of these

56. Physiological antagonist of histamine is: *(Recent Pattern Question 2018)*
- a. Adenosine
- b. Adrenaline
- c. Atropine
- d. Acetylcholine

57. In a first order kinetics area under curve denotes: *(Recent Pattern Question 2018)*
- a. Clearance
- b. Bioavailability
- c. Volume of distribution
- d. Both a and b

58. Adverse drug reaction class B is: *(Recent Pattern Question 2017)*
- a. Predictable side effect
- b. Bizarre effect of a drug
- c. Failure of a drug
- d. Chronic side effect

59. Which of the following is not an example of chronic adverse drug reactions?
- a. Nitrate induced headache
- b. Glucocorticoid induced osteoporosis
- c. Chloroquine induced retinopathy
- d. Amiodarone deposition in cornea

60. After oral administration the fraction of drug reaching the systemic circulation in unchanged form is: *(Recent Pattern Question 2017)*
- a. Elimination
- b. Distribution
- c. Bioavailability
- d. Metabolism

61. Pharmacovigilance is:
- a. Monitoring generic drugs
- b. Monitoring drug efficacy
- c. Monitoring ethical drug
- d. Monitoring adverse effects of drugs

62. Pharmacovigilence is done for:
- a. Pharmacy companies
- b. To monitor potency and efficacy
- c. To monitor adverse effects of drugs
- d. Monitoring ethical drug

63. True about zero order kinetics:
- a. Rate of elimination is independent of plasma concentration
- b. Rate of elimination is dependent on plasma concentration
- c. Clearance of drug is always constant
- d. Half life of drug is constant

64. All drugs are metabolized by acetylation; EXCEPT:
- a. Phenytoin
- b. Isoniazid
- c. Procainamide
- d. Hydralazine

65. Which of the following drug is metabolized by acetylation?
- a. Phenytoin
- b. Isoniazid
- c. Salbutamol
- d. Haloperidol

66. Glucagon acts via:
- a. cAMP
- b. cGMP
- c. Cytoplasmic Ca^+
- d. Intracellular K^+

67. True about highly ionized drug:
- a. Can cross the placental barrier
- b. Well absorbed from intestine
- c. Accumulates in cellular lipids
- d. Excreted mainly by kidneys

68. Which of the following drug is an enzyme inducer?
- a. Rifampicin
- b. Isoniazid
- c. Ketokonazole
- d. Erythromycin

69. All are enzyme inhibitors; EXCEPT:
- a. Carbamazipine
- b. Cimetidine
- c. Valproate
- d. Ketoconazole

70. Which is the best way to manage a patient present with aspirin poisoning?
- a. Make urine acidic with NH_4Cl^-
- b. Make urine alkaline with $NaHCO_3$
- c. Treat with N-acetyl cysteine
- d. Do gastric lavage

71. All of the following act via nuclear receptor; EXCEPT:
- a. Insulin
- b. Vitamin A
- c. PPAR
- d. Thyroxine

72. Which of the following act via ion-channel receptor?
- a. GABA
- b. Androgen
- c. Estrogen
- d. Vitamin A

73. Which of the following drug require therapeutic dose monitoring?
- a. Phenytoin
- b. Warfarin
- c. Metformin
- d. Propanolol

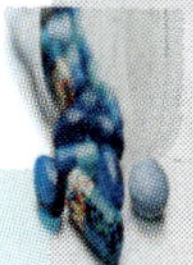

74. Duration of sub-acute toxicity study with animals:
a. 3 months b. 6 months
c. 1 year d. 1½ years

75. For knowing the acute toxicity of a drug, the drug micro doses should be tested on:
a. Two different species b. On rabbit, one rodent
c. Two rabbits d. Two rodents

76. Category X drugs are all; EXCEPT:
a. Warfarin b. Methotrexate
c. Alprazolam d. Thalidomide

77. Number of patients in Phase II clinical trial:
a. 10–100 b. 200–400
c. 1000–2000 d. 2000–4000

78. Patients are first enrolled in this phase of clinical trial:
a. Phase 0 b. Phase I
c. Phase II d. Phase III

79. Pharmacoepidemiology is this phase of clinical trial:
a. Phase 0 b. Phase II
c. Phase IV d. Phase V

80. Which of the following is not a prodrug?
a. Levodopa b. Lisinopril
c. Carbimazole d. Prednisone

81. All are prodrugs; EXCEPT:
a. Minoxidil b. Levodopa
c. Dipivefrine d. Captopril

82. True statement about orphan drugs:
a. Drugs used for orphans
b. Drugs used for rare disease
c. Easily available drugs
d. Drugs with excessive financial benefits

83. What happens to drug after expiry date?
a. Drug has lost its potency
b. Maximum expiry to 3 years from manufacture date
c. Product changes to toxic products
d. Decrease in efficacy

AUTONOMIC NERVOUS SYSTEM & GLAUCOMA

84. A patient with glaucoma and also suffering from Bronchial asthma. Which of the following anti glaucoma drug should be avoided in this patient?
(Most Recent Question June 2022)
a. Timolol b. Pilocarpine
c. Betaxolol d. Brimonidine

85. A person came to emergency with snake bite 8 hours ago. He has already been given 10 vials of antivenom at local hospital. Following is the next step, if patient doesn't recover and signs of neuro paralysis prevails:
(Most Recent Question June 2022)
a. Aspirin b. Neostigmine + Atropine
c. IV Hydrocortisone d. Anti-coagulation therapy

86. Which of the following statement is incorrect?
(Most Recent Question June 2022)
a. Carbamates bind to Ach esterase irreversibly
b. Atropine is used as an antidote of OP poisoning
c. Pralidoxime has its role in reversal of enzyme in carbamate poisoning
d. Atropine is used as an antidote for carbamate poisoning

87. All of the following are side effect of Ritodrine; EXCEPT: *(Most Recent Question June 2022)*
a. Hypoglycemia b. Tachycardia
c. Hypotension d. Tremor

88. A person presented to emergency in comatose state after consuming some unknown poison. Excessive sweating is apparent and on examination there is bradycardia and BP is 80/60 mm Hg. Which of the following is antidote for treatment of this patient?
(Most Recent Question June/Dec 2021)
a. Neostigmine b. Atropine
c. Physostigmine d. N-acetylcysteine

89. A 28-year-old male went to Ladakh. He developed shortness of breath. Which of the following drug will you use for the treatment of mountain sickness at high altitude? *(Most Recent Question June/Dec 2021)*
a. Acetazolamide b. Furosemide
c. Epleronone d. Salbutamol

90. Which of the following is the action of dopamine at low doses? *(Most Recent Question June/Dec 2021)*
a. It increases renal blood flow
b. It causes vasoconstriction
c. It has positive chronotropic action
d. It causes hypertension

91. A lady was stung by many bees. She developed breathing difficulty and hypotension. Drug used for treatment of this condition is? *(Most Recent Question June 2021)*
a. Adrenaline
b. Nor-adrenaline
c. Dopamine
d. Isoprenaline

92. A farmer presented to emergency with garlic odor, pin point pupil and excessive secretions. Which of the following is drug of choice for treatment of this poisoning: *(Most Recent Question June/Dec 2021)*
a. Atropine
b. Flumazenil
c. N–acetylcysteine
d. Oxime

93. A Patient with BPH taking prazosin attended the OPD with recurrent episodes of hypotension. Which drug you will prescribe him now that doesn't cause hypotension?
(Most Recent Question Dec 2019-20)
a. Terazosin b. Doxazosin
c. Tamsulosin d. Alfuzosin

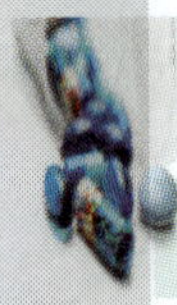

94. Maximum parasympathetic outflow is by which cranial nerve? *(Most Recent Question 2019)*
a. V b. VII
c. IX d. X

95. Long-term use of which of the following drug is most likely associated with development of tremors? *(Most Recent Question 2019)*
a. Propofol b. Salbutamol
c. Betaxolol d. Timolol

96. Which of the following is a long acting bronchodilator? *(Most Recent Question 2019)*
a. Salbutamol b. Terbutaline
c. Adrenaline d. Formoterol

97. Drug of choice for motion sickness: *(Recent Pattern Question 2018-19)*
a. Promethazine b. Ondansetron
c. Cyclizine d. Domperidone

98. Mechanism of action of alpha Methyl-dopa: *(Recent Pattern Question 2018-19)*
a. Alpha 1 agonist
b. Alpha 2 agonist
c. Alpha 1 antagonist
d. Alpha 2 antagonist

99. Which of the following is the action of Pilocarpine? *(Recent Pattern Question 2018-19)*
a. Active mydriatic b. Passive mydriatic
c. Active miotic d. Passive miotic

100. Which of the following agents scan cause recurrent fall in elderly patient with postural hypotension? *(Recent Pattern Question 2018-19)*
a. Methoxamine
b. Prazosin
c. Metformin
d. Acarbose

101. Most sensitive test for organophosphate poisoning: *(Recent Pattern Question 2018-19)*
a. Plasma acetylcholinesterase
b. OP level in blood
c. OP level in urine
d. OP level in lavage

102. In a 2-year-old child refractive error test is done with: *(Recent Pattern Question 2018-19)*
a. 1% atropine ointment b. 1% atropine eye drop
c. Tropicamide 0.5% d. Eucatropine 5%

103. Ritodrine is a: *(Recent Pattern Question 2018)*
a. β_2 agonist b. β_2 antagonist
c. α_1 agonist d. α_1 antagonist

104. Esmolol is a short acting beta blocker because: *(Recent Pattern Question 2018)*
a. It has more plasma protein binding
b. Its plasma hydrolysis by esterases is rapid
c. It has high lipid solubility
d. It has high oral bioavailability

105. Correct about pralidoxime are all; EXCEPT: *(Recent Pattern Question 2018)*
a. It is given slow IV
b. Given effectively in carbamate poisoning
c. It does not cross blood brain barrier
d. Reactivates the AChE enzyme

106. Drug of choice for diabetic diarrhea: *(Recent Pattern Question 2018)*
a. Duloxetine b. Clonidine
c. Domperidone d. Alosetron

107. Botulinum toxin acts on: *(Repeated Frequently)*
a. Inhibition of release of neurotransmitter
b. Post synaptic block
c. At synapse
d. Reuptake inhibitor

108. A farmer presented in OPD clinic with sweating, lacrimation, pin-point pupils with a heart rate of 40/min. Possible diagnosis:
a. Dhatura poisoning
b. Organophosphate poisoning
c. Atropine poisoning
d. Cocaine poisoning

109. A 45 year male presents with delirium, increased body temperature, dryness, dilated pupils and HR 130/min. Possible diagnosis:
a. Carbamate poisoning
b. Organophosphate poisoning
c. Atropine poisoning
d. Cocaine poisoning

110. Anticholinergic side effect is:
a. Salivation b. Dryness
c. Incrased GIT motility d. Sweating

111. Neostigmine used in all; EXCEPT:
a. Myasthenia Gravis b. Curare poisoning
c. Snake bite d. OP poisoning

112. Action of M2 receptor is seen at: *(Recent Pattern Question 2017)*
a. Sphincters: Increase tone
b. Bronchus: Decrease tone
c. Heart: Decrease heart rate
d. Ventricles: Increase force of contraction

113. Methacholine acts mainly as:
a. M1 agonist b. M2 agonist
c. M1 antagonist d. M2 antagonist

114. Tripitramine acts as:
a. M1 agonist b. M2 agonist
c. M1 antagonist d. M2 antagonist

115. Alpha bungaratoxin acts at:
a. Muscarinic receptor agonist
b. Muscarinic receptor antagonist
c. Nicotinic ganglion agonist
d. Neuromuscular junction antagonist

116. All of the following side effects are seen with ipratropium bromide; EXCEPT: ***(Recent Pattern Question 2017)***
a. Urinary incontinence b. Dryness of mouth
c. Irritation in trachea d. Blurred vision

117. Mechanism of action of aminophylline in bronchial asthma: ***(Recent Pattern Question 2017)***
a. Decreasing phosphodiesterase activity
b. Direct action on smooth muscles
c. Releasing catecholamines
d. Stabilizing membrane of mast cells

118. Increased urinary frequency is best managed by: ***(Recent Pattern Question 2016)***
a. Oxybutynin b. Imipramine
c. Alfuzosin d. Bethanechol

119. Which of the following drug is used in urinary retention? ***(Recent Pattern Question 2016)***
a. Bethanechol b. Finasteride
c. Oxybutynin d. Letrozole

120. Which of the following sympathetic receptors acts as vasoconstriction and vasodilatation?
a. Alpha 1 and Alpha 2 b. Alpha 1 and Beta 1
c. Alpha 1 and Beta 2 d. Beta 1 and Beta 2

121. Bronchial calibre is reduced by: ***(Recent Pattern Question 2016)***
a. Beta 2 receptor stimulation
b. Stimulation of sympathetic fibre
c. Stimulation of parasympathetic fiber
d. Alpha 2 receptor stimulation

122. In contrast to epinephrine, norepinephrine does the following:
a. Increase BP, bradycardia b. Increase BP, tachycardia
c. Decrease BP, bradycardia d. Decrease BP, tachycardia

123. Dobutamine mainly act at this receptor:
a. Beta 1 b. Beta 2
c. Alpha 1 d. Alpha 2

124. Midodrine is used in:
a. Hypertension
b. Orthostatic hypotension
c. Increasing cardiac output
d. Decongestant

125. Tachyphylaxis is seen with:
a. Dopamine b. Salbutamol
c. Propranolol d. Haloperidol

126. Longest acting beta adrenergic blocker:
a. Atenolol b. Sotalol
c. Nadolol d. Esmolol

127. Beta-adrenoceptor blocking agent that should be avoided in patients with renal failure is:
a. Atenolol b. Metoprolol
c. Propranolol d. Esmolol

128. Which of the following drug does not produce hypotension during/followed by surgery?
a. Esmolol b. Nadolol
c. Propanolol d. Metoprolol

129. A hypertensive patient who is on beta blockers develops bradycardia and start to sweat whenever he takes the medication. Which beta blocker does not produce such symptoms?
a. Atenolol b. Acebutalol
c. Metoprolol d. Nadolol

130. All of the following beta blockers have intrinsic sympathomimetic activity; EXCEPT:
a. Celiprolol b. Propanolol
c. Pindolol d. Acebutalol

131. β blocker with intrinsic sympathomimetic activity:
a. Nadolol b. Atenolol
c. Pindolol d. Propanolol

132. Which of the following beta blocker is vasodilator?
a. Metoprolol b. Atenolol
c. Propranolol d. Carvedilol

133. Which of following is a non selective alpha blocker?
a. Prazosin b. Tolazoline
c. Terazosin d. Doxazosin

134. Drug with a first dose effect:
a. Yohimbine b. Verapamil
c. Dopamine d. Prazosin

135. Irreversible alpha-1 adrenoreceptor antagonist:
a. Prazosin b. Clonidine
c. Isoprenaline d. Phenoxybenzamine

136. All of the following drugs cause mydriasis; EXCEPT:
a. Pilocarpine b. Epinephrine
c. Atropine d. Phenylephrine

137. All of the following drugs can cause mydriasis; EXCEPT:
a. Atropine b. Phenylephrine
c. Phentolamine d. Tropicamide

138. Shortest acting mydriatics:
a. Atropine b. Homatropine
c. Tropicamide d. Cyclopentolate

139. Treatment of choice for scorpion bite:
a. Anti-venin b. Insulin
c. Steroids d. Atropine

140. Which of the following drug is used for treating overactive bladder?
a. Pirenzepine b. Tolterodine
c. Bethanechol d. Alfuzosin

141. Mechanism of action of Oxybutynin:
a. Cholinergic
b. Anticholinergic
c. Adrenergic
d. Selectively inhibits M2 receptor

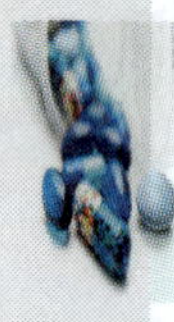

CNS AND PNS

142. A 29-year-old lady, who is a smoker is on nicotine replacement therapy for deaddiction. She now requires alternative therapy for the same, which of the following drug is useful: *(Most Recent Question June 2022)*
a. Flumazenil
b. Acamprosate
c. Varenicline
d. Naltrexone

143. A young male patient who has family history of bipolar disorder in his father, has now come to you in OPD with symptoms of Mania. His genetic testing shows positivity for recessive inheritance of genes involved in mania. Which of the following mood stabilizer can be given to him as most effective treatment?
a. Valproate *(Most Recent Question June 2022)*
b. Lithium
c. Carbamazepine
d. Olanzapine

144. A patient found roadside in an unconscious state having pin point pupil, HR 54/min and BP 90 mmHg. His history reveals he is a drug addict. Which of the following drug he must have consumed?
(Most Recent Question June 2022)
a. Cocaine b. Morphine
c. Amphetamine d. Haloperidol

145. A 70-year-old Parkinson disease patient suffers from constipation after taking anti-Parkinsonian treatment. Which of the following drug may be responsible for above symptoms? *(Most Recent Question June 2022)*
a. Levodopa b. Benztropine
c. Pramipexole d. Metoclopramide

146. Which of the following agent used in rheumatoid arthritis act by opioid and non-opioid receptors?
(Most Recent Question June 2022)
a. Tramadol b. Paracetamol
c. Etoricoxib d. Methotrexate

147. A 25-year-old male presented to emergency with head trauma due to road traffic accident. In hospital, the patient developed seizures. Emergency CT scan revealed widespread cerebral edema. Which of the following is diuretic of choice for cerebral edema in this patient?
(Most Recent Question June/Dec 2021)
a. Mannitol b. Spironolactone
c. Furosemide d. Hydrochlorothiazide

148. A patient developed tachycardia, palpitations, high BP and pupil dilation. Which of the following drug withdrawal can result in above symptoms?
(Most Recent Question June/Dec 2021)
a. Coccaine withdrawal b. Dhatura withdrawal
c. Opioid withdrawal d. Alcohol withdrawal

149. A young boy was brought to the hospital with complaints of few episodes of fast blinking and staring at something for around 20 seconds. ECG shows spike and wave pattern. Which of the following drug should be used for treatment? *(Most Recent Question June/Dec 2021)*
a. Phenytoin b. Sodium valproate
c. Diazepam d. Carbamazepine

150. Which of the following anti-depressant drug acts by inhibiting the reuptake of both serotonin and noradrenaline? *(Most Recent Question June/Dec 2021)*
a. Fluoxetine b. Venlafaxine
c. Phenelzine d. Nortriptyline

151. Which of the following antimicrobials is contraindicated in a patient with seizure disorder?
a. Ampicillin *(Most Recent Question June/Dec 2021)*
b. Imipenem
c. Moxifloxacin
d. Cefixime

152. A patient was given halothane for general anaesthesia. He developed rigidity and hyperthermia. These symptoms are most likely due to which ion:
a. Na^+ *(Most Recent Question June/Dec 2021)*
b. K^+
c. Ca^{2+}
d. Cl^-

153. A patient presented to hospital with road traffic accident. The patient has raised ICP without intracranial hematoma. Which of the following is the preferred drug for the management of this patient?
(Most Recent Question June/Dec 2021)
a. Mannitol b. Prednisolone
c. Glycerol d. Furosemide

154. A drug addict patient presented with agitation and ulceration on skin. The patient had severe itching and scratch marks on the body. On examination there is presence of tachycardia, mydriasis and hypertension. Likely substance responsible for these symptoms is?
(Most Recent Question June/Dec 2021)
a. Cocaine b. Cannabis
c. LSD d. Heroin

155. An elderly male developed the symptoms of dementia and was diagnosed as Alzheimer's disease. Which neurotransmitter level is reduced in this disease?
(Most Recent Question June/Dec 2021)
a. Dopamine b. Acetylcholine
c. Adrenaline d. Serotonin

156. An elderly patient of parkinsonism presented with complaints of resting tremor. Which of the following therapy is not indicated in this patient?
(Most Recent Question Aug 2020)
a. Pramipexole b. Rivastigmine
c. Deep brain stimulation d. Levodopa-carbidopa

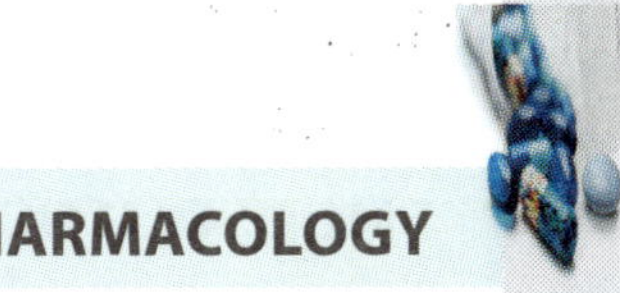

157. Patient presented with facial pain over facial nerve distribution while speaking, chewing, and even on touch. Which drug is to be given for the management of same? *(Most Recent Question Aug 2020)*

a. Lamotrigine b. Carbamazepine
c. Levetiracetam d. Haloperidol

158. A pediatric patient presented in emergency with seizures lasting from last 30 minutes. What will you use immediately to stop the seizures? *(Most Recent Question Aug 2020)*

a. Valproate b. Levetiracetam
c. Diazepam d. Phenobarbitone

159. A Patient with pancreatic cancer is on morphine for pain management. After some time, pain is not relieved as much as before. Possible reason: *(Most Recent Question Aug 2020)*

a. Decreased absorption
b. Opioid receptors desensitization
c. Pain intensity has increased
d. Morphine receptors are upregulated

160. Patient with history of mania. Drug used to control the symptoms: *(Most Recent Question Aug 2020)*

a. Lithium b. Haloperidol
c. Phenytoin d. Lamotrigine

161. Least teratogenic antiepileptic drug in pregnancy is: *(Most Recent Question Dec 2019-20)*

a. Valproate b. Phenytoin
c. Carbamazepine d. Levetiracetam

162. Which of the following anti-epileptic drug has the highest teratogenic potential? *(Most Recent Question 2019)*

a. Valproate b. Carbamazepine
c. Phenytoin d. Lamotrigine

163. A young male presents with reduced sleep, hyperactivity and elevated mood. He has a family history of mania. Which of the following drug is preferred for long-term treatment in this patient? *(Most Recent Question 2019)*

a. Sodium valproate
b. Lithium carbonate
c. Carbamazepine
d. Barbiturates

164. Anti-depressant drug which is used for smoking cessation is? *(Most Recent Question 2019)*

a. Venlafaxine b. Topiramate
c. Bupropion d. Amitriptyline

165. Drug of choice for treatment of Alzheimer's disease is: *(Most Recent Question 2019)*

a. Atropine b. Donepezil
c. Physostigmine d. Fluoxetine

166. Which of the following is an opioid receptor? *(Recent Pattern Question 2018-19)*

a. Epsilon b. Sigma
c. Gamma d. Delta

167. A violent manic patient should not be treated with: *(Recent Pattern Question 2018-19)*

a. Benzodiazepines b. Cognitive therapy
c. Atypical antipsychotics d. Quetiapine

168. All are morphine effects; EXCEPT: *(Recent Pattern Question 2018)*

a. Miosis b. Delayed gastric emptying
c. Respiratory depression d. Hyperalgesia

169. Drug of choice for akathisia: *(Recent Pattern Question 2018)*

a. Lithium b. Fluoxetine
c. Propranolol d. Haloperidol

170. Which is the drug preferred for sleep onset insomnia? *(Recent Pattern Question 2017)*

a. Midazolam b. Lorazepam
c. Ramelteon d. Ritanserin

171. Which of the following is an atypical antipsychotic? *(Recent Pattern Question 2017)*

a. Clozapine b. Chlorpromazine
c. Thioridazine d. Haloperidol

172. Lipodystrophy is caused by which of the following? *(Recent Pattern Question 2017)*

a. Thioridazine b. Fluphenazine
c. Prochlorphenazine d. Clozapine

173. In which drug extra pyramidal side effect is not seen?

a. Haloperidol b. Carbamazepine
c. Chlorpromazine d. Fluphenazine

174. Drug of choice of neuroleptic malignant syndrome:

a. Lorazepam b. Propranolol
c. Dantrolene d. Benzhexol

175. Akathisia is best treated by:

a. Lithium b. Fluoxetine
c. Propanolol d. Haloperidol

176. Which drug has least extrapyramidal symptoms?

a. Haloperidol b. Clozapine
c. Fluphenazine d. Chlorpromazine

177. Which drug has least extrapyramidal symptoms?

a. Aripiprazole b. Loxapine
c. Fluphenazine d. Chlorpromazine

178. Antipsychotic which can cause cataract:

a. Clozapine b. Thioridazine
c. Chlorpromazine d. Quetipaine

179. Atypical antipsychotic with maximum risk of hyperprolactinemia:

a. Risperidone
b. Aripiprazole
c. Olanzapine
d. Sertindole

180. Which of the following drug causes neuroleptic malignant syndrome?

a. Midazolam b. Lorazepam
c. Diazepam d. Haloperidol

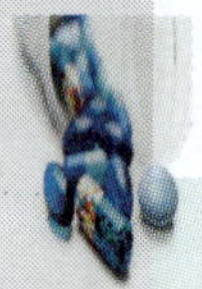

181. Treatment for anxiety attack: *(Recent Pattern Question 2016)*
a. α-blockers b. Diazepam
c. Barbiturates d. Bupropion

182. Which of the following anesthetic agent leads to increase in ICT? *(Recent Pattern Question 2016)*
a. Thiopentone b. Ketamine
c. Propofol d. Sevoflurane

183. True about Benzodiazepine:
a. It is GABA mimetic b. It is GABA facilitator
c. Not a safe drug d. Powerful enzyme inducer

184. Diazepam acts by:
a. GABA mimetic action
b. Exciting CNS
c. GABA facilitator
d. By increasing duration of channel

185. Antidote of benzodiazepine overdose:
a. Flupenthixol b. Fluoxetine
c. Fluvoxamine d. Flumazenil

186. Drug of choice for ADHD:
a. Amphetamine b. Methylphenidate
c. Pemoline d. Modafinil

187. Rivastigmine is given in:
a. Depression b. Alzheimer's disease
c. Schizophrenia d. OCD

188. Which of the following is not used for the prophylaxis of migraine?
a. Propanolol b. Topiramate
c. Verapamil d. Ethosuximide

189. In treatment of Parkinsonism carbidopa is used along with levodopa because:
a. It increases the half life of levodopa by inhibiting its metabolism
b. It inhibits levopda excretion
c. It inhibits peripheral dopa decarboxylase
d. It inhibits central dopa deaminase

190. On-Off phenomenon seen during levodopa therapy is due to:
a. Toxicity of drug
b. As a mild and known side effect of drug
c. Short half life of drug
d. Long half life of drug

191. Antiviral drug amantadine is approved for:
a. Schizophrenia
b. Depression
c. Alzheimer's disease
d. Parkinsonism

192. Ergot derivative used for Parkinson's disease:
a. Emmenagogue b. Benzhexol
c. Bromocriptine d. Ropinirole

193. Anti-Parkinson drug that has the potential to cause retro-peritoneal fibrosis is:
a. Pramipexole b. Bromocriptine
c. Ropinirole d. Levodopa and carbidopa

194. Selegiline acts by:
a. MAO-A inhibition
b. MAO-B inhiition
c. COMT inhibition
d. Dopamine receptor stimulator

195. Which of the following anti epileptic drug act by inhibiting voltage gated sodium channel?
a. Levetiracetam b. Lamotrigine
c. Ethosuximide d. Perampanel

196. True statement about lamotrigine:
a. It acts by blocking NMDA type of glutamate receptors
b. It is a DA agonist used in Parkinson's disease
c. It has Broad spectrum of anti-seizure activity
d. It doesn't have any adverse side effects

197. Drug preferred in absence seizure:
a. Phenytoin b. Sodium valproate
c. Trimethadione d. Ganoxolone

198. Drug preferred in generalized tonic clonic seizure:
a. Phenytoin b. Na^+ Valproate
c. Carbamazepine d. Diazepam

199. A 30-year-old female with partial seizure. Drug of choice:
a. Clonazepam b. Carbamazepine
c. Phenobarbitone d. Lamotrigine

200. Reversible alopecia, weight gain, tremor, Hepatotoxicity is the major side effect of which of the following anti epileptic drug?
a. Valproate b. Lamotrigine
c. Zonisamide d. Phenytoin

201. Which of the following anti epileptic drug causes gum hypertrophy?
a. Phenytoin b. Valproate
c. Topiramate d. Vigabatrin

202. Phenytoin therapy may lead to which of the following:
a. Microcytic anemia
b. Thrombosis
c. Hypercalcemia
d. Folic acid deficiency

203. Vigabatrin acts by:
a. GABA receptor inhibitor
b. Glutamate receptor inhibitor
c. GABA transaminase inhibitor
d. GABA transport inhibitor

204. The recently approved antiepileptic drug lacosamide acts by:
a. Inhibiting synaptic vesicular protein
b. Inhibing CRMP protein
c. Inhibing GABA metabolism
d. Inhibing glutamate release

205. A patient with recent onset primary generalized epilepsy, develops drug reaction and skin rash and neutropenia due to phenytoin sodium. The most appropriate course of action is:
a. Shift to sodium valproate
b. Shift to clonazepam
c. Shift to ethosuximide
d. Restart phenytoin after 2 weeks

206. The antiepileptic drug which causes weight loss:
a. Valproate b. Vigabatrin
c. Topiramate d. Felbamate

207. Drug of choice in acute poisoning of morphine:
a. Naloxone b. Naltrexone
c. Nalmefene d. Methadone

208. Giving intrathecal opioid leads to which side effect? ***(Recent Pattern Question 2017)***
a. Anaphylaxis b. Pruritus
c. Hypotension d. Cardiac arrest

209. All of the following are anti smoking drugs; EXCEPT:
a. Bupropion b. Buspirone
c. Clonidine d. Vareniciline

210. First line therapy in smoking dependence:
a. Nicotine replacement gum
b. Rimonabant
c. Naloxone d. Acute cessation

211. Ebstein anomaly is known teratogenic effect due to this drug:
a. Clozapine b. Phenytoin
c. Lithium d. Lamotrogine

212. Which of the following is SSRI?
a. Desipramine b. Clomipramine
c. Fluvoxamine d. Imipramine

213. Venlafaxine comes under which class of drugs: ***(Recent Pattern Question 2018)***
a. Selective serotonin reuptake inhibitor
b. Serotonergic noradrenergic reuptake inhibitor
c. Tricyclic antidepressant
d. Serotonin receptor antagonist

214. Most common side effect of SSRI:
a. Delayed ejaculation b. Nausea
c. Weight gain d. Insomnia

215. Scopolamine is used mostly in:
a. Hyperemesis gravidarum
b. Vomiting
c. Constipation
d. Motion sickness

216. Disulfiram acts by competitive inhibition of which enzyme?
a. Alcohol dehydrogenase
b. Aldehyde dehydrogenase
c. Alcohol carboxylase
d. Aldehyde carboxylase

217. Mechanism of action of ethanol in methyl alcohol poisoning:
a. Competitively inhibits alcohol Dehydrogenase
b. Selectively inhibits catalase
c. Competitively inhibits lactate dehydrogenase
d. Competitive inhibition of acetaldehyde dehydrogenase

218. All of the following drugs are used in detoxification therapy of chronic alcoholism; EXCEPT:
a. Acamprosate b. Naltrexone
c. Disulfiram d. Flumazenil

219. Which of the following drugs can cause galactorrhea?
a. Bromocriptine b. Pantoprazole
c. Metoclopramide d. Omeprazole

ANTIMICROBIAL AGENTS

220. Which of the following agent is drug of choice in Legionnaire's disease? ***(Most Recent Question June 2022)***
a. Erythromycin b. Azithromycin
c. Vancomycin d. Tigecycline

221. A patient who has just recovered from COVID-19 infection visits your OPD with black discoloration material in nose and posterior part of buccal cavity. He also gives history of using high dose steroid therapy during his treatment of COVID-19. Which of the following is most suitable drug for his treatment? ***(Most Recent Question June 2022)***
a. Fluconazole
b. Amphotericin B
c. Itraconazole
d. Posaconazole

222. A female patient presented with greenish vaginal discharge. Clue cells were present and whiff test was positive in vaginal discharge. What is the drug of choice for this condition? ***(Most Recent Question June/Dec 2021)***
a. Doxycycline b. Metronidazole
c. Ceftriaxone d. Fluconazole

223. A female patient was treated with clindamycin and developed diarrhea most probably pseudomembranous colitis. Which of the following is the likely organism responsible for this? ***(Most Recent Question June/Dec 2021)***
a. Clostridium perfringens
b. Clostridium difficile
c. Clostridium tetani
d. Clostridium septicum

224. Mechanism of action of doxycycline is: ***(Most Recent Question June/Dec 2021)***
a. DNA gyrase inhibitor
b. Cell wall synthesis inhibitor
c. Protein synthesis inhibitor
d. DNA dependent RNA polymerase inhibitor

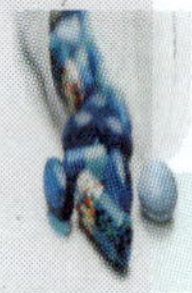

225. A 30-year-old man travelled to Assam. After coming back, he developed fever, Chills and rigors and altered sensorium. The peripheral smear demonstrated the presence of P. falciparum. What is the treatment of choice for this patient? ***(Most Recent Question Dec 2021)***

a. Chlorquine, sulfadoxine pyrimethamine
b. Intravenous artesunate
c. Quinine
d. Primaquine

226. A 35-year-old sexually active female presented with burning micturition and other symptoms of urinary tract infection. Which FQ is least useful in this patient? ***(Most Recent Question Aug 2020)***

a. Ofloxacin b. Moxifloxacin
c. Ciprofloxacin d. Levofloxacin

227. Best treatment for the given condition is: ***(Most Recent Question Dec 2019-20)***

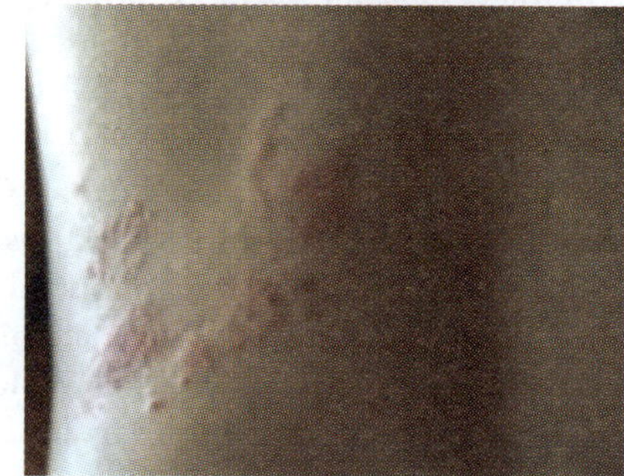

a. Ganciclovir b. Valacyclovir
c. Tenofovir d. Mupirocin

228. Which of the following is the chemoprophylaxis of choice in a person who is on a journey to endemic malarial region? ***(Most Recent Question Dec 2019-20)***

a. Chloroquine b. Quinine
c. Lumefantrine d. Pyrimethamine

229. A lady has taken medication for amoebiasis infection. She drank alcohol in party. She has nausea vomiting and dizziness. Which anti amoebic drug could have led to interaction with alcohol to produce these symptoms? ***(Most Recent Question Dec 2019-20)***

a. Metronidazole b. Nitazoxanide
c. Paromomycin d. Diloxanide

230. A female with 20 weeks pregnancy presents with fever and dysuria. A preliminary diagnosis of cystitis was made. Which of the following drugs will be safe to use for this patient? ***(Most Recent Question 2019)***

a. Ciprofloxacin b. Gentamicin
c. Cotrimoxazole d. Amoxicillin

231. Praziquantel is used for the treatment of: ***(Most Recent Question 2019)***

a. Strongyloidiasis b. Trichomoniasis
c. Schistosomiasis d. Rhinosporidiosis

232. Drug of choice for nasal carriers of MRSA is: ***(Most Recent Question 2019)***

a. Vancomycin b. Teicoplanin
c. Mupirocin d. Linezolid

233. Drug of choice for Enterococcus faecalis: ***(Recent Pattern Question 2018-19)***

a. Cephalexin b. Tetracycline
c. Azithromycin d. Ampicillin

234. Which of the following agent is used for prophylaxis of meningococcal meningitis in pregnancy? ***(Recent Pattern Question 2018-19)***

a. Ceftriaxone b. Rifampicin
c. Ciprofloxacin d. Penicillin G

235. Which of the following is a bacterial protein synthesis inhibitor? ***(Recent Pattern Question 2018-19)***

a. Ceftriaxone b. Streptomycin
c. Nevirapine d. Indinavir

236. In a pregnant female which drug is strictly contraindicated? ***(Recent Pattern Question 2018-19)***

a. Streptomycin b. Isoniazid
c. Cephalosporins d. Penicillin

237. A female patient was treated with antibiotics for chlamydia induced UTI, suddenly presents again with itching/pruritus, vaginal discharge, burning micturition. Which drug should be given? ***(Recent Pattern Question 2018-19)***

a. Ceftriaxone b. Azithromycin
c. Moxifloxacin d. Amphotericin B

238. CYD-TDV Vaccine is used for which of the following infections? ***(Recent Pattern Question 2018-19)***

a. Dengue b. Malaria
c. Yellow fever d. Japanese encephalitis

239. DOC for management of visceral Leishmaniasis: ***(Recent Pattern Question 2018-19)***

a. Parenteral Sodium stibogluconate
b. Liposomal Amphotericin B
c. Miltefosine
d. Pentamidine

240. Preferred drug in UTI: ***(Recent Pattern Question 2018-19)***

a. Fosfomycin b. Trimethoprim
c. Ampicillin d. Moxifloxacin

241. The drug pyronaridine is: ***(Recent Pattern Question 2018)***

a. Antifungal b. Antimalarial
c. Anti-HIV d. PPI drugs

242. Empirical drug of choice for treatment of meningococcal meningitis is: ***(Recent Pattern Question 2018)***

a. Cefoxitin b. Ceftriaxone
c. Cefotetan d. Gentamicin

243. Resistance to ciprofloxacin is due to: ***(Recent Pattern Question 2018)***

a. Transduction b. Transformation
c. Conjugation d. Mutation

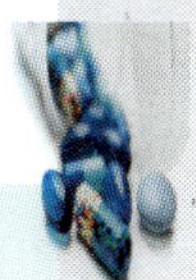

244. Which of the following aminoglycoside is cochleotoxic? ***(Recent Pattern Question 2018)***
a. Kanamycin b. Streptomycin
c. Gentamycin d. Minocycline

245. Following antibiotics inhibit cell wall formation; EXCEPT:
a. Cephalosporin b. Clindamycin
c. Cycloserine d. Vancomycin

246. Which of the following drug acts at 50s ribosome?
a. Stremptomycin b. Tetracycline
c. Quinpristin d. Demeclocycline

247. All of the following penicllins are acid resistant; EXCEPT:
a. Carbenicillin b. Cloxacillin
c. Ampicillin d. Amoxicillin

248. Drug of choice for listeria:
a. Trimethoprim-sulfamethoxazole
b. Ampicillin
c. Chloramphenicol
d. Azithromycin

249. Which of the following drug can cause grey baby syndrome?
a. Tetracycline
b. Chloramphenicol
c. Vancomycin
d. Clindamycin

250. Which of the following antimicrobial agent can result in ototoxicty, nephrotoxicity and redneck syndrome?
a. Methicillin b. Vancomycin
c. Tetracycline d. Chloramphenicol

251. DOC for antibiotic induced colitis:
a. Clindamycin oral b. Metronidazole oral
c. Vancomycin i/v d. Ceftriaxone i/v

252. Vancomycin is used orally for treatment of:
a. Hepatic encephalopathy
b. Pseudomembranous colitis
c. Staphylococcal food poisoning
d. None of the above

253. All of the following drugs are used in MRSA infection; EXCEPT:
a. Vancomycin b. Rifampicin
c. Linezolid d. Nafcillin

254. MRSA is resistant to:
a. Vancomycin b. β lactams
c. Linezolid d. Meropenems

255. Drug which is absolutely contraindicated in pregnancy is:
a. Ceftriaxone b. Chloramphenicol
c. Penicillin d. Azithromycin

256. All antibiotics are safe in pregnancy; EXCEPT:
a. Ciprofloxacin b. Azithromycin
c. Ampicillin d. Cefotaxime

257. Drug of choice for gonorrhea:
a. Azithromycin b. Erythromycin
c. Cefuroxime d. Ceftriaxone

258. Which of the following is a second generation cephalosporin?
a. Cefaclor b. Cephalexin
c. Ceftriaxone d. Cefepime

259. Which of the following β lactams doesn't show cross allergy?
a. Ampicillin b. Cefotaxim
c. Doripenem d. Aztreonam

260. aa-tRNA synthetase inhibitor:
a. Mitomycin- C
b. Mupirocin
c. Metronidazole
d. Methenamine Mandelate

261. The preferred treatment option for primary syphilis is:
a. Injection Benzathine penicillin 2.4 million units IM single dose
b. Injection Benzathine penicillin 2.4 million units IM once a week for 3 weeks
c. Cap. Doxycycline 100 mg orally twice a day for 2 weeks
d. Tab. Azithromycin 2 gm single dose

262. Drug of choice for trachoma:
a. Ceftriaxone b. Azithromycin
c. Erythromycin d. Clarithromycin

263. Side effect of sulfonamide:
a. Thrombocytosis b. Sensorineural hearing loss
c. Crystalluria d. Phototoxicity

264. Ratio of Trimethoprim and Sulfamethoxazole in a Cotrimoxazole tablet: ***(Recent Pattern Question 2016)***
a. 2:1 b. 3:1
c. 5:1 d. 1:5

265. Drug of choice for brucellosis:
a. Chloramphenicol b. Erythromycin
c. Doxycycline d. Cefuroxime

266. Drug of choice for dermatitis herpetiformis:
a. Dapsone b. Rifampicin
c. Ketokonazole d. Azithromycin

267. NOT a fast acting anti- malarial drug:
a. Mefloquine b. Chloroquine
c. Artemisinin d. Pyrimethamine

268. Drug of choice for schistosomiasis:
a. Praziquantel b. Metronidazole
c. Albendazole d. Ivermectin

269. Drug of choice for fasciola hepatica:
a. Praziquantel b. Triclabendazole
c. Ivermectin d. Albendazole

270. Drug of choice for neurocysticercosis:
a. Praziquantel b. Triclabendazole
c. Ivermectin d. Albendazole

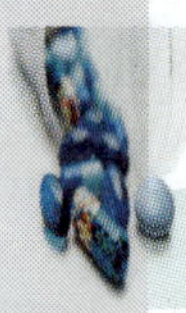

271. **Drug of choice for Taenia Solium:**
   a. Praziquantel b. Triclabendazole
   c. Ivermectin d. Albendazole
272. **Scabies oral drug of choice:**
   a. Permethrin b. Benzyl Benzoate
   c. Ivermectin d. Lindane
273. **Drug of choice for scabies**
   a. Ivermectin
   b. Permethrin
   c. Sulfur
   d. Benzylv benzoate
274. **Drug of choice for tetanus:**
   a. Metronidazole b. Penicillin
   c. Erythromycin d. Clindamycin
275. **Drug of choice for filariasis:**
   a. Metronidazole b. Praziquantel
   c. Ciprofloxacin d. Ivermectin
276. **What is the recommended dose of DEC in filariasis?** ***(Recent Pattern Question 2017)***
   a. 2 mg/kg b. 6 mg/kg
   c. 10 mg/kg d. 20 mg/kg
277. **Which drug is given in combination with DEC for massive reduction of filariasis?** ***(Recent Pattern Question 2017)***
   a. Albendazole
   b. Streptomycin
   c. Pyrimethamine
   d. Tinidazole
278. **Mechanism of action of amphotericin B:**
   a. Cell wall synthesis inhibition
   b. Alters permeability of fungal cell wall
   c. Protein synthesis inhibitor
   d. Act as antibody for fungus
279. **To reduce Amphotericin B toxicity, it is given?** ***(Recent Pattern Question 2017)***
   a. With aminoglycoside
   b. Give intravenous with saline
   c. With 5% dextrose
   d. Liposomal preparation
280. **NOT an adverse effects of amphotericin-B?** ***(Recent Pattern Question 2017)***
   a. Thrombocytopenia
   b. Renal damage
   c. Cholelithiasis
   d. Hepatic damage
281. **Most serious side effects of amphotericin B:**
   a. Hepatic damage b. Renal damage
   c. Cardiotoxicity d. Hypochromic anemia
282. **Which of the following drugs causes acute kidney injury with hypomagnesemia?**
   a. Cyclophosphamide b. Ceftriaxone
   c. Amphotericin-B d. Vancomycin

ANTIVIRALS

283. **A patient from non-endemic area visited a malaria endemic area, and was started on prophylactic therapy of malaria. How long this drug should be continued after leaving from the endemic area?** ***(Most Recent Question Aug 2020)***
   a. 1 week b. 2 weeks
   c. 4 weeks d. 4 months
284. **Dose of oseltamivir for prophylaxis of swine flu in a child aged 3–5 months?** ***(Recent Pattern Question 2018-19)***
   a. 3 mg/kg/day twice daily
   b. 5 mg/kg/day twice daily
   c. 10 mg/kg/day twice daily
   d. 15 mg/kg/day twice daily
285. **Drug not used in CMV retinitis:** ***(Recent Pattern Question 2018)***
   a. Acyclovir
   b. Foscarnet
   c. Ganciclovir
   d. Cidofovir
286. **Drug used in dermatitis herpetiformis are all; EXCEPT:**
   a. Acyclovir b. Colchicine
   c. Dapsone d. Tetracycline
287. **Which of the following is not a protease inhibitor?**
   a. Atazanavir b. Ritonavir
   c. Abacavir d. Indinavir
288. **Reverse transcriptase inhibitor zidovudine is given for:**
   a. HIV b. HBV
   c. HCV d. All of the above
289. **All drugs are used in AIDS; EXCEPT:**
   a. Abacavir b. Ritonavir
   c. Acyclovir d. Tenofovir
290. **Mechanism of action of maraviroc:**
   a. Cyt P 450 inhibitor b. GP 41 inhibitor
   c. CCR5 inhibitor d. GP 120 inhibitor
291. **NRTI which has maximum tendency to cause peripheral neuropathy**
   a. Zidovudine b. Stavudine
   c. Lamivudine d. Didanosine

ANTITUBERCULAR AGENTS

292. **A patient has developed tuberculosis in which mycobacterium is resistant to rifampicin, isoniazid, kanamycin and levofloxacin. This tuberculosis is referred to as:** ***(Most Recent Question June/Dec 2021)***
   a. MDR TB
   b. Rifampicin resistant TB
   c. Extensively resistant TB
   d. Extremely resistant TB

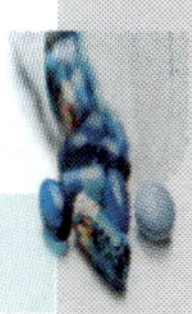

293. Which of the following drug will you omit from the prescription of a patient with XDR tuberculosis in pregnancy? *(Most Recent Question June/Dec 2021)*
a. Kanamycin
b. Ethambutol
c. Moxifloxacin
d. Amoxycillin clavulanic acid

294. Isoniazid is NOT given in: *(Recent Pattern Question 2017)*
a. Renal disease b. Liver disease
c. Diabetes mellitus d. Hypertension

295. If somebody develops resistance to INH, patient will develop simultaneously resistance to which drug? *(Recent Pattern Question 2017)*
a. Streptomycin b. Rifampicin
c. Ethambutol d. Pyrazinamide

296. ATT Drug that kills slowly or intermittently dividing bacteria:
a. Isonizid b. Rifampicin
c. Pyrazinamide d. Streptomycin

297. True statement about action of ethambutol:
a. Exclusive agent against extracellular bacilli
b. Selectively tuberculocidal agent
c. Increase the permeability of cell wall
d. More active on slowly multiplying bacilli

298. Anti TB drug causing optic neuritis:
a. Isoniazid b. Rifampicin
c. Pyrazinamide d. Ethambutol

299. Which of the following anti TB drug is not bactericidal
a. Rifampicin b. Isoniazid
c. Pyrazinamide d. Ethambutol

300. Which of the following anti tubercular drug requires dose adjustment in renal failure:
a. Isoniazid b. Rifampicin
c. Pyrazinamide d. Ethambutol

301. Isoniazid dosage in infants
a. 5 mg/kg PO qday b. 10–15 mg/kg PO qday
c. 300 mg BID d. 300 mg once a week

302. RNA transcription is blocked by this ATT:
a. Rifampicin b. Streptomycin
c. Chloroamphenicol d. INH

303. In patients on isoniazid, which vitamin deficiency is more likely to be seen?
a. Vitamin B9 b. Vitamin B12
c. Vitamin B6 d. Vitamin B3

304. Anti TB drug causing depression and suicidal tendency:
a. Kanamycin b. Cycloserine
c. Streptomycin d. Capreomycin

305. ATT contraindicated in pregnant women
a. Isoniazid b. Rifampicin
c. Streptomycin d. Ethambutol

306. Which anti TB drug is contraindicated throughout the pregnancy:
a. Rifampicin b. Streptomycin
c. Isoniazid d. Ethambutol

307. Ototoxicity caused by:
a. Vancomycin b. Streptomycin
c. Ampicillin d. Rifampicin

308. Dose for tuberculin test:
a. 1 TU b. 2 TU
c. 2.5 TU d. 5 TU

309. ATT drug causing hypothyroidism:
a. Isoniazid b. Ethambutol
c. PAS d. Rifampicin

310. ATT drug causing hyperuricemia:
a. Isoniazid b. Pyrazinamide
c. Streptomycin d. Rifampicin

ANTICANCER DRUGS

311. A patient is suffering from breast cancer is on chemotherapy taking multiple anti-cancer drugs. As cancer is not responding to the low dose therapy there is a need to increases the dose of chemotherapy agents. Which of the following drug requires monitoring of bladder function with the increasing dose?
a. Gemcitabine *(Most Recent Question June 2022)*
b. Cisplatin
c. Methotrexate
d. Ifosfamide

312. A patient was operated for prostate carcinoma and during surgery local metastasis was noted. Which of the following drug this patient should receive? *(Most Recent Question June/Dec 2021)*
a. Leuprolide b. Desmopressin
c. Octreotide d. Tamsulosin

313. Isotope of iodine used for treatment of thyroid cancer is: *(Most Recent Question June/Dec 2021)*
a. I-131 b. I-123
c. I-127 d. I-125

314. Which of the following is used as radiosensitizer in head and neck CA? *(Most Recent Question Aug 2020)*
a. Cisplatin
b. Paclitaxel
c. Amifostine
d. Methotrexate

315. A known patient of cancer, developed infection. He was on anti-cancer therapy. Total leucocyte count was 2000/mm^3. agent preferred for this patient is: *(Most Recent Question Aug 2020)*
a. Romiplostim b. Oprelvekin
c. Filgrastim d. EPO

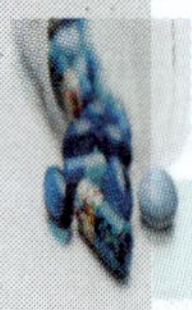

316. Which monoclonal antibody is used in cancer treatment? *(Most Recent Question Dec 2019-20)*
a. Omalizumab b. Denosumab
c. Rituximab d. Methotrexate

317. Most cardiotoxic anti -cancer drug among the following: *(Most Recent Question Dec 2019-20)*
a. Anthracyclines b. Cyclophosphamide
c. Imatinib d. Tamoxifen

318. DOC of anal cancer: *(Recent Pattern Question 2018-19)*
a. Gefitinib b. Eflorinitib
c. 5FU d. Cisplatin

319. Pemetrexed MOA is: *(Recent Pattern Question 2018)*
a. RNA synthesis inhibitor
b. Dihydrofolate reductase inhibitor
c. Dopamine agonist
d. Folate antagonist

320. Folinic acid used in: *(Recent Pattern Question 2018)*
a. Methotrexate toxicity b. Cisplatin toxicity
c. Vincristine toxicity d. 5FU toxicity

321. Which anticancer drug inhibits dihydrofolate reductase? *(Recent Pattern Question 2017)*
a. Vincristine b. Methotrexate
c. Paclitaxel d. Cisplatin

322. Which drug will be preferred in imatinib resistant CML? *(Recent Pattern Question 2017)*
a. Nilotinib b. Infliximab
c. Hydroxyurea d. Gefitinib

323. Breast cancer chemotherapeutic agent that causes osteoporosis:
a. Letrozole b. Nafarelin
c. Tamoxifen d. Leuprolide

324. A 40-year-old lady with breast cancer has undergone MRM and is on Tamoxifen for 1 year. She now presents with bleeding per vaginum 4–5 times. What is the probable cause?
a. Bleeding disorder b. Endometrial cancer
c. Ovarian cancer d. Cervical cancer

325. All are alkylating agents used in chemotherapy; EXCEPT:
a. Melphalan b. Busulfan
c. Cladribine d. Cyclophosphamide

326. All are example of alkylating agents; EXCEPT:
a. Bleomycin b. Busulfan
c. Procarbazine d. Melphalan

327. Alkylating agent used in chemotherapy:
a. Mechlorethamine b. Procarbazine
c. Cyclophosphamide d. All of these

328. True about Cyclophosphamide
a. Antimetabolites b. Alkylating agent
c. Platinum compound d. Topoisomerase inhibitors

329. Which of the following drug is not a purine analogue?
a. 6 Mercaptopurine b. Cladribine
c. Cytarabine d. Fludarabine

330. Mercaptopurine is:
a. Purine analogue b. Nucleoside analogue
c. Pyrimidine analogue d. Anti tumor antibiotics

331. First line chemotherapy for cancer cervix:
a. Cyclophosphamide b. Lomustine
c. Vincristine d. Cisplastin

332. Drug of choice for CML
a. Imatinib mesylate
b. Fludarabine
c. Al trans retinoic acid (for AML 3)
d. Methotrexate

333. Methotrexate mechanism of action:
a. Inhibit dihydrofolate reductase
b. Stimulate dihydrofolate reductase
c. Inhibit tetrahydrofolate reductase
d. Stimulate tetrahydrofolate reductase

334. Antidote for methotrexate toxicity:
a. Folic acid b. Folinic acid
c. Vitamin B d. Thymine

335. Which of the following is not used in treatment for Multiple myeloma:
a. Melphalan b. Thalidomide
c. Zolendronic acid d. Methotrexate

336. Most emetogenic anti CA drug:
a. 5 FU b. Methotrexate
c. Cisplatin d. All of these

337. Most widely used anti CA drug:
a. 5 FU b. Methotrexate
c. Cisplatin d. All of these

338. Which of the following anti neoplastic drug commonly causes hepatotoxicity:
a. 6-mercaptopurine
b. 5-flurouracil
c. Doxorubicin
d. Etoposide

339. Hemorrhagic cystitis is caused by:
a. Procarbazine b. Cisplatin
c. Doxorubicin d. Cyclophosphamide

340. Not used in treatment protocol of hodgkin's lymphoma:
a. Vincristine b. Vinblastine
c. Bleomycin d. Adriamycin

341. Cardiomyopathy is caused by:
a. Actinomycin D b. Doxorubicin
c. Mitomycin C d. Mitoxantrone

342. Which of the following anticancer drug causes hemolytic uremic syndrome?
a. Vincristine b. Vinblastine
c. Cisplatin d. Mitomycin C

343. Chemoradiation was given to a patient. Which drug given will reduce toxicity caused by radiotherapy?
a. Vitamin A b. Gemcitabine
c. Amifostine d. Actinomycin D

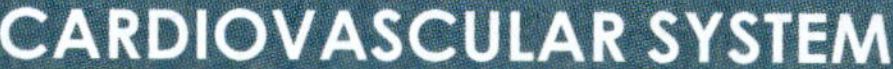

CARDIOVASCULAR SYSTEM

344. What is the best drug treatment of Raynaud's phenomenon? *(Most Recent Question June 2022)*
a. Calcium channel blocker
b. Beta blockers
c. Nitroprusside
d. Prazosin

345. Which of the following is the important and significant side effect of tamoxifen use? *(Most Recent Question June 2022)*
a. Cancer in opposite breast
b. Osteoporosis
c. Endometrial hyperplasia
d. Infertility

346. A patient undergoing spinal surgery developed very high blood pressure of 240/120 mm Hg, which of the following drug is not used in treatment of this patient? *(Most Recent Question June 2022)*
a. IV Esmolol
b. IV Nicardipine
c. IV Nitroprusside
d. IV Mannitol

347. A patient with long history of CHF with maintained ejection fraction and no signs of hypervolemia comes to you with long QRS waves in ECG and cardiac wall hypertrophy. Which of the following drug is best to be started to prolong survival? *(Most Recent Question June 2022)*
a. Digoxin
b. Lisinopril
c. Furosemide
d. Nifedipine

348. Drug used for treatment of pregnancy induced hypertension is: *(Most Recent Question June/Dec 2021)*
a. Alpha methyl dopa
b. Lisinopril
c. Hydralazine
d. Telmisartan

349. A 56-year-old patient who is a known case of hypertension was being treated with antihypertension drugs. He is having chronic cough since 2 weeks. He was started on antimicrobials but cough did not resolve. Which of the following antihypertensive drug may induce chronic cough in this patient? *(Most Recent Question June/Dec 2021)*
a. Lisinopril
b. Minoxidil
c. Propranolol
d. Amlodipine

350. A professor in medical college is teaching students about the adverse effects of a drug. Which of the following drug can cause gynecomastia in men and menstrual irregularities in women? *(Most Recent Question June/Dec 2021)*
a. Spironolactone
b. Propranolol
c. Misoprostol
d. Oxytocin

351. Drug of choice for treatment of digoxin induced ventricular arrhythmias is: *(Most Recent Question June/Dec 2021)*
a. Atropine
b. Lidocaine
c. Amiodarone
d. Procainamide

352. True statement about aliskiren:
a. Safe in pregnancy *(Most Recent Question Aug 2020)*
b. Can increase aldosterone level
c. Contraindicated in diabetes
d. Indirectly increases renin level

353. ACE inhibitor is contraindicated in which of the following condition:
a. Bilateral renal artery stenosis
b. Chronic kidney disease
c. Post myocardial infarction
d. Diabetes mellitus

354. Sublingual nitroglycerine was started in a patient presented with acute chest pain. Mechanism of action of nitroglycerine: *(Most Recent Question Aug 2020)*
a. Stimulate endothelin
b. Releases nitric oxide
c. Calcium channel inhibitor
d. Beta blockade

355. Which of the following drug causes postural hypotension commonly? *(Most Recent Question Dec 2019-20)*
a. ACE inhibitor
b. Beta blocker
c. Alpha blocker
d. Angiotensin receptor blockers

356. Preferred drug for the treatment of ventricular tachycardia is: *(Most Recent Question 2019)*
a. Digoxin
b. Diltiazem
c. Lignocaine
d. Propranolol

357. Gemfibrozil is: *(Recent Pattern Question 2018)*
a. HMG CoA inhibitor
b. PPAR-α activator
c. Inhibit cholesterol synthesis
d. Inhibit cholesterol absorption

358. Mechanism of action of statins is by: *(Recent Pattern Question 2018)*
a. Competitive inhibition
b. Noncompetitive inhibition
c. Uncompetitive
d. Irreversible inhibition

359. Drug of choice for cardiogenic shock: *(Recent Pattern Question 2018)*
a. Dopamine
b. Dobutamine
c. Digoxin
d. Digitoxin

360. Which of the following condition precipitate Digoxin toxicity? *(Recent Pattern Question 2017)*
a. Hypokalemia
b. Hyperkalemia
c. Hypernatremia
d. Hyperphosphatemia

361. All are true statement about digitalis action; EXCEPT:
a. Increases cardiac contraction
b. Pumps sodium inside cell in exchange of Ca^+
c. Increases intracellular calcium
d. Causes bradycardia

362. In a patient with PIH, with BP 150/90, what will be the management ***(Recent Pattern Question 2016)***
a. Lisinopril
b. Labetalol
c. Diuretics
d. CCB

363. Which of the following is not a mechanism of action of Antihypertensive agents?
a. Blockade of alpha adrenergic receptors
b. Blockade of ATP sensitive K^+ channels
c. Blockade of Noradrenaline release
d. Blockade of beta adrenergic receptors

364. Drug not useful in emergency condition in pregnancy:
a. Nifedipine
b. Labetalol
c. Ritodrine
d. Phenobarbitone

365. Which of the following antihypertensive is contraindicated in pregnancy:
a. Beta blockers
b. ACE inhibitors
c. Methyldopa
d. Ca channel blockers

366. All of the following antihypertensive drugs are given in pregnancy; EXCEPT:
a. Methyldopa
b. Labetalol
c. Captopril
d. Nifedipine

367. The drug of choice in scleroderma induced hypertensive crisis is:
a. ACE inhibitors
b. Angiotensin receptor blockers
c. Beta blockers
d. Sodium nitroprusside

368. Drug of choice in supra ventricular tachycardia
a. Adenosine
b. Verapamil
c. Metoprolol
d. Lignocaine

369. Drug of choice for Paroxysmal Supraventricular Tachycardia
a. Digitalis
b. Adenosine
c. Adrenaline
d. Verapamil

370. A Patient who is on anti hypertensive drug develops dry cough. Which of the following drug might be responsible for the condition:
a. Diuretics
b. ACE inhibitors
c. Calcium channel blockers
d. Beta blockers

371. Mechanism of action of statins:
a. Inhibit HMG CoA synthase
b. Stimulate HMG CoA reductase
c. Inhibit HMG CoA reductase
d. Stimulate HMG CoA synthase

372. Not a hypolipidemic drug:
a. Simvastatin
b. Fenofibrate
c. Somatostatin
d. Fluvastatin

373. All of the following anti-arrhythmic drugs are from class Ic; EXCEPT:
a. Encainide
b. Flecainide
c. Tocainide
d. Propafenone

374. Which of the following is an L-type calcium channel blocker:
a. Nifedipines
b. Amlodipines
c. Diltiazem
d. All of these

375. Drug that leads to glucose intolerance:
a. Hydrochlorthiazide
b. ACE inhiitors
c. Verapamil
d. Sulfonylureas

376. Which of the following drug has uricosuric action?
a. Losartan
b. Allopurinol
c. Enalapril
d. Ramipril

377. Angiotensin receptor blockers which attenuate platelet aggregation:
a. Telmisartan
b. Losartan
c. Valsartan
d. Irbesartan

378. Which of the following anti-hypertensives are contraindicated together:
a. CCB & Nitrates
b. Nitrates and β blockers
c. CCB and β blockers
d. CCB and ARB

379. A diabetic patient with hypertension, which drug is preferred:
a. ACE inhibitor
b. Beta blockers
c. CCB
d. Diuretics

ENDOCRINE SYSTEM

380. A 28-year-old female with first trimester pregnancy comes to you in hospital with high level of T3 and T4. Which of the following drug is most appropriate to use? ***(Most Recent Question June 2022)***
a. Carbimazole
b. Propylthiouracil
c. Potassium iodine
d. Propranolol

381. A patient with hyperglycemia and positive ketone bodies in urine comes to you in hospital with altered sensorium. Which of the following drug therapy is most suitable to start? ***(Most Recent Question June 2022)***
a. Metformin
b. Potassium chloride
c. Insulin and IV fluid
d. Ringer lactate

382. Drug combination which is preferred for MTP: ***(Most Recent Question June 2022)***
a. Lupiprostone + Mifepristone
b. Mifepristone + Misoprostol
c. Lubiprostone + Misoprostol
d. Alprostadil + Misoprostol

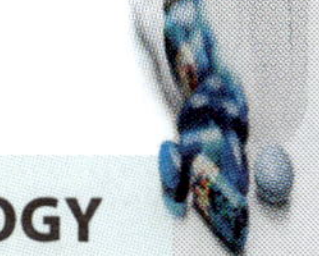

383. In a patient with proliferative diabetic retinopathy, which of the following monoclonal antibodies can be used:
a. Belimumab *(Most Recent Question June 2022)*
b. Bevacizumab
c. Infliximab
d. Rituximab

384. To minimize the HPA axis suppression risk, what is the correct method of administration of prednisolone: *(Most Recent Question June 2022)*
a. Give at night just before bed time
b. Give on alternate days
c. Replace with betamethasone
d. Divide in three doses and give small doses 8 hourly

385. A 30-year-old female presented with gain and cold intolerance. On investigations value of T3 is 70 ng/dl (reference value 100–200 ng/dl) T4 is 3 mcg/dl (reference value 5–12 mcg/dl) and TSH is 20 mIU/L (reference value 0.5–5 mIU/L). Which of the following statement is correct regarding the management of this patient? *(Most Recent Question June/Dec 2021)*
a. Measure T3T4 and TSH after one month
b. Start L–thyroxine (T4) treatment 100 mcg once daily
c. Start L thyroxine (T4) treatment 25 mcg daily and gradually increase
d. Start daily L thyroxine (T4) 100 mcg with liothyronine (T3) 5 mcg

386. A 50-year-old patient of type 2 diabetes mellitus was controlled on oral hypoglycemic drugs. This patient presented to hospital with profuse sweating and dizziness. There was presence of hypoglycemia. Which among the following drugs can result in hypoglycemia in this patient? *(Most Recent Question June/Dec 2021)*
a. Metformin b. Voglibose
c. Vildgliptin d. Glipizide

387. Which of the following anti diabetic drug does not require dose reduction in renal failure?
a. Linagliptin *(Most Recent Question June/Dec 2021)*
b. Sitagliptin
c. Vildagliptin
d. Saxagliptin

388. An old patient presented with complaints of low backache. Serum analysis of PSA level reveals 100 ng/ml. He was diagnosed with prostate cancer. Which of the following agent is indicated for this patient?
a. Goserelin *(Most Recent Question Aug 2020)*
b. Desmopressin
c. Testosterone
d. Somatostatin

389. Which of the following is a Selective estrogen receptor modulator (SERM)? *(Most Recent Question Dec 2019-20)*
a. Tamoxifen b. Rituximab
c. Letrozole d. Trastuzumab

390. The drug of choice for hyperthyroidism in third trimester of pregnancy is: *(Most Recent Question Dec 2019-20)*
a. Carbimazole b. Propylthiouracil
c. Sodium iodide d. Radioactive iodine

391. Mechanism of action of Exenatide in diabetes mellitus is: *(Most Recent Question Dec 2019-20)*
a. It is analogue of GLP released from gut and increase glucose dependent insulin secretion
b. It is DPP–4 inhibitor and result in decreased breakdown of GLP
c. It inhibits SGLT-2 and cause glucosuria
d. It is amylin analogue and decrease glucagon

392. Which among the following is shortest acting steroid? *(Most Recent Question 2019)*
a. Triamcinolone b. Deflazacort
c. Dexamethasone d. Hydrocortisone

393. Insulin of choice for the treatment of diabetes mellitus is: *(Most Recent Question 2019)*
a. Regular Insulin b. NPH insulin
c. Insulin glargine d. Insulin lispro

394. Which of the following is a long acting insulin that never attains a peak concentration in plasma? *(Most Recent Question 2019)*
a. Insulin lispro b. Insulin aspart
c. Insulin glulisine d. Insulin glargine

395. Secretion of prolactin is inhibited by: *(Most Recent Question 2019)*
a. Dopamine b. Nor-adrenaline
c. Adrenaline d. Serotonin

396. Mechanism of action of Exenatide: *(Recent Pattern Question 2018-19)*
a. SGLT inhibitor b. GLP-1 Analogue
c. DPP4 inhibitor d. AMP kinase inhibitor

397. Purpose of adding zinc with insulin: *(Recent Pattern Question 2018-19)*
a. Make the insulin more rapid acting
b. Provide stability in insulin molecule
c. Increase the risk of insulin resistance
d. Prevent insulin from causing hypoglycemia

398. Half-life of parathormone: *(Recent Pattern Question 2018-19)*
a. 4 minutes b. 10 minutes
c. 30 minutes d. 1 hour

399. Which of the following leads to obesity? *(Recent Pattern Question 2018)*
a. Acarbose b. Insulin
c. Sitagliptin d. Pioglitazone

400. Which of the following is a selective estrogen receptor down-regulator? *(Recent Pattern Question 2017)*
a. Flutamide b. Fulvestrant
c. Tamoxifen d. Clomiphene citrate

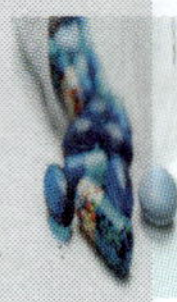

401. Frequency of urine in pregnancy is increased due to:
a. Prostaglandins *(Recent Pattern Question 2016)*
b. Increased progesterone
c. Enlarged uterus pressing on bladder
d. Oxytocin

402. Intermediate acting insulin:
a. Regular insulin b. Glargine
c. Lispro d. NPH

403. Which of the following insulin is rapidly acting?
a. Insulin lispro b. Regular insulin
c. Insulin glargine d. NPH

404. Fastest acting insulin:
a. Insulin aspart b. Insulin Glargine
c. Insulin Lente d. Insulin detemir

405. All are true about Prolactin agonist; EXCEPT:
a. Associated with lactation
b. Stimulate milk production after child birth
c. Dopamine stimulate prolactin production
d. Dopamine inhibit prolactin production

406. Prolactin production is controlled by:
a. Metoclopramide b. Chlorpromazine
c. Dopamine d. None of these

407. MOA of oral hypoglycemic agent
a. Inhibit glucose uptake by skeletal muscle
b. Enhance glucose uptake by skeletal muscle
c. Stimulate glycogenolysis
d. Stimulate gluconeogenesis

408. Antidiabetic drug of choice for obese patients
a. Metformin b. Sulfonylureas
c. Repaglinide d. Acarbose

409. True statement about long term use of tamoxifen:
a. Has no effect on uterine carcinoma
b. Increased risk of heart disease
c. Monitoring of liver enymes is recommended
d. Safer in DVT patients

410. Which of the drug is not used to treat hirsutism:
a. Flutamide b. Finasteride
c. Cyproterone acetone d. Spirinolactone

411. The drug preferred to stop the growth of prostate in a 70-year-old male with Benign hyperplasia of prostate is
a. Spironolactone b. Ketoconazole
c. Finasteride d. Flutamide

AUTACOIDS

412. A patient with bladder cancer on chemotherapy drugs, who is also a known case of CKD, developed tumor lysis syndrome and having very high level of serum uric acid. Which of the following drugs can provide fastest reduction of uric acid level?
(Most Recent Question June 2022)
a. Febuxostat b. Allopurinol
c. Mannitol d. Rasburicase

413. A female patient presented with pain and redness in great toe. Serum uric acid level is 9.6 mg/dl. Apart from prescribing analgesics for relieving pain, the physician prescribed a drug which can decrease the formation of uric acid. Which of the following enzyme is likely to be inhibited by this drug? *(Most Recent Question June 2021)*
a. Xanthine oxidase
b. Thymidylate synthase
c. Phosphpribosyl transferase
d. DHFR

414. Longest acting phosphodiesterase inhibitor among the following drugs is: *(Most Recent Question June 2021)*
a. Sildenafil b. Vardenafil
c. Tadalafil d. Phentolamine

415. Which of the following drug is preferred for closure of ductus arteriosus in a preterm baby with PDA?
a. Aspirin *(Most Recent Question June/Dec 2021)*
b. Ibuprofen
c. Mefenamic acid
d. Paracetamol

416. A patient presented with pain and erythema of great toe. Serum uric acid level was 9.2 mg/dL. She was started on a drug for this condition. The enzyme most likely affected by this drug is: *(Most Recent Question Aug 2020)*
a. Xanthine oxidase
b. Dihydrofolate reductase
c. Phosphodiesterase
d. Thymidylate synthase

417. A patient presented with early morning joint stiffness, for which he was started on an anti-rheumatoid drug. Regular monitoring of visual acuity and fundus examination is required in which disease modifying anti-rheumatoid agent? *(Most Recent Question Aug 2020)*
a. Hydroxychloroquine
b. Methotrexate
c. Sulfasalazine
d. Gold

418. A patient was given a drug for treatment of acute migraine attack. He later developed numbness in tip of thumb and change in color. Which drug could have caused this side effect, and the drug used for the management is:
(Most Recent Question Aug 2020)
a. Sumatriptan and Na^+ nitroprusside
b. Propranolol and Na^+ nitroprusside
c. Dihydroergotamine and Na^+ Nitroprusside
d. Propranolol and Phenoxybenzamine

419. A patient having unilateral headache which is disabling in nature, associated with nausea and vomiting. Which drug can be used to decrease his headache episodes?
(Most Recent Question Dec 2019-20)
a. Propranolol b. Alprazolam
c. Fluoxetine d. Nitrates

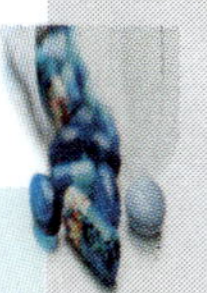

420. All of the following drugs are used for prophylaxis of migraine; EXCEPT: ***(Most Recent Question Dec 2019-20)***
a. Propranolol b. Imipramine
c. Flutamide d. Flunarizine

421. Mechanism of action of allopurinol is: ***(Most Recent Question Dec 2019-20)***
a. Xanthine oxidase inhibition
b. Recombinant uricase
c. Increase uric acid excretion
d. Decrease chemotaxis

422. Most potent opioid is: ***(Most Recent Question Dec 2019-20)***
a. Fentanyl b. Morphine
c. Pentaxocine d. Pethidine

423. Which of the following drug is a selective COX-2 inhibitor? ***(Most Recent Question 2019)***
a. Ketorolac b. Etoricoxib
c. Piroxicam d. Nimesulide

424. Drug of choice for chronic gout is: ***(Most Recent Question 2019)***
a. Allopurinol b. Colchicine
c. Probenecid d. Sulfinpyrazone

425. Most potent analgesic:*(Recent Pattern Question 2018-19)*
a. COX-2 inhibitor b. Remifentanil
c. Morphine d. Sufentanil

426. Paracetamol causes: ***(Recent Pattern Question 2018-19)***
a. Renal failure b. Pancreatic toxicity
c. Neurotoxicity d. Hepatotoxicity

427. What is the impact on foetus in case of Indomethacin used in third trimester? ***(Recent Pattern Question 2018-19)***
a. PDA b. Early closure of PDA
c. VSD d. ASD

428. Zileuton is: ***(Recent Pattern Question 2018)***
a. 5-lipoxygenase inhibitor
b. Cyclooxygenase inhibitor
c. Phospholipase inhibitor
d. Leukotriene receptor antagonist

429. Alcaftadine trial used this concentration of drug: ***(Recent Pattern Question 2018)***
a. 5% b. 1%
c. 0.25% d. 2.5%

430. Phosphodiesterase inhibitor used for erectile dysfunction? ***(Recent Pattern Question 2017)***
a. Sildenafil b. Amrinone
c. Milrinone d. Tamoxifen

431. FDA approved drug Bevacizumab is? ***(Recent Pattern Question 2017)***
a. VEGF 2 inhibitor
b. EGF receptor inhibitor
c. Antibody to VEGF receptor
d. TNF alpha agonist

432. Which of the following drug acts by inhibiting IL-2 activation? ***(Recent Pattern Question 2017)***
a. Cycloserine b. Cyclosporine
c. OKT-3 d. None

433. Sildenafil acts by blocking which enzyme?
a. Phosphodiesterase 3 inhibition
b. Phosphodiesterase 5 inhibition
c. 5 alpha Reductase inhibition
d. Stimulate androgen production

434. Sildenafil is a drug used for erectile dysfunction. It acts by
a. Blocking beta-adrenoceptors
b. Inhibiting phosphodiesterase type 5
c. Inhibiting reuptake of serotonin and nor-adrenaline
d. Selective serotonin reuptake inhibition

435. Side effect of latanoprost:
a. Lacrimation
b. Increased pigmentation of cornea
c. Increased eye lashes hair growth
d. All of the above

436. Which of following prostaglandin analogue is beneficial in glaucoma?
a. PG D2 b. PG E2α
c. PG I2 d. PG F2α

437. Olopatadine is:
a. Mast cell stabilizer
b. Anti- histamine
c. Both mast cell stabilizer and anti histamine
d. None of the above

438. Which of the following is a soft steroid:
a. Betamethasone b. Dexamethasone
c. Prednisolone d. Ciclesonide

439. True about febuxostat:
a. Anti-gout and Xanthine Oxidase inhibitor
b. Purine inhibitor
c. Dose adjustment required in renal impairment
d. Has uricosuric action

440. Drug given for acute gout:
a. Aspirin b. Indomethacin
c. Febuxostat d. Allopurinol

RENAL SYSTEM

441. A known patient of cardiac disease, presented with shown condition (image), and complaints of breathlessness. Which of the following statement is preferred agent used in the treatment of edema for this patient: ***(Most Recent Question Aug 2020)***
a. ACE inhibitor
b. Aldosterone receptor blocker at DCT
c. Na^+ Cl^- transport inhibitor at DCT
d. Na^+ K^+ $2Cl^-$ symptorter inhibitor at loop of henle

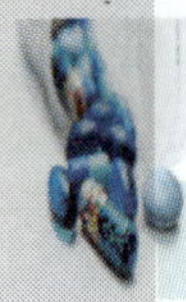

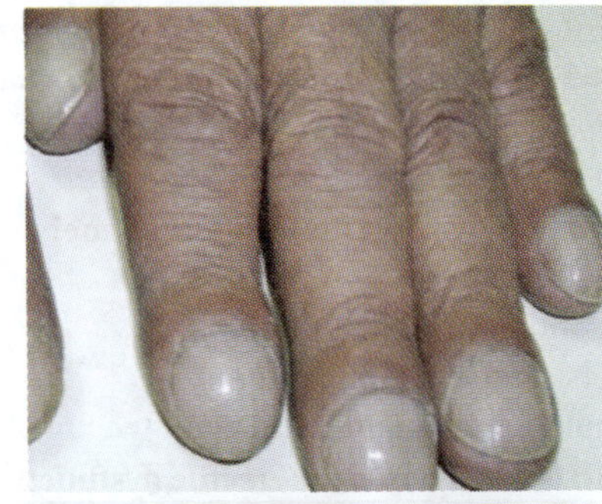

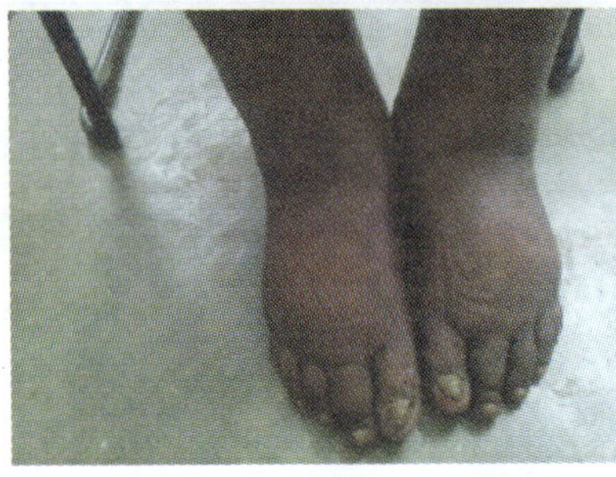

442. Which of the following is a carbonic anhydrase inhibitor? *(Most Recent Question Dec 2019-20)*

a. Hydrochlorothiazide b. Furosemide
c. Acetazolamide d. Mannitol

443. Hydrochlorothiazide works by inhibiting: *(Most Recent Question Dec 2019-20)*

a. Na^+ Cl pump in late DCT
b. Na^+ Cl pump in early DCT
c. Na^+ K^+ 2Cl pump in descending limb of loop of henle
d. Na^+ K^+ 2Cl pump in ascending limb of loop henle

444. Drug of choice for neurogenic diabetes insipidus is: *(Most Recent Question 2019)*

a. Terlipressin b. Desmopressin
c. Chlorthalidone d. Conivaptan

445. DOC for nephrogenic diabetes insipidus: *(Recent Pattern Question 2018)*

a. Mannitol
b. Spironolactone
c. Thiazides
d. Demeclocycline

446. True reason for avoiding diuretics in pregnancy: *(Recent Pattern Question 2017)*

a. Increase vascular resistance
b. Decrease placental circulation
c. Causes maternal distress
d. High risk of birth defects

447. True about acetazolamide: *(Recent Pattern Question 2016)*

a. Increase sodium reabsorption and potassium secretion
b. Carbonic anhydrase inhibitor
c. Acts at ascending limb of loop of Henle
d. Increase aqueous outflow mainly

448. Receptor for vasopressin in collecting duct: *(Recent Pattern Question 2016)*

a. V1 b. V2
c. V3 d. Endothelium

449. Drug used in renal osteodystrophy:

a. Vitamin D b. Calcitriol
c. Calcidiol d. All of these

450. All of the following are potassium sparing diuretic; EXCEPT:

a. Spironolactone b. Triamterene
c. Indapamide d. Amiloride

451. Diuretic of choice for initial management of CKD:

a. Thiazide diuretics b. Loop diuretics
c. K+ sparing diuretics d. Osmotic diuretics

RESPIRATORY SYSTEM

452. A patient suffering from Bronchial asthma comes to you in hospital. All of the following drugs are used in acute exacerbation; EXCEPT: *(Most Recent Question June 2022)*

a. Nebulization by salbutamol
b. Oxygen therapy
c. IV Magnesium sulfate
d. Leukotriene antagonist

453. Which of the following drugs used in emergency management of asthma, does not act by causing bronchodilation? *(Most Recent Question June/Dec 2021)*

a. Salbutamol b. Ipratropium
c. Deriphyllline d. Hydrocortisone

454. Identify the shown image: *(Most Recent Question Aug 2020)*

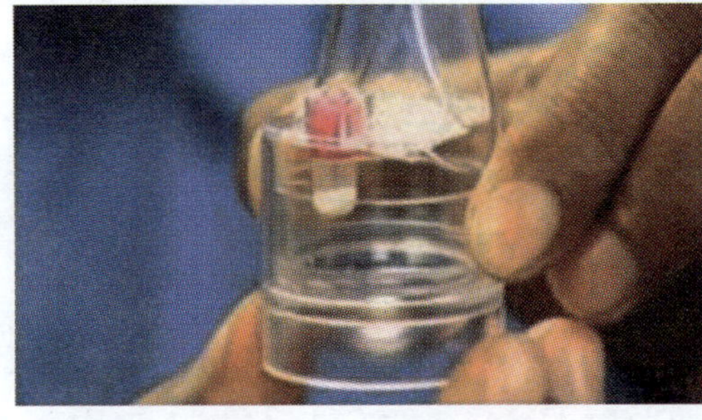

a. Rotahaler b. Spacer
c. Nebulizer d. Metered dose inhaler

455. Which anti -asthma drug is avoided with erythromycin? *(Most Recent Question Dec 2019-20)*

a. Salbutamol b. Ipratropium
c. Theophylline d. Terbutaline

456. DOC for tropical pulmonary eosinophilia: *(Recent Pattern Question 2018)*

a. Albendazole b. Itraconazole
c. Corticosteroid d. DEC

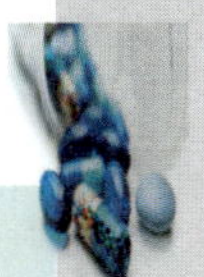

457. All of the following are anti tussives; EXCEPT:
a. Codeine b. Dextromethorphan
c. Ambroxol d. Noscapine

458. Which drug should not be given in acute persistent asthma?
a. Theophylline b. Salbutamol
c. Salmetrol d. Formoterol

459. Which is not useful in persistent severe asthma?
a. Slow acting β2 agonist b. Long acting β2 agonist
c. Inhaled corticosteroids d. High flow oxygen

460. Which is most common side effect of inhaled beclomethasone dipropionate?
a. Pneumonia
b. Oropharyngeal candidiasis
c. Atrophic rhinitis
d. Pituitary adrenal suppression

461. Non-sympathomimetic Bronchodilator preferred in COPD:
a. Ipratropium bromide b. Salmeterol
c. Terbutaline d. Salbutamol

462. Noscapine is an:
a. Antitussive b. Anti emetic
c. Anti dirrheal d. Mucolytics

463. Cough syrup acts by inhibiting?
a. Cough center
b. Respiratory center
c. Breathing center
d. Pulmonary secretion center

464. A 34-year-old man with a long history of asthma is referred to pulmonologist. The physician decides to prescribe zileuton. The mechanism of action of this drug is to:
a. Antagonize Leukotriene D4 receptor
b. Inhibits 5-lipoxygenase
c. Inhibit phosphodiesterases
d. Stimulate P_2 receptors

GIT

465. A tourist has visited an Indian Village and developed mild diarrhea which later on found to be caused by E. coli. Which of the following is the most suitable drug of use in this patient? *(Most Recent Question June 2022)*
a. Loperamide b. Rifaximin
c. Octreotide d. Zinc

466. A patient is taking platinum-based chemotherapy for treatment of ovarian cancer. Which of the following drug should be used to prevent the nausea and vomiting in this patient? *(Most Recent Question June/Dec 2021)*
a. Domperidone b. Promethazine
c. Palonosetron d. Metoclopramide

467. Laxative used in hepatic encephalopathy
(Recent Pattern Question 2018-19)
a. Lactulose b. Sodium picosulfate
c. Lubiprostone d. Bisacodyl

468. Calcium carbonate is used for:
a. Antacid *(Recent Pattern Question 2016)*
b. Renal stone
c. Metabolic alkalosis
d. Renal failure

469. Drug of choice for treatment of NSAID-induced peptic ulcer is:
a. Prostaglandin analogues like Misoprostol
b. H2-receptor antagonists like Ranitidine
c. Proton pump inhibitors like Omeprazole
d. Antacids like $Mg(OH)_2$

470. All of the following are indicated in drug induced vomiting; EXCEPT:
a. Ondansetron
b. Metoclopramide
c. Hyoscine
d. Chlorpromazine

471. Which of the following drug is not effective against chemotherapy induced vomiting?
a. Aprepitant b. Hyoscine
c. Metoclopramide d. Ondansetron

472. All of the following statements about treatment of diarrhea are correct; EXCEPT:
a. Anti-motility drugs are drug of choice for infective diarrhea
b. Loperamide and diphenoxylate are opioids used as anti-motility drugs
c. Diphenoxylate overdose can cause respiratory depression
d. Opioids decrease peristalsis and can be used in diarrhea

HEMATOLOGY AND VITAMINS

473. A 29-year-old female with history of hypercoagulative disorder visiting OPD for anticoagulation treatment. Which of the following drug should be avoided in first trimester of pregnancy?
a. Enoxaparin *(Most Recent Question June 2022)*
b. Unfractionated heparin
c. Warfarin
d. Low molecular weight heparin

474. A patient of myocardial infarction taking anti platelet drug aspirin tablet 325 mg. Which other drug can be added to above treatment to enhance anti platelet activity? *(Most Recent Question June 2022)*
a. Warfarin b. Heparin
c. Clopidogrel d. Dipyridamole

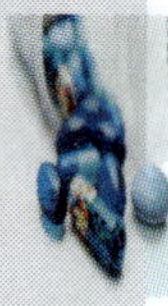

475. Mechanism of action of aspirin in patients suffering from thrombosis: *(Most Recent Question June 2022)*
- a. Fibrinolytics by converting plasminogen to plasmin
- b. Inhibiting conversion of Vit K dependent clotting factors to their active form
- c. Inhibition of cyclo-oxygenase -1 enzyme
- d. P_2Y_{12} receptor inhibitor

476. What is the mechanism of action of tPA? *(Most Recent Question June/Dec 2021)*
- a. Fibrinolysis
- b. Inhibition of factor V and VII
- c. Inhibition of factor III and V
- d. Activation of anti-thrombin III

477. A female patient was taking warfarin for prosthetic heart valves. She became pregnant. What advise will you give regarding use of this drug in early pregnancy? *(Most Recent Question June 2021)*
- a. Continue warfarin without any concern
- b. Continue warfarin but add vitamin K to the therapy
- c. Switch warfarin to heparin
- d. Terminate the pregnancy

478. Vitamin that increases the absorption of iron from stomach is: *(Most Recent Question June/Dec 2021)*
- a. Vitamin A
- b. Vitamin B_{12}
- c. Vitamin C
- d. Vitamin D

479. Mechanism of action of Aspirin
- a. Inhibit PGI2 formation
- b. Inhibit TXA2 formation
- c. Stimulate TXA2 formation
- d. Stimulate platelet aggregation

480. A patient after valve replacement will require follow-up treatment with which of the following: *(Most Recent Question Dec 2019-20)*
- a. Warfarin
- b. ACE inhibitors
- c. Beta blockers
- d. Thiazides

481. Drug contraindicated in porphyria: *(Most Recent Question Aug 2020)*
- a. Isoniazid
- b. Carbamazepine
- c. Thiopentone sodium
- d. Diazepam

482. Child presented in casualty with iron poisoning. Which of the following is the antidote of same? *(Most Recent Question Aug 2020)*
- a. EDTA
- b. BAL
- c. Penicillamine
- d. Deferoxamine

483. Which of the following is an oral direct thrombin inhibitor? *(Most Recent Question Dec 2019-20)*
- a. Dabigatran
- b. Rivaroxaban
- c. Warfarin
- d. Lepirudin

484. Coumarin necrosis occurs due to: *(Recent Pattern Question 2018-19)*
- a. Heparin
- b. Low molecular weight heparin
- c. Warfarin
- d. Clopidogrel

485. Which of the following is a Factor Xa inhibitor? *(Recent Pattern Question 2018-19)*
- a. Apixaban
- b. Argatroban
- c. Fondaparinux
- d. Bivalirudin

486. Neutropenia after chemotherapy is treated by: *(Recent Pattern Question 2018-19)*
- a. Leucovorin
- b. Filgrastim
- c. Ondansetron
- d. Darbepoetin

487. Which among the following is iron chelator? *(Recent Pattern Question 2018)*
- a. EDTA
- b. Deferoxamine
- c. BAL
- d. Dimercaprol

488. What is the mode of action of warfarin? *(Recent Pattern Question 2017)*
- a. Factor Xa inhibitor
- b. Vitamin K antagonist
- c. Activates antithrombin III
- d. Activates factor IX

489. aPTT is done for assessing: *(Recent Pattern Question 2017)*
- a. Warfarin toxicity
- b. LMW heparin
- c. Heparin toxicity
- d. Extrinsic coagulation pathway defect

490. Argatroban acts by inhibiting: *(Recent Pattern Question 2017)*
- a. Factor Xa
- b. Factor IXa
- c. Factor II
- d. Factor IV

491. Anticoagulant of choice in pregnancy: *(Recent Pattern Question 2016)*
- a. Warfarin
- b. Vitamin K
- c. Tranexamic acid
- d. Heparin

492. Which of the following drugs is used in heparin-induced thrombocytopenia? *(Recent Pattern Question 2016)*
- a. Warfarin
- b. Coumarin
- c. Lepirudin
- d. Enoxaparin

493. All of the following are true about Vitamin K; EXCEPT:
- a. Required for synthesis of clotting factors
- b. Hematuria is the first manifestation of deficiency
- c. Used as first line treatment in bleeding conditions
- d. It has a water soluble form also

494. All of following are anti platelet; EXCEPT:
- a. Aspirin
- b. Clopidogrel
- c. Abciximab
- d. Tranexamic acid

495. Aspirin acts by inhibiting the production of:
- a. Prostaglandin
- b. Cytokines
- c. Leukotriene
- d. Thromboxane

496. Mechanism of action of Aspirin:
- a. Inhibit PGI2 formation
- b. Inhibit TXA2 formation
- c. Stimulate TXA2 formation
- d. Stimulate platelet aggregation

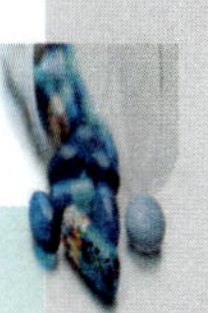

497. Which of the following is not true about Heparin function?

a. Inhibit antithrombin 3
b. Activate antithrombin 3
c. Inhibit factor IIa
d. Inhibit factor Xa

498. True about oral anticoagulant warfarin are all; EXCEPT:

a. Acts in vivo
b. Acts both in vivo and in vitro
c. Interferes with synthesis of Vit K
d. Causes Hematuria

499. All of the following drugs are contraindicated in G6PD; EXCEPT:

a. Ciprofloxacin
b. Primaquine
c. Dapsone
d. Sulfonamide

500. Which of the following drug will cause hemolysis in G6PD patients?

a. Cephalosporins
b. Ampicillin
c. Chloroquine
d. Erythromycin

501. Which of the following is a low molecular weight heparin?

a. Hirudin
b. Enoxaparin
c. Tranexamic acid
d. Lepirudin

502. Low molecular weight heparin mainly affects which factor:

a. Factor X
b. Anti-thrombin
c. Factor Xa
d. Factor IX

503. All of the following are true regarding enoxaparin; EXCEPT:

a. It has higher and predictable bioavailability
b. It act by inhibiting factor IIa mainly
c. Monitoring is not required
d. It has more favorable pharmacokinetics

504. Treatment of choice in severe cystic acne:

a. Isotretinoin
b. Tretinoin
c. Benzoyl peroxide
d. Azelaic acid

505. Vitamin B_{12} is given in severe anemia via which route:

a. I/M
b. IV
c. Oral
d. All of these

506. Antivitamin of biotin:

a. Vitamin B_6
b. Vitamin K
c. Avidin
d. None of these

507. The vitamin which can be used for treatment of hypercholesterolemia is:

a. Thiamine
b. Niacin
c. Pyridoxine
d. Vitamin B_{12}

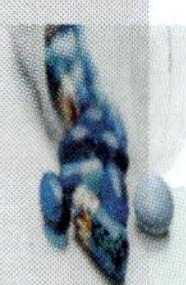

ANSWERS WITH EXPLANATIONS

MOST RECENT QUESTIONS 2023

1. Ans. (d) Fomepizole

Ref: Goodman and Gilman's The Pharmacological Basis of Therapeutics, 14th ed. pg. 521

- The given clinical picture is suggestive of methanol poisoning.
- Antidote for methanol or ethylene glycol poisoning is: Fomepizole.
- **MOA of Fomepizole:** Alcohol dehydrogenase inhibitor
- Alternatively, ethyl alcohol can also be used in this toxicity. It acts by competitive inhibition of methanol metabolism.

Extra Mile

Important antidotes:

Drugs	Antidotes
• Atropine	Physostigmine
• Benzodiazepines	Flumazenil
• Beta-blockers	Glucagon
• Copper	D-penicillamine
• Digoxin	Digibind
• Lead	EDTA/BAL
• Iron	Deferoxamine
• Paracetamol	N-acetylcysteine
• Morphine	Naloxone

2. Ans. (c) Flumazenil

Ref: Goodman and Gilman's The Pharmacological Basis of Therapeutics, 14th ed. pg. 427–434

- Flumazenil is the antidote of benzodiazepines like diazepam, lorazepam, midazolam, etc.
- It is also considered antidote of Z-drugs like zolpidem, zaleplon.

3. Ans. (d) Deferiprone

Ref: Goodman and Gilman's The Pharmacological Basis of Therapeutics, 14th ed. pg. 910

- In a patient with iron toxicity, the management can be decided whether it is acute toxicity or chronic toxicity.
- In acute iron toxicity, injectable chelating agent like **Deferoxamine** is preferred.
- In chronic toxicity like in thalassemia patient with recurrent blood transfusion, oral iron chelator agent like **Deferiprone** or **Deferasirox** is preferred.

4. Ans. (a) Nevirapine for 6 weeks

Ref: Goodman and Gilman's The Pharmacological Basis of Therapeutics, 14th ed. pg. 1252–53

- For prevention of MTCT, it is advised to give Nevirapine to pregnant mother at the onset of labor and do the delivery by elective cesarean section.
- To the newborn, oral Nevirapine 2 mg/kg should be started as soon as possible and continued till 6 weeks.
- After 6 weeks to 1 year, a combination of Zidovudine and Lamivudine will be given. In nonresponsive cases, Raltegravir will be added with the above two-drug therapy.

5. Ans. (a) Inhibits adenosine triphosphate synthase of mycobacteria

Ref: Goodman and Gilman's The Pharmacological Basis of Therapeutics, 14th ed. pg. 1276

- **Bedaquiline** is newly approved antitubercular agent that acts by inhibiting ATP synthase of MTB.
- Other newer agents like **Delamanid** and **Pretomanid** act as mycolic acid synthesis inhibitor.

Extra Mile

- **Ethambutol:** It acts as Arabinosyltransferase inhibitor of MTB. Arabinosyltransferase is an important enzyme required for the polymerization of arabinogalactan, which is an essential constituent of mycobacterium cell wall.
- **Rifampicin:** It is a DNA-dependent RNA polymerase inhibitor.

6. Ans. (b) Fluoxetine

Ref: Goodman and Gilman's The Pharmacological Basis of Therapeutics, 14th ed. pg. 351

- The given clinical picture is suggestive of an adverse drug reaction caused by antidepressant agent like selective serotonin reuptake inhibitors (SSRI).
- Drugs under this class are: Citalopram, Escitalopram, Fluoxetine, Fluvoxamine, Paroxetine, Sertraline.

Side effects of SSRI *(Mn: SSRI)*

- **Serotonin syndrome:** Nausea, vomiting, diarrhea, headache, agitation, anxiety
- **Sexual dysfunction:** Delayed ejaculation, anorgasmia
- Restlessness
- Insomnia

Extra Mile

- Lithium causes side effects like leukocytosis, diabetes insipidus, tremor, hypothyroidism.
- Haloperidol is associated with side effects like extrapyramidal symptoms, hyperprolactinemia.

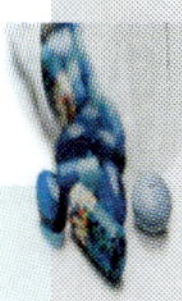

7. Ans. (a) 5-alpha-reductase inhibitor

Ref: Goodman and Gilman's The Pharmacological Basis of Therapeutics, 14th ed. pg. 984–1000

- The given clinical picture is suggestive of BPH.
- Agents used for treatment of BPH are:
  - **Alpha-1 blockers:** Prazosin, Terazosin. They are preferred in patients with history of hypertension with BPH.
  - **Alpha-1A blockers:** Tamsulosin, Silodosin. They are considered DOC for BPH.
  - **5-alpha-reductase inhibitors:** Finasteride, Dutasteride. They inhibit conversion of testosterone to DHT (Dihydrotestosterone). Hence, they can also shrink the size of prostate gland.

8. Ans. (c) Ganciclovir

Ref: Goodman and Gilman's The Pharmacological Basis of Therapeutics, 14th ed. pg. 1211–1459

- The given clinical picture is of patient with CMV retinitis.
- Drugs used for treatment of CMV retinitis are:
  - Ganciclovir, Valganciclovir (Prodrug): DOC. It is available in IV and in implant form.
  - Alternatively, Cidofovir and Foscarnet can also be used.
- **Note:**
  - Aciclovir is DOC in HSV infection. It is ineffective in CMV.
  - Cotrimoxazole is preferred in HIV patients with *Pneumocystis jirovecii* infection
  - Tenofovir is a nucleotide reverse transcriptase inhibitor (NRTI). Used in HIV and HBV.

9. Ans. (a) Phenelzine

Ref: Goodman and Gilman's The Pharmacological Basis of Therapeutics, 14th ed. pg. 113–346

- The given clinical picture of cheese reaction is seen when a tyramine-rich food is given to patients on MAO inhibitor.
- **Example of MAO inhibitors:**
  - MAO-a inhibitors: **Moclobemide**
  - MAO-b inhibitors: **Selegiline, rasagiline, safinamide**
  - Nonselective MAO inhibitors: **Phenelzine, tranylcypromine, isocarboxazid**
- **Examples of tyramine-rich food are:** Cheese, curd, any sweets or food made of milk, soya sauce, fermented meet, banana, beef, red wine, white wine, canned bear.

10. Ans. (c) Tardive dyskinesia

Ref: Goodman and Gilman's The Pharmacological Basis of Therapeutics, 14th ed. pg. 378–79

- Tardive dyskinesia is an EPS seen due to typical antipsychotics like Haloperidol, Droperidol, Flupentixol, Zuclopenthixol
- Other mentioned ADRs are seen with lithium therapy.
- Most common ADR seen with lithium: Tremor

11. Ans. (c) Acetazolamide

Ref: Goodman and Gilman's The Pharmacological Basis of Therapeutics, 14th ed. pg. 562–63

- For the treatment of mountain sickness, preferred agent is carbonic anhydrase inhibitor like **Acetazolamide** is used.
- It causes HCO_3 washout in urine leading to metabolic acidosis and CSF acidosis, which induces hyperventilation → this causes CO2 washout. This prevents altitude sickness.

12. Ans. (b) Nuclear receptor

Ref: Goodman and Gilman's the Pharmacological Basis of Therapeutics, 14th ed. pg. 68–69

- Thyroid hormone acts through nuclear receptor superfamily. Example of nuclear receptor-mediated action is seen with:
  - Thyroxine (T3, T4), Retinoic acid receptor (vitamin A), PPAR (Peroxisome proliferator-activated receptor).
- Examples of ligand-gated receptors are: GABA (a and c), Nicotinic receptor, NMDA, 5HT3
- Examples of GPCR: Alpha-receptor, beta-receptor, muscarinic receptor, dopamine receptor, histamine receptor.
- Examples of enzymatic receptors: Growth hormone, insulin, prolactin, interleukin, interferon.

13. Ans. (a) Prednisolone

Ref: Goodman and Gilman's the Pharmacological Basis of Therapeutics, 14th ed. pg. 1017–20

- For the facial palsy, steroid like prednisolone is preferred.
- Steroid is anti-inflammatory agent, which reduces inflammation and edema around the nerve.

14. Ans. (c) Erythromycin

Ref: Goodman and Gilman's The Pharmacological Basis of Therapeutics, 14th ed. pg. 1144, 1186

- Erythromycin is a macrolide antibiotic, which is effective in gram-positive bacteria, gut anaerobes and in patients allergic to penicillin.
- It is not effective in bacterial vaginosis.

Drugs used for bacterial vaginosis are:

- Metronidazole

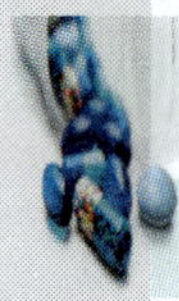

- Tinidazole
- Clindamycin

15. Ans. (d) Levonorgestrel 0.075 mg two tablets within 24 hours

Ref: Goodman and Gilman's The Pharmacological Basis of Therapeutics, 14th ed. pg. 974–75

Emergency contraception:

***Within 72 hours*:**
- LNG (Levonorgestrel) 1.5 mg single dose or 0.75 mg two tablets at interval of 12 hours
- COCP two tablets immediately and two tablets after 12 hours
- Ormeloxifene (SERM)/Centchroman 50 mg two tablets 12 hours apart within 24 hours

***Within 5 days*:**
- IUCD (most effective)
- Ulipristal 30 mg as soon as possible or within 5 days

16. Ans. (a) Type 1

Ref: Goodman and Gilman's The Pharmacological Basis of Therapeutics, 14th ed. pg. 159–60

- Penicillin-induced hypersensitivity is an example of type 1 hypersensitivity reaction (IgE-mediated).
- This ADR is also classified under type B (Bizarre) ADR
- Treatment: Adrenaline 1:1,000; 0.5 mL IM route

17. Ans. (c) Type 3

Ref: Goodman and Gilman's The Pharmacological Basis of Therapeutics, 14th ed. pg. 1268

- Treatment of leprosy using dapsone can induce two types of leprae reaction.
  - Type 1 leprae reaction: Example of HPS reaction type 4
  - Type 2 leprae reaction: Example of HPS reaction type 3
- *Remember rule of 5 (type* ***1*** *lepra reaction is* ***4*** *HPS reaction; type* ***2*** *leprae reaction is* ***3*** *HPS reaction)*
- In any types of leprae reaction, continue the therapy of leprosy and add steroids.

18. Ans. (a) Alpha-adrenergic blockers

Ref: Goodman and Gilman's The Pharmacological Basis of Therapeutics, 14th ed. pg. 269–79

- In the treatment of pheochromocytoma (PCC), the preferred DOC is Phenoxybenzamine (nonselective alpha-blocker).
- To control the intraoperative or postoperative hypertension, same agent is preferred.
- During the therapy of PCC using alpha-blocker, it is mandatory to add beta-blockers with the regimen, to control the cardiac symptoms like palpitation or tachycardia.
- Order of medication: α-blocker then β-blocker

19. Ans. (d) Safer than domperidone in children

Ref: Goodman and Gilman's The Pharmacological Basis of Therapeutics, 14th ed. pg. 1087–88

- Metoclopramide is a D2 blocker, which crosses BBB. It is also associated with extrapyramidal symptoms like dystonia, akathisia, secondary parkinsonism (abnormal posture), hyperprolactinemia.
- There is another D2 blocker like **Domperidone**, which is considered safer than Metoclopramide (not vice versa), because it does not cross BBB.

20. Ans. (a) Cisplatin

Ref: Goodman and Gilman's The Pharmacological Basis of Therapeutics, 14th ed. pg. 1352

- Platinum compound like cisplatin is considered DOC for cervical cancer.
- Cisplatin is DOC in:
- Head and neck CA, Upper GI cancer (esophagus and gastric CA), Cholangiocarcinoma, Bladder cancer, Testicular cancer, ovarian cancer, cervical cancer.
- Other agents that can be used in cervical cancer: 5-FU, Topotecan, Ifosfamide, Paclitaxel.

21. Ans. (c) Nephrotoxicity

Ref: Goodman and Gilman's The Pharmacological Basis of Therapeutics, 14th ed. pg. 1352–53

- Cisplatin is associated with side effects like:
  - Nausea and vomiting
  - Ototoxicity
  - Nephrotoxicity
- Among the given choices, nephrotoxicity is the most important toxicity that is caused by cisplatin. To prevent this toxicity, **Amifostine** is used in addition to chloride diuresis and fluid loading.

22. Ans. (a) 5-fluorouracil

Ref: Goodman and Gilman's The Pharmacological Basis of Therapeutics, 14th ed. pg. 1357–58

- Thymidine is a pyrimidine. Any pyrimidine analog produces deficiency of pyrimidines like cytosine, uracil and thymidine. This leads to deficiency of thymidine in cell and can lead to thymidine-less death of cancer cells.

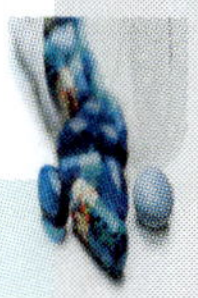

- Pyrimidine analog agents are: **5-Fluorouracil, Capecitabine, Cytarabine, Gemcitabine, Azacitidine.**

23. Ans. (a) Atropine ointment 1%

Ref: Goodman and Gilman's The Pharmacological Basis of Therapeutics, 14th ed. pg. 217–18

- For pediatric patient, preferred mydriatic and cycloplegic agent is a potent antimuscarinic agent like Tropicamide 1% ointment.
- **Note:** Drop is not preferred due to increased risk of atropine fever.
- In adults, preferred mydriatic, cycloplegic agent is Tropicamide > Cyclopentolate.

24. Ans. (c) Related to concept of P-drug

Ref: Khilnani G. The Concept of Personal Drugs in the Undergraduate Pharmacology Practical Curriculum. Indian J Pharmacol. 2008;40:131-2.

- P-drug is Preferred drug/Physician drug, which a physician chooses a drug for a particular condition, according to his expertise.
- Steps and criteria in selecting a P-drug:
  - **Step I:** Define the diagnosis
  - **Step II:** Specify the therapeutic objective
  - **Step III:** Make an inventory of effective groups of drugs
  - **Step IV:** Choose an effective group according to criteria
  - **Step V:** Choose a P-drug

Criteria:

- **Safety:** Possible adverse effects.
- **Tolerability:** Suitability for a patient.
- **Efficacy:** Drug profile.
- **Price:** Always look at the total cost of treatment rather than the cost per unit.

25. Ans. (d) 2 HRZE + 4 HRE

Ref: Goodman and Gilman's The Pharmacological Basis of Therapeutics, 14th ed. pg. 1267, 1279–80

- The first-line treatment of PTB is same in adult and pediatric age group.
- For the first 2 months, HRZE is used as intensive phase treatment. In the next 4 months, HRE is used as continuation therapy.

Definite indications for concomitant steroid therapy in TB include:

- TB meningitis
- Pericarditis
- Addison's disease
- Miliary TB with alveolocapillary block and
- TB uveitis

26. Ans. (a) Xanthine oxidase inhibition

Ref: Goodman and Gilman's The Pharmacological Basis of Therapeutics, 14th ed. pg. 848–49

- The given clinical picture is of gout. Acute cases are treated with NSAIDs, steroids or colchicine.
- Chronic cases of gout can be treated via three ways:
  1. **Decreasing uric acid production:** By inhibiting xanthine oxidase enzyme by drugs like **Allopurinol, Febuxostat**
  2. **Increasing uric acid excretion:** By inhibiting URAT-1 transporter. **Drugs: Probenecid, Lesinurad, Sulfinpyrazone, Benzbromarone**
  3. **Increasing uric acid excretion:** By recombinant uricase which metabolizes uric acid to water-soluble metabolite allantoin. Drugs like **Rasburicase, Pegloticase**

27. Ans. (d) Probenecid

Ref: Goodman and Gilman's The Pharmacological Basis of Therapeutics, 14th ed. pg. 850

- In a patient with chronic gout, uricosuric agents are used to increase the excretion of uric acid by inhibiting reabsorption of uric acid by inhibiting URAT-1 transporter in the renal tubule.
- Drugs under this class are: Probenecid, Lesinurad, Benzbromarone, Sulfinpyrazone.

Extra Mile

- Xanthine oxidase inhibitors used in patient of chronic gout are: **Allopurinol, Febuxostat**
- Recombinant uricase for chronic gout: **Rasburicase, Pegloticase**

28. Ans. (c) Ethambutol

Ref: Goodman and Gilman's The Pharmacological Basis of Therapeutics, 14th ed. pg. 1274–75

- The clinical picture of the patient is suggestive of pulmonary tuberculosis.
- In patients with drug sensitive tuberculosis, first line therapy of 6 month is initiated.
  - **Intensive phase:** 2 months: Isoniazid (H), Rifampicin (R), Pyrazinamide (Z), Ethambutol (E)
  - **Continuation phase:** 4 months: Isoniazid (H), Rifampicin (R), Ethambutol (E)
- Among the given options, ethambutol is the first-line agent that will be used for this patient.

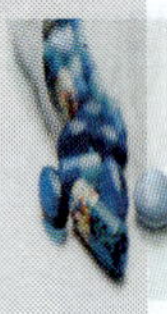

Extra Mile

- **Linezolid:** 2nd-line antibiotic for MDR-TB
- **Treptomycin:** It is an aminoglycoside. Earlier it was used as first line add-on injectable in previously treated tuberculosis patients. As per recent guidelines of NTEP 2020, it is not used nowadays in active management of drug sensitive TB.
- **Levofloxacin** is a fluoroquinolone. Used in MDR TB.

29. Ans. (d) Hydrochlorothiazide

Ref: Goodman and Gilman's the Pharmacological Basis of Therapeutics, 14th ed. pg. 631–32

- The marked site in the tubule is DCT. Diuretics act at this site is thiazide diuretics, which act by inhibiting Na^+–Cl^- cotransporter at the early part of DCT.
- Examples of thiazide diuretics are: Hydrochlorothiazide, Chlorthalidone, Indapamide, Metolazone

30. Ans. (a) Fall in BP upon giving epinephrine in a patient pretreated with phentolamine

Ref: Goodman and Gilman's the Pharmacological Basis of Therapeutics, 14th ed. pg. 252

- Dale's reversal phenomenon/Vasomotor reversal of Dale can be elicited by giving high dose of adrenaline in presence of alpha-blocker.
- Response: Only fall in BP.

CONCEPT OF DALE'S REVERSAL PHENOMENON

- Among sympathetic receptors α1, α2, β1, β2; alpha-1 is more in number, hence shows predominant action on initial dose of epinephrine. Beta-2 is most sensitive receptor, hence shows action at the lesser concentration of epinephrine.
- Epinephrine acts on all sympathetic receptors like alpha and beta. Therefore, at initial dose, there will be increased BP (α1-action), followed by decreased BP (ß2-action). It has biphasic response on BP normally, first increase then decrease.

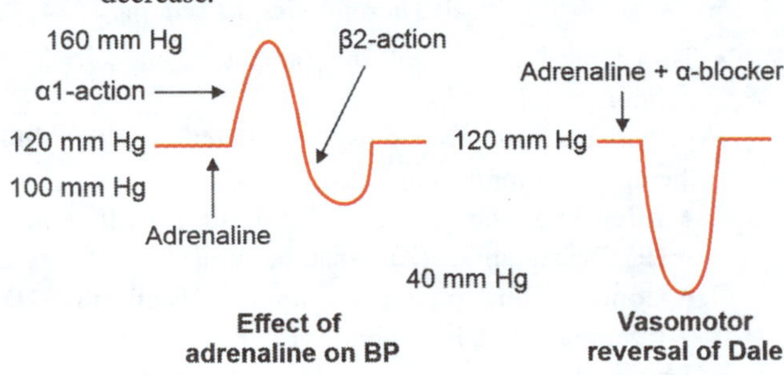

- Epinephrine exposure in presence of alpha-blocker leads to action only on beta-receptor, which causes only fall in BP. This response is called **Dale's Reversal Phenomenon**.

31. Ans. (b) Beta plus alpha-receptor blocker

Ref: Goodman and Gilman's the Pharmacological Basis of Therapeutics, 14th ed. pg. 280–282

- Labetalol is a 3rd-generation beta-blocker, having beta plus alpha-1-blocking property.
- It is the preferred drug for hypertension and hypertensive emergency in pregnancy.
- It is also used in hypertensive emergencies due to its vasodilatory action (by blocking alpha-1 receptor).
- **Note:** It does not cause vasodilation due to its direct action on smooth muscle.

32. Ans. (a) Metoprolol

Ref: Goodman and Gilman's the Pharmacological Basis of Therapeutics, 14th ed. pg. 280–81, 622, 642

- In a patient with chronic congestive heart failure, mortality is mainly due to cardiac remodeling. Drugs reducing the remodeling and hence the mortality are:
  - ACE inhibitors (Lisinopril, Ramipril, etc.)
  - ARBs (Telmisartan, Losartan, etc.)
  - Aldosterone receptor blockers (Spironolactone, Eplerenone)
  - ARNI (ARB—Valsartan + Neprilysin inhibitor—Sacubitril)
  - Beta blockers (Carvedilol, Atenolol) and
  - SGLT 2 inhibitors like Empagliflozin

Note: Other given options in question can be used in patient with heart failure, but has not shown to reduce the mortality.

33. Ans. (b) Norepinephrine

Ref: Goodman and Gilman's The Pharmacological Basis of Therapeutics, 14th ed. pg. 258–59

- The given image shows increased SBP, DBP but reflex bradycardia. This action corresponds to the property of norepinephrine.
- Norepinephrine acts on alpha-1, alpha-2 and beta-1 receptor. This action of drug causes increment in DBP (due to unopposed alpha-1 receptor), which induces reflex bradycardia.

Note:

- Among sympathetic drugs, Norepinephrine is the only agent which causes reflex bradycardia.
- In cardiac transplant patients, reflex action will not be seen. Hence only increase in HR is seen in response to norepinephrine.

34. Ans. (b) Deferoxamine

Ref: Goodman and Gilman's the Pharmacological Basis of Therapeutics, 14th ed. pg. 910, 1524

- In emergency cases of iron overdose, chelator like **Desferrioxamine/Deferoxamine** is used.
- Oral chelator for iron especially in patients those who are on recurrent blood transfusion (e.g., in Thalassemia), we prefer oral agents like **Deferiprone or Deferasirox**.

35. Ans. (b) Pirfenidone

Ref: Rang and Dale's Pharmacology. pg. 400

- Agents which are used to slow down the progression of pulmonary fibrosis are: **Pirfenidone** and **Nintedanib**.
- **Pirfenidone** is a specific agent approved for fibrosis treatment. It acts by reducing fibroblast proliferation, inhibits TGF-beta which is involved in collagen production.
- **Nintedanib** is a tyrosine kinase inhibitor which acts by inhibiting profibrotic mediators like PDGF (Platelet-Derived Growth Factor), FGF (Fibroblast Growth Factor), TGF-beta and VEGF.

Extra Mile

- Example of agents causing pulmonary fibrosis are: Amiodarone, Busulfan, Bleomycin, Cyclophosphamide, Carmustine, Nitrofurantoin, Methotrexate, Gold

36. Ans. (a) Aliskiren

Ref: Goodman and Gilman's the Pharmacological Basis of Therapeutics, 14th ed. pg. 630–31

- In the given image, the arrow marked at angiotensinogen to angiotensin I conversion, which is done by renin.
- Direct Renin inhibitor agent is: **Aliskiren**.
- Note: Renin secretion inhibitor is beta-blocker (Atenolol, Metoprolol).
- Option b: Ramipril is ACE inhibitor.
- Option c: Losartan is ARB.
- Option d: Spironolactone is aldosterone receptor blocker.

37. Ans. (a) Filgrastim

Ref: Goodman and Gilman's the Pharmacological Basis of Therapeutics, 14th ed. pg. 905

- **Filgrastim** is a granulocyte colony stimulating factor (G-CSF), which is used for managing the levels of granulocytes in patients with chemotherapy-induced neutropenia or congenital neutropenia.
- This is given for the purpose of reducing risk of systemic infection.
- Other agents that can be used for same purpose:
  - GM-CSF: **Malgramostim, Regramostim, Sargramostim**
- **Option b:** Darbepoetin-alpha is used for chemotherapy-induced anemia or anemia due to end-stage renal disease
- **Oprelvekin** is an IL-11 agonist used for chemotherapy-induced thrombocytopenia.
- **Romiplostim** is a thrombopoietin receptor agonist used for chemotherapy-induced thrombocytopenia.

38. Ans. (d) Drug A is most efficacious

Ref: Goodman and Gilman's the Pharmacological Basis of Therapeutics, 14th ed. pg. 52–53

- Order of potency: A > B > C > D
- Order of efficacy: B = C > A > D
- Few important observations from the given image:
  - Drug A is most potent and D is least potent.
  - Drug D is least potent and least efficacious.

39. Ans. (c) Gemfibrozil

Ref: Goodman and Gilman's the Pharmacological Basis of Therapeutics, 14th ed. pg. 739–40

- Gemfibrozil is a PPAR-alpha agonist, used in management of hypertriglyceridemia.
- PPAR-alpha acts by nuclear receptor and causes transcription of genes which encodes enzyme LPL (Lipoprotein Lipase). LPL enzyme increases the breakdown of triglycerides. Therefore, this class of drugs is considered best for the treatment of hypertriglyceridemia.
- Other PPAR-alpha agonists: **Clofibrate, Bezafibrate, Fenofibrate**

Extra Mile

- **PPAR-Y agonist:** Pioglitazone, Rosiglitazone. They increase insulin sensitivity and are used in treatment of diabetes mellitus. Rosiglitazone increases risk of cardiac events like M.I.
- **Simvastatin** is HMG-CoA-reductase inhibitor. They are best for reducing LDL.
- **Ezetimibe** is NPC1L1 inhibitor, which inhibits cholesterol absorption from the intestine.
- **Cholestyramine, Colestipol and Colesevelam,** is a bile acid sequestrant. These are safest antidyslipidemic agents in pregnancy and pediatric patients.

40. Ans. (d) Loperamide

Ref: Goodman and Gilman's the Pharmacological Basis of Therapeutics, 14th ed. pg. 1096–97

- **Loperamide** is an opioid which decreases intestine motility and secretion.
- It is used in noninfective diarrhea and in patients with chemotherapy induced diarrhea.
- Note: Atropine is added with opioids while treating diarrhea to reduce the abuse potential and dependency risk of opioids.

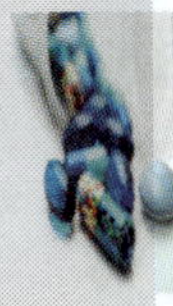

- **Ciprofloxacin** and **Ornidazole** are used in infective diarrhea.

41. Ans. (a) Granisetron + Dexamethasone + Aprepitant

Ref: Goodman and Gilman's the Pharmacological Basis of Therapeutics, 14th ed. pg. 1100, 1102, 1103

- For the management of chemotherapy-induced nausea and vomiting, the preferred agent is 5HT3 antagonist like Ondansetron, Granisetron, Palonosetron.
- Other agents that can be used are:
  - **NK1/Substance P antagonist:** Aprepitant, Rolapitant. It is preferred in chemotherapy-induced delayed nausea and vomiting.
  - **Steroid-like Dexamethasone** also reduces the emesis possibly due to its anti-inflammatory, interaction with 5HT3 and NK1 and NK2 receptors. It also reduces intracranial pressure which adds in alleviating symptoms like nausea and vomiting. Exact mechanism is unclear.
  - **Domperidone** is a D2 antagonist that can be used due to its prokinetic property. But this is not used in combination with another D2 antagonist like Metoclopramide.

42. Ans. (a) Bupropion

Ref: Goodman and Gilman's the Pharmacological Basis of Therapeutics, 14th ed. pg. 349–50, 354

- Antidepressants like SSRI (Escitalopram, Fluoxetine), SNRI (Venlafaxine) and TCA (Imipramine) are associated with sexual side effects like delayed ejaculation, anorgasmia and decreased libido.
- Receptor modulators like Bupropion are not reported with such sexual side effects.

Extra Mile

- **Bupropion** is 5HT receptor modulator with Nicotine receptor partial agonistic property. It is most preferred agent in depressed patient with smoking dependence.

43. Ans. (a) Hemodialysis is not useful in this patient

Ref: Goodman and Gilman's the Pharmacological Basis of Therapeutics, 14th ed. pg. 379–80

- Lithium is considered DOC for management of Mania. It is a drug with narrow therapeutic index and hence TDM is always required with use of lithium.
- If there is toxicity with lithium, preferred treatment modality is hemodialysis.
- **Side effect of lithium** ***(Mn: LITTH)***
  - Leukocytosis
  - Insipidus diabetes
  - Tremor (Fine > Coarse at toxic doses)
  - Teratogenic (can cause Ebstein anomaly if exposed during pregnancy)
  - Hypothyroidism
- **Interaction with lithium and thiazides**
  - Thiazide causes natriuresis. As a compensatory mechanism, there will be increased Na^+ reabsorption along with lithium. Hence with diuretics, there will increase in risk of lithium toxicity.

44. Ans. (b) It acts by inhibiting Vitamin K epoxide reductase which is involved in activation of clotting factor II, VII, IX, X

Ref: Goodman and Gilman's the Pharmacological Basis of Therapeutics, 14th ed. pg. 716

- Dicumarol/Coumadin also known as warfarin acts as competitive inhibitor of vitamin K-dependent factors like 2, 7, 9, and 10.

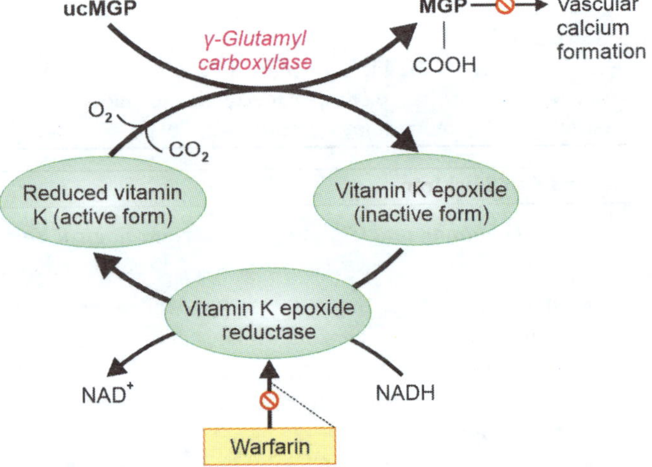

Extra Mile

- Streptokinase is a tissue plasminogen activator (tPA), used as fibrinolytic agent.
- Heparin acts by increasing AT3 activity, which binds to factor IIa and factor Xa.

45. Ans. (b) Liposomal amphotericin B

Ref: Goodman and Gilman's the Pharmacological Basis of Therapeutics, 14th ed. pg. 1312

- In a patient with cryptococcal meningitis, preferred drug is Liposomal Amphotericin B (LAMB).
- Fluconazole is used only after a 2-week IV dose of LAMB which reduces the fungal load.
- 5-Flucytosine is also effective in cryptococcal meningitis. Given as an add-on drug with LAMB.
- Voriconazole is DOC for aspergillosis.

46. Ans. (a) Ratio between a dose producing lethality in 50% and effect in 50%

- Therapeutic index is a measure of safety. It is a ratio between a dose which produces lethality in 50% of experimental population (LD50) and a dose which produces therapeutic effect in 50% experimental population (ED50).

$$\textit{Therapeutic index} = \frac{LD50}{ED50}$$

- Drugs with narrow therapeutic index are unsafe to use. If it is used, TDM is recommended.

GENERAL PHARMACOLOGY

47. Ans. (a) 50% of animal mortality in an experiment after exposure of drug

Ref: Goodman and Gillman 13th ed. pg. 36-37

- LD_{50} is an acronym which stands for Lethal Dose in 50% of experimental population.
- It is a measure of the amount of a substance that is needed to kill half of a test population of animals.
- It is used to measure the acute toxicity of substances, and this type of testing is normally performed with rates and mice.

48. Ans. (b) Physiological

Ref: Goodman Gillman 13th ed. pg. 58-59

- The shown action is an example of physiological antagonism

Types of antagonist:

- **Pharmacological antagonist:** 2 drugs binds to the same receptor and produces opposite response
- **Physiological antagonist:** Two agonists acting at different receptor producing opposite response.
  - **Ex:** Adrenaline is physiological antagonist to Histamine (adrenaline causes bronchodilation and histamine causes bronchoconstriction)
  - Glucagon and Insulin
- **Pharmacokinetic antagonist:** Antagonist action by metabolism and excretion of drug.
  - Ex: Enzyme induction to speed up metabolism
- **Chemical antagonist:** Binds chemically to compound and inactivates it.
- **Ex:** Chelating agents, charcoal (poisoning with iron).

49. Ans. (c) Phase 3

Ref: Goodman and Gillman 13th ed. pg. 6

- Post marketing surveillance is phase IV of clinical trial. Therefore, it starts after phase III clinical trial.
- Phase III clinical trial is therapeutic exploratory and confirmatory trial. After this phase, the pharmaceutical company gets the permission to market the drug with "new drug status".

Rest information on clinical trial is given later in general pharmacology section

50. Ans. (a) Phenytoin

Ref: Katzung 14th ed. pg. 46, 48

- Among the given options, phenytoin is the only agent that follows zero order kinetics.
- **Agents following zero-order kinetics are:**
  - Unfractionated heparin, Phenytoin, Aspirin, Ethanol, Tolbutamide, Theophylline, Warfarin
- **Note:** True zero order kinetics is only followed by alcohol. Rest all other initially follow first order kinetics and at high doses it starts following zero order kinetics.

Extra Mile

First order	Zero order
• If plasma concentration is increased, rate of drug metabolism is also increased	• Drug metabolism doesn't increases upon increasing plasma concentration
• Rate of metabolism is dppt to drug concentration	• Rate of drug metabolism is constant
• Clearance – constant	• Clearance: ippt Pc
• Half life is constant	• Half-life is dppt to plasma concentration

**dppt = directly isp proportional to   ippt = inversely proportional*

51. Ans. (a) Phenytoin

Ref: Katzung 14th ed. pg. 432-33

- Therapeutic drug monitoring (TDM) is monitoring the plasma concentration of that, to avoid toxicity.
- **Conditions for therapeutic drug monitoring:**
  - If drug's effect can not be assessed clinically or via other serum investigations
  - If drug has very narrow therapeutic index
- **Examples of drugs requiring TDM:**
  - Phenytoin, Digoxin, Aminoglycoside, Lithium, Immunosuppressant (Cyclosporin, Tacrolimus), TCA.

52. Ans. (b) Intravenous

- Bioavailability is fraction of unchanged drug reaching the systemic circulation following administration by any route.
- IV route has 100% bioavailability.

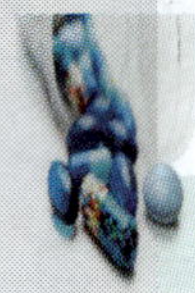

TABLE: Routes of administration, bioavailability, and general characteristics

Route	Bioavailability (%)	Characteristics
Intravenous (IV)	100 (by definition)	Most rapid onset
Intramuscular (IM)	75 to ≤100	Large volumes often feasible; may be painful
Subcutaneous (SC)	75 to ≤100	Smaller volumes than IM; may be painful
Oral (PO)	5 to <100	Most convenient; first-pass effect may be important
Rectal (PR)	30 to <100	Less first-pass effect than oral
Inhalation	5 to <100	Often very rapid onset
Transdermal	80 to ≤100	Usually very slow absorption; used for lack of first-pass effect; prolonged duration of action

53. Ans. (a) Phase 1

- Phase-1 and 0 require healthy human volunteers.

54. Ans. (a) Preclinical stage

Ref: Sharma & Sharma 3rd ed. pg. 101

- **Clinical Trial:** Systemic study of a new drug in human subject to generate data for pharmacological and adverse effects with an aim to determine safety and efficacy.
- The procedures followed during the trial should comply with an elaborate code known as ***"Good clinical practice (GCP)"*** prescribed by international conference on Harmonization.
- GCP provide details about:
  - Designing the trial
  - Collection of the data
  - Recording of information
  - Statistical analysis
  - Documentation and reporting the results of clinical trials

PRECLINICAL EVALUATION PHASE (ANIMAL STUDIES)

- Animals studies are done initially in order to define the pharmacological profile of lead compound
- Aim: Satisfy all requirements that are needed before a compound is considered fit to be tested for first in humans
- It is done according to formal operating code known as *"Good Laboratory Practices"*
- Good laboratory practices ensures reliability and reproducibility of laboratory data and minimises human errors
- Duration of preclinical study: ~2 years
- **Out of 10,000** compounds screened during preclinical phase, only 10 qualify, which are then subjected to clinical trial in humans.

55. (d) All of these

Ref: Goodman & Gillman's 13th ed. pg. 90

- The common antifungal agent ketoconazole is a potent inhibitor of CYP3A4
- Therefore coadministration of ketoconazole with other CYP3A4 inhibitors like anti-HIV drug viral protease inhibitors (ritonavir, indinavir), clarithromycin, itraconazole, nefazodone, and grapefruit juice reduces the clearance of these drugs and increases its plasma concentration and the risk of toxicity. Hence these drugs are not given together.

56. Ans. (b) Adrenaline

Ref: Goodman and Gillman 13th ed. pg. 58

- **Physiological (Functional) antagonism** occurs when two different agents produce opposite effects by acting at the different receptors.
  - Example: Action of histamine and Epinephrine at smooth muscle of bronchus. Histamine causes bronchoconstriction (by acting at H1 receptor) but epinephrine causes bronchodilation (by acting at β2 receptor).

Extra Mile

- **Pharmacological antagonist:** Drug binds at the receptor of agonist and produce no effect, shows no intrinsic activity.
- **Chemical antagonist:** Agent that binds chemically with the agonist. Example: Binding of chelating agent with the meta.

57. Ans. (d) Both a and b

Ref: Goodman and Gillman 13th ed. pg. 22

- **AUC** is the total area under the curve that describes the measured concentration of drug in the systemic circulation as a function of time (from zero to infinity) after its administration.
- AUC represents extent of absorption evaluating the bioavailability of drug from its dosage form and its clearance.

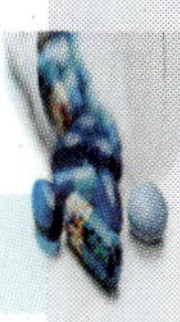

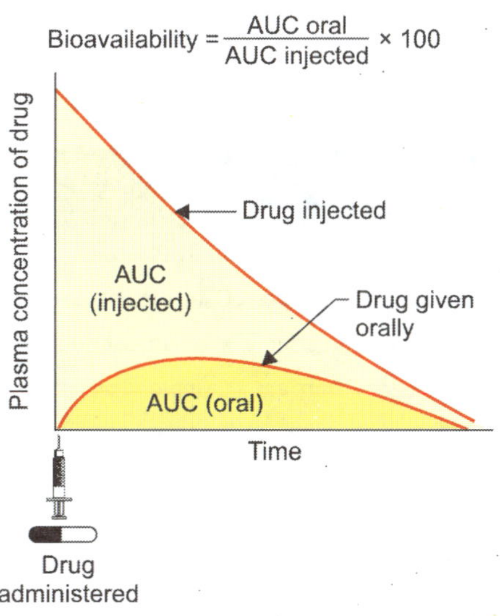

58. Ans. (b) Bizarre effect of a drug

Ref: KD Tripathi, 7th ed. pg. 82

Adverse drug reactions are classified as follows:

Type A (Predictable)	Augmented pharmacological effects: Dose dependent Side effects → at therapeutic dose Toxicity → at high dose Intolerance → toxicity at therapeutic dose
Type B (Unpredictable)	Bizarre effects: **Dose independent** Drug allergy: 4 types Anaphylaxis (type I) Blood cytolysis (type II) Complex (Ag-Ab) mediated reaction (type III) Delayed hypersensitivity (type IV) Idiosyncrasy: Abnormal effect, e.g. CNS depressants causing stimulation
Type C	**Chronic** effects: Duration dependent Adverse effects of prolonged treatment e.g. Corticosteroids causing immunosuppression
Type D	**Delayed effects:** Adverse effects long time after stopping the drug e.g. Carcinogenicity and Mutagenicity by anticancer drugs and radioisotopes
Type E	**End of treatment effects** Adverse effects due to abruptly stopping the drug e.g. withdrawal syndrome of clonidine i.e. rebound hypertension
Type F	**Failure of therapy** Ex: OCP failure Antimicrobial resistance

59. Ans. (a) Nitrate induced headache

Ref: KDT, 7th ed. pg. 82

Note: *Nitrate induced vasodilation and headache occur immediately, these are not chronic adverse drug reactions whereas others are example of type C or chronic ADRs.*

60. Ans. (c) Bioavailability

Ref: KD Tripathi, 7th ed. pg. 16

BIOAVAILABILITY

- Bioavailability is a measure of the fraction of administered dose of a drug that reaches the systemic circulation in the unchanged form.
- **Bioavailability of drug injected IV is 100%,** but is frequently lower after oral ingestion because:
  - The drug may be incompletely absorbed.
  - The absorbed drug may undergo first pass metabolism in the intestinal wall/liver or be excreted in bile.

61. Ans. (d) Monitoring adverse effects of drugs

Ref: KDT, 6th ed. pg. 79

- Pharmacovigilance is the science and activities relating to the ***detection, assessment, understanding and prevention of adverse effects*** or any other possible drug-related problems.
- Recently, its concerns have been widened to include herbals, traditional and complementary medicines, blood products, biologicals, medical devices and vaccines.

62. Ans. (c) To monitor adverse effects of drugs

Please refer to above explanation

63. Ans. (a) Rate of elimination is independent of plasma concentration

Ref: Goodman & Gillman 13th ed. pg. 20

- In pharmacokinetics, drug's clearance, rate of elimination and half life is given by the order of kinetics i.e. by zero order kinetics or first order kinetics.

Zero order kinetics Non-lnear kinetics	First order kinetics (Linear kinetics)
Constant amount of drug is eliminated per unit of time	Constant fraction of drug eliminated per unit of time
Rate of elimination is independent of plasma concentration	Rate of elimination is directly proportional to plasma concentration
Clearance is more at low concentration and less at high concentration	Clearance remains constant

Contd...

Zero order kinetics Non-lnear kinetics	First order kinetics (Linear kinetics)
Half life less at low concentration, more at high concentration	Half life is constant
Only few drugs follow zero order kinetics	Most drugs follow first order kinetics

NOTE: Drugs which follow zero order kinetics: Unfractionated heparin (UFH), Phenytoin, Aspirin, Ethanol, Tolbutamide, Theophylline, Warfarin

Mn: "U Put An End To This War"

Kinetics in a Nutshell:

Zero order	First order
ROE = constant CL α 1/P.C. t½ α PC	ROE α P.C. CL = constant t½ = constant

64. Ans. (a) Phenytoin

Ref: Katzung, 11th ed. pg. 80

ACETYLATION

- Compounds having amino or hydralazine residues are conjugated with the help of N-Acetyl transferase enzyme.
  - If acetylation is slow- increased side effect
  - Fast acetylation- not effective or effectiveness decreases
  - Normal acetylation- effective
- These drugs are remembered as CHIPS-ABC drugs:
  - **Clonazepam** (sedative)
  - **Hydralazine** (anti HTN)
  - **Isoniazid, PAS** (anti TB)
  - **Procainamide** (anti-arrhythmic)
  - **Sulfonamides** (dapsone)
  - **Acebutalol, Amrinone, ASA**
  - **Benzocaine**
  - **Caffeine**
- Phenytoin hydroxylation in liver is carried out by cytochrome P 450.
- **The drugs metabolized by acetylation causes SLE.**

65. Ans. (b) Isoniazid

Ref: KDT, 6th ed. pg. 25

Please refer to above explanation

66. Ans. (a) cAMP

Ref: Katzung, 14th ed. pg. 31

- G-protein receptor for glucagon is Gs which acts via↑Adenylyl cyclase causing ↑ **cAMP.**
- *Refer to above table for detailed explanation.*

67. Ans. (d) Excreted mainly by kidneys

Ref: Katzung, 14th ed. pg. 56; KDT, 6th ed. pg. 16-17

Ionized drugs/hydrophilic drugs	Nonionized drugs/lipophilic drugs
They are water soluble	Lipid soluble
Can not cross epithelial lining	Can cross epithelial lining easily
Poor absorption from intestine	Well absorbed from intestine
Can not cross placental barrier	Can cross placental barrier
Excreted mainly by kidneys	Excreted through faeces, urine, sweat etc.

Extra Mile

When medium is same: Drugs will cross

Example 1: *Acidic* drug will cross acid medium

Acidic drugs like salicylates, barbiturates, etc. are predominantly *unionized* in the acid gastric juice and are absorbed from stomach.

Example 2: Basic drug will cross basic medium.

Basic drugs like morphine, quinine etc. are highly ionized and are absorbed only after reaching small intestine when it gets basic medium.

68. Ans. (a) Rifampicin

Ref: Katzung, 14th ed. pg. 59

- **Enzyme induction** involves microsomal enzyme in liver as well as in other organ.
- It increases the rate of metabolism 2–4 fold. Therefore effect of drug decreases.
- **Enzyme inhibitors** also involves microsomal enzyme.
- It inhibits the microsomal enzyme, which decreases drug metabolism rate and increases duration of drug action.
- Let us take an example of warfarin, which is used as an anti thrombotic agent.
  - **Warfarin + enzyme inducer** = Thrombosis (warfarin metabolism increases and action of warfarin diminishes rapidly and thrombotic condition arises).
  - **Warfarin + enzyme inhibitor** = Bleeding (warfarin metabolism decreases and duration of warfarin action increases and patient develops bleeding tendency)

Drugs which are enzyme inducers and enzyme inhibitors

Enzyme inducers	Enzyme inhibitors
Griseofulvin	Phenylbutazone
Phenytoin	Erythromycin
Rifampicin	Allopurinol, Amiodarone
Smoking	Ciprofloxacin
Carbamazipine	Omeprazole
Phenobarbitone	Cimetidine
Barbiturate	Ketoconazole
DDT	Valproate
Remembered as: GPRS Cell Phone Battery Dead	Mn: PEACOCK Vala

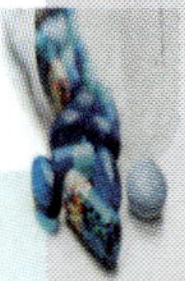

Extra Mile

- Most of the anti epileptic are enzyme inducers except **VALPROATE (an inhibitor)**
- Most of the antimicrobial are enzyme inhibitors except **GRISEOFULVIN (an Inducer)**

69. Ans. (a) Carbamazepine

Ref: Katzung, 14th ed. pg. 59

- Carbamazepine is an enzyme inducer.

Please refer to above explanation.

70. Ans. (b) Make urine alkaline with $NaHCO_3$

Ref: Katzung, 14th ed. pg. 9; KDT, 6th ed. pg. 16

- Aspirin is an acidic drug, it readily crosses any acidic medium. To treat this toxicity, make the urine alkaline with $NaHCO_3$.
- Now, this acidic drug can't be reabsorbed from the basic medium, and it readily gets excreted from the body.

Extra Mile

- In basic drug poisoning like amphetamine, we acidify the urine with NH_4Cl^- to change the medium, which opposes reabsorption and hence excretion.
- N-acetyl cysteine is the DOC for paracetamol poisoning

71. Ans. (a) Insulin

Ref: Goodman & Gillman 13th ed. pg. 851, 809

- Insulin act via enzymatic receptor.
- Ligands that act by intracellular receptors are classified into nuclear and cytoplasmic. All these ligands acts by nuclear transcription but their receptors are either present in nucleus (nuclear receptor) or in cytoplasm (cytoplasmic receptor).
- GRs reside predominantly in the cytoplasm in an inactive form complexed with other proteins. Steroid binding results in receptor activation and translocation to the nucleus
- The GR translocates to the nucleus and induces complex gene expression changes that lead to antiproliferative and apoptotic responses in sensitive cells.

Receptors	Ligands
Nuclear receptors present in nucleus *(Mn: ROAD TRAP Fixed)*	T Thyroxine R Retinoid acid receptor A Vitamin **A** P PPAR (peroxisome proliferator-activated receptor) E Estrogen (Nucleus > Cytoplasm)
Nuclear receptors present in Cytoplasm	All Steroids; mineralocorticoids (Ex: Glucocorticoids, Androgen), Vitamin D
Cell membrane via G protein stimulation	All others like ACTH, LH, GH, FSH

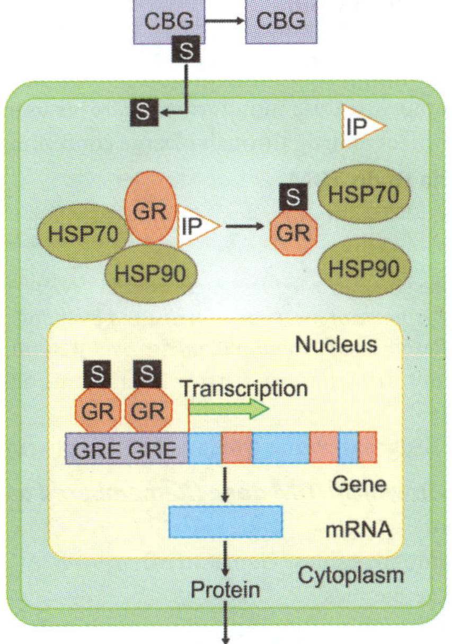

FIGURE: *Intracellular mechanism of action of the GR. The figure shows the molecular pathway by which cortisol (labeled S) enters cells and interacts with the GR to change GR conformation (indicated by the change in shape of the GR), induce GR nuclear translocation, and activate transcription of target*

Extra Mile

(Goodman & Gillman 13th ed.) (Important)

TABLE: Nuclear receptors that induce drug metabolism

Receptor	Ligands
Aryl hydrocarbon receptor (AHR	Omeprazole
Constitutive androstane receptor (CAR)	Phenobarbital
Pregnane X receptor (PXR)	Rifampin
Farnesoid X receptor (FXR)	Bile acids
Vitamin D receptor (VDR)	Vitamin D
Peroxisome proliferator- activated receptor (PPARs)	Fibrates
Retinoic acid receptor (RAR)	*all-trans*-Retinoic acid
Retinoid X receptor (RXR)	9-*cis*-Retinoic acid

72. Ans. (a) GABA

Ref: Goodman & Gillman 13th ed. pg. 851, 809

- Example of receptors acting via ion-channel/Ligand gated receptor:
  - GABA a & c
  - NMDA
  - Nicotinic receptor
  - 5HT3

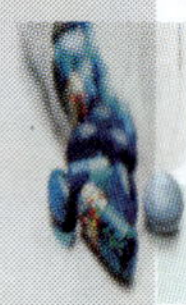

73. Ans. (a) **Phenytoin**

Ref: Katzung, 14th ed. pg. 432; KDT, 6th ed. pg. 34-35

- Therapeutic dose monitoring (TDM) is used to monitor the effect of drug through plasma concentration.

Criteria to do TDM

- When response of drug can't be measured.

Note:

- *Response of warfarin measured by INR.*
- *Response of metformin measured by blood glucose level.*
- *Response of propanolol measured by BP measurement.*

- If any drug having narrow therapeutic index (unsafe drugs).
- If a drug is showing wide variation in pharmacokinetics.

Drugs in which TDM done (Remembered as: DAAALI)

- Digitalis
- Aminoglycosides (Gentamicin)
- Anti epileptics
- Anti Cancer
- Lithium
- Immuno suppressant (Cyclosporine, Tacrolimus, Sirolimus)

TABLE: Therapeutic drug range for some anti-seizure drug

Drug	Reference range
Carbamazepine	4–12
Clobazam	0.03–0.30
Ethosuximide	40–100
Phenytoin	10–20
Phenobarbital	15–40
Valproate	40–100
Lamotrigine	3–15
Levetiracetam	12–46
Oxcarbazepine	5–35
Topiramate	5–20

74. Ans. (a) **3 months**

Ref: Katzung's Pharmacology, 14th ed. pg. 13

Type of test	Approach
Acute toxicity	**Defined as dose that is lethal in approximately 50% of animals and is maximum tolerated dose.** **It requires usually two species, two routes, single dose.**
Subacute toxicity	It requires three doses and two species. **4 weeks to 3 months** may be necessary prior to clinical trial.
Chronic toxicity	It is done in Rodent and non-rodent species for 6 months or longer. Required when drug is intended to be used in humans for prolonged periods. Usually run concurrently with clinical trial.
Carcinogenic potential	**Two years, two species.** It is required when drug is intended to be used in humans for prolonged periods.
Mutagenic potential	Effects on genetic stability and mutations in bacteria (Ames test) or mammalian cells in culture
Investigative toxicology	Determine sequence and mechanisms of toxic action. Discover the genes, proteins, pathways involved. Develop new methods for assessing toxicity.

75. Ans. (a) **Two different species**

Ref: Katzung, 14th ed. pg. 13

Please refer to above table for explanation.

76. Ans. (c) **Alprazolam**

Ref: Goodman & Gillman 13th ed. 1320-21; Katzung's Pharmacology, 10th ed. Ch 60

- Alprazolam comes under "Category D" drugs
- The FDA has established five categories to indicate the potential of a drug to cause birth defects **if used during pregnancy.**
- These categories range from A to X, in increasing order of concern:

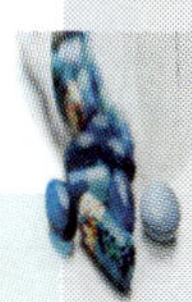

Category A	No risk in controlled human studies	Adequate and well-controlled studies have failed to demonstrate a risk to the fetus in the first trimester of pregnancy (and there is no evidence of risk in later trimesters). *Example drugs:* ***Levothyroxine, Folic Acid, Magnesium Sulfate, Liothyronine***
Category B	No risk in other studies	Animal reproduction studies have failed to demonstrate a risk to the fetus and there are *no adequate and well-controlled studies in pregnant women.* ***Example drugs: Metformin, Hydrochlorothiazide, Cyclobenzaprine, Amoxicillin, PPI*** Should be prescribed only as needed for maternal health.
Category C	Risk not ruled out	Animal reproduction studies have shown an adverse effect on the fetus and there are no adequate and well-controlled studies in humans, but potential benefits may warrant use of the drug in pregnant women despite potential risks. ***Example drugs:Tramadol, Gabapentin, Amlodipine, Trazodone, Prednisone*** Prescribed in pregnancy only when benefit clearly outweighs risk.
Category D	Positive evidence of risk	There is positive evidence of human fetal risk based on adverse reaction data from investigational or marketing experience or studies in humans, but potential benefits may warrant use of the drug in pregnant women despite potential risks. ***Example drugs: Lisinopril, Alprazolam, Losartan, Clonazepam, Lorazepam*** *Not used during pregnancy. Should be prescribed only if absolutely necessary.*
Category X	Contraindicated in pregnancy	Studies in animals or humans have demonstrated fetal abnormalities and/or there is positive evidence of human fetal risk based on adverse reaction data from investigational or marketing experience, and the risks involved in use of the drug in pregnant women clearly outweigh potential benefits. **Example drugs: Atorvastatin, Simvastatin, Warfarin, Methotrexate, Finasteride Thalidomide** Must not be used during pregnancy or in women likely to become pregnant.

77. Ans. (b) 200–400

Ref: Goodman & Gillman 13th ed. pg. 6

TABLE: Clinical Trials and its characteristics

Phase I first in human	Phase II first in patient	Phase III multisite trial	Phase IV postmarketing surveillance
10–100 participants	50–500 participants	A few hundred to a few thousand participants	Many thousands of participants
Usually healthy volunteers; occasionally patients with advanced or rare disease	Patient-subjects receiving experimental drug	Patient-subjects receiving experimental drug	Patients in treatment with approved drug
Open label	Randomized and controlled (can be placebo controlled); may be blinded	Randomized and controlled (can be placebo controlled) or uncontrolled; may be blinded	Open label
Safety and tolerability	Efficacy and dose ranging	Confirm efficacy in larger population	Adverse events, compliance, drug-drug interactions
1–2 years	2–3 years	3–5 years	No fixed duration
US $10 million	US $20 million	US $50–100 million	—
Success rate: 50%	Success rate: 30%	Success rate: 25%–50%	—

- Maximum drug failure occur in this phase: Phase II
- Most important phase of clinical trial: Phase III
- A new drug is launched in market after phase III

Extra Mile

- **Phase 0 trial** is microdosing study, done on normal healthy volunteers. To study the PK/PD of drug by radiolabelling and administering.
- **Phase 5** clinical trial is Pharamcoepidemiology.
- Phase 0 and 1 done on normal healthy volunteers.

78. Ans. (c) Phase II

Ref: Goodman & Gillman 13th ed. pg. 6

Refer to above explanation

79. Ans. (d) Phase V

Ref: Goodman & Gillman 13th ed. pg. 6

Refer to above explanation

80. Ans. (b) Lisinopril

Ref: KDT 6th ed. pg. 24

- Drugs that are administered and then converted to the active drug by biologic processes—inside the body are called a **prodrug.**
- All ACE inhibitors are prodrug EXCEPT **Captopril** and **Lisinopril** (Mn = **ACL**)
- **Other List of prodrugs are (MAMC-PLEADS)**
  - **M**inoxidil, **A**CE inhibitors, **M**ercaptopurine, **C**yclophosphamide, Clopidogrel
  - **P**PI, **L**evodopa, **E**nalapril, **A**lpha methyl dopa, **D**ipivefrine, **S**ulfasalazine, Sulindac

81. Ans. (d) Captopril

Please refer to above explanation

82. Ans. (b) Drugs used for rare disease

Ref: Katzung, 14th ed. pg. 18

- Drugs which are developed specifically for rare diseases are called **orphan drugs.**
- These drugs are difficult to research, develop, and market due to lack of financial benefits.
- Because of this a separate law known as 'The Orphan Drug Act' was passed in 1983.
- **Examples** include deferipirone to treat iron overload in thalasemia patients, N-acetylcysteine to treat paracetamol poisoning, etc.

83. Ans. (d) Decrease in efficacy

Ref: KDT pg. 73

- The food, drug and cosmetics act requires expiry date on all the drugs. Drugs used past the expiry date may lead to suboptimal therapeutic effect due to loss of efficacy.
- Drug and cosmetics act (1940) specifies the life period of drugs (mostly 1–5 years) and the conditions of storage. The expiry of other medicines has to be specified by the manufacturer but cannot exceed 5 years.
- The expiry date doesn't mean that the medicines has actually been found to loss potency or become toxic after it, but simply the quality of the medicine is not assured after the expiry date and the manufacturer is not liable if any harm arises from the use of product.

AUTONOMIC NERVOUS SYSTEM & GLAUCOMA

84. Ans. (a) Timolol

Ref: Goodman and Gillman 13th ed. pg. 216, 1260

- Timolol is non selective beta blocker. This class of drug always has risk of precipitating bronchial asthma.
- Betaxolol is a cardio-selective beta blocker that can be used safely in bronchial asthma patients.
- Other drugs in option like pilocarpine, Brimonidine have no role in bronchial asthma precipitation.

85. Ans. (b) Neostigmine + Atropine

Ref: Goodman and Gillman 13th ed. pg. 168-69

- Snake venom has Nm receptor blocking activity; therefore, Ach cannot act at the neuromuscular junction.
- In a patient with snake bite anti-snake venom is injected in priority. Next line of therapy is Neostigmine.
- Along with neostigmine, atropine is added to reduce the cholinergic symptoms.

86. Ans. (c) Pralidoxime has its role in reversal of enzyme in carbamate poisoning

Ref: Goodman and Gillman 13th ed. pg. 170-71

- Pralidoxime attaches to the anionic site of the Ach esterase enzyme which remains unoccupied in case of OP poisoning. Hence, oximes are effective only in OP poisoning.
- In Carbamate poisoning, both anionic and Esteric sites of Ach esterase are occupied. Therefore, oximes are ineffective in carbamate poisoning.
- **Note:** Atropine can be used as antidote for OP and carbamate poisoning both.

87. Ans. (a) Hypoglycemia

Ref: Goodman and Gillman 13th ed. pg. 201

- Ritodrine is selective β2 agonist, used as uterine relaxant as tocolytic agent.
- **Side effects:**
  - Tremor, tachycardia, tolerance
  - Due to beta 2 stimulation, there can be peripheral vasodilation leading to hypotension and pulmonary edema
  - Hyperglycemia (due to beta 2 stimulation of liver which increases gluconeogenesis and glycogenolysis)

88. Ans. (b) Atropine

Ref: Goodman Gillman 13th ed. pg. 153

- The above-mentioned case is of organophosphate poisoning.
- OP inhibits Acetylcholine esterase enzyme irreversibly, leading to increased level of Ach, which causes all cholinergic symptoms like salivation, lacrimation, Fall in BP, bradycardia, Miosis, etc.
- Antidote of OP and carbamate poisoning is Atropine.

Extra Mile

- Physostigmine, Neostigmine is reversible Ach esterase enzyme inhibitor, they can further worsen the problem.
- NAC is an antidote of paracetamol poisoning.

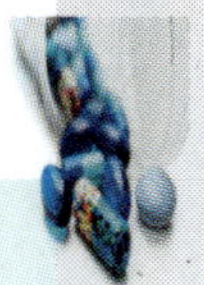

89. Ans. (a) Acetazolamide

- DOC for mountain sickness: Carbonic anhydrase inhibitor (Acetazolamide)

MOA:

- CA inhibitor counteracts the respiratory alkalosis which occurs during ascent to altitude.
- It facilitates the excretion of bicarbonate in the urine. As a result, it slows down acclimatization and helps to prevent high altitude disorders.

90. Ans. (a) It increases renal blood flow

- Dopamine has dose dependent activity on D1, B1 and a1 receptors
- At low dose, D1 receptor causes renal vasodilation, hence increases renal blood flow.
- D1 agonistic action at dose: <2 μg/kg/min
- Beta 1 action at dose: 2–10 μg/kg/min
- Alpha 1 action at dose: >10 μg/kg/min.

91. Ans. (a) Adrenaline

- This is a case of Anaphylactic shock
- DOC for Anaphylactic shock is Adrenaline.
- Route is intramuscular.
- Concentration is 1:1000 (0.5 mL)

92. Ans. (a) Atropine

- This is a case of Organophosphate poisoning. DOC is ATROPINE.
- Flumazenil is DOC of Benzodiazepine poisoning.
- N-acetylcysteine is DOC of Paracetamol poisoning.
- Another example where garlic odor is seen is Arsenic poisoning.

93. Ans. (c) Tamsulosin

Ref: Katzung 14th ed. pg. 159-60

- Prazosin is selective alpha-1 blocker. It is considered as drug of choice in BPH patients with hypertension.
- **Side effect:** Postural hypotension, Retrograde ejaculation
- To counter postural hypotension as side effect, selective alpha-1a blocker like Tamsulosin or Silodosin will be used.
- Alpha 1a subtype is most predominantly present over prostrate, compared to alpha 1b. therefore these drugs has lesser risk of postural hypotension.
- Drug of choice for BPH: **Tamsulosin**

94. Ans. (d) X

- Parasympathetic outflow is from cranial nerve 3, 7, 9, 10 and sacral nerve 2, 3, 4.
- Majority of parasympathetic outflow (~75%) is from vagus nerve (CN-X)

95. Ans. (b) Salbutamol

- Salbutamol is beta-2 agonist, preferred in acute bronchial asthma attack
- Most common side effect associated with the agent is Tremor

96. Ans. (d) Formoterol

- Beta-2 agonists are well known bronchodilators. This includes:
  - Salbutamol, Terbutaline, Formoterol, Salmeterol, Indacaterol, Albuterol etc.
- Among these agents formoterol, salmeterol, Indacaterol are longer acting analogue and are preferred in prophylactic therapy of bronchial asthma and COPD.

97. Ans. (a) Promethazine

Ref: Goodman & Gillman 13th ed. pg. 935

- Drugs that are used as agent of choice for motion sickness are:
  - **Antimuscarinic** agents like Hyoscine and Scopolamine
  - **H1 antagonist drugs** like Promethazine, Diphenhydramine > Buclizine, Cyclizine, etc.
- The anti-motion sickness activity of both these classes becomes more pronounced when combined with ephedrine.
- Both the class of drugs can also be used in Meniere's syndrome.

TABLE: General classification of antiemetic agents

Antiemetic class	Examples	Most effective against
$5HT_3$ receptor antagonists[a]	Ondansetron	Cytotoxic drug-induced emesis
Centrally acting Dopamine receptor antagonists	Metoclopramide Promethazine	
Cannabinoid receptor agonists	Dronabinol nabilone	
Neurokinin receptor antagonists (NK1)	Aprepitant Netupitant	Cytotoxic drug induced emesis (delayed vomiting)
Histamine H_1 antagonists	Cyclizine	Vestibular emesis (Motion sickness)
Muscarinic receptor antagonists	Hyoscine (scopolamine)	

[a] *The most effective agents for chemotherapy induced nausea and vomiting are the 5HT3 antagonists and metoclopramide.*

98. Ans. (b) Alpha 2 agonist

Ref: Goodman & Gillman 13th ed. pg. 203

- Alpha methyldopa is an alpha-2 agonist acts as centrally acting sympatholytic agent

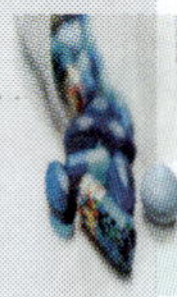

α2 agonist	Uses
Alpha methyldopa	Antihypertensive
Clonidine Tizanidine Moxonidine	Antihypertensive Sedative Analgesics
Apraclonidine Brimonidine	Glaucoma (Decrease aqueous production)
Guanfacine	Antihypertensive ADHD

99. Ans. (c) Active miotic

Ref: Goodman & Gillman 13th ed. pg. 1017

- Pilocarpine is one of the M_3 receptor agonist causing active miosis.
- To understand this concept of active and passive miosis/mydriasis, we need to know the receptors present in eye and its function:

Receptor	M3	α1	Example of drugs
Location	Sphincter pupillae Ciliary muscle	Dilator pupillae/ Radial muscle	
Agonist	Active miosis	Active mydriasis	**M_3 agonist:** Pilocarpine (Active miosis) **α1 agonist:** Dipivefrine (Active mydriasis)
Antagonist	Passive mydriasis	Passive miosis	**M_3 antagonist:** Atropine (Passive mydriasis) **α1 antagonist:** Prazosin (Passive miosis)

100. Ans. (b) Prazosin

Ref: Goodman & Gillman 13th ed. pg. 208-209

- Prazosin is one of the non-selective alpha 1 antagonists used for treatment of hypertension and BPH.
- DOC for HTN + BPH: Prazosin
- DOC for BPH: Silodosin (selective α_{1a} agonist)
- **Side effect:**
  - Marked Postural hypotension (orthostatic/first dose hypotension), syncope → can cause recurrent falls. Therefore, it is given at bedtime
  - Retrograde ejaculation

101. Ans. (a) Plasma acetylcholinesterase

Ref: Goodman & Gillman 13th ed. pg. 170

- The diagnosis of organophosphate poisoning can be made with the help of history of exposure and characteristic cholinergic signs and symptoms.
- In suspected cases of milder or chronic poisoning determination of plasma cholinesterase activities in erythrocytes and plasma establishes the diagnosis. It the most sensitive test.

Extra Mile

- **Symptoms of organophosphate poisoning:**
  - Salivation, Lacrimation, Urination, Diarrhea, GI distress, Emesis, Fasciculation, Bradycardia, Pin point pupil *(Mn: SLUDGE-FBP).*
- **Antidote of OP poisoning:** Atropine (2-4 mg IV or 2 mg IM → repeated every 10–15 minutes till atropinization).
- **AchE reactivators:**
  - **Pralidoxime (2-PAM), Obidoxime:** Action seen peripherally only (1–2 mg IV slow infusion. If symptom persists → repeat the dose)
  - **Diacetylmonoxime (DAM):** Action seen both peripheral and central.

102. Ans. (a) 1% atropine ointment

Ref: KD Tripathi 8th ed. pg. 131

- Atropine 1% ointment is preferred for refractive error test in children below 5 years. It is applied 24 hours and 2 hours before the procedure.
- The shorter acting agents like homatropine, tropicamide and cyclopentolate doesn't produces effective cycloplegia in children (ciliary muscle tone of child is high)
- Ointment is preferred over eye drop as there is increased risk of systemic absorption of eye drop which can cause anticholinergic side effect in child. Example: Hyperthermia, decreased secretion, tachycardia, etc.

Extra Mile

- Cycloplegic agent of choice is adult/elderly: Tropicamide. The protein binding of esmolol is 55%.
- For only fundoscopy/mydriasis, preferred agent is: Phenylephrine (Sympathomimetic)

103. Ans. (a) β_2 agonist

Ref: Goodman & Gillman's 13th ed. pg. 201

- Ritodrine is a β_2-selective agonist that was developed specifically as a uterine relaxant and is used in preterm labor as tocolytic agent.

Other β_2 agonists are:

Short acting	Long acting	Very long acting
• Metaproterenol • Albuterol • Levalbuterol • Pirbuterol • Terbutaline • Isoetharine • Fenoterol • Procaterol	• Salmeterol • Formoterol • Arformoterol	• Indacaterol • Olodaterol • Vilanterol

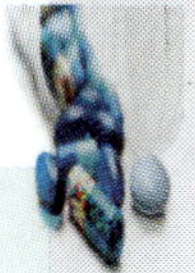

104. Ans. (b) Its plasma hydrolysis by esterases is rapid

Ref: Goodman & Gillman's 13th ed. pg. 216-17

- Esmolol is a β_1-selective antagonist with a rapid onset and a very short duration of action (t½ = 8 minutes).
- The drug is hydrolyzed rapidly by esterases in erythrocytes leading to its short half-life.
- Esmolol is used in urgent settings where immediate onset of β-blockade is warranted so it is given by slow intravenous injection.
- A partial loading dose (500 µg/kg over 1 minute) typically is administered, followed by a continuous infusion of the drug (maintenance dose of 50 µg/kg/min for 4 minutes).

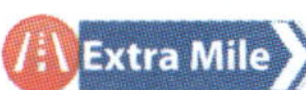

Extra Mile

- The lipid solubility of esmolol is low and has no oral bioavailability so it is given via IV.
- The protein binding of esmolol is 55%.

105. Ans. (b) Given effectively in carbamate poisoning

Ref: Sharma & Sharma 3rd ed. pg. 146-47

- Organophosphate poisoning causes irreversible blockade of AchE enzyme, which causes cholinergic effects on the patients.
- **Symptoms are:** Salivation, lacrimation, urination, diarrhea, GI upset, emsesis, fasciculation, bradycardia, miosis, hypotension, restlessness, tremor, ataxia
- Immediate management is done by atropine.
- Treatment is done by using AChE enzyme reactivating drugs along with atropine.
- AChE reactivating drugs are: Pralidoxime (PAM), obidoxime and Diacetyl=monoxime (DAM).
- Initially, atropine is injected in a dose of 2 mg IV q 10–15 minutes until muscarinic symptoms disappear.
- Thereafter pralidoxime 1–2 g is **given by slow IV infusion** over **15–30 minutes to reactivate AChE**.
- Pralidoxime and obidoxime does not crosses BBB, hence cannot activate AChE inhibited in the brain. Therefore DAM which can cross BBB is used in such cases.

106. Ans. (b) Clonidine

Ref: Sleisenger and Fordtran's Gastrointestinal and Liver Disease, Volume 1; pg. 575

- Diabetic diarrhea is seen in middle aged type 1 poorly controlled diabetic patients and is characterized by intermittent, brown, watery and voluminous stools which is occasionally accompanied by tenesmus.
- In these patients GI adrenergic function is impaired in autonomic neuropathy. Therefore any adrenergic agonist may further stimulate the intestinal absorption of fluid and electrolytes.

Drugs used are:

- **Alpha 2 adrenergic agonist: Clonidine.** Acts as adrenergic antagonist which acts by reversing the peripheral adrenergic resorptive abnormalities.
  - Because of autonomic neuropathies, these patients will not experience postural hypotension.
  - Moreover, clonidine doesn't alter diabetic control or renal function.
- **Somatostatin analogue: Octreotide.** Useful in refractory diabetic diarrhea
- **Codeine, Diphenoxylate with atropine, Loperamide:** Used for symptomatic treatment.

Extra Mile

Anti diarrheal agents

Drugs	Main uses
Tryptophan hydroxylase inhibitor: Telotristat ethyl	Severe diarrhea due to carcinoid tumors
Enkephalinase inhibitor-Racecadotril	Acute diahhrea Safe in children
Octreotide	• Severe secretory diarrhea due to GI tumors • Postgastrectomy dumping syndrome
Crofelemer (plant derived)	HIV/AIDS diarrhea
Alosetron	• Diarrhea-predominant IBS in women
Bile acid sequestrants: Cholestyramine, Colesevelam, Colestipiol	Bile salt induced diarreha
Clonidine	Diabetic diarrhea (DOC)
MOR agonists (µ opioid receptor) • Diphenoxylate, difenoxin, Loperamide	Acute diarrhea Chronic diarrhea Traveler's diarrhea
Antibiotics—empiric therapy • Fluoroquinolone • Ciprofloxacin • Levofloxacin • Norfloxacin • Ofloxacin **Alternative antibiotics** • Azithromycin • Rifaximin	• Acute diarrhea • Traveler's diarrhea • **Azithromycin:** Preferred treatment for children with traveler's diarrhea • **Rifaximin:** Preferred for diarrhea predominant IBS

107. Ans. (a) Inhibition of release of neurotransmitter

Ref: KD Tripathi, 7th ed. pg. 99

- Release of Ach from nerve terminals occurs in small quanta—amount contained in individual vesicles is extruded by exocytosis.

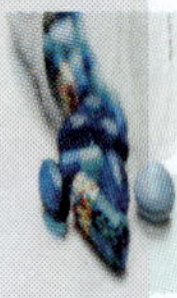

- Two toxins interfere with cholinergic transmission by affecting release:
  - ***Botulinum toxin*** inhibits release of ACh from pre-synapse
  - ***Black widow spider toxin*** induces massive release and depletion
- **Botulinum toxin**
  - Botulinum toxin A and B are highly potent exotoxins produced by ***Clostridium botulinum*** that are responsible for 'botulism' (a type of food poisoning). These neurotoxic proteins cause long-lasting loss of cholinergic transmission by interacting with axonal proteins involved in exocytotic release of Ach.

108. Ans. (b) Organophosphate poisoning

Ref: Katzung Pharamacology, 14th ed. pg. 115

- Organophosphates are irreversible Acetylcholinesterase inhibitor which is well absorbed from the skin, lung, gut, and conjunctiva—thereby making them dangerous to humans and highly effective as insecticides.
- Due to inhibition of acetylcholinesterase enzyme, acetylcholine levels are increased and the patient therefore presents with cholinergic symptoms: ***(Mn: SLUDGE-FB)***
- Salivation, Lacrimation, increased urination, Diarreha, GI distress, Emesis, Faciculation, Bradycardia
- DOC for this poisoning: **ATROPINE**

Extra Mile

OXIMES (Pralidoximes, Di-Acetyl monoxime) are known as AchE enzyme reactivators. These are used only in organophosphate poisoning.
Pin-point pupil is seen in poisoning with: *(Mn: POMP)*
Pontine hemorrhage, Organophosphate, Morphine and Phenol poisoning

109. Ans. (c) Atropine poisoning

Ref: Katzung Pharamacology, 14th ed. pg. 127–28

Refer to above explanation

110. Ans. (b) Dryness

Ref: Katzung'a Pharamacology, 14th ed. pg. 126

- **Anti-cholinergic agent/Muscarinic antagonists** are the class of drugs which competitively inhibit the effect of acetylcholine at muscarinic receptors. Therefore decreasing secretion from glands leading to DRYNESS.
- **Anti-cholinergic side-effect can be remembered by this mnemonic:**
  - Hot as hare: Increased temperature
  - Blind as bat: Mydriasis
  - Dry as bone: Dry mouth, dry eye, dry skin
  - Red as beet: Flushed face
  - Mad as hatter: Delirium

Extra Mile

- Indirect acting Cholinergic agents increases the acetylcholine level by blocking acetylcholine esterase enzyme (Ex: Organophosphate, Carbamate).
- The patient therefore will present with cholinergic symptoms: ***(Mn: SLUDGE-FB)***
  Salivation, Lacrimation, increased urination, Diarrhea, GI distress, Emesis, Fasciculation, Bradycardia
- DOC for this OP poisoning: **ATROPINE**

111. Ans. (d) OP poisoning

Ref: Katzung, 14th ed. pg. 115; KDT, 7th ed. pg. 111

- Neostigmine is a cholinergic agent which act by inhibiting cholinergic esterase enzyme, thereby increasing acetylcholine level at the synapse.
- Ach in eyes causes miosis
- **Uses of Physostigmine:** Atropine/Belladona poisoning
- **Uses of Neostigmine:** Myasthenia Gravis, Snake bite, Curare poisoning, post operative paralytic ileus, reversal of neuromascular blockade.
- **Uses of Rivastigmine:** Alzheimer's disease and parkinsonism
- **DOC for organo-phosphate poisoning:** Atropine

112. Ans. (c) Heart: Decrease heart rate

Ref: Katzung, 14th ed. pg. 127

Cholinergic receptors are:

- **M_1:** The M_1 is primarily a neuronal receptor located in ganglion cells and central neurons, especially in cortex, hippocampus and corpus striatum. It plays a major role in mediating gastric secretion, relaxation of lower esophageal sphincter (LES) caused by vagal stimulation, and in learning, memory, motor functions, etc.
- **M_2:** Cardiac muscarinic receptors are predominantly M_2 and mediate vagal bradycardia. Autoreceptors on cholinergic nerve endings are also M_2 subtype.
- **M_3:** Visceral smooth muscle contraction and glandular secretions are elicited through M_3 receptors, which also mediate vasodilatation through EDRF release. Together the M_2 and M_3 preceptors mediate most of the well-recognized muscarinic actions including contraction of LES.

113. Ans. (b) M2 agonist

Ref: Katzung, 14th ed. pg. 127

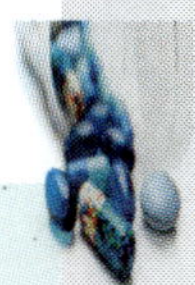

TABLE: Muscarinic receptors

	M1	M2	M3
Site	CNS Stomach	Heart	All remaining
Func:	Gastric secretion CNS excitation	Dec HR	Increase everything
Agonist:	Oxotremorine	Methaholine	Bethanechol
Antagonist	Pirenzepine Telenzepine	Tripitramine	Tolterodine Darifenacin

114. Ans. (d) M2 antagonist

Ref: Sharma & Sharma 3rd ed. pg. 119

Refer to above explanation

115. Ans. (d) Neuromuscular junction

Ref: Sharma & Sharma 3rd ed. pg. 117

- Alpha bungaratoxin is extracted from venom of elapid snake.
- It acts by neuromuscular junction blocking, therefore producing muscular weakness, respiratory failure like symptoms.

TABLE: Nicotinic receptors

	Nn	Nm
Site	At all autonm ganglia, Adrenal medulla	NMJ
Func:	Impulse transmission NE/E secretion	Skeletal ms contraction
Agonist:	Epibatidine, Nicotine, DMPP	Ach, Sch, PTMA
Antagonist:	Hexamethonium Trimethaphan	D- Tubocurarine α- Bungaratoxin

116. Ans. (a) Urinary incontinence

- Ipratropium and Tiotropium is long acting muscarinic antagonist (M3 antagonist).
- Ipratropium bromide, given as inhalation, shows transient local side effects like dry mouth, irritation in trachea and blurred vision.
- Systemic effects like urinary retention are seen, but rare because of poor absorption from GIT and lungs.
- M3 antagonist does not cause incontinence.

117. Ans. (a) Decreasing phosphodiesterase activity

Aminophylline and other methylxanthines act by

- Inhibiting phosphodiesterase enzyme causing – cAMP
- Blocking adenosine receptors
- Releasing Ca^{2+} from sarcoplasmic reticulum in cardiac and skeletal muscles.
- Use–Asthma, COPD, chronic bronchitis

118. Ans. (a) Oxybutynin

Ref: KD Tripathi, 6th ed. pg. 111

- Oxybutynin is a relatively M3 selective muscarinic antagonist which has preferential action on urinary bladder
- It is **indicated in overactive bladder with urinary frequency and urgency.**
- **Drugs which are used in overactive bladder:** ***(remembered as: My SOFTT/BlaDder)***
  - Mirabegron (β3 agonist)
  - Solifenacin
  - Oxybutynin
  - Flavoxate, Fesoterodine
  - Tolterodine, Trospium
  - Darifenacin

  } (M_3 Antagonist) [Solifenacin to Darifenacin]
- **Note: Mirabegron and Vibegron is beta 3 agonist.** Recently approved for overactive bladder. All other drugs are parasympatholytics acting as M3 antagonist

Extra Mile

- Alfuzosin is a selective α1 blocker which is used to treat BPH.
- Bethanechol selectively stimulates M3 receptor present on bladder. It is used in case of atonic bladder (urinary retention).

119. Ans. (a) Bethanechol

Ref: Katzung, 14th ed. pg. 109; KD Tripathi, 6th ed. pg. 111-12

- Bethanechol has mainly muscarinic action without effect on nicotinic receptors and is used to treat urinary retention secondary to general anaesthesia or diabetic neuropathy.
- Bethanechol is totally resistant to hydrolysis by AchE as well as by pseudocholinesterase and hence its t1/2 is very long.
- **Other uses of bethanechol:**
  - To reverse post op or neurogenic bladder atony.
  - To treat GI atony/post op paralytic ileus
  - To treat salivary gland malfunction (xerostomia).
- **Side effects:**
  - Hyperthyroidism, MI (due to risk of developing conduction block), peptic ulcer, asthma exacerbation.

120. Ans. (c) Alpha 1 and Beta 2

Ref: Katzung, 14th ed. pg. 145–47

- Alpha 1 and Beta 2 receptors present at blood vessels causing vasoconstriction and vasodilatation respectively.

TABLE: Sympathetic receptors, their location, function and G protein.

Receptor	Location	Function	G-Protein
α_1	BV, smooth muscle, Salivary glands	Vasoconstriction Increse secretion	Gq
α_2	Presynapse Beta pancreatc cell	Brake/Inhibit NA release Decrease insulin release	Gi
β_1	Heart JG cell	Inc Heart rate Renin release	Gs
β_2	Lungs Smooth muscle Liver	Bronchodilatation Relaxation of smooth muscles Glycogenolysis	Gs
β_3	Adipocyte Detrusor muscle	Lipolysis, thermogenesis Bladder relax	Gs

121. Ans. (c) Stimulation of parasympathetic fiber

Ref: Katzung, 14th ed. pg. 130

- Sympathetic and parasympathetic fibers present widely on the viscera, control their function.
- **Sympathetic fibers** stimulate/constrict heart (increase in HR) and inhibit/Relax all other organs (e.g. Bronchodilation, decreased GI motility, mydriasis, etc.)
  - **Receptor** of sympathetic fibres are: β_1 (present on heart mainly) and β_2 (present on lungs, muscle, liver, etc.)
  - Stimulation of β2 receptor will cause bronchodilation/ Increased bronchial calibre
- **Parasympathetic fibers** inhibit/Relax heart (decreased HR) and stimulate/constrict all other organs (broncho-constriction/**reduced bronchial caliber (bronchoconstriction)**, increased GI motility, miosis, etc.)
  - **Receptors** of parasympathetic fibres are M1, M2 and M3
  - M1 is located mainly in gastric glands and CNS, M2 is located on heart and M3 is located on all other areas like eyes, glands, bladder, instestine, etc.

122. Ans. (a) Increase BP, bradycardia

Ref: Katzung, 14th ed. pg. 141–41; KDT, 6th ed. pg. 122

- Epinephrine (adrenaline) and Norepinephrine (NA) are endogenous catecholamine. These are the hormones responsible for actions like bradycardia and tachycardia by acting on their specific receptors.
- *Systolic blood pressure* (SBP) is *determined by cardiac output* (β_1 *action*). β_1 receptors are present on heart which upon stimulation causes tachycardia.
- *Diastolic BP (DBP) depends on the state of blood vessels.* β2 receptors are present on blood vessels which upon stimulation causes vasodilation → DBP ↓
- Alpha receptors are present on vessel wall, which upon stimulation constricts vessel wall and increase total peripheral resistance → DBP ↑
- *Increased DBP stimulates* baroreceptor mediated release of ACh (reflex action) that decreases heart rate via activation of M2 receptors.
- Reduction in DBP increases central sympathetic outflow and thereby increases heart rate.
- **Note:** NA normally decreases heart rate but if given after a dose of atropine, increase in heart rate will be seen *(reflex action is abolished because of blockage of M2 receptor).*
- Adrenaline acts on α_1, α_2, β_1, β_2 receptors whereas Noradrenaline acts on α_1, α_2, β_1. Which means.
  - Activation of adrenaline causes tachycardia (β_1 action) and NO effect on DBP because action of α_1 and β_2 are neutralized by each other.
  - Activation of NA causes ↑DBP (due to unopposed α_1 action) and reflex bradycardia.

	SBP (β1)	DBP (β2 and α1)	Heart rate		
			Direct	Indirect	Net Effect
Adrenaline/ epinephrine	↑↑	–	↑	–	↑
Noradrenaline/ NE	↑↑	↑↑	↑	↓↓	↓

123. Ans. (a) Beta 1

Ref: Katzung, 14th ed. pg. 149; KDT, 6th ed. pg. 126

- Dobutamine is a relatively selective β1 agonist. Though it acts on both alpha and beta receptors, ***the only prominent action of clinically employed doses is its β1 action, i.e. an increase in force of cardiac contraction and output, without significant change in HR, BP or peripheral resistance.***
- **Use:** Heart failure *(as an ionotrope)*

124. Ans. (b) Orthostatic hypotension

Ref: Katzung's Pharmacology, 14th ed. pg. 149

- Midodrine is a directly acting sympathomimetics *(selective α1 receptor agonist non catecholamines).*

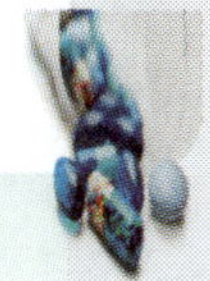

- Primary indication of midodrine is the **treatment of orthostatic hypotension**, typically due to impaired autonomic nervous system function.
- It may also cause hypertension when patient is supine.

Mechanism of Action

- Alpha-1 selective adrenergic agonist; increases peripheral vascular resistance; arteriolar and venous tone increases and results in a rise in sitting, standing, and supine systolic and diastolic blood pressure in patients with orthostatic hypotension.

125. Ans. (b) Salbutamol

Ref: Katzung 11th ed. Ch 2

- Tachyphylaxis is an acute rapid decrease in response to a drug after its administration. It can occur after an initial dose or after a series of small doses.
- Inhalation of an agonist for the beta-2 adrenergic receptor, such as **Salbutamol,** Albuterol (US), is the most common treatment for asthma. ***Polymorphisms of the beta-2 receptor play a role in tachyphylaxis.***
- Increasing the dose of the drug may be able to restore the original response.
- **Drug causing tachyphylaxis: (SAD NET/***Cigarette***)**
  - Salbutamol
  - Amphetamine
  - Dobutamine
  - Nicotine
  - Ephedrine
  - Tyramine

126. Ans. (c) Nadolol

Ref: Katzung Pharma, 14th ed. pg. 162–166

- The β antagonists are rapidly distributed and have large volumes of distribution.
- Most β antagonists have half-lives in the range of 3–10 hours. A major exception is esmolol, which is rapidly hydrolyzed and has a half-life of approximately 10 minutes. *Therefore esmolol is the shortest acting β blocker.*
- **Nadolol** is excreted unchanged in the urine and ***has the longest half-life*** of any available β antagonist (up to 24 hours).
- The half-life of nadolol is prolonged in renal failure. Therefore it is contraindicated in renal failure.
- β blockers which are contraindicated in renal failure are: (*remember as ANS*)
  - Atenolol
  - Nadolol
  - Sotalol

Extra Mile

"ALSO KNOW" ABOUT β BLOCKERS:

- β1 **receptors** are present mainly on heart. Therefore selective β 1 BLOCKERS are for cardiac condition mainly.
- β2 **receptors** are present mainly on respiratory pathway and some on liver, uterus, bladder etc. therefore β2 stimulators are used in conditions like asthma, preterm labor, urinary incontinence etc.
- Most cardioselective β blocker- **NEBIVOLOL**
- Longest acting- **NADOLOL**
- Shortest acting- **LANDIOLOL > ESMOLOL**
- β blockers which is DOC in open angle glaucoma in India-**TIMOLOL**

127. Ans. (a) Atenolol

Ref: Katzung, 14th ed. pg. 179; KDT 6th ed. pg. 140 Table 10.2

128. Ans. (a) Esmolol

Ref: KDT, 6th ed. pg. 147

- Esmolol is an ultra short acting, cardio-selective β blocker devoid of partial agonistic or membrane stabilizing effect.
- It is metabolized by pseudocholineestrase, which is abundant in our body. Thereby making it least likely to cause hypotension followed by or during surgery.
- **It is used in:**
  - Terminating supraventricular tachycardia
  - Episodic atrial fibrillation or flutter
  - Arrhythmia during anaesthesia
  - To reduce BP and HR during cardiac surgery and early treatment of MI.

129. Ans. (b) Acebutalol

Ref: Katzung, 14th ed. pg. 166; KDT, pg. 140

- Some patients are sensitive to beta blockers. They usually develop bradycardia upon intake. Such patients are known as β-blocker sensitive patient.
- However, some beta blockers possess **Intrinsic Sympathomimetic Activity** (ISA) aka partial agonistic activity. For such sensitive patients, beta blockers with partial agonistic activity are preferred.
- These drugs themselves activate β_1 or β_2 receptors sub-maximally.
- **Benefits:**
  - Bradycardia and depression of contractility at rest are not prominent.
  - Withdrawal doesn't exacerbate hypertension or angina.

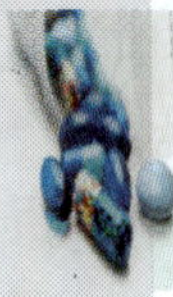

- **Beta Blockers With Partial Agonistic Activity** (*Remembered as* ***Mn.*** *COP Pins CAB*)
  - **C**eliprolol, **O**xprenolol, **P**enbutolol
  - **Pin**dolol
  - **C**arteolol
  - **A**cebutalol, Alprenolol
  - **B**opindolol

130. Ans. (b) Propanolol

Ref: Katzung, 14th ed. pg. 166; KDT, 6th ed. pg. 140

Please refer to above explanation.

131. Ans. (c) Pindolol

Ref: Katzung, 14th ed. pg. 166

Please refer to above explanation.

132. Ans. (d) Carvedilol

Ref: Katzung, 14th ed. pg. 160–164; KDT, 7th ed. pg. 151

- Carvedilol is a third generation beta blocker having blocking property of $\beta_1 + \beta_2 + \alpha_1$.
- It produces peripheral vasodilation due to blocking property of α_1 as well as L type calcium channel blocker.
- Carvedilol also inhibits free radical induced lipid peroxidation.
- Other third generation beta blocker having similar property is Labetalol Bucindolol.

133. Ans. (b) Tolazoline

Ref: KDT, 6th ed. pg. 132

- α_1 receptor is further divided in α_{1A} receptor (present on bladder neck and urethra) and α_{1B} (on blood vessel)
- **Selective α_{1A} blocker:** TAMSULOSIN, SILODOSIN *(causes relaxation of urethra and bladder neck)*

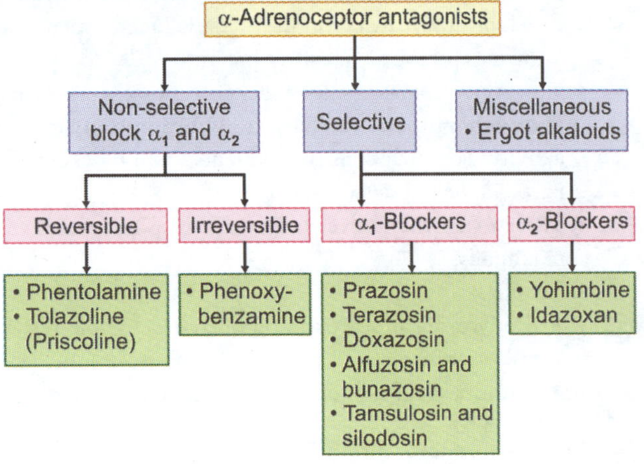

Question Forms

- Hypertensive patient with benign prostatic hyperplasia. What is the DOC: α_1 **selective blocker** (PRAZOSIN/TERAZOSIN/DOXAZOSIN/ALFUZOSIN)
- **Non hypertensive patient with BPH. What is DOC:** TAMSULOSIN (selective α_{1A} blocker)
- Side effect of selective α1 blocker: Postural Hypotension
- DOC for pheochromocytoma- PHENOXYBENZAMINE
- DOC for cheese reaction and clonidine induced rebound hypertension- PHENTOLAMINE, TOLAZOLINE

134. Ans. (d) Prazosin

Ref: Katzung, 14th ed. pg. 159

- **First dose effect** is sudden severe hypotension while changing position from lying to a standing position after first dose intake of alpha blocker, ACE inhibitor.
- Most common class of drug for causing first dose effect: **selective alpha-1 blocker**
- **Selective alpha-1 blocker Drugs**:
  - **Prazosin:** ***Most common among all***
  - Terazosin
  - Doxazosin
  - Alfuzosin
- Other drugs that can cause first dose effect is: Phentolamine, Tolazoline, Phenoxybenzamine.

135. Ans. (d) Phenoxybenzamine

Ref: Katzung, 14th ed. pg. 170

- **Phenoxybenzamine** binds covalently to α receptors, causing **irreversible blockade** of long duration.
- **It is DOC for pheochromocytoma**
- **Examples of reversible α blocker is: Phentolamine, Tolazoline**
- **Clonidine** is α_2 agonist
- **Isoprenaline** is beta agonist (acts at β_1 and β_2)

136. Ans. (a) Pilocarpine

Ref: Katzung, 14th ed. pg. 112

- Agents which dilate the pupillary diameter in order to facilitate fundoscopy are known as mydriatics.
- Eyes are mainly innervated by cholinergic (parasympathetic) nerves which predominantly secrete acetylcholine, which acts at circular iridis muscle causing miosis.
- Stimulation of parasympathetic system constricts pupillary diameter (miosis) while stimulation of sympathetic system dilates pupillary diameter (mydriasis).
- Anticholinergic (e.g. atropine) and sympathomimetic (e.g. phenylephrine) drugs result in mydriasis.

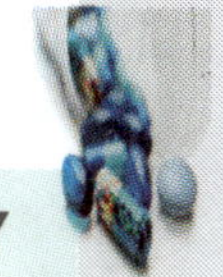

- Pilocarpine is a parasympathomimetic drug, which upon stimulation constricts the pupillary diameter (miosis). Used in treatment of Glaucoma.
- Agents like epinephrine and phenylephrine are sympathomimetic drugs, which acts at radial muscles and causes pupillary dilatation.

137. Ans. (c) Phentolamine

Ref: Katzung, 14th ed. pg. 170

- Phentolamine is an alpha blocker and can cause miosis not mydriasis *(because alpha 1 agonist in the eye causes mydriasis).*
- It causes passive miosis.

138. Ans. (c) Tropicamide

Ref: KDT, 8th ed. pg. 130

- Agents which dilate the pupillary diameter in order to facilitate fundoscopy are known as mydriatics. These are anti-muscarinic class of drugs.

TABLE: Anti-muscarinic drugs used in ophthalmology

Drug	Duration of Effect (days)
Atropine	7–10
Scopolamine	3–7
Homatropine	1–3
Cyclopentolate	1
Tropicamide	0.25 days (6 hrs)

- These agents have mydriatic as well as **cycloplegic action** both.

Extra Mile

- Strongest cycloplegic is: **Atropine**
- Cycloplegic agent of choice in child: **Atropine** 1% ointment (child age group has strong ciliary muscles)
- Cycloplegic agent of choice in adults: **Tropicamide**

139. Ans. (a) Anti-venin

Ref: KDT, 6th ed. pg. 2748

- General time guidelines for the disappearance of symptoms after anti-venom administration are as follows:
  - **Centruroides anti-venom:** Severe neurologic symptoms reverse in 15–30 minutes. Mild-to-moderate neurologic symptoms reverse in 45–90 minutes.
  - **Non-Centruroides anti-venom:** In the first hour, local pain abates. In 6–12 hours, agitation, sweating, and hyperglycemia abate. In 6–24 hours, cardio-respiratory symptoms abate.
- The use of steroids to decrease shock and edema is of unproven benefit.
- Atropine for symptomatic bradycardia.

Remember

- Scorpion venom is composed of neurotoxin cardiotoxin, nephrotoxin, hemolytic toxin, phosphodiesterases, phospholipases, hyaluronidases, glycosaminoglycans, histamine, serotonin, tryptophan, and cytokine releasers.
- *Hence the clinical effects of envenomation are neuromuscular, neuro-autonomic, or local tissue effects.*
- The main targets of scorpion venom are voltage-dependent ion channels, of which sodium channels are mainly affected.
- Alpha blocker like **Prazosin** can also be used for this purpose.

140. Ans. (b) Tolterodine

Ref: KD Tripathi, 8th ed. pg. 129

TOLTERODINE

- This M_3 selective muscarinic antagonist has preferential action on urinary bladder
- It is indicated in overactive bladder with urinary frequency and urgency.

Extra Mile

- Pirenzepine is selective M1 blocker which is an antacid given for PUD.
- Alfuzosin is a selective α1 blocker which is used to treat BPH.
- Bethanechol selectively stimulate M3 receptor present on bladder. It is used in case of atonic bladder (urinary retention).

141. Ans. (b) Anticholinergic

Ref: KDT 8th ed. pg. 129

MOA oxybutynin-cholinergic-*muscarinic* receptor antagonist

- Oxybutynin is a selective M_3 receptor blocker, used to relieve bladder spasm after urologic surgery, eg, prostatectomy.
- It is also used to relieve urinary and bladder difficulties, including frequent urination and inability to control urination, by decreasing muscle spasms of the bladder.
- It competitively antagonizes the M_3 subtypes of the muscarinic acetylcholine receptor.
- **M_3 receptor blockers:** ***Mn:*** *SOFT blaDar*
  - **Solifenacin, Oxybutynin, Flavoxate, Fesoterodine, Tolterodine, Trospium and Darifenacin.**

CNS AND PNS

142. Ans. (c) Varenicline

Ref: Goodman and Gillman 13th ed. pg. 437

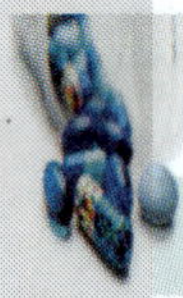

- Varenicline is an anti-smoking drug.
- It has high efficacy and partial agonist for N_N (nicotinic) receptor ($\alpha_3\beta_4$, $\alpha_4\beta_2$) and high efficacy, agonist at α_7 of N_N receptor of Ach.
- Varenicline after binding at the receptor stimulate low-level agonistic activity
- This binding at N_N receptor leads to following effect:
  - Competitively inhibits binding of nicotine
  - Decreases symptoms of nicotine withdrawal
  - Blocks dopaminergic stimulation responsible for reinforcement/pleasure and reward associated with smoking.

143. Ans. (b) Lithium

Ref: Goodman and Gillman 13th ed. pg. 281-82

- This is a case of Mania
- For the treatment of mania the most effective drug is Lithium
- DOC of mania: Lithium
- DOC for prophylaxis of mania: Lithium
- **Drugs effective for mania in patients with bipolar disorder:**
  - Lithium
  - Atypical anti psychotics
  - Carbamazepine
  - Topiramate
  - Valproate (DOC in rapid cycler)

144. Ans. (b) Morphine

Ref: Goodman and Gillman 13th ed. pg. 382-83, 440

- Opioid/Morphine poisoning can present with following symptoms:
  - Hypotension, Bradycardia, Pin point pupil, constipation
- Cocaine poisoning will present with increased BP, tachycardia, mydriasis, nausea, vomiting, chest pain, seizure
- Amphetamine is a CNS stimulant. Its poisoning presents with mydriasis, tremor, increased BP, tachycardia, convulsion and coma
- Haloperidol is typical anti psychotics, act by D2 blockade. Its poisoning presents with extrapyramidal symptoms like dystonia, akathisia and Parkinson like features.

145. Ans. (b) Benztropine

Ref: Goodman and Gillman 13th ed. pg. 291

- The primary aim of therapy for Parkinson's disease is to increase dopamine level or to inhibit acetylcholine by giving centrally acting anti-cholinergic agent. These agents are:
  - Benztropine
  - Benzhexol
  - Trihexyphenidyl
  - Procyclidine
- **Side effects** of centrally acting anti-cholinergic agents are:
  - Blurring of vision, dryness of mouth, constipation, urine retention

146. Ans. (a) Tramadol

Ref: Goodman and Gillman 13th ed. pg. 374

- Tramadol is an opioid analgesic agent.
- It is a weak μ opioid receptor agonist with serotonin norepinephrine reuptake inhibitor.
- **Use:**
  - Mild to moderate pain
  - Labor pain
- **Note:** Tapentadol μ receptor agonist with noradrenaline reuptake inhibitor

147. Ans. (a) Mannitol

Mannitol is an osmotic diuretic preferred in treatment of:

- Cerebral edema
- Increased ICP
- Increased IOP/Glaucoma

Contraindication of osmotic diuretic:

- Active cerebral bleed
- Impending renal failure

148. Ans. (c) Opioid withdrawal

- The symptoms are suggestive of opioid withdrawal. Same can be seen with excitatory phase of cocaine intoxication.
- Opioid usually causes symptoms like constipation, bradycardia, miosis etc. The withdrawal symptoms are usually opposite to the usual effect of opioid.
- Withdrawal symptoms occur after withdrawal of the drug for more than 12 hours and last about a week. Yawning is a common feature. Symptoms are classified into minor, moderate and major.
- Cocaine withdrawal range from moderate to severe dysphoria, depression, anxiety, decreased libido, etc.
- Cannabis does not cause physiological dependence or addiction.
- Alcohol withdrawal present with nausea, vomiting, shaking, restlessness, anxiety, tachycardia, headache, insomnia, etc.

149. Ans. (b) Sodium valproate

- The shown cases describe cases of absence seizure.
- DOC for absence seizure: Ethosuximide
- **Other Drugs used in absence seizure:**
  - Valproate
  - Lamotrigine
  - Clonazepam

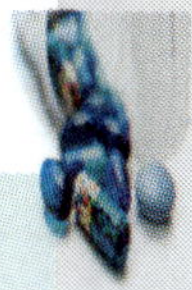

150. Ans. (b) Venlafaxine

- Serotonin Noradrenaline reuptake inhibitor (SNRI), inhibits the reuptake of these two neurotransmitters.
- SNRI drugs are: Venlafaxine, Duloxetine, Milnacipran, Levomilnacipran.

Note:

- Fluoxetine is SSRI.
- Phenelzine is Non selective MAO inhibitor.
- Nortriptyline is a TCA.

151. Ans. (b) Imipenem

- Imipenem can decrease the seizure threshold; therefore, it is epileptogenic in nature.

Drugs that can Lower Seizure Threshold

- Antibiotics
  - Imipenem, penicillins, cephalosporins, metronidazole, isoniazid
- Antihistamines
- Antipsychotics
- Antidepressants
  - Bupropion
  - Tricyclics
- Baclofen
- Fentanyl
- Ketamine
- Lidocaine
- Lithium
- Meperidine
- Propoxyphene
- Theophylline

152. Ans. (c) Ca^{2+}

- This is a case of Malignant hyperthermia can be caused by Halothane, due to overactivity of ryanodine receptor (RyR) mutations, excessive Ca^{++} release from the sarcoplasmic reticulum.
- DOC for malignant hyperthermia: Dantrolene
- Max risk of malignant hyperthermia: Sch
- Local anesthetic agent associated with malignant hyperthermia: Lidocaine.

153. Ans. (a) Mannitol

- Osmotic diuretic is effective in treatment of raised ICP.
- Contraindication for mannitol is active cerebral bleed.

154. Ans. (a) Cocaine

- These are symptoms of cocaine intoxication/Formication.
- It inhibits reuptake of Noradrenaline.

155. Ans. (b) Acetylcholine

- ALZHEIMER'S disease is a neuro degenerative condition. There is degeneration of cholinergic neurons, leading to Associated with depletion of Acetylcholine.
- Symptoms: Memory loss, confusion, inability to learn new things, shortened attention spans
- DOC: Donepezil (Reversible Ach esterase inhibitor).

156. Ans. (b) Rivastigmine

Ref: Goodman and Gillman 13th ed. pg. 333-34

In the parkinsonism treatment, preferred agent is dopaminergic therapy like levodopa in combination with carbidopa (peripheral dopa decarboxylase inhibitor).

- Other drugs used in the management of parkinsons disease are:
  - **Amantadine:** Promote dopamine release, inhibit dopamine uptake and also possess glutamate receptor antagonistic property.
  - **Dopamine receptor agonist:** Pramipexole, Ropinirole, Rotigotine, Apomorphine
- Treatment modality like deep brain stimulation can also be used in conditions like parkinsons disease, OCD, dystonia, essential tremors.
- **Rivastigmine** is a reversible Ach esterase inhibitor, used in treatment of Alzheimer's disease.

157. Ans. (b) Carbamazepine

Ref: Goodman and Gillman 13th ed. pg. 313

- Pain over facial nerve distribution is suggestive of trigeminal neuralgia
- Preferred agent for trigeminal neuralgia or Glossopharyngeal neuralgia: Carbamazepine.
- Other agents that can be used in this condition is: Phenytoin, Ethanol.

158. Ans. (c) Diazepam

Ref: Goodman Gillman 13th ed. pg. 312

- Drug preferred for controlling acute seizure is IV Diazepam.
- DOC for status epilepticus is IV Lorazepam
- While diazepam is an effective agent for treatment of status epilepticus, the effective duration of action of this lipid soluble agent is shortened by its rapid redistribution. Thus, lorazepam is more frequently used; it is less lipid soluble, is more effectively confined to the vascular compartment, and has a longer effective half-life after a single dose

159. Ans. (b) Opioid receptors desensitization

Ref: Goodman Gillman 13th ed. pg. 362

- Due to prolonged or repeated exposure to opioid (over days to weeks), there is decreased effectiveness of the opioid receptor agonist. This is known as tolerance.
- This tolerance is reflected by a reduction in the maximum achievable effect or a right shift in the dose-response curve.
- The development of tolerance to opioids may involve mechanisms of receptor trafficking.

- *Tolerance doesn't develop to symptoms like: Miosis, Constipation and convulsion.*

160. Ans. (a) Lithium

Ref: Goodman and Gillman 13th ed. pg. 294

- Preferred agent for acute attack of mania is: Sedatives (Diazepam/atypical antipsychotics) + Lithium
- Preferred agent for mania: Lithium
- Preferred agent for prophylaxis of mania: Lithium
- **Note:** Carbamazepine is effective for acute mania, but lamotrigine has no role in acute attack of mania.
- All atypical antipsychotics medications with the exception of clozapine, iloperidone, brexpiprazole, and lurasidone, have indications for acute mania, and doses are titrated rapidly close to or at the maximum FDA-approved dose over the first 24–72 hours of treatment.
- Typical antipsychotic drugs are also effective in acute mania, but often are eschewed due to the risk for EPSs.

Extra Mile

TABLE: Comparative efficacy and target serum levels for mood stabilizers

	Acutemania	Prophylaxis	Bipolar depression
Lithium	+++ 1.0–1.5 mEq/L	+++ 0.6–1.0 mEq/L	++ 0.6–1.0 mEq/L
Valproate	+++ 100–120 mEq/L[b]	+++ 60–100 mEq/L	—
Carbamazepine	+ 6–12 μg/mL	++ 6–12 μg/mL	+/– 6–12 μg/mL
Lamotrigine	–	++	++

161. Ans. (d) Levetiracetam

Ref: Katzung 14th ed. pg. 422-23

- Among the given choices, levetiracetam is the least teratogenic anti epileptic drug.
- Hence, DOC for epilepsy in pregnancy: Levetiracetam > Lamotrigine
- **Note:** Valproate has maximum risk of teratogenicity. It is associated with spina bifida.

162. Ans. (a) Valproate

Ref: Katzung 14th ed. pg. 427, 434

- Though all the anti-epileptics have teratogenic potential, Valproate is the most teratogenic among all.
- Treatment with valproate during first trimester is associated with increased risk of neural tube defect including spina bifida, cardiovascular, orofacial and digital abnormalities.
- First trimester exposure with valproate causes 3 fold increased risk of major congenital malformations, most commonly spina bifida (absolute risk: 6–9%).

Extra Mile

- MC congenital defect associated with phenobarbitone exposure: Cardiac defect
- MC congenital defect associated with topiramate exposure: cleft lip and palate (10 fold increased risk)
- Antiseizure drugs with lowest congenital defect risk: Lamotrigine and Levetiracetam
- Antiseizure drug having maximal breast milk secretion: Lamotrigine

163. Ans. (b) Lithium carbonate

Ref: Katzung 14th ed. pg. 524

- Drug of choice for mania is Lithium
- DOC for acute attack of manic episode: Atypical antipsychotics/Benzodiazepines
- Agents that can be used in treatment of Mania: *(Mn: Li ACT Val)*
  - Lithium (DOC)
  - Atypical antipsychotics
  - Carbamazepine
  - Topiramate
  - Valproate

164. Ans. (c) Bupropion

Ref: Katzung 14th ed. pg. 584

- **Book states:** "*The antidepressant Bupropion is approved for nicotine cessation therapy. It is most effective when combined with behavioral therapies*"
- **Note: Topiramate** is approved for decreasing alcohol craving, obesity.

165. Ans. (b) Donepezil

Ref: Katzung 14th ed. pg. 1063

- DOC for Alzheimer's disease: Donepezil (reversible AchEsterase inhibitor)
- Other Ach Esterase inhibitor used in treatment of Alzheimer's disease is Gallantamine, Rivastigmine.

166. Ans. (d) Delta

Ref: Goodman & Gillman 13th ed. pg. 358

Opioid receptors	
Opioid receptor class	**Effects**
MU_1	Euphoria, supraspinal analgesia, confusion, dizziness, nausea, low addiction potential

Contd...

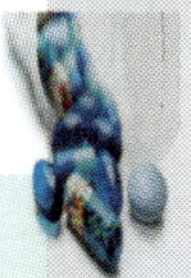

Opioid receptors	
MU_2	Respiratory depression, cardiovascular and gastrointestinal effects, miosis, urinary retention
Delta	Spinal analgesia, cardiovascular depression, decreased brain and myocardial oxygen demand
Kappa	Spinal analgesia, dysphoria, psychomimetic effects, feedback inhibition of endorphin system

Extra Mile

- Sigma (σ) receptor was early identified and was thought to represent a site that accounted for the paradoxical excitatory effects of opiates.
- Agonist binding to the σ receptor is not antagonized by naloxone, and the receptor is not classified as an opiate receptor.

167. Ans. (b) Cognitive therapy

Ref: Goodman & Gillman 13th ed. pg. 281-282

- For acute manic attacks, preferred agents are atypical antipsychotics, benzodiazepines, anticonvulsants (Valproate, carbamazepine), Lithium
- All atypical antipsychotics medications with the exception of clozapine, iloperidone, brexpiprazole, and lurasidone, have indications for acute mania, and doses are titrated rapidly close to or at the maximum FDA-approved dose over the first 24–72 hours of treatment. Typical antipsychotic drugs are also effective in acute mania, but often are eschewed due to the risk for EPSs.

168. Ans. (d) Hyperalgesia

Ref: Goodman & Gillman's 14th ed. pg. 363-64

- Effect of morphine is seen mainly at μ-receptor. Effect on μ-receptor depends on either supraspinal or spinal μ-receptor.
  - **Supraspinal effects:** Physical dependence, euphoria, analgesia, sedation. (PEAS)
  - **Spinal effects:** Constipation, analgesia and respiratory depression. (CAR)
- **Effect of morphine at heart:** No effect at usual dose but at high dose it can cause bradycardia and hypotension.
- **Effect of morphine at eye:** No effect if applied locally. Miosis on systemic intake. Miosis can be worsened to pin point pupil upon systemic morphine toxicity.

Note: Morphine causes analgesia. Hyperalgesia is one of the withdrawal symptoms.

169. Ans. (c) Propranolol

Ref: KDT 8th ed. pg. 471

- **Akathisia** is an extra pyramidal symptom arise mainly due to intake of typical antipsychotics like haloperidol, fluphenazine, etc.
- It is characterized by restlessness, feeling of discomfort and constant purposeless involuntary movement from one place to another.
- **Akathisia is the *most common* extra pyramidal symptom.**

DOC for akathisia: PROPRANOLOL

170. Ans. (c) Ramelteon

Ref: KD Tripathi, 8th ed. pg. 436

- The most common prescription drugs for insomnia incude: Benzodiazepines, nonbenzodiazepines, hypnotics, ramelteon as well as some anti-depressants.

Extra Mile

Types of insomnia, their causes and the drugs used

Insomnia	Causes	Drugs used
Transient insomnia	Lasts less than 7 days Jet lag, Shift work, new place, overnight journey	Rapid onset and short duration of action **Triazolam:** In patients with difficulty going to sleep **Temazepam:** For insomnia caused by inability to stay asleep. Zolpidem, Zoleplon
Short term insomnia	Lasts 1–3 weeks Due to expected but self limiting problems like bereavement, pain, occupational issue.	Flurazepam, Estrazolam, Temazepam Zopiclone, Eszopiclone
Long term insomnia	Lasts > 3 weeks Indicates underlying disease or a personality disorder	Flurazepam, Nitrazepam Intermittent use with a break after every 3rd day

- Benzodiazepines are first-line drugs of choice for short-term management of insomnia, especially for reducing the sleep latency (time to sleep onset).
- Among benzodiazepines, Triazolam is effective in treating individuals who have difficulty going to sleep, while temazepam is useful for insomnia caused by inability to stay asleep.

- Lorazepam, Diazepam and Midazolam is used as preanesthtic drug. It causes high degree of amnesia, has more rapid onset and shorter duration of action.
- *Recently approved Melatonin receptor agonist, Ramelteon is used for sleep onset insomnia, especially in the treatment of circadian disruptions induced by shift work and jet lag.*
- 5HT2 serotonin receptor antagonist, **Ritanserin,** has improved sleep depth and sleep quality.

171. Ans. (a) Clozapine

Ref: KD Tripathi, 7th ed. pg. 440-41

TABLE: Classification of typical vs atypical antipsychotics

Typical/Classical antipsychotics MOA: D2 receptor blocking	• **Phenothiazines:** Chlorpromazine, Thioridazine, Trifluperazine, Fluphenazine, Perphenazine • **Thioxanthenes:** Flupenthixol, Zuclopenthixol, Thiothixene • **Butyrophenones:** Haloperidol, Droperidol, Benperidol, Domperidone
Atypical Antipsychotics **MOA:** 5HT$_{2A}$, D4, D2, α blocking	• Risperidone, Quetiapine, Aripiprazole, Clozapine, Olanzapine, Ziprasidone, Zotepine, Asenapine, Sertidole, Lurasidone

172. Ans. (d) Clozapine

Ref: KD Tripathi, 8th ed. pg. 468

Side effects of Typical vs Atypical

Typical antipsychotics	Atypical antipsychotics
Major side effect: *Extrapyramidal symptoms* • Dystonia: Earliest • Akathisia: MC • Parkinsonism • Neuroleptic malignant syndrome: Most dangerous • Perioral tremors (Rabbit syndrome) • Tardive dyskinesia	***Lipodystrophy syndrome:*** metabolic side effect present with hyperglycemia, hyperlipidemia, weight gain and insulin resistance.

- Among antipsychotics, maximum risk of lipodystrophy syndrome is seen with atypical antipsychotics (MC with CLOZAPINE).
- First antisuicidal drug: Clozapine
- Other side effects of clozapine: **Sedation, Sialorhea, Agranulocytosis**
- DOC for resistant schizophrenia: Clozapine
- Atypical antipsychotics Least commonly associated with lipodystrophy syndrome are **Ziprasidone** and **risperidone**
- Typical antipsychotic with least extra pyramidal symptoms (EPS): **Thioridazine** (low potency drug)
- Atypical antipsychotic with least EPS is clozapina.

173. Ans. (b) Carbamazepine

Ref: KDT 8th ed. pg. 464

- Extra pyramidal side effect or aka Extra pyramidal symptom (EPS) is due to excess blockade of dopamine receptors in basal ganglia, leading to Parkinson like symptoms such as slow movement (bradykinesia), akathisia, stiffness and tremor.
- EPS most commonly seen with the intake of typical antipsychotics, which blocks D2 receptors.

Typical antipsychotics		Important side effect
Strong D2 blocker	Haloperidol- *has maximum risk of EPS* Droperidol	EPS Hyperprolactinemia
Weak D2 blocker	Chlorpromazine Thioridazine – ***has minimum risk of EPS among typicals***	EPS Corneal opacity, Retinal Pigmentation, Decreases seizure threshold
Intermediate D2 blocker	Fluphenazine Pechlorphenazine	

Extrapyramidal Symptoms

- **Dystonia**- earliest EPS which is seen.
  - R_x for dystonia: Diphenhydramine
- **Akathisia**- most common EPS seen.
  Constant purposeless movement from one place to other.
  - ***DOC for Akathisia: PROPANOLOL***
- **Neuroleptic Malignant syndrome:** Severe muscle spasm and high grade fever after intake of anti psychotics.
  - **DOC for NMS:** DANTROLENE
- It is most dangerous type of EPS

174. Ans. (c) Dantrolene

Ref: KDT, 8h ed. pg. 382

- Given the choices,
  DOC for NMS: Dantrolene
- According to recent updates, Bromocriptine is preferred

175. Ans. (c) Propanolol

Ref: KDT, 8th ed. pg. 471

- **Akathisia** is an extra pyramidal symptom that arises mainly due to intake of typical anti psychotics like haloperidol, fluphenazine etc.
- It is characterized by restlessness, feeling of discomfort and constant purposeless involuntary movement from one place to another without any source of anxiety.
- **Akathisia is the *most common* extra pyramidal symptom.**
- DOC for akathisia: **PROPANOLOL.**

176. Ans. (b) Clozapine

Ref: KDT 8th ed. pg. 467

- Among given option Clozapine is the only atypical antipsychotics. As discussed earlier, atypical antipsychtics has less risk of EPS development as compared to typical antipsychotics.
- Overall least risk of EPS among atypicals is: Clozapine

177. Ans. (a) Aripiprazole

Ref: KDT 8th ed. pg. 467

- Among given choice, least risk of EPS among atypicals is: ARIPIPRAZOLE. (Atypical has less EPS risk)
- Typicals always has high EPS.

178. Ans. (d) Quetipaine

- Antipsychotic which is associated with lenticular opacity/Cataract: **Quetiapine**
- Antipsychotic associated with corneal opacity: **Chlorpromazie and Thioridazine**

179. Ans. (a) Risperidone

Ref: KDT, 8th ed. pg. 469

- Atypicals with maximum risk of hyperprolactinemia is: Risperidone
- Most potent atypical antipsychotic: Risperidone
- Atypicals with least risk of EPS: Clozapine
- Atypicals that can cause cardiac arrhythmias: Sertindole, Zotepine
- **Atypicals with maximum risk of obesity: Clozapine, Olanzapine**

180. Ans. (d) Haloperidol

Ref: KDT, 8th ed. pg. 471

Haloperidol is from typical antipsychotic class that is commonly associated with extrapyramidal symptoms like neuroleptic malignant syndrome.

181. Ans. (b) Diazepam

Ref: Katzung's, 11th ed. pg. 462-63

- Anxiety occurvs as a result of mild CNS stimulation which may occur secondary to reduction in GABAergic activity or increase in serotonin activity.
- Therefore, a drug which is used for anxiety is CNS depressant (e.g. Diazepam) or the other which is decreasing serotonin level (e.g. Buspirone, *NOT Bupropion)*.
- **DOC for anxiety attacks: Benzodiazepines**
- **DOC for chronic anxiety disorder: SSRI (Fluoxamine)**
- Anti-serotonergic drugs take around 2 weeks for its therapeutic effect. Hence NOT preferred in acute attack of anxiety.

182. Ans. (b) Ketamine

Ref: Katzung, 11th ed. pg. 437; KDT, 6th ed. pg. 376

- Ketamine is the only intravenous anesthetic that possesses analgesic properties and produces cardiovascular stimulation.
- It causes ***"dissociative anesthesia"*** which is characterized by profound analgesia, immobility, amnesia and feeling of dissociation from one's own body and the surrounding.
- It has bronchodilator effect therefore considered as Induction agent of choice in asthma patient.
- **In addition it also causes:**
  - Hallucination
  - Delusion and illusion
  - Profound analgesia
- **Ketamine increases all pressures like:**
  - BP (hypertension), Heart rate, Cardiac output
  - Intracranial tension (it increases cerebral blood flow)
  - Intraocular pressure (IOP)
- It is contraindicated in intracerebral mass/haemorrhage, MI, schizophrenia, Epilepsy

MOA of Ketamine:

- It acts by blocking NMDA receptor (of glutamate).

Extra Mile

Side effect of other given options:

- **Propofol:** Apnea, Decreases BP and HR
- **Thiopentone:** Laryngospasm, Shivering & Delirium
- **Etomidate:** Adrenocortical suppression

183. Ans. (b) It is GABA facilitator

Ref: KDT, 7th ed. 402, Katzung, 11th ed. pg. 377

- GABA is an inhibitory neurotransmitter.
- Benzodiazepine helps GABA to open the chloride channel. Once Chloride enters, negativity in the neuron increases (hyperpolarized), which leads to depressed neuron.
- It is barbiturate which is GABA mimetic.

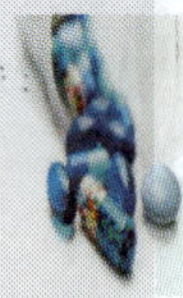

TABLE: Difference between Benzodiazepine and barbiturates

Benzodiazipine	Barbiturates
• Increase FREQUENCY of GABA mediated chloride channel opening • GABA facilitator • Dose response curve: flat • Safe drug • Non-enzyme inducer- no drug interaction • Less amnesia • Antidote: FLUMAZENIL	• Increase DURATION of GABA mediated chloride channel opening • GABA mimetic • Dose-response curve: steep • Unsafe drug • Powerful enzyme inducer; (+)drug interaction • Causes strong amnesia • No antidote available • Treated with forced alkaline diuresis

184. Ans. (c) GABA facilitator

Ref: KDT, 7th ed. 402, Katzung, 11th ed. 377

185. Ans. (d) Flumazenil

- Flumazenil is antidote of benzodiazepine overdose.
- t½ = 60 minutes

186. Ans. (b) Methylphenidate

Ref: KD Tripathi, 6th ed. pg. 470-471 & 126

- **Methylphenidate** acts by releasing NA and DA in brain and is most widely used for attention deficit hyperkinetic disorder because it causes lesser tachycardia and growth retardation as compared to amphetamine.
- It is considered as DOC of ADHD
- **Modafinil**
  - Psychostimulant agent; used most commonly among night-shift (call centre) workers who need alertness and want to keep awake.
  - Increases attention span and improve accuracy compromised by fatigue and sleepiness.
- Considered as first line drug in narcolepsy.
- **Pemoline**
  - It has CNS stimulant actions similar to those of methylphenidate.
  - It can also be used in ADHD, narcolepsy and excessive day-time sleepiness
  - **S/E:** Hepatotoxicity, thus it has limited use
- **Amphetamines**
  - It can also be used in ADHD, but not a drug of choice due to highly abusive tendency.
  - The central effects include alertness, increased concentration an attention spam, euphoria, talkativeness increased work capacity
  - Stimulate respiratory centre and Hunger centre is suppressed.

187. Ans. (b) Alzheimer's disease

Ref: Katzung, 10th ed. Ch 7

- Rivastigmine is a parasympathomimetic drug used for the treatment of mild to moderate dementia of the *Alzheimer's type* and dementia due to Parkinson's disease
- **DOC for alzheimer's disorder**-Donepezil
- **DOC for OCD:** Fluoxetine
- **DOC for parkinsonism:** Levodpa + Carbidopa
- **DOC for drug induced parkinsonism:** Benzhexol (centrally acting anticholinergic)

188. Ans. (d) Ethosuximide

Ref: KD Tripathi, 6th ed. pg. 172 & 406

ETHOSUXIMIDE

- *The most prominent action of ethosuximide is antagonism T type calcium channel → Thereby controlling the seizures like absence seizure. It also raises seizure threshold.*
- *Clinically it is effective only in absence seizures.*

Extra Mile

Drugs used in Prophylaxis of Migraine
- **β Adrenergic blockers:** Propranolol is the **most commonly used** drug for prophylaxis of migraine. It reduces frequency as well as severity of attacks in upto 70% patients. DOC for prophylaxis
- **Tricyclic antidepressants**: amitriptyline has been most extensively tried (25–50 mg at bed time) to reduce migraine attacks.
- **Calcium channel blockers:** Verapamil was found to reduce migraine attacks, but was judged inferior to propranolol.
- Anticonvulsants Valproic acid and gabapentin.
- Topiramate has recently been approved for migraine prohylaxis
- Ethosuximide is the drug used in absent seizure. It has no role in migraine prophylaxis.

189. Ans. (c) It inhibits peripheral dopa decarboxylase

Ref: Katzung, 14th ed. pg. 495

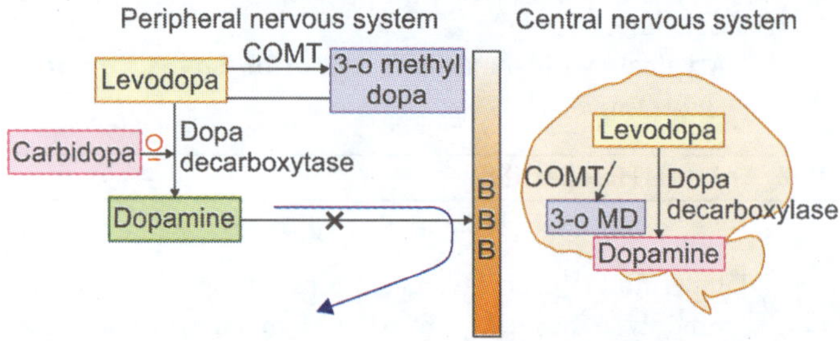

COMT = Catechol othomethyl trasferase,
o MD = Ortho methyl dopa, BBB = Blood brain barrier

- In Parkinsons disease the balance between acetylcholine and dopamine (DA) is dearranged in brain.

- DA is comparatively decreased, making Ach on the higher side.
- **Principle of treatment:**
  - Either increase DA (which is the prime treatment modality), or
  - Decrease the lecel of Ach
- Levodopa can be given for treatment but it is immediately converted to DA in periphery itself by the enzyme dopa decarboxylase and causes varied side effects.
- **Note:** Dopamine cannot cross BBB but levodopa can cross it.
- Carbidopa is peripheral dopa decarboxylase inhibitor. It is always added with levodopa in treatment of Parkinsonism to avoid peripheral conversion of levodopa to carbidopa.

190. Ans. (c) Short half life of drug

Ref: Katzung, 14th ed. pg. 494

- **ON-OFF phenomenon:** unpredictable fluctuation between mobility and immobility
  - **Due to very short t1/2 of Levodopa: 1-2 hrs**
  - **To avoid this it is used along with COMT inhibitor → Entacapone, Tolcapone**

191. Ans. (d) Parkinsonism

Ref: Katzung, 14th ed. pg. 501

- Amantadine is an antiviral for Infuenza A. It has been approved for treatment for Parkinson disease as well.
- Best for early stage PD or if patient not responding to L-Dopa
- **Mechanism of action**
- Facilitate DA release from presynaptic dopaminergic neuron and also Prevents DA uptake
- **Side effect:** Confusion, Hallucination, Ankle edema, Livido reticularis

192. Ans. (c) Bromocriptine

Ref: Katzung, 14th ed. pg. 498; KDT, 6th ed. pg. 167

- Ergots are derived from a fungus *Claviceps purpurea.* Important compounds are:
  - *Ergotamine*
  - *Ergometrine (ergonovine),*
  - *Ergotoxine*
  - ***Bromocriptine***
  - *Methysergide and LSD.*
- These drugs possess partial agonistic and antagonistic effect at 5HT, α and dopaminergic receptors.
- Ergot derivatives *can cause dry gangrene of hand and feet as well as coronary vasospasm.*
- Ergot derivatives are highly specific for migraine pain; they are not analgesic for any other condition.
- **Bromocriptine** is extremely effective in reducing the high levels of prolactin that result from pituitary tumors and has even been associated with regression of the tumor in some cases.
- **Benzhexol** is DOC for drug induced Parkinsonism.
- **Emmenagogues** are herbs which stimulate blood flow in the pelvic area and uterus; some stimulate menstruation.
- **Ropinirole** and pramipexole is a non-ergot derivative drug, and is used in Parkinsonism.

193. Ans. (b) Bromocriptine

Ref: KDT, 6th ed. pg. 167

- **Bromocriptine** and **pergolide** are ergot derivatives and are used in Parkinsonism. All ergot derivatives can cause **retroperitoneal fibrosis,** cardiac and pleural fibrosis. They can also cause digital vasospasm leading to gangrene.
- Newer **nonergot dopamine agonists like pramipexole** and **ropinirole** do not have these limitations (these are **long acting** and **do not cause gangrene**). Adverse known side effect of these drugs is **excessive day time sleepiness**, Gambling habits, increased sexuality.
- Recently approved non ergot ROTIGOTINE is available as transdermal patch.

194. Ans. (b) MAO-B inhibition

Ref: Katzung, 14th ed. pg. 499

- After release of DA in synaptic cleft, it is metabolized either by MAO-b or by COMT (catechol-ortho methyl transferase)
- In order to prevent this metabolism following drugs can be given, which will enhance DA availability:
  - MAO-b inhibitor: Selegiline, Rasagiline, safinamide
  - COMT inhibitor: Entacapone, Tolcapone

Extra Mile

Drugs stimulating DA receptor:
- Ergot Derivative: Bromocriptine, Cabergoline
- Non-Ergot: Pramipexole, Ropinirole, Rotigotine *(available as transdermal patch)*

195. Ans. (b) Lamotrigine

Ref: Katzung, 14th ed. pg. 422

- Abnormal electrical activity in brain is propagated by voltage gated (VG) sodium channel, which is responsible for majority of seizure types.
- Drugs acting by inhibiting VG-Na+ sodium channel: *(Mn: Very Lame Priyanka Chopra Likes it Ruf & Top Zone)*
  - Valproate
  - Lamotrigine

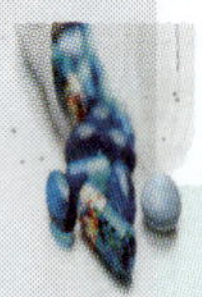

- Phenytoin
- Carbamazepine
- Lacosamide
- Rufinamide
- Topiramate
- Zonisamide
- **Note:** In addition of VG-Na channel blocking action, these drugs also have additional action like N-type calcium channel blockage or by increasing GABAergic activity, etc.

Extra Mile

- Ethosuximide acts by inhibiting T type VG-Ca+ channel blocking.
- Levetiracetam acts by inhibing synaptic vesicular protein inhibition thereby increasing GABA → causing neuronal depression.
- Glutmate receptor inhibitors:
  - **NMDA receptor blocker:** FELBAMATE
  - **AMPA receptor blocker:** PERAMPANEL, TELAMPANEL

196. Ans. (c) It has Broad spectrum of anti-seizure activity

Ref: Lippincott's 5th ed. pg. 186; KDT 6th ed. pg. 409–410

- ***Lamotrigine is effective in a wide variety of seizure types, including partial seizures, generalized seizures, and typical absence seizures and in the Lennox-Gastaut syndrome.***
- **MOA:** Lamotrigine acts by blocking Na^+ channels, T-type Ca^{2+} channels and by increasing GABAergic activity.
- Lamotrigine dosages should be reduced when adding valproate to therapy unless the valproate is being added in a small dose to provide a boost to the lamotrigine serum concentration.
- **Major adverse effect:** Steven Johnson syndrome and toxic epidermal necrolysis, insomnia.
- **Other side effects:** Nausea, drowsiness, dizziness, headache, and Diplopia.

197. Ans. (b) Sodium valproate

Ref: KDT 6th ed. pg. 407–408

- Among options, it is preferred

Uses of Sodium Valproate

- Valproic acid is the drug that can be used for absence seizures.
- It is an alternative/adjuvant drug for GTCS, simple partial seizure and complex partial seizure
- Myoclonic and atonic seizures-control is often incomplete, but valproate is the drug of choice.
- Mania and bipolar illness: As alternative to lithium.
- Valproate has some prophylatic efficacy in migraine.

MOA: Prolongation of Na^+ channel inactivation
Augmentation of release of inhibitory transmitter GABA by inhibiting its degradation

Drugs which can be used for absence seizure:
- Sodium valproate
- Ethusuximide
- Lamotrigine
- Clonazepam.

TABLE: Drug of choice for different seizures

Seizure types	DOC
Absence seizures (petit mal) in children (<2–3 years)	Ethosuximide
Atypical absence seizures	Na+ Valproate
GTCS (Grand mal)	LAMOTRIGINE > Na^+ Valproate
Focal onset/Partial seizure	Carbamazepine
Myoclonic seizures	Na+ Valproate > Lamotrigine
Tonic/Clonic seizures	Na^+ Valproate
Infantile/salam seizure	ACTH
Infantile spasm associated with tuberous sclerosis	Vigabatrin
Febrile seizures/Midazolam (nasal)	Diazepam (per rectal)
Status epilepticus	Lorazepam (IV)
Seizures in eclampsia	Magnesium sulphate
Seizure during pregnancy	LEVETIRACETAM > LAMOTRIGINE
Lennox Gastaut syndrome Dravet syndrome	Na^+ Valproate

198. Ans. (b) Na+ Valproate

Ref: Katzung, 14th ed. pg. 426; KDT, 6th ed. pg. 407-408

- Given the choices the answer will be Na^+ Valproate
- According to Harrison's 19th ed. the current recommendable drug of choice for GTCS is **LAMOTRIGINE > Na^+ Valproate.**

199. Ans. (b) Carbamazepine

Ref: Harrison's, 19th ed. pg. 2552

- **Carbamazepine is DOC** in partial/focal seizure.
- **Harrison states:** *Carbamazepine (or a related drug, oxcarbazepine), lamotrigine, phenytoin, and levetiracetam are currently the drugs of choice approved for the initial treatment of focal seizures, including those that evolve into generalized seizures. Overall they have very similar efficacy, but differences in pharmacokinetics and toxicity are the main determinants for use in a given patient.*

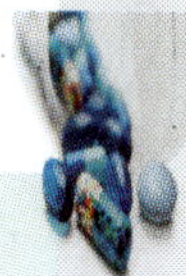

TABLE: Selection of antiepileptic drug

Generalized onset tonic clonic	Focal	Typical absence	Atypical absence, myoclonic, atonic
First-line			
Lamotrigine	Lamotrigine	Valproic acid	Valproic acid
Valproic acid	Carbamazepine	Ethosuximide	Lamotrigine
	Oxcarbazepine	Lamotrigine	Topiramate
	Phenytoin		
	Levetiracetam		
Alternatives			
Zonisamide	Topiramate	Lamotrigine	Clonazepam
Phenytoin	Zonisamide	Clonazepam	Felbamate
Carbamazepine	Valproic acid		Clobazam
Oxcarbazepine	Tiagabine[a]		Rufinamide
Topiramate	Gabapentin[a]		
Phenobarbital	Lacosamide[a]		
Primidone	Exogabine[a]		
Felbamate	Phenobarbital Primidone Felbamate		

[a]As adjunctive therapy

200. Ans. (a) Valproate

Ref: Katzung, 14th ed. pg. 426

TABLE: Important side effects of anti epileptic drugs

Drug	Side effect
Valpraoate	• Fulminant Hepatitis: most grave side effect • Reversible Alopecia, Hepatotoxicity, Weight Gain, Tremor, Pancreatitis, NTD, Thrombocytopenia • PCOS- gender specific side effect
Phenytoin	Gum Hypertrophy: **MC side effect** Hirsutism, Fetal hydantoin syndrome, Megaloblastic anemia
Carbamazepine	Agaranulocytosis: Most serious side effect SJS, Bone marrow suppression, confusion, Ataxia, Blurring of vision
Zonisamide	Renal stone, Amnesia, Drowsiness, wt loss
Topiramate	Renal stone, Somnolence, wt loss
Vigabatrin	Visual acuity decreased, Weight gain
Felbamate	Aplastic anemia, Hepatotoxicity

201. Ans. (a) Phenytoin

Ref: Katzung, 14th ed. pg. 418

- Gum hypertrophy is known side effect of phenytoin.

202. Ans. (d) Folic acid deficiency

Ref: Katzung, 14th ed. pg. 418–19; KDT, 6th ed. 404-405

- Phenytoin is a major epileptic drug which is effective for treatment of partial seizures and generalized tonic-clonic seizures and in the treatment of status epilepticus.
- **MOA:** Phenytoin blocks voltage-gated sodium channels by selectively binding to the channel in the inactive state and slowing its rate of recovery.
- It follows zero order kinetics.
- It can also be used as an anti-arrhythmic drug (class Ib) for the treatment of digitalis induced arrhythmia.
- Use of phenytoin during pregnancy can cause **Fetal hydantoin syndrome** characterized by: hypoplastic phalanges, cleft lip, cleft palate and microcephaly. It occurs due metabolite of phenytoin, ***arene oxide.***
- **Phenytoin decreases folate absorption and increases its excretion →** ***Megaloblastic anemia.***
- Prolonged use of phenytoin can result in gingival hyperplasia **(gum hypertrophy).**
- It can inhibit the insulin release and can cause ***hyperglycemia.***
- **Other adverse effects on long-term use include:** Hirsutism, coarsening of facial features, megaloblastic anemia (treated with folic acid), vitamin D deficiency (rickets and **osteomalacia**), vitamin K deficiency, hyperglycemia (due to inhibition of insulin release), hypersensitivity.

203. Ans. (c) GABA transaminase inhibitor

Ref: Katzung, 14th ed. pg. 431–32

- VIGABATRIN is GABAergic drug acts by inhibiting enzyme GABA transaminase.
- This enzyme inhibition causes increased level of GABA in the neuron.
- **Use:**
  - DOC in infantile spasm + Tuberous sclerosis
  - Simple and complex partial seizure
- Contraindicated in absence seizure, Myoclonic seizure, Pre-existing visual field defect.
- **Side effect:** Visual field defect due to peripheral retinal atrophy, weight gain, amnesia

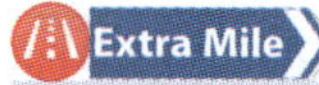

- GABA uptake transport inhibitor: TIAGABINE

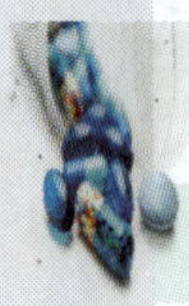

204. Ans. (b) Inhibing CRMP protein

Ref: Katzung, 14th ed. pg. 417

- CRMP is Collapsing Response Mediator Protien, which causes neuronal excitotoxicity by releasing BDNF (Brain Derived Neurotropic Factor).
- The drug Lacosamide acts by inhibiting CRMP protein, thereby causing protective action against neuronal excitotoxicity.

205. Ans. (a) Shift to sodium valproate

Ref: Katzung, 14th ed. pg. 418–19; KDT 6th ed. pg. 405

Hypersensitivity reactions like rashes, DLE, lymphadenopathy and neutropenia require that phenytoin to be stopped and switch to broader spectrum anti-epileptics like valproate.

206. Ans. (c) Topiramate

Ref: Katzung, 14th ed. pg. 427–28

- The only antiepileptic drug which causes weight loss: Topiramate, Zonisamide
- **MOA of topiramate:**
  - VG-Na+ channel blocker
  - Activate GABA receptor
  - Inhibit AMPA receptor *(receptor of Glutamate)*
- **Use:**
  - GTCS, Partial seizure
  - Maintenance therapy of alcohol withdrawal
  - LGS
  - Decreases alcohol craving
- **Side effects:** Urolithiasis, Somnolence

207. Ans. (a) Naloxone

Ref: Katzung, 14th ed. pg. 581

- In acute morphine poisoning the DOC is Naloxone (Opioid antagonist).
- It is short acting and has rapid onset of action. It is given by IV route.
- **Naltrexone**
  - It is a longer acting oral opioid antagonist.
  - Given in long term addiction therapay to prevent relapse.
- **Nalmefene:**
  - Also a naltrexone derivative. Can be given IV.
  - It is recently approved for cholestatic pruritus.

208. Ans. (b) Pruritus

Ref: https://www.ncbi.nlm.nih.gov/pubmed/8706199

- With the increasing utilization of intrathecal and epidural opioids in humans, a wide variety of clinically relevant side effects have been reported.
- The four classic side effects are *pruritus*, nausea and vomiting, urinary retention, and respiratory depression.
- Intrathecal injection has been shown to cause segmental analgesia without affecting other modalities. *It acts in the substantia gelatinosa of dorsal horn to inhibit release of excitatory transmitters from primary afferents carrying pain impulses.* The action appears to be exerted through inter neurons which are involved in the 'gating' of pain impulses. Release of glutamate from primary pain afferents in the spinal cord and its postsynaptic action on dorsal horn neurons is inhibited by morphine.

209. Ans. (b) Buspirone

Ref: Katzung, 14th ed. pg. 584; KDT, 6th ed. pg. 451

BUSPIRONE

- A new class of antianxiety drug.
- Relieves mild-to-moderate generalized anxiety
- The mechanism of anxiolytic action may be dependent on its selective partial agonistic action on 5-HT_{1A} receptors.

The Following Agents can be Used as Anti-Smoking Drugs

- *Vareniciline:*
  - *It is a direct acting nicotinic agonist*
  - *Can be used orally and has a half life of 14–20 hours.*
- *Bupropion: It acts by inhibition of neuronal reuptake of 5-HIT, NE and DA.*
- ***Clonidine:***
  - *It is a very effective drug for reducing the withdrawal effects of nicotine.*
  - *It decreases the craving as well as is useful in insomnia.*
- Nicotine (Gums, Patch, Inhaler)

210. Ans. (a) Nicotine replacement gum

Ref: Katzung, 14th ed. pg. 584

Treatment of smoking dependence:

- **First line:** Nicotine replacement therapy (gum, patch, inhaler).
- **Bupropion and Varenicicline** (Nicotine receptor agonist): Also first line. Considered more effective.
- **2nd line:** Clonidine and Nortryptiline
- **Rimonabant:** Cannabinoid receptor inverse agonist. Withdrawn due to increased depression and suicide risk.

211. Ans. (c) Lithium

Ref: Katzung, 14th ed. pg. 527

- Lithium is DOC in manic disorder.

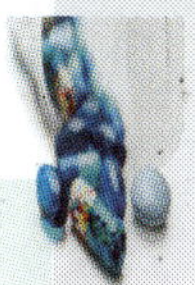

- DOC for prophylaxis of mania: Lithium
- DOC for acute attack of mania: Sedative + Atypical antipsychotics
- DOC for mania in pregnancy: Atypical antipsychotics
- Side effect of lithium *(Mn: LITTH)*
  - **L:** LEUCOCYTOSIS
  - **I:** Insipidus diabetes
  - **T:** Tremors (MC side effect- Coarse tremor);
  - **T:** Teratogenic (Ebstein anomaly)
  - **H:** Hypothyroidism

Extra Mile

Therapeutic Plasma concentration of Lithium
- Acute mania: 1–1.5 mEq/L
- Prophylaxis: 0.6–1 mEq/L
- Toxic plasma conc level: >1.5 mEq/L

212. Ans. (c) Fluvoxamine

Ref: Katzung, 14th ed. pg. 540

- SSRI are selective serotonin reuptake inhibitor. Causing increased level of only serotonin in synaptic cleft.
- DOC in mild to moderate depression
- Drugs are:
  - CITALOPRAM
  - ESCITALOPRAM: **Most specific SSRI**
  - FLUOXETINE: Longest acting (50 hrs)
  - FLUOXAMINE: Shortest acting
  - PAROXETINE
  - SERTRALINE

Extra Mile

- **TCA: Tricyclic Antidepressant**
  - Inhibit reuptake of serotonin, Noradrenaline (NA) and Dopamine (DA)
  - **Drugs are:** Imipramine, Trimipramine, Desipramine, Clomipramine, Nortryptiline, Amitryptilline
- **SNRI: Serotonergic Noradrenergic reuptake inhibitor**
  - Inhibit reuptake of serotonin and NA
  - **Drugs are:** Venlafaxine, Desvenlafaxine, Duloxetine, Milnacipran, Levomilnacipran

213. Ans. (b) Serotonergic noradrenergic reuptake inhibitor

Ref: Goodman & Gillman's 13th ed. pg. 268

- Five medications with a nontricyclic structure that inhibit the reuptake of both 5HT and NE have been approved for use in the US for treatment of depression, anxiety disorders, pain, or other specific conditions. The drugs are:
  - Venlafaxine and its demethylated metabolite desvenlafaxine
  - Duloxetine
  - Milnacipran, and
  - Levomilnacipran

Mn: Vania Duals My Love

214. Ans. (b) Nausea

Ref: Katzung, 14th ed. pg. 546

TABLE: Side effect of antidepressants

Drug	Important side effects
SSRI	**MC side effect: Nausea** Other side effects: • Delayed ejaculation: Now approved for premature ejaculation • Serotonin syndrome • Anorgasmia • Agitation, anxiety, insomnia
TCA	Sedation, weight gain, T wave flattening, QT prolongation, Postural hypotension
SNRI	Serotonin syndrome Insomnia, Tachycardia, Anxiety

215. Ans. (d) Motion sickness

Ref: Katzung's Pharma, 14th ed. pg. 135

- Scopolamine (hyoscine) is a prototypic ***muscarinic receptor antagonist, and*** **is one of the best agents for the prevention of motion sickness.**
- Scopolamine has many effects in the body including decreasing the secretion of fluids, slowing the stomach and intestines, and dilation of the pupils.
- Scopolamine is also used to relieve nausea, vomiting, and dizziness associated with motion sickness and recovery from anesthesia and surgery.

216. Ans. (b) Aldehyde dehydrogenase

Ref: Katzung, 14th ed. pg. 404; KDT, 6th ed. pg. 386

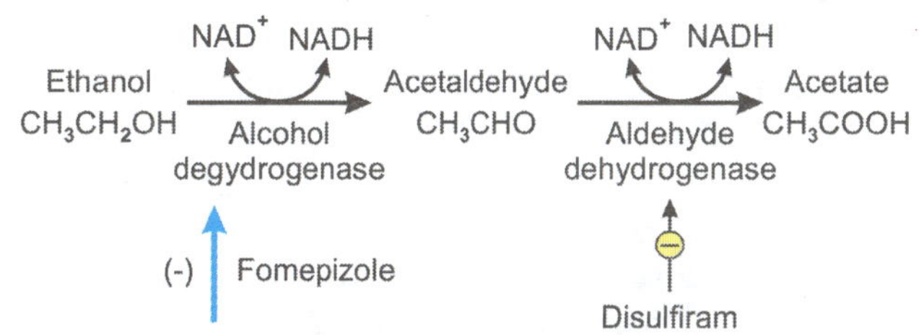

- **Disulfiram is used as an aversion therapy in alcoholics.**
- ***Disulfiram acts by inhibiting aldehyde dehydrogenase.*** If a person still takes alcohol while on disulfiram treatment, alcohol is metabolized as usual, but acetaldehyde accumulates.
- This accumulation of acetaldehyde gives some distressing symptoms like **flushing, burning sensation, throbbing headache, perspiration, dizziness, vomiting, confusion** and **circulatory collapse.**

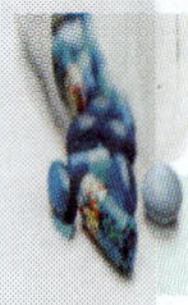

- Therefore, it is recommended only for those alcoholics who are motivated and sincerely desire to leave the habit.
- **Drugs causing disulfiram like reaction:**
  - Griseofulvin
  - Moxalactam
  - Metronidazole
  - Chlorpropamide
  - Cefoperazone
  - Cefotetan
  - Trimethorprim
  - Procarbazine
- **Other drugs that decrease craving for alcohol and smoking: (*remembered as NATO*)**
  - NALTREXONE
  - ACAMPROSATE
  - TOPIRAMATE
  - ONDANSETRON

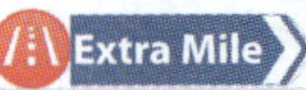

- Drug which inhibits alcohol dehydrogenase- **FOMEPIZOLE**
- Antidote for methanol poisoning: **FOMEPIZOLE > ETHANOL**
- Antidote for ethylene glycol poisoning: **FOMEPIZOLE**

217. Ans. (a) Competitively inhibits alcohol dehydrogenase

Ref: Katzung, 14th ed. pg. 404; KDT, 6th ed. pg. 387

- **Ethanol** acts by competitive inhibition of alcohol dehydrogenase which block further metabolism of methanol into formaldehyde and formic acid. These products also cause retinal damage leading to subsequent blindness.

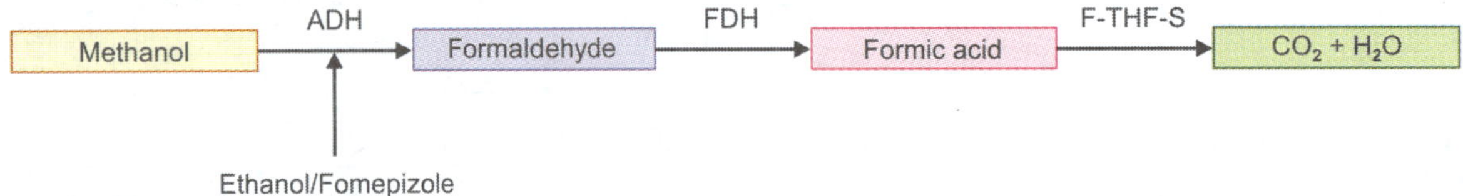

ADH: alcohol dehydrogenase: FDH : formaldehyde dehydrogenase
F-THF-S: 10-formyl tetrahydrofolate synthetase

- **Catalase** is a common enzyme found in nearly all living organisms exposed to oxygen. It catalyzes the decomposition of hydrogen peroxide to water and oxygen
- **Lactate dehydrogenase:** Dummy choice and is present in heart, RBC and is used as marker for malignancy.
- **Acetaldehyde dehydrogenase:** Converts acetaldehyde into acetic acid and is the target for disulfiram which is used to help patients quit alcohol.

Remember

- **Ethanol** is also metabolized by alcohol dehydrogenase and acts as its competitive inhibition. The enzyme's affinity for ethanol is 10-20 times higher than it is for methanol. Given via IV infusion in methanol or ethylene glycol poisoning.
- **Fomepizole** inhibits alcohol dehydrogenase. It is a stronger competitive inhibitor of ADH and, in addition, does not cause hypoglycemia or sedation.
- **Fomepizole** is relatively easier to administer than ethanol. It does not require monitoring of serum concentrations. Hence considered **as drug of choice.**

218. Ans. (d) Flumazenil

Ref: Katzung, 14th ed. pg. 404; KDT, 6th ed. pg. 385

- **Flumazenil is benzodiazepine antagonist. It has no role in alcohol detoxification.**

Alcohol Detoxification

Alcohol can produce physical and psychological dependence. In the treatment of alcohol dependence, major aim is to prevent withdrawal symptoms first and to avoid relapse of addiction thereafter.

- **Benzodiazepines** (chlordiazepoxide and diazepam) are long acting CNS depressant and are given to **prevent withdrawal.**
- **Acamprosate** is an **NMDA antagonist** that can be used for **maintenance therapy of alcohol abstinence.**
- **Naltrexone** is an opioid antagonist that can be used to reduce **alcohol craving.**
- **Disulfiram** can be used in psychologically dependent persons who are motivated to quit alcohol. It is ***contraindicated in physically dependent*** individuals. It produces severe distressing symptoms (like flushing, headache, vomiting, visual disturbances and mental confusion) after intake of alcohol due to accumulation of acetaldehyde.
- **Topiramate and ondansetron** can also *decrease* alcohol craving.

219. Ans. (c) Metoclopramide

Ref: KDT, 6th ed. pg. 643

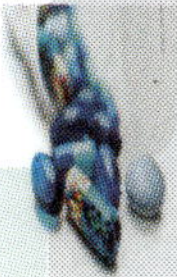

- Galactorrhea is caused by increased level of prolactin.
- Normally, this prolactin is in inhibited state by Dopamine.
- Prolactin is under predominant inhibitory control of hypothalamus through PRIH (Prolactin Release Inhibitory Hormone), which is Dopamine that acts on pituitary lactotrope D2 receptor.
- Dopaminergic agonist like bromocriptine, DA and cabergoline decrease plasma prolactin levels and is used to treat hyperprolactinemia.
- Dopaminergic antagonists like chlorpromazine, haloperidol, **metoclopramide** causes hyperprolactinemia by blocking D2 receptors.

ANTIMICROBIAL AGENTS

220. Ans. (b) Azithromycin

Ref: Goodman and Gillman 13th ed. pg. 1055

- Drug of choice for pneumonia caused by legionella infection is Azithromycin.
- Because of better tissue concentration, single dosing, better tolerability and least drug interaction, azithromycin is preferred than erythromycin.
- **Note:** For atypical infections like Chlamydia, Mycoplasma, atypical mycobacterial infection azithromycin is considered as drug of choice.

221. Ans. (b) Amphotericin B

Ref: Goodman and Gillman 13th ed. pg. 1089-90

- Post covid therapy, risk of opportunistic fungal infection like Mucormycosis is very high. This fungal infection leads to black necrotic lesion. Therefore, it is often termed as black fungus.
- DOC for Mucormycosis is Amphotericin B.
- Other drugs effective in Mucormycosis: Posaconazole, Isavuconazole

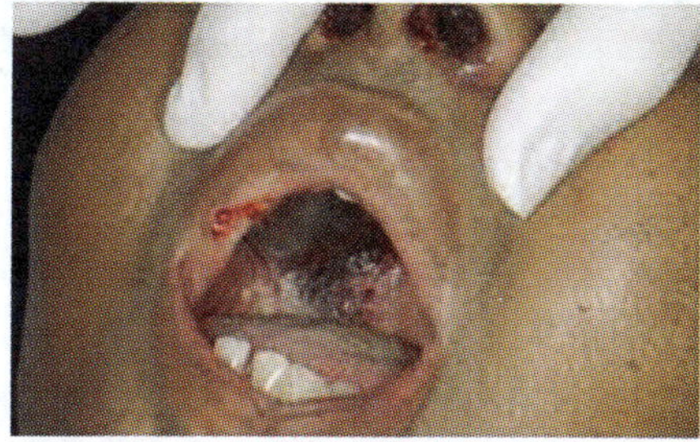

222. Ans. (b) Metronidazole

- The given case is of Bacterial vaginosis, which is caused by organism Gardnerella vaginalis
- DOC is Metronidazole.

223. Ans. (b) Clostridium difficile

- There is maximum risk of pseudomembranous colitis with clindamycin.
- Causative organism is Clostridium difficile.
- Treatment:
  - Mild – Metronidazole
    Moderate/Severe: Fidaxomicin/Vancomycin (PO)

224. Ans. (c) Protein synthesis inhibitor

- Doxycycline is one of the tetracyclines
- **MOA:** 30 s inhibitor → inhibits protein synthesis by interfering with tRNA interaction at A-site.

Extra Mile

- FQ are DNA gyrase inhibitor;
- Example of cell wall inhibitors are: Beta lactams, vancomycin
- Rifampicin act by inhibiting RNA polymerase

225. Ans. (b) Intravenous artesunate

- This is a case of cerebral malaria; treatment initially is started with IV artesunate for 48 hours.
- This is followed by oral artemisinin combination therapy for 3 days.

226. Ans. (b) Moxifloxacin

Ref: Goodman and Gillman 13th ed. pg. 1016-17

- Fluroquinolones are considered as effective drug therapy in urinary tract infection.
- All the fluroquinolones are excreted via kidney, except Moxifloxacin, hence it is not effective in UTI patients.
- Metabolism of moxifloxacin is via hepatic sulfation and glucuronidation. Less than a quarter of systemic moxifloxacin is excreted unchanged via the kidneys, and because high concentrations are not achieved in the urine, it is not recommended for UTIs

Extra Mile

- FQ safer in renal failure: Moxifloxacin
- FQ causing hepatotoxicity: Trovafloxacin (withdrawn) > Moxifloxacin > Pefloxacin
- FQ causing QT prolongation: Ofloxacin, Moxifloxacin, Levofloxacin. Others that can also cause QT prolongation and withdrawn are: Sparfloxacin, Lomefloxacin.

227. Ans. (b) Valacyclovir

Ref: Katzung 14th ed. pg. 865-66

- The shown condition is herpes zoster virus infection.
- Preferred agent for this condition is Valacyclovir.

Note:

- Ganciclovir (option A) is preferred in CMV infection (CMV retinitis, CMV urogenital warts)

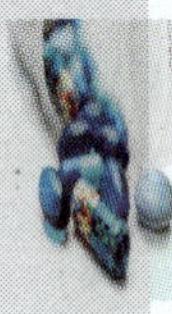

- Tenofovir (option C) is a nucleotide reverse transcriptase inhibitor. It is used in HIV and HBV infection
- Mupirocin (option D): Is used topically for strep pyogens, staph aureus and MRSA nasal carriers.

228. Ans. (a) Chloroquine

Ref: Katzung 14th ed. pg. 918-19

- Among the given options, only chloroquine can be used for treatment and prophylaxis of malaria both.
- Chemoprophylaxis is given to any person travelling to malaria endemic area.
- **Short term prophylaxis (<6 week):** Doxycycline 100 mg/day. Started 2 days prior to journey and continued till 4 weeks after.
- **Long term prophylaxis (> 6 week):** Mefloquine 250 mg/week. Started 2 weeks prior to journey and continued till 4 weeks after.
- If there is any contraindication or unavailability of above drugs, chloroquine can be used as an alternative.

229. Ans. (a) Metronidazole

Ref: Katzung 14th ed. pg. 895-96, 1166

- The given case shows feature of disulfiram like reactions.
- **Drugs causing disulfiram like reaction:**
  - Griseofulvin
  - Metronidazole
  - Cefotetan, Cefoperazone, Cefamandole
  - Moxalactam
  - Procarbazine
  - Chlorpropamide

230. Ans. (d) Amoxicillin

Ref: KDT 8th ed. pg. 1018

Class of Drugs contraindicated in pregnancy and its safer alternative

Class of drug	Contraindicated	Safer alternative
Antibacterials (systemic bacterial infections)	Cotrimoxazole, Fluoroquinolones (X), Tetracycline (X), Doxycycline (X), Chloramphenicol (X) Gentamicin, Streptomycin (X) Kanamycin (X), Tobramycin (X), Clarithromycin, Azithromycin Clindamycin, Vancomycin Nitrofurantoin	Penicillin G, Ampicillin Amoxicillin-clavulanate Cloxacillin, Piperacillin Cephalosporins Erythromycin

Extra Mile

- Sulfonamides (Co-Trimoxazole) if used during pregnancy can lead to kernicterus.
- Aminoglycosides (Gentamicin): Can produce ototoxicity and nephrotoxicity
- Floroquinolones (Ciprofloxacin): Affects growing cartilage and tendon

231. Ans. (c) Schistosomiasis

Ref: Katzung 14th ed. pg. 939

- Drug of choice for all the **flukes** (**trematodes**) is **Praziquantel** except liver fluke, where drug of choice is Triclabendazole or Bithionol.
- Drug of choice for all the **tapeworms** (**cestodes**) is **Praziquantel** except Cysticercosis and Echinococcus where drug of choice is Albendazole.
- Drug of choice for all the **Roundworms (Nematode)** is Albendazole/Mebendazole except Strongyloides, Onchocerca (DOC: Ivermectin) and Filariasis, loa-loa disease (DOC is Diethylcarbamazine).

TABLE: Drugs for the treatment of helminthic infections

Infection organism	Drug of choice	Alternative drugs
Roundworms (nematodes)		
Ascaris lumbricoides (roundworm)	Albendazole or pyrantel pamoate or mebendazole	Ivermectin, piperazine
Trichuris trichiura (whipworm)	Mebendazole or albendazole	Ivermectin, oxantel pamoate drug combinations
Necator americanus (hookworm); *Ancylostoma duodenale* (hookworm)	Albendazole or mebendazole or pyrantel pamoate	
Strongyloides stercoralis (threadworm)	Ivermectin	Albendazole or thiabendazole
Enterobius vermicularis (pinworm)	Mebendazole or pyrantel pamoate	Albendazole
Trichinella spiralis (trichinosis)	Mebendazole or albendazole; add corticosteroids for severe infection	

Contd...

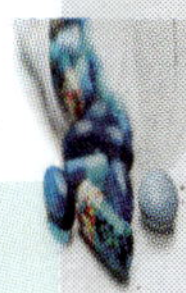

Infection organism	Drug of choice	Alternative drugs
Trichostrongylus species	Pyrantel pamoate or mebendazole	Albendazole
Cutaneous larva migrans (creeping eruption)	Albendazole or ivermectin	Thiabendazde (topical)
Visceral larva migrans	Albendazole	Mebendazole
Angiostrongylus cantonensis	Albendazole or mebendazole	
Wuchereria bancrofti (filariasis); *Brugia malayi* (filariasis); tropical eosinophilia; *Log loa* (loiasis)	Diethylcarbamazine	Ivermectin
Onchocerca volvulus (onchocerciasis)	Ivermectin	
Dracunculus medinensis (guinea worm)	Metronidazole	Thiabendazole or mebendazole
Capillaria philippinensis (intestinal capillariasis)	Albendazole	Mebendazole
Flukes (trematodes)		
Schistosoma haematobium (bilharziasis)	Praziquantel	Metrifonate
Schistosoma mansoni	Praziquantel	Oxamniquine
Schistosoma japonicum	Praziquantel	
Clonorchis sinensis (liver fluke); *Opisthorchis* species	Praziquantel	Albendazole
Paragonimus westermani (lung fluke)	Praziquantel	Bithionol
Fasciola hepatica (sheep liver fluke)	Bithionol or triclabendazole	
Fasciolopsis buski (large intestinal fluke)	Praziquantel or niclosamide	
Heterophyes heterophyes; Metagonimus yokogawai (small intestinal flukes)	Praziquantel of niclosamide	
Tapeworms (cestodes)		
Taenia saginata (beef tapeworm)	Praziquantel or niclosamide	Mebendazole
Diphyllobothrium latum (fish tapeworm)	Praziquantel or niclosamide	
Taenia solium (pork tapeworm)	Praziquantel or niclosamide	
Cysticercosis (pork tapeworm larval stage)	Albendazole	Praziquantel
Hymenolepis nana (dwarf tapeworm)	Praziquantel	Niclosamide nitazoxanide
Echinococcus granulosus (hydatid disease); *Echinococcus multilocularis*	Albendazole	

232. Ans. (c) Mupirocin

Ref: Katzung 14th ed. pg. 1070

- Mupirocin is used for topical treatment of minor skin infection such as impetigo. It is also effective against gram positive cocci including-susceptible and methicillin-resistant strains of staph aureus.
- Intranasal mupirocin ointment is preferred for eliminating nasal carrier of S. aureus
- **MOA:** Inhibits staphylococcal isoleucyl tRNA synthetase.

233. Ans. (d) Ampicillin

Ref: Goodman & Gillman 13th ed. pg. 1036, 1050

- Ampicillin is considered as agent of choice in several infections like:
  - Enterococcus faecalis infection
  - Listeria infection
  - URTI (sinusitis, pharyngitis, otitis media) due to beta haemolytic streptococci
- **Other agents effective against Enterococcus faecalis:** Daptomycin, Linezolid, Tigecycline, Telavancin, Vancomycin, Carbapenems.
- **Agents effective against Enterococcus faecium:** Daptomycin, Linezolid

Extra Mile

- Enterococcus Faecium and Faecalis are highly resistant to aminoglycosides

234. Ans. (a) Ceftriaxone

Ref: Harrison 20th ed. pg. 1112

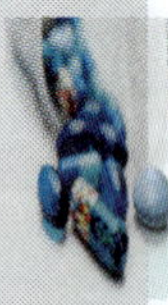

- DOC for meningococcal diseases: Penicillin G
- DOC for meningococcal meningitis: Ceftriaxone
- DOC for Prophylaxis of meningococcal meningitis: Rifampicin
- DOC for prophylaxis of H. influenza meningitis: Rifampicin
- DOC for prophylaxis of meningococcal meningitis in pregnancy: Ceftriaxone
- DOC for listeria: Ampicillin
- **Note:** Rifampicin is known to cross placental barrier, hence avoided (but not contraindicated) in pregnancy.

235. Ans. (b) Streptomycin

Ref: Goodman & Gillman 13th ed. pg. 1039-40

- Streptomycin is one of the aminoglycosides.
- **MOA:**
  - Enters bacteria
  - Binds to 30s ribosomal unit and interferes with initiation of protein synthesis by causing the misreading and premature termination of mRNA translation.
- Other aminoglycosides are: Gentamicin, Tobramycin, Amikacin, Neomycin, Kanamycin, Netilmicin, Paromomycin.

USES OF AMINOGLYCOSIDES (AG)

- **Note:** AG is ineffective against anaerobes.
  - Most commonly used AG: Gentamicin
- Can be used as empirical therapy in majority of infections like UTI, hospital acquired Pneumonia, Meningitis, Peritonitis, Cystic fibrosis, sepsis.
- **Streptomycin:** DOC for tularemia, plague

SIDE EFFECT OF AG

- Ototoxicity
  - **Vestibulotoxicity:** MC due to Streptomycin and gentamicin
  - **Auditory/Cochlear dysfunction:** Irreversible, bilateral, high-frequency hearing loss. MC due to Amikacin, Neomycin, Kanamycin
    - **First symptom of cochlear toxicity:** High pitch tinnitus
- Nephrotoxicity
- Neuromuscular blockade (MC: Neomycin > Kanamycin)

Extra Mile

- Ceftriaxone is a third generation cephalosporin (from β Lactams class → a cell wall inhibitor).
- Nevirapine is one of the anti-retroviral drug from Non-nucleoside reverse transcriptase inhibitors class.
- Indinavir is one of the HIV protease inhibitor.

236. Ans. (a) Streptomycin

Ref: Goodman & Gillman 13th ed. pg. 1045; Harrison 20th ed. pg. 1112

- Streptomycin is highly ototoxic (vestibulotoxic >> Cochleotoxic) and nephrotoxic drug.
- It is strictly contraindicated throughout the pregnancy.

TABLE: Drugs during pregnancy

	Drugs safe in pregnancy	Drugs contraindicated in pregnancy (Safety uncertain)
• **Anti-tubercular**	Isoniazid, Rifampicin, Pyrazinamide, Ethambutol	Streptomycin
• **Antiamoebic**	Diloxanide furoate, paromomycin	Metronidazole, Tinidazole, Quiniodochlor
• **Antimalarial**	Chloroquine, Mefloquine, Proguanil, Quinine (only in 1st trimester)	Primaquine
• **Antifungal**	**Topical:** Clotrimazole, Nystatin, Tolnaftane	Amphotericin B, Fluconazole, Itraconazole, Ketoconazole, Griseofulvin
• **Antiallergies**	Chlorpheniramine, Promethazine	Cetirizine, Loratadine, Fexofenadine
• **Anti bacterials**	Penicillin G, Ampicillin, Amoxicillin-clavulanate, cloxacillin, Piperacillin, Cephalosporins, Erythromycin	Cotrimoxazole, Fluoroquinolones, Tetracycline, Doxycycline, Chloramphenicol, Kanamycin, Tobramycin, Clarithromycin, Vancomycin
• **Antiviral**	–	Ganciclovir, Foscarnet, Amantadine, Vidarabine, a-interferon
• **Anti-retroviral**	Zidovudine, Lamivudine, tenofovir, Nelfinavir, Nevirapine, Saquinavir, Efavirenz	Didanosine, Abacavir, Indinavir, Ritonavir
• **Anti-diabetic**	Insulin (preferably human insulin)	Sulfonylureas, metformin, Acarbose, pioglitazone, Repaglinide
• **Thyroid drugs**	Propylthiouracil	Carbimazole, Radioactive iodine (X), Iodide

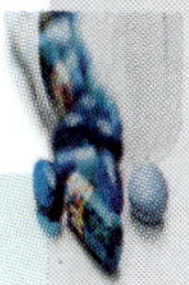

237. Ans. (b) Azithromycin

Ref: Goodman & Gillman 13th ed. pg. 1017

- The patient in the given case has chlamydia induced UTI. The agent that can be preferred for management of such condition is fluroquinolones (FQ).
- **Books state:** *"FQs are more efficacious than trimethoprim-sulfamethoxazole or oral B-Lactams". Moxifloxacin doesn't accumulate in urine and hence NOT approved for treatment of UTI.*
- Fluoroquinolones lack activity for *Treponema pallidum but have activity in vitro against Chlamydia trachomatis and Haemophilus ducreyi.*
- This patient later presented with symptoms of sexually transmitted infection, for which the best option is Azithromycin, single dose is effective.
- **Book states:** *"For chlamydial urethritis/cervicitis, a 7-day course of ofloxacin or levofloxacin is an alternative to a 7-day treatment with doxycycline or a single dose of azithromycin; other available quinolones are NOT effective in these condition"*

238. Ans. (a) Dengue

Ref: Goodman & Gillman 13th ed. pg. 668-69

- CYD-TDV developed by Sanofi Pasteur is a recombinant tetravalent (four-serotype) live attenuated virus vaccine that was first licensed in Mexico in December 2015 for use in individuals 9–45 years of age living in endemic areas.
- However, it is given as a three-dose series on a 0–6-12-month schedule via subcutaneous route.
- It should only be given to individuals with previous history of dengue by any of the 4 serotypes.

Extra Mile

- **Malaria Vaccine:** The RTS, S vaccine is a recombinant protein-based malaria vaccine with AS01 adjuvant against *Plasmodium falciparum* only.It is the first malaria vaccine to be approved in April 2019.
  - The vaccine has been recommended by WHO for pilot introduction in selected areas of 3 African countries

239. Ans. (b) Liposomal Amphotericin B

Ref: Goodman & Gillman 13th ed. pg. 996

- Drug of choice for visceral leishmaniasis: Liposomal Amphotericin B.
  - **Note:** AmpB can be used even during pregnancy
  - **Side effect:** Renal toxicity, hypokalemia, hypomagnesemia
- **Other agents for management of leishmaniasis:**
  - **Sodium stibogluconate:** Given parenterally 20 mg/kg/day for 20 days in cutaneous disease and 28 days in visceral leishmaniasis. Due to increased resistance it has now become obsolete in India. At present oral preparation is available and shows better result.
    - **Side effect:** Pancreatitis, Hepatotoxicity, Bone marrow suppression, haemolytic anemia and renal failure
  - **Pentamidine** can be used in doses of 2–3 mg/kg IV or IM daily or every second day for 4–7 doses to treat cutaneous leishmaniasis.
    - **Side effect:** Nephrotoxic, Hypoglycemia
  - **Miltefosine:** Oral agent. Can be used in visceral and cutaneous leishmaniasis.
    - Only oral preparation available. Teratogenic → Not used in pregnancy

240. Ans. (a) Fosfomycin

- Among the given choices fosfomycin is preferred agent for UTI.
- Recommendations for treatment must be considered in the context of local resistance patterns and national differences in some agents' availability.
- For example, **fosfomycin** and pivmecillinam are not available in all countries but are considered **first-line** options where they are available because they retain activity against a majority of uropathogens that produce extended-spectrum β-lactamases.
  - *Use of **fosfomycin** for UTIs (including complicated infections), particularly for infections caused by multidrug-resistant E. coli.*
- TMP-SMX was earlier recommended as the first-line agent for treatment of uncomplicated UTI, but due to increasing evidence of resistance it is less preferred.
  - ***TMP-SMX** has been recommended as first-line treatment for acute cystitis, and it remains appropriate to consider the use of this drug in regions with resistance rates not exceeding 20%*
- Fluoroquinolones should not be used for uncomplicated cystitis unless no alternatives are available.
  - Most **fluoroquinolones** are highly effective as short-course therapy for cystitis; the exception is moxifloxacin
  - Commonly used for UTI include ciprofloxacin and levofloxacin.
- **Nitrofurantoin** remains highly active against *E. coli* and most non-*E. coli* isolates. *Proteus*, *Pseudomonas*, *Serratia*, *Enterobacter*, and yeasts are all intrinsically resistant to this drug.
  - Resistance to nitrofurantoin remains low compared to TMP-SMX
- In acute cystitis, β-Lactam agents generally are not preferred as well as TMP- SMX or fluoroquinolones.

TABLE: Treatment strategies for acute uncomplicated cystitis

Drug and dose	Estimated clinical efficacy, %	Estimated bacterial efficacy, %	Common side effects
Nitrofurantoin, 100 mg bid × 5–7 day	87–95	82–92	Nausea, headache
TMP-SMX, 1 DS tablet bid × 3 day	86–100	85–100	Rash, urticaria, nausea, vomiting, hematologic abnormalities
Fosfomycin, 3-g single-dose sachet	83-95	78-98	Diarrhea, nausea, headache
Pivmecillinam, 400 mg bid × 3–7 day	55–82	74–84	Nausea, vomiting, diarrhea
Fluoroquinolones, dose varies by agent; 3 day regimen	81–98	78–96	Nausea, vomiting, diarrhea, headache, drowsiness, insomnia
β-Lactams, dose varies by agent; 5–7 day regimen	79–98	74–98	Diarrhea, nausea, vomiting, rash, urticaria

241. Ans. (b) Antimalarial

Ref: Goodman & Gillman's 13th ed. pg. 974

- ***Pyronaridine*** is an antimalarial structurally related to amodiaquine.
- This drug is potent against both *P. falciparum* and *P. vivax and is very well tolerated.*
- It leads to fever resolution in 1–2 days and parasite clearance in 2–3 days.
- It is tested in clinical trials as an adjunct with artemisinin class drugs, has not yet been licensed.

242. Ans. (b) Ceftriaxone

Ref: Harrison 19th ed. pg. 767

- Ceftriaxone is the empirical drug of choice for treatment of meningitis. It is frequently combined with vancomycin.

243. Ans. (d) Mutation

Ref: Goodman & Gillman's 13th ed. pg. 1016

- Ciprofloxacin is one of the fluoroquinolones along with norfloxacin, ofloxacin, levofloxacin, sparfloxacin, etc.
- **MOA of quinolones:** The quinolone antibiotics target bacterial *DNA gyrase* and *topoisomerase IV*.
- The quinolones inhibit gyrase-mediated DNA supercoiling at concentrations that correlate well with those required to inhibit bacterial growth.
- **Mutations of the gene that encodes the A subunit of the gyrase** can confer resistance to these drugs.

244. Ans. (a) Kanamycin

Ref: Goodman & Gillman 13th ed. pg. 1044-45

- All aminoglycosides have the potential to produce reversible and irreversible vestibular, cochlear, renal toxicity and neuromuscular blockade.
- Aminoglycoside-induced ototoxicity may result in irreversible, bilateral, high-frequency hearing loss or vestibular hypofunction.
- A high-pitched tinnitus often is **the first symptom** of cochlear toxicity.
- Drugs like amikacin, neomycin and kanamycin are specifically cochleotoxic > vestibulotoxic.
- Gentamicin, streptomycin is vestiblar > cochleotoxic
- **Tobramycin:** Cochlear = Vestibular toxicity both.

245. Ans. (b) Clindamycin

Ref: KDT 6th ed. pg. 668

- **Lincosamide family** of antimicrobial drugs includes:
  - Clindamycin
  - Lincomycin *(It is obsolete now)*
- **Clindamycin** is among the drugs which act by inhibiting protein synthesis.
- They bind to 50s subunit of ribosome resulting in bacteriostatic inhibition of bacterial protein synthesis.
- It is very effective drug against corynebacterium acne, pneumocycstis carinii and toxoplasma gondii

Drugs which inhibit cell wall formation	Drugs which inhibit protein synthesis
Cycloserine **Vancomycin** Fosfomycin **Beta Lactams** Penicillin Cephalosporin Carbapenem Monolactams **Bacitracin**	• **Tetracycline** *(tRNA inhibitor)* • **Chloramphenicol** *(peptide bond formation inhibitor)* • **Macrolides** (erythro, clarithro, azithro) • **Clindamycin** • **Aminoglycosides** • **Streptogramins** (Quinpristin + Dalfopristin)
*Remembered as: **C**ell **V**all o**F** **B**acteria*	***T**he **C**hild **M**ay **C**limb **A**mino **S**tairs*

246. Ans. (c) Quinpristin

Ref: Sharma & Sharma 3rd ed. pg. 702

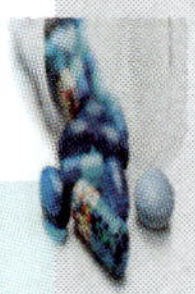

TABLE: Protein synthesis inhibitor drugs acting at 30s and 50s ribosomal unit

Drugs acting by inhibiting 30s ribosome	Aminoglycoside (Streptomycin, Gentamicin, Tobramycin, Kanamycin, Amikacin) Tetracycline (Minocycline, Demeclocyclin, Doxycycline)
Drugs acting by inhibiting 50s ribosome	Streptogramins (Quinpristin & Dalfopristin) Erythromycin (macrolides) Lincosamides (Clindamycin) Linezolid Ketolides (Telithromycin, Cethromycin) Chloramphenicol
*Mn: Buy **AT** 30, **SELL** Karo China in 50*	

247. Ans. (a) Carbenicillin

Ref: Sharma & Sharma 3rd ed. pg. 731

- Some penicillins like PnG, Procaine PnG, Benzathine PnG, Carbenicillin, Ticarcillin, Mezlocillin, Azlocillin, Piperacillin are sensitive to gastric acid degradation.
- Such penicillins are not effecrive orally, and hence are given via parenteral route.

TABLE: Acid Resistant Vs acid Labile penicillins

Acid Resistant penicillin Mn: VODCA BoTal	Acid Labile penicillin Mn: GNM Car Till MAP
• PnV • Oxacillin • Dicloxacillin • Cloxacillin • Ampicillin/Amoxycillin • Bacampicillin • Talampicillin	**Natural penicillins** • Penicillin G • Procaine PnG • Benzathine PnG **Anti-staphylococcal penicillins** • Nafcillin • Methicillin **Antipseudomonal penicillins** • Carbenicillin • Ticarcillin • Mezlocillin • Azlocillin • Piperacillin

248. Ans. (b) Ampicillin

Ref: Goodman & Gillman 13th ed. pg. 1028; Katzung, 9th ed. pg. 1172

- First line drug of choice for listeria species is Ampicillin.
- Second line- TMP-SMZ
- The book states: "Ampicillin or penicillin G (with consideration for addition of gentamicin to both for immunosuppressed patients with meningitis) is the drugs of choice in the management of infections owing to *L. monocytogenes*. The recommended dose of penicillin G is 18–24 million units parenterally per day for at least 2 weeks."

Extra Mile

Listeria along with gropup B streptococci and E.coli is the most common cause of neonatal meningitis.

MOA of ampicillin: Inhibits cell wall synthesis during active multiplication.

First line drug of choice for neonatal meningitis- ampicillin + 3rd gen cephalosporin.

Chloramphenicol is a protein synthesis inhibitor, more specifically it inhibits formation of peptide bond between acceptor and peptide site.

- **Side effect:** Bone marrow suppression
- **Teratogenic S/E- Gray baby syndrome**: Chloramphenicol

249. Ans. (b) Chloramphenicol

Ref: KDT, 6th ed. pg. 717

Antimicrobial drugs	Side effects
Chloramphenicol	Grey baby syndrome Bone marrow suppression
Tetracycline	Teeth discoloration and bone growth suppression Phototoxicity Fanconi syndrome (in case of expired tetracycline) Vestibular dysfunction
Vancomycin	Red man/Red neck syndrome Nephrotoxic and ototoxic
Clindamycin	Pseudomembranous colitis

Extra Mile

VANCOMYCIN: drug of choice for MRSA

Vancomycin NEVER effective against Pseudomonas

β **LACTAMS** never effective against MRSA (except 5th Gen).

AMINOGLYCOSIDE never effective against Anaerobes.

Most common cause of pseudo membranous colitis: **3rd Gen. cephalosporin.**

DOC for pseudo membranous colitis: **VANCOMYCIN (Oral).**

Preferred agent in mild case of pseudomembranous colitis → Metronidazole

250. Ans. (b) Vancomycin

Ref: Katzung, 14th ed. pg. 809; Sharma & Sharma 3rd ed. pg. 742-43; KDT, 6th ed. pg. 732

- Vancomycin is a bactericidal drug acts by cell wall synthesis inhibitor and by damaging cell membrane integrity.
- It is exclusively active against aerobic as well as anaerobic gram positive species such as streptococcus and staphylococci including MRSA.
- Parenterally it is DOC in MRSA, Staph epideermidis infection associated with use of IV catheters or with contibuous peritoneal dialysis.

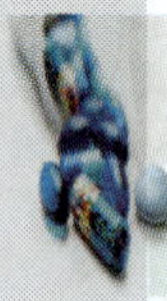

- Orally it is also effective in controlling pseudomembranous colitis not responding to metronidazole (act as local because it is poorly absorbed from GIT).
- **Side effects:**
  - Red neck syndrome (due to histamine release)
  - Ototoxicity, nephrotoxicity, skin rash, reversible neutropenia, etc.

251. Ans. (b) Metronidazole oral

Ref: Katzung's Pharma, 10th ed. Ch 53

- Vancomycin (oral) is now considered as the drug of choice for pseudomembraneous colitis.
- Metronidazole also used for pseudomembraneous colitis in mild cases.
- Ampicillin has been associated with pseudomembranous colitis
- Ceftriaxone is DOC for typhoid/enteric fever. Should be given IV.

Extra Mile

- METRONIDAZOLE is also the drug of choice in the treatment of amebiasis, trichomoniasis, Giardiasis and extraluminal amebiasis.
- For serious pseudomembranous colitis not responding to metronidazole, DOC is Fidaxomicin/Vancomycin (P.O).

252. Ans. (b) Pseudomembranous colitis

Ref: Sharma & Sharma 3rd ed. pg. 742-43; Katzung, 14th ed. pg. 809

Please refer to above explanation for details

253. Ans. (d) Nafcillin

Ref: KD Tripathi, 6th ed. pg. 700 & 708

- Microbes which are resistant to methicillin, are said to be MRSA. Since methicillin is not clinically used nowadays, then if the organism is resistant to Nafcillin and Cloxacillin, they are also said to be MRSA.
- Methicillin is highly penicilinase resistant but not acid resistant.
- MRSA have emerged in many areas. These are insensitive to all penicillinase-resistant penicillins and to other β-lactams as well as to erythromycin, aminoglycosides, tetracylines, etc.
- The drug of choice for these organisms is vancomycin/linezolid, but ciprofloxacin and Rifampicin can also be used.
- Antibiotics effective against Beta lactamase producing bacteria:
  - **Beta lactamase resistant antibiotics:** Cloxacillin, Dcloxacillin, Methicillin and Nafcillin
  - **Beta lactamase inhibitors:** currently there are 3 drugs in this category (and they are added with)
    - Clavulanic acid (+ Amoxycillin)
    - Sulbactam (+ Ampicillin)
    - Tazobactam (+ Piperacillin)

254. Ans. (b) β Lactams

Ref: Sharma & Sharma 3rd ed. pg. 733

- **No β *Lactams* are effective against MRSA, EXCEPT 5th generation cephalosporins like Ceftaroline and Ceftibiprole.**
- **DOC for MRSA:** Vancomycin
- DOC for VRSA: Daptomycin
- Drugs used in VRSA: Quinpristin, Daptomycin, Linezolid

255. Ans. (b) Chloramphenicol

Ref: KD Tripathi, 6th ed. pg. 716 & 909

CHLORAMPHENICOL

- It is a broad-spectrum antibiotic, active against nearly the same range of organisms (gram-positive and negative bacteria, rickettsiae, mycoplasma) as tetracyclines.

Adverse Effects

- Bone marrow depression
- Hypersensitivity reactions
- Grey baby syndrome

TABLE: Choice of drugs for common problems during pregnancy

Drug class (condition)	Unsafe drugs	Safer alternative
Antibacteirals	Fluoroquinolones Tetracycline Doxycycline Chloramphenicol Streptomycin Kananmycin Tobramycin	Penicillin G; Ampicillin Amoxicillin-Clavulanate Cloxacillin, Piperacillin cephalosphorins erythromycin
Antitubercular	Pyrazinamide, Ethambutol Streptomycin	Isoniazid Rifampicin
Anti hypertensives	ACE inhibitors Angiotensin antagonists Diuretics Proanolol and nitroprusside	Methyldopa Hydralazine Atenolol, Metoprolol, pindolol Nifedipine
Anti thyroid drugs	Carbimazole Radio active iodine Iodide	Propylthiouracil (PTU)

256. Ans. (a) Ciprofloxacin

Ref: KDT, 6th ed. pg. 909

- Antibiotics which are safe in pregnancy are remembered as "*PCM*":
  - Penicillin *(PnG, ampicillin etc)*
  - Cephalosporin *(cefotaxime, cefixime etc.)*
  - Macrolides *(erythromycin, azithromycin etc.)*
- *Refer above explanation table.*
- ***Fluoroquinolones (Ciprofloxacin) are contraindicated in pregnancy and below 18 years patient because it effect growing bone and tendon.***

257. Ans. (d) Ceftriaxone

Ref: Katzung, 14th ed. pg. 909; KDT, 6th ed. pg. 706

- Ceftriaxone is a 3rd generation cephalosporin with long duration of action (t½ - 8 hrs.) and with better CSF penetration.
- **Ceftriaxone** is highly effective in a wide range serious infections including bacterial meningitis, typhoid fever, complicated UTI's and STD's like gonorrhea.
- It is first choice drug for single dose therapy of gonorrhea if the penicillinase producing status of organism is not known.
- A single dose of 250 mg IM injection is curative in gonorrhea and in chancroid.
- Drugs which can also be given as first line in case of gonorrhea are:
  - Amoxicillin 3 g oral OR Ampicillin 3.5 g oral-for non penicillinase producing.
  - Ceftriaxone 250 mg IM or Cefuroxime 250 mg IM or Azithromycin 1 g oral single dose- for Penicillinase producing.
- TOC for Gonorrhea → VANCOMYCIN + CEFTRIAXONE

258. Ans. (a) Cefaclor

Ref: Katzung, 14th ed. pg. 804

TABLE: Cephalosporin generations

Drug class	Useful antibacterial spectrum[a]
First generation Cefazolin Cephalexin monohydrate Cefadroxil Cephradine	Streptococci; *Staphylococcus aureus*; some *Proteus, E. coli, Klebsiella*
Second generation Cefaclor Cefuroxime Cefuroxime axetil Cefprozil Cefoxitin Cefotetan Cefmetazole	*Escherichia coli, Klebsiella, Proteus, Haemophilus influenzae, Moraxella catarrhalis*. Not as active against gram-positive organisms as first-generation agents
Third generation Cefotaxime Ceftriaxone Cefdinir Cefditoren pivoxil Ceftibuten Cefpodoxime proxetil Ceftizoxime	*Escherichia coli, Klebsiella, Proteus, Haemophilus influenzae, Moraxella catarrhalis, Citrobacter, Enterobacter, Serratia; Neisseria gonorrhoeae*; activity for *S. aureus, Streptococcus pneumoniae*, and *Streptococcus pyogenes* comparable to first-generation agents. Activity against *Bacteroides* spp. inferior to that of cefoxitin and cefotetan.
Antipseudomonal cephalosporins Ceftazidime	Gram negative activity similar to third generation with addition of activity against *Pseudomonas*; poor activity vs gram-positive organisms
Ceftazidime/avibactam	Expands ceftazidime's against *Pseudomonas* and multidrug-resistant Enterobactericeae, but not against gram-positives
Ceftolozame/tazobactam	Similar to ceftazidime, with enhanced activity against *Pseudomonas* and extended-spectrum β-lactamase-producing Enterobacteriaceae
Fourth generation Cefepime, cefpirome	Comparable to third generation but more resistant to some β-lactamases (especially those of *Pseudomonas* and *Enterobacter*); gram-positive activity similar to cefotaxime
Fifth generation Ceftaroline Ceftobiprole	Similar actvity to 3rd generation but with activity against methicillin resistant *Staphylococcus aureus*

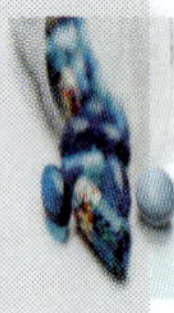

259. Ans. (d) Aztreonam

Ref: KDT, 6th ed. pg. 708

- β lactams contain a β lactam ring and another one is 2nd ring.
- 4 types of β lactams based on 2nd ring:
  - Penicillins *(ampicillin)*
  - Cephalosporins *(cefotaxim)*
  - Carbapenems *(doripenem)*
  - Monobactams *(azteronam)*
- In **monolactams (azteronam)** the 2nd ring is absent, due to which it doesn't show cross allergy with other β lactams.
- Therefore it can be used in patients who are allergic to penicillins.
- It inhibits gram negative enteric bacilli, H. influenza and pseudomonas.
- It doesn't inhibit gram positive cocci or fecal anaerobes.

260. Ans. (b) Mupirocin

Ref: KDT, 6th ed. pg. 733-34

- **Aminoacyl-tRNA synthetases (aaRSs)** are enzymes that catalyze the transfer of amino acids to their cognate tRNA. They play a pivotal role in protein synthesis and are essential for cell growth and survival.
- Mupirocin, a natural product of Pseudomonas fluorescens, is the only aaRS inhibitor approved by the US Food and Drug Administration to this date.
- It is active against gram-positive cocci, including methicillin-susceptible and methicillin-resistant strains of *Staphylococcus aureus*. Mupirocin inhibits staphylococcal isoleucyl tRNA synthetase.
- Mupirocin is indicated for topical treatment of minor skin infections, such as impetigo.

Extra Mile

Methenamine mandelate is the salt of mandelic acid and methenamine and possesses properties of urinary antiseptics. It doesn't treat UTI, but it suppresses.
Mitomycin C is antitumor antibiotics.
Metronidazole, an antibiotic for anaerobes.

261. Ans. (a) Injection Benzathine penicillin 2.4 million units IM single dose

Recommended treatment for syphilis

Stage of syphilis	Treatment	Comment
Early Primary, secondary, or early latent	**Benzathine penicillin G 2.4 MU, IM more**	
Late latent or uncertain duration	Benzathine penicillin G 2.4 million units 1M weekly for 3 wk	
Tertiary without neurophilis	Benzathine penicillin G 2.4 million units N weekly for 3 weeks	Cerebrospinal fluid evaluation recommended in all patients
Neurosyphilis	Aqueous penicillin G 18-24 million units IV daily, given every 3-4 hours or as continuous infusion for 10-14 days	Follow treatment with benzathine penicillin G 2.4 million units 1M weekly for up to 3 weeks

Contd...

262. Ans. (b) Azithromycin

Ref: KDT, 6th ed. pg. 730-31; Katzung, pg. 1172

- Azithromycin is new congener of erythromycin with expanded spectrum and improved pharmacokinetics.
- Because of its higher efficacy, better gastric tolerance and convenient once a day dosing, it is preferred over erythromycin as first line drug of choice for infections such as *(Mn: CHAL MD)*:
  - Chancroid
  - Chlamydia Trachomatis- 1 gm single dose is curative.
  - H. Influenzae
  - Atypical mycobacteria, Atypical pneumonia (by chlamydia)
  - Legionella
  - Moraxella catarrhalis
  - Donovanosis
- Erythromycin and clarithromycin are the macrolides with similar antimicrobial spectrum. But clarithromycin have action against mycobacterium avium complex (MAC), atypical mycobacteria and M. leprae, H.Influenzae, Toxoplasma gondii.

Extra Mile

- **Spiramycin:** Given in treatment of toxoplasma gondii to prevent transmission of infection from mother to fetus.

263. Ans. (c) Crystalluria

Ref: Sharma & Sharma 3rd ed. pg. 715

- Sulfonamides are structural analogue of PABA which enter the synthetic sequence of in place of PABA by competing with the enzyme dihydropteroic acid synthase and forms non-functional analogue of folic acid which is of no use to bacteria.
- Its growth ceases in absence of folic acid, hence these are bacteriostatic drugs.

Classification of sulfonamides:

- **Short acting** (t1/2- 6–9 hrs): Sulfacytine, Sulfadiazine, Sulfasoxazole, Sulfamethizole
- **Intermediate** (t1/2- 1–12 hrs): Sulfamethoxazole, Sulfamoxole

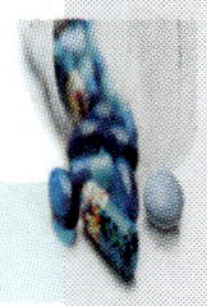

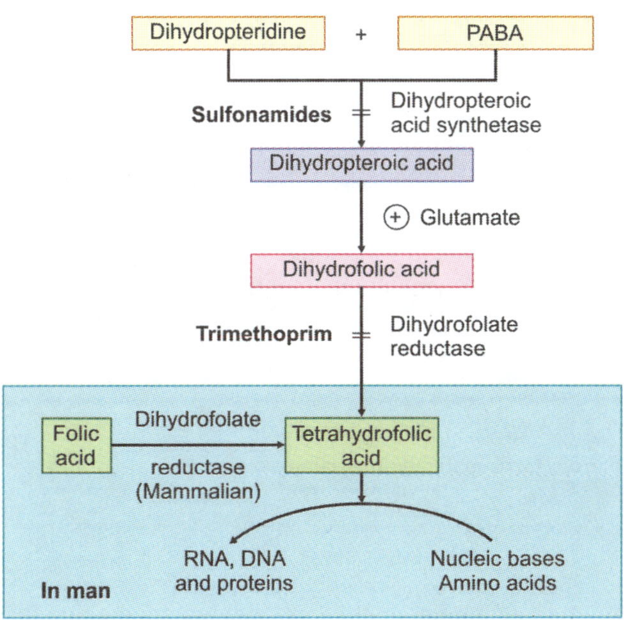

FIGURE: Bacterial Folate synthesis and sites of action of sulfonamides and trimethoprim. Pyrimethamine also inhibits dihydrofolate reductase but preferentially of protozoa

- **Long acting** (t½–7 to 8 days hrs): Sulfadoxine

Side effects (Mn: Karina Cry for ASH)

- Kernicterus in neonates
- Crystalluria and renal toxicity (acetylated metabolites of drug are less soluble in acidic urine)
- **Anemia: Hemolytic anemia in G6PD**
- **SJS: Characterized by mucus ulceration of mouth and genitals**
- Hypersensitivity reaction: Rash at mucocutaneous junction, eosinophilia, Drug fever seen on 7–10th day of treatment.

264. Ans. (d) 1:5

Ref: Sharma & Sharma 3rd ed. pg. 716; Katzung's, 11th ed. pg. 818

- Cotrimoxazole is a combination of Trimethoprim 80 mg and sulfamethoxazole 400 mg.
- Optimal ratio **in drug combination** 1:5–1 Trimethoprim: 5 sulfamethoxazole)
- Ratio of cotrimoxazole **in serum** is 1:20 (1 Trimethoprim: 20 sulfamethoxazole), due to rapid metabolism of trimethoprim and slower metabolism of sulfamethoxazole the ratio changes in plasma.
- A double strength (DS) tablet contains 160 mg Trimethoprim + 800 mg sulfamethoxazole.

Uses:

- UTI
- Prostatitis (since cotrimoxazole gets concentrated in prostatic fluid)
- Typhoid
- Nocardiosis (DOC)
- Pneumocystis carinii induced pneumonia (DOC)

Extra Mile

- Alone these both the drugs shows bacteriostatic action. When combined they become bactericidal.
- **Other combination:** Sulfadoxine (500 mg) + Pyrimethamine (25 mg): Ratio is 20:1
  - Curative in chloroquine resistant P. Falciparum
  - First line in toxoplasmosis

265. Ans. (c) Doxycycline

Ref: Sharma & Sharma 3rd ed. pg. 760

- Doxycycline is from the tetracycline class of drug.
- Tetracyclins are first line DOC in following conditions like
  - Rocky mountain spotted fever
  - Typhus fever
  - Psittacosis
  - Granuloma inguinale
  - Non-specific urethritis (ureaplasma urealyticum)
  - Lyme disease
  - Brucellosis (Brucella abortus)
  - Plague
  - Pasturella abscess

Extra Mile

- First line combination therapy for brucellosis is: Doxycycline and Rifampicin

266. Ans. (a) Dapsone

Ref: Katzung, 14th ed. pg. 1086

- **Dermatitis herpetiformis (DH)** is a chronic blistering skin condition, characterised by blisters filled with a watery fluid.
- DH is neither related to nor caused by herpes virus: the name means that it is a skin inflammation having an appearance similar to herpes.
- It characterized by intensely itchy, chronic papulovesicular eruptions, usually distributed symmetrically on extensor surfaces (buttocks, back of neck, scalp, elbows, knees, back, hairline, groin, or face).
- **Diagnosis** is confirmed by a simple blood test for IgA antibodies, and by a skin biopsy in which the pattern of IgA deposits in the dermal papillae, revealed by direct immunofluorescence, distinguishes it from linear IgA bullous dermatosis and other forms of dermatitis.
- **Treatment:** Dapsone is considered as drug of choice for DH.
- In case of intolerance to dapsone, other drugs which can be used are: Colchicine, Tetracycline, Sulfapyridine.

267. Ans. (d) Pyrimethamine

Ref: KDT, 6th ed. pg. 783

- *The drugs which are erythrocytic schizontocides are used to terminate an episode of malarial fever. They can be divided into:*

Fast-acting high-efficacy drugs	Slow-acting high-efficacy drugs
Chloroquine, amodiaquine, quinine, mefloquine, halofantrine, lumefantrine, atovaquone, artemisinin.	*Pronguanil.* **Pyrimethamine**, *sulfonamides, tetracyclines*
They can be used singly to treat attacks of malarial fever	They are used only in combination for clinical cure

Extra Mile

- DOC for malaria: **Chloroquine** (safe in pregnancy)
- DOC for cerebral malaria: **Artesunate**
- DOC for chloroquine resistant malaria: **ACT**- *artemisinin combination therapy* (artisunate+pyrimethamine + sulfadoxine)
- Fastest acting anti-malarial: **Artimisinin**.
- Safest anti-malarial: **Proguanil**
- Short term prophylaxis of malaria (<6 weeks): **Doxycycline** 100 mg OD (start 2 days before)
- Long term prophylaxis of malaria (>6 weeks): **Mefloquine** 250 mg weekly (start a week before)

268. Ans. (a) Praziquantel

Ref: Katzung, 14th ed. pg. 944; Harrison, 17th ed. pg. 1334

- **Schistosomiasis is a type of infection caused by helminth subtypes that live in fresh water, such as rivers or lakes, in subtropical and tropical regions.**
- Schistosomiasis is also known as bilharzia.
- Symptoms can develop a few weeks after someone is infected by the parasite and include flu-like symptoms, such as a high temperature (fever) above 38°C (100.4°F) and muscle aches, skin rash, cough or urinary symptoms (cystitis, hematuria)

Anti-Helminthic agents

Helminthes	Name	Drug of choice
NEMATODE	Round worm (Ascaris) Pinworm (enterobius vermicularis) Hookworm (N. Americanus, A. duodenale) Whip worm (trichuris trichura) Trichinea worm (trichinella spiralis) Guinea worm (Dracunculus medinensis)	ALBENDAZOLE/MEBENDAZOLE
	Filarial worm (W. Bancrofti, B. Malayi)	DEC/Ivermectin
	Onchocerca volvulus Threadworms (strongyloides stercoralis)	Ivermectin
TREMATODE	Blood fluke (schistosoma japonicum, mansoni & Hematobium) Lung fluke (paragonimus westermani) Liver fluke (fasciola Heaptica) → *DOC:* ***Triclabendazole/Bithionol***	**PRAZIQUANTEL** EXCEPT for fasciola Hepatica (Triclabendazole)
CESTODE	Pork tapeworm (taenia solium) Beef tapeworm (taenia saginata) Fish tapeworm (Diphyllobothrium latum) Dog tapeworm (Echinococcus granulosus) Dwarf tapeworm (Hymenolepis Nana)	**PRAZIQUANTEL/ NICLOSAMIDE**

METRONIDAZOLE is DOC for: Trichomoniasis, Giardiasis, Bacterial vaginosis, Amoebic liver disease, Hydatid disease, Cysticercosis

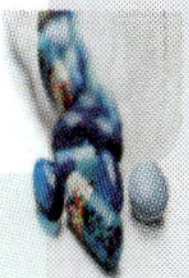

269. Ans. (b) Triclabendazole

Ref: Katzung, 14th ed. pg. 939

- Drug of choice for all trematodes including blood flukes like schistosoma japonicum, mansoni &Hematobium and lung flukes paragonimus westermani is Praziquantel EXCEPT Liver fluke.
- DOC for Liver fluke (fasciola Heaptica) → **Triclabendazole/Bithionol**

270. Ans. (d) Albendazole

Ref: Katzung, 14th ed. pg. 940

Drug of choice for NCC: Albendazole

271. Ans. (a) Praziquantel

Ref: Katzung, 14th ed. pg. 939

- DOC for taenia solium (pork tapeworm) and Taenia saginata (Beef tapeworm) and fish tapeworm is: **PRAZIQUANTEL**

272. Ans. (c) Ivermectin

Ref: Katzung, 14th ed. pg. 939, 1075; KDT, 6th ed. pg. 864

- Scabies is caused by an ectoparasite sarcoptes scabei. It is highly contagious. The mite burrows through the epidermis, laying eggs which form papules that itch intensely.
- Most common site of entry- finger webs.
- **Drugs used are:**
  - **Permethrin 5%:** Broad spectrum and potent insecticide, currently most efficacious.
    - It is DOC for scabies.
    - **MOA:** It causes neurological paralysis in insects by delaying depolarization.
    - Single application needed in most cases.
    - Very less toxicity; 100% cure rate.
  - **Lindane:** Another broad spectrum insecticide. Efficacy lower than permethrin.
    MOA: Kills lice and mites by penetrating through their chitinous cover and affecting the nervous system.
  - **Benzyl benzoate:** Oily liquid with a faint aromatic smell.
    It is applied over face and neck after a bath. A second coat is applied next day which is washed after 24 hours.
  - Crotamiton
  - Sulfur
  - **Ivermectin:** Highly effective in scabies and pediculosis as well. Oral DOC in scabies.
    - It is the only ORALLY administered drug which is used for scabies (ectoparasitosis)
    - A single dose of 0.2 mg/kg has cured almost 90–100% of population.
    - It is contraindicated in children < 5 yrs, pregnant and lactating women.

273. Ans. (b) Permethrin

Ref: Katzung, 14th ed. pg. 1075; KDT, 6th ed. pg. 864

274. Ans. (a) Metronidazole

Must know points for tetanus (8th day illness presenting with lock jaw)

- Penicillin G was considered the drug of choice, but some now consider metronidazole to be superior in this setting. Tetracycline is an alternative for patients who are allergic to penicillin or metronidazole

Tetanus immunoglobulin is used to

- Prevent tetanus and to treat patients with circulating tetanus toxin and provides passive immunity.
- Treat all patients with active tetanus, in combination with other supportive and therapeutic treatments.

275. Ans. (d) Ivermectin

Ref: KDT, 6th ed. pg. 809; Katzung, 14th ed. pg. 939

- Usually *DOC for filariasis is Diethyl carbamazine (DEC).*
- ***Since DEC was not in option, the next drug which comes under first line drug for filariasis is Ivermectin.***
- IVERMECTIN is also considered as drug of choice in following conditions:
  - Strongyloidiasis
  - Onchocerciasis
- PRAZIQUANTEL is drug of choice for:
  - Tapeworm infestation (Taenia saginata, Taenia solium, H. Nana)

276. Ans. (a) 2 mg/kg

Ref: KD Tripathi, 7th ed. pg. 853

Diethylcarbamazine

- It is the first drug for filariasis caused by the nematodes *Wuchereria bancrofti* (90% cases) and *Brugia malayi.*
- Plasma *t1/2* of usual clinical doses is 4–12 hours, depending on urinary pH.
  - Acidic pH: 2–3 hours
  - Alkaline pH: 8–10 hours
- The most important action of DEC appears to be alteration of organelle membranes of the microfilariae promoting cell death.
- The recommended doses in filarisis, Loiasis and Toxocariasis are similar i.e. 50 mg on day 1, 50 mg TDS on day 2, 100 mg TDS on day 3 and then 2 mg/kg TDS for 2–3 weeks.
- It can also be used to treat tropical eosinophilia in a dose of 2 mg/kg TDS for 7 days
- Doses of DEC in chemoprophylaxis:
  - Loiasis 300 mg weekly

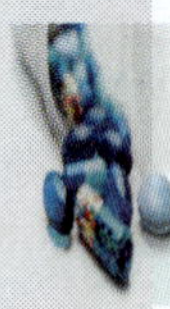

- Filariasis 50 mg monthly
- Yearly treatment with a combination of DEC (2 mg/kg) and **albendazole (400 mg single dose on mass scale has brought down transmission of filariasis by reducing microfilaroma.**

277. Ans. (a) Albendazole

Ref: KD Tripathi, 7th ed. pg. 853

- Yearly treatment with a combination of DEC (2 mg/kg) and **albendazole (400 mg single dose on mass scale has brought down transmission of filariasis by reducing microfilaroma.**
- **Recent** studies have revealed that:
  - 200 mg/day for 8 weeks course of doxycycline eliminated 95% of microfilariae.
  - A combination therapy of Doxycycline and Ivermectin can cause 100% elimination of microfilarie.

278. Ans. (b) Alters permeability of fungal cell wall

Ref: Sharama & Sharma 3rd ed. pg. 781

- Amphotericin binds to fungal cell membrane namely ergosterol and alters the permeability of fungal cell wall by forming pores through which macromolecules like Na^+, K^+, Mg, H^+ leaks out causing fungal cell death.
- Resistance is due to replacement of ergosterol by other steol in fungal plasma membrane.
- Peak antifungal activity of the drug occurs at pH 6.0 to 7.5 and the drug is widely distributed to most tissues EXCEPT CNS.
- Plasma half life: 15 days
- Use:
  - Most commonly used to treat serious fingal infections from yeast or mould group.
  - Superficially can be given to treat candidiasis.
  - **DOC in following conditions:**
    - Invasive aspergillosis (all patients including immunocompromised)
    - Mucormycosis
    - Disseminated histoplasmosis
    - Rapidly progressive coccidiomycosis
    - Rapidly progressive blastomycosis
    - Non AIIDS cryptococcal meningitis
    - Oropharyhgeal and cutaneous candidiasis
    - Kala Azar (liposomal Amp B)

279. Ans. (d) Liposomal preparation

Ref: KD Tripathi, 7th ed. pg. 788

- Amphotericin B can be administered orally (50-100 mg QID) for intestinal moniliasis; also topically for vaginitis, otomycosis.
- **Conventional formulation of AMB (C-AMB)** For systemic mycosis, C-AMB is available as dry powder along with deoxycholate (DOC) for extemporaneous dispersion before use
- It is first suspended in **10** mL water and then diluted to 500 mL with glucose solution ***(saline makes the suspension coarse and should be avoided)***.
- Initially 1 mg test dose is injected IV over 20 minutes. If no serious reaction follows, 0.3 mg/kg is infused over 4–8 hours daily.

Liposomal amphotericin B (small unilamellar vesicles SUV): Consists of 10% AMB incorporated in uniform sized (60–80 nM) unilamellar liposomes made up of lecithin and other biodegradable phospholipids.

The special features of these preparations are:

- They produce milder acute reaction (especially liposomal formulation) on IV infusion.
- They can be used in patients not tolerating infusion of conventional AMB formulation.
- They have lower nephrotoxicity.
- They cause minimal anemia.
- The liposomal preparation delivers AMB particularly to reticuloendothelial cells in liver and spleen especially valuable for Kala Azar and immunocompromised patients.

Extra Mile

AMB combination regimen

- **Amphotericin B + Rifampin or minocycline:** The latter drugs are not themselves antifungal, but enhance the action of amphotericin B.
- **Amphotericin B + Flucytosine:** A shorter course is needed, specially for cryptococcal meningitis, than when amphotericin is used alone.

280. Ans. (c) Cholelithiasis

Ref: Sharma & Sharma 3rd ed. pg. 783

Adverse Drug reactions of Amphotericin B

- The most common, most serious and long term side effect of amphotericin B is Nephrotoxicity (renal tubular necrosis)
- This nephrotoxicity presents with hypokalemia, hypomagnesemia secondary to renal tubular acidosis, azotemia and even irreversible damageif the dose exceeds 5g.
  - In order to prevent the nephrotoxicity, prior hydration with 1L of normal saline is recommended.
  - Liposomal preparation has lesser risk of nephrotoxicity
- Hypochromic normocytic anemia is common and thrombocytopenia and leukopenia although less common but has been noted.

- Intrathecal administration: Arachnoiditis and seizure
- Hepatic impairment and Jaundice
- Infusion related toxicity *(chills, tachypnea, fever, vomiting, hypotemsion, anaphylaxis)*

281. Ans. (b) Renal damage

Ref: Sharma & Sharma 3rd ed. pg. 783

Refer to above explanation for explanation

282. Ans. (c) Amphotericin- B

Ref: Harrison's, 18th ed. Ch. 279

- The most common, most serious and long term side effect of amphotericin B is Nephrotoxicity (renal tubular necrosis)
- This nephrotoxicity presents with hypokalemia, hypomagnesemia secondary to renal tubular acidosis, azotemia and even irreversible damage if the dose exceeds 5 g.
  - In order to prevent the nephrotoxicity, prior hydration with 1L of normal saline is recommended.
  - Liposomal preparation has lesser risk of nephrotoxicity

Note: *Cyclosporine also causes AKI with hypomagnesemia*

ANTIVIRALS

283. Ans. (c) 4 weeks

Ref: Goodman Gillman 13th ed. pg. 977

- **Agents used for malaria prophylaxis:**
  - **Short term prophylaxis (<6 week):** Doxycycline 100 mg/day, 2 days prior to journey till 4 weeks after journey
  - **Long term prophylaxis (>6 week):** Mefloquine 250 mg/week, 2 week prior to journey till 4 weeks after journey.

284. Ans. (a) 3 mg/kg/day twice daily

Ref: Goodman & Gillman 13th ed. pg. 114

- Oseltamivir is one of the Neuraminidase inhibitor effective against influenza A and B.
- It inhibits amantadine- and rimantadine-resistant influenza A viruses and some zanamivir-resistant variants.
  - **Note:** Seasonal influenza H1N1 is resistant to oseltamivir
- **Dose required:**
  - For treatment-Adult: 75 mg twice daily for 5 days. Initiated within 48 hours of onset of illness
  - For Prophylaxis-Adult: 75 mg once daily
  - For pediatric patients dose is according to weight band (given in the table)

TABLE: Recommended dosage and duration of influenza antiviral medications for treatment of chemoprophylaxis

Antiviral agent	Use	Children	Adults
Oral oseltamivir	Treatment (5 days)	• **If younger than 1 year old:** 3 mg/kg/dose twice daily • **If 1 yr or older, dose varies by child's weight:** • 15 kg or less, the dose is 30 mg **twice** a day • >15 to 23 kg, the dose is 45 mg **twice** a day • >23 to 40 kg, the dose is 60 mg **twice** a day • >40 kg, the dose is 75 mg twice a day If child is younger than 3 months old, use of oseltamivir for chemoprophylaxis is not indicated	75 mg twice daily

285. Ans. (a) Acyclovir

Ref: Goodman & Gillman's 13th ed. pg. 1106-7

- Acyclovir's clinical use is limited to herpes viruses. Acyclovir is most active against HSV-1.
- Approximately half as active against HSV-2, and a tenth as potent against VZV and EBV.
- **Book states:** "*Acyclovir is ineffective therapeutically in established CMV infections, but ganciclovir is effective for CMV prophylaxis in immunocompromised patients*".
- EBV-related oral hairy leukoplakia may improve with acyclovir.
- Drugs which can be used in treatment of CMV retinitis are cidofovir, ganciclovir, foscarnet, valaciclovir.
- **DOC for CMV retinitis:** Ganciclovir
- **Fomivirsen** is active against CMV strains **resistant** to ganciclovir, foscarnet, and cidofovir. Fomivirsen is given by intravitreal injection unresponsive to other therapies.

286. Ans. (a) Acyclovir

Ref: Katzung, 11th ed. pg.1468

Please refer to above explanation.

287. Ans. (c) Abacavir

Ref: KDT, 6th ed. pg. 773-74

- Abacavir is a NRTI

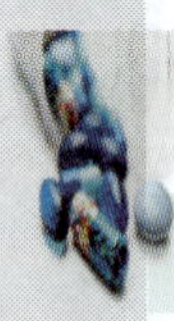

Protease inhibitors *(ends with "navir")*	Nucleoside reverse tanscriptase inhibitor (NRTI)
Indinavir Saquinavir *Ritonavir* *Atazanavir* Nelfinavir Amprenavir Lopinavir	Zidovudine Stavudine Lamivudine Didanosine Emtricitabine Zalcitabine *Abacavir*
Side effect: Lipodystrophy syndrome Minimum side effect seen with: ATAZANAVIR	**Side effect:** acute pancreatitis Peripheral neuropathy Bone marrow suppression and M.I.

Extra Mile

- NRTI which has the maximum risk of acute pancreatitis: DIDANOSINE
- NRTI which has the maximum risk of peripheral neuropathy: STAVUDINE
- **Safest NRTI:** LAMIVUDINE (minimal risk of pancreatitis and peripheral neuropathy)

288. Ans. (a) HIV

Ref: KDT, 6th ed. pg. 770

- ss Viral RNA $\xrightarrow{\text{Reverse trancriptase}}$ ds viral DNA.
- 2 class of reverse transcriptase inhibitors

Neucleoside Reverse Transcriptase Inhibitors (NRTI)	Non-Nucleoside Reverse Transcriptase Inhibitors (NNRTI)
• ZIDOVUDINE • STAVUDINE • DIDANOSINE • LAMIVUDINE • ABACAVIR • ZALCITABINE	• EFAVIRENZ • NEVIRAPINE • DELAVIRDINE *Rememberd as "END"*

Extra Mile

ZIDOVUDINE

- Most commonly used NRTI in the treatment of HIV
- Used as prophylaxis in needle stick injury and to decrease vertical transmission from HIV mother to fetus.
- **Side effect:** Bone marrow suppression.
- Drug of choice for decreasing vertical transmission from HIV mother to fetus: **NEVIRAPINE**
- Safest NRTI: **LAMIVUDINE**
- All NRTI's casues acute pancreatitis and peripheral neuropathy.
  - Maximum risk of acute pancreatitis with: **DIDANOSINE**
  - Maximum risk of peripheral neuropathy with: **STAVUDINE**
- **NRTI** causing aphthous ulcer in mouth: **Zalcitabine (withdrawn)**

289. Ans. (c) Acyclovir

Ref: Katzung, 14th ed. pg. 864–65

- Acyclovir is an acyclic guanosine derivative with clinical activity against HSV-1, HSV-2, and VZV. In vitro activity against Epstein-Barr virus (EBV), cytomegalovirus (CMV), and human herpesvirus-6 (HHV-6).

ANTI-RETROVIRAL DRUGS

- **Nucleoside reverse tanscriptase inhibitor:** Zidovudine, Stavudine, Lamivudine, Didanosine, Emtricitabine, Zalcitabine, ***Abacavir***
- **Nucleotide reverse tanscriptase inhibitor:** ***Tenofovir***
- **Protease inhibitors:** Indinavir, Saquinavir, ***Ritonavir***, Atazanavir, Nelfinavir, Amprenavir, Lopinavir.

290. Ans. (c) CCR5 inhibitor

Ref: Katzung, 14th ed. pg. 872

- Maraviroc is an anti HIV drug which comes under fusion inhibitor category.
- This drug binds to the CCR5 receptor of CD4 cells and inhibits the fusion stage of virus and hence inhibits their speed of replication.
- There are two types of fusion inhibitors:

Drugs which bind to CCR5 receptor of CD4 cells	Drugs which bind to GP 41 subunit of viral envelope
Maraviroc: active against CCR5 receptor of CD4 cell	**Enfuvirtide:** Prevents entry of virus into host cell
Can be given orally	Can only be given in s.c. injection form

291. Ans. (b) Stavudine

Ref: Katzung, 14th ed. pg. 875; KDT, 6th ed. pg. 770

- NRTI's are reverse transcriptase inhibitors, which control the dsDNA formation from ssRNA
- Drugs in the category are: Zidovudine, Stavudine, Didanosine, Lamivudine, Abacavir, Zalcitabine, Emtricitabine
- All NRTI's casues acute pancreatitis, peripheral neuropathy and Lactic acidosis
  - Maximum risk of acute pancreatitis with: **DIDANOSINE**
  - Maximum risk of peripheral neuropathy with: **STAVUDINE**
  - **NRTI** has maximum risk of lactic acidosis: **STAVUDINE**
  - Least toxic NRTI: Emtricitabine

ANTITUBERCULAR AGENTS

292. Ans. (c) Extensively resistant TB

- The given case is of XDR-TB
- XDR TB is defined as resistance with:
  - Rifampicin and Isoniazid
  - Any 1 Fluroquinolones
  - Any 1 second line injectables

Note: In MDR-TB there is resistance with isoniazid and rifampicin.

293. Ans. (a) Kanamycin

- Kanamycin should be avoided due to its teratogenic effect, i.e., ototoxicity.

294. Ans. (b) Liver disease

Ref: KD Tripathi, 7th ed. pg. 767

- INH is hepatotoxic and is avoided in pre-exisintg liver disease
- Isoniazid is an essential component of all anti-tubercular regimens. It is primarily tuberculocidal.
- Fast multiplying organisms are rapidly killed, but quiescent ones are only inhibited.
- The most common mechanism which confers high level INH resistance is by mutation of the catalase-peroxidase *(KatG)* gene.
- INH resistance may also involve mutation in the *inhA* or *kasA genes.*

Adverse effects:

- **Peripheral neuritis** is the most important dose-dependent toxic effects (slow acetylators).
  - Pyridoxine given prophylactically (10 mg/day) prevents the neurotoxicity even with higher doses.
- Hepatitis, a major adverse effect of INH, (seen commonly in fast acetylators) more common in older people and in alcoholics is also a well-known side effect of the drug.
- **Other adverse effects:** Xerostomia, Allergic reactions, decrease seizure threshold.

Extra Mile

- Safest ATT in renal disease patients: Rifampicin
- ATT which has no/least hepatotoxicity: Ethambutol and Streptomycin

295. Ans. (b) Rifampicin

Ref: KD Tripathi, 7th ed. pg. 767

- Rifampicin is considered as effective as isoniazid. This agent is active against slow and intermittently dividing bacterium (spurters).
- If someone develops resistance to INH, they are most likely to develop resistance to rifampicin as well.
- In MDR-TB, there is resistance to INH and rifampicin.
- Gene involved in INH resistance → KatG > inhA Gene.

296. Ans. (b) Rifampicin

Ref: KDT 6th ed. pg. 740-44, Katzung Pharma 14th ed. pg. 845

RIFAMPICIN

- It is a tuberculocidal agent of M. tuberculosis in addition to staph. aureus, pseudomonas, proteus, legionella, etc.
- It has bactericidal action of which covers all subpopulations of TB bacilli, ***but acts best on slowly or intermittently dividing ones as well as on many atypical mycobacteria.***
- Both intracellular and extracellular bacilli are affected.
- **MOA:** It inhibits DNA dependent RNA synthesis
- **Resistance** of rifampicin is due to ***rpoB gene.***
- **Adverse effects:**
  - Hepatoxicity: MC/Major side effect
  - Rifampicin imparts a harmless **orange color to urine,** sweat, tears, and contact lenses *(soft lenses may be permanently stained).*
  - Occasional adverse effects include rashes, thrombocytopenia, and nephritis.
  - It may cause cholestatic jaundice and occasionally hepatitis and flu-like symptoms.

ISONIAZID

- It is primarily tuberculocidal. *Fast multiplying organisms are rapidly killed but quiescent ones are only inhibited.*
- Acts on intracellular as well as extracellular TB bacilli and is equally active in acidic and alkaline medium.
- **MOA:** Inhibit synthesis of mycolic acid, which is a unique fatty acid component of mycobacterial cell wall.
- If given alone, resistance occurs in about 2–3 months
- **Most common mechanism of INH resistance:** Mutation of catalase-peroxidase gene > Mutation of *inh-A* gene.
- **Adverse effects:**
  - **Isoniazid-induced hepatitis** is the most common major toxic effect
  - Peripheral neuropathy is observed in 10–20% of patients
  - Neuropathy is due to a relative pyridoxine (Vit B6) deficiency. Isoniazid promotes excretion of pyridoxine, and this toxicity is readily reversed by administration of pyridoxine.
  - Central nervous system toxicity, which is less common, includes *memory loss, psychosis, and seizures.*

PYRAZINAMIDE

- It is weakly tuberculocidal. PYZ is more lethal to intracellularly located bacilli and to those at sites showing an inflammatory response.
- **MOA:** Resembles that of INH. It inhibits mycolic acid synthesis but by interacting with a different fatty acid synthase encoding gene.
- Resistance of PYZ due to mutation in *pncA gene.*
- **Adverse effects: *Hepatotoxicity***, nausea, vomiting, drug fever, and ***hyperuricemia***

ETHAMBUTOL

- Selectively tubecolostatic agent and clinically as active as streptomycin. *Fast multiplying bacilli are more susceptible* as are many atypical mycobacteria.
- **MOA:** Poorly understood, but it has been found to inhibit arabinosyl transferases involved in arabinogalactan synthesis and to interfere with mycolic acid incorporation in mycobacterial cell wall.
- Resistance of ethambutol due to alteration in the drug target gene- ***emb gene.***
- **Adverse effects:** *Retrobulbar neuritis, resulting in loss of visual acuity and red-green color blindness.*

STREPTOMYCIN

- Tuberculocidal agent, acts only on extracellular bacilli. It penetrates the tubercular cavities but doesn't crosses the CSF. *Has poor action on acidic medium.*
- **Adverse effects:** Ototoxic and nephrotoxic.
- Resistance is due to a point mutation in either the ***rpsL* gene** or ***rrs* gene.**

297. Ans. (c) Increase the permeability of cell wall

Ref: KDT, 6th ed. pg. 742

- Ethambutol inhibits arabinosyl transferases which is involved in cell wall biosynthesis. By inhibiting this enzyme, the bacterial cell wall complex production is inhibited. ***This leads to an increase in cell wall permeability.***

Extra Mile

- ATT acting exclusively on intracellular bacilli: Pyrazinamide
- **ATT acting exclusively on extracellular bacilli: Streptomycin**

298. Ans. (d) Ethambutol

Ref: KDT, 6th ed. pg. 742

- **Side effect of Ethambutol:** Loss of visual acuity/color vision, field defects due to **optic neuritis** is the most important dose and duration of therapy dependent toxicity.

Extra Mile

- Important side effects of antitubercular drugs:
- Peripheral neuropathy (*due to vit B6 deficiency*): ISONIAZID
- Orange color urine- RIFAMPICIN
- Flu-like symptoms- RIFAMPICIN
- Hyperuricemia/gout- PYRAZINAMIDE
- Optic neuritis- ETHAMBUTOL
- Nephrotoxic, Ototoxic, Neuromascular Junction Blocker- STREPTOMYCIN

Other important points to remember about Anti TB drugs:

- *First line anti TB drugs are: **HRZE** (Isoniazid, Rifampicin, Pyrazinamide, Ethambutol)*
- All first line drugs are bactericidal EXCEPT- **Ethambutol** (it is bacteriostatic)
- Most hepatotoxic ATT-**Pyrazinamide**
- 1st line ATT with exclusive intracellular action-**Pyrazinamide**
- 1st line ATT with exclusive extracellular action-**Streptomycin**
- Which anti TB drugs are NOT hepatotoxic-**Ethambutol and Streptomycin.**

- It should not be used in children below 6 years of age because these young patients may not be able to report visual impairment.

299. Ans. (d) Ethambutol

Ref: KDT, pg. 742

- Ethalmbutol is selectively tuberculostatic and clinically as active as Streptomycin.

TABLE: 1st Line ATT Drugs action on bacteria and hepatoxicty

Drug	Bactericidal/ Bacteristatic	Hepatotoxicity
Isoniazid	Cidal	+
Rifampicin	Cidal	+
Pyrazinamide	Cidal	++++
Ethambutol	STATIC	- No
Streptomycin	Cidal	- No

300. Ans. (d) Ethambutol

Ref: Katzung's Pharmacology, 14th ed. pg. 846

- **Dose of Ethambutol:** 15-25 mg/kg OD dose.
- About 20% drug is excreted in feces and 50% in urine in unchanged form.
- ***Ethambutol accumulates in renal failure, and the dose should be reduced by half if creatinine clearance is less than 10 mL/min.***
- **Side effect:** Most common serious adverse event is retro-bulbar neuritis, resulting in loss of visual acuity and ***red green color blindness*** *(Patient develop BLUE VISION).*

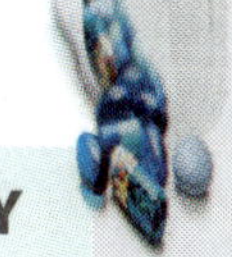

- It can also cause hyperuricemia and peripheral neuritis.
- **It is also Contraindicated** in children as they are unable to report loss of visual acuity and red-green color discrimination.

301. Ans. (a) 5 mg/kg PO qday

Ref: Katzung, 14th ed. pg. 843; KD Tripathi, 6th ed. pg. 746

TABLE: Recommended doses of antitubercular drug

DRUG	Daily dose			
	mg/kg	For >50 kg	mg/kg	For >50 kg
Isoniazid (H)	5 (4–6)	300 mg	10 (8–12)	600 mg
Rifampin (R)	10 (8–12)	600 mg	10 (8–12)	600 mg
Pyrazinamide (Z)	25 (20–30)	1500 mg	35 (30–40)	2000 mg
Ethambutol (E)	15 (15–20)	1000 mg	30 (25–35)	1600 mg

302. Ans. (a) Rifampicin

Ref: KDT, 7th ed. pg. 768

MOA OF IMPORTANT ATT

- **Streptomycin**- inhibit protein synthesis
- **Chloroamphenicol**- inhibit protein synthesis by inhibiting transpeptidation
- **Rifampicin**- inhibit DNA dependent RNA synthesis by inhibiting RNA polymerase
- **INH & Pyrazinamide:** inhibits mycolic acid, a component of mycobacterial cell wall
- **Ethambutol:** Inhibit incorporation of mycolic acid into bacterial cell wall by inhibiting arabinosyl transferase, thus weakening the wall.

303. Ans. (c) Vitamin B_6

Ref: KDT, 6th ed. pg. 740-41

- For patients who are on isoniazid; peripheral neuropathy is observed in 10–20% of patients given dosages greater than 5 mg/kg/day but is infrequently seen with the standard 300 mg adult dose.
- Pyridoxine (Vit B_6), 25–50 mg/day, is recommended for those with conditions predisposing to neuropathy, an adverse effect of isoniazid.
- Note: *Isoniazid as a single agent is also indicated for treatment of latent tuberculosis. The dosage is 300 mg/day (5 mg/kg/day) or 900 mg twice weekly for 9 months.*

304. Ans. (b) Cycloserine

Ref: KDT, 6th ed. pg. 744; Katzung's Pharma, 14th ed. pg. 847

- **Cycloserine (Cys)** is a 2nd line ATT. It is a chemical analogue of D-alanine:
- Cycloserine being cell wall inhibitior is tuberculostatic in nature and inhibits some other gram-positive bacteria, E. coli, Chlamydia also.
- **MOA:** it inhibits bacterial cell wall synthesis by inactivating the enzymes which recemize L-alanine and link two D-alanine residues.
- The dosage of cycloserine in tuberculosis is **0.5–1 g/day** in two divided doses.
- **Adverse effect:** The CNS toxicity of Cys is high-sleepiness, headache, tremor, depression and **psychosis**.
- **Use:** MDK. TB.

Extra Mile

- 2nd line ATT, Kanamycin, Amikacin, Capreomycin have similar side effect of ototoxicity and nephrotoxicity, same as streptomycin (1st line ATT).
- *Capreomycin, can induce electrolyte abnormalities.*

305. Ans. (c) Streptomycin

Ref: KDT, 6th ed. pg. 743-44

- Streptomycin has been assigned to pregnancy category D by the FDA.
- Streptomycin crosses the placenta; reported cord concentrations have been equal to or less than the mother's serum concentration.
- **There are reports of fetal eighth cranial nerve damage with subsequent bilateral deafness**. Most authorities, including the Centers for Disease Control and the American Thoracic Society, *discourage the use of streptomycin during pregnancy due to the risk of fetal ototoxicity.*
- Note: Streptomycin is no longer an ATT drug

306. Ans. (b) Streptomycin

Ref: KDT 6th ed. pg. 743-744

Please refer to above explanation

307. Ans. (b) Streptomycin

Please refer to above explanation.

308. Ans. (d) 5 TU

Ref: Essentials of TB Diagnosis Children, 3rd ed. pg. 325

309. Ans. (c) PAS

Ref: 2008 WHO Guidelines for Programmatic Management or Drug Resistant Tuberculosis

- Second line ATT like PAS (para amino salicylic acid) and ethionamide can lead to hypothyroidism. Exact mechanism is poorly understood.

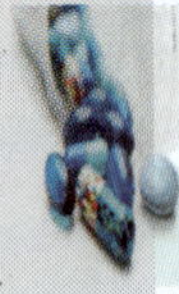

- PAS also causes adverse reactions like GI upset, hepatotoxicity, Hypersensitivity.

310. Ans. (b) Pyrazinamide

Ref: Katzung, 14th ed. pg. 846; KDT, 6th ed. pg. 742

Pyrazinamide Microsomal deaminase Pyrazinoic acid (POA) → 5-hydroxypyrazinoic acid

- Pyrazinamide is hydrolyzed by microsomal deaminase to pyrazinoic acid (POA) and then hydroxylated to 5-hydroxypyrazinoic acid by xanthine oxidase for excretion by the kidneys.
- ***Pyrazinamide is a first line antitubercular drug that can cause hyperuricemia (secondary to inhibition of uric acid secretion in the kidney) and hepatotoxicity.***
- This hyperuricemia leads to arthralgia due to competitive inhibition of xanthine oxidase by POA. ***It should not be stopped if hyperuricemia develops***
- *Ethambutol also produces hyperuricemia due to interferance with urate excretion.*

ANTICANCER DRUGS

311. Ans. (d) Ifosfamide

Ref: Goodman and Gillman 13th ed. pg. 1172

- Ifosfamide is associated with side effects like hemorrhagic cystitis.
- One of the metabolites of Ifosfamide is acrolein, which causes bladder toxicity. It can cause bladder side effects like hemorrhagic cystitis, hematuria and bladder fibrosis.
- Upon increasing dose the toxic effect over bladder can increase therefore, it is recommended to monitor the bladder function.

312. Ans. (a) Leuprolide

- Leuprolide is a GnRH analogue. If given in continuous dosing, it act as antagonist (due to feedback mechanism).
- In advanced prostatic cancer, leuprolide is preferred.
- **Uses of leuprolide:**
  - Endometriosis
  - Fibroids
  - Precocious puberty

Extra Mile

- **Desmopressin:** It is ADH analogue. Used as DOC for central diabetes insipidus
- **Octreotide:** It is a somatostatin analogue (act as an antagonist of GH). Used in gigantism, carcinoid tumor, esophageal variceal bleed.
- **Tamsulosin:** It is an alpha 1a antagonist. Used for DOC for BPH

313. Ans. (a) I-131

- I-131 is used in treatment of thyroid cancer, hyperthyroidism.
- It is contraindicated in patients younger than 35 years and in pregnant females.
- I-123 is used for diagnosing thyroid related diseases.

314. Ans. (a) Cisplatin

Radiosensitizing anti cancer drugs are:
- Cisplatin
- Mitomycin-c
- 5-FU
- Gemcitabine: A very potent radiosensitizer and should not be used with radiotherapy.
- Hydroxyurea

315. Ans. (c) Filgrastim

- During anti-cancer therapy, bone marrow suppression is common, which include leucopenia as well, that can result in systemic bacterial infection.
- In the given case, a leucocyte count of 2000/mm^3, is indicative of decreased leucocyte count (leucopenia), and require therapy with granulocyte colony stimulating factor (G-CSF).
- Filgrastim is one of stimulant that can increase the leucocyte.

Extra Mile

- **ROMIPLSTIM:** It is platelet stimulant. Used in chemo induced thrombocytopenia or ITP.
- **Oprelvekin:** IL-11 agonist. Also used for chemo induced thrombocytopenia or ITP.
- **EPO:** Used in anemia due to end stage renal disease or chemo induced anemia.

316. Ans. (c) Rituximab

Ref: Katzung 14th ed. pg. 652

- Among the given choices, rituximab is the only monoclonal antibody (MAB) used in cancer therapy like non-Hodgkin's lymphoma, CLL etc.
- Rituximab targets CD20 B Lymphocytes.
- Depletion of B lymphocytes reduces inflammation by decreasing the presentation of antigens to T lymphocytes and inhibiting the secretion of proinflammatory Cytokines
- It used in various malignant and non-malignant conditions.
- **Uses of rituximab:**
  - CLL
  - Rheumatoid arthritis
  - Idiopathic thrombocytopenic purpura

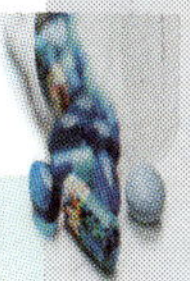

- SLE
- Non-Hodgekins lymphoma

Note:

- Omalizumab (option A) is MAB against IgE. It is used for bronchial asthma
- Denosumab (option B) is MAB against RANK ligand and prevents activation of osteoclast. It is used in osteoporosis.
- Methotrexate (option D) is DHFR inhibitor (NOT a MAB) used in multiple conditions like rheumatoid arthritis, psoriasis, as immunosuppressant and in some cancers like choriocarcinoma, osteosarcoma, etc.

317. Ans. (a) Anthracyclines

Ref: Katzung 14th ed. pg. 964-65

- Anthracyclines are cell cycle non-specific anti-cancer drugs. It is one of the anti-tumor antibiotics.
- **Drugs under anthracyclines are:**
  - Doxorubicin
  - Daunorubicin
  - Epirubicin
  - Valrubicin
- **Side effect:** Cardiotoxicity, Nausea, Vomiting, Alopecia, Bone marrow suppression.
- **Upon HPE of heart:** Vacuolar degeneration of myofibrils.

318. Ans. (c) 5FU

Ref: SRB 5th ed. pg. 987

Chemoradiation is the preferred treatment of anal cancer. 5FU is the preffered drug. Initially radiation is given for 3 weeks to the perenium and pelvis. This is followed by chemotheraphy using 5FU and mitomycin C.

319. Ans. (b) Dihydrofolate reductase inhibitor

Ref: Goodman & Gillman's 13th ed. pg. 1179

- Pemetrexed is a most recent folate analogue which is avidly transported into cells via the reduced folate carrier and is converted to its metabolite (PGs- Polyglutamate) that inhibit Thymidylate synthase and glycine amide ribonucleotide transformylase, as well as DHFR. (Dihydrofolate Reductase)
- It is even more potent than methotrexate.
- Like MTX, it induces p53 and cell-cycle arrest, but this effect does not depend on induction of p21.
- **Use:** It has activity against ovarian cancer, mesothelioma, and adenocarcinomas of the lung.
- Other effects and side effects are similar to methotrexate like myelosuppression, GI toxicity. The toxicity can be attenuated with folate and vitamin B_{12} supplementation.

Extra Mile

- A newer congener, **pralatrexate**, is more effectively taken up and polyglutamated than MTX and is approved for treatment of CTCL peripheral T cell lymphoma.
- Pramipexole is an antiparkinsonism drug which is a dopamine agonist.

320. Ans. (a) Methotrexate toxicity

Ref: Goodman & Gillman's 13th ed. pg. 1177

- Folic acid is an essential dietary factor which is converted to FH4 by DHFR enzyme and provide methyl groups for the synthesis of precursors of DNA.
- Folic acid analogues such as MTX interfere with FH4 metabolism, thereby inhibiting DNA replication.
- **Adverse effects:** Myelosuppression, GI toxicity.
- **Folinic acid (Leucovorin)** can reverse toxic effects; used as "rescue" in high-dose therapy.
- *Glucarpidase*, a methotrexate-cleaving enzyme, is approved to treat toxicity.

321. Ans. (b) Methotrexate

Ref: K.D. Tripathi, 6th ed. pg. 823

- Methotrexate is one of the oldest and highly efficacious antineoplastic drugs
- **MOA:** It inhibits dihydrofolate reductase (DHFRase)- blocking the conversion of dihydrofolic acid (DHFA) to tetrahydrofolic acid (THFA) which is an essential coenzyme required for one carbon transfer reactions in de novo purine synthesis and amino acid interconversions.
- **DHFRase inhibitors are:** methotrexate, Pemetrexed, Pralatrexate

Extra Mile

- Vincristine is a mitotic spindle formation inhibitor
- Paclitaxel is a spindle breakdown inhibitor
- Cisplatin is a platinum based compound.

322. Ans. (a) Nilotinib

Ref: KD Tripathi, 7th ed. pg. 870

- **Nilotinib** It is a second generation Bcr-Abl, PDGF-receptor β and c-kit receptor tyrosine kinase inhibitor with **20-50 fold higher affinity for these kinases than imatinib.** Thus, it can overcome resistance to imatinib due to Bcr-Abl mutation and is effective in chronic CML nonresponsive to imatinib.
- It is only 30% bioavailable orally, but absorption is improved by food. It is also useful in accelerated phase of CML. Thus, it is an alternative drug in imatinib non-tolerant or resistant cases of CML, and has now been used as a first-line drug as well.

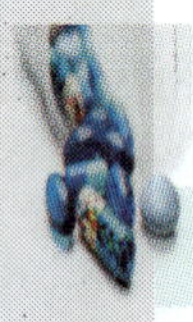

323. Ans. (a) Letrozole

Ref: Katzung, 14th ed. pg. 739; KDT, 6th ed. pg. 305

- Adrenal cortex mainly produces androgen, and this androgen in females is converted to estrogen with the help of enzyme aromatase.
- Androgen $\xrightarrow{\text{Aromatase}}$ Estrogen
- Excess formation of estrogen exposes a person to develop breast CA and on the other hand also protect females from osteoporosis *(estrogen is protective in bone).*
- A class of breast cancer drugs called aromatase inhibitors decreases the body's production of estrogen, at a level where there is nearly total estrogen deprivation in body.
- But at the same time it decreases bone mineral density and increase the risk of fractures in postmenopausal women.
- **Aromatase inhibitors include:** Letrozole, Anastrazole, and Exemestane.
- Letrozole is currently recommended as the first line therapy in case of advanced breast CA.
- **S/E:** Hot flushes, nausea, diarrhea, dyspepsia and thinning of hair and most commonly bone loss (osteoporosis)

Extra Mile

- **Tamoxifen** is a selective estrogen receptor modulator (SERM). It is beneficial in breast, bone and blood cancer.
- Side effect: Tamoxifen increases risk of endometrial CA.
- Only pulsatile exposure to GnRH induces LH/FSH secretion, while continuous exposure desensitizes pituitary which results in loss of GnRH release.

GnRH Agonist	GnRH Antagonist
Given in continuous manner for the treatment of breast CA, prostate CA, and precocious puberty. Drugs are: • Leuprolide • Nafarelin • Goserelin • Busurelin	Given in any manner/pulsatile manner for the treatment of infertility and hypogonadism. **Drugs are:** • Ganirelix • Letrorelix • Abarelix • Cetrorelix
Causes flare up reaction	Doesn't cause flare up reaction

324. Ans. (b) Endometrial cancer

Ref: KDT, 6th ed. pg. 304-5

- Tamoxifen is selective estrogen receptor modulator (SERM).
- It is having agonistic activity at uterine endometrium.

TABLE: Action of Tamoxifen

Agonistic activity	Antagonistic activity
Uterus: causes proliferation of endometrium → ***can cause vaginal bleeding*** *as seen in the case*	Breast CA
Bone: decrease resorption	Blood vessels
Lipid profile: decrease LDL without affecting HDL → decrease risk of CAD	

325. Ans. (c) Cladribine

Ref: KDT, pg. 819-20; Katzung, 14th ed. pg. 958–961

- ***Alkylating agents*** have cytotoxic and radiomimetic actions. They are mainly cell cycle non-specific, i.e. act on dividing as well as resting cells.
- Cross-linking of DNA appears to be of major importance to the cytotoxic action of alkylating agents, and replicating cells are most susceptible to these drugs.
- **Drugs are:**

Alkylating agents- cell cycle-nonspecific agents	Antimetabolites- cell cycle-specific agents
Nitrogen mustard • *Cyclophosphamide* • Ifosfamide • Mechlorethamine • *Melphalan* • Chlorambucil	**Folic acid antagonist:** Methotrexate **Purine analogues** • 6 Mercaptopurine • 6 thioguanine • Cladribine • Fludarabine
Drugs acting by Methylation • Procarbazine • Dacarbazine • Temozolomide	***Pyrimidine analogues*** • Capecitabin • Gemcitabin • Cyatarabine and 5 FU
Nitrosoureas • Carmustine • Lomustine • Semustine • Streptozocin **Miscellaneous** • Busulfan • Altretamine • Thiotepa • Trabectadin	

326. Ans. (a) Bleomycin

Ref: KDT, 819-20, 26; Katzung, 14th ed. pg. 951

- **Bleomycin:** This is a mixture of closely related glycopeptides antibiotics having potent antitumour activity.
- It is highly effective in testicular tumour and squamous cell carcinoma of skin, oral cavity, head and neck, genitourinary tract and esophagus.

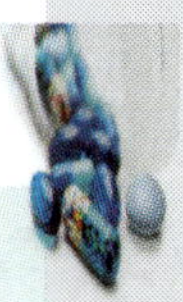

- **Side effect:** pulmonary fibrosis and myelosuppression.
- *Please refer to above explanation for more details of alkylating agents.*

327. Ans. (d) All of these

Ref: KDT, pg. 819-20; Katzung, 11th ed. pg. 1280

Please refer to above explanation.

328. Ans. (b) Alkylating agent

Ref: Katzung, 14th ed. pg. 951; KDT, pg. 819-820

- Cyclophosphamide is the most widely used alkylating agent.
- It is an inactive compound. Transformation into active metabolite occurs in liver, and a wide range of anti tumor action is exerted.
- It has prominent immunosuppressant property, so it has been particularly utilized in bone marrow transplantation. In other organ transplants it is employed only as a reserve drug.
- **Drugs of different category are:**

Alkylating agents	Antimetabolites	Platinum compound	Topoisomerase inhibitors
Cyclophosphamide Ifosfamide Mechlorethamine *Melphalan* *Busulfan* Procarbazine **Nitrosourea** Carmustine Lomustine Semustine	**Folic acid antagonist** Methotrexate **Purine analogues** 6 Mercaptopurine 6 thioguanine ***Cladribine*** Fludarabine **Pyrimidine analogues** Capecitabin Gemcitabin **Cyatarabine** and 5 FU	Cisplatin Carboplatin Oxaliplatin	**TOPOISOMERASE- I** Irinotecam **TOPOISOMERASE-II** Etoposide Anthracycline Doxorubicin Daunorubicin

329. Ans. (c) Cytarabine

Ref: Katzung, 14th ed. pg. 951; KDT, 6th ed. pg. 820

- Cytarabine is pyrimidine analogue

Please refer to above explanation.

Extra Mile

- DOC for hairy cell leukemia- **CLADRIBINE**
- DOC for CLL- **FLUDARABINE**
- DOC for pancreatic CA- **GEMCITABINE**
- 6 Mercaptopurine metabolized by- **XANTHINE OXIDASE**
- **DOC** for choriocarcinoma- **METHOTREXATE**

330. Ans. (a) Purine analogue

Ref: Katzung, 14th ed. pg. 960; KDT, 6th ed. pg. 820

- Mercaptopurine is synthetic purine used in cancer chemotherapy.
- Use: Childhood acute leukemia.

331. Ans. (d) Cisplastin

Ref: KDT, 6th ed. 832; Katzung, 14th ed. pg. 956, 957

- Cisplatin is considered as first line chemotherapy in cervix CA and is very effective in metastatic testicular and ovarian carcinoma.
- Cisplatin is a platinum coordination complex that is hydrolyzed intracellularly to produce a highly reactive moiety which causes cross linking of DNA by platinum compound.
- The primary binding site is the N7 of guanine, but covalent interaction with adenine and cytosine also occurs.
- Cyclophospahmide, lomustine and vincristine is considered as the 2nd line drugs for the carcinoma of cervix.

Extra Mile

- Most emetogenic anti CA drug: **CISPLATIN**
- Specific side effect of cisplatin: Nephrotoxicity and Ototoxicity.
- Nitrosoureas like Lomustine can cross BBB and is considered as DOC for brain tumor like Glioma.
- Most common marrow sparing anti CA drug- **VINCRISTINE**

332. Ans. (a) Imatainib mesylate

Ref: KD Tripathi, 6th ed. pg. 828 & 832

IMATINIB

- DOC for CML & GIST - Imatinib Mesylate
- It inhibits the tyrosine protein kinases in chronic myeloid leukaemia (CML) cells and and c-kit receptor found in gastrointestinal stromal tumour (GIST).
- Adverse effects are fluid retention, edema, vomiting, abdominal pain, myalgia and liver damage

TABLE: Drugs of choice for some commonly asked malignancies

Malignancy	First line drugs
Chronic Lymphatic leukaemia	Fludarabine
Chronic Myeloid leukaemia	Imatinib
Hairy cell leukemia	CLADRIBINE
Multiple myeloma	Bortezomib > Melphalan
Choriocarcinoma	Methotrexate
Prostate carcinoma	Bicalutamide/Flutamide

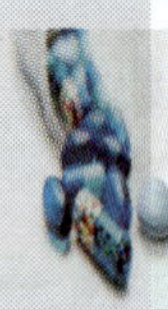

333. Ans. (a) Inhibit dihydrofolate reductase

Ref: Katzung, 14th ed. pg. 957; KD Tripathi, 6th ed. pg. 823

METHOTREXATE (MTX)

$$\text{DHFA} \xrightarrow{\text{DHF Rase}} \text{THFA}$$

- Methotrexate is a highly efficacious antineoplastic drug which inhibits dihydrofolate reductase (DHFRase) enzyme- blocking the conversion of dihydrofolic acid (DHFA) to tetrahydrofolic acid (THFA).
- This conversion is essential for formation of an essential coenzyme required for one carbon transfer reactions in denovo purine synthesis and amino acid interconversions.
- Methotrexate has cell cycle specific action kills cells in S phase; primarily inhibits DNA synthesis.

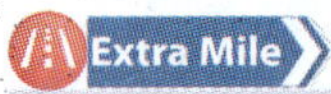

Drug of choice for Mtx toxicity: FOLINIC ACID.

334. Ans. (b) Folinic acid

Ref: Katzung, 14th ed. pg. 957; KDT, 6th ed. pg. 823

- *The toxicity of Mtx can not be overcome by folic acid, because it will not be converted to the active coenzyme form.however folinic acid rapidly reverses the effect.*
- *Thymidine also counteracts the Mtx toxicity.*
- *Refer to above explanation.*

335. Ans. (d) Methotrexate

Ref: Katzung, 14th ed. pg. 955, 957; KDT, 6th ed. pg. 823

- **Methotrexate** is an antimetabolite which act by inhibiting Dihydro folate Reductase.
- It is DOC for Choriocarcinoma, and is also considered among the first line drugs in Breast CA, testicular tumors, cervix CA and osteogenic sarcoma.
- Mtx is NOT indicated in MM.
- **Melphalan** is very effective in multiple myeloma and has been used in advanced ovarian cancer.
- First line drugs of multiple myeloma: Melphalan, Prednisolone, Cyclophosphamide.
- **Thalidomide** was used previously for morning sickness but later withdrawn due to severe teratogenic effects (phocomelia).
- It has been re-introduced due to its immunomodulatory and anti-cancer properties. It has been approved for multiple myeloma and erythema nodosum leprosum and is being tried for myelodysplastic syndrome, melanoma, Bechet disease, HIV associated ulcers and graft versus host disease.
- **Zolendronic acid:** It is a *bisphosphonate* indicated for the treatment of bony metastases and multiple myeloma.

336. Ans. (c) Cisplatin

Ref: Katzung, 14th ed. pg. 956; KDT, 6th ed. pg. 828

- **Cisplatin** is a platinum coordination complex that is hydrolyzed intracellularly to produce a highly reactive moiety which causes cross linking of DNA by platinum compound.
- It is a highly emetic drug. Antiemetics are routinely administered before infusing cisplatin.
- **DOC for cisplatin induced vomiting**: Ondansetron
- **Major s/e of cispltin:** Ototoxicity and nephrotoxicity.

337. Ans. (c) Cisplatin

Ref: Katzung 14th ed. pg. 956, 957

- **Cisplatin** is a widely used anti cancer drug.
- It has major antitumor activity in a broad range of solid tumors including
  - Non-small cell and small cell lung cancer
  - Esophageal and gastric cancer
  - Head and neck cancer and
  - Genitourinary cancers, particularly testicular, ovarian, and bladder cancer.
- When used in combination regimens with vinblastine and bleomycin or etoposide and bleomycin, cisplatin-based therapy has led to the cure of nonseminomatous testicular cancer.

Extra Mile

5-FU is a pyrimidine analogue used in colorectal cancer.
Methotrexate is considered as DOC for choriocarcinoma.

338. Ans. (a) 6-mercaptopurine

Ref: Katzung, 14th ed. pg. 960–61; KDT, 6th ed. pg. 820

- 6 mercaptopurine (6-MP) is a purine analogue which is metabolized by xanthine oxidase
- It is a competitive inhibitor of DNA.
- Allopurinol is NOT given along with 6-MP because allopurinol inhibits xanthine oxidase enzyme, which leads to increased toxicity due to accumulation of xanthine.

Anti-neoplastic drugs	Their side effect
Cyclophosphamide, ifosphamide	Hemorrhagic cystitis
Procarbazine	Disulfiram like reaction
Bleomycin, busulfan	Pulmonary fibrosis
Vincristine, vinblastine	Peripheral neuropathy
Cisplatin	Ototoxicity, Nephrotoxicity
6Mercaptopurine, 6Thioguanine	Hepatotoxicity
Doxorubicin, Daunorubicin	Cardiotoxic

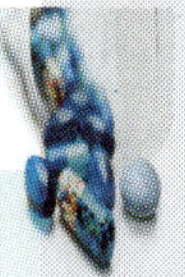

339. Ans. (d) Cyclophosphamide

Ref: Katzung, 14th ed. pg. 988; KDT, 6th ed. pg. 822

- **Cyclophosphamide** is a prodrug and is activated by hepatic biotransformation to aldophosphamide which is degraded to ***acrolein.*** This end product acrolein is responsible for hemorhagic cystitis, which is considered as the adverse side effect of cyclophosphamide.
- *This adverse effect can be controlled by* ***Mesna*** *(mercapto ethane sulfonic acid).*
- **Note:** Cyclophosphamide is DOC for Wegener's granulomatosis (*granulomatosis with polyangiitis*)
- *All natural anticancer products can cause bone marrow suppression EXCEPT bleomycin and vincristine.*

340. Ans. (a) Vincristine

Ref: Katzung, 14th ed. pg. 970; Harrison, 17th ed. pg. 699

Preferred regimen for Hodgkins and Non-hodgkins lymphoma

Hodgkins lymphoma *(ABVD)*	Non-hodgkin's lymphoma
A: Adriamycin (Doxorubicin) **B:** Bleomycin **V:** Vinblastine **D:** Dacarbazine	**R:** Rituximab **C:** Cyclophosphamide **H:** Hydroxdaunorubicin (doxorubicin) **O:** Oncovin (*vincristine*) **P:** Prednisolone

341. Ans. (b) Doxorubicin

Ref: Katzung, 14th ed. pg. 964–65; KDT, 6th ed. pg. 826-27

- **Doxorubicin** and daunorubicin are anti-tumor antibiotics. Activity of Daunorubicin is limited to acute leukemia while doxorubicin is effective in several solid tumors.
  - **MOA:** Cause breaks in DNA strands by activating topoisomerse II and generating quinolone type free radicals.
  - Doxrorubicin and daunorubicin both these antibiotics produce cardiotoxicity as a unique adverse effect.
- **Actinomycin D (Dactinomycin)** It is a very potent antineoplastic drug, highly efficacious in Wilms' tumour and rhabdomyosarcoma
  - Prominent adverse effects are vomiting, stomatitis, diarrhoea, erythema and desquamation of skin, alopecia and bone marrow depression
- **Mitoxantrone:** Recently introduced analogue of doxorubicin with lower cardiotoxicity, probably because it does not produce quinine type free radicals. Though cardiomyopathy can occur, major toxicity is marrow depression and mucosal inflammation.
- **Mitomycin C:** This highly toxic drug is used only in resistant cancers of stomach, cervix, colon, rectum, bladder, etc.
  - Bone marrow and GIT are the primary targets of toxicity.

342. Ans. (d) Mitomycin C

Ref: KDT, 6th ed. pg. 827

- After 8–10 months of start of mitomycin-C treatment, the drug leads to endothelial damage
- The Renal lesions seen are similar to those seen in idiopathic HUS and include arteriolar fibrin thrombi, expanded sub-endothelial zones in glomerular capillary walls.
- HUS can be seen with: Mitomycin C, Gemcitabine

343. Ans. (c) Amifostine

Ref: Cancer Medicine 6th ed. pg. 595

TABLE: Radiosensitizers vs Radiation protection agent

Radiosensitizers	Radiation protection agent
Actinomycin Gemcitabine Hydroxyurea Metronidazole Misonidazole 5-FU Mitomycin Paclitaxel	Amifistone GM-CSF TL-1

CARDIOVASCULAR SYSTEM

344. Ans. (a) Calcium channel blocker

Ref: Goodman and Gillman 13th ed. pg. 499

- Nifedipine, diltiazem, amlodipine, and felodipine appear to provide symptomatic relief in Raynaud disease
- Some studies indicated that prazosin can decrease the incidence of digital vasospasm in patients with Raynaud disease; however, its relative efficacy as compared with Ca^{2+} channel blockers is not known

345. Ans. (c) Endometrial hyperplasia

Ref: Goodman and Gillman 13th ed P 811-812

- Tamoxifen is a SERM (Selective Estrogen Receptor Modulator) which is widely used in management of ER+ve breast carcinoma.
- It is agonistic activity over bones, liver, uterine endometrium.
- Hence, it can cause endometrial hyperplasia.

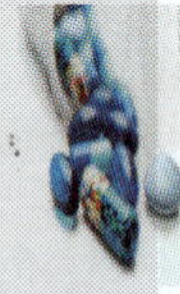

- In addition, it can also be utilized in osteoporosis management and prophylaxis due to its agonistic activity over bone where it increases the osteoblastic activity.
- Due to its agonistic activity in liver, it can increase the lipid metabolism, hence it can reduce the LDL activity.

346. Ans. (d) IV Mannitol

Ref: Goodman and Gillman 13th ed. pg. 452-53

- IV Mannitol is an osmotic diuretic. It can be used in treatment of glaucoma, cerebral edema, dialysis disequilibrium syndrome
- **Drugs used in hypertensive emergency:**
    - Nicardipine- DOC
    - Clevidipine, Clinidipine
    - Hydralazine
    - Labetalol, Esmolol
    - Na^+ Nitroprusside
    - Fenoldopam

347. Ans. (b) Lisinopril

Ref: Goodman and Gillman 13th ed. pg. 483

- In a patient with chronic congestive heart failure, cardiac remodeling is seen as compensatory mechanism.
- The cardiac remodeling, leads to mortality. Drugs reducing cardiac remodeling are:
    - **ACE inhibitor:** Captopril, Lisinopril. It is the most effective agent in cardiac remodeling
    - **ARB's:** Telmisartan, Losartan, Candesartan
    - **Aldosterone receptor antagonist:** Spironolactone, Eplerenone
    - **ARNI:** Valsartan + Sacubitril
    - **Beta blockers:** (Low dose) This class of drug has shown to reverse the cardiac remodeling.

348. Ans. (a) Alpha methyl dopa

- Among the given choices, drug which is preferred for pregnancy induced hypertension is Alpha Methyl dopa.
- **Note:**
    - DOC for hypertension in pregnancy: Labetalol
    - DOC for hypertensive emergency in pregnancy: Labetalol
    - **Anti-hypertensives safer in pregnancy:***(Mn: Lady Hardinge Medical College)*
        - Labetalol
        - Hydralazine
        - Alpha methyldopa, Clonidine
        - CCB's (DHP's- Ex: Amlodipine)
        - Cardio selective beta blockers
    - **Anti-Hypertensives contraindicated in pregnancy:** *(Mn: Avoid DNB)*
        - ACE inhibitors (- PRILS), ARBs (- SARTAN)
        - Diuretics
        - Na+ Nitroprusside, Non-DHP's (Verapamil)
        - Beta blockers (Non-Selective)

349. Ans. (a) Lisinopril

- Lisinopril is an ACE inhibitor, which increases level of Bradykinin level
- Increased bradykinin is known to cause dry cough and angioedema like symptoms.

Side effects of ACE inhibitors:

- Angioedema
- Dry Cough
- Elevated K+
- Orthostatic hypotension
- Cholestatic hepatotoxicity
- Dysgusea

350. Ans. (a) Spironolactone

- Spironolactone is an aldosterone receptor antagonist, which is utilized in resistant hypertension and chronic CHF.
- Its metabolite Canrenone, 7 alpha spirolactone, is a known androgen receptor antagonist, which causes gynecomastia, decreased libido.

351. Ans. (b) Lidocaine

- Lidocaine is DOC for treatment of digoxin induced ventricular arrhythmia.
- It is a class Ib anti arrhythmic drug.
- Atropine is used for bradyarrhythmia. It can also be used.
- Amiodarone should be avoided in digoxin induced arrhythmia as amiodarone can increase the plasma level of Digoxin and precipitates digoxin toxicity.

352. Ans. (d) Indirectly increases renin level

Ref: Goodman Gillman 13th ed. pg. 486

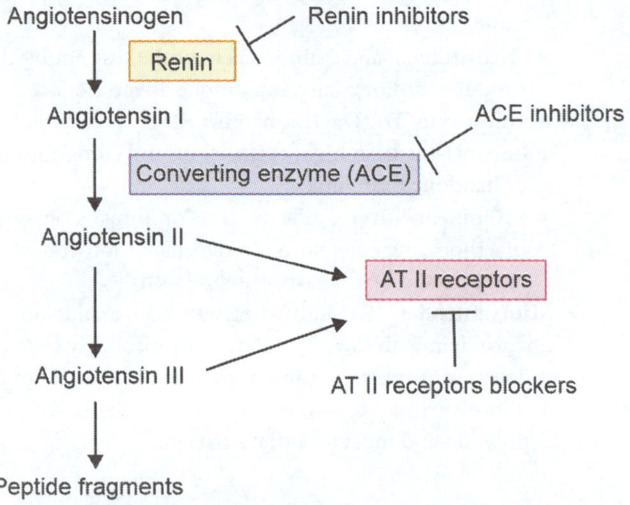

- Aliskiren is one of the renin inhibitors
- It is contraindicated in pregnancy, like other RAAS inhibitors due risk of fetal malformation.
- RAAS inhibitors are preferred in diabetes, not contraindicated.

Note: *Renin secretion inhibitor – β-blocker*

353. Ans. (a) Bilateral renal artery stenosis

Ref: Katzung's Pharmacology, 14th ed. pg. 188

- Patients with B/L renal artery stenosis or patients with single kidney having renal artery stenosis will develop renal failure if treated with ACEI.
- In stenosis there is reduced GFR, and body manage the adequate GFR by angiotensin II mediated efferent arteriole constriction to maintain the renal perfusion. In such patients, Inhibition of ACE can induce acute renal insufficiency.

354. Ans. (b) Releases nitric oxide

- Nitroglycerine act as source of nitric oxide, which increases cGMP level which causes dephosphorylation of myosin light chain and the reduction of intracellular calcium → causes relaxation of smooth muscles and causes vasodilation.

355. Ans. (c) Alpha blocker

Ref: Katzung 14th ed. pg. 184

- Among the given choices, alpha blockers are more commonly associated with postural hypotension.
- Drugs under alpha blockers are:
  - Selective alpha 1 blocker: Prazosin, terazosin, Doxazosin, Alfuzosin
  - Non-selective alpha blocker: Phentolamine, Tolazoline, Phenoxybenzamine
- **Side effect of alpha blockers:**
  - Postural hypotension
  - Retrograde ejaculation

Note: *Among the given choices, ACE inhibitors can also cause postural hypotension initially. But it is more commonly associated with alpha blockers.*

356. Ans. (c) Lignocaine

Ref: Katzung 14th ed. pg. 241

- **Lidocaine** is one of the local anaesthetics having anti-arrhythmic properties (Class 1B)
- It has low incidence of toxicity and high degree of effectiveness in arrhythmias associated with acute MI.
- Used only by IV route (t1/2: 1–2 hours)
- **MOA:** Blocks inactivated sodium channels
- **Use:**
  - DOC for termination of ventricular tachycardia and prevention of ventricular fibrillation
  - DOC for digoxin induced arrhythmia.
- It has least cardiotoxicity among sodium channel blockers.
- **Side effect:**
  - Depress myocardial contractility (can cause hypotension in heart failure patients)
  - **MC side effect:** Neurologic- Paresthesias, tremor, nausea, light headedness, hearing disturbances, slurring of speech and seizure episodes.

357. Ans. (b) PPAR-a activator

Ref: Goodman & Gillman's 13th ed. pg. 6 13-14

Gemfibrozil

- Gemfibrozil, a PPARα activator, classified under hypolipidemic drugs, fibrates.
- The PPAR family is composed of three members: α, β and γ.
- PPARα is the target for the fibrate class of drugs, including the widely prescribed *gemfibrozil* and *fenofibrate*.
- Exact mechanism how the fibrates lower lipoprotein levels, or raise HDL levels, remains unclear.
- Fibrates bind to PPARα and:
  - Reduce triglycerides through PPARα-mediated stimulation of fatty acid oxidation
  - **Increased LPL synthesis** would enhance the clearance of triglyceride-rich lipoproteins.
  - **Reduced expression of apo C-III** which serves as an inhibitor of lipolysis and receptor-mediated clearance, would enhance the clearance of VLDLs.
- Fibrate-mediated increases in HDL-C are due to PPARα stimulation of apo A-I and apo A-II expression, which increases HDL levels.
- Fenofibrate is more effective than gemfibrozil at increasing HDL levels.

Extra Mile

- PPARγ is the target for the thiazolidinedione class of anti-type 2 diabetic drugs, including rosiglitazone and pioglitazone. PPARγ does not induce xenobiotic metabolism.
- Ezetimibe inhibits intestinal cholesterol absorption.
- HMG-CoA inhibitor are statins (For example, simvastatin, rosuvastatin, etc.)

358. Ans. (a) Competitive inhibition

Ref: Goodman & Gillman's 13th ed. pg. 609

- Statins exert their major effect—reduction of LDL levels—through a mevalonic acid–like moiety that **competitively** inhibits HMG-CoA reductase, which is the rate limiting enzyme in the cholesterol biosynthesis.
- **Drugs are** atorvastatin, rosuvastatin, fluvastatin, lovastatin, pravastatin, simvastatin, pitavastatin.

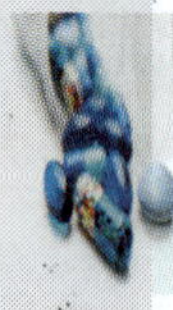

Extra Mile

- Food increases absorption of statins
- Statins are most active at night, so given at night except rosuvastatin and atorvastatin which are longest acting statins.

359. Ans. (b) Dobutamine

- DOC for cardiogenic shock: Dobutamine
- DOC in Acute heart failure: Dobutamine

360. Ans. (a) Hypokalemia

Ref: KD Tripathi, 7th ed. pg. 496

- Electrolyte imbalance like hypokalemia, hypomagnesemia and hypercalcemia increases the risk of digoxin toxicity.
- Hypo K^+ increases digoxin binding with Na^+K^+ ATPase, hence increases digoxin toxicity risk.
- Hyper K^+ increases the risk of asshythmia.

Extra Mile

Digoxin

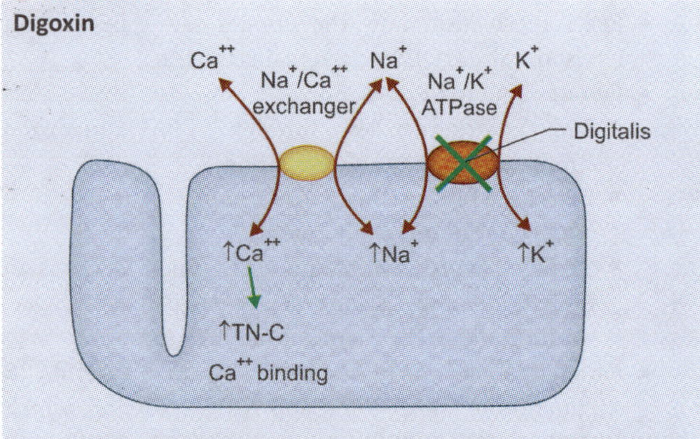

1. Inhibition of NA+/K ATPase pump by digitalis
2. Increased NA+ concentration inside the cell
3. Increased exchange of Na+ for Ca++
4. Increased intracellular Ca++
5. Increased influx of Ca++ from sarcoplasmic reticulum
6. Increased contractility of cardiac muscle

361. Ans. (b) Pumps sodium inside cell in exchange of Ca+

Ref: Katzung, 14th ed. pg. 217–18

- In normal situation, Na-Ca+ exchanger pumps out Ca^+ in exchange of Na^+. But after bloking action of Digoxin, the direction of exchanger channel is reversed causing Pumping out Na^+ in exchange with Ca^+ from outside.
- This accumulated Ca^+ intracellular acts at sarcoplasmic reticulum and causes release of more calcium → Ionotropic action

362. Ans. (b) Labetalol

Ref: Katzung, 14th ed. pg. 183

- CCBs and Diuretics are contraindicated in pregnancy for blood pressure management.
- In this given scenario, anti hypertensive will be started for patient's PIH management.
- Drug preferred in pregnancy induced hypertension: Labetalol (DOC)
- DOC for hypertensive emergency in pregnancy: Labetalol

363. Ans. (b) Blockade of ATP sensitive K+ channels

Ref: Katzung, 14th ed. pg. 175–76

- K^+ channel openers (minoxidil, diazoxide) are used as antihypertensives and not the channel blockers. Blockers of ATP sensitive K^+ channels like sulfonylureas are used in diabetes mellitus.
- **Antihypertensive drugs can act by the following mechanisms:**
  - **Diuretics:** Thiazides and loop diuretics
- DOC for hypertension: Thiazide Diuretics
  - **Vasodilators: These have different mechanisms like**
    - NO releasers e.g. sodium nitroprusside and hydralazine
    - K^+ channel openers e.g. minoxidil, Diazoxide
    - Ca^+ channel blockers e.g. amlodipine, Nifedipine, Verapamil, Diltiazem
    - D1 agonist e.g. fenoldopam
  - **Sympathetic blockers:** These can have following mechanisms
    - Ganglion blockers e.g. trimethaphan
    - Adrenergic neuron blockers e.g. guanethidine
    - Alpha 2 agonists e.g. clonidine, alpha methyldopa
    - Receptor blockers like alpha and beta blockers
  - **Renin angiotensin system blockers:** These include:
    - Renin inhibitors e.g. Enalkiren, Remikiren
    - ACE inhibitors e.g. Enalapril, Captopril, Lisinopril
    - Angiotensin receptor blockers e.g. Losartan, Telmisartan
    - Aldosterone antagonists e.g. Spironolactone, Eplerenone

364. Ans. (a) Nifedipine

Ref: Katzung, 14th ed. pg. 203–204; KDT, pg. 323

- Nifedipine is a calcium channel blocker which is used as an alternative drug for premature labor.
- Influx of calcium ions plays an important role in uterine contractions. CCB's reduce tone of myometrium and oppose contractions.
- These drugs, especially Nifedipine can postpone labor only if started early enough.
- In emergency situation, Ritodrine (β2 selective agonist) is considered as the drug of choice to suppress preterm labor.

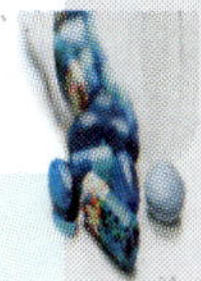

Extra Mile

- **Drug of choice for hypertension in pregnancy:** LABETALOL
- **Drug of choice for epilepsy in pregnancy:** Levetiracetam
- DOC for status eclampticus in pregnancy → phenobarbitone

365. Ans. (b) ACE inhibitors

Ref: KDT, 6th ed. pg. 553

Antihypertensive to be avoided during pregnancy	Antihypertensive safer during pregnancy
• ACE inhibitors (Ex- captopril, enelapril etc.) • Angiotensin antagonist (losartan, telmisartan)	• Hydralazine • Methyldopa • Atenolol • Metoprolol
• Thiazide diuretics (Ex- hydrochlorthiazide) • Furosemide • Propanolol • Nitroprusside	• *Labetalol- DOC* • Nifedipine • Prazosin and Clonidine

Drugs and their Respective Risk

- **Diuretics:** Tend to reduce blood volume; increase risk of placental infarcts, fetal wastage, still birth.
- **ACE inhibitors, AT1 antagonists:** Growth retardation and fetal damage risk.
- **Propanolol:** Causes low birth weight, neonatal hypoglycemia and bradycardia.
- **Nitroprusside:** Contraindicated in eclampsia.

366. Ans. (c) Captopril

Ref: KDT, 6th ed. pg. 553

Please refer to above explanation.

367. Ans. (a) ACE inhibitors

Ref: Katzung, 14th ed. pg. 187–188

- ACE inhibitors are drug of choice for scleroderma induced hypertensive crisis. Other important points and side effects about ACE inhibitors can be remembered as:
  C - Cough
  A - Angioedema
  P - Prodrugs (EXCEPT captopril and Lisinopril)
  T - Taste disturbances
  O - Orthostatic hypotension (when combined with diuretics)
  P - Pregnancy (contraindicated)
  R - bilateral Renal artery stenosis (contraindicated)
  I - Increased K^+ (contraindicated)
  L - Lower the formation of Ang II (Mechanism)

368. Ans. (b) Verapamil

Ref: Katzung, 14th ed. pg. 246

- Supra ventricular tachycardia is a condition presenting as rapid heart rhythm originating at or above the AV node. SVT can be contrasted with the potentially more dangerous ventricular tachycardias- rapid rhythms that originate within the ventricular tissue.
- Calcium channel blockers have well-documented efficacy in hypertension and supraventricular tachyarrhythmias.
- SA and AV nodal tissues, which are mainly composed of slow response cells, are affected markedly by verapamil, moderately by diltiazem, and much less by dihydropyridines.
- *Thus, verapamil and diltiazem decrease atrioventricular nodal conduction and are effective in the management of supraventricular tachycardia.*

Extra Mile

DOC for paroxysmal supra ventricular tachycardia: **ADENOSINE**
DOC for SVT: **VERAPAMIL**
DOC for Atrial Fibrillation: **Esmolol**
DOC for digitalis induced ventricular arrhythmia: **LIGNOCAINE**

369. Ans. (b) Adenosine

Ref: Katzung, 14th ed. pg. 246; KD Tripathi, 6th ed. pg. 509 & 518

- Paroxysmal supraventricular tachycardia (PSVT) is sudden onset episodes of atrial tachycardia (rate 150–200/min) with 1: 1 atrioventricular conduction
- An attack of PSVT can be terminated by IV injection of verapamil, diltiazem, esmolol or digoxin; ***but most cardiologists now prefer adenosine.***
- Adenosine has a very short t ½ in blood (~ 10 sec)
- Almost complete elimination occurs in a single passage through coronary circulation.

370. Ans. (b) ACE inhibitors

Ref: KDT, 6th ed. pg. 484

- Angiotensin converting enzyme normally helps in conversion of angiotensin I to angiotensin II, which acts as a vasoconstrictor in case of hypovolemia.
- In addition to that, ACE also helps in breakdown of bradykinin.
- When ACE inhibitors (captopril) are given, it inhibits ACE and in addition inhibits breakdown of bradykinin also, which leads to accumulation of bradykinin level in body.
- This increased level of bradykinin presents with Dry cough, rashes, urticaria and angioedema.

Other side effects of ACE inhibitors	Contraindications of ACE (–)	Safe alternative of ACE (–)
Hypotension Hyperkalemia Fetal growth retardation	Pregnancy Bilateral Renal artery stenosis Hyperkalemia	Angiotensin receptor blocker is a safe alternative in case of cough, angioedema.

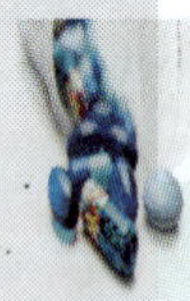

Extra Mile

- Why ACEI is contraindicated in bilateral renal stenosis
  - Patients with B/L renal artery stenosis or patients with single kidney having renal artery stenosis will develop renal failure if treated with ACEI.
  - In stenosis there is reduced GFR, and body manage the adequate GFR by angiotensin II mediated efferent arteriole constriction to maintain the renal perfusion. In such patients, Inhibition of ACE can induce acute renal insufficiency.

371. Ans. (c) Inhibit HMG CoA reductase

Ref: KDT 6th ed. pg. 614

- **HMG-CoA Reductase Inhibitors (statins):** This class of compound is the most efficacious and best tolerated hypolipidaemic drugs.
- **MOA:** Competitively inhibit conversion of HMG-CoA to mevalonate by the enzyme HMG-CoA reductase.
- **Drugs (Statins):** Lovastatin, Simvastatin, Pravstatin, Atorvasttin, Rosuvastatin

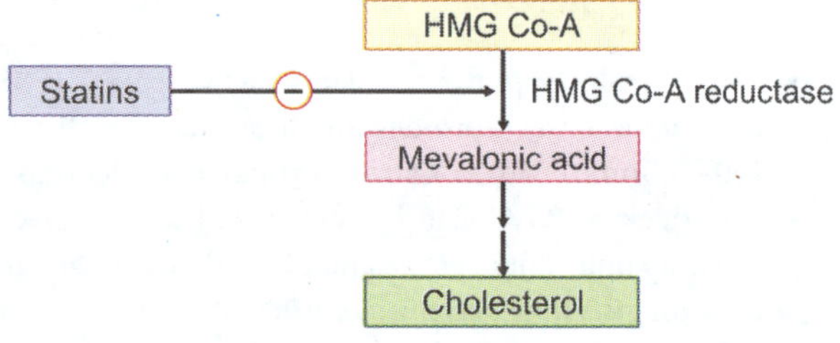

Extra Mile

- All statins are given at night except: Rosuvastatin, Atorvastain (can be given at anytime)
- Major side effects of statins: Myopathy
- Most potent statin: Pitavastain

372. Ans. (c) Somatostatin

Ref: KDT, 6th ed. pg. 235

SOMATOSTATIN

- Somatostatin inhibits the secretion of GH, TSH and prolactin by pituitary, insulin and glucagon by pancreas and most importantly. It inhibits most of G.I secretions gastrin and HCl.
- It can be used in controlling esophageal varices and bleeding peptic ulcer.
- Drugs like *simvastatin*, atorvastatin, *fluvastatin*, lovastatin and rosuvastatin are statins, which are hypolipidemic drugs. They act by inhibiting HMG-CoA Reductase.
- *Fenofibrate* are from fibrates category, which has maximum triglyceride lowering activity.

Extra Mile

- Statins end with *"vastatin"*
- Maximum LDL lowering activity is by: STATINS
- Longest acting statin: ROSUVASTATIN

373. Ans. (c) Tocainide

Ref: KDT, 6th ed. pg. 511

TABLE: Anti arrhythmic drugs

Class	Actions	Drugs
I- (Na^+#)	(Na^+ channel blockers)	
	Ia: Na^++K^+ channel blocking property	Quinidine, Procainamide, Disopyramide
	Ib: Na^+# & K^+ channel opening property	Tocainide, Lidocaine, Phenytoin, Mexiletine
	Ic: no effect on K^+ channel	Flecainide , Encainide, Propafenone, Mericizine
II- (β#)	Antiadrenergic agents (β blockers)	Propranolol, Esmolol, (Sotalol is Class III mainly)
III- (K#)	Agents widening AP (Prolong repolarization and ERP)	Ibutilide, Sotalol, Bretylium, Amiodarone, Dronadarone, Dofetilide
IV- (Ca+#)	Calcium channel blockers	Verapamil, Diltiazem
V	Drugs with other mechanism of actions	Magnesium (**DOC** in torsades de pointes) Atropine: DOC for Bradycardia a and AV Block Digoxin Adenosine: DOC for PSVT

Note: *Class IA agents also have Class III property; propranolol has Class I action as well; sotalol and bretylium have both class II and class III actions.*

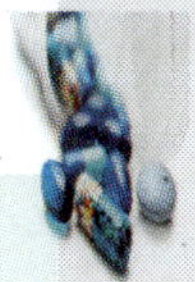

374. Ans. (d) All of these

Ref: KDT 6th ed. pg. 528

TABLE: Types of calcium channel blocker

	L-Type (long lasting current)	T-Type (transient current)	N-Type (neuronal)
Locations and function	Excitation–contraction coupling in cardiac and smooth muscle SA, A-V node: Conductivity Endocrine cell: Hormone release Neurons: transmitter release	Sa node-pacemaker activity "T" current and repetitive spikes in thalamic and other neurons Endocrine cells hormone release Certain arteries constriction	Only on Neurons in CNS, sympathetic and myenteric plexuses transmitter release
Blocker (drugs)	**DHP's:** Amlodipines, Nifedipine **Non- DHP:** Diltiazem, verapamil	Mibefradil, flunarizine, ethosuximide Trimethadione	ω- conotoxin

375. Ans. (a) Hydrochlorthiazide

Ref: KDT, 6th. pg. 274

Drugs causing glucose intolerance (hyperglycemia)		
Glucocorticoids	Diazoxide	Clozapine
Thiazides		β adrenergic agonist
Phenytoin	Protease inhibitors	Thyroid hormone
Pentamidine	β-IFN	Nicotinic acid

Note:
- Sulfonylureas are oral hypoglycemic agents. They cause hypoglycemia.
- ACE inhibitors also cause hypoglycemia.
- Other agents causing hypoglycemia: Quinine, Pentamidine, Octreotide, Insulin.

376. Ans. (a) Losartan

Ref: KDT, 6th ed. pg. 488

- Losartan has a uricosuric effect in hypertensive patients, and causes a decrease in serum uric acid levels by 20% to 25%.
- Losartan acts by inhibiting the urate/lactate exchanger and urate/chloride exchanger in the proximal convoluted tubule and leads to uricosuria.
- Allopurinol reduces approximately 30% decrease in serum uric acid, resulting from the ability of allopurinol to inhibit xanthine oxidase, the enzyme responsible for the oxidation of purine to uric acid.

377. Ans. (b) Losartan

Ref: KDT, 6th ed. pg. 488

ANGIOTENSIN RECEPTOR BLOCKERS

- These are orally active AT 1 receptor antagonists which include **losartan, candesartan, valsartan, telmisartan and irbesartan.**
- **Losartan** is a competitive antagonist and inverse agonist of A-II, 10,000 times more selective for AT1 than AT2 receptor.
- It does not block any other receptor or ion channel, EXCEPT **Thromboxane A2 receptor**, which is responsible for its platelet anti-aggregatory property attenuation.

Extra Mile

- Telmisartan has PPAR-Y agonist action which can increase sensitivity to insulin. Therefore preferred in diabetics.

378. Ans. (c) CCB and β blockers

Ref: KDT, 6th ed. pg. 553

- Verapamil or diltiazem (CCB's) with β blockers are avoided because they may cause marked bradycardia and A-V block.
- Nitrates are used in conditions like CHF, Angina pectoris, MI, and Diffuse esophageal spasm. It can be given in combination with CCBs or β blockers.

Other antihypertensive combinations to be avoided:
- An α or β adrenergic blocker with clonidine: An apparent antagonism of clonidine action has been observed.
- **Nifedipine with diuretic:** Synergism between these two is still unproven.
- Methydopa with clonidine or any two drugs of same class.
- ACE inhibitor with ARB

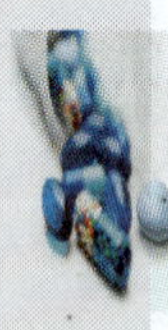

379. Ans. (a) ACE inhibitor

Ref: Harrison's, 18th ed. Ch 344

- In a diabetic patient, hypertension can accelerate complications of DM, particularly cardiovascular disease and nephropathy. In these patients ACE inhibitor is preferred. It slows down the progression of diabetic nephropathy.
- ***American Diabetic Association recommends that all patients with diabetes and hypertension be treated with an ACE inhibitor or an ARB.***
- Subsequently, agents that reduce cardiovascular risk (beta blockers, thiazide diuretics, and calcium channel blockers) should be incorporated into the regimen.

ENDOCRINE SYSTEM

380. Ans. (b) Propylthiouracil

Ref: Goodman and Gillman 13th ed. pg. 796-97

- Anti-thyroid DOC in first trimester: PTU
- Anti-Thyroid DOC in 2nd–3rd trimester: Methimazole/Carbimazole
- **Note:** Carbimazole/Methimazole exposure in first trimester can lead to aplasia cutis/scalp defect.

381. Ans. (c) Insulin and IV fluid

Ref: Goodman and Gillman 13th ed. pg. 873

- The given case is of diabetic keto-acidosis (DKA)
- Diabetic ketoacidosis (DKA) is defined as an acute metabolic disorder, which is characterized by an increased presence of circulating ketones, and the development of ketoacidosis in the presence of hyperglycemia. This syndrome occurs as a result of insulin deficiency

Treatment of DKA

- IV 0.9% saline infusion
- Correction of hypokalemia
- IV insulin (as long as serum potassium is ≥3.3 mEq/L [3.3 mmol/L])
- Rarely IV sodium bicarbonate (if pH <7 after 1 hour of treatment)

382. Ans. (b) Mifepristone + Misoprostol

Ref: Goodman and Gillman 13th ed. pg. 816

- The preferred agent for MTP is Mifepristone + Misoprostol
- Mifepristone (an anti progestin), in combination with misoprostol or other PGs, is available for the termination of early pregnancy.
- When mifepristone is used to produce a medical abortion, a PG (Ex: Misoprostol) is given 48 hours after the antiprogestin to further increase myometrial contractions and ensure expulsion of the detached blastocyst
- Misoprostol also causes cervical ripening with softening and dilation of the cervix.
- The dosage is mifepristone 200 mg orally followed 1–3 days later by misoprostol 800 mcg (4 tablets of 200 mcg) vaginally

383. Ans. (b) Bevacizumab

Ref: Goodman and Gillman 13th ed. pg. 1218

- Bevacizumab is humanized monoclonal IgG1 antibody that targets VEGF
- **Use:**
  - Wet macular degeneration, Proliferative diabetic retinopathy (Intravitreous)
  - Colorectal CA, Non small cell lung CA and Glioblastoma

384. Ans. (b) Give on alternate days

Ref: Goodman and Gillman 13th ed. pg. 855

- Exogenous steroid, can lead to HPA axis suppression. To diminish the HPA axis suppression, following steps are taken:
  - Intermediate action preparations (Prednisone or Prednisolone) should be given in the morning as a single dose.
  - Alternate day therapy with same glucocorticoids
  - Pulse therapy with higher glucocorticoid doses

385. Ans. (c) Start L thyroxine (T4) treatment 25 mcg daily and gradually increase

- The given case is of hypothyroidism on the basis of lab parameters and clinical symptoms.
- In the management of such patient, we never start the treatment with high dose. It is always started with low dose and then we proceed slowly according to the patients need.
- Treatment of hypothyroidism is always started with T4, since its long acting.
- T3 is utilized in management of acute hypothyroid emergencies like myxedema coma

386. Ans. (d) Glipizide

- **Hypoglycemia** is always increases sympathetic drive, which can lead to symptoms like tremor, tachycardia, sweating.
- **Among the** given choices, Glipizide (a Sulfonyurea) is known to cause hypoglycemia.
- **Metformin, an** AMP kinase agonist, is the safest oral

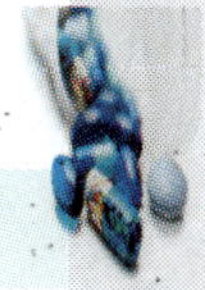

hypoglycemic agent. It is not associated with hypoglycemia
- **Voglibose,** an alpha glucosidase inhibitor in intestine. It is also not associated with hypoglycemia
- **Vildagliptin,** a DPP4 inhibitor also doesn't cause hypoglycemia

387. Ans. (a) Linagliptin

- Gliptins are DPP IV inhibitors.
- All the gliptins are excreted *via* renal route except Linagliptin, which is excreted *via* hepatic route.
- Therefore, linagliptin is safe in renal failure patients, and doesn't require dose adjustment.

388. Ans. (a) Goserelin

Ref: Goodman Gillman 13th ed. pg. 1243

The shown case history is pointing towards prostate cancer.
Agents used for prostate cancer are:
- **GnRH agonist** (continuous manner → act as antagonist): Goserelin, Histrelin, Triptorelin, nafarelin
- **GnRH antagonist:** Degarelix, Cetrorelix
- **Non steroidal androgen receptor antagonist:** Enzalutamide: Bicalutamide, Flutamide, Nilutamide, Apalutamide, Darolutamide
- **Spindle breakdown inhibitor:** Docetaxel
- **Topoisomerase II inhibitor:** Etoposide

389. Ans. (a) Tamoxifen

Ref: Katzung 14th ed. pg. 724

- Selective estrogen receptor modulator (SERM) are non-steroidal drugs used for management of breast cancer. Agents under this class are: Tamoxifen, Droloxifene, Toremifene, Raloxifene.
- These agents have agonistic and antagonistic action over estrogen receptor (ER).
- **Tamoxifen is:**
  - **ER antagonist at:** Breast, blood vessels
  - **ER agonist at:** Pituitary, Liver, Uterus, Bone
  - **Tamoxifen** increases risk of endometrial CA
- **Raloxifene** has ER antagonistic activity at breast, agonistic effect over bone and neutral effect over uterus. Therefore, it doesn't increase the risk of endometrial CA

390. Ans. (a) Carbimazole

Ref: Katzung 14th ed. pg. 693-94

Treatment of Hyperthyroidism in Pregnancy

- **1st trimester:** PTU
- **2nd – 3rd trimester:** Carbimazole/Methimazole
- Exposure to methimazole/carbimazole in first trimester leads to teratogenicity like:
  - Fetal goiter, Aplasia cutis, Choanal atresia, Esophageal atresia, Scalp defect *(Mn: FACES)*
- **Carbimazole is prodrug of methimazole**

391. Ans. (a) It is analogue of GLP released from gut and increase glucose dependent insulin secretion

Ref: Katzung 14th ed. pg. 762

- **Exentatide** is one of the GLP1 agonist, which increases insulin secretion from beta cell of the pancreas. Other GLP1 agonists are:
  - Liraglutide (inj- SC route)
  - Semaglutide (PO route)

Extra Mile

- **DPP4 inhibitors are:** Sitagliptin, Saxagliptin, Linagliptin, Vildagliptin
- **SGLT2 inhibitors:** Canagliflozin, Dapagliflozin, Empagliflozin
- **Amylin analogue:** Pramlintide

392. Ans. (d) Hydrocortisone

Classification of steroids

Short acting: (8–12 hours)	• Cortisone • Hydrocortisone
Intermediate acting (12–36 hours)	• Fludrocortisone • Prednisone • Prednisolone • Methylprednisolone
Long acting (36–72 hours)	• Triamcinolone • Dexamethasone • Betamethasone

393. Ans. (a) Regular Insulin

Ref: Katzung 14th ed. pg. 753

- **Regular insulin** is a short-acting, soluble crystalline zinc insulin
- Hypoglycemic effect appears within 30 minutes after subcutaneous injection, peaks at about 2 hours, and lasts for 5–7 hours.
- For very insulin-resistant subjects who would otherwise require large volumes of insulin solution, a U500 preparation of human regular insulin is available both in a vial form and a disposable pen
- **IV infusion:** Used in treatment of diabetic ketoacidosis

394. Ans. (d) Insulin glargine

Ref: Katzung 14th ed. pg. 755

- **Insulin glargine** is a soluble, "peakless" (i.e. having broad concentration plateau), long acting insulin analogue.
- Onset: 1–1.5 hours. Duration of action: 11–24 hours.

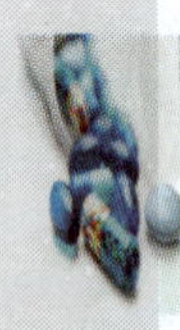

TABLE: Summary of bioavailability characteristics of the insulins

Insulin preparations	Onset of action	Peak action	Effective duration
Insulins lispro, aspart, glulisine	5–15 minutes	1–1.5 hours	3–4 hours
Human regular	30–60 minutes	2 hours	6–8 hours
Technosphere inhaled insulin	5– 15 minutes	1 hour	3 hours
Human NPH	2–4 hours	Flat	~24 hours
Insulin detemir	0.5–1 hours	Flat	17 hours
Insulin degludec	0.5–1.5 hours	Flat	>42 hours

395. Ans. (a) Dopamine

- Dopamine keeps inhibitory control over prolactin.
- This explains the reason behind hyperprolactinemia in psychotic patients who are treated with dopamine antagonists.
- Dopamine agonists (bromocriptine, cabergoline) therefore are used in treatment of hyperprolactinemia, acromegaly.

396. Ans. (b) GLP-1 Analogue

Ref: Goodman & Gillman 13th ed. pg. 877

- **GLP-1 analogue drugs are:** Exenatide, Liraglutide, Albiglutide, Dulaglutide, Lixisenatide
- These agents activate the GLP-1 receptor → Increased insulin biosynthesis and release
- These agents are resistant to degradation by DPP4 enzyme → Has extended activity following injection.
- **Side effect:** Nausea, vomiting, Pancreatitis

TABLE: Properties of insulin secretagogues

Class generic name	Daily dosage (mg)	Duration of action (hours or dosing frequency)
Sulfonylureas		
Glimepiride	1–8	24
Glipizide	5–40	12–18
Glipizide (extended release)	5–20	24
Glyburide	1.25–20	12–24
Glyburide (micronized)	0.75–12	12–24
Nonsulfonylureas (Meglitinides)		
Nateglinide	180–360	2–4
Repaglinide	0.5–16	2–6
GLP-1 Agonists		
Albiglutide	30–50	Weekly
Dulaglutide	0.75–1.5	Weekly
Exenatideb	2	Weekly

Contd...

Class generic name	Daily dosage (mg)	Duration of action (hours or dosing frequency)
Liraglutide	0.6–1.8	Daily
Lixisenatide	0.010–0.020	Daily
Dipeptidyl Peptidase–4 Inhibitors		
Alogliptin	25	Daily
Linagliptin	5	Daily
Saxagliptin	2.5–5	Daily
Sitagliptin	25–100	12–16
Vildagliptin	50–100	Twice daily

397. Ans. (b) Provide stability in insulin molecule

Ref: KD Tripathi 8th ed. pg. 286

- The insulin molecules namely regular human insulin and NPH insulin/lente is clear at neutral pH and exist as dimers that assemble into hexamers in the presence of two zinc ions. This provides stability in the insulin.
  - Become cloudy after adding zinc
- These hexamers are furthers stabilized by phenolic compounds like phenol and meta-cresol.
- Zinc is also necessary for proper processing, storage and secretion of insulin and also protect against Beta cell loss.
- Studies have shown that zinc manages the behaviour of amylin (a protein secreted from beta cell) to help slow down carbohydrate absorption. Unmanaged amylin can form clumps that interfere with insulin secretion.
- Since zinc is so closely tied to insulin functioning, its deficiency is associated with poor beta cell function and higher incidence of insulin resistance.

Extra Mile

Lente insulin (Insulin-zinc suspension): Two types of insulin-zinc suspensions have been produced.

- The one with large particles is crystalline and practically insoluble in water (ultralente). It is long-acting.
- The other has smaller particles and is amorphous (semilente), is short-acting. Their 7:3 ratio mixture is called 'Lente insulin' and is intermediate-acting

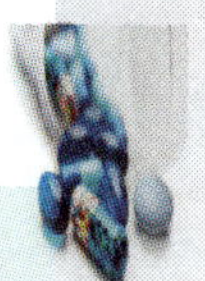

398. Ans. (a) 4 minutes

Ref: Sharma & Sharma 3rd ed. pg. 625

- Parathyroid hormone is a 84 amino acid compound which is responsible for calcium homeostasis in body.
  - Acts over osteoblast → Stimulate osteoclast → Bone resorption
- Principle factor regulating parathyroid hormone synthesis and release: Hypocalcemia
- Rapidly metabolized in liver and kidney
- Plasma half-life: 2–4 minutes

Endocrine organ	Hormones	Basic structure	Half-life
Hypothalamus	Hypothalamic releasing hormones	Small: 3 to 44 amino acid peptides	1–2 min
Pituitary	"Trophic" hormones	Large glycoproteins	20 min. – 3 hrs
Thyroid	Calcitonin	32 AA	10–30 min.
Parathyroid	PTH–parathyroid hormone	84 AA	4 min.
Pancreas	Insulin, glucagon (major)	–51 AA/29 AA	5–8 min./ negligible
Adipose tissue	Leptin	167 AA	30 min.
Kidney	Renin, erythro-poietin	340 AA/193 AA	15 min.
Liver	IGF-1	153 AA	12–15 hrs.
Heart	ANP/BNP	28 AA/32 AA	2 min./20 min.

399. Ans. (b) Insulin

Ref: Sharma & Sharma 3rd ed. pg. 636

- Insulin in diabetes facilitates glucose uptake (through GLUT-4) and increases intracellular glucose oxidative metabolism.
- Insulin decreases glycogenolysis, increases lipogenesis, decreases lipolysis, increases FA synthesis and triglyceride formation and storage. It also blunts lipolytic action if aderenaline, growth hormone and glucagon.
- Thus insulin lowers the blood glucose levels by promoting the glucose utilization and suppressing its production.

Extra Mile

- Acarbose, miglitol and voglibose is from α-glucosidase inhibitor group. Alpha glucosidase usually facilitates digestion of complex starch, oligosaccharides, monosaccharides. If they are inhibited the sugar moiety will not be absorbed, reducing the sugar level.
- **Side effect:** Flatulence, diarrhea, abdominal pain.
- Pioglitazone can cause increase in weight gain, which is attributed to fluid retention and edema.

400. Ans. (b) Fulvestrant

Ref: KD Tripathi, 7th ed. pg. 313

- **Fulvestrant** is the first member of a distinct class of estrogen receptor (ER) ligands called 'selective estrogen receptor down-regulators' (SERDs) or 'pure estrogen antagonists' that has been introduced for the treatment of metastatic ER positive breast cancer in postmenopausal women which has stopped responding to tamoxifen.
- In contrast to tamoxifen, it inhibits ER dimerization so that ER interaction with DNA is prevented and receptor degradation is enhanced. The ER is thus downregulated resulting in more complete suppression of ER responsive gene function. This feature along with its higher ***affinity*** for the ER probably accounts for its efficacy in tamoxifen resistant cases.
- Fulvestrant is administered as (250 mg) monthly IM injections in the buttock. It is slowly absorbed and has an elimination *t1/2* of more than a month.

Extra Mile

Clomiphene citrate binds to both ER-alpha and ER-beta and acts as pure estrogen antagonist
Tamoxifen is selective estrogen receptor modulator
Flutamide is selective antagonist of androgen receptor.

401. Ans. (a) Prostaglandins

Ref: Anatomy and Physiology, Ch 27, Development and Inheritance pg. 832

The text states: *"Rising estrogen and oxytocin during pregnancy, stimulate the production of prostaglandins in endometrium. These prostaglandins further stimulate smooth muscle contractions, thereby increasing frequency of urination and late in pregnancy cause spasms in uterine musculature."*

402. Ans. (d) NPH

Ref: Sharma & Sharma 3rd ed. pg. 641; KDT, 6th ed. pg. 259

Insulin type	Onset of action (hr.)	Duration of action (hr)
Ultrashort (Rapid Acting) Insulin Lispro Insulin Aspart Insulin Gluilisine	15 – 30 minutes	3–5 hrs
Short acting Regular insulin	30–60 minutes	6–8 hrs
Intermediate acting Insulin lente Neutral protamine hagedorn (NPH)/Isophane insulin	**1–2 hrs**	**16–20 hrs**
Long Acting Insulin Glargine Insulin Detemir Insulin Degludec	**2–4 hrs**	**16–24 hrs** **Degludec: >24 hours**
Inhaled insulin (Afreeza) (Human insulin)-**Liquid form**	**5–10 minutes**	**3 hours**

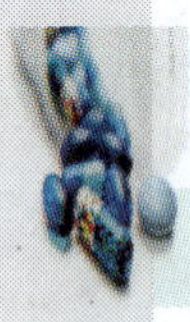

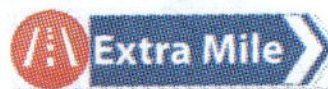

Most common side effect of insulin: Hypoglycemia
DOC for Diabetic ketoacidosis (DKA): Regular insulin

403. Ans. (a) Insulin lispro

Ref: KDT 6th ed. pg. 259

Please refer to above explanation.

404. Ans. (a) Insulin aspart

- Ultrashort acting insulins are the fastest acting ones.
- Onset of action within 15–30 minutes and duration of action is 3–5 hours.

405. Ans. (c) Dopamine stimulate prolactin production

Ref: KDT, 6th ed. pg. 235-236

- Prolactin is produced from anterior pituitary and is associated with lactation.
- Prolactin is under predominant inhibitory control of hypothalamus through PRIH (Prolactin Release Inhibitory Hormone), which is Dopamine that acts on pituitary lactotrope D2 receptor.
- Dopaminergic agonist like bromocriptine, DA, cabergoline decrease plasma prolactin levels and is used to treat hyperprolactinemia
- Dopaminergic antagonists like chlorpromazine haloperidol, metoclopramide causes hyperprolactinemia by blocking D2 receptors.
- A progressive increase in prolactin occurs during pregnancy, peaking at term. After childbirth, this dopamine is inhibited and prolactin now stimulates milk production.

Extra Mile

Milk production is stimulated by: Prolactin (remember production by prolactin).
Milk secretion is stimulated by: Oxytocin
DOC for hyperprolactinemia: Bromocriptine

406. Ans. (c) Dopamine

Ref: KDT, 6th ed. pg. 235-236

- Prolactin is under predominant inhibitory control of hypothalamus through PRIH (Prolactin Release Inhibitory Hormone), which is **Dopamine** that acts on pituitary lactotrope D2 receptor.
- A progressive increase in prolactin occurs during pregnancy, peaking at term. After childbirth, this dopamine is inhibited and prolactin now stimulates milk production.

407. Ans. (b) Enhance glucose uptake by skeletal muscle

Ref: KDT, 6th ed. pg. 267

OHA drugs	Mechanism of action
Metformin and thiazolidinediones	Inhibition of hepatic gluconeogenesis Enhance glucose uptake in skeletal muscle
Sulfonylureas and ripaglinde	Stimulate insulin release from pancreas
Acarbose	Decrease absorption of glucose from intestine

408. Ans. (a) Metformin

Ref: KDT, 6th ed. pg. 267

METFORMIN

- Metformin is an antidiabetic drug from biguanides category.
- They improve lipid profile, hence considered as DOC for DM in obese patients.
- **MOA:**
  - Increase peripheral utilization of glucose
  - Inhibit hepatic gluconeogenesis
- Metformin never causes hypoglycemia.
- Recent report says, metformin is weight neutral drug.
- Another drug from Biguanides is *Phenformin*, which is withdrawn, because it causes lactic acidosis.
- **Sulfonylureas** causes a brisk release of insulin from pancreas which stimulate the functional receptors for the intake of glucose. They cause weight gain
  - They can cause hypoglycemia.
  - Preferred in thin patients with DM
- **Repaglinide** has same MOA as sulfonylureas, but it is short acting.
  - Used to control sudden rise of glucose after meal.
- **Acarbose** act by inhibiting G.I. absorption of sugar.
  - **s/e:** Can cause osmotic diarrhea.

Extra Mile

- Safest sulfonylureas: Tolbutamide (safer in elderly also)

*Remembered as: **MOST**- Metformin for Obese; Sulfonylureas for Thin.*

409. Ans. (c) Monitoring of liver enymes is recommended

Ref: KDT, 6th ed. pg. 304-5

- Tamoxifen is a SERM that acts as antagonist at estrogen receptors in the breast. It decreases the risk of contralateral breast cancer and is approved for primary prevention of breast cancer in women at high risk.

Adverse Effects of Tamoxifen Therapy

- Hot flashes
- Menstrual irregularities,
- Endometrial hyperplasia
- Cataract
- *Hepatotoxicity*
- Development of fatty liver: Due to an idiosyncratic reaction to a metabolite of the medication
- Steatohepatitis: Minor serum aminotransferase elevations, ***monitoring of serum enzymes during long term tamoxifen therapy is often recommended.***

410. Ans. (b) Finasteride

Ref: KDT, 6th ed. pg. 294

- Hirsutism is male pattern hair growth in females. For example: Moustache, beard, chest hair.
- **Finasteride** is a 5α-reductase inhibitor. By inhibiting 5α-reductase it prevents conversion of testosterone to DHT by the type II isoenzyme, resulting in a decrease in serum DHT levels by about 65–70% and in prostate DHT levels by up to 85–90%.
- Decreasing the amount of DHT leads to increased hair regrowth and slower hair loss. Hair growth on other parts of the body is not affected by finasteride.
- **USES:** This medication is used to treat male pattern baldness (androgenetic alopecia) at the crown and in the middle of the scalp. Can also be used in treatment of BPH.
- **Flutamide:** Androgen receptor antagonist. Studies have shown that it is helpful in treatment of hirsutism. Can also be used in treatment of BPH.
- **Spironolactone:** Antialdosterone antiandrogenic compound, used in the treatment of hirsutism.
- **Cyproterone acetate:** A progestin that also has strong antiandrogenic action.

Drugs causing Hirsutism

Mn: MAD COP

- Minoxidil
- Androgen
- Dizoxide
- Cyclosporine
- OCP's
- Phenytoin

411. Ans. (c) Finasteride

Ref: Katzung 14th ed. pg. 1085

- Most of the actions of testosterone are mediated by its conversion to DHT by 5-alpha reductase. Important amongst these are growth of prostate, male pattern baldness and hirsutism in females.
- **Finasteride and dutasteride** are 5-alpha reductase inhibitors useful in the treatment of BPH, male pattern baldness and hirsutism by reducing the production of DHT.

Note: *Flutamide and Nilutamide act as antagonists of androgen receptors. These are useful for the treatment of prostatic carcinoma. Flutamide can cause gynaecomastia and reversible liver damage.*

AUTACOIDS

412. Ans. (d) Rasburicase

Ref: Goodman and Gillman 13th ed. pg. 705

Rasburicase is a recombinant uricase, which reduces uric acid more effectively than allopurinol.

In the given case scenario, where the uric acid level is high due to tumor lysis syndrome, Rasburicase is most preferred drug.

413. Ans. (a) Xanthine oxidase

- This is case of gout. Drug that decreases production of uric acid, act by inhibiting xanthine oxidase.
- To inhibit Xanthine oxidase Allopurinol is used, i.e., DOC for chronic gout.

414. Ans. (c) Tadalafil

- Phosphodiesterase inhibitors are used for:
  - Erectile dysfunction/Impotence
  - Pulmonary hypertension
- Most commonly used PDE5 inhibitory is Sildenafil.
- Longest acting PDE5 inhibitor is Tadalafil.
- **Half life of PDE5 inhibitors:**
  - Sildenafil: 4 hours
  - Vardenafil: 5–6 hours
  - Tadalafil: 17 hours

415. Ans. (b) Ibuprofen

- NSAIDs are used to close the ductus arteriosus.
- Drugs:
  - Ibuprofen (safest)
  - Indomethacin
  - Aspirin

416. Ans. (a) Xanthine oxidase

Ref: Goodman and Gillman 13th ed. pg. 703

- In the shown case, high uric acid level and pain and erythema in great toe is indicative of gout.
- DOC for management of chronic gout is Allopurinol, which act by inhibiting xanthine oxidase enzyme.

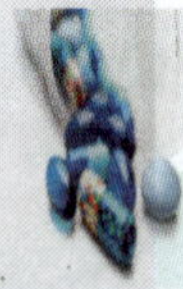

- **Drugs used in chronic gout:**
  - **Xanthine oxidase inhibitor:** Allopurinol, Febuxostat
  - **Uricosuric agent:** Probenecid, Benzbromarone, Lesinurad, Sulfinpyrazone
  - **Uric acid metabolism:** Rasburicase, Pegloticase (convert purine to water soluble metabolite, allantoin → easily excreted).

417. Ans. (a) Hydroxychloroquine

Ref: Goodman and Gillman 13th ed. pg. 1256

- HCQ is known to cause, early onset maculopathy, which causes reduction in visual acuity.
- Fundoscopy reveals typical bulls eye maculopathy, which is an irreversible side effect of the drug.
- Other given drugs in option, are also DMARD's, and can be used in rheumatoid arthritis.

Extra Mile

Drugs causing ocular side effects

Drugs	Ocular side effects
Amiodarone	• Vortex keratopathy (corneal microdeposits)
Sildenafil	• Cyanopsia
Digoxin	• Xanthopsia
Tamoxifen	• Crystalline maculopathy/pigmentary retinopathy
Vigabatrin	• Visual field constriction
Ethambutol, Chloramphenicol	• Toxic optic neuropathy (progressive central scotoma)
Topical steroid	• Glaucoma
Systemic steroids	• Cataract
Thioridazine	• Retinal pigmentation

418. Ans. (c) Dihydroergotamine and Na+ Nitroprusside

Ref: Goodman Gillman 13th ed. pg. 233-34

- Ergot derivatives like Dihydroergotamine, Bromocriptine is associated with fibrotic reaction, that can cause gangrene like situation in this patient.
- Ergotamine is therefore not a preferred agent in migraine
- Agent that can be used in management of such condition is vasodilators like calcium channel blockers (DHP's), Na^+ Nitroprusside, alpha blockers.

Extra Mile

- DOC for migraine: Sumatriptan ($5HT_{1B/D}$ agonist)
- DOC for prophylaxis of migraine: Propranolol

419. Ans. (a) Propranolol

Ref: Katzung 14th ed. pg. 168, 291

- The shown case is possibly is of migraine patient.
- Drug of choice for prophylaxis of migraine is: Propranolol.
- Drug of choice for migraine treatment: Triptans (Sumatriptan, Rizatriptan, Naratriptan, Frovatriptan).

Agents used for prophylaxis of migraine:

- Beta blockers (Propranolol, Metoprolol, Timolol)
- Divalproex Na^+
- Verapamil
- TCA (Amitriptyline, Nortriptyline)
- Valproate
- Topiramate
- Botulinum toxin
- Methysergide

GRP antagonist

- Rimegepant
- Olcegepant
- Ubrogepant

420. Ans. (c) Flutamide

Ref: Katzung 14th ed. pg. 744

- Flutamide is a non-steroidal antiandrogen agent used in metastatic prostate cancer, treatment of hirsutism, juvenile nasopharyngeal angiofibroma.
- **Agents used for migraine prophylaxis:**

  Please refer to above explanation

421. Ans. (a) Xanthine oxidase inhibition

Ref: Katzung 14th ed. pg. 661-62

- **Allopurinol** is DOC for chronic gout.
- MOA of Allopurinol: Xanthine oxidase inhibitor
- **Note:**
  - **Recombinant uricase:** Rasburicase, Pegloticase
  - **Uricosuric agent:** Probenecid, Benzbromarone, Lesinurad

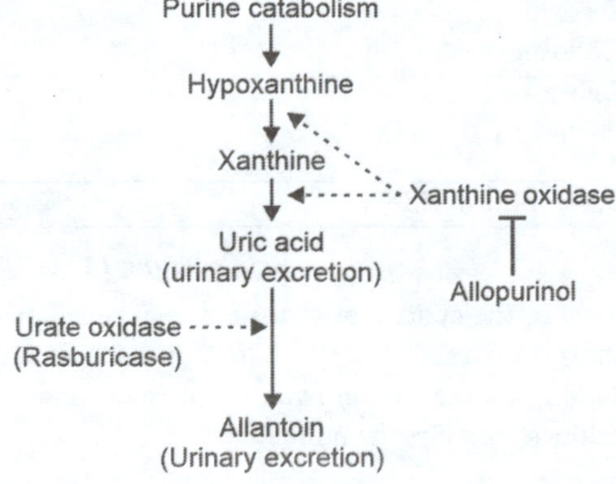

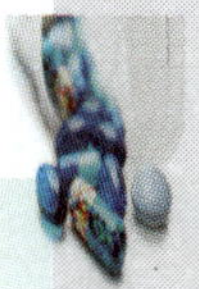

422. Ans. (a) Fentanyl

Ref: Katzung 14th ed. pg. 567-68

- Among the given choices, fentanyl is the most potent opioid, which is around 100 times more potent than morphine.
- Overall, most potent opioid is: Sufentanyl (1000 times more potent than morphine).

423. Ans. (b) Etoricoxib

Ref: Katzung 14th ed. pg. 323, 647

TABLE: Non-steroidal anti-inflammatory drugs classification

Selective COX-2 Inhibitor (Coxibs)	Non-selective COX-1 and 2 inhibitor
• Celecoxib • Etoricoxib • Valdecoxib • Rofecoxib • Parecoxib	• Indomethacin • Ibuprofen • Naproxen • Piroxicam • Aspirin • Ketoprofen

424. Ans. (a) Allopurinol

Ref: Katzung 14th ed. pg. 661

- DOC for chronic gout/period between acute gout attacks: Allopurinol
- MOA: Xanthine oxidase inhibitor
- When initiating allopurinol therapy, colchicine or NSAID should be used until steady-state serum uric acid is normalized or decreased to less than 6 mg/dL and they should be continued for 6 months or longer.
- **Initial dose:** 50–100 mg/day
- **Side effect:**
  - Precipitation of gout (that's why initially given with NSAIDS or colchicine)
  - GI intolerance (N/V/D)
  - Peripheral neuritis and necrotizing vasculitis
  - Bone marrow suppression → Aplastic anemia
  - Hepatotoxicity and interstitial nephritis
  - Maculopapular rash and exfoliative dermatitis
  - Cataract

Extra Mile

- DOC for acute gout attack: Probenecid (NSAID except Aspirin)
- **Febuxostat:** Also a xanthine oxidase inhibitor. Used in patients with intolerance to allopurinol or not responding to it.
- **Uricosuric agents like Probenecid, Sulfinpyrazone, Lesinurad** can also be used in treatment of gout especially when allopurinol or febuxostat is contraindicated.

425. Ans. (d) Sufentanil

Ref: Goodman & Gillman 13th ed. pg. 376

- Fentanyl citrate and sufentanil citrate are congeners of fentanyl and are considered as potent analgesics
- After systemic delivery:
  - Fentanyl is about 100 times more potent than morphine
  - Sufentanil is about 1000 times more potent than morphine
- Time to peak analgesic effect after IV administration: ~5 minutes
- These drugs are well known to be used as epidural analgesic.

426. Ans. (d) Hepatotoxicity

Ref: Goodman & Gillman 13th ed. pg. 696

- Paracetamol/Acetaminophen is a non-selective COX inhibitor
- **Use:** Analgesic and antipyretic agent. Preferred in patients where aspirin is contraindicated
- **Usual dose:** 325–650 mg every 4–6 hours. Maximum FDA recommended dose is 4 g/day
- Peak plasma concentration: 30–60 minutes
- **Half-life:** 2 hours
- Metabolism of acetaminophen in liver by:
  - Hepatic conjugation with glucuronic acid (~60%)
  - Sulfuric acid (~35%)
  - Cysteine (~3%);
  - CYP mediated N-hydroxylation to form NAPQI (*N*-acetyl-*p*-benzoquinone imine)
- Note: NAPQI is one of the highly reactive intermediate metabolite of acetaminophen metabolism. This usually reacts with sulfhydryl groups is GSH → rendered harmless.
- In hepatotoxicity condition GSH level depleted.

SIDE EFFECTS

- The most serious acute adverse effect of over dosage of acetaminophen is a potentially fatal hepatic necrosis.
- Due to hepatotoxicity there is saturation of glucuronide and sulfate conjugation and increasing amounts undergo CYP-mediated *N*-hydroxylation to form excess of NAPQI (it accumulates due to depletion of GSH).
- The highly reactive NAPQI causes enzymatic dysfunction, produces oxidative stress and apoptosis.
- In adults hepatotoxicity may occur after ingestion of single dose of 10–15 g. Doses of 20–25 g is potentially fatal.

TREATMENT OF ACETAMINOPHEN TOXICITY:

- Activated charcoal within 4 hours of ingestion decreases absorption by 50–90%
- **N-acetylcysteine:** antidote of choice for acetaminophen toxicity. It acts by detoxifying NAPQI by:
  - Repleting GSH stores
  - Conjugate directly with NAPQI by serving as a GSH substitute

Extra Mile

In Paracetamol Toxicity:
- Liver enzyme abnormalities typically peak 72–96 hours after ingestion
- **Biopsy:** Centrilobular necrosis with sparing of the periportal area
- **Other side effects:** Renal tubular necrosis and Hypoglycemic coma

427. Ans. (b) Early closure of PDA

Ref: Goodman & Gillman 13th ed. pg. 690, 697

- Indomethacin is a potent nonselective inhibitor of COX enzyme. It is considered 20 times more potent than aspirin
- Patency of ductus arteriosus is due to prostaglandin
- Exposure of COX inhibitor (indomethacin) in 3rd trimester causes pre-mature closure of ductus arteriosus.

Extra Mile

- An IV formulation of indomethacin is approved for closure of persistent patent ductus arteriosus in premature infants.

428. Ans. (a) 5-lipoxygenase inhibitor

Ref: Goodman & Gillman's 13th ed. pg. 740-41

- In the pathway of leukotriene synthesis where phospholipase cleaves the phospholipid of cell membrane to form arachidonic acid, steroids can inhibit this particular synthesis.

Phospholipase A2
Phospholipid ------------------------→ Arachidonic acid
(–) Steroids

- Further the arachidonic acid is metabolized to form leukotriene and prostaglandin with the help of 5'LOX and COX enzyme respectively.

Drugs acting at different sites:

- **PLA2 inhibitor:** Steroids
- **LOX inhibitor:** Zileuton
- **Receptor inhibitor:** Montelukast, zafirlukast, pranlukast

429. Ans. (c) 0.25%

- ALCAFTADINE is a H_1 receptor antagonist, and can be used for allergic conjunctivitis
- The trial done for alcaftadine used 0.25% solution.
- **The trial states:** *"When Alcaftadine was tested against placebo and olopatadine, only Alcaftadine 0.25% was shown to have a clinically significant reduction in conjunctival redness scores 7 and 15 minutes after administration"*

430. Ans. (a) Sildenafil

Ref: KD Tripathi, 7th ed. pg. 303

- Sildenafil is an orally active drug for treatment of ED. Sildenafil acts by selectively inhibiting PDE-5, causing increase in cGMP and enhancing Nitric Oxide action on corpus cavernosum.
- Amrinone and Milrinone are PDE-3 inhibitor and are also called inodilators. They are used in CHF.
- Tamoxifen is a selective estrogen receptor modulator, used in breast cancer.

431. Ans. (c) Antibody to VEGF receptor

Ref: KD Tripathi, 7th ed. pg. 871

- ***Bevacizumab*** It is a humanized **monoclonal antibody that binds VEGF-A** and hinders its access to the VEGF receptor, interrupting angiogenic signalling.
- Combined with 5-FU, bevacizumab is used in metastatic colorectal cancer. Added to conventional chemotherapy, it improves survival in metastatic non-small cell lung cancer, breast cancer, clear cell renal carcinoma and glioblastoma. Bevacizumab is administered by IV infusion every 2–3 weeks.
- Adverse effects are–rise in BP, arterial thromboembolism leading to heart attack and stroke, vessel injury and hemorrhages, heart failure, proteinurea, gastrointestinal perforations, and healing defects.

Extra Mile

- Epidermal growth factor (EGF) receptor inhibitors are: Gefitinib and Erlotinib. Mostly used in non-small cell lung cancer
- Example of VEGF 2 receptor inhibitor is sunitinib. It is used in metastatic RCC and GIST.

432. Ans. (b) Cyclosporine

- Cyclosporine and Tacrolimus are immunosuppressants, specifically inhibit antigen stimulated activation & proliferation of helper T-cells as well as expression of various cytokines including IL-2 by inhibiting calcineurin.
- **Other immunomodulators are:**
  - **IL 1 receptor inhibitor:** Anakinra
  - **IL 6 Receptor inhibitor:** Tocilizumab
  - **Co-Stimulation inhibitor:** Abatacept, Bilatacept
  - **TNF-α inhibitor:** Adalimumab, Certolizumab, Etanercept, Infliximab, Golimumab

433. Ans. (b) Phosphodiesterase 5 inhibition

Ref: KD Tripathi, 6th ed. pg. 294-295

- Sildenafil, Tadalafil and vardenafil are selective PDE-5 inhibitors effective in erectile dysfunction.
- **5α-REDUCTASE INHIBITOR**
  - **Finasteride** is competitive inhibitor of the enzyme 5α-reductase which converts testosterone into more active dihydrotestosterone responsible for androgen

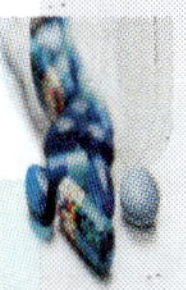

action in many tissues including prostate gland and hair follicles.
  - Used in treatment of BPH
- **Flutamide:** A nonsteroidal drug having specific antiandrogenic, but no other hormonal activity.
  - Used in prostate CA

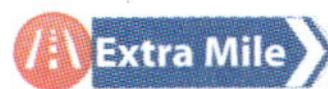

Tadalafil is the **longest acting** phosphodiesterase inhibitor.

434. Ans. (b) Inhibiting phosphodiesterase type 5

435. Ans. (c) Increased eye lashes hair growth

Ref: KDT, 6th ed. pg. 147

- Latanoprost is a prostaglandin analogue. It is stable long acting PGF2α derivative which is used for glaucoma.
- **MOA:** It works by increasing aqueous humor outflow.
- Other drugs act by similar mechanism: **Travoprost, bimatoprost**
- **Side effect:**
  - Latanoprost may increase the brown pigmentation in iris **(NOT corneal pigmentation)**, changing eye color to brown: Heterochromia iridis
  - It may also cause eyelashes to grow longer and thicker and darken in color
  - **Other side effects:** Stinging, burning, itching, swelling of the eye, redness of the eyelids, dry eyes.

436. Ans. (d) PG F2α

Ref: KD Tripathi, 6th ed. pg. 146 -47

- Low concentration of $PGF_{2\alpha}$ lowers intraocular tension without inducing ocular inflammation.
- It acts by increasing unveoscleral outflow.
- Latanoprost is a $PGF_{2\alpha}$ derivative. It has shown efficacy similar to timolol and the effect is well sustained over long-term. Therefore it has become the first choice drugs of glaucoma in developed countries.

Extra Mile

- PGE_2, PGI_2 TXA_2 has no role in glaucoma treatment.
- PGE_2 cause vasodilatation in most, but not all, vascular beds.
- PGI_2 is uniformly vasodilatory and is more potent hypotensive than PGE_2
- TXA_2 consistently produces vasoconstriction.

437. Ans. (c) Both mast cell stabilizer and antihistamine

Ref: Clinical Oculor Pharmacology, 1st ed. pg. 257

- **Olopatadine hydrochloride** is an antihistamine (as well as anticholinergic and mast cell stabilizer)
- It is used as eye drop to treat itching associated with allergic conjunctivitis.
- Side effects include headache, eye burning and/or stinging, blurred vision, dry eyes, foreign body sensation, hyperemia, keratitis and taste perversion.

438. Ans. (d) Ciclesonide

Ref: KDT, 6th ed. pg. 226

- **Hard steroids may include:** Difluprednate ophthalmic emulsion, Budesonide, prednisolone, betamethasone and dexamethasone.
- **Soft steroids may include** ***(Mn: CFL)*****:** Ciclesonide, Fluorometholone, Loteprednol etabonate
- **Ciclesonide:** Is an inhaled corticosteroid indicated for the maintenance treatment of asthma and as prophylactic therapy in adult and adolescent patients aged 12 years and older
- The soft steroids fluorometholone and loteprednol 0.5% are ideal for treatment of an acute inflammatory episode in dry eye.

439. Ans. (a) Anti-gout and Xanthine Oxidase inhibitor

Ref: Katzung's Pharmacology, 14th ed. pg. 662–63

- Febuxostat is a non-purine inhibitor of xanthine oxidase and thereby reduces the formation of xanthine and uric acid and is useful in management of gout.
- It is 80% absorbed following oral administration and extensively metabolized in the liver.
- All of the drug and its metabolites appear in the urine although less than 5% appears as unchanged drug. Because it is highly metabolized to inactive metabolites, no dosage adjustment is necessary for patients with renal impairment.

440. Ans. (b) Indomethacin

Ref: Katzung, 14th ed. pg. 648

- Primary gout is seen due to decreased uric acid excretion
- Secondary gout can be secondary to any cause causing hyperuricemia.
- **DOC for acute gout:** NSAID-DOC (Indomethacin), Colchicine and corticosteroids
  - **Colchicine** is fastest acting. It is NOT an anti-inflammatory drug but it specifically suppresses gout inflammation.
  - Not preferred over NSAID because of its side effects of GI upset.
- All NSAIDS can be given in acute gout EXCEPT aspirin as it competes with tubular excretion of uric acid leading to Hyperuricemia.
- **Probenecid:** Has uricosuric action
- **DOC for chronic gout:** Allopurinol

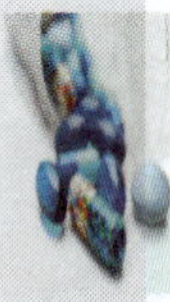

RENAL SYSTEM

441. Ans. (d) Na$^+$ K$^+$ 2Cl$^-$ symptorter inhibitor at loop of henle

Ref: Goodman and Gillman 13th ed. pg. 453

- The history of patient and shown image where clubbing and pedal edema are seen, is indicative of congestive heart failure.
- Preferred agent to reduce the congestion is loop diuretics, which acts by Na$^+$K^{+2}Cl blockade at thick ascending limb of loop of henle.

Extra Mile

- Ionotropic agent of choice in acute CHF: Dobutamine
- Other drugs used in heart failure:
  - Inotrope like: Dopamine, Dopexamine, Isoprenaline
  - PDE3 inhibitor (Inodilator): Amrinone, Milrinone, Enoximone
  - Cardiac glycoside: Digoxin
  - Vasodilators: Hydralazine, Sodium Nitroprusside.

442. Ans. (c) Acetazolamide

Ref: Katzung 14th ed. pg. 260-61

- Among the given options, Acetazolamide is the carbonic anhydrase (CA) inhibitor
- **Other agents under CA inhibitor:** Dorzolamide, Brinzolamide, Dichlorphenamide, Methazolamide
- **Site of action of CA inhibitor:** Proximal convoluted tubule

443. Ans. (b) Na$^+$ Cl pump in early DCT

Ref: Katzung 14th ed. pg. 264-65

- Hydrochlorthiazide is a thiazide diuretic, act at distal convoluted tubule by inhibiting Na$^+$ Cl$^-$ cotransporter in early part of DCT.
- **Other thiazide diuretics are:** Chlorthalidone, Indapamide, Metolazone
- **Thiazide diuretics** are preferred in hypertension and nephrogenic diabetes insipidus management.
- **Note:** Loop diuretics act at thick ascending limb of loop of Henle by inhibiting Na$^+$K$^+$2Cl cotransporter.

444. Ans. (b) Desmopressin

Ref: Katzung 14th ed. pg. 682

- Desmopressin is a long acting synthetic analogue of vasopressin
- DOC for neurogenic/pituitary diabetes insipidus: Desmopression
- **Note:** Desmopressin is also used for treatment of Hemophilia A and von Willebrand disease, nocturnal enuresis.

Extra Mile

- DOC for nephrogenic diabetes insipidus: Thiazide diuretics
- Conivaptan and Tolvaptan: Vasopressin receptor antagonist. DOC for SIADH (Syndrome of Inappropriate Anti Diuretic Hormone). Also approved to be used in heart failure for free water clearance and in hyponatremia.

445. Ans. (c) Thiazides

Ref: Goodman & Gillman's 13th ed. pg. 466

- Nephrogenic DI may be congenital or acquired. Causes can be:
  - Hypercalcemia, hypokalemia, postobstructive renal failure, Li+, foscarnet, clozapine, demeclocycline, and other drugs can induce nephrogenic DI.
- Thiazide *diuretics* reduce the polyuria of patients with DI and often are used to treat nephrogenic DI.
- **DOC for central diabetes insipidus:** Desmopressin (V2 receptor agonist)
- **DOC for nephrogenic diabetes insipidus:** Thiazide diuretics.
- **DOC for lithium induced diabetes insipidus:** Amiloride

446. Ans. (b) Decrease placental circulation

Ref: http://www.ncbi.nlm.nih.gov/pmc/articles/PMC 2628835

- Diuretics causes massive fluid loss via urine, which causes decreased volume and thereby decreases placental circulation. This might compromise fetal blood supply.
- Option A: Diuretics do not increase vascular resistance, instead it decreases the resistance.
- Option C: No maternal distress. However fetal stress is a possibility
- Option D: There have been few reported cases of birth defects associated with diuretic use.

447. Ans. (b) Carbonic anhydrase inhibitor

Ref: Katzung's, 11th ed. pg. 416

- **Acetazolamide** is a carbonic anhydrase inhibitor which acts on the proximal tubule of nephron.
- **In kidney,** it inhibits H$^+$ secretion and HCO_3 reabsorption, which inturn reduces sodium reabsorption.
- In eye, it reduces the aqueous formation by limiting generation of bicarbonate ion in ciliary epithelium.

448. Ans. (b) V2

Ref: Katzung's 11th ed. p-658–659

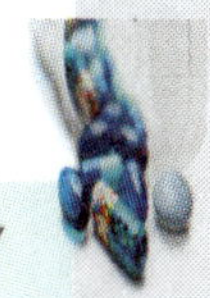

TABLE: Vasopressin receptor location and functions

Receptor	Localization	Functions	
V1a	Vascular smooth muscle Platelets Hepatocytes Myometrium	Vasoconstriction, myocardial hypertrophy Platelet aggregation Glycogenolysis Uterine contraction	
V1b*	Anterior pituitary	ACTH release	
V2	Basolateral membrane collecting tubule	Insertion of AQP2 water channels into apical membrane, induction of AQP2 synthesis	Free water reabsorption
	Vascular endothelium Vascular smooth muscle	vWF and factor 8 release Vasodilatation	
*Termed V3 in some classification schemes.			

TABLE: Hormones from posterior pituitary

Antidiuretic hormone (ADH)/ Vasopressin	Increase water reabsorption by the kidneys and cause vasoconstriction and increased blood pressure. Acts on V2 receptor. **Note:** V1b is also known as V3 receptor
Oxytocin	***Stimulates milk ejection*** from breasts and uterine contractions

449. Ans. (d) All of these

Ref: Katzung, 14th ed. pg. 775–776

- Vitamin D has been used in treating renal osteodystrophy
- In mild forms of malabsorption, vitamin D should suffice to raise serum levels of 25(OH)D into the normal range. Many patients with severe disease do not respond to vitamin D.
- Calcitriol and **Calcidiol** have been used successfully in treatment of renal osteodystrophy and intestinal osteodystrophy.

450. Ans. (c) Indapamide

Ref: KDT, 6th ed. pg. 540

Indapamide is a thiazide diuretic

Diuretic class	Drugs	MOA	Site of action
Osmotic diuretic	Mannitol	Inhibit water and solute reabsorption	All part of tubule, but mainly proximal tubule
Loop diuretics	Furosemide Torsemide	Inhibit Na^+-K^+-$2Cl^-$ co-transport	Thick ascending loop of henle
Thiazide diuretic	Hydrochlorthiazide Benzthiazide Chlorthalidone Indapamide	Inhibit Na^+- Cl^- co-transport	Distal tubule
K^+ sparing diuretic	Spironolactone Triamterene Amiloride	Decrease Na^+ reabsorption Decrease K^+ secretion	Collecting tubule
Carbonic anhydrase inhibitor	Acetazolamide	Inhibit H^+ secretion and HCO_3 reabsorption, which reduces Na^+ reabsorption	Proximal tubule

451. Ans. (a) Thiazide diuretics

Ref: KDT, 6th ed. pg. 540

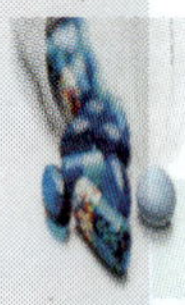

- **Drugs under thiazide diuretics:** Hydrochlorthiazide, chlorthalidone, bendroflumethiazide, indapamide and metazolone.
- **Thiazide diuretics act on DCT by blocking Na^+ Cl channel**
- In cases of initial management of CKD *(stage 1 & 2)*, thiazide diuretics is preferred and is considered as drug of choice, preferably Metazolone *(has anti-hypertensive action)* and indapamide.
- Patients with stages 1 and 2 are comparatively higher than the advanced stages.
- *However, thiazide diuretics are NOT given if serum creatinine is more than 2.5 or GFR is less than 60 ml/min.*
- Thiazide diuretics have limited utility in stages 3–5 CKD, such that administration of loop diuretics, including furosemide, bumetanide, or torsemide, may also be needed. *(Harrison's 18th ed. Ch 280)*
- The combination of loop diuretics with metolazone, which inhibits the sodium chloride co-transporter of the distal convoluted tubule, can help effect renal salt excretion. Ongoing diuretic resistance with intractable edema and hypertension in advanced CKD may serve as an indication to initiate dialysis.

Indapamide is longer acting and more potent than hydrochlorthiazide. It is *effective as an antihypertensive at lower doses than those required for the diuretic effect* (due to its direct vasodilatory action). It also produces less metabolic adverse effects (hypokalemia, hyperglycemia, hyperuricemia etc.) and can be used as an antihypertensive in diabetic patients (whereas other thiazides are contra-indicated).

RESPIRATORY SYSTEM

452. Ans. (d) Leukotriene antagonist

Ref: Goodman and Gillman 13th ed. pg. 741

- Leukotriene antagonist like Montelukast, Zafirlukast can be used in allergic conditions like allergic rhinitis and in prophylaxis of bronchial asthma.
- It is not used in acute bronchial asthma attack.
- Book states: *"In patients with severe asthma who are not controlled on high doses of ICS and LABA, anti-LTs do not appear to provide any additional benefit"*

453. Ans. (d) Hydrocortisone

- Steroids in bronchial asthma act by inhibiting PL-A2, and produces anti-inflammatory effect.
- Steroids do not cause bronchodilation. However, they increase the sensitivity of beta 2 receptors for salbutamol.
- Other agents like salbutamol, ipratropium and deriphyllin has Bronchodilating property.

454. Ans. (a) Rotahaler

- The shown device is known as rotahaler, which is used for delivering dry powder, in conditions like bronchial asthma and COPD.

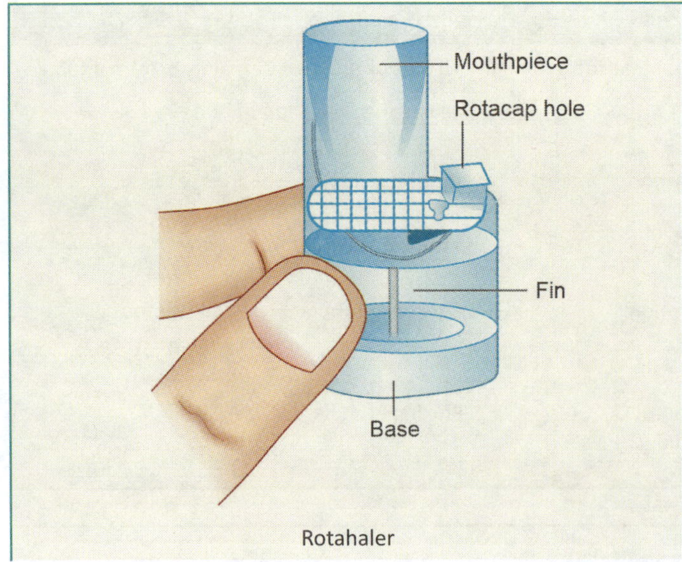

Rotahaler

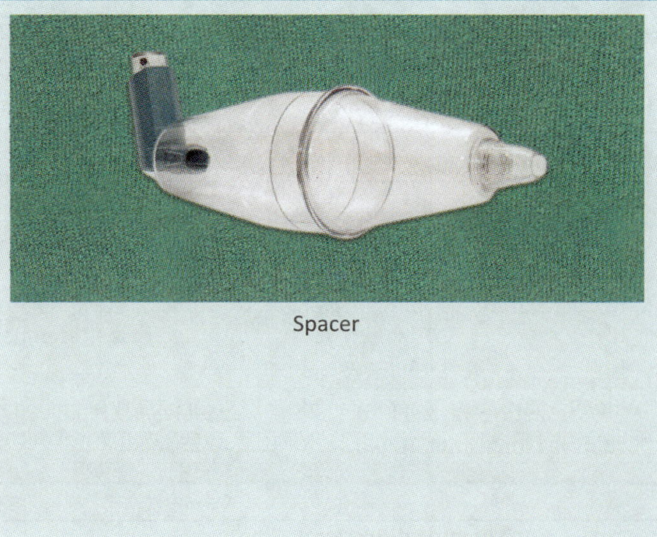

Spacer

Contd...

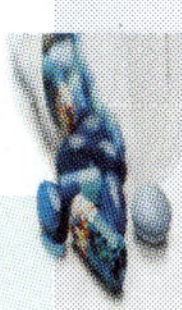

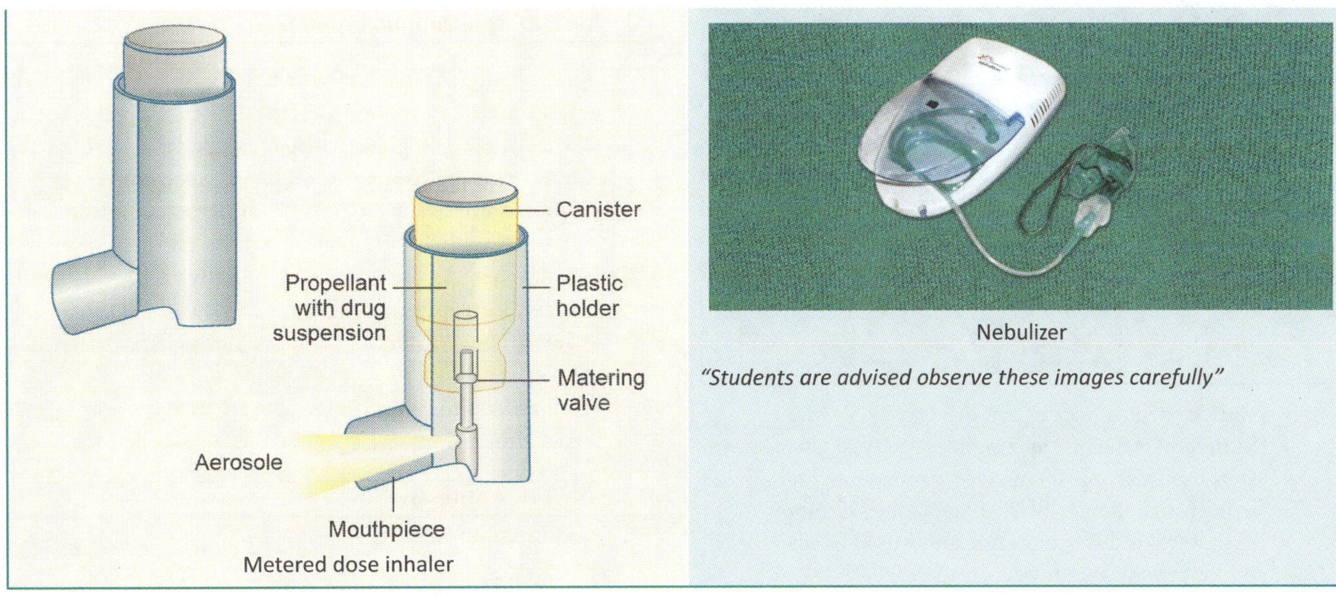

Metered dose inhaler

Nebulizer

"Students are advised observe these images carefully"

455. Ans. (c) Theophylline

Ref: Katzung 14th ed. pg. 352, 1172

- Erythromycin is an enzyme inhibitor and it will increase the risk of toxicity of drugs following zero order kinetics.
- Theophylline is one of the methylxanthines, used in bronchial asthma, follows zero order kinetics.

Clinical effects of theophylline intoxication

Clinical		Laboratory
CNS	Agitation, hyperreflexia, tremor, ataxia, seizures	Hypercalcemia Hypokalemia
GI	Nausea, vomiting, diarrhea, abdominal	Metabolic acidosis with respiratory alkalosis
CV	Sinus tachycardia, hypotension, volume depletion, supraventricular tachycardia, ventricular tachycardia, cardiac arrest	
Pulm	Tachypnea	

456. Ans. (d) DEC

Ref: Harrison's 19th ed. pg. 422, 1687

- Eosinophilia is the presence of >500 eosinophils per μL of blood and is common in many settings besides parasite infection.
- **Common causes of eosinophilia are:**
  - Allergic reaction to drugs (Iodides, aspirin, sulfonamides, nitrofurantoin, penicillins, and cephalosporins).
  - Allergies such as hay fever, asthma, eczema, serum sickness, allergic vasculitis, and pemphigus are associated with eosinophilia.
  - Collagen vascular disease like rheumatoid arthritis.
- Tropical eosinophilia is usually caused by filarial infection.
- Tropical eosinophilia due to *Wuchereria bancrofti* or *Brugia malayi* occurs most commonly in Southern Asia, Africa, and South America.
- **Drug of choice:** Diethylcarbamazine.

457. Ans. (c) Ambroxol

Ref: KDT 6th ed. pg. 214

- Ambroxol is a metabolite of bromhexine having mucolytic action.
- Antitussives are drugs that act in the CNS to raise the threshold of cough centre.
- Since antitussives aim to control rather than eliminate cough they are used only for dry unproductive cough or if cough is unduly tiring, disturbs sleep or is hazardous.

Mucolytics	Antitussives
Bromhexine Ambroxol Acetylcysteine Carbocisteine	Opioids Codeine Pholcodeine Nonopioids Noscapine Dextromethorphan Chlophedianol

458. Ans. (c) Salmetrol

Ref: KDT 6th ed. pg. 218

- β_2 agonist is the drug of choice for acute attack of bronchial asthma.
- Other β_2 Agonists

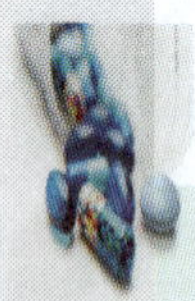

SABA (Short acting β2 agonist)	Salbutamol Terbutaline	Used for acute attack of BA
LABA (Long acting β_2 agonist)	**Salmeterol**-slow onset of action, long duration of action **Formeterol**-fast onset of action, long duration of action **Indacaterol**-fast OOA and long DOA	Used for prophylaxis of BA

- **DOC** for acute attack of asthma: SALBUTAMOL
- **Salmeterol** is the first long acting selective β_2 agonist with slow onset of action. It is used as maintenance therapy and for nocturnal therapy BUT not for acute symptoms.
- **Formeterol** is fast acting and can be used in acute attack and for prophylaxis as well.
- **Theophylline** is a phosphodiesterase inhibitor. In acute attack sustained release oral form can be given.

459. Ans. (a) Slow acting β_2 agonist

Ref: KD Tripathi, 6th ed. pg. 227

TABLE: Treatment of choice

Severe asthma	Status asthmaticus/ refractory asthma
• Continuous symptoms; activity limitation; frequent exacerbations/ hospitalization • Regular high dose inhaled steroid + • Inhaled long-acting β_2 agonist (salmeterol) twice daily • Rescue treatment with short acting inhaled β_2 agonist	• Any patient of asthma has the potential to develop acute severe asthma which may be lifethreatning. • Hydrocortisone hemisuccinate 100 mg • Nebulized salbutamol + ipratropium bromide • High flow humidified oxygen inhalation • Salbutamol/terbutaline in order to reach smaller bronchi

460. Ans. (b) Oropharyngeal candidiasis

- Most of the side effects of steroids are mainly hoarseness, orophyrangeal candidiasis, decreased growth in children with adrenal suppression.
- The plausible explanation is that since these drugs are inhaled, they avoid the first pass metabolism that orally administered steroids undergo and hence have preponderance to cause the usual manifestations of steroid toxicity.

461. Ans. (a) Ipratropium bromide

Ref: Katzung Pharmacology, 10th ed. Ch 10

- Ipratropium bromide is an anti-cholinergic agent/ Muscarinic antagonists which competitively inhibit the effect of acetylcholine at muscarinic receptors.
- **Ipratropium** appears to be at least as effective in patients with COPD that includes a partially reversible component. A longer-acting, selective anti-muscarinic agent, **tiotropium,** is DOC for COPD.
- **Salbutamol and terbutaline** are β_2 agonist, used in acute cases of asthma.
- **Salmetrol is slow acting** β_2 agonist, used for prophylaxis of asthma.

462. Ans. (a) Antitussive

Ref: KDT, 6th ed. pg. 215

- Forceful expulsion of air from lungs due to pulmonary irritation is called coughing. It can be productive or non-productive.
- **Antitussive** is a class of drug which ***relieves coughing by suppressing cough center.*** These drugs are mainly used for dry cough. Examples of antitussives are:
  - **Opioids:** Codeine, Phalcodeine, Ethylmorphine
  - **Non-Opioids:** NOSCAPINE, Dextromethorphan
- **Expectorants** are class of drugs that increase bronchial secretion or reduce its viscosity (mucolytics). They are mainly used in productive cough. Examples of expectorants are:
  - **Mucolytics:** Bromhexeine, Ambroxol
  - **Bronchial secretion enhancers:** Guaiphenisine, sodium or potassium citrate.

463. Ans. (a) Cough center

Please refer to above explanation.

464. Ans. (b) Inhibits 5-lipoxygenase

- Leukotrienes are biochemical mediators that contribute to asthma symptoms
  - Contracting airway smooth muscle
  - Increasing vascular permeability and mucus secretion
  - Attracting and activating airway inflammatory cells
- **Zileuton is a 5-lipoxygenase inhibitor that decreases leukotriene production,** and zafirlukast and montelukast are cysteinyl leukotriene receptor antagonists.
- They are useful to prevent asthma attacks and cause modest improvements in lung function. They lessen the need for β_2-agonist rescue therapy.

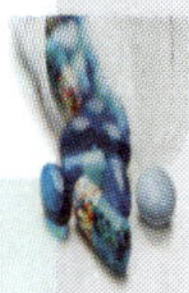

GIT

465. Ans. (a) Loperamide

Ref: Goodman and Gillman 13th ed. pg. 931-32

- The given case is a patient of Traveler's diarrhea.
- Loperamide is an opioid, which reduces the intestinal motility and it remains the antimotility agent of choice for traveler's diarrhea.
- In addition to its anti-peristaltic effect, it has also been shown to increase the intestinal absorption of fluid and electrolytes.
- When used as sole therapy, loperamide provides relief for mild to moderate diarrhea (up to five loose stools per day with or without mild cramping pain), in comparison to either a placebo or bismuth subsalicylate.

Extra Mile

- Rifaximin is an agent used in irritable bowel syndrome
- Octreotide can be used in secretary diarrhea
- Zinc is a supplemental/add-on drug given in infective diarrhea and secretary diarrhea along with other drugs.

466. Ans. (c) Palonosetron

- DOC for chemo induced nausea and vomiting: 5HT3 antagonist (Ondansetron, Granisetron).
- DOC for chemo induced delayed vomiting: NK1 antagonist: Aprepitant, Rolapitant, Netupitant

467. Ans. (a) Lactulose

Ref: Goodman & Gillman 13th ed. pg. 928, 940

USES OF LACTULOSE

- Constipation caused by opioids
- Idiopathic chronic constipation
- Lactulose also used to treat hepatic encephalopathy

LACTULOSE IN HEPATIC ENCEPHALOPATHY

- Impaired liver function/severe liver disease are unable to detoxify the ammonia coming from colon which is produced by colonic bacterial metabolism of fecal urea.
- The drop in luminal pH that accompanies hydrolysis to short-chain fatty acids in the colon results in "trapping" of the ammonia by its conversion to the polar ammonium ion.
- Combined with the increase in colonic transit, this therapy significantly lowers circulating ammonia levels. The therapeutic goal in this condition is to give sufficient amounts of lactulose (usually 20–30 g three to four times per day) to produce two to three soft stools a day with a pH of 5–5.5.

468. Ans. (a) Antacid

Ref: Katzung's, 14th ed. pg. 1089

- This medication is used to treat symptoms caused by too much stomach acid such as heartburn, upset stomach, or indigestion.
- It is an antacid that works by lowering the amount of acid in the stomach.
- It can also be used in renal osteodystrophy with hyperphosphatemia, hypocalcemia and osteoporosis like conditions.
- It can cause metabolic alkalosis (Milk-alkali syndrome)

469. Ans. (c) Proton pump inhibitors like Omeprazole

Ref: KDT, 6th ed. pg. 632

- Proton pump inhibitors (PPIs) are the drugs of choice for peptic ulcer disease (PUD) due to any etiology (even NSAID induced).
- PPIs are also the agents of choice for gastroesophageal reflux disease (GERD) and Zollinger Ellison Syndrome (ZES).
- **Misoprosotol:** Specific agent for NSAID induced ulcer.

470. Ans. (c) Hyoscine

Ref: KD Tripathi, 6th ed. pg. 641, 642, 644, 646

HYOSINE

- It is the most effective drug for motion sickness.
- Suitable only for short brisk journies.
- It act by blocking conduction of nerve impulses in the pathway leading from the vestibular apparatus to the vomiting centre and is *not effective in vomiting of other etiologies.*

ONDANSETRON

- It is considered as the drug of choice for drug induced vomiting.
- Used mainly to control cancer chemotherapy induced vomiting.
- Effective in postoperative nausea and vomiting as well.

METOCLOPRAMIDE

- It is an effective and popular drug for many types of vomiting like: Postoperative, drug induced, disease associated (especially migraine), radiation sickness, etc.

CHLORPROMAZINE

- These are from typical antipsychotic having potent antiemetic action; act by blocking D2 receptors in the CTZ.

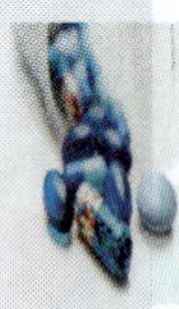

- They have broad spectrum antiemetic action effective in:
  - Drug induced and postanaesthetic nausea and vomiting
  - Diease induced vomiting
  - Malignancy associated and cancer chemotherapy induced vomiting
  - Radiation sickness vomiting and morning sickness.

471. Ans. (b) Hyoscine

Ref: KDT, 6th ed. pg. 646-47

472. Ans. (a) Anti-motility drugs are drug of choice for infective diarrhea

Ref: KDT, 6th ed. pg. 664

- All Anti-motility drugs are contraindicated in infective diarrhea. These are indicated only in non-infective secretory diarrhea.

Extra Mile

- Loperamide is a non-addictive over the counter anti-diarrheal drug.
- **Diphenoxylate** is an opioid but has addictive potential if used for prolonged periods. It is always given in combination **with atropine to prevent the abuse** (atropine will produce dry mouth and other anticholinergic side effects).
- Opioids are used as anti-motility drugs used in secretory diarrhea.

HEMATOLOGY AND VITAMINS

473. Ans. (c) Warfarin

Ref: Goodman and Gillman 13th ed. pg. 594

- Warfarin is an anticoagulant which act as competitive inhibitor of vitamin K dependent factors.
- Exposure of warfarin in first trimester can lead to Fetal warfarin syndrome/Contradi Syndrome. It is characterized by features like: Nasal Hypoplasia, Chondrodysplasia puncta, bone and cartilage defect.

Anti-coagulants use in Pregnancy (ACC/AHA Guidelines):

- **Week 0–12:** Heparin
- **Week 13–36:** Warfarin
- **Week >36:** Switch to heparin/LMWH
- **Onset of labor:** Stop heparin
- **If normal delivery:** Start LMWH after 6 hours
- **If caesarean delivery:** Start LMWH after 24 days
- **After 7 days post-partum:** Switch to warfarin

474. Ans. (c) Clopidogrel

Ref: Goodman and Gillman 13th ed. pg. 597

- In patients with myocardial infarction, dual anti platelet therapy with aspirin and P_2Y_{12} inhibitor like clopidogrel or prasugrel has shown to have better efficacy.
- Studies shows that the combination of clopidogrel plus aspirin is superior to aspirin alone for prevention of recurrent ischemia in patients with unstable angina.
- The current guidelines recommend use of dual anti platelet therapy for 12 months in all patients with acute coronary syndrome.

475. Ans. (c) Inhibition of cyclo-oxygenase -1 enzyme

Ref: Goodman and Gillman 13th ed. pg. 596

- The anti-platelet activity of aspirin act by inhibiting COX_1 enzyme
- Option a: Fibrinolytic agents are tPA: Streptokinase
- Option b: Vitamin K dependent factors inhibitor: Warfarin
- Option d: P_2Y_{12} inhibitors are Clopidogrel, Prasugrel

476. Ans. (a) Fibrinolysis

- tPA like streptokinase, Urokinase are fibrinolytic agent, act by activating plasminogen to plasmin which causes fibrinolysis.

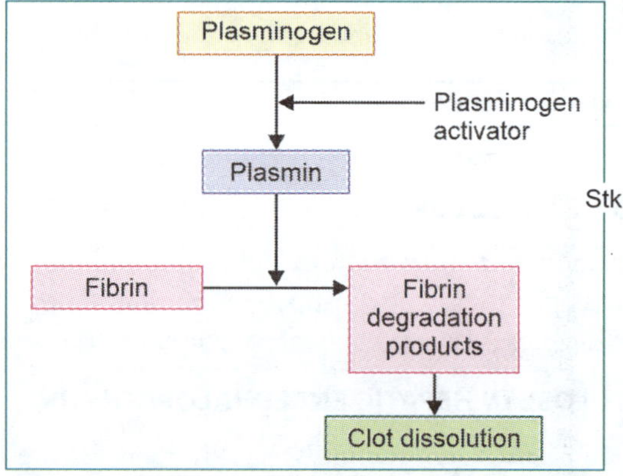

477. Ans. (c) Switch warfarin to heparin

- Warfarin is teratogenic agent. Therefore, it is contraindicated in first trimester in pregnancy.
- Warfarin leads to contradi syndrome/fetal warfarin syndrome where there is bone and facial defect like nasal septum and cartilage defect.
- So, it is advised for the patient to stop warfarin and switch to heparin.
- AHA guidelines discussed above

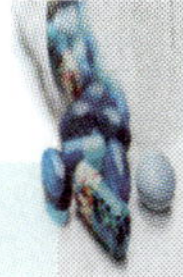

478. Ans. (c) Vitamin C

- Absorption of iron is increased at acidic pH. Ascorbic acid provides the acidic pH needed for absorption of iron.
- **Factors increasing absorption of iron:**
  - Acid
  - Vitamin C
- **Factors decreasing absorption of iron:**
  - Phytates
  - Oxalates
  - Tannates

479. Ans. (b) Inhibit TXA2 formation

Ref: KDT, 6th ed. pg. 609; Katzung, 14th ed. pg. 620

- ASPIRIN has an antiplatelet effect by inhibiting the production of thromboxane.
- Thromboxane, normally helps in platelet aggregation.
- TXA_2 formation is suppressed even at very low doses **of aspirin.**
- Aspirin acts as COX inhibitor. It doesn't inhibit PGI_2 formation.
- TEUROTROBAN–TXA_2 receptor antagonist.

480. Ans. (a) Warfarin

Ref: Katzung 14th ed. pg. 614-15

- After valve replacement, anti-coagulant like warfarin is started to avoid any thrombotic episode.
- Warfarin is an oral anti-coagulant, used for prophylactic purposes, NOT in emergencies.
- **Example of prophylactic uses are:**
  - Prevention of venous thrombosis and associated pulmonary embolism
  - Prevention of thromboembolism in patients with prosthetic heart valves
  - Prevention of thrombosis during atrial fibrillation
- Note: Warfarin act by inhibiting Vitamin K dependent clotting factors (factor 2, 7, 9, 10)

481. Ans. (c) Thiopentone sodium

Ref: Goodman and Gillman 13th ed. pg. 392

- Barbiturates are contraindicated in porphyria.
- Barbiturate induces ALA synthase, which is the rate limiting enzyme in porphyrin synthesis)

Extra Mile

- Drugs that can precipitate Acute intermittent porphyria:
  - Phenytoin, Primidone
  - Rifampicin
  - OCP
  - Barbiturate
  - Sulphonamide

482. Ans. (d) Deferoxamine

Ref: Goodman Gillman 13th ed. pg. 1313

ACUTE IRON TOXICITY

- Seen mainly in young child with at least 10 tablets ingestion
- **Symptoms:** Necrotizing gastroenteritis with vomiting, abdominal pain, and bloody diarrhea followed by shock, lethargy, and dyspnea.
- **Treatment:**
  - Whole bowel irrigation
  - **Deferoxamine** (IV)- chelating agent → promote its excretion
  - Note: Activated charcoal is ineffective
  - **Oral: DEFERIPRONE** and **DEFERASIROX- can be used in t/t of Hemochromatosis, iron overload in thalassemia**

483. Ans. (a) Dabigatran

Ref: Katzung 14th ed. pg. 618

Thrombin Inhibitors

- **Indirect: Act by targeting thrombin by increasing the activity of AT3 ~ 1000 times**
  - Heparin, LMWH (Enoxaparin, Dalteparin, Tinzaparin, Parnaparin)
  - Preferred Route: S.C.
- **Direct: By targeting thrombin directly**
  - Inj: (Hirudin, Lepirudin, Bivalirudin, Argatroban, Melagatran)
  - Oral: Dabigatran
  - Note: Antidote of dabigatran toxicity: **Idarucizumab**

484. Ans. (c) Warfarin

Ref: Goodman & Gillman 13th ed. pg. 593-94

- Warfarin (one of coumarin derivative) is an oral antagonist acts by antagonizing vitamin K dependent factors.
- Vitamin K dependent clotting factor: II, VII, IX, X
- Vitamin K dependent anticlotting factors: Protein C and Protein S
- Warfarin is administered as a racemic mixture of *S*- and *R*-warfarin.
- *S*-Warfarin is 3- to 5-fold more potent than *R*-warfarin and is mainly metabolized by CYP2C9.
- Because of the long t½ of coagulation factors, the anti-thrombotic action of warfarin is achieved in 4–5 days

SIDE EFFECTS

- Bleeding: Most common side effect (risk high if INR >4)
- Birth defect and abortion if administered during pregnancy (fetal warfarin syndrome)

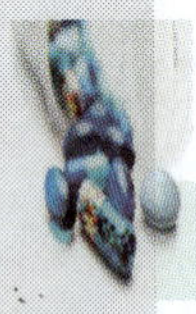

- **Skin necrosis/Coumarin necrosis:** Can occur 3–10 days after initiation of warfarin. Usually due to protein C and S deficiency
- Purple toe syndrome-blue tinged discoloration of plantar surface and side of toes, that blanches with pressure. Can occur 3–8 weeks after initiation of therapy.

485. Ans. (a) Apixaban

Ref: Goodman & Gillman 13th ed. pg. 595

- Factor Xa inhibition results in reduced thrombin generation → suppression of platelet generation and fibrin formation.
- Factor Xa inhibitor drugs are: Rivaroxaban, Apixaban, Edoxaban
- Dose of apixaban: 5 mg BD
- **Use:**
  - Stroke prevention in patients with atrial fibrillation
  - Deep vein thrombosis, Pulmonary embolism
  - Postoperative thromboprophylaxis is patients undergoing hip/knee surgery
- Contraindicated for stroke prevention in patients with mechanical heart valve
- **Side effects:**
  - **Bleeding**- MC side effect. Incidence 50% lesser than warfarin induced bleeding except GI bleed.
    - (GI bleed: Apixaban, Rivaroxaban > Warfarin)
- **Antidote:** Andexanet Alfa, Ciraparantag

486. Ans. (b) Filgrastim

Ref: Goodman & Gillman 13th ed. pg. 756

- Filgrastim is G-CSF (Granulocyte Colony Stimulating Factor)
- The principal action of filgrastim is the stimulation of CFU-G to increase neutrophil production
- Forms of G-CSF are now available, including two longer-acting pegylated forms, pegfilgrastim and lipegfilgrastim.
- **Use:**
  - Severe neutropenia after autologous hematopoietic stem cell transplantation
  - Neutropenia after high dose cancer chemotherapy
  - Congenital neutropenia
  - Neutropenia of any other cause
- **Dose:** 1–20 μg/kg/day via IV or subcutaneous route
- **Side effect:** Mild-to-moderate bone pain

487. Ans. (b) Deferoxamine

Ref: Goodman & Gillman's 13th ed. pg. 63, 1314

- Iron chelating agent is: Deferoxamine

TABLE: Antidotes of different poisoning

Poisoning indication(s)	Antidote
Acetaminophen	Acetylcysteine
Organophosphorus and carbamate pesticides	Atropine sulfate
Drug-induced dystonia	Benztropine
Na^+ channel blocking drugs	Bicarbonate, sodium
Neuroleptic malignant syndrome	Dantrolene
Ca^{2+} channel blocking drugs, fluoride	Calcium gluconate or chloride
Valproate hyperammonemia	Carnitine
Malignant hyperthermia	Dantrolene
Iron	Deferoxamine
Cardiac glycosides	Digoxin immune Fab
Drug-induced dystonia	Diphenhydramine
Lead, mercury, arsenic	Dimercaprol (BAL)
Lead	EDTA, $CaNa_2$
Methanol, ethylene glycol	Fomepizole/Ethanol
Benzodiazepines	Flumazenil
β adrenergic antagonists	Glucagon hydrochloride
Cyanide	Hydroxocobalamin hydrochloride
Hyperkalemia	Insulin (High dose)
Methotrexate	Leucovorin calcium
Methemoglobinemia	Methylene blue
Opioids	Naloxone hydrochloride
Sulfonylurea-induced hypoglycemia	Octreotide acetate
Carbon monoxide	Oxygen, hyperbaric
Copper	D-Penicillamine
Anticholinergic syndrome	Physostigmine salicylate
Isoniazid seizures	Pyridoxine hydrochloride
Coumarin, indanedione	Vitamin K_1 (Phytonadione)

488. Ans. (b) Vitamin K antagonist

Ref: KD Tripathi, 7th ed. pg. 620, 621

- Warfarin and its congeners act as anticoagulants only in vivo (body), NOT in vitro (lab).
- It acts by inhibiting Vitamin K. Due to overdose, hematuria is the *first manifestation* noted.
- Dose monitoring is done by INR
- Antidote of warfarin overdose: Vitamin K

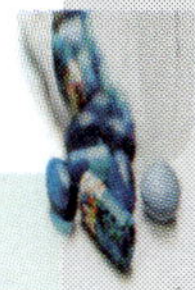

489. Ans. (c) Heparin toxicity

Ref: KD Tripathi, 7th ed. pg. 618-620

PT (Prothrombin Time)	aPTT (Activated Partial Thromboplastin Time)
• Assess activity of extrinsic coagulation pathway. • Used when on warfarin treatment. • WePT: Warfarin for extrinsic; PT value assessed.	• Assess activity of intrinsic coagulation pathway. • Used while on heparin treatment. • ***HINT: Heparin for Intrinsic; aPTT value assessed.***

490. Ans. (c) Factor II

Ref: KD Tripathi, 7th ed. pg. 620

- Direct thrombin inhibitors are a class of medication that act as anticoagulants (delaying blood clotting) by **directly inhibiting the enzyme thrombin (factor II).**
- **Argatroban** is a synthetic non-peptide compound which **binds reversibly to the catalytic site of thrombin,** but not to the substrate recognition site.
- Administered by IV infusion, it can be used in place of lepirudin for short-term indications in patients with heparin-induced thrombocytopenia.
- **Other direct thrombin inhibitors are:**
  - PARENTERAL ROUTE: **Lepirudin, Bivaluridin, Desirudin**
  - Oral rote: **Dabigatran**
- Note: Heparin is indirect thrombin inhibitor which acts by antithrombin 3 mediated inhibition of factor IIa and Xa.

491. Ans. (d) Heparin

Ref: KD Tripathi, 6th ed. pg. 597

- Heparin is a powerful and instantaneously acting anticoagulant, effective both in vivo and in vitro.
- It acts indirectly by *activating* plasma antithrombin III
- The heparin -AT III complex then binds to clotting factors of the intrinsic and common pathways (Xa, IIa, IXa, XIa, XIIa and XIIIa) and inactivates them.
- **Heparin is the anticoagulant of choice in pregnancy**
- Warfarin on the other hand is effective only in vivo (body). It acts by inhibiting vitamin K.

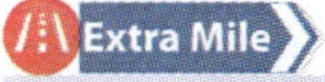

Heparin is monitored by aPTT
Low molecular heparin inhibits factor X_a only. It does not require monitoring because of consistent bioavailability.
Antidote for heparin overdose: Protamine Sulfate.
Warfarin monitoring is done by: INR
Antidote of warfarin overdose: Vitamin K.
TOC for warfarin induced bleeding: FFP

492. Ans. (c) Lepirudin

Ref: Katzung's, 11th ed. pg. 593-594

- Heparin is a powerful and instantaneously acting anticoagulant, effective both in vivo and in vitro.
- It acts indirectly by *activating* plasma antithrombin III
- The heparin -AT III complex then binds to clotting factors of the intrinsic and common pathways (Xa, IIa, IXa, XIa, XIIa and XIIIa) and inactivates them.
- **HIT syndrome** is a condition which arises as a potential side effect of heparin use where heparin binds with platelet factor 4 and causes thrombocytopenia *(usually seen 3–4 days after heparin use).*
- **To treat this condition, direct thrombin inhibitors are used. Drugs under direct thrombin inhibitors are: Lepirudin, bivalirudin, hirudin, dabigatran, argatroban, melagatran.**

Extra Mile

- Enoxaparin: It is low molecular weight heparin
- Warfarin is oral anticoagulant, which act by inhibiting vitamin K dependent clotting factors (Factor II, VII, IX, X).

493. Ans. (c) Used as first line treatment in bleeding conditions

Ref: KDT, 6th ed. pg. 594, 595

VITAMIN K

- It is a fat-soluble dietary principle required for the synthesis of clotting factors.
- ***Action:*** Vit. K acts as a cofactor at a late stage in the synthesis of coagulation proteins prothrombin, factors VII. IX and X.
- ***Utilization:*** Fat-soluble forms-absorbed from the intestine via lymph; while water-soluble forms are absorbed directly into portal blood.
- **Vitamin K has 3 forms:**
  - K_1- fat soluble: Phytonadione
  - K_2- fat soluble: Menaquinone, Acetomenaphthone
  - K_3- water soluble: *Menadione sod. Bisulfate and Diphosphate*
- ***Use:*** vit K is used in prophylaxis (NOT as first line treatment)and treatment of bleeding due to deficiency of clotting factors in the following situations:
  - *Dietary deficiency*
  - *Prolonged antimicrobial therapy*
  - *Obstructive jaundice or malabsorption syndrome*
  - *Liver disease (cirohosis, viral hepatitis)*
  - *Newborns*
  - *Overdose of oral anticoagulants*

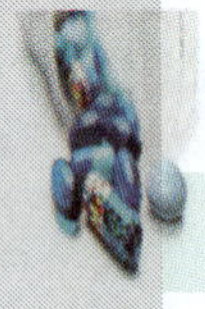

- In case of bleeding disorders, stop the anticoagulant immediately and fresh frozen plasma is recommended.

494. Ans. (d) Tranexamic acid

Ref: KDT, 6th ed. pg. 608

- Antiplatelet drugs interfere with platelet function and are useful in prophylaxis of thromboembolic disorders.
- Platelets express several glycoprotein (GP) receptors on their surface like GP IIa/IIIb.
- These receptors are not exposed normally, but once exposed due to some injury they make the platelets sticky.
- Upon injury thromboxane A2 (TXA2) and ADP produced, which expose the sticky receptors (GP IIa/IIIb) that crosslinks the platelets, inducing aggregation.
- Prostacyclin (PGI2) synthesized in the intima of blood vessel is an inhibitor of TXA2. Normally, a balance between PGI2 and TXA2 is required to control thrombus formation.

TABLE: Antiplatelet drugs and their target of inhibition

Antiplatelet drugs	Target of inhibition
Aspirin	Inhibit TXA2
Clopidogrel and Ticlodipine	Inhibit ADP irreversibly by binding with P2Y12 receptor
Cangrelor, Ticagrelor	Inhibit ADP reversibly
Abciximab Tirofiban Eptifibatide	Inhibit GP IIb/IIIa

Extra Mile

Fibrin is associated with clotting. Agents which lyse this fibrin is known as Fibrinolytics.
Overdose of fibrinolytic agents causes results in excessive intravascular fibrinolysis resulting in bleeding.
Tranexamic acid is a specific antidote for fibrinolytic agents.
Antifibrinolytic drugs are:

- Epsilon Amino Caproic acid (EACA)
- Tranexamic acid

495. Ans. (d) Thromboxane

Ref: KDT, 6th ed. pg. 609; Katzung, 9th ed. pg. 446

Thromboxane helps in platelet aggregation.

- TXA_2 formation is suppressed at very low doses **of aspirin.**
- Aspirin blocks thromboxane formation by inhibiting COX activity by enzyme COX1 and TX- synthase irreversibly.

496. Ans. (b) Inhibit TXA2 formation

Ref: KDT, 6th ed. pg. 609; Katzung 9th ed. pg. 446

Please refer to above explanation

497. Ans. (a) Inhibit antithrombin 3

Ref: KD Tripathi, 6th ed. pg. 597

- Heparin is a powerful and instantaneously acting anticoagulant, effective both in vivo and in vitro.
- It acts indirectly by *activating* plasma antithrombin III. Antithrombin mediated inhibition of factor IIa and Xa mainly.
  - The heparin –AT III complex then binds to clotting factos of the intrinsic and common pathways (Xa, IIa, IXa, XIa, XIIa and XIIIa) and inactivates them.
- Warfarin on the other hand effective only in vivo (body). it act by inhibiting vitamin K.

Extra Mile

Heparin is monitored by aPTT (*remembered as HINT:* ***Heparin-Intrinsic***)
Low molecular heparin inhibits factor X_a only. It doesn't require monitoring because of consistent bioavailability.
Antidote for heparin overdose: **Protamine Sulfate.**
Warfarin monitoring is done by: **INR**
Antidote of warfarin overdose: **Vitamin K.**

498. Ans. (b) Acts both in vivo and in vitro

- Oral anticoagulant is warfarin. It is used only in vivo (body), not in vitro (lab).
- Warfarin is not used to store blood.
- It acts by inhibiting Vitamin K. Due to overdose, hematuria is the first manifestation noted.
- Dose monitoring is done by INR.
- Antidote of warfarin overdose: Vitamin K

PT (Prothrombin Time)	aPTT (activated Partial Thromboplastin Time)
Assess activity of Extrinsic coagulation pathway Used when on warfarin treatment ***WePT: Warfarin for extrinsic; PT value assessed.***	Assess activity of Extrinsic coagulation pathway. Used while on heparin treatment. ***HINT: Heparin for Intrinsic; aPTT value assessed.***

499. Ans. (a) Ciprofloxacin

Ref: KDT, 6th ed. pg. 64

- G_6PD is an enzyme present on RBC membrane provides strength to RBC which can counteract free radicals and oxidizing stress of drugs.
- In absence of G6PD enzyme, these cells can't bear the stress and results in Hemolysis.

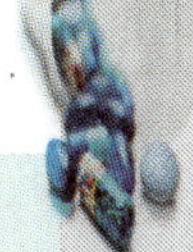

- **Drugs causing Hemolysis in G_6PD deficiency patients are:**
  - Anti malarials (Primaquine, chloroquine)
  - Antibiotic (Nitrofurantoin, Furazolidone)
  - Sulfonamide (dapsone)
  - Fava beans
- **Ciprofloxacin** is one of the quinolones, effective against G+ and G- including pseudomonas.
- It is contraindicated in pregnancy and children below 18 years of age because it effects growing bone and tendons.
- Ciprofloxacin is considered as oral DOC for enteric fever.
- DOC for enteric fever: Ceftriaxone

500. Ans. (c) Chloroquine

Ref: KDT 6th ed. pg. 64

Please refer to above explanation

501. Ans. (b) Enoxaparin

- Enoxaparin is a low molecular weight heparin.
- It acts by inhibiting factor Xa mainly (Xa >> IIa).
- LMWH usually doesn't need monitoring because of consistent bioavailability.
- **Drugs under LMWH:**
  - Enoxaparin
  - Dalteparin
  - Tinzaparin
  - Reviparin

Extra Mile

Hirudin along with Lepirudin and Bivalirudin is an anticoagulant which is act by direct thrombin (factor IIa) inhibition.
Tranexamic acid is an anti-fibrinolytic agent.

502. Ans. (c) Factor Xa

Ref: KD Tripathi, 6th Ed. pg. 597-598

- Low molecular heparin inhibits factor Xa mainly, having some action at factor IIa as well. It doesn't require monitoring because of consistent bioavailability.
- Heparin is a powerful and instantaneously acting anticoagulant, effective both in vivo and in vitro.
- It acts indirectly by *activating* plasma antithrombin III
- The heparin –AT III complex then binds to clotting factors of the intrinsic and common pathways (Xa, IIa, IXa, XIa, XIIa and XIIIa) and inactivates them.
- Warfarin on the other hand is effective only in vivo (body). It acts by inhibiting vitamin K.

Note:

- Fondaparinaux is synthetic LMWH acts exclusively at factor Xa.

503. Ans. (b) It act by inhibiting factor IIa mainly

Ref: KDT, 6th ed. pg. 599-600

- Low molecular weight heparin, Enoxaparin, inhibits only factor Xa mainly (Xa >> IIa) whereas unfractionated heparin inhibits both factor IIa and factor Xa (IIa >> Xa).

504. Ans. (a) Isotretinoin

Ref: Katzung, 11th ed. pg. 1308, 1455; KDT, pg. 854

- **13-*cis*-Retinoic acid (Isotretinoin) is an analogue of vitamin A.** It is used for the treatment of severe cystic acne
- Isotretinoin (Accutane) is a synthetic retinoid currently restricted to the treatment of severe cystic acne that is refractory to standard therapies.
- It appears to act by inhibiting sebaceous gland size and function.
- Half life- 10–20 hours.
- **Common side effect:** Hypervitaminosis A, dryness of skin and mucous membrane.
- **Teratogenic effect:** Extremely high risk of CNS, face, ear, and other malformations. Risk is equal throughout all the three trimester.

Extra Mile

- **Al-trans vitamin A (Tretinoin):** Effective topical agent in the treatment of acne vulgaris. It is a potent comedolytic and stimulate epidermal cell turnover, resulting in peeling.
- **Benzoyl peroxide** is an effective topical agent in the treatment of acne vulgaris
- MOA of benzoyl peroxide- its antimicrobial activity against *P acnes* and to its peeling and comedolytic effects.
- **Azelaic acid** effective in the treatment of acne vulgaris.
- MOA of azelaic acid-antimicrobial activity against *P acnes* as well as an in vitro inhibitory effect on the conversion of testosterone to dihydrotestosterone.

505. Ans. (a) I/M

Ref: KDT, 6th ed. pg. 588

VITAMIN B12

- Present in two forms: Cyanocobalamin and hydroxocobalamin.
- Dietary sources: Liver, kidney, sea fish, egg yolk, meat and cheese.
- Only vegetable source: Legumes (pulses)
- Daily requirement: 1–2 μg/day. In cases of pregnancy and lactation: 3–5 μg/day.

Manifestation of Deficiency

- **Megaloblastic anemia**- the first manifestation.
  - Hypersegmented neutrophils and giant platelets.

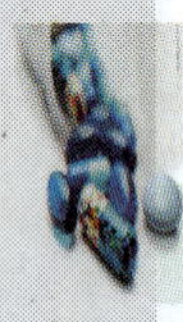

- **SACD:** subacute combined degeneration of spinal cord; peripheral neuritis, paresthesias.
- **Glossitis, GI disturbance:** Damage to epithelial structures.

Preparation Dose and Administration

- **Cynocobalamin:** 35 μg/5 mL liquid; 100, 500, 1000 μg Inj.
- **Hydroxycobalamin:** 500, 1000 μg Inj.
- **Methylcobalamin:** 0.5 mg tab.
- In case of severe anemia (like pernicious anemia), Vitamin B_{12} should be given by IM or deep s.c (but not by IV) injection.
- Parenteral administration is necessary to bypass the defective absorptive mechanism.
- Hydroxycobalamin has been preferred for parenteral use because of better retention.

506. Ans. (c) Avidin

Ref: KD Tripathi, 6th ed. pg. 876

BIOTIN

- Biotin is a sulfur containing organic acid found in egg yolk, liver, nuts and many other articles of food.
- It is well absorbed from intestine and excreted mainly unchanged in urine.
- **Avidin,** a heat labile protein in egg white, binds and prevents the absorption of biotin.

507. Ans. (b) Niacin

Ref: KDT, 6th ed. pg. 875

- Lipids that are liberated from adipose tissue are used to build very-low-density lipoproteins (VLDL) in the liver, which are precursors of low-density lipoprotein (LDL)
- Because niacin blocks the breakdown of fats, it causes a decrease in free fatty acids in the blood and, as a consequence, decreases the secretion of VLDL and cholesterol by the liver.
- When niacin is added to statins, it reduces carotid intima-media thickness, a marker of atherosclerosis.

PATHOLOGY

5

MOST RECENT QUESTIONS 2023

1. All are features of irreversible injury; except:
(Most Recent Question July 2023)

a. Pyknotic nucleus
b. Blebs formation
c. Karyolysis
d. Densities in mitochondria

2. Ferroportin is inhibited by:
(Most Recent Question July 2023)

a. IL-1
b. TNF-alpha
c. IL-6
d. TGF-beta

3. Chronic inflammatory mediator is:
(Most Recent Question July 2023)

a. IL-1
b. IL-6
c. TNF-alpha
d. TGF-beta

4. If disease is getting transmitted from grandmother to mother, then the chances of disease getting transferred to next generation are: *(Most Recent Question July 2023)*

a. 25%
b. 50%
c. 75%
d. 100%

5. If both parents are suffering from beta-thalassemia trait, then the chances of child being diseased are:
(Most Recent Question July 2023)

a. 25%
b. 50%
c. 75%
d. 100%

6. Pattern of inheritance shown in the following pedigree is: *(Most Recent Question July 2023)*

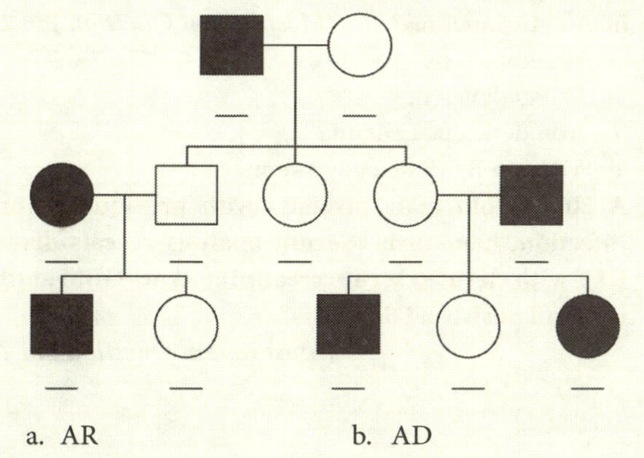

a. AR
b. AD
c. XLR
d. XLD

7. An adult patient presents with fatigue, pallor. Routine blood investigation shows low RBC count, low Hb, MCV 60 fl, MCH 20 pg. Diagnosis is:
(Most Recent Question July 2023)

a. Vitamin B_{12} deficiency
b. ACD
c. Sideroblastic anemia
d. IDA

8. Primary effusion lymphoma is caused by:
(Most Recent Question July 2023)

a. HHV-8
b. HIV-1
c. Hepadnavirus
d. HIV-2

9. 30-year-old patient presents with purpura, renal impairment, hemoptysis and recurrent upper respiratory infection. c-ANCA positivity is seen. Possible diagnosis is: *(Most Recent Question July 2023)*

a. Goodpasture's syndrome
b. MPA
c. Churg-Strauss syndrome
d. Wegener's granulomatosis

10. Lab report of patient shows HBsAg positive, IgM anti-HBc Ab positive. He came to the hospital for some other illness but these viral markers are found to be positive. This indicates that patient has:
(Most Recent Question July 2023)

a. Acute Hep B
b. Chronic Hep B
c. Persistent infection
d. HIV-1

11. A patient presented with ascites, peripheral edema and deranged LFT. The gross specimen of liver is shown. What is the most likely cause?
(Most Recent Question July 2023)

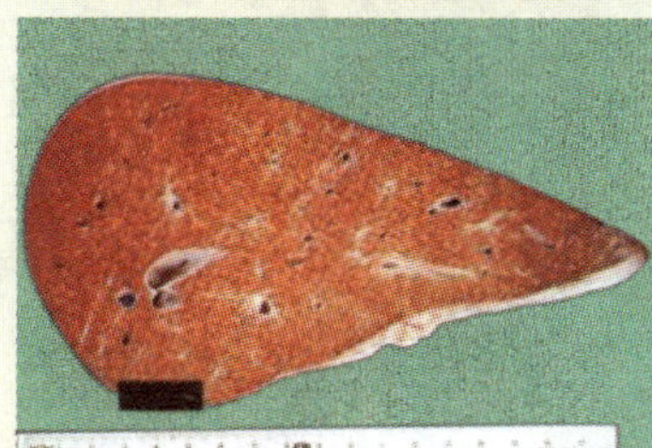

a. Alcoholic liver disease
b. Chronic hepatitis
c. CV congestion
d. Hepatic cirrhosis

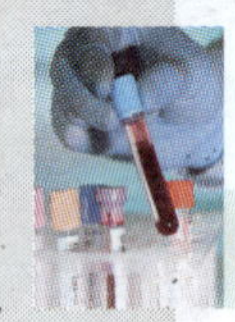

12. Child presents with hematuria (20 RBC/HPF), RBC casts, edema. There was evidence of deranged RFT as well. Possible diagnosis is:
(Most Recent Question July 2023)

a. FSGS
b. PSGN
c. MCD
d. IgA nephropathy

13. Patient presents with hypertension, palpitations and sweating. Aldosterone levels were found to be elevated and potassium levels were low. Possible diagnosis is:
(Most Recent Question July 2023)

a. Pheochromocytoma
b. Cushing's disease
c. Conn's syndrome
d. Pituitary adenoma

14. Most common brain tumor in adults is:
(Most Recent Question July 2023)

a. Medulloblastoma
b. Meningioma
c. Retinoblastoma
d. Glioblastoma

15. An adult female presents with headache. Radiological investigations revealed frontal dural-based tumor. Which of the following will you most likely observe in the same? ***(Most Recent Question Jan 2023)***

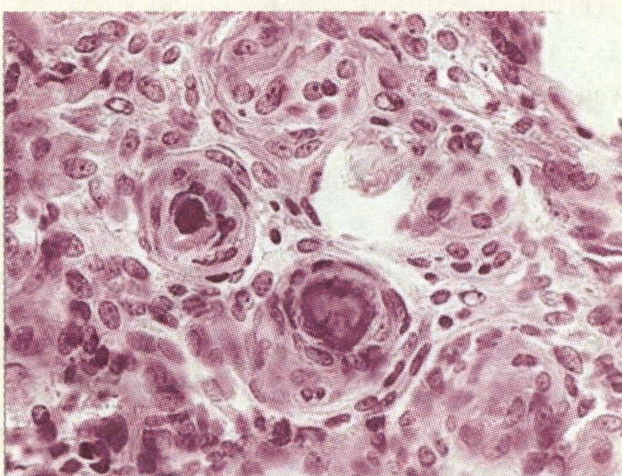

a. Pseudorosette
b. Psammoma bodies with whirling of tumor cells
c. Fried egg appearance
d. True rosette

16. A patient died due to MI. Which stain is used to see the infarct portion of heart?
(Most Recent Question Jan 2023)

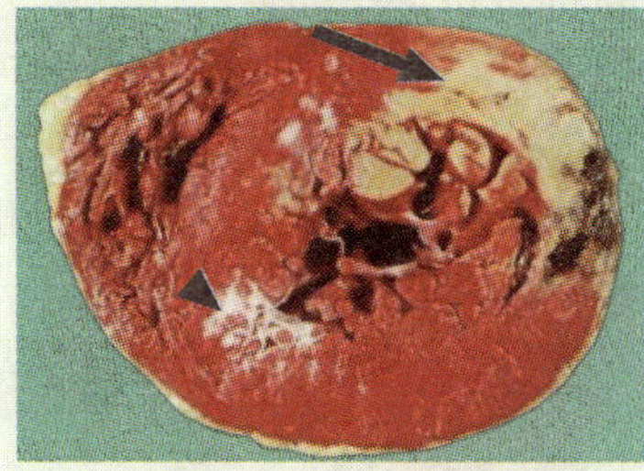

a. Congo red
b. Masson's trichrome
c. Triphenyltetrazolium chloride
d. Prussian blue

17. A 5-year-old boy presented with periorbital and pedal edema as well as ascites. Upon electron microscopy, effacement of podocytes was seen. Identify the given condition: ***(Most Recent Question Jan 2023)***

a. Minimal change disease
b. FSGS
c. IgA nephropathy
d. Nephrotic syndrome

18. A 70-year-old male with hip pain and lytic lesions in the hip bone. Serum calcium levels were raised. Given image represents: ***(Most Recent Question Jan 2023)***

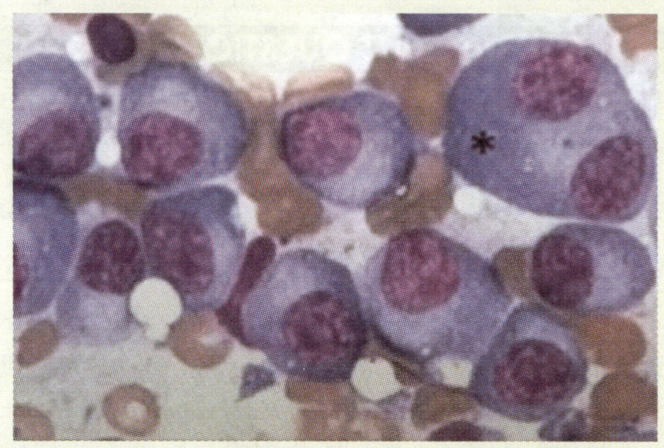

a. Plasma cell leukemia
b. ALL
c. AML
d. Multiple myeloma

19. Which of the following cast is composed of Tamm-Horsfall protein? ***(Most Recent Question Jan 2023)***

a. RBC cast
b. WBC cast
c. Hyaline cast
d. Waxy cast

20. Tzanck smear is used for the diagnosis of:
(Most Recent Question Jan 2023)

a. HSV-1 and 2
b. HIV
c. Hepatitis B
d. All of these

21. Splenectomy is indicated in which of the following hemolytic anemias? ***(Most Recent Question Jan 2023)***

a. Hereditary spherocytosis
b. G6PD deficiency
c. Iron deficiency anemia
d. Vitamin B_{12} deficiency anemia

22. A 20-year-old male presents with previous history of infection, hematuria. Serum analysis reveals deranged KFT with elevated serum creatinine. Anti-GBM antibody is found positive. Diagnosis is:
(Most Recent Question Jan 2023)

a. GPS
b. PSGN
c. MPGS
d. IgA nephropathy

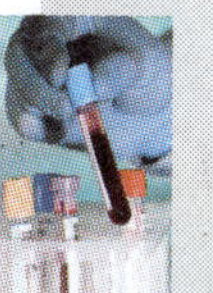

23. A 60-year-old patient presents with throbbing unilateral headache and nodular thickening along with temporal artery. Microscopic examination reveals giant cells and granuloma. What is the most likely diagnosis? ***(Most Recent Question Jan 2023)***

a. Takayasu arteritis b. Temporal arteritis
c. Buerger's disease d. HSP

24. Which of the following is marker for intestinal inflammation? ***(Most Recent Question Jan 2023)***

a. Fecal lactoferrin b. TTG
c. IL-3 d. All of these

25. A 50-year-old chronic smoker presents with intermittent claudication of the legs. Initially the pain was experienced during activity and later on at rest also. What is this also known as? ***(Most Recent Question Jan 2023)***

a. Takayasu arteritis
b. Temporal arteritis
c. Buerger's disease/TAO
d. HSP

26. A young boy presents with a small round cell tumor of the eye. Diagnosis is: ***(Most Recent Question Jan 2023)***

a. Retinosarcoma b. Neuroblastoma
c. Ewing's sarcoma d. Retinoblastoma

CELL INJURY AND INFLAMMATION

27. Dystrophic calcification is seen in: ***(Most Recent Question June 2022)***

a. Hyperparathyroidism
b. Atherosclerosis
c. Vitamin D disorder
d. Lymphoreticular malignancy

28. Which of the following molecules are required for adhesion of leukocyte to vascular endothelial cells in acute inflammation? ***(Most Recent Question Dec 2021)***

a. PECAM-1 b. Selectins
c. Integrin d. Fibronectin

29. A patient undergoes a surgery on the anterior chest wall. Post-surgery he notices a lesion having itching and present within the margins of the wound in the pre-sternal area. What is the most likely diagnosis? ***(Most Recent Question Dec 2021)***

a. Lipoma b. Keloid
c. Hypertrophic scar d. Normal granulation tissue

30. What is the location of lactate dehydrogenase inside the cell? ***(Most Recent Question Dec 2020)***

a. Nucleus b. Cytoplasm
c. Mitochondria d. Ribosomes

31. Lysosomal enzymes are presented in: ***(Most Recent Question Dec 2020)***

a. Cytosol b. Mitochondria
c. Endoplasmic reticulum d. Nucleus

32. An 83-year-old man shows presence of perinuclear pigment in the cardiac muscle fibers. What is the nature of pigment? ***(Most Recent Question Dec 2020)***

a. Hemosiderin b. Lipofuscin
c. Melanin d. Iron

33. Macrophages play an important role in phagocytosis and chronic inflammation. Which of the following cells perform the same function in the liver? ***(Most Recent Question Aug 2020)***

a. Merkel cell b. Hofbauer cell
c. Kupffer cell d. Stellate cells

34. A patient died of myocardial infarction and his heart was taken out and immersed in a solution. The normal area of the heart turned brick red whereas infarcted portion turned white. Which of the following can be the likely component of the solution? ***(Most Recent Question Aug 2020)***

a. Formalin
b. Triphenyl tetrazolium chloride
c. Ethanol
d. Glutaraldehyde

35. Which among the following ions is important in cell injury? ***(Most Recent Question Dec 2019)***

a. Calcium b. Sodium
c. Potassium d. Chloride

36. Stellate granuloma is found in: ***(Recent Pattern Question 2018-19)***

a. Cat scratch disease b. Leprosy
c. Coccidomycosis d. Histoplasmosis

37. Which proteoglycan is involved in process of healing? ***(Recent Pattern Question 2018-19)***

a. Chondroitin sulphate b. Dermatan sulphate
c. Keratan sulphate d. Syndecan

38. Secondary healing mechanism is: ***(Recent Pattern Question 2018-19)***

a. Granuloma formation b. Scab formation
c. Granulation tissue d. Neovascularization

39. Rolling of leucocytes on endothelial cells is mediated by: ***(Recent Pattern Question 2018)***

a. Selectins b. Integrins
c. Transferrin d. PECAM-1

40. Liquefactive necrosis is seen in which of the following? ***(Recent Pattern Question 2018)***

a. Kidney b. Heart
c. Cerebrum d. Intestine

41. P53 regulates which phase of cell cycle? ***(Recent Pattern Question 2018)***

a. G1S b. G2
c. G2M d. S

42. Pro-apoptotic gene and anti-apoptotic gene belong to which gene family? ***(Recent Pattern Question 2017)***

a. p53 b. Bcl
c. BRAF d. Rb

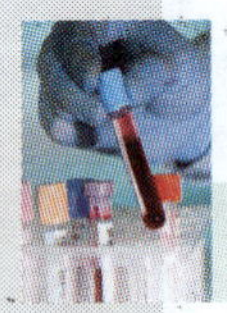

43. Colliquative necrosis is seen in? *(Recent Pattern Question 2017)*
a. Arthus phenomenon b. Malignant hypertension
c. Tuberculoma d. Lung abscess

44. DNA synthesis is seen in which phase of cell cycle? *(Recent Pattern Question 2017)*
a. Resting phase b. Synthetic phase
c. Mitotic phase d. Premitotic phase

45. Which of the following is an opsonin? *(Recent Pattern Question 2017)*
a. C3a b. C3b
c. C5a d. C5b

46. Councilman bodies are formed due to process of ____? *(Recent Pattern Question 2017)*
a. Necrosis b. Cirrhosis
c. Apoptosis d. Necroptosis

47. Stellate shaped granuloma is seen in? *(Recent Pattern Question 2017)*
a. Sarcoidosis b. Cat scratch
c. Crohn's disease d. Tuberculosis

48. Which of the following helps in cell to cell adhesion? *(Recent Pattern Question 2016)*
a. Interleukins b. Interferons
c. E- Cadherin d. Matrix metallo proteinase

49. A reversible change occurring in which a mature cell type is replaced by another mature cell, is called:
a. Dysplasia b. Metaplasia
c. Hyerplasia d. Hypertrophy

50. A patient who was previously with good muscle mass, now presents with decreased muscle mass. There is history of RTA which led him to be bedridden for 6 months. This decrease in muscle mass is best explained by:
a. Metaplasia b. Dysplasia
c. Hypertrophy d. Atrophy

51. A pregnant uterus is an example of:
a. Metaplasia b. Dysplasia
c. Atrophy d. Hypertrophy

52. In individuals who donate one lobe of the liver for transplantation, the remaining organ soon grows back to its original size. This is an example of which adaptive mechanism?
a. Hypertrophy
b. Atrophy
c. Hyperplasia
d. Metaplasia

53. Apoptosis is:
a. Internally controlled, programmed cell death
b. Externally controlled, programmed cell death
c. Internally controlled, programmed enzyme degradation
d. Externally controlled, programmed karyolysis

54. All are true about apoptosis; EXCEPT:
a. Considerable apoptosis may occur in a tissue before it becomes apparent in histology
b. Apoptotic cells appear as round mass of the intensely eosinophilic cytoplasm with dense nuclear chromatin fragments
c. Apoptosis of cells induce inflammatory reaction
d. Condensation of chromatin

55. All are true about apoptosis; EXCEPT:
a. Inflammation is present
b. Chromosomal breakage
c. Clumping of chromatin
d. Cell shrinkage

56. Light microscopic characteristic feature of apoptosis is:
a. Intact cell membrane
b. Eosinophilic cytoplasm
c. Nuclear moulding
d. Condensation of the nucleus

57. Apoptosis is inhibited by:
a. Bcl-2 b. Bax
c. Bad d. P53

58. In apoptosis, protein hydrolysis is due to activation of:
a. Caspases b. Upases
c. Transglutaminase d. Catalase

59. Caspases are associated with which of the following?
a. Hydropic degeneration b. Collagen hyalinization
c. Embryogenesis d. Fatty degeneration

60. Caspases are involved in?
a. Necrosis b. Apoptosis
c. Atherosclerosis d. Inflammation

61. Earliest feature of reversible cell injury is:
a. Amorphous densities b. Ribosomal detachment
c. Hydropic swelling d. Bleb formation

62. All of the following statements are true regarding reversible cell injury; EXCEPT:
a. Diminished generation of ATP
b. Formation of blebs in the plasma membrane
c. Condensation of nuclear chromatin
d. Detachment of ribosomes from the granular endoplasmic reticulum

63. Which of the following type of necrosis is most commonly associated with ischemic injury:
a. Coagulative necrosis b. Casseous necrosis
c. Liquiefactive necrosis d. Fat necrosis

64. Internucleosomal cleavage of DNA is characteristic of?
a. Reversible cell injury b. Irreversible cell injury
c. Necrosis d. Apoptosis

65. Integrins include receptor; EXCEPT?
a. Fibronectin
b. Glycoprotein on platelet surface
c. Leukocyte adhesion molecule
d. Platelet derived growth factor

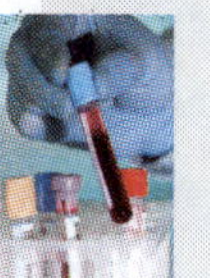

66. Exudation of plasma and leucocytes in acute inflammation is from?
a. Venules b. Capillaries
c. Arterioles d. Arterioles and capillaries

67. Dystrophic calcification is seen in?
a. Rickets b. Hyperparathyroidism
c. Atheromatous plaque d. Vitamin A intoxication

68. Digestion of foreign material by a neutrophil or macrophage during phagocytosis is mainly due to?
a. Complement b. Hydrogen peroxide
c. Kinins d. Lysosomal enzymes

69. Which of the following is a peroxisomal free radical scavenger?
a. Superoxide dismutase b. Glutathione peroxidase
c. Catalase d. All of these

70. Which among the following is the hallmark of acute inflammation?
a. Vasoconstriction
b. Stasis
c. Vasodilation and increase in permeability
d. Leukocyte margination

71. Which of the following is not an inflammatory mediator?
a. Tumor necrosis factor b. Myeloperoxidase
c. Interferons d. Interleukin

72. All of the following host tissue responses can be seen in acute infection; EXCEPT:
a. Exudation b. Vasodilation
c. Margination d. Granuloma formation

73. Oxygen dependent killing is done through?
a. NADPH oxidase b. Superoxide dismutase
c. Catalase d. Glutathione peroxidase

74. Which of the following is required for post-translational modification?
a. Vitamin B_{12} b. Biotin
c. Beta-carotene d. Vitamin C

75. Cell swelling is seen in all; EXCEPT:
a. Infection b. Malignancy
c. Calcification d. Hypoxia

76. Fat necrosis occurs at all sites; EXCEPT:
a. Pancreas b. Liver
c. Breast d. Peritoneum

77. Morphological changes seen in chronic non-specific inflammation include an increase in:
a. Neutrophils, lymphocytes and liquiefactive necrosis
b. Neutrophils, macrophages and fibrosis
c. Lymphocytes, plasma cells and fibrosis
d. Giant cells, macrophages and coagulative necrosis

78. Foci of granulomatous inflammation show all of the following; EXCEPT?
a. Eosinophils b. Epithelioid cells
c. Fibrosis d. Lymphocytes

79. All are true about white infarcts; EXCEPT:
a. Edema is present
b. Occurs in organs with end arterial supply
c. Well-defined margins
d. Coagulative necrosis

HEMODYNAMICS

80. Which is the most abundant plasma protein?
a. Albumin b. Globulin
c. Fibrinogen d. Bence jones protein

81. Testing for which of the following infection is not done before giving blood transfusion?
(Most Recent Question June 2022)
a. HIV 1, 2 b. Hep B
c. Hep C d. Hep A

82. A chronic cigarette smoker presented with pain and black necrotic fingers as shown. What is the most likely diagnosis is? *(Most Recent Question Dec 2021)*

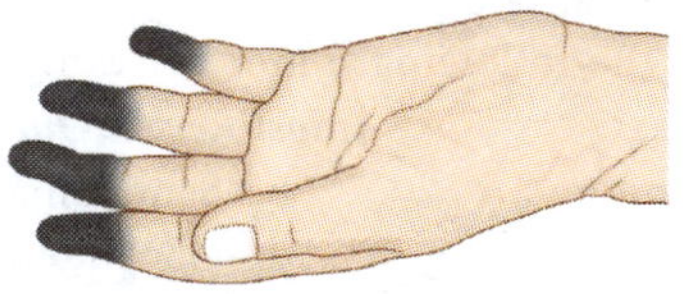

a. Berger's disease b. Thrombo-angitis obliterans
c. Fournier gangrene d. Deep vein thrombosis

83. Supra – Vital staining is used for:
(Most Recent Question June 2021)
a. Schnuffer dots b. Heinz bodies
c. Acanthocytes d. Pappenheimer bodies

84. All are true about components of Virchow's triad; EXCEPT:
a. Vasculitis b. Stasis in veins
c. Turbulence in artery d. Increased protein C

85. All are true about arterial thrombosis; EXCEPT:
a. Retrograde growth b. Line of Zahn
c. White thrombus
d. Complete lumen obstruction

86. Which is the most common site of arterial embolization?
a. Brain b. Kidney
c. Mesentery d. Lower extremities

87. Chicken fat appearance is seen in:
a. Antemortem clots b. Postmortem clots
c. Fat necrosis d. Fibrinoid necrosis

88. All of the following are true in respect of angioneurotic edema; EXCEPT:
a. It is caused by deficiency of complement proteins
b. It is more common in females
c. It manifests as pitting edema
d. It is an autosomal dominant disorder

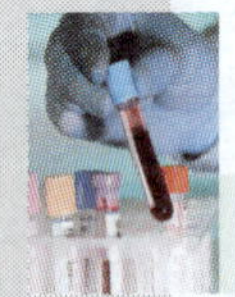

89. Hypersensitivity angiitis is seen in?
a. SLE
b. Polyarteritis Nodosa
c. Henoch Schonlein purpura
d. Burgers disease

NEOPLASIA

90. A 65-year-old man presents with hypercalcemia and deranged KFT. Workup shows Hb is low, TLC is elevated and X-ray skull shows multiple lytic lesions. Comment on diagnosis: ***(Most Recent Question June 2022)***
a. Hyperparathyroidism b. Multiple myeloma
c. Grave's disease d. Renal tubular acidosis

91. Which of the following subtype of breast cancer has best prognosis? ***(Most Recent Question Dec 2021)***
a. Luminal A
b. Luminal B
c. HER 2+ve
d. Triple negative breast cancer

92. Which of the following tumor arises from all the three germ layers? ***(Most Recent Question Dec 2021)***
a. Teratoma b. Seminoma
c. Sex-cord tumors d. Choristoma

93. 40-year-old man having a well circumscribed testicular swelling and undergoes orchiectomy which on further evaluation has OCT4 + tissue. The most likely diagnosis is? ***(Most Recent Question Dec 2021)***
a. Seminoma b. Testicular torsion
c. Teratoma d. Yolk sac tumor

94. A child presented with leukocoria and strabismus. What is the likely diagnosis? ***(Most Recent Question Dec 2021)***

a. Rhabdomyosarcoma b. Retinoblastoma
c. Congenital cataract d. Neuroblastoma

95. What is the likely diagnosis of the given condition? ***(Most Recent Question Dec 2020)***

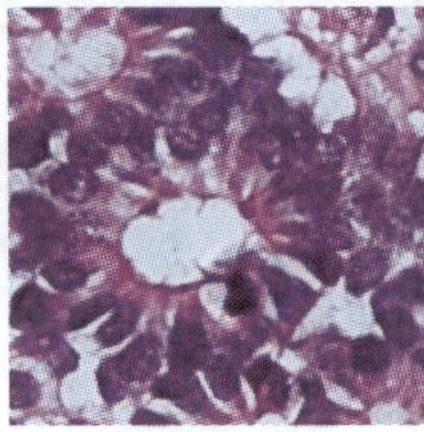

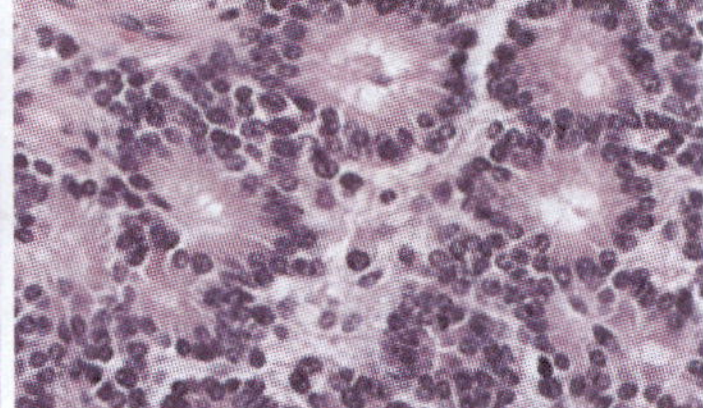

a. Retinoblastoma b. Medulloblastoma
c. Ewing's sarcoma d. Neuroblastoma

96. A child presents with difficulty in eating due to jaw swelling and enlarged cervical lymph nodes. Lymph node biopsy report is shown below. What is the clinical diagnosis? ***(Most Recent Question Dec 2020)***

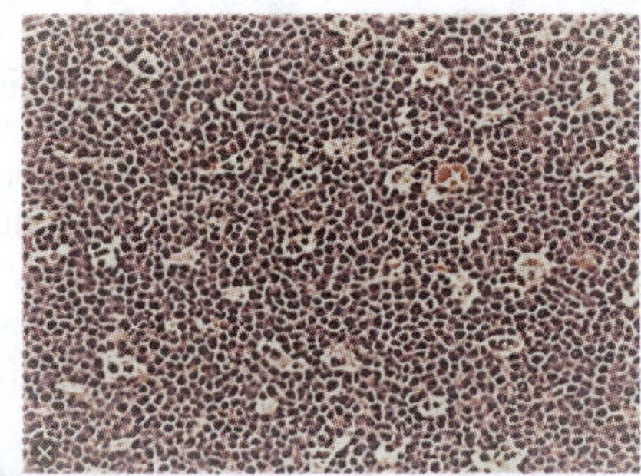

a. Hodgkin disease b. Infectious mononucleosis
c. Kikuchi disease d. Burkitt lymphoma

97. A 60-year-old male presents with low backache. X-ray LS spine shows osteoblastic changes. What is the clinical diagnosis? ***(Most Recent Question Dec 2020)***
a. Multiple myeloma b. Pott spine
c. Carcinoma prostate d. Renal cell carcinoma

98. Which of the following is a tumor marker of pancreatic cancer? ***(Most Recent Question Aug 2020)***
a. CEA b. CA15-3
c. NSE d. AFP

99. Which of the following contributes to the immortality of cancer cells? ***(Most Recent Question Aug 2020)***
a. Topoisomerase b. Telomerase
c. RNA polymerase d. Helicase

100. A patient presented with development of seizures for which the CT guided biopsy was done. The histopathology reported presence of psammoma bodies as shown in the image. Which of the following is the most likely diagnosis of this patient? ***(Most Recent Question Aug 2020)***

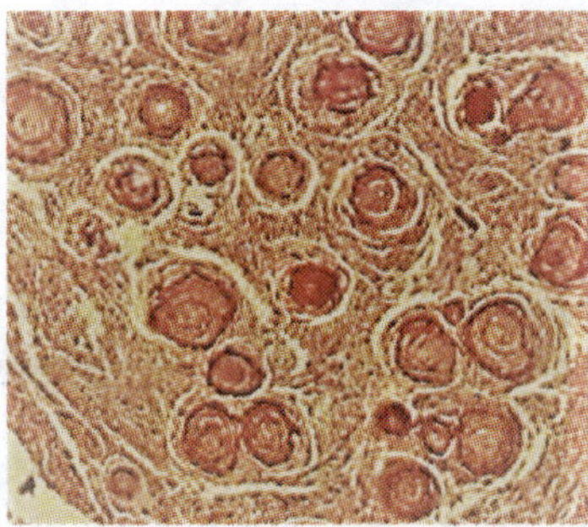

a. Astrocytoma b. Ependymoma
c. Meningioma d. Medulloblastoma

101. Which is the most common tumor of mediastinum? ***(Most Recent Question Dec 2019)***
a. Thymoma b. Lymphoma
c. Neurogenic tumor d. Pericardial cyst

102. Which of the following is an embryonic neural tumor? ***(Most Recent Question Dec 2019)***

a. Fibrous astrocytoma
b. Neuroglioma
c. Ependymoma
d. Medulloblastoma

103. Most common anterior mediastinal tumour? ***(Recent Pattern Question 2019)***

a. Thymoma
b. Neurofibroma
c. Pericardial cyst
d. Bronchogenic cyst

104. Which of the following is true about Anaplasia? ***(Recent Pattern Question 2018-19)***

a. Loss of cohesion between cells
b. Loss of differentiation
c. Change of epithelium types
d. Benign and fully reversible

105. Cell that can form any other cell in the body is called: ***(Recent Pattern Question 2018-19)***

a. Totipotent
b. Multipotent
c. Pluripotent
d. Lineage stem cells

106. Hyaline globules are seen in all; EXCEPT: ***(Recent Pattern Question 2018)***

a. Hepatoblastoma
b. Yolk Sac tumor
c. Teratoma
d. Hepatocellular carcinoma

107. Which is the most common tumor associated with superior vena cava syndrome? ***(Recent Pattern Question 2018)***

a. Lung cancer
b. Lymphoma
c. Metastasis
d. Thyroid cancer

108. Which is the most common cancer which results in death? ***(Recent Pattern Question 2018)***

a. Oral cancer
b. Breast cancer
c. Prostate cancer
d. Lung cancer

109. Which of the following shows breast necrosis and calcification? ***(Recent Pattern Question 2018)***

a. Comedo subtype of DCIS
b. Cribriform subtype of DCIS
c. Colloid carcinoma
d. Lobular carcinoma in situ

110. Mucosal melanosis and hamartomatous polyps are seen in: ***(Recent Pattern Question 2018)***

a. Peutz-Jeghers syndrome
b. Cronkhite Canada syndrome
c. Familial adenomatous polyposis
d. Hereditary non polyposis colonic cancer

111. Jumping gene is known as? ***(Recent Pattern Question 2017)***

a. Transposon
b. Retroposon
c. Insertion sequence
d. Integron

112. Which is correct about non-seminomatous germ cell tumour? ***(Recent Pattern Question 2017)***

a. Spreads via lymphatics
b. Testicular contour distorted
c. Prognosis better than germ cell tumour
d. Radiosensitive

113. Warthin tumour is? ***(Recent Pattern Question 2017)***

a. Adenolymphoma
b. Pleomorphic adenoma
c. Mucoepidermoid carcinoma
d. Acinic cell carcinoma

114. Loss of polarity is a feature of: ***(Recent Pattern Question 2017)***

a. Metaplasia
b. Dysplasia
c. Necroptosis
d. All of these

115. L-myc leads to? ***(Recent Pattern Question 2017)***

a. Burkitt lymphoma
b. Neuroblastoma
c. Oat cell cancer
d. GIST

116. Which of the following Cancer is not due to infectious etiology? ***(Recent Pattern Question 2017)***

a. Small cell cancer of lung
b. H.C.C
c. Naso-pharyngeal cancer
d. MALToma

117. Most common middle mediastinal tumour? ***(Recent Pattern Question 2017)***

a. Bronchogenic cyst
b. Pericardial cyst
c. Neurofibroma
d. Lymphoma

118. The lesion shown below is caused by? ***(Recent Pattern Question 2017)***

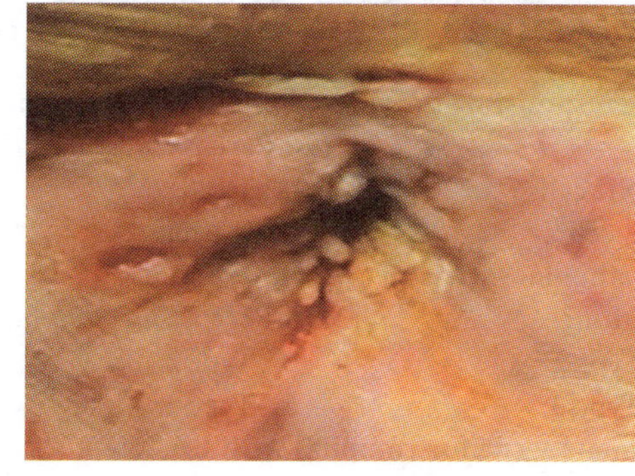

a. HPV
b. HSV
c. HIV
d. EBV

119. In a FAP patient which is an important CA risk? ***(Recent Pattern Question 2016)***

a. Retinoblastoma
b. Brain tumour
c. Colorectal CA
d. Prostate CA

120. Esophageal irradiation causes damage by ***(Recent Pattern Question 2016)***

a. Decreasing secretion
b. Glandular dysplasia
c. Stricture formation
d. Glandular hypertrophy

121. Oncocytes are seen in all of the following, EXCEPT:

a. Pituitary
b. Thyroid
c. Pancreas
d. Thymus

122. Tumor marker for mesotheliomas is?

a. Desmin
b. Keratin
c. Vimentin
d. Alpha-feto protein

123. Tongue cancer NOT seen with?

a. Alcohol
b. Smoking
c. Chewing tobacco
d. Apthous ulcer

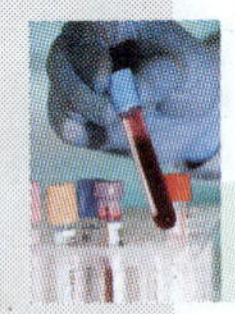

124. Most radiosensitive tumour is:
a. Ewing's sarcoma
b. Seminoma
c. Osteosarcoma
d. Osteoid osteoma

125. Radiation exposure during infancy has been linked to which of the following carcinoma?
a. Breast
b. Melanoma
c. Thyroid
d. Lung

126. UV radiation has which of the following effects on the cells?
a. Prevents formation of pyrimidine dimers
b. Stimulates formation of pyrimidine dimers
c. Prevents formation of purine dimers
d. All of the above

127. The most radiosensitive cells are:
a. Neutrophils
b. Lymphocytes
c. Erythrocytes
d. Megakaryocytes

128. The following parasitic infections predispose to malignancies?
a. Paragonimus westermani
b. Guinea worm infection
c. Clonorchiasis
d. Ancyclostoma

IMMUNITY AND HYPERSENSITIVITY

129. Cells responsible for chronic graft rejection are: *(Most Recent Question June 2022)*
a. NK cells
b. T cells
c. B cells
d. Plasma cells

130. Myasthenia gravis is which type of hypersensitivity reaction? *(Most Recent Question June 2022)*
a. Type 1
b. Type 2
c. Type 3
d. Type 4

131. A female went for camping with her friends. She had a bee sting which resulted in edema, redness on face and difficulty in breathing. What is the type of mechanism responsible for this type of reaction? *(Most Recent Question June 2022)*
a. Cytotoxic
b. Immune complex mediated
c. Cell mediated
d. IgE mediated

132. Rh incompatibility is _____ type of hypersensitivity reaction? *(Most Recent Question Dec 2021)*
a. Type I
b. Type II
c. Type III
d. Type IV

133. A child got stung by a honey- bee while playing. After that the child presented with hypotension, edema, breathlessness. Which of the following antibody is responsible for this? *(Most Recent Question Dec 2021)*
a. IgA
b. IgG
c. IgE
d. IgM

134. A child presented with thymic hypoplasia, decreased immunity and hypocalcemia. He also has tetralogy of fallot. What is the diagnosis? *(Most Recent Question Dec 2021)*
a. Di-George syndrome
b. SCID
c. Wiskott-Aldrich syndrome
d. Bruton disease

135. The cell given in lymph node biopsy below shows origin from which of the following cell lines? *(Most Recent Question Dec 2020)*

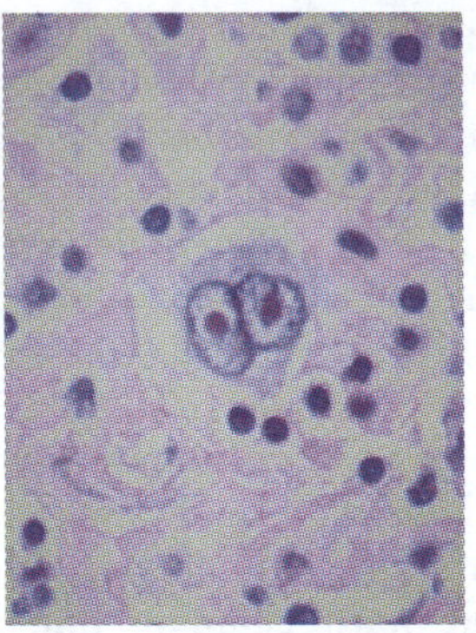

a. B cells
b. CD4 cells
c. NK cell
d. CD8 cell

136. A 55-year-old patient presented with difficulty in breathing and rashes after ingesting sea food. He has shown similar reaction in the past following consumption of the same food items. Which of the following hypersensitivity reaction is present in this case? *(Most Recent Question Dec 2020)*
a. Type 1
b. Type 2
c. Type 3
d. Type 4

137. A 47-year-old female presented with arthralgia, difficulty in swallowing food and gritty feeling in the eyes. She is also found to be having increased titers of ANA. Which of the following is the likely diagnosis? *(Most Recent Question Dec 2020)*
a. Sjögren's syndrome
b. Rheumatoid arthritis
c. Serum sickness
d. SLE

138. An elderly diabetic male patient underwent kidney transplantation from his twin brother. The type of grafting is: *(Most Recent Question Dec 2020)*
a. Allograft
b. Isograft
c. Xenograft
d. Autograft

139. Which of the following is the molecule required for presentation of the antigens by an antigen presenting cell to the TH2 cell? *(Most Recent Question Aug 2020)*
a. Toll like receptor
b. MHC
c. G protein coupled receptor
d. Lectin receptor

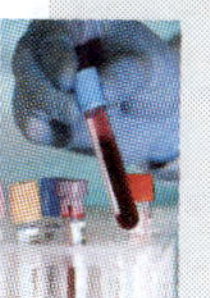

140. A boy presents in the emergency because of development of allergy due to pollen inhalation. Which of the following cells is important in the pathogenesis of this condition? *(Most Recent Question Aug 2020)*

a. NK cell b. Neutrophils
c. Helper T cell d. Cytotoxic T cell

141. Which of the following is not a component of Systemic Inflammatory Response Syndrome? *(Most Recent Question Dec 2019)*

a. Temperature b. Heart rate
c. Respiratory rate d. Blood pressure

142. Acute graft rejection occurs within: *(Recent Pattern Question 2019)*

a. Few hours b. <1 month
c. <6 months d. 6–12 months

143. Type II Hypersensitivity is seen in: *(Recent Pattern Question 2019)*

a. Pernicious anaemia b. Serum sickness
c. Arthus phenomenon d. Pathergy phenomenon

144. Which of the following is a causative agent of Farmer's Lung? *(Recent Pattern Question 2019)*

a. Thermophilic Actinomycetes
b. Aspergillus Fumigatus
c. Actinobacter
d. Aspergillus Flavus

145. First line of defence against tumour and virus? *(Recent Pattern Question 2019)*

a. NK cell
b. T cell
c. Histiocyte
d. Macrophage

146. Xenograft is: *(Recent Pattern Question 2018-19)*

a. Graft across species
b. Graft from same species
c. Graft from same individual
d. Graft from same organ

147. Which of the following is a Type 2 Hypersensitivity reaction? *(Recent Pattern Question 2018-19)*

a. Chronic Kidney Rejection episode
b. Autoimmune Hemolytic anaemia
c. Arthus reaction
d. Mitsuda reaction

148. Acute graft rejection occurs within? *(Recent Pattern Question 2018-19)*

a. Minutes b. Days to weeks
c. >6 weeks to 6 months d. >6 months

149. Neonatal lupus is screened by which antibody? *(Recent Pattern Question 2018)*

a. Anti-Ro
b. Anti-smith
c. Antiribonucleoprotein antibody
d. Antiphospholipid antibody

150. Class MHC 2 antigen attaches to: *(Recent Pattern Question 2017)*

a. CD4 b. CD8
c. CD16 d. CD34

151. Which is not an antibody mediated hypersensitivity reaction? *(Recent Pattern Question 2017)*

a. Type 1 b. Type 2
c. Type 3 d. Type 4

152. Which is a flow cytometric B cell marker? *(Recent Pattern Question 2017)*

a. CD 2 b. CD 3
c. CD 7 d. CD 19

153. Caplan syndrome is characterised by? *(Recent Pattern Question 2017)*

a. Pneumoconiosis with HLA B27
b. Pneumoconiosis with reactive arthritis
c. Pneumoconiosis with progressive massive fibrosis
d. Pneumoconiosis with rheumatoid arthritis

154. HLAB27 is maximally associated with: *(Recent Pattern Question 2017)*

a. Rheumatoid arthritis b. Ankylosing spondylitis
c. Rieter syndrome d. Psoriasis

155. Which is the first line of defence in viral infection? *(Recent Pattern Question 2017)*

a. B lymphocyte b. Macrophages
c. T lymphocytes d. Large granular lymphocyte

156. TH1 is involved in which type of hypersensitivity? *(Recent Pattern Question 2017)*

a. Type1 b. Type 2
c. Type 3 d. Type 4

157. Which of the following is an example of Type 3 hypersensitivity *(Recent Pattern Question 2016)*

a. Asthma b. Contact dermatitis
c. SLE d. AIHA

158. Which is true about type II hypersensitivity reaction? *(Recent Pattern Question 2016)*

a. Immune complex mediated
b. Antigen – antibody mediated
c. Arthus phenomenon
d. Granulomatous reaction

159. Highest molecular weight immunoglobulins are *(Recent Pattern Question 2016)*

a. IgG b. IgA
c. IgM d. IgD

160. Primary immune response is by which cell?

a. B cell b. T cell
c. B and T cell both d. Complement mediated

161. Steven Johnson Syndrome is seen with what kind of hypersensitivity reaction?

a. Type 1 b. Type 2
c. Type 3 d. Type 4

162. Patch test is what type of hypersensitivity?
a. Type 1
b. Type 2
c. Type 3
d. Type 4

163. Which of these is not an antigen presenting cell?
a. Bipolar cells
b. Dendritic cell
c. Follicular dendritic cell
d. Tissue macrophages

164. Which interleukin is associated with growth of natural killer cells?
a. IL-2
b. IL-7
c. IL-8
d. IL-13

165. In graft rejection, which type of HLA is involved?
a. MHC class I
b. MHC class II
c. MHC class III
d. MHC class IV

166. HLA-B27 is associated with:
a. Osteoarthritis
b. Sjgren syndrome
c. Behçet disease
d. Reiter's syndrome

167. Nitro-blue tetrazolium test is done for?
a. Chronic glomerulonephritis
b. Chronic granulomatous disorder
c. Acute granulomatous disease
d. Chediak Higashi syndrome

168. C1 is controlled by:
a. Magnesium
b. Manganese
c. Phosphate
d. Calcium

169. Which among the following is not an autoimmune disease?
a. Myasthenia gravis
b. Systemic lupus erythematosus
c. Grave's disease
d. Sickle cell disease

170. Tuberculin test is which type of hypersensitivity?
a. Type 1
b. Type 2
c. Type 3
d. Type 4

HEMATOLOGY

171. A 10-year-old child brought in with history of repeated blood transfusions in the past. Mother is presently worried about her son, since earlier he was maintaining good grades in class but now from past few months his grades are deteriorating, and he remains lethargic and extremely pale. His blood investigations show crescent shaped red Blood Cells. What should be the next step in management in this patient?

(Most Recent Question June 2022)

a. IV antibiotics
b. Blood transfusion
c. Normal saline
d. Observation

172. A child visited the hospital with his mother with complaints of severe fatigue, lethargy, pallor and irritation. He is a known case of IDA. He is on oral iron supplements. After reviewing the child doctors are planning to start with IV iron supplementation. What test should be done next?

(Most Recent Question June 2022)

a. TIBC
b. Ferritin
c. Hb value
d. Hematocrit

173. A 60-year-old man presents with 2-month history of weakness and pallor. Per abdomen shows moderate splenomegaly. Peripheral blood shows Hb = 10 gm/dl, leukocytosis and platelet 3 lac/cu. mm. P. smear shows metamyelocytes 15%, Promyeloblasts 30%, Myeloblast 45 %. Which of the following is the diagnosis?

(Most Recent Question June 2022)

a. ALL
b. CLL
c. CML
d. AML

174. A patient is suffering from iron deficiency anemia. What stain shall be used on Bone marrow specimen to confirm the iron stores depletion?

(Most Recent Question June 2022)

a. Alizarin red
b. Methylene blue
c. Prussian blue
d. Von Kossa

175. Macrocytic anemia will be seen in:

(Most Recent Question June 2022)

a. Sideroblastic anemia
b. Anemia of chronic disease
c. Thalassemia
d. Chronic liver disease

176. Which of the following causes S.C.I.D?

(Most Recent Question Dec 2021)

a. Deficiency of adenosine deaminase
b. Deficiency of tyrosine kinase
c. Vitamin B_{12} deficiency
d. Folate deficiency

177. Child with anemia having MCV 76fl. He is not responding to any medication and has history of getting repeated blood transfusions. Which of the following is next line of investigation?

(Most Recent Question Dec 2021)

a. Hemoglobin electrophoresis
b. Osmotic fragility test
c. Serum ferritin levels
d. Folate levels

178. Child with anemia having MCV 80-100fl and is not responding to any medication. Which of the following is next line of investigation?

(Most Recent Question Dec 2021)

a. Hemoglobin electrophoresis
b. Osmotic fragility test
c. Serum ferritin levels
d. Coombs test

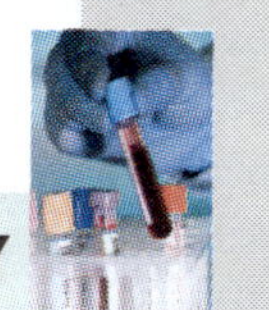

179. A 50-year-old man presented with gum bleeding and fatigue. His peripheral smear shows marked leukocytosis with 70% cells showing MPO positivity. What is the diagnosis? ***(Most Recent Question Dec 2020)***

a. AML b. CML
c. CLL d. ALL

180. Based on the given peripheral smear, which of the following is most likely diagnosis? ***(Most Recent Question Dec 2020)***

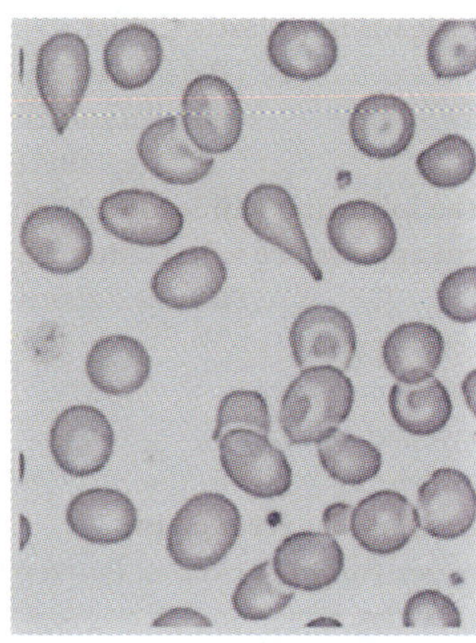

a. Iron deficiency anemia b. Thalassemia major
c. Myelofibrosis d. Myelodysplastic syndrome

181. A 10-year-old boy presented with a swollen knee after suffering a trauma. Which of the following is the likely condition seen in this patient? ***(Most Recent Question Dec 2020)***

a. Von Willebrand disease
b. Factor 8 deficiency
c. Immune thrombocytopenia
d. Vitamin K deficiency

182. A 3-year-old child is having progressive anemia. On examination splenohepatomegaly is noted with malar eminence prominence. Peripheral smear is shown here. The clinical diagnosis is: ***(Most Recent Question Dec 2020)***

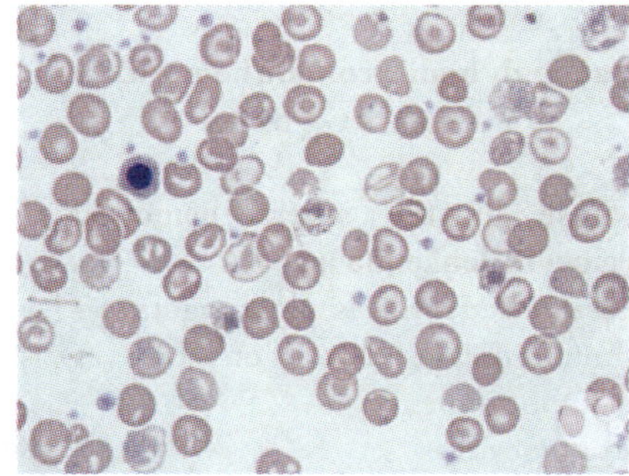

a. Thalassemia b. Iron deficiency anemia
c. Sideroblastic anemia d. Lead poisoning

183. Owl eye appearance of cells in urine microscopic examination of post kidney transplant patient is a feature of: ***(Most Recent Question Dec 2020)***

a. CMV b. EBV
c. HL d. NHL

184. A 4-year-old child presents with development of fever, petechial spots and complaint of fatigue. He is also having presence of pallor, hepatosplenomegaly as well as sternal tenderness. The clinical situation described above is most consistently associated with which of the following? ***(Most Recent Question Aug 2020)***

a. AML b. ALL
c. CLL d. CML

185. An old man underwent a bone marrow examination which revealed the presence of the finding shown in the image. What is the likely diagnosis of the affected individual? ***(Most Recent Question Aug 2020)***

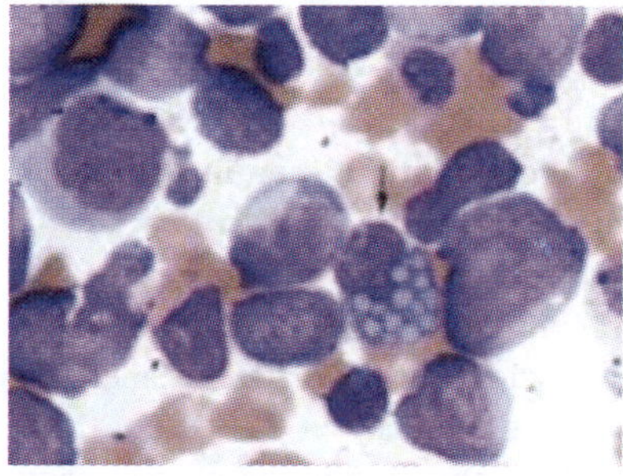

a. Multiple myeloma b. ALL
c. Tuberculosis d. Sickle cell disease

186. An elderly patient presents with complaint of fatigue in the lower back and presence of headache for last few weeks. Lab investigations revealed elevated value of ESR and his radiograph revealed the presence of multiple punched out lesions in the skull. Which of the following is the best investigation for this patient? ***(Most Recent Question Aug 2020)***

a. Serum electrophoresis showing IgG
b. Serum levels of CA15-3
c. Whole body PET scan
d. CT head with contrast

187. Comment on the diagnosis. ***(Recent Pattern Question 2019)***

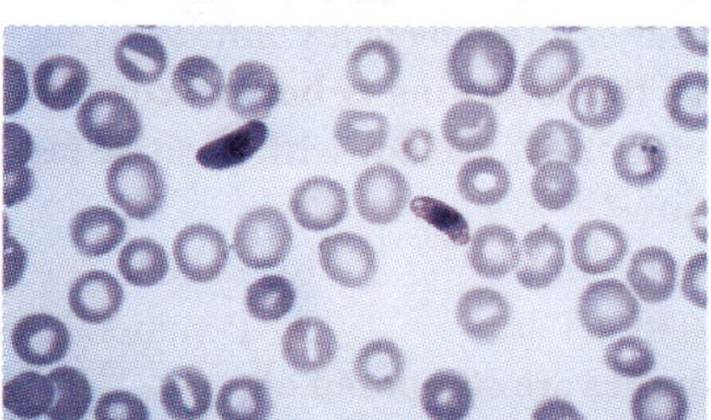

a. Malaria b. Hereditary spherocytosis
c. G6PD deficiency d. Babesia

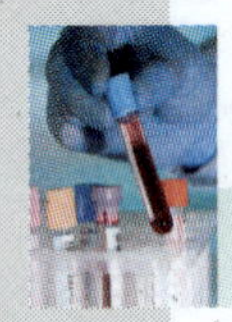

188. Which of the following interfere with iron absorption? ***(Recent Pattern Question 2019)***

a. Vitamin C b. Phytates
c. Oxalate d. Myoglobin

189. Most sensitive indicator for Iron deficiency anaemia? ***(Recent Pattern Question 2019)***

a. Serum Ferrtin
b. TIBC
c. Percentage saturation of transferrin
d. Bone marrow iron

190. Correct about of Anaemia of chronic disease ***(Recent Pattern Question 2019)***

a. High ferritin
b. Increased percentage of saturation of transferrin
c. High transferrin
d. High serum iron

191. All are reduced in Iron deficiency anaemia; EXCEPT: ***(Recent Pattern Question 2018-19)***

a. T.I.B.C
b. Percentage saturation of transferrin
c. Hemoglobin
d. Ferritin

192. Which type of anemia is seen in patients of rheumatoid arthritis? ***(Recent Pattern Question 2018)***

a. Normocytic and hypochromic anemia
b. Microcytic and hypochromic anemia
c. Normocytic and normochromic anemia
d. Macrocytic anemia

193. Which of the following is the correct sequence of early erythropoiesis in a developing fetus? ***(Recent Pattern Question 2018)***

a. Yolk sac, bone marrow and liver
b. Yolk sac, liver and bone marrow
c. Liver, bone marrow and yolk sac
d. Bone marrow, yolk sac and liver

194. WHO cut off for diagnosis of anemia in nonpregnant female is < _______? ***(Recent Pattern Question 2018)***

a. 07 g% b. 10 g%
c. 11 g% d. 12 g%

195. Which of the following tests is to be done to screen a lady with family history of thalassemia? ***(Recent Pattern Question 2018)***

a. Hb A2 Levels
b. NESTROFT
c. High performance liquid chromatography
d. P. smear and reticulocyte count

196. Which of the following is best to confirm diagnosis of thalassemia trait in a lady with positive family history of thalassemia?

a. Elevated HbA2 b. Reticulocytosis
c. NESTROFT d. Peripheral Smear

197. Heinz bodies are composed of: ***(Recent Pattern Question 2017)***

a. DNA b. RNA
c. Iron d. Denatured haemoglobin

198. Positive coombs test is seen in which haemolytic anaemia? ***(Recent Pattern Question 2017)***

a. SLE b. PAN
c. TTP d. HUS

199. Arsenic is used in treatment of? ***(Recent Pattern Question 2017)***

a. A.M.L
b. C.M.L
c. Myeloproliferative disease
d. A.L.L

200. Which virus leads to Aplastic Crisis? ***(Recent Pattern Question 2017)***

a. Pox virus b. Parvo virus B19
c. Hepatitis A d. Hepatitis B

201. Which of the following will lead to X-ray appearance of crew hair cut appearance with Gamma Gandy bodies? ***(Recent Pattern Question 2017)***

a. Sickle cell anaemia
b. Hereditary spherocytosis
c. Acute myeloid leukemia
d. Osteoporosis

202. Gamma gandy bodies are seen in? ***(Recent Pattern Question 2017)***

a. Portal hypertension
b. Plasma cell dyscaria
c. Plasma cell leukemia
d. Primary sclerosing cholangitis

203. Rosenthal syndrome occurs due to deficiency of: ***(Recent Pattern Question 2017)***

a. Factor 2 b. Factor 5
c. Factor 9 d. Factor 11

204. Which of the following is a B-cell disease ***(Recent Pattern Question 2016)***

a. Amyloidosis b. Multiple myeloma
c. ALL d. Mycosis fungoides

205. Lacunar Reed Sternberg cell is found in which type of Hodgkin's lymphoma? ***(Recent Pattern Question 2016)***

a. Mixed cellularity b. Lymphocyte rich
c. Nodular sclerosis d. Lymphocyte depleted

206. JAK –2 mutation is seen in:

a. Polycythemia vera b. I.T.P
c. C.M.L d. C.M.M.L

207. Gamma Gandy bodies contain hemosiderin and _______?

a. Na^+ b. Ca^{++}
c. Mg^{++} d. K^+

208. The cause of the severe hemorrhage in acute promyelocytic leukemia is?

a. Disseminated intravascular coagulation
b. Immune complex deposits on blood vessels
c. Thrombocytopenia
d. Thrombocytosis

209. Which is the most common Hodgkin's lymphoma?

a. Nodular sclerosis b. Mixed cellularity
c. Lymphocyte depleted d. Lymphocyte rich

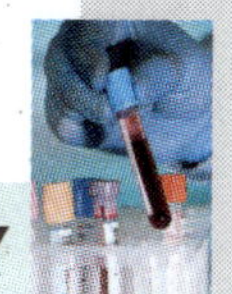

210. Which is the percentage of blasts in AML?
a. 8% b. 15%
c. 20% d. 25%

211. Presence of >10% plasma cells with no lytic lesion and M protein in serum is seen in:
a. Smoldering myeloma
b. Multiple myeloma
c. Monoclonal Gammopathy of unknown significance
d. Nonsecretory myeloma

212. Langerhans cell CD marker is?
a. CD1 b. CD2
c. CD4 d. CD56

213. RBC contains?
a. Iron b. Folic acid
c. Vitamin C d. Biotin

214. Leucopenia is NOT seen in?
a. New born
b. Starvation
c. Enteric fever
d. Viral or protozoal infection

215. Prevalence of Burkitt's lymphoma is highest in?
a. Australia b. Africa
c. Asia d. America

216. Reticulocytosis is NOT seen in:
a. Thalassemia b. Hereditary spherocytosis
c. Chronic renal failure d. Sickle cell anemia

217. GLUT present on surface of RBC?
a. GLUT 1 b. GLUT 2
c. GLUT 3 d. GLUT 4

218. Splenectomy is useful in which of the following:
a. Chronic ITP b. Sickle cell anemia
c. Tuberculosis d. Good pasture syndrome

219. Extrinsic pathway of clotting factors is measured by:
a. Prothrombin time
b. Activated partial thromboplastin time
c. Bleeding time
d. Clotting time

220. Which of following viruses cause hemolysis of red blood cells?
a. Rubella b. Human parvo virus B19
c. Measles d. Dengue virus

221. G6PD helps in maintaining the integrity of RBC by:
a. Controlling oxidative stress on RBC
b. Controlling reduction stress on RBC
c. Maintaining flexibility of cell membrane
d. Component of electron transport chain

222. Low TIBC is seen in:
a. Anemia of chronic disease
b. Iron deficiency anemia
c. Fanconi anemia
d. Aplastic anemia

223. Comment on type of anemia in peripheral smear:

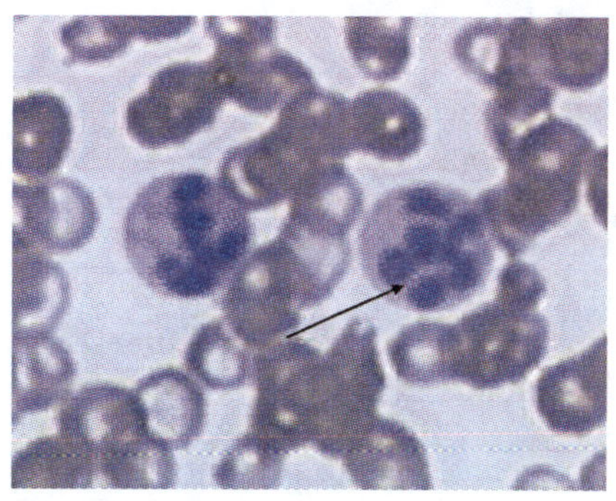

a. Pernicious anemia
b. Iron deficiency anemia
c. Sickle cell anemia
d. Hereditary spherocytosis

224. Fetal hemoglobin has features which of these?
a. Most susceptible to denaturation by acid
b. Resistant to denaturation by alkali
c. By 20 weeks 90% of fetal Hb is HbF
d. It has 2 alpha and 2 beta chains

225. Which is the life span of transfused RBC?
a. 30 days b. 45 days
c. 60 days d. 120 days

226. Schistocytes are seen in:
a. HUS b. HSP
c. Abetalipoproteinemia d. Myelofibrosis

227. All are seen in thalassemia major; EXCEPT:
a. Transfusion dependency
b. Splenoheptatomegaly
c. Ineffective erythropoiesis
d. Macrocytic anemia

228. Low iron & low TIBC is seen in:
a. Anaemia of chronic disease
b. Sideroblastic anaemia
c. Iron deficiency anaemia
d. Aplastic anemia

229. Reticulocytes are stained with:
a. Brilliant cresyl blue b. Sudan black
c. Warthin starry d. Hemotoxylin-eosin stain

230. Which is the storage form of iron:
a. Transferrin b. Ferritin
c. Hepcidin d. Ferroportin

231. Which is the most common type of Hodgkin's lymphoma?
a. Nodular sclerosis
b. Mixed cellularity
c. Lymphocyte predominant
d. Lymphocyte depleted

232. Which is the most common ALL subtype?
a. Pre B cell
b. Pre T cell
c. T cell
d. B cell

233. All cause Reticulocytosis; EXCEPT:
a. Aplastic anemia
b. Thalassemia
c. Sickle cell anemia
d. Chronic blood loss

234. Hodgkins lymphoma is caused by:
a. EBV b. CMV
c. HHV6 d. HHV8

235. Which of the following leukemia almost never develops after radiation?
a. Acute myeloblastic leukemia
b. Chronic myeloid leukemia
c. Acute lymphoblastic leukemia
d. Chronic lymphocytic leukemia

236. Which is the most common defectively produced antibody in multiple myeloma?
a. IgG
b. IgM
c. IgA
d. IgD

CARDIOVASCULAR PATHOLOGY

237. A normal individual underwent an evaluation of his cardiac tissue. Which isoform of lactate dehydrogenase is predominant in the cardiac tissue? *(Most Recent Question Aug 2020)*
a. LDH1 b. LDH2
c. LDH3 d. LDH4

238. Berry aneurysm most commonly occurs due to: *(Recent Pattern Question 2019)*
a. Endothelial injury of vessel due to HTN
b. Intimal elastic lamina layer defect
c. Endothelial layer defect
d. Adventitia defect

239. Most sensitive and specific marker for MI is: *(Recent Pattern Question 2019)*
a. Troponin I b. Cytokeratin
c. Myoglobin d. CPK- MM

240. Antecedent diagnosis of Group A streptococcal infection in Acute rheumatic fever can be made by: *(Recent Pattern Question 2019)*
a. AS0 b. CRP
c. ESR elevation d. Low C3 levels

241. Most common cardiac defect in Down syndrome is: *(Recent Pattern Question 2019)*
a. Endocardial cushion defect
b. Ventricular septal defect
c. Perpheral pulmonic stenosis
d. Anomalous origin of left coronary artery from pulmonary artery (A.L.C.A.P.A)

242. Histopathological finding 12 hours after ischemic injury to heart is? *(Recent Pattern Question 2018-19)*
a. Karyorrhexis of myocytes
b. Neocapillary invasion of myocytes
c. Hyper-eosinophilia of myocytes
d. Coagulation necrosis of myocytes

243. Which of the following is the correct description for type of heart lesion seen in patients of rheumatic arthritis? *(Recent Pattern Question 2018)*
a. Osler's nodes b. McCallum patch
c. Floppy valves d. Myxomatous degeneration

244. Which is the most common cause of death in rheumatic heart disease? *(Recent Pattern Question 2017)*
a. Cardiac failure
b. Bacterial endocarditis
c. Mural thrombus
d. Coronary insufficiency

245. Which is the earliest histopathological change in myocardial infarction? *(Recent Pattern Question 2017)*
a. Stretching and waviness of fibers
b. Neutrophilic infiltration
c. Coagulative necrosis
d. Fibrovascular response

246. Most common primary cardiac tumour? *(Recent Pattern Question 2017)*
a. Myxoma b. Rhabdomyoma
c. Rhabdomyosarcoma d. Angiosarcoma

247. Which is the first organ to be affected in left ventricular failure?
a. Lungs b. Liver
c. Kidney d. Brain

248. Which of the following is pathognomonic for rheumatic fever?
a. Aschoff nodules
b. Anitschkow cells
c. McCallum's patch
d. Vegetations along the cusps

249. All are true about myocardial response and changes to myocardial infarction; EXCEPT?
a. Neutrophilic infiltrates in first 48 hours
b. Loss of contractility within 2 minutes
c. Reversible injury within 20–40 minutes
d. Waviness of fibres at border of infarct

250. All are complications of atherosclerosis; EXCEPT?
a. Ulceration b. Thrombosis
c. Embolism d. Necrosis

251. Which is incorrect about Buerger's disease?
a. Ischemia of nerves
b. Deep vein thrombosis
c. Segmental inflammation
d. Superficial thrombophlebitis

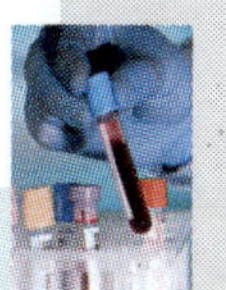

252. Why is Troponin C not used for MI diagnosis?
a. Troponin C binds to calcium
b. Troponin C is present in both cardiac and smooth muscle
c. Troponin C is present in both cardiac and skeletal muscle
d. It elevates late after onset of MI

253. Postmortem findings of myocardial infarction are all; EXCEPT:
a. Coagulative necrosis
b. Glycogen depletion
c. Granulation with type 4 collagen
d. Loss of nuclei

254. The most common primary neoplasm of the heart in adults is?
a. Lipoma b. Myxoma
c. Papillary fibroelastoma d. Rhabdomyoma

255. Which is the most common cardiac tumor?
a. Myxoma b. Rhabdomyosarcoma
c. angiosarcoma d. Metastasis

256. Which is the most common site of rhabdomyoma?
a. Left atrium b. Right atrium
c. Left ventricle d. Right ventricle

257. Which is the most common cardiac valve tumor?
a. Myxoma b. Rhabdomyoma
c. Papillary fibroelastoma d. Secondaries

258. Tree bark like calcification in chest X-ray is seen in?
a. Syphilitic aneurysm b. Aorto-Arteritis
c. Neurofibromatosis d. Atherosclerosis

259. Exudate in rheumatic fever is?
a. Serous b. Purulent
c. Fibrinous d. Myxomatous

260. Fibrinoid necrosis may be observed in all of the following; EXCEPT?
a. Malignant hypertension
b. Polyarteritis nodosa
c. Diabetic glomerulosclerosis
d. Aschoff's nodule

261. Polyarteritis Nodosa (PAN) typically involves which of the following?
a. Large elastic arteries
b. Small- or medium-sized muscular arteries
c. Arterioles
d. Capillaries

262. Medial calcification is seen in?
a. Atherosclerosis
b. Arteriolosclerosis
c. Monckeberg's sclerosis
d. Dissecting aneurysm

263. All are examples of medium vessel vasculitis; EXCEPT?
a. Classic PAN
b. Kawasaki disease
c. Buerger disease
d. SLE

LUNGS

264. A 45-year patient working in a factory for past 20 years presents with breathlessness. HRCT chest shows pleural thickening and fibrosis. Diagnosis is:
(Recent Pattern Question 2019)
a. Asbestosis
b. Coal worker pneumoconiosis
c. Silicosis
d. Berylliosis

265. Curschmann spirals are characteristic of which of the following airway disease?
a. Chronic bronchitis b. Emphysema
c. Atelectasis d. Bronchial asthma

266. Simmond focus in tuberculosis is seen in?
a. Brain b. Lungs
c. Liver d. Blood vessels

267. All are true about chronic bronchitis; EXCEPT:
a. Increased Reid's index
b. Submucosal gland hypertrophy
c. Eosinophilic infiltration of airways
d. Bronchorrhea

268. All are true about silicosis; EXCEPT:
a. Egg shell calcification
b. Nodular fibrosis
c. Bloody pleural effusion
d. Quartz is the main form implicated in pathogenesis

269. Kveim test is used for diagnosis of?
a. Sarcoidosis b. Sicca syndrome
c. Scleroderma d. C.R.E.S.T. syndrome

270. Schaumann body is seen in cases of:
a. Silicosis b. Asbestosis
c. Sarcoidosis d. Anthracosis

271. Which is the most common clinical presentation of sarcoidosis?
a. Pleural plaque b. Hilar lymphadenopathy
c. Pulmonary fibrosis d. Interstitial calcification

272. Lung cancer is most commonly associated with?
a. Silicosis b. Berylliosis
c. Asbestosis d. Anthracosis

273. Which is the most common type of lung cancer?
a. Small cell lung cancer b. Large cell lung cancer
c. Squamous cell cancer d. Adenocarcinoma

274. Which is the most common lung cancer in females?
a. Squamous cell CA b. Adenocarcinoma
c. Small cell lung CA d. Large cell CA

275. Which is the most aggressive lung CA?
a. Squamous cell CA b. Adenocarcinoma
c. Small cell lung CA d. Large cell CA

276. Azzopardi effect is seen in:
a. Squamous cell CA b. Adenocarcinoma
c. Small cell lung CA d. Large cell CA

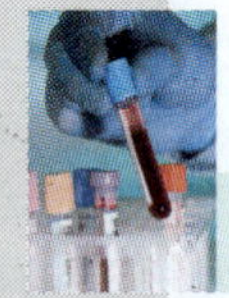

277. Which is the most common cancer associated with asbestosis?
a. Mesothelioma
b. Adenocarcinoma lung
c. Squamous cell cancer of lung
d. Large cell cancer lung

KIDNEY

278. Urine examination of a middle-aged man shows Bence Jones proteins. On X-ray Skull multiple lytic lesions are seen. Which of the following protein factions is elevated in this condition? ***(Most Recent Question June 2022)***
a. Alpha– globulin b. Beta1 – Globulin
c. Gamma – Globulin d. Beta2 – Globulin

279. A 8-year-old child develops sore throat and couple of weeks later he has periorbital edema and passage of cola-colored urine. Which of the following most closely fits in the description provided?
(Most Recent Question Dec 2021)
a. Minimal change disease
b. F.S.G.S
c. IgA Nephropathy
d. Post streptococcal glomerulonephritis

280. A 56-year-old diabetic patient has chronic renal failure, and is undergoing hemodialysis. Which of the following amyloid is most likely to get deposited?
(Most Recent Question Dec 2020)
a. AA b. A beta
c. A beta 2 d. A cal

281. A patient has been diagnosed with a solid cancer of the bowel. He also experienced massive proteinuria after few months of initial diagnosis of cancer. Which of the following is a likely cause for the development of the urinary finding? ***(Most Recent Question Aug 2020)***
a. Focal segmental glomerulosclerosis
b. Minimal change disease
c. Membranous glomerulopathy
d. MPGN

282. An 8-year-old patient presents with abdominal pain, rashes on legs and difficulty in walking. First differential diagnosis is: ***(Most Recent Question Dec 2019)***

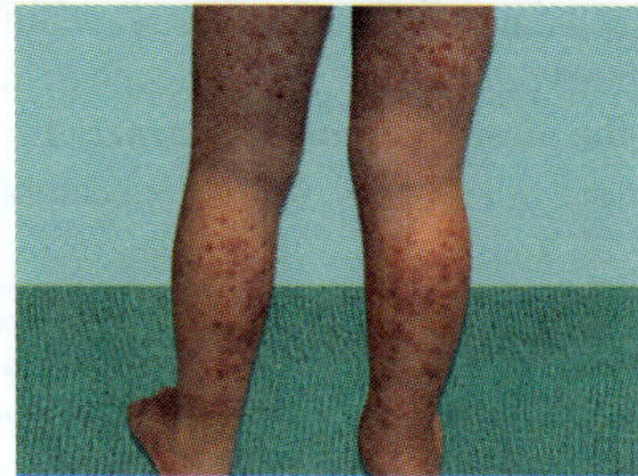

a. IgA nephropathy b. HSP
c. Meningococcemia d. PSGN

283. Which of these is a Nephritic syndrome?
(Recent Pattern Question 2019)
a. Minimal change disease
b. Membranous Glomerulopathy
c. Post infectious Glomerulonephritis
d. Focal segmental glomerulosclerosis

284. Most characteristic finding of diabetic nephropathy?
(Recent Pattern Question 2019)
a. Kimmelstiel-Wilson disease
b. Diffuse glomerulosclerosis
c. Focal segmental glomerulosclerosis
d. Armanni-Ebstein change

285. Most characteristic feature of diabetic nephropathy:
(Recent Pattern Question 2018-19)
a. Kimmelstiel-Wilson change
b. Armanni-Ebstein change
c. Focal segmental glomerulosclerosis
d. Membrano proliferative glomerulonephritis

286. Fatty change is seen in? ***(Recent Pattern Question 2017)***
a. Brain b. Kidney
c. Adrenal d. Bladder

287. The presence of sub-epithelial humps on electron microscopic examination of kidney biopsy is seen in?
(Recent Pattern Question 2017)
a. PSGN
b. Chronic glomerulonephritis
c. Crescentic glomerulonephritis
d. Membranous glomerulopathy

288. Crescent formation is seen in?
(Recent Pattern Question 2017)
a. FSGS b. MGN
c. RPGN d. PSGN

289. Adult polycystic kidney disease is:
(Recent Pattern Question 2016)
a. Autosomal recessive b. Autosomal dominant
c. X-linked recessive d. X-linked dominant

290. Owl eye inclusions in urine are seen in:
(Recent Pattern Question 2016)
a. EBV b. HSV-1
c. HSV-2 d. CMV

291. Hydropic degeneration of the renal tubular epithelium occurs in:
a. Chronic alcoholism
b. Carbon tetrachloride poisoning
c. Excessive renal sodium loss
d. Hypokalemia

292. Podocytes are seen in:
a. Bowman's capsule
b. Proximal convoluted tubule
c. Distal convoluted tubule
d. Collecting tubule

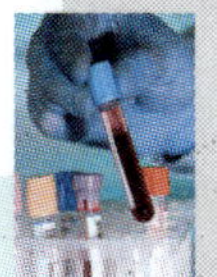

293. Maximum endocapillary proliferation is seen in:
a. Membranous glomerulonephritis
b. Mesangioproliferative glomerulonephritis
c. Focal segmental glomerulonephritis
d. Post streptococcal GN

294. Wire loop lesions are seen in:
a. SLE
b. Diabetic nephropathy
c. Benign nephrosclerosis
d. Wegener's granulomatosis

295. The drug which causes renal papillary necrosis is:
a. Acetophenetidin b. Gentamicin
c. Gold d. Methicillin

296. Which of the following statement is incorrect about ADPKD?
a. Autosomal dominant
b. Chromosome 4 and 16 are involved
c. Cysts in liver and pancreas
d. Bilateral kidney transplantation

297. WBC cast is seen in:
a. Pyelonephritis b. Glomerulonephritis
c. Chronic renal failure d. Hyaline cast

298. RBC cast is seen in:
a. Minimal change disease
b. Renal vein thrombosis
c. Bladder schistomiasis
d. Rapidly progressive glomerulonephritis

299. Which is the most common glomerulonephritis associated with HIV?
a. Focal segmental glomerulosclerosis
b. Diffuse glomerulosclerosis
c. Membranoproliferative glomerulonephritis
d. Crescentic glomerulonephritis

300. Which of the following is true about complications of hemodialysis?
a. A beta amyloid deposition
b. Cardiovascular complications
c. Renal rickets
d. Metabolic acidosis

301. Which is the most common malignant tumor of kidney:
a. Papillary carcinoma b. Papillary adenoma
c. Renal cell CA d. Wilm's tumor

302. Which is the most common risk factor for RCC?
a. Urinary tract infection b. Renal calculi
c. Smoking d. Hypertension

303. Which is the RCC with best prognosis?
a. Clear cell CA b. Papillary CA
c. Medullary CA d. Chromophobe

304. Which is the most common type of RCC associated with dialysis?
a. Clear cell CA b. Papillary CA
c. Medullary CA d. Chromophobe

305. Which is the most common type of RCC?
a. Papillary CA b. Clear cell CA
c. Medullary CA d. Chromophobe

306. Which of the following organ is least likely to be affected in cases of ADPKD?
a. Brain b. Heart
c. Liver d. Lung

307. Which is the most common organ associated with polycystic disease?
a. Brain b. Heart
c. Liver d. Lung

308. Which is the least common cause of death in case of polycystic disease?
a. Coronary heart disease b. Infection
c. Berry aneurysm rupture d. Pancreatic cyst

LIVER

309. A 30-year-old female presents with a history suggestive of chronic liver disease. Liver biopsy shows Hepatocytes with ground glass appearance. Comment on the diagnosis:
(Most Recent Question June 2022)
a. Hepatitis B b. Rotor syndrome
c. Hemochromatosis d. Hepatitis A

310. A 22-year-old has history of recurrent episodes of jaundice. Labs show elevated unconjugated hyperbilirubinemia with normal liver enzymes. Diagnosis is?
(Most Recent Question June 2022)
a. Crigler-Najjar syndrome
b. Dubin Johnson syndrome
c. Rotor syndrome
d. Gilbert syndrome

311. A known case of diabetes mellitus came to the hospital with pigmentation of skin over the arms. He is also found out to be suffering from micronodular cirrhosis. On liver biopsy iron deposits are seen. Comment on the diagnosis. ***(Most Recent Question June 2022)***
a. Alpha 1 anti-trypsin deficiency
b. Hemochromatosis
c. Wilson's disease
d. Alcoholic hepatitis

312. The following serological status is noted in a patient: HbsAg positive and HbeAg positive. Diagnosis is:
a. Acute viral hepatitis ***(Recent Pattern Question 2019)***
b. Chronic viral hepatitis
c. Acute viral hepatitis with infectivity
d. Remote infection

313. Chronic viral hepatitis is seen with:
(Recent Pattern Question 2019)
a. HBV b. HCV
c. HDV d. HEV

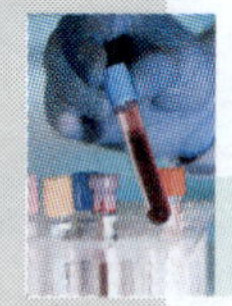

314. Mallory hyaline bodies are seen in:
(Recent Pattern Question 2017)
a. Acute viral hepatitis b. Wilson disease
c. Fulminant hepatitis d. All of these

315. Conjugated hyperbilirubinemia is seen in?
(Recent Pattern Question 2017)
a. Criggler Najar type 1 b. Criggler Najar type 2
c. Gilbert syndrome d. Dubin Johnson syndrome

316. Pathologic changes or clinical manifestations which occur in patients with primary hemochromatosis include all of the following; EXCEPT?
a. Congestive heart failure
b. Diabetes mellitus
c. Testicular atrophy
d. Photosensitivity dermatitis

317. Elevated alpha-fetoprotein is seen in all; EXCEPT?
a. Hepatocellular cancer b. Colonic cancer
c. Tuberculoma d. Pancreatic cancer

318. Unconjugated hyperbilirubinemia is seen in:
a. Rotor's syndrome
b. Crigler-Najjar syndrome
c. Dubin Johnson syndrome
d. All of the above

319. Which of the following hereditary hyperbilirubinemia is autosomal dominant?
a. Dubin Johnson syndrome
b. Rotor syndrome
c. Crigler-Najjar syndrome type I
d. Crigler-Najjar syndrome type II

320. Which of the following hereditary hyperbilirubinemia is most fatal?
a. Dubin Johnson syndrome
b. Rotor syndrome
c. Crigler–Najjar syndrome type I
d. Crigler–Najjar syndrome type II

321. "Onion skin" fibrosis of bile duct is seen in:
a. Primary biliary cirrhosis
b. Primary sclerosing cholangitis
c. Extrahepatic biliary fibrosis
d. Congenital hepatic fibrosis

322. The complications of gallstones include all of the following; EXCEPT:
a. Adenocarcinoma of ampulla of Vater
b. Acute intrahepatic cholangitis
c. Acute pancreatitis
d. Gangrenous cholecystitis

323. Most common tumor of liver is:
a. Cavernous hemangioma
b. Hepatocellular carcinoma
c. Adenoma
d. Metastasis

324. What accumulates in the space of Disse in cirrhosis?
a. Collagen type 1 & 4 b. Collagen type 2 & 3
c. Collagen type 1 & 3 d. Collagen type 2 & 4

325. Which of the following is not a function of liver?
a. Production of albumin b. Detoxification of ammonia
c. Production of vitamin K d. Metabolism of drugs

326. Which of the following is a thorium induced tumor?
a. Renal cell carcinoma b. Lymphoma
c. Angiosarcoma of liver d. Astrocytoma

GASTROINTESTINAL TRACT

327. A middle-aged lady presents with abdominal pain and diarrhea. Her intestinal biopsy demonstrated villous atrophy and serum has presence of anti – TTG antibodies. Which of the following is the most likely diagnosis in her? ***(Most Recent Question Dec 2021)***
a. Celiac sprue b. Topical sprue
c. Whipple disease d. Ulcerative colitis

328. A patient who undergoes a gastrectomy is most likely to develop which of the following deficiencies?
(Most Recent Question June 2021)
a. Folic acid b. Pyridoxine
c. Thiamine d. Cobalamin

329. A 30-year-old woman is having progressive dysphagia. On examination she has thickening of oral mucosa and leather like skin. She is also hypertensive and has limited exercise capacity due to lung fibrosis. Which of the following is the possible diagnosis?
(Most Recent Question Dec 2020)
a. Peutz-Jeghers syndrome b. Postcricoid dysphagia
c. Achalasia cardia d. Scleroderma

330. Which of the following is implicated is the development of angiosarcoma of the liver?
(Most Recent Question Aug 2020)
a. Copper b. Zinc
c. Arsenic d. Iron

331. A 2-year-old child presents with diarrhea and failure to thrive. The finding on upper GI endoscopy is shown in the image. What is the correct etiology of this presentation?
(Most Recent Question Dec 2019)

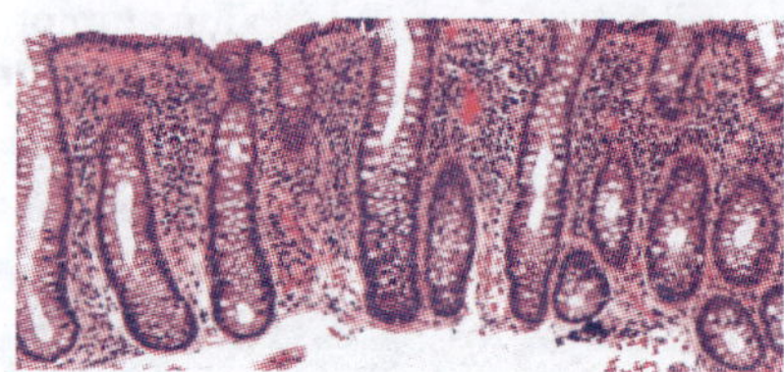

a. Anti-tissue transglutaminase antibody
b. Antimitochondrial antibody
c. Anticentromere antibody
d. Antitopoisomerase antibody

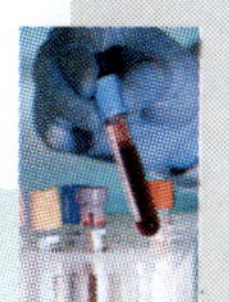

332. Whipple's disease is caused by: *(Recent Pattern Question 2019)*
- a. Bacteria
- b. Virus
- c. Protozoa
- d. Helminths

333. Whipple's is disease is caused by: *(Recent Pattern Question 2018)*
- a. Bacteroides
- b. Acinetobacter
- c. H. pylori
- d. Tropheryma whippelii

334. Which of the following is called chronic hypertrophic gastritis? *(Recent Pattern Question 2017)*
- a. Type A gastritis
- b. Type B gastritis
- c. Menetrier's disease
- d. Type AB gastritis

335. Serpiginous ulcers with deep fissures are seen in? *(Recent Pattern Question 2017)*
- a. Crohn's disease
- b. Ulcerative colitis
- c. Neutropenic colitis
- d. Amoebic dysentery

336. Duodenal villous atrophy is seen in: *(Recent Pattern Question 2016)*
- a. Crohn's disease
- b. Ulcerative colitis
- c. Celiac disease
- d. Cystic fibrosis

337. Pseudo-pancreatic cyst secretes:
- a. Lipase
- b. Amylase
- c. Trypsin
- d. Ptylin

338. An increased incidence of pancreatitis is associated with all of the following, EXCEPT:
- a. Alcoholism
- b. Cholelithiasis
- c. Chlorothiazide therapy
- d. Hypertension

339. Hyperplasic gastric polyps are most likely to be found in association with which one of the following conditions?
- a. Gastric carcinoma
- b. Familial polyposis syndrome
- c. Chronic gastritis
- d. Crohn's disease

340. Anti-parietal cell antibodies are found in patients with?
- a. Good-pasture syndrome
- b. Primary biliary cirrhosis
- c. Wegener granulomatosis
- d. Pernicious anemia

341. All are true about GIST, EXCEPT:
- a. Most common mesenchymal tumour of GIT
- b. C-kit (CD117) positive
- c. Originate from interstitial cells of Cajal
- d. Majority seen in duodenum

342. All are true about amoebiasis, EXCEPT:
- a. Flask shaped ulcers
- b. Disease affects caecum and ascending colon
- c. Anchovy pus in liver
- d. Coagulative necrosis

343. All are true about familial adenomatous polyposis, EXCEPT:
- a. APC gene on chromosome 5
- b. Mutation in nucleotide excision base repair gene
- c. Colorectal cancer develops in 100% patients before the age of 30 years
- d. Prophylactic polypectomy is recommended as standard therapy

344. Which is the most likely to be associated with type A gastritis?
- a. Decreased growth of luminal bacteria
- b. Decreased chances of gastric carcinoma
- c. Decreased plasma concentration of gastrin
- d. Increased MCV of RBC

345. Which type of gastric carcinoma has the best prognosis?
- a. Linitis plastic
- b. Polypoidal growth
- c. Ulcerative
- d. Superficial spreading

346. All are seen in Crohn's disease, EXCEPT:
- a. Poor perianal hygiene
- b. Stricture formation
- c. Crypt abscess
- d. Rectum is commonly involved

347. Radiation given to oesophagus will lead to:
- a. Fibrosis of oesophagus
- b. Thinning of mucosal layer
- c. Volcano ulcer in esophagus
- d. Strawberry appearance of mucosa

348. Which is the most common tumor of the spleen?
- a. Hemangioma
- b. Lymphoma
- c. Angiosarcoma
- d. Metastasis

349. Which is the most common site of lymphoma?
- a. Duodenum
- b. Pancreas
- c. Mesenteric lymph nodes
- d. Stomach

350. Which of the following is not associated with Crohn's disease?
- a. Pseudo-polyps
- b. Fistula
- c. Malignancy
- d. Perineal sepsis

351. Which antibody is suggestive of diagnosis of ulcerative colitis?
- a. p-ANCA
- b. c-ANCA
- c. a.M.A
- d. a. N.A

CENTRAL NERVOUS SYSTEM

352. Which of the following disease shows the presence of deposition of Tau protein? *(Most Recent Question Dec 2020)*
- a. CJD
- b. Rabies
- c. Parkinson's disease
- d. Alzheimer's disease

353. Which of the following disease shows deposition of PrP^{SC} protein in neuronal cytoplasm? *(Most Recent Question Dec 2020)*
- a. Variant Creutzfeldt-Jacob disease
- b. Rabies
- c. Parkinson's disease
- d. Alzheimer's disease

354. Most common site of Brain metastasis is: *(Recent Pattern Question 2019)*
- a. Lung cancer
- b. Head and neck cancer
- c. Prostate cancer
- d. Breast cancer

355. Which enzyme protects the brain from free radical injury?
a. Myeloperoxidase b. Superoxide dismutase
c. MAO d. Hydroxylase

356. Negri bodies are found in:
a. Cerebellum b. Hypothalamus
c. Hippocampus d. Brain stem

357. Lewy's body is seen in:
a. Alzheimer's b. Rabies
c. Parkinsonism d. Multi infarct dementia

358. Ubiquitin deposit in neurons is seen in:
a. Huntington's chorea b. Pick's disease
c. Cortical dementia d. AIDS related dementia

359. Glioma Retinae is:
a. Retinoblastoma b. Meningioma
c. Optic nerve glioma d. Giant cell astrocytoma

ENDOCRINE SYSTEM

360. A patient presents with the presence of a thyroid swelling and weight loss. The cervical lymphadenopathy report of the patient suggested the presence of cells with Orphan Annie-eye nuclei. Which of the following is a likely diagnosis for this patient?
(Most Recent Question Aug 2020)
a. Follicular thyroid cancer
b. Medullary thyroid cancer
c. Papillary thyroid cancer
d. Anaplastic thyroid cancer

361. Which is not seen in Tumour lysis Syndrome?
(Recent Pattern Question 2019)
a. Hypophosphatemia b. Hypocalcemia
c. Hyperuricemia d. Hyperkalemia

362. Comment on the diagnosis for SAP normal, PTH normal, Vitamin D3 normal with elevated serum Calcium values? ***(Recent Pattern Question 2019)***
a. Vitamin D intoxication b. Hyperparathyroidism
c. Multiple myeloma d. Nutritional rickets

363. Which of the following is correct about MEN 2 A Syndrome? ***(Recent Pattern Question 2018-19)***
a. Parathyroid adenoma b. Pituitary adenoma
c. Pancreas adenoma d. Cavernous angioma

364. Pheochromocytoma produces all, EXCEPT:
(Recent Pattern Question 2018-19)
a. Nor-epinephrine
b. Secretin
c. Vasoactive intestinal polypeptide
d. Calcitonin

365. Which of the following is not directly related to Hashimoto's thyroiditis?
a. Hypothyroidism b. Slow onset
c. Neuropathy d. Autoimmune disease

366. Amyloid stroma is seen with:
a. Papillary carcinoma Thyroid
b. Medullary carcinoma Thyroid
c. Follicular carcinoma Thyroid
d. Anaplastic carcinoma Thyroid

367. Which is the most common cause of death in a diabetic patient?
a. Cardiac b. Renal
c. Hypoglycemia d. Infection

368. Hyperparathyroidism is seen in all, EXCEPT:
a. MEN I b. MEN IIA
c. MEN IIB d. Parathyroid hyperplasia

369. All are included in MEN-IIB; EXCEPT?
a. Pheochromocytoma
b. Hyperparathyroidism
c. Mucosal neuroma
d. Marfanoid habitus

370. Which is incorrect about Neuroblastoma?
a. Most common abdominal tumor in infants
b. X-ray abdomen shows calcification
c. Can show spontaneous regression
d. Urine contains 5 H.I.A.A.

371. Which is characteristic histo-pathological feature of kidney in DM?
a. Nodular sclerosis b. Fibrin cap
c. Papillary necrosis d. Diffuse glomerulosclerosis

372. Psamomma bodies are seen in:
a. Papillary carcinoma thyroid
b. Medullary carcinoma thyroid
c. Follicular carcinoma thyroid
d. Anaplastic carcinoma

373. Orphan Annie eye nucleus is seen in:
a. Papillary thyroid cancer b. Follicular Lymphoma
c. Hurthle cell tumor d. Paraganglioma

374. Which is produced by Phaeochromocytoma in M.E.N 2A Sipple syndrome?
a. Epinephrine
b. Nor epinephrine
c. Dopamine
d. 5- H.I.

375. Pseudo-myxoma peritonei occur due to?
a. Dysgerminoma
b. Brenner's tumor
c. Theca cell tumor
d. Mucinous cystadenosarcoma

GENETICS

376. NF – 1 presenting as café-au lait spots follows which pattern of inheritance:
a. AD b. AR
c. XLR d. XLD

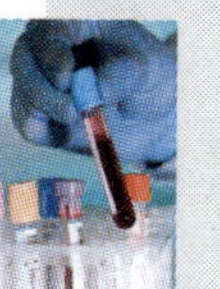

377. A couple is trying to have a child for the past 2 years, and after multiple unsuccessful trials they went for respective examination. Investigation of female came out to be absolutely normal but male shows presence of gynecomastia, small testis and scanty pubic hairs. He had a history of antisocial behavior during school days. Most probably he has: *(Most Recent Question June 2022)*

a. Williams syndrome
b. Noonan syndrome
c. Klinefelter syndrome
d. Marfan syndrome

378. Neural tube defects shows which pattern of inheritance?

a. AD
b. AR
c. XLD
d. Multifactorial

379. Pattern of inheritance seen with a disease inherited from grandmother to father and then father to his son. *(Most Recent Question June 2022)*

a. AD
b. AR
c. XLR
d. XLD

380. ATP7B gene mutation is associated with: *(Most Recent Question June 2021)*

a. Menke disease
b. Hemochromatosis
c. Wilson disease
d. Huntington disease

381. Joint and Skin hyperextensibility and laxity is seen in: *(Most Recent Question June 2021)*

a. Ehler Danlos syndrome
b. Marfan Syndrome
c. Cutix laxa
d. Osteopetrosis

382. Comment on the diagnosis? *(Most Recent Question Dec 2020)*

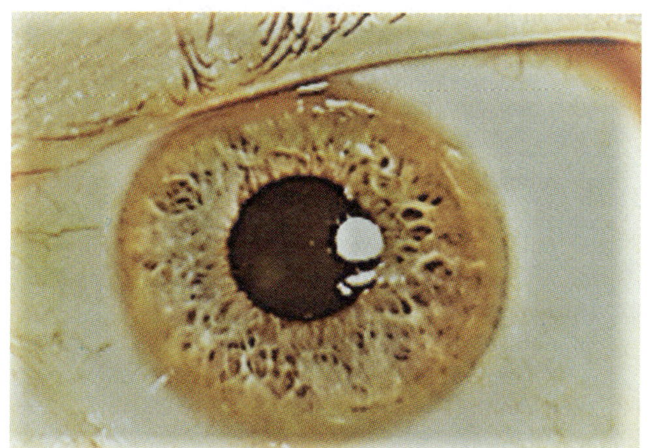

a. NF-1
b. Arcus senilis
c. Wilson disease
d. Myotonic dystrophy

383. Comment on the diagnosis: *(Most Recent Question Dec 2020)*

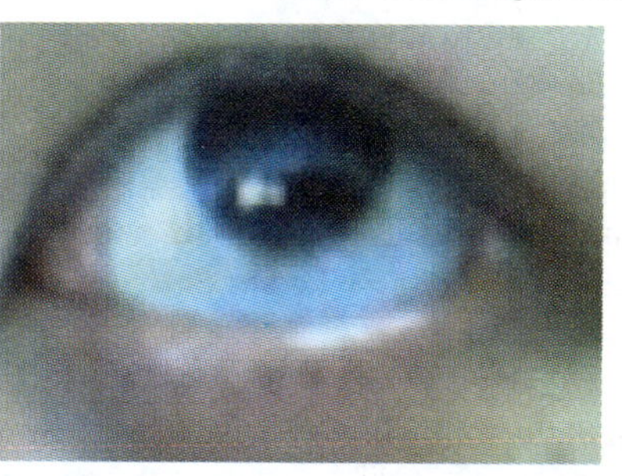

a. Scurvy
b. Osteogenesis imperfecta
c. Rickets
d. Paget's disease

384. Comment on the diagnosis from the following Karyotype? *(Most Recent Question Aug 2020)*

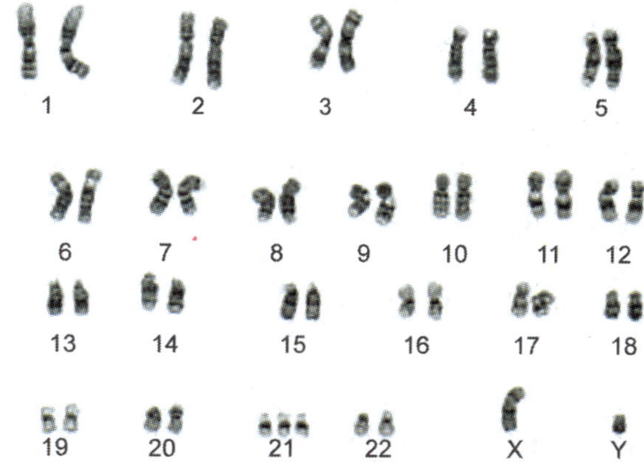

a. Down syndrome
b. Turner syndrome
c. Klinefelter syndrome
d. Edward syndrome

385. A patient has been diagnosed with a condition due to a DNA repair gene defect. He is having mottled hyper-pigmentation on the skin and high risk for development skin cancers as per the physician. Which of the following is a likely enzyme defect in the patient? *(Most Recent Question Aug 2020)*

a. Helicase
b. Nucleotide excision repair defect
c. ATN gene
d. MSH gene

386. Which of the following is the mode of inheritance in a patient suffering from Red green colour blindness? *(Most Recent Question Aug 2020)*

a. Autosomal dominant
b. Autosomal recessive
c. X-linked dominant
d. X-linked recessive

387. A 17-year-old girl is brought with complaints of short height, amenorrhea with widely spaced hypoplastic nipples. What is correct about Karyotyping for this case? *(Most Recent Question Dec 2019)*

a. 45 X0
b. 46 XXY
c. 47 XXX
d. 46 XY

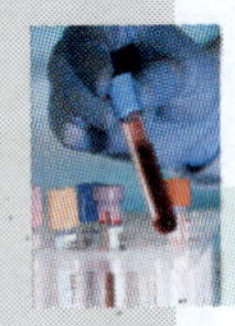

388. Which of the following disease has XLR pattern of inheritance? ***(Recent Pattern Question 2018-19)***
a. Hurler Syndrome
b. Thalassemia
c. Hereditary Spherocytosis
d. G6PD

389. Consanguinity is seen with which pattern of inheritance? ***(Recent Pattern Question 2018-19)***
a. AR
b. AD
c. XLR
d. XLD

390. Which of the following is regarded as outward expression of gene? ***(Recent Pattern Question 2018)***
a. Phenotype
b. Proteomics
c. Genotype
d. Anticipation

391. Which of the following has a polygenic pattern of inheritance? ***(Recent Pattern Question 2018)***
a. Diabetes mellitus
b. Familial hypercholesterolemia
c. G6PD
d. Resistant rickets

392. BRCA 1 is located on which chromosome? ***(Recent Pattern Question 2017)***
a. Chromosome 13q21
b. Chromosome 17q21
c. Chromosome 17q23
d. Chromosome 13q23

393. The defect Marfan syndrome is: ***(Recent Pattern Question 2017)***
a. Fibrillin 1
b. Fibrillin 2
c. Fibrillin 3
d. Fibrillin 4

394. Klinefelter syndrome genotype is: ***(Recent Pattern Question 2017)***
a. 45XO
b. 46XXY
c. 47XYY
d. 47XXY

395. Which of the following is responsible for the lesion shown in the image?

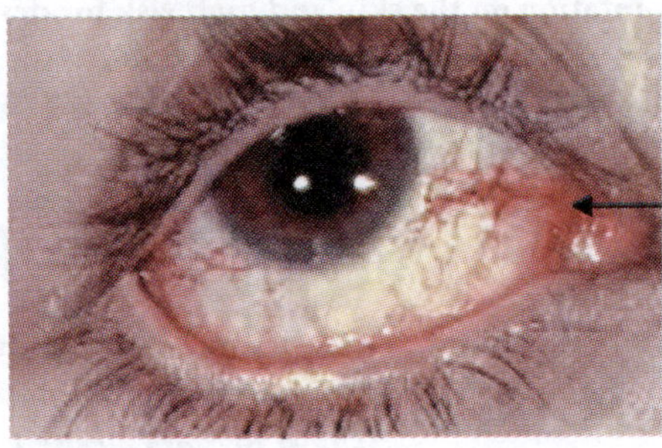

a. 11q (14-15)
b. 11q(22-23)
c. 13q14
d. Inv 16

396. Which is correct about autosomal recessive condition, in case of one homozygous and one heterozygous parent?
a. 50% carrier and 50% affected
b. 25% carrier and 75% affected
c. 75% carrier and 25% affected
d. 50% carrier and 25% affected

397. Karyotyping is useful in diagnosis of:
a. Autosomal recessive disorders
b. X-linked recessive disorders
c. Chromosomal abnormalities
d. Biochemical abnormalities

398. Anticipation is seen in:
a. Translocation
b. Chromosome breaking
c. Trinucleotide - repeat expansion
d. Mitochondrial mutation

399. Hereditary retinoblastomas develop due to abnormality in which of the following chromosome?
a. 13ql4
b. 13pl4
c. 14pl3
d. 14ql3

400. A 22-year-old man has features of arm span greater than height, subluxed lenses, flattened and dilation of the aortic bulb. Which is the most likely diagnosis?
a. Ehlers-Danlos syndrome
b. Marfan syndrome
c. Werner's syndrome
d. Laurence-Moon-Biedl syndrome

401. Shortest chromosome is:
a. Chromosome 1
b. Chromosome 13
c. Chromosome 21
d. Chromosome 22

402. Autoimmune thyroiditis is seen with:
a. Down syndrome
b. Marfan syndrome
c. Louis Barr syndrome
d. Edward syndrome

403. All are true about Lyon's hypothesis; EXCEPT:
a. Only one of X chromosomes is genetically active
b. Only X chromosome from the mother undergoes pyknosis
c. Inactivation occurs on 16th day of embryonic life
d. Gene Xist causes gene silencing

404. Preferential expression of gene depending on parent of origin is called:
a. Genomic imprinting
b. Mosaicism
c. Chimerism
d. Cloning

405. All are true about F.I.S.H; EXCEPT:
a. Can detect numeric abnormalities of chromosomes
b. Can detect complex translocation of chromosomes
c. Can be performed on prenatal samples
d. All of the above

406. Sickle cell anemia is:
a. Autosomal recessive
b. Autosomal dominant
c. X-linked recessive
d. X-linked dominant

407. Duchene-muscular dystrophy is:
a. Autosomal dominant
b. Autosomal recessive
c. X-linked dominant
d. X-linked recessive

408. Which of the following is autosomal recessive?
a. Albinism
b. Duchenne muscular dystrophy
c. Marfan's syndrome
d. Incontinentia pigmentia

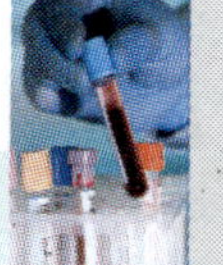

409. Which of the following is XLR?
a. Cystic fibrosis
b. Hemophilia
c. Hereditary spherocytosis
d. Neurofibromatosis

410. Which of the following is an X-linked dominant disorder?
a. Vitamin D resistant rickets
b. Familial hypercholesterolemia
c. Red green color blindness
d. Achondroplasia

411. Which is false about Hurler syndrome?
a. X-linked
b. Mental retardation
c. Joint stiffness
d. Coarse facial features

412. Which is true about Down syndrome?
a. Decrease in AFP
b. Increase in AFP
c. Increase in hCG
d. Increased progesterone

413. Alpha feto-protein is decreased in:
a. Down syndrome
b. Marfan's syndrome
c. Omphalocele
d. Turner syndrome

414. BRCA 1 gene is located on which chromosome?
a. Chromosome 13
b. Chromosome 17
c. Chromosome 19
d. Chromosome 21

415. All are familial breast cancer gene is all, EXCEPT:
a. BRCA1
b. P53
c. P16
d. PTEN

416. Klinefelter syndrome is:
a. 47 XXXY
b. 47XXY
c. 47 XX
d. 47 XY

417. Cat eye syndrome is seen with?
a. Retinoblastoma
b. Chromosome 22 defect
c. Zonular cataract
d. Cridu-chat syndrome

RESPIRATORY SYSTEM

418. A 60-year-old man complains of new onset dyspnea for last one year. Occupation history reveals he was working at construction site before retirement. Which of the following is the most probable diagnosis?
(Most Recent Question Dec 2021)
a. Silicosis
b. Asbestosis
c. Anthracosis
d. Byssinosis

419. A man working as a mason in Kota stone factory in Rajasthan has his Chest X-ray finding of 'Snow-storm'. Which of the following may have contributed to the same?
(Most Recent Question Dec 2021)
a. Silicosis
b. Asbestosis
c. Anthracosis
d. Baggasosis

420. Meig's Syndrome presents as:
(Most Recent Question Dec 2021)
a. Triad of ascites, pleural effusion and benign ovarian tumor
b. Triad of ascites pleural effusion and malignant ovarian tumor
c. Triad of ascites pleural effusion and HCC
d. Triad of ascites pleural effusion and squamous cell cancer SCC

421. A worker in cardboard factory is at risk of development of which of following disease?
(Most Recent Question June 2021)
a. Byssinosis
b. Bagassosis
c. Asbestosis
d. Anthracosis

422. Most common malignancy seen in a patient with Asbestosis: ***(Most Recent Question June 2021)***
a. Mesothelioma
b. Adenocarcinoma
c. Small cell
d. Squamous cell

423. Most common cause of atypical pneumonia?
(Recent Pattern Question 2019)
a. Mycoplasma pneumoniae
b. Klebsiella pneumoniae
c. Hemophilus influenzae
d. Chylamydia

424. Which organ is involved in Good-pasture syndrome?
(Recent Pattern Question 2018-19)
a. Liver
b. Adrenals
c. Kidney
d. Brain

425. Not a feature of bronchial asthma:
(Recent Pattern Question 2018-19)
a. Thickening of bronchial wall
b. Increase in number of goblet glands
c. Hypertrophy of smooth muscle
d. Increased IgE

426. Which of the following condition is characterized by presence of hyaline deposits in alveolar walls?
(Recent Pattern Question 2018)
a. Interstitial lung disease
b. Asthma
c. Hyaline membrane disease
d. Chronic bronchitis

427. Asthma is associated with:
a. IL-1
b. IL-2
c. IL-4
d. IL-6

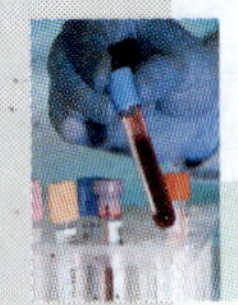

ANSWERS WITH EXPLANATIONS

MOST RECENT QUESTIONS 2023

1. Ans (b) Blebs formation

Ref: Robbins Basic Pathology, 10th ed. pg. 37, 40

- Irreversible cell injury is characterized by changes that cannot be reversed, leading to cell death. Various features are associated with irreversible injury.
- **Blebs formation:** This is a feature of reversible injury, not irreversible injury. Blebs are small, bubble-like protrusions on the cell surface that occur due to cytoskeletal changes and alterations in membrane integrity.
- In irreversible injury, the nucleus undergoes changes such as pyknosis, where the nucleus becomes shrunken, darkly stained, and densely aggregated. This indicates irreversible cell damage.
- **Karyolysis** refers to the dissolution of the nucleus due to enzymatic degradation of chromatin. It is also an irreversible change.
- **Densities in mitochondria** refer to the presence of electron-dense materials within mitochondria, which can indicate mitochondrial damage. Mitochondrial changes are associated with irreversible injury.

2. Ans (c) IL-6

Ref: Robbins and Cotran Pathologic Basis of Disease, 10th ed. pg. 658, 659, 848

- **Ferroportin** is a protein involved in iron transport. Its activity is regulated by hepcidin, a peptide hormone.
- Hepcidin synthesis is induced by interleukin-6 (IL-6) during inflammation. Hepcidin binds to ferroportin, leading to its degradation and decreased iron transport.
- **IL-1** is involved in the acute phase response and inflammation but is not the primary regulator of ferroportin.
- Tumor necrosis factor-alpha **(TNF-alpha)** contributes to inflammation and immune responses, but its role in ferroportin regulation is not as significant as IL-6.
- Transforming growth factor-beta **(TGF-Beta)** has various roles, including in tissue repair and fibrosis, but its direct influence on ferroportin is limited compared to IL-6.

3. Ans (d) TGF-beta

Ref: Robbins and Cotran Pathologic Basis of Disease, 10th ed. pg. 658, 659

- Chronic inflammation is characterized by the persistent presence of inflammatory cells and mediators in tissues.
- **TGF-β** is a key mediator of chronic inflammation. It promotes, fibrosis, which is a feature of chronic inflammation.

Extra Mile

- **Interleukin-1 (IL-1) TNF-α** are an important mediator of acute inflammation and fever but is also involved in chronic inflammation.
- **Note:** IFN Gamma is also a mediator for chronic inflammation.

4. Ans (b) 50%

Ref: Robbins and Cotran Pathologic Basis of Disease, 10th ed. pg. 144

- In an autosomal dominant condition, only one copy of the mutated gene is needed to cause the disease. This means that if the grandmother has the mutated gene, there is a 50% chance that she will pass it to her daughter. And if the daughter has the mutated gene, there is a 50% chance that she will pass it to her child.

5. Ans (a) 25%

Ref: Robbins and Cotran Pathologic Basis of Disease, 10th ed. pg. 641, 644, 1232

- Beta-thalassemia is an autosomal recessive condition. This means that both parents need to have the mutated gene in order for the child to have the disease. If both parents have the trait, there is a 25% chance that each child will have the disease.
- Both parents may have the trait, but neither one has the disease. However, there is a 25% chance that each child will inherit the mutated gene from both parents and have the disease.

6. Ans (a) AR

Ref: Robbins and Cotran Pathologic Basis of Disease, 10th ed. pg. 144

- Pedigree analysis is used to understand the inheritance pattern of genetic traits within families.
- The pedigree represents an autosomal recessive inheritance pattern.

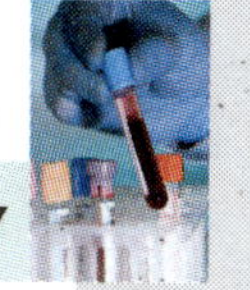

- This is indicated by the presence of affected individuals in multiple generations (horizontal transmission), often skipping generations, and parents of affected individuals being carriers (heterozygous) rather than affected.

7. Ans (d) IDA

Ref: Harrison's Principles of Internal Medicine, 21st ed. pg. 749-750

- Anemia refers to a decrease in the number of red blood cells or a decrease in hemoglobin concentration, leading to reduced oxygen-carrying capacity.
- The clinical scenario of fatigue, pallor, low RBC count, low Hb, and microcytic hypochromic red blood cells (MCV 60 fl, MCH 20 pg) is characteristic of iron deficiency anemia (IDA).
- Microcytic anemia indicates small red blood cells.
- Vitamin B_{12} deficiency (Option a): This condition leads to megaloblastic anemia, characterized by macrocytic red blood cells.
- ACD (Anemia of chronic disease) (Option b): ACD is typically normocytic normochromic anemia with low iron levels due to chronic inflammation.
- Sideroblastic anemia (Option c): This involves defective heme synthesis and can lead to microcytic or normocytic anemia.

8. Ans (a) HHV-8

Ref: Rook's Textbook of Dermatology, 9th ed. pg. 26.61, 26.62, 103.15, 103.16

- Primary effusion lymphoma (PEL) is a rare type of non-Hodgkin lymphoma that is associated with human herpesvirus-8 (HHV-8), also known as Kaposi's sarcoma-associated herpesvirus (KSHV).
- HHV-8 is responsible for the development of primary effusion lymphoma, particularly in individuals with compromised immune systems, such as those with HIV/AIDS.
- HIV-1 (Option b) and HIV-2 (Option d): While these viruses are associated with immunodeficiency, they are not the direct cause of primary effusion lymphoma.
- Hepadnavirus (Option c): This virus, such as hepatitis B virus, is not linked to primary effusion lymphoma.

9. Ans (d) Wegener's granulomatosis

Ref: Robbins and Cotran Pathologic Basis of Disease, 10th ed. pg. 514

- Wegener's granulomatosis, now referred to as granulomatosis with polyangiitis (GPA), is a type of autoimmune vasculitis that primarily affects small blood vessels in the respiratory tract and kidneys.
- The clinical scenario of purpura on the skin, renal impairment, hemoptysis (coughing up blood), and respiratory infection, along with the presence of C-ANCA (cytoplasmic antineutrophil cytoplasmic antibodies), is consistent with Wegener's granulomatosis (GPA).
- **Goodpasture's syndrome** involves lung and kidney damage due to antibodies attacking basement membranes. It does not typically present with purpura.
- **MPA** is a systemic vasculitis that often affects the kidneys and lungs. It shares some similarities with GPA but does not always involve granulomatous inflammation.
- **Churg-Strauss syndrome** is characterized by eosinophil-rich inflammation and affects multiple organs, including the respiratory tract, heart, and nervous system.

10. Ans (a) Acute Hep B

Ref: Harrison's Principles of Internal Medicine, 21st ed. pg. 2565-66, 2576, 2592-99

- The presence of specific viral markers in blood can help diagnose different stages of hepatitis B virus (HBV) infection.
- HBsAg (Hepatitis B surface antigen) and IgM anti-HBc antibodies (IgM antibodies against the core antigen) indicate acute hepatitis B infection.
- The presence of these markers suggests an active infection.

11. Ans (c) CV congestion

Ref: Robbins and Cotran Pathologic Basis of Disease, 10th ed. pg. 857, 861-63

- The gross image of the liver in this case shows centrilobular congestion (Nutmeg liver). This is a type of congestion that occurs in the central part of the liver lobules.
- It is caused by an increase in pressure in the hepatic veins, which are the veins that drain blood from the liver.
- This condition can be caused by heart failure, where the backflow of blood due to compromised heart function leads to congestion in the central veins of the liver.
- Alcoholic liver disease, chronic hepatitis and hepatic cirrhosis typically show signs of hepatocellular damage and fibrosis rather than central vein congestion.

12. Ans (b) PSGN

Ref: Robbins Basic Pathology, 10th ed. pg. 907-09, 918

- The clinical presentation of hematuria (red blood cells in urine), RBC casts, edema, and deranged renal function, along with the presence of PSGN (Poststreptococcal glomerulonephritis), indicates acute PSGN.
- This type of glomerulonephritis often follows streptococcal infections and is characterized by immune complex deposition.

Extra Mile

- **MCD** is a cause of nephrotic syndrome, characterized by heavy proteinuria, but it does not typically involve hematuria and RBC casts.
- **FSGS** can also cause nephrotic syndrome, but it is characterized by scarring of the glomeruli rather than immune complex deposition.
- **IgA nephropathy**, also known as Berger's disease, is characterized by IgA immune complex deposition and can cause hematuria, but it is not usually associated with RBC casts.

13. Ans (c) Conn's syndrome

Ref: Harrison's Principles of Internal Medicine, 21st ed. pg. 2964, 2965

- Conn syndrome, also known as primary hyperaldosteronism, involves excessive production of aldosterone by the adrenal glands, leading to increased sodium retention and potassium loss.
- The clinical scenario of hypertension, palpitations, sweating, elevated aldosterone levels, and hypokalemia is consistent with Conn's syndrome.
- Elevated aldosterone levels contribute to sodium retention, which in turn leads to hypertension and potassium loss.

Other options:

- **Pheochromocytoma** is a tumor of the adrenal medulla that produces excess catecholamines, causing symptoms like palpitations and sweating. However, it is not associated with aldosterone-related electrolyte imbalances.
- **Cushing's disease** involves excessive cortisol production due to pituitary adenomas. It does not directly affect aldosterone levels or potassium levels.
- **Pituitary adenomas** can cause various hormonal imbalances, but they are not directly associated with the clinical picture described.

14. Ans. (b) Meningioma

Ref: CMDT 2023, pg. 997

Current Medical Diagnosis and Treatment (CMDT) states that one-third of all primary intracranial neoplasms are meningiomas, one-quarter are gliomas and the remainder are pituitary adenomas.

15. Ans (b) Psammoma bodies with whirling of tumor cells

Ref: Robbins and Cotran Pathologic Basis of Disease, 10th ed. pg. 46

- Based on the given image and scenario, the diagnosis is meningioma where psammoma bodies are found. As many as 90% of meningiomas are benign and noncancerous. Psammoma bodies are foci of dystrophic calcification.

Conditions where psammoma bodies are found:

1. Papillary thyroid carcinoma
2. Papillary serous carcinoma of the endometrium
3. Serous cystadenocarcinoma of the ovary
4. Melanotic schwannoma
5. Meningioma
6. Mesothelioma

16. Ans (c) Triphenyltetrazolium chloride

Ref: Robbins and Cotran Pathologic Basis of Disease, 10th ed. pg. 35

- Myocardial infarction can be demonstrated by Triphenyltetrazolium chloride with tris HCl buffer or by Nitroblue tetrazolium dye test in an unfixed and fresh heart by immersing the slices of heart from suspected area or different areas of heart in these chemical dyes.
- **Interpretation:**
  - Healthy viable heart muscle will stain deep red from the cardiac lactate dehydrogenase.
  - Areas of infarctions/necrosis will be pale.

17. Ans (a) Minimal change disease

Ref: Robbins and Cotran Pathologic Basis of Disease, 10th ed. pg. 914

- The given scenario is suggestive of Minimal change disease. It is a kidney disorder that can lead to nephrotic syndrome. Nephrotic syndrome is a group of symptoms that include protein in the urine, low blood protein levels in the blood, high cholesterol levels, high triglyceride levels, and swelling.
- Light microscopy of renal biopsy specimens from patients with MCD shows minimal to no change; however, electron microscopy reveals the effacement of podocyte foot processes. Immunofluorescent staining of biopsy specimens is negative, and no immune complexes are evident.

18. Ans (d) Multiple myeloma

Ref: Robbins and Cotran Pathologic Basis of Disease, 10th ed. pg. 914

- Multiple myeloma (MM) or plasma cell myeloma is a cancer of plasma cells, a type of white blood cell that

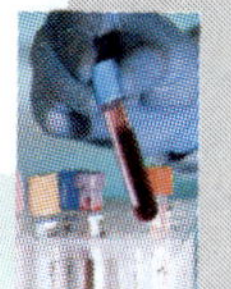

normally produces antibodies. Often, no symptoms are noticed initially. As it progresses, bone pain, anemia, kidney dysfunction, and infections may occur. Complications may include amyloidosis.

- Multiple myeloma is diagnosed based on blood or urine tests finding abnormal antibodies, bone marrow biopsy finding cancerous plasma cells, and medical imaging finding bone lesions. Another common finding is high blood calcium levels.

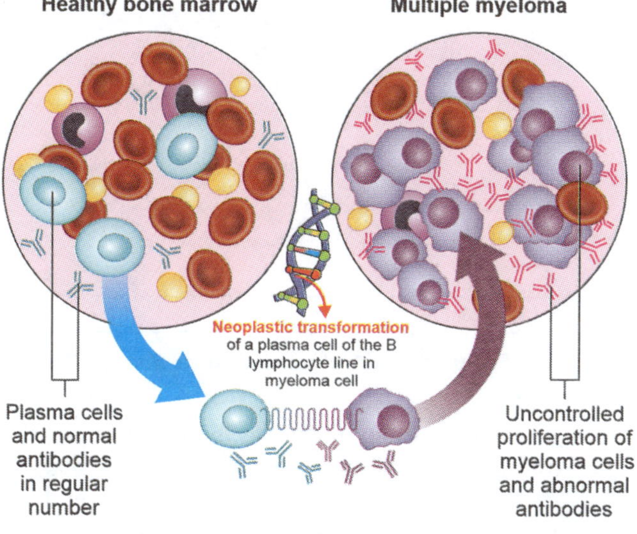

19. Ans (c) Hyaline cast

***Ref:* Robbins and Cotran Pathologic Basis of Disease, 10th ed. pg. 914**

- Hyaline casts are the simplest and most common type of urinary cast. Urinary casts are microscopic clusters of urinary particles, such as cells, fat bodies, or microorganisms, wrapped in a protein matrix and found in the urine.
- "The hyaline cast is made of Tamm-Horsfall protein—the most abundant protein in the urine."

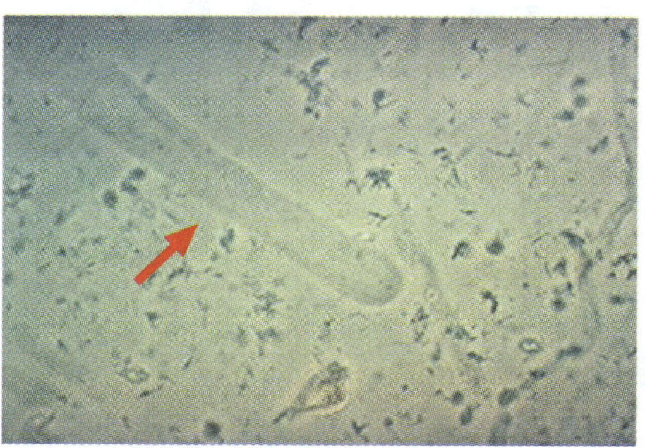

20. Ans (a) HSV-1 and 2

***Ref:* Robbins and Cotran Pathologic Basis of Disease, 10th ed. pg. 1162**

- The Tzanck smear is a quick and reliable tool for the evaluation of various erosive and vesiculobullous skin lesions.
- Tzanck cells (acantholytic cells) are found in:
  - Herpes simplex
  - Varicella and herpes zoster
  - Pemphigus vulgaris
  - Cytomegalovirus

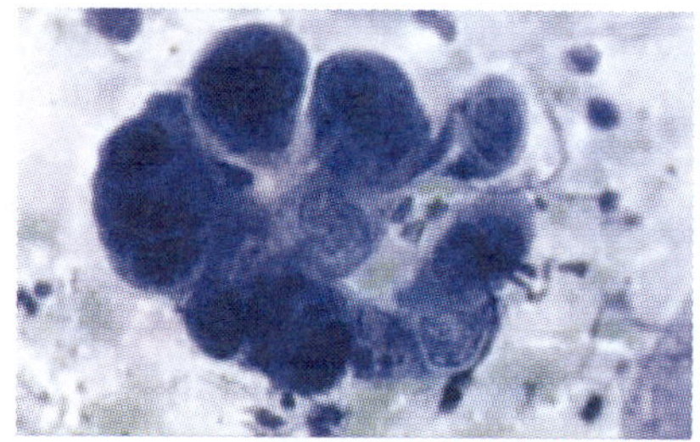

21. Ans (a) Hereditary spherocytosis

***Ref:* Robbins and Cotran Pathologic Basis of Disease, 10th ed. pg. 640**

Splenectomy is the definitive treatment for Hereditary spherocytosis (HS). Except in the unusual autosomal recessive variant of HS, splenectomy usually eliminates hemolysis and the associated signs and symptoms.

Other options:

- **G6PD deficiency:** The main treatment for G6PD deficiency is avoidance of oxidative stressors. Rarely, anemia may be severe enough to warrant a blood transfusion.
- **Iron deficiency anemia:** It is treated by iron supplements. Either oral or parental or IV.
- **Vitamin B_{12} deficiency anemia:** It is treated by B_{12} supplementation or IM injection of cyanocobalamin.

22. Ans (a) GPS

***Ref:* Robbins and Cotran Pathologic Basis of Disease, 10th ed. pg. 913**

- Goodpasture's syndrome (GPS) or antiglomerular basement membrane disease is a rare autoimmune disease in which antibodies attack the basement membrane in lungs and kidneys, leading to bleeding from the lungs, glomerulonephritis, and kidney failure.
- It is thought to attack the alpha-3 subunit of type IV collagen, which has therefore been referred to as Goodpasture's antigen. Goodpasture syndrome may quickly result in permanent lung and kidney damage, often leading to death.

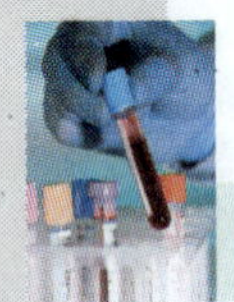

- It is treated with medications that suppress the immune system such as corticosteroids and cyclophosphamide, and with plasmapheresis, in which the antibodies are removed from the blood.

23. Ans (b) Temporal arteritis

Ref: Robbins and Cotran Pathologic Basis of Disease, 10th ed. pg. 511

- The given scenario is suggestive of giant cell arteritis (GCA), also called temporal arteritis.
- It is an inflammatory autoimmune disease of large blood vessels.
- Symptoms may include headache, pain over the temples, flu-like symptoms, double vision, and difficulty opening the mouth.
- Complications can include blockage of the artery to the eye with resulting blindness, as well as aortic dissection, and aortic aneurysm. GCA is frequently associated with polymyalgia rheumatica.

Physical examination:

- Palpation of the head reveals prominent temporal arteries with or without pulsation.
- The temporal area may be tender.
- Decreased pulses may be found throughout the body.
- Evidence of ischemia may be noted on fundal examination.
- Bruits may be heard over the subclavian and axillary arteries.

Laboratory tests:

- Erythrocyte sedimentation rate, an inflammatory marker, >60 mm/hour (normal 1–40 mm/hour).
- C-reactive protein, another inflammatory marker, may be elevated.
- Liver function tests (LFTs) are abnormal particularly raised alkaline phosphatase (ALP).
- Platelets may also be elevated.

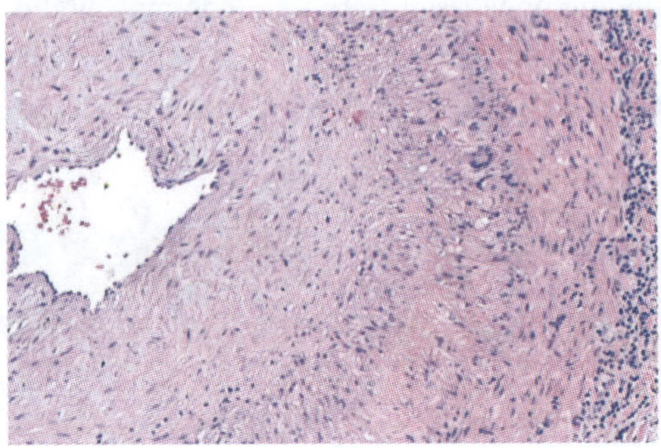

24. Ans (a) Fecal lactoferrin

Ref: Robbins and Cotran Pathologic Basis of Disease, 10th ed. pg. 83

- An elevated lactoferrin level in the stool indicates that inflammation is likely present and active in the digestive tract but does not indicate either its location or cause. In general, the degree of elevation is associated with the severity of the inflammation.

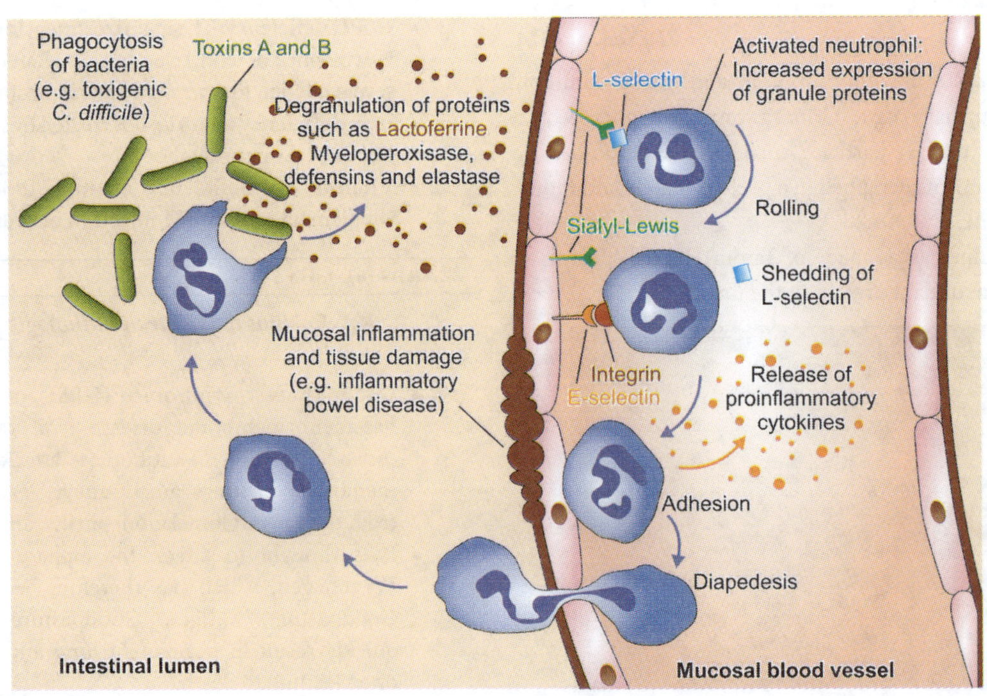

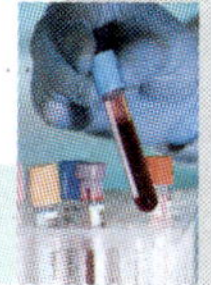

25. Ans (c) **Buerger's disease/TAO**

Ref: Robbins and Cotran Pathologic Basis of Disease, 10th ed. pg. 515

- Buerger's disease (also known as thromboangiitis obliterans, TAO) affects blood vessels in the body, most commonly in the arms and legs. Blood vessels swell, which can prevent blood flow, causing clots to form. This can lead to pain, tissue damage, and even gangrene (the death or decay of body tissues). It is commonly found in smokers.

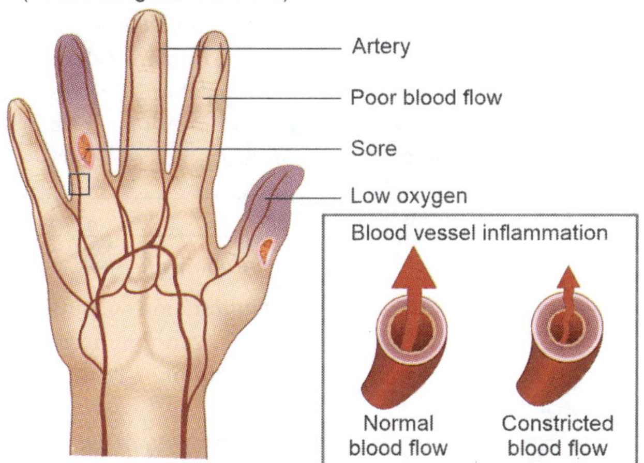

26. Ans (d) **Retinoblastoma**

Ref: Robbins and Cotran Pathologic Basis of Disease, 10th ed. pg. 1324

- Small round blue cell tumor is a group of malignant neoplasms that have a characteristic appearance under the microscope, i.e., consisting of small round cells that stain blue on routine H&E stained sections.

Tumors that belong to this group are:

- Desmoplastic small round cell tumor
- Ewing's sarcoma
- Neuroblastoma
- Medulloblastoma
- Rhabdomyosarcoma
- Synovial sarcoma
- Carcinoid tumor
- Mesothelioma
- Small cell lung cancer
- Wilms' tumor
- Retinoblastoma
- Small cell lymphoma
- Hepatoblastoma
- Merkel cell carcinoma
- Mesenchymal chondrosarcoma

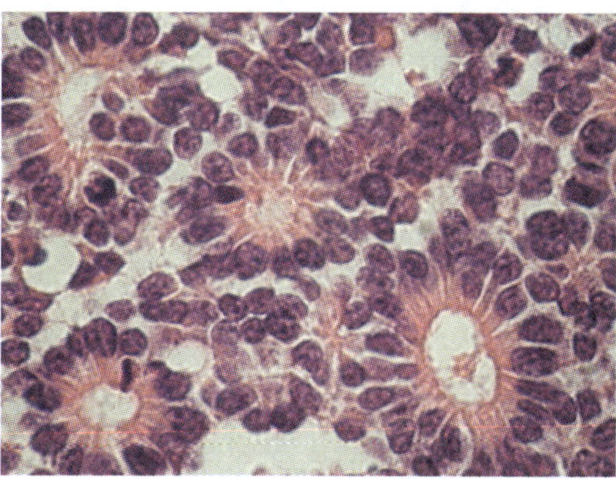

CELL INJURY AND INFLAMMATION

27. Ans. (b) **Atherosclerosis**

Ref: Pocket Companion to Robbins pg. 58

- Option A and C will cause increased calcium levels and metastatic calcification.
- Option B has calcification in tunica intima of blood vessel and is example of dystrophic calcification that occurs in damaged tissues.
- Option D is a broad term that includes all 4 types of leukemia and 2 types of lymphomas.

28. Ans. (c) **Integrin**

Ref: Robbins and Cotran Review of Pathology E-Book pg. 4

Integrins are heterodimeric proteins consisting of alpha and beta subunits. These glycoproteins are expressed on the surface of leukocytes, where they can mediate leukocyte-endothelial cell adhesion within a few minutes after an inflammatory stimulus.

29. Ans. (c) **Hypertrophic scar**

Ref: Final Edge by Deepak Marwah pg. 352

Hypertrophic scar	Keloid
Itching not present or mild	Severe itching and worsens after 1 year
Never crosses boundaries of original incision	Extends to normal tissues and has claw like lesions
Occurs at original site of incision and has minimal vascularity	Occurs at vaccination sites, injection and incision sites and piercing sites
Occurs due to hypertrophy of mature fibroblasts with minimal blood vessels	*Immature fibroblasts with immature blood vessels and exhibits high tendency to recur and collagen bundles are absent*

30. Ans. (b) Cytoplasm

Reference: Robbins 10th ed. pg. 827

- LDH is a cytoplasmic enzyme that is present in almost all tissues but at high concentrations in muscle, liver, and kidney.
- Red blood cells also contain moderate concentrations of this enzyme.

Extra Mile

- If LDH-1 is found to be greater than LDH-2, it indicates myocardial infarction, and is called 'flipped' ratio of LDH-1/LDH. The increase in LDH persists for approximately ten days. It increases at 12 hours and peaks at 24-48 hours. It is the last of all biomarkers to rise in MI.
- Increased LDH-5 in serum is seen with muscular dystrophy
- An increase in LDH-3 is associated with the massive destruction of platelets as in pulmonary embolism.

31. Ans. (a) Cytosol

Ref: Ganong 26th ed. pg. 37

Lysosomes are present in Cytoplasm. The interior of lysosome is more acidic (Approx. pH = 5.0) than cytoplasm and is used to destroy endocytosed bacteria as well as worn out cell components. The acidic pH is maintained by proton pump.

32. Ans. (b) Lipofuscin

Ref: Robbins 10th ed. pg. 77

- Lipofuscin/Lipochrome is the wear and tear pigment that is composed of polymers of lipids and phospholipids complexed with protein. It is derived via lipid peroxidation of polyunsaturated lipids of intracellular membrane. It is a telltale sign of free radical injury and lipid peroxidation.
- It is seen in cells undergoing slow and regressive changes in the liver and heart of aging patients or patients with severe malnutrition and cancer cachexia.

33. Ans. (c) Kupffer cell

Ref: Robbins 10th ed. pg. 827

- Kupffer cells are the security system and belong to mononuclear macrophage system. They are attached to luminal phase of endothelial cells that are adjacent to hepatocytes.
- Option A, Merkel cells are found in skin and are mechanoreceptors. They exist in clusters at the stratum basale closely related to nerve endings. Option B is found in placenta.
- Option D, Stellate cells are found in space of Disse between the hepatocytes and sinusoidal endothelial cells and are responsible for producing the majority of extracellular matrix.

34. Ans. (b) Triphenyl tetrazolium chloride

Ref: Robbins 10th ed. pg. 548

Triphenyl tetrazolium chloride is the stain that imparts brick red color to intact noninfarcted myocardium with intact LDH activity.
Since the dehydrogenases leak out from damaged membranes of dead cells it results in an unstained pale zone.

35. Ans. (a) Calcium

Ref: Robbins 10th ed. pg. 119

Irreversible form of cell damage is primarily dependent upon mitochondrial calcium accumulation. The resultant mitochondrial calcium uptake and overload, results in mitochondrial permeability transition and cell death.

36. Ans. (a) Cat scratch disease

Ref: Robbins E-Book, pg. 462

- Cat-scratch disease is a manifestation of infection by *Bartonella henselae* characterized by necrotizing granulomatous inflammation exhibiting a *characteristic stellate shape.*

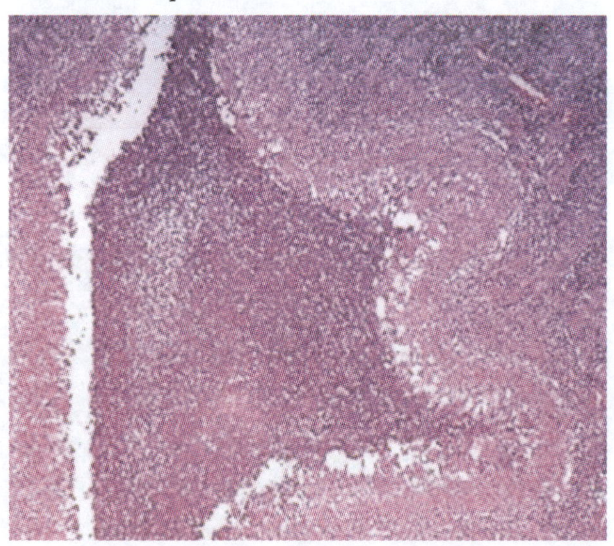

37. Ans. (d) Syndecan

Ref: Robbins E-book, pg. 22-23

- Choice A, B and C are Glycosaminoglycans and hence are ruled out.
- Proteoglycans have core proteins or glycoproteins with large GAG side-chains and they participate in cell-cell and cell-matrix interactions, cell proliferation, and migration associated with wound healing.

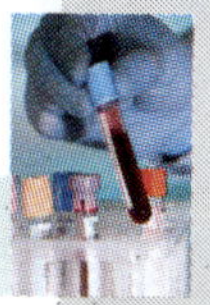

- Proteoglycans involved in wound healing are:

> - Small leucine-rich Proteoglycans
> - Glypicans
> - Versican-isoform
> - Perlecan
> - Syndecans-1 and syndecans-4

38. Ans. (c) Granulation tissue

Ref: Robbins E-book, pg. 95

- Secondary healing is where a full-thickness wound is allowed to close and heal. It results in an inflammatory response that is more intense than with primary wound healing.
- In addition, a larger quantity of *granulation tissue is fabricated because of the need for wound closure.*
- Secondary healing results in pronounced contraction of wounds. Fibroblastic differentiation into myofibroblasts, which resemble contractile smooth muscle, is believed to contribute to wound contraction. These myofibroblasts are maximally present in the wound from the 10th – 21st days.

39. Ans. (a) Selectins

Ref: Robbins 9th ed. pg. 75-78

TABLE: Three phases of leucocyte recruitment at the sites of inflammation

Leukocyte adhesion to endothelium	Transmigration of diapedesis	Chemotaxis of leukocytes
• **Margination:**Q Leukocyte flow peripherally along endothelial surface at inflamed site (normal location—axial)	• Leukocyte migration through endothelium	• Leukocytes migration in the tissues toward the site of injury is called as chemotaxis
• **Rolling**Q (transient adhesion) of leucocytes to endothelium—mediated by **selectins** {leukocytes (L-selectinQ, endothelium (E-selectin)Q, and on platelest and endothelium (P-selectin)}Q	• Mediated by CD31 or **PECAM-1 (platelet endothelial cell adhesion molecule)**Q	**Examples:** **Exogenous chemo attractants**— bacterial products **Endogenous chemo attractants**— IL-8, C5a and leukotriene B4 (LTB4)Q
• **Firm adhesion**Q of leucocytes of endothelium— brought about by **integrins**		

40. Ans. (c) Cerebrum

Ref: Robbins 9th ed. pg. 41-44

Liquefactive/colliquative necrosis occurs due to digestion of dead cells and results in transformation of tissue into liquid viscous mass. The most common site involved is central nervous system.

41. Ans. (a) G1S

Ref: Robbins 9th ed. pg. 25-26, 292-293

- The guardian of genome mediates cell cycle arrest. It occurs in *late G1 phase* and is caused by p53 dependent transcription of CDK1.
- This prevents phosphorylation of RB essential for cells to enter G1 phase.
- Such a pause in cell cycling is welcome as it gives some breathing time for cells to repair the DNA damage.

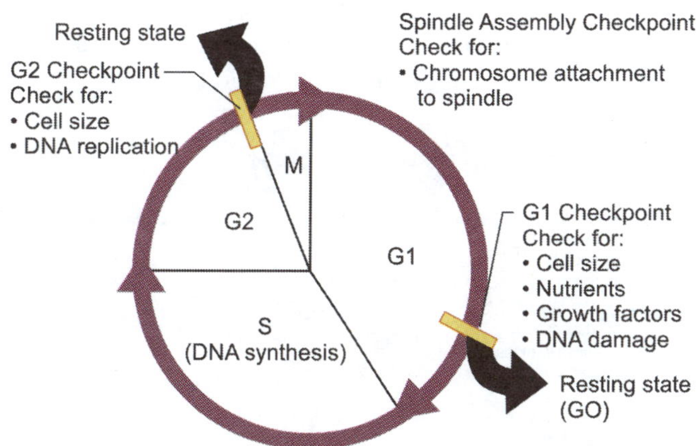

FIGURE: Various check points in cell division cycle

42. Ans. (b) Bcl

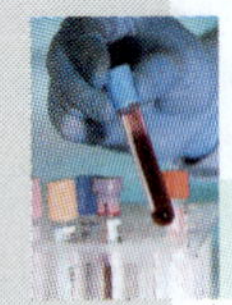

- The major mechanism of intrinsic mitochondrial pathway of apoptosis is by pro- and anti-apoptotic members of *bcl* proteins.
- Bcl protein was first detected on B cell lymphoma and hence its name.
- It is located on mitochondrial inner membrane and regulates cell growth and cell death.
- Pro-apoptotic mechanisms can damage mitochondrial membranes and allow leakage of cytochrome C into the cytoplasm. Cytochrome C is the life-line of intact mitochondria.

Growth promoter/antiapoptotic proteins	Proapoptotic proteins
Bcl-2, Bcl-X and Mcl-1	Bim, Bad and Bid

43. Ans. (d) Lung abscess

Liquefaction or colliquative necrosis also occurs commonly due to ischaemic injury and bacterial or fungal infection but hydrolytic enzymes in tissue degradation have a dominant role in causing semi-fluid material. The *common examples are infarct brain and abscess cavity.*

44. Ans. (b) Synthetic phase

- Cell cycle is defined as the sequence of events that causes cell division.
- It consists of following phases:
  - G1 phase (Presynthetic growth)
  - S phase (DNA synthesis)
  - G2 (Premitotic growth), and
  - M phase (mitotic).
  - Quiescent cells that are not actively cycling are said to be in the G0 state. Cells can enter G1 either from the G0 quiescent cell pool, or after completing a round of mitosis, as for continuously replicating cells.

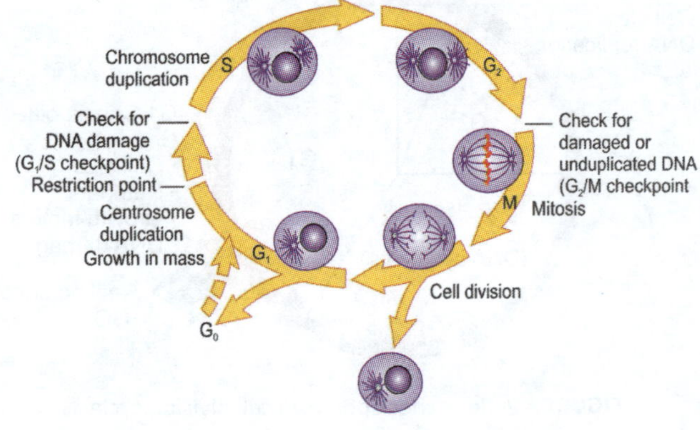

45. Ans. (b) C3b

- *The C3b molecules act as opsonins*; they bind covalently to the pathogen and thereby target it for destruction by phagocytes equipped with receptors for C3b.
- Anaphylatoxins, or complement peptides, are fragments (C3a, C4a and C5a) that are produced as part of the activation of the complement system.

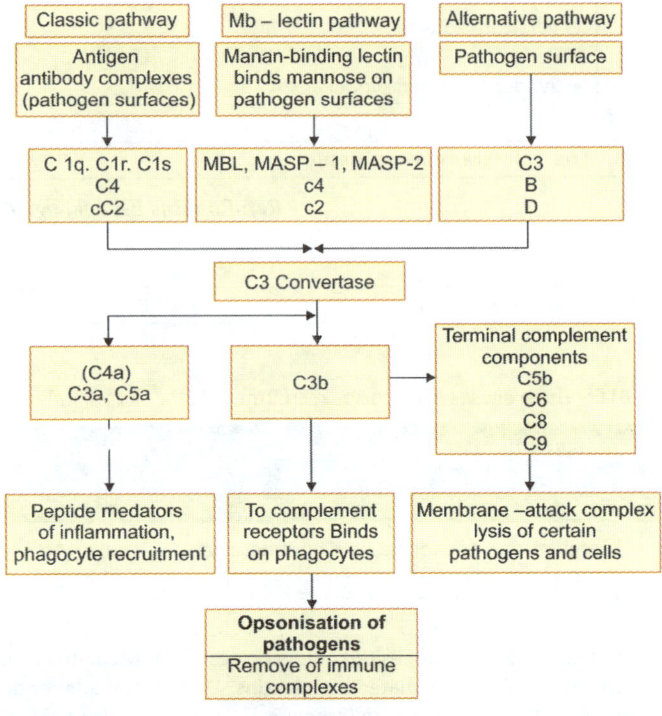

46. Ans. (c) Apoptosis

The councilman bodies are formed due to process of apoptosis in viral hepatitis.

Important pathological process associated with apoptosis:

- Tumours exposed to chemotherapeutic agents
- Graft versus host disease
- Rejection episodes
- Depletion of CD4 cells in AIDS
- Prostatic atrophy after orchidectomy
- Alzheimer's disease
- MI (20% necrosis and 80% apoptosis)

Important physiological processes with apoptosis

- Organised cell destruction during formation of embryo
- Endometrial shedding, regression of lactating breast
- Involution of thymus
- Normal cell destruction followed by replacement proliferation such as intestinal epithelium

47. Ans. (b) Cat scratch

Necrotising noncaseating granulomas are present in cat Scratch disease caused by Bartonella Henselae. The granulomas show *stellate microabscess* surrounded by palisading histiocytes.

Stellate shaped granuloma

Caseating and noncaseating Granuloma

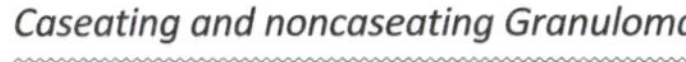

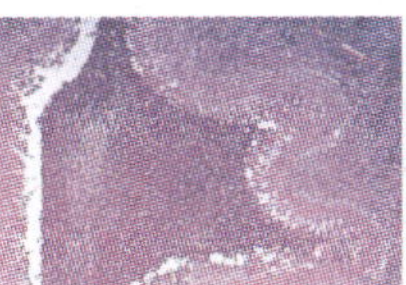

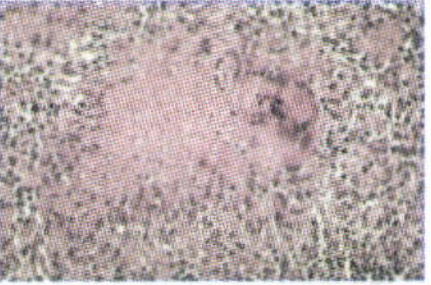

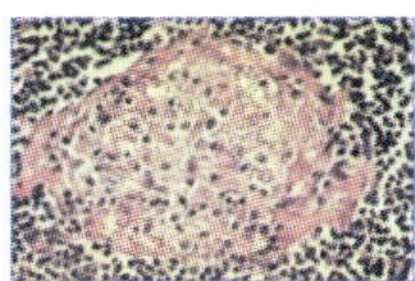

Cat scratch disease | Caseating granulomas TB, sarcoidosis | Noncaseating

48. Ans. (c) E-cadherin

Ref: Robbin's Pathology, 9th ed. pg. 307

- Normal epithelial cells are tightly glued to each other and the ECM by a variety of adhesion molecules.
- E-cadherin, a cell surface protein, maintains intercellular adhesiveness serving to hold the cells together and relay signals between the cells.
- In several epithelial tumors, including adenocarcinomas of the colon, stomach, and breast, E-cadherin function is lost.

Extra Mile

- TNF and IL-1 (interleukins) serve critical roles in leukocyte recruitment by promoting adhesion of leukocytes to endothelium and their migration through vessels.
- Interferons are inflammatory cytokines.
- Matrix metalloproteinase (MMP) regulate tumor invasion by:
  - Remodelling insoluble components of the basement membrane and interstitial matrix
  - By releasing ECM-sequestered growth factors.

49. Ans. (b) Metaplasia

Ref: Robbin's Pathology, 9th ed. pg. 37

- **Metaplasia** is an ***adaptive response*** of a cell in response to stress.
- It is a reversible change in which a ***differentiated (mature) cell type is replaced by another differentiated cell type.***
- ***It can be of two types:***
  - **Epithelial metaplasia**
    - **Squamous metaplasia:** MC seen in respiratory tract (in response to smoking) where columnar epithelium is replaced by squamous epithelium.
    - **Glandular metaplasia:** Metaplasia of squamous epithelium into columnar (glandular) epithelium. Example Barret's esophagus (metaplasia of stratified squamous epithelium of esophagus is replaced by intestinal-like columnar cells).
  - Connective tissue metaplasia:
    - One type of connective tissue is replaced by another.
    - **Example: Myositis ossificans.**

Extra Mile

- **Hypertrophy:** Increased cell **size** in response to increase in workload. It occurs in tissues incapable of cell division.
- **Hyperplasia:** increase in cell number in response to growth factors or hormones.
- **Atrophy:** Decrease in cell and organ size as a result of disuse or decreased nutrient supply.

50. Ans. (d) Atrophy

Ref: Robbin's Pathology, 9th ed. pg. 36

- Prolonged disuse of muscle can cause atrophy of muscle leading to decreased muscle mass in this patient (*atrophy of disuse*).

Other Causes of Atrophy can be:

- Loss of innervation (denervation atrophy)
- Diminished blood supply (ischemic/senile atrophy)
- Inadequate nutrition
- Loss of endocrine stimulation
- Pressure

51. Ans. (d) Hypertrophy

Ref: Robbin's Pathology, 9th ed. pg. 34

- **Hypertrophy refers to an increase in the size of cells,** that results in an increase in the size of the affected organ.
- The most common stimulus for hypertrophy of muscle is increased workload.
- A gravid uterus is an example of hypertrophy and hyperplasia both, but mainly hypertrophy.
- **Robbin's 9th ed. pg. 34 states:** "The massive physiologic growth of the uterus during pregnancy is a good example of hormone-induced enlargement of an organ that results mainly from hypertrophy of muscle fibers".
- Breast enlargement at puberty and at pregnancy is also an example of hypertrophy and hyperplasia both.

52. Ans. (c) Hyperplasia

Ref: Robbin's Pathology, 9th ed. pg. 36

- In individuals who donate one lobe of the liver for transplantation, the remaining cells proliferate so that the organ soon grows back to its original size. This is a classic example of compensatory hyperplasia.

53. Ans. (a) Internally controlled, programmed cell death

Ref: Robbin's Pathology, 9th ed. pg. 52

- Apoptosis is internally controlled, programmed cell death

Salient Features of Apoptosis:

- No inflammation
- Cell shrinkage
- Formation of apoptotic bodies

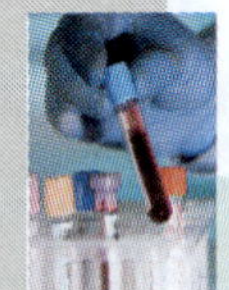

Example

- **Physiological:** Embryogenesis, organogenesis, Menstruation
- **Pathological:** Acute viral hepatitis—Councilman bodies.

54. Ans. (c) Apoptosis of cells induce inflammatory reaction

Ref: Robbin's Pathology, 9th ed. pg. 52-53

Remember Important Features of Apoptosis:

- Formation of cytoplasmic blebs and apoptotic bodies
- *Cell shrinkage:* The cells are smaller in size and the cytoplasm is dense
- *Chromatin condensation:* This is the most characteristic feature of apoptosis
- Absence of inflammation
- Gel electrophoresis of DNA shows 'step ladder pattern'.

55. Ans. (a) Inflammation is present

Ref: Robbin's Pathology, 9th ed. pg. 52-55

Since in apoptosis the dead cell is rapidly cleared, before its contents have leaked out, therefore cell death by this pathway does not elicit an inflammatory reaction in the host.

56. Ans. (d) Condensation of the nucleus

Ref: Robbin's Pathology 9th ed. pg. 53-54

The Morphologic Features Characteristic of Apoptosis include:

- *Cell shrinkage:* The cell is smaller in size having dense cytoplasm and the organelles are tightly packed.
- *Chromatin condensation:* This is the *most characteristic feature of apoptosis.*
- Formation of cytoplasmic blebs and apoptotic bodies.

57. Ans. (a) Bcl-2

Ref: Robbin's Pathology, 9th ed. pg. 53-54

- Apoptosis is inhibited by anti-apoptosis genes which are mostly Bcl family genes.
  - **Example:** Bcl-2, Bcl-X, Bcl-XL
- **Pro**-apoptotic genes: they initiate and are involved in apoptosis.
  - **Example:** BAD, BIM, BAX, BAK
- **P53 is a tumor suppressor gene and it causes apoptosis when there is excess DNA damage which cannot be repaired**

58. Ans. (a) Caspases

Ref: Robbin's Pathology, 9th ed. pg. 53-54

- **Caspases**, or *c*ysteine-*asp*artic prote*ases* are a family of cysteine proteases that play essential roles in apoptosis, necrosis, and inflammation.
- Caspases are essential in cells for apoptosis, or programmed cell death, in development and most other stages of adult life, and have been termed "executioner" proteins for their roles in the cell.
- Some caspases are also required in the immune system for the maturation of lymphocytes.

59. Ans. (c) Embryogenesis

Ref: Robbin's Pathology, 9th ed. pg. 53-54

- Caspases are cysteine proteases and are critical for the process of apoptosis. Physiologically, apoptosis is required to eliminate the cells no longer required and to maintain a steady number of various cell populations in tissues.
- The programmed cell death (apoptosis) is required at the time of different processes in embryogenesis like implantation, organogenesis, developmental involution and metamorphosis.

60. Ans. (b) Apoptosis

Ref: Robbin's Pathology, 9th ed. pg. 53-54

Caspases are present in normal cells as inactive proenzymes and when they are activated they cleave proteins and induce apoptosis. These are cysteine proteases.

61. Ans. (c) Hydropic swelling

Ref: Robbin's Pathology, 9th ed. pg. 40

REVERSIBLE CELL INJURY

- Cell swelling

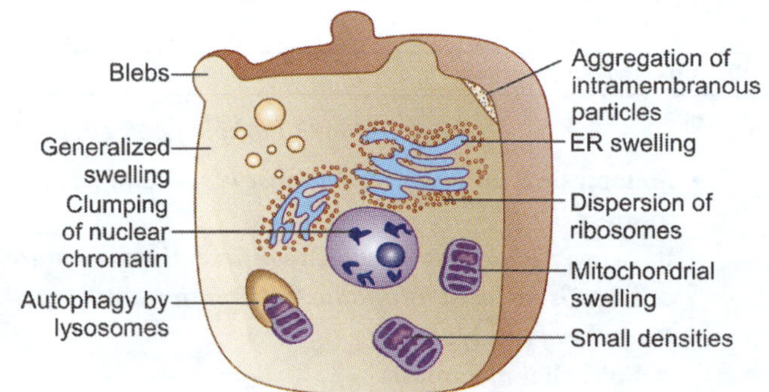

- Detachment of ribosomes from granular endoplasmic reticulum
- Dissociation of polysomes into monosomes.
- Plasma membrane blebbing, blunting, villous distortion, myelin figures, mitochondrial swelling, rarefaction.
- Nuclear disaggregation of granular and fibrillar elements.

62. Ans. (c) Condensation of nuclear chromatin

Ref: Robbin's Pathology, 9th ed. pg. 40

Refer to the explanation of the above question

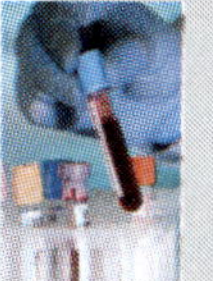

63. Ans. (a) Coagulative necrosis

Ref: Robbin's Pathology, 9th ed. pg. 41-43, 50

COAGULATIVE NECROSIS

- This pattern of necrosis is typically seen in hypoxic environments, such as infarction.
- Coagulative necrosis occurs primarily in tissues such as the kidney, heart and adrenal glands.
- ***Severe ischemia most commonly causes coagulative necrosis.***
- Coagulation occurs as a result of protein denaturation, causing the albumin in protein to form a firm and opaque state.
- It is characterized by the formation of a gelatinous (gel-like) substance in dead tissues in which the architecture of the tissue is maintained, and can be observed by light microscopy.

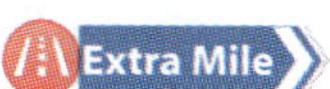

Extra Mile

LIQUEFACTIVE NECROSIS

- It is characterized by the digestion of dead cells to form a viscous liquid mass. This is typical of bacterial, or sometimes fungal, infections because of their ability to stimulate an inflammatory response.
- The necrotic liquid mass is frequently creamy yellow due to the presence of dead leukocytes and is commonly known as pus.
- Hypoxic infarcts in the brain presents as this type of necrosis, because the brain contains little connective tissue but high amounts of digestive enzymes and lipids, and cells therefore can be readily digested by their own enzymes.

CASEOUS NECROSIS

- It can be considered a combination of coagulative and liquefactive necroses, typically caused by mycobacteria, fungi and some foreign substances.
- **The necrotic tissue appears as white and friable,** like **clumped cheese.**
- Microscopic examination shows **amorphous granular debris** enclosed within a distinctive inflammatory border. Granuloma has this characteristic.

FAT NECROSIS

- It is specialized necrosis of fat tissue, resulting from the action of activated lipases on fatty tissues such as the pancreas.
- In the pancreas it leads to acute pancreatitis, a condition where the pancreatic enzymes leak out into the peritoneal cavity, and liquefy the membrane by splitting the triglyceride esters into fatty acids through fat saponification.
- Calcium, magnesium or sodium may bind to these lesions to produce a chalky-white substance. The calcium deposits are microscopically distinctive and may be large enough to be visible on radiographic examinations. To the naked eye, calcium deposits appear as gritty white flecks.

Contd...

Fibrinoid necrosis is a special form of necrosis usually caused by **immune-mediated vascular damage.** It is marked by complexes of antigen and antibodies, sometimes referred to as "immune complexes" deposited within arterial walls together with fibrin.

64. Ans. (d) Apoptosis

Ref: Robbin's Pathology, 9th ed. pg. 52-53

The inter nucleosomal cleavage of DNA into oligonucleosomes (in multiples of 180-200 base pairs) is brought about by Ca^{+} and Mg^{2+} dependent endonucleases and is characteristic of apoptosis.

65. Ans (d) Platelet derived growth factor

Ref: Robbin's Pathology, 9th ed. pg. 52-53

Integrin superfamily consists of proteins that promote cell to cell, or cell to matrix adhesion. In contrast, selectins promote only cell to cell adhesion.

The Extracellular Domain Binds to:

- Matrix glycoproteins
- Adhesions molecules on other cells
- Activated complement components

66. Ans. (a) Venules

Ref: Robbin's Pathology, 9th ed. pg. 73-74

- Post capillary venules are an important point of interchange between the lumen of the vessels and the surrounding tissue.
- Moreover both vascular leakage and leucocyte exudation occur preferentially in venules in many types of inflammation.

67. Ans. (c) Atheromatous plaque

Ref: Robbin's Pathology, 9th ed. pg. 65-66

- Atheromatous plaque would have dead cells, so there is presence of dystrophic calcification.

68. Ans. (d) Lysosomal enzymes

Ref: Robbin's Pathology, 9th ed. pg. 81, 94

- The polymorphonuclear leukocyte (PMN) (Neutrophil) is particularly important in acute inflammation. The PMNs contain lysosomes.
- These granules contain several potent lytic enzymes which make it possible for these cells to destroy many types of bacteria and to liquefy the cell fragments resulting from tissue injury.
- The formation of hydrogen peroxide within neutrophils contributes to the bactericidal effect of these cells, as does the presence of superoxide, myeloperoxidase, and *halide ion.*

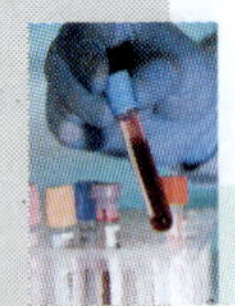

69. Ans. (d) All of these

Ref: Robbin's Pathology, 9th ed. pg. 48

- Catalase is present in peroxisomes and decomposes H_2O_2 into O_2 and H_2O.
- Superoxide dismutase is found in many cell types and converts superoxide ions to H_2O_2. This group includes both manganese-superoxide dismutase, which is localized in mitochondria, and copper-zinc-superoxide dismutase, which is found in the cytosol.
- Glutathione peroxidase also protects against injury by catalyzing free radical breakdown.

70. Ans. (c) Vasodilation and increase in permeability

Ref: Robbin's Pathology, 9th ed. pg. 73

- Hallmark of acute inflammation is ***increased vascular permeability*** leading to the escape of protein-rich exudate into the extravascular tissue, causing edema.

71. Ans. (b) Myeloperoxidase

Ref: Robbin's Pathology, 9th ed. pg. 82-83

Myeloperoxidase (MPO) is an enzyme present in primary (or azurophilic) granules of the neutrophils. In the presence of a halide such as $C1^-$, MPO converts H_2O_2 to HOCl (hypochlorous radical) during the process of respiratory burst.

72. Ans. (d) Granuloma formation

Ref: Robbin's Pathology, 9th ed. pg. 97

- Granuloma formation is characteristic of chronic granulomatous inflammation and is not seen in acute inflammation.
- Vasodilation, increase in permeability, exudation, margination, rolling etc. are seen in acute inflammation.

73. Ans. (a) NADPH oxidase

Ref: Robbin's Pathology, 9th ed. pg. 79

- The generation of reactive oxygen intermediates is due to the rapid activation of an enzyme; NADPH oxidase which is involved in oxygen dependent killing.
- Catalase, superoxide dismutase and glutathione peroxidase are free radical scavengers that prevent oxygen mediated injury.

74. Ans. (d) Vitamin C

Ref: Robbin's Pathology, 9th ed. pg. 8

- As the collagen molecule is produced, it undergoes many changes, termed post-translational modifications.
- These modifications take place in the Golgi compartment of the ER.
- Collagen, like most proteins that are destined for transport to the extracellular spaces for their function or activity, is produced initially as a larger precursor molecule called procollagen.
- Procollagen contains additional peptides at both ends that are unlike collagen. On one end of the molecule, called the amino terminal end, special bonds called disulfide bonds are formed among three procollagen chains and ensure that the chains line up in the proper alignment. This step is called registration. Once registration occurs, the three chains wrap around each other forming a string-like structure.
- One of the first modifications to take place is the very critical step of hydroxylation of selected proline and lysine amino acids in the newly synthesized procollagen protein.

75. Ans. (c) Calcification

Ref: Robbin's Pathology, 9th ed. pg. 40-41, 65

- Cellular swelling may occur due to cellular hypoxia, which damages the sodium-potassium membrane pump; it is reversible when the cause is eliminated.
- Cellular swelling is the first manifestation of almost all forms of injury to cells.
- On microscopic examination, small clear vacuoles may be seen within the cytoplasm; these represent distended and pinched-off segments of the endoplasmic reticulum.
- This pattern of non-lethal injury is sometimes called hydropic change or vacuolar degeneration.
- The ultrastructural changes of reversible cell injury include: Blebbing blunting, distortion of microvilli, loosening of intercellular attachments, mitochondrial changes, dilation of the endoplasmic reticulum.

76. Ans. (b) Liver

Ref: Robbin's Pathology, 9th ed. pg. 50-51

- In fat necrosis the enzyme lipase releases fatty acids from triglycerides.
- The fatty acids then complex with calcium to form soaps. These soaps appear as white chalky deposits.
- It is usually associated with trauma of the pancreas or acute pancreatitis.
- It can also occur in the breast, the salivary glands, neonates after a traumatic delivery but rarely in peritoneum.

77. Ans. (c) Lymphocytes, plasma cells and fibrosis

Ref: Robbin's Pathology, 9th ed. pg. 93

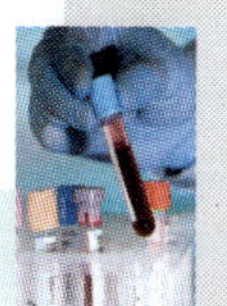

78. Ans. (a) Eosinophils

Ref: Robbin's Pathology, 9th ed. pg. /97

- A special form of chronic inflammation is seen in response to tissue invasion by *Mycobacterium tuberculosis*.
- Macrophages and multinucleated giant cells accumulate about the organisms, and fibrous tissue form about these small focal lesions or tubercles.
- This combination of macrophages and fibrosis is granulomatous inflammation.
- Epithelioid cells and multinucleated Langhans giant cells are present. The former are derived from macrophages and the latter by cytoplasmic fusion of macrophages.
- These lesions may heal by scarring and become calcified, or they undergo caseation necrosis.

79. Ans. (a) Edema is present

Ref: Robbin's Pathology, 9th ed. pg. /130

White infarct	Red infarct
• Occurs in solid organs with end arterial circulation • Occurs in solid organs • Have well-defined margins • Edema is **absent**	• Occurs in organs with **dual blood supply** • Venous occlusion leads to red infarct, like in ovarian torsion • Ill-defined haemorrhagic margins • Edematous tissues

All infarcts are wedge shaped and have features of ischemic coagulative necrosis.

HEMODYNAMICS

80. Ans. (a) Albumin

Ref: Ganong 26th ed. pg. 552

- Albumin is the most abundant protein in the blood and accounts for about 50 percent of all plasma proteins. It gets synthesized by the liver and secreted immediately without storage.
- The physiological regulators of albumin are the colloid osmotic pressure and nutritional status.
- Fibrinogen is least abundant protein in the blood.

81. Ans. (d) Hep A

Ref: Harrison 21st ed. pg. 896

- Blood should be mandatorily tested for minimum of following infections before infusion: Hepatitis B, Hepatitis C, HIV, Syphilis and Malaria.
- Hepatitis A spreads via feco-oral route.

82. Ans. (b) Thrombo-angitis obliterans

Ref: Bailey and Love 21st ed. pg. 967

- TAO presents with digital gangrene due to arteriosclerosis of distal pulses.
- Option A presents with hematuria after a sore throat and is leading cause of Glomerulonephritis. Option C involves scrotal skin. Option D is seen after prolonged immobilization and leads to limb swelling.

83. Ans. (b) Heinz bodies

Ref: Robbins and Cotran Pathology 2020 E-Book pg. 215

- Supravital staining is used for RBC inclusions that are not well visualized with Romanowsky dyes.
- Heinz bodies appear as small round inclusions within the red cell body in case of G6PD deficiency and are visualized more clearly with supravital staining (e.g., with new methylene blue, crystal violet or bromocresol green).

84. Ans. (d) Increased protein C

Ref: Robbin's Pathology, 9th ed. pg. 122

Virchow's triad (in thrombosis) includes:

1. Endothelial injury
2. Stasis or turbulent blood flow
3. Hypercoagulability

Vasculitis	Vasculitis implies endothelial injury and is important for thrombus formation in coronary circulation.
Stasis in veins	Contributes to venous thrombosis
Turbulence in artery	Contributes to arterial thrombosis
Increased protein C	Protein C deficiency contributes to blood hyperviscosity whereas increased protein C would lead to bleeding

85. Ans. (d) Complete lumen obstruction

Ref: Robbin's Pathology, 9th ed. pg. 124-125

Arterial thrombus	Venous thrombus
• Associated with active blood flow leading to endothelial injury	Stasis of blood
• Grows in retrograde manner	Antegrade growth from point of attachment
• **Line of Zahn** is produced by alternating pale layers of platelets mixed with fibrin and darker layers containing more cells	Line of Zahn is absent
• **Incomplete lumen obstruction** leading to ischemia and organ infarction	**Complete vessel occlusion**

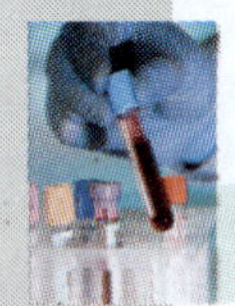

86. Ans. (d) Lower extremities

Ref: Robbin's Pathology, 9th ed. pg. 124-126

- *The site of arterial emboli is the heart and major site of embolization are lower extremities Brain > intestines > kidneys, etc.*
- **Most common site for venous thrombosis is deep leg veins below the knees**
- Most of pulmonary emboli arise in deep leg veins above (femoral veins) the level of the knee.

87. Ans. (b) Postmortem clots

Ref: Robbin's Pathology, 9th ed. pg. 125

- Postmortem clots may have a yellow appearance at upper end and red at the lower. These are sometimes called "chicken fat" clots. The surface is still shiny and smooth indicating a clot, not a thrombus.
- The yellow portion represents clotted plasma and the red cells have settled out and clotted at the bottom of the clot.

88. Ans. (c) It manifests as pitting edema

Ref: Robbin's Pathology, 9th ed. pg. 1162

- Angio-neurotic edema is a localized nonpitting edema involving deeper layers of the skin and subcutaneous tissue. It is an autosomal dominant clinical condition caused by **deficiency of C1 inhibitor protein** (a complement regulatory protein) and associated with elevated levels of bradykinin. It is more common in females.
- Diagnosis of hereditary angioedema is suggested by the presence of lack of pruritus and urticarial lesions, prominence of recurrent gastrointestinal attacks of colic and episodes of laryngeal edema. The levels of complement proteins C1 is normal but levels of C2 and C4 are depleted.
- Danazol is the drug which can be used for hereditary angioedema.

89. Ans. (c) Henoch Schonlein purpura

Ref: Robbin's Pathology, 9th ed. pg. 506, 510

Cutaneous small-vessel vasculitis (also known as "Cutaneous leukocytoclastic angiitis and "Hypersensitivity angiitis") is an inflammation of small blood vessels, characterized clinically by palpable purpura.

Subtypes of Small-Vessel Vasculitis Include:

- Henoch-Schonlein purpura
- Acute hemorrhagic edema of infancy
- Urticarial vasculitis
- Cryoglobulinemic vasculitis

NEOPLASIA

90. Ans. (b) Multiple myeloma

Ref: Harrison 21st ed. pg. 871

- Features of CRAB like HyperCalcemia, **R**enal failure, **A**nemia and **B**ony lytic lesions point to diagnosis as Multiple myeloma.
- Option A leads to hypercalcemia and lytic lesions but does not have renal failure
- Option C presents with features of hyperthyroidism and option D leads to metabolic acidosis.

91. Ans. (a) Luminal A

Ref: SRB Manual of Surgery pg. 553

The classification of four molecular subtypes of breast cancer

Subtypes	ER	PR	HER 2
Luminal A	+	+/–	–
Luminal B	+	+/–	+/–
HER2+	–	–	+
TNBC	–	–	–

- Luminal A subtype breast cancer, even in associated with high-risk features, generally has an excellent prognosis.

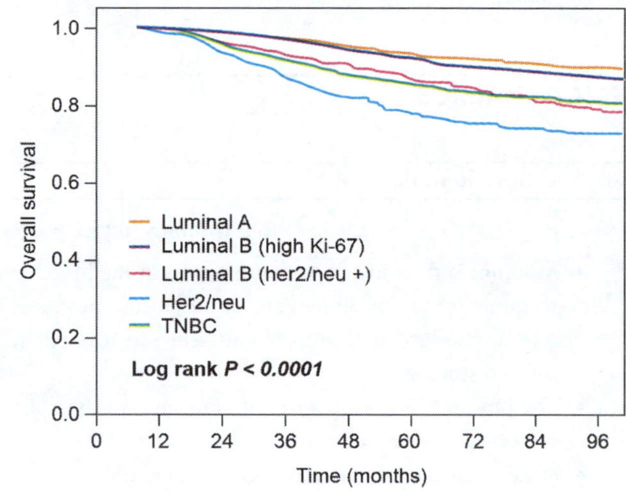

92. Ans. (a) Teratoma

Ref: Robbins Basic Pathology E-Book pg. 991

- Teratoma is a germ cell tumor that is derived from all the three germ layers. It contains immature or fully formed tissue, including teeth, hair, bone and muscle.

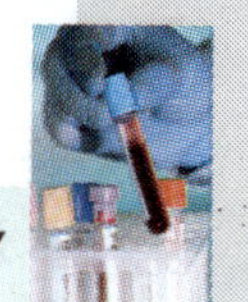

- Option D is presence of normal tissue at an abnormal site like Meckel diverticulum or chocolate cyst of ovary in endometriosis.

93. Ans. (a) Seminoma

Ref: Robbins and Cotran Review of Pathology E-Book pg. 327

- OCT4 is an octamer-binding transcription factor expressed in undifferentiated pluripotent cells including germ cells and embryonic stem cells.
- Seminoma is the most common pure GCT in the testis and accounts for 35% to 50% of all testicular tumors. The mean age of patients is approximately 40 years.
- Most seminomas are discovered as painless testicular masses. Grossly, seminoma is usually well circumscribed and homogenous.

94. Ans. (b) Retinoblastoma

Ref: AK Khurana Ophthalmology pg. 317

- Retinoblastoma presents as leukocoria/ white pupil.
- Direct interference of the normal red reflex from opacities and abnormalities occurring anywhere from the cornea through to the posterior pole can create the leukocoric reflex. Like in the image shown, the white retinal mass seen in retinoblastoma creates leukocoria.
- Option A presents with orbital mass. Option C is usually bilateral. Option D presents with abdominal lump in neonates and intra-abdominal calcification.

95. Ans. (a) Retinoblastoma

Ref: Robbins 10th ed. pg. 1377

The image shows small round cells with Hyperchromatic nuclei surrounding a clear lumen and are called Flexner-Wintersteiner Rosettes.

Flexner-Wintersteiner	Homer wright rosettes	Perivascular pseudorosettes
Retinoblastoma	**PNM: Mnemonic** **P**ineoblastoma **N**euroblastoma **M**edulloblastoma	Ependymoma
Tumor cells Lumen formed by cell borders and cytoplasmic extensions. There will be no basement membrane	Tumor cells Pale neuropil (dense feltwork of interwoven cytoplasmic processes of nerve cells and neuroglial cells)	Tumor cells Neuropil projecting towards a central blood vessel

96. Ans. (d) Burkitt lymphoma

Ref: Harrison 20th ed. pg. 774

- The clinching point for diagnosis is starry sky appearance on lymph node biopsy in a child with jaw swelling. This is a feature of Burkitt lymphoma.
- The slide shows tightly packed immature intensely basophilic cells with some areas in between showing scattered macrophages phagocytizing cell debris and apoptotic cells.
- Option A is ruled out as Reed Sternberg cells are not seen.
- Option B is ruled out as history of sore throat and splenomegaly is not present
- Option C is ruled out as it presents with painless cervical lymphadenopathy with necrosis, karyorrhectic debris, and the presence of the typical cell types, namely crescentic histiocytes and plasmacytoid monocytes.

97. Ans. (c) Carcinoma prostate

Ref: Harrison 20th ed. pg. 624-25

- The presence of osteoblastic changes in LS spine indicates metastasis from carcinoma prostrate.
- Option A has bony lytic lesions. Option B shows focal reduction in joint space with development of gibbus. Option D also has lytic lesions and is ruled out.

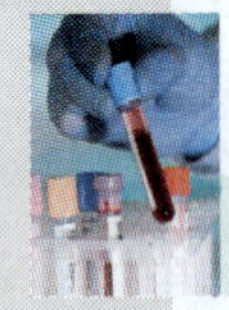

98. Ans. (a) CEA

Ref: Robbins 10th ed. pg. 345

Option B is for recurrence of breast cancer. Option C is for neuroblastoma and small cell cancer lung. Option D is for HCC and nonseminomatous germ cell tumours.

Tumor markers	Tumor types
Hormones	
Human chorionic gonadotropin	Trophoblastyic tumors, nonseminomatous testicular tumors
Calcitonin	Medullary carcinoma of thyroid
Catecholamine and metabolites	Pheochromocytoma and related tumors
Oncofetal antigens	
α-fetoprotein	Liver cell cancer, nonseminomatous germ cell tumors of testis
Lineage-specific proteins	
Immunoglobulins	Multiple myeloma and other gammopathies
Prostate-specific antigen and prostate-specific membrane antigen	Prostate cancer
Mucins and other Glycoproteins	
CA-125	Ovarian cancer
CA-19-9	Colon cancer, pancreatic cancer
CA-15-3	Breast cancer
Cell-free DNA markers	
EGFR mutants in serum	Lung cancer
TP53, APC, RAS mutants in stool and serum	Colon cancer
TP53, RAS mutants in stool and serum	Pancreatic cancer
TP53, RAS mutants in sputum and serum	Lung cancer
TP53 mutants in urine	Bladder cancer

99. Ans. (b) Telomerase

Ref: Robbins 10th ed. pg. 967

- Telomerase is the enzyme responsible for maintenance of the length of telomeres by addition of guanine-rich repetitive sequences. Telomerase activity is exhibited in gametes and stem and tumor cells.
- DNA polymerase is not capable to completely copy DNA at the very ends of chromosomes; therefore, approximately 50 nucleotides are lost during each cell cycle, which results in gradual telomere length shortening. Critically short telomeres cause senescence, following crisis, and cell death.
- However, in tumor cells the system of telomere length maintenance is activated. Besides catalytic telomere elongation, independent telomerase functions can be also involved in cell cycle regulation.
- Inhibition of the telomerase catalytic function and resulting cessation of telomere length maintenance will help in restriction of tumor cell replication potential.

100. Ans. (c) Meningioma

Ref: Robbins 10th ed. pg. 1300

The image shows round lamellated calcified lesion called psammoma bodies in brain biopsy specimen. The patient has an intracranial space occupying lesion, called Meningioma. This lamellated concentric calcification occurs around necrotic tumor cells and is an example of dystrophic calcification.

> Psamomma bodies are seen in (Mnemonic- **PSM-A**)
> - **P**apillary thyroid carcinoma
> - **P**apillary serous carcinoma of endometrium
> - **S**erous cystadenoma of ovary
> - **M**eningioma
> - **M**esothelioma

101. Ans. (c) Neurogenic tumor

Ref: Robbins 10th ed. pg. 724

The most prevalent tumor of mediastinum is neurogenic tumor located in posterior mediastinum. Kindly avoid controversy on this question and the answer given here has been verified from multiple textbooks.

102. Ans. (d) Medulloblastoma

Ref: Robbins 10th ed. pg. 1298

The leading embryonal neoplasm is medulloblastoma which accounts for 20% of pediatric brain tumors.

103. Ans. (a) Thymoma

Ref: Bailey and Love, 26th ed. pg. 868

Most common anterior mediastinum tumour is thymoma. Choice B is seen in posterior mediastinum. Choice C and D are found in middle mediastinum.

Anterior mediastinum
Thymoma
Lymphoma
Germ cell tumor

Middle mediastinum
Cystic lesions
Lymphoma
Mesenchymal tumors

Superior mediastinum
Lymphoma
Thyroid
Parathyroid

Posterior mediastinum
Neurogenic tumors
Cystic lesions
Mesenchymal tumours

104. Ans. (b) Loss of differentiation

Ref: Robbins E-book, pg. 192

- Anaplasia implies reversion of cells to a more primitive or undifferentiated form. In another words, there is complete loss of differentiation of normal cell.

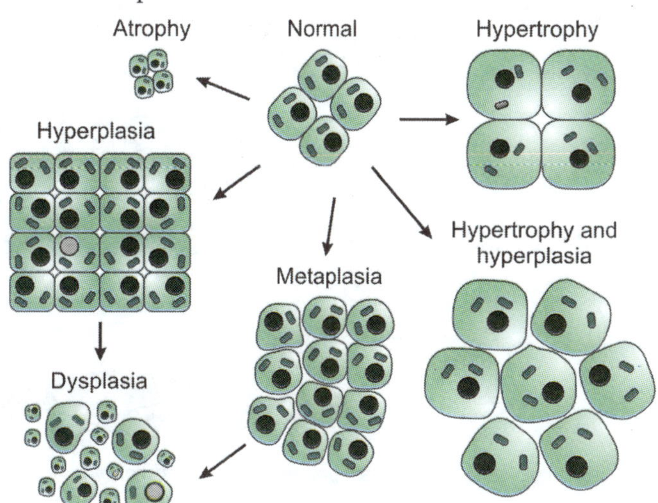

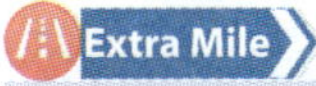
Extra Mile

Metaplasia	Dysplasia
Conversion of a mature, differentiated cell into another form of a mature cell type, often following injury or insult	Development of abnormal types of cells within a tissue, which may signify a stage preceding the development of cancer
Conversion in cell type	Change in the phenotype of cells or a tissue
Occurs in various types of tissues	Mainly occurs in the epithelium
An adaptive process that occurs due to an external stimulus	Occurs due to the alternation of genetic material
A reversible process	An irreversible process
Does not lead to the formation of cancer	May cause cancer

105. Ans. (a) Totipotent

Ref: Robbins E-book, pg. 25-26

- **Totipotent cells** can form all the cell types in a body, **plus** the extraembryonic, or placental, cells. Embryonic cells within the first couple of cell divisions after fertilization are the only cells that are totipotent.
- **Pluripotent cells** can give rise to all of the cell types of the three germ cell layers; embryonic stem cells are considered pluripotent.
- **Multipotent cells** can develop into more than one cell type, but are more limited than pluripotent cells; adult stem cells and cord blood stem cells are considered multipotent.

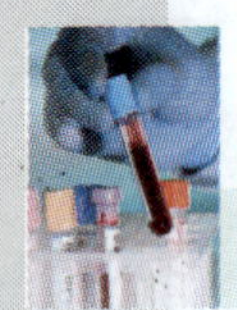

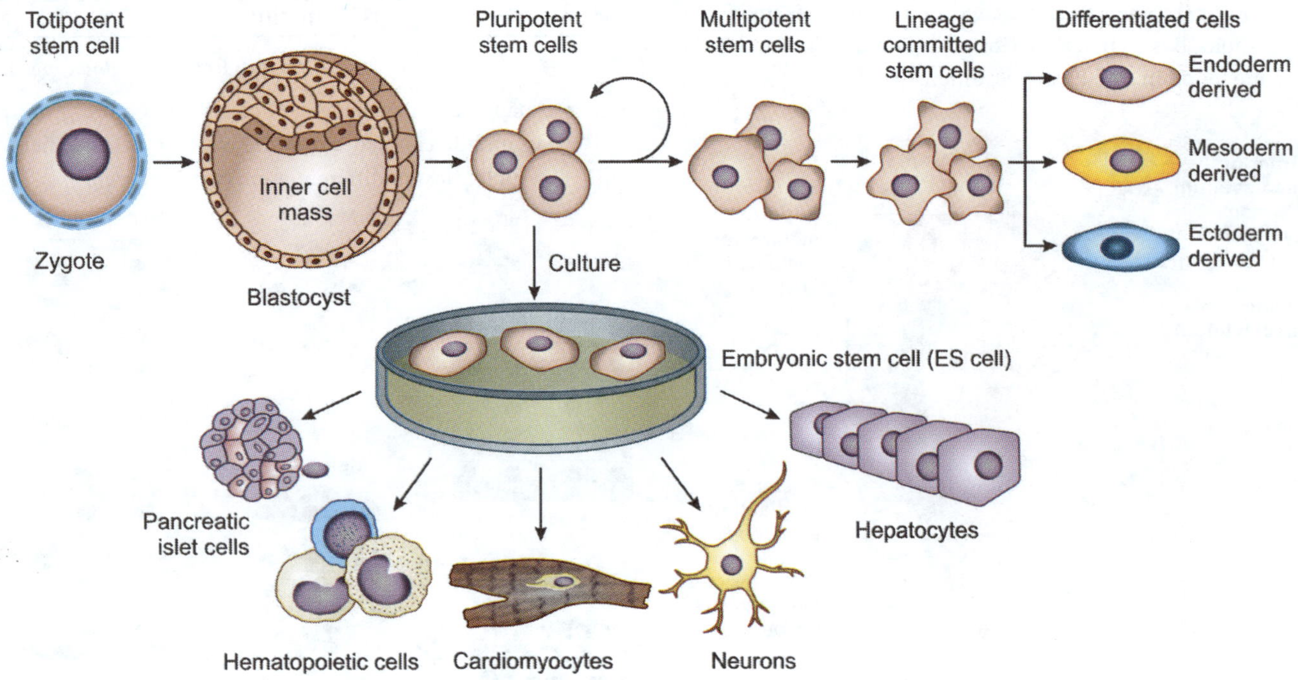

106. Ans. (c) Teratoma

Ref: Robbins 9th ed. pg. 977

All tumors that produce α-fetoprotein have hyaline globules. These are eosinophilic round bodies found in following causes:

Malignant causes	Benign causes
• Yolk sac tumor • Hepatocellular carcinoma • Clear cell carcinoma • Kaposi sarcoma • Choroid plexus carcinoma • Adenoid cystic carcinoma	• Meningioma • Pleomorphic adenoma • α-1 anti-trypsin deficiency

107. Ans. (a) Lung cancer

Ref: Harrison 19th ed. pg. 1987

- SVC syndrome leads to severe reduction in venous return from head, neck and upper extremities and the causes are:

Malignant	Benign
Lung cancer	Central line catheter
Lymphoma	Pacemaker leads
Metastasis	Defibrillator leads

108. Ans. (d) Lung cancer

Ref: Harrison 19th ed. pg. 467

- The most common cancer leading to death in both males and females.
- The prevalence of carcinoma lung as contributor to death in males is 28% as compared to prostate cancer as 10%.
- The prevalence of carcinoma lung as contributor to death in females is 26% compared to breast cancer as 15%.

Distribution of *Cancer releted deaths*

Male (%)		Female(%)	
Lung	28	Lung	26
Prostate	10	Breast	15
Colorectal	8	Colorectal	9
Pancreas	7	Pancreas	7

Extra Mile

GLOBOCAN 2020 mentions female Breast cancer as most commonly diagnosed cancer. The same data is present on WHO website lung cancer remains the leading cause of cancer death.

109. Ans. (a) Comedo subtype of DCIS

Ref: Robbins E-book, pg. 743

- The distinctive *comedo-subtype is characterized by extensive central necrosis.*
- This produces necrotic tissue with tooth paste consistency.
- Calcifications are frequently encountered in DCIS due to *calcification of necrotic tissue and are easily picked up by mammography.*

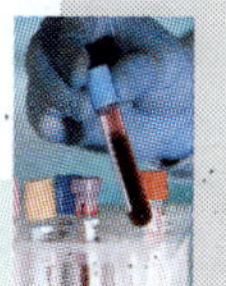

- Cribriform subtype of DCIS is a low grade tumor and hence necrosis in not seen.
- Colloid carcinoma produces abundant mucin both intracellularly and extracellularly.
- LCIS tends to be bilateral and may not be detected on mammography as it does *not* produce calcification.

110. Ans. (a) Peutz-Jeghers syndrome

Ref: Harrison 19th ed. pg. 240

- Peutz-Jeghers syndrome is characterized by dark brown spots on lips, buccal mucosa, nose and around eyes. There is concomitant intestinal polyposis. The most common location of polyps is in jejunum.
- It is an autosomal dominant disorder with STK11 mutation.
- The malignant potential of polyps ranges from never to rare transformation.

111. Ans. (a) Transposon

- Transposons, also called jumping genes, are pieces of DNA that move readily from one site to another.
- They move either within or between the DNAs of bacteria, plasmids and bacteriophages in a manner, that plasmid genes can become part of the chromosomal complement of genes.
- Interestingly, when transposons transfer to a new site, it is usually a copy of the transposon that moves, while the original remains in situ (like photocopying).
- Transposons can code for metabolic or drug resistance enzymes and toxins. They may also cause mutations in the gene into which they insert or alter the expression of nearby genes.
- In contrast to plasmids or bacterial viruses, transposons cannot replicate independently of the recipient DNA. More than one transposon can be located in the DNA for example, resistance genes. Thus, transposons can jump from:
  - The host genomic DNA to a plasmid
  - One plasmid to another
  - A plasmid to genomic DNA.
- An *insertion sequence* is a short DNA sequence that acts as a simple transposable element. Insertion sequences have two major characteristics: they are small relative to other transposable elements (generally around 700 to 2500 bp in length) and only code for proteins implicated in the transposition activity (they are thus different from other transposons, which also carry accessory genes such as antibiotic resistance genes.

112. Ans. (b) Testicular contour distorted

TABLE: Distinguishing features of seminomatous (SGCT) and non-seminomatous (NSGCT) germ cell tumours of testis

Features	SGCT	NSGCT
Primary tumor	Large confined to testis for sufficient time, testicular contour retained	Similar at times indistinct: Testicular contour may be distorted
Metastasis	Generally to regional lymph nodes	Haematogenous spread early
Response to radiation	Radiosensitive	Radio-resistant
Serum markers	hCG: generally low levels	hCG, AFP, or both high levels
Prognosis	Better	Poor

113. Ans. (a) Adenolymphoma

- Warthin's tumour is called papillary cystadenoma lymphomatosum or adenolymphoma.
- It is a *benign tumour* of parotid comprising 8% of all parotid tumours seen in men from 4th to 7th decades of life.
- A common *wrong answer* from most candidates is pleomorphic adenoma. It is the most common tumour of the parotid.
- Most common malignant salivary gland tumour is mucoepidermoid carcinoma.

114. Ans. (b) Dysplasia

Loss of polarity implies loss of architectural orientation of cells which is seen in dysplasia.

TABLE: Differences between metaplasia and dysplasia

Feature	Metaplasia	Dysplasia
Definition	Change of one type of epithelial or mesenchymal cell to another type of adult epithelial or mesenchymal cell	Disordered cellular development may be accompanied with hyperplasia or metaplasia
Types	Epithelial (squamous columnar) and mesenchymal (osseous, cartilaginous)	Epithelial only
Tissues affected	Most commonly affects bronchial mucosa, uterine endocervix; other mesenchymal tissues (cartilage, arteries)	Uterine cervix, bronchial mucosa

Contd...

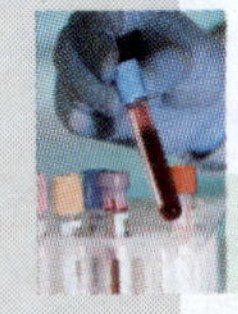

Feature	Metaplasia	Dysplasia
Cellular changes	Mature cellular development	Disordered cellular development (pleomorphism, nuclear hyperchromasia, mitosis, loss of polarity)
Natural history	Reversible on withdrawal of stimulus	May regress on removal of inciting stimulus, or may progress higher grades of dysplasia or carcinoma in situ

115. Ans. (c) Oat cell cancer

c-myc	Burkitt's lymphoma
L-myc	Lung cancer
N-myc	Neuroblastoma
KIT (CD117)	Gastrointestinal stromal tumors

116. Ans. (a) Small cell cancer of lung

H.C.C	Hepatitis B virus
Nasopharyngeal cancer	EBV
MALToma	*H. pylori*

117. Ans. (d) Lymphoma

TABLE: Mediastinal tumor & masses

Anterior	Middle	Posterior
MC Thymoma • Lymphoma	MC Lymphoma	Neurogenic tumors – neuroblastoma/ ganglioneuroblastoma/ ganglioneuroma
Metastatic CA Thyroid lesions	Bronchopulmonary of foregut malformations – bronchogenic cyst, oesophageal duplication Pericardialcyst	Lymphoma Bronchogenic cyst Gastroenteric hernia
Teratoma		Spinal tumors–PNET
Thymic infiltration – leukaemia/ lymphoma/ histiocytosis		Trauma–vertebral haematoma

118. Ans. (a) HPV

Human papillomavirus (HPV) which is the most common sexually transmitted infection, is a cause of anal dysplasia and cancer.

The approximately 40 HPV subtypes that can cause anogenital infections are divided into:

1. **Low-risk types (e.g. types 6 and 11)** that cause anal warts (condyloma acuminata)
2. **High-risk types (e.g. types 16, 18 and 33)** that can cause anal dysplasia and cancer.

HPV infection is associated with cervical, vulvar, vaginal, and penile cancers, and some patients have HPV-related dysplasia or cancer in multiple sites. Approximately 90% of anal cancers are attributable to HPV infection.

119. Ans. (c) Colorectal CA

Ref: Robbins Pathology, 9th ed. pg. 809

- Familial adenomatous polyposis (FAP) is an autosomal dominant disorder in which patients develop numerous colorectal adenomas as teenagers.
- **Robbins states: "Colorectal adenocarcinoma develops in 100% of untreated FAP patients, often before age 30 and nearly always by age 50"**
- As a result, prophylactic colectomy is the standard therapy for individuals carrying *APC* mutations. Colectomy prevents colorectal cancer, but patients remain at risk for neoplasia at other sites.
- **FAP is also associated with a variety of extraintestinal manifestations:**
  - Congenital hypertrophy of the retinal pigment epithelium
  - Gardner syndrome and
  - Turcot syndrome

120. Ans. (c) Stricture formation

Ref: Harrisons, 19th ed. pg. 532

TABLE: Some etiologic factors associated with squamous cell cancer of the esophagus

- Excess alcohol consumption
- Cigarette smoking
- Other ingested carcinogens
  - Nitrates (converted to nitrites)
  - Smoked opiates
  - Fungal toxins in pickled vegetables
- Mucosal damage from physical agents
  - Hot tea
  - Lye ingestion
  - Radiation-induced strictures
  - Chronic achalasia
- Esophageal web with glossitis and iron deficiency (i.e., Plummer-Vinson or Paterson-Kelly syndrome)
- Congenital hyperkeratosis and pitting of the palms and soles (i.e. tylosis palmaris et plantaris)
- Dietary deficiencies of selenium, molybdenum, zinc, and vitamin A

TABLE: Some etiologic factors associated with adenocarcinoma of the esophagus

- Chronic gastroesophageal reflux
- Obesity
- Barrett's esophagus
- Male gender
- Cigarette smoking

121. Ans. (d) Thymus

- Oncocytes have been found to arise in various glandular and secretory epithelia. In the head and neck area, oncocytic change has been noted in numerous organs such as: the **salivary glands, pituitary, thyroid, parathyroid, nasal cavities, sinuses, ocular caruncle, lacrimal glands, buccal mucosa, Eustachian tube and the larynx.** They have also been **called oxyphilic cells, Askanazy cells and Hurthle cells in the thyroid gland.**
- The parotid gland is the most common site where oncocytic changes may occur, usually at the ductal or acinar cell level.

122. Ans. (b) Keratin

Ref: Robbin's Pathology, 9th ed. pg. 724

- *Keratin expression is helpful in determining epithelial origin in anaplastic cancers.*
- ***Tumors that express keratin include** carcinomas, mesotheliomas, thymomas, sarcomas and trophoblastic neoplasms.*
- *Furthermore, the precise expression pattern of keratin subtypes allows prediction of the origin of the primary tumor when assessing metastases.*

123. Ans. (d) Apthous ulcer

Ref: Robbin's Pathology 9th ed. pg. 728-730; Sternberg's Diagnostic Surgical Pathology, 5th ed. pg. 777

- Most cases of tongue CA are associated with lifestyle habits of smoking and drinking, tobacco chewing.
- **Most significant etiologic agent is tobacco.**
- Alcohol appears to act synergistically with tobacco as either a co-carcinogen (increasing the risk) or a promoter (decreasing the lag time) of neoplastic transformation.
- The neoplasm most often develops as an area of leukoplakia, chronic ulcer, or erythroplakia on the **lateral aspect of the middle one-third of the tongue.**

124. Ans. (a) Ewing's sarcoma

Ref: Robbin's Pathology, 9th ed. pg. 1203

HIGHLY RADIOSENSITIVE TUMOURS = W.E.L.M.S

- Wilms
- Ewing tumour
- Lymphoma
- Malignant myeloma
- Seminoma

125. Ans. (c) Thyroid

Ref: Robbin's Pathology, 9th ed. pg. 109

- The most radio-sensitive organ sites in children in the order of sensitivity are thyroid, breasts, bone marrow and brain.
- Exposure to ionizing radiation in first 2 decades predisposes a person for development of papillary CA.

126. Ans. (b) Stimulates formation of pyrimidine dimers

Ref: Robbin's Pathology, 9th ed. pg. 324-25

- The carcinogenicity of UV-B light is attributed to the formation of pyrimidine dimers in DNA. This type of DNA damage is repaired by nucleotide excision repair pathway.
- In patients with Xeroderma Pigmentosum, defective DNA repair is illustrated by appearance of high frequency of cancers.

127. Ans. (b) Lymphocytes

Ref: Robbin's Pathology, 9th ed. pg. 325-26

- The most radiosensitive blood cell is lymphocyte as it has a large nucleus.
- The least radiosensitive blood cell is platelets.

128. Ans. (c) Clonorchiasis

Ref: Robbin's Pathology, 9th ed. pg. 874-75

- **Clonorchis Sinesis:** Cholangiocarcinoma
- **Schistosoma Hematobium:** Squamous cell cancer of urinary bladder
- **Schistosoma Japonicum:** Colorectal cancer

IMMUNITY AND HYPERSENSITIVITY

129. Ans. (b) T cells

Ref: Robbins Pathology E-Book, 2013 pg. 137

- Histopathological change of interstitial fibrosis, tubular atrophy and arteritis is seen in Chronic allograft rejection
- T cells are central in the rejection of grafts. The rejection reaction consists of the sensitization stage and the effector stage.
- Sensitization stage: CD4 and CD8 T cells, via their T-cell receptors, recognize the allo-antigens expressed on the cells of the foreign graft
- Effector stage: CD4-positive T cells initiate macrophage-mediated delayed type hypersensitivity responses and provide help to B cells for antibody production.

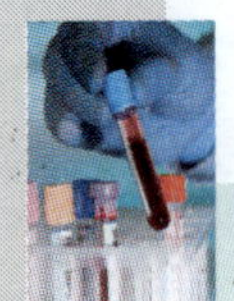

130. Ans. (b) Type 2

Ref: Robbins and Cotran 2020 E-Book pg. 1226

Myasthenia gravis is an autoimmune disease with antibodies blocking Ach receptors. Hence it is an example of type 2 hypersensitivity.

Extra Mile

Myasthenia Gravis: According to latest data is type 5 hypersensitivity reaction > type 2 hypersensitivity reaction. Both are autoimmune but cell death occurs in type 2 and does not occur in type 5 hypersensitivity.

131. Ans. (d) IgE mediated

Ref: Robbins and Cotran Atlas 2020, E-Book pg. 166

Bee sting results in release of histamine and can cause IgE mediated anaphylaxis. This explains the redness on face and difficulty in breathing in this patient.

132. Ans. (b) Type II

Ref: Robbins and Cotran Review of Pathology E-Book pg. 67

- Rh incompatibility is an example of type II hypersensitivity. Rh negative mother will become sensitized to Rh positive RBC due to feto-maternal leak. The result is production of IgM class of antibodies that do not cross the placenta. Hence first baby is unaffected.
- However, if second pregnancy is also Rh positive, the IgG class of antibodies will be produced. They can cross the placenta and enter fetus and cause extensive destruction of RBC of fetus. The resultant severe anemia will cause CHF in the fetus and called as immunogenic hydrops fetalis.

133. Ans. (c) IgE

Ref: Robbins and Cotran Review of Pathology E-Book pg. 57

Bee sting results in release of histamine and can cause IgE mediated anaphylaxis. This explains the redness on face and difficulty in breathing in this patient.

134. Ans. (a) Di-George syndrome

Ref: Robbins and Cotran Review of Pathology E-Book pg. 71

- Hypocalcemia indicates parathyroid gland hypoplasia. The combination of parathyroid gland and thymic hypoplasia indicates Di-George syndrome.
- It is a defect of pharyngeal pouch system and is caused by heterozygous chromosomal deletion at 22q11.2.
- Co-truncal cardiac abnormality seen is TOF.
- SCID occurs due to adenosine deaminase defect that result in defective T cell function.
- Bruton agammaglobulinemia/ X-linked agammaglobulinemia is an inherited immunodeficiency disorder. It is characterized by the absence of mature B cells which in turn leads to severe antibody deficiency and recurrent infections.

135. Ans. (a) B cells

Ref: Robbins 10th ed. pg. 612

- The image shows typical owl eye appearance of Neoplastic giant Reed Sternberg cell seen in case of HL. It is derived from germinal center and postgerminal center B cells.
- Owl eye appearance is due to prominent nucleoli inside nucleus.
- Activation of transcription factor NF-Kβ is a common event that turns on genes that are believed to promote the growth and survival of RS Cells.

136. Ans. (a) Type 1

Ref: Robbins 10th ed. pg. 214

- Hemodynamic collapse, rash, pruritus and bronchospasm are seen in Type 1 hypersensitivity reaction that is common with sea food, drugs, insect bites, bee sting or any pharmaceutical product including vaccines. The resultant laryngeal edema explains the breathing difficulty in this patient.
- Option B is seen with mismatched Blood transfusion or Rh incompatibility.
- Option C presents as rash and complements mediated damage to skin, blood vessels, kidneys and joints.
- Option D is cell mediated delayed hypersensitivity seen with Mantoux test, lepromin test, patch test and pathergy test.

137. Ans. (a) Sjögren's syndrome

Ref: Harrison 20th ed. pg. 2561

- The difficulty in swallowing dry food items like chips or biscuits points to deficient saliva production. Gritty sensation below eyes indicates deficient tear production from lacrimal glands.
- The presence of anemia of chronic disease and anti Ro antibody helps in reaching diagnosis of Sjögren's syndrome.
- Option B involves small joints of hands and resultant deformities
- Option C presents with fever and rash
- Option D presents with musculoskeletal complaints with rash, anemia and renal compromise.

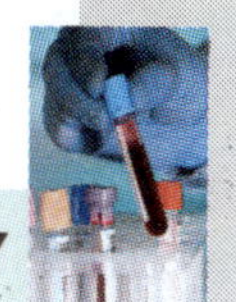

138. Ans. (b) Isograft

Ref: Robbins 10th ed. pg. 234

Type of graft	Donor
Allograft	First degree relatives
Isograft	Monozygotic twins
Xenograft	Across species like pig heart valves
Autograft	Self-body tissue like in burns and Hodgkin's lymphoma

139. Ans. (b) MHC

Ref: Robbins 10th ed. pg. 204

MHC molecules are present on surface of antigen presenting cells. When the antigen attaches to MHC I molecule it will activate CD4 cells while antigen attachment to MHC II molecule will activate CD8 cells. By limiting the specificity of T cells for peptides displayed by cell surface MHC molecules, the immune system ensures that T cells see only antigens which are derived from microbes or from proteins ingested by cells.

140. Ans. (c) Helper T cell

Ref: Robbins 10th ed

The patient is developing type 1 hypersensitivity reaction. The antigen will activate T4 cells that in turn will produce cytokines responsible for systemic response like wheezing, sneezing and cough.

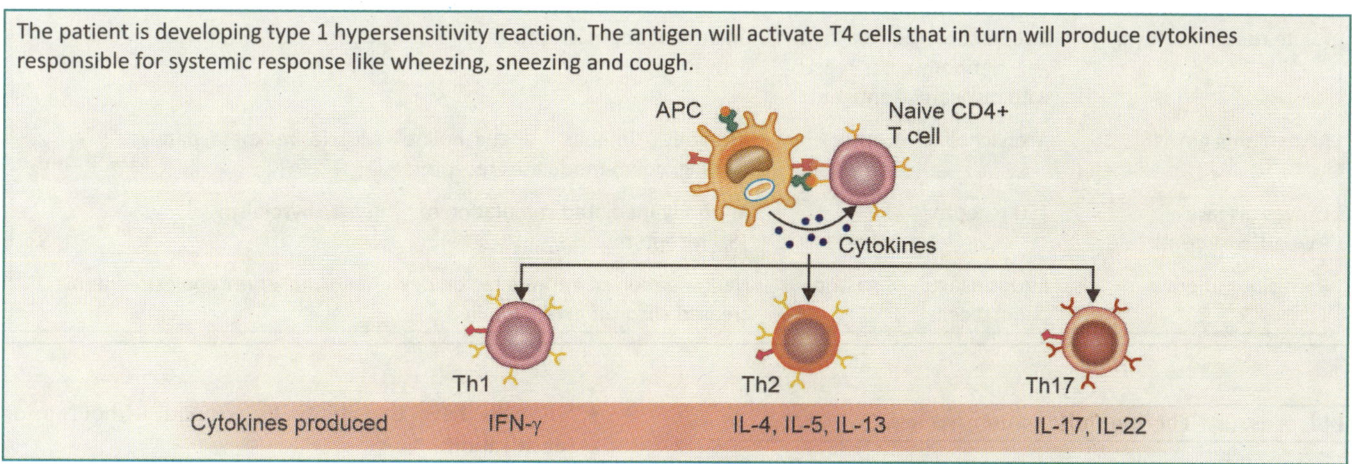

141. Ans. (d) Blood pressure

Ref: Bailey and Love 27th ed. pg. 1223

Criteria for SIRS are considered to be met if at least 2 of the following 4 clinical findings are present:

- Temperature higher than 38°C (100.4°C) or lower than 36°C (98.8°F)
- Heart rate (HR) higher than 90 beats/min
- Respiratory rate (RR) higher than 20 breaths/min or arterial carbon dioxide tension ($PaCO_2$) lower than 32 mm Hg
- White blood cell (WBC) count higher than 12,000/μL or lower than 4000/μL or with 10% immature (band) forms

Rejection stage	Pathogenesis	Time course
Hyperacute	Antibody mediated due to pre-existing antibodies, resulting in complement activation and thrombosis	Minutes to hours
Acute	Acute cellular rejection due to activated lymphocytes Humoral rejection due to antidonor antibodies produced after transplant	First 6 months
Chronic	Antibody and cell-mediated rejection	Months to years

142. Ans. (c) <6 months

Ref: Bailey and Love: 26th ed. pg. 1410

143. Ans. (a) Pernicious anaemia

Ref: Robbins Pathology E-Book, pg. 139

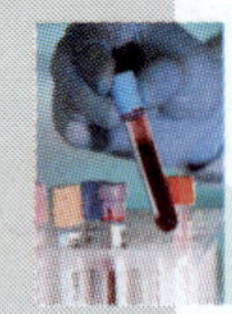

- Pernicious anaemia is associated with anti-parietal cell antibodies and is an example of type 2 hypersensitivity reaction.
- Choice B and C are type 3 hypersensitivity reactions.
- Choice D is type 4 hypersensitivity phenomenon.

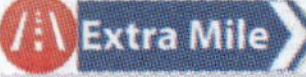

Disease	Target antigen	Mechanisms of disease	Clinicopathologic manifestations
Autoimmune hemolytic anemia	Red blood cell membrane proteins	Opsonization and phagocytosis of red blood cells	Hemolysis. anemia
Autoimmune thrombocytopenic purpura	Platelet membrane proteins (GpIIb:IIIa integrin)	Opsonization and phagocytosis of platelets	Bleeding
Pemphigus vulgaris	Proteins in intercellular junctions of epidermal cells (desmogleins)	Antibody-mediated activation of proteases, disruption of intercellular adhesions	Skin vesicles (bullae)
Vasculitis caused by ANCA	Neutrophil granule proteins. presumably released from activated neutrophils	Neutrophil degranulation and inflammation	Vasculitis
Goodpasture syndrome	Protein in basement membranes of kidney glomeruli and lung alveoli	Complement- and Fc receptor—mediated inflammation	Nephritis. lung hemorrhage
Acute rheumatic fever	Streptococcal cell wall antigen: antibody cross-reacts with myocardial antigen	Inflammation. macrophage activation	Myocarditis. arthritis
Myasthenia gravis	Acetylcholine receptor	Antibody inhibits acetylcholine binding. down-modulates receptors	Muscle weakness, paralysis
Graves disease (hyperthyroidism)	TSH receptor	Antibody-mediated stimulation of TSH receptors	Hyperthyroidism
Pernicious anemia	Intrinsic factor of gastric parietal cells	Neutralization of intrinsic factor, decreased absorption of vitamin B_{12}	Abnormal erythropoiesis. anemia

144. Ans. (a) Thermophilic actinomycetes

Ref: Harrison 20th ed. pg. 1970

Farmer's lung is a hypersensitivity pneumonitis which is caused by thermophilic actinomycetes. The same organism grows on sugarcane dust and is the antigen leading to Bagassosis.

Disease	Antigen	Source
Farming/Food Processing		
Farmer's lung	Thermophilic Actinomycetes	Grain, moldy hay, silage Sugarcane
Bagassosis	Thermophilic actinomycetes	

145. Ans. (a) NK cell

Ref: Robbins review E-book, pg. 67

- NK cells have the ability to respond without prior sensitization.
- They carry receptors for MHC class I molecules which inhibit their lytic function. When expression of class I MHC molecules is reduced on a cell surface by viral interference, inhibitory receptors on NK cells do not receive a signal and the targeted cells is destroyed.
- NK cells have CD16, Fc receptor that allows them to bind to opsonised cells and lyse them. This is a form of type II hypersensitivity with antibody mediated disease.

146. Ans. (a) Graft across species

Ref: CMDT 2018, pg. 157

- Autologous graft (autograft): Within an individual, auto transplantation
- Syngeneic graft (syngraft, isograft): Identical twins, isotransplantation
- Allogeneic graft (allograft, homograft): Non-identical, allotransplantation

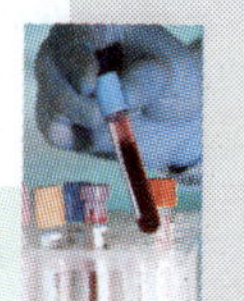

- Xenogeneic graft (heterologous graft, heterograft): Between species, xenotransplantation

147. Ans. (b) Autoimmune Hemolytic anaemia

Ref: Robbins E-book, pg. 135

- Choice A is type of type 4 Hypersensitivity reaction.
- Choice C is type of type 3 Hypersensitivity reaction.
- Choice D is type of type 4 Hypersensitivity reaction.

148. Ans. (b) Days to weeks

Ref: Robbins E-book, pg. 164

- Acute rejections appear within days or weeks and hence choice B is correct.
- Choice C is a close choice but it mentions only after 6 weeks of graft deployment while acute rejection can occur earlier as well.
- **Acute rejection is mediated by T cells and antibodies that are activated by alloantigens in the graft.** It occurs within days or weeks after transplantation, and is the principal cause of early graft failure. It also may appear suddenly months or even years later, after immunosuppression is tapered or terminated. Based on the role of T cells or antibodies, acute rejection is divided into two types, although in most rejecting grafts, both patterns are present

149. Ans. (a) Anti-Ro

Ref: Nelson 20th ed. pg. 1152

In SLE, Anti-Ro antibody can easily cross the placenta and damage the A-V node of the developing fetus. This leads to the baby being born with *complete heart block*. Right from day 0 of life the presentation is bradycardia and syncope. The baby may have a *malar rash* in butterfly distribution. This is called as neonatal lupus.

Antismith antibody	Most specific test for SLE
Antiribonucleoprotein antibody	Leads to psychosis in SLE
Antiphospholipid antibody	APLAS leading to recurrent abortions

150. Ans. (a) CD4

- Class I MHC antigens have loci as HLA-A, HLA-B and HLA-C. CD8+ (i.e. T suppressor) lymphocytes carry receptors for class I MHC: These cells are used to identify class I antigens on them.
- Class II MHC antigens have single locus as HLA-D. These antigens have further 3 loci: DR, DQ and DP. Class II MHC is identified by 8 cells and CD4+ (i.e. T helper) cells.
- Class III MHC antigens are some components of the complement system (C2 and C4) coded on HLA complex but are not associated with HLA expression and are not used in antigen identification.
- In view of high polymorphism of class I and Class II genes, they have a number of alleles on loci numbered serially like HLA-A 1, HLA-A 2, HLA-A3 etc.
- MHC antigens present on the cell surface help the macrophage in its function of recognition of bacterial antigen, i.e. they help of identify self from foreign and accordingly present the foreign antigen to T cells (CD4 + or CD8+) or to B cells.

151. Ans. (d) Type 4

TABLE: Comparative features of four types of hypersensitivity reactions

Feature	Type 1 (Anaphylactic, atopic	Type 2 (Antibody – mediated, cytotoxic)	Type 3 (Immune – complex, arthus reaction)	Type 4 (Delayed T cell – mediated)
Definition	Rapidly developing immune response in a previously sensitised person	Reaction of humoral antibodies that attack cell surface antigens and cause cell lysis	Results from deposition of antigen antibody complexes of tissues	Cell-mediated slow and prolonged response
Peak action time	15–30 minutes	15–30 minutes	Within 6 hours	After 24 hours
Mediated by	IgE antibodies	IgG or IgM antibodies	IgG, IgM antibodies	**Cell mediated**
Etiology	Genetic basis, pollutants, viral infections	HLA – linked, exposure to foreign tissues/ cells	Persistence of low grade infection, environmental anti-gens, autoimmune process	Cutaneous antigens

152. Ans. (d) CD 19

- B cell markers are CD 19, 20, 21 and 23.
- T_H cell markers are CD 4, 3, 7, 2
- T_C cell markers are CD 8, 3, 7, 2
- NK cell markers are CD 2, 16, 56

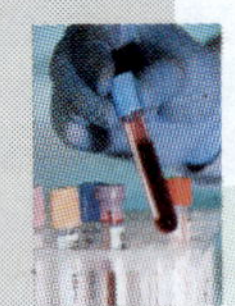

153. Ans. (d) Pneumoconiosis with rheumatoid arthritis

- Progressive massive fibrosis of pneumoconiosis in association with *rheumatoid arthritis is known as Caplan syndrome.*
- Unlike lesions caused by progressive massive fibrosis, which congregate in the upper lobes, these lesions known as Caplan lesions tend to coalesce in the peripheral lung fields.

154. Ans. (b) Ankylosing spondylitis

Clinical Associations with HLA – B27	
Disorder	**HLA –B27 (%)**
Ankylosing spondylitis	90
Reactive arthritis (Reither's syndrome)	40–80
Juvenile SpA	70
Inflammatory bowel disease	35-75
Psoriatic arthritis With spondylitis With peripheral arthritis	 50 15
Undifferentiated SpA	70
Acute anterior uveitis	50
Aortic insufficiency, heart block	80

155. Ans. (d) Large granular lymphocyte

- *The natural killer cells are called as large granular lymphocytes and are responsible for A.D.C.C (Antibody dependant cell cytotoxicity).* This mechanism is particularly effective against viruses and tumour cells.
- NK cells are a part of natural or innate immunity and recognise antibody coated cells. Thus they bring about killing of target cells directly.

156. Ans. (d) Type 4

- *Delayed type of hypersensitivity is mediated by T cell dependant effector mechanisms involving both CD4+ TH1 cells and CD8 Cytotoxic T cells.*
- Antibodies do not play a role in type IV hypersensitivity reactions. The activated TH1 cells release Cytokines that will cause accumulation and activation of macrophages which will cause local damage.
- *TH 2 cells release IL-4 and are involved in Type 1 Hypersensitivity reaction.*

157. Ans. (c) SLE

Ref: Chapter 5; Robbins, 8th ed.

TABLE: Hypersensitivity reactions

Type I (IgE mediated)	Type II (IgG, IgM and complement mediated)
• Eczema • Hay fever • Asthma atopy • Urticaria • Anaphylactic shock • Acute dermatitis • *Prausnitz Kustner (PK) reaction* • *Casoni's test*	• Blood transfusion reactions • Erythroblastosis fetalis • AIHA or thrombocytopenia or agranulocytosis • Pemphigus vulgaris • Good pasture syndrome • Bullous pemphigoid • Pernicious anemia • Acute rheumatic fever • Graves disease • Myasthenia gravis
Type III (IgG, IgM, complement and leucocyte mediated)	**Type IV (Cell mediated)**
• Local–Arthus reaction • Systemic-serum sickness • Schick test • Polyarteritis nodosa (PAN) • **SLE** • Acute viral hepatitis • Penicillamine toxicity • Hyperacute graft rejection • **Type 2** lepra reaction (ENL) • Hypersensitivity pneumonitis • Infective endocarditis • Henoch schonlein purpura	• Tuberculin test • Lepromin test • Sarcoidosis • Tuberculosis • Contact dermatitis • Granulomatous inflammatin • **Type I lepra reaction** • ***Patch test*** • Temporal arteritis • **Graft rejection** • Fairleys test • Frie's test

158. Ans. (b) Antigen – antibody mediated

Type II or Cytotoxic Hypersensitivity depends on the abnormal production of IgG or IgM directed against tissue antigens or a normal reaction to foreign antigens expressed on host cells. There are three main mechanisms of injury in Type II reactions:

- Activation of complement followed by complement mediated lysis or phagocytosis and removal by leukocytes
- Antibody dependent cellular cytotoxicity
- Inactivation of a biologically active molecule

159. Ans. (c) IgM

Ref: Ananthanarayan and Paniker's, 8th ed. pg. 100

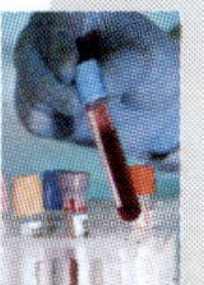

TABLE: Immunoglobulins and their salient features

Immunoglobulins	Salient features
IgG	• **Most abundant Ig,** makes as about 80% • Marker of chronic infection • Only Ig that can cross placenta
IgA	• 2nd most abundant, 10–13% • Found in glandular secretion like saliva, tear, ileum, and mucosal secretion like bronchial secretion
IgM	• 5–8% of total Ig; aka pentameric Ig and **has highest molecular weight** • First Ig to be synthesized by fetus (20 weeks AOG) • Marker of acute infection
IgD	• Present mostly intravascular • Serve as recognition receptor for antigens
IgE	• Mostly extravascular in distribution • Highly elevated levels in case of type-I HPS reaction • Produced chiefly in the linings of respiratory and intestinal tracts

TABLE: Immunoglobulin and their effective valency

Antibody	Effective valency
• IgM	5
• IgG	2
• IgD	2
• IgE	2
• IgA	2,4

Extra Mile

- Ig having maximum molecular weight: **IgM**
- **First antibody produced by newborn: IgM**
- All immunoglobulins are heat stable except: **IgE**
- Ig present in **breast milk: IgA**
- Ig with **maximum half-life: IgG**
- Ig with **minimum half-life: IgE**
- Ig having **maximum serum concentration**: **IgG**
- Ig having **least serum concentration: IgE**

160. Ans. (a) B cells

Ref: Robbin's Pathology, 9th ed. pg. 187, 191

PRIMARY COMPLEMENT IMMUNE RESPONSE

- The first exposure to a foreign antigen, a lag phase occurs in which no antibody is produced, *but activated B cells are differentiating into plasma cells.* The lag phase can be as short as 2–3 days, but often is longer, sometimes as long as weeks or months.
- The amount of antibody produced is usually relatively low.
- Over time, antibody level declines to the point where it may be undetectable.
- The first antibody produced is manily IgM (although small amounts of IgG are usually also produced).

161. Ans. (d) Type 4

Ref: Chapter 55, Harrison, 19th edition

Clinical Features of Severe Cutaneous Drug Reactions

Diagnosis	Mucosal lesions	Typical skin lesions
Stevens-Johnson syndrome	Erosions usually at two or more sites	Small blisters on dusky purpuric macules or atypical targets; rare areas of confluence; detachment ≤10% of body surface area
Toxic epidermal necrolysis	Erosions usually at two or more sites	Individual lesions like those seen in Stevens-Johnson syndrome; confluent erythema; outer layer of epidermis separates readily from basal layer with lateral pressure; large sheet of necrotic epidermis; total detachment of >30% of body surface area

TABLE: Classification of adverse drug reactions based on immune pathway

Hypersensitivity type	Key pathway	Adverse drug reaction type
Type I	IgE	Urticaria, angioedema, anaphylaxis
Type II	IgG-mediated cyto-toxicity	Drug induced hemolysis
Type III	Immune complex	Vasculitis, serum sickness, drug-induced lupus
Type IV b	T lymphocyte-mediated eosinophil inflammation	Tuberculin skin test, contact dermatitis
Type IV c	T lymphocyte-mediated cytotoxic lymphocyte inflammation	Drug-induced hypersensitivity syndrome Morbiliform eruption
Type IV d	T lymphocyte-mediated neutrophil inflammation	Acute generalized exanthematous pustulosis

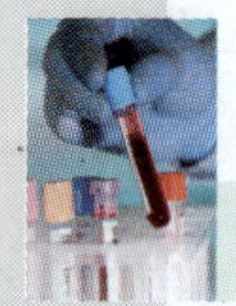

162. Ans. (d) Type 4

Ref: Robbin's Pathology, 8th ed. ch. 5

163. Ans. (a) Bipolar cells

Ref: Robbin's Pathology 9th ed. pg. 191-192: Pocket Companion to Robbin's Pathology, 8th ed. pg. 119

T cells cannot be activated by soluble antigens. Therefore presentation of processed antigen by **antigen presenting cells** is required for activation of T cells.

Important Antigen Presenting Cells are:

- Macrophage
- B cells
- Dendritic cells **(most potent APCs)**
- Langerhans cells

Bipolar cell is a type of neuron which has two extensions. Bipolar cells are specialized sensory neurons for the transmission of special senses. As such, they are part of the sensory pathways for smell, sight, taste, hearing and vestibular functions.

164. Ans. (a) IL-2

Ref: Robbin's Pathology, 9th ed. pg. 192-93

Salient Features of NK Cell

- Growth factor for NK cell-**IL2** (proliferate in response to IL2) and **IL-15.**
- NK cell activity is augmented by interferon
- They secrete perforin which results in formation of transmembrane pore resulting in cell death
- Cytotoxic against virus infected cells, tumour cells, transplanted foreign cells
- Its activity is neither antibody dependent nor MHC restricted.
- Component of innate immunity.
- NK cells + for-CD 16, CD56

165. Ans. (a) MHC class I

Ref: Robbin's Pathology, 9th ed. pg. 231, 232

- In transplantation immunology, the major impact in graft loss comes from the effects of HLA-B and -DR antigens
- The histocompatibility antigens [human leukocyte antigens (HLA)] are cell surface antigens that induce as response leading to rejection of allografts
- The principal physiologic function of the cell surface histocompatiblity molecules is the bind peptide fragments foreign proteins for presentation to antigen specific T cells.
- The histocompatibility antigens are encoded by a closely linked multiallelic cluster of genes: Mix histocompatibility complex (MHC) or human leukocyte antigens complex (HLA complex)
- HLA complex of genes is located on the short arm of chromosome 6.
- It consists of three separate clusters of genes:

TABLE: HLA Complex (MHC complex)

Class I	Class II	Class III
• Comprising A, B and C loci • Responsible for graft rejection and cell mediated cytolysis • Found on the surface of all nucleated cells and platelets	• 'D' region → DR, DQ, DP • Responsible for • Graft versus host response • Mixed leucocyte reaction • Found only on cells of the immune system	• **Complement region encodes** • C_2 and C_4 • Properdin factor B • Heat shock protein • TNF – α and β • Enzyme 21-hydroxylase

Remember

Histocompatibility Reactions

Graft versus host disease	Host versus graft disease (Graft rejection)
• HLA class II is primarily involved • T-helper cells (CD-4)	• HLA class I is primarily involved • Cytotoxic T cell (CD-8)

166. Ans. (d) Reiter's syndrome

Ref: Robbin's Pathology, 9th ed. pg. 116, 787

In addition to its association with ankylosing spondylitis, HLA-B27 is implicated in other types of seronegative spondyloarthropathy

- Reactive arthritis (Reiter's syndrome)
- Acute anterior uveitis and iritis
- Psoriatic arthritis
- Ulcerative colitis associated spondyloarthritis

167. Ans. (b) Chronic granulomatous disorder

Ref: Robbin's Pathology, 9th ed. pg. 237-238

Nitro blue tetrazolium is used in a diagnostic test, particularly for chronic granulomatous disease. When there is an NADPH oxidase defect, the phagocyte is unable to make reactive oxygen species or radicals required for bacterial killing. As a result, bacteria may thrive within the phagocyte. The higher the blue score, the better the cell is at producing reactive oxygen species.

168. Ans. (d) Calcium

Ref: Robbin's Pathology, 9th ed. pg. 89, 238

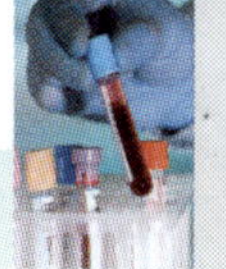

- The initial enzyme of complement pathway, C1, is a complex formed through a calcium-dependent association between two reversibly interacting subunits, C1q and C1r2s2.
- In the absence of an immune response, approximately 70% of C1 exists as a complex between these two subunits.

169. Ans. (d) Sickle cell disease

Ref: Robbin's Pathology, 9th ed. pg. 211-15, 635

- Sickle cell disease is a genetic condition which is characterized by mutation in beta globin chain of hemoglobin **(glutamic acid is replaced with valine in the 6th position of beta chain).**
- Other given choices like SLE, Grave's and MG are all autoimmune conditions.

170. Ans. (d) Type 4

Ref: Robbin's Pathology, 9th ed. pg. 208-209

HEMATOLOGY

171. Ans. (b) Blood transfusion

Ref: Harrison 21st ed. pg. 758

- Crescent shaped RBCs point to sickle cell anemia. During extensive hemolysis of these rigid sickle shaped RBC the child is anemic and needs another blood transfusion.
- Even if child presented with bone pain or abdominal pain due to sickling crisis, Blood transfusion should be given.
- Option A and D are dummy choices and are ruled out.
- Option C, IV fluids are given in sickling crisis patients depending on level of dehydration of patient.

172. Ans. (b) Ferritin

Ref: Harrison 21st ed. pg. 749-750

- Since the child has not responded to oral iron supplementation which is likely due to side effects of oral iron intake, hence a baseline serum ferritin must be done before starting parenteral iron to compare and check for response.
- Option A will remain elevated till Iron levels normalize but objective is not to normalize serum iron but build iron stores as well.
- Option C and D will be low but do not tell information about levels of iron stores.

173. Ans. (c) CML

Ref: Harrison 21st ed. pg. 821

AML has maturational arrest and only myeloblasts are found in bone marrow and peripheral smear. The presence of metamyelocytes 15%, Promyeloblasts 30%, Myeloblast 45% indicates shift to left and is a feature of CML. ALL and CLL are ruled out as they would have lymphoblasts in circulation.

174. Ans. (c) Prussian blue

Ref: Robbins and Cotran Review of Pathology, E-Book pg. 287

Alizarin red	Calcium
Methylene blue	Dye to demonstrate presence of bacteria and cell structures. It is a cationic stain (positively charged blue dye); and binds to negatively charged parts of the cells, such as nucleus
Prussian blue	Iron
Von Kossa	Calcium

175. Ans. (d) Chronic liver disease

Ref: Robbins E-Book 2014 pg. 128

- CLD disease leads to defective lipoprotein formation. This affects RBC membrane formation and leads to macrocyte formation.
- Option A and C leads to microcytic hypochromic anemia.
- Option B leads to normocytic normochromic anemia.

176. Ans. (a) Deficiency of adenosine deaminase

Ref: Robbins and Cotran Review of Pathology E-Book pg. 71

- SCID is most commonly due to an X-linked mutation of the gene coding for the γ chain that leads to deficiency of adenosine deaminase.
- Adenosine deaminase deficiency leads to an accumulation of toxic purine degradation by-products, most potently affecting lymphocytes.
- Hence Antibody production is severely impaired even when mature B cells are present, because of the lack of T-cell help. NK cells, a component of innate immunity, are variably affected.

177. Ans. (a) Hemoglobin electrophoresis

Ref: Harrison 21st ed. pg. 761

Since the child is having microcytic anemia and history of repeated BT, provisional diagnosis is Thalassemia. The next investigation to be ordered is Hemoglobin electrophoresis.

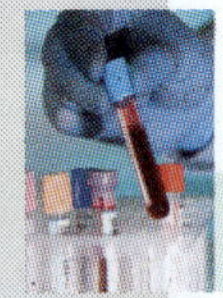

178. Ans. (d) Coombs test

Ref: Harrison 21st ed. pg. 781

Since child is having normocytic anemia and not responding to any conventional treatments, a provisional diagnosis of autoimmune hemolytic anemia is kept. The next best investigation for AIHA is Direct coomb's test.

179. Ans. (a) AML

Ref: Harrison 20th ed. pg. 743

The bone marrow aspiration with more than 20% MPO positive immature cells points to acute leukemia with myeloid origin. MPO is the hallmark enzyme of myeloid lineage and can be detected by cytochemical staining, immunohistochemistry or flow cytometry.

- Option A presents with massive splenomegaly with FISH showing t(9:22) translocation.
- Option C presents with cervical lymphadenopathy with autoimmune hemolytic anemia.
- Option D presents in children with hepatosplenomegaly and lymphoblasts and Immunophenotyping shows terminal deoxynucleotidyl transferase (**TdT**) positivity.

180. Ans. (c) Myelofibrosis

Ref: Robbins 10th ed. pg. 626

- The peripheral smear shows tear drop shape RBCs which are seen in myelofibrosis.
- Option A shows microcytic hypochromic cells with anisocytosis and poikilocytosis.
- Option B shows target cells
- Option D may show a Cytopenia in single or multiple cell lines. Morphologic abnormalities are often observed in the granulocytes. These can include bilobed or unsegmented neutrophils (called pseudo Pelger-Huet abnormality) or hypersegmentation on the nuclei (6-7 lobes) similar to megaloblastic disease. Other abnormalities such as giant hypogranular platelets and megakaryocytes with nuclei called as pawn ball megakaryocytes may be seen on peripheral smear.

181. Ans. (b) Factor 8 deficiency

Ref: Harrison 20th ed. pg. 831

- Joint swelling is a common feature of clotting factor 8 deficiency.
- Option A is the most common bleeding disorder and presents with recurrent nosebleeds and hematomas. Prolonged bleeding from trivial wounds, oral cavity bleeding, and excessive menstrual bleeding are common. Gastrointestinal bleeding rarely occurs.
- Option C and D usually present with excessive bleeding post minor surgery.

182. Ans. (a) Thalassemia

Ref: Harrison 20th ed. pg. 696

- Anemia with splenohepatomegaly points to evidence of extramedullary haematopoiesis. The peripheral smear shows target cells. This points to diagnosis as thalassemia.
- Malar prominence due to bone marrow expansion is also a feature of thalassemia.
- Option A does not have organomegaly.
- Option B should have pappenheimer bodies in peripheral smear. Splenohepatomegaly is not seen in Sideroblastic anemia.
- Option D is a cause of Sideroblastic anemia.

183. Ans. (a) CMV

Ref: Robbins 10th ed. pg. 365

Owl eye appearance is seen in infected kidney tubular cells due to CMV and leads to graft failure. The prominent intranuclear basophilic inclusions spanning one half of nuclear diameter are usually set off from the nuclear membrane by a clear halo.

184. Ans. (b) ALL

Ref: Robbins 10th ed. pg. 601

Key word in the MCQ that points out Acute Leukemia is sternal tenderness. This coupled with age of the child, organomegaly and features of bleeding and infection is suggestive of Acute Lymphoblastic Leukemia. ALL is the leading cancer seen in children.

185. Ans. (a) Multiple myeloma

Ref: Robbins 10th ed. pg. 613

At 3 o'clock position, the peripheral smear shows Mott cells, the cytoplasm of which shows accumulation of incomplete light chains. These intracytoplasmic inclusions are called Russel Bodies.
Option B would show lymphoblasts with TDT positivity
Option C would show NCNC anemia and Option D would show Sickle RBC.

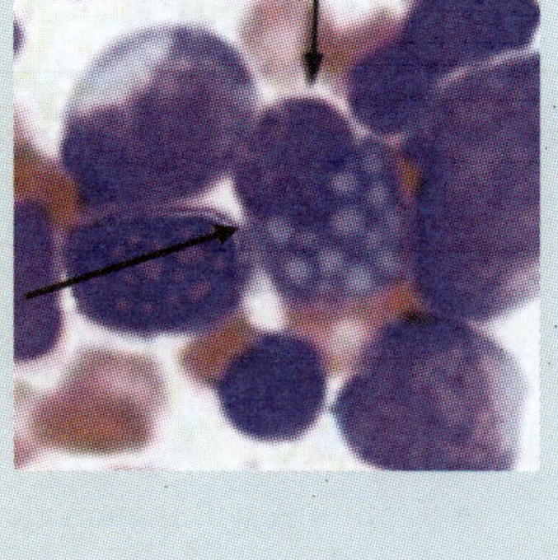

186. Ans. (a) Serum electrophoresis showing IgG

Ref: Robbins 10th ed. pg. 613

- Low backache in geriatric age group with multiple lytic lesions in skull favours diagnosis of Multiple myeloma. Since the condition has overproduction of incomplete

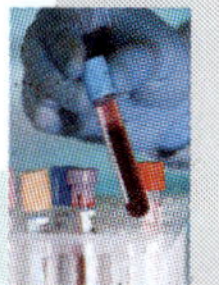

light chains it leads to hyperviscosity. The screening test for multiple myeloma is serum electrophoresis.

- Option B is used to monitor breast cancer treatment and disease recurrence.
- Option C is used to diagnose distant metastasis.
- Option D will not have utility in diagnosis of multiple myeloma as the lytic lesions in rain drop configuration have already been picked up using a X-ray skull.

187. Ans. (a) Malaria

Ref: Manson Tropical diseases: 23rd ed. pg. 1237

The peripheral smear shows banana-shaped gametocyte of falciparum malaria.

188. Ans. (b) Phytates

Ref: Harrison 20th ed. pg. 684

Iron deficiency is a major world health problem, that is, to a great extent, caused by poor iron absorption from the diet. Several dietary factors can influence this absorption. Absorption enhancing factors are ascorbic acid and meat, fish and poultry; inhibiting factors are plant components in vegetables, tea and coffee (e.g., polyphenols, phytates), and calcium.

189. Ans. (a) Serum Ferrtin

Ref: CMDT 2019, pg. 512

- Low ferritin levels < 2 ng/mL is a highly reliable indicator of reduced iron stores. Serum ferritin can increase in response to inflammation and hence normal or elevated ferritin level does not exclude diagnosis of IDA.
- As iron deficiency progresses iron levels will be less than 30 mcg/dL and transferrin levels rise to compensate.
- The elevated transferrin leads to lower saturation to <15%.

190. Ans. (a) High ferritin

Ref: CMDT 2019, pg. 512

- Anemia of chronic disease leads to release of Hepcidin from the liver.
- Hepcidin leads to inhibition of release of iron from stores leading to stores/ferritin being normal to increased since consumption is reduced.
- TIBC shows an inverse relation to serum ferritin always and hence is reduced.

Variable	Anemia of chronic disease	Iron-deficiency anemia
Iron	Reduced	Reduced
Transferrin	Reduced to normal	Increased
Transferrin saturation	Reduced	Reduced
Ferritin	Normal to increased	Reduced
Soluble transferrin receptor	Normal	Increased
Ratio of soluble transferrin receptor to log ferritin	Low (<1)	High (>2)
Cytokine levels	Increased	Normal

Contd...

191. Ans. (a) T.I.B.C

Ref: Robbins E-book, pg. 454

Iron deficiency anaemia has all parameters reduced except Total iron binding capacity.

	Iron deficiency anemia
Hematocrit	↓ to ↓↓↓
MCV	↓ to ↓↓↓
MCHC	↓
Serum iron	↓ to ↓↓↓
Serum TIBC	Normal to ↑
Serum ferritin	↓ to ↓↓
Stainable iron in marrow	Absent
Reticulocytes	Normal to ↓

192. Ans. (c) Normocytic and normochromic anemia

Ref: Robbins 9th ed. pg. 652

- Rheumatoid arthritis leads to development of anemia of chronic disease.
- A more common presentation of anemia of chronic disease is normocytic normochromic anemia. In late presentation microcytic hypochromic anemia is noted.

193. Ans. (b) Yolk sac, liver and bone marrow

Ref: Robbins 9th ed. pg. 579-580

- Erythropoiesis starts in the yolk sac at 2 weeks of gestation and leads to production of embryonic hemoglobin.
- It shifts to liver spleen at 14 weeks of gestation and leads to production of fetal hemoglobin.
- At birth the hematopoiesis shifts to the bone marrow. The major hemoglobin at birth is fetal hemoglobin.

194. Ans. (d) 12 g%

Ref: Robbins 9th ed. pg. 630-631

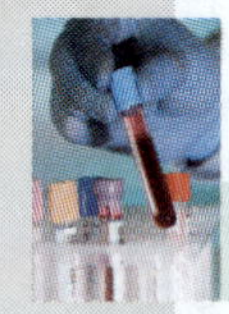

TABLE: Hemoglobin levels to diagnose anemia at sea level (g/L)±

Population	Non-anemia*	Anemia*		
		Mild	Moderate	Severe
Children 6–59 months of age	110 or higher	100–109	70–99	Lower than 70
Children 5–11 years age	115 or higher	110–114	80–109	Lower than 80
Children 12–14 years of age	120 or higher	110–119	80–109	Lower than 80
Nonpregnant women (15 years of age and above)	120 or higher	110–119	80–109	Lower than 80
Pregnant women	110 or higher	100–109	70–99	Lower than 70
Men (15 years of age and above)	130 or higher	110–129	80–109	Lower than 80

195. Ans. (b) NESTROFT

Ref: Textbook of hematology Dr. Tejender Singh 2nd ed. pg. 90-92, Hemoglobinopathies by Anupam Sachdev 1st ed. pg. 100

Initial screening test for diagnosis of β-thalassemia carriers is NESTROFT. The naked eye single tube osmotic fragility test is based on osmotic fragility using 0.36% buffered saline.

Procedure

- Two test tubes labeled as Buffered saline (2 mL) and distilled water 2 mL) are taken and a drop of water is added to each of tubes, which is left undisturbed for half an hour at room temperature. Following this contents of the tube are shaken and held against a white paper on which a thin black line is drawn.

Interpretation

- The line is clearly visible through the DW tube and if the same is seen in Buffered saline tube, it indicates that the test is negative.

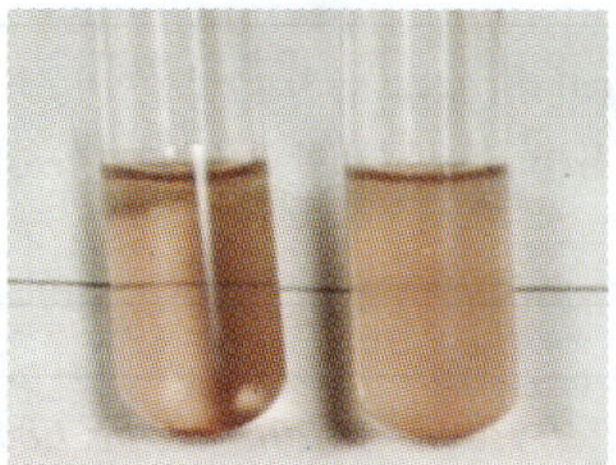

Ditilled water Buffered saline

Positive NESTROFT

Distilled water Buffered saline

Negative NESTROFT

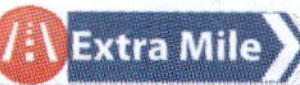

Extra Mile

- Thalassemia syndrome is the most common genetic syndrome worldwide.
- IOC for thalassemia is β globin gene sequencing >> HPLC >> Hb electrophoresis.

196. Ans. (a) Elevated HbA2

Ref:Robbins 9th ed. P 640

- Quantification of HbA2 and Hb variant via HPLC gives an accurate estimate of HbA2 levels
- Values of HbA_2 >3.5% with reduced RBC indices are indicative of β-thalassemia carriers.
- The earlier cut off of HbA2 >3% must be interpreted with caution as per current guidelines.

Extra Mile

Hemoglobin	Structure	Levels at birth	Levels in adults	Comments
A	$\alpha_2\beta_2$	20–25%	97%	Reaches adult levels by 1 year of age
A_2	$\alpha_2\delta_2$	0.5%	2.5%	Elevated in β thalassemia trait
F	$\alpha_2\gamma_2$	75–80%	<1%	Reaches adult levels by 1 year of age
HbH	β_4	15–20% in HbH disease	NA	HbH produces heinz bodies in the erythocytes and hemolysis
HB Bart	γ_4	100% in hydrops fetalis, 15–25% in HbH disease	NA	Increase in carriers of α thalassemia trait at birth

NA = not applicable.

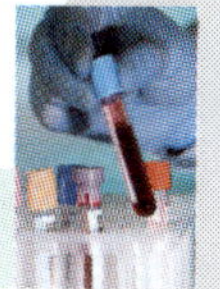

197. Ans. (d) Denatured haemoglobin

Summary of Inclusions in RBCs

Howell jolly bodies	DNA
Basophilic stippling	RNA remnants
Siderotic granules/pappenhiemer bodies	Iron
Heinz bodies	Denatured Haemoglobin

198. Ans. (a) SLE

Positive coombs test is seen in autoimmune haemolytic anaemia caused by SLE.
The remaining three choices of the question are examples of microangiopathic haemolytic anaemia.

TABLE: Causes of Microangiopathic Haemolytic Anemia

Thrombocytic thrombocytopenic purpura
Haemolytic uremic syndrome
Disseminated intravascular coagulation
Infections: Gram–negative septicaemia
Snake bites
Hemolytic transfusion reactions
Obstetric complications: Abruptio placentae, amniotic fluid embolism, retained dead fetus, eclampsia
Malignant hypertension
Immunologic disorders: Vasculitis
Polyarteritis nodosa

199. Ans. (a) A.M.L

- Arsenic trioxide is used in management of *M3 AML/ Acute Pro-myelocytic Leukemia. Also used is A.T.R.A (Al-trans- Retinoic acid).*
- Acute Pro-Myelocytic Leukemia has high risk of early hemorrhagic death due to disseminated intravascular coagulation and hyperfibrinolysis. The prognosis of APL has improved dramatically following the introduction of all-trans retinoic acid (ATRA) and its combination with anthracycline-based chemotherapy during induction and consolidation
- Arsenic trioxide and A.T.R.A are considered in frail or elderly patients. This combination can also be used in patients who are unable to tolerate anthracycline-based therapy.

200. Ans. (b) Parvo virus B19

- Hepatitis B, C and D can lead to aplastic anaemia. In contrast Parvo virus B19 leads to a transient bone marrow illness called aplastic crisis.
- Parvovirus B19 (B19V) is a single-stranded DNA virus of the family Parvo-viridae and genus Erythrovirus.
- It has a unique tropism for human erythroid progenitor cells. The virus requires the P blood antigen receptor (also known as globoside) to enter the cell.

201. Ans. (a) Sickle cell anaemia

Gamma-Gandy bodies (GGB) are siderotic nodules present in the spleen.

Causes of Gamma Gandy bodies are:

1. Portal hypertension
2. Sickle cell anaemia
3. Acquired hemochromatosis
4. Paroxysmal nocturnal hemoglobinuria
5. Angio-sarcoma.

202. Ans. (a) Portal hypertension

203. Ans. (d) Factor 11

- Rosenthal syndrome is Factor XI deficiency/Haemophilia C/Plasma thromboplastin antecedent deficiency.
- These patients will experience severe bleeding after dental extractions. FXI deficiency is inherited in an autosomal recessive pattern.

204. Ans. (c) ALL

Ref: Robbins, 9th ed. pg. 590

Acute Lymphoblastic Leukemia/Lymphoma

- **Acute lymphoblastic leukemia/lymphomas (ALLs) are neoplasms composed of immature B (pre-B) or T (pre-T)cells, which are referred to as *lymphoblasts*.**
- About 85% are B-ALLs, which typically manifest as childhood acute "leukemias."
- The less common T-ALLs tend to present in adolescent males as thymic "lymphomas."
- **ALL is the most common cancer of children.**

Extra Mile

- **Multiple myeloma** is a plasma cell neoplasm commonly associated with lytic bone lesions, hypercalcemia, renal failure, and acquired immune abnormalities.
- **Amyloidosis** is a disorder characterized by the extracellular deposits of misfolded proteins that aggregate to form insoluble fibrils.
- **Mycosis fungoides/Sezary syndrome** is a disorder of helper T cells among adults. Patients present with cutaneous patches, plaques, nodules or generalized erythema.

205. Ans. (c) Nodular sclerosis

Ref: Harsh Mohan, 7th ed. pg. 350

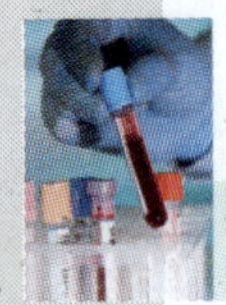

TABLE: Type of Hodgkin's lymphoma

Nodular sclerosis	Most common type of Hodgkin lymphoma	Lacunar Reed-Sternberg cell variants in a mixed inflammatory background; broad sclerotic bands of collagen usually also present	$CD15^+$, $CD30^+$ Reed-Stemberg cells	Most common in young adults, often arises in the mediastinum cervical lymph nodes
Mixed cellularity type	Second most common form of Hodgkin lymphoma	Frequent classic Reed-Sternberg cells in a mixed inflammatory background	$CD15^+$, $CD30^+$, Reed-Stemberg cells	Most common in men, more likely to present at advanced stages than the **nodular sclerosis** type EBV+ in 70% of cases

206. Ans. (a) Polycyathemia vera

Ref: Robbin's Pathology, 9th ed. pg. 616

JAK-2 Mutation is seen in:

1. Polycythemia vera
2. Primary myelofibrosis
3. Essential thrombocytosis

207. Ans. (b) Ca^{++}

208. Ans. (a) Disseminated intravascular coagulation

Ref: Robbin's Pathology, 9th ed. pg. 317-18, 612, 663

- Acute promyelocytic leukemia (APL) is characterized by more severe hemorrhagic phenomena than those of other acute leukemias.
- The hemorrhagic diathesis results from disseminated intravascular coagulation.
- About 40% of patients with APL have a chromosomal abnormality with translocation from the long arm of 17 to 15 (t 15q;17q)
- The patient may present with massive ecchymoses, hematuria, epistaxis, or meno-metrorrhagia.

209. Ans. (a) Nodular sclerosis

Ref: Robbin's Pathology, 9th ed. pg. 606-607

Hodgkin's Disease
Nodular lymphocyte
Predominant Hodgkin's disease
Classical Hodgkin's disease
Nodular sclerosis Hodgkin's disease
Lymphocyte-rich classic Hodgkin's disease
Mixed-cellularity Hodgkin's disease
Lymphocyte-depletion Hodgkin's disease

Contd...

210. Ans. (c) 20%

Ref: Nelson 18th ed. ch. 495

- The characteristic feature of AML is that >20% of bone marrow cells on bone marrow aspiration or biopsy touch preparations constitute a fairly homogeneous population of blast cells, with features similar to those that characterize early differentiation states of the myeloid-monocyte-megakaryocyte series of blood cells. The most common classification of the subtypes of AML is the FAB system.

TABLE: French-American-British (FAB) classification of acute myelogenous leukemia

Subtype	Common name
M1	Acute myeloblastic leukemia without maturation
M2	Acute myeloblastic leukemia with maturation
M3	Acute promyeloblastic leukemia
M4	Acute myelomonocytic leukemia
M5	Acute monocytic leukemia
M6	Erythro leukemia
M7	Acute megakaryocytic leukemia

211. Ans. (a) Smoldering myeloma

Ref: Harrison, 19th ed. pg. 715

TABLE: Diagnostic criteria for multiple myeloma

MONOCLONAL Gammopathy of Undetermined Significance is defined by the presence of three criteria:
- Serum monoclonal M protein (M-protein) concentration **<3 g/dL**
- Bone marrow plasma cell concentration **<10%**
- No evidence of end organ damage

Smoldering MM is present when
- Serum M protein concentration is **>3 g/dL**
- Bone marrow plasma cell concentration is **>10%**
- No evidence of end-organ damage.

Symptomatic myeloma is present when
- M-protein **≥30 g/L**
- Bone marrow clonal cells **≥10%**
- Must have evidence of ROTI (end-organ damage) that can be attributed to the plasma cell proliferative process; manifested by CRAB (calcium, renal failure, anemia, and bone lesions).

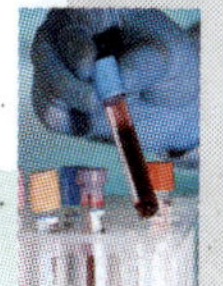

212. Ans. (a) CD1

Ref: Robbin's Pathology, 9th ed. pg. 590

- Langerhans cells are characterized by two types of markers: an ultrastructural marker, the **Birbeck granule** and different membrane markers: **HLA-D antigens, T4 antigen, and some of the CD1 antigens.**
- These antigens which are specific for the epidermal Langerhans cells, are not expressed by the other epidermal cells. Three CD1 antigens are biochemically defined on human thymocytes, they display a glycoprotein chain non covalently attached to beta-2-microglobulin.

213. Ans. (a) Iron

Ref: Robbin's Pathology, 9th ed. pg. 631, 649

214. Ans. (d) Viral or protozoal infection

Ref: Robbin's Pathology, 9th ed. pg. 582-83

- Leucocytosis is seen with viral infections on account of increase in number of natural killer cells.

Leucopenia MNEMONIC _ VINDICATE

V- Vascular causes like MI
I- Infection like sepsis
N- Neoplasm like CLL
D-
I- DRUG INTOXICATION like lithium
C- Congenital like DOWN
A- Autoimmune like polyarteritis nodosa.
T- Trauma
E - Endocrinologic causes like cushing's disease

215. Ans. (b) Africa

Ref: Robbin's Pathology, 9th ed. pg. 588

- Globally, Burkitt lymphoma (BL) is endemic in certain regions of equatorial Africa and other tropical locations between latitudes 10° south and 10° north. Incidence in these areas of endemic disease is 100 per million children.
- Epstein-Barr virus (EBV) infection is found in nearly all areas. In endemic areas, there seems to be a correlation with the geographic distribution of endemic malaria.
- Malaria infection also probably plays a role in the pathogenesis of BL, as it can lead to inhibition of EBV-specific immune response. The exact mechanism of EBV-mediated lymphomagenesis, however, is not well understood, but evidence exists for a significant interaction between viral and cellular microRNA (miRNA) interfering with normal gene expression and translation. EBV can be detected in 25–40% of immunodeficiency-associated cases.

216. Ans. (c) Chronic renal failure

Ref: Robbin's Pathology, 9th ed. pg. 631-35, 638

- The same question was asked in different exams with different choices.
- Choices a, b, d are examples of hemolytic anemias and hence the answer by exclusion is chronic renal failure.
- CRF has low erythropoietin levels due to less production and has normocytic normochromic anaemia.

217. Ans. (a) GLUT 1

Ref: Harrison's, 19th ed. pg. 2402

Basic Rule

- **GLUT 1 and 3** = Everywhere in body (for Basal Absorption of Glucose) including RBC
- **GLUT 2** = In liver and pancreas
- **GLUT 4** = In muscle and adipose

Energy-yielding metabolism in erythrocytes depends on a constant supply of glucose from the blood plasma, where the glucose concentration is maintained at about 5 mm. Glucose enters the erythrocyte by facilitated diffusion via a specific glucose transporter, at a rate about 50,000 times greater than un-catalyzed transmembrane diffusion.

218. Ans. (a) Chronic ITP

Ref: Robbin's Pathology, 9th ed. pg. 658-59

- Splenectomy may be done in patients with chronic ITP, as platelets which have been bound by antibodies are taken up by macrophages in the spleen (which have Fc receptors).
- Durable remission following splenectomy is achieved in 60–65% of ITP cases, less so in older subjects. However, the use of splenectomy to treat ITP has diminished since the development of steroid therapy and other pharmaceutical remedies.

Remember

Drug treatment in ITP

- *Steroids* and steroid sparing agents
- ***Anti-D:*** Suitable for Rh-positive, non-splenectomized patients is intravenous administration of Rho(D) immune globulin. Following administration, anti-D-coated red blood cell complexes saturate Fcγ receptor sites on macrophages, resulting in preferential destruction of red blood cells, therefore sparing antibody-coated platelets.
- ***Romiplostim:*** A thrombopoiesis stimulating Fc-peptide fusion protein that is administered by subcutaneous injection.

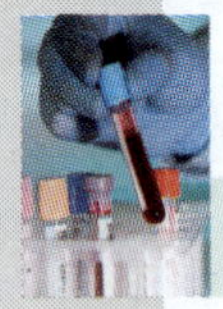

- ***Eltrombopag*** is an orally-administered agent with an effect similar to that of romiplostim. It too has been demonstrated to increase platelet counts and decrease bleeding in a dose-dependent manner.

219. Ans. (a) Prothrombin time

Ref: Robbin's Pathology, 9th ed. pg. 116-18

Prothrombin time	Extrinsic pathway	Factor 5/7
Activated partial thromboplastin time	Intrinsic pathway	Factor 8
Bleeding time	Platelet function and platelet count	Platelet function and count

220. Ans. (b) Human parvo virus B19

Ref: Robbin's Pathology, 9th ed. pg. 635-36

- Human parvo virus B19 is responsible for aplastic crisis that can be life threatening in cases of sickle cell anaemia and hereditary spherocytosis. It is treated with blood transfusion.
- **Remember:** Parvovirus infection in pregnant women is associated with hydrops fetalis due to severe fetal anemia, sometimes leading to miscarriage or stillbirth. The risk of fetal loss is about 10% if infection occurs before pregnancy week 20 (*especially between weeks 14 and 20*), but minimal after then.

221. Ans. (a) Controlling oxidative stress on RBC

Ref: Robbin's Pathology, 9th ed. pg. 634

- G6PD helps in neutralizing the effect of oxidative stress on the RBC.
- Oxidative stress is induced by drugs like primaquine and hence in patients of G6PD there is accelerated hemolysis (intravascular during the hemolytic episode) resulting in hemoglobinuria and passage of shockingly black urine by the patient.

222. Ans. (a) Anemia of chronic disease

Ref: Robbin's Pathology, 9th ed. pg. 652

- In anemia of chronic disease, in response to inflammatory cytokines, the liver produces increased amounts of hepcidin.
- Hepcidin in turn causes increased internalisation of ferroportin molecules on cell membranes *which prevents release from iron stores.*
- Since stores of iron are un-utilized, serum ferritin is increased. TIBC levels are inverse of serum ferritin.
- Low serum iron and low ferritin levels with an elevated TIBC are diagnostic of iron deficiency.

223. Ans. (a) Pernicious anemia

Ref: Robbin's Pathology, 9th ed. pg. 647-648

- Since **hypersegmented neutrophils** are seen with oval RBC the answer is pernicious anemia.

224. Ans. (b) Resistant to denaturation by alkali

Ref: Robbin's Pathology, 9th ed. pg. 635

- Fetal blood contains fetal hemoglobin composed of **two alpha and two gamma subunits.**
- This difference in composition gives the different types of hemoglobin different chemical properties.
- Fetal hemoglobin is resistant to alkali (basic) denaturation, whereas adult hemoglobin is susceptible to such denaturation. Therefore, exposing the blood specimen to sodium hydroxide (NaOH) will denature the adult but not the fetal hemoglobin. The fetal hemoglobin will appear as a pinkish color under the microscope while the adult hemoglobin will appear as a yellow-brownish color.

225. Ans. (c) 60 days

Ref: Harrison, 18th ed. /ch. 113

- Life span of transfused RBC is **60–80** days
- Life span of fetal RBC = 100 days
- Life span of neutrophil = 6 hours
- Life span of neutrophil in tissues = 6 days
- Life span of platelets = 5–7 day
- Life span of transfused platelets = 2–3 days

226. Ans. (a) HUS

Ref: Robbin's Pathology, 9th ed. pg. 644

Characteristic of Schistocytes/Helmet Cells

- Fragmented part of a red blood cell.
- Irregularly shaped, jagged, and have two pointed ends
- Does not have central pallor.

Seen in

- Hemolytic uremic syndrome
- Thrombotic thrombocytopenic purpura
- Disseminated intravascular coagulation

227. Ans. (d) Macrocytic anemia

Ref: Robbin's Pathology, 9th ed. pg. 638

- Thalassemia major presents before 1 year of age with severe anemia which necessitates packed RBC transfusions every 2–3 months. The child is said to be transfusion dependent as survival is decided by RBC being transfused.

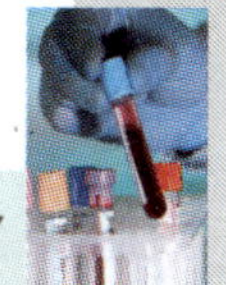

- The ineffective erythropoiesis in bone marrow results in shift of hematopoiesis to liver and the bone marrow. Hence the liver and spleen enlarge in size. But the net result is defective microcytes being produced. The type of anaemia is *microcytic hypochromic anaemia.*
- **Remember: Causes of macrocytic anaemia: "ABCDEF":**
  - Alcohol + liver disease
  - B_{12} deficiency
  - Compensatory reticulocytosis (blood loss and hemolysis)
  - Drug (cytotoxic and AZT)/Dysplasia (marrow problems)
  - Endocrine (hypothyroidism)
  - Folate deficieny/Fetus (pregnancy)

228. Ans. (a) Anemia of chronic disease

Ref: Robbin's Pathology 9th ed. pg. 652

Parameter	Iron deficiency anemia	Sideroblastic anemia	Anemia of chronic disease
Serum iron	Low	High	**Low**
Serum ferritin	Low	High	**High**
T.I.B.C	Increased	Decreased	**Low**

229. Ans. (a) Brilliant cresyl blue

Ref: Robbin's Pathology, 9th ed. pg. 631-32

- Reticulocytes are immature red blood cells, typically composing about 1% of the red cells in the human body. They develop and mature in the red bone marrow and then circulate for about a day in the blood stream before developing into mature red blood cells. Like mature red blood cells, reticulocytes do not have a cell nucleus. **They are called reticulocytes because of a reticular (mesh-like) network of ribosomal RNA that becomes visible under a microscope with certain stains.**
- **The most common supravital stain used is methylene blue or brilliant cresyl blue**, which makes it possible to see the reticulofilamentous pattern of ribosomes.
- By counting the number of such cells the rate of red blood cell formation can be determined, providing an insight into bone marrow activity and anemia.

230. Ans. (b) Ferritin

Ref: Robbin's Pathology, 9th ed. pg. 650

- ***Ferritin is the storage and transferrin is the transport form of iron.***
- Hepcidin is released by liver in setting of anemia of chronic disease. Ferroportin is a transmembrane protein that transports iron from the inside of a cell to the outside of it.
- **Remember:** Ferroportin is inhibited by hepcidin, which binds to ferroportin and internalises it within the cell. This results in the retention of iron within cells, and a reduction in iron levels within the plasma. This is especially significant in enterocytes which are shed at the end of their lifespan where ferroportin is expressed on the basolateral membranes. The extra iron retained within them is not only prevented from entering the bloodstream but ends up being excreted into the faeces. ***Hepcidin is thus the "master regulator" of human iron metabolism.***
- In the setting of anemia, low serum ferritin is the most specific lab test for iron deficiency anemia. However, it is less sensitive, since its levels are increased in the blood by infection or any type of chronic inflammation, and these conditions may convert what would otherwise be a low level of ferritin from lack of iron, into a value in the normal range. For this reason, low ferritin levels carry more information than those in the normal range. ***Low ferritin may also indicate hypothyroidism, vitamin C deficiency or celiac disease.***

231. Ans. (a) Nodular sclerosis

Ref: Robbin's Pathology, 9th ed. pg. 607-610

TABLE: Types of Hodgkins lymphoma

Nodular sclerosis	***It is the most common subtype*** and is composed of large tumor nodules showing scattered lacunar classical RS cells set in a background of reactive lymphocytes, eosinophils and plasma cells with varying degrees of collagen fibrosis/sclerosis
Mixed cellularity	***Most common format seen in India;*** also the most common in HIV positive patients. Biopsy shows classic Reed Sternberg cells Normal lymphocyte Reed-sternberg cell

Contd...

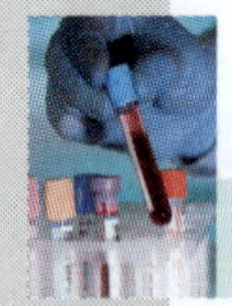

Lymphocyte depleted	*It is a rare subtype*, composed of large numbers of often pleomorphic RS cells with only few reactive lymphocytes which may easily be confused with diffuse large cell lymphoma. Many cases previously classified within this category would now be reclassified under anaplastic large cell lymphoma
Lymphocyte rich	Good/best prognosis
Nodular lymphocytic predominant	Expresses CD_{20}, and is classified as a form of non-classical Hodgkin's.

- Microscopic examination of the lymph node biopsy reveals complete or partial effacement of the lymph node architecture by scattered large malignant cells known *as* ***Reed–Sternberg cells*** admixed within a reactive cell infiltrate composed of variable proportions of lymphocytes, histiocytes, eosinophils, and plasma cells.
- The Reed–Sternberg cells are identified as large often bi-nucleated cells with prominent nucleoli and an unusual $CD45^-$, CD30+, $CD15+/^-$ immunophenotype. In approximately 50% of cases, the Reed–Sternberg cells are infected by the Epstein–Barr virus.
- Characteristics of classic Reed–Sternberg cells include large size (20–50 micrometres), abundant, amphophilic, finely granular/homogeneous cytoplasm; two mirror-image nuclei ***(owl eyes)*** each with an eosinophilic nucleolus and a thick nuclear membrane (chromatin is distributed close to the nuclear membrane).

232. Ans. (a) Pre B cell

Ref: Robbin's Pathology, 9th ed. pg. 590-93

- ***Most common subtype of ALL is L1 according to older classification and Pre B cell variety by the latest WHO classification.***
- The recent WHO International panel on ALL recommends that the FAB classification be abandoned, since the morphological classification has no clinical or prognostic relevance. It instead advocates the use of the immunophenotypic classification:
- Acute lymphoblastic leukemia/lymphoma.
  - Synonyms: Former Fab L1/L2

Precursor B Acute Lymphoblastic Leukemia/ Lymphoma. Cytogenetic Subtypes

1. t(12;21)(p12,q22)
2. t(1;19)(q23;p13)
3. t(9;22)(q34;q11)
4. t(V,11)(V;q23)

Precursor T Acute Lymphoblastic Leukemia/Lymphoma

- Burkitt's leukemia/lymphoma. Synonyms: Former FAB L3
- Biphenotypic acute leukemia

233. Ans. (a) Aplastic anemia

Ref: Robbin's Pathology, 9th ed. pg. 631

- **Aplastic anemia is characterized by destruction of bone marrow and thereby reduction in pluri-potent stem cells and their progeny.** *Henceforth the production of reticulocytes is less.*
- Thalassemia and sickle cells are hemolytic anemias having extra-vascular hemolysis and thereby reticulocytosis.
- In chronic blood loss the loss of RBC provoke the bone marrow to be more aggressive and release reticulocytes in circulation.
- **Remember:** Reticulocytopenia may be a result of viral Parvovirus B19 infection, which invades and destroys red blood cell precursors and halts the red cell production.

234. Ans. (a) EBV

Ref: Robbin's Pathology, 9th ed. pg. 588-90, 606

EBV	Nasopharyngeal cancer, Burkitt lymphoma, Hodgkins and non-Hodgkin lymphoma; Infectious mononucleosis (Paul Bunnel test).
CMV	CMV retinitis
HHV 6	Primary effusion lymphoma
HHV 8	Kaposi sarcoma

235. Ans. (d) Chronic lymphocytic leukemia

Ref: Robbin's Pathology, 9th ed. pg. 324-325

Cancers associated with radiation: • ALL, AML, CML • Thyroid cancer • Breast cancer • Lung cancer • Bladder, ovarian cancer
Cancers not seen with radiation: • CLL • Hodgkin's lymphoma • Prostate cancer, testis cancer and cervical cancer

236. Ans. (a) IgG

Ref: Robbin's Pathology, 9th ed. pg. 598-99

- The over production of light chains of IgG is the most common abnormality in multiple myeloma. In Waldenstrom cryoglobulinemia, IgM is overproduced.
- Most common presentation of multiple myeloma is anemia > bone pain.
- Least common presentation of multiple myeloma is hyperviscosity

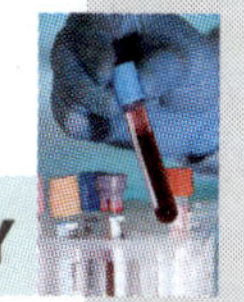

- Investigation of choice for multiple myeloma is bone marrow biopsy
- Screening test for multiple myeloma is serum electrophoresis showing M spike
- Most common cause of death in multiple myeloma is infections
- Most common cause of kidney damage in multiple myeloma is hypercalcemia.

CARDIOVASCULAR PATHOLOGY

237. Ans. (a) LDH1

Ref: Robbins 10th ed. pg. 553

- LDH-1: Present primarily in cardiac myocytes and erythrocytes.
- LDH-2: Present mostly in white blood cells.
- LDH-3: Present in highest quantity in lung tissue.
- LDH-4: Highest amounts found in pancreas, kidney, and placenta.
- LDH-5: Highest amounts found in liver and skeletal muscle.
- In blood, LDH-2 is > than LDH-1 value, but in cardiac tissue LDH-1 is prodominant

238. Ans. (b) Intimal elastic lamina layer defect

Ref: Harrison 20th, ed. pg. 2084

As an aneurysm develops, it typically forms a neck with a dome. The length of the neck and the size of the dome vary greatly and are important factors in planning neurosurgical obliteration or endovascular embolization.

- The arterial internal elastic lamina disappears at the base of the neck. The media thins, and connective tissue replaces smooth-muscle cells. At the site of rupture (most often the dome), the wall thins, and the tear that allows bleeding is often ≤0.5 mm long.
- Aneurysm size and site are important in predicting risk of rupture. Those >7 mm in diameter and those at the top of the basilar artery and at the origin of the posterior communicating artery are at greater risk

239. Ans. (a) Troponin I

Ref: Harrison 20th ed. pg. 384

Cardiac specific markers of myocardial damage include quantitative determination of CK-MB, Troponin I and Troponin T. Troponins can become elevated by 3 hours. The circulating values remain elevated up to a week.

240. Ans. (a) ASO

Ref: Nelson 20th ed. pg. 1333

Because other illnesses may closely resemble Acute rheumatic fever, antecedent group A Streptococcal Infection is needed whenever possible. The tests are:

- Increasing or rising Anti-Streptolysin O titer or other streptococcal antibodies indicates recent streptococcal infection
- A Positive throat Culture
- A Positive Rapid group streptococcal carbohydrate antigen test in a child

Extra Mile

TABLE: Guidelines for the Diagnosis of Initial or Recurrent Attack of Rheumatic Fever (Jones Criteria, Updated 2015)

Major manifestations	Minor manifestations	Supporting evidence of antecedent group a streptococcal infection
Carditis Polyarthritis Erythema marginatum Subcutaneous nodules Chorea	Clinical features: Arthralgia Fever Laboratory features: Elevated acute phase reactants: Erythrocyte sedimentation rate C-reactive protein Prolonged P-R interval	Positive throat culture or rapid streptococcal antigen test Elevated or increasing streptococcal antibody titer

241. Ans. (a) Endocardial cushion defect

Ref: Nelson 20th ed. pg. 2165

Syndrome	Features
CHROMOSOMAL DISORDERS Trisomy 21 (Down syndrome) Trisomy 21 p (cat eye syndrome) Trisomy 18 Trisomy 13	Endocardial cushion defect, VSD, ASD Miscellaneous, total anomalous pulmonary venous return VSD, ASD, PDA, coarctation of aorta, bicuspid aortic or pulmonary valve VSD, ASD, PDA, coarctation of aorta, bicuspid aortic or pulmonary valve

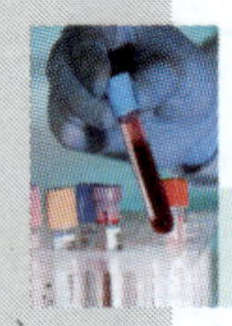

242. Ans. (c) Hyper-eosinophilia of myocytes

Ref: Robbins E-book, pg. 853

HISTOPATHOLOGICAL CHANGES AFTER MI

- First half an hour no changes are seen, which is followed by glycogen depletion and development of waviness of fibers.
- Between 12- and 24-hours H*yper-eosinophilia* of the cytoplasm of myocytes as assessed by hematoxylin-eosin staining is characteristic of myocardial damage.
- *Neutrophil infiltration* is present by 24 hours at the border areas.
- As the infarct progresses between 24 and 48 hours*, coagulation necrosis* is established, with various degrees of nuclear pyknosis, early karyorrhexis, and karyolysis.
- The myocyte striations are preserved and the sarcomeres elongate. The border areas show prominent neutrophil infiltration by 48 hours.
- At 3-5 days, the central portion of the infarct shows loss of myocyte nuclei and striations; in smaller infarcts, neutrophils invade the infarct and fragment, resulting in more *severe karyorrhexis* (nuclear dust).
- By 5-7 days, *macrophages and fibroblasts begin to appear* in the border areas.
- By 1 week, neutrophils decline and *granulation tissue is established with neocapillary invasion* and lymphocytic and plasma cell infiltration.

Time frame	Light microscopy
0–6 hours	No change, stretching and waviness of fibres
6–12 hours	Coagulative necrosis begins with neutrophilic infiltration
48–72 hours	Coagulative necrosis is complete
3rd–7th day	Initiation of resorption of necrosed fibres and fibrovascular response
3rd week	Necrosed muscles removed and in growth of fibrocollagenous tissue.

243. Ans. (b) McCallum patch

Ref: Robbins 9th ed. pg. 557-59

- Acute rheumatic mitral valvulitis leads to chordal elongation and defective cooptation of valve leaflets.
- This leads to a posterolaterally directed jet of mitral regurgitation which is directed towards an area of fibrotic thickening on posterior left atrial wall.
- This *fibrotic thickening in left atrium is called McCallum patch.*

244. Ans. (a) Cardiac failure

Rheumatic endocarditis leads to death most commonly due to cardiac failure.

Causes of Mortality in RHD (Decreasing Incidence wise):

- CHF
- Bacterial endocarditis
- Cerebral embolism of left atrial appendage
- Coronary insufficiency

245. Ans. (a) Stretching and waviness of fibers

246. Ans. (a) Myxoma

- The most common primary tumour of the heart is myxoma. It constitutes 50% of all primary cardiac tumours.
- Most common site is left atrium.
- Most common tumour of heart is metastasis from lung cancer.

247. Ans. (a) Lungs

Ref: Robbin's Pathology, 9th ed. pg. 529-30

- In left ventricular failure, the pooling of blood in lungs will lead to development of pulmonary edema which causes hypoxia and findings of dysnea, orthopnea, pink frothy sputum and death. Hence, lungs are immediately affected following LVF.
- Subsequently due to low BP the kidneys shall be affected and in severe LVF brain perfusion shall also be affected.

248. Ans. (a) Aschoff nodules

Ref: Robbin's Pathology, 9th ed. pg. 558

- The pathognomonic feature of rheumatic fever is *aschoff nodules*. They are the foci of eosinophilic staining collagen surrounded by *T-lymphocytes*, plasma cells and plump macrophages called Anitschkow cells.
- The Anitschkow cells have abundant cytoplasm and central round to ovoid nucleus in which chromatin has wavy ribbon fashion because of which they are called *caterpillar cells*
- The involvement of endocardium by aschoff nodules along the line of closure of valves leads to improper closure of leaflets. This leads to *leakage of blood which hits the free wall of left atria* and leads to *Macullum's patch.*

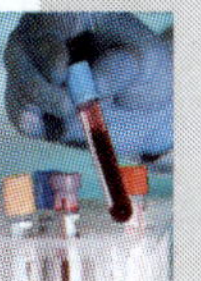

249. Ans. (c) Reversible injury within 20–40 minutes

Ref: Robbin's Pathology, 9th ed. pg. 540-41

TABLE: Evolution of Morphological Changes in MI

Time	Gross findings	Light microscopy
0–30 minutes	None	None
30 minutes–4 hours	None	Waviness of fibres at border
4–12 hours	Occasional dark mottling	Beginning of coagulative necrosis, oedema, haemorrhage
12–24 hours	Dark mottling	Ongoing coagulative necrosis, marginal band contraction necrosis and beginning of neutrophilic infiltration

TABLE: Myocardial response

Feature	Time
Cessation of aerobic respiration or onset of ATP depletion	Seconds
ATP reduced to 50% of normal	10 minutes
Irreversible cell injury	20–40 minutes
Microvascular injury	>1 hour

250. Ans. (d) Necrosis

Ref: Robbin's Pathology, 9th ed. pg. 512-15

TABLE: Complications of Atherosclerosis and their Importance

Aneurysm formation	Aortic aneurysm >5.5 cm can rupture
Calcification	Dystrophic calcification
Ulceration	Increases thrombus formation
Thrombosis	Occlusion of coronary arteries
Embolism	Erosion of plaque

251. Ans. (b) Deep vein thrombosis

Ref: Robbin's Pathology, 9th ed. pg. 512-15; Robbins, 8th ed. pg. 517

- Buerger disease is associated with HLA B-5 and HLA-A9.
- In thromboangiitis obliterans there is acute and chronic segmental inflammation of vessels with thrombosis in the lumen
- Typically, the thrombus contains microabscesses with a central focus of neutrophils surrounded by inflammation
- Later, the inflammatory process extends into contiguous veins and nerves and in time all the arteries, veins and nerves become encased in fibrous tissue, a characteristic that is very rare with vasculitis.

252. Ans. (b) Troponin C is present in both cardiac and smooth muscle

Ref: Harrison, 19th ed. pg. 265e-7

- Troponins of cardiac origin are regulatory proteins that control the calcium mediated interaction of Actin and Myosin.
- The troponin complex consists of three subunits: Troponin T, which binds to Tropomyosin and facilitates contractions; Troponin I, which binds to Actin and inhibits Actin/Myosin interaction; and Troponin C, which binds the calcium ions.
- The amino acid sequence of the skeletal and cardiac isoforms of Troponin T and Troponin I are sufficiently dissimilar and therefore detectable by monoclonal antibody assay.
- *Troponin C is not used clinically because both cardiac and smooth muscles share Troponin C isoforms.*

253. Ans. (c) Granulation with type 4 collagen

Ref: Robbin's Pathology, 9th ed. pg. 540-43

Time	Gross examination	Histopathology (light microscopy)
0–0.5 hours	None	None
0.5–4 hours	None	Glycogen depletion, as seen with a PAS stain Possibly waviness of fibers at border
4–12 hours	Sometimes dark mottling	Initiation of coagulation necrosis Edema Hemorrhage
12–24 hours	Dark mottling	Ongoing coagulation necrosis Karyopyknosis Hypereosinophilia of myocytes Contraction band necrosis in margins Beginning of neutrophil infiltration

Contd...

Time	Gross examination	Histopathology (light microscopy)
1–3 days	Infarct center becomes yellow-tan	Continued coagulation necrosis Loss of nuclei and striations Increased infiltration of neutrophils to interstitium
3–7 days	Hyperemia at border Softening yellow-tan center	Beginning of disintegration of dead muscle fibers Necrosis of neutrophils Beginning of macrophage removal of dead cells at border
7–10 days	Maximally soft and yellow-tan Red-tan margins	Increased phagocytosis of dead cells at border Beginning of granulation tissue formation at margins
10–34 days	Red-gray and depressed borders	Mature granulation tissue with type I collagen
2–8 weeks	Gray-white granulation tissue	Increased collagen deposition Decreased cellularity
More than 2 months	Completed scarring	Dense collagenous scar formed

254. Ans. (b) Myxoma

Ref: Robbin's Pathology, 9th ed. pg. 575-76

- **MC tumor of heart:** Secondaries
- MC site of primary for cardiac secondaries: Lungs
- Most common **primary** neoplasm of heart in **adult: Myxoma**
- Most common **primary** neoplasm of heart in **child: Rhabdomyoma**
- Most common **malignant** cancer of heart in adults: Angiosarcoma
- Most common **malignant** cancer of heart in children: Rhabdomyosarcoma
- Myxoma is a soft mass, consisting of edematous connective tissue irregularly covered by thrombus, commonly attached to the endocardium by a pedicle, and hanging free into a cavity, **usually the left atrium. (MC site of myxoma: Left atrium)**
- It may block the mitral orifice, producing a murmur similar to that of mitral stenosis.
- Embolism from the surface of the neoplasm or an overlying thrombus is common.
- The papillary fibroelastoma is very rare and occurs on heart valves. **Therefore most common cardiac valve tumor is papillary fibroelastoma.**

Extra Mile

- *MC site of myxoma: Left atrium*
- MC site of rhabdomyoma: *Left ventricle*
- Myxoma is MC seen in **females**
- **MC age group of myxoma:** 3rd– 6th decade

255. Ans. (d) Metastasis

Ref: Robbin's Pathology, 9th ed. pg. 575-76

Please refer to above explanation

256. Ans. (c) Left ventricle

Ref: Robbin's Pathology 9th ed. pg. 575-76

Please refer to above explanation

257. Ans. (c) Papillary fibroelastoma

Ref: Robbin's Pathology, 9th ed. pg. 575-77

Please refer to above explanation

258. Ans. (a) Syphilitic aneurysm

Ref: Harrison, 19th ed. pg. 1638

- Syphilitic aortitis, an inflammatory aortitis involving the ascending aorta, sinuses of Valsalva and the aortic valve, is observed most commonly in patients older than 50 years.
- Syphilitic aortitis is associated with aortic insufficiency, ascending aortic aneurysms, and a positive serologic test for syphilis. In these patients, angina resulting from occlusion of the ostia of the coronary vessels also can be present.
- Calcification occurs in a linear pattern along the ascending aorta.
- On gross specimen examination, the aorta has been described as revealing a "tree-bark" appearance.

259. Ans. (c) Fibrinous

Ref: Robbin's Pathology, 9th ed. pg. 557-56

An exudate is any fluid that filters from the circulatory system into lesions or areas of inflammation.

Types of Exudate

Purulent or suppurative exudate consists of plasma with both active and dead neutrophils, fibrinogen, and necrotic parenchymal cells. This kind of exudate is consistent with more severe infections, and is commonly referred to as pus.

Contd...

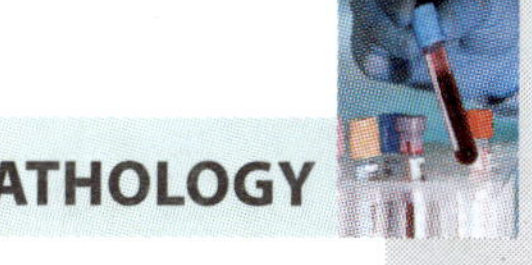

Fibrinous exudate is composed mainly of fibrinogen and fibrin. It is characteristic of rheumatic carditis, but is seen in all severe injuries such as strep throat and bacterial pneumonia. Fibrinous inflammation is often difficult to resolve due to the fact that blood vessels grow into the exudate and fill the space that was occupied by fibrin. Often, large amounts of antibiotics are necessary for resolution.
Catarrhal exudate is seen in the nose and throat and is characterized by a high content of mucus.
Serous exudate (sometimes classified as serous transudate) is usually seen in mild inflammation, with little protein content. Its consistency resembles that of serum, and can usually be seen in certain disease states like tuberculosis.

260. Ans. (c) Diabetic glomerulosclerosis

Ref: Robbin's Pathology, 9th ed. pg. 509-510, 558

Fibrinoid necrosis is a distinctive morphological pattern of cell injury characterized by deposition of fibrin like proteinaceous material in walls of arteries. Areas of fibrinoid necrosis appear as smudgy eosinophilic regions with obscured underlying cellular details.

Fibrinoid necrosis is seen in:
- Malignant hypertension
- Vasculitis like PAN
- Acute rheumatic fever

261. Ans (b) Small- or medium-sized muscular arteries

Ref: Robbin's Pathology, 9th ed. pg. 506-507

- PAN typically involves small- to medium-sized muscular arteries. In contrast, large arteries and the aorta are involved in Takayasu arteritis.
- Small arteries and arterioles are involved in a number of other diseases, including systemic lupus erythematosus.
- Active lesions in PAN demonstrate a neutrophilic infiltration of the involved vessel wall with thrombosis and segmental, fibrinoid necrosis. Intermittent healing produces fibrosis of the arterial wall and intimal thickening, which may lead to obstruction and infarction.
- Aneurysmal dilations may arise as a result of asymmetrical involvement. Although the lesions in PAN resemble other immune mediated vascular lesions, the exact etiology of the disorder has not been elucidated.
- PAN generally affects middle-aged men and has a poor prognosis, although steroids may be beneficial.

262. Ans. (c) Monckeberg's sclerosis

Ref: Robbin's Pathology, 9th ed. pg. 491

- Monckeberg's arteriosclerosis, also called medial calcific sclerosis, is a form of arteriosclerosis or vessel hardening, where *calcium deposits form in the middle layer* of the walls of medium sized vessels *(the tunica media)*
- It is usually more benign than other forms of arteriosclerosis because it does not cause narrowing of the lumen, but can still be associated with important medical conditions. Monckeberg's arteriosclerosis is most commonly found in the radial or ulnar arteries causing "pipestem" arteries, which will present as a bounding pulse.
- It is associated with trophic foot ulceration and peripheral artery occlusive disease.
- Its presence predicts risk of cardiovascular events and leg amputation in diabetic patients.

263. Ans. (d) SLE

Ref: Robbin's Pathology, 9th ed. pg. 506, 509-10

Large vessel vasculitis	Medium vessel vasculitis	Small vessel vasculitis
• Giant cell arteritis • Takayasu's arteritis	• Classic PAN • Kawasaki • Buerger disease	**Immune complex mediated** • **SLE** • HSP • Cryoglobulin vasculitis • Good pasture syndrome **Pauci- immune** • Wegener's granulomatosis • Microscopic polyangitis • Churg Strauss syndrome

LUNGS

264. Ans. (a) Asbestosis

Ref: Harrison 20th ed. pg. 691: Robbins 9th ed. pg. 1978

Pleural thickening and calcification are a feature of asbestosis. The history of occupational exposure further helps in diagnosis

265. Ans. (d) Bronchial asthma

Ref: Robbin's Pathology, 9th ed. pg. 682

Findings in Bronchial Asthma in Broncho-Alveolar Lavage or in Sputum
- **Curschmann spirals**, is a finding in bronchial asthma which may result from extrusion of mucus plugs from subepithelial mucous gland ducts or bronchioles.
- **Charcot-Leyden crystals:** It is composed of an eosinophilic protein called **galectin-10.**

The other characteristic histologic findings of asthma, collectively called "airway remodeling" include:
- Airway wall thickenig
- An increase in the size of the submucosal glands and number of airway goblet cells

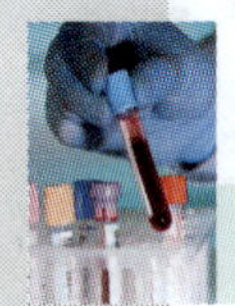

- Subbasement membrane fibrosis (*due to deposition of type I and III collagen*)
- Increased vascularity
- Hypertrophy and/or hyperplasia of the bronchial wall muscle

266. Ans. (c) Liver

Rich focus	Cortex of brain
Simon focus	Healed site of primary infection at lungs apex
Simmond focus	Liver
Weigart focus	Intima of blood vessels

267. Ans. (c) Eosinophilic infiltration of airways

Ref: Robbin's Pathology, 9th ed. pg. 678-679

- Chronic bronchitis is characterised by **lymphocytic infiltration** of airways coupled with submucosal gland hypertrophy
- **Reid's index** is ratio of mucus gland layer thickness to thickness of wall between epithelium and cartilage. Normal value is 0.4 and is increased in chronic bronchitis
- Bronchorrhea is due to low grade infection since the ciliated columnar epithelium and Muco-ciliary clearance is compromised.

Extra Mile

- **Earliest feature of chronic bronchitis:** Mucus hypersecretion in large airways
- Reid index increased in chronic bronchitis **(*normal = 0.4*)**

268. Ans. (c) Bloody pleural effusion

Ref: Robbin's Pathology, 9th ed. pg. 688-690

- Silicosis is a nodular fibrosing disease due to inhalation of silica, and is the most common chronic occupational disease in world.
- Mostly the form implicated is Quartz.
- Involvement of upper lobes of the lungs
- **CXR:** shows presence of **egg shell calcification**
- Polarised microscopy shows presence of birefringent silica particles

269. Ans. (a) Sarcoidosis

Ref: Harrison, 19th ed. pg. 2210

The **Kveim-Siltzbach test** is a skin test used to detect sarcoidosis, where part of a spleen from a patient with known sarcoidosis is injected into the skin of a patient suspected to have the disease. If noncaseating granulomas are found (4–6 weeks later), the test is positive.

270. Ans. (c) Sarcoidosis

Ref: Robbin's Pathology, 9th ed. pg. 693

- Schaumann body is laminated concretions of calcium and protein, which is a characteristic finding of sarcoidosis.

Findings of Sarcoidosis:

- Non-necrotizing granulomas
- Asteroid body
- Schaumann body

Extra Mile

Sarcoidosis

- **MC clinical presentation of sarcoidosis: Bilateral hilar lymphadenopathy (90% of cases) > Eye**
- **Sarcoidosis MC seen in patients below 40 years (F > M)**
- **Marker of disease activity: TNF concentration in broncho-alveolar fluid**
- **Mikulicz syndrome:** Bilateral sarcoidosis of parotid, sub-maxillary and sublingual gland.

271. Ans. (b) Hilar lymphadenopathy

Ref: Robbin's Pathology, 9th ed. pg. 692-93

272. Ans. (c) Asbestosis

Ref: Robbin's Pathology, 9th ed. pg. 690-92

- Sufferers may experience severe dyspnea (shortness of breath) and are at an increased risk for certain malignancies, including lung cancer but especially mesothelioma.
- ***The most common anatomical site for mesothelioma is the pleura,*** but it can also arise in the peritoneum, the pericardium or the tunica vaginalis.
- Most people who develop mesothelioma have worked in jobs where they inhaled or ingested asbestos fibers, or were exposed to airborne asbestos dust and fibers in other ways. Washing clothes of a family member who worked with asbestos also creates a risk for developing mesothelioma.
- *Unlike lung cancer, there seems to be **no** association between mesothelioma and tobacco smoking*, but smoking greatly increases the risk of other asbestos-induced cancers.

Extra Mile

- Anthracosis is a pneumoconiosis, which is seen among coal workers.
- There is no association between anthracosis and development of tuberculosis or lung cancer.

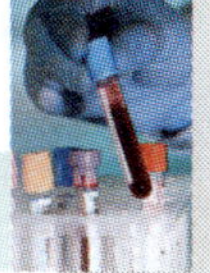

273. Ans. (d) Adenocarcinoma

Ref: Robbin's, 9th ed. pg. 714–15

According to Robbins 9th ed. the frequency of major lung cancer and their proportion are:

- Adenocarcinoma (38%)
- Squamous cell carcinoma (20%)
- Small cell carcinoma (14%)
- Large cell carcinoma (3%)
- Other (25%)

Extra Mile

LUNG CA

- MC CA causing death: lung CA
- MC risk factor for lung CA: Smoking
- Peak age for development for lung CA: 50–60's
- MC lung cancer in females: Adenocarcinoma
- Most aggressive type of lung CA: Small cell lung CA
- Lung CA MC associated with paraeoplastic syndrome: Small cell lung CA
- Lung CA associated with smoking: Squamous cell CA and small cell lung CA
- Centrally located lung CA: Squamous cell CA and small cell lung CA
- Peripherally located lung CA: Adenocarcinoma and large cell CA

274. Ans. (b) Adenocarcinoma

Ref: Robbin's, 9th ed. pg. 714–15

275. Ans. (c) Small cell lung CA

Ref: Robbin's Pathology, 9th ed. pg. 717

- **Small cell carcinoma** is a highly malignant tumor with a strong relationship to cigarette smoking.
- **Around** 1% occurs in nonsmokers.
- They are the most aggressive of lung tumors, metastasizing widely and are always fatal.

276. Ans. (c) Small cell lung CA

Ref: Robbin's Pathology, 9th ed. pg. 717

- **Azzopardi effect** is basophilic staining of vascular walls due to encrustation by DNA from necrotic tumor cells.
- It is seen in small cell lung carcinoma.

277. Ans. (b) Adenocarcinoma lung

Ref: Robbin's Pathology, 9th ed. pg. 690-92

- The answer has been triple checked from standard textbooks and is a denocarcinoma.
- *Mesothelioma is mentioned as associated with asbestosis but not most common.*

KIDNEY

278. Ans. (c) Gamma – Globulin

Ref: Harrison 21st ed. pg. 871

- Multiple myeloma has excessive production of incomplete light chains of antibodies which are being excreted in urine and are called Bence jones proteins.
- Antibodies belong to gamma globulin faction of proteins.

279. Ans. (d) Post streptococcal glomerulonephritis

Ref: Pocket Companion to Robbins pg. 909

The patient has infection with nephritogenic strains of streptococcus which leads to sore throat. The immune complex formation leads to damage to glomerulus and causes cola color urine. Option B does not have cola color urine. Option C is seen in adults. Option D presents with hematuria after URTI.

280. Ans. (c) A beta 2

Ref: Robbins 10th ed. pg. 269

- Beta 2 microglobulin is a component of MHC class I molecules and is not excreted via the filter of dialysis membrane. The levels rise in the body and get deposited in or around the joints or soft tissues of patients. It can lead to two manifestations, Dialysis dementia and Carpal tunnel syndrome.
- Option A is associated with multiple myeloma, option B with Alzheimer's disease and option D with medullary carcinoma thyroid.

281. Ans. (c) Membranous glomerulopathy

Ref: Harrison 20th ed. pg. 2144

The two pointers to the diagnosis as option A, MGN are:

1. Malignancy associated Nephrotic Syndrome is membranous Glomerulopathy
2. Leading cause of nephrotic syndrome in geriatric population is membranous Glomerulopathy
   - Option B is ruled out as it presents with hematuria and Hypertension along with proteinuria.
   - Option C is the leading cause of nephrotic syndrome in young adults

282. Ans. (b) HSP

Ref: Robbins 10th ed. pg. 923

- The image shows purpura visible on calves and backside of thighs. This along with abdominal pain and arthralgia points to first Differential diagnosis of Henoch-Schonlein purpura. It is an IgA mediated vasculitis affecting skin, joints and viscera.

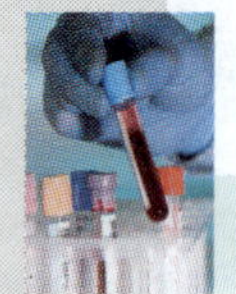

- Option A presents with microscopic hematuria.
- Option C presents with fever and rash all over the body with low platelet count.
- Option D presents with hematuria with hypertension post sore throat or skin infection caused by group A beta hemolytic streptococcus infection.

283. Ans. (c) Post infectious glomerulonephritis

Ref: Harrison 20th ed. pg. 2137

- Choices A, B and D present as Nephrotic syndrome
- Post infectious Glomerulonephritis occurs after skin and throat infection with particular M types of streptococci.
- Post streptococcal glomerulonephritis due to impetigo develops 2-6 weeks after skin infection and 1–3 weeks after streptococcal pharyngitis. The renal biopsy shows subepithelial deposits which appear as humps.

284. Ans. (a) Kimmelstiel-Wilson disease

Ref: Robbins basic pathology , E-Book, pg. 781

- Nodular glomerulosclerosis is also called inter-capillary glomerulosclerosis or Kimmelstiel-Wilson disease.

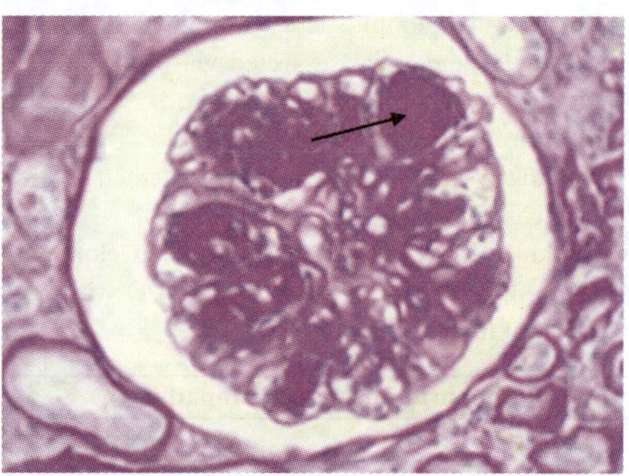

- It presents as ovoid, spherical, laminated hyaline masses in periphery of the glomerulus. It is PAS+ and finally obliterates the glomerular tuft.
- It is specific for diabetes mellitus, membranoproliferative glomerulonephritis, light chain disease and amyloidosis.

285. Ans. (a) Kimmelstiel-Wilson change

Ref: Robbins E-Book, pg. 781

- The characteristic finding of Diabetic nephropathy is Kimmelstein Wilson change and is also referred as nodular glomerulosclerosis.
- Most common light microscopy finding is diffuse diabetic glomerulopathy. Large acellular accumulations also may be observed within these areas. These are circular on section and are known as the Kimmelstiel-Wilson lesions/nodules.
- *Armani-Ebstein change* consists of deposits of glycogen in the tubular epithelial cells (pars straight of proximal convoluted tubule and loop of Henle).

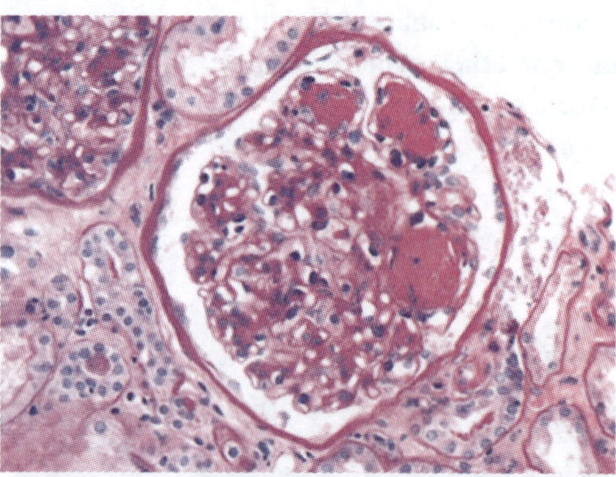

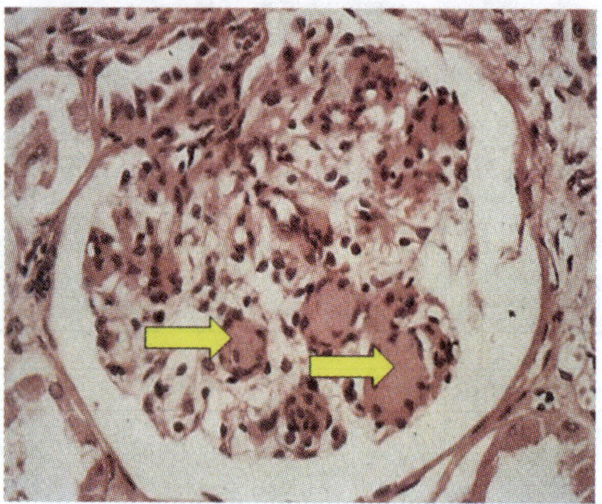

286. Ans. (b) Kidney

- *Fatty change is particularly common in the liver but may occur in other non – fatty tissues as well, e.g. in the heart, skeletal muscle, kidneys (lipoid nephrosis or minimum change disease) and other organs.*
- Fatty change, steatosis or fatty metamorphosis is the intracellular accumulation of neutral fat within parenchymal cells.
- It includes, now abandoned, terms of fatty degeneration and fatty infiltration because fatty change neither necessarily involves degeneration nor an infiltration. The deposit is in the cytosol and represents and absolute increase in the intracellular lipids.

287. Ans. (a) PSGN

- The presence of lumpy bumpy appearance due to sub-epithelial deposits is a characteristic appearance in PSGN.
- The Sub-epithelial spikes on electron microscopy are a feature of membranous glomerulopathy.

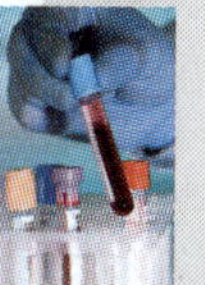

288. Ans. (c) RPGN

Type	Clinical features	Pathogenesis	Pathology	
			LM	EM
Acute GN	Acute nephrotic syndrome	Immune complex disease (local or circulating)	Diffuse proliferation, leucocytic infiltration	Subepithelial deposits (humps)
RPGN	Acute renal failure	(i) Type I: Anti GBM type (ii) Type II: Immune complex type (iii) Type III: Pauci-immune RPGN	Proliferation crescents[Q]	(i) Linear deposits along GBM (ii) Subepithelial deposits (iii) No deposits
Minimal change disease	Nephrotic syndrome (higher selective proteinuria)	Reduction of normal negative charge on GBM Cell-mediated mechanism	Normal glomeruli, lipid vacuolation in tubules	Loss of foot processes, no deposits
Membranous GN	Nephrotic syndrome	Immune complex disease (local)	Diffuse thickening of capillary wall	Subepithelial deposits (Spikes)
Membrano-Proliferative GN	Nephrotic syndrome	Type I: Immune complex disease Type II: Dense deposit disease (alternate pathway activation) Type III: Rare, with systemic disease and drugs	Lobular proliferation of mesangial cells increased mesangial matrix, double contour of GBM called as tram track appearance	Type I: Subendothelial deposits Type II: Dense intramembranous deposits Type III: Subendothelial and subepithelial deposits

289. Ans. (b) Autosomal dominant

Ref: Robbin's Pathology, 9th ed. pg. 946

- **ADPKD** is autosomal dominant—Polycystic kidney disease.
- Occurs due to mutation in PKD 1 and PKD 2 gene
- MC type of mutation: PKD 1. (80–85%)
- **Pathological feature:** Large multcystic kidney. It also involves commonly:
  - MC: Liver-Polycystic liver disease (40%)
  - Heart: Mitral valve prolapse (20–25%)
  - Brain: Berry aneurysm

290. Ans. (d) CMV

Ref: Harsh Mohan, 7th ed. pg. 175

Cytomegalic cells in vivo (presumed to be infected epithelial cells) are two to four times larger than surrounding cells and often contain an 8–10 μm intranuclear inclusion that is eccentrically placed and is surrounded by a clear halo, producing an "owl's eye" appearance.

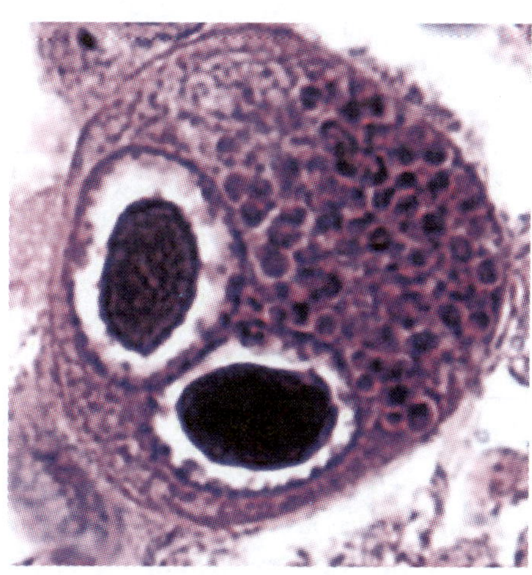

Smaller granular cytoplasmic inclusions are demonstrated occasionally. Cytomegalic cells are found in a wide variety of organs, including the salivary gland, lung, liver, kidney, intestine, pancreas, adrenal gland, and central nervous system

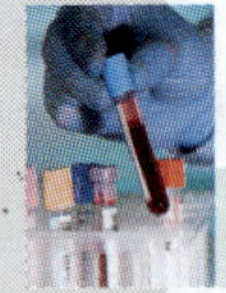

291. Ans. (d) Hypokalemia

Ref: Robbin's Pathology, 9th ed. pg. 1127, 1143

- Hydropic (vacuolar) degeneration results from a more severe degree of water imbibition into the cell cytoplasm.
- It occurs in some severe bacterial infections with high fever, certain types of poisoning, and hypokalemia.
- Potassium is drawn from cells and replaced by sodium and water in large amounts.
- In its most striking form, hydropic degeneration involves the renal tubular epithelium.

292. Ans. (a) Bowman's capsule

Ref: Robbin's Pathology, 9th ed. pg. 900-901

- Podocytes (or visceral epithelial cells) are cells in the Bowman's capsule in the kidneys that wrap around the capillaries of the glomerulus.
- The Bowman's capsule filters blood, holding back large molecules such as proteins, and passing through small molecules such as water, salts, and sugar, as the first step in forming urine.

293. Ans. (d) Post streptococcal GN

Ref: Robbin's Pathology, 9th ed. pg. 909-910

- PSGN is characterized by enlarged hyper-cellular glomeruli.
- There is also swelling of endothelial cells & combination of proliferation, swelling, leukocyte infiltration obliterates capillary lumen.
- Endo-capillary proliferation is also seen in MPGN

294. Ans. (a) SLE

Ref: Robbin's Pathology, 9th ed. pg. 221-225

Sub-endothelial deposits create a homogeneous thickening of the capillary wall called wire loop lesion, which can be seen by means of light microscopy when they are extensive. They usually reflect active disease.

295. Ans. (a) Acetophenetidin

Ref: Robbin's Pathology, 9th ed. pg. 423. 936t

- *Renal papillary necrosis due to phenacetin is a gradual process with slow loss of renal function.*
- The most common cause of renal papillary necrosis is diabetic glomerulopathy.

296. Ans. (d) Bilateral kidney transplantation

Ref: Robbin's Pathology, 9th ed. pg. 945-947

- The kidney transplantation is always unilateral. The left kidney is preferred for transplantation and is deployed in right iliac fossa.
- The most common extra-hepatic manifestation of polycystic kidney disease is hepatic cysts.
- ADPKD is autosomal dominant gene which is genetically heterogeneous with two genes identified: PKD1 (chromosome region 16p13.3; around 85% cases) and PKD2 (4q21; around 15% cases)

297. Ans. (a) Pyelonephritis

Causes of WBC casts	Causes of RBC Casts
• Acute pyelonephritis • Interstitial nephritis • Lupus nephritis	• Acute glomerulonephritis • Goodpasture syndrome • Lupus nephritis • Renal infarction • Right sided heart failure • Renal vein thrombosis • Polyarteritis Nodosa

298. Ans. (d) Rapidly progressive glomerulonephritis

Ref: Robbin's Pathology, 9th ed. pg. 912-915

- RBC casts are a feature of glomerular damage. Normally <3 RBC/HPF are going to leak. But in case of glomerular damage the number of RBC in urine will exceed the limit mentioned above and these RBC get impinged on tamm-horsfall protein. The resultant RBC casts can be seen under microscopic examination of urine.
- Bladder schistomiasis will cause hematuria and eosinophiluria.
- Renal vein thrombosis is a complication of severe dehydration and causes a painful enlarged kidney with hematuria.
- *Minimal change disease is the most common cause of nephritic syndrome and causes proteinuria.*

Extra Mile

Different Renal Casts and conditions where they are seen:

- **Hyaline cast: MC type;** seen in normal individuals in dehydration or vigorous exercise
- **Muddy brown cast:** Seen in acute tubular necrosis
- **RBC casts:** Nephritic syndrome
- **Fatty casts:** Pathognomonic for high urinary protein nephrotic syndrome.
- **White blood cell casts:** Pyelonephritis

299. Ans. (a) Focal segmental glomerulosclerosis

Ref: Robbin's Pathology, 9th ed. pg. 918-920

Depending on the cause, focal segmental glomerulosclerosis is broadly classified as:

- Primary, when no underlying cause is found; usually presents as nephrotic syndrome

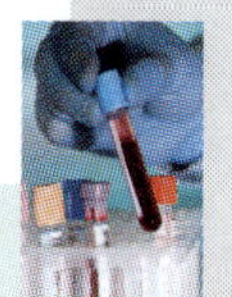

- Secondary, when an underlying cause is identified; usually presents with kidney failure and proteinuria. *This is actually a heterogeneous group including numerous causes such as Infections such as HIV (known as HIV-Associated Nephropathy)*

Other Causes of FSGS

- Toxins and drugs such as heroin and pamidronate
- Chronic pyelonephritis
- VUR

300. Ans. (b) Cardiovascular complications

- Hypotension is the most common acute complication of hemodialysis.
- Numerous factors appear to increase the risk of hypotension, including excessive ultrafiltration with inadequate compensatory vascular filling, impaired vasoactive or autonomic responses, osmolar shifts.
- A beta 2 amyloid deposition is seen in dialysis dementia and thus rules out choice A.
- Metabolic acidosis is treated with dialysis and thus rules out choice D.
- Cardiovascular disease constitutes the major cause of death in patients with ESRD.
- Cardiovascular mortality and event rates are higher in dialysis patients than in patients post-transplantation, although rates are extraordinarily high in both populations.

301. Ans. (c) Renal cell CA

Ref: Robbin's Pathology, 9th ed. pg. 952

- Robbins 9th ed. States: "by far the **most common malignant tumor is renal cell carcinoma**, followed by Wilms tumor, which is found in children.
- Incidence of RCC is: 85%
- M > F (2:1)
- Most of the RCC are **sporadic** > AD (familial)

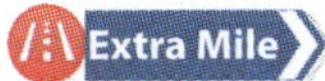
Extra Mile

KIDNEY CA *(extract from Robbins 9th ed.)*

- MC benign tumor of kidney: Renal papillary adenoma
- MC malignant tumor of kidney: RCC > Wilm's tumor
- MC kidney tumor associated with tuberous sclerosis: Angiomyolipoma
- MC type of RCC: Clear cell CA (70–80%)
- MC type of renal CA associated with dialysis: Papillary CA
- MC renal CA associated with sickle cell trait: Medullary CA
- Renal CA having best prognosis: Chromophobe type

302. Ans. (c) Smoking

Ref: Robbin's Pathology, 9th ed. pg. 953

Robbins states: "Tobacco is the most significant risk factor. Cigarette smokers have double the incidence of renal cell carcinoma".

Risk factors for RCC:

- **MC risk factor: Smoking**
- **Obesity (F > M), Hypertension, asbestos exposure, CKD, tuberous sclerosis**
- **VHL (Von Hippel-Lindau syndrome):** Around half to 2/3rd of the patients with VHL develop renal cyst and bilateral RCC.

303. Ans. (d) Chromophobe

Ref: Robbin's Pathology, 9th ed. pg. 954

304. Ans. (b) Papillary CA

Ref: Robbin's Pathology, 9th ed. pg. 952-54

305. Ans. (b) Clear cell CA

Ref: Robbin's Pathology, 9th ed. pg. 952-54

306. Ans. (d) Lung

Ref: Robbins, 9th ed. pg. 946

Please refer to Explanation of Question 194.

307. Ans. (c) Liver

Ref: Robbins, 9th ed. pg. 946

308. Ans. (d) Pancreatic cyst

Ref: Robbins, 9th ed. pg. 946

Since pancreas is among the least commonly involved organs, the cause of death will also be less as compared to other mentioned conditions.

Cause of death in case of PKD *(according to Bailey 26th ed. and Robbins 9th ed.)*

- **MC cause of death:** Chronic renal failure
- Coronary/hypertensive heart disease: ~40% of cases
- Infection: 25% of cases
- Rupture of berry aneurysm: ~15% of cases

LIVER

309. Ans. (a) Hepatitis B

Ref: Clinical Hepatology by Dancygier pg. 219

- "Ground-glass" hepatocytes are liver cells which have eosinophilic granular, glassy cytoplasm on light microscopy.

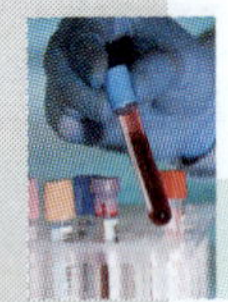

- It is a histological hallmark of chronic hepatitis B virus infection and contains surface antigens in the proliferated endoplasmic reticulum. Different types of ground glass hepatocytes are recognized at different hepatitis B virus replicative stages.

310. Ans. (d) Gilbert syndrome

Ref: Robbins E-book 2021 pg. 289

- Option A presents in pediatric age group and leads to kernicterus in neonates.
- Since patient is having unconjugated hyperbilirubinemia, option B and C are ruled out.
- Gilbert syndrome presents with episodic jaundice and common triggers are fasting, hemolytic reactions, febrile illnesses, menstruation, and physical exertion.
- *Gilbert's syndrome* is marked by the impaired conjugation of bilirubin due to reduced bilirubin UDPGT activity (typically 10–35% of normal). Unlike both Crigler-Najjar syndromes, Gilbert's syndrome is very common. The reported incidence is 3–7% of the population.

311. Ans. (b) Hemochromatosis

Ref: Harrison 21st ed. pg. 3233

- Combination of hyperpigmentation with liver cirrhosis and pancreatic damage leading to diabetes mellitus leads to diagnosis as hemochromatosis.
- Option A leads to pan-acinar emphysema and cirrhosis.
- Option C presents with liver cirrhosis and basal ganglia damage.
- Option D presents with RUQ pain and derangement of SGOT.

312. Ans. (c) Acute viral hepatitis with infectivity

Ref: Harrison 20th ed. pg. 2350

- The presence of HBeAg indicates replication of virus and high infectivity of the patient.
- Choice A requires HBsAg positivity with IgM anti HbcAg positivity
- Choice B requires HBsAg positivity with IgG anti HbcAg positivity
- Choice D will have only IgG anti- HBcAg indicating past infection.

313. Ans. (b) HCV

Ref: CMDT 2019, pg. 698

- Most common cause of chronic viral hepatitis is Hepatitis C
- Leading cause of transfusion of associated hepatitis is Hepatitis B.
- Leading cause of fulminant viral hepatitis is hepatitis D (superinfection).
- Leading cause of Fulminant viral hepatitis in pregnancy is hepatitis E.

314. Ans. (b) Wilson disease

Mallory hyaline bodies are eosinophilic intracytoplasmic inclusions seen in peri-nuclear location with swollen and ballooned hepatocytes.

Causes of Mallory hyaline bodies are:

- Primary biliary cirrhosis
- Indian childhood cirrhosis
- Cholestatic syndrome
- Wilson disease
- Intestinal bypass surgery
- Focal nodular hyperplasia
- Hepatocellular carcinoma

315. Ans. (d) Dubin Johnson syndrome

TABLE: Causes of Hereditary Hyperbilirubinemia

Unconjugated hyperbilirubinemia	Conjugated hyperbilirubinemia
Gilbert disease (defect in ligandin leading to defective uptake of unconjugated hyperbilirubinemia)	Dubin Jonhson syndrome (Black Liver due to deposition of epinephrine).
Criggler Najar syndrome (absent UDPGT activity) Type 1: More severe due to complete absence enzyme Type 2: Less severe due to partial absence of enzyme	Rotor syndrome (Milder variant of Dubin Johnson but liver texture and color are normal).

316. Ans. (d) Photosensitivity dermatitis

Ref: Robbin's Pathology, 9th ed. pg. 650-651, 847-849

PRIMARY HEMOCHROMATOSIS

In the skin, hemosiderin deposits occur in the dermis around sweat glands, and there is also an increase in melanin deposition in the epidermis.(Bronzing of skin)

- The pancreas is usually slightly enlarged, firm, and deeply pigmented. (Type 1 Diabetes Mellitus)
- The liver is usually enlarged, rusty red or ochre in color, and nodular and lobules are separated by dense fibrous tissue (Pigmentary cirrhosis)
- Restrictive cardiomyopathy

317. Ans. (c) Tuberculoma

ALPHA-FETO PROTEIN (AFP)

- It is a glycoprotein synthesized normally early in fetal life by the yolk sac, fetal liver and fetal GIT.

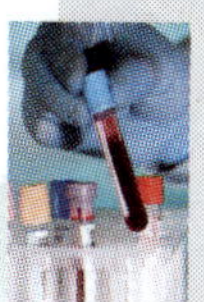

AFP is raised in:
- Hepatocellular carcinoma
- Lung cancer
- Colon cancer
- Pancreatic cancer
- Non-seminoma germ cell tumor of testis
- Cirrhosis and hepatitis
- Pregnancy

318. Ans (b) Crigler-Najjar Syndrome

Ref: Robbins Pathology, 9th ed. pg. 853-54

- In **Crigler-Najjar Syndrome** due to absence of UDP glucoronyltransfersase enzyme, conjugation of bilirubin is not possible and this results in elevation of unconjugated bilirubin to very high levels in the first 24 hours of life of neonate.

TABLE: Hereditary hyperbilirubinemias

Disorder	Inheritance	Detects in bllirubin metabolism	Liver pathology	Clinical course
Crigler-Najjar syndrome type I	Autosomal recessive	Absent UGT 1A1 activity	None	Fatal in neonatal period
Crigler-Najjar syndrome type II	Autosomal dominant with variable penetrance	Decreased UGT1A1 activity	None	Generally mild, occasional kemicterus
Gilbert syndrome	Autosomal recessive	Decreased UGT1A1 activity	None	Innocuous
Conjugated hyperbilirubinemia				
Dubin-Johnson syndrome	Autosomal recessive	Impaired biliary excretion of bilirubin glucuronides due to mutation in caralicular multidrug resistance protein 2 (MRP2)	Pigmented cytoplasmic globules	Innocuous
Rotor syndrome	Autosomal recessive	Decreased hepatic uptake and storage Decreased biliary excretion	None	Innocuous
UGT1A1, Uridine diphosphate glucoronosyltransferase family, peptide A1				

319. Ans. (d) Crigler-Najjar syndrome type II

Ref: Robbins Pathology, 9th ed. pg. 853-54

320. Ans. (c) Crigler-Najjar syndrome type I

Ref: Robbins Pathology, 9th ed. pg. 853-54

321. Ans. (b) Primary sclerosing cholangitis

Ref: Robbin's Pathology, 9th ed. pg. 860

PRIMARY SCLEROSING CHOLANGITIS

- Leads to obstructive jaundice leading to elevation of serum transaminases, gamma glutamyl transferase and alkaline phosphatase
- Typical *onion skin* fibrosis of bile ducts
- Percutaneous transhepatic cholangiography demonstrates irregularity and beading of the hepatic and common bile ducts in three patients.

Extra Mile

- Onion skin appearance in kidney seen in hyperplastic arteriosclerosis
- Onion skin like lesions due to arteritis seen in Lyme's and SLE
- Onion skin fibrosis around bile ducts seen in PSC
- Onion skin pattern of deposition of reactive bone in ewing's sarcoma
- Onion bulb appearance in sural nerves seen in CIDP **due to recurrent demyelination and remyelination**

322. Ans. (a) Adenocarcinoma of ampulla of Vater

The complications of gallstones include gangrenous cholecystitis by pressure on the mucosa and blood vessels in an acutely inflamed gallbladder

- Cholangitis by blocking the major biliary ducts and allowing bacteria to ascend into the liver
- Obstructive jaundice by blocking the common duct
- Acute pancreatitis by blocking the ampulla of Vater or a major pancreatic duct
- Gallstone ileus.

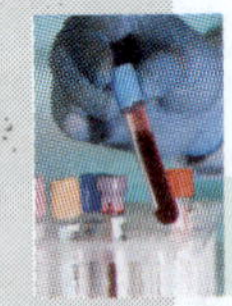

323. Ans. (d) Metastasis

Ref: Harrison, 19th ed. pg. 544

- Most common tumor of liver is metastasis
- Most common benign tumor of liver is cavernous hemangioma
- Most common cause of hepatocellular cancer is hepatitis B.

324. Ans. (c) Collagen type 1 & 3

Ref: Robbin's Pathology, 9th ed. pg. 823-824

- In cirrhosis, types I and III collagen and other ECM components are deposited in the space of Disse. In advanced fibrosis and cirrhosis, fibrous bands separate nodules of hepatocytes throughout the liver.
- In the normal liver, extracellular matrix (ECM) consisting of interstitial collagens (fibril-forming collagens types I, III, V, and XI) is present only in the liver capsule, in portal tracts, and around central veins. The liver has no true basement membrane; instead, a delicate framework containing type IV collagen and other proteins lies in the space between sinusoidal endothelial cells and hepatocytes (the space of Disse).

325. Ans. (c) Production of vitamin K

Ref: Robbin's Pathology, 9th ed. pg. 821

- **Vitamin K is produced by the bacteria of gut** and is used by liver for gamma carboxylation of factor 2/7/9/10.
  - Liver produces albumin which falls in liver cirrhosis producing ascites/edema.
  - Ammonia is combined with carbon dioxide to produce urea which in turn is excreted by the liver.
  - The cytochrome P450 is responsible for metabolism of drugs.

326. Ans. (c) Angiosarcoma of liver

Ref: Harrison, 19th ed. pg. 2027

Agents Leading to Angiosarcoma of Liver

- Arsenic
- Thorotrast (Liberates Alpha particles)
- Vinyl chloride

GASTROINTESTINAL TRACT

327. Ans. (a) Celiac sprue

Ref: Robbins and Cotran Review of Pathology E-Book pg. 268

- The presence of anti-Tissue transglutaminase antibodies and villous atrophy indicates celiac sprue. It occurs due to allergy to gluten/gliadin component of cereals like barley. Rye, oats and wheat.
- Option B occurs due to recurrent infection with gram negative organisms. Option C occurs with intracellular bacteria called as Tropheryma whipelli. Option D is associated with p-ANCA

328. Ans. (d) Cobalamin

Ref: Robbins and Cotran Pathology 2021 E-Book pg. 652

In event of gastrectomy intrinsic factor deficiency will make the person develop Vitamin B_{12} deficiency.

329. Ans. (d) Scleroderma

Ref: Harrison 20th ed. pg. 2553

- The key word in the question is leather like skin which is seen in scleroderma. The esophageal wall fibrosis explains the progressive dysphagia.
- The fibrosis of blood vessels will increase peripheral resistance and cause systemic hypertension.
- Fibrosis of pulmonary artery will cause PAH which causes limitation of exercise capacity. This is worsened further when lung fibrosis ensues
- Option A presents with hamartomatous polyps and mucosal melanosis
- Option B presents with dysphagia with iron deficiency anemia and koilonychia. It is alternate name for Plummer Vinson syndrome
- Option C presents with megaesophagus, megacolon and mega heart.

330. Ans. (c) Arsenic

Ref: Bailey and Love 27th ed. pg. 146

A spectrum of liver lesions has also been attributed to chronic arsenic exposure.

- Angiosarcoma liver
- Cirrhosis
- Hepatocellular carcinoma
- Hepatoportal sclerosis

Extra Mile

Must know agents incriminated in causing cancers

Inhaled particles		Asbestos	Mesothelioma
		Wood dust	Paranasal sinus cancers
Chemicals	Environmental pollutants/ chemicals used in industry		Angiosarcoma (vinyl chloride) Bladder cancer (aniline dyes, vulcanisation of rubber) Lung, nasal cavity (nickel)

Contd...

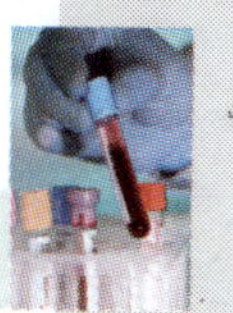

			Skin (arsenic) Lung (beryllium, cadmium, chromium) All sites (dioxins)
	Medical	Alkylating agents used in cytotoxic chemotherapy	Leukaemia Lymphoma Lung cancer
		Immunosuppressive treatment	Kaposi's sarcoma
		Stilboestrol	Adenocarcinoma of vagina in daughters of treated mothers
		Tamoxifen	Endometrial cancer
Fungal and plant toxins	Aflatoxins		Hepatoma
Obesity/lack of physical exercise			Breast Endometrium Kidney Colon Esophagus

331. Ans. (a) Anti-tissue transglutaminase antibody

Ref: Robbins 10th ed. pg. 787

The histology image shows blunting of villi in the child with failure to thrive. This is seen in celiac sprue. Screening test is anti-tissue transglutaminase antibody.

Option A is seen in primary biliary cirrhosis. Option B is seen with CREST syndrome and option C is seen with systemic sclerosis.

332. Ans. (a) Bacteria

Ref: CMDT 2019, pg. 647

Whipple's disease is caused by Tropheryma whipelli which is an intra-cellular rod shaped gram positive bacteria found in macrophages of the gut. The lamina propria of gut harbours macrophages inside which these bacteria are demonstrated using PAS stain. The small intestinal malabsorbtion occurs in these patients leading to osmotic diarrhea. The investigation of choice is Small intestinal mucosal biopsy/Duodenal biopsy.

333. Ans. (d) Tropheryma whippelii

Ref: Harrison 19th ed. pg. 1092-93

- Whipple's disease is a malabsorption syndrome caused by Tropheryma whippelii. It is an intracellular bacteria found in gut macrophages.

Mnemonic: *WHIPPLE*
Weight loss
Hyperpigmentation
Infection with Tropheryma whippelii
PAS positive granules in macrophages
Polyarthritis
Lymphadenopathy
Steatorrhea

Extra Mile

IOC for Whipple's disease is small intestinal biopsy.
Most common *heart valve* involved in Whipple's disease is aortic valve.
CNS features are in form of cognition defect like progressive dementia.
MC extraintestinal manifestation of Whipple's disease is CNS feature of dementia.
Current treatment is ceftriaxone for 2 weeks and oral doxycycline for 1 year.

334. Ans. (c) Menetrier's disease

- Menetrier's disease has chronic hypertrophic gastritis with foveolar cell hyperplasia. The rugosities of stomach are enlarged with atrophy of parietal cells.
- Type A gastritis is autoimmune gastritis and has body-fundus involvement.
- Type B gastritis is *H. pylori* related and involves the antrum. It is also called hyper-secretory gastritis.
- Type AB gastritis affects the mucosal region of A as well as B types and is overall the most common type of gastritis in all age groups.

335. Ans. (a) Crohn's disease

Serpiginous ulcers are features of Crohn's Disease. Pseudopolyps are seen in ulcerative colitis.

Feature	Crohn's disease	Ulcerative colitis
Distribution	Segmental with skip areas	Continuous without skip areas
Location	Commonly terminal ileum and/or ascending colon	Commonly rectum, sigmoid colon and extending upwards
Extent	Usually involves the entire thickness of the affected segment of bowel wall	Usually superficial, confined to mucosal layer
Ulcers	Serpiginous ulcers may develop into deep fissures	Superficial mucosal ulcers without fissures

Contd...

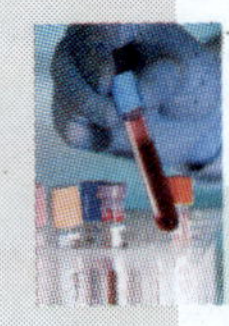

Feature	Crohn's disease	Ulcerative colitis
Pseudo-polyps	Rarely seen	Commonly present
Fibrosis	Common	Rare
Shortening	Due to fibrosis	Due to contraction of muscularis

336. Ans. (c) **Celiac disease**

Ref: Robbins, 9th ed. pg. 783

HPE Findings of Celiac Disease

- Biopsy specimens from the second portion of the duodenum or proximal jejunum, which are exposed to the highest concentrations of dietary gluten, are **generally diagnostic in celiac disease.**
- The histopathology is characterized by increased numbers of intraepithelial CD8+ T lymphocytes (**intraepithelial lymphocytosis**), crypt hyperplasia, and **villous atrophy.**

337. Ans. (b) **Amylase**

Ref: Sabiston, 19th ed. pg. 1524-1525, 1531; Schwartz, 9th ed. pg. 1200-1203; Bailey, 26th ed. pg. 1133-1134

PSEUDOPANCREATIC CYST

- A chronic collection of pancreatic fluid surrounded by a non-epithelialized wall of granulation tissue and fibrosis
- Pseudo-cysts account for 75% of cystic lesions of the pancreas.
- MC complication of chronic pancreatitis.

> - Located anywhere from the mediastinum to the scrotum
> - Found most often in the lesser sac or anterior para-renal space
> - Traumatic pseudocysts tend to occur anterior to the body of the gland
> - Chronic pancreatitis pseudocysts are commonly located within the substance of the gland

- Alcohol is the MC cause of pancreatitis related pseudo-cysts

Diagnosis

- No definitive laboratory findings are available to establish a diagnosis of pancreatic pseudocyst.
- ***Elevated serum amylase and lipase concentrations may occur in half of these patients.***
- *Persistently elevated amylase after resolution of acute pancreatitis should prompt investigation for a pseudocyst.*
- CECT abdomen is investigation of choice for diagnosis of a pancreatic pseudocyst.

338. Ans. (d) **Hypertension**

Ref: Robbin's Pathology, 9th ed. pg. 884-86

- Acute pancreatitis is seen chiefly in males after age 40 and often associated with obesity and alcoholism.
- In about 50% of the cases, gallstones are also present.
- Pancreatitis occurs in about 10% of cases of hyperparathyroidism.
- Long term thiazides can also contribute to development of pancreatitis.
- In some cases calculi resulting from the hypercalcemia of hyperparathyroidism develop in pancreatic ducts and lead to obstruction and inflammation.

339. Ans. (c) **Chronic gastritis**

Ref: Robbin's Pathology, 9th ed. pg. 763, 804

- Gastric polyps are not common.
  When they occur, they are usually hyperplastic polyps consisting of hyperplastic mucosal epithelium over an inflamed edematous stroma.
- They are most often seen in association with the chronic mucosal damage found in chronic gastritis.

340. Ans. (d) **Pernicious anemia**

Ref: Robbin's Pathology, 9th ed. pg. 764

- Antiparietal cell antibodies are found in patients with pernicious anemia.
- The antineutrophilic cytoplasmic antibodies are found in patients with Wegener granulomatosis.
- Wegener granulomatosis may also present with pulmonary and renal involvement but will have associated upper respiratory tract findings, e.g, sinusitis and sinus abscesses.

341. Ans. (d) **Majority seen in duodenum**

Ref: Robbin's Pathology, 9th ed. pg. 775-76

- Majority of gastrointestinal stromal tumours originate from *stomach.* The cell of origin is interstitial cell of Cajal which are present in muscularispropria.
- The useful marker is c-kit (CD 117) detectable in 95% of patients.
- PET scan is the imaging modality of choice
- Treatment is tyrosine kinase inhibitors like imatinib mesylate.

342. Ans. (d) **Coagulative necrosis**

Ref: Robbin's Pathology, 9th ed. pg. 795-96

- The typical flask shaped ulcer in amoebiasis is due to liquefactive necrosis affecting caecum and ascending colon and rectum.

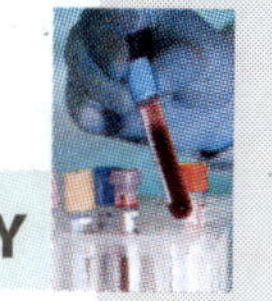

- Once the infection spreads hematogenously from the gut to the liver it results in generation of liver abscess which has presence of anchovy sauce pus.

343. Ans. (d) Prophylactic polypectomy is recommended as standard therapy

Ref: Robbin's Pathology, 9th ed. pg. 809

- In FAP as many as >100 polyps may be present in colon, and anyone of these can turn malignant any day, hence *prophylactic colectomy* is recommended as standard treatment.
- Most of the polyps are tubular polyps. In *attenuated FAP* (30 Polyps) are seen in proximal colon.
- The defect is in APC gene on chromosome 5, due to mutation in nucleotide excision base excision repair gene.

Extra Mile

- ***Turcot Syndrome:*** Adenomatous colonic polyposis +CNS tumours (2/3 medulloblastomas and 1/3 are gliomas)
- ***Gardener syndrome:*** Intestinal polyps + Epidermal cysts + Fibromatosis + Osteomas

344. Ans. (d) Increased MCV of RBC

Ref: Robbin's Pathology, 9th ed. pg. 764

Type A gastritis is autoimmune gastritis. The antiparietal cell antibodies lead to decreased intrinsic factor production. This leads to decreased absorption of vitamin B_{12} and resultant increased MCV.

345. Ans. (d) Superficial spreading

Ref: Robbins's Pathology, 9th ed. pg. 772-73

346. Ans. (d) Rectum is commonly involved

Ref: Robbin's Pathology, 9th ed. pg. 798-99

- *Crohn's disease can lead to formation of perianal fistula which leads to poor perianal hygiene.*
- The stricture formation seen in Crohn's disease occurs due to transmural inflammation.
- Most common part of GIT involved is ileum in Crohn's disease and rectum is spared.

Extra Mile

- *Fecal lactoferrin* is a highly sensitive and specific marker for detecting intestinal inflammation.
- *Fecal calprotectin* levels correlate well with histological inflammation and predict relapses and detect pouchitis.

347. Ans. (b) Thinning of mucosal layer

- The normal esophageal mucosa undergoes continuous cell turnover and renewal. Acute radiation esophagitis is primarily due to effects on the basal epithelial layer. This causes a thinning of the mucosa, which can progress to denudation.
- Acute toxicity is manifested clinically as dysphagia, odynophagia, and substernal discomfort, and usually occurs within two to three weeks after the initiation of radiation therapy (RT). Patients may describe a sudden, sharp, severe chest pain radiating to the back.

348. Ans. (a) Hemangioma

Ref: Robbin's Pathology, 9th ed. pg. 625

- Most common tumor of spleen is **hemangioma**
- Most common malignant tumor of spleen is **lymphoma**
- Most common malignant non-lymphoid tumor of spleen is **angiosarcoma**

349. Ans. (d) Stomach

Ref: Robbin's Pathology, 9th ed. pg. 773

- MALT lymphoma (MALToma) is a form of lymphoma involving the mucosa-associated lymphoid tissue (MALT), frequently of the stomach, but virtually any mucosal site can be afflicted. It is a cancer originating from B cells in the marginal zone of the MALT, and is also called extranodal marginal zone B cell lymphoma.
- Gastric MALT lymphoma is frequently associated (72–98%) with chronic inflammation as a result of the presence of *Helicobacter pylori.*

350. Ans. (a) Pseudo-polyps

Ref: Robbin's Pathology, 9th ed. pg. 798

- Pseudo-polyps are seen in ulcerative colitis. An **inflammatory pseudopolyp** is an island of normal colonic mucosa which only appears raised because it is surrounded by atrophic tissue (denuded ulcerative mucosa).
- It must be distinguished from inflammatory polyps, which are regions of inflamed and elevated mucosa surrounded by granular mucosa.

351. Ans. (a) p-ANCA

Ref: Robbin's Pathology, 9th ed. pg. 600

- p-ANCA, or Perinuclear Anti-Neutrophil Cytoplasmic Antibodies, show a perinuclear staining pattern. It is directed against myeloperoxidase.
- It is fairly specific, but not sensitive for ulcerative colitis, so is not useful as a sole diagnostic test. When measured together with Anti-saccharomyces cerevisiae antibodies (ASCA), p-ANCA has been estimated to have a specificity of 97% and a sensitivity of 48% in differentiating patients with ulcerative colitis from normal controls.

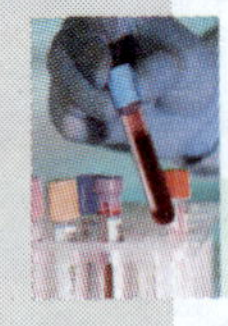

- It is also seen in about 50% of cases of Churg-Strauss syndrome
  - Primary sclerosing cholangitis
  - Microscopic polyangiitis
  - Focal necrotising and crescentic glomerulonephritis
  - Rheumatoid arthritis

CENTRAL NERVOUS SYSTEM

352. Ans. (d) Alzheimer's disease

Ref: Robbins 10th ed. pg. 1276

CJD	PrP^{SC} protein in neuronal Cytoplasm
Rabies	Negri bodies in cerebellum and Ammon horn of hippocampus
Parkinson's disease	Lewy Bodies in neuronal cytoplasm
Alzheimer disease	Tau protein in microtubular associated protein in axons that contributes to neurofibrillary tangles

353. Ans. (a) Variant Creutzfeldt-Jacob disease

Ref: Robbins 10th ed. pg. 1276

CJD	PrP^{SC} protein in neuronal cytoplasm. The disease is commonly seen in patients who have consumed beef of infected animals suffering from Bovine spongiform encephalopathy.
Rabies	Negri bodies in cerebellum and Ammon horn of hippocampus
Parkinson's disease	Lewy Bodies in neuronal cytoplasm
Alzheimer disease	Tau protein in microtubular associated protein in axons that contributes to neurofibrillary tangles

354. Ans. (a) Lung cancer

Ref: Bailey and Love 26th ed. pg. 614

The leading cause of brain metastasis is lungs > Breast > Melanoma

TABLE Tissue of origin for brain metastases (approximate)

Origin	Percentage
Lung	40
Breast	15
Melanoma	10
Renal/GU	10
Other Unknown	25

355. Ans. (b) Superoxide dismutase

Ref: Robbin's Pathology, 9th ed. pg. 48, 80

- Antioxidant enzymes include glutathione peroxidase, SOD and catalase.
- Deficiency of SOD 1 gene may result in motor neuron disorder.

356. Ans. (c) Hippocampus

Ref: Robbin's Pathology, 9th ed. pg. 277

- **Negri bodies** are eosinophilic, sharply outlined, pathognomonic inclusion bodies (2–10 μm in diameter) ***found in the cytoplasm of certain nerve cells containing the virus of rabies, especially in Ammon's horn of the hippocampus.***
- They are also found in the cells of the medulla and various other ganglia. Negri bodies can also be found in the neurons of the salivary glands, tongue, or other organs. Staining with Mann's, giemsa, or Sellers stains can permit differentiation of rabies inclusions from other intracellular inclusions. With these stains, Negri bodies appear magenta in color and have small (0.2 μm to 0.5 μm), dark-blue interior basophilic granules.
- Histologic examination of tissues from clinically rabid animals show Negri bodies in about 50% of the samples; in contrast, the dFA test shows rabies antigen in nearly 100% of the samples.

Extra Mile

Some other important bodies
- Lewy bodies: Parkinson's disease
- Russel bodies: multiple myeloma
- Mallory bodies: Alcoholism
- Donovan bodies: Leishmaniasis
- Heinz bodies: G-6-PD
- Howell jolly bodies: Sickle cell anemia
- Councilman bodies: yellow fever

357. Ans. (c) Parkinsonism

Ref: Robbin's Pathology, 9th ed. pg. 1294-95

Lewy body is an eosinophilic cytoplasmic inclusion consisting of a dense core surrounded by a halo of 10-nm-wide radiating fibrils, the primary structural component of which is alpha-synuclein. It is seen in Parkinsonism, Dementia with lewy bodies, shy dragger syndrome.

Alzheimer disease	Hirona bodies/neurofibrillary tangles
Rabies	Negri bodies
Parkinsonism, dementia with lewy bodies	Lewy bodies
Pick bodies	Picks disease

358. Ans. (a) Huntington's chorea

Ref: Robbin's Pathology, 9th ed. pg. 1297-98

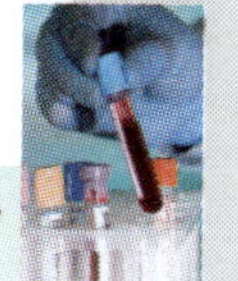

- The neuropathology of Huntington's disease consists of prominent neuronal loss and gliosis in the caudate nucleus and putamen.
- *Intraneuronal inclusions containing aggregates of ubiquitin and the mutant protein huntingtin are found in the nuclei of affected neurons.*
- HD is caused by an increase in the number of polyglutamine (CAG) repeats (>40) in the coding sequence of the Huntington gene located on the short arm of chromosome 4.

359. Ans. (a) Retinoblastoma

Ref: Robbin's Pathology, 9th ed. pg. 1339; Dorland Medical Dictionary

- Glioma retinae is a congenital blastoma occurring in both hereditary and sporadic forms and is composed in tumour arising from embryonic retinal cells.
- It appears in one or both eyes in children under 5 years of age and is usually diagnosed initially by a bright white pupillary reflex (Leucocoria). It is caused by germline or somatic mutations or both, in both the alleles of retinoblastoma gene (Rb1)

ENDOCRINE SYSTEM

360. Ans. (c) Papillary thyroid cancer

Ref: Bailey and Love 27th ed. pg. 816

The Histology slide shows thyroid follicles lined with cells with large empty looking Nuclei called "Orphan Annie eye nuclei". This is a feature of papillary cancer of thyroid. Papillary cancer of thyroid spreads via lymphatics and that explains the cervical lymphadenopathy.

361. Ans. (a) Hypophosphatemia

Ref: Harrison 20th ed. pg. 519

- Hyperphosphatemia can be caused by the release of intracellular phosphate pools by lysis of tumour cells.
- It produces a reciprocal depression in serum calcium, which causes severe neuromuscular irritability and tetany.
- Deposition of calcium phosphate in the kidney and hyperphosphatemia may cause renal failure. Potassium is the principal intracellular cation, and massive destruction of malignant cells may lead to hyperkalemia.
- The break-down of DNA from nucleus will produce urate crystals that will block kidney tubules and lead to urate nephropathy.

362. Ans. (c) Multiple myeloma

Ref: CMDT 2019, pg. 546

Vitamin D3 intoxication	Ruled out as serum vitamin D3 levels are elevated
Hyperparathyroidism	Ruled out as PTH are elevated
Multiple Myeloma	Myeloma cells produce IL-6 leading to enhanced osteoclastic activity. SAP hence remains normal while the enhanced osteoclastic activity leads to increased serum calcium values.
Nutritional rickets	Leads to low calcium and less vitamin D3 levels

363. Ans. (a) Parathyroid adenoma

Ref: Harrison 20th ed. pg. 2747

MEN 2A is called Sipple syndrome and includes the following

- Medullary carcinoma thyroid (MC of all of these)
- Pheochromocytoma
- Parathyroid adenoma

The defect lies on chromosome 10 and *RET* proto-oncogene is responsible.

Extra Mile

MEN 2B (also known as MEN 3)	MTC (>90%) Pheochromocytoma (>50%) Associated abnormalities (40–50%) • **M**ucosal neuromas • **M**arfanoid habitus • **M**edullated corneal nerve fibers • **M**egacolon	MEN 4 (12p13)	**P**arathyroid adenoma **P**ituitary adenoma **R**eproductive organ tumors

364. Ans. (b) Secretin

Ref: Harrison 20th ed. pg. 2741

- Pheochromocytomas can produce *calcitonin, opioid peptides, somatostatin, corticotropin, and vasoactive intestinal peptide.*
- Corticotropin hypersecretion causes Cushing syndrome, and vasoactive intestinal peptide overproduction leads to watery diarrhea.
- Calcitonin is also produced by medullary carcinoma of thyroid which is related to Pheochromocytoma.

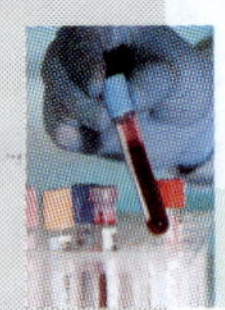

365. Ans (c) Neuropathy

Ref: Robbin's Pathology, 9th ed. pg. 1086-87

- Hashimoto's thyroiditis or chronic lymphocytic thyroiditis is an autoimmune disease in which the thyroid gland is gradually destroyed by a variety of cell and antibody mediated immune processes.
- Physiologically, antibodies against thyroid peroxidase and/or thyroglobulin cause gradual destruction of follicles in the thyroid gland. Accordingly, the disease can be detected clinically by looking for these antibodies in the blood. It is also characterized by invasion of the thyroid tissue by leukocytes, mainly T-lymphocytes. It is associated with non-Hodgkin lymphoma.

366. Ans. (b) Medullary carcinoma thyroid

Ref: Robbin's Pathology, 9th ed. pg. 1099

MEDULLARY CARCINOMA THYROID

- Accounts for approximately 7% of malignant tumour of thyroid
- It arises from ultimo-branchial bodies (from the para-follicular C cells derived from thyroid follicles).
- *It contains amyloid stroma*
- Familial medullary carcinomas occur in 25% of patients (Marfanoid habitus, Amyloid disease also occur in patients with familial medullary cancer).
- Medullary carcinoma occurs in association with (MEN 2A) syndrome.
- All patients with medullary carcinoma of thyroid should be screened for RET mutated gene.
- Medullary Carcinoma thyroid secretes calcitonin, this *does not cause hypocalcemia* but causes diarrhea.

367. Ans. (a) Cardiac

Ref: Robbin's Pathology, 9th ed. pg. 1115

- *Cardiovascular insufficiency and cerebrovascular accidents are the most common causes of mortality.* The impact of cardiovascular disease can be gauged by its involvement in as many as 80% of deaths of type 2 diabetics; in fact, diabetics have a 3 to 7.5 times greater incidence of death from cardiovascular causes than nondiabetic populations.
- The hallmark of cardiovascular disease is *accelerated atherosclerosis* of the large and medium-sized arteries (i.e., macrovascular disease).

368. Ans. (c) MEN IIB

Ref: Robbin's Pathology, 9th ed. pg. 1137

MEN type 1
- Parathyroid hyperplasia or adenoma
- Islet cell hyperplasia, adenoma, or carcinoma
- Pituitary hyperplasia or adenoma
- Other, less common manifestations: foregut carcinoid, pheochromocytoma, subcutaneous or visceral lipomas

MEN IIA
- Medullary Thyroid Cancer (MTC)
- Pheochromocytoma
- Parathyroid hyperplasia or adenoma

MEN IIB (Now called as MEN 3)
- MTC
- Pheochromocytoma
- Mucosal and gastrointestinal neuromas
- Marfanoid features

369. Ans. (b) Hyperparathyroidism

Please refer to above explanation

370. Ans. (d) Urine contains 5H.I.A.A

Ref: Robbin's Pathology, 9th ed. pg. 476

- ***Neuroblastoma (NB) is the most common extracranial solid cancer in childhood and the most common cancer in infancy.***
- Neuroblastoma is one of the few human malignancies known to demonstrate spontaneous regression from an undifferentiated state to a completely benign cellular appearance.
- *The most common location for neuroblastoma to originate (i.e., the primary tumor) is the adrenal glands.* This occurs in 40% of localized tumors and in 60% of cases of widespread disease.
- Neuroblastoma can also develop anywhere along the sympathetic nervous system chain from the neck to the pelvis.
- N-myc oncogene amplification within the tumor is a common finding in neuroblastoma. The degree of amplification shows a bimodal distribution: either 3- to 10-fold, or 100- to 300-fold. The presence of this mutation is highly correlated to advanced stages of disease
- Since it originates from chromaffin cells, in about 90% of cases of neuroblastoma, elevated levels of catecholamines or their metabolites are found in the urine or blood. Catecholamines and their metabolites include dopamine, homovanillic acid (HVA), and/or vanillyl mandelic acid (VMA)

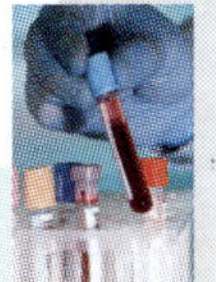

371. Ans. (d) Diffuse glomerulosclerosis

Ref: Robbin's Pathology, 9th ed. pg. 111

- Diabetic nephropathy is a common cause of end-stage renal disease worldwide. It is characterised by diffuse or nodular glomerulosclerosis, afferent and efferent hyaline arteriolosclerosis, and tubulointerstitial fibrosis and atrophy.
- **Note:** *HPS finding of HIV nephropathy- Focal segmental glomerulosclerosis (FSGS)*

372. Ans. (a) Papillary carcinoma thyroid

Ref: Robbin's Pathology, 9th ed. pg. 1095

- Psammoma bodies are associated with the papillary histo-morphology and are thought to arise from:
  1 The infarction and calcification of papillae tips
  2 Calcification of intra-lymphatic tumor thrombi
- ***Psammoma bodies are commonly seen in certain tumors such as:***
  - **Papillary thyroid carcinoma**
  - Papillary renal cell carcinoma
  - Ovarian papillary serous cyst-adenocarcinoma
  - Endometrial adenocarcinomas (Papillary serous carcinoma ~3%-4%)
  - Meningiomas, in the central nervous system
  - Peritoneal and Pleural Mesothelioma
  - Somatostatinoma
  - Prolactinoma
  - Mesothelioma

373. Ans. (a) Papillary thyroid cancer

Ref: Robbin's Pathology, 9th ed. pg. 1095-96

Orphan Annie Eye Nucleus is Seen in

- Papillary carcinoma thyroid
- Polymorphous low grade adenocarcinoma
- Hashimoto Thyroiditis
- Grave's disease
- Nodular goiter

374. Ans. (a) Epinephrine

Ref: Robbin's Pathology, 9th ed. pg. 1134-36

- *Phaeochromocytoma size <5 cm and associated with MEN 2A can produce epinephrine due to sufficient methyl transferase enzyme.*
- However if phaeochromocytoma is >5 cm or is an extradrenal phaeochromocytoma due to absence of methyl transferase enzyme, produces only nor-epinephrine.

375. Ans. (d) Mucinous cystadenosarcoma

Ref: Robbin's Pathology, 9th ed. pg. 1027

- Pseudomyxoma peritonei (PMP) is a clinical condition caused by cancerous cells (mucinous adenocarcinoma) that produce abundant mucin or gelatinous ascites.
- The primary tumor appears to arise from the MUC2 expressing goblet cells and most commonly from these cells in the appendix. The K-Ras and p53 genes may be involved in the oncogenesis. It may be diagnosed with a range of conditions.
- *While the majority of these cases are where it associated with appendiceal carcinomas other conditions may also be found, peritoneal carcinomas, several mucinous tumors (mucinous adenocarcinoma, mucinous cystadenoma, and mucinous cystadenocarcinoma).*

GENETICS

376. Ans. (a) AD

Ref: Pocket companion to Robbins E-Book pg. 117

Neurofibromatosis-1 is an autosomal dominant disorder characterized by multiple café au lait macules, intertriginous freckling, multiple cutaneous neurofibromas, and learning disability or behavior problems.

Extra Mile

NF-1: associated with optic glioma and Pheochromocytoma
NF-2 : associated with acoustic neuroma

377. Ans. (c) Klinefelter syndrome

Ref: Nelson 20th ed. pg. 2650

- The key words are gynecomastia with features of hypogonadism like small testis and scanty pubic hair in a male patient showing antisocial behavior. This is seen in Klinefelter syndrome.
- Option A presents with idiopathic hypercalcemia and supravalvular aortic stenosis.
- Option B looks like Turner syndrome and has pulmonic stenosis.
- Option D has tall person with arm span > height and aortic dissection.

378. Ans. (d) Multifactorial

Ref: Nelson 20th ed. pg. 2802

Neural tube defects account for the largest proportion of congenital anomalies of the CNS and result from failure of

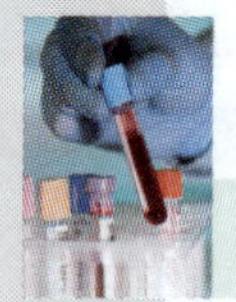

the neural tube to close spontaneously between the 3rd and 4th week of in utero development. Although the precise cause of NTDs remains unknown, evidence suggests that many factors, including hyperthermia, evidence suggests that many factors, including hyperthermia, drugs (valproic acid), malnutition, low red cell folate levels, chemicals, maternal obesity or diabetes, and genetic determinants (mutations in folate-responsive or folate-dependent enzyme pathways) can adversely affect normal development of the CNS from the time of conception.

379. Ans. (a) AD

Ref: Robbins and Cotran Pathological basis of Disease: 2020 E-Book pg. 145

Since all the three generations are affected irrespective of gender it points to autosomal dominant disorder. The point against XLR is that grandmother is also affected. In XLR females are not affected and are carriers.

380. Ans. (c) Wilson disease

Ref: Robbins and Cotran Pathology 2020 E-Book pg. 231

- ATP7A mutation on X- chromosome results in development of Menke's disease with Copper deficiency.
- ATP7B mutation on chromosome 13 results in development of Wilson disease with Copper excess.

381. Ans. (a) Ehler Danlos syndrome

Ref: Robbins and Cotran Pathology 2020 E-Book pg. 187

- Ehlers-Danlos syndrome is a connective tissue disorder characterized by of skin hyperextensibility, joint hypermobility, and vascular fragility.
- Joint dislocations, musculoskeletal pain, atrophic scars, easy bleeding, vessel/viscera rupture, severe scoliosis, and obstetric complications may occur.
- These manifestations are secondary to abnormal collagen, with specific molecular defects in types I, III, and V collagen

382. Ans. (c) Wilson disease

Ref: Harrison 20th ed. pg. 2982

The image shows brownish ring in periphery of cornea and is KF ring which is a characteristic feature seen in Wilson disease. It is called hepatolenticular degeneration.

383. Ans. (b) Osteogenesis imperfecta

Ref: Nelson 20th ed. pg. 3381

The image shows blue sclera which is a characteristic feature of Osteogenesis imperfecta.

384. Ans. (a) Down syndrome

Ref: Robbins 10th ed. pg. 166

Notice the trisomy of 21st chromosome which helps in identifying Down Syndrome

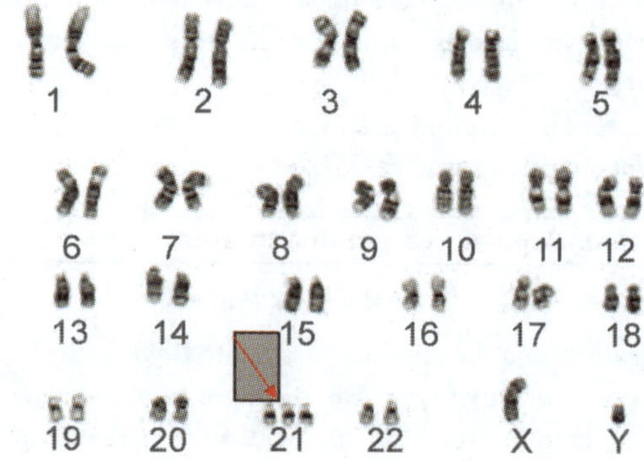

385. Ans. (b) Nucleotide excision repair defect

Ref: Robbins 10th ed. pg. 1148

- The diagnosis of the patient based on mottled hyperpigmentation, increased risk of skin cancer and DNA Repair defect is Xeroderma pigmentosum.
- The pattern of inheritance in Xeroderma pigmentosum is AR and gene involved is XPA on chromosome 9q22.
- These patients can develop SCC and melanoma.
- Option A is related to premature aging in Werner syndrome
- Option C is related to ataxia telangiectasia
- Option D is related to Colon cancer.

386. Ans. (d) X-linked recessive

Ref: Robbins 10th ed. pg. 146

System	Disease
Musculoskeletal	Duchenne muscular dystrophy
Blood	Hemophilia A and B Chronic granulomatous disease Glucose-6-phosphate dehydrogenase deficiency
Immune	Agammaglobulinemia Wiskott-Aldrich syndrome
Metabolic	Diabetes insipidus Lesch-Nyhan syndrome
Nervous	Fragile X syndrome

387. Ans. (a) 45 X0

Ref: Robbins 10th ed. pg. 171

The features of short height with amenorrhea and widely spaced hypoplastic nipples are seen in Turner syndrome.

388. Ans. (d) G6PD

Ref: CMDT 2019, pg. 521

- Glucose-6-phosphate dehydrogenase (G6PD) deficiency is an *XLR enzyme defect* that causes episodic hemolytic anemia because of the decreased ability of red blood cells to deal with oxidative stresses. G6PD deficiency leads to excess oxidized glutathione (hence, inadequate levels of reduced glutathione) that forces hemoglobin to denature and form precipitants called *Heinz bodies*.

389. Ans. (a) AR

Ref: Robbins E-book, pg. 246

- Marriage amongst cousins/close relatives is called as consanguinity.
- The high consanguinity rates, could induce the expression of autosomal recessive diseases, including very rare or new syndromes.

390. Ans. (a) Phenotype

Ref: Robbins 8th ed. pg. 136-37

Phenotype	Physical appearance ascribed to a particular genetic make-up
Proteomics	Measurement of all proteins expressed in a cell or tissue
Genotype	Genetic composition describing number of chromosomes
Anticipation	Increase in severity of disease with successive generations

391. Ans. (b) Familial hypercholesterolemia

Ref: CMDT 2017, pg. 1212

Disease with Polygenic Pattern of Inheritance

- Hypertension
- Diabetes mellitus
- Gout
- Schizophrenia
- Bipolar disorder

392. Ans. (b) Chromosome 17q21

- The Cytogenetic Location of BRCA1 gene is 17q21.31, which is the long (q) arm of chromosome 17 at position 21.31
- Cytogenetic Location: 13q13.1, which is the long (q) arm of chromosome 13 at position 13.1
- BRCA1- and BRCA2-associated hereditary breast and ovarian cancer syndrome (HBOC) is characterized by an increased risk for female and male breast cancer, ovarian cancer (includes fallopian tube and primary peritoneal cancers).

393. Ans. (a) Fibrillin 1

- Fibrillin is the major component of extracellular microfibrils and is widely distributed in connective tissue throughout the body.
  - *Mutations in the fibrillin-1 (FBN1) gene, on chromosome 15q21.1, have been found to cause Marfan syndrome, a dominantly inherited disorder characterised by clinically variable skeletal, ocular, and cardiovascular abnormalities.*

394. Ans. (d) 47XXY

395. Ans. (b) 11q(22-23)

- The image shows dilated blood vessels in the sclera which is called telangiectasia. It is seen in *Ataxia-telangiectasia*.
- The gene for ataxia-telangiectasia has been localized to band 11q22-23.
- The main abnormalities on physical examination are ocular and cutaneous telangiectasia and neurologic symptoms (ataxia and abnormal eye movements present in virtually all cases) and choreo-athetosis.

396. Ans. (a) 50% carrier and 50% affected

Ref: Harsh Mohan, 7th ed. pg. 255

397. Ans. (c) Chromosomal abnormalities

Ref: Robbin's Pathology, 9th ed. pg. 158

Karyotyping is the study of chromosomes and is used in cytogenetics to study the chromosomal abnormalities. After arresting the cells in metaphase the chromosomes are examined to check for:

- *Change in Number of chromosomes - To detect abnormalities in chromosome numbers such as aneuploidy (trisomy, tetrasomy), polyploidy.*

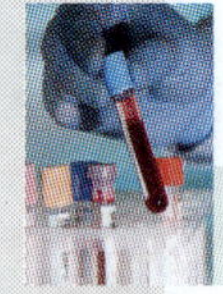

- *For detection of structural chromosomal anomalies such as translocation, deletions, inversion of chromosomes.*

398. Ans. (c) Trinucleotide - repeat expansion

Ref: Robbin's Pathology, 9th ed. pg. 168

- Anticipation is a phenomenon where by the symptoms of a genetic disorder become apparent at an earlier age as it is passed to next generation. In most cases, an increased severity of symptoms is also noted.
- In triplet nucleotide repeat mutation, the DNA fragment is unstable and tends to expand further during cell division.

So, in successive generations the expanded repeat increases and the manifestations of disease may worsen or may be observed at an earlier age; this phenomenon is referred to as anticipation.

399. Ans. (a) 13q l4

Ref: Robbin's Pathology, 9th ed. pg. 1339

• Wilm's tumor-Aniridia complex (WAGR syndrome)	11 p 13 part of (deletion of short arm of chromosome)
• Retinoblastoma	13q 14.11 (deletion of part of long arm of chromosome 13)
• Prader-Willi syndrome Angelman syndrome	15q 11-13 (deletion of part of long arm of chromosome 15)
• DiGeorge's syndrome Velo-Cardio-facial syndrome	22q11 (deletion of part of long arm of chromosome -22)

400. Ans. (b) Marfan syndrome

Ref: Robbin's Pathology, 9th ed. pg. 144

- The presentation in the question is of a patient with Marfan syndrome.
- Marfan syndrome is caused by a mutation in a single allele of the fibrillin gene (FBN1).
- The gene product is a major component of elastin-associated microfibrils. Long, thin extremities; ectopic lentis; and aortic aneurysms are the classical triad.
- Mutations in the FBN2 gene can also cause Marfan syndrome, but without aneurysms.

401. Ans. (c) Chromosome 21

Ref: Robbin's Pathology, 9th ed. pg. 158

- In karyotyping the image of stained chromosome pairs in metaphase stage is arranged in order of decreasing length.
- **Chromosome 21 is the smallest human Autosome.**
- Chromosome 1 is the largest chromosome.

402. Ans. (a) Down syndrome

Ref: Robbin's Pathology, 9th ed. pg. 161

Autoimmune Thyroiditis is Seen with

- Down syndrome
- Turner syndrome
- Congenital rubella syndrome
  - Autoimmune thyroiditis is *not* seen with Marfan's Syndrome.
  - Louis Barr syndrome is known as ataxia telangiectasia. It characterised by deficiency of IgA with increased incidence of lympho-reticular malignancy.
  - Edward syndrome is eighteen trisomy which is characterised by clenched hand and *overlapping of fingers* where the index finger of the neonate overlaps third finger and fifth finger overlaps the fourth finger.

403. Ans. (b) Only X chromosome from the mother undergoes pyknosis

Ref: Robbin's Pathology, 9th ed. pg. 164

Lyon hypothesis is:

- Only one of the X chromosome is genetically active
- Other X chromosome which can be of paternal or maternal origin undergoes pyknosis and is rendered inactive.
- Inactivation of either paternal or maternal X chromosomes occurs at random among the cells of blastocyst by about 16th day of embryonic life
- Inactivation of X is because of a gene called Xist which causes gene silencing DNA methylation.

404. Ans. (a) Genomic imprinting

Ref: Robbin's Pathology, 9th ed. pg. 172-173

Preferential expression of an allele depending on parental origin is genomic imprinting.

- **Prader wili syndrome:** Deletion of paternal chromosome 15
- **Angelman syndrome:** Deletion of maternal chromosome 15
- **Beckwith weidmann syndrome:** Have two paternal but no maternal copies of chromosome 11
- **Albright's hereditary osteodystrophy:** Mutation in Gs alpha subunit leading to short stature, brachydactyl and PTH resistance only when mutation is inherited from the mother.

405. Ans. (d) All of the above

Ref: Robbin's Pathology, 9th ed. pg. 177-178

- FISH can be performed in prenatal samples, like samples obtained by amniocentesis, Cordocentesis, chorionic villus sampling or umbilical cord blood, peripheral blood lymphocytes.
- Since it does not need dividing cells, it is extremely useful for rapid diagnosis

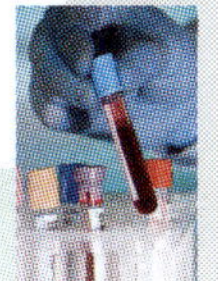

Advantages of FISH

- Can detect numerical abonormalities of chromosomes like aneuploidy
- It can detect minor micro-deletions
- Can detect complex translocations
- For gene amplification analysis
- For mapping of recently isolated genes to their chromosomal locus

406. Ans. (a) Autosomal recessive

Ref: Robbin's Pathology, 9th ed. pg. 141

AUTOSOMAL DOMINANT

- One mutated copy of the gene in each cell is sufficient for a person to be affected by an autosomal dominant disorder.
- Autosomal dominant disorders tend to occur in every generation of an affected family.
- Associated diseases can be remembered as *"DOMINANT"*

D= Dystrophy Myotonic.
O- Ostogenesis Imperfecta.
M- Marfan's syndrome.
I- Intermittent Porphyria.
N- Noonan's Syndrome.
A- Adult Polycystic Kidney, Achondroplasia.
N- Neurofibromatosis.
T- Tuberous sclerosis.

AUTOSOMAL RECESSIVE

- Two mutated copies of the gene are present in each cell when a person has an autosomal recessive disorder.
- Autosomal recessive disorders are typically not seen in every generation of an affected family.
- **Diseases can be remembered as *"ABCDEFGH SPW"*:**

A- Albinism, Alpha 1 Antitrypsin Deficiency
B-Beta Thalassemia
C-Cystic Fibrosis, CGD, CAH
D-Deafness(SNHL), Dubin Johnson
E-Enzyme Deficiencies (Glycogen Storage And Lysosomal Storage)
F-Friedrich's Ataxia, Fanconi Anemia
G- Galactosemia
H-Hemochromatosis, Hurler syndrome
S-Sickle Cell Disease
P-Phenylketonuria
W-Wilson's disease

X-LINKED DOMINANT

- X-linked dominant disorders are caused by mutations in genes on the X chromosome.
- *Females are more frequently affected than males,* and the chance of passing on an X-linked dominant disorder differs between men and women.
- Families with an X-linked dominant disorder often have both affected males and affected females in each generation. *A characteristic of X-linked inheritance is that fathers cannot pass X-linked traits to their sons (no male-to-male transmission).*
- Ex: hypophosphatemic rickets, also called vitamin D-resistant rickets.

X-LINKED RECESSIVE

- X-linked recessive disorders are also caused by mutations in genes on the X chromosome.
- *Males are more frequently affected than females*, and the chance of passing on the disorder differs between men and women.
- Families with an X-linked recessive disorder often have affected males, but rarely affected females, in each generation.
- A characteristic of X-linked inheritance is that fathers cannot pass X-linked traits to their sons (no male-to-male transmission).
- **Diseases under this are:**
  - G6PD
  - Duchenne muscular dystrophy
  - Hemophilia A

407. Ans. (d) X-linked recessive

Ref: Robbin's Pathology, 9th ed. pg. 142

408. Ans. (a) Albinism

Ref: Robbin's Pathology, 9th ed. pg. 141

409. Ans (b) Hemophilia

Ref: Robbin's Pathology, 9th ed. pg. 142

"Less hCG is Detected Clinically in A Woman"

- Lesch-Nyhan syndrome
- Hemophilia, Hunter's syndrome
- Chronic granulomatous disease
- G6PD deficiency
- Duchenne muscular dystrophy
- Color blindness
- Agammaglobulinemia
- Wiskott-Aldrich syndrome

410. Ans. (a) Vitamin D resistant rickets

Ref: Robbin's Pathology, 9th ed. pg. 142

Vitamin D resistant rickets	PHEX gene. X-linked dominant
Familial hypercholesterolemia	Autosomal dominant
Red green colour blindness	X-linked recessive
Achondroplasia	Autosomal dominant

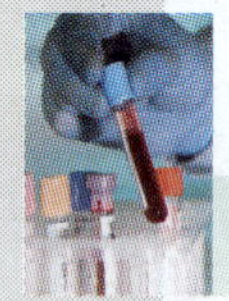

411. Ans. (a) X-linked

Ref: Robbin's Pathology, 9th ed. pg. 155

- HURLER syndrome is autosomal recessive while HUNTER SYNDROME is X linked recessive
- HURLER syndrome is marked by progressive deterioration, hepatosplenomegaly, dwarfism and unique facial features. There is a progressive mental retardation, with death frequently occurring by the age of 10 years
- Hurler is due to defective IUDA gene, which has been mapped to the 4p16.3 site on chromosome 4. The gene is named IUDA because of its iduronidase enzyme protein product.

412. Ans. (a) Decrease in AFP

Ref: Robbin's Pathology, 9th ed. pg. 161, Nelson, 18th ed. ch. 81

AFP	UE3	hCG	Associated conditions
Low	Low	High	Down syndrome
Low	Low	Low	Trisomy 18 (Edward's syndrome)
High	n/a	n/a	Neural tube defects (like spina bifida that may have associated increased levels of acetylcholinesterase in the amniotic fluid), omphalocele, gastroschisis, multiple gestation triplets, or an underestimation of gestational age.

413. Ans. (a) Down syndrome

Ref: Nelson, 18th ed. ch. 81

414. Ans. (b) Chromosome 17

Ref: Robbin's Pathology, 9th ed. pg. 291

- The BRCA2 **gene** is **located** on chromosome 13 and encodes over 3000 amino acids. It appears that BRCA2 plays an important role in male breast cancer.
- *The human BRCA1 gene is located on the long (q) arm of chromosome 17*

415. Ans. (c) P16

Ref: Robbin's Pathology, 9th ed. pg. 1054-55

- Genes called BRCA1, BRCA2, TP53 or PTEN are linked with breast cancer.
- *P16 plays an important role in cell cycle regulation by decelerating cell progression from G1 phase to S phase, and therefore acts as a tumor suppressor that is implicated in the prevention of cancers, notably melanoma, oropharyngeal squamous cell carcinoma, cervical cancer, and esophageal cancer.*

416. Ans. (b) 47XXY

Ref: Robbin's Pathology, 9th ed. pg. 165

417. Ans. (b) Chromosome 22 defect

Ref: Harrison, 19th ed. pg. 83e-6

- Cat Eye Syndrome is a rare condition caused by the short arm (p) and a small section of the long arm (q) of human Chromosome 22 being present three (trisomic) or four times (tetrasomic) instead of the usual two times.
- The term "Cat Eye" syndrome was coined because of the particular appearance of the vertical colobomas in the eyes of some patients. Preauricular skin tags and/or pits constitute the most consistent features and suggest the presence of a supernumerary bisatellited marker chromosome 22 derived from duplication of the CES critical region.
- ***Please do not confuse with "Cat eye reflex" of retinoblastoma in which there is an abnormal appearance of the pupil, called leukocoria.***
- Other signs and symptoms include deterioration of vision, a red and irritated eye with glaucoma, and faltering growth or delayed development. Some children with retinoblastoma can develop a squint. Retinoblastoma presents with advanced disease in developing countries and eye enlargement is a common finding.

RESPIRATORY SYSTEM

418. Ans. (b) Asbestosis

Ref: Robbins and Cotran Review of Pathology E-Book pg. 2192

Asbestosis can develop many years after patient has had exposure. In all other occupational disorders breathlessness occurs while they are exposed to dust at workplace. Like in byssinosis we have Monday chest tightness or anthracosis patient would be feeling breathless while at his workplace. In this case the presentation has occurred at post retirement age.

419. Ans. (a) Silicosis

Ref: Harrison 21st ed. pg. 2192

Key word is "snow-storm appearance" on CXR which is seen in silicosis. Option B leads to coin shadow. Option C leads to progressive massive fibrosis. Option D presents as Monday chest tightness.

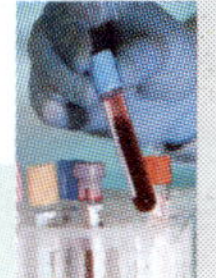

420. Ans. (a) Triad of ascites, pleural effusion and benign ovarian tumor

Ref: Harrison 21st ed. pg. 2199

Meig Syndrome presents with ascites, right sided pleural effusion, and benign ovarian tumor like fibroma, thecoma.

421. Ans. (b) Bagassosis

Ref: Textbook of Community Medicine by Rajvir Bhalawar pg. 1069

Sugar cane fiber is used to make cardboard and paper. The fungus that grows in it is called Thermophilic actinomyces. Inhalation of spores of it will lead to development of shortness of breath in patient. If person leaves the job, symptoms will remit but long term damage will cause lung fibrosis.

422. Ans. (b) Adenocarcinoma

Ref: Harrison 21st ed. pg. 2167-68

Most common cancer seen in a patient with asbestosis is Adenocarcinoma of lung. Mesothelioma is associated with asbestosis but is *not* most common.

423. Ans. (a) Mycoplasma pneumoniae

Ref: Harrison 20th ed. pg. 910

- Atypical bacterial pneumonia is caused by atypical organisms that are not detectable on Gram stain and cannot be cultured using standard methods.
- The most common organisms are Mycoplasma pneumoniae, Chlamydophila pneumoniae, and Legionella pneumophila. Atypical bacterial pneumonia generally is characterised by a symptom complex that includes headache, low-grade fever, cough, and malaise.
- CAP is caused by pneumococcus. If question asks about etiology of hospitalized patient of CAP the answer is still pneumococcus. Do not confuse with organism causing hospital acquired pneumonia which is caused by Staphylococcus aureus.

Extra Mile

TABLE Microbial causes of community-acquired pneumonia, by site of care

	Hospitalized Patients	
Outpatients	Non-ICU	ICU
Streptococcus pneumoniae Mycoplasma pneumonlae Haemophllus influenzae	*S. pneumonlae M. pneumoniae Chiamydla pneumoniae H. influenzae*	*S. pneumoniae Staphylococcus aureus Legionella spp. Gram-negative bacilli*

424. Ans. (c) Kidney

Ref: Robbins E-Book, pg. 519

Good pasture disease is a term used to describe glomerulonephritis, with or without pulmonary hemorrhage, and the presence of circulating anti–glomerular basement membrane (anti-GBM) antibodies

425. Ans. (a) Thickening of bronchial wall

Ref: Robbin E-book, pg. 502-504

- Increased numbers of goblet cells (goblet cell hyperplasia) is part of airway remodelling in asthma.
- The remodelling also includes epithelial proliferation, thickening of the reticular basement membrane, increased bronchial vascularity and hypertrophy of smooth muscle and submucosal glands.
- *Thickening of bronchial wall is seen in bronchiectasis.*

426. Ans. (c) Hyaline membrane disease

Ref: Robbins 9th ed. pg. 672

The immature lungs in hyaline membrane disease show eosinophilic hyaline membranes in alveoli, alveolar ducts and terminal bronchioles.

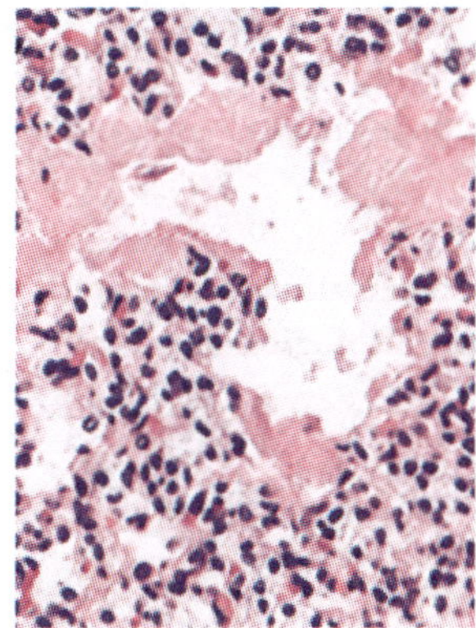

The membranes contain necrotic epithelial cells admixed with extravasated plasma proteins.

427. Ans. (c) IL-4

Ref: Robbin's Pathology, 9th ed. pg. 204

- Asthma is a chronic allergic inflammatory disease, the initiation and progression of which is dependent on the cytokines interleukin IL-4 and IL-13 acting through related receptor complexes.
- Disease pathogenesis is affected by intracellular signaling pathways that couple primarily to specific motifs within the intracellular domain of the IL-4 receptor alpha chain, a subunit that is common to the IL-4 and IL-13 receptor complexes.

MICROBIOLOGY AND PARASITOLOGY

6

MOST RECENT QUESTIONS 2023

1. **A patient presented with infective endocarditis 6 months after prosthetic valve implantation. What may be the etiological agent?** ***(Most Recent Question July 2023)***
   a. *Staphylococcus epidermidis*
   b. *Pseudomonas aeruginosa*
   c. *Streptococcus viridans*
   d. *Staphylococcus aureus*
2. **Patient developed diarrhea after seafood consumption. Organism exhibits Kanagawa phenomenon. Choose the correct etiological agent.** ***(Most Recent Question July 2023)***
   a. *Vibrio cholerae*
   b. *Vibrio parahaemolyticus*
   c. *E. coli*
   d. *C. jejuni*
3. **Farmer with traumatic ulcer in eye, septate hyphae seen in microscopy. Etiological agent is:** ***(Most Recent Question July 2023)***
   a. *Mucor*
   b. *Pseudomonas*
   c. *Staphylococcus aureus*
   d. *Aspergillus*
4. **Patient with diarrhea, stool microscopy revealed pathogen exhibits falling leaf motility with four pairs of flagella. What is the causative agent?** ***(Most Recent Question July 2023)***
   a. *Giardia lamblia*
   b. *Entamoeba histolytica*
   c. *Balantidium coli*
   d. *E. coli*
5. **A neonate is admitted with the features of meningitis. Bacteria isolated from cerebrospinal fluid (CSF) is bacitracin-resistant. Choose the correct pathogen.** ***(Most Recent Question July 2023)***
   a. GBS   b. GAS
   c. *Listeria*   d. *E. coli*
6. **Corneal scraping obtained from a patient presented with hydrophobia. Choose the best test:** ***(Most Recent Question July 2023)***
   a. RT-PCR
   b. Serum viral load
   c. Antibody detection by ELISA
   d. Antigen detection by ELISA
7. **All the following associated with exotoxins; except:** ***(Most Recent Question July 2023)***
   a. HUS
   b. Toxic shock syndrome
   c. Meningitis
   d. Pseudomembranous colitis
8. **Pencil-shaped macroconidia are seen in:** ***(Most Recent Question July 2023)***
   a. *Trichophyton*   b. *Microsporum*
   c. *Epidermophyton*   d. *Aspergillus*
9. **Which of the following antibodies/immunoglobulins are found in the highest concentration in blood/serum?** ***(Most Recent Question Jan 2023)***
   a. IgA   b. IgG
   c. IgM   d. IgD
10. **The cells that participate in inflammation known as macrophages are known by what name in the liver:** ***(Most Recent Question Jan 2023)***
    a. Hofbauer cells   b. Kupffer cells
    c. Mesangial cells   d. Monocytes
11. **Rheumatoid arthritis occurs due to:** ***(Most Recent Question Jan 2023)***
    a. Type 2 hypersensitivity
    b. Autoimmunity
    c. Type 1 hypersensitivity
    d. Immunodeficiency
12. **A patient develops runny nose, wheezing several times a year. These features are due to degranulation of which of the following?** ***(Most Recent Question Jan 2023)***
    a. Neutrophils   b. Monocytes
    c. Mast cells   d. Eosinophils

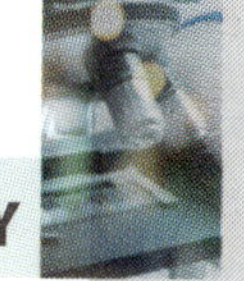

13. A person who met with a road traffic accident recently had undergone grafting using patient's own tissue as shown in the image. Identify the graft from the following list: ***(Most Recent Question Jan 2023)***

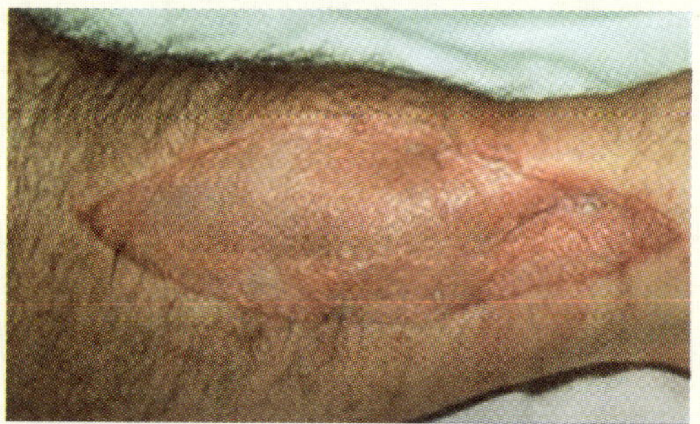

a. Autograft
b. Allograft
c. Xenograft
d. Isograft

14. Tzanck smear as shown in the image is used in the diagnosis of: ***(Most Recent Question Jan 2023)***

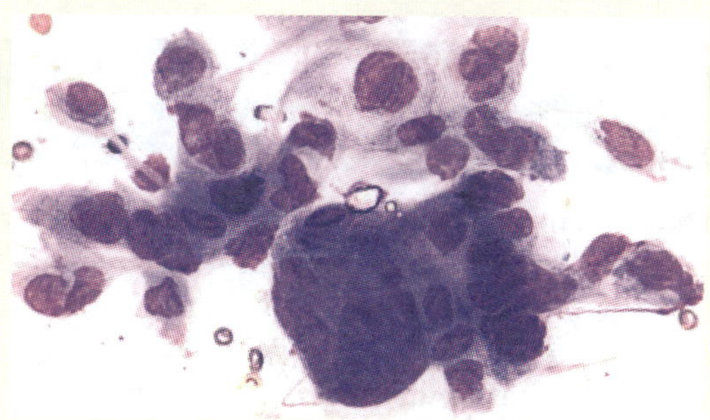

a. HIV
b. HPV
c. HDV
d. HSV

15. A patient presented with painful blisters on the trunk involving a dermatome as shown in the image. What is the most likely organism implicated in causing it? ***(Most Recent Question Jan 2023)***

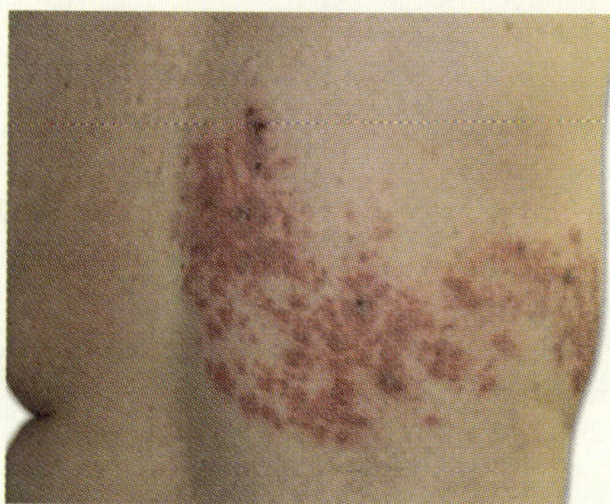

a. Chicken pox
b. Measles
c. Molluscum contagiosum
d. Varicella zoster

16. Inclusion body of a virus is shown in the image. It is indicative of which of the following infections? ***(Most Recent Question Jan 2023)***

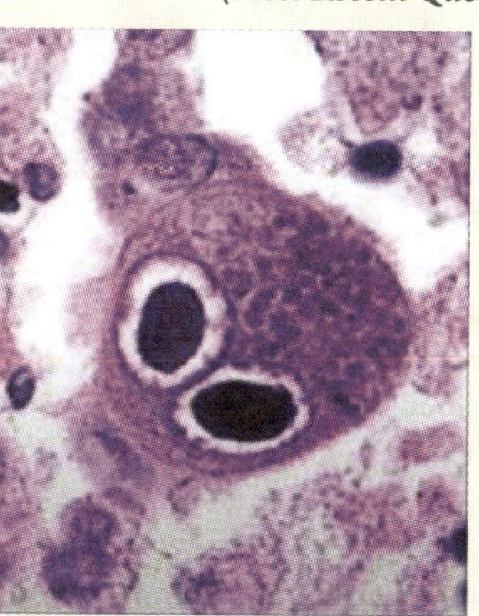

a. Measles virus
b. Rabies virus
c. Cytomegalovirus
d. Herpes virus

17. A patient presents with GI distress, on inquiry patient informed he usually eats food outside. Which of the following hepatitis can develop following this? ***(Most Recent Question Jan 2023)***

a. Hepatitis A
b. Hepatitis B
c. Hepatitis C
d. Hepatitis D

18. A child presented with maculopapular rash that begins behind the ears then spreads to face and rest of the body. History revealed fever, conjunctivitis and runny nose that developed few days back. Most likely diagnosis is: ***(Most Recent Question Jan 2023)***

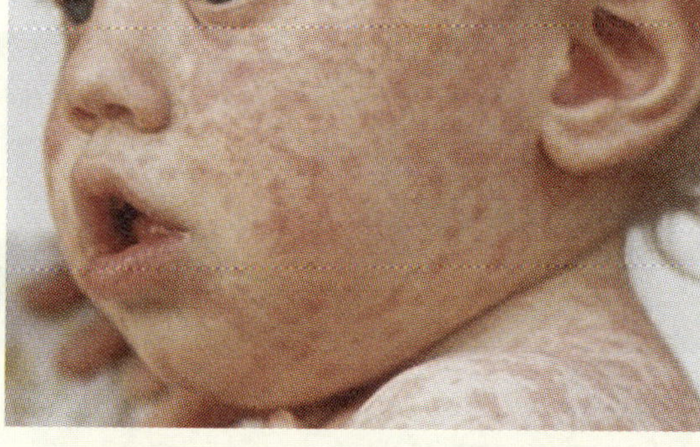

a. Exanthema subitum
b. Chicken pox
c. Measles
d. Erythema infectiosum

19. Which of the following dimorphic fungus can cause subcutaneous infection? ***(Most Recent Question Jan 2023)***

a. *Histoplasma capsulatum*
b. *Paracoccidioides brasiliensis*
c. *Sporothrix schenckii*
d. *Coccidioides immitis*

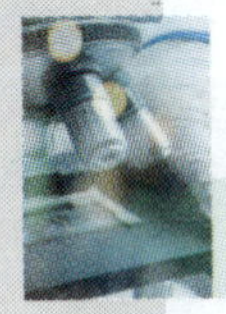

20. A forest worker recently had a trauma following which he is presented with a verrucous growth on the feet. Which of the following is the most likely infection? *(Most Recent Question Jan 2023)*

a. Mycetoma
b. Botryomycosis
c. Sporotrichosis
d. Chromoblastomycosis

21. A female is presented with foul-smelling vaginal discharge. Wet mount was prepared and the microscopy of the discharge reveals motile trophozoites. What is the most likely infection? *(Most Recent Question Jan 2023)*

a. Bacterial vaginosis
b. Vulvovaginal candidiasis
c. Trichomoniasis
d. Chlamydia

22. Which of the following parasite that takes entry through feet? *(Most Recent Question Jan 2023)*

a. *Enterobius*
b. *Strongyloides*
c. *Ascaris*
d. *Trichuris*

23. An unconscious patient is found to have fever, sweating and severe paleness. What is the most likely diagnosis of the presentation? *(Most Recent Question Jan 2023)*

a. Encephalitis
b. Pyogenic meningitis
c. TB meningitis
d. Cerebral malaria

24. An adult male who is a truck driver having multiple sexual partners presented with a painless ulcer on genitalia. What is the investigation to be performed? *(Most Recent Question Jan 2023)*

a. Gram stain
b. Dark-field microscopy
c. Whiff test
d. p24 antigen test

25. A truck driver with past history of genital ulcers is presented with the following lesion as shown in the image. What is the most likely diagnosis? *(Most Recent Question Jan 2023)*

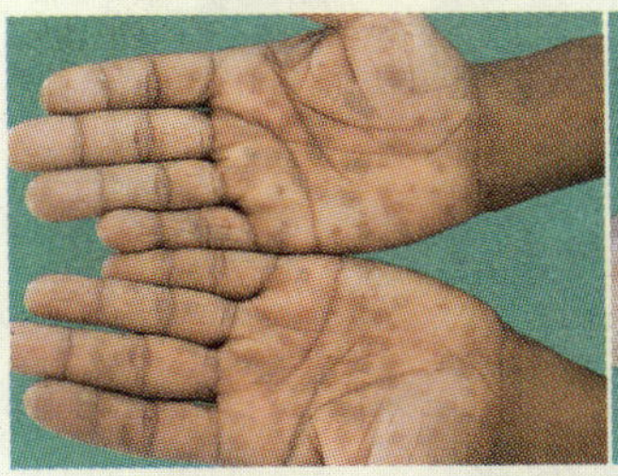
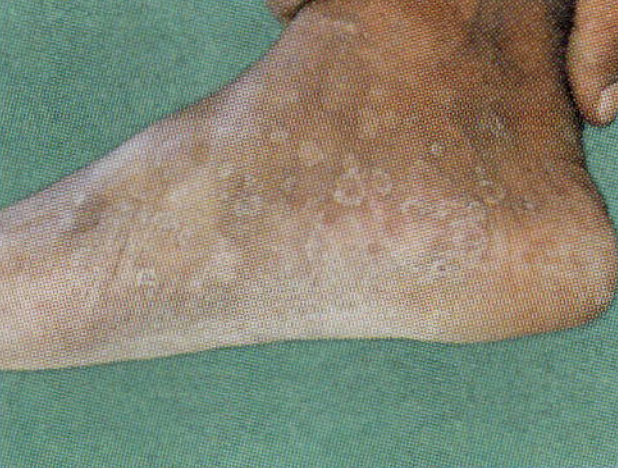

a. Primary syphilis
b. Secondary syphilis
c. Hand-foot-mouth disease
d. Kawasaki disease

26. A male working in a cattle farm is presented with a skin lesion on the forearm. Gram stain of the causative agent showed purple brick-shaped organisms with spores in the center. Which is the most likely agent? *(Most Recent Question Jan 2023)*

a. *Brucella abortus*
b. *Pseudomonas aeruginosa*
c. *Bacillus anthracis*
d. *Clostridium perfringens*

27. A chronic smoker presents with high fever cough, confusion and diarrhea. CXR reveals bilateral lung infiltrates. A sputum sample was collected and Gram stain reveals gram-ve organism. Which is the most likely agent? *(Most Recent Question Jan 2023)*

a. *Mycoplasma pneumoniae*
b. *Klebsiella pneumoniae*
c. *Legionella pneumophila*
d. *Streptococcus pneumoniae*

28. Culture media that is helpful in differentiating lactose fermenters vs. non-lactose fermenters: *(Most Recent Question Jan 2023)*

a. MacConkey's agar
b. Chocolate agar
c. Blood agar
d. Potassium tellurite agar

29. Which of the following agent is used in plasma sterilization? *(Most Recent Question Jan 2023)*

a. Ethylene oxide
b. Vaporized H_2O_2
c. Aldehydes
d. Glutaraldehyde

GENERAL MICROBIOLOGY, MEDIA, TESTING

30. Which organism cannot be grown on an artificial culture media? *(Most Recent Question June 2022)*

a. S. aureus
b. M. tuberculosis
c. M. leprae
d. Strep. Pneumonia

31. Which of the following is used in blood spillage? *(Most Recent Question June 2022)*

a. Isopropyl alcohol
b. Phenol
c. Sodium hypochlorite
d. Hydrogen peroxide

32. Cotton swabs are discarded in which bin? *(Most Recent Question June/Dec 2021)*

a. Red
b. Yellow
c. Blue
d. Black

33. Mode of transmission to bacteria through bacteriophage is by? *(Most Recent Question Dec 2020)*

a. Transformation
b. Transduction
c. Translation
d. Conjugation

34. A bacterium which can sustain 80°C is classified as: *(Most Recent Question Aug 2020)*

a. Thermophilic
b. Mesophilic
c. Cycrophilic
d. Halophilic

35. DNA transfer in bacteria via phage is: *(Recent Pattern Question 2018-19)*

a. Conjugation
b. Transduction
c. Transformation
d. Translation

36. Sporulation occurs in this phase of bacterial growth curve: *(Recent Pattern Question 2018-19)*

a. Stationary phase
b. Lag phase
c. Log phase
d. Decline phase

37. Glutaraldehyde is used for all of the following; EXCEPT: *(Recent Pattern Question 2018)*

a. Bronchoscope b. Thermometer
c. Proctoscopes d. Endoscopic tubes

38. Most potent disinfectant: *(Recent Pattern Question 2018)*

a. 70% alcohol b. Glutaraldehyde
c. Povidone-iodine d. Sodium hypochlorite

39. Sporulation is seen in which phase of bacterial growth phase? *(Recent Pattern Question 2017)*

a. Lag phase b. Log phase
c. Stationary phase d. Decline phase

40. Cold sterilization is done by: *(Recent Pattern Question 2017)*

a. Steam b. Ionizing radiation
c. Infra red d. UV

41. Metachromatic granules can be stained by: *(Recent Pattern Question 2016)*

a. Albert stain b. Gram stain
c. Gram-negative stain d. Prussian blue

42. Most important limitation/drawback of Tuberculin test is: *(Recent Pattern Question 2016)*

a. False negative cases
b. Can't differentiate between latent and active TB
c. Does not differentiate between primary TB and miliary TB
d. Can't screen the latent TB

43. Lysogenic conversion is *(Recent Pattern Question 2016)*

a. Integration of host bacterial nucleic acid to phage
b. Integration of phage nucleic acid to host bacteria genome
c. Bacterial mechanism to cause antigenic shift
d. Bacterial method to acquire resistance

44. Mesophilic organism grows at: *(Recent Pattern Question 2016)*

a. –20 to 7°C b. 10 to 20°C
c. 25 to 40°C d. 55 to 80°C

45. Yellow bag is destroyed by: *(Recent Pattern Question 2016)*

a. Incineration b. Autoclave
c. Hot air oven d. Steam sterilization

46. Incineration is done for: *(Recent Pattern Question 2016)*

a. Human body parts b. Syringes
c. Body fluids d. Gloves

47. Grease, dusting powder and paraffin are sterilized by: *(Recent Pattern Question 2016)*

a. Gamma radiation b. Sunlight
c. Dry heat sterilization d. Autoclave

48. Gram Stain is a:

a. Simple stain b. Differential stain
c. Negative stain d. None of these

49. Method of choice for sterilization of liquid paraffin:

a. Flaming b. Moist heat
c. Autoclave d. Hot air oven

50. Hot air oven efficiency is best checked by which bacteria:

a. Stearothermophillus b. Bacillus subtilis
c. Clostridium tetani d. Streptococcus

51. Prion is best destroyed by

a. Autoclaving at 135 degrees
b. Hot air oven at 160 degrees
c. Hydrogen peroxide
d. Sodium hypochlorite

52. Which of the following culture medium is made by adding Agar:

a. Solid medium b. Liquid medium
c. Selective medium d. Transport medium

53. Agar is added to Broth medium:

a. To make the medium liquid
b. To make the medium solid
c. To provide extra nutrition to grow
d. None of the above

54. Which of the following bacteria is isolated with Cetrimide agar?

a. Clostridium perfringens
b. Clostridium tetani
c. Pseudomonas aeruginosa
d. E. coli

55. Thayer martin agar medium is for:

a. N. Meningitis b. Pseudomonas
c. Clostridium d. Trypanoma pallidum

56. Which of the following is best for diagnosing genital TB?

a. PCR b. Montoux
c. LJ medium d. ZN staining

57. In Robertson cooked meat media, meat color will change to:

a. Pink b. Red
c. Blue d. No color change

58. Mac Conkey medium is an example of:

a. Selective media b. Differential media
c. Enriched media d. Transport media

59. All of the following are examples of Indicator media; EXCEPT:

a. Blood agar b. Eosin methylene blue
c. MacConkey d. Stuart media

60. Stain used in preparation of AFB smear:

a. Giemsa stain b. Loeffler's stain
c. Ziehl-Neelson stain d. India ink stain

61. Weil Felix reaction is what type of agglutination reaction:

a. Slide agglutination b. Tube agglutination
c. Passive agglutination d. Direct agglutination

62. Which of the following is an example of precipitation reaction:

a. Coomb's Test
b. Counter current immune-electrophoresis
c. Weil-Felix Test
d. Widal Test

63. Which of the following test is an example of tube agglutination test:
- a. Blood grouping
- b. Vibrio cholera serotyping
- c. Widal test
- d. ANA

64. In prokaryotes, which of the following is present:
- a. Nucleolus
- b. ER
- c. Golgi bodies
- d. Muramic acid

65. Lancefield classification is done on the basis of:
- a. C -substance
- b. Glycoprotein O
- c. Muramic acid
- d. Antibiotic resistance

66. Which of the following protein is attached to surface of bacteria and phagocytized?
- a. Antigen
- b. Antibody
- c. C-Reactive protein
- d. Propendin

67. All of the following methods are used for the diagnosis of HIV infection in a 2 month old child; EXCEPT:
- a. DNA PCR
- b. Viral culture
- c. HIV Elisa
- d. P24 antigen assay

68. Paul Bunnel test is used for diagnosis of:
- a. Chicken pox
- b. Yellow fever
- c. Genital Herpes
- d. Infectious mononucleosis

BACTERIOLOGY

69. Cat scratch disease is caused by: ***(Most Recent Question June 2022)***
- a. Bartonella henselae
- b. Toxoplamosis
- c. B. Quintana
- d. B. Bacilliformis

70. A patient comes to the emergency with history of IV drug abuse and developed infection. Which of the following is the most likely cause? ***(Most Recent Question June 2022)***
- a. Strep. Viridians
- b. S. Aureus
- c. E. coli
- d. Enterobacterium faeca

71. Which of the following is the causative agent for the given clinical picture? ***(Most Recent Question June 2022)***

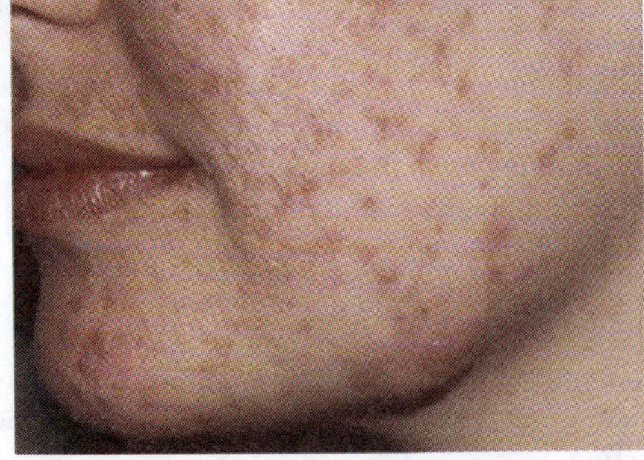

- a. Propionibacterium acne
- b. Actinomyces
- c. Fifidobacterium
- d. Mobiluncus

72. A patient came to the emergency complaining of fever, neck rigidity and pain since night. Analysis showed elevated protein. Identify the diagnosis? ***(Most Recent Question June 2022)***
- a. Bacterial meningitis
- b. TB meningitis
- c. Viral meningitis
- d. Fungal meningitis

73. A patient presented with multiple episodes of bloody diarrhea. On investigations of blood sample enterochemorrhagic strain of *E. coli* was isolated. On which of the following media this organism can be cultured? ***(Most Recent Question June/Dec 2021)***
- a. TCBS
- b. Selenite F broth
- c. Flobertson cooked mead media
- d. Sorbitol MacConkey agar

74. Tumbling motility is seen in: ***(Most Recent Question June/Dec 2021)***
- a. Vibrio
- b. Listeria
- c. Proteus
- d. Treponema pallidum

75. Gram positive alpha hemolytic cocci with catalase negative and optochin resistant causing endocarditis? ***(Most Recent Question June/Dec 2021)***
- a. Streptococcus pneumoniae
- b. Streptococcus agalactiae
- c. Staphylococcus epidermidis
- d. Streptococcus sanguis

76. A child presented with complaint of dysphagia, cough, and greyish white membrane over the tonsils. Which of the following is causative organism? ***(Most Recent Question June/Dec 2021)***

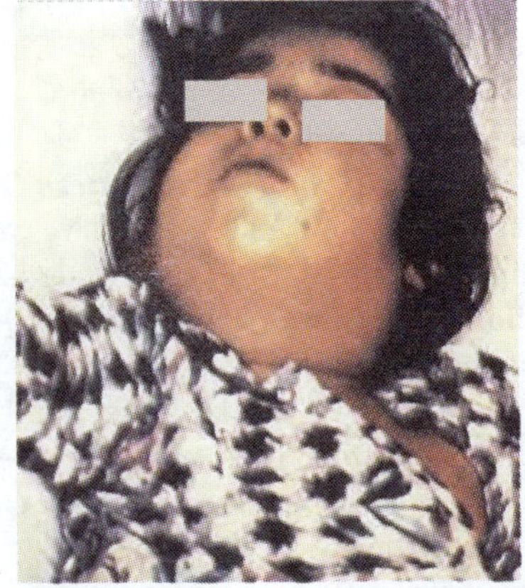

- a. Clostridium
- b. C. diphtheria
- c. Candida
- d. Pneumococcus

77. Cost effective method to test for syphilis in village with poor resource? ***(Most Recent Question June/Dec 2021)***
- a. Dark field
- b. Immunofluorescence
- c. Culture
- d. Simple microscopy

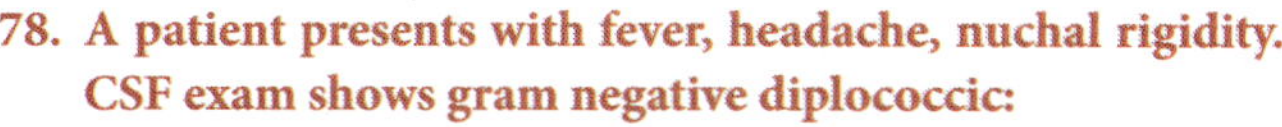

78. A patient presents with fever, headache, nuchal rigidity. CSF exam shows gram negative diplococcic:
(Most Recent Question June/Dec 2021)

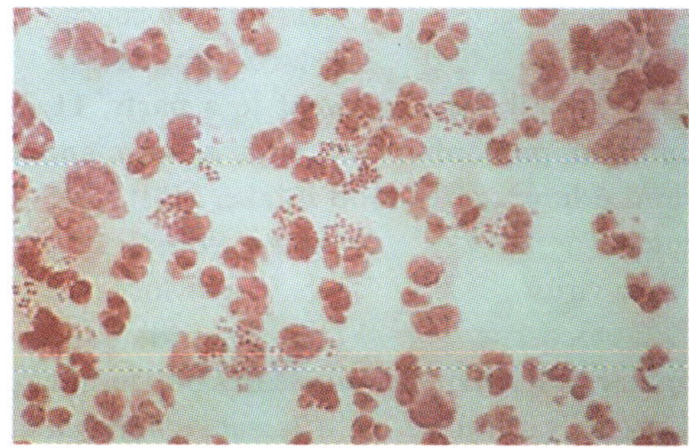

a. Neisseria meningitis
b. Streptococcus pneumoniae
c. Haemophilus influenzae
d. Staphylococcus aureus

79. A 5-year-old child presents with fever, respiratory distress, inspiratory stridor. Thumb- print sign is noted on radiography. What is the most common agent causing the problem: ***(Most Recent Question June/Dec 2021)***

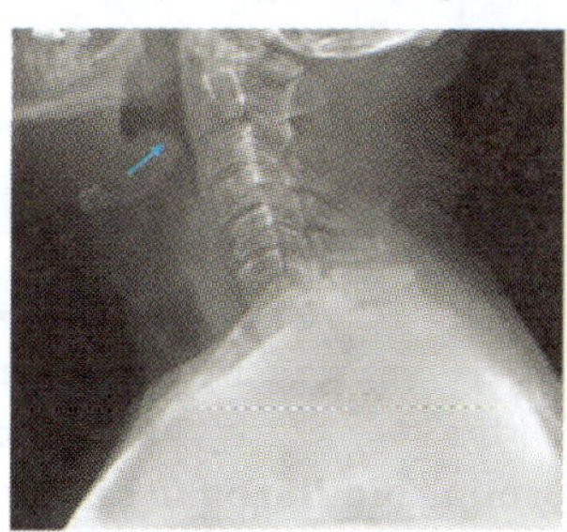

a. Streptococcus pneumoniae
b. Haemophilus influenzae B
c. Parainfluenza virus
d. Staphylococcus aureus

80. Which of the following doesn't form membrane:
(Most Recent Question June/Dec 2021)

a. Diphtheria b. Infectious mononucleosis
c. Ludwig's angina d. Staphylococcus aureus

81. A patient presents with fever, prostration and rash on extremities. Which of the following is the etiological agent? ***(Most Recent Question Dec 2020)***

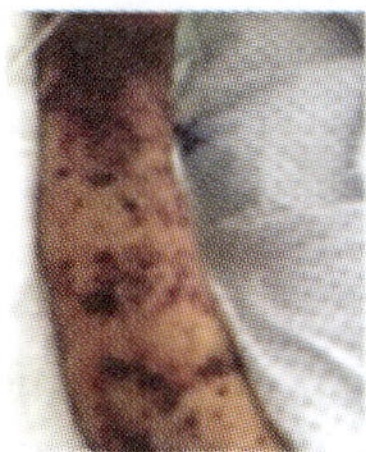

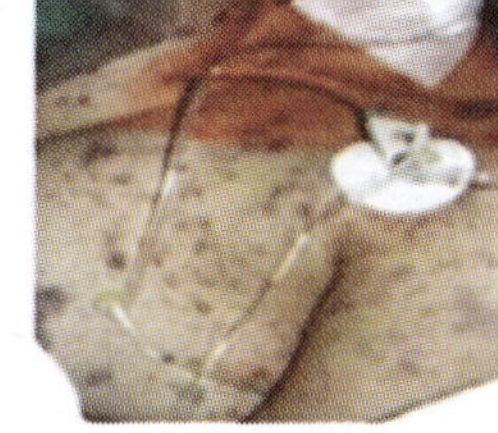

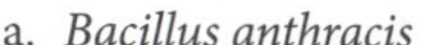

a. *Bacillus anthracis* b. *N. meningitidis*
c. *Francisella tularensis* d. *Moraxella catarrhalis*

82. Identify the given non spore forming bacteria?
(Most Recent Question Dec 2020)

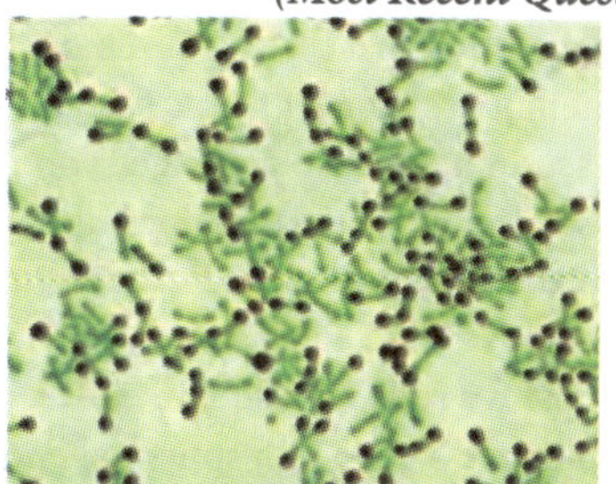

a. Clostridium difficile b. Clostridium perfringens
c. Clostridium tetani
d. Corynebacterium diphtheria

83. A patient presents with following findings. What will be the media used to diagnose this condition?
(Most Recent Question Aug 2020)

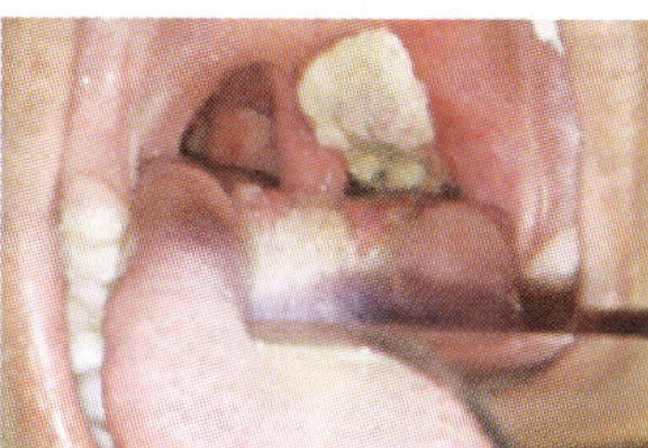

a. Loffler's serum slope b. Lowenstein Jensen
c. Cary blair d. Chocolate agar

84. A 45-year-old patient who was recently got denture fixed, presented with following lesions that bleed on scraping. Causative agent for this condition?
(Most Recent Question Aug 2020)

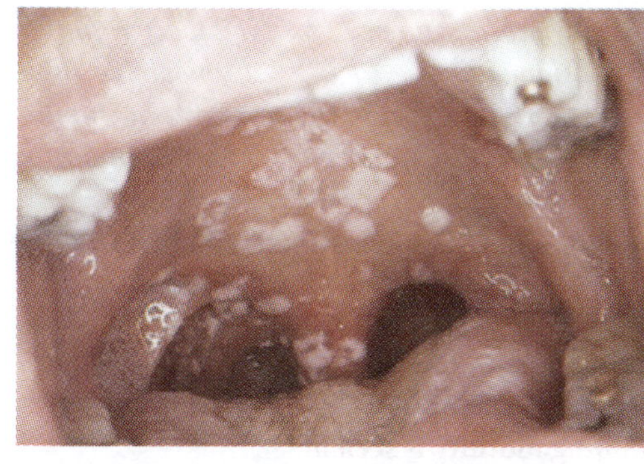

a. Diphtheria b. Candida
c. Strep mutans d. Staph aureus

85. Bacterial vaginosis is caused by all; EXCEPT:
(Most Recent Question Aug 2020)

a. Gardenerella b. Mobilincus
c. Proteus d. Coccobacillus

86. The causative agent for duodenal ulcer is:
(Most Recent Question Aug 2020)

a. *Shigella* b. *E. coli*
c. *H. pylori* d. *Lactobacilli*

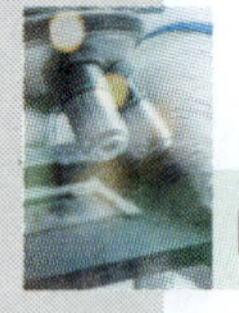

87. Which is correct about Diptheria membrane? *(Recent Pattern Question 2019)*
a. Grey membrane that bleeds on removal
b. Grey membrane that does not bleed on removal
c. Grey pseudomembrane that bleeds on removal
d. Grey pseudomembrane that does not bleed on removal

88. Bacillus Anthrax is: *(Recent Pattern Question 2018-19)*
a. Gram positive cocci in cluster
b. Gram positive rods with square ends
c. Gram positive bacilli with spherical ends
d. Gram negative cocci in cluster

89. Which of the following is the most likely cause in a case of granuloma with positive AFB? *(Recent Pattern Question 2018-19)*
a. Cat scratch disease b. Trench fever
c. Leprosy d. Syphilis

90. Legionnaire disease causes? *(Recent Pattern Question 2018-19)*
a. Respiratory disease b. U.T.I
c. Retroperitoneal fibrosis d. Acute gastroenteritis

91. When should you perform Widal test in a case of Typhoid? *(Recent Pattern Question 2018-19)*
a. 1st week b. 2nd week
c. 3rd week d. 4th week

92. Which of the following is anaerobic non-acid fast bacilli? *(Recent Pattern Question 2018)*
a. Tuberculosis b. Listeria
c. Nocardia d. Actinomyces

93. Which of the following is a capnophilic bacteria? *(Recent Pattern Question 2018)*
a. *Staphylococcus aureus* b. *Mycobacterium*
c. *Clostridium* d. *Haemophilus influenzae*

94. Anton test is done for: *(Recent Pattern Question 2017)*
a. Klebsiella b. Listeria monocytogenes
c. Proteus mirabilis d. Nisseria

95. Diphtheria toxin acts by: *(Recent Pattern Question 2017)*
a. Inhibiting glucose synthesis
b. Inhibiting protein synthesis
c. Promoting acetylcholine release
d. Altering cyclic GMP levels

96. Tumbling motility is seen in: *(Recent Pattern Question 2017)*
a. Listeria monocytogenes b. C. Jejuni
c. Trichomonas d. Gonococcus

97. "Fish in stream" appearance is seen in? *(Recent Pattern Question 2017)*
a. Hemophilus ducreyi b. Proteus
c. Mycoplasma d. V. Cholerae

98. Pontiac fever is caused by? *(Recent Pattern Question 2017)*
a. Rickettsia rickettsii b. Brucella
c. Legionella d. Moraxella

99. A 30-year-old patient presented with fever, headache and vomiting. He had splenectomy few years ago. Most probable organism? *(Recent Pattern Question 2017)*
a. Meningococcus b. Pneumococcus
c. E. Coli d. C. Diptheriae

100. Out of 20 children that went to a party, 11 developed abdominal pain, diarrhea with nausea and vomiting around 6 hours after food intake. Most likely causative agent: *(Recent Pattern Question 2017)*
a. Rota virus b. Staphylococcus
c. Streptococcus d. Clostridium perfringens

101. Secondary bacterial pneumonia in a post-influenza patient is most likely due to? *(Recent Pattern Question 2017)*
a. Staphylococcus aureus b. Moraxella
c. Listeria d. Klebsiella

102. Corynebacterium diphtheria is *(Recent Pattern Question 2016)*
a. Gram-positive cocci b. Gram-positive bacilli
c. Gram-negative cocci d. Gram-negative bacilli

103. Which of the following is the most severe form of Diptheria *(Recent Pattern Question 2016)*
a. Nasal
b. Cutaneous
c. Nasophyranx
d. Laryngophyranx

104. McFadyean reaction is seen in: *(Recent Pattern Question 2016)*
a. Yersinia pestis b. Clostridium perfringens
c. Bacillus anthrax d. Staphylococcus aureus

105. Organism forming biofilm on in catheter? *(Recent Pattern Question 2016)*
a. Staph epidermis b. Acinetobacter baumannii
c. Meningococci d. Mycobacterium

106. Staph. epidermis has become important due to *(Recent Pattern Question 2016)*
a. Biofilm formation
b. Virulence
c. Wide spectrum antibiotics
d. Novobiocin resistance

107. During examination of skin smears in leprosy test result was 1+ to 2+. How many oil fields should be surveyed *(Recent Pattern Question 2016)*
a. 10 b. 25
c. 50 d. 100

108. In an oil immersion field 1-10 acid fast bacilli were seen per 10 field. It indicates *(Recent Pattern Question 2016)*
a. + b. ++
c. +++ d. Scanty

109. Which disease occurs after eating uncooked meat *(Recent Pattern Question 2016)*
a. Bacillus anthrax b. Brucella
c. Trichosis d. TB

110. Yersinia pestis is transmitted by:
a. Flea *(Recent Pattern Question 2016)*
b. Rodent
c. Mite
d. Sandfly

111. Gram negative anaerobic bacteria use this method of gene transfer:
a. Transduction b. Conjugation
c. Translation d. Transformation

112. Method of bacterial gene transfer where viruses play role:
a. Transduction b. Conjugation
c. Translation d. Transformation

113. During the lag phase of bacterial growth curve, there is:
a. Increase in number b. Increase in metabolic rate
c. Increase in size d. Decreased metabolic rate

114. CLO test is done for:
a. HPV b. Salmonella typhi
c. HIV d. H. pylori

115. Tumbling motility is seen in:
a. Yersinia b. Listeria
c. Proteus d. Pseudomonas aeruginosa

116. Which of the following is a kidney shaped bacteria:
a. Campylobacter jejuni
b. Corynebacterium Diphtheriae
c. Meningococci
d. Gonococci

117. Granuloma in lymph nodes seen is in all infections; EXCEPT:
a. TB b. Sarcoidosis
c. Staph Aureus d. Hemophilus ducreyi

118. Which of the following organisms causes fastest food poisoning:
a. Staph. Aureus b. Clostridium Perfringens
c. Bacillus Cereus d. Vibrio cholerae

119. A Person ate some milk products in a party and after 6 hours started vomiting. Which organism is most likely the cause:
a. Bacillus cereus b. Clostridium perfringens
c. Staphylococcus d. Clostridium botulism

120. Food poisoning 2 hours after intake of food is caused by?
a. Salmonella typhi
b. Bacillus cereus
c. Staphylococcus aureus
d. Clostridium

121. How does staph aureus become resistant to methicillin:
a. Heat shock protein
b. Protein A
c. Transpeptidase
d. Protein C

122. Organism responsible for toxicity due to Chinese fried rice:
a. Staph. Aureus b. B. Cereus
c. Salmonella d. Shigella

123. The following are true about Bacillus Cereus induced diarrhea; EXCEPT
a. Can be transmitted by parenteral route
b. The enterotoxins are not resistant to acidic contents of the stomach
c. It is caused by enterotoxins
d. It is usually associated with fried rice or chinese food which is reheated

124. Incubation period of salmonella:
a. 7–21 days b. 2–5 days
c. 14–21 days d. 0–60 days

125. Rice watery stool is a common indicative of which organism?
a. Vibrio cholerae O1
b. Vibrio cholerae O139
c. Vibrio vulnificus
d. Shigella

126. Which of the following is most likely cause of a child presenting with fever and diarrhea?
a. EPEC b. ETEC
c. EHEC d. EIEC

127. Which organism causes haemolytic uremic syndrome?
a. Neisseria b. Salmonella
c. Pseudomonas d. E. coli

128. HUS is caused by:
a. EIEC b. EPEC
c. ETEC d. EHEC

129. Traveller's diarrhea is caused by:
a. EIEC b. EPEC
c. ETEC d. EHEC

130. Anti-microbials are given with which type of diarrhea:
a. Traveller's diarrhea b. Rotavirus
c. Secretory diarrhea d. Osmotic diarrhea

131. Which is the staphyloccocal toxin which is responsible for food poisoning?
a. Beta Exotoxin
b. Enterotoxin
c. Alpha Exotoxin
d. Toxic Shock Syndrome Toxin (TSST-1)

132. Which of the following contains single flagella?
a. Treponema Pallidum b. Escherichia Coli
c. Vibrio cholerae d. Heliobacter Pylori

133. Clostridium difficile can be spread through all; EXCEPT:
a. Oral - fecal route b. Direct
c. Hand to hand contact d. Needles

134. All of the following organisms cause gas gangrene; EXCEPT:
a. Clostridium Difficile b. Clostridium Welchi
c. Clostridium Septicum d. Clostridium Perfringens

135. Necrotizing enteritis is caused by:
a. Clostridium tetani b. Clostridium difficile
c. Clostridium perfringens d. Clostridium septicum

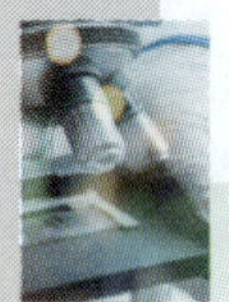

136. Gas gangrene is caused by:
a. Clostridium perfringens b. Bacillus cereus
c. Helicobater pylori d. Treponema pallidum

137. Fournier gangrene is caused by:
a. Cl. Welchi b. Proteus
c. Streptococcus d. Mixed infection

138. Anchovy Sauce pus/chocolate brown pus is the clinical feature of:
a. Amoebic liver abscess b. Pyogenic liver abscess
c. Peritoneal abscess d. Hydatid liver

139. A patient presents with signs of pneumonia. The bacterium obtained from sputum was a Gram positive cocci which showed alpha hemolysis on sheep agar. Which of the following test will help to confirm the diagnosis:
a. Bile solubility b. Coagulase test
c. Bacitracin test d. CAMP test

140. Energy store of cell is:
a. Adenosine monophosphate
b. Adenosine diphosphate
c. Adenosine triphosphate
d. Adenosine quadriphosphate

141. Most common cause of Pneumatocele:
a. Streptococcus pneumoniae
b. Haemophilus influenza
c. Serratia marcescens
d. Staphylococcus aureus

142. Child presented with cystic fibrosis and Bronchorrhea. Which group of organism is appropriate causative agent:
a. Staph. Aureus, H. influenza, Pseudomonas
b. Streptococcus pneumonia, Klebsiella, H. Influenza
c. H.Influenza, Klebsiella, staph aureus
d. Strep.Pneumoniae, H.Influenza, Klebsiella

143. Streptococcus pyogenes can be checked by which drug disc diffusion method?
a. Bacitracin b. Polymycin
c. Optochin d. None of these

144. Chronic burrowing ulcer is caused by:
a. Peptostreptococcus
b. Strep.pyogenes
c. Anaerobic streptococci
d. Microaerophilic streptococci

145. Which of the following is common with Streptococcus infection?
a. Cellulitis b. Gangrene
c. Pyoderma d. UTI

146. All are true about Entamoeba Histolytica; EXCEPT:
a. Cyst are 4 nucleated
b. Cyst are 8 nucleated
c. Trophozoites colonise in the colon and rectum
d. The chromatid bodies are stained by iron hematoxylin

147. Which of the following is a non motile bacteria?
a. Klebsiella pneumoniae b. Helicobacter pylori
c. Vibrio Cholerae d. E. coli

148. Miliary shadow on X-ray is seen in all; EXCEPT:
a. TB
b. Loeffler's pneumonia
c. Klebsiella
d. Varicella pneumonia

149. True about Bubonic plague:
a. An infection of the lung
b. An infection of blood stream
c. An infection of lymph nodes
d. All of the above

150. Site where Neisseria Meningitidis bacteria harbour normally?
a. Skin b. Genitals
c. Nasopharynx d. Lower GIT

151. Which of the following is gram negative diplococci:
a. Cornynebacterium Diphtheriae
b. Neisseria Meningitidis
c. Streptococcus pneumoniae
d. Staphylococcus

152. Neisseria meningitidis possesses following virulent factors; EXCEPT:
a. Capsule
b. Lipo-oligosaccharide(LOS)
c. β lactamase
d. IgA protease cation

153. Which one of the following microbe, found in ear discharge, has a high predilection for meningitis
a. H. influenza
b. Moraxella species
c. Staphylococcus aureus
d. Streptococcus pneumoniae

154. Which one of the following organisms is the most frequent cause of acute pyogenic meningitis in adults:
a. Streptococcus pneumoniae
b. Neisseria meningitis
c. Haemophilus influenza
d. Listeria monocytogenes

155. Meningococcal vaccine not used for:
a. Serotype A b. Serotype B
c. Serotype C d. Serotype Y

156. Air crescent sign seen in infection due to:
a. Staphylococcus b. Streptococcus
c. Diphtheria d. Aspergillus

157. Incubation period of diphtheria:
a. 2-3 days b. 5-7 days
c. 14-15 days d. 21 days

158. Calymmatobacterium is:
a. Gram negative b. Gram positive
c. Acid fast d. Non-acid fast

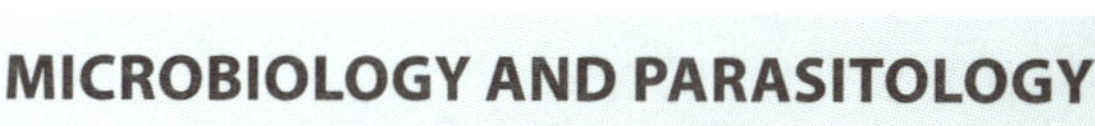

159. Prolonged salmonella septicemia is caused by:
a. S. Enteritidis
b. S. Typhimurium
c. S. Typhi
d. S. Cholerae-suis

160. Draughtsman appearance of colonies is seen with:
a. Streptococcus
b. Pneumococcus
c. Staphylococcus
d. Menngococcus

161. A 3-year-old boy fell down and injured his leg while he was playing on ground. After a few days, there is crepitus felt from injured area, what could be the probable causative organism?
a. Corynebacterium Diphtheriae
b. Pseudomonas Aeruginosa
c. Clostridium Tetani
d. Clostridium Welchii

162. Drum stick appearance is characteristic of:
a. Corynebacterium diphtheriae
b. Clostridium tetani
c. Neisseria meningitides
d. Strep Pneumoniae

163. Drugs indicated in MRSA infection are all; EXCEPT:
a. Vancomycin
b. Teicoplanin
c. Linezolid
d. Imipenem

164. True about Aspergillosis?
a. Angioinvasive
b. Oto-mycosis
c. Occur in asthmatics
d. All of these

165. Not a common cause of community acquired pneumonia; EXCEPT:
a. Staphylococci
b. Mycoplasma
c. Chlamydia pneumonia
d. Streptococci

166. Leptospirosis is caused by:
a. Dog urine
b. Mosquito
c. Rat urine
d. Cat urine

167. Blood culture of a patient shows growth of gram positive cocci which are catalase positive and coagulase negative. The patient was on a CVP line last week. The most likely etiological agent is?
a. Staphylococcus aureus
b. Staphylococcus epidermidis
c. Streptococcus pyogenes
d. Enterococcus faecalis

168. Which of the following parasite causes myocarditis?
a. Trichuris trichura
b. Ancyclostoma duodenale
c. Taenia solium
d. Trichenella spiralis

VIROLOGY

169. Which of the following is tested before blood transfusion? *(Most Recent Question June 2022)*
a. Hep B
b. Hep A
c. HIV/HIV2
d. Hep C

170. Reinfection with which of the following virus can lead to more severe disease with complications?
(Most Recent Question June/Dec 2021)
a. Dengue
b. Rabies
c. Measles
d. Mumps

171. HIV (Immunocompromised) patient presents with diarrhea. What is the most common causative organism: *(Most Recent Question June/Dec 2021)*

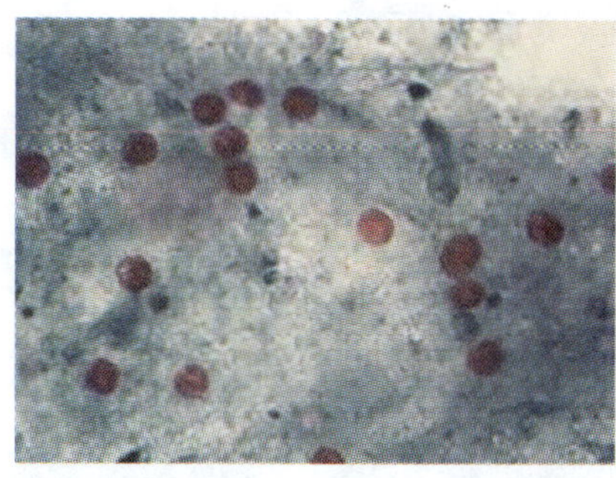

a. Cryptosporidium parvum
b. Rotavirus
c. Giardia lamblia
d. Adenovirus

172. Identify the organism
(Most Recent Question June/Dec 2021)

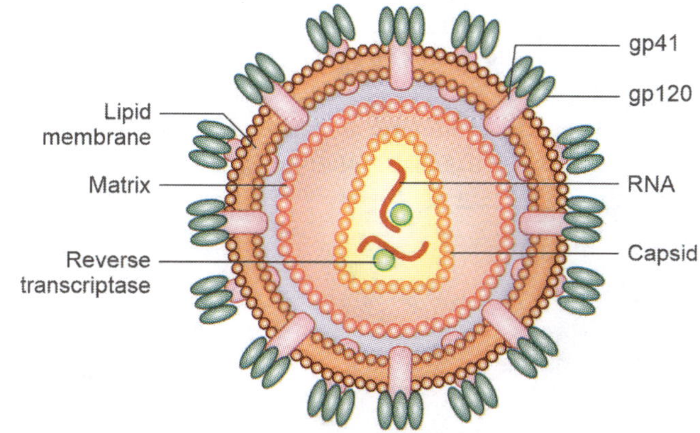

a. HIV
b. Herpes
c. Hepatitis B
d. Adenovirus

173. What is being amplified in RT-PCR for COVID-19?
(Most Recent Question Dec 2020)
a. DNA
b. RNA
c. MPO
d. Cytosolic proteins

174. A 5-year-old child came into OPD with fever, rashes on the body. There were rashes on the axilla and flexor surface with various macules, papules and vesicles. Rashes and blisters are in different stages and non-uniform. Most probable diagnosis?
(Most Recent Question Dec 2020)
a. Chicken pox
b. Smallpox
c. Epstein Barr virus
d. Measles

175. Child presents with sores in the mouth and a rash on the hands and feet as shown in the image below. What is the causative organism for it? *(Most Recent Question Dec 2020)*

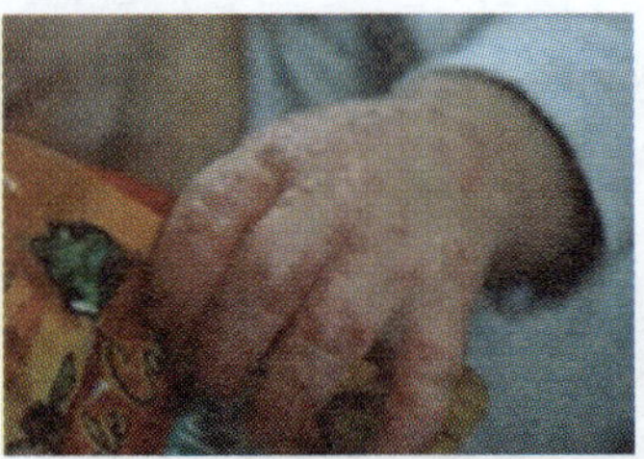
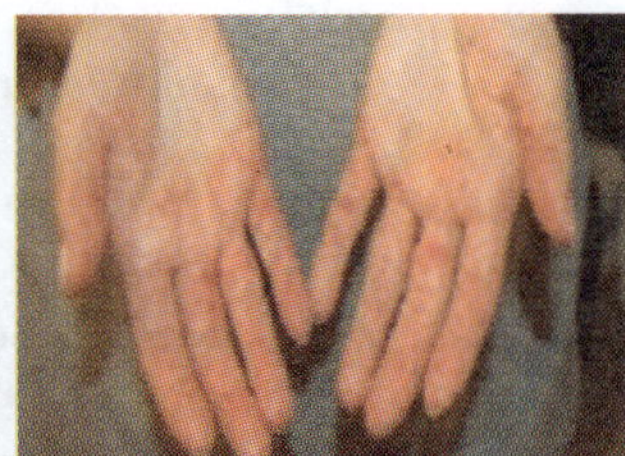
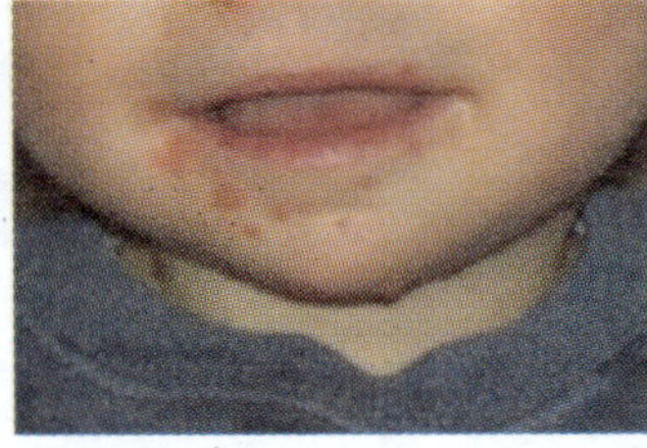
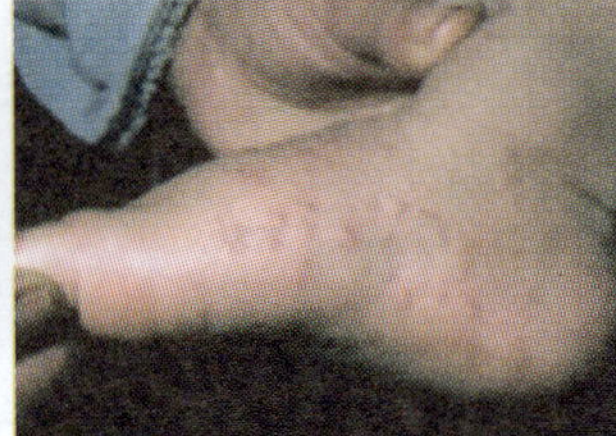

a. Coxsackievirus A16
b. Pox virus
c. Herpes virus
d. Human papilloma virus

176. Doctor working in ICU is complaining of loss of smell. Next best test to go for *(Most Recent Question Dec 2020)*

a. Nasopharyngeal swab for RT PCR
b. Rapid antigen test
c. IgM Antibody to SARS-Cov 2
d. CXR

177. Child presents with fever and pleomorphic rash as shown in the image. Diagnosis? *(Most Recent Question Aug 2020)*

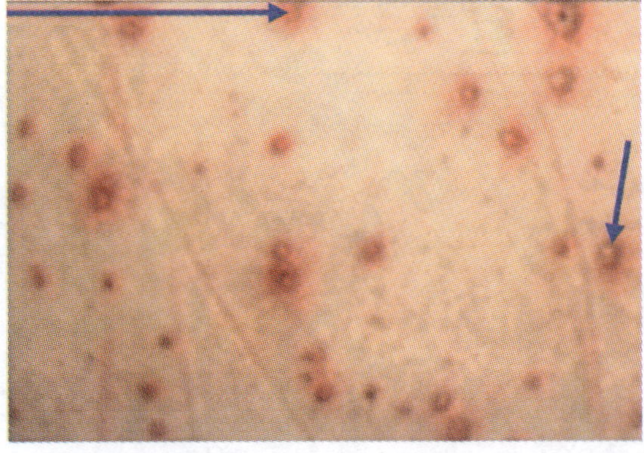

a. Chicken pox
b. Small pox
c. Measles
d. Rubella

178. A 5-year-old child presents with cough, runny nose and conjunctivitis. The physician notices small white lesion inside patient's mouth. Next day red rash started on face and then covered the trunk part of the body. What is the most likely diagnosis? *(Most Recent Question Aug 2020)*

a. Chicken pox
b. Small pox
c. Measles
d. Rubella

179. Identify the microorganism: *(Most Recent Question Aug 2020)*

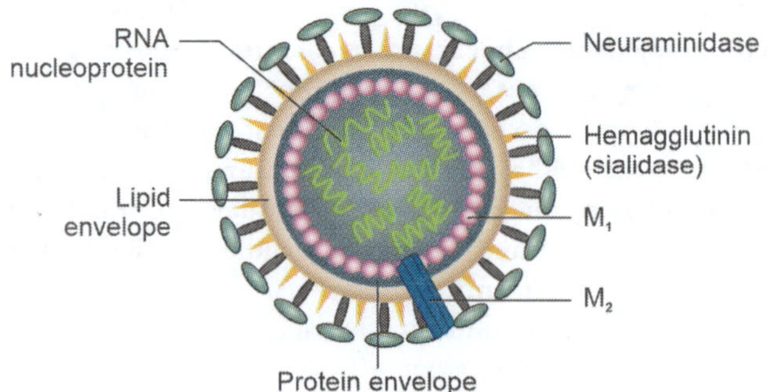

a. Influenza virus
b. Corona virus
c. Rheo virus
d. Rabies virus

180. Rapid diagnosis of rabies is made with: *(Recent Pattern Question 2018-19)*

a. Rabies virus specific antibodies
b. Inoculation in mouse
c. Skin biopsy with fluorescent antibody testing
d. Corneal impression smear

181. Most common infectious cause of haemolysis: *(Recent Pattern Question 2018-19)*

a. *E. coli* 0157
b. Malaria
c. Parvovirus B19
d. Bartonella henselae

182. Which of the following virus is from Herpes virus family? *(Recent Pattern Question 2018-19)*

a. Rubella
b. Measles
c. Rabies
d. EBV

183. Molluscum contagiosum is a ________________: *(Recent Pattern Question 2018-19)*

a. Adenovirus
b. Flavi virus
c. Rubi virus
d. Pox virus

184. Which of the following is an RNA virus? *(Recent Pattern Question 2017)*

a. Hepatitis B virus
b. Hepatitis C virus
c. Herpes virus
d. Adenovirus

185. Hand foot mouth disease is caused by: *(Recent Pattern Question 2017)*

a. Enterobius
b. Coxsackie
c. Adenovirus
d. Prion disease

186. Which is true about rota virus infection? *(Recent Pattern Question 2017)*

a. Vaccine preventable disease
b. Can be treated by saline infusion
c. Predominates in summer season
d. Has high mortality rate

187. Intracytoplasmic inclusion body is seen in: *(Recent Pattern Question 2017)*

a. HSV
b. Polio
c. Rabies
d. Yellow fever

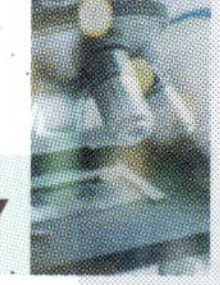

188. A patient presented with fever, cervical lymphadenopathy and night sweats four weeks after unprotected sexual contact. Next investigation: ***(Recent Pattern Question 2016)***

a. p24 b. ELISA
c. CD4 d. HIV PCR

189. m-RNA to C-DNA is made by

a. Reverse transcriptase b. DNA polymerase
c. RNA polymerase d. DNA Ligase

190. Intracytoplasmic and Intranuclear inclusion body is seen in:

a. Measles b. Mumps
c. Rabies d. Yellow fever

191. Intra nuclear inclusion body is exclusively seen in:

a. Rabies virus b. Pox virus
c. Measles virus d. Herpes virus

192. Which among the following disease is transmitted by virus:

a. Molluscum contagiosum b. Taenia capitis
c. Rhinosporodiosis d. Impetigo

193. Molluscum contagiosum is a:

a. Bacteria b. Fungus
c. Virus d. Parasite

194. Which of the following disease acts by Reverse transcriptase action:

a. HTLV- I b. HIV
c. Both A and B d. Hepatitis C

195. Hemagglutination is caused by which organism:

a. Influenza virus b. Mumps
c. Adenovirus d. Parvovirus

196. Which of the following is not caused by virus:

a. Rocky mountain spotted fever
b. KFD
c. Dengue
d. Yellow fever

197. Most common cause of common cold/coryza is?

a. Influenza virus b. Adenovirus
c. RSV d. Rhinovirus

198. Duffy antigen is a receptor for?

a. P. Falciparum b. P. Ovale
c. P. Vivax d. P. Malariae

199. Human papilloma virus is a:

a. RNA virus b. DNA virus
c. Both d. None of these

200. Jarisch Herxheimer (J-H) reaction is commonly seen in

a. Primary syphillis b. Secondary syphilis
c. Late congenital syphilis d. Latent syphilis

201. Intermediate host for Rabies is?

a. Human b. Rat
c. Dogs d. Cats

202. True about chicken pox:

a. Incubation period 2-3 days.
b. Vesicobullous rash
c. Vesicobullous rash
d. Spare palm & sole

MYCOLOGY AND PARASITOLOGY

203. A patient is presented with some unknown fungal infection. On H&E staining, there is presence of sclerotic bodies having a muriform cell appearance. Which is the possible condition? ***(Most Recent Question June 2022)***

a. Histoplasmosis
b. Chromoblastomycosis
c. Coccidiodomycosis
d. Candida albicans

204. Which organism does not have cystic stage? ***(Most Recent Question June 2022)***

a. Trichomonas
b. Ancylostoma duodenale
c. Giardia lamblia
d. Entamoeba histolytica

205. A patient resident of Bihar came to the OPD with history of diabetes and complaining of multiple sinus draining in foot as shown in the image below. Identify the condition? ***(Most Recent Question June 2022)***

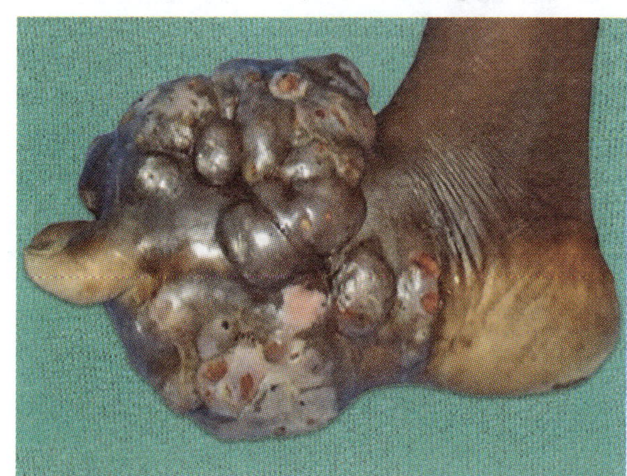

a. Madura foot
b. Gas gangrene
c. Chronic bacterial osteomyelitis
d. Osteosarcoma

206. A pt. presented with multiple asymptomatic scaly patches varying in color from white to tan to brown to pink. On potassium hydroxide wet mount spaghetti and meat ball appearance is seen. Which of the following is causative organism for this disease? ***(Most Recent Question June/Dec 2021)***

a. Tinea corporis b. Malassezia furfur
c. Sporotrichosis d. Blastomycosis

207. LGV/Granuloma inguinale is caused by: ***(Most Recent Question June/Dec 2021)***

a. T. pallidum
b. Chlamydia
c. Herpes simplex
d. Klebsiella granulomatis

QUESTIONS

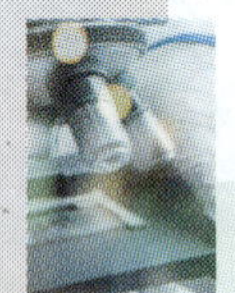

208. Identify the organism:
(Most Recent Question June/Dec 2021)

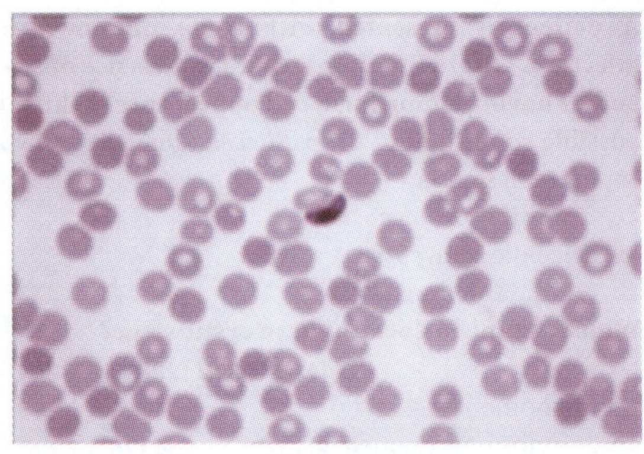

a. P falciparum b. P wave
c. P knowlesi d. P malariae

209. Which of the following is strongly associated with mucomycosis? ***(Most Recent Question June/Dec 2021)***

a. Diabetic ketoacidosis b. Pregnancy
c. Pneumocystis d. Histoplasmosis

210. A lady presented with foul smelling greyish white discharge and whiff test was positive. On examination following cells were seen as shown in image given below. Identify the causative organism and drug of choice:
(Most Recent Question June/Dec 2021)

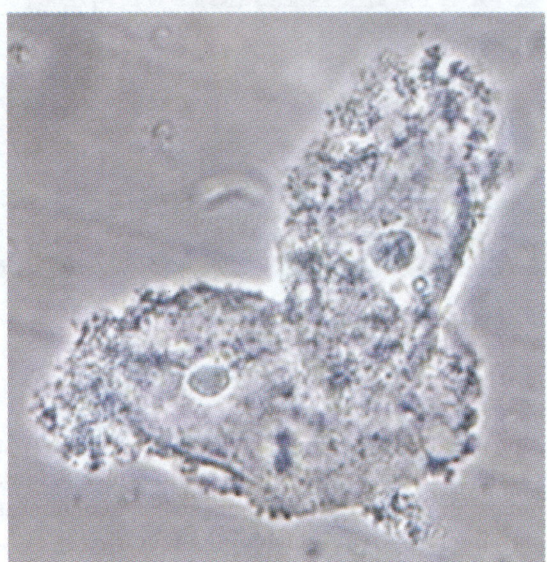

a. Candida, fluconazole
b. Trichomonas, metronidazole
c. Gardnerella vaginalis, metronidazole
d. Bonococci. Doxycycline

211. Which can cause condyloma acuminata?
(Most Recent Question June/Dec 2021)

a. HPV 1.6 b. HPV16,18
c. HPV 31,33 d. HPV 6,11

212. Post covid patient with history of diabetes presents with black eschar, orbital swelling and proptosis. What is the most probable diagnosis?
(Most Recent Question June/Dec 2021)

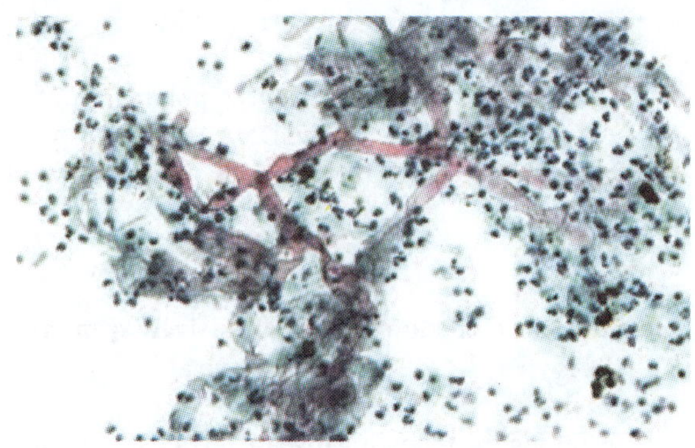

a. Mucormycosis b. Aspergillus
c. Pseudomonas d. Acanthamoeba

213. Identify this organism causing diarrhea
(Most Recent Question June/Dec 2021)

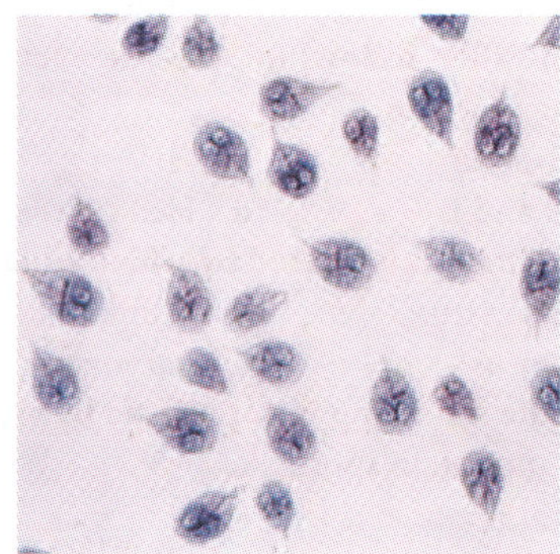

a. Rotavirus b. Giardia lamblia
c. Cryptosporidium d. Adenovirus

214. Identify the egg as shown in image below?
(Most Recent Question Dec 2020)

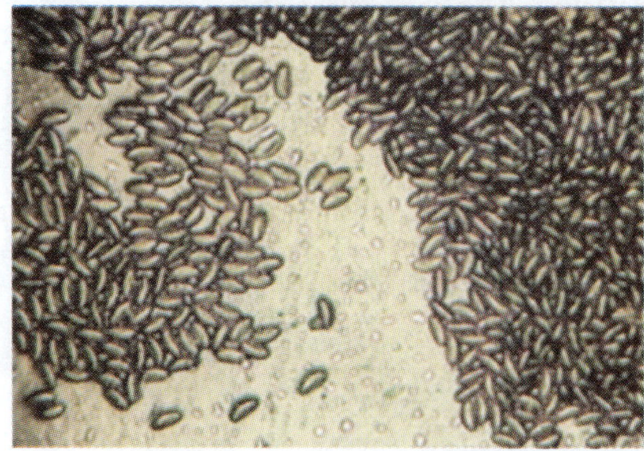

a. Trichuris trichura b. Enterobius vermicularis
c. Ankylostoma d. Ascaris

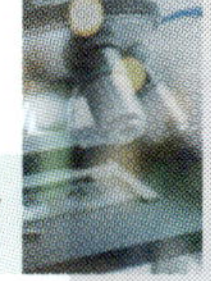

215. A 30-year-old patient with history of travel of Ohio in USA shows the following Bronchoalveolar lavage smear characteristics with lactophenol cotton blue staining. He has developed possible infection with?

(Most Recent Question Dec 2020)

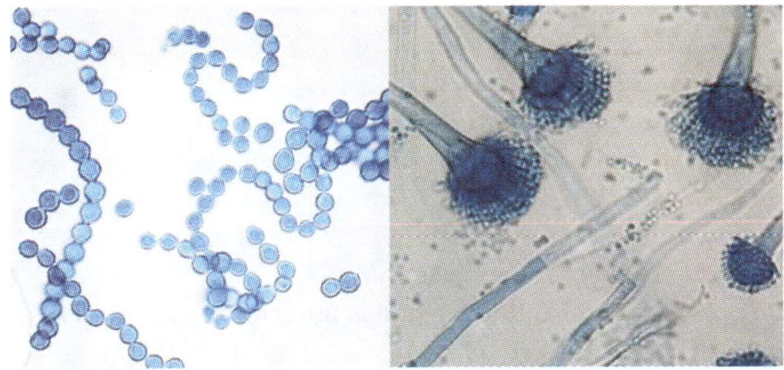

a. Coccidioidomycosis
b. Histoplasma
c. Blastomyces
d. Cryptococcus

216. A 35-year-old patient presented with recurrent episodes of colicky abdominal pain and diarrhea. No history of fever. Stool sample was given for investigation and showed the following image. Possible diagnosis?

(Most Recent Question Dec 2020)

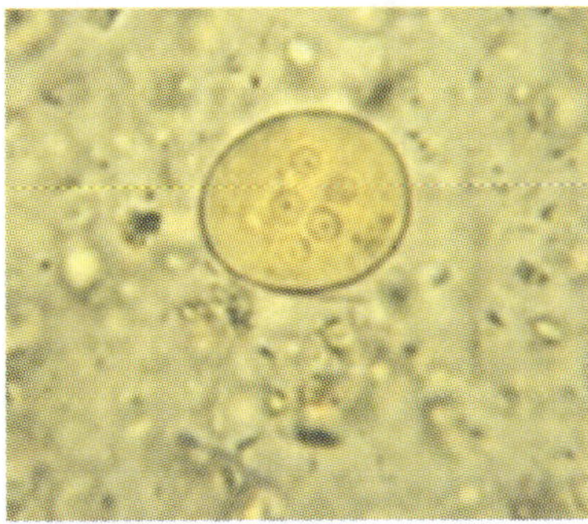

a. *E. histolytica* b. *E. coli*
c. *Giardia lambia* d. *Shigella*

217. Identify the parasite as shown in photo:

(Most Recent Question Dec 2020)

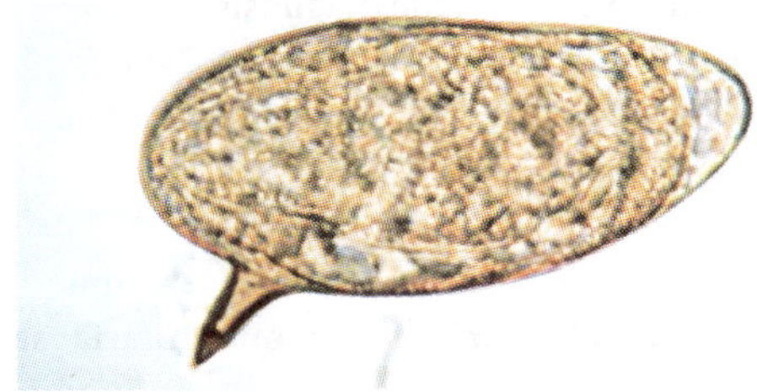

a. Fasciola hepatica
b. Schistosoma japonicum
c. Schistosoma mansoni
d. Schistosoma hematobium

218. Identify the parasite as shown in this image:

(Most Recent Question Aug 2020)

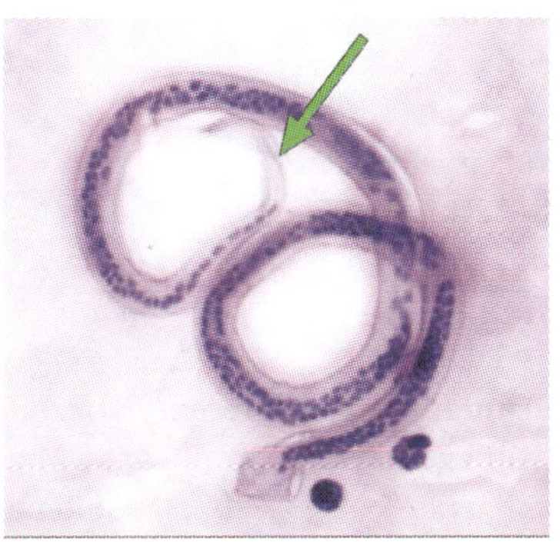

a. Brugia malayi b. Wuchereria bancrofti
c. Taenia solium d. Taenia saginatum

219. Most sensitive test for microfilariae:

(Most Recent Question Aug 2020)

a. DEC challenge test
b. Immunofluorescence test
c. Thick films
d. Membrane filter concentration technique

220. Kala-azar cannot occur at an altitude of:

(Most Recent Question Aug 2020)

a. 400 meters b. 500 meters
c. 600 meters d. 200 meters

221. NIH swab is used for: ***(Most Recent Question Aug 2020)***

a. Pin worm b. Whip worm
c. Round worm d. Schistosomiasis

222. Smallest cestode among the following:

(Most Recent Question Aug 2020)

a. H. Nana b. Schistosoma
c. T. Saginata d. T. Solium

223. Identify the given image:

(Most Recent Question Aug 2020)

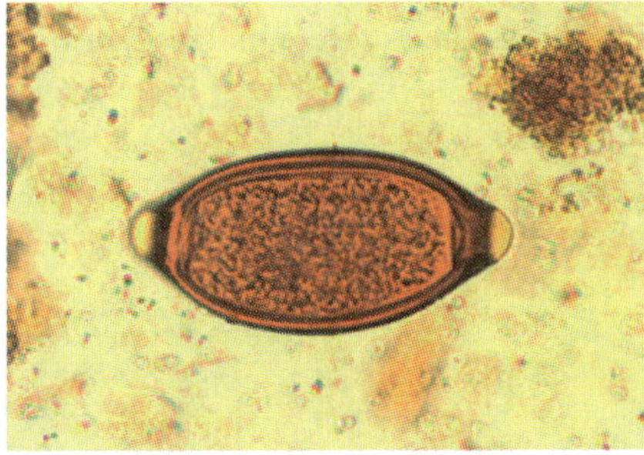

a. Taenia solium b. Trichuris spiralis
c. Trichuris trichura eggs d. Wuchereria bancrofti

224. A patient presented with some unknown fungal infection. Microscopic examination revealed brown coloured spherical fungi with septate hyphae. Possible condition: ***(Recent Pattern Question 2018-19)***

a. Histoplasmosis b. Chromoblastomycosis
c. Coccidiodomycosis d. Candida albicans

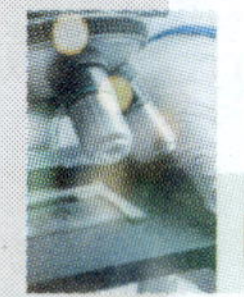

225. Which is correct about larval stage of Taenia solium? ***(Recent Pattern Question 2018-19)***
   a. Larva currens
   b. Cysticercosis cellulose
   c. Cutaneous larva migrans
   d. Visceral larva migrans

226. Germ tube test is done for: ***(Recent Pattern Question 2018)***
   a. Chlamydia   b. *Candida albicans*
   c. Bacterial vaginosis   d. *Neisseria gonorrhoeae*

227. Microsporum involves: ***(Recent Pattern Question 2018)***
   a. Skin, hair and nails   b. Skin and hair
   c. Skin and nails   d. Hair and nails

228. Pulmonary eosinophilia is seen due to which of the following infection? ***(Recent Pattern Question 2018)***
   a. Ancylostoma   b. Trichinella
   c. Filaria   d. Roundworm

229. Which parasite lives in bladder plexus? ***(Recent Pattern Question 2018)***
   a. *Schistosoma*   b. *Fasciola*
   c. *Ascaris*   d. *Echinococcus*

230. What is true about Echinococcus Granulosus? ***(Recent Pattern Question 2017)***
   a. Definitive host in humans
   b. Accidental intermediate host in humans
   c. Intermediate host in dogs
   d. Definitive host in snails

231. Which plasmodium infection has predilection for attacking old RBCs? ***(Recent Pattern Question 2017)***
   a. Plasmodium Vivax   b. Plasmodium Ovale
   c. Plasmodium malariae   d. Plasmodium Falciparum

232. Mature spherules in sputum sample is seen in which of the following? ***(Recent Pattern Question 2017)***
   a. Staphylococcus   b. Streptococcus
   c. Coccidioidomycosis   d. Aspergillus

233. Which parasite causes severe malabsorption syndrome? ***(Recent Pattern Question 2016)***
   a. Giardiasis
   b. Hook worm
   c. Ascariasis
   d. Amoebiasis

234. Definitive host of ascariasis ***(Recent Pattern Question 2016)***
   a. Dog   b. Man
   c. Pig   d. Monkey

235. All are cestodes; EXCEPT ***(Recent Pattern Question 2016)***
   a. Treponema pallidum
   b. Echinococcus
   c. Taenia solium
   d. Taenia saginata

236. Kerion is a
   a. Bacteria   b. Prion
   c. Virus   d. Fungus

237. Which of the following method is used in the rapid identification of Candida:
   a. Culture in solid   b. Germ tube method
   c. Growing in an animal   d. Culture in liquid

238. KOH mount is done for:
   a. Bacterial vaginosis   b. Candida
   c. Syphilis   d. Chancroid

239. Lyme disease is caused by:
   a. Borrelia vincenti   b. Borrelia Burgdorferi
   c. Borrelia Recurrentis   d. Treponema Pertenue

240. Groove sign is seen in
   a. Chancroid   b. Syphilis
   c. Granuloma inguinale   d. LGV

241. Which of the following fungal infection is a leading cause of corneal ulcer?
   a. Trichophyton   b. Aspergillus
   c. Mucor   d. Sprothrix

242. Enterobius vermicularis commonly resides in:
   a. Duodenum   b. Ileum
   c. Appendix and cecum   d. Sigmoid colon

243. Which parasite multiplies in appendix and blocks lumen?
   a. Pin worm   b. Strongyloides stercoralis
   c. Round worm   d. Hook worm

244. All are true about Toxocariasis; EXCEPT?
   a. Dogs and foxes are the host of toxocara canis
   b. Causes visceral larva migrans
   c. Causes cutaneous larva migrans
   d. Hypereosinophilia is a significant finding

245. Cutaneous larva migrans is caused by-
   a. Trichinella
   b. Ancylostoma braziliense
   c. Angiostrongylus cantonensis
   d. Toxocara canis

246. All are TRUE regarding filariasis; EXCEPT:
   a. Involves lymphatic system
   b. Caused by wucheria bancrofti
   c. Man is an intermediate host
   d. DEC is used in treatment

247. A person was bitten by an infected louse and developed a disease. What is the probable diagnosis?
   a. Scrub typhus   b. Epidemic typhus
   c. Endemic typhus   d. Indian Tick typhus

248. Tape worm is found mainly in
   a. Liver   b. Stomach
   c. Caecum   d. Ileum & jejunum

249. In which stage of filariasis are microfilaria seen in peripheral blood:
   a. Acute adenolymphangitis stage
   b. Tropical eosinophilia
   c. Chyluria
   d. Elephantiasis

250. Ova in stool are not of diagnostic significance in:
a. Ankylostoma
b. Entrobius
c. Strongyloides
d. Trichuris

251. Example of Zoonoses are all; EXCEPT:
a. Plague
b. Rabies
c. Taeniasis
d. Brucellosis

252. A 20 year old man presents with swelling of left lower limb and hydrocoele. All of the following may be the causative agent; EXCEPT:
a. Brugia malayi
b. Brugia timoria
c. Wuchereria bancrofti
d. Onchocerca volvulus

IMMUNOLOGY AND MISCELLANEOUS

253. Rh-ve mother had Rh+ve child. This Rh incompatibility is which type of hypersensitivity reaction?
(Most Recent Question June/Dec 2021)
a. Type 1
b. Type 2
c. Type 3
d. Type 4

254. Which of the following immunoglobulins is a pentamer:
(Most Recent Question June/Dec 2021)

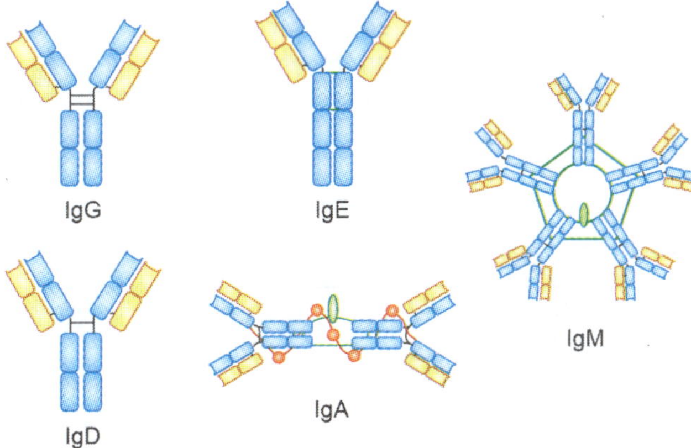

a. IgM
b. IgA
c. IgE
d. IgG

255. A lady got stung by a bee after which she develops shock. What is the substance that is most importantly related to the patients presentation:
(Most Recent Question June/Dec 2021)
a. Histamine
b. Leukotrienes
c. Bradykinin
d. Complement

256. A Pregnant women got bitten by a rabid dog. What is the management ***(Most Recent Question June/Dec 2021)***
a. Active immunity (vaccine) + rabies immunoglobulin + local treatment
b. Active immunity (vaccine)
c. Rabies immunoglobulin
d. Local treatment

257. Which antibody is seen in recent infection?
(Most Recent Question Aug 2020)
a. IgM
b. IgG
c. IgE
d. IgD

258. N. meningitis can be due to deficiency of this complement system: ***(Recent Pattern Question 2018-19)***
a. C1–C4 deficiency
b. C5–C9 deficiency
c. C3 deficiency
d. C2 deficiency

259. Classical complement activated by:
(Recent Pattern Question 2018-19)
a. C1
b. C3 convertase
c. IgA
d. Ag – Ab complex

260. In normal immune system, the epithelioid cells are derived from: ***(Recent Pattern Question 2018)***
a. TH1
b. TH2
c. Macrophages
d. TH19

261. Meningococcal meningitis is seen with which of the following complement deficiency?
(Recent Pattern Question 2018)
a. C1q
b. C2
c. C4
d. C5

262. All of the following are true about bacteriophage; EXCEPT: ***(Recent Pattern Question 2017)***
a. It is a bacteria
b. It helps in transduction
c. It imparts toxigenicity by lysogenic conversion
d. It can cause drug resistanc

263. IgM is:
a. Monomer
b. Dimer
c. Pentamer
d. Tetramer

264. First antibody produced by newborn?
a. IgA
b. IgG
c. IgE
d. IgM

265. Immunoglobulin found in bronchial secretion:
a. IgA
b. IgG
c. IgM
d. IgE

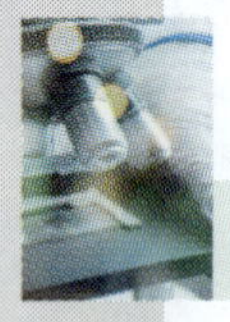

ANSWERS WITH EXPLANATIONS

MOST RECENT QUESTIONS 2023

1. Ans. (a) *Staphylococcus epidermidis*

- *Staphylococcus epidermidis*, a coagulase-negative staphylococcus, is the most common cause of prosthetic valve endocarditis (PVE).
- PVE is an infection of the heart valves or other structures in the heart that occurs after a prosthetic valve has been implanted.
- It is usually caused by bacteria that enter the bloodstream during surgery or during a procedure that involves the heart.

2. Ans. (b) *Vibrio parahaemolyticus*

- *Vibrio parahaemolyticus* is a gram-negative bacterium that is found in marine environments. It can cause diarrhea, vomiting, and abdominal cramps in humans after consumption of contaminated seafood.
- The bacterium produces a toxin called the Kanagawa toxin, which is responsible for the symptoms of the infection.
- **The Kanagawa phenomenon**—a characteristic hemolysis pattern on blood agar. This phenomenon stems from a thermostable direct hemolysin produced by the bacterium, contributing to its pathogenesis and virulence. It is not seen with *E. coli, C. jejuni* or *V. cholerae.*

3. Ans. (d) *Aspergillus*

- The etiological agent of traumatic ulcer in the eye with septate hyphae is most likely *Aspergillus.*
- *Aspergillus* is a fungus that is commonly found in soil and decaying organic matter.
- It can cause a variety of infections in humans, including keratitis, a corneal ulcer.
- Septate hyphae are characteristic of *Aspergillus,* and they can be seen in microscopy of corneal scraping.

4. Ans. (a) *Giardia lamblia*

- *Giardia lamblia* is a protozoan parasite that has four pairs of flagella. These flagella help the parasite to move in a characteristic "falling leaf" motion.
- *Giardia lamblia* is the most common cause of parasitic diarrhea in the world. It is found in contaminated water, food, and soil.
- The parasite is ingested by drinking contaminated water or eating contaminated food.
- The parasite attaches to the walls of the small intestine and causes inflammation.

Note:

- ***Entamoeba histolytica*:** Another protozoan parasite that causes diarrhea but it lacks flagella.
- ***Balantidium coli*:** A ciliated protozoan that causes diarrhea, but is less common than *Giardia.*
- ***E. coli*:** A bacterium that can cause diarrhea, but it does not have flagella.

5. Ans. (a) GBS

- Group B streptococcus (GBS) is a common cause of neonatal meningitis.
- It is also the most common cause of early-onset sepsis in newborns.
- GBS is bacitracin-resistant.
- Neonates can acquire GBS during childbirth, leading to potential infection.
- GBS infections in neonates can be severe, causing meningitis and sepsis.

Note:

b. **GAS (Group A streptococcus):** Less commonly associated with neonatal meningitis.
c. ***Listeria*:** Typically, susceptible to bacitracin and causes meningitis in neonates, but it is not as common as GBS.
d. ***E. coli*:** It can cause neonatal meningitis but it is not typically bacitracin-resistant.

6. Ans. (a) RT-PCR

- RT-PCR is a sensitive and specific test to detect viral genetic material.
- Hydrophobia is a classic symptom of rabies infection. Detecting rabies virus RNA using RT-PCR is effective for diagnosis.
- The test identifies viral genetic material in corneal scraping.
- It confirms rabies infection swiftly, enabling appropriate management.

7. Ans. (c) Meningitis

- Exotoxins are toxic substances released by certain bacteria as part of their growth and metabolism. These toxins can cause various diseases when they come into contact with the host.
  - **Hemolytic uremic syndrome (HUS),** Toxic shock syndrome (TSS), and Pseudomembranous colitis are all conditions associated with exotoxins. HUS is often caused by Shiga toxin-producing bacteria, such as *E. coli.*
  - TSS is associated with toxins produced by *Staphylococcus aureus* and *Streptococcus pyogenes.*

- Pseudomembranous colitis is caused by *Clostridium difficile*, which produces toxins that damage the intestinal lining.
- **Meningitis**, on the other hand, is typically caused by bacterial invasion of the meninges (the protective membranes covering the brain and spinal cord) and is not primarily associated with the action of exotoxins.
- Instead, it involves the direct presence and growth of bacteria within the cerebrospinal fluid.

8. Ans. (a) *Trichophyton*

- Pencil-shaped macroconidia are seen in the genus *Trichophyton*. These macroconidia are spindle-shaped and have tapering ends. They are produced in chains on the hyphae of the fungus.
- *Trichophyton* is a genus of fungus that causes a variety of skin infections, including tinea pedis (athlete's foot), tinea cruris (jock itch), and tinea corporis (ringworm).

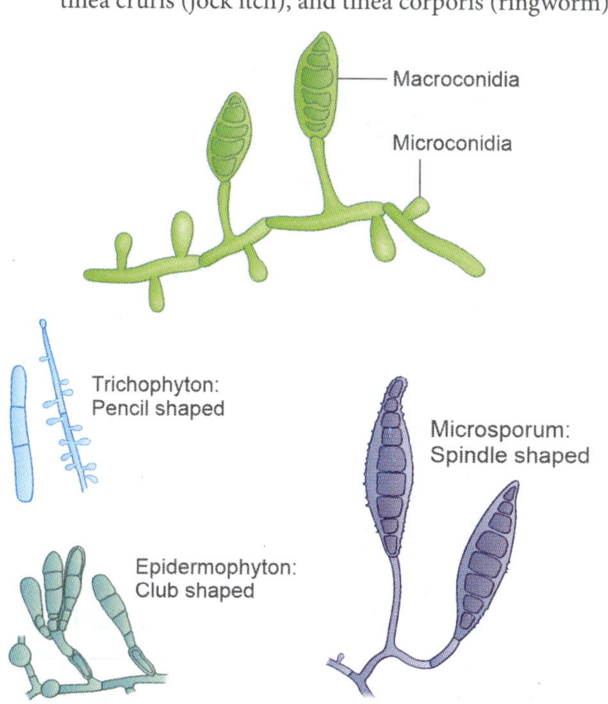

- ***Microsporum*** produces teardrop/spindle-shaped macroconidia.
- ***Epidermophyton*** produces clavate (club-shaped) macroconidia.
- ***Aspergillus*** produces septate hyphae, but does not produce macroconidia.

9. Ans. (b) IgG

Ref: Ananthanarayan and Paniker's Textbook of Microbiology, 10th ed. pg. 98

- IgG antibodies are found in the highest concentration in blood/serum and play a critical role in long-term immunity. They can cross the placenta and provide passive immunity to the fetus.
- IgA antibodies are mainly found in body secretions such as saliva, tears, and breast milk.
- IgM antibodies are the first antibodies produced during an immune response.

10. Ans. (b) Kupffer cells

Ref: Ananthanarayan and Paniker's Textbook of Microbiology, 10th ed. pg. 139

- Kupffer cells are specialized macrophages found in the liver.
- They play a crucial role in the immune response against pathogens and foreign substances in the liver.
- Kupffer cells are responsible for phagocytosing and clearing microorganisms, cellular debris, and toxins from the blood.
- Their presence in the liver helps to maintain its overall immune function and homeostasis.
- **Hofbauer cells** are involved in fetal development and immune regulation within the placental environment.
- **Mesangial cells** are located in the renal glomeruli and play a role in the structural support and filtration function of the kidney.
- **Monocytes** are circulating immune cells that can differentiate into macrophages when they migrate to different tissues, including the liver.

Extra Mile

- Macrophages in CNS: Microglial cell
- Macrophages in connective tissue: Histiocytes
- Macrophages in skin: Langerhans cell

11. Ans. (b) Autoimmunity

Ref: Harrison's Principles of Internal Medicine, 20th ed. pg. 2854

- Rheumatoid arthritis is an autoimmune disease characterized by chronic inflammation of the joints.
- In the case of rheumatoid arthritis, the immune system targets the synovium, which is the lining of the joints, leading to inflammation, pain, and joint damage.

12. Ans. (c) Mast cells

Ref: Ananthanarayan and Paniker's Textbook of Microbiology, 10th ed. pg. 100

- The degranulation of mast cells releases histamine, which is responsible for the development of symptoms such as runny nose and wheezing.

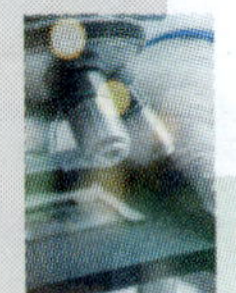

- When mast cells degranulate in response to triggers such as allergens or irritants, histamine is released, leading to symptoms like nasal congestion, wheezing, and itching.

13. Ans. (a) Autograft

Ref: Ananthanarayan and Paniker's Textbook of Microbiology, 10th ed. pg. 185

- An autograft refers to the transplantation of tissue from one part of the body to another within the same individual.
- In the given scenario, where the patient's own tissue was used for grafting, it indicates an autograft.
- Autografts are advantageous as they minimize the risk of rejection since the tissue is from the patient's own body.

Extra Mile

- An **allograft** involves the transplantation of tissue between individuals of the same species but with different genetic backgrounds.
- A **xenograft** involves the transplantation of tissue from one species to another.
- An **isograft** involves the transplantation of tissue between genetically identical individuals, such as identical twins.

14. Ans. (d) HSV

Ref: Ananthanarayan and Paniker's Textbook of Microbiology, 10th ed. pg. 476

- Tzanck smear is a microscopic test used in the diagnosis of viral infections, particularly those caused by herpes viruses.
- It involves collecting a sample from a skin lesion, staining it, and examining it under a microscope.
- In the case of HSV infection, Tzanck smear typically reveals multinucleated giant cells with intranuclear inclusions, known as Tzanck cells. This finding is indicative of HSV infection.

Extra Mile

- **HIV** is typically diagnosed using serological tests that detect antibodies or viral nucleic acids.
- **HPV** is commonly diagnosed through visual inspection, Pap tests, or specific HPV DNA tests.
- **HDV** infection is typically diagnosed by detecting specific antibodies or viral RNA.

15. Ans. (d) Varicella zoster

Ref: Ananthanarayan and Paniker's Textbook of Microbiology, 10th ed. pg. 478

- The image provided in the question shows a dermatomal distribution of painful blisters on the trunk, which is indicative of herpes zoster, commonly known as shingles.
- Herpes zoster is caused by the reactivation of the Varicella-zoster virus (VZV), the same virus that causes chicken pox.
- The characteristic appearance of a vesicular rash following a specific dermatomal pattern suggests VZV as the most likely organism implicated in causing the condition.
- **Note:** A lesion of chicken pox is filled with clear fluid and molluscum contagiosum lesion is umbilicated.

16. Ans. (c) Cytomegalovirus

Ref: Ananthanarayan and Paniker's Textbook of Microbiology, 10th ed. pg. 518

- The inclusion body shown in the image is characteristic of CMV infection. CMV is a member of the Herpesviridae family and commonly causes infections in immunocompromised individuals.
- The presence of large, intranuclear inclusion bodies, known as **owl's eye** or cytomegalic inclusion bodies, is a hallmark of CMV infection.

17. Ans. (a) Hepatitis A

Ref: Ananthanarayan and Paniker's Textbook of Microbiology, 10th ed. pg. 545

- In the given scenario, the patient's gastrointestinal (GI) distress following the consumption of food outside suggests a possible foodborne infection.
- Hepatitis A virus (HAV) and hepatitis E are commonly transmitted through the fecal-oral route, often associated with contaminated food or water.
- It causes acute hepatitis characterized by symptoms such as nausea, vomiting, abdominal pain, and jaundice.
- Therefore, the patient's symptoms and history are consistent with hepatitis A infection.
- **Note:** Hepatitis B and hepatitis C are transmitted through blood transfusion, sexual contact or needle prick injury. Hepatitis D infection requires coinfection with hepatitis B.

18. Ans. (c) Measles

Ref: Ananthanarayan and Paniker's Textbook of Microbiology, 10th ed. pg. 518

- The presentation of a maculopapular rash that begins behind the ears and then spreads to the face and rest of the body, accompanied by fever, conjunctivitis, and runny nose, is characteristic of measles.
- Measles, also known as rubeola, is a highly contagious viral infection caused by the measles virus. The rash typically appears a few days after the onset of fever and other symptoms.

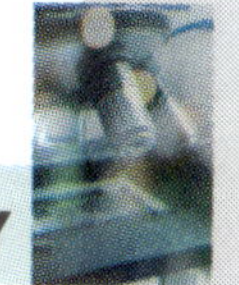

Extra Mile

- **Exanthema subitum,** also known as roseola infantum or sixth disease, is a viral infection caused by human herpesvirus 6 (HHV6) or human herpesvirus 7 (HHV7). It is characterized by a high fever followed by a rash, but the rash usually appears after the fever subsides and does not start behind the ears.
- Chicken pox, caused by the varicella-zoster virus (VZV), presents with a generalized vesicular rash that typically starts on the trunk and spreads to the face and limbs.
- Erythema infectiosum, also known as fifth disease, is a viral infection caused by parvovirus B19. It is characterized by a slapped cheek appearance followed by a lacy rash on the extremities.

19. Ans. (c) *Sporothrix schenckii*

Ref: Ananthanarayan and Paniker's Textbook of Microbiology, 10th ed. pg. 606

- Among the options provided, *Sporothrix schenckii* is the dimorphic fungus that can cause subcutaneous infections.
- Sporotrichosis is a chronic fungal infection that usually occurs through traumatic inoculation of the fungus into the skin.
- It typically presents as a localized cutaneous lesion that progresses along lymphatic channels, forming nodules and ulcers.
- *Sporothrix schenckii* exists in a mold form in the environment and converts to a yeast form in host tissues.

Extra Mile

- ***Histoplasma capsulatum*** is a dimorphic fungus that causes histoplasmosis, primarily a systemic infection involving the lungs.
- ***Paracoccidioides brasiliensis*** is another dimorphic fungus that causes paracoccidioidomycosis, a systemic mycosis primarily affecting the lungs and mucous membranes.
- ***Coccidioides immitis*** is the causative agent of coccidioidomycosis (Valley fever), which primarily affects the respiratory system.

20. Ans. (d) Chromoblastomycosis

Ref: Ananthanarayan and Paniker's Textbook of Microbiology, 10th ed. pg. 605

- The presentation of a verrucous growth on the feet in a forest worker following trauma is most likely indicative of chromoblastomycosis.
- Chromoblastomycosis is a chronic fungal infection caused by several dematiaceous fungi, such as *Fonsecaea* and *Cladophialophora* species.
- It typically occurs after traumatic inoculation of the fungus into the skin, leading to the development of slowly progressive, wart-like lesions.

Extra Mile

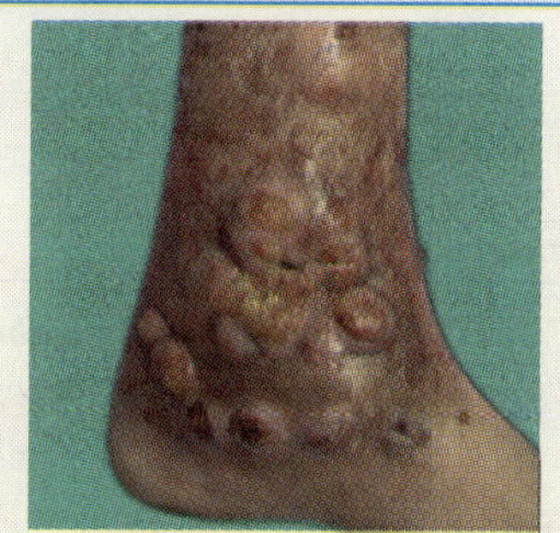

Mycetoma/Madura foot with multiple draining sinus

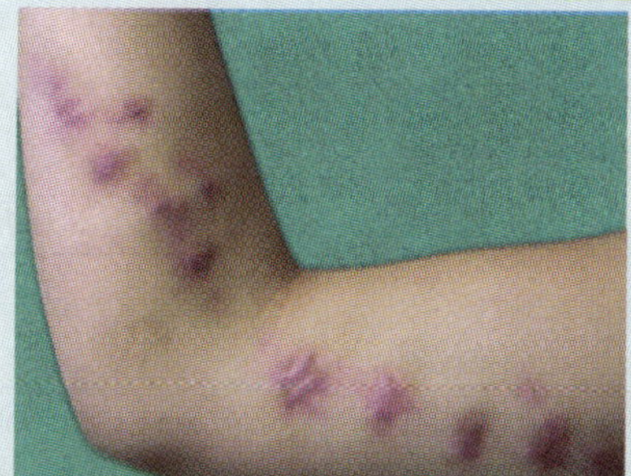

Sporotrichosis

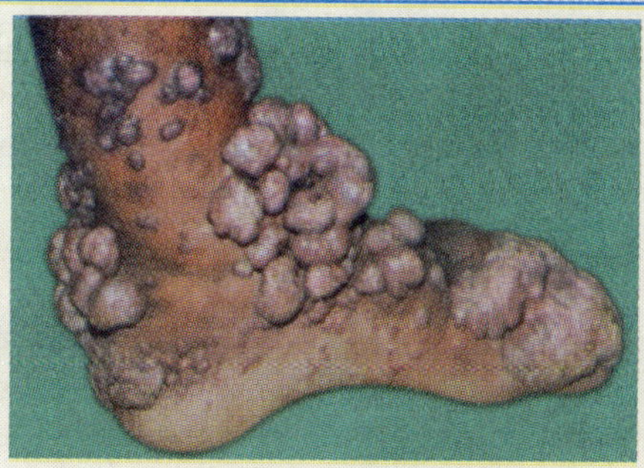

Chromoblastomycosis

21. Ans. (c) Trichomoniasis

Ref: Rook's Textbook of Dermatology, 9th ed. pg. 30

- Trichomoniasis is a common sexually transmitted infection caused by the protozoan parasite *Trichomonas vaginalis.*
- Trichomoniasis is characterized by symptoms such as foul-smelling vaginal discharge, itching, and irritation.
- The presence of motile trophozoites on wet mount microscopy is a characteristic finding of *Trichomonas vaginalis.*

Extra Mile

- Bacterial vaginosis (Option a) is caused by an imbalance in vaginal bacteria and is typically associated with a shift in the normal vaginal flora.

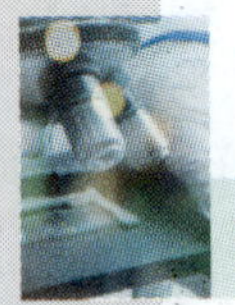

- Vulvovaginal candidiasis (Option b) is caused by an overgrowth of *Candida* species, typically *Candida albicans*, and does not exhibit motile trophozoites.
- Chlamydia (Option d) is caused by the bacterium *Chlamydia trachomatis* and is not associated with motile trophozoites.

22. Ans. (b) *Strongyloides*

Ref: Ananthanarayan and Paniker's Textbook of Microbiology, 10th ed. pg. 238

- *Strongyloides* is a genus of parasitic roundworms that can infect humans.
- *Strongyloides* larvae can penetrate the skin, typically through bare feet, when in contact with contaminated soil or water.
- *Enterobius* (Option a) is the pinworm that causes enterobiasis and does not enter the body through the feet.
- *Ascaris* (Option c) is the roundworm that causes ascariasis, and its larvae are not known to penetrate the skin.
- *Trichuris* (Option d) is the whipworm that causes trichuriasis, and its larvae do not enter through the feet.

23. Ans. (d) Cerebral malaria

Ref: Ananthanarayan and Paniker's Textbook of Microbiology, 10th ed. pg. 72

- Cerebral malaria is a severe and potentially life-threatening form of malaria caused by the parasite *Plasmodium falciparum*.
- It is characterized by symptoms such as high fever, sweating, and severe anemia leading to paleness.
- Encephalitis (Option a) refers to inflammation of the brain and can cause symptoms such as headache, confusion, and neurological deficits but is not specific to malaria.
- Pyogenic meningitis (Option b) is a bacterial infection of the meninges and presents with symptoms such as fever, neck stiffness, and altered mental status.
- TB meningitis (Option c) is a form of meningitis caused by *Mycobacterium tuberculosis* and presents with symptoms such as neck rigidity, headache, fever, and neurological deficits.

24. Ans. (b) Dark-field microscopy

Ref: Ananthanarayan and Paniker's Textbook of Microbiology, 10th ed. pg. 232

- Dark-field microscopy is the investigation of choice for diagnosing syphilis.
- Syphilis is a sexually-transmitted infection caused by the bacterium *Treponema pallidum*.
- Dark-field microscopy allows for the visualization of the motile spirochetes in the ulcer discharge, confirming the diagnosis of syphilis.
- **Gram stain** (Option a) is not suitable for visualizing *Treponema pallidum* due to its thin structure and lack of Gram stain uptake.
- The **Whiff test** (Option c) is used to diagnose bacterial vaginosis.
- **p24 antigen test** (Option d) is used for detecting the presence of the p24 protein of the human immunodeficiency virus (HIV).

25. Ans. (b) Secondary syphilis

Ref: Ananthanarayan and Paniker's Textbook of Microbiology, 10th ed. pg. 233

- The lesion shown in the question is characteristic of secondary syphilis.
- Secondary syphilis is a stage of syphilis that occurs several weeks to months after the initial infection.
- It is characterized by a variety of symptoms, including a maculopapular rash, typically involving the palms and soles.
- Primary syphilis (Option a) refers to the initial stage of syphilis and is characterized by the presence of a painless ulcer called a chancre.
- Hand-foot-mouth disease (Option c) is a viral infection caused by Coxsackievirus or Enterovirus and typically presents with sores in the mouth, hands, and feet.
- Kawasaki disease (Option d) is an acute febrile illness primarily affecting children and is characterized by symptoms such as fever, rash, conjunctivitis, and changes in the lips and oral mucosa.

26. Ans. (c) *Bacillus anthracis*

Ref: Ananthanarayan and Paniker's Textbook of Microbiology, 10th ed. pg. 371

- The description of purple brick-shaped organisms with spores in the center is characteristic of *Bacillus anthracis*, the causative agent of anthrax.
- Anthrax is primarily a disease of animals, especially herbivores, like cattle, sheep, and goats.
- Humans can acquire anthrax through contact with infected animals or their products.
- The spores of *Bacillus anthracis* can survive in the soil for a long time and can cause infection when they enter the body through breaks in the skin.

27. Ans. (c) *Legionella pneumophila*

Ref: Ananthanarayan and Paniker's Textbook of Microbiology, 10th ed. pg. 252

- The clinical presentation of a chronic smoker with high fever, cough, confusion, and diarrhea, along with bilateral lung infiltrates on CXR, is suggestive of *Legionella* pneumonia.
- *Legionella* pneumonia is caused by the gram-negative bacterium *Legionella pneumophila*.
- It is commonly associated with water sources, such as hot water tanks, cooling towers, and air conditioning systems.
- Legionella pneumonia often presents with severe pneumonia and can cause extrapulmonary manifestations, including diarrhea and confusion.
- *Mycoplasma pneumoniae* (Option a) is a common cause of community-acquired pneumonia but does not typically present with diarrhea or confusion.
- *Klebsiella pneumoniae* (Option b) is another gram-negative bacterium associated with pneumonia, especially in immunocompromised individuals, but it does not cause diarrhea.
- *Streptococcus pneumoniae* (Option d) is a gram-positive bacterium and a common cause of community-acquired pneumonia, but it does not typically cause diarrhea or confusion.

28. Ans. (a) MacConkey's agar

Ref: Ananthanarayan and Paniker's Textbook of Microbiology, 10th ed. pg. 42

- **MacConkey's agar** is a selective and differential culture medium commonly used in microbiology laboratories.
- It contains crystal violet and bile salts, which inhibit the growth of gram-positive bacteria and allow the growth of gram-negative bacteria.
- MacConkey's agar also contains lactose as a carbohydrate source and pH indicators (neutral red or crystal violet).
- Lactose fermenters, such as *Escherichia coli*, ferment lactose, producing acid that causes the colonies to appear pink or red on MacConkey's agar.
- Non-lactose fermenters, such as *Salmonella* and *Shigella* species, do not ferment lactose and produce colorless colonies.
- **Chocolate agar (Option b)** is an enriched medium used for the cultivation of fastidious organisms like *Haemophilus influenzae*.
- **Blood agar (Option c)** is a general-purpose medium used for the cultivation of a wide range of organisms and does not differentiate lactose fermenters from non-lactose fermenters.
- **Potassium tellurite agar (Option d)** is used for the selective isolation of *Corynebacterium diphtheriae*, the causative agent of diphtheria, and does not differentiate lactose fermenters from non-lactose fermenters.

29. Ans. (b) Vaporized H_2O_2

Ref: Ananthanarayan and Paniker's Textbook of Microbiology, 10th ed. pg. 37

- Plasma sterilization, also known as low-temperature sterilization, is a method used to sterilize heat-sensitive medical equipment and instruments.
- In this process, vaporized hydrogen peroxide (H_2O_2) is commonly used as the sterilizing agent.
- The H_2O_2 is converted to plasma state by applying a high-frequency electric field, creating a plasma of reactive species.
- The reactive species, including free radicals and ions, have sterilizing properties and effectively kill microorganisms.
- **Ethylene oxide** (Option a) is another agent used for low-temperature sterilization, but it is not specific to plasma sterilization.
- **Aldehydes** (Option c), such as formaldehyde and glutaraldehyde, are commonly used as disinfectants and sterilant but are not specifically associated with plasma sterilization.

GENERAL MICROBIOLOGY, MEDIA, TESTING

30. Ans. (c) M. leprae

Ref: Ananthanarayana and Panicker's Textbook of Microbiology, 10th ed. pg. 371, 372

- It has not been possible thus far to cultivate lepra bacilli either in bacteriological media or in tissue culture.
- It was discovered that lepra bacilli could multiply in the footpads of mice kept at a low temperature (20°C).

31. Ans. (c) Sodium hypochlorite

Ref: Ananthanarayana and Panicker's Textbook of Microbiology, 10th ed. pg. 37

- Sodium hypochlorite is a disinfectant widely used in the hospitals at different concentrations.
- It is mainly used in blood spillage.

32. Ans. (b) Yellow

Ref: Ananthanarayana and Panicker's Textbook of Microbiology, 10th ed. pg. 657

- The cotton swabs used for disinfection would be discarded in yellow bin.

33. Ans. (b) Transduction

Ref: Ananthanarayan and Paniker's Textbook of Microbiology, 10th ed. pg. 68

- **Transduction**, a process of genetic recombination in bacteria in which genes from a host cell (a bacterium) are incorporated into the genome of a bacterial virus

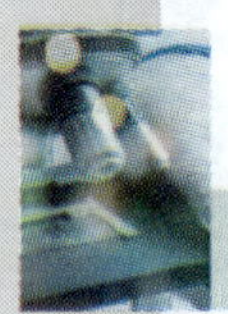

(bacteriophage) and then carried to another host cell when the bacteriophage initiates another cycle of infection.

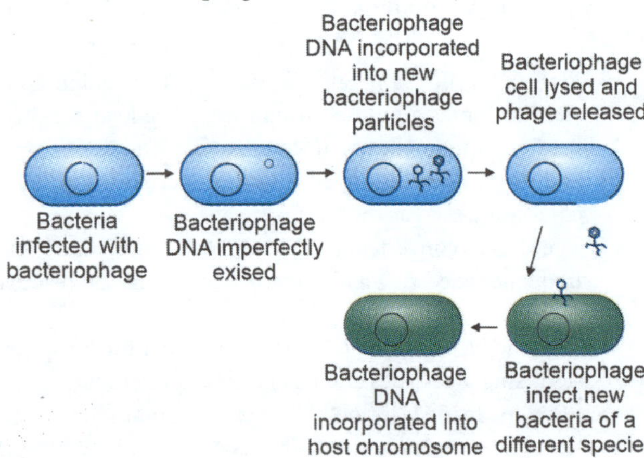

34. Ans. (a) Thermophilic

- A thermophile is an organism—a type of extremophile—that thrives at relatively high temperatures, between 41 and 122°C (106 and 252°F).
- Many thermophiles are archaea. Thermophilic eubacteria are suggested to have been among the earliest bacteria.

35. Ans. (b) Transduction

Ref: Textbook of Microbiology by Surinder Kumar, pg. 93 Microbiology by Ananthanarayan and Paniker, 8th ed., pg. 60

Some bacteria also transfer genetic material between cells via following ways:

- **Transduction:** Transfer of genetic material from one bacterium to another by a bacteriophage is known as transduction
  - Most widespread mechanism of gene transfer among prokaryotes
- **Transformation:** Transfer of genetic material through the agency of free DNA
- **Conjugation:** DNA is transferred through direct cell contact. Gram negative anerobes like E. Coli, Bacteroides, Porphyromonas, and Fusobacterium use this method of gene transfer

Extra Mile

- Bacteriophages are viruses that parasitize bacteria
- Most bacteriophages carry their genetic information (the phage genome) as a length of double-stranded DNA coiled up inside a protein coat.
- **Lysogenic conversion:** Phage DNA integrated in bacterial chromosome as prophase → replicated stably as part of host cell chromosome → transferred to daughter cell.

Contd...

- **In other words:** *"This process by which the prophage DNA confers genetic information to a bacterium is called lysogenic or phage conversion."*
- **Note:** In transduction, phage acts only as a vehicle carrying bacterial genes from one cell to another but in lysogenic conversion the phage DNA itself is the new genetic element.

36. Ans. (a) Stationary phase

Ref: Microbiology by Ananthanarayan and Paniker, 8th ed. pg. 24

PHASES OF BACTERIAL GROWTH CURVE

LAG PHASE

- No appreciable increase in number but there is **increase in size of the cells**
- Accumulation of enzymes and metabolic intermediates
- **Maximum cell size** is obtained at the end of lag phase

LOG PHASE

- Also called **exponential phase**
- Number of cells increase exponentially
- Cells are **small and stain uniformly**
- Increase in metabolic rate

STATIONARY PHASE

- Viable **count of cells remain stationary** as an equilibrium exists between dying cells and newly formed cells
- Cells are viable and show **irregular staining** due to intracellular storage granules
- **Sporulation occurs at this stage**
- Production of antibiotics and exotoxins

PHASE OF DECLINE

- **Population** of cells **decrease** due to cell death
- **Involution forms** are common

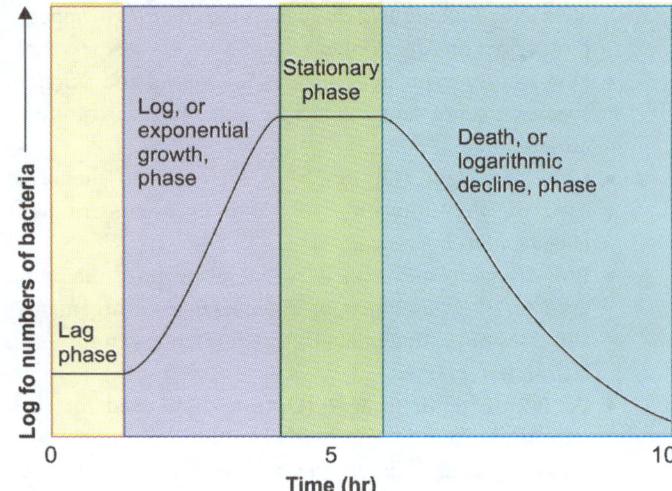

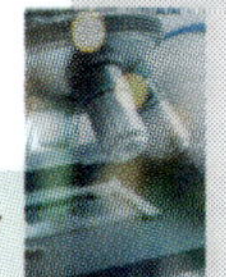

37. Ans. (b) Thermometer

Ref: Textbook of Diagnostic Microbiology, E-book, pg. 67

- **High level of disinfectant:** 2% glutaraldehyde for 20 minutes for all instruments coming in contact with mucous membrane. Like bronchoscope, proctoscope, endoscopic tubes, etc.
- **Intermediate level of disinfectant:** Phenol or alcohol is used to disinfect thermometer.
- **Low level of disinfectant:** Lysol for floors and fabrics.

38. Ans. (d) Sodium hypochlorite

Ref: Textbook of Diagnostic Microbiology, E-book, pg. 68

- After repeated vitro studies, it is confirmed that the most potent disinfectant is hypochlorite, which disclosed the lowest minimum bactericidal concentration against various micro-organisms, when compared with iodine tincture and chlorhexidine.
- Sodium hypochlorite is proved to be efficient even at very low concentration surface disinfectant (0.1, 0.5% to 1% blood spill) and the action is achieved very rapidly (within 30–60 minutes).

39. Ans. (c) Stationary phase

Ref: Ananthanarayan, 8th ed. pg. 24

40. Ans. (b) Ionizing radiation

Ref: Ananthanarayan's Microbiology, 8th ed. pg. 35

- Cold sterilization is a process in which sterilization is carried out at low temperature with the help of chemicals, radiations, membranes.
- Ionizing radiation such as X-rays, gamma rays and cosmic rays, cause no appreciable increase in temperature in this method, it is referred to as cold sterilization.

41. Ans. (a) Albert stain

Ref: Ananthnarayan, 9th ed. MedPub

- **Albert stain** is a type of differential stain used for staining the volutin granules also known as Metachromatic granules found in *Corynebacterium diphtheriae*.
- The name metachromatic is because of its property of changing color, i.e. *when stained with blue stain they appear red in colour. When grown in Loffler's slopes, C. diphtheriae produces large number of granules.*

Extra Mile

- **Stains used for C. Diphtheriae:**
  - Ponders stain
  - Albert stain
  - Neisser stain
  - Loeffler methylene blue

42. Ans. (b) Can't differentiate between latent and active TB

Ref: Harrisons, 19th ed. pg. 1114; Lange Microbiology by Jawetz, Ch 8

- The skin test with tuberculin PPD (TST) is most widely used in screening for latent tuberculosis.
- It has very low sensitivity and specificity and is **unable to discriminate between latent TB and active disease.**
- **False negative reactions** are common in immunosuppressed patients and in those with overwhelming TB.
- **False-positive reactions** may be caused by infections with non-tuberculous mycobacteria and by BCG vaccination.

43. Ans. (b) Integration of phage nucleic acid to host bacteria genome

Ref: PubMed

- Lysogenic conversion is characterized by **integration of the bacteriophage nucleic acid into the host bacterium's genome.**
- Once the genetic material of phage bacteria is introduced, the host bacterium continues to live and reproduce normally.
- The genetic material of the bacteriophage, called a prophage, can be transmitted to daughter cells at each subsequent cell division, and a later event (such as UV radiation or the presence of certain chemicals) can release it, causing proliferation of new phages via the lytic cycle.
- For example, a number of strains of the diphtheria bacillus acquire the capacity to form diphtheria toxin immediately after penetration of the phage into the cell and retain that capacity until the moment of the cell's dissolution (lysis).

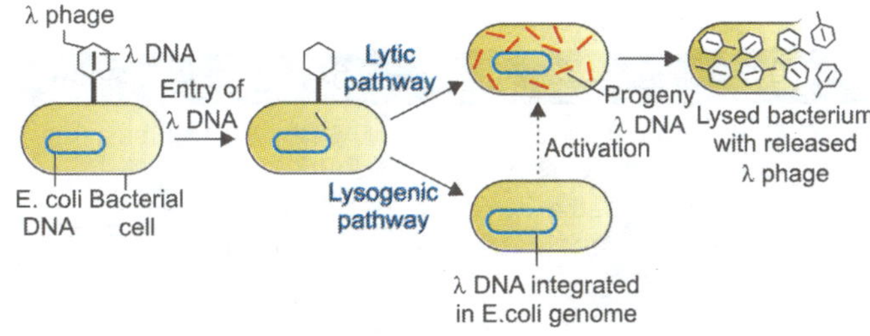

44. Ans. (c) 25 to 40°C

Ref: Ananthnarayan, 9th ed. ch-1

Organisms on the basis of their growth at different temperature:

- **Psychrophilic:** (below 20°C)
- **Psychrotrophs:** (important cause of food spoilage)
- **Mesophilic:** (25–40°C)
- **Thermophilic:** (55–80°C)

45. Ans. (a) Incineration

Ref: PubMed

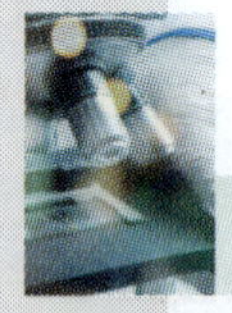

Cat.	Type of Bag/Container used	Type of waste	Treatment/disposal options
Yellow	Non-chlorinated plastic bags Separate collection system leading to effluent treatment system	• Human anatomical waste • Animal anatomical waste • Soiled waste • Expired or discarded medicines • Chemical waste • Microbiological and other clinical lab waste • Chemical liquid waste	Incineration of Plasma pyralysis or deep burial
Red	Non-chlorinated plastic bags or containers	Contaminated waste (Recyclable) tubing, bottles, intravenous tubes and sets, catheters, urine bags, syringes (without needles) gloves	Auto/Micro/Hydro and then sent for recycling not be sent to landfill
White/Translucent	Puncture, leak, tamper proof containers	Waste sharps including metals	Auto or Dry Heat Sterlization followed by shredding or multilation or encapsulation
Blue	Cardboard boxes with blue colored marking	Glassware	Disinfection or auto/Micro/hydro and then sent for recycling

46. Ans. (a) Human body parts

Ref: Please refer to above explanation

47. Ans. (c) Dry heat sterilization

Ref: Ananthnarayan, 9th ed. PubMed

- Heat sterilization is considered as the most reliable method of sterilization.
- It can be done by 2 methods
  - Dry heat
  - Moist heat

Dry heat	Moist heat
Mechanism of killing: • Killing effect is due to protein denaturation, oxidative damage and the toxic effect of metabolite	**Mechanism of killing:** • Is due to protein denaturation and coagulation
Methods and its use: • **Flaming:** for loop wire, searing spatulas • Incineration: ▪ Contaminated cloth ▪ Pathological waste ▪ Anatomical remains • **Hot air oven** ▪ All glass syringes and glass wares ▪ **Liquid paraffin** ▪ **Dusting powder** ▪ Swabs ▪ Scalpel, foreceps, scissors ▪ Fat and grease	**Methods and use:** • **Pasteurization** ▪ Holder method ▪ Flash method • **Autoclaving (steam sterilization):** *121°C x 15 min at 15 psi. Used for:* ▪ Culture media ▪ Aprons, dressing ▪ Surgical instruments except sharps ▪ **Gloves** ▪ Catheter ▪ Sputum

TABLE: Radiation used for sterilization

Ionizing radiation (aka cold sterilization)	Nonionizing radiation
Methods: • **Photon irradiation (γ):** Most commonly used among radiation sterilization • Electron irradiation (β) **Uses:** Used for heat sensitive materials like: • Plastic disposables • Bone and tissue grafts • Adhesive dressings • **Catgut suture**	**Methods:** • **Infrared rays:** Used for prepacked items like catheters and syringes • **UV Radiation:** Operation theatre, Laboratories

48. Ans. (b) Differential stain

Ref: Microbiology by Ananthanarayan and Paniker, 8th ed. pg. 15

DIFFERENTIAL STAIN

- These are positive stain, which divide bacterial population into two different groups by imparting two different colors
  - **Gram Stain:** It is the **most common staining method of bacteriology**. It stains cell wall of bacteria.
    - **Gram positive** appears blue
    - **Gram negative** appears pink/red
  - **Z-N stain** is used to distinguish acid fast bacteria and non-acid fast bacteria.
    - Presence of mycolic acid is responsible for the acid-fast nature of bacteria.

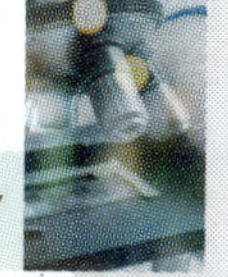

49. Ans. (d) Hot air oven

Ref: Microbiology by Ananthanarayan and Paniker, 8th ed. pg. 31

- **Flaming:** In this method the articles should be sterilized on the hot flame of Bunsen burner.
- **Hot air oven:** It is also called *dry heat sterilizer.*

Note: The articles should be sterilized at the temperature 160°C for 2 hours or 150–170°C for 1 hour.

  - Glass ware like test tube, pipette, flask and glass syringes, fixed oil glycerin, liquid paraffin, propylene glycol and zinc oxide etc. can be sterilized by this method.
- **Auto clave:** This type of sterilization is done by steam heat under pressure.
  Use: Glass ware, surgical dressing, rubber, gloves, surgical instrument are sterilized by this method.

50. Ans. (b) Bacillus subtilis

Ref: Textbook of Microbiology S. Kumar/14

- Hot air oven is dry heat sterilization technique used most commonly to sterilize glassware and metal items.
- *Sterility check* is done for each and every lot to enhance quality of sterilization. For this purpose the *biological indicator organism bacillus subtilis is used.*
- Non pathogenic clostridium tetani can also be used to check the efficiency *(Bacillus subtilis > Non-pathogenic clostridium tetani).*
- **Note:** ***Stearothermophillus is used to check efficiency of autoclave.***

51. Ans. (a) Autoclaving at 135 degrees

Ref: Microbiology by Ananthanarayan and Paniker, 8th ed. pg. 32

- Prions are best destroyed by autoclave at 135 degree for one hour.

52. Ans. (a) Solid medium

Ref: Microbiology by Ananthanarayan and Paniker, 8th ed. pg. 39-40

GROWING BACTERIAL CULTURES IN LIQUID NUTRIENT BROTH

- Nutrient broth is a liquid bacterial growth medium made of powdered beef extract and short chains of amino acids that have been dissolved in water.
- Liquid medium is convenient to use for growing bacteria in test tubes, and can reveal information about the oxygen requirements of bacteria growing within.
- Bacteria that require oxygen will grow close to the water's surface, and bacteria that cannot tolerate the presence of oxygen will grow at the bottom of the test tube.

GROWING BACTERIAL CULTURES ON SOLID MEDIA

- *Broth media can be made solid by adding agar,* a gel like polysaccharide extracted from red algae.
- Broth with about 1.5% agar added will be liquid when heated, but solid at room temperature, making it easy to pour into a vessel, such as a Petri dish or test tube when hot.
- The solution then becomes solid once cooled.

53. Ans. (b) To make the medium solid

- *Broth media can be made solid by adding agar,* a gel like polysaccharide extracted from red algae.
- Broth with about 1.5% agar added will be liquid when heated, but solid at room temperature, making it easy to pour into a vessel, such as a Petri dish or test tube when hot.
- The solution then becomes solid once cooled.

54. Ans. (c) Pseudomonas aeruginosa

Ref: Microbiology by Ananthanarayan and Paniker, 8th ed. pg. 317

- Pseudomonas is isolated from feces or other samples by using selective media such as cetrimide agar.
- E.Coli is cultured in Mac-conkey media
- Clostridium tetani grows on ordinary media and is improved by blood and serum.
- Clostridium perfringens grows on blood agar plate.

55. Ans. (a) N. Meningitis

Ref: Microbiology by Ananthanarayan and Paniker, 8th ed. pg. 225, 227

- Thayer martin medium is selective medium for N. Meningitis.

56. Ans. (c) LJ medium

Ref: Harrison, 19th ed. pg. 1110

- Harrison states: *"In genitourinary TB - **culture** of 3 morning urinary specimen yields a definitive diagnosis in 90% cases. LJ medium is most common solid medium used for culture.*
- Prevalence of GU TB= **10–15%**
- **MC c/o:** Urinary frequency, dysuria, nocturia, hematuria, and flank or abdominal pain.
- **Diagnosis:** Culture of three morning urine specimens-definitive diagnosis in nearly 90% patient.
- **Other test:** IV pyelography, abdominal CT, MRI-may show deformities and obstructions
- **Suggestive findings:** Calcifications and ureteral strictures

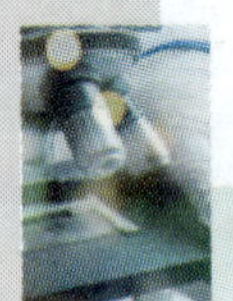

- **Complication:**
  - **Female:** Affects the fallopian tubes and the endometrium and may cause infertility, pelvic pain, and menstrual abnormalities.
  - **Diagnosis** requires biopsy or culture of specimens obtained by dilation and curettage.
  - **Male**- affects the epididymis, producing a slightly tender mass that may drain externally through a fistulous tract; orchitis and prostatitis may also develop.
- **Rx:** Genitourinary TB **responds well to chemotherapy**.

57. Ans. (a) Pink

Ref: Microbiology by Ananthanarayan and Paniker, 8th ed. pg. 47

- Color change in Robertson cooked meat media depends on clostridial organism:
  - **Clostridium perferingens (Saccarolytic activity):** color turns to **pink** *(Mn: P-P)*
  - **If Clostridium tetani (Proteolytic activity):** colour turns to **black**

Note: *Robertson cooked meat medium is most widely used fluid medium for culture of anaerobes.*

58. Ans. (b) Differential media

Ref: Microbiology by Ananthanarayan and Paniker, 8th ed. pg. 40

DIFFERENTIAL MEDIA (NEUTRAL RED)

- It distinguishes one microorganism type from another growing on the same media.
- This type of media is used for the detection of microorganisms and by molecular biologists to detect recombinant strains of bacteria.
- **Examples of differential media include:**
  - Blood agar
  - Eosin methylene blue (EMB)
  - *MacConkey (MCK)*
  - Mannitol salt agar (MSA) Staph

Extra Mile

- **Mac Conkey agar** is a culture medium designed to grow Gram-negative bacteria and differentiate them for lactose fermentation and lactose non-fermenter.
- It consists of Peptone, Lactose, Agar neutral red and E. coli klebsiella Na taurocholate shows up lactose fermenters as PINK COLONIES
- Non lactose Fermenters are colorless. Shigella, Salmonella profess

59. Ans. (d) Stuart media

Ref: Microbiology by Ananthanarayan and Paniker, 8th ed. pg. 40, 43

DIFFERENTIAL MEDIA

- It is also known as differential media which distinguishes one microorganism type from another growing on the same media.
- This type of media is used for the detection of microorganisms and by molecular biologists to detect recombinant strains of bacteria.
- Examples of differential media include:
  - Blood agar
  - Eosin methylene blue (EMB)
  - MacConkey (MCK)
  - mannitol salt agar (MSA)

TRANSPORT MEDIA

Examples of Transport Media Include

- Thioglycolate broth for strict anaerobes
- **Stuart transport medium** - a non-nutrient soft agar gel containing a reducing agent to prevent oxidation, and charcoal to neutralize
- Certain bacterial inhibitors- for gonococci, and buffered glycerol saline for enteric bacilli.
- Venkat-Ramakrishnan (VR) medium for *V. cholerae*.

60. Ans. (c) Ziehl-Neelson stain

Ref: Microbiology by Ananthanarayan and Paniker, 8th ed. pg. 352

- Z-N stain is used to distinguish acid fast bacteria and non-acid fast bacteria.
- Presence of mycolic acid is responsible for the acid-fast nature of bacteria.
- For the diagnosis and control of tuberculosis Sputum microscopy is the most reliable single method.
- Preparation of smear is from the thick purulent part of the sputum. They are the dried, heated fixed and stained by the Ziehl-Neelsen technique.
- The *smear is then covered with strong carbol fuchsin* and gently heated for 5–7 minutes, without letting the stain boil and become dry.
- *Wash the slide* with water and *decolourise* it with 20% sulphuric acid, followed by 95% ethanol for two minutes.
- Smear is then *counterstained* with Loeffler's methylene blue, 1% picric acid or 0.2% malachite green for one minute.
- Now, under the *oil immersion objective*, acid fast bacilli are seen as bright red rods while the background is blue, yellow or green depending on the counterstain used.
- At least 10,000 acid fast bacilli should be present per ml of sputum for them to be readily demonstrable in direct smears.

61. Ans. (b) Tube agglutination

Ref: Microbiology by Ananthanarayan and Paniker, 8th ed. pg. 108

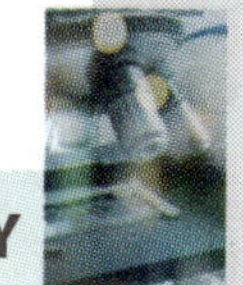

TABLE: Agglutination tests and their uses

Agglutination test	Used mainly for
Direct agglutination test	Determination of blood group Bacterial agglutination test for serotyping & serogrouping. **Eg: Vibrio Cholera, Salmonella Sp.**
Slide agglutination test	Used for serotyping of salmonella **VDRL for syphillis**
Tube agglutination test	Aka standard agglutination test. Used for serological diagnosis of typhoid, brucellosis and typhus fever. **Ex: Widal Test, *Weil felix reaction*, and Kahn test**
Passive agglutination test	Rheumatoid factor **ANA for SLE** Antibody to Trichenella spiralis and antibody to group A strep.

62. Ans. (b) **Counter current immune-electrophoresis**

Ref: Microbiology by Ananthanarayan and Paniker, 8th ed. pg. 104

TABLE: Common precipitation tests and their examples

Precipitation test	Example
Ring test	**Ascoli thermoprecipitin test (anthrax)** and grouping of streptococci by **Lancefield technique**
Slide test	**VDRL test** for syphilis
Tube test	**Kahn test** for syphilis
Immunodiffusion tests	**Elek test** for toxigenicity of diphtheria bacilli
Electroimmuno diffusion	**Counter current immune-electrophoresis** and rocket electrophoresis

63. Ans. (c) **Widal test**

Ref: Microbiology by Ananthanarayan and Paniker, 8th ed. pg. 108

AGGLUTINATION TEST

- It is a blood test used to identify unknown antigens.
- Blood with the unknown antigen is mixed with a known antibody and whether or not agglutination occurs helps to identify the antigen.
- *Refer to above explanation of Q 61.*

64. Ans. (d) **Muramic acid**

Ref: Microbiology by Ananthanarayan and Paniker, 8th ed. pg. 10, 63, 425

- All the above options except muramic acid are membrane bound organelles which are absent in prokaryotes and only present in eukaryotes.
- Muramic Acid is one of the important components of the peptidoglycan wall present in the cell wall of prokaryotic cells.

65. Ans. (a) **C -substance**

Ref: Microbiology by Ananthanarayan and Paniker, 8th ed. pg. 205, 673

- Lancefield classification is a grouping system for beta hemolytic bacteria based on the polysaccharide in their cell walls, C – substance (carbohydrate), which is antigenic. So this classification is serologic.

66. Ans. (b) **Antibody**

Ref: Microbiology by Ananthanarayan and Paniker, 8th ed. pg. 102-103

- Antibody is attached to the surface of bacteria for opsonization, which further get phagocytized.

67. Ans. (c) **HIV Elisa**

Ref: Microbiology by Ananthanarayan and Paniker, 8th ed. pg. 570, 576

- ELISA HIV measures antibodies against the virus. These antibodies are of IgG type and can cross the placenta. Hence a baby born to HIV positive lady will test HIV positive on day 0 of life and may continue till these antibodies are cleared by the baby's immune system. The clearance may take 12-18 months and therefore Babies born to HIV lady may be false positive till the age mentioned.
- However DNA PCR or viral culture or p24 antigen positive on first few days of life is indicative of perinatal transmission rate of the virus which is 30%

Extra Mile

- The pernnatal transmission rate can be reduced by at least 50% in case single dose nevirapine given to the mother and to the baby within 72 hours. Breast feeding is indicated in baby born to HIV positive patient.

68. Ans. (d) **Infectious mononucleosis**

Ref: Microbiology by Ananthanarayan and Paniker, 8th ed. pg. 476

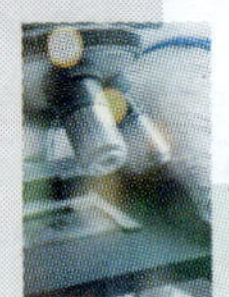

Infectious mononucleosis is diagnosed by Paul Bunnel test.

Revision of Key Points About Infectious Mononucleosis
- **Ebstein Barr virus** is causative for infectious mononucleosis.
- Infectious mononucleosis is called a **glandular fever**
- Clinical features include fever, lymphadenopathy, sore throat and presence of abnormal lymphocytes in blood.
- **Monospot test** is also used for diagnosis of infectious mononucleosis,
- Patients develop skin rash if they consume an antibiotic like **ampicillin**

EBV is also **oncogenic** in nature because it causes **B cell clonal activation.**

BACTERIOLOGY

69. Ans. (a) Bartonella henselae

Ref: Ananthanarayana and Panicker's Textbook of Microbiology, 10th ed. pg. 420

- A febrile illness with lymphadenopathy following a cat scratch had been known for long under the name 'cat scratch disease'.
- Symptoms typically include a non-painful bump or blister at the site of injury and painful and swollen lymph nodes.

70. Ans. (b) S. aureus

Ref: Ananthanarayana and Panicker's Textbook of Microbiology, 10th ed. pg. 204

- Staphylococcus aureus is the single most common cause of bacterial infection among drug users.
- Persons who inject drugs are at increased risk of developing Staphylococcus aureus bacteremia.

71. Ans. (a) Propionibacterium acne

Ref: Ananthanarayana and Panicker's Textbook of Microbiology, 10th ed. pg. 274

- Propionibacterium acnes is a gram-positive human skin commensal that prefers anaerobic growth conditions and is involved in the pathogenesis of acne
- Acne often debuts during changes in hormonal levels in pre-teens; however, it is also very common as an adult-onset condition, often associated with hormonal fluctuation during the menstrual cycle and pregnancy.

72. Ans. (b) TB meningitis

Ref: Ananthanarayana and Panicker's Textbook of Microbiology, 10th ed. pg. 677

- Neutrophils (x 10^6/L) - Usually <100 (but may be normal) Table to different TB/viral/bacterial meningitis

CSF Picture

Type	Cell	Protein	Glucose	Others
Normal	0-5 All Lymphocyte	20–40 mg/dL	50–70 mg/dL	Clear sterile
Acute Bacterial	↑↑ (100–10000) mostly neutrophils	↑ 100–200 mg/dL But not more than 500 mg/dL	↓ <40 mg/dL	Turbid, culture may be positive
Tubercular	↑ Lymphocyte in early week of infection. Later neutrophil elevated.	↑↑ 100–500 mg/dL may be even in gm/dL	↓ <40 mg/dL	AFB ZN stain ⊕ TB PCR cobweb formation ⊕
Aseptic viral	↑ (100–1000) mostly lymphocyte	↑ 50–200 mg/dL	Normal	Culture sterile

- Lymphocytes (x 10^6/L) - 50–1000 (but may be normal)
- Protein (g/L) - 1–5 (but may be normal)
- Glucose (CSF: blood ratio) - <0.3

73. Ans. (d) Sorbitol MacConkey agar

Ref: Ananthanarayana and Panicker's Textbook of Microbiology, 10th ed. pg. 41

- Sorbitol MacConkey Agar is a selective, differential medium, used for the isolation of pathogenic Escherichia coli in a laboratory setting.

74. Ans. (b) Listeria

Ref: Jawetz, Melnick and Adelberg's Medical Microbiology, 28th ed. pg. 339

- Tumbling motility is one of the useful characteristics of Listeria monocytogenes.
- This can be helpful to identify the causative pathogen along with Gram staining before the confirmatory microbiological examination.

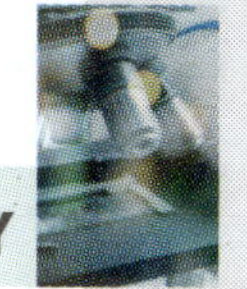

75. Ans. (d) Streptococcus sanguis

Ref: Ananthanarayana and Panicker's Textbook of Microbiology, 10th ed. pg. 220

CATALASE NEGATIVE STREPTOCOCCUS

- γ (No hemolysis) → Enterococcus
- α (Partial hemolysis) → S. pneumonia, viridans streptococcus
- β (Complete hemolysis) → S. pyogenes, S. agalactiae

CATALASE POSITIVE STREPTOCOCCUS

- Streptococcus sanguinis, S. oralis, and S. gordonii cause endocarditis in patients with damaged heart valves and reach the bloodstream mainly from the mouth, as a result of dental procedures, such as tooth extraction.
- Streptococcus sanguinis is Gram positive alpha hemolytic cocci with catalase negative and optochin resistant.

76. Ans. (b) C. diphtheria

Ref: Ananthanarayana and Panicker's Textbook of Microbiology, 10th ed. pg. 673

- Diphtheria is a serious bacterial infection of the nose and throat caused by the Corynebacterium diphtheriae.
- Marked swellings of cervical lymph nodes (lymphadenitis) and swelling of the surrounding soft-tissue give rise to the characteristic "bull-neck" appearance.
- Most common complications are myocarditis and neuritis. Formation of pseudomembrane (bleeds on removal)

77. Ans. (a) Dark field

Ref: Ananthanarayana and Panicker's Textbook of Microbiology, 10th ed. pg. 683

- Dark field microscopy is the most specific and sensitive technique to diagnose syphilis when an active chancre or condyloma lata is present.
- This technique allows for a presumptive diagnosis of syphilis even before antibodies have developed.

78. Ans. (a) Neisseria meningitis

Ref: Ananthanarayana and Panicker's Textbook of Microbiology, 10th ed. pg. 230

- Neisseria meningitidis, often referred to as meningococcus, is a diplococcal, Gram-negative bacterium that can cause meningitis and other forms of meningococcal disease.

79. Ans. (a) Streptococcus pneumoniae

Ref: Ananthanarayana and Panicker's Textbook of Microbiology, 10th ed. pg. 335; https://radiopaedia.org/articles/thumb-sign-epiglottitis-1

- The thumb sign in epiglottitis is a manifestation of an oedematous and enlarged epiglottis which is seen on lateral soft-tissue radiograph of the neck, and it suggests a diagnosis of acute infectious epiglottitis.

80. Ans. (c) Ludwig's angina

Ref: Ananthanarayana and Panicker's Textbook of Microbiology, 10th ed. pg. 214; https://www.ncbi.nlm.nih.gov/books/NBK482354/

- Ludwig angina is a type of bacterial infection that occurs in the floor of the mouth, under the tongue.
- It often develops after an infection of the roots of the teeth (such as tooth abscess) or a mouth injury.
- It is polymicrobial in nature.

81. Ans. (b) *N. meningitidis*

Ref: Harrison 20th ed. pg. 1118

- The image shows multiple petechiae and purpura on extremities and buttocks of patient. Coupled with abrupt onset fever and prostration, meningococcemia would be first differential diagnosis.
- Option A presents with eschar formation.
- Option C presents with ulcer on hand/foot at site of tick bite and regional lymph node enlargement with high grade fever.
- *Option D, M. catarrhalis* causes a large proportion of cases of lower respiratory tract infections in elderly patients with chronic obstructive pulmonary diseases and chronic bronchitis and frank pneumonia.

82. Ans. (d) Corynebacterium diphtheria

Ref: Ananthanarayan and Paniker's Textbook of Microbiology, 10th ed. pg. 242

- Corynebacterium diphtheriae is a Gram-positive nonmotile, club-shaped bacillus. Strains growing in tissue, or older cultures in vitro, contain thin spots in their cell walls that allow decolorization during the Gram stain and result in a Gram-variable reaction.
- Slender rods
- Clubbing at both ends
- Pleomorphic
- Non capsulated
- Granules are composed of polymetaphosphate
- Staining with Loeffler's methylene blue show bluish purple metachromatic granules, with purple bodies.

83. Ans. (a) Loffler's serum slope

Ref: Ananthanarayan and Paniker's Textbook of Microbiology, 10th ed. pg. 242

- The image shows features of faucial diphtheria. The swab from the lesion is plated on Loeffler serum slope, for early detection of corynebacterium.

- Due to its serum content, Loeffler medium can be used for the determination of proteolytic activities of microorganisms.
- The gray-white surface of the medium provides an excellent background for the detection and observation of colonial pigmentation.

84. Ans. (b) Candida

Ref: Ananthanarayan and Paniker's Textbook of Microbiology, 10th ed. pg. 615

- Oral candidiasis is an opportunistic infection of the oral cavity often caused by the overgrowth of Candida, a yeast-like fungus commonly found in the gastrointestinal tract of humans, as normal skin flora and in mucous membranes.
- It presents as whitish thrush on mucous membranes, which usually bleeds on scaping.

85. Ans. (c) Proteus

- Bacterial vaginosis is a type of vaginal inflammation caused by the overgrowth of bacteria naturally found in the vagina, which upsets the natural balance. Women in their reproductive years are most likely to get bacterial vaginosis, but it can affect women of any age.
- **Caused by:**
  - Gardenerella
  - Mobilincus
  - Coccobacillus

86. Ans. (c) *H. pylori*

- Among the given organisms, H. Pylori is the causative organism for peptic ulcer disease in more than 80-90% of the patients with PUD.
- Infection with H. Pylori impairs the protective mechanisms of GIT against low pH and digestive enzymes → leading to mucosal ulceration

87. Ans. (c) Grey pseudomembrane that bleeds on removal

Ref: Nelson 20th ed. pg. 2018

- Development of a localized or coalescing pseudomembrane can occur in any portion of the respiratory tract in case of Diptheria.
- The pseudomembrane is characterized by the formation of a dense, grey debris layer composed of a mixture of dead cells, fibrin, RBCs, WBCs, and organisms.
- *Removal of the membrane reveals a bleeding, oedematous mucosa.* The distribution of the membrane varies from local (e.g., tonsillar, pharyngeal) to widely covering the entire tracheobronchial tree.

88. Ans. (b) Gram positive rods with square ends

Ref: Textbook of Microbiology by Surinder Kumar, pg. 282; Lange Microbiology, Ch 12

- The genus *bacillus* includes large aerobic, gram-positive rods occurring in chains.
- Principle pathogen of bacillus species is bacillus anthracis (causes anthrax) and bacillus cereus (food poisoning).
- Anthrax is primarily a disease of herbivores—goats, sheep, cattle, horses, etc.
- In humans anthrax is acquired by:
  - Injured skin: Cutaneous anthrax
  - Mucous membrane: Gastrointestinal anthrax
  - Inhalation of spores: Inhalational anthrax (Woolsorter's disease)

Morphology:

- The typical cells, measuring 1 × 3–4 μm, have **square ends** and are arranged in long chains; spores are located in the center of the non-motile bacilli
- **Culture:** Round colonies with "cut-glass" appearance in transmitted light

Laboratory test:

- **Specimen:** Pus, Blood or sputum
- **Smear:** shows chain of large gram positive rods
- **Blood agar plates:** shows non-hemolytic gray to white colonies with rough texture and ground glass appearance.
- **Nutrient agar:** Medusa head appearance/comma shaped outgrowth from the colonies.
  - Long chain of bacilli resembles locks of matted hair under the low power microscope.
- **Gelatin stab:** Inverted fir tree appearance.

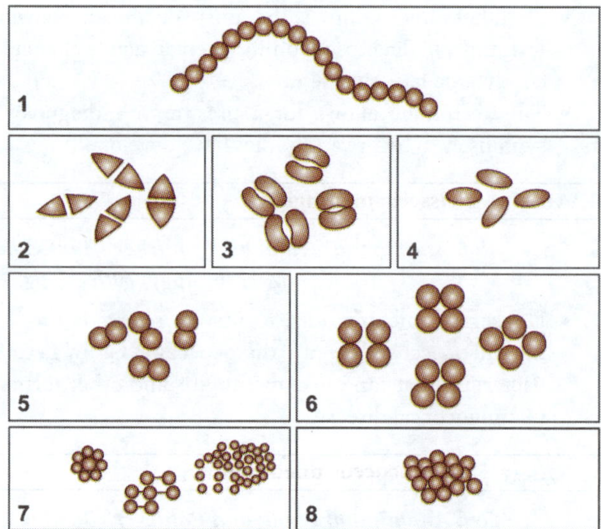

1

2

3

Arrangement of bacteria: A. Cocci: 1. Streptococci 2. Pneumococci 3. Gonococci 4. Meningococci 5. Neisseria catarrhalis 6. Gaffkya tetragena 7. Sarcina 8. Staphylococci; B. Bacilli: 1. Bacilli in cluster 2. Bacilli in chains (B. anthrax) 3. Diplobacilli (K. pneumoniae)

Extra Mile

- **Bacillus anthracis**
  - It is the first pathogenic bacterium to be observed under the microscope
  - First communicable disease shown to be transmitted by inoculation of infected blood
  - First bacterium used for the preparation of **an attenuated vaccine** by Pasteur was *B. anthracis.*

89. Ans. (c) Leprosy

Ref: Textbook of Microbiology by Surinder Kumar, pg. 328

- Choice A has a stellate granuloma while choice D has a gumma. Hence both are ruled out. Choice B is a rickettsial disease
- Choice C leprosy is a chronic granulomatous disease
- A lepromatous leprosy patient develops numerous nodular skin lesions **(lepromata)** on face, ear lobes, hands, feet and less commonly trunk.
- It shows AFB positive bacilli.
- Skin Biopsy shows: Many macrophages, seen as large foamy cells packed with AFB
- **Microscopy of lepromatous leprosy**
  - Smears are stained by Ziehl-Neelsen method using 5 percent instead of 20 percent sulphuric acid for decolorization. Acid-fast bacilli (AFB) arranged in parallel bundles within macrophages

The smears are graded, based on the number of bacilli as follows:

No AFB in 100 O/F → Neg
1–9 AFB/100 O/F → Scanty
10–99 AFB/ 100 O/F → 1+
1–10 AFB/O/F → 2+
>10 AFB/O/F → 3+

90. Ans. (a) Respiratory disease

Ref: Harrison 20th ed. pg. 1138

- The bacterium L. pneumophila leads to legionnaire disease.
- The most common form of transmission of Legionella is inhalation of contaminated aerosols produced in conjunction with water sprays, jets or mists.
- It has 2 distinct clinical syndromes: Legionnaires disease, which most often manifests as severe pneumonia accompanied by multisystemic disease, and Pontiac fever, which is an acute, febrile, self-limited, viral-like illness

91. Ans. (b) 2nd week

Ref: Harrison 20th ed. pg. 1176

AMNESTIC RESPONSE

- Widal test should be done in *second week* of presentation of a case of typhoid. It is a serological test with patient showing H and/or O titres greater than or equal to 1:160 and typhoid-like symptoms is strongly suggestive of diagnosis of typhoid fever. *False positive widal is seen in case of malaria.*
- The criterion standard for diagnosis of typhoid fever has long been culture isolation of the organism. In the first week bone marrow culture or blood culture should be done.
- Bone marrow aspiration and blood are cultured in a selective medium (e.g., 10% aqueous oxgall) or a nutritious medium (e.g., tryptic soy broth) and are incubated at 37°C for at least 7 days.

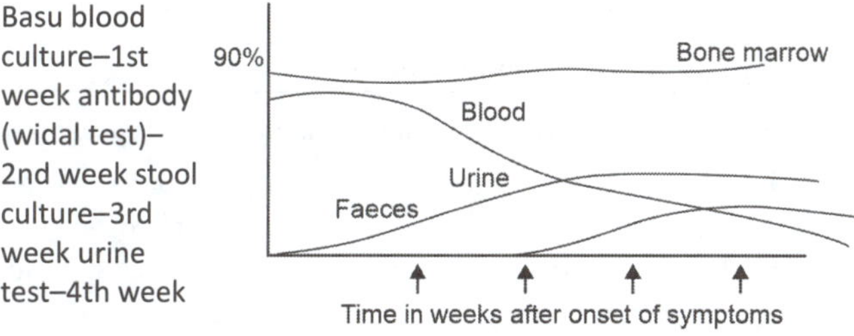

92. Ans. (d) Actinomyces

Ref: Textbook of Diagnostic Microbiology, E-book, pg. 505

- **Nocardia:** Aerobe, acid fast
- **Actinomyces:** Anerobe, non-acid-fast bacilli
- **Tuberculosis:** Aerobic, acid fast
- **Listeria:** Facultative anaerobe, Gram-positive, non-acid-fast

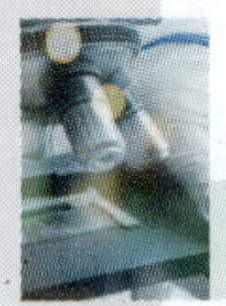

93. Ans. (d) *Haemophilus influenzae*

Ref: Textbook of Diagnostic Microbiology, E-book, pg. 14

- **Capnophilic bacteria:** Organisms which thrive on the high concentration of CO_2. They require ~5–10% of CO_2. For example, *Haemophilus influenzae, Neisseria.*
- **Facultative anaerobe:** These are capable of growing under both aerobic and anaerobic conditions. For example, *Staphylococcus aureus.*
- **Obligate anaerobe:** These organisms grow only under non-oxygen environment. Oxygen is toxic for these organisms. For example, *Clostridium.*
- **Obligate aerobe:** There is absolute requirement of oxygen for survival for this type of organism. For example, *Mycobacterium.*

94. Ans. (b) Listeria monocytogenes

Ref: Ananthnarayan and Paniker's Textbook of Microbiology, 8th ed. pg. 395

- The Anton test is used in the identification of *L. monocytogenes*; instillation of a culture into the conjunctival sac of a rabbit or guinea pig causes severe keratoconjunctivitis within 24 hours.
- Experimental inoculation in rabbits causes marked monocytosis, hence the name monocytogenes. Monocytosis is a feature of human listeriosis also.

95. Ans. (b) Inhibiting protein synthesis

Ref: Ananthanarayan's Microbiology, 8th ed. pg. 234

- The diphtheria toxin causes damage to eukaryotic cells and tissues by inhibition of protein synthesis in the cells.
- Although the toxin is responsible for the lethal symptoms of the disease, the virulence of C. diphtheria cannot be attributed to toxigenicity alone, since a distinct invasive phase apparently precedes toxigenesis.

96. Ans. (a) Listeria monocytogenes

Ref: Handbook of Zoonoses, 2nd ed. pg. 322

- Listeria monocytogenes is Gram-positive, nonspore forming rod shaped bacteria with rounded ends.
- The organisms occasionally appear in a palisade arrangement, along with some V or Y forms.
- It is motile via one to six peritrichous flagella and exihibits characteristic tumbling motility.
- Tumbling motility can be seen best microscopically using cultures grown in tryptose broth incubated at 20°C. The organism is weakly motile at 37°C.

97. Ans. (d) V. Cholerae

Ref: Ananthnarayan and Paniker's Textbook of Microbiology, 8th ed. pg. 302

- *In stained films of mucus flakes from acute cholera cases,* the vibrios are seen arranged in parallel rows, described by Koch as the '*fish in stream*' appearance.
- "School of Fish" appearance is seen in H. ducreyi.
- Vibrios are Gram-negative, rigid, curved rods that are actively motile by means of a polar flagellum. The name 'vibrio' is derived from the characteristic vibratory motility/darting motility
- The cholera vibrio is a short, curved, cylindrical rod, about 1.5 × 0.2-0.4 µm in size, with rounded or slightly pointed ends. The cell is typically **comma shaped.**
- Aside from *V. cholera*, darting motility is also seen in Campylobacter.

98. Ans. (c) Legionella

Ref: Ananthnarayan and Paniker's Textbook of Microbiology, 8th ed. pg. 400

- Pontiac fever was named for Pontiac, Michigan, where the first case was recognized. It caused by various species of **Gram-negative bacteria in the genus *Legionella.***
- It is a milder, non-fatal, influenza like illness with fever, chills, myalgia and headache.
- Pontiac fever resolves spontaneously and often goes undiagnosed.
- Both Pontiac fever and the more severe Legionnaire's disease are caused by the same bacteria, Leginonella Pneumophila but Pontiac fever does not include pneumonia.

Extra Mile

Legionnaire's disease:
- Can be either epidemic or sporadic.
- **Incubation period:** 2–10 days
- Presents with fever, non-productive cough and dyspnea. If untreated it rapidly progresses to pneumonia.

99. Ans. (b) Pneumococcus

Ref: Ananthnarayan and Paniker's Textbook of Microbiology, 8th ed. pg. 219-220

- The pathogen that most commonly causes sepsis in patients who have undergone splenectomy, as well as in children with sickle cell disease, is S. pneumoniae (pneumococcus).
- Asplenic patients are at risk for rapidly progressive septicemia and death. Such patients should be vaccinated against pneumococci, H. influenzae type b, meningococci, and influenza virus, and if fever develops, they should receive empirical antimicrobial therapy immediately.
- Mortality among patients with post-splenectomy sepsis can be as high as 50%. Most commonly caused by *Streptococcus pneumoniae*, this infection often has a sudden onset and a fulminant course.

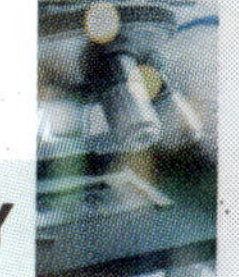

100. Ans. (b) Staphylococcus

Bacterial Food Poisoning

Incubation period, organism	Symptoms	Common sources
1–6 H		
Staphylococcus aureus	Nausea, vomiting, diarrhea	Ham, poultry, potato or egg salad, mayonnaise, cream pastries
Bacillus cereus	Nausea, vomiting, diarrhea	Fried rice
8–16 H		
Clostridium perfringens	Abdominal cramps, diarrhea (vomiting rare)	Beef, poultry, legumes, gravies
B. cereus	Abdominal cramps, diarrhea (vomiting rare)	Meats, vegetables, dried beans, cereals
> 16 H		
Vibrio cholerae	Watery diarrhea	Shellfish
Enterotoxigenic *Escherichia coli*	Watery diarrhea	Salads, cheese, meats,water
Enterohemorrhagic *E.coli*	Bloody diarrhea	Ground beef, roast beef, salami, raw milk, raw vegetables, apple juice
Salmonella spp.	Inflammatory diarrhea	Beef, poultry, eggs, dairy products
Campylobacter jejuni	Inflammatory diarrhea	Poultry, raw milk
Shigella spp	Dysentery	Potato or egg salad, lettuce, raw vegetables
Vibrio parahaemolyticus	Dysentery	Mollusks, crustaceans

101. Ans. (a) Staphylococcus aureus

- Staphylococcus aureus is the most common cause of postinfluenza secondary bacterial pneumonia.
- It most often affects the elderly patients.

102. Ans. (b) Gram-positive bacilli

Ref: Harrisons, 19th ed. pg. 978

- *C. diphtheriae* is a **Gram-positive bacillus that is unencapsulated, nonmotile, and nonsporulating.**
- The bacteria have a characteristic club-shaped bacillary appearance and typically form clusters of parallel rays, or *palisades*, that are referred to as **"Chinese characters."**

103. Ans. (d) Laryngopharynx

Ref: Harrisons, 19th ed. pg. 978

- Diptheria is a nasopharyngeal and skin infection caused by *Corynebacterium diphtheriae*. Toxigenic strains of *C. diphtheria* produce a protein toxin that causes systemic toxicity, myocarditis, and polyneuropathy.
- The toxigenic strains cause pharyngeal diphtheria, while the non-toxigenic strains commonly cause cutaneous disease.
- **Harrisons states:** *"Respiratory/pharyngeal form of diphtheria is from notiable diseases, while cutaneous diphtheria is NOT."*
- **Most severe form of diphtheria:** Laryngeal

104. Ans. (c) Bacillus anthrax

Ref: Harrisons, 19th ed. pg. 261e2

- **McFadyean reaction** is a special staining reaction, demonstrating a pink capsule around a blue cell, after staining with methylene blue, which is used as a presumptive diagnosis for **anthrax** in a blood smear.
- Anthrax is caused by *B. anthracis*, a Gram-positive, nonmotile, spore-forming rod that is found in soil and predominantly causes disease in herbivores such as cattle, goats, and sheep.

105. Ans. (a) Staph epidermis

Ref: Harrisons, 19th ed. pg. 145e-4

- Many bacterial, fungal, and protozoal species have the ability to grow in multicellular masses called biofilms.
- These masses are biochemically and morphologically quite distinct from the free-living individual cells referred to as *planktonic cells.*
- Growth in biofilms leads to altered microbial metabolism, production of extracellular virulence factors, and decreased susceptibility to antimicrobial agents, biocides, and host defense molecules and cells.
- **Examples of bacterial organisms forming biofilm:**
  - P. aeruginosa, staphylococci and other pathogens growing on implanted medical devices, and dental pathogens growing on tooth surfaces to form plaque
  - **S. epidermis** – on Prosthetic valve, IV catheter
  - **Strep Mutans/sanguinis** – on Dental plaques
  - **Pseudomonas** – Cystic fibrosis, contact lens
  - **Strep. viridans** – Endocarditis
  - **Non-typable H. influenza**- Otitis. Media

106. Ans. (a) Biofilm formation

- S. epidermis is a pathogenic organism which affects interventions like catheter, canula.
- It is an organism which can form biofilm.
- It is novobiocin sensitive.

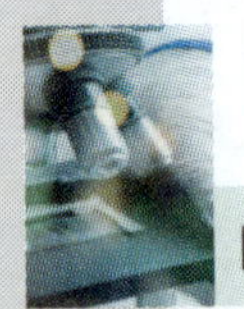

107. Ans. (d) 100

108. Ans. (b) ++

Ref: PubMed; http://www.hrsa.gov/hansensdisease/diagnosis/skinsmears.html

Refer to above explanation of Q. 89

109. Ans. (a) Bacillus anthrax

Ref: Harrisons, 19th ed. pg. 261e-2

- **There are three major clinical forms of anthrax:**
  - Gastrointestinal, cutaneous, and inhalational.
  - **Gastrointestinal anthrax** typically results from the **ingestion of contaminated meat.**
  - **Cutaneous anthrax** typically begins as a papule following the introduction of spores through an opening in the skin. This papule then evolves to a painless vesicle followed by the development of a coal-black, necrotic eschar.
  - **Inhalational anthrax is the** form most likely to be responsible for death in the setting of a bioterrorist attack.

110. Ans. (a) Flea

Ref: Harrisons, 19th ed. pg. 1070

- Plague is a systemic zoonosis caused by ***Yersinia pestis.***
- It predominantly affects small rodents in rural areas of Africa, Asia, and the Americas and is usually **transmitted to humans by an arthropod vector (the flea).**
- Sometimes, infection follows contact with animal tissues or respiratory droplets.
  - The genus *Yersinia* comprises **gram-negative bacteria** of the family Enterobacteriaceae (gamma proteobacteria).

111. Ans. (b) Conjugation

Ref: Microbiology by Ananthanarayan and Paniker, 8th ed. pg. 60

112. Ans. (a) Transduction

Ref: Microbiology by Ananthanarayan and Paniker, 8th ed. pg. 61, 63

113. Ans. (c) Increase in size

Ref: Microbiology by Ananthanarayan and Paniker, 8th ed. pg. 24

Refer to above explanation of Q. 36

114. Ans. (d) H. pylori

Ref: Internet Source

- The rapid urease test also known as the Campylobacter like organism (CLO) test is **done for H. pylori** *in which the conversion of urea to ammonia and carbon dioxide by the urease enzyme present in the H. pylori is tested.*
- The Typhidot or dot ELISA is a test for the rapid diagnosis of S. typhi giving the separate identification of IgG and IgM antibodies whereas Widal test tests for specific antibody titres.
- Antigen tests which are EIA (Enzyme immunoassay) and Rapid HIV antibody test are used for detecting specific HIV antibodies and PCR (Polymerase Chain Reaction Test) is used for detecting genetic material of HIV.

115. Ans. (b) Listeria

Ref: Microbiology by Ananthanarayan and Paniker, 8th ed. pg. 226, 395

Listeria is the bacteria that is classically associated with tumbling motility.

Swarming Motility	Proteus
Gliding Motility	P. Aeruginosa, Mycoplasma
Darting Motility	Campylobacter, Vibrio Cholera
Falling Leaf Motility	Giardia
Shooting Star Motility	Vibrio
Cork Screw Motility	T. Pallidum
Lashing motility	Borrelia

116. Ans. (d) Gonococci

Ref: Microbiology by Ananthanarayan and Paniker, 8th ed. pg. 227

TABLE: Various Shapes of Bacteria

Shape	Associated bacteria
• Club Shape	Cornyebacteria
• Lanceolate	Pneumococci
• Half Moon/Lens	Meningococci
• Kidney Shape	Gonnococci
• Comma	Vibrio And Campylobacter

117. Ans. (c) Staph Aureus

Ref: Robbin's, 9th ed.

Diseases Characterized by Granulomas

- **Tuberculosis:** The granulomas of tuberculosis tend to contain necrosis ("caseating tubercules"), but non-necrotizing granulomas may also be present.

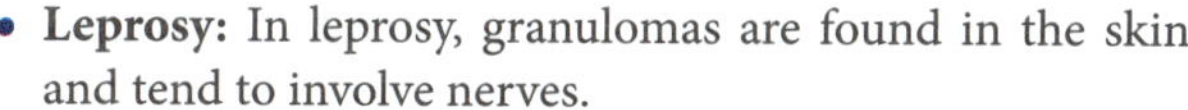

- **Leprosy:** In leprosy, granulomas are found in the skin and tend to involve nerves.
- **Sarcoidosis:** is a disease of unknown cause characterized by non-necrotizing ("non-caseating") granulomas in multiple organs and body sites, most commonly the lungs and lymph nodes within the chest cavity.
- **Hemophilus Ducreyi** causes chancre. It presents with painful genital ulcer with painful lymphadenopathy
- **Staph aureus** infections like pyoderma, abscess, HAP, food poisoning etc doesn't involve lymph nodes.

118. Ans. (a) Staph. aureus

Ref: Harriosn 18th ed./128, Microbiology by Ananthanarayan and Paniker, 8th ed. pg. 198

Refer to above explanation of Q. 117

119. Ans. (c) Staphylococcus

Ref: Harrison, 18th ed. pg. 128, Microbiology by Ananthanarayan and Paniker, 8th ed. pg. 198

- **Staphylococcus** causes food poisoning by enterotoxin A, due to intake of milk or milk products.
  - It is a preformed, heat stable enterotoxin, which stimulate the vagus nerve causing vomiting as main and first symptom.
  - I.P. < 6 hours
- *Outbreaks following picnics where potato salad, mayonnaise, and cream pastries have been served offer classic examples of staphylococcal food poisoning.*
- **Bacillus cereus** is an important cause of food poisoning, isolated from soil, vegetables, milk cereals, meat etc.
- It produces 2 types of food poisoning:

Diarrhea type- main symptom	Emetic type- main symptom
• Associated with wide range of food intake including meat, puddings etc. • I.P. 8-16 hrs • Occurs due to heat labile enterotoxin	• *Associated with intake of Chinese fried rice* • I.P. 1-5 hrs • Due to pre-formed, heat stable toxin

- **Clostridium perfringens** causes gastroenteritis after intake of infected meat or meat products. I.P. - 8-16 hours.
- **Clostridium botulism** causes food poisoning due to consumption of canned food. I.P. 1 to 3 days.

120. Ans. (c) Staphylococcus aureus

Ref: Microbiology by Ananthanarayan and Paniker 8th ed. pg. 198, Harrison's 18th ed./Ch 128

- Among the given options staph aureus has the shortest incubation period (1-6 hrs).

Please refer to above explanation for more details

121. Ans. (c) Transpeptidase

Ref: Microbiology by Ananthanarayan and Paniker, 8th ed. pg. 197, 201-202

Resistance develops due to alteration in transpeptidase (penicillin binding protein) on which all beta lactam antibiotics act. Hence MRSA is resistant to all β-lactam antibiotics.

122. Ans. (b) B. Cereus

Ref: Microbiology by Ananthanarayan and Paniker, 8th ed. pg. 247, 654

As indicated in the table above, the common source of B. cereus is fried rice . Refer above explanation for details.

123. Ans. (a) Can be transmitted by parenteral route

Ref: Microbiology by Ananthanarayan and Paniker, 8th ed. pg. 247, 654

124. Ans. (a) 7-21 days

Ref: Microbiology by Ananthanarayan and Paniker, 8th ed. pg. 293

- I.P of salmonella is 3–21 days
- **Features of Typhoid-Step ladder pyrexia, Rash (rose spot)** relative bradycardia, hepatospenomegaly, epistaxis
- **Complication**-Intestinal perforation and GI hemorrhage most common complication, seen during 3rd and 4th week.

125. Ans. (a) Vibrio cholerae O1

Ref: Microbiology by Ananthanarayan and Paniker, 8th ed. pg. 302-305

- ***Though the various strains of cholera may present with rice watery diarrhea, the classic rice watery diarrhea is usually associated with strains O1 and strain O139.***
- *In these strains the more common strain to find is strain O1.*

126. Ans. (a) EPEC

Ref: Microbiology by Ananthanarayan and Paniker, 8th ed. pg. 276 & 277

ENTEROPATHOGENIC E. COLI/ENTEROADHERENT E. COLI (EPEC)

- It causes diarrhoea in infants and children usually occuring as institutional out breaks.
- In infantile enteritis, it does not produce enterotoxin, nor are they invasive,
- The bacilli are seen in to be adherent to the mucosa of the upper small intestine and cause disruption of the brush border microvilli.

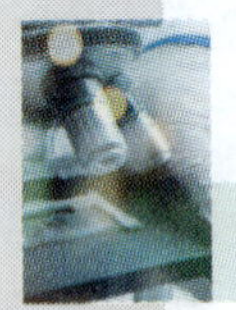

- These strains can be identified by their adhesion to HEP - 2 cells.

ENTEROTOXIGENIC E. COLI (ETEC)

- **It causes traveller's diarrhoea [ETEC is the most common cause of traveller's diarrhea].**
- It produces enterotoxins. They can produce heat labile toxin (LT) or heat stable toxin or both.
- Toxin production alone may not lead to illness. The strain should first be able to adhere to intestinal mucosa.
- This adhesiveness is medicated by *fimbria! or colonisation factor antigen (CFA).*

ENTEROINVASIVE E. COLI (EIEC)

- They themselves resemble shigella and their infection resembles shigellosis *(remember: Shiga like toxin is elaborated by enterohemorrhagic E. coli).*
- These strains are *non motile, do not ferment lactose or ferment it late* with acid without producing any gas.
- They produce mild diarrhoea to frank dysentry and occur in adult as well as in children.
- They have been termed enteroinvasive because they have the capacity to invade intestinal epithelial cells in vivo and penetrate HeLa or HEP - 2 cells in tissue culture.
- This ability of penetration is plasmid determined which codes for outer membrane antigens called the 'virulence marker antigen' (VMA). The detection of plasmid can be diagnostic.
- For laboratory diagnosis of EIEC, the *sereny test* used to be employed.

ENTERO-HEMORRHAGIC E. COLI OR VEROTOXIGENIC E. COLI

- These strains produce verocytotoxin (VT) or **shiga like toxin (SLT)**
- They can cause mild diarrhoea to fatal hemorrhagic colitis.
- This toxin also acts on vascular endothelium to promote the synthesis of coagulation factor VIII, vWF which triggers platelet aggregation.
- They can cause hemolytic uremic syndrome particularly in young children and the elderly.
- **0157 : H 7 is the most prominent serotype of EHEC, associated with HUS**, but 06, 026, 055, 091, 0103, 0111, 0113 and OX3 have also been associated with this syndrome.
- The primary target for VT is vascular endothelium.
- Laboratory diagnosis of VTEC diarrhea is established by demonstration of the bacilli or VT in feces directly or in culture.

ENTEROAGGREGATIVE E COLI (EACE)

- They have been associated with persistent diarrhea, especially in developing countries.
- In vitro they appear aggregated in a 'stacked brick' formation in Hep-2 cells.

127. Ans. (d) *E. coli*

Ref: Microbiology by Ananthanarayan and Paniker, 8th ed. pg. 276-77

- Hemoltic uremic syndrome (HUS) is a **type 3 hypersensitivity reaction** associated with small vessel vasculitis.
- Organisms causing HUS is E.Coli (particularly EHEC) and shigella dysentriae.

128. Ans. (d) EHEC

Ref: Ananthanaryan, 8th ed. pg. 276 & 277

Please refer to above explanation

129. Ans. (c) ETEC

Ref: Microbiology by Ananthanarayan and Paniker, 8th ed. pg. 276 & 277

Please refer to above explanation

130. Ans. (a) Traveller's diarrhea

Ref: Harrison 19th ed./727, Ananthanarayan 9/e 279

- **Antimicrobials are given for Traveller's diarrhea.**
- **Standard regimen is a 3-day course of a quinolone taken twice daily.**
- The current approach to self-treatment of travellers' diarrhea for the typical short-term traveller is to carry three once-daily doses of an antibiotic and to use as many doses as necessary to resolve the illness.
- If neither high fever nor blood in the stool accompanies the diarrhea, **loperamide** should be taken in combination with the antibiotic; studies have shown that this combination is more effective than an antibiotic alone and does not prolong illness.
- **Prophylaxis- bismuth subsalicylate**- widely used but only ~60% effective.
- For certain individuals (e.g., athletes, persons with a repeated history of travelers' diarrhea, and persons with chronic diseases), a single daily dose of a **quinolone, azithromycin, or rifaximin during travel of <1 month's duration** is 75–90% efficacious in preventing travellers' diarrhea.
- **Causes of travellers' diarrhea– Enterotoxigenic E coli is most common cause.**
- **Other causes**- Enteroaggrative E coli, Salmonella, Shigella, Vibrio, Campylobacter etc.

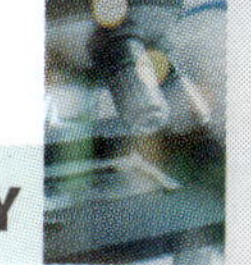

131. Ans. (b) Enterotoxin

Ref: Microbiology by Ananthanarayan and Paniker, 8th ed. pg. 198-199

- Enterotoxins are responsible for food poisoning and are produced when Staphylococcus Aureus grows in carbohydrate and protien foods. There are multiple types of enterotoxins (A-E, G-I, K-M) and these are usually superantigens.
- The alpha toxin is a potent hemolysin which acts on a broad spectrum of cell membranes, including RBC's.
- The beta toxin degrades spingomyelin and is also toxic for many types of cells.
- TSST-1 is the same as enterotoxin F and is therefore also a superantigen and is associated with fever, shock multisystem involvement and a desquamative skin rash.

132. Ans. (c) Vibrio cholerae

Ref: Microbiology by Ananthanarayan and Paniker, 8th ed. pg. 302-305

- Vibrio Cholerae is the organism with a single flagellum. Bacteria with a single flagellum are called monotrichous. Lophotrichous bacteria have multiple flagella located at the same end of the bacteria (or a few sites) such as Helicobacter Pylori.
- *Endoflagella are spirochetes flagella which is not external to the bacteria* but present within the cell from end to end of the cell providing rigidity to the cell and giving it the **corkscrew movement.**

Amphitrichous bacteria	A. fecalis
Peritrichous bacteria	E. coli
Endoflagella	Spirochetes

133. Ans. (d) Needles

Ref: Microbiology by Ananthanarayan and Paniker, 8th ed. pg. 251, 263, 634

- The organism is carried by about 3% of the general population and about 30% of the hospitalised patients in their gastrointestinal tract.
- It is usually transmitted by the feco-oral route and direct contact and hand to hand transmission are important modes of transmission in the hospitalized patients.
- *Clostridium difficile causes pseudomembranous colitis.*

134. Ans. (a) Clostridium Difficile

Ref: Microbiology by Ananthanarayan and Paniker, 8th ed. pg. 251, 263, 634

- Gas gangrene is myonecrosis caused by bacterial infection which can further lead to toxemia and shock. It is noticed by the black sores and crepitus caused by gas (nitrogen is the predominant gas component (74.5%), followed by oxygen (16.1%).
- **Clostridium microbes which cause gas gangrene are:**
  - Clostridium perfringens/welchi
  - Clostridium septicum
  - Clostridium Novyi
- *Clostridium Difficile causes acute enterocolitis.*
- *In a diabetic patient, the more likely pathogen of gas gangrene is Klebsiella pneumonia.*

Extra Mile

- Clostridium microbe that causes tetanus: Clostridium tetani
- Clostridium microbe that causes food poisoning:
  - **Perfringens type A-** Gastroenteritis
  - **Perfringens type C-** Necrotising enteritis
  - **Botulinum-** Botulism
  - **Difficle-** Acute colitis

135. Ans. (c) Clostridium perfringens

Ref: Microbiology by Ananthanarayan and Paniker, 8th ed. pg. 251-252

136. Ans. (a) Clostridium perfringens

Ref: Microbiology by Ananthanarayan and Paniker, 8th ed. pg. 251-52

Please refer to above explanation.

137. Ans. (d) Mixed infection

Ref: Microbiology by Ananthanarayan and Paniker, 8th ed. pg. 226, 270-75

- Fournier gangrene, is defined as a polymicrobial necrotizing fasciitis of the perineal, perianal, or genital area.
- In the majority of cases Fournier gangrene is a mixed infection caused by both aerobic and anaerobic bacteria.

Causal Agents

- Wound cultures from patients with Fournier gangrene reveal that it is a polymicrobial infection with an average of 4 isolates per case.
- *Escherichia coli is the predominant aerobe, and Bacteroides* is the predominant anaerobe that causes Fournier's gangrene
- Other common microflora include the following:
  - *Proteus*
  - *Staphylococcus*
  - *Enterococcus*
  - *Streptococcus*
  - *Pseudomonas*
  - *Clostridium*
  - *Klebsiella*

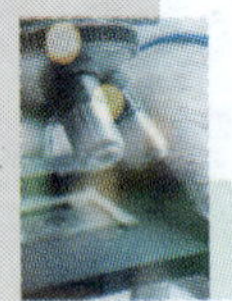

138. Ans. (a) Amoebic liver abscess

Ref: Microbiology by Ananthanarayan and Paniker, 8th ed. pg. 595, 625

AMOEBIC LIVER ABSCESS

- It is a liver abscess caused by Entamoeba histolytica
- It is common in tropical countries.
- It exists in vegetative form outside the body and is spread by the faeco-oral route.
- Presents with Pain in the right hypochondrium, fever, Profuse sweating and rigors, loss of weight etc.
- Investigation of choice: Ultrasound abdomen
- DOC: Metronidazole

139. Ans. (a) Bile solubility

Ref: Microbiology by Ananthanarayan and Paniker, 8th ed. pg. 206,218,219

- Organism causing respiratory tract infection (pneumonia) and alpha hemolysis is pneumococci.
- Two tests are commonly employed for distinguishing pneumococci from other alpha-hemolytic streptococci :
  1. *Optochin sensitivity*
  2. *Bile solubility*

140. Ans. (c) Adenosine triphosphate

- ATP is a nucleotide derived from adenosine that occurs in muscle tissue.
- It is the major source of energy for cellular reactions
- Energy is stored in the cell in form of ATP (Adenosine triphosphate)

141. Ans. (d) Staphylococcus aureus

Ref: Harrisons's, 19th ed.

- Pulmonary pneumatoceles are thin-walled, air-filled cysts that develop within the lung parenchyma.
- They can be single emphysematous lesions but are more often multiple, thin-walled, air-filled, cystlike cavities.
- Pneumatoceles are generally observed soon after the development of pneumonia and can be observed on the initial chest radiograph.
- *They are commonly caused by Staphylococcus aureus.*
- Other agents also causes pneumatocele including:
  - *Streptococcus pneumonia*
  - H. influenza,
  - E. coli
  - Group A streptococci
  - *Serratia marcescens*
  - Klebsiella pneumoniae, adenovirus, and tuberculosis.
- Noninfectious etiologies include hydrocarbon ingestion, trauma, and positive pressure ventilation.

142. Ans. (a) Staph. Aureus, H. influenza, Pseudomonas

Ref: Harrison's, 19th ed. pg. 145e3-e5

Most common cause of pulmonary infection in Cystic fibrosis.

Age group	MC Organism
Children	Staph Aureus
Adolescent &adult	Pseudomonas aeroginosa
Overall	Pseudomonas aeroginosa

143. Ans. (a) Bacitracin

Ref: Microbiology by Ananthanarayan and Paniker, 8th ed. pg. 201, 206-07, 2012

- The various species of Streptococcus can be checked by various drug disks which is indicated as whether it is sensitive or resistant to the drug.
- S. pyogenes is bacitracin sensitive.
- S. agalactiae is bacitracin resistant.
- S. pneumoniae is inhibited by optochin.
- S. viridans is not inhibited by optochin.

144. Ans. (c) Anaerobic streptococci

Ref: Microbiology by Ananthanarayan and Paniker, 8th ed. pg. 635-36

- Chronic burrowing ulcer is also known as Meleney's synergistic hospital gangrene.
- It is caused by a mixed pattern of organisms like: *anaerobic streptococci*, coliforms, Staphyolococci, Bacteroides etc.

145. Ans. (a) Cellulitis

Ref: Microbiology by Ananthanarayan and Paniker, 8th ed. pg. 205

SKIN AND SOFT TISSUE INFECTION BY STREPTOCOCCUS

1. **Erysipelas**-diffuse infection involving the superficial lymphatics
2. **Impetigo**-superficial infection of skin (pyoderma)
3. **Cellulitis**-cellulitis is caused mainly by hemolytic streptococci. It specifically affects the dermis and subcutaneous fat.
4. **Lymphangitis**

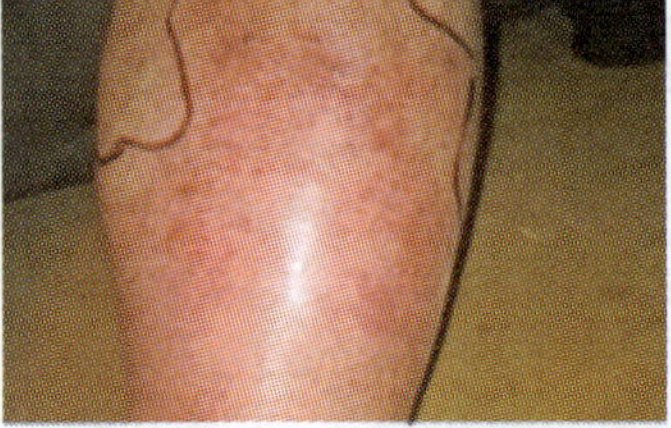

- **Gangrene-type of ischemic necrosis**
  - **Dry gangrene:** Arterial obstruction
  - **Wet gangrene:** Venous obstruction
- **Pyoderma** is most commanly caused by Staph Aureus

146. Ans. (b) Cyst are 8 nucleated

Ref: Microbiology by Ananthanarayan and Paniker, 8th ed. pg. 625, 626

- Cyst of E. histolytical is **quadri-nucleate (4 nuclei)**
- Chromatid bodies are seen as refractile oblong bars with rounded ends in leprations with normal saline and as black when stained with iron-haematoxylin.
- Trophozoites colonize cecum and ascending colon, sigmoid colon, rectum and appendix in decreasing order of frequency.

147. Ans. (a) Klebsiella pneumoniae

Ref: Microbiology by Ananthanarayan and Paniker, 8th ed. pg. 278, 707

- All the bacteria in the list except Klebsiella pneumoniae have flagella (or endoflagella) which gives them the property of motility.

148. Ans. (c) Klebsiella

Ref: Microbiology by Ananthanarayan and Paniker, 8th ed. pg. 278, 707

149. Ans. (c) An infection of lymph nodes

Ref: Microbiology by Ananthanarayan and Paniker, 8th ed. pg. 322-25

- In human beings plague occurs in three major forms:
  - ***Bubonic plague:*** *Infection of the lymph nodes*
  - **Pneumonic plague:** Infection of the lungs
  - **Septicemic plague:** Infection of the blood
- Bubonic Plague is caused by the bacteria *Yersinia pestis* from enterobacteriaceae family.
- Rodents, such as rats, carry the disease. It is spread by their fleas.
- People can get the plague when they are bitten by a flea that carries the plague bacteria from an infected rodent.
- After an **incubation period of 2–5 days, the lymph node** draining the site of entry of bacillus become infected.
- As the plague bacillus usually enters through flea bites on the legs, the inguinal nodes are involved and hence the name "bubonic" (*bubon means groin*).

150. Ans. (c) Nasopharynx

Ref: Microbiology by Ananthanarayan and Paniker, 8th ed. pg. 224-25; K. Park 20th ed. pg. 150,151

- **N. Meningococci are capsulated *Gram negative diplococci***
- **Reservoir for N. Meningitides**-Human nasopharynx is only reservoir of meningococcus. (N.meningitidis)
- **Most important source**- carriers are the most imp source, not clinical cases.
- They are arranged in pairs with adjacent sides flattened—7 *half moon shaped.*
- **Transport medium—Stuart's medium.**
- **Blood agar, chocolate agar and Muller-Hinton agar** are the media commonly used for culturing meningococci.
- **Age group**- 3 month-5 years
- **Serotype**- total 13, out of which serotype A,B,C are most important
  - **Serotype A**- Epidemics
  - **Serotype B**- Both epidemic and local out breaks
  - **Serotype C**- Local out breaks
- Chemoprophylaxis has been suggested for close contacts.
- Is DOC for prophylaxis.
- Ceftriaxone > ciprofloxacin > Rifampicin

151. Ans. (b) Neisseria Meningitidis

Ref: Microbiology by Ananthanarayan and Paniker, 8th ed. pg. 224-25

MENINGOCOCCI

- **Meningococci are *Gram negative diplococci***
- Strep. Pneumoniae is a gram positive diplococci.
- Corynebacterium Diphtheriae is Gram positive bacillus. They are non-motile, non-sporing and non-acid fast.
- Staphylococcus are Gram positive cocci. They are also non-motile, non-spore forming, non-acid fast.

152. Ans. (c) β lactamase

Ref: Microbiology by Ananthanarayan and Paniker, 8th ed. pg. 224-26

- **Lipo-oligosaccharide** (**LOS**) is a component of the outer memberane of N. meningitidis which acts as an endotoxin which is responsible for septic shock and hemorrhage due to the destruction of red blood cells.
- Other virulence factors include a polysaccharide capsule which prevents host phagocytosis and aids in evasion of the host immune response; and fimbriae which mediate attachment of the bacterium to the epithelial cells of the nasopharynx.
- **Beta-lactumases are enzymes (and not virulence factors) produced by some bacteria and are responsible for their resistance to beta-lactam antibiotics like penicillins and carbapenems**

153. Ans. (d) Streptococcus pneumoniae

Ref: Dhingra, 5th ed. pg. 61, 81

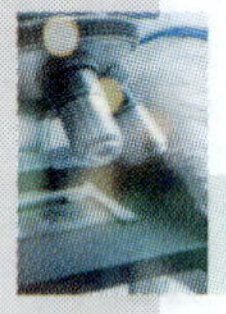

- **Meningitis** is the **commonest intracranial complication** of otitis media.
- In infants and children, otogenic meningitis usually follows acute otitis media while in adults, it is due to chronic middle ear infection.
- Most common organisms in infants and children are **Streptococcus pneumonia (30%)**, *H. influenza* (20%), and Moraxella catarrhalis (12%). Other organisms include Strep pyogenes, Staph aureus and Pseudomonas.
- Strep. Pneumoniae is also the most common cause of pyogenic meningitis in adults.

154. Ans. (a) Streptococcus pneumoniae

Ref: Dhingra, 5th ed. pg. 61, 81

155. Ans. (b) Serotype B

Ref: Microbiology by Ananthanarayan and Paniker, 9th ed. pg. 230

- Effective vaccines prepared from purified group A, C, Y, W-135 menigococcal capsular polysaccharide.
- Immunity is group specific.
- Good immunity after single dose, in older children and adults but little value in age <3 years.
- Takes 10–14 days for immunity to develop.
- Vaccine may be monovalent (A or C) or polyvalent (A-C, A-C-Y)
- **There is no group B vaccine available at present.**

156. Ans. (d) Aspergillus

Ref: Microbiology by Ananthanarayan and Paniker, 8th ed. pg. 659 -660

- Air crescent sign/meniscus sign appears as crescent of air in intrapulmonary cavity.
- It is formed due to angio-invasive aspergillosis. Although indolent with few or no symptoms, fatal hemoptysis can occur.

Extra Mile

- **Aspergillus fumigatus** is the most common cause of aspergillosis.
- Most common type of fungal infection of nose and paranasal sinuses is due to: Aspergillus.
- Most common fungus causing allergy is: Aspergillus.
- Aspergillus has septate hyphae that branch typically at 45°C (V shaped).
- Non septate hyphae with *obtuse branching*- **Rhizopus/mucor**

157. Ans. (a) 2–3 days

Ref: Harrison's, 18th ed. Ch 138

Harrison's states: *"The incubation period for respiratory diphtheria is 2–5 days; however, disease can develop as long as 10 days after exposure"*

Types of Diphtheria Infections are:

1. **Faucial (tonsillar pharyngeal):** Commonest type, grey with white pseudomembrane and cervical lymphadenopathy (bull neck) + toxemia
2. **Laryngeal:** Most severe form
3. **Nasal:** Mildest form
4. **Cutaneous form:** Only non toxigenic strain, punched-out ulcer
5. **Other form:** Conjuctival, otic, genital

158. Ans. (a) Gram negative

Ref: Microbiology by Ananthanarayan and Paniker, 8th ed. pg. 396-97

- **Calymmatobacterium Granulomatis** is known by another name: Klebsiella Granulomatis.
- It is non-motile bacteria containing **gram-negative**, pleomorphic rods that cause granulomatous lesions in humans, especially in the inguinal region.
- It causes **granuloma inguinale** aka Donovanosis, which is a contagious sexually transmitted disease occurring predominantly in tropical areas and characterized by deep purulent ulcers on or near the genital organs.
- Encapsulated bacilli called Donovan bodies (*macrophage) in which these bacilli multiply.*
- Bacteria stained at the ends, known as bipolar staining or *safety pin appearance or telephone hand appearance.*
- Granuloma inguinale is treated with streptomycin or with broad-spectrum antibiotics.

159. Ans. (d) S. Cholerae suis

Ref: Microbiology by Ananthanarayan and Paniker, 8th ed. pg. 300

- S. Cholera suis can cause septicemic disease with focal suppurative lesions, such as osteomyelitis, deep abscesses, endocarditis, pneumonia and meningitis

160. Ans. (b) Pneumococcus

Ref: Microbiology by Ananthanarayan and Paniker, 8th ed. pg. 19, 63, 193

- *Due to alpha hemolysis, colonies of pneumococci resemble colonies of Str. viridans.*
- On further incubation the colonies of pneumococci become flat with raised edges and central umbonation, so that concentric rings are seen on the surface when viewed from above seems as draughtsman appearance or Carrom coin appearance.

161. Ans. (d) Clostridium Welchii

Ref: Microbiology by Ananthanarayan and Paniker, 8th ed. pg. 643, 655, 249-54

- Clostridium Welchii is also known as Clostridium perfringens.
- It is the most common bacterial agent which causes gas gangrene.
- Gas gangrene results in tissue necrosis, putrefaction of tissues, and gas production.
- It is caused primarily by Clostridium perfringens alpha toxin, usually after a injury or trauma.
- These gases form bubbles in muscle and produce characteristic smell of decomposing tissue.
- The local spread of gases under tissue produces Crepitations when pressed on it.
- *Crepitations: Sound of snow crushing*
- After rapid and destructive local spread (which can take hours), systemic spread of bacteria and bacterial toxins may result in death.

162. Ans. (b) Clostridium tetani

Ref: Microbiology by Ananthanarayan and Paniker, 8th ed. pg. 249-54

- There are species of Clostridium that bears terminal spores which appears as drumstick shaped under microscope.
- ***Clostridium tetani*** is a gram positive obligate anaerobe which is the causative agent of tetanus, bears spores which are spherical, terminal and twice the diameter of vegetative cells. This gives it a drumstick appearance upon viewing under microscope.

Bacteria	Appearance
• Clostridium tetani	Drumstick appearance
• **Corynebacterium diphtheria**	Chinese letter pattern
• Neisseria meningitides	D- shaped
• N. Gonorrhea	Kidney shaped appearance
• Strep Pneumoniae	Flame shaped appearance

163. Ans. (d) Imipenem

Ref: Harrison's 19th ed.

- Microbes which are resistant to methicillin are said to be MRSA.
- Methicillin is highly penicilinase resistant but not acid resistant.
- MRSA have emerged in many areas. These are insensitive to all penicillinase-resistant penicillins and to other β-lactams as well as to erythromycin, aminoglycosides, tetracylines, etc.
- The drug of choice for these organisms is vancomycin, but ciprofloxacin and Rifampicin can also be used.
- Drug of choice for V.R.S.A is Daptomycin > Linezolide.
- **IMIPENEM** is an extremely potent and broad-spectrum β-lactam antibiotic whose range of activity includes *gram positive cocci, Enterobacteriaceae, Ps. Aeruginosa, Listeria as well as anaerobes like Bact. Fragilis and Cl. difficile.*

164. Ans. (d) All of these

Ref: Microbiology by Ananthanarayan and Paniker, 8th ed. pg. 613

ASPERGILLOSIS

- *Aspergillus fumigatus* is the most common cause of aspergillosis.
- Aspergillus is a mould with septate *branching* hyphae. Ability of A. fumigatus to grow at 45° C helps to distinguish it from other species.
- Mode of transmission: Inhalation of Aspergillus spores (Conidia).
- *The commonest human disease caused by aspergillus is: otomycosis.*
- *Aspergillus infection in neutropenic patient is characterized by hyphae invasion of blood vessels, thrombosis, necrosis and hemorrhagic infarction.*
- **Clinical manifestations**
  - *Allergic bronchopulmonary aspergillosis* occurs in patients with preexisting asthma or cystic fibrosis.
  - *Endobronchial saprophytic pulmonary aspergillosis (Aspergilloma)* in a patient with prior chronic lung disease, such as tuberculosis, sarcoidosis, bronchiectasis or histoplasmosis
  - *Invasive aspergillosis* develops as an acute pneumonic process with or without dissemination in the immuno-compromised patients (most common among patients with acute leukemia and recipient of tissue transplants.
    - CT finding: *Halo sign and crescent sign*
  - *Allergic sinusitis* may take three forms :
    - A fungal ball may form.
    - Chronic fibrosing granulomatous inflammation
    - Allergic fungal sinusitis
  - *Aspergillosis in AIDS*
    - Most commonly infect lung
    - CD4 + cell count is < 50/μL
    - Most common radiologic finding is bilateral diffuse or focal pulmonary infiltrates with a tendency to cavitate.

165. Ans. (a) Staphylococci

Ref: Microbiology by Ananthanarayan and Paniker, 8th ed. pg. 199-200

- *Staphylococci causes hospital acquired pneumonia.*
- **Community-acquired pneumonia** (**CAP**) is pneumonia acquired infectiously from normal social contact (that is, in the community).
- The most important infection in newborns is caused by *Streptococcus agalactiae*, also known as Group B Streptococcus or GBS. It causes >50% of cases of CAP in the first week of life.
- *Streptococcus pneumoniae is the most common cause of community acquired acute pneumonia in adults.* It is the most common cause of *lobar pneumonia*

Causes of Pneumonia

In infants	In adults
Group B Streptococcus	• *Streptococcus pneumoniae*
Streptococcus	• *Hemophilus influenza*
Pneumoniae	• *Escherichia coli*
Escherichia coli	• *Klebsiella pneumoniae*
Klebsiella pneumoniae	• *Influenza, Paranifluenza and RSV virus*

166. Ans. (c) Rat urine

Ref: Microbiology by Ananthanarayan and Paniker, 8th ed. pg. 381-83

- **Leptospirosis** is caused by infection with bacteria of the genus *Leptospira* and affects humans as well as other animals.
- One of the zoonotic infection, which transmits from animals to human
- Leptospirosis is transmitted by the urine of an infected animal like rat, mice or moles and is contagious as long as the urine is still moist.

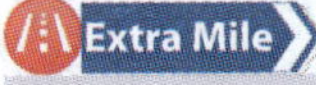

Extra Mile

Doxycycline 200–250 mg once a week used as prophylaxis

167. Ans. (b) Staphylococcus epidermidis

Ref: Microbiology by Ananthanarayan and Paniker, 8th ed. pg. 655, 679

STAPHYLOCOCCUS

- Gram positive cocci, coagulase and Catalase positive: Staphylococcus aureus
- Gram positive cocci, *Coagulase negative*: Staphylococcus epidermidis and saprophyticus.
- Staph. Epidermis infect most commonly through artificial device like: IV canula, Prosthetic device, shunts and implants.
- MCC of catheter associated blood stream infection: Staph. Epidermis
- MC organism causing prosthetic valve endocarditits: Coagulase negative Staphylococcus.

168. Ans. (d) Trichenella spiralis

Parasitic infections associated with eosinophilic myocarditis:

PROTOZOA

- Trypanosoma cruzi (Chagas disease)
- Toxoplasma gondii (Toxoplasmosis)

METAZOA

- *Trichenella spiralis*
- Toxocara canis
- Echinococcus granulosus (Hydatid cyst)
- Schistosomiasis

VIROLOGY

169. Ans. (a) Hep B

Ref: Ananthanarayana and Panicker's Textbook of Microbiology, 10th ed. pg. 545, 546

- HBV is a bloodborne virus and the infection is transmitted by parenteral, sexual and perinatal modes.
- All blood is screened for hepatitis B, as well as other blood-borne viruses such as HIV and hepatitis C.

170. Ans. (a) Dengue

Ref: Ananthanarayana and Panicker's Textbook of Microbiology, 10th ed. pg. 529

- Dengue viruses are spread to people through the bite of an infected Aedes species. Once a person has been infected with one strain, their body will build up an immunity to only that strain of the virus.
- This means that a person can become infected with dengue fever another 3 times in their life.
- Moreover, each dengue fever reinfection is much more dangerous than the previous infection.
- DEN 1 followed by DEN 2 causes severe disease.

171. Ans. (a) Cryptosporidium parvum

Ref: Ananthanarayana and Panicker's Textbook of Microbiology, 10th ed. pg. 577

- Cryptosporidium is a protozoan and an obligate intracellular parasite that causes the diarrheal disease cryptosporidiosis infection that affects patients with HIV/AIDS. It can be visualized by using modified ZN stain.

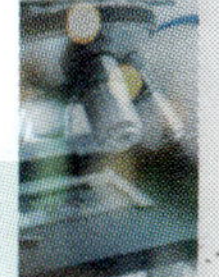

172. Ans. (a) HIV

Ref: Ananthanarayana and Panicker's Textbook of Microbiology, 10th ed. pg. 577

- HIV is a round, ball-shaped virus. It has two single strands of RNA for its genome.
- It has a protective envelope, which comes from the host cell's membrane.
- The proteins gp120 and gp41 help HIV enter a cell to infect it.
- The viral matrix helps anchor the envelope proteins to the rest of the virus particle.

173. Ans. (a) DNA

Ref: CDC. gov

RT-PCR catalyses the synthesis of c DNA copy of RNA present in COVID-19/SARS CoV 2 genome. This DNA is subsequently amplified. The number of amplifications required to generate a critical threshold value will depend on RNA load present in nasopharyngeal sample of patient.

174. Ans. (a) Chicken pox

Ref: Ananthanarayan and Paniker's Textbook of Microbiology, 10th ed. pg. 477

- **The early (prodromal) symptoms** in adolescents and adults are nausea, loss of appetite, aching muscles, and headache. This is followed by the characteristic rash or oral sores, malaise, and a low-grade fever that signal the presence of the disease.
- **In children** the illness is not usually preceded by prodromal symptoms, and the first sign is the rash or the spots in the oral cavity. The rash begins as small red dots on the face, scalp, torso, upper arms and legs; progressing over 10–12 hours to small bumps, blisters and pustules; followed by umbilication and the formation of scabs.
- Commonly visible evidence of the disease develops in the oral cavity and tonsil areas in the form of small ulcers which can be painful or itchy or both; this enanthem (internal rash) can precede the exanthem (external rash) by 1 to 3 days or can be concurrent.
- These symptoms of Chicken pox appear 10 to 21 days after exposure to a contagious person.

175. Ans. (a) Coxsackievirus A16

Ref: Ananthanarayan and Paniker's Textbook of Microbiology, 10th ed. pg. 498

- Hand-foot-and-mouth disease — a mild, contagious viral infection common in young children — is characterized by sores in the mouth and a rash on the hands and feet. Hand-foot-and-mouth disease is most commonly caused by a coxsackievirus A16.

Symptoms Include

- Fever
- Sore throat
- Painful, red, blister-like lesions on the tongue, gums and inside of the cheeks
- A red rash, without itching but sometimes with blistering, on the palms, soles and sometimes the buttocks
- Irritability in infants and toddlers
- Loss of appetite

176. Ans. (a) Nasopharyngeal swab for RT PCR

Ref: Ananthanarayan and Paniker's Textbook of Microbiology, 10th ed. pg. 456

- Smell and taste disorders are reported very frequently and at an early stage in the evolution of the infectious disease caused by the SARS-CoV-2. These symptoms could be sensitive and specific to establish the condition of the infection, and may suggest the flow of decisions as to further therapy. So, RT-PCR molecular assays for SARS-CoV-2 detection is done.

177. Ans. (a) Chicken pox

Ref: Ananthanarayan and Paniker's Textbook of Microbiology, 10th ed. pg. 477

- The classic symptom of Chicken pox is a rash that turns into itchy, fluid-filled blisters that eventually turn into scabs.
- The rash may first show up on the chest, back, and face, and then spread over the entire body, including inside the mouth, eyelids, or genital area.

178. Ans. (c) Measles

Ref: Ananthanarayan and Paniker's Textbook of Microbiology, 10th ed. pg. 518

- The pick up point in question is rash starting from face and extending to trunk. This is seen with measles. The white lesion noticed inside the mouth by physician was koplik spots.
- The classic symptoms of measles include a four-day fever (the 4 D's) and the three C's—cough, coryza (head cold, fever, sneezing), and conjunctivitis (red eyes)—along with a maculopapular rash.
- Fever is common and typically lasts for about one week; the fever seen with measles is often as high as 40°C (104°F).

179. Ans. (a) Influenza virus

- The shown viral structure having neuraminidase, hemagglutinin etc. is of influenza virus.

Identify the other viral structures:

Corona virus

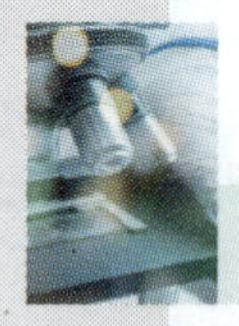

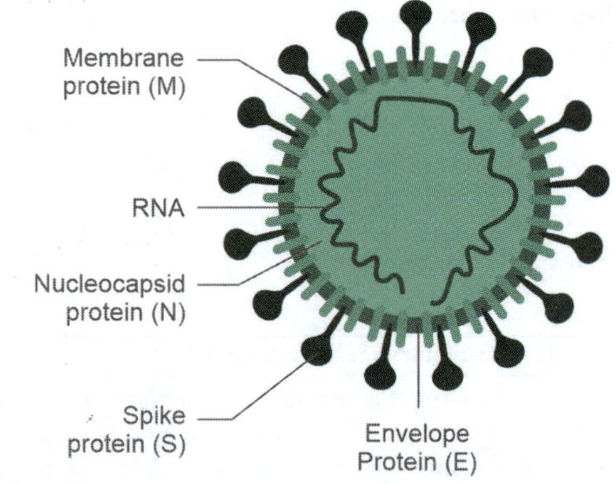

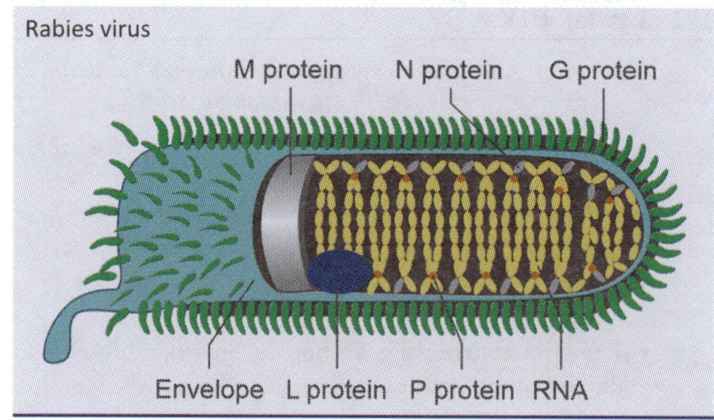

Extra Mile

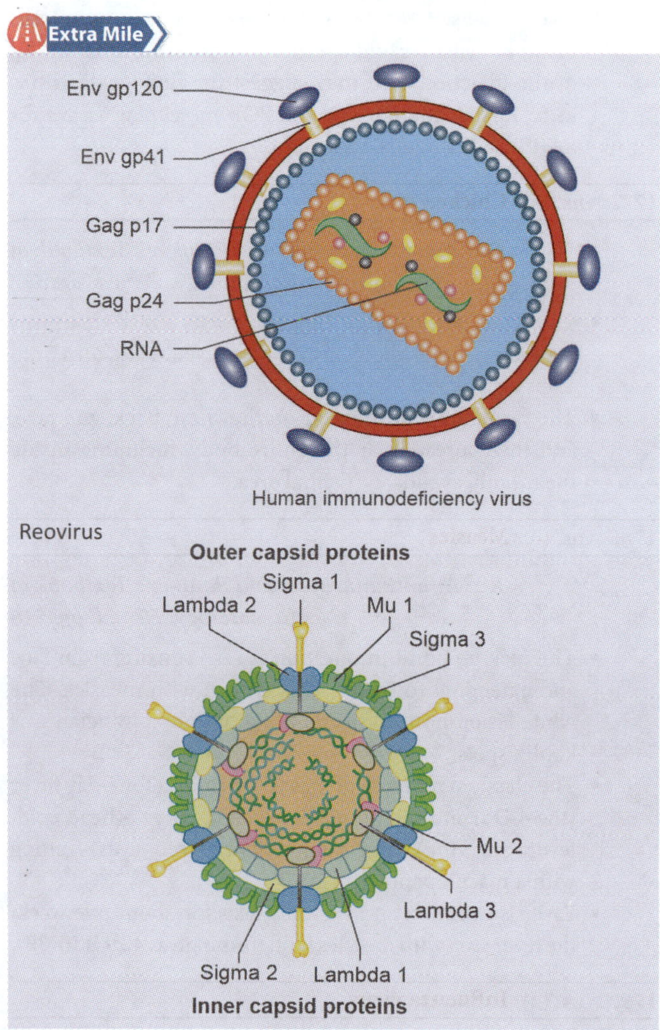

Contd...

180. Ans. (c) Skin biopsy with fluorescent antibody testing

Ref: Textbook of Microbiology by Surinder Kumar, pg. 592

Laboratory tests of rabies

IMMUNOFLUORESCENCE TEST

- Performed on samples of saliva, serum, spinal fluid, and skin biopsies of hair follicles at the nape of the neck.
- **Rabies Antigens by Immunofluorescence:**
  - MC method used for demonstration of rabies virus.
  - Specimen used are corneal smears and skin biopsy (from face or neck) or saliva ante mortem, and brain post-mortem.
- **Serology**
  - Rabies antibodies can be detected in the serum and CSF of the patient by ELISA
- **RT-PCR (Reverse Transcription- Polymerase Chain Reaction)**
  - Can detect rabies virus in saliva and in skin biopsy samples

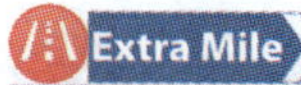
Extra Mile

Laboratory Diagnosis of Rabies (in animals)

Immunofluorescence Test

- Highly reliable and the best test available for the rapid diagnosis of rabies viral antigen in infected specimens.
- Can establish diagnosis within a few hours.
- Examination of salivary glands by immunofluorescence is useful
- **Note:** Fluorescent antibody titers in clinical rabies have been well in excess of 1:10,000, a feature which helps to distinguish between rabies and vaccine reaction.

Contd...

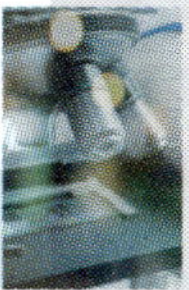

HPE
- Definitive pathologic diagnosis of rabies. Demonstration of Negri bodies in hippocampus or the spinal cord is characteristic.
- MC used method if immunofluorescence is NOT available. A negative negri bodies doesn't rule out the infection

Corneal Test
- Rabies virus antigen can be detected in live animals in corneal impressions or in frozen sections of skin biopsies by the fluorescent antibody test. *A negative test doesn't rule out possibility of infection.*

181. Ans. (a) E. coli 0157

Ref: Textbook of Microbiology by Surinder Kumar, pg. 749

- ***E. coli* 0157: H7** is the infectious cause of haemolytic uremic syndrome, Haemorrhagic colitis
- **Parvovirus B19:** Is known to cause aplastic crisis in chronic haemolytic anemia
- **Bartonella henselae:** Cat – scratch disease, Bacillary angiomatosis

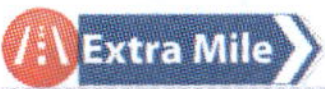

Extra Mile
- **Ebola virus:** Ebola hemorrhagic fever
- **Hantaan virus:** Hemorrhagic fever with renal syndrome
- **Guanarito virus:** Venezuelan hemorrhagic fever
- **Sabia virus:** Brazilian hemorrhagic fever

182. Ans. (d) EBV

Ref: Textbook of Microbiology by Surinder Kumar, pg. 536

- Ebstein barr virus is from herpes family, HHV 4.

TABLE: Classification of human herpes viruses

Subfamily	Virus	Primary target cell	Site of latency	Mode of spread
A. Alphaherpesvirinae				
Human herpesvirus 1	Herpes simplex type 1	Mucoepithelial cell	Neuron	Close contact
Human herpesvirus 2	Herpes simples type 2	Mucoe pithelial cells	Neuron	Close contact (sexually transmitted disease)
Human herpesvirus 3	Varicella-zoster virus	Muco epithelial cells	Neuron	Respiratory and close contact
B. Betaherpesvirinae				
Human herpesvirus 5	Cytome galovirus	Monocyte, lymphocyte, and epithelial cells	Monocyte, lymphocyte,	Close contact, transfusions, tissue transplant, and congenital
Human herpesivirus 6	Herpes lymphotropic virus	T cells	T cells	Respiratory and close contact
Human herpesvirus 7	Human herpesvirus 7	T cells	T cells	
Gamma herpesvirinae				
Human herpesvirus 4	Epstein-barr virus	B cells and epithelial cells	B cell	Saliva (kissing disease)
Human herpesvirus 8	Kaposi's sarcoma-related virus	Lymphocyte and other cells		Close contact (sexual)

Extra Mile
- **Rabies** virus is from the Rhabdoviridae family *(Genus: Lyssa virus; serotype 1)*
- **Rubella** is from family Togaviridae (*Genus: Rubivirus*).
- **Measles (Rubeola)** virus is a paramyxovirus, from Morbillivirus family.

183. Ans. (d) Pox virus

Ref: Textbook of Microbiology by Surinder Kumar, P 534

- **Molluscum contagiosum** virus is a pox virus, which causes a contagious, benign epidermal tumor that occurs in humans only.
- **Lesion:** small, pink, papular, warty, pearl-like benign tumors of the face, arm, back and buttocks.

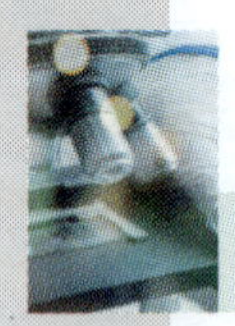

TABLE: Poxviruses causing disease in humans

Genus	Virus	Primary host	Disease
Orthopoxvirus	Variola	Humans	Smallpox (now eliminated)
	Vaccinia	Humans	Localized lesion; used for smallpox vaccination
	Buffalopox	Water buffalo	Human infections rate; localized lesion
	Monkeypox	Rodents, monkeys	Human infections rate; generalized disease
	Cowpox	Cows	Human infections rare; localized ulcerating lesion
Parapoxvirus	Orf	Sheep	Human infections rare; localized lesion
	Pseudocowpox	Cows	
	Bovine popular stomatitis	Cows	
Mollusapoxvirus	Molluscum contagiosum	Humans	Many benign skin nodules
Yatapoxvirus	Tanapox	Monkeys	Human infections rare; localized lesion
	Yabapox	Monkeys	Human infections very rare and accidental; localized skin tumors

184. Ans. (b) Hepatitis C virus

Ref: Ananthnarayan and Paniker's Textbook of Microbiology, 8th ed. pg. 545

DNA and RNA virus

DNA virus	RNA virus
• Pox virus: *Largest virus* • Parvovirus: *Smallest virus* • Adenovirus • Papovavirus • Hepadna virus • Herpes virus	• Rotavirus: *Only double stranded RNA virus* • Orthomyxovirus • Reovirus • Bunya virus • Arena virus • Hepatitis A, C, D, E virus • Picorna, polio, coxsackie, echo and entero virus.

185. Ans. (b) Coxsackie

Ref: Ananthnarayan and Paniker's Textbook of Microbiology, 8th ed. pg. 489

Coxsackie viruses produce a variety of clinical syndromes in humans ranging from trivial to fatal infections:

1. **Herpangina (vesicular pharyngitis)** is a common clinical manifestation of coxsackie Group A infection in children. It is a severe febrile pharyngitis, with headache, vomiting and pain in the abdomen.
2. **Aseptic meningitis** may be caused by most Group A and all Group B viruses. A maculopapular rash may be present. The disease may sometimes occur as epidemic.
3. **Hand, Foot and Mouth Disease (HFMD)** was identified in 1960 as an exanthematous fever affecting mainly young children, characterized by clusters of papulovesicular lesions on the skin and oral mucosa. It occurs as sporadic cases and as outbreaks.
4. Epidemic pleurodynia or **Bornholm disease** *(so called because it was first described on the Danish island of Bornholm)* is a febrile disease with stitch-like pain in the chest and abdomen, caused by Group B viruses.
5. Myocarditis and pericarditis in the newborn, associated with high fatality may be caused by Group B viruses.
6. Fulminant diabetes and orchitis
   - **Transplacental** and neonatal transmission has been demonstrated with **Coxsackie B viruses.**

186. Ans. (b) Can be treated by saline infusion

Ref: Ananthnarayan and Paniker's Textbook of Microbiology, 8th ed. pg. 557-58

- Rotaviruses are the commonest cause of diarrhea in infants and children over the world and account for about half the cases of children hospitalized for diarrhea.
- It occurs throughout the year but **predominates in winter months,** when the virus may be detected in most of the patients. It sometimes produces large epidemics of diarrhea in winter.
- Rotavirus diarrhea is usually seen in children below the age of five years, but is **most frequent between 6 and 24 months of age**.
- Mode of spread: fecal-oral route.
- Incubation period: 2–3 days.
- Vomiting and diarrhea occur with little or no fever. Stools are usually greenish yellow or pale, with no blood or mucus. The **disease is self-limited** and recovery occurs within 5–10 days. **Mortality is low. Rehydration with O.R.S. is all the treatment needed.**
- Rotavirus vaccines are given orally before the age of 6 months.

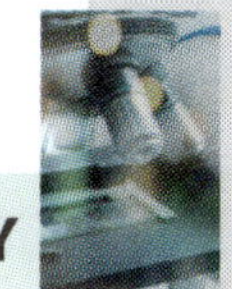

187. Ans. (c) Rabies

- **Inclusion bodies** are nuclear or cytoplasmic aggregates of stainable substances, usually proteins. They typically represent sites of viral multiplication in a bacterium or a eukaryotic cell and usually consist of viral capsid proteins.

Examples of viral inclusion bodies

Intracytoplasmic	Intranuclear	Intracytoplasmic + Intranuclear
• **Negri bodies** in Rabies • **Guarnieri bodies** in Small pox • **Henderson-Peterson bodies** in Molluscum contagiosum	• **Cowdry type A in Herpes simplex virus** and Varicella zoster virus and Torres bodies in Yellow fever • **Cowdry type B** in Polio and adenovirus	• **Warthin finkeldey bodies** in *Measles* and SSPE.

188. Ans. (a) p24

Ref: PubMed

- This is a possible suspicion of HIV infection.
- p24 antigen is a **viral protein** that makes up most of the viral core.
- Serum concentrations of **p24 antigen are high in the first few weeks after infection**; tests sensitive to p24 antigen are therefore useful for diagnosing very early infection when antibody levels are still low.

189. Ans. (a) Reverse transcriptase

Ref: Microbiology by Ananthanarayan and Paniker, 9th ed. pg. 574-75

- cDNA is created from mRNA with use of **reverse transcriptase.** First formed is single stranded DNA and then double stranded DNA.

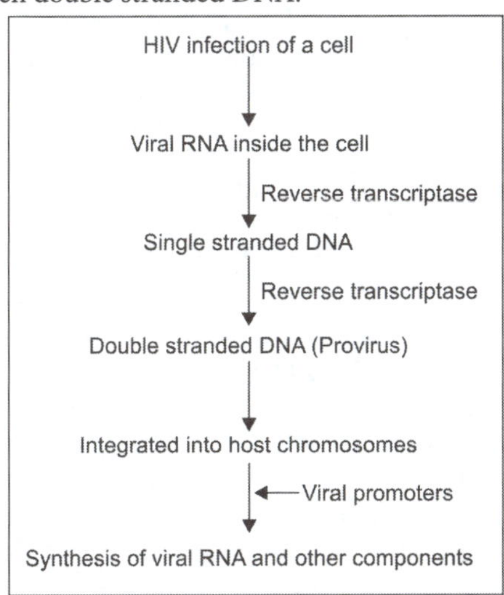

190. Ans. (a) Measles

Ref: Microbiology by Ananthanarayan and Paniker, 8th ed. pg. 444, 453

Refer to above explanation

191. Ans. (d) Herpes virus

Ref: Microbiology by Ananthanarayan and Paniker, 8th ed. pg. 444, 453

Please refer to above explanation

192. Ans. (a) Molluscum contagiosum

- Contagiosum is a viral infection of skin which is caused by a virus, *the moluscum contagiosum virus*, from pox virus family.
- The virus is contagious through direct contact.
- The virus also can be spread by sexual contact and can occur in people with compromised immune systems.

193. Ans. (c) Virus

Ref: Microbiology by Ananthanarayan and Paniker, 8th ed. pg. 443, 445

Please refer to above explanation

194. Ans. (c) Both A and B

Ref: Microbiology by Ananthanarayan and Paniker, 8th ed. pg. 569-70

- **Reverse transcriptase (RNA-directed DNA polymerase):** catalyzes the transcription of retrovirus RNA into DNA.
- Reverse transcriptase is central to the infectious nature, which causes HIV infection in humans which leads to AIDS, and
- Human T-cell lymphotrophic virus I (HTLV-I), which causes adult T-cell leukemia and tropical spastic paraparesis.

195. Ans. (a) Influenza virus

Ref: Microbiology by Ananthanarayan and Paniker, 8th ed. pg. 429

- A large number of viruses agglutinate erythrocytes from different species by the process known as Hemagglutination.
- Hemagglutination of influenza virus is due to presence of hemagglutinin spikes on the surface of virus.
- Viruses causing Hemagglutination are:
  - Influenza Virus
  - Rubella
  - RhinoVirus
  - Parainfluenza Virus
  - EnteroVirus
  - Reo Virus
  - *Measles*
  - Coxsackie Virus
  - *Rabies*
  - Toga Virus
  - Echo Virus

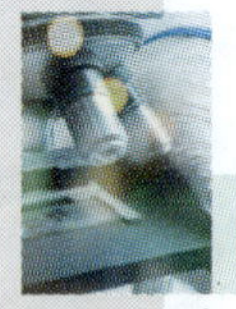

196. Ans. (a) Rocky mountain spotted fever

Ref: Microbiology by Ananthanarayan and Paniker, 8th ed. pg. 406, 408, 413

Disease	Causative agent
RMSF *(Rocky Mountain Spotted Fever)*	*R. Rickettsii*
Kyasanur forest disease	*Group B togavirus (Flavivirus)*
Dengue	*Arbovirus* 4 serotypes (Den- 1, 2, 3, 4)
Yellow fever	*Flavivirus fibricus*

197. Ans. (d) Rhinovirus

Ref: Microbiology by Ananthanarayan and Paniker, 8th ed. pg. 490

- Common cold is a viral infection of the upper respiratory tract. The most commonly implicated viruses are:
  1. Rhinovirus: most common cause (30–80%), a type of Picornavirus
  2. Human coronavirus ~15%
  3. Influenza viruses 10–15%
  4. Adenoviruses 5%
  5. Other viruses include: Human parainfluenza virus, human respiratory syncytial virus, and enteroviruses.

198. Ans. (c) P. vivax

Ref: Microbiology by Ananthanarayan and Paniker, 8th ed. pg. 694

- **Duffy antigen/chemokine receptor** (DARC) also known as **CD234,** is a protein that in humans is encoded by *DARC* gene.
- The Duffy antigen is located on the surface of red blood cells.
- The Duffy antigen protein is also the *receptor for the human malarial parasites Plasmodium vivax.*
- Polymorphisms in this gene are the basis of the Duffy blood group system.

Clinical Significance of Duffy Antigen

- **Asthma:** There appears to be a correlation with both total IgE levels and asthma and mutations in the Duffy antigen.
- **Malaria:** On erythrocytes the Duffy antigen acts as a receptor for invasion by the human malarial parasites *P. vivax* and *P. knowles*.
- *Duffy negative individuals whose erythrocytes do not express the receptor are believed to be resistant to merozoite invasion.*
- **HIV infection:** The absence of the DARC receptor appears to increase the susceptibility to infection by HIV. HIV-1 appears to be able to attach to erythrocytes via DARC
- **Lung transplantation:** The Duffy antigen has been implicated in lung transplantation rejection.
- **Multiple myeloma:** An increased incidence of Duffy antigen has been reported in patients with multiple myeloma compared with healthy controls
- **Pneumonia:** The Duffy antigen is present in the normal pulmonary vascular bed. Its expression is increased in the vascular beds and alveolar septa of the lung parenchyma during suppurative pneumonia.
- **Prostate cancer:** Experimental work has suggested that DARC expression inhibits prostate tumor growth. The reasons for this increased risk are not known.
- **Sickle cell anemia:** Duffy antigen-negative individuals with sickle cell anaemia tend to suffer from more severe organ damage than do those with the Duffy antigen.

199. Ans. (b) DNA virus

Ref: Microbiology by Ananthanarayan and Paniker, 8th ed. pg. 549

- **Human papillomavirus** (**HPV**) is a DNA virus from the papovavirus family that is capable of infecting humans.
- Usually it causes no symptoms in most people, but some types can cause warts (verrucae), while others can in a minority of cases lead to cancers of the cervix, vulva, vagina, penis, oropharynx and anus.
- HPV has been linked with an increased risk of cardiovascular disease.
- In addition, HPV 16 and 18 infections are a cause of a unique type of oropharyngeal (throat) and cervix cancer.

DNA and RNA virus

DNA virus	RNA virus
• Pox virus: *Largest virus* • Parvovirus: *Smallest virus* • Adenovirus • Papovavirus • Hepadna virus • Herpes virus	• Rotavirus: *Only double stranded RNA virus* • Orthomyxovirus • Reovirus • Buniya virus • Arena virus • Hepatitis A, C, D, E virus • Picorna, polio, cocksackie, echo and entero virus.

200. Ans. (b) Secondary syphilis

Ref: Microbiology by Ananthanarayan and Paniker, 8th ed. pg. 378

- The Jarisch-Herxheimer reaction is classically associated with penicillin treatment of syphilis.
- It is believed to be caused by the release of endotoxin-like substances when large numbers of *Treponema pallidum* are killed by antibiotics.
- It has also been documented in tick-borne rickettsial diseases like Lyme disease and relapsing fever where the infecting organism is also a spirochete.

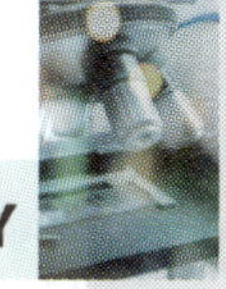

- The reaction can be expected *in 50% of primary syphilis, **90% of secondary syphilis,** and in 25% of early latent infection,* but is very rare in late syphilis.
- It has been suggested that it is more severe in patients with HIV

201. Ans. (c) Dogs

Ref: Microbiology by Ananthanarayan and Paniker, 8th ed. pg. 112, 174, 427

202. Ans. (d) Spare palm & sole

- **IP of chicken pox**-10-21 days
- Infectious period is 2 days before to 5 days after the onset of rash. The rash is maculo-papulo-vesicular rash.
- **Rash is symmetrical and centripetal**, mainly on trunk, pleomorphic, **spare palm and sole**
- *Portal of entry of virus-respiratory tract or conjunctiva*
- Rash appear on the day the fever starts

MYCOLOGY AND PARASITOLOGY

203. Ans. (b) Chromoblastomycosis

Ref: Ananthanarayana and Panicker's Textbook of Microbiology, 10th ed. pg. 605

- In Chromoblastomycosis, Histologically, the lesions show the presence of the fungus as round Or irregular, dark brown, yeast-like bodies with septae, called sclerotic bodies.

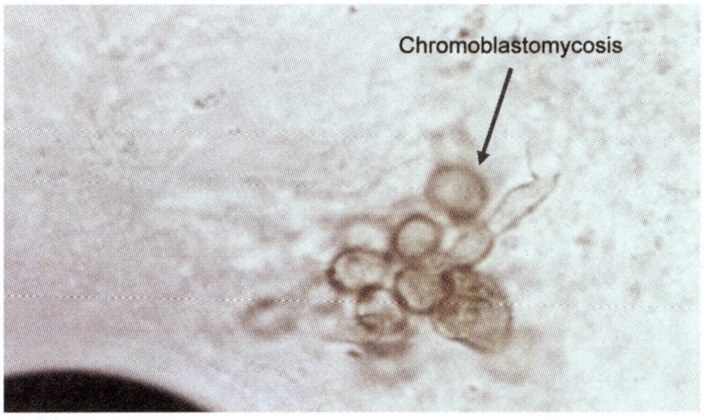

204. Ans. (a) Trichomonas

Ref: Ananthanarayana and Panicker's Textbook of Microbiology, 10th ed. pg. 682

- In trichomoniasis, pus cells and motile trophozoites of Trichomonas vaginalis are seen. There is no cyst formed.

205. Ans. (a) Madura foot

Ref: Ananthanarayana and Panicker's Textbook of Microbiology, 10th ed. pg. 398

- It is a chronic granulomatous infection.
- Characterized by the development of indurated swellings, mainly in the connective tissue, suppuration and the discharge of 'sulphur granules'.
- The lesion often points towards the skin, leading to multiple discharging sinuses.

206. Ans. (b) Malassezia furfur

Ref: Ananthanarayana and Panicker's Textbook of Microbiology, 10th ed. pg. 600

- Malassezia furfur of the skin causes hypopigmented or hyperpigmented macular lesions along the trunk of the body.
- Malassezia furfur is believed to be the causative agent in various dermatological disorders including Pityriasis versicolor, and Seborrheic dermatitis.
- Malassezia is present as a combination of both short pseudohyphae and spores, the light microscopic appearance of which is referred to as "spaghetti and meatballs" pattern.

207. Ans. (d) Klebsiella granulomatis

Ref: Ananthanarayana and Panicker's Textbook of Microbiology, 10th ed. pg. 683

- Granuloma inguinale (donovanosis) is a genital ulcerative disease caused by the intracellular gram-negative bacterium Klebsiella granulomatis (formerly known as Calymmatobacterium granulomatis).

208. Ans. (a) P falciparum

Ref: Ananthanarayana and Panicker's Textbook of Microbiology, 10th ed. pg. 80; https://www.cdc.gov/dpdx/malaria/index.html

- Plasmodium falciparum is a protozoan parasite, one of the species of Plasmodium that cause malaria in humans.
- It is transmitted by the female Anopheles mosquito. Gametocytes of Plasmodium falciparum are crescent- or sausage-shaped, and are usually about 1.5 times the diameter of an RBC in length.

209. Ans. (a) Diabetic ketoacidosis

Ref: Ananthanarayana and Panicker's Textbook of Microbiology, 10th ed. pg. 614

- Mucormycosis involving the oral cavity is one such entity that presents as necrosis of bone in immunocompromised patients.

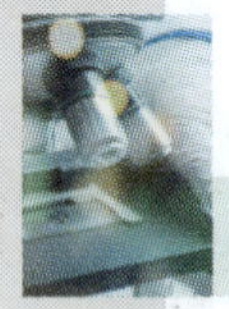

- Mucormycosis is an opportunistic fungal infection that mainly affects the patients with uncontrolled diabetes mellitus.

210. Ans. (c) Gardnerella vaginalis, metronidazole

Ref: Ananthanarayana and Panicker's Textbook of Microbiology, 10th ed. pg. 682

- Gardnerella vaginalis commonly is associated with bacterial vaginosis.
- Treatment is generally directed against the anaerobic flora and consists of metronidazole, tinidazole or clindamycin for 5 to 7 days.

211. Ans. (d) HPV 6,11

Ref: Ananthanarayana and Panicker's Textbook of Microbiology, 10th ed. pg. 557

- Condyloma acuminata refers to anogenital warts caused by human papillomavirus (HPV).
- The most common strains of HPV that cause anogenital warts are 6 and 11.
- HPV is a double-stranded DNA virus primarily spread through sexual contact.

212. Ans. (a) Mucormycosis

Ref: Ananthanarayana and Panicker's Textbook of Microbiology, 10th ed. pg. 614

- Fungal infections, including mucormycosis, aspergillosis and invasive candidiasis, have been reported in patients with severe COVID-19 or those recovering from the disease and have been associated with severe illness and death.
- Outpatient use of systemic corticosteroids/other immunomodulating drugs for mild or moderate patients with COVID-19 should be avoided.

213. Ans. (b) Giardia lamblia

Ref: Ananthanarayana and Panicker's Textbook of Microbiology, 10th ed. pg. 579

- Giardia duodenalis aka Giardia intestinalis and Giardia lamblia, is a flagellated protozoa
- Giardia that colonizes the small intestine, causing a diarrheal condition known as giardiasis.

214. Ans. (b) Enterobius vermicularis

- The given stool preparation shows low magnification view of clusters of eggs of pinworm infection, also known as enterobiasis.
- The most common symptom is itching in the anal area. This can make sleeping difficult. The period of time from swallowing eggs to the appearance of new eggs around the anus is 4–8 weeks.

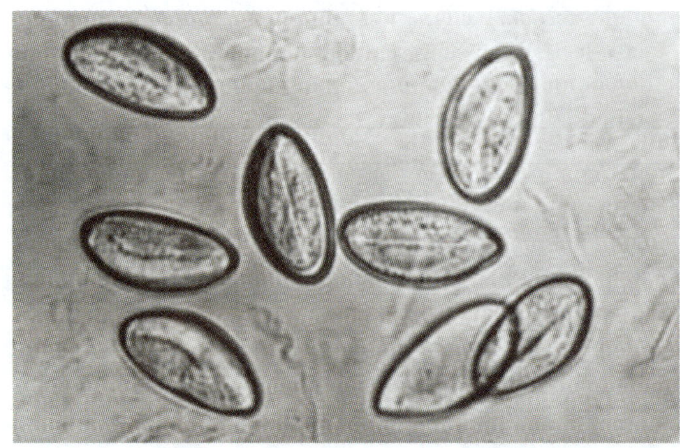

215. Ans. (b) Histoplasma

Ref: Ananthanarayan and Paniker's Textbook of Microbiology, 10th ed. pg. 610

- Histoplasmosis is a type of lung infection. It is caused by inhaling Histoplasma capsulatum fungal spores.
- These spores are found in soil and in the droppings of bats and birds.
- This fungus mainly grows in the central, southeastern, and mid-Atlantic states of USA.

216. Ans. (a) *E. histolytica*

Ref: Ananthanarayan and Paniker's Textbook of Microbiology, 10th ed. pg. 684

- The cyst in fecal sample is of *E. histolytica*, having around 4 nuclei in the mature cyst.

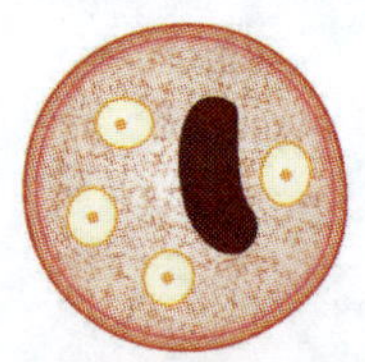

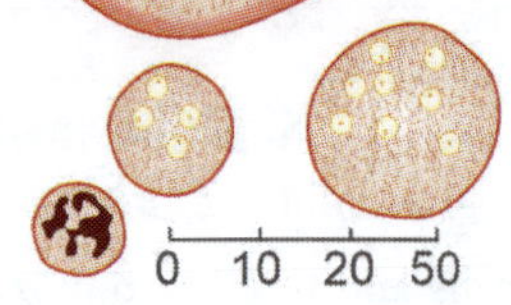

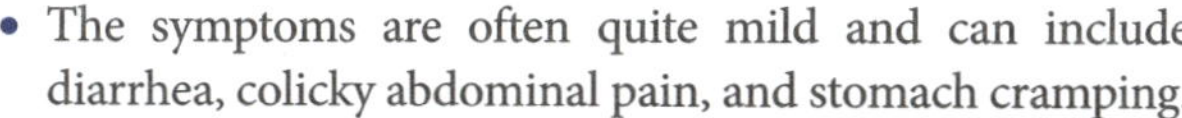

- The symptoms are often quite mild and can include diarrhea, colicky abdominal pain, and stomach cramping.
- Amebic dysentery is a severe form of amebiasis associated with stomach pain, bloody stools, and fever.

217. Ans. (c) Schistosoma mansoni

- Schistosoma mansoni is a water-borne parasite of humans, and belongs to the group of blood flukes (Schistosoma).
- The adult lives in the blood vessels (mesenteric veins) near the human intestine. It causes intestinal schistosomiasis (similar to S. japonicum, S. mekongi, S. guineensis, and S. intercalatum).
- Clinical symptoms are caused by the eggs. As the leading cause of schistosomiasis in the world, it is the most prevalent parasite in humans. It is classified as a neglected tropical disease.

Extra Mile

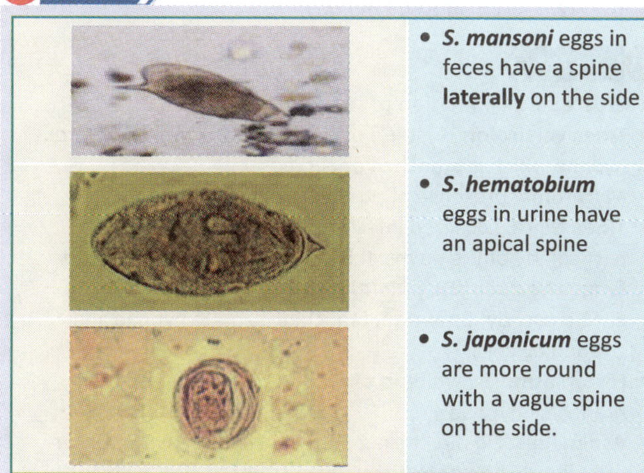

218. Ans. (b) Wuchereria bancrofti

- Wucheria bancrofti is a dioecious worm, and it exhibits sexual dimorphism.
- The adult worm is long, cylindrical, slender, and smooth with rounded ends. It is white in color and almost transparent. The body is quite delicate, making removing it from tissues difficult. It has a short cephalic or head region connected to the main body by a short neck, which appears as a constriction.
- The anal region is an elaborate structure consisting of 12 pairs of papillae. The female worm is 60 millimeters to 100 millimeters long and 300 micrometers wide, nearly three times larger in diameter than the male. Its tail gradually tapers and becomes rounded at the tip.
- Females are ovoviviparous and can produce thousands of juveniles known as microfilariae.

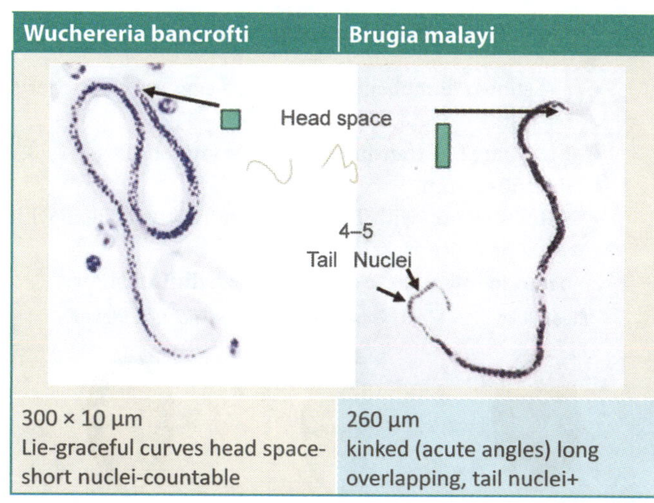

219. Ans. (d) Membrane filter concentration technique

- Membrane filters have a known uniform porosity of predetermined size (generally 0.45 µm) sufficiently small to trap microfilariae. Using the membrane filter technique, sample is passed through the membrane using a filter funnel and vacuum system. Any organisms in the sample are concentrated on the surface of the membrane.

220. Ans. (c) 600 meters

- Kala-azar or Visceral leishmaniasis (VL) is a disease of low altitude (approximately 500 meters mean sea level).

221. Ans. (a) Pin worm

- NIH swab is used for diagnosis of pin worm.
- Eggs of worm are often deposited in large number on the perianal skin at the night.
- They can be demonstrated by scraping this area by NIH swab in the morning before taking bath. It is repeated for 3 consecutive days.
- It is spread over glass and examined using microscope.

222. Ans. (a) H. Nana

- Hymenolepis Nana (H. Nana) is also known as dwarf tapeworm, which is found throughout the world.
- It is the smallest tapeworm infecting humans.

  Characteristics of this worm are:
  - **Scolex:** Armed rostellum
  - **Eggs:** With 4–8 polar filaments
  - **Infective stage:** Eggs
  - **Intermediate host:** Fleas, floor beetles
  - **Definitive host:** Man

223. Ans. (c) Trichuris trichura eggs

- The shown dumbbell/barrel shaped eggs are of Trichuris Trichura.
- It has plug like translucent polar prominences
- **Size:** 50–54 um
- **Note:** Infection with Trichuris trichura is associated with rectal prolapse as well

Learn to identify these eggs of these helminths:

Liver fluke

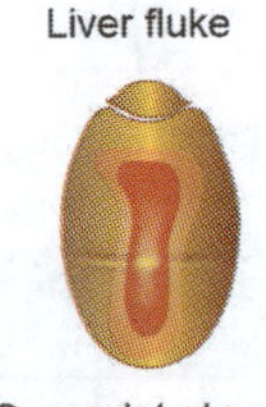

Operculated egg

Pinworm

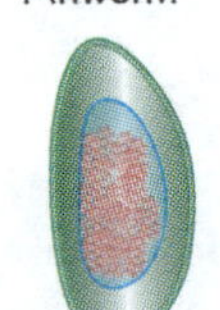

Plano convex

Trichuris trichiura

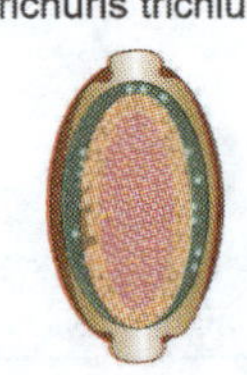

Bipolar plugs

Ascarid

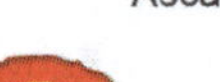

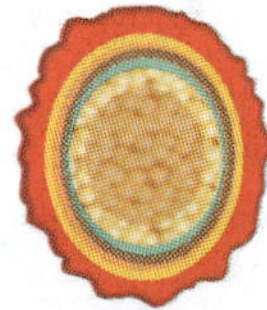

Fertilized

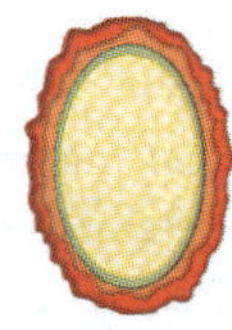

Unfertilized

224. Ans. (b) Chromoblastomycosis

Ref: Textbook of Microbiology by Surinder Kumar, pg. 659

- The fungal hyphae are broken down into smaller sections/compartment by septa → septate hyphae
  - Example: Apergillus
- If there is no septation/compartment → Non-septate (Coenocytic)
  - Mucor, Zygomycetes

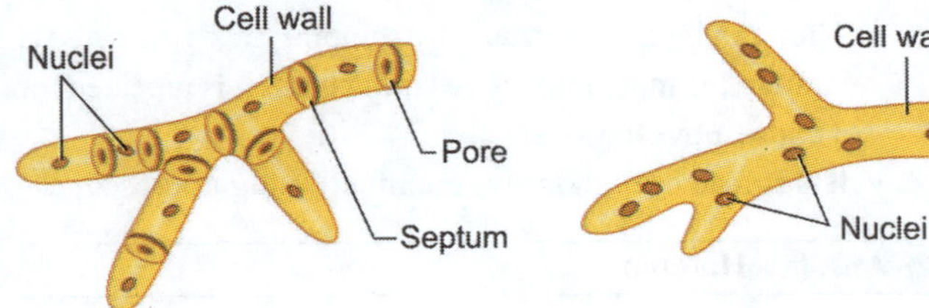

Chromoblastomycosis

- It is one of the subcutaneous mycosis.
- Characterized by: Crusted, warty lesions in limbs
- **Cause:** Soil inhabiting fungi of the family Dematiaceae.

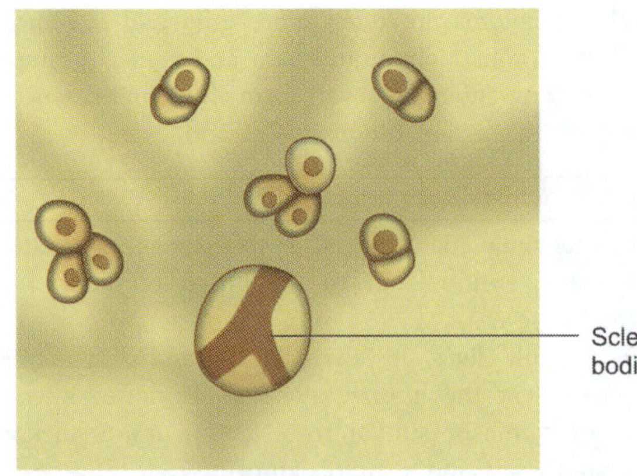

Laboratory Diagnosis

- Microscopically dark fungal elements on skin scraping or pus
- Histologically, it shows fungus having round or irregular, dark brown, yeast-like bodies with septae, called *sclerotic cells (seen on KOH mount).*

Extra Mile

Microscopic examination of some fungi

- **Tinea versicolor:** cluster of round yeast cell with short, stout hyphae which is branched or curved
- **Mycetoma:** presence of pus in draining sinus
- **Tinea Nigra:** Localized infection of the stratum corneum, particularly of the palms. It is caused by the dematiaceous fungus ***Hortaea (Exophiala) werneckii.***
  - **Microscopy:** Brownish, branched, septate hyphae and budding cells
- **Histoplasmosis:** white to tan fluffy colony with septate branching hyphae
- **Aspergillus:** On direct examination of sputum with KOH or calcofluor white or in histologic sections → non-pigmented septate mycelium, with dichotomous branching.
- **Coccidiodomycosis:** Large number of barrel shaped anthropores, characteristically alternate with smaller intervening empty cells.
- **Candida albicans:** Culture colonies are creamy white, smooth and with yeast odour. Identified by production of germ tube test.

225. Ans. (b) Cysticercosis cellulose

Ref: Lange Microbiology, Ch 46

- The larval stage of taenia solium is Cysticercus cellulose, which lives in pig or in human tissues causing human cysticercosis.

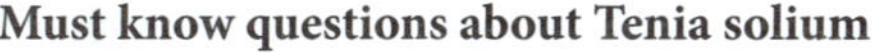

Must know questions about Tenia solium:

- **Life span:** >25 years; Cysticercus survives 5–6 years in human body
- **Final host:** Man
- **Intermediate host:** Pig/Man
- **Infective stage:** Cysticercus and Egg
- **Source of infection:** Consuming raw/undercooked pork
- **Inhabitation site:**
  - Adult org: In human intestine
  - Cysticercus: In tissues

226. Ans. (b) ***Candida albicans***

Ref: Textbook of Diagnostic Microbiology, E-book, pg. 634

- A germ tube test is a diagnostic test in which a sample of fungal spores are suspended in serum and examined by microscopy. It is particularly indicated for colonies of white or cream color on fungal culture.
- A positive germ tube test is strongly indicative of *Candida albicans*. This test also helps to differentiate between *Candida albicans* and *non-albicans Candida* (germ tube test negative).

227. Ans. (b) Skin and hair

Ref: Textbook of Diagnostic Microbiology, E-book, pg. 607

- **Trichophyton:** Skin, hair, nail
- **Epidermophyton:** Skin, nail
- **Microsporum:** Skin, hair

228. Ans. (c) Filaria

Ref: Harrison 19th ed. pg. 1420

- Tropical or pulmonary eosinophilia is due to microfilaria in lung. There is no microfilaria in blood.
- It is characterized by coughing, asthmatic attacks and enlarged spleen.
- **DOC:** Diethylcarbamazine

229. Ans. (a) ***Schistosoma***

Ref: Harrison 19th ed. pg. 605

***Schistosoma* has 3 species mainly and resides in:**

- *S. mansoni:* Resides in mesenteric veins draining sigmoido-rectal region
- *S. japonicum:* Resides in mesenteric veins draining the ileocecal region
- *S. haematobium:* Bladder plexus
- *Fasciola:* Liver fluke (*Fasciola hepatica*)
- Paragonimus westermani: *Lung fluke*

230. Ans. (b) Accidental intermediate host in humans

Ref: Textbook of surgical gastroenterology pg. 767, PK mission ed 2016

Human echinococcosis is a zoonotic disease that is caused by parasites, namely tapeworms of the genus *Echinococcus*.

Transmission

- *E. granulosus* requires two host types, a definitive host and an intermediate host.
- The definitive host of this parasite are dogs
- Intermediate host are most commonly sheep, however, cattle, horses, pigs, goats, and camels are also potential intermediate hosts.
- Humans can also be an *intermediate host* for *E. granulosus*, however this is uncommon and therefore *humans are considered an accidental intermediate host.*

231. Ans. (c) Plasmodium malariae

Ref: Harrison's, 19th ed. pg. 1371

- *P. vivax*, *P. ovale*, show a marked predilection for young RBCs
- *P. malariae* has predilec tion for old RBCs
- *P. falciparum* can invade erythrocytes of all ages and may be associated with very high levels of parasitemia.

TABLE: Characteristics of plasmodium species infecting humans

	Finding of indicated species			
Characteristic	**P. falciparum**	**P. vivax**	**P. ovale**	**P. malariae**
Duration of intrahepatic phase (days)	5.5	8	9	15
Number of merozoites released per infected hepatocyte	30,000	10,000	15,000	15,000
Duration of erythrocytic cycle (hours)	48	48	50	72
Red cell preference	Younger cell (but can invade cells of all ages)	Reticulocytes and cells up to 2 weeks old	Reticulocytes	**Older cells**
Morphology of RBC and parasites	Usually only ring forms; banana-shaped game-tocytes, (*Maurer dots*)	Irregularly shaped large rings and trophozoites; enlarged erythrocytes; (Schuffner's dots)	Infected erythocytes, enlarged and oval with tufted end; (James dots)	Band or rectangular forms of trophozoites common (Ziemann's dot)
Ability to cause relapses	No	Yes	Yes	No

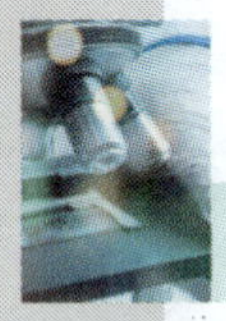

232. Ans. (c) Coccidioidomycosis

Ref: Atlas of Infectious diseases: Fungal Infection, pg. 33

- Mature spherule in sputum sample is seen in coccidiodomycosis.
- Coccidioidomycosis may present with a syndrome of erythema nodosum, fever, and conjunctivitis. Serious complications include cavitating lung lesions or meningitis.

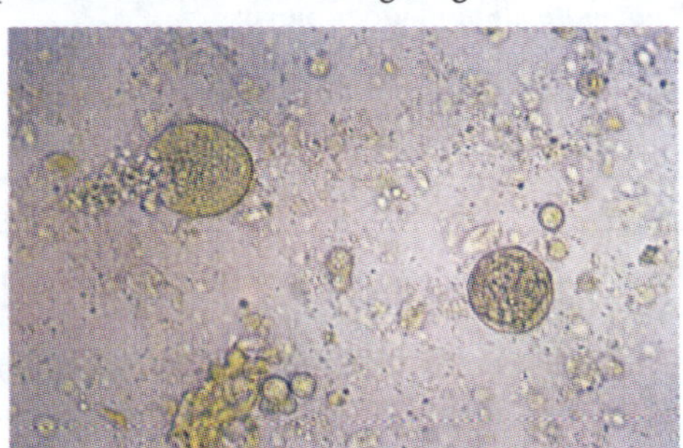

FIGURE: Potassium hydroxide (KOH) preparation of sputum. *The chitin in the spherule cell wall is resistant to digestion by KOH, whereas host cells in sputum are not*. Two mature spherules are evident in the figure, one of which has ruptured and is releasing endospores. Although KOH is not a sensitive test, the finding of spherules in a sputum specimen is diagnostic of coccidioidomycosis.

- Coccidioides *immitis* grows readily on routine culture media. Unlike other dimorphic fungi, colonies usually are visually apparent within 3 to 5 days. On solid media, the fungus appears as a nonpigmented mold. Unlike specimens obtained from patients. *C limitis* growing in culture is highly infectious and represents an extreme laboratory hazard.

233. Ans. (a) Giardiasis

Ref: Harrisons, 19th ed. pg. 1946

Giardiasis

- **Mode of transmission:** Fecal-oral
- **Incubation period:** 7–10 days
- **Signs/symptom:**
  - Chronic diarrhea, abdominal pain, bloating, nausea, flatus due to postinfectious irritable bowel syndrome or **protein losing enteropathy**; postinfection fatigue
- **Diagnosis:** Fecal, **string test**, or duodenal aspirate microscopy; stool antigen assay
- **Treatment:** Metronidazole for ongoing infection; no specific antiparasitic therapy for postinfectious syndromes.
- **Note:** Hookworm infection can cause iron deficiency anemia

Important causes of Malabsorption Syndrome *(Table from Harrison's 19th ed)*

Impaired mucosal absorption/mucosal loss or defect	
• Crohn's disease • Amyloidosis • Scleroderma • Lymphoma • Eosinophilic enteritis • Mastocytosis • Tropical sprue	• Celiac disease • Collagenous sprue • Whipple's disease • Folate and vitamin B_{12} deficiency • **Infections—giardiasis**

234. Ans. (b) Man

Ref: Harrisons, 19th ed. pg. 1413

- *Ascaris lumbricoides*is the largest intestinal nematode **parasite of humans,** reaching up to **40 cm** in length.
- **Humans are definitive host** of ascaris
- **Clinical disease arises** from **larval migration in the lungs** or effects of the adult worms in the intestines.
- **Clinical Features:**
  - Around, ~9–12 days after egg ingestion, patients may develop an irritating non-productive cough and burning substernal discomfort that is aggravated by coughing or deep inspiration.
  - Eosinophilia develops during this symptomatic phase and subsides slowly over weeks.
  - Chest X-rays may reveal evidence of eosinophilic pneumonitis **(Loffler's syndrome),** with rounded infiltrates a few millimeters to several centimeters in size.
- **Treatment:** Mebendazole (DOC)

235. Ans. (a) Treponema pallidum

Ref: Harrisons, 19th ed. pg. 1146; table 245e1

- Cestodes are helminthes. **Example of cestodes:**

Cestodes	Intermediate host	Definitive host
Taenia solium	Pig	Man
Taenia saginata	Beef	Man
Echinococcus granulosus	Man, camels and sheep	Dog
Echinococcus multilocularis	Rodents and humans	Foxes, dogs and cats
H. nana	Man	Man
D. latum	Cyclops, fresh water fish	Man

Note: *Treponema pallidum is a spirochete*

236. Ans. (d) Fungus

Ref: Microbiology by Ananthanarayan and Paniker, 8th ed. pg. 605

- **Kerion** is the result of the host's response to a **fungal** ringworm infection of the hair follicles of the scalp and beard accompanied by secondary bacterial infection.

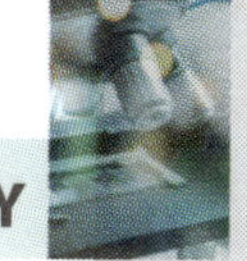

- It is usually caused by Zoophilic dermatophytes like *Trichophyton verrucosum* and *T. mentagrophytes.*
- **Treatment:** *Oral Griseofulvin is the treatment of choice.*

237. Ans. (b) Germ tube method

Ref: Microbiology by Ananthanarayan and Paniker, 8th ed. pg. 607-608

- A **germ tube test** is a diagnostic test in which a sample of fungal spores are suspended in serum and examined by microscopy for the detection of any germ.
- It is particularly indicated for colonies of white or cream color on fungal culture, where a *positive germ tube test is strongly indicative of Candida albicans*

238. Ans. (b) Candida

Ref: Microbiology by Ananthanarayan and Paniker, 8th ed. pg. 601; Greenwood, 16 ed. pg. 570

- For direct microscopy of tissue infected with fungus, 10% KOH is used. KOH digests cells and other tissue material, enabling fungus elements to be seen clearly.
- **Special stains for fungus:** PAS, methanamine silver
- **Culture media for fungus:**
  - Sabouraud's glucose agar (MC)
  - Corn meal agar
  - Czapek-dox medium
  - Culture medium are supplemented with chloramphenicol- to suppress bacterial contamination.
  - **Temp:** 22°–30°C

239. Ans. (b) Borrelia Burgdorferi

Ref: Microbiology by Ananthanarayan and Paniker, 8th ed. pg. 377, 379, 381

- Causal agent of lyme disease: Borrelia Burgdorferi *(I.P. 3 to 30 days)*
  - Vector: Ticks
- **Lyme disease occurs in 3 stages:**
  - **Stage 1:** Localized infection, appears an annular skin lesion (Erythema Migrans)
  - **Stage 2:** Disseminated infection, now with headache, fever, arthralgia, myalgia and lymphadenopathy.
  - **Stage 3:** Persistent infection, presents with chronic arthritis, encephalopathy, and acrodermatitis.

Extra Mile

- **Borrelia vincenti:** ulcerative gingivostomatitis or oropharyngitis (*Vincent's Angina*)
- **Borrelia Recurrentis:** Louse borne relapsing fever
- **Treponema carateum:** Causes Pinta
- **Treponema Pertenue:** Causes Yaws
- **Treponema Pallidum:** Syphilis

240. Ans (d) LGV

Ref: Microbiology by Ananthanarayan and Paniker, 8th ed. pg. 417, 420

GROOVE SIGN

- Large, hard, fixed, and extremely tender lymph nodes in the groin above and below the inguinal ligament, with a groove along the ligament characteristic of lymphogranuloma venereum.
- LGV caused by Chlamydia trachomatis
- **DOC:** Doxycycline.
- **DOC in pregnancy:** Erythromycin

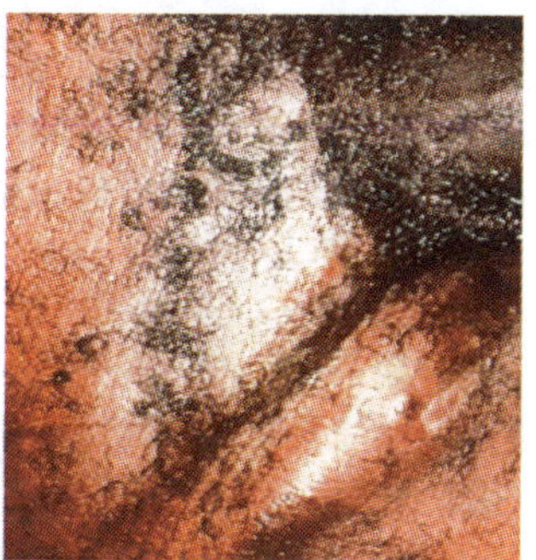

Classification of Chlamydia Trachomatis

- **A, B, Ba, C:** Trachoma conjunctivitis
- **D to K:** Inclusion conjunctivitis
- **L1, L2, L3:** LGV

Extra Mile

- Chlamydia are obligate intracellular parasites, therefore cannot be cultured on non-living artificial media. Isolation of chlamydia can be done by inoculation into:
  - Tissue culture (cell culture, Mc coy cells)- **Most preferred.**
  - Embryonated eggs particularly in yolk

241. Ans. (b) Aspergillus

Ref: Microbiology by Ananthanarayan and Paniker, 8th ed. pg. 613, 659-60

- Fungal infections of the cornea are secondary to injury, bacterial infection and treatment with antibacterial agents and steroids. LASIK and agricultural occupation predispose too.
- Occur most often in hot climates.
- *Aspergillus and Fusarium* are the most common isolates in fungal keratitis worldwide.

242. Ans. (c) Appendix and cecum

Ref: Manson's tropical Diseases, 22nd ed. pg. 1516

- The life cycle of Enterobius vermicularis begins with eggs being ingested. The eggs hatch in the duodenum.
- The emerging pinworm larvae grow rapidly and migrate through the small intestine towards the colon

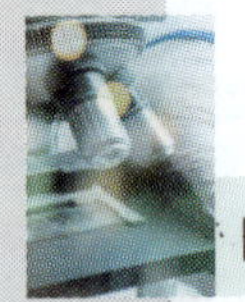

- The male and female pinworms mate in the ileum.
- The gravid female pinworms settle in *the ileum, caecum, appendix,* and *ascending colon,* where they attach themselves to the mucosa and ingest colonic contents.

243. Ans. (c) Round worm

Ref: Manson's Tropical Diseases, 22nd ed. pg. 1516

- Older literature indicates that the pin worm is the parasite which multiples in the appendix and blocks the lumen causing appendicitis. Although new data indicates that the most common parasite in the appendix is the round worm or Ascaris lumbricoides.

244. Ans. (c) Causes cutaneous larva migrans

Ref: Manual of Family Practice, pg. 622

- Toxocara canis can cause visceral tarva migrans leading to hepatitis and pneumonitis. It can also lead to vision loss due to ocular larva migrans.
- The life cycle of Toxocara canis occurs in dogs and humans acquire the injectionas accidental hosts.

245. Ans. (b) Ancylostoma braziliense

Ref: Atlas of Clinical Microbiology Vol. II/Ch. 19

- Cutaneous larva migrans caused by Ancyclostoma braziliensie is the most common tropically acquired dermatosis. Using their proteases, larvae/penetrate through follicles, fissures or intact skin.

246. Ans. (c) Man is an intermediate host

Ref: Manson's Tropical Diseases, 22nd ed. pg. 1477

For filarial parasite	For malarial parasite
• Man: Definitive host • Mosquito: Intermediate host	• Man: Intermediate host • Mosquito: Definitive host

LYMPHATIC FILARIASIS

- Lymphatic filariasis is caused by W. Bancrofti, B. Malayi and B. Timori.
- Man is definitive host and mosquito acts as intermediate host.
- Microfilariae resides in the blood and adult worm in the lymphatics.
- The principal pathologic changes result from inflammatory damage to the lymphatics, which is caused by adult worms and not by microfilariae.

Clinical Manifestations

1. Asymptomatic or subclinical microfilaremia
2. Acute adenolymphangitis
3. Hydrocele
4. Chronic lymphatic disease

Diagnosis

- A definitive diagnosis can be made only by detection of parasite.
- Assays for circulating antigens of W. bancrofti permit the diagnosis of microfilaremic and nonmicrofilaremic infection. Tests are:
  - ELISA
  - Rapid-format immunochromatographic card test.
  - Ultrasound in conjuction with Doppler techniques may result in the identification of motile adult worms: ***Filarial dance sign.***
- **Treatment:** ***Diethylcarbamazine: Drug of choice.***

247. Ans. (b) Epidemic typhus

Ref: Microbiology by Ananthanarayan and Paniker, 8th ed. pg. 410

Rickettsial Diseases

Disease	Cause	Vector
Epidemic typhus	R. Prowazeki	Louse
Endemic typhus	R. Typhii	Rat flea
Scrub Typhus	R. Tsutsugamushi	Trombiculid mite
Indian tick typhus	R. conori	Tick
RMSF	R. Ricketsii	Tick
Trench fever	Rochalimaea Quintana	Louse
Q fever	Coxiella burnetii	None but rarely soft tick

248. Ans. (d) Ileum & jejunum

Ref: Chatterjee, 12th ed. pg. 116

- Tapeworm infection can also be caused by eating raw or undercooked meat from an animal or a fish that has the larval form of the tapeworm cysts in its muscle tissue.
- Once ingested, the larvae then develop into adult tapeworms in the small intestine (jejunum and ileum).

TAPEWORMS

- Taenia saginata: The beef tape worm
- Taenia solium: The pork tape worm
- *Habitat of tapeworms: Small intestine (upper jejunum)*
- Definitive host: Man
- **Intermediate host:** Cattle (cow or buffalo) for T. Saginata Pig for T. Solium.

249. Ans. (a) Acute adenolymphangitis stage

- **Filariasis** is caused by thread-like nematodes, which are transmitted by black flies and mosquitoes.
- The adult worms, which usually stay in lymphatics, release early larval forms known as microfilariae into the

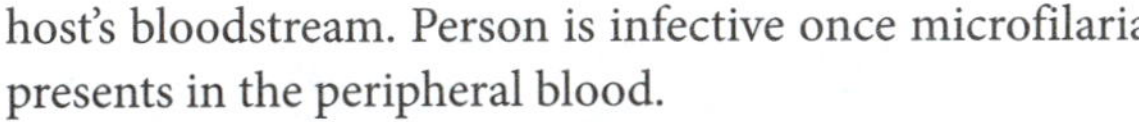

host's bloodstream. Person is infective once microfilaria presents in the peripheral blood.

- This inflammatory phase is characterised by Lymphangitis, lymphadenitis and adenolymphangitis.
- It lasts for a few days, then subsides spontaneously & recurs at irregular intervals for a period of weeks to months.
- These circulating microfilariae can be taken up with a blood meal by the arthropod vector; in the vector, they develop into infective larvae that can be transmitted to a new host.
- Filariasis is diagnosed in microfilaraemic cases primarily through direct observation of microfilariae in the peripheral blood.
- **Remember:** *W. bancrofti is nocturnally periodic i.e. micro filariae are scarce in peripheral blood by day and increase at night.*

250. Ans. (c) Strongyloides

Ref: Jawetz, Melnick, & Adelberg's Medical Microbiology, 24th ed.

- Ova/egg in stool is not required for diagnosis of Strongyloides. Larva is seen in stool infected with Strongyloides.
- In the other given cases like ankylostoma, Enterobius, and trichuris if ova/egg is seen, it indicates infestation of that parasite.

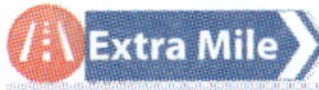

Extra Mile

- *Shape of Trichuris trichura egg: Barrel shaped*

251. Ans. (c) Taeniasis

Ref: Harrison's, 18th ed. Ch 159

- Zoonosis are infectious diseases of animals that can naturally be transmitted to humans.
- **Plague** is a systemic **zoonosis** caused by *Yersinia pestis* ***(gram negative).*** It predominantly affects small rodents in rural areas of Africa, Asia, and the Americas and is usually transmitted to humans by an arthropod vector (the flea).
- **Rabies** is a zoonotic infection that occurs in a variety of mammals throughout the world except in Antarctica and on some islands. Rabies virus is a member of the family Rhabdoviridae. Rabies virus is a lyssavirus that infects a broad range of animals and causes serious neurologic disease when transmitted to humans.
- **Brucellosis** is a bacterial zoonosis transmitted directly or indirectly to humans from infected animals, predominantly domesticated ruminants and swine.
- **TAENIASIS** is a tapeworm infection to humans. Taenia saginata (beef tapeworm) and Taenia Solium (pork tapeworm).

252. Ans. (d) Onchocerca volvulus

Ref: Diagnostic Medical Parasitology, 3rd ed. pg. 275, Park, 19th ed. pg. 221

- **Onchocerca volvulus** results in **river blindness** and subcutaneous nodules.
- "Lymphatic filariasis" covers infection with three closely related nematode worms - **W. Bancrofti, B. Malayi and B. timoria.**
- All three infections are transmitted to **man** by the bites of infective mosquitoes.
- All three parasites have basically similar life cycles in man- adult worms living in lymphatic vessels whilst their offspring, the microfilariae circulate in peripheral blood and are available to infect mosquito vectors when they come to feed.

Extra Mile

- **Diethylcarbamazine (DEC)** is the drug of choice for filariasis.
- **Ivermectin** is the drug of choice for **Onchocerca volvulus**

IMMUNOLOGY AND MISCELLANEOUS

253. Ans. (b) Type 2

Ref: Ananthanarayana and Panicker's Textbook of Microbiology, 10th ed. pg. 194

- Rh factor incompatibility between mother and fetus can also cause a type II hypersensitivity hemolytic reaction, referred to as hemolytic disease of the newborn (HDN).
- Type II hypersensitive reactions involve antibody-mediated destruction of cells.

254. Ans. (a) IgM

Ref: Ananthanarayana and Panicker's Textbook of Microbiology, 10th ed. pg. 98

- Soluble immunoglobulin M (IgM) forms a pentamer containing a joining (J) chain polypeptide.
- While IgM pentamer has various immune functions, it also behaves as a carrier of circulating apoptosis inhibitor of macrophage.

255. Ans. (a) Histamine

Ref: Ananthanarayana and Panicker's Textbook of Microbiology, 10th ed. pg. 166

- Chemicals such as histamine are released that cause the tissue around the bite or sting to swell, turn red, itch and be painful.
- Applying ice to the site may provide some mild relief

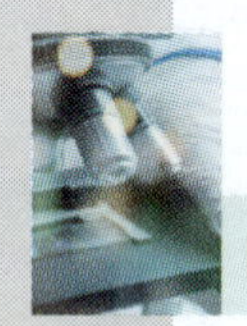

256. Ans. (a) Active immunity (vaccine) + rabies immunoglobulin + local treatment

Ref: Ananthanarayana and Panicker's Textbook of Microbiology, 10th ed. pg. 541; https://www.ncbi.nlm.nih.gov/pmc/articles/PMC4163280/

- Rabies is a fatal infectious disease and rabies post-exposure prophylaxis is the method of choice for prevention of human rabies.
- Any pregnant woman who is bitten by a rabid dog is at risk. They need proper post-exposure management.
- Vaccination is not contraindicated in pregnancy and breast feeding.
- Rabies pre-exposure and post-exposure prophylaxis

Rabies vaccines
Post-exposure prophylaxis IM schedule: • 5 dose Essen regime (1-1-1-1-1) on day 0, 3, 7, 14 and 28. • 3 dose regime (2-1-1) on day 0, 7 and 21. **Post-exposure prophylaxis ID schedule:** • 2 site- Thai red cross regimen (2-2-2-0-2) on day 0, 3, 7 and 28. **Post-exposure for previously vaccinated:** • IM or ID on day 0 and 3.
Pre-exposure prophylaxis: • IM or ID day 0, 7, 21 or 28.

257. Ans. (a) IgM

Ref: Ananthanarayan and Paniker's Textbook of Microbiology, 10th ed. pg. 100

- **Immunoglobulin M (IgM):** Found mainly in blood and lymph fluid, this is the first antibody the body makes when it fights a new infection.
- **In chronic infection IgG** antibody is seen
- **Immunoglobulin E (IgE):** Normally found in small amounts in the blood. There may be higher amounts when the body overreacts to allergens or is fighting an infection from a parasite.

258. Ans. (b) C5-C9 deficiency

Ref: Textbook of Microbiology by Surinder Kumar, pg. 262

- Meningococcal disease is favoured by deficiency of the terminal complement components (C5-C9).

TABLE: Human genetic deficiencies of complement components and associated diseases

Complement deficiency	Association with disease
C1 inhibitor	Hereditary angioneurotic edema
C1r	Systemic lupus erythematosus-like disease, frequently fatal from overwhelming infection
C2	Increased susceptibility to infections
C3	Recurrent bacterial infections
C4	Systemic lupus erythematosus-like disease
C5	Recurrent infections–lupus-like disease
C6, C7, C8	Recurrent infections: Disseminated gonococcal infections
C9	Not more susceptible to disease than other individuals in the general population
Factor 1	Low C3 levels with recurrent bacterial infections

Contd...

259. Ans. (d) Ag – Ab complex

Ref: Textbook of Microbiology by Surinder Kumar, pg. 142

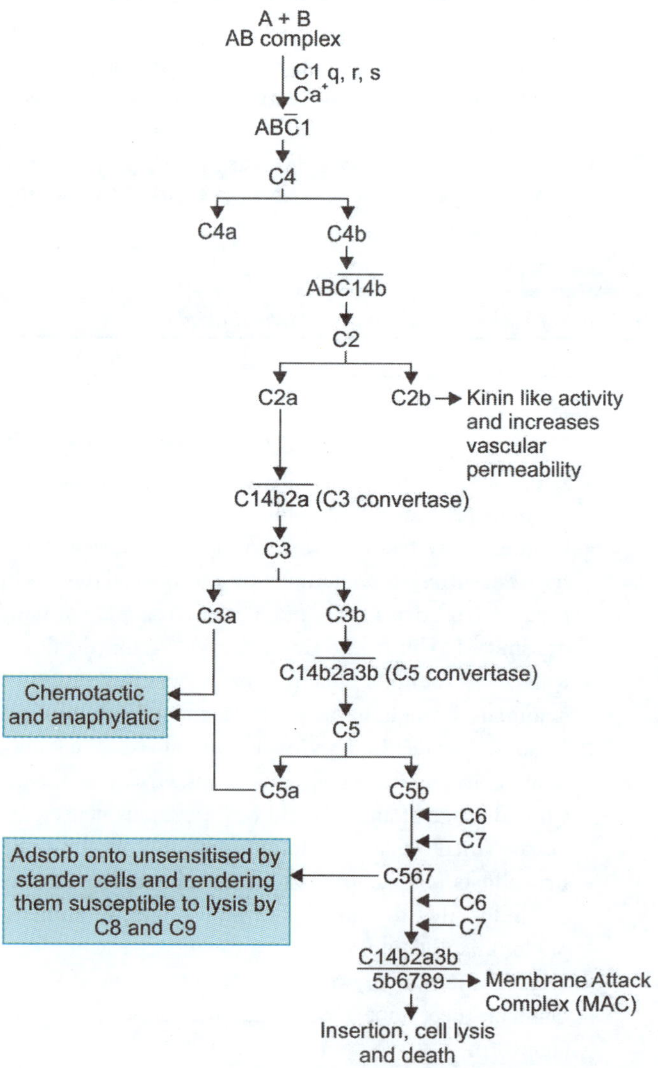

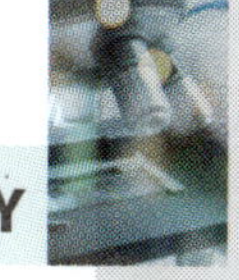

- The classical pathway is so called because it was the first one identified. Steps involved are as follows:
  - Antigen-Antibody binding: first step is the binding of C1 to the antigen-antibody complex → activation of C1s
  - Production of C3 convertase
  - Production of C5 convertase
  - Formation of membrane attack complex (MAC).

260. Ans. (c) Macrophages

Ref: Robbins Basic Pathology, E-book, pg. 85

- Epithelioid cells are defined as cells that resemble epithelial cells (keratinocytes). They have large oval, pale, vesicular nuclei and abundant eosinophilic cytoplasm.
- The best-known epithelioid cells are those *derived from macrophages* within granulomas, but tumor cells can also be described as epithelioid. Immunostaining may be needed to identify the type of epithelioid cell.

MOST COMMON LESIONS WITH EPITHELIOID CELLS

- Granulomas
- Squamous cell carcinoma
- Spitz nevus (spindle and epithelioid cell nevus)
- Melanoma

261. Ans. (d) C5

Ref: Harrison 19th ed. pg. 997

- Meningococcal disease is associated with terminal complement deficiency (C5–C9) which forms the membrane attack complex. Hence the bactericidal activity is reduced in this condition and increases susceptibility to invasive meningococcal infection *up to 600 times.*

262. Ans. (a) It is a bacteria

- **Bacteriophages are viruses that infect bacteria**. It helps in transduction and not transformation.
- **It imparts toxigenicity by lysogenic conversion e.g.** toxin production by diphtheria bacillus due to presence of prophage beta.
- Penicillinase resistance in Staphylococcus is a **classical example of plasmid mediated drug resistance transmitted by transduction or bacteriophage.**

Extra Mile

- Transformation is bacterial gene transfer through the agency of free DNA as shown by Griffith in the experiments of **Pneumococci with mice. Transformation plays no role in transfer of drug resistance.**

263. Ans. (c) Pentamer

Ref: Anatnayayan, 9/ed. pg. 98

Antibody	Effective valency
IgM	5
IgG	2
IgD	2
IgE	2
IgA	2,4

Extra Mile

- **Ig** having maximum molecular weight: **IgM**
- **First antibody produced by newborn: IgM**
- All immuniglobulin are heat stable EXCEPT: **IgE**
- Ig present in **breast milk: IgA**
- Ig with **maximum half life: IgG**
- **Ig crosses placenta**: **IgG**
- Ig with **minimum half life: IgE**
- Ig having **maxilum serum concentration: IgG**
- Ig having **least serum concentration: IgE**

264. Ans. (d) IgM

Ref: Microbiology by Ananthanarayan 9th ed./98-99

- First antibody produced by newborn is IgM at 20 weeks age of gestation.
- Immunoglobulin that can cross placenta: IgG_1
- Immunoglobulin that is present in breast milk: IgA

265. Ans. (a) IgA

Ref: Microbiology by Ananthanarayan and Paniker, 8th ed. pg. 100

TABLE: Immunoglobulins and their salient features

Immuno-globulins	Salient features
IgG	**Most abundant Ig,** consists of about 80% Marker of chronic infection Only Ig that Can cross placenta (IgG_1 subtype)
IgA	2nd most abundant, 10-13% Found in glandular secretion like saliva, tear, ileum, and mucosal secretion like bronchial secretion
IgM	5–8% of total Ig; aka pentameric Ig. First Ig to be synthesized by fetus (20 weeks AOG) Marker of acute infection
IgD	Present mostly intravascular Serve as recognition receptor for antigens
IgE	Mostly extravascular in distribution Highly elevated levels in case of type-I HPS reaction *Produced chiefly in the linings of respiratory and intestinal tracts*

FORENSIC MEDICINE

7

MOST RECENT QUESTIONS 2023

1. **A 10-year-old boy will have _____permanent and ___ temporary teeth.** *(Most Recent Question July 2023)*
   a. 20, 4 b. 16, 8
   c. 12, 8 d. 12, 12
2. **Identify the plant.** *(Most Recent Question July 2023)*

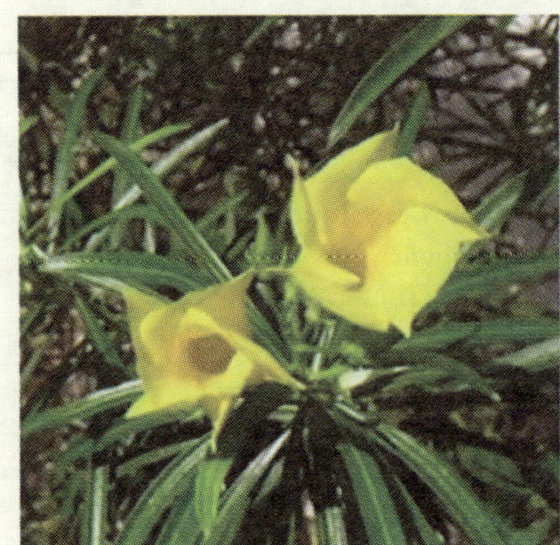

   a. Nerium odorum b. Cascabela thevetia
   c. Aconite d. Cerbera odollam
3. **A dead body is brought for postmortem examination with stellate-shaped gunshot wound and muzzle impression print. What can be the distance?** *(Most Recent Question July 2023)*
   a. Close range
   b. Contact shot
   c. Intermediate range
   d. Distant range
4. **A dead body is recovered from a river. The body has signs of antemortem drowning, and also has multiple cuts on flexor aspect of arm. What can be the cause of these wounds?** *(Most Recent Question July 2023)*
   a. Self-inflicted wound
   b. Active self-defense wound
   c. Postmortem artifact
   d. Passive self-defense wound
5. **MTP can be done up to 24 weeks for:** *(Most Recent Question July 2023)*
   a. Contraceptive failure
   b. Rape victim
   c. Congenital malformation
   d. Social indications
6. **Patient died and relatives said he had a tattoo, but it was not visible on autopsy. Which is the best location of check for the evidence of tattoo?** *(Most Recent Question July 2023)*
   a. Spleen b. Artery
   c. Lymph node d. Liver
7. **Police recovers beheaded skull. The relatives of a missing person give the photographs of missing person to police. These two samples can be analyzed with which technique?** *(Most Recent Question July 2023)*
   a. Fingerprint b. DNA fingerprint
   c. Superimposition d. Cheiloscopy
8. **In a case of road traffic accident presented with EDH. Where will be impact of collision?** *(Most Recent Question July 2023)*
   a. Pterion b. Angle of mandible
   c. Lambdoid suture d. Any of the above
9. **Inquest in the case of death in police custody is done by:** *(Most Recent Question Jan 2023)*
   a. Jail Superintendent
   b. Executive Magistrate
   c. Police Inspector
   d. Superintendent of Police
10. **A public witness was ordered by court to come and record his evidence in court. This is considered:** *(Most Recent Question Jan 2023)*
   a. Oral evidence b. Hearsay evidence
   c. Subpoena d. Circumstantial evidence
11. **Just before death, a person made efforts to save himself which led to contraction of one group of muscles and primary relaxation was absent. This can lead to:** *(Most Recent Question Jan 2023)*
   a. Rigor mortis b. Cadaveric spasm
   c. Algor mortis d. Livor mortis

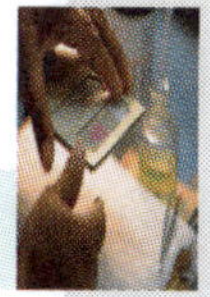

12. Nothing is an offense done by a person under unsoundness of mind, if he is not able to understand nature and consequences of his act and what he is doing is wrong in law. This is according to which law of insanity?

(Most Recent Question Jan 2023)

a. McNaughten's rule   b. Durham law
c. Current's rule   d. Irresistible impulse test

13. Study of death in all its aspects is called:

(Most Recent Question Jan 2023)

a. Thanatology   b. Thanatopraxis
c. Disinterment   d. Molecular death

14. Cherry red postmortem hypostasis is seen in:

(Most Recent Question Jan 2023)

a. Hydrogen sulfide   b. Yellow phosphorus
c. Carbon monoxide   d. Hydrogen cyanide

15. Which of the following is not a blood stain analysis test:

(Most Recent Question Jan 2023)

a. Barberio's test
b. Teichmann's test
c. Takayama (Hemochromogen) test
d. Spectroscopy

16. All of the following are signs and symptoms of acute cocaine poisoning during stage of excitement; except:

(Most Recent Question Jan 2023)

a. Feeling of well-being
b. Tingling or numbness in hands and feet
c. Pupils dilated and rapid pulse and sweating
d. Cocaine bugs

17. Homicidal smothering and traumatic asphyxia are causes of death in: *(Most Recent Question Jan 2023)*

a. Burking   b. Bansdola
c. Mugging   d. Garotting

AUTOPSY & IDENTIFICATION

18. During autopsy the following finding is noted. This finding is clinically suggestive of:

(Most Recent Question June/Dec 2021)

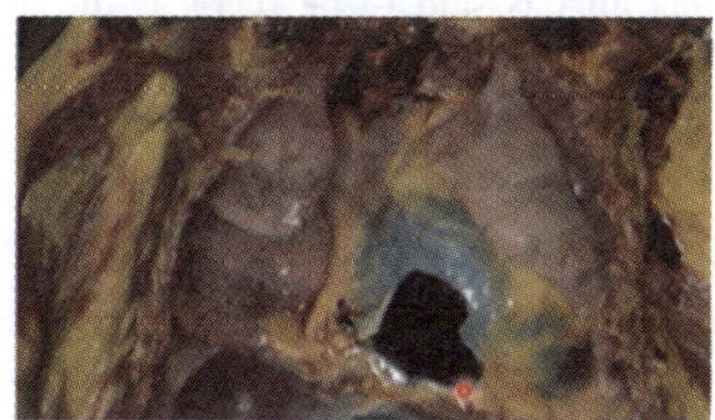

a. Congenital pulmonary hypoplasia
b. Cardiac tamponade
c. Pulmonary embolism
d. Pulmonary artery aneurysm

19. Examination of a stain sample under microscope crystals were seen as shown in image. These crystals are formed in which of the following test?

(Most Recent Question June/Dec 2021)

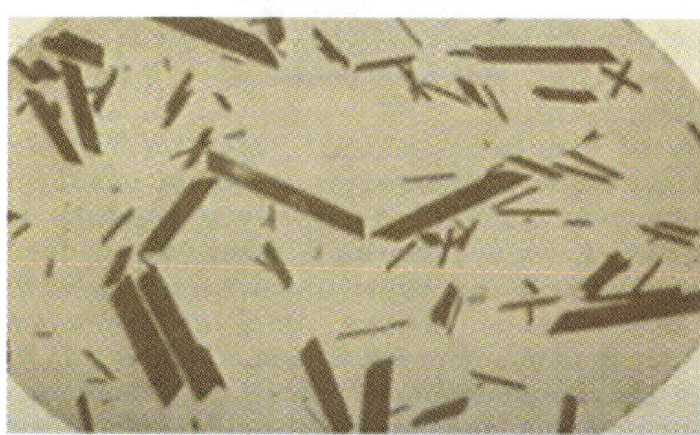

a. Barberios test
b. Teichman's test
c. Takayama test
d. Spectroscopy test

20. Cherry red color post-mortem staining is associated with which poisoning event:

(Most Recent Question June/Dec 2021)

a. H_2S b. Nitrate
c. Carbon monoxide   d. Hydrogen cyanide

21. A person died due to starvation. Which is correct in such case during autopsy:

(Most Recent Question June/Dec 2021)

a. Enlarged heart   b. Enlarged stomach
c. Distended gallbladder   d. Expanded lungs

22. In Barberios test, yellow color needle shaped crystals are seen under microscope. This is done to detect which stain *(Most Recent Question June/Dec 2021)*

a. Sputum   b. Semen
c. Blood   d. CSF

23. Identify the fingerprint pattern shown in image:

(Most Recent Question Aug 2020)

a. Loop   b. Whorl
c. Arch   d. Composite

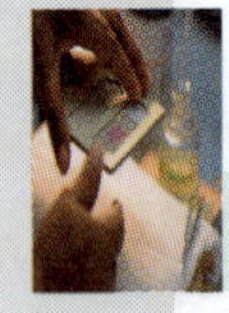

24. Microscopic crystals as shown is seen in which test: *(Most Recent Question Aug 2020)*

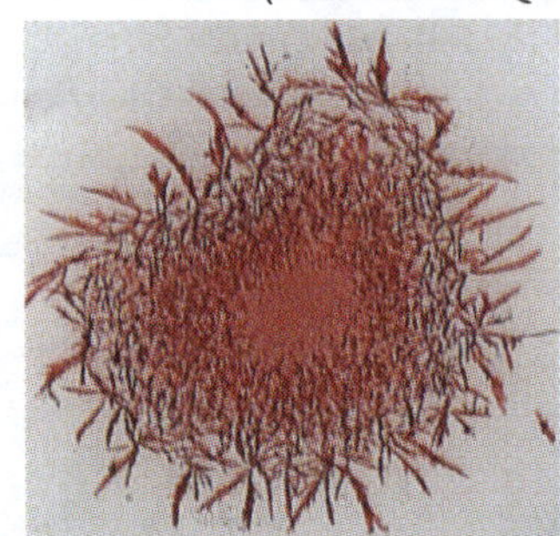

a. Teichmann test b. Florence test
c. Barberio test d. Takayama test

25. A case of road traffic accident was brought for autopsy. Findings were, Stiff neck, stiff upper and lower limbs. Primary relaxation was absent. This is suggestive of: *(Most Recent Question Dec 2019-20)*

a. Rigor mortis b. Cadaveric spasm
c. Heat stiffness d. Cold stiffness

26. A dead fetus was found in a water canal. The crown heal length was found to be 25 cm. distinct fingernails visible with minimum hair growth. Approximate age of fetus is: *(Most Recent Question Dec 2019-20)*

a. 3 months b. 5 months
c. 7 months d. 9 months

27. Gender assessment in a 12-year-old child is best done by: *(Most Recent Question Dec 2019-20)*

a. Skull b. Femur
c. Hip bone d. Mandible

28. For autopsy of stomach, incision of choice is given along: *(Most Recent Question 2019)*

a. Lesser curvature b. Greater curvature
c. Vertical d. Pylorus

29. Study of birth defects is called: *(Recent Pattern Question 2018-19)*

a. Teratology b. Tetralogy
c. Anthropology d. Parturitology

30. Confirmatory test of blood stain: *(Recent Pattern Question 2018-19)*

a. Kastle meyer test b. Haemin crystal test
c. Spectroscopic test d. Orthotoluidine test

31. Gustafson method of age estimation by teeth utilizes: *(Recent Pattern Question 2018-19)*

a. Number of tooth
b. Transparency of root
c. Height and weight of teeth
d. Structural feature of enamel

32. Which of the following is used for biometric evaluation? *(Recent Pattern Question 2018)*

a. Iris b. Pupil
c. Lens d. Cornea

33. 21st tooth erupts at: *(Recent Pattern Question 2018)*

a. 5 years b. 8 years
c. 10 years d. 12 years

34. Cephalic index 75–80 is seen in: *(Recent Pattern Question 2018)*

a. Mongols b. Aryans
c. Negros d. Chinese

35. Stack's formula for age determination from teeth is used in: *(Recent Pattern Question 2017)*

a. Infants
b. Adults
c. Between 25 and 50 years of age
d. > 50 years of age

36. Boyde's method is useful for age estimation of: *(Recent Pattern Question 2017)*

a. Dead infant b. Adult
c. Toddler d. School going child

37. The antero-posterior diameter of the skull is minimum in:

a. Brachycephaly b. Dolicocephaly
c. Plagicephaly d. Trigonocephaly

38. Mongols are:

a. Dolicocephalic b. Mesaticephalic
c. Brachycephalic d. Anglocephalic

39. Palatoprints used for identification of human beings are usually taken from:

a. Anterior part of palate b. Posterior part of palate
c. Lateral part of palate d. Middle part of palate

40. Breslau's second life test detects changes in which of the following organs:

a. Brain
b. Lung
c. Heart
d. Stomach and small intestine

41. Raygat's test is used for testing function maturity of:

a. Small intestine b. Kidney
c. Lungs d. Heart

COURT OF LAW AND IPC

42. Grievous hurt is said to be there, if the person is in severe body pain/unable to follow ordinary pursuits for minimum how many days/week *(Most Recent Question June 2022)*

a. 16 days b. 18 days
c. 20 days d. 25 days

43. In court of law, examination of a witness is being done to develop new or old facts and to try to weaken the evidence by showing that evidence was biased inaccurate inconsistent by a lawyer during which of the following: *(Most Recent Question June 2022)*

a. Direct examination b. Cross examination
c. Redirect examination d. Court room examination

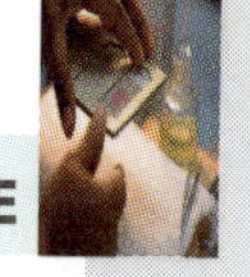

44. A patient died because of doctor negligence but some other factors also were the reason of his death. This type of malpractice is known as:

(Most Recent Question June 2022)

a. Contributory negligence
b. Res ipsa loquitor
c. Volenti non fit injuria
d. Respondeat superior/Novus actus interveniens

45. A physician referred a patient to a radiologist. Some person known to radiologist later visited the physician with a thank you letter and money packet. Which is true regarding above situation.

(Most Recent Question June/Dec 2021)

a. Doctor should be punished under IPC law
b. Medical dichotomy
c. Association of a Physician
d. Covering

46. Judicial hanging is a method of execution of a condemned criminal. Cause of death in such case is mostly due to: *(Most Recent Question June/Dec 2021)*

a. Vagal inhibition
b. Cervical vertebral fracture
c. Asphyxia
d. Cerebral hypoxia

47. A person has committed a criminal offence, caught by police and later brought to a criminal court but the court directs police to transfer the case to juvenile courts if it was proved that accused is of ___________ year age:

(Most Recent Question June/Dec 2021)

a. 21　　b. 17
c. 25　　d. 19

48. In an unconscious patient with head injury requiring emergency surgery, if there are no relatives to give consent, the doctor should

(Most Recent Question June/Dec 2021)

a. Operate without consent
b. Should not operate
c. Wait for the arrival of relatives
d. Take consent from the person who brought the patient

49. A 17-year-old girl was kidnapped. Police caught the accused and brought him to police station. After some time, the accused was found dead. Inquest in this case will be done by: *(Most Recent Question Aug 2020)*

a. Coroner　　b. Judicial magistrate
c. Police　　d. Medical examiner

50. Under what circumstances dying declaration (DD) given by a person of sound mind becomes invalid:

(Most Recent Question Aug 2020)

a. If victim survives after recording DD
b. DD was half recorded
c. DD not signed by the dying person
d. If DD recorded by doctor

51. McNaughton's rule, IPC in India is:

(Most Recent Question Dec 2019-20)

a. IPC 82　　b. IPC 84
c. IPC 87　　d. IPC 85

52. Which IPC section is related to medical negligence?

(Most Recent Question Dec 2019-20)

a. 300　　b. 302
c. 304-A　　d. 304 – B

53. A female after 4 years of marriage died and one note was from her mentioning that she was tortured for dowry. In this case inquest will be done by:

(Most Recent Question Dec 2019-20)

a. Police
b. Village headman
c. Magistrate
d. Judge

54. Grounds of divorce are all; EXCEPT:

(Most Recent Question 2019)

a. Impotency　　b. Frigidity
c. Mental retardation　　d. Poverty

55. IPC for causing abortion without women's consent:

(Most Recent Question 2019)

a. 312　　b. 313
c. 314　　d. 315

56. Before dying declaration, the role of a doctor is:

(Most Recent Question 2019)

a. To assess compos mentis
b. To record statement even in presence of magistrate
c. Cross examines the person
d. Put person under oath before declaration

57. McNaughton rule is for:

(Recent Pattern Question 2018-19)

a. Civil responsibility of insane
b. Criminal responsibility of insane
c. Capacity of witness
d. Testamentary capacity

58. Which of the following is related to legal responsibility of insane person: *(Recent Pattern Question 2018-19)*

a. Hasse's rule　　b. Curren's rule
c. Morrison rule　　d. Rule of nine

59. True about summon to medical examiner for criminal case: *(Recent Pattern Question 2018-19)*

a. Under penalty document
b. Issued by magistrate
c. Conduct money paid along with summon
d. Punishable under IPC Sec 87

60. First class magistrate is selected by

(Recent Pattern Question 2017)

a. State government
b. Chief justice of supreme court
c. Chief justice of high court
d. Governor

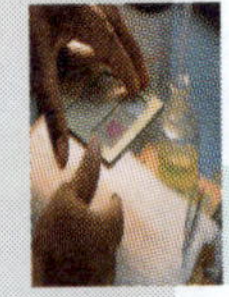

61. Investigation of custody death is done by: *(Recent Pattern Question 2017)*
a. Medical officer
b. Magistrate
c. Constable
d. Sub-inspector

62. Which of these following is an example of a leading question? *(Recent Pattern Question 2016)*
a. How did you get cuts on T-shirt
b. Cause of injury
c. Whether it is caused by knife
d. Size of incised wound

63. Inquest of dowry death is done by:
a. Magistrate b. Police
c. Medical officer d. Sub-inspector

64. Dowry death investigation is done by:
a. Magistrate b. Sub-inspector
c. Police d. Medical officer

65. IPC 321:
a. Grievous hurt b. Hurt
c. Punishment of hurt d. Voluntarily causing hurt

66. Punishment for Rape is not less than
a. 5 years b. 7 years
c. 10 years d. 20 years

67. Hurt is defined by IPC:
a. 317 b. 319
c. 320 d. 321

68. Grevious hurt is defined under IPC
a. 320 b. 302
c. 300 d. 376

69. Criteria for grievous hurt are all; EXCEPT:
a. Endanger to life
b. Privation to eye/sight
c. Permanent disfiguration of face
d. Injured person admitted in hospital for 21 days

70. Adultery comes under IPC section
a. 497 b. 498
c. 375 d. 376

71. Infanticide comes under which section
a. 83 b. 315
c. 299 d. 317

72. Death due to bodily injury caused by husband or his relative after marriage is punished under IPC:
a. 304 b. 304 A
c. 304 B d. 498 A

73. Cruel behavior towards wife by husband, family members or his relatives comes under which IPC section:
a. 498 A b. 304
c. 304 A d. 304 B

74. Extending the hanging for pregnant women comes under which CrPC:
a. Section 413 b. Section 414
c. Section 419 d. Section 416

75. Which of the following is not illegal in India:
a. Bestiality b. Masturbation
c. Buccal coitus d. Indecent assault

TOXICOLOGY

76. Toxicity of the venom of king cobra is: *(Most Recent Question June/Dec 2021)*
a. Musculo toxic b. Neurotoxic
c. Vasculotoxic d. Not defined

77. A chronic alcoholic with history of 25 years of alcoholism suddenly left alcohol. After 72 hours which of the following is seen as withdrawal feature: *(Most Recent Question June/Dec 2021)*
a. Wernicke's encephalopathy
b. Tremors
c. Seizures
d. Delirium tremens

78. A 40-year-old patient presents win casualty with lacrimation, diarrhea, congested eyes, tachycardia and hypertension. Which of the following should be suspected? *(Most Recent Question June/Dec 2021)*
a. Cocaine withdrawal b. Cannabis withdrawal
c. Opium withdrawal d. Dhatura poisoning

79. A 35-year-old patient comes to casualty with history of unknown poisoning by some seed/drug. On examination patient presented with dilated pupil, dry mouth and decreased secretions. Which poisoning should the you suspect. *(Most Recent Question June /Dec 2021)*
a. Cocaine b. Heroin
c. Cannabis d. Dhatura

80. A 40-year-old patient was brought by police in unconscious state to casualty with history of unknown poisoning. On examination patient had needle track ulcers over upper limbs. Patient had increased blood pressure, increased heart rate and respiratory rate of 30/minutes. Which poisoning should you suspect: *(Most Recent Question June/Dec 2021)*
a. Cocaine b. Heroin
c. Cannabis d. LSD

81. Identify the method of solvent abuse: *(Most Recent Question Aug 2020)*

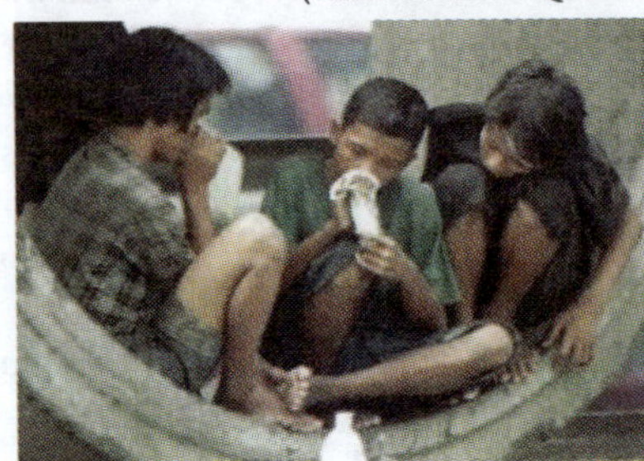

a. Bagging b. Huffing
c. Glading d. Sniffing

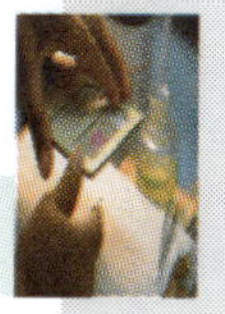

82. A patient is brought to casualty with history of snake bite with features as shown. During the course of treatment the patient expires. The accused snake is brought by relatives as shown in image. What will be the caused of death in this case? *(Most Recent Question Aug 2020)*

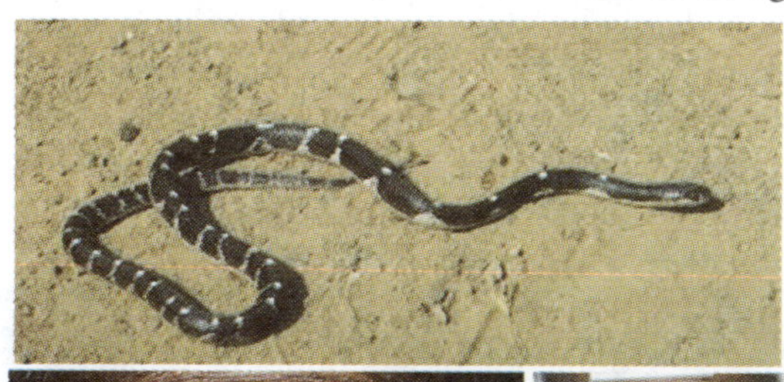

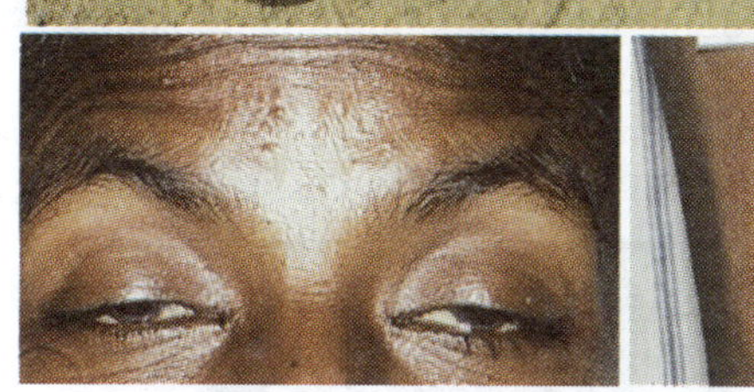

a. Shock b. Respiratory paralysis
c. Coagulopathy d. Renal failure

83. Rotten egg odor is associated with: *(Most Recent Question Aug 2020)*

a. Arsenic b. Hydrogen sulphide
c. Aluminum phosfide d. Phosphorus

84. Antidote is be used iron poisoning is: *(Most Recent Question Aug 2020)*

a. BAL b. EDTA
c. Deferoxamine d. Trientine

85. Which of the following produces catecholamine storm as seen with scorpion sting? *(Most Recent Question Dec 2019-20)*

a. Spider b. Tick
c. Sea urchin d. Ciguatera

86. Poisoning caused by bullet retained in body is: *(Most Recent Question Dec 2019-20)*

a. Lead b. Phosphorus
c. Nitro cellulose d. Iron

87. A patient was found to have pink colored skin and mucosa, bitter almond smell from breath and frothy discharge. Case of death in this patient: *(Most Recent Question Dec 2019-20)*

a. Cyanide poisoning b. CO poisoning
c. H_2S poisoning d. Datura poisoning

88. A farmer with pinpoint pupils, increased secretions and urination. What is the most likely diagnosis? *(Most Recent Question Dec 2019-20)*

a. Organophosphate poisoning
b. Opioid poisoning
c. Alcohol poisoning
d. Atropine poisoning

89. The toxin extracted from the poisonous plant shown in image is: *(Most Recent Question Dec 2019-20)*

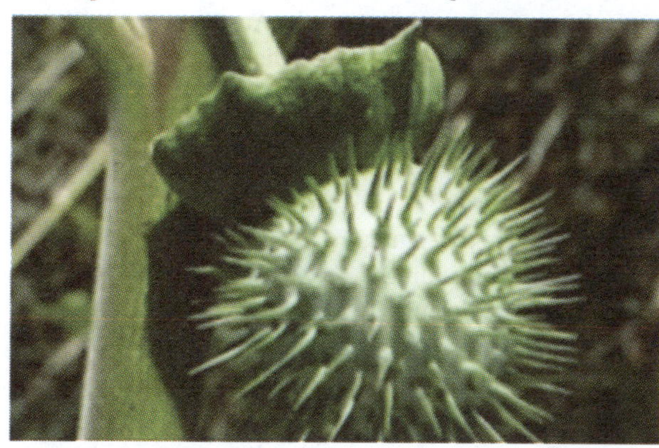

a. Cocaine b. Hyoscine
c. Thiamine d. Tetrahydrocannabinol

90. Gastric lavage is contraindicated in: *(Recent Pattern Question 2018-19)*

a. Organo-phosphosphate poisoning
b. Hydrocarbons
c. Bicarbonate
d. PCM toxicity

91. Wall scraping is used in treatment of which poisoning: *(Recent Pattern Question 2018-19)*

a. Oxalic acid b. Sulphuric acid
c. Carbolic acid d. Phenol

92. Aconite poisoning is mainly caused by: *(Recent Pattern Question 2017)*

a. Fruit b. Leaf
c. Root d. Bark

93. Heroin is which type of derivative of opium? *(Recent Pattern Question 2017)*

a. Natural b. Semi-natural
c. Synthetic d. Semi-synthetic

94. Binocellate mark is seen in which snake? *(Recent Pattern Question 2017)*

a. Cobra b. Viper
c. Sea scale viper d. Krait

95. Cherry red discoloration is seen in which poisoning? *(Recent Pattern Question 2017)*

a. Nickel b. Carbon monoxide
c. Phosphorus d. Cyanide

96. Which of the following is a cyanide poisoning antidote? *(Recent Pattern Question 2017)*

a. Sodium dantrolene b. Sodium thiosulfate
c. Sodium valprotate d. Sodium formaldehyde

97. Cyanide poisoning antidote: *(Recent Pattern Question 2017)*

a. Hydroxocobalamin b. Sodium chloride
c. Sodium bicarbonate d. Sodium gluconate

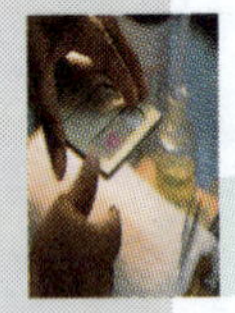

98. Acrodynia is associated with:
a. Lead b. Mercury
c. Zinc d. Arsenic

99. Maximum damage to the esophagus is caused by:
a. Acid b. Alkali
c. Organophosphate d. Kerosene

100. In which of the following poisoning CSF is required to be preserved:
a. Alcoholic poisoning
b. Arsenic poisoning
c. Copper poisoning
d. Organophosphorous poisoning

101. Which of the following is NOT used in organophosphate poisoning?
a. Charcoal b. Atropine
c. Oximes d. PAM

102. Gastric lavage is contraindicated in which poisoning:
a. Kerosene b. Alcohol
c. Organophosphate d. Lead

103. To which of following a person gets easily tolerated and addicted?
a. Tobacco b. Caffeine
c. Cannabis d. Alcohol

104. Antidote for phosphorus poisoning:
a. Atropine b. Calcium gluconate
c. Copper sulphate d. Physostigmine

105. All are true about arsenic poisoning; EXCEPT:
a. Aldrich mees line on nails
b. Mimics tetanus
c. Rain drop pigmentation on body
d. Hyperkeratosis of palms and soles

106. Rain drop appearance is seen in which poisoning:
a. Arsenic b. Lead
c. Mg d. Tin

107. Miosis is caused by all; EXCEPT:
a. Opiates b. Organophosphates
c. Pontine hemorrhage d. Cyanide

108. Treatment of choice in cyanide poisoning is:
a. Sodium chloride b. Sodium carbonate
c. Sodium thiosulfate d. Atropine

109. Sea snake venom is mostly:
a. Hepatotoxic b. Neurotoxic
c. Haemolytic d. Myotoxic

110. Bitten by krait. Manifestation would be:
a. Neurotoxic b. Myotoxic
c. Vasculotoxic d. Cardiotoxic

111. Blood alcohol level while driving mg%:
a. 10 b. 20
c. 30 d. 40

112. Hooch' tragedy is due to:
a. Ethyl alcohol b. Methyl alcohol
c. Ethylene glycol d. Cannabis

113. Which of the following is NOT a form of cannabis:
a. Bhang b. Charas
c. Cocaine d. Ganja

114. A narcotic abuse case presents with jet black tongue. The most likely cause is:
a. Cannabis toxicity b. Alcohol poisoning
c. LSD poisoning d. Cocaine poisoning

115. Vitriolage can be done by which of the plant:
a. Croton tigilum b. Arbus precagtorius
c. Bhilawanol d. Calotropes

BURNS AND DROWNING

116. A body was recovered within few minutes of death and following condition was noted. This is commonly associated with: ***(Most Recent Question June/Dec 2021)***

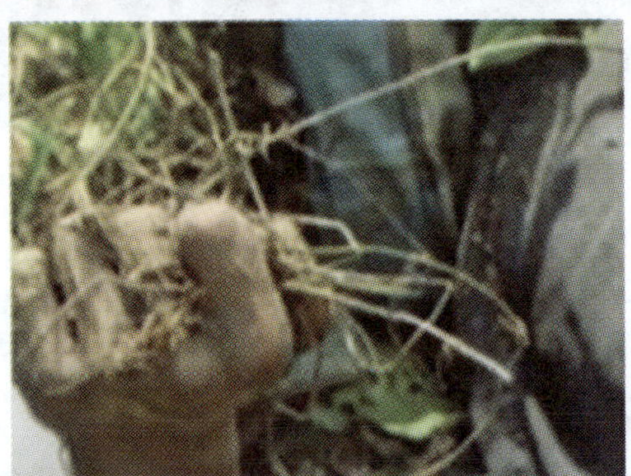

a. Torture b. Poisoning
c. Drowning d. Sudden death

117. In case of Asphyxial death due to hanging how, will you comment upon whether person was suspended from more or less than his height:
(Most Recent Question June/Dec 2021)
a. Hyperextended neck
b. Transverse mark over neck
c. Accessibility of suspension point
d. Tightness of ligature

118. In the investigation of severe burn body, which of the following sample is taken for identification:
(Recent Pattern Question 2019)
a. Blood b. Hair
c. Teeth d. Bone

119. Gettler test is done in: ***(Recent Pattern Question 2017)***
a. Burn
b. Drowning
c. Hanging
d. Strangulation

120. Mesohalophilic diatoms live in:
(Recent Pattern Question 2017)
a. Brackish water b. Sea water
c. Fresh water d. Sewer water

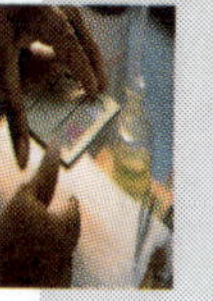

121. Most conclusive sign of ante-mortem death due to burns
(Recent Pattern Question 2016)
a. Heat hyperemia
b. Heat fracture
c. Presence of carboxyhemoglobin
d. Absence of line of redness

122. Most common cause of death in drowning:
a. Electrolyte imbalance
b. Pneumonia
c. Cardiac arrest
d. Vasovagal shock

123. In case of cold water drowning death is due to
a. Vagal stimulation
b. Vagal inhibition
c. Hypervolemia
d. Ventricular fibrillation

124. Most common feature indicative of Antemortem drowning:
a. Washerwomen feet
b. Pugilistic attitude
c. Clenched fist
d. Cyanosis

125. Paltauff haemorrhage is seen in:
a. Drowning
b. Suffocation
c. Throttling
d. Burns

126. Presence of diatoms in bone marrow are characteristic of which of the following?
a. Putrefaction
b. Drowning
c. Strangulation
d. Throttling

127. Pugilistic attitude is seen in:
a. Drowning
b. Burns
c. Lightening
d. Hanging

128. Degloving injury involve:
a. Avulsion of subcutaneous layer with fat
b. Erosion of skin with muscle
c. Peeling of the skin
d. Necrosis of muscle

129. Crocodile skin is seen in:
a. Drowning
b. High voltage electric burns
c. Neck ligature
d. High temperature water burns

130. Lichenburg flower is a classical finding in which of the following:
a. Lightening stroke
b. Electrical injuries
c. Joule burn
d. Scald burn

131. Scald burns can be caused by:
a. Molten metal
b. Electric burns
c. High temperature liquids
d. Lightening stroke

132. Which of the following is seen in antemortem burns:
a. Decreased alkaline phosphatase
b. Cl– increased & albumin decreased in vesicles
c. Presence of carbonaceous deposits in respiratory tract
d. Dull base of blister

133. In case of burning fire in a closed room, death occurs due to:
a. CO_2 poisoning
b. CO poisoning
c. Cardiac fauilre
d. Respiratory failure

IMPOTENCY, SEXUAL PERVERSION AND SEXUAL OFFENCES

134. Sexual pleasure obtained by getting hurt by opposite sex is called as: *(Most Recent Question June 2022)*
a. Masochism
b. Sadism
c. Transvestism
d. Exhibitionism

135. Excessive sexual desire in male is known as:
(Most Recent Question June/Dec 2021)
a. Satyriasis
b. Masochism
c. Voyeurism
d. Nymphomania

136. Sexual gratification through obscene telephone calls is:
(Most Recent Question Aug 2020)
a. Scopophilia
b. Scoptophilia
c. Scatologia
d. Voyeurism

137. Stains over clothes when examined showed yellow color needle shape crystals. Examined stain is of:
(Most Recent Question Dec 2019-20)
a. Sputum
b. Semen
c. Blood
d. CSF

138. Lesbianism is also known as:
(Recent Pattern Question 2018)
a. Machoism
b. Tribadism
c. Nymphomania
d. Transsexualism

139. In an eligible couple, the age of woman is:
(Recent Pattern Question 2017)
a. 18–45 years
b. 18–49 years
c. 21–45 years
d. 15–49 years

140. Statutory rape is considered below the age
(Recent Pattern Question 2016)
a. 16 years
b. 18 years
c. 20 years
d. 22 years

141. Impotent quoad is seen in:
a. Inability of the male to beget children and in the female, the inability to conceive children
b. An individual who may be impotent with any particular woman but not with others
c. Inability of a person to perform sexual intercourse
d. Inability to start or maintain the sexual arousal pattern in the female

142. A posthumous child is:
a. Still born
b. Child born after father's death
c. Child born after mother's death
d. Fictitious child claimed by a women as her own

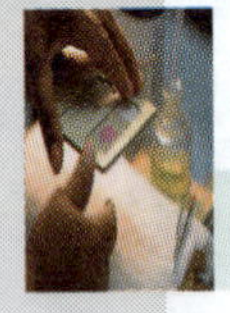

143. A female forges to have a child, whereas she doesn't have. It is:
a. Cheating
b. Posthumous child
c. Suppositious child
d. Superstitious child

144. A child who is born to an unmarried women:
a. Posthumous child
b. Illegitimate child
c. Suppositious child
d. Fictitious child

145. Most important cause of impotence:
a. Male factor
b. Female factor
c. Psychogenic
d. Anatomical

146. Which of the following is not a crime:
a. Rape
b. Sodomy
c. Incest
d. Indecent Assault

147. Hymen in false virgin is:
a. Annular
b. Elastic
c. Imperforate
d. Semilunar

148. All of the following are paraphilias; EXCEPT:
a. Bestiality
b. Frotteurism
c. Sadomasochism
d. Bisexuality

149. Frotteurism is:
a. Sexual satisfaction by contact with articles of opposite sex like hanky, sandals, clothes
b. Sexual satisfaction by rubbing the genitalia with the body of the person of other sex
c. Sexual gratification by exposing one's genitalia
d. Sexual satisfaction by watching the sexual act

150. Frotteurism:
a. Pleasure in watching intercourse
b. Pleasure in using article of opposite sex
c. Pleasure in touching opposite sex
d. Pleasure in wearing opposite sex clothes

151. A person who gets satisfaction by watching others indulged in sexual activity:
a. Voyeurism
b. Frotteurism
c. Fetischism
d. Exihibitionism

152. A 24-year-old male is convinced to be a female, is diagnosed as:
a. Transvestism
b. Transsexualism
c. Homosexualism
d. Undinism

153. Incessant sexual desire in males:
a. Satyriasis
b. Nymphomania
c. Vaginismus
d. Quoad hoc

154. Florence test is used for
a. Blood
b. Semen
c. Urine
d. Albumin

155. The seminal stains shows fluorescence when examined under the filtered ultraviolet light, this property of seminal stains is due to presence of:
a. Choline
b. Spermine
c. Sperm
d. Enzymes

156. Identification of semen is done by:
a. Haemochromogen test
b. Barberios test
c. Guaiacum test
d. Leuco malachite green test

157. Saliva is tested by:
a. Amylase
b. Ortho-toluidine
c. Acid phosphatase
d. Tetra-methyl-Benzidine

INJURY/GUNSHOT INJURY/FIREARM INJURY/STAB WOUND

158. Artificial bruise can be differentiated from true bruise by which of the following:
(Most Recent Question June 2022)
a. Presence of vesicles
b. Colour change noted with time
c. Diffuse irregular margins
d. No itching

159. In an injury it is noted under microscope that hair bulbs were crushed. Most likely the injury is:
(Most Recent Question June 2022)
a. Abrasion
b. Incised wound
c. Lacerated wound
d. Stab wound

160. Lucid interval is mostly associated with:
(Most Recent Question June/Dec 2021)
a. Epidural hemorrhage
b. Subdural hemorrhage
c. Subarachnoid hemorrhage
d. Intracerebral hemorrhage

161. Finding in the image shown is suggestive of:
(Most Recent Question June/Dec 2021)

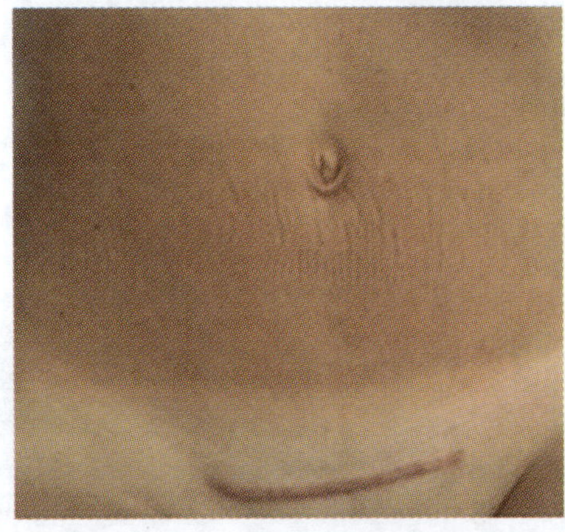

a. Scar
b. Tattoo
c. Mole
d. Ligature mark

162. Gutter fracture of skull bone is associated with impact by: ***(Most Recent Question June/Dec 2021)***
a. Sharp object
b. Blunt object
c. Fall from height
d. Bullet

163. A dead body comes with neck wound having clean cut margins, with vertebral bone disruptions. What type of wound is this? ***(Most Recent Question Aug 2020)***
a. Incised
b. Chop
c. Lacerated
d. Stab

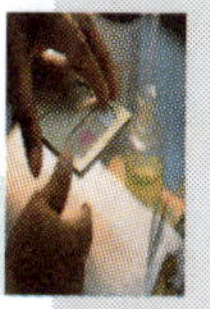

164. A cricketer got hit by ball and fainted. After sometime he regained consciousness and fainted again. This phenomenon is mostly associated with?

(Most Recent Question Dec 2019-20)

a. EDH b. SDH
c. SAH d. Intracerebral hemorrhage

165. A gunshot case brought for autopsy shows an entry wound with inverted margins and surrounded by tattooing, burning and singeing of hairs is not noted. What is the range of firearm weapon?

(Most Recent Question Dec 2019-20)

a. Contact b. Near
c. Distant d. 2 meters

166. After injury hair bulbs are seen crushed under microscopy. Probable type of wound:

(Most Recent Question Dec 2019-20)

a. Abrasion b. Laceration
c. Stab injury d. None

167. Entry wound kind of depression will be seen in:

(Most Recent Question Dec 2019-20)

a. Inversion b. Eversion
c. Pond's fracture d. Depression

168. Organ injured commonly in seat belt injury:

(Most Recent Question 2019)

a. Mesentery b. Spleen
c. Liver d. Lungs

169. Gun powder in hand during gun-shot residue testing is collected using: *(Recent Pattern Question 2018)*

a. Paraffin wax b. Benzidine
c. Acid phosphatase d. Sulfur

170. Lacerated looking incised wounds are seen at:

(Recent Pattern Question 2017)

a. Cheek prominence b. Scrotum
c. Shin d. Forehead

171. Yellow color of bruise is seen due to:

(Recent Pattern Question 2017)

a. Biliverdin in one day b. Biliverdin in 14 day
c. Bilirubin on 4th day d. Bilirubin on 9th day

172. In a large bruise, color changes begins from:

(Recent Pattern Question 2017)

a. From the center
b. From the periphery
c. All at same time
d. Little lateral from the main site of bruise

173. Oblique bullet injury causes which type of wound

(Recent Pattern Question 2016)

a. Oval b. Round
c. Stellate d. Keyhole

174. Teeth bite marks are which type of abrasion:

a. Pressure abrasion
b. Contusions
c. Graze abrasion
d. Linear abrasion

175. Brush burn is a:

a. Linear abrasion
b. Pressure abrasion
c. Graze abrasion
d. Contusion

176. Whiplash injury is damage to

a. Skull
b. Spine
c. Rib cage
d. Long bones

177. Bruise is bluish-black in color after:

a. 24 hour
b. 2 day
c. Few days
d. Few months

178. True about Countre-coup injury:

a. Injury located towards the impact
b. Injury common in stationary head
c. Injury common in moving head
d. All of the above

179. Which of the following is not seen in black gun powder of Bullet:

a. Sulphur
b. Charcoal
c. Potassium
d. Nitrocellulose

180. True statement about Tandem bullet:

a. Bullet that rotates in end on end during its motion
b. Bullet which travel in irregular fashion
c. Bullet that first hits some other object along the way
d. Two bullets are ejected one after the other

181. Tailing of wound suggests:

a. Direction of injury b. Weapon used
c. Type of wound d. Surface of weapon

182. Which of the following is NOT associated with stabbing injury:

a. Point wound b. Puncture wound
c. Perforation d. Chopping

183. Tentative cuts are seen in:

a. Suicide b. Homicide
c. Accidental cut d. Traumatic cut

184. 'Flaying' is seen in which type of laceration?

a. Split b. Stretch
c. Avulsion d. Tears

ABORTION, THANATOLOGY AND HANGING

185. As per MTP act 2021 opinion of two doctors is need for:

(Most Recent Question June 2022)

a. 12-20 weeks pregnancy b. 20-24 weeks pregnancy
c. 12-24 weeks pregnancy d. 20-26 weeks pregnancy

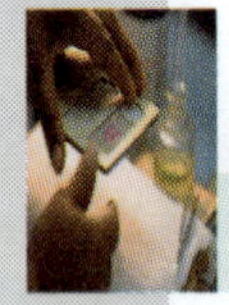

186. A dead body as shown in image was brought for autopsy. Odor in such case will be: ***(Most Recent Question June/Dec 2021)***

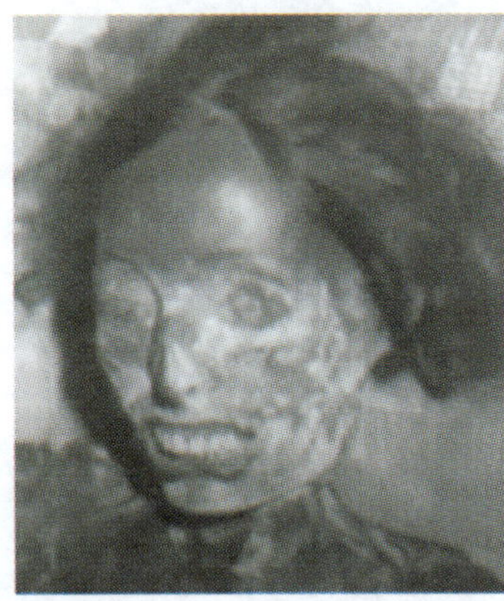

a. Ammoniacal b. Bitter almond
c. Burnt rope d. Odorless

187. With regards to fetal death classification lung is dipped in water in which test: ***(Most Recent Question Aug 2020)***

a. Foderes test b. Ploquets test
c. Hydrostatic test d. Wredin's test

188. A person was found dead in bushes with tied arms. Cyanosis of nails noted with scratches over face, neck and chin. All of the following are correct in this case; EXCEPT? ***(Most Recent Question Dec 2019-20)***

a. Case of homicide b. Asphyxia
c. Case of suicide d. Throttling/smothering

189. True about a Posthumous child: ***(Most Recent Question Dec 2019-20)***

a. Child born to unmarried couple
b. Child born after death of father
c. After death of mother during delivery
d. After death of both parents

190. A female faked pregnancy and presented a real child to blackmail a guy. Which is correct about this case? ***(Most Recent Question Dec 2019-20)***

a. Supposititious child b. Spurious child
c. Superfecundation d. Superfetation

191. Presence of cut injuries in scrotum is suggestive of: ***(Most Recent Question Dec 2019-20)***

a. Suicidal b. Accidental
c. Homicidal d. Genocidal

192. Rule which describes the cadaveric rigidity and sequential onset of rigor mortis: ***(Recent Pattern Question 2018-19)***

a. Curren's rule b. Nysten's rule
c. Hasse's rule d. Durham rule

193. Which cavity should be opened first in the suspicion of hanging? ***(Recent Pattern Question 2018)***

a. Thorax b. Head
c. Abdomen d. Neck

194. Specific gravity of unrespired lung: ***(Recent Pattern Question 2018)***

a. 0.94 b. 1.2
c. 0.75 d. 1.04

195. Respired lung weight as compared to body weight is: ***(Recent Pattern Question 2018)***

a. 1/10 b. 1/20
c. 1/35 d. 1/70

196. Person identification can be done by: ***(Recent Pattern Question 2017)***

a. Proctoscopy b. Colposcopy
c. Chelioscopy d. Endoscopy

197. A diabetic patient develops DVT and PE. Leading cause of death I(a) in medical certificate is? ***(Recent Pattern Question 2017)***

a. Pulmonary embolism b. DVT
c. DM d. Renal failure

198. Which of the following is more dangerous in causing spinal damage? ***(Recent Pattern Question 2017)***

a. Hyperextension of the neck
b. Hyperflexion of the neck
c. Both hyperflexion and hyperextension of the neck
d. None can cause spinal damage

199. Wilful MTP is allowed up to how many weeks in India ***(Recent Pattern Question 2016)***

a. 12 weeks b. 20 weeks
c. 28 weeks d. 32 weeks

200. Which of the following points towards female skull differentiating from male ***(Recent Pattern Question 2016)***

a. Mastoid bigger
b. Prominent frontal emience
c. Orbit square with round edges
d. Prominent jaw

201. All are correct about MTP; EXCEPT:

a. Only qualified medical practitioner is allowed to perform it
b. Medical assistant can perform in absence of gynecologist
c. Husband's consent is not required
d. Can be done upto 20 weeks

202. Which of the following statement is true about MTP:

a. Consent of one doctor is enough upto 14 weeks
b. Husband's consent for MTP is must
c. Make sure to lodge a police complaint in case of MTP due to rape
d. Age proof is generally not required

203. A doctor can do MTP after practicing or assisting how many MTPs:

a. 22 b. 20
c. 12 d. 25

204. In case of typical hanging, position of knot is at:

a. Occiput b. Angle of mandible
c. Below the chin d. Side of neck

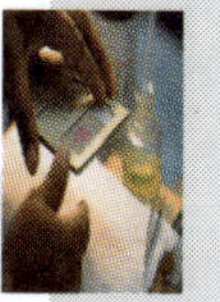

205. On examination a dead guy was found a ligature mark on neck. According to police, the person's leg were touching the ground while hanging. You suspected death due to partial hanging. This death is due to weight of around:

a. 1.15 kg b. 2.20 kg
c. 3.10 kg d. 4.50 kg

206. A 28 year female committed suicide. On the site it was noticed that her feet was not touching the ground. Which of the following shows its suicidal and not homicidal:

a. Ligature mark continuous around the neck
b. The position of the knot at the angle of mandible
c. Saliva dribbling to the opposite side of the knot
d. Red congested face

207. Le-facies expression is due to

a. Hanging b. Strangulation
c. Throttling d. Café coronary

208. All are strangulation; EXCEPT:

a. Burking b. Throttling
c. Garrotting d. Mugging

209. Burking is a method of:

a. Homicidal smothering and traumatic asphyxia
b. Suicidal smothering and traumatic asphyxia
c. Accidental smothering and choking
d. Choking and traumatic asphyxia

210. Overlying leads to death due to

a. Strangulation b. Suffocation
c. Mugging d. Choking

211. Postmortem rigidity disappears first in:

a. Upper limbs b. Neck
c. Lower limbs d. Eyelids

212. On postmortem examination, stiffening of muscles is observed in a burn deceased. This indicates that the person is exposed to intense heat above what temperature?

a. 30°C b. 40°C
c. 50°C d. 60°C

213. In asphyxia, the organ to be dissected last is:

a. Neck b. Head
c. Thorax d. Abdomen

FORENSIC PSYCHIATRY

214. A chronic alcoholic comes to casualty in disoriented state, agitation, tremors after 2 days of sudden alcohol withdrawal. Probable diagnosis will be:

a. Hangover *(Most Recent Question Aug 2020)*
b. Delirium tremens
c. Wernicke's encephalopathy
d. Korsakoff psychosis

215. A person got agitated, fainted and lost consciousness at airport. A bag full of enema and laxative was recovered from him. During treatment X-ray abdomen showed as picture as shown. All of the following are true in this scenario; EXCEPT? *(Most Recent Question Dec 2019-20)*

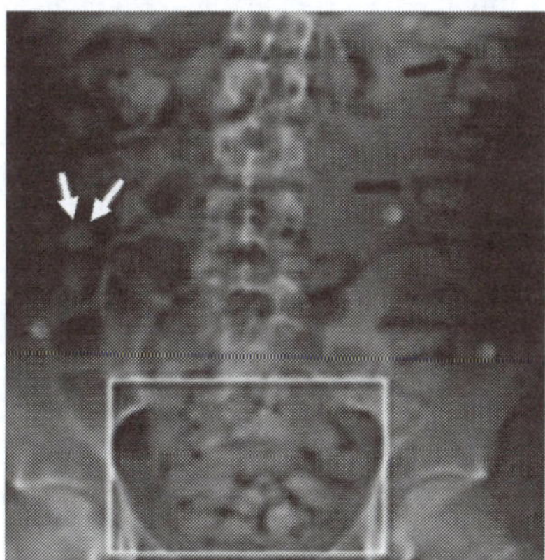

a. Abdominal CT scan is indicated
b. The person is malingering
c. He is at risk of poisoning
d. It's a case of body packer syndrome

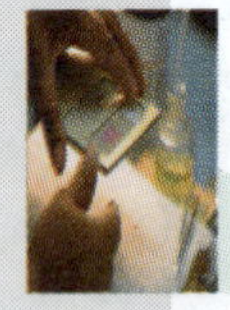

ANSWERS WITH EXPLANATIONS

MOST RECENT QUESTIONS 2023

1. Ans. (a) 20, 4

Ref: VV Pillay. Textbook of Forensic Medicine and Toxicology, 18th ed. pg. 76

- There are two sets of teeth:
  - **Temporary (deciduous/milk) teeth:** These are twenty in number, i.e. four incisors, two canines and four molars in each jaw.
  - **Permanent teeth:** These are thirty-two in number, i.e. 4 incisors, 2 canines or cuspids, 4 premolars or bicuspids and 6 molars in each jaw.
- At the age of 6, a child has 20 temporary teeth already and 4 molars are erupted. Therefore, at the age of 6, a child has 24 teeth (20 temporary and 4 permanent). This number remains constant from 6 to 11 years as temporary teeth are being replaced by permanent ones.
- Canines will be replaced in 11th year only, which makes 4 temporary teeth till age 10.
- At the age of 10 years, permanent teeth like 1st molar, central incisor, lateral incisor, 1st premolar and 2nd premolar are erupted in 4 quadrants of teeth, which makes it 20 permanent teeth and 4 temporary ones.

Eruption of Teeth

Permanent Teeth Eruption	
Average age of Eruption (Years)	**Teeth** *Mn*: **Mummy Is In Pain, Papa Can Make Medicine**
6	1st molar
7	Incisor (Central)
8	Incisor (Lateral)
9	1st premolar
10	2nd premolar
11	Canine
12–14	2nd molar
17–25	3rd molar

2. Ans. (b) *Cascabela thevetia*

Ref: VV Pillay. Textbook of Forensic Medicine and Toxicology, 18th ed. pg. 578

- *Cascabela thevetia*/Yellow oleander is a poisonous plant native throughout Mexico and in Central America, and cultivated widely as an ornamental. It is a relative of Nerium oleander, giving it a common name yellow oleander.
- It contains cardiac glycosides. Antidotes for treatment include atropine and digoxin immune fabs (antibodies) and treatment may include oral administration of activated charcoal.

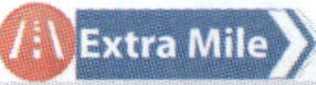

The other important plants

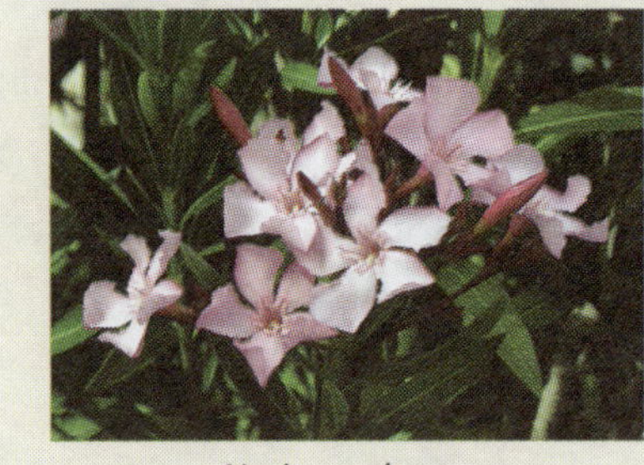

Nerium odorum

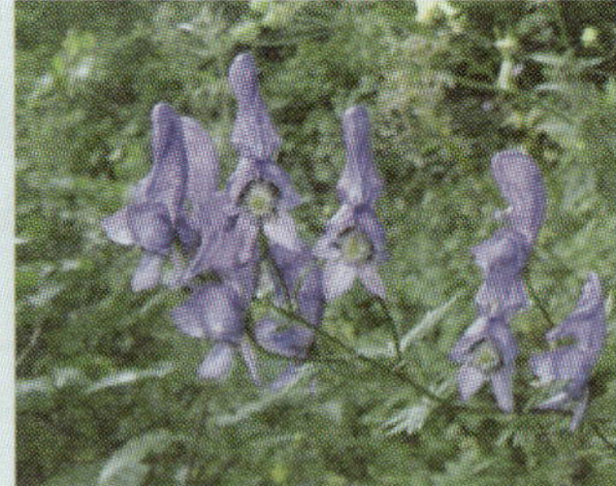

Aconite

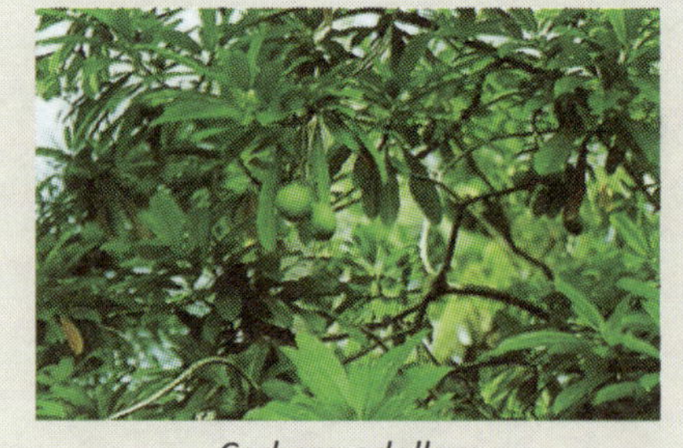

Cerbera odollam

3. Ans. (b) Contact shot

Ref: VV Pillay. Textbook of Forensic Medicine and Toxicology, 18th ed. pg. 225

- A contact shot is a gunshot wound incurred while the muzzle of the firearm is in direct contact with the body at the moment of discharge.

Contact shots are often the result of close-range gunfights, suicide, or execution.

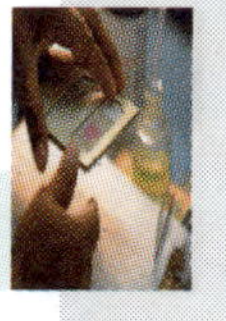

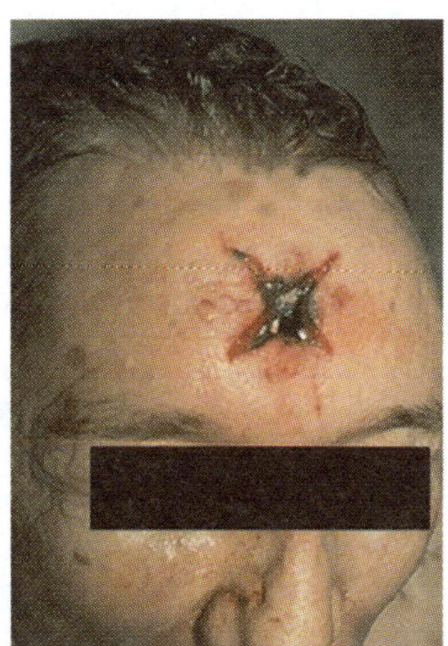

Range of Fire:

Range	Inches (barrel to skin)	Physical properties
• Contact	0	Soot, seared skin, triangular tears
• Close	0–6	Soot, abrasion collar (may be obscured by soot)
• Intermediate	<48	Tattooing, abrasion collar
• Distant or indeterminate	Any distance	Abrasion collar (intermediate objects will prevent soot and gunpowder from contacting the skin)

4. Ans. (b) Active self-defense wound

Ref: VV Pillay. Textbook of Forensic Medicine and Toxicology, 18th ed. pg. 298

- Defense wounds are caused by immediate and instinctive reaction of the victim to save himself. They are classified into two types:
  - **Active defense wound:** Caused when the victim tries to grasp the weapon.
  - **Passive defense wound:** Caused when the victim raises the hands, arms or legs to defend himself.
- **Option a:** Self-inflicted wounds (fabricated, fictitious or forged injuries). Injuries inflicted by oneself or by some other in agreement with him/her.
- **Option c:** A postmortem artifact is any change caused in the body after death that is likely to lead to misinterpretation of medically significant antemortem findings. It is introduced in the period between death and autopsy or during autopsy.

5. Ans. (b) Rape victim

Ref: VV Pillay. Textbook of Forensic Medicine and Toxicology, 18th ed. pg. 389

The MTP Act 1971 and
The MTP Amendment Act 2021

	MTP Act 1971	The MTP Amendment Act 2021
Indications (Contraceptive failure)	Only applies to married women	Unmarried women are also covered
Gestational age limit	20 weeks for all indications	24 weeks for rape survivors Beyond 24 weeks for substantial fetal abnormalities
Medical practitioner opinions required before termination	One RMP till 12 weeks Two RMPs till 20 weeks	One RMP till 20 weeks Two RMPs 20–24 weeks Medical board approval after 24 weeks
Breach of the woman's confidentiality	Fine up to Rs1000	Find and/or imprisonment of 1 year

6. Ans. (c) Lymph node

Ref: VV Pillay. Textbook of Forensic Medicine and Toxicology, 18th ed. pg. 177

- Migration of tattoo pigment particles from the dermis to lymph nodes can mimic other disease processes at surgery and on imaging. The technique can be used in autopsy when tattoo is not visible.

7. Ans. (c) Superimposition

Ref: VV Pillay. Textbook of Forensic Medicine and Toxicology, 18th ed. pg. 472

- Craniofacial superimposition is a technique used in the field of forensic anthropology to assist in the analysis of an unknown skull. The process involves superimposing an image of the recovered skull over an antemortem image of the suspected individual.
- **Option a:** Fingerprint analysis has been used to identify suspects and solve crimes for more than 100 years, and it remains an extremely valuable tool for law enforcement. One of the most important uses for fingerprints is to help investigators link one crime scene to another involving the same person.

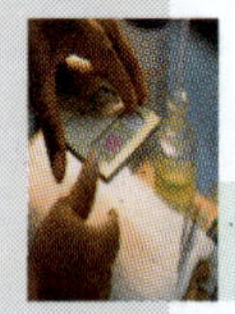

- **Option b:** DNA fingerprinting is a laboratory technique used to determine the probable identity of a person based on the nucleotide sequences of certain regions of human DNA that are unique to individuals.
- **Option d:** Cheiloscopy deals with the identification of humans based on lip traces. The lip print of every person is unique.

8. Ans. (a) Pterion

Ref: VV Pillay. Textbook of Forensic Medicine and Toxicology, 18th ed. pg. 452

- The pterion is the region where the frontal, parietal, temporal, and sphenoid bones join. It is located on the side of the skull, just behind the temple.

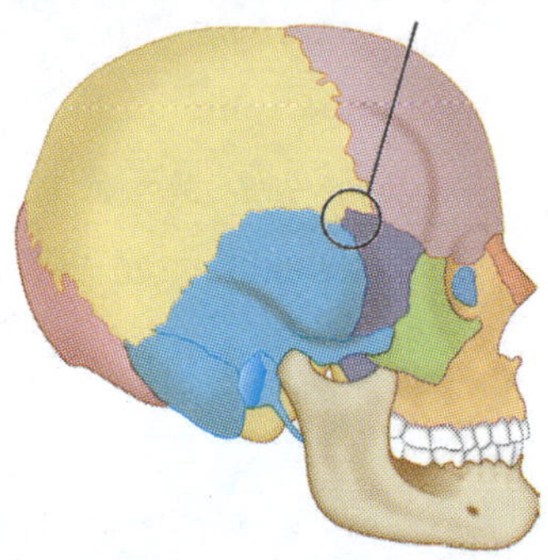

- It is considered as the weakest part of the skull. The anterior division of the middle meningeal artery runs underneath the pterion.
- A traumatic blow to the pterion may rupture the middle meningeal artery causing an epidural hematoma (EDH). The pterion may also be fractured indirectly by blows to the top or back of the head that place sufficient force on the skull to fracture the pterion.

9. Ans. (b) Executive Magistrate

Ref: VV Pillay. Textbook of Forensic Medicine and Toxicology, 18th ed. pg. 2

- In India, an inquest in the case of death in police custody is usually conducted by an Executive Magistrate.
- The Executive Magistrate is a judicial officer who has the authority to conduct inquiries, issue warrants, and perform other judicial functions.
- The role of the Executive Magistrate in this context is to investigate the circumstances surrounding the death and determine whether any foul play or negligence was involved.

10. Ans. (a) Oral evidence

Ref: VV Pillay. Textbook of Forensic Medicine and Toxicology, 18th ed. pg. 11

- When a court orders a witness to come and record their evidence in court, it typically refers to the witness providing their testimony orally. Oral evidence is the spoken testimony given by a witness under oath in a court proceeding. It involves the witness presenting their first-hand knowledge or observations of the events relevant to the case.
- In legal proceedings, oral evidence is often considered more reliable than hearsay evidence, which is second-hand information or statements made by others. Hearsay evidence is generally excluded because it can be less trustworthy and may not allow for cross-examination of the original speaker.

11. Ans. (b) Cadaveric spasm

Ref: VV Pillay. Textbook of Forensic Medicine and Toxicology, 18th ed. pg. 171

- Cadaveric spasm, also known as instantaneous rigor, is a phenomenon where a person's muscles undergo sudden and involuntary contraction just before or at the moment of death. It occurs when the body is in extreme stress or undergoing intense physical exertion right before death.
- In the given scenario, the person's efforts to save themselves triggered the contraction of one group of muscles. The absence of primary relaxation refers to the fact that the muscles did not relax immediately after the contraction, which is a characteristic feature of cadaveric spasm.

Extra Mile

- Rigor mortis is the stiffening of the body's muscles that occurs several hours after death due to chemical changes in the muscle tissues.
- Algor mortis refers to the cooling of the body after death.
- Livor mortis refers to the pooling and settling of blood in the dependent parts of the body, causing discoloration.

12. Ans. (a) McNaughten's rule

Ref: VV Pillay. Textbook of Forensic Medicine and Toxicology, 18th ed. pg.110

- The statement provided is in line with the principles established by the McNaughten's rule, which is a legal test for determining insanity in criminal cases. The McNaughten's rule, named after the case of Daniel McNaughten in 1843, sets forth the following criteria for establishing the defense of insanity:
  1. The accused must have been suffering from a mental disorder at the time of the offense.
  2. Due to the mental disorder, the accused must not have understood the nature and consequences of their actions.

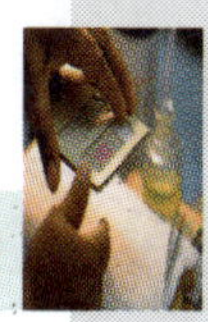

3. The accused must not have known that what they were doing was wrong in a legal or moral sense.

- According to the McNaughten's rule, if accused persons meet these criteria, they are considered legally insane and cannot be held criminally responsible for their actions.

13. Ans. (a) Thanatology

Ref: VV Pillay. Textbook of Forensic Medicine and Toxicology, 18th ed. pg. 146

- Thanatology is a multidisciplinary field that encompasses the scientific, psychological, social, and cultural aspects of death and dying.
- It involves the examination and exploration of various topics related to death, including the processes of dying, grief and bereavement, cultural practices and rituals surrounding death, the psychological impact of death on individuals and society, and the ethical considerations associated with end-of-life care.

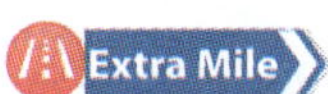

Extra Mile

- Thanatopraxis/Embalming is the technique used to preserve and expose mortal remains with utmost care.
- Disinterment is the act of digging corpse out of the ground.

14. Ans. (c) Carbon monoxide

Ref: VV Pillay. Textbook of Forensic Medicine and Toxicology, 18th ed. pg. 547

- Cherry red postmortem hypostasis is commonly associated with carbon monoxide (CO) poisoning.
- In cases of CO poisoning, a distinct cherry red coloration can be observed. CO is a toxic gas that binds strongly to hemoglobin. This binding creates a bright red or cherry red appearance in the affected tissues, including the skin. A phenomenon quite similar to livor mortis.
- The cherry red coloration in CO poisoning is most notable in areas with a high concentration of blood vessels, such as the lips, cheeks, and nail beds.

15. Ans. (a) Barberio's test

Ref: VV Pillay. Textbook of Forensic Medicine and Toxicology, 18th ed. pg. 68

- **Barberio's test:** It is used for detection of spermine in the sample. Few drops of Barberio's reagent is added to the sample. It produces needle-shaped, yellow color crystals of sperm.
- **Teichmann's test:** It is used to detect the presence of hemoglobin in a stain or sample. It involves adding a small amount of the stain or sample to a microscope slide, mixing it with a reagent (e.g., hydrogen peroxide), and observing the formation of characteristic rhomboid-shaped crystals under a microscope.
- **Takayama (Hemochromogen) test:** It is used to detect the presence of blood in a sample. It involves adding a sample to a test tube along with reagents such as pyridine and sodium hydroxide → mixture heated; and if blood is present, a bluish-purple color develops due to the formation of hemochromogen.
- **Spectroscopy:** It is the most delicate and reliable test for detecting the presence of blood in both recent and old stains. Less than 0.1 mg. of blood is sufficient. It is most sensitive test.

16. Ans. (d) Cocaine bugs

Ref: VV Pillay. Textbook of Forensic Medicine and Toxicology, 18th ed. pg. 624

- During the stage of excitement in acute cocaine poisoning, several signs and symptoms may manifest. These include:
  a. **Feeling of well-being:** Cocaine can induce a sense of euphoria, leading to an intense feeling of happiness or well-being
  b. **Tingling or numbness in hands and feet** due to peripheral vasoconstriction
  c. **Pupils dilated and rapid pulse and sweating**
- "Cocaine bug" is not a recognized sign or symptom of acute cocaine poisoning. It may refer to a hallucination or delusional parasitosis, where individuals experiencing cocaine intoxication may have a sensation of insects crawling on or under their skin. This perception is known as formication and is seen mainly in the chronic addicts.

17. Ans. (a) Burking

Ref: VV Pillay. Textbook of Forensic Medicine and Toxicology, 18th ed. pg. 345

- Homicidal smothering and traumatic asphyxia are causes of death associated with a criminal method known as "Burking."
- The method of Burking involves forcibly smothering or compressing the chest and abdomen of a victim, thereby obstructing their airway and preventing normal breathing. The weight or pressure applied to the victim's body restricts their ability to inhale, leading to asphyxia and subsequent death.

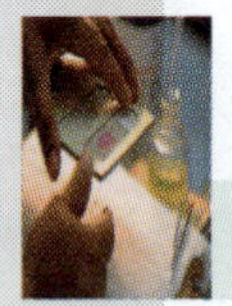

Extra Mile

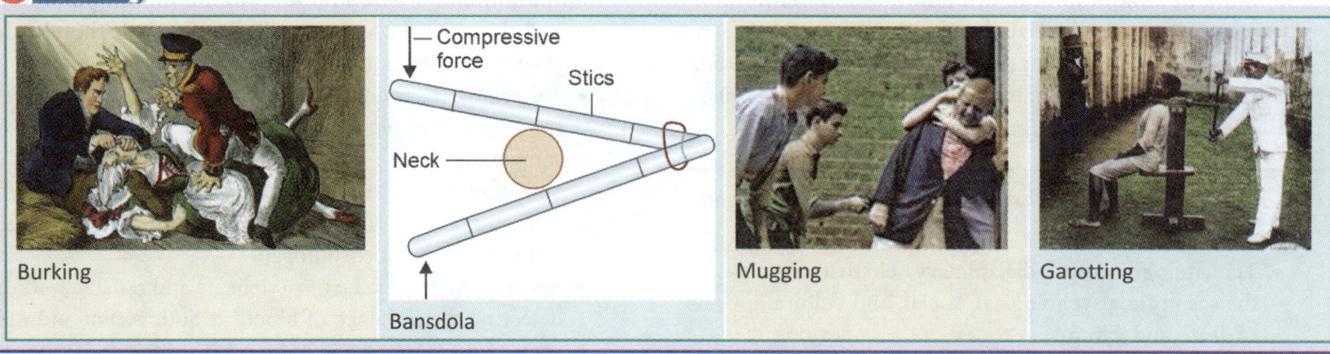

AUTOPSY & IDENTIFICATION

18. Ans. (b) Cardiac tamponade

Ref: Essentials of Forensic Medicine and Toxicology by Dr KS Narayan Reddy 34th ed. pg. 253

- The photograph demonstrates a gush of blood-stained fluid upon opening the pericardial layer during an autopsy, which is suggestive of cardiac tamponade.
- Cardiac tamponade is excessive accumulation of fluid or blood in the pericardial space.
- Around 200 to 300 ml of blood can cause death by increasing intra-pericardial pressure and producing progressive compression to heart and leads to decompensated heart failure.
- It is usually associated with myocardial infarction with rupture of wall, blunt chest and abdominal trauma and penetrating or perforating injuries to the heart.
- Normal volume of pericardial fluid is 10–50 mL.

19. Ans. (b) Teichman's test

Ref: Essentials of Forensic Medicine and Toxicology by Dr KS Narayan Reddy 34th ed. pg. 155

- The photograph demonstrates microscopic slide showing yellowish-red rhombic crystals of haemin or haematin chloride arranged single or in clusters. It is a positive finding of Teichmann's test
- Teichmann's test also known as haemin Crystal Test, is a type of microchemical test for detection of blood. Such tests are based on the property of haeme (iron) part of haemoglobin to form characteristic-coloured crystals with certain reagents.
- Other microchemical test include Takayama test also known as Haemochromogen crystal test where pink feather crystals of haemochromogen or reduced alkaline haematin arranged in clusters, sheaves, etc.

20. Ans. (c) Carbon monoxide

Ref: Essentials of Forensic Medicine and Toxicology by Dr KS Narayan Reddy 34th ed. pg. 151, 578

- **Cherry red** post-mortem staining is seen in carbon monoxide poisoning. It is due to the formation of carboxy-hemoglobin (COHb). It can be seen with concentration of 30 to 40 % COHb.
- Bluish-green post-mortem lividity is seen in H2S poisoning.
- Chocolate or copper brown post-mortem lividity is seen in poisoning by nitrites, potassium chlorate, potassium bicarbonate, nitrobenzene, acetanilide, bromates, and aniline.
- Bright red post-mortem lividity is seen in hydrocyanic acid poisoning.
- Dark brown or yellow post-mortem lividity is seen in phosphorous poisoning.

21. Ans. (c) Distended gallbladder

Ref: Essentials of Forensic Medicine and Toxicology by Dr KS Narayan Reddy 34th ed. pg. 314

- Distended gall bladder with bile is an autopsy finding of death due to starvation.
- Other specific findings include, oedema around joints, pressure sores, brittle hair and nails, absence of fat in omentum, reduction in size and weight of all organs except brain (pale and soft), brown atrophy of heart etc.

22. Ans. (b) Semen

Ref: Essentials of Forensic Medicine and Toxicology by Dr KS Narayan Reddy 34th ed. pg. 406

- A **Barberio's test** is done to detect the presence of **semen**.
- A saturated aqueous or alcoholic solution of picric acid when added to spermatic fluid produces yellow needle-shaped rhombic crystals of spermine picrate.

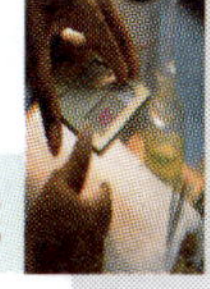

The reaction probably depends on the presence of prostatic secretion.

- **Other tests for sperm detection include:**
  - Florence test
  - Acid phosphatase test
  - Creatine phosphokinase test
  - Immunological methods
  - Choline and spermine test (thin layer chromatography).

23. Ans. (c) Arch

Ref: Review of Forensic Medicine and Toxicology, Gautam Biswas, 3rd ed. pg. 85

- The shown fingerprint in image is arch type of fingerprint.
- Most common type of fingerprint: Loop

TYPES OF FINGERPRINT PATTERN

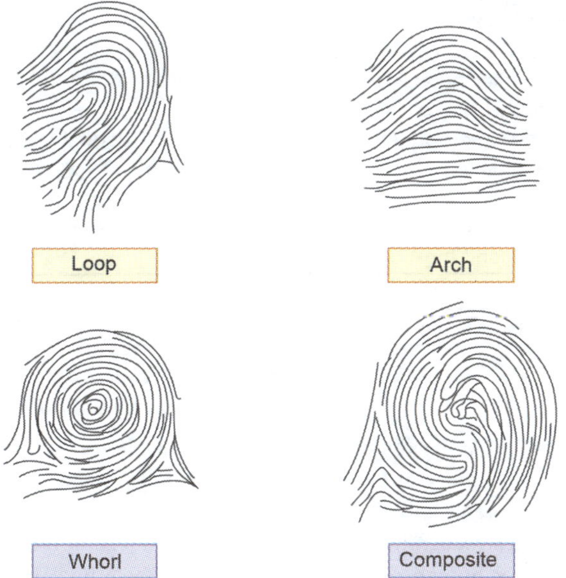

24. Ans. (d) Takayama test

Ref: Review of Forensic Medicine and Toxicology by Gautam Biswas, 3rd ed. pg. 424

- A takayama test, also known as hemochromogen crystal assay, is used to determine if blood is present in a sample of interest. This assay is used by experimenters, or investigators of crime scenes, to confirm if an unknown **sample indeed contains blood**.
- These crystals will **appear pink feathery** when viewed under a microscope. A lack of crystal formation signals to experimenter that no blood is present within the sample, and iron is not present to allow the reaction to occur.

25. Ans. (b) Cadaveric spasm

Ref: Review of Forensic Medicine and Toxicology by Gautam Biswas, 4th ed. pg. 150-152

- Cadaveric spasm is a condition in which the muscles of the body that were in a state of contraction immediately before it continue to be so after death.
- It is different from Rigor mortis, as in cadaveric spasm primary relaxation is absent and it mostly indicates sudden death as in trauma and associated with excitement, fatigue or exhaustion.
- Heat stiffness is seen when the body is subjected to high temperature and the muscle proteins coagulate. It is not associated with the road traffic accident, same is the case of cold stiffening.

26. Ans. (b) 5 months

Ref: Review of Forensic Medicine and Toxicology by Gautam Biswas, 4th ed, pg. 329

- Length of the fetus at different age is:
  - At 3 months approximately 9 cm
  - At 5 months approximately 25 cm
  - At 7 months approximately 35 cm and
  - At 9 months approximately 45 cm
- Moreover at 5 months the nails are distinct and minimum hair growth on scalp is seen.
- In a 9-month-old fetus the scalp is covered with dark hair which is not the case here.
- The lanugo hair starts to be visible on the body from 16 weeks. Hence the most appropriate answer is five months.

27. Ans. (c) Hip bone

Ref: Review of Forensic Medicine and Toxicology by Gautam Biswas, 4th ed. pg. 71

- Recognizable sex differences appear after puberty except in the pelvis.
- For this reason, the gender assessment in a 12-year-old boy can be best done by the pelvis of the hip bone with accuracy of 95% in gender assessment.
- Male pelvis is massive with prominent muscular markings and large acetabulum whereas the female pelvis is less massive with the smaller acetabulum.

28. Ans. (b) Greater curvature

Ref: Forensic Medicine and Toxicology by RN Karmakar pg. 327-28

- Stomach autopsy is done to examine any food particle, its state of digestion, smell, color, character or presence of any foreign/suspicious body. This is very important if determining time of death is a major factor.
- For doing autopsy of stomach, double ligature is applied and the stomach is opened along greater curvature (from cardiac to pylorus).

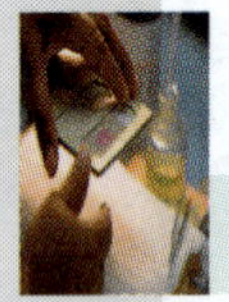

29. Ans. (a) Teratology

Ref: PubMed

- Teratology is the science that studies the causes of structural, functional, behavioral and metabolic disorders present at birth (congenital malformation). It includes:
  - Size
  - Arrangement
  - Composition of any organ or part of the body
- **Classification of anomalies:**
  - **Genetic/Chromosomal:** AR, X-linked, Down syndrome, Turner syndrome
  - Teratogenic agent or environmental (~10% of congenital anomalies)
    - **Physical:** External traumatic injuries
    - Radiation/atomic explosion
    - Chemical agent like thalidomide, anticonvulsants, alcohol, smoking
    - **Infectious agents:** German measles, CMV, HSV, Syphilis
    - **Antigens:** Rh factor

30. Ans. (c) Spectroscopic test

Ref: The Essentials of FSM by KS Narayan Reddy, 31st ed. pg. 405-407

TESTS OF BLOOD STAIN

- **Spectroscopic test:** Most specific/confirmatory method for blood stain test
- **Kastle-Meyer/Phenolpthalein test:** Color produced is Pink Purple.
- **Microchemical test:** Based on RBC content of blood.
- **Takayama's test:** Hb converted to Haemochromogen crystal. Salmon pink feathery haemochromogen crystals are obtained.
- **Teichmann's Haemin crystal test:** Hb converted into Hemin/Hematin crystals. Brown rhombic haemic crystal are seen
- **Benzidine test**
  - Best preliminary test as it detects blood present in dilution of 1 in 3 lakhs.
  - **Color produced:** Deep Blue
  - *Not used because it is a potential carcinogen.*

31. Ans. (b) Transparency of root

Ref: Forensic Medicine and Toxicology by Rabindra Nath Karmakar, pg. 11

GUSTAFSON METHOD

- Used for age determination, when teeth eruption is complete (after age 17–25 years)

It has 6 criteria:

- **Degree of attrition:** Wear and tear due to mastication. Not very reliable
- **Degree of periodontitis:** With age → regression of gum and periodontal tissue. It can be due to disease of gum or lack of oral hygiene. So not reliable also
- Degree of secondary dentine formation
- Degree of cementum apposition (gradual thickening of cementum following changes in position of teeth at the end of root).
- Degree of root resorption
- **Degree of root transparency/translucency** (due to mineral deposition in dentine canal → gradually becomes translucent but the dentine tissue become transparent due to osteoporosis). ***It is most dependable criteria.***

Extra Mile

- Modified Gustafson's is Daliz's formula
- **Stack's formula:** For age estimation of infant and children from the height and weight of teeth.
- **Boyde's method:** Age estimation from the structural feature of enamel
- **Lamendin method:** Uses 2 criteria gingival and root transparency for age estimation. Gives better result than Gustafson's method.

32. Ans. (a) Iris

Ref: Guide to Biometric Reference Systems and Performance Evaluation, pg. 25

- Iris is the only internal organ available for acquisition. Its information, richness and stability make it a very suitable and efficient biometric modality.
- Iris recognition is reported as the most reliable biometrics for human recognition and it is suitable for large scale identification purposes.
- It is already being used in government programs, border or restricted areas access control.

33. Ans. (b) 8 years

Ref: Pediatric Otolaryngology, Volume 2, pg. 1170

- A child has a total of 20 primary teeth by age of 3 years:
  - 10 in the maxillary arch
  - 10 in the mandibular arch
- Subsequently permanent dentition starts at 6 yrs (21st Tooth). Hence choice A cannot be the answer. The correct answer is 8 yrs.
- As the permanent teeth erupt, a mixed dentition results, giving rise to mixed dentition *(combination of primary and permanent teeth)* between ages of 6 years and 12 years.
- The early mixed dentition is characterized by the eruption of the permanent maxillary and mandibular incisors and

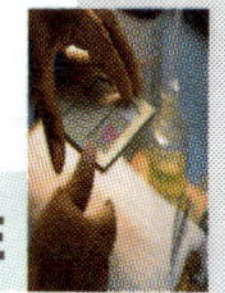

first molar teeth, with concurrent exfoliation of their primary counterparts.

- After these teeth have erupted, dental development becomes quiescent during what is known as the intertransitional period, from age 9 to 11. During this time, no further permanent teeth erupt.
- By the age of 13 years, adolscents have 28 permanent teeth.

TABLE: Initiation and eruption timing of the permanent dentition

Tooth	Initiation (Month)	Eruption (Year)
Maxilla		
Central incisor	5–5.25 *in utero*	7–8
Lateral incisor	5–5.25 *in utero*	8–9
Canine	5.5–6 *in utero*	11–12
First premolar	Birth	10–11
Second premolar	7.5–8	10–12
First molar	3.5–4 *in utero*	10–12
Second molar	8.5–9	12–13
Third molar	3.5–4 (years)	17–25
Mandible		
Central incisor	5–5.25 *in utero*	6–7
Lateral incisor	5.25 *in utero*	7–8
Canine	5.5–6 *in utero*	9–11
First premolar	Birth	10–12
Second premolar	7.5–8	11–12
First molar	3.5–4 *in utero*	6–7
Second molar	8.5–9	11–13
Third molar	3.5–4 (years)	17–25

34. Ans. (d) Chinese

Ref: Principles of Forensic Medicine & Toxicology, 2017 ed. Bardale, pg. 92

Cephalic index: A number expressing the ratio of the maximum breadth of a skull to its maximum length. Range of cephalic index are as follows:

- **Dolicocephalic:** 70–75. For example, Pure Aryans, Negroes, aborigines
- **Mesaticephalic:** 75–80. For example, Europeans and Chinese
- **Brachycephalic:** 80–85. For example, Mongols
- **Hyperbrachycephalic:** >85.

35. Ans. (a) Infants

Ref: KS Narayana Reddy's 'The Essentials of Forensic Medicine and Toxicology'; 29/e, pg. 64-65

Stack's Method

- Stack evolved a method to know the age of infants from the weight and height of the erupting teeth of the child.
- This method can be based on both the deciduous and permanent teeth during their eruptive phase.

36. Ans. (a) Dead infant

Ref: KS Narayana Reddy's 'The Essentials of Forensic Medicine and Toxicology'; 29/e, pg. 64-65

Boyde's Method

- Cross-striations develop in the enamel of the teeth, till the complete formation of the enamel.
- They represent daily incremental lines.
- The age of an individual can be calculated in terms of days by counting the number of lines from the neonatal line onwards.
- Neonatal line is formed very soon after birth and can be seen in about 2–3 weeks or by electron microscopy within 1–2 days after birth.
- ***It is useful*** to estimate the age of a dead infant.

37. Ans. (a) Brachycephaly

Ref: KS Narayana Reddy's 'The Essentials of Forensic Medicine and Toxicology'; 29/e, pg. 54

Types of skull *(Mn: DuMB)*	Cephalic index	Race
Dolicho-cephalic (long headed)	70–75	Pure Aryans, Aborigines, Negroes
Mesaticephalic (medium headed)	75–80	Europeans and Chinese
Brachycephalic (short headed)	80–85	Mongols

Note: $\text{Cephalic index} = \frac{\text{Maximum breadth of skull}}{\text{Maximum length of skull}} \times 100$

Note: Anteroposterior diameter of the skull is maximum in dolichocephalic and minimum in brachycephalic

38. Ans. (c) Brachycephalic

Ref: KS Narayana Reddy's 'The Essentials of Forensic Medicine and Toxicology'; 29/e, pg. 54

39. Ans. (a) Anterior part of palate

Ref: KS Narayana Reddy's 'The Essentials of Forensic Medicine and Toxicology'; 29/e, pg. 80

Palatoprints

- Harrison Allis suggested study of palate prints for identification.
- The structural details like the rugae are individual-specific and permanent **In the anterior part of the palate**
- The palatoprints can be used in the same way as fingerprints.
- **Thomas and Kurtze** have classified Palatoprints based on characteristics of rugae:

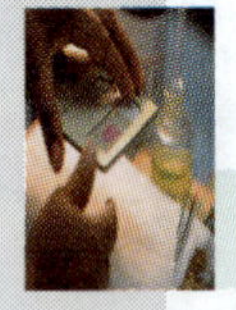

- Primary rugae: 5–10 mm or >10 mm
- Secondary rugae: 3–5 mm
- Tertiary rugae: <3 mm

40. Ans. (d) Stomach and small intestine

Ref: KS Narayan Reddy's 'The Essentials of Forensic Medicine and Toxicology'; 26/e, pg. 381

Breslau's Second Life Test

- Air is swallowed into the stomach during respiration.
- The stomach and intestines are removed after tying double ligature at each end.
- They float in water if respiration has taken place, otherwise they sink.
- This is known as Breslau's second life test.
- This test is not of much value as air may be swallowed by child in attempting to free the air-passages of fluid obstruction in cases of stillbirth.
- It is useless when there is decomposition.

41. Ans. (c) Lungs

Tests for lung functional maturity/Lung chances in fetus after respiration

- **Hydrostatic test (Raygat's test):** Respired air remains in the lunge as residual air which cannot be removed after death. Hence lungs floats in water.
- **Static test or Fodere's test**—Weight of lung before (30–40 g) and after respiration (60–66 gm) is measured. The increase in weight of lung is due to increased blood flow.
- **Ploucquet's test**—weight of lung ***is doubled after respiration.***

  Before respiration –1/70 of body wt.

  After respiration –1/35 of body wt.

COURT OF LAW AND IPC

42. Ans. (c) 20 days

Ref: The Essentials of Forensic Medicine and Toxicology, 33rd ed. pg. 292

Any of the following injuries are grievous:

- Emasculation
- Permanent privation of sight of either eye
- Permanent privation of hearing of either ear
- Privation of any member or joint
- Destruction or permanent impairing of the power of any member or joint.
- Permanent disfiguration of the head or face
- Fracture or dislocation of a bone or tooth
- Any hurt which endangers life, or which causes the victim to be in severe bodily pain, or unable to follow his ordinary pursuits for a period of twenty days or three weeks.

43. Ans. (b) Cross examination

Ref: The Essentials of Forensic Medicine and Toxicology, 33rd ed. pg. 14

- The examination of witness by the adverse party shall be called his Cross-Examination.
- In law, cross-examination is the interrogation of a witness called by one's opponent. The purpose of cross-examination is not simply to attack an adversary, but to strengthen your own case.
- The objective of cross-examination is to check the credibility of the witness. It is one of the principle tests which the law has devised for the ascertainment of the truth, and it is certainly one of the most efficacious.

44. Ans. (a) Contributory negligence

Ref: The Essentials of Forensic Medicine and Toxicology, 33rd ed. pg. 39

- Contributory negligence is any unreasonable conduct, or absence of ordinary care on the part of the patient, or his personal attendant, which combined with the doctor's negligence, contributed to the injury complained of, as a direct, proximate cause and without which the injury would not have occurred.

45. Ans. (b) Medical dichotomy

Ref: Essentials of Forensic Medicine and Toxicology by Dr KS Narayan Reddy 34th ed. pg. 27

- Medical dichotomy is also known as fees splitting. A physician shall not give or receive any gift, gratuity, commission or bonus for the referring/recommending or procuring any patient for medical, surgical or other treatment, which is against medical ethics and is considered as a professional misconduct.
- Here the doctor can be punished by only the medical council, by either issuing him a warning notice or professional death sentence.

Extra Mile

- **Association** is tying up with manufacturing firms such as drugs/chemicals, apparatus, or instruments used in the treatment of patient for personal benefit.
- **Covering** is appointing unqualified persons in professional matters.

46. Ans. (b) Cervical vertebral fracture

Ref: Essentials of Forensic Medicine and Toxicology by Dr KS Narayan Reddy 34th ed. pg. 323

- In judicial hanging the knot is placed beneath the chin or in the sub-mental position. At the time of execution,

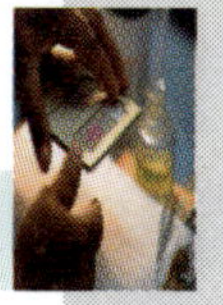

the person is dropped through the trap door, it leads to sudden jerk of head and the maximum force will be at the point opposite to the position of knot.

- This causes fracture-dislocation usually at the level of the second and third, or third and fourth cervical vertebrae, resulting in damage of cervical cord or rupture of brain stem leading to instantaneous death.
- Asphyxia, cerebral hypoxia, cerebral venous congestion and vagal inhibition are the cause of death in hanging and ligature strangulation. The commonest being a combination of asphyxia and venous congestion.

47. Ans. (b) 17

***Ref:* Essentials of Forensic Medicine and Toxicology by Dr KS Narayan Reddy 34th ed. pg. 79**

- According to the Juvenile Justice (Care and protection of children) Act, 2000 **"juvenile or boy"** means a person (boy or girl) who has not completed 18 years of age.
- "Juvenile in conflict with law" would mean a juvenile alleged to have committed an offence and not completed 18 years of age on the date of commission of such an offence as per Juvenile Justice care and protection of children amendment bill, 2006.

48. Ans. (a) Operate without consent

***Ref:* Essentials of Forensic Medicine and Toxicology by Dr KS Narayan Reddy 34th ed. pg. 50**

- Informed consent is necessary prior to surgery except in emergency situations. Here the Doctor is performing the surgery in good faith and for the benefit of patient.
- Hence the Doctor cannot be held liable as per section 88 IPC.
- **Section 88** of IPC says "Act not intended to cause death, done by consent in good faith for person's benefit.

49. Ans. (b) Judicial magistrate

***Ref:* Review of Forensic Medicine and Toxicology, Gautam Biswas, 3rd ed. pg. 44**

CONDITIONS IN WHICH INQUEST IS DONE BY MAGISTRATE

Judicial Magistrate

- Death in police custody
- Death in police firing
- Death in police interrogation

Executive Magistrate

- Death in mental asylum
- Dowry death
- Exhumation

50. Ans. (a) If victim survives after recording DD

***Ref:* Review of Forensic Medicine and Toxicology, Gautam Biswas, 3rd ed. pg. 49**

- If the victim survives after giving dying declaration, then it will not be considered.
- But, it has corroborative value and the victim will be called to give oral evidence.

51. Ans. (b) IPC 84

***Ref:* Forensic Medicine and Toxicology by Rabindra Nath Karmakar, pg. 566**

- The Indian counterpart of McNaughton's rule is IPC Sec 84.
- According to this rule: *"Nothing is offence which is done by a person, who at the time of doing it, is, by reason of unsoundness of mind, incapable of knowing the nature of act or that he was doing what is either wrong or contrary to law"*

52. Ans. (c) 304-A

- **IPC 304:** Culpable homicide not amounting to murder
- **IPC 304 A:** Causing death by medical negligence
- **IPC 304 B:** Dowry death

53. Ans. (c) Magistrate

- Within 7 years of marriage, Bodily injury caused by husband or relative, which lead to death comes under Dowry death and punished under IPC 304 B.
- Inquest in such condition is done by magistrate.

54. Ans. (d) Poverty

***Ref:* Forensic Medicine and Toxicology by RN Karmakar pg. 370**

- Poverty is not a ground for divorce
- **Impotence** can be ground for divorce. A wife can sue for marriage dissolution on grounds of husband's impotency, given that the 2 facts are proved:
  - Husband was impotent at the time of marriage
  - Husband continues is to be impotent till the filing of suit

Grounds for divorce:

- Adultery
- Cruelty
- Desertion
- Impotency
- Forced conversion of religion
- Communicable venereal diseases, incurable disease like leprosy, incurable mental disorder and insanity
- Either of spouse not alive or not seen for more than 7 years
- Frigidity (an example of mental cruelty)

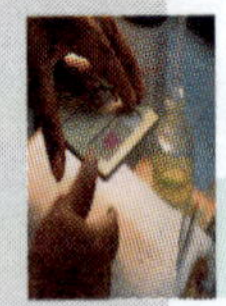

55. Ans. (b) 313

Ref: Forensic medicine and toxicology by RN Karmakar pg. 532

- Artificial abortion if justifiable, is not a criminal offence (MTP Act)
- IPC 312–316 describes criminal artificial abortion
  - **IPC–312:** With mother's consent
  - **IPC–313:** Without mother's consent
  - **IPC–314:** Death of mother during procedure

56. Ans. (a) To assess compos mentis

Ref: Forensic medicine and toxicology by RN Karmakar, P 259

- Dying declaration (Sec 32 IEA) is written or oral statement of a person (who is dying due to some unlawful act), relating to the cause of his death.
- The statement is recorded by magistrate, or if the condition is serious, the doctor or any other person can record the statement in absence of magistrate.
- If the person survives, he is called to give oral evidence and the dying declaration becomes useless.
- **Role of a doctor in dying declaration:**
  - Assess the condition of the patient
  - Arrange for dying declaration and send call for magistrate
  - Certify the compos mentis (mental soundness of person)- major role
  - Record dying declaration in absence of magistrate

Extra Mile

Differences between dying declaration and dying deposition

Dying declaration	Dying deposition (more superior than dying declaration)
• Recorded by magistrate, doctor or even a common person	• Recorded only by magistrate
• Person NOT put under oath (it is believed that a dying person does not lie)	• Person is put under oath
• Person is NOT cross examined	• The person is cross examined
• Accepted in India under sec 32 IEA (Indian Evidence Act)	• Not accepted in India

57. Ans. (b) Criminal responsibility of insane

Ref: Forensic Medicine and Toxicology by Rabindra Nath Karmakar, pg. 566

- McNaughton rule explains the criminal responsibility of insane, which says if a person commits crime, the person will be held guilty but considering the unsoundness of mind he/she not punished as per the verdict given by the jury of England. This theory is NOT acceptable in India.
- The Indian counterpart of McNaughton's rule is IPC Sec 84.
- According to this: *"Nothing is offence which is done by a person, who at the time of doing it, is, by reason of unsoundness of mind, incapable of knowing the nature of act or that he was doing what is either wrong or contrary to law"*

58. Ans. (b) Curren's rule

Ref: Forensic Medicine and Toxicology by Rabindra Nath Karmakar, pg. 566

Other Rules Regarding Fixing up Criminal Responsibility

- **Durham's rule (1954):** A person is not criminally held responsible if his unlawful act was the product of mental disease or defect.
- **Curren rule (1961):** An accused person will not be criminally responsible if at the time of committing the act, he did not have the capacity to regulate his conduct to the requirement of law, as a result of mental disease or defect.
- **American law institute rest (1970):** A person is not held responsible for his criminal conduct if at the time of commission of such criminal conduct he lacks substantial capacity to appreciate the wrongfulness of his conduct to the requirement of law, resulting from mental disease or defect.
  However, repeated criminal conduct does not alone prove such abnormality
- **Irresistible impulse test (New Hampshire Doctrine):** An accused person will not be held criminally responsible, even when he knows the nature and quality of his act and that it is wrong, but he is incapable of restraining himself from committing it due to destruction of his free will to control him as a result of the mental disease.

Extra Mile

- **Hasse's rule:** To calculate the fetal age. As per this rule up to 5th month IUL, square root of the length of fetus is the age in months.
- **Morrison rule:** To know the fetal length. As per this rule, after 5th month, age in lunar month multiplied by 5 is the length of fetus.

59. Ans. (a) Under penalty document

Ref: Forensic Medicine and Toxicology by Rabindra Nath Karmakar, pg. 314

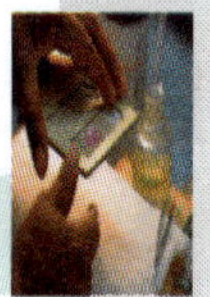

Summon/Subpoena (Sub = under; Poena = Penalty)

- A written document issued by court, compelling the attendance of witness for giving evidence in relation to a particular case, with a warning NOT to be absent without proper ground and after attendance not to leave the court without proper permission under penalty.
- **Two types of summons:**
  - **Subpoena Ad testificandum:** To given evidence in court
  - **Subpoena Duces Tecum:** To produce some document in the court (CrPC Sec 91)
- **Punishment for non-compliance**
  - **Civil case:** Liable to pay damages
  - **Criminal case:** Arrest warrant issued compelling attendance **(CrPC 87)**. Later on may be ordered for punishment either in form of fine or even imprisonment **(IPC Sec 174)**
- **Conduct money:** Money paid to witness as expense of attending the court
  - **Civil case:** Paid along with summon
  - **Criminal case:** Not paid to witness, but court will pay the expenses as per Govt. rule
    - For government employees, paid by employer

60. Ans. (a) State Government

- **Courts of Judicial Magistrate of First Class** are at the second lowest level of the Criminal Court structure in India. According to the Section 11 of the Criminal Procedure Code, 1973 (CrPc), a Court of Judicial Magistrate of First Class may be **established by the State Government** in consultation with the High Court of the respective state at such places in the district and in any number by a notification.
- According to Section 29 of the CrPc, a Judicial Magistrate of First Class may pass a sentence of imprisonment for a term not exceeding three years, or of fine not exceeding ten thousand rupees or of both.

61. Ans. (b) Magistrate

Magistrate Inquest: Court of Trail

- Usually conducted by DM, SDM or Executive Magistrate (i.e. collector, Deputy Collector or Tahsildar)
- Magistrate inquests are usually done in following circumstances:
  - **Dowry death**, i.e. unnatural death within 7 years of marriage
  - Death in prison
  - Death in police custody or interrogation or during police firing
  - Death in any psychiatric hospital
- Exhumation, i.e. digging out of an already buried body is also done upon order of magistrate.

62. Ans. (c) Whether it is caused by knife

Ref: Review of Forensic medicine by Sumit Seth pg. 248-49

- During a court trial, questions are put to the witness by the public prosecutor or the defence lawyer.
- A leading question is one the answer of which is desired in only YES or NO. **Examples of leading question:**
  - Whether you were present at the crime site?
  - Did you see this person at crime site?
  - Is this the knife you saw at crime site?
  - Whether the accused was holding knife or gun?
- The other options like *"how did you get cuts on T-Shirt; cause of injury, size of incised wound"*needs explanatory answer and cannot be answered in yes or no.
- Leading question can only be asked by **defence lawyer in cross examination. (Recent exam 2018)**
- A leading question is NOT allowed in chief examination by public prosecutor *(EXCEPT when the witness is hostile)*
- **Note:** Leading question has been classified under 141 IEA (Indian Evidence Act)

63. Ans. (a) Magistrate

Ref: The Essentials of FSM by KS Narayan Reddy 31st ed. pg. 5, 272

Inquest: Inquiry into the cause of death

- **Police Inquest**
  - *Most common type of inquest in India*
  - Investigating officer usually is sub inspector or officer not below the rank of (senior) head constable.

Magistrate Inquest: Court of Trail

- Usually conducted by DM, SDM or Executive Magistrate (i.e. collector, Deputy Collector or Tahsildar)
- Magistrate inquests are usually done in following circumstances:
  - **Dowry deaths** i.e. unnatural deaths within 7 years of marriage
  - Death in prison
  - Death in police custody or interrogation or during police firing
  - Death in any psychiatric hospital
- Exhumation i.e. digging out of an already buried body also done upon order of magistrate.

Coroner's Inquest: Court of Inquiry

- Coroner is an advocate, attorney, pleader, or first class magistrate with 5 years experience or metropolitan magistrate
- Coroner court is a court of inquiry & accused need not be present.

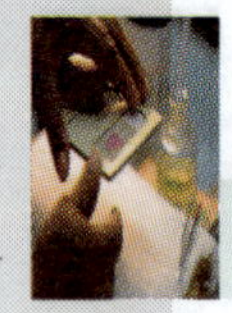

- Coroner court can't impose fine or punishment; but it can punish those guilty of contempt of his court when the offence is committed in the premises of his court (i.e. city limit only)
- *In India it was practiced in Mumbai, Kolkata. But now abolished.*

64. Ans. (a) Magistrate

Ref: The Essentials of FSM by KS Narayan Reddy, 31st ed. pg. 5, 272

Please refer to above explanation.

65. Ans. (d) Voluntarily causing hurt

Ref: The Essentials of FSM by KS Narayan Reddy, 31st ed. pg. 270-71

TABLE: Some Important IPC sections and their definitions

INDIAN PENAL CODE (IPC):
CRIMINAL PROCEDURE CODE (CrPC):

IPC Section	Definition
Sec 82	A child under 7 years is incapable of committing an offence. Not applicable to railway act.
Sec 83	A child >7 &< 12 is presumed to be mature enough to be capable of committing an offence.
Sec 84	Act of a person of unsound mind is not liable (McNaughten's rule)
Sec 85	Act of a person who's intoxicated against will.
Sec 87	A person less than 18 years cannot give valid consent to suffer any harm which may result from an act not intended or not known to cause death or grievous hurt. E.g. consent for wrestling contest
Sec 88 to 93	Legal protection to medical doctors. Sec 89 – a child < 12 years cannot give valid consent to suffer any harm which can occur by an act done in good faith or for its benefit e.g. consent for operation
CrPC 174	Police inquest
CrPC 176	Magistrate's inquest
Sec 179	Punishment for refusal to answer question by the police
Sec 191	Definition of perjury
Sec 193	Punishment for perjury
Sec 197	Issuing false certificate (3–7 years of punishment)
Sec 201	Disappearance of evidence (2 years of punishment)
Sec 297	Trespassing of burial place, Necrophilia, Necrohagia
Sec 299	Definition of Culpable homicide
Sec 300	Murder
Sec 302	Punishment for murder/infanticide
Sec 304	Culpable homicide not amounting to murder
Sec 304 A	Causing death by negligence
Sec 304 B	Dowry death
307	Attempt to murder
308	Attempt to culpable homicide
309	Attempt to suicide
Sec 317	Exposure and Abandonment of child <12 years
Sec 318	Concealment of birth by secret disposal of dead body
Sec 319	Hurt
Sec 320	Grievous hurt
Sec 321	***Voluntarily causing hurt***
Sec 322	***Voluntarily causing grievous hurt***
Sec 323	**Punishment for voluntary causing hurt**
Sec 324	**Voluntary causing hurt by dangerous weapon/means**
Sec 325	Punishment for voluntarily causing grievous hurt
Sec 326	Punishment for voluntarily causing grievous hurt by a dangerous weapon/means
Sec 351	Assault
Sec 354	Assault to outrage the modesty of a woman
Sec 375	Definition of rape
Sec 376	Punishment of rape
Sec 377	Unnatural sexual offence
Sec 497	Adultery

Contd...

66. Ans. (c) 10 years

Ref: The essentials of FSM by KS Narayan Reddy, 31st ed. pg. 384-85

- **IPC for rape:** 375
- **IPC punishment of rape:** 376. This IPC states that whoever commits rape shall be punished with imprisonment for a term of not less than 10 years, which may extend to imprisonment for life, and shall also be liable to fine.
- Punishment for Rape
  - **376–A:** If resulting in death or vegetative state (cortical death)
    - Punishment up to 20 years to death sentence
  - **376–B:** Sexual intercourse by husband during separation (on wife's complaint)
    - Punishment– 2–7 years
  - **376–C:** Sexual intercourse by person in authority
    - Punishment– 5–10 years
  - **376–D:** Gang Rape
    - Punishment– 20 years to life imprisonment
  - **376–E:** Repeat offenders
    - Punishment– Life imprisonment to death sentence.

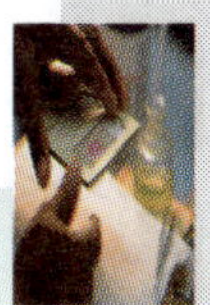

67. Ans. (b) 319

Ref: The Essentials of FSM by KS Narayan Reddy, 31st ed. pg. 384-85

Please refer to above table.

68. Ans. (a) 320

Ref: The Essentials of FSM by KS Narayan Reddy, 31st ed. pg. 384-85

Please refer to above table.

69. Ans. (d) Injured person admitted in hospital for 21 days

Ref: Legal Apptitude and Legal Reasoning for the Clat by Bhardwaj A. pg. 36

Section for grievous hurt: IPC 320

The book states: "*the mere fact that the injured remained in hospital for 20 days would not be enough to conclude that he was unable to follow his ordinary pursuits during that. Continuance of severe body pain for 20 days or disability to follow one's avocation for 20 days constitutes grievous hurt*"

Criteria

- Emasculation
- Permanent privation of the sight of either eye
- Permanent privation of hearing of either ear
- Privation of any joint or permanent impairment of the power of any member of joint
- Permanent disfiguration of head or face
- Fracture or dislocation of bone or tooth
- Any hurt which endangers life or which causes the sufferer to be admitted during the span of 20 days in severe body pain or unable to follow his ordinary pursuits.

70. Ans. (a) 497

Ref: The Essentials of FSM by KS Narayan Reddy, 31st ed. pg. 24

Please refer to above table.

71. Ans. (b) 315

Ref: The Essentials of FSM by KS Narayan Reddy, 31st ed. pg. 408

- **IPC Section 315 and 316** discusses the offence of foeticide and infanticide.
- If a person commits an act with the intention of preventing the child from being born alive or an act that results in the death of the child after birth, that person is committing foeticide/infanticide as long as they do not do it in the interest of the mother's health or life.
- **Section 317** states that is it a crime against children, if their mother or father expose or leave a child in a place with the intention of abandonment.
- **Sections 82 and 83** of the IPC states: A child who commits a crime and is below the age of seven is not considered to have committed a crime.
- **Section 299:** Culpable homicide

72. Ans. (c) 304 B

Ref: The Essentials of FSM by KS Narayan Reddy, 31st ed. pg. 272

Dowry Death

- Bodily injury caused by husband or relative, which lead to death comes under Dowry death and punished under IPC 304 B.
- **IPC section 304 B states:** Whenever any death of a woman is caused by any burns or bodily injury or occurs otherwise than under normal circumstances within seven years of her marriage and it is shown that soon before her death she was subjected to cruelty or harassment by her husband or any relative of her husband for, or in connection with, any demand for dowry, such death shall be called "dowry death" and such husband or relative shall be deemed to have caused her death.
- Whoever commits dowry death shall be punished with imprisonment for a term which shall not be less than **seven years and it may extend to life time imprisonment.**

73. Ans. (a) 498 A

Ref: The Essentials of FSM by KS Narayan Reddy, 31st ed. pg. 272-73

- Cruel behavior towards wife by husband or his relatives punished by IPC 498 A.
- **IPC section 498 A** states that whosoever being husband or relative subject women to cruelty shall be punished with imprisonment of upto 3 years with or without fine.

74. Ans. (d) Section 416

Ref: The Essentials of FSM by KS Narayan Reddy, 31st ed. pg. 5-6, 314-15

Section 416: If a woman sentenced to death is found to be pregnant, the High Court shall order the execution of the sentence to be postponed, and may, if it thinks fit, commute the sentence to imprisonment for life.

Section 413. Execution of order passed under Section 368: When a case submitted to the High Court for the confirmation of a sentence of death, the Court of Session receives the order of confirmation or other order of the

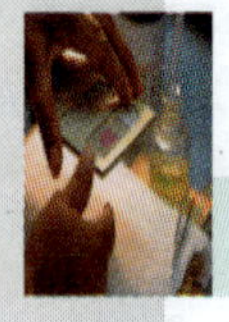

High Court thereon, it shall cause such order to be carried into effect by issuing a warrant or taking such other steps as may be necessary.

Section 414. Execution of sentence of death passed by High Court: When a sentence of death is passed by the High Court in appeal or in revision, the Court of Session shall, on receiving the order of the High Court, cause the sentence to be carried into effect by issuing a warrant.

Section 419. Direction of warrant for execution: Every warrant for the execution of a sentence of imprisonment shall be directed to the officer in charge of the jail or other place in which the prisoner is, or is to be, confined.

75. Ans. (b) Masturbation

Ref: The essentials of FSM by KS Narayan Reddy, 31st ed. pg. 404

- Masturbation is an offence only when practiced openly; Ex: In telephone booth, lavatories.

TOXICOLOGY

76. Ans. (b) Neurotoxic

Ref: Essentials of Forensic Medicine and Toxicology by Dr KS Narayan Reddy 34th ed. pg. 520

- King cobra belongs to the class Elapidae, the constituent of their venom is Neurotoxic.
- Other snakes belong to Elapidae class include Krait, Mambas, Tiger snake, Taipan, Death adder, Copper head snakes and Coral snakes.

Extra Mile

- **Musculotoxic** venom is seen in Sea Snakes
- **Vasculotoxic** venom is seen in Viper snakes due to the presence of hemolysins which cause disruption of endothelial cell functions.

77. Ans. (d) Delirium tremens

Ref: Essentials of Forensic Medicine and Toxicology by Dr KS Narayan Reddy 34th ed. pg. 539

- **Delirium Tremens** results from the long-continued action of the alcohol on the brain.
- It typically begins 72 to 96 hours after the withdrawal of alcohol.
- There is an acute attack of insanity in which the main symptoms are coarse muscular tremors of face, tongue and hands, insomnia, restlessness, loss of memory, psychomotor agitation, confusion, violent behaviour etc.
- It is considered unsoundness of mind, not intoxication, hence the person will not be liable for any acts during such episodes.

78. Ans. (c) Opium withdrawal

Ref: Essentials of Forensic Medicine and Toxicology by Dr KS Narayan Reddy 34th ed. pg. 563

- The symptoms are suggestive of Opium withdrawal. Same can be seen with excitatory phase of cocaine intoxication.
- Opioid usually causes symptoms like constipation, bradycardia, miosis etc. The withdrawal symptoms are usually opposite to the usual effect of opioid (like diarreha, tachycardia, mydriasis).
- Withdrawal symptoms occur after withdrawal of the drug for more than 12 hours and last about a week. Yawning is a common feature. Symptoms are classified into minor, moderate and major.
- **Minor:** Dilated pupils, piloerection, yawning etc.
- **Moderate:** Restlessness, insomnia, hypertension etc.
- **Major:** Vomiting, diarrhoea, hypotension etc.
- Death may be so rapid that the needle may still be found in the vein, when the body is discovered.

Extra Mile

- Cocaine withdrawal range from moderate to severe dysphoria, depression, anxiety, decreased libido, etc.
- Cannabis does not cause physiological dependence or addiction.

79. Ans. (d) Dhatura

Ref: Essentials of Forensic Medicine and Toxicology by Dr KS Narayan Reddy 34th ed. pg. 557

- The symptoms are highly suggestive of datura fastuosa poisoning. The active principle is hyoscine, hyoscyamine and traces of atropine.
- Peripheral effects are predominant and result from anticholinergic (parasympatholytic) action.
- **Signs and symptoms includes (8 D's):**
  - Dryness of mouth, dysphagia, dilated pupils, dry-hot skin, drunken gait, delirium, drowsiness, death due to respiratory failure.
- 1st stage of Cocaine intoxication is stage of excitement, symptoms mainly include restlessness, rapid pulse, dilated pupils etc. 2nd stage of depression includes (within an hour or less) symptoms such as feeble respiration, profuse perspiration, collapse, hypertension, anxiety leading to paranoia etc.

Extra Mile

- Heroin is a semisynthetic narcotic derived from opium. Heroin provides intense euphoria for several minutes followed by sedation for an hour.
- Cannabis sativa intoxication produces psychiatric and physical symptoms.

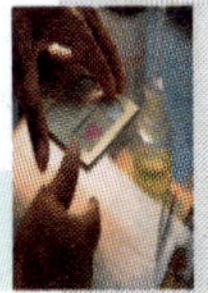

80. Ans. (a) Cocaine

Ref: Essentials of Forensic Medicine and Toxicology by Dr KS Narayan Reddy 34th ed. pg. 560

- Increased blood pressure, heart rate and respiratory rate is due to the action of cocaine on sympathetic system. Other symptoms include hyperactivity, hyperthermia and mydriasis.
- Cocaine is a powerful stimulant of CNS for a short time, followed by depression. The euphoric effect depends on the release of neurotransmitters. Its action is somewhat like that of amphetamine.

Extra Mile

- **Heroin** is a semisynthetic derivative of Morphine. Intense euphoria lasts for minutes followed by sedation for about one hour, and the effects are completely lost in 3 to 6 hours.
- **LSD** (lysergic acid diethylamide) comes under the class of psychedelics (hallucinogens). They produce an alteration in environmental awareness while the individual maintains the capacity to recognise that what he is experiencing is not real.

81. Ans. (a) Bagging

Ref: Review of Forensic Medicine and Toxicology, Gautam Biswas, 3rd ed. pg. 622

TECHNIQUES FOR INHALATION

- **Sniffing:** Inhalation of fumes from the liquid in an open container.
- **Bagging:** Placing the chemical in a bag and then putting it over the face.
- **Huffing:** Applying the chemical to a cloth/rag and then inhaling it by covering nose and mouth with the cloth/rag.
- **Glading:** Inhaling the aerosols from air freshner

82. Ans. (b) Respiratory paralysis

Ref: Review of Forensic Medicine and Toxicology, Gautam Biswas, 3rd ed. pg. 527, 528

First image shows a snake with head barely distinguishable from neck and paired transverse bands. These are features of common krait. The patient has developed envenomation from krait (Bungarus species) as evident from bilateral ptosis.

Signs and symptoms of krait bite are:

- Abdominal pain
- Ptosis
- Dysarthria
- Dysphagia
- Chest pain
- Quadriparesis
- Respiratory paralysis and death may occur

83. Ans. (b) Hydrogen sulphide

Ref: Review of Forensic Medicine and Toxicology, Gautam Biswas, 3rd ed. pg. 469

TABLE: Smell due to various poisons

S. No.	Poison	Odor
1.	Phosphorus, heavy metal poisoning (arsenic, selenium, thallium), parathion, malathion, alphos	Garlic-like
2.	Ethanol, methyl or propyl alcohol, chloroform, nitrites, acetone	Sweet and fruity
3.	Paraldehyde, choloral hydrate	Acrid
4.	H_2S, mercaptans, disulfrum	Rotten eggs
5.	HCN	Bitter almond
6.	Carbolic acid	Phenolic
7.	Organophosphates	Kerosene-like
8.	Zinc phosphide	Fishy
9.	Methyl salicylates	Oil of wintergreen
10.	Marijuana	Burnt rope, hemp

84. Ans. (c) Deferoxamine

Ref: Review of Forensic Medicine and Toxicology, Gautam Biswas, 3rd ed. pg. 476

Deferoxamine is used as antidote for:

- Acute iron poisoning
- Hemochromatosis
- Transfusional chronic iron overload

S. No.	Toxic agent	Specific antidote
1.	Acetaminophen	N-acetyl cysteine
2.	Anticholinergics (e.g. dhatura, atropine)	Physostigmine
3.	Anticholinesterases (e.g. OPCs)	Atropine and pralidoxime (2-PAM)
4.	Benzodiazepines	Flumazenil
5.	CO	Oxygen, hyperbaric oxygen
6.	Cyanide	Sodium nitrite, sodium thiosulfate
7.	Heavy metals (lead, mercury, iron) and arsenic	Specific chelating agents
8.	Methanol, ethylene glycol	Ethanol or fomepizole
9.	Opioids	Naloxone
10.	Snake venom	Specific antivenin

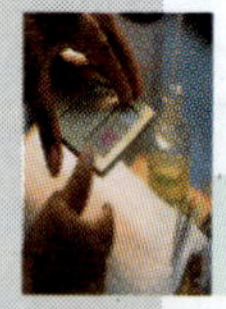

85. Ans. (a) Spider

Ref: Review of Forensic Medicine and Toxicology by Gautam Biswas, 4th ed. pg. 540-41

- Most scorpion and spider stings cause only local pain and swelling and respond to local measures such as cold compresses and wound care. A number of species, however, possess potent venom and can cause significant envenomation.
- The Venom stimulates the autonomic nervous system and release massive amounts of catecholamines causing a catecholamine storm and it may even cause neurotoxicity. There could be nausea, vomiting, restlessness blurred vision, profuse sweating, cyanosis coma and respiratory depression.
- In children death may occur due to cardiac failure.

Extra Mile

- A **sea urchin sting** may present with: Weakness, muscle aches, shock, paralysis, intense fatigue
- **Ciguatera poisoning** may present with: Nausea, vomiting, itching, tingling, headache, vertigo

86. Ans. (a) Lead

Ref: Review of Forensic Medicine and Toxicology by Gautam Biswas, 4th ed. pg. 218

- Bullets are made of soft metal which is usually lead with varying amount of antimony and/or tin added to provide hardness.
- Therefore, if the bullet is retained in the body the most likely poisoning is that of lead.
- Lead intoxication (plumbism) from retained bullets has rarely been reported but may be fatal if unrecognized.
- Bullets lodged within joint spaces or pseudocysts are more likely to develop this complication, although patients with retained missiles in other locations may also be at risk.

87. Ans. (a) Cyanide poisoning

Ref: Review of Forensic Medicine and Toxicology by Gautam Biswas, 4th ed. pg. 591-92

- The pink colored skin is due to increased hemoglobin saturation because cyanide blocks the utilization of oxygen at tissue level. Moreover the almond smell from the breath is highly suggestive of hydrogen cyanide which is a highly toxic chemical and generates Cyanide (CN-).
- There is also corrosive acid on the mouth throat and stomach.

88. Ans. (a) Organophosphate poisoning

- Cholinergic symptoms are all feature of organophosphate (OP) poisoning.
- Patients with organophosphate poisoning present with: Salivation, Lacrimation, Urination, Diarrhea, GI distress, Emesis, Fasciculation and bradycardia.
- DOC for OP poisoning: Atropine

89. Ans. (b) Hyoscine

- The shown plant in the image is: Datura stramonium, known by the common names Jimsonweed, Angel's trumpet, Devil's Weed, Thorn apple, Tolguacha, Jamestown weed, stinkweed, datura.
- It contains tropane alkaloids that are sometimes used as a hallucinogen.
- The active ingredients are atropine, **hyoscyamine** and **scopolamine** which are classified as deliriants, or anticholinergics

90. Ans. (b) Hydrocarbons

Ref: Harrison's 20th ed. pg. 3306

CONTRAINDICATION OF GASTRIC LAVAGE

- Hydrocarbon and petroleum distillate
- Caustic or corrosive poisoning-due to increased risk of gastric perforation and aspiration pneumonitis.
- Uncontrolled convulsion- due to increased risk of aspiration
- Comatose patients-compromised/unprotected airway
- Cardiac arrhythmias
- Recent upper GI surgery
- Combative patients or those who refuse- absolutely contraindicated

Extra Mile

TABLE: Contraindications of gastric lavage

Absolute contraindications	Relative contraindications
• Alkali	• Kerosene or volatile poisoning
• Mineral acid	• Strychinine
• Vegetable acids	• Hypothermia
• Organic acids except carbolic acid	• Bleeding disorder

91. Ans. (a) Oxalic acid

Ref: Forensic Medicine and Toxicology by Rabindra Nath Karmakar, pg. 79

- Oxalic acid is a colorless organic compound with a wide-range of use in cleaning and bleaching applications

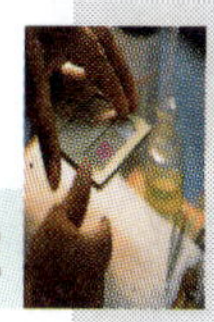

- Oxalic acid poisoning is the accidental or intentional intake of oxalic acid or oxalic acid compound

SIGNS AND SYMPTOMS

- Vomiting
- Burning pain in throat, mouth
- Swelling of mouth and tongue- inability to speak clearly
- Skin burns/blister formation
- Red, watery eyes

TREATMENT

- The immediate administration of an antidote: Lime and chalk (precipitated chalk or saccharate solution of lime).
- They can be scraped off the wall, whitewashed fences, or ceilings, crushed egg shells, mixed with milk/water and given.
- Emesis to remove unabsorbed poison
- Demulcent drink to protect gastric mucosa
- IV 10% Calcium gluconate—to treat hypocalcemia

92. Ans. (c) Root

- Although entire plant is poisonous, the **root is most potent.**
- *Dry root* is conical or tapering, shows bases of the broken rootlets and shriveled with longitudinal wrinkles.
- **NO odor, Sweet taste** (mitha bish)

Mechanism of Action

- Aconitine binds with the voltage-dependent sodium-ion channels.
- Aconitine first stimulates and then paralyzes the peripheral terminations of sensory, secretory and motor nerves

93. Ans. (d) Semi-synthetic

OPIUM/AFIM

- Heroin (brown Sugar/Junk): **Semi-synthetic derivative of opium**
- Juice from **unripe capsule** of Papaver Somniferum (poppy) contains opioid alkaloids
- Poppy seeds are used for cooking and are non-toxic
- **Poison of choice for suicide:** As it produces painless death.
- **Pinpoint pupil,** respiratory depression.
- Marquis test: to detect opium
- **Antidote:** *Naloxone sodium*
- Treatment for morphine withdrawal: Methadone
- Along with routine viscera, Brain, blood and bile to be preserved.
- **Speedball** is the use of *cocaine with morphine or heroin*

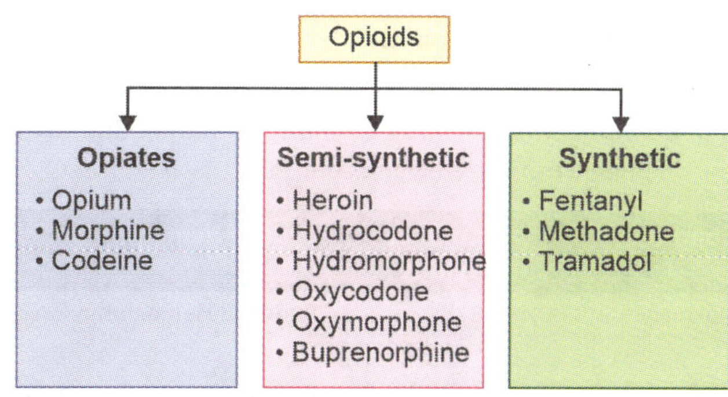

94. Ans. (a) Cobra

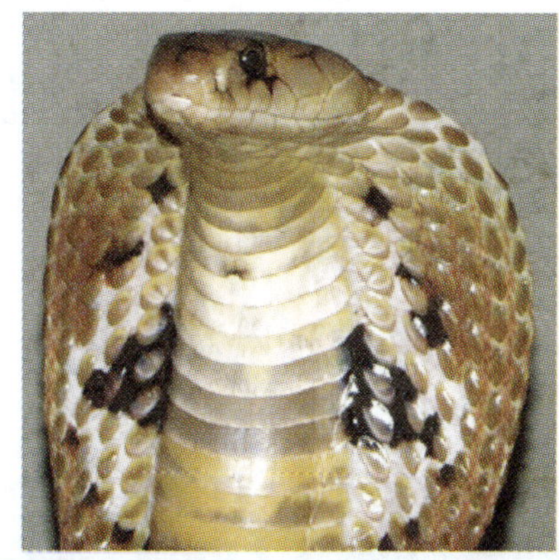

Appearance	Poisonous snakes	Nonpoisonous snakes
Habit	Nocturnal	**Not** specific
Head scales	Usually small	Usually large
	3 exceptions (Poisonous snakes with large head scales) Pit Vipers Cobra Krait **Pit viper** pit below the eye **Cobra** 3rd labial touches eye and nasal shields **Krait:** 4 infralabials scales below mouth and 4th being largest	
Belly scales	Large and cover the entire breadth of belly	Small, not covering the entire belly
Distal scales	Single row	Double row
Tail	Compressed	Noncompressed
Fangs	Long and canalized, like hypodermic needle	Short or small grooved
Bite mark	**Two fang marks**	**Small teeth marks**

95. Ans. (b) Carbon monoxide

- The color of livor mortis depends on the type of hemoglobin
- Normally, the lividity is bluish or purple due to the presence of deoxyhemoglobin.

Conditions	Color of lividity	Type of hemoglobin
Normal	Blue purplish	Reduced Hemoglobin
Carbon monoxide Burns	Cherry red Bright red	Carboxyhemoglobin and increased oxygen content in blood **(Anemic anoxia)**
Cyanide	Bright red	Cyanide inhibits cytochrome oxidase and decreased O_2 utilization by tissues. **(Histotoxic anoxia)** Increased oxygen content in blood
Hypothermia/ Refrigeration	Pink	Oxygen retention in cutaneous blood by cold air
NaCl/Nitrite/ Nitrate/aniline Potassium chlorate	Chocolate Brown	Methemoglobin **(meth Hb)**
Septic abortion	Bronze	**Due to** Cl. Perfringens
Hydrogen sulphide	Green	**Sulfhemoglobin**

96. Ans. (b) Sodium thiosulfate

TABLE: Poisoning and their Antidote

Poisoning	Antidote/treatment
Oxalic acid (ink remover)	Calcium gluconate
Phosphorus	Copper sulphate
Organophosphorus	Atropine
Dhatura	Physostigmine
Arsenic	BAL, DMSA
Mercury	BAL, DMSA
Lead (Plumbism)	EDTA, DMSA
Alcohol	Ethyl alcohol
Opium (Afeem)	Naloxone
Heroine/Brown sugar/ Junk/ Smack	Amyl nitrite
Bhang/Ganja/Charas	Diazepam
Strychinine	Diazepam
Copper	EDTA, penicillamine desferrioxamine
Cyanide	• Hydroxocobalamin. If not available then Na^+ thiosulphate/Na^+ nitrite can be used • **GASTRIC LAVAGE:** *5% of sodium thiosulphate,* sodium nitrite.

97. Ans. (a) Hydroxocobalamin

Hydrocyanic acid (Cyanide poisoning)

- CYANOGEN/PRUSSIC ACID is colorless, **odor *resembling bitter almond.***
- **Cause of death in cyanide poisoning:**
  - Cytotoxic and histo-toxic anoxia.
  - Corrosive effect on the mucous membrane, when inhaled instantaneous death is the result.

Treatment

- **ANTIDOTE:** Hydroxocobalamin
- **GASTRIC LAVAGE:** *5% of sodium thiosulphate,* sodium nitrite.

98. Ans. (b) Mercury

Ref: The Essentials of FSM by K.S. Narayan Reddy, 31st ed. pg. 505

MERCURY POISONING (HYDRAGYRISM)

- Vapours of mercuric compounds are poisonous because it will be absorbed in the systemic circulation.
- Mercuric compounds being soluble are more poisonous than mercurous (less soluble) compounds.

Clinical Presentation of Mercury Poisoning (Remembered as MEATS)

- **Mercuria lentis:** Brownish deposition of mercury on anterior lens.
- **Membranous colitis**
- **Erethism:** Characterized by shyness, irritability, tremors, loss of memory & insomnia.
- **Acrodynia (Pink disease):** Generalized pinkish body rash starting from tips of fingers & toes
  - **Characterized by 5 P's:** Pinkish, Puffy, Painful, Paresthetic hands and feet with Peeling of skin.
- **Tremors:** Also known as *Danbury tremors, hatter's or glass-blower's shake*
- **Salivation & gingivitis**: excessive salivation associated with metallic taste, gingivitis, loosening of teeth and ***blue-black line on gums.***

Extra Mile

TABLE: Different metallic poisoning and their effect on hair and skin

Poisoning	Color of Hair & Skin
Arsenic (As)	• Yellow color of skin, hair & mucous membrane • Milk rose (Brownish pigmentation)/Rain drop pigmentation • BLACK FOOT DISEASE
Copper (Cu)	• Jaundiced skin • Green-blue skin, hair & perspiration • Green – purple line on gums

Contd...

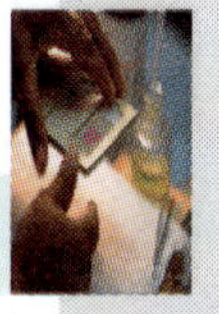

Mercury (Hg)	• Blue-black line on gums with jaw necrosis and loosening of tooth • Brown deposits on anterior lens capsule (mercuria lentis) • Acrodynia (pink disease)
Lead (Pb)	• Blue stippled burtonian line on gums, especially on upper jaw.

Other Features of Mercury Poisoning

- Proximal Convoluted Tubule necrosis
- Prevalence of abortions are common
- **Minimata disease** is an organic mercury poisoning due to consumption of fish poisoned by mercury.

99. Ans. (b) Alkali

Ref: The Essentials of FSM by K.S. Narayan Reddy, 31st ed. pg. 499

- Maximum damage to the esophagus is caused by ingestion of alkali as compared to acid.
- Alkali causes Liquifactive necrosis which is more damaging than coagulative necrosis caused by acid.
- Liquifactive necrosis is caused by hydrolytic enzymes. It attracts WBC which leads to bacterial infection and Pus formation. It can cause CNS ischemia also.
- Acid causes coagulative necrosis due to coagulation of proteins. Coagulative necrosis is seen in all organs of body except brain.
- MCC of coagulative necrosis is hypoxia.

100. Ans. (a) Alcoholic poisoning

Ref: The Essentials of FSM by K.S. Narayan Reddy, 31st ed. pg. 540-41

- In case of alcohol poisoning, CSF as much as can be withdrawn is required to be preserved.
- Preservative used is Na/K- Fluride and K-Oxalate.
  - Fluoride is added to CSF for alcohol estimation.

Extra Mile

TABLE: Poisoning and Organ preserved

Poisoning	Organ preserved
Strychnine poisoning	Spinal cord (entire length)
Pesticides and Insecticides poisoning	Fat
CO, Cyanide, Organophosphates, Opiates, Barbiturates, Alkaloids and Strychnine poisoning *(Mn: COOBAS)*	Brain
Arsenic, Radium and Thalium poisoning *(Mn: ART)*	Bone

101. Ans. (a) Charcoal

Ref: The Essentials of FSM by K.S. Narayan Reddy, 31st ed. pg. 485-86

ORGANOPHOSPHORUS

- **Alkyl phosphate:** Malathion (bug killer)
- **Aryl phosphate:** Parathion; Diazinon (Tik 20)
- Absorbed by inhalation, through skin, mucous membrane & gastro intestinal tract.
- **MOA:** It irreversibly inhibits acetylcholine esterase enzyme, which subsequently leads to increase in acetylcholine in body and patient presents with cholinergic symptoms.

Clinical Features

- Increases all secretions of body (eg: increased sweating, salivation, urination, diarrhea, emesis).
- Stimulate bronchial asthma
- Miosis
- Bradycardia
- Irritability, confusion and fine tremors.

Investigation

- **RBC cholinesterase:** Most popular and most commonly used.
- Plasma cholinesterase

Treatment

- **Antidote:** Atropine
- Atropine (antidote) is highly effective in counteracting peripheral muscarinic effects, and higher doses are required to antagonize CNS effects.
- It is not effective against nicotinic actions.
- Cholinesterase reactivators like DAM (Di Acetyl Monoxime), PAM (Pralidoxime iodide) action is most marked at nicotinic site.
- Oximes should be started as early as possible preferably withing 24 hours before phosphorylated enzyme has undergone aging & become resistant to hydrolysis
- Oximes do not cross BBB. It directly detoxify OPC.
- *Note: Activated charcoal is used in case of cyanide poisoning.*

102. Ans. (a) Kerosene

Ref: The Essentials of FSM by K.S. Narayan Reddy, 31st ed. pg. 551

TABLE: Contraindications of Gastric Lavage

Absolute contraindications	Relative contraindications
• Alkali • Mineral acid • Vegetable acids • Organic acids **except carbolic acid**	• **Kerosene or volatile poisoning** • Strychinine • Hypothermia • Bleeding disorder

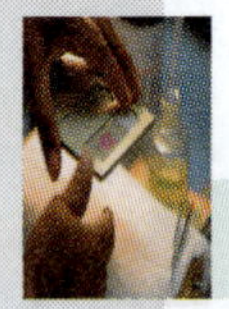

103. Ans. (a) Tobacco

Ref: The Essentials of FSM by K.S. Narayan Reddy, 31st ed. pg. 577

- Among the given options, tobacco is the substance which is most commonly used in India and also persons can easily get addicted and can tolerate this agent.

104. Ans. (c) Copper sulphate

Ref: The Essentials of FSM by K.S. Narayan Reddy, 31st ed. pg. 512-13

- *White phosphorus is toxic while Red phosphorus is non-toxic*
- **Phosphorus poisoning presents with Phossy jaw, Garlicky mucosa.**
- Garlicky mucosal odor is also seen in Celphos and Arsenic poisoning.
- **Antidote:** Copper sulphate

105. Ans. (b) Mimics tetanus

Ref: The Essentials of FSM by K.S. Narayan Reddy, 31st ed. pg. 501–502

Arsenic Poisoning Features

- It is the most commonly used homicidal poison.
- Presents with Haemorrhagic gastroenteritis and necrosis of intestinal mucosa.
- **It mimics Cholera** NOT tetanus ***(Strychinine mimics tetanus).***
- Diarrhea accompanied by tenesumus and anal irritation.
- **Arsenic poisoning is also characterized by:**
  - Black foot disease
  - Red velvety mucosa upon PM
  - *Rain drop pigmentation on body*
  - Reinsch test or maRsh test- used to test the arsenic
- They deposited on skin, hair and nail because they contain keratin, hence it is preserved.
- Hyperkeratosis on palms and soles.
- **Fatal dose:** 0.1–0.2 gm.
- On nails specific lines seen known as: **Aldrich Mees Line**
- **Upon chronic poisoning**
  - Sensory motor polyneuropathy causing tingling, numbness and paresis
  - Encephalopathy
- **Antidote:** BAL, Succimer.

106. Ans. (a) Arsenic

Ref: The Essentials of FSM by K.S. Narayan Reddy, 31st ed. pg. 501-502

Please refer to above explanation.

107. Ans. (d) Cyanide

Ref: The Essentials of FSM by K.S. Narayan Reddy, 31st ed. pg. 588-89

HYDROCYANIC ACID (CYANIDE POISONING)

- CYANOGEN/PRUSSIC ACID is colorless, with an odor ***resembling bitter almond.***
- Hydrocyanic acid, a colorless volatile liquid found in fruits like peach, plum, bitter almond.
- Cyanides (white powder) used in photography, electroplating, fumigation of ship.
- It is Cytochrome oxidase and Carbonic anhydrase inhibiter.
- **Cause of death:**
  - Cytotoxic and histo-toxic anoxia.
  - Corrosive effect on the mucous membrane, when inhaled leads to instantaneous death.

Signs and Symptoms

- Headache, giddiness, convulsion, seizure
- **Dilated & fixed pupil**
- Smell of bitter almond and froth at the mouth
- Cyanosed face, clenched jaw
- Respiratory failure leads to death

Fatal dose: 60 mg of pure acid or 60 drops of crude oil of bitter almond or 200 mg of KCN

Treatment

- **ANTIDOTE:** Hydroxocobalamin.
- **GASTRIC LAVAGE:** *5% of sodium thiosulphate,* sodium nitrite.

PM: BRICK RED blood due to cyano-meth Hb.
(Brain, Lung, Blood, Urine, Vomitus are preserved.)

108. Ans. (c) Sodium thiosulfate

Ref: The Essentials of FSM by K.S. Narayan Reddy, 31st ed. pg. 588-89

109. Ans. (d) Myotoxic

Ref: The Essentials of FSM by K.S. Narayan Reddy, 31st ed. pg. 524

TABLE: Snakes and their respective poisoning

Snake	Type of poisoning
Vipers	Vasculotoxic, Hemotoxic
Sea snakes	Myotoxic
Cobra, Krait	Neurotoxic

110. Ans. (a) Neurotoxic

Ref: The Essentials of FSM by K.S. Narayan Reddy 31st ed. pg. 523

Please refer to above explanation.

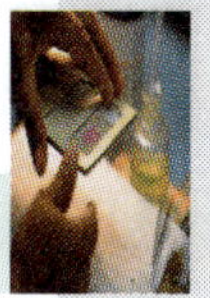

111. Ans. (c) 30

Ref: The Essentials of FSM by K.S. Narayan Reddy, 31st ed. pg. 530-40

- **30 mg%- Normal limit for drink and drive**
- 80 mg%- Nystagmus
- 150 mg%- Muscle incoordination
- 400 mg%- Coma

112. Ans. (b) Methyl alcohol

Ref: Internet Source

- Methyl alcohol poisoning is referred to as HOOCH tradegy. It is converted in the body to formaldehyde which is toxic to retina, leading to blindness. Concomitant high anion gap metabolic acidosis results in mortality.
- The latest hooch tragedy was in Mumbai in June, 2015 and in Cuttack, Odissa in 2012.

113. Ans. (c) Cocaine

Ref: The Essentials of FSM by K.S. Narayan Reddy, 31st ed. pg. 562-63

- Cannabis and its products contain (–) D-9 TetraHydroCoannabinol (Δ9-THC).
- It is obtained from Indian hemp plant known as cannabis Sativa.
- Different parts of this plants give different products:
  - Dried leaves: **Bhang**
  - Dried female inflorescence: **Ganja**
  - Resinous extract of stem: **Charas/Hashish**
  - Marijuana/Marihuana: Other name for cannabis
- In case of cannabis abuse there is an episode of acute violent behavior for which the person claims amnesia. This is known as **Run Amok.**

Extra Mile

TABLE: Commonly abused substances and their characteristic clinical feature

Substance	Characteristic clinical feature		
Cocaine	Magnus symptoms *(cocaine bugs or Tactile hallucination)* **Black tongue and teeth**		
Cannabis	• Run Amok	• Amotivation syndrome	• Flash backs
Alcohol	• Mc-Evan's sign	• Morbid jealousy	
LSD	• Bad Trips	• Flash backs	
Amphetamine	Paranoid hallucinatory syndrome (like paranoid schizophrenia)		
Phencyclidine (Angel dust)	Dissociative anesthesia		

114. Ans. (d) Cocaine poisoning

Ref: The Essentials of FSM by K.S. Narayan Reddy, 31st ed. pg. 564-65

115. Ans. (c) Bhilawanol

Ref: The Essentials of FSM by K.S. Narayan Reddy, 31st ed. pg. 517

Semi carpus anacardium (*bhilawanol* or marking nut): Juice applied to the skin produces irritation, painful blisters, followed by itching and eczematous eruption. Lesions formed resemble bruise which ulcerate and slough.

Active principles: *Bilawanol* and *semicarpol*

- Used by washermen as marking ink on clothes
- Used to produce artificial bruise
- Used as abortifacient by an abortion stick

BURNS AND DROWNING

116. Ans. (c) Drowning

Ref: Essentials of Forensic Medicine and Toxicology by Dr KS Narayan Reddy 34th ed. pg. 155

- The photograph demonstrates the phenomenon of Cadaveric spasm where, grass/weed firmly grasped in the hands of a victim died due to drowning, which indicates that the victim was alive on entering the water body.
- Cadaveric spasm also known as instantaneous rigor or cataleptic rigidity. It is the persistence of contraction of muscles after death may be due to the failure of the chemical processes required for active muscular relaxation to occur during molecular death.

117. Ans. (c) Accessibility of suspension point

Ref: Essentials of Forensic Medicine and Toxicology by Dr KS Narayan Reddy 34th ed. pg. 322

- The accessibility of suspension point should be noted by measuring the height from ground to hanging point (suspension point), and height of support such as chair, table etc. to reach the suspension point.

118. Ans. (c) Teeth

Ref: PubMed

- In severely burnt body, dental data is most helpful in identification.

119. Ans. (b) Drowning

- Gettler test is done to distinguish between freshwater drowning and salt water drowning.
- It is done by measuring the chloride difference of right and left side of heart. A difference of >25% is considered as significant.

120. Ans. (a) Brackish water

- Oligohalophilic diatoms live in fresh water.
- Polyhalophilic diatoms live in sea water.
- **Mesohalophilic diatoms** live in brackish water (water midway in salinity between freshwater and seawater)

121. Ans. (c) Presence of carboxyhemoglobin

Ref: Textbook of Forensic Medicine And Toxicology: Principles And Practice by Vij, pg. 221

TABLE: Difference between antemortem burns vs postmortem burns

Features	Antemortem Burns	Postmortem Burns
Line of redness	Present around the injured burn area	Not so
Vesicles	Contain serous fluid with **high proportion of albumin and chloride**	Contain air mostly. If fluid present it comprises of very little albumin and no chlorides
Base of blister	**Red and inflamed**	*Dull, dry, hard and yellow*
Inflammation evidence	Inflammatory edema and repair processes; (+) Leucocyte Inflitration	No such changes noticed
Presence of carbonaceous deposits/soot in the respiratory tract	**PRESENT.** *Indicates death from suffocation following antemortem burn*	Not present
Presence of Carboxyhemoglobin	Present ***(its highly suggestive and diagnostic)***	Absent
Enzymatic activity	Time related **increase** in enzymatic activity: • **Immediate:** Tissue Cathepsin • **At 2 hours:** Leucine Aminopeptidase • **At 3 hours:** Acid Phosphatase • **At 4 hours:** Alkaline Phosphatase	Never noticed

122. Ans. (c) Cardiac arrest

Ref: The Essentials of FSM by K.S. Narayan Reddy, 31st ed. pg. 339-40

DROWNING

- In most of the cases it is accidental.

Types of Drowning

- Wet drowning
  - Most common form of drowning.
  - In this type water is withheld in lungs.
  - **Cause of death in wet drowning: Cardiac Arrest**
  - In fresh water death is earlier compared to sea water. Fresh water causes hemodilution and due to hemodilution there is hyperkalemia which causes ventricular fibrillation.
  - In case of sea water, death is little later, because sea water causes hemoconcentration in body, which leads to Hypernatremia and as a result death due to bradycardia.
- **Dry drowning**
  - In this type of drowning, water in not inside the lung.
  - Death is due to Reflex Laryngospasm.
- **Delayed drowning/Near Drowning**
  - This is also known as post immersion syndrome.
  - Resuscitation after drowning and death after 24 hours.
  - **Cause of death:**
    - Metabolic acidosis
    - Pneumonia
    - Electrolyte imbalance.
- **Hydrocution/Immersion syndrome**
  - Drowning in extreme cold water.
  - **Cause of death:** Vaso-vagal shock (VVS).

123. Ans. (b) Vagal inhibition

Ref: The essentials of FSM by KS Narayan Reddy, 31st ed. pg. 342

- **Cause of death in drowning:**
  - **Asphyxia:** Cause of death in sea water drowning. Inhalation of fluid causes obstruction to the air passages which leads to respiratory and circulatory failure due to anoxia.
  - **Ventricular fibrillation: MCC of death in fresh water drowning.** Death may occur in 3-5 minutes from a combination of anoxia and electrolyte imbalance which might lead to ventricular tachycardia and fibrillation.
  - **Vagal Inhibition:** MCC of death in icy cold water, drunkenness, high emotion or excitement.
  - **Exhaustion**
  - **Injuries**

Extra Mile

- Fatal period:
  - **Death in fresh water:** 4–5 minutes
  - **Death in salt water:** 8–10 minutes

124. Ans. (c) Clenched fist

Ref: The essentials of FSM by KS Narayan Reddy, 31st ed. pg. 344

- Presence of gravel, grass. etc firmly grasped in hand due to cadaveric spasm strongly suggest that person was alive when drowned as it indicates the struggle of person for life.

TABLE: Postmortem signs of drowning

Pathognomic Signs: Indicates antemortem drowning	Non Specific signs
External • Fine copious white leathery froth from mouth, nose and air passage which increases on chest pressure. • Weeds, grass, mud etc in tightly clenched hand: A very definite sign. **Internal** • Water in stomach and intestine and middle ear • **Diatoms** in brain and bone marrow of long bones.	• Cutis anserine or goose skin • Washer woman hand and feet • Paltauf (subpleural, pectechial) haemorrhage • Emphysema aqousum

125. Ans. (a) Drowning

Ref: The essentials of FSM by KS Narayan Reddy, 31st ed. pg. 344

- Paltauff haemorrhage is subpleural, pectechial haemorrhage. It is shiny, pale pink or bluish red and may be minute or 3 5 cm in diameter, seen in case of drowning.
- During drowning there is more powerful inspiratory efforts which causes air entry to lungs with water and foam which makes the lungs heavy and increased pressure inside. This causes forced expiration which causes rupture of alveolar walls that may present subpleurally and is referred as paltauff haemorrhage.
- ***Paltauff haemorrhage most commonly occur in lower lobes of lung.***

Extra Mile

- Other important findings of drowning:
  - Emphysema aquosum
  - Oedema aquosum
  - Diatoms (microscopic unicellular or colonial algae)
  - Washerwomen hand/feet
  - Cutis anserine or goose skin

126. Ans. (b) Drowning

Ref: The Essentials of FSM by K.S. Narayan Reddy, 31st ed. pg. 346

127. Ans. (b) Burns

Ref: The Essentials of FSM by K.S. Narayan Reddy, 31st ed. pg. 299

- Pugilistic attitude is seen in case of burns.
- It is also known as Boxing or fencing attitude.
- Pugilistic attitude is due to coagulation of proteins other than those affected by rigor mortis.
- It is seen in both antemortem as well as postmortem burns.

Extra Mile

- **Most common finding of antemortem drowning:** Clenched Fist.
- In case of Lightning: Branching tree pattern seen.

128. Ans. (c) Peeling of the skin

Ref: The Essentials of FSM by K.S. Narayan Reddy, 31st ed. pg. 296-98; Internet source

An injury most commonly to an extremity or digit in which the skin and subcutaneous tissue are separated from the deeper tissue layers thereby depleting its blood supply and increasing the risk of tissue necrosis.

129. Ans. (b) High voltage Electric burns

Ref: The Essentials of FSM by K.S. Narayan Reddy, 31st ed. pg. 308-309

ELECTRICAL INJURIES

- **JOULE BURN:** contact electrical and endogenous burn.
- **CROCODILE FLASH BURN:** high voltage burn.
- Multiple lesions due to 'ARC EFFECT'.
- **Cause of Death**- ventricular fibrillation.
- Current pearls and wax drops seen on autopsy.

130. Ans. (a) Lightening stroke

Ref: The Essentials of FSM by K.S. Narayan Reddy, 31st ed. pg. 310-311

- **Lightening stroke:** It is an electrical discharge from the cloud to the earth.
- **Classical finding:** FILLIGREE BURN/ LITCHENBURG'S FLOWERS: Superficial, irregular, thin resembling the branches of a tree also known as arborescent burn.
- Most common site is shoulder flanks. *(Cause is staining of tissues with Hb along the path of current.)*

131. Ans. (c) High temperature liquids

Ref: The Essentials of FSM by K.S. Narayan Reddy, 31st ed. pg. 305

Scalds: Cause . by application of liquid above 60°C or steam. Skin becomes sodden and bleach. Clothes are wet but do not burn.

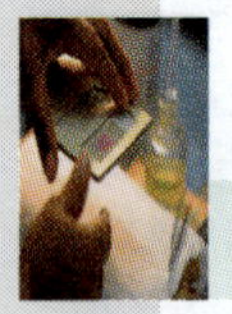

132. Ans. (c) **Presence of carbonaceous deposits in respiratory tract**

Ref: Textbook of Forensic Medicine And Toxicology: Principles And Practice by Vij pg. 221

TABLE: Difference between antemortem burns vs postmortem burns

Features	Antemortem Burns	Postmortem Burns
Line of redness	Present around the injured burn area	Not so
Vesicles	Contain serous fluid with **high proportion of albumin and chloride**	Contain air mostly. If fluid present it comprises of very little albumin and no chlorides
Base of blister	**Red and inflamed**	*Dull, dry, hard and yellow*
Inflammation evidence	Inflammatory edema and repair processes; (+) Leucocyte Inflitration	No such changes noticed
Presence of carbonaceous deposits/soot in the respiratory tract	**PRESENT.** *Indicates death from suffocation following antemortem burn*	Not present
Presence of Carboxyhemoglobin	Present (its highly suggestive and diagnostic)	Absent
Enzymatic activity	Time related **increase** in enzymatic activity: **Immediate**: Tissue Cathepsin **At 2 hrs:** Leucine Aminopeptidase **At 3 hrs:** Acid Phosphatase **At 4 hrs: Alkaline Phosphatase**	Never noticed

133. Ans. (b) **CO poisoning**

Ref: The essentials of FSM by KS Narayan Reddy, 31st ed. pg. 582

IMPOTENCY, SEXUAL PERVERSION AND SEXUAL OFFENCES

134. Ans. (a) **Masochism**

Ref: The Essentials of Forensic Medicine and Toxicology, 33rd ed. pg. 431

- Masochism is behavior in which someone gets sexual pleasure from their own pain or suffering.

135. Ans. (a) **Satyriasis**

Ref: Essentials of Forensic Medicine and Toxicology by Dr KS Narayan Reddy 34th ed. pg. 358

- Satyriasis is excessive sexual desire seen in men.
- Nymphomaniac is excessive sexual desire seen in women.
- Masochism or passive algolagnia is sexual gratification obtained or increased by the suffering of pain (self).
- This condition is the opposite of Sadism (active algolagnia), where sexual gratification is obtained by inflicting pain upon the partner.
- Voyeurism or Scotophilia is obtaining gratification by observing an unsuspecting person who is naked, in the process of disrobing, or engaged in sexual activity etc. Most often, the victim is a stranger.

136. Ans. (c) **Scatologia**

Ref: Review of forensic medicine and toxicology, Gautam biswas, 3rd ed. pg. 397

- **Scatologia**, also called **Coprolalia**, deviant sexual practice in which sexual pleasure is obtained through the compulsive use of obscene language. The affected person commonly satisfies his desires through obscene telephone calls, usually to strangers.

Different Sexual Perversion: refer to the table given later

137. Ans. (b) **Semen**

Ref: Review of Forensic Medicine and Toxicology by Gautam Biswas, 4th ed. pg. 437

- The yellow needle shaped crystals are of spermine picrate and the test performed is the Barberio's test—which is a presumptive chemical examination for semen.
- In this test the alcoholic solution of picric acid is added to dried seminal stain which produces the characteristic crystals as described above. It depends on the presence of spermine from prostatic secretions.

138. Ans. (b) **Tribadism**

Ref: Principles of Forensic Medicine & Toxicology, 2017 ed. Bardale, pg. 316

- **Lesbianism/tribadism:** Gratification of sexual desire of a woman by a woman.
- **Masochism:** Pleasure on receiving painful stimulus from sexual partner.
- **Nymphomania:** Excess sexual desire in female.
- **Transsexualism:** A gender identity that is inconsistent with or not culturally associated with their assigned sex and desire to permanently transition to the gender with which they identify.

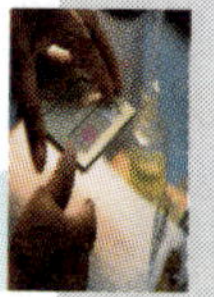

139. Ans. (d) 15–49 years

Eligible Couples

For the purpose of family welfare, an eligible couple is the one who is currently married and the wife is in the reproductive phase, i.e. of age 15–49 years. There are nearly 180 such couples per 1000 population on average in India. All these are targeted for family welfare activities. Those with two or more children are targeted for sterilization and with fewer children for spacing methods such as condom, pills and IUDs.

140. Ans. (b) 18 years

Ref: https://www.ageofconsent.net/world/India

The Age of Consent in India is **18 years old**. The age of consent is the minimum age at which an individual is considered legally old enough to consent to participation in sexual activity. Individuals aged 17 or younger in India are not legally able to consent to sexual activity, and such activity may result in prosecution for **statutory rape** or the equivalent local law.

141. Ans. (b) An individual who may be impotent with any particular woman but not with others

Ref: The Essentials of FSM by K.S. Narayan Reddy, 31st ed. pg. 357-58

- **IMPOTENCE:** Inability of a person to perform sexual intercourse. *It cannot be placed as a defense for rape.*
- **STERILITY:** Inability of the male to beget children and in the female, the inability to conceive children.
- **FRIGIDITY:** Inability to start or maintain the sexual arousal pattern in the female.
- **QUOAD:** An individual who may be impotent with any particular woman but not with others.

142. Ans. (b) Child born after father's death

Ref: The Essentials of FSM by K.S. Narayan Reddy, 31st ed. pg. 369

- **Posthumous child:** Child born after father's death, the mother being conceived by the said father.
- **Suppositious child:** Fictitious child claimed by a women as her own, a women may pretend pregnancy & deliver and later produce a living child as her own or substitute a living male child for a dead child or for a living female child born for her.
- **Spurious or phantom child (pseudocyesis):** Usually seen in women nearing menopause or younger women with an intense desire for children.

143. Ans. (c) Suppositious child

Ref: The Essentials of FSM by K.S. Narayan Reddy, 31st ed. pg. 370; Forensic Medicine By P.V. Guhara, pg. 230

- **A suppositious child** is one produced by a women whom claims it as her own whereas in actual fact it is not her child. A women may substitute a living male child for a dead or living female child born of her or may feign pregnancy and delivery and later produce a living child.
    - *Suppositious child also known as fraudulent offspring*
- **Posthumous child** is a child born after the death of the father in a legally married couple.

144. Ans. (b) Illegitimate child

Ref: The Essentials of FSM by K.S. Narayan Reddy, 31st ed. pg. 369-70; Principles of Forensic Medicine and Toxicology By Rajesh Bardale / 364

- A child is born to a couple who are not married legally is considered to be **illegitimate or a bastard.**

Conditions for being illegitimate or bastard if:

- The child is born out of wedlock OR
- Birth of child is not within a competent period after the cessation of the relationship of a man and wife OR
- Born within wedlock when procreation by the husband is not possible because of congenital or acquired malformation or disease.

145. Ans. (c) Psychogenic

Ref: The Essentials of FSM by K.S. Narayan Reddy, 31st ed. pg. 356-58

- Impotence is inability to perform sexual acticity.
- It is applied to male only
- Most important cause of impotence is: **Psychogenic**
- *If psychogenic cause is ruled out then male factor should be tested next*
- ***Note:*** *FRIGIDITY: Impotency which is seen in females*

146. Ans. (c) Incest

Ref: The Essentials of FSM by K.S. Narayan Reddy, 31st ed. pg. 398

- Incest is Sexual intercourse with close relative. It is not considered as crime in India.
- Other acts like rape, sodomy and indecent actions are considered as crime in India and are punished as and according to law.
    - **Rape:** Punished under IPC 376
    - **Adultery:** Under IPC 497
    - **Sodomy or any other un-natural sexual activity:** punished under IPC 377
    - **Grievous hurt or Indecent assault:** Punished under IPC 320.

147. Ans. (b) Elastic

Ref: The essentials of FSM by KS Narayan Reddy, 31st ed. pg. 365-66

- The presence of unruptured hymen is a presumption, BUT IS NOT AN ABSOLUTE PROOF OF VIRGINITY.
- This makes the diagnosis of virginity difficult. With an intact hymen there are: TRUE VIRGINS and FALSE VIRGIN.
- **References states:** *"Hymen may not be ruptured even after repeated acts of coitus if it is loose, lax, folded and* ***elastic*** *or thick, tough and fleshy which permits displacement, distortion and stretching without rupture"*

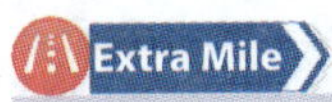
Extra Mile

- **MC type of hymen:** Semilunar/Crescentic.

148. Ans. (d) Bisexuality

Ref: The Essentials of FSM by K.S. Narayan Reddy, 31st ed. pg. 402-403

- **Paraphilias:** Abnormal & unorthodox sex play by using unusual objects or parts are know as paraphilia eg. Sadomasochism, Transvestism, Bestiality, Frotteurism, Homosexuality etc.
- **Bisexuality** means hermaphrodite; an individual with both ovary & testis & external genitals of both sexes.

TABLE: Different paraphilias/perversion

Sexual perversion	Mode of sexual pleasure
Sadism	Pleasure in giving pain to sexual partner
Masochism	Pleasure on receiving painful stimulus from sexual partner
Bondage	Sadism + masochism are found together
Fetischism	Sexual gratification by article of opposite sex
Frotteurism	Sexual gratification by contact. Ex: rubbing genitalia on another person
Exhibitionism	Satisfaction in exhibition of genitals with or without mastutbation
Transvestism/ Eonism	Pleasure in wearing clothes of opposite sex
Uranism	Sexual gratification by fingering, fellatio, cunnilingus etc.
Buccal coitus or Sin of Gomorrah	**Fellatio** is oral stimulation of penis by male or female **Cunnilingus** is oral stimulation of female genitals
Voyeurism/ Scotophilia	Also known as Peeping tom Desire to watch sexual intercourse or to observe genitals of others
Trolism	Extreme degree of voyeurism. Ex: A perverted husband enjoy watching his wife having sexual intercourse with another man.
Urolangia/ Coprophilia	Sexual excitement by sight or odor of urine or faeces.
Tribadism/ Lesbianism	Gratification of sexual desire of a women by another women
Sodomy or Buggery of Greek Love	• Anal sex • Gerantophilia –when passive agent is adult • Paederasty – when the passive agent is young boy (catamite)
Incest	Sexual intercourse with close relative
Bestiality	Sexual intercourse by a human being with a lower animal

Contd...

149. Ans. (b) Sexual satisfaction by rubbing the genitalia with the body of the person of other sex

Ref: The Essentials of FSM by K.S. Narayan Reddy, 31st ed. pg. 404

- **Frotteurism:** Rubbing the genitalia with the body of the person of other sex for sexual satisfaction.
- *Refer to above explanation.*

150. Ans. (c) Pleasure in touching opposite sex

Ref: The Essentials of FSM by K.S. Narayan Reddy, 31st ed. pg. 404

Please refer to above explanation.

151. Ans. (a) Voyeurism

Ref: The essentials of FSM by KS Narayan Reddy, 31st ed. pg. 403-404

152. Ans. (a) Transvestism

Ref: The Essentials of FSM by K.S. Narayan Reddy, 31st ed. pg. 403

TRANSVESTISM/EONISM (trans = opposite; vista = clothing): Whole personality is dominated by the desire of being identified with the opposite sex.

153. Ans. (a) Satyriasis

Ref: The essentials of FSM by KS Narayan Reddy, 31st ed. pg. 357

- **Satyriasis:** Excessive sexual desire in males
- **Nymphomania:** Excessive sexual desire in females
- **Vaginismus** is one of the causes of female sterilization. It is spasmodic contraction of vagina due to hyperaesthesia.
- **Quoad hoc:** Individual impotent with one particular women, but NOT with others.

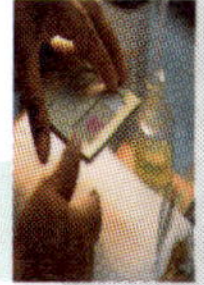

154. Ans. (b) Semen

Ref: The Essentials of FSM by K.S. Narayan Reddy, 31st ed. pg. 405

Tests for Detection of:

Seminal Stain *(Mnemonic- "Creat Acid Fast Bacilli')*
- **Acid phosphatase test:** To detect Aspermia cases
- **Barberios test:** To detect Spermine (yellow needle shaped spermine picrate)
- **Creatine phosphokinase test:** For old seminal stain
- **Florence test:** Choline crystals of semen shows fluoroscence when examined *(Rhombotic crystals of choline iodide)*
- **Most specific test for seminal stain:** Isoenzyme LDH assay
- **For dry seminal stain:** UV rays used

Blood Benzidine test
- Best preliminary test as it detects blood present in dilution of 1 in 3 lakhs.
- Color produced: Deep Blue
- Not used because it is a potential carcinogen.

Kastle-Mayer/Phenolpthalein test- color produced is Pink Purple.

Microchemical test: Based on RBC content of blood.
- **Takayama's test:** Hb converted to Haemochromogen crystal.
  - Salmon pink feathery haemochromogen crystals are obtained.
- **Teichmann's Haemin crystal test:** Hb converted into Hemin/Hematin crystals.
  - Brown rhombic haemic crystal are seen
- **Spectroscopic test:** Most specific/confirmatory method for blood stain test
- Thin layer chromatography (TLC)
- Electrophoresis

Note: Test to distinguish human vs. animal blood- Precipitin Test.

155. Ans. (a) Choline

Ref: The Essentials of FSM by K.S. Narayan Reddy, 31st ed. pg. 405-406

Please refer to above explanation.

156. Ans. (b) Barberios test

Ref: The Essentials of FSM by K.S. Narayan Reddy, 31st ed. pg. 405

Please refer to above explanation.

157. Ans. (a) Amylase

• Amylase	Saliva
• Ortho-toluidine	Blood
• Acid phosphatase	Semen
• Tetra-methyl-Benzidine	Blood

INJURY/GUNSHOT INJURY/FIREARM INJURY/ STAB WOUND

158. Ans. (a) Presence of vesicles

Ref: The Essentials of Forensic Medicine and Toxicology, 33rd ed. pg. 189

- Artificial bruises or false bruises or fake bruises are reproduced over the body mainly for the purpose of malingering. They are produced by rubbing of irritant substances on the skin.
- It is irregular in shape, well defined, regular and covered with vesicles. It is seen in the surrounding skin due to the irritants.

159. Ans. (c) Lacerated wound

Ref: The Essentials of Forensic Medicine and Toxicology, 33rd ed. pg. 190

- A laceration is a pattern of injury in which blunt forces result in a tear in the skin and underlying tissues. The hallmark of lacerations is the presence of tissue bridging.
- Furthermore, in a lacerated wound hair and hair bulbs are crushed. Margins are irregular, ragged and uneven and their ends are pointed or blunt.

160. Ans. (a) Epidural hemorrhage

Ref: Essentials of Forensic Medicine and Toxicology by Dr KS Narayan Reddy 34th ed. pg. 243

- Lucid interval is the period of time between regaining consciousness after a short period of unconsciousness.
- In a head injury case, Initial unconsciousness could be due to the cerebral concussion, and patient regain consciousness after a short period.
- The advancing extradural hemorrhage starts exerting pressure on to the brain. Hence the patient becomes confused, appear to be drunk and later advances to sleep and coma.

161. Ans. (a) Scar

Ref: Essentials of Forensic Medicine and Toxicology by Dr KS Narayan Reddy 34th ed. pg. 88

- The given photograph demonstrates old healed scar present over the pubic region.
- A scar is a fibrous tissue covered by epithelium without hair follicles, sweat glands or pigment, produced from the healing of a wound.
- Injury to the dermis produces a scar, while superficial injuries involving only the epidermis do not produce a scar. Scars are permanent hence used as a feature of identification of an individual.

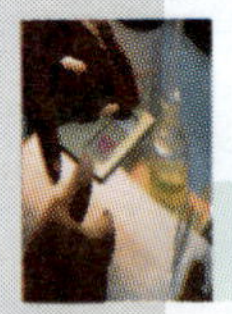

Extra Mile

- **Tattoo marks** are designs made manually in the upper epidermis of skin using needles dipped in coloring matter.
- **Moles or Nevi** are type of skin growth they often appear as small, dark brown spots and are caused by clusters of pigmented cells
- **Ligature mark** is an example of pressure abrasion (crushing or friction abrasions) produced by the crushing of superficial layers of the epidermis by the ligature material.

162. Ans. (d) Bullet

Ref: Essentials of Forensic Medicine and Toxicology by Dr KS Narayan Reddy 34th ed. pg. 218, 231

- Bullets may graze or rub the top and sides of the cranium without entering it. In such cases, entry and exit wounds are found on the scalp about 2 to 3 cm apart, while the skull between the two wounds shows an oval or elongated gutter-like depression, producing a gutter fracture.
- It is almost always associated with oblique bullet wounds. They are usually accompanied by irregular, depressed fracture of the inner table of the skull. The dura mater and brain may be torn.

163. Ans. (b) Chop

Ref: Review of Forensic Medicine and Toxicology, Gautam Biswas, 3rd ed. pg. 195

- Wound with clean cut margin is chop wound.
- A laceration is a wound that occurs when skin, tissue, and/or muscle is torn or cut open. Lacerations may be deep or shallow, long or short, and wide or narrow.
- Most lacerations are the result of the skin hitting an object, or an object hitting the skin with blunt force producing extensive bruising and laceration of deeper tissue, it is called crush injury.

164. Ans. (a) EDH

Ref: Review of Forensic Medicine and Toxicology by Gautam Biswas, 4th ed. pg. 255

- The phenomena described in the question is a classic **lucid interval** which is associated with extradural hemorrhage.
- In subdural hemorrhage the clinical course is less well defined and in subarachnoid hemorrhage it varies greatly.
- A lucid interval is the period of time between regaining consciousness after a short period of unconsciousness, resulting from a head injury and deteriorating after the onset of neurologic signs and symptoms caused by that injury.

165. Ans. (b) Near

Ref: Review of Forensic Medicine and Toxicology by Gautam Biswas, 4th ed. pg. 225-26

- Firearm bonds can be classified as close shot (contact) wounds, near shot wounds or distant wounds.
- Close shot or flame range wounds lie within 2 to 3 inches and there is evidence of burning, singeing, blackening and tattooing of the skin in and around the entry wound.
- In distant shot there is no evidence of burning, singeing, blackening or tattooing.
- In this case there is tattooing present along with inverted edges which is **characteristic of a near shot wound**.

166. Ans. (b) Laceration

Ref: Review of Forensic Medicine and Toxicology by Gautam Biswas, 4th ed. pg. 202

- Hair bulbs are crushed in a laceration injury
- Laceration is the result of a shearing force and causes deeper skin tearing, through the epidermis and sometimes through the dermis and/or subcutaneous tissues.
- Lacerations most commonly occur where underlying bone is prominent – classically at the orbital margins.
- The most significant difference that can distinguish between lacerations and incised wounds is that incised wounds have clean distinct edge.

167. Ans. (a) Inversion

Ref: Review of Forensic Medicine and Toxicology by Gautam Biswas, 4th ed. pg. 242

- In ponds fracture there is a smooth concave depression without a fracture line (occurring in children).
- In depressed fracture the portion of the fractured bone is driven inwards to a distance equivalent to the thickness of the skull table.
- Entry wound kind of depression is seen inversion. It will not be seen in eversions there the fragment is elevated above the skull table (or surface).

168. Ans. (a) Mesentery

Ref: Forensic medicine and toxicology by RN Karmakar pg. 204

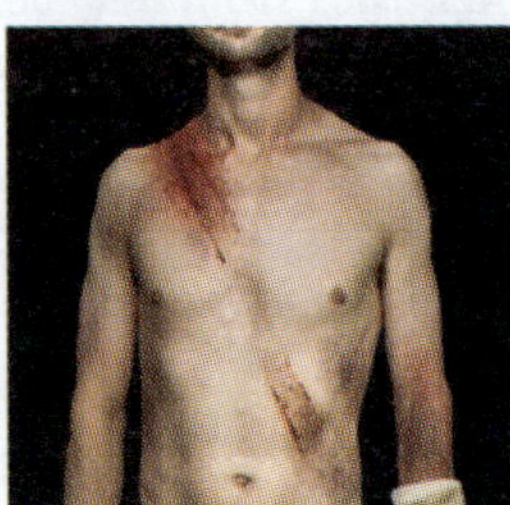

- Seat belt is usually worn diagonally across the chest, and fastened on across the opposite side, lower lateral abdominal region.
- Seat belt injury occur when there is sudden halt of a moving car. It results into following injury:
  - Abrasion, contusion and hematoma of lower abdomen
  - More commonly, laceration, avulsions or perforation of mesentery or gas filled intestine and also injury to the vertebral column, particularly lumbar vertebra
  - Rupture of abdominal organs (like liver, spleen, pancreas and cecum) due to compression.
- These injuries are collectively known as seat belt syndrome.

169. Ans. (a) Paraffin wax

Ref: ***Principle of Forensic Medicine & Toxicology, 2017 ed. Bardale, pg. 217,***

- **The basic formula for black powder:**
  - A mixture of saltpeter (potassium nitrate), charcoal and sulfur.
  - Later versions of gunpowder contain these same basic ingredients, but the overall chemistry evolved to include modifications that produced "smokeless gunpowder," **Cordite**, which eliminated the sulfur.
  - Other advances added materials such as nitrocellulose (guncotton) and glycerol trinitrate (nitroglycerin).
- Gunshot residue, or simply GSR, is a means of testing for the presence of certain materials on the hands and clothing of a subject in hopes of determining that this individual may have discharged a firearm.
- Gunshot residue contains burned particles (potassium nitrite) and some unburned particles (potassium nitrate), and criminal investigators collected these particles by **applying melted paraffin wax to a subject's hands**. Upon removal of the wax cast, a reagent containing diphenylamine and sulfuric acid was applied to the cast. The development of blue specks was indicative of the presence of nitrates.

170. Ans. (b) Scrotum

- *Lacerated looking incised wound* is seen at area where there is loose skin. For example scrotum and axilla.
- *Incised looking lacerated wounds* are seen at area where there is bony prominences. For example forehead, shin, etc.

171. Ans. (d) Bilirubin on 9th day

Ageing or Dating of Bruise

- As bruises heal, there is a gradual destruction and removal of the extravasated blood. Color change *starts at the periphery and extends inwards to the center.*
- *It follows this order:*

Red (Oxyhemoglobin)

Blue (Deoxyhemoglobin)

Brown/violet (Hemosiderin) by day 5

Green (Hematoidin/biliverdin) – day 5 to 7

↓

Yellow (Bilirubin) – after day 7

172. Ans. (b) From the periphery

- A large bruise takes longer time to heal than a smaller bruise. The color changes begin at the periphery first.
- A large old bruise may contain all possible colors seen in a bruise – from purple in the center to yellow at the edges.

173. Ans. (d) Keyhole

Ref: Forensic medicine, Clinical and Pathological aspect by Jason, Anthony and Williams. pg. 161

- If a bullet strikes the skull at an oblique, shallow angle, a characteristic defect may occur. This defect is often referred to as "keyhole defect" based on its resemblance to an old fashioned wooden door keyhole.
- **Graze wound** occurs when a bullet strikes the skin at a shallow angle and passess across the skin almost parallel to the skin surface, abrading the skin without penetrating the body. Abrasion produced is elongated, ovoid to elliptical in shape.
- **In tangential gunshot wound** bullet strikes the skin at a shallow angle, but penetrates into subcutaneous tissue, lacerating the tissue before exiting at a point separate from entry. The entry and exit wound appear as crescent shaped abrasion.

Extra Mile

TABLE: Wounds from shot gun suggesting range

Shape of wound	Distance
Cruciate or stellate shaped	Contact over bone
Oval shaped	Up to 30 cm
Rat hole wound	30–100 cm
Satellite wound	More than 2 meters
Individual pellets	Over 4 meters

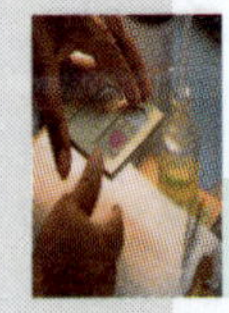

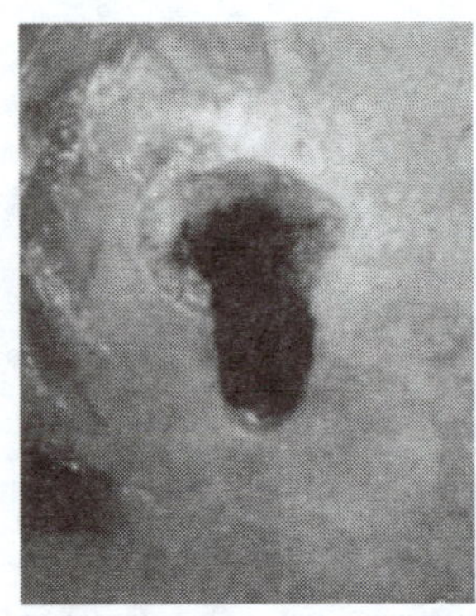

174. Ans. (a) Pressure abrasion

Ref: The Essentials of FSM by KS Narayan Reddy, 31st ed. pg. 166-67

- **Abrasion:** An injury involving superficial layers of skin & is caused by friction between skin & some rough object. It is of 3 types:

Scratch	Graze	Imprint/Pressure/ Contact abrasion
• Produced by sharp object as pin • Direction of injury is indicated by sharp edge initially & heaped up epithelium at end	• Also known as Friction or brush burn • Produced when broad surface of skin slides against rough surface	• Also known as Patterned abrasion • Produced as a result of direct impact or pressure with some object. • **Example:** Ligature mark in hanging & strangulation; nail & thumb mark in throttling; **teeth mark in biting**; tire marks in accident etc.

175. Ans. (c) Graze abrasion

Ref: The Essentials of FSM by KS Narayan Reddy, 31st ed. pg. 166-67

- Brush burn or friction burn is seen in graze abrasion.
- Produced when broad surface of skin slides against rough surface.

176. Ans. (b) Spine

Ref: The essentials of FSM by KS Narayan Reddy, 31st ed. pg. 246

- Fracture of spine need not injure the cord, but the cord is rarely injured without associated fractures of the vertebral column. **"Whiplash injury"** is an exception to this rule. This injury sustained commonly by the occupants of the front seat. When the vehicle comes to a sudden stop, there is forward thurst which produces acute hyperflexion but this converted into acute hyperextension as the forehead strikes the windscreen which causes injury to the cervical column.

177. Ans. (b) 2 days

Ref: The Essentials of FSM by K.S. Narayan Reddy, 31st ed. pg. 169-70

TABLE: Color changes of bruise according to duration and systemic causes

Color	Duration	Due to
Red	Day 0	Hemoglobin (fresh blood)
Blue	1 day	Deoxygenated hemoglobin
Bluish Black/ Dark Blue to Brown	2-4 days	Hemosiderin
Green	5-7 days	Biliverdin/Haematoidin
Yellow	7-10 days	Bilirubin
Normal color	14-15 days	Pigment removed by phagocytes

Note: *These color changes are not seen in subconjunctival hemorrhage which is being kept oxygenated by air. It is red at first then becomes yellow and finally disappears.*

178. Ans. (c) Injury common in moving head

Ref: The Essentials of FSM by KS Narayan Reddy 31st ed. pg. 233; Reddy's Essentials of Forensic Medicine & Toxicology 23 ed. pg. 205

- Coup & Countre coup lesions are most commonly seen in brain.
- Remember countre coup injury this way:
  - When a body is in motion, brain is also in motion in same direction.
  - A sudden stop, puts the body in static condition, but the brain is still in motion, and hits the skull leading to injury known as coup injury, brain then again hits on the opposite side causing countrecoup injury.

TABLE: Differences between coup and countre coup injury

Coup	Countre-coup
• Means that the injury is located towards the side of impact/injury. • It results directly by the impacting force • Seen MC in stationary condition	• Means that the lesion is present in an area opposite the side of impact/injury. • It results due to sudden hitch of a moving head. • Seen MC in moving head

179. Ans. (d) Nitrocellulose

Ref: The essentials of FSM by KS Narayan Reddy, 31st ed. pg. 197-98

Gun powders can be of two types and is made of:

Black gun powder	Smokeless powder
Consists of: • Potassium nitrate 75% • Sulphur 10% • Charcoal 15%	Consists of: • *Nitrocellulose* (single base; gun cotton) • Nitroglycerine + Nitrocellulose • Nitroglycerine + Nitrocellulose + Nitroguanidine (triple base)

180. Ans. (d) Two bullets are ejected one after the other

Ref: The Essentials of FSM by K.S. Narayan Reddy, 31st ed. pg. 213

- **Tandem or Piggyback bullet** are the bullets ejected one after the other, when the first bullet having been stuck in the barrel, fails to leave the barrel & is ejected when the next bullet is fired.

Extra Mile

TABLE: Different types of bullet movements

Term	Feature
Yawning Bullet	Bullet which travel in an irregular fashion instead of travelling straight and cause a key hole entry wound.
Ricochet bullet	Bullet strikes some intervening object first, and then after ricocheting & rebounding from this hits the object.
Dum dum Bullet	A jacketed bullet with its nose cut off to expose the core and it expands on impact
Tumbling B.	One that rotates in end on end during its motion.
Souvenir Bullet	A bullet left in body for long time & it gets surrounded by dense fibrous tissue
Gutter wound	Bullet strikes the skull but does not enter and travel in soft tissue and form an elongated gutter like depression
Bullet gaze/slap	Bullet that does not perforate the skin, but produces only friction wound

181. Ans. (a) Direction of injury

Ref: The essentials of FSM by KS Narayan Reddy, 31st ed. pg. 178

- Tailing of wound is one of the characteristics of the incised wound which indicates the direction in which the cut was made.
- Incised wounds are deeper at the beginning as more pressure is exerted at this point (head of wound). Towards the end of the cut the wound becomes increasingly shallow, till finally as the knife leaves the tissues, the skin alone is cut. This is known as tailing of wound.

182. Ans. (d) Chopping

Ref: The essentials of FSM by KS Narayan Reddy, 31st ed. pg. 182-83

- Stab wound is produced when force is delivered along long axis of narrow or a pointed object, such as knife, dagger, sword, chisel, screw driver etc into the depth of the body.
- It can present as point wound, puncture wound or perforation.
- **Chop wound/slash wound** are deep gaping wound caused by a blow with the sharp cutting edge with a heavy weapon like axe, sword, chopper or meat cleaver.

183. Ans. (a) Suicide

Ref: The essentials of FSM by K.S. Narayan Reddy, 31st ed. pg. 180

- Tentative cuts/Hesitation marks are multiple small superficial cuts seen in cases where there is a trial of suicide.
- MC site for tentative cuts are: **Forearm**

184. Ans. (c) Avulsion

Ref: KS Narayana Reddy's 'The Essentials of Forensic Medicine and Toxicology'; 29/e, pg. 171

Avulsion (Shearing Laceration)

- The shearing and grinding force by a weight, such as heavy vehichle wheel passing over a limb may produce separation of the skin from the underlying tissues over a relatively large area. This is called 'flaying'.
- The underlying muscles are crushed and the bones may be fractured.
- The separated skin may show abrasions from the rotating frictional effect of the tyre, but one portion is still in continuity with the adjacent skin.

ABORTION, THANATOLOGY AND HANGING

185. Ans. (b) 20-24 weeks pregnancy

Ref: The Essentials of Forensic Medicine and Toxicology, 33rd ed. pg. 401, 402

- According to the MTP (Amendment) Act 2021, for abortions up to 20 weeks, one doctor's approval is needed, for 20–24 weeks of the gestation period, opinion of two medical practitioners is necessary.
- Earlier, the law required one doctor for up to 12 weeks and two for between 12 and 20 weeks.

186. Ans. (d) Odorless

Ref: Essentials of Forensic Medicine and Toxicology by Dr KS Narayan Reddy 34th ed. pg. 163

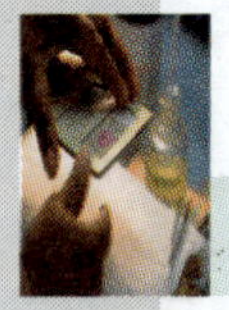

- The image demonstrates findings of mummification. Mummification is a late post-mortem change, where in drying and shriveling of the cadaver occurs due to dehydration or evaporation of water from the body. Hence there will be no possible odor produced from the body.

Extra Mile

- **Bitter almond** smell is associated with Cyanide poisoning
- **Burnt rope smell** is associated with marijuana intoxication
- **Garlicky odor** is associated with Arsenic, Selenium, Thallium and Aluminum phosphide poisoning.

187. Ans. (c) Hydrostatic test

Ref: Review of forensic medicine and toxicology, Gautam Biswas, 3rd ed. pg. 327

- The lung float test, also called the hydrostatic test or docimasia, is a controversial autopsy procedure used in determining whether lungs have undergone respiration.
- It has historically been employed in cases of suspected infanticide to help determine whether or not an infant was stillborn. In the test, lungs that float in water are thought to have been aerated, while those that sink are presumed to indicate an absence of air.

188. Ans. (c) Case of suicide

Ref: Review of Forensic Medicine and Toxicology by Gautam Biswas, 4th ed, pg. 177-78

- This cannot be a case of suicide. This is probably a case of manual strangulation (throttling) or smothering as on postmortem examination there is cyanosis of nails which suggest asphyxia.
- It may also be associated with cyanosis and congestion of the face (not mentioned in question).
- Also the scratch marks over face neck and chin can indicate fingertip bruising and nail scratch abrasions which further point towards homicide.
- It may be of the assailants or of the victim's own fingernails while he was trying to free himself from the attacker's grip.

189. Ans. (b) Child born after death of father

Ref: Review of Forensic Medicine and Toxicology by Gautam Biswas, 4th ed. pg. 369

- A posthumous birth is the birth of a child after the death of a biological parent. A person born in these circumstances is called a posthumous child or a posthumously born person.
- Posthumous birth has special implications in law, potentially affecting the child's citizenship and legal rights, inheritance, and order of succession.
- Most instances of posthumous birth involve the birth of a child after the death of its father, but the term is also applied to infants delivered shortly after the death of the mother.

190. Ans. (a) Supposititious child

Ref: Review of Forensic Medicine and Toxicology by Gautam Biswas, 4th ed, pg. 369

- Supposititious children are fraudulent offspring. This situation arises when an heir is required and a suitable baby might be procured and passed off as genuine.
- Women may pretend pregnancy and delivery and later produce a living child as her own or she may actually have a female child or a male child and exchange them for another child of another gender.
- This is done mostly for obtaining money or property.

191. Ans. (c) Homicidal

Ref: Review of Forensic Medicine and Toxicology by Gautam Biswas, 4th ed. pg. 205

- Suicidal cut injuries on the scrotum are very painful to produce and usually are on accessible areas of the body, therefore they are least likely.
- Accidental injury will be likely seen on the exposed part of the body (usually around the hands). Therefore, the most likely cause of the cut injury is homicidal only.
- Cut wound on nose, ears and genitals are usually homicidal and may result from sexual jealousy by angry lover husband or wife.

192. (b) Nysten's rule

Ref: Forensic Medicine: Clinical and Pathological Aspects, pg. 101

- Nysten's rule describes that rigor mortis doesn't start in all muscles simultaneously. It can be used for rough estimation of time since death.
- The law states: *"the rigidity in humans begins in mandibular joint then in trunk and neck, followed by upper extremities and then lower extremities. It follows the same order during resolution".*
- The development of rigor mortis is thus descending.

193. Ans. (b) Head

Ref: APC Essentials of Forensic Medicine By Anil Aggarwal pg. 143

- In suspected cranial injury, neck and chest should be opened first. It decompresses the CVS draining the blood in chest cavity.
- While in suspected neck trauma/hanging, **cranial cavity is opened first** to drain out blood from head.

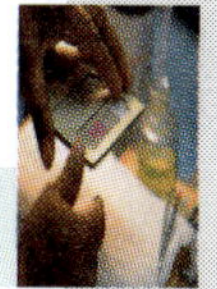

A bloodless field is thus created in the neck which prevents artifactual hemorrhages occurring in the neck.

- The **neck should be opened or dissected last** in case of death due to asphyxia/hanging.
- This is because the neck structure show marked congestion and suffusion of blood along with petechial hemorrhage in cases of asphyxia, therefore in an already congested neck it becomes sometimes difficult to distinguish a bruise on neck from congestion.
- Therefore, the neck needs to be drained of blood by opening the other structures like head, thorax, abdomen first to have a clear field devoid of artifacts.

194. Ans. (d) 1.04

Ref: Guide to Forensic Medicine & Toxicology, pg. 157

TABLE: Difference between respired and unrespired lung

Character	Unrespired lung	Respired lung
Weight in relation to body weight	1/70	1/35
Specific gravity	1.04	0.94
Color	Uniform, reddish	Mottled/marbled appearance

195. Ans. (c) 1/35

Ref: Textbook and Principles of Forensic Medicine by Bardale, pg. 357

Character	Unrespired lungs	Respired lungs
Weight in relation to body weight	1/70	1/35
Volume	Small	Large and covers the heart
Consistency	Liver like: Dense firm noncrepitant	Soft, spongy, elastic, crepitant
Extension	Up to the level of 4th and 5th rib	Up to the level of 6th and 7th rib
Specific gravity	1.04	0.94
Margin	Sharp	Rounded
Color	Uniform reddish	Mottled/marbled appearance
Air vesicle	Not inflated	Inflated
Section	Little froth less blood exudates on pressure	Abundant frothy blood exudates
Breslow life test	Whole or part sinks	Expanded
Microscopy	Cuboidal lining	Squamous epithelium
Blood vessel	Less patent	More patent

196. Ans. (c) Chelioscopy

Ref: Textbook of forensic medicine and toxicology by R N Karmakar pg. 358

Chelioscopy is the study of furrows or grooves present on the lips.

Le Moyne Snyder (1950) pointed out that the pattern of the furrows on the lips like finger prints are also individualistic and the prints left over glass, wine bottles, cup, saucer, fruit, cloth, paper, love letters may help in identification. Later on *Santosh* classified the furrows or the grooves of the lips into simple and compound types and further subdivided into 6 types.

Kazvo Suzuki and Yasvo Tsuchihashi (1970) classified lip prints as follows (Figs)

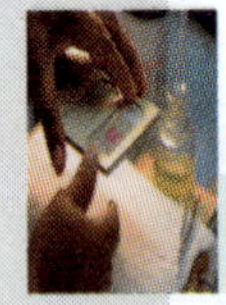

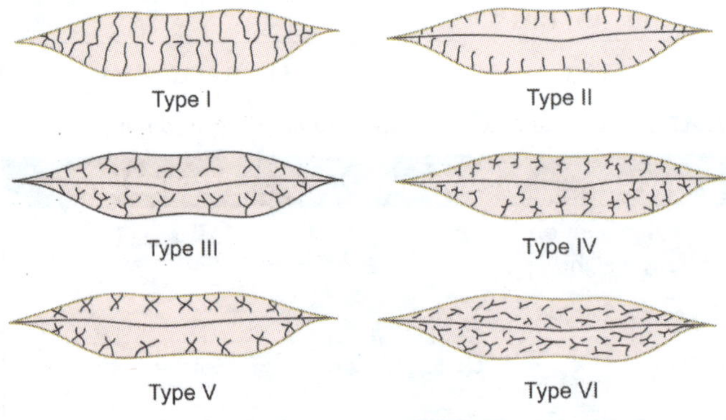

FIGURES: Types of lip-prints

- Type-I (Long vertical type)—Grooves running vertically for whole length
- Type-II (Short vertical type)—Grooves running vertically for partial length
- Type-III (Branching type)—Grooves are branched.
- Type-IV (Diamond type)—Grooves are intersected
- Type-V (Reticular type)—Grooves are reticulated
- Type-VI (Non-specific type)—Irregular having no specific pattern

197. Ans. (a) Pulmonary embolism

- In death certificate, 1A is the immediate cause of death. Like in this example, diabetic patient developed DVT, which leads to pulmonary embolism. The pulmonary embolism is the immediate cause of death.
- Line 1c is known as essence of death certificate.
- Given below is an example of death certificate:

Cause of death the disease or condition thought to be the underlying cause should appear in the lowest completed line of part I		
I	(a) *Disease or condition leading **directly** to death*	Intraperitoneal hemorrhage
	(b) *Other disease or condition, if any, **leading to** I*(a)	Ruptured metastatic deposit in liver
	(c) *Other disease or condition, If any, leading to I*(b)	Primary adenocarcinoma of ascending colon
II	*Other significant conditions* **Contributing to death** *but not Related to the disease or Condition causing it*	Non–insulin dependent diabetes mellitus

The colon cancer on line I (c) led directly to the liver metastases on line I (b), which ruptured, causing the fatal hemorrhage on I (a). Adenocarcinoma of the colon is the underlying cause of death

198. Ans. (a) Hyperextension of the neck

Hyperextension is more dangerous because flexion is protected by the contraction of strong posterior neck muscles.

199. Ans. (b) 20 weeks

Medical Termination is permitted up to 20th week.

- Indications of MTP:
  - **Social:** Failure of contraceptives in a married woman (till 20 weeks).
  - **Eugenic:** Fetus with serious physical or mental abnormalities diagnosed by a medical board
  - **Therapeutic:** If continuation of pregnancy endangers mother life (can be done anytime).
  - **Humanitarian:** If pregnancy is the outcome of rape allowed upto 24 weeks.

Important Points about MTP Act 1971:

- Only a qualified registered practitioner can perform it. Chief Medical Officer of district is empowered to certify that a doctor can perform it.
- *A medical practitioner should have performed **25 cases of MTP** in a recognized hospital*
- The operation should be performed either in a Government hospital or a place recognized by government.
- Non government institutions authorized by chief medical officer can also perform MTP.
- *Consent of husband is **not** required, however written consent of the women or her guardian (if she is minor or mentally ill) is required*
- Abortion can't be performed at the husband's request, if the woman is not willing.
- **No age proof is required**
- If the woman was raped, it's not necessary to lodge a police complaint
- Professional secrecy should be maintained
- If the duration of pregnancy is upto 20 weeks, opinion of single doctor is required
- Between 20 and 24 weeks, two doctors should provide opinion that there is an indication.
- Termination can be performed by any of the doctor

MTP (Amendment) Act 2021

- MTP is permitted till 24 weeks only in case of surviors
- If failure of contraception, MTP is permitted upto 20 weeks
- If substantid fetal abnormality, MTP can be done even after 24 weeks.

Opinion

- For MTP upto 20 weeks – 1 RMP
- For 20–24 weeks – 2 RMP

200. Ans. (b) Prominent frontal emience

Ref: Review of Forensic medicine by Sumit Seth pg. 5-6

TABLE: Important identification differences between male and female

		Male	Female
Skull	**General appearance**	Larger, heavier	Smaller, lighter, smooth
	Capacity:	1500–1550 cc	Capacity: 1350–1400 cc
	Forehead:	Steeper, less rounded	Vertical, round
	Orbits	**Square,** relatively smaller	Rounded, relatively larger
	Frontal eminence	Small	**Large**
	Mastoid	Large, round, blunt	Small, smooth, pointed
	Rest all structure	Larger, broader	Relatively small, less prominent
Mandible	**General**	Larger and thicker	Smaller and thinner
	Chin	Square	Rounded
	Angle of body and ramus	Less obtuse (125°), prominent, everted	More obtuse, not prominent, inverted
Pelvis	**General**	Deep funnel	Flat bowl
	Framework	Massive, tougher, narrow, tough	Less massive, smooth
	Preauricular sulcus	Not frequent, shallow, narrow	Frequent, deep, broad
	Obturator foramen	Large, OVAL with base upwards	Small, triangular with apex forward
	Greater sciatic notch	Smaller, narrower, deeper	Larger, Wider, shallower
	Subpubic angle	V shaped, 70–75°	U-shaped, 75–90°
	Corpobasal index of sacrum	More in males	Less in female

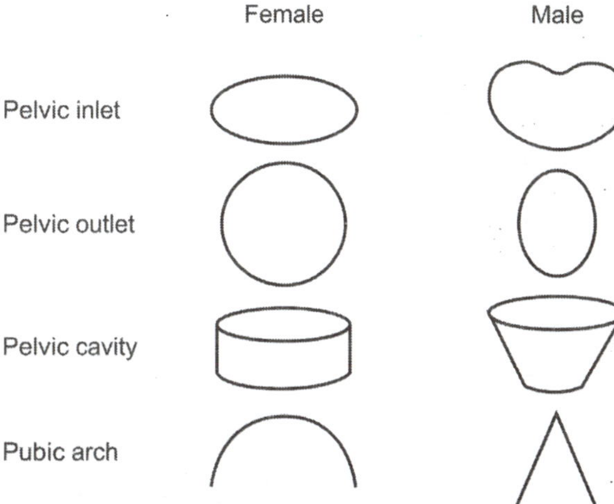

FIGURES: Comparison of male and female pelvis

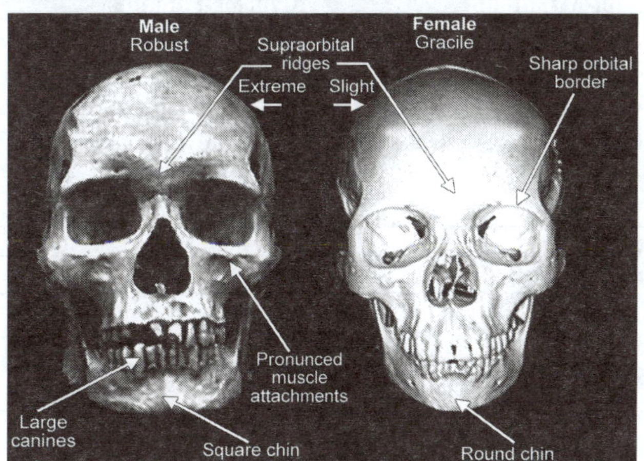

FIGURES: Comparison of male and female skullls

201. Ans. (b) Medical assistant can perform in absence of gynecologist

Ref: The Essentials of FSM by K.S. Narayan Reddy, 31st ed. pg. 374-75

Please refer to above explanation of Q. 156.

202. Ans. (d) Age proof is generally not required

Ref: The Essentials of FSM by K.S. Narayan Reddy, 31st ed. pg. 374-75

- Please read the question carefully. After reading the options of this question, we generally get a tendency to mark among option A to C.
- Please read the last option carefully, it's given as if it has no significance. But actually that's the correct answer.
- In case of MTP, age proof is not required.
- *Please refer to the previous answer for detailed explanation.*

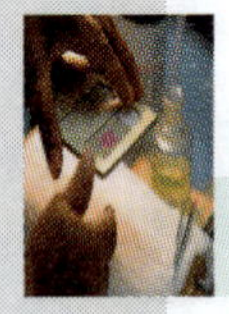

203. Ans. (d) 25

Ref: The Essentials of FSM by K.S. Narayan Reddy, 31st ed. pg. 374-375

Please refer to above explanation.

204. Ans. (a) Occiput

Ref: The Essentials of FSM by K.S. Narayan Reddy, 31st ed. pg. 314-15

HANGING

- A form of violent asphyxia as a result of suspension of the body by a ligature round the neck the constricting force being the weight of body.

TABLE: Type of Hanging according to position of Knot

Typical Hanging	Atypical Hanging
• Knot of ligature should be at the nape of neck on the back (Occiput). • 'V' shape above thyroid cartilage • Eg: suicide hanging	• At any site other than the nape of neck • ***Most common site is near on angle of mandible*** • No V- shape • Eg: Judicial hanging

205. Ans. (d) 4.50 kg

Ref: The Essentials of FSM by K.S. Narayan Reddy, 31st ed. pg. 314-18

- Upon hanging the death can either be cervical bone fracture or can be secondary to vascular occlusion.
- ***In case of partial hanging some part of body touching the ground. Therefore weight responsible for death is weight of head, which is nearly equal to 4–5 kg.***
- There are 4 important vascular structures in neck which can bear weight of upto:
  - **Jugular vein: 2 kg**
  - Carotid artery: 5 kg
  - Tracheal artery: 15 kg
  - Vertebral artery: 20-30 kg.

TABLE: Type of Hanging according to degree of suspension

Complete hanging	Incomplete (partial) hanging
• Body is fully suspended & no part of body touches the ground • Constricting force is weight of body	• The lower part of body is in touch with ground • Weight of head acts as constricting force

206. Ans. (c) Saliva dribbling to the opposite side of the knot

Ref: Textbook of Forensic Medicine and Toxicology: Principles and Practice by Vij/162

TABLE: Difference between Hanging and Strangulation by ligature

Trait	Hanging	Strangulation by ligature
Manner of death	Mostly suicidal	Homicidal
Face	Pale, No petechiae	**Red congested,** marked petechiae
Bleeding	Bleeding from nose, mouth and ears not common	Common
Saliva	Often dribbles out of mouth	Very rare
Ligature	Oblique, Non-continuous, placed high up in the neck between chin and larynx	Horizontal or trans-verse, continuous round the neck, low down in the neck below or across the thyroid
Abrasion and Echhymosis around the edge of ligature	Rare	Common
Larynx and trachea fracture	Rare That too in Judicial hanging	Comparatively more common

Note: *Position of knot in suicidal hanging is at the nape of neck. In Judicial hanging position of knot mostly is at the angle of mandible.*

207. Ans. (a) Hanging

Ref: The Essentials of FSM by KS Narayan Reddy, 31st ed. pg. 319

- Le facies sympathique is an expression which is seen in cases of antemortem hanging.
- When the ligature knot presses on cervical sympathetic, the eyes on the same side may remain open and its pupil dilated. This particular finding is known as le facies sympathique.

208. Ans. (a) Burking

Ref: The essentials of FSM by KS Narayan Reddy, 31st ed. pg. 335

- **Strangulation** is a form of asphyxia which is caused by constriction of the neck by a ligature without suspending the body. It can be several types:
  - **Bansdola:** One bamboo stick at back of neck and other at the front of neck. Both ends tied with rope which causes death of the victim.
  - **Garotting:** Victim is attacked from behind with a rope over the neck.

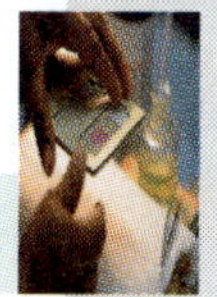

   - **Mugging:** Strangulation caused by holding the neck of the victim in the bend of the elbow.
- **Suffocation is** a form of asphyxia, which is caused by deprivation of oxygen, either due to lack of oxygen in environment or from obstruction of air passages at the level of nose and mouth.
- **Forms of suffocation asphyxia:**
   - **Burking** is a method of homicidal **smothering and traumatic asphyxia.**
   - **Smothering:** form of asphyxia caused by closing the external respiratory orifices either by hand or other means
   - **Gagging:** Asphyxia by forcing cloth into the mouth.
   - **Overlaying:** Asphyxia due to compression of chest. Ex: Mother overlied on infant.
   - **Choking:** Asphyxia by obstruction of air passages, usually between the pharynx and bifurcation of trachea. Almost always accidental.
   - **Café coronary:** Alcoholic who is grossly intoxicated dies while having meal. Death occurs due to sudden heart attack. High blood alcohol content anesthesizes the gag reflex.

209. Ans. (a) Homicidal smothering and traumatic asphyxia

Ref: The essentials of FSM by KS Narayan Reddy, 31st ed. pg. 335

Please refer to above explanation.

210. Ans. (b) Suffocation

Ref: The Essentials of FSM by KS Narayan Reddy, 31st ed. pg. 335

Please refer to above explanation.

211. Ans. (d) Eyelids

Ref: The Essentials of FSM by K.S. Narayan Reddy 31st ed. pg. 140-43, 147; Reddy's, 27th pg. 142

Order of appearance and disappearance (in sequence)
- Heart (left chamber in 1 hour)
- Eyelids (3-4 hours)
- Face muscles
- Neck and trunk
- Upper extremities
- Legs
- Small muscle of finger and toes (last to be affected, 11–12 hours)

Extra Mile

- Postmortem rigidity lasts for **18-36 hours in** summer and 24–48 hours in winter.
- Postmortem rigidity disappear in the same order as that of the appearance

212. Ans. (d) 60°C

Ref: AK Gupta's 'Essentials of Forensic medicine & Toxicology' 4/e, pg. 96

- When temperature of flame is 65 degree Celsius or above, body is rigid with limbs flexed known as pugilistic or Fencing posture ***due to coagulation of albumin constituents of muscles (Boxer's posture in defence).***
- But this is not always a true ante-mortem phenomenon as heat stiffening can occur after death due to postmortem bums.

213. Ans. (a) Neck

Ref: Forensic Medicine and Toxicology' by RN Karmakar

Bloodless dissection of neck is to be done in asphyxia.

FORENSIC PSYCHIATRY

214. Ans. (b) Delirium tremens

Ref: Review of Forensic Medicine and Toxicology, Gautam Biswas, 3rd ed. pg. 547

- **Delirium tremens** is the most severe symptom of sudden alcohol withdrawal in chronic alcoholics.

Causes
- Sudden excess or sudden withdrawal of alcohol.
- Long continual ingestion of alcohol.
- Shock due to severe trauma, e.g. fracture in a chronic alcoholic.
- Acute infections, like pneumonia or influenza in a chronic alcoholic.

215. Ans. (b) The person is malingering

Ref: Review of Forensic Medicine and Toxicology by Gautam Biswas, 4th ed. pg. 546

- This seems to be a case of body packer. His symptoms are consistent with his condition. Therefore malingering will be least likely option here.
- A body packer is someone who carries drugs such as heroin or cocaine, packed in rubber or plastic, in his/her body in order to smuggle them.
- These people can present with symptoms that vary from mild abdominal complaints to respiratory insufficiency and even death.
- Physical examination and additional radiology tests are helpful for the diagnosis. Any packages can usually be seen on a plain abdominal X-ray. Detailed information on the number of drug packages, their exact location in the gastrointestinal tract and complications, such as small intestine obstruction or perforation, can be derived from a CT scan. Loss of consciousness can be explained by rupture of bag and absorption of contents into systemic circulation.

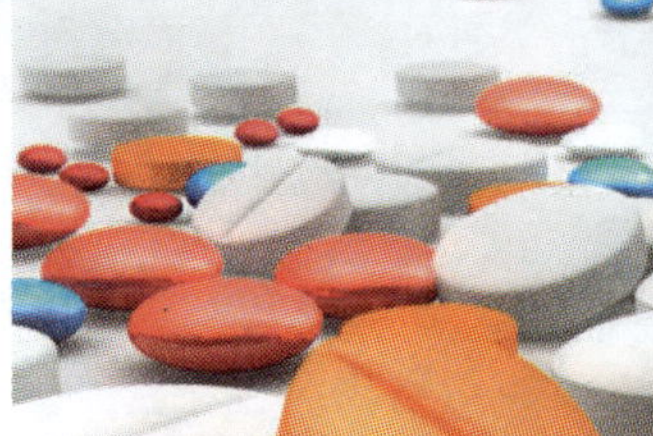

PREVENTIVE AND SOCIAL MEDICINE (PSM)

8

MOST RECENT QUESTIONS 2023

1. What are the delivery criteria in a type A PHC? *(Most Recent Question July 2023)*

a. <20 deliveries/month
b. Equal to 10 deliveries/month
c. Equal to 30 deliveries/month
d. <30 deliveries/month

2. Which of the following is direct cause of maternal death? *(Most Recent Question July 2023)*

a. Embolism
b. Pre-eclampsia
c. Anemia
d. Diabetes

3. 6 × 6 × 6 strategy under Anemia Mukt Bharat includes all, EXCEPT: *(Most Recent Question July 2023)*

a. Beneficiaries
b. Intervention
c. Coordination/ministries
d. Institutional mechanism

4. Which of the following is NOT included under Anemia Mukt Bharat program: *(Most Recent Question July 2023)*

a. Folic acid
b. Iron
c. Anti helminthic
d. Antibiotics

5. Labeled arrow in the given image of rule of halves for hypertension indicates? *(Most Recent Question July 2023)*

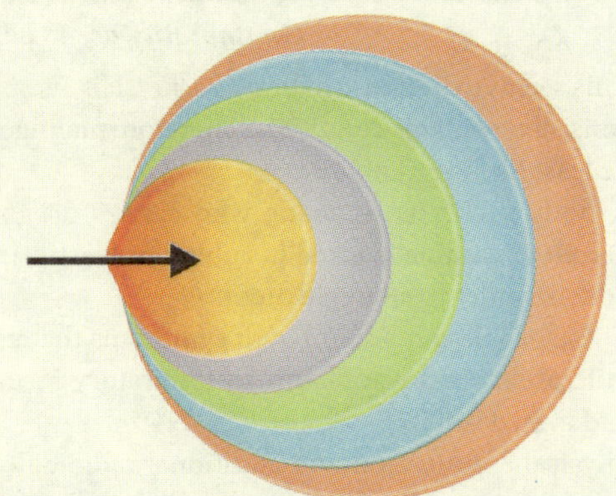

a. Inadequately treated
b. Adequately treated
c. Diagnosed and treated
d. Undiagnosed hypertension

6. Total number of live births/1000 woman in reproductive age group? *(Most Recent Question July 2023)*

a. Total fertility rate
b. Age specific fertility rate
c. General fertility rate
d. Net reproductive rate

7. Which of the following statement is correct about triage? *(Most Recent Question July 2023)*

a. Red – Ambulatory
b. Yellow - Stable need observation
c. Black – Minor injuries
d. Green – Life threatening

8. What will be the dose of vitamin A for 1–6-year-old in endemic area? *(Most Recent Question July 2023)*

a. 2 lakh IU orally every 6 months
b. 1 lakh IU for 6 months orally
c. 2 lakh IU for 6 weeks
d. 2 lakh IU for 1 year

9. Which of the following is not included in Urban health care? *(Most Recent Question July 2023)*

a. PHC
b. CHC
c. District Hospital
d. Subcenter

10. In an experiment, 39 was highest number but was mistaken for 93. What will it affect? *(Most Recent Question July 2023)*

a. Mean will remain same
b. Median will increase
c. Mean, median both increase
d. Mean will increase, median will remain the same

11. Which international agency helps in construction of sanitary latrines (Toilet building) in India? *(Most Recent Question July 2023)*

a. USAID
b. CURE
c. REDCROSS
d. FORD

12. At what age of gestation a pregnant woman with a family history of diabetes to her mother should be screened for her diabetes? *(Most Recent Question July 2023)*

a. 20 weeks
b. 36 weeks
c. At 1st visit
d. 24–28 weeks

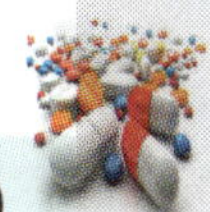

13. Identify the graph: *(Most Recent Question July 2023)*

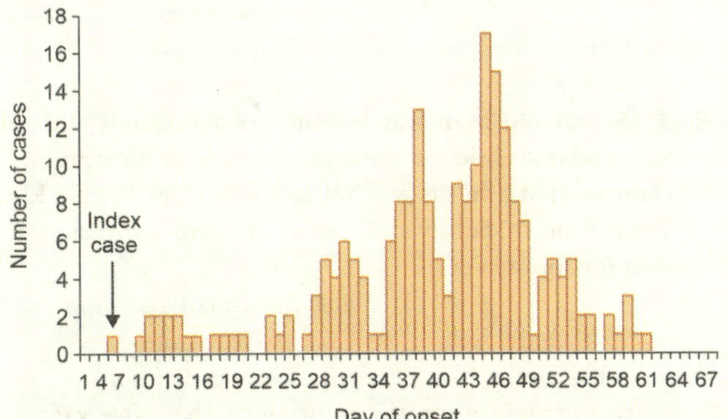

a. Point source single exposure epidemic
b. Common source, continuous exposure epidemic
c. Common source single exposure
d. Propagated epidemic

14. A 10-year-old girl came for a health checkup and diagnosed with malnutrition. She doesn't go to school. Which of the following program will benefit her? *(Most Recent Question July 2023)*

a. Rashtriya Bal Swasthya Karyakram
b. Janani Suraksha Yojna
c. Mid-Day Meal
d. Navjat Shishu Karyakram Yojna

15. Which of the following assess chronic malnutrition for height for age? *(Most Recent Question July 2023)*

a. Stunting
b. Wasting
c. Constitutional growth delay
d. Congenital growth delay

16. Criterion of mid-arm circumference in Shakir's tape for severe acute malnutrition is? *(Most Recent Question July 2023)*

a. < 11.5 b. < 12.5
c. < 13.5 d. < 14.5

17. In an HIV patient, co-infected with TB, which of the following is investigation of choice to diagnose TB: *(Most Recent Question July 2023)*

a. Culture
b. Chest x-ray
c. CBNAAT
d. Culture in liquid medium

18. Which of the following combination is correct regarding the disposal of an expired tablet? *(Most Recent Question July 2023)*

a. Red bag – Hydroclaving
b. Blue bag – incineration
c. Yellow bag – incineration
d. Yellow bag – burial

19. School Health Program comes under this program?

a. Ayushman Bharat *(Most Recent Question July 2023)*
b. RBSK (Rashtriya Bal Swasthya Karyakram)
c. RKSK (Rashtriya Kishore Suraksha Karyakram)
d. NSSK (Navjaat Shishu Surakhsa Karyakram)

20. According to SDG proposed goals toward 2030, what is the target for the maternal mortality ratio? *(Most Recent Question July 2023)*

a. Less than 18 b. Less than 20
c. Less than 22 d. Less than 70

21. Which of the following is not included in Ayushman Bharat Scheme? *(Most Recent Question July 2023)*

a. 5 lakh per family per year is given
b. 10 lakh per family per year is given
c. Health and wellness center
d. Includes economically weaker section

22. A 32-year male presented to emergency ward following crush injury of hand. He had received last TT injection at age of 25 years. Wound cleaning is already done. What is next management? *(Most Recent Question July 2023)*

a. TT only b. Td only
c. TT with Ig d. Td with Ig

23. Anthrax is which category bioterrorism? *(Most Recent Question July 2023)*

a. A b. B
c. C d. D

24. In a patient is on OCP, the risk of which cancer decreased: *(Most Recent Question July 2023)*

a. Endometrial b. Cervical cancer
c. Breast cancer d. Oral cavity cancer

25. Known case of HIV with CD4 count <50 he is at risk of which infection? *(Most Recent Question July 2023)*

a. Candida
b. S. aureus
c. MAC
d. Pneumocystis Jiroveci Pneumonia

26. According to STEP approach, which of the following is NOT included: *(Most Recent Question July 2023)*

a. Blood pressure b. Blood group
c. Blood lipid d. Blood sugar

27. Which system is involved in this condition? *(Most Recent Question July 2023)*

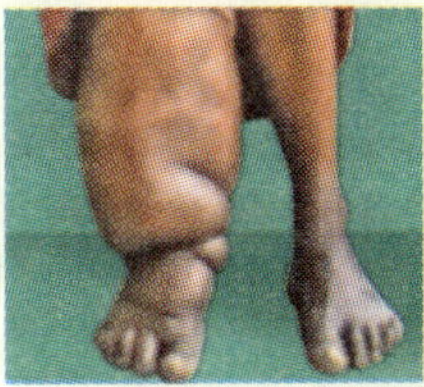

a. Arterial b. Venous
c. Lymphatics d. Nervous

28. A child presenting to clinic with history of cough, coryza, conjunctivitis and fever. On examination rash is seen which arises behind ear and spreading all over chest, back and abdomen. What is diagnosis:

(Most Recent Question July 2023)

a. Measles b. Dengue
c. Rubella d. Chikungunya

29. A patient presenting with loss of cold sensation followed by hot, touch and pain. Diagnosis is:

(Most Recent Question July 2023)

a. TB b. Leprosy
c. HIV d. CANDIDA

30. A 3 Year baby presented with diarrhea. On examination baby is severely dehydrated, lethargic high respiratory rate, BP 80/60. Fluid given for management:

(Most Recent Question July 2023)

a. ORS 100 ml/kg 4 hrs b. ORS 100 ml/kg 6 hrs
c. I/V infusion with NS d. RL

31. Protein requirement of 55 kg female:

(Most Recent Question July 2023)

a. 45 gm b. 54 gm
c. 65 gm d. 55 gm

32. Per capita space in school should be?

(Most Recent Question Jan 2023)

a. >10 sq. ft b. >15 sq. ft
c. >5 sq. ft d. >20 sq. ft

33. The frontal anterior incisors of child who had white patches on them turned brown following over supplementation of which of the following?

(Most Recent Question Jan 2023)

a. Vitamin A b. Fluorine
c. Chlorine d. Riboflavin

34. Tobacco control law is which level of prevention:

(Most Recent Question Jan 2023)

a. Primary level prevention
b. Primordial level prevention
c. Secondary level prevention
d. Tertiary level prevention

35. Handwashing during Covid -19 is what type of prevention? *(Most Recent Question Jan 2023)*

a. Primary level prevention
b. Primordial level prevention
c. Secondary level prevention
d. Tertiary level prevention

36. Giving class in a village for wound dressing after a dog bite is which mode of communication?

(Most Recent Question Jan 2023)

a. Lecture
b. Flashcard
c. Demonstration
d. Group discussion

37. Eligible couple register is maintained at which level?

(Most Recent Question Jan 2023)

a. CHC b. PHC
c. Sub center d. Ground level

38. A 35-year-old man was leaving for a vacation with his wife and one child. At the same time his brother and wife came to visit him his brother and wife came to visit him. What type of family did you come across during your visit for the survey?

(Most Recent Question Jan 2023)

a. Extended family b. Nuclear family
c. Joint family d. Third generation

39. Doctor explaining to the community that after vaccination it won't lead to impotency. What type of barrier is this: *(Most Recent Question Jan 2023)*

a. Environmental barrier b. Psychological barrier
c. Physical barrier d. Cultural barrier

40. After vasectomy, for how many weeks a person should use barrier method? *(Most Recent Question Jan 2023)*

a. 3–4 weeks b. 6–8 weeks
c. 12–20 weeks d. 20–24 weeks

41. What is the denominator of infant mortality rate?

(Most Recent Question Jan 2023)

a. 100 total births
b. 1000 total live birth
c. 100,000 live births
d. Total live births weighing over 1000 grams at birth

42. Infectivity is also known as?

(Most Recent Question Jan 2023)

a. Secondary attack rate b. Case fatality rate
c. Serial interval d. Incubation

43. A patient came with grade 3 dog bite and previous history of prophylaxis for monkey bite have completed 4 weeks ago. What is next step of management?

(Most Recent Question Jan 2023)

a. Wound cleaning + IgM + rabies serum
b. Wound cleaning + rabies vaccination 0, 3
c. Wound cleaning + rabies vaccination 0,3,7
d. Only wound cleaning with running water

44. Which oil is preferred to decrease the risk of coronary artery disease? *(Most Recent Question Jan 2023)*

a. Omega -3 fatty acid
b. Omega -6 fatty acids
c. Omega -9 fatty acids
d. Saturated fatty acid

45. Essential components of RCH program in India include all of the following EXCEPT:

(Most Recent Question Jan 2023)

a. Safe motherhood
b. Woman education and empowerment
c. Children and newborn care
d. Screening and treatment for STD/RTI

46. In a demographic cycle, highest birth rate is seen in? *(Most Recent Question Jan 2023)*
a. Stage I b. Stage II
c. Stage III d. Stage IV

CONCEPT OF HEALTH AND DISEASE

47. Which indicator is used for comparison of life expectancy between two countries *(Most Recent Question June 2022)*
a. HDI b. HPI
c. DALY d. PQLI

48. Burden of disease in a society is best indicated by? *(Most Recent Question June/Dec 2021)*
a. Incidence b. Prevalence
c. Case fatality rate d. Daly

49. All of following are principles of primary health care; EXCEPT: *(Most Recent Question Aug 2020)*
a. Community participation
b. Appropriate facility
c. Intersectoral coordination
d. Equitable distribution

50. A doctor is teaching an intern about knee reflex demonstration. What type of learning is this? *(Most Recent Question Dec 2019-20)*
a. Cognitive learning b. Affective learning
c. Psychomotor learning d. None of these

51. Identify the logo given in the image below: *(Most Recent Question Dec 2019-20)*

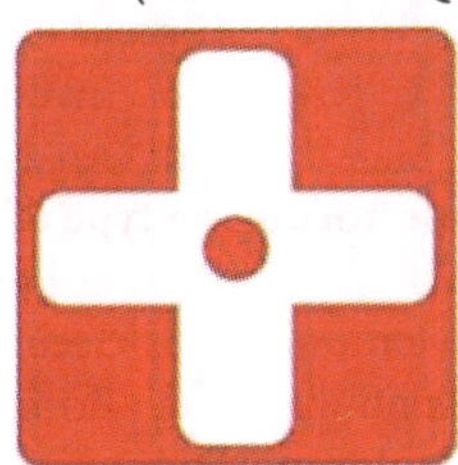

a. First aid
b. Red cross
c. Suraksha clinic
d. Allopathic clinic practitioners

52. True about PQLI *(Recent Pattern Question 2016)*
a. Literacy rate, birth rate, life expectancy at birth
b. Life expectancy at 1 year, IMR, literacy rate
c. Life expectancy at birth, income, literacy rate
d. Soon to be replaced by GNP

53. Father of public health:
a. Tuberculosis b. Cholera
c. Malaria d. Plague

54. PQLI lies between:
a. 0 and 1 b. 0 and 10
c. 0 and 100 d. 1 and 10

55. Which of the following is true about Human Development Index:
a. Maternal mortality rate b. IMR
c. Life expectancy-birth d. Life expectancy- 1 year

56. HDI consists of all; EXCEPT:
a. Real GDP per capita income
b. Life expectancy at birth
c. Mean year of schooling and expected year of schooling
d. Range 0–100

57. Human development index value is:
a. 0–1 b. 0–100
c. Any number d. No number

58. Not included in PQLI is:
a. Income b. Literacy
c. Life expectancy at age 1 d. Infant mortality

59. Image of iceberg phenomenon with value of 12 cases mentioned above the surface, 20 at the surface, 50 beneath the surface. Which disease has following pattern:
a. Tuberculosis b. Measles
c. Rabies d. Tetanus

60. In iceberg phenomenon, the submerged part represents:
a. Undiagnosed cases in community
b. Diagnosed cases in community
c. Clinical cases that physician sees
d. Clinical cases that investigator sees

61. Changes in occurrence of a disease over a long period of time:
a. Secular trend b. Cyclic trends
c. Seasonal trends d. Epidemic

62. Disease recurring after many years:
a. Secular trends b. Cyclic trend
c. Seasonal trend d. Propagated epidemics

63. A disease condition like influenza pandemics occurs every 10 years. Which trend is reflected here?
a. Secular trend b. Epidemic
c. Seasonal trend d. Cyclic trend

64. Accidents happening during weekends is:
a. Cyclic trends b. Seasonal trends
c. Secular trends d. Point source epidemic

65. Which of following defines ability of organism to cause infection:
a. Pathogenicity b. Infectivity
c. Antigenicity d. Virulence

STUDY DESIGNS AND PREVENTIVE MEASURES

66. If counseling and screening for TB in a HIV patient is done in ICTC clinic as per NACO guidelines, what is the level of prevention *(Most Recent Question June 2022)*
a. Primordial b. Primary
c. Secondary d. Tertiary

67. Relative risk is estimation from
(Most Recent Question June 2022)
a. Case control study b. Cohort study
c. Cross sectional study d. RCT

68. In a study, a doctor wants to check the incidence of some disease in workers band managers after sound exposure for 1 year between exposed and non-exposed group. Which study design is used?
(Most Recent Question June/Dec 2021)
a. Cohort study b. Case control study
c. Ecological study d. Experimental study

69. A doctor is doing a clinical trial in which there is error in clinical overreporting of disease in one group. The selection bias removal can be done by?
(Most Recent Question June/Dec 2021)
a. Matching b. Stratification
c. Blinding d. Randomization

70. Best quantitative method to study previous research studies is: *(Most Recent Question June/Dec 2021)*
a. Systematic reviews b. Meta-analysis
c. Surveys d. Group interviews

71. A man came for checkup after his father had a cerebrovascular accident due to hypertension. What type of prevention? *(Most Recent Question Aug 2020)*
a. Primordial b. Primary
c. Secondary d. Specific protein

72. A researcher was conducting study in relation of Depression associated with history of social medial usage. One group had social medial users with depression and another group had social media users without depression. Which type of study design is used?
(Most Recent Question Aug 2020)
a. Cohort study b. Case control study
c. Cross sectional study d. Random sampling

73. A research study is being conducted on patients in rehabilitation where impact of addiction among young adults was assessed on their subsequent divorce. Among two groups of study subject, divorced and non-divorced, history of alcohol/drug use was assessed. What kind of study was done? *(Most Recent Question Dec 2019-20)*
a. Cohort study b. Case control study
c. RCT d. Descriptive study

74. There is a group of 200 Hypertensive patients. First group of 100 patients follow medical advice whereas second group of 100 patients follow lifestyle advice. There is test for both the groups after 3 months. Which of the following is best test for significance of compare blood pressure levels in both the groups?
(Most Recent Question Dec 2019-20)
a. Paired student's t-test
b. Unpaired student's t-test
c. Fischer test
d. Chi-square test

75. On Republic Day, a camp was organized and people were screened for Hypertension by checking BP and for diabetes by checking their BMI and blood sugar level, which level of prevention is this?
(Most Recent Question Dec 2019-20)
a. Primary b. Primordial
c. Secondary d. Tertiary

76. In Africa vaccination was given in an epidemic outbreak area for a specific disease but due to shortage of vaccines, mass chemoprophylaxis treatment was given to people who were not diseased. Which type of prevention is this?
a. Specific protection
b. Health promotion
c. Early diagnosis and treatment
d. Rehabilitation

77. True about Quarantine: *(Most Recent Question 2019)*
a. Restriction of movement of infected patient
b. Restriction of movement of healthy contact of an infectious disease
c. Movement restricted for shortest incubation period
d. Isolation of diseased person

78. Framingham study is: *(Recent Pattern Question 2018)*
a. Prospective cohort b. Retrospective cohort
c. Case control study d. Cross sectional study

79. Incidence can be calculated by:
(Recent Pattern Question 2018)
a. Cohort study b. Case control study
c. Cross sectional study d. Retrospective cohort

80. Hospital patient admission rate differs in different hospitals with different disease. This causes which type of bias? *(Recent Pattern Question 2016)*
a. Subject bias b. Investigator bias
c. Berkesonian bias d. Analyser bias

81. Fetal cardiac monitoring is a type of:
(Recent Pattern Question 2016)
a. Primary prevention b. Secondary prevention
c. Tertiary prevention d. Primordial prevention

82. Relative risk calculation is done for:
(Recent Pattern Question 2016)
a. Cohort study b. Case control study
c. Cross sectional study d. Ecological study

83. What is true about double blind trial?
a. Patient getting double treatment
b. Patient does not know that he is a part of clinical trial
c. Patient is getting both placebo and medication
d. Patient does not know what is he getting

84. Randomization is:
a. It brings bias in study group, therefore avoided
b. It is the procedure by which participants are allocated into groups usually called 'study' and 'control' group
c. It ensures that investigator has full control over allocation of participants to study or control group
d. It is done usually before entering in the study and then consent is taken

85. 'Primordial Prevention' means:
a. Preventive action taken prior to onset of disease
b. Prevention of emergence of risk factors of the disease
c. Prevention of disease from causing complication
d. Early detection of disease by screening

86. Immunization is which type of prevention?
a. Primordial b. Primary
c. Secondary d. Tertiary

87. Polio vaccine is which type of prevention:
a. Primary b. Secondary
c. Tertiary d. Primordial

88. All of the following are true regarding primary prevention; EXCEPT:
a. Immunization
b. Specific protection
c. Early diagnosis and treatment
d. Contraceptives

89. Screening of cervical cancer is which level of prevention?
a. Primordial b. Primary
c. Secondary d. Tertiary

90. Vaccine is what level of prevention:
a. Primordial b. Primary
c. Secondary d. Tertiary

91. Tracking of blood pressure is which type of prevention:
a. Primordial b. Primary
c. Secondary d. Tertiary

92. All of the following comes under primary prevention; EXCEPT:
a. Pap smear b. Helmets
c. Contraception d. Vaccines

93. PAP smear is an example of:
a. Early diagnosis and treatment
b. Health promotion
c. Specific protection
d. Disability limitation

94. Desk provided with table top to prevent neck problems is an example of:
a. Primordial prevention b. Primary protection
c. Specific protection d. Disability limitation

95. Patient is on psychotherapy, what is the level of prevention:
a. Primordial b. Primary
c. Secondary d. Tertiary

96. Iodized salt is given in an area endemic to goiter. Type of prevention:
a. Health promotion
b. Specific protection
c. Primordial prevention
d. Treatment

97. IFA supplementation is an example of:
a. Primordial b. Specific protection
c. Secondary d. Tertiary

98. Tracking of BP implies:
a. BP increase with age
b. BP decreases with age
c. BP of normotensive becomes hypertensive
d. BP of hypertensive remains hypertensive

99. Best for prevention of risk factor:
a. Primordial prevention
b. Primary prevention
c. Secondary prevention
d. Tertiary prevention

EPIDEMIOLOGY, SCREENING AND VACCINES

100. In measles epidemic, 7-month-old child was given measles vaccine. When should the next dose of measles vaccine be given? ***(Most Recent Question June 2022)***
a. Give booster at 16 months
b. 9 months
c. Give boost at 9–16 months
d. Booster at 9 month
e. At preschool age

101. Vaccines given at birth to a baby ***(Most Recent Question June 2022)***
a. Pentavalent MR, HIB
b. BCG OPV, MR
c. BCG, OPV, Hepatitis B
d. BCG, IP, Hepatitis B

102. When is the first dose of hepatitis B vaccine given to neonate? ***(Most Recent Question June 2022)***
a. At birth b. 6 weeks
c. 2 months d. 6 months

103. Number of maternal deaths due to pregnancy related process expressed per 100000 live births is known as: ***(Most Recent Question June/Dec 2021)***
a. Maternal mortality rate
b. Maternal mortality ratio
c. Maternal mortality proportion
d. Adult lifetime risk of maternal death

104. HPV vaccine is based on: ***(Most Recent Question June/Dec 2021)***
a. E1, E2 b. E6, E7
c. E 7 d. L1, L2

105. Heat sensitive substance/device present on the vaccine to monitor its viability is: ***(Most Recent Question June/Dec 2021)***
a. MMV b. MVM
c. VVM d. MVV

106. Father of epidemiology is:
a. Hippocrates b. John Snow
c. Ambroise Pare d. Rudolf Virchow

107. Father of Medicine:
a. John Snow b. Edward Jenner
c. Louis Pasteur d. Hippocrates

108. Which of the following set is termed as epidemiological triad?
a. Endemic, epidemic and outbreaks
b. Agent, host and environment
c. Incidence, prevalence and disease load
d. Agent, man and disease

109. Which of the following is indicative of severity/lethality of disease? *(Most Recent Question Aug 2020)*
a. Proportional mortality rate
b. Case specific death rate
c. Case fatality rate
d. Total deaths due to that disease

110. Long term changes/sequelae of a disease are seen in: *(Most Recent Question Aug 2020)*
a. Secular trend of a disease
b. Cyclical trend of a disease
c. Disease changing its traits according to herd immunity in the population
d. Disease changing the symptoms as per seasons

111. A screening test is used for a disease in a population. In the image shown below what does B-C represents *(Most Recent Question Dec 2019-20)*

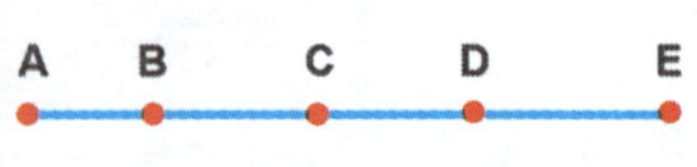

A = Disease onset
B = First possible detection
C = Critical point
D = Usual time of diagnosis
E = Final outcome

a. Lead time b. Screening time
c. Incubation period d. Latent period

112. Sample registration system does not include: *(Most Recent Question Dec 2019-20)*
a. Maternal mortality rate
b. Infant mortality rate
c. Crude birth rate
d. Crude death rate

113. Mortality is taken into consideration in: *(Most Recent Question Dec 2019-20)*
a. Gross reproductive rate (GRR)
b. Net reproduction rate (NRR)
c. Total fertility rate (TFR)
d. Complete family size

114. Prevalence is associated with: *(Most Recent Question Dec 2019-20)*
a. Sensitivity
b. Specificity
c. Positive predictive value
d. Accuracy

115. Yellow fever vaccine is valid for: *(Most Recent Question Dec 2019-20)*
a. Life long b. 10 years
c. 5 years d. 20 years

116. BCG is diluted with: *(Most Recent Question 2019)*
a. NS b. DW
c. RL d. Distilled water

117. Vaccine storage at level of PHC? *(Recent Pattern Question 2018-19)*
a. Walk in freezer b. Walk in coolers
c. Ice line refrigerator d. Cold boxes

118. In a baby who is on steroids, live vaccine can be given after: *(Recent Pattern Question 2018-19)*
a. 2 weeks b. 4 weeks
c. 6 weeks d. 10 weeks

119. All of the following live vaccines are contraindicated in pregnancy; EXCEPT: *(Recent Pattern Question 2018)*
a. Yellow fever b. BCG
c. Rubella d. OPV

120. Food poisoning is an example of: *(Recent Pattern Question 2018)*
a. Point source epidemic
b. Propagated source epidemic
c. Common source epidemic
d. Pandemic

121. Diabetes, hypertension or CAD screening should be started after: *(Recent Pattern Question 2018)*
a. 30 b. 35
c. 45 d. 55

122. Neonatal tetanus prevention is best done by: *(Recent Pattern Question 2018)*
a. Tetanus toxoid
b. Tetanus immunoglobulin
c. Metronidazole
d. Penicillin

123. True about incidence: *(Recent Pattern Question 2018)*
a. Total number of cases in a community
b. Number of at risk patients
c. Number of new cases
d. Number of deaths in community

124. Only vaccine given to adults *(Recent Pattern Question 2018)*
a. DPT b. dT
c. MMR d. OPV

125. In a case of epidemic, 3 villages are affected simultaneously with typhoid cases. Upon study it is found that one milk man is going to all these 3 villages. Identify the type of epidemic: *(Recent Pattern Question 2017)*
a. Point source
b. Common source, propagative
c. Common source, multiple exposure
d. Common source, continuous exposure

126. When some people develop a disease after exposure from a primary case, it is known as: *(Recent Pattern Question 2017)*
a. Incidence b. Prevalence
c. Lead time d. Secondary attack rate

127. In situation of an epidemic investigation, what is the medical officer's first role/first to do:
(Recent Pattern Question 2017)
a. Hypothesis formulation
b. Find out at risk population
c. Find out about number of cases
d. Verification of diagnosis

128. Net reproduction rate is defined as:
(Recent Pattern Question 2017)
a. Number of live birth in the reproductive age group of a female
b. Average number of children born to a married woman
c. Average number of girls born to a woman assuming no mortality
d. Number of girls born to a woman during her lifetime assuming mortality

129. If net reproduction rate is desired to be 1, what should be the couple protection rate:
(Recent Pattern Question 2017)
a. 42　　b. 60
c. 70　　d. 82

130. Lung cancer patients: 300 smokers and 300 nonsmokers, 10 year history taken. What can be calculated?
(Recent Pattern Question 2017)
a. Prevalence　　b. Incidence
c. RR　　d. Odds ratio

131. What is the recommended dose for human rabies immunoglobulin (Ig) in 4-month-old child?
(Recent Pattern Question 2016)
a. 20 IU/kg　　b. 30 IU/kg
c. 40 IU/kg　　d. 50 IU/kg

132. What is the measles vaccine dose?
(Recent Pattern Question 2016)
a. 0.1 cc　　b. 0.5 cc
c. 0.01 cc　　d. 1.0 cc

133. Reconstructed Japanese encephalitis vaccine at 2–8 degrees can be stored up to how many years?
(Recent Pattern Question 2016)
a. 1　　b. 2
c. 3　　d. 4

134. True about sentinel surveillance:
(Recent Pattern Question 2016)
a. Includes notifiable cases
b. Done through evaluation of sub centre reports
c. Done by anganwadi worker
d. Increase reporting bias

135. Varicella zoster immunization is given to all; EXCEPT:
(Recent Pattern Question 2016)
a. Contacts with varicella zoster
b. To the newborn and pregnant female who was exposed 6 week before delivery
c. All HIV positive patients
d. Patients with varicella zoster

136. In a population of 5000, number of new cases of TB is 500; old cases in the same population are 150. What is the prevalence of TB:
a. 9%　　b. 12%
c. 13%　　d. 18%

137. First case which comes to the notice of investigator is:
a. Index case　　b. Initial case
c. Primary case　　d. Secondary case

138. First case in community is known as:
a. Index case　　b. Initial case
c. Primary case　　d. Secondary case

139. Quarantine is:
a. Separation for the period of communicability of infected person from others
b. Limitation of freedom of movement of well person or animals till incubation period of disease
c. Identification of source of infection and factors influencing its spread in community
d. Notification of disease to local health authority to put control measures on it

140. Disease seen all over the world:
a. Endemic　　b. Epidemic
c. Pandemic　　d. Sporadic

141. Point source epidemic is:
a. Gradual rise and gradual fall in number of cases
b. Sharp rise and sharp fall in number of cases
c. Sharp rise and fall is interrupted by secondary waves
d. Gradual rise and fall is interrupted by secondary waves

142. Period between infected host to appearance of 1st symptom
a. Incubation period　　b. Serial interval
c. Communicable period　　d. Latent period

143. Period of disease initiation to disease detection is known as:
a. Window period　　b. Generation time
c. Lead time　　d. Latent period

144. Number of live birth per 1000 women in the reproductive age is:
a. Net reproductive rate　　b. Total fertility rate
c. Gross reproduction rate　　d. General fertility rate

145. General fertility rate:
a. Average number of children born to a women in her reproductive life span
b. Annual number of live births per 1000 married women during reproductive age
c. Total number of girl child born to a female
d. Total number of boy child born to a female

146. Average number of girls born to woman experiencing current fertility pattern is denoted by:
a. Net reproductive rate　　b. Total fertility rate
c. Gross reproduction rate　　d. General fertility rate

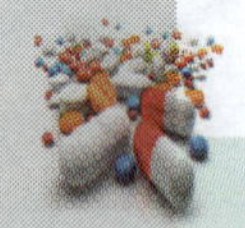

147. Maternal mortality rate is expressed as:
a. 1000 live births b. 100,000 live births
c. 1000 pregnancies d. 100 pregnancies

148. Which of the following is true about cohort study?
a. Disease to risk factor study
b. Effect to cause
c. NOT associated with attributable risk
d. Associated with antecedent causation

149. Disadvantage of case control study when compared to cohort study:
a. Easy to carry out
b. Rapid and inexpensive
c. Cannot measure cause to effect
d. Useful in rare diseases

150. Cross-sectional study is associated with:
a. Indicates prevalence b. Incidence
c. Positive predictive value d. Relative risk

151. Cohort study can determine all; EXCEPT:
a. Prevalence b. Incidence
c. Relative risk d. Exposure

152. True statement about PPV is:
a. It increases with prevalence
b. It decreases with prevalence
c. No relation with prevalence
d. Increases incidence

153. Sensitivity is used to calculate:
a. True negative b. False positive
c. True positive d. False negative

154. Components of epidemiological triad are all; EXCEPT
a. Environment b. Agent
c. Host d. Pathogenesis

155. Predictive value indicating positive test in a screening modality is calculated by:
a. TP/TP + FP × 100 b. TN/TN + FN × 100
c. TP/TP + FN × 100 d. TN/FP + TN × 100

156. Specificity formula:
a. TP/TP + FP × 100 b. TN/TN + FN × 100
c. TP/TP + FN × 100 d. TN/FP + TN × 100

157. Important "great divide year" after which the added population exceeds that of previous decade:
a. 1957 b. 1921
c. 1951 d. 1957

158. All are true about case control study; EXCEPT:
a. Attribute risk b. Measurement of exposure
c. Matching d. Odd's ratio

159. All of the following vaccines are contraindicated in pregnancy; EXCEPT:
a. Measles
b. Rubella
c. BCG
d. Tetanus

160. Yellow fever vaccination becomes effective after how many days of vaccination:
a. 5 days b. 10 days
c. 10 weeks d. 10 months

161. All of the following are true for yellow fever; EXCEPT:
a. Caused by vector aedes
b. Incubation period of 3–6 days
c. One attack gives life long immunity
d. Validity of vaccination certification begins immediately after vaccination

162. Postexposure prophylaxis schedule of rabies vaccine in a previously immunized person:
a. Day 0, 3, 7, 14, 21,90
b. Day 0, 3, 7, 14, 28, 90
c. Day 0, 3
d. Day 0, 7, 14

163. Pre-exposure schedule in rabies vaccine?
a. Day 0, 3, 7, 14, 28, 90 b. Day 0, 3, 7, 14, 21, 90
c. Day 0, 7, 28 d. Day 0, 7, 21

164. Live attenuated vaccine can be given to:
a. Children under 8 years
b. HIV patients
c. Patients on steroids
d. Patients on radiation

165. Toxoids are prepared from:
a. Exotoxins b. Biotoxins
c. Both d. None

166. Japanese encephalitis vaccine is:
a. Live attenuated b. Inactivated toxoid
c. Cellular fractions d. Combined

167. Strain of Varicella zoster vaccine is:
a. Nakayama b. DANISH 1331
c. Jeryll Lynn d. Oka

168. Reverse cold chain is used for:
a. Transportation of vaccines to laboratory to check its potency
b. Carrying stool samples of polio patients from Primary Health Centre (PHC) to laboratory
c. Transportation of outdated vaccines from PHC to district hospital
d. Transportation of vaccines from camps to sub center

169. Which of the following vaccines does not provide herd immunity:
a. Hepatitis A b. Rabies
c. Measles d. Diphtheria

170. Naranjo algorithm is used for:
a. Environmental factors effecting drug
b. Para-meteric based data evaluation
c. Calculating adverse drug reaction
d. Demographic factor affecting drugs action

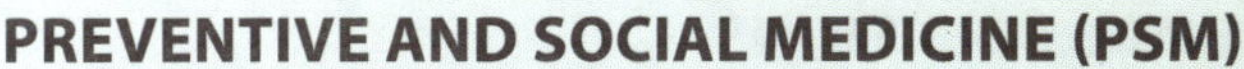

COMMUNICABLE AND NONCOMMUNICABLE DISEASE

171. All tests done before blood transfusion; EXCEPT: *(Most Recent Question June 2022)*

a. Hepatitis A
b. Hepatitis B
c. HIV 1,2
d. Hepatitis C

172. In 14th century during outbreak of plague quarantine of ship sailors was done for? *(Most Recent Question June/Dec 2021)*

a. 60 days
b. 7 days
c. 14 days
d. 40 days

173. Color coded STD kit used for female with lower abdominal pain? *(Most Recent Question June/Dec 2021)*

a. Kit 7 – black
b. Kit 5 – red
c. Kit 4 – blue
d. Kit 6 – yellow

174. A child presented with swelling on face and also with swelling in scrotum. He cannot chew properly/open mouth. This condition is possibly a complication of? *(Most Recent Question June/Dec 2021)*

a. Measles
b. Mumps
c. Rubella
d. Diphtheria

175. Causative organism of donovanosis (Granuloma inguinale) is: *(Most Recent Question June/Dec 2021)*

a. T. pallidum
b. Chlamydia trachomatis
c. Herpes simplex
d. Klebsiella granulomatis

176. Secondary/Re infection of this virus cause severe disease due to antibody response? *(Most Recent Question June/Dec 2021)*

a. Rabies virus
b. Dengue virus
c. Measles virus
d. Polio virus

177. Following disease has highest mortality after clinical manifestations develop *(Most Recent Question June/Dec 2021)*

a. H1N1 influenza
b. NIPAH
c. Ebola
d. Rabies

178. Which of the following can be transmitted trans-placentally and can cause microcephaly: *(Most Recent Question June/Dec 2021)*

a. Rubella virus
b. Zika virus
c. CMV
d. Parvo virus

179. Life cycle image of an organism is given below. Identify it. *(Most Recent Question June/Dec 2021)*

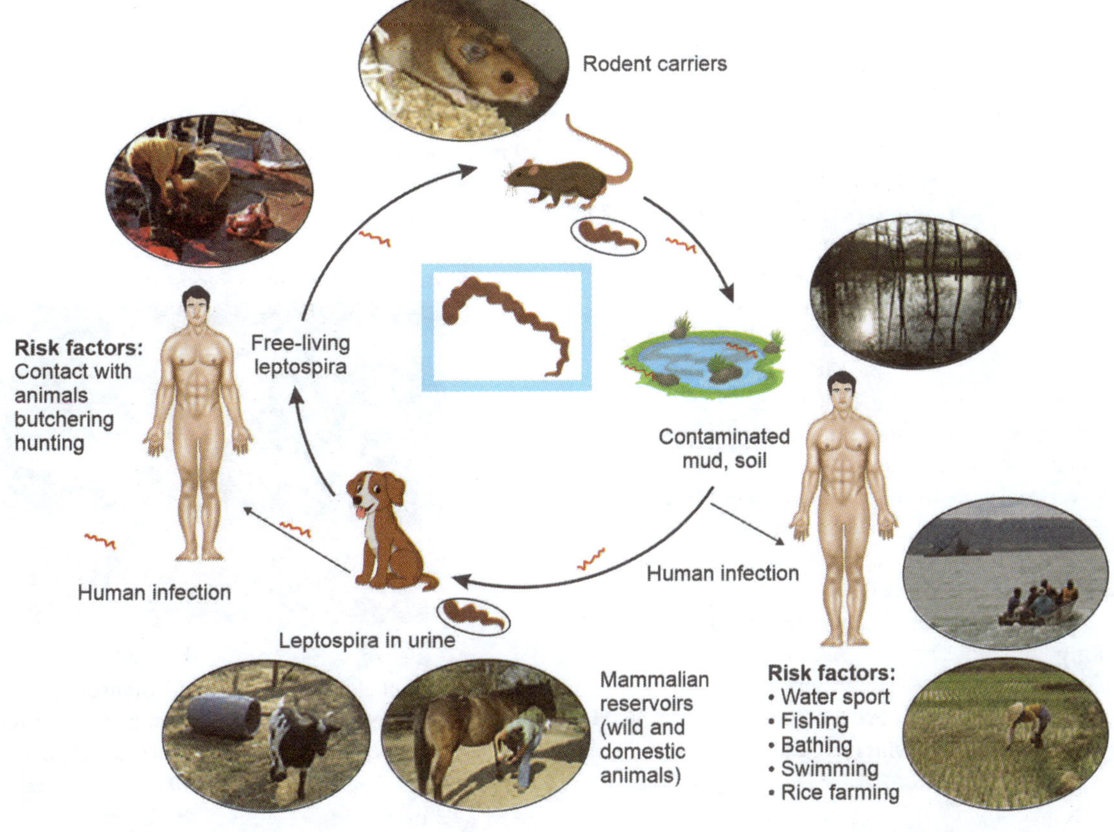

a. Hanta virus
b. Leptospirosis
c. Yersinia peptis
d. Rickettsia

180. A child reported to a PHC with runny nose and fever since last 3 days. Rash started on face and then covered the trunk. What's the most likely diagnosis? ***(Most Recent Question Aug 2020)***

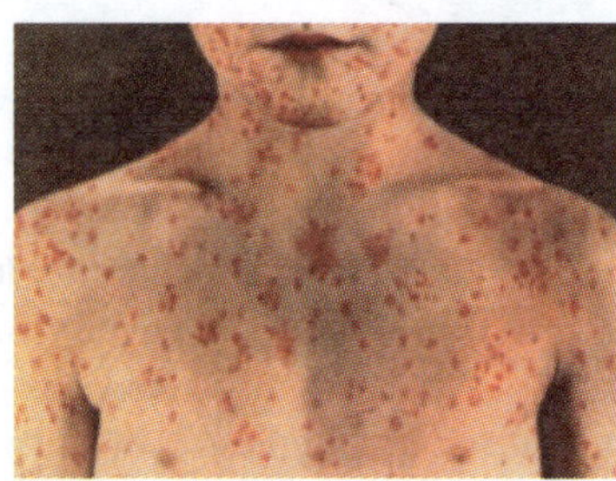

a. Measles b. Chicken pox
c. Mumps d. Rubella

181. First investigation for a suspected case of pulmonary TB: ***(Most Recent Question Aug 2020)***

a. Chest X-ray
b. Sputum smear examination
c. CBNAAT
d. Liquid culture

182. First investigation for TB diagnosis in PLHIV (Persons Living with HIV): ***(Most Recent Question Aug 2020)***

a. Chest X-ray
b. Sputum smear examination
c. CBNAAT
d. Liquid culture

183. In ORS, Sodium is given along with Glucose for: ***(Most Recent Question Aug 2020)***

a. Reducing secretions b. Osmosis
c. Facilitative diffusion d. Co-Transport

184. SARS is caused by novel variant of: ***(Most Recent Question Dec 2019-20)***

a. Pox virus b. Toga virus
c. Coronavirus d. Lyssa virus

185. STD kit color for female with vaginitis ***(Most Recent Question Dec 2019-20)***

a. Kit 1 Grey b. Kit 2 Green
c. Kit 3 White d. Kit 4 Blue

186. A health worker nurse got an accidental prick with HIV+ needle. Parameter used to test for confirmatory diagnosis is ***(Most Recent Question Dec 2019-20)***

a. ELISA b. P24 antigen
c. Western blot assay d. PCR

187. Vector of Zika virus disease is: ***(Most Recent Question Dec 2019-20)***

a. Sandfly b. Aedes aegypti
c. Culex d. Anopheles

188. A person comes with right eye 6/60 and left eye 3/60. He shall be categorized into which type of blindness? ***(Most Recent Question Dec 2019-20)***

a. Manifest b. Social
c. Economic d. No blindness

189. Disease spread by the shown vector is all; EXCEPT: ***(Most Recent Question Dec 2019-20)***

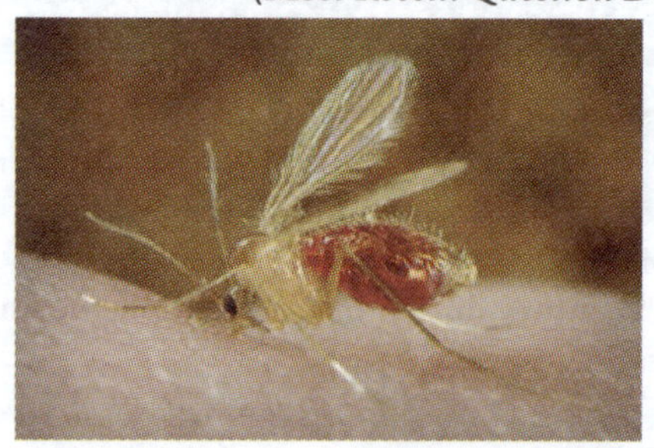

a. Kala azar b. Oriental sore
c. Chagas disease d. Cutaneous leishmania

190. N95 mask is used for: ***(Most Recent Question Dec 2019-20)***

a. Respiratory droplets b. Aerosol
c. In general d. Pollution

191. Subacute sclerosing panencephalitis is a rare and dangerous complication of:

a. Measles b. Mumps
c. Rubella d. Varicella

192. Amplifier host of Japanese encephalitis: ***(Most Recent Question 2019)***

a. Pig b. Dogs
c. Cats d. Birds

193. According to WHO, which one is a notifiable disease? ***(Most Recent Question 2019)***

a. Yellow fever b. Polio
c. Influenza d. Malaria

194. Amount of sodium in ORS as per WHO: ***(Most Recent Question 2019)***

a. 65 mmol/L b. 75 mmol/L
c. 20 mmol/L d. 100 mmol/L

195. Identify the mosquito: ***(Recent Pattern Question 2018-19)***

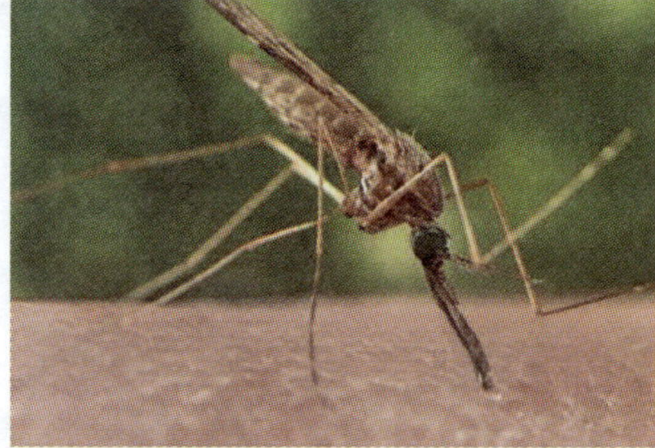

a. Culex b. Aedes
c. Anopheles d. Mansonia

196. In a case of measles, postexposure immunoglobulin can be given within how many days after exposure: ***(Recent Pattern Question 2018-19)***

a. 3 days b. 7 days
c. 10 days d. 14 days

197. In a case of cholera period of isolation is for _____days? *(Recent Pattern Question 2018-19)*

a. 7 days
b. 7–14 days
c. 3–4 weeks
d. 1–2 months

198. How much is the daily iodine requirement of a 3–5 months old child? *(Recent Pattern Question 2018-19)*

a. 150–200 mcg/day
b. 100–120 mcg/day
c. 200–400 mcg/day
d. >400 mcg/day

199. Advantage of adding zinc with ORS: *(Recent Pattern Question 2018-19)*

a. Reduces infection
b. Antispasmodic
c. Reduces duration of diarrhea
d. Enhance sodium absorption

200. Which of the following disease transmission does not require vector? *(Recent Pattern Question 2018-19)*

a. RMSF
b. Q fever
c. Scrub typhus
d. Trench fever

201. Correct about lepromin test: *(Recent Pattern Question 2018-19)*

a. Differentiates from TB
b. Example of type 2 Hypersensitivity reaction
c. Test result can be read after 24 hours
d. Classify the type of leprosy

202. Corrcct about initiating treatment in an adult patient with AIDS: *(Recent Pattern Question 2018-19)*

a. CD4 count <200/cu.mm required for initiation of treatment
b. CD4 count <350/cu.mm required for initiation of treatment
c. CD4 count <500/cu.mm required for initiation of treatment
d. No cut off of CD 4 count required for initiation of treatment

203. Cattle and sheep livestock is natural host for which of the following? *(Recent Pattern Question 2018)*

a. Crimean-Congo fever
b. Dengue
c. KFD
d. Yellow fever

204. True about chicken pox infection: *(Recent Pattern Question 2018)*

a. Centrifugal distribution
b. Centripetal distribution
c. Severe prodromal symptoms
d. Involves mainly extensor surface

205. Which is the most common clinical feature of Tularemia? *(Recent Pattern Question 2018)*

a. Fever
b. Headache
c. Lymphadenopathy
d. Diarrhea

206. Quintan fever is caused by: *(Recent Pattern Question 2018)*

a. Rickettsia typhi
b. Bartonella
c. Coxiella burnetti
d. Rickettsia conorii

207. Culex mosquito is a vector for: *(Recent Pattern Question 2018)*

a. Chikungunya fever
b. Dengue fever
c. Japanese encephalitis
d. Malaria

208. What is the color of RTI/STI kit number 6? *(Recent Pattern Question 2017)*

a. Grey
b. Yellow
c. Red
d. Black

209. Black RTI kit is used in: *(Recent Pattern Question 2017)*

a. Urogenital infection
b. Genital ulcer
c. Cervicitis
d. Inguinal bubo

210. Which cancer is preventable by vaccine? *(Recent Pattern Question 2016)*

a. Ovarian CA
b. Cervix CA
c. Breast CA
d. Uterus CA

211. Incubation period for cholera: *(Recent Pattern Question 2016)*

a. 1–7 days
b. Few hours to 5 days
c. 2 weeks
d. 4 weeks

212. All of the following are WHO notifiable diseases; EXCEPT:

a. Cholera
b. Chicken pox
c. Plague
d. Yellow fever

213. Which of the following diseases are notifiable to WHO in Geneva under the International Health Regulations?

a. Plague, polio and malaria
b. Cholera, influenza and yellow fever
c. Cholera, plague and polio
d. Cholera, plague and yellow fever

214. Chicken pox is infective:

a. 2 days before and 2 days after rash appearance
b. 2 days before and 5 days after rash appearance
c. 4 days before and 4 days after rash appearance
d. 4 days before and 5 days after rash appearance

215. Which has lowest incubation period?

a. Mumps
b. Influenza
c. Measles
d. Chicken pox

216. Nosocomial infections are those which develop:

a. 24 hours after hospitalization
b. Within 48 hours of hospitalization
c. After 48 hours of hospitalization
d. After 7 days of hospitalization

217. Cycle that is seen in RBCs in malaria:

a. Sexual
b. Sporogony
c. Exogenous
d. Endogenous

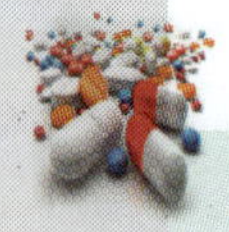

218. Following is not caused by virus:
- a. Rocky mountain spotted fever
- b. KFD
- c. Dengue
- d. Yellow fever

219. Which of the following is transmitted by mites?
- a. Endemic typhus
- b. Epidemic typhus
- c. Trench fever
- d. Scrub typhus

220. Which of the following is not transmitted by aedes mosquito:
- a. Bancroftian filariasis
- b. Yellow fever
- c. Dengue fever
- d. Chikungunya fever

221. Subacute Sclerosing Pan Encepahalitis (SSPE) is a late complication of:
- a. Measles
- b. Mumps
- c. Rubella
- d. Chickenpox

222. Spread of TB in a community or prevelance of TB infection is estimated by:
- a. Tuberculin test
- b. AFB smear
- c. Chest X-ray
- d. Mantoux test

223. Tuberculosis diagnosis in India is based on:
- a. Sputum smear microscopy
- b. Sputum culture examination
- c. Mantoux test
- d. Chest X-ray

224. Test to differentiate MTB from leprosy:
- a. AFB smear
- b. Culture
- c. Mantoux test
- d. Chest X-ray

225. Sputum positive TB patients should be isolated at least for:
- a. 2 weeks
- b. 3 weeks
- c. 4 weeks
- d. 6 weeks

226. Sputum positive patient who should be quarantined:
- a. Pregnant women
- b. Old people
- c. Children above 6 years
- d. Children below 6 years

227. Intermediate host of rabies is:
- a. Man
- b. Dog
- c. Cow
- d. Rat

228. Leptospirosis is transmitted by:
- a. Fecal oral route
- b. Aerosol route
- c. Infected rat's urine
- d. Milk

229. Single drug treatment recommended for Trachoma control in India is:
- a. Azithromycin
- b. Tetracycline
- c. Erythromycin
- d. Penicillin

230. Not a component of SAFE strategy for control of Trachoma:
- a. Surgery
- b. Antibiotics
- c. Facial cleanliness
- d. Education

231. Pneumonic plague transmission route:
- a. Mice
- b. Tick
- c. Inhalation
- d. Flea

232. Plague is transmitted by all; EXCEPT?
- a. X. Cheopsis
- b. X. Astia
- c. Pulex irritans
- d. Culex

233. Ebola virus is spread by:
- a. Tics
- b. Inhalation from person to person
- c. Air droplet
- d. Through contact of body fluids

234. A village affected with epidemic of cholera, what is the 1st step which should to be taken in the village to decrease the chances of death from cholera:
- a. Safe water supply and sanitation
- b. Cholera vaccination to all individuals
- c. Primary Chemoprophylaxis
- d. Treat everyone in the village with tetracycline

235. Reverse smoking causes:
- a. Carcinoma lip
- b. Carcinoma hard palate
- c. Carcinoma soft palate
- d. Carcinoma lung

236. Which of the following increases the risk of lung CA?
- a. Amount of smoking/day
- b. Length of cigarette
- c. Duration of smoking
- d. All of the above

NATIONAL HEALTH PROGRAMS & POLICIES

237. All health care providers are working at village level; EXCEPT? *(Most Recent Question June 2022)*
- a. ANM
- b. AWW
- c. Trained Dais
- d. ASHA

238. Which of the following is a home-based pregnancy test kit provided by GOI *(Most Recent Question June/Dec 2021)*
- a. NIKSHAY
- b. NISCHAY
- c. Free days
- d. Nayi pahel

239. In rural areas, patients don't have insurance. But under ESI, registered medical practitioners can give the following service to the beneficiary? *(Most Recent Question June/Dec 2021)*
- a. Sickness benefit
- b. Direct pattern medical benefit
- c. Indirect pattern medical benefit
- d. Extended sickness benefit

240. WHO definition of blindness is: *(Most Recent Question Aug 2020)*
- a. <1/60 in better eye
- b. <1/60 in worse eye
- c. <3/60 in better eye
- d. <3/60 in worse eye

241. If you are posted as a Medical officer in an area under NVBDCP, and you will be advised to spray Malathion for malaria prophylaxis. What could be the probable decision you will take regarding frequency of Malathion spray? *(Most Recent Question Aug 2020)*

a. Once very fortnight
b. Once every 3 months
c. Twice every 3 months
d. Once every month

242. A country is developing an outbreak of a notifiable disease. What's the probable time within which one should report it to WHO? *(Most Recent Question Aug 2020)*

a. 6 hours b. 12 hours
c. 24 hours d. 48 hours

243. Training is given to an ANM worker. Now you have to check her ability to do immunization. You are the medical officer. She is having cotton, lunch box and syringe-needle after immunization of a child. Which of the following is true about their disposal? *(Most Recent Question Dec 2019-20)*

a. Syringe with needle in translucent black container
b. Used vial in translucent white container
c. Cotton swab in Yellow bag
d. Food waste in blue box

244. One ASHA worker in rural areas is designated for how much population? *(Most Recent Question Dec 2019-20)*

a. 1000 b. 3000
c. 5000 d. 2000

245. Under ESI, after certification by Medical Officer, Beneficiaries get 70% wages for 3 months under *(Most Recent Question Dec 2019-20)*

a. Medical benefit b. Sickness benefit
c. Disablement benefit d. Dependents' benefit

246. Which of the following are included in NPCDCS? *(Most Recent Question Dec 2019-20)*

a. Bronchial asthma, Hypertension, CVD
b. Diabetes, hypertension, Bronchial asthma
c. CVD, Diabetes, bronchial asthma
d. CVD, Cancer, Diabetes, Stroke

247. Which of the following is not correct about Urban Malaria scheme? *(Recent Pattern Question 2018-19)*

a. Comprise vector control by intensive Anti-larval measure
b. Includes all urban areas with more than 50,000 population
c. Areas with annual parasite index of 2 are included
d. Includes area with slide positivity of more than 10 cases per 10,000 smears

248. Blood smear for malaria is collected by: *(Recent Pattern Question 2018-19)*

a. Male MPW b. Medical officer
c. ASHA d. Health assistant

249. Sputum for AFB is collected at village level by: *(Recent Pattern Question 2018-19)*

a. Medical officer b. Anganwadi worker
c. Health worker male d. Health assistant

250. Active surveillance of malaria is done by: *(Recent Pattern Question 2018-19)*

a. Anganwadi workers b. Multipurpose worker
c. ASHA d. Medical officer

251. Suraksha clinic is for: *(Recent Pattern Question 2018-19)*

a. NVBDCP b. RTI/STD
c. Blood transfusion safety d. Women safety

252. Ujjawala Scheme is for: *(Recent Pattern Question 2018-19)*

a. Drug abuser rehabilitation
b. Blind persons rehabilitation
c. Online tracking of AIDS positive patients
d. Child trafficking

253. Under vision 2020: In a school eye screening program, a teacher checks vision of a student will refer to which centre: *(Recent Pattern Question 2018-19)*

a. Service centre b. Training centre
c. Centre for excellence d. Vision centre

254. HIV sentinel surveillance not done in which population? *(Recent Pattern Question 2018-19)*

a. Migrant labourer b. Street children
c. Truck driver d. Transgenders

255. Programs included in NRHM is/are: *(Recent Pattern Question 2018)*

a. National vector borne disease control program
b. Revised national tuberculosis control program
c. Iodine deficiency disorder control program
d. All of the above

256. Which of the following is not emphasized in school health services? *(Recent Pattern Question 2018)*

a. Dental caries b. Infectious diseases
c. Malnutrition d. Lung infections

257. Which of the following is not the work responsibility of ASHA? *(Recent Pattern Question 2018)*

a. Immunization and contraception counseling
b. Delivery at home
c. Provide primary medical care for minor ailments
d. Promote construction of household toilets

258. True about incentives given to ASHA worker in Janani Suraksha Yojna: *(Recent Pattern Question 2018)*

a. 400 INR to ASHA and 1000 INR to mother in rural area in high performing states
b. 400 INR to ASHA and 1000 INR to mother in rural area in low performing states
c. 400 INR to ASHA and 1000 INR to mother in urban area high performing states
d. 400 INR to ASHA and 1000 INR to mother in Urban area low performing states

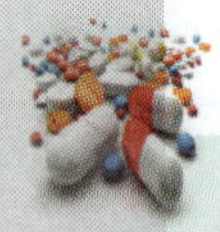

259. An IQ of 55 comes in which category: ***(Recent Pattern Question 2017)***

a. Profound b. Mild
c. Moderate d. Idiot

260. 1 male health worker, 1 female health worker should be present at each PHC. This is given by which committee? ***(Recent Pattern Question 2016)***

a. Jungalwalla Committee
b. Kartar Singh Committee
c. Bhore Committee
d. Mudaliar Committee

261. All are true about national mental heath program; EXCEPT:

a. Inpatient service b. Outpatient service
c. Complete hospitalization d. Emergency service

262. Regarding mental health program, which statement is true?

a. Started in 1951 b. Started in 1987
c. Started in 1987 d. Started in 1999

263. Cafeteria approach is related with which of the following?

a. National rural health mission
b. National surveillance program for communicable diseases
c. Reproductive and child health program
d. National vector borne disease control programme

264. Maximum recommended number of students in a school class room:

a. 30 b. 35
c. 40 d. 50

265. NOT included in immunization schedule:

a. Kala-azar b. Polio
c. Hepatitis d. BCG

266. In national vector borne disease control program which disease is not included?

a. Malaria b. Yellow fever
c. Japanese encephalitis d. Kala-azar

PREVENTIVE OBSTETRICS, PEDIATRICS AND GERIATRICS

267. Maternal death according to WHO is: ***(Most Recent Question June 2022)***

a. Antenatal to 2 weeks after delivery
b. Antenatal to 6 weeks after delivery
c. Delivery to 6 weeks post partum
d. Delivery to 2 weeks post partum

268. Most common cause of blindness among children in India: ***(Most Recent Question June/Dec 2021)***

a. Cataract b. Glaucoma
c. Vitamin A deficiency d. Refractive errors

269. Minimum antenatal visits according to WHO: ***(Most Recent Question June/Dec 2021)***

a. 10 b. 8
c. 4 d. 5

270. To prevent neural tube defect in a woman with history of NTD, dose of folic acid to be given to woman is: ***(Most Recent Question June/Dec 2021)***

a. 0.1 mg b. 0.4 mg
c. 1 mg d. 4 mg

271. Vitamin K at birth is given to prevent: ***(Most Recent Question June/Dec 2021)***

a. Hypocalcemia
b. Hypokalemia
c. Anemia
d. Hemorrhagic disease of newborn

272. All are true about colostrum; EXCEPT: ***(Most Recent Question June/Dec 2021)***

a. Contain High sugar and fat
b. Thick and yellow color (deep lemon color)
c. Has High IgA
d. Has High amino acids and minerals

273. For a pregnant female, minimum number of antenatal visits required are: ***(Most Recent Question Aug 2020)***

a. 3 b. 4
c. 5 d. 6

274. Breast feeding should be continued for minimum how many months? ***(Most Recent Question Dec 2019-20)***

a. 6 months b. 2 months
c. 12 months d. 5 months

275. Which test is done at sub centre during pregnancy? ***(Most Recent Question 2019)***

a. USG b. Haemoglobin
c. OGTT d. Triple test

276. For doctor to practise MTP minimum number of MTP to be performed is ***(Recent Pattern Question 2018-19)***

a. 10 b. 25
c. 50 d. 100

277. How much additional calories per day is required in a pregnant lady: ***(Recent Pattern Question 2018-19)***

a. 350 kcal b. 550 kcal
c. 650 kcal d. 520 kcal

278. Most common cause of LBW in India: ***(Recent Pattern Question 2018-19)***

a. Short gestational age
b. Intrauterine growth retardation
c. Maternal diabetes mellitus
d. Genetic cause

279. According to WHO, all are true about reduced osmolarity ORS (in mmol/L); EXCEPT: ***(Recent Pattern Question 2018)***

a. Glucose – 90 b. Na – 75
c. Potassium – 20 d. Citrate – 10

280. Iron required in lactation: *(Recent Pattern Question 2017)*
a. 300 mg/day b. 400 mg/day
c. 20 mg/day d. 100 mg/day

281. Total calories (kcal/day) required for a Female with sedentary activity: *(Recent Pattern Question 2017)*
a. 1900 b. 2200
c. 2500 d. 2800

282. Total osmolarity of reduced osmolality ORS: *(Recent Pattern Question 2017)*
a. 215 mmol/L b. 220 mmol/L
c. 225 mmol/L d. 245 mmol/L

283. Most common indirect cause of maternal mortality:
a. Anemia b. Sepsis
c. Hemorrhage d. Obstructed labor

284. Obstetric care will mostly affect:
a. Infant mortality rate
b. Early neonatal mortality rate
c. Late neonatal mortality rate
d. Perinatal mortality rate

285. Registration of birth should be done:
a. Within 15 days b. After 21 days
c. Before 21 days d. Within 30 days

286. According to Integrated Management of Neonatal And Childhood Illness, color used in triage for home management
a. Red b. Green
c. Black d. Yellow

287. Best agent for diarrhea is:
a. Cotrimoxazole b. Metronidazole
c. ORS d. Ringer lactate

288. Exclusive breast feeding is up to:
a. 6 weeks b. 6 months
c. 9 Months d. 1 year

289. Infant mortality rate does not include:
a. Post neonatal mortality b. Early neonatal mortality
c. Perinatal mortality d. Late neonatal mortality

NUTRITION AND HEALTH

290. A 30-year-old male is presents with chief complains of diarrhea, ascites, knee edema. He reports that his family eats food cooked with mustard oil. Identify the condition? *(Most Recent Question June 2022)*
a. Neurolathyrism b. Epidemic dropsy
c. Endemic ascites d. Alfatoxicosis

291. People of a community are consuming Khesari Dal for last few years. Lathyrism prevention step in community are all; EXCEPT: *(Most Recent Question June 2022)*
a. DEC b. Ban the crop
c. Vitamin C d. Toxin removal

292. Which nutrient is deficient in breast milk? *(Most Recent Question June 2022)*
a. Vitamin A b. Vitamin K
c. Vitamin B d. Pantothenic acid

293. High content of sodium is found in: *(Most Recent Question June/Dec 2021)*
a. Cereals b. Green leafy vegetables
c. Loaf of bread d. Conned soup

294. Which of the following food has the lowest glycemic index? *(Most Recent Question June/Dec 2021)*
a. Papaya b. Potato
c. Sweet corn d. Watermelon

295. A maize eater case presents with dermatitis diarrhea. Mental issues present. Diagnosis is? *(Most Recent Question June/Dec 2021)*
a. Riboflavin deficiency
b. Thiamine deficiency (beri beri)
c. Pellagra
d. Osteomalacia

296. Poor man with gum bleeding as shown in image. This is seen due to deficiency of: *(Most Recent Question June/Dec 2021)*

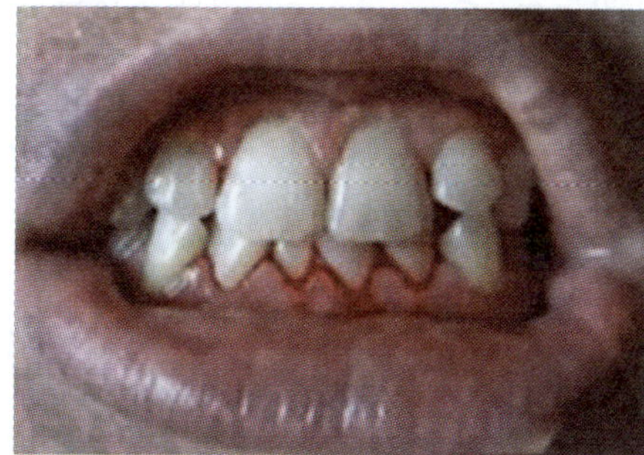

a. Vitamin A b. Vitamin C
c. Vitamin E d. Vitamin D

297. Highest thermic effect is seen in *(Most Recent Question June/Dec 2021)*
a. Carbohydrate diet b. Protein diet
c. Fat diet d. Vitamin diet

298. Least Iron content is present in: *(Most Recent Question Aug 2020)*
a. Beans b. Milk
c. Spinach d. Liver

299. Best index for calculation of nutrient value of protein *(Most Recent Question 2019)*
a. Serum albumin concentration
b. Arm-muscle circumference
c. Creatinine-height index
d. Serum transferrin level

300. Best index for measurement health indicator in society: *(Most Recent Question 2019)*
a. Under 5 mortality rate b. Infant mortality rate
c. Child death rate d. Maternal mortality rate

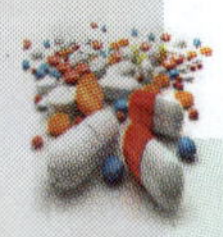

301. Which of these has the max natural source of vitamin A? *(Most Recent Question 2019)*
a. Carrot
b. Halibut liver oil
c. Cod fish oil
d. Cow milk

302. According to WHO, marker for obesity index is: *(Most Recent Question 2019)*
a. Quetelet index
b. Chandler index
c. Pearl index
d. Sullivan's index

303. As compared to cow milk, the protein content of human milk is:
a. 3–4 times more than cow milk
b. 3–4 times less than cow milk
c. Double than cow milk
d. Same as cow milk

304. Nowadays which is the most common pasteurization method? *(Most Recent Question 2019)*
a. Holder (vat) method
b. Ultra high temperature method
c. High temperature and short time method
d. Low temperature and long time method

305. Waist to hip ratio that increases risk of cardiovascular disease is: *(Recent Pattern Question 2018-19)*
a. >0.80 in male
b. >0.80 in female
c. >0.85 in male
d. >0.85 in female

306. Which of the following food adulteration can lead to beriberi? *(Recent Pattern Question 2018-19)*
a. Maize
b. Sorghum
c. Undermilled rice
d. Polished rice

307. True about low glycemic index food: *(Recent Pattern Question 2018-19)*
a. Reduced peak and rapid absorption
b. Reduced peak and prolonged absorption
c. High peak and fast absorption
d. High peak and prolong absorption

308. The glycemic index for glucose is: *(Recent Pattern Question 2018)*
a. 0.5
b. 1
c. 1.5
d. 2

309. Plant source with highest protein: *(Recent Pattern Question 2017)*
a. Black gram
b. Dry peas
c. Soyabean
d. Bengal gram

310. What is the dose of iron and folic acid given till 5 years? *(Recent Pattern Question 2017)*
a. 20 mg iron with 0.1 mg FA
b. 20 mg iron with 0.2 mg FA
c. 50 mg iron with 0.5 mg FA
d. 100 mg iron with 0.5 mg FA

311. Total calories (kcal/day) required for a male with moderate activity *(Recent Pattern Question 2017)*
a. 2230
b. 2730
c. 2900
d. 3500

312. How many calories are there in 100 mL breast milk? *(Recent Pattern Question 2017)*
a. 65
b. 75
c. 80
d. 100–110

313. RDA Vitamin B12 in pregnancy: *(Recent Pattern Question 2017)*
a. 1.2 mcg
b. 1.5 mcg
c. 0.8 mcg
d. 0.2 mcg

314. Epidemic dropsy is caused by this toxin: *(Recent Pattern Question 2016)*
a. BOAA
b. Sanguinarine
c. Alkaloid
d. Ergot

315. In first 6 months of lactation how much extra calories are required by the lactating mother?
a. 150 kcal
b. 350 kcal
c. 600 kcal
d. 650 kcal

316. All of the following statements are true with regard to a reference Indian adult woman; EXCEPT:
a. She is healthy
b. She is between 20–39 years of age
c. She may be engaged in 8 hours of moderately active work in a day
d. She weighs 60 kg

317. In Xeropthalmia, what is X1B:
a. Conjunctival xerosis
b. Bitot's spot
c. Corneal xerosis
d. Corneal ulcer

318. Secondary sign noted for xerophthalmia according to WHO:
a. Conjuctival xerosis
b. Corneal xerosis
c. Bitot spots
d. Night blindness

319. Xerophthalmia is a public health problem if bitot's spot incidence is:
a. 0.1%
b. 1%
c. 0.5%
d. 5%

320. According to prevalence criteria for determining xerophthalmia problems given by WHO, following are true for an endemic area:
a. Bitot spot 5% poluation of under 6 years
b. Conjuctival xerosis 1%
c. Conjuctival ulcers 0.05%
d. Night blindness 1%

321. Trace element is what percent of bodyweight:
a. 0.001%
b. 0.01%
c. 0.1%
d. 1%

322. Protein daily requirement is:
a. <1 g/kg
b. 2 g/kg
c. 3 g/kg
d. 4 g/kg

323. Which of the following vitamin is not an antioxidant?
a. Vitamin A
b. Vitamin B
c. Vitamin C
d. Vitamin E

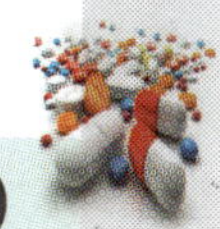

324. Pellagra is caused by deficiency of:
a. Thiamine
b. Niacin
c. Biotin
d. Ascorbic acid

325. All are features of kwashiorkor; EXCEPT:
a. Irritability b. Edema in lower limb
c. Increase appetite d. Apathy

326. Toxin of epidemic dropsy is:
a. BOAA b. Sanguinarine
c. Alkaloid d. Ergot

327. All are tests of pasteurization of milk efficiency; EXCEPT:
a. Methylene blue reductase test
b. Phosphatase test
c. Standard plate count
d. Coliform count

328. Refrigerated breast milk can be kept for:
a. 6 hours b. 10 hours
c. 12 hours d. 24 hours

329. Methionine is a limiting amino acid in:
a. Cereals b. Maize
c. Wheat d. Pulses

330. What is the biological value of egg protein?
a. 80 b. 90
c. 100 d. 120

331. Vitamin D is high in:
a. Human milk b. Cow's milk
c. Green vegetables d. Egg

332. Which of the following is a rich source of vitamin D?
a. Milk b. Shark liver oil
c. Halibut liver oil d. Cod liver oil

333. Vitamin D is found in:
a. Iron b. Milk
c. Meat d. Fish liver oil

334. Physiologically most active form of vitamin D is:
a. Calciferol b. Calcidiol
c. Ergocalciferol d. Calcitriol

335. Most essential fatty acid is:
a. Linoleic acid b. Linolenic acid
c. Arachidonic acid d. All of the above

336. All are essential fatty acids; EXCEPT:
a. Linoleic acid b. Linolenic acid
c. Arachidonic acid d. Glutamic acid

337. Hypothyroidism is associated with deficiency of:
a. Iron b. Iodine
c. Zinc d. Fluorine

338. Chronic malnutrition is assessed by:
a. Weight/height
b. Height/age
c. Weight/age
d. Mid arm circumference

ENVIRONMENT AND HEALTH

339. Association between Social factors and disease causation is described by: *(Most Recent Question June 2022)*
a. Sociology b. Social pathology
c. Society d. Culture

340. People went camping for a week. Best method of disposal of waste: *(Most Recent Question June 2022)*
a. Compositing b. Dumping
c. Burial d. Manure pit

341. A couple brought their son to the doctor. They were worried because their son likes to eat food from multinational companies. What will we call this shift from consumption of traditional natural foods to western fast foods? *(Most Recent Question June/Dec 2021)*
a. Food transition b. Social pathology
c. Acculturation d. Demographic change

342. Rabies -free state in India is: *(Most Recent Question Dec 2019-20)*
a. Sikkim
b. Jammu and Kashmir
c. Andaman and Nicobar islands
d. Rajasthan

343. Urban HEART is: *(Most Recent Question Dec 2019-20)*
a. Urban Health Equity Assessment and Response Tool
b. Urban Health evaluation Assessment and response Tool
c. Urban health Equity Assessment and Response Technique
d. Urban Health Evaluation Assessment and Response Technique

344. Horrock's apparatus is used for: *(Recent Pattern Question 2018)*
a. Measuring the hardness of water
b. Surveillance of drinking water quality
c. Calculating bleaching powder dose for water disinfection
d. Calculating mid arm circumference in malnutrition

345. Hospital infection is known as *(Recent Pattern Question 2016)*
a. Opportunistic infection
b. Nosocomial infection
c. Viral infection
d. Health care infection

346. For hookworm to be a major public health problem, chandler's index should be more than:
a. 100 b. 200
c. 250 d. 300

347. Chandler's index is:
a. Number of hookworm larva per gram of stool
b. Number of hookworm eggs per gram of stool
c. Number of hookworm per gram of stool
d. Number of E. coli in a water sample

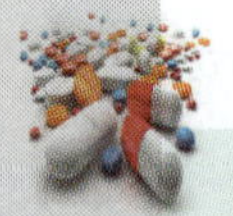

348. Chandler's index is associated with:
a. Hook worm b. Pin worm
c. Round worm d. Guinea worm

349. Soiling index is used to monitor:
a. Water pollution b. Air pollution
c. Soil pollution d. All of the above

350. The indicator agents to determine fecal pollution of drinking water is:
a. Proteus species
b. Coagulase-negative staphylococcus
c. Klebsieila species
d. E. coli

351. In India, at least how many meters away the sanitary well should be located from likely source of contamination:
a. 10 meters b. 15 meters
c. 50 meters d. 75 meters

FAMILY PLANNING AND CONTRACEPTION

352. What is the content present in given contraceptive image? ***(Most Recent Question June 2022)***

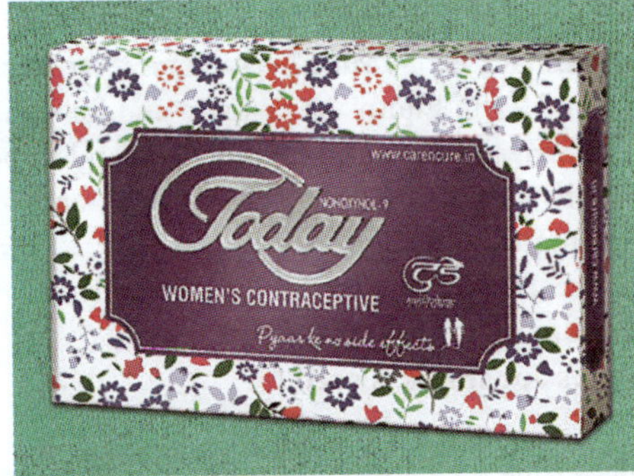

a. LNG b. Ethinyl estradiol
c. Nonoxynol 9 d. EE+LNG

353. After 6 weeks delivery, a P1L1 females desires contraception for at least 3 years. Which one is the best option? ***(Most Recent Question June 2022)***
a. POP b. OCP
c. Copper T d. Condom

354. Which of the following is NOT an Absolute contraindication of IUD: ***(Most Recent Question June/Dec 2021)***
a. Unexplained uterine bleeding
b. Previous ectopic pregnancy history
c. PID
d. Small size fibroid

355. All are true about vasectomy (NSV); EXCEPT: ***(Most Recent Question June/Dec 2021)***
a. Recanalization possible
b. Use contraceptive for 3 months
c. Sterility soon after vasectomy
d. Permanent method of contraception

356. Identify the contraceptive shown in the photograph given below: ***(Most Recent Question Aug 2020)***

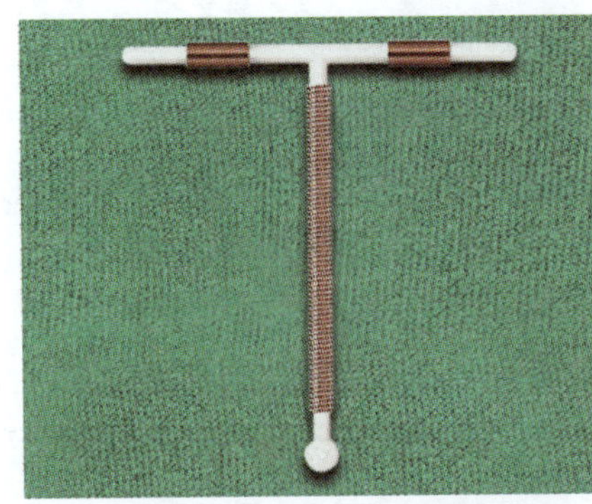

a. CuT 7 b. CuT220B
c. CuT 380A d. NOVA-T

357. A male underwent Vasectomy and after 3 months his wife got pregnant. What advice should have been given to him post-vasectomy? ***(Most Recent Question Aug 2020)***
a. Abstinence for 3 months after the procedure
b. Usage of barrier methods for 3 months after the procedure
c. OCPs usage for 1 month
d. Female condom usage for 1 months

358. A women who is lactating came to OPD 6 weeks after delivery, for check -up and to get advice for the contraception. Which of the following is not advised? ***(Most Recent Question Dec 2019-20)***
a. Combined OCP b. Norplant
c. IUCD d. Mini pill

359. A 22 years old low socioeconomic female worker present within 8 hours of sexual assault on 13th day of cycle and asked for emergency contraception. What will be your advice? ***(Most Recent Question Dec 2019-20)***
a. LNG 1.5 milligram
b. Misoprostol 800 mcg stat
c. Mifepristone 3 doses
d. OCP from 1st day of next cycle

360. Spermicidal cream which is used in contraceptives: ***(Most Recent Question Dec 2019-20)***
a. Gossypol b. Nonoxynol – 9
c. Centchroman d. Clomiphene

361. Target couple is: ***(Most Recent Question Dec 2019-20)***
a. Couple with 3 children
b. Couple using contraception
c. Currently married couple where the wife is in reproductive age (15-49 year)
d. Couple that is eligible for practicing family planning

362. Highest Contraceptive failure: ***(Recent Pattern Question 2018-19)***
a. Implant b. IUCD
c. Spermicide d. OCP

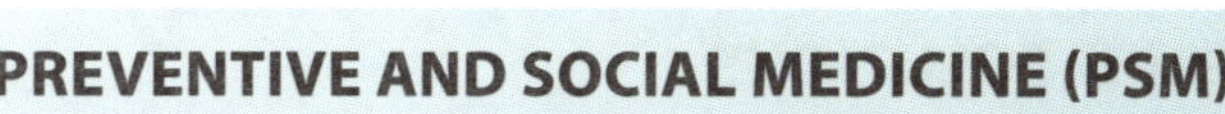

363. Unmet need for contraceptive means:
- a. Contraception desired ***(Recent Pattern Question 2018)***
- b. Sexually inactive female
- c. Family planning in those who are not using any contraception
- d. Women younger than 25 years

364. Definition of pearl index is: ***(Recent Pattern Question 2017)***
- a. Failure rate in 100 couple
- b. Failure rate in 1000 couple
- c. Failures per 100 women years of exposure
- d. Failures per 1000 women years of exposure

365. 100 females used contraceptive for 1 year. There is 1 failure (HWY). How much is the accidental pregnancy rate? ***(Recent Pattern Question 2017)***
- a. 0.01
- b. 1
- c. 1.5
- d. 2.0

366. Best contraceptive for a lactating female:
- a. Barrier
- b. Triphasic pill
- c. Combined OCP
- d. Progesterone only pill

367. Mechanism of action of combined OCP pills:
- a. Prevent fertilization
- b. Prevent release of ovum from ovary
- c. Prevent implantation of fertilized ovum
- d. Reduce sperm motility

368. OCPs give protection against:
- a. STDs
- b. Breast cancer
- c. Ovarian cancer
- d. Hepatocellular carcinoma

369. Best time to screen in Breast self examination (BSE) technique is:
- a. Just before the menstruation
- b. Just after the menstruation
- c. During ovulation
- d. 2–3 days post-ovulation

370. True about pearl index:
- a. Population study
- b. Family planning
- c. Contraceptive methods
- d. Contraceptive failure

371. Failure rate of pomoroy's technique of sterilization?
- a. 0.1%
- b. 0.5%
- c. 1%
- d. 5%

DEMOGRAPHY AND HEALTH

372. Identify image ***(Most Recent Question June 2022)***

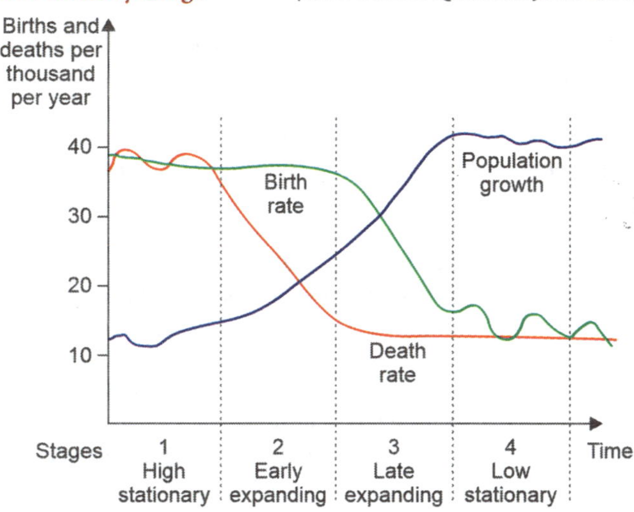

- a. Population cycle
- b. Demographic transition model
- c. Disaster management cycle
- d. Planning cycle

373. In a European country birth rate is below death rate with no population addition (no new birth is reported but deaths are continuously happening) what does it indicate? ***(Most Recent Question June 2022)***
- a. Low stationary
- b. High stationary
- c. Declining
- d. Late expanding

374. True statement with respect to population pyramid ***(Most Recent Question June 2022)***
- a. As the height increases life expectancy decreases
- b. Base denotes fertility
- c. Broad base means more no of working population
- d. Middle part indicates > male than females

375. In a population of 10000 the sex ratio is more than 1000. What is the correct option from below? ***(Most Recent Question June/Dec 2021)***
- a. Males less than 5000
- b. Females less than 5000
- c. Males less than 500
- d. Females more than 500

376. A married couple has 1 child birth recently. They belong to which phase of family cycle? ***(Most Recent Question June/Dec 2021)***
- a. Formation
- b. Extension
- c. Complete extension
- d. Contraction

377. Registration of births to married couples on state and national levels is done by?
- a. Census ***(Most Recent Question June/Dec 2021)***
- b. National family health survey
- c. Civil registration system
- d. National medical commission

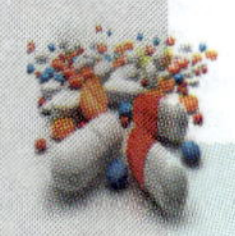

378. Mid-year population is taken on: *(Most Recent Question Aug 2020)*

a. 1st September b. 1st November
c. 1st April d. 1st July

379. Which of the following is NOT constrained by Time or existing resources? *(Most Recent Question Aug 2020)*

a. Vision b. Target
c. Goal d. Mission

380. Delphi technique used for collective opinion of: *(Most Recent Question Aug 2020)*

a. Population b. Group
c. Community d. Individual

381. Sustainable development goals is designed by: *(Most Recent Question Dec 2019-20)*

a. UNICEF b. United Nations
c. WHO d. Government of India

382. Death registration has to be done in: *(Recent Pattern Question 2018-19)*

a. 7 days b. 14 days
c. 21 days d. 28 days

383. Which of the following is true about population attributable risk: *(Recent Pattern Question 2018-19)*

a. $\text{PAR} = \dfrac{\text{Incidence among exposed}}{\text{Incidence among non-exposed}}$

b. $\text{PAR} = \dfrac{\text{Incidence among exposed-incidence among non exposed}}{\text{Incidence among exposed}} \times 100$

c. $\text{PAR} = \dfrac{\text{Incidence among non-exposed} - \text{incidence among exposed}}{\text{Incidence among total population}} \times 100$

d. $\text{PAR} = \dfrac{\text{Incidence among total population} - \text{incidence among non-exposed}}{\text{Incidence among total population}} \times 100$

384. In which of the following mortality is considered: *(Recent Pattern Question 2018-19)*

a. Total fertility rate
b. Net reproduction rate
c. Gross reproduction rate
d. General fertility rate

385. Birth rate reduced and death rate reduced. Population is in which stage: *(Recent Pattern Question 2017)*

a. 1 b. 2
c. 4 d. 5

386. Which is not a demographic indicator? *(Recent Pattern Question 2016)*

a. Social Mobility
b. Mortality
c. Life expectancy
d. Emigration

387. Numerator of dependency ratio is:

a. Population >10 years and <65 years
b. Population <15 years and >65 years
c. Population < 10 years- and >60 years
d. Population >15 years and >60 years

388. Age pyramid of India is:

a. Broad at base and narrow at apex
b. Broad from base to apex
c. Broad at apex and narrow at base
d. Spindle shaped

389. All of the following are true regarding confounding factor; EXCEPT:

a. It is associated with exposure under investigation
b. It is distributed equally in study and control groups
c. It is associated both with exposure and disease
d. It is removed by matching in case control study

390. Area under standard normal curve on area between two standard deviation on either side of mean is:

a. 68.3% b. 85.2%
c. 95.4% d. 99.7%

391. In a standard, normal curve, between three standard deviations on either side of mean will cover approximately

a. 68.3% values b. 94.2% values
c. 95.4% values d. 99.7% values

392. Growth curve of country like India, true is:

a. Tapering at top b. Tapering at bottom
c. Bulging in middle d. Widening of base

393. Range of kuppu swami scale for upper middle class:

a. 26–29 b. 16–25
c. 16–26 d. 26–30

DISASTER MANAGEMENT, DISINFECTION AND BMW MANAGEMENT

394. Blood bag is discarded in which color bag? *(Most Recent Question June 2022)*

a. Red b. Yellow
c. White d. Blue

395. Which colored bag is used to dispose cotton swab contaminated with blood? *(Most Recent Question June/Dec 2021)*

a. Black b. Red
c. Blue d. Yellow

396. In a train accident there were 74 dead, 64 were severely injured, 20 moderately injured and 32 mildly injured. Color coding in Triage highest to lowest category is: *(Most Recent Question Aug 2020)*

a. Green – Yellow -Red – Black
b. Black – Red – Yellow – Green
c. Black – yellow – Red – Green
d. Red – Yellow – Green – Black

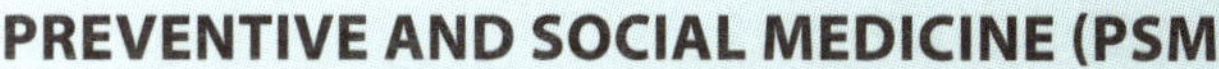

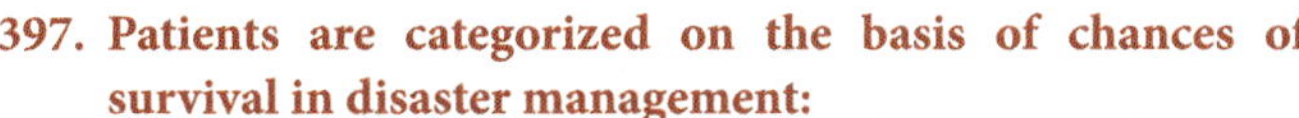

397. Patients are categorized on the basis of chances of survival in disaster management:
(Most Recent Question Dec 2019-20)
a. Triage b. Tagging
c. Mitigation d. Surge capacity

398. Most common reported disease in post disaster period:
(Most Recent Question 2019)
a. Acute gastroenteritis
b. Pneumonia
c. Leptospirosis
d. Malnutrition

399. Best method for waste disposal when suitable land available: *(Recent Pattern Question 2018-19)*
a. Burial b. Dumping
c. Controlled tipping d. Composting

400. Human anatomical wastes are disposed of in a ______ bag? *(Recent Pattern Question 2018-19)*
a. Yellow b. Red
c. Black d. Blue

401. Most important step to be taken before disaster:
(Recent Pattern Question 2018-19)
a. Response and rehabilitation
b. Response and mitigation
c. Response and preparedness
d. Mitigation and preparedness

402. First step to be taken postdisaster:
(Recent Pattern Question 2018-19)
a. Response and mitigation
b. Response and rehabilitation
c. Reconstruction and mitigation
d. Mitigation and preparedness

403. Which ministry will be responsible for rehabilitation postdisaster? *(Recent Pattern Question 2018-19)*
a. Ministry of HRD
b. Ministry of Home affairs
c. Ministry of Agriculture
d. Ministry of water and forest

404. In a triage black color is for:
(Recent Pattern Question 2018)
a. Immediate resuscitation required
b. Ambulatory patients
c. Unsalvageable
d. Highest priority patients

405. Body fluids and fetuses are classified under this category of waste: *(Recent Pattern Question 2018)*
a. Infectious waste b. Pathological waste
c. Genotoxic waste d. Humanized waste

406. Disaster management day:
a. 2nd week of November b. 2nd week of October
c. 4th week of October d. 4th week of November

407. Who will be in-charge in case of disaster management?
a. PHC b. Sub centre
c. CHC d. District hospital

408. During massive disaster what should be done first:
a. Search and rescue, first aid
b. Triage
c. Stabilization of victims
d. Hospital treatment and redistribution of patients to hospitals if necessary

409. In a disaster management triage, patients who need surgery within 24 hours, are categorized under which color category:
a. Red b. Green
c. Yellow d. Black

410. Which is the color of highest priority in emergency triage?
a. Red b. Yellow
c. Black d. White

411. Gamma rays are used for sterilization of:
a. Catheters b. Canulas
c. Syringes d. All of the above

412. Autoclaving is not useful for disposal of:
a. Surgical dressings b. Metallic instruments
c. Petri dishes d. Liquid paraffin

413. Hot air oven can be used to sterilize all; EXCEPT:
a. Scalpels
b. Glassware
c. Plastic Syringes
d. Dressings

HEALTH PLANNING, CARE AND MANAGEMENT IN INDIA

414. All facilities provided at CHC; EXCEPT:
(Most Recent Question June 2022)
a. Specialist present like surgeon
b. Blood storage facility present
c. 1st referral unit
d. Intensive neonatal unit

415. A woman 25–45 years, 8th pass, married/divorced belongs to the same village community, with well communication skill/leadership quality. Selected by village personnel. She is eligible to work as:
(Most Recent Question June/Dec 2021)
a. Trained dai
b. Anganwadi worker
c. Accredited social health activist
d. Auxiliary midwife

416. For the population of 10,000, trench method sanitary landfill pit of depth 2 meter is to be constructed. How much land area is required per year?
(Most Recent Question June/Dec 2021)
a. 4 acres b. 3 acres
c. 2 acres d. 1 acre

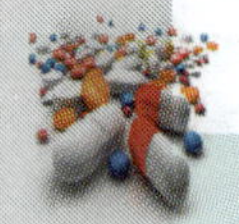

417. NITI Aayog has replaced:
(Most Recent Question Dec 2019-20)
a. National Board of Examinations (NBE)
b. National Institute of Health and Family welfare (NIHFW)
c. Medical council of India (MCI)
d. National Planning Commission (NPC)

418. Which agency collects data and publishes large scale surveys continuously regarding morbidity, family planning, vital events?
a. AIIMS *(Most Recent Question Dec 2019-20)*
b. Central Bureau of Health
c. National Sample Survey
d. Sample Registration system

419. Main focus on UNICEF is on:
(Most Recent Question Dec 2019-20)
a. Child health b. Nutritional health
c. Mental health d. Social health

420. Population covered by PHC in plains:
(Recent Pattern Question 2018-19)
a. 20,000 b. 30,000
c. 50,000 d. 80,000

421. Which is correct about Kartar Singh Committee?
a. No private practice *(Recent Pattern Question 2017)*
b. Multi-purpose worker scheme
c. ROME scheme
d. Equal pay for equal work

422. As per norms pharmacist and lab technician are suggested per how much population?
(Recent Pattern Question 2017)
a. 5000 b. 10,000
c. 15,000 d. 20,000

423. In a District hospital, the requirement of special new born care beds is? *(Recent Pattern Question 2017)*
a. 6 b. 10
c. 16 d. 20

424. Number of visits to be carried out by ASHA in a home delivery *(Recent Pattern Question 2016)*
a. 3 b. 4
c. 6 d. 7

425. Under RNTCP, rural lab covers how much population in plains *(Recent Pattern Question 2016)*
a. 5000
b. 20,000–30,000
c. 1 lakh
d. 1 lakh to 5 lakh

426. Which of the following is NOT an element of PHC:
a. Water chlorination
b. Maternal health care
c. Sanitation
d. Equity of distribution

427. A health care system which is appropriate to everyone whether the service is needed at all in relation to essential human needs, can be accessible to everyone, available to everyone as first level of health care and the cost can be affordable by everyone is:
a. Primary health care b. Secondary health care
c. Tertiary health care d. Basic health care

428. All are true about principles of primary health care; EXCEPT?
a. Community participation
b. Intersectoral co-ordination
c. Unequitable distribution
d. Appropriate technology

429. Not evaluated in clinical evaluation of pneumonia at PHC:
a. Respiratory rate b. Inability to feed
c. Oxygen saturation d. Chest indrawing

430. Population covered by CHC:
a. 5000 b. 20,000
c. 30,000 d. 100,000

431. 1st referral unit is:
a. PHC b. CHC
c. Subcenter d. District hospital

432. Beds in CHC:
a. 20 b. 30
c. 40 d. 60

433. National Rural Health Mission was established in:
a. 1993 b. 1995
c. 2005 d. 2010

434. Multipurpose worker scheme was implemented in India with the recommendation of:
a. Bhore Committee b. Kartar Singh Committee
c. Srivastava Committee d. Jungalwalla Committee

435. Asha worker works for ___ population:
a. 3000 b. 1000
c. 5000 d. 400

436. All are true about ASHA are all; EXCEPT:
a. Selected by village panchayat/Gram Sabha
b. Trained by ANM
c. Minimum class 4 passed
d. Comes under NRHM 2005–2012

437. ASHA is located at:
a. Subcentre b. PHC
c. CHC d. Village

438. All of the following are true about Accredited Social Health Activist (ASHA); EXCEPT:
a. Is a mental health worker
b. Is a basic sanitation activist
c. Is deployed for one thousand population
d. Arranges escort/accompanies pregnant women/children requiring admission/treatment

439. Functions of female multipurpose health worker includes:
a. Visit 4 sub-centers/month
b. Collection of blood sample
c. Conduct 50% delivery
d. Chlorination of water

440. A female multipurpose worker should be able to detect all of the following; EXCEPT:
a. Mal-presentation
b. Renal disease
c. Anemia
d. Hydramnios

441. A female multipurpose health worker does not work in:
a. Distribution of condoms
b. Birth/death statistics
c. Active malaria surveillance
d. Immunization of mothers

442. Amount of cereals provided to children under the mid-day meals in schools is:
a. 50 grams b. 100 grams
c. 150 grams d. 75 grams

443. Mid-day meal programme provides
a. 1/3 calories, 1/3 proteins b. 1/3 calories, 1/2 proteins
c. 1/2 calories, 1/3 proteins d. 1/2 calories,1/2 proteins

444. BMI obesity starts:
a. 25 b. 30
c. 35 d. 40

445. Body mass index is calculated by:
a. (Weight in kg/Height in meters^2)
b. (Weight in kg/Height in meters^3)
c. (Weight in kg^2)/Height in meters^2)
d. (Weight in kg^2 × Height in meters^2)

446. Least common cause of neonatal mortality in India:
a. Prematurity b. Birth injuries
c. Low birth weight d. Asphyxia

447. ICDS include children up to age of ______________years
a. 3 b. 5
c. 6 d. 14

448. Baby Friendly Hospital Initiative was launched in the year
a. 1981 b. 1991
c. 1993 d. 1997

449. All of the following are features of baby friendly hospitals; EXCEPT:
a. Breast feeding is initiated within half an hour of normal delivery
b. No pacifiers and teats are given
c. No advertisements, promotional material or free products for infant feeding are allowed
d. Infants are kept in the nursery for first 24 hours

450. Which of the following seen in block?
a. Panchayat samiti b. Panchayat sabha
c. Gram sabha d. Gram samiti

451. Community development is block comprises of:
a. 70 villages and 70,000 population
b. 100 villages and 1,00,000 population
c. 500 villages and 5,00,000 population
d. 1000 villages and 10,00,000 population

OCCUPATIONAL HEALTH

452. While working on a machine a person lost both of his hands. Due to this he is unable to write and lost his job. Identify the most appropriate term for this condition, where he lost his job: *(Most Recent Question June 2022)*
a. Disease b. Impairment
c. Disability d. Handicap

453. Which of the following is correct about school health guidelines? *(Most Recent Question Aug 2020)*
a. Minimum area 5 sq ft per student
b. Minus type desk
c. Can allot 60 students per classroom
d. Light coming from front of the class

454. A factory worker had history of frequent exposure to groundnuts, subsequently he develops Hepatocellular carcinoma. Most likely exposure association is: *(Most Recent Question Aug 2020)*
a. Ergot toxin b. Aflatoxin
c. Sanguinarine d. Pyrrolizidine alkaloids

455. A medical officer examines workers in mines and diagnosed Silicosis. What should be his comments? *(Most Recent Question Aug 2020)*
a. It is reversible once we remove the cause
b. It takes 6–10 years to develop
c. Fibrotic changes in the lungs of the patient can be reversed
d. TB screening should be done at regular intervals

456. Anthracosis is caused by: *(Most Recent Question Dec 2019-20)*
a. Silica b. Asbestos
c. Coal dust d. Sugar cane waste

457. Green house gas includes *(Recent Pattern Question 2016)*
a. CO_2, ozone, methane b. Only ozone
c. Ozone, methane only d. Methane, CO

458. Maximum permissible dose of radiation exposure for general human beings is:
a. 0.5 Rad per person per year
b. 5 Rad per person per year
c. 50 Rad per person per year
d. 5 Rem per person

459. Acceptable noise level (in decibels) for Hospital wards is:
a. 20–35 b. 35–45
c. 45–55 d. 50–60

460. Absbestosis is associated with which cancer:
a. Lung cancer b. Liver cancer
c. Colon cancer d. Stomach cancer

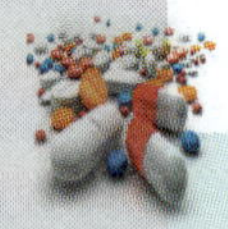

461. Mesothelioma is seen in which type of pneumoconiosis:
a. Anthracosis
b. Byssinosis
c. Asbestosis
d. Silicosis

462. Bagassosis is the name given to occupational disease of lung caused by inhalation of
a. Silica
b. Cotton dust
c. Sugarcane dust
d. Asbestos

463. All are FALSE about Lead Poisoning; EXCEPT:
a. CPU >100 mcg/L indicates exposure to lead
b. Greatest source is drinking water from lead pipes
c. Stippling of basophils is a significant finding
d. Can cause Blue Line on gums

464. One of the following symptoms is NOT caused by inorganic lead poising:
a. Anemia
b. Insomnia
c. Pallor
d. Burtonian line

465. Nausea, Vomiting, Blue line on gums, Wrist/foot drops, Pallor, Colic are manifestations of poisoning due to:
a. Mercury
b. Arsenic
c. Organic lead
d. Inorganic lead

466. True about ESI act 1948:
a. Applicable on educational institutions also
b. Employer : Employee contribution is 1.75:4.75%
c. Maternity benefit for 3 months
d. Benificiaries are those income with >15000/month

467. In which of the following management techniques, interpretation is done in terms of finding out cost effectiveness:
a. Cost effective analysis
b. Cost benefit analysis
c. System analysis
d. Network analysis

468. Critical path is shown by:
a. Time
b. Money
c. Man power
d. Proper sequence

469. In a baby ward, temperature should be:
a. 27°–29°C
b. 29°–31°C
c. 32°–33°C
d. 33°–35°C

DISINFECTION AND MISCELLANEOUS

470. A nurse spilled blood on floor. Which of the following is used to disinfect it: ***(Most Recent Question Aug 2020)***
a. 70% Ethyl alcohol
b. Glutaraldehyde
c. 1% sodium hypochlorite
d. Cresol

471. Maximum level disinfectant property is seen with: ***(Most Recent Question Dec 2019-20)***
a. Phenol
b. Glutaraldehyde
c. Lysol
d. Cetrimide

472. Recycling, tubing and recyclable catheters will be disposed in which bag according to biomedical waste management? ***(Most Recent Question Dec 2019-20)***
a. Red
b. Blue
c. Yellow
d. White

473. Kyoto protocol is for: ***(Most Recent Question Dec 2019-20)***
a. Water sanitization
b. Food and nutrition
c. To reduce greenhouse gas emission
d. Water chlorination

474. Worms and bugs attached to clothing of a person is called as: ***(Most Recent Question Dec 2019-20)***
a. Infection
b. Infestation
c. Contamination
d. Contagion

475. Inertization is: ***(Most Recent Question 2019)***
a. Reducing organic and combustible waste to inorganic
b. Burning biomedical waste
c. Biomedical waste converted into harmless
d. Recycling of waste for re-use

476. In chlorination of water, the main disinfecting action is due to
a. Hypochlorite ions
b. Hydrogen ions
c. Hydrochloric acid
d. Hypochlorous acid

477. Residual chlorine is detected by:
a. Horrock's test
b. Polarimeter
c. Ortho toluidine test
d. Chromatography

478. In Nalgonda technique:
a. Lime is added after bleaching powder
b. Alum is added after lime
c. Lime is added after alum
d. Bleaching powder is added before lime

479. Hardy Weinberg law indicates all; EXCEPT:
a. States that genotype frequencies in a population remain constant or are in equilibrium from generation to generation unless specific disturbing influences are introduced
b. Hardy Weinberg law states that population is static
c. Factors influencing gene pool include mutation, natural selection, population movements(assertive mating), public health measures
d. Natural selection is a process where harmful genes are not eliminated from the gene pool and genes favorable to individual are not passed onto offspring

480. In 1935 students were admitted to a college where height and weight was taken. Based on previous data a study was conducted in 1977 in same population to determine how many will develop CAD in 1986. This study is known as:
a. Experimental
b. Cohort
c. Retrospective cohort
d. Mixed cohort

481. Biological environmental changes are recurrent. What is to be done to reduce error
 a. Standardization
 b. Excessive training of examiner
 c. Using 2 examiner
 d. Repeated measurement

BIOSTATISTICS

482. Best measure of central tendency for skewed data, too high and too low values are present in community wide range of values reported in a community is measured by: *(Most Recent Question June 2022)*
 a. Mean
 b. Median
 c. Mode
 d. Standard deviation

483. How would you demonstrate balance diet to uneducated patient's relatives and family pictorially? *(Most Recent Question June/Dec 2021)*
 a. Pie chart
 b. Histogram
 c. Pictogram
 d. Component bar graph

484. What is the percentage of ISD in the given graph: *(Most Recent Question June/Dec 2021)*

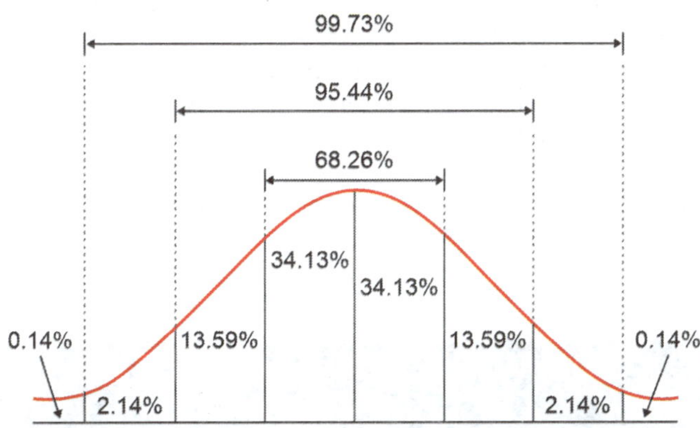

 a. 68.3%
 b. 75.4%
 c. 98.5%
 d. 99.7%

485. Discrete probability distribution that describes probability of given number of events occurring in a fixed interval of time is known as: *(Most Recent Question June/Dec 2021)*
 a. Normal probability distribution
 b. Gaussian distribution
 c. Poisson's distribution
 d. Binomial distribution

486. Difference between lowest and highest in data distribution is known as: *(Most Recent Question June/Dec 2021)*
 a. Quartile range
 b. Range
 c. Coefficient of variation
 d. Variance

487. Identify the statistical diagram shown below: *(Most Recent Question Aug 2020)*

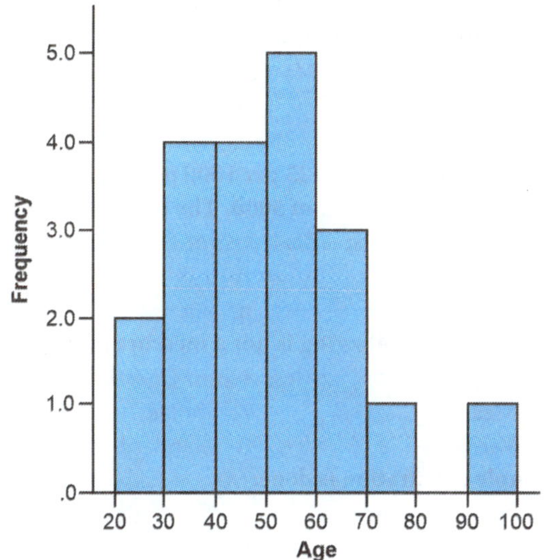

 a. Bar diagram
 b. Histogram
 c. Frequency polygon
 d. Scatter diagram

488. A researcher did study on staff, nurses and JRs doing yoga (divided into male and female). Yoga shows 25% decreased risk of infections. Which is the best to test the significance of the result? *(Most Recent Question Aug 2020)*

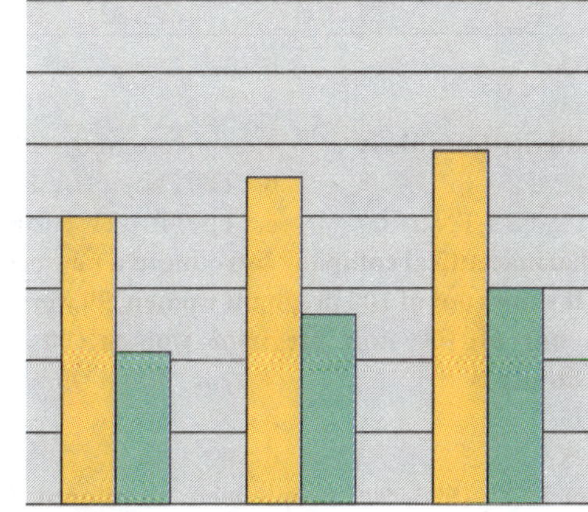

 a. ANOVA
 b. Chi square test
 c. Z test
 d. Correlation

489. In different types of graphs, secular trend of a disease is best represented by: *(Most Recent Question Aug 2020)*
 a. Line diagram
 b. Bar graph
 c. Box and whiskers plot
 d. Stem leaf plot

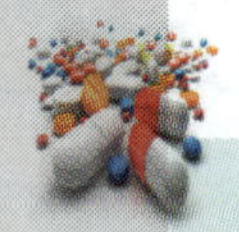

490. Calculate Neonatal mortality rate from the data given. Total live births were 4000. Total deaths among day 0-7 babies = 40, day 7-28 = 40, more than one month age = 40 and in utero (perinatal) = 40. *(Most Recent Question Dec 2019-20)*

a. 10 b. 20
c. 30 d. 40

491. Newborn birth rate is 25 per 1000 population in a village with total population of 5000. The total number of pregnancies per year is: *(Most Recent Question Dec 2019-20)*

a. 125 b. 138
c. 145 d. 250

492. Which of the following is not a measure of dispersion? *(Most Recent Question Dec 2019-20)*

a. Mean b. Range
c. Variance d. Standard error

493. Sample registration is done: *(Recent Pattern Question 2018)*

a. Every 3 months b. Every 6 months
c. Every 9 months d. Every 12 months

494. Pictoral diagram of frequency distribution is: *(Recent Pattern Question 2018)*

a. Histogram b. Scatter diagram
c. Pie chart d. Bar chart

495. Calculate odds ratio from the given table: *(Recent Pattern Question 2017)*

	Disease	Non diseased
Exposure	33	53
Non exposed	2	27
	35	82

a. 32 b. 8.4
c. 88.4 d. 11.4

496. Sensitivity formula is *(Recent Pattern Question 2016)*

a. TP/TP + FP × 100 b. TN/TN + FN × 100
c. TP/TP + FN × 100 d. TN/FP + TN × 100

497. A pharmaceutical company introduced a new pregnancy kit. It shows out of 100 pregnant women, 99 were positive and out of 100 non pregnant women, 90 negative. Sensitivity is *(Recent Pattern Question 2016)*

a. 95 b. 97
c. 98 d. 99

498. From 1970–1995, 500 people were monitored. Exposed to smoking 400, Non-exposed 100. Out of 400 exposed 50 developed the lung cancer and out of 100 non exposed 5 developed the lung cancer. Calculate relative risk: *(Recent Pattern Question 2016)*

a. 1.2 b. 2.5
c. 12.5 d. 1.5

499. In a hospital 10 babies were born in a day, each weighs 2.7 kg. what is the probable standard deviation:

a. 0.00 b. 0.27
c. 2.7 d. 27

500. All are true about Chi-square test; EXCEPT:

a. Non parametric test
b. Degree of freedom is calculated by (c – 1)(r – 1)
c. Used to test significance of association between two quantitative data
d. Used for non-Gaussian distribution

501. In a 4 × 5 table for Chi-square test, what is the degree of freedom?

a. 20 b. 16
c. 12 d. 9

502. Correlation coefficient of 1.76 indicates

a. Positive correlation b. Highly positive correlation
c. Absence of correlation d. Wrong calculation

503. Which is the best method of central tendency that is used to show quantitative variable:

a. Mean b. Median
c. Mode d. Box and whisker

504. Frequently occurring value in a series is known as

a. Average b. Median
c. Mean d. Mode

505. A smoker states that he has been smoking for 6 years. In the first year he was taking up to 5 sticks per day only. In the next 3 years he increased it to half pack per day. In the 5th year, his habits worsened to 1 pack per day. In the last year he stated that his daily sticks consumption is 2 packs per day. Select the correct statement:
Mean, median and mode of number of sticks are:

a. 16, 10, 15 b. 16, 10, 10
c. 10, 10, 15 d. 16, 10, 15

506. Calculate the mean & mode of the given values: 2, 2, 3, 4, 4, 4, 4, 5, 5, 7, 8, 8, 9

a. 4 and 5 b. 5 and 4
c. 5 and 9 d. 9 and 5

COMMUNICATION FOR HEALTH EDUCATION

507. 4–8 speakers interact in from of a large group of audience to talk about a topic. There is no specific agenda, no set speech and no order of speaking. At the end there is interaction with audience? *(Most Recent Question June 2022)*

a. Panel discussion b. Group discussion
c. Symposium d. Workshop

508. Best method of teaching villagers about ORS is: *(Most Recent Question June/Dec 2021)*

a. Lecture b. Role play
c. Demonstration d. Flash cards

509. As a medical officer of a PHC, you want to talk and discuss some health-related issue with antenatal mothers. How many members will you include in a group discussion? *(Most Recent Question June/Dec 2021)*

a. 4–6 b. 3–5
c. 6–12 d. 12–15

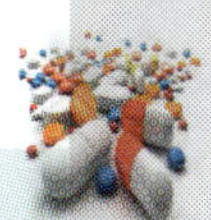

ANSWERS WITH EXPLANATIONS

MOST RECENT QUESTIONS 2023

1. Ans. (a) <20 deliveries/month

Ref: Park's Textbook of Preventive and Social Medicine, 25th ed. pg. 693

Types of PHCs

- **Type A PHC:** PHC with delivery load of less than 20 deliveries in a month.
- **Type B PHC:** PHC with delivery load of 20 or more deliveries in a month.

Extra Mile

- **Type A CHC:** <100 deliveries/month
- **Type B CHC:** >100 deliveries/month

2. Ans. (a) Embolism

Ref: Park's Textbook of Preventive and Social Medicine, 25th ed. pg. 510

Direct causes of maternal death	Indirect causes of maternal death
• Post partum hemorrhage: MC direct cause in India	• Anemia: MC indirect cause
• Thromboembolism	• Heart disease
• Hypertensive crisis	• Diabetes
• Dystocic childbirth	• HIV/AIDS
• Infection/Sepsis	• Malaria
• Complication to abortion	
• Allergy to anesthesia	

3. Ans. (c) Coordination/ministries

Ref: Park's Textbook of Preventive and Social Medicine, 25th ed. pg. 680

- The 6x6x6 strategy under Anemia Mukt Bharat, implies six age groups **beneficiaries**, six **interventions** and six **institutional mechanisms**.
- The strategy focuses on ensuring supply chain, demand generation and strong monitoring using the dashboard for addressing anemia, both due to nutritional and non-nutritional causes.

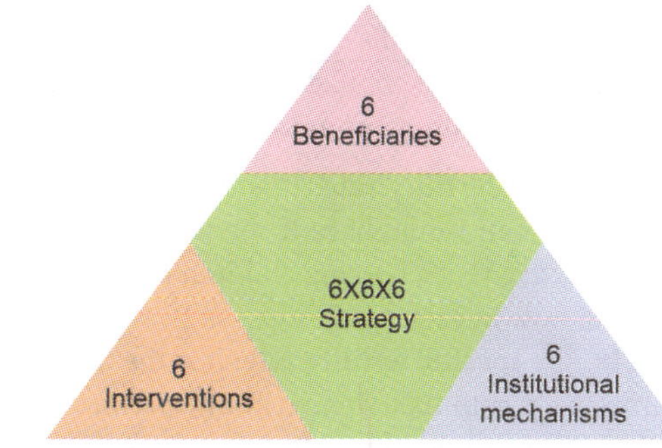

4. Ans. (d) Antibiotics

Ref: Park's Textbook of Preventive and Social Medicine, 25th ed. pg. 680

- Antibiotics are not part of Anemia Mukt Bharat
- The Anemia Mukt Bharat strategy is a universal strategy and will focus on the following interventions:
  - Prophylactic Iron and Folic Acid supplementation
  - Deworming by Albendazole twice a year
  - Behavior Change Communication Campaign (Solid Body, Smart Mind) focusing on four key behaviors.
  - Fortification of food with iron
  - Digital hemoglobin measurement
  - Focus on other cause of anemia (Example: Malaria, Thalassemia)

5. Ans. (b) Adequately treated

Ref: Park's Textbook of Preventive and Social Medicine, 25th ed. pg. 403

- Rule of Half, explain the status of hypertension in society.
- Outer-most circle denotes the whole community and inner most circle denote the adequately treated ones.

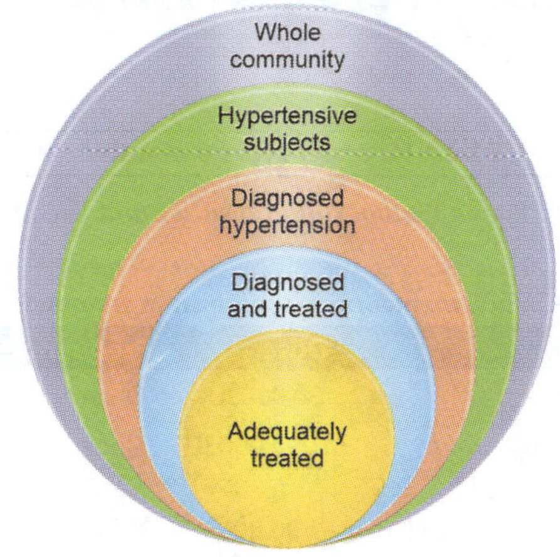

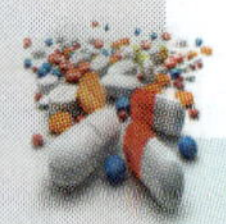

6. Ans. (c) General Fertility Rate

Ref: Park's Textbook of Preventive and Social Medicine, 25th ed. pg. 539

$$= \frac{\text{No. of live births during the year}}{\text{Midyear female population aged 15–49 years in the same area and year}} \times 1000$$

Option a: Total fertility rate: It is the average number of children a woman would have if she were to pass through her reproductive years, bearing children at the same rate as the woman now in each age group.

Option b: Age specific fertility rate: It is the number of the live births in a year to 1000 women in any specified age-group.

Option d: Net reproduction rate: It is defined as the number of daughters a new-born girl will bear during her lifetime, assuming fixed age specific fertility and mortality rates.

Gross reproduction rate: Number of girl live birth per female in age group of 15-49 years.

7. Ans. (b) Yellow - Stable need observation

Ref: Park's textbook of Preventive and Social Medicine, 25th ed. pg. 856

Triage color coding:

Red	• Patient requires immediate treatment • E.g. suicide attempt via poisoning, hanging, or self-inflicted trauma
Yellow	• Patient is stable at the moment and is not in any immediate danger, but will require observation • E.g. passive suicidal ideation, command hallucinations
Green	• Patients who will require medical treatment at some point, once more critical injuries have been treated • E.g. drug refill for anti-depressant or anti anxiety medications
Black	• For those who are already decreased, or for patients whose injuries are so extensive that they will not be able to survive, given the level of care available

8. Ans. (a) 2 lakh IU orally every 6 months

Ref: Park's Textbook of Preventive and Social Medicine, 25th ed. pg. 672

Vit-A supplementation for children in endemic areas

Age	Dose	Frequency
<6 months	50,000 IU	Once
6–11 months or weight <8 kg	1,00,000 IU	Once
1–5 years or weight >8 kg	2,00,000 IU	Every 6 months till 5 years of age

9. Ans. (d) Subcenter

Ref: Park's Textbook of Preventive and Social Medicine, 25th ed. pg. 513

- The subcenter is the peripheral outpost of the Indian healthcare system. One subcenter caters to the healthcare needs of 5000 population in general and 3000 population in hilly, tribal and backward areas.
- Inclusions in urban health care (From base to top).

Inclusions in UHC	Population that it caters
• Mahila Arogya Samiti	150–500
• ASHA	1000–2500
• ANM	10,000
• Urban PHC	50,000
• Urban CHC	2.5 lakh

10. Ans. (d) Mean will increase, median will remain the same

Ref: Park's Textbook of Preventive and Social Medicine, 25th ed. pg. 908

- There are three measures of central tendency, namely mean, median and mode.
- Mean is the average value and is statistically the best measure of central tendency.
- Median is the middle value when the data set is arranged in ascending or descending order.
- Mode is the highest occurring value
- When 39 is mistaken for 93, mean value will increase; median remains same.

11. Ans. (d) FORD

Ref: Park's Textbook of Preventive and Social Medicine, 25th ed. pg. 817

- American automobile major, **Ford Motor** Company has announced that it is funding $200,000 (Rs 1.26 crore), for supporting two international social projects that aim to improve health and sanitation conditions in India and Mexico, as part of the Bill Ford Better World Challenge (BFBWC).
- Main works by this foundation is:
  - Making sanitary latrines
  - NIHAE: National Institution for health Administration and Education
  - Calcutta drainage system

Extra Mile

- The **USAID Global Health Supply Chain Program**-Procurement and Supply Management (GHSC-PSM) project enhances the health care experience in the communities we serve through transformative supply chain solutions.

Contd...

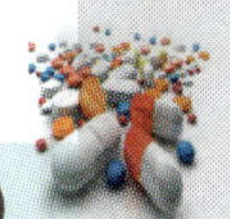

- **CURE International** is a global nonprofit network of children's hospitals that provide surgical care in a compassionate, gospel-centered environment.

12. Ans. (d) 24–28 weeks

- Screening for GDM is usually done at 24-28 weeks of gestation because insulin resistance increases during the second trimester and glucose levels rise in women who do not have the ability to produce enough insulin to adopt this resistance.

Ref: Park's Textbook of Preventive and Social Medicine, 25th ed. pg. 421

13. Ans. (d) Propagated epidemic

Ref: Park's Textbook of Preventive and Social Medicine, 25th ed. pg. 73

- **Propagated (or progressive source) epidemic:** A single index case who infected a number of other individuals. One or more of the people infected in the initial wave infected a group of people who become the second wave of infection. So here transmission is person-to-person, rather than from a common source. Propagated epidemic curves usually have a series of successively larger peaks, which are one incubation period apart. For example, COVID-19 cases, SARS
- **Point source outbreaks (epidemics)** involve a common source, such as contaminated food or an infected food handler, and all the exposures tend to occur in a relatively brief period. Consequently, point source outbreaks tend to have epidemic curves with a rapid increase in cases followed by a somewhat slower decline, and all of the cases tend to fall within one incubation period.
- **Continuous common source epidemics** may also rise to a peak and then fall, but the all the cases do not occur within the span of a single incubation period. This implies that there is an ongoing source of contamination.

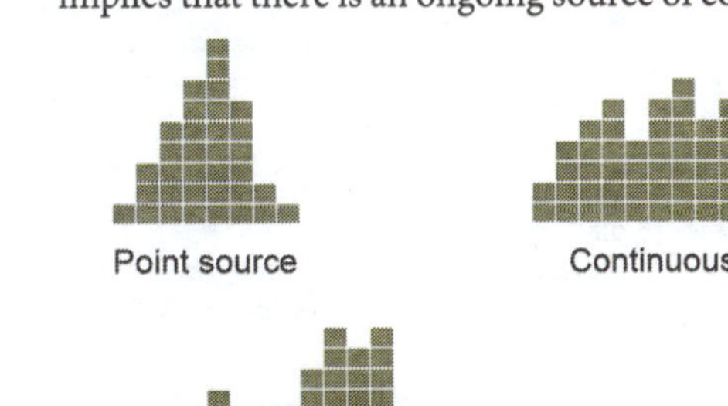

Point source

Continuous source

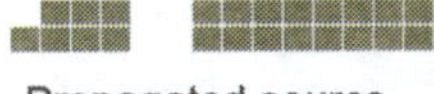

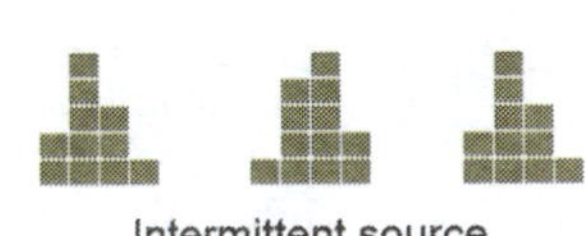

Propagated source

Intermittent source

14. Ans. (a) Rashtriya Bal Swasthya Karyakram

- **Rashtriya Bal Swasthya Karyakram (RBSK)** is an initiative aimed at screening children from 0 to 18 years for the 4 Ds - Defects at birth, Diseases, Deficiencies and Development Delays including Disabilities. Children diagnosed with illnesses shall receive follow up including surgeries at Govt and Pvt Hospital level, free of cost under NHM.
- **Janani Suraksha Yojana (JSY)** is a safe motherhood intervention under the National Rural Health Mission (NHM). It is being implemented with the objective of reducing maternal and infant mortality by promoting institutional delivery among pregnant women.
- **The Mid-Day Meal Scheme** is a school meal program in India designed to better the nutritional standing of school-age children nationwide. The scheme has been renamed as POSHAN Scheme.
- **Navjaat Shishu Suraksha Karyakram (NSSK)** aims to train medical personnel in basic newborn care and resuscitation.

Ref: Park's Textbook of Preventive and Social Medicine, 25th ed. pg. 498

15. Ans. (a) Stunting

Ref: Park's Textbook of Preventive and Social Medicine, 25th ed. pg. 696

- Child **stunting** refers to a child who is too short for his or her age (<-2SD) and is the result of chronic or recurrent malnutrition. Stunting is a contributing risk factor to child mortality and is also a marker of inequalities in human development.
- Option b: **Wasting** is an indicator of acute malnutrition. It indicates recent and severe weight loss, because a person has not had enough food to eat and/or they have had an infectious disease, such as diarrhea, which has caused them to lose weight.
- Option c: **Constitutional delay** of growth and puberty is a transient state of hypogonadotropic hypogonadism associated with prolongation of childhood phase of growth, delayed skeletal maturation, delayed and attenuated pubertal growth spurt, and relatively low insulin-like growth factor-1 secretion.

16. Ans. (a) <11.5

Ref: Park's Textbook of Preventive and Social Medicine, 25th ed. pg. 604

- **Severe Acute Malnutrition (SAM)** is defined by very low weight-for-height/length (Z- score below -3 SD of the median WHO child growth standards), or a mid-upper arm circumference < 115 mm, or by the presence of nutritional edema.

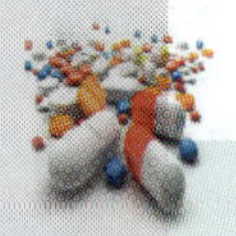

- When Shakir tape is wrapped around the arm, the measuring point overlaps one of the colored zones toward the other end of the tape:
- **Green (>13.5 cm)** indicates normal or acceptable nutrition;
- **Yellow (>12.5–13.5 cm)** indicates borderline nutrition;
- Red (<12.5 cm) indicates malnutrition.

17. Ans. (c) CBNAAT

Ref: Park's Textbook of Preventive and Social Medicine, 25th ed. pg. 188

- IOC for diagnosing cases of tuberculosis in HIV, COVID-19, Diabetes, previously treated TB, pediatric TB case is diagnosed with CBNAAT.
- Culture in liquid medium is gold standard for diagnosing TB in HIV patient.

18. Ans. (c) Yellow bag– incineration

Ref: Park's textbook of Preventive and Social Medicine, 25th ed. pg. 849

- Expired tablets, blood bag, etc. are disposed in yellow bag and it is treated by incineration.
- Red bag is treated with autoclaving followed by recycling.
- Blue bag contains metallic instrument and implant. These are treated with autoclave then recycled.

Details on BMW management has been discussed in further questions

19. Ans. (a) Ayushman Bharat

Ref: Park's Textbook of Preventive and Social Medicine, 25th ed. pg. 963

- School health program comes under PHC and Ayushman Bharat

20. Ans. (d) Less than 70

Ref: Park's Textbook of Preventive and Social Medicine, 25th ed

- **SDG Targets to be achieved by 2030**
  - MMR should be Less than 70 per 100,000 live births
  - Neonatal Mortality rate should be Less than 12 per 1000
  - Under 5 mortalities rates should be less than 25 per 1000
  - Reduce premature cardiovascular death to 1/3rd
  - Eliminate HIV, TB, Malaria

21. Ans. (b) 10 lakh per family per year is given

Ref: Park's textbook of Preventive and Social Medicine, 25th ed. pg. 515

- 'Prime Minister's People's Health Scheme', Ayushman Bharat PM-JAY lit. 'Live Long India Prime Minister's People's Health Scheme';) is a national public health insurance scheme of the Government of India that aims to provide free access to health insurance coverage for low-income earners in the country.
- It offers coverage of up to Rs.5 lakh per family per year for secondary and tertiary hospitalization care.

22. Ans. (a) TT only

Ref: Park's textbook of Preventive and Social Medicine, 25th ed. pg. 338

- In the given case of crush injury (dirty wound), there is history of TT intake 7 years back. In this case, we will give TT only.
- However, if the history of TT intake is beyond 10 years, immunoglobulin should be added with TT.

Tetanus prophylaxis in wound management:

History of tetanus immunization	Clean, minor wounds	All other wounds
• Uncertain or <3 doses	TT	TT+TIG
• 3 or more doses	If > 10 yrs. since last dose, give TT	If > 5yrs since last dose, give TT

23. Ans. (a) A

Ref: Park's Textbook of Preventive and Social Medicine, 25th ed. pg. 523

Categories of bioterrorism:

	Criteria	Examples
Category A	High mortality, disseminate easily, needs special action	*Bacillus, Anthracis, Yersinia pestis, Variola major, Francisella tularensis, Filoviruses and Arenaviruses family*
Category B	Moderately easy to disseminate, moderate morbidity	*Brucella species, Salmonella species, Escherichia coli 0157:H7, Vibrio cholerae, Alphaviruses family*
Category C	Easily produced, potential for high morbidity and mortality	*Mycobacterium tuberculosis* Nipah virus, Hantavirus*

24. Ans. (a) Endometrial

Ref: Park's textbook of Preventive and Social Medicine, 25th ed. pg. 414

- OCP increases the risk of: Breast and Cervix
- OCP decreases the risk of: Ovarian cancer, Endometrial cancer, colorectal cancer

25. Ans. (c) MAC

Ref: Park's textbook of Preventive and Social Medicine, 25th ed. pg. 371

- Among persons with HIV, MAC infection is most commonly seen among those with a CD4 count <50 cells/microL. Dramatic declines in the rate of new MAC cases accompanied the use of prophylaxis against MAC infection early in the epidemic, and more recently, the widespread use of effective antiretroviral therapy.

Extra Mile

CD4 count	Risk of infection
<50	Disseminated MAC CMV retinitis CNS lymphoma Histoplasmosis
200	Pneumocystis Toxoplasmosis Cryptosporidiosis Coccidiomycosis
500	Bacterial infection Herpes simplex, TB, candidiasis, Kaposi's sarcoma, Hairy Leukoplakia

26. Ans. (b) Blood group

Ref: Park's textbook of Preventive and Social Medicine, 25th ed. pg. 391

- The WHO STEP wise approach is used to know high risk population for non-communicable disease. It utilizes:
  - Behavioral and Psychological factors (alcohol habits, smoking, exercise, diet)
  - Physical factors (BP, BMI, Age)
  - Hormonal or Biological (RBS, Lipid profile, thyroid profile)

27. Ans. (c) Lymphatics

Ref: Park's Textbook of Preventive and Social Medicine, 25th ed. pg. 295

- The shown image is of filariasis, which resides in lymphatics, hence the name lymphatic filariasis
- Lymphatic filariasis is caused by infection with parasites classified as nematodes (roundworms) of the family Filariodidea.
- Lymphatic filariasis blocks the lymphatic system and can lead to the abnormal enlargement of body parts, causing pain, severe disability.

28. Ans. (a) Measles

Ref: Park's Textbook of Preventive and Social Medicine, 25th ed. pg. 159

- Measles is a highly contagious, vaccine-preventable infectious disease caused by measles virus.
- The classic symptoms of measles include a four-day fever (the 4 Ds) and the three Cs—cough, coryza (head cold, fever, sneezing), and conjunctivitis (red eyes)—along with a maculopapular rash.
- Fever is common and typically lasts for about one week; the fever seen with measles is often as high as 40°C.
- IP: 10-14 days

Option b: Clinical features of dengue include: Headache, Retro-orbital pain, Myalgia. Arthralgia/bone pain, Rash, Bleeding manifestations

Option c: Clinical features of rubella include: Mild fever of 102°F (38.9°C) or lower, Headache, Stuffy or runny nose, Red, itchy eyes, Enlarged, tender lymph nodes at the base of the skull

Option d: Clinical features of Chikungunya include: Fever, Joint pain, Headache, Muscle pain, Joint swelling, Rash

29. Ans. (b) Leprosy

Ref: Park's Textbook of Preventive and Social Medicine, 25th ed. pg. 342

- A patient with leprosy presents with:
  - Hypopigmented patches
  - Loss of touch (earliest: light touch affected)
  - Presence of thickened nerve (MC: Ulnar nerve)
  - Positive Zn stain

30. Ans. (d) RL

Ref: Park's textbook of Preventive and Social Medicine, 25th ed. pg. 563

Fluid in severe dehydration due to gastroenteritis:

- The first portion of the intravenous fluid, preferably isotonic Ringer's lactate (30 mL/kg), is to be given very rapidly, and the remaining 70 mL/kg to complete rehydration is given more slowly over 2.5 to 5 hours, depending on the child's age.

31. Ans. (a) 45 gm

Ref: Park's textbook of Preventive and Social Medicine, 25th ed. pg. 666

- According to the Dietary Reference Intake report for macronutrients, a sedentary adult should consume 0.8 grams of protein per kilogram of body weight, or 0.36 grams per pound.
- That means that the average sedentary man should eat about 56 grams of protein per day, and the average woman should eat about 46 grams.
- For a 55kg female: $55 \times 0.8 = 44$

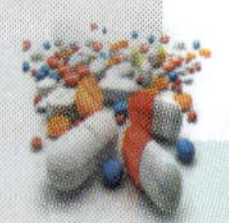

32. Ans. (a) >10 sq. ft

Ref: Park's Textbook of Preventive and Social Medicine 25th ed. pg. 664

- Per capita space in school should be greater than 10 sq. ft per student.
- Sufficient space is important to ensure the comfort and well-being of students, allowing them to move freely and engage in various activities.
- Adequate space also helps in preventing overcrowding and the spread of infectious diseases in school settings.

33. Ans. (b) Fluorine

Ref: Park's Textbook of Preventive and Social Medicine 25th ed. pg. 733

- Over-supplementation of fluorine can lead to dental fluorosis, which is characterized by white or brownish patches on the teeth, particularly on the enamel of the anterior incisors.
- Excessive intake of fluoride, whether through drinking water, dietary sources, or supplements, can cause fluorosis, affecting the appearance and strength of tooth enamel.

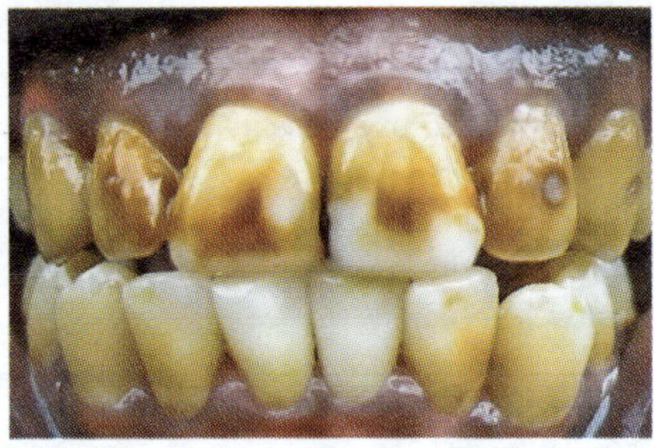

Extra Mile

Vitamin A
- Excessive intake can cause symptoms like nausea, vomiting, blurred vision, bone pain, hair loss, and skin changes. High doses during pregnancy can increase the risk of birth defects and liver toxicity.

Chlorine
- High levels can irritate the respiratory system, causing coughing, wheezing, and chest tightness.
- Prolonged exposure can result in skin and eye irritation, and there may be potential cancer risks associated with long-term exposure.

Riboflavin
- Overconsumption may cause gastrointestinal disturbances such as diarrhea and stomach cramps.
- It can increase sensitivity to light and interfere with certain laboratory test results.

34. Ans. (a) Primary level prevention

Ref: Park's Textbook of Preventive and Social Medicine 25th ed. pg. 870

- Tobacco control law is a primary level prevention measure.
- Primary prevention focuses on preventing the onset of a disease or condition and aims to promote health and prevent the occurrence of risk factors.
- Tobacco control laws, such as ban on smoking in public places and restrictions on tobacco advertising, are implemented to reduce the prevalence and initiation of smoking, thereby preventing tobacco-related diseases and promoting public health.

Extra Mile

- **Primordial level prevention:** Primordial prevention refers to preventing the emergence of risk factors in a population or community.
- **Secondary level prevention:** Secondary prevention aims to detect and treat diseases in their early stages to prevent further progression.
- **Tertiary level prevention:** Tertiary prevention focuses on reducing the impact of a disease or condition and preventing disability or complications.

35. Ans. (a) Primary level prevention

Ref: Park's Textbook of Preventive and Social Medicine 25th ed. pg. 870

- Handwashing during Covid-19 is a primary level prevention measure.

Detailed discussion given above

36. Ans. (c) Demonstration

Ref: Park's Textbook of Preventive and Social Medicine 25th ed. pg. 901

- Giving a class in a village for wound dressing after a dog bite involves demonstrating the proper technique of wound dressing to the community members.
- Demonstration is a form of communication that involves showing how to perform a task or skill.
- In this context, demonstrating wound dressing techniques allows the community members to visually learn and understand the correct procedure.

Extra Mile

- **Lecture:** A lecture typically involves oral presentation and information sharing without practical demonstrations.
- **Flashcard:** Flashcards are visual aids that present information or prompts for learning.
- **Group discussion:** Group discussion involves interactive communication among participants.

37. Ans. (c) Sub center

Ref: Park's Textbook of Preventive and Social Medicine 25th ed. pg. 973

- The Eligible Couple (EC) register is maintained at the sub center level in the Indian healthcare system.
- The EC register is an important tool for tracking and providing family planning services. It helps in maintaining records of eligible couples, their contraceptive choices, and the provision of family planning methods.
- Sub centers are the peripheral healthcare facilities that provide primary healthcare services in rural areas, making them an appropriate level for maintaining the EC register.

Extra Mile

- **Community Health Centre (CHC):** CHCs are higher-level healthcare facilities that serve as referral centers for primary healthcare facilities.
- **Primary Health Centre (PHC):** PHCs are intermediate-level healthcare facilities that provide primary healthcare services to a defined population.
- **Ground level:** "Ground level" is not a specific healthcare facility or level in the healthcare system.

38. Ans. (a) Extended family

Ref: Park's Textbook of Preventive and Social Medicine 25th ed. pg. 773

- The scenario describes an extended family.
- An extended family includes relatives beyond the nuclear family (parents and children). It involves the inclusion of additional family members such as grandparents, aunts, uncles, cousins, etc.
- In the given scenario, the presence of the man's brother and wife along with his own wife and child indicates the presence of extended family members.

Extra Mile

- **Nuclear family:** A nuclear family consists of parents and their children without additional extended family members.
- **Joint family:** A joint family includes multiple generations living together and sharing common resources. It typically involves the presence of parents, children, grandparents, and sometimes uncles, aunts, and cousins.
- **Third generation:** Third generation does not specifically define a type of family structure.

39. Ans. (d) Cultural barrier

Ref: Park's Textbook of Preventive and Social Medicine 25th ed. pg. 952

- The doctor's explanation addressing the misconception that vaccination leads to impotency indicates a cultural barrier.
- Cultural barriers are based on beliefs, values, and norms within a specific culture or community that can influence perceptions and acceptance of certain practices, including vaccination.
- In this case, the misconception regarding vaccination and impotency is rooted in cultural beliefs, and the doctor is addressing this barrier through education and communication.

Extra Mile

- **Environmental barrier:** Environmental barriers refer to physical or structural factors that impede access or implementation of health interventions.
- **Psychological barrier:** Psychological barriers are related to individuals' thoughts, emotions, or attitudes that may hinder acceptance or understanding of health information.
- **Physical barrier:** Physical barriers are tangible obstacles that restrict the accessibility of healthcare services or interventions.

40. Ans. (c) 12–20 weeks

Ref: Park's Textbook of Preventive and Social Medicine 25th ed. pg. 877

- After vasectomy, it is recommended for the patient to use a barrier method of contraception for a period of 12-20 weeks or until confirmed azoospermia (absence of sperm in the semen).
- This period allows sufficient time for any remaining sperm to be cleared from the reproductive system before considering the patient as sterile.
- It is important to ensure the effectiveness of the vasectomy procedure and prevent unintended pregnancies during this period.

41. Ans. (b) 1000 total live birth

Ref: Park's Textbook of Preventive and Social Medicine 25th ed. pg. 641

- The denominator of the infant mortality rate is the number of live births.
- The infant mortality rate (IMR) is a measure of the number of deaths among infants (under one year of age) per 1,000 live births.
- To calculate the IMR, the number of infant deaths is divided by the number of live births, and the result is multiplied by 1,000 to express it as a rate per 1,000 live births.
- The denominator represents the population at risk of infant mortality, which is the number of live births.

42. Ans. (a) Secondary attack rate

Ref: Park's Textbook of Preventive and Social Medicine 25th ed. pg. 156

- **Infectivity** is a term used to describe the ability of an infectious agent (e.g., virus, bacteria) to cause infection in susceptible individuals.

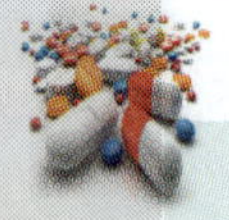

- It refers to the capacity of the agent to produce clinical illness or infection in contacts who are exposed to the primary case.
- Another term used to measure infectivity is the secondary attack rate, which represents the proportion of susceptible individuals who develop infection after exposure to an infectious case.

Extra Mile

- **Case fatality rate:** Case fatality rate is the proportion of individuals diagnosed with a specific disease who die from that disease.
- **Serial interval:** Serial interval refers to the time interval between the onset of symptoms in a primary case and the onset of symptoms in secondary cases.
- **Incubation:** Incubation period is the time interval between exposure to an infectious agent and the appearance of clinical symptoms in the infected individual.

43. Ans. (b) Wound cleaning + rabies vaccination 0, 3

Ref: Park's Textbook of Preventive and Social Medicine 25th ed. pg. 319

- Class 3 dog bite refers to a severe bite that has caused deep tissue damage, multiple puncture wounds, or injury to vital areas.
- In this scenario, the next step of management involves thorough wound cleaning to reduce the risk of infection. Cleaning the wound with soap and water is essential.
- Following wound cleaning, the patient should receive post-exposure prophylaxis (PEP) for rabies, which involves administering rabies vaccine on days 0, 3.
- Two doses should be enough as the patient has been completely vaccinated < 6 months ago.
- This schedule helps stimulate an immune response against the rabies virus and prevent the development of rabies.

44. Ans. (a) Omega -3 fatty acid

Ref: Park's Textbook of Preventive and Social Medicine 25th ed. pg. 413

- Omega-3 fatty acids have been extensively studied and shown to have numerous health benefits, particularly in reducing the risk of coronary artery disease (CAD).
- These fatty acids, found in fatty fish like salmon, mackerel, and sardines, as well as in flaxseeds and walnuts, have anti-inflammatory properties and help lower triglyceride levels, reduce blood clotting, and improve overall heart health.
- Regular consumption of omega-3 fatty acids, either through dietary sources or supplements, is recommended to decrease the risk of CAD.

45. Ans. (b) Woman education and empowerment

Ref: Park's Textbook of Preventive and Social Medicine 25th ed. pg. 507

- The RCH program in India aims to improve maternal and child health outcomes and promote reproductive health services.
- The essential components of the RCH program include:
  - Safe motherhood
  - Children and newborn care
  - Screening and treatment for sexually transmitted diseases (STDs) and reproductive tract infections (RTIs).
- While woman education and empowerment are crucial for overall health and well-being, they are not explicitly listed as a component of the RCH program.

46. Ans. (a) Stage I

Ref: Park's Textbook of Preventive and Social Medicine 25th ed. pg. 530

- The demographic cycle refers to the different stages of population growth in a country or region.
- In Stage I (High stationary) of the demographic cycle, both the birth rate and death rate are high, resulting in slow population growth. This is usually associated with pre-industrial societies with limited access to healthcare and high fertility rates.
- Stage I is seen when a country is economically most weak.
- India is presently in stage 3 of demographic cycle.

Extra Mile

S. no.	Stages	Characteristics
1.	First stage (High stationary)	High birth rate and high death rate
2.	Second stage (Early expanding)	Death rate begins to decline and birth rate remains the same
3.	Third stage (Late expanding)	Death rate decline further and birth rate start declining
4.	Fourth stage (Low stationary)	Birth rate rapidly falls and becomes equal to death rate.
5.	Fifth stage (Stage of decline)	Death rate is higher than the birth rate

CONCEPT OF HEALTH AND DISEASE

47. Ans. (a) HDI

Ref: Park Textbook of Preventive and Social Medicine, 25th ed. pg. 17

- The Human Development Index (HDI) is a measurement system used by the United Nations to evaluate the level of individual human development in each country.

48. Ans. (d) Daly

Ref: K. Park 25th ed. pg. 26

- DALY is a measure of overall disease burden, expressed as a number of years lost due to ill-health, disability or early death.

49. Ans. (b) Appropriate facility

Ref: Park, 25th ed. pg. 951

Principles of primary health care:
- Equitable distribution
- Community participation
- Intersectoral coordination
- Appropriate technology

50. Ans. (c) Psychomotor learning

Ref: Park, 23rd ed. pg. 891

Psychomotor learning is the relationship between cognitive functions and physical movement and is demonstrated by physical skills such as movement, coordination, manipulation, dexterity, grace, strength, speed—actions which demonstrate the fine or gross motor skills, such as use of precision instruments or tools and attention is given to the learning of coordinated activity involving the arms, hands, fingers, and feet, while verbal processes are not emphasized.

51. Ans. (c) Suraksha clinic

Ref: K. Park, 25th ed. pg. 457

- The shown logo is of suraksha clinic
- NACO has branded the STI/RTI services as **"Suraksha Clinic"**, and has developed a communication strategy for generating demand for these services

Extra Mile

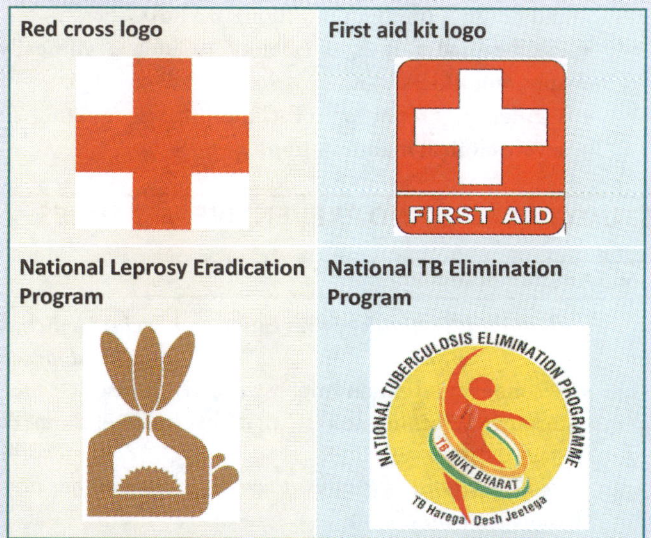

52. Ans. (b) Life expectancy at 1 year, IMR, literacy rate

Ref: K. Park, 23rd ed. pg. 17

TABLE: Comparison between PQLI and HDI

PQLI (Physical Quality of Life Index)	HDI (Human Development Index)
Literacy rate	Knowledge
Infant mortality rate	Income
Life expectancy (at 1 year)	Life expectancy (@ birth)
Range: 0 and 100	Range: 0 and +1
Value in India: **65**	**0.633**

Extra Mile
- *Range of correlation coefficient: –1 to +1*

53. Ans. (b) Cholera

Ref: K. Park, 23rd ed. pg. 5

- **Father of public Health:** John Snow, identified Cholera
- Father of modern epidemiology: John Snow
- Father of Medicine/first true epidemiologist: Hippocrates.

54. Ans. (c) 0 and 100

Ref: K. Park, 23rd ed. pg. 17

Physical Quality of Life Index (PQLI)	Human Development Index (HDI)
Literacy rate	Knowledge
Infant mortality rate	Income
Life expectancy (at 1 year)	Life expectancy (@ birth)
Range: 0 and 100	Range: 0 and +1
Value in India: 65	**0.633**

Extra Mile
- Range of correlation coefficient: –1 to +1

55. Ans. (c) Life expectancy - birth

Ref: K. Park, 23rd ed. pg. 17

Please refer to above table

56. Ans. (d) Range 0–100

Ref: K. Park, 23rd ed. pg. 17

Refer to above explanation

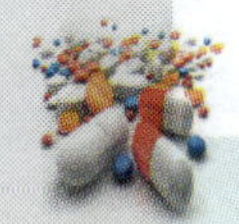

57. Ans. (a) 0–1

Ref: K. Park, 23rd ed. pg. 17

- The HDI value ranges between 0 to 1.
- This value for a country shows the distance that it has already travelled towards maximum possible value of 1 and also allows comparisons with other countries.

58. Ans. (a) Income

Ref: K. Park 23rd ed. pg. 17

Components/Indicators of PQLI

- Literacy rate
- Infant mortality rate
- Life expectancy at age 1 year

59. Ans. (a) Tuberculosis

Ref: K. Park, 23rd ed. pg. 39, 135

- **Iceberg phenomenon** can be compared to a disease in community.
- **Floating tip of iceberg** (visible portion): Clinical cases that physicians sees in community. It can be detected by diagnostic tests.
- **Submerged part** (hidden portion): Are the latent, undiagnosed cases and carriers. It is detected by screening test by an epidemiologist.
- **Water surface** (demarcation line): Demarcation between apparent and inapparent disease.
- **Iceberg phenomenon of a disease is NOT shown by:**
  - Rabies
  - Tetanus
  - Measles
  - Rubella

60. Ans. (a) Undiagnosed cases in community

Ref: K. Park, 23rd ed. pg. 39, 135; K. Park, 21st ed. pg. 37

61. Ans. (a) Secular trend

Ref: K. Park, 23rd ed. pg. 66, 21st ed. pg. 61,62

Time Distribution of Disease

- **Secular trend:** It implies changes in occurrence of a disease over a period of long time, generally several years or decade.
  - **Ex:** Polio, Diphtheria, Pertusis are the diseases which are reducing in India in fast few decades; and diseases like DM, Obesity and hypertension has increased in past few decades.
- **Epidemic:** Short term fluctuation of a disease occur in few days, week, or months. E.g. food poisoning, Bhopal gas tragedy.

Periodic Fluctuation

- **Cyclic trends:** Some diseases occur in cycles spread over a period of time which means days, weeks, months, or years. Non-infectious condition may also show periodic fluctuations *ex: automobile accidents in US are more frequent on weekends, esp: Saturday*. Other examples can be measles occurring every 2–3 years, Rubella every 6–9 years, influenza pandemics at intervals of 7–10 years (due to antigenic variations)
- **Seasonal trend:** It is seasonal variation/fluctuation in occurrence of a disease. The seasonal variation of disease occurence may be related to environmental condition like humidity, rainfall, temperature.
- Example: Measles and varicella in early spring season, upper respiratory infection in incidence increases in winter, gastroenteritis increases in summer.

62. Ans. (a) Secular trends

Ref: K. Park, 23rd ed. pg. 66, 21st ed. pg. 62

Please refer to above explanation

63. Ans. (d) Cyclic trend

Ref: K. Park, 23rd ed. pg. 66, 21st ed. pg. 62

64. Ans. (a) Cyclic trends

Ref: K. Park, 23rd ed. pg. 65-66, 21st ed. pg. 61,62

Please refer to above explanation

65. Ans. (b) Infectivity

Ref: K. Park, 23rd ed. pg. 36

- **Infectivity:** This is ability of an infectious agent to invade and multiply (produce infection) in a host.
- **Pathogenicity:** It is the ability to induce **clinically apparent illness.**
- **Virulence:** Proportion of clinical cases resulting in **severe clinical manifestation.**

STUDY DESIGNS AND PREVENTIVE MEASURES

66. Ans. (c) Secondary

Ref: Park Textbook of Preventive and Social Medicine, 25th ed. pg. 48

- Secondary prevention emphasizes early disease detection through screening test so that the treatment can be started early.

More detailed discussion about level of prevention has been given later in this chapter

67. Ans. (b) Cohort study

Ref: Park Textbook of Preventive and Social Medicine, 25th ed. pg. 83

- Relative risk is a ratio of the probability of an event occurring in the exposed group versus the probability of the event occurring in the non-exposed group.
- Relative risk can be directly determined in a cohort study by calculating a risk ratio (RR).

68. Ans. (a) Cohort study

Ref: K. Park 25th ed. pg. 78

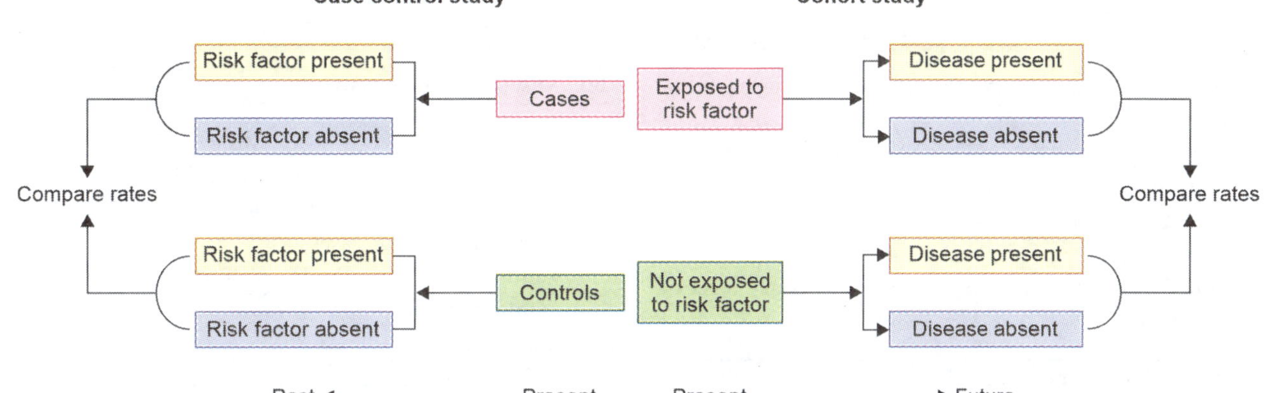

69. Ans. (d) Randomization

Ref: K. Park 25th ed. pg. 90

- Randomisation is a statistical procedure by which participants are allocated into groups usually called "study" and "control" groups, to receive or not to receive an experimental preventive or therapeutic procedure.
- It is an attempt to eliminate "bias" and allow for comparability.

70. Ans. (b) Meta-analysis

Ref: K. Park 25th ed. pg. 86

- Meta analysis is a quantitative, formal, epidemiological study design used to systematically assess the results of previous research to derive conclusions.

71. Ans. (c) Secondary

Ref: Park, 25th ed. pg. 48

- This is an example of **secondary prevention**. As in secondary prevention level, we try to detect a disease early, identify risks and try to prevent the disease and its symptoms from progressing.
- The man is at high risk of development of cardiac illness due to family history.
- All the screenings are under secondary level of prevention.

72. Ans. (b) Case control study

Ref: Park, 25th ed. pg. 79

- Case control study involves two populations - cases and controls. In case control studies, the unit is the individual rather than the group. The focus is on a disease or some other health problem that has *already developed*.

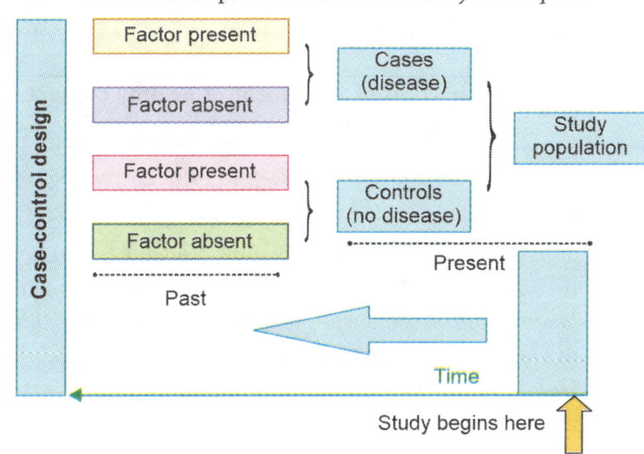

73. Ans. (b) Case control study

Ref: K. Park, 25th ed. pg. 75

- A case–control study is a type of observational study in which two existing groups differing in outcome are identified and compared on the basis of some supposed causal attribute.
- A case–control study is a retrospective, Effect to cause, Disease to risk factor andOutcome to exposure aka TROHOC study.

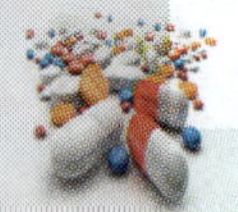

74. Ans. (b) Unpaired student's t-test

Ref: Statistical and Behavioral Sciences, 2nd ed. pg. 376

- An unpaired t-test (also known as an independent t-test) is a statistical procedure that compares the averages/ means of two independent or unrelated groups to determine if there is a significant difference between the two.

75. Ans. (c) Secondary

Ref: K. Park, 25th ed. pg. 46, 384-86

- All screening and diagnostic tests are secondary level of prevention
- Secondary prevention is a method to detect and address an existing disease prior to the appearance of symptoms.
- Examples: Screening of hypertension and cancer screenings
- **Note:** Treatment measures are also secondary level of prevention

76. Ans. (a) Specific protection

Ref: K. Park, 25th ed. pg. 110

- Specific protection targets a type or group of diseases and complements the goals of health promotion
- Health-promotional activities do not target a specific disease or condition but rather promote health and well-being on a very general level.

77. Ans. (b) Restriction of movement of healthy contact of an infectious disease

Ref: K. Park 25th ed. pg. 132

- **Quarantine** is defined as: *"The limitation of freedom of movement of such well persons who are exposed to communicable disease for a period of time no longer than the longest usual incubation period of the disease, in such manner as to prevent effective contact with those not so exposed."*
- **Isolation** on the other hand is separation of infected person from others for the period of communicability.

78. Ans. (a) Prospective cohort

Ref: K. Park 23rd ed. pg. 80

- The Framingham heart study was initiated in 1948 by US public health service to study the relationship between number of risk factors (like BP, smoking, serum cholesterol, obesity) and subsequent development of cardiovascular disease.
- Study was done in town of Framingham for 20 years in view of the slow development of heart disease.
- It is an example of prospective cohort study.

79. Ans. (a) Cohort study

Ref: K. Park 23rd ed. pg. 65

- Incidence and relative risk is accurately calculated by cohort study.
- It is a type of analytical or observational study used for hypothesis testing, also called TROHOC study prospective study/forward looking study/*cause to effect study*/exposure to outcome study/*risk factor to disease study* incidence study follow-up study.
- Prevalence is determined by cross sectional studies.

80. Ans. (c) Berkesonian bias

Ref: K. Park, 23rd ed. pg. 73-74

- Berkesonian bias is a type of study bias that arises because of the different rates of admission to hospitals for people with different diseases.
- It is termed after Dr. Joseph Berkeson who recognized this problem.

81. Ans. (b) Secondary prevention

Ref: K. Park, 23rd ed.

- Fetal cardiac monitoring is a screening test to detect any fetal distress in utero.
- *All screening and diagnostic tests are secondary level of prevention.*

TABLE: Levels of prevention

Level of prevention	Timing	Mode of prevention	Example
Primordial	Before emergence of risk factor	–	• Preventing obesity • Practising healthy lifestyle
Primary	Risk factor present but no disease yet	*By health promotion and specific protection*	• ***All vaccines*** • Contraceptives • Mosquito nets/ repellants/DDT • Chemoprophylaxis
Secondary	When disease has probably started	*By early diagnosis and treatment*	• All screening and diagnostic tests • Treatment measures • *BP monitoring*
Tertiary	Disease in progression	*By disability limitation and rehabilitation.*	• Physiotherapy • Crutches in polio

82. Ans. (a) Cohort study

Ref: K. Park, 23rd ed. pg. 78

- Relative risk is the ratio of disease among exposed and disease among non exposed. It is also known as risk ratio.
- RR = incidence of disease among exposed/Incidence of disease among non-exposed
- It is a direct measure of strength of association between suspected cause and effect.

83. Ans. (d) Patient does not know what is he getting

Ref: K. Park, 23rd ed. pg. 83

- In **double blind trial**, neither patient nor the doctor are aware of group allocation and the treatment received. Patient is either getting placebo or the drug.
- All the clinical trials must take an informed consent regarding the same from the participants.

Extra Mile

- **SINGLE BLIND TRIAL:** It is planned in such a way that participant is not aware whether he belong to the study group or control group.
- **TRIPLE BLIND TRIAL:** In this type of trial, the participant, the investigator and the person analyzing the data are all "blind" (not aware)
- **Note: Double blinding is most commonly used method when blind trial is conducted.**

84. Ans. (b) It is the procedure by which participants are allocated into groups usually called 'study' and 'control' group

Ref: K. Park, 23rd ed. pg. 82, 21st ed. pg. 78

- Randomization is "heart" of a control trial. It is a statistical procedure by which the participants are allocated into groups usually called "study" and "control" group.
- It is an attempt to eliminate bias and allow comparability.
- By doing this it is ensured that investigator has NO control over allocation of participants to study or control group. THIS REMOVES SELECTION BIAS.
- RANDOMIZATION is done only after the participant has entered the study, i.e., after having been qualified for the trial and has given his informed consent to participate in the study.

85. Ans. (b) Prevention of emergence of risk factors of the disease

Ref: K. Park, 23rd ed. pg. 41, 370

- Primordial prevention refers to prevention of development of risk factors in countries or population groups where they are yet to appear.
- For instance, adult health problems like obesity, hypertension etc. take root in childhood, when lifestyles like smoking, eating patterns, physical exercise are formed
- As part of primordial prevention, efforts are made to discourage high risk children, adolescents and young adults from adopting harmful lifestyles. The primary intervention is through individual and mass education.

86. Ans. (b) Primary

Ref: K. Park, 23rd ed. pg. 41, 370-73

- All vaccines/immunization are primary level of prevention.
- *BCG vaccine used for treatment of bladder CA is secondary level of prevention.*

Extra Mile

TABLE: Level of prevention with their modes and example

Level of prevention	Timing	Mode of prevention	Example
Primordial	Before emergence of risk factor	–	• Practising healthy lifestyle • Preventing obesity
Primary	Risk factor present but NO disease yet	By health promotion and specific protection	• ***All vaccines*** • Contraceptives • Mosquito nets/repellants/DDT • Chemoprophylaxis
Secondary	When Disease has probably started	By early diagnosis and treatment	• ***All screening and diagnostic tests.*** • Treatment measures • *BP monitoring*
Tertiary	Disease in progression:	By disability limitation and rehabilitation.	• Physiotherapy • Crutches in polio

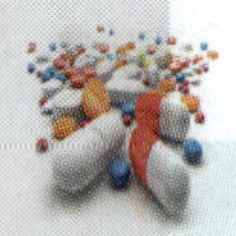

87. Ans. (a) Primary

Ref: K. Park, 23rd ed. pg. 41, 370-74

88. Ans. (c) Early diagnosis and treatment

Ref: K. Park, 23rd ed. pg. 41, 370-74

- Early diagnosis and treatment comes under secondary level of prevention.

Please refer to above explanation

89. Ans. (c) Secondary

Ref: K. Park, 23rd ed. pg. 41, 370-74

- *All screening and diagnostic tests and treatment measures come under secondary level of prevention.*
- *Refer to previous explanation.*

90. Ans. (b) Primary

Ref: K. Park, 23rd ed. pg. 41, 370-74

- All vaccines/immunization are primary level of prevention.
- *Refer to above table.*

91. Ans. (c) Secondary

Ref: K. Park, 23rd ed. pg. 41, 376

- Tracking of blood pressure helps in early diagnosis of hypertension.
- Hence comes in secondary level of prevention.

92. Ans. (a) Pap smear

Ref: K. Park, 23rd ed. pg. 41, 385

- **Primary prevention** is the action taken prior to the onset of disease which removes the possibilities of disease occurrence.
- **Modes of intervention:**
  - Health promotion
  - Specific protection
- It is applicable for "risk factors are present but disease has not yet taken place"
- *Pap smear is a screening test, which comes under secondary level of prevention.*

93. Ans. (a) Early diagnosis and treatment

Ref: K. Park, 23rd ed. pg. 41, 370

- Pap smear is a screening test for cervical cancer. It is an example of secondary level of prevention. The mode of secondary level of prevention is by early diagnosis and treatment.

94. Ans. (c) Specific protection

Ref: K. Park, 23rd ed. pg. 41, 370

- ***Specific prevention of neck problem before onset of disease.***
- Desk provided with table top, probably decrease the risk of developing neck problems like cervical spondylosis etc.
- This is primary level of prevention done by specific protection.

95. Ans. (c) Secondary

Ref: K. Park, 23rd ed. pg. 41, 370-73

- Any treatment measure comes under secondary level of prevention.
- *Refer to above explanation*

96. Ans. (b) Specific protection

Ref: K. Park, 23rd ed. pg. 41, 370-73

- Iodised salt is given in an area which has risk of developing goiter. This is a primary level of prevention done by specific protection.
- Primordial prevention is done before the emergence of risk factor.

97. Ans. (b) Specific protection

Ref: K. Park, 23rd ed. pg. 41

- IFA supplement is a chemoprophylaxis given during pregnancy for anemia. It comes under primary level of prevention which is implemented under specific protection.

98. Ans. (d) BP of hypertensive remains hypertensive

Ref: K. Park 23rd ed. pg. 374

Park 23rd/P 374 States:

If BP of a person is tracked from early childhood to adult life then those individuals whose blood pressure was initially high in the distribution, would probably continue in the same "track".

99. Ans. (a) Primordial prevention

Ref: K. Park, 23rd ed. pg. 41, 21st ed. pg. 39-40

- Primordial level of prevention is defined as prevention of emergence or development of risk factors in countries or population groups in which disease entity is not yet appeared, or population group which are not yet exposed.
- **Modes of intervention:**
  - Individual education
  - Mass education
- ***Primordial level is considered as best level of prevention for non-communicable diseases***

EPIDEMIOLOGY, SCREENING AND VACCINES

100. Ans. (b) 9 months

Ref: Park Textbook of Preventive and Social Medicine, 25th ed. pg. 136

The Indian Academy of Pediatrics (IAP) recommends the next dose measles vaccine at 9 months of age in an epidemic.

101. Ans. (c) BCG, OPV, Hepatitis B

Ref: Park Textbook of Preventive and Social Medicine, 25th ed. pg. 136

At birth

- BCG, 0.1 mL (0.05 mL for <1 month age), Intradermal, Left upper arm
- OPV, 2 drops,
- Hep-B (birth dose), 0.5 mL, Intramuscular, Anterolateral side of mid-thigh – LEFT (k/a Birth dose)

102. Ans. (a) At birth

Ref: Park Textbook of Preventive and Social Medicine, 25th ed. pg. 136

- Hepatitis B Birth dose at birth or as early as possible within 24 hours.

103. Ans. (b) Maternal mortality ratio

Ref: K. Park 25th ed. pg. 510

Statistical Measures of Maternal Mortality
Maternal mortality ratio (MMR) Number of maternal death during a given time period per 100000 live births during the same time period
Maternal mortality rate (MMRate) Number of maternal deaths in a given period per 100000 women of reproductive age during the same time period
Adult lifetime risk of maternal death The probability that a 15-year-old women will die eventually from a maternal cause
The proportion of maternal deaths among deaths of women of reproductive age (PM) The number of maternal deaths in a given time period divided by the total deaths among women aged 15–49 years

104. Ans. (b) L1, L2

Ref: K. Park 25th ed. pg. 113

- HPV vaccines are based on hollow virus like particles assembled from recombinant HPV coat proteins. The natural virus capsid is composed of two proteins, L1 and L2.
- Examples of HPV vaccines are Gardasil and Cervarix.

105. Ans. (c) VVM

Ref: K. Park 25th ed. pg. 121

- **Vaccine vial monitors** are the only temperature monitoring devices that routinely accompany vaccines throughout the entire supply chain.
- It is a chemical indicator label attached to the vaccine container. It records its cumulative heat exposure through a gradual change in color.

106. Ans. (b) John Snow

Ref: K. Park, 23rd ed. pg. 5-6

- Father of public Health: Cholera
- *Father of modern epidemiology: John Snow*
- Father of Medicine/first true epidemiologist: Hippocrates.

107. Ans. (d) Hippocrates

Ref: K. Park, 23rd ed. pg. 5-6

Refer to above answer

108. Ans (b) Agent, host and environment

Ref: K. Park, 23rd ed. pg. 33-34, Park, 19th pg. 30

A broad concept of disease causation that synthesized the basic factors of agent, host and environment (see adjacent figure) This model—agent, host and environment--has been in use for many years. It helped epidemiologists to focus on different classes of factors, especially with regard to infectious diseases

Epidemiological triad

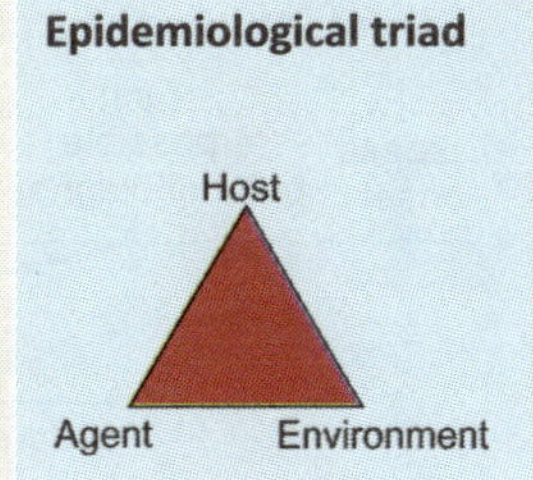

109. Ans. (c) Case fatality rate

Ref: Park, 25th ed. pg. 25

- Case fatality rate measures the risk of persons dying from a certain disease within a given time period.
- Case fatality rate is calculated as number of deaths from a specific disease during a specific time period divided by number of cases of the disease during the same time period, usually expressed as per 100.

Case Fatality Rate

$$\frac{\text{Number of deaths}}{\text{Number of all cases}} \times 100\% = \text{Case Fatality Rate (CPR)}$$

- The case fatality rate is used to link mortality to morbidity. One function of the case fatality rate is to measure various aspects or properties of a disease such as its pathogenicity, severity or virulence.

110. Ans. (a) Secular trend of a disease

Ref: Park, 25th ed. pg. 74

- **"Secular trend"** implies changes in the occurrence of disease (i.e., a progressive increase or decrease) over a **long period of time, generally several years or decades.** Although it may have short-term fluctuations imposed on it, a secular trend implies a consistent tendency to change in a particular direction or a definite movement in one direction.
- Examples include coronary heart disease, lung cancer and diabetes which have shown a consistent upward trend in the developed countries during the past 50 years or so, followed by a decline of such diseases as tuberculosis, typhoid fever, diphtheria and polio.

111. Ans. (b) Screening time

Ref: K. Park, 25th ed. pg. 145

- **Screening time:** First possible point of diagnosis to first critical diagnosis (B to C in image)
- **Lead time:** First possible point of diagnosis to usual time of diagnosis (B to D in image)
- **Incubation period:** Time period between infection to first symptom
- **Latent period:** Time interval between when an individual is infected and when he/she becomes capable of infecting other susceptible individual.

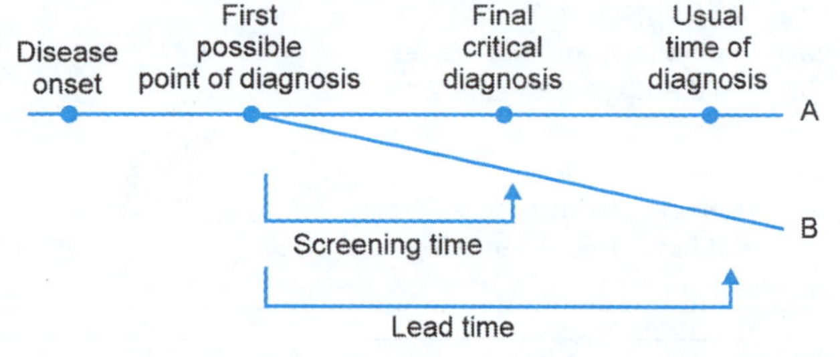

112. Ans. (a) Maternal mortality rate

Ref: K. Park, 25th ed. pg. 596

- Sample Registration System (SRS) was initiated in 1964–65 to provide national as well as state level reliable estimates of fertility and mortality.

Includes

- Crude Birth Rate (CBR)
- Crude Death Rate (CDR)
- Natural Growth Rate
- Infant Mortality Rate (IMR)

113. Ans. (b) Net reproduction rate (NRR)

Ref: K. Park, 25th ed. pg. 523

- **Net Reproduction Rate (NRR):** Number of daughters a newborn girl will bear during her lifetime assuming fixed age-specific fertility and mortality rates.
- NRR = 1: Each generation of women is exactly reproducing itself
- *To achieve NRR = 1: Couple Protection Rate (CPR) should be >60%.*

114. Ans. (c) Positive predictive value

Ref: K. Park, 25th ed. pg. 60

- Prevalence: Is total current (Old + New) cases in a given population over a point or period of time.
  Prevalence = Incidence × Mean duration of the disease (P = I × D)
  - Prevalence describes balance between incidence, mortality and recovery. As prevalence increases, positive predictive value increases and negative predictive value decreases.
  - Incidence reflects causal factors
  - Duration reflects the prognostic factors

115. Ans. (a) Life long

Ref: K. Park, 25th ed. pg. 300

- The vaccine is administered subcutaneously at the insertion of deltoid in a single dose of 0.5 ml irrespective of age.
- **Immunity begins to appear on the 7th day and lasts for more than 35 years, and possibly for life.**
- **WHO recommends revaccination after 10 years for international travel**

Extra Mile

- Yellow Fever Vaccine:– Live attenuated, lyophilized (Freeze dried) vaccine
- Strain: 17D strain (Chick Embryo grown)
- Cold chain Temperature: – 30° to + 5°C Reconstitution with Diluent
- YF vaccine is the only Live vaccine that can be administered in Pregnancy (if there is risk of exposure).
- Yellow Fever Vaccine and Cholera Vaccine cannot be given together: Maintain a gap of 3 weeks or more between them.

116. Ans. (a) NS

Ref: K. Park 25th ed. pg. 213

- For reconstituting the vaccine, normal saline is recommended as diluent (distilled water can cause irritation)
- Reconstituted vaccine can be used up to 3 hours and left over should be discarded
- A satisfactory injection should produce a wheal of 5 mm in diameter.

117. Ans. (c) Ice line refrigerator

Ref: K. Park 25th ed. pg. 118-19

TABLE: Cold chain equipment

Storage	Transportation
Electrical • Walk in cooler • Walk in freezer • Ice line refrigerator (ILR) • Domestic refrigerator • Deep freezer	• Refrigerated vaccine • Insulated vaccine van • Cold box • Vaccine carrier: Used to carry 16–20 vials • Day carriers: Used to carry 6–8 vials. Two fully frozen ice packs are used
Solar • Solar refrigerator battery drive • Solar refrigerator direct drive **Nonelectrical** • Cold box • Vaccine carrier	**Note:** • The risk of cold chain failure is greatest at sub-centre and village level • Therefore, vaccines are NOT stored at sub centre level and must be supplied on the day of use

TABLE: Differences between all the equipment

Equipment	Temperature	Used for storing	Installed at
Walk in cooler	Maintain + 2 to + 8°C	Store all vaccines like BCG, HepB, DPT, Pentavalent, IPV, TT	• **Govt medical store depots** • **State and regional vaccine stores**
Walk in freezer	(–15 to – 25°C)	• For bulk storage of OPV vaccine • Preparation of frozen ice packs for vaccine transportation	**National, regional and state vaccine stores**
Deep freezer	(–15 to – 25°C)	• Store OPV vaccine for 3 months • Freezing ice packs	District level and sub district level
Ice line refrigerator (ideal for safe storage of vaccine)	(+2 to + 8°C)	• For vaccines like OPV, BCG, Measles and JE stored at the bottom of basket • DPT, TT, Hep B, IPV, pentavalent and Diluents—kept in upper part of basket	Large size ILR: District and sub district level Small size ILR: **PHC**
Domestic refrigerator	(+2 to + 8°C)	• Placement of vaccine in the refrigerator with freezer on top is as follows: • **Top shelf:** Measles, BCG, OPV, Rota virus • **Middle shelf:** DPT, Pentavalent, TT, IPV, Hep-B, JE • **Bottom shelf:** Ice packs filled with water and in door of refrigerator	Used for storage vaccine at private clinics and nursing homes
Cold boxes	Fully frozen ice packs are used. Kept at bottom and sides	Used for transportation of vaccines	Supplied to all **peripheral centres**

118. Ans. (b) 4 weeks

Ref: K. Park 25th ed. pg. 111; www.immunize.org/askexperts/precautions-contraindications.asp

- Book states: *"Live vaccines should not be administered to persons with immune deficiency diseases or to persons whose immune system is suppressed because of leukaemia, lymphoma, malignancy or because of therapy with corticosteroids, alkylating agent, anti-metabolites and radiation"*
- The immunosuppressive effect of corticosteroid may vary.
- As dose of 2 mg/kg or 20 mg/day for 2 weeks or more raise concern about safety of vaccination with live vaccines like MMR, varicella etc.
- It is recommended to wait for 1 month after discontinuation of steroid therapy before administering a live vaccine virus.
- **Note:** Inactivated vaccines and toxoids can be used administered to all immunocompromised patients in usual doses and schedules.

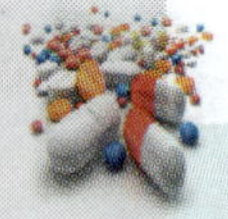

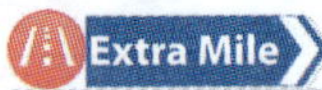

Extra Mile

- Pregnancy is also a contraindication for live vaccines.
- When two live vaccines are required, they should be given either simultaneously at different sites or with an interval of atleast 3 weeks

119. Ans. (a) Yellow fever

Ref: K. Park 23rd ed. pg. 283

Contraindications of Yellow Fever Vaccines

- Children aged <9 months for routine immunization (or <6 months during an epidemic)
- Pregnant women (except during outbreak)
- People with severe egg protein allergy
- People with severe immunodeficiency caused by HIV/AIDS.

120. Ans. (a) Point source epidemic

Ref: K. Park 23rd ed. pg. 64-65

Types of Epidemics

- **Point source or single exposure epidemics:**
  - Sharp rise and sharp fall in number of cases
  - Clustering of cases in narrow spectrum of time
  - All cases develop within one incubation period of disease.
  - **Ex: Food poisoning, measles, chicken pox, *Bhopal gas tragedy***
- **Common source, continuous or repeated exposure epidemics:**
  - Sharp rise in number of cases
  - Fall in number of cases is interrupted by secondary waves/peaks
  - **Ex: Contaminated well in a village, sex worker in a gonorrhea outbreak**
- **Propagated epidemics:**
  - Gradual rise and gradual fall over a long time (tail off)
  - Usually infectious in origin and results from person to person transmission
  - Transmission continues till number of susceptibles is depleted or they are no longer exposed to infected individuals
  - **Ex: Hep A, Polio, HIV, Tuberculosis**

Extra Mile

- **Endemic:** Constant presence of a disease in a defined geographical area.
- **Pandemic:** Epidemic affecting a large population, occurring over a large geographical area.
- **Sporadic:** Scattered cases. They are widely separated in space and time and show little or no connection.

121. Ans. (c) 45

Ref: K. Park 23rd ed. pg. 360, 395

- Diabetes, hypertension and coronary artery diseases are among the diseases with high mortality.
- **Book states:** *"CHD is responsible for 30–50%" of deaths in diabetics over the age of 40 years.*
- *"Target population for screening diabetes are those from age group 40 and above"*

122. Ans. (a) Tetanus toxoid

Ref: K. Park 23rd ed. pg. 311-312

- Tetanus occurring in newborn is known as neonatal tetanus. However it is acquired more commonly during the active age i.e., 5–40 years.
- Infants usually contract the disease during the birth, when delivered in a nonaseptic condition, especially when the umbilical cord is cut with the unclean instrument or when the umbilical stump is dressed with ashes, soil or cow dung.
- No age is immune unless protected by previous immunization.
- *The immunity resulting from 2 injections from tetanus toxoid is highly effective and lasts for several years.*

Prevention of Neonatal Tetanus

- **Active immunization:** Tetanus is best prevented by active immunization with tetanus toxoid. It stimulates the production of the protective antitoxin. Two preparations are available:
  - **Combined vaccine:** DPT.
    - Offered routinely to infants under expanded immunization program.
    - 3 doses of vaccine given starting at 6 weeks of age in a gap of 4–8 weeks
  - **Monovalent vaccine:**
    - Plain or fluid (formal) toxoid
    - Tetanus vaccine, adsorbed
- **Passive immunization**
  - Temporary protection can be provided by an injection of human tetanus hyperimmunoglobulin or ATS. It is the prophylactic to be used.
  - **Dose:** 250 IU for all ages.

123. Ans. (c) Number of new cases

Ref: K. Park 23rd ed. pg. 60

Incidence

Incidence rate is defined as "the number of NEW cases occurring in a defined population during a specified period of time". It is given by the formula:

$$\text{Incidence} = \frac{\text{Number of new cases of specific disease during a given time period}}{\text{Population at-risk during that period}} \times 100$$

For example, if there had been 500 new cases of an illness in a population of 30,000 in a year, the incidence rate would be:
= 500/30,000 × 1000
= 16.7 per 1000 per year

124. Ans. (b) dT

Ref: K. Park 23rd ed. pg. 162

- **Book states:** *"For immunizing children over 12 years of age and adults, the preparation of choice is dT, which is adult type of diphtheria tetanus vaccine"*
- This preparation contains no more than 2 L of diphtheria toxoid per dose, as compared to 25 L in the ordinary DPT vaccine.
- Administration of dT vaccine to adults is carried out in 2 doses at an interval of 4–6 weeks, followed by booster 6–12 months after second dose.

125. Ans. (d) Common source, continuous exposure

Ref: K. Park, 23rd ed. pg. 65

- **EPIDEMIC:** Sudden occurrence and rise of a particular health related behaviour/events which is in excess of "expected occurrence"
- **Common source, continuous or repeated exposure epidemics:**
  - Sharp rise in number of cases
  - Fall in number of cases is interrupted by secondary waves/peaks
  - **Ex: Contaminated well in a village, Sex worker in a gonorrhea outbreak**

126. Ans. (d) Secondary attack rate

Ref: K. Park, 23rd ed. pg. 100

- **Secondary attack rate** is defined as "the number of exposed persons developing the disease within the range of incubation period, following exposure to the primary case." It is given by the formula:

$$\text{SAR} = \frac{\text{No. of exposed person developing the disease within range of incubation period}}{\text{Total no. of exposed/susceptible contacts}}$$

127. Ans. (d) Verification of diagnosis

Ref: K. Park, 23rd ed. pg. 131

In case of investigating an epidemic, an orderly procedure or the following practical guidelines should be followed:

- **Verification of diagnosis:** It is the first step in epidemic investigation
- **Confirmation of existence of epidemic:** It is the next step to confirm if epidemic exists. It is done by comparing the disease frequencies during the same period of previous years.
- Defining the population at risk
- Rapid search for all cases and their characteristics
- Data analysis
- Hypothesis formulation
- Testing of hypothesis
- Ecological factor evaluation
- Further investigation of population at risk
- Writing the report

128. Ans. (d) Number of girls born to a woman during her lifetime assuming mortality

Ref: K. Park, 23rd ed. pg. 488-89

- **Net Reproduction Rate (NRR):** Net Reproduction Rate (NRR) is denied as the number of assuming fixed age-specific fertility and mortality rates (21).
  NRR is a demographic indicator. NRR of 1 is equivalent to attaining approximately the 2-child norm.
- **General Fertility Rate (GFR):** It is the "number of live births per 1000 women in the reproductive age-group (15–44 or 49 years) in a given year".

$$\text{GFR} = \frac{\text{Number of live births in an area during the year}}{\text{Mid-year female population age 15-44 (or 49) in the same area in same year}} \times 1000$$

  General fertility rate is a better measure of fertility than the crude birth rate because the denominator is restricted to the number of women in the child–bearing age, rather than the whole population. The major weakness of this rate is that not all women in the denominator are exposed to the risk of childbirth.
- **General Marital Fertility Rate (GMFR):** It is the "number of live births per 1000 married women in the reproductive age group (15–44 or 49) in a given year".

$$\text{GMFR} = \frac{\text{Number of live births in an year}}{\text{Mid-year married female population in the age-group 15-49 years}} \times 1000$$

- **Total fertility rate (TFR):** Total fertility rate represents the average number of children a woman would have if she were to pass through the women now in each age group.
- **Total marital fertility rate:** Average number of children that would be born to a married woman if she experiences the current fertility pattern throughout her reproductive span.
- **Gross reproduction rate (GRR):** Average number of girls that would be born to a woman if she experiences the current fertility pattern throughout her reproductive span (15–44 or 49 years), assuming no mortality.

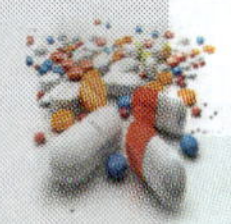

129. Ans. (b) 60

Ref: K. Park, 23rd ed. pg. 493

Couple Protection Rate (CPR)

- **Couple protection rate** (CPR) is an indicator of the prevalence of contraceptive practice in the community. It is defined as the per cent of eligible couples effectively protected against childbirth by one or the other approved methods of family planning, viz. sterilization, IUD, condom or oral pills.
- Sterilization accounts for over 60% of effectively protected couples. Demographers are of the view that the **demographic goal of NRR = 1 can be achieved only if the CPR exceeds 60%.**

130. Ans. (d) Odds ratio

- The *given scenario is a retrospective study*, also known as case control study. It is better known to calculate the odd's ratio.
- Prevalence is better given by cross sectional study.
- Incidence and relative risk is accurately calculated by cohort study.

131. Ans. (a) 20 IU/kg

Ref: K. Park, 23rd ed. pg. 280

- Rabies Ig for passive immunization is administered only once, preferably at, or as soon as possible after the initiation of post exposure vaccination.
- Beyond 7th day after the first dose, rabies Ig is not indicated
- The dose of human rabies Ig is 20 IU/kg body weight.
- The dose of equine Ig and F (ab') 2 products, is 40 IU/kg body weight.

132. Ans. (b) 0.5 cc

Ref: K. Park, 23rd ed. pg. 148

- Only live attenuated vaccines are recommended for use.
- The vaccine is presented as freeze-dried product. Before use, the lyophilized vaccine is reconstituted with sterile diluent.
- **Each dose of 0.5 cc** contains ≥ 1000 viral infective units of the vaccine strain.

Extra Mile

- Reconstituted measles vaccine **loses 50% of its potency after 1 hour at 20°C.**
- It **loses almost all potency after 2 hour at 37°C.**
- The vaccine is sensitive to light, hence **kept in colored glass vials.**
- After reconstitution, the vaccine must be **stored in the dark at 2–8°C and used within 4 hours.**

133. Ans. (c) 3

Ref: http://www.who.int/immunization_standards/vaccine_quality/pq266_je_1dose_biologicale/en/; K. Park 23rd ed. pg. 481

- JE vaccine can be stored at 2–8° C for up to 3 years (shelf life)
- Similarly, Rabies vaccines prequalified by WHO, do not contain preservatives, such as thiomersal. The shelf life of these vaccines is ≥3 years, provided they are stored at +2 to +8° C and protected from sunlight.

134. Ans. (a) Includes notifiable cases

Ref: K. Park, 23rd ed. pg. 40

- **Surveillance** is defined as "the continuous scrutiny of the factors that determines the occurrence and distribution of disease and other conditions of ill health"
- **The main objectives of surveillance are:**
  - To provide information about new and changing trends in the health status of a population.
  - To provide timely warning of public health disasters so that intervention can be mobilized.
  - To provide feedback which may be expected to modify the policy of the system itself and lead to redefinition of objectives.

Sentinel Surveillance:

- A method to identify the "missing cases" (by usual surveillance).
- **The** sentinel surveillance data is extrapolated to the entire population to estimate the disease prevalence in total population.
- **This** system provides more valuable and detailed information that could be obtained from traditional notification system *(e.g. Subcenter reports).*
- Advantage:
  - **Reporting bias is minimized** and feedback information to the providers is simplified
- **Done by whom?**
  - Sentinel surveillance agencies
  - Competent physicians (or institutions) in selected areas

135. Ans. (d) Patients with varicella zoster

Ref: K. Park, 23rd ed. pg. 145

Varicella Zoster Immunoglobulin (VZIG)

- VZIG given within 72 hours of exposure, has been recommended for prevention of chicken pox in exposed susceptible individuals particularly in immunosuppressed patients. These include:
  - Person with congenital cellular immunodeficiency
  - Susceptible persons receiving immunosuppressive therapy

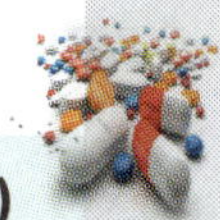

- Persons with HIV/AIDS
- Susceptible and exposed persons, in particular pregnant women
- Newborns
- Premature infants of low birth weight

- **Note:** VZIG has no role in established disease
- **Dose of VZIG:** 12.5 units/kg up to max of 625 units
- **Since VZIG appears to bind the varicella vaccine, the two should not be given together.**

136. Ans. (c) 13%

Ref: K. Park, 23rd ed. pg. 61

- Prevalence is calculated as

$$\frac{\text{No. of new cases + no of old cases}}{\text{Total Population}} \times 100$$

- Therefore prevalence = $\frac{500 + 150}{5000} \times 100$
- Prevalence = 13%

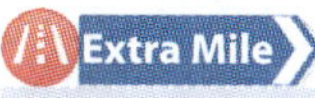

Extra Mile

- *Prevalence is a Proportion*
- *Incidence is a Rate*

137. Ans. (a) Index case

Ref: K. Park 23rd ed. pg. 95

- **Index case:** In epidemiology, first case of a disease in a group which is **seen** by an investigator or which brought to the attention of the clinician. ***It is not always the primary case.***
- **Primary case:** ***First case of communicable disease introduced into the population unit being studied.***
- **Secondary case:** All case who develop from primary case
- **Incubation period:** Entry of organism till 1st sign/ symptom
- **Median incubation:** Time period for 50% case to occur

138. Ans. (c) Primary case

Ref: K. Park, 23rd ed. pg. 95, 21st ed. pg. 91

- **Index case:** First case which comes to attention of investigator.
- **Primary case:** First case of communicable disease introduced into the population unit being studies.
- **Secondary case:** Cases which arise due to contacts with primary case.

139. Ans. (b) Limitation of freedom of movement of well person or animals till incubation period of disease

Ref: K. Park, 23rd ed. pg. 120, 21st ed. pg. 111

- **QUARANTINE** is defined as **Limitation of freedom of movement of such well person or domestic animals who are exposed to a communicable disease for a longer period of time, not longer than the longest usual incubation period of the disease.** This effectively prevents the contact with those who are not exposed, thereby reduces chances of possible transmission.
- **ISOLATION** is separation for the period of communicability of INFECTED person or animals from others in order to reduce direct or indirect transmission.
- **Epidemiological investigations** Identification of source of infection and factors influencing its spread in community
- **Notification:** Notification of an infectious disease to local health authority to put control measures on it.

140. Ans. (c) Pandemic

Ref: K. Park, 23rd ed. pg. 93, 21st ed. pg. 88-89

- **Endemic:** Constant presence of a disease or an infectious agent within a given geographical area or a population group.
- **Epidemic:** Sudden occurrence and rise of a particular health related behaviour/event which is in excess of "expected occurrence".
- **Sporadic:** Scattered cases, which occur irregularly, haphazardly from time to time. These cases are few and separated widely in space and time that they show little or no connection with each other, nor a recognizable common source of infection.
- **Pandemic:** An epidemic usually affecting a large proportion of population, occurring over a wide geographic area such as a section of nation, the entire nation, a continent or the world.

141. Ans. (b) Sharp rise and sharp fall in number of cases

Ref: K. Park, 23rd ed. pg. 64, 93

Types of Epidemics

- **Point source or single exposure epidemics**
  - Sharp rise and sharp fall in number of cases
  - Clustering of cases in narrow spectrum of time
  - All cases develop within one incubation period of disease.
  - **Ex: Food poisoning, measles, chicken pox, *Bhopal gas tragedy***

Extra Mile

- **Endemic:** Constant presence of a disease in a defined geographical area
- **Pandemic:** Epidemic affecting a large population, occurring over a large geographical area.
- **Sporadic:** Scattered cases. They are widely separated in space and time and shows little or no connection.

142. Ans. (a) Incubation period

Ref: K. Park, 23rd ed. pg. 100

- **Incubation period:** Interval between infection of host of appearance of 1st symptom.
- **Generation time:** The interval of time between receipt of infection by a host and a **maximal infectivity** of the host ***(Generation time = Incubation period)***
- **Serial interval:** The gap in time between the onset of primary case and secondary case is called serial interval.
- **Communicable period:** Time during which an infectious agent may be transferred directly or indirectly from an infected person to another person, from an infected animal to a person or vice versa including arthropods.
- **Latent period:** The period from disease **initiation to disease detection**.

143. Ans. (d) Latent period

Ref: K. Park, 23rd ed. pg. 99, 21st ed. pg. 94

- In infectious diseases the term incubation period is used, which is equivalent to latent period in non-infectious diseases.
- **Latent period** is defined as "the period from disease initiation to disease detection"

144. Ans. (d) General fertility rate

Ref: K. Park, 23rd ed. pg. 488

- **General fertility rate** is the annual number of live births per 1000 married women of child bearing age (15-49 years).
- **Total fertility rate** average number of children born to a women in her reproductive life span.
- **Gross reproduction rate** is total number of girl children born to a female. It is half of the TFR.
- **Net reproduction rate** is total number of girl children born to a female, taking into account their mortality.

145. Ans. (b) Annual number of live births per 1000 married women during reproductive age

Ref: Park's, 21st ed. pg. 451

Please refer to above explanation

146. Ans. (c) Gross reproduction rate

Ref: K. Park, 23rd ed. pg. 488-89

147. Ans. (b) 100,000 live births

Ref: K. Park, 23rd ed. pg. 25, 557

- Maternal Mortality Rate (MMR) is expressed as per 100,000 live births.
- $\text{MMR} = \dfrac{\text{No. of maternal deaths in a given year}}{\text{Total no. of live births in the same year}} \times 100{,}000$
- MMR is a RATIO
- **MCC of MMR in India:** Post-partum hemorrhage
- **MC direct cause of MMR:** PPH
- **MC indirect cause of MMR:** Anemia
- **Maternal death:** Death of mother anytime during pregnancy/labor or **within 42 days** of termination of pregnancy.

148. Ans. (d) Associated with antecedent causation

Ref: K. Park, 23rd ed. pg. 75

COHORT STUDY

- Is a type of analytical or observational study used for hypothesis testing, also called as TROHOC study/ prospective study/forward looking study/*cause to effect study*/exposure to outcome study/*risk factor to disease study*/incidence study/follow up study.
- **Strength of association of prospective study is given by:**
  - **Relative risk:** Incidence exposed/incidence among non exposed
  - **Attributable risk =**

$$\frac{\text{incidence among exposed - incidence among non-exposed}}{\text{Inidence among exposed}} \times 100$$

- **Population attributable risk =**

$$\frac{\text{incidence among total - incidence among non-exposed}}{\text{Inidence among total}} \times 100$$

- Classical example of cohort study is FRAMINGHAM HEART STUDY which is an antecedent study.
- Other examples include DOLLS AND HILLS which is an example of prospective study on smoking and lung cancer.

149. Ans. (c) Cannot measure cause to effect

Ref: K. Park, 23rd ed. pg. 75-76

- *"Cause to effect"* study is done only in Cohort study. In case- control study, study is done from *"effect to cause"*.

Comparison Between Cohort Study and Case Control Study

Cohort study	Case control study
• Time consuming	• Less time consuming
• Expensive	• Relatively cheaper
• Chance of loss of follow up is high	• No loss of follow up
• NOT useful for rare diseases	• Useful for rare diseases
• It has ethical issues	• NO ethical issues
• Calculate incidence and relative risk (more accurate)	• Calculate Odd's ratio

Contd...

Cohort study	Case control study
• Cohort study is also known as: ▪ Prospective study ▪ *Cause to effect study* ▪ Exposure to outcome study ▪ Incidence study ▪ Follow up study	• Case control study is also known as: ▪ Retrospective study ▪ Effect to cause study ▪ Outcome to exposure study ▪ Case reference study

150. Ans. (a) Indicates prevalence

Ref: K. Park, 23rd ed. pg. 75-77

Cross sectional study is the simplest form of observational epidemiological study which is based on single examination of a cross section of a population at one point of time, results of sample are then projected to the whole population

Advantages

- Provides prevalence of a disease
- Provides a whole picture of population at one point of time
- More useful for chronic disease

Disadvantages

- Tells about distribution of a disease rather than the etiology
- Establishment of time sequence of a disease is not possible
- Provides little information of a natural history and incidence of a disease

151. Ans. (a) Prevalence

Ref: K. Park, 23rd ed. pg. 75-77, 21st ed. pg. 71-72

- Prevalence is determined by cross sectional studies.

152. Ans. (a) It increases with prevalence

Ref: K. Park, 23rd ed. pg. 140-141

POSITIVE PREDICTIVE VALUE

- Ability of screening test to identify correctly all those who have disease out of all those who test positive on a screening test.
- It depends upon sensitivity, specificity and prevalence of a disease in a population
- PPV of a screening is directly proportional to prevalence of disease
- **If Prevalence of a disease increases in a population, PPV increase for the screening test.**

PPV=TP/TP+FP x 100

- PPV α Prevalence

153. Ans. (c) True positive

Sensitivity: Defined as ability of a screening test to identify all those who have disease (Cases/True Positive)

$$\text{Sensitivity} = \frac{a}{(a+c)} \times 100 = \frac{TP}{(TP+FN)} \times 100$$

154. Ans. (d) Pathogenesis

The causative factors of disease include AGENT, HOST, ENVIRONMENT. These 3 are referred as Epidemiological triad. Interaction of these 3 factors is required for development of disease.

155. Ans. (a) TP/TP + FP × 100

SENSITIVITY	$\frac{TP}{TP+FN} \times 100$	PREDICTIVE VALUE OF A NEGATIVE TEST	$\frac{TN}{TN+FN} \times 100$
SPECIFICITY	$\frac{TN}{FP+TN} \times 100$	% OF FALSE NEGATIVES	$\frac{FN}{TP+FN} \times 100$
PREDICTIVE VALUE OF A POSITIVE TEST	$\frac{TP}{TP+FP} \times 100$	% OF FALSE POSITIVES	$\frac{FP}{FP+TN} \times 100$

156. Ans. (d) TN/FP + TN × 100

Ref: K. Park, 23rd ed. pg. 139-140, 21st ed. pg. 113

- Specificity is defined as ability of a test to identify correctly those who do not have the disease i.e. "true negatives"

$$Specificity = \frac{\text{True Negative}}{\text{False Positive + True Negative}} \times 100$$

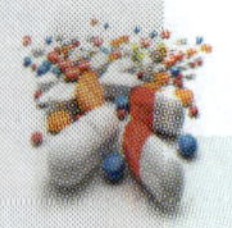

157. Ans. (b) 1921

Ref: Internet Source

The year **1921** is a "**year of the great divide**" in the demographic history of India when mortality started to decline leading to acceleration in the rate of population growth. During the next three decades (1921–51) the rate of population growth continued at a level of over one per cent per annum. It is going increasingly since then. Hence the year 1921 is rightly called the demographic divide or year of great divide.

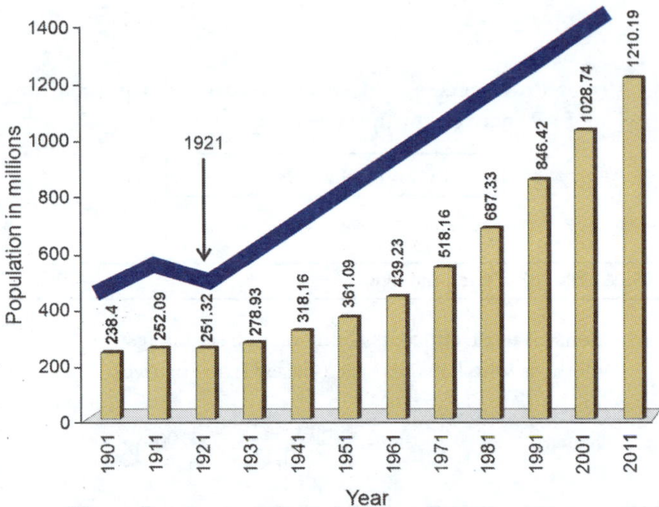

Impact of economic growth in an economy will generally have the following impact on the population:

- High birth rate and High death rate – Leads to low population growth (under-developed economy).
- *High birth rate and Low death rate: Leads to High population growth (developing economy)*
- Low birth rate and Low death rate: Leads to Low population growth (developed economy).
- In countries where children are regarded as assets, the rate of birth will be high, however due to low economic growth the health services will be poorer leading to high death rates also. E.g. India
- Once the country achieves certain level of economic growth over a period of time, the health services would become accessible to people, which would lead to high rate of birth and low rate of death.
- Once a good level of economic growth and literacy rate is achieved, the people will tend to have less children, leading to low rate of birth and low rate of death.

158. Ans. (a) Attribute risk

Ref: K. Park, 23rd ed. pg. 71-72

Case control study is often called retrospective study.

The 4 Basic Steps of Case Control Study

- Matching
- Measurement of exposure
- Selection of cases and controls
- Analysis and interpretation (relative risk)

$$\textit{Relative Risk} = \frac{\text{Incidence among exposed}}{\text{Incidence among non-exposed}}$$

159. Ans. (d) Tetanus

Ref: K. Park, 23rd ed. pg. 312

- All live and meningococcal vaccines are C/I in pregnancy EXCEPT: **YF and OPV**
- Measles, rubella and BCG are live vaccines while Tetanus is from toxoid category.
- Remember, these live vaccines can't cross the placenta
- These vaccines are still contraindicated because pregnancy is an immune-compromised state, they might harm mother.

Vaccines Indicated During Pregnancy

- Killed
- Toxoids (*tetanus*)
- Cell fraction (Hep A, Hep B)
- OPV and YF

160. Ans. (b) 10 days

Ref: K. Park, 23rd ed. pg. 121, 283

- Yellow fever vaccine certificate becomes valid **after** 10 days of vaccination and valid upto lifetime.
- Immunity of yellow fever vaccination coverage: **10 days-lifetime.**
- Quarantine period of yellow fever: **6 days** (maximum I.P of YF)

161. Ans. (d) Validity of vaccination certification begins immediately after vaccination

Ref: K. Park, 23rd ed. pg. 121, 283

162. Ans. (c) Day 0, 3

Ref: K. Park, 23rd ed. pg. 279-80

Rabies vaccines
Post-exposure prophylaxis IM schedule: • 5 dose Essen regime (1-1-1-1-1) on day 0, 3, 7, 14 and 28. • 3 dose regime (2-1-1) on day 0, 7 and 21. **Post-exposure prophylaxis ID schedule:** • 2 site- Thai red cross regimen (2-2-2-0-2) on day 0, 3, 7 and 28. **Post-exposure for previously vaccinated:** • IM or ID on day 0 and 3.
Pre-exposure prophylaxis: • IM or ID day 0, 7, 21 or 28.

163. Ans. (c) Day 0, 7, 28

Ref: K. Park, 23rd ed. pg. 279-80

- Pre-exposure schedule in rabies vaccine is on day 0, 7, 28.

Please refer to above table

164. Ans. (a) Children under 8 years

Ref: K. Park, 23rd ed. pg. 103, 21st ed. pg. 28

- Live vaccines are prepared from live (generally attenuated) organisms. Generally live vaccines are more potent then killed vaccines. In case of administration of live vaccines usually require single dose except polio vaccine which require 3 doses.
- Live vaccines are usually contraindicated in persons with immunodeficiency disorders or persons with leukemia, lymphoma, malignancies, or because of therapy with alkylating agents, corticosteroids, radiotherapy, antimetabolite drugs.
- Pregnancy is the another contraindication unless risk of infection exceeds the risk of harm to the fetus.

165. Ans. (a) Exotoxins

Ref: K. Park, 23rd ed. pg. 105

166. Ans. (a) Live attenuated

Ref: K. Park, 23rd ed. pg. 286-87

- JE vaccine is a live attenuated vaccine. It is available in killed vaccine form also.
- **Strain:** SA 14-14-2- live
  Nakayama strain-killed
- *One dose of JE vaccine is given at 16–24 months of age.*

Extra Mile

- **MC live vaccine used:** BCG
- **MC killed vaccine used:** Pertusis
- **All live vaccines are contra-indicated in pregnancy EXCEPT:** YF and OPV

Live Vaccine	Killed	Toxoids	Cell fraction	Combined
• BCG • OPV *(sabin)* • MMR • Yellow fever • Live J.E. • Live H1N1 • Live cholera	Hep A Hep B Pertusis IPV *(salk)* Rabies Meningococcal Killed J.E. Killed H1N1	Diphtheria Tetanus	Hep B Meningococcal HiB Pneumococcal	DPT MMR

167. Ans. (d) Oka

Ref: K. Park, 23rd ed. pg. 143

Vaccines and their Associated Strain

Vaccine	Strain
• Anti HIV	Ankara strain *(under trial)*
• Anti-malarial	Lytic cocktail (SPF 66)
• BCG	DANISH 1331
• Japanese Encephalitis	Nakayama Strain (killed) SA 14-14-2 (live) currently used
• Killed H1N1	California strain
• Measles	Edmonston strain
• Mumps	Jeryll Lynn Strain
• Rabies	Fixed viral strain
• Rubella	RA 27/3 strain
• Varicella	**Oka strain**
• Yellow fever	17 D strain

168. Ans. (b) Carrying stool samples of Polio patients from Primary Health Centre (PHC) to laboratory

Ref: K. Park 23rd ed. pg. 109-110, 19th ed. pg. 99

- **WHO indicators of AFP surveillance and laboratory performance:** It has several indicators, including Stool specimens for isolation of a non-polio enterovirus (Target > 10%).
- The indicator of quality of **"reverse cold chain"** (which means that **the specimen has been maintained at <8°C during transportation from field to laboratory continuously)** and how well laboratory has been able to perform routine isolation of enteroviruses.

Revising Concept and Key Points of 'Cold Chain'

- **Cold chain** is a system of storage and transport of vaccines at low temperature from the **manufacturer to the actual vaccination site**
- The cold chain system is necessary because vaccine failure may result due to non strict temperature controls
- **Polio** is the most sensitive to heat, requiring storage at minus 20°C.
- Vaccines which must be stored in the **freezer compartment** are: **Polio and measles.**
- Vaccines which must be stored in the **COLD PART but never allowed to freeze** are: Typhoid, DPT, tetanus toxoid, DT, BCG and diluents.

169. Ans. (b) Rabies

Ref: K. Park, 23rd ed. pg. 102, 21st ed. pg. 97

- Herd immunity is the level of resistance of a community or a group of people to a particular disease.

Vaccines which DO NOT provide herd protection	Vaccines which provide herd protection	
• Tetanus • *Rabies* • Japanese encephalitis • Hepatitis B • Yellow fever	• **Diphtheria** • Pertussis • **Measles** • Mumps • **Hepatitis A** • Polio	Small pox Rubella Meningococcal vaccine Rota virus vaccine H. influenza and pneumococcal V

170. Ans. (c) Calculating adverse drug reaction

- The **Naranjo algorithm**, **Naranjo Scale**, or **Naranjo Nomogram** is a questionnaire designed by Naranjo *et al.* for determining the likelihood of whether an adverse drug reaction is actually due to the drug rather than the result of other factors.
- Probability is assigned via a score termed definite, probable, possible or doubtful. Values obtained from this algorithm are sometimes used in peer reviews to verify the validity of author's conclusions regarding adverse drug reactions. It is also called the Naranjo scale or Naranjo score.

Scoring
• ≥ 9 = definite ADR
• 5–8 = probable ADR
• 1–4 = possible ADR
• 0 = doubtful ADR

COMMUNICABLE AND NONCOMMUNICABLE DISEASE

171. Ans. (a) Hepatitis A

Ref: Park Textbook of Preventive and Social Medicine, 25th ed. pg. 230

- WHO recommends that, at a minimum, screening of all blood donations should be mandatory for the following infections and using the following markers:
  - HIV-1 and HIV-2: Screening for either a combination of HIV antigen-antibody or HIV antibodies
  - Hepatitis B: Screening for hepatitis B surface antigen (HBsAg)
  - Hepatitis C: Screening for either a combination of HCV antigen-antibody or HCV antibodies
  - Syphilis (*Treponema pallidum pallidum*): Screening for specific treponemal antibodies.

172. Ans. (d) 40 days

Ref: US Department of Health and Human Services, cdc. gov website

- The practice of quarantine began during 14th century in an effort to protect coastal cities from plague epidemic.
- Ships arriving in Venice from infected ports were required to stop at anchor for 40 days before landing. This practice was called quarantine.

173. Ans. (d) Kit 6 – yellow

Ref: K. Park 25th ed. pg. 360

Refer to STI table for more details. Color kit 6 (Yellow) is used for lower abdominal pain.

174. Ans. (b) Mumps

Ref: K. Park 25th ed. pg. 165

- Mumps is a generalized virus infection. It is characterized by pain and swelling in either one or both parotid glands but may also involve the sublingual and submandibular glands.
- It may also affect testes (leading to orchitis), pancreas, CNS, ovaries, restate, etc.

175. Ans. (d) Klebsiella granulomatis

Ref: K. Park 25th ed. pg. 360

- Donovanosis is also known as granuloma inguinale. The first manifestation, appearing after 3–40 days incubation period, is usually a small Papule which ruptures to form a granulomatous lesion that is characteristically pain free and bleeds readily on contact, often elevated above the level of surrounding skin.
- Its causative organism is Klebsiella granulomatis.

176. Ans. (b) Dengue virus

Ref: K. Park 25th ed. pg. 270

- There are 4 dengue virus serotypes which are designated as DENV—1, DENV—2, DENV—3 and DENV—4.
- Secondary infection with dengue serotype 2 or multiple infection with different serotypes lead to severe form of dengue.
- The first infection sensitizes the patient, while the second infection with different serotype appears to produce immunological catastrophy.

177. Ans. (d) Rabies

Ref: who.int

- Rabies is a vaccine-preventable, zoonotic, viral disease. Once clinical symptoms appear, rabies is virtually 100% fatal.

- In up to 99% of cases, domestic dogs are responsible for rabies virus transmission to humans.
- It is spread to people and animals through bites or scratches, usually via saliva.

178. Ans. (b) Zika virus

Ref: K. Park 25th ed. pg. 301

- Zika virus is a mosquito borne flavivirus that is transmitted through the bite of an infected mosquito from the Andes genus.
- Transmission from an infected mother to her baby during pregnancy or around the time of birth is also seen.

179. Ans. (b) Leptospirosis

Ref: K. Park 25th ed. pg. 318

- Leptospirosis is essentially animal infection by several serotypes of leptospirosis.
- Leptospirosis are excreted in the urine of infected animals for a long time, often for an entire lifetime in case of rodents.
- Infection may spread from wild animals to domestic livestock and then to humans.

180. Ans. (a) Measles

Ref: Park, 25th ed. pg. 160

- Clinically measles is characterized by fever and catarrhal symptoms of the upper respiratory tract (coryza, cough), followed by a typical rash.
- In the eruptive phase of infection, a typical dusky-red, macular or maculopapular rash which begins behind the ears and spreads rapidly in a few hours over the face and neck, and extends down the body taking 2 to 3 days to progress to the lower extremities.

181. Ans. (b) Sputum smear examination

Ref: Park, 25th ed. pg. 201

- All presumptive TB will undergo sputum smear examination. Two specimens are collected (spot-early morning or spot-spot).
- If the first smear is positive and the patient is not at the risk of drug resistant TB, he will be categorized as microscopically confirmed TB (sensitivity status not known).
- If the first smear is negative, CXR may be considered and if reported as suggestive of TB, the 2nd sample will be subjected to smear and CBNAAT simultaneously.
- Based on CBNAAT results, patient will be categorized as microbiologically confirmed drug sensitive TB.

182. Ans. (c) CBNAAT

Ref: Park, 25th ed. pg. 202

- Among patients of HIV, risk of tuberculosis infection is extremely high.
- CBNAAT is the first investigation for diagnosing tuberculosis in these patients.
- Please follow the flow chart given below:

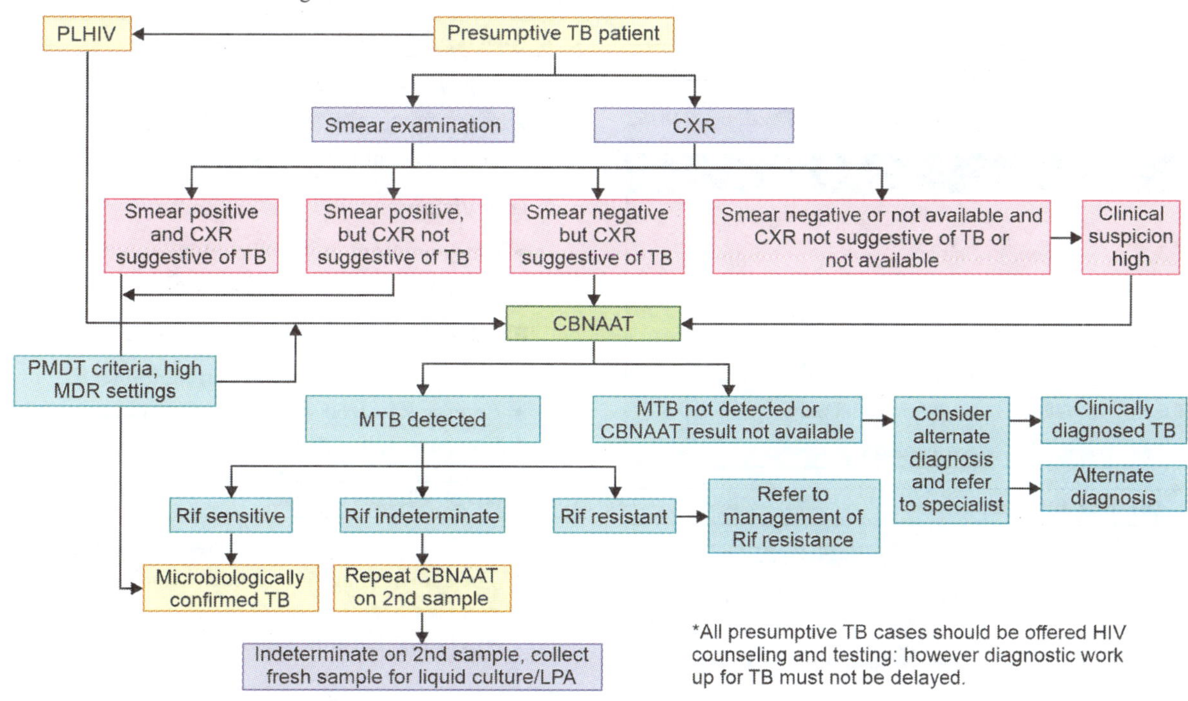

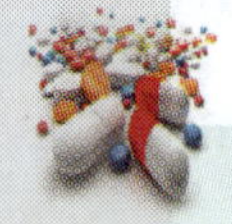

183. Ans. (d) Co-Transport

Ref: Park, 25th ed. pg. ??

- ORS works because of the Sodium Glucose Co-Transport System.
- The jejunum contains SGLT-1 transporter proteins.
- If 2:1 ratio of Na^+ and glucose is consumed, SGLT-1 actively transports both across epithelial wall.
- Osmotic imbalance is created and water is immediately pulled into vascular system.

Extra Mile

Contents of ORS

Reduced osmolarity ORS	grams/liter	Reduced osmolarity ORS	mmol/liter
Sodium chloride	2.6	Sodium	75
Glucose, anhydrous	13.5	Chloride	65
Potassium chloride	1.5	Glucose, anhydrous	75
Trisodium citrate dihydrate	2.9	Potassium	10
Total Weight	**20.5**	**Total Osmolarity**	**245**

184. Ans. (c) Coronavirus

Ref: K. Park, 25th ed. pg. 184

- Severe acute respiratory syndrome (SARS) is a viral respiratory disease caused by a SARS-associated coronavirus. SARS is an airborne virus and can spread through small droplets of saliva in a similar way to the cold and influenza.
- It was the first severe and readily transmissible new disease to emerge in the 21st century and showed a clear capacity to spread along the routes of international air travel.

185. Ans. (b) Kit 2 Green

Ref: K. Park, 25th ed. pg. 348-52

KIT	Color
KIT 1	Grey: Urethral discharge, cervicitis
KIT 2	Green: Vaginitis
KIT 3	White: Genital ulcers
KIT 4	Blue Genital ulcers
KIT 5	Red: Genital ulcers
KIT 6	Yellow: Lower abdominal pain
KIT 7	Black: Scrotal Swelling

186. Ans. (b) P24 antigen

Ref: K. Park, 25th ed. pg. 368

For early detection of HIV infection RT PCR HIV RNA >p24 antigen is best. The latest 4th generation E.I.A incorporates both p24 antigen and antibodies to HIV-1&2.

187. Ans. (b) Aedes aegypti

Ref: K. Park, 25th ed. pg. 293

- Vector of zika virus is aedes aegypti

Extra Mile

- **Aedes:** Yellow fever, dengue fever, rift Nile valley fever, chikungunya fever
- **Culex:** Wuchereria Bancrofti, (filariasis), west Nile virus, Japanese encephalitis
- **Sandfly:** Leishmaniasis

188. Ans. (c) Economic

Ref: K. Park, 25th ed. pg. 419; AK Khurana, 5th ed. pg. 484

- WHO definition of blindness: Visual acuity of <3/60 in better eye with best possible correction

Low Vision

- Category 1 <6/18–6/60 Low Vision
- Category 2 <6/60–3/60 **Economic Blindness**

Blindness

- Category 3 <3/60–1/60 Social Blindness
- Category 4 <1/60 – PL+ Manifest Blindness
- Category 5 PL – Absolute Blindness

189. Ans. (c) Chagas disease

Ref: K. Park, 25th ed. pg. 321

- The shown image is of sandfly which can act as vector of disease transmission for:
  - Visceral Leishmaniasis (Kala Azar) – Leishmania Donovan's

- Cutaneous Leishmaniasis (Oriental Sore) – Leishmania tropica
- Mucocutaneous Leishmaniasis – Leishmania braziliensis
- Chagas disease is caused by *T. cruzi*, which is transmitted by insect vector triatoma infestans

190. Ans. (a) Respiratory droplets

Ref: K. Park, 25th ed. pg. 127-31

- N95 respirators and surgical masks are examples of personal protective equipment that are used to protect the wearer from airborne particles and from liquid respiratory droplets contaminating the face.

191. Ans. (a) Measles

Ref: K. Park, 25th ed. pg. 160, 563

- MC complication of measles in young children: otitis media.
- SSPE (Subacute Sclerosing Pan Encephalitis) is complication of measles: 7 per million cases of Measles
- Usually occurs 7–10 years after initial infection.

192. Ans. (a) Pig

Ref: K. Park 25th ed. pg. 311

- JE is a mosquito borne encephalitis caused by a group B arbovirus (Flavivirus) and transmitted by Culicine mosquitoes.
- JE has several extrahuman hosts
  - Pig → Mosquito → Pig
  - Ardeid bird → Mosquito → Ardeid bird
- Disease transmitted to man by infected host. Man is incidental dead-end host.
- Infected pigs do not show any symptom. They are considered as amplifier host
- Cattles and Buffaloes: Mosquito attractants
- Domestic animal which shows signs of encephalitis due to JE virus infection: Horse.

193. Ans. (a) Yellow fever

Ref: K. Park 25th ed. pg. 904

- At the international level, following diseases are notifiable to WHO in Geneva, under the International Health Regulations (IHR).
- According to IHR, yearly data of notification should be detailed by age and sex,
- **Notifiable diseases are:**
  - Cholera, Plague, Yellow fever, as per WHO
  - Relapsing fever, louse borne typhus, polio, influenza, malaria, rabies and salmonellosis as per international surveillance.

194. Ans. (b) 75 mmol/L

Ref: K. Park 25th ed. pg. 247

TABLE: Composition of reduced osmolarity ORS

Constituent	Amount (mmol/L)
• Sodium	75
• Glucose, Anhydrous	75
• Chloride	65
• Potassium	20
• Citrate	10
Total	**245**

195. Ans. (c) Anopheles

Identification features of Anopheles mosquito

- Spotted wings
- When at rest, inclined at an angle of 45° to the surface
- No buzzing sound

TABLE: Difference between Anopheles and Aedes mosquito

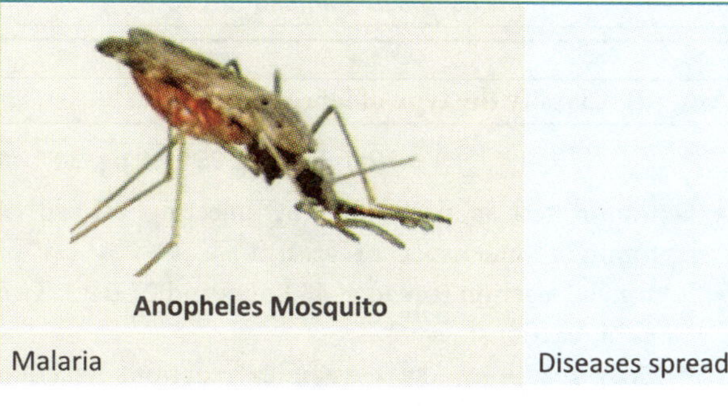 Anopheles Mosquito		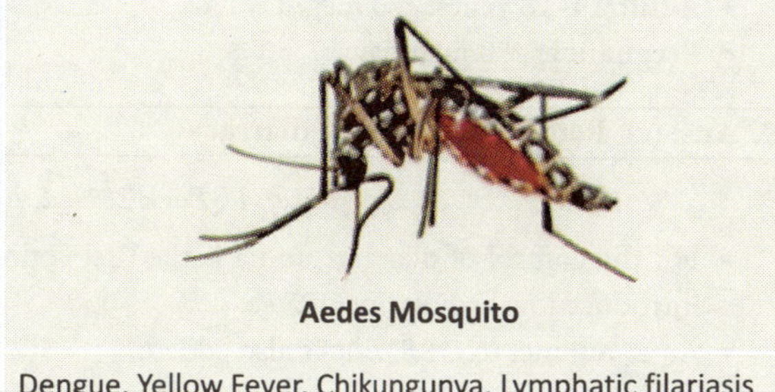 Aedes Mosquito
Malaria	Diseases spread	Dengue, Yellow Fever, Chikungunya, Lymphatic filariasis

Contd...

Pregnant females	Which mosquitoes bite?	Pregnant females
Night	When do they bite?	Day
With abdomen sticking upwards	Resting position	Lies parallel to resting surface
Predominantly rural	Location	Predominantly urban
Bodies of water	Breeding ground	Shallow water surfaces

196. Ans. (a) 3 days

Ref: K. Park 25th ed. pg. 162

- Apart from vaccine, measles can be prevented by administration of immunoglobulin early in the incubation period.
- **Dose:** 0.25 mL/kg
- It should be given within 3–4 days of exposure
- These persons who are passively immunized should be given live measles vaccine 8–12 weeks later

197. Ans. (b) 7–14 days

Ref: K. Park 25th ed. pg. 253

- Infection of cholera is dose dependent. Infection occurs when the number of vibrio ingested exceeds the dose that is infective for individual.
- To produce clinical disease 10^{11} organisms required.
- **Note:** An infected person can excrete 10-20 L of fluid, which contain 10^7–10^9 vibrios per mL.
- A case of cholera is infectious for a period of 10–14 days
- Convalescent carriers are infectious for 2–3 weeks.
- A chronic carrier state may last from a month up to 10 years or more.

198. Ans. (b) 100–120 mcg/day

Ref: K. Park 25th ed. pg. 681, PubMed

Requirement of iodine in child age group:
- **7–12 month:** 110 mcg/day
- **1–8 years:** 90 mcg/day
- **9–13 years:** 120 mcg/day
- **Adult/14–18 years:** 150 mcg/day
- **Pregnancy:** 250 mcg/day

199. Ans. (c) Reduces duration of diarrhea

Ref: K. Park 25th ed. pg. 489

- For the control of diarrhea, India is the first country to introduce low osmolarity ORS.
- As an adjunct to ORS, zinc is also added.
- Addition of zinc results in reduction of the number and severity of episodes and duration of diarrhea.

200. Ans. (b) Q fever

Ref: K. Park 25th ed. pg. 328

- **Q fever** differs from other rickettsial infection. There is no arthropod involved in its transmission to man.
- **Transmission can be due to:**
  - Inhalation of infected dust contaminated by urine or faeces of diseased animal or through aerosol *(most important route: Respiratory route).*
  - Through abrasion, conjunctiva or ingestion of contaminated food such as meat, milk and milk products
- I.P.: 2–3 weeks
- **Clinical feature:** Acute onset fever, chills, general malaise, headache. NO rash or local lesion. The infection can cause: Pneumonia, hepatitis, encephalitis.
- **DOC:** Doxycycline

Extra Mile

Rickettsial diseases, their Agents and insect vectors

Disease	Rickettsial agent	Insect vectors
Epidemic typhus	*R. prowazekii*	Louse
Endemic typhus	*R. typhi*	Flea
Scrub typhus	*R. tsutsugamushi*	Mite
Indian tick typus	*R. conorii*	Tick
Rocky mountain spotted fever	*R. rickettsii*	Tick
Rickettsial pox	*R. akari*	Mite
Q fever	*C. burnetii*	
Trench fever	*Rochalimaea quintana*	Louse

201. Ans. (d) Classify the type of leprosy

Ref: K. Park 25th ed. pg. 347-48

- Lepromin test is performed by injecting 0.1 ml of lepromin in inner aspect of forearm
- Routinely, reaction is read at 48 hours and 21 days. Two types of reactions:
  - **Early reaction:** Aka **Fernandez reaction.** Reaction is evidenced by redness and induration at the site of

inoculation. Size >10 mm after 48 hours is considered positive
- **Early reaction** indicates if a person has been previously sensitized by exposure to and infection by leprosy bacilli.
- It is described as **delayed hypersensitivity reaction (type IV)** to soluble constituents of leprosy bacilli.

- **Late reaction: Aka Mitsuda reaction:** Become apparent 7–10 days after injection. Evaluate after 21 days. Reaction is said to be positive if there is nodule >5 mm at the site of inoculation
  - **Late reaction** is induced by bacillary component of the antigen. It indicates cell mediated immunity

- **Value of lepromin test:**
  - **Lepromin test** is NOT a diagnostic test
  - **Drawbacks:** Positives result in non-cases and negative result in lepromatous and near-lepromatous cases.
  - A useful tool in evaluating the immune status of leprosy patients (cell mediated immunity).
  - It is of considerable value in confirming the results classification and cases of leprosy on clinical and bacteriological ground.
  - In other words the test is widely used as an aid to classify the type of disease.

202. Ans. (d) No cut off of CD 4 count required for initiation of treatment

Ref: K. Park 25th ed. pg. 380-81

TABLE: When to start ART

When to start in adult (>19-year-old)	ART should be initiated in all adults living with HIV, regarding of WHO clinical stage and at any CD4 cell count.
	As a priority. ART should be initiated in all adults with severe or advanced HIV clinical disease (WHO clinical stage 3 or 4) and adults with a CD4 count ≤350 cells/mm³.
When to start ART in pregnant and breast-feeding women	ART should be initiated in all pregnant and breastfeeding women living with HIV, regardless of WHO clinical stage and at any CD4 cell count and continued lifelong.
When to start ART in adolescents (10–19 years of age)	ART should be initiated in all adolescents living with HIV, regardless of WHO clinical stage and at any CD4 cell count (conditional recommendation). As priority, ART should be initiated in all adolescents with severe or advanced HIV clinical disease (WHO clinical stage 3 or 4) and adolescents with a CD4 count ≤ 350 cells/mm³.
When to start ART in children younger than 10 years of age	ART should be initiated in all children living with HIV, regardless of WHO clinical stage or at any CD4 cell count. • Infants diagnosed in the first year of life • Children living with HIV 1 year old to less than 10 years old (conditional recommendation).
	As a priority, ART should be initiated in all children <2 years of age or children younger than 5 years of age with WHO clinical stage 3 or 4 or CD count ≤750 cells/mm³ or CD4 percentage <25% and children 5 years of age and older with WHO clinical stage 3 or 4 or CD4 count ≤350 cells/mm³.
Timing of ART for adults and children with TB	ART should be started in all TB patients living with HIV regardless of CD4 count. TB treatment should be initiated first, followed by ART as soon as possible within the first 8 weeks of treatment. HIV-positive TB patients with profound immunosuppression (e.g. CD4 counts less than 50 cells/mm³) should receive ART within the first two weeks of initiating TB treatment.
	ART should be started in any child with active TB disease as soon as possible and within 8 weeks following the initiation of antituberculosis treatment regardless of the CD4 cell count and clinical stage.

203. Ans. (a) Crimean-Congo fever

Ref: PubMed

- Host of Crimean-Congo hemorrhagic fever is cattle like cows and sheep.

Crimean-Congo hemorrhagic fever (CHF) is caused by infection with a tick-borne virus (Nairovirus) in the family *Bunyaviridae*. The disease was first characterized in the crimea in 1944 and given the name Crimean hemorrhagic fever.

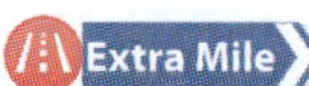

- **Host of KFD:** Small mammals like squirrels and rats are main reservoirs. Monkeys are amplifying host.
- **Monkeys and forest mosquitoes** are the reservoir of the Yellow fever.

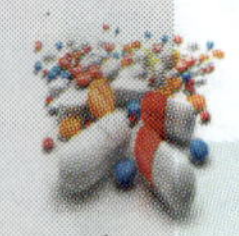

204. Ans. (b) Centripetal distribution

Ref: K. Park 23rd ed. pg. 145

TABLE: Differences between smallpox and chicken pox

Smallpox	Chicken pox
• ***Incubation:*** *About 12 days* (Range: 7–17 days)	About 15 days (Range 7–12 days)
• ***Prodromal symptoms:*** Severe	Usually mild
• ***Distribution of rash:***	
• Centrifugal	• Centripetal
▪ Palms and soles frequently involved	▪ Seldom affected
▪ Axilla usually free	▪ Axilla affected
▪ Rash predominant on extensor surfaces and bony prominences	▪ Rash mostly on flexor surfaces
• ***Characteristics of the rash:***	
▪ Deep-seated	▪ Superficial
▪ Vesicles multilocular and umbilicated	▪ Unilocular dew-drop like appearance
▪ Only one stage of rash may be seen at one time	▪ Rash pleomorphic i.e. different stages of the rash evident at one given time, because rash appears in successive crops
▪ No area of inflammation is seen around the vesicles	▪ An area of inflammation is seen around the vesicles
• ***Evolution of rash:***	
▪ Evolution of rash is slow, deliberate and majestic, passing through definite stages of macule, papule, vesicle and pustule	▪ Evolution of rash is very rapid
▪ Scabs begin to form 10–14 days after the rash appears	▪ Scabs begin to form 4–7 days after the rash appears
• ***Fever:***	
▪ Fever subsides with the appearance of rash, but may rise again in the pustular stage (secondary rise of fever)	▪ Temperature rises with each fresh crop of rash

205. Ans. (c) Lymphadenopathy

Ref: Harrison's 19th ed. pg. 1067-68

- Tularemia is a zoonosis caused by *Francisella tularensis.*
- Humans of any age, sex, or race are universally susceptible to this systemic infection.
- It is primarily a disease of wild animals and persists in contaminated environments, ectoparasites, and animal carriers.
- *F. tularensis* is a class A bioterrorism agent. With rare exceptions, tularemia is the only disease produced by *F. tularensis*—a small (0.2 μm by 0.2–0.7 μm), gram-negative, pleomorphic, nonmotile, non-spore-forming bacillus. Bipolar staining results in a coccoid appearance.
- **Incubation period:** 2–10

Clinical Manifestations

- Tularemia often starts with a sudden onset of fever, chills, headache, and generalized myalgias and arthralgias.

TABLE: Clinical presentation of tularemia

	Rate of occurrence, %	
Sign or symptom	**Children**	**Adults**
Lymphadenopathy	96	65
Fever (>38.3°C of >101°F)	87	21
Ulcer/eschar/papule	45	51
Myalgias/arthralgias	39	2
Headache	9	5
Cough	9	5
Pharyngitis	43	–
Diarrhea	43	–

206. Ans. (b) Bartonella

Ref: K. Park 23rd ed. pg. 302

- **Quintan fever or Trench fever** (also known as "five-day fever" and "urban trench fever") is a moderately serious disease transmitted by body louse.
- It is caused by **Bartonella Quintana** (found in the stomach of the body louse).
- The disease is limited to central Europe.

Extra Mile

- *Rickettsia conorii* causes Indian tick typhus
- *Coxiella burnetti* causes Q fever
- Epidemic typhus is caused by Louse
- *Rickettsia typhi* causes Murine typhus (flea borne typhus).

207. Ans. (c) Japanese encephalitis

Ref: K. Park 23rd ed. pg. 284-85

- Japanese encephalitis (JE) is a mosquito borne infection, caused by group B arbovirus (Flavivirus) and transmitted by culex mosquito.
- Disease is transmitted by man by the bite of infected mosquito. Man is incidental dead end host.

- Major host for JE: Pigs.
- Infected pigs do not show any overt symptom but circulate the virus so that mosquitoes get infected and transmit the virus to man. Therefore pigs are also considered as amplifier host.
- Cattles and buffaloes are mosquito attractants.
- **Mosquito vectors of JE:**
  - Culex tritaeniorhynchus (common)
  - Culex vishnui (common)
  - Culex gelidus

Extra Mile

Disease	Vector
Chikungunya fever	Aedes mosquito
KFD	Ticks
Malaria	Anopheles mosquito • **An. Culicifacies:** For rural areas • **An. Stephensi:** For urban areas
Dengue	*Aedes aegypti* *Aedes albopictus*

208. Ans. (b) Yellow

Ref: K. Park, 23rd ed. pg. 438

- NACO has branded the STI/RTI (sexually transmitted infection/Reproductive tract infection) as "suraksha clinic" and has developed a communication strategy for generating demand for these services.
- Prepacked STI/RTI color coded kits have been provided for free supply to all designated STI/RTI clinics.

TABLE: RTI/STI color kits under NACP/RCH/NRHM

Contents of the STI/RTI drug kits			
STI/RTI syndromic diagnosis	Name of the kit prescribed	Color coding of the kit	Contents of the kits (name of the drugs)
Urethral discharge (UD) Cervicitis (CD) Ano-rectal Discharge (ARD) Presumptive Treatment (PT)	Kit-1	Gray	1 tablet of Azithromycin (1 gram) 2 tablets of Azithromycin (500 mg): If chlamydia Cefixime 400 mg single dose: If gonococcal
Vaginitis (VD)	Kit-2	Green	1 table of secnidazole (2 gram)/2 tablets of secnidazole (1 gram) & fluconazole (150 mg)
Genital Ulcer-Disease Non-Herpetic (GUD-NH)	Kit-3	White	Injection Benzathine penicillin (2.4 MU) + 1 tablet azithromycin (1 gram)
Genital Ulcer-Disease Non-Herpetic (GUD-NH)- for patient allergic to penicillin	Kit-4	Blue	28 tablets/capsules of Doxycycline (100 mg) and 1 tablet of azithromycin (1 gram)
Genital Ulcer-Disease-Herpetic (GUD-H)	Kit-5	Red	21 tablets of Acyclovir (400 mg)
Lower Abdominal Pain (LAP/PID)	Kit-6	Yellow	1 tablet of cefixime (400 mg) 28 tablets of Metronidazole (400 mg) 28 tablets of Doxycycline (100 mg)
Inguinal bubo (IB)/Scrotal swelling	Kit-7	Black	42 tablets of Doxycyline (100 mg) and 1 tablet of Azithromycin (1 gram)

209. Ans. (d) Inguinal bubo

Please refer to above explanation

210. Ans. (b) Cervix CA

Ref: PubMed

- Among the given options, only cervix cancer can be prevented by vaccine.
- The most common causative agent of cervix CA is HPV (6, 11, 16, 18). HPV 16 and 18 has maximum risk.
- Vaccine is protective against either: 2, 4 or 9 types of HPV.
- Three HPV vaccines have Food and Drug Administration (FDA) approval in the US
- Cervarix *(provides protection against HPV 16, 18)* is for girls only, while Gardasil *(against 6, 11, 16, 18)* and Gardasil 9 can be used for both girls and boys. Gardasil 9 offers girls protection against more strains of HPV that can cause cervical cancer.
- The HPV vaccine is **recommended for girls and boys ages 11 or 12,** although it can be given as early as age 9. It is ideal for girls and boys to receive the vaccine before they have sexual contact and are exposed to HPV.

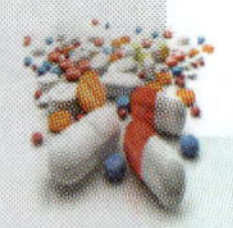

211. Ans. (b) Few hours to 5 days

Ref: K. Park 23rd ed. pg. 230

- Incubation period of cholera is **few hours** to **5 days**, but **commonly 1–2 days**.

212. Ans. (b) Chicken pox

Ref: K. Park, 23rd ed. pg. 143, 841, 21st ed. pg. 780

- **The following diseases are notifiable to WHO in Geneva:**
  - Cholera
  - Plague
  - Yellow fever
- In addition to these a few others like: Louse borne typhus, relapsing fever, Polio, Influenza, malaria, rabies and salmonellosis are subject to international surveillance.

213. Ans. (d) Cholera, plague and yellow fever

Ref: K. Park, 23rd ed. pg. 841-42, 21sted. pg. 780

214. Ans. (b) 2 days before and 5 days after rash appearance

Ref: K. Park, 23rd ed. pg. 143

- Chicken pox is infective 2 days before appearance of rash and 5 days after rash disappearance
- Measles is infective 4 days before appearance of rash and 5 days after rash disappearance
- *Mnemonic: Rule of 25 and 45*
  - *2–5: Chicken pox*
  - *4–5: Measles*

215. Ans. (b) Influenza

Ref: K. Park, 23rd ed. pg. 153

Disease	Causative organism	Incubation period
Mumps	RNA Myxo virus	14–21 days
Influenza	Orthomyxo virus	18–72 hours
Measles (rubeola)	RNA Paramyxo virus	10–14 days
Chicken pox	Human Herpes virus 3	14–16 days

216. Ans. (c) After 48 hours of hospitalization

Ref: K. Park, 23rd ed. pg. 94, 359

- Nosocomial infections are hospital acquired infections.
- It is considered nosocomial if it develops **after a minimum of 48 hours of hospitalization.**
- *Most common organism responsible for nosocomial infection:* ***Staph. Aureus.***

217. Ans. (d) Endogenous

Ref: K. Park 23rd ed. pg. 255-57

TABLE: Cycle of plasmodium in humans

Pre-erythrocytic
- Development of sporozoites in liver
- Liberate merozoites known as "Cryptozoites"
- No clinical sign/symptoms; sterile blood.

Erythrocytic
- Parasite resides inside RBCs **(endogenous);** passes through the stages of Trophozoite, schizont, Merozoite.
- Multiplication of parasite leads to clinical signs/symptoms now

Gametogony
- Few merozoites develop in RBCs of spleen and bone marrow to form gametocytes

Exo-erythrocytic
- Persist in liver
- Seen in P. vivax and P. ovale.
- Causes relapse of vivax and ovale malaria

218. Ans. (a) Rocky mountain spotted fever

Ref: K. Park, 23rd ed. pg. 299-300

TABLE: Diseases, their causative agents and vectors

Disease	Causative agent	Vector
RMSF *(Rocky Mountain Spotted Fever)*	*R. Rickettsii*	Tick
Kyasanur forest disease (KFD) aka monkey disease	*Group B togavirus (Flavivirus)*	Hard tick (in India); Soft tick (outside India)
Dengue	*Arbovirus* 4 serotypes (Den- 1,2,3,4)	Aedes Aegypti
Yellow fever	*Flavivirus fibricus*	Aedes Aegypti

219. Ans. (d) Scrub typhus

Ref: K. Park, 23rd ed. pg. 299-300, Park's, PSM, 20/ 262

Rickettsial Diseases, their Agents and Insect Vectors

Disease	Rickettsial agent	Insect vectors
Epidemic typhus	*R. prowazekii*	Louse
Endemic typhus	*R. typhi*	Flea
Scrub typhus	*R. tsutsugarnushi*	Mite
Indian tick typhus	*R. conorii*	Tick
Rocky mountain spotted fever	*R. rickettsii*	Tick
Rickettsial pox	*R. akari*	Mite
Q fever	*C. burnetii*	
Trench fever	*Rochalimae aquintana*	Louse

- DOC for rickettsial infection: **Doxycycline**

220. Ans. (a) Bancroftian filariasis

Ref: K. Park, 23rd ed. pg. 270-71, Park, 20th pg. 262

Bancroftian filariasis is transmitted by Culex Mosquito.

Anopheles (Sophisticated mosquito)	Culex (nuisance mosquito)	Aedes (tiger mosquito)	Mansonoides
Malaria	• Japanese encephalitis • West nile fever • *Bancroftian filariasis* • Viral arthritis	• Yellow fever • Rift valley fever • Chikangunya fever • Dengue • Dengue haemorrhagic fever	Brugian filariasis

221. Ans. (a) Measles

MEASLES

- Caused by RNA paramyxovirus
- **I.P.: 10–14 days.**
- Pathognomonic feature: **Koplik's spot** (on Buccal mucosa opposite 2nd molar)
- **Most common complication** of measles in **young children: Otitis Media**
- Late/rare complication of measles: **SSPE.**

Extra Mile

- Late complication of mumps: Orchitis
- Most common late complication of chicken pox: Shingles
- Complication of rubella infection in pregnancy: *Congenital Rubella Syndrome*
  - ***Triad of CRS***
    - *Sensorineural deafness*
    - *Congenital heart defect (PDA most commonly)*
    - *Cataract*

222. Ans. (a) Tuberculin test

Ref: K. Park, 23rd ed. pg. 185

- **Tuberculin Test** is the only way of estimating the prevalence of infection in a community.
  - A positive test indicates past or present infection by *Mycobacterium tuberculosis.*
  - Remember: A positive tuberculin test is NOT a confirmatory diagnostic of MTB.
- **Sputum smear examination** (Z-N stain) by direct microscopy is the diagnostic choice for TB case detection.
- Chest X-ray is a supportive diagnostic test for TB.
- **Montoux test** is also a screening test for TB. A positive test indicates current or past infection.

223. Ans. (a) Sputum smear microscopy

Ref: K. Park, 23rd ed. pg. 176-77

- **Sputum smear examination** (Z-N stain) by direct microscopy is the diagnostic choice for TB case detection in India.
- **Chest X-ray** is a supportive diagnostic test for TB.
- **Montoux test** is also a screening test for TB. A positive test indicates current or past infection with any of the mycobacterium species.

224. Ans. (b) Culture

Ref: K. Park, 23rd ed. pg. 176-177, 183

- **Sputum smear examination** (Z-N stain) by direct microscopy to check acid fast bacilli is the diagnostic of choice for TB case detection in India.
- Lepsrosy is caused by M. Leprae and is diagnosed by clinical examination.
- ***All mycobacterial infections are acid fast. So, MTB and M.Leprae can't be differentiated by AFB smear.***
- Culture has better sensitivity and M.TB infection can be differentiated from other mycobacterial infection by culture.

225. Ans. (c) 4 weeks

Ref: K. Park, 23rd ed. pg. 181-182

226. Ans. (d) Children below 6 years

Ref: K. Park, 23rd ed. pg. 182-84

- **About national TB program, if a person is smear positive for TB:**
  - All the family who is in close contact with the patient is given prophylaxis
  - Children under age 6 is given prophylaxis

Note: *India's Revised National Tuberculosis Control Programme (RNTCP) recommends screening of all household contacts of smear-positive pulmonary tuberculosis (PTB) cases for tuberculosis (TB) disease, and 6-month isoniazid preventive therapy (IPT) for asymptomatic **children aged <6 years.***

227. Ans. (b) Dog

Ref: K. Park, 23rd ed. pg. 276-77

- Rabies is caused by Lyssa virus type 1
- **Types of rabies virus:** Street virus and fixed virus
- **I.P.:** 4 days to 3–8 weeks or upto years in some cases
- ***Intermediate host:*** *Dog*
- **Dead end host:** Humans

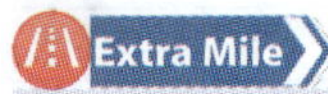

- *Rat bite or Human bite doesn't cause rabies.*

228. Ans. (c) Infected rat's urine

Ref: K. Park, 23rd ed. pg. 291-92

- *Leptospirosis* is caused by infection with bacteria of the genus *Leptospira* and affects humans as well as other animals.
- One of the zoonotic infection, which transmits from animals to human
- Leptospirosis is transmitted by the urine of an infected animal like rat, mice or moles and is contagious as long as the urine is still moist.

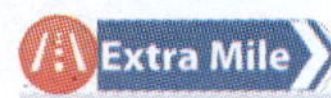

- Doxycycline 200–250 mg once a week used as prophylaxis.

229. Ans. (a) Azithromycin

Ref: K. Park, 23rd ed. pg. 308-309

- Trachoma is caused by *C. Trachomatis.*
- I.P.- 5-12 days
- **SAFE** strategy used for control of trachoma
  - **S:** Surgery
  - **A:** Antibiotic
  - **F:** Face wash
  - **E:** Environment
- DOC for Trachoma: **Azithromycin** > tetracycline

Extra Mile

- Please don't confuse between SAFE strategy and Safe delivery strategy.
  - *Safe delivery strategy is used for prevention of neonatal Tetanus.*
  - Neonatal tetanus is aka 8th day disease (I.P.- 8 days)
- **DOC for Ricketsial diseases:** *Doxycycline*

230. Ans. (d) Education

Ref: K. Park, 23rd ed. pg. 308-209

Please refer to above explanation

231. Ans. (c) Inhalation

Ref: K. Park, 23rd ed. pg. 292-94

- **Pneumonic plague**, a severe type of lung infection
- It is one of three main forms of plague, all of which are caused by the bacterium *Yersinia pestis.*
- Primary pneumonic plague results from inhalation of fine infective droplets and can be transmitted from human to human without involvement of fleas or animals.

232. Ans. (d) Culex

Ref: K. Park, 23rd ed. pg. 292-93

- The commonest and most effective vector of plague is rat flea x.cheopsis.
- Others are X. Astia, X. Brasiliensis and Pulexirritans.
- Culex is a vector of lymphatic filariasis and Japanese encephalitis *(culex tritaeniorhynchus).*

233. Ans. (d) Through contact of body fluids

Ref: K. Park, 23rd ed. pg. 356

- Incubation period of ebola virus **2–21 days**
- According to WHO *"Ebola then spreads through human-to-human transmission via direct contact (through broken skin or mucous membranes) with the blood, secretions, organs or other bodily fluids of infected people, and with surfaces and materials (e.g. bedding, clothing) contaminated with these fluids."*

234. Ans. (a) Safe water supply and sanitation

Ref: K. Park, 23rd ed. pg. 232-33

- Cholera is an acute diarrheal disease caused by *Vibrio cholerae.*
- I.P.- 1–2 days
- **First step in epidemic of cholera: Verification of diagnosis**
- **First line treatment of choice:** Water and electrolyte replacement because most death in cholera is due to hypovolemic shock.
- In the given question, safe water supply and sanitation should be the 1st step to decrease mortality from cholera.

Extra Mile

- Stool appearance of cholera: "*Rice watery stool*"
- **Chemoprophylaxis of cholera:** Tetracycline 500 mg BID for 5 days.
- **Drug of choice for cholera:**
  - **Adults:** Doxycycline 300 mg stat.
  - **Children:** Azithromycin 20 mg/kg, single dose
  - **Pregnant Female:** Azithromycin 1 gm, single dose

235. Ans. (b) Carcinoma hard palate

Ref: K. Park, 21st ed. pg. 357-58

- In eastern coastal regions of Andhra Pradesh epidermoid **carcinoma of hard palate** is most common. It is linked with habit of reverse smoking of cigar *(chutta),* i.e., smoking with burning end inside the mouth.

236. Ans. (d) All of the above

Ref: K. Park, 21st ed. pg. 360

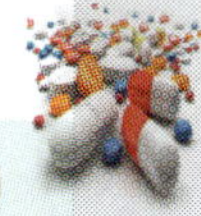

- Recent studies have shown that smoking increases the risk of lung cancer by 8.6% as compared to non smokers.
- **The risk is strongly related to:**
  - Number of cigarette smoked
  - Age of starting to smoke
  - Mode of smoking
  - Nicotine and tar content
  - Length of cigarette
- One study in India has proved that there is no difference between the tar and nicotine delivery of the filter and non-filter cigarettes smoked in India. Therefore a **filter gives NO protection to Indian smokers.** The "king-size" filter cigarettes deliver more tar and nicotine than ordinary cigarette.

NATIONAL HEALTH PROGRAMS & POLICIES

237. Ans. (a) ANM

Ref: Park Textbook of Preventive and Social Medicine, 25th ed. pg. 564

- ANMs works at health sub-centers. The sub-center is a small village-level institution that provides primary health care to the community.
- The sub-center works under the Primary Health Centre (PHC).
- Health workers like ASHA, AWW, Trained Dais Work at Village Level.

238. Ans. (b) NISCHAY

Ref: K. Park 25th ed. pg. 575

- The simple way to confirming the first trimester is to conduct a urine examination using a pregnancy test kit.
- The kit detects pregnancy on the basis on the basis of presence of human chorionic gonadotropin hormone in the urine.
- The government of India has made **"Nischay"** pregnancy test kit available across the country. This kit is distributed by ASHA.

239. Ans. (c) Indirect pattern medical benefit

Ref: K. Park 25th ed. pg. ??

- ESI Act is passed in 1948. It is an important measure of social security and health insurance in India.
- It provides certain cash and medical benefits to industrial employees in case of illness, maternity and employment injury.
- Medical benefit is provided either directly through the agency of ESI hospitals and dispensaries, or indirectly through a panel of private medical practitioners appointed as "insurance medical practitioners".

240. Ans. (c) <3/60 in better eye

Ref: Park, 25th ed. pg. 430

Distance Vision Impairment

- Mild - Presenting visual acuity worse than 6/12
- Moderate: Presenting visual acuity worse than 6/18
- Severe: Presenting visual acuity worse than 6/60
- Blindness: Presenting visual acuity worse than 3/60

241. Ans. (b) Once every 3 months

Ref: Park, 25th ed. pg. 833

- Adult mosquitoes are most commonly controlled by spraying houses with residual insecticides. DDT is the insecticide of choice and dosages of 1–2 grams of pure DDT per sq. metre are applied 1–3 times a year to walls and other surfaces where mosquitoes rest.
- In areas where DDT resistance is encountered, malathion and propoxur and to a lesser extent gamma-HCH (lindane) are recommended.

Toxicants suitable against malaria vectors as residual spray applications

Toxicant	Dosage in g/m²	Average duration of effectiveness (months)
DDT	1 to 2	6 to 12
Lindane	0.5	3
Malathion	2	3
OMS–33	2	3

242. Ans. (c) 24 hours

Ref: WHO.int, Park, 25th ed. pg. 803

- Notifiable disease must be reported to WHO within 24 hours of diagnosis

243. Ans. (c) Cotton swab in Yellow bag

Ref: K. Park, 25th ed. pg. 828

- Soiled waste like items contaminated with blood, and fluids, including cotton, dressings, soiled plaster casts, linen, beddings are all disposed in a yellow plastic bag and the treatment includes incineration or deep burial
- Syringe with needle is discarded in white/translucent puncture proof container
- Glassware including medicine vials is discarded in blue box

244. Ans. (a) 1000

Ref: K. Park, 25th ed. pg. 934

Health personnel	Norm suggested for population
Health Assistant	1 per 30,000
Nurse	1 per 5000
Pharmacist	1 per 10,000
Lab technician	1 per 10,000
ASHA	1 per 1000
Trained dai/ TBA	1 per 1000
Village health guide (VHG)	1 per 1000

245. Ans. (b) Sickness benefit

Ref: K. Park, 25th ed. pg. 852

Benefits of ESI Act

- Medical benefit: Full medical care
- Sickness benefit: 70% of the average daily wages and is payable for 91 days (in any continuous period of 365 days).
- Temporary disablement benefit: 90% of the average daily wages till recovery.
- Permanent disablement benefit: 90% of wages for loss of earning as worked out by a medical board.

246. Ans. (d) CVD, Cancer, Diabetes, Stroke

Ref: National Programs of India, Dr. J. Kishore, ed. pg. 8

- National Program for Prevention and Control of Cancer, Diabetes, CVD and Stroke (NPCDCS).

The NPCDCS Program has Two Components

- Cancer
- Diabetes, CVDs and Stroke.

247. Ans. (d) Includes area with slide positivity of more than 10 cases per 10,000 smears

Ref: K. Park 25th ed. pg. 429, 286

- The urban malaria scheme was launched in 1971 to reduce or interrupt malaria transmission in urban areas.
- It is currently protecting 130 million population from malaria and other mosquito borne diseases
- It comprises of following methodologies:
  - Vector control by intensive antilarval measure and drug treatment
  - Prevention of mosquito breeding in domestic and peri domestic areas by using larvivorous fish in water bodies
  - Use of larvicides in water bodies
- The expert committee on malaria had recommended the inclusion of:
  - All urban areas with more than 50,000 population
  - Slide positivity rate of **5% and above**
  - Areas with annual parasitic index ≥2 per 1000 per year have been classified as high risk areas, and thereby eligible for vector control.

248. Ans. (a) Male MPW

Ref: K. Park 25th ed. pg. 973

Work responsibilities for health worker male/male MPW (Multi-purpose worker)

- Malaria surveillance activities
- Collect thick and thin blood smears on glass slide from a case having fever
- Identify cases of Japanese encephalitis, filariasis, kala azar
- Identify persons 15 years and above with prolonged cough and take sputum smear and supervise the TB patients to take regular treatment (DOTS-MDT)
- Identify suspects of leprosy patients, blindness all cases including cataract suspects
- Administer vaccine under expanded program on immunization
- Spread awareness and educate public on family planning and distribution of conventional contraceptives
- Identify cases of diarrhea, dysentery, jaundice, whooping cough, diphtheria, encephalitis, acute eye infection and notify to health assistant. Give ORS and educate community about preventive measures
- Maintain record of birth, death and other diseases like TB, leprosy, malaria cases

249. Ans. (c) Health worker male

Ref: K. Park 25th ed. pg. 973

- Collection of sputum from TB suspected patients and making smear is job responsibility of health worker-male.
- Under RNTCP they need to:
  - Identify persons >15 years with prolonged cough and haemoptysis. Take their sputum smear and refer them to PHC for further investigations.
  - Check whether all cases of TB are taking regular medication or not and motivate them to do so.
  - Assist ASHA and village health volunteers to carry out DOTS activities.

250. Ans. (b) Multipurpose worker

Ref: K. Park 25th ed. pg. 449

- Aim of malaria surveillance program:
  - Target controlled interventions in high transmission areas and assess their impact
  - Early detection of outbreaks

- The active surveillance (active case detection) is done by multipurpose worker/ANM in rural areas with blood smears
- Passive case detection is done in fever cases by ASHA/ peripheral health volunteer.
- Best method of diagnosis with maximum sensitivity and specificity: Microscopy
- Method of choice for malaria diagnosis in remote areas/tribal, inaccessible rural areas: RDT kit (Rapid Diagnostic Test).

251. Ans. (b) RTI/STD

Ref: K. Park 25th ed. pg. 472

- According to STD control program, STD control is linked to HIV/AIDS control as behaviour leading to both are same
- HIV is transmitted more easily in presence of STD
- NACO, therefore has branded the Sexually Transmitted Infection (STI)/Reproductive Tract Infections (RTI) services as **Suraksha clinic, and has developed** a communication strategy for generating demand for these services.
- Prepacked STI/RTI color coded kits are provided at all state AIDS control societies. The kits are:
  - **Kit 1:** Grey—For urethral discharge, anorectal discharge and cervicitis
  - **Kit 2:** Green—for vaginitis
  - **Kit 3:** White—for genital ulcers—non herpitic
  - **Kit 4:** Blue—for genital ulcers—non herpitic in patient allergic to penicillin
  - **Kit 5:** Red—for genital ulcers—herpitic
  - **Kit 6:** Yellow—for lower abdominal pain
  - **Kit 7:** Black—for Inguinal bubo

252. Ans. (d) Child trafficking

Ref: K. Park 25th ed. pg. 645

- In India, Ujjawala scheme was launched to combat child trafficking by the ministry of women and child development on 4th December 2007.
- Scheme has 5 provisions for victims trafficked for commercial sexual exploitation:
  - **Prevention:** Formation of community vigilance group, adolescents group, awareness creations and organizing work-shops
  - **Rescue:** Safe withdrawal of victims from exploitation place
  - **Reintegration:** Of victims into society
  - **Rehabilitation:** By providing them safe shelter, medical care, basic amenities, legal aid, vocational training and employment
  - **Repatriation:** Provide support to cross border victims for their safe repatriation to their country of origin

253. Ans. (a) Service centre

Ref: K. Park 25th ed. pg. 474

Vision 2020: The Right to Sight

- A global initiative to reduce avoidable (preventable and curable) causes of blindness by year 2020.
- The plan has the following features:
  - Target diseases are cataract, refractive error, childhood blindness, corneal blindness, glaucoma, diabetic retinopathy
  - The proposed 4 tier structure includes:
    - Center of excellence (20)
    - Training centers (200)
    - Service centers (2000)
    - Vision centers (20,000)
- The shown **image** depicts the proposed structure for primary, secondary and tertiary eye care (referral from base to apex)

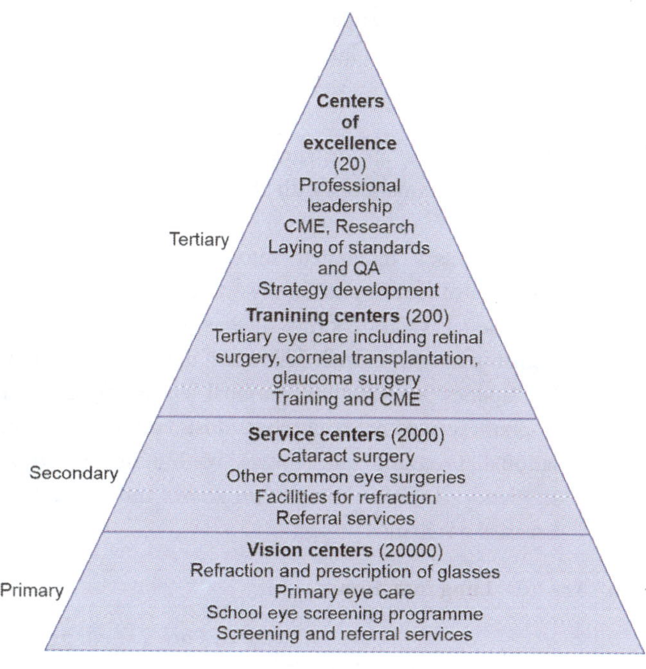

254. Ans. (b) Street children

Ref: K. Park 25th ed. pg. 373

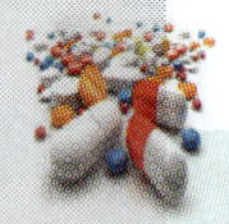

Key population affected with HIV in India

- The HIV epidemic in India is driven by sexual transmission, which accounts for 86% of new infection in 2017.
- The following population is mainly affected, which needs sentinel surveillance:
  - **Female sex workers:** in 2017, ~1.6% were found to be living with AIDS
  - **IV drug abusers:** Major route of HIV transmission in north-east states. In 2017, 6.3% of HIV drug abusers are found to be living with AIDS
  - **Hijras/transgenders:** Prevalence in 2017 was found to be 3.1%
  - **Migrant labourers:** An estimated 7.2 million migrant workers in India, of whom 0.2% are living with HIV
  - **Truck drivers:** NACO estimated 0.2% of truck drivers are living with HIV in 2017–18. They are considered as bridge population for HIV transmission since they often have unprotected sex with high risk groups as well as their regular sex partners.

255. Ans. (d) All of the above

Ref: K. Park 23rd ed. pg. 449

- The main aim of NRHM is to provide accessible, affordable, accountable, effective and reliable primary health care, and bridging the gap in rural health care through creation of a cadre of Accredited Social Health Activist (ASHA).
- The mission is an instrument to integrate multiple vertical programs alongwith their funds at the district level.
- The programs integrated into NRHM are existing programs of health and family welfare including RCH II: national vector borne disease control programs against malaria, filarial, kala-azar dengue fever/DHF and Japanese encephalitis; national leprosy eradication program; revised national tuberculosis control program; national program for control of blindness; iodine deficiency disorder control program, and integrated disease surveillance project.

256. Ans. (d) Lung infections

Ref: K. Park 23rd ed. pg. 579

- School health services is an economical and powerful means of raising community health, especially in future generations.
- It is based on the local health problems of school child and vary from one place to another.
- **According to surveys, the main emphasis of school health fall in following categories:**
  - Malnutrition
  - Infectious diseases
  - Intestinal parasites
  - Diseases of the skin, eye and ear
  - Dental caries
- **Objectives of school health service**
  - Promotion of positive health
  - Prevention of diseases
  - Early diagnosis, treatment and follow up of defects
  - Awakening health consciousness in children
  - Provision of healthful environment

257. Ans. (b) Delivery at home

Ref: K. Park 23rd ed. pg. 449-450

- ASHA is a health activist in the community, who creates awareness on health. Her responsibilities are as follows:
  - Create awareness and information on nutrition, basic sanitation, hygienic practices and the need for timely utilization of health and family welfare services.
  - Counsel the women for safe delivery, breastfeeding, immunization, contraception and prevention of common infections including STI's.
  - Facilitate the services available at anganwadi, subcenter, PHC.
  - Escort/accompany pregnant women and children requiring treatment/admissions to the nearest health center.
  - Act as depot holder for essential provisions being made available to every habitation like ORS powder, iron and folic acid tablet, chloroquine, disposable delivery kits, OCP's, condoms etc.
  - Provide primary medical care for minor ailments like diarrhea, fever and first aid for minor injuries. Also provide DOTS under RNTCP.
  - To inform about the birth and death in her village or any unusual health problems/outbreaks in the community.
  - To promote construction of household toilets under total sanitation campaign.

258. Ans. (d) 400 INR to ASHA and 1000 INR to mother in Urban area low performing states

Ref: K. Park 23rd ed. pg. 455

- The scale of assistance under the scheme from 2012–2013 for encouraging safe delivery at the health institutions is as follows:

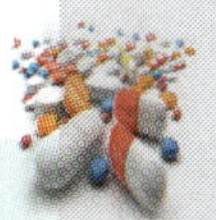

Rural area				Urban area		
Category	Mother's package	ASHA's package*	Total ₹	Mother's package	ASHA's package**	Total ₹
LPS	1400	600	2000	1000	400	1400
HPS	700	600	1300	600	400	1000

Abbreviations: LPS, low performing states; HPS, high performing states

* ASHA incentive of ₹600/- in rural areas includes ₹300/- for ANC component and ₹300/- for accompanying pregnant woman for institutional delivery.

** ASHA incentive of ₹400/- in urban area includes ₹200/- for ANC component and ₹200/- for accompanying pregnant woman for institutional delivery.

259. Ans. (b) Mild

Ref: K. Park, 23rd ed. pg. 582

TABLE: Categories of mental retardation

Mental Status	IQ Range
Normal IQ	>70
Mild mental retardation	50–70
Moderate MR	35–49
Severe MR	20–34
Profound MR	Below 20

260. Ans. (b) Kartar Singh Committee

Ref: K. Park, 23rd ed. pg. 874-75

- **Kartar Singh Committee:** Recommended multipurpose worker scheme. Kartar singh committee recommended:
  - **Current ANM** to be replaced by the newly designated "female health worker" and present day basic health workers, malaria surveillance workers, family planning health assistants to be replaced by "male health workers"
- **Bhore Committee recommendation:**
  - Integration of preventive and curative services at all administrative levels
  - **Short-term program:** Each PHC should cater to a population of 40,000 with a secondary health centre to serve as a supervisory, coordinating and referral institution
  - **Long-term program aka 3 million plan:** Setting up a 75 bedded primary health unit for each 10,000 to 20,000 population; and secondary health unit with 650 bedded hospital, again regionalized around district hospital with 2500 beds
  - **Major change in medical education** which includes 3 month training in preventive and social medicine to prepare **"social physicians".**
- **Srivastava Committee**
  - Group on medical education and manpower.
  - Recommended bands of para-professionals and semi-professional health worker.
  - ROME (Reorientation of Medical Education) scheme.
  - Village Health Guide scheme.
  - 3-Tier rural health infrastructure
- **Jungalwalla committee**
  - Equal pay for equal work
  - No private practice
- **Mudaliar committee:** Health survey and planning committee

261. Ans. (c) Complete hospitalization

Ref: K. Park, 23rd ed. pg. 473-74

Community Mental Health Programme Include Essential Elements

- Inpatient services
- Outpatient service
- Partial hospitalization
- Emergency services
- Diagnostic services
- Precare and after care services including foster home placement and home visiting
- Education services
- Training
- Research and evaluation

262. Ans. (c) Started in 1987

Ref: K. Park, 23rd ed. pg. 473-74

- National Mental Health Program: **1982**
- National Family Planning Program: **1952**
- National Aids Control Program: **1987**
- National Anti Malaria Program: **1999**

263. Ans (c) Reproductive and child health program

Ref: K. Park, 23rd ed. pg. 452, Park, 19th ed. pg. 392

- India's family welfare program seeks to promote on a voluntary basis, responsible and planned parenthood with the "two child norm" male, female or both through **'cafeteria approach'**, that is **an independent choice of family planning methods, best suited for the couples.**

264. Ans. (c) 40

Ref: K. Park 23rd ed. pg. 804-805

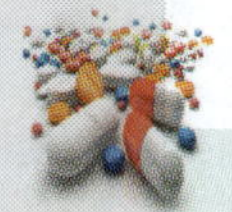

265. Ans. (a) Kala-azar

Ref: K. Park, 21st ed. pg. 113

- Indian Academy of Pediatrics (IAP) approved following vaccines (Kala Azar is NOT included in schedule)
- **Following vaccines are approved by IAP:** Polio, hepatitis, BCG, DPT, Hib, MMR, TT, typhoid.

266. Ans. (b) Yellow fever

Ref: K. Park, 21st ed. pg. 380

- The National Vector Borne Disease Control Programme (NVBDCP) is implemented for the prevention and control of vector borne diseases such as: Malaria, Filariasis, kala-azar, Japanese encephalitis, Dengue and Chikunguniya.
- Yellow fever is NOT a part of NVBDCP.

PREVENTIVE OBSTETRICS, PEDIATRICS AND GERIATRICS

267. Ans. (b) Antenatal to 6 weeks after delivery

Ref: Park Textbook of Preventive and Social Medicine, 25th ed. pg. 610

- A maternal death is defined as a death while pregnant or within 42 days of the end of pregnancy, from any cause related to or aggravated by the pregnancy.

268. Ans. (c) Vitamin A deficiency

Ref: K. Park 25th ed. pg. 431

- The most common causes of blindness in developed countries are accidents, glaucoma, diabetes, vascular diseases like hypertension, cataract.
- In India, the most common cause of blindness being responsible for 50–80% of all blindness.
- Vitamin A deficiency is responsible for most childhood blindness in India.

269. Ans. (b) 8

Ref: K. Park 25th ed. pg. 575.

WHO ANC model recommends 8 antenatal visits.

- 1 in 1st trimester up to 12 weeks
- 2 in 2nd trimester at 20 weeks and 26 weeks
- 3 in 3rd trimester at 30, 34, 36, 38, 40 weeks.

270. Ans. (d) 4 mg

Ref: Institute of Medicine (US). Dietary Reference Intakes for Thiamine, Riboflavin, Niacin, Vitamin B6, Folate, Vitamin B12, Pantothenic Acid, Biotin, and Choline. Washington (DC): National Academies Press (US); 1998

- All women who can become pregnant should get 400 mcg of frolic acid each day, in addition to consuming food with folate for a varied diet, to lower the chance of having a baby with neural tube defect.

271. Ans. (d) Hemorrhagic disease of newborn

Ref: K. Park 25th ed. pg. 675

- Newborn infants tend to be deficient in vitamin K due to minimal stores of prothrombin at birth and lack of an established intestinal flora.
- Soon after birth, all infants or those at increased risk should receive a single IM dose of a vitamin K preparation to prevent hemorrhagic disease of newborn.

272. Ans. (a) Contain High sugar and fat

Ref: K. Park 25th ed. pg. 585

- The first milk which is called **colostrum** is the most suitable food for the baby during this early period because it contains a high concentration of protein and other nutrient the body needs **except** high sugar and fat.

273. Ans. (b) 4

Ref: Park, 25th ed. pg. 575

Antenatal care (ANC) is defined as, care given to pregnant female by skilled health care professional, in order to ensure health and safety of both pregnant mother and baby.

- Components of ANC:
  - Risk identification
  - Prevention and management of pregnancy related diseases
  - Health education and health promotion
- Ideally ANC begin soon after conception and continue throughout the pregnancy.
- Antenatal visits (total ~ 13):
  - Once a month during first 7 months
  - Twice a month in 8th month
  - Once a week thereafter
- Minimum 4 antenatal visits recommended:
  - 1st visit: Within 12 weeks, preferable as soon as pregnancy is suspected (for pregnancy registration and first ANC check up)
  - 2nd visit: Between 14 and 26 weeks
  - 3rd visit: Between 28 and 34 weeks
  - 4th visit: Between 36 weeks and term

Extra Mile

- Registration of pregnancy is the responsibility of ANM, that should be done within 12 weeks.

274. Ans. (a) 6 months

Ref: K. Park, 25th ed. pg. 542, 565

- Exclusive breast feeding is recommended till 6 months.

275. Ans. (b) Hemoglobin

Ref: K. Park 25th ed. pg. 961

- At sub-centre laboratory examinations that are given are:
  - Urine test for pregnancy confirmation
  - Hemoglobin estimation
  - Urine and albumin and sugar

276. Ans. (b) 25

Ref: K. Park 25th ed. pg. 557

MTP Act 1971

- **Conditions for MTP:**
  - **Medical:** Where continuation of pregnancy might endanger mother's life
  - **Eugenic:** There is high risk of child being born with serious physical or mental abnormalities
  - **Humanitarian:** Where pregnancy is outcome of rape
  - **Socio-economic:** Social or economic environment that could lead to risk of injury to the health of mother
  - **Failure of contraceptive devices:** Where pregnancy is as a result of contraceptive method failure
- In case the woman is under 18 years or a lunatic of any age—a written consent of guardian is necessary
- **Who can perform?**
  - **If pregnancy below 12 weeks:** A registered medical practitioner having experience in OBG
  - **If >12 weeks – 20 weeks:** Opinion of two registered medical practitioner is necessary
- **Where to be performed:** Established hospitals or a place approved by government or any non-government institution after obtaining license from chief medical officer of district.

MTP Rules 1975

- **Approval of boards:** According to new rules the chief medical officer of district is empowered to certify if the doctor has necessary training in gynaecology and obstetrics to do abortions. Application to certification boards is NOT required.
- **Qualification required:**
  - If assisted an RMP of an approved institution in performance of **25 cases** of MTP or
  - 6 months of house manship in OBG or
  - MD in OBG or
  - 3 years of practice in OBG for those doctors registered before 1971 MTP Act
  - 1 year of practice in OBG for those doctors registered after 1971 MTP Act

277. Ans. (a) 350 kcal

Ref: K. Park 25th ed. pg. 690-91

- The energy requirement of women is increased over and above their normal requirement in following conditions:
  - **Pregnancy:** + 350 kcal/day throughout pregnancy
  - **Lactation:** + 600 kcal/day during first 6 months and +520 kcal/day during next 6 months.

Extra Mile

TABLE: Energy requirement of indians at different ages

Age group	Remarks	(kcal/day)
Man	Sedentary work Moderate work Heavy work	2,320 2,730 3,490
Woman	Sedentary work Moderate work Heavy work Pregnant woman Lactation	1,900 2,230 2,850 +350 +600 +520
Infants	0-6 months 6-12 months	500 670
Children	1-3 years 4-6 years 7-9 years	1,060 1,350 1,690

278. Ans. (b) Intrauterine growth retardation

Ref: K. Park 25th ed. pg. 587

Low birth weight

- Defined as birth weight of less than **2.5 kg,** regardless of gestational age
- The birth weight of an infant is the single most important determinant of its chances of survival, healthy growth and development.
- Two main groups of low birth weight:
  - **Premature born (short gestation):** MC in developed countries where population of low birth weight is less
  - **Fetal growth retardation:** MC in countries (like India) where proportion is high. It is considered as the most common cause of low birth weight in India.

Extra Mile

- Apart from birth weight, babies can be classified in 3 groups according to gestational age:
  - **Preterm:** Born before 37 weeks of gestation (<259 days)
  - **Term:** Born between 37–42 weeks (259–293 days)
  - **Post-term:** Born at 42 completed week or any time after (≥294 days)

Contd...

- **Preterm babies are further classified as:**
  - **Extremely preterm:** (<28 weeks)
  - **Very preterm** (28 to <32 weeks)
  - **Moderate to late preterm** (32–37 weeks)
- Birth weight >4 kg is considered as overweight
- **Average birth weight in India:** 2.8 kg.

279. Ans. (a) Glucose – 90

Ref: K. Park 23rd ed. pg. 224

- In reduced osmolarity ORS, content of glucose is 75 mmol/L

Composition of reduced osmolarity ORS	
Reduced osmolarity ORS	**Grams/Liter**
• Sodium chloride	2.6
• Glucose, anhydrous	13.5
• Potassium chloride	1.5
• Trisodium citrate, dehydrate	2.9
• Total weight	20.5
Reduced osmolarity ORS	**mmol/Liter**
• Sodium	75
• Chloride	65
• Glucose, anhydrous	75
• Potassium	20
• Citrate	10
• Total osmolarity	245

280. Ans. (c) 20 mg/day

Ref: K. Park, 23rd pg. 636

- **Park states:** *"Iron required during lactation is 21 mg/day"*

281. Ans. (a) 1900

Ref: K. Park, 23rd ed. pg. 634

TABLE: Energy requirements of Indians at different ages

Age group	Remarks	(kcal/day)
Man	Sedentary work **Moderate work** Heavy work	2,320 **2,730** 3,490
Woman	**Sedentary work** Moderate work Heavy work Pregnant woman Lactation	**1,900** 2,230 2,850 +350 +600 +520
Infants	0–6 months 6–12 months	500 670
Children	1–3 years 4–6 years 7–9 years	1,060 1,350 1,690

Contd...

282. Ans. (d) 245 mmol/L

Ref: K. Park, 23rd ed. pg. 224

Composition of reduced osmolarity ORS

Reduced osmolarity ORS	Grams/Liter
• Sodium chloride • Glucose, anhydrous • Potassium chloride • Trisodium citrate, dehydrate	2.6 13.5 1.5 2.9
Total weight	**20.5**
Reduced osmolarity ORS	**mmol/liter**
• Sodium • Chloride • Glucose, anhydrous • Potassium • Citrate	75 65 75 20 10
Total osmolarity	**245**

283. Ans. (a) Anemia

- **Most common Indirect cause of maternal mortality in India:** Anemia
- **Most common cause of maternal mortality in India: Post** partum hemorrhage (PPH)
- **Most common direct cause of MMR**: PPH

Direct maternal mortality	Indirect maternal mortality
• It results from obstetric complication of pregnant state (pregnancy, labor and puerperium) from interventions or incorrect treatment.	• It results from previous existing disease or disease that develops during pregnancy.
• **Ex:** PPH, obstructed labor, sepsis	• Anemia, HTN, gestational DM, epilepsy

284. Ans. (d) Perinatal mortality rate

Ref: K. Park, 23rd ed. pg. 563-64

- **Perinatal period** is from 28th week age of gestation to 7th day of newborn life.
- Perinatal mortality rate includes late fetal deaths and early neonatal deaths.

- A better obstetric care will be able to diagnose any fetal stress which will result in early intervention, which will certainly help in delivering a healthy baby.
- Therefore an obstetric will mostly affect Perinatal mortality rate.

285. Ans. (c) Before 21 days

Ref: K. Park, 23rd ed. pg. 840-41

Registration of Some Vital Events

- Birth: Before 21 days
- Death: Before 21 days
- Marriage: Before 30 days

286. Ans. (b) Green

Ref: Park's PSM, 21st ed. pg. 414

- According to Integrated Management of Neonatal and Childhood Illness (IMNCI), childhood morbidity and mortality is caused by diarrhea, ARI, malaria, malnutrition etc.
- Conditions are classified according to severity, and treatment action taken according to color code triage:
  - **Red:** Urgent referral after pre-referral treatments.
  - **Yellow:** Treat at outpatient health facility (treat local infection, give oral drugs, advise care-taker)
  - ***Green:*** *Home management* (advise care-taker on how to give oral drugs, when to approach immediately, follow up etc.)

287. Ans. (c) ORS

Ref: K. Park, 23rd ed. pg. 224, 453

- WHO recommends ORS as the best measure in diarrhea for preventing the complications that may arise due to water and electrolyte loss.
- Metronidazole can be used as supportive therapy. It controls thc anaerobic infection of GI.

288. Ans. (b) 6 months

Ref: K. Park, 23rd ed. pg. 508, 530-33

Exclusive breast feeding: 0–6 month and should be continue upto 2 years

289. Ans. (c) Perinatal mortality

Ref: K. Park, 23rd ed. pg. 567, 19th pg. 449 fig 9

$$\text{IMR} = \frac{\text{Number of death of children less than 1 year of age in a year}}{\text{Number of live births in the same year}} \times 1000$$

Perinatal Mortality Rate (PMR)

$$\text{PMR} = \frac{\text{[Late fetal deaths (28 weeks gestation and more) + early neonatal deaths (first week) in one year]}}{\text{Live births in the same year}} \times 100$$

Perinatal Mortality Rate (PMR)=

$$\frac{\text{Late fetal deaths + Early neonatal deaths}}{\text{Late fetal deaths + live births}} \times 100$$

Where Late fetal means 28 weeks gestation or more; Early neonatal means first week

NUTRITION AND HEALTH

290. Ans. (b) Epidemic dropsy

Ref: Park Textbook of Preventive and Social Medicine, 25th ed. pg. 714

- Consumption of adulterated mustard oil (Brassica nigra) with argemone oil (Argemone mexicana) even for a short duration leads to a clinical condition known as Epidemic dropsy.
- Sanguinarine and dehydrosanguinarine are two major toxic alkaloids of Argemone oil, which cause widespread capillary dilatation, proliferation and increased capillary permeability.

291. Ans. (a) DEC

Ref: Park Textbook of Preventive and Social Medicine, 25th ed. pg. 713, 714

- Beta-oxalyl-amino-L-alanine acid (BOAA), an excitatory neurotoxin and glutamate agonist, has been identified as the constituent of the chickling pea responsible for Lathyrism.
- Eating the chickling pea with grain having high concentrations of Sulphur-based amino acids reduces the risk of lathyrism if grain is available. Boiling in water or repeated steeping in hot water and discarding the extracts can detoxify the seeds. Eating with antioxidants can be protective.

292. Ans. (b) Vitamin K

Ref: Park Textbook of Preventive and Social Medicine, 25th ed. pg. 675

- Overall, human breast milk has been found to be low in certain nutrients: vitamin D, iodine, iron, and vitamin K.
- Breast milk contain adequate amount of vitamin B complex

293. Ans. (c) Loaf of bread

Ref: The US Federal Food, Drug and Cosmetic Act, Section 201, Chapter II, (gg)

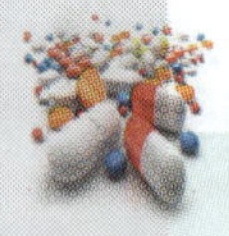

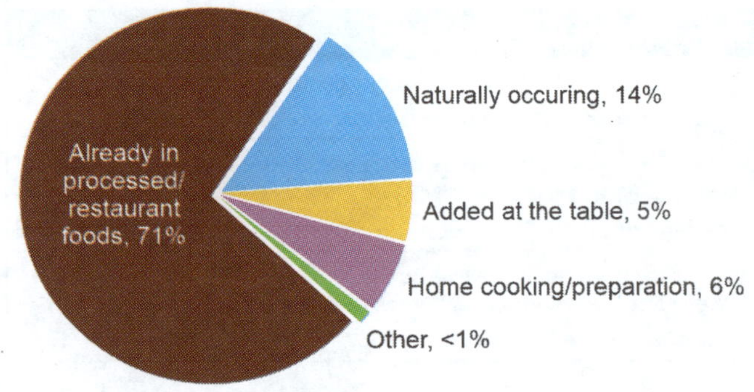

294. Ans. (a) Papaya

Ref: K. Park 25th ed. pg. 671

Classification	GI range	Examples
Low GI	55 or less	Most fruit and vegetables (except potatoes, watermelon and sweet corn). Whole grains, pasta foods, beans, lentils
Medium GI	56–69	Sucrose, basmati rice, brown rice
High GI	70 or more	Corn flakes, baked potato, some white rice varieties (e.g. jasmine), white bread, candy bar and syrupy foods.

295. Ans. (c) Pellagra

Ref: K. Park 25th ed. pg. 676

- Pellagra is caused due to niacin deficiency. The disease is characterised by 3D's — diarrhea, dermatitis and dementia. In addition glossitis and stomatitis.
- Mental changes may also occur which include depression, irritability and delirium.

296. Ans. (b) Vitamin C

Ref: K. Park 25th ed. pg. 678

- Vitamin C deficiency causes scurvy, the signs of which are swollen and bleeding gums, subcutaneous bruising or bleeding into the skin or joints, delayed wound healing anaemia and weakness.

297. Ans. (b) Protein diet

Ref: K. Park 25th ed. pg. 666

- Protein has the highest Thermidor effect and can increase your metabolic rate by 15–30%.
- Carbohydrates increase your metabolic rate by 5–10%, and fats increase it by just 0–3%

298. Ans. (b) Milk

Ref: Park, 25th ed. pg. 680

- Foods rich in heme-iron are liver, meat, poultry and fish.
- The iron content of milk is low in all mammalian species.
- Iron content of breast milk averages less than 0.2 mg/dl, and it is well utilized.
- Foods containing non-heme iron are those of vegetable origin, e.g., cereals, green leafy vegetables, legumes, nuts, oilseeds, jaggery and dried fruits.
- In fact, milk reduces iron absorption.
- Milk is also a poor source of vitamin C

299. Ans. (a) Serum-albumin concentration

Ref: K. Park 25th ed. pg. 667

- To assess the state of protein nutrition, multiple tests have been suggested. These include:
  - Serum albumin concentration, Arm-muscle circumference, Creatinine-height index, Serum transferrin level.
- At present, the best measure of the state of protein nutrition is serum-albumin concentration.
  - **Normal:** >3.5 g/dL
  - **Mild malnutrition:** <3.5 g/dL
  - **Severe malnutrition:** 3 g/dL
- Serum albumin and transferrin assess the ability of liver to synthesize protein.

300. Ans. (b) Infant mortality rate

Ref: K. Park 25th ed. pg. 25

- IMR is the ratio of deaths under 1 year of age in a given year to the total number of live births in the same year.
- It is usually expressed as a rate per 1000 live births
- It is one of the most universally accepted indicators of health status not only of infants, but also of whole population and of the socio-economic conditions under which they live.
- In addition IMR is also a sensitive indicator of the availability, utilization and effectiveness of health care, particularly perinatal care.

301. Ans. (b) Halibut liver oil

Ref: K. Park 25th ed. pg. 672

Vitamin A is widely distributed in animal and plant foods.

- In animal food it is present as preformed vitamin A (Retinol). Ex in: Liver, egg, butter, cheese, fish and meat.
  - 1 mcg of retinol = 1 RE (Retinol Equivalents)
- In plant foods as provitamins (carotenes). Ex in green leafy vegetables (cheapest source), fruits like mango, papaya, carrots

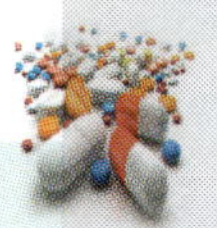

TABLE: Retinol content of some foods

Food products	Retinol Equivalents (RE) (mcg/100 gram)		
Halibut liver oil	900,000	Carrot	1,167
Cod liver oil	18,000	Spinach	607
Liver Ox	16,500	Amaranth	515
Margarine	900	Mango ripe	313
Butter	825	Papaya	118
Egg	140	Tomato	85
Cow milk	38	Orange	25

302. Ans. (a) Quetelet index

Ref: K. Park 25th ed. pg. 429

- For assessment of obesity, WHO has given the Body Mass Index formula, also known as Quetelet index.
- $\text{BMI} = \dfrac{\text{Weight (in kg)}}{\text{Height (in m}^2)}$

Other indices are:

- $\text{Ponderal index} = \dfrac{\text{Weight (in cm)}}{\text{Cube root of body weight (kg)}}$
- Broca index = Height in cm — 100
- $\text{Corpulence index} = \dfrac{\text{Actual weight}}{\text{Desirable weight}}$
  - This shouldn't exceed 1.2

Extra Mile

- **Pearl index:** Measures contraceptive failures
- **Chandler index:** Used for measurement of hookworm infestation as public health problem
- **Sullivan's Index** is measurement of Disability Free Life Expectancy

303. Ans. (b) 3–4 times less than cow milk

Ref: K. Park 25th ed. pg. 591-92

- Human milk has low protein content. It is ***around 3 times less than cow's milk*** and lower than the most mammals.
- Vitamin D is present in human milk (earlier it was believed that human milk was deficient in vitamin D)
- In human breast milk vitamin A and C content is more than cow's milk
- Iron absorption and bioavailability of human milk is more (70%) as more compared to cow's milk (30%)
- Human milk is more rich in copper, selenium and cobalt, as compared to cow's milk.

TABLE: Comparison between breast milk during the 1st month of lactation and unprocessed cow milk

Constituent	Breast milk (g/L)	Cow milk (g/L)
Proteins	11	33
• Casein	4	28
• Soluble protiens	7	5
▪ Lactalbumin	3.5	1.5–1.8
▪ Beta-lactaglobulin	0	3.7
▪ Lactotransferrin	1–2	0.2–0.5
▪ Immunoglobulin	1–2	0.5
▪ Lysozyme	0.5	Traces
Non-protein: Nitrogenous substances	0.32	0.32
Lipids	35	35
• Linoleic acid	3.5	1
Carbohydrates	70	50
▪ Lactose	62	50
▪ Nitrogenous oligosaccharides	8	0
Minerals:	2	8
• Ca (Calcium)	0.33	1
• P (Phosphorus)	0.15	1
• Fe (Iron)	0.4–1.5 mg	0.3–0.5 mg
Vitamins		
• C60 mg	20 mg	
• D50 IU	25 IU	
Energy	640–720 kcal	650 kcal
	2670–3000 kJ	2717 kJ

304. Ans. (c) High temperature and short time method

Ref: K. Park 25th ed. pg. 711

- HTST method, also known as High Temperature and Short Time method.
  - Milk is rapidly heated to 72°C, held at that temperature for not less than 15 seconds and then rapidly cooled to 4°C
  - **Book states:** "*This is the most widely used method* now"
  - Large amount of milk can be pasteurized by HTST method

305. Ans. (d) >0.85 in female

Ref: K. Park 25th ed. pg. 429

- Waist circumference is measured at the mid-point between lower border of rib and iliac crest. It correlates closely to BMI and waist to hip ratio.

- Changes in waist circumference reflects changes in risk factor of cardiovascular disease and other chronic diseases.
- Increased risk of metabolic complications with **waist circumference:**
  - Men ≥102 cm
  - Women ≥88 cm
- Waist hip ratio is calculated by waist circumference measurement divided by hip measurement.
- **Waist hip ratio** that increases the risk of cardiovascular disease:
  - Men: **>1**
  - Women: **>0.85**

306. Ans. (d) Polished rice

Ref: K. Park 25th ed. pg. 675

- Beri-Beri occurs as a result of thiamine deficiency.
- Thiamine is usually lost from rice during process of milling, washing and cooking of rice.
- This is the reason peoples are advised to avoid highly polished rice and consume parboiled and under milled rice.
- Thiamine is also destroyed in toast and in cereals cooked with baking soda.

Extra Mile

- Thiamine deficiency can lead to: Beri-Beri and Wernicke's encephalopathy
- Beri-Beri occur in 3 main forms:
  - **Dry Beri-Beri:** Characterized by nerve involvement (peripheral neuritis)
  - **Wet Beri-Beri:** Aka cardiac Beri-Beri. Heart involvement
  - **Infantile Beri-Beri:** Seen in infants between 2–4 months. Occur secondary to thiamine deficient mother breast feeding.

307. Ans. (b) Reduced peak and prolonged absorption

Ref: K. Park 25th ed. pg. 670

- **Glycemic index (GI)** of a food is defined by the area under 2 hours blood glucose response curve (AUC) following the ingestion of a fixed portion of test carbohydrate (usually 50 g) as a proportion (%) of the AUC of the standard (either glucose or white bread).
- Food can be of low glycemic index or high glycemic index:
  - **Low glycemic index:** Food products having soluble and insoluble fibers, which favour slow release of sugar into small intestine and slow absorption into blood (reduced peak and prolonged absorption rate).
  - **High glycemic index:** Foods with readily digestible and absorbable sugar (high peak and rapid absorption)

Classification	GI range	Examples
Low GI	55 or less	Most fruit and vegetables (except potatoes, watermelon and sweet corn), whole grains, pasta foods, beans lentils
Medium GI	56–69	Sucrose, basmati rice brown rice
High GI	70 or more	Corn flakes, baked potato, some white rice varieties (e.g jasmine), White bread, candy bar and syrupy foods.

308. Ans. (b) 1

Ref: K. Park 23rd ed. pg. 613–14

- Glycemic index (GI) of a food is defined by the area under 2 hours blood glucose response curve (AUC) following the ingestion of a fixed portion of test carbohydrate (usually 50 g) as a proportion (%) of the AUC of the standard (either glucose or white bread).
- A value of 100 represents the standard, an equivalent amount of pure **glucose**.
- Food can be of low glycemic index or high glycemic index:
  - **Low glycemic index:** Food products having insoluble fibers, which favor slow release of sugar into small intestine and its absorption into blood.
  - **High glycemic index:** Foods with readily digestible and absorbable sugar.

309. Ans. (c) Soyabean

Ref: K. Park, 23rd pg. 628

TABLE: Nutritive value of pulses (values/100 g)

Pulses	Energy (kcal)	Proteins (g)
Bengal gram	360	17.1
Black gram	347	24.0
Red gram	335	22.3
Soyabean	432	43.2
Green gram	348	24.5
Peas dry	315	19.7
Horse gram	321	22.0

310. Ans. (a) 20 mg iron with 0.1 mg FA

Ref: K. Park, 23rd pg. 620, 624

311. Ans. (b) 2730

Ref: K. Park, 23rd ed. pg. 634

Please refer to above explanation

312. Ans. (a) 65

Ref: K. Park, 23rd ed. pg. 630

TABLE: Nutritive value of milks compared (value per 100 g)

	Buffalo	Cow	Goat	Human
Fat (g)	6.5	4.1	4.5	3.4
Protein (g)	4.3	3.2	3.3	1.1
Lactose (g)	5.1	4.4	4.6	7.4
Calcium (mg)	210	120	170	28
Iron (mg)	0.2	0.2	0.3	
Vitamin C (mg)	1	2	1	3
Minerals (g)	0.8	0.8	0.8	0.1
Water (g)	81.0	87	86.8	88
Energy (kcal)	117	67	72	65

313. Ans. (a) 1.2 mcg

Ref: K. Park, 23rd ed. pg. 620

Vitamin B_{12}

- Vitamin B_{12} is complex organo-metallic compound with a cobalt atom. The preparation which is therapeutically used is cyanocobalamin, which is relatively cheap.

Source: Good sources are liver, kidney, meat, fish, eggs, milk and cheese. Vitamin B_{12} is not found in foods of vegetable origin. It is also synthesized by bacteria in colon.

Deficiency: Vitamin B_{12} deficiency is associated with megaloblastic anaemia (pernicious anaemia), demyelinating neurological lesions in the spinal cord.

REQUIREMENT

Intake values recommended by ICMR (2010) are as below:

Population group	Per day requirement
a. Normal adults	1 mcg
b. Pregnancy	1.2 mcg
c. Lactation	1.5 mcg
d. Infants & children	0.2 mcg

314. Ans. (b) Sanguinarine

Ref: K. Park, 23st ed. pg. 658

- **Epidemic dropsy** is caused by contamination of mustard oil with Argemone oil *(seeds of argemone Mexicana seeds closely resemble that of mustard oil)*
- Toxin which is contained in argemone oil is ***Sanguinarine***
- This sanguinarine interferes with oxidation of Pyruvic acid, which leads to accumulation of pyruvic acid in blood.
- This may cause non-inflammatory edema of lower limbs, diarrhea, dyspnea and even cardiac failure and death.

315. Ans. (d) 650 kcal

Ref: DC Dutta, 8th ed. pg. 174

Dutta states: A healthy mother will produce **about 500–800 mL of milk a day** to feed her infant. This requires about **700 kcal/day** for the mother, which must be made up from diet or from her body store. For this purpose a store of about 5 kg of fat during pregnancy is essential to make up any nutritional deficit during lactation.

Extra Mile

- Iron need during lactation is 1 mg/day.
- Daily requirement of calcium during pregnancy and lactation averages 1–1.5 g.

316. Ans (d) She weighs 60 kg

Ref: Park, 19th pg. 501-2

- 60 kg weight is of Indian reference man and not woman

TABLE: Summary of Indian reference man and woman

An Indian reference man	An Indian reference woman
• Between **18 and 29 years** of age	• Between **18 and 29 years of age**
• **Weighs 60 kg** • **Height = 1.73**	• **Healthy** and **weighs 55 kg.** • **Height = 1.61**
• Free from disease and physically fit for active work.	• Engaged for **8 hours** in general household work, in light industry or in other moderately active work.
• Employed for 8 hours in occupation that usually involves moderate activity	• Spends 4–6 hours sitting or moving around only through light activity
• Spends 8 hours in bed, 4–6 hours sitting and moving around and 2 hours in walking and in active recreation or household duties	• Spends 2 hours in walking or in active recreation or in household duties

317. Ans. (b) Bitot's spot

Ref: K. Park, 23rd ed. pg. 615, 641

- **Xeropthalmia:** All the ocular manifestation of Vitamin A deficiency.
- First clinical sign of Vitamin A deficiency: *Conjunctival Xerosis*
- First clinical symptom of vitamin A deficiency: *Night blindness*

WHO Classification of Xeropthalmia

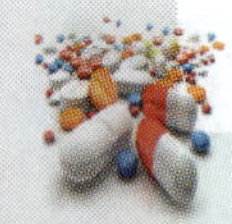

CLASS	SIGNS
X1A	Conjunctival xerosis
X1B	Conjunctival xerosis with bitot's spot
X2	Corneal xerosis
X3A	Corneal xerosis with ulceration
X3B	Keratomalacia

318. Ans. (c) Bitot spots

Ref: K. Park, 23rd ed. pg. 606, 615, 641

- First clinical sign: Conjuctival xerosis
- First clinical symptom: Night blindness
- *Refer to above table.*

319. Ans. (c) 0.5%

Ref: K. Park, 23rd ed. pg. 615, 641

Criteria and Prevalence for Determining Xerophthalmia Severity:

Criteria	Prevalence at risk
• Night blindness	>1%
• Bitot's spot	>0.5%
• Corneal xerosis/keratomalacia	>0.01%
• Corneal ulcer	>0.05%
• Serum retinol	>5%

- *Refer to previous answer for WHO classification of Xerophthalmia*

320. Ans. (d) Night blindness 1%

Ref: K. Park, 23rd ed. pg. 615, 641, 899

Please refer to above explanation.

321. Ans. (b) 0.01%

Ref: K. Park, 23rd ed. pg. 625

- Minerals form only 5 percent of the typical human diet but are essential for normal health and function.
- **Trace elements (or trace minerals)** are usually defined as minerals that are required in amounts between 1 to 100 mg/day by adults or make up less than 0.01 percent of total body weight.
- **Macrominerals** are defined as minerals that are required by adults in amounts greater than 100 mg/day or make up ***less than 1 percent of total body weight***.
- **Ultra-trace minerals** generally are defined as minerals that are required in amounts less than 1 mg/day.

322. Ans. (a) <1 g/kg

Ref: K. Park, 21st ed. pg. 563

- According to Indian medical council recommendation the daily protein requirement is <1 g/kg body weight (0.83 g).
- Assessment of protein nutritional status is done by: arm muscle circumference, the creatinine-height index, serum albumin and transferrin, total body nitrogen etc.
- Best measure of the state of protein nutrition is: Serum albumin concentration (should be more than 3.5 g/dL)

323. Ans. (b) Vitamin B

Ref: K. Park, 23rd ed. pg. 626

- Antioxidants are substances which are both nutrients and non-nutrients.
- These antioxidants reduce the toxic effects of reactive oxygen species and nitrogen species which are generated during physiological or pathological conditions and result in oxidant damage
- **Vitamins which acts as antioxidants are *remembered as ACE*:** vitamin A, C and E
- Other vitamins which acts as anti-oxidants are: Selenium, Glutathione
- **Non-nutrient products that also act as anti-oxidants are**: Plant phenols, Flavonoids, Coumarins, caffeic, benzyl isothiocyanates, gallic and ellagic acid.
- Vitamin B is not an antioxidant.

324. Ans. (b) Niacin

Ref: K. Park, 23rd ed. pg. 619

- Pellagra is caused by deficiency of Vitamin B3 *(Niacin)*.
- It is seen commonly in maize eating populations because maize is deficient in tryptophan which is usually converted to niacin.
- Therefore maize eaters develop deficiency of Niacin which ultimately leads to pellagra.
- **4 D's associated to Pellagra:**
  - Diarrhea
  - Dermatitis
  - Dememntia
  - Death
- In severe cases of pellagra *Casal's Necklace* is seen which is a scaly pigmented rash around neck, seems like necklace.

325. Ans. (c) Increase appetite

Ref: K. Park, 23rd ed. pg. 639-40

TABLE: Features of Kwashiorkor and Marasmus

Features	Marasmus	Kwashiorkor
Muscle wasting	Obvious	Hidden by fat and edema
Edema	None	Present in lower legs and face
Mental changes	Quiet and apathic	Irritable, Moaning and apathic
Weight	*Very low*	*Low to Normal*
Appetite	Good	Poor
Hepatomegaly	None	Present, due to fat deposition
Hair changes	Seldom	Sparse, silky *"flag sign"*

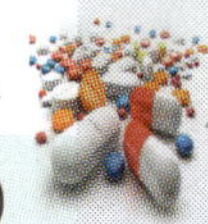

326. Ans. (b) Sanguinarine

Ref: K. Park, 23st ed. pg. 658

- **Epidemic dropsy is** caused by contamination of mustard oil with Argemone oil *(seeds of argemone Mexicana seeds closely resembles to that of mustard oil)*
- Toxin which is contained in argemone oil is **Sanguinarine**
- This sanguinarine interferes with oxidation of Pyruvic acid, which leads to accumulation of pyruvic acid in blood.
- This may cause non-inflammatory edema of lower limbs, diarrhea, dyspnea and even cardiac failure and death.

327. Ans. (a) Methylene blue reductase test

Ref: K. Park, 23rd ed. pg. 655

There are 3 tests to check the efficiency of milk pasteurization:

- **Phosphatase test:** *Most widely used method.* Phosphatase enzyme present in raw milk is degraded upon heating. If found in pasteurized milk, it indicates inadequate pasteurization or addition of raw milk.
- **Standard plate count:** To determine the bacteriological quality of pasteurized milk. 30,000 bacterial count per ml of pasteurized milk is the standard value in most western countries.
- **Coliform count:** Coliform organisms are completely destroyed by pasteurization and therefore, their presence in pasteurized milk is an indication of improper pasteurization or post pasteurization contamination.

Extra Mile

- Pasteurization of milk is by following methods:
  - **Holder Method/vat method:** 63°C × 30 min- most commonly used method
  - **Flash Method:** 72°C × 15 sec
  - **UHT method (ultra high temp):** 125°C for 2–3 secs, rapidly cooled and bottled ASAP

328. Ans. (d) 24 hours

- Refrigerated milk can be kept for around 24 hours
- At Room temperature: Upto 6 to 8 hour
- In Freezer: 3 months

329. Ans. (d) Pulses

Ref: K. Park, 23rd ed. pg. 628

- Pulses contain 20–25% of protein, which is considered more than eggs, fish, meat products. However the quality of protein in pulses is inferior to that of meat products.
- Soyabean contains 40% of protein
- Pulses protein are poor in **methionine** and to a lesser extent in **cysteine.**
- Amino acid rich in pulses: **Lysine**

Extra Mile

TABLE: Food products and their limiting amino acid

Food item	Limiting amino acids
Pulses	Methionine and Cysteine
Cereals	Threonine and Lysine
Maize	Tryptophan and Lysine

330. Ans. (c) 100

Ref: K. Park, 23rd ed. pg. 630

Biological value [BV] is a measure of the proportion of absorbed protein from a food which becomes incorporated into the proteins of the organism's body.

TABLE: Biological value of Proteins in several food products

- **Whole egg: 100**
- Cow milk: 91
- Beef: 80
- Casein: 77
- Soy: 74
- Wheat gluten: 64

331. Ans. (d) Egg

Ref: K. Park, 23rd ed. pg. 617

- Given these options, the correct answer will be egg which contains 1.25 to 1.5 μg/100 gm.

TABLE: Compare the sources of vitamin D from different dietry sources

Dietary sources	Vitamin D content (μg/100 g)
Halibut liver oil	500–10,000
Cod fish liver oil	200–750
Shark liver oil	30–100
Fish fat	5–30
Eggs	**1.25–1.5**
Butter	0.5–1.5
Milk, whole	0.1

Extra Mile

- **Richest source of Vitamin D:** Halibut fish liver oil > codfish liver oil > shark liver oil
- Human milk is a poor source of vitamin D.
- Cow's milk is poor in Vitamin C and Iron.
- Vitamin D and Vitamin B_{12} has no plant source.

332. Ans. (c) Halibut liver oil

Ref: K. Park, 23rd ed. pg. 617

- **Richest source of Vitamin D:** Halibut fish liver oil > codfish liver oil > shark liver oil

333. Ans. (d) Fish liver oil

Ref: K. Park, 23rd ed. pg. 617

Please refer to above explanation

334. Ans. (d) Calcitriol

Ref: K. Park, 23rd ed. pg. 617

- Vitamin D has 3 forms:
  - D1: Calciferol
  - D2: Ergocalciferol
  - ***D3: Calcitriol - most potent/active form, synthesized by sunlight. Also found in fish liver oil and animal fats***

335. Ans. (a) Linoleic acid

Ref: K. Park, 23rd ed. pg. 609-10

- **Essential fatty acid are**
  - Linoleic acid: *Most essential fatty acid*
  - Linolenic acid
  - Arachidonic acid
  - Eicosapentanoic acid
  - DHA
- **Richest source of essential fatty acid:** Safflower oil
- **Richest source of saturated fatty acid:** Coconut oil
- **Richest source of MUFA:** Groundnut oil.

336. Ans. (d) Glutamic acid

Ref: K. Park, 23rd ed. pg. 609-10

Refer to previous explanation.

337. Ans. (b) Iodine

- Iodine deficiency leads to hypothyroidism which manifests as goiter.
- Due to hypothyroidism, thyroid cells try to compensate it by hyperplasia and hypertrophy of thyroid gland cells (goiter).
- Iron deficiency leads to Microcytic anemia (IDA).
- Zinc deficiency may manifest with *acrodermatitis enteropathica.*
- Fluorine deficiency/excess manifests with dental caries.

Extra Mile

- *Optimum level of fluorine in drinking water: 0.5–0.8 mg per liter.*

338. Ans. (b) Height/age

Ref: K. Park, 23rd ed. pg. 640; Nelson's Pediatrics, 18th ed. Ch 43

The nutritional indices commonly calculated for young children are:

- **Weight for height** – an index used to measure wasting or acute malnutrition; (WHAM)
- **Height for age** – an index used to measure stunting or chronic malnutrition; (HA-CM)
- **Weight for age** – an index used to measure underweight (or wasting and stunting combined). (WASW)
- **Mid arm circumference** is a specific indicator of wasting or acute malnutrition.

ENVIRONMENT AND HEALTH

339. Ans. (b) Social pathology

Ref: Park Textbook of Preventive and Social Medicine, 25th Ed. pg. 729

- In the modern context, the term social pathology is also used to describe the relation between disease and social conditions.

340. Ans. (c) Burial

Ref: Park Textbook of Preventive and Social Medicine, 25th ed. pg. 853

- There are two options of disposing of compost while camping and that is to either bury your food scraps or take them home.
- Burial is the best method for disposal of waste while camping

341. Ans. (c) Acculturation

Ref: K. Park 25th ed. pg. 728

- Acculturation is referred to "culture contact". It is defined as assimilation to a different culture.
- It is the process of learning and incorporating the values, beliefs, language, customs, dietary habits, activity levels and substance use.

342. Ans. (c) Andaman and Nicobar islands

Ref: K. Park, 25th ed. pg. 296

- The Islands of Andaman and Nicobar and Lakshadweep have been reported to be rabies free from time immemorial. Recently, a survey of the islands of Andaman and Nicobar and Lakshadweep was done between July and August 2003 to assess their rabies free status.

- It was revealed that these islands continue to remain rabies free.

343. Ans. (a) Urban Health Equity Assessment and Response Tool

Ref: K. Park, 25th ed. pg. 528-31

Urban HEART: Urban Health Equity Assessment and Response Tool.

- Health services accessibility.
- Outcome and process assessment (Health care).
- Consumer participation.
- Socioeconomic factors.
- National health programs.
- Urban health. I. WHO Centre for Health Development

344. Ans. (c) Calculating bleaching powder dose for water disinfection

Ref: K. Park 23rd ed. pg. 728

Book states: *"Horrock's water testing apparatus is designed to find out the dose of bleaching powder required for disinfection of water".*

345. Ans. (b) Nosocomial infection

Ref: K. Park, 23rd ed. pg. 94

- Nosocomial infection is defined as infection acquired by patient while in a hospital or other health care facility.
- Infection occurs more than 48 hours after admission
- It denotes a new disorder, unrelated to patients primary condition
- Examples: UTI, surgical wound infection.
- **Sources of infection can be:**
  - **Patients** with viral infection (measles, viral hepatitis, influenza), skin infections, UTI and respiratory infection.
  - **Hospital staff** viz doctors, nurses, ward boys
  - **Environment:** Hospital environment viz dust, bed clothes, furniture, sinks, etc.

346. Ans. (d) 300

Ref: K. Park, 23rd ed. pg. 243-44

- **Chandler's index** is also known as Endemic index.
- It is defined as average number of hookworm eggs per gram of stool for the entire community.
- >300 eggs per gram of stool denotes important public health problem.

TABLE: Interpretation of chandler's index:

Average No. of eggs/g of stool	Interpretation
• < 200	No significance
• 200–250	Potential danger
• 250–300	Minor public health problem
• >300	Major public health problem

347. Ans. (b) Number of hookworm eggs per gram of stool

Ref: K. Park, 23rd ed. pg. 243-44

- **Chandler's index** is also known as Endemic index.
- It is defined as average number of hookworm eggs per gram of stool for the entire community.
- *Refer to above table for interpretations.*

348. Ans. (a) Hook worm

Ref: K. Park, 23rd ed. pg. 243-44

Please refer to above explanation

349. Ans. (b) Air pollution

Ref: Park, 23rd ed. pg. 736

Indicators of Air Pollution

- **Smoke or Soiling index:** A known volume of air is filtered through a white filter paper under specified conditions and the stain is measured by photoelectric meter. Smoke concentration is estimated and expressed as micrograms/cubic metre of air as an average level over a period of time.
- **Sulphur dioxide:** This gas is a major contaminant in many urban and industrial areas. Its concentration is estimated in all air pollution surveys. ***So, it is the best indicator of air pollution***
- **Grit and dust measurement:** Deposit gauges collect grit, dust and other solids. There are analysed monthly.
- **Coefficient of haze:** A factor used, particularly in the USA in assessing the amount of smoke or other aerosol in air.
- **Air pollution index:** It is an arbitrary index which takes into account one or more pollutants as a measure of the severity of pollution.

350. Ans (d) *E. coli*

Ref: Park, 23rd ed. pg. 720-21

- Ideally, drinking water shouldn't contain any organism known to be pathogenic.
- The primary bacterial indicator recommended as a bacteriological indicator is the **coliform group** of organisms as a whole. These include both fecal and non-fecal organisms.
- Typical example of the fecal group is **E. coli** ***(single best indicator)*** and of the non-faecal group, ***Klebsiella aerogens.***

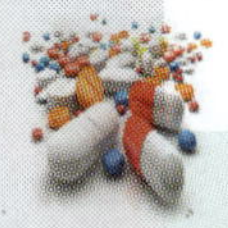

Reasons why coliform organisms are chosen as indicators of fecal pollution rather than the water borne pathogens directly:

- Constant presence of coliform organisms in great abundance in human intestine. These organisms are foreign to potable water. Therefore their presence is looked upon as evidence of fecal contamination.
- They are easily detected by culture methods
- Longer survival as compared to other water borne pathogens
- They have greater resistance to the forces of natural purification, as compared to water borne pathogens

Other Indicators Include

- **Faecal streptococci:** Faecal streptococci regularly occur in faeces, but in much smaller numbers than E. coll. Their presence is regarded as important **confirmatory evidence of recent faecal pollution of water.**
- **Cl. perfringens:** They also occur regularly in faeces and their spores are capable of surviving in water for a longer time than organisms of the coliform group. So, **the presence of spores in the absence of the coliform group**, suggests that faecal contamination occurred at **some remote time**.

351. Ans. (b) 15 meters

Ref: K. Park, 23rd ed. pg. 709, Park, 19th pg. 465

- The safe distance between the latrine and a source of water supply will depend upon the porosity of the soil, level of ground water, its slope and direction of flow. In general, it may be stated, that latrines of any kind should not be *located within 15 m* (50 ft) from a source of water supply, and should be at a lower elevation to prevent the possibility of bacterial contamination of the water supply.

FAMILY PLANNING AND CONTRACEPTION

352. Ans. (c) Nonoxynol 9

Ref: Park Textbook of Preventive and Social Medicine, 25th ed. pg. 546

- Today contraceptive pills are a specially shaped, soft pessary that is inserted deep in the vagina, 10 Minutes before the intercourse.
- It belongs to the class of medicines called spermicidal contraceptives used to prevent pregnancy.
- It contains Non-oxynol 9.

353. Ans. (c) Copper T

Ref: Park Textbook of Preventive and Social Medicine, 25th ed. pg. 547

- A copper IUD is a small device with a fine copper wire wrapped around a plastic frame.
- It's placed inside the uterus to prevent pregnancy. It can prevent pregnancy for up to 10 years after insertion.

354. Ans. (d) Small size fibroid

Ref: K. Park 25th ed. pg. 548

Contraindications of IUD:

- **Absolute**- a) suspected pregnancy b) pelvic inflammatory disease c) vaginal bleeding of undiagnosed etiology d) cancer of the cervix, uterus or amnesia and other pelvic tumours e) previous ectopic pregnancy.
- **Relative**- a) anemia b) menorrhagia c) history of PID since last pregnancy d) purulent cervical discharge e) distortion's of the uterine cavity due to congenital malformations, fibroids f) unmotivated person.

355. Ans. (c) Sterility soon after vasectomy

Ref: K. Park 25th ed. pg. 560

- In vasectomy, it is customary to remove a piece of vas at least 1 cm after clamping. The cut ends are lighted and then folded back on themselves and sutured into position, in this way cut ends face opposite to each other.
- This will prevent recanalization. But spontaneous recanalization is possible in vas deference post damage.
- It is important to note that vasectomy does not produce immediate sterilization. It is a permanent method of contraception. In some cases it takes around 3 month to complete sterilization effect.

356. Ans. (c) CuT 380A

Ref: Park, 25th ed. pg. 547

Types of IUD

- Non-medicated
- Medicated
- Both are usually made of polyethylene or other polymers; in addition, the medicated or bioactive IUDs release either metal ions (copper) or hormones (progestogens). The non-medicated or inert IUDs are often referred to as first generation IUDs.
- The copper IUDs comprise the second and the hormone-releasing IUDs the third generation IUDs. The medicated IUDs were developed to reduce the incidence of side-effects and to increase the contraceptive effectiveness.
- In India, under the National Family Welfare Programme, Cu-T-200 B is being used. From the year 2002, Cu-T-380 A has been introduced in the programme

357. Ans. (b) Usage of barrier methods for 3 months after the procedure

Ref: Park, 25th ed. pg. 600

Post-operative Advice

- The patient should be told that he is not sterile immediately after the operation; at least 30 ejaculations may be necessary before the seminal examination is negative.
- To use contraceptives until aspermia has been established.
- To avoid taking bath for at least 24 hours after the operation.
- To wear a T-bandage or scrotal support (langot) for 15 days and to keep the site clean and dry.
- To avoid cycling or lifting heavy weights for 15 days; there is, however, no need for complete bed rest.
- To have the stitches removed on the 5th day after the operation.

358. Ans. (a) Combined OCP

Ref: K. Park, 25th ed. pg. 528

Contraindications for Use of Combined Oral Contraceptive pills:

- Age > 40 years and Smoking and age > 35 years
- Breast and genital cancers
- History of thromboembolism
- Cardiac abnormalities
- Congenital hyperlipidemia
- Undiagnosed abnormal uterine bleeding
- Pregnancy
- Nursing mothers (0–6 months)
- Chronic renal disease
- Epilepsy
- Amenorrhea

359. Ans. (a) LNG 1.5 milligram

Ref: K. Park, 25th ed. pg. 535

- Post-coital contraception is advocated as an emergency method; for example, after unprotected intercourse, rape or contraceptive failure. It is recommended within 72 hours of an unprotected intercourse. In India Levonorgestrel 0.75 mg tablet is approved for emergency contraception.
- It is used as one tablet of 0.75 mg within 72 hours of unprotected sex and the 2nd tablet after 12 hours of 1st dose.

360. Ans. (b) Nonoxynol – 9

Ref: K. Park, 25th ed. pg. 528

- Nonoxynol-9 (N-9) is a typical surfactant used as a vaginal spermicide.
- Spermicides are locally acting non-hormonal contraceptives.
- When present in the vagina during intercourse, they damage or kill sperms without eliciting systemic effects.

361. Ans. (d) Couple that is eligible for practicing family planning

Ref: K. Park, 25th ed. pg. 527

- The term target couple was applied to couples who have had 2–3 living children, and family planning was largely directed to such couples.
- The definition of a target couple has been gradually enlarged to include families with one child or even newly married couples with a view to develop acceptance of the idea of family planning from the earliest possible stage.

362. Ans. (c) Spermicide

Ref: K. Park 25th ed. pg. 550-54

- Contraceptive failure is measured by pearl index.

$$PI = \frac{\text{Total accidental pregnancy}}{\text{Total month of exposure}} \times 1200$$

- Spermicide is a chemical method of contraception usually used with vaginal sponge. It has highest contraceptive failure (highest pearl index).
- No spermicide is effective alone for contraception, therefore they are best used with barrier methods.
- Commonly used modern spermicides are "surface – active agents" → which attach themselves to spermatozoa and inhibits oxygen uptake → Sperms killed.
- Failure rate of different forms of contraception are as follows:

Contraceptive method	Failure rate (Pearl index- per 100 women years -HWY)
OCP	0.1–0.5
IUCD	0.2–3.0 (**Mirena/LNG-20:** 0.2 per 100 women)
Subdermal implant/Norplant	0.7
Centchroman/Saheli	1.83–2.84
Condoms	Male: 2–14 Female: 5–21
Diaphragm	6–12
Vaginal sponge/Today	Nulliparous: 9–20 Parous: 20–40

- **Main drawbacks of spermicide:**
    - High failure rate
    - Must be used immediately before intercourse
    - Difficulty in application
    - Lots of messiness and mild burning sensation

363. Ans. (c) Family planning in those who are not using any contraception

Ref: K. Park 23rd ed. pg. 511

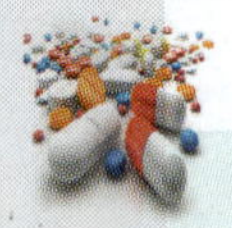

- Many women who are sexually active would prefer to avoid becoming pregnant, without using any methods of contraception neither by their partner.
- These womens are considered to have an "unmet need" for family planning.
- Concept is usually applied and limited to married women only, however it can be applied to sexually active fecund women.

Unmet Need

Unmet need for family planning is defined as the percentage of women of reproductive age, either married or in a union who want to stop or delay childbearing but are not using any method of contraception.

$$\text{Unmet need for family planning} = \frac{\text{Women of reproductive age (15–49) who are married or in a union and who have an unmet need for family planning}}{\text{Total number of women of reproductive age (15–49) who are married or in a union}}$$

- **Most common reasons for unmet needs are:**
    - Inconvenient or unsatisfactory services
    - Lack of information
    - Contraceptives side effect fears
    - Opposition from husband or relatives
- According to national family health survey, it is most commonly seen in women below 20 years (almost entirely for spacing the birth).
- It is higher in rural areas than in urban areas.

364. Ans. (c) Failures per 100 women years of exposure

Ref: K. Park, 23rd ed. pg. 510

- **Pearl index** is used to measure the contraceptive efficacy/ contraceptive failure.
- It is defined as the number of failures per 100 women-years (HWY) of exposure. It is given by the formula:

$$\text{Failure rate per HWY} = \frac{\text{Total accidental pregnancies}}{\text{Total months of exposure}} \times 1200$$

365. Ans. (a) 0.01

Ref: K. Park, 23rd ed. pg. 510

- Failure rate is 1 HWY; Total month of exposure is 12. We have to find out the number of accidental pregnancies.
- Putting the values in pearl index formula:

$$\text{Failure rate per HWY} = \frac{\text{Total accidental pregnancies}}{\text{Total months of exposure}} \times 1200$$

$$1 = \frac{x}{12} \times 1200$$

$$12 = 1200\,x$$

Therefore, $x = \frac{12}{1200} = \mathbf{0.01}$

366. Ans. (d) Progesterone only pill

Ref: K. Park, 23rd ed. pg. 503

Please refer to above explanation

367. Ans. (b) Prevent release of ovum from ovary

Ref: K. Park, 23rd ed. pg. 501

- Combined oral contraceptive pills act by inhibiting ovulation by suppressing the release of gonadotropins.
- Continuous progesterone by OCPs which give negative feedback to GnRH, which decreases LH release and upto some extent FSH release also.
- This prevents LH surge and as a result inhibits ovulation.

368. Ans. (c) Ovarian cancer

Ref: K. Park, 23rd ed. pg. 501-502

Beneficial Effects of OCPs

- Ovarian CA
- PID
- Ectopic pregnancy
- Endometrial CA

369. Ans. (b) Just after the menstruation

Ref: K. Park, 23rd ed. pg. 389-90

- **Breast self-examination** (BSE) is a screening method used in an attempt to detect early breast cancer. The method involves the woman herself looking at and feeling each breast for possible lumps, distortions or swelling.
- **For pre-menopausal** women, the most commonly recommended time is just after the end of menstruation, because the breasts are least likely to be swollen and tender at this time.
- **For postmenopausal,** women or these having irregular cycles might do a self-exam once a month regardless of their menstrual cycle.

370. Ans. (d) Contraceptive failure

Ref: Park's PSM, 23rd ed. pg. 510

- Pearl index is used to measure the contraceptive efficacy/ contraceptive failure.
- It is defined as the number of failures per 100 women-years (HWY) of exposure.

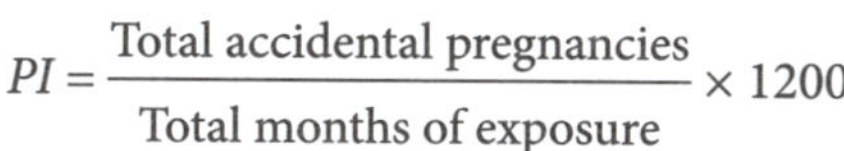

$$PI = \frac{\text{Total accidental pregnancies}}{\text{Total months of exposure}} \times 1200$$

- Another method used to measure contraceptive failure/efficacy is *life table analysis.*
- Life table analysis: Calculates failure rates for each month of use.

371. Ans. (a) 0.1%

Ref: K. Park, 23rd ed. pg. 494-96

- Pomoroy's technique is the most popular method of ligation.
- Failure Rate: 0.1–0.3%
- *Failure rate of vasectomy: 0.15 per HWY*

DEMOGRAPHY AND HEALTH

372. Ans. (b) Demographic transition model

Ref: Park Textbook of Preventive and Social Medicine, 25th ed. pg. 530

- Demographic Transition Model refers to the transition from high birth and high death rates to low birth and low death rates regime as a country develops from a pre-industrial to an industrialized economic system.

The four stages of the demographic transition model:

- **Stage 1: High fluctuating**
  Birth Rate and Death rate are both high. Population growth is slow and fluctuating.
- **Stage 2: Early expanding**
  Birth Rate remains high. Death Rate is falling. Population begins to rise steadily.
- **Stage 3: Late expanding**
  Birth Rate starts to fall. Death Rate continues to fall. Population is rising.
- **Stage 4: Low fluctuating**
  Birth Rate and Death Rate both low. Population is steady.

373. Ans. (c) Declining

Ref: Park Textbook of Preventive and Social Medicine, 25th ed. pg. 530

- According to demographic model, when the birth rate is less than death rate or when no new birth is reported and death is continuously happening, the population goes into decline phase.
- A population decline in humans is a reduction in a human population size.

374. Ans. (b) Base denotes fertility

Ref: Park Textbook of Preventive and Social Medicine, 25th ed. pg. 532

- This population pyramid is wide at the base, which means there are a large proportion of young people in the country.
- A wide base suggests high birth rate. Narrow base shows low birth rate as small numbers of children are born.

375. Ans. (a) Males less than 5000

Ref: K. Park 25th ed. pg. 534.

- Sex ratio is defined as "the number of females per 1000 males."

$$\frac{\text{Male population}}{\text{Female population}} \times 1000$$

376. Ans. (b) Extension

Ref: K. Park 25th ed. pg. 739.

Basic model of nuclear family life cycle

Phases of family life cycle	Events characterizing	
Description	**Beginning**	**End**
• Formation	• Marriage	• Birth of 1st child
• Extension	• Birth of first child	• Birth of last child
• Complete extension	• Birth of last child	• 1st child leaves home
• Contraction	• 1st child leaves home	• Last child leaves home parents
• Complete contraction	• Last child has left home parents	• 1st spouse dies
• Dissolution		• Death of surviour

377. Ans. (c) Civil registration system

Ref: K. Park 25th ed. pg. 903

- Registration of vital events is the precursor of health statistics.
- The Civil Registration System (CRS) is defined as a unified process of continuous, permanent, compulsory and universal recording of the vital events and characteristics thereof, as per legal requirements in the country.
- In India, the Civil Registration System covers registration of births and deaths.

378. Ans. (d) 1st July

Ref: Park, 25th ed. pg. 63

- Arithmetic mean of the population on 1 January and on 31 December of a year is used to calculate annual rates.
- Mid-year population or mean population, is regarded as the population on July 1 and is assumed to be the point

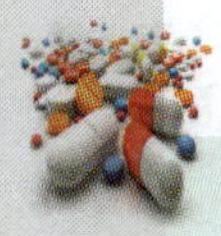

at which half of the changes in the population during the year have occurred.

- It is used to calculate, crude birth rate and crude death rate.
- Example: Crude birth rate

$$= \frac{\text{Total number of births} \times 1000}{\text{Total mid year population (as on 1}^{\text{st}}\text{ July)}}$$

379. Ans. (c) Goal

Ref: Park, 25th ed. pg. 931

- GOAL is defined as the ultimate desired state towards which objectives and resources are directed. Unlike objectives and targets, goals are not constrained by time or existing resources, nor are they necessarily attainable.

380. Ans. (b) Group

Ref: Park, 25th ed. pg. ??

- The Delphi method is a structured communication technique. It is a process used to arrive at a group opinion or decision by surveying a panel of experts. Experts respond to several rounds of questionnaires, and the responses are aggregated and shared with the group after each round.
- Delphi method is highly used in collective intelligence.

381. Ans. (b) United Nations

Ref: K. Park, 25th ed. pg. 963

- The Sustainable Development Goals (SDGs), also known as the Global Goals, were adopted by all United Nations Member States in 2015 as a universal call to action to end poverty, protect the planet and ensure that all people enjoy peace and prosperity by 2030.
- The 17 SDGs are integrated—that is, they recognize that action in one area will affect outcomes in others, and that development must balance social, economic and environmental sustainability.

382. Ans. (c) 21 days

Ref: K. Park 25th ed. pg. 903

- According to Central Birth and Death Registration Act 1969:
  - The time limit for registration of vital events like births and death is 21 days
  - Late fee is imposed in case of default
  - From October 2018, Aadhar number is must for registration of death
- **Lay reporting of health information:** Collection of information (birth and death), its use and its transmission to other levels of the health system by the non-professional health worker (like village health guide).

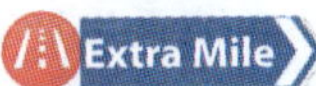

- **Registration of marriage:** Within 30 days

383. Ans. (d) $\text{PAR} = \frac{\text{Incidence among total population} - \text{incidence among non-exposed}}{\text{Incidence among total population}} \times 100$

Ref: K. Park 25th ed. pg. 86

- **Population – attributable risk is** incidence of disease (or death) in total population minus the incidence of disease (or death) among those who were NOT exposed to the suspected causal factor divided by incidence among total population.
- **Use:** It provides an estimate of the amount by which the disease could be reduced in that population if the suspected factor is eliminated or modified.

Extra Mile

$$\text{Relative risk} = \frac{\text{Incidence among exposed}}{\text{Incidence among non-exposed}}$$

$$\text{Attributable risk} = \frac{\text{Incidence among exposed} - \text{incidence among non exposed}}{\text{Incidence among exposed}} \times 100$$

384. Ans. (b) Net reproduction rate

Ref: K. Park 25th ed. pg. 539–540

- **Net Reproduction Rate (NRR):** No. of daughters a newborn girl will bear during her life time ***assuming fixed age specific fertility and mortality rates.***
  - It is a demographic indicator
  - NRR of 1 is equivalent to attaining approximately the 2-child norm.
  - If NRR <1, the reproductive performance of the population is said to be below replacement level.
- **Total Fertility Rate:** it is the average number of children a woman would have if she were to pass through her reproductive years bearing children at the same rates as the women now in each age group.
- **Gross Reproduction Rate:** Average number of girls that would be born to a woman if she experiences the current fertility pattern throughout her reproductive span (15–44 or 49 years), assuming no mortality.
- **General Fertility Rate:** It is the number of live birth per 1000 women in reproductive age group (15–44 or 49 years) in a given year

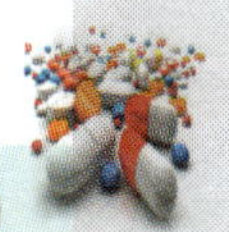

- GFR = $\frac{\text{No. of live births in an area during a year}}{\text{Mid year female population of age 15–44 (or 49) years}} \times 1000$

385. Ans. (c) 4

Ref: K. Park, 23rd ed. pg. 479

Demographic Cycle

The history of world population since 1650 suggests that there is a demographic cycle of 5 stages through which a nation passes:

- **First stage (High stationary):** This stage is characterized by a **high birth rate and a high death rate** which cancel each other and the population remains stationary.
- **Second stage (Early expanding):** The **death rate begins to decline, while the birth rate remains unchanged**. Many countries in South Asia, and Africa are in this phase. Birth rates have increased in some of these countries possibly as a result of improved health conditions, and shortening periods of breastfeeding.
- **Third stage (Late expanding):** The death rate declines still further, and the birth rate tends to fall. The population continues to grow because births exceed deaths. **India has entered this phase.**
- **Fourth stage (Low stationary):** This stage is characterized by a **low birth and low death rate** with the result that the population becomes stationary.
- **Fifth stage (Declining):** The population begins to decline because birth rate is lower than the death rate.

386. Ans. (d) Emigration

Ref: K. Park 23rd ed. pg. 481

- Demographic characteristics provide an overview of its population size, composition, territorial distribution and changes therein and the **components of changes such as: Nativity, mortality, social mobility.**
- Demographic indicators have been divided into 2 parts:
  - **Population statistics:** Include indicators that measures the population size, sex ratio, density and dependency ratio
  - **Vital statistics:** Include indicators such as birth rate, death rate, natural growth rate, life expectancy at birth, mortality and fertility rates.

387. Ans. (b) Population <15 years and >65 years

Ref: K. Park 23rd ed. pg. 484

- Dependency ratio is the proportion of persons above 65 years of age and children below 15 years of age who are considered to be dependent on economically productive age group (15-64).

$$\textit{Dependency Ratio} = \frac{\text{Persons} < 15 \text{ years} + > 65 \text{ years}}{\text{Persons between 15 and 65 years}}$$

- Dependency ratio of India is 62 per 100 or 0.62. This means 62 non-earning peoples in India are dependent on 100 earning population.

388. Ans. (a) Broad at base and narrow at apex

Ref: K. Park 23rd ed. pg. 482

389. Ans. (b) It is distributed equally in study and control groups

Ref: K. Park 23rd ed. pg. 72

390. Ans (c) 95.4%

Ref: K. Park 23rd ed. pg. 849

- The standard normal curve is a smooth, bell shaped, perfectly symmetrical curve, based on infinitely large number of observations.
- The area between 2 standard deviations on either side of the mean will cover most of the values i.e. ~95%.

The normal distribution or 'normal curve' is an important concept in statistical theory. In a normal curve:

- The area between one standard deviation on either side of the mean will include approximately 68% of values in the distribution.
- The area between two standard deviations will cover approx 95% of the values.
- The area between two standard deviations will cover approx 99.7% of the values

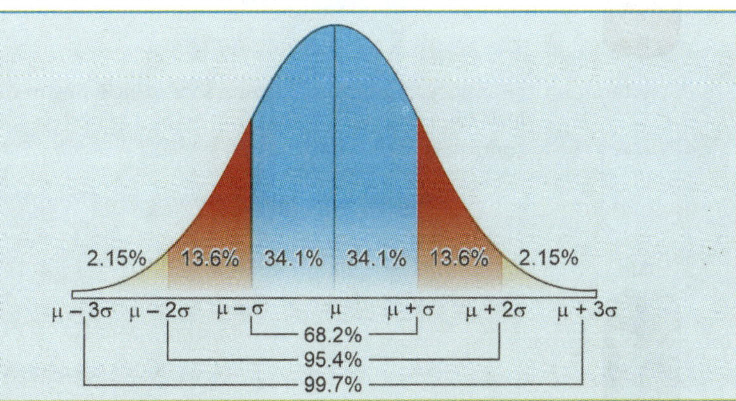

More About Standard Curve

- The standard normal curve is a smooth, **bell-shaped, perfectly symmetrical curve**
- It is based on an infinitely large number of observations.
- The **total area of the curve is 1**
- Its **mean is zero**
- Its **standard** deviation is 1
- The mean, median and mode all coincide

391. Ans. (d) 99.7% values

Ref: K. Park, 23rd ed. pg. 848-49

392. Ans. (a) Tapering at top

Ref: K. Park, 23rd ed. pg. 848-49

393. Ans. (b) 16–25

Ref: K. Park, 23rd ed. pg. 690

MODIFIED KUPPUSWAMI SCALE: Scale of socio-economic status of urban families, includes Education status of head, occupation status of head, Income per capita.

Total score of 3 components	Socioeconomic class
• 26–29	Upper
• 16–25	Upper-middle
• 11–15	Lower-middle
• 05–10	Upper-lower
• <5	Lower

DISASTER MANAGEMENT, DISINFECTION AND BMW MANAGEMENT

394. Ans. (b) Yellow

Ref: Park Textbook of Preventive and Social Medicine, 25th ed. pg. 853

- Blood bag is discarded in yellow color bag.
- More information about waste disposal is given later in this chapter

395. Ans. (d) Yellow

Ref: K. Park 25th ed. pg. 853

Cat.	Type of Bag/ Container used	Type of Waste	Treatment/Disposal Option
Yellow	Non-chlorinated plastic bags Separate collection system leading to effluent treatment system	• **Human anatomical waste** • **Animal anatomical waste** • **Soiled waste** • **Expired or discarded medicines** • **Chemical waste** • **Micro, Bio-t and other clinical lab waste** • **Chemical liquid waste**	Incineration or plasma Pyrolysis or deep burial*
Red	Non-chlorinated plastic bags or containers	**Contaminated waste (Recyclable)** tubing, bottles, intravenous tubes and sets, catheters, urine bags, syringes (without needles) and gloves	Auto/Micro/Hydro and then sent for recycling. Not be sent to landfill
White	(Translucent) puncture, leak, tamper proof containers	**Waste sharps including metals**	Auto or dry heat sterilization followed by shredding or mutilation or encapsulation
Blue	Cardboard boxes with blue colored marking	**Glassware**	Disinfection or auto/micro/hydro and then sent for recycling

396. Ans. (d) Red – Yellow – Green – Black

Ref: Park, 25th ed. pg. 857

Triage System

- Red indicates high priority treatment or transfer,
- Yellow signals medium priority,
- Green indicates ambulatory patients and
- Black for dead or moribund patients.

397. Ans. (a) Triage

Ref: K. Park, 25th ed. pg. 833-34

- **Triage:** Consists of rapidly classifying the injured 'on the basis of severity of their injuries and likelihood of their survival' with prompt medical intervention.
- Triage yields best results when carried out at the site of disaster.
- **Triage sieve:** Quick survey to separate the dead and the walking from the injured.
- **Triage sort:** Remaining casualties are assessed and allocated to categories.
- **Triage system:** Most commonly uses four color code system:
  - Red (Highest Priority): Immediate resuscitation or limb/life saving surgery in next 6 hours.
  - Yellow (High Priority): Possible resuscitation or limb/life saving surgery in next 24 hours.
  - Green (Low Priority): Minor illness/Ambulatory patients.
  - Black (Least Priority): Dead and moribund patients.

Note: *Tagging: Is the procedure where identification, age, place of origin, triage category, diagnosis and initial treatment are tagged on to every victim of disaster through a Color Coding.*

398. Ans. (a) Acute gastroenteritis

Ref: K. Park 25th ed. pg. 858

- **Book states:** *"most commonly reported disease in post-disaster period is outbreak of gastroenteritis".*

399. Ans. (c) Controlled tipping

Ref: K. Park 25th ed. pg. 814

- **Book states:** *"Controlled tipping or sanitary landfill is the most satisfactory method of refuse disposal where suitable land is available"*
- **Three methods of controlled tipping:**
  - **The trench method:** Preferred where level ground is available. The refuse is compacted in long trench (6–10 feet deep, 12–36 feet wide) and covered with excavated earth.
  - **The ramp method:** Preferred where terrain in moderately sloping
  - **The area method:** Used for filling land depressions, disused quarries and clay pits. The refuse uniformly consolidated in layers up to 2–2.5 m (6–8 ft). Each layer is sealed with mud (12 inches/30 cm thick).

Extra Mile

Other methods of refuse disposal

- **Dumping:** Easy method for disposal of dry waste. Refuse is dumped (as open) in low lying areas usually as a method of land reclamation. It is the most insanitary method that creates public health hazard (WHO expert committee).
- **Incineration:** Disposal of refusal hygienically by burning or incineration. Method of choice where suitable land is NOT available. Best for hospital and industrial waste.
- **Composting:** Method of combined disposal of refuse and night soil or sludge. Best and cultivation and soil. Methods of composting:
  - **Bangalore method** (Anaerobic method)
  - **Mechanical composting** (Aerobic composting)
- **Manure pits:** Done by digging manure pits by individual house hold. Preferred in rural areas where system of refuse collection and disposal is not systematic. Refuse is converted into manure in 5-6 months → used in field.
- **Burial:** Preferred for small camps. Refuse is disposed in a small trench (1.5 m wide and 2 m deep). It is covered with 20–30 cm of earth every day. Can be taken out after 6 month and used in field.

400. Ans. (a) Yellow

Ref: K. Park 25th ed. pg. 853

TABLE: Biomedical waste management

Color Category	Type of biomedical waste	Treatment options
Yellow	• Human and Animal anatomical waste • Soiled waste (with blood, body fluid)	Incineration/Deep burial Nonchlorinated chemical disinfection
	• Expired/Discarded/cytotoxic medicine • Chemical waste • Chemical liquid waste • Discarded linen, mattress, beddings contaminated with blood or body fluids	

Contd...

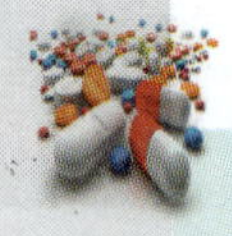

Color Category	Type of biomedical waste	Treatment options
Red	• Recyclable contaminated waste ▪ Disposable items such as tubes, bottles, IV sets, urine bags, syringes without needle, gloves	Autoclaving or microwaving/ hydroclaving followed by shredding
White/Translucent *(puncture/leak proof container)*	• Waste sharps including metals: Needles, blades or any contaminated sharp object	Autoclaving or dry heat sterilization followed by shredding and mutilation
Blue	• Glassware: Included medicine vials except those contaminated with cytotoxic waste • Metallic body implants	Disinfection (by soaking waste with detergent and sodium hypochlorite)/ Autoclaving/ Microwaving/ Hydroclaving

401. Ans. (d) Mitigation and preparedness

Ref: K. Park 25th ed. pg. 857, 859

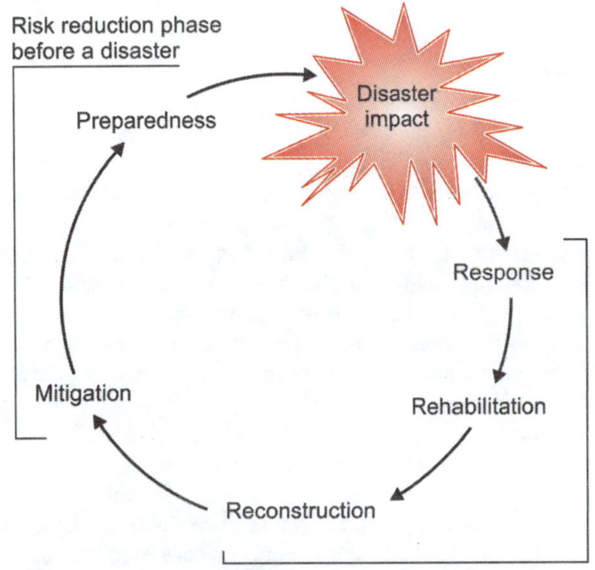

- There are 3 fundamental aspects of disaster management (as seen in disaster cycle):
  - Disaster response
  - Disaster preparedness
  - Disaster mitigation
- Before the disaster the most important steps are mitigation and preparedness of disaster
- **Emergency prevention and mitigation** involves measures designed to either prevent hazard or to lessen the effect of emergencies. It also reduces the medical causalities drastically. It includes:
  - Flood mitigation works
  - Appropriate land use planning
  - Improved building codes
  - Reduction and protection of vulnerable population and structures
- **Disaster preparedness:**
  - It is a long-term development activities whose goals are to strengthen the overall capacity and capability of a country to manage efficiently all types of emergency
  - **Objective:** To ensure that all resources, systems are in place to provide prompt effective assistance to disaster victims thus facilitating relief measures and rehabilitation of services
- **Cornerstone of emergency preparedness programme:** Community members, resources, organizations and administration.

402. Ans. (b) Response and rehabilitation

Ref: K. Park 25th ed. pg. 857

- After the disaster the first step is **response in first few hours** in order to manage the mass casualties.
- This is further divided into:
  - **Search, rescue and first aid** (most immediate help comes from an uninjured survivor)
  - **Field care:** Most injured ones are converged spontaneously to health facilities using any form of transport
  - **Triage:** Rapidly classifying the injured on basis of severity of injury.
    - Highest priority is given to victim whose immediate or long term prognosis is dramatically affected by simple intensive care
    - **Lowest priority:** Moribund patients
    - **Most accepted triage method:** 4 color coded system:
      - **Red:** High priority treatment or transfer
      - **Yellow:** Mdium priority
      - **Green:** Ambulatory patients
      - **Black:** Dead or moribund patients
  - **Tagging:** Victims should be tagged with name, age, place of origin, triage category, diagnosis and initial treatment
  - Identification and removal of dead from disaster scene

- **Rehabilitation and reconstruction:**
  - The final phase in a disaster should lead to restoration of the pre-disaster condition. This is done by:
  - **Water supply:** First priority of ensuring water quality is chlorination (increase residual chlorine level to about 0.2–0.5 mg/L)
  - Food safety
  - Basic sanitation and personal hygiene
  - Vector control

403. Ans. (b) Ministry of Home Affairs

Ref: K. Park 25th ed. pg. 862

- The overall coordination of disaster management vests with ministry of Home affairs
- Top-level decision making committee:
  - Cabinet committee on security
  - National crisis management committee
- Agency responsible for preparation of disaster management plans and its execution at national level: The National Disaster Management Authority
- Health management in a disaster is under: Ministry of Health and family welfare (a special wing under it-Emergency Medical Relief Wing)

Extra Mile

- **World disaster reduction day:** Second Wednesday of October
- **Execution of relief work in case of natural disasters:** The state government

404. Ans. (c) Unsalvageable

Ref: PubMed

- In a disaster management, categorization of victims are done on the basis of likelihood of survival.

TABLE: Triage color code and their significance

Category	Color	Remarks/steps
Category 1	**Red**	**Highest priority**—patient immediate resuscitation or life-saving surgery (0 to 6 hours)
Category 2	Yellow/ blue	High possible resuscitation or life saving surgery (within 6 to 24 hours)
Category 3	Green	Ambulatory/low minor injuries; non-life threating
Category 4	Black	Dead, Moribund; least priority/ unsalvagable

405. Ans. (b) Pathological waste

Ref: K. Park 23rd ed. pg. 789

TABLE: Classification of health care waste

Waste category	Description and examples
Infectious waste	Waste suspected to contain pathogens e.g. laboratory culture; waste from isolation wards; tissues (swabs), materials, or equipments that have been in contact with infected patients; excreta.
Pathological waste	Human tissues or fluids e.g. body parts; blood and other body fluids; fetuses.
Sharps	Sharp waste e.g. needles; infusion sets; scalpels; knives; blades; broken glass.
Pharmaceutical waste	Waste containing pharmaceuticals e.g. pharmaceuticals that are expired or no longer needed: items contaminated by or containing pharmaceuticals (bottles, boxes)
Genotoxic waste	Waste containing substances with genotoxic properties e.g. waste containing cytostatic drugs (often used in cancer therapy): genotoxic chemicals.
Chemical waste	Waste containing chemical substances e.g. laboratory reagents; film developer; disinfectants that are expired or no longer needed; solvents.
Wastes with high content of heavy metals	Batteries; broken thermometers; blood-pressure gauges; etc.
Pressurized containers	Gas cylinders, gas cartridges aerosol cans
Radioactive waste	Waste containing radioactive substances e.g. unused liquids from radiotherapy or laboratory research; contaminated glassware, packages, or absorbent paper; urine and excreta from patients treated or tested with unsealed radionucleides; sealed sources.

406. Ans. (b) 2nd week of October

Ref: K. Park 23rd ed. pg. 795

- **WORLD DISASTER REDUCTION DAY:** 2ND WEDNESDAY IN MONTH OF OCTOBER
- **24TH OCTOBER:** UN DAY
- **25TH NOVEMBER:** INT'L DAY FOR ELIMINATION OF VIOLENCE AGAINST WOMEN

407. Ans. (d) District hospital

Ref: K. Park, 23rd ed. pg. 795-96

- There are 3 fundamental aspects of disaster management:
  - Disaster response
  - Disaster preparedness, and
  - Disaster mitigation

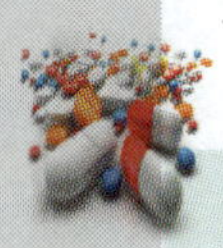

- District hospital take role in case of disasters like earth quake, flood etc.

408. Ans. (a) Search and rescue, first aid

Ref: K. Park, 23rd ed. pg. 795-97

- The management of mass casualties (massive disaster) can be further divided into:
  - Search and rescue, first aid,
  - Triage
  - Stabilization of victims,
  - Hospital treatment and redistribution of patients to hospitals if necessary.
- Foremost step for disease prevention and control in post disaster phase is chlorination of all the water bodies. Most practical and effective strategy of disease prevention is "supplying safe drinking water and proper disposal of excreta.

409. Ans. (c) Yellow

Ref: K. Park, 23rd ed. pg. 795-97

- In a disaster management, categorization of victims are done on the basis of likelihood of survival.

TABLE: Triage color code and their significance

Category	Color	Remarks/steps
Category 1	Red	**Highest priority-** patient immediate resuscitations or life-saving surgery (0–6 hr)
Category 2	Yellow	High priority resuscitation or life saving surgery (within 6–24 hr)
Category 3	Green	Ambulatory/low minor injuries; non-life threating
Category 4	Black	Dead, Moribund; least priority

410. Ans. (a) Red

Ref: K. Park, 23rd ed. pg. 795-97

411. Ans. (d) All of the above

Ref: K. Park 23rd ed. pg. 127-128

- Gamma radiation is used for sterilizing plastics, syringes, swabs, culture plates, catheter, rubber, oils, greases and metal foils.

412. Ans. (d) Liquid paraffin

Ref: K. Park, 23rd ed. pg. 128

- **Autoclaving** is a method of disinfection mainly used for surgical dressings, instruments, laboratory wares, media and pharmaceutical products.
- Principle: Steam + High pressure (~30 psi) and temperature 121°C.
- Efficiency test of autoclaving: spores of *Bacillus Stearothermophillus.*

413. Ans. (c) Plastic syringes

Ref: K. Park, 23rd ed. pg. 127-28

HOT AIR OVEN

- Holding period of 160 C x 1 hour
- Used for forceps, glasswares, scissors, scalpels, glass syringes, swabs and few pharmaceutical products like liquid paraffin, fats, grease.

HEALTH PLANNING, CARE AND MANAGEMENT IN INDIA

414. Ans. (d) Intensive neonatal unit

Ref: Park Textbook of Preventive and Social Medicine, 25th ed. pg. 967

- At CHC, intensive neonatal unit is not established
- Special newborn care units (SNCUs) have been established at district hospitals and sub- district hospitals with annual delivery load more than 3000 to provide care for sick newborns, that is, all type of neonatal care except assisted ventilation and major surgeries.

415. Ans. (c) Accredited social health activist

Ref: K. Park 25th ed. pg. 959

- ASHA must be resident of the village-a woman (married/widow/divorced) preferably in the age group of 25 to 45 years with formal education upto eight class, having communication skill and leadership qualities.

416. Ans. (d) 1 acre

Ref: K. Park 25th ed. pg. 821

- There are two types of trench latrines— Shallow and deep.
- **Shallow trench latrine** — this is simply a trench dug with ordinary tools. The trench is 30 cm wide and 90–150 cm deep. It's length depends on the number of users: 3–3.5 m are necessary for 100 people. The shallow trench is a rudimentary arrangement for a short period (up to one week).
- **Deep trench latrine** — this type is intended for camps of longer duration, from a few weeks to months. The trench is 1.8 to 2.5 m deep and 75–90 cm wide. Other requirements are same as for shallow trench latrine. Almost 1 acre land is required for 10,000 people

417. Ans. (d) National Planning Commission (NPC)

Ref: K. Park, 25th ed. pg. 913

- Government of India has established NITI Aayog (National Institution for Transforming India) to replace Planning Commission on 1st January 2015. It will seek to provide a critical directional and strategic input into the development process.
- NITI Aayog will emerge as a "think-tank" that will provide Governments at the central and state levels with relevant strategic and technical advice across the spectrum of key elements of policy.

418. Ans. (c) National Sample Survey

- The National Sample Survey (NSS) is one of the oldest continuing household sample surveys in the developing world. The survey included information on land utilization, prices of essential commodities, and daily wages of skilled and unskilled laborers at the village level.
- At the household level, data was obtained on demographic characteristics as well as land ownership, cultivation, and utilization.

419. Ans. (a) Child health

Ref: K. Park, 25th ed. pg. 962

UNICEF's GOBI Campaign to Encourage 4 Strategies for a 'Child Health Revolution'

- G: Growth Charts
- O: Oral Rehydration
- B: Breast Feeding.
- I: Immunizations for TB, Polio, Diphtheria, Pertussis, Tetanus and Measle.

420. Ans. (b) 30,000

Ref: K. Park 25th ed. pg. 964

Health Care Unit	Population covered	
	Plain	Hilly/Tribal/Backward
CHC	120,000	80,000
PHC	30,000	20,000
MPW	5000	3000
AWW	400-800	300-800
ASHA/VHG/TBA	1000	One ASHA per habitation

421. Ans. (b) Multi-purpose worker scheme

Ref: K. Park, 23rd ed. pg. 874-75

- **Kartar Singh Committee:** Recommended multi-purpose worker scheme. Kartar Singh Committee recommended:
  - **Current ANM** to be replaced by the newly designated "female health worker" and present day basic health workers, malaria surveillance workers, family planning health assistants to be replaced by "male health workers"

422. Ans. (b) 10,000

Ref: K. Park, 23rd ed. pg. 900

TABLE: Suggested norms for health personnel

Personnel category	Norms suggested
Nurses	1 per 5000
Health worker male and female	1 per 5000 in plain 1 per 3000 in tribal and hilly areas
Trained dai	One for each village
Health assistant (male and female)	1 per 30,000 in plain 1 per 20,000 in tribal and hilly areas
Pharmacist	1 per 10,000
Lab technician	1 per 10,000
ASHA	1 per 1000

423. Ans. (c) 16

The guidelines are from India New Born Action Plan 2014

Special New Born Care Unit (SNCU)

- It should be present in all district and sub-district hospitals.
- It comprises 12 beds and 4 beds for rooming in purposes
- The unit provides care for sick newborns >1800 g and routine new born care except ventilator services.

New Born Stabilization Unit (NBSU)

- It should be present in all CHC and FRU
- It comprises 4 beds and 2 beds for rooming in purposes.
- The unit aims to stabilize the sick new-borns before referral and manage baby >1800 g with jaundice, sepsis and hypothermia.

New Born Care Corner (NBCC)

- It should be present at all points where delivery will occur including PHC and subcenter.
- It comprises minimum one bed.
- Objective is to provide immediate care at birth, feeding support and immediate referral.

424. Ans. (d) 7

Ref: Park's, 23rd ed. pg. 449-50

- ASHA will make visits to all newborns according to specified schedule up to 42 days of life. The scheduled visits are as follows:

- **Six visits** in case of **institutional delivery**: Day 3, 7, 14, 21, 28, 42
- **Seven visits** in case of **home delivery:** Day 1, 3, 7, 14, 28, 42
- **Five visits** in case of **caesarean delivery** (mother discharged after 5–6 days): **Day** 7, 14, 21, 28, 42

425. Ans. (c) 1 lakh

Ref: K. Park, 23rd ed. pg. 428

- Designated microscopy centre (DMC): The most peripheral laboratory under RNTCP network is DMC which serves a population of around **100,000 in plains** and **50,000 in tribal and hilly areas.**

426. Ans. (d) Equity of distribution

Ref: K. Park, 23rd ed. pg. 891

- PHC is Primary Health Care outlined by Alma Ata in 1978.
- It is defined as essential health care, which is characterized by 4 A's
  - Acceptable *(it should be acceptable by everyone)*
  - Accessible *(it should be accessible by everyone)*
  - Available *(it should be available to everyone)*
  - Affordable *(it should be affordable to everyone)*

TABLE: Elements of PHC (Primary Health Care) (remembered as ELEMENTS)

E	Essential drugs
L	Locally endemic disease prevention and control
E	EPI (Expanded program of immunization)
M	MCH (Maternal and child Health care including family planning)
E	Education
N	Nutrition
T	Treatment of common ailments
S	Safe water supply and sanitation

- Equity of distribution is NOT an element of PHC, but it is one of the principles/pillars of the PHC.
- ***4 Principles/Pillars of Primary Health Care:***
  - Equitable distribution
  - Community participation
  - Intersectoral coordination
  - Appropriate technology.

427. Ans. (a) Primary health care

Ref: K. Park, 23rd ed. pg. 891-92

Please refer to above explanation

428. Ans. (c) Unequitable distribution

Ref: K. Park, 23rd ed. pg. 891-92

Please refer to above explanation.

429. Ans. (c) Oxygen saturation

Ref: K. Park, 23rd ed. pg. 904-905

430. Ans. (d) 100,000

Ref: K. Park, 23rd ed. pg. 907

- **CHC** is community health Centre. It covers 120,000 population in plain areas and 80,000 population in hilly areas.
- Since, 120,000 is not in option, 100,000 is the closest and best answer.

Extra Mile

- PHC is considered as *Primary level of health care* is. It is considered as *1st level of contact.*
- CHC is considered as *secondary level of health care* and *first referral unit.*
- *Tertiary level of health* care is delivered through medical colleges and hospitals.

Health Care Unit	Population covered	
	Plain	Hilly/Tribal/Backward
CHC	120,000	80,000
PHC	30,000	20,000
MPW	5000	3000
AWW	400–800	300–800
ASHA/VHG/TBA	1000	

431. Ans. (b) CHC

Ref: K. Park 23rd ed. pg. 907

Please refer to above explanation

432. Ans. (b) 30

Ref: K. Park 23rd ed. pg. 907

- **PHC level: 4 to 6 bed** and staff 15 and 1 MBBS and medical officer
- **CHC level: 30 beds** and 30 staff including 7 doctors MD/MS/OBS/GYNE/ PEDIA/ OPTHA/ANES/PSM
- **Sub center level: zero bed** and 3 staff. MPW *(1 male and 1 female)*/ ANM *(auxillary nurse midwife).*

433. Ans. (c) 2005

Ref: K. Park, 23rd ed. pg. 448

- National Rural Health Mission (NRHM) was established in 2005.
- Goal of NRHM is to provide every village in the country with a trained female community health activist: **ASHA** *(Accredited Social Health Activist).*

Other Important Health Programmes of India

- National Tuberculosis Programme (NTP): 1962
- Revised National TB Control Programme (RNTCP): 1993
- National AIDS Control Programme (NACP): 1987
- National Malaria Control Programme (NMCP): 1953
- National Leprosy Control Program: 1955
- Integrated Child Development Services scheme (ICDS): 1975
- National Programme for Control of Blindness (NPCB): 1976

434. Ans. (b) Kartar Singh Committee

Ref: K. Park, 23rd ed. pg. 874

- **Kartar Singh Committee:** Recommended multi-purpose worker scheme
- **Bhore Committee:** Health survey and development
- **Srivastava Committee**
  - Group on medical education and manpower.
  - Recommended bands of para-professionals and semi-professional health worker.
  - ROME (Reorientation of Medical Education) scheme.
  - Village Health Guide scheme.
  - 3-Tier rural health infrastructure
- Jungalwalla committee
  - Equal pay for equal work
  - No private practice

435. Ans. (b) 1000

Ref: K. Park, 23rd ed. pg. 449, 21st ed. pg. 407

- ASHA is Accredited Social Health Activist.
- One ASHA works for **1000 population.**
- In tribal, hilly and desert areas, the norm is one ASHA per habitation.

Impact Indicators of ASHA

- Infant mortality rate
- Child malnutrition rate
- Number of TB/leprosy case detection as compared to previous year.

Extra Mile

ASHA
- **ASHA** must be the resident of the village preferably in the **age group of 25–45 years**.
- Minimum **education** required for ASHA: **8TH pass**
- ASHA is selected by village panchayat/Gram Sabha
- ASHA comes under national Rural Health Mission (NRHM): 2005–2012
- Act as bridge between village and ANM (Auxiliary Nurse midwife)
- Training of ASHA is done by ANM and AWW for a **minimum duration of 23 days**.

Extra Mile

- One multi-purpose worker (MPW) is for: **5000 population**
- One village health guide (VHG) is for: **1000**
- One Anganwadi worker (AWW) is for: **400–800**

436. Ans. (c) Minimum class 4 passed

Ref: K. Park, 23rd ed. pg. 449-50, s 21st ed. pg. 407

- ***Minimum education required for ASHA: 8th pass***
- *Please refer to above explanation for more details.*

437. Ans. (d) Village

Ref: K. Park, 23rd ed. pg. 449-50

438. Ans. (a) Is a mental health worker

Ref: K. Park, 23rd ed. pg. 449-50

439. Ans. (c) Conduct 50% delivery

Ref: K. Park, 23rd ed. pg. 903-904

- The Female Health Workers are expected to provide comprehensive primary health care to the community.
- The range of services they are expected to provide under Multi purpose Health Worker (MPW) scheme is very wide and encompasses promotive, preventive and curative services including conducting around 50% of deliveries, *anemic mothers and other pregnancy related issues.*
- **Visit:** At least *one visit, once in two months* to each household in the area allotted.
- *Collection of blood samples are functions of MPW male.*
- Female health workers have no role in the process of chlorination or disinfection of water.

440. Ans (b) Renal disease

Ref: K. Park, 23rd ed. pg. 903, 196th pg. 754

- Renal disease cannot be picked up by a health worker unless it is responsible for alteration of the urine grossly.
- *Please refer to above explanation*

441. Ans. (c) Active malaria surveillance

Ref: K. Park, 23rd ed. pg. 903-904

442. Ans. (d) 75 grams

Ref: K. Park, 23rd ed. pg. 661, 20th 575

A Midday School Meal

Foodstuffs	g/day/child
• Cereals and millets	75
• Pulses	30
• Oils and fats	8
• Leafy vegetables	30
• Nonleafy vegetables	30

Principles of Mid Day Meal Programme

- The meal should be a *supplement and not a substitute to the home diet*
- The meal should supply at least **one-third of the total energy** requirement, and **half of the protein** need
- The cost of the meal should be *reasonably low*
- The meal should be such that it can be prepared *easily in schools*; no complicated cooking process should be involved.
- As far as possible, *locally available foods should be used*; this will reduce the cost of the meal, and the menu should be frequently changed to avoid monotony.

443. Ans. (b) 1/3 calories, 1/2 proteins

Ref: K. Park, 23rd ed. pg. 661-62

- Mid-day meal program is also known as National Program of Nutritional Support to primary education.
- The main advantage of this program is to influence more children towards schools in order to improve the literacy.
- This meal only act as a supplement and NOT as a substitute to home diet.
- *This meal should provide 1/3 of the total calories requirement and ½ of the total protein requirement.*

444. Ans. (b) 30

Ref: K. Park, 23rd ed. pg. 399-400

- BMI is Body Mass Index, aka Quetlet's Index.
- It is calculated as: BMI = weight (kg)/height $(m)^2$

Classification	BMI
Underweight	<18.5
Normal BMI	18.5–24.99
Overweight/pre-obese	25–29.99
Obesity • Grade I • Grade II • Grade III	>30.0 • 30–34.99 • 35–39.99 • ≥40

445. Ans. (a) (Weight in kg/Height in meters^2)

Ref: K. Park, 23rd ed. pg. 399-400

446. Ans. (b) Birth injuries

Ref: K. Park, 23rd ed. pg. 564

- **Most common cause of neonatal mortality in India** is preterm birth.
- A preterm child is more likely to be low birth weight and premature, which contribute to neonatal mortality rate.
- Death due to Birth injuries are there, but it is relatively very less as compared to prematurity, low birth weight and asphyxia.

447. Ans. (c) 6

Ref: K. Park, 23rd ed. pg. 590,661, 21st ed. pg. 545, 611

- **ICDS** is Integrated Child Development Services which was started in 1975.
- This program include a strong supplementary nutrition component in form of Vitamin A prophylaxis and iron & folic acid distribution.
- The workers at village level who deliver the services are called *Anganwadi workers.*

Beneficiaries of ICDS

- Preschool children below 6 years.
- Adolescent girls 11 to 18 years old.
- Pregnant and lactating mothers.
- 15–49 years reproductive age women

448. Ans. (b) 1991

Ref: K. Park, 23rd ed. pg. 540-41

- The **Baby Friendly Hospital Initiative (BFHI,** is programme of the World Health Organization and UNICEF.
- *Main goal of this initiative is to improve infant and young child nutrition by promoting breast feeding.*
- This includes helping the mother *initiate breast-feeding within the **first hour** of birth in normal delivery* and 4 hours following caesarean section
- It also aims at improving the care of pregnant women, mothers and newborns at health facilities that provide

maternity services for protecting, promoting and supporting breastfeeding.
- No advertisement promotional material or free products for infant feeding should be allowed in the facility.

449. Ans. (d) Infants are kept in the nursery for first 24 hours

Ref: K. Park, 23rd ed. pg. 540-541

450. Ans. (a) Panchayat samiti

Ref: K. Park, 23rd ed. pg. 881-82

- **Panchayat Samiti** is a local government body at the tahsil level in India. It works for the villages of the tahsil that together are called a **Development Block**.
- The Panchayat Samiti is the link between the Gram Panchayat and the zila parishad.

Note:
- ***Gram Sabha** has been envisaged as the foundation of the Panchayati Raj system. A village having population not less than 1500 forms Gram Sabha and every adult of the village is member of Gram Sabha. These members of gram sabha can elect members of gram panchayat.*

451. Ans (b) 100 villages and 1,00,000 population

Ref: Park's PSM, 20 pg. 783, 784

"Under the community development programme, the rural areas of the country have been organized into Community Development Blocks —each Block comprising approximately **100 villages and a population of one lakh.**"

OCCUPATIONAL HEALTH

452. Ans. (d) Handicap

Ref: Park Textbook of Preventive and Social Medicine, 25th ed. pg. 50

As the person is not able to fulfill his role in the society, he will be considered as handicap.
- **Impairment** – any loss or abnormality of psychological, physiological or anatomical structure or function.
- **Disability** – any restriction or lack of ability to perform an activity in the manner or within the range considered normal for a human being.
- **Handicap** – the result when an individual with impairment cannot fulfill a normal life role.

453. Ans. (b) Minus type desk

Ref: Park, 25th ed. pg. 634

Healthful School Environment

- **Location:** The school should normally be centrally situated with proper approach roads and at a fair distance from busy places and roads, cinema houses, factories, railway tracks and market places. The school premises should be properly fenced and kept free from all hazards.
- **Site:** The site should be on suitable high land, and not subject to inundation or dampness and can be properly drained. The School Health Committee (1961) had recommended that 10 acres of land be provided for higher elementary schools and 5 acres for primary schools with an additional one acre of land per 100 students. In congested areas, the nearest public park or playground should be made available to the students.
- **Structure:** Nursery and secondary schools, as far as possible, be single storied. Exterior walls should have a minimum thickness of 10 inches and should be heat resistant.
- **Classroom:** Verandahs should be attached to classrooms. No classroom should accommodate more than 40 students. Per capita space for students in a classroom should not be less than 10 sq. ft.
- **Furniture:** Furniture should suit the age group of students. It is desirable to provide single desks and chairs. **Desks should be of "minus" type.** Chairs should be provided with proper back-rests, with facilities for desk-work.
- **Doors and windows:** The windows should be broad with the bottom sill, at a height of 2'–6" from the floor level; combined door and window area should be at least 25 per cent of the floor space; windows should be placed on different walls for cross-ventilation; the ventilators should not be less than 2 per cent of the floor area.
- **Color:** Inside color of the classroom should be white and should be periodically white-washed.
- **Lighting:** Classrooms should have sufficient natural light, preferably from the left, and **should not be from the front.**
- **Water supply:** There should be an independent source of safe and potable water supply, which should be continuous, and distributed from the taps.
- **Eating facilities:** Vendors other than those approved by the school authorities should not be allowed inside school premises; there should be a separate room provided for mid-day meals.
- **Lavatory:** Privies and urinals should be provided - one urinal for 60 students and one latrine for 100 students. Arrangements should be separately made for boys and girls.

454. Ans. (b) Aflatoxin

Ref: Park, 25th ed. pg. 713

- Aflatoxin, a food contaminant produced by the fungi *Aspergillus flavus* and *Aspergillus parasiticus*, is a known human carcinogen and hepatotoxic that has been shown to be a causative agent in the pathogenesis of hepatocellular carcinoma

455. Ans. (d) TB screening should be done at regular intervals

Ref: Park, 25th ed. pg. 221

People who are at increased risk of TB because of biological and behavioral factors that compromise immune system:

- Live with HIV
- Have diabetes or silicosis
- Undergoing immunosuppressive therapy
- Undernourished
- Use tobacco
- Suffer from alcohol-use disorders
- Inject drugs.

456. Ans. (c) Coal dust

Ref: K. Park, 25th ed. pg. 843

List of Pneumoconiosis

- Silicosis – silicon dust
- Anthracosis – Coal dust
- Asbestosis – Asbestosis dust
- Byssinosis – Cotton fibre
- Bagassosis – Molasses (sugarcane)
- Farmers lung – Mould hay

457. Ans. (a) CO_2, ozone, methane

Ref: Inventory of US greenhouse gas emissions and sinks, 1990-1994 By United States Environmental Protection Agency

- A **greenhouse gas** is a gas in an atmosphere that absorbs and emits radiation within the thermal infrared range. This process is the fundamental cause of the greenhouse effect.
- **The primary greenhouse gases in Earth's atmosphere** are **water vapor, carbon dioxide, methane, nitrous oxide,** and **ozone (O_3).**
- Chlorofluorocarbons (CFCs), Hydrofluorocarbons (HFCs) and other compounds such as perfluorinated carbons are also green house gases.
- Without greenhouse gases, the average temperature of Earth's surface would be about –18°C (0°F), rather than present average of 15°C (59°F).

458. Ans. (b) 5 Rad per person per year

Ref: K. Park, 23rd ed. pg. 804

- Maximum permissible radiation exposure for general population: 5 Rad (0.5 Rem) per person per year.
- Maximum permissible radiation exposure for workers: 50 Rad (5 Rem) per person per year.
- Greatest source of radiation outside house: Extra-terrsetrial cosmic rays.
- Greatest source of radiation inside house: TV
- Greatest man-made source of radiation: X-ray

Extra Mile

- *Permissible sound level in hospital wards: 20–35 decibel.*
- *Maximum tolerable sound level: <85 decibel*
- *Permanent hearing loss at: >100 decibel*
- *Tympanic membrane ruptures at: 150–160 decibel.*

459. Ans (a) 20–35

Ref: K. Park, 23rd ed. pg. 741-42, 19th pg. 599

Acceptable noise levels (dBA)		
Residential:	Bed room Living room	25 40
Commercial:	Office Conference Restaurants	35–45 40–45 40–60
Industrial:	Workshop Laboratory	40–60 40–50
Educational:	Class room Library	30–40 35–40
Hospitals:	**Wards**	**20–35**

460. Ans. (a) Lung cancer

Ref: K. Park, 23rd ed. pg. 807

- Asbestosis occurs due to long duration (>10 years) exposure to asbestos.
- This may lead to pulmonary fibrosis, carcinoma of bronchus, mesothelioma of pleura/peritoneum and GIT cancer.

Other Important Occupational Cancer

Agent	Associated cancer
Asbestosis	Mesothelioma
Arsenic	Skin, lung, liver CA
Benzene	Leukemia
Benzidine	Bladder CA
Silica	Lung CA
Wood dust	Nasal sinus

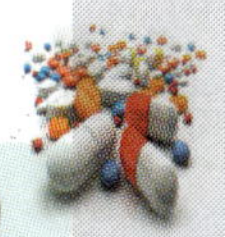

- *Most common occupational cancer: Skin CA (75%), mainly squamous cell CA.*

461. Ans. (c) Asbestosis

Ref: K. Park, 23rd ed. pg. 807

- Pneumoconiosis occurs due to occupational exposure to dust.
- Dust particle of size 0.5–3 microns are most dangerous, as they can reach the interior of lungs easily.
- Most common pneumoconiosis associated with Mesothelioma and lung cancer: **Asbestosis**.
- Most common pneumoconiosis: **Silicosis**

TABLE: Other important pneumoconiosis to remember

Disease	Exposure source
• Silicosis	Silica dust
• Anthracosis	Coal dust
• Asbestosis	Asbestos dust
• Bagassosis	Sugarcane dust (*thermoactinomyces sacchari*)
• Byssinossis	Cotton fibre
• Siderosis	Iron dust

462. Ans. (c) Sugarcane dust

Ref: K. Park, 23rd ed. pg. 807

463. Ans. (d) Can cause Blue Line on gums

Ref: K. Park, 23rd ed. pg. 807-808

- Lead poisoning is known as Plumbism.
- This is most commonly seen among painters, therefore also known as Painter's colic.
- *Most common source of lead poisoning: Petrol*
- Most common mode of lead poisoning: Inhalation

Clinical Finding of lead poisoning:

- *Burtonian line: Blue line on gums*
- Facial pallor: First and most consistent sign (always present).
- Lead colic: Constipation/diarrhea
- Wrist drop/foot drop
- Encephalopathy

Investigation of Pb Poisoning:

- CPU: Coproporphyrin in Urine is a useful *screening test- > **150: exposure to lead***
- Amino Levulinic Acid (ALAU), lead levels in blood and urine: *Diagnostic test.*
- Upon PBS, ***basophilic stippling of RBC's*** and *Microcytic Hypochromic anemia* seen.
- DOC for Pb poisoning: **EDTA**

464. Ans. (b) Insomnia

Ref: K. Park, 23rd ed. pg. 807-808

- Insomnia is caused by organic lead poisoning.
- Organic lead poisoning causes CNS side effects while Inorganic lead poisoning causes non-CNS side effects.

Due to organic lead (CNS effects)	Due to inorganic lead (Non-CNS effects)
• Insomnia • Mental confusion • Headache • Delirium	• Facial pallor: *earliest and most consistent sign.* • Anemia: Microcytic Hypochromic • RBC's stippling • Burtonian Line on upper gums • Lead Colic: constipation *(or copper)* • Lead Palsy (wrist + foot drop)

465. Ans. (d) Inorganic lead

Ref: K. Park, 23rd ed. pg. 807-808

Please refer to above explanation

466. Ans. (c) Maternity benefit for 3 months

Ref: K. Park, 23rd ed. pg. 8015-16

- ESI (The Employees State Insurance) Act 1948 covers the social security and health insurance in India.
- ESI NOT applicable on: *(MERD)*
  - Mines
  - *Education*
  - Railways
  - Defence
- *The employer contributes 4.75% and employee contributes 1.75 % of total wage bill.*
- *It covers all employees getting wages upto 15,000 per month.*
- *Maternity benefit for a duration of 12 weeks (3 months).*
- Sickness benefits payable upto 91 days and extended sickness benefit payable for upto 2 years.

467. Ans. (c) System analysis

Ref: K. Park, 23rd ed. pg. 872

- **Cost effective analysis** is a management technique where benefits are stated in terms of results achieved. Eg: No. of life saved.
- **Cost benefit analysis** is a management technique where benefits are stated in terms of money.
- **System analysis** is a management technique of ***finding out the cost effectiveness*** of the available alternatives.
- **Network analysis** is the graphic plan of all events and activities to be completed in order to reach an end objective. 2 types of network analysis technique:
  - **PERT** (Programme Evaluation and Review Technique): Arrow diagram representation of event.
  - **CPM** (Critical Path Method): The longest path.

468. Ans. (a) Time

Ref: K. Park, 23rd ed. pg. 872

- **Network analysis** is the graphic plan of all events and activities to be completed in order to reach an end objective. 2 types of network analysis technique:
  - **PERT** *(Programme Evaluation and Review Technique):* An arrow diagram representing the logical sequence in which events must take place. It aids in planning scheduling and monitoring the project.
  - **CPM** *(Critical Path Method):* The longest path of the network. If any activity in the critical path is delayed, entire project will be delayed.

469. Ans. (b) 29–31°C

DISINFECTION AND MISCELLANEOUS

470. Ans. (c) 1% sodium hypochlorite

- Blood spills are disinfected using 1% sodium hypochlorite
- Hypochlorites are the most widely used chlorine disinfectant, available as:
  - Solid: Sodium hypochlorite
  - Liquid: Calcium hypochlorite
- House bleach is the most prevalent chlorine products, which is an aqueous solution of 5.25-6.15% of sodium hypochlorite

Extra Mile

- **Cresol:** It is an excellent coal-tar disinfectant. 3–10 times more powerful than phenol

471. Ans. (b) Glutaraldehyde

Ref: K. Park, 25th ed. pg. 136-38

- Among the given options glutaraldehyde has maximum disinfectant property.
- Glutaraldehyde is used for sterilization of:
  - Endoscopes and bronchoscope
  - Metal instruments
  - Corrugated rubber anaestetic tubes
  - Mask
- A solution of 2% glutaraldehyde (cidex) required immersion of 20 minutes for disinfection and 6 to 10 hours for sterilization.

472. Ans. (a) Red

Ref: K. Park, 25th ed. pg. 830

- Wastes generated from disposable items such as tubing, bottles, intravenous tubes and sets, catheters, urine bags, syringes (without needles and fixed needle syringes) and vaccutainers with their needles cut) and gloves are disposed in Red colored non-chlorinated plastic bags or containers.

473. And. (c) To reduce greenhouse gas emission

Ref: K. Park, 25th ed. pg. 771-774

Kyoto Protocol

- This protocol has been started on 16th Feb 2005
- Targeted reductions in transmissions of Greenhouse gases such as Carbondioxide, Methane, Nitrous oxide, Sulphurhexafluoride, Perfluorocarbons, Chlorofluoro-carbons.

474. Ans. (c) Contamination

Ref: K. Park, 25th ed. pg. 98

Contamination

The presence of an infectious agent

- On a body surface
- On or in clothes, beddings, toys, etc.
- On or in surgical instruments or dressings, or other inanimate articles or
- In substances like water, milk and food.

475. Ans. (c) Biomedical waste converted into harmless

Ref: K. Park 25th ed. pg. 851

- Inertization is a method of disposal of biomedical waste.
- It involves mixing the waste with cement or other substances before disposal, in order to minimize the risk of toxic substances contained in the wastes migrating into the surface water or ground water.

Extra Mile

- **Incineration:** It is high temperature dry oxidation process, that reduces organic and combustible waste into inorganic incombustible matter and results in a very significant reduction of waste- volume and weight

476. Ans. (d) Hypochlorous acid

Ref: K. Park, 23rd ed. pg. 714-15

CHLORINATION OF WATER

- **Disinfecting action of chlorine in water is mainly due to hypochlorous acid (HOCl).**
- Hypochlorite ions has minor role in disinfection.
- Compared to UV rays or ozone, only Chlorine has residual germicidal effect.

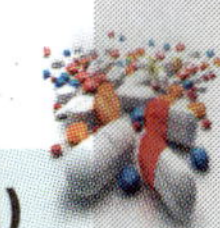

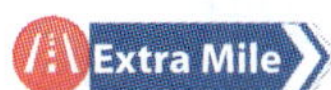

Extra Mile

- **Chlorine has no effect on:**
  - Bacterial spores, protozoal cysts and helminthic ova
  - Viral agents of Hepatitis A, Polio are also resistant at normal doses.
- **Horrock's apparatus:** Cl_2 demand (to measure Cl_2 required for water disinfection)

477. Ans (c) Ortho toluidine test

Ref: K. Park, 23rd ed. pg. 715, 19th pg. 578

- **Orthotolidine arsenite test** - used for testing residual chlorine at the end of **one hour contact.**
- If the "free" residual chlorine level is less than 0.5 mg/litre, the chlorination procedure should be repeated before any water is drawn.
- Wells are best **disinfected at night** after the day's draw off.
- During epidemics of cholera, wells should be disinfected every day

Extra Mile

- **Horrock's Apparatus** is used for **estimating the chlorine demand of the well water** and calculate the amount of bleaching powder required to disinfect the well.
- Roughly, **2.5 grams of good quality bleaching powder** would be required to disinfect **1,000 litres** of water. Bleaching powder contains **33% available chlorine**
- The **hypochlorous acid** is the most effective form of chlorine for **water disinfection.**
- Chlorine acts best as a disinfectant when the **pH of water is around 7.**
- The **standard prescribed** for chloride is **200 mg/L**
- **The maximum permissible level is 600 mg/L**

478. Ans. (b) Alum is added after lime

Ref: K. Park, 23rd ed. pg. 714-15

- Nalgonda Technique is utilized for defluorination of water.
- Sequence of components added for defluorination is: *(LAB)*
  - Lime
  - Alum
  - Bleaching powder

479. Ans. (d) Natural selection is a process where harmful genes are not eliminated from the gene pool and genes favorable to individual are not passed onto offspring.

According to Hardy Weinberg law genes are passed on to the offsprings in a gene pool.

480. Ans. (d) Mixed cohort

481. Ans. (d) Repeated measurement

BIOSTATISTICS

482. Ans. (b) Median

Ref: Park Textbook of Preventive and Social Medicine, 25th ed. pg. 910

- For distributions that have outliers or are skewed, the median is often the preferred measure of central tendency.

483. Ans. (a) Pie chart

Ref: K. Park 25th ed. pg. 909

- Charts and diagrams are useful methods of presenting simple statistical data. They create a powerful impact on the imagination of people.
- In pie charts areas of a circle are compared. The area of each segment depends upon the angle.
- Pie charts are extremely popular with the ordinary people, but not with experts and professionals who consider them inferior to bar charts.

484. Ans. (a) 68.3%

485. Ans. (c) Poisson's distribution

Ref: K. Park 25th ed. pg. 912

- The normal distribution or "normal curve" is an important concept in statistical theory
- In probability theory and statistics, the **Poisson distribution** is a discrete probability distribution that expresses the probability of a given number of events occurring in a fixed interval of time or space if these events occur with a known constant mean rate and independently of the time since the last event

486. Ans. (b) Range

Ref: K. Park 25th ed. pg. 911

- The range is far the simplest measure of dispersion. It is defined as the difference between the highest and lowest figures in a given sample.

487. Ans. (b) Histogram

Ref: Park, 25th ed. pg. 908

- A histogram is a graphical representation that organizes a group of data points into user-specified ranges. It is similar in appearance to a bar graph.

- The histogram condenses a data series into an easily interpreted visual by taking many data points and grouping them into logical ranges or bins.

488. Ans. (b) Chi square test

Ref: Park, 25th ed. pg. 915

- Chi-square (X^2) Test offers an alternate method of testing the significance of difference between two proportions.
- It has the advantage that it can also be used when more than two groups are to be compared. For example, a research group is interested in whether or not the yoga and risk of certain infection are related for a population.

489. Ans. (a) Line diagram

Ref: Park, 25th ed. pg. 909

- The secular trend describes the occurrence of disease over a prolonged period, usually years. So, line graph is best for presentation of secular trend of a disease as line diagrams are used to show the trend of events with the passage of time.

490. Ans. (b) 20

Ref: K. Park, 25th ed. pg. 600

- Neonatal mortality rate (NNMR): Number of neonatal deaths per 1000 live births in that year.
- **Neonatal period:** The first 4 weeks of a child's life (after birth)

Neonatal mortality rate =

$$\frac{\textit{(total neonatal death in a given year)}}{\textit{(total number of live births in same years)}} \times 1000$$

$$\text{Neonatal mortality rate} = \frac{80}{4000} \times 1000$$

Neonatal mortality rate = 20

491. Ans. (b) 138

Ref: K. Park, 25th ed. pg. 559

- Birth rate = 25/1000 population
- Population under the sub-center = 5000
- Therefore, expected number of live births = (25 × 5000)/1000 = 125 births
- Correction factor (pregnancy wastage) = 10% of 125 = say 13
- Therefore, total no. of expected pregnancies in a year = 125 + 13 = 138

492. Ans. (a) Mean

Ref: K. Park, 25th ed. pg. 884

- Mean is a measure of central tendency.
- Mean (Average): is obtained as sum of all values divided by the no. of values.
- Formula for mean =

$$\overline{X} = \frac{X_1 + X_2 + X_3 \ldots X_N}{N}$$

Where
$\overline{X}$ = the mean
X_1 = the first value
X_2 = the second value
X_3 = the third value
X_N = the last value
N = the number of values

493. Ans. (b) Every 6 months

Ref: K. Park 23rd ed. pg. 841

Sample Registration System (SRS)

Since civil registration is deficient in India, a Sample Registration System (SRS) was initiated in the mid-1960s to provide reliable estimates of birth and death rates at the National and State levels. The SRS is a dual-record system, consisting of continuous enumeration of births and deaths by an enumerator and an independent survey every 6 months by an investigator-supervisor. The half-yearly survey, in addition to serving as an independent check on the events recorded by the enumerator, produces the denominator required for computing rates.

The SRS now covers the entire country. It is a major source of health information.

494. Ans. (a) Histogram

Ref: K. Park 23rd ed. pg. 845

Histogram

It is a pictorial diagram of frequency distribution. It consists of a series of blocks (Figure). The class intervals are given along the horizontal axis and the frequencies along the vertical axis. The area of each block or rectangle is proportional to the frequency. The figure is the histogram of the frequency distribution of blood pressure in females 45–64 years.

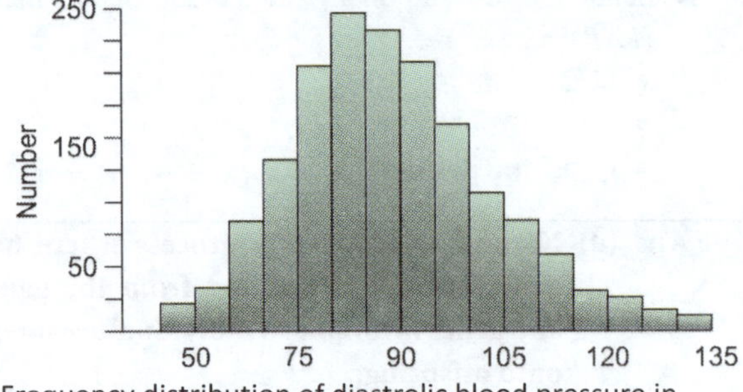

Frequency distribution of diastrolic blood pressure in females aged 45–64 years

495. Ans. (b) 8.4

Ref: K. Park, 23rd ed. pg. 65

- An odds ratio (OR) is a measure of association between an exposure and an outcome. The OR represents the odds that an outcome will occur given a particular exposure, compared to the odds of the outcome occurring in the absence of that exposure.
- $OR = \frac{a \times d}{b \times c} = \frac{33 \times 27}{53 \times 2} = \mathbf{8.4}$

496. Ans. (c) TP/TP + FN × 100

Sensitivity: Defined as ability of a screening test to identify all those who have disease (cases/True positive)

$$\text{Sensitivity} = \frac{a}{(a + c)} \times 100 \quad = \frac{TP}{(TP + FN)} \times 100$$

497. Ans. (d) 99

	Pregnant	Non-Pregnant
Positive test	99	10
Negative test	1	90

$$\text{Sensitivity} = \frac{a}{(a + c)} \times 100 \quad = \frac{99}{99 + 1} \times 100 = \mathbf{99}$$

498. Ans. (b) 2.5

Ref: K. Park, 23rd ed. pg. 78

- RR = incidence of disease among exposed/ Incidence of disease among non-exposed

	Disease (+)	Disease (–)	Total
Exposed	50	350	400
Non- exposed	5	95	100

- Putting the value in formula = 50/400 ÷ 5/100
 = 50/400 × 100/5
 = 2.5

499. Ans. (a) 0.00

Ref: K. Park, 23rd ed. pg. 848

- Standard deviation is the deviation from the mean value.
- 10 babies were born, each weighs 2.7 kg, which gives a mean value of 2.7, indicating there is no deviation from the mean value.
- Hence the answer will be 0 (zero)
- *Standard deviation is also known as root mean square deviation.*

500. Ans. (c) Used to test significance of association between two quantitative data

Ref: K. Park, 23rd ed. pg. 852

- Chi-square test is used to test significance of association between two *QUALITATIVE* data.
- It is used for non-Gaussian distribution.
- This test is a non-parametric test of significance.
- Degree of freedom used in chi- square test is calculated by (c-1) (r-1)

501. Ans. (c) 12

Ref: K. Park, 23rd ed. pg. 852

- **Degree of freedom:** It is the no. of observations in a dataset that can freely vary once the parameters have been estimated.
- It is used in *chi-square test and t-test.*
- ***DOF***: *(c-1) (r-1), where c is no. of columns and r is no. of rows.*
- In the given question there are 4 columns and 5 rows.
- Therefore (4-1) (5-1) gives **12.**

502. Ans. (d) Wrong calculation

Ref: K. Park, 23rd ed. pg. 852-53

- Correlation coefficient (r) is used to find out if there is any significant relationship between two variables (e.g.: x and y) or not.
- Correlation coefficient (r) tends to lie between –1.0 to +1.0 (-1 < r < +1)
  - *If r = + 1:* Strong positive association between two variables
  - *If r = 0:* No association between two variables
  - *If r = –1:* Strong negative association

503. Ans. (a) Mean

Ref: K. Park, 23rd ed. pg. 847-88

- Best measure of central tendency: **MEAN**
- Best measure of central tendency for NOMINAL data: **MODE**
- Best measure of central tendency for ORDINAL data: **MEDIAN**
- Best measure of central tendency foe metric/quantitative data: **MEAN**

504. Ans. (d) Mode

Ref: K. Park, 23rd ed. pg. 847-88

THE MODE

- The mode is the commonly occurring value in a distribution of data. It is the most frequent item or the most fashiionable" value in a series of observations. For example, the diastolic blood pressure of 20 individuals was:

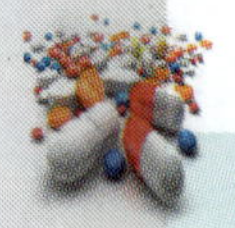

85, 75 79, 71, 95, 75, 75, 77, 75, 90
71, 75, 79, 95, 75, 77, 84, 75, 81, 75

- The mode or the most frequently occurring value is 75.

505. Ans. (b) 16, 10, 10

Ref: K. Park, 23rd ed. pg. 847-88

- Patient is smoker from last 6 years.
- In the first year 5 sticks per day; in the 2nd, 3rd and 4th year it is 10 sticks per day; in 5th year 20 sticks per day and in 6th year 40 sticks per day.

Therefore, mean = $\frac{5 + 10 + 10 + 10 + 20 + 40}{6}$

= 15.83, which is rounded as **16**

- Median is middle value in ascending order. Since, it has two middle value,

$\frac{10 + 10}{2} = \mathbf{10}$

- Mode is most repeated/frequent value, which is 10, repeated 3 times.
- *Therefore the mean, median and mode will be 16, 10, 10 respectively.*

506. Ans. (b) 5 and 4

Ref: Park, 22nd ed. pg. 789-90

Mean = $\Sigma\frac{X}{n}$

Therefore, mean =

$\frac{2 + 2 + 3 + 4 + 4 + 4 + 4 + 5 + 5 + 7 + 8 + 8 + 9}{13}$ = 65/13

Mean = 5

- Mode is most repeated/frequent value, which is 4, repeated 4 times.
- *Therefore the mean, mode will be 5 and 4 respectively.*

COMMUNICATION FOR HEALTH EDUCATION

507. Ans. (a) Panel discussion

Ref: Park Textbook of Preventive and Social Medicine, 25th ed. pg. 928

- A panel discussion is a specific format used in a meeting, conference, or convention. It is a live, in-person or virtual discussion about a specific topic amongst a selected group of experts who share differing perspectives in front of an audience.
- The main purpose of a panel discussion is for the panelists to share their wisdom and provide insights to create real value and takeaways for the audience.

508. Ans. (c) Demonstration

Ref: K. Park 25th ed. pg. 247

- According to WHO, Oral Rehydration Therapy can be safely and successfully used in treating acute diarrheal diseases due to all etiologies, in all age groups, and in all countries.
- The aim of oral fluid therapy is to prevent dehydration and reduce mortality.
- Mothers should be **demonstrated** how to administer ORS solution to their children. It is best for a demonstration to be given by a nurse or by a health worker.

509. Ans. (c) 6–12

Ref: K. Park 25th ed. pg. 927

- A group is an aggregation of people interacting in a face-to-face situation.
- For effective group discussion, the group should comprise not less than 6 and not more than 12 members.
- The participants are all seated in a circle, so that each is fully visible to all the others.

MEDICINE

9

MOST RECENT QUESTIONS 2023

1. A 33-year-old woman is being evaluated for excessive daytime sleepiness and forgetfulness which have been present for the past 1 year. She has a short neck and her BMI is 43, her BP is 170/98 mm Hg. In an awake state, ABG shows pO_2 70 mm Hg, pCO_2 53 mm Hg, HCO_3 33 mmol/L. What is the most likely diagnosis?

(Most Recent Question July 2023)

a. Obesity hypoventilation syndrome
b. Central sleep apnea
c. Narcolepsy
d. Obstructive sleep apnea

2. All of the following will show hypokalemia; except:

(Most Recent Question July 2023)

a. RTA 1
b. RTA 2
c. RTA 4
d. Ureterosigmoidostomy

3. A 10-year-old child is brought with a 2-week history of not feeding well and excessive irritability. On examination, neck stiffness is present. His sister has taken treatment for pulmonary TB. In work-up, LP was performed. Which of the following is likely to be found in CSF?

(Most Recent Question July 2023)

a. Lymphocytosis, low sugar and high protein
b. Lymphocytosis, high sugar and high protein
c. Neutrophils, low sugar and low protein
d. Neutrophils, low sugar and high protein

4. A 50-year-old patient with lung cancer presents with breathlessness and light headedness. On lung auscultation bronchial breath sounds are heard on the left infero-scapular region along with focal area of dullness. Diagnosis is?

(Most Recent Question July 2023)

a. Cardiac Tamponade
b. Pleural effusion
c. Constrictive pericarditis
d. Pneumothorax

5. A 50-year-old patient diagnosed with pneumonia develops increasing breathlessness. Percussion note is stony dull in left infra-axillary and inframammary and infra scapular areas. On lung auscultation, reduced intensity of breath sounds are heard in the same areas mentioned above. Diagnosis is:

(Most Recent Question July 2023)

a. Cardiac tamponade
b. Pleural effusion
c. Pneumothorax
d. Pneumomediastinum

6. $ABCD_2$ scoring includes all of the following parameters; except: *(Most Recent Question July 2023)*

a. Age
b. Hypertension
c. History of stroke
d. Diabetes mellitus

7. A 60-year-old man presents with sudden onset right-sided hemiparesis for the last 3 hours. BP is 200/100 mm Hg. NCCT head is shown as follows. All of the following are to be done for management; except:

(Most Recent Question July 2023)

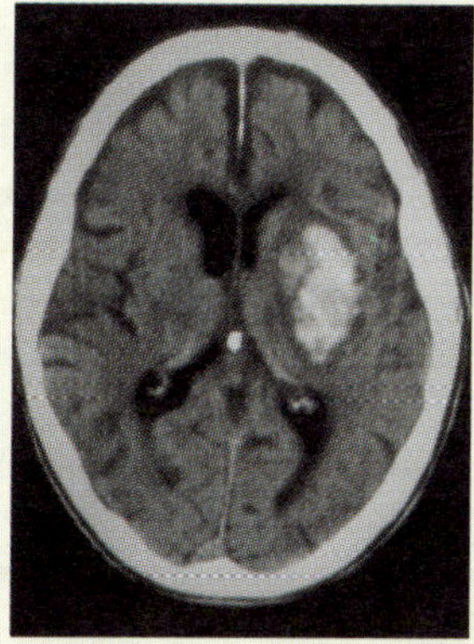

a. Thrombolysis
b. BP control
c. Edema management
d. Elective Hyperventilation

8. A 60-year-old patient is diagnosed with acute ischemic stroke and advised thrombolysis with alteplase. The weight of the patient is 80 kg. How much dose (in mg) should be given stat? *(Most Recent Question July 2023)*

a. 8
b. 10
c. 12
d. 15

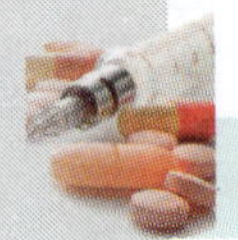

9. A 50-year-old man presents with involuntary hand movements along with development of cognitive and emotional problems. Which of the following medical disorders is the likely diagnosis?

(Most Recent Question July 2023)

a. Parkinsonism b. Friedreich ataxia
c. Alzheimer's disease d. Huntington Chorea

10. Which of the following JVP findings is expected to be seen in a patient with muffled heart sounds, hypotension and raised JVP? ***(Most Recent Question July 2023)***

a. Absent x descent b. Absent y descent
c. C waves are enlarged d. A waves are absent

11. A 65-year-old man is brought to the hospital with complaints of suddenly not making any sense while speaking, and using nonsensical grammar, though he can speak quickly. He could communicate effectively prior to this. Which of the following defect is present in this patient? ***(Most Recent Question July 2023)***

a. Motor aphasia b. Anomic aphasia
c. Fluent aphasia d. Conduction aphasia

12. Scissoring gait will occur due to increased firing in which of the following nerve? ***(Most Recent Question July 2023)***

a. Superior Gluteal nerve
b. Inferior gluteal nerve
c. Obturator nerve
d. Femoral nerve

13. In a patient diagnosed with dialysis dementia which deposition is seen in cerebral cortex?

(Most Recent Question July 2023)

a. Amyloid beta-2 microglobulin
b. Amyloid beta macroglobulin
c. Amyloid transthyretin
d. Amyloid Beta

14. Antibody seen in acute inflammatory demyelinating polyneuropathy (AIDP) will belong to which class?

(Most Recent Question July 2023)

a. IgG b. IgM
c. IgE d. IgA

15. Which of the following is correct about Wolff-Parkinson-White (WPW) syndrome?

(Most Recent Question July 2023)

a. Short PJ interval
b. Broad QRS interval
c. Tall Tented T waves
d. Prolonged PR interval

16. A 40-year woman presents with difficulty in eating due to persistent dry mouth. She also has grittiness in eyes due to dry eyes. On examination, dental caries is noted with enlarged cervical lymph nodes. Possible diagnosis is: ***(Most Recent Question July 2023)***

a. MCTD b. Sarcoidosis
c. Sjogren Syndrome d. Wegener's Granulomatosis

17. A 70-year-old man presents with low back pain and progressive pallor. On work up, KFT is deranged, LFT is normal with normal level of albumin, but gamma globulins are disproportionately increased. X-ray spine shows multiple lytic lesions. Which of the following is the cell of origin of the diagnosis of this patient?

(Most Recent Question July 2023)

a. Lymphocyte b. Plasma cell
c. Histiocytes d. Monocytes

18. A patient had an RTA and is brought with bradycardia along with high BP. GCS is less than 8. Next step in management is: ***(Most Recent Question July 2023)***

a. Urgent CT head b. Intubate and IPPV
c. Thrombolysis d. IV Fluids

19. A patient presented with pedal edema, raised JVP till mandible and ascites. What is the most likely diagnosis?

(Most Recent Question July 2023)

a. Cardiac failure b. Renal failure
c. Liver failure d. Brain injury

20. Calcitonin is a marker of which malignancy?

(Most Recent Question July 2023)

a. Papillary thyroid cancer
b. Follicular thyroid cancer
c. Medullary thyroid cancer
d. Anaplastic thyroid cancer

21. A 60-year-old bedridden patient develops sudden onset breathlessness and chest pain. CTPA was done. Which noninvasive imaging modality will be useful to find the etiology of this presentation?

(Most Recent Question July 2023)

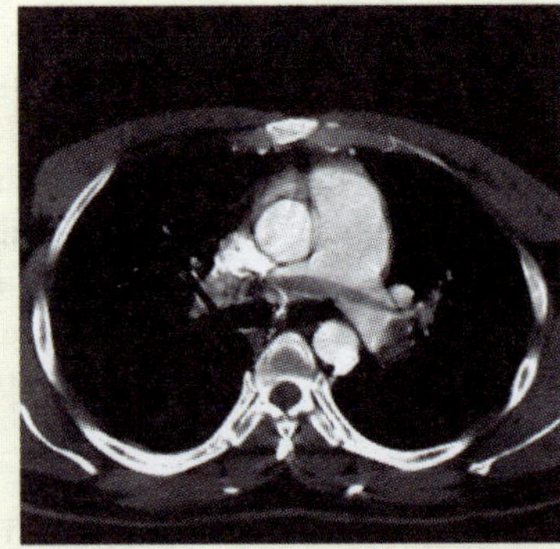

a. D dimer b. MRA
c. Coagulogram d. Ultrasound/Doppler

22. A 23-year-old patient presents with a history of fatigue and passage of smoky urine. On m/e, 20 dysmorphic RBC/HPF, 2-4 RBC/HPF and no bacteria are noted. Dipstick shows 2+ proteinuria. What is the most likely diagnosis? ***(Most Recent Question July 2023)***

a. Minimal change disease b. Acute glomerulonephritis
c. UTI d. Bladder calculi

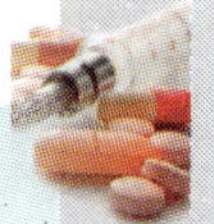

23. An elderly male patient with history of COPD, HTN and diabetes mellitus is on multiple drugs. Which of the following criteria are used to avoid use of certain drugs in these patients? *(Most Recent Question July 2023)*

a. Beers Criteria b. Duke's Criteria
c. Light Criteria d. Jones Criteria

24. Which of the following drugs is least useful in management of patients with Thalamic Dejerine Roussy syndrome? *(Most Recent Question July 2023)*

a. Analgesics b. TCA
c. Gabapentin d. Cannabinoids

25. Which of the following will help in making a definitive diagnosis of bronchial asthma? *(Most Recent Question July 2023)*

a. Only basis of patient history
b. FEV1 showing increment of more than 15% after giving a bronchodilator
c. Focal Wheezing sound
d. HRCT chest

26. A 20-year-old male who is an intravenous drug user presents with fever for the last one week (38.5°C). On work up, TLC is 20000/mm³, blood culture report is pending, and spots are noted on fundus examination. How many minor Duke criteria are satisfied for diagnosis of infective endocarditis? *(Most Recent Question July 2023)*

a. 0 b. 1
c. 2 d. 3

27. Reversibility of airflow obstruction in asthma is defined as FEV1 change pre and post bronchodilator to be: *(Most Recent Question July 2023)*

a. >10% b. >12%
c. >18% d. >20%

28. A 30-year-old female presents with recurrent episodes of epistaxis and perennial runny nose. She has been passing cola-color urine off and on. Recently for work up of hemoptysis, multiple cavitary lesions were noted in both lungs. Which of the following tests would help in confirming diagnosis of this condition? *(Most Recent Question July 2023)*

a. p-ANCA b. c-ANCA
c. Anti GBM d. dsDNA

29. A pregnant woman is having excessive bleeding after her delivery. Her husband says that she has had excessive bleeding earlier also after a dental extraction 5 years ago. No history of easy bruising or joint swelling is present. PT is normal with deranged aPTT and BT. Which of the following is correct about the diagnosis of this patient? *(Most Recent Question July 2023)*

a. Deficiency of factor 8 b. Deficiency of factor 9
c. Deficiency of factor 7 d. Deficiency of vWF

30. A 40 kg female patient admitted in hospital for past one week for alcoholism is currently having multiple episodes of seizures. On work up, serum sodium is 120 mEq/L. Calculate the total correction to be given to this patient. *(Most Recent Question July 2023)*

a. 100
b. 200
c. 300
d. 400

31. A 37-year-old woman presented with recurrent episodes of pain and pressure sensation behind her left eye. The orbital pain was associated with intermittent proptosis. The symptoms and signs worsened due to exercise and Valsalva maneuvers. Diagnosis is: *(Most Recent Question July 2023)*

a. Orbital varices
b. Orbital dermoid
c. Orbital metastasis
d. Caroticocavernous fistula

32. What can be given to eat in celiac sprue? *(Most Recent Question July 2023)*

a. Sooji/Semolina b. Oats
c. Poha/Pulao d. Wheat

33. An elderly patient presents with focal seizures. CT shows multiple-ring enhancing granulomas. Which of the following is not to be given immediately in the next 24 hours? *(Most Recent Question July 2023)*

a. Steroids b. Anti edema treatment
c. Seizure control d. Antihelminthic treatment

34. A patient is being taken to the hospital for anaphylaxis in a fully equipped ambulance after a honey-bee sting. Which of the following is correct about its management? *(Most Recent Question July 2023)*

a. Injection adrenaline IM 1:1000 dilution
b. Injection adrenaline IM 1:1000 dilution, repeat again if no response, till patient reaches hospital
c. Injection adrenaline IV 1:10,000 dilution
d. Urgent intubation to secure the airway

35. Giant v wave in JVP is seen in? *(Most Recent Question Jan 2023)*

a. Tricuspid regurgitation b Patent ductus arteriosus
c. Dilated Cardiomyopathy d. Aortic regurgitation

36. A 60-year-old man has been on bed rest for 10 days. He develops sudden onset breathlessness and chest pain. Which of the following is the best investigation? *(Most Recent Question Jan 2023)*

a. ECG
b. CT Pulmonary angiography
c. Echocardiography
d. D-Dimer assay

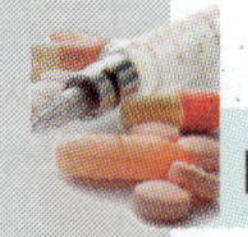

37. A child presents with fever for the last 14 days with neck rigidity. LP is done and it shows 75% mononuclear cells with CSF sugar = 50 mg (Blood sugar 100 mg/dL) and protein is 3000 mg/dL. CXR of patient shows upper lobe involvement with hilar lymph node enlargement. Diagnosis is: ***(Most Recent Question Jan 2023)***

a. Bacterial meningitis b. Viral meningitis
c. Fungal meningitis d. TB meningitis

38. A patient presents with distended neck veins that increase on inspiration. On further examination, regular pulse is noticed which tends to disappear on deep inspiration. There is no parasternal heave or murmur. S3 heart sound is present. Diagnosis is: ***(Most Recent Question Jan 2023)***

a. Tricuspid Stenosis
b. Aortic regurgitation
c. Constrictive pericarditis
d. Pulmonary artery hypertension due to COPD

39. A young patient develops a bout of acute dysentery. He subsequently develops bilateral ascending quadriplegia. Pain and proprioception sensation are preserved. First differential diagnosis is: ***(Most Recent Question Jan 2023)***

a. GBS b. Transverse myelitis
c. Polymyositis d. M. Gravis

40. A 6-year-old child presents with one-day history of high-grade fever, loss of consciousness, severe pallor and up-going plantar. Hypoglycemia was seen in lab work up. Diagnosis is: ***(Most Recent Question Jan 2023)***

a. TB meningitis b. Bacterial meningitis
c. Cerebral malaria d. Fungal meningitis

41. The most common cause of death in diabetic ketoacidosis is: ***(Most Recent Question Jan 2023)***

a. Dehydration
b. Cerebral edema
c. Hypokalemia
d. Sepsis

42. Which is not included in qSOFA score?

a. Serum lactate (>100 mmol/L)
b. RR (>22/min)
c. GCS score <15 (altered mental status)
d. SBP (<100 mm Hg)

43. Which of the following is least responsible for invasive hematogenous candidiasis? ***(Most Recent Question Jan 2023)***

a. Lower Limb Vascular Surgery
b. Indwelling urine catheter
c. Neutropenia
d. Prolonged steroid usage

44. Drug which decreases mortality in CHF is: ***(Most Recent Question Jan 2023)***

a. Metoprolol b. Furosemide
c. Prazocin d. Torsemide

45. Select the correct components of Child-Pugh score. ***(Most Recent Question Jan 2023)***

a. Encephalopathy, ascites, albumin, Bilirubin and PT
b. Encephalopathy, albumin, Bilirubin, Globulin and PT
c. Encephalopathy, albumin, SGOT, Bilirubin and aPTT
d. Encephalopathy, albumin, Bilirubin, Globulin and aPTT

46. A 70-year-old smoker presents with high-grade fever, cough and confusion with diarrhea. CXR shows bilateral infiltrates in both lower lung fields. On sputum gram stain, no organisms were detected. Na = 126 mEq/L, AST-62, ALT 56, RBS -112 mg/dL and serum Bilirubin 0.8 mg%. Which of the following organisms is responsible? ***(Most Recent Question Jan 2023)***

a. Streptococcus b. Legionella
c. Pneumocystis Jiroveci d. Klebsiella

47. Which of the following is the cause of exudative pleural effusion? ***(Most Recent Question Jan 2023)***

a. Cardiac failure b. Liver cirrhosis
c. Nephrotic syndrome d. Rheumatoid arthritis

48. A child has developed recurrent lung infections with thickened sputum and CXR shows bronchial wall thickening. He has been suffering from steatorrhea since birth. Which of the following is first differential diagnosis? ***(Most Recent Question Jan 2023)***

a. Cystic Fibrosis
b. Alpha 1 anti-trypsin deficiency
c. Hyaline membrane disease
d. Malabsorption syndrome

49. A 70-year-old man presents with right hip pain and back pain. Work up shows Hb = 8 g%, Serum calcium = 12 mg% and Serum creatinine = 2.5 mg/dL. Bone marrow biopsy shows 60% plasma cells. Diagnosis is:

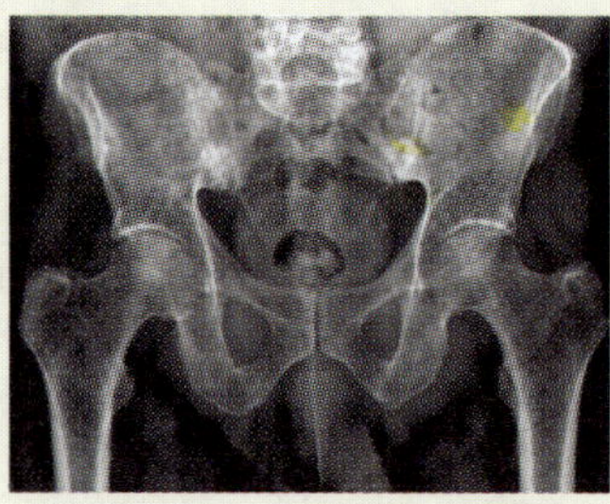

a. Multiple myeloma b. CML
c. AML d. ALL

50. A 20-year-old patient developed URTI infection and 10 days later presents with periorbital edema with RBC in urine and 800 mg protein/g of urinary creatinine. BP = 140/90 mm Hg and C3 levels are reduced. Anti-DNA-ase antibody is present. Diagnosis is:

a. Nephrotic syndrome b. Good pasture syndrome
c. Minimal change disease d. PSGN

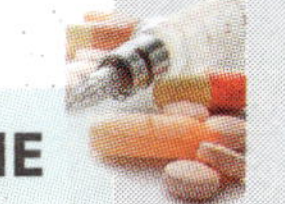

51. A female has difficulty in standing up from squatting position, cannot comb her hair and has violaceous heliotrope rash around upper eye lid. The presentation is of which of the following conditions?
(Most Recent Question Jan 2023)

a. Polymyositis
b. Dermatomyositis
c. SLE
d. Scleroderma

52. HIV positive patient presents with cryptococcal meningitis. Treatment is:
(Most Recent Question Jan 2023)

a. High dose Fluconazole
b. LAMB
c. High dose Fluconazole with flucytosine
d. Voriconazole

53. Which of the following tumor leads to hyperglycemia, necrolytic migratory erythema with depression?
(Most Recent Question Jan 2023)

a. Insulinoma
b. Glucagonoma
c. VIPoma
d. Somatostatinoma

54. Secretory diarrhea with hypokalemia and hypovolemia is commonly seen in which pancreatic tumor?
(Most Recent Question Jan 2023)

a. Insulinoma
b. Glucagonoma
c. VIPoma
d. Somatostatinoma

55. IOC for pancreatic neuroendocrine tumor is:
(Most Recent Question Jan 2023)

a. Gallium 68 Dotatate PET
b. MRI
c. Multi detector CT
d. Ultrasonogram

56. The most common cause of Cushing's syndrome in a 68-year-old male is: *(Most Recent Question Jan 2023)*

a. Ectopic ACTH production
b. Ectopic CRH production
c. Adrenal Carcinoma
d. Pituitary microadenoma

57. HRCT chest showing small nodules in upper lobes of lungs with ground glass appearance with thickened intralobular and interlobular septa is seen in which of the following occupational lung diseases?
(Most Recent Question Jan 2023)

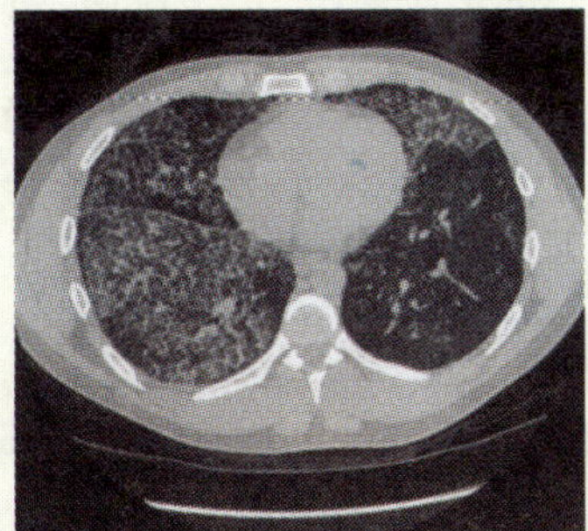

a. Silicosis
b. Anthracosis
c. Asbestosis
d. Bagassosis

58. A postmenopausal woman presents with knee pain. Joint aspiration was done and shows needle-shaped negatively birefringent crystals in polarized microscopy. The diagnosis is: *(Most Recent Question Jan 2023)*

a. Gout
b. Pseudo-gout
c. Osteoarthritis
d. Rheumatoid arthritis

59. Which is correct about cryptic TB?
(Most Recent Question Jan 2023)

a. Positive skin tuberculin test and positive CXR
b. Negative skin tuberculin test and normal CXR
c. Positive skin tuberculin test and normal CXR
d. Negative skin tuberculin test and positive CXR

60. Patient presents with hemoptysis and hematuria. Anti-GBM antibody is seen. Diagnosis is:
(Most Recent Question Jan 2023)

a. SLE
b. Goodpasture syndrome
c. FSGS
d. PAN

61. A 35-year-old young female has a sudden onset of severe headache which she describes as "Never ever had a headache as bad as this one". She is nonhypertensive but nondiabetic and has nuchal rigidity. Probable diagnosis is: *(Most Recent Question Jan 2023)*

a. SAH
b. Chronic migraine
c. Meningitis
d. Encephalitis

62. Which of the following is correct for management of the condition shown in CT chest?
(Most Recent Question Jan 2023)

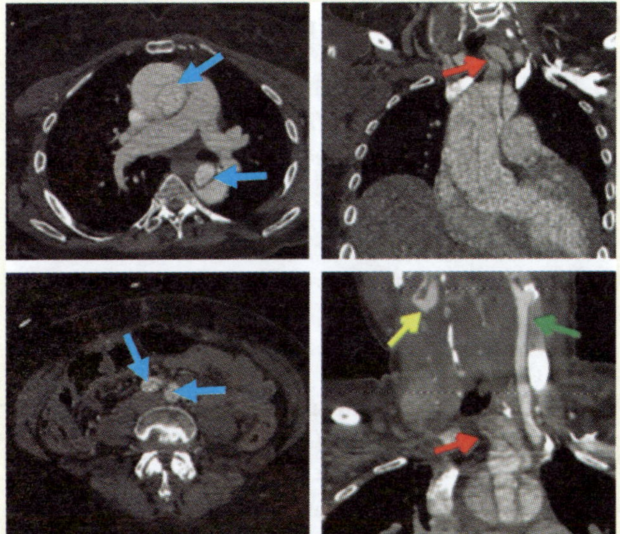

a. Control hypertension and immediate surgery
b. Wait and Watch
c. Perform MRI
d. IV NTG Drip

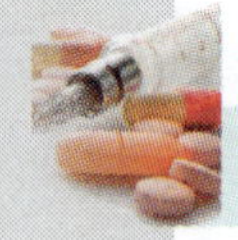

63. A 40-year-old man with 15-year history of smoking ten cigarettes per day presents with an episode of mild hemoptysis. Chest X-ray shows a 3 cm upper lobe mass near the pleura. Which is the next best step for management of this patient?

(Most Recent Question Jan 2023)

a. CT guided Biopsy b. Bronchoscopy
c. Sputum Cytology d. Sputum for AFB

64. Which of the following is a feature of Gaisbock syndrome? ***(Most Recent Question Jan 2023)***

a. Absolute leukocytosis
b. Relative/apparent erythrocytosis
c. Hypotension
d. Thrombocytosis

65. A female presents with history of taking OCP and headache for the last 6 months which worsens on recumbent position and improves as day progresses. Fundus examination shows papilledema. There is no focal neurological deficit. MRI shows raised ICP. What is the probable cause? ***(Most Recent Question Jan 2023)***

a. Pseudotumor cerebri b. Chronic migraine
c. Temporal arteritis d. M. Gravis

66. After recovery from COVID-19, a patient presents with tingling and numbness in finger. He admits to use of excess of multivitamin therapy during COVID-19 illness episode. Which of the following is the cause of this presentation? ***(Most Recent Question Jan 2023)***

a. Hypervitaminosis D b. Hypervitaminosis B6
c. Cobalamin toxicity d. Folic acid excess

67. A patient presents with ptosis, muscle weakness which increases at the end of day and gets relieved with Neostigmine. Diagnosis is:

(Most Recent Question Jan 2023)

a. Lambert Eaton syndrome
b. Myasthenia gravis
c. Duchenne muscular dystrophy
d. Amyotrophic lateral sclerosis

68. The most common cause of elective splenectomy is:

(Most Recent Question Jan 2023)

a. Acute ITP b. Hereditary spherocytosis
c. G6PD d. Hairy cell leukemia

69. Preferred management of acromegaly is:

(Most Recent Question Jan 2023)

a. Somatostatin analogue intravenous
b. Lanreotide Depot formulation
c. Terlipressin Nasal Spray
d. IV Octreotide

70. Which is a feature of hemolysis?

(Most Recent Question Jan 2023)

a. Decreased LDH b. Decreased haptoglobin
c. Reticulocytopenia d. Conjugated bilirubin

71. A patient presents with abdominal pain episodes and recurrent renal stones. In work up for X-ray, hands show evidence of brown tumor. Which imaging should be performed to determine the etiology of this presentation? ***(Most Recent Question Jan 2023)***

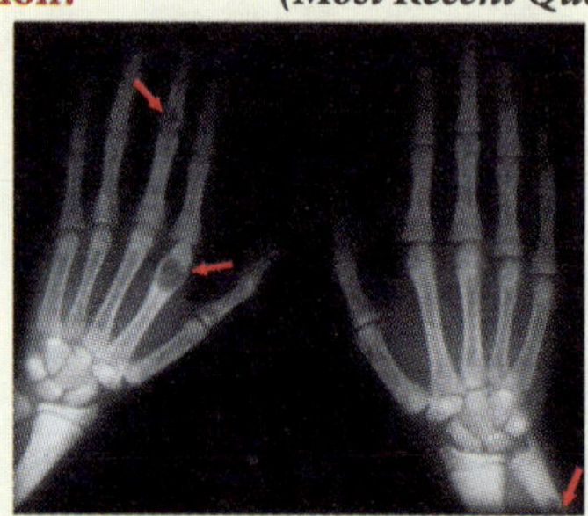

a. PET-CT b. USG
c. Tc 99 Sestamibi Scan d. X-ray

72. Which device will give FiO2 of 0.25 to 0.45 in a stable patient with normal inspiratory reserve?

(Most Recent Question Jan 2023)

a. Simple mask b. Venturi mask
c. Partial rebreathing mask d. Nasal cannula

73. All are superior mediastinal tumors; except:

(Most Recent Question Jan 2023)

a. Thymoma b. Parathyroid tumor
c. Thyroid swelling d. Neurogenic tumors

74. A 60-year-old patient presents with throbbing unilateral headache, nodular thickening along the temporal artery. Biopsy of vessels shows giant cells and granulomatous vasculitis. The likely diagnosis is:

(Most Recent Question Jan 2023)

a. Takayasu arteritis b. Temporal arteritis
c. Buerger's disease d. HSP

75. A 19-year-old patient presents with icterus for a few days after extensive workout in a gym. LFT shows elevated unconjugated serum Bilirubin, normal AST, normal ALT and normal SAP. Past medical history is significant for evidence of recurrent episodes of jaundice since birth. Diagnosis is: ***(Most Recent Question Jan 2023)***

a. Dubin Johnson b. Gilbert Syndrome
c. Crigler-Najjar Type 1 d. Crigler-Najjar Type 2

76. An HIV positive patient develops lung infection. His CD4 count is 50 cells/mm3 and sputum shows acid-fast organism. Which of the following organisms is responsible? ***(Most Recent Question Jan 2023)***

a. MAI b. P. Jiroveci
c. Nocardia d. Streptococcus

77. A smoker had blood-tinged sputum while coughing. On workup, chest X-ray was normal. Which of the following is the next procedure done?

(Most Recent Question Jan 2023)

a. Bronchoscopy b. Repeat CXR
c. CT chest d. Sputum test

78. A man presents with 18-year history of exposure to asbestos. Which of the following is most likely to develop in this patient? ***(Most Recent Question Jan 2023)***

a. Lung granuloma
b. Mesothelioma
c. Idiopathic pulmonary fibrosis
d. Pulmonary TB

CARDIOLOGY

79. Comment on ECG findings shown. ***(Most Recent Question June 2022)***

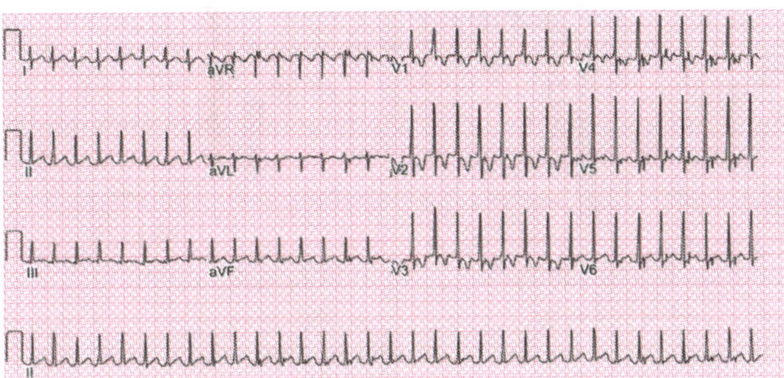

a. Ventricular fibrillation
b. PSVT
c. Ventricular tachycardia
d. Atrial fibrillation

80. A patient complains of palpitations. On examination Irregularly irregular radial pulse is present and ECG shows absent P wave. Which of the following condition is likely? ***(Most Recent Question June 2022)***

a. Atrial fibrillation
b. PSVT
c. Ventricular tachycardia
d. Ventricular fibrillation

81. You saw a guy collapse in a case of roadside accident and started giving CPR. Rescue team has arrived. Which of the following is correct about your options? ***(Most Recent Question June 2022)***

a. Continue five rounds of CPR @ 30:2 followed by application of AED
b. Continue CPR while team applies AED Paddles
c. Stop CPR and let them apply paddles
d. Handover the patient and leave

82. Dullness to percussion and decreased breath sounds near the base of left lung infra-scapular location is seen in which of the following conditions? ***(Most Recent Question June 2022)***

a. Cardiac tamponade
b. Chronic constrictive pericarditis
c. Pulmonary embolism
d. Left sided pleural effusion

83. Hypotension 80/40 mm Hg, diminished/smooth heart sounds with absent y descent in JVP is seen in: ***(Most Recent Question June 2022)***

a. Constrictive pericarditis
b. Acute pericarditis
c. Cardiac failure
d. Cardiac tamponade

84. J wave is seen in: ***(Most Recent Question June 2022)***

a. Hypothermia
b. Heat stroke
c. High altitude pulmonary edema
d. Drowning

85. A child came with profuse sweating and light headedness. What does D indicate in ABCDE? ***(Most Recent Question June 2022)***

a. Dehydration
b. Diarrhea
c. Disability
d. Dementia

86. A 70-year-old patient presents with sudden onset chest pain. ECG shows which of the following? ***(Most Recent Question Dec 2021)***

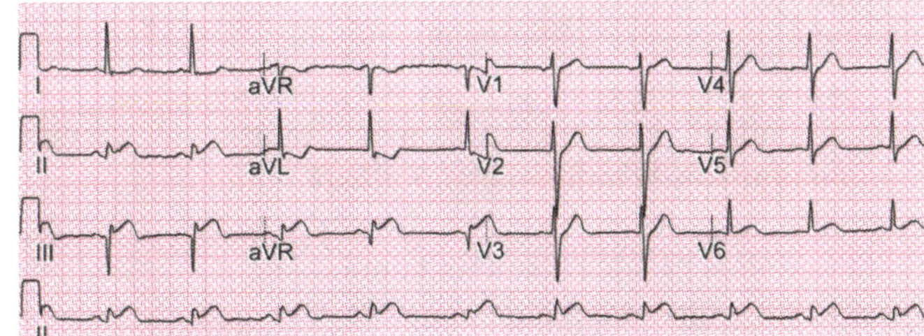

a. Anterior wall MI
b. Inferior wall MI
c. Pericarditis
d. Posterior wall MI

87. MBBS student was asked to diagrammatically represent cardiac axis deviation in a patient. The following schemata shown represents? ***(Most Recent Question Dec 2021)***

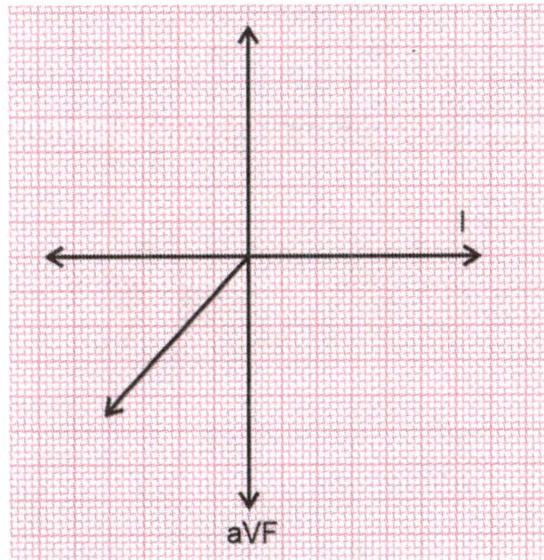

a. Right ventricular hypertrophy
b. Left ventricular hypertrophy
c. Biventricular hypertrophy
d. Normal axis

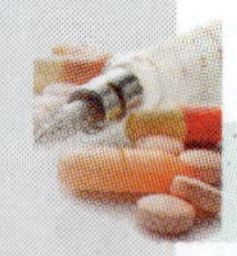

88. An 18-year-old female patient with recurrent infections of respiratory tract. ECG was given:

(Most Recent Question Dec 2021)

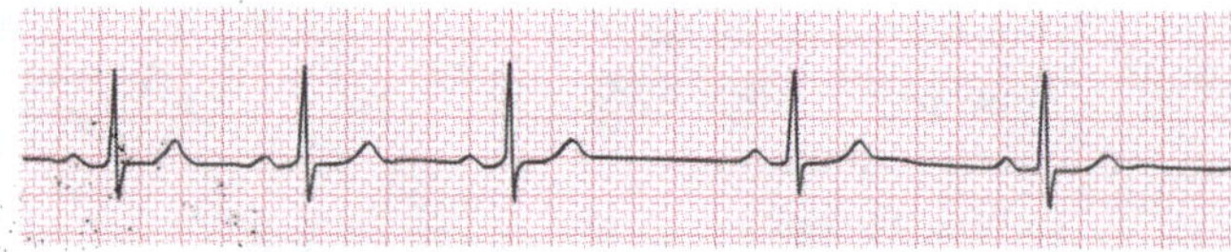

a. Wolf Parkinson white syndrome
b. Atrial flutter
c. Atrial fibrillation
d. Sinus arrhythmia

89. Best treatment for unconscious middle aged in patient in the ambulance shall be which of the following?

(Most Recent Question Dec 2021)

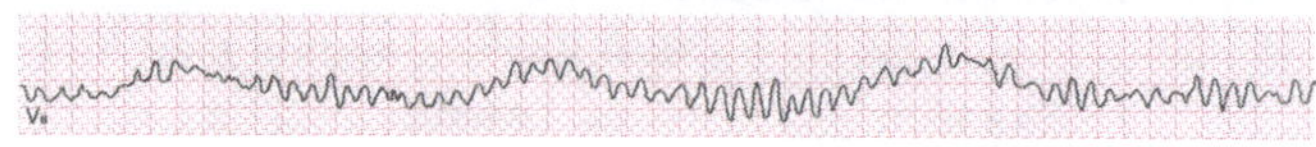

a. Take to ICU
b. Start CPR and defibrillation
c. Carotid sinus massage
d. Observation

90. Tall T waves, wide QRS and prolonged PR interval is seen in? ***(Most Recent Question Dec 2021)***

a. Hypokalemia
b. Hyperkalemia
c. Hyponatremia
d. Hypernatremia

91. A patient has presented with features of cardiac tamponade. Which is a true finding?

(Most Recent Question Dec 2021)

a. Pulsus paradoxus is always present
b. Kussmaul sign is always present
c. Tall A wave is present
d. Jugular veins column is visibly distended without pulsations

92. Correct position of sites of auscultation of heart valves is:

(Most Recent Question Dec 2021)

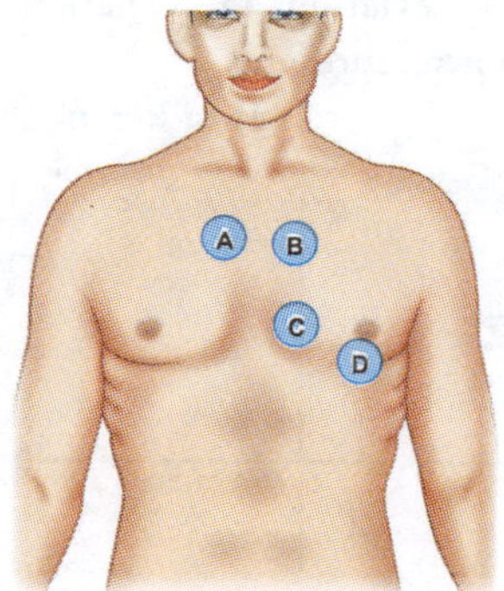

a. A = Pulmonic, B = Aortic, C = Mitral area, D = Tricuspid area
b. A = Aortic, B = Pulmonic, C = Tricuspid area, D = Mitral area
c. A = Pulmonic, B = Aortic, C = Tricuspid area, D = Mitral area
d. A = Mitral, B = Aortic, C = Mitral area, D = Pulmonic area

93. A young male had no symptoms, but auscultation reveals wide fixed split S2. The clinical diagnosis is:

(Most Recent Question Dec 2021)

a. ASD
b. VSD
c. TOF
d. BAV

94. Which murmur is shown here?

(Most Recent Question Dec 2020)

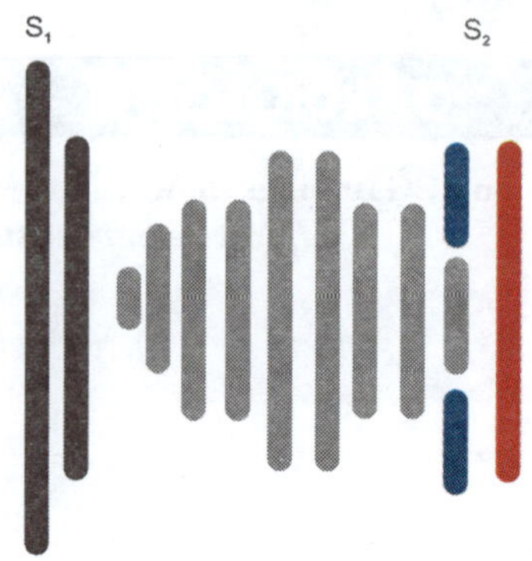

a. Ejection systolic
b. Pan systolic
c. Early diastolic
d. Mid diastolic

95. Comment on the diagnosis in the patient with rapid X and Y descent in JVP with following CXR?

(Most Recent Question Dec 2020)

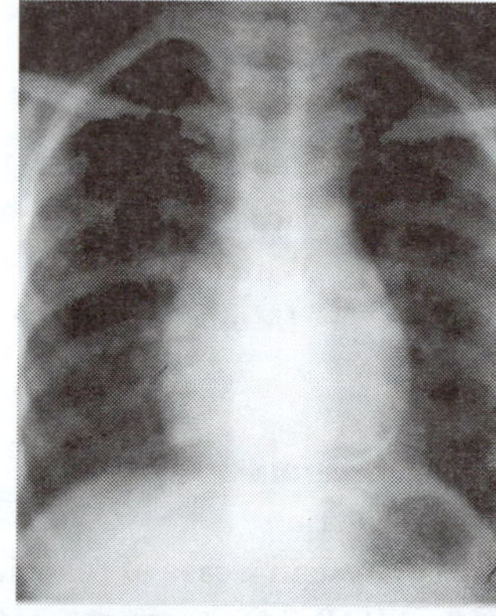

a. Cardiac tamponade
b. Constrictive pericarditis
c. Dilated cardiomyopathy
d. Hypertrophic cardiomyopathy

96. A 70-year-old man presents with complaints of breathlessness and occasional episodes of chest pain. General physical examination shows a high volume pulse and BP of 150/70 mm Hg. On cardiovascular examination the apex beat is displaced 1.5 cm lateral to mid clavicular line. On auscultation diastolic murmur is heard. What is the diagnosis?

(Most Recent Question Dec 2020)

a. Aortic insufficiency
b. Mitral insufficiency
c. Pulmonary insufficiency
d. Tricuspid insufficiency

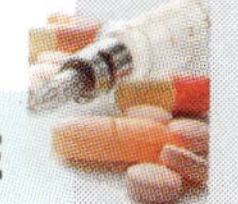

97. The following image shows:

(Most Recent Question Dec 2020)

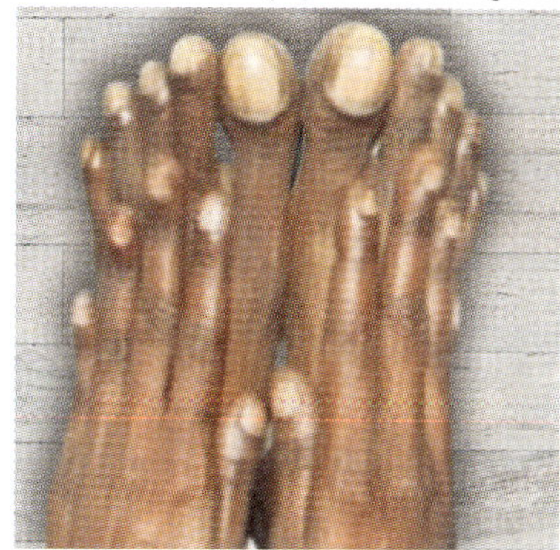

a. Clubbing
b. Cyanosis
c. Raynaud phenomenon
d. Pallor

98. Patient with previous history of MI three years ago now presents with gradual increase in breathlessness on climbing stairs. On examination, S1 is loud with S3 being heard with a bell. Which of the following is the correct diagnosis? *(Most Recent Question Dec 2020)*

a. Pericarditis
b. Pulmonary embolism
c. LV aneurysm
d. Congestive heart failure

99. A 30-year-old patient of valvular heart disease presents with fever for last 2 weeks. On physical examination the following features are noticed in this patient. Which of these will be the abdomen examination finding of this patient? *(Most Recent Question Aug 2020)*

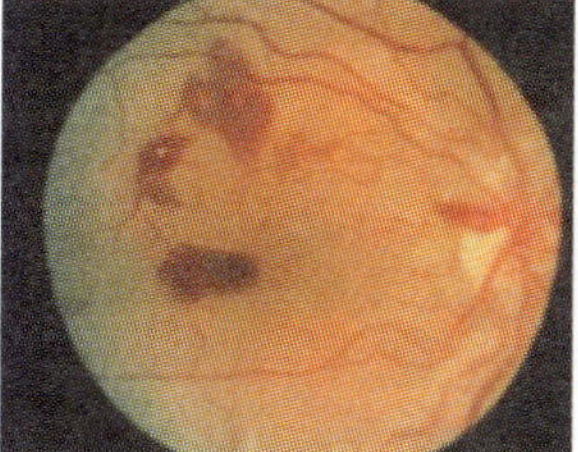

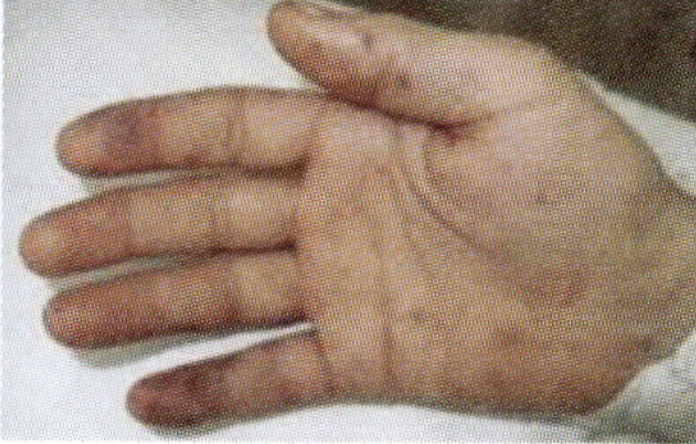

a. Ascites
b. Portal Hypertension
c. Splenomegaly
d. Renal artery Bruit

100. A 70-year-old man collapsed in his house and was rushed to the hospital. On arrival his ECG tracing was as shown below. Which of the following is the best intervention for this patient? *(Most Recent Question Aug 2020)*

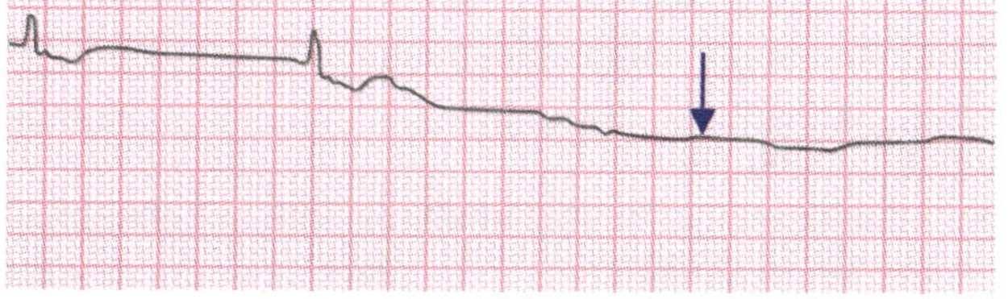

a. Use of Automated external defibrillator
b. Injection of Vasopressin 40 IU
c. Injection of adrenaline 1 mg IV
d. Injection of atropine 0.5 mg IV

101. An elderly patient with Hypertension fell down in his bathroom. His BP was 220/110 on admission. Which of the following statements is correct about this patient?

(Most Recent Question Aug 2020)

a. Start anti platelet drugs
b. Platelets are transfused even if the platelet count is not low
c. Reduce the BP to <120
d. Putamen is the most common site

102. A 70-year-old man has recurrent episodes of exertional syncope and recurrent episodes of chest pain on climbing stairs. He was diagnosed as a case of valvular aortic stenosis. Which of the following is the radiological finding of XRC of this patient?

(Most Recent Question Aug 2020)

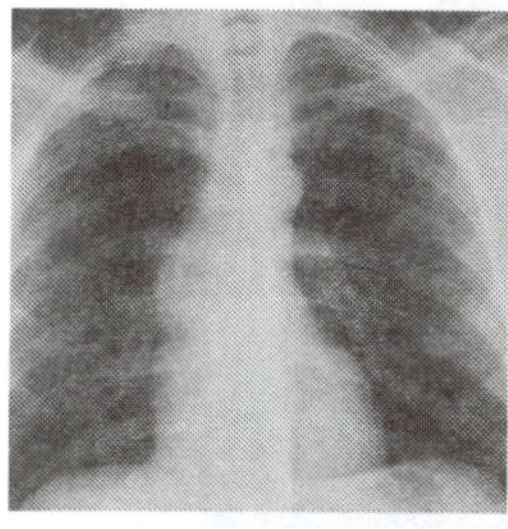

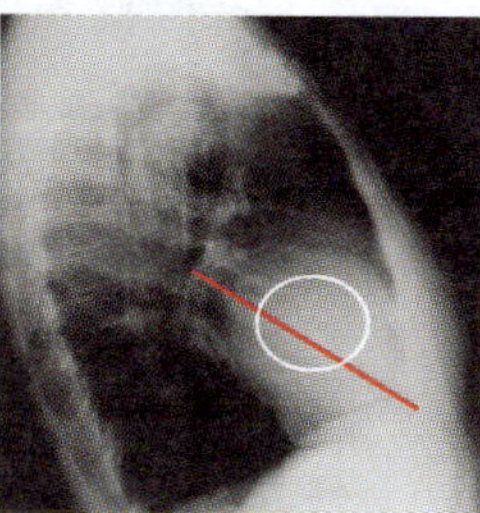

a. Dilated aortic Root
b. Double atrial shadow
c. Widening of anterior mediastinum
d. Post stenotic dilatation of aorta

103. A 50-year-old man presents with recurrent episodes of chest pain on exertion. He is diagnosed as a case of chronic stable angina. On routine monitoring BP is found to be consistently elevated. Which of the following is the best drug for management of this patient?

(Most Recent Question Aug 2020)

a. Enalapril
b. Amlodipine
c. Metoprolol
d. Thiazides

104. What is the impression from the following CXR?

(Most Recent Question Aug 2020)

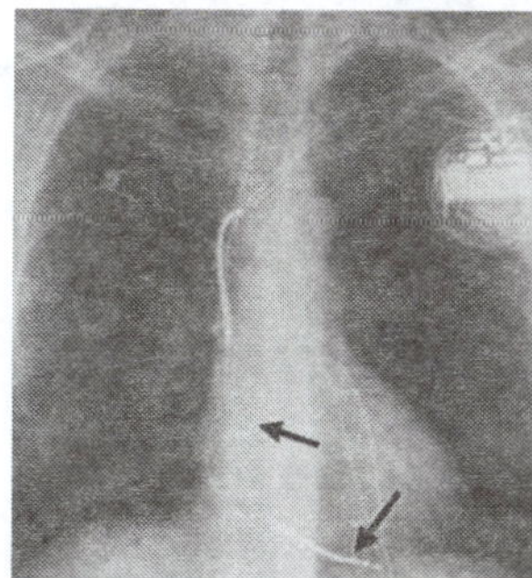

a. Chemo-port device
b. Pacemaker
c. Artifact
d. Travel tract for bypassing accessory pathway

105. A young woman presents as shown below, and these complaints are triggered by cold temperatures or emotional stress. Episodes usually affect the fingers and toes along with numbness and pain in the affected areas. There is no underlying comorbidity in the patient. Comment on the diagnosis.

(Most Recent Question Aug 2020)

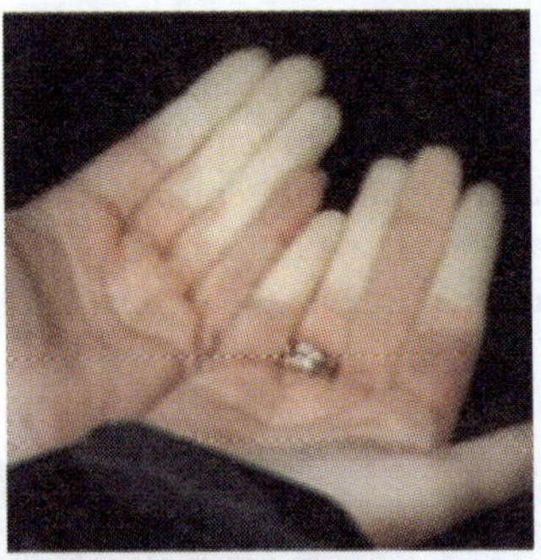

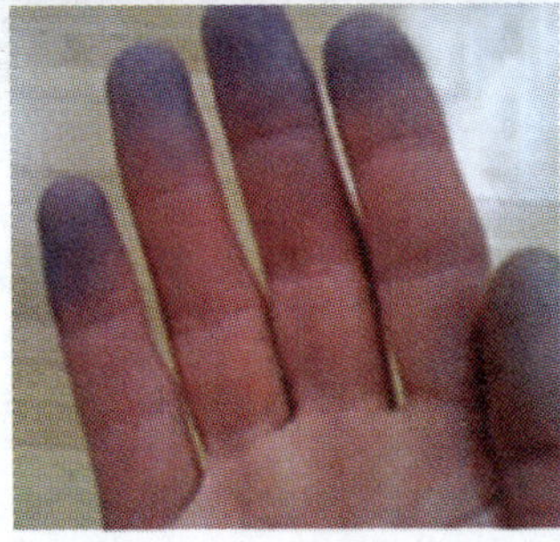

a. Primary Raynaud phenomenon
b. Secondary Raynaud phenomenon
c. Harlequin sign
d. Ainhum

106. A 60-year-old woman who is a known case of lung cancer is having shortness of breath. On examination her neck veins are engorged showing gross elevation of JVP, Heart sounds are distant and breath sounds appear reduced on left side infra-scapular area. CXR is done and is shown below. Comment on the diagnosis of the patient.

(Most Recent Question Aug 2020)

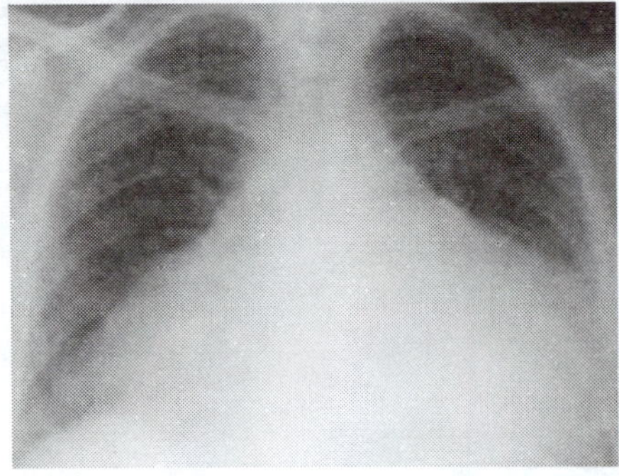

a. Cardiac Tamponade
b. Congestive heart failure
c. Bilateral pleural effusion
d. SVC Syndrome

107. In the given tracing shown below, HV interval denotes:

(Most Recent Question Aug 2020)

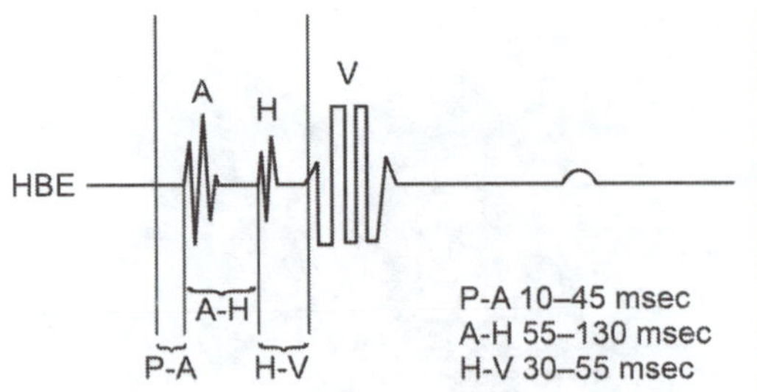

a. AV intranodal conduction
b. Septal Activation of bundle of His
c. Antegrade conduction from Bundle of His to bundle branches
d. Retrograde conduction from Bundle to His to Purkinje fibers

108. A 50-year-old lady with Hypertension was admitted with breathlessness in supine position and palpitations for last 4 days. On physical examination her heart rate is 120/min with congested neck veins. Per abdomen shows liver palpable 3 cm below costal margin. The finding shown in the image below is?

(Most Recent Question Aug 2020)

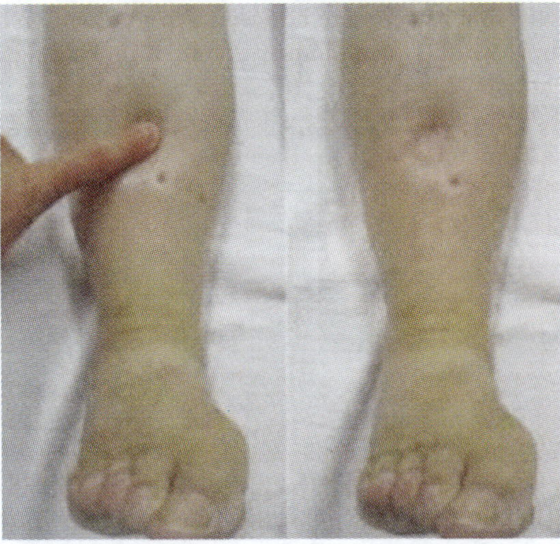

a. Deep vein thrombosis
b. Superficial venous thrombophlebitis
c. Pitting Pedal edema
d. Lymphedema

109. All are true about steps followed in management of ventricular fibrillation; EXCEPT? ***(Most Recent Question 2019)***

a. CPR cycle duration is 2 minutes
b. Chest compressions at 100-120/min
c. Start CPR followed by immediate defibrillation
d. Intravenous access followed by Immediate defibrillation

110. Comment on the diagnosis.

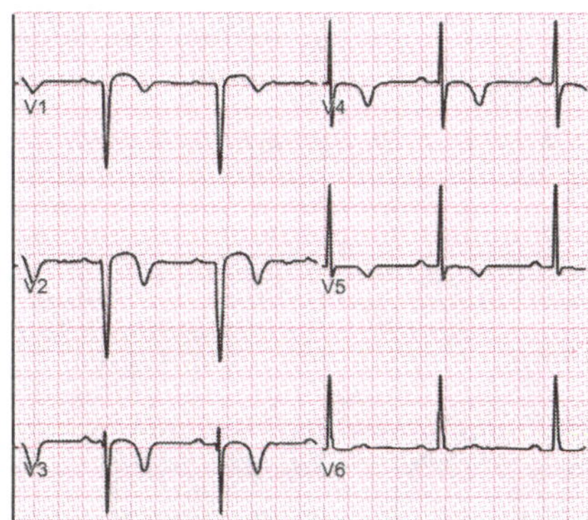

a. Prinzmetal angina
b. Myocardial ischemia
c. Pulmonary embolism
d. Hyperkalemia

111. Which of the following is used for management of this 65-year-old patient with respiratory distress? Bedside Echo shows an Ejection fraction of 35%. ***(Most Recent Question 2019)***

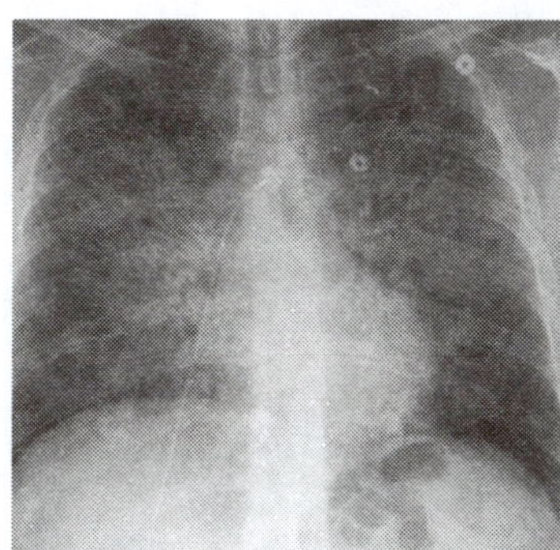

a. Lasix, nitrates and sacubitril-valsartan
b. Lasix, norepinephrine and sacubitril-valsartan
c. Lasix, nitrates and morphine
d. Lasix, ACEI and digoxin

112. Which of the following leads to a continuous murmur?

a. Peripheral Pulmonic stenosis
b. Severe Pulmonary artery hypertension
c. Type A aortic dissection
d. Rupture of cardiac chamber

113. Which is true about Postural Hypotension? ***(Most Recent Question 2019)***

a. Decrease in systolic blood pressure 20 mm Hg within 6 minutes of postural change
b. Decrease in systolic blood pressure 20 mm Hg within 3 minutes of postural change
c. Decrease in diastolic blood pressure 20 mm Hg within 6 minutes of postural change
d. Decrease in diastolic blood pressure 20 mm Hg within 3 minutes of postural change

114. A 60-year-old female presents with left sided weakness for more than one hour and left sided facial weakness with BP of 160/100 mm Hg. CT is normal. What is the next best step? ***(Most Recent Question 2019)***

a. Start thrombolysis
b. Give loading dose of aspirin and clopidogrel
c. Only manage BP
d. No intervention required

115. Best management of a hemodynamically stable patient with ECG showing Broad QRS complex with antidromic tachycardia is: ***(Recent Pattern Question 2018-19)***

a. Oral Verapamil
b. Oral Beta-blocker
c. Cardioversion
d. Intravenous Procainamide

116. Which of these is not done in Wolf Parkinson White syndrome? ***(Recent Pattern Question 2018-19)***

a. Treadmill
b. Holter monitoring
c. Oral beta blocker
d. Procainamide

117. Which of the following is not correct about defibrillation? ***(Recent Pattern Question 2018-19)***

a. Easy for untrained person
b. Decrease in success rate with delay in initiation
c. Improves prognosis
d. 1-minute gap between 2 shocks

118. Modified Duke's criteria are used for diagnosis of? ***(Recent Pattern Question 2018-19)***

a. Infective endarteritis
b. Infectious mononucleosis
c. Inflammatory myopathy
d. Infective endocarditis

119. Which of the following shall be seen with use of a small size BP cuff? ***(Recent Pattern Question 2018-19)***

a. False elevation of BP
b. Falsely low value of BP
c. Cancels the effect of calcified arteries
d. Increases trans-arm impedance

120. Which of the following is a cardioprotective lipid? ***(Recent Pattern Question 2018-19)***

a. LDL
b. HDL
c. VLDL
d. Chylomicrons

121. Rescue P.C.I is done for which of the following? ***(Recent Pattern Question 2018-19)***

a. Persistent chest pain with ST elevation >30 minutes after thrombolysis
b. Persistent chest pain with ST elevation >60 minutes after thrombolysis
c. Persistent chest pain with ST elevation >90 minutes after thrombolysis
d. Persistent chest pain with ST elevation for >120 minutes after thrombolysis

122. Which of the following condition should *not* be considered if JVP rises on deep inspiration? *(Recent Pattern Question 2018)*

a. Constrictive pericarditis
b. Restrictive cardiomyopathy
c. Complete heart block
d. Atrial fibrillation

123. The PR interval in ECG denotes *(Recent Pattern Question 2018)*

a. Atrial depolarization only
b. Atrial depolarization with A-V conduction
c. Ventricular depolarization and ventricular repolarization
d. Atrial depolarization with atrial repolarization

124. Which of the following is not associated with pulmonary artery hypertension? *(Recent Pattern Question 2018)*

a. Interstitial lung disease
b. Left ventricular hypertrophy
c. Mitral stenosis
d. Cor-pulmonale

125. A patient presents with pedal edema with Water-hammer pulse. What is the diagnosis? *(Recent Pattern Question 2017)*

a. B_1 deficiency
b. B_3 deficiency
c. B_6 deficiency
d. B_{12} deficiency

126. Which is correct about the ECG finding of hypocalcemia? *(Recent Pattern Question 2017)*

a. Prolonged QT
b. Tall tented T wave
c. Prolonged PR
d. Narrow QRS

127. Which is the preferred bypass graft used in CABG? *(Recent Pattern Question 2017)*

a. Internal mammary artery
b. Great saphenous vein
c. Short saphenous vein
d. Gastro-epiploic artery

128. Wide fixed Split S2 is seen in? *(Recent Pattern Question 2017)*

a. PDA
b. ASD
c. TOF
d. VSD

129. What is the earliest change in ECG in case of hyperkalemia? *(Recent Pattern Question 2017)*

a. Tall tented T wave
b. Inverted P
c. Prolonged QRS
d. T wave inversion

130. Which rhythm disorder is shown in this ECG? *(Recent Pattern Question 2017)*

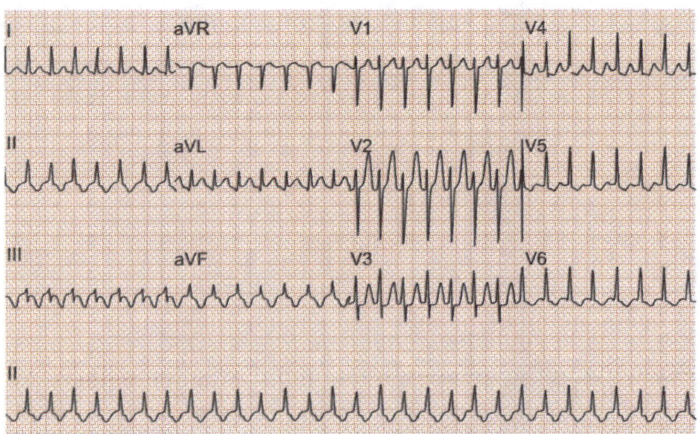

a. Ventricular fibrillation b. PSVT
c. Atrial fibrillation d. Atrial flutter

131. Which is incorrect about the ECG shown below? *(Recent Pattern Question 2017)*

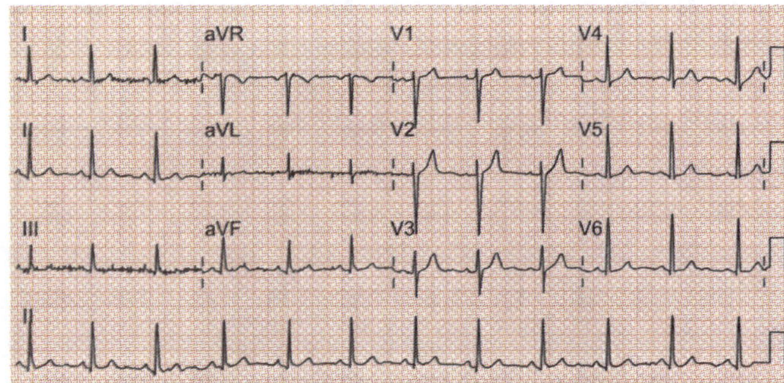

a. QT = 0.04 sec b. PR = 0.16 sec
c. QRS = 0.10 sec d. P wave = 0.12 sec

132. The ECG finding shown below is due to which of the following drugs? *(Recent Pattern Question 2017)*

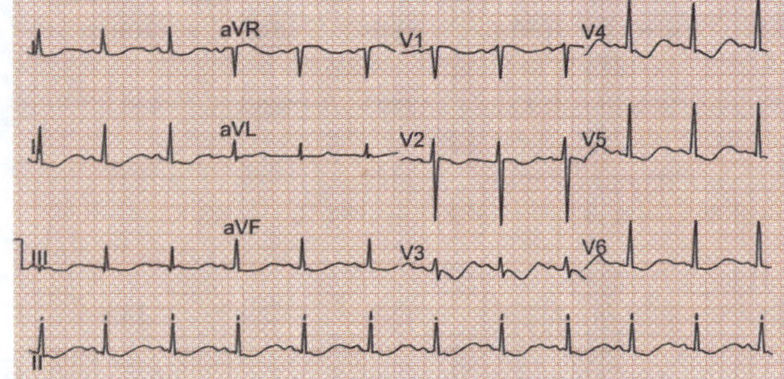

a. Diuretics b. A.R.B
c. A.C.E inhibitors d. Beta blockers

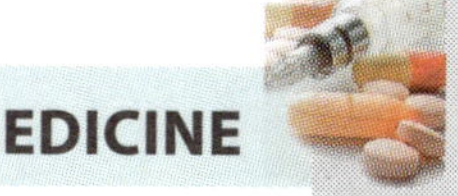

133. Which of the following is correct about the image shown below? ***(Recent Pattern Question 2017)***

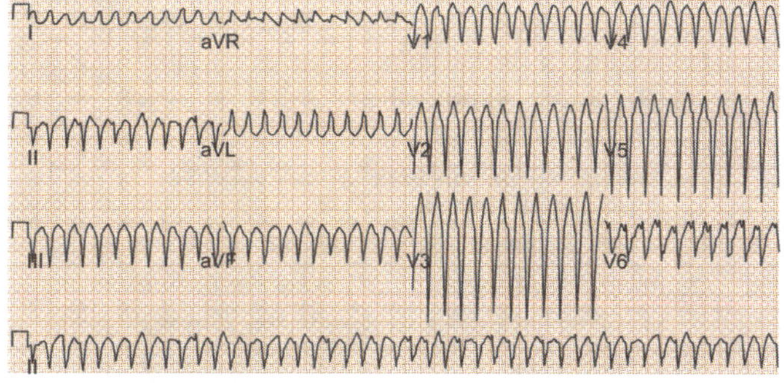

a. Atrial fibrillation b. Atrial flutter
c. PSVT d. VT

134. During CPR when is vasopressin given? ***(Recent Pattern Question 2016)***

a. No role
b. Use every 3 minutes
c. First line drug of choice
d. Given along with adrenaline

135. Which antiarrhythmic drug is given in post resuscitation arrhythmia? ***(Recent Pattern Question 2016)***

a. Lignocaine b. Magnesium sulfate
c. Amiodarone d. Atropine

136. In JVP y descent is absent and X wave is prominent? This suggests:

a. Restictive cardiomyopathy
b. Cardiac tamponade
c. Constrictive pericarditis
d. Right ventricular failure

137. Digitalis is used in mitral stenosis when patient develops?

a. Atrial fibrillation
b. Right ventricular failure
c. Acute pulmonary edema
d. Myocarditis

138. Murmur heard in aortic stenosis?

a. Right 2nd intercostal, low pitch murmur
b. Apex, low pitch murmur
c. Left Sternal area, low pitch murmur
d. Pan-systolic murmur, high pitch murmur

139. In coarctation of aorta, site of rib notching is?

a. Superior to rib b. Inferior to rib
c. At sternum d. At Vertebra

140. Cardiac marker earliest to rise in MI?

a. CPK MB b. LDH
c. SAP d. Troponin I

141. Hypotension with muffled heart sounds and congested neck veins is seen in?

a. Cardiac tamponade
b. Pericardial effusion
c. Constrictive pericarditis
d. Acute congestive heart failure

142. Which of the following is given to decrease Serum Triglycerides?

a. Fibrates b. Statins
c. Ezetimibe d. Niacin

143. In a patient there is dyspnea in upright position which is relieved in supine position. Diagnosis?

a. Tachypnea
b. Orthopnea
c. Paroxysmal nocturnal dyspnea
d. Platypnea

144. Which is the best way to differentiate between stable angina and NSTEMI?

a. ECG
b. Cardiac-biomarker
c. Trans thoracic Echocardiography
d. Multi uptake gated Acquisition scan

145. Duroziez's sign is seen in?

a. Aortic regurgitation b. Aortic stenosis
c. Mitral stenosis d. Mitral regurgitation

146. Which of the following is a diagnostic criteria for Rheumatic fever?

a. Oral ulcer b. Malar rash
c. Erythema Marginatum d. Morning stiffness

147. Organism leading to hospital acquired infective endocarditis?

a. Staph aureus
b. Klebsiella
c. Streptococcus pneumoniae
d. Meningococcus

148. Etiology of Dressler syndrome is?

a. Viral b. Autoimmune
c. Idiopathic d. Toxin mediated

149. Rib notching is seen in?

a. Coarctation of aorta
b. Hypertension
c. Fibromuscular dysplasia
d. Aortic dissection

150. A 60 year old female with family history of premature coronary artery disease has a DBP = 100 mm Hg on two consecutive occasions. Best treatment is?

a. Rest b. Sedative
c. Anti-hypertensive drugs d. Error in BP machine

151. A 65-year-old male had MI one year ago. Now the same patients presents with hypertension. Which of the following drug is best suited for this patient?

a. Clonidine b. Thiazide
c. Metoprolol d. Lisinopril

152. Resistant hypertension is defined as?

a. Resistance to 2 or more anti hypertension drugs
b. Resistance to 3 or more anti-hypertensive drugs including thiazides
c. Resistance to aldosterone
d. Resistance of Angiotension II receptors

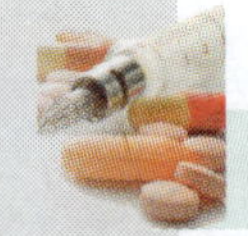

153. An 8-year-old girl, collapsed while playing and died. CXR given below. Which of the following is unlikely to be an etiology of this event?

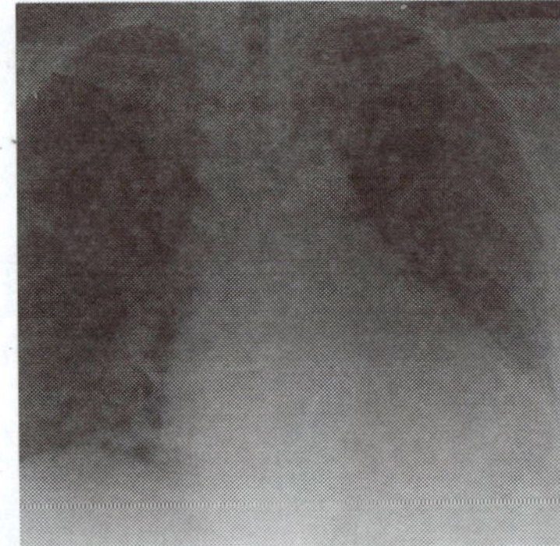

a. Stroke b. Cardiomyopathy
c. Arrhythmia d. Shock

154. If a person is having ventricular tachycardia, extra systoles correspond to which of following?
a. P wave b. QRS complex
c. T wave d. R wave

155. Internal jugular vein pressure determines pressure of:
a. RA b. RV
c. LA d. LV

156. Hyaline atherosclerosis is seen in:
a. Benign hypertension b. Malignant hypertension
c. Diabetic nephropathy d. Analgesic nephropathy

157. Maccallum patch in rheumatic heart disease is seen in?
a. Right atrium b. Left atrium
c. Right ventricle d. Left ventricle

158. Canon A wave is seen in:
a. Atrial fibrillation b. Complete heart block
c. Ventricular fibrillation d. Mobitz 1 heart block

159. Aortic dissection is seen in?
a. Takayasu disease b. Atherosclerosis
c. Syphilis aortitis d. Marfan syndrome

160. Incorrect about conduction system of heart:
a. SAN is dominant pacemaker
b. AVN exhibits conduction delay of 0.1 sec
c. Purkinje fibres have the slowest conduction
d. Left fascicle divides into anterior and posterior fascicle

161. A wave in JVP is absent in:
a. Atrial fibrillation b. Heart block
c. Tricuspid regurgitation d. Complete heart block

162. Canon a waves are seen in:
a. Atrial fibrillation b. Junctional tachycardia
c. Constrictive pericarditis d. Cardiac tamponade

163. Severe mitral stenosis is identified by:
a. Loud S1
b. Loud opening snap
c. Duration of mid-diastolic murmur
d. Intensity of mid-diastolic murmur

164. What would you do immediately after identification by ECG of patient going into cardiac arrest?
a. Give epinephrine b. Check for breathing
c. Check for pulse d. Chest compressions

165. P wave in ECG is due to:
a. Ventricular depolarization
b. Atrial repolarization
c. Ventricular repolarization
d. Atrial depolarization

166. Initial ECG change in Hyperkalemia is?
a. Tall tented T waves b. PR prolongation
c. qRS widening d. ST segment depression

167. Incorrect about Dressler syndrome is?
a. Post MI pericarditis
b. Post MI pleuritis
c. Autoimmune
d. Treatment with steroids is necessary

168. Most common cause of aortic dissection:
a. Syphilis b. Hypertension
c. Marfan syndrome d. Cystic medial necrosis

169. Marker specific for myocardial infarction:
a. Troponin I b. Troponin C
c. CPK–MB d. LDH

170. All are used for secondary prevention of MI; EXCEPT:
a. Aspirin b. Statins
c. Beta blockers d. Warfarin

171. Reverse split S2 is seen in
a. Aortic stenosis b. Mitral stenosis
c. Pulmonary artery hypertension
d. Pulmonic stenosis

172. ECG finding of Hyperkalemia:
a. T wave inversion b. ST depression
c. P pulmonale d. Wide QRS complex

173. Coronary artery disease is associated with all; EXCEPT:
a. Chylamydia b. Poor dental hygiene
c. Smoking d. Alcohol

174. Pericardical cyst is seen at:
a. Cardiophrenic angle b. Middle mediastinum
c. Posterior mediastinum d. Lingula

175. Snow man appearance or figure of 8 appearance is seen in?
a. Total anomalous pulmonary venous connection
b. Transposition of great arteries
c. Tetralogy of fallot
d. Tricuspid atresia

176. Which of the following is a cause of wide pulse pressure:
a. Aortic stenosis b. Aortic regurgitation
c. Mitral stenosis d. Tricuspid stenosis

177. Canon a wave is seen in?
a. Junctional rhythm b. Atrial fibrillation
c. Atrial flutter d. Ventricular fibrillation

178. Most common cause of unilateral pedal edema?
a. Pregnancy b. Lymphedema
c. Venous insufficiency d. Milroy disease

179. Which of the following is primary defect in HOCM?
a. Systolic dysfunction b. Diastolic dysfunction
c. Valvular dysfunction d. Rhythm defects

180. According to revised guidelines of American heart association, which of the following drugs is not recommended in cardiac arrest?
a. Adrenaline b. Atropine
c. Amiodarone d. Vasopressin

181. A Patient presented with deficiency of thiamine. What could be possible outcome:
a. Delayed wound healing b. Cardiac abnormality
c. Memory loss d. Gingival bleeding

182. After intake of NSAID tablet a lady complains of difficulty in breathing and appearance of bee hives. Pulse rate is 100 and BP is 90/60 mm Hg. Diagnosis is:
a. Massive pulmonary embolism
b. Neurogenic shock
c. DIC
d. Anaphylaxis

183. Which is the best investigation best to confirm diagnosis of anaphylaxis?
a. Ig A levels b. Ig D levels
c. Serum tryptase d. Serum precipitins

184. MCC of abdominal aortic aneurysm?
a. Idiopathic b. Trauma
c. Atherosclerosis d. Arteriosclerosis

185. A 1-year-old male child is having a Heart Rate 40/min, BP 90/60. His serum Potassium = 6.5. What is the next best management?
a. Ipratropium b. Adrenaline
c. Sodium bicarbonate d. Calcium chloride

186. Mortality in primary cardiac amyloidosis develops over?
a. 3–6 months b. 6–12 months
c. 12–18 months d. 24–36 months

187. Which is best for plaque morphology in atherosclerosis?
a. CCTA b. Echocardiography
c. ECG d. Coronary angiography

NEUROLOGY

188. Which of the following is seen in Hypoglossal nerve injury? ***(Most Recent Question June 2022)***
a. Tongue deviation to contralateral side
b. Tongue deviation to same side
c. Backward falling of tongue
d. Inability in tongue protrusion

189. A person brings his father who was became unconscious while working in hot sun in 44 degrees C in June afternoon presents to hospital with heat exhaustion/heat stroke. Which of the following will not be seen? ***(Most Recent Question June 2022)***
a. Headache b. Hyperthermia
c. Hypotension d. Pin-point pupils

190. A female patient presents with fever for past 3 days and cannot touch neck to chest. LP was done, and CSF findings are: ***(Most Recent Question June 2022)***
Opening pressure = increased
Appearance = White cloudy
Cells = Neutrophils predominantly seen
CSF Sugar = 15 mg/dL
Protein = 100 mg/dL
a. Bacterial meningitis b. Tubercular meningitis
c. Viral meningitis d. Fungal meningitis

191. A person on a mountain at 5000 m is having headache, dizziness and cerebral edema. Which of the following is responsible for development of high-altitude cerebral edema? ***(Most Recent Question June 2022)***
a. Desaturation b. Increased blood pressure
c. Altered mentation d. Retinal hemorrhage

192. Young male 25 years of age presents with Ptosis which is worse in the evening and shows improvement in the morning. The patient complains of exertional fatigue. Work up with ice pack test shows relief in ptosis. Diagnosis is? ***(Most Recent Question June 2022)***
a. Huntington chorea
b. Amyotrophic lateral sclerosis
c. External Opthalmoplegia d. M. Gravis

193. A known hypertensive patient is brought to ER with Palpitations and SOB. On examination BP = 210/120 mm Hg with development of encephalopathy. All of the following can be given; EXCEPT? ***(Most Recent Question June 2022)***
a. IV Mannitol b. IV Nicardipine
c. IV Esmolol d. IV sodium nitroprusside

194. The GCS of RTA patient is 10. This implies ***(Most Recent Question June 2022)***
a. Mild TBI b. Moderate TBI
c. Severe TBI d. Patient is dead

195. Young patient developed sudden onset fever and agitated behavior for 2 days. No meningeal signs were noted. EEG shows periodic focal Temporal lobe spikes. CSF shows 40 cells with 90% lymphocytes and 10% neutrophils with normal CSF Sugar and slight elevation protein. Which of the following should be started in the patient? ***(Most Recent Question Dec 2021)***
a. ATT b. Acyclovir
c. Ceftriaxone d. Amphotericin B

196. A 45-year-old male with HbA1c = 8% comes to ER with hemiplegia 8 hours prior to consult. NCCT head shows intracerebral bleed. BP = 198/110 mm Hg. Which of the following intervention is best scheduled for this patient? ***(Most Recent Question Dec 2021)***
a. t-PA
b. IV Labetalol
c. Sublingual nifedipine
d. Observation and monitoring

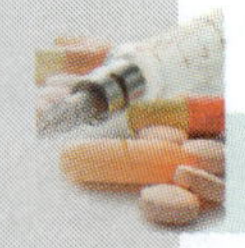

197. A young female patient presents with complaints of worst headache of her life. NCCT head shows evidence of which of the following? *(Most Recent Question Dec 2021)*

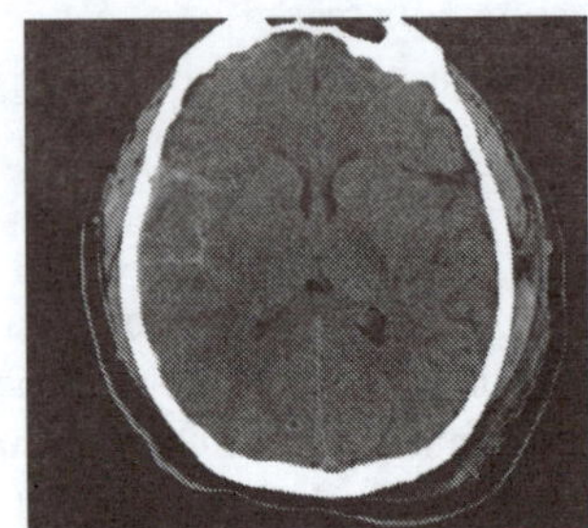

a. Encephalitis b. Meningitis
c. SAH d. SDH

198. Patient has had RTA and his GCS = 9/15. There is no external site of bleeding visible. IVF fluid resuscitation was done, and patient is still hypotensive. Which of the following is least likely cause of this presentation? *(Most Recent Question Dec 2021)*

a. Subdural hematoma b. Hemothorax
c. Splenic rupture d. Retroperitoneal bleed

199. Comment on diagnosis based on schematic diagram showing neurological deficits in a patient: *(Most Recent Question Dec 2021)*

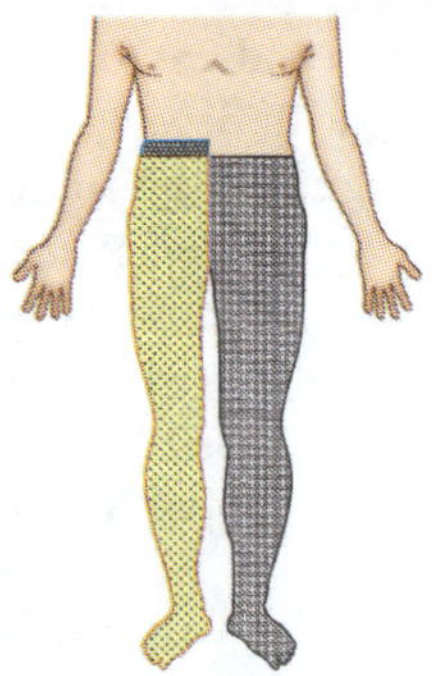

a. Gullian barre syndrome
b. Wallenberg syndrome
c. Brown Sequard syndrome
d. Millard Gubler syndrome

200. A patient was asked to copy the clock face made by the physician. The image on right is made by the patient. Which is correct about this image? *(Most Recent Question Dec 2020)*

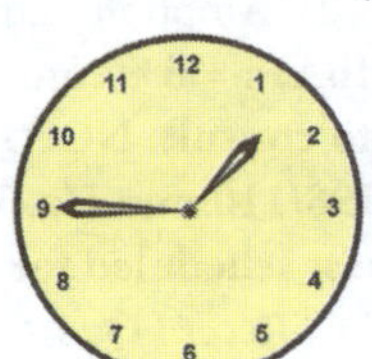

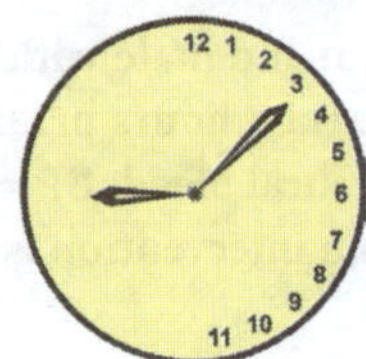

a. Apraxia b. Agraphia
c. Hemianopia d. Hemi-neglect

201. A 30-year-old man presents with repeated myoclonic jerks and dementia. Which is the most probable etiology? *(Most Recent Question Dec 2020)*

a. Vascular dementia b. AD
c. V-CJD d. Huntington chorea

202. A 60-year-old woman presents with weakness in right arm for a duration of four hours. The weakness gradually became lesser and resolves. She is a known case of Hypertension and BMI is elevated. Which of the following is the probable diagnosis of this case? *(Most Recent Question Aug 2020)*

a. Transient ischemic attack
b. Compressive Neuropathy
c. Transverse Myelitis
d. Stroke

203. A 40-year-old man is brought to the ER with LOC following RTA. GCS is 8/15 and CT head was performed. Which of the following is the diagnosis?

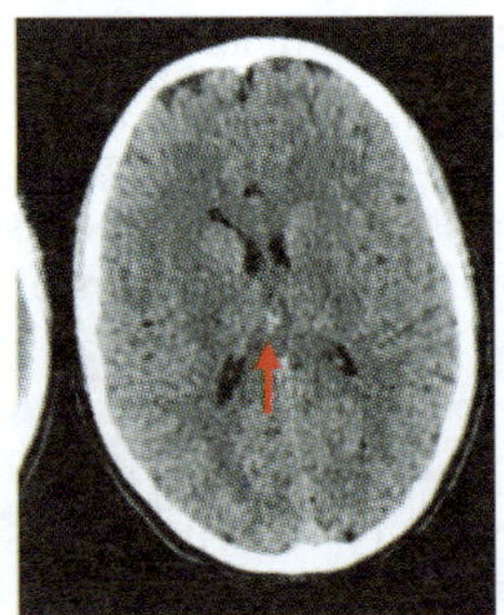

a. SAH
b. SDH
c. Cerebral amyloid angiopathy
d. Diffuse axonal injury

204. A 60-year-old patient has right sided homonymous hemianopia with macular sparing. Localize the neurological site of lesion in this patient. *(Most Recent Question Aug 2020)*

a. Optic chiasma b. Optic tract
c. Medial geniculate body d. Occipital cortex

205. A 30-year-old alcoholic had his last drink 48 hours ago. He develops anger and rage attacks and appears unable to identify faces of family members and can see inanimate objects. He has been brought to the ER. What is your diagnosis? *(Most Recent Question Aug 2020)*

a. Delirium tremens b. Alcoholic hallucinosis
c. Korsakoff psychosis d. Wernicke's encephalopathy

206. A patient had RTA and was put on mechanical ventilation. He is opening his eyes on verbal command. He moves all his limbs spontaneously. What will be his GCS score? *(Most Recent Question 2019)*

a. 9T b. 10T
c. 11T d. 12T

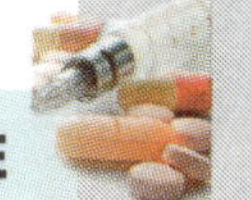

207. Postural tremors are seen in all; EXCEPT: *(Most Recent Question 2019)*

a. Alcohol withdrawal b. Essential tremors
c. Generalized paresis d. Physiological tremors

208. Ipsilateral 3rd nerve palsy with crossed hemiplegia is a feature of? *(Most Recent Question 2019)*

a. Weber syndrome b. Benedikt syndrome
c. Wallenberg syndrome d. Horner syndrome

209. A 60-year-old male diabetic and hypertensive patient was found unconscious in the morning. On examination pulse rate is 120/min, BP = 160/100 mm Hg and bilateral extensor plantars are elicited. What is the next step to be done for management? *(Most Recent Question 2019)*

a. Order CT scan
b. Check blood glucose
c. Give intravenous mannitol
d. Immediately reduce BP with antihypertensives

210. Which of the following is not a feature of Parkinson disease? *(Recent Pattern Question 2018-19)*

a. Hypophonia b. Freezing
c. Rigidity d. Diplopia

211. Normal deep tendon reflexes with muscle weakness is seen in? *(Recent Pattern Question 2018-19)*

a. M. Gravis b. G.B.S
c. Transverse myelitis d. Traumatic neuritis

212. Reversible dementia is seen in? *(Recent Pattern Question 2018-19)*

a. B_{12} deficiency
b. Acute inflammatory demyelinating polyneuropathy
c. Creutzfeldt Jacob disease
d. Pick's disease

213. Extensor plantar reflex on pinching gastrocnemius muscle is called? *(Recent Pattern Question 2018-19)*

a. Gower sign b. Homan sign
c. Oppenheim reflex d. Gordon reflex

214. Which is the most common cranial nerve involved in raised ICP? *(Recent Pattern Question 2018-19)*

a. Abducens b. Trochlear
c. Trigeminal d. Facial

215. Which of the following is not seen in Horner syndrome? *(Recent Pattern Question 2018-19)*

a. Mydriasis b. Ptosis
c. Anhidrosis d. Enopthalmos

216. Painless burn in hand is seen in: *(Recent Pattern Question 2018)*

a. SLE b. Syringomyelia
c. Mononeuritis multiplex d. Diabetes mellitus

217. Prosopagnosia is: *(Recent Pattern Question 2018)*

a. Inability to read
b. Inability to write
c. Anosmia
d. Inability to recognize face

218. Wernicke's encephalopathy is due to deficiency of: *(Recent Pattern Question 2018)*

a. Thiamine b. B_6
c. Niacin d. B_{12}

219. Which of the following manifestation is seen in metabolic encephalopathy? *(Recent Pattern Question 2018)*

a. Motor aphasia
b. Sensory aphasia
c. Conduction aphasia
d. Anomic aphasia

220. Which of these is the best for management of methanol poisoning? *(Recent Pattern Question 2018)*

a. Acamprosate b. Fomepizole
c. Disulfiram d. Naltrexone

221. All are examples of upper motor neuron lesion; EXCEPT: *(Recent Pattern Question 2018)*

a. Prion disease b. Multiple sclerosis
c. Anterior horn cell disease d. Tuberous sclerosis

222. What is the most common cause of meningitis in young adults? *(Recent Pattern Question 2017)*

a. Listeria b. Strep pneumonia
c. Neisseria meningitis d. Group B streptococcus

223. What is seen in complete transection of spinal cord? *(Recent Pattern Question 2017)*

a. Loss of bladder control
b. Loss of temperature regulation
c. Hemianaesthesia
d. Hemiparesis

224. Which of the following is not lost on the same side in hemi-section of the spinal cord? *(Recent Pattern Question 2017)*

a. Position sense b. Thermal sense
c. Vibration sense d. Tactile discrimination

225. Pendular knee jerk is seen in lesion at____________? *(Recent Pattern Question 2017)*

a. Cerebellum b. Basal ganglia
c. Tectum d. Uncus

226. Unconscious proprioception is carried by? *(Recent Pattern Question 2017)*

a. Dorsal column
b. Spinocerebellar pathways
c. Anterior spinothalamic tract
d. Rubro-spinal pathway

227. In which of the following will EMG show decremental response? *(Recent Pattern Question 2017)*

a. M. Gravis
b. Lambert-Eaton syndrome
c. Guillain-Barrē syndrome
d. Botulinism

228. Most common cause of headache? *(Recent Pattern Question 2016)*

a. Tension headache
b. Cluster headache
c. Migraine
d. Raised intra-cranial tension

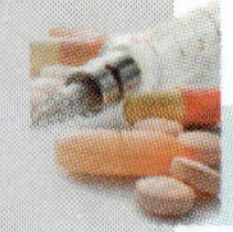

229. **Which of the following is the correct Miller Fisher syndrome triad?** ***(Recent Pattern Question 2016)***
   a. Global confusion, areflexia, ataxia
   b. Ophthalmoplegia, ataxia, areflexia
   c. Ophthalmoplegia, areflexia, aphasia
   d. Global confusion, areflexia, aphasia
230. **CT head of a patient shows?** ***(Recent Pattern Question 2016)***

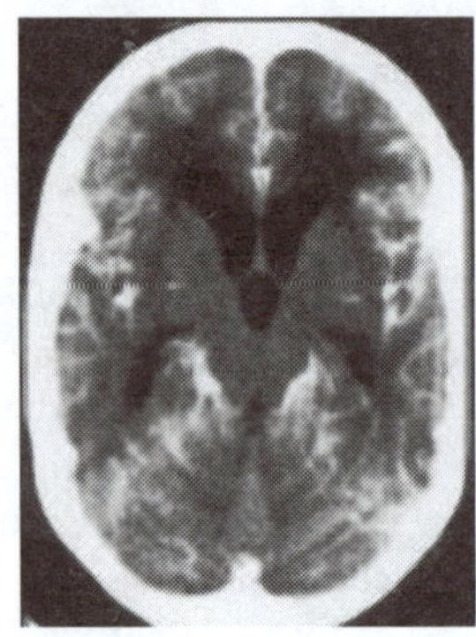

   a. Neurosarcoidosis b. SAH
   c. TB meningitis d. Intraparenchymal bleed
231. **Treatment of post-lumbar puncture headache?** ***(Recent Pattern Question 2016)***
   a. Codeine b. Dantrolene
   c. Caffeine d. Diazepam
232. **Best treatment for glioblastoma multiforme?** ***(Recent Pattern Question 2016)***
   a. Chemotherapy b. Radiation
   c. Excision with radiation d. Stereotactic surgery
233. **Axillary freckling is seen in?** ***(Recent Pattern Question 2016)***
   a. Neurofibromatosis b. Tuberous sclerosis
   c. Ichthyosis vulgaris d. Von Hippel-Lindau
234. **True about chorea?** ***(Recent Patter Question 2016)***
   a. Semi-purposive and rhythmic movements
   b. Slow and uniform movement
   c. Slow writhing movement
   d. Semi-purposive and non-repetitive, randomly distributed movements
235. **Which tract damage leads to loss of pain and temperature?** ***(Recent Pattern Question 2016)***
   a. Lateral spinothalamic tract
   b. Ventral spinothalamic tract
   c. Lateral corticospinal pathway
   d. Dorsal column
236. **Lesion of which tract leads to loss of voluntary skilled movements?** ***(Recent Pattern Question 2016)***
   a. Corticospinal tract
   b. Rubrospinal tract
   c. Tectospinal tract
   d. Lateral spinothalamic pathway
237. **Log roll positioning is done for?**
   a. Spine injury evaluation ***(Recent Pattern Question 2016)***
   b. Relieve compression on back
   c. Perform rapid sequence intubation
   d. Perform peritoneal lavage
238. **Kernohan-Woltman sign is?** ***(Recent Pattern Question 2016)***
   a. Medial displacement of midbrain
   b. Lateral displacement of midbrain
   c. Upper displacement of pons
   d. Downward displacement of pons
239. **Which is true about uncal herniation?** ***(Recent Pattern Question 2016)***
   a. 3rd nerve involvement b. 4th nerve involvement
   c. 6th nerve involvement d. 7th nerve involvement
240. **A lady cannot speak but can tell by writing. Which of the following brain areas is affected?**
   a. Broca's area b. Wernicke's area
   c. Paracentral lobule d. Insula
241. **Nucleus ambiguus is located in?**
   a. Medulla b. Pons
   c. Midbrain d. Paracentral lobule
242. **Wernicke's area is located in:**
   a. Superior temporal gyrus b. Inferior temporal gyrus
   c. Post-central gyrus d. Angular gyrus
243. **Glasgow coma scale = 3 indicates?**
   a. Death b. Severe disability
   c. Coma d. Brain death
244. **Glasgow coma scale score of M_4 represents?**
   a. Withdrawal on flexion b. Decorticate posturing
   c. Decerebrate posturing d. Localise pain
245. **A patient after alcoholic drink fell asleep in chair overnight with hanging arm and develops Saturday Night Palsy. Which of the following best describes the clinical manifestations?**
   a. Neuropraxia b. Axonotmesis
   c. Neurotmesis d. Necroptosis
246. **CSF glucose compared to blood glucose is of ______ concentration in blood?**
   a. <30% b. 30–60%
   c. 60–80% d. 40–50%
247. **A 32-year-old AIDS positive female presented with headaches and nuchal stiffness. On lumbar puncture examination clear CSF was obtained with leucocytes >100/cu.mm. India ink staining was positive. The most probable diagnosis is?**
   a. Candida meningitis b. Tubercular meningitis
   c. Cryptosporidium d. Cryptococcus meningitis
248. **A man has acute onset of paraplegia with symmetrical bilateral areflexia. Diagnosis is:**
   a. Acute transverse myelitis
   b. Subacute combined degenerative disorder
   c. Guillian Barre syndrome
   d. Poliomyelitis

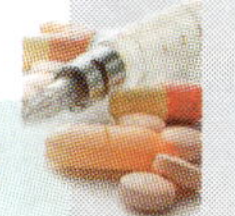

249. Boxers present with:
a. Epidural hemorrhage
b. Subdural hemorrhage
c. Sub arachnoid hemorrhage
d. Intra ventricular hemorrhage

250. All of the following are causes of primary headache; EXCEPT:
a. Migraine b. Tension headache
c. Cluster headache d. Sinusitis

251. DOC for listeria meningitis:
a. Ampicillin b. Cefotaxime
c. Cefotriaxone d. Ciprofloxacin

252. DOC for Herpes simplex encephalitis:
a. Acyclovir
b. Inosine prabonex
c. Intravenous immunoglobulins
d. Amphotericin B

253. SSPE is seen in?
a. Rubella b. Mumps.
c. Measles d. Chicken pox

254. All are seen in Horner syndrome; EXCEPT:
a. Ptosis b. Miosis
c. Hyperhidrosis d. Enophthalmos

255. Which is not a part of lower motor neuron:
a. Anterior nerve root b. Peripheral ganglia
c. Peripheral nerve d. Anterior horn cell

256. Most common brain tumor?
a. Astrocytoma b. Glioblastoma Multiforme
c. Meningioma d. Ependymoma

257. Increased intra-cranial tension leads to?
a. Hyotension and tachycardia
b. Hypertension and tachycardia
c. Hypertension and bradycardia
d. Hypotension and bradycardia

258. In increased intracranial pressure which is the first cranial nerve to be affected first?
a. 3rd b. 4th
c. 5th d. 6th

259. A road traffic accident patient in the casualty is comatose with unilaterally dilated pupil. The NCCT of the patient shows a Lesion peripherally present with concavo – convex border. What is the probable diagnosis?
a. Sub-dural hematoma
b. Epi-dural hematoma,
c. Sub-arachnoid hemorrhage
d. Intra-parenchymal bleeding

260. Extradural hemorrhage on NCCT is visualized as?
a. Hyperdense biconvex b. Hypodense biconcave
c. Hyperdense biconcave d. Hypodense biconvex

261. The submerged part of cerebral cortex is?
a. Insula b. Broadman area
c. Corpus callosum d. Piriform sulcus

262. Investigation of choice for sub-arachnoid hemorrhage is:
a. NCCT b. MRI
c. CECT d. MRA

263. Wernicke's aphasia is characterized by all; EXCEPT:
a. Non fluent speech b. Poor comprehension
c. Poor repetition d. Para-phasia

264. Most common benign brain tumor?
a. Meningioma b. Oligodendroglioma
c. Ependymoma d. Medulloblastoma

265. Lewy bodies are seen in:
a. Parkinsonism b. Alzheimer's disease
c. Huntington chorea d. All of above

266. Least chances of seizures are seen with?
a. Hypoglycemia b. Hypocalcemia
c. HIV encephalopathy d. Neuro-cysticercosis

267. A patient presents with headache and nuchal rigidity. Lumbar puncture was performed and CSF shows normal protein and normal glucose with clear CSF. Microscopic examination of CSF showed 50 lymphocytes/cu.mm with lymphocytic pleocytosis. What is the diagnosis?
a. Bacterial meningitis b. Viral meningitis
c. TB meningitis d. Aseptic meningitis

268. Which of the following is not seen in tubercular meningitis?
a. Evidence of old pulmonary lesions or a miliary pattern is found on chest radiography
b. Culture of CSF is diagnostic in majority of cases and remains the gold standard.
c. It is seen most often in young children but also develops in adults.
d. Cerebrospinal fluid reveals a low leukocyte count.

269. CSF finding in Gullian Barre syndrome is?
a. Normal cells with increased protein
b. Increased protein with normal cells
c. Normal cells and normal protein
d. Increased cells with low sugar

270. Which is the earliest symptom of Parkinson's disease?
a. Tremors b. Rigidity
c. Bradykinesia d. Chorea

271. Which of the following is *not* a feature of Parkinsonism?
a. Chorea b. Recurrent falls
c. Tremors d. Freezing

272. Earliest feature of parkinsonism?
a. Anosmia b. Rigidity
c. Postural instability d. Freezing

273. Which of the following is not the feature of upper motor neuron disease?
a. Hypotonia b. Spasticity
c. Weakness of muscles d. Superficial reflex absent

274. Incorrect about LMN defect?
a. Flaccid paralysis b. Muscular hypertrophy
c. Hypo-reflexia d. Superficial reflex present

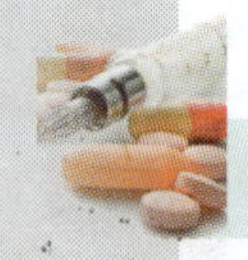

275. Right 12th nerve damage leads to:
- a. Tongue deviation to left on protrusion
- b. Tongue deviation to right on protrusion
- c. Nasal twang to voice
- d. Scanning speech defects

276. Which of the following tests are helpful in diagnosing neural tube defect?
- a. Acetyl choline esterase in the amniotic fluid
- b. Alpha-ketoglutarate in the amniotic fluid
- c. Glutamate in the amniotic fluid
- d. Beta hydroxyl butyrate in the amniotic fluid

277. Protein deposited in Alzheimer's disease is:
- a. Tau protein
- b. Alpha synuclein protein
- c. Huntington protein
- d. Protein 14.3.3

278. Unilateral ptosis is not seen in?
- a. Myasthenia gravis
- b. Thyroid ophthalmopathy
- c. Marfan syndrome
- d. Pancoast tumor

279. A patient after an accident was unconscious. On physical examination there was unilateral papillary dilatation. Possible reason for the same is?
- a. Uncal herniation
- b. Tonsillar herniation
- c. Cingulate herniation
- d. Transcalvarial herniation

280. Most common site of brain hemorrhage is?
- a. Putamen
- b. Internal capsule
- c. Ventral pons
- d. Cerebellum

281. Investigation of choice for myasthenia gravis?
- a. Single fiber E.M.G
- b. Muscle biopsy
- c. Nerve conduction velocity
- d. Anti-acetylcholine receptor antibody

282. CSF is absorbed by:
- a. Choroid plexus
- b. Sub-arachnoid granulations
- c. Dura matter
- d. Pia matter

283. Incorrect about dementia pugilistica:
- a. Seen in boxers
- b. Difficulty in gait
- c. Decreased cognition
- d. Nystagmus

284. Most common cause of cerebro vascular accident:
- a. Infection
- b. Hemorrhage
- c. Embolism
- d. Aortic dissection

285. Korsakoff psychosis is seen in:
- a. Thiamine deficiency
- b. Riboflavin deficiency
- c. Niacin deficiency
- d. Cyanacobalamin deficiency

286. Two point discrimination test exhibits maximum sensitivity in?
- a. Shin
- b. Toes
- c. Finger pads
- d. Soles

287. A patient presented with right sided hemiplegia while on warfarin. Which of the following will be the initial investigation of choice?
- a. Chest X-ray
- b. CT-scan
- c. MRI
- d. PET-scan

288. Hemiballismus is due to lesion in:
- a. Ipsilateral caudate nucleus
- b. Contralateral sub-thalamic lesion
- c. Contralateral Putamen
- d. Ipsilateral sub-thalamic lesion

289. Pontine stroke is due to involvement of?
- a. Basiliar artery
- b. Middle cerebral artery
- c. Middle meningeal artery
- d. Anterior communicating artery

290. Which vessel does not contribute to circle of Willis:
- a. Middle cerebral artery
- b. Anterior cerebral artery
- c. Posterior cerebral artery
- d. Internal carotid artery

291. Duret hemorrhage is?
- a. Traumatic brain hemorrhage in contre-coup injury
- b. Adrenal hemorrhage in water house friderichsen
- c. Brain hemorrhage due to tear of basiliar artery branches
- d. Petechial hemorrhages in fat embolism

292. Which of the following is not a feature of Wernicke's encephalopathy:
- a. Global confusion
- b. Ophthalmoplegia
- c. Ataxia
- d. Aphasia

293. Broca's aphasia is characterized by:
- a. Non-fluent aphasia
- b. Word salad
- c. Anomia
- d. Apraxia

294. Which of the following cranial nerve is first compressed in unruptured berry aneurysm?
- a. 3rd nerve
- b. 4th nerve
- c. 5th nerve
- d. 6th nerve

295. Which of the following is not a test for integrity of 7th and 9th nerve:
- a. Position of uvula
- b. Palate symmetry
- c. Taste
- d. Tongue protusion

296. Cranial Nerve 8 palsy causes all; EXCEPT:
- a. Loss of gag reflex
- b. Vertigo
- c. Motion sickness
- d. Tinnitus

297. A patient is unable to solve mathematical calculations, which part of his brain is damaged?
- a. Temporal lobe
- b. Frontal lobe
- c. Parietal lobe
- d. Occipital lobe

298. Asymetrical Ptosis is seen in?
- a. Myasthenia gravis
- b. Thyroid myopathy
- c. Drug induced myopathy
- d. Duchenne's muscular dystrophy

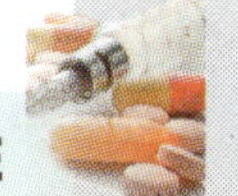

299. Cut off for T.I.A definition?

a. 12 hours b. 24 hours
c. 48 hours d. 36 hours

300. What are nitrergic neurons:

a. Postganglionic neurons releasing nitric oxide
b. 1st order neurons releasing nitric oxide
c. Post ganglionic neurons releasing substance P
d. 1st order neurons releasing calcitonin gene related peptide

301. Stenosis of aqueduct of sylvius results in?

a. Enlargement of lateral ventricles
b. Enlargement of fourth ventricle
c. Enlargement of lateral and third ventricle
d. Enlargement of lateral and fourth ventricle

ENDOCRINOLOGY

302. Necrolytic migratory erythema is seen in: *(Most Recent Question June 2022)*

a. Insulinoma b. Glucagonoma
c. Somatostatinoma d. VIPoma

303. What is the treatment of Hyperthyroidism in first trimester? *(Most Recent Question June 2022)*

a. PTU b. Carbimazole
c. Methimazole d. Lugol's Iodine

304. A 25-year-old male who is trying to have a baby for last 2 years is found to have azoospermia. Physical examination shows scattered pubic hair with Gynecomastia and hypogonadism Diagnosis is? *(Most Recent Question June 2022)*

a. Klinefelter Syndrome b. Turner Syndrome
c. Down syndrome d. Edward syndrome

305. A known case of sarcoidosis presents with nausea and vomiting. Serum Calcium level – 12.5 mg%. Which of the following is least useful for this patient? *(Most Recent Question Dec 2021)*

a. Mineralocorticoids b. Bisphosphonates
c. Glucocorticoids d. Normal Saline

306. A 65-year-old male presented with weakness, lethargy, excessive cold intolerance and slow ankle jerk. On TFT. TSH =16 mU/L (normal: 0.4–4.0 mU/L) and T4 = 0.3 ng/dL (normal: 0.6–1.6 ng/dL) and T3 = 70 pg/dL (normal: 230–619 pg/dL). What would be the most appropriate management? *(Most Recent Question Dec 2021)*

a. Start levothyroxine at 100 microgram and decrease the dose gradually
b. Start levothyroxine at 25 microgram and increase the dose gradually
c. Start levothyroxine at 25 microgram and decrease the dose gradually
d. Give Liothyronine and Levothyroxine simultaneously

307. Patient has palpitations and episodic Hypertension and diaphoresis. Which of the following tests must be done to identify? *(Most Recent Question Dec 2021)*

a. Urinary Metanephrine and VMA
b. Urinary 5HIAA
c. Urinary HVA levels
d. Urinary Chromogranin A levels

308. GH hormone levels is high but IGF-1 levels are low. Diagnosis is? *(Most Recent Question Dec 2021)*

a. GH receptor defect b. GH Levels deficiency
c. GHRH deficiency d. GnRH deficiency

309. While doing preop check up for cataract surgery you notice that a patient has lemon yellow tint of skin and the following tongue appearance. This would occur due to? *(Most Recent Question Dec 2021)*

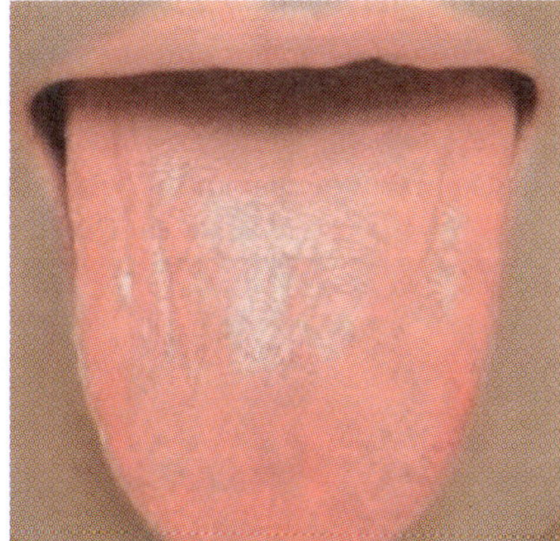

FIGURE: Darken skin of person

a. Vitamin B_{12} deficiency b. Vitamin C deficiency
c. Carnitine deficiency d. Vitamin B_1 deficiency

310. A patient presents with head, hand enlargement with gynecomastia and lactation. Where is the tumor located? *(Most Recent Question Dec 2020)*

a. Anterior pituitary
b. Posterior pituitary
c. Hypothalamus
d. Adrenal gland

311. What is the likely diagnosis of this case? *(Most Recent Question Dec 2020)*

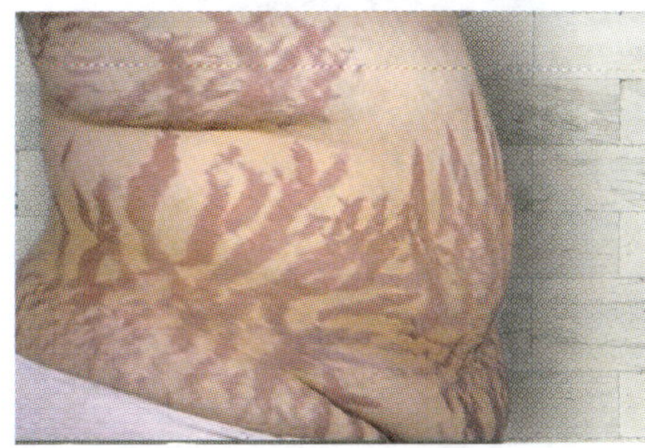

a. Cushing syndrome b. PCOD
c. Acromegaly d. Conn syndrome

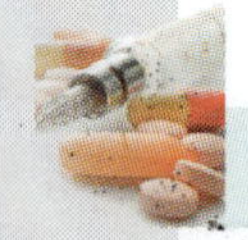

312. A DM patient will develop which macrovascular complication after 20 years? *(Most Recent Question Dec 2020)*

a. Retinopathy
b. Neuropathy
c. Coronary artery disease
d. Nephropathy

313. A 35-year-old recently divorced male is suffering from palpitations, headache and diaphoretic episodes on recurrent basis. He has visited the psychiatrist multiple times. What should be the next best step for management of this case? *(Most Recent Question Aug 2020)*

a. He should visit psychologist instead of psychiatrist
b. Check for catecholamines levels to rule out pheochromocytoma
c. Check for hyperthyroidism
d. Increase dose of anti-anxiety medication

314. A 45-year-old lady was diagnosed with ovarian tumor. She was lost to follow up but now the same patient has presented with gross abdominal distention and the following test is being performed in the OPD by the physician. Comment on the finding being elicited? *(Most Recent Question Aug 2020)*

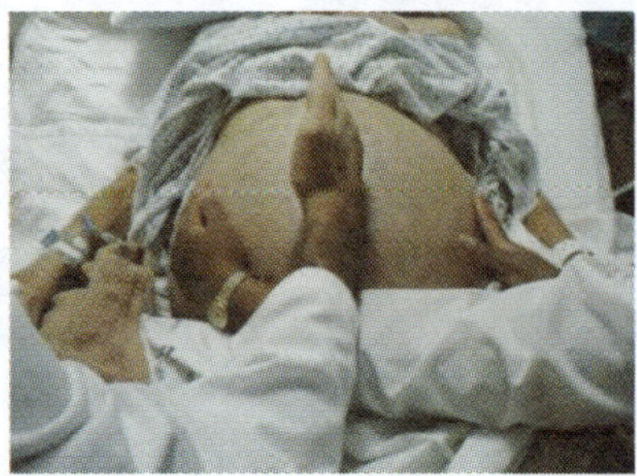

a. Fluid thrill
b. Shifting dullness
c. Puddle sign
d. Hingorani sign

315. A 35-year-old woman presented with complaints of palpitations and weight loss. On examination sinus tachycardia is present, and the following lesion was noticed on the shin of the patient. What is the clinical diagnosis? *(Most Recent Question Aug 2020)*

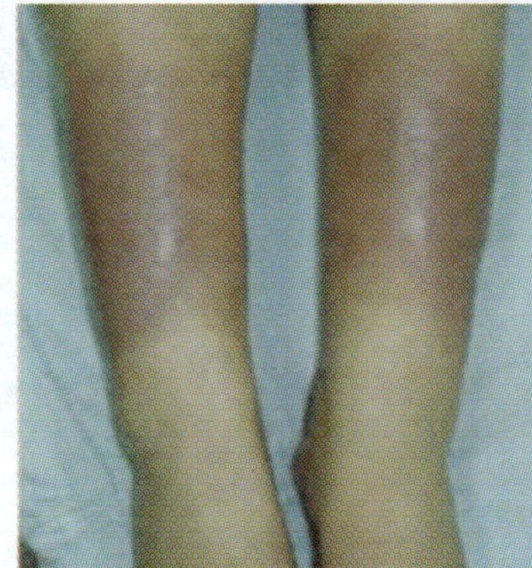

a. Hypothyroidism
b. Hyperthyroidism
c. Filariasis
d. Milroy disease

316. Most common cause of fulminant diabetes is? *(Most Recent Question 2019)*

a. Viruses
b. Diabetic Ketoacidosis
c. Non-ketotic hyperosmolar coma
d. Autoimmunity

317. Most common joint involved in diabetes is seen is? *(Most Recent Question 2019)*

a. Ankle
b. Knee
c. Shoulder
d. Foot

318. Which type of Insulin is used to manage a case of Diabetic ketoacidosis? *(Most Recent Question 2019)*

a. Regular
b. Lispro
c. Glargine
d. Aspart

319. Slow onset of action and lack of peak is seen with? *(Most Recent Question 2019)*

a. Glargine
b. Lispro
c. Regular
d. NPH

320. Most common characteristic physical finding of prolactinoma after galactorrhea is? *(Most Recent Question 2019)*

a. Bitemporal hemianopia
b. Anovulatory cycles
c. Amenorrhea
d. Infertility

321. An 18-year-old boy appears for army medical. On medical check-up his FBS = 120 and PP = 140 and HbA1c = 6.1%. What is the diagnosis? *(Most Recent Question 2019)*

a. Impaired glucose tolerance
b. Type 2 diabetes mellitus
c. Type 1 diabetes mellitus
d. Normal

322. Fulminant diabetes mellitus is seen in? *(Recent Pattern Question 2018-19)*

a. Diabetic ketoacidosis
b. Coxsackie B virus
c. Non-Ketotic hyperosmolar coma
d. Autoimmune pancreatitis

323. In a newly diagnosed case of sick child with Type 1 diabetes mellitus (DM), insulin was given. Which of the following will increase? *(Recent Pattern Question 2018)*

a. pH
b. Breathing rate
c. Glucosuria
d. Urine osmolality

324. All of the following syndromes are seen with obesity; EXCEPT:

a. Prader-Willi syndrome
b. Cushing syndrome
c. Laurence Moon-Biedl syndrome
d. Carcinoid syndrome

325. Which of the following is associated with elevated alkaline phosphate, low calcium with low phosphate? *(Recent Pattern Question 2018)*

a. Paget's disease
b. Osteoporosis
c. Primary hyperparathyroidism
d. Vitamin D deficiency

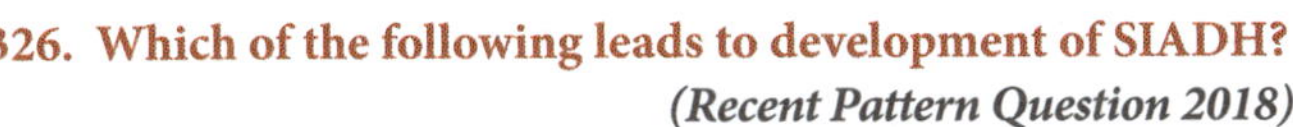

326. Which of the following leads to development of SIADH? ***(Recent Pattern Question 2018)***

a. Head trauma b. Pituitary adenoma
c. Lithium d. All of the above

327. Which of the following is seen in secondary thyrotoxicosis but not in Grave's disease? ***(Recent Pattern Question 2017)***

a. Lid retraction b. Lid lag
c. Exophthalmos d. Atrial fibrillation

328. A 15-year-old Type I DM patient presents to O.P.D. When should you recommend the patient to come for follow-up visits for microvascular complications evaluation? ***(Recent Pattern Question 2017)***

a. 1 year b. 5 years
c. 10 years d. 20 years

329. Nephrognic DI occurs due to defect in?

a. Na-K ATPase b. SGLT-2
c. Aquaporin 1 d. Aquaporin 2

330. Which is the gene involved in pathogenesis of Type 1 Diabetes mellitus? ***(Recent Pattern Question 2017)***

a. CTLA-4 b. ABCD1
c. HNF-1 Alpha d. HNF-4 Alpha

331. Which is the most common tumor of pituitary? ***(Recent Pattern Question 2017)***

a. Non-functioning adenoma
b. Prolactinoma
c. ACTH producing adenoma
d. Oncocytoma

332. Which chromosome is responsible for most common type of MODY? ***(Recent Pattern Question 2017)***

a. Chromosome 11 b. Chromosome 12
c. Chromosome 13 d. Chromosome 14

333. Which is not a diabetic patient? ***(Recent Pattern Question 2016)***

a. FBS = 136 mg% b. 2 hour value = 180 mg%
c. HbA1c = 7% d. RBS > 210 mg%

334. Cause of death in diabetic ketoacidosis? ***(Recent Pattern Question 2017)***

a. Cerebral edema b. Dehydration
c. Electrolyte imbalance d. Central pontine myelinosis

335. Hyperpigmentation is seen with excess of which hormone?

a. FSH b. LH
c. TSH d. ACTH

336. Female with blood sugar of 600 mg% and sodium of 110 mEq. Insulin was given, what will happen to serum sodium levels?

a. Sodium increase b. Sodium decrease
c. Sodium unaffected d. Relative sodium deficiency

337. Which is most common type of Diabetic neuropathy?

a. Sensory polyneuropathy b. Autonomic neuropathy
c. Radiculopathy d. Myelopathy

338. Lady 45 years of age presents with decreased oestrogen level, increased testosterone and temporal hair recession. Diagnosis is?

a. Osteoporosis
b. Rheumatoid arthritis
c. P.C.O.D
d. Granulosa theca cell tumor

339. Which of the following present with hypothyroidism?

a. Struma ovarii b. Grave's disease
c. Myasthenia gravis d. Toxic multinodular goiter

340. Earliest finding in Diabetic nephropathy is:

a. Shrunken kidney is hallmark
b. Fibrin Caps
c. Elevated Creatinine Clearance
d. Urine albumin > 30 mg/gm of urinary creatinine

341. Aldosterone is secreted by:

a. Pituitary b. Zona glomerulosa
c. Zona fasciculata d. Adrenal medulla

342. Glucose fever is related with:

a. Glucagonoma b. Parathyroid adenoma
c. Insulinoma d. Addison disease

343. All are seen in Addison's disease; EXCEPT:

a. Hyponatremia b. Hyperkalemia
c. Hypotension d. Metabolic alkalosis

344. In prolactinoma most common symptom other than galactorrhea is?

a. Bitemporal hemianopia b. Amennorhea
c. Thyroid dysfunction d. Headache

345. Turner syndrome presents with which heart defect?

a. Patent ductus arteriosus b. Atrial septal defect
c. Coarctation of aorta d. Ventricular septal defect

346. Rib notching is found in all the following; EXCEPT:

a. Neurofibromatosis b. Coarctation of aorta
c. Taussig bing operation d. Hypoparathyroidism

347. All are true about Hyperthyroidism; EXCEPT:

a. Anxiety b. Palpitations
c. Tachycardia d. Weight gain

348. Obesity in children is seen in:

a. Adrenal insufficiency
b. Pseudo-hypo-parathyroidism
c. Prader Willi syndrome
d. Soto syndrome

349. True about obesity?

a. Seen mostly in females
b. Prevalence decrease upto 40 years of age
c. No genetic predisposition
d. Smoking is a risk factor

350. Which is the best indicator for short term control (2–3 weeks) of blood glucose?

a. Serum fructosamine b. HbA1c
c. Blood sugar d. Urine sugar

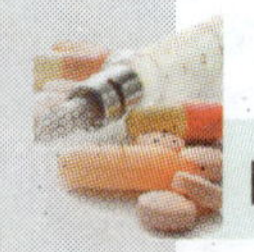

351. Post Prandial capillary glucose should be__________ mg/dl for adequate diabetes control:
a. <100 mg/dL b. <140 mg/dL
c. <180 mg/dL d. <200 mg/dL

352. All are true about Diabetes insipidus; EXCEPT:
a. Low urine osmolality
b. Dilutional hyponatremia
c. Water deprivation test is used for diagnosis
d. Polyuria

353. All are correct about SIADH; EXCEPT:
a. Normal KFT
b. Low uric acid
c. Relative hypernatremia
d. Normal BP with gain of water

354. Whipple's triad is useful for diagnosis of:
a. Insulinoma b. Glucagonoma
c. Somatostatinoma d. V.I.Poma

355. Best test for diagnosis of Carcinoid tumor:
a. 24-hour urinary 5H.I.A.A.
b. 24-hour catecholamines
c. 24-hour vaniylmandelic acid levels
d. 24-hour metanephrine levels

356. Which of the following is produced by carcinoid tumor?
a. G.A.B.A b. Serotonin
c. Epinephrine d. Norepinephrine

357. Most reliable marker for hypothyroidism:
a. T3
b. T4
c. TSH
d. Thyroxine binding globulin

358. Wolf Chaikoff effect is due to:
a. Iodine deficiency b. Excessive iodine
c. Iodine metabolism defect d. TPO enzyme deficiency

359. Which of the following is not a feature of thyrotoxicosis?
a. Palpitation b. Anxiety
c. Weight loss d. Menorrhagia

360. Proptosis not seen in?
a. Grave's disease b. Sarcoidosis
c. Pituitary Apoplexy d. Myxedema

361. All are true about Plummer Vinson syndrome; EXCEPT?
a. Glossitis b. Lower esophageal web
c. Anemia d. Premalignant condition

362. All of following are seen in GH deficiency; EXCEPT:
a. Hyperglycemia b. Stunting
c. Delayed bone age d. High pitched voice

363. Vitamin D deficiency has all; EXCEPT:
a. Hypocalcemia b. Increased SAP
c. Increased PTH d. Hyperphosphatemia

364. Which of the following finding shall be seen in patient with hyper-parathyroidism?
a. Hypophosphatemia b. Hyperphosphatemia
c. Hypermagnesemia d. Hypomagnesemia

365. All are features of hyper-parathyroidism; EXCEPT:
a. Increase serum calcium
b. Decreased serum phosphate
c. Diarrhea
d. Nephrocalcinosis

366. Secretory diarrhea is caused by all; EXCEPT?
a. Medullary thyroid tumor b. Carcinoid Tumor
c. Celiac sprue d. Glucagonoma

367. Chorionic villus sampling is done for all; EXCEPT?
a. Downs b. Trisomy 21
c. Phenylketonuria d. Gastrochisis

368. Congenital adrenal hyperplasia due to 11 beta hydroxylase deficiency presents with all; EXCEPT?
a. Metabolic acidosis
b. Hypokalemia
c. Virilization
d. Hypertension

HEMATOLOGY

369. A family member is volunteering for Blood donation for a person with RTA. Before giving Blood transfusion, which of the following is not tested for?
(Most Recent Question June 2022)
a. HIV 1 and HIV2 b. Hepatitis B
c. Hepatitis A d. Hepatitis C

370. A 60-year-old man presents with 2-month history of weakness and pallor. Per abdomen shows moderate splenomegaly. Peripheral blood shows Hb = 10 gm/dL, leukocytosis and platelet 3 lac/cu. mm. P. smear shows metamyelocytes 15%, Promyeloblasts 30%, Myeloblast 45 %. Which of the following is the diagnosis?
(Most Recent Question June 2022)
a. ALL b. CLL
c. CML d. AML

371. A 60-year-old man presents with complaints of early satiety, progressive pallor and chronic abdominal pain for 6 months. Hb = 10 gm%, DLC shows basophilia and Platelet count = 6 lac/cu.mm. Bone marrow aspiration done shows band cells, myelocytes = 15%, Metamyelocytes = 20% and mature blasts of 9%. Which of the following is responsible for this presentation?
(Most Recent Question Dec 2021)
a. t(8:14) b. t(9:22)
c. t(2:8) d. t(8:22)

372. In a patient with Myeloma defining events, the next investigation to be done for diagnosis is:
a. FDG-PET-CT *(Most Recent Question Dec 2021)*
b. Bone scan
c. Serum electrophoresis
d. Somatostatin Receptor Scintigraphy

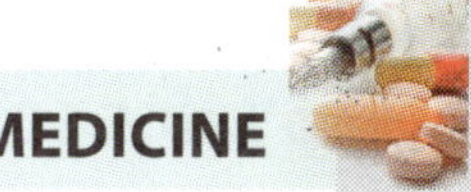

373. A 1-year-old boy fell down while playing with his sister and developed a big swelling on left knee joint. Which of the following is the possible etiology of this presentation? ***(Most Recent Question Dec 2020)***

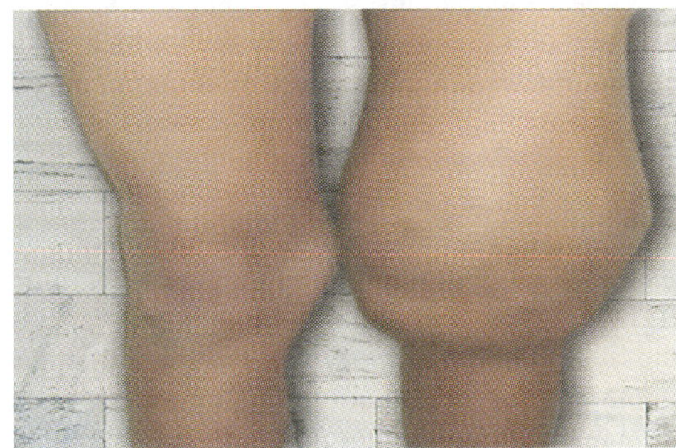

a. Von Willebrand disease
b. Factor 8 level deficiency
c. Glanzmann Thromboasthenia
d. Para – Hemophilia

374. A young girl presents with continuous menstrual bleed for 10 days on her first ever menses at the onset of menarche. Which test must be done in this case for evaluation? ***(Most Recent Question Dec 2020)***

a. Blood coagulation profile
b. Vitamin K levels
c. LFT
d. PFA-100

375. A 3-year-old child is suffering from progressive anemia. On examination spleno – hepatomegaly is noted with malar eminence prominence. Peripheral smear is shown here. The clinical diagnosis is? ***(Most Recent Question Dec 2020)***

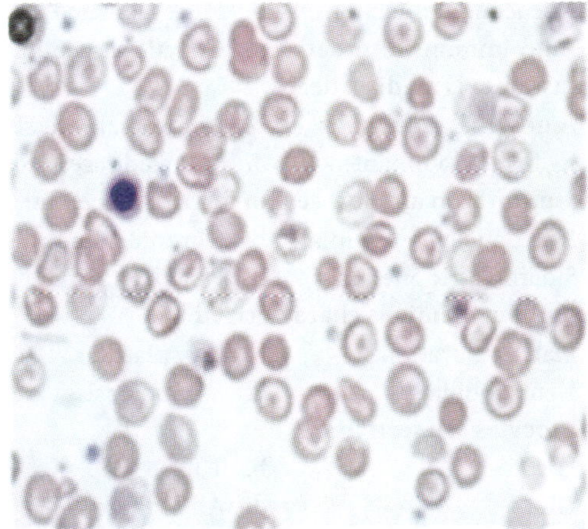

a. Thalassemia
b. Iron deficiency anemia
c. Sideroblastic anemia
d. Lead poisoning

376. Amyloid protein deposition seen in a patient undergoing recurrent hemodialysis is? ***(Most Recent Question Dec 2020)***

a. A beta
b. A-beta 2
c. A -Cal
d. AL

377. A young woman is having recurrent headaches and visual blurring episodes. Work up shows grossly elevated platelet count with normal WBC and RBC count. Possible diagnosis is? ***(Most Recent Question Dec 2020)***

a. Polycythemia vera
b. CML
c. Essential thrombocytosis
d. Myelofibrosis

378. A 50-year-old patient presented with gingival bleed and recurrent infection. Per abdomen examination shows hepato-splenomegaly. On peripheral smear large blasts with distorted N:C ratio were noted and 70% cells were found to be MPO positive. What is the diagnosis? ***(Most Recent Question Dec 2020)***

a. CML
b. AML
c. CLL
d. ALL

379. A child presents with difficulty in eating due to jaw swelling and enlarged cervical lymph nodes. Lymph node biopsy report is shown below. What is the clinical diagnosis? ***(Most Recent Question Dec 2020)***

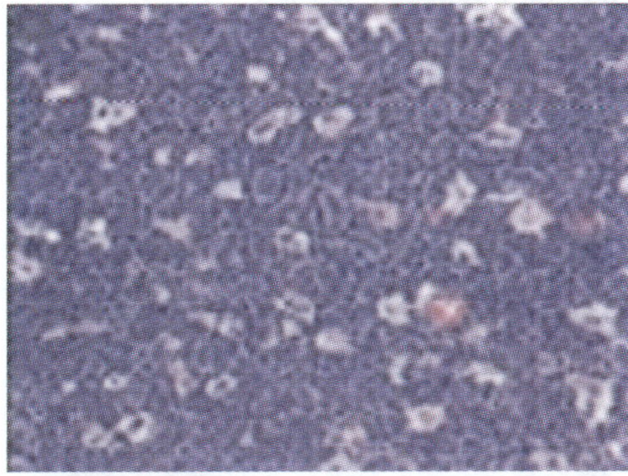

a. Hodgkin disease
b. Infectious mononucleosis
c. Kikuchi disease
d. Burkitt lymphoma

380. Comment on the diagnosis of peripheral smear shown below. ***(Most Recent Question Dec 2020)***

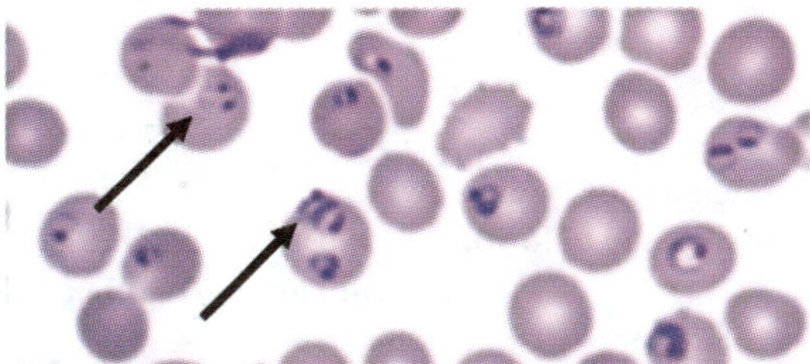

a. Dohle bodies
b. Falciparum malaria
c. Plasmodium vivax
d. Heinz bodies

381. An elderly chronic alcoholic patient presented to the OPD. The following findings were noted in the patient. What is the best investigation to be done in this patient? *(Most Recent Question Aug 2020)*

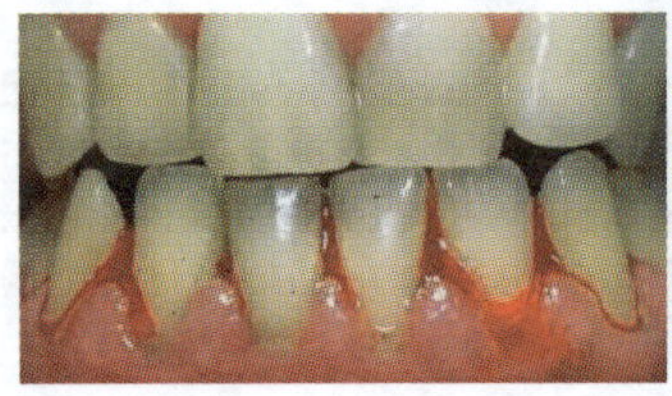
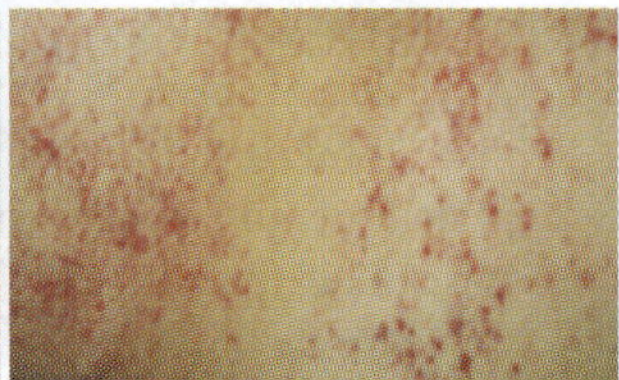

a. Plasma ascorbate levels
b. Factor 8 assay
c. RBC transketolase activity
d. Thrombin time

382. A 12-year-old girl has developed Acute ITP and is managed with steroids. There is recurrence of low platelet count once steroids were stopped. On current physical examination there are no petechiae or any physical evidence of bleeding. Which is the next line of treatment? *(Most Recent Question Aug 2020)*

a. Continue steroids as long they are effective
b. Splenectomy is required
c. Wait and watch as self-resolution will occur in most cases of acute ITP in children
d. Rho Immunoglobulin IV

383. The coagulogram of this patient shows increased Prothrombin time, activated partial thromboplastin time with platelet count of 1.2 Lacs/cu mm. The diagnosis is? *(Most Recent Question 2019)*

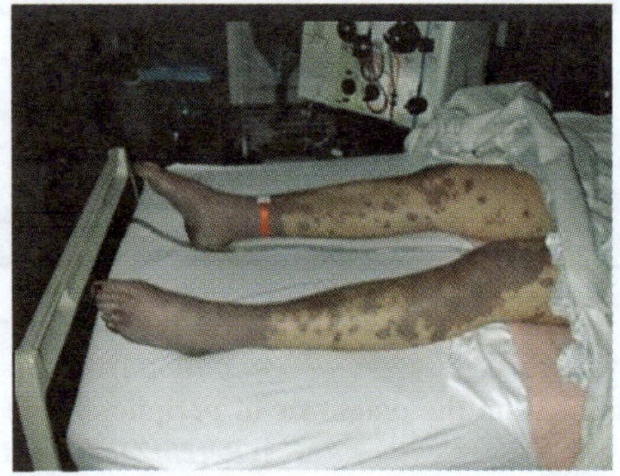

a. Henoch-Schonlein purpura
b. Porphyria
c. D.I.C
d. Acute ITP

384. Which of the following test is used for diagnosis of DIC? *(Recent Pattern Question 2018-19)*

a. Fibrin degradation products
b. Activated partial thromboplastin time
c. Prothrombin time
d. D- Dimer assay

385. In sickle cell crisis bone pain is due to: *(Recent Pattern Question 2018)*

a. Bone infarction
b. Osteoporosis
c. Osteomalacia
d. Periosteal reaction

386. A 35-year-old patient shows abnormal Schilling test. Antibiotics were given for 5 days which results in normalization of Schilling test. What is the diagnosis of the patient? *(Recent Pattern Question 2018)*

a. Bacterial overgrowth syndrome
b. Chronic pancreatitis
c. Atrophic gastritis
d. Ileocecal TB

387. HTLV-1 is associated with which disease: *(Recent Pattern Question 2016)*

a. AML
b. NHL
c. Adult T cell leukemia
d. AML

388. In cobalamin deficiency which is not seen?

a. Microcytic anemia
b. Long tract signs
c. Loss of proprioception
d. Rhomberg sign

389. Adult with progressive pallor, hyper-segmented neutrophils and MCV>100 shows?

a. Hereditary spherocytosis
b. Megaloblastic anemia
c. Dimorphic anemia
d. Thalassemia

390. Poikilocytosis and anisocytosis is seen in?

a. Megaloblastic anemia
b. Iron deficiency anemia
c. Nutritional deficiency anemia
d. Hereditary spherocytosis

391. 2-year-old child with ALL, which of the following has the best prognosis?

a. Age between 1 and 10 years
b. TLC >1 lac
c. Petechiae
d. t(9:22)

392. Blood transfusion associated acute lung injury occurs due to?

a. Nosocomial infections
b. HLA mediated
c. Auto-immune disorder
d. Genetic susceptibility

393. Thalassemia is an disorder?

a. Autosomal dominant
b. Autosomal recessive
c. X-linked dominant
d. X-linked recessive

394. Low serum iron and low serum ferritin is seen in:

a. Iron deficiency anemia
b. Chronic kidney disease
c. Sideroblastic anemia
d. Fanconi anemia

395. Thrombocythemia is characterized by:

a. Platelet elevation
b. Low platelets
c. Neutrophilia
d. Monocytosis

396. Schistocytes are seen in:

a. HUS
b. TTP
c. DIC
d. All of these

397. Correct about vitamin-K deficiency is?

a. Associated thrombocytopenia with prolonged bleeding
b. Deficiency is rarely seen, except in infants
c. Factor X is first to be affected
d. Warfarin causes Vitamin K deficiency

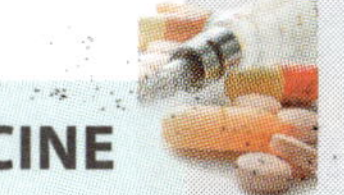

398. Hemolytic anemia is associated with the following gall stones:
a. Pigmented b. Mixed
c. Cholesterol d. None

399. A 60-year-old industrial worker presents with shortness of breath for the past week. Blood withdrawn shows thick brownish red color. Diagnosis?
a. Sickle cell anemia b. Hemolytic anemia
c. Meth-hemoglobinemia d. G-6-P-deficiency

400. All are true about cross-matching of blood; EXCEPT:
a. Mandatory in all cases except emergency
b. Recipient serum is tested against donor packed cells
c. Donor serum is tested against recipient packed cells
d. Involves visible agglutination

401. Bleeding time is increased in all; EXCEPT:
a. Dengue hemorrhagic fever
b. Von willebrand disease
c. Chronic liver disease
d. Bernard soulier syndrome

402. Blood is stored at blood bank at:
a. +4°C b. –4°C
c. + 24°C d. –60°C

403. Which of following is a myelo-proliferative disease?
a. Acute lymphatic leukemia
b. Acute myeloid leukemia
c. Chronic myeloid leukemia
d. Chronic lymphocytic leukemia

404. Which organism causes infection after splenectomy:
a. H. Influenzae b. Staph aureus
c. E. coli d. Klebsiella

405. Drug of choice in chronic myeloid leukemia:
a. Imitanib mesylate b. Fludarabine
c. Cladribine d. Pentostatin

406. Philadelphia chromosome refers:
a. Long arm of chromosome 9 and long arm of chromosome 22
b. Short arm of chromosome 9 and short arm of chromosome 22
c. Short arm of chromosome 9 and long chromosome 22
d. Long arm of chromosome 9 and short arm of chromosome 2

407. All are seen in Thalassemia major; EXCEPT
a. Macrocytic anemia b. Transfusion dependency
c. Hepato-splenomegaly d. Target cells

408. Which of the following is *not* a hyper-coagulable state
a. Pregnancy b. MI
c. Abruptio-placentae d. Cirrhosis

409. Elective splenectomy is done in
a. Hereditary spherocytosis
b. G6PD
c. Beta thalassemia
d. Sickle cell anemia

410. Priapism can be due to?
a. C.M.L b. Myelo-fibrosis
c. A.I.H.A. d. Thrombocytopenia

411. Hairy cell leukemia is
a. B cell tumor
b. T cell tumor
c. NK cell tumor
d. All of the above

GASTROINTESTINAL TRACT

412. Chronic alcoholic patient with C.L.D presents with sudden onset hematemesis. Which of the following is the most likely cause? *(Most Recent Question June 2022)*
a. Mallory Weiss syndrome
b. Esophageal bleeding varices
c. Perforation peptic ulcer
d. Boerhaave syndrome

413. A patient is identified as having a tumor in Ileum, leading to urinary 5HIAA being elevated. Diagnosis is?
a. Carcinoid tumor *(Most Recent Question June 2022)*
b. Neuroblastoma
c. Leiomyoma
d. Chromaffinoma

414. CLD patient presented to OPD with fever and gross abdominal distention. On abdominal examination tenderness is elicited. Ascitic fluid reveals presence of 500 cells/cu.mm. Which is the next best step?
(Most Recent Question Dec 2021)
a. Large volume paracentesis
b. IV albumin plus midodrine
c. IV Octreotide
d. IV ceftriaxone

415. The following Barium swallow shows:
(Most Recent Question Dec 2021)

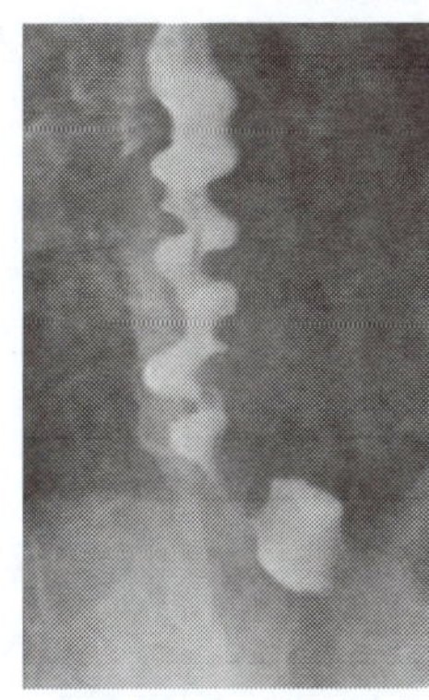

a. Diffuse esophageal spasm
b. Achalasia cardia
c. Cancer Esophagus
d. Pulsion diverticulum

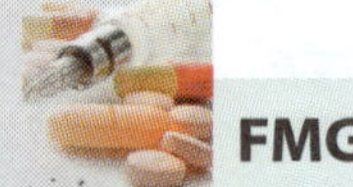

416. In a boarding school multiple kids eating from the same canteen have simultaneously developed symptoms of poor oral intake, jaundice and abdominal pain. Which of the following is the test to be done in them?
(Most Recent Question Dec 2020)

a. IgM HAV b. Ig G HAV
c. IgM HBV d. Ig G HBV

417. Comment on the diagnosis.
(Most Recent Question Dec 2020)

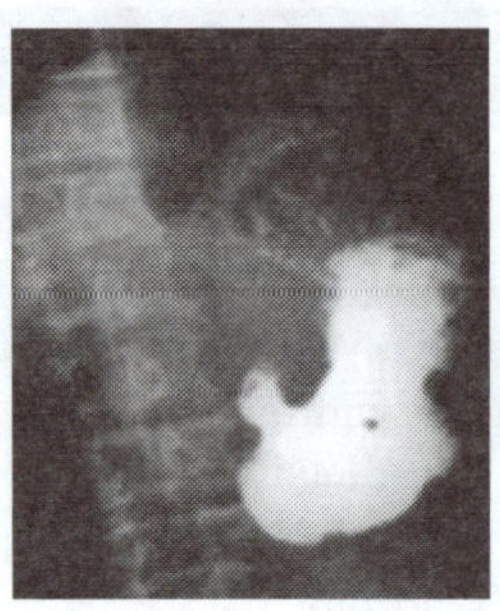

a. Portal gastropathy b. Pyloric stenosis
c. Esophageal varices d. Menetrier's disease

418. A 60-year-old man has presented with chronic projectile vomiting and significant weight loss. Which of the following electrolyte abnormality is seen in this patient?
(Most Recent Question Aug 2020)

a. Hypokalemic hypochloremic Metabolic alkalosis with Hyponatremia
b. Hypokalemic hypochloremic Metabolic alkalosis with Hypernatremia
c. Hypokalemic hypochloremic Metabolic alkalosis with Hypercalcemia
d. Hypokalemic hypochloremic Metabolic alkalosis with Hypomagnesemia

419. A 35-year-old patient with ulcerative colitis develops ulcer on the anterior compartment of the leg. Comment on the diagnosis of patient.
(Most Recent Question Aug 2020)

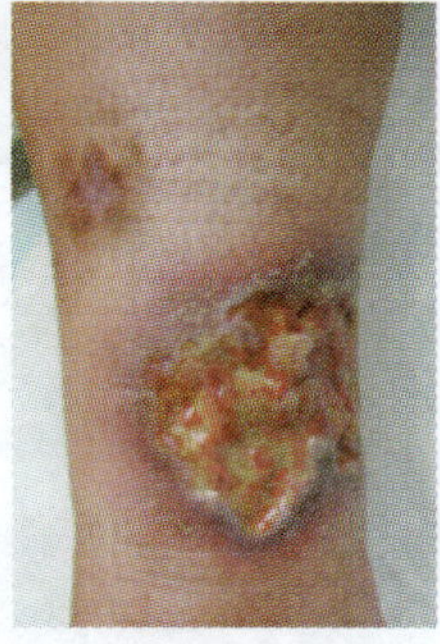

a. Venous ulcer
b. Erythema migrans
c. Erythema nodosum
d. Pyoderma gangrenosum

420. A 3-year-old child presents with steatorrhea, weight loss and features of malabsorption. Which test is done for confirmation of diagnosis? *(Most Recent Question 2019)*

a. Small intestinal mucosal biopsy
b. Fecal elastase
c. Benedict's test for reducing substances
d. Rectal mucosal suction biopsy

421. Which of the following is correct about cancer developing in Ulcerative colitis? *(Recent Pattern Question 2018-19)*

a. Not a premalignant condition
b. Incidence dependant on smoking history
c. Directly related to duration of disease
d. Increased risk in younger patients

422. Initial treatment for management of mild to moderate Crohn's disease is: *(Recent Pattern Question 2018)*

a. Mesalamine
b. Infliximab
c. Budesonide
d. Sulfasalazine

423. Which of the following is true about carcinoid tumor?

a. Occurs along structures derived from foregut
b. Presentation is hypertension and diaphoresis
c. Intestinal carcinoids are of high malignant potential
d. Best diagnosed by elevated urinary vanillylmandelic acid levels

424. Carcinoid tumor leads to increase in levels of?

a. 5-Hydroxy tryptamine ***(Recent Patter Question 2017)***
b. 5-Hydroxyindole acetic acid
c. Homovanillic acid
d. Vaniyl mandelic acid

425. Gastric cancer is caused by

a. Squamous metaplasia ***(Recent Pattern Question 2016)***
b. Blood group O
c. Intestinal metaplasia
d. Intestinal hyperplasia

426. Most common site of GIST?
(Recent Pattern Question 2016)

a. Stomach b. Jejunum
c. Ileum d. Colon

427. A lady presented with IDA and malabsorption. Most accurate test for diagnosis is?
(Recent Pattern Question 2016)

a. Antiendomysial antibody
b. Anti-tissue transglutaminase antibody
c. Antiepidermal tissue transglutaminase antibody
d. Antimitochondrial antibody

428. A patient presents with sensory ataxia and patchy loss of papilla on tongue, the first investigation to be done is?

a. B_{12} levels ***(Recent Pattern Question 2016)***
b. Punch biopsy of terminal ileum
c. Brush biopsy of terminal ileum
d. Serum iron studies

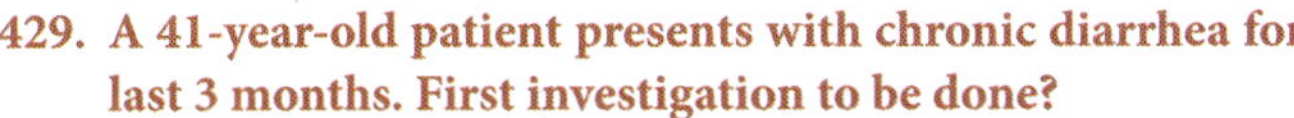

429. A 41-year-old patient presents with chronic diarrhea for last 3 months. First investigation to be done? *(Recent Pattern Question 2016)*

a. D-xylose absorption
b. Intestinal biopsy
c. Tissue transglutaminase antibody
d. Schilling's test

430. Patient presents with loss of tongue papilla. Hemoglobin = 9.5 gm% and MCV = 100 fl? *(Recent Pattern Question 2016)* **First investigation to be performed is?**

a. B_{12} estimation
b. Brush biopsy
c. Folic acid levels
d. Incision biopsy

431. Cushing ulcer is seen in? *(Recent Pattern Question 2016)*

a. Stomach
b. Duodenum
c. Jejunum
d. Ileum

432. Most common site of carcinoid tumor is?

a. Appendix
b. Ileum
c. Stomach
d. Rectum

433. A 45-year-old male is brought to casualty after a night party with complaints of epigastric pain, penetrating towards back. Which is the best for diagnosis?

a. Serum lipase
b. CPK-MB
c. ALP
d. Gamma- GGT

434. GERD is best diagnosed by?

a. 24-hour pH Monitoring
b. Upper GI endoscopy
c. Barium meal follow through
d. Barium Swallow

435. Which cereal is not to be given in celiac sprue?

a. Wheat
b. Maize
c. Corn
d. Rice

436. In ulcerative colitis, which is *not* true about malignancy?

a. Metaplasia
b. Low grade dysplasia
c. High grade dysplasia
d. Pleomorphism

437. Iron is absorbed from:

a. Duodenum with fast clearance
b. Jejunum with fast clearance
c. Ileum with low clearance
d. Bone marrow

438. Enteric fever on fourth day is best diagnosed by:

a. Stool test
b. Widal test
c. Urine test
d. Blood culture

439. Which of the following is seen on the image?

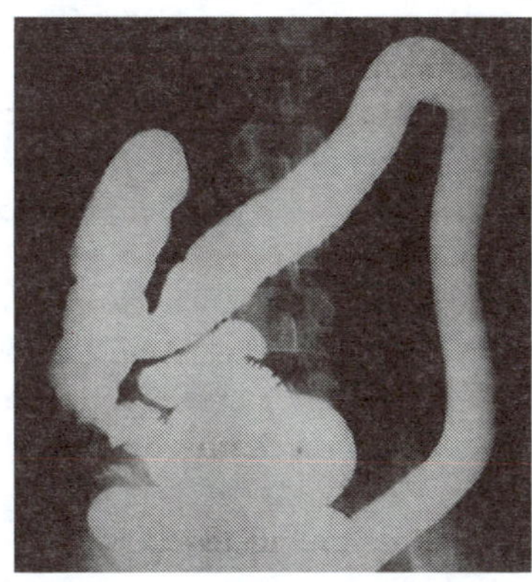

a. Barium enema = Pipe stem colon
b. Double contrast enema= Apple core appearance
c. Barium enema = Pseudo-polyps
d. Double contrast enema = Thumb printing sign

440. Which of the following is the most probable diagnosis of this X-ray abdomen?

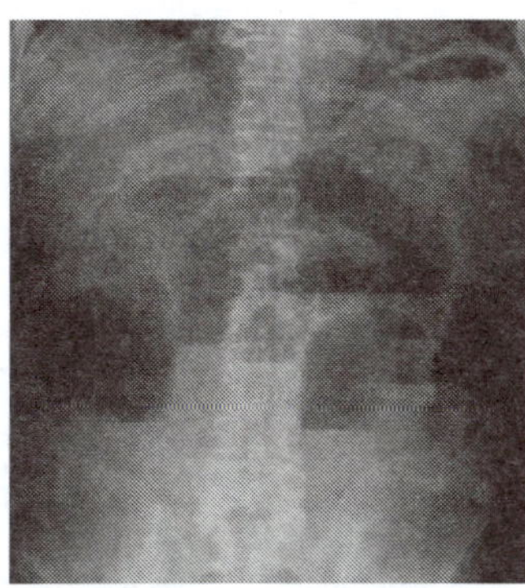

a. Gas under diaphragm- Peritonitis
b. Multiple air fluid level- Adhesions and bands
c. Bird beak – Volvulus
d. Normal X-ray PA view

441. Diagnosis:

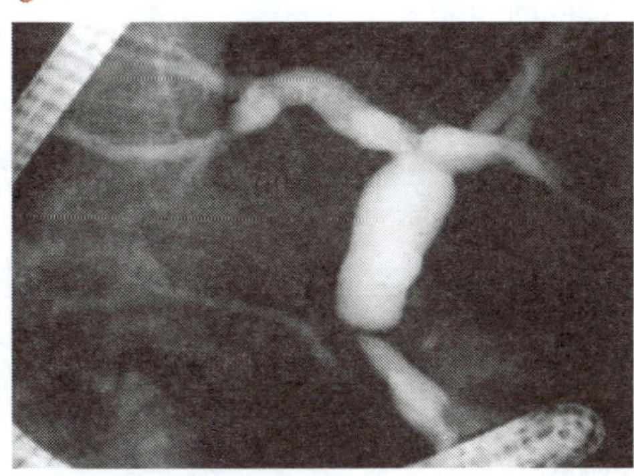

a. CBD dilatation on ERCP
b. CBD dilatation on PTC
c. Cystic duct dilation on ERCP
d. Cystic duct ectasia on ERCP

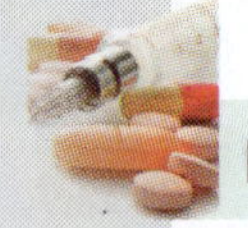

442. IOC for G.E.R.D:

a. 24-hour pH monitoring b. Upper G.I. endoscopy
c. Ultrasound d. X-ray abdomen

443. Aspirin is given in management of which cancer:

a. Pancreatic cancer b. Liver cancer
c. Colon cancer d. Stomach cancer

444. Cobble stoning of colon is seen in?

a. Crohn's disease b. Ulcerative colitis
c. Ischemic colitis d. Amoebic colitis

445. Which of the following is not true about Crohn's disease?

a. It can involve stomach and duodenum also
b. Skip lesion
c. All layers of intestine are involved
d. Invasion of lymph nodes seen

446. Which of the following is least likely to be seen with Crohn's disease:

a. Skip lesions b. Fistula
c. Toxic megacolon d. Transmural involvement

447. In which of the following conditions smoking is protective?

a. Ulcerative colitis
b. Crohn's disease
c. SLE
d. Alzheimer's

448. Barrett's esophagus causes which cancer:

a. Adenocarcinoma
b. Squamous cell CA
c. Carcinoid tumor
d. Esophageal leiomyoma

449. H. pylori causes all; EXCEPT:

a. Peptic ulcer
b. Maltoma
c. Carcinoid tumor
d. Gastric CA

450. Traveler diarrhea is caused by?

a. Campylobacter
b. Aeromonas
c. Actinobacillus
d. Cryptosporidium

HEPATOLOGY

451. Comment on this serological report of a hepatitis B patient ***(Most Recent Question Aug 2020)***

Ig G Anti HBc	Positive
HBsAg	Negative
HBeAg	Negative
Anti HBs	Positive

a. Acute hepatitis B, High infectivity
b. Chronic hepatitis B, High infectivity
c. Chronic hepatitis B, low infectivity
d. Previous infection with hepatitis B

452. A 40-year-old patient came to OPD with symptoms of excessive sleepiness and lethargy all the time. On physical examination the clinical features depicted in the images were seen. Per abdominal examination shows no free fluid in abdomen. Liver and spleen are not palpable. He tells of regular Alcohol consumption. Which is the most probable diagnosis? ***(Most Recent Question Aug 2020)***

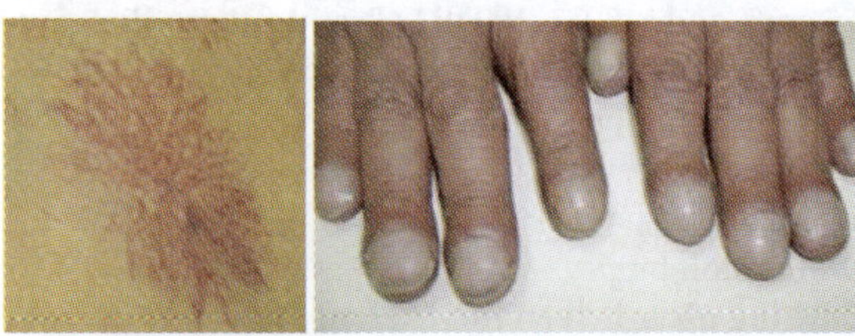

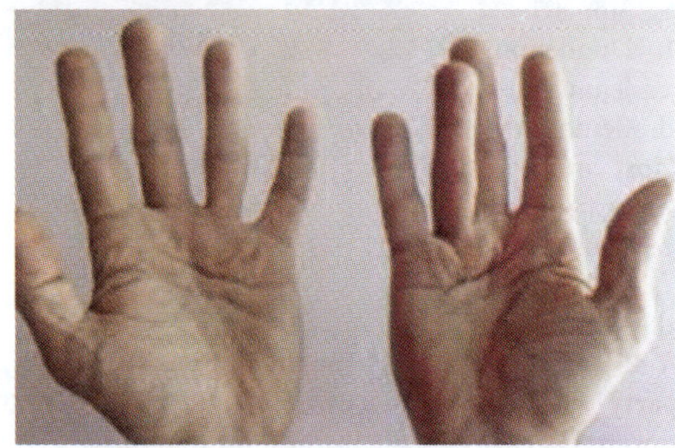

a. Hepatolenticular degeneration
b. Decompensated alcoholic cirrhosis
c. Portal hypertension
d. Budd chiari syndrome

453. Prophylactic CNS radiation is given for which of the following cancers? ***(Most Recent Question Aug 2020)***

a. Liver cancer
b. Lung cancer
c. Prostate cancer
d. Breast cancer

454. A 5-year-old boy has presented with multiple episodes of hematemesis. On admission his vitals are stable and splenomegaly is noted. The mother tells that at birth the boy had developed jaundice and an exchange transfusion procedure had been performed in the same hospital. What is the diagnosis? ***(Most Recent Question Aug 2020)***

a. Budd Chiari Syndrome b. Sinusoidal fibrosis
c. Portal vein thrombosis d. Non cirrhotic portal Fibrosis

455. Which of the following is not a component of Child Pugh classification? ***(Recent Pattern Question 2018-19)***

a. SGOT b. Bilirubin
c. Albumin d. Prothrombin time

456. Not a prehepatic cause of portal HTN? ***(Recent Pattern Question 2018-19)***

a. Budd Chiari syndrome b. Banti disease
c. Portal vein thrombosis d. Pyelophlebitis

457. Fatty liver with hepatomegaly is seen in: *(Recent Pattern Question 2018)*
- a. Marasmus
- b. Metabolic syndrome
- c. Wilson disease
- d. Nutmeg liver

458. Which is the best investigation for Wilson disease? *(Recent Pattern Question 2017)*
- a. KF ring
- b. Urine copper
- c. Serum copper
- d. Liver copper

459. Steatosis is due to: *(Recent Pattern Question 2016)*
- a. Triglycerides
- b. LDL
- c. VLDL
- d. Cholesterol

460. Central regulator of iron metabolism is: *(Recent Pattern Question 2016)*
- a. Transferrin
- b. Ferritin
- c. Ferroportin
- d. Hepcidin

461. In Wilson disease which of the following is useful?
- a. Iron
- b. Zinc
- c. Copper
- d. Selenium

462. In hemochromatosis, all are seen; EXCEPT:
- a. Hippocampal sclerosis
- b. Damage to Pancreas
- c. Hyperpigmentation of skin
- d. Restrictive cardiomyopathy

463. Most common chronic viral illness is caused by:
- a. Hepatitis A
- b. Hepatitis B
- c. Hepatitis C
- d. Hepatitis D

464. Palmar erythema in liver failure is due to:
- a. Coagulopathy
- b. Hyperbilirubinemia
- c. Hyperammonemia
- d. Estrogen

465. A man presented with (+) fever, chills and jaundice. Diagnosis:
- a. Acute Cholecystitis
- b. Acute cholangitis
- c. Choledocholithiasis
- d. Acute viral hepatitis

466. Fulminant liver disease is defined as encephalopathy, coagulopathy developing within how many weeks?
- a. 2 weeks
- b. 3 weeks
- c. 4 weeks
- d. 8 weeks

467. Most common cause of Fulminant hepatitis in pregnancy
- a. Hep B
- b. Hep C
- c. Hep D
- d. Hep E

468. Best marker for maternal to child transfer of hepatitis B virus?
- a. HBcAg
- b. HBxAg
- c. HBeAg
- d. IgM Anti- HBcAg

469. Spironolactone is most useful in?
- a. Cardiac Hypertrophy
- b. Cirrhotic ascites
- c. Exudative pleural effusion
- d. Renal artery stenosis

470. Raised Intra-abdominal pressure to consider abdominal compartment syndrome is?
- a. 0-12 mm Hg
- b. >12 mm Hg
- c. >20 mm Hg
- d. >30 mm Hg

471. Trans-esophageal echocardiography is better over trans-thoracic echocardiography in?
- a. Evaluation of left ventricle
- b. Evaluation of left atria and left Atrial appendage thrombus
- c. Evaluation of Pericardial fluid
- d. Evaluation of commissural fusion

472. Select the best answer from the picture of temperature charting of patient with history of constipation for over 2 weeks

Date	1st week							2nd week							3rd week							4th week			
Day of disease	1	2	3	4	5	6	7	8	9	10	11	12	13	14	15	16	17	18	19	20	21	22	23	24	25

Pulse	Temp.
170	108
160	107
150	106
140	105
130	104
120	103
110	102
100	101
90	100
80	99
70	98
60	97
50	96
40	95
Respirations	
Stools	

Temperature
Pulse

- a. Enteric fever
- b. Brucellosis
- c. Relapsing fever
- d. Hodgkin lymphoma

RHEUMATOLOGY

473. Comment on the cause of this presentation: *(Most Recent Question Dec 2021)*

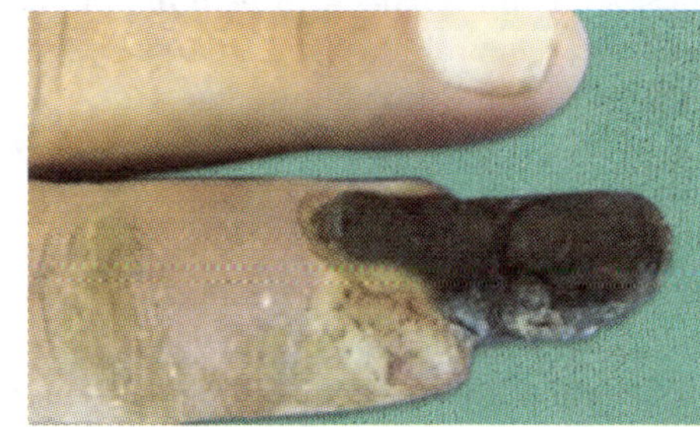

- a. Raynaud phenomenon
- b. Buerger's disease
- c. Fournier gangrene
- d. Ainhum

474. A young female complaints of feeling weakbess in blinking of eye, diplopia and having dysphagia. The symptoms are increased at end of day. The most likely diagnosis is? *(Most Recent Question Dec 2021)*
- a. Patterson kelly
- b. Thyroid disease
- c. M. Gravis
- d. Scleroderma

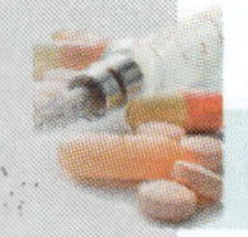

475. Comment on the image shown below:

(Most Recent Question Dec 2020)

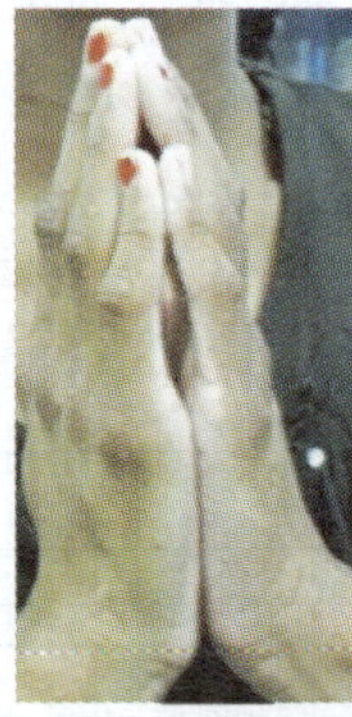

a. Prayer sign b. Phalen sign
c. Tinel sign d. Schamroth sign

476. A 47-year-old female with joint pains has difficulty in swallowing dry food and has gritting sensation below eyes. She has NCNC anemia with increased ESR, positive ANA, Anti Ro antibody. What is the diagnosis?

(Most Recent Question Dec 2020)

a. Sjogren syndrome b. Rheumatoid arthritis
c. Serum sickness d. SLE

477. A 30-year-old woman is suffering from progressive dysphagia. On examination she has thickening of oral mucosa and leather like skin. She is also hypertensive and has limited exercise capacity due to lung fibrosis. Which of the following is the possible diagnosis?

(Most Recent Question Dec 2020)

a. Peutz Jehgers syndrome b. Post cricoid dysphagia
c. Achalasia cardia d. Scleroderma

478. An obese woman presents with pain in both knee joints and can hear sound of click from knee joint while walking. What is the probable diagnosis?

(Most Recent Question Dec 2020)

a. RA b. AS
c. Reiter syndrome d. Osteoarthritis

479. A 30 year old female patient presented with pain in joints of hand with rash on dorsum of hand with extensive skin induration and skin tightening. Comment on the diagosis. *(Most Recent Question Aug 2020)*

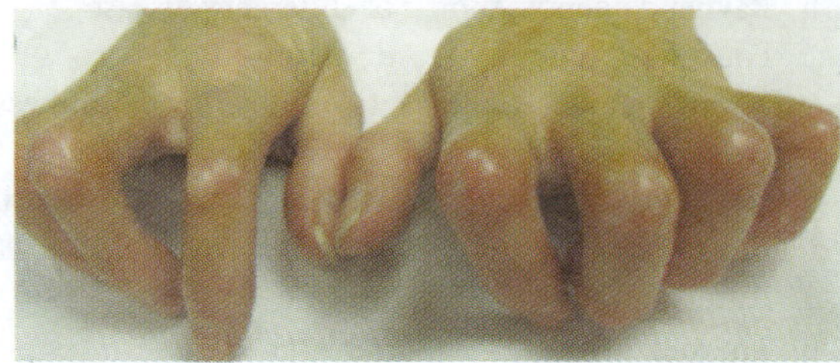

a. Rheumatoid arthritis b. Psoriatic arthritis
c. Osteoarthritis d. Scleroderma

480. A 60-year-old male patient presented with severe low back pain. Labs show a grossly elevated ESR, X-ray skull shows multiple punched out lesions. Which is the most important investigation to be done for this case?

(Most Recent Question Aug 2020)

a. Serum acid phosphatase
b. CT head with contrast
c. PET scan
d. Serum electrophoresis

481. Most common pulmonary manifestation of SLE:

a. Shrinking Lung syndrome
b. Pleuritis *(Most Recent Question 2019)*
c. Intra alveolar hemorrhage.
d. Interstitial inflammation

482. Which of the following cannot be diagnosed without positive ANA? *(Most Recent Question 2019)*

a. SLE b. Sjogren Syndrome
c. Drug induced lupus d. Scleroderma

483. Correct about Rheumatoid nodules?

(Recent Pattern Question 2018-19)

a. Tender, located on extensor surface and seen with arthritis
b. Non-tender, located on extensor surface and seen with arthritis
c. Non-tender, located on flexor surface and seen with arthritis
d. Tender, located on flexor surface and seen with arthritis

484. Which of the following is the best investigation for acute gout? *(Recent Pattern Question 2018)*

a. Serum uric acid b. Uric acid in synovial fluid
c. Uric acid in urine d. Anti CCP antibodies

485. Pulseless disease is: *(Recent Pattern Question 2017)*

a. Takayasu's arteritis
b. Raynaud phenomenon
c. Coarctation of aorta
d. Wegener's granulomatosis

486. Best Lab test for rheumatic fever?

(Recent Pattern Question 2016)

a. ASO b. CRP
c. Anti DNASe B d. Anti phospholipid

487. What is the effect of rheumatoid arthritis on the lung?

a. DL_{CO} normal *(Recent Pattern Question 2016)*
b. CXR is normal
c. Exudative pleural effusion
d. Flow volume pattern showing a obstructive pattern

488. In which of causes of oral ulcer, Auto-antibodies are not seen?

a. Behçet disease b. SLE
c. Pemphigus d. Celiac disease

489. Which antibody is incriminated in causing Henoch Schonlein Purpura?

a. IgA b. IgG
c. IgM d. IgD

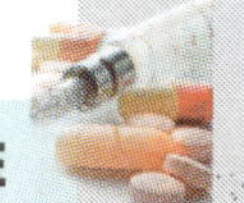

490. LE cells are seen in:
a. SLE b. Dermatomyositis
c. Sickle cell anemia d. Scleroderma

491. Wegener's granulomatosis is diagnosed by:
a. P-ANCA b. c-ANCA
c. m-ANCA d. A.N.A

492. Antibody in Goodpasture syndrome:
a. Lupus anticoagulant b. Anti-GBM antibody
c. Anti-Ro antibody
d. Anti- mitochondrial antibody

493. Which of the following condition does not cause multiple painful ulcers on tongue?
a. TB b. Sarcoidosis
c. Herpes d. Behçet's disease

494. Wrong about Duchenne muscular dystrophy is?
a. Pseudo-hypertrophy of calf muscles
b. Gower sign positive
c. Death occurs due to pneumonia
d. Female is symptomatic

495. Gower's sign is seen in
a. Duchenne muscular dystrophy
b. Congenital myopathy
c. Gullian barre syndrome
d. All of the above

496. Joint usually not involved in Rheumatoid arthritis?
a. D.I.P b. P.I.P
c. M.C.P d. Wrist

497. Correct about Wegener Granulomatosis is?
a. Both lung and kidney are involved
b. p-ANCA is positive
c. Seen with inflammatory bowel disease
d. Nongranulomatous vasculitis

498. All are seen in rheumatoid arthritis; EXCEPT:
a. Deformities
b. Mononeuritis multiplex
c. Peri-articular osteoporosis
d. Sero-negative arthritis

499. Which of the following is seen in sarcoidosis:
a. Hypercalcemia b. Hypocalcemia
c. Hyperphosphatemia d. Hypophosphatemia

500. Sequela of rheumatic heart disease in a 5 year old child is:
a. Mitral stenosis b. Mitral regurgitation
c. Tricuspid stenosis d. Tricuspid regurgitation

501. Which of the following is not a major Criteria for rheumatic fever?
a. Carditis b. Arthritis
c. Syndenham chorea d. ASO titer

502. All are major criteria for rheumatic fever; EXCEPT:
a. Pancarditis b. Chorea
c. Deforming arthritis d. Subcutaneous nodules

503. All of the following are Jones criteria; EXCEPT:
a. Elevated ASO titers b. History of sore throats
c. Increased PR interval d. Arthritis

504. Which one of the following is not associated with anti (Ro) SSA antibody
a. Rheumatoid arthritis b. Sicca syndrome
c. Sarcoidosis d. Ankylosing spondylitis

505. Anti RO bodies are present in all; EXCEPT:
a. SLE
b. Sjogren syndrome
c. Neonatal lupus
d. Mixed connective tissue disorder

506. In Henoch schonlen purpura Ig and complement involved:
a. IgG, C 3 b. IgA, C 3
c. IgA, C 1 d. IgG, C 1

507. Which of these doesn't present with granulomatous Vasculitis?
a. Polyarteritis nodosa b. Wegener's
c. Churg strauss syndrome
d. Microscopic polyangitis

508. Martel sign is seen in?
a. Gout b. Ankylosing spondylitis
c. Osteoarthritis d. Rheumatoid arthritis

509. Lady presents with joint pain in both knees and low grade fever off and on. On examination she has a rash on sun exposed parts. Clinical diagnosis?
a. SLE b. Rheumatoid arthritis
c. Photo-dermatitis d. Porphyria

510. In long standing rheumatoid arthritis which will be seen?
a. Milk alkali syndrome b. Nephrolithiasis
c. Paradoxical aciduria d. Secondary amyloidosis

511. Rheumatoid arthritis is seen with?
a. HLA DR3 b. HLA DR4
c. HLA DR 27 d. HLA B 27

512. Gold is used for management of?
a. Ankylosing Spondylitis b. Rheumatoid arthritis
c. Psoriatic arthritis d. Rheumatic arthriitis

RESPIRATORY SYSTEM

513. A male smoker patient who has difficulty in swallowing is most likely to develop which of the following? *(Most Recent Question June 2022)*
a. Squamous cell cancer
b. Adenocarcinoma
c. Bronchoalveolar carcinoma
d. Large cell cancer

514. Comment on ABG report: pH = 7.28, pCO_2= 80 mm Hg and HCO_3= 28 mEq/L? *(Most Recent Question June 2022)*
a. Respiratory alkalosis
b. Respiratory acidosis
c. Metabolic acidosis
d. Metabolic alkalosis

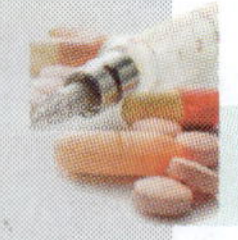

515. A patient presents with complaints of morning time productive cough that is yellow that increases on turning from left to right side. Which of the following lung diseases is likely to be present?

(Most Recent Question June 2022)

a. Lung cancer
b. Bronchiectasis
c. Bronchial asthma
d. Pulmonary embolism

516. A patient is having sudden exacerbation of dyspnea and can't talk. On chest auscultation prolonged expiration is noted. ABG report shows pH= 7.3, PCO_2= 68 mm Hg, HCO_3 = 43 meq/L. Which of the following intervention should be done in this child?

(Most Recent Question Dec 2021)

a. Intravenous soda bicarbonate
b. Ammonium chloride
c. NIV
d. Fluid resuscitation

517. 45-year-old patient presents with fever, weight loss and occasional hemoptysis. Diagnosis is?

(Most Recent Question Dec 2021)

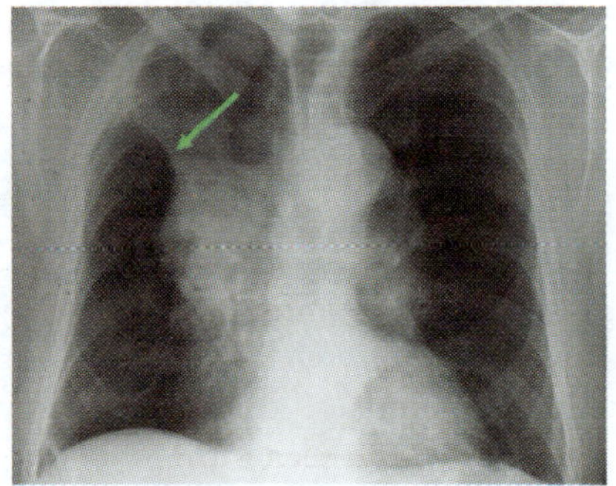

a. TB
b. Bronchogenic carcinoma
c. Mesothelioma
d. Aspergillus

518. A 40-year-old man presents with shortness of breath. On examination clubbing with bi-basiliar crepitations on auscultation is noted. Spirometry shows FEV1 = 60% with FEV1/FVC ratio of 0.9 with no response to bronchodilator. Diagnosis?

(Most Recent Question Dec 2021)

a. Chronic bronchitis
b. Bronchiectasis
c. Pulmonary fibrosis
d. Bronchogenic carcinoma

519. X-ray finding of COVID-19?

(Most Recent Question Dec 2021)

a. Ground glass opacities along the periphery
b. Apical coin shadow
c. Apical consolidation
d. Peripheral reticular opacities

520. Patient of COPD is on Salmeterol and still has dyspnea on exertion. What drug will be given next?

(Most Recent Question Dec 2021)

a. Systemic steroids
b. Roflumilast
c. Tiotropium
d. Hydrocortisone

521. Baby turns blue at birth that resolves on crying. What should be done next? ***(Most Recent Question Dec 2021)***

a. Intubation
b. Oropharyngeal Airway
c. C-PAP
d. Tracheostomy

522. Patient underwent surgery after fracture neck of femur. After 5 days he developed with sudden onset breathlessness. Diagnosis is:

(Most Recent Question Dec 2021)

a. Venous thrombo-embolism
b. Air embolism
c. Systemic embolism
d. Fat embolism

523. Investigations for Pulmonary embolism:

(Most Recent Question Dec 2021)

a. CTPA
b. CECT chest
c. Doppler
d. USG

524. A smoker presents with occasional bouts of cough and progressive shortness of breath. CXR was done followed by bronchoscopy. Which of the following is the likely etiology? ***(Most Recent Question Dec 2020)***

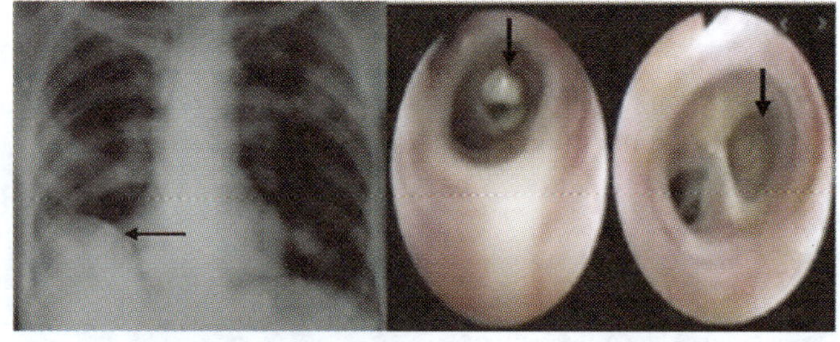

a. Pulmonary tuberculosis
b. Hydatid cyst
c. Bronchogenic carcinoma
d. Aspergillosis

525. Pleural effusion was tapped and pleural fluid protein was found to be 2.4 gm% while serum protein was 6 gm%. Pleural fluid LDH is 50 U/L while serum LDH is 200 U/L. What is the likely etiology of pleural fluid?

(Most Recent Question Dec 2020)

a. TB
b. CHF
c. Rheumatoid arthritis
d. Malignancy

526. On Post-operative day 2, routine X-ray of patient was performed. The patient is not complaining of any respiratory distress and is comfortable in hospital bed. On auscultation bilateral equal air entry is heard. What is the next step in the management of the patient?

(Most Recent Question Aug 2020)

a. Wait and watch and give supplemental oxygen if required
b. Perform needle thoracotomy urgently
c. Do a thoracostomy with wide bore tube and under water seal
d. Perform elective intubation and positive pressure ventilation

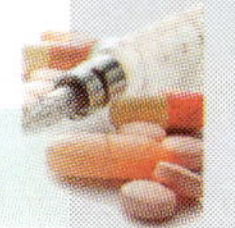

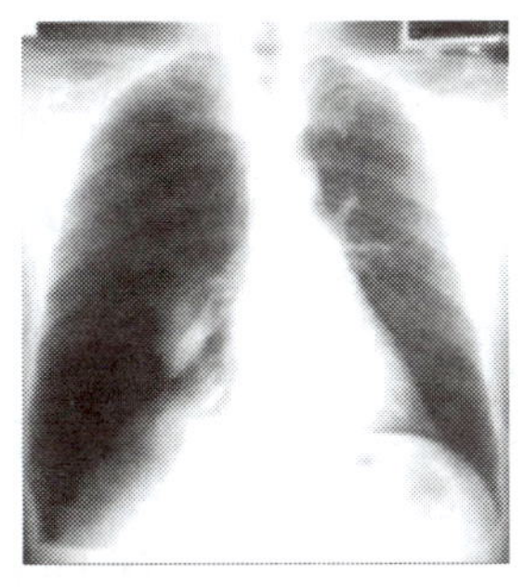

527. A 30-year-old woman has presented with complaints of fever for 3 days with SOB. On examination bronchial breathing is heard on right mammary area with normal air entry bilaterally. Comment on the diagnosis.
(Most Recent Question Aug 2020)

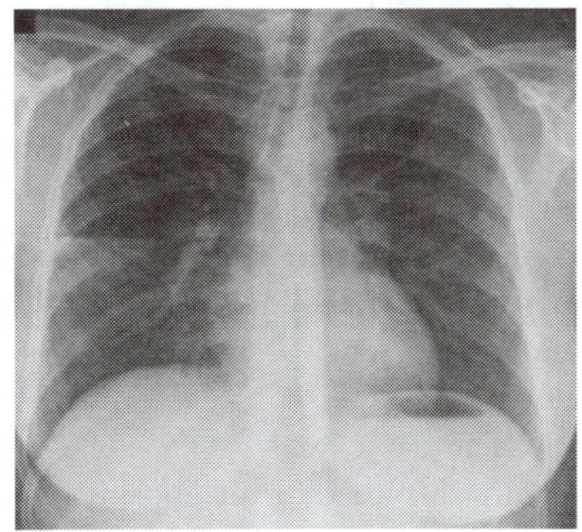

a. Right lower lobe pneumonia
b. Right middle lobe pneumonia
c. Right sided hydropneumothorax
d. Right sided Hydrothorax

528. Comment on the diagnosis of the Flow volume curve shown below: ***(Most Recent Question Aug 2020)***

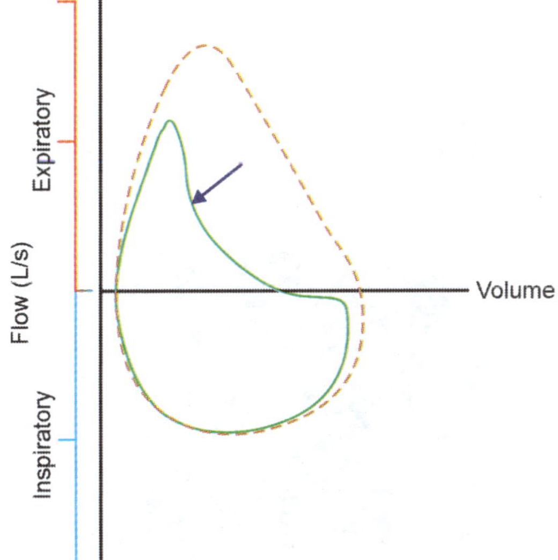

a. COPD
b. Interstitial lung disease
c. Retrosternal Goiter
d. Tracheal stenosis

529. A 28-year-old pregnant female presents with prolonged labor. Which Arterial Blood gas abnormality is expected to be present in this case?
(Most Recent Question Aug 2020)

a. Respiratory acidosis
b. Respiratory alkalosis
c. Metabolic acidosis
d. Metabolic alkalosis

530. A 30-year-old car driver was involved in an accident. He is brought to ER with complaints of breathlessness. On physical examination vitals are PR-110/min, BP = 90/60 mm Hg and temp of 37 degrees. Extensive bruising is noticed on right side of chest. An urgent bedside CXR was performed. ***(Most Recent Question Aug 2020)***

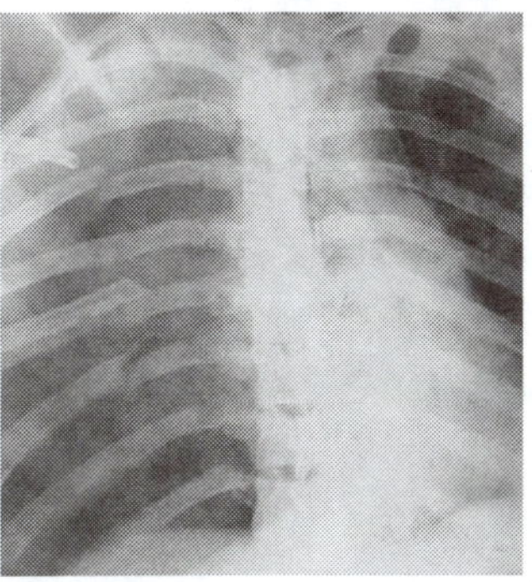

What is the best management of this case?

a. Thoracotomy
b. Thoracostomy
c. Elective intubation and PPV
d. Fluid resuscitation

531. A 30-year-old man who works in a glass factory presents with complaints of progressive shortness of breath on exertion. He is predisposed to development of which of the following? ***(Most Recent Question Aug 2020)***

a. Histoplasmosis
b. Tuberculosis
c. Mesothelioma
d. Pleural calcification

532. All are true about Allergic Bronchopulmonary aspergilloma; EXCEPT: ***(Recent Pattern Question 2018-19)***

a. Distal bronchiectasis
b. Increased in bronchial gland secretions
c. Increased Ig E
d. Seen in asthmatics

533. On putting a Subclavian vein catheter, a patient has developed sudden onset severe respiratory distress. Clinical diagnosis is? ***(Recent Pattern Question 2018-19)***

a. Pneumothorax
b. Sepsis
c. A.R.D.S
d. Nosocomial pneumonia

534. Which is correct about transudative pleural effusion?
(Recent Pattern Question 2018)

a. Pleural fluid protein to serum protein ratio <0.5
b. Pleural fluid LDH to Serum LDH >0.6
c. Pleural Fluid LDH more than 2/3 of upper reference limit for serum LDH
d. Pleural fluid sugar to blood sugar ratio >0.5

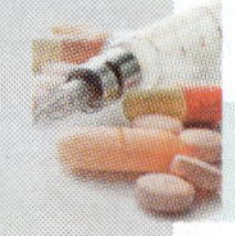

535. Which of the following is seen in COAD?
a. Chronic bronchitis *(Recent Pattern Question 2018)*
b. Follicular bronchiolitis
c. Desquamative pneumonitis
d. Chemical pneumonitis

536. A 26-year-old patient presents with a history suggestive of tuberculosis. On examination he has pleural effusion. All of the following parameters will be used for analysis of pleural fluid; EXCEPT: *(Recent Pattern Question 2017)*
a. Gene XPERT b. LDH
c. Albumin d. ADA

537. A 2 year malnourished child presents with fever, weight loss, tachypnea. CXR of the patient is shown below. What is the best treatment? *(Recent Pattern Question 2017)*

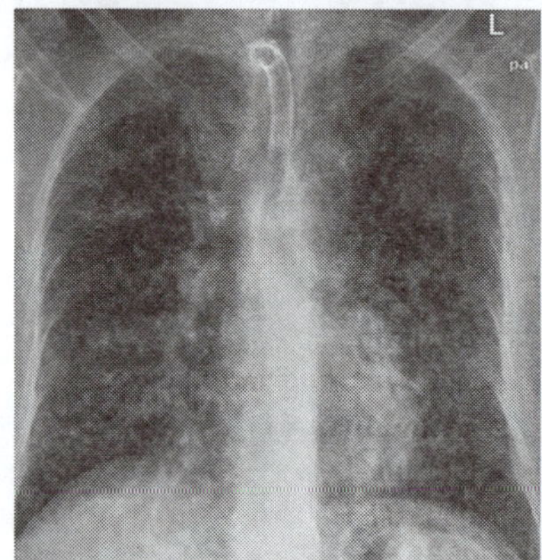

a. A.T.T
b. A.T.T plus steroids
c. Chloramphenicol
d. Clarithromycin + amoxicillin

538. Leukostasis syndrome affects which organ? *(Recent Pattern Question 2016)*
a. Liver b. Spleen
c. Kidney d. Lung

539. Drainage of hemothorax is done best through which space? *(Recent Pattern Question 2016)*
a. 2nd intercostal space b. 5nd paravertebral space
c. 5th midaxillary space d. 7th midaxillary space

540. Shock lung synonym is used for? *(Recent Pattern Question 2016)*
a. COPD b. Alveolar proteinosis
c. ARDS d. HMD

541. Pneumatocele is caused by? *(Recent Pattern Question 2016)*
a. Staphylococcus aureus
b. Streptococcus pyogenes
c. Hemophilus parainfluenzae
d. Mycoplasma pneumoniae

542. Hospital acquired pneumonia is treated by? *(Recent Pattern Question 2016)*
a. Azithromycin b. Doxycycline
c. Levofloxacin d. Vancomycin

543. A patient develops fracture of shaft of femur. On day 3, he develops respiratory distress and decrease SPO_2 and petechiae. Probable diagnosis is? *(Recent Pattern Question 2016)*
a. Hypostatic pneumonia b. Hemolytic pneumonia
c. Crush syndrome d. Fat embolism

544. Biot breathing is seen in:
a. Flail chest b. Uremia
c. High altitude d. Lesion in the brain

545. Which is the best test to be done for Pulmonary embolism?
a. D Dimer Assay
b. MRI
c. Ventilation perfusion scan
d. CT with IV contrast

546. Which of the following patients will not be able to respond to increased carbon dioxide levels?
a. Narcotic over-dosage
b. Obesity
c. Pulmonary edema
d. Type 1 respiratory failure

547. In HIV positive patient with pneumocystis jiroveci infection, which of the following is used for prevention?
a. Azithromycin
b. Acyclovir
c. Levofloxacin
d. Sulfomethoxazole and trimethoprim

548. Pop-corn calcification is seen with?
a. Pulmonary Hamartoma
b. Aspergillosis
c. Broncho-Alveolar cancer
d. Pulmonary Embolism

549. ARDS is characterised by all; EXCEPT?
a. Decreased surfactant
b. Alveolar transudate
c. Decreased lung compliance
d. pAO_2/ FiO_2 ratio <200

550. A 45-year-old with trauma presents after 4 hours with cheek swelling and urine not passed. On examination crepitus is palpated with periorbital swelling. What is your diagnosis?

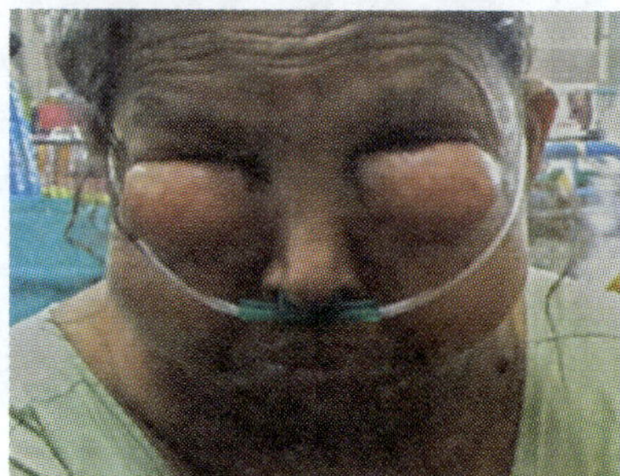

a. Renal shut down b. Lung laceration
c. Gas gangrene d. Base of skull fracture

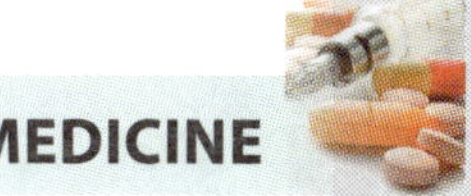

551. All are true about Aspirin sensitive asthma; EXCEPT:
- a. Nasal polyposis
- b. Treatment with inhaled corticosteroids
- c. Rhinosinusitis
- d. Increased prostaglandins

552. In a patient with COPD, best management option is?
- a. Quit smoking
- b. Bronchodilators
- c. Low flow oxygen
- d. Mucolytics

553. In a patient with smoking history, which is important?
- a. Duration of smoking
- b. Number of smoking
- c. Brand of Cigarette
- d. Filter of cigarette

554. Hyperventilation leads to?
- a. Increased CO_2
- b. Decreased CO_2
- c. Increased DL_{CO}
- d. Decreased PO_2

555. What is the diagnosis of CXR shown?

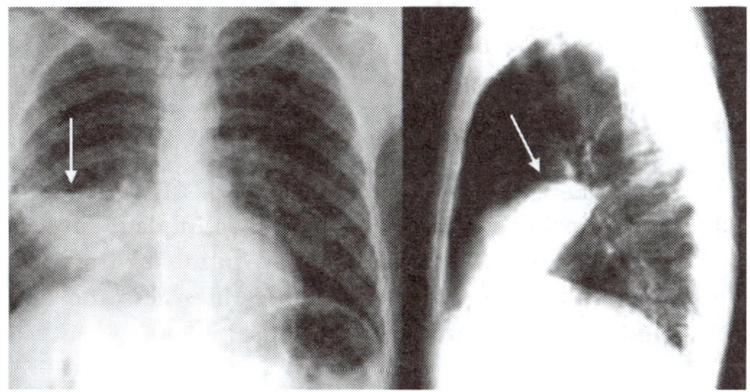

- a. Viral pneumonia
- b. Bacterial pneumonia
- c. Fungal pneumonia
- d. TB

556. Female patient with bilateral hilar lymphadenopathy and joint pain. ACE levels are elevated. Diagnosis is?
- a. Sarcoidosis
- b. Silicosis
- c. Hodgkin's lymphoma
- d. Non Hodgkin's lymphoma

557. Mesothelioma is most commonly caused by?
- a. Asbestosis
- b. Silicosis
- c. Anthracosis
- d. Coal workers pneumoconiosis

558. Oxygen (30–50%) is *not* given in:
- a. COPD
- b. Pneumonia
- c. Minimal pleural effusion
- d. Severe asthma

559. Which of the following is due to chronic smoking:
- a. Centri-acinar emphysema
- b. Panacinar emphysema
- c. Irregular emphysema
- d. Mixed variety

560. Mottling of lungs is seen in?
- a. Silicosis
- b. histoplasmosis
- c. ARDS
- d. Nocardia

561. Which is correct regarding the CXR?

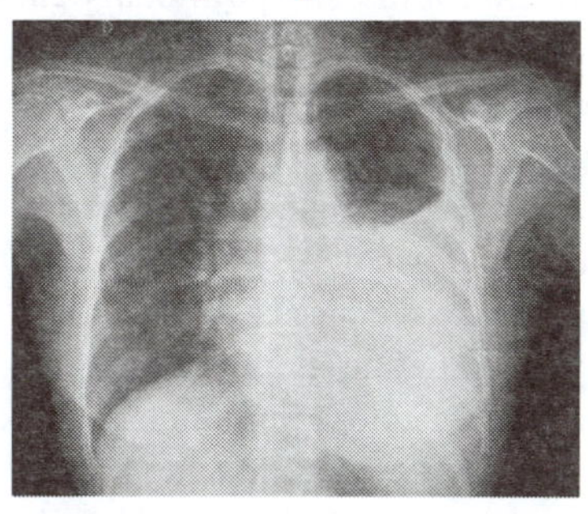

- a. Pleural thickening
- b. Segmental collapse
- c. Ellis curve
- d. Hypertranslucency

562. Diagnosis on CXR is?

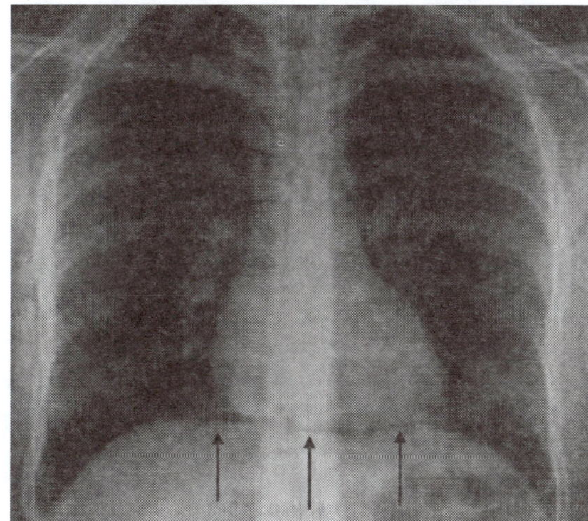

- a. Congenital diaphragmatic hernia
- b. Bochdalek hernia
- c. Pneumothorax
- d. Pneumo-mediastinum

563. CURB 65 criteria includes all; EXCEPT:
- a. Age is always more than or equal to 65 years
- b. Respiratory rate more than 30/min
- c. Systolic blood pressure is more than 90 mm Hg
- d. BUN level is more than >7 mmol/L

564. Most common type of emphysema
- a. Panacinar emphysema
- b. Irregular emphysema
- c. Centriacinar emphysema
- d. Paraseptal emphysema

565. Emphysema presents with all; EXCEPT:
- a. Cyanosis
- b. Barrel shaped chest
- c. Associated with smoking
- d. Type 1 respiratory failure

566. In case of Pulmonary embolism, Right ventricle hypokinesia and decreased urine output, which Drug therapy is most helpful:
- a. Thrombolytic
- b. LMW heparin
- c. Warfarin
- d. Heparin

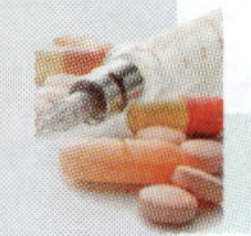

567. Best treatment for massive pulmonary embolism:
a. Intravenous tissue plasminogen activator
b. Heparin
c. Pulmonary thromboembolectomy
d. Low molecular weight heparin + warfarin

568. What is the full form of ARIA?
a. Allergic rhinitis induced asthma
b. Allergic rhinitis and its impact on asthma
c. Allergy rheumatology immunology and asthma
d. Acetlycholine receptor inducing activity

569. Pneumatocele is commonly caused by:
a. Streptococcus pneumoniab. Haemophilus ducreyi
c. Serratia marcescens
d. Klebsiella pneumonia

570. Finger in glove sign is seen in?
a. Pulmonary alveolar proteinosis
b. Pneumocystis carinii
c. Tuberculosis
d. Bronchocele

571. Aspergillosis can present with all; EXCEPT:
a. Lung cavity
b. Ear infection
c. Normal component in sputum
d. Rhinocerebral involvement

572. Allergic broncho-pulmonary Aspergillosis presents with all; EXCEPT:
a. Eosinophiluria
b. Occurs in asthmatics
c. Brownish plugs in sputum
d. Central bronchiectasis

573. Central bronchiectasis is seen with
a. Cystic adenomatoid malformation
b. Cystic fibrosis
c. Broncho carcinoma
d. Tuberculosis

574. IOC for Bronchiectasis:
a. HRCT scan
b. Spiral CT
c. Bronchoscopy
d. Pulmonary angiography

575. Miliary shadow on X-ray is seen in all; EXCEPT:
a. Tuberculosis
b. Loeffler's pneumonia
c. Klebsiella
d. Varicella pneumonia

576. TB causes all; EXCEPT:
a. Conjunctivitis
b. Uveitis
c. Lymphadenopathy
d. Addison disease

577. Congenital tuberculosis affects which organ the most
a. Brain
b. Liver
c. Kidney
d. Lungs

578. Which drugs are not used in severe persistent Asthma:
a. Short acting beta 2 agonist
b. Oral corticosteroids
c. Long acting beta 2 agonist
d. Inhaled high dose Steroids

579. Most common cause of community acquired pneumonia?
a. Pneumococcus
b. Streptococcus pyogenes
c. Staph. Aureus
d. Mycoplasma

580. Unipolar flagellated organsim that causes pneumonia
a. Pseudomonas
b. Mycoplasma
c. Aeromonas
d. Klebsiella pneumonia

581. Which of the following is not true in obstructive lung disease?
a. $FEV_1 \downarrow$
b. TLC $\downarrow$
c. FVC $\downarrow$
d. Reduced timed vital capacity

582. Which of the following is the common cause of respiratory failure Type 2?
a. COPD
b. Acute asthma
c. ARDS
d. Pneumonia

583. A 65-year-old lady suddenly dies 7 days after a surgery of femur fracture suddenly dies while having lunch in the ward. What would be the most likely cause:
a. Calf vein thrombosis
b. Pulmonary embolism
c. Myocardial infarction
d. Choking on food

584. A 65-year-old woman after total knee implant surgery complains of calf pain and swelling in the leg from last 2 days. Later she complains of breathlessness and dies suddenly in the ward. Probable cause?
a. Pulmonary embolism
b. Myocardial infarction
c. Stroke
d. ARDS

585. Westermark sign is seen in:
a. Pulmonary embolism
b. Pulmonary sequestration
c. Pulmonary alveolar proteinosis
d. Pneumothorax

586. Mean pulmonary artery pressure is:
a. 15 mm Hg
b. 8 mm Hg
c. 25 mm Hg
d. 10 mm Hg

587. What is not correct about smoking?
a. Nicotine causes increase in blood sugar
b. It reduces anxiety due to release of beta endorphins
c. Acts a psychostimulant
d. Acts on alpha 2 beta 4 nicotinic receptor

588. A 65-year-old man presented with hemoptysis and stage 3 clubbing. The probable diagnosis of the patient is?
a. Non small cell lung Ca
b. Small cell cancer of lung
c. Tuberculosis
d. Sarcoidosis

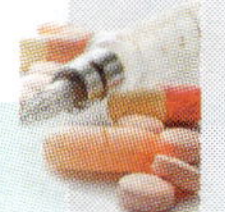

589. The following CXR shows

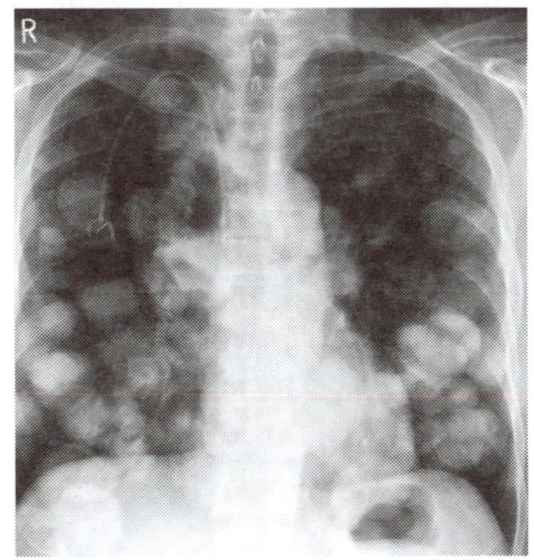

a. Metastasis to lungs b. Pneumothorax
c. Pneumatocele d. Bronchial adenoma

590. Look at the image of popcorn on CXR. In which condition is this seen?

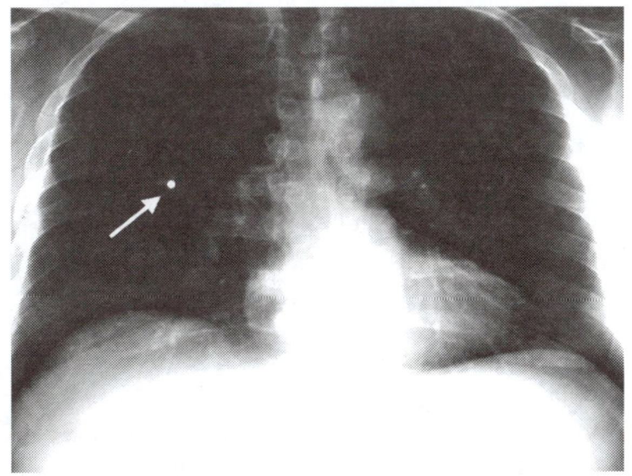

a. TB b. Metastasis
c. Pulmonary hamartoma d. Carcinoid tumor

591. ARDS includes all; EXCEPT?

a. Hypoxia
b. Alveolar Transudate
c. Non cardiogenic pulmonary edema
d. Normal P.C.W.P

592. Which component of cigarette smoke is responsible for CAD?

a. Nicotine
b. Tar
c. Polycyclic aromatic hydrocarbons
d. Benzene

593. Smoking causes all cancers; EXCEPT:

a. Liver cancer b. Oral cancer
c. Kidney cancer d. Bladder cancer

594. Water test is done for?

a. Pneumothorax b. Diabetic insipidus
c. Peritonitis d. Bladder injury

595. Hypersensitivity pneumonitis is consistent with the following findings; EXCEPT:

a. Decreased DLCO
b. Precipitating antibodies to causative antigens
c. Granuloma on lung biopsy
d. Eosinophilic alveolitis

596. Drug of choice for treatment of type 2 Brittle Asthma is

a. β-adrenergic agonist
b. Inhaled corticosteroids
c. Antileukotrines DM
d. Subcutaneous epinephrine

597. All of the following criteria are required for diagnosis of obesity hypoventilation syndrome; EXCEPT:

a. Hypertension
b. Sleep disorder breathing
c. BMI ≥30 kg/m^2
d. $PaCO_2$ ≥45 mm Hg

598. The following CXR shows

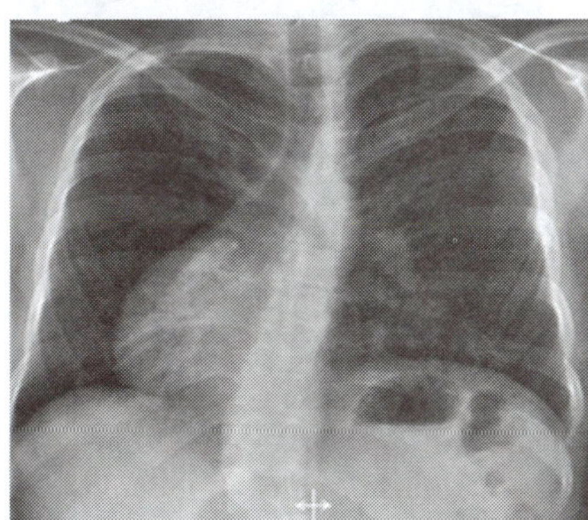

a. Dextrocardia b. Pneumothorax
c. Pneumomediastinum d. Pulmonary hamartoma

599. The CXR shows:

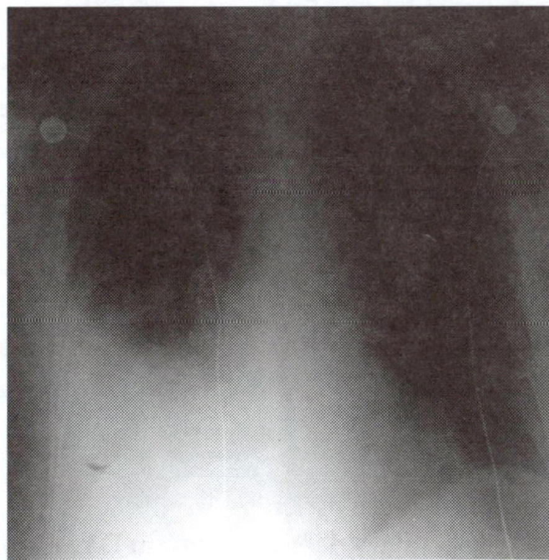

a. Meniscus sign
b. Consolidation lower lobe
c. Bilateral pneumothorax
d. Pulmonary artery hypertension

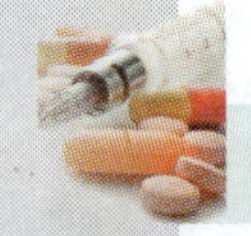

NEPHROLOGY

600. A 50-year-old patient presents with Palpitations, episodic headache and sweating episodes. Work up shows small left sided supra renal mass. Which of the following would be done for confirmation? *(Most Recent Question June 2022)*

a. Urinary Vanillylmandelic acid levels
b. Blood 5HIAA levels
c. Urine Myoglobin
d. Stool trypsin levels

601. A 35-year-old female presented with a one -year history of neglected dysuria, hesitancy, supra-pubic pain and intermittent hematuria. Comment on the diagnosis with the help of this X-ray pelvis. *(Most Recent Question Dec 2020)*

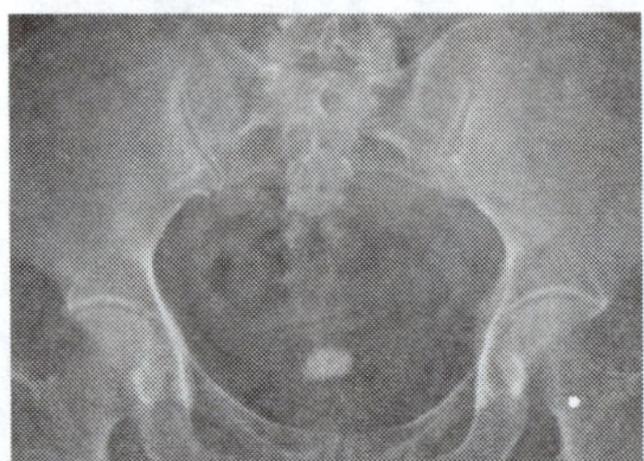

a. Bladder stone b. Prostate calcification
c. Bladder cancer d. Womb stone

602. A 3-year-old child presents with peri-orbital edema, foamy urine and dipstick examination of urine sample shows 4+ proteinuria. Which of the following drugs will be useful for management of this condition? *(Most Recent Question Dec 2020)*

a. Azathioprine b. Prednisolone
c. Cyclophosphamide d. Cyclosporine

603. An elderly patient presents with signs of moderate dehydration and urine osmolality is found to be extremely low. Which of the following is the possible etiology? *(Most Recent Question Dec 2020)*

a. SIADH b. ADPKD
c. Diabetes insipidus d. RTA

604. An elderly patient with malignancy develops hematuria. Dipstick performed on urine sample shows 4+ proteinuria. Which of these is the possible diagnosis of this patient? *(Most Recent Question Aug 2020)*

a. MGN b. MPGN
c. FSGS
d. Diffuse Glomerulosclerosis

605. What is the primary defect in vitamin D resistant rickets? *(Most Recent Question Aug 2020)*

a. Defective phosphate absorption from gut
b. Phosphate wasting from proximal renal tubule
c. Defective Calcium absorption from gut
d. Calcium wasting from proximal renal tubules

606. A 25-year-old male patient is having loose stools 18 times per day and his urine frequency is reduced to < 400 ml per day. What will be the correct finding of this patient? *(Most Recent Question Aug 2020)*

a. Urine sodium >40
b. Kidney biopsy showing Glomerular sclerosis
c. Hyperosmolar urine
d. Post renal azotemia

607. A 6-year-old child weighs 12 kg. The urine output of the child is only 0.4 ml/kg/ hour for last 12 hours and serum creatinine has shown a doubling over the baseline. What is stage of AKI by KDIGO criteria? *(Most Recent Question Aug 2020)*

a. 1 b. 2
c. 3 d. 4

608. A girl is having honey crust lesions on face which was diagnosed by her paediatrician as impetigo. She has now been brought to your hospital with facial puffiness and not eating well. When you work up the patient, which of the following will be the most common finding encountered in this case?

a. RBC in urine *(Most Recent Question Aug 2020)*
b. Nephrotic range proteinuria
c. Derangement of liver enzymes
d. Focal Neurological deficit

609. What is the most common cause of death in patients of G6PD deficiency? *(Recent Pattern Question 2018)*

a. Low oxyhemoglobin values
b. Acute renal failure
c. Sequestration crisis
d. Low oxygen affinity

610. Which of the following is correct about urinary loss in Fanconi syndrome? *(Recent Pattern Question 2017)*

a. Bicarbonate, uric acid and amino-acids
b. Bicarbonate, chloride and amino acids
c. Bicarbonate, sugar and potassium
d. Bicarbonate, uric acid and potassium

611. Which is the Gold standard investigation for Renal Artery Stenosis? *(Recent Pattern Question 2017)*

a. DTPA b. MRA
c. Doppler d. Contrast arteriography

612. Nephrotic syndrome is associated with? *(Recent Pattern Question 2017)*

a. Goodpasture disease
b. Membranoproliferative glomerulonephritis
c. Membranous glomerulopathy
d. Berger disease

613. Broad casts are seen in: *(Recent Pattern Question 2016)*

a. Chronic renal failure
b. Chronic glomerulonephritis
c. Minimal change disease
d. Membranous nephropathy

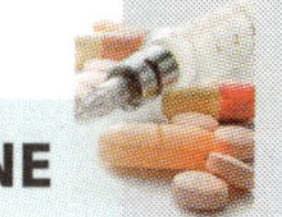

614. Streptococcal skin infection is followed by episode of hematuria and hypertension. All are needed for diagnosis; EXCEPT? ***(Recent Pattern Question 2016)***
a. Serum C3 b. ASO
c. Anti DNA-ase B d. CRP

615. Salt losing nephritis is? ***(Recent Pattern Question 2016)***
a. Interstitial nephritis b. Glomerulonephritis
c. Lupus nephritis d. IgA nephropathy

616. Cockroft gault formula is used for calculation of ***(Recent Pattern Question 2016)***
a. GFR b. Microalbuminuria
c. Serum anion gap d. Urinary anion gap

617. A 70-year-old patient develops pneumonia and sepsis and has renal failure with BP 70/50. Best drug used is? ***(Recent Pattern Question 2016)***
a. Adrenaline b. Phenylephrine
c. Norepinephrine d. Ephedrine

618. All are true about most common cause of nephrotic syndrome in children; EXCEPT?
a. It is not associated with hypertension
b. Minimal change disease, occurs in children <10 year
c. Massive Proteinuria >3.5 gm%/24 Hours
d. Low Complement Levels

619. Drug helpful in Chronic kidney disease?
a. Beta blocker b. Amlodipine
c. ACE inhibitor d. Telmisartan

620. Which of the following will have high chance of developing contrast nephropathy?
a. Diabetic nephropathy
b. Hypertension
c. Malignant hypertension
d. Hypertensive Glomerulosclerosis

621. Patient on insulin in CKD stage 4. What is the dose adjustment of insulin required?
a. Increased insulin b. Decreased insulin
c. Normal insulin d. Add DPP-4 inhibitors

622. Which of the following helps most in nephrolithiasis?
a. Low sodium diet b. Low calcium diet
c. High sodium diet d. Low citrate diet

623. Absolute indication for hemodialysis is?
a. Hypertension b. Hypokalemia
c. Pericarditis d. Metabolic alkalosis

624. Most common cause of glomerulonephritis?
a. P.S.G.N
b. Diabetes mellitus
c. Autosomal dominant Polycystic kidney disease
d. Crescentric Glomerulonephritis

625. All are true about GFR; EXCEPT?
a. 30-40% decrease after 70 years of age
b. Best estimated by Creatinine clearance
c. CKD is defied as GFR < 30 ml/min/1.73 m^2 for 4 weeks
d. GFR is dependent on height in children

626. Membranous Glomerulopathy is seen in?
a. Diabetes b. HTN
c. Renal failure d. Malignancy

627. Positive dipstick for RBC with Red color urine and clear supernatant after centrifugation is due to:
a. Porphyria b. Hematuria
c. Hemolysis d. Rhabdomyolysis

628. RBC cast is present in:
a. Acute tubular nephritis b. Acute glomerulonephritis
c. Acute Pyelonephritis d. Acute interstitial nephritis

629. Oliguric renal failure is due to all; EXCEPT:
a. Diabetic nephropathy b. Fanconi syndrome
c. Multiple myeloma d. Aminoglycosides

630. Which of the following Microorganism is incriminated in infection after Hemodialysis?
a. Chlamydia b. Gram-positive organisms
c. Acid-Fast d. Anaerobes

631. Episodic microscopic to gross hematuria is seen in:
a. IgA nephropathy b. Minimal change disease
c. Chronic renal failure d. Nephritic syndrome

632. Xantho-granulomatous infection is caused by:
a. Nephrolithiasis b. Urinary obstruction
c. Proteus Mirabilis d. All of the above

633. Hypokalemia is seen in:
a. RTA-I b. RTA-II
c. RTA-III d. RTA-IV

634. Acute renal failure results in:
a. Hyperkalemic alkalosis b. Hypokalemic alkalosis
c. Hyperkalemic acidosis d. Hypokalemic acidosis

635. All of the following causes acute renal failure; EXCEPT:
a. Pyelonephritis b. Snakebite
c. Rhabdomyolysis d. Analgesic nephropathy

636. Which of these is correct about Struvite stones?
a. Present in alkaline urine
b. Most common kidney disease
c. Are Calcium pyrophosphate stones
d. Most common kidney stones

637. All are seen in Nephrotic syndrome; EXCEPT:
a. Atherosclerosis b. Thrombo-embolism
c. Hypertension d. Lipiduria

638. Red cell cast are more common with
a. Acute tubular necrosis b. Nephrotic syndrome
c. Nephritic syndrome d. Interstitial nephritis

639. Interstitial nephritis is common with
a. NSAID b. Black water fever
c. Rhabdomyolysis d. Tumor lysis syndrome

640. Which of the following does not cause Polyuria:
a. Interstitial nephritis
b. Hypokalemia
c. A.D.H insufficiency
d. Rhabdomyolysis

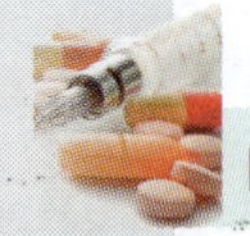

641. Triad of Hematuria, hypertension and edema are a feature of?
- a. Acute glomerulonephritis
- b. Acute pyelonephritis
- c. Chronic glomerulonephritis
- d. Renal cell carcinoma

642. Type of glomerulopathy in HIV positive patient is?
- a. Focal segmental glomerulosclerosis
- b. Diffuse glomerulosclerosis
- c. Membranous glomerulopathy
- d. Mesangio-proliferative glomerulonephritis

643. Hemodialysis can be performed for long periods from the same site due to?
- a. Arteriovenous fistula reduces bacterial contamination of site
- b. Arteriovenous fistula results in arterialization of vein
- c. Arteriovenous fistula reduces chances of graft failure
- d. Arteriovenous fistula facilitates small bore needles for high flow rates

644. Chronic hemodialysis in ESRD patient is done?
- a. Once per week
- b. Twice per week
- c. Thrice per week
- d. Daily

INFECTION

645. A child from low socio-economic strata is brought with complaints of fever and abnormal behavior for last 3 months. The child is in altered sensorium for past one week. On examination neck rigidity is seen with CSF showing increased lymphocytes, glucose=30mg% and proteins 300 mg%. What is the diagnosis? ***(Most Recent Question Dec 2020)***
- a. Viral meningitis
- b. Fungal meningitis
- c. Tubercular meningitis
- d. N. Meningitidis

646. A nurse developed a prick from a HIV positive patient. She is very anxious and asks you which test will be done for quick/early identification of transmission of HIV infection to her? ***(Most Recent Question Dec 2020)***
- a. 3rd generation ELISA
- b. Western blot
- c. EIA P24 antigen
- d. CD4: CD8 ratio

647. A 30-year patient from Middle East country comes to your clinic with complaints of fever with night sweats for last one month with musculoskeletal pain and difficulty in walking. Per abdomen examination is normal. Which of the following is the possible etiological agent? ***(Most Recent Question Dec 2020)***
- a. West Nile virus disease
- b. Infectious mononucleosis
- c. Brucellosis
- d. Tularemia

648. A 2 year old male child presents with recurrent UTI episodes which on culture are found to be due to E. coli. Which of the following test is to be done to determine the etiology of the disease? ***(Most Recent Question Dec 2020)***
- a. USG
- b. Voiding cystourethrogram
- c. Retrograde ureterography
- d. Urine culture

649. A 35-year-old HIV patient came with fever and neck rigidity. CSF examination shows the following organism. What is the diagnosis? ***(Most Recent Question Dec 2020)***

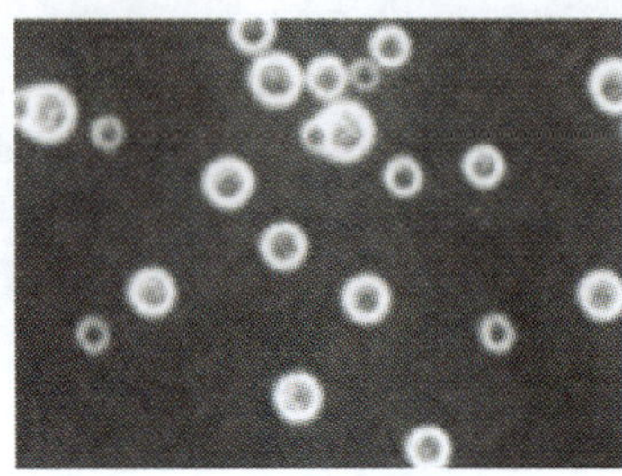

- a. Cryptococcus
- b. Toxoplasma
- c. Pneumococcus
- d. Meningococcus

650. A 30-year-old AIDS Positive male patient has developed fever, vomiting and meningismus. Which of the following tests will help in rapid diagnosis of Cryptococcal meningitis? ***(Most Recent Question Aug 2020)***
- a. India ink preparation of CSF
- b. Blood Lateral flow assay for cryptococcal antigen
- c. Blood culture
- d. CSF Cultures

651. Which of the following is a good prognosis determining step in septic shock? ***(Recent Pattern Question 2018-19)***
- a. Adequate IVF
- b. Adequate vasopressor
- c. Adequate IVF plus vasopressor
- d. Time between hypotension and introduction of antibiotic

652. Rapid diagnosis of rabies is made with? ***(Recent Pattern Question 2018-19)***
- a. Skin biopsy with fluorescent antibody testing
- b. Rabies virus specific antibodies
- c. Inoculation in mouse
- d. Corneal impression smear

653. Recurrent Neisseria meningitis episodes are caused by deficiency of? ***(Recent Pattern Question 2018-19)***
- a. C5-C9 deficiency
- b. IgA deficiency
- c. CD4 cell deficiency
- d. Perforin deficiency

654. In fever of unknown origin, how many times blood sample should be drawn? ***(Recent Pattern Question 2018-19)***
- a. 2
- b. 3
- c. 4
- d. 5

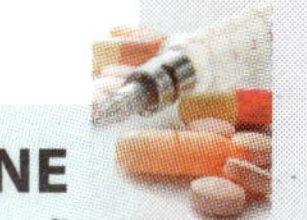

655. A 6-year child presents with low grade fever for 7 days and on examination has enlarged cervical lymph nodes with a palpable spleen tip. He was given ampicillin followed by development of extensive rash all over the body. Diagnosis is? *(Recent Pattern Question 2018-19)*

a. Infectious mononucleosis
b. Scarlet fever
c. Kawasaki
d. Hodgkin's Lymphoma

656. Correct about initiating treatment in AIDS patient *(Recent Pattern Question 2018-19)*

a. No cut off of CD4 count required for initiation of treatment
b. CD4 count < 200/cu.mm required for initiation of treatment
c. CD4 count <350/cu.mm required for initiation of treatment
d. CD4 count <500/cu.mm required for initiation of treatment

657. Which of the following is correct about differential leucocyte count in late catarrhal stage of pertussis? *(Recent Pattern Question 2018)*

a. Neutropenia b. Eosinophilia
c. Monocytosis d. Lymphocytosis

658. Which is the drug of choice for prophylaxis of meningococcal meningitis in pregnancy: *(Recent Pattern Question 2018)*

a. Penicillin b. Ceftriaxone
c. Rifampicin d. Ampicillin

659. In a diagnosed lepromatous leprosy patient, the treatment was started. After intake of drug skin lesions and fever develop within few days. Which type of hypersensitivity reaction leads to this manifestation? *(Recent Pattern Question 2018)*

a. Type 4 b. Type 3
c. Type 2 d. Type 1

660. What is the incubation period of hepatitis B? *(Recent Pattern Question 2018)*

a. 1–30 days b. 15–45 days
c. 45–180 days d. 2 weeks–6 months

661. Which of the following is an initial presentation of HIV infection when ART is not started? *(Recent Pattern Question 2018)*

a. Primary CNS lymphoma
b. Kaposi sarcoma
c. Bacterial pneumonia
d. Extrapulmonary tuberculosis

662. The most important parameter to monitor dengue hemorrhagic fever is? *(Recent Pattern Question 2017)*

a. Platelet count b. Hemoglobin
c. Total leukocyte count d. Hematocrit

663. Causative agent for hand-foot-mouth disease is? *(Recent Pattern Question 2017)*

a. Enterovirus b. Coxsackie
c. Adenovirus d. Hepatitis C

664. Empirical antibiotic regimen in suitable community acquired pneumonia in previously healthy adults? *(Recent Pattern Question 2016)*

a. Amoxicillin + Clavulanate b. Azithromycin
c. Ceftriaxone d. Moxifloxacin

665. Mad cow disease is due to?

a. Protein misfolding b. Bacterial
c. Viral d. Spirochete

666. Sputum smear is diagnostic if?

a. >25 neutrophils and >10 squamous epithelial cells
b. <25 neutrophils and <10 squamous epithelial cells
c. >25 neutrophils and <10 squamous epithelial cells
d. <25 neutrophils and >10 squamous epithelial cells

667. Meningitis bacteria are normally present in?

a. Nasopharynx b. Skin
c. Genitals d. Lower G.I.T

668. Quadrivalent Meningococcal vaccine is not used for?

a. Serotype A b. Serotype B
c. Serotype C d. Serotype Y

FLUIDS AND ELECTROLYTES

669. A young adult presents with gastric outlet obstruction and vomiting. Which of the following fluid will be used? *(Most Recent Question June 2022)*

a. RL b. NS
c. 5% Dextrose in water d. 20 % Dextrose in water

670. A 8-month-old child with diarrhea was given potassium correction to patient, K value is not improving and floppiness in child is noted. Which of the following is responsible for this presentation? *(Most Recent Question Dec 2021)*

a. Magnesium deficiency b. Calcium deficiency
c. Albumin deficiency d. Sodium deficiency

671. A Soldier after patrolling duty is showing altered behavior. He is dehydrated and sweating in extremely warm atmosphere. What should be done? *(Most Recent Question Dec 2021)*

a. Wash limb with cold water and put on fan
b. Put Feet in Ice water bucket
c. Inj Prochlorperazine
d. Put wet cloth immersed with 25°C water on body and put on fan

672. A 25-year-old guy was involved in a road traffic accident. Which of the following Intravenous fluid is not given to this patient? *(Most Recent Question Dec 2020)*

a. 5% dextrose b. Hypertonic saline
c. Normal saline d. Ringer lactate

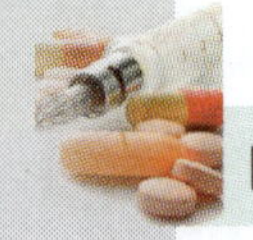

673. A patient underwent hysterectomy and developed abdominal distention and pain 3 days postoperatively. Which electrolyte imbalance will be seen?
(Most Recent Question Dec 2020)
a. Hyponatremia b. Hypernatremia
c. Hypokalemia d. Hyperkalemia

674. A young man with blunt abdominal trauma arrives in shock. Which one of the cannulas shown below can be used for rapid transfusion of blood products?
(Most Recent Question Dec 2020)

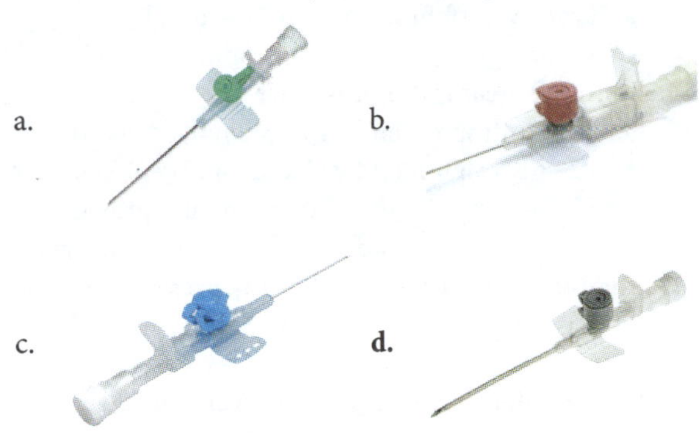

675. Which of these has no role in treatment of dangerous hyperkalemia? ***(Recent Pattern Question 2018)***
a. Injecting calcium chloride
b. Salbutamol
c. Hemodialysis
d. IV soda-bicarbonate

676. High anion gap acidosis is seen in all; EXCEPT:
(Recent Pattern Question 2018)
a. Lactic acidosis b. Diarrhea
c. Acute renal failure d. Salicylate poisoning

677. Anion gap is increased in all; EXCEPT:
(Recent Pattern Question 2018)
a. Renal tubular acidosis b. Diabetic ketoacidosis
c. Acute tubular necrosis d. Ethylene glycol poisoning

678. In which of the following condition is blood osmolality increased: ***(Recent Pattern Question 2018)***
a. Diarrhea b. SIADH
c. Psychogenic polydipsia d. Cerebral toxoplasmosis

679. Which is correct about a female with chronic vomiting?
(Recent Pattern Question 2018)
a. Hypokalemic hypochloremic metabolic alkalosis
b. Hypokalemic hyperchloremic metabolic alkalosis
c. Hypokalemic hypochloremic metabolic acidosis
d. Hypokalemic hyperchloremic metabolic acidosis

680. Normal anion gap is seen in?
(Recent Pattern Question 2017)
a. Renal tubular acidosis b. Diabetic Keto-acidosis
c. Hyper-alimentation d. Acute tubular necrosis

681. Increased anion gap is seen in?
(Recent Pattern Question 2017)
a. Starvation b. Renal tubular acidosis
c. Diarrhea d. Fistula

682. In a patient who was brought to casualty after RTA with pulse rate 108, SBP 80. Which fluid is to be given ideally?
a. Plasma b. Normal saline
c. Blood d. 5% dextrose

683. All are seen in Hypokalemia; EXCEPT?
a. U wave in ECG b. Tall T wave in ECG
c. ST Depression d. Prolonged QU interval

684. Which of the following presents with hypokalemia and metabolic acidosis?
a. Diarrhea b. Vomiting
c. Nasogastric suction d. Conn's syndrome

685. Seborrheic dermatitis, cellulitis, alopecia and apathy is seen in?
a. Pyridoxine deficiency b. Biotin deficiency
c. Riboflavin deficiency d. Vitamin A deficiency

686. Normal anion gap is seen in:
a. Diabetic ketoacidosis b. Chronic renal failure
c. Renal tubular acidosis d. Methanol toxicity

687. Normal anion gap is seen in:
a. Diabetic ketoacidosis b. Lactic acidosis
c. Starvation ketoacidosis d. Renal tubular acidosis

688. Widened anion gap is caused by all; EXCEPT:
a. Lactic acidosis b. Diarrhea
c. Diabetic keto-acidosis d. Methanol poisoning

689. Hypernatremia causes all; EXCEPT:
a. Seizure
b. Increased plasma osmolality
c. Brain hemorrhage
d. Central pontine myelinosis

690. Chvostek's sign is elicited by:
a. Facial nerve stimulation by tapping over the parotid
b. BP cuff in arm for 5 minutes
c. Tapping over extensor pollicis brevis
d. Tapping over flexor retinaculum

691. Which can be given immediately in hemorrhagic stroke?
a. Packed RBC b. Colloids
c. Blood transfusion d. Hypertonic fluids

692. Women working in hot environment & drinking lots of water without intake of salts are liable to develop
a. Heat hyperpyrexia b. Heat cramps
c. Heat stroke d. Heat encephalopathy

693. Hypocalcemia will *not* lead to?
a. Bone fractures b. Tetany
c. QT prolongation d. Osteoporosis

694. After Road traffic accident a patient presented to casualty with vitals showing BP of 90/60 mm Hg with heart of 56 bpm. Which kind of shock occurs?
a. Cardiogenic b. Neurogenic
c. Distributive d. Hypovolemic shock

695. Which of the following hormone has shortest half life?
a. Renin b. Cortisol
c. Aldosterone d. Norepinephrine

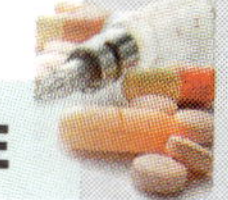

ANSWERS WITH EXPLANATIONS

MOST RECENT QUESTIONS 2023

1. Ans. (a) Obesity hypoventilation syndrome

Ref: Harrison 21st ed. pg. 2203

- BMI >40 indicates morbid obesity. Extreme fat in chest wall limits chest expansion and explains the low pO_2 and the build-up of CO_2 in this patient. Carbon dioxide depresses the brain and hence, the excessive sleepiness of patient can be explained. Diagnosis is obesity hypoventilation syndrome.
- Option b will present with feeling of suffocation and breathlessness on sleeping as respiratory drive is depressed in central sleep apnea.
- Option c will have excessive daytime sleepiness but will have build-up of carbon dioxide/respiratory acidosis.
- Option d has lots of snoring and apneic episodes which are not given in the history of this patient.

2. Ans. (c) RTA 4

Ref: CMDT 2023, pg. 885

- RTA 4 has resistance of aldosterone and hence, potassium and hydrogen cannot be excreted. This explains metabolic acidosis with hyperkalemia. In all other varieties of RTA, potassium leaks from kidney tubules and causes hypokalemia.
- Ureterosigmoidostomy is a diversion procedure done in patients with cancer of urinary bladder. Urine diverted to colon causes diarrhea and hypokalemia.

3. Ans. (a) Lymphocytosis, low sugar and high protein

Ref: Harrison 21st ed. pg. 1117

Child is having signs of meningeal irritation and contact with case of TB. Hence, findings of TB meningitis are to be selected. Since the process is slow and develops over couple of weeks, the usual cells seen at diagnosis are lymphocytes. The proteins are grossly elevated forming a cob -web coagulum in the test tube in which the sample is collected. CSF sugar is always reduced due to inflammatory process. Correct answer is option a.

4. Ans. (a) Cardiac Tamponade

Ref: Harrison 21st ed. pg. 2020

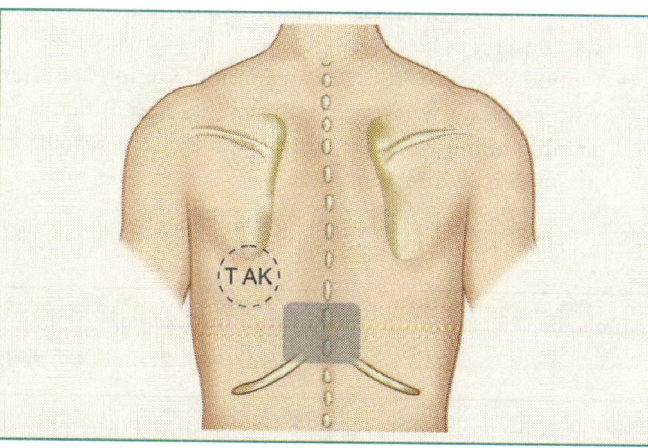

Lung malignancy can be spread to the heart causing malignant pericardial effusion and cardiac tamponade if undetected. The mass effect of this pericardial effusion falls on left lower lobe leading to lung consolidation. This explains bronchial breathing at left infero-scapular region and is called Ewart's sign. The lightheadedness of patient can be explained due to low BP caused by cardiac tamponade.
Pleural effusion presents with reduced is entry and stony dull percussion note and is hence ruled out.

5. Ans. (b) Pleural effusion

Ref: Harrison 21st ed. pg. 2198

Pneumonia patient is having reduced air entry in left side with percussion note of stony dullness indicating development of parapneumonic effusion.
Option a will have low BP with Ewart's sign. It is seen usually with malignant pericardial effusion/cardiac tamponade. Option c is ruled out as it has absent air entry and absent breath sounds. Option d (pneumomediastinum) will have auscultatory finding of Hamman crunch sign.

6. Ans. (c) History of stroke

Ref: Harrison 21st ed. pg. 3344

$ABCD_2$ score is used to predict the chances of development of stroke in a patient presenting with transient ischemic attack. Option c is wrong as it is not the history of stroke but clinical features of stroke that are taken into consideration.

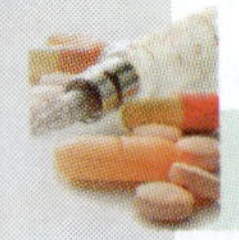

	Parameter	Score
A Age	≥60 years	1
B Blood pressure	Systolic ≥140 mm Hg or diastolic ≥90 mm Hg	1
C Clinical	Unilateral weakness Speech problem, no weakness Any other	2 1 0
D Duration	≥60 min 10–59 min <10 min	2 1 0
D Diabetes	Yes	1

7. Ans. (a) Thrombolysis

Ref: Harrison 21st ed. pg. 3351

The image shows a left-sided hyperdensity in NCCT head in area of lenticular nucleus and internal capsule. This explains the right-sided hemiparesis. Thrombolysis is contraindicated in hemorrhagic stroke as it has side effect of bleeding. Another pointer is elevated BP of 200/100 mm Hg.

8. Ans. (a) 8

Ref: Harrison 21st ed. pg. 3337

- Dose used is 0.9 mg/kg to maximum of 90 mg. 10% of this is given as bolus and remainder over 60 minutes.
- Hence, in this case, total dose will be $0.9 \times 80 = 72$ mg, of which 10%, i.e., 7.2 mg will be given as bolus. Hence, the closest answer is option a, i.e., 8 mg.

9. Ans. (d) Huntington Chorea

Ref: Harrison 21st ed. pg. 3375

- A combination of involuntary hand movements and cognitive issues points to Huntington chorea.
- Option a will present after 60 years of age with resting tremors and bradykinesia, which is essential for diagnosis, but which is not described in the question.
- Option b will have sensory ataxia with extensor plantar.
- Option c presents with dementia and does not have involuntary hand movements.

10. Ans. (b) Absent y descent

Ref: Harrison 21st ed. pg. 2022

- Muffled heart sounds with hypotension and raised JVP indicate Beck's triad of cardiac tamponade. Due to high intrapericardial pressure, ventricular filling is impaired and leads to absent y descent.
- Option a is seen in tricuspid regurgitation. Option c is dummy choice as there is no such medical term of large C waves. Option d is seen in atrial fibrillation.

11. Ans. (c) Fluent aphasia

Ref: Harrison 21st ed. pg. 196

- The patient can speak fluently, this implies Broca's area is not involved. The patient is talking jargon, as mentioned in the question - using nonsensical grammar and not making any sense. This implies damage to Wernicke's area.
- This area is for comprehension and understanding of speech. Involvement causes patient to coin new terms which is called word salad or jargon speech. The correct answer is fluent aphasia which is also called receptive dysphasia.
- Option a is seen in Broca area lesion. Option b is seen with metabolic encephalopathy and implies difficulty in naming an object. Option d has problem in repetition, but understanding is normal.

12. Ans. (c) Obturator nerve

Ref: Harrison 21st ed. pg. 3281

Scissoring gait is seen in children with spastic cerebral palsy and is an upper motor neuron lesion. UMN causes adductor muscle spasm. Nerve supply of adductor muscles is obturator nerve.

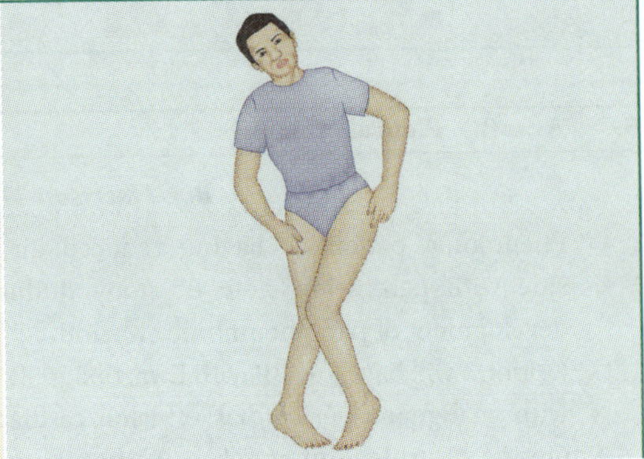

Inferior gluteal nerve injury leads to denervation of the ipsilateral gluteus maximus muscle and causes *lurching gait*. This results from the weakening or absence of an ipsilateral hip extension. Clinically, patients may also report wasting of the ipsilateral gluteus maximus muscle and loss of the defined shape to the affected buttock.	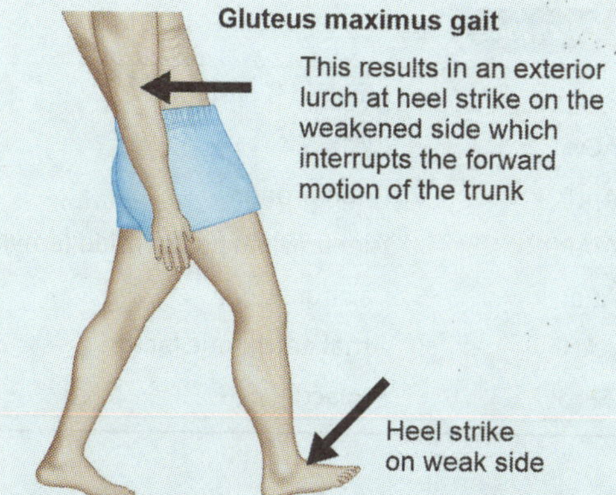
Superior gluteal nerve injury leads to denervation of gluteus medius and minimus and leads to Trendelenburg sign.	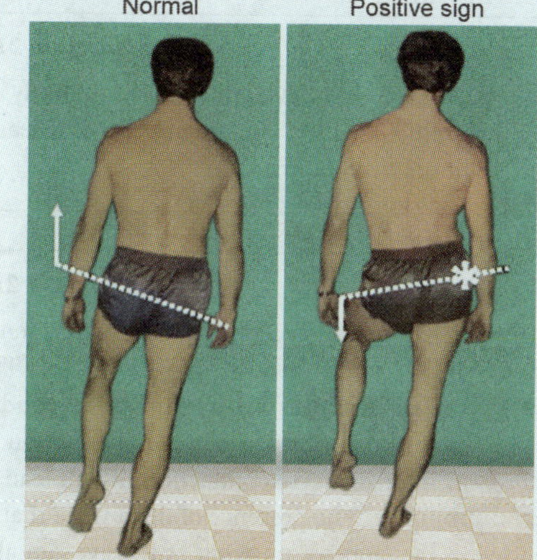
Hand knee gait is seen in poliomyelitis due to quadriceps wasting.	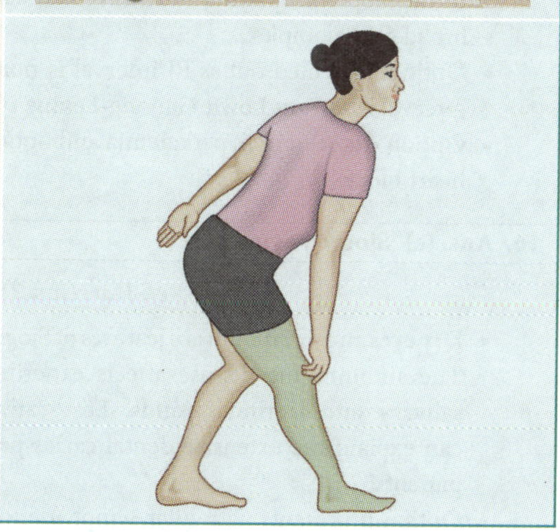

13. Ans. (a) Amyloid beta-2 microglobulin

Ref: Harrison 21st ed. pg. 303

Abeta$_2$	Dialysis dementia
Abeta	Alzheimer's disease Cerebral amyloid angiopathy
ATTR	Familial amyloid polyneuropathy

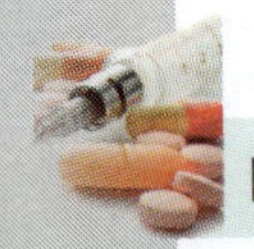

Extra Mile

Aβ	Amyloid β protein	Alzheimer's disease; Down's syndrome
ACys	Cystain C	Cerebral amyloid angiopathy
AprP	Prion protein	Spongiform encephalopathies
AIAPP	Islet amyloid polypeptide (amylin)	Diabetes-associated
ACal	Calcitonin	Medullary carcinoma of the thyroid
AANF	Atrial natriuretic factor	Atrial fibrillation
APro	Prolactin	Endocrinopathy

14. Ans. (a) Ig G

Ref: Harrison 21st ed. pg. 3505

AIDP/GBS has IgG Anti GM1 antibody that leads to polyradiculopathy. The progression of disease can be from 12 hours to 48 hours.

15. Ans. (b) Broad QRS interval

Ref: Harrison 21st ed. pg. 1896

- WPW has an accessory pathway that sends the current of SA node directly into ventricles. The current in ventricles travels via inter-myocyte conduction instead of Purkinje fibers. Since the conduction will be slower in inter-myocyte conduction, it will lead to broad QRS complex. The presence of delta wave that causes change in the slope of upswing of R wave can also explain the broad QRS complex.
- Option a is ruled out as PJ interval is normal. Short PJ interval is seen in Lown-Ganong-Levine syndrome.
- Option c is seen in hyperkalemia and option d is seen in heart blocks.

16. Ans. (c) Sjogren Syndrome

Ref: Harrison 21st ed. pg. 2358

- Dry eyes and dry mouth are features of Sjogren syndrome. The autoimmune disease affects exocrine glands, like salivary and lacrimal glands. Less saliva production can explain the extensive dental caries present in these patients.
- Option b presents with hilar lymphadenopathy. Option d presents with recurrent epistaxis, hemoptysis and hematuria.

17. Ans. (b) Plasma cell

Ref: Harrison 21st ed. pg. 870

Keyword is gamma globulins which are disproportionately elevated with CRAB features in the form of pallor, deranged KFT and bony lytic lesions. Only hypercalcemia is not given but the remaining features point to etiology of multiple myeloma. The cell of origin is plasma cell.

18. Ans. (b) Intubate and IPPV

Ref: Harrison 21st ed. pg. 2270

GCS less than 8 implies patient is in coma and has impaired airway reflexes. This implies air way control in the form of elective intubation is mandatory. The presence of bradycardia with hypertension indicates Cushing reflex seen in raised ICP.

19. Ans. (a) Cardiac failure

Ref: Harrison 21st ed. pg. 1817

Elevated JVP indicates cardiac injury. RVF can explain pedal edema and ascites that will take some time to develop.

20. Ans. (c) Medullary thyroid cancer

Ref: Harrison 21st ed. pg. 2138

Calcitonin is a tumor marker for medullary carcinoma of thyroid.

21. Ans. (d) Ultrasound/Doppler

Ref: Harrison 21st ed. pg. 2138

- CTPA shows a saddle embolus and diagnosis is pulmonary thromboembolism. Noninvasive test to be performed is ultrasound/Doppler of lower extremity veins as source of clot can be determined.
  - D-Dimer is a screening test that is performed before doing CTPA. The question is not related to screening but to finding the etiology of pulmonary thromboembolism.

22. Ans. (b) Acute glomerulonephritis

Ref: Harrison 21st ed. pg. 2096

- The keyword in MCQ is passage of smoky urine and presence of dysmorphic RBC which indicates glomerular

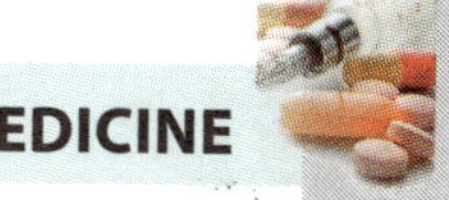

bleeding. Correct answer is acute glomerulonephritis. 2+ proteinuria implies sub-nephrotic proteinuria which is seen with glomerulonephritis.

- Option a will have foamy urine and 4+ proteinuria with amount exceeding 3.5 gram per day. Option c will have fever with burning micturition and cloudy urine with a large number of WBCs in urine. Option d will have hematuria but eumorphic RBC would be present.

23. Ans. (a) Beers Criteria

Ref: 5-minute Clinical Consult 2020, pg. 399

Since multiple medications are prescribed for various illnesses in old age, the chances of drug interactions are higher. Hence, Beers criteria are used to evaluate inappropriate medication usage in older adults.

Duke's criteria	Infective Endocarditis
Light's criteria	Pleural effusion to differentiate exudate vs transudate
Jones criteria	Rheumatic fever

24. Ans. (a) Analgesics

Ref: CMDT 2023, pg. 999

Thalamic Dejerine Roussy syndrome occurs due to ischemic stroke damaging the thalamus. The patient complains of burning pain on contralateral side of body as if someone poured burning water on the extremities. Since it is a neuropathic pain, analgesics would not work in this situation.

25. Ans. (b) FEV1 showing increment of more than 15% after giving a bronchodilator

Ref: Harrison 21st ed. pg. 2138

- Asthma is a reversible airway disorder characterized by improvement in FEV1 by > 12 percent after using a bronchodilator. Hence, option b is correct.
- Option d is used for diagnosis of diseases, like ILD, pneumoconiosis, bronchiectasis. Only history and wheezing in chest cannot be the basis for any diagnosis.

26. Ans. (d) 3

Ref: Harrison 21st ed. pg. 1025-26

Minor Duke criteria satisfied in the question stem are:

- IV drug user
- Fever >38.5°C
- Spots on fundus examination

Modified duke criteria for the diagnosis of endocarditis	
Major criteria	Two separate positive blood cultures with microorganisms typical for infective endocarditis (*viridans streptococci, streptococcus bovis*, HACEK group, *staphylococcus aureus, enterococci*)
	Echocardiographic evidence of endocardial involvement (typical valvular lessions: Vegetations, abscess, or partial dehiscence of a prosthetic valve)
Minor criteria	Predisposition: Predisposing heart condition or IV drug use
	Temperature >38°C
	Vascular phenomena: Major arterial emboli, septic pulmonary infarcts, mycotic aneurysm, intracranial hemorrhage, conjunctival hemorrhage, Janeway lesions
	Immunological phenomena: Glomerulonephritis, Osler nodes, Roth spots, rheumatoid factor
	Microbiological evidence: Positive blood culture but not meeting major criterion, or serologic evidence of active infection with organism consistent with infective endocarditis
For the diagnosis of endocarditis to be made, the following must be present: • 2 major criteria • 1 major criterion and 3 minor criteria • 5 minor criteria	

27. Ans. (b) >12%

Ref: Harrison 21st ed. pg. 2138

Definition of reversibility of airflow obstruction in bronchial asthma is change of FEV1 >12 percent before and after use of salbutamol.

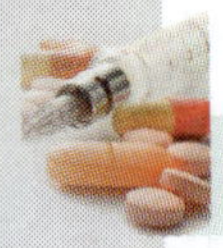

28. Ans. (b) c-ANCA

Ref: Harrison 21st ed. pg. 2806

The question stem has three main pointers that indicate vasculitis as a possible etiology of presentation:

- Upper respiratory tract involvement: Epistaxis
- Lower respiratory tract involvement: Hemoptysis and multiple cavitary lesions
- Kidney involvement: Hematuria
  - The combination of three features points to diagnosis of Wegener's Granulomatosis/Granulomatosis with Angiitis. The antibody responsible for this vasculitis is c-ANCA.
  - Option a is used for diagnosis of microscopic polyangiitis.
  - Option c is used for diagnosis of Goodpasture syndrome which has combination of features of hemoptysis and hematuria, but upper respiratory tract involvement is not seen. Option d is seen in systemic lupus erythematosus.

29. Ans. (d) Deficiency of vWF

Ref: Harrison 21st ed. pg. 909

- History of excessive bleeding after delivery and dental extraction in past point to bleeding disorder. Options a and b are seen in males in pediatric age group.
- Since prothrombin time is normal, option c is ruled out. The history is classical for Von Willebrand disease where a female patient will present with history of excessive bleeding after any procedure. Coagulogram shows normal prothrombin time with increased aPTT and bleeding time. Absence of spontaneous bruising or joint bleeding in past further helps in excluding options a and b.

30. Ans. (d) 400

Ref: CMDT 2023, page no 879

Total sodium deficit = Total body water × (140 – actual value)

= 40 kg × 0.5 × (140 – 120) = 40 × 0.5 × 20 = 400 mEq

In acute onset hyponatremia, hyponatremia can be corrected at the rate it fell; but in chronic hyponatremia, the rate of correction should be a maximum of 8 mEq/ day.

31. Ans. (a) Orbital varices

Ref: Parson Diseases of Eye 2019 ed. pg. 444

Orbital varices are venous malformations that consist of low-pressure plexuses causing them to be asymptomatic. They can cause intermittent proptosis which can be induced by increasing the orbital pressure by Valsalva, coughing, or straining. Options b and c would not be affected by Valsalva.

Option d is complication of cavernous sinus thrombosis where eyeball will pulsate with every beat of heart.

32. Ans. (c) Poha/Pulao

Ref: Harrison 21st ed. pg. 2463

Maize and rice (Poha, Pulao) can be given to patients with celiac sprue. Sooji/semolina is derived from wheat. BROW (Barley, Rye, Oats, Wheat) cereals are contraindicated in celiac sprue.

33. Ans. (d) Antihelminthic treatment

Ref: Harrison 21st ed. pg. 1119–1120

- Antihelminthic treatment is delayed in NCC patients by 48-72 hours. Immediate steps are directed at managing vasogenic cerebral edema, which causes focal seizures in the patient. Hence, dexamethasone is given to reduce cerebral edema. Initially phenytoin infusion and later Carbamazepine must be given to control focal seizures.
- Killing the worms directly will worsen the inflammation in brain and increase seizure frequency.

34. Ans. (b) Injection adrenaline IM 1:1000 dilution, repeat again if no response, till patient reaches hospital

Ref: Harrison 21st ed. pg. 2727

Preferred route of administration in anaphylaxis initially is intramuscular undiluted and should be repeated if no response, since absorption will be erratic due to low perfusion of tissues. Correct answer is option b. IV adrenaline can be used in ICU setting. Intubation with laryngeal edema would not be possible.

INTUBATION IS FRAUGHT WITH HAZARD

- Airway manipulation may worsen swelling.
- Laryngeal edema will often preclude the use of a laryngeal mask airway.
- In severe angioedema, orotracheal intubation may simply be impossible.
- There is a high risk of hemodynamic collapse following intubation: Start epinephrine and give fluid beforehand
- Indications for epinephrine any of the following:
  - Airway involvement.
  - Breathing difficulty.
  - Circulation (hypotension).
  - 2 organs involved (e.g., vomiting + urticaria).
- Dosing:
  - If IM is faster 0.5 mg IM, repeat q5min for up to three cumulative doses if needed (then, if needed, transition to epinephrine infusion.)
  - If IV faster:

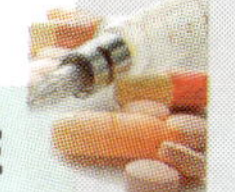

- Anaphylaxis due to intravenous medication or bee sting usually begins within <30 minutes.
  - Initiation of reaction immediately following exposure is a poor prognostic sign
- Anaphylaxis due to food or oral medication usually begins within a few hours.
- Among patients who die, the time between *exposure* and *death* is:
  - ~5 minutes for iatrogenic anaphylaxis (e.g., IV medication induced)
  - ~15 minutes for insect venom anaphylaxis.
  - ~30 minutes for food anaphylaxis.

35. Ans. (a) Tricuspid regurgitation

Ref: Harrison 21st ed. pg. 1817

- v wave occurs in isovolumetric relaxation when blood begins to fill in atrial chambers. The jets of blood of tricuspid regurgitation will add up and lead to extra volume of blood in atrial chambers causing large v wave.
- Option b leads to continuous murmur and heart failure in neonates.
- Option c leads to dicrotic pulse and chronic congestive heart failure.
- Option d is ruled out as it is left-sided lesion causing left ventricular failure.

36. Ans. (b) CT Pulmonary angiography

Ref: Harrison 21st ed. pg. 2095

- Prolonged immobilization will lead to deep vein thrombosis and increased chances of clot formation in soleal veins. The embolization of this clot into pulmonary artery will explain the sudden onset breathlessness in the patient. Chest pain can be explained by pleural infarction. CTPA is the investigation of choice for pulmonary embolism.
- Option a may show sinus tachycardia or S1Q3T3 pattern that is not specific for pulmonary thromboembolism.
- Option c will show right ventricular failure in this condition but not diagnose the etiology. We need to demonstrate occlusion of pulmonary artery by CTPA to confirm the diagnosis.
- Option d is the screening tool for identification of pulmonary embolism and DVT.

37. Ans. (d) TB meningitis

Ref: Harrison 21st ed. pg. 1117

- Two-week history of fever with nuchal rigidity points to infectious etiology. LP shows mononuclear cell increase with low sugar, and gross increase in protein points to TB meningitis.
- Option a will have an increase in polymorphonuclear cells in CSF.
- Option b will have normal sugar levels in CSF.
- Option c occurs in immunocompromised patients and does not have gross increase of proteins.

38. Ans. (c) Constrictive pericarditis

Ref: Harrison 21st ed. pg. 2024

Distended neck veins that increase on inspiration imply Kussmaul sign. Options a and b are both ruled out due to the presence of murmur. Option d will have loud P2 due to pulmonary artery hypertension.

The answer is option c, constrictive pericarditis, which is further supported by pulse disappearing on deep inspiration, i.e., Pulsus paradoxus.

Extra Mile

Pulsus Paradoxus plus Kussmaul sign = Constrictive pericarditis
Pulsus Paradoxus with nonpulsatile elevated JVP= Cardiac Tamponade

39. Ans. (a) GBS

Ref: Harrison 21st ed. pg. 3505

The clinical course of acute dysentery followed by ascending paralysis favors diagnosis as GBS.

- Option b will have sensory level with root pains plus bladder/bowel involvement.
- Option c will cause proximal muscle weakness in a young female.
- Option d will present with diplopia and asymmetrical ptosis with diurnal variation.

40. Ans. (c) Cerebral malaria

Ref: Harrison 21st ed. pg. 979

- Option a is ruled out as it develops over couple of weeks with nuchal rigidity.
- Option b is ruled out as pallor is not seen and it develops over a couple of days instead of extremely fast deterioration in one day as seen in the given case.
- Option d is seen with immunocompromised state.
- The diagnosis is cerebral malaria that will cause high-grade fever with altered sensorium and UMN signs with hemolysis component explaining sudden onset pallor.

41. Ans. (b) Cerebral edema

Leading cause of death in DKA as per OP Ghai is cerebral edema, though some sources mention dehydration. The reason for this is rapid fluid shifts across the brain and damage to the blood-brain barrier by acidosis. Dehydration will occur only if medical care is not provided on time or is inadequate.

42. Ans. (a) Serum lactate (>100 mmol/L)

Ref: Harrison 21st ed. pg. 2238

SIRS criteria (two or more)	qSOFA criteria (two or more)
36 > Temperatrue >38	Systolic blood pressure <100 mm Hg
Respiratory rate >22/min	Respiratory rate >20/min
Heart rate >90 bpm	Glasgow Coma Scale ≤14
4000 > White cell count >12,000	

43. Ans. (a) Lower Limb Vascular Surgery

Ref: Harrison 21st ed. pg. 1672

TABLE: Well-recognized factors and conditions predisposing to hematogenously disseminated candidiasis

Antibacterial agents	Abdominal and thoracic surgery
Indwelling intravenous catheters	Cytotoxic chemotherapy
Hyperalimentation fluids	Immunosuppressive agents for organs transplantation
Indwelling urinary catheters	Respirators
Parenteral glucocorticoids	Myeloperoxidase deficiency
Severe burns	Neutropenia
CARD9 deficiency (central nervous system)	Low birth weight (neonates) diabetes

44. Ans. (a) Metoprolol

Ref: Harrison 21st ed. pg. 1946

Beta blockers are the major mortality reducing agents used in congestive heart failure. They will reduce oxygen consumption of heart. Furosemide and Torsemide are high ceiling diuretics which will reduce pulmonary edema and produce symptomatic relief. Option c is used in the patients suffering from hypertension.

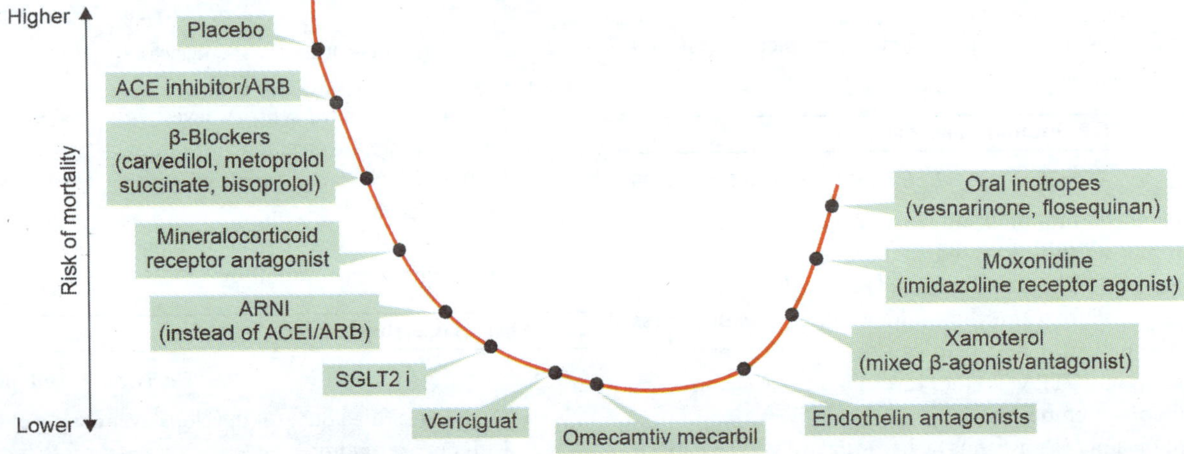

Progressive decline in mortality with angiotensin-converting enzyme (ACE) inhibitors or angiotensin receptor blockers (ARBs) or angiotensin receptor-neprilysin inhibitors (ARNIs), beta blockers, mineralocorticoid receptor antagonists, sodium-glucose cotransporter-2 (SGLT-2) inhibitors, and balanced vasodilators

45. Ans. (a) Encephalopathy, ascites, albumin, Bilirubin and PT

Ref: CMDT 2023, page 706

Child-Pugh score is used to assess severity of cirrhosis and assess need for registration of orthotopic liver transplantation. Components are BA_3T (Bilirubin, Albumin, Ascites, Asterixis and Prothrombin time).

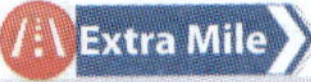

MELD Score: Model for end stage liver disease is also used to assess need for orthotopic liver transplantation and predict mortality in percentage. Components are Bilirubin, INR, S. Creatinine.

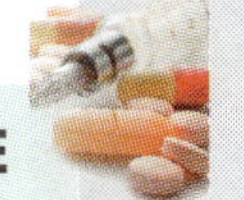

46. Ans. (b) Legionella

Ref: Harrison 21st ed. pg. 1254

- The keywords are bilateral infiltrates in both lungs indicating pneumonia. The presence of hyponatremia (Na = 126 mEq/L) indicates atypical pneumonia. Legionella pneumophila leads to SIADH and causes excess water reabsorption. This explains hyponatremia seen in this patient.
- Option a is the leading cause of lobar pneumonia and does not present with diarrhea.
- Option c occurs in AIDS positive patients and causes pneumonia when CD4 count less than 200 cells/mm^3. Option d is common in alcoholics and produces reddish brown sputum.

47. Ans. (d) Rheumatoid arthritis

Ref: Harrison 21st ed. pg. 2198

- Rheumatoid arthritis is an inflammatory condition which leads to fibrin-rich exudative pleural effusion.
- Option a will cause increase in hydrostatic pressure that leads to transudative pleural effusion. Options b and c lead to reduced serum albumin and reduced oncotic pressure causing transudative pleural effusion.

48. Ans. (a) Cystic Fibrosis

Ref: Harrison 21st ed. pg. 2176

- A combination of recurrent lung infections and steatorrhea points to cystic fibrosis. CF leads to increased viscosity of body fluids. Thick lung secretions lead to failure of mucociliary escalator and increased incidence of lung infections. Thick pancreatic secretions lead to reduced level of serum amylase and hence, sugar remains unabsorbed. This will cause osmotic diarrhea. Reduced lipase will lead to steatorrhea.
- Option b leads to pan-acinar emphysema and cirrhosis. Option c presents in neonatal age group and leads to respiratory distress. Option d cannot explain recurrent lung infections.

49. Ans. (a) Multiple myeloma

Ref: Harrison 21st ed. pg. 870

- The keyword is bone marrow biopsy showing plasma cells > 60% pointing to cause as multiple myeloma. The plasma cells lead to release of cytokines that cause lytic lesions in bones. Bone marrow colonization by plasma cells leads to lesser production of RBC and resultant anemia. The overproduction of light chains blocks kidney tubules and leads to renal failure.
- CML presents with massive splenomegaly and leukocytosis. AML and ALL lead to anemia, bleeding from mucosa and hepatosplenomegaly. AML occurs in adults and ALL in children commonly.

50. Ans. (d) PSGN

Ref: Harrison 21st ed. pg. 337

Presence of subnephrotic proteinuria with hypertension after recovery from a URTI indicates post infectious glomerulonephritis. Confirmation of diagnosis is with Anti-DNA-ase antibody.

Options a and c will have proteinuria >3.5 g/day. Option b presents hematuria with hemoptysis.

51. Ans. (b) Dermatomyositis

Ref: CMDT 2023, page 842

- The female patient has proximal muscle weakness leading to difficulty in getting up from squatting position.
- Skin manifestation of heliotrope rash makes diagnosis of dermatomyositis.
- Option a will not have skin manifestations. Option c will have malar rash with photosensitivity and arthritis. Option d will have Raynaud phenomenon with dysphagia and pulmonary artery hypertension.

52. Ans. (b) LAMB

Ref: Harrison 21st ed. pg. 946

The drug of choice for cryptococcal meningitis is liposomal amphotericin-B. Option a is used after completing 2 weeks intravenous course of LAMB and is given for next 10 weeks orally.

Option d is used for management of aspergillosis.

53. Ans. (b) Glucagonoma

Ref: Harrison 21st ed. pg. 665

Necrolytic migratory erythema is characteristic dermatitis involving intertriginous areas, especially groin and buttocks.

54. Ans. (c) VIPoma

Ref: Harrison 21st ed. pg. 665

Vasoactive intestinal polypeptide causes secretory diarrhea with hypokalemia. Option a will cause hypoglycemic episodes. Option b will cause impaired glucose tolerance. Option d will present with diabetes mellitus, cholelithiasis, steatorrhea, abdominal pain and obstructive jaundice.

55. Ans. (a) Gallium 68 Dotatate PET

Ref: Harrison 21st ed. pg. 667

The order of answer shall be Gallium-68 Dotatate PET-CT > CT/MRI > Somatostatin receptor scintigraphy.

56. Ans. (d) Pituitary microadenoma

Ref: Harrison 21st ed. pg. 2960

TABLE: Causes of cushing's syndrome

Causes of cushing's syndrome	Female: Male ratio	%
ATCH-Dependent Cushing's		**90**
Cushing's disease (=ACTH-producing pituitary adenoma)	4:1	75
Ectopic ACTH syndrome (due to ACTH secretion by bronchial or pancreatic carcinoid tumors, small-cell lung cancer, medullary thyroid carcinoma, pheochromocytoma, and others)	1:1	15
ACTH-Independent Cushing's	**4:1**	**10**
Adrenocortical adenoma		5–10
Adrenocortical carcinoma		1
Rare causes: Macronodular adrenal hyperplasia; primary pigmented nodular adrenal disease (micro-and/or macronodular); McCune-Albright syndrome		<1

57. Ans. (a) Silicosis

Ref: Harrison 21st ed. pg. 2169

- CT chest showing multiple small nodules with diffuse ground appearance with *thickened intralobular and interlobular septa* producing polygonal shapes called crazy paving is seen in silicosis.
- CXR chest showing lower lung field linear opacities, irregular heart border and ground glass appearance of CXR is seen in asbestosis.
- *If in this question, lower lobe was mentioned with no mention of interlobular septa involvement, then answer will be asbestosis.*

58. Ans. (a) Gout

Ref: Harrison 21st ed. pg. 3251

- Keywords are negatively birefringent crystals on polarized microscopy which is seen with monosodium urate. Knee joint can also be involved in gout.
- Option b (pseudo-gout) commonly involves knee joint but will have positively birefringent crystals on polarized microscopy.
- Option c is a degenerative joint disease due to old age. Option d is seen in young females with small joint involvement like PIP, MCP and wrist joint involvement bilaterally.

59. Ans. (b) Negative skin tuberculin test and normal CXR

Ref: Semantic Scholar

Cryptic Miliary TB

This is unusual presentation seen in the elderly and characterized by:

- Age over 60 years.
- Intermittent low-grade fever
- Unexplained weight loss and general debility.
- Hepatosplenomegaly in 25–50%.
- Normal chest X-ray.
- Negative tuberculin skin test.
- Blood dyscrasia: Leukemoid reaction, pancytopenia
- Confirmation by biopsy (granulomas and/or AFB demonstrated) of liver of bone marrow.

60. Ans. (b) Goodpasture syndrome

Ref: Harrison 21st ed. pg. 2281

A combination of hemoptysis and hematuria points to etiology as Goodpasture syndrome. The anti-basement membrane antibody damages blood vessels as well as alveolar and glomerular lining.

61. Ans. (a) SAH

Ref: Harrison 21st ed. pg. 3353

The case presentation mentions "Worst headache of my life" kind of description by the patient. The presence of nuchal rigidity, headache and sudden onset points to diagnosis as subarachnoid hemorrhage. Option b presents with pulsating headache and does not have nuchal rigidity. Options c and d should have fever present.

62. Ans. (a) Control hypertension and immediate surgery

Ref: Harrison 21st ed. pg. 2106

CT chest shows Tennis ball appearance of aortic dissection. The leading cause of tear in aorta is uncontrolled hypertension. Hence, option a is best for management. Option b will cause expiry of patient. Option c will not give any additional information about diagnosis. Option d will help in lowering of BP and reduce pulmonary edema but emergency surgical repair is the best way for management.

63. Ans. (a) CT guided Biopsy

Ref: Harrison 21st ed. pg. 270

Since the patient is having a peripheral lung tumor, CT guided transthoracic biopsy will be used for tissue diagnosis. Option b (bronchoscopy) will be used for central lung cancer.

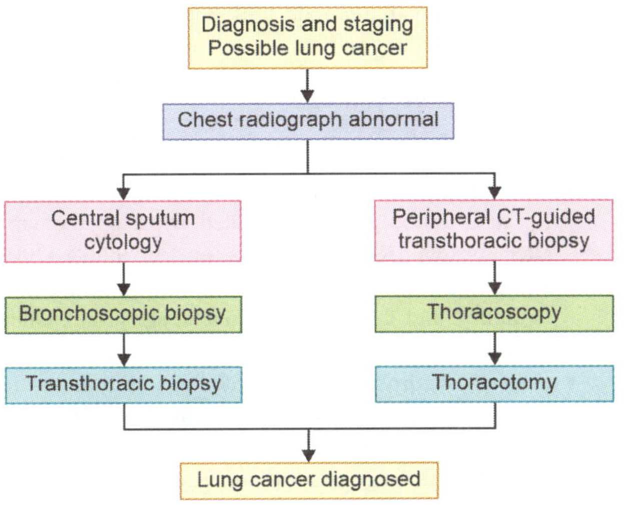

64. Ans. (b) Relative/apparent erythrocytosis

Ref: Harrison 21st ed. pg. 439

Polycythemia vera	JAK 2 mutation	Excess production of RBC due to clonal expansion of normoblasts
Secondary polycythemia	Hypoxia due to COPD or cyanotic heart disease	Excess production of RBC due to increased erythropoietin levels
Gaisbock syndrome/Relative polycythemia	Volume depletion due to excess diuretics	RBC count is increased due to reduced plasma concentration

65. Ans. (a) Pseudotumor cerebri

Ref: Harrison 21st ed. pg. 2937

The keywords papilledema and raised ICP narrow down the diagnosis to pseudotumor cerebri. It is caused by use of OCP, excess vitamin A, steroid withdrawal and leads to features of raised ICP.

Option b leads to pulsatile headache. Option c presents with jaw claudication and temporal headache. Option d presents with ptosis and diurnal variation of symptoms.

66. Ans. (b) Hypervitaminosis B6

Ref: Harrison 21st ed. pg. 3493

Excess use of vitamin B6 leads to neurotoxicity by causing cell death in dose-dependent fashion. Paradoxically symptoms associated with vitamin B6 toxicity are similar to those with vitamin B6 deficiency. A patient will experience peripheral sensory neuropathy. Most commonly, this causes numbness in a stocking-glove distribution over the extremities.

67. Ans. (b) Myasthenia gravis

Ref: Harrison 21st ed. pg. 3511

Ptosis with diurnal variation of symptoms and relief with acetylcholinesterase inhibitors are features of Myasthenia Gravis. Option a presents with arm and leg weakness with areflexia and is commonly associated with lung cancer. Option c presents with Gower sign and pseudohypertrophy of calf muscles. Option d presents with asymmetrical arm weakness progressing over years and features of both LMN and UMN lesion.

68. Ans. (b) Hereditary spherocytosis

Ref: Harrison 20th ed. pg. 780–907

Acute ITP	Steroids TPO-RA and Rituximab
Chronic ITP	ITP can resolve spontaneously in adults. So splenectomy should only be done as last resort.
Hereditary spherocytosis	Severe case: elective splenectomy at 4-6 years Moderate case: delay splenectomy till puberty Mild case: avoid splenectomy
G6PD	Avoid drugs that trigger hemolysis
Hairy cell leukemia	Cladribine

69. Ans. (b) Lanreotide Depot formulation

Ref: Harrison 21st ed. pg. 2913

The main objective is to shrink the pituitary tumor for which long-acting form of octreotide called Lanreotide is used. Options a, c and d are used in bleeding esophageal varices.

70. Ans. (b) Decreased haptoglobin

Ref: Robbins and Cotran, E-Book, pg. 215

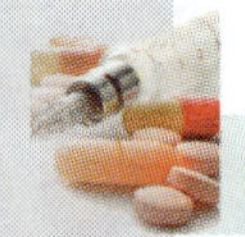

Hemolysis will cause LDH to rise. Free hemoglobin will bind to haptoglobin. Consumption of haptoglobin explains decreased haptoglobin. Hemolysis leads to reticulocytosis and elevated unconjugated hyperbilirubinemia.

71. Ans. (c) Tc 99 Sestamibi Scan

Ref: Harrison 21st ed. pg. 2984:

The presence of lytic lesion in metacarpal bones and renal stones, result implies elevated serum calcium and elevated PTH. To locate parathyroid tumor, "sestamibi scan" is done. Another keyword is brown tumor which indicates hyperparathyroidism.

72. Ans. (d) Nasal cannula

Delivery of Oxygen

Class	Device	Oxygen flow (L/min)	Approx FiO_2	Comments
Variable delivery	Nasal prongs	2 4 6	28% 35% 45%	Stable patients only
	Semi-rigid (Hudson mask)	5 6 8 10 12	35% 50% 55% 60% 65%	Low cost Frequently Used Not accurate at controlling FiO_2

73. Ans. (d) Neurogenic tumors

Ref: Robbins and Cotran E-book, 2021 ed.

TABLE: Mediastinal tumors and other masses

Superior mediastinum Lymphoma Thymoma Thyroid lesions Metastatic carcinoma Parathyroid tumors
Anterior mediastinum Thymoma Teratoma Lymphoma Thyroid lesions Parathyroid tumors
Posterior mediastinum Neurogenic tumors (schwannoma, neurofibroma) Lymphoma Gastroenteric hernia
Middle mediastinum Bronchogenic cyst Pericardial cyst Lymphoma

74. Ans. (b) Temporal arteritis

Ref: Harrison 21st ed. pg. 2811

- Keyword is nodular thickening of temporal artery which is seen in temporal/giant cell arteritis. It is a leading cause of vasculitis in geriatric population and is an extra-cranial cause of headache. Temporal artery supplies the skin of scalp and narrowing will cause ischemia of scalp which is perceived as headache by the patient.
- Option a involves subclavian arteries and leads to arm claudication. Option c leads to intermittent claudication and causes gangrene of toes. Option d presents as extensor purpura on buttocks or back of thighs.

75. Ans. (b) Gilbert Syndrome

Ref: Harrison 21st ed. pg. 2559

- Most common inherited liver disease is Gilbert disease. It causes jaundice (unconjugated hyperbilirubinemia) after unexplained physical stress or drug intake. Option a is ruled out as it causes increase in conjugated bilirubin. Options c and d present in neonatal age group. Gilbert disease has a benign course and does not need treatment.
- Gilbert syndrome is inherited in an autosomal recessive manner. Uridine diphosphoglucuronate-glucuronosyltransferase 1A1 (UG1A1) is important for converting unconjugated to conjugated bilirubin and is defective in this condition.

76. Ans. (a) MAI

Ref: Harrison 21st ed. pg. 1404

Keyword is acid fast bacilli and CD4 count less than 100 narrows down diagnosis as Mycobacterium avium-intracellulare (MAI).

Common opportunistic infection in AIDS Patients

CD4 count <500 cells/mm^3	Mycobacterium Tuberculosis
CD4 count <200 cells/mm^3	Pneumocystis Jiroveci
CD4 count <100 cells/mm^3	Cerebral toxoplasmosis
D4 count <50 cells/mm^3	CMV Retinitis Mycobacterium avium-intracellulare

77. Ans. (c) CT chest

Ref: Harrison 21st ed. pg. 270

- CT chest needs to be performed to identify the source and location of source of hemoptysis. Option a (bronchoscopy) would be done after CT scan. Repeat CXR would not provide any new information. Option d is not done. Along with CXR, complete blood count, serum creatinine and coagulogram are done.

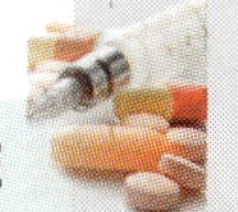

- In massive hemoptysis, first step is to protect airways, especially contralateral lung with selective bronchus intubation. The treatment of choice for massive hemoptysis is bronchial artery embolization.

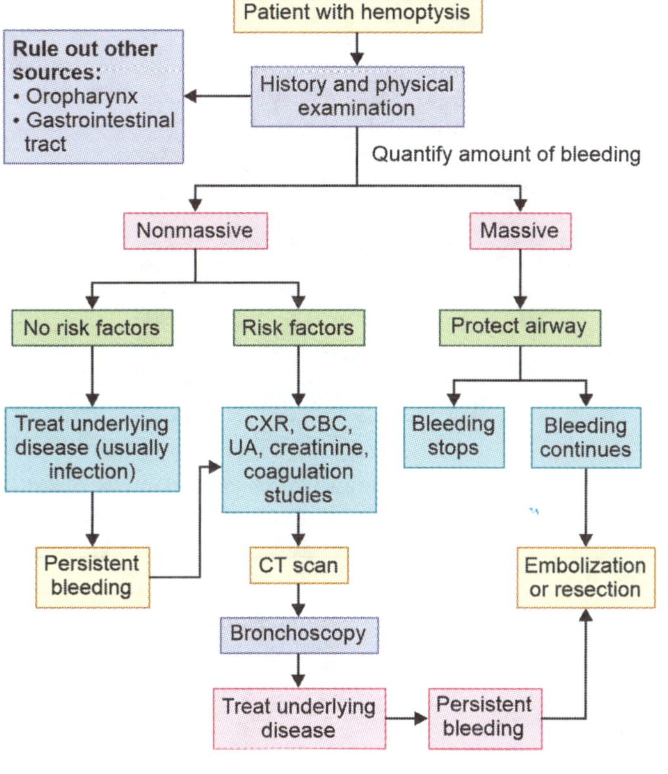

78. Ans. (b) Mesothelioma

Ref: Harrison 21st ed. pg. 2167

The most characteristic cancer seen in asbestosis is mesothelioma. The most common cancer seen in patients with asbestosis is adenocarcinoma of lung.

CARDIOLOGY

79. Ans. (b) PSVT

Ref: Harrison 20th ed. pg. 1890

The ECG shows narrow complex tachycardia with heart rate of approximately 200bpm. P waves are not visible and global ST depression is seen in all leads. This can be explained by sudden increase in oxygen consumption of heart due to re-entry phenomenon of PSVT.

80. Ans. (a) Atrial fibrillation

Ref: Harrison 20th ed. pg. 1903

The word is irregularly irregular radial pulse which is a characteristic feature of atrial fibrillation. Absent P wave can be explained by SAN activity being suppressed by ectopic foci activity in left atrium in these patients.

81. Ans. (b) Continue CPR while team applies AED Paddles

Ref: AHA 2020 Update

- The main component of BLS is deployment of AED to terminate tachyarrhythmia.
- Option a is wrong because if we wait for five rounds 10 minutes would have passed by and person would be brain dead. One round/cycle of CPR = 2 minutes
- Option c is wrong as CPR should never be stopped while other tasks like putting an IV line or putting paddles of AED is being done
- Option d is wrong as it is applicable in case of a bystander CPR where a non-medico is giving CPR. He should vacate his position and let a trained person handle the case.

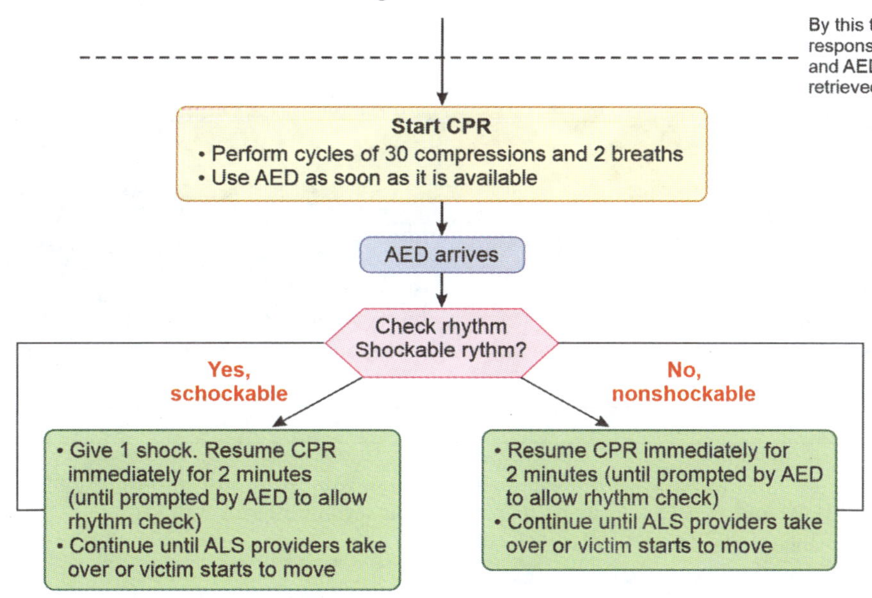

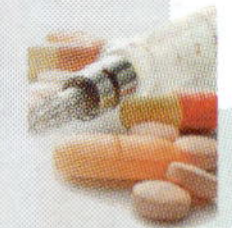

82. Ans. (a) Cardiac tamponade

Ref: Harrison 21st ed. pg. 2020

The logic is that the base of left lung is compressed by massive pericardial effusion. Therefore, when you examine below the angle of left scapula it leads to patch of dullness and increased vocal fremitus.

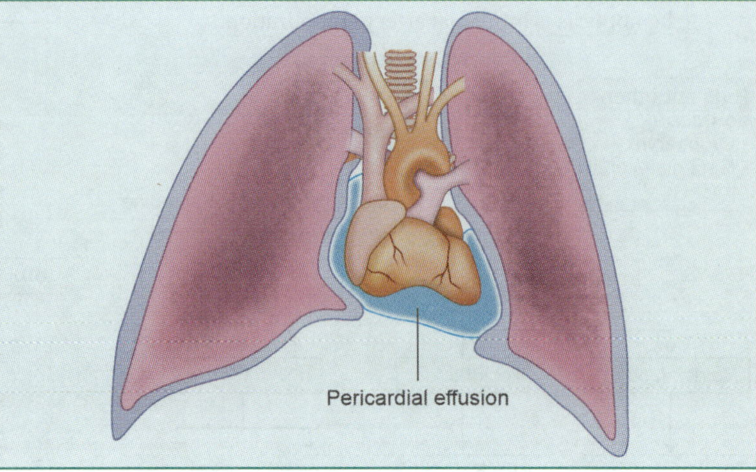

83. Ans. (d) Cardiac tamponade

Ref: Harrison 21st ed. pg. 2022

Traditionally we use the term muffled heart sounds for cardiac tamponade. But in this question the term used was smooth/ diminished heart sounds. The classical features of Beck's triad, hypotension with diminished heart sounds help in diagnosis. The third component of elevated JVP was given as absent y descent. The reason for absent y descent is elevated end diastolic pressure to increased intrapericardial space pressure that hampers filling of heart chambers.

84. Ans. (a) Hypothermia

Ref: Harrison 21st ed. pg. 3632

ECG finding of Hypothermia shows a J wave at the start of ST segment along with PR prolongation and broadening of qRS complex.

85. Ans. (c) Disability

Ref: AHA 2020 Guidelines

- The Airway, Breathing, Circulation, Disability, Exposure (ABCDE) approach is applicable in all clinical emergencies for immediate assessment and treatment.
- It would involve checking for AVPU which is an acronym for **'Alert', 'Voice', 'Pain', 'Unresponsive'** status apart from checking pupillary size and response to light.

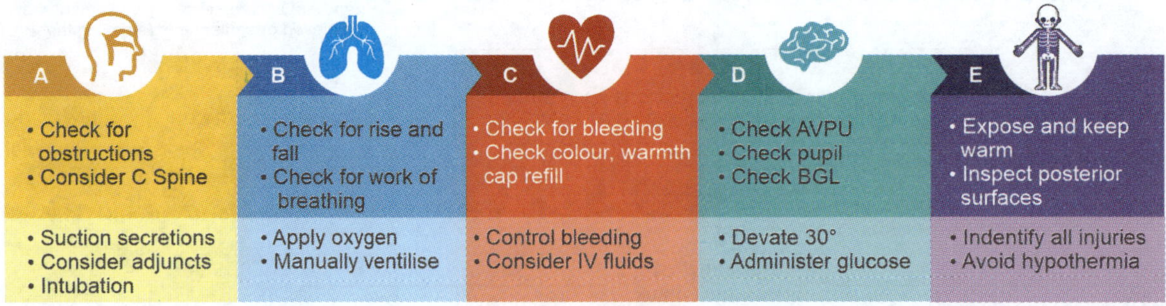

86. Ans. (b) Inferior wall MI

Ref: Harrison 21st ed. pg. 2053

- ECG shows ST Elevation in lead II, III and aVF. Heart rate is 60 bpm which is seen in inferior wall MI
- Option a will show ST segment changes in lead I, aVL, V1 to V4.

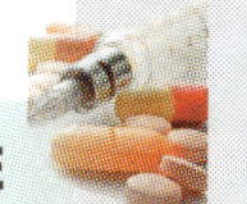

- Option c will show ST segment changes in all the leads of ECG
- Option d will show ST segment changes in lead V7 to V9.

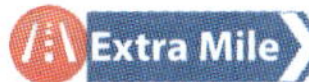

A 70-year-old man presents with vomiting and central chest pain. O/E bradycardia is present with BP = 90/60 mm Hg. cTnI is elevated to 99th Centile of URL. Diagnosis is?

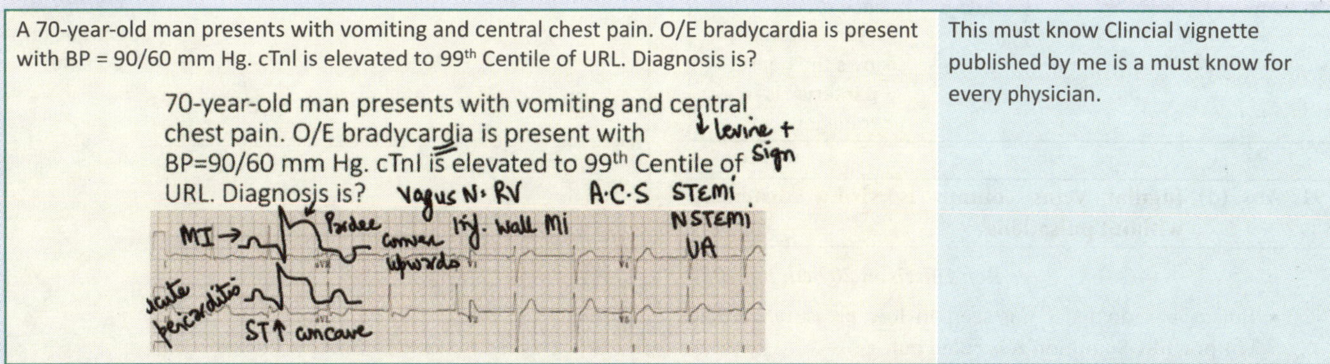

This must know Clincial vignette published by me is a must know for every physician.

87. Ans. (a) Right ventricular hypertrophy

Ref: Harrison 21st ed. pg. 1825

The vector points in right lower quadrant and is seen in cases of right ventricular enlargement.

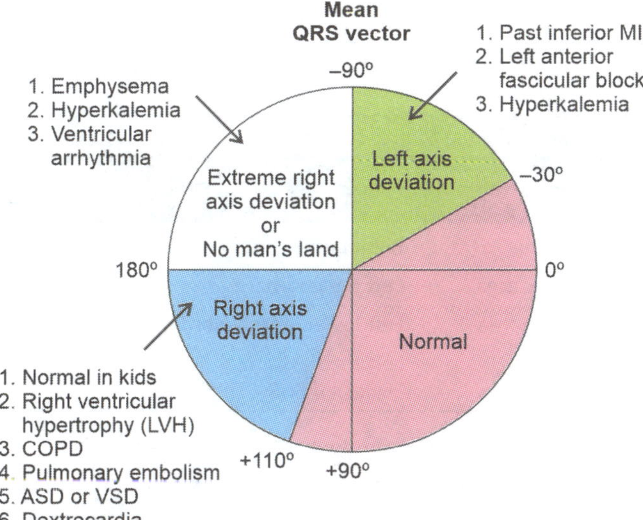

88. Ans. (d) Sinus arrhythmia

Ref: Ganong 25th ed. pg. 527

The ECG shows variation in RR interval, but P waves are present before each qRS complex. This is seen in sinus arrythmia.

- Atrial Fibrillation is ruled out as P wave is present preceding each qRS complex
- Atrial flutter is ruled out as saw tooth waves are not present
- W.P.W has delta waves and is a rare condition.

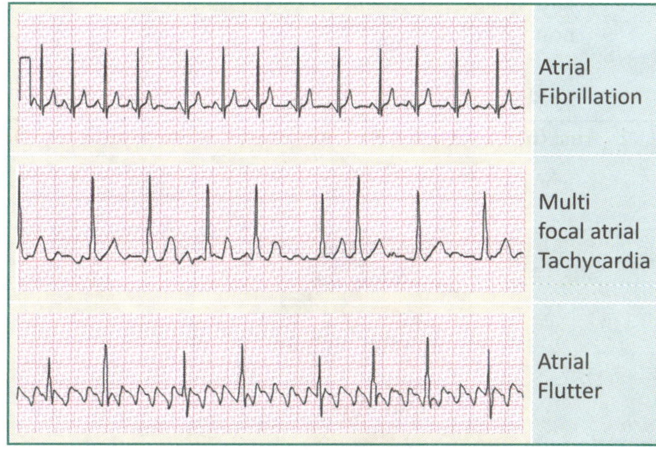

89. Ans. (b) Start CPR and defibrillation

Ref: Harrison 21st ed. pg. 1929

The ECG shows ventricular fibrillation. The ventricles are twitching and to re-establish the SAN dominance defibrillation will be required. Since getting an AED into action will take time, CPR must be started while other team member fixes the paddles of AED.

90. Ans. (b) Hyperkalemia

Ref: Harrison 20th ed. pg. 1829-30

- Option a is ruled out as it leads to T wave inversion and ST depression
- Option c and d leads to fluid shift across the brain and causes cerebral edema.

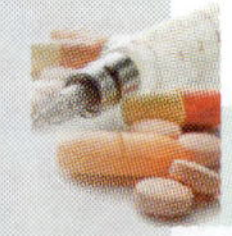

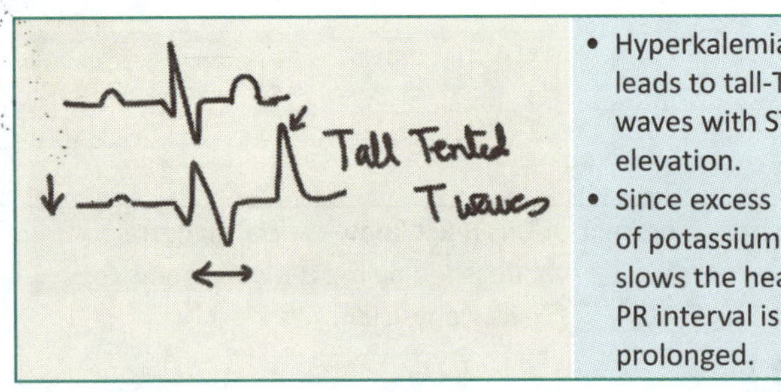

- Hyperkalemia leads to tall-Tented waves with ST elevation.
- Since excess of potassium slows the heart, PR interval is prolonged.

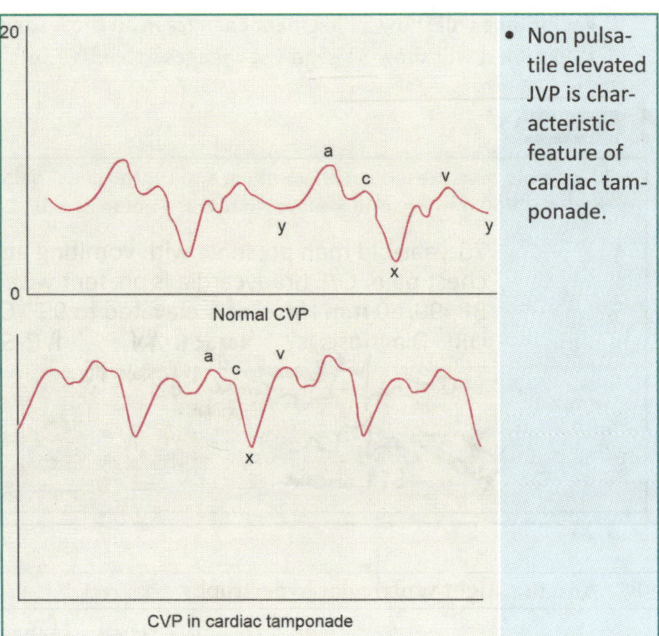

- Non pulsatile elevated JVP is characteristic feature of cardiac tamponade.

91. Ans. (d) Jugular veins column is visibly distended without pulsations

Ref: Harrison 20th ed. pg. 2021

- Pulsus paradoxus is not seen in low pressure cardiac tamponade. So option A is ruled out.
- Kussmaul sign is absent in cardiac tamponade. So option B is ruled out.
- Tall a wave is seen in tricuspid stenosis. Cardiac tamponade has absent y descent option d is correct as nonpulsatile elevated JVP is seen in cardiac tamponade.

92. Ans. (b) A= Aortic, B= Pulmonic, C= Tricuspid area, D= Mitral area

Ref: Harrison 20th ed. pg. 1820

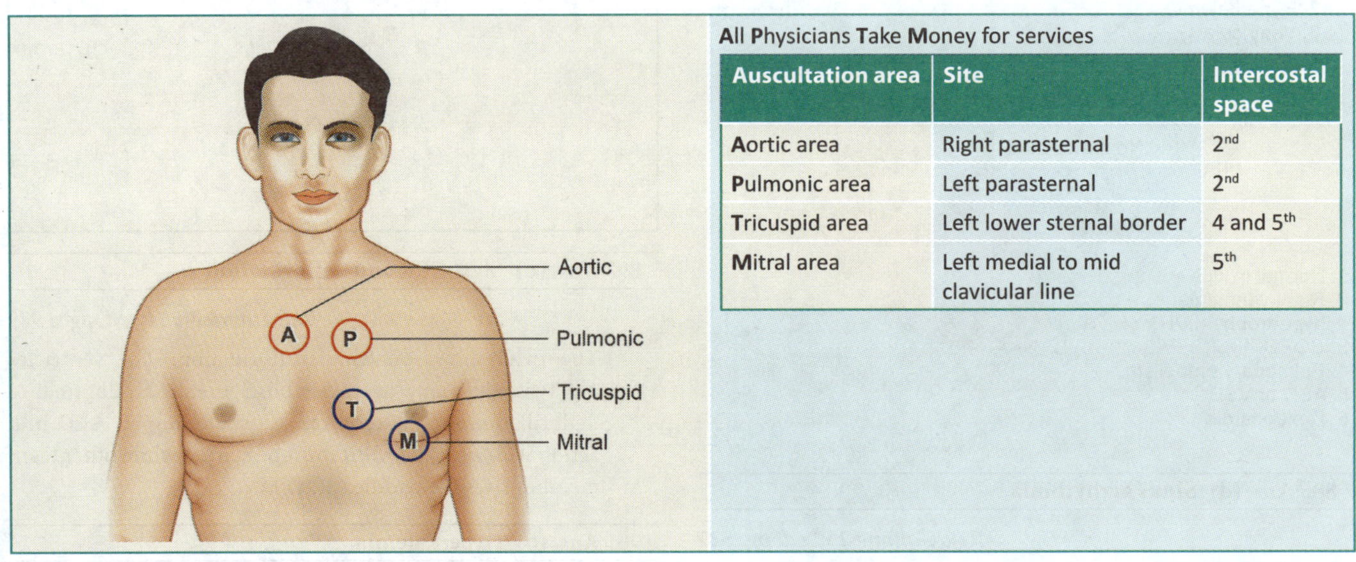

All Physicians Take Money for services

Auscultation area	Site	Intercostal space
Aortic area	Right parasternal	2nd
Pulmonic area	Left parasternal	2nd
Tricuspid area	Left lower sternal border	4 and 5th
Mitral area	Left medial to mid clavicular line	5th

93. Ans. (a) ASD

Ref: Harrison 20th ed. pg. 1819

Wide fixed split S2 is seen in ASD. Option b has wide variable split S2. Option d has single S2. Option d is bicuspid aortic valve that leads to Aortic stenosis. It leads to narrow split S2.

94. Ans. (a) Ejection systolic

Ref: Harrison 20th ed. pg. 1673

- The murmur in the image begins after ejection click, peaks in middle of systole and ends at S2. This is a feature of ejection systolic murmur.
- In pansystolic murmur the intensity of murmur does not change and remains constant, all through systole.

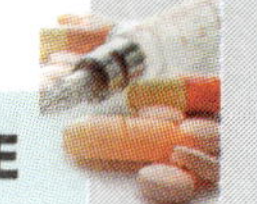

- In early diastolic murmur which starts after S2 the intensity drops in early part of diastole
- In mid diastolic murmur which starts after S2 the murmur peaks in middle of diastole and then drops in intensity.

95. Ans. (b) Constrictive pericarditis

Ref: Harrison 20th ed. pg. 1845-46

- Rapid X and Y descent is a feature of constrictive pericarditis. The given CXR shows *normal* CT ratio and *calcification* around cardiac borders which appears well delineated.
- Option a, c and d are ruled out as they will have increased CT ratio.

96. Ans. (a) Aortic insufficiency

Ref: Harrison 20th ed. pg. 1673

- The displacement of apex beat to left indicates pathology in left side of heart. This rules out options c and d.
- The presence of high-volume pulse and diastolic murmur helps in confirming diagnosis as Aortic insufficiency.
- Mitral insufficiency is ruled out as it shows pansystolic murmur

97. Ans. (a) Clubbing

Ref: Macloed's Clinical Examination E-book, pg. 50

The image shows convexity of nails/parrot beak appearance which is seen in clubbing. The color of tips of extremities is normal ruling out Option b, c and d.

98. Ans. (d) Congestive heart failure

Ref: Harrison 20th ed. pg. 1766

- Since patient had MI previously, he would have developed cardiac damage. He is now having features suggestive of pulmonary edema and S3. This indicates development of Chronic CHF.
- Option a presents with chest pain at rest with pericardial friction rub
- Option b presents with breathlessness with wide split S2
- Option c presents with low cardiac output and clot formation in aneurysm that can embolise the brain. It would require Echo for diagnosis and cannot be commented on physical findings alone.

99. Ans. (c) Splenomegaly

Ref: Harrison 20th ed. pg. 923

- Clinical history of undiagnosed fever in a known case of Valvular heart disease points to differential diagnosis of Infective endocarditis. The first image shows presence of Roth spots on fundus examination. The second image shows erythematous macules in palms known as Janeway lesions.
- Infective endocarditis leads to shower of infective emboli into systemic circulation. This can lead to splenic abscess formation and resultant splenomegaly. It is a complication and *not* a diagnostic criterion.
- To confirm the diagnosis modified Duke criteria will be used.

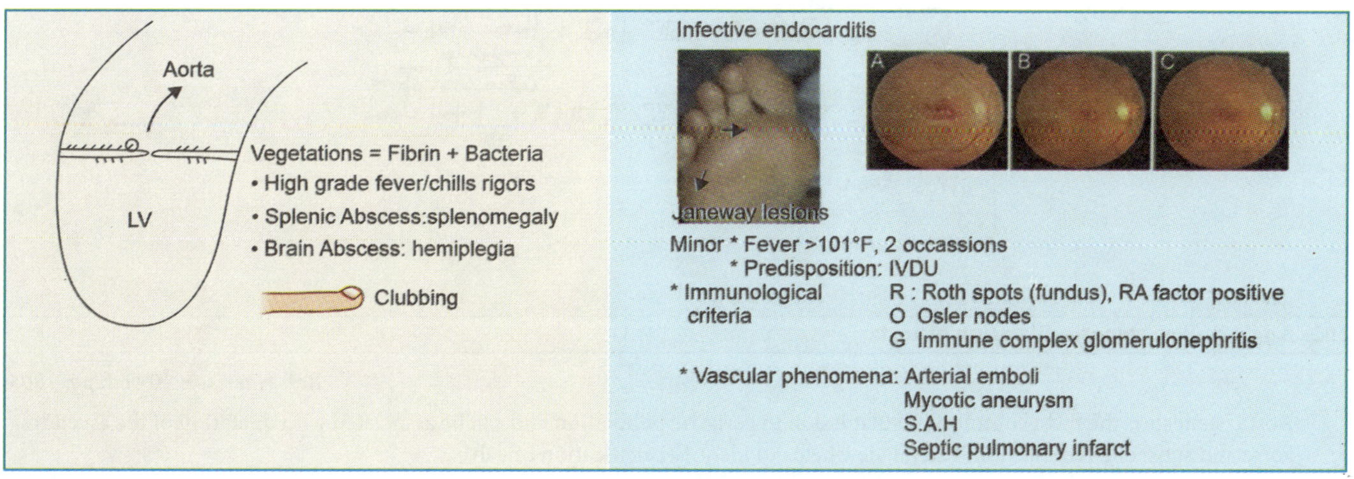

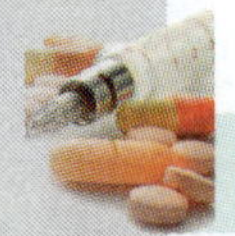

100. Ans. (c) Injection of adrenaline 1 mg IV

Ref: Harrison 20th ed. pg. 2064

- The ECG shows asystole or cardiac arrest. 1 mg shot of adrenaline is required to stimulate the SAN and restart the heart on a priority.
- Option a is used in shockable rhythm like ventricular tachycardia and ventricular fibrillation. Asystole shown in the ECG is an example of non-shockable rhythm.
- Option b has no role in current resuscitation protocol.
- Option d is used in management of symptomatic bradycardia.

Shockable rhythm	Non shockable rhythm
Ventricular fibrillation	Asystole (1:10000) ↑↑↑ Adrenaline
Ventricular tachycardia	Pulseless electrical activity

V.fib

Pulseless electrical activity → Hypovolemia, hypothermia, T.pneumothorax

101. Ans. (d) Putamen is the most common site

Ref: Harrison 20th ed. pg. 3092

- Option a is ruled out as antiplatelet drugs can worsen CNS bleed in first 24 hours of hemorrhagic stroke. NCCT head is required urgently to differentiate ischemic stroke and hemorrhagic stroke.
- Option b is ruled out as there is no role of platelet transfusion in CNS bleed due to Hypertensive crisis.
- Option c is ruled out as fast reduction of BP is not indicated in CNS events. Immediate lowering of BP will cause worsening of brain perfusion.
- Option d is correct as Putamen is the most common site of brain hemorrhage.

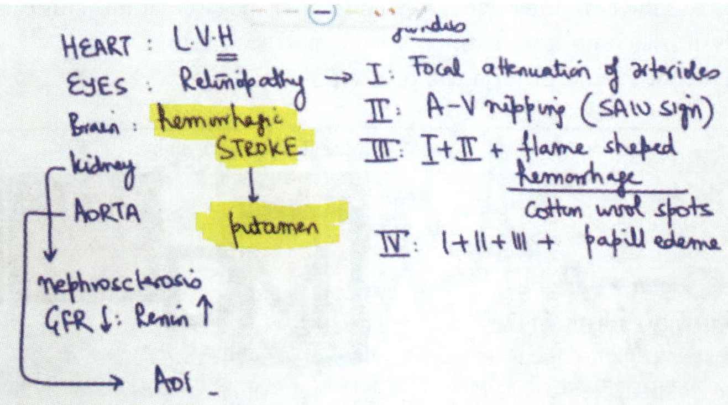

102. Ans. (d) Post stenotic dilatation of aorta

Ref: Harrison 20th ed. pg. 1805

Aortic stenosis is the most common valvular lesion in geriatric population and can be associated with dilatation of the ascending aorta and subsequent dissection. Lateral view helps to identify calcification of valve.

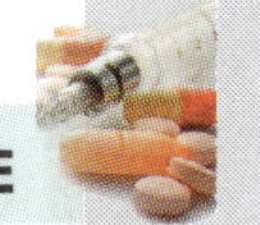

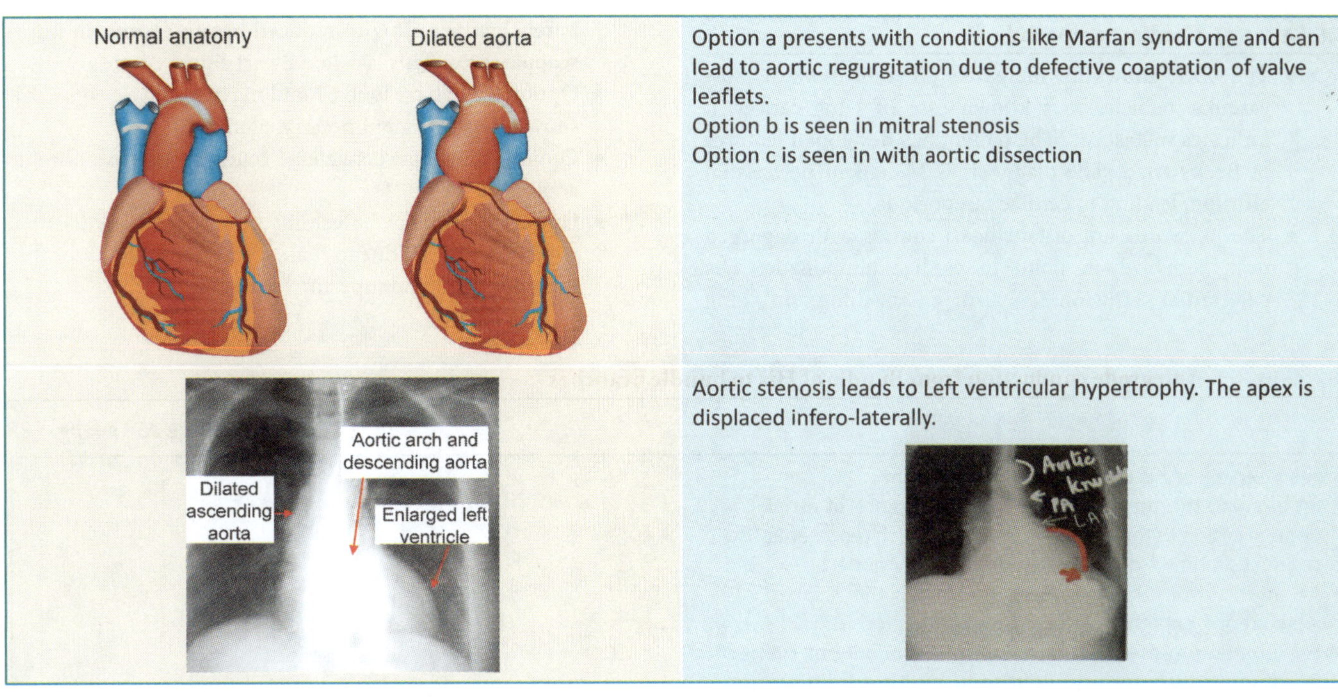

103. Ans. (c) Metoprolol

Reference: Harrison 20th ed. pg. 1583

- The *major mortality reducing drug* in patients of chronic stable angina is Beta blockers. Metoprolol is the most widely studied drug in these patients. It reduces oxygen consumption of heart and helps in improving efficiency of ventricular function.
- Option a is also a mortality reducing drug in hypertensive patients with chronic stable angina
- Option b is used in chronic stable angina only if beta blockers are contraindicated. They have disadvantage of casing pedal edema and hence dose titration is required.
- Option d has disadvantage of causing derangement of lipid profile and glucose levels.

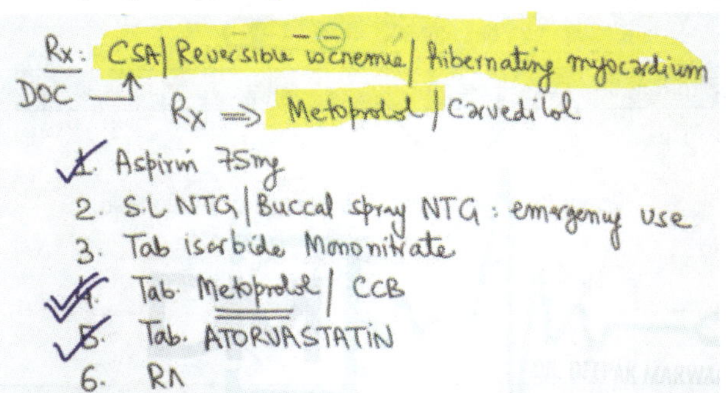

104. Ans. (b) Pacemaker

Ref: Radiology Essentials E-book, 2020 ed. pg. 67

- Notice the two wires, one going to Atrium and other to the ventricle, from the device whose job is to control the heart rate. This device is a pacemaker.
- Option a, Chemo-port is used to deliver chemotherapy directly into subclavian vein. This avoids the superficial thrombophlebitis and extravasation related problems seen with peripheral vein infusion.
- Option d can be mapped out using electrophysiological studies using special electrodes and leads. It cannot be seen on plain Chest X-ray.

105. Ans. (a) Primary Raynaud phenomenon

Ref: Harrison 20th ed. pg. 2552

- The image shows color change in finger tips from white to blue and finally red. Diagnosis is primary Raynaud phenomenon since *no cause/etiology* has been found.
- In case Raynaud phenomenon is associated with autoimmune diseases like SLE, Dermatomyositis, Rheumatoid arthritis, Scleroderma then we call it secondary Raynaud phenomenon.
- 'Harlequin sign' is characterised by asymmetric flushing and sweating of the face, representing localised ipsilateral autonomic dysfunction, due to a cervical sympathetic deficit located at the preganglionic or postganglionic level on the non-flushing side.
- Ainhum is manifestation of peripheral arterial disease that leads to auto- amputation of toes in Africans.

106. Ans. (a) Cardiac tamponade

- The CXR shows an increased CT ratio with narrow vascular pedicle. In a known case of Lung cancer, it indicates metastasis. The patient has developed features of Beck's triad. The diagnosis is Malignant pericardial effusion, leading to cardiac tamporiode.
- The keywords are distant heart sounds with engorged neck veins which point to cardiac tamponade. The pericardial effusion is also encroaching on lung parenchyma leading to reduced breath sounds in infra-scapular area. This is called Ewart sign.
- Option a will have loud S1 and narrow split S2 with CXR showing bat wing pulmonary edema
- Option b will have bilateral blunting of costophrenic angle
- Option d will have flushing of face and mediastinal widening in CXR due to mass effect like lung tumor that is compressing the superior vena cava.

107. Ans. (c) Antegrade conduction from Bundle of His to bundle branches

Ref: Ganong 25th ed. pg. 527

Three intervals of His Bundle Electrocardiogram

- PA interval, the time from the first appearance of atrial depolarization to the A wave in the HBE, which represents conduction time from the SA node to the AV node
- AH interval from the A wave to the start of the H spike, which represents the AV nodal conduction time
- HV interval represents conduction in the bundle of His and the bundle branches. HV interval, the time from the start of the H spike to the start of the QRS deflection in the ECG, which represents conduction in the bundle of His and the bundle branches.

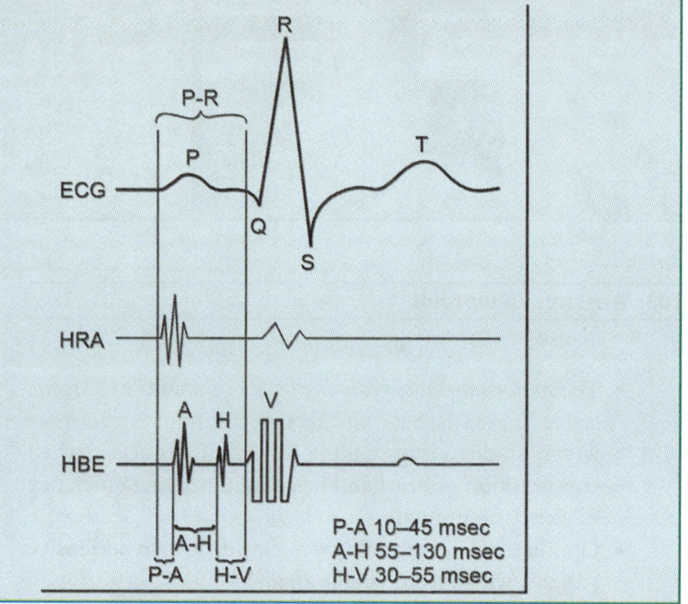

108. Ans. (c) Pitting Pedal edema

Ref: Macloeds Clinical Examination E-book, pg. 59

The image shows presence of pitting pedal edema. The etiology is described in the question as congestive heart failure.

109. Ans. (d) Intravenous access followed by Immediate defibrillation

Ref: Harrison, 20th ed. pg. 2064

One cycle of CPR is for 2 minutes and chest compressions are given@100-120/min. intravenous access is done after defibrillation and not before. Hence Choice d is wrong.

Ventricular fibrillation of pulseless ventricular tachycardia

Chest compressions at 100–120/min immediate defibrillation and resume CPR for 2 minutes

↓ No ROSC

2 minutes of chest compressions/ventrilation and repeat shock

↓ No ROSC

Continue chest compressions, IV or IO access, advanced airway
Epinephrine 1 mg 3–5 minutes
Repeat shock

↓ No ROSC

I.V. amiodarone 300 mg (may repeat 150 mg), continue CPR repeat shock

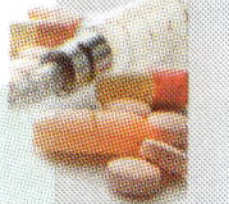

110. Ans. (b) Myocardial ischemia

Ref: Harrison, 20th ed. pg. 1680

The ECG shows heart rate of 70/min with T wave inversion noted in leads V1 to V4. This indicates possible myocardial ischemia. Choice a and d are ruled out as there is no ST elevation. Pulmonary embolism leads to $S_1Q_3T_3$ pattern and in this case limb leads are not seen.

111. Ans. (c) Lasix, Nitrates and morphine

Ref: Harrison, 20th ed. pg. 1771

The CXR shows evidence of bat wing edema which is seen with Acute decompensated CHF which is managed by LMNOP: Lasix, Morphine, Nitrates, Oxygen and Positioning of the patient.

112. Ans. (a) Peripheral Pulmonic stenosis

Ref: Harrison, 20th ed. pg. 1674

Continuous murmurs are seen in:
1. Peripheral pulmonic stenosis
2. Coarctation of aorta
3. Patent ductus arteriosus
4. Rupture of sinus of Valsalva
5. Mammary souffle
6. Venous Hum

113. Ans. (b) Decrease in systolic blood pressure 20 mm Hg within 3 min of postural change

Ref: AHA clinical Cardiac Consult pg. 280

Orthostatic hypotension is defined as decrease of BP >20 mm Hg systolic and Diastolic >10 mm Hg accompanied with symptoms of cerebral hypoperfusion.

114. Ans. (a) Start thrombolysis

Ref: Harrison, 20th ed. pg. 3081, 3087

The patient has presented with features of right sided cortical stroke leading to focal deficits on the left side.
How to Interpret the normal CT head given in the question?

> Hemorrhagic stroke is ruled out
> - Most importantly *CT scan showing no hemorrhage* or edema >1/3 of MCA territory *is an indication for thrombolysis* (Table 420-1 20th edition Harrison)

- In this scenario, the patient is treated as a case of ischemic stroke and managed with thrombolysis. The cut off for management of Thrombolysis is >4.5hours from symptom onset.
- *The closest choice is choice B which is used for management of Transient Ischemic attack. As per the definition of TIA symptoms resolve within 24 hours and most cases within one hour (Page 3087). TIA usually resolves before presenting to the physician.*
- Choice c, BP should not be lowered in CNS events as it mantains brain perfusion. Only if BP is >185/110 mm Hg that lowering of BP should be done before initiating thrombolysis.

115. Ans. (d) Intravenous Procainamide

Ref: Harrison, 20th ed. pg. 1741

Anti-dromic tachycardia implies conduction via the accessory pathway in Wolf Parkinson White syndrome and retrograde conduction via the bundle of His. DOC for management of acute episode in WPW is procainamide and to prevent episodes of fast conduction flecainide is given. Since patient is hemodynamically stable DC shock is ruled out.

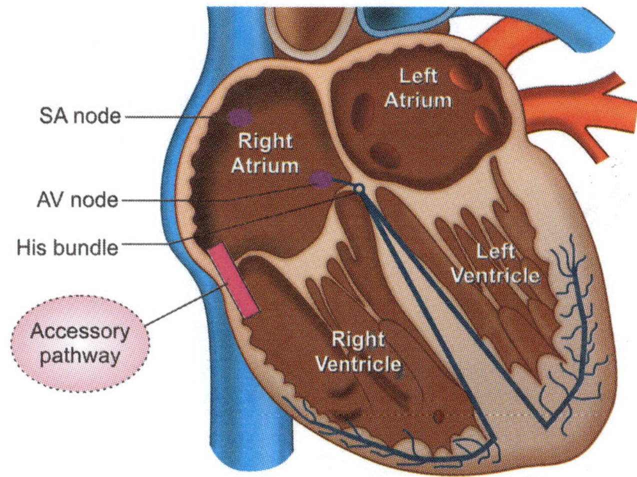

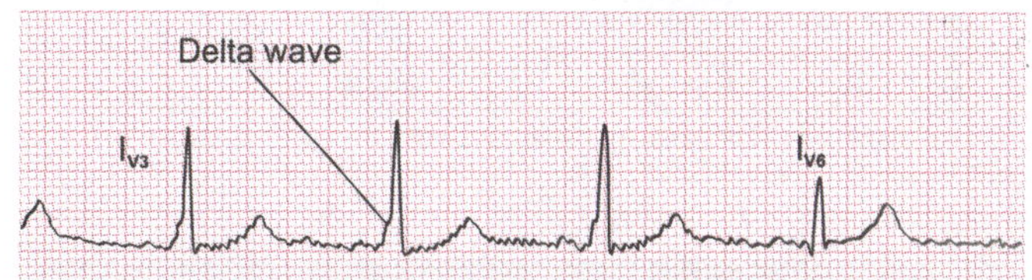

116. Ans. (a) Treadmill

Ref: Harrison, 20th ed. pg. 1742

- Wolf Parkinson White syndrome has an accessory pathway called Bundle of Kent that bypasses the normal conduction system in the heart. The faster conduction in these patients leads to complaints of tachycardia, dizzy spells and recurrent syncopal episodes.
- Choice b is correct as for these patients Holter monitoring (continuous ECG monitoring using a device worn by the patient for 24 hours) should be done to identify the tendency for arrythmias.
- Choice c is correct as Beta blockers can control the fast beating ventricular rate.

- Choice d is correct as Procainamide slows the conduction via bundle of Kent leading to current to go via normal route and termination of a tachycardia episode.

117. Ans. (d) 1-minute gap between 2 shocks

Ref: AHA 2015 Guidelines

The time lag between two Defibrillation shocks is 2 minutes during which CPR is continued at a rate of 30:2.

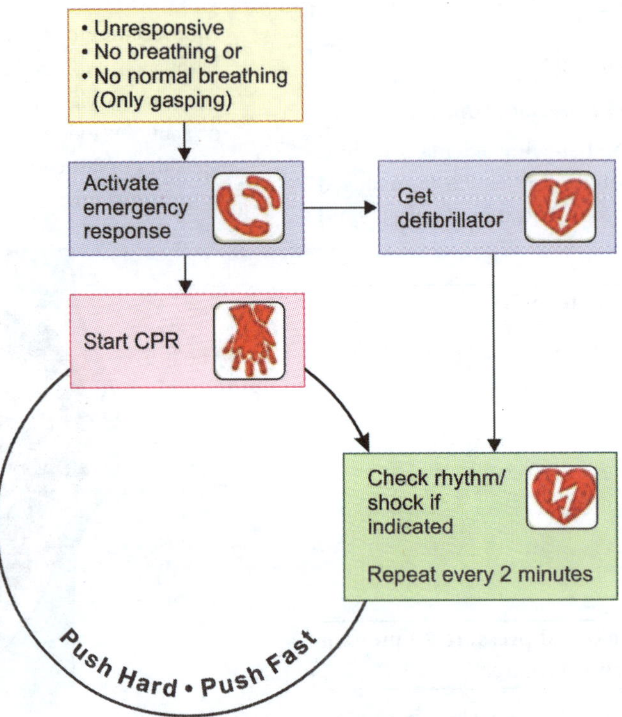

FIGURE: Simplified adult BLS algorithm

118. Ans. (d) Infective endocarditis

Ref: Harrison 20th ed. pg. 925

Major Criteria

- Blood culture positive for IE
  - Typical microorganisms consistent with IE from separate blood cultures
    - Viridans streptococci; *Streptococcus bovis*, HACEK group, *Staphylococcus aureus*, or
    - Community-acquired enterococci, in the absence of a primary focus
  - Microorganisms consistent with IE from persistently positive blood cultures, defined as follows:
    - At least two positive blood cultures of blood samples drawn > 12 hours apart; or
    - All of three or a majority of ≥4 separate cultures of blood (with first and last sample drawn at least 1 h apart)
  - Single positive blood culture for *Coxiella burnetii* or antiphase I IgG antibody titer >1:800
- Evidence of endocardial involvement
- Echocardiogram positive for IE (TEE recommended in patients with prosthetic valves, rated at least "possible IE" by clinical criteria,or complicated IE [paravalvular abscess]; TTE as first test in other patients), defined as follows:
  - Oscillating intracardiac mass on valve or supporting structures, in the path of regurgitant jets, or implanted material in the absence of an alternative anatomic explanation; or
  - Abscess; or
  - New partial dehiscence of prosthetic valve
- New valvular regurgitation (worsening or changing or pre-existing murmur not sufficient)

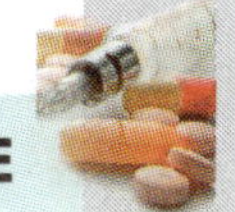

Minor criteria
• Predisposition, predisposing heart condition or injection drug use • Fever, temperature >38°C • Vascular phenomena, major arterial emboli, septic pulmonary infarcts, mycotic aneurysm, intracranial hemorrhage, conjunctival hemorrhages, and janeway lesions • Immunologic phenomena: Glomerulonephritis, Osler nodes, Roth's spots and rheumatoid factor • Microbiological evidence: Positive blood culture but does not meet a major criterion as noted previously (excluding single positive cultures for coagulase-negative staphylococci and organisms that do not cause endocarditis) or serologic evidence of active infection with organisms consistent with IE • Echocardiographic minor criteria eliminated

119. Ans. (a) False elevation of BP

Ref: AHA BP Measurement Guidelines

During BP recording the cuff should cover 80% of arm circumference. In case the BP cuff is undersized it will over estimate the BP value while an over sized cuff will under estimate the actual BP values.

American Heart Association guidelines for in-clinic blood pressure measurement

Recommendation	Comments
Patient should be seated comfortably, with back supported, legs uncrossed, and upper arm bared.	Diastolic pressure is higher in the seated position, whereas systolic pressure is higher in the supine position
	An unsupported back may increase diastolic pressure; crossing the legs may increase systolic pressure
Patient's arm should be supported at heart level.	If the upper arm is below the level of the right atrium, the readings will be too high; if the upper arm is above heart level, the readings will be too low.
	If the arm is unsupported and held up by the patient, pressure will be higher.
Cuff bladder should encircle 80 percent or more of the patient's arm circumference.	An undersized cuff increases errors in measurement
Mercury column should be deflated at 2 to 3 mm per second.	Deflation rates greater than 2 mm per second can cause the systolic pressure to appear lower and the diastolic pressure to appear higher

120. Ans. (b) HDL

Ref: Harrison, 20th ed. pg. 1851

High density lipoprotein plays a role in reverse cholesterol transport from tissues and is cardioprotective in nature.

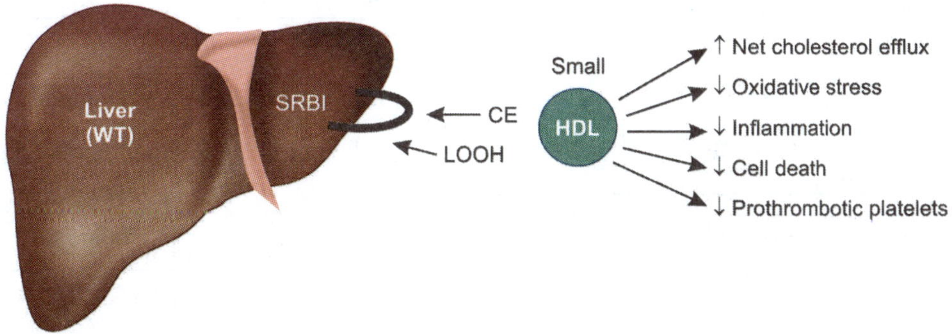

121. Ans. (c) Persistent Chest pain with ST elevation >90 minutes after thrombolysis

Ref: Harrison, 20th ed. pg. 1879

Rescue PCI should be done in case of failure of reperfusion which is defined as Persistent Chest pain and ST segment elevation >90 minutes.

Extra Mile

Primary PCI is done in cases of STEMI and should have a door to device time of less than 90 minutes.
Delayed PCI is done in cases of NSTEMI and has no time guidelines unlike above subtypes.
PCI with drug eluting stents is used in cases of single and double vessel disease in case of chronic stable angina.
Window period for thrombolysis in STEMI is 12 hours

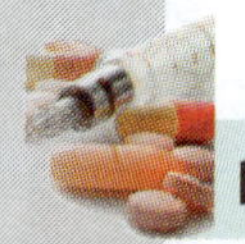

122. Ans. (d) Atrial fibrillation

Ref: Harrison 19th ed. pg. 444

- Normally JVP falls with inspiration.
- Choice a, Constrictive pericarditis is characterized by presence of calcification around the ventricles. Hence the compliance of heart is reduced and it cannot accommodate blood. This leads to elevated JVP on inspiration.
- Choice b, restrictive cardiomyopathy is characterized by poor heart function and leads to reduced compliance of heart. This explains the rise of JVP with inspiration.
- Choice c, complete heart block is characterized by no conduction at level of AV nodes. This leads to A:V dissociation and presence of giant a waves on JVP. Hence JVP will rise with inspiration. (Watch my video "Frog Sign" on youtube to see real life case).
- Choice d is characterized by twitching of atria and *absence of a waves on JVP*. Hence JVP cannot rise on inspiration.

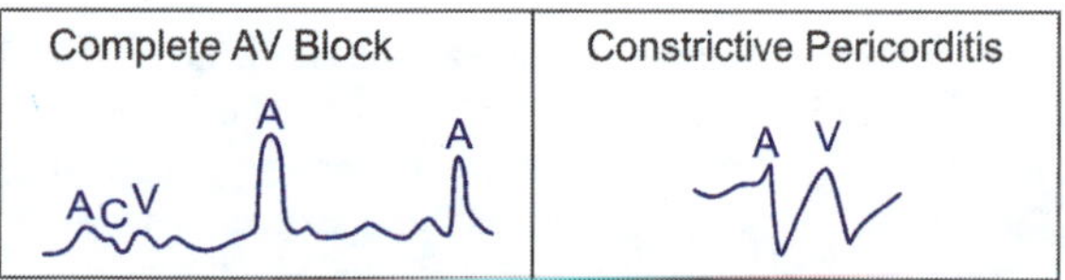

123. Ans. (b) Atrial depolarization with A-V conduction

Ref: Harrison 19th ed. pg. 1451

P wave	Atrial depolarization
PR interval	Atrial depolarization and AVN conduction
Q	Septal activation
QRS	Ventricular depolarization
QT	Ventricular repolarization plus ventricular repolarization

124. Ans. (b) Left ventricular hypertrophy

Ref: Harrison 19th ed. pg. 1658-59

- Pulmonary artery hypertension is due to constriction of pulmonary bed secondary to chronic hypoxia.
- Interstitial lung disease leads to lung shrinkage, and mitral stenosis due to pulmonary edema leads to hypoxia. Hence PAH will develop.
- Cor-pulmonale is right sided heart failure due to pulmonary artery hypertension. Leading cause of Cor-pulmonale is COPD.

125. Ans. (a) B_1 deficiency

Water hammer pulse is seen in high output cardiac failure caused by wet beri-beri. The development of CHF can explain the pedal/periorbital edema of the patient.

126. Ans. (a) Prolonged QT

QT interval shows an inverse relation with values of calcium and magnesium.

Must know information about QT interval

- 360–440 msec (9–10 small, squares)
- Measured in lead II or V5–V6

QT prolongation	QT shortening
• *Hypocalcemia* • Hypomagnesemia • Hypokalemia (prolonged QU interval) • Class IA and III drugs • Subarachnoid hemorrhage • Long QT syndrome • Romano ward syndrome	• *Hypercalcemia* • Digoxin • Congenital short QT syndrome

127. Ans. (a) Internal mammary artery

Long-term patency rates are considerably higher for internal mammary and radial artery implantations than for saphenous vein grafts. In patients with left anterior descending coronary artery obstruction, survival is better when coronary bypass involves the internal mammary artery rather than a saphenous vein.

128. Ans. (b) ASD

PDA	Narrow split S2
ASD	Wide fixed S2
TOF	Single S2
VSD	Wide variable split S2

129. Ans. (a) Tall tented T wave

The earliest ECG finding of hyperkalemia is tall tented T wave.

Serum potassium	ECG changes
5.5–6.5 mM	Tail peaked T waves
6.5–7.5 mM	Loss of P waves
7–8 mM	Wide, qRS, PR prolongation
>8 mM	Sine wave pattern

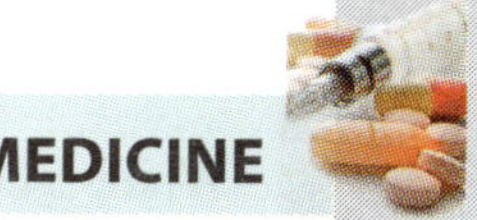

Treatment

Intervention	Lowering of potassium	During	Comments
Calcium gluconate or calcium chloride	No change in potassium levels	Effect starts in 1–3 minutes and lasts for 30–60 minutes	Reduces excitability of heart and is the drug of choice
Insulin drip (**most effective drug** to lower K^+ concentration)	0.5–1.5 mmol/L	4–6 hours	Redistribution of potassium by sending potassium inside cells
Parenteral or nebulized salbutamol	0.5–1.0 mmol/L	Full effect takes up to 24 hours	Sorbitol in enema omitted in post-operative patients due to increased incidence of sorbital-induced colonic necrosis
Hemodialysis		(**Most effective method** to lower potassium)	Refractory life threatening hyperkalemia failing to respond to conventional measures

130. Ans. (b) PSVT

- The heart rate is 150 bpm
- Axis is normal
- P waves are absent with narrow complex QRS
- ST segment depression is noted in lead II
- The diagnosis is PSVT

131. Ans. (a) QT = 0.04 sec

Normal QT interval is 360–440 milli-seconds (Average 400 msec). The QT interval is written wrongly as 0.04 seconds where as it is 0.4 seconds.

132. Ans. (a) Diuretics

- The heart rate is about 70 bpm and axis is normal.
- P, PR interval and QRS complex is of normal duration.
- Lead II and chest lead V3 shows T wave inversion with presence of U waves suggestive of hypokalemia.
- Choice b and c lead to Hyperkalemia and tall tented T waves whereas in the ECG given the T waves are inverted.
- Choice d is ruled out as bradycardia is not present.

133. Ans. (d) Ventricular Tachycardia (VT)

The image shows a broad complex QRS with heart rate of 200 min suggestive of diagnosis of ventricular tachycardia.

134. Ans. (a) No role

Ref: AHA 2020 Guidelines

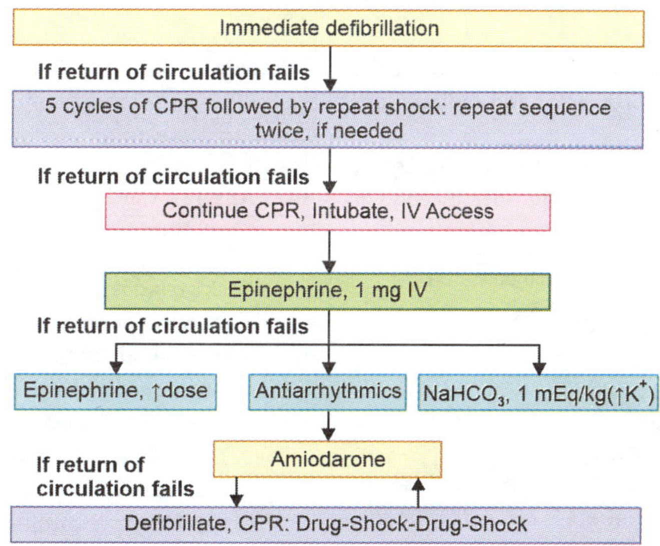

135. Ans. (c) Amiodarone

Ref: AHA 2020 Guidelines

Refer to explanation of above question

136. Ans. (b) Cardiac tamponade

Ref: Harrison, 19th ed. pg. 1573

JVP Findings

JVP Waves	Findings Constrictive pericarditis	Findings Cardiac tamponade
X wave	Prominent	Prominent
Y wave	Prominent	Absent[Q]

137. Ans. (a) Atrial fibrillation

Ref: Harrison, 19th ed. pg. 1487-88

- Beta blockers, nondihydropyridine calcium channel blockers (e.g., verapamil or diltiazem), and digitalis glycosides are useful in slowing the ventricular rate of patients with AF.
- In patients in atrial fibrillation, digitalis is used to *slow* ventricular rate. A rapid ventricular rate in mitral stenosis shortens diastole, thereby reducing left ventricular filling, which, in turn, further increases left atrial pressure and reduces cardiac output.

138. Ans. (a) Right 2nd intercostal, low pitch murmur

Ref: Harrison, 19th ed. pg. 144B

- Aortic stenosis is the most common cause of a mid-systolic murmur in an adult.
- *The murmur of AS is low to medium pitch and rasping or harsh in character.*
- It is usually loudest to the right of the sternum in the second intercostal space (aortic area) and radiates into the carotids.
- Mid-systolic murmurs begin at a short interval after S_1, end before S_2, and are usually crescendo-decrescendo in configuration.

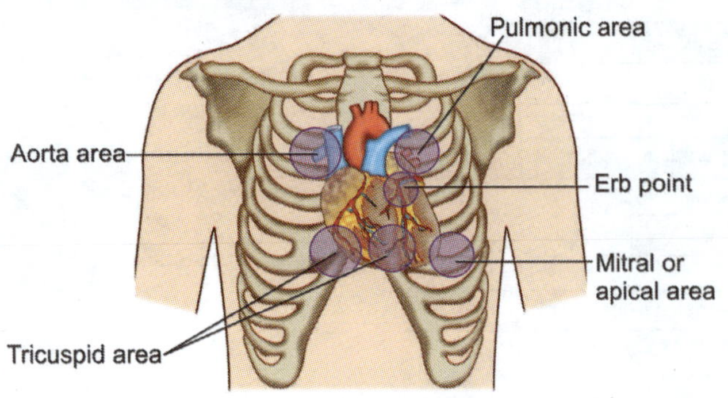

139. Ans. (b) Inferior to rib

Causes of inferior rib notching	Causes of superior rib notching
• Arterial: Aortic coarctation, aortic thrombosis, pulmonary-oligemia/AV malformation, Blalock Taussig shunt, Tetralogy of fallot, absent pulmonary artery and pulmonary stenosis. • Venous: AV Malfomations of chest wall, superior vena cava or other central venous obstruction. • Neurogenic: Intercostal neuroma, Neurofibromatosis type 1, poliomyelitis. • Osseous: Hyperparathyroidism, Thalassemia	• Poliomyelitis • Osteogenesis Imperfecta • Neurofibromatosis • Marfan's syndrome • Collagen vascular disease • Hyperparathyroidism.

140. Ans. (d) Troponin I

Ref: Braunwald, 8th ed. Table 50-4

Biomarker	Range of Times to Initial Elevation (hr)	Mean Time to Peak Elevations (Nonreperfused)	Time to Return to Normal Range
Frequently Used in Clinical Practice			
MB-CK	4–6	24 hours	48–72 hours
cTnl	3	24 hours	5–10 days
cTnT	3	12 hours–2 days	5–14 days
Infrequently Used in Clinical Practice			
Myoglobin	1–4	6–7 hours	24 hours

141. Ans. (a) Cardiac Tamponade

Ref: Harrison, 18th ed. chapter 238

Beck's triad is a collection of three medical signs associated with acute cardiac tamponade, an emergency condition wherein fluid accumulates around the heart and impairs its ability to pump blood. The signs are:

1. *Low arterial blood pressure*
2. *Distended neck veins*
3. *Distant, muffled heart sounds.*

Constrictive pericarditis can present with hypotension and congested neck veins but muffled heart sounds are not present. Auscultatory finding heard is pericardial shock.

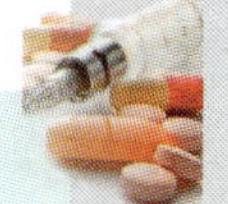

142. Ans. (a) Fibrates

Ref: Harrison, 19th ed. pg. 2449

- The *fibrates, or fibric acid derivatives,* act in part to stimulate the activity of peroxisome proliferator-activated receptors (PPARs), which are involved in fatty acid breakdown. *The main action of fibrates is to lower triglyceride levels (by 35 to 50 percent). Fibrates also raise serum high density lipoprotein (HDL) by 15 to 25 percent. Fibrates are the drugs of choice when treating isolated elevated triglycerides.*
- *Niacin,* fibrates, and prescription omega-3 fatty acids are approved for the treatment of patients with hypertriglyceridemia.
- *Statins* (or HMG-CoA reductase inhibitors) are a class of cholesterol lowering drugs that inhibit the enzyme HMG-CoA reductase which plays a central role in the production of cholesterol.
- *Ezetimibe* inhibits the absorption of cholesterol from the small intestine and decreases the amount of cholesterol normally available to liver cells, leading them to absorb more from circulation and thus lowering levels of circulating cholesterol.

143. Ans. (d) Platypnea

Ref: Harrison, 19th ed. pg. 1992

- Platypnea-orthodeoxia is a striking clinical syndrome characterized by *dyspnea and deoxygenation accompanying a change to a sitting or standing from a recumbent position.*
- In orthopnea (reverse findings are seen) the dysnea is seen in supine position and reduces in sitting position. It is usually due to acute CHF and bilateral diaphragmatic hernia.

Causes of Platypnea

- ASD or PFO with position-dependent shunting
- Other Cardiac conditions
  - Atrial Myxoma[Q]
  - Constrictive pericarditis
  - Aortic aneurysm
- Pulmonary
  - Multiple pulmonary emboli
  - Pulmonary emphysema
  - Radiation-induced bronchial stenosis
  - Hepatopulmonary syndrome[Q]
  - Amiodarone toxicity of the lungs
  - Pulmonary A-V communications
  - Fat embolism syndrome

144. Ans. (b) Cardiac Biomarkers

Ref: Harrison, 19th ed. pg. 1580

- The cardiac troponins, are elevated in case of NSTEMI.
- However in chronic Stable angina the symptoms arise on exertion/emotion or post-prandially and have characteristic ST segment depression on exercise testing. Cardiac biomarkers are *normal* as no cell death occurs in this case.

145. Ans. (a) Aortic regurgitation

Ref: Harrison, 19th ed. pg. 411

Duroziez's sign is seen in severe aortic regurgitation, *gradual pressure over the femoral artery leads to a systolic and diastolic bruit.* The systolic murmur is heard best when the proximal femoral artery is compressed and the diastolic when the distal femoral artery is compressed.

146. Ans. (c) Erythema Marginatum

Ref: Harrison, 19th ed. pg. 2149

Morning stiffness is seen in Rheumatoid arthritis, while the question is on Rheumatic fever. Erythema Marginatum is a major Jones criteria for diagnosis of Rheumatic Fever.

Revised Jones criteria (2015 update)	
A. Diagnosis	
For all patient populations with evidence of preceding gas infection Initial ARF – 2 Major or 1 major plus 2 minor Recurrent ARF- 2 Major or 1 major and 2 minor or 3 minor	
B. What are major criteria?	
Low-risk populations	**Moderate-and high-risk population**
• Carditis ▪ Clinical and/or subclinical carditis	• Carditis ▪ Clinical and/or subclinical carditis
• Arthritis ▪ Polyarthritis only	• Arthritis ▪ Monoarthritis or polyarthritis ▪ Polyarthralgia
• Chorea	• Chorea
• Erythema marginatum	• Erythema marginatum
• Subcutaneous nodules	• Subcutaneous nodules
C. What are the minor criteria	
Low-risk populations	**Moderate-and high-risk population**
• Polyarthraigia	• Monoarthralgia
• Fever ($\geq$38.5°)	• Fever ($\geq$38°C)
• **ESR$\geq$60 mm** in 1st hour and/or CRP $\geq$3.0 mg/d	• **ESR$\geq$30** mm/h and /or CRP $\geq$3.0
• Prolonged PR interval, after accounting for age variability (unless carditis is a major criterion) in all population	

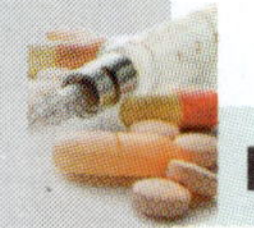

147. Ans. (a) Staphylococcus aureus

Ref: Harrison, 19th ed. pg. 816

- Overall *S. aureus* infection is the most common cause of IE, including Prosthetic Valve Endocarditis, acute Infective Endocarditis, and IVDA(Intravenous drug Abuse) Infective Endocarditis.
- The mortality rate of *S. aureus* IE is 40–50%.

148. Ans. (b) Autoimmune

- Post-MI pericarditis following myocardial infarction is called Dressler syndrome and is an *autoimmune process.*
- *It also seen* as an unusual complication after percutaneous procedures such as coronary stent implantation, after implantation of epicardial pacemaker leads and trans-venous pacemaker leads,and following blunt trauma,stab wounds,and heart puncture.

149. Ans. (a) Coarctation of aorta

Ref: Harrison, 19th ed. pg. 1525

- Coarctation of Aorta is most common cause of rib notching. It Usually involves the posterior 4th - 8th Ribs.
- *Collateral flow* bypassing the aortic constriction to reach the abdomen and lower extremities comes almost entirely from the two *subclavian arteries* via the thyrocervical, costocervical, and *internal mammary arteries* and their subdivisions to the *posterior intercostals* and then into the descending aorta.
- The large volume of blood traversing this route, and increased pulsation of the *intercostal arteries*, leads to erosion of lower border of ribs.

150. Ans. (c) Anti- hypertensive drugs

Ref: Harrison, 19th ed. pg. 1622

This is a case of Atherosclerotic cardiovascular disease with diastolic hypertension which can be a presentation of essential hypertension. Hence to reduce the diastolic overload of the heart, anti- hypertensive drugs are required for this case.

Extra Mile

Causes of Isolated Diastolic Hypertension are

- Essential hypertension
- Hypothyroidism
- Cushing syndrome

151. Ans. (d) Lisinopril

Ref: Harrison, 19th ed. pg. 1623, 18th ed. ch. 247

- *ACEIs* attenuate the development of left ventricular hypertrophy, improve symptomatology and risk of death from CHF, and *reduce morbidity and mortality rates in post-myocardial infarction patients.*
- *Similar benefits in cardiovascular morbidity* and mortality rates in patients with CHF have been *observed with the use of ARBs.*
- ACEIs provide better coronary protection than do calcium channel blockers, whereas calcium channel blockers provide more stroke protection than do either ACEIs or beta blockers.

152. Ans. (b) Resistance to 3 or more anti-hypertensive drugs including thiazides

Ref: Harrison, 18th ed. chapter 247

- *Resistant hypertension* refers to patients with blood pressures persistently >140/90 mm Hg despite taking three or more antihypertensive agents, including a diuretic, in a reasonable combination and at full doses.
- Resistant or difficult-to-control hypertension is more common in patients >60 years than in younger patients.
- Resistant hypertension may be related to:
  - "Pseudoresistance" (high office blood pressures and lower home blood pressures), nonadherence to therapy
  - Identifiable causes of hypertension (including obesity and excessive alcohol intake

153. Ans. (d) Shock

Ref: Harrison, 18th ed. chapter 233 and 238

- The CXR shows increased CT ratio which points to probable diagnosis of Dilated cardiomyopathy
- Patients dilated cardiomyopathy are predisposed to development of arrhythmia.
- Since atrial fibrillation is common, embolic stroke can occur and can lead to development of sudden death.

154. Ans. (b) QRS complex

Ref: Harrison, 19th ed. pg. 1489

- The origin of premature beats/ ventricular extra systoles in the ventricle at sites remote from the Purkinje network produces slow ventricular activation and a wide QRS complex that is typically >140 ms in duration.
- Ventricular premature complexes are common and increase with age and the presence of structural heart disease.

155. Ans. (a) Right atrium (RA)

Ref: Chapter 227, Harrison, 18th ed.

NORMAL JVP = 5–8 CM OF WATER

- Elevated JVP is indicative of right sided CHF

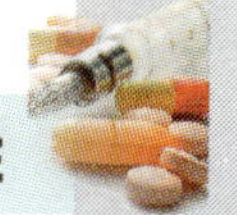

- Kussmaul sign is seen in constrictive pericarditis
- *Kussmaul sign is not seen in cardiac tamponade*
- Canon a waves are seen AV dissociation/ventricular tachycardia/junctional tachycardia

156. Ans. (a) Benign hypertension

Ref: Robbins, 8th ed. chapter 10

- **Hyaline arteriolosclerosis,** the vascular lesion associated with hypertension, is both more prevalent and more severe in diabetics.
- It takes the form of an *amorphous, hyaline thickening of the wall* of the arterioles, which causes narrowing of the lumen.
- It is encountered frequently in elderly patients, whether normotensive or hypertensive, hyaline arteriolosclerosis is more generalized and more severe in patients with hypertension.

157. Ans. (b) Left atrium

Ref: Robbins, 8th ed. Chapter 11

Mural endocardial lesions can be seen as *MacCallum* plaques in rheumatic heart disease. These plaques appear as map-like areas of thickened, roughened, and wrinkled part of the endocardium in the left atrium. They are *caused by regurgitant jets of blood flow, due to incompetence of the mitral valve.*

158. Ans. (b) Complete heart block

Ref: Harrison, 18th ed. chapter 227

- The 'a' wave reflects right atrial contraction and occurs just after the electrocardiographic P wave, preceding the first heart sound (S_1).
- The *a* wave is not present with atrial fibrillation.
- Canon *a* wave occurs with
  1. Atrioventricular (AV) dissociation/complete heart block due to right atrial contraction against a closed tricuspid valve.
  2. Wide complex tachycardia like ventricular tachycardia
  3. Junctional tachycardia rhythm

159. Ans. (d) Marfan syndrome

Ref: Harrison, 19th ed. pg. 2512

- Etiology of an aneurysm may affect the incidence of dissections. Atherosclerosis, when advanced, typically results 4 in medial and adventitial fibrosis, which hampers the development of dissections. *Dissections are common in Marfan syndrome, idiopathic T.A.A (thoracic aorta aneurysm).*

160. Ans. (c) Purkinje fibres have the slowest conduction

Ref: Harrison, 19th ed. pg. 265e-12

- Purkinje fibers have the fastest speed of conduction of 4 m/secs.
- The dominant pacemaker is the SAN due to its automaticity and the lowest RMP of all the pacemakers.

161. Ans. (a) Atrial fibrillation

Ref: Harrison, 19th ed. pg. 1443-1444

- A wave in JVP is due to atrial contraction. In atrial fibrillation, since the atria are twitching, the power of atria is reduced to a level that a wave would be absent.
- Heart block will have large a waves.
- Tricuspid Regurgitation has absent x and large v waves.
- Constrictive Pericarditis has a large y descent.

162. Ans. (b) Junctional tachycardia

Ref: Harrison, 19th ed. pg. 1480

Atrial fibrillation	Absent 'a' waves
Junctional tachycardia	The AVN node becomes the dominant pacemaker and simultaneously depolarizes the Atria and ventricles. Hence the AV valves might not be open and hence the atria will contract against the closed AV valves resulting in very large a waves
Constricitive pericarditis	Due to impaired compliance of ventricles, rapid ventricular filling occurs leading to steep y
Cardiac tamponade	Absent y waves

163. Ans. (c) Duration of mid-diastolic murmur

Ref: Harrison, 19th ed. pg. 1539

- Severity of mitral Stenosis implies that the mitral valve orifice has become smaller in size. This implies that the blood will take longer time to go from left atrium to left ventricle. This implies the LENGTH Of murmur will increase.

164. Ans. (d) Chest compressions

Ref: Harrison, 19th ed. pg. 1768

- According to AHA 2020 guidelines, the basic life support entails C_A_B and a shift from ABC protocol. Therefore the first thing to be done is chest compressions@100 times per minute. The depth of sternal depression should be 2 inches (5 cm)
- ALSO remember that in Advance cardiac life support the drugs used are epinenphrine, and amiodarone. ATROPINE has been withdrawn from management of cardiac arrest.

165. Ans. (d) Atrial depolarization

ECG finding	Significance
P wave	Atrial Depolarization
QRS	Ventricular depolarization
T wave	Ventricular repolarization
U wave	Delayed repolarization of papillary muscles
PR interval	Spread of impulse from SAN to AVN
ST segment	Iso-electric segment

166. Ans. (a) Tall tented T waves

Ref: Harrison, 19th ed. pg. 310

Serum potassium >5.5 mEq/L is associated with repolarization abnormalities:

- Peaked T waves (usually the earliest sign of hyperkalemia) **Serum potassium >6.5 mEq/L is associated with progressive paralysis of the atria.**
- P wave widens and flattens
- PR segment lengthens
- P waves eventually disappear

Serum potassium >7.0 mEq/L is associated with conduction abnormalities and bradycardia:

- Prolonged QRS interval with bizarre QRS morphology
- High-grade AV block with slow junctional and ventricular escape rhythms, followed by sine wave appearance.

Serum potassium level of >8.0–9.0 mEq/L causes cardiac arrest due to:

- Asystole
- Ventricular fibrillation

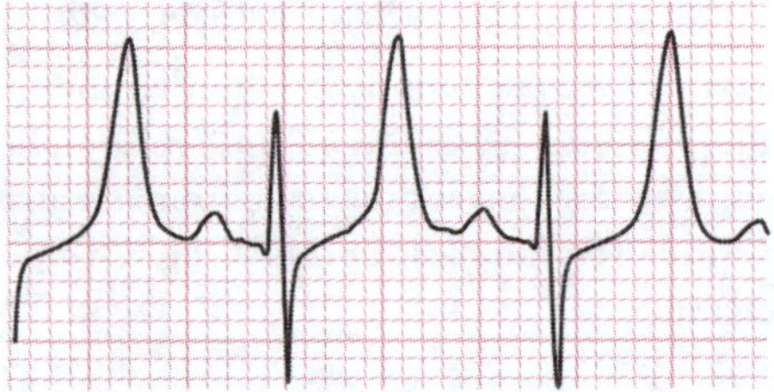
Tall tented T waves

167. Ans. (d) Treatment with steroids is necessary

- Dressler syndrome is post MI pericarditis/Pleuritis and is characterized by autoimmunity causing damage to the heart. The resultant inflammation causes chest pain in these patients upto 6 weeks of a preceding myocardial inflammation. The investigations show ECG evidence of pericarditis with ST elevation with concavity in upwards direction. The CPKMM levels are normal. The treatment of these patients shall be aspirin 650 mg TID.

168. Ans. (b) Hypertension

Ref: Harrison, 19th ed. pg. 1640

- *70% cases of aortic dissection occur due to hypertension.* The tear occurs in tunica media and causes a tearing pain in the chest with maximum intensity in interscapular area. The IOC for aortic dissection is trans-esophageal echocardiography > MRI chest.
- Marfan syndrome also can present with aortic dissection, which in fact is the leading cause of death in these patients. Syphilis involves the arch of aorta and causes an aneurysm that can rupture any day.

169. Ans. (a) Troponin I

Ref: Harrison, 19th ed. pg. 1600

- The best test for diagnosis of MI is troponin I which can be quantified as value more than 0.04 ng/dl after 3 hours of onset of myocardial infarction.

170. Ans. (d) Warfarin

Ref: AHA 2020 update: Secondary prevention of MI

- Aspirin and clopidogrel have been shown to reduce mortality due to MI.
- Statins regress atherosclerosis and β blockers due to oxygen conserving action will prevent future episode of MI.
- Warfarin is not routinely used in post MI Patients.

171. Ans. (a) Aortic stenosis

Ref: Harrison pg. 19th ed. pg. 1529

- Reverse split S2 implies aortic valve closes very late to a level that it closes after the pulmonic valve closure (Normally aortic valve closes first and then pulmonic valve).
- ***This occurs in severe aortic stenosis*** where the valvular obstruction makes the work of left ventricle harder. The longer ejection time leads to delayed closure of aortic valve. Due to this delayed closure the split becomes narrowed
- *In mitral stenosis loud S1 is seen. In pulmonary artery hypertension loud P2 is seen. In pulmonic stenosis single S2 is seen.*

172. Ans. (d) Wide QRS complex

Ref: Harrison, 19th ed. pg. 310

ECG Findings of Hyperkalemia

- The first ECG finding in hyperkalemia is tall tented T waves followed by slowing of depolarization of heart.
- This results in prolonged PR interval with QRS widening.
- Subsequently the P waves start becoming smaller.

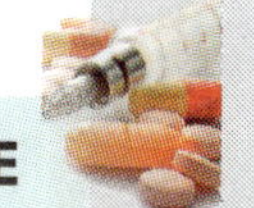

- Sine wave pattern leading to ventricular fibrillation/ diastolic arrest of heart.

173. Ans. (d) Alcohol

Ref: Harrison, 19th ed. pg. 95e-5

- Alcohol in mild amounts has been shown to have beneficial effect on heart. All of you would have heard and read about benefits of red wine.
- Studies have shown chylamydia as incriminating factor for atherosclerosis and so does poor dental hygiene.

174. Ans. (a) Cardiophrenic angle

Ref: Harrison, 19th ed. pg. 1719

Most common site of pericardial cyst is cardiophrenic angle.

Extra Mile

- ***Anterior mediastinal** tumors are **thymoma, lymphoma, pheochromocytoma,***
- **Posterior mediastinal tumors are neurogenic tumors** (20% of mediastinal tumors).
- **Middle mediastinal tumors are** pericardial cyst, bronchogenic cyst, thyroid mass, tracheal tumors.

175. Ans. (a) Total anomalous pulmonary venous connection

Ref: Nelson, 18th ed./ch 431

Conditions	Radiological findings
Total anomalous pulmonary venous connection	Figure of 8 or snowman heart
Transposition of great arteries	Egg on side appearance
TOF	Boot shaped heart
Ebstein anomaly	Box shaped heart

176. Ans. (b) Aortic regurgitation

Ref: Harrison, 19th ed. pg. 1534

Pulse pressure is SBP – DBP. In aortic stenosis or mitral stenosis SBP is low leading to reduction of pulse pressure. In tricuspid stenosis since the blood flow into right side of heart is reduced, so is left side inflow and therefore reduction in SBP.

Other Changes in Pulse Pressure Include

- Increased pulse pressure: Aortic regurgitation, Aortic sclerosis
- Decreased pulse pressure: Aortic stenosis, Mitral stenosis
- Increased diastolic pressure: Mitral stenosis
- Decreased diastolic pressure: Aortic regurgitation, Patent ductusarteriosus

Causes of wide pulse pressure

- Atherosclerosis
- Arteriovenous fistula
- **Chronic aortic regurgitation**
- Thyrotoxicosis
- Fever
- Anemia
- Pregnancy
- Anxiety
- Heart block
- Aortic dissection
- Endocarditis
- Raised intracranial pressure

177. Ans. (a) Junctional rhythm

Ref: Harrison, 19th ed. pg. 1443-44

- In Junctional rhythm the inherent AV node is the dominant pacemaker that causes simultaneous activation of atria and ventricles. Normally the Atria contract before the ventricles. Therefore in JUNCTIONAL RHYTHM atria will contract against the closed tricuspid and mitral valves leading to a very large a wave referred to as canon a waves.

REMEMBER *the traditional question on canon a waves is related to complete heart block.*

JVP findings	Conditions
Absent a waves	Atrial fibrillation
Canon a waves	Complete heart block , junctional rhythm, A-V dissociation
Large a waves	Tricuspid stenosis,pulmonic stenosis, pulmonary artery hypertension.

178. Ans. (c) Venous insufficiency

Ref: Harrison, 19th ed. pg. 253

- Edema is defined as a palpable swelling caused by an increase in interstitial fluid volume. The most likely cause of leg edema in patients over age 50 is venous insufficiency.
- The most important cause of unilateral pedal edema is also venous insufficiency which must be evaluated using a Doppler exam.

179. Ans. (b) Diastolic dysfunction

Ref: Harrison, 19th ed. pg. 1568

- HOCM stands for Hypertrophic Obstructive Cardiomyopathy.
- It is characterized by diastolic dysfunction, attributed to the hypertrophy, fibrosis, and intraventricular gradient when present.
- Asymmetrical septal hypertrophy and hypertrophy of left ventricular wall leads to decrease in LV cavity size.

Clinical Features

1. Dyspnea (MC symptom)
2. Effort intolerance

3. Sub endocardial ischemia leading to angina
4. Sudden death in HOCM is seen in young male players due to ischemic *ventricular fibrillation.*
5. Narrow split S_2 is seen.

Treatment

- Propranolol (decrease heart rate, decrease O_2 consumption) and Verapamil

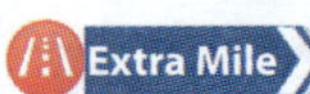

Drugs C/I in HOCM: Furosemide, ACE Inhibitors, Digoxin, NTG as they will all decrease pre-load, which will lead to decrease flow to right and then left side of heart leading to Decreased SBP

180. Ans. (b) Atropine

Ref: AHA 2020 Guidelines; Management of Cardiac Arrest

181. Ans. (b) Cardiac abnormality

Ref: Harrison, 19th ed. pg. 96e-1t

- **Vitamin B1** deficiency causes Beri-Beri which is of two types- WET BERI-BERI having cardiac failure and DRY BERI-BERI causing CNS problems like Wernicke encephalopathy and Korsakoff psychosis.
- Gingival bleeding and delayed wound healing (choice a) is seen with scurvy. Memory loss is seen with niacin deficiency.

182. Ans. (d) Anaphylaxis

Ref: Harrison 19th ed. pg. 2116

The life-threatening anaphylactic response of a sensitized human appears within minutes after systemic exposure to specific antigen and is manifested by:

- Respiratory distress due to laryngeal edema
- Intense bronchospasm
- Vascular collapse, or by shock without antecedent respiratory difficulty.
- Cutaneous manifestations exemplified by pruritus and urticaria with or without angiedema are characteristic of such systemic anaphylactic reactions.
- Gastrointestinal manifestations include nausea, vomiting, crampy abdominal pain, and diarrhea.

183. Ans. (c) Serum tryptase

Ref: Harrison 19th ed. pg. 2116

- *Elevations of tryptase levels in serum implicate mast cell activation in a systemic reaction and are particularly informative for anaphylaxis* with episodes of hypotension during general anesthesia or when there has been a fatal outcome.
- However, because of the short half-life of tryptase, elevated levels are best detected within 4 hours of a systemic reaction
- Immunoassays using purified antigens can demonstrate the presence of specific IgE in the serum of patients with anaphylactic reactions, and intracutaneous skin testing may be performed after the patient has recovered to elicit a local wheal and flare in response to the putative antigen.

184. Ans. (c) Atherosclerosis

Ref: Harrison 19th ed. pg. 1639

- Abdominal aortic aneurysms <4.0 cm may affect 1–2% of men older than 50 years.
- *At least 90% of all abdominal aortic aneurysms >4.0 cm are related to atherosclerotic disease, and most of these aneurysms are below the level of the renal arteries.*
- Abdominal aortic aneurysm commonly produces no symptoms. It is detected on routine examination as a palpable, pulsatile, expansile, and non-tender mass.
- Some patients complain of strong pulsations in the abdomen; others experience pain in the chest, lower back, or scrotum. Aneurysmal pain is usually a harbinger of rupture and represents a medical emergency.

185. Ans. (d) Calcium chloride

Ref: Harrison, 19th ed. pg. 312

- In a clinical setting of hyperkalemia in 1 year old child, cardiac arrhythmias associated with hyperkalemia *include sinus bradycardia, sinus arrest, slow idioventricular rhythms, ventricular tachycardia, ventricular fibrillation, and asystole.*
- Intravenous calcium serves to protect the heart while measures are taken to correct hyperkalemia.
- Calcium raises the action potential threshold and reduces excitability without changing the resting membrane potential. By restoring the difference between the resting and threshold potentials, calcium reverses the depolarization blockade caused by hyperkalemia.
- *The recommended dose of treatment of hyperkalemia is 10 mL of 10% calcium gluconate (3–4 mL of calcium chloride), infused intravenously over 2–3 minutes with cardiac monitoring.*
- The effect of the infusion starts in 1–3 min and lasts 30–60 min; the dose should be repeated if there is no change in ECG findings or if they recur after initial improvement.

186. Ans. (c) 12–18 months

Ref: Harrison, 19th ed. pg. 1567

- Amyloid involvement of the heart is seen, especially in the elderly population.

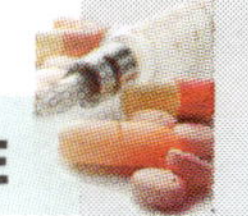

- Recent data suggests that life expectancy has increased from 6 to 16–20 months in the most common subtype, AL amyloid.
- Gold standard diagnostic test for restrictive cardiomyopathy is right-ventricular biopsy, which demonstrates positivity for Congo Red staining.

187. Ans. (a) CCTA

Ref: Harrison, 19th ed. pg. 270e-4

- *Coronary lesions prone to rupture* and subsequent development of MI have different morphology compared with stable plaques, and *can be evaluated by CCTA* to identify vulnerable plaques before they lead to clinical events.
- Coronary angiography is used to detect percentage of blockage in coronary artery.

NEUROLOGY

188. Ans. (b) Tongue deviation to same side

Ref: Macloed's Clinical examination, 2018 ed. pg. 133

The main feature of LMN lesion of hypoglossal nerve leads to ipsilateral deviation of tongue to the site of lesion.
In contrast the supranuclear lesions occur at the cerebral cortex, the corticobulbar tract of the internal capsule, cerebral peduncles, or the pons. Supranuclear lesions cause the tongue to protrude away from the nerve because of predominant neural crossing for upper motor neurons.

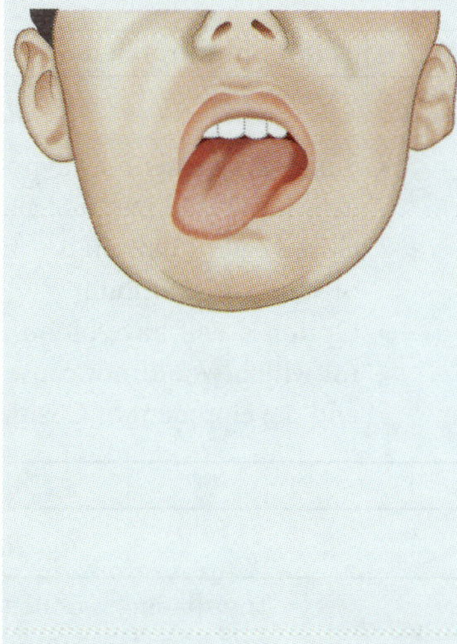

189. Ans. (d) Pin-point pupils

Ref: Harrison 21st ed. pg. 3637

Heat stroke occurs when there is a total loss of thermos regulatory functions. Features are tachypnea, tachycardia, hypotension and widened pulse pressure with disorientation and weakness. Sympathomimetic features will predominate and would cause pupillary dilatation.

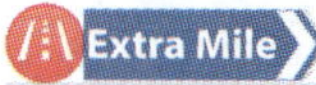

Triad of heart stroke
- Exposure to heat stress
- CNS dysfunction
- Core temperature of >40.5°C

190. Ans. (a) Bacterial meningitis

Ref: Harrison 21st ed. pg. 1102

- In a clinical settting of fever with nuchal rigidity and turbid CSF showing predominantly neutrophils and low CSF sugar(normal CSF sugar= 2/3rd of Blood sugar), Acute bacterial meningitis is confirmed.
- Option b has predominant lymphocytes with straw color CSF.
- Option c has normal CSF sugar and is hence ruled out.
- Option d, Fungal meningitis occurs in patients with reduced immunity.

191. Ans. (a) Desaturation

Ref: Harrison 21st ed. pg. 3617

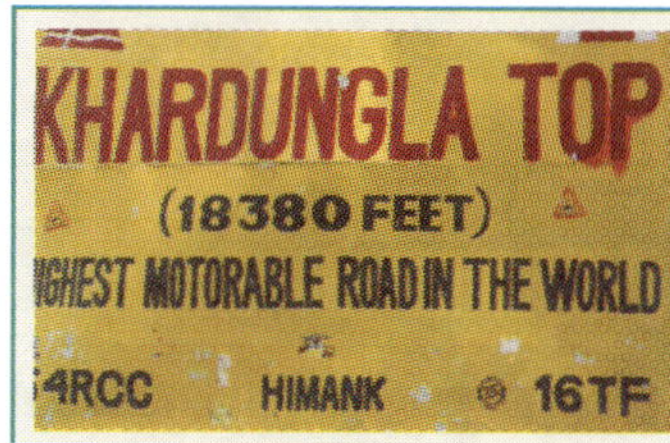

The reason for development of high-altitude cerebral edema is hypobaric hypoxia resulting in desaturation. The manifestation is altered mentation/bizarre behavior and coma.

192. Ans. (d) M. Gravis

Ref: Harrison 21st ed. pg. 3510

- The main key word is diurnal variation of neurological symptoms with ptosis being worse in evening and relieved in morning. Ice pack test has now replaced Tensilon test to diagnose myasthenia gravis.
- Option a presents with dementia and chorea.
- Option b has gradual onset asymmetrical motor weakness developing over years and does not show any diurnal variation in symptoms.

193. Ans. (a) IV Mannitol

Ref: Harrison 21st ed. pg. 2087

The patient is having hypertensive crisis. This would require lowering of BP by 25% within minutes to 2 hours or to a BP of 160/100–110 mm Hg. This can be accomplished by Nicardipine or nitroprusside. The advantage of using esmolol is to counterbalance the reflex tachycardia that would occur in these patients. There is no role of mannitol in patients with Hypertensive emergencies.

Preferred Parenteral Drugs for Selected Hypertensive Emergencies

Hypertensive encephalopathy	Nitroprusside, nicardipine, labetalol
Malignant hypertension (when IV therapy is indicated)	Labetalol, nicardipine, nitroprusside, enalaprilat

Contd...

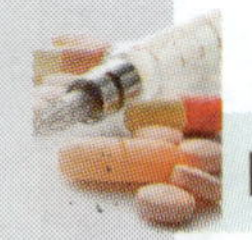

Stroke	Nicardipine, labetalol, nitroprusside
Myocardial infarction/unstable angina	Nitroglycerin, nicardipine, labetalol, esmolol
Acute left ventricular failure	Nitroglycerin, enalaprilat, loop diuretics
Aortic dissection	Nitroprusside, esmolol, labetalol
Adrenergic crisis	Phentolamine, nitroprusside

194. Ans. (b) Moderate TBI

Ref: Harrison 21st ed. pg. 3456

Severity	GCS*	LOC	PTA
Mild	13–15	<20 min-1 hour	<24 hours
Moderate	9–12	1–24 hours	24 hours- <7 days
Severe	3–8	>24 hours	>7 days

GCS: Glasgow coma scale
LOC: Loss of consciousness
PTA: Posttraumatic amnesia
*The Glasgow coma scale (GCS) is the most commonly used scale to

195. Ans. (b) Acyclovir

Ref: Harrison 21st ed. pg. 1106

- Short history points to bacterial/viral etiology of CNS infecton. Absence of nuchal rigidity rules out meningitis.
- CSF finding of lymphocytosis and normal sugar points to viral encephalitis.
- The leading cause is herpes simplex-1 that has prediliction to damage temporal lobe of brain. Supportive of this is EEG finding of periodic temporal spikes.
- Hence patient should be started empirically on acyclovir.
- Option a is used in TB meningitis. Option c in acute bacterial meningitis. Option d is used for fungal meningitis.

196. Ans. (b) IV Labetalol

Ref: Harrison 20th ed. pg. 3349

- Option a thrombolysis will Contraindicated in hemorrhagic stroke.
- Option c causes sudden unpredictable fall of BP and can worsen brain infarction.
- Option d is ruled out as High BP needs to be managed in this case to value of 160/90 mm Hg. Recent trials have shown that acute and rapid lowering of BP to less than 140 mm Hg have better functional outcome.

197. Ans. (c) SAH

Ref: Harrison 20th ed. pg. 3354

The image shows blood in Slyvian fissure which is characteristic feature of SAH. The phrase "Worst headache of my life/Thunderclap headache" is another important pointer.

198. Ans. (a) Subdural hematoma

Ref: Harrison 20th ed. pg. 2428

- Since the patient is hypotensive with no evidence of external bleeding, internal bleed must be present in closed cavity. Option b, c and d imply closed cavity bleed of substantial amount.
- Option a will have blood amount usually less than 100 ml which would not cause shock unresponsive to bleed and development of Cushing reflex will cause BP to rise.

199. Ans. (c) Brown Sequard syndrome

Ref: Harrison 20th ed. pg. 2187

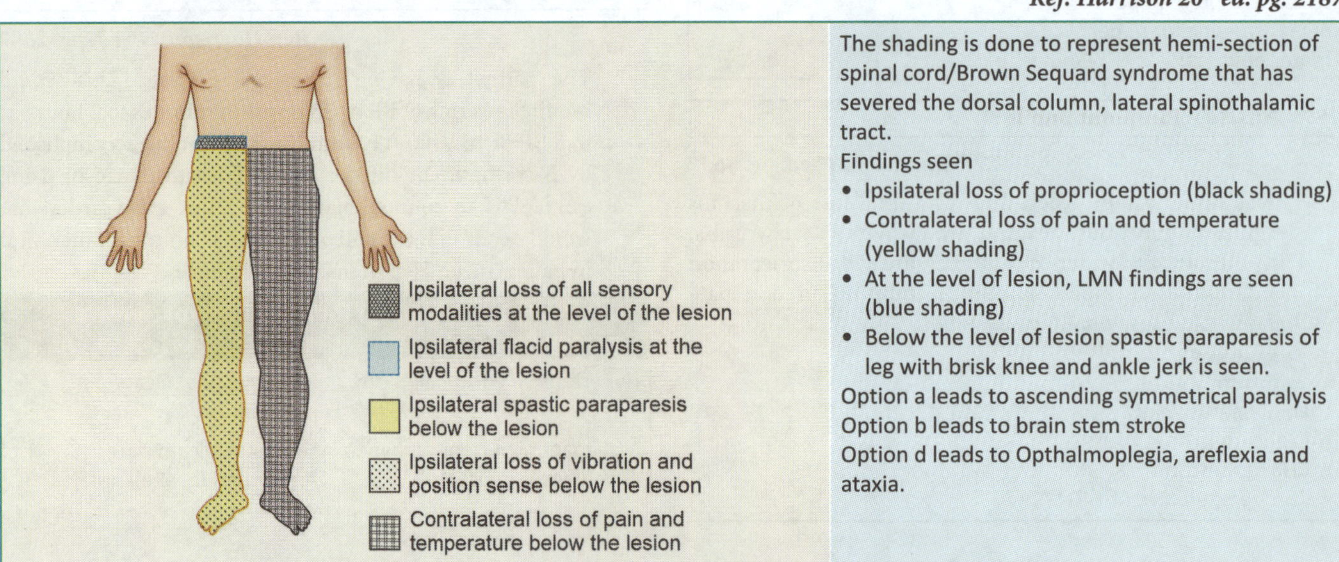

The shading is done to represent hemi-section of spinal cord/Brown Sequard syndrome that has severed the dorsal column, lateral spinothalamic tract.

Findings seen
- Ipsilateral loss of proprioception (black shading)
- Contralateral loss of pain and temperature (yellow shading)
- At the level of lesion, LMN findings are seen (blue shading)
- Below the level of lesion spastic paraparesis of leg with brisk knee and ankle jerk is seen.

Option a leads to ascending symmetrical paralysis
Option b leads to brain stem stroke
Option d leads to Opthalmoplegia, areflexia and ataxia.

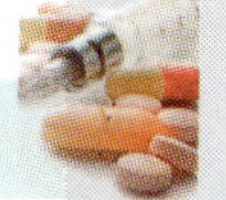

200. Ans. (a) Apraxia

Ref: Strokeengine.ca

The Clock-Drawing Test is a simple and effective cognitive test used to assess cognitive dysfunction, particularly for dementia followed by. Loss of visuospatial skills called as apraxia.

Major visuospatial errors seen on the CDT given in image

1. Right/Left reversal
2. Omitting one half of the clock

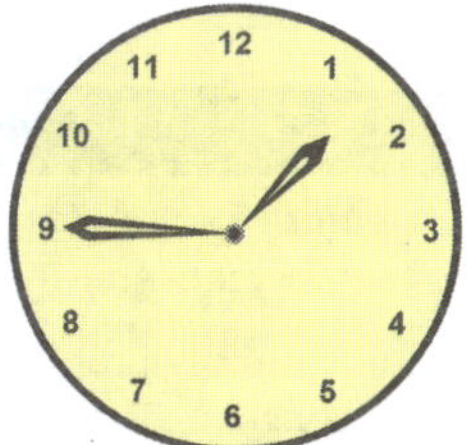

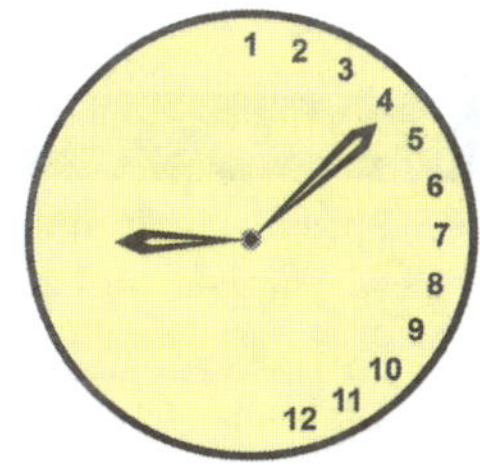

201. Ans. (c) V-CJD

Ref: Harrison 20th ed. pg. 3149

- Dementia in young age with myoclonic jerks is seen with CNS infection in patients consuming tainted beef products. The prion particles ingested are small enough to cross blood brain barrier and result in neurodegeneration. This presentation is called as variant creutzfeldt Jacob disease.
- Option a presents with dementia in patients with atherosclerotic risk factors.
- Option b is seen in old age only
- Option d presents with chorea and not myoclonic jerks.

202. Ans. (a) Transient ischemic attack

Ref: Harrison 20th ed. pg. 3087

- Since the neurological features have resolved they indicate the presence of TIA. Stroke features would not resolve by themselves.
- Transient ischemic attack is a warning symptom of stroke where the neurological features resolve by themselves in 24 hours and neuro imaging is normal.
- Option b presents with radicular pain and focal weakness. Important cause can be disc prolapse that presses on nerve roots.
- Option c presents with ascending flaccid paralysis with sensory level and bladder/Bowel involvement.
- Option d has been ruled out as features of stroke can cause incapacitation and debility.

203. Ans. (d) Diffuse axonal injury

Ref: Bailey and Love 27th ed. pg. 336

- The image shows punctuate hyperdensities in post head injury patient in coma. This favors diagnosis as diffuse axonal injury.
- Option a is ruled out as it produces blood in Sylvian fissure. Option b presents with concavo-convex hyperdensity. Option c leads to weakening of wall of blood vessels causing intraparenchymal bleeding.

204. Ans. (d) Occipital cortex

Ref: Harrison 20th ed. pg. 162-63

Sparing of the macula is encountered frequently in infarction of the occipital lobes due to PCA occlusion. Macular sparing may be caused by collateral vascular supply to the macular region or by the very large macular representation in the occipital cortex.

205. Ans. (a) Delirium tremens

Ref: Harrison 20th ed. pg. 3282

- Agitation, global confusion, disorientation, hallucinations, fever, hypertension, diaphoresis, autonomic hyperactivity and profound global confusion are hallmark of Delirium Tremens.
- Alcoholic hallucinosis is a ruled out as it is characterized by predominantly auditory hallucinations that occur either during or after a period of heavy alcohol consumption.

206. Ans. (a) 9T

Ref: Harrison 20th ed. pg. 3183 and NCBI Bookshelf

- Opening eyes on command = 3
- Moving limbs/obeying commands = 6
- Intubated = T
- The total score is 9T

The maximum score in intubated patient can be 10T and minimum as 2T.

Extra Mile

Glasgow coma scale- P

The GCS-P is calculated by subtracting the Pupil Reactivity Sore (PRS) from the Glasgow Coma Scale (GCS) total score:

- GCS-p GCS - PRS
- The Pupil Reactivity Sore is calculated as follows:

Pupils unreactive to light - Pupil Reactivity Score

- Both pupils - 2
- One pupil - 1
- Neither pupil - 0

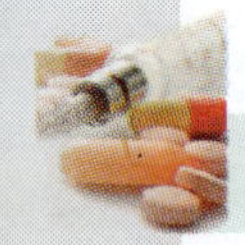

207. Ans. (c) Generalized paresis

Ref: 5-minute Neurology, Consult ed. pg. 32

Postural tremor occurs when limb is positioned against gravity. It is seen in choices A, B and D. General **paresis** is a late manifestation of neurosyphilis and is characterized by delusion of grandiosity.

Mnemonic

P: Personality
A: Affect
R: Reflexes (Hyperactivity)
E: Argyll Robertson Pupil
S: Sensorium (hallucinations, delusions)
I: Intellect deterioration
S: Speech defects

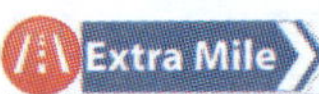

Extra Mile

Classification of tremors and their characteristics and treatment

TABLE: Classification of tremors and their characteristics and treatment

Type of Tremor	Frequency	Occurrence	Etiology
Postural tremor	5–9 Hz	When limb is positioned against gravity	Physiologic tremor, essential tremor, alcohol or drug withdrawal, metabolic disturbances, psychogenic tremor
Rest tremor	3–6 Hz	When limb is fully supported against gravity and the muscles are not voluntarily activated	Parkinson's disease, multiple system atrophy, progressive supranuclear palsy, rubral tremor, psychogenic tremor
Action tremor	3–10 Hz	During any type of movement	Cerebellar lesions, rubral tremor, psychogenic tremor

208. Ans. (a) Weber syndrome

Ref: Harrison 20th ed. pg. 191

Weber syndrome occurs due to occlusion of posterior cerebral artery P1 segment. It leads to compromise of oculomotor nerve and crus cerebri. Due to involvement of crus cerebri corticospinal pathway is affected. Since the corticospinal pathway crosses over at the lower border of medulla contralateral hemiplegia occurs.

Brain stem stroke always leads to crossed hemiplegia.

209. Ans. (b) Check blood glucose

Ref: Harrison, 20th ed. pg. 2072

- Choice c is ruled out since no features of raised ICP are given.
- Choice d is ruled out since BP lowering is done in case of CNS events if the BP >185/110 mm Hg. Moreover, CT is required for diagnosis of a CNS event. At lower BP values, reducing BP would be counterproductive and can lower Brain perfusion.
- Now, we have to choose between the two choices CT scan and blood glucose.
- As per the algorithm of management of an unconscious patient, blood sugar levels should be checked first.
- In any unconscious patient of diabetes mellitus, status of blood sugar should be assessed immediately as hypoglycemia/hyperglycemia would change the line of management.
- Once these two possibilities are ruled out then CT head is to be performed to rule out a CNS event.
- Page 2072: 20th edition of Harrison quotes "the studies most useful in diagnosis of coma are chemical-toxicologic analysis of blood and urine followed by Cranial CT/MRI, EEG and CSF examination".

210. Ans. (d) Diplopia

Ref: Harrison, 19th ed. pg. 3120

- Due to rigidity of vocal cords patient speaks slowly and cannot raise his voice. This is choice a hypophonia/soft voice.
- Choice b is correct as patient of PD cannot start a movement like a normal person.
- Choice c is correct and when it involves upper limb it is called cog wheel rigidity and lower limb involvement is called lead pipe rigidity.

Cardinal features	Other motor features	Nonmotor features
Bradykinesia Rigidity Resting Tremor Gait disturbance/ postural instability	Micrographia Masked facies Reduced eye blink Soft voice Freezing	Anosmia Mood disorders, e.g., depression Sleep disturbances Autonomic disturbances Cognitive impairment/dementia

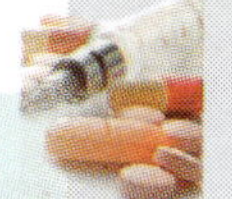

211. Ans. (a) M. Gravis

Ref: Harrison, 20th ed. pg. 3233

- The presence of muscle weakness/fatiguability with *normal reflexes* is a feature of M. Gravis. Due to lesser number of receptors available at NMJ and rundown presynaptic release of Ach, decremental response to repetitive nerve stimulation is a *hallmark* feature of this disease.
- Guillain barre has segmental demyelination of spinal cord and presents with ascending symmetrical paralysis with areflexia.
- Transverse myelitis also presents with ascending paralysis and areflexia due to spinal cord involvement.
- Traumatic neuritis is a LMNL and leads to flaccidity and areflexia.

212. Ans. (a) B_{12} deficiency

Ref: Harrison, 20th ed. pg. 152

- The question is framed to check whether the student is aware of vitamin deficiencies that lead to reversible dementia. These are B1, B12 and nicotinic acid.
- Choice b Acute inflammatory demyelinating polyneuropathy presents as ascending symmetrical flaccid paralysis and is also called Guillain Barre syndrome.
- Choice c is a prion disease and presents as dementia with myoclonic jerks and leads to neuro-degeneration.
- Choice d leads to frontotemporal dementia with inappropriate aggressive behavior.

213. Ans. (d) Gordon reflex

Ref: Oxford Handbook of Neurology, 2nd ed. pg. 605

- Gordon reflex is an alternative method of eliciting the Balbinski sign. It presents as extensor plantar response when the calf muscle is squeezed. The clinical sign is used to determine whether a lesion of the pyramidal tract exists. The Gordon reflex is closely associated with the Babinski, Chaddock, and Oppenheim reflexes.
- Choice a is seen in Duchene muscular dystrophy
- Choice b is seen in deep vein thrombosis
- Choice c is alternative method eliciting an extensor plantar by providing *tactile stimulus on shin.*

Alternative methods of eliciting Babinski sign

214. Ans. (a) Abducens

Ref: Harrison, 20th ed. pg. 192

The abducens nerve has the longest subarachnoid course and is therefore the most common cranial nerve involved in case of raised ICP. It is also the most common nerve involved in post lumbar puncture or spinal anesthesia.

Extra Mile

- Cranial nerve with longest intracranial route is trochlear nerve
- Only cranial nerve with crossed origin/only one with dorsal origin is trochlear nerve
- Cranial nerve with longest intra-osseous route is facial
- Cranial nerve with longest route overall is Vagus

215. Ans. (a) Mydriasis

Ref: Harrison 20th ed. pg. 541

Due to damage to sympathomimetic fibers, mydriasis cannot occur in Horner syndrome. It is usually caused by lung cancer which is then called Pancoast tumor of superior sulcus tumor.

Features of Horner syndrome: Mnemonic: SAMPLE

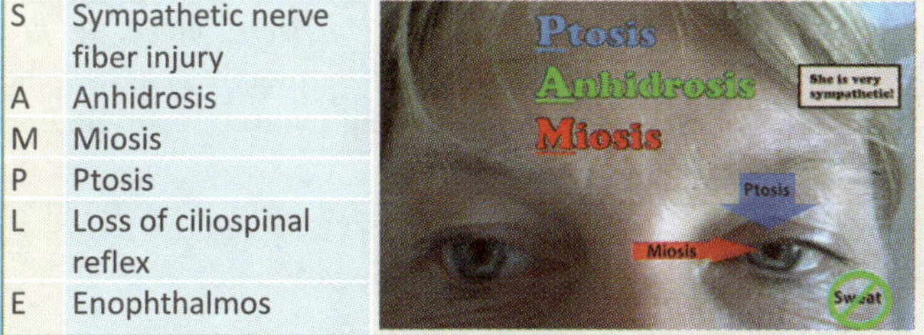

S	Sympathetic nerve fiber injury
A	Anhidrosis
M	Miosis
P	Ptosis
L	Loss of ciliospinal reflex
E	Enophthalmos

216. Ans. (b) Syringomyelia

Ref: Harrison 19th ed. pg. 2654

- Syringomyelia is characterized by dilatation of syrinx leading to compression of lateral spinothalamic pathways.
- This leads to sensory loss in hands that leads to *painless burn* which is not appreciated by the patient.
- Muscle wasting in the lower neck, shoulders, arms and hands with asymmetric or absent reflexes in arms represents expansion of cavity in gray matter of cord.
- Diabetes mellitus leads to neuropathic ulcers involving the sole of foot.
- Mononeuritis multiplex leads to multiple peripheral neuropathies like carpal tunnel syndrome, tarsal tunnel syndrome, meralgia paresthetica occurring simultaneously.

Extra Mile

- Expansion of syrinx can lead to involvement of descending tract of trigeminal nerve leading to cough induced headache.
- Characteristic feature of syringomyelia is dissociative anesthesia.
- IOC for syringomyelia is MRI spine

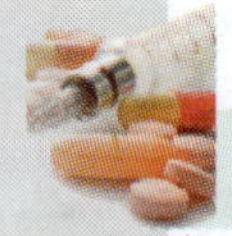

217. Ans. (d) Inability to recognize face

Ref: Harrison 19th ed. pg. 182

Prosopagnosia is inability to recognize familiar faces including self-image in the mirror. The affected person can identify a face as a face or a car as a car but cannot tell the person or model of car.

The *lesion* lies in occipitotemporal area.

218. Ans. (a) Thiamine

Ref: Harrison 19th ed. pg. 2607

Wernicke' encephalopathy is manifestation of Dry beriberi.

Extra Mile

- Clinical features are (G.O.A) Global Confusion, ophthalmoplegia and ataxia.
- 1st clinical feature to respond to IV thiamine treatment is ophthalmoplegia.
- 1st to be initiated is intravenous thiamine followed by dextrose.
- Dextrose infusion will first lead to worsening of neurological features
- Best test for thiamine deficiency is serum thiamine levels >> RBC transketolase activity

219. Ans. (d) Anomic aphasia

Ref: Harrison 19th ed. pg. 178

Metabolic encephalopathy leads to anomic aphasia. The presentation is difficulty in naming an object, word finding pauses, and impaired spelling.

Motor aphasia	Lesion in Broca's area
Sensory aphasia	Lesion in Wernicke's area
Conduction aphasia	Lesion in arcus fasciculus

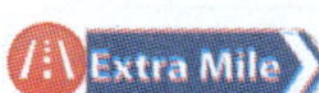

Anomic aphasia is also seen in:
1. Alzheimer's disease
2. Head trauma
3. Metabolic encephalopathy—Uremic encephalopathy, ammonia intoxication

220. Ans. (b) Fomepizole

Ref: Harrison 19th ed. pg. 473 e-12

Methanol causes ethanol like CNS depression and increased serum osmolality. Formic acid leads to retinal toxicity and manifests as clouding, spots and blindness.

MANAGEMENT

- Gastric aspiration
- Sodium bicarbonate
- High dose folinic acid
- Fomepizole is the DOC and helps in management of high anion gap metabolic acidosis
- Ethanol can be used in absence of fomepizole and is given via nasogastric tube
- Hemodialysis for enhancing methanol elimination and shortening duration of treatment.

221. Ans. (c) Anterior horn cell disease

Ref: Harrison: 19th ed. pg. 154

- Anterior horn cell disease involves motor neuron in the ventral horn of spinal cord and hence is an example of lower motor neuron disease.
- Prion particles infect the neurons and lead to corticospinal pathway damage.
- Multiple sclerosis is pure white matter disease characterized by plaques.
- Tuberous sclerosis has subependymal nodules in periven-tricular location. It presents as epilepsy since birth.

222. Ans. (b) Strep pneumoniae

TABLE: Causative agents of meningitis age wise

Neonate	Group B streptococcus (India) Klebsiella > E. coli
Child	Pneumococcus
Adult	Pneumococcus
Adult (epidemic)	Meningococcus

223. Ans. (a) Loss of bladder control

Complete Cord Transection Syndrome

Complete cord transection syndrome results in complete loss of all sensibility and voluntary movement below the level of the lesion. It can be caused by fracture dislocation of the vertebral column, by a bullet or stab wound, or by an expanding tumor. The following characteristic clinical features will be seen after the period of spinal shock has ended:

- *Bilateral lower motor neuron paralysis and muscular atrophy in the segment of the lesion.* The result from damage to the neurons in the anterior gray column (i.e lower motor neuron) and possibly from damage to the nerve roots of the same segment.
- *Bilateral spastic paralysis below the level of the lesion.* A bilateral Babinski sign is present, and depending on the level of the segment of the spinal cord damaged, bilateral loss of the superficial abdominal and cremaster reflex occurs. All these signs are caused by an interruption of the corticospinal tract on both side of the cord.
- *Bilateral loss of the sensations below the level of the lesion.* The loss of pain, temperature, and light touch sensations is caused by section of the lateral and anterior spinothalamic tracts on both sides.
- *Bladder and bowel functions are no longer under voluntary control, since all the descending autonomic fibers have been destroyed.*

224. Ans. (b) Thermal sense

Hemisection of spinal cord is called Brown Sequard syndrome.

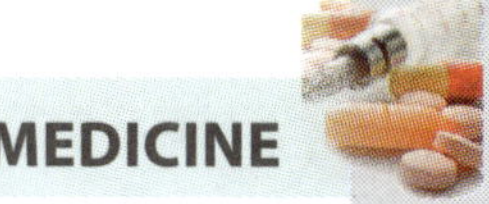

Manifestation of Brown Sequard Syndrome

- *Interruption of the lateral corticospinal tracts*—Ipsilateral spastic paralysis below the level of the lesion and Babinski sign ipsilateral to the lesion (abnormal reflexes and Babinski sign may not be present in acute injury)
- *Interruption of posterior white column*—Ipsilateral loss of tactile discrimination, as well as vibratory and position sensation, below the level of the lesion
- *Interruption of lateral spinothalamic tracts*—Contralateral loss of pain and temperature sensation. This usually occurs 2–3 segments below the level of the lesion

225. Ans. (a) Cerebellum

- Pendular knee jerk is seen in cerebellar lesions
- DTR are normal in basal ganglia damage.
- Hung up reflexes are seen in chorea.
- Hung up ankle jerks are seen in hypothyroidism

Must know points about cerebellar lesions

- Scanning speech: The words are broken into syllable components (Dysarthria).
- Nystagmus
- Hypotonia
- Pendular knee jerk
- Truncal ataxia:
  - Positive Romberg sign, with *eye open*
- Tests for coordination shows incoordination:
  There will be dysmetria and dyssynergia in the following tests:
  - Finger nose test
  - Balaney's past pointing test
  - Knee heel test
  - Dysdiadochokinesia
- Intention tremor.
- Ataxic gait (Reeling gait)

Site of lesion

- **Cerebellar vermis:** The midline structure is concerned for posture and equilibrium. Lesion at this site causes truncal and gait ataxia.
- **Cerebellar hemispheres:** The smooth conduction of movement (by co-ordinated contraction and relaxation of muscles is controlled by cerebellum. ***Lesion in cerebellar hemisphere produces ipsilateral signs***.

226. Ans. (b) Spinocerebellar pathways

- *Unconscious proprioception* is the sensation of limb and joint position and range and direction of limb mediated by *(spinocerebellar pathways and serves as a back up to)* the dorsal column medial lemniscal system.
- Unconscious proprioception involves acquisition and maintenance of skilled motor activities such as walking speaking writing, swallowing, unconscious proprioception.
- *The spinocerebellar pathways, unlike the other sensory pathways follow a two-order neuronal system and do not directly project the cortex.*
- The system consists of three second order fiber tracts ventral spinocerebellar, dorsal spinocerebellar and cuneocerebellar.

227. Ans. (a) M. Gravis

- In M. Gravis, the fundamental defect is a decrease in the number of available AChRs at the postsynaptic muscle membrane. These changes result in decreased efficiency of neuromuscular transmission.
- Therefore, although ACh is released normally, it produces small end-plate potentials that may fail to trigger muscle action potentials.
- The amount of ACh released per impulse normally declines on repeated activity (termed *presynaptic rundown*).
- This mechanism accounts for the decremental response to repetitive nerve stimulation seen on electrodiagnostic testing.

228. Ans. (a) Tension headache

- Overall the *most common cause of headache is tension headache.*
- Episodic tension headache is usually associated with a stressful event. This headache type is of moderate intensity, self-limited, and usually responsive to non-prescription drugs.
- Chronic tension headache often recurs daily and is associated with contracted muscles of the neck and scalp. This type of headache is bilateral and usually occipitofrontal.
- Most common cause of secondary headache is systemic infection
- Rare cause of primary headache is cluster headache
- Rare cause of secondary headache is brain tumor.

229. Ans. (b) Ophthalmoplegia, ataxia, areflexia

Miller Fisher syndrome presents as:

- Rapidly evolving ataxia
- Areflexia of limbs without weakness
- Ophthalmoplegia often with pupillary paralysis

The MFS variant accounts for <5% of all cases of G.B.S and is strongly associated with antibodies to the ganglioside GQ1b.

230. Ans. (c) TB meningitis

- Contrast-enhanced computed tomography shows tuberculous meningitis demonstrating acute hydrocephalus and meningeal enhancement. Notice the dilated lateral ventricles.

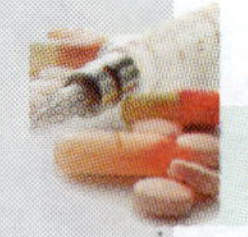

- Diagnostic triad of tubercular meningitis:
  - Basal exudates
  - Infarcts
  - Hydrocephalus

Must know points for tubercular meningitis

- The combination of unrelenting headache, stiff neck, fatigue, night sweats, and fever with a *CSF lymphocytic pleocytosis and a mildly decreased glucose concentration* is highly suspicious for tuberculous meningitis.
- If there is a pellicle in the CSF or a *cobweb-like clot* on the surface of the fluid, AFB can best be demonstrated in a smear of the clot or pellicle

231. Ans. (c) Caffeine

Post-lumbar puncture headache usually resolves without specific treatment:

1. Care is largely supportive with oral analgesics like acetaminophen, nonsteroidal anti-inflammatory drugs and anti emetics.
2. Patients may obtain relief by lying in a comfortable (especially a recumbent or head-down Trendelenburg) position.
3. For some patients, beverages with caffeine can provide temporary pain relief.
4. *For patients with persistent pain, treatment with IV caffeine (500 mg in 500 mL saline administered over 2 hours) is effective.*
5. Alternatively, an epidural blood patch accomplished by injection of 15 mL of autologous whole blood is usually effective.
6. Some clinicians reserve epidural blood patch for patients who do not respond to caffeine, while others prefer to use blood patch as initial management for unremitting post-LP symptoms.

232. Ans. (c) Excision with radiation

- These are highly infiltrative tumors, and the areas of increased T2/FLAIR signal surrounding the main tumor mass contain invading tumor cells.
- Treatment involves *maximal surgical resection followed by partial-field external beam radiotherapy* (6000 cGy in thirty 200-cGy fractions) with concomitant temozolomide, followed by 6–12 months of adjuvant temozolomide.

233. Ans. (a) Neurofibromatosis

NF-1 is diagnosed when *any two of the following seven signs* are present:

1. Six or more café au-lait macules. *Café au-lait spots are the hallmark of neurofibromatosis and are present in almost 100% of patients.*
2. *Axillary or inguinal freckling*[Q] consisting of multiple hyperpigmented areas 2–3 mm in diameter.
3. Two or more iris Lisch nodules. Lisch nodules are hamartomas located within the iris and are best identified by a slit-lamp examination.
4. Two or more neurofibromas or one plexiform neurofibroma.
5. Osseous lesion such as sphenoid dysplasia (which may cause pulsating exophthalmos) or cortical thinning of long bones with or without pseudoarthrosis.
6. Optic gliomas are present in ≈15% of patients with NF-1.
7. First degree relative with NF-1.

234. Ans. (d) Semi-purposive and non-repetitive, randomly distributed movements

Lesion	Manifestations	Lesion seen in
Chorea	State of *excessive*, spontaneous movements, *irregularly timed, non-repetitive*, randomly distributed and abrupt in character.	Caudate
Atheotosis	Because of the slowness, the movements have a writhing (i.e. squirming, twisting, or snakelike) appearance	Globus pallidus
Hemiballismus	Very severe form of chorea in which the movements have a *violent, flinging quality*. Ballism has been defined as "continuous, violent, coordinated involuntary activity involving the axial and proximal appendicular musculature such that the limbs are flung about.	Subthalamic nucleus

235. Ans. (a) Lateral spinothalamic tract

Important tracts

Posterior/Dorsal column	Joint position, vibration and pressure
Lateral spinothalamic tract	Pain and temperature
Ventral spinothalamic	Pressure, touch
Lateral corticospinal/ pyramidal pathways	Distal limb movements
Vestibulospinal and tectospinal tract	Axial and proximal limb movements

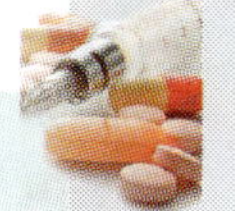

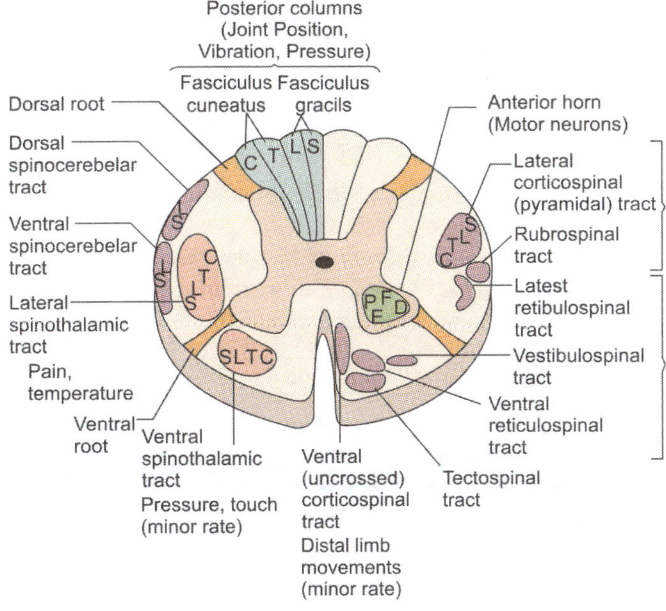

236. Ans. (a) Corticospinal tract

- The corticospinal tract (along with the corticobulbar tract) is the primary pathway that carries the motor commands that underlie voluntary movement.
- The **lateral corticospinal tract** is responsible for the control of the distal musculature and the **anterior corticospinal tract** is responsible for the control of the proximal musculature.
- A particularly important function of the lateral corticospinal tract is the fine control of the digits of the hand.
- The corticospinal tract is the only descending pathway in which some axons make synaptic contacts directly onto alpha motor neurons.
- This direct cortical innervation presumably is necessary to allow the powerful processing networks of the cortex to control the activity of the spinal circuits that direct the exquisite movements of the fingers and hands.

237. Ans. (a) Spine injury evaluation

- *Log rolling* is a method of turning patients to either inspect their backs for *spine injury evaluation* especially in sports related injuries. It will also help to put the patient on long spinal board.
- To log roll a patient, *there should be a minimum of four people*. The *objective is to keep the whole spine in alignment*. To achieve it the cervical spine is stabilized and the patient is moved with the neck, shoulders and pelvis kept in the same plane.

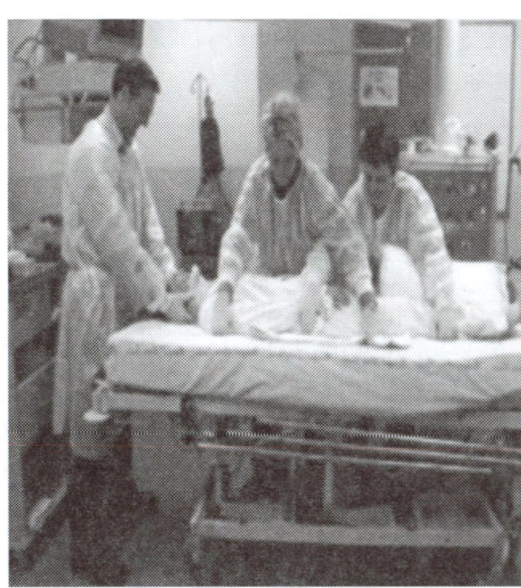

238. Ans. (b) Lateral displacement of midbrain

- *Lateral displacement of the midbrain may compress the opposite cerebral peduncle*
- *This produces an ipsilateral Babinski's sign and ipsilateral hemiparesis*
- Normally in CNS lesion the hemiparesis and Babinski sign is bilateral
- This unusual fact is called as Kernohan-Woltman sign.
- Herniation may also compress the anterior and posterior cerebral arteries as they pass over the tentorial reflections, with resultant brain infarction

239. Ans. (a) 3rd nerve involvement

Ref: Harrison, 19th ed. pg. 1772

- *Uncal transtentorial* herniation refers to impaction of the anterior medial temporal gyrus (the uncus) into the tentorial opening just anterior to and adjacent to the midbrain.
- *The uncus compresses the third nerve as it traverses the subarachnoid space, causing enlargement of the ipsilateral pupil (putatively because the fibers subserving parasympathetic pupillary function are located peripherally in the nerve).*

240. Ans. (a) Broca's area

Ref: Harrison, 19th ed. pg. 177

- Broca's area damage is called **expressive aphasia** (non-fluent aphasia).
- Pattern has loss of the ability to produce language (spoken or written).
- Patient has insight to his problem and is frustrated.
- *Remember: Broca is broke. Speaks broken words.*
- Damage to paracentral lobule would lead to loss of control over urination and lead to urge incontinence.

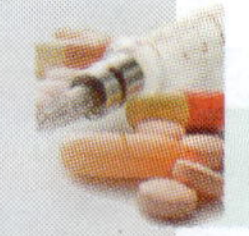

- Damage to insula leads to loss of hand eye coordination and loss of social skills.

241. Ans. (a) Medulla

Ref: Ganong, 25th ed. pg. 525

- *Nucleus ambiguus is a group of large motor neurons, situated deep in the medullary reticular formation.*
- *The nucleus ambiguus contains the cell bodies of nerves that innervate the muscles of the soft palate, pharynx, and larynx which are strongly associated with speech and swallowing.*

242. Ans. (a) Superior temporal gyrus

Ref: Harrison, 19th ed. pg. 177

- Wernicke's area is located in the posterior section of the superior temporal gyrus (STG) in the dominant cerebral hemisphere (which is the left hemisphere in about 95% of right handed individuals and 60% of left handed individuals).
- Damage caused to Wernicke's area results in receptive, fluent aphasia. This means that the person with aphasia will be able to fluently connect words, but sentences will lack meaning.

243. Ans. (b) Severe disability

Ref: Harrison, 19th ed. chapter 370

- *Patients scoring 3 or 4 have an 85% chance of dying or remaining vegetative.*
- Glasgow come scale of <8 indicates coma.
- The minimum score in glasgow coma scale is 3 (severe disability) and maximum score is 15.

244. Ans. (a) Withdrawl on flexion

Ref: Chapter 370: Harrison, 19th ed.

Best motor response (M)	
Obeys	6
Localizes	5
Withdraws (flexion)	4
Abnormal flexion posturing	3
Extension flexion posturing	2
Nil	1

245. Ans. (a) Neuropraxia

Ref: Maheshwari, 5th ed. pg. 69

- In most cases of compressive radial neuropathy, the type of injury is a "neuropraxia" that does not involve damage to the axon.
- Neuropraxia is classified as a *transient conduction block of motor or sensory function without neuronal degeneration*. Therefore, despite decreased motor function, patients with neuropraxia are able to regain normal neurologic function within several weeks to months.
- Posture-induced radial neuropathy, known as *Saturday night palsy*, occurs because of compression of the radial nerve.

	Neurotmesis	Axonotmesis	Neurapraxia
Pathological			
Anatomical continuity	May be lost	Preserved	Preserved
Essential damage	Complete disorganisation, Schwann sheaths preserved[Q]	Nerve fibres interrupted	Selective demyellnation of larger fibres, no degeneration of axons[Q]
Clinical			
Motor paralysis	Complete	Complete	Complete
Muscle atrophy	Progressive	Progressive	Very little
Sensory paralysis	Complete	Complete	Usually much sparing
Autonomic paralysis	Complete	Complete	Usually much sparing
	Electrical phenomena		
Nerve conduction distal to the lesion	Absent	Absent	Absent
Fibrillation	Present	Present	Occasionally detectable
Recovery			
Surgical repair	Essential	Not necessary	Not necessary

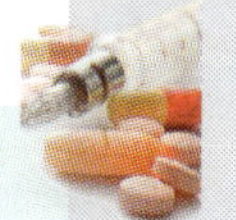

246. Ans. (c) 60–80%

Ref: Harrison 18th edition, chapter 381

- The glucose level in CSF is proportional to the blood glucose level and corresponds to 60–70% of the concentration in blood.

Hypoglycorrhachia (low CSF glucose levels) can be caused by

- CNS infections
- Inflammatory conditions
- Subarachnoid hemorrhage
- Hypoglycemia
- Impaired glucose transport, increased CNS glycolytic activity
- Metastatic carcinoma.

CSF glucose levels can be useful in distinguishing among causes of meningitis as more than 50% of patients with bacterial meningitis have decreased CSF glucose levels while patients with viral meningitis usually have normal CSF glucose levels.

247. Ans. (d) Cryptococcus meningitis

Ref: Harrison 18th edition, Chapter 189

- *C. neoformans* is the leading infectious cause of *meningitis* in patients with AIDS[Q]
- It is the initial AIDS-defining illness in <2% of patients and generally occurs in patients with CD4+ T cell counts <100/μL[Q]
- Most patients present with a picture of subacute meningoencephalitis with fever, nausea, vomiting, altered mental status, headache, and meningeal signs.
- The CSF profile may be normal or may show only modest elevations in WBC or protein levels and decrease in glucose. The opening pressure in the CSF is usually elevated.
- **The diagnosis of cryptococcal meningitis is made by the detection of cryptococcal antigen in CSF by lateral flow assay or ELISA or India ink staining of CSF sample.** Blood cultures for fungus are often positive. A biopsy may be needed to make a diagnosis of CNS cryptococcoma.
- Treatment is with IV amphotericin B[Q] 0.7 mg/kg daily, or liposomal amphotericin 4–6 mg/kg daily, with flucytosine 25 mg/kg qid for at least 2 weeks and, if possible, until the CSF culture turns negative. This is followed by fluconazole 400 mg/d PO for 8 weeks, and then fluconazole 200 mg/d until the CD4+ T cell count has increased to >200 cells/uL for 6 months in response to cART.

248. Ans. (c) Gullian Barre syndrome

Ref: Harrison, 18th ed. Chapter 386

The symmetrical nature of disease favors diagnosis of Guillain-Barre syndrome. The absence of sensory symptoms also makes Transverse myelitis an unlikely diagnosis.

	Poliomyelitis	Guillain-Barre syndrome	Transverse myelitis
Fever	Present; may be biphasic	May have a prodromal illness	May have a prodromal illness
Symmetry Sensations	Asymmetric Intact; may have diffuse myalgias	Symmetrical Variable	Symmetrical Impaired below the level of the lesion
Respiratory insufficiency	May be present	May be present	May be present
Cranial nerves	Affected in bulbar and bulbospinal variants	Usually affected	Absent
Radicular signs	May be present	Present	Absent
Bladder, bowel complaints	Absent	Transient; due to autonomic dysfunction	Present
Nerve conduction	May be abnormal	Abnormal	Normal
Cerebrospinal fluid	Lymphocytic pleocytosis; normal or increased protein	Albumino-cytologic dissociation	Variable
MRI spine	Usually normal	Usually normal	Characteristic

249. Ans. (b) Subdural hemorrhage

Ref: Harrison, 18th ed. chapter 378

- Boxing is a violent sport in which every participant accepts the risk of brain damage or death. This sport has been linked to acute neurological injury and chronic brain damage. The *most common life-threatening injury encountered by its participants is subdural hematoma* (SDH), and the most feared consequence of chronic insult to the nervous system is dementia pugilistica, or punch drunkenness.

250. Ans. (d) Sinusitis

Ref: Harrison, 18th ed. chapter 14

Primary Headache		Secondary Headache	
Type	%	Type	%
Tension –Type	69	Systemic infection	63
Migraine	16	Head injury	4
Idiopathic stabbing	2	Vascular disorders	1
Extertional	1	Subarachnoid hemorrhage	<1
Cluster	0.1	Brain tumor	0.1

251. Ans. (a) Ampicillin

Ref: Harrison, 18th ed. chapter 139

252. Ans. (a) Acyclovir

Ref: Harrison, 18th ed. chapter 381

253. Ans. (c) Measles

Ref: Harrison, 18th ed. chapter 192

254. Ans. (c) Hyperhidrosis

Ref: Harrison, 18th ed. chapter 370

Horner syndrome (Horner's syndrome) results from an interruption of the sympathetic nerve supply to the eye and is characterized by the *classic triad* of *miosis* (i.e., constricted pupil), *partial ptosis*, and *loss of hemifacial sweating* (i.e., anhidrosis)

(Mnemonic: PERFECT M.E.A.L) Clinical features of Horner syndrome

Ptosis
Miosis
Enophthalmos (pseudo)
Anhidrosis
Loss of ciliospinal reflex

ANATOMY OF HORNER SYNDROME

- *First-order central sympathetic fibers arise from the posterolateral hypothalamus,* descend uncrossed through the midbrain and pons, and terminate in the intermediolateral cell column of the spinal cord at the level of C8-T2 (ciliospinal center of Budge).
- *Second-order preganglionic pupillomotor fibers exit the spinal cord at the level of T1 and enter the cervical sympathetic chain,* where they are in close proximity to the pulmonary apex and the subclavian artery. (association with pancoast tumor)
- *The third-order pupillomotor fibers ascending along the internal carotid artery* enter the cavernous sinus.

255. Ans. (b) Peripheral ganglia

Ref: Harrison, 18th ed. chapter 374

Lower motor neurons are motor neurons located in either the *anterior grey column, anterior nerve roots* or the *cranial nerve nuclei of the brainstem and cranial nerves with motor function*

Lower motor neurons are classified based on the type of muscle fiber they innervate:

- Alpha motor neurons innervate extrafusal muscle fibers, the most numerous type of muscle fiber and the one involved in muscle contraction.
- Beta motor neurons innervate intrafusal fibers of muscle spindles with collaterals to extrafusal fibers
- Gamma motor neurons innervate intrafusal muscle fibers, which together with sensory afferents compose muscle spindles. These are part of the system for sensing proprioception

256. Ans. (c) Meningioma

Ref: Harrison, 18th ed. chapter 379

- Meningiomas are the most common primary brain tumor, accounting for approximately 32% of the total.
- Overall most common Brain tumor is metastases arising from hematogenous spread from a lung primary.
- The most common sources of brain metastases are lung, breast carcinoma and melanoma.
- **Remember: Metastasis > Meningioma>Astrocytoma.**

257. Ans. (c) Hypertension and Bradycardia

Ref: Harrison, 18th ed. chapter 25

- Cushing's reflex is a *hypothalamic response* to brain ischemia wherein the sympathetic nervous system is activated which causes increased peripheral vascular resistance with a *subsequent increase in BP.*

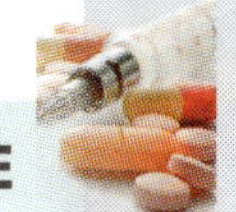

- The *increased BP then activates the parasympathetic nervous system* via carotid artery baroreceptors, *resulting in vagal-induced bradycardia.*
- The brain ischemia that leads to cushings reflex is usually due to the poor perfusion that results from increased ICP due to head bleeds or mass lesions.
- Cushing's reflex leads to the clinical manifestation of Cushing's triad.
- *Cushing's triad = hypertension, bradycardia, and irregular respirations (Cheyne-Stokes breathing).*
- Cushing's triad signals *impending danger of brain herniation*, and thus, the need for decompression. Consider administering mannitol, hyperventilation, and elevation of the head of bed as temporizing measures

258. Ans. (d) 6th

Ref: Harrison, 19th ed. pg. 209

- In raised intracranial tension the cranial nerves afflicted are the ones which have long intracerebral courses leading to false localizing signs. *Since the 6th cranial nerves emerges straight forwards from the brainstem , while others originate obliquely ,the nerve is more liable to the mechanical effects of backward brainstem displacement by ICSOL.*
- Neurological signs have been described as "false localizing" if they reflect dysfunction distant or remote.

259. Ans. (a) Sub-dural hematoma

Lesions	NCCT finding
Sub dural hematoma	Concavo-convex bleed hyper-density
Extra dural hemorrhage	Biconvex /flame shaped hyper-density
Sub arachnoid hemorrhage	Intra-ventricular bleed/blood in slyvian fissure
Intra–parenchymal bleed	Mostly a lesion or hyper-density in basal ganglia secondary to hypertension

260. Ans. (a) Hyperdense biconvex

Ref: Harrison's 17th ed. Ch 364

- **Extradural hemorrhage:** Bleeding occurs between skull and duramatter. Bleeding occurs due to the rupture of Middle meningeal artery. Lucid Interval (Consciousness between two periods of unconsciousness) exists.
- In NCCT it shows hyperdensity which has bi-convex or flame shaped appearance.
- **Treatment:** Burr hole surgery.
- **Subdural hemorrhage:** Occurs due to rupture of Cortical bridging veins. ***In NCCT it shows concavo-convex or sickle shaped bleed.***

261. Ans. (a) Insula

Ref: Textbook of Anatomy Vol. 3 by Vishram singh, pg. 391

- *Insula is called Island of Reil or central lobe.*
- The word insula means hidden. *The insula is the submerged portion of cerebral cortex in the floor of lateral sulcus.*
- The insulae are involved in consciousness and play a role in diverse functions usually linked to emotion or the regulation of the body's homeostasis. These functions include perception, motor control, self-awareness, cognitive functioning, and interpersonal experience.

262. Ans. (a) NCCT

Ref: Harrison, 19th ed. pg. 1785

- The basic rule for intracranial hemorrhage is to perform NCCT Head.
- Remember MRI is recommended for ICH >>48 hours.
- NCCT Brain in SAH, shows accumulation of blood in slyvian fissure.
- Drug of choice for management of SAH is nimodipine 60 mg TDS for 3 weeks with complete bed rest.
- Neurosurgical consult is required in case of development of hydrocephalus.

263. Ans. (a) Non fluent speech

Ref: Harrison, 19th ed. pg. 177-178

- **Wernicke's area in the brain (Brodmann area 22) is present** in the posterior part of the superior temporal gyrus of the dominant hemisphere.
- People with (Wernicke's area damage) **receptive** aphasia are **unable to understand language in its written or spoken form, and even though they can speak with normal grammar, syntax, rate, and intonation, they cannot express themselves meaningfully using language.**
- A patient with Wernicke's aphasia can and may speak a great deal, but he or she confuses sound characteristics, **producing *"word salad"* in extreme cases.**
- **Paraphasia** is seen in people with wernicke's area damage and it presents like **a syllable from later in the word replaces a syllable from earlier in the word - "papple" for apple or "lelephone" for telephone. Similarly patient might use the word "plants" for "pants"**

Extra Mile

- Wernicke's Area is for understanding of speech = hence lesion results in receptive dysphasia
  Broca's Area for expression = hence lesion results in non-fluent aphasia.

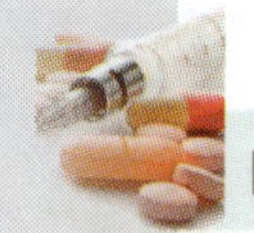

264. Ans. (a) Meningioma

Ref: Harrison, 19th ed. pg. 599-600

- Most malignant brain tumor is Glioma (subtype – astrocytoma)
- Most common brain tumor overall is metastasis to brain (oat cell cancer/breast cancer/malignant melanoma)
- *Most common benign brain tumor is Meningioma*
- IOC for brain tumor is gadolinium enhanced MRI

265. Ans. (a) Parkinsonism

Ref: Harrison, 19th ed. pg. 2606

- Lewy bodies are intra-neuronal inclusion bodies in Parkinsonism and in Dementia with lewy body (D.L.B).
- *Hirona bodies are seen in Alzheimer's disease. **The intra-neuronal inclusions in AD are known as neurofibrillary tangles.***

266. Ans. (c) HIV encephalopathy

Ref: Harrison, 19th ed. pg. 1263

- HIV leads to asymptomatic neurocognitive impairment or HIV-associated dementia.
- Hypoglycemia can lead to neuroglucopenia and seizures
- Hypocalcemia/Tetany leads to larynospasm. The resultant hypoxia can lead to seizures.
- NCC leads to intracranial calcification and leads to seizures.

267. Ans. (b) Viral meningitis

Ref: Harrison, 19th ed. pg. 890

- *The key word in the diagnosis of patient is lymphocytic pleocytosis.* Pleocytosis means a dimorphic cell population where first neutrophils and later lymphocytes are predominant".
- Harrison states that "**As a rule, a lymphocytic pleocytosis with a low glucose concentration should suggest fungal or tuberculous meningitis, or noninfectious disorders (e.g., sarcoid, neoplastic meningitis)". Where as in this question CSF sugar is normal. Hence the answer is viral meningitis.**
- **Viral meningitis** has typical profile of **lymphocytic pleocytosis (25–500 cells/L), a normal protein concentration (20–80 mg/dL), a normal glucose concentration,** and a normal or mildly elevated opening pressure (100–350 mm H_2O).

CSF	Normal	Acute bacterial meningitis	Tubercular meningitis	Viral meningitis	Gullian -Barre syndrome	Fungal meningitis
Pressure	50–180 mm H_2O	Increased	Increased	Increased	Normal	Elevated
Color	Clear	**Turbid**	Straw	**Clear**	Normal	Normal
Cells	0–4 lymphocytes/ cu.mm	>1000	>100	>25	Normal	25–500
Sugar	2/3rd of blood sugar	Decreased	Decreased	Normal	Normal	Low
Protein	15–45 mg %	Increased	Increased	Increased	Increased *(albumin-cytological disassociation)*	Normal/elevated

268. Ans. (d) Cerebrospinal fluid reveals a low leukocyte count

Ref: Harrison 19th ed. / 898-99

Refer to above table

- Tubercular meningitis is seen most often in young children but also develops in adults, especially those infected with HIV.
- Tubercular meningitis results from the hematogenous spread of primary or post primary pulmonary TB.
- The disease often presents subtly as headache and slight mental changes after a prodrome of weeks of low-grade fever, malaise, anorexia, and irritability.
- *In general, examination of cerebrospinal fluid (CSF) reveals a high leukocyte count (up to 1000/μL), usually with a predominance of lymphocytes but sometimes with a predominanc of neutrophils in the early stage; a protein content of 1-8 g/L (100-800 mg/dL); and a low glucose concentration.*
- Culture of CSF is diagnostic in up to 80% of cases and remains the gold standard. Polymerase chain reaction has a sensitivity of up to 80%, but rates of false-positivity reach 10%.
- Imaging studies (CT and MRI) may show hydrocephalus and abnormal enhancement of basal cisterns or ependyma.

269. Ans. (a) Normal cells with increased protein

Ref: Harrison, 19th ed. pg. 2694

Refer to above table

- The characterized feature of GBS is albumino-cytological dissociation, characterized by elevated proteins due to autoimmunity while the cell count remains perfectly normal.
- A normal CSF protein level does not rule out GBS, however, as the level may remain normal in 10% of patients. CSF protein may not rise until 1–2 weeks after the onset of weakness.
- Normal CSF cell counts may not be a feature of GBS in HIV-infected patients. CSF pleocytosis is well recognized in HIV-associated GBS.

270. Ans. (a) Tremors

Ref: Harrison 19th ed. pg. 2609

- In the early presentation, about 70% patients experience a slight tremor in the hand or foot on one side of the body, or less commonly in the jaw or face. The tremor consists of a shaking or oscillating movement, and usually appears when a person's muscles are relaxed, or at rest, hence the term "resting tremor".
- The tremor of PD can be exacerbated by stress or excitement, sometimes attracting unwanted notice.
- Resting tremor is the earliest and most common symptom of Parkinson's disease.
- The most debilitating feature is Akinesia.
- Non motor symptoms precede motor symptoms.

271. Ans. (a) Chorea

Ref: Harrison 19th ed. pg. 2609

Chorea occurs due to lesion of caudate nucleus whereas the disease process in parkinsonism afflicts the substantia nigra.

Cardinal features	Other motor features	Non motor features
• Bradykinesia • Rest tremor • Rigidity • Gait disturbance/postural instability	• Micrographia • Masked facies (Hypomimia) • Reduced eye blink • Hypo-phonia/soft voice • Dysph*agia* • *Freezing*	• **Anosmia-earliest feature** • Sensory disturbances (e.g., pain) • Mood disorders (e.g., depression) • Sleep disturbances • **Autonomic disturbances** ▪ Orthostatic hypotension ▪ Gastrointestinal disturbances ▪ Genitourinal disturbances ▪ Sexual dysfunction • Cognitive impairment/Dementia

- Parkinson's disease (PD) is the second msot common neurodegenerative disease, exceeded only by Alzheimer's disease (AD)

272. Ans. (a) Anosmia

Ref: Harrison, 19th ed. pg. 2609

Non-motor symptoms may precede motor symptoms of Parkinson's diagnosis by years. The most recognizable early symptoms include:

- Loss of sense of smell, constipation
- REM behavior disorder
- Mood disorders
- Orthostatic hypotension

Subsequently Motor Features Appear

- Tremors (resting 4–6 Hz)
- Rigidity
- Bradykinesia
- Good Response to levodopa

273. Ans. (a) Hypotonia

Ref: Ganong, 25th ed. pg. 110, 233

	LMN	UMN	Extra pyramidal damage
TONE	Decreased tone/flaccidity	Increased spasticity	Decreased rigidity
DTR	Areflexia	Brisk reflex	Normal
SPECIAL FEATURES	Fasciculations + wasting	Babinski's sign + No wasting	Chorea, atheosis, hemiballismus
Superficial reflex	Present	Absent	–
EXAMPLE	Motor neuron disease	Cerebral malaria	Punch drunk syndrome

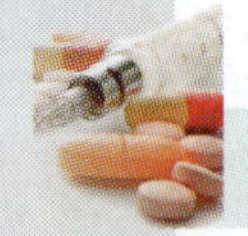

274. Ans. (b) Muscular hypertrophy

Please refer to above explanation

275. Ans. (b) Tongue deviation to right on protrusion

Ref: Harrison, 19th ed. Ch 367

Following a lesion of the hypoglossal nucleus or nerve

- ATROPHY of the muscles of the IPSILATERAL one-half of the tongue occurs.
- FASCICULATIONS (tiny, spontaneous contractions) can be seen.
- *Upon protrusion, the tongue will deviate TOWARD the side of the lesion (i.e., same side).* This is due to the unopposed action of the genioglossus muscle on the normally innervated side of the tongue (the genioglossus pulls the tongue forward).
- The corticobulbar input to the hypoglossal nucleus arises from motor cortex and is predominantly CROSSED. Thus, a lesion in motor cortex will result in deviation of the tongue toward the opposite side or CONTRALATERAL to the lesion.

276. Ans. (a) Acetyl choline esterase in the amniotic fluid

Ref: Nelson 18th ed. / ch. 592

- Failure of closure of the neural tube allows excretion of fetal substances (α–fetoprotein, acetylcholinesterase) into the amniotic fluid, serving as biochemical markers for a neural tube defect. Prenatal screening of maternal serum for AFP in the 16th to 18th wk of gestation is an effective method for identifying pregnancies at risk for fetuses with neural tube defects in utero.

277. Ans. (a) Tau protein

Ref: Harrison, 19th ed. pg. 172t, 175

- Pathologies and dementias of the nervous system such as Alzheimer's disease can result when *tau proteins* become defective and no longer stabilize microtubules properly.
- *Alpha synuclein protein* is seen in parkinsonism.
- *Huntington protein* is related to Huntington disease related to chromosome 4. Protein 14.3.3 is related to prion disease like variant Creutzfeldt Jakob disease.

278. Ans. (b) Thyroid ophthalmopathy

Ref: Harrison, 19th ed. pg. 2294-95

- The question is on unilateral ptosis whereas thyroid ophthalmopathy has PROPTOSIS.
- In myasthenia gravis, due to anti-Ach-receptor blocking antibodies there is ptosis which can be unilateral or asymmetrical which will again appear unilateral.
- Marfan syndrome has congenital Ptosis.
- Pancoast tumor causes horner syndrome in which unilateral sympathetic chain is compressed leading to Ptosis, Miosis, Anhidrosis, Enophthalmos and loss of Cilio-spinal reflex.

279. Ans. (a) Uncal herniation

Ref: Harrison, 19th ed. pg. 1772

- In uncal or mid brain herniation, the raised ICT compresses the same side third cranial nerve while it originates from Edinger-Westphal nucleus. This causes ptosis, diplopia and divergent squint. The reason for unconsciousness can be damage to reticular activating system in the midbrain.

280. Ans. (a) Putamen

Ref: Harrison, 19th ed. pg. 2582

- Most common site of brain hemorrhage is Putamen.
- Intraparenychmal hemorrhage is most lethal and has mortality rate of 40%.
- The IOC is NCCT. For management BP must be controlled which is to maintain a target BP of 160/90.

281. Ans. (a) Single Fiber E.M.G

Ref: Harrison, 19th ed. pg. 442e-6

- *Single fiber E.M.G is the investigation of choice* for myasthenia gravis and shows a decremental response
- Antiacetylcholine receptor blocking antibody TITER is the most specific test for diagnosis of myasthenia gravis. Also remember that *Tensilon test is a screening test* for myasthenia gravis. False positive tensilon test can be seen in motor neuron disease.

282. Ans. (b) Subarachnoid granulations

Ref: Harrison, 19th ed. pg. 443e-4

- *CSF is produced by the choroid villi* in the lateral ventricles and third ventricles. The CSF flows via aqueduct of slyvius to the 3rd ventricle and then via foramen of Munro to the 4th ventricle. The CSF emerges out of Foramen of Luschka and Magendie and accumulates at the base of the skull in basal cisterns.
- *This CSF is then reabsorbed via the arachnoid granulations back into the blood stream.*
- The CSF is produced at a rate of 20 mL per hour and reabsorbed at the same rate. The total amount of CSF at any point of time is 150 mL.

283. Ans. (d) Nystagmus

Ref: Harrison, 19th ed. pg. 2608

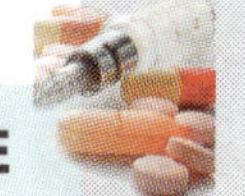

- Dementia pugilistica is seen in athletes who participate in body contact sport like martial arts, boxing etc.
- Repeated blows to the head of the athlete over entire career span of the boxer can lead to cortical damage and Parkinson like features. *(Best example to remember this is Muhammad Ali, the greatest boxer of all times, suffers from dementia pugilistica).*
- Nystagmus is not a clinical feature of this disease and is rather seen with vestibular diseases or cerebellar lesions.

284. Ans. (c) Embolism

Ref: Bringham Intensive Review of Internal Medicine 2nd ed. pg. 888

- Most common type of stroke is ischemic stroke caused by non rheumatic atrial fibrillation leading to clots from atria to embolise to brain.

285. Ans. (a) Thiamine deficiency

Ref: Harrison, 19th ed. pg. 2607, 2724

There are six Major Symptoms of Korsakoff's Syndrome

1. Anterograde amnesia
2. Retrograde amnesia
3. Severe memory loss
4. Confabulation
5. Minimal content in conversation
6. Lack of insight or Apathy

Thiamine is essential for the carboxylation of pyruvate and deficiency during this metabolic process is thought to cause damage to the medial thalamus and mammillary bodies of the posterior hypothalamus as well as generalized cerebral atrophy. These brain regions are all parts of the limbic system, which is involved in emotion and memory.

286. Ans. (c) Finger pads

Ref: De Jong Neurological Examination, 7th ed. pg. 542

- Two-point discrimination is the ability to discern that two nearby objects touching the skin are truly two distinct points, not one. It is often tested with two sharp points during a neurological examination and is assumed to reflect how finely innervated an area of skin is.
- The maximum sensitivity for this test is in lips and finger tips which can be remembered as the most sensitive areas in the body.

287. Ans. (b) CT-scan

Ref: Harrison, 19th ed. pg. 2582

- For evaluation of bleeding in the brain the preferred investigation is CT scan. The bleeding in the brain shows up as hyper-density on CT scan.

288. Ans. (b) Contralateral subthalamic lesion

Ref: Harrison, 19th ed. pg. 2623

Lesion	Manifestation
Caudate nucleus	Contralateral chorea
Globus pallidus	Contralateral atheotosis
Sub-thalamic nucleus	Contralateral hemiballismus
Cerebellum	Ipsilateral intentional tremors
Internal capsule	Contra-lateral hemiplegia with hemi-anesthesia
Ventral pons	Locked in syndrome

289. Ans. (a) Basiliar artery

Ref: Harrison, 19th ed. pg. 2573

Basiliar artery occlusion	Pontine stroke
Middle cerebral artery	Contralateral hemiplegia
Anterior cerebral artery	Spastic paraplegia
Posterior cerebral artery	Midbrain stroke like weber syndrome
Vertebral artery	Medullary stroke

290. Ans. (a) Middle cerebral artery

Ref: Gray's Anatomy, 40th ed. pg. 246

- The Circle of Willis is a part of the cerebral circulation and is composed of the following arteries:
  - Anterior cerebral artery (left and right)
  - Anterior communicating artery
  - Internal carotid artery (left and right)
  - Posterior cerebral artery (left and right)

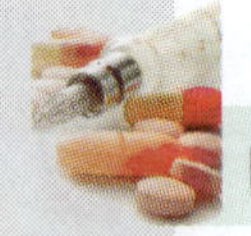

- Posterior communicating artery (left and right) ***The basilar artery and middle cerebral arteries, supplying the brain, are not considered part of the circle.***

291. Ans. (c) Brain hemorrhage due to tear of basiliar artery branches

Ref: Radiology Review Manual, 7th ed. pg. 234

- The classical appearance of a Duret hemorrhage is located in the midline near the ponto-mesencephalic junction.
- Often however, these hemorrhages can be multiple or even extend into the cerebellar peduncles.
- Usually it is seen in patients with severe herniation for 12–24 hours prior to death.

292. Ans. (d) Aphasia

Ref: Harrison, 19th ed. pg. 2724

The classic triad of symptoms found in Wernicke's encephalopathy is:

- Global Confusion
- Ophthalmo-plegia (Most commonly affecting the lateral rectus muscle).
- Ataxia

For diagnosis: Thiamine can be measured using an erythrocyte transketolase activity assay or by activation by measurement of in vitro thiamine diphosphate levels.

293. Ans. (a) Nonfluent aphasia

Ref: Harrison, 19th ed. pg. 177-78

- Broca's area is present in inferior frontal gyrus and is responsible for fluency, syntax and expression of speech and damage to this area causes loss of ability to express self and thereby development of nonfluent aphasia.
- Word salad is seen in patients with damage to Wernicke's area (Area responsible for comprehension).
- Anomia is seen in global aphasia where both Broca and Wernicke area are damaged.
- Apraxia is seen in patients with damage to non dominant parietal lobe.

294. Ans. (a) 3rd nerve

Ref: Harrison, 19th ed. pg. 1784–85

- Most common cranial nerve affected in unruptured berry aneurysm is the 3rd cranial nerve which will present as ipsilateral ptosis, and strabismus.

295. Ans. (d) Tongue protusion

Ref: Harrison, 19th ed. pg. 2537–38

Functions of the Glossopharyngeal Nerve

- Receives general sensory fibers from the tonsils, the pharynx, the middle ear and the posterior 1/3 of the tongue.
- Receives visceral sensory fibers from the carotid bodies, carotid sinus.
- Receives special sensory fibers from the posterior one-third of the tongue.
- Supplies parasympathetic fibers to the parotid gland via the otic ganglion.
- Supplies motor fibers to stylopharyngeus muscle, the only motor component of this cranial nerve.
- Contributes to the pharyngeal plexus.

Testing of 9th Nerve

1. Testing the gag reflex using a wooden spatula
2. Asking the patient to swallow or cough
3. Evaluating for speech impediments.
4. Test the posterior one-third of the tongue with bitter and sour substances to evaluate for impairment of taste.

296. Ans. (a) Loss of gag reflex

Ref: Harrison, 19th ed. pg. 2537-38

Damage to the vestibulocochlear nerve may cause the following symptoms:

- Hearing loss
- Vertigo
- False sense of motion
- Loss of equilibrium (in dark places)
- Nystagmus
- Motion sickness
- Gaze-evoked tinnitus

The gag reflex has the following pathway

- The sensory limb is mediated predominantly by CN IX (glossopharyngeal nerve)
- The motor limb by CN X (Vagus nerve).

The gag reflex involves a brisk and brief elevation of the soft palate and bilateral contraction of pharyngeal muscles evoked by touching the posterior pharyngeal wall.

297. Ans. (c) Parietal lobe

Ref: Harrison, 19th ed. pg. 209

Performing Mathematical calculations is a function of parietal lobe. Damage to the left hemisphere of this lobe will result in problems in mathematics, long reading, writing, and understanding symbols. The parietal association cortex enables individuals to read, write, and solve mathematical problems.

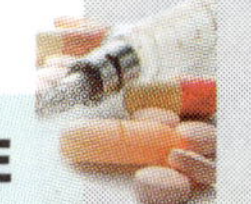

298. Ans. (a) Myasthenia gravis

Ref: Harrison, 19th ed. pg. 2701

- Myasthenia gravis is characterized by eye muscle weakness, ptosis and diplopia. In contrast all myopathies have proximal weakness (exception being Myotonic dystrophy).

299. Ans. (b) 24 hours

Ref: Harrison, 19th ed. pg. 2568, 17th ed. Ch. 364

- The standard definition of TIA requires that all neurologic signs and symptoms resolve within 24 hours regardless of whether there is imaging evidence of new permanent brain injury; stroke has occurred if the neurologic signs and symptoms last for >24 hours.

300. Ans. (b) 1st order neurons releasing nitric oxide

Ref: Vascular Medicine, 3rd ed. pg. 84

301. Ans. (c) Enlargement of lateral and third ventricle

Ref: Harrison, 19th ed. pg. 174

- Aqueduct of slyvius connects the third ventricle to the fourth one. Therefore the obstruction to this area will not only cause enlargement of third ventricle but will also dilate the lateral ventricles proximal to the obstruction.

ENDOCRINOLOGY

302. Ans. (b) Glucagonoma

Ref: Harrison 20th ed. pg. 665

The characteristic dermatologic feature of Glucaganoma is necrolytic migratory erythema. It is characterized by rash/erosion and bullae in intertriginous and periorofacial sites.

Extra Mile

Mnemonic for Glucaganoma: **4D**
1. **D**ermatosis
2. **D**iabetes/Impaired glucose tolerance
3. **D**eep Vein thrombosis risk and depression
4. **D**iarrhea (less common feature)

303. Ans. (a) PTU

Ref: Harrison 21st ed. pg. 2942

The DOC of Grave disease is Carbimazole but it is not used in first trimester due to risk of teratogenicity like aplasia cutis. PTU is highly protein bound and is not transferred to the fetus and is hence preferred in pregnancy.

304. Ans. (a) Klinefelter Syndrome

Ref: Harrison 21st ed. pg. 3050

- Gynecomastia with small testis and hypogonadism in a male patient is a feature of Klinefelter syndrome.
- Option b will be a short stature female patient.
- Option c and d will have pediatric presentation.

305. Ans. (a) Mineralocorticoids

Ref: Harrison 21st ed. pg. 3184

Sarcoidosis is a cause of steroid responsive hypercalcemia. Since hypercalcemia has the potential to cause systolic arrest of heart, it must be dealt aggressively. Steps to be followed are:
1. Normal saline with Furosemide drip
2. IV Ibandronate (Drug of choice)
3. Calcitonin Nasal Spray
4. IV hydrocortisone

306. Ans. (b) Start levothyroxine at 25 microgram and increase the dose gradually

Ref: Harrison 21st ed. pg. 2936,
Bailey and Love, Textbook of Surgery 27th ed. pg. 807

Since TSH is elevated and T4 and T3 are reduced it implies primary hypothyroidism. In patient with no residual thyroid function starting dose is 100–150 micrograms. However in this case since T3 and T4 are being produced starting dose would be 25 μg/day.

Levothyroxine Dosage

For	Initial dose	May be adjusted in
Adults	1.6 mcg/kg daily	4–6 weeks
Adults over 50, or with Cardiovascular Disease	12.5 to 25 mcg daily	6–8 weeks
Severe & Longstanding Hypothyroidism	12.5 to 25 mcg daily	2–4 weeks

307. Ans. (a) Urinary Metanephrine and VMA

Ref: Harrison 20th ed. pg. 2977

Episodic hypertension, palpitations and diaphoresis makes you suspect catecholamines excess/pheochromocytoma. The test used to diagnose is 24-hour urinary fractionated Metanephrine levels >>24 hour urinary vaniyl mandelic acid levels.

308. Ans. (a) GH receptor defect

Ref: Harrison 20th ed. pg. 2899

- Option b and c will cause GH deficiency and are ruled out. Option d is gonadotropin releasing

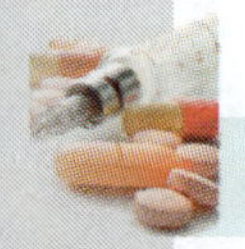

hormone deficiency. Answer by exclusion is Option a which is laron syndrome

- Laron syndrome is a congenital disorder characterized by marked short stature with defect in GH *receptor defect*. It is associated with normal or high serum growth hormone (GH) and low serum insulin-like growth factor-1 (IGF-I) levels which **fail to rise after exogenous GH administration.**

309. Ans. (a) Vitamin B_{12} deficiency

Ref: Short cases in Clinical Medicine by Abdullah, pg. 112

- Strict vegan, lemon yellow tint of skin and atrophic glossitis point to vitamin B_{12} deficiency.
- The image shows atrophic glossitis/smooth tongue which occurs due to atrophy of filiform papillae. It has a multifactorial etiology.
- Atrophy may be associated with xerostomia, pernicious anemia, iron-deficiency anemia, pellagra, or syphilis; may be accompanied by painful burning sensation; may be an expression of erythematous candidiasis and respond to antifungal treatment.

310. Ans. (a) Anterior pituitary

Ref: Harrison 20th ed. pg. 2678-79

- Head size and hand size enlargement point to the etiology of acromegaly/gigantism. The cells involved are somatrophs or somato-lactotrophs.
- Somatolactotrophs produce excess of growth hormone as well as prolactin. This explains the concomitant gynecomastia and galactorrhea occurring in the patient. The tumor is located in anterior pituitary.

311. Ans. (a) Cushing syndrome

Ref: Harrison 20th ed. pg. 2725

- The image shows purple striae on flanks and anterior abdominal wall. The diagnosis to be considered is Cushing Syndrome.
- Option b will produce acanthosis nigricans which has hyperpigmentation in neck folds and axilla.
- Option c is associated with skin tags.
- Option d does not have any associated skin findings.

312. Ans. (c) Coronary artery disease

Ref: Harrison 20th ed. pg. 2875

Diabetic macroangiopathy	Diabetic microangiopathy
• Coronary artery disease • Peripheral arterial disease	• Neuropathy • Nephropathy • Retinopathy

313. Ans. (b) Check for catecholamines levels to rule out pheochromocytoma

Ref: Harrison 20th ed. pg. 2740

- Palpitations, headache and diaphoretic episodes (PHD mnemonic) helps you understand the possibility of pheochromocytoma. Initial presentation can mimic anxiety neurosis as explained in the video lecture snapshot.
- Option b is ruled out as it has weight loss and heat intolerance with physical finding of pretibial myxedema.
- Option d is ruled out as anxiety presents with patient worrying over trivial matters. Symptoms like palpitations, shortness of breath and chest pain are rarely found in anxiety.

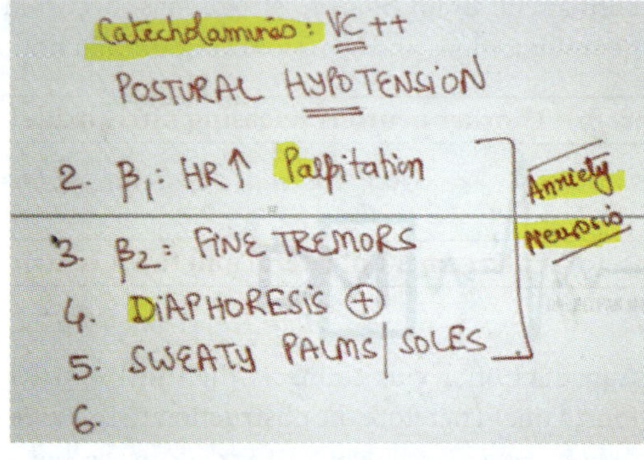

314. Ans. (a) Fluid thrill

Ref: Harrison 20th ed. pg. 283

- The gross abdominal distention is picked up while testing for fluid thrill that develops in massive ascites.
- When the physician will flick over the distended flanks on one side the turbulence set up in ascitic fluid will be perceived on the hand placed on contralateral flank.
- The physician's assistant has kept his hand in the middle to reduce chances of transmission of impulse via subcutaneous fat in abdominal wall.
- Option b is ruled out as patient has to be turned to one side for eliciting shifting dullness.
- Option c is done to determine minimally detectable ascitic fluid >100 mL.
- Option d is used to differentiate ovarian tumor in pregnancy as two discrete masses will be felt. One would be the gravid uterus and second would be the ovarian tumor.

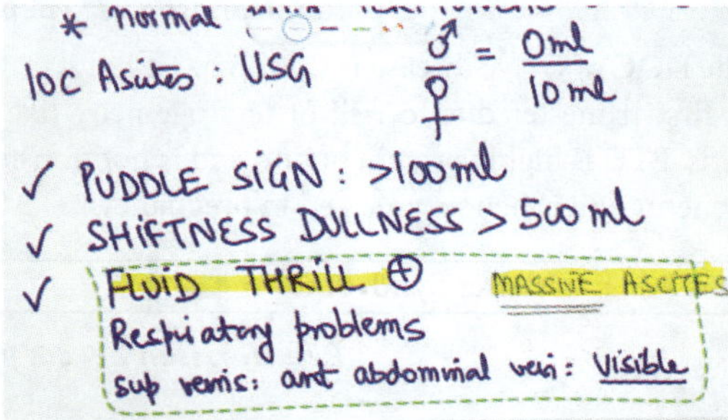

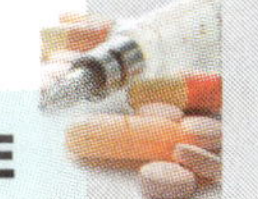

315. Ans. (b) Hyperthyroidism

Ref: Harrison 20th ed. pg. 2703

- The image shows pretibial myxedema which is a characteristic feature of Grave's disease.
- Option a is ruled out due to presence of weight loss and sympathomimetic symptoms
- Option c leads to lymphedema of legs and genitals
- Option d is present since birth with lymphedema.

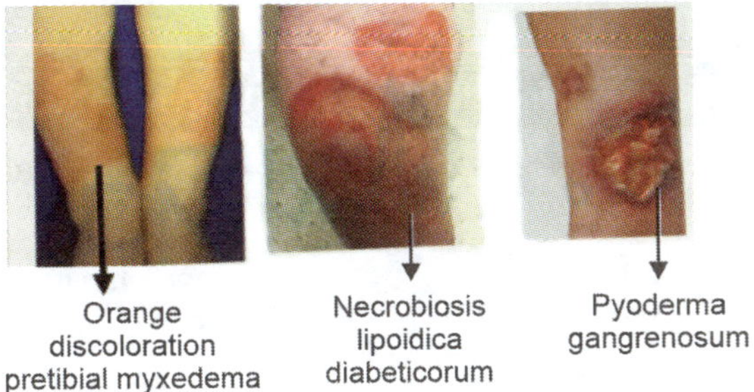

316. Ans. (a) Viruses

Ref: Harrison 20th ed. pg. 2851

The leading cause of fulminant diabetes is viral insult that damages the beta cells of pancreas and can lead to development of type 1 diabetes mellitus.

317. Ans. (d) Foot

Ref: Harrison 20th ed. pg. 2642

- The distribution of joint involvement in diabetic neuropathy is tarsal and tarsometatarsal joints of foot.
- In tabes dorsalis knees, hips and ankles are most commonly affected
- In syringomyelia, Glenohumeral joint, elbow and wrist are involved.

Extra Mile

TABLE: Disorders associated with neuropathic joint disease

Diabetes mellitus	Amyloidosis
Tabes dorsalis	Leprosy
Meningomyelocele	Congenital indifference to pain
Syringomyelia	Peroneal muscular atrophy

318. Ans. (a) Regular

Ref: CMDT 2019, pg. 1256

- Immediately after initiation of fluid replacement, regular insulin can be given intravenously in loading dose of 0.1 unit/kg as a bolus to prime the tissue insulin receptors.
- Subsequently IV infusion of insulin at 0.1 units/kg/hr are continuously infused or given hourly as an intramuscular injection is sufficient to replace the insulin deficit in most patients.

319. Ans. (a) Glargine

Ref: CMDT 2019, pg. 1238

Glargine is called peak-less insulin. It acts after 0.5 hour and has a flat curve with effective duration of 24 hours.

Insulin preparations	Onset of action	Peak action	Effective duration
Insulins lispro, aspart,[1] glulisine	5–15 minutes	1–1.5 hours	3–4 hours
Human regular	30-60 minutes	2 hours	6–8 hours
Human NPH	2–4 hours	6–7 hours	10–20 hours
Insulin glargine	0.5–1 hour	Flat	~24 hours
Insulin determir	0.5–1 hour	Flat	17 hours
Insulin degludec	0.5–1.5 hours	Flat	More than 42 hours
Technosphere inhaled insulin	5–15 minutes	1 hour	3 hours

[1]Insulin aspart formulated with niacinamide has ~10 minutes faster onset of action.

320. Ans. (a) Bitemporal hemianopia

Ref: Harrison, 20th ed. pg. 2676

Physical findings most commonly encountered in patients with hyperprolactinemia are galactorrhea and, in the case of prolactinomas, visual-field defects. Choices B, C and D are not physical findings but symptoms.

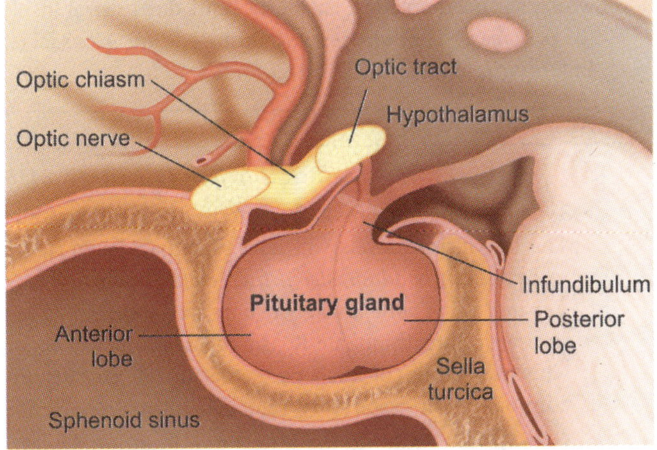

Notice the position of optic chiasma with respect to anterior pituitary in the line diagram shown here.

321. Ans. (a) Impaired glucose tolerance

Ref: Harrison, 20th ed. pg. 2850

Value given	Normal value	Interpretation
120 mg%	<100 mg%	Elevated
140 mg%	<140 mg%	Border line
6.1%	<5.6%	Elevated to Impaired glucose tolerance range
Please note that normal HbA1c is <5.6% and values of 5.7 to 6.4% is impaired glucose tolerance.		

Type of diabetes	Normal glucose tolerance	Hyperglycemia: Pre-diabetes: Impaired fasting glucose or impaired glucose tolerance	Diabetes mellitus: Not insulin requiring	Diabetes mellitus: Insulin required for control	Diabetes mellitus: Insulin required for survival
Type 1 Type 2 Specific types Gestational diabetes Time (years)					
FPG	<5.6 mmol/L (100 mg/dL)	5.6–6.9 mmol/L (100–125 mg/dL)	≥7.0 mmol/L (126 mg/dL)		
2-h PG	<7.8 mmol/L (140 mg/dL)	7.8–11.0 mmol/L (140–199 mg/dL)	≥11.1 mmol/L (200 mg/dL)		
HbA1C	<5.6%	5.7–6.4%	≥6.5%		

322. Ans. (b) Coxsackie B virus

Ref: Harrison, 20th ed. pg. 2851

Fulminant diabetes is an autoimmune form of diabetes which has been noted in Japan. It occurs due to viral insult to pancreas. The viruses incriminated are Coxsackie, Enterovirus and rubella.

323. Ans. (a) pH

Ref: Harrison 19th ed. pg. 2418

- Type 1 diabetes mellitus is characterized by insulinopenia. The low insulin levels will lead to ketoacidosis. *Hence when insulin is administered the ketone production will stop and pH of patient will rise to normal values.*
- Increase in breathing rate/Kussmaul breathing will occur with worsening of diabetic ketoacidosis. On insulin administration respiratory rate will normalize. Hence choice B is wrong.
- On insulin administration glucose levels will come back to normal and glucosuria will disappear. Hence choice C is wrong.
- Due to solute diuresis (sugar rich urine) in diabetes mellitus urine osmolality is >300 mOsm. It will normalize on treatment. Hence Choice D is wrong.

324. Ans. (d) Carcinoid syndrome

Ref: Harrison 19th ed. pg. 415e-2

Carcinoid syndrome presents with diarrhea and flushing episodes. It does not cause obesity.

Feature	Syndrome: Prader-Willi	Syndrome: Laurence-Moon-Biedl
Inheritance	Sporadic; two-thirds have defect	Autosomal recessive
Stature	Short	Normal; infrequently short
Obesity	• Generalized • Moderate to severe • Onset 1–3 years	• Genera-lized • Early onset, 1–2 years
Craniofacies	• Narrow bifrontal diameter • Almond shaped eyes[Q] • Strabismus-V-shaped mouth • High-arched palate	Not distinctive

325. Ans. (d) Vitamin D deficiency

Ref: Harrison 19th ed. pg. 2494 and 426e-2

- Choice A, Paget's disease has increased bone remodeling leading to disproportionate rise of SAP with *normal* serum calcium and phosphate.
- Choice B, osteoporosis has *normal* values of calcium, phosphate and SAP.
- Choice C, primary hyperparathyroidism leads to *increase* in value of serum calcium due to increased bone resorption. The increased PTH leads to loss of phosphate in urine of patient leading to *low* phosphate levels.
- Choice D, vitamin D deficiency leads to low serum calcium values. The resultant low calcium leads to secondary increase of PTH. This increased PTH explains the urinary loss of phosphate and low phosphate levels. The increased bone turnover leads to elevated SAP. Hence in this condition *both calcium and phosphate are low and SAP is elevated.*

326. Ans. (a) Head trauma

Ref: Harrison 19th ed. pg. 2281

Syndrome of Inappropriate Anti-Diuretic Hormone is seen with following CNS causes:

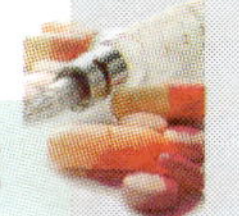

1. Head trauma
2. Amyotrophic lateral sclerosis
3. Agenesis of corpus callosum
4. *Brain abscess*
5. *Cerebral toxoplasmosis*
6. Delirium tremens
7. GBS
8. Hydrocephalus/*Tubercular meningitis*
9. Multiple sclerosis
10. *Bronchial adenoma, Ca lung, carcinoid tumor*

Note: *Important causes are italicized*

327. Ans. (d) Atrial fibrillation

Ref: Page 469, SRB Surgery, 5th ed.

TABLE: Differences in primary and secondary thyrotoxicosis

	Primary (Grave's disease)	Secondary
Neck swelling	Diffuse smooth bilateral involvement	Large nodular involvement
Eye signs and exophthalmos	More common	Not seen
Cardiac features	Resting tachycardia	Atrial fibrillation
Age group	Young	Older
Presentation	Entire gland is overactive and no pre-existing goiter is present	The inter-nodular tissues are overactive and it occurs in setting of pre-existing multinodular goiter.

328. Ans. (b) 5 years

ADA recommends the following ophthalmologic examination schedule:

1. Individuals with *type 1 DM* should have an initial eye examination *within 5 years of diagnosis*
2. Individuals with *type 2 DM* should have an initial eye examination *at the time of diabetes diagnosis*
3. Women with DM who are pregnant or contemplating pregnancy should have an eye examination prior to conception and during the first trimester
4. If eye exam is normal, repeat examination in 2–3 years may be appropriate.

Screening guidelines for other complications

1. The ADA recommends *annual screening for distal symmetric neuropathy* beginning with the initial diagnosis of diabetes and annual screening for autonomic neuropathy 5 years after diagnosis of type 1 DM and at the time of diagnosis of type 2 DM.

Contd...

2. An annual microalbuminuria measurement (albumin-to-creatinine ratio in spot urine) is advised in individuals with type 1 or type 2 DM *Screening for microalbuminuria should commence 5 years after the onset of type 1 DM and at the time of diagnosis of type 2 DM.*
3. Regardless of protein excretion results, the GFR should be estimated using the serum creatinine in all patients on an annual basis.

329. Ans. (d) Aquaporin 2

The defect in nephrogenic DI is in the collecting duct where V2 receptor/aquaporin-2 receptors are exhibiting resistance. An important cause of receptor resistance is lithium.

330. Ans. (a) CTLA-4

Ref: Harrison, 19th ed. pg. 2403

- Polymorphism in promoter region of insulin gene, CTLA-4 contributes to susceptibility to type 1 diabetes mellitus.
- The most common cause of type 1 diabetes mellitus is autoimmunity. Most patients have DR3 and/or DR4 haplotype.
- Haplotype DQA1*0301 is strongly associated with type 1 DM
- Concordance of type 1 DM in identical twin is 40–60%
- Chances of type 1 DM if single parent has type 1 DM is only 3–4%.

331. Ans. (a) Nonfunctioning adenoma

Ref: Page 2265, Harrison:19th ed. and pg. 611: UICC Manual of Oncology, 2015 edition

- The majority of pituitary adenomas (33–40%) are clinically non-functioning and produce no distinct clinical hypersecretory syndrome.
- Most of them arise from gonadotrope cells and may secrete small amounts of alpha- and beta-glycoprotein hormone subunits or, very rarely, intact circulating gonadotropins.
- The most common secretory adenoma is prolactinoma.
- The least common secretory adenoma is TSH secreting tumors. The UICC manual of oncology 2015 edition mentions it as rare (<1%). This is followed by LH/FSH secreting tumor whose prevalence is mentioned as 1%.

332. Ans. (b) Chromosome 12

The most common type of MODY is MODY3 and is due to defect on chromosome number 12. The gene involved is HNF-1 alpha.

MODY, caused by mutations in:
1. HNF–4α (MODY1)
2. Glucokinase (MODY2)
3. HNF–1α (MODY3)
4. IPF–1 (MODY4)
5. HNF–1 β (MODY5)
6. Neuro D1 (MODY6)

333. Ans. (b) 2 hour value = 180 mg%

TABLE: Criteria for the Diagnosis of Diabetes Mellitus

• Symptoms of dilabetes plus random blood glucose concentration ≥11.1 mmol/L (200 mg/dL) or
• Fasting plasma glucose ≥7.0 mmol/L (126 mg/dL) or
• A1C >6.5% or
• Two-hour plasma glucose ≥11.1 mmol/L (200 mg/dL) during an oral glucose tolerance test

334. Ans. (a) Cerebral edema

- The Major nonmetabolic complication of DKA therapy is cerebral edema, which most often develops in children as DKA is resolving.
- Precipitating events leading to D.K.A:
  1. Infection
  2. Myocardial infarction
  3. Venous thrombosis
  4. Upper gastrointestinal bleeding
  5. Acute respiratory distress syndrome

335. Ans. (d) ACTH

Ref: Harrison, 19th ed. pg. 401e-4

The precursor molecule of ACTH is pro-opio-melanocortin (P.O.M.C). This P.O.M.C breaks down to produce ACTH and MSH (melanocyte stimulating hormone). In conditions like primary addison disease P.O.M.C is elevated. The resultant increase in MSH leads to hyperpigmentation.

336. Ans. (a) Sodium increase

Ref: Harrison, 18th ed. / ch 344

- In hyperosmolar coma seen with diabetes mellitus, Serum sodium concentration is usually decreased because of the osmotic flux of water from the intracellular to the extracellular space in the presence of hyperglycemia.
- Hence *sodium* and *blood sugar follow inverse relation* in diabetes mellitus

Extra Mile

Diagnostic criteria for nonketotic hyperglycaemic hyperosmotic syndrome (HHS)

- Profound dehydration (decreased skin turgor, postural changes in blood pressure and pulse rate)
- Neurological symptoms (ranging from mental confusion to coma)
- Plasma glucose levels >600 mg/dL (36 mmol/L)
- Plasma osmolality (Posm) >310 mOsm/kg
- Arterial pH >7.3
- Plasma bicarbonate levels >15 mmol/L
- Normal anion gap (<14 mEq/L)
- Absence of ketones

337. Ans. (a) Sensory polyneuropathy

Ref: Harrison, 19th ed. pg. 2426, 2682

- *Most common form of diabetic neuropathy is distal symmetric polyneuropathy.*
- *Most frequently presents with distal sensory loss.*
- Symptoms may include a sensation of numbness, tingling, sharpness, or burning that begins in the feet and spreads proximally.
- Neuropathic Pain typically involves the lower extremities, is usually present at rest, and worsens at night.
- Physical examination reveals sensory loss, loss of ankle reflexes, and abnormal position sense.

338. Ans. (c) P.C.O.D.

Ref: Harrison 19th ed. pg. 331, 332

- Testosterone is the most important androgen in both men and women.
- In women, testosterone is produced primarily through peripheral conversion of androstenedione (50 percent) with the remainder of production concentrated in the ovary (25 percent) and adrenal cortex (25 percent).
- ***In women, abnormally high levels of testosterone have been associated with hirsutism and polycystic ovary syndrome.***
- Granulosa-theca cell tumors, more commonly known as granulosa cell tumors, belong to the sex cord–stromal category.
- They commonly *produce estrogen*, and estrogen production often is the reason for early diagnosis.

339. Ans. (c) Myasthenia Gravis

Ref: Harrison, 18th ed. chapter 386, table 386-3

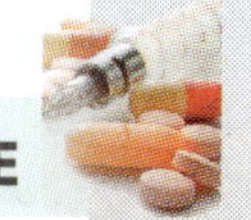

Disorders associated with Myaesthenia Gravis

Disorders of the thymus: Thymoma, thymic hyperplasia
Other autoimmune disorders: Hashimoto's thyroiditis, Graves' disease, rheumatoid arthritis, lupus erythematosus, skin disorders, family history of autoimmune disorder

340. Ans. (d) Urine albumin > 30 mg/gm of urinary creatinine

Ref: Harrison, 18th ed. chapter 44

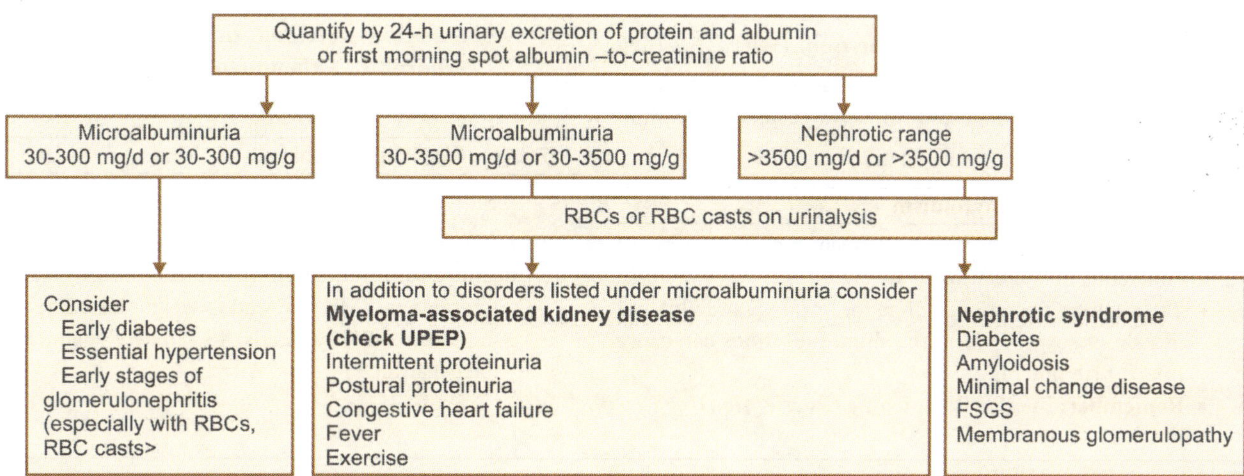

341. Ans. (b) Zona glomerulosa

Ref: Harrison's, 18th ed. Ch 336

- Adrenal gland is divided into adrenal cortex and adrenal medulla, the cortex is further sub-divided into 3 parts, listing them from outside to inside for production of different hormones.
- **Zona Glomeruosa:** Mineralocorticoids
- **Zona Fasciculata:** Glucocorticoids
- **Zona Reticuaris:** Sex Steroids

Extra Mile

Aldosterone	: ↑Conn's ↓ Addisons
Cortisol	: ↑Cushing syndrome
Sex Sterioids hyperplasia	: ↑Congenital adrenal ↓Hypogonadism
Medulla Tumor	: Pheochromocytoma

342. Ans. (d) Addison disease

Ref: Journal, Indian Academy of Clinical Medicine, Vol. 13, No. 1 Jan-March, 2012, pg. 72-3

- *It is known that if glucose infusion is given without glucocorticoid in patients with Addison's disease, they may develop high fever (glucose fever). The exact reason is not specified in textbooks.*

343. Ans. (d) Metabolic alkalosis

Ref: Harrison, 19th ed. pg. 2324

- Addison disease in India is most commonly caused by tuberculosis.

Clinical Features of Addison's

1. Hypotension
2. Salt wasting and salt craving
3. Hypotension fatigue dizziness/ pre-syncope
4. Hyponatremia
5. Hyperkalemia[Q]
6. Metabolic acidosis[Q]
7. Hyperpigmentation-on palmar creases/sole creases/ previous scars/areola/oral cavity

Investigations

- Non contrast CT abdomen for adrenal damage
- Investigation of choice- Cosyntropin test (ACTH stimulation test)

Treatment

- Drug of choice is hydrocortisone (life-long support)
- If asked DOC of Addisonian crisis: i.v. hydrocortisone

Remember metabolic alkalosis is seen with CONN syndrome.

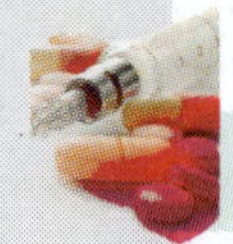

344. Ans. (b) Amennorhea

Ref: Harrison, 19th ed. pg. 2267

- Most common symptom in females with prolactinoma (after galactorrhea) is menstrual - abnormalities.
- Most common symptom in men is: Loss of libido followed by headache.

345. Ans. (c) Coarctation of aorta

Ref: Harrison, 19th ed. pg. 1620

The most common congenital cardiac malformations in Turner syndrome is Bicuspid Aortic valve and Coarctation of Aorta.

346. Ans. (d) Hypoparathyroidism

- The inferior notching of ribs is seen due to pulsation of collaterals in coarctation of aorta.
- Taussig bing operation is done for tetralogy of fallot and is a shunt surgery where the shunt pulsations can cause inferior rib notching.
- **Remember:** Inferior rib notching ***(Roesler sign)***

1. Enlarged collateral vessels -Coarctation of the aorta
2. Interrupted aortic arch
3. Subclavian artery obstruction-Takayasu disease
4. Blalock-Taussig shunt: Involves only upper 2 rib spaces
5. AVM of the chest wall
6. SVC obstruction with enlarged venous collaterals
7. Neurogenic tumors - schwannoma (usually single)
8. Neurofibromatosis type 1 (rarely can be superior if neurofibroma is very large)
9. **Superior notching of ribs is seen in Marfan syndrome, rheumatoid arthritis, SLE and hyperparathyroidism.**

347. Ans. (d) Weight gain

Ref: Harrison, 19th ed. pg. 152

- T3 and T4 have sympatho-mimetic activity and they affect basal metabolic rate. Hence in thyrotoxicosis the increase in BMR will lead to weight loss. The sympatho-mimetic activity leads to anxiety palpitations and tachycardia.

348. Ans. (c) Prader Willi syndrome

Ref: Harrison, 19th ed. pg. 415e-4

Adrenal insufficiency	Salt and water loss leads to weight loss
Pseudo-hypoparathyroidism	PTH receptor defect leads to hypocalcemia and hyperphosphatemia
Soto syndrome	• Soto's syndrome aka cerebral gigantism is a rare genetic disorder characterized by excessive physical growth during the first 2 to 3 years of life. Obesity is however not seen. • Patients with Soto's syndrome tend to be large at birth and are often taller, heavier, and have macrocephaly.

PRADER WILLI SYNDROME

- Neonatal hypotonia with normal growth immediately after birth
- Small hands and feet, mental retardation
- Hypogonadism
- Some have partial deletion of chromosome 15 and loss of paternally expressed genes
- Hyperphagia leading to severe childhood obesity; ghrelin paradoxically elevated.

349. Ans. (d) Smoking is a risk factor

Ref: Harrison, 19th ed. pg. 2392

- The prevalence of obesity is same for men and women at 36%.
- Prevalence increases with age.
- Genetic pre-disposition plays an important role.
- Smoking predisposes to obesity.

BMI (kg/m²)	Weight status	BMI percentile for children	Weight status
<18.5	Underweight	<5th percentile	Underweight
18.5–24.9	Normal weight	5th–84th percentile	Normal weight
25–29.9	Overweight	85th–94th percentile	At risk for overweight
30–34.9	Obese	≥95th percentile	Overweight
35–39.9	Moderately obese		
40–49.9	Morbid obesity		
≥50	Super morbid obesity		

350. Ans. (a) Serum fructosamine

Ref: Evidence Based Diabetes Care, 2nd ed. pg. 229

- Serum fructosamine is a retrospective test that determines fluctuations in blood sugar in the previous 2–3 weeks.

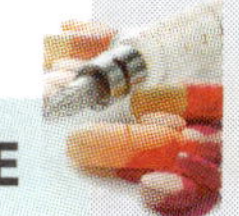

- In contrast glycosylated hemoglobin gives fluctuations in blood sugar value over the previous 6-8 weeks.
- **Also remember:** Severity of bronze diabetes is determined by GLYCATED albumin.

351. Ans. (c) <180 mg/dL

Ref: Harrison, 18th ed. ch. 344

TABLE: Treatment goal for adults with diabetes

Parameters	Goal
HbA1C	<7%
Preprandial capillary plasma glucose	70–130 mg/dL
Peak post prandial capillary plasma glucose	<180 mg/dL
Blood pressure	<130/80
LIPIDS	
LDL	<70 mg/dL
HDL	>40 mg/dL in men >50 mg/dL in women
Triglycerides	<150 mg/dL

352. Ans. (b) Dilutional hyponatremia

Ref: Harrison, 19th ed. pg. 303-304

- Diabetes insipidus has either low levels of vasopressin or it is not able to act. Therefore these patients pass a large amount of dilute urine(Polyuria and resultant polydipsia develops). The result is that due to loss of water from body these patients will develop relative hypernatremia.
- ***The diagnostic test is water deprivation test***

Drugs

- NEUROGENIC diabetes inspidus is treated with desmopressin nasal spray.
- Nephrogenic diabetes inspidus is treated with thiazide diuretics.
- **Remember:** Dilutional hyponatremia is seen with S.I.A.D.H.

353. Ans. (c) Relative hypernatremia

Ref: Harrison 19th ed. pg. 2280

- SIADH is characterized by gain of water and hence dilutional hyponatremia sets in. The gain of water explains low uric acid.
- Since in SAIDH most of the water is reabsorbed via the CD, the low urine output prompts a physician to possibility of renal parenchymal disorder for which KFT must be done and must be normal to consider diagnostic possibility of SIADH.

354. Ans. (a) Insulinoma

Ref: Harrison, 19th ed. pg. 569

- Whipple's triad is used for diagnosis of insulinoma. The findings seen are:
  1. Fasting hypoglycemia (sympathomimetic symptoms)
  2. Relief of symptoms with oral/IV sugar
  3. Rebound hypoglycemia
- IOC for insulinoma is 72 hour prolonged fasting test[Q]
- Imaging modality is P.E.T scan[Q]
- ***Drug of choice is diazoxide***

355. Ans. (a) 24-hour urinary 5H.I.A.A.

Ref: Harrison, 19th ed. pg. 564-65

- **5-HIAA is the major urinary metabolite of serotonin, a ubiquitous bioactive amine.** Serotonin, and consequently 5-HIAA, are produced in excess by most carcinoid tumors, especially those producing the carcinoid syndrome of flushing, hepatomegaly, diarrhea, bronchospasm, and heart disease.

356. Ans. (b) Serotonin

Ref: Harrison, 19th ed. pg. 564-65

- Argentaffin cells in Carcinoid produce 5HT derivatives like serotonin. Epinephrine and norepinephrine are produced by chromaffin cells which are seen in phaeochromocytoma.

357. Ans. (c) TSH

Ref: Harrison, 19th ed. pg. 2289

- Best test for diagnosis of hypothyroidism is T.S.H (Thyroid Stimulating Hormone).
- TSH can also be used for monitoring response to treatment.

358. Ans. (b) Excessive iodine

Ref: Harrison, 19th ed. pg. 2285, 2297

- Excess iodide transiently inhibits thyroid iodide organification, a phenomenon known as the *Wolff-Chaikoff effect.*
- Thyroid hormone synthesis becomes excessive as a result of increased iodine exposure (Jod-Basedow phenomenon which is opposite of Wolf Chaikoff effect.)
- Iodine deficiency increases thyroid blood flow and upregulates the iodine trapping, stimulating more efficient iodine uptake.
- Ingestion of excess thyroid hormone or thyroid tissue is known as thyrotoxicosis factitia. In the first and second statements of this explanation iodine intake was affected but in Throtoxicosis factitia is due to the ingestion of hormone.

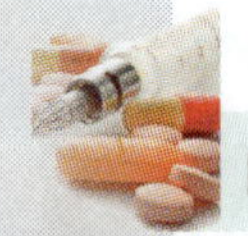

359. Ans. (d) Menorrhagia

Ref: Harrison, 19th ed. pg. 2293

- Thyrotoxicosis is characterized by increased sympathomimetic action causing palpitations, anxiety and increased BMR causing weight loss. *The menstrual abnormality in Grave's disease is oligo-menorrhea.*
- REMEMBER. Weight gain with menorrhagia is seen in hypothyroidism.
- Weight gain with hirusutism with oligomenorrhea is seen in Cushing syndrome.

360. Ans. (d) Myxedema

Ref: Harrison, 19th ed. pg. 2289

Choices	Logic
Grave's	Cytokines appear to play a major role in thyroid-associated ophthalmopathy. There is infiltration of the extraocular muscles by activated T cells; the release of cytokines such as IFN-alpha and TNF results in fibroblast activation and increased synthesis of glycosaminoglycans that trap water, thereby leading to characteristic muscle swelling
Sarcoidosis	Approximately 20% of patients with ophthalmic findings of sarcoid have soft tissue involvement of the orbit or lacrimal gland and present as a mass lesion with proptosis, ptosis, or ophthalmoplegia
Pituitary apoplexy	Pituitary adenoma if a Macro-adenoma or is associated with pituitary apoplexy can lead to Proptosis

361. Ans. (b) Lower esophageal web

Ref: Harrison, 19th ed. pg. 237

- Plummer Vinson syndrome is a premalignant condition characterized by *upper esophageal web* plus *Koilonchyia* and *iron deficiency anemia*. These patients also complain of a burning sensation on the tongue and oral mucosa, and atrophy of lingual papillae produces a smooth, shiny, red dorsum of the tongue.

362. Ans. (a) Hyperglycemia

Ref: Harrison 19th ed. pg. 2257–58

- From late in the first year until mid teens, poor growth and/or shortness is the hallmark of childhood GH deficiency.
- It tends to be accompanied by delayed physical maturation so that bone maturation and puberty may be delayed by several years.
- Severe GH deficiency in early childhood also results in slower muscular development, so that gross motor milestones may be delayed.
- Some severely GH-deficient children have recognizable, cherubic facial features characterized by maxillary hypoplasia and forehead prominence. These children have a high pitched voice and are stunted. *GH deficiency is associated with hypoglycemia.* In contrast gigantism or acromegaly is associated with impaired glucose tolerance.

363. Ans. (d) Hyperphosphatemia

Ref: Harrison 19th ed. /96e-7

- Vitamin D deficiency will lead to Hypocalcemia. This will result in secondary increase in PTH.
- This PTH will now act on proximal convoluted tubule to *cause loss of phosphate*. The increased bone turnover will cause increase in serum alkaline phosphate.
- Important calcium/phosphate and SAP fluctuations which are asked (especially those in bold).

Condition	Rickets	Hyperparathyroidism	Osteoporosis[Q]	Paget disease	Chronic renal failure[Q]
Serum calcium	Less	Increased	**Normal**	Normal	**Less**
Serum phosphate	Less	Less	**Normal**	Normal	**Increased**
SAP	Increased	Increased	Normal	Disproportionate Increased	**Increased**
PTH	Increasing	Increased	**Normal**	Normal	**Increased**

364. Ans. (a) Hypophosphatemia

Refer to above table

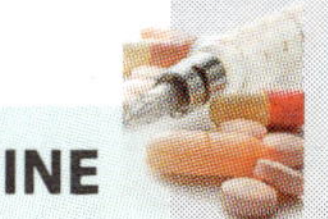

365. Ans. (c) Diarrhea

Ref: Harrison, 19th ed. pg. 2342

- Hyperparathyroidism leads to increase PTH. PTH increases serum calcium by increasing dietary absorption of vitamin D3. It also ensures that the proximal convoluted tubule start loosing phosphate in urine leading to decreased serum phosphate.
- The increase serum calcium leads to deposition in kidney parenchyma forming calcium phosphate stones. The increased level of calcium also leads to constipation. Therefore abdominal pain are a feature of hyperparathyroidism. Renal Colic is due to stones and severe constipation. *Diarrhea is not seen with hypercalcemia/hyperparathyroidism.*

366. Ans. (c) Celiac sprue

Ref: Harrison, 19th ed. pg. 570

- In Secretory diarrhea, the epithelial cells' ion transport processes are turned into a state of active secretion. In celiac sprue, malabsorbtion of sugar occurs. This unabsorbed sugar leads to osmotic gradient and draws in water leading to osmotic diarrhea.

Causes of Secretory Diarrhea

- The most common cause of acute-onset secretory diarrhea is a bacterial infection of the gut.
- Features of secretory diarrhea include a high purging rate, a *lack of response to fasting*, and a normal stool ion gap (i.e., 100 mOsm/kg or less), indicating that nutrient absorption is intact.

Causes of Secretory diarrhea
1. Zollinger Ellison syndrome
2. VIPoma
3. Glucagonoma
4. Insulinoma

367. Ans. (d) Gastrochisis

Ref: Chapter 96: Intrauterine Diagnosis of Fetal Disease, Nelson 18th ed.

- All structural defects can be best picked up by antenatal ultrasound whereas chromosomal and genetic aberrations can be picked up by chorionic villus sampling.
- Chorionic villi are tiny finger-shaped growths found in the placenta. The genetic material in chorionic villus cells is the same as that in the baby's cells.
- During CVS, a sample of the chorionic villus cells is taken for biopsy. The chorionic villus cells are checked for problems. The procedure is generally done late in the first trimester, most often between the 10th and 12th weeks.

368. Ans. (a) Metabolic acidosis

Ref: Harrison, 19th ed. pg. 2327

11 beta hydroxylase deficiency, is characterized by:

- Mineralocorticoid excess and hence hypertension can be seen
- *Mineralocorticoid excess leads to hypokalemia and metabolic alkalosis.*
- Glucocorticoid deficiency leads to hypoglycemia plus excess of ACTH leads to hyperpigmentation around genitals
- Excess of adrenal androgens leads to Virilization.

Variant	Gene	Impact on steroid synthesis	Diagnostic marker in serum (and urine)
21-Hydroxylase deficiency (21OHD)	*CYP21A2*	Glucocorticoid deficiency, mineralocorticoid deficiency, adrenal androgen excess	17-Hydroxyprogesterone
11-Hydroxylase deficiency (11OHD)	*CYP11B1*	*Glucocorticoid deficiency, mineralocorticoid excess, adrenal androgen excess*	*11-Deoxycortisol*
17-Hydroxylase deficiency (17OHD)	*CYP17A1*	Glucocorticoid deficiency, mineralocorticoid excess, androgen deficiency	11-Deoxycorticosterone
3-Hydroxysteroid dehydrogenase deficiency	*HSD3B2*	Glucocorticoid deficiency, mineralocorticoid deficiency, adrenal androgen excess	17-Hydroxypregnanolone

HEMATOLOGY

369. Ans. (c) Hepatitis A

Ref: Harrison 21st ed. pg. 896

Blood should be mandatorily tested for minimum of following infections before infusion:
- Hepatitis B, Hepatitis C, HIV, Syphilis and Malaria.
- Hepatitis A spreads via feco-oral route.

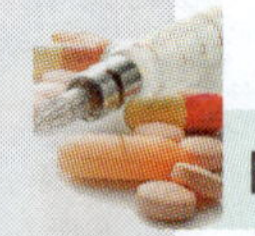

370. Ans. (c) CML

Ref: Harrison 21st ed. pg. 821

AML has maturational arrest and only myeloblasts are found in bone marrow and peripheral smear. The presence of metamyelocytes 15%, Promyeloblasts 30%, Myeloblast 45 % indicates shift to left and is a feature of CML. ALL and CLL are ruled out as they would have lymphoblasts in circulation.

371. Ans. (b) t(9:22)

Ref: Harrison 20th ed. pg. 820

- Bone marrow aspiration shows shift to left with presence of myelocytes, metamyelocytes and myeloblasts. This is a feature of Chronic myeloid leukemia. In all other leukemias maturational arrest occurs and only single cell type will be predominant in bone marrow. CML occurs due to balanced translocation t(9:22) that leads to bcr-abl mutation.
- Option a, c and d is seen with Burkitt lymphoma that presents in African children with jaw swelling and lymph node biopsy showing starry sky appearance.

372. Ans. (a) FDG-PET-CT

Ref: Harrison 20th ed. pg. 876

To identify bony lytic lesions and their extent PET-CT is recommended.

Investigation to Evaluate End-Organ Damage
Hemogram to assess for anemia
Chemistry panel for renal function and calcium
Skeletal survey to evaluate bone lesions
PET/CT or MRI if smoldering MM or solitary plasmacytoma with no other MDE or extramedullary disease

373. Ans. (b) Factor 8 level deficiency

Ref: Harrison 20th ed. pg. 831

- Joint swelling is a common feature of clotting factor 8 deficiency.
- Option a is the most common bleeding disorder and presents with recurrent nosebleeds and hematomas. Prolonged bleeding from trivial wounds, oral cavity bleeding, and excessive menstrual bleeding are common. Gastrointestinal bleeding rarely occurs.
- Option c and d usually present with excessive bleeding post minor surgery.

374. Ans. (d) PFA-100

Ref: Harrison 20th ed. pg. 827

- Since the patient is having excessive vaginal bleeding during menses, high index of suspicion for diseases with platelet malfunction like Bernard Soulier syndrome and Glanzmann thrombasthenia must be considered.
- Bernard Soulier syndrome is a defect in platelet adhesion due to a problem with GPIb/IX/V complex on the surface of the platelets.
- Glanzmann thromboasthenia is a genetic platelet disorder in which the platelets have qualitative or quantitative deficiencies of the fibrinogen receptor $\alpha IIb\beta 3$ leading to defective aggregation of platelets
- Both of these tests can be easily identified using PFA-100 test.

375. Ans. (a) Thalassemia

Ref: Harrison 20th ed. pg. 696

- Anemia with spleno-hepatomegaly points to evidence of extramedullary hematopoiesis. The peripheral smear shows target cells. This points toward diagnosis as thalassemia.
- Malar prominence due to bone marrow expansion is also a feature of thalassemia.
- Option a does not have organomegaly.
- Option b should have pappenheimer bodies in peripheral smear. Spleno-hepatomegaly is not seen in Sideroblastic anemia
- Option d is a cause of Sideroblastic anemia.

376. Ans. (b) A-beta 2

Ref: Harrison 19th ed. pg. 2479

- Beta 2 microglobulin is too large to be filtered across the dialysis machine filter and tends to accumulate in patients undergoing recurrent hemodialysis.
- The accumulation in brain tends to cause these patients to develop dementia and is called dialysis dementia. The accumulation in carpal tunnel compresses the median nerve.
- Option a is associated with Alzheimer disease. Option c is associated with medullary carcinoma of thyroid. Option d is associated with multiple myeloma.

377. Ans. (c) Essential thrombocytosis

Ref: Harrison 20th ed. pg. 737

- Gross elevation of platelet count will lead to hyper-viscosity and increase thrombogenic potential. The sluggish flow associated with hyper-viscosity will explain recurrent headaches and visual blurring episodes. The diagnosis is essential thrombocytosis associated with mutations in JAK2 (V617F, MPL and CALR manifested clinically by overproduction of platelets without a definable cause.

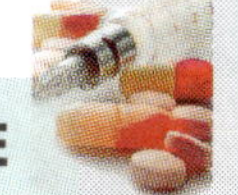

- Option a will have tremendous rise of RBC and WBC as well while in the given case, they are normal.
- Option b shows shift to left with low NAP Scores.
- Option d shows pancytopenia with Spleno-hepatomegaly.

378. Ans. (b) AML

Ref: Harrison 20th ed. pg. 743

The bone marrow aspiration with more than 30% MPO positive immature cells points to acute Leukemia with myeloid origin. MPO is the hallmark enzyme of myeloid lineage and can be detected by cytochemical staining, immunohistochemistry or flow cytometry.

- Option a presents with massive splenomegaly with FISH showing t(9:22) translocation.
- Option c presents with cervical lymphadenopathy with autoimmune hemolytic anemia.
- Option d presents in children with hepatosplenomegaly and lymphoblasts and Immunophenotyping shows terminal deoxynucleotidyl transferase (**TdT**) positivity.

379. Ans. (d) Burkitt lymphoma

Ref: Harrison 20th ed. pg. 774

- The clinching point for diagnosis is starry sky appearance on lymph node biopsy in a child with jaw swelling. This is a feature of Burkitt lymphoma.
- The slide shows tightly packed immature intensely basophilic cells with some areas in between showing scattered macrophages phagocytizing cell debris and apoptotic cells.
- Option a is ruled out as Reed Sternberg cells are not seen.
- Option b is ruled out as history of sore throat and splenomegaly is not present
- Option c is ruled out as it presents with painless cervical lymphadenopathy with necrosis, karyorrhectic debris, and the presence of the typical cell types, namely crescentic histiocytes and plasmacytoid monocytes.

380. Ans. (b) Falciparum malaria

Ref: Harrison 20th ed. pg. 882

- The peripheral smear shows multiple ring stages visualized in RBCs which is characteristic of Falciparum malaria.
- Option a is seen inside neutrophils and not RBC
- Option c will have single ring per RBC
- Option d will require supravital stains for diagnosis.

381. Ans. (a) Plasma ascorbate levels

Ref: Harrison 20th ed. pg. 829

- Alcoholic patients can have nutritional deficiencies. Bleeding gums with petechiae point to scurvy in the patient. The best test for these patients is plasma ascorbate levels.
- Option b is used for diagnosis of Hemophilia A.
- Option c is used for diagnosis of thiamine deficiency in alcoholics. Option c is deranged in alcoholics due to reduced production of clotting factors.

382. Ans. (c) Wait and watch as self-resolution will occur in most cases of acute ITP in children

Ref: Harrison 20th ed. pg. 826

- Patients of ITP can relapse with mild concurrent infections. If there is no evidence of bleed or petechiae, gradual resolution is the rule.
- Option a would cause steroid toxicity.
- Option b would be the answer if multiple relapses occur with evidence of severe thrombocytopenia.
- Option d is used in Rh positive patients with acute ITP with steroids when platelet count is <5K/cu.mm.

383. Ans. (c) D.I.C

Ref: CMDT 2019, pg. 563

As per the question:

Prothrombin time	Increased
Activated partial thromboplastin time	Increased
Platelet count	Reduced (Normal = 1.5–4.5 Lac/cu.mm)
Interpretation	Consumption of clotting factors and platelets seen in Disseminated intravascular coagulation.

- Choice a has non thrombocytopenic purpura due to complement mediated damage to blood vessels. Platelet count is normal in HSP.
- Choice b has recurrent abdominal pain with photo-sensitivity but no bleeding
- Choice d has only low platelet count with normal PT and aPTT

384. Ans. (a) Fibrin degradation products

Ref: Harrison, 20th ed. pg. 835

- Fibrin and fibrinogen degradation product (FDP) testing is commonly used to diagnose disseminated intravascular coagulation (DIC).
- The reference range of FDP levels is less than 10 mcg/mL. Level of more than 40 mg/mL is considered critical.
- Choice b and c are deranged in multiple conditions like haemophilia and chronic liver disease and hence are not diagnostic of DIC.
- Choice d, D- Dimer assay is used as a screening test for pulmonary embolism.

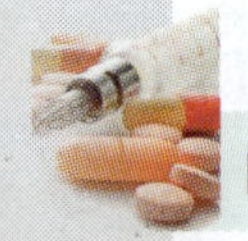

Fibrinolytic system and its regulation

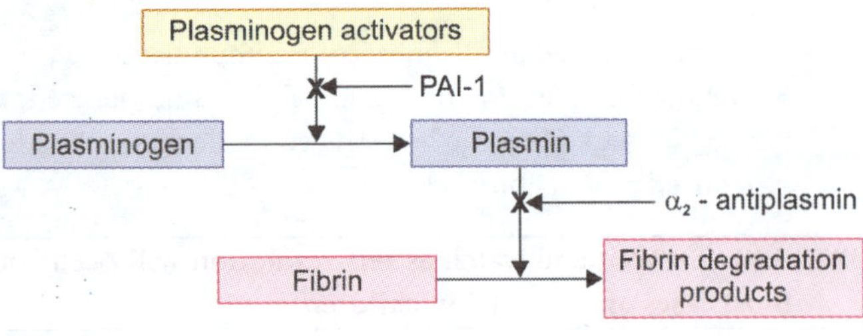

385. Ans. (a) Bone infarction

Ref: Harrison, 19th ed. pg. 634

- Sickle cell anemia leads to development of sickling episodes. This leads to vaso-occlusive crisis and bone infarction involving mainly long bones.
- The *hand foot syndrome* is caused by painful infarcts of digits and dactylitis.
- The vaso-occlusive crisis/painful crisis develop suddenly and lead to pain anywhere in the body lasting for weeks.
- Spleen is also destroyed by these cumulative small infarcts by 18–36 months of age.

386. Ans. (a) Bacterial overgrowth syndrome

Ref: Harrison 19th ed. pg. 350e-1

- Schilling test helps in determining etiology of vitamin B_{12} deficiency.
- Bacterial overgrowth syndrome occurs due to growth of *large intestinal microbiota flora* like bacteroides to *multiply in small intestine.*
- Hence after a course of antibiotics when the flora will die, normal B_{12} absorption can take place and Schilling's test will become normal.

TABLE: Differential results of the Schilling's test in several diseases associated with cobalamin malabsorption

	58Co-labeled cobalamin	With intrinsic factor	With pancreatic enzymes	After 5 days of antibiotics
Pernicious anemia	Reduced	Normal	Reduced	Reduced
Chronic pancreatitis	Reduced	Reduced	Normal	Reduced
Bacterial overgrowth	Reduced	Reduced	Reduced	Normal
Ileal disease	Reduced	Reduced	Reduced	Reduced

- In chronic pancreatitis, test will become normal with addition of pancreatic supplements.
- In atrophic gastritis, IF supplementation will normalize the Schilling's test.
- If in spite of antibiotics, IF supplementation and pancreatic enzymes the test remains abnormal, it indicates presence of ileal mucosal disease.

387. Ans. (c) Adult T cell leukemia

Human T cell linked virus is related to development of:
- Adult T cell leukaemia
- Tropical spastic paraparesis

Clinical Picture for Adult T cell Leukemia

1. Rapidly progressive skin lesions that mimic mycosis fungoides
2. Pulmonary involvement
3. Hypercalcemia
4. Lymphocytosis with cells containing lobulated or "flower-shaped" nuclei
5. Serum levels of CD25 can be used as a tumor marker. *The cumulative lifetime risk of developing ATL is 3% among HTLV-1 infected patients*

Extra Mile

HTLV-I infection is transmitted in three ways:
- Mother to child, especially via breast milk
- Sexual activity
- Blood via contaminated transfusions or contaminated needles.

The virus is most commonly transmitted perinatally. Compared with HIV, which can be transmitted in cell-free form, HTLV-I is less infectious, and its transmission usually requires cell-to-cell contact.

388. Ans. (a) Microcytic anemia

Ref: Harrison, 19th ed. pg. 640, 645

B12 deficiency is characterised by:
- Loss of vibratory and position sense (Rhomberg sign)
- Abnormal gait
- Dementia
- Impotence
- Loss of bladder and bowel control
- Macrocytic anemia

389. Ans. (b) Megaloblastic anemia

Ref: Harrison, 19th ed. pg. 81e-3f

The presence of macrocytes with hyper segmented neutrophils confirms the answer as megaloblastic anemia.

390. Ans. (b) Iron deficiency anemia

Ref: Harrison, 19th ed. pg. 627–28

- Initially the anemia is normocytic normochromic and subsequently hypochromic and microcytic. There is mild to moderate anisocytosis (variation in size) and poikilocytosis (Variation and shape).
- The long, thin elliptocytes of iron deficiency are sometimes referred to as pencil cells.
- Target cells are uncommon and anisochromasia is characteristic. There are two features that can be useful in making the distinction from thalassaemia trait.

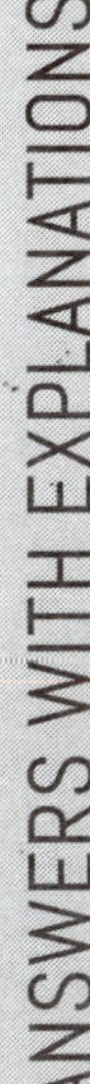

- Subsequently there is a fall in the MCV and the MCH and, when it is measured by a sensitive technique, a fall in the MCHC as well.

391. Ans. (a) Age between 1 and 10 years

Ref: Harrison, 19th ed. pg. 699-700

Prognostic factor in acute lymphoblastic leukemia

Excellent prognosis	• t(12;21) and TEL-AML1 fusion • Hyperdiploidy and trisomy of specific chromosomes (4, 10 and 17) is associated with an excellent prognosis. • Age >1 years and <10 years
Dismal prognosis	• t(9;22) or Philadelphia chromosome and BCR-ABL fusion • Hypodiploidy with chromosome number <45 is associated with a poor prognosis • Age >10 years • WBC >50,000/cu.mm^3 • CNS leukemia at presentation

392. Ans. (b) HLA mediated

Ref: Harrison, 18th ed. Chapter 113

- Transfusion-Related Acute Lung Injury (TRALI) is a syndrome characterized by acute respiratory distress following transfusion.
- *TRALI usually results from the donor plasma that contains high-titer anti-HLA antibodies that bind recipient leukocytes.*
- The leukocytes aggregate in the pulmonary vasculature and release mediators that increase capillary permeability.
- Testing the donor's plasma for anti-HLA antibodies can support this diagnosis.
- The implicated donors are frequently multiparous women, and transfusion of their plasma component should be avoided.
- All plasma-containing blood products have been implicated including rare reports of IVIG and cryoprecipitate.
- *Symptoms of TRALI typically develop during, or within 6 hours of a transfusion.* Patients present with the rapid onset of dyspnea and tachypnea. There may be associated fever, cyanosis, and hypotension and clinical exam reveals non-cardiogenic pulmonary edema.

393. Ans. (b) Autosomal recessive

Ref: Harrison, 18th ed. Chapter 104

THALASSEMIA SYNDROMES

- The thalassemia syndromes are inherited disorders of alpha- or beta-globin biosynthesis and have autosomal recessive inheritance.
- The *most common genetic mutation* in thalassemia arises from mutations that derange splicing of the mRNA precursor or prematurely terminate translation of the mRNA.
- Investigation of choice is high performance liquid chromatography
- Treatment of choice is allogenic bone marrow transplantation
- For survival in thalassemia major recurrent packed RBC transfusions are given initially.

394. Ans. (a) Iron deficiency anemia

Ref: Chapter 104: Harrison, 18th ed.

Disease	Serum iron	Serum ferritin	TIBC
Iron deficiency anemia	Decreased	Decreased	Increased
Chronic kidney disease (anemia is due to deficiency of erythropoietin)	Normal	Normal/ decreased if lost in urine due to kidney pathology	Normal
Sideroblastic anemia	Increased	Increased	Decreased
Fanconi anemia (congenital aplastic anemia)	Normal	Normal	Normal

395. Ans. (a) Platelet elevation

Ref: Harrison, 18th ed. chapter 115

Essential thrombocytosis (primary thrombocythemia) is a nonreactive, *chronic myeloproliferative disorder* in which sustained megakaryocyte proliferation leads to an increase in the number of circulating platelets.

396. Ans. (d) All of the above

Ref: Harrison's, 17th ed. Ch. 109

- Schistocytes are fragmented part of a red blood cells which are typically irregularly shaped, jagged, and have two pointed ends. A true schistocyte does not have central pallor. *They are sometimes referred to as **"helmet cells"**.*
- The presence of schistocytes on the peripheral blood smear suggests red blood cell injury from damaged endothelium ***and is a characteristic feature of microangiopathic hemolytic anemia.***

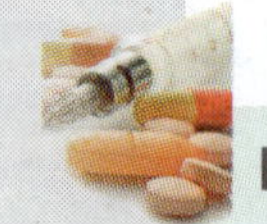

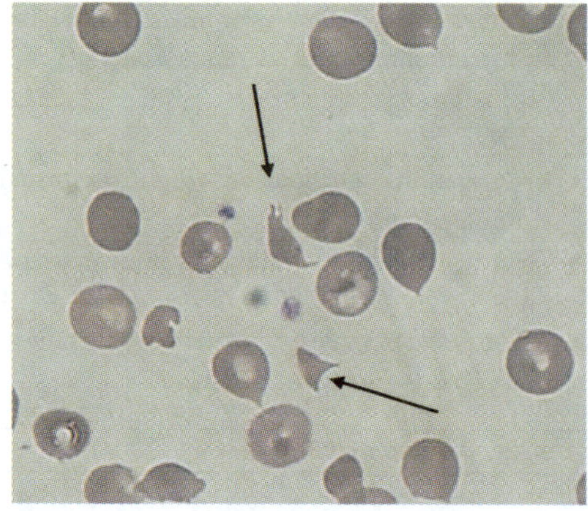

- Microangiopathic hemolytic anemia is an infrequent cause of Coombs-negative intravascular hemolytic anemia, and its causes include:
  1. ***Thrombotic thrombocytopenic purpura***
  2. ***Hemolytic uremic syndrome***
  3. ***Disseminated intravascular coagulation***
  4. Valvular prosthesis

397. Ans. (b) Deficiency is rarely seen, except in infants

Ref: Harrison, 19th ed. pg. 96e-8

- Vitamin-K is a fat soluble compound. It promotes blood clotting by increasing hepatic biosynthesis of prothrombin and other coagulation factors.
- The best sources are green leafy vegetables, liver, cheese, butter and egg yolk. *Deficiency, usually seen only in neonates, in disorders of absorption or during antibiotic therapy is characterized by hemorrhage.*
- *Warfarin acts by inhibiting Vitamin K*, and does not causes deficiency of the same.
- Factor VII is the first to reduce, since it has shortest half life.

398. Ans. (a) Pigmented

Ref: Harrison, 19th ed. pg. 2078

- Pigmented gall stones have composition of Calcium Bilirubinate and are seen in hemolytic anemia like hereditary spherocytosis, sickle cell anemia.

399. Ans. (c) Meth-hemoglobinemia

Ref: Harrison, 19th ed. pg. 636

- Sickle cell anemia has a pediatric presentation.
- Hemolytic anemia will cause pallor and not brown discoloration of blood.
- In G6PD in event of intravascular hemolysis the hemoglobinuria will cause a black urine. Therefore by exclusion the answer is meth-hemoglobinemia.

400. Ans. (c) Donor serum is tested against recipient packed cells

Ref: Harrison, 19th ed. pg. 138e-2

Cross-matching blood is performed prior to a blood transfusion in order to *determine if the donor's blood is compatible with the blood of an intended recipient*, or to identify matches for organ transplantation.

401. Ans. (c) Chronic liver disease

Ref: Harrison, 19th ed. pg. 405

- Dengue hemorrhagic fever has thrombocytopenia so bleeding time is increased.
- Von wilebrand disease has deficiency of vWf which acts as an adhesive and glues the platelet to the damaged vessel wall. Hence the platelets are not able to glue on to the bleeding site and the bleeding time is increased.
- Bernard soulier is a platelet function defect of Ib/IIa receptor defect which leads to defective platelet adhesion and thereby an increased bleeding time.
- In chronic liver disease, the clotting factor 7 (shortest half life) depletes very fast leading to prolongation of PROTHROMBIN TIME.

402. Ans. (a) +4°C

Ref: Harrison, 19th ed. pg. 138e-6

Blood is stored in blood bank at 4 degrees Celsius. This results in decrease in metabolic rate of RBC and their cellular requirements. Hence the advantage is that the shelf life of blood in blood bank is 21–42 days. *(Average of 35 days as best answer in MCQ).*

- Cryoprecipitate is stored at minus 20°C.
- In contrast platelets are stored in blood bank at room temperature with average of +20°–24°C.

403. Ans. (c) Chronic myeloid leukemia

Ref: Harrison, 19th ed. pg. 672

The following are Myelo-proliferative disorders:

1. Polycythemia vera
2. Chronic myeloid leukemia
3. Essential thrombocytosis
4. Myelofibrosis
5. Systemic mastocytosis
6. Chronic eosinophilic leukemia

404. Ans. (a) H. influenzae

Ref: Harrison, 19th ed. pg. 484, 652

- Spleen protects from capsulated organisms and hence protects from infection from organisms like *Pneumococcus, Meningococcus, Hemophilus influenzae.*

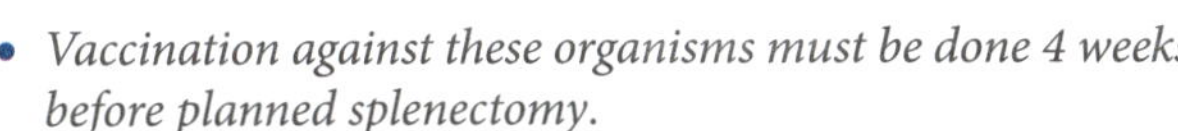

- *Vaccination against these organisms must be done 4 weeks before planned splenectomy.*

405. Ans. (a) Imatinib mesylate

Ref: Harrison, 19th ed. pg. 102e-3

- *Imatinib mesylate is an inhibitor of tyrosine kinase which is used for treatment of the following cancers*
  - Chronic myeloid leukemia
  - Gastro-intestinal stromal tumors
  - Systemic mastocytosis

406. Ans. (a) Long arm of chromosome 9 and long arm of chromosome 22

Ref: Harrison, 19th ed. pg. 101e-3

- The exact chromosomal defect in Philadelphia chromosome is a *translocation*, between the long arms of chromosome 22 and 9. The result is that a fusion gene is created by *juxta positioning* the *Abl1 gene on chromosome* 9 (region q34) to a *part of the BCR ("breakpoint cluster region") gene on chromosome 22 (region q11).*
- The significance of knowing this information is that this chromosome defect causes activation of an enzyme by the name of tyrosine kinase which provides energy to the cancer cells to divide uncontrollably.

407. Ans. (a) Macrocytic anemia

Ref: Harrison, 19th ed. pg. 637

- Thalassemia major is a hemolytic anemia where defective RBC's are produced resulting in transfusion dependency since the defective RBC's are destroyed by the spleen. *These defective RBC in blood circulation are referred to as target cells on a peripheral smear.*
- The type of anemia seen is referred to as ***Microcytic Hypochromic anemia***.
- The Hematopoiesis that occurs in liver and spleen in these patients is referred to as extramedullary hematopoiesis and is responsible for spleno-hepatomegaly in these patients.

408. Ans. (d) Cirrhosis

Ref: Harrison, 19th ed. pg. 739

- In cirrhosis of the liver the production of all clotting factors will be reduced and therefore in these patients bleeding diathesis is seen.
- In pregnancy the elevated fibrinogen levels will lead to hyper-coagulable state.
- In abruption placentae the retro-placental clot formation implies the same hypercoagualability.
- In MI the preceding plaque fissure results in development of increased clotting tendency.

409. Ans. (a) Hereditary spherocytosis

Ref: Harrison, 19th ed. pg. 651

- In hereditary spherocytosis, the RBCs have a tendency to be trapped and destroyed in splenic sinusoids. The main features of this disease include anemia, reticulocytosis, jaundice, and splenomegaly. Hence elective splenectomy would be the treatment of choice for this condition.

410. Ans. (a) C.M.L.

Ref: Harrison, 19th ed. pg. 324, 634

Priapism is characterized by prolonged, painful and irreducible erection, not resulting in ejaculation. It is an emergency with a poor prognosis, as the risk of impotence is 50%.

Causes of Priapism

- Sickle cell anemia
- Chronic myelogenous leukemia, Chronic lymphocytic leukemia, and acute lymphoblastic leukemia. The hyper-leukocytosis leads to increased viscosity of blood and resultant priapism
- Drugs

411. Ans. (a) B cell tumor

Ref: Harrison 19th ed. pg. 706

- Hairy cell leukemia is a B cell tumor disease that presents in older males.
- Usual presentation involves pancytopenia with splenomegaly.
- The malignant cells appear to have *"hairy" projections* on light and electron microscopy and show a characteristic staining pattern with *tartrate-resistant acid phosphatase*.
- *Bone marrow* is typically not able to be aspirated, and *biopsy shows a pattern of fibrosis.*
- Patients with this disorder are prone to unusual infections, including infection by Mycobacterium avium intracellulare, and to vasculitic syndromes.
- Hairy cell leukemia is responsive to chemotherapy with interferon, pentostatin, or *cladribine, with the latter being the usually preferred treatment.*

GASTROINTESTINAL TRACT

412. Ans. (b) Esophageal bleeding varices

Ref: Harrison 21st ed. pg. 311

- Option a is seen in an alcoholic after binge drinking.
- Option b is a more logical conclusion as Bleeding esophageal varices are a known complication of CLD and presents with sudden onset hematemesis.
- Option c presents with rebound tenderness and rigidity of anterior abdominal wall.
- Option d will cause subcutaneous emphysema.

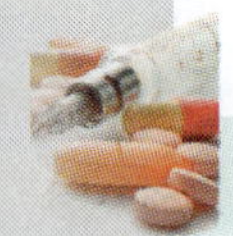

413. Ans. (a) Carcinoid tumor

Ref: Harrison 21st ed. pg. 2987

- Carcinoid tumor produces 5HT derivatives like Serotonin and histamine. The breakdown of these results in 5 Hydroxy indole acetic acid levels to spike.
- Option b and d originate from chromaffin cells and lead to excess of urinary Vanillylmandelic acid levels.

414. Ans. (d) IV ceftriaxone

Ref: Harrison 20th ed. pg. 2632

- The presence of neutrophils in ascitic fluids indicates infection called spontaneous bacterial peritonitis. This occurs in patients of refractory ascites.
- Antibiotics like third generation cephalosporins should be started on priority. For prevention Norfloxacin should be started.
- Option a is done for massive ascites. Option b is used for Hepatorenal syndrome. Option c is used for bleeding esophageal varices.

415. Ans. (a) Diffuse esophageal spasm

Ref: Harrison 20thed. pg. 2428

The barium swallow shows segmentations in esophagus due to non-coordinated peristalsis seen in Diffuse esophageal spasm. Option b will produce pencil tip appearance. Option c will produce irregular filling defect called rat tail appearance. Option d is another name for Zenker diverticulum.

416. Ans. (a) IgM HAV

Ref: Harrison 20th ed. pg. 2349

The development of jaundice in multiple patients simultaneously who are eating food from a common source points to food contamination with hepatitis A.
The best way to identify an infection is to pick up IgM class of antibodies. The abdominal pain would be right upper quadrant discomfort caused by stretching of liver capsule due to inflammation of liver.

417. Ans. (b) Pyloric stenosis

Ref: Bailey and Love 27th ed. pg. 1117

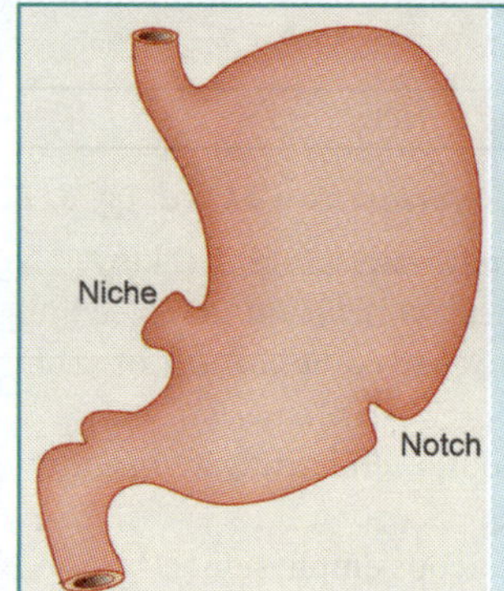

The image shows barium meal study in which *niche and notch* appearance is seen in stomach. This is seen in patients with pyloric stenosis.
Option a and C are visualized with endoscopy showing dilated vessels.
Option d is visualised with endoscopy showing hyperplasia of stomach rugosities. The classical description is "cerebriform appearance of stomach rugosities".

418. Ans. (a) Hypokalemic hypochloremic Metabolic alkalosis with Hyponatremia

Ref: Harrison 20th ed. pg. 315

- Patients with chronic vomiting will loose HCL leading to hypochloremia.
- The loss of water from body due to recurrent episodes of vomiting leads to dehydration and stimulation of RAAS.
- The high aldosterone activity leads to potassium and hydrogen ions loss in the urine. This causes hypokalemic alkalosis.
- Hypovolemic hyponatremia is observed in patients with GIT losses.

419. Ans. (d) Pyoderma gangrenosum

Ref: Harrison 20th ed. pg. 2268

- The image shows a purple rimmed ulcer on the shin with pouting granulation tissue which is the leading dermatological complication seen in patients of IBD and is known as pyoderma gangrenosum.
- Option a is usually located above medial malleolus and shows hyperpigmentation of skin.
- Option b is tick bite seen in Lyme's disease
- Option c is seen on shins in patients of sarcoidosis.

420. Ans. (a) Small intestinal mucosal biopsy

Ref: Harrison, 20th ed. pg. 2253

- The clinical presentation given is of malabsorbtion syndrome and is confirmed with small intestinal mucosal biopsy.
- Choice b allows the diagnosis or exclusion of pancreatic exocrine insufficiency, which can be caused by chronic pancreatitis, cystic fibrosis, pancreatic tumor.
- Choice c is done for picking up sugar in stool of osmotic diarrhea patient.
- Choice d is done for Hirschsprung's disease.

421. Ans. (c) Directly related to duration of disease

Ref: Harrison, 20th ed. pg. 2275

- The risk of neoplasia in UC is increased with *duration* and *extent of disease.*
- Incidence is 2% at end of 10 years and a huge 18% at end of 30 years. The risk is 1.5-2 times higher than general population.
- Choice a is wrong as UC is a premalignant condition.
- Choice b is wrong as smoking has no bearing on development of colorectal cancer in ulcerative colitis.
- Choice d is wrong as disease should be present for long duration to lead to development of malignancy. Annual biopsy is recommended for patients with extensive colitis persisting for 10–12 years.

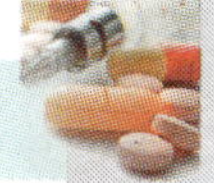

422. Ans. (c) Budesonide

Ref: Harrison: 19th ed. pg. 1963

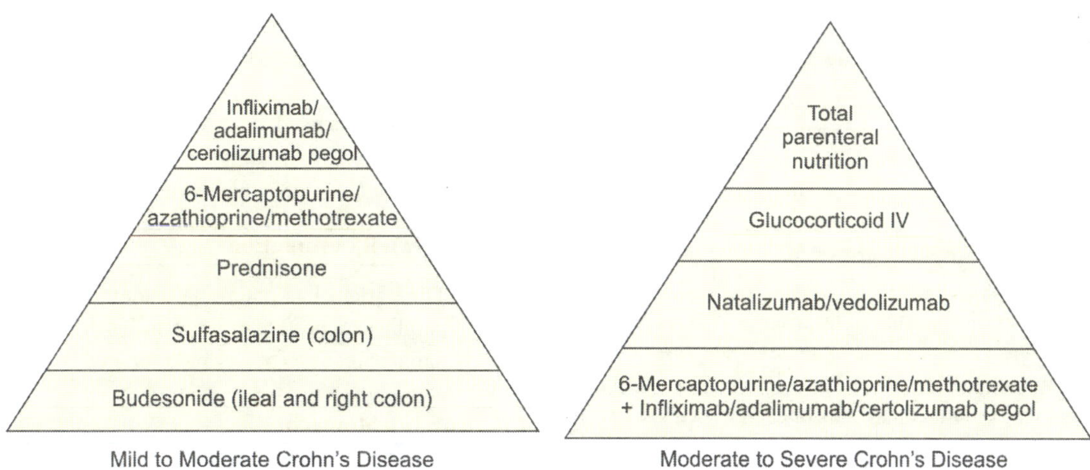

423. Ans. (a) Occurs along structures derived from foregut

Ref: Harrison 19th ed. pg. 537

- Carcinoid tumor can occur at sites derived from foregut, midgut and hindgut.
- The most common site is bronchus which is derived from foregut.
- In the GIT, common sites are ileum, rectum and appendix.
- Most intestinal carcinoids are asymptomatic and are of *low* malignant potential.
- Bronchial carcinoid can *present* as flushing episodes with secretory diarrhea.
- Elevated VMA levels are found in neuroblastoma and *not pheochromocytoma*[Q].

424. Ans. (b) 5-Hydroxyindole acetic acid

Carcinoid tumor produces 5HT derivatives like serotonin and histamine. The degradation of these leads to elevated levels of Urinary 5-Hydroxyindole acetic acid.

Investigations used for Diagnosis

1. Urinary 5-HIAA levels
2. Plasma neuropeptide K
3. Serum chromogranin A

Must know points about carcinoid tumor

Name	Biologically Active Peptide(s) Secreted	Tumor location in GIT	Malignant, %	Associated with Multiple Endocrine Neoplasia	Main symptoms/signs
Carcinoid syndrome	Serotonin Tachykinins, Prostaglandins	Midgut (75–87%)[Q] Foregut (2–33%) Hindgut (1–8%) Unknown (2–25%)	95–100	Rare	Diarrhea (32–84%)[Q] Flushing (63–75%) Pain (10–34%) Asthma (4–18%) Heart disease (11–41%)

425. Ans. (c) Intestinal metaplasia

- Serial endoscopic examinations of the stomach in patients with atrophic gastritis have documented replacement of the usual gastric mucosa by intestinal type cells. This process of *intestinal metaplasia* may lead to cellular atypia and eventual neoplasia.
- Gastric cancer is associated with blood group A.
- Gastric adenocarcinomas may be subdivided into two categories: a *diffuse type*, in which cell cohesion is absent,

so that individual cells infiltrate and thicken the stomach wall without forming a discrete mass; and an *intestinal type*, characterized by cohesive neoplastic cells that form gland like tubular structures.
- Diffuse cancers have defective intercellular adhesion, mainly as a consequence of loss of expression of E-cadherin.

426. Ans. (a) Stomach

- Up to 70% of GIST arise in the stomach and remaining in small bowel.
- Most exhibit an exophytic growth pattern growing across the bowel wall.
- Mucosal ulceration occurs in large aggressive tumors.
- It is the *most common mesenchymal neoplasm of the gastrointestinal tract.*
- It arises from the intestinal cells of cajal which are called pacemaker cells of intestine.
- They express *cKIT (CD117)* which is a tyrosine kinase growth factor receptor
- Imatinib mesylate is used for treatment.

427. Ans. (b) Anti-tissue transglutaminase antibody

- Anti T.T.G antibodies have higher sensitivity and specificity for diagnosis of celiac sprue as compared to anti endomyosial antibody
- *Choice C, antiepidermal tissue transglutaminase antibody is seen in Dermatitis herpetiformis* which is a papulo-vesicular eruption caused by ingestion of gluten. It is characterized by the deposition of IgA in the dermal papillae.
- *Choice D,* antimitochondrial antibody is seen in primary biliary cirrhosis.

428. Ans. (a) B_{12} levels

- Cobalamin deficiency may cause a bilateral peripheral neuropathy or degeneration (demyelination) of the posterior and pyramidal tracts of the spinal cord. This explains the presence of sensory ataxia in the patient.
- The patchy loss of papillae points to diagnosis of geographical tongue consistent with vitamin B_{12} deficiency. Hence cobalamin/B_{12} estimation should be done.
- Cobalamin can measured by an automated enzyme-linked immunosorbent assay (ELISA). Normal serum levels range from 118–148 pmol/L (160–200 ng/L). In patients with megaloblastic anemia due to cobalamin deficiency, the level is usually <74 pmol/L (100 ng/L).

429. Ans. (b) Intestinal biopsy

Ref: Harrison, 19th ed. pg. 1938

- *A small intestinal biopsy is essential in evaluation of a patient with documented steatorrhea or chronic diarrhea lasting for >3 months.*
- Endoscopy is done and is a preferred method for obtaining biopsy material from proximal small intestinal mucosa.
- **Choice A** is ruled out due to false negative D-xylose test and ease of obtaining small intestinal biopsy after endoscopy.
- **Choice C** is used for evaluation of celiac sprue and is not the first test to be done.
- **Choice D** is not available in United States or India.

430. Ans. (a) B_{12} estimation

- The patient has macrocytic anemia with loss of tongue papillae suggestive of vitamin B_{12} deficiency. The loss of papillae leads to beef/y bald tongue.

431. Ans. (a) Stomach

- Cushing's ulcer is a gastroduodenal ulcer produced by elevated intracranial pressure caused by an intracranial tumor, head injury or other space-occupying lesion.
- The ulcer, usually single and deep, may involve the esophagus, stomach, and duodenum.
- Increased intracranial pressure may affect different areas of the hypothalamic nuclei or brainstem leading to overstimulation of the vagus nerve or paralysis of the sympathetic system. Both of these circumstances increase secretion of gastric acid and the likelihood of ulceration of gastroduodenal mucosa.

432. Ans. (b) Ileum

Ref: Harrison, 18th ed. Table 350-3

Site	Percentage of site
Bronchus, lung, trachea	27.9
Midgut	
Jejunum	1.8
Ileum	14.9
Meckel's diverticulum	0.5
Appendix	4.8
Colon	8.6
Liver ovary	0.4
Testis	1.0
Hindgut	<0.1
Rectum	13.6

433. Ans. (a) Serum lipase

Ref: Harrison, 19th ed. pg. 2100

- The cardinal symptom of acute pancreatitis is abdominal pain, which is characteristically dull, boring, and steady.
- *Elevated lipase levels are more specific to the pancreas than elevated amylase levels. Lipase levels remain high for 12 days. In patients with chronic pancreatitis (usually*

caused by alcohol abuse and question mentions that the patient is back from a party), lipase levels may be elevated in the presence of a normal serum amylase level

- Usually, the pain is sudden in onset and gradually intensifies in severity until reaching a constant ache.
- *The pain radiates directly through the abdomen to the back in approximately one half of cases.*
- Fever (76%) and tachycardia (65%) are common abnormal vital signs; hypotension may be noted
- Abdominal tenderness, muscular guarding (68%), and distention (65%) are observed in most patients; bowel sounds are often diminished or absent because of gastric and transverse colonic ileus; guarding tends to be more pronounced in the upper abdomen
- Lipase has a slightly longer half-life and its abnormalities may support the diagnosis if a delay occurs between the pain episode and the time the patient seeks medical attention.

434. Ans. (a) 24-hour pH monitoring

Ref: Harrison 19th ed. pg. 261-2

- Ambulatory 24-hour pH monitoring is the criterion standard in establishing a diagnosis of GERD, with a sensitivity of 96% and a specificity of 95%. It quantifies the gastresophageal reflux and allows a correlation between the symptoms of reflux and the episodes of reflux.
- However the diagnosis can be established on basis of Upper Gastrointestinal endoscopy with esophageal manometry.
- Esophageal pH <4.0, for 4 hrs/day is diagnostic of GERD.

435. Ans. (a) Wheat

Ref: Harrison, 19th ed. pg. 1940

- Coeliac disease is caused by a reaction to gliadin found in wheat, oats, rye and Barley. Upon exposure to gliadin, there is production of anti-tissue transglutaminase antibody which cross-reacts with small-bowel tissue, causing an inflammatory reaction.
- This leads to villous atrophy and leads to osmotic diarrhea.

436. Ans. (a) Metaplasia

Ref: Robbins, 8th ed. chapter 15

- Categories in ulcerative colitis, include indefinite for dysplasia, low-grade dysplasia, and high-grade dysplasia. It may be difficult to distinguish dysplasia from the reactive/reparative atypia that occurs after periods of disease activity.
- These diagnoses must be made with caution, because the implications for the patient are serious. Low-grade dysplasia warrants consideration for colectomy, whereas high-grade dysplasia or carcinoma is an indication for colectomy
- Dysplasia is defined as an unequivocal neoplastic alteration of colonic epithelium. It may consist of architectural disorganization of colonic crypts, cytologic atypia (including nuclear hyperchromasia), pseudostratification, pleomorphism, clumped chromatin, and prominent nucleoli, with increased mitotic activity, particularly in the upper portion of the crypts.

437. Ans. (a) Duodenum with fast clearance

Ref: Harrison, 18th ed. Chapter 103

- *Iron absorbed from the diet from the duodenum or released from stores circulates in the plasma bound to transferrin.*
- *The turnover of transferrin-bound iron is very rapid typically 60–90 min.*
- Because almost all of the iron transported by transferrin is delivered to the erythroid marrow, the clearance time of transferrin-bound iron from the circulation is affected most by the plasma iron level and the erythroid marrow activity.
- When erythropoiesis is markedly stimulated, the pool of erythroid cells requiring iron increases and the clearance time of iron from the circulation decreases. The half-clearance time of iron in the presence of iron deficiency is as short as 10–15 minutes.

438. Ans. (d) Blood culture

Ref: Harrison 18th ed. Chapter 153

- The definitive diagnosis of enteric fever requires the isolation of *S.* typhi or *S.* paratyphi from blood, bone marrow, other sterile sites, rose spots, stool, or intestinal secretions.

For diagnosis in the first week

- Sensitivity of **blood culture** is only 40–80%, probably because of high rates of antibiotic use in endemic areas and the small quantities of *S. typhi* (i.e., <15 organisms/mL).
- **Bone marrow culture** is 55–90% sensitive, and, unlike that of blood culture, its yield is not reduced by up to 5 days of prior antibiotic therapy.
- Culture of **intestinal secretions (best obtained by a noninvasive duodenal string test)** can be positive despite a negative bone marrow culture.

439. Ans. (a) Barium enema-Pipe stem colon

Ref: Internal Medicine Guide 2e/36

Lead pipe appearance of colon is the classical barium enema finding in chronic ulcerative colitis. There is complete loss of haustral markings in the diseased section of colon, and the organ appears smooth walled and cylindrical.

440. Ans. (b) Multiple air fluid level- Adhesions and bands

Ref: Manual of Emergency Medicine, 5th ed. pg. 247

- In X-ray you can see that due to intestinal obstruction secondary to adhesions or bands, the loops proximal to the point of obstruction will become dilated and fluid-filled and are usually greater than 2.5–3 cm in size
- Loops of small bowel in a *step-ladder* configuration from the left upper to the right lower quadrant are seen.
- Mostly fluid-filled loops of bowel may demonstrate a *string-of-beads sign* caused by the small amount of visible air in those loops.

441. Ans. (a) CBD dilatation on ERCP

Ref: Cleveland Internal Medicine Case Reviews, 5th ed. pg. 93

You can see the endoscope in left top half and right 5 o' clock position which is radiopaque. It is advanced into D2 from where the ampulla of vater is located. The probe is advanced and dye injected which shows dilatation of whole biliary tree. A stricture is also noted proximal to which the biliary pathway is advanced.

442. Ans. (a) 24-hour pH monitoring

Ref: Harrison, 19th ed. pg. 261-62

- 24-hour pH monitoring is done for GERD.
- Components of 24-hour pH monitoring:
  - Percent total time pH <4
  - Percent upright time pH <4
  - Percent supine time pH <4
  - Number of reflux episodes
  - No. of reflux episodes in 5 minutes
  - Longest reflux episode (minutes)

Remember: This method is also used for detection of *laryngesophageal reflux* that causes asthma, laryngospasm.

443. Ans. (c) Colon cancer

Ref: Gastrointestinal Oncology, 2nd ed. pg. 24

- Aspirin has been shown to reduce the risk of colorectal cancer in latest studies in JAMA in September 2013. How it works is a matter of research but has shown a reduction in mortality.

444. Ans. (a) Crohn's disease

Ref: Harrison, 19th ed. pg. 1951–52

CD is a transmural process. Endoscopically, aphthous or small superficial ulcerations characterize mild disease; in more active disease, stellate ulcerations fuse longitudinally and transversely to demarcate islands of mucosa that frequently are histologically normal.

This "cobblestone" appearance is characteristic of CD, both endoscopically and by barium radiography

Ulcerative colitis	Crohn disease
Only colon involved	Panintestinal
Continuous inflammation extending proximally from rectum	Skip-lesions with intervening normal mucosa
Inflammation in mucosa and submucosa only	Transmural inflammation
No granulomas	Noncaseating granulomas
Perinuclear ANCA (pANCA) positive	ASCA positive
Bleeding (common)	Bleeding (uncommon)
Fistulae (rare)	Fistulae (common)

445. Ans. (d) Invasion of lymph nodes seen

Ref: Harrison, 19th ed. pg. 1951

- Crohn's disease is an inflammatory bowel disease in which all the layers of intestine are involved. It involves both the small as well as large intestine.
- Most common part involved is the ileo-caecal area and skip lesions are common with normal areas interspersed. Invasion of lymph nodes is a feature of malignancy and can be easily excluded.

446. Ans. (c) Toxic megacolon

Ref: Harrison's, 17th ed. Ch. 289

- Crohn's disease is a chronic, recurrent disease characterized by patchy transmural inflammation involving any segment of the gastrointestinal tract from the mouth to the anus ***but most common site is Ileum.***
- Crohn's disease is one of the two main forms of Inflammatory bowel disease and is also known as Granulomatous colitis.
- ***Earliest manifestation is Apthous ulcers.***
- Skip lesions, stricture formation, string sign of kantor is also seen.
- **Hallmark feature of crohn's** is fistula formation.
- **Cobble stone appearance is seen** on X-ray.
- **Note:** *Toxic mega colon can be seen in Crohn's disease but more commonly is seen in Ulcerative colitis.*

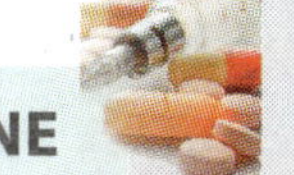

447. Ans. (a) Ulcerative colitis

Ref: Harrison 19th ed. pg. 1952-53

EPIDEMIOLOGY OF IBD

	Ulcerative colitis	Crohn's disease
Male/female ratio	1:1	1.1–1.8:1
Smoking	May prevent disease	May cause disease
Oral contraceptives	No increased risk	Odds ratio 1.4
Appendectomy	Protective	Not protective
Monozygotic twins	6% concordance	58% concordance
Dizygotic twins	0% concordance	4% concordance

448. Ans. (a) Adenocarcinoma

Ref: Harrison's, 17th ed. Ch. 286

- Metaplastic columnar epithelium develops during healing of erosive esophagitis with continued acid reflux since columnar epithelium is more resistant to acid-pepsin damage than is squamous epithelium.
- The metaplastic epithelium has different epithelial types, including goblet cells and columnar cells.
- Finding intestinal metaplasia with goblet cells in the esophagus is diagnostic of Barrett's esophagus; this type of mucosa is thought to be at risk of cancer

449. Ans. (c) Carcinoid tumor

Ref: Harrison 19th ed. pg. 1039-1040

- *H. pylori* is gram negative bacteria, non sporing, micro aerophilic, extra cellular bacteria. *H. pylori* releases urease enzyme which converts urea to ammonia. Ammonia stimulates G cells of stomach which inturn stimulates parietal cells and cause secretion of HCl à Hyperchlorydia. This acid travels into stomach & duodenum and causes **peptic ulcers**.
- H. pylori is a type I carcinogen, which, if present in stomach for long term can cause cancer called MALTOMA (Mucosa Associated Lymphoid Tumor), which is a B-type NHL.

Extra Mile

- MC site of duodenal ulcer in duodenum: D1
- Peptic ulcer refractory to PPI treatment is seen in Zollinger Ellison Syndrome
- IOC for *H. pylori*: Urea breath test > Urease test
- Urea breath test: Test for eradication of infection

450. Ans. (a) Campylobacter

Ref: Harrison, 19th ed. pg. 266

- Diarrhea, the leading cause of illness in travelers, is usually a short-lived, self-limited condition; however, 40% of affected individuals need to alter their scheduled activities, and another 20% are confined to bed.
- The most frequently identified pathogens causing travelers' diarrhea are
  1. Toxigenic *Escherichia coli* and Enteroaggregative *E. coli (Most common but not in choices)*
  2. In Southeast Asia *Campylobacter* infections appear to predominate
  3. *Salmonella*, *Shigella*
  4. Rotavirus
  5. Norovirus has caused numerous outbreaks on cruise ships
  6. Except for giardiasis, parasitic infections are uncommon causes of travelers' diarrhea.
- A growing problem for travelers is the development of antibiotic resistance among many bacterial pathogens. Examples include strains of *Campylobacter* resistant to quinolones and strains of *E. coli*, *Shigella*, and *Salmonella* resistant to trimethoprim-sulfamethoxazole

HEPATOLOGY

451. Ans. (d) Previous infection with hepatitis B

Ref: Harrison 20th ed. pg. 2347

- Option a is ruled out as IgM Anti Hbc is absent
- Option b is ruled out HbsAg is negative and HBeAg is negative. HBeAg is used to diagnose high infectivity.
- Option c is ruled out HbsAg is negative
- This patient has a previous remote infection with hepatitis B and due to good immunological response was able to clear the surface antigen from blood to below the threshold for detection by conventional kit.

Hepatitis B serological interpretation

HBsAg	Anti-HBs	Anti-HBcAg	HBeAg	Anti-Hbe	Interpretation
+	–	IgM	+	–	Acute hepatitis B, high infectivity
+	–	IgG	+	–	Chronic hepatitis B, high infectivity
+	–	IgG	–	+	Late acute or chronic hepatitis B, low infectivity HbeAg-negative ("precore–mutant") hepatitis B (chronic or, rarely, acute)
+	+	+	+/–	+/–	• HBsAg of one subtype and heterotypic and Hbs (common) • Process of seroconrversion from HBsAg to anti-HBs (rare)
		IgM	+/–	+/–	• Acute hepatitis B • Anti-HBc window
		IgG		+/–	• Low–level hepatitis B carrier • Hepatitis B remote past

	HBsAg	Anti HBs	Anti HBc	HBc Ag
A.H infectivity ↑	+	–	IgM	+
C.H	+	–	IgG	+
Recovery	–	+	IgG	–
Vaccinated	–	+	–	–
Gap period	–	–	+ IgM	–

452. Ans. (b) Decompensated alcoholic cirrhosis

Ref: Harrison 20th ed. pg. 2400

- The first image shows spider angioma in an alcoholic patient with cirrhosis. The second image shows Clubbing and the third image shows Dupuytren's contracture.
- Since liver is shrunken it is not palpable. Absence of splenomegaly makes portal hypertension unlikely. Since the patient is having excessive sleepiness, possibility of hepatic encephalopathy development should be kept. The patient should be evaluated for presence of asterixis and blood ammonia levels.
- Option a is ruled out as it indicated Wilson disease which presents in second decade of life.
- Option c is ruled out as esphageal varices, splenomegaly and ascites are not present.
- Option d presents with sudden onset right upper quadrant pain with ascites.

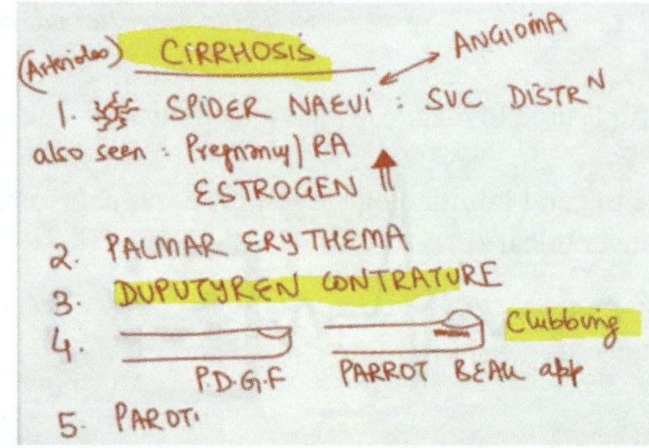

453. Ans. (b) Lung cancer

Ref: Harrison 20th ed. pg. 553

- Prophylactic cranial irradiation is considered for all patients having SCLC. SCLC is the leading cause of metastasis to brain.
- In pediatrics leading cause of CNS metastasis is Acute lymphoblastic leukaemia for which CNS irradiation and intrathecal methotrexate are used.

454. Ans. (c) Portal vein thrombosis

Ref: Nelson Textbook of Pediatrics 20th ed. pg. 1975

- The combination of clinical findings of Hematemesis and splenomegaly points to diagnosis of portal hypertension.
- Now since child underwent exchange transfusion for neonatal jaundice it implies vascular access was taken via umbilical vein. Umbilical vein catheterization carries the inherent risk of causing portal vein thrombosis.
- Once portal vein thrombosis occurs pressure in splenic vein will rise and cause congestive splenomegaly.
- Later due to rising pressure in portal vein portal systemic collaterals will develop in the form of esophageal varices. The rupture of esophageal varices explains the first line of the question as to why the child had hematemesis.

455. Ans. (a) SGOT

Ref: Harrison, 20th ed. pg. 2337

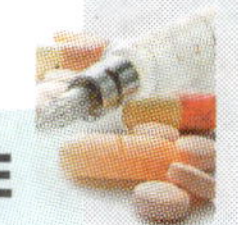

Child Pugh Classification

Points	1	2	3
Encephalopathy	None	Minimal	Advanced (coma)
Ascites	Absent	Controlled	Refractory
Bilirubin (mmol/L)	<34	34–51	>51
Albumin (g/L)	>35	28–35	<28
Prothrombin (sec)*	<4	4–6	>6

*International normalized ratio

Note: *The Child-Pugh score is calculated by adding the scores for the five factors and can range from 5 to 15. The resulting Child-Pugh class can be A (a score of 5–6), B (7–9), or C (≥10). Decompensation indicates cirrhosis, with a Child-Pugh score of ≥7 (class B). This level has been the accepted criterion for listing a patient for liver transplantation*

456. Ans. (a) Budd Chiari syndrome

Ref: Harrison, 20th ed. pg. 2410

Budd chiari syndrome leads to occlusion of hepatic veins and leads to post hepatic cause of portal hypertension.

Pre-hepatic causes	Hepatic causes	Post hepatic causes
Portal vein thrombosis Splenic vein thrombosis Massive splenomegaly (Banti's syndrome)	**Presinusoidal** • Schistosomisis • Congenital hepatic fibrosis **Sinusoidal** • Cirrhosis–many causes • Alcoholic hepatitis **Postsinusoidal** • Hepatic sinusoidal obstruction (venoocclusive syndrome)	**Posthepatic** • Budd-Chiari syndrome • Inferior vena caval webs • Cardiac causes ▪ Restrictive cardiomyopathy ▪ Constrictive pericarditis ▪ Severe congestive heart failure

- Choice b, Banti's disease is fibro-congestive splenomegaly and is a pre-hepatic cause of portal HTN
- Choice c and d are also prehepatic causes of portal hypertension.

Extra Mile

Clinical Features of portal Hypertension

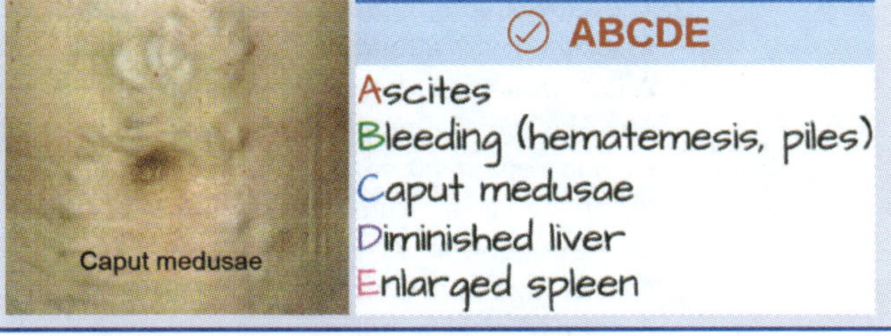

457. Ans. (b) Metabolic syndrome

Ref: Harrison, 19th ed. pg. 2452

Metabolic syndrome is the most common cause of non-alcoholic fatty liver disease.

It is a lifestyle disease characterized by centripetal obesity, increased blood pressure, impaired glucose tolerance and hypertriglyceridemia.

CAUSES OF NONALCOHOLIC FATTY LIVER

1. *Metabolic syndrome*[Q] *(MC cause)*
2. Reye syndrome
3. Pregnancy
4. Drugs
5. Kwashiorkor

458. Ans. (d) Liver copper

Investigations for Wilson disease and their relative importance

Test	Usefulness
Serum ceruloplasmin	+
KF rings	++
24-h urine Cu	+++
Liver Cu	++++

459. Ans. (a) Triglycerides

The intracellular triglyceride accumulation is expressed histologically as microvesicular steatosis.

460. Ans. (d) Hepcidin

Ref: Chapter 162, Goldman and Cecil Textbook of Medicine, 24th ed.

- Hepcidin is a 25 amino acid peptide and central regulator of iron homeostasis through its effects on iron homeostasis through its effects on intestinal absorption, macrophage recycling of iron from senescent RBC and iron metabolism from hepatic stores. Thus hepcidin affects all major sites of iron metabolism.
- Hematopoiesis occurs in marrow cords, essentially loose arrangement of cells in dilated sinus area between the arterioles that feed the bone and the venous sinus that returns blood to efferent veins. Erythropoiesis occurs in erythroid islands.

461. Ans. (b) Zinc

Ref: Harrison, 18th ed. Chapter 360

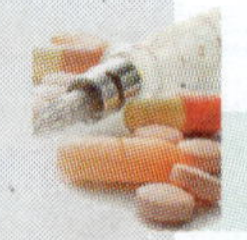

Disease status	First choice
Initial hepatic	
Hepatitis or cirrhosis without decomposition	Zinc
Hepatic decompensation	
Mild	Trientine and zinc
Moderate	Trientine and zinc
Severe	Hepatic transplantation
Initial neurologic/psychiatric	Tetrathiomolybdate and zinc
Maintenance	Zinc

462. Ans. (a) Hippocampal sclerosis

Ref: Harrison, 18th ed. Chapter 357

Organs Involved in Hemochromatosis are:

- Liver (first organ to be affected) = 95%
- Excessive skin pigmentation
- Diabetes mellitus (bronze diabetes)
- Arthropathy
- Cardiac involvement (restrictive cardiomyopathy)
- Pituitary involvement (leading to hypopituitarism and hypogonadism) = mentioned in textbook as endocrine involvement.

463. Ans. (c) Hepatitis C

Ref: Harrison, 18th ed. Chapter 306

- Chronic hepatitis follows acute hepatitis C in 50–70% of cases; chronic infection is common even in those with a return to normal in aminotransferase levels after acute hepatitis C, *adding up to an 85% likelihood of chronic HCV infection after acute hepatitis C.*

464. Ans. (d) Estrogen

Ref: Harrison, 18th ed. chapter 311

- The hyperdynamic circulatory state of portal hypertension is associated with a dilated, vascular periphery. *This is driven by an excess of systemic nitric oxide and estrogen.*
- When these telangectasias occur in the palms, it frequently manifests as a diffuse Palmar erythema.
- This is because the skin on the thenar and hypothenar prominences is thicker and the ectatic vessels are deeper within the dermis.
- Ectatic blood vessels commonly form, and are often noted atop the chest, neck and face. These are referred to as 'spider telangectasias' because they fill centrifugally (like legs of a spider) after the center is blanched.
- Palmar erythema can also be seen in pregnancy, polycythemia, thyrotoxicosis, rheumatoid arthritis, excema, psoriasis and even normal individuals

Extra Mile

Signs of Liver Cell Failure

1. The liver and spleen may be enlarged, with the liver edge being firm and nodular
2. Scleral icterus
3. Palmar erythema
4. Spider angiomas
5. Parotid gland enlargement
6. Digital clubbing
7. Muscle wasting, or the development of edema and ascites.
8. Men may have decreased body hair and gynecomastia as well as testicular atrophy, which may be a consequence of hormonal abnormalities or a direct toxic effect of alcohol on the testes.
9. In women with advanced alcoholic cirrhosis, menstrual irregularities usually occur, and some women may be amenorrheic.

465. Ans. (b) Acute cholangitis

Ref: Harrison, 18th ed. Chapter 311

Acute cholangitis	• The characteristic presentation of acute cholangitis involves biliary ***pain, jaundice, and spiking fevers with chills*** (Charcot's triad). • ERCP with endoscopic sphincterotomy is safe and the preferred initial procedure for both establishing a definitive diagnosis and providing effective therapy. • Blood cultures are frequently positive, and leukocy-tosis is typical.
Acute cholecystitis	• Attack of biliary pain that progressively worsens. Approximately 60–70% of patients report having experienced prior attacks that resolved spontaneously. • As the episode progresses, however, the pain of acute cholecystitis becomes more generalized in the right upper abdomen, which may radiate to right shoulder.
Acute viral hepatitis	This is the closest differential diagnosis and is ruled out because of the following points mentioned below. • The *prodromal symptoms like* anorexia, nausea and vomiting, fatigue, malaise, arthralgias, myalgias, headache, photophobia, pharyngitis, cough, and coryza may precede the onset of jaundice by 1–2 weeks. • The nausea, vomiting, and anorexia are frequently associated with alterations in olfaction and taste. • A *low-grade fever* between 38° and 39°C (100°–102°F) is more often present in hepatitis A and E than in hepatitis B or C, except when hepatitis B is heralded by a serum sickness–like syndrome. • Dark urine and clay-colored stools may be noticed by the patient from 1–5 days before the onset of clinical jaundice

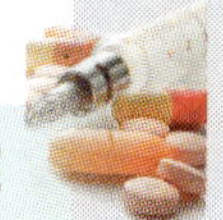

466. Ans. (d) 8 weeks

Ref: Harrison, 19th ed. pg. 2018

- It is sub-divided into "*fulminant hepatic failure*", which *requires onset of encephalopathy within 8 weeks* and Sub-fulminant which leads to encephalopathy after 8 weeks but before 26 weeks.
- Acute liver failure is a broad term that encompasses both fulminant and subfulminant.

467. Ans. (d) Hep E

Ref: Harrison, 19th ed. pg. 152e-2t, 0215

- Most common cause of fulminant hepatitis in pregnancy is HEV
- Most common cause of viral hepatitis in India overall = Hepatitis A
- Most common cause of blood transfusion associated hepatitis = HBV
- Most common viral hepatitis in India in children= HAV
- Most common viral hepatitis in India in adults= HEV
- Most common cause of FULMINANT hepatic failure= toxins> Hepatitis D.

468. Ans. (d) IgM anti- HBcAg

Ref: Harrison, 19th ed. pg. 2017-18

- In most cases, serologic markers of infection and antigenemia appear 1–3 mo after birth, suggesting that transmission occurred at the time of delivery; virus contained in amniotic fluid or in maternal feces or blood may be the source.
    - Most common mode of acquisition, is during delivery.
    - In case the body is exposed to virus, the immune system of baby will produce IgM anti HBc.
    - Anti-HBc is the most valuable single serologic marker of acute HBV infection because it is present almost as early as HBsAg and continues to be present later in the course of the disease when HBsAg has disappeared

469. Ans. (b) Cirrhotic ascites

Ref: Harrison, 19th ed. pg. 286-87

- Diuretics that block aldosterone receptors in the distal convoluted tubule are preferred because of the presence of hyperaldosteronism in patients with cirrhosis.
- Spirinolactone is useful in CHF but not in hypertrophy of heart. It is also useful in transudative pleural effusion
- ACE inhibitors and CCB are used is renal artery stenosis.

470. Ans. (c) >20 mm Hg

- Intra-abdominal hypertension is defined as a pressure over 12 mm Hg in adults. However, if the pressure continues to rise over 20 mm Hg and organs begin to fail, the syndrome has now progressed to the end stage of the highly fatal process termed abdominal compartment syndrome.
- **Causes of primary (acute) abdominal compartment syndrome include the following:**
    - Penetrating trauma
    - Intraperitoneal hemorrhage
    - Pancreatitis
    - External compressing forces (debris from a motor vehicle collision or after a explosion)
    - Pelvic fracture
    - Rupture of abdominal aortic aneurysm
    - Perforated peptic ulcer

IAP can be easily monitored by measuring bladder pressure. Measurement of intraluminal bladder pressure

471. Ans. (b) Evaluation of left atria and left Atrial appendage thrombus

Ref: Harrison, 19th ed. pg. 270e-2

- Trans-esophageal echocardiography is better than trans-thoracic echocardiography as it is better able to evaluate the left Atrial thrombus and left Atrial appendage. Therefore in patients of atrial fibrillation of long standing duration for evaluation of clots in left atrium, trans-esophageal echocardiography is done.

472. Ans. (a) Enteric fever

Ref: Harrison, 19th ed. pg. 1050-51

Clinical features of Typhoid fever begin 7–14 days after ingestion

- Fever pattern is stepwise, characterized by a rising temperature over the course of each day that drops by the subsequent morning.
- Over the course of the first week of illness, gastrointestinal manifestations of the disease develop. These include diffuse abdominal pain and tenderness and, in some cases, fierce colicky right upper quadrant pain.
- The individual then develops a dry cough, dull frontal headache, delirium, and an increasingly stuporous malaise.
- The patient develops rose spots, which are salmon-colored, blanching, truncal, Maculo-papules usually 1–4 cm wide and fewer than 5 in number; these generally resolve within 2–5 days.

RHEUMATOLOGY

473. Ans. (b) Buerger's disease

Ref: Bailey and Love, Textbook of Surgery 27th ed. pg. 967

Digital gangrene is a feature of Thromboangitis obliterans/ Buerger's disease. Option a leads to color change in tip of finger from white to blue to red. Option c involves the scrotum. Option d is idiopathic condition seen in Blacks leading to Digital gangrene. Since it is rare condition it has been ruled out in this image based spotter.

474. Ans. (c) M. Gravis

Ref: Harrison 20th ed. pg. 2977

- Weakness of eye muscles and chewing muscles with diurnal variation of symptoms points to M.Gravis.
- Option a will have coexistent IDA and koilyonychia. Option b will have heat intolerance and weight loss.
- Option d presents with Raynaud phenomenon and skin tightening.

475. Ans. (a) Prayer sign

Ref: William's Endocrinology 14th ed. pg. 1495

- The image shows limited joint mobility and flexion deformity in the little finger. This is seen in long standing diabetes mellitus and is characterized by hand stiffness resulting from flexion contractures of the fingers and thickened, tight, waxy skin.
- Option b and c are seen with entrapment neuropathy. Option d is seen with clubbing of fingers.

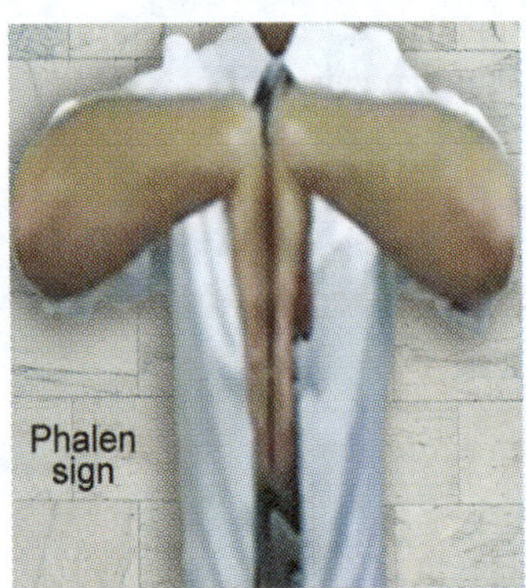

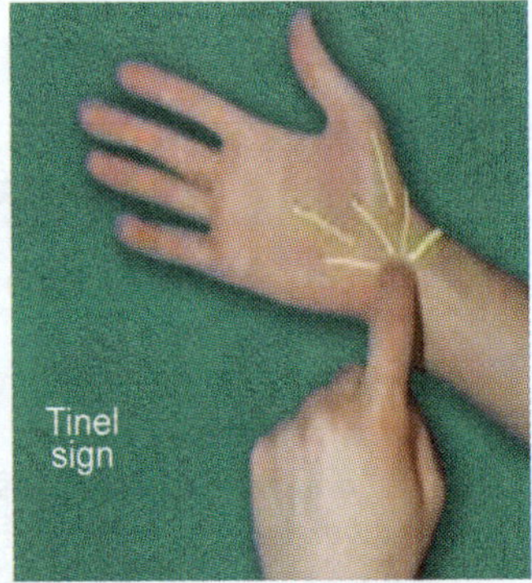

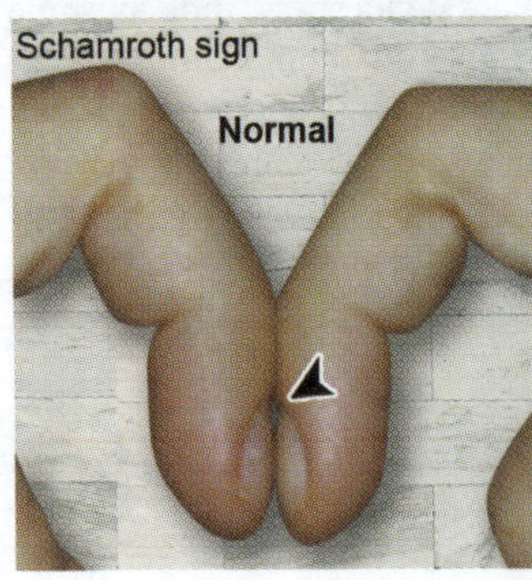

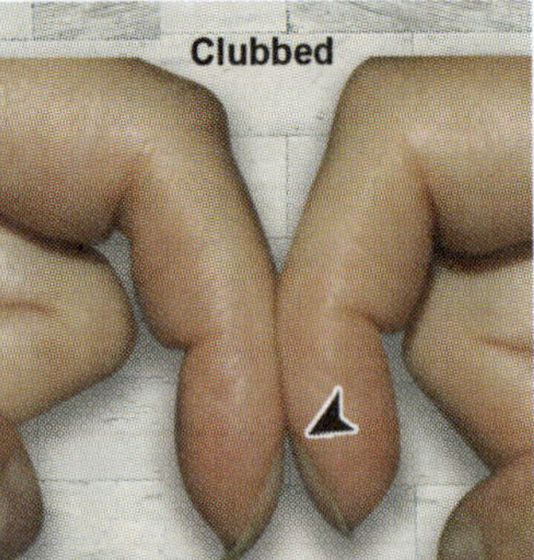

476. Ans. (a) Sjogren syndrome

Ref: Harrison 20th ed. pg. 2561

- The difficulty in swallowing dry food items like chips or biscuits points to deficient saliva production. Gritty sensation below eyes indicates deficient tear production from lacrimal glands.
- The presence of anemia of chronic disease and anti Ro antibody helps in reaching diagnosis of Sjogren syndrome.
- Option b involves small joints of hands and resultant deformities
- Option c presents with fever and rash
- Option d presents with musculoskeletal complaints with rash, anemia and renal compromise.

477. Ans. (d) Scleroderma

Ref:: Harrison 20th ed. pg. 2553

- The key word in the question is leather like skin which is seen in scleroderma. The esophageal wall fibrosis explains the progressive dysphagia.
- The fibrosis of blood vessels will increase peripheral resistance and cause systemic hypertension.
- Fibrosis of pulmonary artery will cause PAH which causes limitation of exercise capacity. This is worsened further when lung fibrosis ensues
- Option a presents with hamartomatous polyps and mucosal melanosis
- Option b presents with dysphagia with iron deficiency anemia and koilonychia. It is the alternate name for Plummer Vinson syndrome
- Option c presents with mega-esophagus, mega-colon and mega-heart.

478. Ans. (d) Osteoarthritis

Ref: Harrison 20th ed. pg. 2628

- Joint pain from OA is primarily activated related and occurs in weight bearing joints. As disease progresses pain becomes continuous and buckling of knee may occur.
- The mechanical stress and biochemical changes in cartilage can cause the joint to crackle and crunch. The crepitus produced will alarm the patient and he/she will seek your medical advice.
- In case of reduced joint space, deformity at knee joint and physical incapacitation of patient, total knee replacement is suggested.
- Option a involves small joints of hand in young female. Option b involves sacroiliac joint in young male. Option c is seen after unprotected sexual exposure and leads to uveitis, conjunctivitis, arthritis, urethritis and keratoderma blennorrhagicum.

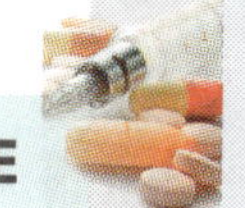

479. Ans. (d) Scleroderma

Ref: Harrison 20th ed. pg. 2552

Notice the contractures in fingers with skin tightening which is a feature of scleroderma.

Rheumatoid arthritis	Psoriatic arthritis	Scleroderma
RA will have extensive deformities and extensor rheumatoid nodules.	Notice the DIP involvement with nail changes. Rash here points to lesion of psoriasis.	Skin induration/tightening is the keyword for cracking this question.

480. Ans. (d) Serum electrophoresis

Ref: Harrison 20th ed. pg. 797

- Low back pain in old man with lytic punched out lesions in X-ray skull indicates first differential diagnosis as multiple myeloma. Since the condition causes production of excess amount of positively charged proteins, the serum osmolality tends to rise. The screening test for diagnosis of this hyper-viscosity syndrome is serum electrophoresis. The technique will determine increased protein as light chain of IgG.
- Option a is increased in prostate cancer.
- Option b is not required as there is no CNS Lesion and lytic lesions in skull have already been picked up by X-ray skull.
- Option c is not required as hematological malignancy is diagnosed with bone marrow biopsy.

481. Ans. (b) Pleuritis

Ref: Harrison, 20th ed. pg. 2520

The most common lung manifestation of SLE is pleuritis with or without pleural effusion. It may respond to NSAIDS or may require steroids. Life threatening manifestations include interstitial inflammation and shrinking lung syndrome.

482. Ans. (a) SLE

Ref: Harrison, 20th ed. pg. 2518

- ANA> reference value is the first immunological manifestation mentioned in SLICC criteria for diagnosis of SLE. It is not a criterion for diagnosis of the remaining rheumatological diseases mentioned in choices b, c and d.
- This test is positive in 95% cases at the onset of disease and the remaining patients turn positive within one year of disease onset.
- ANA testing using immuno-fluorescent antibodies is more reliable than ELISA.

483. Ans. (b) Non-tender, located on extensor surface and seen with arthritis

Ref: Harrison, 20th ed. pg. 2528-2529

Rheumatic nodules are the most common extra-articular feature of rheumatoid arthritis and consists of non-tender nodules on extensor surface of joints.

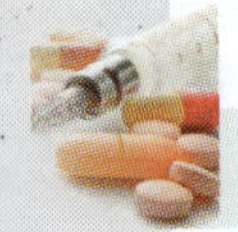

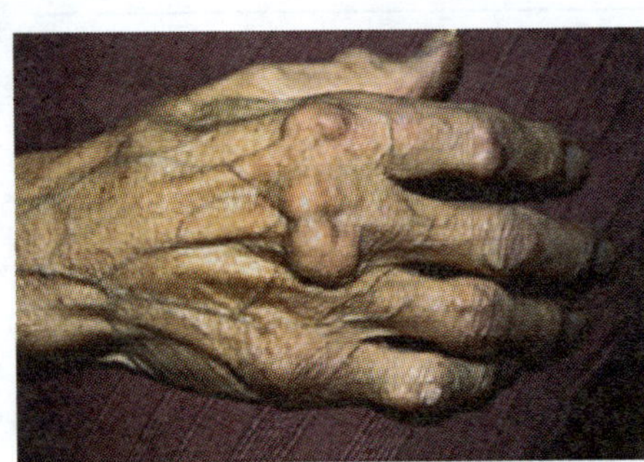

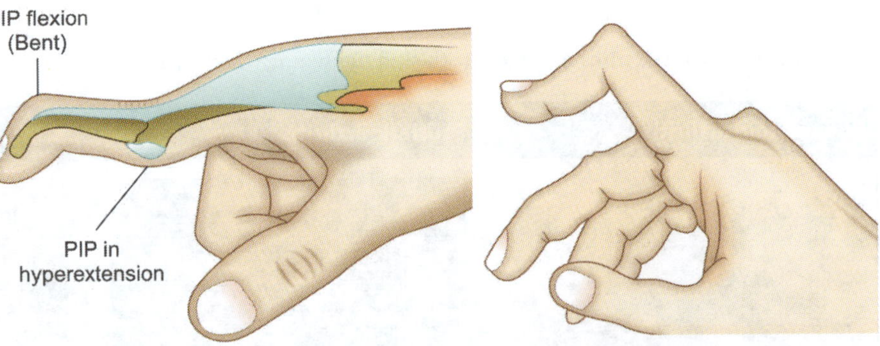

484. Ans. (b) Uric acid in synovial fluid

Ref: Harrison 19th ed. pg. 2223

- Since 50% of patients with acute gouty attack have normal serum uric acid levels, the best test to confirm the diagnosis is joint aspiration uric acid crystals.
- Under microscope, needle shaped MSU crystals are seen both intracellularly and extracellularly.
- With compensated polarized light, crystals are brightly birefringent with negative elongation.
- The clinical presentation is dramatic with overnight development of red inflamed 1st MTP joint.
- Anti CCP antibodies are used for diagnosis of rheumatoid arthritis.

485. Ans. (a) Takayasu's arteritis

Diagnosis of Takayasu's arteritis should be suspected strongly in a patient who develops:

1. A decrease or absence of peripheral pulses, this disease is hence called pulseless disease
2. Unequal blood pressure between left and right arm

Extra Mile

Clinical Manifestations of Takayasu's Arteritis

Artery	Percent of arteriographic abnormalities	Potential clinical manifestations
Subclavian	93	Arm claudication, Raynaud's phenomenon
Common carotid	58	Visual changes, syncope, transient ischemic attacks, stroke
Abdominal aorta	47	Abdominal pain, nausea, vomiting
Renal	38	Hypertension, renal failure

3. Arterial bruits.
   - It is an inflammatory and stenotic disease of medium- and large-sized arteries characterized by a strong predilection for the aortic arch and its branches. For this reason, it is often referred to as the *aortic arch syndrome*
   - *Most common vessel involved is left subclavian artery followed by common carotid artery.*
   - The diagnosis is confirmed by arteriography

486. Ans. (a) ASO

- Evidence of an antecedent Group A Streptococcal infection is usually based on elevated or increasing serum antistreptococcal antibody titers.
- *As most cases do not have a positive throat swab culture or rapid antigen test, serologic evidence is usually needed.*
- *The most common serologic tests are the antistreptolysin O (ASO) and anti-DNase B (ADB) titers*
- If only a single antibody is measured (usually antistreptolysin O), only 80–85% of patients with acute rheumatic fever have an elevated titer.

487. Ans. (c) Exudative pleural effusion

Lung Disease in Rheumatoid Arthritis

- Most common pulmonary manifestation is pleural involvement leading to pleural friction rub and effusion. This is due to inflammatory breakdown of pulmonary nodules.
- *Pleural effusions tend to be exudative with increased numbers of monocytes and neutrophils.*
- Interstitial lung disease. Pulmonary function testing shows a restrictive pattern (e.g. reduced total lung capacity) with a reduced diffusing capacity for carbon monoxide (DLCO).
- Caplan's syndrome is characterized by the development of nodules and pneumoconiosis following silica exposure.

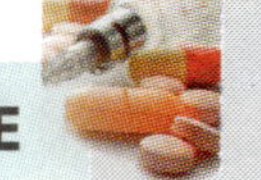

488. Ans. (a) Behçet's disease

Ref: Harrison, 19th ed. pg. 2194

- Although Behçet's disease is classified among the vasculitides laboratory diagnostic does not include regularly autoantibodies associated with vascular manifestations of systemic autoimmune diseases.
- The autoantigens for pemphigus vulgaris and pemphigus foliaceus are desmoglein 3 and desmoglein 1, respectively.
- *The anti-desmoglein 1 antibodies in pemphigus foliaceus and anti-desmoglein 3 antibodies in pemphigus vulgaris are pathogenic.*
- *Anti-tissue transglutaminase antibodies are pathognomonic for celiac disease.*
- Anti- nuclear antibody is seen in SLE
- Causes of Apthous Ulcers:

Infections:
- Viral (Herpes, CMV, EBV, HIV)
- Fungal (Candida)
- Bacterial (Vincent's infection, syphilis)

Dermatological:
- Pemphigus, pemphigoid, lichen planus

Drug:
- Chemotherapy drugs
- Erythema multiforme, Stevens-Johnson syndrome

Systemic diseases:
- Behcet's syndrome, SLE

Nutritional:
- Vitamin deficiency (Vitamin B and C), iron deficiency

Neoplasia:
- Leukemia, squamous cell carcinoma, Kaposi's sarcoma

Gastrointestinal:
- Crohn's disease, celiac disease

Traumatic
- Dentures

Chemical or thermal burns:
- Corrosives, hot liquids

489. Ans. (a) IgA

Ref: Harrison, 18th ed. Chapter 326

- The Presumptive pathogenic mechanism for Henoch-Schönlein purpura is immune-complex deposition.
- IgA is the antibody class most often seen in the immune complexes and has been demonstrated in the renal biopsies of these patients.
- A number of inciting antigens have been suggested including upper respiratory tract infections, various drugs, foods, insect bites, and immunizations.

490. Ans. (a) SLE

Ref: Harrison, 18th ed. chapter 319

- An LE cell is a neutrophil or macrophage that has phagocytized (engulfed) the denatured nuclear material of another cell
- LE cell testing was once performed to diagnose systemic lupus erythematous (SLE) but has been replaced for this purpose by antinuclear antibody testing.
- The LE cell reaction is positive in 50%–75% of individuals with acute disseminated lupus.
- Positive reactions are also seen in rheumatoid arthritis, chronic hepatitis (lupoid), scleroderma, dermatomyositis, polyarteritis nodosa, acquired hemolytic anemia, and Hodgkin disease.

491. Ans. (b) c-ANCA

Ref: Harrison, 18th ed. Chapter 326:

- c-ANCA = Wegener granulomatosis/Granulomatosis with angitis
- p-ANCA
  - Microscopic polyangitis
  - Primary sclerosing cholangitis
  - Churg strauss syndrome

The terminology of *cytoplasmic ANCA* (cANCA) refers to the diffuse, granular cytoplasmic staining pattern observed by immunofluorescence microscopy when serum antibodies bind to indicator neutrophils. Proteinase-3, a 29-kDa neutral serine proteinase present in neutrophil azurophilic granules, is the major cANCA antigen.

492. Ans. (b) Anti-GBM antibody

Ref: Harrison, 18th ed. Chapter 283

- Patients who develop autoantibodies directed against glomerular basement antigens frequently develop a glomerulonephritis termed *antiglomerular basement membrane (anti-GBM) disease.* When they present with lung hemorrhage and glomerulonephritis, they have a pulmonary-renal syndrome called *Goodpasture's syndrome.*

Extra Mile

- Good's syndrome is a Thymoma with immunodeficiency
- It is a cause of combined B and T cell immunodeficiency in adults.
- The clinical characteristics of Good's syndrome are increased susceptibility to bacterial infections with encapsulated organisms and opportunistic viral and fungal infections.
- The most consistent immunological abnormalities are hypogammaglobulinaemia and reduced or absent B cells.

493. Ans. (b) Sarcoidosis

Ref: Harrison, 19th ed. pg. 237, 417

Painful ulcers in mouth

- Apthous ulcers
- Denture stomatitis
- Tuberculosis
- Carcinoma tongue
- Behcet disease
- Thermal burns
- Herpes
- Arsenic poisoning

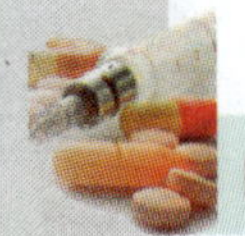

494. Ans. (d) Female is symptomatic

Ref: Harrison, 19th ed. pg. 462e-5

- Duchenne's muscular dystrophy is an X-linked recessive condition where boys suffer from disease while girls are carriers. **The protein defective is dystrophin** due to defect of dystrophin gene on chromosome Xp.21.
- Boys present between 3-5 years of age with clumsy gait and history of recurrent falls. The gait is peculiar and is known as **waddling gait**. Most children become wheel chair bound by 12–15 years of age. **Gower sign** is a characteristic feature characterized by child getting up gradually.
- On physical examination pseudo-hypertrophy (called so because of the physical appearance) but actually has fat deposition around the muscles. The weakness of respiratory muscles results in **recurrent pneumonia that ultimately results in mortality.**

Investigations

1. CPK MM
2. EMG and nerve conduction velocity
3. Muscle biopsy and western blot analysis of tissue specimen

495. Ans. (a) Duchenne muscular dystrophy

Please refer to above question

496. Ans. (a) D.I.P

Ref: Harrison, 19th ed. pg. 2142

- Rheumatoid arthritis characteristically causes swelling of small joints in the hand like the P.I.P, M.C.P and the wrist joint bilaterally.
- Isolated D.I.P joint involvement is seen in psoriatic arthropathy.
- D.I.P joint involvement is also seen with osteo-arthritis but the involvement is with pain at the base of thumb. Knee joint is the commonest joint involved in these patients.

497. Ans. (a) Both lung and kidney are involved

Ref: Harrison, 19th ed. pg. 2183-84

According to the American College of Rheumatology accepted classification criteria for Wegener's, two or more positive criteria have a sensitivity of 88.2% and a specificity of 92.0% of describing Wegener's.

- **Nasal or oral inflammation:**
  - Painful or painless oral ulcers or
  - Purulent or bloody nasal discharge
- **Lungs:** Abnormal chest X-ray with:
  - Nodules,
  - Infiltrates or
  - Cavities
- **Kidneys:** Urinary sediment with:
  - Microhematuria or
  - Red cell casts
- ***Biopsy:*** *Granulomatous inflammation*
  - Within the arterial wall or
  - In the perivascular area

498. Ans. (d) Sero-negative arthritis

Ref: Harrison, 19th ed. pg. 2136

- Patients of rheumatoid arthritis harbor an antibody by the name of anti – C.C.P (cycliccitrulline phosholipid antibodies).
- The rheumatoid nodules in these patients can compress on various peripheral nerves leading to mono-neuritis multiplex. The joints are damaged with peri-articular erosions and osteoporosis.
- ***The characterstic joint involvement is P.I.P, M.C.P and the wrist joint bilaterally.***

Seronegative arthritis is a broad term and included within he group are the entities psoriatic arthritis, Reiter's syndrome, enteropathic arthritis, reactive arthritis, ankylosing spondylitis, undifferentiated seronegative arthritis, Whipple's disease, arthritis associated with pustular acne, post-intestinal bypass arthritis, and several forms of HIV associated arthritis.

499. Ans. (a) Hypercalcemia

Ref: Harrison, 19th ed. pg. 313, 2208

- Hypercalcemia is seen with sarcoidosis as the granulomas present in this disease synthesize vitamin D_3. This increases the amount of absorption of calcium from the intestine and leads to hypercalcemia.

500. Ans. (b) Mitral regurgitation

- In rheumatic heart disease, the damage to chordae tendinae by inflammatory aschoff nodules results in development of mitral regurgitation in pediatric presentation.
- The most common valve involvement >18 years of age is mitral stenosis
- Remember that pulmonic valve is not involved in rheumatic etiology

501. Ans. (d) ASO titer

Ref: Harrison, 19th ed. pg. 2151

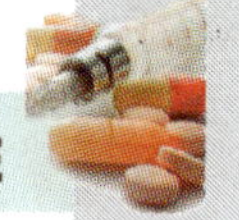

Modified Jones Criteria

Low-risk populations	Moderate-and high-risk populations
• Carditis ▪ Clinical and/or subclinical carditis	• Carditis ▪ Clinical and/or subclinical carditis
• Arthritis ▪ Polyarthritis only	• Arthritis ▪ Monoarthritis or polyarthritis ▪ Polyarthralgia
• Chorea	Chorea
• Erythema marginatum	Erythema marginatum
• Subcutaneous nodules	Subcutaneous nodules

Minor Criteria

Low-risk populations	Moderate and high-risk populations
• Polyarthralgia	Monoarthralgia
• Fever (≥38.5°)	Fever (>38°C)
• ESR >60 mm in 1st hour	ESR ≥30 mm/hr and/or CRP ≥3.0
• Prolonged PR interval, after accounting for age variability (unless carditis is a major criterion) in all population.	

Supporting evidence of a preceding streptococcal infection within the last 45 days	• Elevated or rising antistreptolysin O or other streptococcal antibody, or • A positive throat culture, or • Rapid antigen test for group A streptococcus, or • Recent scarlet fever

502. Ans. (c) Deforming arthritis

Ref: Harrison, 19th ed. pg. 2151

Please refer to above question

The arthritis in rheumatic arthritis is migratory polyarthritis involving the large joints and is NON erosive arthritis.

503. Ans. (b) History of sore throats

Ref: Harrison, 19th ed. pg. 2151

Refer above

- History of sore throats is not a component of Jones criteria.

504. Ans. (d) Ankylosing spondylitis

Ref: Harrison 19th ed. pg. 377e-5

- **SSA autoantibodies** (also called **anti-Ro**, or the combination **anti-SSA/Ro** or **anti Ro/SSA autoantibodies**) are anti-nuclear auto-antibodies that are associated with many autoimmune diseases, such as systemic lupus erythematosus, neonatal lupus and primary biliary cirrhosis. Also, they are often present in Sjögren's syndrome and sarcoidosis as well.
- Presence of Anti-SSA/Ro in pregnant women with SLE is associated with an increased risk of neonatal lupus Erythematosus in the child.

505. Ans. (d) Mixed connective tissue disorder

Ref: Harrison, 19th ed. pg. 2165

- Anti-Rho or SS-A antibodies are seen in SLE, Sjogren syndrome and can be transmitted across the placenta resulting in neonatal lupus which presents as complete heart block.
- *Mixed connective tissue disorder is associated with U1 R.N.P. (Ribo-Nucleo-protein antibody).*

506. Ans. (b) IgA, C 3

Ref: Harrison, 19th ed. pg. 2190

- Henoch Schonlein purpura is a small-vessel vasculitis in which complexes of immunoglobulin A (IgA) and C3 are deposited on arterioles, capillaries, and venules.
- As with IgA nephropathy, serum levels of IgA are high in HSP.
- IgA nephropathy has a predilection for young adults while HSP is more predominant among children. Further, IgA nephropathy typically only affects the kidneys while HSP is a systemic disease.
- HSP involves the skin and connective tissues, scrotum, joints, gastrointestinal tract and kidneys.
- **Investigation:** IgA levels high, platelet count normal and skin biopsy (IOC).
- **Treatment:** Steroids

507. Ans. (d) Microscopic polyangitis

Ref: Harrison, 19th ed. pg. 2186

- MPA is characterized by pauci-immune, necrotizing, small vessel vasculitis without clinical or pathological evidence of granulomatous inflammation
- The family of vasculitic granulomatoses comprise
  1. Wegener's granulomatosis[Q]
  2. Churg-Strauss syndrome[Q]
  3. Polyarteritis nodosa[Q]
  4. Bronchocentric granulomatosis
  5. Giant cell arteritis[Q]
  6. Systemic lupus erythematosus.

508. Ans. (a) Gout

Ref: Harrison, 19th ed. pg. 2233–34

- In approximately 40% of cases, *the gouty erosions have a raised margin or lip that radiologically is referred to as Martel's hook or Martel's Sign.* No loss of bone density is expected.

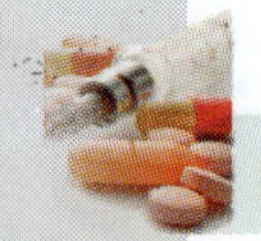

- The osteological signs of gout can be located on the joint surfaces, around the joint itself, or even at a distance from the joint.
- Lesions from gout have a diagnostic appearance on radiographs that radiologists refer to as a "punched out" appearance, and which can be seen as crescent-shaped erosions, with smooth, well remodelled margins, on dry bone
- Lesions vary in size, are usually rounded or oval, and may have a sclerotic border.

509. Ans. (a) SLE

Ref: Harrison, 19th ed. pg. 2126-27

The diagnosis is based on joint pain in fever with rash and photosensitivity. Rheumatoid arthritis involves the small joints symmetrically and does not have presence of Rash.

The diagnostic criteria for SLE are as follows:

- Rash Fixed erythema, over the Malar Eminences
- Erythematous circular raised patches with adherent keratotic scaling and follicular plugging; atrophic scarring may occur
- Photosensitivity Exposure to UV light causes rash
- Oral ulcers Includes oral and nasopharyngeal ulcers
- Synovitis/Non-erosive arthritis of two or more peripheral joints
- Serositis: Pleuritis or pericarditis documented by ECG or rub or evidence of effusion
- Renal disorder Proteinuria >0.5 g/day or 3+, or cellular casts
- Neurologic disorder Seizures or psychosis without other causes
- Hematologic disorder Hemolytic anemia or leukopenia
- Immunological criteria like positive CRP, low C3, ELISA cardiolipin antibody
- ANA positivity

510. Ans. (d) Secondary amyloidosis

Ref: Harrison, 19th ed. pg. 719, 723, 2458

- Reactive amyloid A (AA) amyloidosis, one of the most severe complications of RA, is a serious, potentially life-threatening disorder caused by deposition of AA amyloid fibrils in multiple organs. These AA amyloid fibrils derive from the circulatory acute-phase reactant serum amyloid A protein (SAA), and may be controlled by treatment
- The introduction of biological therapies targeting specific inflammatory mediators revolutionised the treatment of rheumatoid arthritis (RA). Targeting key components of the immune system allows efficient suppression of the pathological inflammatory cascade that leads to RA symptoms and subsequent joint destruction.
- Milk alkali syndrome occurs due to abuse of calcium containing anta-acids leading to hypercalcemia

511. Ans. (b) HLA DR 4

Ref: Harrison, 19th ed. pg. 372e-1

HLA allele	Diseases with increased risk
HLA-B27[Q]	Ankylosing spondylitis Post-gonococcal arthritis Acute anterior uveitis
HLA-B47	21-hydroxylase deficiency
HLA-DR2[Q]	Systemic lupus erythematosus
HLA-DR3	Autoimmune hepatitis Primary Sjogren syndrome Diabetes mellitus type 1 Systemic lupus erythematosus
HLA-DR4[Q]	Rheumatoid arthritis Diabetes mellitus type 1
HLA-DR3 and – DR4[Q] combined	Diabetes mellitus type 1
HLA-DQ2 and HLA-DQB	Celiac disease

512. Ans. (b) Rheumatoid arthritis

Ref: Harrison, 19th ed. pg. 2144-45

- *Minocycline, gold salts, enicillamine, azathioprine, and cyclosporine have all been used for the treatment of RA with varying degrees of success; however, they are used sparingly now due to their inconsistent clinical efficacy or unfavorable toxicity profile.*

Drugs used in Rheumatoid arthritis

1. Hydroxychloroquine–preferred in pregnancy
2. Lefluonomide
3. Methotrexate–preferred drug
4. Abatacept
5. Anakinra
6. Rituximab

RESPIRATORY SYSTEM

513. Ans. (a) Squamous cell cancer

Ref: Harrison 21st ed. pg. 595

Lung cancer seen in smoker is usually Small cell carcinoma or squamous cell carcinoma. Option b and c mean the same and are seen in nonsmokers. Option d is also seen in non-smoker and presents with paraneoplastic manifestation of gynecomastia.

514. Ans. (b) Respiratory acidosis

Ref: Harrison 21st ed. pg. 367

Since pH is low, acidosis is present. Elevated carbon dioxide levels indicate respiratory etiology. Bicarbonate is on higher side of normal and indicates compensation process has started.

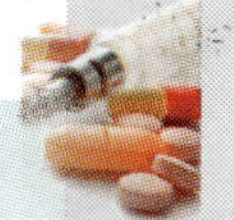

515. Ans. (b) Bronchiectasis

Ref: Harrison 21st ed. pg. 2174

- The clinical history of purulent(yellow) bronchorrhea with postural variation indicates a reservoir of pus in large airways. This is seen in Bronchiectasis which is characterized by destruction and dilatation of large airways.
- Option a can have airway destruction and infection but has associated features like hemoptysis and cachexia.
- Option c does not have postural variation of bronchorrhea.
- Option d is seen after DVT.

516. Ans. (c) NIV

Ref: Harrison 20th ed. pg. 2188

- Prolongation of expiration and sudden onset breathlessness point to etiology as COPD/ Asthma. pH is low implying acidosis. CO_2 is high implying respiratory cause. Bicarbonate is elevated owing to compensation by kidney.
- NIV/Non-invasive ventilation using tight fitting face mask is best intervention for acute exacerbation of COPD.
- Option a is used for metabolic acidosis. Option b is used for metabolic alkalosis. Option d is used in cases of hypovolemic shock.

517. Ans. (b) Bronchogenic carcinoma

Ref: Harrison 20th ed. pg. 599

- Chest X-ray shows right upper lobe collapse with mediastinal widening. The clinical findings of hemoptysis and weight loss point to lung cancer as first differential diagnosis.
- Option a, TB will cause cavitation. Lung collapse can also occur in TB but mediastinal widening is less likely.
- Option c causes pleural plaque calcification
- Option d causes lung cavitation or central bronchiectasis.

518. Ans. (c) Pulmonary fibrosis

Ref: Harrison 20th ed. pg. 2192

- Chronic bronchitis presents with rhonchi and does not have clubbing. Also FEV1/FVC ratio is <0.7. So, Option a is ruled out.
- Normal timed vital capacity is equal or greater than 0.8.
- Bronchiectasis presents with purulent bronchorrhea and shortness of breath. Clubbing is seen but FEV1/FVC ratio should be reduced. Hence, Option b is ruled out
- Pulmonary fibrosis presents with shortness of breath with bi-basiliar crepitations. FEV1 is less but time vital capacity (FEV1/FVC) is normal or increased.
- Option d presents with finding of mass effect with cachexia, hemoptysis, malignant pleural effusion and/or Horner syndrome

519. Ans. (a) Ground glass opacities along the periphery

Ref: Harrison 20th ed. pg. 2977

COVID-19 causes GGO in lung periphery. Option b is seen with asbestosis. Option c can occur with TB or any bacterial pneumonia. Option d is seen with Interstitial lung disease.

520. Ans. (c) Tiotropium

Ref: Harrison 20th ed. pg. 2187

COPD patients are started initially on LABA. If improvement does not occur then LAMA is added. Hence, answer is Option c.

521. Ans. (b) Oropharyngeal Airway

Ref: Harrison 20th ed.

- Central cyanosis in a baby when quiet and resolves on crying is characteristic of bilateral choanal atresia.
- Since babies are obligatory nose-breathers' cyanosis would be present when child is quiet.
- The immediate management would be to put in an oro-phyrangeal airway that makes the baby resort to mouth breathing till trans-nasal airway repair is done.

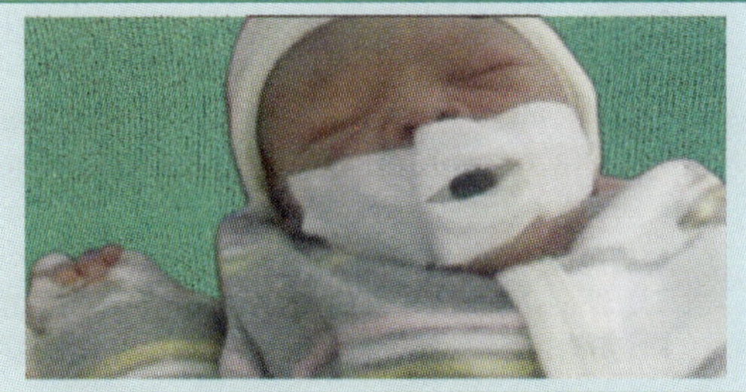

522. Ans. (a) Venous thrombo-embolism

Ref: Harrison 20th ed. pg. 2097

- Prolonged immobilization after fracture femur predisposes to Deep vein thrombosis. The clots from soleal veins can travel retrogradely and lead to pulmonary thromboembolism.
- Option b presents after trauma to jugular vein or post op Neuro-surgery.
- Option c occurs with cardiac lesions like infective endocarditis where vegetations can embolize to systemic circulation.
- Option d occurs trauma to long bones but needs GURD Criteria for diagnosis. There is no mention of CNS features like coma, axillary rash, petechiae, icterus etc in the case.

523. Ans. (a) CTPA

Ref: Harrison 20th ed. pg. 2097

The best way to demonstrate presence of clot in pulmonary artery is CT pulmonary angiography.

524. Ans. (b) Hydatid cyst

Ref: Harrison 20th ed. pg. 1644

- CXR shows a circumscribed shadow in right lower lung field. Bronchoscopy shows a large white mass encroaching into the bronchus. This is a feature of Hydatid cyst.
- Humans are accidental intermediate hosts of Echinococcus granulosus and cysts are found in liver followed by lungs.
- Option a is ruled out as it involves the apex of lungs.
- Option c will cause an ill-defined mass producing a mass effect. Most of lung cancers are not seen on Chest X-ray.
- Option d requires serological testing to detect precipitins against the aspergillus.

525. Ans. (b) CHF

Ref: Harrison 20th ed. pg. 2006

- In pleural effusion, light's criteria are used to identify transudate vs exudate
- Pleural fluid Protein/Serum protein = 2.4/ 6 = 0.4 (for exudate should be > 0.5)
- Pleural fluid LDH/Serum LDH = 50/200 = 0.4 (for exudate should be > 0.6)
- Since both the values are lesser than the cut off for exudate, the patient is having transudative etiology.
- Option a, c and d have exudative etiology and hence are ruled out.

526. Ans. (a) Wait and watch and give supplemental oxygen if required

Ref: Harrison 20th ed. pg. 2009

- The CXR shows presence of small pneumothorax. Since the patient is not having any respiratory distress wait and watch policy is to be followed and high flow oxygen supplementation is required if sp02 falls.
- Option b is done only if hemodynamic compromise occurs in tension pneumothorax. Option c is done as definitive treatment for tension pneumothorax/ Empyema.
- Option d is done for flail chest leading to type 2 respiratory failure.

Rx:
Cyanosis (+) ⇒ IC drainage Tube 5ICS MAL + (−) suction bag
Cyanosis (−) ⇒ Needle aspiration
<25% lung collapse : supplement O_2
25-50% " : needle aspiration
50% " or central cyanosis

527. Ans. (b) Right middle lobe pneumonia

Ref: Harrison 20th ed. pg. 911

There is no blunting of CP angle that rules out both options c and d. The opacity shows right middle zone pneumonia.

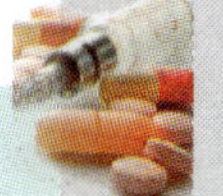

528. Ans. (a) COPD

Ref: Harrison 20th ed. pg. 1947

Notice the concavity in the expiration part of flow volume curve. This indicates obstructive pattern which is suggestive of diagnosis of COPD.

Asthma/ COPD

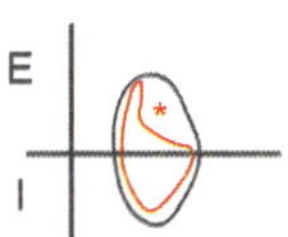

Restrictive lung disease

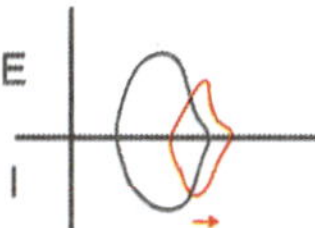

Left shift of curve

Retrosternal goiter

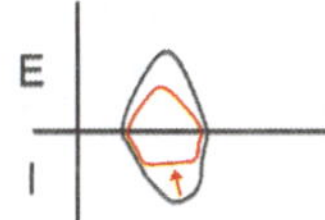

Tracheal stenosis

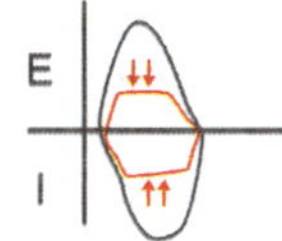

529. Ans. (b) Respiratory alkalosis

Ref: pg. 315: Harrison 20th ed.

- The respiratory rate is increased in prolonged labor due to maternal exhaustion. This leads to carbon dioxide washout and less production of protons. The patient will develop respiratory alkalosis.
- Respiratory acidosis occurs when there is respiratory muscle paralysis due to magnesium toxicity.
- Metabolic acidosis occurs when patient goes into shock due to PPH
- Metabolic alkalosis occurs due to hyperemesis gravidarum or as a blood transfusion complication.

530. Ans. (c) Elective intubation and PPV

Ref: Bailey and Love 27th ed. pg. 368

- The image shows a flail chest sustained by the patient post MVA and is best managed with elective ventilation and positive pressure ventilation to overcome respiratory acidosis caused by hypoventilation.
- Option a is done to remove a lung tumor. The chest is opened up to take access.
- Option b is when Chest tube is inserted in pleural space to evacuate pus/blood or air. The term is used while managing empyema, hemothorax or pneumothorax.

531. Ans. (b) Tuberculosis

Ref: Harrison 20th ed. pg. 1246

- Since the patient is working in the glass industry, he is predisposed to development of silicosis. Patients with silicosis have tendency to develop pulmonary tuberculosis.
- Option a is seen in explorers or trekkers who happen to enter caves with bat infestation.
- Option c and d are ruled out as they are seen in patients with asbestosis.

532. Ans. (a) Distal bronchiectasis

Ref: Harrison 20th ed. pg. 1535

Allergic bronchopulmonary aspergilloma is related to development of *Central bronchiectasis.*

It is seen in asthmatics and is associated with increase of IgE.

Predisposing conditions
- Bronchial asthma, cystic fibrosis

Obligatory criteria
- Elevated serum total IgE levels (>1000 IU/ml)
- Elevated serum IgG and/or IgE against *A. fumigatus*

Other criteria (at least three of five)
- Immediate type I reaction to *A. fumigatus* antigen
- Presence of serum *A. fumigatus* precipitins
- Transient and/or permanent chest radiographic opacities
- Eosinophil count >1000 cells/*ml* in peripheral blood
- Central bronchiectasis on HRCT chest

533. Ans. (a) Pneumothorax

Ref: Harrison, 20th ed. pg. 853

Leading cause of respiratory distress post subclavian central line access is puncture of lung leading to traumatic pneumothorax.

COMPLICATIONS OF CENTRAL VENOUS CATHETERIZATION

Immediate

- Bleeding
- Arterial puncture
- Arrhythmia
- Air embolism
- Thoracic duct injury (with left SC or left IJ approach)
- Catheter malposition
- Pneumothorax or hemothorax

Delayed

- Infection
- Venous thrombosis, pulmonary emboli
- Catheter migration
- Myocardial perforation
- Nerve injury

534. Ans. (a) Pleural fluid protein to serum protein ratio <0.5

Ref: Harrison 19th ed. pg. 1716

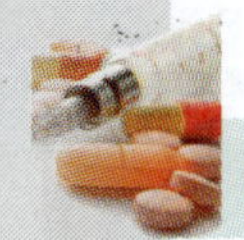

To differentiate between exudative and transudative pleural effusion, the following criteria known as *Light's criteria* is used:

1. Pleural fluid protein/serum protein >0.5
2. Pleural fluid LDH/Serum LDH >0.6
3. Pleural fluid LDH more than 2/3rd the upper normal limit for serum

Exudative pleural effusion meets at least one of the given criteria while transudative meets none.

535. Ans. (a) Chronic bronchitis

Ref: Harrison 19th ed. 1701

- Chronic obstructive airway disease leads to development of damage to ciliated columnar epithelium. The resultant stasis promotes low grade infection leading to bronchorrhea. This manifestation is called chronic bronchitis.
- Follicular bronchiolitis is due to hyperplasia of bronchial associated lymphoid tissue (BALT) seen due to collagen vascular disease and immune deficiency states. It mainly involves the lower lobes of lung.
- Desquamative pneumonitis is interstitial lung disease in smokers. It leads to development of pulmonary fibrosis.
- Chemical pneumonitis is due to aspiration of stomach acid and is also known as Mendelson syndrome.

536. Ans. (c) Albumin

- Pleural effusion in TB could be a presentation of primary TB due to sub-pleural location of Gohn's focus or can present as extra-pulmonary TB.
- Gene XPERT is a nucleic acid amplification based test which in a matter of few hours can tell if MTB is present and can also determine resistance.
- The values of LDH are taken in Light's criteria for pleural effusion to determine exudative nature of the fluid
- Adenosine deaminase has 90% sensitivity and 92 % specificity for determining the tubercular nature of fluid.
- The question is based on common sense that albumin values in serum and ascitic fluid are evaluated in patients of ascites.

537. Ans. (a) A.T.T

The CXR shows a miliary picture and ATT must be initiated. Since the child is malnourished and is having Miliary TB, his cell mediated immunity is already reduced. Hence steroids would be contraindicated in this case. The antibiotics would be useful in bacterial pneumonia which is ruled out due to radiological picture.

538. Ans. (d) Lung

Ref: Wintrobe's Clinical Hematology, 13th ed. pg. 1583

- It is seen with hyperleucocytosis with WBC count > 10^5/cu. mm. *Leukostasis affects pulmonary and brain circulation*. The presence of dysnea, tachypnea, lethargy and slurred speech is characteristic.
- WBC counts are in excess of 100,000/cu.mm and lead to leukostatic plugging of the capillaries followed by endothelial damage to blood vessels.
- The mortality occurs due to respiratory failure, intracranial hemorrhage and coma.
- The low PO_2 is due to increased consumption of oxygen by leucocytes.
- It is common with acute leukemia subtypes like acute promyelocytic leukemia, acute monocytic leukemia and T cell type of ALL.
- Treatment is leukapheresis

539. Ans. (c) 5th midaxillary space

- The 5th intercostal space in the mid-axillary line is generally used for most situations. This area is commonly known as the "safe triangle", bordered by the anterior border of latissimus dorsi, the lateral border of the pectoralis major, a line superior to the horizontal level of the nipple and an apex below the axilla.

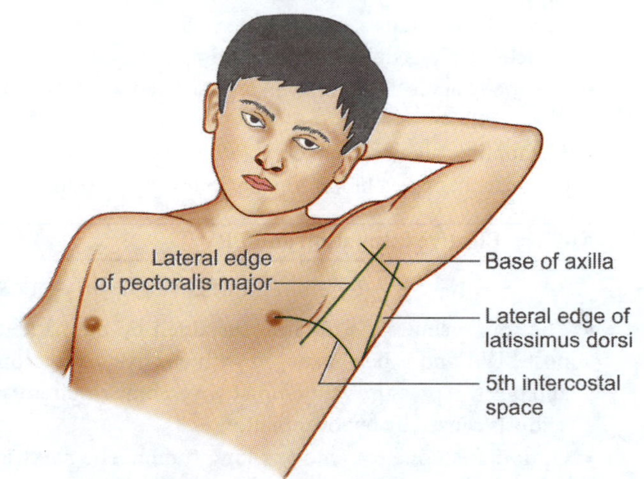

540. Ans. (c) ARDS

Shock Lung/ ARDS is a clinical syndrome caused by diffuse alveolar capillary and epithelial damage. There is usually rapid onset of life-threatening respiratory insufficiency, cyanosis, and severe arterial hypoxemia that is refractory to oxygen therapy and that may progress to multisystem organ failure. The histologic manifestation of ARDS in the lungs is known as *diffuse alveolar damage*.

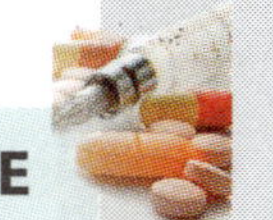

541. Ans. (a) **Staphylococcus aureus**

- *S. aureus* is a cause of serious respiratory tract infections in newborns and infants; these infections present as shortness of breath, fever, and respiratory failure.
- Chest X-ray may reveal pneumatoceles (shaggy, thin-walled cavities). Pneumothorax and empyema are recognized complications of this infection.

542. Ans (c) **Levofloxacin**

Ref: Harrison, 20th ed. pg. 963

Empirical Antibiotic Treatment of Health Care-Associated Pneumonia

The antibiotics recommended with no risk factors for gram negative pathogens are Piperacillin/tazobactam cefepime or levofloxacin

543. Ans. (d) **Fat embolism**

- In the clinical setting of fracture of long bone and subsequent respiratory distress and development of petechiae satisfies GURD criteria for diagnosis of fat embolism.

The criteria for diagnosing fat embolism are as follows:

Major criteria

- Symptoms and radiologic evidence of respiratory insufficiency
- Cerebral sequelae unrelated to head injury or other conditions
- Petechial rash

Minor criteria are as follows:

- Tachycardia (heart rate >110 beats/min)
- Pyrexia (temperature >38.5°C)
- Retinal changes of fat or petechiae
- Renal dysfunction
- Jaundice
- Acute drop in hemoglobin level
- Sudden thrombocytopenia
- Elevated erythrocyte sedimentation rate
- Fat microglobulinemia

544. Ans. (d) **Lesion in the brain**

Biot's Breathing: Biot's Breathing is characterized by irregularly irregular breathing with sudden apnea and is seen in CNS lesions and is a sign of increased intracranial pressure.

Kussmaul's Respiration. Kussmaul Breathing is deep rapid respiration in metabolic acidosis and is classically associated with diabetic ketoacidosis

Cheyne-Stokes Respiration. Cheyne-Stokes Respiration is one of increasingly deep respiration followed by a steady diminution of breathing until an apneic episode occurs in neurologic diseases with raised ICP. Obesity may be present. Some patients will show pupillary dilation with rapid breathing and pupillary contraction with apnea.

Contd...

The differential diagnoses are

- CNS disease
- CHF
- Pneumonia
- Carbon monoxide poisoning
- Medications (e.g., morphine).

Apneustic Breathing. Apneustic breathing is seen in severely ill patients with coma. The patient holds his or her breath at the end of inspiration until the Hering-Breuer (carotid body) reflex initiates exhalation. This breathing pattern suggests pontine disease.

545. Ans. (d) **CT with IV contrast**

Ref: Harrison, 19th ed. pg. 1633-64

- A definitive diagnosis of PE depends on visualization of an intraluminal filling defect in more than one projection.
- *Chest CT with contrast has become the main test for diagnosis replacing the older invasive pulmonary angiography.*
- Catheter-based diagnostic testing is used in case of an unsatisfactory chest CT and those patients where catheter-directed thrombolysis or embolectomy is planned.

546. Ans. (a) **Narcotic over-dosage**

- Narcotics cause CNS depression and lead to inability of respiratory centre to respond to increasing carbon dioxide levels.
- Abnormalities of central respiratory drive and reduced central respiratory drive will decrease minute ventilation.

Causes of Reduced Respiratory Drive

- Sedative drugs
- Altered drug metabolism (hepatic/renal failure)
- Iatrogenic drug overdose.
- Head injury, raised intracranial pressure and central nervous system infection
- Severe hypercapnia or hypoxaemia can also depress the respiratory center
- Inadequate ventilation may be caused by reduced respiratory drive, an increase in dead space or an increase in CO_2 production.

547. Ans. (d) **Sulfomethoxazole and trimethoprim**

Ref: Harrison, 19th ed. pg. 492

- Prophylaxis with trimethoprim-sulfamethoxazole prevents many opportunistic infections, including infection with *P. carinii, Toxoplasma gondii,* and community-acquired respiratory, gastrointestinal, and urinary tract pathogens.
- Intolerance of TMP-SMZ is common; desensitization is useful less often in transplant patients than in patients with AIDS.

548. Ans. (a) Pulmonary hamartoma

Ref: Harrison, 19th ed. pg. 515-16

- Popcorn calcification is virtually diagnostic on chest radiographs for *pulmonary hamartoma.*
- It characteristically appears as well-defined, solitary pulmonary nodules; they may show varying patterns of calcification, including an irregular popcorn, stippled, or curvilinear pattern, or even a combination of all 3 patterns.

549. Ans. (b) Alveolar transudate

Ref: Harrison, 19th ed. pg. 1736-38

- *ARDS is characterised by high protein pulmonary edema and an exudate.* The natural history of ARDS is marked by three phases—exudative, proliferative, and fibrotic—each with characteristic clinical and pathologic features.
- The presence of alveolar and interstitial fluid and the loss of surfactant can lead to a marked reduction of lung compliance.
- Without an increase in end-expiratory pressure, significant alveolar collapse can occur at end-expiration, impairing oxygenation.
- In most clinical settings, positive end-expiratory pressure (PEEP) is empirically set to minimize FiO_2 and maximize $PaO_{2.}$
- Diagnostic Criteria for ALI AND ARDS

Oxygena-tion	Onset	Chest radiograph	Absence of Left Atrial Hypertension
ALI: PaO_2/FIO_2≤300 mm Hg	Acute	Bilateral alveolar or interstitial infiltrates	PCWP ≤18 mm Hg or no clinical evidence of increased left atrial pressure
ARDS: PaO_2/FIO_2≤ 200 mm Hg	Acute	Bilateral alveolar or interstitial infiltrates	PCWP ≤18 mm Hg or no clinical evidence of increased left atrial pressure

550. Ans. (b) Lung laceration

- The image shows presence of subcutaneous empysema which is also hinted in line 2 of the question where it mentions crepitus is palpated.
- Chest trauma, a major cause of subcutaneous emphysema, can cause air to enter the skin of the chest wall from the neck or lung.
- Most students mark it as renal shut down which is not the answer because it would not happen within 4 hour of trauma insult.
- Gas gangrene will again take time to develop and would lead to development of crepitus in the injured part.

Causes of Subcutaneous Emphysema

- Trauma to parts of the respiratory system other than the lungs, such as rupture of a bronchial tube, may also cause subcutaneous emphysema
- May also occur with fractures of the facial bones, neoplasms, during asthma attacks.

When the alveoli of the lung are ruptured, as occurs in pulmonary laceration, air may travel beneath the visceral pleura (the membrane lining the lung), to the hilum of the lung, up to the trachea, to the neck and then to the chest wall.

551. Ans. (d) Increased prostaglandins

Ref: Harrison, 19th ed. pg. 1680

- Aspirin-sensitive asthma is associated with severe rhinosinusitis and recurrent nasal polyposis.
- The complex pathogenesis of aspirin-sensitive asthma involves chronic eosinophilic inflammatory changes, with evidence of increased mast cell activation.
- Aspirin-sensitive asthma is an underdiagnosed condition affecting up to 20% of the adult asthmatic population.
- It is associated with more severe asthma,requires increased use of inhaled and oral corticosteroids, more presentations to hospital and a risk of life- threatening reactions with aspirin.
- The cyclo-oxygenase pathways play a major role in the respiratory reactions that develop after aspirin ingestion.

552. Ans. (c) Low flow oxygen

Ref: Harrison, 19th ed. pg. 1707, 1740

- In COPD, Ventilation/perfusion matching leads to under-ventilated lung which usually has low oxygen content. This leads to localized vasoconstriction limiting blood flow to that lung tissue.
- Supplemental oxygen abolishes this constriction, leading to improved ventilation/perfusion matching.
- High flow oxygen is not tolerated as it leads to crusting, dryness and epistaxis.
- The treatment is guided by PaO_2 which should be maintained at 60 mm Hg or so (SaO_2 of 85-90%). During the period of exercise, sleep or other activities, the flow rate may be increased by another 1–2 L/min.
- While continuous therapy is required for patients who show hypoxaemia at rest, intermittent treatment during specific periods may be used for patients who demonstrate intermittent hypoxaemia

553. Ans. (a) Duration of smoking

Though this is a highly debatable topic most serach results and discussion with faculty and google books (IASLC Textbook of Prevention and Early Detection of Lung

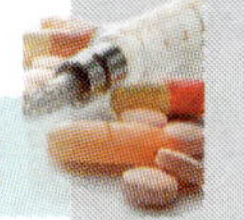

Cancer) mention *duration of smoking* to be more important that the number of cigarettes smoked.

554. Ans. (b) Decreased CO_2

Ref: Harrison, 19th ed. pg. 1731-32

- Hyperventilation leads to carbon dioxide washout. It is usually a feature of type 1 respiratory failure.
- *Type 1 respiratory failure is defined as a low level of oxygen in the blood (hypoxemia) without an increased level of carbon dioxide in the blood (hypercapnia), and the $PaCO_2$ may be normal or low.*
- It is typically caused by a ventilation/perfusion (V/Q) mismatch; the volume of air flowing in and out of the lungs is not matched with the flow of blood to the lungs. The basic defect in *Type 1 respiratory failure* is failure of oxygenation characterized by:

P_aO_2	Decreased (<60 mm Hg)
P_aCO_2	Normal or Decreased (<50 mm Hg)
$P_{A\text{-}a}O_2$	Increased

555. Ans. (b) Bacterial pneumonia

The image in PA view shows well defined homogenous opacity suggestive of lobar pneumonia.

556. Ans. (a) Sarcoidosis

Ref: Harrison, 19th ed. pg. 2206

Löfgren syndrome symptoms consist of fever, bilateral hilar lymphadenopathy (BHL), and polyarthralgias

557. Ans. (a) Asbestosis

Ref: Harrison, 19th ed. pg. 1689

- Working with asbestos is the most common risk factor for mesothelioma.
- Indeed, the relationship between asbestos and mesothelioma is so strong that many consider mesothelioma a "signal" or "sentinel" tumor.
- In rare cases, mesothelioma has also been associated with irradiation of the chest or abdomen, intrapleural thorium dioxide (thorotrast) as a contrast medium, and inhalation of other fibrous silicates.

558. Ans. (c) Minimal pleural effusion

Ref: Harrison, 18th ed. Chapter 252 and 267

- Severe asthma and pneumonia will require supplemental oxygen so are ruled out.
- Low flow oxygen is mainstay of therapy for Chronic bronchitis.
- Pleural effusion will not be benefitted by supplemental oxygen as lung parenchyma is not involved.

559. Ans. (a) Centri-acinar emphysema

Ref: Harrison, 19th ed. pg. 1701

- Centri-acinar lesions are more common in smokers and severe in the upper lobes, particularly in the apical segments.
- In severe centriacinar emphysema the distal acinus also becomes involved, and so, as noted, the differentiation from panacinar emphysema becomes difficult.

560. Ans. (a) Silicosis

Ref: Chapter 256: Harrison, 18th ed.

Causes of Miliary Mottling

- Miliary tuberculosis
- Fungal infections
- Varicella pneumonia
- Metastases–miliary metastases like thyroid carcinoma, renal cell carcinoma, breast cancer
- Sarcoidosis
- Pneumoconioses
- *Silicosis*
- Coal workers pneumoconiosis
- Pulmonary haemosiderosis
- Hypersensitivity pneumonitis
- Langerhans cell histiocytosis (LCH)
- Pulmonary alveolar proteinosis

561. Ans. (c) Ellis curve

Ellis curve is seen in pleural effusion. It has a S shaped border in axilla where fluid accumulates in pleural cavity. You can see the transverse border of fluid on right lung field in this X-ray. Pneumonia does not have a sharp border.

562. Ans. (d) Pneumo-mediastinum

In the area of arrows a *continuous diaphragm sign* is noted. Normally diaphragm is seen below lungs only. This kind of presentation is noted in pneumo-mediastinum.

563. Ans. (c) Systolic blood pressure is more than 90 mm Hg

Ref: Harrison's, 17th ed. Ch. 251

- CURB 65 also known as the CURB criteria is a clinical prediction rule that has been validated for predicting mortality in Community Acquired Pnemonia.
- **The CURB-65 criteria includes five variables:**
  - Confusion
  - Urea >7 mmol/L
  - Respiratory rate ≥30/min
  - **Blood pressure, systolic ≤90 mm Hg or diastolic ≤60 mm Hg; and**

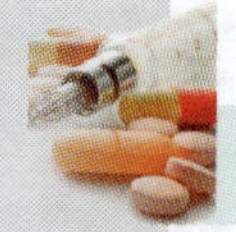

- Age ≥65 years
- Each criteria has one point which predicts the mortality in CAP.
  - **Score 0:** 30-day mortality rate is 1.5%- can be treated outside the hospital.
  - **Score 2:** 30-day mortality rate is 9.2%, and patients should be admitted to the hospital.
  - **Score 3:** Mortality rates are 22% overall; these patients may require admission to an ICU.

564. Ans. (c) Centriacinar emphysema

Ref: Harrison, 19th ed. pg. 1701

Emphysema: The abnormal permanent enlargement of air spaces distal to the terminal bronchioles, accompanied by the destruction of the walls and without obvious fibrosis. It begins in the respiratory bronchioles and spreads peripherally.

> SMOKING CAUSES intake of TAR which causes ↑ marcrophages in alveolar region. These macrophages secrete enzyme Elastase which causes autodigestion of elastin → leading to ↓ elasticity → Emphysema

Centriacinar emphysema is MOST COMMON FORM.

- Associated with smoking
- Usually seen in apices
- ***Causes type-I respiratory failure: 3pO$_2$, 3pCO$_2$***
- ***MOST RELIABLE radiographic sign: Flattening of the diaphragm***
- **Symptoms:** Persistent cough, Dyspnea, Wheezing, Chest pain, Fever.
- **Upon examination:**
  - Increased RR
  - BARREL SHAPED CHEST (AP diameter > transverse)
  - No cyanosis
  - Pink puffers

Extra Mile

- Panlobular emphysema: Involves entire acinus UNIFORMLY.
- Paraseptal emphysema: Involves only distal acinus *(alveolar ducts and sac). Found near pleura and can result in pneumothorax.*
- Irregular or cicatricial: Can be either of them.

565. Ans. (a) Cyanosis

Ref: Harrison, 19th ed. pg. 1664f

- Emphysema is characterized by damage to respiratory bronchioles ***leading to bleb formation***. The air gets trapped in the lungs causing hypoxia. However these patients do not have cyanosis and are called as ***PINK PUFFERS.***
- *Cigarette smoking is the most common cause of emphysema* and the type seen is known as centri-acinar emphysema. ***These patients develop type 1 respiratory failure*** and the resultant hypoxia causes a ***barrel shaped chest in*** these patients.

566. Ans. (a) Thrombolytic

Ref: Harrison, 19th ed. pg. 1634-35

- Anticoagulation with heparin has long been the standard treatment for normotensive patients with pulmonary embolism. By preventing clot propagation, heparin allows endogenous fibrinolysis to occur, with eventual resolution of thromboemboli. Presumably through this mechanism, heparin therapy has been shown to significantly reduce both the incidence of recurrent pulmonary embolism and patient mortality.
- However in the absence of an absolute contraindication, patients with pulmonary embolism induced hypotension or shock are usually treated with thrombolytic agents. The three thrombolytic agents used in treatment of pulmonary embolism- ***streptokinase, urokinase and recombinant tissue-type plasminogen activator(rt-PA).***

567. Ans. (a) Intravenous tissue plasminogen activator

Ref: Harrison, 19th ed. pg. 1634-35

- Massive pulmonary embolism is best managed by thrombolysis using tissue plasminogen activator.
- In case thrombolysis is contraindicated then in these patient fogarthy catheter removal of clot in pulmonary artery would be done.
- In submassive pulmonary embolism heparin is used. Chronic pulmonary embolism leading to pulmonary-hypertension (known as *chronic thromboembolic hypertension*) is treated with a surgical Procedure known as a pulmonary thromboendarterectomy

568. Ans. (b) Allergic rhinitis and its impact on asthma

ARIA stands for Allergic Rhinits and its impact on asthma. It is a set of guidelines for allergic rhinitis.

569. Ans. (a) Streptococcus pneumonia

- Pneumatocoele often occur as a sequela to acute pneumonia, commonly caused by Staphylococcus aureus.
- Pulmonary pneumatoceles are thin-walled, air-filled cysts that develop within the lung parenchyma. They can be single emphysematous lesions but are more often multiple. **Also occur with other agents, including Streptococcus pneumoniae,** Haemophilus influenzae, Escherichia coli, group Astreptococci, Serratia marcescens, Klebsiella pneumoniae, adenovirus, and tuberculosis.". Pneumatocele formation is associated with hyperimmunoglobulin E syndrome (Job syndrome).

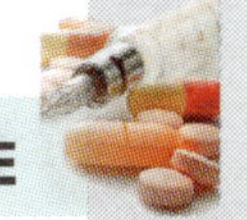

570. Ans. (d) Bronchocele

- *A bronchocele is a mucous-filled dilated bronchi surrounded by aerated lung.*
- CT chest can identify a bronchocele as a tubular intrapulmonary opacity distinct from vascular shadows
- Their appearance is similar to a "finger in glove"or the shape of the letters V or Y.

571. Ans. (d) Rhinocerebral involvement

Ref: Harrison, 19th ed. pg. 489, 1346

- Rhino-cerebral involvement is seen with mucormycosis in diabetics.
- A rapidly invasive Aspergillus infection in the lungs often causes cough, fever, chest pain, and difficulty breathing. Cavity in lungs in usually caused by A niger. A. fumigatus can be a normal component of sputums

572. Ans. (a) Eosinophiluria

Ref: Harrison, 19th ed. pg. 1346-47

- A.B.P.A allergic brochopulmonary Aspergillosis is hypersensitivity to the antigens on cell wall of aspergillus fumigatus. The clinical profile is an asthmatic patient presenting with passage of browinish plugs in the sputum.
- CXR shows fleeting pulmonary opacities and absolute eosinophil count is increased. Eosinophilia is a feature of asthma anyway but not eosinophiluria
- HRCT shows presence of Central bronchiectasis.
- Treatment of choice for ABPA is steroids.
- **Remember:** Eosinophiluria is a feature of allergic interstitial nephritis.

573. Ans. (b) Cystic fibrosis

Ref: Harrison, 19th ed. pg. 1681, 1686

- Central Bronchiectasis is a classical finding in allergic Bronchopulmonary aspergilloma. It is also documented to be present in cystic fibrosis.
- The cardinal diagnostic tests include an elevated serum level of total IgE (usually >1000 IU/mL), a positive skin-prick test to A. fumigatus extract, or detection of Aspergillus-specific IgE and IgG (precipitating) antibodies.

574. Ans. (a) HRCT scan

Ref: Harrison, 19th ed. pg. 308e-3f, 1694

- The best test to evaluate the destruction and dilatation of large airways which are filled with pus in Bronchiectasis is HRCT
- CT angiography is preferred for pulmonary embolism
- Pulmonary angiography is done for lung sequestration and is gold standard for pulmonary embolism.

575. Ans. (c) Klebsiella

Ref: Harrison, 19th ed. pg. 1108

- Military mottling or snow storm appearance on CXR is seen in Disseminated TB, Loffler pneumonia, silicosis and chicken pox pneumonia
- Klebsiella causes pneumonia and CXR shows bulging fissure sign due to accumulation of pus in interlobar fissure.

576. Ans. (b) Uveitis

Ref: Harrison, 19th ed. pg. 1112, 1119

- Phlyctenular conjunctivitis occurs as hypersensitivity to tuberculosis bacteria.
- Tubercular lymphadenitis is the most common form of extra-pulmonary TB
- Most common cause of Addison disease in India is tuberculosis though on global scale it is autoimmunity being the leading cause.

577. Ans. (b) Liver

- Congenital transmission usually occurs from a lesion in the placenta through the umbilical vein.
- The tubercle bacilli first reach the fetal liver, where a primary focus with periportal lymph node involvement may occur.
- The bacilli in the lung usually remain dormant until after birth, when oxygenation and pulmonary circulation increase significantly.

578. Ans. (b) Oral corticosteroids

Ref: Harrison, 19th ed. pg. 1676

- Severe persistent asthma is managed with L.A.B.A., inhaled high dose steroids and S.A.B.A. as when required Oral steroids are given in very severe persistent asthma.

579. Ans. (a) Pneumococcus

Ref: Harrison 19th ed. pg. 805

Infection	Causative organism
Lobar pneumonia/community acquired pneumonia	Pneumococcus
Nosocomial pneumonia	Staph. aureus
HIV associated pneumonia	P. jiroveci
Meningitis adults (sporadic)	Pneumococcus
Meningitis adults (epidemic)	Neisseria meningitides

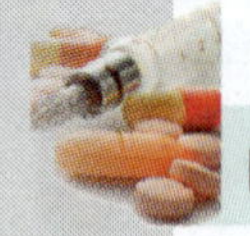

580. Ans. (a) Pseudomonas

Ref: Harrison, 19th ed. pg. 1044-45

- *Pseudomonas aeruginosa is a Gram-negative, aerobic, rod-shaped and polar-flagella bacterium with unipolar motility.*
- The coliforms and proteus are gram negative bacteria and only klebsiella is non-flagellated.
- Furthermore, it is an opportunistic pathogen responsible for ventilator-acquired pneumonia (VAP). VAP due to P. aeruginosa is usually multidrug-resistant and associated with severe infection and increased mortality.

581. Ans. (b) TLC↓

Ref: Harrison, 19th ed. pg. 306e-2f

Parameter	Obstructive	Restrictive
FEV1	Reduced	Reduced
TLC	Normal/increased	Reduced
FVC	Reduced	Reduced
FEV1/FVC ratio	Reduced	Normal/increased
Residual volume	Increased	Decreased

582. Ans. (a) COPD

Ref: Harrison, 19th ed. pg. 1731-32

Type 2 respiratory failure occurs as a result of alveolar hypoventilation and results in the inability to eliminate carbon dioxide effectively.

- Increased resistive loads e.g., bronchospasm in COPD
- Loads due to reduced lung compliance [e.g., alveolar edema, atelectasis, intrinsic positive end-expiratory pressure).
- Diminished CNS drive to breathe due to drug overdose, brainstem injury, sleep-disordered breathing, and hypothyroidism.
- Reduced strength can be due to impaired neuromuscular transmission (e.g., myasthenia gravis, Gullian-Barré syndrome, amyotrophic lateral sclerosis, phrenic nerve injury).
- Respiratory muscle weakness (e.g., myopathy, electrolyte derangements, fatigue).
- Loads due to reduced chest wall compliance (e.g., pneumothorax, pleural effusion, abdominal distention), and loads due to increased minute ventilation requirements (e.g., pulmonary embolus with increased dead space fraction, sepsis).

583. Ans. (b) Pulmonary embolism

Ref: Harrison, 19th ed. pg. 1631

- The first clinical diagnosis for this case presentation is PE since Venous thromboembolism (VTE), which encompasses deep venous thrombosis (DVT) and pulmonary embolism (PE), is one of the three major cardiovascular causes of death, along with myocardial infarction and stroke.
- ***Fracture of femur will lead to immobilization for a long period. Hence PE is all the more likely in this setting.***
- Sudden cardiac death is defined as natural death due to cardiac causes in a person who may or may not have previously recognized heart disease but in whom the time and mode of death are unexpected.

584. Ans. (a) Pulmonary embolism

Ref: Harrison's, 19th ed. pg. 1631

- *PE is the most common preventable cause of death among hospitalized patients.PE and DVT occurring after total hip or knee replacement is currently taken as unacceptable, and steps are taken to prevent it by giving subcutaneous fondaparinux.*
- For patients who have DVT, the most common history is a cramp in the lower calf that persists for several days and becomes more uncomfortable as time progresses. For patients who have PE, the most common history is unexplained breathlessness.

585. Ans. (a) Pulmonary embolism

On chest radiography, the Westermark Sign is a wedge shaped opacity due to pulmonary infarction.

Other Signs in Pulmonary Embolism

- Palla Sign
- Hampton Hump Sign
- IOC – Spirometry
- **Gold Standard IOC** – Pulmonary Angiography

586. Ans. (a) 15 mm Hg

- Pulmonary arterial pressure is about 15 mm Hg, and the pulmonary arterial systolic and diastolic pressures are about 25 and 10 mm Hg, respectively. Pulmonary venous pressure is about 8 mm Hg.

587. Ans. (d) Acts on alpha 2 beta 4 nicotinic receptor

Ref: Harrison, 19th ed. pg. 507, 1705

Average cigarette provides 1 mg of nicotine

- Nicotine's mood-altering effects are different by report: in particular it is both a stimulant and a relaxant. First causing a release of glucose from the liver and epinephrine from the adrenal medulla, it causes stimulation.
- By reducing the appetite and raising the metabolism, some smokers lose weight as a consequence. Nicotinic receptors are known as *alpha 4 beta 2 receptors.*

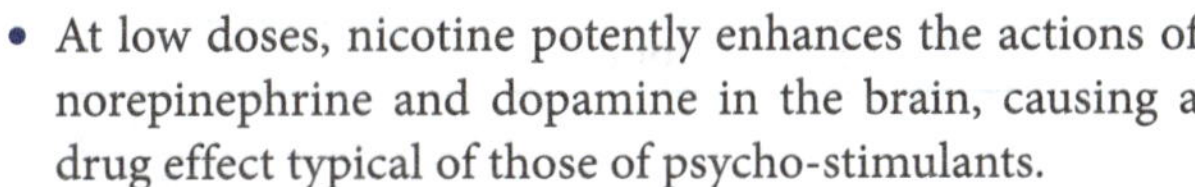

- At low doses, nicotine potently enhances the actions of norepinephrine and dopamine in the brain, causing a drug effect typical of those of psycho-stimulants.

588. Ans. (a) Non small cell lung Ca

Ref: Harrison, 19th ed. pg. 510-511

- Most common cause of hemoptysis is tuberculosis but at 65 years of age it is more likely a presentation of lung cancer.
- Lung cancers can cause hemoptysis but clubbing is seen with non small cell cancer of the lung only. Remember that *clubbing is absent in small cell cancer of the lung.*

589. Ans. (a) Metastasis to lungs

- Metastatic malignant neoplasms are the most common form of secondary lung tumors. Lung metastases are identified in 30–55% of all cancer patients, though prevalence varies based on the type of primary cancer.
- Chest radiography (CXR) is the initial imaging modality used in the detection of suspected pulmonary metastasis in patients with known malignancies. Chest CT scanning without contrast is more sensitive than CXR
- *The most common radiographic pattern of pulmonary metastasis is the presence of multiple nodules, ranging in size from 3 mm to 15 cm or more.*
- *The nodules are more common in the lung bases (owing to higher blood flow than upper lobes) and in the outer third of the lungs in the subpleural region.*
- They are approximately spherical and of varying sizes. Nodules of same size are believed to originate at the same time, in a single shower of emboli from the primary tumor. Nodules that are smaller than 2 cm are usually round and have smooth margins. Larger nodules are lobulated and have irregular margins; they may become confluent with adjacent nodules, resulting in a conglomerate multinodular mass.

590. Ans. (c) Pulmonary hamartoma

- Pulmonary hamartomas, the most common benign tumors of the lung, are the third most common cause of solitary pulmonary nodules.
- Pulmonary hamartomas are usually asymptomatic and are typically discovered as an incidental coin lesion on a routine chest radiograph.
- *On chest X ray pulmonary hamartomas appear as well defined, solitary pulmonary nodules with varying patterns of calcification, including an irregular popcorn, stippled portion. Popcorn calcification is virtually diagnostic.*

591. Ans. (b) Alveolar Transudate

Ref: Harrison, 19th ed. pg. 1736

- ARDS is characterized by *type 1 respiratory failure* which has only hypoxia but the value of CO_2 is normal. ARDS has non cardiogenic pulmonary edema with normal PCWP.
- PCWP (Normal is 8–12 mm Hg) is increased in Cardiogenic pulmonary edema.
- Alveolar Transudate is seen in cardiogenic pulmonary edema. ARDS is non cardiogenic in origin.

592. Ans. (d) Benzene

Ref: Harrison, 19th ed. pg. 447t, 663

Cigarette smoke product	Effects on human body
Aceta-aldehyde/anabasine	Addictive
Benzene	Carcinogenic + Cardio-toxic + reproductive potential toxicity
Benzopyrine	Carcinogenic
Carbon monoxide	Reproductive potential toxicity
Vinyl chloride	Carcinogenic

593. Ans. (a) Liver cancer

- Smoking DOES NOT cause liver cancer and primary brain cancer.
- Kidney and bladder cancer are associated with smoking.

594. Ans. (a) Pneumothorax

A very surprising question included in medicine as nothing is mentioned about this test in most books.

In cases of spontaneous pneumothorax air leaks into the pleural cavity. This air may be reabsorbed but leaves behind a bronchopleural fistula which on autopsy can be picked by "water test".

This is not a clinical test but done by forensic team post mortem.

Please don't confuse with:

- **Water loading test** is done for SIADH
- **Water deprivation test** is done for diabetes insipidus.

595. Ans. (d) Eosinophilic alveolitis

Ref: Harrison, 19th ed. pg. 1681

Hypersensitivity pneumonitis is seen in conditions like Bagassosis, Farmer's lung. It is a type IV hypersensitivity reaction with normal eosinophil count. The granulomatous involvement of lung explains a reduced DL_{CO}.

596. Ans. (d) Subcutaneous epinephrine

Ref: Harrison, 19th ed. pg. 1680

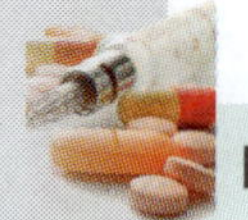

597. Ans. (a) Hypertension

Ref: Harrison, 19th ed. pg. 1724-25

598. Ans. (a) Dextrocardia

- Situs solitus is the normal position, and situs inversus is the mirror image of situs solitus.
- Cardiac situs is determined by the atrial location.
- **In situs inversus:**
  - Morphologic right atrium is on the left, and the morphologic left atrium is on the right.
  - Normal pulmonary anatomy is also reversed so that the left lung has 3 lobes and the right lung has 2 lobes.
  - Liver and gallbladder are located on the left
  - Spleen and stomach are located on the right.

599. Ans. (a) Meniscus sign

The CXR shows pleural effusion as both Costophrenic and *Cardiophrenic angles are obliterated in a CXR and also notice the smooth concavity of fluid rising up in a S shape.* This differentiates from pneumonia.

NEPHROLOGY

600. Ans. (a) Urinary Vanillylmandelic acid levels

Ref: Pocket Companion to Robbins, pg. 700

- The features of palpitations, headache and sweating point to possibility of pheochromocytoma.
- The supra renal location also confirms the same. The best way to diagnose pheochromocytoma is plasma fractionated Metanephrine levels > Urinary free metanephrine levels> urinary Vanillylmandelic acid levels.
- Option b is used for diagnosis of Carcinoid tumor.
- Option c is a dummy choice and Option d is done for confirming pancreatic exocrine insufficiency.

601. Ans. (a) Bladder stone

Ref: Harrison 20th ed. pg. 1434

- X-ray pelvis shows a well-defined radio-opaque shadow opposite shadow of coccyx. This is a bladder stone.
- Option b has minimal calcification to be seen on X-ray. Option c would require a cystoscopy with biopsy for diagnosis.
- Option d is a calcified fibroid and would be seen in post-menopausal woman while our patient is in younger age group.

602. Ans. (b) Prednisolone

Ref: Nelson 20th ed. pg. 2521

Presence of 4+ proteinuria and periorbital edema in a child points to diagnosis as minimal change disease. It responds well to steroids and is called steroid responsive nephrotic syndrome.

603. Ans. (c) Diabetes insipidus

Ref: Harrison 20th ed. pg. 2685

- In cases of moderate dehydration, urine osmolality should be increased and urine should be concentrated.
- However, Diabetes insipidus patients develop polydipsia and polyuria. The urine osmolality is low either due to deficiency of ADH or resistance to ADH.
- The reason for dehydration can be explained by limited access to water in old age due to debilitation like cardiac disease, pedal edema, diabetic foot ulcers or stroke.
- Option a presents with concentrated urine. Option b presents with flank pain and incidental hypertension. Option d presents with salt wasting and metabolic acidosis.

604. Ans. (a) MGN

Ref: Harrison 20th ed. pg. 2144

The two pointers to the diagnosis as Option a, MGN are:

1. Malignancy associated Nephrotic Syndrome is membranous Glomerulopathy
2. Leading cause of nephrotic syndrome in geriatric population is membranous Glomerulopathy
   - Option b is ruled out as it presents with hematuria and Hypertension along with proteinuria.
   - Option c is the leading cause of nephrotic syndrome in young adults whereas the case given is of geriatric age group.

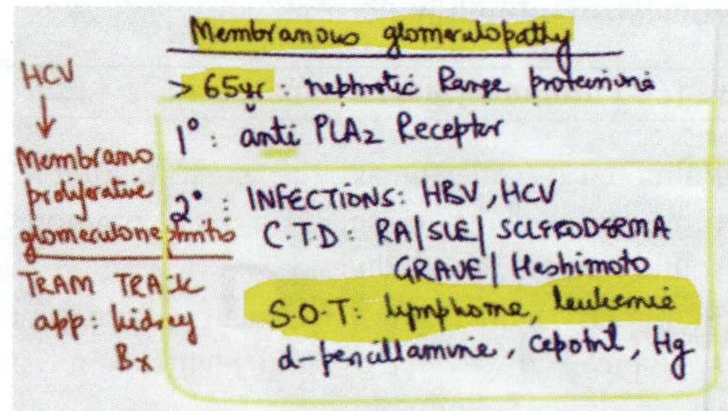

605. Ans. (b) Phosphate wasting from proximal renal tubule

Ref: Nelson 20th ed. pg. 598

Vitamin D resistant rickets occurs due to defect of PHEX gene that leads to phosphate wasting from PCT. This phosphate wasting weakens the bone matrix and predisposes to development of bony deformities

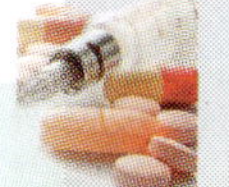

606. Ans. (c) Hyperosmolar urine

Ref: Harrison 20th ed. pg. 297

- Diarrhea and development of oliguria point to severe hypovolemia and resultant pre-renal subtype of AKI. This definitely rules out Option d.
- Option a is ruled out high urinary sodium is seen in renal subtype of AKI where tubules are damaged leading to salt wasting.
- Option b is ruled out glomeruli are under-perfused and not having fibrosis. Kidney biopsy is not done in oliguric phase of AKI. First management has to be done. Moreover, fibrosis is seen in chronic phase of kidney injury.
- Option c is correct as urine is concentrated in case of under-perfusion of kidneys.

607. Ans. (b) 2

Ref: KDIGO 2012 Guidelines

ACUTE KIDNEY INJURY

Stg	S. CREATININE	Urine output	
I	1.5–1.9 Times ↑	< 0.5 ml/kg/hr	6 hr
II	2.0 – 2.9 Times ↑	– same	12 hr
III	> 3.0 Times	< 0.3 ml/kg/hr	24 hr

608. Ans. (a) RBC in urine

Ref: Harrison 20th ed. pg. 2137

The child has developed renal failure leading to volume overload and resultant facial puffiness. This is due to immune complex mediated glomerulonephritis. It occurs after few weeks of pyoderma causes by GABHS. This is a classic presentation of PSGN and will cause hematuria with hypertension and sub nephrotic proteinuria.

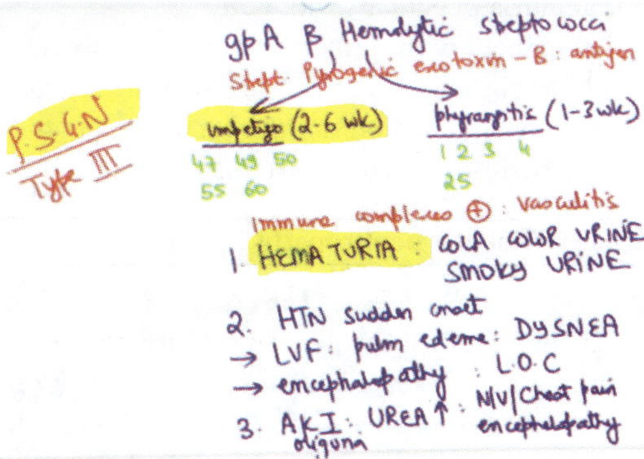

609. Ans. (b) Acute renal failure

Ref: Harrison 19th ed. pg. 656

- The *most serious threat* in adult patients of G6PD is development of *acute renal failure.*
- In G6PD, acute hemolytic anemia episode occurs due to exposure to fava beans, infections and drugs. *Due to intravascular hemolysis, hemoglobinuria occurs and causes tubular blockage.* The patient passes dark urine and develops jaundice. The peripheral smear shows bite cells and supravital stain reveals *Heinz bodies.*
- Sequestration crisis is encountered in sickle cell anemia.

610. Ans. (a) Bicarbonate, uric acid and amino-acids

Bicarbonate	Urinary bicarbonate loss leads to bicarbatonuria and explains the metabolic acidosis seen in Fanconi's syndrome
Uric acid	Urinary uric acid is derived from tubular secretion, possibly from the S2 segment of the proximal tubule. Overall, 98–100% of filtered urate is reabsorbed; 6–10% is secreted, ultimately appearing in the final urine.
Amino acid	Aminoaciduria is a feature of Fanconi syndrome

611. Ans. (d) Contrast arteriography

- DTPA scan showing decreased uptake on affected side with damaged kidney contributing less than 40% of total kidney function is used for diagnosis of RAS.
- Doppler ultrasound of the renal arteries produces reliable estimates of renal blood flow velocity and offers the opportunity to track a lesion over time. Positive studies usually are confirmed at angiography, whereas false-negative results occur frequently, particularly in obese patients.
- Gadolinium-contrast magnetic resonance angiography offers clear images of the proximal renal artery but may miss distal lesions. An advantage is the opportunity to image the renal arteries with an agent that is not nephrotoxic.
- **Contrast arteriography is the "gold standard" for evaluation and identification of renal artery lesions.**

612. Ans. (c) Membranous glomerulopathy

Nephrotic range massive proteinuria	*Intermediate*	Nephritic syndrome hematuria, decreased GFR
FSGS Membranous glomerulopathy Minimal change disease	Membranoproliferative GN Focal proliferative GN IgA nephropathy Idiopathic SLE (Lupus Nephritis) Cryglobulinemia	Diffuse proliferative GN Crescentic GN

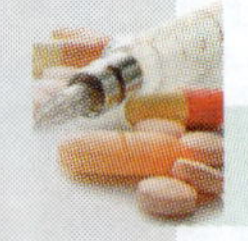

613. Ans. (a) Chronic renal failure

- Broad casts are seen in chronic renal failure and occur due to dilated tubules of enlarged nephrons that have undergone compensatory hypertrophy in response to reduced renal mass (i.e. chronic renal failure).

614. Ans. (d) CRP

- The clinical diagnosis is post-streptococcal glomerulonephritis.
- The antistreptolysin (ASO), antinicotinamide adenine dinucleotidase (anti-NAD), antihyaluronidase (AHase), and anti–DNAse B are commonly positive after pharyngitis and anti–DNAse B and AHase titers are more often positive following skin infections
- Most patients have marked depression of serum hemolytic component CH50 and serum concentrations of C3
- The decrease in C3 concentration typically occurs before the increase in ASO titers
- Urine sediment has red blood cells, red blood cell casts, white blood cells, granular casts, and, rarely, white blood cell casts
- Dysmorphic red blood cells indicative of glomerular hematuria can usually be detected by performing phase-contrast microscopy.

615. Ans. (a) Interstitial nephritis

- Salt losing nephritis is an interstitial nephritis associated with hyponatremia and hypovolemia.
- Glomerulonephritis follows a skin infection or a pyoderma and presents with hypertension and hematuria with sub-nephrotic proteinuria.
- Lupus nephritis presents with hematuria and hypertension in SLE patients and shows wire loop lesions.
- IgA nephropathy is the most common cause of hematuria and presents after 48 hours of a respiratory tract infection.

616. Ans. (a) GFR

Cockcroft-Gault formula is used for calculation of GFR

Creatinine Clearance (mL/min) =

$$\frac{[140 - \text{age (years)} \times \text{weight (kg)} \times [0.85 \text{ if female}]}{72 \times \text{serum creatinine}}$$

617. Ans. (c) Norepinephrine

Ref: Harrison, 19th ed. pg. 1761

Septic Shock Management

- Initial management of hypotension should include the administration of IV fluids, typically beginning with 1–2 L of normal saline over 1–2 hours.
- To avoid pulmonary edema, the central venous pressure should be maintained at 2–10 cm H_2O.
- The urine output rate should be kept at >0.5 mg/kg/h by continuing fluid administration; a diuretic such as furosemide may be used if needed.
- In about one-third of patients, hypotension and organ hypoperfusion respond to fluid resuscitation; a reasonable goal is to maintain a mean arterial blood pressure of >65 mm Hg (systolic pressure >90 mm Hg).
- *If these guidelines cannot be met by volume infusion, vasopressor therapy is indicated. Titrated doses of norepinephrine or dopamine should be administered through a central catheter.*

618. Ans. (d) Low complement levels

Ref: Harrison, 19th ed. pg. 1841

- Nephrotic syndrome is kidney disease with proteinuria, hypoalbuminemia, and edema. Nephrotic-range proteinuria is 3 grams per day or more. On a single spot urine collection, it is 2 g of protein per gram of urine creatinine.
- *Signiticantly low C3 levels are indicative of acute Glomerulonephritis.*
- The most common form of nephrotic syndrome in children, minimal change disease presents with normal C_3 levels. Congenital and hereditary focal glomerulosclerosis may result from mutations of genes that code for podocyte proteins, including nephrin, podocin, or the cation channel 6 protein

619. Ans. (c) ACE inhibitor

Ref: Harrison, 19th ed. pg. 2478-79

- ACE inhibitors may slow the progression of renal disease in CRF.
- ACE inhibitor therapy generally lowers systemic blood pressure, does not alter renal function and decreases proteinuria in patients with CRF.
- The reduction in proteinuria appears to be variable and may depend on pre-treatment glomerular haemodynamics and/or the activity of the renin-angiotensin-aldosterone system.

620. Ans. (a) Diabetic nephropathy

Ref: Harrison, 18th ed. chapter 279

- Iodinated contrast agents used for cardiovascular and CT imaging are a leading cause of AKI. The risk of AKI, or "contrast nephropathy," is negligible in those with normal renal function but increases markedly in the setting of chronic kidney disease, particularly diabetic nephropathy.
- The most common clinical course of contrast nephropathy is characterized by a rise in SCr beginning

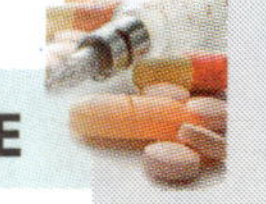

24–48 hours following exposure, peaking within 3–5 days, and resolving within 1 week.

- Contrast nephropathy is thought to occur from a combination of factors
  - Hypoxia in the renal outer medulla due to perturbations in renal microcirculation and occlusion of small vessels
  - Cytotoxic damage to the tubules directly or via the generation of oxygen free radicals, especially since the concentration of the agent within the tubule is markedly increased
  - Management is with N-acetylcysteine and brisk diuresis.

621. Ans. (b) Decreased insulin

Ref: Harrison, 18th ed. Chapter 344

- Exogenous insulin is normally metabolized by the kidney. However, when there is impairment of kidney function, the half-life of insulin is prolonged because of lower levels of degradation.
- This necessitates *insulin dose reduction.*
- **Also remember:** The clearance of both sulfonylureas and its metabolites is highly dependent on kidney function. In patients with Stage 3-5 CKD, first-generation sulfonylureas should be avoided. Of the second-generation sulfonylureas, glipizide is recommended because its metabolites are not active, and there is a lower potential for development of hypoglycemia.

622. Ans. (a) Low sodium diet

Ref: Harrison, 19th ed. pg. 1870-71

- Because calcium and sodium compete for reabsorption in the renal tubules, excess sodium intake and consequent excretion result in loss of calcium in the urine. High-sodium diets are associated with greater calcium excretion in the urine.
- Calcium intake in patients with kidney stones should be normal with adequate water intake.

623. Ans. (c) Pericarditis

Ref: Harrison, 19th ed. pg. 1810, 1822

Absolute indication for hemodialysis is uraemic pericarditis followed by uraemic encephalopathy

Indications for emergency dialysis is AEIOU

- **A** cidosis, especially if severe (pH < 7.2 and refractory to HCO_3 or unable to give HCO_3 due to volume overload) or symptomatic (arrhythmias).
- **E** lectrolytes, especially potassium with EKG changes. Temporize with Ca, D50, insulin, bicarb, kayexalate.
- **I** ngestions, especially those that cause renal failure such as salicylates or ethylene glycol.
- **O**verload, i.e. volume overload causing pulmonary edema. Temporize with nitrates and mega doses of Lasix (160–200 mg IV) – push slowly to avoid ototoxicity.
- **U** remia, i.e. confusion, pericarditis, seizures, platelet dysfunction with severe bleeding, intractable N/V.

When to start dialysis in CKD?

- Dialysis should be instituted whenever the glomerular filtration rate (GFR) is <15 mL/min and there is one or more of the following: symptoms or signs of uraemia, inability to control hydration status or blood pressure or a progressive deterioration in nutritional status.
- In any case, dialysis should be started before the GFR has fallen to 6 mL/min/1.73m^2, even if optimal pre-dialysis care has been provided and there are no symptoms.

624. Ans. (a) P.S.G.N

Ref: Harrison, 19th ed. pg. 1837

- Acute post-streptococcal glomerulonephritis (PSGN) is the most common type of acute GN out of the options provided. Acute nephritic syndrome is the most serious and potentially devastating form of the various renal syndromes.
- Most often, the patient is a boy, aged 2–14 years, who suddenly develops puffiness of the eyelids and facial edema in the setting of a post-streptococcal infection. The urine is dark and scanty, and the blood pressure may be elevate.
- Rapidly progressive glomerulonephritis (RPGN) is defined as any glomerular disease characterized by extensive crescents (usually >50%) as the principal histologic finding and by a rapid loss of renal function (usually a 50% decline in the glomerular filtration rate [GFR] within 3 mo) as the clinical correlate.

625. Ans. (c) CKD is defined as GFR < 30 ml/min/1.73 m^2 for 4 weeks

Ref: Harrison, 19th ed. pg. 290-91

- CKD is defined as GFR < 60 mL/min/1.73 m^2 *for 12 weeks/3 months. Hence choice C is wrong.*
- The average rate of decline varies, but it averages about 0.8 mL/min/1.73 m^2/year after age of 30 years. The decline accelerates after about age 65 to 70.
- In terms of GFR ranges for specific ages, an average 85-year-old male would be expected to have a glomerular filtration rate around 55–60 mL/min/1.73 m^2, depending on his GFR at age 30. *Hence choice A is seen.*
- Choice b is correct.

$$C_{CR} = \frac{U_{CR} \times V}{P_{CR}}$$

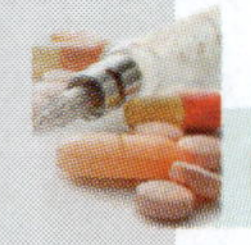

626. Ans. (d) Malignancy

Ref: Harrison, 18th ed. chapter 283

Cause of Membranous Glomerulopathy

Autoimmune diseases	Infectious diseases	Malignancy
Ankylosing spondylitis Dermatomyositis Hashimoto MCTD Rheumatoid arthritis Sjögren SLE Scleroderma	Filariasis Hepatitis B Hepatitis C Leprosy Malaria Syphilis	Carcinoma (solid organ)[Q] Leukemia Lymphoma Melanoma
Drugs Captopril[Q] Gold Lithium Penicillamine Probenecid	***Miscellaneous*** De novo in renal allografts Kimura disease Sarcoidosis Sickle cell disease	

627. Ans. (b) Hematuria

Ref: Harrison, 19th ed. pg. 1804-05

Both myoglobinuria and hematuria have positive blood test on urine dipstick. Evaluate color of supernatant after centrifugation of urine. Since RBC will settle down, it will cause clear supernatant.

628. Ans. (b) Acute glomerulonephritis

Ref: Harrison, 18th ed.

Nephritic syndrome	Hematuria, RBC casts Azotemia, oliguria Edema, hypertension
Chronic renal failure	• Azotemia for >3 months • Prolonged symptoms or signs of uremia • Symptoms or signs of renal osteodystrophy • Kidneys reduce in size bilaterally • Broad casts in urinary sediment
Nephrotic syndrome	• Proteinuria > 3.5 g per 1.73 m^2 per 24 h • Hypoalbuminemia • Edema • Hyperlipidemia

629. Ans. (d) Aminoglycosides

Ref: Harrison, 18th ed. Chapter 280

Aminoglycosides lead to development of non-oliguric renal failure.

Common Causes of Chronic Kidney Disease (Decreasing Order of Prevalence)

- Diabetic glomerular disease
- Glomerulonephritis
- Hypertensive nephropathy
- Primary glomerulopathy with hypertension
- *Vascular and ischemic renal disease (Multiple myeloma due to Bence jones proteins and hypercalcemia)*
- Autosomal dominant polycystic kidney disease
- *Other cystic and tubulointerstitial nephropathy (fanconi syndrome)*

630. Ans. (b) Gram-positive organisms

Ref: Harrison, 18th ed. chapter 281

- Hemo-dialysis (HD) catheter-related bloodstream infections (CRBSIs) are a major complication of long-term catheter use in HD. *Gram positive organism are seen followed by gram negative organisms.*
- Similarly in peritoneal dialysis, the clinical presentation typically consists of pain and cloudy dialysate, often with fever and other constitutional symptoms. The most common culprit organisms are gram-positive cocci, including *Staphylococcus,* reflecting the origin from the skin. Gram-negative rod infections are less common; fungal and mycobacterial infections can be seen in selected patients, particularly after antibacterial therapy.
- In cases where peritonitis is due to hydrophilic gram negative rods (e.g., *Pseudomonas* sp.) or yeast, antimicrobial therapy is usually not sufficient, and *catheter removal is required to ensure complete eradication of infection.* Non-peritonitis catheter-associated infections (often termed *tunnel infections*) vary widely.

631. Ans. (a) IgA nephropathy

Ref: Harrison's, 17th ed. Ch. 277

- IgA nephroathy also known as Bergers disease. IgA antibodies get deposited in mesangial cells and cause dysfunction of mesangial cells and ***lead to microscopic/ gross hematuria.***
- It is classically characterized by episodic nature and is one of the most common forms of glomerulonephritis worldwide.
- The two most common presentations of IgA nephropathy are recurrent episodes of macroscopic hematuria during or immediately following an upper respiratory infection in children (Henoch-Schönlein purpura) or asymptomatic microscopic hematuriamost often seen in adults.

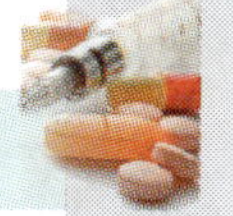

- **Minimal change disease** or lipoid nephrosis is the most common nephrotic syndrome in children. Presence of abnormal T-cell release cytokines and cause damage to visceral cell damage i.e., effacement of podocyte which leads to massive proteinuria.
- **In PSGN** the classic presentation is an acute nephritic picture with hematuria, pyuria, red blood cell casts, edema, hypertension, and oliguric renal failure, which may be severe enough to appear as RPGN.

632. Ans. (d) All of the above

Ref: Urologic Emergencies: A Practical Approach, pg. 117-118

- Xantho-granulomatous pyelonephritis (XGP) is the end result of severe, chronic infection of the kidney, seen in ~ 0.6 to 1.4% of renal inflammations.
- ***The combination of urinary obstruction, nephrolithiasis, and UTI are important elements in the development of XGP.***
- ***Infection is usually secondary to E.coli, or Proteus Mirabilis.***
- Most patients present with recurrent fevers and urosepsis, anemia, and a painful renal mass.
- *Microscopically, there are granulomas and lipid-laden macrophages around the abscess.*

633. Ans. (a) RTA-1

Ref: Harrison, 19th ed. pg. 332e-7t

- There are three forms of renal tubular acidosis (RTA). Types 1 and 2 may be acquired or primary whereas the ***most common form, type 4 RTA,*** is usually acquired in association with moderate renal dysfunction and is ***characterized by hyperkalemia.***

TYPE-I Distal RTA (dRTA)

- In this type of RTA kidneys are unable to acidify the urine to pH <5.5 in the presence of systemic metabolic acidosis or after acid loading as a result of *impaired hydrogen ion secretion* or bicarbonate reabsorption in the distal nephron.
- **Other features are: HYPOKALEMIA**, hypocitraturia, hypercalciuria, nephrocalcinosis, and/or nephrolithiasis. Chronic untreated acidosis may cause rickets or osteomalacia.

TYPE-II Proximal RTA (pRTA)

- It is the result of *impaired bicarbonate reabsorption in* the proximal tubular where the bulk of filtered bicarbonate is recovered. It is most often secondary to various autoimmune, drug-induced, infiltrative, or other tubulopathies or a result of tubular injury from inherited diseases.
- **Clinical features are:** Hyperphosphaturia, hyperuricosuria, hypercalciuria, nonselective amino aciduria and glycosuria.

634. Ans. (c) Hyperkalemic acidosis

Ref: Harrison, 19th ed. pg. 1808, 1810

- Acute kidney injury will cause inability to excrete H^+ and K^+ both leading to hyperkalemic acidosis.
- The acidosis seen is high anion gap metabolic acidosis.

635. Ans. (d) Analgesic nephropathy

Ref: Harrison, 19th ed. pg. 1861

- AKI is a serious complication of snakebites by the viperidae family.
- Pyelonephritis can be hematogenously acquired and cause extensive necrosis of kidney parenchyma.
- Crush injury or Rhabdo-myolysis can result in myoglobinuria causing blockage of kidney tubules and resultant acute tubular necrosis.

Remember: Analgesic nephropathy causes chronic interstitial nephritis and presents with chronic kidney disease.

636. Ans. (a) Present in alkaline urine

Ref: Harrison, 19th ed. pg. 1871

- These struvite stones are also known as triple-phosphate stone.

Two Conditions Must Coexist for the Formation of Struvite Calculi

- Alkaline urine (pH >7.2)
- The presence of ammonia in the urine.

637. Ans. (c) Hypertension

Ref: Harrison, 19th ed. pg. 1841

Essential Features of Diagnosis of Nephrotic Syndrome are:

- Proteinuria >3.5 g/24 hours period
- Hypo-albuminaemia <2.5 gm%
- Edema –peri-orbital edema- pedal edema

Non Essential Features are:

- Hyperlidemia- increased cholesterol and increased triglycerides
- Lipiduria
- Loss of protein C/S/AT III in urine leading to hypercoagulable state.
- **Hypertension as a feature is mainly seen with NEPHRITIC syndrome.** *(Remember Nephritic syndrome has inflammation of kidney blood vessels resulting in vasculitis, reduction in GFR and increase in BP.)*

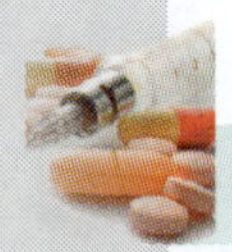

638. Ans. (c) Nephritic syndrome

Ref: Robbins, 8th ed. / Ch. 14

The presence of red blood cells within the cast is always pathological, and is strongly indicative of glomerular damage, which can occur in

- Glomerulonephritis like P.S.G.N, acute glomerulonephritis, R.P.G.N
- Vasculitis, including Wegener's granulomatosis, systemic lupus erythematosus or Goodpasture's syndrome.
- Renal infarction
- Subacute bacterial endocarditis.
- RBCs may appear normally shaped, swollen by dilute urine (in fact, only cell ghosts and free hemoglobin may remain), or crenated by concentrated urine.
- The presence of dysmorphic RBCs in urine suggests a glomerular disease such as a glomerulonephritis. Dysmorphic RBCs have odd shapes as a consequence of being distorted via passage through the abnormal glomerular structure.

639. Ans. (a) NSAID

Ref: Harrison, 19th ed. pg. 1856

Choices B,C,D lead to acute tubular necrosis and hence by exclusion the answer is A.

Causes of Acute Interstitial Nephritis

- Drugs like beta lactams, quinolones, NSAID, COX-2 inhibitors, phenytoin, valproate and P.P.I
- Infections like streptococcus, staphylococcus
- Connective tissue disorder like SLE, Sjogren
- Light chain nephropathy
- Urate nephropathy

Causes of Chronic Interstitial Nephritis

- V.U.R
- Sickle cell disease
- Hypokalemic nephropathy

640. Ans. (d) Rhabdomyolysis

Ref: Harrison, 19th ed. pg. 1804

- Interstitial nephritis is characterized by tubular damage leading to polyuria.
- Rhabdomyolysis leads to myoglobinuria and blockage of kidney tubules and subsequent reduction of urine output.

641. Ans. (a) Acute glomerulonephritis

Ref: Robbins, 8th ed. Chapter 14

- Acute glomerulonephritis is characterized by kidney vasculitis and resultant GFR reduction. This causes high renin hypertension to develop in a patient & lead to edema. The swelling presents first in Periorbital area followed by swelling around genitals and then swelling around the feet.
- Acute pyelonephritis is characterized by fever, accelerated heart rate, painful urination, abdominal pain radiating to the back, nausea, and tenderness at the costo-vertebral angle on the affected side
- Chronic glomerulonephritis is bilaterally shrunken kidneys.
- Renal cell carcinoma is characterized by unilaterally enlarged kidneys, painless Hematuria.

642. Ans. (a) Focal segmental glomerulosclerosis

Ref: Robbins, 8th ed. Chapter 14

- HIV nephropathy is associated with development of focal segmental glomerulosclerosis. (Also seen with reflux nephropathy). ***It is also the commonest cause of nephrotic syndrome in adults.***

643. Ans. (b) Arteriovenous fistula results in arterialization of vein

Ref: Harrison, 19th ed. pg. 1822-23

- The fistula, graft, or catheter through which blood is obtained for hemodialysis is often referred to as a *dialysis access*.
- A native fistula created by the anastomosis of an artery to a vein (e.g., the Brescia-Cimino fistula, in which the cephalic vein is anastomosed end-to-side to the radial artery) results in arterialization of the vein.
- This facilitates its subsequent use in the placement of large needles (typically 15 Gauge) to access the circulation.
- Fistulas have the highest long-term patency rate of all dialysis access options
- The most important complication of arteriovenous grafts is thrombosis of the graft and graft failure, principally due to intimal hyperplasia at the anastomosis between the graft and recipient vein.
- Many patients undergo placement of an arteriovenous graft (i.e., the interposition of prosthetic material, usually polytetrafluoroethylene, between an artery and a vein) or a tunneled dialysis catheter

644. Ans. (c) Thrice per week

Ref: Harrison, 19th ed. pg. 1823

For the majority of patients with ESRD, between 9 and 12 hours of dialysis are required each week, usually divided into three equal sessions.

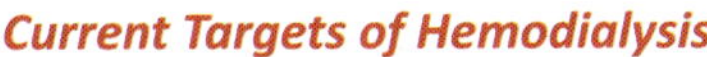

Current Targets of Hemodialysis

- Urea reduction ratio (the fractional reduction in blood urea nitrogen per hemodialysis session) of >65–70%.
- Body water–indexed clearance x time product (KT/V) above 1.2 or 1.05.

Remember: Hypotension is the most common acute complication of hemodialysis. Since the introduction of bicarbonate-containing dialysate, dialysis-associated hypotension has become less common. The management of hypotension during dialysis consists of discontinuing ultrafiltration, the administration of 100–250 mL of isotonic saline or 10 mL of 23% saturated hypertonic saline, or administration of salt-poor albumin.

INFECTION

645. Ans. (c) Tubercular meningitis

Ref: Harrison 20th ed. pg. 1011

- The presence of CSF lymphocytosis with gross elevation of protein (Up to 10 times above normal value of 15-45 mg%) points to Tubercular etiology.
- The development of neurological features over months also helps to rule out bacterial and viral etiology which present over couple of days.
- Fungal meningitis is seen in immunocompromised patients like those who are having AIDS or are on high dose steroids.

646. Ans. (c) EIA P24 antigen

Ref: Harrison 20th ed. pg. 1424

- 3rd generation ELISA test will take >3 weeks to turn positive. Hence for early diagnosis either a NAAT/ PCR or p24 antigen can be used.
- The latest 4th generation EIA solves the problem by combining antibodies to HIV with detection of p24 antigen as well.

Window period infection to detection

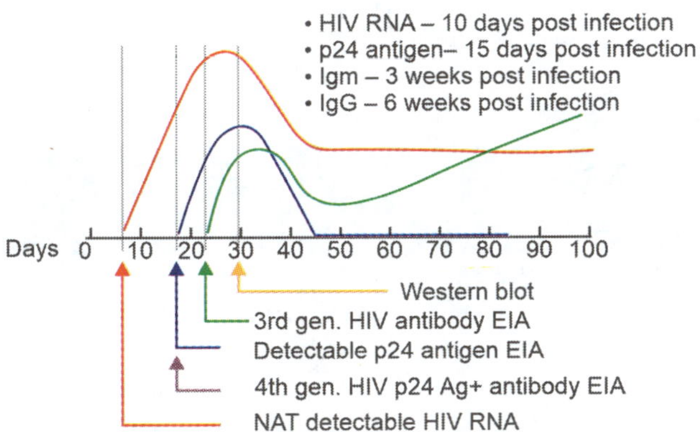

- Note the time frames when these important tests turn positive. Also note that if the choices of question include 4th generation ELISA then it would be the answer with remaining choices being the same.
- For **early identification** of infection acquirement, the sequence to be answered is HIV RNA >4th generation EIA which includes detection of p24 antigen > IgM Antibody HIV > Western Blot

647. Ans. (c) Brucellosis

Ref: Harrison 20th ed. pg. 1193

Option a will have features of encephalitis and is ruled out.
Option b presents in young adults with fever, pharyngitis and splenomegaly.
Option d will present with abrupt onset fever for few days with ulcer at site of tick bite and local regional lymphadenopathy.
The nationality of patient implying endemicity with long duration of fever and musculoskeletal pain makes Brucellosis as possible differential
Overall presentation of brucellosis fits one of three patterns

1. Febrile illness that resembles typhoid
2. Fever and mono-arthritis typically of hip or knee in young child
3. Endemic zone (Middle East like Egypt, Iraq, Syria) patient with fever and difficulty in walking to the clinic.

648. Ans. (b) Voiding cystourethrogram

Ref: Nelson 20th ed. pg. 2556

Recurrent UTI episodes in a male child point to possible etiology of posterior urethral valves. They can be best visualized during a voiding cystourethrogram.

649. Ans. (a) Cryptococcus

Ref: Harrison 20th ed. pg. 1527

The leading cause of meningitis in AIDS Positive patient is Cryptococcus neoformans. The image shows India ink preparation showing capsulated organisms.

650. Ans. (b) Blood Lateral flow assay for cryptococcal antigen

Ref: Harrison 20th ed. pg. 1527

- The leading cause of meningitis in AIDS Positive patients is Cryptococcal meningitis.
- The cryptococcal antigen lateral flow assay is a recently developed dipstick sandwich immunochromatographic assay that has shown equivalent or superior overall sensitivity compared to that of enzyme immunoassay (EIA) and latex agglutination tests and has demonstrated good individual sensitivity for the capsular polysaccharide glucuronoxylomannan (GXM) of all four *C. neoformans* serotypes

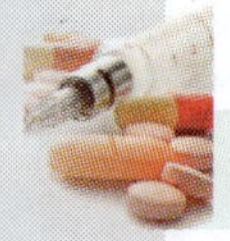

- Option a is ruled out India ink preparation has less sensitivity and is dependent on experience of doctor/ technician evaluating the slide.
- The question can be solved by exclusion as rapid test is always positive for antigen-based test and does not matter whether it is CSF or Blood/serum/plasma based.
- Option c and D are ruled out as culture techniques take days to give conclusive report.

651. Ans. (c) Adequate IVF plus vasopressor

Ref: Harrison, 20th ed. pg. 2050

Saline or balanced crystalloids and nor-epinephrine should be started to obtain a MAP of 65 mm Hg. Vasopressor support is must in patients of septic shock. The preferred vasopressor is nor epinephrine in septic shock and *not* dopamine.

652. Ans. (a) Skin biopsy with fluorescent antibody testing

Ref: Harrison, 20th ed. pg. 1488

- Direct fluorescent antibody testing with rabies virus specific antibodies is highly sensitive and specific for detection of rabies virus antigen in tissues. This test can be easily applied to skin biopsy and brain tissue samples.
- Choice b is ruled out as brain is an immune privileged site, serum antibodies may not develop until late in the disease.
- Choice c is not done . Choice d is an outdated method . Corneal impression is obtained by pressing the surface of sterile glass slide gently but firmly onto the cornea.

653. Ans. (a) C5-C9 deficiency

Ref: Harrison, 20th ed. pg. 1124

The importance of humoral immunity in defence against N. meningitidis infection is best demonstrated by predisposition of persons deficient in terminal component of complement deficiency (C5-C9).

654. Ans. (b) 3

Ref: Harrison, 20th ed. pg. 115

Three consecutive negative blood cultures is mandatory in definition of F.U.O

Definition of fever of unknown origin

- Fever ≥ 38.3°C (≥101°F) on at least two occasions
- Illness duration of ≥3 weeks
- No known immunocompromised state
- Diagnosis that remains uncertain after a thorough history-taking, physical examination, and the following obligatory investigations: Determination of erythrocyte sedimentation rate (ESR) and C-reactive protein (CRP) level; platelet count; leukocyte count and differential; measurement of levels of hemoglobin, electrolytes, creatinine, total protein, alkaline phosphatase, alanine aminotransferase, aspartate aminotransferase, lactate dehydrogenase, creatine, kinase, ferritin, antinuclear antibodies, and rheumatoid factor, protein electrophoresis; urinalysis; blood cultures (n = 3); urine culture; chest X-ray; abdominal ultrasonography; and tuberculin skin test (TST) or interferon γ release assay (IGRA).

655. Ans. (a) Infectious mononucleosis

Ref: Harrison, 20th ed. pg. 1358

- The key word in the question is development of rash after being given ampicillin. Infectious mononucleosis presents as low-grade fever in first 2 weeks of illness. Most common clinical sign is Lymphadenopathy and pharyngitis. Gradually the spleen enlarges. The morbilliform rash on arms and trunk develops both in patients exposed to penicillin derivatives and those who are not exposed to penicillin. *Atypical lymphocytosis is the blood picture with deranged LFT. Most cases are self-limited.*
- Choice b is ruled out as it responds to ampicillin and does not develop after its administration.
- Choice c should have desquamation with mucocutaneous manifestations.
- Choice d does not have a rash and can't be diagnosed on short history of 7 days

656. Ans. (a) No cut off of CD4 count required for initiation of treatment

Ref: www.who.int

The latest guidelines are in favor of initiating ART among all adults living with HIV regardless of WHO clinical stage or at any CD4 cell count.

Extra Mile

2014 CDC Case definition for HIV infection among adolescents and adults

Stage	CD4 Count	CD4%	Clinical evidence
Stage 0	Early HIV infection		
Stage 1	≥500 cells/mm³	≥26	No AIDS-defining condition
Stage 2	200-499 cells/mm³	14–25	No AIDS-defining condition
Stage 3	<200 cells/mm³	<14	*or* Documentation of AIDS-defining condition

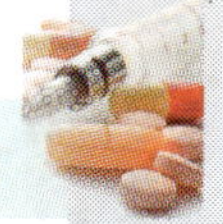

657. Ans. (d) Lymphocytosis

Ref: Harrison 19th ed. pg. 1023

Absolute lymphocytosis occurs during *late catarrhal and paroxysmal phases* of pertussis. It correlates with severity of disease.

TABLE: Case definition of pertussis

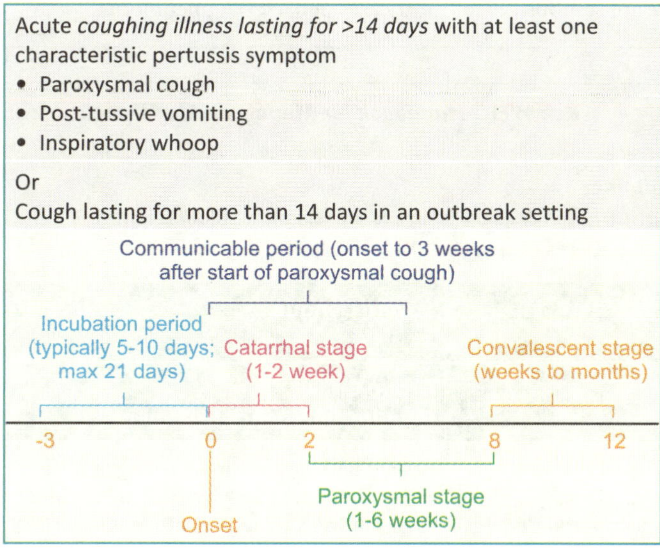

Acute *coughing illness lasting for >14 days* with at least one characteristic pertussis symptom
- Paroxysmal cough
- Post-tussive vomiting
- Inspiratory whoop

Or
Cough lasting for more than 14 days in an outbreak setting

658. Ans. (b) Ceftriaxone

Ref: Harrison 19th ed. pg. 1003

- *Ceftriaxone* used as a single IM or IV injection is highly effective in carriage eradication and can be *used for all ages and in pregnancy.*
- Ciprofloxacin or ofloxacin is administered by mouth and is not in recommended in pregnancy. It is given to household contacts.
- Rifampicin is no longer an optimal agent as it fails to eradicated carriage in 15–20% of cases.

659. Ans. (b) Type 3

Ref: Davidson 22nd ed. pg. 347; Harrison 19th ed. pg. 1125

- The clinical diagnosis of the patient is *type 2 lepra reaction*. The pathogenesis of type 2 lepra reaction is *type 3 hypersensitivity reaction.*
- Type 2 lepra reaction/Erythema Nodosum Leprosum occur *exclusively in patients with lepromatous end of leprosy* spectrum. The most common clinical features are crops of painful erythematous papules that resolve spontaneously in few days to weeks. Concomitant fever, lymphadenitis, neuritis and anemia may develop.
- Type 1 lepra reaction occurs in half of patients with border line forms of leprosy but *not* in patients with pure lepromatous disease. The type of hypersensitivity reaction is type 4 hypersensitivity.

660. Ans. (c) 45–180 days

Ref: Pink Book 2018, CDC Guidelines; Harrison 19th ed. pg. 2006

TABLE: The ABCs of Hepatitis

	Hepatitis A	Hepatitis B	Hepatitis C
Routes of transmission	Ingestion of fecal matter, even in microscopic amounts, from: • Close person-to-person contact with an infected person • Sexual contact with an infected person • Ingestion of contaminated food or drinks	Contact with infectious blood, semen, and other body fluids primarily through: • Birth to an infected mother • Sexual contact with an infected person • Sharing of contaminated needles, syringes, or other injection drug equipment	Contact with blood of an infected person primarily through: • Sharing of contaminated needles, syringes, or other injection drug equipment Less commonly through: • Sexual contact with an infected person
Incubation period	15–50 days (Average: 28 days)	45–160 days (Average: 120 days)	14–180 days (Average: 45 days)
Symptoms of acute infection	**Symptoms of all types of viral hepatitis are similar and can include one or more of the following:** • Fever • Fatigue • Loss of appetite • Nausea • Vomiting • Abdominal pain • Gray-colored bowel movements • Joint pain • Jaundice		

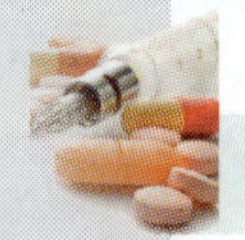

661. Ans. (c) Bacterial pneumonia

Ref: Harrison 19th ed. pg. 1250

- Pulmonary disease is the most frequent complication of HIV infection.
- *The most common manifestation of pulmonary disease is pneumonia.*
- Three of the 10 most common AIDS defining illnesses are recurrent bacterial pneumonia, tuberculosis and *P. jiroveci* pneumonia.
- Encapsulated organisms like *S. pneumoniae and H. influenzae* are responsible for most cases of bacterial pneumonia.

662. Ans. (d) Hematocrit

Ref: WHO Handbook for Management of Dengue Fever

- For monitoring patients of severe dengue hematocrit is performed.
- *A rising hematocrit indicates development of dengue shock syndrome*
- *A falling hematocrit indicates bleeding and need for platelet transfusion in case the platelets are less than 10,000/cu.mm.*
- Hematocrit values can be used to monitor fluid resuscitation in patients of dengue.

Dengue without warning signs	Dengue with warning signs		Severe Dengue
Group A **May be sent home**	**Group B** **Referred for in –hospital care**		**Group C** **Require emergency treatment**
Patients who do not have warning signs **AND** Who are able: • To tolerate adequate volume of oral fluids • To pass urine at least once every 6 hours	Patient with any of the following features: • Co-existing conditions such as pregnancy, infancy, old age, diabetes mellitus • Social circumstances such as living alone, living far from hospital	Or Existing warming signs: • Abdominal pain or tenderness • Persistent vomiting • Clinical fluid accumulation • Mucosal bleeding • Lethargy/restlessness • Liver enlargement >2 cm • Laboratory: Increase in Hct	Patient with any of the following features • Severe plasma leakage with shock and/or fluid accumulation with respiratory distress • Severe bleeding • Severe organ impairment
Laboratory tests • Full blood count • Haematocrit	**Laboratory tests** • Full blood count • Haematocrit		**Laboratory tests** • Full blood count • Haematocrit • Other organ function tests as indicated

663. Ans. (b) Coxsackie

- Hand-foot-and-mouth disease (HFMD) is an acute viral illness that presents as a vesicular eruption in the mouth, but it can also involve the hands, feet, buttocks, and/or genitalia.
- *Coxsackie virus A type 16 (CVA16) is the etiologic agent involved in most cases of HFMD*, but the illness is also associated with coxsackie virus A5, A7, A9, A10, B2, and B5 strains.
- Initially, macular lesions appear on the buccal mucosa, tongue, and/or hard palate. These mucosal lesions rapidly progress to vesicles that erode and become surrounded by an erythematous halo.

664. Ans. (b) Azithromycin

Previously healthy and no antibiotics received in past 3 months	Comorbidities or antibiotics received in past 3 months
Macrolide like clarithromycin or azithromycin Doxycycline	Respiratory fluroquinolone like moxifloxacin Beta lactam like Amoxicillin/Clavulanate plus a macrolide

665. Ans. (a) Protein misfolding

Ref: Harrison, 19th ed. pg. 444e-9

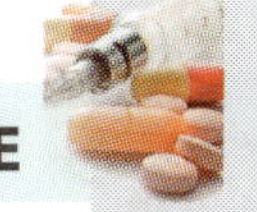

- When a prion enters a healthy organism, it induces existing, properly folded proteins to convert into the misfolded prion form. In this way, the prion acts as a template to guide the misfolding of more proteins into prion form.
- All known mammalian prion diseases are caused by the prion protein, PrP. The endogenous, properly folded form is denoted PrP^C (for **Common** or **Cellular**), whereas the disease-linked, misfolded form is denoted as PrP^{Sc} (for **Scrapie**, after one of the diseases first linked to prions and neurodegeneration.)
- The precise structure of the prion is not known, though they can be formed by combining PrP^C, polyadenylic acid, and lipids in a Protein Misfolding Cyclic Amplification (PMCA) reaction

666. Ans. (c) >25 neutrophils and <10 squamous epithelial cells

Ref: Harrison, 19th ed. pg. 806

- Expectorated sputum is necessarily contaminated by upper respiratory secretions as it passes through the oropharynx and mouth.
- When examining the Gram stain of such a specimen, the examiner should determine whether it is mostly purulent material from the lung or mainly saliva.
- Since squamous epithelial cells line the upper airway but not the tracheo-bronchial tree, their presence indicates that upper airway secretions have contaminated the specimen to some degree.
- *Several criteria have been proposed for determining that a sputum specimen is not excessively contaminated with oropharyngeal flora and is therefore acceptable for culture.*
- *For example:*
  - *Fewer than 10 squamous epithelial cells per field when viewed through a low-power (10x) lens (total magnification 100x) and more than 25 neutrophils per low-power field, or- a ratio of neutrophils to epithelial cells greater than 5:1*
- Even if the specimen conforms to those standards, the patient doesn't necessarily have pneumonia.
- That diagnosis depends upon clinical and radiographic information. Patients with viral bronchitis, chronic obstructive lung disease, or tracheal intubation, for example, can have purulent sputum with a predominant organism in the absence of infection of the lung parenchyma.
- In some clearly satisfactory sputum specimens collected from patients with pneumonia due to a single organism (e.g., *Streptococcus pneumoniae*), not only is the infecting organism visible with Gram stain, but often small numbers of other types of bacteria are also present.
- A common mistake is to conclude that the Gram stain shows "mixed flora" and therefore does not help establish a diagnosis.

667. Ans. (a) Nasopharynx

Ref: Harrison's, 19th ed. pg. 997, 999

- *The natural habitat and reservoir for meningococci is the mucosal surfaces of the human nasopharynx and, to a lesser extent, the urogenital tract and anal canal.*
- Approximately 5-10% of adults are asymptomatic nasopharyngeal carriers, but that number increases to as many as 60-80% of members of closed populations (e.g., military recruits in camps).
- The modes of infection include direct contact or respiratory droplets from the nose and throat of infected people.
- The incubation period averages 3–4 days (range 1–10 days), which is the period of communicability.
- Bacteria can be found for 2-4 days in the nose and pharynx and for up to 24 hours after starting antibiotics

668. Ans. (b) Serotype B

Ref: Harrison, 19th ed. pg. 1002

- *There are currently three vaccines available in the USA to prevent meningococcal disease, all quadrivalent in nature, targeting serogroups A, C, W-135, and Y.*
- Meningococcal polysaccharide or conjugate vaccines provide no protection against serogroup B disease and MenB vaccines provide no protection against serogroup A, C, W or Y disease. For protection against all 5 serogroups of meningococcus it is necessary to receive both vaccines.
- Only recently vaccine targeting serogroup B has also been created and is *protein* based.

Trade name	Type of vaccine	Serogroups included	Year licensed	Approved ages
Menveo	Conjugate	A, C, W, Y	2010	2 months-55 years
Men Hibrix	Conjugate	C, Y, and Hib	2012	6 weeks-18 months
Tru-menba	Protein	B	2014	10-25 years
Bexsero	Protein	B	2015	10-25 years

FLUIDS AND ELECTROLYTES

669. Ans. (b) NS

Ref: Harrison 21st ed. pg. 366-67

Patients with multiple vomiting episodes will develop dehydration. This leads to activation of RAAS system and increased aldosterone values. Increased Aldosterone leads to increased urinary loss of potassium and hydrogen and causes Hypokalemic Alkalosis. The fluid of choice for correction of metabolic alkalosis is Normal Saline.

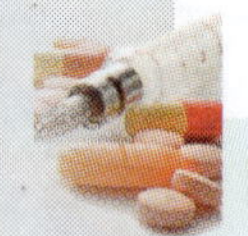

670. Ans. (a) Magnesium deficiency

Ref: Harrison 20th ed. pg. 3186

- Hypomagnesemia leads to less firing of Neuromuscular end plate. Hence weak muscle contraction occurs and explains floppiness seen in magnesium deficient state.
- Hypomagnesemia coexists with hypokalemia in malnourished children due to combination of less dietary intake and GI losses.
- Hence Magnesium should be given parenterally in PEM children who manifest weakness/ floppiness even after potassium correction.

671. Ans. (d) Put wet cloth immersed with 25°C water on body and put on fan

Ref: Harrison 20th ed. pg. 3637

- The soldier is suffering from heat hyper-pyrexia. Covering him with a wet bed sheet and placing a fan in front will cause evaporative losses from the body and will bring down the core temperature.
- Use of ice-cold water or ice will cause peripheral vasoconstriction and cause extreme rise of body temperature.

672. Ans. (a) 5% dextrose

Ref: Bailey and Love 27th ed. pg. 336

In patients with raised ICP, hypotonic fluids like 5% dextrose are contraindicated as they will cause further increase in swelling of brain and will cause deterioration. Rather we need to use hypertonic saline and mannitol.

673. Ans. (c) Hypokalemia

Ref: Harrison 20th ed. pg. 306

The leading electrolyte imbalance contributing to postoperative ileus is hypokalemia. Option a and B lead to development of seizures. Option d affects cardiac conduction and can lead to diastolic arrest.

674. Ans. (d)

Ref: Understanding Anaesthetic Equipment and Procedures E-book, 2018 ed. pg. 343

For rapid transfusion of blood products 14–16G cannula is used. Orange is widest bore but can be put only by a person trained in ATLS. Else a grey cannula is used.

675. Ans. (d) IV soda-bicarbonate

Ref: Harrison 19th ed. pg. 311

- Intravenous bicarbonate has *no role in management of hyperkalemia.* It should not be given in the form of intravenous bolus of undiluted ampoules due to risk of development of hypernatremia. Slow infusion in concomitant metabolic acidosis helps by a *delayed drop* over 4–6 hours.
- Calcium chloride is given to antagonize the effect of potassium on the heart.
- β_2 agonists are useful in case of dangerous hyperkalemia and have additive effect on insulin drip.
- Hemodialysis is the *most effective method* to treat hyperkalemia.

Extra Mile

The most effective drug required to treat dangerous hyperkalemia is *insulin* drip

676. Ans. (b) Diarrhea

Ref: Harrison, 19th ed. pg. 317

ANION GAP

Increased	Normal	Decreased
KULT **K**etoacidosis **U**remia **L**actic acidosis **T**oxins—ethylene glycol and methyl alcohol poisoning	**DR FUSE** **D**iarrhea **R**enal tubular acidosis type 1, 2, 4 **F**istula **U**reterosigmoidostomy	Multiple myeloma Nephrotic syndrome

677. Ans. (a) Renal tubular acidosis

Ref: Harrison 19th ed. pg. 317

Refer to explanation of above question.

678. Ans. (a) Diarrhea

Ref: Harrison 19th ed. pg. 2275

- In choice B, extra ADH will lead to gain of water and low plasma osmolality. Same would happen in compulsive water drinking in choice C.
- Cerebral toxoplasmosis leads to SIADH and gain of water.
- Diarrhea will lead to water loss and *hemoconcentration* which can explain increased blood osmolality.

679. Ans. (a) Hypokalemic hypochloremic metabolic alkalosis

Ref: Harrison: 19th ed. pg. 322

- The repeated vomiting episodes lead to loss of hydrochloric acid. The resultant dehydration triggers activation of RAAS system.
- The elevated aldosterone level lead to excess urinary loss of potassium and hydrogen.
- The resultant manifestation is called hypochloremic hypokalemic metabolic alkalosis.

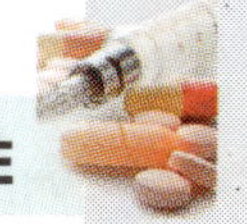

Extra Mile

- Hypokalemic metabolic acidosis is seen in diarrhea with dehydration.
- Hyperkalemic metabolic acidosis is seen with ureterosigmoidostomy.

680. Ans. (a) Renal tubular acidosis

Normal anion gap (hyperchloremic acidosis)	
GI HCO_3 –loss	Colostomy Diarrhea Enteric fistulas Ileostomy Use of ion-exchange resins
Urologic procedures	Uretero-sigmoidostomy Uretero-ileal conduit
Renal HCO_3 –loss	Tubulo-interstitial disease Renal tubular acidosis, types 1, 2, and 4
Ingestions	$CaCl_2$ Mg sulfate
Parenteral infusion	Arginine lysine Ammonium chloride
Other	Hypoaldosteronism Hyperkalemia Toluene

681. Ans. (a) Starvation

Causes of high anion gap	
Cause	**Examples**
Ketoacidosis	Diabetes Chronic alcoholism undernutrition Fasting
Lactic acidosis (from physiologic processes)	Shock Primary hypoxia due to lung disorders Seizures
Lactic acidosis (from exogenous toxins)	Carbon monoxide Cyanide Iron Isoniazid Toluene
Renal failure	–
Toxins metabolized to acids	Alcohol Methanol Ethylene glycol Paraldehyde Salicylates
Rhabdomyolysis	–

682. Ans. (b) Normal saline

Ref: Harrison, 19th ed. pg. 1749-50

- *In controlled hemorrhagic shock (CHS)*, where the source of bleeding has been occluded, fluid replacement is aimed toward normalization of hemodynamic parameters.
- *In uncontrolled hemorrhagic shock (UCHS),* in which the bleeding has temporarily stopped because of hypotension, vasoconstriction, and clot formation, fluid treatment is aimed at restoration of radial pulse or restoration of sensorium or obtaining a blood pressure of 80 mm Hg by aliquots of 250 mL of lactated Ringer's solution (hypotensive resuscitation).
- *Crystalloid is the first fluid of choice for resuscitation. Immediately administer 2 L of isotonic sodium chloride solution or lactated Ringer's solution in response to shock from blood loss.* Fluid administration should continue until the patient's hemodynamics become stabilized. Because crystalloids quickly leak from the vascular space, each liter of fluid expands the blood volume by 20-30%; therefore, 3 L of fluid needs to be administered to raise the intravascular volume by 1 L.
- Alternatively, colloids restore volume in a 1:1 ratio. Currently available colloids include human albumin, hydroxy-ethyl starch products (mixed in either 0.9% isotonic sodium chloride solution or lactated Ringer's solution), or hypertonic saline-dextran combinations.

683. Ans. (b) Tall T waves in ECG

Ref: Harrison, 19th ed. pg. 307, 310

- *The earliest electrocardiogram (ECG) change associated with hypokalemia is a decrease in the T-wave amplitude.*
- As potassium levels decline further, ST-segment depression and T-wave inversions are seen, while the PR interval can be prolonged along with an increase in the amplitude of the P wave.
- The U wave is described as a positive deflection after the T wave, often best seen in the mid-precordial leads (e.g., V_2 and V_3). When the U wave exceeds the T-wave amplitude, the serum potassium level is <3 mEq/L.
- In severe hypokalemia, T- and U-wave fusion with giant U waves masking the smaller preceding T waves becomes apparent on the ECG.
- A pseudo-prolonged QT interval may be seen, which is actually the QU interval with an absent T wave.

Severe hypokalemia can also cause a variety of tachyarrhythmias, including ventricular tachycardia/ fibrillation and rarely atrioventricular block.

684. Ans. (a) Diarrhea

Ref: Harrison, 18th ed. Chapter 45

Diarrhea	Loss of potassium in stool and hypoperfusion of tissues explains the presence of lactic acid leading to metabolic acidosis
Vomiting	Loss of acid in vomiting leads to metabolic alkalosis
Nasogastric suction	Same as above
Conn syndrome	Hyperaldosteronism will promote acid loss leading to metabolic alkalosis.

Extra Mile

Must know causes of metabolic acidosis = K.U.L.T

K = ketoacidosis due to starvation or diabetic complications
U = uremia
L = Lactic acidosis
T = Toxins (methyl alcohol, ethylene glycol)

685. Ans. (b) Biotin deficiency

Ref: Harrison, 18th ed. Chapter 74

Seborrheic dermatitis is seen with following vitamin deficiency
1. Niacin
2. Riboflavin
3. Pyridoxine
4. Biotin

- Niacin deficiency has 3D = diarrhea, dementia and dermatitis (Not in the choices).
- Vitamin A deficiency has night blindness and eye signs and therefore is ruled out
- Riboflavin deficiency is diagnosed by Magenta tongue, angular stomatitis, seborrhea, cheilosis but does not have alopecia and apathy.
- In adults, biotin deficiency results in mental changes (depression, hallucinations), paresthesia, anorexia, and nausea. A scaling, *seborrheic,* and erythematous rash may occur around the eyes, nose, and mouth as well as on the extremities.
- In infants, biotin deficiency presents as hypotonia, lethargy, and *apathy*. In addition, infants may develop *alopecia and a characteristic rash* that includes the ears.

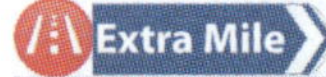

Nutrient	Clinical finding
Thiamine	Beriberi: neuropathy, muscle weakness and wasting, cardiomegaly, edema, ophthalmoplegia confabulation
Riboflavin	Magenta tongue, angular stomatitis, seborrhea, cheilosis
Niacin	Pellagra: Pigmented rash of sun-exposed areas, bright red tongue, diarrhea, apathy, memory loss, disorientation
Vitamin B6	Megaloblastic anemia, atrophic glossitic, depression, ↑homocysteine
Vitamin B12	Megaloblastic anemia, loss of vibratory and position sense, abnormal gait, dementia, impotence, loss of bladder and bowel control, ↑ homocysteine, ↑ methylmolonic acid

686. Ans. (c) Renal tubular acidosis

Ref: Harrison's, 17th ed. Chapter 48

- **Anion gap:** The anion gap is the difference between primary measured cations (sodium Na^+ and potassium K^+) and the primary measured anions (chloride Cl^- and bicarbonate HCO_3^-) in serum.
- So we take value of sodium and from it subtract the value of chloride and bicarbonate.
- **Value of Normal anion gap** = 10–12 mmol/L

AG calculated as follows: $AG = Na^+ - (Cl^- + HCO_3^-)$

Normal anion gap (Mn: FUSED CAR)	Increased anion gap (Mn: MUDPILES)	Decreased anion gap (Mn: BPH-M)
F- Fistula pancreatic	**M** - Methanol	Bromide intoxication
U- Ureterosigmoidostomy	**U** - Uremia	Plasma cell dyscrasia
S- Small bowel fistula	**D** - DKA/AKA/SKA *(diabetic/alcoholic/starvation)*	Hypoalbuminemia
E- Extra chloride	**P** - Paraldehyde/ phenformin	Monoclonal protein
D- Diarrhea	**I** - Iron / INH	
C- Carbonic anhydrase Inhibitor *(acetazolamide)*	**L** - Lactic acidosis	
A- Adrenal insufficiency	**E** - Ethylene glycol	
R- Renal tubular acidosis	**S** - Salicylates	

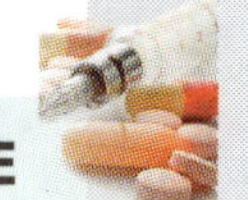

687. Ans. (d) Renal tubular acidosis

Please refer to above explanation

688. Ans. (b) Diarrhea

Please refer to above explanation

689. Ans. (d) Central pontine myelinosis

Ref: Harrison's, 17th ed. Ch. 334

- Normal serum sodium concentration: 135–145 mEq/L. Hypernatremia is defined as a sodium concentration >145 mEq/L.
- All patients with hypernatremia have hyperosmolality, unlike hyponatremic patients who can have a low, normal, or high serum osmolality.
- Altered mental status is the most common manifestation, ranging from mild confusion and lethargy to deep coma.
- Hyperthermia, delirium, seizures, and coma may be seen with severe hypernatremia (i.e., sodium >158 mEq/L). Symptoms in the elderly may not be specific; a recent change in consciousness is associated with a poor prognosis.
- The sudden shrinkage of brain cells in acute hypernatremia may lead to ***parenchymal or subarachnoid hemorrhages***.
- **Central pontine myelinolysis** *presents most commonly as a complication of treatment of patients with profound, life threatening* ***hyponatremia*** *(if hypertonic saline is given too rapidly in a patient* in whom hyponatremia has been present for >24–48 hours*)*.

690. Ans. (a) Facial nerve stimulation by tapping over the parotid

Ref: Harrison, 19th ed. pg. 315

- Hypocalcemia/Tetany is characterized by irritability of nerves. This can be elicited by tapping over the facial nerve when it is entering into the parotid gland. This will cause twitching of facial musculature. The sign is referred to as Chvostek sign.

691. Ans. (d) Hypertonic fluids

Ref: Harrison, 19th ed. pg. 1779

Hypertonic 3% saline can be used in Raised ICT

- Osmotic therapy (ie, mannitol, hypertonic saline), barbiturate, anesthesia, and neuromuscular blockage, along with concomitant monitoring of intracranial pressure with intracranial pressure monitor is generally required in order to maintain adequate cerebral perfusion pressure of greater than 70 mm Hg.

692. Ans. (b) Heat cramps

Ref: Harrison, 19th ed. pg. 479e-2

Heavy sweating causes heat cramps,especially when the water is replaced without also replacing salt or potassium.

693. Ans. (d) Osteoporosis

Ref: Harrison, 19th ed. pg. 2494-95

- **Osteoporosis** is not due to hypocalcemia but is due to imbalance between the osteoclastic activity and osteoblastic activity
- The IOC for osteoporosis is DEXA scan while the DOC is bisphosphonates along with calcitonin nasal spray.
- Hypocalcemia can cause rickets in children or osteomalacia in adults in which the weakened bone is susceptible to fracture.
- If serum calcium becomes less than 7 mg% then it causes tetany.
- The QT interval in ECG is inversely related to calcium levels in the blood.

694. Ans. (b) Neurogenic

Ref: Harrison, 19th ed. pg. 1750

- In road traffic accident case there can be poly-trauma which can damage the spine as well. The damage to thoracic spine can destroy the sympatho-mimetic outflow to the heart causing bradycardia with hypotension.

In this question if *tachycardia was given with hypotension, the answer would be hypovolemic shock* secondary to damage to organs like liver and spleen.

695. Ans. (d) Norepinephrine

Ref: Harrison, 19th ed. pg. 444e-3t

Molecule	Half life
Renin	80 minutes
Cortisol	100 minutes
Aldosterone	<20 minutes
Nor epinephrine	2–2.5 minutes
Epinephrine	2–3 minutes

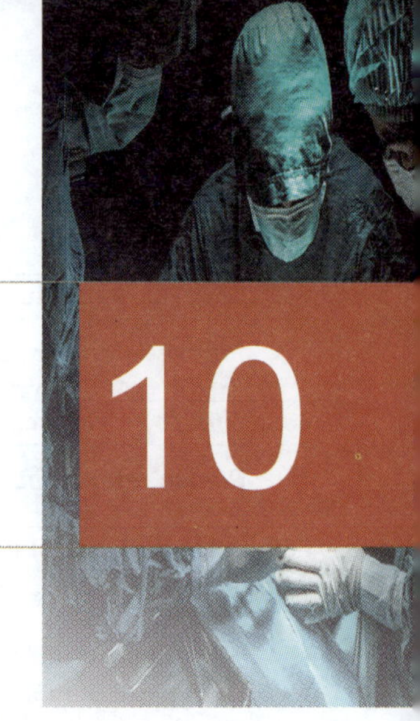

SURGERY

10

MOST RECENT QUESTIONS 2023

1. A 65-year-old patient presents with progressive anemia and fatigue. Which of the following is usual protocol for screening for colon cancer in this patient? ***(Most Recent Question July 2023)***

a. Flexible sigmoidoscopy
b. Colonoscopy
c. Barium enema
d. Fecal occult blood

2. A 65-year-old man developed a burn injury 5 years ago. He has recently developed this lesion in the same area. What is the probable diagnosis? ***(Most Recent Question July 2023)***

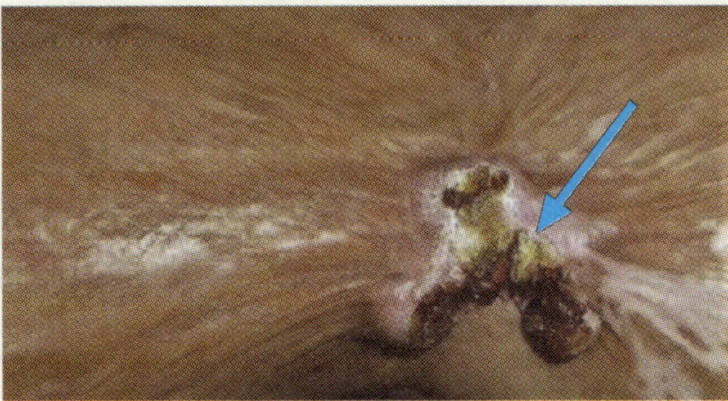

a. Marjolin's ulcer
b. Venous ulcer
c. Arterial ulcer
d. Infected burn wound

3. Which material is the mesh used for Lichtenstein repair of hernia? ***(Most Recent Question July 2023)***

a. Polyglycolic acid
b. Polypropylene
c. Polyacrylamide
d. Polyglactin

4. A 65-year-old patient presents with complaints of nonprogressive dysphagia with halitosis. He says that he develops regurgitation of food items eaten in earlier meals and recent episodes occurred even when he was lying in supine position. What is the first differential diagnosis of this patient? ***(Most Recent Question July 2023)***

a. Achalasia cardia
b. Pulsion diverticulum
c. Esophageal cancer
d. Bronchiectasis

5. A 67-year-old man presents after undergoing Billroth II gastrectomy operation with complaints of diarrhea 20 minutes after meals. What should be the initial management? ***(Most Recent Question July 2023)***

a. Small frequent meals based on fat and protein
b. Reverse Billroth II to Billroth I procedure
c. Insulin plus glucose
d. PPI plus amoxicillin

6. Identify the instrument shown in the given image: ***(Most Recent Question July 2023)***

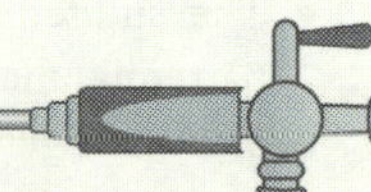

a. Veress needle
b. Sprotte needle
c. Quincke needle
d. Hasson's cannula

7. Involvement of which of the following leads to this clinical presentation? ***(Most Recent Question July 2023)***

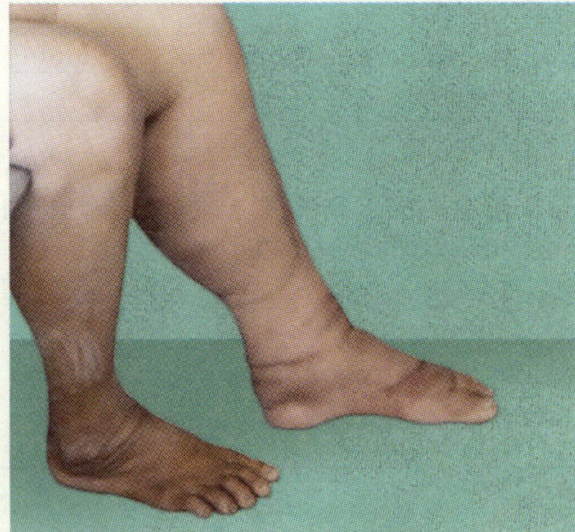

a. Arteries
b. Veins
c. Lymphatics
d. Nerves

8. A patient with inflammatory breast cancer involving 2/3rd of breast surface and peau d'orange appearance is in which stage? ***(Most Recent Question July 2023)***

a. T4a
b. T4b
c. T4c
d. T4d

9. A patient is suffering from diarrhea, dermatitis, alopecia, rash involving face, perineum and delayed wound healing after a minor surgery. This can be explained by deficiency of which of the following?

(Most Recent Question July 2023)

a. Zinc
b. Magnesium
c. Niacin
d. Vitamin C

10. Identify the maneuver shown here:

(Most Recent Question July 2023)

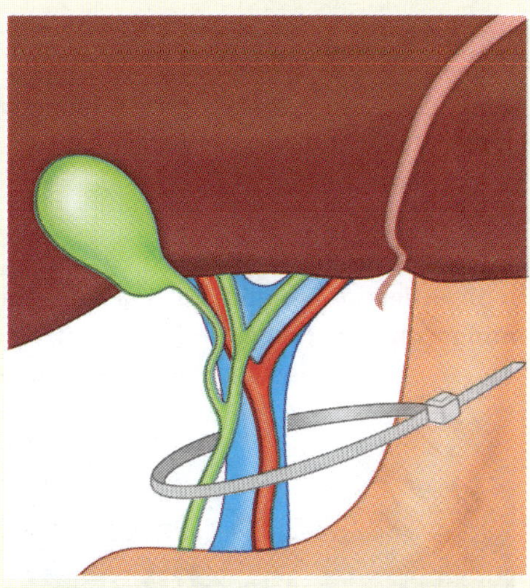

a. Kocher maneuver
b. Pringle maneuver
c. Cattell maneuver
d. Mattox maneuver

11. Which of the following is not a layer of esophagus?

(Most Recent Question July 2023)

a. Mucosa
b. Submucosa
c. Serosa
d. Muscularis

12. Identify the following image:

(Most Recent Question July 2023)

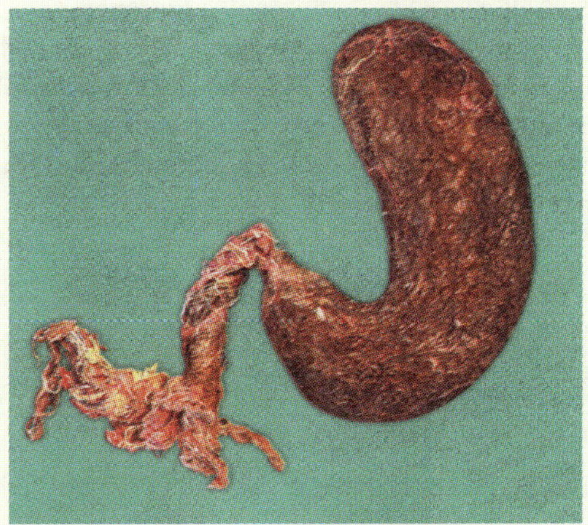

a. Trichobezoar
b. Phytobezoar
c. Lactobezoar
d. Gangrene of stomach

13. A 30-year-old patient says that a pre-existing lesion as shown has suddenly increased in size in last 6 months. Diagnosis is: ***(Most Recent Question July 2023)***

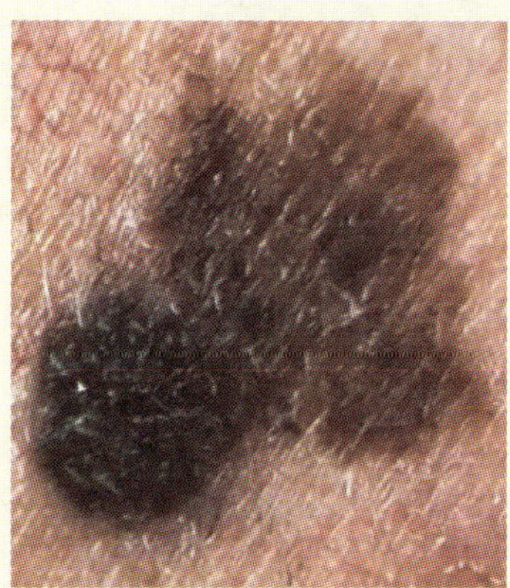

a. Basal cell carcinoma
b. Squamous cell carcinoma
c. Melanoma
d. Junctional melanocytic nevus

14. A 25-year-old male presents with midline swelling in neck that measures 2 × 2 cm in size and moves upward on swallowing and tongue protrusion. What is the treatment of choice of this condition?

(Most Recent Question July 2023)

a. Sistrunk operation
b. Commando operation
c. Local irradiation
d. Radioiodine ablation

15. Which is the most common fluid preferred for managing intraoperative fluid loss?

(Most Recent Question July 2023)

a. Normal saline
b. Ringer lactate
c. Blood
d. Colloids

16. A 45-year-old patient admitted in ICU is having sudden onset respiratory distress. CXR is shown here. Diagnosis is: ***(Most Recent Question July 2023)***

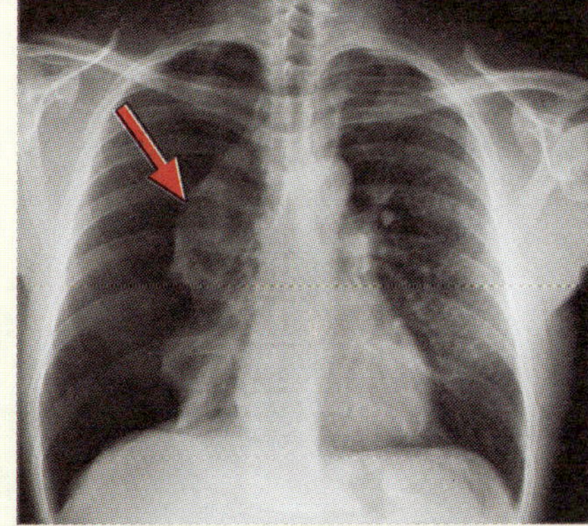

a. Pneumothorax
b. Pleural effusion
c. ARDS
d. Cardiogenic pulmonary edema

17. **Child is having cystic swelling in floor of mouth which is bluish red in color for past 5 years. It shows positive transillumination. Diagnosis is:** *(Most Recent Question July 2023)*
   a. Pleomorphic adenoma b. Dermoid cyst
   c. Ranula d. Cystic hygroma
18. **For staging of intestinal cancer, which of the following should be considered?** *(Most Recent Question July 2023)*
   a. Lymph node involvement
   b. Depth of invasion
   c. Metastasis
   d. Size of tumor
19. **A 65-year-old female underwent radiation therapy for recurrence of breast cancer. Two weeks later she is having odynophagia, nausea and vomiting. She says her weight has reduced further. Which of the following is responsible for this presentation?** *(Most Recent Question July 2023)*
   a. Radiation esophagitis b. Esophageal candidiasis
   c. Achalasia d. Pseudoachalasia
20. **Which of the following conditions is depicted in the given CT image?** *(Most Recent Question July 2023)*

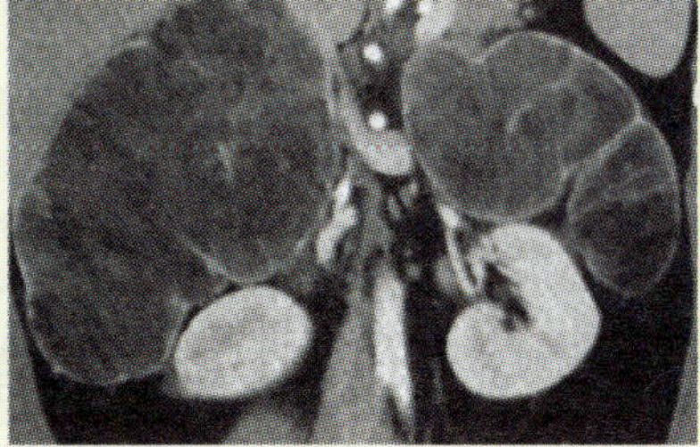

   a. Cirrhosis
   b. Hepatocellular cancer
   c. Renal cell cancer
   d. Congenital adrenal hyperplasia
21. **Which of the following is the preferred treatment in this condition in a patient with RTA?** *(Most Recent Question July 2023)*

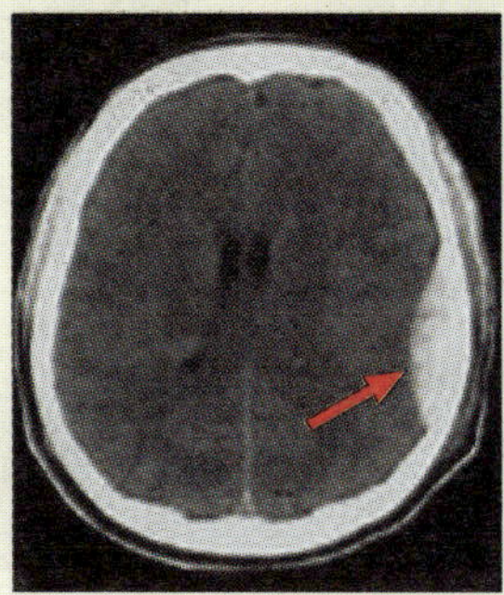

   a. Elective hyperventilation
   b. Craniotomy with evacuation
   c. Anticoagulants
   d. Conservative management
22. **A 20-year-old patient presents with complaints of palpitations, daily headaches which are found to be due to hypertension and diaphoresis. Workup shows elevated metanephrine values. Which of the following is preferred imaging modality for this patient?** *(Most Recent Question July 2023)*
   a. MIBG scan b. MRI abdomen
   c. Sestamibi scan d. CT chest
23. **A 30-year-old male has suffered an open manhole injury and presents with blood at the meatus. Which of the following is most likely injury in this patient?** *(Most Recent Question July 2023)*
   a. Rupture of bulbar urethra
   b. Rupture of membranous urethra
   c. Rupture of prostatic urethra
   d. Rupture of penile urethra
24. **Which investigation should be done for this patient presenting with recurrent episodes of flank pain?** *(Most Recent Question July 2023)*

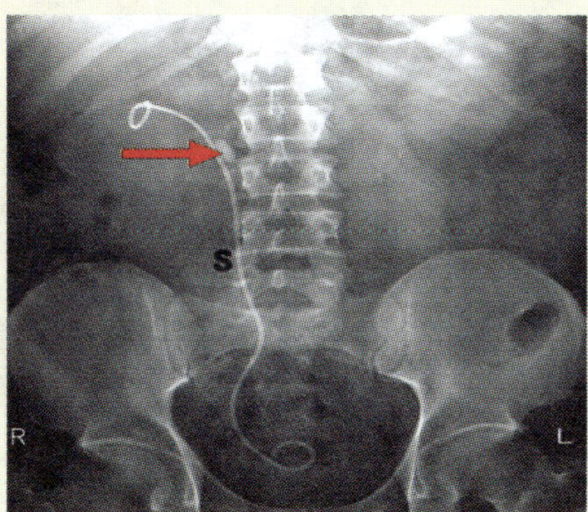

   a. Double J-stent b. Nephrostomy tube
   c. PCNL d. Cystostomy
25. **A 30-year-old patient presented with severe abdominal pain in the emergency. CT abdomen is scheduled but delayed as the patient was hypotensive. The following findings were noted on the abdominal wall. What is the diagnosis of this patient?** *(Most Recent Question July 2023)*

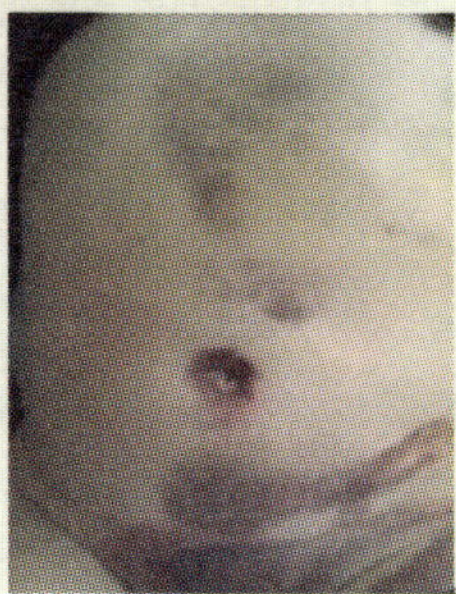

   a. Acute pancreatitis b. Fat necrosis
   c. Necrotizing fasciitis d. Pseudo-obstruction colon

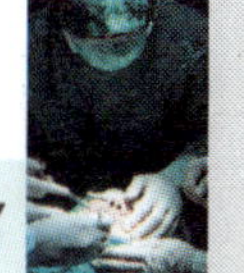

26. Which of the following is correct site for doing needle thoracentesis? *(Most Recent Question July 2023)*
   a. Upper border of lower rib
   b. Lower border of upper rib
   c. Middle part of intercostal space
   d. Upper part of intercostal space

27. Which of the following statements is correct about triage? *(Most Recent Question July 2023)*
   a. Red - Ambulatory
   b. Yellow - Stable need observation
   c. Black - Minor injuries
   d. Green - Life threatening

28. Which of the following is the cause of constriction of esophagus at 23 cm from the incisors? *(Most Recent Question Jan 2023)*
   a. Cricopharyngeal sphincter
   b. Left bronchus
   c. Right bronchus
   d. Aortic arch

29. Which of the following is not a component of qSOFA? *(Most Recent Question Jan 2023)*
   a. Serum lactate >2 mmol/L
   b. RR >22
   c. GCS <15
   d. SBP <100 mm Hg

30. Which of the following is the cause of the condition given here in the image? *(Most Recent Question Jan 2023)*

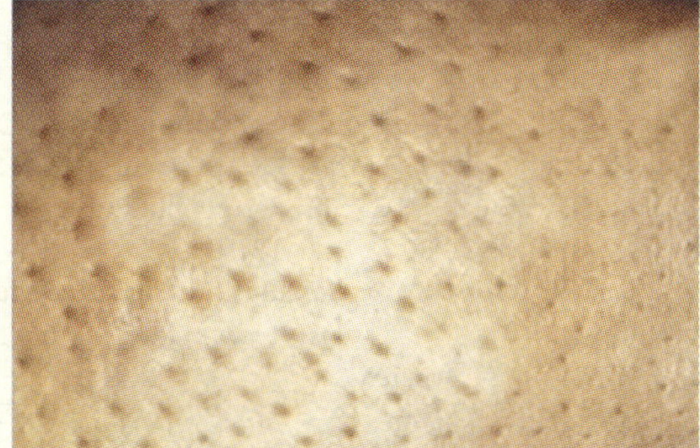

   a. Superficial dermal lymphatics
   b. Deep dermal lymphatics
   c. Artery
   d. Chest wall fixation

31. Genetic testing for mutation in BRCA1 and BRCA2 genes should be checked in all; except: *(Most Recent Question Jan 2023)*
   a. Men with breast cancer
   b. Woman with breast cancer diagnosed after 50 years of age
   c. Bilateral breast cancer
   d. Breast and ovarian cancer

32. A 4-year-old female was brought to emergency department with complaint of accidental ingestion of coin while playing. Child is having drooling and cannot even drink water. A chest X-ray of the child is given here. Which of the following will be the management for this patient? *(Most Recent Question Jan 2023)*

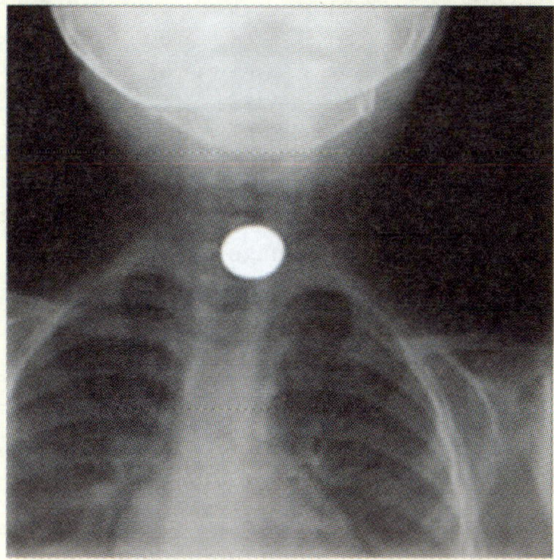

   a. Esophagoscopy   b. Bronchoscopy
   c. Heimlich maneuver   d. Wait and watch

33. A patient came to OPD with complaints of pus discharge and pain in perianal region. After further investigation, the diagnosis of fistula-in-ano was made. Gold standard investigation for diagnosis of fistula-in-ano is: *(Most Recent Question Jan 2023)*
   a. MRI   b. CT
   c. X-ray   d. Endoanal ultrasound

34. All of the following are true regarding the condition in the image given here; except: *(Most Recent Question Jan 2023)*

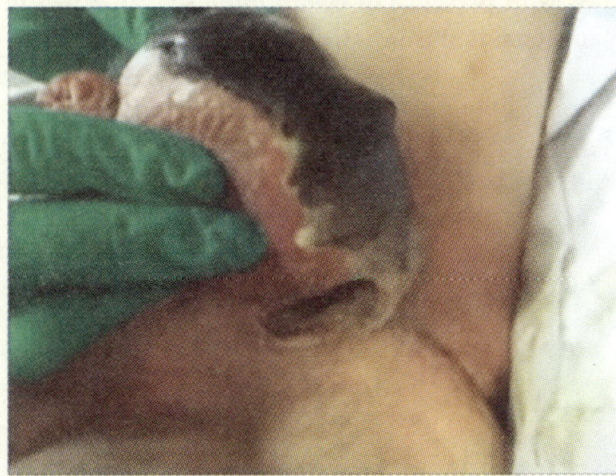

   a. Necrosis of perineum
   b. Scrotal support
   c. Increased incidence in diabetics
   d. Polymicrobial etiology

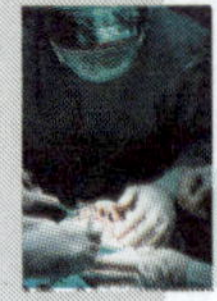

35. Identify the instrument shown in the image:
(Most Recent Question Jan 2023)

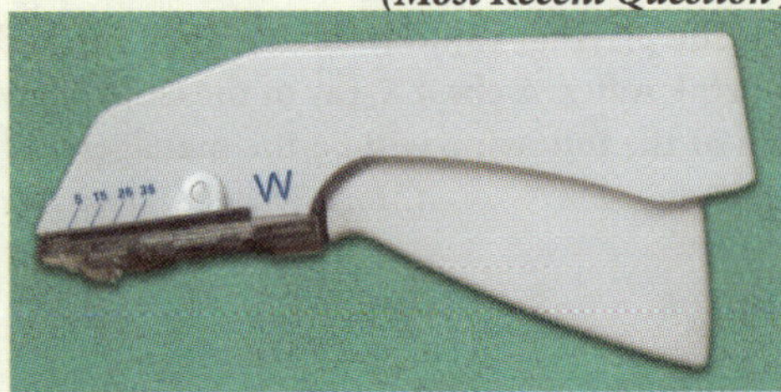

a. Linear stapler
b. Circular stapler
c. Curved stapler
d. Skin stapler

36. Which of the following is the best description of the type of graft as shown in the image?
(Most Recent Question Jan 2023)

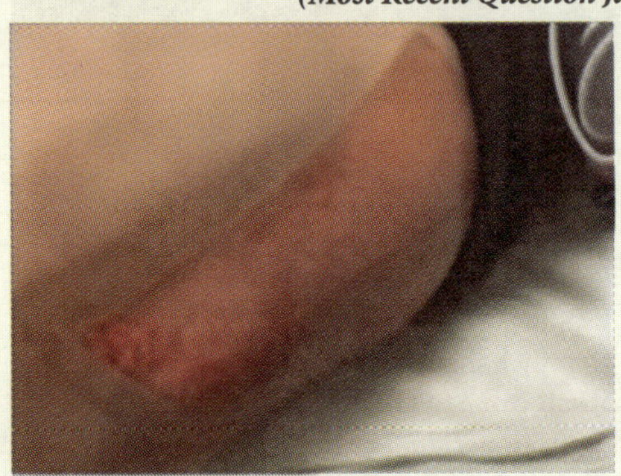

a. Xenograft
b. Allograft
c. Autograft
d. Isograft

37. A 27-year-old male presented to surgery OPD with complaints of dragging sensation in groin which causes problems in daily commuting to work. There is a mass felt near the right side of the inguinal region as shown in the image. On examination, it is found to be expansile mass with presence of cough impulse. What will be the management of this patient?
(Most Recent Question Jan 2023)

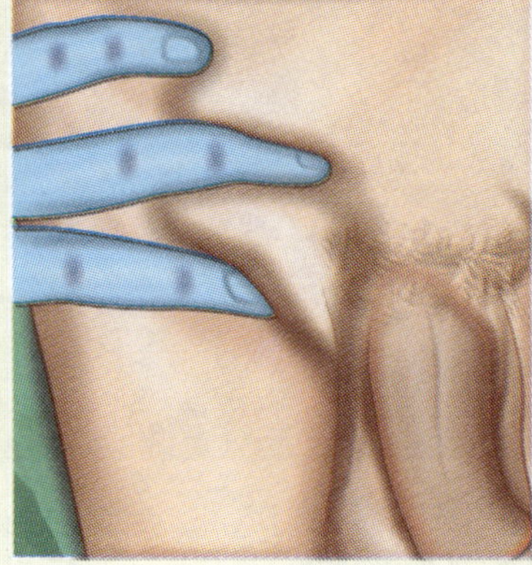

a. Hernioplasty
b. Herniotomy
c. Wait and watch
d. Herniorrhaphy

38. Which of the following is the gold standard treatment of choice for varicose veins?
(Most Recent Question Jan 2023)

a. Thermal ablation
b. Stripping procedure
c. Subfascial endoscopic perforator surgery
d. Phlebectomy

39. A 25-year-old male met with a bike accident and was brought to the emergency department by his relatives. On examination, he is beginning to develop features of hypovolemic shock and his urine output has started to decrease. Which of the following is the likely stage of shock in this patient? ***(Most Recent Question Jan 2023)***

a. Class I
b. Class II
c. Class III
d. Class IV

40. A 67-year-old male patient is a known case of testicular carcinoma and presented to the hospital for follow-up. Which of the following Lymph node is the 1st to be involved in a case of metastasis?
(Most Recent Question Jan 2023)

a. Iliac LN
b. Paracaval LN
c. Inguinal LN
d. Para-aortic LN

41. A 50-year-old woman presented to the hospital with complaint of mass felt in the right breast with visible ulceration of breast. On examination, the 5 cm stony hard mass is palpated with axillary node involvement. What will be the TNM staging of this patient?
(Most Recent Question Jan 2023)

a. cT3a N1 M0
b. cT4b N1 M0
c. pT3a N1 M0
d. pT4b N1 M0

42. Which of the following is not a component of Child-Turcotte-Pugh score? ***(Most Recent Question Jan 2023)***

a. Total bilirubin
b. Serum albumin
c. Ascites
d. aPTT

43. Which of the following organism is the causative agent of gas gangrene? ***(Most Recent Question Jan 2023)***

a. Clostridium perfringens
b. *Clostridium septicum*
c. Clostridium novyi
d. *Clostridium difficile*

44. Which of the following is not used as a graft in the CABG? ***(Most Recent Question Jan 2023)***

a. LIMA
b. Great saphenous vein
c. Radial artery
d. Intercostal artery

45. A 36-year-old female patient had recently undergone laparotomy. What will be the feature of wound dehiscence seen in this patient? ***(Most Recent Question Jan 2023)***

a. Serosanguineous discharge
b. Rebound Tenderness
c. Hypotension
d. Severe abdominal pain

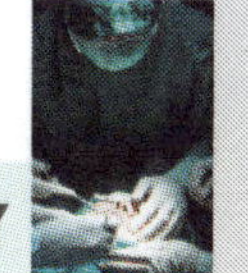

46. A 55-year-old male was brought to the emergency department with history of fall from stairs. On examination, the patient has a head injury. A Non-contrast Computed Tomography (NCCT) head was done for this patient which is shown here. Which of the following is the most likely diagnosis? ***(Most Recent Question Jan 2023)***

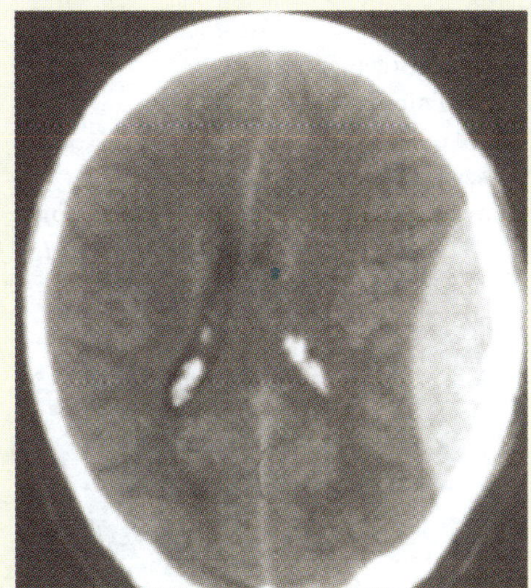

a. EDH
b. SAH
c. ICH
d. SDH

47. Which of the following will not have bilateral hydronephrosis? ***(Most Recent Question Jan 2023)***

a. Phimosis
b. Posterior urethral valve
c. Urethral stricture
d. Retrocaval ureter

48. Which of the following is the treatment of the condition shown in the image? ***(Most Recent Question Jan 2023)***

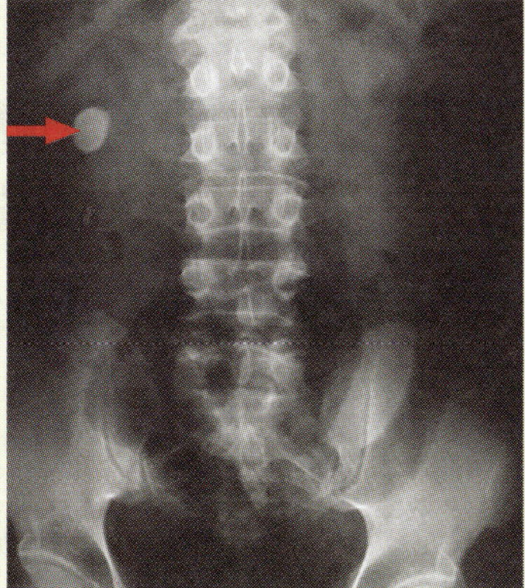

a. ESWL
b. PCNL
c. Ureteroscopy
d. Reassurance to the patient

49. A CT image of a patient is given here. What is the most likely diagnosis? ***(Most Recent Question Jan 2023)***

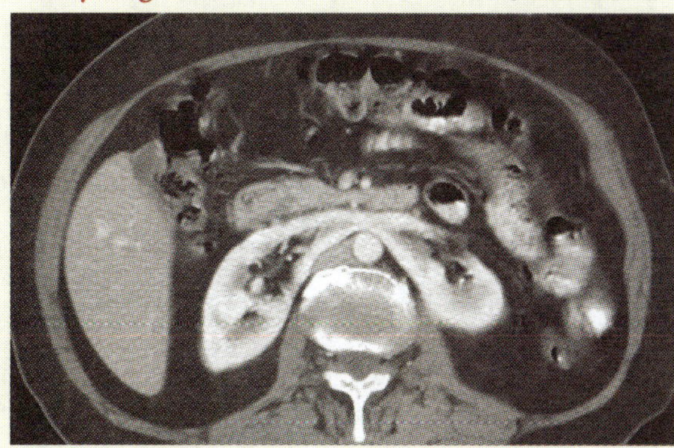

a. Hydronephrosis
b. Horseshoe kidney
c. Polycystic kidney
d. Renal cell cancer

50. Which of the following procedure has least chance of recurrence of duodenal ulcer? ***(Most Recent Question Jan 2023)***

a. Gastrectomy
b. Gastroenterostomy
c. Selective Vagotomy and drainage
d. Highly selective vagotomy

51. Which of the following is a universal feature in all types of shock? ***(Most Recent Question Jan 2023)***

a. Decrease in tissue perfusion
b. Reduced Peripheral resistance
c. Decrease in RR
d. Cold extremities

52. A 54-year-old male patient is presented to surgery OPD with complaint of lesions in the buccal mucosa as shown here. He has a history of chewing pan masala for more than 30 years. What can be done in this patient for management? ***(Most Recent Question Jan 2023)***

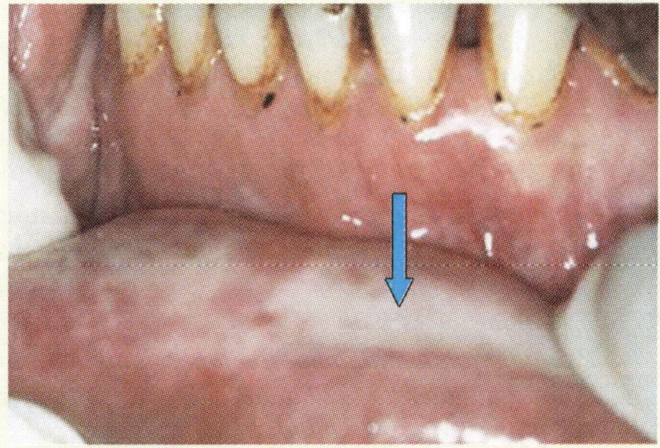

a. Local surgical excision/release
b. Reassure the patient
c. Sclerotherapy
d. Vitamin supplementation

53. A homosexual man complains of painful defecation and prolapsing mass from anus, which does not reduce and has foul-smelling discharge. On examination, cauliflower-like mass was seen. On biopsy, diagnosis of squamous cell carcinoma was made. Which of the following is the preferred treatment option? *(Most Recent Question Jan 2023)*

a. Abdominoperineal resection
b. Chemotherapy
c. Chemoradiation
d. Radiotherapy

54. The condition shown in the image is due to nonfusion of: *(Most Recent Question Jan 2023)*

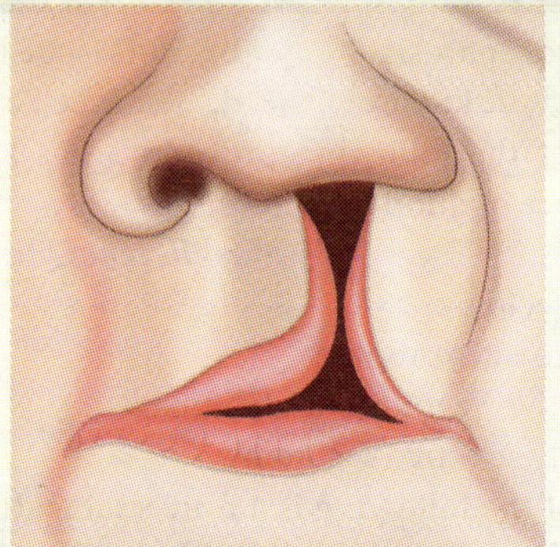

a. Medial nasal process and maxillary process
b. Lateral nasal process and maxillary process
c. Maxillary process and mandible
d. Palatine process

55. A diabetic patient developed DVT along with necrolytic erythema migrans. What is the most likely cause? *(Most Recent Question Jan 2023)*

a. Glucagonoma
b. Gastrinoma
c. Insulinoma
d. Somatostatinoma

56. Increased tone of LES is due to: *(Most Recent Question Jan 2023)*

a. Decreased substance P in LES
b. Decreased Ach receptors in LES
c. Decreased NO in LES
d. Absent Meissner's plexus in esophagus

57. All of the following are correct about neuroblastoma; except: *(Most Recent Question Jan 2023)*

a. Lymphatic spread
b. Early lung metastasis
c. Treatment is chemotherapy followed by surgery
d. Most common intra-abdominal malignancy in children

58. Which of the following is not true about IHPS? *(Most Recent Question Jan 2023)*

a. Presents with nonbilious vomiting
b. USG is 100% sensitive to detect IHPS
c. Caused by hypertrophy of inner longitudinal muscles
d. Occurs in first born male

59. Select the correctly matched options: *(Most Recent Question Jan 2023)*

a. EDH: Pinpoint pupil
b. Penetrating injury to eustachian tube: CSF otorrhea
c. Liver injury: Kehr's sign
d. Mastoid bruising: Skull base fracture

60. Most important risk factor for acute mastitis is: *(Most Recent Question Jan 2023)*

a. Breast engorgement
b. Cracked nipple
c. Failure of lactation
d. Massage

61. Which nerve is damaged in this presentation? *(Most Recent Question Jan 2023)*

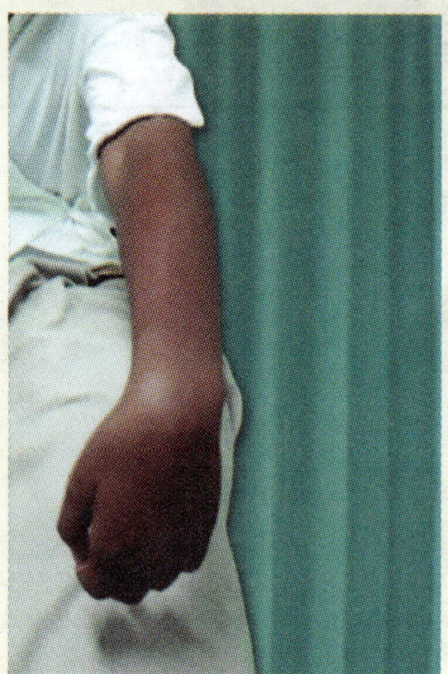

a. Radial nerve
b. Ulnar nerve
c. Median nerve
d. Axillary nerve

GASTROINTESTINAL TRACT

62. A chronic alcoholic patient who was suffering from C.L.D, presented with hematemesis. What can be the most appropriate cause of hematemesis? *(Most Recent Question June 2022)*

a. Esophageal varices
b. Mallory Weiss tear
c. Boerhaave syndrome
d. Peptic ulcer disease

63. A sick child is brought to your ER with bilious vomiting. What will be the most appropriate test to diagnose the condition? *(Most Recent Question June 2022)*

a. Barium swallow
b. Barium meal
c. Barium meal follow through
d. CECT of abdomen

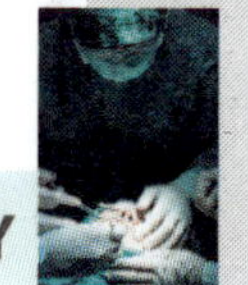

64. Identify the pathology in the newborn baby as shown in the image. ***(Most Recent Question June 2022)***

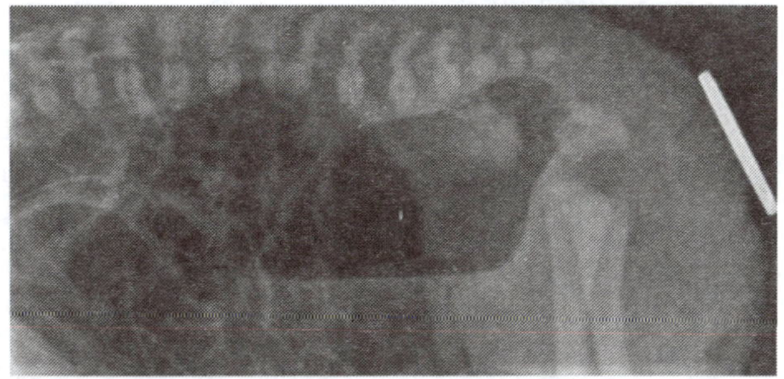

a. Meningocele
b. Congenital megacolon
c. Imperforate anus
d. Pyloric stenosis

65. Best investigation for GERD: ***(Most Recent Question June 2022)***

a. 24-hour ambulatory pH monitoring
b. Upper GI endoscopy
c. CECT
d. MRI

66. A patient has undergone surgery as shown in the image. After the operation, after 30 minutes of taking the meal patient develops pallor, dizziness and sweating. Diagnosis is: ***(Most Recent Question June 2022)***

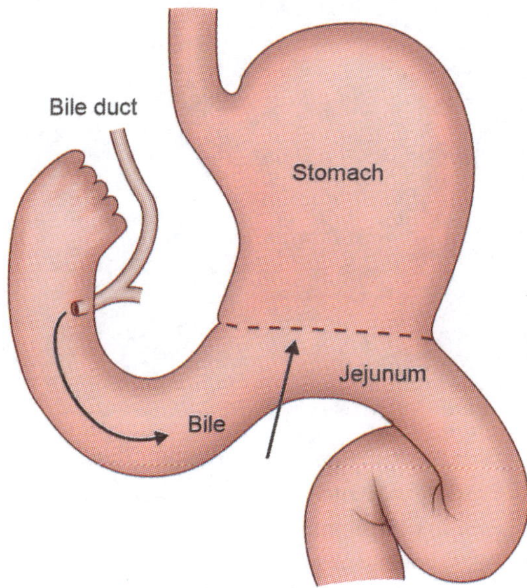

a. Reflux gastritis
b. Dumping syndrome
c. Post vagotomy diarrhea
d. Frey's syndrome

67. Identify the pathology in the image given. ***(Most Recent Question June 2022)***

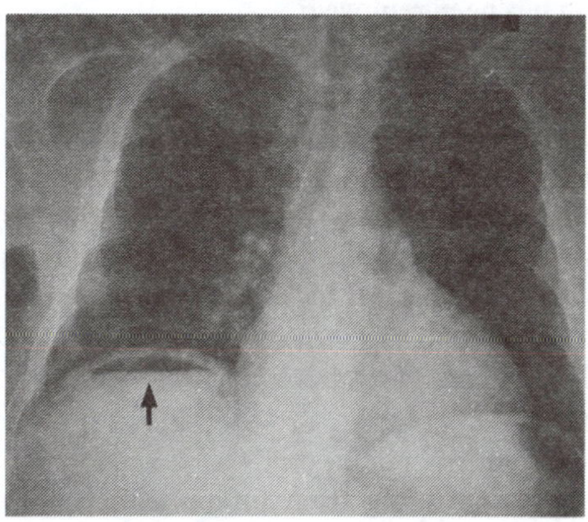

a. Acute pancreatitis
b. Liver abscess
c. Acute cholecystitis
d. Hollow viscus perforation

68. This is the specimen removed from stomach of a young female patient. You should now send this patient for which consult? ***(Most Recent Question June 2022)***

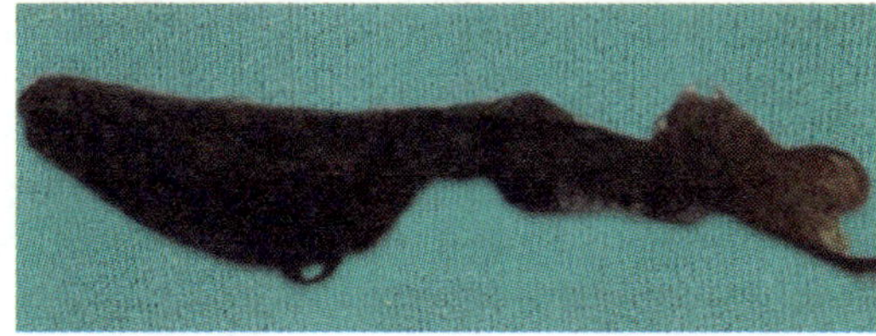

a. Pediatrician
b. Psychiatrist
c. Cardiologist
d. Dermatologist

69. A 35-year-old female presented to emergency with upper abdominal pain radiating to back. On X-ray, colon cut-off sign was seen. What is the diagnosis? ***(Most Recent Question Dec. 2021)***

a. Acute pancreatitis
b. Acute appendicitis
c. Acute cholecystitis
d. Chronic pancreatitis

70. A patient presented with the symptoms of dysphagia, retrosternal pain, and regurgitation of food items eaten the day before. What is the diagnosis? ***(Most Recent Question Dec. 2021)***

a. Patterson Kelly syndrome
b. Achalasia cardia
c. Esophageal diverticula
d. Reflux esophagitis

71. A 50-year-old female who had total gastrectomy 10 years ago, presented with neurological symptoms. Which of the following type of anemia is most likely to be seen in this patient? ***(Most Recent Question Dec. 2021)***

a. Iron deficiency anemia
b. Megaloblastic anemia
c. Hemolytic anemia
d. Aplastic anemia

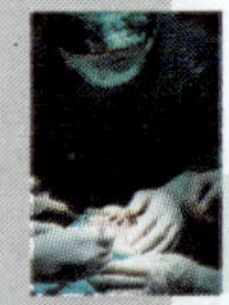

72. Which of the following vitamin deficiency will be seen in a female with Crohn's disease, in whom the terminal ileum has been removed?

(Most Recent Question Dec. 2021)

a. Vitamin B_{12} deficiency b. Vitamin C deficiency
c. Vitamin K deficiency d. Niacin deficiency

73. A 40-year-old patient presented with passage of mucus and blood in the stool. On sigmoidoscopy, inflammation was seen, mainly in the rectum. On biopsy, crypt abscess was detected. What is the most probable diagnosis?

a. Ulcerative colitis *(Most Recent Question Dec. 2021)*
b. Irritable bowel syndrome
c. Crohn's disease
d. Pseudomembranous colitis

74. A patient suffering from inflammatory bowel disease presented with peritonitis following ileal perforation. Exploratory laparotomy was done. Which of the following should be preferred?

(Most Recent Question Dec. 2021)

a. Ileostomy followed by definitive surgery later
b. Ileal pouch anal anastomosis
c. Resection of diseased segment with anastomosis with normal segment
d. Right hemicolectomy with ileo-transverse anastomosis

75. A patient is taking broad spectrum antibiotics for a long period of time presented with diarrhea. Which of the following is causative organism for this?

(Most Recent Question Dec. 2021)

a. Clostridium botulinum
b. Clostridium tetani
c. Clostridium difficile
d. Clostridium perfringens

76. A 7-week pregnant female presented to emergency with pain in right lower abdomen. On USG, acute appendicitis was diagnosed. What is the best management?

(Most Recent Question Dec. 2021)

a. Ochsner-Sherren regime
b. Emergency appendectomy
c. Termination of pregnancy
d. Give antibiotics and wait till second trimester

77. A 5-year-old child was brought to the hospital with the history of constipation. Even after taking prescribed stool softeners, child was able to pass stool one per in a week. Mother also tells that when the child was born he passed greenish stool only after 48 hours of birth. Which of the following should be done in this child?

(Most Recent Question Dec. 2021)

a. Ask the mother to give high fiber diet
b. Plain X-ray abdomen
c. Barium enema and anorectal manometry
d. Surgical treatment

78. Short chain fatty acids are absorbed in:

a. Stomach *(Most Recent Question Dec. 2021)*
b. Small intestine
c. Cecum
d. Large intestine

79. A patient presented in the emergency with pain in the right iliac fossa. The patient was clinically stable for 2 days, but then his symptoms started worsening. He was offered the treatment of extraperitoneal drainage. What would be the most likely pathology in this patient?

a. Perinephric abscess *(Most Recent Question June 2021)*
b. Appendicular abscess
c. Rupture ectopic pregnancy
d. Acute cholecystitis

80. An elderly woman who did not eat food for the last 2 days presented with bilious vomiting. X-ray abdomen is shown below. Diagnosis is:

(Most Recent Question June 2021)

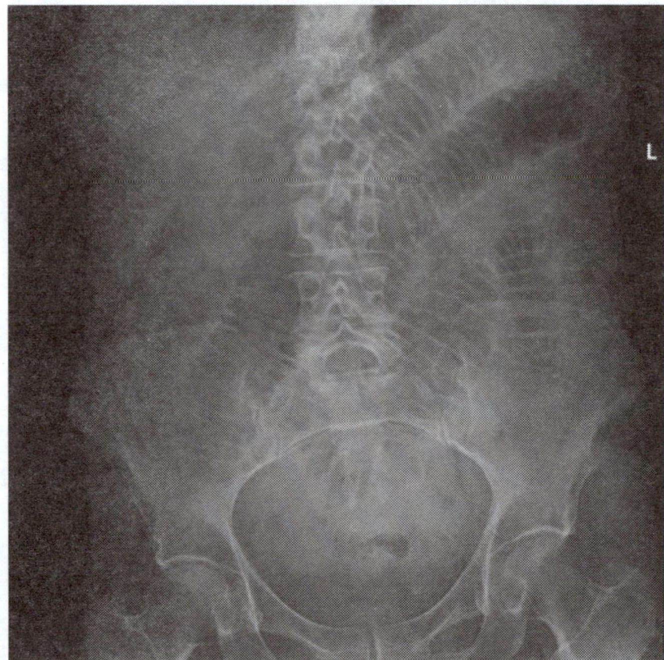

a. Distal obstruction in the small intestine
b. Proximal obstruction in the small intestine
c. Pseudo obstruction
d. Distal colonic obstruction

81. What is the site of maximum pain in acute appendicitis?

(Most Recent Question June 2021)

a. McBurney's point
b. Flank region
c. Right upper abdomen
d. Umbilicus

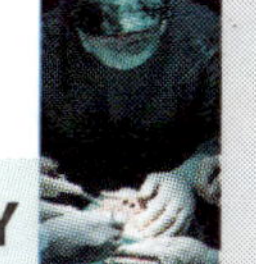

82. What is the diagnosis on the basis of image given below? ***(Most Recent Question Dec 2020)***

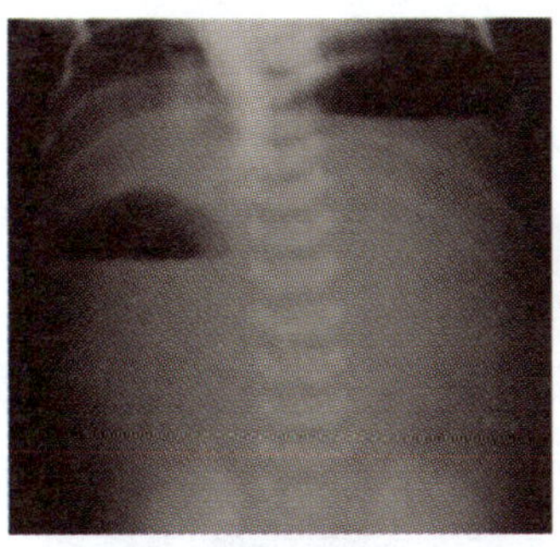

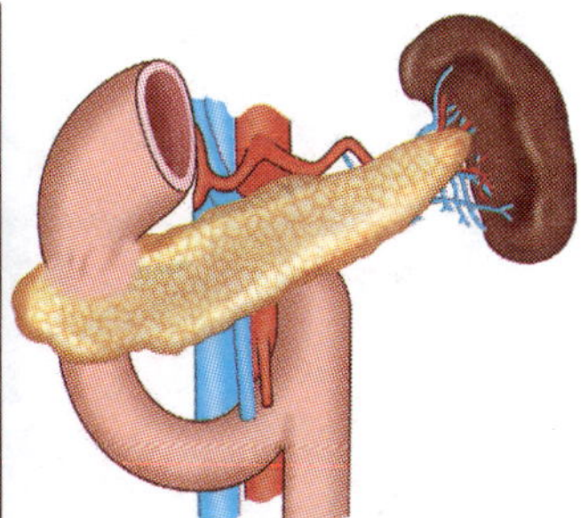

a. Pancreas divisum
b. Annular pancreas
c. Duodenal atresia
d. Hypertrophic pyloric stenosis

83. The chest X-ray of a 4-day-old neonate having respiratory distress with a scaphoid abdomen is given below. What is the diagnosis? ***(Most Recent Question Dec 2020)***

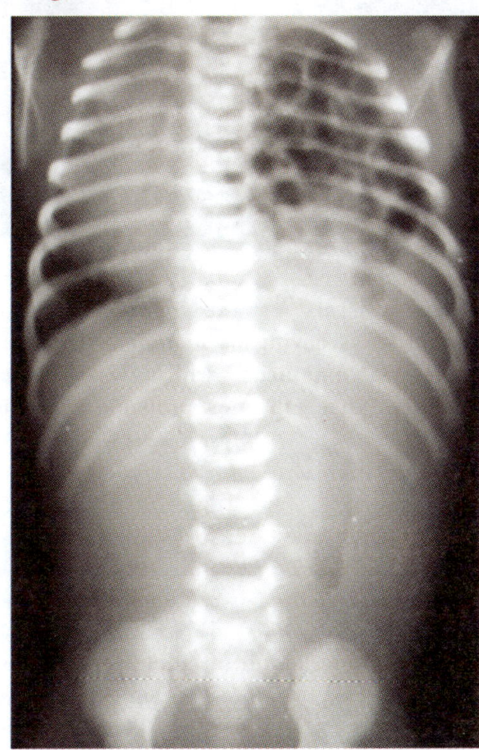

a. Pneumonia
b. Bochdalek hernia
c. Hiatus hernia
d. Pneumothorax

84. A 3-week-old male child was brought to the emergency with multiple episodes of non bilious vomiting. Barium meal image is given below. What is the diagnosis? ***(Most Recent Question Dec 2020)***

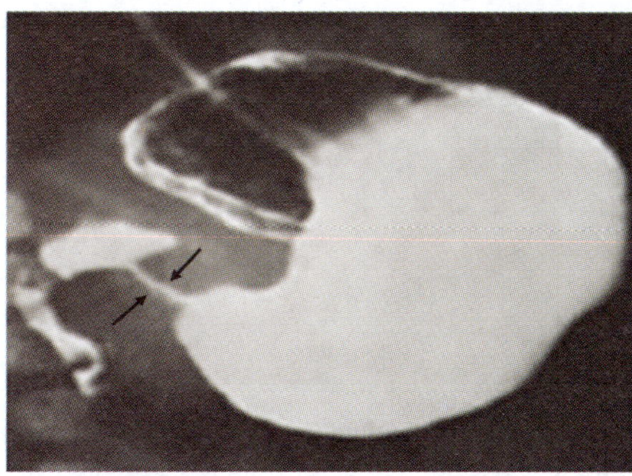

a. Duodenal atresia
b. Congenital hypertrophic pyloric stenosis
c. Annular pancreas
d. Gastric ulcer

85. The given postoperative X-ray abdomen is shown below. What is the most common electrolyte abnormality that can cause this condition? ***(Most Recent Question Dec 2020)***

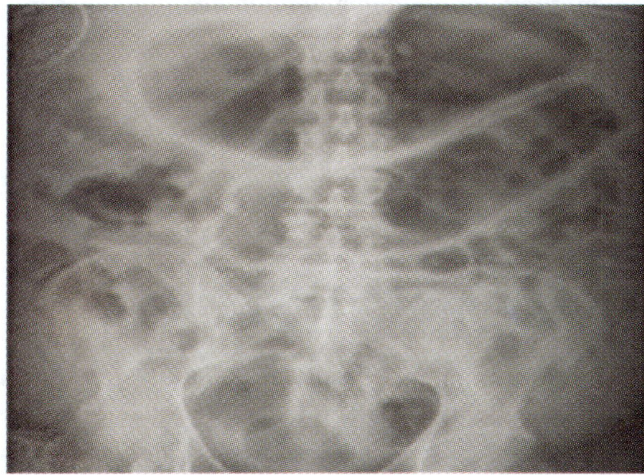

a. Hypokalemia
b. Hyperkalemia
c. Hyponatremia
d. Hypernatremia

86. A 25-year-old young female presented with abdominal swelling. The swelling was moving perpendicular to the line of attachment of mesentery. What is the most probable diagnosis? ***(Most Recent Question Dec 2020)***

a. Spigelian hernia
b. Peritoneal cyst
c. Pseudocyst of pancreas
d. Chylolymphatic cyst

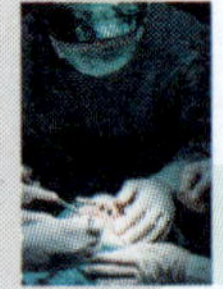

87. While performing surgery on a 2-year-old child for acute appendicitis, the structure given in the image was found, 2 feet proximal to ileocecal junction. It was measuring 2 inches in length. What is the diagnosis?
(Most Recent Question Dec 2020)

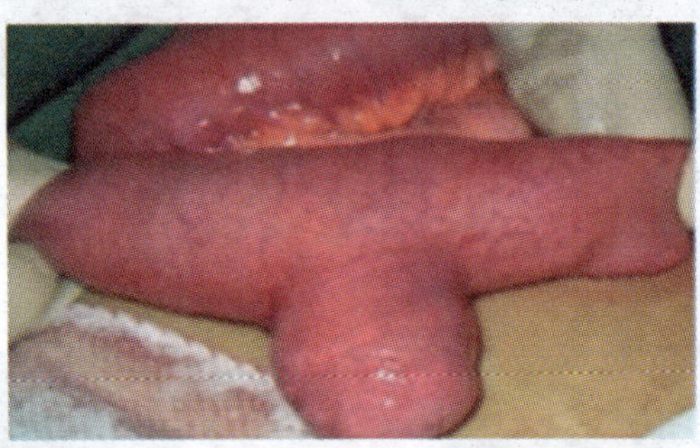

a. Meckel's diverticulum
b. Appendicitis
c. Sarcoma
d. Zenker's diverticulum

88. What is the name of stoma created after surgery for colon cancer, whose image is given below?
(Most Recent Question Dec 2020)

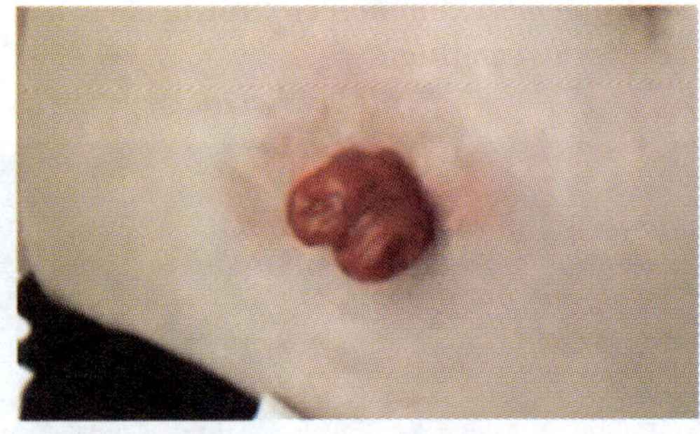

a. Loop colostomy b. End colostomy
c. Loop ileostomy d. End ileostomy

89. A patient has been complaining of wetting of underwear with profuse purulent discharge even after multiple cleaning attempts. What is the most probable diagnosis?
(Most Recent Question Dec 2020)

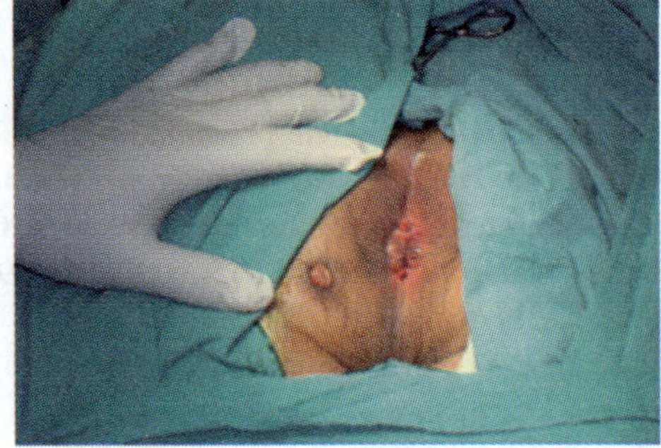

a. Pilonidal cyst b. Perianal abscess
c. Hemorrhoids d. Anal fistula

90. What is the diagnosis on the basis of image given below?
(Most Recent Question Dec 2020)

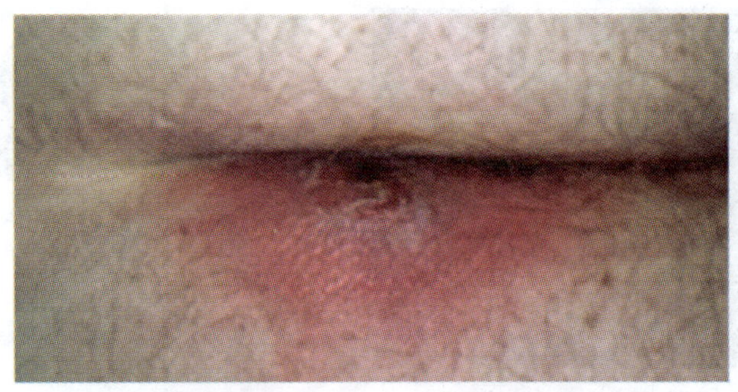

a. Perianal abscess b. Anorectal fistula
c. Haemorrhoids d. Pilonidal sinus

91. What is the diagnosis on the basis of image given below?
(Most Recent Question Dec 2020)

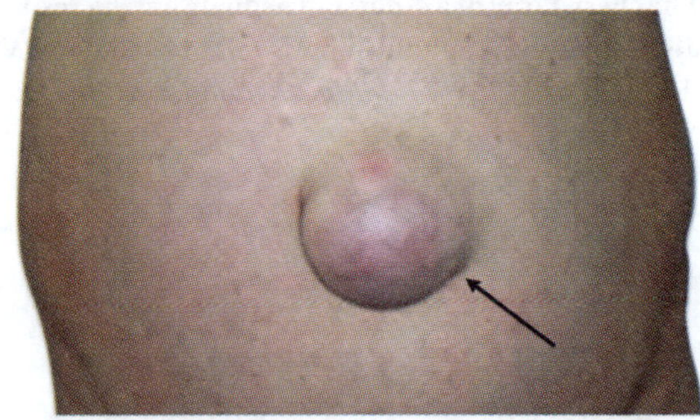

a. Umbilical hernia b. Paraumbilical hernia
c. Epigastric hernia d. Inguinal hernia

92. A newborn was having herniation of liver and small intestine via umbilicus, which was covered with membranes. What is the most probable diagnosis?
(Most Recent Question Dec 2020)

a. Epigastric hernia b. Ectopia vesicae
c. Omphalocele d. Gastroschisis

93. Dohlman operation is done for?
(Most Recent Question Dec 2020)

a. Pharyngeal pouch b. Esophageal web
c. Anal stenosis d. Schatzki ring

94. Specific tumor marker for carcinoma pancreas is:
(Most Recent Question Aug 2020)

a. CA19-9
b. CEA
c. Neuron -specific enolase
d. AFP

95. Which of the following is the characteristic feature associated with Barrett's esophagus?
(Most Recent Question Aug 2020)

a. Squamous metaplasia
b. Gastric metaplasia with goblet cells
c. Intestinal metaplasia with goblet cells
d. Severe dysplasia

96. The given image of barium swallow suggests the diagnosis of: ***(Most Recent Question Aug 2020)***

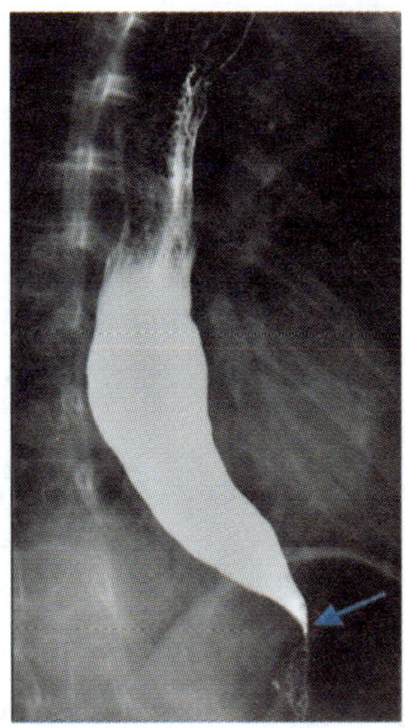

a. Achalasia cardia
b. Diffuse esophageal spasm
c. Nutcrackers esophagus
d. Carcinoma esophagus

97. A 35-year-old obese man underwent Laparoscopic Nissen's fundoplication of GORD. 6 hours post-operatively he feels fine and is stable. Which of the following is the most appropriate step in management of this patient? ***(Most Recent Question Aug 2020)***

a. Monitor vitals hourly
b. Insert chest tube and monitor hourly drain
c. Perform ABG serially
d. Respiratory muscles and lower limb physiotherapy

98. What is the diagnosis based on the given image of barium enema? ***(Most Recent Question Aug 2020)***

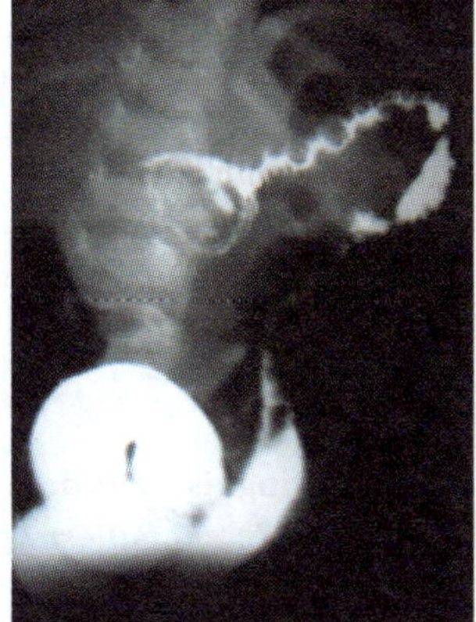

a. Hirschsprung's disease
b. Sigmoid volvulus
c. Carcinoma colon
d. Intussusception

99. A resected appendix specimen is shown below. Patient had raised serum chromogranin levels. The diagnosis is: ***(Most Recent Question Aug 2020)***

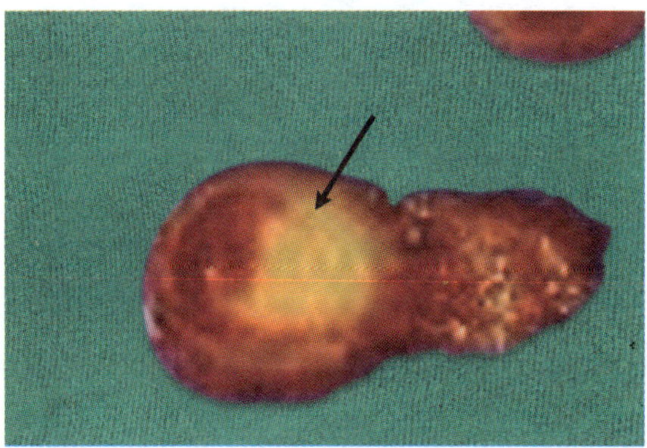

a. Mucocele
b. Mucinous cystadenocarcinoma
c. Adenocarcinoma with signet cell appearance
d. Carcinoid tumor

100. Which of the following is not the incision used for appendicectomy? ***(Most Recent Question Aug 2020)***

a. Kocher's incision
b. Rutherford Morrison incision
c. Lanz incision
d. Grid-iron incision

101. Which of the following is not done in a case of Fissure in ano? ***(Most Recent Question Aug 2020)***

a. Sitz bath
b. Topical calcium channel blockers
c. Proctoscopy
d. High fiber diet

102. A 20-year-old female diagnosed with adenocarcinoma stomach and on examination following lesion is seen. Diagnosis is: ***(Most Recent Question Dec 2019)***

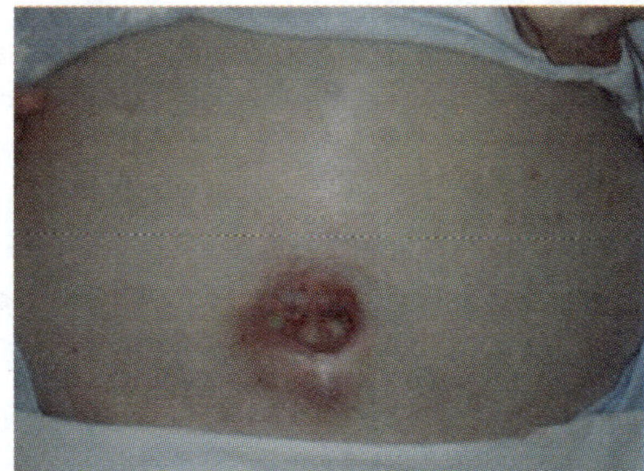

a. Sister Mary Joseph nodule
b. Busacca nodule
c. Infected umbilical hernia
d. Lisch nodule

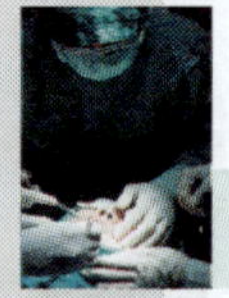

103. A child of 6 months was presented with following presentation. What is the management protocol? *(Most Recent Question Dec 2019)*

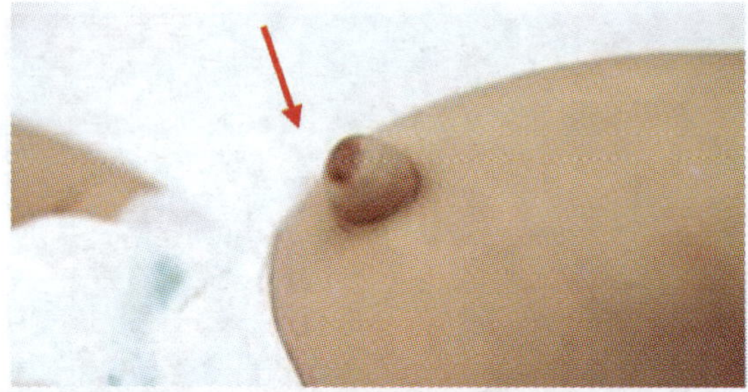

a. Surgery if persistence beyond 2 years of age even if asymptomatic
b. Surgery if persistence beyond 5 years of age only if symptomatic
c. Immediate surgery
d. Hernioplasty

104. A 28-year-old alcoholic patient walks to hospital with the complaints of multiple episodes of vomiting and chest pain after binge drinking. On per abdomen examination release sign is noted. X-ray abdomen in standing position shows pneumoperitoneum. The most probable reason for this presentation is: *(Most Recent Question Dec 2019)*

a. Boerrhave syndrome
b. Tension pneumothorax
c. PUD perforation
d. Mallory Weiss tear

105. Triad of abdominal pain, fever and jaundice is called: *(Most Recent Question Dec 2019)*

a. Charcot's triad
b. Saint's triad
c. Virchow triad
d. Murphy's triad

106. A 32-year-old man presented with fever and pain in upper right hypochondrium after food intake. Investigation of choice: *(Most Recent Question Dec 2019)*

a. CECT
b. Ultrasound
c. MRI
d. HRCT

107. All of the following are true about Crohn's disease; EXCEPT: *(Most Recent Question Dec 2019)*

a. Recurrence is more common
b. Rectum is involved
c. Serpiginous ulcers are formed
d. Transmural involvement

108. A 7-day-old infant presents with bilious vomiting and gross abdominal distention with absent bowel sounds. X-ray abdomen shows multiple gas filled loops. Diagnosis is: *(Most Recent Question 2019)*

a. Hirschsprung disease
b. Congenital Hypertrophic pyloric stenosis
c. Duodenal atresia
d. Malrotation of gut

109. Meconium ileus is a presentation seen in which of the following diseases? *(Most Recent Question 2019)*

a. Mucoviscidosis
b. Hirschsprung disease
c. Ileal atresia
d. Congenital aganglionosis

110. Which is the first investigation to be done in case of Neonate presenting with frothiness in mouth and dyspnea? *(Most Recent Question 2019)*

a. Bronchoscopy with injection of methylene blue
b. NG Tube insertion and CXR to check position of tube
c. CT chest
d. Endoscopy

111. Seat Belt injury leads to: *(Most Recent Question 2019)*

a. Splenic laceration
b. Splenic contusion
c. Gut ischemia
d. Mesenteric adenitis

112. What is the location of Killian dehiscence? *(Most Recent Question 2019)*

a. Below Superior constrictor
b. Below Inferior constrictor
c. Below cricopharyngeal muscle
d. Below upper 1/3rd of smooth muscle of oesophagus

113. MC immediate complication of splenectomy: *(Recent Pattern Question 2018-19)*

a. Hemorrhage
b. Fistula
c. Bleeding from gastric mucosa
d. Pancreatitis

114. Best treatment strategy for Anal cancer: *(Recent Pattern Question 2018-19)*

a. Chemoradiation
b. Surgery
c. Radiation
d. Chemotherapy

115. Which is false about Crohn's disease? *(Recent Pattern Question 2018-19)*

a. No occurrence after surgery
b. Aphthous ulcer
c. Skip lesions
d. Fistula formation

116. Which of the following is not done in Carcinoma oesophagus? *(Recent Pattern Question 2018-19)*

a. Biopsy
b. pH-metry
c. CT chest
d. PET scan

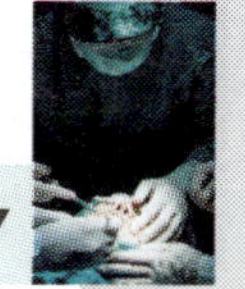

117. A 30-year-old man presents with a four days history of right iliac fossa pain. USG image is shown below. Which is the best management algorithm?

(Recent Pattern Question 2018-19)

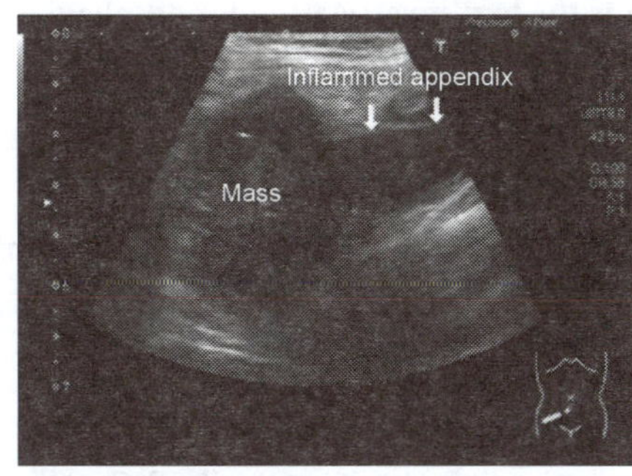

a. Ochsner-Sherren regimen
b. Urgent appendectomy
c. Extraperitoneal drainage and parenteral antibiotics
d. Per cutaneous drainage and parenteral antibiotics

118. Comment on the diagnosis of a film shown of a 65-year-old man with acute abdomen.

(Recent Pattern Question 2018-19)

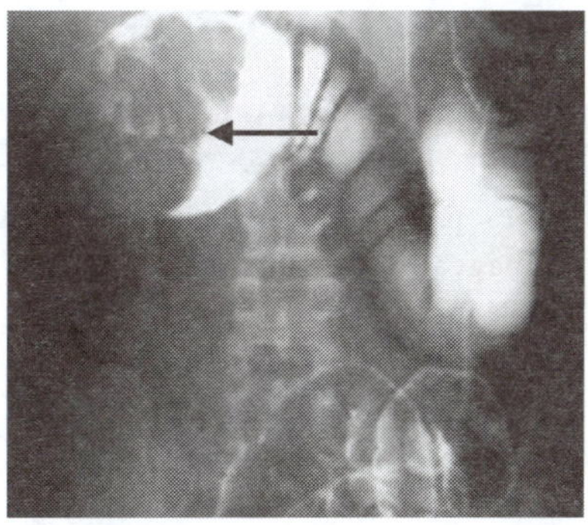

a. Ileocolic intussusception
b. Sigmoid volvulus
c. Toxic megacolon
d. Colocolic intussusception

119. Surgery is indicated in Ulcerative Colitis in all; EXCEPT:

(Recent Pattern Question 2018-19)

a. Toxic megacolon b. Colonic perforation
c. Colonic obstruction d. Refractory fistula

120. Which is the most common site of the carcinoma of the esophagus? ***(Recent Pattern Question 2018)***

a. Lower 1/3rd b. Middle 1/3rd
c. Upper 1/3rd d. GE junction

121. A 9-month-old child presents with excessive cry, right iliac fossa sausage lump and blood in stools. What is the best treatment? ***(Recent Pattern Question 2018)***

a. IVF-antibiotic-NG tube
b. IVF-antibiotic-air enema
c. IVF-antibiotics-barium enema
d. IVF-antibiotics-warm saline enema

122. Metastatic liver disease is found in _____% of patients undergoing surgery for primary colorectal cancer?

(Recent Pattern Question 2018)

a. 10% b. 15%
c. 33% d. 75%

123. Which is the most common cause of hypergastrinemia?

a. Postvagotomy ***(Recent Pattern Question 2018)***
b. Regular use of PPI
c. Resection of small intestine
d. Atrophic gastritis

124. What prefix symbol is used to describe the administration of neo-adjuvant treatment given in colorectal cancer?

(Recent Pattern Question 2017)

a. h b. p
c. y d. z

125. A 20-year-old patient presents with RIF pain and fever. USG is shown in image. Diagnosis is:

(Recent Pattern Question 2017)

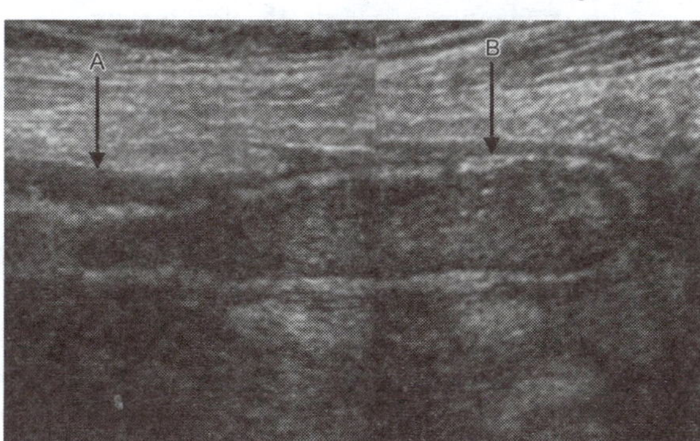

a. Acute appendicitis
b. Intussusception
c. Volvulus
d. Intestinal obstruction

126. Gastric outlet obstruction leads to:

(Recent Pattern Question 2017)

a. Hypochloremic metabolic alkalosis
b. Hyperchloremic metabolic acidosis
c. Hypernatremic metabolic alkalosis
d. Hyponatremic metabolic acidosis

127. Dysphagia lusoria is due to:

(Recent Pattern Question 2017)

a. Aberrant blood vessel
b. Esophageal diverticulum
c. Duodenal obstruction
d. Gastric outlet obstruction

128. Which is the most common site of origin of peritoneal deposits? ***(Recent Pattern Question 2016)***

a. Stomach cancer
b. Colorectal cancer
c. Pancreatic cancer
d. Ovarian cancer

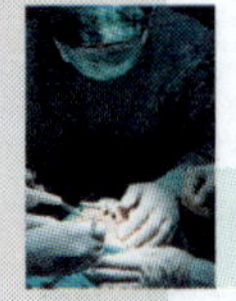

129. What does the arrow in the given CT abdomen show? *(Recent Pattern Question 2016)*

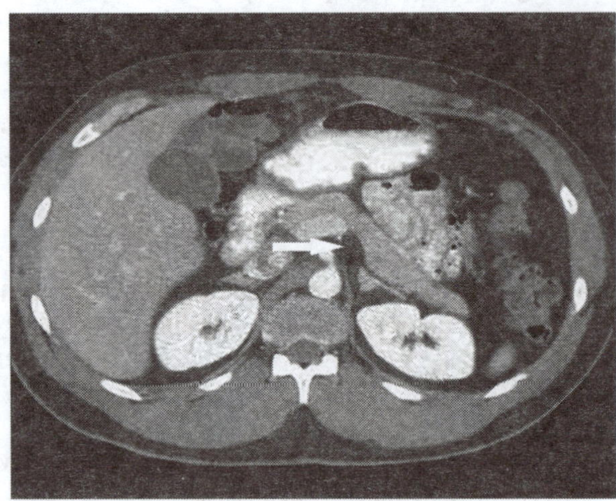

a. Left adrenal gland b. Pancreas
c. Lesser omentum d. Epiploic foramen

130. Which of the following is associated with Gardner syndrome? *(Recent Pattern Question 2016)*

a. Retinoblastoma b. Neuroblastoma
c. Desmoid tumor d. Dermoid cyst

131. Hypertrophic pyloric stenosis presents at: *(Recent Pattern Question 2016)*

a. 3 day b. 3 weeks
c. 3 month d. 3 years

132. A 40-year-old chronic alcoholic presents with distended abdomen, hematemesis and fresh blood in stool. On examination huge ascites and distended veins over abdominal wall are noted. Most likely cause of hematemesis is: *(Recent Pattern Question 2016)*

a. Esophagitis
b. Esophageal varices
c. Esophageal cancer
d. Erosion of gastroduodenal artery

133. A 30-year-old known alcoholic presents to the emergency with massive Upper GIT bleeding. On examination pulse = 110/min and BP = 80/60. First step to be taken is: *(Recent Pattern Question 2016)*

a. Cold saline lavage
b. Immediate BT
c. Transfer for urgent sclerotherapy
d. Large bore cannula for IVF

134. Which is the rarest position of appendix? *(Recent Pattern Question 2016)*

a. Retro-caecal b. Post-ileal
c. Pre-ileal d. Para-caecal

135. Which is the best way to diagnose lower small intestine obstruction? *(Recent Pattern Question 2016)*

a. Pain abdomen b. Multiple air fluid levels
c. Profuse bilious vomiting d. Feculent vomiting

136. What is the location of first constriction of esophagus from the incisor tooth?

a. 15 cm b. 18 cm
c. 25 cm d. 40 cm

137. Which is the best investigation for dysphagia?

a. Enteroscopy
b. Barium swallow
c. Barium enema
d. Barium meal follow through

138. What is incorrect about Zenker's diverticulum?

a. Regurgitation of previous day food
b. Halitosis
c. Located at killian's triangle
d. Metabolic alkalosis

139. Achalasia Cardia presents with all; EXCEPT:

a. Halitosis
b. Regurgitation of previous day's food
c. Dysphagia (liquids > solids)
d. Corkscrew esophagus

140. Achalasia cardia presents with all; EXCEPT:

a. Increased lower esophagus sphincter tone
b. Normal peristalsis
c. Dilatation proximally
d. Malignancy

141. Dysphagia mainly for liquids is seen with:

a. Achalasia cardia b. Zenker diverticulum
c. Barrett's esophagus d. Diffuse esophageal spasm

142. Lower esophageal sphincter tone is due to:

a. Vasoactive intestinal peptide
b. Nitrous oxide
c. Acetylcholine
d. Pancreatic polypeptide

143. Pseudo-achalasia is seen with:

a. Chagas disease b. Scleroderma
c. Tumor infiltration d. Diffuse esophageal spasm

144. Which Metaplasia occurs in lower esophagus in a smoker?

a. Gastric metaplasia
b. Goblet cells intestinal metaplasia
c. Esophageal metaplasia
d. Intestinal dysplasia

145. Which of the following is more prone to Carcinoma?

a. Barrett esophagus b. Boerhaave syndrome
c. Mallory Weiss tear d. Esophageal varices

146. Scoring of esophageal reflux is done by:

a. Ranson score b. Gleason score
c. Alvarado score d. De meester scoring

147. Which is the best investigation for detecting esophageal perforation?

a. CXR b. CT chest
c. Upper G.I. endoscopy d. CT chest with contrast

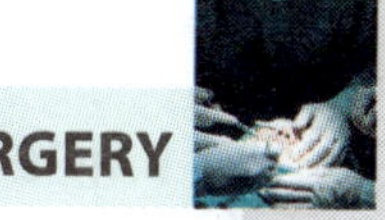

148. Para-esophageal hernia is best diagnosed by:
- a. Chest X-ray
- b. Barium study
- c. CT scan
- d. Endoscopic ultrasound

149. To differentiate malignancy from benign lesion in GIT. What is the investigation of choice?
- a. USG
- b. Biopsy
- c. Endoscopy
- d. P.E.T scan

150. Dysphagia lusoria is due to:
- a. Aberrant right subclavian artery
- b. Aberrant left subclavian artery
- c. Aberrant internal carotid artery
- d. Aberrant innominate artery

151. Boerhaave syndrome is:
- a. Spontaneous Rupture of esophagus
- b. Traumatic rupture of esophagus
- c. Tear at gastro-esophageal junction
- d. Foreign body esophagus

152. Which is the most important factor for development of appendicitis and its complications?
- a. Bacterial proliferation
- b. Age
- c. Increased dietary fiber
- d. Bowel lumen obstruction

153. Mc-burney's point is:
- a. 1/3rd distance from left anterior superior iliac spine
- b. 2/3rd distance from the anterior superior iliac spine
- c. 1/3rd distance from the umbilicus to ASIS
- d. 1/3rd distance from right anterior superior spine

154. A 25-year-old young male presented with a tender mass in right iliac fossa. On physical examination he has pain and fixed flexed hip. Diagnosis is:
- a. Psoas abscess
- b. Appendicitis
- c. Amoeboma
- d. Ileocaecal TB

155. Which is the best guide to finding appendix intra operatively?
- a. Locate ileo-ceacal junction
- b. Locate the blind tube of appendix
- c. Locate the anterior taenia of the caecum
- d. Locate the mesenteric supply

156. Identify the structure shown in the given picture

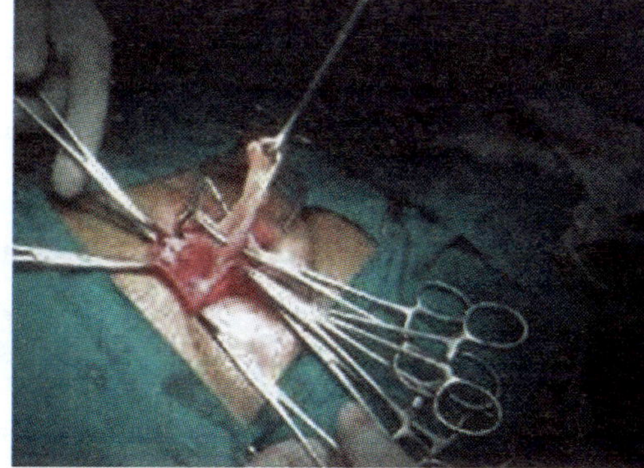

- a. Appendix
- b. Meckel diverticulum
- c. Diverticulosis
- d. Ligament of Treitz

157. What will be the location of appendix in silent appendix?
- a. Pelvic
- b. Preileal
- c. Retrocaecal
- d. Pelvic

158. MANTREL score is done for:
- a. Acute appendicitis
- b. Acute pancreatitis
- c. Acute cholecystitis
- d. Acute salpingitis

159. In a child which of the following diseases is misdiagnosed as appendicitis?
- a. Gastroenteritis
- b. Lymphadenitis
- c. Intussusception
- d. All of these

160. Ochsner sherren regimen is used for management of:
- a. Appendicular mass
- b. Appendicular abscess
- c. Appendicitis
- d. Peritonitis following appendicitis

161. What is true about Carcinoid tumor?
- a. Always benign
- b. Kulchitsky cell tumor
- c. Present with paroxysmal hypertension
- d. Punch biopsy is diagnostic

162. Carcinoid tumor is seen most commonly in?
- a. Ileum
- b. Rectum
- c. Appendix
- d. Duodenum

163. What is incorrect about peritonitis?
- a. Most common cause is P.U.D
- b. Bile causes more damage than blood in peritoneum
- c. X-ray abdomen shows Gas under diaphragm
- d. Absence of free gas rules out peritonitis

164. Which is the most common organism seen in gastrointestinal perforation peritonitis?
- a. Staph aureus
- b. Pneumococcus
- c. Anaerobic streptococcus
- d. Coagulase-negative staphylococci

165. Non-intestinal peritonitis in females is caused by:
- a. E. coli
- b. Klebsiella
- c. Chlamydia
- d. Bacteroides

166. Which is the most common tumor of retro-peritoneum?
- a. Stroma
- b. Sarcoma
- c. Teratoma
- d. Retro-teratoma

167. Which is the most common presentation of retroperitoneal tumor?
- a. Abdominal pain
- b. Hydronephrosis
- c. Constipation
- d. Abdominal lump

168. Adult patient developing intussusception is due to?
- a. Carcinoid tumor
- b. Mesenteric insufficiency
- c. Villous adenoma
- d. Bariatric surgery

169. All are true about intestinal obstruction radiographically; EXCEPT?
- a. Supine abdominal film is done
- b. More than 2 air fluid levels
- c. Small intestine dilation >3 cm
- d. Pneumatosis intestinalis

170. Best treatment protocol of a enterogenic cyst?
a. Enucleation
b. Resection with intestine part
c. Aspiration with marsupialization
d. Observe

171. On removing whole colon (total colectomy) what will be the most common complication?
a. Anastomotic leak
b. Dyselectrolytemia
c. Death
d. Fulminant sepsis

172. Which of the following is NOT seen in pyloric stenosis:
a. Projectile vomiting
b. Paradoxical aciduria
c. Bilious vomiting
d. Metabolic acidosis

173. Congenital pyloric stenosis presents with?
a. Hypokalemic metabolic acidosis
b. Hypokalemic metabolic alkalosis
c. Hyperkalemic metabolic acidosis
d. Hyperkalemic metabolic alkalosis

174. In Hypertrophic pyloric stenosis, which of the following is seen?
a. Metabolic acidosis
b. Metabolic alkalosis
c. Metabolic alkalosis with paradoxical bicarbonaturia
d. All of the above

175. Which of the following polyp is least likely to turn malignant?
a. Inflammatory polyp
b. Familial adenomatous polyposis
c. Hamartomatous polyp
d. Hyperplastic polyp

176. All are surgical indications in Crohn's disease; EXCEPT:
a. Colonic obstruction
b. Refractory fistula
c. Massive hemorrhage
d. Toxic megacolon

177. A child is passing blood with act of defecation. The probable diagnosis is
a. Juvenile rectal polyp
b. Adenomatous polyposis
c. Rectal ulcer
d. Post Surgery

178. Earliest complication of ileostomy is:
a. Obstruction
b. Necrosis
c. Diarrhea
d. Prolapse

179. Post resection of terminal ileum, deficiency of which of the following vitamins is seen along with Steatorrhea?
a. B_{12}
b. B_9
c. C
d. B_6

180. Denver shunt is used in:
a. Ascites
b. Dialysis
c. Raised ICP
d. Headache

181. ROME criteria is for?
a. IBS
b. Colonic cancer
c. Ulcerative colitis
d. Colonic hemangioma

182. What is the cause of chronic tropical pancreatitis?
a. Parasitic infection
b. Malnutrition
c. Idiopathic
d. Genetic

183. Severity of pancreatitis can be best assessed by:
a. Serial Serum amylase
b. Stool trypsin levels
c. RANSON Score
d. ARDS development

184. Which is not included in APACHE score?
a. Serum bilirubin
b. GCS score
c. pH of blood
d. Age of patient

185. What is the most common complication after ERCP?
a. Acute pancreatitis
b. Pseudopancreatic cyst
c. Chronic pancreatitis
d. Necrotizing pancreatitis

186. Lisch nodule is seen in:
a. Neurofibromatosis
b. Multiple endocrine neoplasia 2A
c. Turcot syndrome
d. Familial adenomatous polyposis

187. In case of annular pancreas, what is the surgery of choice?
a. Duodeno-duodenostomy
b. Duodenojejunostomy
c. Pancreato-jejunostomy
d. Porto-enterostomy

188. Not a early post-operative complication of splenectomy is:
a. Thrombocytosis
b. Splenosis
c. Sub diaphragmatic abscess
d. Pulmonary complications

189. Which of the following is a side effect of vagotomy?
a. Delayed gastric emptying
b. Gastric atony
c. Diarrhea
d. All of these

190. Pseudo obstruction of intestine is also known as
a. Hartmann's syndrome
b. Ozili's syndrome
c. Ogilvie's syndrome
d. Mirizzi syndrome

191. What is the most common site of gastric ulcer?
a. Duodenal cap
b. Lesser curvature
c. Second part of duodenum
d. Greater curvature

192. Posterior perforation of ulcer in Antral canal will lead to fluid deposition in:
a. Greater Omentum
b. Right Sub-phrenic abscess
c. Sub-hepatic space
d. Lesser sac

193. Purtscher's Retinopathy is due to:
a. Acute pancreatitis
b. Chronic pancreatitis
c. Meckel's diverticulum
d. Diverticulitis

194. What is the etiology of type-A gastritis?
a. Hypersensitivity reaction I
b. Autoimmune
c. Bacterial
d. Viral

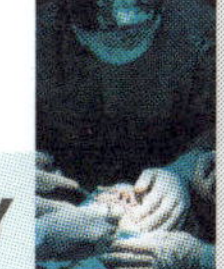

195. What is the most common location of lymphoma in the GIT?

a. Stomach b. Ileum
c. Mesentery d. Colon

196. Sister Mary Joseph nodule is commonly seen with:

a. Ovarian CA b. Colon CA
c. Pancreatic CA d. Stomach CA

197. Krukenburg tumor originates from:

a. Liver b. Stomach
c. Ovary d. Gallbladder

198. Angiodysplasia is seen in:

a. Stomach of adult b. Jejunum of a child
c. Left side of the colon d. Right side of the colon

199. Which of the following is not a type of mesenteric cyst?

a. Mesothelial b. Enterogenous
c. Chylolymphatic d. Epidermoid

200. What is the most common type of mesenteric cyst?

a. Simple (mesothelial cyst)
b. Chylolymphatic cyst
c. Enterogenous
d. Dermoid

201. Immunoproliferative lymphoma presents with:

a. Obstruction b. Peritonitis
c. Chronic diarrhea d. Tenesmus

202. Which of following is used for initial management of rectal prolapse in children?

a. Digital positioning
b. Transanal surgery
c. Injection sclerotherapy
d. Resection rectopexy

203. Which is not a cause of acute anal pain?

a. Thrombosed hemorrhoids
b. Acute anal fissure
c. Fistula in ano
d. Perianal abscess

204. Which of the following is seen in case of fistula in ano?

a. Purulent discharge with bleeding
b. Serous discharge with bleeding
c. Painful bleeding with constipation
d. Painless bleeding with constipation

205. Goodsall's rule in fistula in ano is used for distinguishing:

a. High and low fistula
b. Anterior and posterior fistula
c. External and internal fistula
d. Lateral and medial fistula

206. Which is the most common cancer of anus?

a. Adenocarcinoma b. Squamous cell CA
c. Basal cell CA d. Melanoma

207. Which is the most common cancer of anus?

a. Squamous b. Basaloid
c. Cuboidal d. Cloacogenic

208. Anal cancer is associated with:

a. Human papilloma virus b. EBV
c. HTLV-1 d. Polyoma virus

209. What is the most common site of metastases of carcinoma rectum?

a. Lung b. Liver
c. Brain d. Vertebra

210. The following image shows

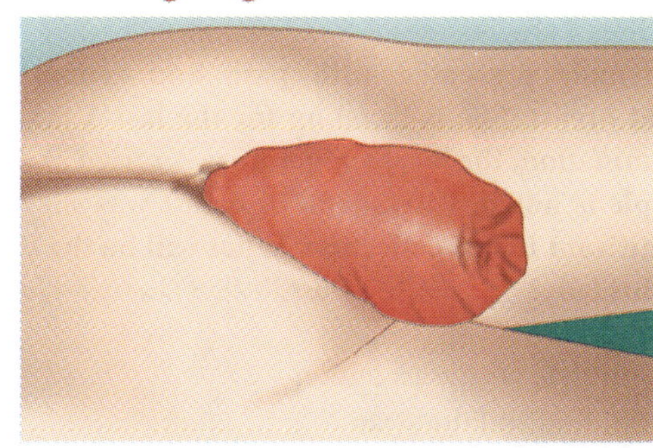

a. Rectal prolapse b. Fistula in ano
c. Perianal abscess d. Rectal cancer

211. MC complication after hemorrhoidectomy:

a. Prolapse b. Urine retention
c. Fecal incontinence d. Bleeding

212. What is incorrect about anal canal?

a. 1/3rd above dentate line and 2/3rd below the dentate line
b. Extraperitoneal
c. Anoderm is painful
d. Keratinization

213. What is true about Ischiorectal fossa boundaries?

a. Anterior border is formed by inferior fascia of urogenital diaphragm.
b. Superior border is formed by Gluteus Maximus
c. Lateral border is formed by Levator Ani
d. Posterior border is formed by obturator internus muscle.

214. What is the diagnosis?

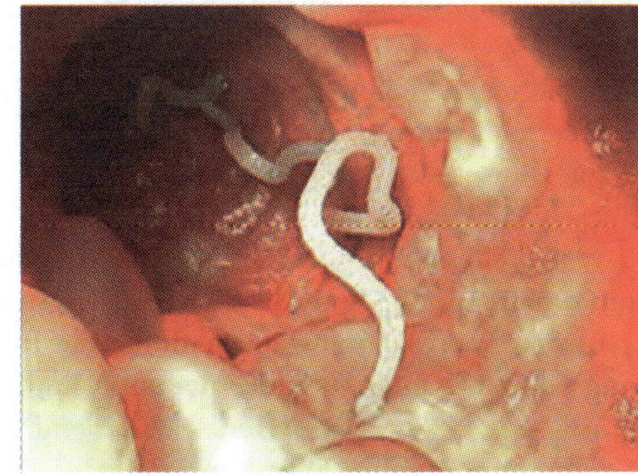

a. Perforation by Ascariasis
b. Volvulus by Ascariasis
c. Ascending cholangitis by Ascariasis
d. Solitary ascariasis in the bowel

BREAST

215. A 30-year-old lady presents with mobile breast lump which she describes as breast mouse. Most likely diagnosis: ***(Most Recent Question June 2022)***

a. Phyllodes tumor
b. Fibroadenoma
c. Invasive ductal carcinoma
d. Breast abscess

216. A female presented with pain and redness of the right breast. She is lactating for the last 3 months. On examination, the local temperature is raised and cracked nipple is noted. Ultrasound of breast was suggestive of significant liquid collection. What will be the treatment in this lady? ***(Most Recent Question June 2022)***

a. Antibiotics
b. Multiple needle aspiration
c. Incision and drainage
d. Breast support

217. A lady presented with breast lump in the lower outer quadrant of the breast which was histologically confirmed as an invasive breast cancer of no special type. Which of the following has better prognosis? ***(Most Recent Question June 2022)***

a. Mucinous breast cancer
b. Overexpression of Her–2 neu gene
c. High mitotic index
d. Axillary lymph node involvement

218. Which of the following breast cancer has the best prognosis? ***(Most Recent Question Dec. 2021)***

a. Triple negative breast cancer
b. Luminal A
c. Her–2 neu
d. Luminal B

219. A 25-year-old female presented with history of painful, red, fluctuant 2 cm mass in the right breast after 3 days of delivery. On ultrasound, collection was present. Which of the following is the most appropriate management? ***(Most Recent Question Dec. 2021)***

a. Antibiotics and follow-up for 3 days
b. Hot fermentation
c. Express the milk every three hours
d. Incision and drainage

220. A 32-year-old female presented to OPD with 2 cm single, asymptomatic mobile lump in the right breast, noticed by patient on breast self-examination. The lump was diagnosed to be benign. What advice will you give to the patient? ***(Most Recent Question Dec. 2021)***

a. Observation + regular follow-up
b. Excision + histology
c. Biopsy
d. Give danazol

221. In the pathological examination of breast cancer, signet-ring were found. What can be the likely diagnosis? ***(Most Recent Question June 2021)***

a. Ductal carcinoma *in situ*
b. Lobular carcinoma
c. Invasive ductal carcinoma NOS
d. Phyllodes tumor

222. A 30-year-old patient presented to OPD with the left sided breast lump. On examination, it was hard and irregular in shape but mobile over the chest wall. What is the most probable diagnosis? ***(Most Recent Question Dec 2020)***

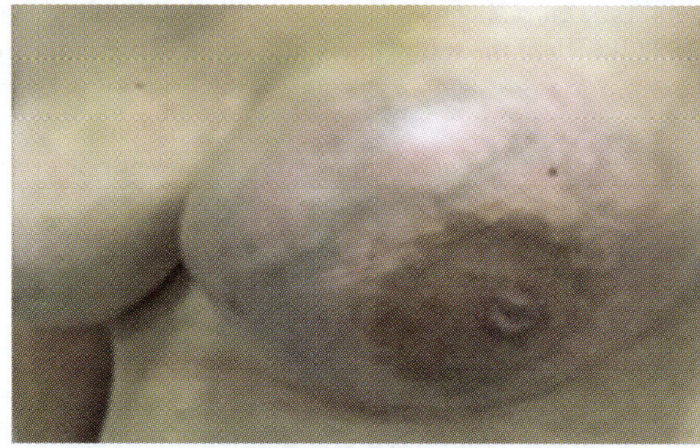

a. Breast abscess
b. Breast cancer
c. Phyllodes tumor
d. Fibroadenoma

223. After breast cancer surgery, patient developed following abnormality. Which of the following is the possible reason? ***(Most Recent Question Dec 2020)***

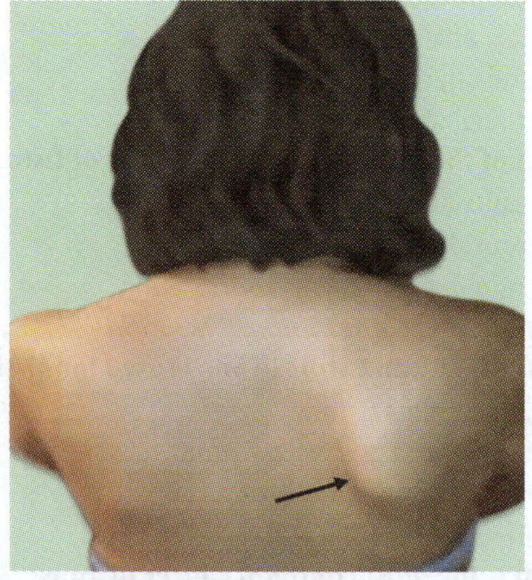

a. Injury to long thoracic nerve
b. Paralysis of latissimus dorsi muscle
c. Paralysis of deltoid muscle
d. Paralysis of suprascapular nerve

224. In a patient with solitary thyroid swelling, what is the first investigation the surgeon should advice before planning thyroid surgery? *(Most Recent Question Aug 2020)*

a. TFT
b. FNAC
c. Biopsy
d. Ultrasound

225. A lactating female presented with complaints of pain in one breast. On examination, the affected breast was tender and engorged. Baby refused to feed from the affected breast. What is the preferred treatment option? *(Most Recent Question Aug 2020)*

a. Antibiotics only
b. NSAIDs
c. Warm compresses
d. Incision and drainage with antibiotics

226. Which patient has better prognosis in breast cancer? *(Most Recent Question Dec 2019)*

a. Luminal A
b. Luminal B
c. Triple negative
d. Her2+

227. Dye for Sentinel Lymph node biopsy is injected in which of the following sites? *(Recent Pattern Question 2018-19)*

a. Axilla
b. Tail of spence
c. Nipple
d. Areola

228. Correct description about Paget's disease of breast? *(Recent Pattern Question 2018-19)*

a. Eczema of skin of nipple
b. Eczema of skin of areola
c. Mastitis carcinomatosis
d. Atrophic scirrhous carcinoma

229. MC benign breast tumor? *(Recent Pattern Question 2018-19)*

a. Fibroadenoma
b. Fibroadenosis
c. D.C.I.S
d. Phyllodes tumor

230. Breast triple assessment contains all; EXCEPT? *(Recent Pattern Question 2018-19)*

a. Clinical examination
b. Axillary Sampling
c. USG
d. FNAC and biopsy

231. Which of the following is not an indication for Fibro-adenoma surgery? *(Recent Pattern Question 2018)*

a. Patient's decision
b. Size more than 5 cm
c. Complex type
d. Recurrence

232. In a breast lump of 4 cm no nodal metastasis is present. Which is the stage of breast cancer? *(Recent Pattern Question 2018)*

a. Stage I
b. Stage II
c. Stage III
d. Stage IV

233. Peau d'orange appearance in breast cancer is seen with which stage of cancer? *(Recent Pattern Question 2017)*

a. T4A
b. T4B
c. T4C
d. T4D

234. Breast cancer more than 5 cm is defined as stage_____ *(Recent Pattern Question 2017)*

a. T1
b. T2
c. T3
d. T4

235. What is the diagnosis of the mammography report in a 30-year-old woman with breast lump felt on self-examination of breast? *(Recent Pattern Question 2017)*

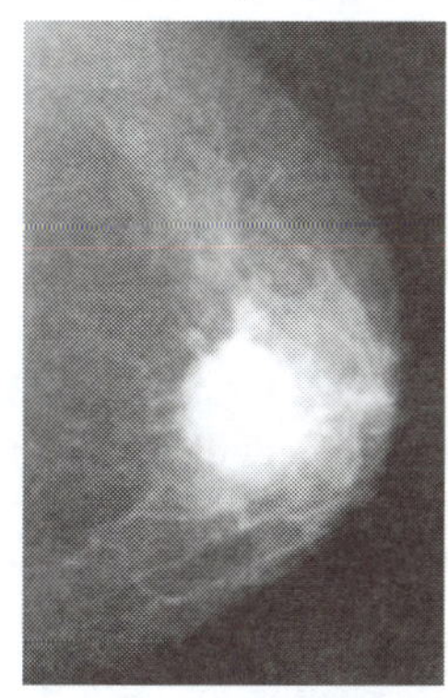

a. Fibroadenoma
b. Breast cancer
c. Fibroadenosis
d. Brodie's Serocystic disease

236. Which is the most common quadrant for carcinoma Breast? *(Recent Pattern Question 2016)*

a. Lower outer
b. Lower inner
c. Upper outer
d. Upper inner

237. Which is the most common Familial Breast cancer gene? *(Recent Pattern Question 2016)*

a. BRCA1
b. BRCA 2
c. Li-Fraumeni syndrome
d. STK 11

238. Skin of nipple and areola drains to which lymph node? *(Recent Pattern Question 2016)*

a. Anterior axillary
b. Supra-clavicular
c. Central
d. Infra-clavicular

239. A 25-year-old female presents with a breast lump and green discharge from inverted nipples. What is the first differential diagnosis? *(Recent Pattern Question 2016)*

a. Duct ectasia
b. Mastitis
c. Carcinoma
d. Paget's disease

240. Young female with painless, mobile lump of 4 cm in a breast. What is the diagnosis?

a. Breast abscess
b. Breast cyst
c. Fibroadenoma
d. Peau d'orange

241. Which breast cancer involves both breasts?

a. Lobular carcinoma
b. Mucoid carcinoma
c. Ductal carcinoma
d. Ductal carcinoma in situ

242. A biopsy of the opposite breast is considered in which of the following types of breast carcinoma?

a. Comedo carcinoma
b. Medullary carcinoma
c. Mucinous carcinoma
d. Lobular carcinoma

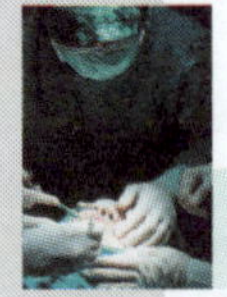

243. What is correct regarding Peau d'orange in breast carcinoma?
a. Infiltration of cooper's ligament with cancer cells
b. Infiltration of skin of breast with cancer cells
c. Associated with lobular carcinoma of breast
d. Good prognosis

244. Tissue diagnosis of Breast lump in pregnant lady is made by?
a. FNAC b. Core cut biopsy
c. Mammography d. MRI

245. Which is the next investigation to be done for painful breast lump in a lactating woman?
a. Mammography b. USG
c. MRI d. FNAC

246. All are true about Paget's disease of breast; EXCEPT?
a. It is often bilateral
b. Crusting of areola skin
c. Lumpectomy is performed usually
d. Paget cells are positive for HER2/neu

247. In breast conservative surgery the healthy margin excised is typically?
a. 1 cm b. 2 cm
c. 3 cm d. 4 cm

248. A 35 year pregnant female came to your clinic with lump as shown in the image. What will be the initial screening method?

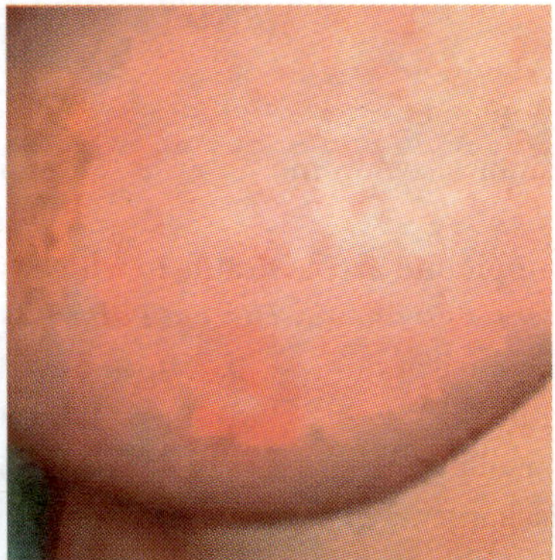

a. USG b. MRI
c. Mammogram d. FNAC

249. Breast cancer is called stage 4 when there is?
a. Involvement of chest wall b. Satellite lesion
c. Ulceration of surface skin d. Spreads to adrenal gland

250. As per AJCC breast cancer staging T4 is:
a. Distant metastasis
b. Satellite lesions
c. Spread to contralateral axillary lymph nodes
d. Sentinel lymph node involvement

251. Which is the most important prognostic factor for carcinoma breast?
a. HER2/Neu b. Histology grade
c. Tumor staging d. Tumor growth rate

252. What is the probable diagnosis?

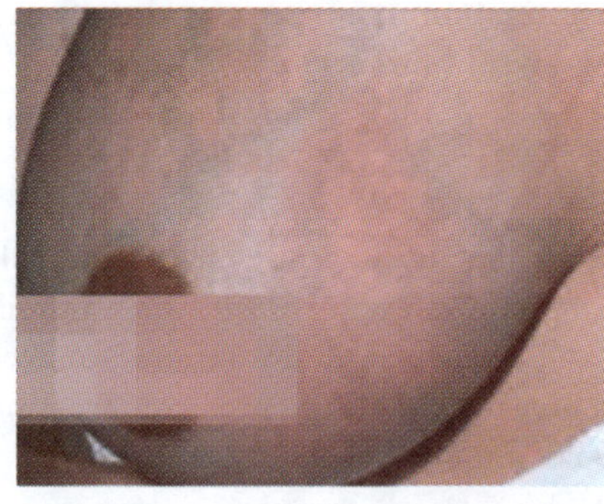

a. Mastitis b. Mondor disease
c. Cystosarcoma phyllodes d. Paget disease

253. Sentinel node biopsy is done for all; EXCEPT:
a. Colon carcinoma b. Ocular cancer
c. Breast cancer d. Malignant melanoma

254. Stage of 3 cm breast cancer involving 4 axillary lymph nodes
a. Stage I b. Stage II
c. Stage III d. Stage IV

255. A 28-year-old female presents with infiltrating breast carcinoma with 1 cm hard lump. T1-N0-M0. What is the best treatment?
a. Radical mastectomy
b. Simple mastectomy
c. Extended radical mastectomy
d. Super radical mastectomy

THYROID AND SALIVARY GLANDS

256. A 65-year-old male presented with weakness, lethargy, excessive cold intolerance and slow ankle jerk. On TFT. TSH = 16 mU/L (normal: 0.4-4.0 mU/L) and T4 = 0.3 ng/dL (normal: 0.6–1.6 ng/dL) and T3 = 70 pg/dL (normal: 230 - 619 pg/dL). What would be the most appropriate management? ***(Most Recent Question Dec. 2021)***
a. Start levothyroxine at 100 microgram and decrease the dose gradually
b. Start levothyroxine at 25 microgram and increase the dose gradually
c. Start levothyroxine at 25 microgram and decrease the dose gradually
d. Give Liothyronine and T4 drug simultaneously

257. A 23-year-old male presented with High BP along with profuse sweating and headache. Which initial investigation should be done in this case? ***(Most Recent Question Dec. 2021)***
a. 24 hours urinary metanephrines
b. 24 hours urinary 5HIAA
c. 24 hours urinary HVA
d. 24 hours urinary chromogranin A levels

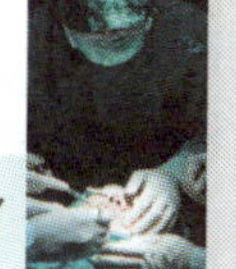

258. A patient presented with the presence of a thyroid swelling and weight loss. The physician found presence of cervical lymphadenopathy. Total thyroidectomy with radical lymph node dissection was performed. Histopathology report of the resected specimen is shown below. Which of the following is the most likely diagnosis?

(Most Recent Question Aug 2020)

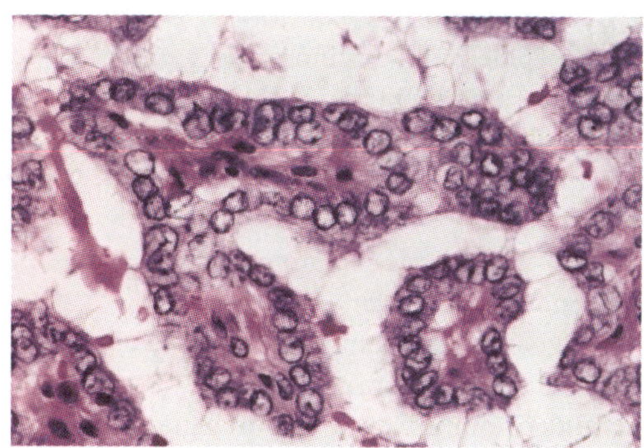

a. Papillary carcinoma thyroid
b. Follicular carcinoma thyroid
c. Medullary carcinoma thyroid
d. Anaplastic carcinoma thyroid

259. A 35-year-old women presented with complains of palpitations and weight loss on examination, sinus tachycardia is present and the following lesion was noticed on the shin of the patient. What is the clinical diagnosis?

(Most Recent Question Aug 2020)

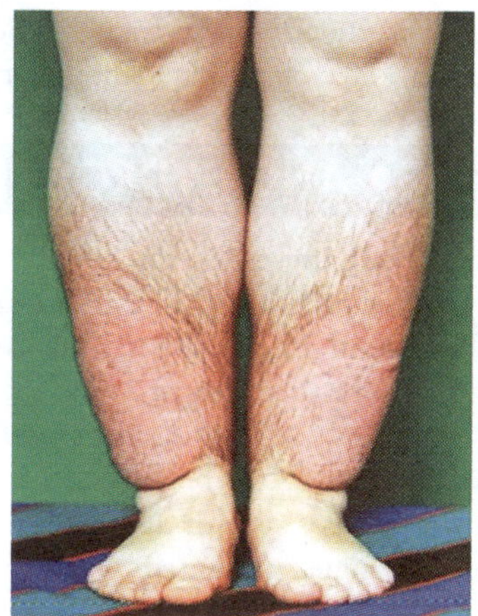

a. Hypothyroidism
b. Hyperthyroidism
c. Filariasis
d. Milroy's disease

260. A 27-year-old woman presents with 26 weeks of gestation with a thyroid lesion which is found to be papillary carcinoma of thyroid. Which is the best treatment for this patient? ***(Most Recent Question 2019)***

a. Thyroid ablation using radioactive Iodine
b. Total thyroidectomy
c. Observation
d. Hemi-thyroidectomy

261. Sebaceous cyst is not seen in?

(Recent Pattern Question 2018-19)

a. Back
b. Soles
c. Scalp
d. Scrotum

262. Patient complains of painless swelling over the face with difficulty in swallowing. The appearance of face is shown. The probable diagnosis is:

(Recent Pattern Question 2018-19)

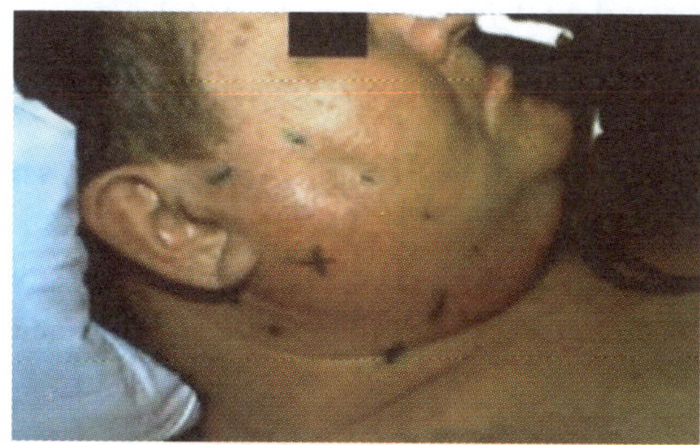

a. Acute parotitis
b. Cancer of parotid gland
c. Angioedema of face
d. Acute Sialpadenitis

263. A 35-year-old lady has presented with a 6-month painless fluctuant, non-transilluminant swelling with a thin watery discharge. Clinical diagnosis is:

(Recent Pattern Question 2019)

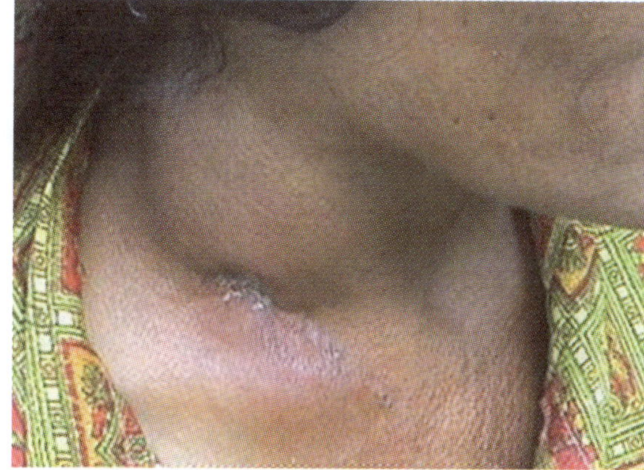

a. Branchial Cyst
b. Secondaries
c. TB
d. Lymphoma

264. Lid lag sign is also known as:

(Recent Pattern Question 2018)

a. Stellwag's sign
b. Von Graefe's sign
c. Dalrymple sign
d. Mobius sign

265. Which is the most common malignancy of the endocrine system?

a. Thyroid cancer
b. Pancreatic cancer
c. Pituitary adenoma
d. Adrenal malignancy

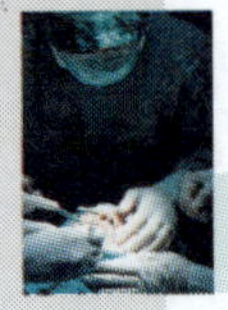

266. Which of the following is the most useful investigation for thyroid function?
a. TSH b. T3
c. T4 d. Thyroglobulin

267. Papillary carcinoma of thyroid is spread via?
a. Lymphatic b. Hematogenous
c. Local spread d. All of these

268. Which iodine isotope is used for thyroid ablation?
a. Iodine 131 b. Iodine 123
c. Iodine 213 d. Iodine 132

269. Which is the most common nerve to be damaged in thyroid surgery?
a. Recurrent laryngeal nerve
b. Inferior laryngeal nerve
c. External branch of superior laryngeal nerve
d. Internal branch of superior laryngeal nerve

270. Which is the tumor marker for medullary carcinoma of thyroid?
a. Albumin b. TSH
c. Thyroglobulin d. Calcitonin

271. Which cancer arises from C-cells of thyroid?
a. Follicular b. Anaplastic
c. Papillary d. Medullary

272. Which thyroid cancer is associated with radiation exposure?
a. Medullary b. Papillary
c. Follicular d. Anaplastic carcinoma

273. Which thyroid tumor has the best prognosis?
a. Papillary b. Follicular
c. Anaplastic d. Medullary

274. A male patient with euthyroid state presents with the following condition. What is the diagnosis?

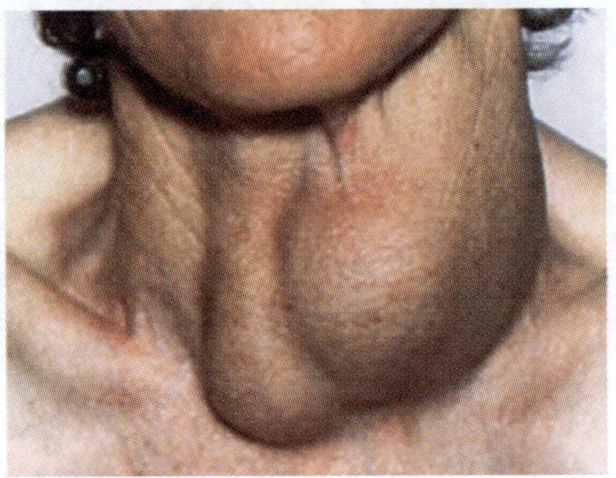

a. Thyroglossal cyst b. Multiple nodular goiter
c. Solitary thyroid nodule d. Toxic nodular goiter

275. FNAC can diagnose all of the following thyroid lesions; EXCEPT
a. Anaplastic carcinoma b. Papillary carcinoma
c. Follicular carcinoma d. Medullary carcinoma

276. Which of the following is not a landmark of facial nerve during superficial parotidectomy?
a. Tragus
b. Mastoid process
c. Posterior belly of digastric muscle
d. Zygomatic bone

277. Which is the most common parotid gland tumor?
a. Warthin's tumor
b. Mucoepidermoid carcinoma
c. Pleomorphic adenoma
d. Adenoid cystic carcinoma

278. Nerve invasion is seen in which type of parotid carcinoma?
a. Muco-epidermoid carcinoma
b. Adenoid cystic carcinoma
c. Malignant mixed tumors
d. Acinic cell carcinoma

279. Warthin's tumor is tumor of which gland?
a. Parotid gland b. Submandibular gland
c. Lingual gland d. Minor salivary glands

280. Most commonly salivary gland fistula starts from which gland?
a. Parotid gland b. Salivary gland
c. Submandibular glands d. Sublingual glands

281. Salivary gland stone is formed most commonly in:
a. Submandibular gland b. Mandibular gland
c. Sublingual gland d. Parotid gland

282. What is the surgery of choice for pleomorphic adenoma?
a. Superficial parotidectomy b. Total parotidectomy
c. Radical parotidectomy d. Radiotherapy

HERNIA AND HYDROCELE

283. A 14-year-old boy presented to the OPD. His scrotum was empty on the left side. On clinical examination, the left testis as found in the superficial inguinal pouch. What is the most likely diagnosis?
(Most Recent Question June 2022)
a. Cryptorchidism b. Left undescended testis
c. Left ectopic testis d. Retractile testis

284. A 25-year-old male presented with vague dragging sensation in the scrotum. On clinical examination, a bag of worm feel was noted in the scrotum on the left side. However, the left testis was normal. What can be the likely diagnosis? ***(Most Recent Question June 2022)***
a. Left hydrocele b. Inguinal hernia
c. Epididymoorchitis d. Left varicocele

285. What is the pathological grading used for prostate cancer? ***(Most Recent Question June 2022)***
a. Bloom Richardson b. Gleason's
c. Fuhrman nuclear grading d. Ranson Score

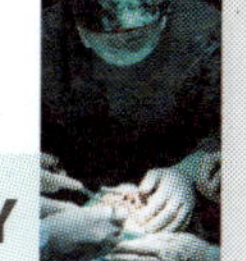

286. Which of the following isotope is used in the treatment of prostate cancer? *(Most Recent Question June 2022)*
a. I-131 b. I-125
c. I-123 d. I-121

287. A patient presented with herniation of intestine loop which passes along the spermatic cord and reaches till the cremaster muscle. What is the type of hernia? *(Most Recent Question Dec. 2021)*
a. Femoral hernia b. Indirect inguinal hernia
c. Direct inguinal hernia d. Obturator hernia

288. A 5-month-old baby was brought to the hospital with bilateral undescended testis. What is the most appropriate treatment? *(Most Recent Question Dec. 2021)*
a. Immediate orchidopexy
b. Wait and watch for spontaneous resolution
c. GnRH for one month and if no descent then surgical treatment
d. Wait for 2 years

289. A 40-year-old male patient presented with testicular swelling and one mass over supraclavicular area and one over the umbilical region. What is the diagnosis?
a. Testicular tumor *(Most Recent Question Dec. 2021)*
b. Testicular torsion
c. Spermatocele
d. Acute epididymo-orchitis

290. A 30-year-old male patient presented with scrotal enlargement. On Work-up, LDH was significantly raised with normal alpha-feto protein and hCG. Histopathology is shown below. What is the most likely diagnosis? *(Most Recent Question Dec. 2021)*

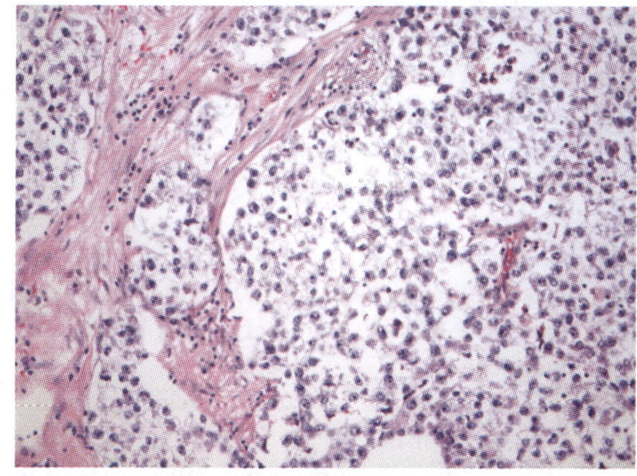

a. Teratoma b. Seminoma
c. Choriocarcinoma d. Yolk sac tumor

291. Three testicle appearance is seen in: *(Most Recent Question Dec. 2021)*
a. Acute epididymo-orchitis
b. Vaginal hydrocele
c. Spermatocele
d. Testicular torsion

292. A 50-year-old patient felt heaviness in the left scrotum. He was suspecting he has developed cancer, so he came to the emergency department. There was no pain or tenderness. Transillumination test was negative. What is the most likely diagnosis? *(Most Recent Question Dec. 2021)*
a. Acute epididymo-orchitis
b. Vaginal hydrocele
c. Varicocele
d. Testicular torsion

293. Which of the following viruses is responsible for causing Orchitis? *(Most Recent Question June 2021)*
a. Adeno virus b. Herpes virus
c. Polio virus d. Mumps virus

294. An elderly male is having metastasis in the lumbar vertebra and pelvic bone. What is the most likely diagnosis in this patient? *(Most Recent Question June 2021)*
a. Testicular cancer b. Lung cancer
c. Colon cancer d. Prostate cancer

295. In a newborn baby with empty scrotum, testis was found to be lying close to the peritoneum. Which of the following may help in the testis reaching into the scrotum? *(Most Recent Question June 2021)*
a. GnRH analogues
b. Testosterone
c. Cold compresses
d. Manually bring the testis down to the bottom of the scrotum

296. Deep inguinal ring is a defect in: *(Most Recent Question Aug 2020)*
a. External oblique muscle aponeurosis
b. Transversus abdominis muscle aponeurosis
c. Internal oblique muscle aponeurosis
d. Fascia transversalis

297. A boy in the gym lifted the equipment and suddenly felt pain in the groin. He came to the hospital. On examination, swelling was felt in left inguinal canal. What should be the next step? *(Most Recent Question Aug 2020)*
a. NSAIDs and send the patient home
b. Immediate exploration
c. FNAC and USG
d. Coconut bandage to hold the swelling up

298. A patient with irreducible groin hernia was brought to the emergency. What should be the next step? *(Most Recent Question Aug 2020)*
a. Exploratory laparotomy
b. Attempt Reduction followed by elective surgery
c. Attempt Reduction in emergency surgery
d. Attempt reduction under local anesthesia

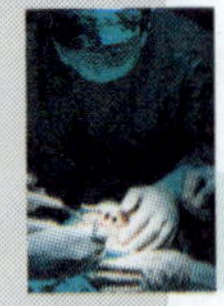

299. In a newborn male baby mother found empty scrotum. On examination, left testis is in inguinal region and right testis is in perineum. Which of the following is correct? ***(Most Recent Question Aug 2020)***

a. Right testis is undescended and left testis is ectopic
b. Left testis is undescended and right testis is ectopic
c. Both testes are undescended
d. Both testes are ectopic

300. Identify the abnormal condition given below. ***(Most Recent Question Dec 2019)***

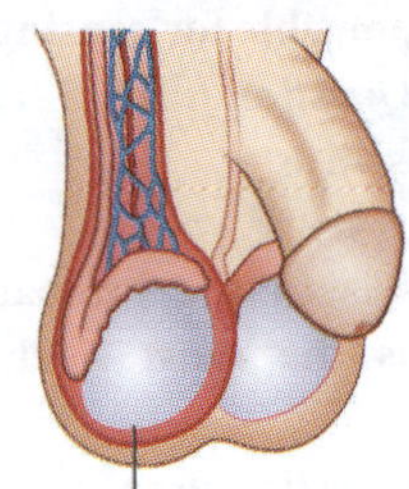
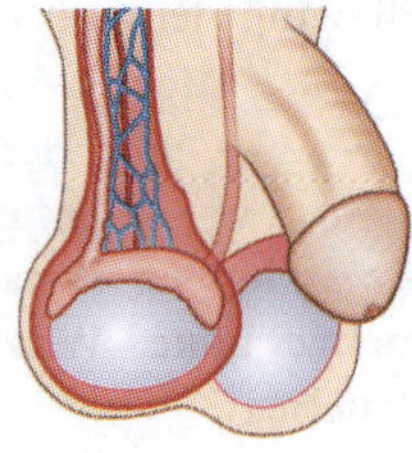
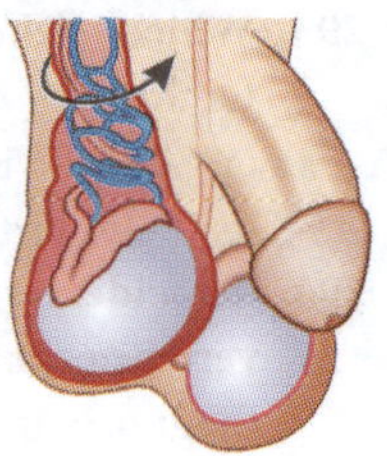

a. Testicular torsion   b. Hydrocele
c. Varicocele   d. Testicular atrophy

301. Bell clapper testis predisposes to? ***(Recent Pattern Question 2018-19)***

a. Torsion testis   b. Varicocele
c. Cancer of testis   d. Hydrocele

302. In NYHUS classification which of these is called Type 3A hernia? ***(Recent Pattern Question 2018)***

a. Femoral   b. Direct
c. Indirect   d. Pantaloons

303. A 40-year-old patient was being operated for direct hernia. During surgery two sacs were seen. The diagnosis is? ***(Recent Pattern Question 2016)***

a. Pantaloons hernia   b. Richter hernia
c. Spigelian hernia   d. Littre hernia

304. A 30-year-old obese male patient presents with complete inguinal hernia and on examination doughy consistency is felt with dull note on percussion. This suggests that the contents of the hernia sac contain: ***(Recent Pattern Question 2016)***

a. Omentum   b. Large intestine
c. Small intestine   d. Encysted ascitic fluid

305. Deep inguinal ring is a defect in aponeurosis of:

a. External oblique muscle of abdomen
b. Internal oblique muscle of abdomen
c. Transverse abdominis muscle
d. Transversalis fascia

306. A 3-year-old child presents with red scrotal swelling which shows self resolution by next day morning and is maximum in evening with positive transillumination test. What is the diagnosis?

a. Scrotal abscess   b. Congenital hydrocele
c. Secondary abscess   d. Infantile hydrocele

307. Hydrocele in a child is managed by:

a. Herniotomy   b. Plication of sac
c. Eversion of sac   d. Inversion of sac

308. What is not true about hernia in children?

a. Conservative Management till patient is asymptomatic
b. Hernia treatment is done with herniotomy
c. Absorbable mesh is not used
d. Long standing hernia decreases chances of incarceration

309. The content of Littre's hernia is?

a. Omentum
b. Bladder
c. Meckel's diverticulum
d. Part of circumference of intestine

310. A 15-year-old male presents with pain in inguinal area and lower abdomen. On examination tenderness over a non-reducible swelling with negative cough impulse is noted. What is the diagnosis?

a. Strangulated hernia   b. Testicular torsion
c. Scrotal abscess   d. Femoral hernia

311. Femoral hernia presents:

a. Below and lateral to pubic tubercle
b. Above and medial to pubic tubercle
c. Below and medial to pubic tubercle
d. Above and lateral to pubic tubercle

312. All are true about femoral hernia; EXCEPT?

a. Common in nulliparous women
b. Lockwood infra-inguinal approach is used
c. Cough impulse is present
d. Higher incidence of strangulation than inguinal hernia

313. Which hernia has the highest rate of strangulation?

a. Direct inguinal hernia   b. Indirect inguinal hernia
c. Femoral hernia   d. Incisional hernia

314. Which of the following hernia presents as emergency?

a. Direct inguinal hernia   b. Indirect inguinal hernia
c. Femoral hernia   d. Incisional hernia

315. Double sac hernia is known as:

a. Richter hernia   b. Cooper's hernia
c. Littre's hernia   d. Spigelian hernia

316. A patient has direct inguinal hernia. On operation intra-operative indirect inguinal hernia is seen. What is the diagnosis?

a. Maydl's hernia   b. Velpeau hernia
c. Petit hernia   d. Saddle bag hernia

317. Meckel's diverticulum forms wall in case of which type of hernia?

a. Ritcher's hernia   b. Spigelian hernia
c. Cooper's hernia   d. Littre's hernia

318. Spigelian hernia is:

a. Hernia through petit triangle
b. Hernia passing through obturator canal
c. Hernia through linea alba
d. Hernia at level of arcuate line

319. What is the location of bochdaleck hernia?

a. Posterolateral b. Anteroposterior
c. Anterolateral d. Posteromedial

320. A 25-year-old male presents with fever and red, swollen scrotum. Upon examination testis is felt separate from epididymis because of marked swelling in epididymis. What is the diagnosis?

a. Testicular torsion b. Fournier's gangrene
c. Epididymo orchitis d. Testicular cancer

UROLOGY

321. A 1½-year-old child is having problem with urination for the last 3 months. You have introduced a contrast dye from the urethra to visualize and understand the problem. Name this investigation most likely? *(Most Recent Question June 2022)*

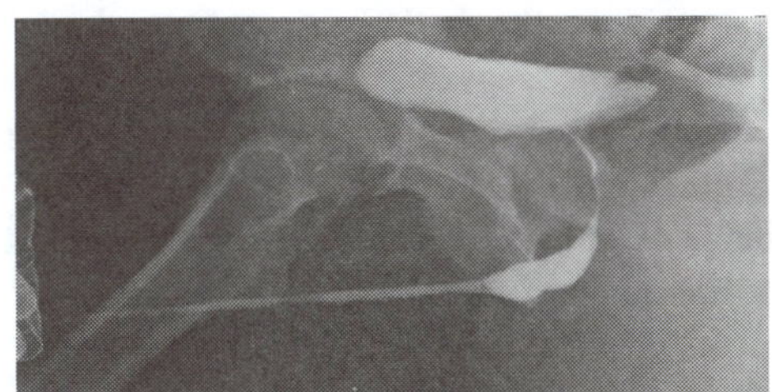

a. Micturating cystourethrogram
b. Retrograde urethrogram
c. Antegrade pyelography
d. Retrograde pyelography

322. Which of the following pathology will have irregular margins of the urinary bladder with the organism found around the ureteric orifice? *(Most Recent Question June 2022)*

a. Tuberculosis
b. Schistosomiasis
c. Transitional cell bladder carcinoma
d. Papilloma urinary bladder

323. The internal opening in the fistula in Ano usually begins from: *(Most Recent Question Dec. 2021)*

a. Mucocutaneous junction
b. Crypt at dentate line
c. Anal verge
d. Anorectal junction

324. A 47-year-old man presented with a renal mass on the lower pole of right kidney with 7 × 5 × 3 cm size. What is the preferred treatment option? *(Most Recent Question Dec. 2021)*

a. Partial nephrectomy b. Total radical nephrectomy
c. ESWL d. Radiotherapy

325. Which of the following is the most common type of renal stone? *(Most Recent Question Dec. 2021)*

a. Triple phosphate b. Uric acid
c. Cysteine d. Calcium oxalate

326. Whitaker test is done in: *(Most Recent Question Dec. 2021)*

a. Posterior urethral valves
b. Hydronephrosis to compare abdominal and urinary bladder pressure
c. Ureterocele
d. Benign prostatic hyperplasia

327. A patient was operated for benign prostatic hyperplasia. On evaluation, carcinoma prostate was detected. On further work up patient was found to have metastasis. Which of the following drug should be used for the management? *(Most Recent Question Dec. 2021)*

a. Cisplatin b. Adriamycin
c. Leuprolide d. BCG

328. A 35-year-old woman was brought to the hospital with history of continuous dribbling of urine with normal voiding pattern. What is the most likely cause? *(Most Recent Question Dec. 2021)*

a. Posterior urethral valve
b. Ureteric opening distal to external urinary sphincter
c. Urinary tract infection
d. Vesicoureteric reflux

329. A 54-year-old multiparous female presents with leakage of urine while coughing or laughing. This is called: *(Most Recent Question Dec. 2021)*

a. Vesicovaginal fistula b. Urethrovaginal fistula
c. Urge incontinence d. Stress incontinence

330. 80-year-old male presented with a ballotable mass in the left flank region. On examination painless hematuria is documented on urine microscopy. Most likely cause in this patient: *(Most Recent Question June 2021)*

a. Hydronephrosis b. Pyelonephritis
c. Renal cell carcinoma d. Polycystic kidney disease

331. What is the diagnosis on the basis of image given below? *(Most Recent Question Dec 2020)*

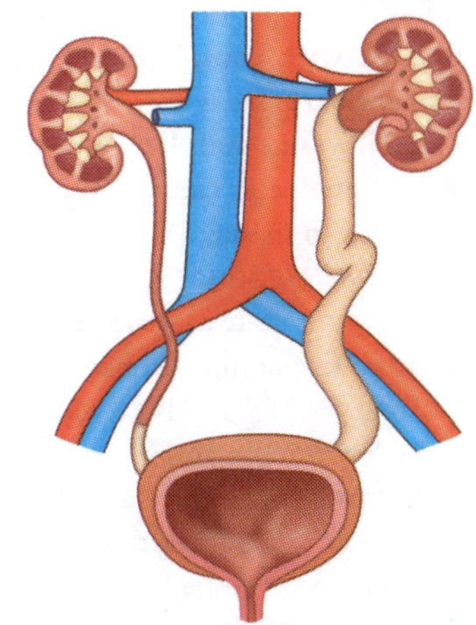

a. Ectopic ureter b. Ureterocele
c. Duplication d. Bifid ureter

332. A patient of RTA with pelvic fracture was brought to the emergency. On evaluation proximal membranous urethra was found to be injured. What is the immediate management? ***(Most Recent Question Dec 2020)***

a. Suprapubic cystostomy b. Laparotomy
c. Foleys catheterization d. Emergency repair

333. What is the diagnosis on the basis of image given below? ***(Most Recent Question Dec 2020)***

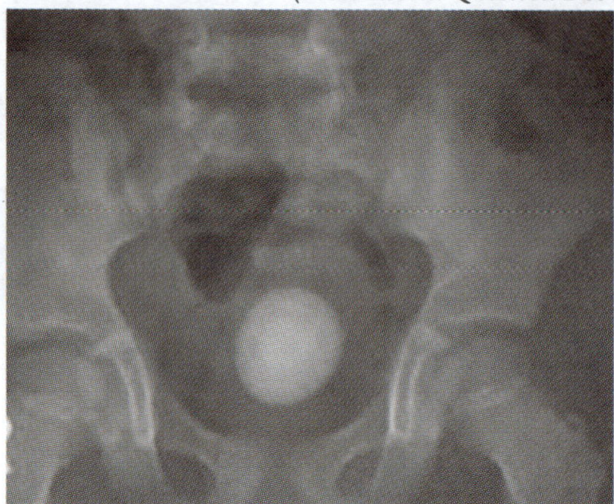

a. Prostatic stone b. Bladder stone
c. Schistosomiasis d. Ureteric stone

334. A patient presented to OPD with complaints to severe pain during erection and abnormal curvature of penis for the last 6 months. What is the most probable diagnosis? ***(Most Recent Question Dec 2020)***

a. Peyronie's disease b. Paraphimosis
c. Balanoposthitis d. Priapism

335. A young guy comes to your OPD with the complaint that he develops pain in penis during erection and cannot have sex. Which is the likely diagnosis? ***(Most Recent Question Dec 2020)***

a. Paraphimosis b. Phimosis
c. Hypospadias d. Peyronie's disease

336. A patient present with complaints of palpitations. On examination, her heart rate is 110/min and BP = 140/100 mm Hg. She tells you that her mother has recently expired due to Renal cell cancer. Which investigation would you perform to manage this case? ***(Most Recent Question Aug 2020)***

a. Serum hydroxy indole acetic acid levels
b. Serum hydroxy-tryptamine levels
c. 24 hours urinary V.M.A levels
d. 24 hours urinary fractionated metanephrines

337. Which of the following is false related to renal stones? ***(Most Recent Question Aug 2020)***

a. Most common type of stone is triple phosphate
b. Stone can be removed via ureter
c. Most of the renal stones can be removed by ESWL
d. Stones <5 mm can be managed conservatively

338. What is the diagnosis based on the given image of IVP? ***(Most Recent Question Aug 2020)***

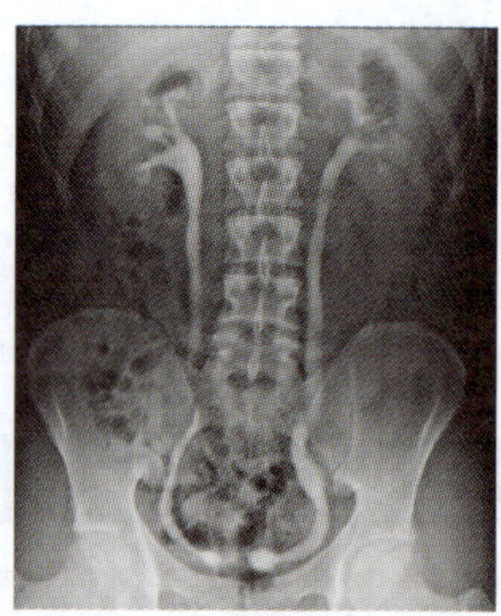

a. Ureterocele b. Ectopic ureteric orifice
c. PUJ obstruction d. Posterior urethral valve

339. After alcohol consumption, patient went to bathroom and slipped in the bathroom and developed pain in the suprapubic region. On examination, abdominal distention was present without suprapubic bulge. Heart rate and blood pressure was normal. What is the most probable diagnosis? ***(Most Recent Question Aug 2020)***

a. Membranous urethral injury
b. Acute urinary retention
c. Intraperitoneal bladder rupture
d. Extraperitoneal bladder rupture

340. A 60-year-old patient presented to OPD with excruciating low backache not responding to pain killer tablets. His PSA levels are 100 ng/ml and MRI spine shows lytic lesions at L5-S1. DRE shows asymmetrically enlarged stony hard prostate. Which of the following drug is indicated for the treatment? ***(Most Recent Question Aug 2020)***

a. Somatostatin b. Goserelin
c. Terlipressin d. Testosterone

341. A male infant who was brought with urinary retention was found to have bilateral hydronephrosis. There was history of recurrent urinary tract infections. What is the probable diagnosis? ***(Most Recent Question Aug 2020)***

a. PUJ obstruction b. Posterior urethral valves
c. Horse shoe kidney d. Retrocaval ureter

342. A 62-year-old female has kidney stone and treated with PCNL. After 2 days she again comes to OPD with chills and fever. What is the complication? ***(Most Recent Question Dec 2019)***

a. Bacterial sepsis b. Acute pancreatitis
c. Splenic injury d. Ureteric stricture

343. Prostatic cancer mostly seen in which part of prostate gland? ***(Most Recent Question Dec 2019)***

a. Posterior b. Lateral
c. Medial d. Anterior

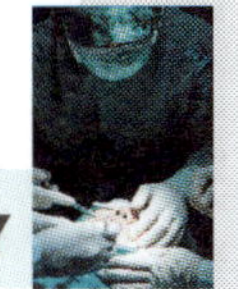

344. In kidney transplantation donor organ will be placed at which site? *(Most Recent Question Dec 2019)*
a. Left Kidney fossa
b. Right Iliac fossa
c. Retroperitoneal space
d. Retropubic space

345. A 40-year-old man is suffering from heaviness in scrotum. A bag of worms feel is observed on scrotal examination and the swelling is seen to reduce in supine position. What is the best treatment? *(Most Recent Question 2019)*
a. Suction drainage b. Varicocelectomy
c. Jaboulay procedure d. Herniotomy

346. Which of these is the best for management of a 3cm stone in renal pelvis without evidence of hydronephrosis? *(Recent Pattern Question 2018-19)*
a. ESWL b. PCNL
c. Antegrade pyeloplasty d. Retrograde pyeloplasty

347. Germ cell tumor not seen in males: *(Recent Pattern Question 2018-19)*
a. Choriocarcinoma b. Seminoma
c. Sertoli cell tumor d. Teratoma

348. Cut off for diagnosis of Priapism is? *(Recent Pattern Question 2018-19)*
a. 1 hours b. 2 hours
c. 3 hours d. 4 hours

349. A person could not pass urine after suffering from pelvic fracture. On examination vitals are stable but bladder is not palpable. What is the probable diagnosis? *(Recent Pattern Question 2018)*
a. Membranous urethra rupture
b. Bulbar urethra rupture
c. Recto-urethral injury
d. Intraperitoneal rupture of bladder

350. The kidney stone whose development is insensitive to pH of urine is: *(Recent Pattern Question 2018)*
a. Calcium oxalate b. Triple phosphate
c. Uric acid d. Cystine

351. A 60-year-old smoker male patient presents with painless gross hematuria for 1 day. IVU shows 1.2 cm filling defect at the lower pole of infundibulum. Which is the next best investigation to be done? *(Recent Pattern Question 2018)*
a. Cystoscopy b. Urine cytology
c. USG abdomen d. DMSA scan

352. A 70-year-old man after TURP for BPH develops seizures in postoperative state. What is the diagnosis? *(Recent Pattern Question 2018)*
a. Water intoxication
b. Anesthetic over-dosage
c. Mismatched blood transfusion
d. Malignant hyperthermia

353. What does the following image show? *(Recent Pattern Question 2017)*

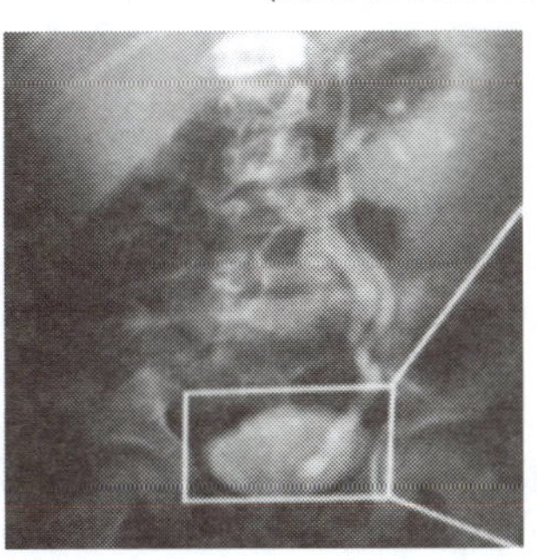

a. Misplaced Cu-T 380Ag b. Fecolith
c. Ureterocele d. Appendicolith

354. What is the best treatment for metastatic advanced prostate carcinoma? *(Recent Pattern Question 2017)*
a. T.U.R.P b. Androgen ablation
c. Chemotherapy d. Radical prostatectomy

355. Seminoma spreads by? *(Recent Pattern Question 2016)*
a. Hematogenous route b. Direct route
c. Lymphatics d. Directly by spermatic cord

356. In a person if testis cancer is suspected, which test is to be done first? *(Recent Pattern Question 2016)*
a. Scrotal USG b. MRI
c. FNAC d. PET/CT

357. A 28-year-old patient from Bihar presents with on and off pain in right scrotum and then gradual onset swelling develops over the duration of 2 years. Trans illumination test is positive. Top of testis can be reached. The probable diagnosis is? *(Recent Pattern Question 2016)*
a. Right hydrocele
b. Right inguinal hernia
c. Right epididymal cyst
d. Right encysted hydrocele of cord

358. A 50-year-old patient complains of pain and swelling in right side scrotum for two days. He tells that this swelling has been gradually increasing in size with a dragging sensation for 2 years. On examination there is a large inguinoscrotal irreducible swelling with extreme tenderness and redness. What is the probable diagnosis? *(Recent Pattern Question 2016)*
a. Right hydrocele
b. Right strangulated inguinal hernia
c. Right testicular torsion
d. Right pyocele

359. A young boy 18 years of age presents with pain in groin for 2 days. On examination the testis seems high and cremasteric reflex is absent. Elevation of testis worsens the pain. What is the probable diagnosis? *(Recent Pattern Question 2016)*
a. Right testicular torsion
b. Right strangulated hernia
c. Right inguinal hernia
d. Right epididymo-orchitis

360. Which is the most common type of renal stone?
a. Calcium oxalate b. Triple phosphate
c. Struvite stone d. Urate stone

361. Which renal stone is radiolucent?
a. Uric acid b. Calcium oxalate
c. Triple phosphate d. Calcium phosphate

362. Stag horn calculi associated with proteus infection are:
a. Uric acid stones b. Triple phosphate stones
c. Calcium oxalate stones d. Cystine stones

363. Alkaline urine is seen in:
a. Uric acid stone b. Oxalate stone
c. Triple phosphate stone d. Cystine stone

364. What is the cause of urinary retention?
a. Vaginal fibroid b. Cervical fibroid
c. Uterine fibroid d. Subserosal fibroid

365. What is the most useful investigation for calculus in ureteric colic?
a. CECT b. NCCT
c. USG d. X-ray

366. Transitional cell carcinoma is seen in
a. Prepuce b. Testis
c. Prostate d. Urinary bladder

367. Which is the most common tumor of urinary bladder?
a. Squamous cell cancer b. Carcinosarcoma
c. Transitional cell cancer d. Clear cell cancer

368. What is the most common clinical presentation of bladder cancer?
a. Painful urinary stasis b. Painless urinary stasis
c. Painful hematuria d. Painless hematuria

369. What is the most common clinical subtype of transitional cell carcinoma of bladder?
a. Local Metastatic b. Distant metastasis
c. Superficial d. Deep

370. All are true about transitional cell cancer of urinary tract; EXCEPT:
a. Bladder is a frequent site
b. Most common risk factor is smoking
c. Females and males are equally affected
d. Vitamin A is effective against bladder CA

371. Rupture of urethra above the deep perineal pouch causes urine retention in which region?
a. Medial aspect of thigh
b. Scrotum
c. True pelvis only
d. Anterior abdominal wall

372. Which amongst following is the most common cause of UTI?
a. Instrumentation b. Urethral diverticulum
c. Bladder stones d. Pregnancy

373. Spider leg sign on IVP suggests?
a. Renal stone b. Polycystic kidney
c. Hypernephroma d. Hydronephrosis

374. Adder head appearance on IVP is seen in
a. Ureteral duplication
b. Ureterocele
c. Ureteric hypoplasia
d. Polycystic kidneys

375. Reinke's crystals are seen in?
a. Leydig cells
b. Sertoli cells
c. Curschmann spirals
d. Creola bodies

376. Which is the most common testicular tumor?
a. Seminoma
b. Teratoma
c. Sertoli cell tumor
d. Chorio-CA

377. Which is the first lymph node involved in lymph node metastasis in testicular tumor?
a. Inguinal b. Para aortic
c. External iliac d. Internal iliac

378. Which is the most specific marker for prostate cancer?
a. P.S.A b. P.A.P
c. Transrectal USG d. N.S.E

379. What is incorrect about PSA?
a. Liquefaction of seminal coagulum
b. Produced by both normal cells and malignancy
c. Increased with prostatitis
d. Persists in blood even after prostatectomy

380. A 70-year-old man with prostate cancer was given radiotherapy. The recurrence of the cancer is monitored biochemically by
a. Androgens levels
b. Prostate specific antigen and carcino-embryonic antigen
c. Prostate specific antigen only
d. ALP and CEA

381. Three glass urine test with first glass specimen of urine showing threads is diagnostic of
a. Urethritis
b. Prostatitis
c. Cystitis
d. Epididymitis

382. Prostate cancer spreads to the vertebral column via?
a Bateson plexus
b Inferior hypogastric plexus
c Superior hypogastric plexus
d All of the above

383. What is the indication for Radical prostatectomy?
a. Localized prostate cancer, life expectancy < 10 years
b. Localized prostate cancer, life expectancy > 10 years
c. Locally advanced prostate cancer, life expectancy < 10 years
d. Locally advanced disease with extension to lateral pelvic fascia

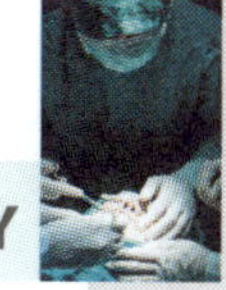

384. Which of the following is correct about the image given below?

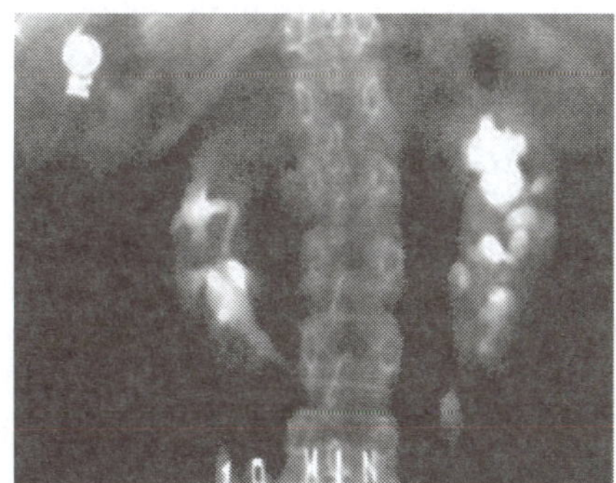

a. Horse shoe kidney
b. Undescended left kidney
c. Congenital absent left kidney
d. Papillary carcinoma

385. The given picture shows

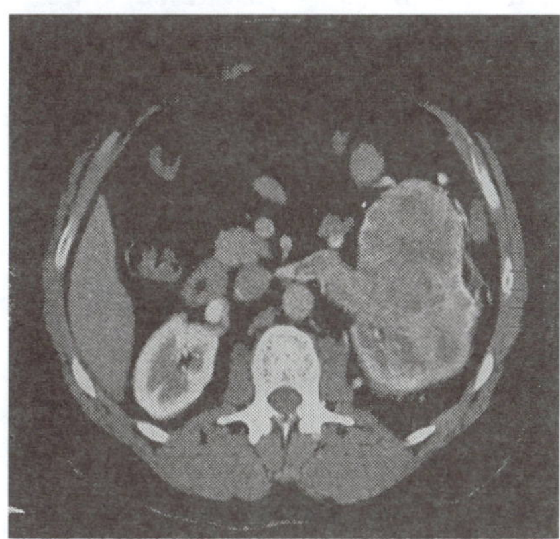

a. Renal cell cancer
b. Hydronephrosis
c. Polycystic kidneys
d. Nephrolithiasis

386. What does the given picture show?

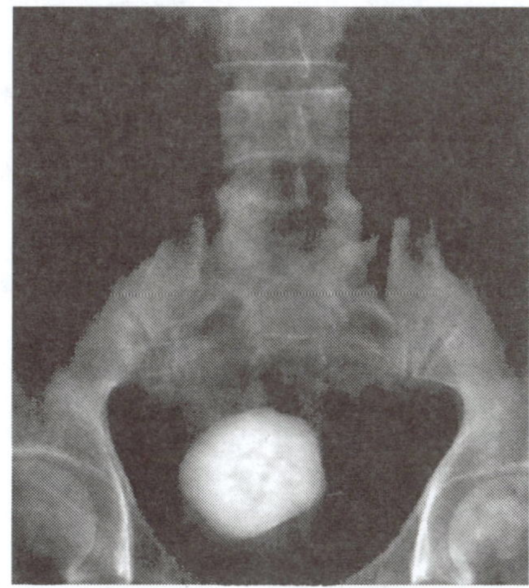

a. Foreign body
b. Bladder stone
c. Bladder diverticulum
d. Fecolith

387. What is the probable diagnosis?

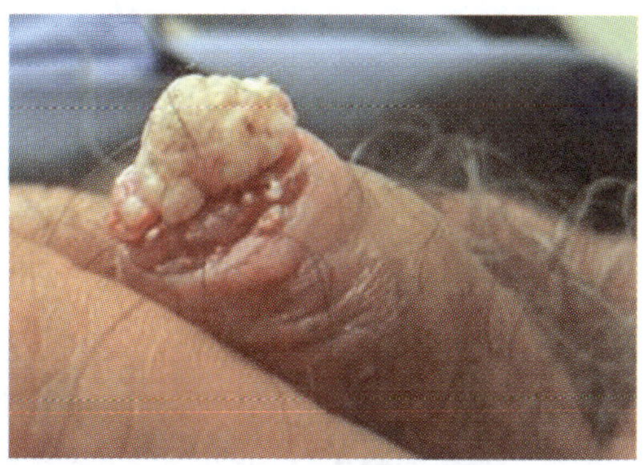

a. Chancroid
b. Carcinoma penis
c. Chancre
d. Bowen disease

388. In carcinoma penis tumor staging, stage III involves:

a. Shaft of penis
b. Inguinal lymph node metastasis operable
c. Inguinal lymph node metastasis inoperable
d. Confined to prepuce

389. A 5-year-old child pulls penis skin while urinating. Upon examination there is erythema and edema over the prepuce. What is the diagnosis?

a. Hypospadias
b. Urethral Stone
c. Posterior urethral valve
d. Phimosis

390. Chordee is associated with:

a. Epispadias
b. Hypospadias
c. Phimosis
d. Posterior urethral valve

391. The treatment of balanitis xerotica obliterans (BXO) is

a. Chemotherapy
b. Circumcision
c. Radiotherapy
d. Partial amputation of penis

392. Which is a major cause of death in renal transplant patients?

a. Uremia
b. Malignancy
c. Rejection
d. Infection

HEPATOBILIARY SYSTEM

393. A 50-year-old patient who has undergone cholecystectomy few days back presented with upper abdominal pain. MRCP was done which showed evidence of bile-leak from the cystic duct stump. Patient is hemodynamically stable. Which of the following should be done in the management of this patient?

a. CECT ***(Most Recent Question June 2022)***
b. ERCP and stenting
c. Exploratory laparotomy
d. Conservative treatment with antibiotics

394. Which of the following is a type III choledochal cyst?
(Most Recent Question June 2022)

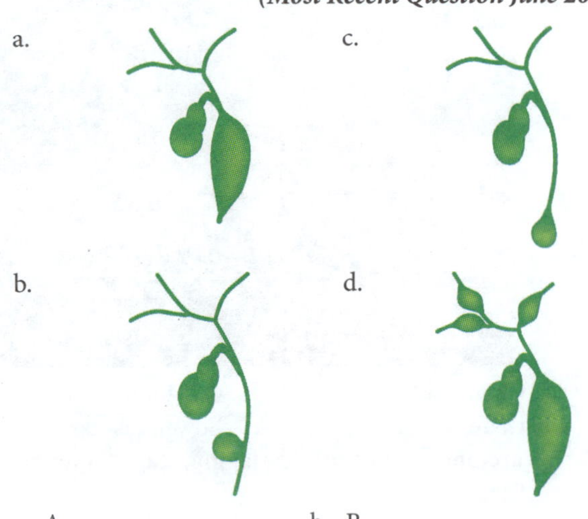

a. A
b. B
c. C
d. D

395. A 30-year-old female was incidentally diagnosed with gall bladder polyp of 0.5 cm on ultrasound. Patient was asymptomatic. What is the next step in the management? ***(Most Recent Question Dec. 2021)***
a. Laparoscopic cholecystectomy
b. Open cholecystectomy
c. CECT abdomen
d. Reassure the patient and follow-up

396. What do you expect in a patient after gallbladder removal? ***(Most Recent Question Dec. 2021)***
a. Weight loss
b. Steatorrhea
c. Hypoglycemia
d. High cholesterol

397. A patient underwent laparoscopic cholecystectomy for gallbladder stone. After operation, patient was sent home on the same day. Patient came back on another day with complaints of right upper quadrant pain. Liver function test was done and it was normal. WBC count was 13000/ Cu.mm. What is the most probable diagnosis?
(Most Recent Question Dec. 2021)
a. Bile leak at site
b. CBD stone
c. Acute pancreatitis
d. Right lobar pneumonia

398. A patient with chronic liver disease presents with history of hematemesis and melena. On endoscopy, esophageal varices were present. On the day of evaluation, repeat bleeding occurred and the patient died. What is the most likely cause of death?
(Most Recent Question Dec. 2021)
a. Esophageal varices bleeding
b. Hypovolemic shock
c. Cardiogenic shock
d. Neurogenic shock

399. A chronic liver disease patient presented to OPD with pain and tenderness all over the abdomen. Ascitic fluid examination revealed neutrophils. 500/mm^3. What is the next best step? ***(Most Recent Question Dec. 2021)***
a. IV ceftriaxone
b. Large fluid paracentesis
c. IV albumin plus midodrine
d. IV octreotide

400. A patient presented with pain in the right hypochondrium. Blood investigations showed AST-22 IU/L and ALT-27 IU/L. Serum bilirubin levels = 5mg%, also ALP-200 mg%. What should be the initial investigation in this patient?
a. USG abdomen ***(Most Recent Question June 2021)***
b. CECT abdomen
c. Hepatitis A and Hepatitis E markers
d. HIDA scan

401. A pregnant woman underwent ultrasound during follow-up. The incidental finding is given in the image. What is the diagnosis? ***(Most Recent Question Dec 2020)***

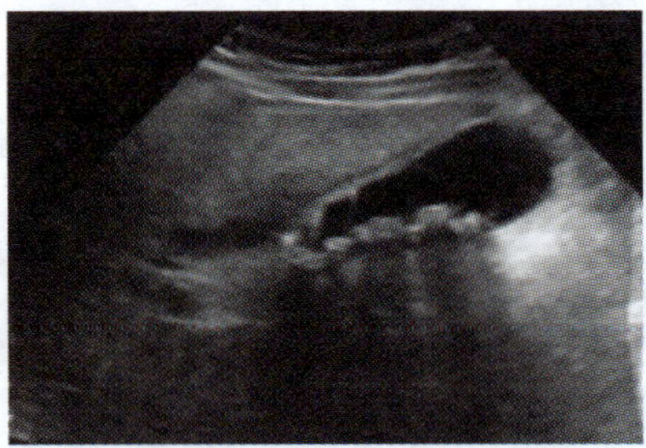

a. Simple hepatic cyst
b. Multiple gallstones
c. Amoebic liver abscess
d. Renal stone

402. Gallstone impinging on the cystic duct with dilatation of the common hepatic duct suggests the diagnosis of:
(Most Recent Question Dec 2020)
a. Mirizzi's syndrome
b. Acute cholecystitis
c. Cholesterolosis
d. Porcelain gallbladder

403. A 45-year-old male patient presented with abdominal pain and hepatomegaly. Ultrasound image is given below. What is the most probable diagnosis?
(Most Recent Question Aug 2020)

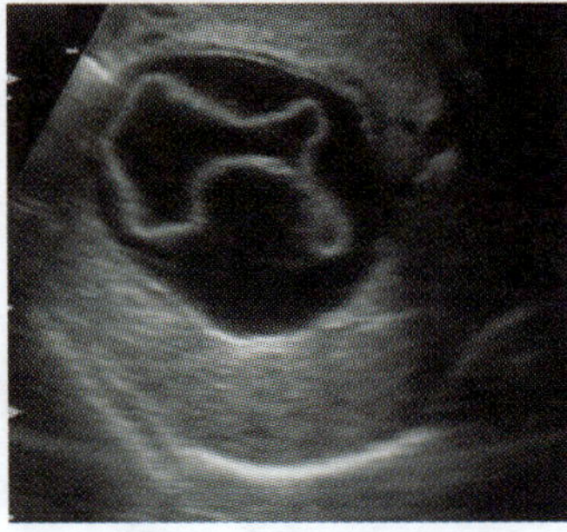

a. Hydatid cyst
b. Amebic liver abscess
c. Pyogenic liver abscess
d. Simple hepatic cyst

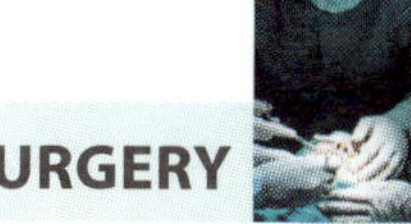

404. Which of the following is implicated in the development of angiosarcoma of the liver? *(Most Recent Question Aug 2020)*

a. Copper b. Zinc
c. Arsenic d. Iron

405. The image of gall bladder specimen is given below. What is the most probable diagnosis? *(Most Recent Question Aug 2020)*

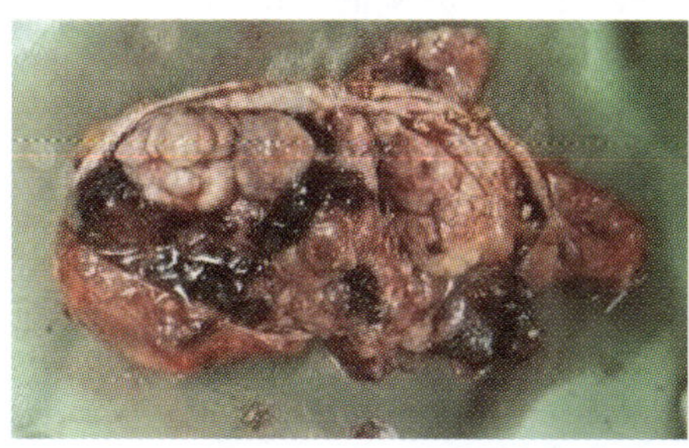

a. Carcinoma gall bladder b. Mixed gall bladder stone
c. Gall bladder polyp d. Strawberry gall bladder

406. A 6-year-old child is brought with high fever with rigors for 5 days with pain in right hypochondrium. On examination patient is anicteric and tenderness is noted in Right upper quadrant. What is best investigation for this case? *(Recent Pattern Question 2018-19)*

a. USG
b. Serology
c. SGOT/ LFT
d. Contrast CT scan

407. AFP is a tumor marker for which of the following? *(Recent Pattern Question 2018-19)*

a. HCC b. RCC
c. Oncocytoma d. Chordoma

408. Comment on the image shown below. *(Recent Pattern Question 2018-19)*

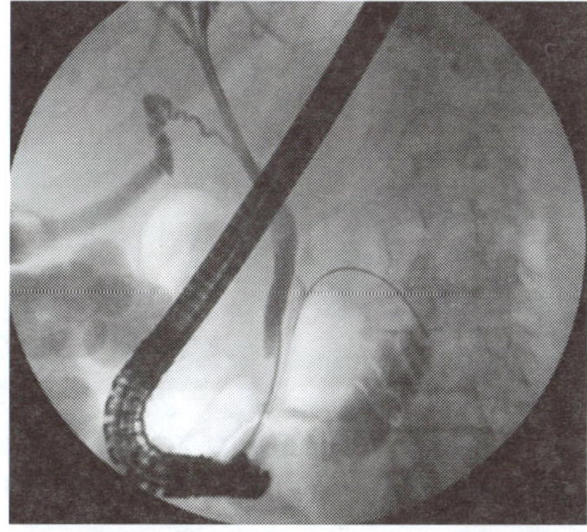

a. Percutaneous Transhepatic cholangiogram
b. T tube cholangiogram
c. E.R.C.P
d. HIDA scan

409. Which of the following is correct about Zollinger Ellison syndrome? *(Recent Pattern Question 2018)*

a. Associated with MEN1
b. Most common site is stomach
c. Best test for diagnosis is pentagastrin test
d. Metastasis to adjacent gut

410. Which ligament is compressed in the Pringle maneuver? *(Recent Pattern Question 2017)*

a. Hepatoduodenal ligament
b. Gastroduodenal ligament
c. Gastrohepatic ligament
d. Lienorenal ligament

411. A patient comes with RUQ pain. The USG image shows? *(Recent Pattern Question 2017)*

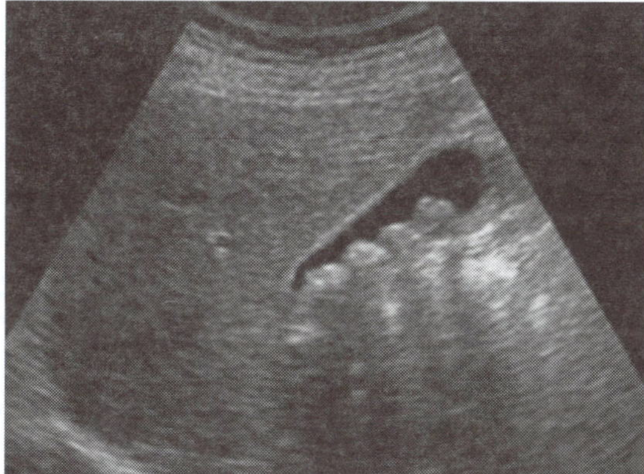

a. Cholelithiasis b. Cholecystitis
c. Cholangiocarcinoma d. Porcelain Gallbladder

412. A 28-year-old man from Bihar develops right hypochondriac pain. USG shows 5 × 5 × 4 cm abscess in left lobe of liver. Hydatid serology is negative. What is the treatment? *(Recent Pattern Question 2016)*

a. Anti –Amoebic drugs
b. Aspiration + Anti amoebic drugs
c. Catheter drainage + Anti amoebic drugs
d. Percutaneous aspiration and infusion of scolicidal agents

413. Aflatoxin leads to? *(Recent Pattern Question 2016)*

a. Liver cancer b. Hepatic adenoma
c. Bladder cancer d. Retinoblastoma

414. What is the ideal management of a hemodynamically unstable patient with suspected liver injury? *(Recent Pattern Question 2016)*

a. Inotropic support
b. Exploratory Laparotomy
c. Rapid transfusion of fresh blood
d. Rapid infusion of iv crystalloids

415. A 40-year-old patient is having high grade fever associated with abdominal pain in right upper quadrant, with hepatomegaly and liver dullness on percussion. What is the clinical diagnosis?

a. Pyogenic liver abscess b. Amoebic liver abscess
c. Hydatid cyst d. Neoplastic growth

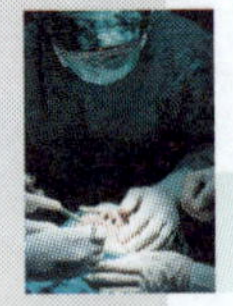

416. Anchovy sauce pus is seen in:
a. Amoebic liver abscess
b. Pyogenic liver abscess
c. Hydatid cyst
d. Cold abscess

417. A patient has obstructive jaundice. USG can tell all of the following; EXCEPT?
a. Number of stones in CBD
b. Peritoneal deposits
c. Size of liver
d. Extrahepatic versus intrahepatic causes

418. The organism associated with fish consumption which causes carcinoma gallbladder
a. Clonorchis sinensis
b. Gnathostoma
c. Stronglyoidosis cantonensis
d. H. diminuta

419. A 30-year-old lady presents with fever and pain in right hypochondrium with presents breath catch up upon palpation. What is the clinical diagnosis?
a. Acute pancreatitis
b. Acute cholecystitis
c. Acute appendicitis
d. Acute mediastinitis

420. Charcot triad is used for
a. Acute cholangitis
b. Acute cholecystitis
c. Cholelithiasis
d. Gall bladder CA

421. Murphy sign is seen in:
a. Acute appendicitis
b. Acute cholecystitis
c. Acute pancreatitis
d. Acute cholangitis

422. Which of the following is Not associated with elevation of Right hemi-diaphragm:
a. Amebic abscess
b. Pyogenic abscess
c. Cholecystitis
d. Sub diaphragmatic abscess

423. Liver biopsy is indicated for diagnosis/evaluation of all; EXCEPT?
a. Autoimmune hepatitis
b. Storage disorders
c. Hemangioma
d. Hepatocellular carcinoma

424. Which is the most common benign liver tumor?
a. Hemangioma
b. Hepatocellular carcinoma
c. Hepatoma
d. Secondaries

425. Pringle's maneuver is mainly used to control bleeding from
a. IVC
b. Hepatic artery
c. Cystic artery
d. Hepatic vein

426. What is the true color of cholesterol stone?
a. Black
b. Dark yellow
c. Brown
d. Pale yellow

427. In Hemolytic anemia which stones are commonly seen?
a. Pigment stone
b. Cholesterol stone
c. Mixed stone
d. All of these

428. Aspirin protects against all; EXCEPT?
a. MI
b. Stroke
c. Colorectal cancer
d. Liver cancer

HEAD AND NECK

429. What severity of head injury does Glasgow coma scale of 10 denote? *(Most Recent Question June 2022)*
a. Mild
b. Moderate
c. Severe
d. Moribund

430. Which of the following types of esophageal cancer is most likely to the present with progressive difficulty in swallowing and weight loss? *(Most Recent Question June 2022)*
a. Adenocarcinoma
b. Small cell carcinoma
c. Transitional cell carcinoma
d. Squamous cell carcinoma

431. Which of the following is the most appropriate treatment for the given condition? *(Most Recent Question Dec. 2021)*

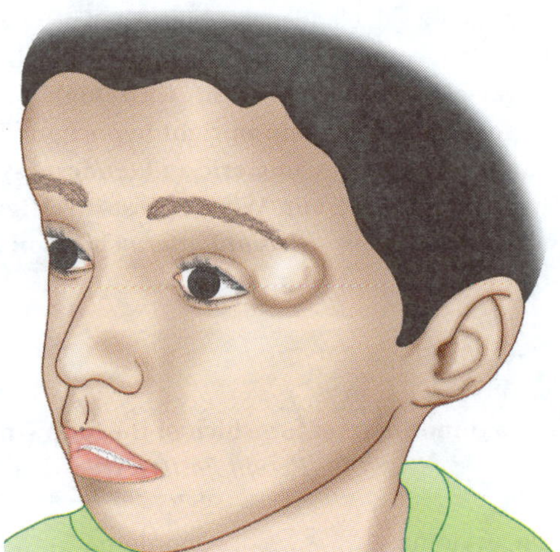

a. Sclerotherapy
b. Incision and drainage
c. Radiotherapy
d. Surgical excision

432. In case of type 3 branchial fistula, the internal opening is located in which part of pharynx? *(Most Recent Question Dec. 2021)*
a. Pyriform sinus
b. Tonsillar fossa
c. External auditory canal
d. Cricopharyngeus muscle

433. Cleft lip results from: *(Most Recent Question June 2021)*
a. Failure of fusion of maxillary and median nasal process
b. Failure of fusion of 2 palatine shelves
c. Separation of the nasal septum and vomer from the palatine processes
d. Anteroposterior orientation of muscles responsible for closure of velopharynx

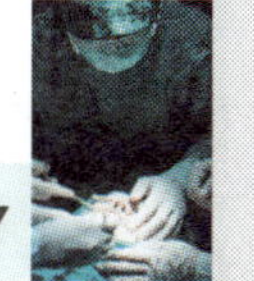

434. What is the preferred management of the given condition in the image? ***(Most Recent Question Dec 2020)***

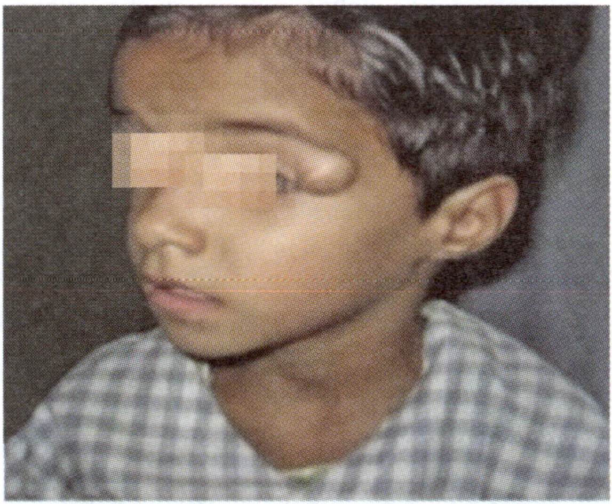

a. Surgical excision
b. Intralesional steroids
c. Chemotherapy
d. Radiotherapy

435. A player after head injury with ball, became unconscious and fell on the ground. All other teammates came to help him, suddenly he got-up and starting playing again. After some time, player suddenly fell on the ground. What is the type injury?
(Most Recent Question Dec 2020)

a. Extradural hematoma
b. Subdural hematoma
c. Diffuse axonal injury
d. Subarachnoid hemorrhage

436. The image of patient after a lifesaving procedure is given. Identify the procedure?
(Most Recent Question Dec 2020)

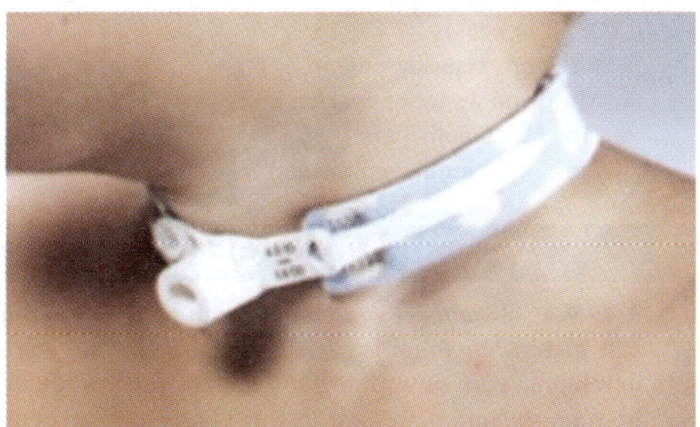

a. Nasotracheal intubation
b. Needle cricothyrodotomy
c. Endotracheal intubation
d. Tracheostomy

437. A patient presented with neck swelling with purulent discharge, whose image is given below. What is the diagnosis? ***(Most Recent Question Dec 2020)***

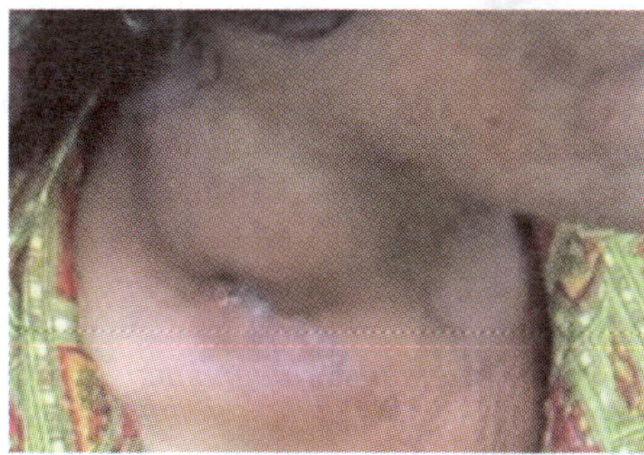

a. Cystic hygroma
b. Collar stud abscess
c. Brachial fistula
d. Thyroglossal cyst

438. A 65-year-old man patient presents with pulsatile swelling in the neck below the angle of jaw. It produces an outward expansile impulse. Which of the following is the most probable diagnosis?
(Most Recent Question Dec 2020)

a. Normal phenomenon
b. Parapharyngeal abscess
c. Carotid body tumor
d. Cystic hygroma

439. Which of the following statement is correct about ranula? ***(Most Recent Question Aug 2020)***

a. Mainly a retention cyst
b. Characteristic Translucent
c. Related to submandibular gland
d. Diagnosed by FNAC

440. All are premalignant conditions of oral cavity; EXCEPT:
(Recent Pattern Question 2018-19)

a. Chronic hyperplastic candidiasis
b. Oral submucosal fibrosis
c. Oral lichen planus
d. Leukoplakia

441. Comment on the diagnosis of this 60 year old man.
(Recent Pattern Question 2018-19)

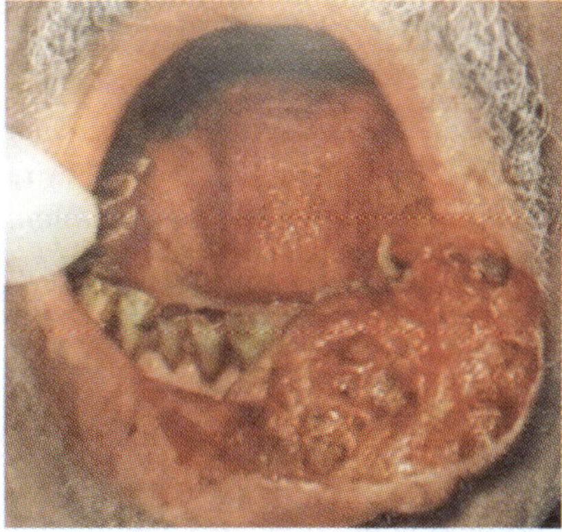

a. Basal cell Cancer
b. Plunging Ranula
c. Epulis
d. SCC of lip

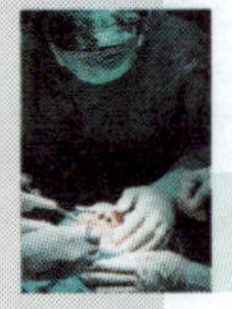

442. MC subtype of Rodent ulcer is? *(Recent Pattern Question 2018-19)*
a. Superficial spreading b. Acral lentiginous
c. Nodulocystic d. Pigmented

443. Which among the following is the cause of submucosal fibrosis? *(Recent Pattern Question 2018)*
a. Alcohol b. Candidiasis
c. Betel nut chewing d. Pan leaf chewing

444. Which nerve is involved in thoracic outlet syndrome? *(Recent Pattern Question 2017)*
a. Pain and paraesthesia in axillary nerve distribution
b. Pain and paraesthesia in median nerve distribution
c. Pain and paraesthesia in radial nerve distribution
d. Pain and paraesthesia in ulnar nerve distribution

445. Pott puffy tumor is seen at: *(Recent Pattern Question 2017)*
a. Frontal bone b. Temporal bone
c. Occipital bone d. Sphenoid bone

446. Cranio-pharyngioma is a brain tumor arising from? *(Recent Pattern Question 2016)*
a. Rathke pouch b. Neurohypophysis
c. Posterior pituitary d. Median eminence

447. A biker develops a head injury and non-contrast CT scan shows presence of Lentiform hemorrhage. What is the diagnosis? *(Recent Pattern Question 2016)*
a. Extradural bleeding
b. Subdural bleeding
c. Intraparenchymal bleeding
d. Intraventricular bleeding

448. Metastasis to neck lymph nodes is from?
a. Breast cancer
b. Nasopharyngeal cancer
c. Adrenal carcinoma
d. Stomach cancer

449. What is the most common malignant brain tumor?
a. Astrocytoma b. Glioblastoma multiforme
c. Oligodendroglioma d. Ependymoma

450. Stereotactic radiotherapy is used for treatment of?
a. Brain tumor b. Lung carcinoma
c. Cervical cancer d. Renal carcinoma

451. Which of the following tumors is cured by radiation?
a. Rhabdomyosarcoma b. Neuroblastoma
c. Chloroma d. Seminoma

452. Which is the most common secondary malignancy in retinoblastoma?
a. Ewing's sarcoma b. Osteosarcoma
c. Chondrosarcoma d. Rhabdomyosarcoma

453. All are seen in Trotters' triad; EXCEPT:
a. Unilateral conductive hearing loss
b. Ipsilateral earache and facial pain
c. Ipsilateral paralysis of the soft palate
d. Seen with juvenile nasopharyngeal angiofibroma

454. What is true about tongue cancer?
a. Most common type is adenocarcinoma
b. Cervical lymph node metastasis is universally present
c. MC site is on Lateral margin
d. Slurring of speech is a common complaint

455. What is the most common site of tongue cancer?
a. Base of tongue
b. Tip of tongue
c. Lateral margin of tongue
d. Posterior attachment of tongue

456. What is your diagnosis?

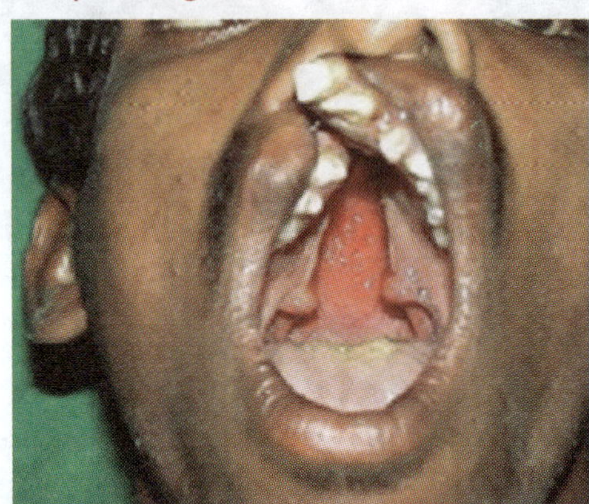

a. Cleft lip b. Cleft palate
c. Cleft lip and palate d. Bifid uvula

457. Secretory sinus in neck, moving upon deglutination:
a. Branchial sinus b. Pilonidal cyst
c. Thyroglossal fistula d. Sublingual dermoid cyst

458. A newborn has a swelling in neck due to soft cystic mass with transillumination test positive. What is the diagnosis?
a. Potato tumor b. Branchial cyst
c. Cystic hygroma d. Carotid body tumor

459. All of the following are true regarding cystic hygroma; EXCEPT
a. Brilliantly transilluminant
b. Mostly on posterior neck region
c. Lined by endothelium
d. Lined by columnar epithelium

VASCULAR SURGERY

460. A 45-year-old smoker complains of calf pain on walking 400 meters. In follow-up visits he says that he starts developing pain on walking 100 meters only. Gradually he starts having pain even during sleeping, thereby he prefers to sleep with legs dangling which makes him feel better. What is the most likely pathology in this patient? *(Most Recent Question June 2022)*
a. Venous claudication b. Neurological claudication
c. Sciatica d. Rest pain

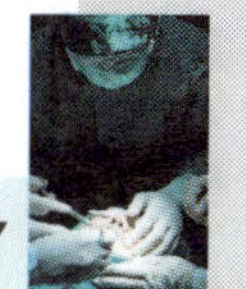

461. Which of the following is used in the treatment for a female has color change of digits as white, blue and red on cold exposure? *(Most Recent Question June 2022)*

a. CCB
b. Beta blockers
c. Alpha blockers
d. NSAID

462. A male patient with history of smoking presented with black necrotic index finger as shown below. What is the diagnosis? *(Most Recent Question Dec. 2021)*

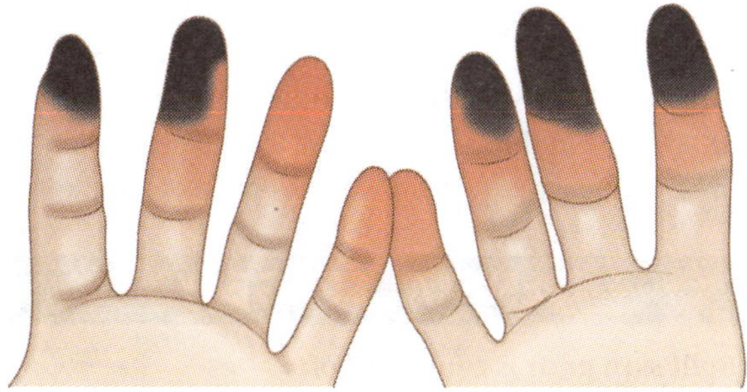

a. Ainhum
b. Raynaud's phenomenon
c. Fournier's gangrene
d. Buerger's disease

463. A 50-year-old female underwent total hip replacement after fracture of the neck of femur, for which she developed breathlessness and was brought to the emergency. What is the most likely cause of this condition? *(Most Recent Question Dec. 2021)*

a. Venous thromboembolism
b. Air embolism
c. Systemic embolism
d. Fat embolism

464. Which of the following is the investigation of choice for pulmonary embolism? *(Most Recent Question Dec. 2021)*

a. Ultrasound
b. CECT chest
c. Doppler
d. CT angiography

465. What is the origin of ulcer, given in the image? *(Most Recent Question Dec 2020)*

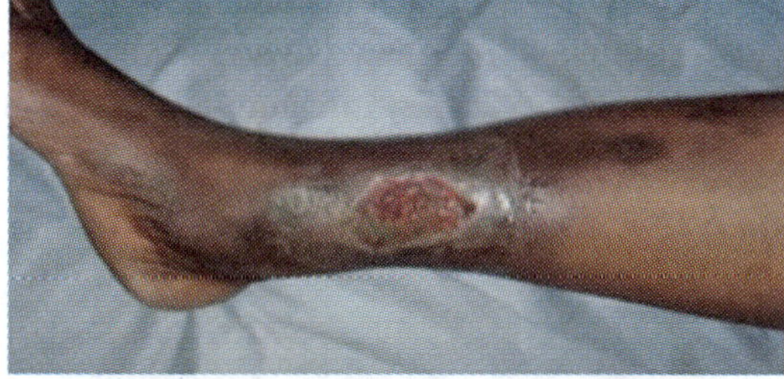

a. Venous ulcer
b. Arterial ulcer
c. Diabetic ulcer
d. Pressure ulcer

466. A bed ridden patient developed low -grade fever, pain in the calf region and pedal edema. It is related to: *(Most Recent Question Dec 2020)*

a. Cellulitis
b. DVT
c. Necrotizing fasciitis
d. Varicose vein

467. A 60-year-old patient presents with restricted ambulation and prolonged bed rest due to acute lumbago presented with severe pain in left leg below the knee. On examination discoloration of left calf with significantly increased girth is noted. What is the clinical diagnosis? *(Most Recent Question Dec 2020)*

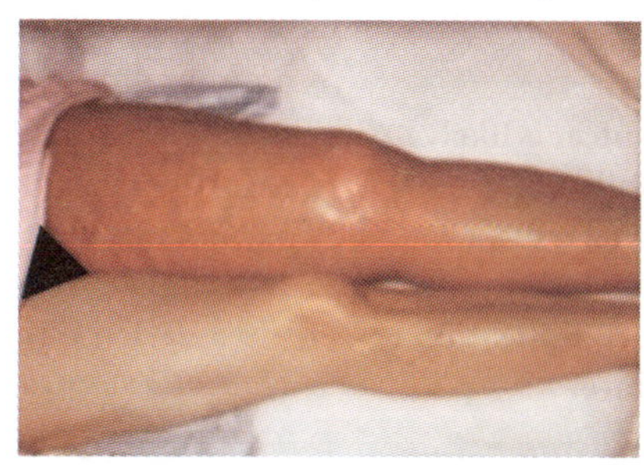

a. Acute lymphangitis
b. Superficial migratory thrombophlebitis
c. Deep vein thrombosis
d. Milroy disease

468. A patient had Blunt injury to his calf during a hit and run accident. On examination, there was pain on passive stretching and distal pulses were feeble. What is the most probable diagnosis? *(Most Recent Question Aug 2020)*

a. Compartment syndrome
b. Necrotizing fasciitis
c. Buerger's disease
d. DVT

469. Correct about cellulitis is? *(Most Recent Question Dec 2019)*

a. Nonsuppurative and noninvasive
b. Suppurative and invasive
c. Nonsuppurative and invasive
d. Suppurative and invasive

470. Long term diabetic patient walked barefoot few miles on hot sand. He developed blisters on feet and legs What is the most probable diagnosis? *(Most Recent Question Dec 2019)*

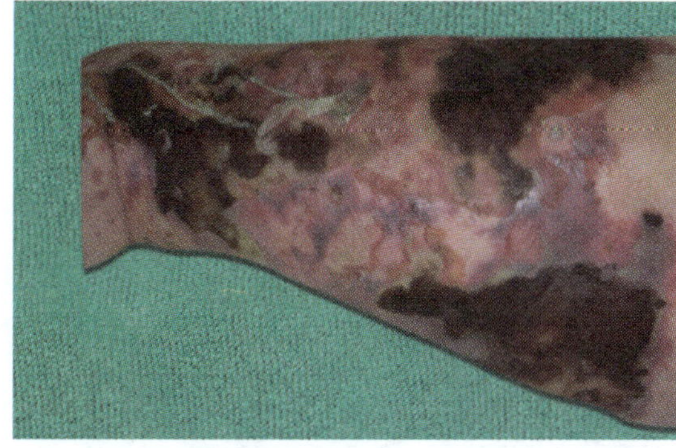

a. Diabetic foot
b. Burn
c. Necrotizing fasciitis
d. Chilblains

471. A patient of varicose veins came to hospital; intern was on duty. Which test he shall perform to evaluate for saphenofemoral incompetence.
(Most Recent Question Dec 2019)
a. Brodie Trendelenberg test I
b. Brodie Trendelenburg test II
c. Perthe's test
d. Thomas test

472. Which ulcer is likely to develop in a long standing chronic venous ulcer? ***(Most Recent Question 2019)***
a. Marjolin ulcer
b. Apthous ulcer
c. Bazin ulcer
d. Arterial ulcer

473. Which complication is seen after Varicose vein stripping procedure? ***(Most Recent Question 2019)***
a. Neuralgia
b. Deep vein thrombosis
c. Acrocyanosis
d. Telangiectasia

474. Most common complication of below knee stripping of Varicose veins is: ***(Recent Pattern Question 2018-19)***
a. Haemorrhage
b. Thromboembolism
c. Neuralgia
d. Infection

475. Which is the most common site of peripheral aneurysm?
(Recent Pattern Question 2018)
a. Femoral artery
b. Radial artery
c. Popliteal artery
d. Brachial artery

476. Intermittent claudication is defined as pain __________?
(Recent Pattern Question 2018)
a. At rest
b. On first step of walking
c. Relieved on standing still
d. Increase on limb dependency

477. Which of the following is the best management for radiation induced occlusive disease of carotid artery?
(Recent Pattern Question 2018)
a. Low dose aspirin
b. Carotid angioplasty and stenting
c. Carotid endarterectomy
d. Carotid bypass procedure

478. All of the following result after chronic edema to legs; EXCEPT?
a. Marjolin's ulcer
b. Thickening of skin
c. Soft tissue infections
d. Varicose veins

479. Buerger disease affects which layers of artery?
a. Tunica media
b. Tunica adventitia
c. Tunica intima
d. All of the above

480. All are true about Buerger disease; EXCEPT:
a. Ulnar artery and peroneal arteries involved
b. Nerve involvement present
c. Small acral vessels of limb involvement causes hypohidrosis
d. Phlebitis migrans

481. Patient presents with varicose vein with sapheno-femoral incompetence with normal perforators. The best management plan is:
a. Endovascular striping
b. Sclerotherapy
c. Sapheno-femoral flush ligation
d. Saphenofemoral flush ligation with stripping

482. Thromboangitis obliterans involves?
a. Arteries
b. Veins
c. Nerves
d. All of these

483. Hoffman Tinel sign is seen in?
a. Deep vein thrombosis
b. Nerve regeneration
c. Pulmonary embolism
d. Upper motor neuron lesion

GENERAL SURGERY

484. Split skin graft is composed of:
(Most Recent Question June 2022)
a. Only epidermis
b. Epidermis and partial dermis
c. Epidermis and deep dermis
d. Epidermis, dermis and subcutaneous fat

485. A 30-year-old lady after fire-works accident presented with burns from the neck down to the lower back. What will be the preferred sequence of treatment?
(Most Recent Question June 2022)
a. First debridement then resuscitation then grafting
b. First debridement then grafting and then resuscitation
c. First resuscitation then grafting and then debridement
d. First resuscitation then debridement and then grafting

486. Which of the following is the best method for hair removal to avoid surgical site infection?
(Most Recent Question June 2022)
a. Shaving site with razor the morning of operation
b. Hair clippers inside the operation theater
c. Shaving site with a razor the night before operation
d. Depilatory creams before the operation

487. A patient suffered from injury 3 days ago following which he was brought to tertiary care hospital. What would be the initial treatment in this patient?
(Most Recent Question June 2022)

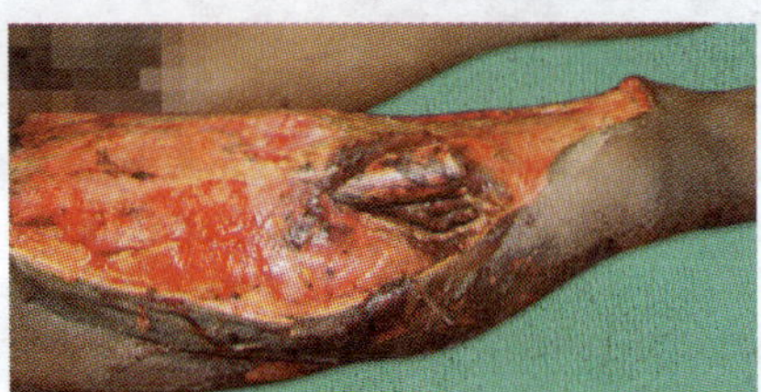

a. Debridement and rotational advancement flap closure
b. Debridement and primary closure
c. Amputation
d. Debridement and hyperbaric oxygen

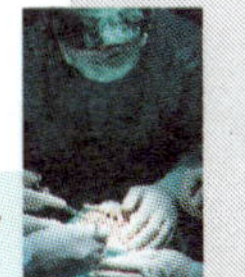

488. Which of the following incisions is cosmetically preferred for appendicectomy? *(Most Recent Question June 2022)*

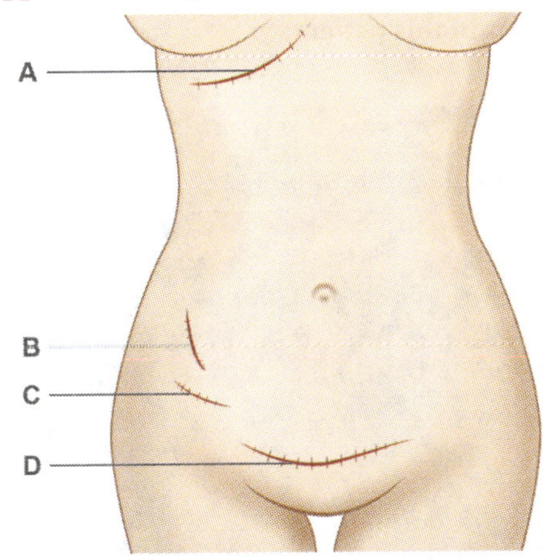

a. A
b. B
c. C
d. D

489. A 60-year-old female presented in a state of shock and abdominal distension she has history of prolonged use of NSAIDs. Chest X-ray is given below. Identify the condition. *(Most Recent Question Dec. 2021)*

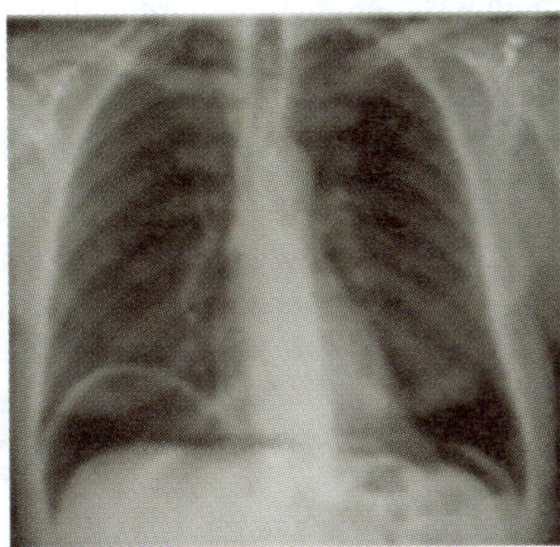

a. Pneumothorax
b. Pleural effusion
c. Hydropneumothorax
d. Perforation of peptic ulcer

490. What is the cause of cannon ball appearance on chest X-ray as shown below? *(Most Recent Question Dec. 2021)*

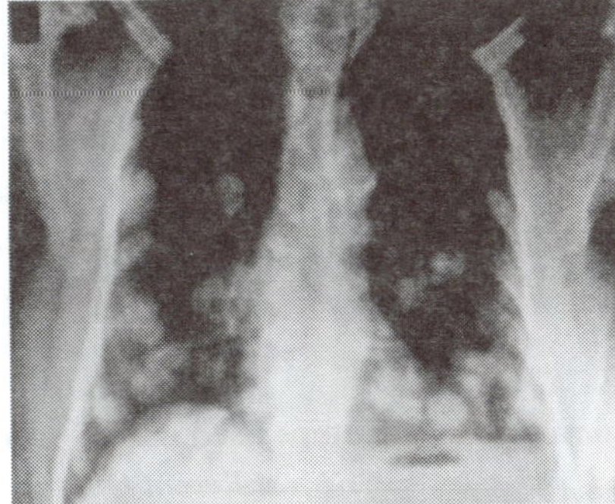

a. Tuberculosis
b. Carcinoma lung
c. Lung metastasis
d. Fungal infection

491. Popcorn calcification on chest X-ray is seen in: *(Most Recent Question Dec. 2021)*

a. Pulmonary hamartoma
b. Bronchogenic carcinoma
c. Aspergilloma
d. Mesothelioma

492. A 50-year-old patient presented with history of chronic cough, occasional hemoptysis and weight loss. Golden "S" sign was seen on the chest X-ray. What is the diagnosis? *(Most Recent Question Dec. 2021)*

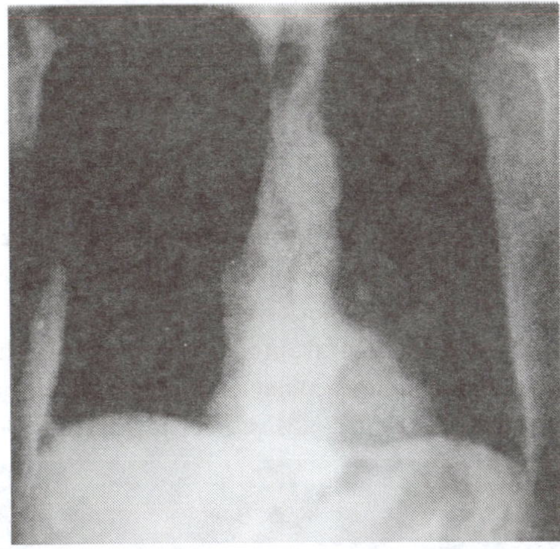

a. Tuberculosis
b. Bronchogenic carcinoma
c. Mesothelioma
d. Aspergilloma

493. A child was brought to emergency by the mother with difficulty in swallowing for the past few hours. The child was able to speak. X-ray was taken. Identify the location of foreign body. *(Most Recent Question Dec. 2021)*

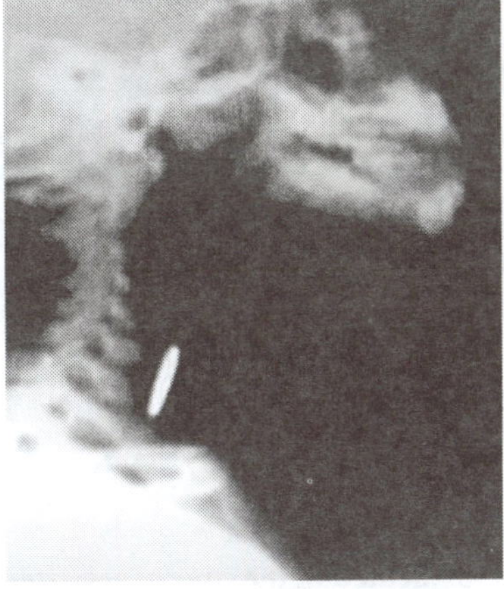

a. Esophagus
b. Trachea
c. Mediastinum
d. Artifact of X-ray

494. Pressure sores are formed when the pressure is above: *(Most Recent Question Dec. 2021)*

a. 5 mm Hg
b. 10 mm Hg
c. 20 mm Hg
d. 30 mm Hg

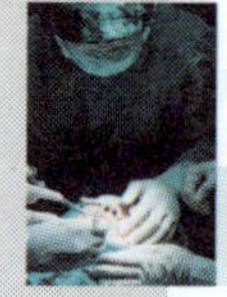

495. After resection of a lipoma over neck region, the patient developed an elevated scar within the operative site with itching sensation. What is the diagnosis? ***(Most Recent Question Dec. 2021)***

a. Hypertrophic scar
b. Stich granuloma
c. Granulomatous scar
d. Keloid

496. A patient of RTA was brought to the emergency with BP of 80/90 mm Hg. FAST was positive. Fluid resuscitation was done but the patient was not improving. What is the next best step? ***(Most Recent Question Dec. 2021)***

a. Observation
b. CECT
c. Diagnostic laparoscopy
d. Exploratory laparotomy

497. A trauma patient was brought to the emergency. There was raised JVP, cold clammy skin, heart sounds were not audible clearly and neck veins were engorged. Patient died in the hospital and autopsy was done, which showed the following image. What is the most likely cause of death in this patient? ***(Most Recent Question Dec. 2021)***

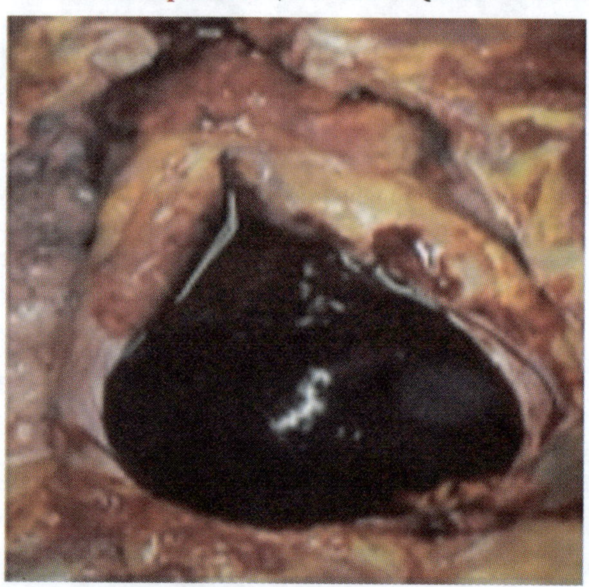

a. Cardiac tamponade
b. Fat necrosis
c. Hemothorax
d. Intestinal perforation

498. A patient presented in the emergency after head trauma. On examination, he was able to open his eyes on painful stimuli, shows withdrawal movement and used inappropriate words. What is the Glasgow coma score of this patient? ***(Most Recent Question June 2021)***

a. E3M5V4
b. E2M3V3
c. E1M3V3
d. E2M3V2

499. A chronic smoker presented to the emergency. His X-ray chest was done which showed the following. Probable diagnosis in this patient: ***(Most Recent Question June 2021)***

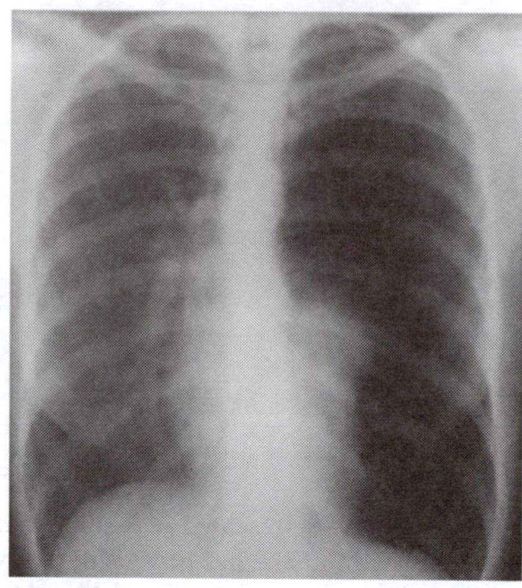

a. Pneumothorax
b. Tension pneumothorax
c. Hemothorax
d. Hydropneumothorax

500. What is the probable cause of the condition shown in the given X-ray? ***(Most Recent Question June 2021)***

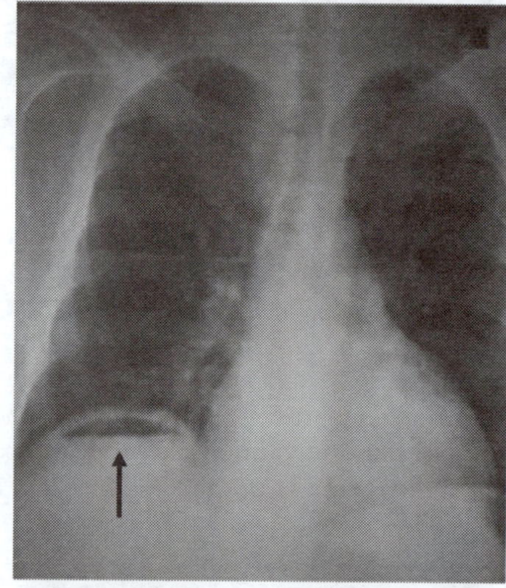

a. Pleural effusion
b. Perforation peritonitis
c. Sigmoid volvulus
d. Intestinal obstruction

501. Radioisotope used in thyroid cancer treatment: ***(Most Recent Question June 2021)***

a. I 131
b. 99 Tc
c. 89 St
d. 133 Cs

502. Most common radioisotope used in PET scan: ***(Most Recent Question June 2021)***

a. 18F
b. 13C
c. 14 C
d. All of these

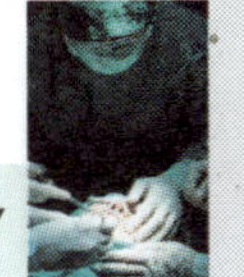

503. A patient of injury to right side of the chest presented to emergency. The patient's chest X-ray is given below. What is the preferred treatment option?

(Most Recent Question Dec 2020)

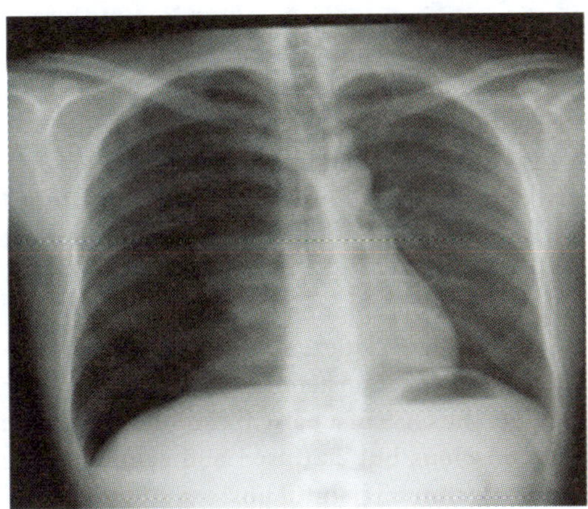

a. Chest tube insertion on left side
b. Conservative management
c. Chest tube insertion on right side
d. Thoracotomy

504. The patient developed this lesion over chest after 6 months of surgery. What is the diagnosis?

(Most Recent Question Dec 2020)

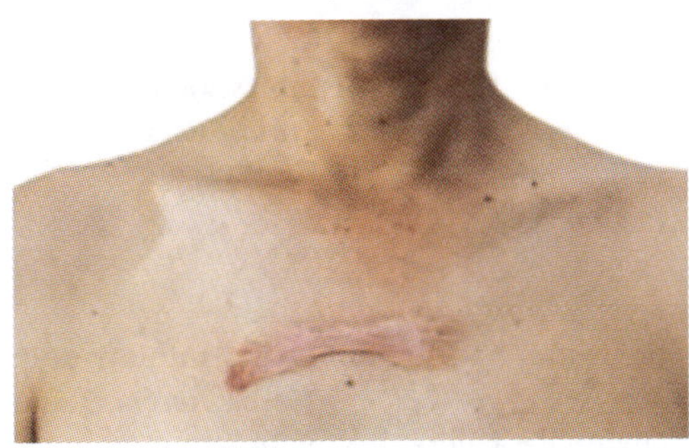

a. Atrophic scar b. Keloid
c. Hypertrophic scar d. Contracture

505. Which of the following fluid should not be given in the patient with head injury?

(Most Recent Question Dec 2020)

a. Normal saline b. Hypertonic saline
c. Ringer lactate d. 5% dextrose

506. What kind of shock is seen in the patient with profuse bleeding per rectum with cold clammy extremities and CVP of 2 cm H_2O? ***(Most Recent Question Dec 2020)***

a. Cardiogenic b. Neurogenic
c. Hypovolemic d. Distributive

507. Best method to check for the correct placement of central venous catheter?

a. Measure $PaCO_2$ b. Measure pH
c. Chest X-ray d. Temperature

508. A patient was brought to the emergency. Immediate and fast crystalloid IV transfusion has to be done. Which color IV cannula should be used for giving the fluids?

(Most Recent Question Dec 2020)

a. Blue b. Pink
c. Orange d. Green

509. What is the diagnosis on the basis of image given below?

(Most Recent Question Dec 2020)

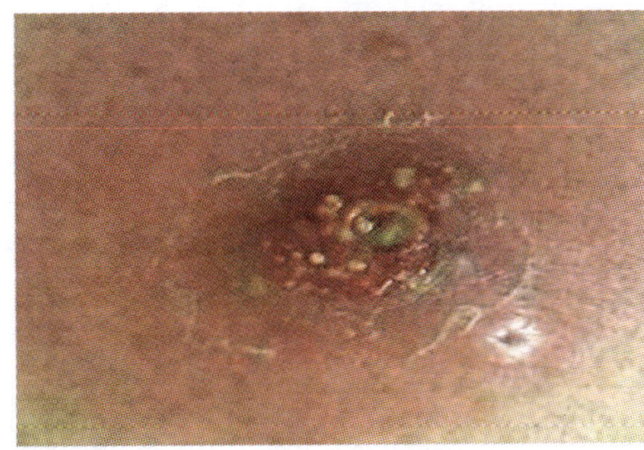

a. Cellulitis b. Folliculitis with abscess
c. Erysipelas d. Carbuncle

510. Which fluid should be given in severe head injury?

(Most Recent Question Dec 2020)

a. 5% dextrose b. Normal saline
c. Hypertonic saline d. Ringer lactate

511. A 30-year-old patient presents with acute abdomen. X-ray abdomen was done in standing position. Which of the following is correct about management of this condition? ***(Most Recent Question Dec 2020)***

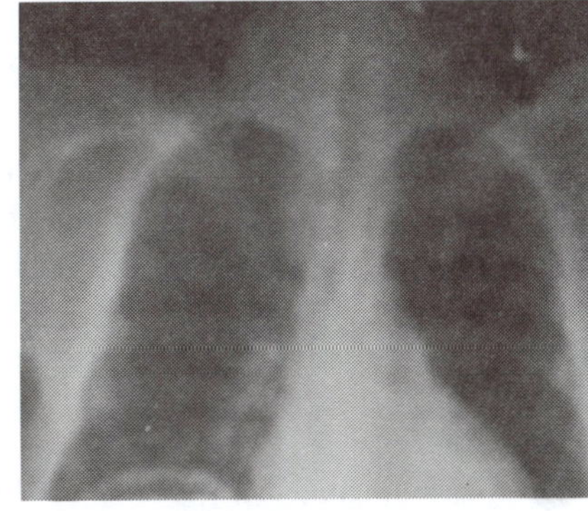

a. Drain the peritoneal fluid
b. X-ray guided drainage of peritoneal accumulation
c. Exploratory laparotomy
d. Insert flatus tube and perform barium studies

512. In a train accident, there were 74 dead, 64 were severely injured, 20 moderately injured and 32 mildly injured. Color-coding in triage highest to lowest category is:

(Most Recent Question Aug 2020)

a. Green – Yellow – Red – Black
b. Yellow – Red – Green – Black
c. Black – Yellow – Red – Green
d. Red – Yellow – Green – Black

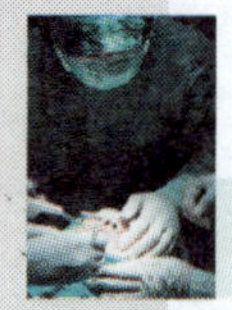

513. Mandatory exploration is required in the injuries of which zones of retroperitoneum:

(Most Recent Question Aug 2020)

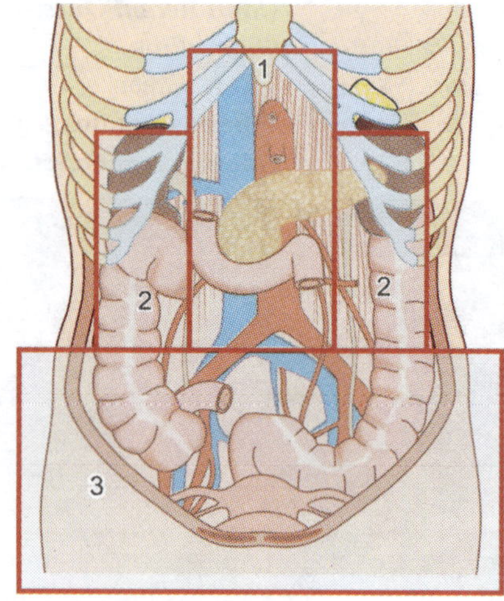

a. 1
b. 2
c. 3
d. 1 and 3

514. A 40-year-old patient with femur fracture develops respiratory distress on second day of admission to orthopedics department. CXR shows multiple pulmonary infiltrates. The most probable clinical diagnosis is:

(Most Recent Question Dec 2019)

a. Fat embolism
b. Pulmonary embolism
c. Air embolism
d. Tropical pulmonary eosinophilia

515. A 20-year-old man presented to emergency department after falling from motorbike. The investigation of choice should be? ***(Most Recent Question Dec 2019)***

a. CECT
b. MRI
c. NCCT
d. MRI

516. Which of the following components of ALVARADO score has a value assigned as 2?

(Most Recent Question Dec 2019)

a. Elevated body temperature
b. Leukocytosis
c. Shift to left
d. Migratory RIF pain

517. Patient categorization on the basis of chances of survival in disaster management is called____?

(Most Recent Question Dec 2019)

a. Mitigation
b. Tagging
c. Surge capacity
d. Triage

518. A patient presented to emergency after RTA with multiple rib fractures. He is conscious, speaking single words. On examination, respiratory rate was 40/min and BP was 90/40 mm Hg. What is the immediate next step?

(Most Recent Question 2019)

a. Urgent IV fluid administration
b. Intubate the patient
c. Chest–ray
d. Insert needle in 2nd intercostal space

519. Correct procedure of inserting Nasogastric tube is.

(Most Recent Question 2019)

a. Supine with neck flexed
b. Supine with neck extended
c. Sitting with neck flexed
d. Sitting with neck extended

520. Calculate the GCS of a patient exhibiting eye opening on pain, conscious but confused and cannot tell time and exhibits flexion on painful noxious stimuli to the arm.

(Most Recent Question 2019)

a. 8
b. 9
c. 10
d. 11

521. Most appropriate management of recurrent keloid is:

(Most Recent Question 2019)

a. Excisional surgery
b. Intramarginal excision followed by radiation
c. Cryosurgery
d. Silicone gel sheeting

522. Which of the following is not scanned by FAST USG?

(Most Recent Question 2019)

a. Pericardium
b. Pleural cavity
c. Spleen
d. Liver

523. Prophylactic antibiotics to minimise SSI are given______________? ***(Most Recent Question 2019)***

a. 60 minutes before skin incision
b. 1-3 hours before skin incision
c. At time of surgical incision
d. Night before surgery for peaking of effect

524. Which procedure is done in case of Ranula management?

(Most Recent Question 2019)

a. Incision and drainage
b. Aspiration
c. Excision
d. Sclerosant injection

525. Which of the following is best for diagnosis of pheochromocytoma? ***(Most Recent Question 2019)***

a. 24-hour urinary Vaniyll Mandelic acid
b. 24-hour urinary Fractionated Metanephrine
c. 24-hour Urinary Hydroxy indole acetic acid
d. 24-hour Urinary Hydroxy tryptamine

526. Comment on the diagnosis?
(Most Recent Question 2019)

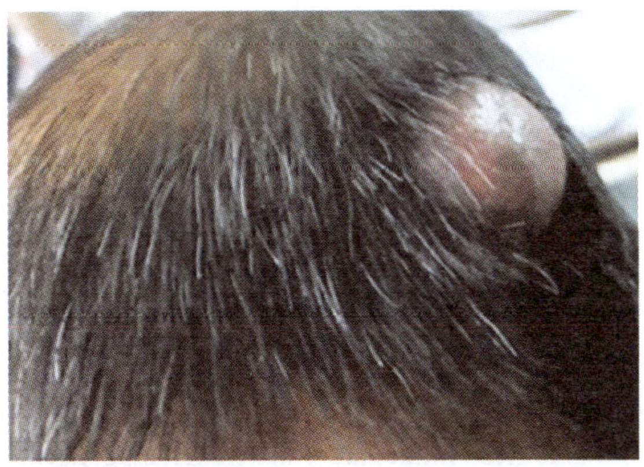

a. Sebaceous cyst b. Implantation dermoid
c. Angular dermoid d. Lipoma

527. Comment on the diagnosis *(Most Recent Question 2019)*

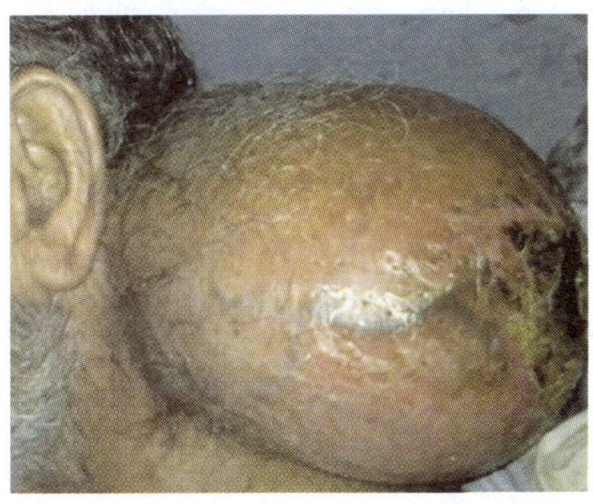

a. Lipoma b. Encephalocele
c. Cystic hygroma d. Lymphadenopathy

528. Which organ has highest chances of Graft rejection response? *(Most Recent Question 2019)*

a. Cornea b. Gut
c. Liver d. Skin

529. In hypovolemic shock which organ should be assessed for determining under-perfusion?
(Most Recent Question 2019)

a. Kidney b. Heart
c. Lung d. Liver

530. Which of the following is not a hospital acquired infection? *(Recent Pattern Question 2018-19)*

a. S.S.I b. S.T.D
c. U.T.I d. Pneumonia

531. Amount of blood loss in class III circulatory failure/ Haemorrhagic shock? *(Recent Pattern Question 2018-19)*

a. <15% b. 15-30%
c. 30-40% d. >40%

532. Identify the lesion shown.
(Recent Pattern Question 2018-19)

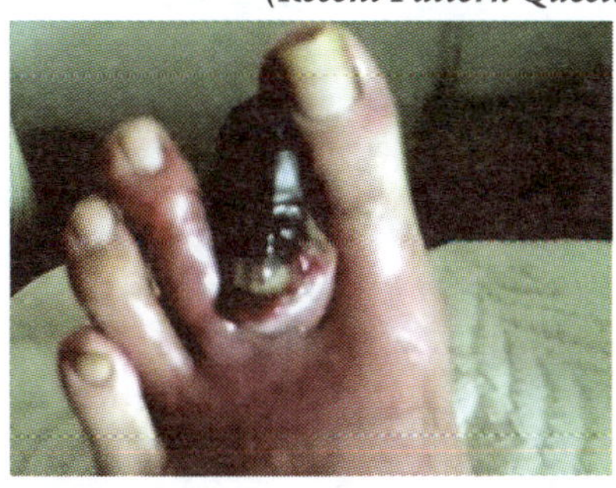

a. Wet gangrene b. Dry gangrene
c. Frost bite d. Ainhum

533. The following patient has presented after chest trauma. On examination crepitus is felt. The clinical diagnosis is?
(Recent Pattern Question 2018-19)

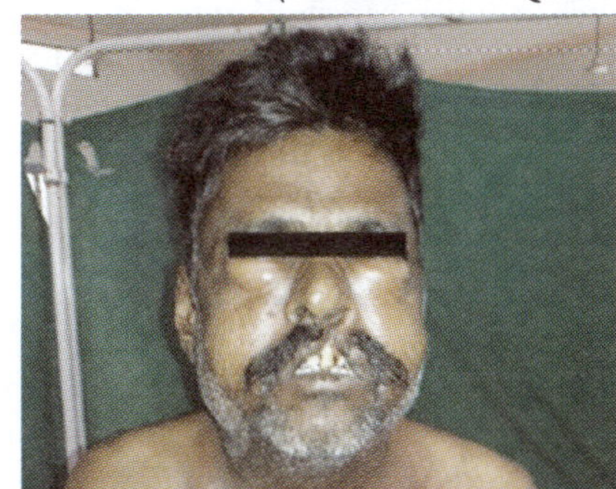

a. Subcutaneous Emphysema
b. Gas gangrene
c. Acute tubular necrosis
d. SVC syndrome

534. What is the GCS for a brain dead patient?
(Recent Pattern Question 2018)

a. 3 b. 5
c. 6 d. 8

535. A 50 kg patient has 40% burn of the body surface area. BP 90/60 mm Hg. Calculate the ringer lactate solution to be given for first 8 hours of fluid:
(Recent Pattern Question 2018)

a. 1 L b. 2 L
c. 4 L d. 8 L

536. Which is the best method to administer oxygen in case of burns of airways? *(Recent Pattern Question 2018)*

a. Elective intubation b. Mask
c. Nasal prongs d. Tracheostomy

537. In which of the following conditions is Fogarthy catheter used? *(Recent Pattern Question 2017)*

a. Acute limb ischemia
b. Tube thoracotomy with underwater seal
c. Suprapubic drainage of bladder
d. Total parenteral nutrition

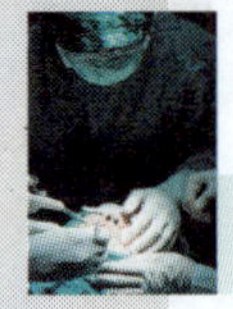

538. Which of the following needle is used to suture skin? *(Recent Pattern Question 2017)*
a. Cutting needle b. Reverse Cutting needle
c. Round body needle d. Straight needle with eye

539. Shock index is defined as? *(Recent Pattern Question 2017)*
a. Pulse rate/BP b. BP/Pulse rate
c. CVP/PCWP d. PCWP/CVP

540. Which is used to control bleeding? *(Recent Pattern Question 2017)*
a. Pressure b. Packing
c. Position d. All of these

541. What is the preferred fluid used in burns after 24 hours? *(Recent Pattern Question 2017)*
a. Ringer lactate
b. Colloids
c. Hypertonic saline
d. Switch to oral or parenteral nutrition

542. A patient presents with knife stab wound to the Lower neck. Pulse rate is 110/min with BP = 100/70 mm Hg. Which is the next step? *(Recent Pattern Question 2017)*
a. Immediate wound exploration
b. Formal wound exploration in OT in GA
c. Put stent to prevent pneumothorax
d. Urgent angiography

543. A patient with abdominal trauma is brought to casualty. On examination the vitals are stable with no evidence of peritonitis. Next best step is? *(Recent Pattern Question 2017)*
a. Urgent exploratory laparotomy
b. CT Abdomen
c. F.A.S.T
d. Diagnostic peritoneal lavage

544. Class I haemorrhagic shock is caused by __________ml loss of blood. *(Recent Pattern Question 2017)*
a. 750 b. 1000
c. 1500 d. 2000

545. Fogarthy catheter is used in which of the following? *(Recent Pattern Question 2017)*
a. Acute limb ischemia
b. Suprapubic catheterization of Urinary bladder
c. Deflating sigmoid volvulus
d. Coronary stenting

546. A patient underwent inguinal lymph node dissection and drain was placed. On 10th day severe bleeding occurs. What type of bleeding is this? *(Recent Pattern Question 2016)*
a. Reactionary hemorrhage b. Secondary
c. Primary d. Tertiary

547. A 25-year-old Patient with abdominal trauma presents with Hypovolemic shock, and is unresponsive to crystalloids. What is the next step? *(Recent Pattern Question 2016)*
a. Albumin b. Colloids
c. Blood transfusion d. Immediate laparoscopy

548. Which is the best parameter to monitor Hypovolemic shock? *(Recent Pattern Question 2016)*
a. Urine output b. Respiratory rate
c. Blood pressure d. Pulse rate

549. A 25-year-old patient presents in emergency with abdominal trauma. Why is FAST done? *(Recent Pattern Question 2016)*
a. Detection of pericardial fluid accumulation
b. Detection of bowel lacerations
c. Detection of Mesenteric Tear
d. Detection of aortic transection

550. Increased cardiac output is seen in which shock?
a. Septic shock b. Anaphylaxis
c. Neurogenic d. Hemolysis

551. What is given immediately in hemorrhagic shock?
a. Packed RBC b. Colloids
c. Crystalloids d. Isotonic fluids

552. Plasma expanders are most useful in which shock?
a. Septic shock b. Vasovagal shock
c. Neurogenic shock d. Cardiogenic shock

553. Neurogenic shock is caused by:
a. Burns b. Dehydration
c. Hemorrhage d. Anesthesia

554. Which is the preferred fluid in a poly-traumatic patient with shock?
a. Ringer lactate b. Normal saline
c. Dextran d. Dextrose-normal saline

555. Which is the first fluid of choice in Hypovolemic shock?
a. Dextran b. Normal saline
c. Dextrose normal saline d. Hartmann solution

556. All are criteria for Systemic inflammatory response syndrome in children; EXCEPT:
a. Tachycardia b. Hypotension
c. Fever d. Leukocytosis

557. A new born boy has lumbosacral meningomyelocele and is awaiting surgical repair. The sac is best protected with sterile gauze piece soaked with
a. Mercurochrome b. Tincture benzoin
c. Methylene blue d. Normal saline

558. In 1 mL of 0.9%, normal saline content of Na is:
a. 0.1 mEq b. 0.3 mEq
c. 0.5 mEq d. 10 mEq

559. In 1 mL of 3 percent saline what is the quantity of sodium?
a. 0.5 mEq b. 1 mEq
c. 10 mEq d. 50 mEq

560. In IV fluid what percentage of energy is supplied by glucose when patient is on total parenteral nutrition?
a. 20 b. 30
c. 40 d. 50

561. According to "rule of 9". What is the percentage of burn in hand?
a. 1% b. 5%
c. 9% d. 14%

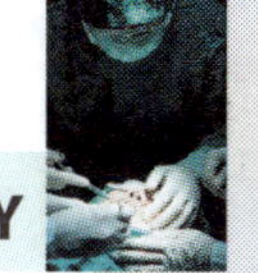

562. What is the % Body surface area involved in burns of the perineum?
a. 1% b. 3%
c. 5% d. 9%

563. What is the best solution for burns?
a. NS 0.9% b. Ringer's lactate
c. 25% dextrose d. Colloid

564. All are given for management of burns; EXCEPT?
a. Hypotonic solutions b. Albumin
c. 25% dextrose d. Hartmann solution/ATLS

565. What is the first fluid preferred in a burn patient?
a. Crystalloids b. Colloids
c. Any of above d. Both of above

566. All are true about a burn patient; EXCEPT:
a. Hematemesis is an early complication
b. For Head and neck burn exposure treatment done
c. Stridor can be present
d. Most common infection is by pseudomonas

567. What is the cause of death in 70% burns patient in whom enteral feeding is not given:
a. Dehydration b. Malnutrition
c. Electrolyte imbalance d. Bacterial infection

568. A burn patient is brought to emergency. Upon examination he was found dead. What could be the possible cause?
a. Sepsis b. Hypoxia
c. Malnutrition d. Hypovolemia

569. Which is true about burn?
a. Above 5% of surface area must be involved to produce shock
b. Inhaled hot gas will not cause supraglottic airway burn and laryngeal edema.
c. Early elective intubation is safest
d. If oral fluids are to be used, salt must be avoided

570. What is correct about 3rd degree burns?
a. Erythema and painful
b. Erythema and painless
c. Painless and cherry red
d. Painful and cherry red

571. Which virus causes infection in burn patients?
a. HSV b. CMV
c. EBV d. VZV

572. What is the cause of death in burns?
a. Sepsis b. Shock
c. Dyselectrolytemia d. ARDS

573. Burns present as all of the following; EXCEPT
a. Sepsis b. Shock
c. Acute kidney injury d. Air embolism

574. Middle area of face fracture (le-fort fracture) is characterized by all; EXCEPT
a. Proptosis b. Lengthening of face
c. Enopthalmos d. Ecchymosis

575. In Brown-Sequard syndrome ipsilateral loss will be of?
a. Pain b. Temperature
c. Tactile discrimination d. Proprioception

576. Blow out injury with ptosis occurs due to damage to:
a. Zygomatic arch
b. Orbital floor
c. Sphenoid bone
d. Palantine and maxillary bones

577. Fournier gangrene is caused by:
a. Clostridium welchii
b. Clostridium septicum
c. Anaerobic Streptococcus
d. Bacillus subtilis

578. Continuous burrowing ulcer is caused by?
a. Streptococcus viridans
b. Streptococcus pyogenes
c. Staphylococcus aureus
d. Microaerophilic streptococcus

579. All of the following are released/increased in surgical stress; EXCEPT:
a. ADH b. Insulin
c. ACTH d. Cortisol

580. All are true about Keloid; EXCEPT:
a. May be familial b. Arises on sternum
c. Subsides over time d. Hyperkeratotic

581. Which organ is most commonly affected by blunt trauma to abdomen?
a. Spleen b. Intestine
c. Liver d. Mesentery

582. Wound dehiscence occurs after how many days following surgery?
a. 2–4 days b. Within 2 days
c. 5–12 days d. >2 weeks

583. What does split thickness of skin graft mean?
a. Is a skin graft including the epidermis and part of the dermis
b. Is a skin graft including the epidermis and complete dermis
c. Is a skin graft including part of the epidermis and part of the dermis
d. Is a skin graft including part of epidermis and whole of the dermis

584. What is a xenograft:
a. Transplantation of organs from a 1st degree relative
b. Transplantation of organs from unrelated donor
c. Transplantation of tissues from self
d. Transplantation of living tissues/organs from one species to another

585. Fibrosis is seen in all; EXCEPT:
a. Marjolin's ulcers b. Buruli ulcer
c. Venous ulcer d. Peptic ulcer

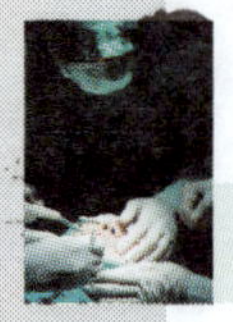

586. Carcinoma developed in a scar is called:
a. Sarcoma
b. Adenocarcinoma
c. Dermoid tumor
d. Marjolin's ulcer

587. Osteomyelitis first occurs in:
a. Metaphysis
b. Epiphysis
c. Diaphysis
d. All of these

588. Clean and small wound heals by?
a. Primary intention
b. Secondary intention
c. Tertiary intention
d. All of these

589. Female patient with injury on her scalp, hair was shaved and sutures were put. On which day sutures should be removed?
a. 8-10 days
b. 2 weeks
c. 3 weeks
d. 1 month

590. What is incorrect about Laparoscopy?
a. Smaller incisions
b. Minimal postoperative pain
c. Trocar injury in patients with low body mass index
d. Recovery time is longer

591. A guy driving a car fast suddenly slams on the brakes. He was wearing a seat belt. The organ most likely to be affected is:
a. Liver
b. Spleen
c. Mesentery
d. Kidney

592. A motor cyclist after multiple trauma is having hypoventilation. What is the cause?
a. Damage to respiratory centre
b. Damage to respiratory apparatus
c. Both a and b
d. None of the above

593. What is the best investigation for a hemodynamically stable patient with blunt abdominal trauma?
a. CECT abdomen
b. MRI abdomen
c. Diagnostic Peritoneal lavage
d. FAST

594. Painful lockjaw is seen in all of the following; EXCEPT?
a. Tetany
b. Temporomandibular joint abscess
c. Mandibular abscess
d. Odontogenic pulp abscess

595. What is the most common site of basal cell carcinoma in lips?
a. Upper lip
b. Central 1/3
c. Lower lip
d. Commissures

596. Fracture of neck of fibula leads to which nerve injury?
a. Common peroneal nerve
b. Obturator nerve
c. Genitofemoral nerve
d. Posterior tibial nerve

597. What is the most common Nosocomial infection acquired by a patient undergoing surgery?
a. S.I.R.S
b. Surgical site infection
c. Pneumonia
d. Catheter based infection

598. Upon aspiration in supine position, food particle goes most commonly to?
a. Right lower lobe superior basal
b. Right lower lobe postero basal
c. Left lower lobe superior basal
d. Left lower lobe postero basal

599. What is the management of Epidermoid Carcinoma?
a. 5FU + external beam radiation
b. Mitomycin + External beam radiation
c. External beam Radiation
d. Surgery + Imiquimod

600. In TNM staging, N = ?
a. Nature of tumor
b. Number of tumors
c. Number of lymph nodes involved
d. Metastasis

NEUROLOGY

601. A patient presented to emergency with complaints of headache. Patient described it as the worst headache of his life. CT image is given below. What is the diagnosis?
(Most Recent Question Dec. 2021)

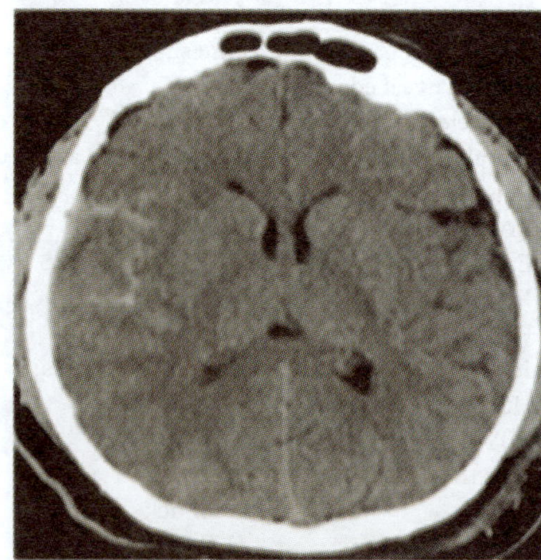

a. Extradural hemorrhage
b. Subdural hemorrhage
c. Migraine
d. Subarachnoid hemorrhage

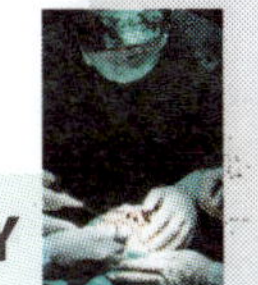

602. A 55-year-old woman working in the office, suffered a head trauma after a road traffic accident. Which of the following is associated with lucid interval?
(Most Recent Question Dec. 2021)

a. Acute subdural hemorrhage
b. Chronic subdural hemorrhage
c. Subarachnoid hemorrhage
d. Extradural hemorrhage

603. A 50-year-old man was brought to emergency after road traffic accident. He was diagnosed with cerebral edema. Which of the following drug should be used?
(Most Recent Question Dec. 2021)

a. Steroids
b. Mannitol
c. Acetazolamide
d. Glycerol

604. Battle sign is: *(Most Recent Question Dec. 2021)*

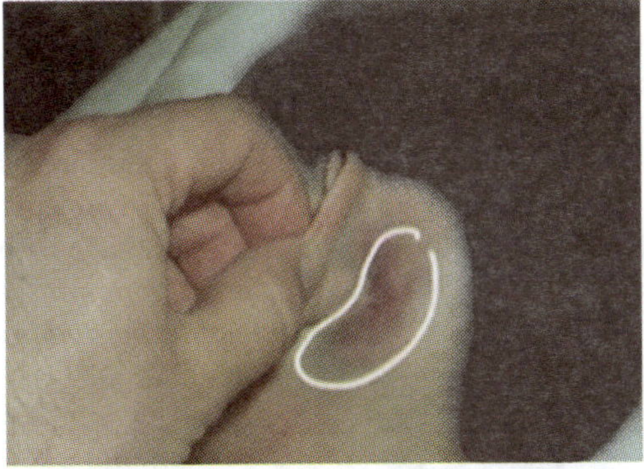

a. Bruising on mastoid
b. CSF rhinorrhea
c. Periorbital ecchymosis
d. Acute mastoiditis

605. A patient suffered from road traffic accident 6 hours ago before he was brought to the emergency with altered sensorium. His Glasgow coma score was 12. CT scan of head was done which is as shown below. He is most likely suffering from: *(Most Recent Question June 2021)*

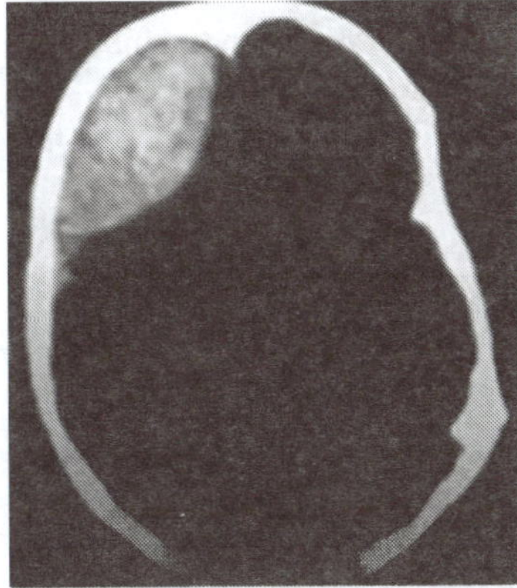

a. Subdural hematoma
b. Extradural hematoma
c. Subarachnoid hemorrhage
d. Intracerebral hematoma

606. A 50-year-old patient presented with development of intractable seizures. CT Head shows intracranial space occupying lesion for which a CT guided biopsy was done. The histopathology reported presence of psammoma bodies. Which of the following is the most likely diagnosis of this patient?
(Most Recent Question Aug 2020)

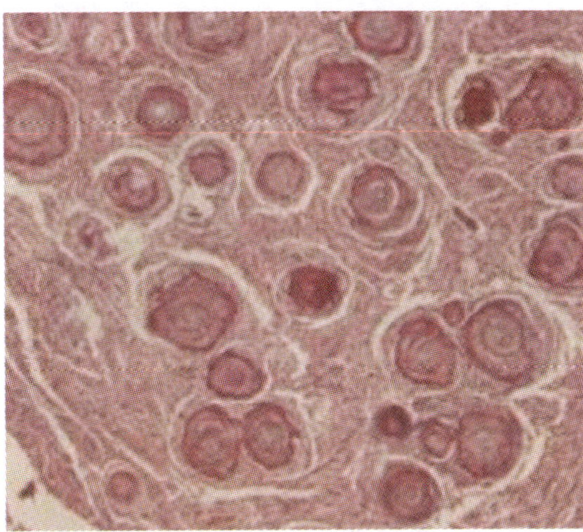

a. Astrocytoma
b. Ependymoma
c. Meningioma
d. Medulloblastoma

607. A 40-year-old man is brought to emergency with loss of consciousness following RTA. GCS is 8/15 and patient was having decerebrate rigidity. MRI head was performed and the image is given below. Which of the following is the diagnosis? *(Most Recent Question Aug 2020)*

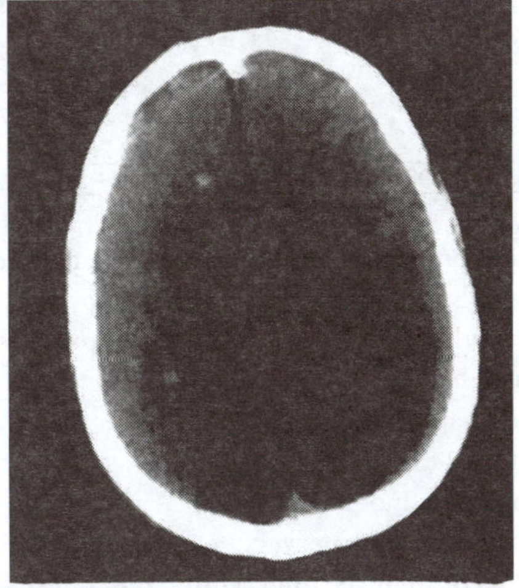

a. Subarachnoid hemorrhage
b. Subdural hemorrhage
c. Cerebral amyloid angiopathy
d. Diffuse axonal injury

MISCELLANEOUS

608. What should be the best treatment in a patient who presented in the emergency with respiratory distress and was noticed having dilated neck veins? CXR is shown below: *(Most Recent Question June 2022)*

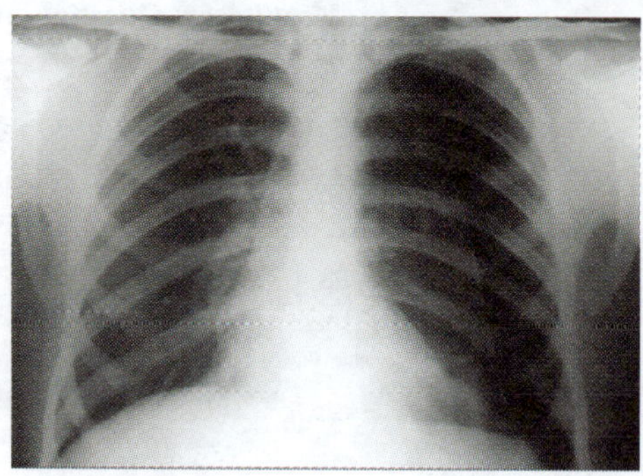

a. Endotracheal intubation
b. Needle Thoracostomy
c. Tracheostomy
d. Thoracocentesis

609. Patient has undergone surgical procedure for a lung pathology where his pre-operative and post operative chest-X-rays are shown below. What can be the likely diagnosis in this patient? *(Most Recent Question June 2022)*

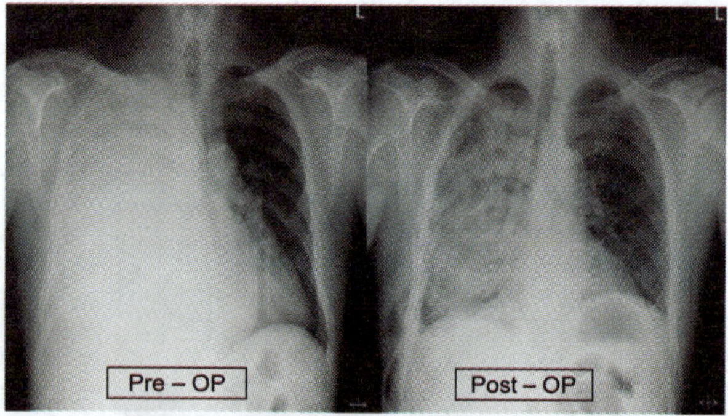

a. Right pneumothorax
b. Left pneumothorax
c. Right Empyema
d. Left empyema

610. Best results in Coronary artery bypass grafting are obtained by: *(Most Recent Question June 2022)*

a. Long saphenous vein
b. Internal mammary artery
c. Poly tetra fluoro ethylene
d. Gastroepiploic artery

611. An elderly male is undergoing renal transplantation. He received the graft from the twin brother this graft is known as: *(Most Recent Question Dec 2020)*

a. Autograft
b. Isograft
c. Allograft
d. Xenograft

612. What is the name of given instrument? *(Most Recent Question Dec 2020)*

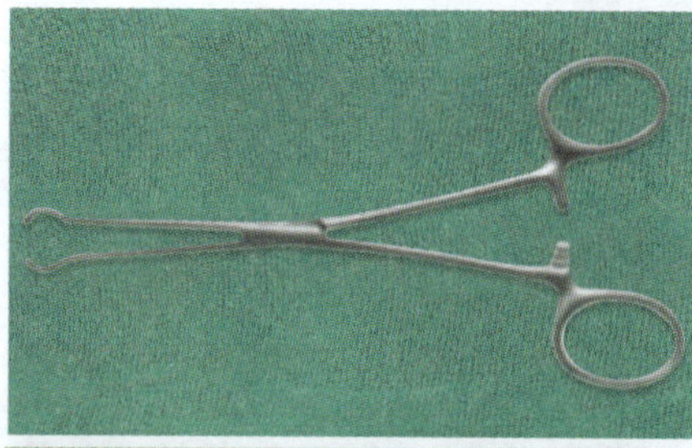

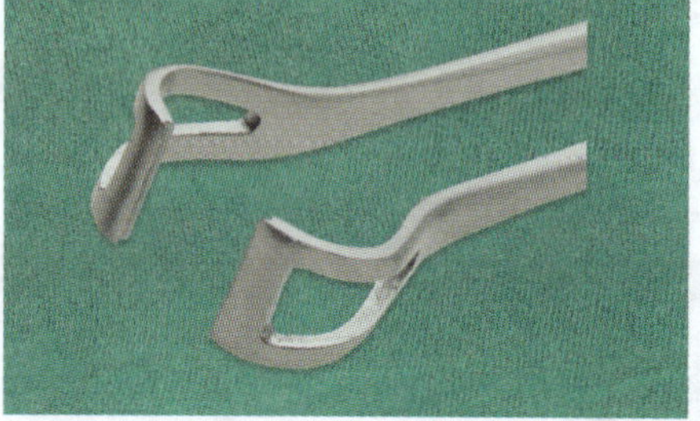

a. Ovum forceps
b. Allis tissue forceps
c. Sponge holding forceps
d. Babcock's forceps

613. Identify the condition shown in the image which has been progressively increasing for last 6 months. *(Most Recent Question Aug 2020)*

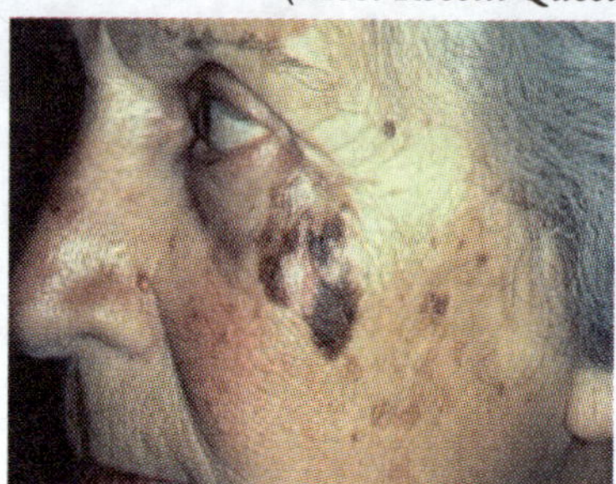

a. Basal cell carcinoma
b. Squamous cell carcinoma
c. Malignant melanoma
d. Nevus

614. Cutaneous horn as shown in the image is associated with which of the following skin cancer? *(Most Recent Question Aug 2020)*

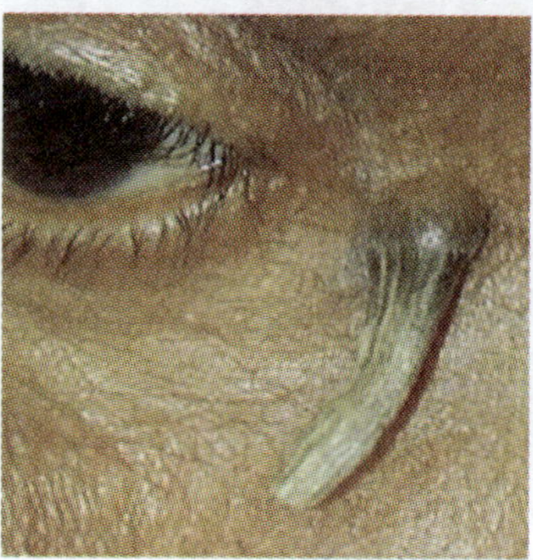

a. Basal cell carcinoma
b. Squamous cell carcinoma
c. Malignant melanoma
d. Actinic keratosis

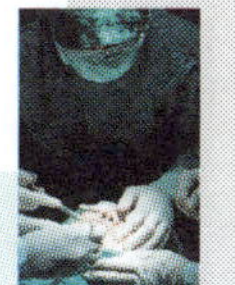

615. Comment on the diagnosis from the image shown below of a patient from rural India?
(Most Recent Question Aug 2020)

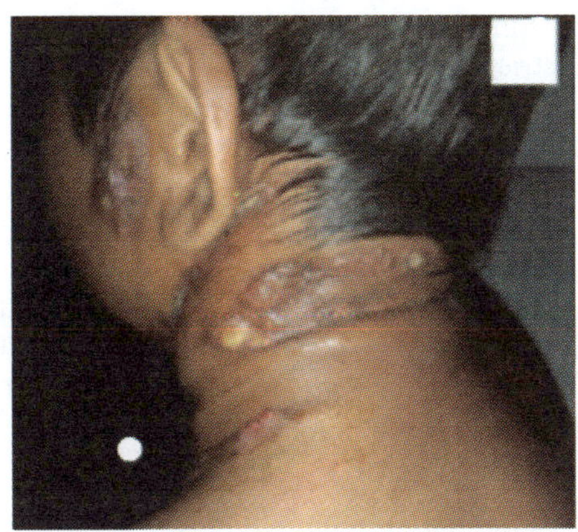

a. Cervical lymphadenopathy with occult primary
b. Castleman disease
c. Scrofuloderma
d. Reactive lymphadenopathy

616. Which of the following organism is responsible for causing this lesion shown on the face of patient?
(Most Recent Question Aug 2020)

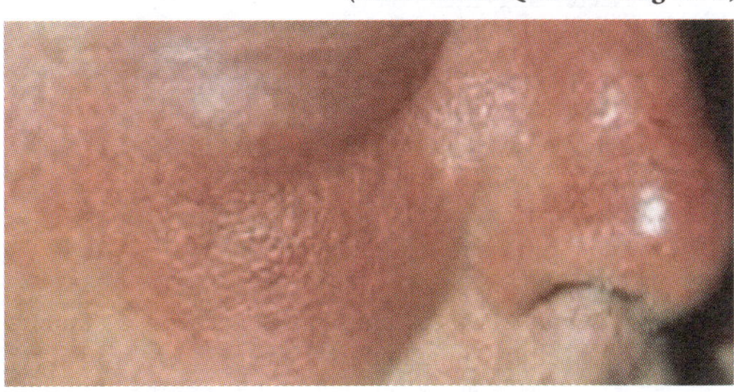

a. Streptococcus
b. Staphylococcus
c. Bacteroides
d. Fungus

617. A lady with 50% TBSA burn with involvement of dermis and subcutaneous tissue came to emergency department. Burns will be classified as:
(Most Recent Question Dec 2019)

a. 1st degree
b. 2nd degree superficial
c. 2nd degree deep
d. 3rd degree burn

618. Rodent ulcer is seen in? *(Most Recent Question Dec 2019)*

a. Squamous cell ca
b. Rhinophyma
c. Basal cell cancer
d. Adenocarcinoma

619. Most common oral cancer
(Most Recent Question Dec 2019)

a. Squamous cell ca
b. Adenocarcinoma
c. Transition cell ca
d. Mucoepidermoid

620. Identify the condition shown in image:
(Most Recent Question Dec 2019)

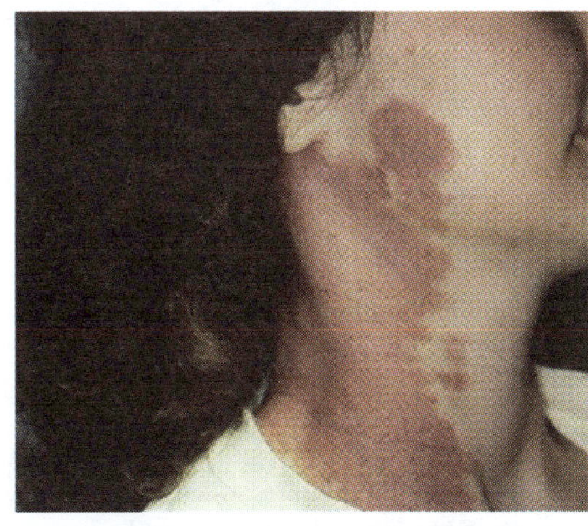

a. Port wine stain
b. Strawberry nevus
c. Erythema multiforme
d. Exanthem Nodosum

621. Which Instrument is shown below?
(Most Recent Question 2019)

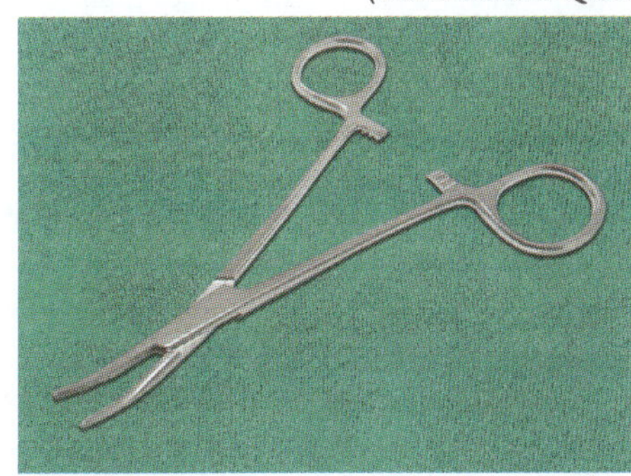

a. Artery forceps
b. Kocher forceps
c. Allis forceps
d. Babcock forceps

622. Which instrument is shown below?
(Most Recent Question 2019)

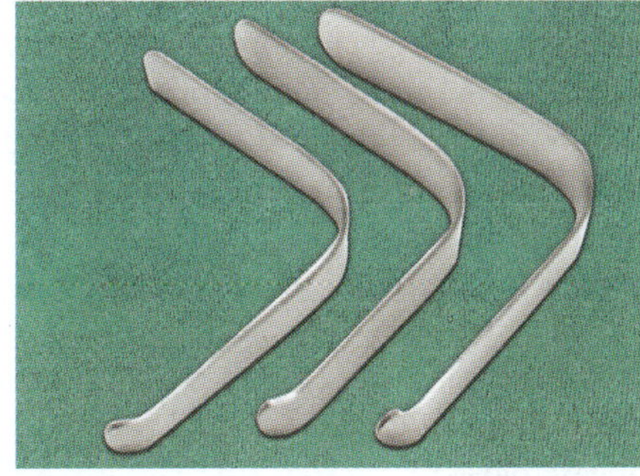

a. Tongue depressor
b. Doyen retractor
c. Self-retaining retractor
d. Langenbeck's retractor

623. In TNM staging T indicates.
(Recent Pattern Question 2017)

a. Size of tumor
b. Nodal metastasis
c. Distant metastasis
d. Depth of invasion

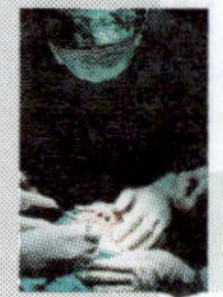

624. A 65-year-old patient presents with low backache and low grade fever. X-ray spine shows.
(Recent Pattern Question 2017)

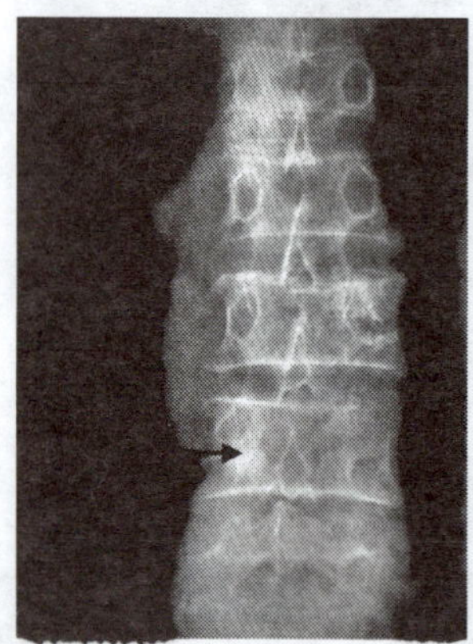

a. Osteomyelitis b. Osteomalacia
c. Hypoparathyroidism d. Metastasis

625. What is correct regarding descent of testes during fetal stage?
a. Gestational age 1–7 months in abdomen
b. Gestational age 1–7 months in inguinal canal
c. Gestational age 7–9 months in scrotum.
d. Gestational age lies in 7–9 months in abdomen.

626. Which is not a derivative of midgut?
a. Appendix
b. Jejenum
c. Ascending colon
d. Descending colon

627. All are true about amoebic liver abscess; EXCEPT?
a. Sterile pus
b. Amoebae reach the right lobe > left lobe
c. Intercostal tenderness
d. Hepatocellular jaundice

628. A 30-year-old patient presents with pain in right hypochondrium for 5 days with soft and tender liver and intercostal tenderness. He complains of catch in breath on inspiration and has a non productive cough. On examination the lung fields are clear, patient looks pale and emaciated. What is the probable diagnosis?
a. Amoebic liver abscess
b. Pyogenic live abscess
c. Hydatid cyst
d. Hepatic adenoma

629. Strawberry Gallbladder is seen in?
a. Cholesterolosis
b. Porcelain Gall bladder
c. Mirizzi syndrome
d. Wegener's granulomatosis

630. All are features of Saint's triad; EXCEPT?
a. Gall stones b. Diverticulitis
c. Hiatus hernia d. Cholesterosis

631. Bent inner tube sign is seen in
a. Volvulus
b. Intussusception
c. Intestinal obstruction
d. Gastric antral vascular ectasia

632. Bird beak sign on barium enema is seen in?
a. Achalasia cardia
b. Sigmoid volvulus
c. Carcinoma esophagus
d. Carcinoma sigmoid colon

633. All are common causes of ileal obstruction; EXCEPT:
a. Adhesions b. Obstructed hernia
c. Stricture d. Hirschsprung's disease

634. What is the most common site of GIST?
a. Stomach b. Liver
c. Kidney d. Brain

635. What is the most common site of lymphoma of GIT?
a. Stomach b. Duodenum
c. Ileum d. Colon

636. The most common cause of intestinal obstruction in infants is:
a. Intussusception
b. Congenital bands
c. Necrotising enterocolitis
d. Sigmoid volvulus

637. The vessel which needs to be ligated in a patient with a bleeding peptic duodenal ulcer is:
a. Left gastroepiploic artery
b. Gastroduodenal artery
c. Left gastric artery
d. Superior Pancreatico-duodenal artery

638. All the following are True regarding FAST-EXCEPT:
a. It cannot reliably exclude injury in penetrating trauma
b. It detects free fluid in the abdomen or pericardium
c. It is accurate in detecting <50 mL of free blood
d. It is focused abdominal sonar for trauma

639. Wolfe Graft is:
a. Thin split thickness graft
b. Medium thickness split thickness skin graft
c. Full thickness skin graft
d. Thick split thickness skin graft

640. Pringle maneuver may be required for treatment of?
a. Bleeding Esophageal Varices
b. Mesenteric Ischemia
c. Injury to Tail of Pancreas
d. Liver Laceration

641. Optional timing of administration of prophylactic antibiotic for surgical patients is:
a. One hour prior to induction of anaesthesia
b. At the induction of anaesthesia
c. Any time during the surgical procedure
d. One hour after induction

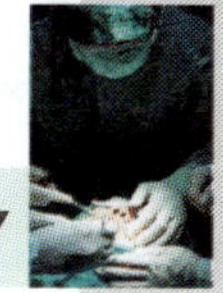

642. What is the raw material used in nylon suture?

a. Polyester polymer
b. Polyamide polymer
c. Polyethylene terephthalate
d. Polybutylene terephthalate

643. All the following statements are true regarding torsion of testis; EXCEPT

a. Anatomical abnormality is unilateral and contralateral testis should not be fixed
b. Prompt exploration and twisting & fixation is the only way to save the torted testis
c. Most common between 10 & 25 years of age
d. Inversion of testis is the most common predisposing cause

644. 'Fifth vital sign' commonly elicited by anaesthesiologists on surgical patients is:

a. FiO_2
b. Pain
c. Blood pressure
d. Core temperature

645. The most common cancer of oral cavity is

a. Adenocarcinoma
b. Melanoma
c. Sarcoma
d. Squaous cell carcinoma

646. Barrett's esophagus is diagnosed by

a. Squamous metaplasia
b. Intestinal metaplasia
c. Squamous dysplasia
d. Intestinal dysplasia

647. Boerhaave's syndrome is due to?

a. Drug induced esophagus perforation
b. Corrosive injury
c. Spontaneous perforation
d. Gastroesophageal reflux disease

648. Which one of the following is not a treatment of Gastroesophageal Variceal hemorrhage?

a. Sclerotherapy
b. Sengstaken tube
c. Trans-jugular intrahepatic Porta-caval shunt
d. Gastric freezing

649. "Limey bile" is?

a. Present in the CBD
b. Thin and clear
c. Like toothpaste emulsion in the gallbladder
d. Bacteria rich

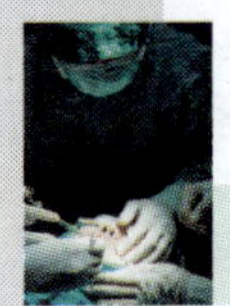

ANSWERS WITH EXPLANATIONS

MOST RECENT QUESTIONS 2023

1. Ans. (d) Fecal occult blood

Ref: Bailey and Love's Short Practice of Surgery, 26th ed. pg. 1090, 1334

Fecal occult blood testing of people aged 60–69 years is recommended as screening program. Fecal hematin has a peroxidase-like activity which is detected by this test. Studies have shown a 15–20% reduction in colorectal cancer-related mortality in the screened population. Flexible sigmoidoscopy is also used, but due to invasive nature it has less acceptability.

2. Ans. (a) Marjolin's ulcer

Ref: Bailey and Love's Short Practice of Surgery, 27th ed. pg. 984

The image shows an ulcer development in healed burn (notice the contractures). This is the presentation of Marjolin's ulcer. It is a well-differentiated squamous cell cancer.

3. Ans. (b) Polypropylene

Ref: Bailey and Love's Short Practice of Surgery, 26th ed. pg. 1032

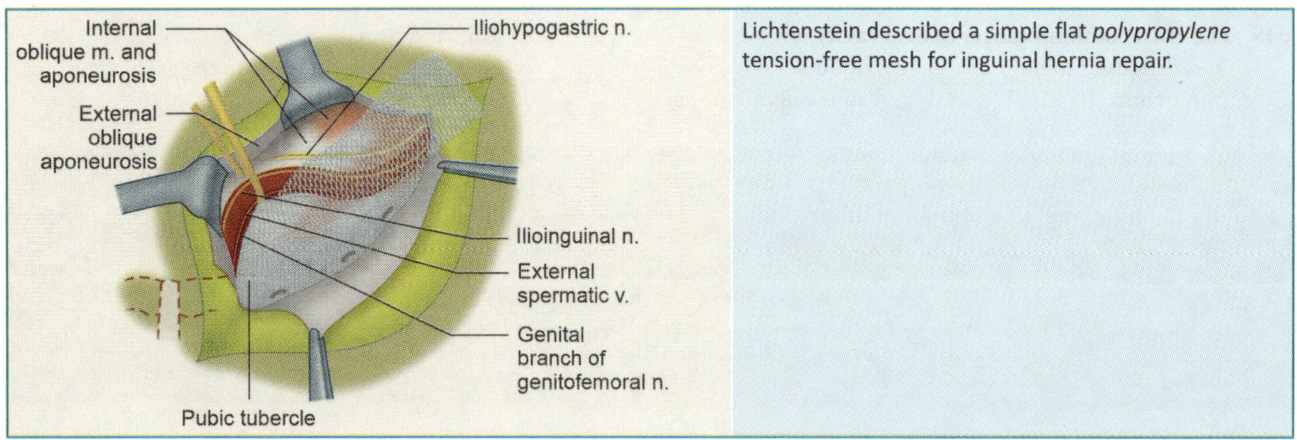

Lichtenstein described a simple flat *polypropylene* tension-free mesh for inguinal hernia repair.

4. Ans. (b) Pulsion diverticulum

Ref: Bailey and Love's Short Practice of Surgery, 27th ed. pg. 1101

Option a, Achalasia cardia has progressive dysphagia and occurs in young female patient. Recurrent pneumonia episodes are more common. Option c, Esophageal cancer has progressive dysphagia with severe weight loss leading to cachexia. Option d, Bronchiectasis presents with purulent bronchorrhea. Diagnosis is Pulsion diverticula.

5. Ans. (a) Small frequent meals based on fat and protein

Ref: Bailey and Love's Short Practice of Surgery, 27th ed. pg. 1184

The clinical presentation is of early dumping syndrome which can be resolved with small frequent meals high on protein and fat. It occurs as small bowel is filled with contents from the stomach leading to sudden high osmotic load delivered to gut. This causes sequestration of fluid from circulation into gut leading to diarrhea.

FEATURES OF EARLY AND LATE DUMPING

	Early	Late
Relation to meals	Almost immediate	Second hour after meal
Durations of attack	30–40 minutes	30–40 minutes
Relief	Lying down	Food
Aggravated by	More food	Exercise
Major symptoms	Epigastric fullness, sweating, light-headness, tachycardia, colic, sometimes diarrhea	Tremor, faintness, prostration

6. Ans. (a) Veress needle

Ref: Bailey and Love's Short Practice of Surgery, 27th ed. pg. 1202

The image shows Veress needle that is used for creating pneumoperitoneum with carbon dioxide prior placing the trocar.

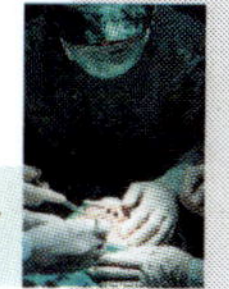

7. Ans. (c) Lymphatics

Ref: Bailey and Love's Short Practice of Surgery, 27th ed. pg. 1013

The image shows nonpitting edema in both feet seen in lymphedema caused by Lymphatic filariasis.

8. Answer: (d) T4d

Ref: www.ajronline.org/breast cancer staging

T4a	Extension to chest wall (does not include pectoralis muscle invasion only)	
T4b	Ulceration, ipsilateral satellite skin nodules, or skin edema-including peau d'orange.	
T4c	Both the above	
T4d	Inflammatory ca	

9. Ans. (a) Zinc

Ref: Harrison's 21st ed. pg. 2532

The presence of diarrhea with dermatitis at specific sites like face and perineum points to zinc deficiency.

Zinc is a micronutrient that is essential to human health. Zinc plays a manor role in regulating every phase of the wound healing process; ranging from membrane repair, oxidative stress, coagulation, inflammation and immune defence, tissue re-epithelialization, angiogenesis, to fibrosis/scar formation.

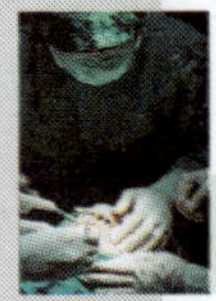

10. Ans. (b) Pringle maneuver

Ref: Harrison's 21st ed. pg. 374

- The image shows a soft clamp placed on the portal triad to reduce the arterial and portal venous inflow into the liver and is called Pringle maneuver. However, it does not control the backflow from IVC and hepatic veins.
- Pringle maneuver indications are:
  - Halt hemorrhage and find the source of bleeding in liver trauma, allowing time for repair
  - In the setting of hepatic resection of benign and malignant lesions, it can be used to control bleeding.
- Option a, **Kocher maneuver** is the dissection of the lateral peritoneal attachments of the duodenum to allow inspection of the duodenum, pancreas, and other retroperitoneal structures over to the great vessels.
- Option c, **Cattell maneuver** is mobilization of the ascending colon to the midline.
- Option d, **Mattox maneuver** is mobilization of the descending colon to the midline to expose the abdominal aorta.

11. Ans. (c) Serosa

Ref: Bailey and Love's Short Practice of Surgery, 27th ed. pg. 1067

Unlike the rest of gut, esophagus has no serosa which rather facilitates easier spread of esophageal cancer as compared other GI malignancies.

12. Ans. (a) Trichobezoar

Ref: Bailey and Love's Short Practice of Surgery, 27th ed. pg. 1142

The image shows Trichobezoar/hairball which is exclusively found in young female psychiatric patients due to pathological ingestion of hair which remains undigested in stomach. Diagnosis is usually made on Endoscopy.

13. Ans. (c) Melanoma

Ref: Bailey and Love's Short Practice of Surgery, 26th ed. pg. 609

- The lesion shows pre-existing nevus which is showing vertical growth in form of nodularity as well as horizontal spread. Cumulative ultraviolet radiation (UVR) exposure in white-skinned races increased the risk.
- Option a, Basal cell carcinoma is common in elderly males, has pearly rolled out margins, occurs on face and is called rodent ulcer. Option b, Squamous cell carcinoma will not have pigmentation as visible in the image. Option d, Junctional melanocytic nevus would be considered only if the lesion had not increased in size. They are light to dark macules 1–10 mm in diameter located on sun-exposed parts of body and are benign proliferators of melanocytes.

14. Ans. (a) Sistrunk operation

Ref: Bailey and Love's Short Practice of Surgery, 26th ed. pg. 755

Midline neck swelling that moves up with tongue protrusion is thyroglossal cyst. Treatment is Sistrunk operation which includes excision of whole thyroglossal tract. The procedure involves removal of the body of hyoid bone and suprahyoid tract. Option b, commando operation is done for cancer of tongue. Option c, Local irradiation is done for Hodgkin lymphoma. Option d, Radioiodine ablation is done for Graves' disease.

15. Ans. (a) Normal saline

Ref: uptodate.com

- Normal saline (NS) and Ringer lactate are preferred crystalloids for managing intraoperative fluid loss.
- In most clinical settings, normal saline is the choice of fluid for many indications for fluid resuscitation, maintenance, or as a solvent for medication delivery except burns, cholera and metabolic acidosis.

Extra Mile

- Excess of NS can cause hyperchloremic acidosis.
- Ringer lactate with blood products will bind to citrate in additive solution of whole blood.
- Hypotonic fluids like 5% dextrose will worsen cerebral edema.

16. Ans. (a) Pneumothorax

Ref: Bailey and Love's Short Practice of Surgery, 26th ed. pg. 919

Chest X-ray (CXR) shows collapsed lung on right side with tracheal shift to left. The right side has absent vascular markings in comparison with left side. These features point to the development of pneumothorax.

17. Ans. (c) Ranula

Ref: Bailey and Love's Short Practice of Surgery, 26th ed. pg. 779

The bluish cystic swelling in floor of mouth is called Ranula. It is a mucous extravasation cyst that arises from sublingual gland. It can resolve spontaneously but can require surgery. Incision and drainage (I&D) can result in recurrence. Option a, Pleomorphic adenoma is derived from parotid gland and will present as jaw swelling. Option b, Dermoid cyst is midline swelling. Option d, Cystic hygroma arises in posterior triangle of neck.

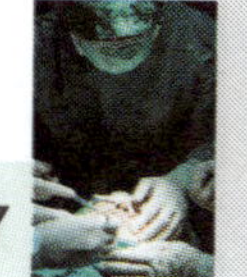

18. Ans. (b) Depth of invasion

Ref: Bailey and Love's Short Practice of Surgery, 26th ed. pg. 1090, 1334

For all GI malignancies, the most important determinant of extent of disease is depth of invasion by cancer cells.

19. Ans. (a) Radiation esophagitis

Radiation esophagitis is a side effect for patients undergoing radiation for malignancies, usually for lung, breast, and other thoracic cancers due to its close proximity. Usual manifestations occur within 3–4 weeks of receiving radiation.

20. Ans. (d) Congenital adrenal hyperplasia

Ref: Bailey and Love's Short Practice of Surgery, 26th ed. pg. 844

- CT abdomen shows distorted kidney on left side and above it is cerebriform appearance of adrenal glands which is visible in congenital adrenal hyperplasia.
- Since liver is not in the image, option a and b cannot be commented on. The mass is bilateral and above the kidneys making renal cell carcinoma (RCC) unlikely.

21. Ans. (b) Craniotomy with evacuation

Ref: Bailey and Love's Short Practice of Surgery, 26th ed. pg. 334

The non-contrast CT (NCCT) scan of the head shows lenticular hyperdensity which is seen with extradural hemorrhage. Management is craniotomy with evacuation of hematoma to reduce the midline shift and intracranial pressure.

22. Ans. (b) MRI abdomen

Ref: Bailey and Love's Short Practice of Surgery, 26th ed. pg. 845

The clinical diagnosis of patient is pheochromocytoma. The imaging modality to be done initially is MRI abdomen. MIBG scan is done if biochemical evidence of tumor is present in the form of elevated metanephrines but MRI abdomen is normal. MRI is preferred since Contrast media used in CT scan can trigger paroxysms.

23. Ans. (a) Rupture of bulbar urethra

Ref: Bailey and Love's Short Practice of Surgery, 26th ed. pg. 1479

Rupture of anterior urethra	Rupture of posterior urethra
Trauma to *bulbous urethra* due to fall astride projectile object like cycling, manhole cover, gymnasium	Trauma to *membranous and/or prostatic urethra* after pelvic fracture sustained in RTA.
a. Penile urethra b. Bulbar urethra c. Membranous urethra d. Prostatic urethra	a. Penile urethra b. Bulbar urethra c. Membranous urethra d. Prostatic urethra

Contd...

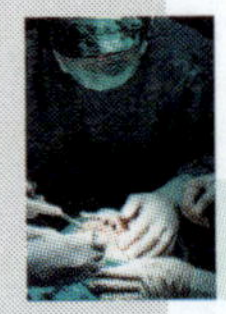

Rupture of anterior urethra	Rupture of posterior urethra
Presentation Blood at the meatus perineal hematoma *Retention of urine* Tell patient not to pass urine else extravasation occurs.	*Presentation* Difficulty in passing urine Blood at the meatus Extravasation of urine to scrotum, perineum and abdominal wall and hence bladder is empty.
PR examination shows normal prostate.	PR examination shows floating prostate

24. Ans. (a) Double J-stent

Ref: Bailey and Love's Short Practice of Surgery, 26th ed. pg. 1452

A kidney, ureter, and bladder (KUB) X- ray shows a right-sided renal calculus and double J pigtail ureteric stent that can help in relieving ureteric obstruction.

25. Ans. (a) Acute pancreatitis

Ref: Bailey and Love's Short Practice of Surgery, 26th ed. pg. 1225

- The image shows bruising around umbilicus (Cullen sign) and spreading from flanks to midline (Grey Turner sign) indicating extravasated pancreatic enzymes. The patient is having acute abdomen due to acute pancreatitis.
- Cullen sign can be seen in ruptured ectopic pregnancy as well.

26. Ans. (a) Upper border of lower rib

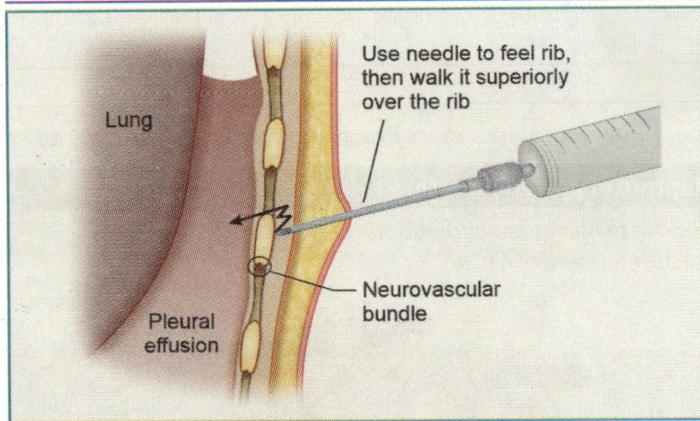

The intercostal neurovascular bundle is located along the lower edge of each rib.

Hence the needle must be placed on upper edge of lower rib in intercostal space *to avoid injury to the neurovascular bundle.*

Alternatively, it can be said that pleural tapping should be done from lower part of intercostal space.

27. Ans. (b) Yellow - Stable need observation

Red	• Patient requires immediate treatment • E.g. suicide attempt via poisoning, hanging, or self-inflicted trauma
Yellow	• Patient is stable at the moment and is not in any immediate danger, but will require observation • E.g. passive suicidal ideation, command hallucinations
Green	• Patients who will require medical treatment at some point, once more critical injuries have been treated • E.g. drug refill for antidepressant or antianxiety medications
Black	• For those who are already decreased, or for patients whose injuries are so extensive that they will not be able to survive, given the level of care available

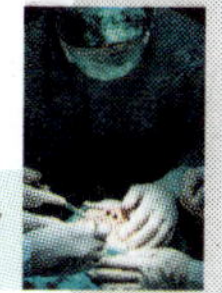

28. Ans. (d) Aortic arch

Ref: Gray's Anatomy, 42nd ed. pg. 1057

NATURAL CONSTRICTIONS OF ESOPHAGUS

Site	Vertebral level	Distance from central incisor
Cricopharynx	C 6	15 cm
Aortic arch	T 4	23 cm
Lt main bronchus	T 5	28 cm
Esophageal hiatus	T 10	40 cm

29. Ans. (a) Serum lactate >2 mmol/L

Ref: Harrison's 21st ed. pg. 2238

Criterion		
Altered mental status GCS <15	No	Yes
Respiratory rate ≥22	No	Yes
Systolic BP ≤100	No	Yes

3 points qSOFA score	**High risk** qSOFA scores 2–3 are associated with a 3–14 fold increase in hospital mortality. Assess for evidence of organ dysfunction with blood testing including serum lactate and calculation of the full SOFA score.

30. Ans. (a) Superficial dermal lymphatics

Ref: Bailey and Love's Short Practice of Surgery, 27th ed. pg. 879

The image shows peau d'orange appearance of surface of breast and is caused by involvement of superficial dermal lymphatics leading to cutaneous lymphatic edema. When the infiltrated skin is tethered by sweat ducts, it cannot swell leading to orange skin. Occasionally, the same phenomenon is seen over a chronic abscess.

31. Ans. (b) Woman with breast cancer diagnosed after 50 years of age

BRCA2 is associated with male breast cancer and is located on chromosome 13q. Hence option a is correct. Option c, Bilateral breast cancer represents 2–11% of all breast cancers and can be associated with BRCA1, BRCA2 mutations. Option d is associated with BRCA1. The correct answer is option b which is presentation of sporadic breast cancer due to p53 mutation.

Risk factors for having a harmful BRCA1 or BRCA2 mutation

PERSONAL RISK FACTORS

- Breast cancer diagnosed at a young age (<50 years)
- History of ovarian cancer, certain types of breast cancer, or both
- Cancer in both breasts
- 1 or more relatives diagnosed with breast cancer at a young age (<50 years), 1 relative diagnosed with ovarian cancer, or 2 or more relatives diagnosed with breast or pancreatic cancer
- Ashkenazi Jewish ancestry and at least 1 close relative diagnosed with breast, ovarian, or pancreatic cancer

FAMILY RISK FACTORS

- 2 or more relatives diagnosed with breast cancer at a young age (<50 years)
- A male relative diagnosed with breast cancer
- A relative diagnosed with both ovarian cancer and breast cancer or with cancer in both breasts
- A relative diagnosed with ovarian cancer
- A relative identified as having BRCA1 or BRCA2 mutations

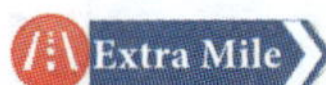

Familial breast cancer	BRCA1; BRCA2	D	Breast cancer Ovarian cancer Papillary serous carcinoma of the peritoneum Prostate cancer	Screening mammography; pelvic ultrasound; PSA (in males) Prophylactic mastectomy; prophylactic opphorectomy

32. Ans. (a) Esophagoscopy

Since the child is symptomatic, esophagoscopy is indicated. If the child was asymptomatic, then the answer would be wait and watch.

The majority of ingested foreign bodies (80–90%) pass through the gastrointestinal tract spontaneously and without complications. Impaction, perforation, or obstruction often occur at areas of physiological narrowing or angulations. *Areas of physiological narrowing include the upper esophageal sphincter, aortic arch, left main stem bronchus, lower esophageal sphincter, pylorus, ileocecal valve, and anus; the duodenal sweep is a physiological angulation.* Once foreign bodies have traversed the esophagus, most objects pass within 4–6 days, or in worse case in up to 4 weeks. Generally, objects greater than 2–2.5 cm in diameter will not pass through the pylorus or ileocecal valve and objects longer than 5–6 cm will not pass through the duodenal sweep.

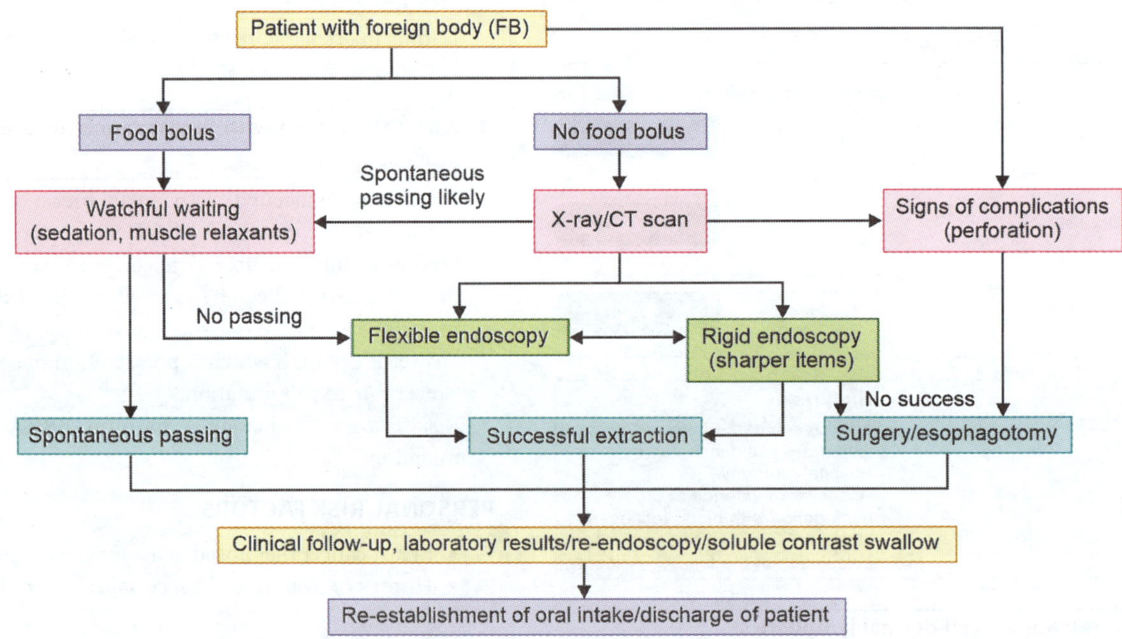

* Up to 14–16 cm from the alignment cervical esophagotomy more than 16 cm from the alignment thoracic esophagotomy

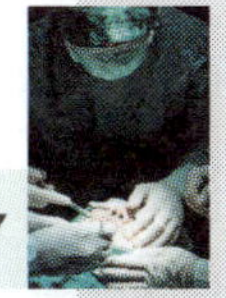

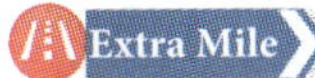

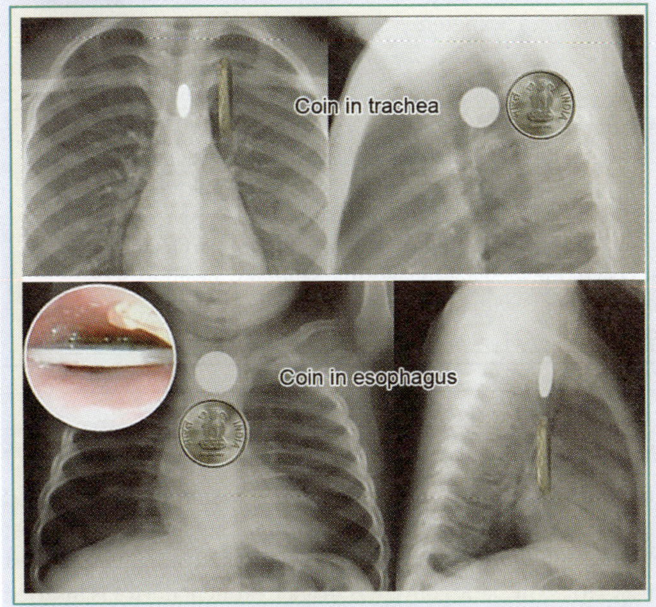

33. Ans. (a) MRI

Ref: Bailey and Love's Short Practice of Surgery, 28th ed. pg. 1365

Magnetic resonance imaging (MRI) allows precise definition of the fistulous track and identification of secondary fistulas or abscesses. It provides accurate information for appropriate surgical treatment, decreasing the incidence of recurrence and allowing side effects such as fecal incontinence to be avoided.

34. Ans. (b) Scrotal support

Ref: Bailey and Love's Short Practice of Surgery, 27th ed. pg. 1509

The image shows Fournier gangrene of scrotum where testis is spared. It is polymicrobial infection of soft tissues of perineum, external genitals and perianal region. It is a form of necrotizing fasciitis which leads to exposure of scrotal contents. It can occur after minor injuries or procedures in perineal areas. Concomitant illness like diabetes mellitus and alcoholism can be triggered. There is no role of scrotal support in management of this patient.

35. Ans. (d) Skin stapler

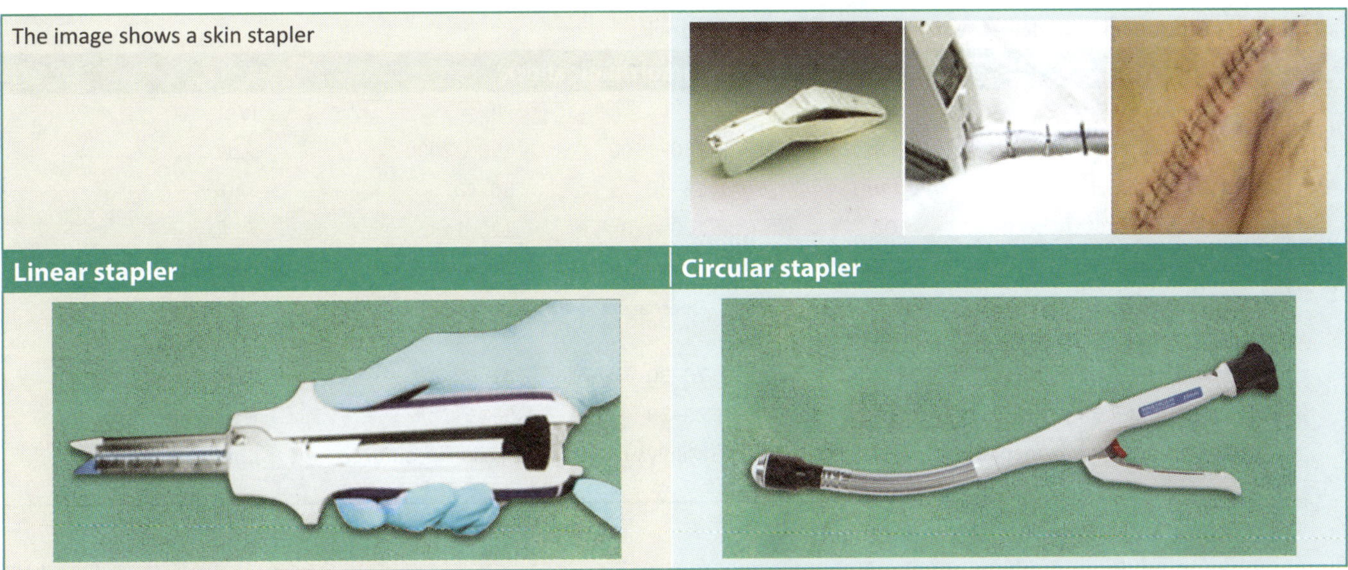

36. Ans. (c) Autograft

Ref: Bailey and Love's Short Practice of Surgery, 28th ed. pg. 634

The image shows skin grafting from thigh and is an example of autograft. Xenograft is across species like pig heart valves or pig heart, allograft is across first-degree relatives, like kidney transplantation and isograft is across monozygotic twins where rejection is unlikely as DNA is identical.

37. Ans. (a) Hernioplasty

Ref: Bailey and Love's Short Practice of Surgery, 28th ed. pg. 1032

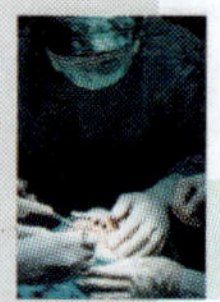

The image shows an indirect inguinal hernia in an adult which is causing the symptoms. The preferred method of management is hernioplasty. It involves herniotomy (removal of hernial sac) plus reinforcement of posterior wall of inguinal canal with a tension-free synthetic mesh. If it was a child, the answer would be option b, Herniotomy.

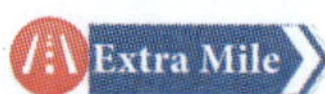

Inguinal hernia repairs may be divided into the following three general types:

1. Herniotomy (removal of the hernial sac only) - This, by itself, is adequate for an indirect inguinal hernia in children in whom the abdominal wall muscles are normal; formal repair of the posterior wall of the inguinal canal is not required
2. Herniorrhaphy (herniotomy plus repair of the posterior wall of the inguinal canal) - This may be suitable for a small hernia in a young adult with good abdominal wall musculature; the Bassini and Shouldice repairs are examples of herniorrhaphy
3. Hernioplasty (herniotomy plus reinforcement of the posterior wall of the inguinal canal with a synthetic mesh) - This is required for large hernias and hernias in middle-aged and elderly patients with poor abdominal wall musculature; the Lichtenstein tension-free mesh repair is an example of hernioplasty

38. Ans. (a) Thermal ablation

Ref: Bailey and Love's Short Practice of Surgery, 27th ed. pg. 977

Endothermal ablation technologies replaced surgical ligation and stripping as the gold standard treatment once randomised trials demonstrated that the were marginally safer, have extremely high technical efficacy, offer superior quality of life post procedure (with a rapid recovery) and equivalent improvements in quality of life in the longer term. The techniques are cost effective as they can be performed as an outpatient under local anesthetic. The basic concept is that a treatment device is inserted into the incompetent axial vein percutaneously.

39. Ans. (b) Class II

Ref: ATLS guidelines

Urine output begins to decrease in class II hemorrhagic shock.

Class of hemorrhagic shock				
	I	II	III	IV
Blood loss (nil.)	Up to 750	750–1500	1500–2000	>2000
Blood ID5s (% blood volume)	Up to 15	15–30	30–40	>40
Paw rate (per minute)	<100	100–120	120–140	>140
Blood pressure	Normal	Normal	Decreased	Decreased
Pulse pressure (rn m Hg)	Normal or increased	Decreased	Decreased	Decreased
Respiratory rate (per minute)	14–20	20–30	33–40	>35
Urine output In-IL/hr	>30	20–30	5–15	Negligible
Central nervous system/mental status	Slightly anxious	Mildly anxious	Anxious, confused	Confused, lethargic

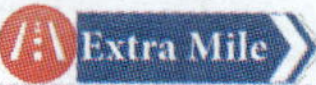

LETHAL TRIAD AND ACUTE COAGULOPATHY OF TRAUMA/SHOCK

The lethal triad is:

- Hypothermia
- Coagulopathy
- Acidosis

These three factors both cause, and contribute to, **acute coagulopathy of trauma/shock (ACoTS)** which leads to, and result from, major hemorrhage.

- They feed off one another, such that bleeding begets more bleeding.
- This is the theoretical rationale for damage control resuscitation.

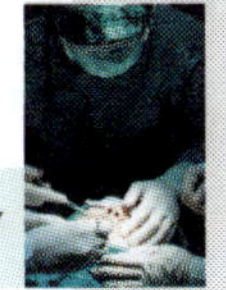

40. Ans. (d) Para-aortic LN

- The primary lymphatic drainage (ipsilateral metastasis) from the left testis is in the following order: *Para-aortic*, preaortic, left common iliac, and left external iliac nodes.
- The primary lymphatic drainage (ipsilateral metastasis) from the right testis is in the following order: *Interaortocaval*, precaval, preaortic, paracaval, right common iliac, and right external iliac nodes.

41. Ans. (b) cT4b N1 M0

Breast tumor of any size involving the chest wall is T4. Involvement of ipsilateral axillary Lymph nodes is N1. Since this is a clinical finding hence prefix c will be used.

T4a	Extension to chest wall (does not include pectoralis muscle invasion only)	Tumor size **T**	Tumor size <2 cm T1	Tumor size 2–5 cm T2	Tumor size > 5 cm T3	Tumor extends to skin or chest wall T4
T4b	Ulceration, ipsilateral satellite skin nodules, or skin edema-including peau d'orange	Lymph nodes **N**	**NO** No lymph node metastasis	**N1** Metastasis to ipsilateral, movable, axillary LNs	**N2** Metastasis to ipsilateral fixed, axillary, or IM LNs	**N3** Metastasis to infraclavicular/ supraclvicular LN, or to axillary and IM LNs
T4c	a+b	Metastasis **M**	**MO** No distant metastasis	**M1** Distant metastasis		
T4d	Inflammatory ca					

42. Ans. (d) aPTT

Prothrombin time/International normalized ratio is component of Child-Pugh score. Components of score are BA3PT: Bilirubin, albumin, ascites, asterixis and PT.

43. Ans. (a) *Clostridium perfringens*

Ref: Bailey and Love's Short Practice of Surgery, 27th ed. pg. 44

44. Ans. (d) Intercostal artery

Ref: CMDT 2023, pg. 901

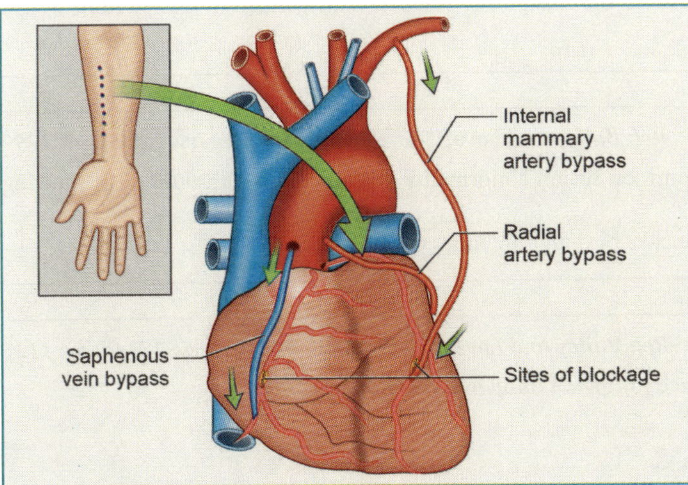

Grafts using one or both internal mammary arteries (usually to the left anterior descending artery or its branches) provide the best long-term results in terms of patency and flow. Segments of the saphenous vein (or, less optimally, other veins) or the radial artery interposed between the aorta and the coronary arteries distal to the obstructions are also used. One to five distal anastomoses are commonly performed.

45. Ans. (a) Serosanguineous discharge

Ref: Bailey and Love's Short Practice of Surgery, 27th ed. pg. 297

Wound dehiscence is disruption of any or all of the layers in a wound. Dehiscence may occur in up to 3% of abdominal wounds and is very distressing to the patient.

Wound dehiscence most commonly occurs from the fifth to the eighth postoperative day when the strength of the wound is at its weakest. It may herald an underlying abscess and usually presents with a serosanguineous discharge. The patient may have felt a popping sensation during straining or coughing. Most patients will need to return to the operating theater for resuturing. In some patients, it may be appropriate to leave the wound open and treat with dressings or vacuum-assisted closure (VAC) pumps.

46. Ans. (a) EDH

Ref: Bailey and Love's Short Practice of Surgery, 27th ed. pg. 333

The image shows a left-sided lenticular hyperdensity which is characteristic feature of Extradural hemorrhage.

47. Ans. (d) Retrocaval ureter

Ref: Bailey and Love's Short Practice of Surgery, 27th ed. pg. 1402

Retrocaval ureter is when right ureter passes behind the IVC instead of lying on its right side. This can lead to obstruction of right ureter causing right-sided hydronephrosis. The remaining causes will obstruct urine flow to affect both ureters.

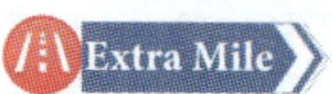

Causes of Bilateral hydronephrosis

A. Congenital
- Congenital stricture of external urethral meatus, pin-hole meatus.
- Congenital posterior urethral valve.

B. Acquired
- BPH
- Carcinoma prostate
- Postoperative bladder neck scarring
- Inflammatory/traumatic urethral stricture
- Phimosis
- Carcinoma cervix
- Bladder carcinoma

Retrocaval Ureter

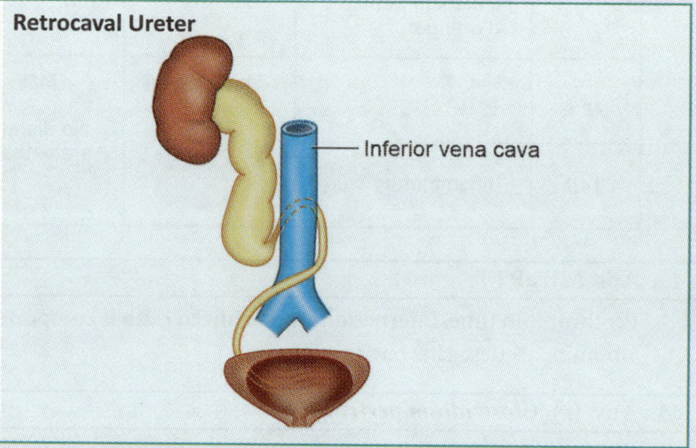

48. Ans. (b) PCNL

Ref: Bailey and Love's Short Practice of Surgery, 27th ed. pg. 1409

The X-ray KUB shows a large shadow on the right side at position of renal pelvis. The best management of kidney stone >2 cm is PCNL.

49. Ans. (b) Horseshoe kidney

Ref: Bailey and Love's Short Practice of Surgery, 27th ed. pg. 1399

- The image shows horseshoe kidney which is the most common fusion abnormality of the kidney with 90% cases showing fusion at the lower pole.
- In case both the upper and lower poles fuse, it is called pancake or doughnut kidney.

50. Ans. (d) Highly selective vagotomy

Ref: Bailey and Love's Short Practice of Surgery, 27th ed. pg. 1121

Operative mortality, side effects and incidence of recurrence following duodenal ulcer operations.

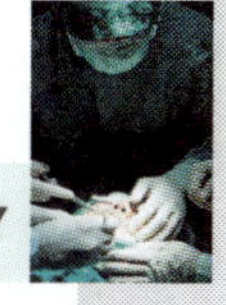

Operation	Operative mortality (%)	Significant side effects (%)	Recurrent ulceration (%)
Gastrectomy	<1–2	<20–40	1–4
Gastroenterostomy alone	<1	<10–20	50
Trurical vagotorny and drainage	<1	<10–20	2–7
Selective vagotomy and drainage	<1	<10–20	5–10
Highly selective vagotomy	<0.2	<5	2–10
Trurical vagotorny and antrectomy	<1	<10–20	1

51. Ans. (a) Decrease in tissue perfusion

Ref: Bailey and Love's Short Practice of Surgery, 27th ed. pg. 17

- Cold extremities are seen in all types of shock except warm subtype of septic shock where bounding pulses and warm extremities can be seen.
- Hence option d is ruled out. Shock causes increased peripheral resistance and increased rate of breathing.
- Universal feature of all types of shock is underperfusion of tissues.

52. Ans. (a) Local surgical excision/release

Ref: Bailey and Love's Short Practice of Surgery, 27th ed. pg. 763

The image shows lesions of oral submucous fibrosis seen due to use of pan masala, areca nut with or without alcohol. Surgical excision/release and reconstruction can lead to short-term benefit, though recurrence will occur at the same site. Cessation of use will halt progression but will not cause improvement.

53. Ans. (c) Chemoradiation

Ref: Bailey and Love's Short Practice of Surgery, 27th ed. pg. 1371

Primary treatment of SCC of anal canal is chemoradiotherapy/Combined modality therapy called Nigro regimen. It is a combination of 5-fluorouracil with mitomycin-C or cisplatin. Local staging is done by MR scanning and PET-CT helps in determining spread. Small marginal tumors are treated by local excision.

54. Ans. (a) Medial nasal process and maxillary process

Ref: Bailey and Love's Short Practice of Surgery, 27th ed. pg. 686

Cleft lip (CL) and cleft palate (CP) are the most common congenital orofacial deformities. A combination of genetic predisposition and in-utero exposure to teratogens (nicotine, alcohol, antiepileptic drugs) can arrest the fusion of the facial processes required for normal facial development. Failure of fusion of the maxillary prominence with the medial nasal prominence causes cleft lip (CL). Failure of fusion of the palatine prominences causes cleft palate (CP).

55. Ans. (a) Glucagonoma

Ref: Bailey and Love's Short Practice of Surgery, 27th ed. pg. 849

Necrolytic migratory erythema (dermatitis) with diabetes mellitus and depression is seen with pancreatic neuroendocrine tumor called glucagonoma.

56. Ans. (c) Decreased NO in LES

Ref: CMDT 2023, pg. 618

Nitric oxide (NO) is a vasodilator and lower levels will cause spasm/increased tone of LES. In achalasia, there appears to be denervation of esophagus resulting primarily from loss of NO producing inhibitory neurons in myenteric plexus.

57. Ans. (b) Early lung metastasis

Ref: Bailey and Love's Short Practice of Surgery, 27th ed. pg. 138

- Option a is correct. Neuroblastoma commonly shows metastasis to lymph nodes, bones and liver and raise urinary catecholamines.
- Option c is correct as small, localized tumors are excised while advanced tumors have surgery after chemotherapy.
- Option d is correct since it presents as abdominal or paravertebral mass. Hence answer by exclusion is option b.

58. Ans. (c) Caused by hypertrophy of inner longitudinal muscles

Ref: Bailey and Love's Short Practice of Surgery, 27th ed. pg. 127

Infantile hypertrophic pyloric stenosis (IHPS) occurs due to hyperplasia and hypertrophy of the pyloric inner circular

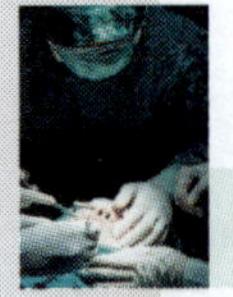

muscle fibers. It presents in first born male with nonbilious vomiting. Diagnosis is confirmed with Ultrasound showing target sign/cervix sign.

Extra Mile

Infantile hypertrophic pyloric stenosis
- Most commonly affects boys aged 2–8 weeks
- Projectile vomiting after feeds
- Test feed or ultrasound to confirm the diagnosis
- Gastric peristalsis can be seen and an 'olive' felt
- Hypochloremic metabolic alkalosis must be corrected before surgery
- Pyloromyotomy splits the hypertrophied muscle leaving the mucosa intact

59. Ans. (d) Mastoid bruising: Skull base fracture

Ref: Bailey and Love's Short Practice of Surgery, 27th ed. pg. 332

- Skull base fracture causes *battle sign* of mastoid bruising.
- EDH will have ipsilateral mid-dilated pupil with sluggish reaction to light called Hutchinson pupil. Pinpoint pupils are seen in pontine hemorrhage and opioid overdosage.
- CSF otorrhea occurs after fracture of petrous part of temporal bone.
- Kehr's sign is seen with splenic rupture.

60. Ans. (b) Cracked nipple

Ref: Bailey and Love's Short Practice of Surgery, 27th ed. pg. 865

Cracked nipple is the usual forerunner of acute infective mastitis. The nipple should be rested for 24–48 hours, and breast emptied with breast pump. Failure to detect or neglect results in acute mastitis.

61. Ans. (a) Radial nerve

Ref: Bailey and Love's Short Practice of Surgery, 27th ed. pg. 443

The image shows wrist drop and the nerve involved is radial nerve.

GASTROINTESTINAL TRACT

62. Ans. (a) Esophageal varices

Ref: Harrison 21st ed. pg. 311

Option a is seen after binge drinking in an alcoholic and needs protracted retching which was not given in the question. Option b is more logical conclusion as Bleeding esophageal varices are a known complication of CLD and presents with sudden onset hematemesis. Option c presents with rebound tenderness and rigidity of anterior abdominal wall. Option d will cause subcutaneous emphysema.

63. Ans. (d) CECT of abdomen

Ref: Bailey and Love, 27th ed. pg. 866

The leading cause of bilious vomiting in neonates is malrotation of gut > Duodenal atresia as per Nelson textbook of pediatrics. In setting of obstruction barium would not be done and CECT abdomen shows a swirling whirlpool sign.

Although typically innocuous as a contrast medium, barium sulfate is an insoluble salt that can precipitate and worsen intestinal obstruction. Option a is done for Esophageal disorders. Option b for stomach pathology. Option c will be answered as gold standard for midgut Volvulus but in the scenario given CT abdomen would be faster and give more anatomical details to the operating surgeon.

Contraindications to Barium Meal:

- Complete bowel obstruction
- Suspected perforation
- Paralytic ileus
- Very ill patient
- Recent GI surgery

64. Ans. (c) Imperforate anus

Ref: Bailey and Love, 27th ed. pg. 1346

The image shows a coin placed at buttocks of child as a radiological marker. The child is placed in prone lateral X-ray to demonstrate the distal most segment of large bowel and then to differentiate whether it is low or high type of anal atresia. This is not an invertogram where the child is kept inverted which taking the X-ray image.

65. Ans. (a) 24-hour ambulatory pH monitoring

Ref: Bailey and Love, 27th ed. pg. 1071

Best for detection of GERD is 24-hour pH monitoring. Diagnostic criteria is documentation of esophageal pH of Less than 4 for >4.2% of time per day of recording is diagnostic.

Extra Mile

Dee-meester scoring is done to grade severity of GERD

66. Ans. (b) Dumping syndrome

Ref: Bailey and Love, 27th ed. pg. 1123

- An operation in which the pylorus is removed, bypassed, or destroyed increases the rate of gastric emptying. Duodenal feedback inhibition of gastric emptying is lost after a bypass procedure.

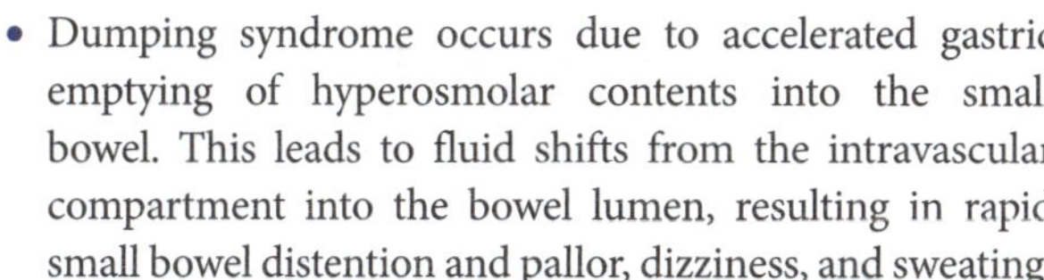

- Dumping syndrome occurs due to accelerated gastric emptying of hyperosmolar contents into the small bowel. This leads to fluid shifts from the intravascular compartment into the bowel lumen, resulting in rapid small bowel distention and pallor, dizziness, and sweating.
- Option d results in gustatory sweating and flushing due to salivary gland surgery.

67. Ans. (d) Hollow viscus perforation

Ref: Bailey and Love, 27th ed. pg. 1125

The image shows Gas under diaphragm diagnostic of perforation peritonitis. Option A would present with colon cut off sign. Option b and c would require an Ultrasound for evaluation.

68. Ans. (b) Psychiatrist

Ref: Bailey and Love, 27th ed. pg. 1142

Trichobezoars are concretions of hair in stomach which are usually found in young psychiatric females. These patients often deny eating their own hair which is called trichophagy. It is caused by the pathological ingestion of hair, which remains undigested in the stomach. These patients would need a psychiatric consult.

69. Ans. (a) Acute pancreatitis

Ref: Bailey and Love, Textbook of Surgery, 27th ed. pg. 1017

In acute pancreatitis, a person has a sudden onset of pain in the center of upper abdomen. The pain may intensify and become severe, and it may spread into the back.

The colon cut-off sign is seen with acute pancreatitis, secondary to the inflammation extending to the splenic flexure via the phrenicocolic ligament.

70. Ans. (c) Esophageal diverticula

Ref: Bailey and Love, Textbook of Surgery, 27th ed. pg. 1101

An esophageal diverticulum is a pouch that protrudes outward in a weak portion of the esophageal lining.

- This pocket-like structure can appear anywhere in the esophageal lining between the throat and stomach.
- The symptoms of esophageal diverticula include difficulty in swallowing with a feeling of food caught in the throat, retrosternal pain, and regurgitation with coughing after meals.

71. Ans. (b) Megaloblastic anemia

Ref: Bailey and Love, Textbook of Surgery, 27th ed. pg. 1124

Nutritional anemias resulting from a vitamin B12, folate or iron deficiency are common in people who have had a gastrectomy.

- Megaloblastic anemia following gastrectomy is due to the total absence or inadequate secretion of intrinsic factor and is manifested by megalobastic changes in bone marrow, blood cells, and other proliferative cells.

72. Ans. (a) Vitamin B12 deficiency

Ref: Bailey and Love, Textbook of Surgery, 27th ed. pg. 1241

Ileocecal Resection removes diseased tissue of terminal ileum, which is often severely affected by Crohn's disease.

- Massive ileal resections result in an inability to reabsorb dietary fluid and jejunal secretions and are associated with impairment of absorption of vitamin B12, bile salts, and fatty acids.

73. Ans. (a) Ulcerative colitis

Ref: Bailey and Love, Textbook of Surgery, 27th ed. pg. 1267

Ulcerative colitis is a chronic inflammatory bowel disease in which abnormal reactions of the immune system cause inflammation and ulcers on the inner lining of large intestine.

- It commonly involves the rectum and may extend in a proximal and continuous fashion to involve other parts of the colon.
- Patients with mainly distal disease may have constipation accompanied by frequent discharge of blood and mucus.
- Crypt abscesses occur when inflammatory cells accumulate within crypts of the gastrointestinal system.

74. Ans. (a) Ileostomy followed by definitive surgery later

Ref: Bailey and Love, Textbook of Surgery, 27th ed. pg. 1270

Temporary defunctioning protective ileostomy in moribund cases of peritonitis due to ileal perforation is a lifesaving procedure.

- Thereafter, the patient is managed with antibiotics and continued postoperative care.
- Definitive surgery is planned later once all the complications are effectively managed.

75. Ans. (c) Clostridium difficile

Ref: Bailey and Love, Textbook of Surgery, 27th ed. pg. 1273

Clostridium difficile is the main cause of nosocomial infectious diarrhea and the causative agent of antibiotic-associated colitis.

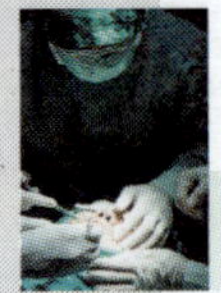

- Antibiotic use may result in diarrhea through different mechanisms, including osmotic diarrhea, and colonization and overgrowth of toxin-secreting Clostridium difficile.
- Clostridium difficile is a Gram-positive, spore-forming anaerobic bacillus.
- Spores of C difficile can survive for long periods on inanimate objects (resisting heat, acid and antibiotics), a major reason why this bacterium can cause such problems within healthcare settings.

76. Ans. (b) Emergency appendectomy

Ref: Bailey and Love, Textbook of Surgery, 27th ed. pg. 1308

Appendicitis in pregnancy is one of the most common non-obstetric surgical diseases during pregnancy.

- Due to unspecific symptoms associated with normal pregnancy such as abdominal pain, nausea and vomiting, appendicitis in pregnant women is very difficult to diagnose.
- Appendiceal rupture occurs more frequently in pregnant individuals, especially in the third trimester. Therefore, Emergency appendectomy is always planned.

77. Ans. (c) Barium enema and anorectal manometry

Ref: Bailey and Love, Textbook of Surgery, 27th ed. pg. 1278

The given clinical scenario is suggestive of Hirschsprung disease.

- Hirschsprung disease is a congenital condition characterized by absence of ganglion cells at rectosigmoid junction usually. This presents as delayed passage of meconium and constipation subsequently.
- In Hirschsprung disease, the affected section of intestine cannot contract normally. Therefore, barium enema and anorectal manometry are ordered.
- Anorectal manometry detects the relaxation reflex of the internal sphincter after distention of the rectal lumen. This normal inhibitory reflex is presumed absent in patients with Hirschsprung disease.

78. Ans. (d) Large intestine

Ref: Bailey and Love, Textbook of Surgery, 27th ed. pg. 1259

Short chain fatty acids (SCFA) have distinct physiological effects: they contribute to shaping the gut environment, influence the physiology of the colon, they can be used as energy sources by host cells and the intestinal microbiota and they also participate in different host-signaling mechanisms.

SCFA are absorbed in the large intestine.

79. Ans. (b) Appendicular abscess

Ref: Bailey and Love, Textbook of Surgery, 27th ed. pg. 1312

Failure of resolution of an appendix mass or continued spiking pyrexia usually indicates that there is pus within the phlegmonous appendix mass.

Ultrasound or abdominal CT scan may identify an area suitable for the insertion of a percutaneous drain. This procedure may be rarely unsuccessful and in that case laparotomy though a midline incision is indicated.

80. Ans. (a) Distal obstruction in the small intestine

Ref: Bailey and Love, Textbook of Surgery, 27th ed. pg. 1285

Plain abdominal radiographs are used as a screening tool for bowel obstruction.

- The main findings include dilated bowel loops (see 3-6-9 rule) with or without the presence of fluid levels.
- Erect chest radiographs can also be used to screen for complicating perforation.

81. Ans. (a) McBurney's point

Ref: Bailey and Love, Textbook of Surgery, 27th ed. pg. 1301

McBurney's point refers to the point on the lower right quadrant of the abdomen at which tenderness is maximal in cases of acute appendicitis

- Acute appendicitis is characterized by the inflammation, infection, or swelling of the appendix.
- The sign is seen in a vast majority of individuals with appendicitis.

82. Ans. (b) Annular pancreas

Ref: Bailey and Love 27th ed. pg. 1219

- The X-ray shows double bubble appearance of duodenal atresia. This can occur due to annular pancreas. It occurs due to failure of complete rotation of ventral pancreatic bud development so that a ring of pancreatic tissue surrounds the second or third part of duodenum.
- In some cases, it may not cause atresia but duodenal stenosis. The treatment is bypass duodenoduodenostomy. This entire presentation is common in children with Down syndrome.

83. Ans. (b) Bochdalek hernia

Ref: Bailey and Love, 27th ed. pg. 938-39

The CXR shows loops of bowel in chest wall. This is presentation of Congenital diaphragmatic hernia which

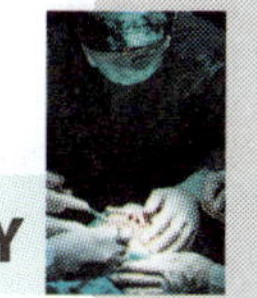

occurs due to congenital defect in diaphragm. This herniation of bowel into chest cavity is called as Bochdalek hernia. It occurs posteriorly in the diaphragm due to failure of pleuroperitoneal membrane closure in utero. Scaphoid abdomen is explained by herniation of abdominal contents into chest cavity.

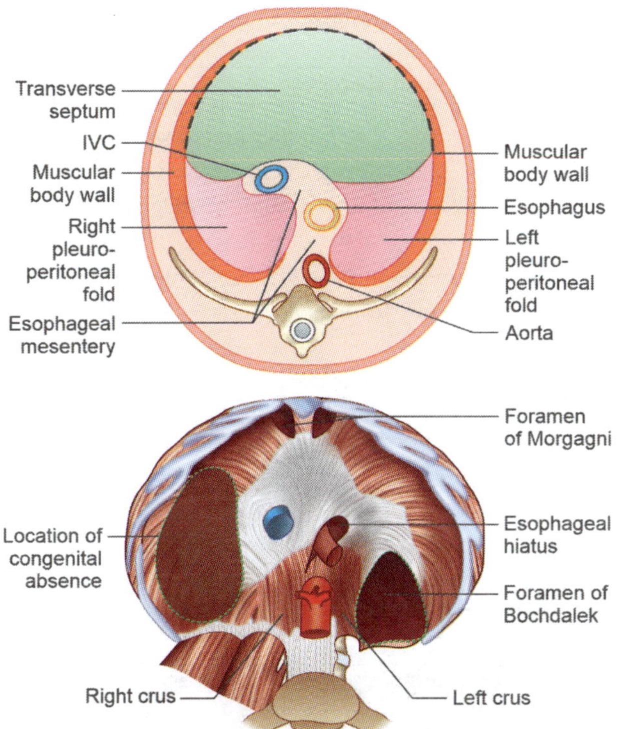

84. Ans. (b) Congenital hypertrophic pyloric stenosis

Ref: Bailey and Love 27th ed. pg. 128

Nonbilious vomiting in a neonate with minimal passage of contrast *via* pylorus confirms diagnosis as congenital hypertrophic pyloric stenosis. The condition is common in first born boys. Nowadays for diagnosis ultrasound is done.

85. Ans. (a) Hypokalemia

Ref: Bailey and Love 27th ed. pg. 1297

X-ray abdomen shows dilated bowel loops diagnostic of ileus. The leading electrolyte abnormality responsible is hypokalemia. The resultant stasis leads to accumulation of fluid and gas in the bowel associated with distention, vomiting, absence of bowel sounds and absolute constipation.

86. Ans. (d) Chylolymphatic cyst

Ref: Bailey and Love 27th ed. pg. 1062

The key word is abdominal swelling that is mobile in single direction i.e. perpendicular to line of attachment of mesentery. The diagnosis is mesenteric cyst. It is of two types as shown in the image.

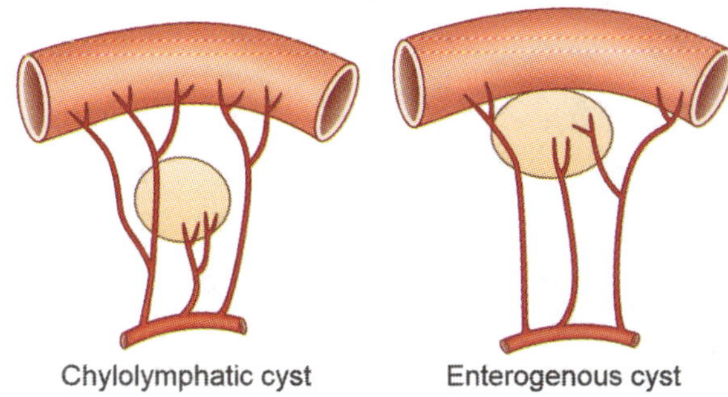

Extra Mile

Tillaux's traid helps us in diagnosis of Mesenteric cyst during physical examination:

This triad consists of:

- Fluctuant swelling (cyst) near the umblicus.
- It moves freely in direction vertical on the attachment of mesentery
- It is dull surrounded by a zone of resonance and traversed by band of resonance.

87. Ans. (a) Meckel's diverticulum

Ref: Bailey and Love 27th ed. pg. 1252

The postoperative specimen shows a diverticulum on anti-mesenteric margin which is following the rule of 2 (2 feet from ileocaecal junction and measuring 2 inches in length). The diagnosis is Meckel diverticulum.

Extra Mile

Most common malformation of mid gut is Meckel's Diverticulum

Rule of 2

<2 years of age

2× more common in males

2% of population

2 feet proximal to ileocecal valve

2 inches in length

2% adults symptomatic

2 ectopic tissues present (gastric and pancreatic)

88. Ans. (c) Loop ileostomy

Ref: Bailey and Love 27th ed. pg. 1556

The image shows a stoma with two openings in right iliac fossa of the patient. The RIF location helps in determining it is ileostomy and the presence of two stomas help in determining it is loop ileostomy. In case single opening was present here then the answer would have been end ileostomy.

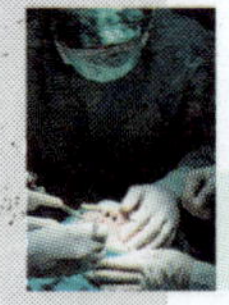

Extra Mile

Notice the location of various similar nature procedures

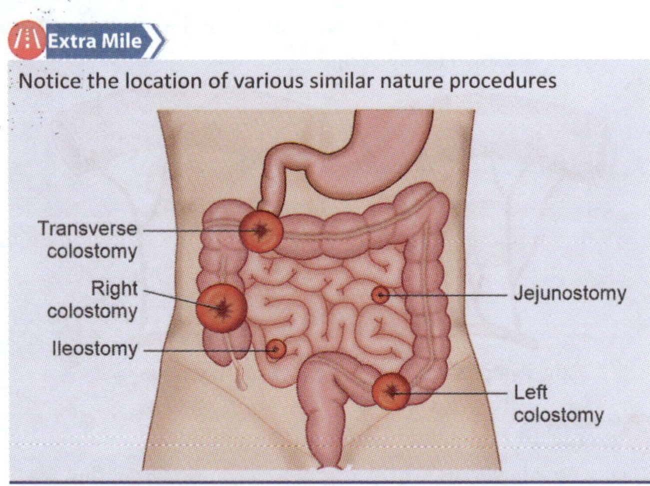

- The per operative image shows anal orifice and an external orifice near the thumb of visible hand of surgeon. This external orifice is of anal fistula which is causing soiling of undergarments of patient and poor perianal hygiene.
- Pilonidal sinus is ruled out because of location which is between the gluteal cleft.

89. Ans. (d) Anal fistula

Ref: Bailey and Love 27th ed. pg. 1363

90. Ans. (a) Perianal abscess

Ref: Bailey and Love 27th ed. pg. 1362

The image shows extensive redness with evidence of suppuration around anus leading to diagnosis of perianal abscess.

Option b is ruled out as no visible external opening is seen.

Option c leads to hematochezia with/without visible thrombosed vein

Option d is seen at gluteal cleft

91. Ans. (b) Paraumbilical hernia

Ref: Bailey and Love 27th ed. pg. 1029

- The image shows herniation of contents via anterior abdominal wall and part of umbilicus in an adult patient. This is a paraumbilical hernia.
- Option a is seen in babies and involves only the umbilicus. Majority will self-resolve by 3 years of age. Option c and d can be excluded by location.

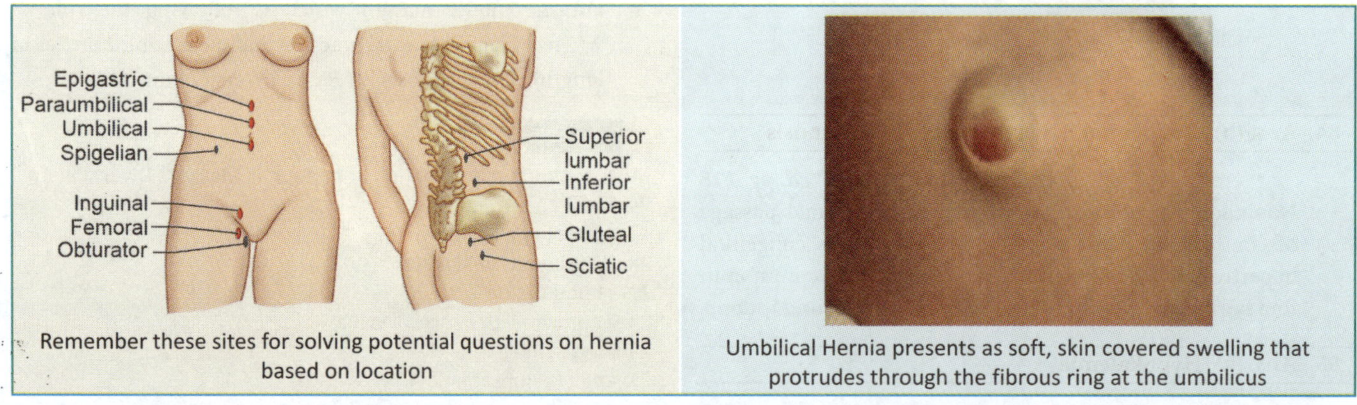

Remember these sites for solving potential questions on hernia based on location

Umbilical Hernia presents as soft, skin covered swelling that protrudes through the fibrous ring at the umbilicus

92. Ans. (c) Omphalocele

Ref: Nelson Pediatrics 20th ed. pg. 975

Features	Omphalocele	Gastroschisis
Site of the defect	Central umbilical	Right paraumbilical
Sac	Always present	Never present
Anomalies of rotation and fixation	Present	Present
Gender	More frequent in females	Equal
Associated anomalies	Frequent (heart anomalies)	Rare
Intestinal atresia	Rare	Up to 10%

Contd...

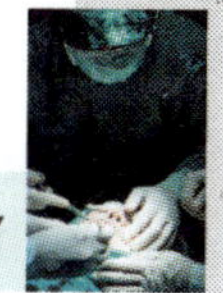

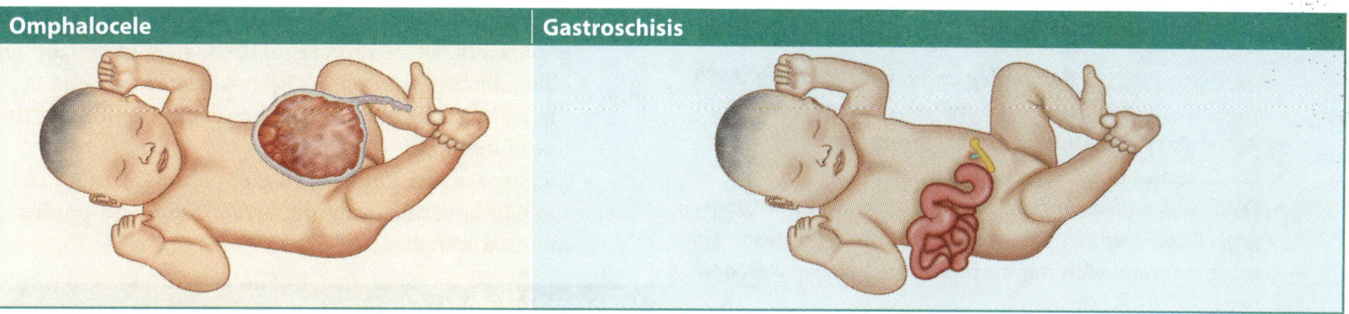

93. Ans. (a) Pharyngeal pouch

Ref: Sabiston E-book, pg. 1020

Dohlman operation is an endoscopic diverticulotomy procedure done for Zenker's diverticulum. The procedure is palliative one as it widens the mouth of diverticulum making the retention of food items less likely.

94. Ans. (a) Ca 19-9

Ref: Bailey and Love 27th ed. pg. 1235

- Radioimmunoassay for Carbohydrate antigen Ca 19.9 is secreted by pancreatic cancer cells. It is not sensitive or specific but baseline values should be done and can be used specially for identifying any recurrence.
- Option b is tumor marker for Colonic Cancer
- Option c is tumor marker for neuroblastoma and small cell cancer of lung
- Option d is tumor marker for HCC and Non seminomatous germ cell tumor of testis.

95. Ans. (c) Intestinal metaplasia with goblet cells

Ref: Bailey and Love 27th ed. pg. 1115

Reflux esophagitis leads to irritation of esophageal mucosa and change of epithelium from squamous to columnar with goblet cells. This replacement is called as Intestinal metaplasia

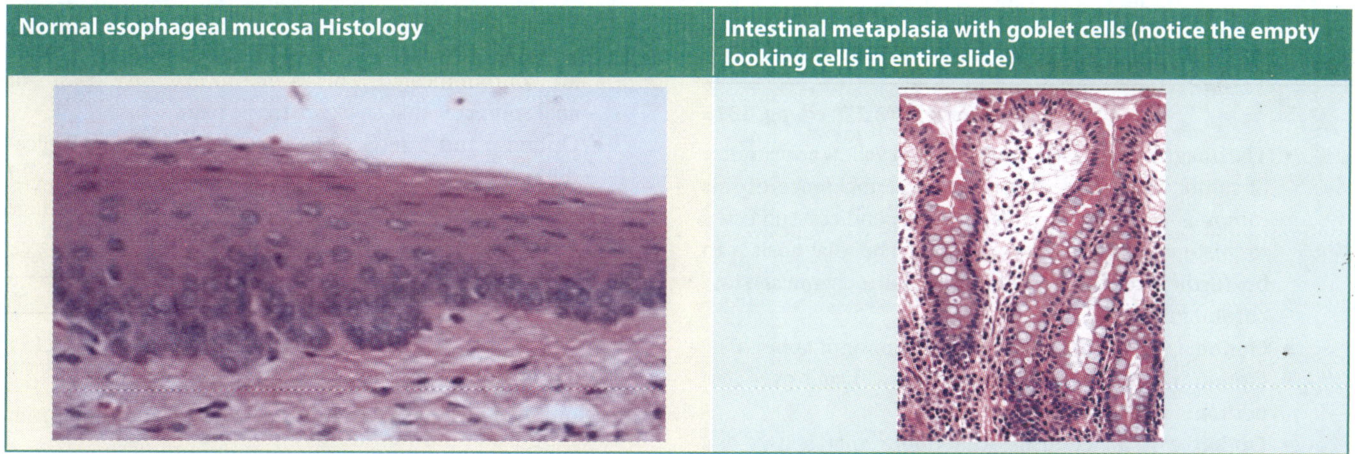

96. Ans. (a) Achalasia cardia

Ref: Bailey and Love 27th ed. pg. 1095

The barium meal shows tapering of contrast at lower part of esophagus. This is due to increased tone of LES and aperistalsis in lower 1/3rd of esophagus. It is called Bird beak appearance and is seen in Achalasia Cardia.

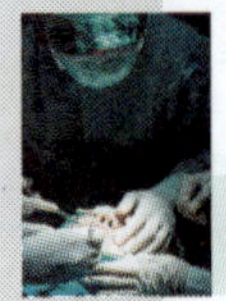

97. Ans. (a) Monitor vitals hourly

Ref: Bailey and Love 27th ed. pg. 1080

Complication of Laparoscopic procedure range from:

- Respiratory acidosis due to CO_2 absorption
- Low Cardiac output and hypotension
- DVT and pulmonary embolism (It can occur with any procedure leading to prolonged immobilization. So more common with routine procedure than laparoscopic ones)

Therefore, vital monitoring must be done for next 24 hours to pick up any of these complications. Long term complications seen with total fundoplication can be dysphagia and gas bloat syndrome due to overcorrection. This would prevent patient from belching and feeling of fullness after a short meal.

98. Ans. (d) Intussusception

Ref: Bailey and Love 27th ed. pg. 1289

- The barium meal follow-through shows claw sign which is diagnostic of ileo-colic Intussusception. However nowadays the diagnosis is made by CT abdomen which has the highest sensitivity for diagnosis of this condition. CT shows a target or sausage shaped soft tissue mass.
- Option a is ruled out as it presets in neonates with failure to pass meconium.
- Option b on barium enema will show bird beak defect. Do not confuse with bird beak in barium swallow in achalasia.
- Option c is diagnosed with colonoscopic biopsy

99. Ans. (d) Carcinoid tumor

Ref: Bailey and Love 27th ed. pg. 1315

- The image shows a well circumscribed yellow appearance of tumor in appendix specimen. The incidence of this tumor is once in every 300-400 appendices subjected to histopathological examination. The diagnosis can be further confirmed by immunohistochemical stain chromogranin B.
- Option a will appear as large Cystic tumor of appendix.
- Option b is an epithelial tumor that will spill over into peritoneum and produce mucin.
- Option c is an epithelial cell tumor that shows will show metastasis and spread to adjacent areas while the specimen shows localized tumor.

100. Ans. (a) Kocher's incision

Ref: Bailey and Love 27th ed. pg. 1309

- Kocher's incision is used for open cholecystectomy. Option b, c and d are used for appendectomy.
- Rutherford Morrison incision is useful if the appendix is paracecal or retrocecal or fixed. It is essentially an oblique muscle cutting incision with its lower end over the Mcburney's point. All the layers are divided in the line of incision.
- Mcburneys incision is a muscle splitting incision. Lanz incision is cosmetically the best incision and produces minimal scarring.

Important incisions to be practiced

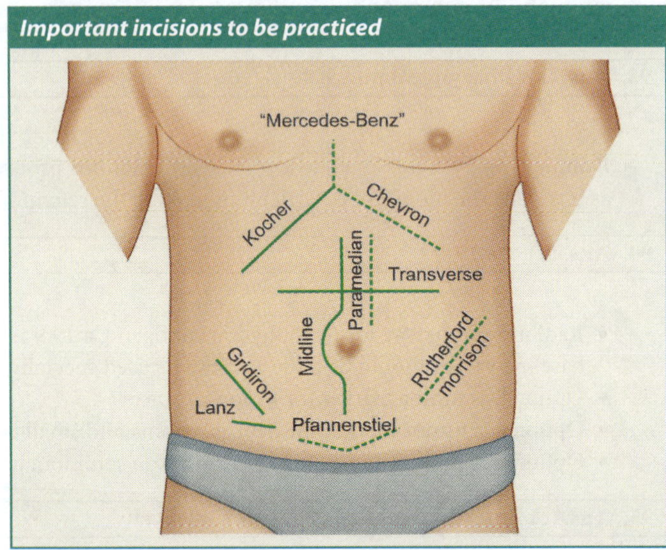

101. Ans. (c) Proctoscopy

Ref: Bailey and Love 27th ed. pg. 1350-1

- Fissure in ano will cause extensive spasm of anal sphincter and both digital exploration and proctoscopy are contraindicated. This is due to extensive spasm of anal sphincter that causes extreme pain.
- Option a and b reduce the spasm of sphincter. Topical diltiazem and GTN relax the sphincter. Option d will make the stool soft and will reduce the further damage to sphincter.

102. Ans. (a) Sister Mary Joseph nodule

Ref: Bailey and Love 27th ed. pg. 1135

- The image shows Sister Mary Joseph Nodule on the umbilicus which is seen in cases of advanced stomach cancer.
- Option b is seen on iris in granulomatous uveitis. There is no herniation of abdominal contents visible. Option d is seen on iris in NF-1.

103. Ans. (a) Surgery if persistence beyond 2 years of age even if asymptomatic

Ref: Bailey and Love 27th ed. pg. 1037

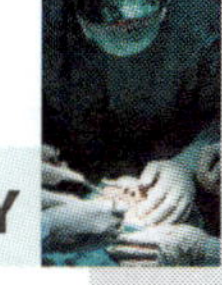

Asymptomatic umbilical hernia is managed conservatively under 2 years of age. 95% resolve spontaneously. If hernia persists beyond age of 2 years it is unlikely to resolve and surgical repair is indicated.

104. Ans. (c) PUD perforation

Ref: Bailey and Love 27th ed. pg. 1050

- The main point in the question is development of pneumoperitoneum/gas under diaphragm. This can be explained by perforation of a peptic ulcer in this alcoholic. Positive release sign implies rebound tenderness which is a feature of Perforation peritonitis. Binge drinking followed by multiple vomiting was incidental events.
- However in the same case presentation if the gas was above the diaphragm (continuous diaphragm sign) then the diagnosis will change to Boerhaave syndrome.

105. Ans. (a) Charcot's triad

Ref: Bailey and Love 27th ed. pg. 1168

- The triad of RUQ pain/tenderness with jaundice and fever/rigors is called Charcot triad and is seen in ascending cholangitis. The diagnosis is confirmed by USG showing dilated bile ducts and obstructive pattern seen on LFT.
- Option b has presence of hiatus hernia, cholelithiasis and colonic diverticulosis.
- Option c has venous stasis, activation of blood coagulation and vein damage. It is seen with Deep vein thrombosis.
- Option d has lower RIF pain with nausea/vomiting and fever. It is seen in acute appendicitis.

106. Ans. (b) Ultrasound

Ref: Bailey and Love 27th ed. pg. 1199

Since patient is having pain in RUQ after food intake, the first Differential diagnosis is cholelithiasis. Confirmation of diagnosis will require Ultrasound for diagnosis. If the same patient develops fever with leukocytosis then diagnosis is acute calculous cholecystitis.

107. Ans. (b) Rectum is involved

Ref: Bailey and Love 27th ed. pg. 1243

Rectum is involved more commonly in UC while it is spared in CD. The Inflammatory nature of disease ensure it has waxing and waning course with flare ups/ recurrences. CD leads to full thickness involvement of entire GIT. The damage occurs in form of deep serpiginous ulcers that break through the serosal side and lead to fistula formation.

108. Ans. (d) Malrotation of gut

Ref: Bailey and Love 26th ed. pg. 1994

- Choice a presents with delayed passage of meconium and is ruled out.
- Choice b presents with non-bilious vomiting and is ruled out.
- Choice c presents with bilious vomiting and does not have any abdomen distention. X-ray abdomen shows double bubble appearance.
- Choice d presents with bilious vomiting and abdominal distention and multiple gas filled loops.

109. Ans. (a) Mucoviscidosis

Ref: Nelson 20th ed. pg. 1802

- Meconium ileus occurs primarily in new-born infants with cystic fibrosis which is also called mucoviscidosis.
- It is an exocrine gland defect of chloride transport that results in abnormally viscous secretions. The distal 20–30 cm of ileum is collapsed and filled of pale stool.
- The proximal bowel is dilated and filled with thick meconium that resembles sticky syrup or glue. The peristalsis fails to propel this viscid material forward and becomes impacted in the ileum.

110. Ans. (b) NG Tube insertion and CXR to check position of tube

Ref: Nelson 20th pg. 1783

- The clinical diagnosis of this neonate with frothing and bubbling at the mouth and nose is esophageal atresia.
- The symptoms worsen with episodes of feeding and aspiration of gastric contents if fistula is present
- In setting of early onset respiratory distress, inability to pass a nasogastric or orogastric tube suggests esophageal atresia.
- *Plain X-ray will show a coiled feeding tube lying in esophageal pouch and air distended stomach.*
- Choice a bronchoscopy with methylene blue is injected into endotracheal tube and dye is observed in oesophagus during forced inspiration to detect orifice of fistula in TEF.
- Choice c and d are not recommended for diagnosis of esophageal atresia.
- Esophagogram can detect a H type of defect shown.

Types of Tracheo-esophageal Fistula

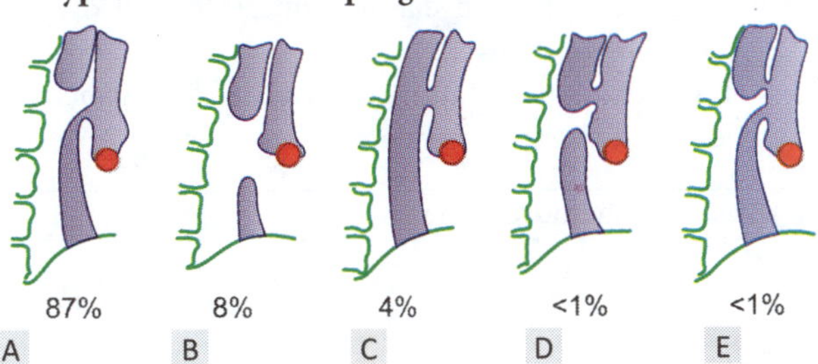

111. Ans. (c) Gut ischemia

Ref: Bailey and Love: 26th ed. pg. 882

Mesenteric tears usually occur due to the shearing force applied on the mesentery, which happens while the movable intestines continue moving with the same speed of the car, although the car is decelerated by the act of the brakes (described in physics as the inertia). These tears can be so trivial that a frank intestinal ischemia would not be apparent immediately. The abdominal wall ecchymosis may lead to misdiagnosis as soft tissue injury.

112. Ans. (b) Below Inferior constrictor

Ref: Bailey and Love 26th ed. pg. 1018

The Killian's dehiscence is located *below inferior constrictor muscle* and above cricopharyngeal muscle. Laimer's triangle lies below cricophyrageus and above longitudinal muscle of esophagus

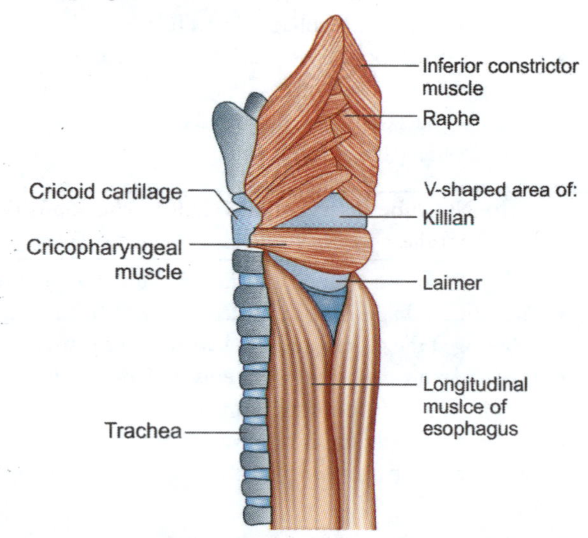

113. Ans. (a) Hemorrhage

Ref: Bailey 27th ed. pg. 1186

- Immediate complication is bleeding due to slippage of ligature.
- Gastric dilatation and gastric mucosal damage leading to hematemesis are uncommon complications.
- Fistula can develop due to damage to wall of greater curvature of stomach.
- Damage to tail of pancreas can lead to pancreatitis, localised abscess formation.

114. Ans. (a) Chemoradiation

Ref: SRB 5th ed. pg. 987 and Bailey 26th ed. pg. 1266

- The primary management of anal cancer is by chemoradiotherapy also called Combined Modality Therapy (C.M.T).
- Initially radiotherapy for 3 weeks 3000 rads are given for 3 weeks to the perineum and pelvis.
- The chemotherapy includes a combination of 5FU with mitomycin C or cisplatin.

115. Ans. (a) No occurrence after surgery

Ref: SRB 5th ed. pg. 894

Crohn's disease can recur even after surgical procedures unlike ulcerative colitis where total proctocolectomy cures the disease. Choice B, C and D are characteristic features of Crohn's disease.

TABLE: Difference between Crohn's disease and ulcerative colitis

Crohn's disease	Ulcerative colitis
It affects ileum and often colon but can involve any part of GIT–rectal sparing is common	It affects rectum and colon from distal to proximal
Full thickness–transmural disease	It affects mucosa and submucosa–not deeper
Skin lesions are typical	Skip lesions are not observed
Granulomatous lesion on histology–deep ulcers; pseudopolyps are not found	Not a granulomatous lesion–superficial ulcers, pseudopolyps are present
Stricture and fistula are common	Narrowing can occur but not very common
Anal fissure and perianal abscess are more common	Fissure and perianal disease can occur but not as common as in Crohn's disease
May mimic appendicitis	Will not mimic appendicitis
Bleeding is not common	Bleeding is common
Fever is common	Fever is uncommon
Mass in RIF is common	Mass is not a common feature
Anal pathology very common	Anal pathology is rare
Discontinuous segmental asymmetrical colitis	Continuous mucosal disease–colitis
Toxic megacolon is rare	Toxic megacolon is common
Normal vascular pattern	Distorted vascular pattern
Fistula is very common	Fistula is uncommon
Recurrence is common after resection	Total proctocolectomy cures the disease

116. Ans. (b) pH-metry

Ref: SRB 5th ed. pg. 806-807

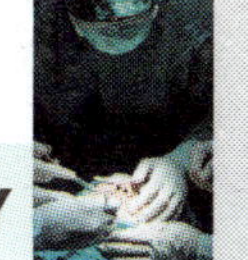

Biopsy will be done for diagnosis while CT chest will let us know the extent of spread of cancer. PET scan is done to evaluate response to therapy. It will also help to know involvement of lymph nodes which may be involved but are not picked up on a CT scan. *There is no role of pH monitoring in diagnosis or determining prognosis of carcinoma esophagus.*

117. Ans. (a) Ochsner-Sherren regimen

Ref: SRB 5th ed. pg. 946

The image shows an appendicular mass where nature has already contained the infection. If disturbed it will cause fecal fistula. Hence a conservative approach will be followed.

MANAGEMENT PROTOCOL OF APPENDICULAR MASS

- Use conservative Ochsner-Sherren regime:
  - IV fluid
  - NGT
  - Analgesics
  - Antibiotics–parenteral
  - Mark the limits of the mass on the abdominal wall using a skin pencil
  - Monitor-vital sign, size of the mass, input/output chart
  - Clinical improvement is expected in 24–48 hours

118. Ans. (d) Colocolic intussusception

Ref: SRB 5th ed. pg. 932

The image shows a barium enema showing a claw sign and haustrations point to etiology of colocolic intussusception. The geriatric age group also point to the presentation of same.

Ileocolic intussusception	Sigmoid volvulus	Toxic megacolon
The classic meniscus sign can be seen as an abrupt cut off of barium flow at junction of colon and ileum.	The image shows inner tube bent sign diagnostic of sigmoid volvulus. It is called as coffee bean sign and occurs due to anticlockwise rotation of sigmoid colon	Notice the hugely dilated colonic loops suggestive of toxic megacolon. There is **no** meniscus sign/ Claw sign visualised

119. Ans. (d) Refractory fistula

Ref: Harrison 20th ed. pg. 2274

Fistula formation is a feature of Crohn's disease. Choices A, B and C will necessitate surgery.

INDICATIONS OF SURGERY IN ULCERATIVE COLITIS

Ulcerative Colitis
Intractable disease
Fulminant disease
Toxic megacolon
Colonic perforation
Massive colonic hemorrhage
Extracolonic disease
Colonic obstruction
Colon cancer prophylaxis
Colon dysplasia or cancer

120. Ans. (b) Middle 1/3rd

Ref: SRB 5th ed. pg. 805

In spite of the controversy about the topic, the correct answer is middle 1/3rd.

Location of cancer esophagus	Incidence
Middle 1/3rd	50%
Lower 1/3rd	33%
Upper 1/3rd	17%

Extra Mile

Esophageal Cancer

- Barrett esophagus predisposes to development of adenocarcinoma.
- Most Common gross presentation is fungating—cauliflower appearance.
- Recent onset dysplasia is the most common presentation; though for dysphagia to develop 2/3rd of lumen should be obliterated.
- Shouldering sign/irregular filling defect is seen on fluoroscopy in barium meal.
- Biopsy is done for histopathological diagnosis and CT chest for staging.

121. Ans. (b) IVF-antibiotic-air enema

Ref: Nelson 20th ed. pg. 2624; Bailey and Love 26th ed. pg. 116

- The clinical presentation is of intussusception and needs urgent hydrostatic reduction.

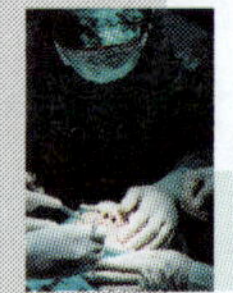

- Three methods are available for reduction of intussusception by hydrostatic pressure
  - Air enema
  - Microbarium sulfate solution
  - Warm saline
- The complications of all of three methods are gut perforation.
- *Gut perforation rate is least with air enema* provided that the pressure is kept below 120 cm of water above the level of buttocks. Hence, Bailey mentions this method before others and thus this is the best answer.
- The success rate of radiological hydrostatic reduction under fluoroscopy or ultrasonic guidance is approximately 80–95.

122. Ans. (c) 33%

Ref: Bailey and Love 26th ed. pg. 1164

- Colorectal cancer is the third most common cancer in the world and liver is the most common site of metastasis. The spread occurs *via* the portal circulation.
- *Metastatic liver disease is found in* ***one third*** *of patients having surgery for primary colorectal cancer.*
- 50% *will develop* metastasis in case of colorectal carcinoma in due course of time which leads to death.
- Resection and intra-arterial chemotherapy using 5 FU are therapeutic modalities.

123. Ans. (b) Regular use of PPI

Ref: Harrison 19th ed. pg. 568

PPI are widely available and supression of acid production will lead to elevation of gastrin levels.

Causes of Hypergastrinemia:

- Regular use of PPI
- Atrophic gastritis/pernicious anemia
- Zollinger Ellison syndrome
- Menetrier's disease

124. Ans. (c) y

Selected Additional Descriptors Encountered in the TNM Classification

m Symbol	The suffix m, in parentheses, is used to indicate the presence of multiple primary tumors at a single site
y Symbol	In those cases in which classification is performed during or following multimodality therapy. The eTNM or pTNM category is identified by a y prefix **This convention should typically be used following neoadjuvant therapies and may be most applicable to induction chemotherapy**
r Symbol	*Recurrent* tumors, when classified after a disease free interval, are identified by the prefix r
R-Classification	The absence of presence of *residual* tumor after treatment is described by the symbol R as follows RX: Presence of residual tumor cannot be assessed R0: No residual tumor R1: Microscopic residual tumor R2: Macroscopic residual tumor

Contd...

125. Ans. (a) Acute appendicitis

The clinical history and USG image is diagnostic of appendicitis. The appendix lumen is dilated >6 mm and wall is hyperechoic.

Sonographic criteria for acute appendicitis	CT criteria for acute appendicitis
Non compressible appendix of size >6 mm AP diameter Hyperechoic thickened appendix wall >2 mm: Target sign Appendicolith Interruption of submucosal continuity Peri-appendicular fluid	Thickened caecum funnelling contrast into the orifice of appendix called arrow head sign. Thickened meso-appendix Appendicular phlegmon Fecolith

126. Ans. (a) Hypochloremic metabolic alkalosis

- The repeated vomiting episode leads to loss of stomach acid and leads to hypochloraemia.
- Due to fluid loss renal blood flow falls which explains the positive stimulus for RAAS system.
- The increase aldosterone leads to urinary loss of hydrogen and potassium.
- Hence, GOO leads to *hypochloraemic hypokalemic metabolic alkalosis.*

127. Ans. (a) Aberrant blood vessel

- Dysphagia lusoria is due to aberrant right subclavian artery. *It is also called arteria lusoria, and is one of the most common intrathoracic arterial anomalies.*
- Although mostly asymptomatic, the retroesophageal and retrotracheal course of the lusorian artery might result in:

- Unspecific thoracic pain
- Dysphagia
- Dyspnea
- Arterio-esophageal fistula with hematemesis
- Arterio-tracheal fistulae with haemoptysis
- Aneurysmal formation with risk of rupture

128. Ans. (d) Ovarian cancer

Ref: Grainger & Allison's Diagnostic Radiology 6th ed. pg. 714

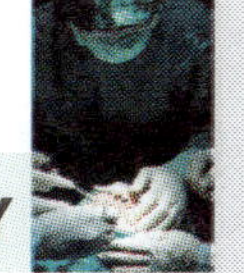

Peritoneal seeding is a common mechanism of metastatic dissemination in advanced gynecological malignancy and GIT malignancy

Peritoneal Carcinomatosis

Site of primary	Percentage
Ovarian cancer	71%
Gastric cancer	17%
Colorectal cancer	10%

- Do remember that if only GIT malignancies are mentioned then the answer is Stomach cancer
- The most common seeding site is pouch of Douglas

More aggressive neoplasms exhibit peritoneal deposits closer to primary tumor.

129. Ans. (b) Pancreas

Remember the marking shown in CT scan Abdomen as this is a favourite question with National Board.

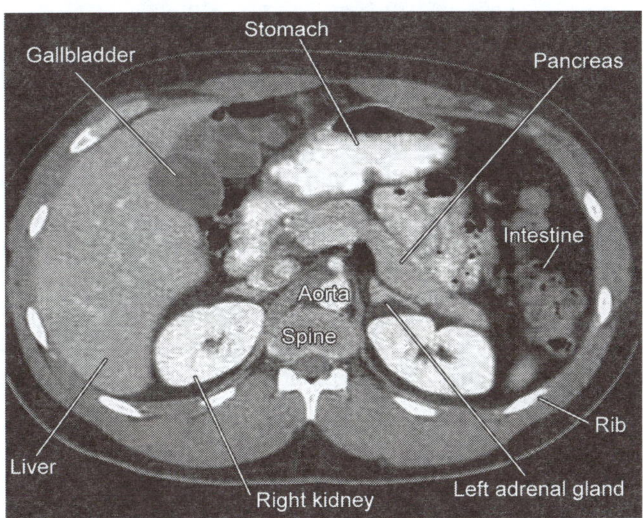

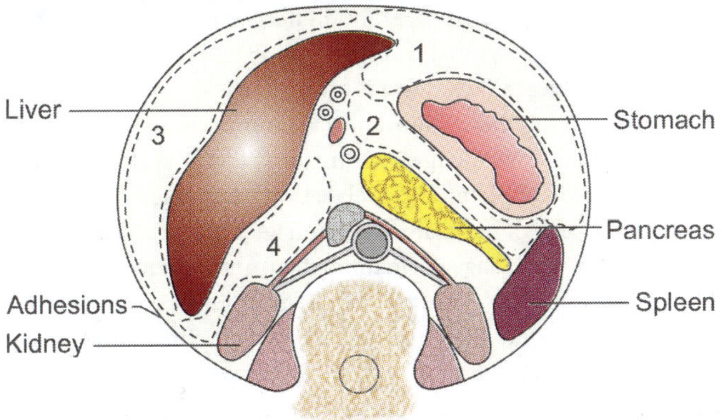

130. Ans. (c) Desmoid tumor

Gardner syndrome is occurrence of familial adenomatous polyposis (FAP) with the extra-colonic manifestations. The polyps in FAP can develop adenocarcinoma colon and hence prophylactic colectomy is performed. Other features seen are:

1. *Desmoids* or osteomas can cause parietal lumps, obstruction, and bleeding.
2. *Dental abnormalities* may develop and may result in jaw pain.
3. *Epidermoid cysts* may develop, but they manifest as only cosmetic defects.
4. *Gastric polyps* may manifest as epigastric pain or bleeding.
5. *Duodenal polyps* may cause pain, bleeding, or jaundice, whereas ileal polyps may cause obstruction.
6. *Thyroid carcinoma* (papillary carcinoma) may manifest as a neck mass, hoarseness of voice.

Mnemonic

DAISY POTS

Desmoid tumor of abdomen

Polyps

Osteomas

Thyroid cancer

Sebaceous cysts

131. Ans. (b) 3 weeks

Ref: Bailey, 26th ed. pg. 113

- *Infantile hypertrophic pyloric stenosis (IHPS) presents with non-bilious projectile vomiting between 2 and 8 weeks of age and is only rarely seen after 13 weeks.*
- It is easily distinguished from many other serious causes of vomiting, such as infections because the baby is particularly hungry.
- The non-bilious nature is stressed here to contrast the condition with the bilious vomiting of the potentially life-threatening malrotation and volvulus seen occasionally in neonates.

132. Ans. (b) Esophageal varices

Ref: Bailey, 25th ed. pg. 1043-44

The presence of ascites and dilated veins are suggestive of portal hypertension in a chronic alcoholic. Since patient presents with hematemesis it indicates bleeding esophageal varices for which octreotide infusion should be started with aggressive resuscitation.

133. Ans. (d) Large bore cannula for IVF

Ref: Bailey, 26th ed. pg. 16-17

- The probable clinical diagnosis is portal hypertension with varices
- Volume resuscitation is initiated through *large-bore intravenous lines* with rapid infusion of either isotonic saline (although care must be taken to avoid hyperchloremic

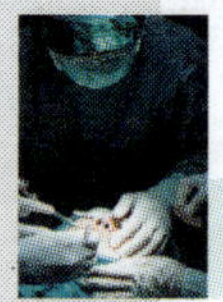

acidosis from loss of bicarbonate buffering capacity and replacement with excess chloride) or a balanced salt solution such as Ringer's lactate (being cognizant of the presence of potassium and potential renal dysfunction).

134. Ans. (b) Post-ileal

Ref: Bailey, 26th ed. pg. 1199

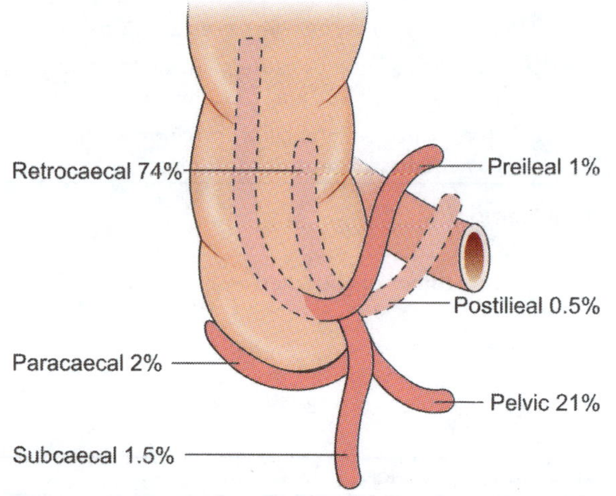

Most common positon of appendix is Retro-caecal 74%
Least common position of appendix is Post-ileal variety

135. Ans. (b) Multiple air fluid levels

Ref: Bailey, 26th ed. pg. 1189

- In intestinal obstruction, fluid levels appear later than gas shadows as it takes time for gas and fluid to separate.
- These are most prominent on an erect film. In adults, two inconstant fluid levels–one at the duodenal cap and the other in the terminal ileum–may be regarded as normal.

136. Ans. (a) 15 cm

Bailey and Love, 26th ed. ch. 62/982

The esophagus has 3 constrictions in its vertical course, as follows:

- **The first constriction is at 15 cm from the upper incisor teeth**, where the esophagus commences at the cricopharyngeal sphincter; this is the narrowest portion of the esophagus and approximately corresponds to the sixth cervical vertebra
- **The second constriction is at 25 cm from the upper incisor teeth,** where it is crossed by the aortic arch and left main bronchus.
- **The third constriction is at 40 cm from the upper incisor teeth,** where it pierces the diaphragm; the lower esophageal sphincter (LES) is situated at this level.

137. Ans. (b) Barium swallow

Ref: Bailey & Love, 26th ed. pg. 989

- Dysphagia is difficulty in swallowing. The cause can be esophageal in origin.
- The motility disorders are best evaluated with esophageal manometry.
  - **Barium swallow:** For esophageal diseases
  - **Barium meal follow through:** Small intestine pathology.
  - **Barium enema:** Colonic and rectal diseases

138. Ans. (d) Metabolic alkalosis

Ref: Bailey & Love, 26th ed. pg. 1018

- In Zenker's diverticulum, the contents of stomach are not lost and therefore metabolic alkalosis cannot occur. *Loss of stomach acid in lieu of reverse peristalsis in chronic vomiting leads to metabolic alkalosis.* When there is excessive pressure within the lower pharynx, the weakest portion of the pharyngeal wall balloons out, forming a diverticulum. Uncoordinated swallowing, impaired relaxation of the cricopharyngeus muscle leads to an increase in pressure within the distal pharynx, so that its wall herniates through the point of least resistance (Killian's triangle).
- Best investigation for Zenker diverticulum is barium swallow and best treatment is surgical resection.

139. Ans. (d) Corkscrew esophagus

Ref: Bailey & Love, 26th ed. pg. 1014

- Corkscrew esophagus is seen in diffuse esophageal spasm and not in achalasia cardia.
- **Diffuse esophageal spasm** is a condition in which uncoordinated contractions of the esophagus occur. These spasms do not propel food effectively to the stomach. It can cause dysphagia, regurgitation and chest pain.
- **Esophageal achalasia** is an esophageal motility disorder involving the smooth muscle layer of the esophagus and the lower esophageal sphincter (LES). It is characterized by incomplete LES relaxation, increased LES tone, and lack of peristalsis of esophagus. Diagnosis is reached with esophageal manometry and barium swallow radiographic studies. Permanent relief is brought by Esophageal dilatation and surgical cleaving of the muscle (Heller myotomy).

140. Ans. (b) Normal peristalsis

Ref: Bailey & Love, 26th ed. Ch. 62/1014

- Achalasia is a rare disease caused by loss of inhibitory ganglion cells within the esophageal myenteric plexus

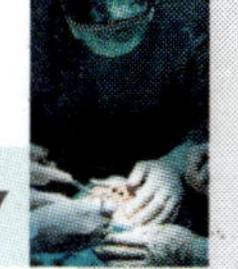

- It leads to a hypertensive lower oesophageal sphincter (LES) which fails to relax on swallowing.
- *Long-standing achalasia is characterized by progressive dilatation and sigmoid deformity of the esophagus with hypertrophy of the LES.*

Clinical Presentation

- **Progressive dysphagia is the most common presenting symptom. It generally concerns initially liquids and later both liquids and solids from the outset.**
  - **Dysphagia**: Liquids > Solid
- The second most common symptom is the regurgitation of undigested food during or shortly after a meal.

Investigation

- **Screening: Barium study-Bird beak appearance**
- **IOC:** Manometry

Treatment

- **Medical management:**
  - Calcium channel blockers
  - Nitrates
  - Botulinum toxin *(injected into the LES under endoscopic guidance)*
- **Surgical management:**
  - **Harrison states:** *"The only durable therapies for achalasia are **pneumatic dilatation** and **Heller myotomy.**"*
  - **Surgery of choice: Heller's myotomy**

141. Ans. (a) Achalasia cardia

Please refer to above explanation

142. Ans. (c) Acetylcholine

Ref: Bailey & Love, 26th ed. pg. 988

There are two types of control of LES via the Myenteric plexus:

- Excitatory (cholinergic) ganglionic neurons
- Inhibitory (nitric oxide) ganglionic neurons

Functionally, inhibitory neurons mediate Deglutitive lower esophageal sphincter (LES) relaxation and the sequential propagation of peristalsis.

143. Ans. (c) Tumor infiltration

Ref: Bailey & Love, 26th ed. pg. 1014

- Tumor infiltration, most commonly seen with carcinoma in the gastric fundus or distal esophagus can mimic idiopathic achalasia.
- The resultant "pseudoachalasia" accounts for up to 5% of suspected cases and is more likely with advanced age, abrupt onset of symptoms (<1 year), and weight loss. Hence, endoscopy should be part of the evaluation of achalasia.

144. Ans. (b) Goblet cells intestinal metaplasia

Ref: Sabiston, 19th ed. pg. 1033-36

- Metaplasia of lower esophagus is usually seen in BARRETT'S Esophagus. This condition arises due to severe reflux esophagitis.
- MC type of metaplasia seen in columnar epithelium is intestinal epithelium ***(Intestinal metaplasia).***
- Barrett's esophagus requires both endoscopically visible segment of columnar lining of distal esophagus and *intestinal metaplasia showing goblet cells on biopsy*
- Barret's esophagus is a Premalignant condition for adenocarcinoma

145. Ans. (a) Barrett esophagus

Ref: Bailey & Love, 26th ed. ch. 62/1000

- Barrett's metaplasia, endoscopically recognized by tongues of reddish mucosa extending proximally from the gastroesophageal junction or histopathologically by the finding of specialized columnar metaplasia*(intestinal type with goblet cells),* is associated with at least a 20-fold increased risk for development of **esophageal development of adenocarcinoma.**

146. Ans. (d) De meester scoring

Ranson score	Acute pancreatitis
Gleason score	Prostate cancer
Alvarado score	Acute appendicitis
De meester score	GERD

147. Ans. (d) CT chest with contrast

Ref: Bailey & Love, 26th ed. pg. 989

- Esophageal perforation causes pleuritic retrosternal pain that can be associated with pneumomediastinum and subcutaneous emphysema.
- Mediastinitis is a major complication of esophageal perforation, and prompt recognition is key to optimizing outcome.
- CT of the chest is most sensitive in detecting mediastinal air, but water soluble contrast (diatrizoate meglumine) will help in determining extravasation.
- *Esophageal perforation is confirmed by a CT with contrast usually Gastrografin followed by thin barium.*
- Treatment includes nasogastric suction and parenteral broad-spectrum antibiotics with prompt surgical

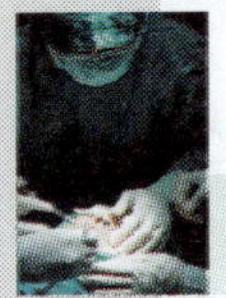

drainage and repair in noncontained leaks. Conservative therapy with NPO status and antibiotics without surgery may be appropriate in cases of minor instrumental perforation that are detected early.

148. Ans. (b) Barium study

Ref: Bailey & Love, 26th ed. ch. 62/1003

- The symptoms of rolling hernia are mostly due to twisting and distortion of the oesophagus and stomach.
- Dysphagia is common. Chest pain may occur from distension of an obstructed stomach. Classically, the pain is relieved by a loud belch.
- Strangulation, gastric perforation and gangrene can occur.
- The hernia *may be visible* on a plain radiograph of the chest as a gas bubble, often with a fluid level behind the heart.
- ***A barium meal is the best method of diagnosis.***
- Symptomatic rolling hernias nearly always require surgical repair as they are potentially dangerous.

149. Ans. (b) Biopsy

Ref: Chapter 91: Harrison, 18th ed.

- Taking multiple biopsies increases the yield. Cytologic examination of tumor brushings complements standard biopsies and should be performed routinely.
- The extent of tumor spread to the mediastinum and para-aortic lymph nodes should be assessed by CT scans of the chest and abdomen and by endoscopic ultrasound.
- Positron emission tomography scanning provides a useful assessment of resectability, offering accurate information regarding spread to mediastinal lymph nodes

150. Ans. (a) Aberrant right subclavian artery

Ref: Bailey & Love, 26th ed. pg. 1022

- During development of aortic arch, if the proximal portion of the right fourth arch disappears instead of distal portion, *the right subclavian artery* will arise as the last branch of aortic arch and is called as aberrant right subclavian artery.
- It then courses behind the esophagus (or rarely in front of esophagus, or even in front of trachea) to supply blood to right arm. This *causes pressure on esophagus and results in dysphagia*. It can sometimes result in upper gastrointestinal tract bleeding

151. Ans. (a) Spontaneous rupture of the esophagus

Ref: Bailey & Love, 26th ed. pg. 992

- Oesophageal rupture in Boerhaave syndrome is thought to be the result of a *sudden rise in internal esophageal pressure produced during vomiting, as a result of neuromuscular incoordination* causing failure of the cricopharyngeus muscle to relax. The syndrome is commonly associated with the consumption of excessive food and/or alcohol as well as eating disorders such as bulimia.
- The *most common anatomical location of the tear in Boerhaave syndrome is at left postero-lateral wall of the lower third of the oesophagus*, 2–3 cm before the stomach
- The most common cause of oesophageal perforation is iatrogenic, which occurs in cervical part of oesophagus.

152. Ans. (d) Bowel lumen obstruction

Ref: Bailey & Love, 26th ed./ch 75 pg. 1201

- Obstruction of the appendix lumen has been widely held to be important, and some form of luminal obstruction, either by a faecolith or a stricture, is found in the majority of cases
- Obstruction of the appendiceal lumen seems to be essential for the development of appendiceal gangrene and perforation.

153. Ans. (d) 1/3 rd distance from the right anterior superior spine

Ref: Bailey & Love, 26th ed. pg. 1203

McBurney's point is the name given to the point over the right side of the abdomen that is *one-third of the distance from the anterior superior iliac spine to the umbilicus* . This point roughly corresponds to the most common location of the base of the appendix where it is attached to the cecum.

154. Ans. (b) Appendicitis

Ref: Bailey & Love, 25th ed. pg. 1208

- The most common symptom of appendicitis is abdominal pain. Typically, symptoms begin as periumbilical or epigastric pain migrating to the right lower quadrant (RLQ) of the abdomen.
- *Patients of appendicitis usually lie down, flex their hips, and draw their knees up to reduce movements* and to avoid worsening their pain. Later, a worsening progressive pain along with vomiting, nausea, and anorexia are described by the patient.
- The duration of symptoms is less than 48 hours in approximately 80% of adults but tends to be longer in elderly persons and in those with perforation.

Clinical Signs in Apppendicitis

- **Rovsing sign** (RLQ pain with palpation of the LLQ): Suggests peritoneal irritation

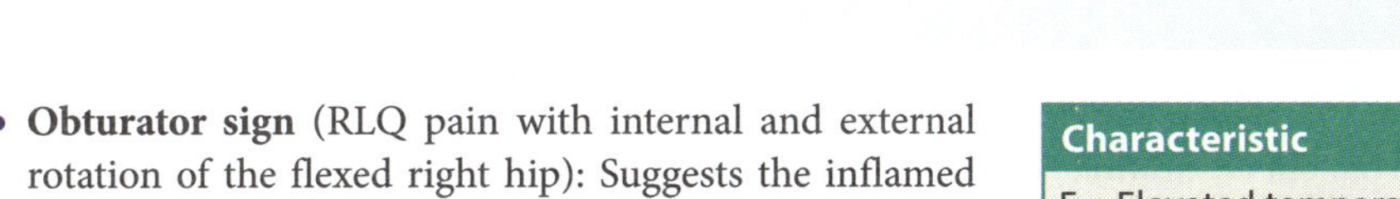

- **Obturator sign** (RLQ pain with internal and external rotation of the flexed right hip): Suggests the inflamed appendix is located deep in the right hemipelvis
- **Psoas sign** (RLQ pain with extension of the right hip or with flexion of the right hip against resistance): Suggests that an inflamed appendix is located along the course of the right psoas muscle
- **Dunphy sign** (sharp pain in the RLQ elicited by a voluntary cough): Suggests localized peritonitis
- **Markle sign** (pain elicited in a certain area of the abdomen when the standing patient drops from standing on toes to the heels with a jarring landing): Has a sensitivity of 74%

155. Ans. (c) Locate the anterior taenia of the caecum

Ref: Bailey & Love, 26th ed. ch. 75/1204

- *Three taeniae coli of the caecum, fuse to form the outer longitudinal muscle coat of the appendix.*
- *During operation, this can be used to find an elusive appendix, as gentle traction on the taeniae coli, particularly the anterior taenia, will lead the operator to the base of the appendix.*

156. Ans. (a) Appendix

Ref: Bailey & Love, 26th ed. ch. 75/1204

- *The base of the appendix can be identified during surgery by following the convergence of the taeniae coli toward the inferior portion of the cecum, forming a continuous muscular layer surrounding the appendix.*

The position of the appendicular tip is inconstant and can be situated in the following locations:

- **Retrocecal (65%)** – rigidity is often absent, and even application of deep pressure may fail to elicit tenderness **(Silent appendix)**
- Descending pelvic (31%)
- Transverse and retrocecal (2.5%)
- Ascending, paracecal, and preileal (1%)
- Ascending, paracecal, and postileal (0.4%)

157. Ans. (c) Retrocaecal

Ref: Bailey & Love, 26th ed. Ch 75/1204

158. Ans. (a) Acute appendicitis

Characteristic	Score
M = Migration of pain to the RLQ	1
A = Anorexia	1
N = Nausea and vomiting	1
T = Tenderness in RLQ	2
R = Rebound pain	1
E = Elevated temperature	1
L = Leukocytosis	2
S = Shift of WBCs to the left	1
Total	10
RLQ = right lower quadrant; WBCs = white blood cells	

159. Ans. (d) All of these

Infants	Pre-school Children	School Children
Pyloric Stenosis	Intussusceptions, Meckel's Diverticulitis, Acute Gastroenteritis	The most common mimicker of appendicitis in this population is mesenteric lymphadenitis
Adults	**Women in their childbearing years**	**Elderly**
Pyelonephritis, Colitis Diverticulitis	(Higher incidence of false-positive diagnoses in this group) Pelvic Inflammatory Disease (PID), Tubo-Ovarian Abscess, Ruptured Ovarian Cyst Or Ovarian Torsion, And Ectopic Pregnancy.	Diverticulitis Bowel Obstruction Malignancies Of The G.I Tract & Reproductive System Perforated Ulcers Cholecystitis

160. Ans. (a) Appendicular mass

Ref: Bailey & Love, 26th ed. pg. 1211

- The appendix that is acutely inflamed may perforate and later wall off from the peritoneal cavity by omentum and adjacent bowel loop to form a tender, palpable right iliac fossa mass. It is a common surgical pathology which occurs in about 2–6% of patients who presented with acute appendicitis. The initial school of thought regards this condition to be managed conservatively, with the famous one being the Ochsner-Sherren regimen. The idea behind this is that, surgery would be hazardous and increase the mortality rate.
- The conservative management of appendicular mass can be summarized by mnemonic "ABCDEF" which is
  - **A:** Analgesic, Antibiotic, antipyretic
  - **B:** Bed rest
  - **C:** Charting (vital sign, size of the mass)
  - **D:** Diet (Keep Nil by Mouth)
  - **E:** Exploratory laparotomy
  - **F:** Fluid maintenance

Three methods are proposed for management of appendicular mass which are:

- Conservative management
- Interval appendectomy

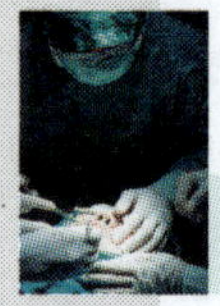

- Early surgical intervention. The selection of methods depends on surgeon preference and patient's condition.

161. Ans. (b) Kulchitsky cell tumor

Ref: Harrison, 18th ed. ch. 350

- Carcinoid tumors arise from argentaffin cells of the crypts of Lieberkühn.
- They are found in distal duodenum to the ascending colon, which are embryologically derived from the midgut.
- *More than **50% of intestinal carcinoids are found in the distal ileum,** with most congregating close to the ileocecal valve.*
- Most intestinal carcinoids are asymptomatic and of low malignant potential, but invasion and metastases may occur, leading to the carcinoid syndrome.
- **Carcinoid tumors are classified as**
  - Typical carcinoid [Kulchitsky cell carcinoma producing 5-HIAA]
  - Atypical carcinoid [producing 5 Hydroxy tryptophan]
- It can be benign or malignant and presents with secretory diarrhea and flushing.
- **Diagnosis** is made by Octreoscan and urinary 5 H.I.A.A (Hydroxy-indole- acetic acid) levels.
- **Drug of choice** is Octreotide.

162. Ans. (a) Ileum

Ref. Harrison, 18th ed. ch. 350

Most common site of carcinoid Tumor: Bronchus>ileum >Rectum> appendix

163. Ans. (d) Absence of free gas rules out peritonitis

- The peritoneum, which is a sterile environment, reacts to various pathologic stimuli with a fairly uniform inflammatory response.
- *Primary peritonitis* is most often spontaneous bacterial peritonitis (SBP) caused by chronic liver disease. *Secondary peritonitis* is by far the *most common form of peritonitis* encountered in clinical practice and is most commonly due to PUD. *Tertiary peritonitis* often develops in the absence of the original visceral organ pathology usually in setting of immunocompromised status.
- Chemical (sterile) peritonitis may be caused by irritants such as bile, blood, barium, or other substances or by transmural inflammation of visceral organs (e.g. Crohn disease) without bacterial inoculation of the peritoneal cavity. However *bile being alkaline has more irritation than blood.*
- Free air is present in most cases of anterior gastric and duodenal perforation but is much less frequent with perforations of the small bowel and colon and is unusual with appendiceal perforation. Upright films are useful for identifying free air under the diaphragm (most often on the right) as an indication of a perforated viscus.

Remember

- The free gas appears about 1-2 hours after the perforation of bowel
- *Absence of free gas in the peritoneal cavity does not necessarily exclude presence of perforation as it is absent in approximately 25% cases of perforated duodenal ulcer.*

164. Ans. (c) Anaerobic streptococcus

Ref: Harrison, 19th ed. pg. 972

MICROORGANISMS IN PERITONITIS

Gastrointestinal Sources

- *Escherichia coli*
- *Streptococci(anaerobic)*
- *Bacteroides*
- *Clostridium*
- *Klebsiella pneumoniae*

Other Sources

- *Chlamydia trachomatis*
- *Neisseria gonorrhoeae*
- *Haemolytic streptococci*
- *Staphylococcus*
- *Streptococcus pneumonia*
- *Mycobacterium tuberculosis* and other spp.
- Fungal infections

165. Ans. (c) Chlamydia

Ref: Harrison, 19th ed. pg. 972

Paths to Peritoneal Infection

- Gastrointestinal perforation, e.g., perforated ulcer, appendix, diverticulum
- Transmural translocation (no perforation), e.g., pancreatitis, ischaemic bowel
- Exogenous contamination, e.g. drains, open surgery, trauma
- *Female genital tract infection, e.g., pelvic inflammatory disease with chlamydia*
- Haematogenous spread (rare), e.g., septicaemia

166. Ans. (b) Sarcoma

Ref: Bailey and Love, 26th ed. ch. 61/985

- One third of malignant tumors that arise in the retroperitoneum are sarcomas, and approximately 15% of soft tissue sarcomas arise in the retroperitoneum.
- Retroperitoneal sarcomas are malignant tumors arising from mesenchymal cells, which are usually located in muscle, fat, and connective tissues. Retroperitoneal sarcomas have varying clinical courses depending on their histologic subtype and grade.

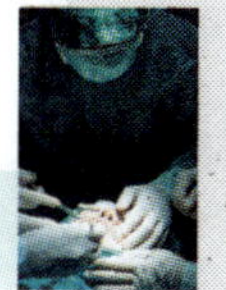

167. Ans. (d) Abdominal lump

Ref: Bailey and Love, 26th ed. ch. 61/985

- Primary retroperitoneal neoplasms are an extremely rare group of tumors (lymphoma is not included in the definition). **The most common type is soft tissue sarcoma (90%).**
- The commonest age range for presentation is around 40–50 years.
- *Sarcomas that arise in the retroperitoneum most commonly present as an abdominal mass, often without other symptoms.*
- Early satiety, gastrointestinal obstruction or bleeding, lower extremity swelling, or pain are among the first symptoms leading to the discovery of a retroperitoneal sarcoma.
- **Investigation:** CT is the most commonly used tool. MRI can be used for further differentiation, but histology is always required. Percutaneous biopsy may be undertaken and for assessment of tumor grade.

168. Ans. (c) Villous adenoma

Ref: Bailey & Love, 26th ed. pg. 1184

ADULT INTUSSCEPTION

- Bowel intussusception in adults is considered a rare condition, accounting for 1–5% of bowel obstruction.
- Adult cases of intussusception are associated with a lead point which is:
  1. Polyp
  2. Submucosal lipoma
  3. Inflammatory bowel disease
  4. Postoperative adhesions
  5. Meckel's diverticulum
  6. Villous adenoma
  7. Metastatic neoplasms
  8. Iatrogenically, due to the presence of intestinal tubes, jejunostomy feeding tubes or after gastric surgery.

Most common cause of pediatric intussusception is Meckel's diverticulum>polyp.

169. Ans. (d) Pneumatosis intestinalis

Ref: Bailey & Love, 26th ed. pg. 1189

- Plain film radiographs of the abdomen in supine position can be helpful in diagnosing small bowel obstruction.
- An upright chest radiograph is best for ruling out free air under the diaphragm.
- Signs of small bowel obstruction include:
  - Bowel dilatation proximal to the site of obstruction, air–fluid levels
  - Paucity of large bowel gas, bowel wall thickening
  - A fixed loop
  - Ground glass appearance signifying intraluminal fluid.
  - Although the cecum may dilate greatly in chronic obstruction without rupturing, perforation should be suspected whenever this portion of the colon is greater than 10 cm in diameter.
  - Step ladder pattern of air fluid levels.

170. Ans. (b) Resection with intestine part

Ref: Bailey & Love, 26th ed. pg. 903

- Enterogenous cyst arises from either a diverticulum of the mesentric border of the intestine that has become sequestrated from the intestinal canal during embryonic life or from a duplication of the intestine.
- An enterogenous cyst has a thicker wall than a chylolymphatic cyst and is lined by mucous membrane, sometimes ciliated.
- The content is mucinous and is either colorless or yellowish brown as a result of past haemorrhage. The muscle in the wall of an enteric duplication cyst and the bowl with which it is in contact have a common blood supply, *consequently removal of the cyst always entails resection of the related portion of intestine.*

171. Ans. (a) Anastomotic leak

Ref: Bailey & Love, 26th ed. pg. 1150; Advances in Minimally Invasive Surgery, 2nd ed. pg. 250

Anastomotic leak is one of the most dreaded early complications of colorectal surgery. The incidence of anastomotic leak following colectomy is generally reported between 2 and 6%. Anastomotic leaks present in one of three ways:

1. Asymptomatic leak
2. Subtle insidious leak
3. Dramatic early leak

The *asymptomatic leak* is incidentally found during endoscopic or radiographic studies. The incidence of radiographically detected leaks is 4–6 times higher than clinically detected leaks. The *subtle insidious leak* can present peri-operatively with nonspecific signs and symptoms common in the post operative period, and occur 5–14 days following surgery. The *dramatic early leak* can present with any combination of acute abdominal pain, distention, fever, tachycardia, diffuse peritonitis, oliguria, or shock within several days of surgery.

172. Ans. (c) Bilious vomiting

Ref: Sabiston, 19th ed. pg. 1841

- In HPS, hypertrophy of the circular muscle of the pylorus results in constriction and obstruction of the gastric outlet.

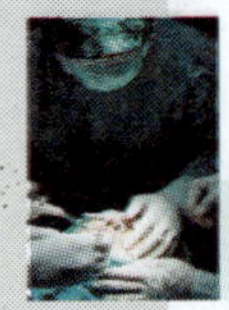

- Most commonly clinical presentation is seen between 3–6 weeks of life
- ***Clinical features:***
- *Projectile nonbilious vomiting*
- Visible gastric peristalsis may be seen as a wave of contraction from the left upper quadrant to the epigastrium
- The infants usually feed vigorously between episodes of vomiting
- **Typical electrolyte abnormality: Hypochloremic, hypokalemic, metabolic alkalosis with paradoxical aciduria.**
- **Remember:** Hypokalemic metabolic acidosis is seen with diarrhea.

Why metabolic alkalosis and paradoxical aciduria?

- Loss of stomach contents will lead to dehydration. This will trigger the R.A.A.S system into an overdrive and lead to release of aldosterone. Since aldosterone leads to potassium and hydrogen loss in the DCT of the kidney, patient will develop hypokalemic metabolic alkalosis and aciduria (paradoxically)

173. Ans. (b) Hypokalemic metabolic alkalosis

Ref: Bailey & Love, 26th ed. ch. 63/1023

174. Ans. (b) Metabolic alkalosis

Please refer to above explanation

175. Ans. (d) Hyperplastic polyp

Ref: Bailey & Love, 26th ed. pg. 1224

Inflammatory polyp	Seen in ulcerative colitis and crohn's disease, and can turn malignant
Familial adenomatous polyposis	• <1% of all colorectal cancers. • Autosomal dominant • > 100 colorectal adenomas, caused by germ-line mutations of the tumor suppressor gene APC
Hamartomatous polyp	They are growths, like tumors found in organs as a result of faulty development. Hamartomatous polyps are seen in Peutz-Jegher Syndrome or Juvenile Polyposis Syndrome.
Hyperplastic polyp	Most common colonic polyps • Quite small • Composed of cells showing dysmaturation and hyperplasia • *No neoplastic potential, but some might have adenomatous changes and should be excised for histopathology.*

176. Ans. (d) Toxic megacolon

Ref: Bailey & Love, 26th ed. pg. 1156

Indications for Surgery in Crohn's Disease

- **Small Intestine**
  - Stricture and obstruction unresponsive to medical therapy
  - *Massive hemorrhage*
  - *Refractory fistula*
  - Abscess
- **Colon and rectum**
- **Intractable disease**
  - Fulminant disease
  - Perianal disease unresponsive to medical therapy
  - Refractory fistula
  - *Colonic obstruction*
  - Cancer prophylaxis
  - Colon dysplasia or cancer

177. Ans. (a) Juvenile rectal polyp

Ref: Bailey & Love, 26th ed. pg. 1224

The most common cause of bleeding per rectum in children is juvenile rectal polyp up to adolescence age. Though in infants and young children (up to 1 year) the cause is anal fissure.

178. Ans. (b) Necrosis

Ref: Bailey & Love, 26th ed. pg. 1150

Complications of Ileostomy

Stoma necrosis may occur in the early postoperative period and usually is caused by skeletonizing the distal small bowel and/or creating an overly tight fascial defect.

179. Ans. (a) B_{12}

Ref: Harrison, 18th ed. ch. 294

- Post resection of ileum, vitamin B_{12} deficiency is seen.
- Steatorrhea is fat malabsorption leading to malodorous stools. Fat malabsorption leads to deficiency of vitamin A, D, E, K.

180. Ans. (a) Ascites

Ref: Bailey & Love, 26th ed. pg. 980

- A peritoneo-venous shunt (also called Denver shunt) is a shunt which drains peritoneal fluid from the peritoneum into veins, usually the internal jugular vein or the superiorvena cava.
- It is sometimes used in patients with refractory ascites.

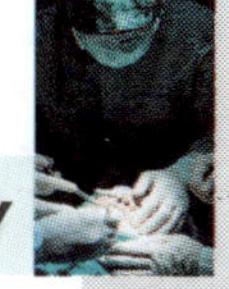

- It is a long tube with a non-return valve running subcutaneously from the peritoneum to the internal jugular vein in the neck, which flows ascitic fluid to pass directly into the systemic circulation.

181. Ans. (a) IBS

Ref: Bailey & Love, 26th ed. pg. 1179

The Rome criteria is a system developed to classify the functional gastrointestinal disorders (FGIDs), disorders of the digestive system in which symptoms cannot be explained by the presence of structural or tissue abnormality, based on clinical symptoms. *Some examples of FGIDs include irritable bowel syndrome, functional dyspepsia, functional constipation, and functional heart burn.*

182. Ans. (b) Malnutrition

Ref: Bailey & Love, 26th ed. pg. 1134

CHRONIC TROPICAL PANCREATITIS

- Most common cause of chronic pancreatitis is alcohol intake
- *Non alcoholic form of chronic pancreatitis* prevalent in the tropics like Africa, Asia and India
- Diabetic stage of the disease referred to as fibrocalculous pancreatic diabetes
- **Etiology:** Malnutrition, cyanogens toxicity (present in insufficiently processed cassava), antioxidant def. and genetic factors
- **Classical triad:** Steatorrea, diabetes, abdominal pain
- **Main treatment:** Management of diabetes
- **Main cause of death:** Complications of diabetes (MC diabetic nephropathy)

183. Ans. (c) RANSON Score

Ref: Bailey & Love, 26th ed. pg. 1128

RANSON CRITERIA

At Admission

- Age in years >55 years
- White blood cell count >16000 cells/mm^3
- Blood glucose >10 mmol/L (>200 mg/dL)
- Serum AST >250 IU/L
- Serum LDH >350 IU/L

Within 48 hours

- Serum calcium <2.0 mmol/L (<8.0 mg/dL)
- Hematocrit fall >10%
- Oxygen (hypoxemia PO_2 <60 mm Hg)
- BUN increased by 1.8 or more mmol/L (5 or more mg/dL) after IV fluid hydration
- Base deficit (negative base excess) >4 mEq/L
- Sequestration of fluids >6 L

Alternatively, Pancreatitis severity can be assessed by any of the following:

- APACHE II score ≥8
- **CT scan:** Substantial pancreatic necrosis (at least 30% glandular necrosis according to contrast-enhanced CT)

184. Ans. (a) Serum bilirubin

Ref: Bailey & Love, 26th ed. pg. 1128

APACHE score is: Acute Physiology and Chronic Health Evaluation

The APACHE II point score is calculated from 12 routine physiological measurements:

- Age
- Temperature (rectal)
- Mean arterial pressure
- pH arterial
- Heart rate
- Respiratory rate
- Sodium (serum)
- Potassium (serum)
- Creatinine
- Hematocrit
- White blood cell count
- Glasgow Coma Scale

Extra Mile

- Now APACHE III is also available. The APACHE III is used to produce an equation predicting hospital mortality after the first day of ICU treatment.
- **There are 4 components:** Age, Major disease category (reason for ICU admission), Acute (current) physiology, and Prior site of healthcare (e.g. hospital floor, emergency room, etc.)

185. Ans. (a) Acute pancreatitis

Ref: Schwartz's, 9th ed. pg. 1352

Complications of ERCP

1. ***Pancreatitis is the most common ERCP complication.*** Transient increase in serum pancreatic enzymes may occur in as many as 75% of patients.
2. Most ERCP-associated *bleeding* is intraluminal, although intra-ductal bleeding can occur.
3. *Post-ERCP cholangitis.*
4. Cardiopulmonary complications
5. Duodenal hematoma
6. Colonic perforation
7. Cardiopulmonary complications

186. Ans. (a) Neurofibromatosis

- **Neurofibromatosis type 1**/von Recklinghausen disease caused by inherited gene, the NF1 gene codes for the protein neurofibromin.

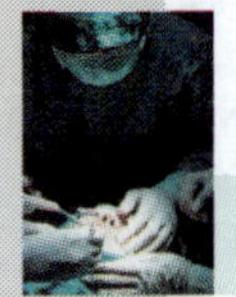

- Patients with neurofibromatosis develop café-au-lait spots, and benign and malignant tumors of the nervous system.
- Benign nervous system involvement includes neurofibromas, and the malignant include peripheral nerve sheath tumor.
- *They can also develop distinctive eye lesions called Lisch nodules, which are iris hamartomas*
- The *most common cause of death is CNS tumors.*

Extra Mile

- Turcot syndrome is characterized by intestinal polyposis and CNS tumors: Most commonly glioblastoma or medulloblastoma
- MEN2A sipple consists of parathyroid adenoma, medullary carcinoma thyroid, phaeochromocytoma.

187. Ans. (a) Duodeno-Duodenostomy

Ref: Bailey & Love, 26th ed. pg. 1194

- Duodenal atresia and stenosis are treated surgically. In patients with duodenal obstruction, a duodenoduodenostomy is the most commonly performed procedure.
- *A duodenojejunostomy is now rarely performed due to its higher risk of long-term complications.*
- Presenting symptoms and signs are the result of high intestinal obstruction. Duodenal atresia is typically characterized by onset of vomiting within hours of birth. While vomitus is most often bilious, it may be non-bilious because 15% of defects occur proximal to the ampulla of Vater.

188. Ans. (b) Splenosis

Ref: Bailey & Love, 26th ed. pg. 1095-96

Complications of Splenectomy:

- Intraoperative complications:
  - Pancreatic injury
  - Hemorrhage
  - Bowel injury: Colon and stomach
  - Diaphragmatic injuries
- Early post op complications
  - *Pulmonary: Atelectasis, pleural effusion, pneumonitis*
  - *Sub phrenic abscess*
  - Thrombocytopenia and *thrombotic complications*
  - Wound problems
  - Ileus
- Late post op complications:
  - Over whelming post splenectomy infection
  - Splenosis

Splenosis occurs due to seeding of peritoneal cavity with splenic tissue which recruits local blood supply.

189. Ans. (d) All of these

Post Vagotomy Complications:

1. **Post vagotomy diarrhea:**
   - About 30% or more of patients suffer from diarrhea after gastric surgery.
2. **Post vagotomy gastric atony:**
   - After vagotomy, gastric emptying is delayed. This is true for both truncal and selective vagotomies but not in the case of highly selective or parietal cell vagotomy.
   - With selective or truncal vagotomy, patients lose antral pump function and therefore have a reduction in their ability to empty solids
3. **Incomplete Vagal Transaction:**
   - It predisposes the patient to the possible development of recurrent ulcer formation. The type of vagotomy performed influences the likelihood of this problem.
   - In highly selective vagotomy, incomplete vagotomy is rarely a problem because of the meticulous dissection required during this procedure.

190. Ans. (c) Ogilvie's syndrome

Ref: Bailey & Love, 26th ed. pg. 1198

- Pseudo-obstruction of the colon is called as ogilvie's syndrome which is characterized by distention of the colon, with signs and symptoms of colonic obstruction, in the absence of an actual physical cause of the obstruction.
- Mirizzi syndrome is a gallstone becoming impacted in cystic duct or neck of gallbladder causing compression of CBD and resultant obstructive Jaundice.

191. Ans. (b) Lesser curvature

Ref: Bailey & Love, 26th ed. pg. 1034

Most peptic ulcers are caused by *H. pylori* or NSAIDs with lesser curvature being the most common site of gastric ulcer and duodenal cap being the site of duodenal ulcer.

192. Ans. (d) Lesser sac

Ref: Bailey & Love, 26th ed. pg. 1041

Posterior perforation of peptic ulcer leads to escape of contents to enter into lesser sac *via* foramen of Winslow. Posterior gastric ulcers may erode into the lesser sac behind the stomach. The lesser sac behind the stomach is a potential space and is less effective in sealing off a posteriorly situated gastric ulcer eroding through the wall of the stomach.

193. Ans. (a) Acute pancreatitis

Ref: Bailey & Love, 26th ed. ch. 313

- Purtscher-like retinopathy is seen in:

1. Acute pancreatitis
2. Fat embolization
3. Amniotic fluid embolization
4. Preeclampsia
5. Hemolysis
6. Elevated liver enzymes, and low platelets (HELLP) syndrome; and vasculitic diseases, such as lupus.

- The findings of white lesions in the retina associated with intraretinal and pre-retinal hemorrhages and papillitis are due to lymphatic extravasation from trauma. These lesions are known as Purtscherflecken (larger infarcts of the retinal capillary bed) and cotton-wool spots (small retinal microinfarcts at the level of the nerve fiber layer).
- No proven treatment exists for Purtscher retinopathy that occurs after traumatic injury.

194. Ans. (b) Autoimmune

Ref: Bailey & Love, 26th ed. pg. 1031

- *Autoimmune metaplastic atrophic gastritis is an autoimmune disease that attacks parietal cells, resulting in hypochlorhydria and reduced production of intrinsic factor. Consequences include atrophic gastritis, B_{12} malabsorption, and, frequently, pernicious anemia. Risk of gastric adenocarcinoma increases 3-fold. Diagnosis is by endoscopy. Treatment is with B_{12}.*
- Type B, or antral-predominant, gastritis is caused by *H. pylori* infection.
- The number of *H. pylori* organisms decreases dramatically with progression to gastric atrophy, and the degree of inflammation correlates with the level of these organisms.
- Early on, with antral-predominant findings, the quantity of *H. pylori* is highest and a dense chronic inflammatory infiltrate of the lamina propria is noted, accompanied by epithelial cell infiltration with Polymorphonuclear leukocytes

195. Ans. (a) Stomach

- Primary **gastric lymphoma** is an uncommon condition, accounting for less than 15% of gastric malignancies and about 2% of all lymphomas. However, the stomach is a very common extranodal site for lymphomas (lymphomas originating somewhere else with metastasis to stomach). It is also the most common source of lymphomas in the gastrointestinal tract.

196. Ans. (d) Stomach CA

Ref: Bailey & Love, 26th ed. ch. 63/1050

- Tumor of the stomach may spread via the abdominal cavity to the umbilicus (Sister Joseph's nodule).
- The ovaries may sometimes be the sole site of transcoelomic spread (Krukenberg's tumors).

197. Ans. (b) Stomach

Ref: Bailey & Love, 26th ed. ch. 63/1050

198. Ans. (d) Right side of the colon in adults

Ref: Bailey & Love, 26th ed. ch. 69/1171

- *Angiodysplasia is a degenerative lesion of previously healthy blood vessels found most commonly in the cecum and proximal ascending colon.*
- 77% of angiodysplasias are located in the cecum and ascending colon, 15% are located in the jejunum and ileum, and the remainder are distributed throughout the alimentary tract. These lesions typically are non-palpable and small (<5 mm).
- **Angiodysplasia is the most common vascular abnormality of the GI tract.** After diverticulosis, it is the second leading cause of lower GI bleeding in patients older than 60 years.

199. Ans. (d) Epidermoid

Ref: Schwartz, 9th ed. pg. 1277, Sabiston, 19th ed. pg. 1104-05

Types of mesenteric cysts	Features
1. Chylolymphatic cyst 2. Simple (mesothelial cyst) 3. Enterogenous 4. Urogenital remnant 5. Dermoid	MC age for mesenteric cyst-2nd decade of life MC in women **C/F**: painless abdomen swelling>recurrent attack of abdomen pain without vomiting>acute abdomen (torsion, rupture discharge, infection)
Diagnosis of mesenteric cyst	**CT scan** is IOC
Chylolymphatic mesenteric cyst	**Most common type** • Arise from misplaced lymphatic tissue • Located at mesentry of ileum • Thin walled, with clear fluid (pic above) • Unilocular, solitary • Blood supply independent
Treatment of choice	**Chylolymphatic- Enucleation** **Enterogenous- Resection and anastomosis**

200. Ans. (b) Chylolymphatic cyst

Ref: Schwartz, 9th ed./1277, Sabiston 19th ed./1104-05

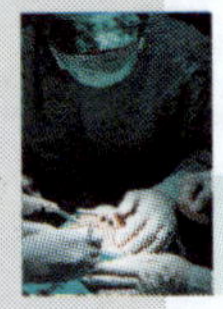

201. Ans. (c) Chronic diarrhea

- *Immunoproliferative small intestinal disease* (IPSID) is a B cell tumor.
- The presentation includes chronic diarrhea, steatorrhea associated with vomiting and abdominal cramps.
- IPSID presents with intestinal secretions of an abnormal IgA that contains a shortened heavy chain and is devoid of light chains.
- The clinical course is one of exacerbations and remissions, with death due to malnutrition and wasting or the development of a lymphoma.

202. Ans. (a) Digital positioning

Ref: Bailey & Love, 26th ed. pg. 1220

- Patients who present with a prolapsed rectum should undergo manual reduction. Conservative management is appropriate in selected patients. Treatment should be directed to the underlying cause. After treating the underlying cause, conservative management is usually successful.
- The prolapsed bowel may be grasped with lubricated gloved fingers and pushed back in with gentle steady pressure. If the bowel has become edematous, firm steady pressure for several minutes may be necessary to reduce the swelling and allow for reduction. If the prolapse immediately recurs, it may be reduced again and the buttocks taped together for several hours.
- However, if the prolapse persists after an adequate trial of medical therapy (usually a period of months), surgical intervention may be required. Pain, excoriations, and rectal bleeding are considered indications for surgical treatment.

203. Ans. (c) Fistula in ano

Ref: Bailey & Love, 26th ed. pg. 1259

Causes of Acute Anal Pain

1. Thrombosed hemorrhoids
   - **External hemorrhoids** are located distal to the dentate line and are covered with anoderm. Because the anoderm is richly innervated, thrombosis of an external hemorrhoid **may cause significant pain.**
2. Acute anal fissure
   - Characteristic symptoms include tearing pain with defecation and hematochezia (usually described as blood on the toilet paper)
3. Perianal abscess
   - Severe anal pain is the most common presenting complaint. Walking, coughing, or straining can aggravate the pain.

Fistula in ano presents with

Patients usually complain of intermittent purulent discharge (which may be bloody). Schwartz's 9th ed and oxford textbook of surgery do not mention pain as a feature of fistula in ano

204. Ans. (a) Purulent discharge with bleeding

Ref: Bailey & Love, 26th ed. pg. 1259

- A fistula in ano is an abnormal tract with external opening in the perianal area and communicates with the rectum or anal canal by an identifiable internal opening. Fistulas arise as a result of cryptoglandular infection with resultant perirectal abscess.
- The patient may present with recurrent perianal abscesses or with a bloody and purulent discharge.

205. Ans. (b) Anterior and posterior fistula

Ref: Bailey & Love, 26th ed. pg. 1260

- Goodsall's rule used to *indicate the likely position of the internal opening* according to the position of the external opening(s).
- The site of the internal opening may be felt as a point of induration or seen as an enlarged papilla. Whenever possible, it is important to determine by examination the level of the internal opening in relation to the levator mechanism.
- Goodsall's law indicates that fistulas with an *anterior external opening, drain directly into the anus at the dentate line*, and those with a posterior external opening take a curved course to enter the anal canal in the midline.

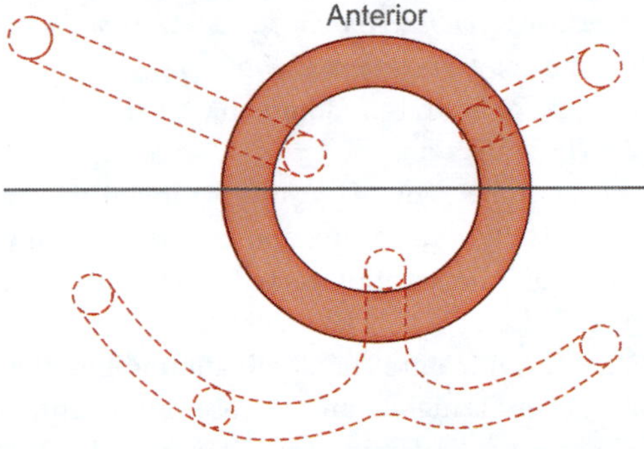

206. Ans. (b) Squamous cell CA

Ref: Sabiston, 19th ed. pg. 1405-06

CARCINOMA ANAL CANAL

- Carcinomas arising proximal to the (dentate line) pectinate line are known as ***basaloid,*** *cuboidal*, or *cloacogenic* tumors; ***about one-third of anal cancers have this histologic pattern.***
- Malignancies arising distal to the pectinate line have **squamous histology,** ulcerate more frequently, and **constitute 55% of anal cancer**
  - **MC type of CA anal canal:** Squamous cell CA > BCC > Melanoma
  - Median age at diagnosis: 60 years
  - **MC symptom:** Bleeding PR
  - **MC site of metastasis:** Lung
  - **MC site of LN metastasis:** Inguinal LNs

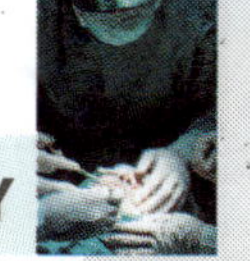

Clinical Features of anal Canal CA

- Most patients present with rectal bleeding and pain
- Patients are frequently misdiagnosed as having a benign anorectal condition such as hemorrhoids.
- **Additional symptoms:** Incontinence, change in bowel habits, pelvic pain, and rectovaginal or rectovesical fistulas are ominous.

Diagnosis: IOC for diagnosis of CA anal canal: Proctoscopy with biopsy.

Treatment

- **Nigro regimen:** Chemoradiation is the treatment of choice.
- **Chemotherapy regime:** 5-FU + Mitomycin, Cisplatin
- More than 80% are cured by chemoradiation. If any residual tumor is left behind after chemoradiation, APR is performed.

207. Ans. (a) Squamous

Ref: Bailey & Love, 26th ed. pg. 1267

208. Ans. (a) Human papilloma virus

Ref: Bailey & Love, 26th ed. pg. 1266

- The development of anal cancer is associated with infection by human papilloma virus.
- The infection may lead to:
  - Anal warts (condyloma acuminata)
  - Anal intraepithelial neoplasia
  - Squamous cell carcinoma.
- The risk for anal cancer is increased among homosexual males.
- Anal cancer risk is increased in both men and women with AIDS, because of their immunosuppressed state

209. Ans. (b) Liver

Ref: Bailey & Love, 26th ed. pg. 1226

- Cancers of the colon spread to regional lymph nodes or to the liver through the portal venous circulation.
- *The liver represents the most frequent visceral site of metastasis.*
- Colorectal cancer rarely spreads to the lungs, supraclavicular lymph nodes, bone, or brain without prior spread to the liver.

210. Ans. (a) Rectal prolapse

Ref: Bailey & Love, 26th ed. pg. 1220

- The image shows a rectal prolapse which is a sliding hernia through a defect in the pelvic fascia.

211. Ans. (b) Urine retention

Ref: Bailey & Love, 26th ed. pg. 1256

- Urinary retention is a common complication following hemorrhoidectomy and occurs in 10% to 50% of patients. Many factors are thought to contribute to urinary retention following hemorrhoidectomy, with pain being a major contributor.
- Bleeding is often minor and can be stopped with local pressure.
- Chronic complications include:
  - Poor wound healing
  - Abscess
  - Healing
  - Anal stenosis

212. Ans. (a) 1/3rd above the dentate line and 2/3rd below the dentate line

Ref: Bailey & Love 26th ed./1237

- The anal canal is completely extraperitoneal.
- The length of the (surgical) anal canal is about 4 cm (range, 3–5 cm), with *two thirds of this being above the dentate line and one third below the dentate line (the anatomical anal canal).*
- The epithelium of the (anatomical) anal canal is called anoderm. It is pigmented and keratinised.
- In anatomy texts, the rectum changes to the anal canal at the dentate line. *For surgeons, however, the demarcation between the rectum above and the anal canal below is the anorectal ring.*
- The anorectal ring is situated about 5 cm from anus. At the anorectal angle, the rectum turns backwards to continue as the anal canal.

213. Ans. (a) Anterior border is formed by inferior fascia of urogenital diaphragm.

Ref: IB Singh Anatomy, 2nd ed./fig. 25.12

<table>
<tr><td colspan="2">ANTERIOR
• Fascia of Colles covering the Transversus perinei superficialis
• Inferior fascia of the urogenital diaphragm</td><td colspan="2">POSTERIOR
• Gluteus maximus
• Sacrotuberous ligament</td></tr>
<tr><td colspan="2">LATERAL
• Tuberosity of the ischium
• Obturator internus muscle
• Obturator fascia</td><td>SUPERIOR
• Levator ani
INFERIOR
• Skin</td><td>MEDIAL
• Levator ani
• Sphincter ani externus muscle
• Anal fascia</td></tr>
</table>

214. Ans. (d) Solitary ascariasis in the bowel

Ref: Bailey & Love, 26th ed. pg. 71

- The image shows a round worm in the bowel.
- While roundworms most commonly reside in the jejunal and ileal lumen, on occasion they may migrate into the duodenum and ampullary orifice.

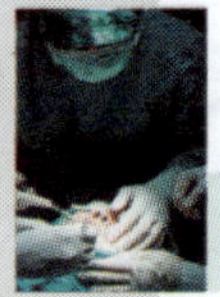

- While intestinal obstruction is more common in children, adults experience allergic reactions more frequently.

BREAST

215. Ans. (b) Fibroadenoma

Ref: Bailey and Love, 27th ed. pg. 868

The key words are breast mouse and mobility of breast lump. Both point to the most common benign breast tumor called fibroadenoma. Option a leads to bosselated appearance of breast. Option c will cause breast mass adherent to chest wall. Option d presents with fever and redness of breast surface.

216. Ans. (c) Incision and drainage

Ref: pg. 866, Bailey and Love 27th ed.

The key words are cracked nipple and pain, redness of breast which point to etiology as breast abscess. It would be managed with incision and drainage. Option a is ruled out as antibiotics have poor penetration in setting of abscess. Option b will be a traumatizing experience for the patient. Option d will be suitable for breast engorgement.

217. Ans. (a) Mucinous breast cancer

Ref: Bailey and Love, 27th ed. pg. 872

- Mucinous breast cancer is rare subtype but shows better prognosis with 10 year survival rate of 90%.
- The most common histological type of breast cancer is an invasive carcinoma of no special type, previously known as invasive ductal carcinoma, not otherwise specified (IDC, NOS).
- Option b is wrong as HER2 gene amplification is associated with shorter disease-free and shorter overall survival in breast cancer.
- Option c implies higher tumor load and shorter survival.
- Option d implies spread of cancer and shorter survival

218. Ans. (b) Luminal A

Ref: Bailey and Love, Textbook of Surgery, 27th ed. pg. 872

Luminal type A has better prognosis than other breast cancer subtypes.

- Luminal A has high hormone receptor expression (ER > PR), negative HER2 expression, and a low proliferation rate, properties that contribute to its better prognosis.

219. Ans. (d) Incision and drainage

Ref: Bailey and Love, Textbook of Surgery, 27th ed. pg. 866

The clinical scenario is suggestive of a breast abscess.

- Treatment of an abscess is primarily through incision and drainage (I and D).
- Smaller abscesses (<5 mm) may resolve spontaneously with the application of warm compresses and antibiotic therapy.
- Larger abscesses will require I and D as a result of an increase in collection of pus, inflammation, and formation of the abscess cavity, which lessens the success of conservative measures.

220. Ans. (a) Observation + regular follow-up

Ref: Bailey and Love, Textbook of Surgery, 27th ed. pg. 865

Young female presenting with asymptomatic mobile lump is characteristic feature of Fibroadenoma.

- The traditional management options available to women diagnosed with a fibroadenoma include observation or surgical excision.
- Most fibroadenomas may be managed conservatively without surgery, but those masses that are symptomatic or increasing in size may require surgical excision.

221. Ans. (b) Lobular carcinoma

Ref: Bailey and Love, Textbook of Surgery, 27th ed. pg. 872

In signet-ring cell carcinoma of the breast, which was recognized as a distinct clinicopathologic variant of lobular carcinoma, more than 20% of the malignant cells appear as signet rings formed by mucin-positive intracytoplasmic vacuoles.

222. Ans. (c) Phyllodes tumor

Ref: Bailey and Love 27th ed. pg. 870

- Notice the Bosselated appearance of breast with gross asymmetry as compared to contralateral breast. The diagnosis is phyllodes tumor. Notice the growth causing tortuous dilated veins on breast surface.
- Option a is ruled out as it always warm to touch with erythema of overlying skin.
- Option b is ruled out cancer is always fixed to adjacent tissues while the question mentions it to be mobile.
- Option d is ruled out as it does have bosselated appearance and is firm and regular in shape.

223. Ans. (a) Injury to long thoracic nerve

Ref: Sabiston 20th ed. pg. 820

- The image shows winging of scapula. This occurs due to intraoperative damage to long thoracic nerve.

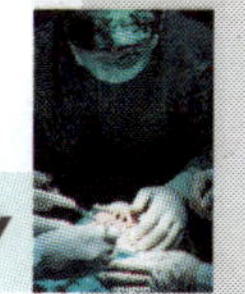

- This nerve supplies the serratus anterior muscle which fixes the scapula to chest wall. The damage to this nerve will lead to muscle weakness and resultant deficit of winging of scapula.
- The second most common nerve damaged intra-op during breast surgery is thoracodorsal nerve leading to paralysis of Latissimus dorsi muscle.

224. Ans. (a) TFT

Ref: Bailey and Love 27th ed. pg. 808

- The first investigation to be performed in solitary thyroid swelling is to determine thyroid status- Euthyroid versus hypo/hyperthyroid.
- The best imaging modality for Solitary thyroid swelling is Ultrasound.
- However, investigation of choice is USG guided FNAC.

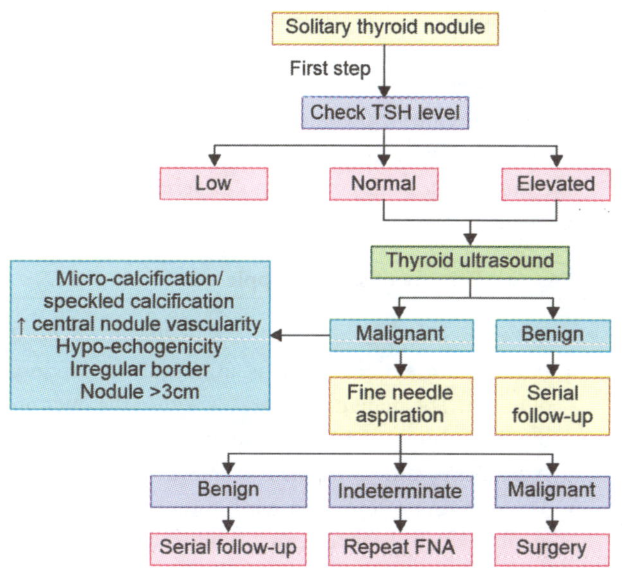

225. Ans. (d) Incision and drainage with antibiotics

Ref: Bailey and Love 27th ed. pg. 866

The clinical history is diagnostic of breast abscess which would require incision and drainage along with antibiotic coverage with cloxacillin

226. Ans. (a) Luminal A

Ref: Bailey and Love 27th ed. pg. 872

Luminal A subtype has better prognosis in Carcinoma Breast. It is low grade and grow slowly. The Four molecular subtypes of breast cancer. In some books a fifth type is given as miscellaneous. In contrast Triple negative/Basal like molecular subtype is highly aggressive.

Subtype	Pathology	Prevalence	Characteristics
Luminal A	ER and/or PR + HER 2– Low Ki67 Grade 1–2	30–70%	• Best prognosis • Fairly high survival rates • Fairly low recurrence rates
Luminal B	• ER and/or PR + • HER2+ or HER2– and high Ki67 • Higher tumor grade • Larger tumor size • More often node+	10–20	• Prognosis good, but • Survival not as high as luminal
Triple negative (basal-like)	ER and PR– HER2–	15–20%	• Aggressive • Poorer prognosis in first 5 years
HER2 type	ER and PR– Typically HER2+	5–15%	• Younger age • Outcome improved with introduction of anti-HER2 agents

227. Ans. (d) Areola

Ref: SRB 5th ed. pg. 543

Sentinel lymph node is localised by pre-operative (within 12 hours) or perioperative injection of isosulfan vital blue or 99m TC radioisotope labelled albumin *near the tumor or into subdermal plexus around the nipple*. Marker will pass into the sentinel node which can be visually detected as blue staining or with hand held gamma camera. It is biopsied with small incision made directly overt it. Frozen section biopsy or touch imprint cytology is done for presence of malignant cells.

Combined approach using Radioisotope Peritumoral injection is done on day of surgery and perioperative injection of patent blue dye in sub-areolar region is used nowadays.

228. Ans. (a) Eczema of skin of nipple

Ref: SRB 5th ed. pg. 533

- Paget's disease of the nipple is an intraductal carcinoma of breast. The malignancy spreads within the duct up to the skin of nipple and down into the substance of breast. It mimics eczema of nipple and areola.
- The disease presents as a hard nodule underneath the areola which later ulcerates and causes destruction of nipple. It contains large ovoid clear Paget cells with malignant features.
- Choice c, mastitis carcinomatosis is alternative name for inflammatory carcinoma and is the most aggressive breast cancer.
- Choice d is seen in elderly females and is a slow growing tumor with better prognosis.

229. Ans. (a) Fibroadenoma

Ref: SRB 5th ed. pg. 516

The most common benign encapsulated tumor of breast is called as fibroadenoma. It is classified as hyperplasia of single lobule of breast. On mammography is shows a popcorn calcification. Excision is via sub-mammary or circumareolar incision.

230. Ans. (b) Axillary sampling

Ref: SRB: 5th ed. pg. 545

Axillary sampling is done after axillary incision and 10–15 nodes are removed for sampling. It is not done now. Triple assessment technique includes choices A, C and D

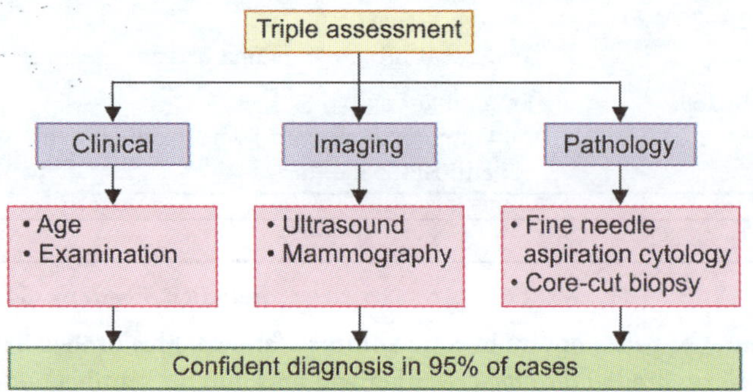

231. Ans. (a) Patient's decision

Ref: SRB 5th ed. pg. 517

Indications for surgery in Fibroadenoma are:

1. Size >3 cm
2. Multiple
3. Giant type
4. Recurrence
5. Cosmesis
6. Complex type

- *Fibroadenoma which is small (size <3 cm), single lesion and patient's age <30 years can be left alone with regular follow-up with USG at 6 monthly interval.*
- 30% fibroadenomas may disappear or reduce in size over 2–4 years.
- Complex fibroadenoma is a variant of typical fibroadenoma with fibrocystic changes, apocrine metaplasia, cyst formation, sclerosing adenosis. It occurs in old age and occasionally may turn malignant.
- Juvenile fibroadenoma which occurs at young age never turns malignant.

232. Ans. (b) Stage II

Ref: Harrison 19th ed. pg. 540

- Since size of tumor is 4 cm, it belongs to T2 stage.
- On account of no nodal involvement or distal metastasis the TNM status is T2N0M0. Hence it is stage IIA as per the staging giving below.

Stage Groups

Stage	TNM status
0	Tis N0 M0
IA	T1/T1 mi N0 M0
IB	T0/T1 mi M0 T1/T1 mi N1 mi M0
IIA	T0 N1 M0 T1 N1 M0 T2 N0 M0
IIB	T2 N1 M0 T3 N0 M0
IIIA	T0 N2 M0 T1 N2 M0 T2 N2 M0 T3 N1 M0 T3 N2 M0
IIIB	T4 N0 M0 T4 N1 M0 T4 N2 M0
IIIC	Any T N3 M0
IV	Any T any N M1

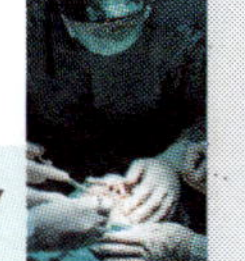

233. Ans. (b) T4B

THE TNM STAGING OF CARCINOMA BREAST (AJCC 7TH EDITION, 2010 PAGE 539: SRB)

T1- Tumor less than 2 cm (20 mm)
T1 mi – Microinvasion 1 mm or less in greatest dimension
T1a – 1–5 mm
T1b – 5–10 mm
T1c – 10–20 mm
T2 – 20–50 mm in greatest dimension
T3 - > 50 mm in greatest dimension
T4 – Any size with direct extension to the chest wall or skin or both.
T4a – Tumor of any size extending into the chest wall, not including only pectoralis muscle invasion/adhesion (Chest wall means ribs, intercostal muscles and serratus anterior but not pectoral muscles).
T4b – *Ulceration or ipsilateral satellite nodules and/or oedema including peaud'orange of the skin which don't meet the criteria for inflammatory carcinoma.*
T4c – T4a and T4b.
T4d – Inflammatory carcinoma

234. Ans. (c) T3

Refer to the explanation of the above question.

235. Ans. (b) Breast cancer

The mammography image shows *mass lesion with surrounding area micro-calcification* diagnostic of a breast cancer. The popcorn lesion will appear as a discrete lesion.

236. Ans. (c) Upper outer

Ref: Bailey, 26th ed. pg. 811

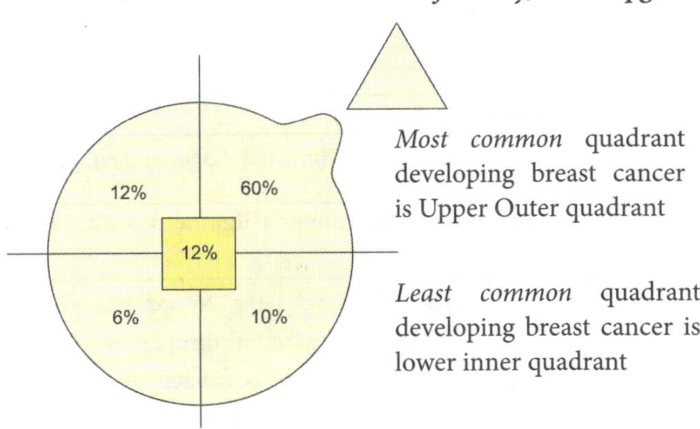

Most common quadrant developing breast cancer is Upper Outer quadrant

Least common quadrant developing breast cancer is lower inner quadrant

237. Ans. (a) BRCA1

Ref: Harsh Mohan Text book of Pathology, 7th ed. pg. 207

Incidence of sporadic, familial and hereditary breast cancer

BRCA1	45%
BRCA2	35%
STK11	<1%
Sporadic breast cancer	65–75%
Familial breast cancer	20–30%
Hereditary breast cancer	5–10%

238. Ans. (a) Anterior axillary

Ref: Chapter 44: Vishram Singh Anatomy: Volume 1

- Deep lymphatics drain the breast parenchyma and skin of nipple and areola.
- The Nipple and areola drains to the sub-areolar lymphatic plexus of Sappey.
- *Most of this drainage occurs to anterior axillary group of lymph nodes.*

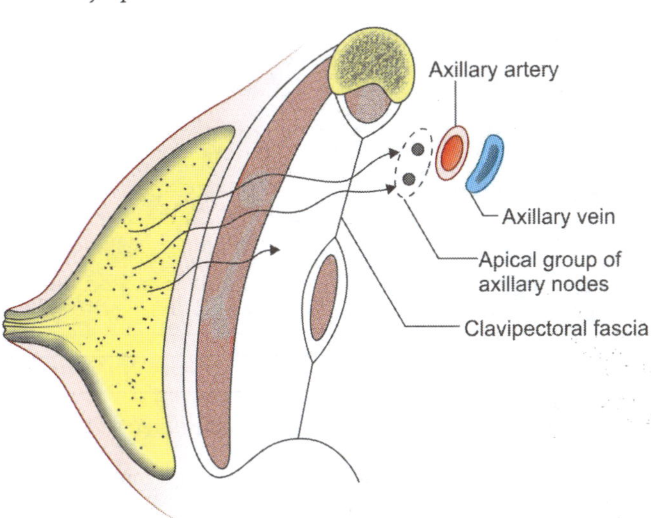

239. Ans. (a) Duct ectasia

Ref: Bailey, 26th ed. pg. 802

Causes of breast discharge

Discharge from the surface
• Paget's disease • Skin diseases (eczema, psoriasis) • Rare causes (e.g. chancre)
Discharge from a single duct
• Blood-stained

Contd...

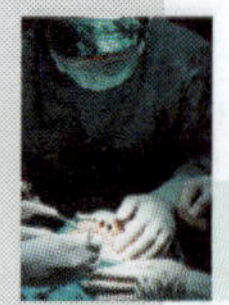

Discharge from the surface
Intraduct papilloma Intraduct carcinoma Duct ectasia
• Serous (any color)
Fibrocystic disease Duct ectasia Carcinoma
Discharge from more than one duct
• Blood-stained
Carcinoma Ectasia Fibrocystic disease
• Black or green
Duct ectasia
• Purulent
Infection
• Serous
Fibrocystic disease Duct ectasia Carcinoma
• Milk:
Lactation Rare causes (hypothyroidism, pituitary tumor)

240. Ans. (c) Fibroadenoma

Ref: Sabiston, 19th ed. pg. 827

- Fibroadenoma aka Breast mouse is the most common benign tumor of breast.
- It is MC seen in young age group females (15–30 years)
- Clinically, it is slow growing, painless solitary mass, which is mobile in nature *(that's why known as breast mouse).*
- **IOC:** FNAC
- **Upon mammography:** Popcorn calcification

241. Ans. (a) Lobular carcinoma

Ref: Sabiston, 19th ed. pg. 842, Bailey, 26th ed. pg. 809

LOBULAR CARCINOMA BREAST SALIENT FEATURES

- Mostly Multi-centric and **bilateral**
- Histological hallmark: *Indian file pattern* due to the tendency of tumor cells to invade in linear strand.
- Presenting feature-Breast mass with ill-defined margins
- Cellular feature- cytoplasmic mucoid globule
- *Neighbourhood calcification*-calcification in LCIS typically occurs in adjacent tissues. *It is a unique feature* and adds to diagnosis.

BREAST CANCER- AT A GLANCE

MC cancer in women (Worldwide) MC cancer in women in urban area (India)	
• MC arise from TDLU (terminal duct lobular unit) • **MC type-** Invasive ductal • **MC malignant type-** inflammatory breast CA • **MC Site-** upper outer quadrant • MC Site of metastasis is bone (osteolytic) lumbar vertebra>femur>thoracic vertebrae. • **MC Cause of death-** metastatic disease i.e. malignant pleural effusion • 2nd Most common cause of cancer death in women *(1st is lung in both sexes)*	

Evaluation/Diagnosis by triple assessment-
• Clinical
• Imaging (Mammography/USG)
• Histopathology
  ▪ **1st initial Investigation is FNAC**
  ▪ **Best/gold standard test-** HPE after biopsy
  ▪ **USG-** for young patient
  ▪ **MRI-** Patient with breast implant condition
  ▪ **PET scan-** For recurrence
  ▪ **Mammography:** For older patient
  ▪ **Mammography:** IOC for micro-calcification	

BIRADS	**Breast imaging reporting and data system** 0-incomplete assessment 1-Negative **2-Benign** 3-Probably benign 4-Suspicious 5-Highly suggestive of malignancy **6-Malignant**

242. Ans (d) Lobular carcinoma

Ref: Bailey & Love, 26th ed. pg. 809

243. Ans. (a) Infiltration of cooper's ligament with cancer cells

Ref: Bailey & Love, 26th ed. pg. 798, 808

- The term implies appearance of dimpled texture of an orange peel. Peau d'orange is caused by *cutaneous lymphatic edema*, which causes swelling.
- The *ligaments of Cooper* are hollow conical projections of fibrous tissue filled with breast tissue; the apices of the cones are attached firmly to the superficial fascia and thereby to the skin overlying the breast. These ligaments account for the dimpling of the skin overlying a carcinoma and can also explain nipple retraction.

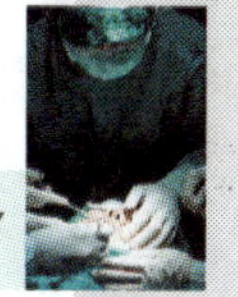

244. Ans. (b) Core cut biopsy

Ref: Sabiston, 10th ed. pg. 830-31

- Since the question asks about tissue diagnosis and NOT screening, the best option will be core-cut biopsy/True-cut biopsy.
- For screening FNAC is preferred.
- **Mammography** is considered as IOC in patients >40 years with breast condition. Since the above given patient is pregnant, mammography will NOT be preferred.
- **USG:** Initial investigation for palpable lesions in women <35 years. But it is Not useful in screening
- **MRI** is indicated in patients with breast implant.

Biopsy Techniques for Breast Lesions

Technique	Advantages	Disadvantages
FNAC	Rapid painless inexpensive No incision prior to selection of local therapy	Does not distinguish invasive from in situ cancer Marker (ER, PR, HER) not routinely available. Requires experienced cytopathologist
True –cut (core-cut) Biopsy	Rapid, relatively painless, inexpensive. No incision Can be read by any pathologist. Markers (ER, PR, HER-2) routinely available	False-negative results, incomplete lesions characterization can occur

245. Ans. (b) USG

Ref: Bailey & Love, 26th ed. pg. 527

- *Breast abscess* is highly probable in this lactating patient. Ultrasonography is used to distinguish solid from cystic structures and to direct needle aspiration for abscess drainage.
- Ultrasound is the imaging method of choice for the majority of women aged < 40 years and during pregnancy and lactation.
- Breast MRI does not form part of the initial imaging assessment of patients in the symptomatic breast disease.

246. Ans. (a) It is often bilateral

Ref: Bailey & Love, 26th ed. pg. 810

Paget disease of the breast is a malignant condition with appearance of eczema, with skin changes involving the nipple of the breast. *Symptoms usually only affect one breast.* Symptoms may include:

Skin	The first symptom is usually an eczema-like rash. Later, the skin may become flaky or scaly.
Discharge	Straw-colored or bloody.
Sensation	Burning sensation usually occurs in more advanced stages, when serious destruction of the skin often prompts the patient to consult. In more advanced stages, the disease may cause tingling and pain.
Nipple changes	May turn inwards
Breast changes	Lump in the breast with redness, oozing and crusting.

Contd...

- Immunohistochemistry allows definitive diagnosis of mammary PD. Paget cells can be demonstrated by immune-histochemical methods using several antibodies to cell surface and cytoplasmic markers (e.g., low-molecular-weight keratins found in simple epithelia, EMA, ***HER2/neu***, polyclonal pCEA+).
- Paget's disease of the breast is a type of cancer of the breast. Treatment usually involves a lumpectomy or mastectomy to surgically remove the tumor. Chemotherapy and/or radiotherapy may be necessary, but the specific treatment often depends on the characteristics of the underlying breast cancer.

247. Ans. (a) 1 cm

Ref: Bailey & Love, 26th ed. pg. 813

The amount of breast tissue excised with the lesion may vary with the clinical situation, but is typically 5 mm to 10 mm in all directions. Breast-conserving surgery (BCS): BCS may consist of removal of the tumor with a 1 cm margin of normal tissue (wide local excision) or a more extensive excision of a whole quadrant of the breast (quadrantectomy).

248. Ans. (a) USG

Ref: Scwartz, 10th ed. pg. 527

- The development of a dominant mass during pregnancy or lactation should never be attributed to hormonal changes.
- Breast cysts can be differentiated from solid echogenic abnormalities and will also be used to guide FNAC, core needle biopsy. *In the pregnant lady with breast lump ultrasound will be done initially*, and is a first line investigation modality.
- A dominant mass must be treated with the same concern in a pregnant woman as any other. Breast cancer develops in 1 in every 3000–4000 pregnancies.
- **Differential diagnosis of breast mass in pregnant and lactating patient:**
  1. Breast cancer
  2. Fibroadenoma
  3. Lactating adenoma
  4. Galactocele
  5. Fibrocystic changes

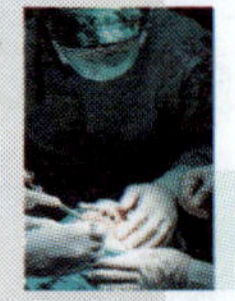

249. Ans. (d) Spreads to adrenal glands

Ref: Schwartz, 10th ed. pg. 532

- Involvement of chest wall by the cancer, satellite lesions and skin ulceration *constitute stage T4 by TNM staging.*
- Stage 4 of breast cancer can be any T stage, any nodal Stage, but is always M1 stage which is spread to distant organs.
- Do not mix up T_4 with stage 4 as both are fundamentally separate concepts.

250. Ans. (b) Satellite lesions

Ref: Schwartz, 10th ed. pg. 532

To	No evidence of primary tumor
TIS	Carcinoma in situ
T1	Tumor ≤2 cm
T1a	Tumor >0.1 cm but ≤0.5 cm
T1b	Tumor >0.5 but < 1 cm
T1c	Tumor >1 cm but ≤2 cm
T2	Tumor >2 cm but ≤5 cm
T3	Tumor >5 cm
T4	Extension to chest wall, inflammation, satellite lesions, ulcerations

251. Ans. (c) Tumor staging

Ref: Schwartz, 10th ed. pg. 535

- The most important prognostic variable is tumor staging with *Nodal status>Tumor size>Histological grade*
- The breast cancer markers that are most important in *determining therapy* are estrogen receptor, progesterone receptor and HER-2/neu.
- *Tumor growth rate* correlates with early relapse. S-phase analysis using flow cytometry is the most accurate measure.
- *Histologic classification* of the tumor has also been used as a prognostic factor. Tumors with a poor nuclear grade have a higher risk of recurrence than tumors with a good nuclear grade.
- *Molecular changes in the tumor* are also useful. Tumors that overexpress *erbB2* (HER2/neu) or have a mutated p53 gene have a worse prognosis.

252. Ans. (a) Mastitis

Ref: Bailey & Love, 26th ed. pg. 805, 810

Notice the fullness in lateral quadrant with erythema of overlying skin, diagnostic of Mastitis

Mondor disease	• It involves thrombophlebitis of the superficial veins of the breast and anterior chest wall. • It sometimes occurs in the arm and is known as axillary web syndrome • Patients with this disease often have abrupt onset of superficial pain, with possible swelling and redness of a limited area of their anterior chest wall or breast.
Cystosarcoma phyllodes	• Phyllodes tumors are a fibro-epithelial tumor composed of an epithelial and a cellular stromal component. • They may be considered benign, borderline, or malignant depending on histologic features including stromal cellularity, infiltration at the tumor's edge, and mitotic activity. • All forms of phyllodes tumors are regarded as having malignant potential. They are also known as ***serocystic disease of Brodie.***
Paget disease	• Patients with mammary Paget disease (PD) present with a relatively long history of an eczematous skin lesion or persistent dermatitis in the nipple and adjacent areas • *Since in this pic areola is blurred and visible areola appears normal, Paget's is ruled out.*

253. Ans. (b) Ocular cancer

Ref: Bailey & Love, 26th ed. pg. 813

- The **sentinel lymph node** is the **first lymph node** or group of nodes draining a cancer. In case of established cancerous dissemination it is postulated that the sentinel lymph node/s is/are the target organs primarily reached by metastasizing cancer cells from the tumor.
- ***The main uses of sentinel lymph node biopsy are in breast cancer and malignant melanoma surgery****. Other cancers which have been investigated with this technique are penile cancer, urinary bladder cancer, prostate cancer, testicular cancer and renal cell cancer.*

254. Ans. (c) Stage III

Since the size of the tumor given is 3 cm, it will be stage T2
Since the number of lymph nodes involved is 4 axillary lymph nodes the stage will be N2
Distant metastasis stage Mo
Stage I and IV are easily ruled out. Stage II has nodal stage 1 (N_1)
Stage III has nodal stage 2 (N_2)

Brief Description of the Terms

Tis: In situ	N0: No regional lymph nodes involved	M0: No metastasis
T0: Not evident clinically	N1: Ranging from micromeatses to <3 axillary lymph nodes involvement.	M1: Presence of metastasis

Contd...

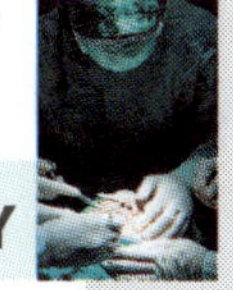

T1: Tumor size 0.1 cm-2.0 cm	N2: Axillary lymph nodes ranging from 3–9 or involvement of intermarry group of lymph nodes	
T2: 2 cm – 5 cm	N3: >10 axillary lymph-nodes involved or clinically detected inter mammary group of lymph nodes	
T3: >5 cm		
T4: Involvement of chest muscle, skin and ulceration.		

255. Ans. (b) Simple mastectomy

Ref: Sabiston, 19th ed. pg. 849-853

- According to staging given in question, this is a case of stage 1 breast CA for which simple mastectomy is preferred.

Types of mastectomy	
Simple or Total mastectomy	Removal of breast tissue, nipple-areola complex, and skin
Extended simple mastectomy	Simple mastectomy + removal of level I axillary LNs.
Modified radical mastectomy	Removes all breast tissue and skin, nipple areola complex, pectoralis major and minor muscles and the level, I, II and III axillary LNs,
Extended radical mastectomy	Radical mastectomy + Removal or internal mammary, LNs
Super radical mastectomy	Radical mastectomy+Removal of internal mammary, mediastinal and supraclavicular LNs

THYROID AND SALIVARY GLANDS

256. Ans. (b) Start levothyroxine at 25 microgram and increase the dose gradually

Ref: Harrison 21st ed. pg. 2936; Bailey and Love, Textbook of Surgery, 27th ed. pg. 807

Since TSH is elevated and T4 and T3 are reduced it implies primary hypothyroidism.

In patient with no residual thyroid function starting dose is 100–150 micrograms. However in this case since T3 and T4 are being produced starting dose would be 25 μg per day

TABLE: Levothyroxine dosage

For	Initial dose	May be adjusted in
Adults	1.6 mcg/kg daily	4–6 weeks
Adults over 50, or with cardiovascular disease	12.5 to 25 mcg daily	6–8 weeks
Severe and longstanding hypothyroidism	12.5 to 25 mcg daily	2–4 weeks

257. Ans. (a) 24 hours urinary metanephrines

Ref: Bailey and Love, Textbook of Surgery, 27th ed. pg. 840

This is a suspected case of Pheochromocytoma.

- Pheochromocytoma is a rare, catecholamine-producing tumor with preferential localization in the adrenal gland presenting with severe, often therapy-resistant hypertension, sweating, pallor, anxiety attacks, and headache.
- The diagnosis of pheochromocytomas largely depends on detecting elevated catecholamines or catecholamines metabolites in the blood and urine.
- Plasma fractionated metanephrine and urinary free metanephrine tests are used for biochemical confirmation of diagnosis.

258. Ans. (a) Papillary carcinoma thyroid

Ref: Bailey and Love 27th ed. pg. 816

The Histology slide shows thyroid follicles lined with cells with large empty looking Nuclei called as "Orphan Annie eye nuclei". This is a feature of papillary cancer of thyroid. It shows lymphatic spread which explains the cervical lymphadenopathy and radical neck dissection that was performed.

259. Ans. (b) Hyperthyroidism

Ref: Bailey and Love, 27th ed. pg. 1006

- The image shows pretibial myxedema which is seen in patients with grave's disease. Hence answer is hyperthyroidism. Sympathomimetic symptoms given in the question give more credibility to diagnosis.
- Myxedema is seen in both hypo and hyperthyroidism but pretibial myxedema is seen in Grave's disease.

260. Ans. (b) Total thyroidectomy

Ref: Bailey and love 26th ed. pg. 766

- Thyroidectomy during pregnancy has not been associated with adverse maternal or neonatal outcomes. There are no indications for termination of pregnancy.

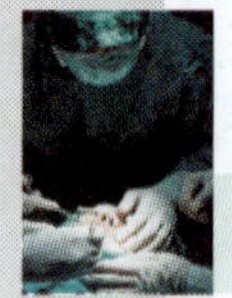

- Whenever possible, the operation should be performed during the second trimester or after delivery.
- *Thyroid cancer, the most common endocrine malignancy, is often detected in young female patients.* About 10% of thyroid cancers occurring during the reproductive years are diagnosed during pregnancy or in the early post-partum period.
- *Patients with large, locally aggressive or metastatic differentiated thyroid cancer require total thyroidectomy with excision of adjacent structures.* Along with this, nodal surgery is done followed by radioiodine ablation with long term TSH suppression.
- Choice a is ruled out since radioactive iodine is not used in pregnancy
- Choice d is ruled out since total thyroidectomy is done for cancer.

261. Ans. (b) Soles

Ref: SRB: 5th ed. pg. 78

- Sebaceous cyst is a retention cyst which occurs due to blockage of duct of sebaceous gland causing a cystic swelling.
- It is commonly seen on scrotum, face and scalp but *not seen in palms and soles as there are no sebaceous glands.*

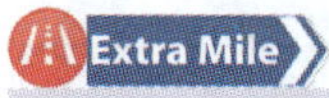

Multiple sebaceous cysts on scrotum is called as strawberry scrotum.

262. (b) Cancer of parotid gland

Ref: Bailey and Love: 26th ed. pg. 732

The image shows a parotid mass with marking of indelible ink. The painless mass rules out choice a and d while Choice c involves mainly the lips and tongue. The patient is having a parotid tumor and needs an urgent MRI to evaluate the mass followed by FNAC.

263. (c) TB

Ref: Bailey and Love: 25th ed. pg. 700

The image shows a large swelling extending in both anterior and posterior triangle of neck with an orifice of a *fistulous tract* with some excoriation and inflammation.

Features in favor of TB are:
- Indian patient
- Long standing history
- Location of large abscess overlapping both anterior and posterior triangle of neck
- Non-transilluminant fluctuant swelling.
- Normal overlying skin of abscess

- In contrast Branchial cyst is a *transilluminant fluctuant swelling* in upper or mid 1/3rd of sternocleidomastoid containing cholesterol crystals. The site of orifice is lower 1/3rd of neck on anterior border of sternocleidomastoid. The internal orifice of branchial fistula is present on posterior faucial pillar behind the tonsil. *The cyst becomes red and infected* before a fistula develops *while in this case no evidence of any infection is seen as overlying skin is normal.*
- Choice b secondaries is ruled out as they would show a progressive increase and do not have any draining fistula. Same logic is valid for ruling out choice d, Lymphoma.

264. Ans. (b) Von Graefe's sign

Ref: SRB 5th ed. pg. 470

Lid lag sign or Von Graefe's sign is inability of upper eyelid to keep pace with the eyeball when it looks downwards to follow the examiner's finger.

Extra Mile

Eye signs are common in primary thyrotoxicosis.
1. **Lid retraction:** Here upper eyelid is higher than normal; lower eyelid is in normal position. It is due to *sympathetic overactivity* causing spasm of involuntary smooth muscle part of the levator palpebrae superioris (*Muller's muscle*). It is a sign of thyrotoxicosis, not a sign of exophthalmos.
2. **Dalrymple's sign:** Upper eyelid retraction, so visibility of upper selera.
3. **Stellwag's sign:** Absence of normal blinking—so *staring look. First sign to appear.* It is due to widening of palpebral fissure due to lid retraction and also due to contraction of voluntary part of levator palebrae superioris muscle.
4. **Joffroy's sign:** Absence of wrinkling on forehead when patient looks up (frowns) with head is bent down/flexed position.
5. **Moebius sign:** It is lack of convergence of eyeball. Defective convergence is due to lymphocytic infiltration of inferior oblique and rectus muscles in case of primary thyrotoxicosis. There will be diplopia.
6. **Rosenbach's sign:** Tremor of closed eyelids

265. Ans. (a) Thyroid cancer

Ref: Harrison, 18th ed. pg. 341

- Thyroid carcinoma is the most common malignancy of the endocrine system.
- Differentiated tumors, such as papillary thyroid cancer (PTC) or follicular thyroid cancer (FTC), are often curable, and the prognosis is good for patients identified with early-stage disease.
- In contrast, anaplastic thyroid cancer (ATC) is aggressive, responds poorly to treatment, and is associated with a bleak prognosis.

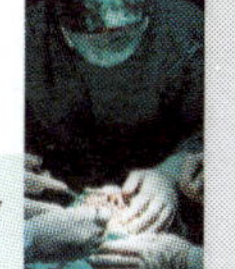

266. Ans. (a) TSH

Ref: Harrison, 19th ed. pg. 341

Best thyroid function test is *TSH as it helps in differentiating between primary and secondary thyrotoxicosis*. The change of TSH values also indicate the improvement in medical condition of the patient. For example after resection of a pituitary adenoma secreting excess of TSH, the values of TSH will come back towards normal.

267. Ans. (a) Lymphatic

Ref: Bailey & Love, 26th ed. pg. 765

- Lymphatic spread is common for papillary carcinoma thyroid whereas follicular carcinoma thyroid spreads via the blood stream. In papillary carcinoma thyroid, total thyroidectomy is performed and approximately 4-6 weeks after surgical thyroid removal, patients must have radioiodine therapy to detect and destroy any metastasis and residual tissue in the thyroid.

268. Ans. (a) Iodine 131

Ref: Bailey & Love, 26th ed. pg. 768

269. Ans. (c) External branch of superior laryngeal nerve

Ref: SRB, 5th ed. pg. 493; Bailey & Love, 26th ed. pg. 762

- Injury to external branch of SLN in vocal is more common because to proximity to cord superior thyroid artery. This leads to loss of tension.

270. Ans. (d) Calcitonin

Ref: Bailey and Love, 26th ed. ch. 51/764

- Medullary thyroid cancer is a rare form of thyroid cancer and accounts for 3 to 10% of all thyroid cancers. It grows from specialized thyroid cells called *parafollicular cells.*
- **Parafollicular cells-C-cells**; specialized thyroid cells that secrete calcitonin and play a major role in diagnosis of medullary thyroid cancer.
- Calcitonin is a tumor marker and remember there is no hypocalcemia in medullary carcinoma of thyroid.

271. Ans. (d) Medullary

Ref: Bailey and Love, 26th ed. ch. 5/741

Medullary thyroid cancer grows from specialized thyroid cells called *parafollicular* C-cells which are specialized thyroid cells that secrete calcitonin and play a major role in medullary thyroid cancer.

272. Ans. (b) Papillary

Ref: Bailey & Love, 26th ed. pg. 763-64

- Ionizing radiation can cause genetic mutations leading to malignant transformation.
- This association is much stronger for thyroid cancer than for other malignancies, and radiation is the only well-established environmental risk factor for thyroid malignancy.
- The risk of developing thyroid cancer after exposure to radiation is greater in those exposed during childhood and increases with higher doses of radiation delivered to the thyroid. This is true for exposure to ionizing radiation given for medical purposes and for environmental exposures.
- *The association with radiation is much stronger for papillary than for follicular cancer.*

273. Ans. (a) Papillary

Ref: Bailey & Love, 26th ed. pg. 765-66

THYROID MALIGNANCY

- Papillary carcinoma thyroid (PTC) has excellent prognosis (10 years survival rate >90%)
- **MC type-** Papillary Thyroid CA (PTC)
- Among people exposed to external radiation-PTC
- Lateral aberrant thyroid- PTC
- Psammoma bodies-PTC
- Orphan Annie nuclei-PTC
- Intranuclear inclusion/pseudo inclusion-PTC
- **Most reliable feature for PTC diagnosis-** nuclear feature, i.e. orphan Annie nuclei.
- Diagnosis by –FNAC
- **Treatment:** Total or near total thyroidectomy
- Most common thyroid cancer in *iodine sufficient* persons - PTC

274. Ans. (b) Multiple nodular goiter

Ref: Bailey & Love, 26th ed. pg. 749

- Notice the multiple enlarged lobes of this multiple nodular goiter which represents a spectrum of disease ranging from a single hyper-functioning nodule (toxic adenoma) within a multi-nodular thyroid to a gland with multiple areas of hyper function.
- Thyroglossal cyst is ruled out as it is present in midline.
- The answer should not be given as toxic nodular goiter because we cannot comment on thyrotoxicosis status of patient as eye signs etc. are not visible or given and the question also mentions a EUTHYROID status of the patient.

275. Ans. (c) Follicular carcinoma

Ref: Bailey & Love, 24th/785, Schwartz, 8th/1420

- FNAC is unable to distinguish benign follicular lesions from follicular carcinoma. Large follicular tumors (>4 cm) in older men are more likely to be malignant.
- **FNAC is the investigation of choice for solitary thyroid nodules.**
- It cannot distinguish between a follicular Adenoma and a Follicular Carcinoma *as this distinction is dependent not on cytology but on histological criteria such as capsular and vascular invasion.* It therefore cannot be used to diagnose follicular carcinomas.

276. Ans. (d) Zygomatic bone

- Surgical landmarks to the facial nerve include the tympanomastoid suture line, the tragal pointer, and the posterior belly of the digastric muscle.
- The *tympanomastoid suture line* lies between the mastoid and tympanic segments of the temporal bone and is approximately 6–8 mm lateral to the stylomastoid foramen. The main trunk of the nerve can also be found midway between (10 mm posteroinferior to) the cartilaginous *tragal pointer* of the *external auditory canal* and the posterior belly of the digastric muscle.

277. Ans. (c) Pleomorphic adenoma

Ref: Bailey & Love, 26th ed. pg. 732

PLEOMORPHIC ADENOMA

- Overall most common tumor of salivary gland
- MC benign salivary gland tumor
- MC tumor of major salivary glands
- MC site is parotid tail (superficial lobe).

Extra Mile

- 2nd MC benign tumor of parotid gland: **Warthin's tumor**
- MC malignant tumor of parotid gland: **Mucoepidermoid CA**
- 2nd MC malignant tumor of parotid gland: **Adenoid cystic CA**

278. Ans. (b) Adenoid cystic carcinoma

Ref: Bailey & Love, 26th ed. pg. 733

- *The adenoid cystic carcinoma is characterized by propensity to spread along nerves.*
- Tumor may be present for more than 10 years and then suddenly infiltrate the adjacent tissues extensively.
- Tumor has affinity for growth along perineural planes.
- Lung metastases are most frequent.

279. Ans. (a) Parotid gland

Ref: Bailey & Love, 26th ed. pg. 733

WARTHIN TUMOR

- *An exclusive tumor of parotid gland*
- Second most common benign parotid tumor (5%)
- Most common *bilateral benign neoplasm of the parotid*
- Marked male as compared to female predominance
- Occurs later in life (sixth and seventh decades)
- Presents as a lymphocytic infiltrate and cystic epithelial proliferation
- May represent heterotopic salivary gland epithelial tissue trapped within intra-parotid lymph nodes
- Incidence of bilaterality and multi-centricity of 10%
- Malignant transformation rare.

280. Ans. (a) Parotid gland

Ref: Schwartz, 10th ed. pg. 600

- MC cause of salivary gland fistula is parotid gland surgery.
- A parotid fistula is a communication through which saliva is discharged.
- Various forms of treatment have been described for parotid gland fistula, including tympanic neurectomy with or without chorda tympani section, radiotherapy and even completion of the parotidectomy.

281. Ans. (a) Submandibular gland

Ref: Bailey and Love, 26th ed. ch. 50/732

- Salivary gland stone (sialolithiasis) is due to duct obstruction, which further lead to calcification.
- This calcification further causes secondary bacterial invasion which leads to **SIALADENITIS**
- **Most common organism associated with sialadenitis: Staph. aureus and Strep. viridans**
- **Most common salivary gland associated with sialolithiasis: submandibular gland *(80 %) > Parotid gland (20%)***
- A stone located in the collecting duct or within the gland may be managed by either endoscopic retrieval, lithotripsy or, least likely, surgical removal.
- Sialography is usually required to identify the stone.
- Parotid duct stones are usually radiolucent and rarely visible on plain radiography. They are frequently located at the confluence of the collecting ducts or located in the distal aspect of the parotid duct adjacent to the parotid papilla.

282. Ans. (a) Superficial parotidectomy

Ref: Bailey & Love, 26th ed. pg. 733-34

Treatment of Choice for Pleomorphic Adenoma

- **In parotid gland:** Superficial parotidectomy
- **In other salivary glands:** Excision of the affected gland

Extra Mile

Indications or radiotherapy in salivary gland tumors	
• High grade tumors • Cervical LN metastasis • Large primary lesions	• Perineural invasion • Bone invasion

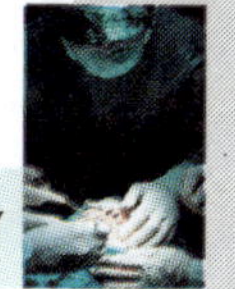

HERNIA AND HYDROCELE

283. Ans. (c) Left ectopic testis

Ref: Bailey and Love, 27th ed. pg. 1498

The common sites for ectopic testes include:

- Superficial inguinal pouch which lies anterior to external oblique aponeurosis. *Don't confuse with superficial inguinal ring.*
- Perineum
- Opposite side of the scrotum
- Femoral canal

Ectopic testis	Undescended testis
Abnormally located testis away from normal path of descent	Abnormally located testis within normal path of descent

284. Ans. (d) Left varicocele

Ref: Bailey and Love, 27th ed. pg. 1501

- Option a presents with cystic swelling of testis with positive transillumination test
- Option b presents as an expansile mass with cough impulse positive
- Option c presents with acute scrotum. The diagnosis is varicocele is based on key word bag of worms in a testis swelling.

285. Ans. (b) Gleason's

Ref: Bailey and Love, 27th ed. pg. 1469

Bloom richardson grading	Breast cancer
Gleason scoring	Prostrate cancer
Fuhrman nuclear grading	Renal cell cancer
Ranson score	Acute pancreatitis

286. Ans. (b) I-125

Ref: Bailey and Love, 27th ed. pg. 1473

Iodine-125 low dose rate brachytherapy is an effective modality to administer a high dose to the prostate while minimizing toxicities for the adjacent organs at risk. Also used is Palladium-103.

287. Ans. (b) Indirect inguinal hernia

Ref: Bailey and Love, Textbook of Surgery, 27th ed. pg. 1023

- The keyword in favor of diagnosis as Indirect inguinal hernia is the "passage of the sac along the spermatic cord".
- In contrast, direct inguinal hernia is protrusion of abdominal contents through the transversalis fascia within Hesselbach's triangle.

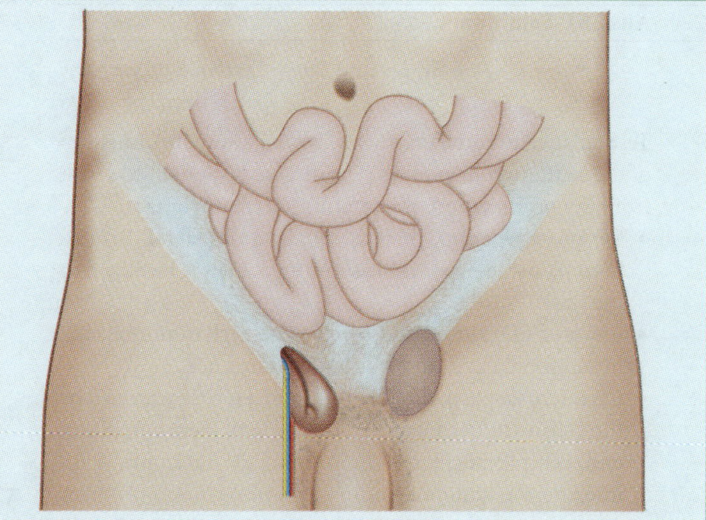

- Indirect inguinal hernias are the most common type of groin hernia. Indirect inguinal hernias occur when abdominal content such as fat or bowel pushes down along the inguinal canal.
- All indirect inguinal hernia passes through the inguinal canal or the groin and the visible bulge in the groin is the first symptom.
- Indirect inguinal hernias are more likely to cause bowel obstruction than direct inguinal hernias. This is because the inguinal canal, can be narrow. The narrow area enlarges as the canal travels downward. The narrow area can strangulate the tissue which is further herniated down the canal.

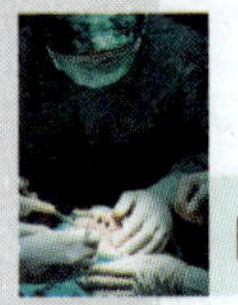

288. Ans. (c) GnRH for one month and if no descent then surgical treatment

Ref: Bailey and Love, Textbook of Surgery, 27th ed. pg. 1498

A palpable undescended testis ideally requires a day-case orchidopexy between 6 and 12 months of age.

- Initial use of gonadotropin releasing hormone stimulates the pituitary to secrete luteinizing hormone which in turn stimulates the Leydig cells of the testicle to produce testosterone and thereby initiate descent.

289. Ans. (a) Testicular tumor

Ref: Bailey and Love, Textbook of Surgery, 27th ed. pg. 1506

The case is having Troisier sign of left supra-clavicular lymphadenopathy which is seen with malignant spread of cancer. Hence, answer is option a.

- Testicular cancer is the most common solid malignancy affecting males between the ages of 15 and 45.
- Signs and symptoms of testicular cancer include: A lump or enlargement in either testicle or a feeling of heaviness in the scrotum.
- When testicular cancer spreads, it most commonly spreads to the lung and the lymph nodes of the chest, pelvis, and the base of the neck. More advanced stages may have spread to the liver and bones.

290. Ans. (b) Seminoma

Ref: Bailey and Love, Textbook of Surgery, 27th ed. pg. 1506

Testicular seminoma originates in the germinal epithelium of the seminiferous tubules. The disease is thought to result from the proliferation of immature spermatogonia.

- On physical exam, there is usually a unilateral, firm to hard palpable mass in the scrotum, which is localized to the testis.
- Elevated LDH levels are correlated to high tumor burden in seminoma and possibilities of recurrence.
- On microscopic pathology, seminoma is characterized by the cells with fried egg appearance with clear cytoplasm and central nucleus with prominent nucleolus, with interspersed lymphocytes.

291. Ans. (c) Spermatocele

Ref: Bailey and Love, Textbook of Surgery, 27th ed. pg. 1504

Spermatoceles are also known as spermatic cysts. They are fluid-filled masses, often painless, and they grow near the testicles.

A spermatocele presents as a cyst distinct from the testis that can trans illuminate or feel like a third testicle on physical examination.

292. Ans. (c) Varicocele

Ref: Bailey and Love, Textbook of Surgery, 27th ed. pg. 1501

Option a presents with fever and pain which is not present in this case.

- Option b has positive transillumination test and is hence, ruled out.
- Option d presents as acute scrotum.
- Varicocele is an enlargement of the veins within the scrotum that holds the testicles. These veins transport oxygen-depleted blood from the testicles. These veins are called the pampiniform plexus.
- A feeling of heaviness or dragging in the scrotum is the characteristic feature of varicocele.

293. Ans. (d) Mumps virus

Ref: Bailey and Love, Textbook of Surgery, 27th ed. pg. 786

Mumps is the most common cause of acute painful parotid swelling and predominantly affects children. It is spread via airborne droplets of infected saliva.

Complications of mumps are orchitis, oophoritis, pancreatitis, sensorineural deafness and meningoencephalitis are rare, but are more likely to occur in adults.

294. Ans. (d) Prostate cancer

Ref: Bailey and Love, Textbook of Surgery, 27th ed. pg. 1378

Prostatic carcinoma is the most common malignant tumor in men. The disease frequently presents with osteoblastic lesions in lumbo-sacral spine due to spread *via* Bateson plexus.

Prostate cancer can spread by local invasion, lymphatic spread or by Hematogenous metastases.

295. Ans. (a) GnRH analogues

Ref: Bailey and Love, Textbook of Surgery, 27th ed. pg. 125

The GnRH and hCG combination is an effective therapy for undescended testes located at and beyond the external inguinal ring and should be the first treatment choice because of its noninvasiveness.

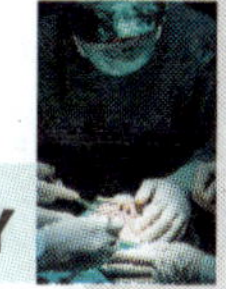

296. Ans. (d) Fascia transversalis

Ref: page 1029: Bailey and Love 27th ed. pg. 1029

Deep inguinal ring lies in transversalis fascia just deep to abdominal muscles. The ring lies midway between the anterior superior iliac spine and pubic tubercle approximately 2-3 cm above femoral artery pulse in the groin.

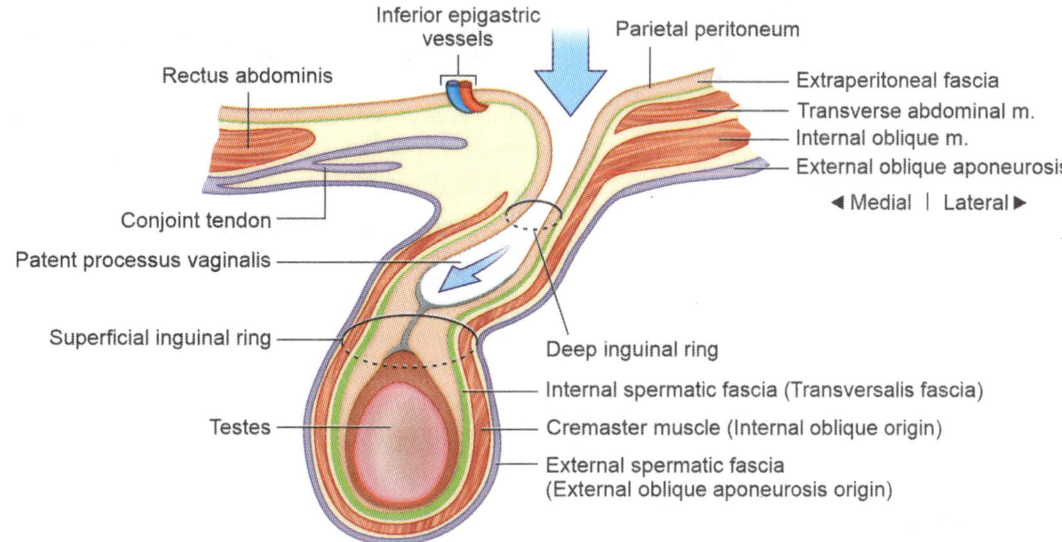

297. Ans. (a) NSAIDs and send the patient home

Ref: Bailey and Love 27th ed. pg. 1026

Strenuous sports and physical activity, particularly weight-lifting, can cause inguinal hernia. The patient at the moment would be managed conservatively with NSAIDS and would undergo an elective repair at a later date. Emergency surgery for hernia is done only if it becomes strangulated.

298. Ans. (b) Attempt Reduction followed by elective surgery

Ref: Bailey and Love 27th ed. pg. 1024

- Since hernia has become irreducible it has become liable for development of complications like strangulation. Hence an elective repair is recommended. The chances of strangulation however less in inguinal hernia as compared to femoral hernia.
- For an acutely incarcerated hernia without bowel present, the manual reduction can be attempted. Sedation may be necessary if this area is particularly painful for the patient. The patient should be supine, and Trendelenburg may help reduce incarcerated groin hernias. Gentle pressure on the hernia itself from all sides will help the hernia reduce intra-abdominally. Ice helps reduce acute inflammation of the hernia sac.

299. Ans. (b) Left testis is undescended and right testis is ectopic

Ref: Bailey and Love 27th ed. pg. 1497

The left testis in inguinal region is in normal path of descent and hence is undescended testis while right testis is at abnormal site in perineum and hence is ectopic.

300. Ans. (a) Testicular torsion

Ref: Bailey and Love 27th ed. pg. 1500

- The image shows bell clapper testis due to high investment of tunica vaginalis. Normally testis is anchored such that testis cannot rotate.
- The contraction of cremaster muscles with abdominal wall muscles in response to mechanical, sexual or thermic stimulus can result in testis torsion.
- Torsion of testis is seen in boys just before puberty primarily due to enlargement of hydatid in response to gonadotropins. A hydatid of Morgagni is an embryological remnant found in upper pole of testis or epididymis. The pain increases over couple of day and torted testis can be seen as blue dot sign.

301. Ans. (a) Torsion testis

Ref: SRB 5th ed. pg. 1018

- The bell clapper deformity allows the testicle to twist spontaneously on the spermatic cord since the long axis of the testicle is oriented transversely rather than cephalocaudal.
- This congenital abnormality is present in approximately 12% of males and is bilateral in 40% of cases.

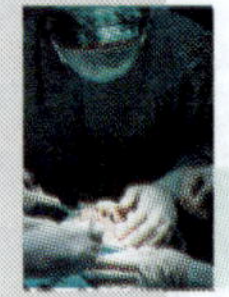

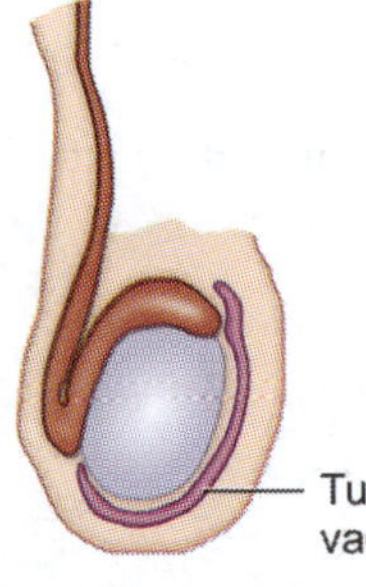

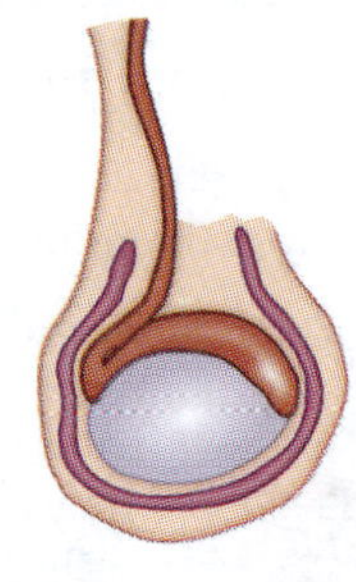

- Torsion occurs as the testicle rotates between 90° and 180°, compromising blood flow to and from the testicle. Complete torsion usually occurs when the testicle twists 360° or more; incomplete or partial torsion occurs with lesser degrees of rotation.

302. Ans. (b) Direct

Ref: SRB 5th ed. pg. 754

In NYHUS classification, type 3A hernia is direct inguinal hernia.

Type 1: Indirect hernia with normal deep ring
Type 2: Indirect hernia with dilated deep ring
Type 3: Posterior wall defect
  3A: Direct hernia
  3B: Pantaloon hernia
  3C: Femoral hernia
Type 4: Recurrent hernia

303. Ans. (a) Pantaloons hernia

Ref: Bailey, 25th ed. pg. 956

Site of primary	Percentage
Pantaloon hernia	The pantaloons hernia is the simultaneous occurrence of a direct and an indirect hernia. The pantaloons hernia causes two bulges that straddle the inferior epigastric vessels
Ritcher hernia	Richter's hernia is a hernia at any site through which only a portion of the circumference of a bowel wall, usually the jejunum, incarcerates or strangulates. Because the entire lumen is not compromised, symptoms of bowel obstruction can be absent, despite gangrene of the strangulated portion
Spigelian hernia	Spigelian hernia are herniations through the semilunar line, which is the lateral margin of the rectus muscle. At or just below the junction with the semicircular line of Douglas, unlike groin hernias, these hernias lie cephalad to the inferior epigastric vessels. The tight aponeurotic defect predisposes them to incarceration.
Littre hernia	Any groin hernia that contains a Meckel's diverticulum is Littre's hernia. This type of hernia is usually incarcerated or strangulated.

304. Ans. (a) Omentum

Ref: Bed Side Clinics in Surgery: ed. pg. 552: 2014

The clinical finding of doughy feel suggest diagnosis of omentocele.

Comparison of enterocele and omentocele

Omentocele	Enterocele
Doughy feel	Soft elastic feel
Dull note on percussion	Reduction with gurgling sound and resonant percussion note
Absent bowel sounds	Presence of bowel sounds

Other Findings of Hernia

- Expansile impulse on cough
- Reducibility indicates uncomplicated hernia
- Deep ring occlusion test since congenital hernia occurs through the deep ring
- Whether possible to get above the swelling, to differentiate scrotal or inguino-scrotal swelling
- Soft elastic feel with resonant note and audible bowel sounds suggests presence of enterocele.

305. Ans. (d) Transversalis fascia

Ref: Bailey & Love, 26th ed. pg. 955

- Deep inguinal ring is the opening in the *transversalis fascia* through which the ductus deferens and gonadal vessels (or round ligament in the female) enter the inguinal canal.
- Located midway between anterior superior iliac spine and pubic tubercle, it is bounded medially by the lateral umbilical fold (inferior epigastric vessels) and inferiorly by the ilio-pubic tract. Indirect inguinal hernias exit the abdominal cavity through the deep inguinal ring.

306. Ans. (b) Congenital hydrocele

Ref: Bailey & Love, 26th ed. pg. 1382

- The key word of question is positive transillumination test, which narrow down the diagnosis to hydrocele.
- Hydrocele is an accumulation of fluid in layers of tunica vaginalis.
- **Vaginal hydrocele:** MC type. Accumulation of fluid within tunica vaginalis layers
- **Congenital hydrocele:**
  - It is due to patent processus vaginalis which allows peritoneal fluid to move freely.
  - Size of hydrocele fluctuates usually related to activity
  - **Treatment:** Herniotomy

307. Ans. (a) Herniotomy

Ref: Bailey and Love, 26th ed. ch. 79/1382

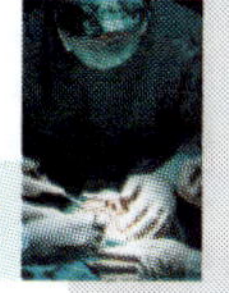

- Congenital hydroceles *are treated by herniotomy* if they do not resolve spontaneously
- **Lord's operation** is suitable when the sac is reasonably thin-walled. There is minimal dissection and the risk of haematoma is reduced.
- Eversion of the sac with placement of the testis in a pouch prepared by dissection in the fascial planes of the scrotum is an alternative **(Jaboulay's procedure)**
- Aspiration of the hydrocele fluid is simple, but the fluid always reaccumulates within a week or so. It may be suitable for men who are unfit for scrotal surgery

308. Ans. (a) Conservative Management till patient is asymptomatic

- Most of the pediatric patients with an inguinal hernia have indirect inguinal hernia.
- Inguinal hernias *do not spontaneously heal and must be surgically repaired because of the ever-present risk of incarceration.*
- *In patients with a long-standing history of inguinal hernia, the repeated protrusion of abdominal contents through the inguinal canal enlarges the internal and external rings, reducing the risk of incarceration and strangulation. This makes repair more difficult and recurrence more likely*

309. Ans. (c) Meckel's diverticulum

Ref: Bailey & Love, 26th ed. pg. 1170

- When Meckel's diverticulum forms the content of hernia, it is known as Littre's hernia.

310. Ans. (a) Strangulated hernia

Ref: Sabistan, 19th ed. pg. 1127

- Strangulation occurs more often in patients who have a partially reducible or an irreducible hernia
- Indirect inguinal hernias strangulate more commonly, the direct variety not so often because of the wide neck of the sac.
- **MC constricting agent:** Neck of the sac > External inguinal ring in children > Adhesions within the sac.
- **MC contents:** Small intestine > Omentum

Clinical features of strangulated inguinal Hernia

1. Sudden onset inguinal pain
2. Generalized abdomen pain
3. Tense and extremely tender hernia
4. Discoloration of overlying skin with a reddish or bluish tinge
5. There is no expansile cough impulse.

311. Ans. (a) Below and lateral to pubic tubercle

Ref: Bailey and Love, 26th ed, ch. 60/960

- The femoral hernia appears **below and lateral to the pubic tubercle** and lies in the upper leg rather than in the lower abdomen. Inadequate exposure of this area during routine examination leads to failure to detect the hernia.
- The hernia often rapidly becomes irreducible and loses any cough impulse due to the tightness of the neck. It may only be 1–2 cm in size and can easily be mistaken for a lymph node

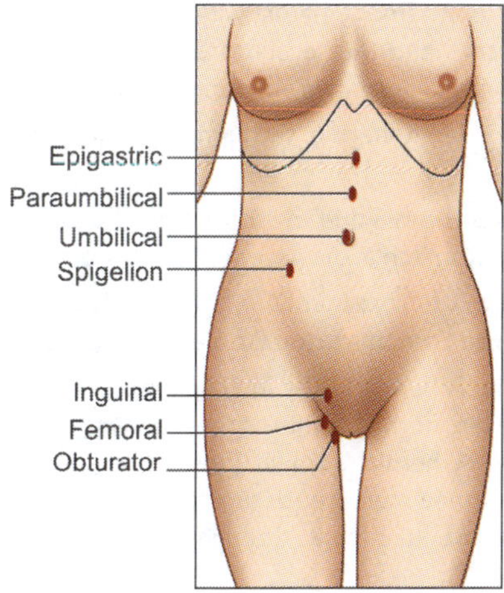

312. Ans. (c) Cough impulse is present

Ref: Bed Side Clinics in Surgery; Makhan Lal Saha, pg. 49

- **Femoral hernias** occur just below the inguinal ligament, when abdominal contents pass through a naturally occurring weakness called the femoral canal. The femoral hernia follows the tract below the inguinal ligament through the femoral canal. The canal lies medial to the femoral vein and lateral to the lacunar (Gimbernat) ligament. *Because femoral hernias protrude through such a small defined space, they frequently become incarcerated or strangulated*
- Femoral hernias are uncommon variety accounting for only 3% of all hernias.
- Femoral hernias mostly develop in women because of the wider bone structure of the female pelvis.
- The *cough impulse is not seen in femoral hernia.* Lockwood infra-inguinal approach is used in repair.

313. Ans. (c) Femoral hernia

Ref: Bailey & Love, 26th ed. Ch. 60/960

- High risk of strangulation is seen with femoral hernia as it has lacunar ligament (Gimbernat's) medially. This is a strong curved ligament with a sharp unyielding edge which impedes reduction of a femoral hernia.
- 50% of cases present as an emergency

314. Ans. (c) Femoral hernia

Please refer to above explanation

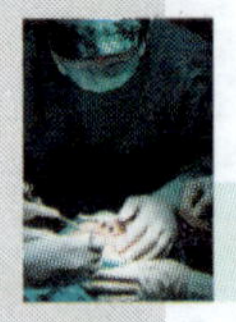

315. Ans. (b) Cooper's hernia

Ref: Sabiston, 19th ed. pg. 1126-27

HERNIAS AT A GLANCE

Amyand's hernia: Containing the appendix vermiformis within the hernia sac

Cooper's hernia: A femoral hernia with two sacks, the first being in the femoral canal, and the second passing through a defect in the superficial fascia and appearing almost immediately beneath the skin.

Epigastric hernia: A hernia through the linea alba above the umbilicus.

Hiatus hernia: A hernia due to "short oesophagus" — insufficient elongation — stomach is displaced into the thorax

Littre's hernia: A hernia **involving a Meckel's diverticulum. It** is named after the French anatomist Alexis Littré

Lumbar hernia: A hernia in the lumbar region (not to be confused with a lumbar disc hernia), contains the following entities:
Petit's hernia: A hernia through Petit's triangle (inferior lumbar triangle). It is named after French surgeon Jean Louis Petit.
Grynfeltt's hernia a hernia through Grynfelt-Lesshaft triangle (superior lumbar triangle).

Maydl's hernia: Two adjacent loops of small intestine are within a hernial sac with a tight neck. The intervening portion of bowel within the abdomen is deprived of its blood supply and eventually becomes necrotic.

Morgagni hernia: A type of hernia where abdominal contents pass into the thorax through a weakness in the diaphragm

Obturator hernia: Hernia through obturator canal.

Pantaloon hernia (Saddle Bag hernia): A **combined direct and indirect hernia**, when the hernial sac protrudes on either side of the inferior epigastric vessels.

Paraumbilical hernia: A type of umbilical hernia occurring in adults

Perineal hernia: A perineal hernia protrudes through the muscles and fascia of the perineal floor. It may be primary but usually is acquired following perineal prostatectomy, abdominoperineal resection of the rectum, or pelvic exenteration.

Richter's hernia: A hernia involving only one sidewall of the bowel, which can result in bowel strangulation leading to perforation through ischaemia without causing bowel obstruction or any of its warning signs.

Sliding hernia: Occurs when an organ drags along part of the peritoneum, or, in other words, the organ is part of the hernia sac. The colon and the urinary bladder are often involved. The term also frequently refers to sliding hernias of the stomach.

Sciatic hernia: This hernia in the greater sciatic foramen most commonly presents as an uncomfortable mass in the gluteal area. Bowel obstruction may also occur. This type of hernia is only a rare cause of sciatic neuralgia.

Velpeau hernia: A hernia in the groin in front of the femoral blood vessels

316. Ans. (d) Saddle bag hernia

Ref: Sabiston, 19th ed. pg. 1126-27

Please refer to above explanation

317. Ans. (d) Littre's hernia

Ref: Sabiston, 19th ed. pg. 1126-27

318. Ans. (d) Hernia at the level of arcuate line

Ref: Bailey and Love, 26th ed. ch. 60/966

Spigelian hernia
- Spigelian hernia herniates through the spigelian fascia, *which is the aponeurotic layer between the rectus abdominis muscle medially, and the semilunar line laterally.*
- **Always occur at or above the arcuate line** because of the lack of posterior rectus sheath. These are inter-parietal hernias, ***which penetrate between the muscles of the abdominal wall;*** therefore, there is often no notable swelling.

319. Ans. (a) Posterolateral

Ref: Bailey & Love, 26th ed. pg. 871-72

- Bochdalek's hernia is the most common form of diaphragmatic hernia, occurring in approximately 1 in 2500 births and twice as often in males as in females.
- *Bochdalek's hernia results from failure of normal development of the posterolateral diaphragm during embryogenesis.*
- Separation of the developing thoracic and abdominal cavities occurs during the eighth week of gestation, when the opening between the chest and abdomen (the pleuroperitoneal canal) closes. A congenital diaphragmatic hernia results when the pleuroperitoneal membrane fails to form.
- Most Bochdalek's hernias occur on the left side, allowing protrusion of the abdominal viscera into the chest. The herniated bowel passes through the defect, filling the chest cavity and causing hypoplasia of the left lung and a shift of mediastinal structures to the right side. It is not uncommon for other abnormalities to be associated with Bochdalek's hernia; these may include neural tube defects and cardiovascular abnormalities
- The left-sided Bochdalek hernia occurs in approximately 85% of cases. Left-sided hernias allow herniation of both the small and large bowel and intraabdominal solid organs into the thoracic cavity.
- In right-sided hernias (13% of cases), only the liver and a portion of the large bowel tend to herniate. Bilateral hernias are uncommon and are usually fatal

Remember

- The 3 basic types of congenital diaphragmatic hernia include the posterolateral Bochdalek hernia (occurring

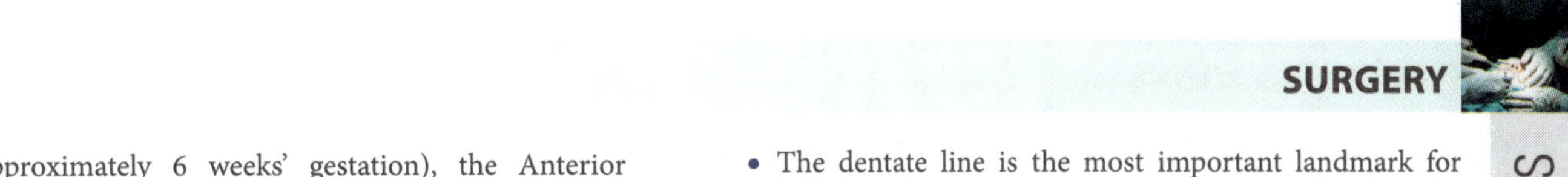

at approximately 6 weeks' gestation), the Anterior Morgagni hernia, and the hiatus hernia.

320. Ans. (c) Epididymo orchitis

Ref: Bailey & Love, 26th ed. pg. 1384

ACUTE EPIDIDYMO ORCHITIS

- Inflammation of the epididymis and testis, from an ascending infection from the lower urinary tract.
- *Initially epididymis is involved, after that there is involvement of testis.*
- ***Most cases of epididymitis in men younger than 35 years are due to sexually transmitted organisms [C. trachomatis (MC) and N. gonorrhoe]***
- In children and older men this is due to urinary pathogens such as E. coli.
- *Patient presents with fever, swollen, red and tender scrotum.*
- *The epididymis and testis are swollen (Thickened cord with reactive hydrocoele).*
- **Urine analysis** typically demonstrates WBCs and bacteria in the urine or urethral discharge
- **Scrotal USG** showing enlarged epididymis with increased blood flow with reactive hydrocoele.

Extra Mile

- Testicular torsion is commonly seen in pre-pubertal age group (10–25 years). Patients usually presents with sudden agonizing pain.

UROLOGY

321. Ans. (b) Retrograde urethrogram

Ref: Bailey and Love, 27th ed. pg. 1481

- The key word of dye introduced from urethra is sufficient to solve this question as option b.
- Option a will show reflux in ureters while the image shows only the bladder and urethra.
- Option c and d will show kidney parenchyma.

322. Ans. (a) Tuberculosis

Ref: Bailey and Love, 27th ed. pg. 1443

The description of diminutive and narrow urinary bladder by examiner implies Thimble bladder which is seen with TB Bladder.

323. Ans. (b) Crypt at dentate line

Ref: Bailey and Love, Textbook of Surgery, 27th ed. pg. 1345

The anatomic anal canal begins at the dentate line and ends at the anal verge.

- The dentate line is the most important landmark for understanding the epithelium of the anal canal.
- Fistula-in-ano is a tract connecting the anal canal to the perianal skin, often occurs following anorectal abscess. The internal opening in the fistula in ano usually begins from the crypt at dentate line.

324. Ans. (b) Total radical nephrectomy

Ref: Bailey and Love, Textbook of Surgery, 27th ed. pg. 1420

Renal masses include a diverse group of tumors comprised benign masses, indolent cancers, and more aggressive cancers. Over 90% of kidney cancers are renal cell carcinoma (RCC).

- While advances have been made in systemic therapies, the mainstay of treatment for the localized renal mass remains surgical resection, either *via* radical nephrectomy (RN) or partial nephrectomy (PN).
- Radical Nephrectomy remains the gold standard treatment for the localized renal mass in any patient with tumor size ≥7 cm.
- Partial nephrectomy is now the preferred treatment for many people with early-stage kidney cancer. It is often done to remove single small tumors (<4 cm) size.

325. Ans. (d) Calcium oxalate

Ref: Bailey and Love, Textbook of Surgery, 27th ed. pg. 1405

The presence of calcium oxalate crystals is very common and generally has little clinical significance.

- They are found in urine with a pH between 6.0 and 7.0.
- The formation of calcium oxalate crystals can be caused by a combination of factors including decreased urine volume or a diet rich in oxalates (cabbage, rhubarb, spinach, tropical fruits, etc.) or calcium (dairy products).

326. Ans. (b) Hydronephrosis to compare abdominal and urinary bladder pressure

Ref: Bailey and Love, Textbook of Surgery, 27th ed. pg. 1412

The Whitaker test, a urodynamic study, combined with antegrade pyelography is used to evaluate persistent upper urinary tract dilatation after operative correction of obstruction.

- This test will differentiate patients with residual or recurrent obstruction from those with dilatation secondary to permanent changes in the musculature.
- It is useful in evaluating patients with questionable ureteropelvic or ureterovesical junction obstruction, or primary defects in the ureteral musculature.

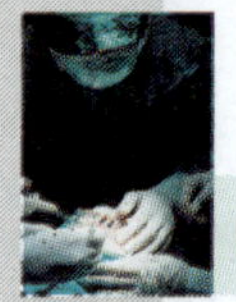

327. Ans. (c) Leuprolide

Ref: Bailey and Love, Textbook of Surgery, 27th ed. pg. 156

Prostate cancer is among the most common cancers in men worldwide.

- Currently treatment with luteinizing hormone–releasing hormone (LHRH) agonists is the predominant form of androgen deprivation therapy (ADT) and has become the standard of care for metastatic prostate cancer.
- Leuprolide is an established luteinizing hormone–releasing hormone (LHRH) agonist used as first-line treatment in advanced prostate cancer.

328. Ans. (b) Ureteric opening distal to external urinary sphincter

Ref: Bailey and Love, Textbook of Surgery, 27th ed. pg. 1429

Option a is present in pediatric age-group in boys and presents with poor urinary flow and is hence, ruled out.

- Absence of fever and dysuria rules out option c.
- Option d is a cause of UTI in children.
- Leakage from fistulae or upper tract duplication with an ectopic ureter is leading cause of continuous urinary dribbling.
- This occurs when there is a ureteric fistula or an ectopic ureter associated with a duplex system opening into the urethra beyond the urethral sphincter in females or into the vagina.
- The history is diagnostic, and IVU or ultrasonography may reveal the upper pole segment, which is often poorly functioning.
- Treatment is by excision of the aberrant ureter and portion of kidney.

329. Ans. (d) Stress incontinence

Ref: Bailey and Love, Textbook of Surgery, 27th ed. pg. 1375

Stress incontinence is involuntary urinary leakage which occurs when the intra-abdominal pressure rises.

- This is most common in females who have had vaginal deliveries and have small-volume urinary leakage associated with activity such as coughing, laughing, sneezing or exercising.

330. Ans. (c) Renal cell carcinoma

Ref: Bailey and Love, Textbook of Surgery, 27th ed. pg. 1416

The classic triad of flank pain, painless hematuria, and flank mass is characteristic of renal cell carcinoma.

- Option a is a complication of obstructive uropathy.
- Option b presents with costovertebral tenderness.
- Option d presents with flank pain and hypertension.

331. Ans. (b) Ureterocele

Ref: Bailey and Love 27th ed. pg. 1401

The image shows left sided cystic outpouching of distal ureter into the urinary bladder and is feature of ureterocele.

332. Ans. (a) Suprapubic cystostomy

Ref: Bailey and Love 27th ed. pg. 1481

- Initial emergent treatment is to maintain hemodynamic stability and drainage of the urinary bladder, often with placement of a suprapubic catheter (SPT) and primary endoscopic realignment of the urethra if possible.
- Immediate urethral repair is relatively contraindicated because life-threatening injuries must be corrected first in any trauma algorithm.
- Urethral repair should be undertaken after the patient has stabilized, when hemorrhage is less of a concern. If open repair is planned, it is better to allow the pelvic hematoma to subside prior to the procedure.

333. Ans. (b) Bladder stone

Ref: Bailey and Love 27th ed. pg. 1434

- The image shows X-ray pelvis with radio-opaque shadow diagnostic of bladder stone.
- Option a will be too small and would be much inferior in location
- Option c can't be visualized on X-ray and size rules out option d.

334. Ans. (a) Peyronie's disease

Ref: Bailey and Love 27th ed. pg. 1490

- Peyronie's disease is characterized by curvature in the penile shaft that is often preceded by painful erections and accompanied by an area of fibrosis.
- The characteristic angulation is frequently associated with erectile dysfunction, either as a result of buckling of the penile shaft with intromission or because of a lack of rigidity distal to the area of associated fibrosis. This lack of rigidity seems to be the result of compromise to the distal penile blood supply.
- Remaining options do not have any curvature in penis and hence are ruled out.

335. Ans. (d) Peyronie's disease

Ref: Bailey and Love 27th ed. pg. 1490

- Patients with Peyronie's disease develop a fibrous scar tissue on the penis which causes curved, painful erections. The fibrosis and curvature both affect the normal filling of blood in the penis during an erection.

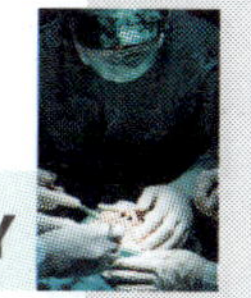

- In option a the skin of prepuce once retracted cannot be pulled back and leads to swelling of glans penis.
- Option b is present since birth and leads to poor urinary stream.
- Option c will cause ammoniacal dermatitis of scrotum due to ventrally placed urethral opening.

336. Ans. (d) 24 hours urinary fractionated metanephrines

Ref: Bailey and Love 27th ed. pg. 1418

Family history of mother died due to RCC gives us a hint of VHL gene mutation. Patients who may have inherited this VHL gene mutation can develop pheochromocytomas. The clinical features of sympathomimetic stimulation also point to excess catecholamines. Hence 24-hour urinary metanephrine levels will help to screen for pheochromocytoma.

Tumor associated with VHL gene (3p 25–26)	• Haemangioblastoma • Pancreatic neuroendocnine tumors • Pheochromocytoma • Renal cysts • Pancreatic cysts • Ovary cystadenoma • Epididymal cystadenoma

- Option a and b is used to evaluate for typical carcinoid and atypical carcinoid respectively. Option c is used to evaluate for neuroblastoma.

337. Ans. (a) Most common type of stone is triple phosphate

Ref: Bailey and Love 27th ed. pg. 1407

- Option a is false as MC kidney stone is calcium oxalate. Triple phosphate stones are struvite/Staghorn calculi formed secondary to alkaline pH of urine induced by proteus mirabilis infection.
- Option b is correct as ureteroscopic removal of large stones can be done.
- Option c is correct as renal stones less than 2 cm can be removed by Extracorporeal shock wave lithotripsy.
- Option d is correct as caliber of ureter is 5mm and stones less than 5mm may be passed spontaneously or with diuresis.

338. Ans. (a) Ureterocele

Ref: Bailey and Love 27th ed. pg. 1401

The given IVP shows bilateral cobra head appearance of distal ureter diagnostic of ureterocele.

339. Ans. (c) Intraperitoneal bladder rupture

Ref: Bailey and Love 27th ed. pg. 1425

- Option a presents with blood at the meatus and inability to pass urine.
- Option b will lead to severe pubic area pain with fully distended bladder leading to suprapubic bulge. The bulge is not present in this case and hence this option is ruled out
- Option c will lead to rupture of bladder and spill of urine into peritoneal space. That explains the abdominal distention develop in the case. If the urine is sterile, features of peritonitis may not develop.
- Option d is ruled out as it occurs with fracture pelvis and produces suprapubic tenderness and swelling.

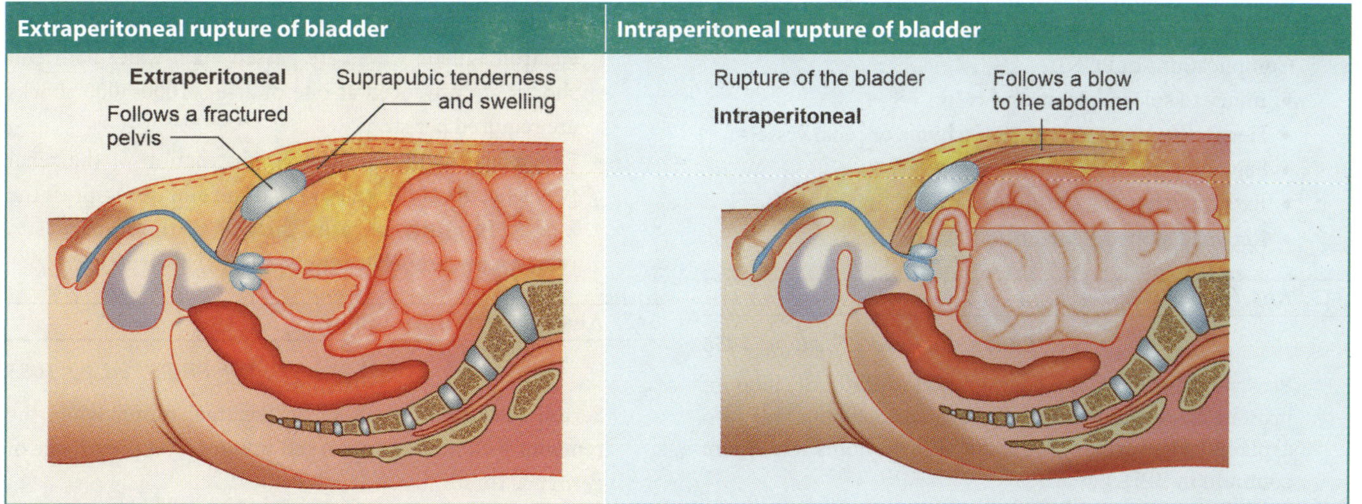

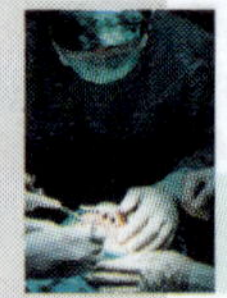

340. Ans. (b) Goserelin

Ref: Bailey and love 27th ed. pg. 1474

- Prostate cancer is a testosterone dependent cancer. In advanced prostate cancer, Goserelin is given parenterally. It is a gonadotropin releasing hormone (GnRH) agonist which will ultimately cause an inhibition of testosterone production.
- Normal PSA levels are <4.0 ng/mL while in this case the values are 25X of normal with metastasis to spine that can explain the low backache.
- Option a and c are ruled out as they are used for management of portal hypertension.

Extra Mile

Recently agents such as enzalutamide (a second generation androgen receptor blocker), degarelix (an LHRH antagonist), abiraterone (a drug that blocks the production of testoster one from its precursors) and taxane chemotherapy have all been shown to promote survival in metastatic prostate cancer

341. Ans. (b) Posterior urethral valves

Ref: Bailey and Love 27th ed. pg. 1477

- Posterior urethral valves will cause obstructive uropathy. Most of time it is picked up antenatally as it leads to bilateral hydronephrosis. If USG is not done or it is not picked up then the presentation is of neonate with recurrent UTI, uremia and renal failure as given in this case.
- Option a and d can be unilateral and hence Bilateral hydronephrosis will not be present.

342. Ans. (a) Bacterial sepsis

Ref: Bailey and Love 27th ed. pg. 1409

Urosepsis and bacteremia can be seen in patients with kidney stones and any diagnostic or therapeutic instrumentation done in these patients.

Complications of PCNL

- Injury to spleen, pleura and colon
- Hemorrhage from renal parenchyma or renal vessels
- Sepsis
- Extravasation due to rupture of collecting system
- Retained stone fragments

343. Ans. (a) Posterior

Ref: Bailey and Love 27th ed. pg. 1456

Prostate cancer arises commonly in posterior lobe of prostate while BPH involves the median lobes. This also explains why urinary obstructive symptoms are more common in BPH.

344. Ans. (b) Right Iliac fossa

Ref: Bailey and Love 27th ed. pg. 1549-50

The new kidney is placed in right iliac fossa where it gets its blood supply from the internal iliac artery. The donor renal vein is anastomosed end to side to external iliac vein. While the vascular anastomosis is being done, the kidney is kept cold with application of topical ice.

345. Ans. (b) Varicocelectomy

Ref: Bailey and Love 26th ed. pg. 1381

The clinical diagnosis of patient is varicocele. The key word is bag of worms feel on scrotal examination. When examined in the erect position, the scrotum on the affected side hangs lower than normal, and on palpation, with the patient standing, the varicose plexus feels like a bag of worms. There may be a cough impulse.

MANAGEMENT

- Operation is not indicated for an asymptomatic varicocele.
- When the discomfort is significant, then embolisation of the gonadal veins is the usual first line intervention.
- If this is not possible, or if the varicocele recurs (as it does in around 20 per cent after embolisation), then *surgical ligation of the testicular veins/* Varicocelectomy is the appropriate treatment.

346. Ans. (b) PCNL

Ref: SRB 5th ed. pg. 1017

- Kidney stone of size more than 2.5 cm in size is treated with percutaneous nephrolithotomy. In contrast Extracorporeal shock wave lithotripsy is used for stones of size less than 2.5 cm. The piezo-ceramic electromagnetic waves are passed via a water bath and shocks are produced at rate of 2/sec. 1000-4000 shocks are required per stone.
- Pyeloplasty is the surgical reconstruction of the renal pelvis (a part of the kidney) to drain and decompress the kidney. In nearly all cases, the goal of the surgery is to relieve a ureteropelvic junction (UPJ) obstruction.

347. Ans. (c) Sertoli cell tumor

Ref: SRB 5th ed. pg. 1083

Sertoli cell tumor is a sex cord stromal tumor while the remaining choices are germ cell tumors. The prevalence of germ cell tumor is 95%.

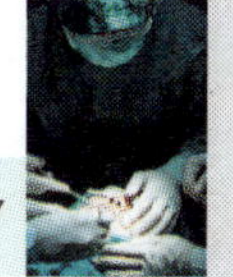

Germ cell tumors	Sex cord stromal tumors
• Seminoma • Spermatocytic seminoma • Embryonal carcinoma Polyembryoma • Embryonal carcinoma and teratoma ('teratocarcinoma') • Teratoma Mature Immature With malignant transformation • Choriocarcinoma • Yolk sac tumor	• Leydig cell tumor • Serto cell tumor • Granulosa cell tumor • Mixed forms

348. Ans. (c) 3 hours

Ref: SRB 5th ed. pg. 1063 and American Urological Association Guidelines

Priapism is a persistent penile erection that continues beyond 4 hours and is unrelated to, sexual stimulation. Typically, only the corpora cavernosa are affected.

Subtypes of priapism include:

- Ischemic (veno-occlusive, low flow) priapism is a nonsexual, persistent erection characterized by little or no cavernous blood flow and abnormal cavernous blood gases (hypoxic, hypercarbic, and acidotic). Ischemic priapism is an emergency.

Contd...

- Non-ischemic (arterial, high flow) priapism is a nonsexual, persistent erection caused by unregulated cavernous arterial inflow. Typically the penis is neither fully rigid nor painful. Antecedent trauma is the most commonly described etiology.
- Stuttering (intermittent) priapism is a recurrent form of ischemic priapism in which unwanted painful erections occur repeatedly with intervening periods of detumescence.

349. Ans. (a) Membranous urethra rupture

Ref: SRB 5th ed. pg. 1037 and 1052

- The patient has pelvic fracture which resulted in trauma to membranous and/or prostatic urethra. This is called *posterior urethral rupture.*
- The presentation will be blood at meatus with inability to pass urine.
- There is extravasation of urine to scrotum, perineum and abdominal wall which explains why bladder is empty.
- This extravasation of urine is called extraperitoneal extravasation of urine.
- *Intraperitoneal rupture of bladder* is seen due to kick on abdomen and leads to diffuse abdominal pain, distention and features of peritonitis as urine leaks into peritoneal space. Vitals will reveal presence of shock. X-ray abdomen will show ground glass appearance. Emergency laparotomy is required with bladder repair.

TABLE: Comparison of anterior and posterior urethra rupture

Rupture of anterior urethra	Rupture of posterior urethra
Trauma to *bulbous urethra* due to fall astride projectile object like cycling, manhole cover, gymnasium	Trauma to *membranous and/or prostatic urethra* after pelvic fracture sustained in RTA.
d c b a a. Penile urethra b. Bulbar urethra c. Membranous urethra d. Prostatic urethra	d c b a a. Penile urethra b. Bulbar urethra c. Membranous urethra d. Prostatic urethra

Contd...

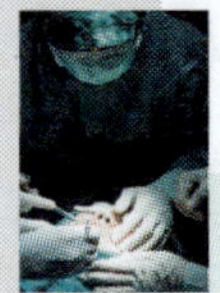

Rupture of anterior urethra	Rupture of posterior urethra
Presentation • Blood at the meatus • Perineal hematoma • *Retention of urine* • Tell patient not to pass urine else extravasation occurs.	*Presentation* • Difficulty in passing urine • Blood at the meatus • Extravasation of urine to scrotum, perineum and abdominal wall and hence bladder is empty.
• PR examination shows normal prostate.	• PR examination shows *floating prostate*.

@Note anterior urethra is undersurface and posterior urethra is dorsal surface.

350. Ans. (a) Calcium oxalate

Ref: Harrison 19th ed. pg. 964

- The normal urinary pH is 5.8–6.2.
- Persistent urinary pH <5.5 *(acidic urine)* leads to development of uric acid and cystine stones.
- Persistent urinary pH >7.2 *(alkaline urine)* leads to development of struvite stone.
- Urine pH >7.5 *(alkaline urine)* leads to development of calcium phosphate stone.
- Calcium oxalate stones development is *independent of urinary pH* and is due to idiopathic hypercalciuria.

Extra Mile

- Increasing urine pH > 6.2 can dramatically increase uric acid solubility. Hence urinary alkalization is done with potassium citrate. Also give allopurinol.
- For calcium phosphate stones keep pH of urine between 6.2 and 6.5.
- For cystine stones keep pH > 7.0 by urinary alkalization.

351. Ans. (a) Cystoscopy

Ref: SRB 5th ed. pg. 1025

- The age of patient, clinical presentation of painless gross hematuria points to etiology as bladder tumor.
- The IVU finding can be explained by the fact that bladder tumor could have *obstructed the ureteric orifice leading to hydronephrosis*.
- Infundibulum in kidney is the area between the calyx and renal pelvis. The filling defect is due to hydronephrosis.
- Cystoscopy must be done for tissue diagnosis of bladder tumor and resection.
- MRI pelvis should be done to check for invasion and pelvic wall extension.
- DMSA scan is done to evaluate for location of scar in pyelonephritis.

352. Ans. (a) Water intoxication

Ref: Bailey 26th ed. pg. 1349

- Water intoxication is postoperative complication of TURP.
- The absorption of water into the circulation at the time of transurethral resection can give rise to CCF, hyponatremia and hemolysis. These features can mimic stroke
- Nowadays this is rarely seen due to use of isotonic glycine during irrigation post TURP.

353. Ans. (c) Ureterocele

- The image shows a characteristic cobra/adder head appearance of an ureterocele with contrast filling the bladder. The bladder outline is normal.

354. Ans. (b) Androgen ablation

Guidelines for Management of Prostate Cancer

- For advanced disease process, androgen ablation is used. It can be achieved with bilateral capsular orchiectomy or drugs
- Drugs like LHRH agonist and androgen blocking agents like flutamide, bicalutamide are used.
- Radiotherapy is used for bone secondaries. Chemotherapeutic drug used is docetaxel.

Prostate Cancer Treatment Guidelines

Treatment by Recurrence Risk

Clinically localized	Therapy
• T3a • Gleason score 8–10 • PSA > 20 ng/mL	• Radiation therapy + Androgen deprivation therapy (2–3 years) • Radial prostatectomy + Pelvic lymph node dissection (in select patients)

Locally advanced	Therapy
T3b–T4 with any Gleason score	• Radiation therapy + Androgen deprivation therapy (2–3 years) • Radiation therapy + Brachytherapy +/– Androgen deprivation therapy (4 to 6 months) • Radical prostatectomy + Pelvic lymph node dissection (in select patients) • Androgen deprivation therapy (in select patients)
Metastatic	**Therapy**
Any T, N1, M0	• **Androgen deprivation therapy** • **Radiation therapy + Androgen deprivation therapy (2–3 years)**
Any T, N, M1	• **Androgen deprivation therapy**

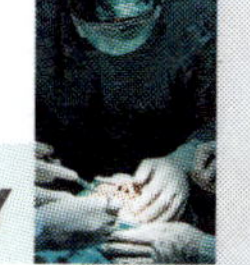

355. Ans. (c) Lymphatics

Ref: Bailey, 26th ed. pg. 1385

- *Seminomas metastasise mainly via the lymphatics and haematogenous spread is uncommon.*
- The lymphatic drainage of the testes is to the para-aortic lymph nodes near the origin of the gonadal vessels.
- The contralateral para-aortic lymph nodes are sometimes involved by tumor spread, but the inguinal lymph nodes are affected only if the scrotal skin is involved.

There are a number of histological types of non-seminomatous germ cell tumors (NSGCT), which may coexist within a single tumor:

- Embryonal carcinoma. Highly malignant tumors that occasionally invade cord structures.
- Yolk sac tumor. Tumors with this component secrete alpha fetoprotein (AFP)
- Choriocarcinoma. Often produces human chorionic gonadotropin (HCG).This is a highly malignant tumor that metastasizes early via both the lymphatics and the bloodstream
- Teratoma. These tumors contain more than one cell type with components derived from ectoderm, endoderm

356. Ans. (a) Scrotal USG

Ref: Bailey, 26th ed. pg. 1386-87

- *The diagnosis of testicular cancer is confirmed by ultrasound scanning of the testis which is also able to assess the contralateral testis.*
- It is a mandatory test in all suspected cases of testicular tumor.
- Chest X-ray is used to detect Canon Ball metastasis
- CT scan chest and abdomen is used to detect metastasis
- Measure the levels of tumor markers which are raised in around 50% of cases.
- *Rise in AFP* is seen in around 50–70% of NSGCTs
- *Rise in HCG* is seen in 40–60% of NSGCTs and around 30% of seminomas.
- When raised, these markers are used to monitor the response to treatment. The mean serum half-lives of AFP and HCG are 5–7 days and 2–3 days, respectively, and reassessment of the markers following orchidectomy can indicate whether all the tumor tissue has been removed.

357. Ans. (a) Right hydrocele

Findings in favour of diagnosis of Hydrocele-

- Translucent swelling with positive trans-illumination test
- Possible to 'get above the swelling' on examination of the scrotum
- The swelling usually surrounds the testis and epididymis such that they may become impossible to palpate separately.
- Be wary of an acute hydrocele in a young man since there may be a testicular tumor.
  - *Choice b:* Right inguinal hernia is ruled out as top of testis can be reached
  - *Choice c:* Epididymal cysts are present *bilaterally* and arc *present behind the testis* whereas he patient is having a unilateral swelling.
  - *Choice d: Encysted hydrocele of the cord* is a smooth oval swelling near the spermatic cord, which is liable to be mistaken for an inguinal hernia. The swelling moves downwards and becomes less mobile if the testis is pulled gently downwards.
  - Ascites should be considered if the swellings are bilateral.

358. Ans. (d) Right pyocele

- *The difference in this question from the previous question would be development of an acute on chronic presentation.*
- Scrotal pyoceles are purulent collections within the potential space between the visceral and parietal tunica vaginalis surrounding the testicle.
- The presentation of scrotal pyoceles is subacute onset of pain and swelling, which may mimic other pathology.
- The imaging modality of choice to diagnose a scrotal pyocele is ultrasound.
- Internal echoes within the pyocele fluid collection typically represent cellular debris.
- Other sonographic findings include loculations, septae, and fluid-fluid or air-fluid levels in the tunica vaginalis external to the testicle.
- By contrast, a hydrocele will appear on ultrasound as a simple fluid with an anechoic region that collects anterior and lateral to the testis. If the fluid contains internal echoes on ultrasound, the diagnosis of hematocele (most common in the setting of trauma) or pyocele may be made.
- Fournier's gangrene is the most concerning complication of a scrotal pyocele.

359. Ans. (a) Right testicular torsion

Ref: Bailey, 26th ed. pg. 1379

- Testicular torsion is most common between 10 and 25 years of age

Clinical Findings

- Sudden agonising pain in the groin and the lower abdomen.
- Feels nauseated and may vomit.
- The testis seems high and the tender twisted cord can be palpated above it.
- The cremasteric reflex is lost.
- *Elevation of the testis reduces the pain in epididymo-orchitis and makes it worse in torsion.*
- *Inversion of the testis is the most common predisposing cause.*

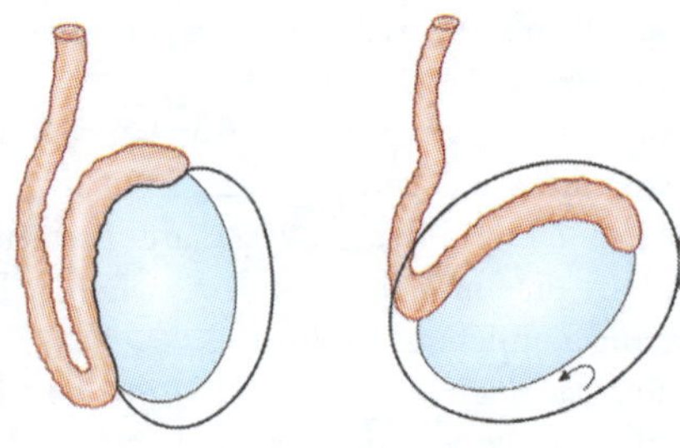

360. Ans. (a) Calcium oxalate

Ref: Bailey and Love, 26th ed. pg. 1292

Types of Renal Stones (Urolithiasis):

1. **Calcium stones (75–85%)**
   - Made of **calcium oxalate.**
2. **Struvite stone/Triple phosphate stone (15% of cases)**
   - Formed mainly after infection by urea splitting bacteria **(Proteus and some staphylococci) which cause alkaline urine** lead to precipitation of phosphate crystals.
   - Causes Staghorn calculi, which occupy large position of renal pelvis.
3. **Uric acid stone**
   - Common in patients with hyperuricemia.
   - Cause: Urine of pH less than 5.5 (uric acid is insoluble in acidic urine) à leading to saturation
   - It is radiolucent stone.
4. **Cystine stone**
   - Due to genetic defect in renal absorption of amino acid cysteine à leading to cystinuria.
5. **Xanthine stones due to xanthinuria**

361. Ans. (a) Uric acid

Radiolucent kidney stones mnemonic **L.U.X**
RadioLucent stones are Uric acid and Xanthine stones

362. Ans. (b) Triple phosphate stones

Ref: Bailey & Love, 26th ed. Ch 75/1292

363. Ans. (c) Triple phosphate stone

Ref: Bailey & Love, 26th ed. Ch 75/1292

364. Ans. (b) Cervical fibroid

- The distribution of myoma/Fibroid in the body of the uterus is broadly classified as follows (Figure):
- Intramural (interstitial) 75%
- Submucous 15%
- Subserous 10%
- The majority of myomas arise in the uterus. Tumors can therefore be classified as uterine and extrauterine.
- The uterine growth is further divided into those that arise from the body and those that arise from the cervix.

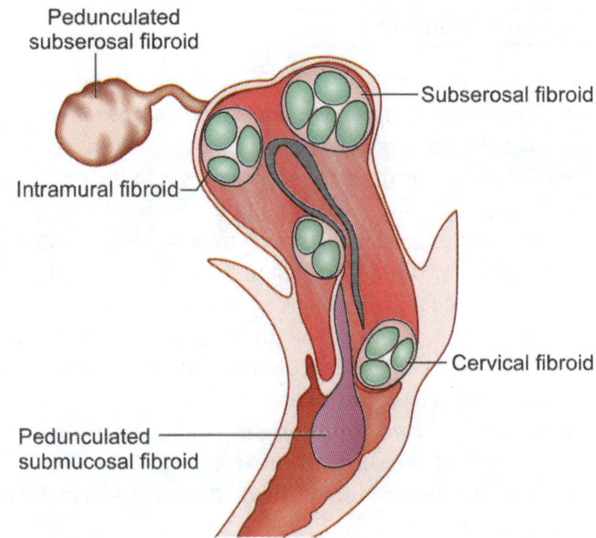

FIGURE: Varieties of submucous fibroid. Various anatomical sites of fibromyomas

Cervical Fibroid

- Cervical fibroid is a single fibroid encountered in 1% of all fibroids. It may develop as a central, anterior, posterior fibroid or grow laterally in the broad ligament.

Symptoms

- A cervical fibroid exerts pressure on the bladder, ureter and in rare cases on the rectum. A woman may feel a lump in the lower abdomen. **During pregnancy, it can cause retention of urine**. Obstructed Labor occurs if the cervical fibroid lies below the presenting part.

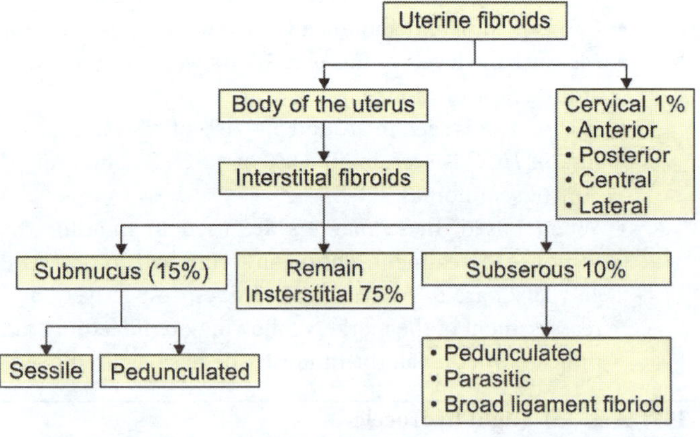

365. Ans. (b) NCCT

Ref: Bailey & Love, 26th ed. pg. 1293

- *Helical computed tomography (CT) scanning without radiocontrast enhancement is now the standard radiologic procedure for diagnosis of nephrolithiasis.*

- The advantages of CT include detection of uric acid stones in addition to the traditional radiopaque stones, no exposure to the risk of radiocontrast agents, and possible diagnosis of other causes of abdominal pain in a patient suspected of having renal colic from stones.
- Ultrasound is not as sensitive as CT in detecting renal or ureteral stones.

366. Ans. (d) Urinary bladder

Ref: Bailey & Love, 26th ed. pg. 1330-35

- Transitional cell epithelium lines → the urinary tract from the renal pelvis to the ureter, urinary bladder, and the proximal two-thirds of the urethra.
- **Transitional cell carcinoma:** Cancers can occur at any point mentioned above:
  - **90% of malignancies develop in the bladder**
  - 8% in the renal pelvis
  - 2% in the ureter or urethra.

Extra Mile

- Bladder cancer is the **fourth (4th)** most common cancer in men and the **thirteenth (1 + 3 = 4)** in women.
- **Among urothelial tumors-**95% are **transitional cell in origin**.
- **Polychronotropism**-urothelial tumors exhibit polychronotropism, which is the tendency to recur over time in new locations in the urothelial tract.
- Most imp risk factor- **Cigarette smoking**
- **Other-**aniline dyes, drugs phenacetin, external beam radiation. Chronic cyclophosphamide, *Schistosoma haematobium* (a parasite-cause both Scc and Tcc)
- Vitamin A - protective.
- 3 clinical subtypes-
  - **Superficial** (75%)
  - Invade muscle (20%)
  - Metastatic (5%)
- Clinical presentation
  1. **Hematuria** (painless)- Most common presentation (80–90% of cases)
  2. Irritative bladder symptoms such as dysuria, urgency, or frequency of urination occur in 20-30% of patients with bladder cancer.
- **MC site of lymphatic metastasis: Pelvic lymph nodes (obturator MC)**
- **MC site of hematogenous spread**- **LIVER > LUNG**
- **Diagnosis–** diagnosis and initial staging is made **by cystoscopy and TUR.**
  - Newer, voided urine assays (i.e., bladder tumor antigen [BTA-Stat, BTA-TRAK], NMP-22, fibrin/fibrinogen degradation products [FDP]) are being used for the detection and surveillance of urothelial carcinoma.
- **Management**-cystoscopy and TUR or biopsy
- Further management depends on stage, grade, size, multiplicity, recurrecnce pattern
- Drugs for intravesical chemo- **Mitomycin, Thiotepa, Epirubicin, BCG (most effective)**

367. Ans. (c) Transitional cell cancer

Ref: Bailey & Love, 26th ed. pg. 1330-35

368. Ans. (d) Painless hematuria

Ref: Bailey & Love, 26th ed. pg. 1330-35

369. Ans. (c) Superficial

Ref: Bailey & Love, 26th ed. pg. 1330-35

370. Ans. (c) Females and males are equally affected

Ref: Bailey & Love, 26th ed. pg. 1330-35

Epidemiological studies have shown protective effect of Vitamin A on bladder cancer.

371. Ans. (c) True pelvis only

Ref: Bailey & Love 26th ed. pg. 1361

The prostate has been avulsed from the membranous urethra secondary to fracture of the pelvis. Extravasation occurs above the triangular ligament and is peri-prostatic and perivesical area of the pelvis.

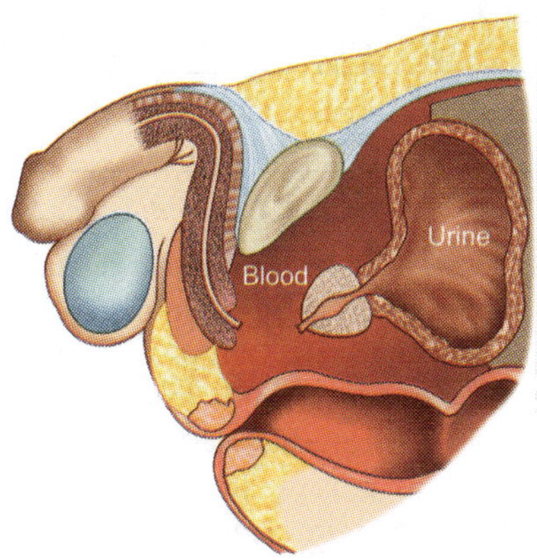

372. Ans. (a) Instrumentation

Ref: Harrison, 18th ed. pg. 288

- Urethral catheterization is the single most important predisposing factor in the development of nosocomial urinary tract infection. Cystoscopy may be followed by a transient bacteremia.
- *The most important risk factor for bacteriuria is the presence of a catheter.* Eighty percent of nosocomial UTIs are related to urethral catheterization, while 5-10% are related to genitourinary manipulation. Catheters inoculate organisms into the bladder and promote colonization by providing a surface for bacterial adhesion and causing mucosal irritation.

373. Ans. (b) Polycystic kidney

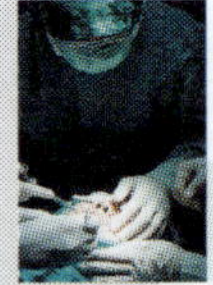

Extra Mile

- **Driven snow appearance** - Pindborg's tumor
- **Sunray appearance** - Osteogenic Sarcoma, Ewing Sarcoma
- **Floating Water Lily sign -** Lung Hydatid, Echinococcus
- **Popcorn calcification -** Pulmonary Hamartoma
- **Honeycomb appearance** - RA, Scleroderma, Interstitial Lung Disease
- **Egg shell calcification** - Sarcoidosis, Silicosis, Lymphoma, T.B., Histoplasmosis
- **Spring water cyst** = Pluero Pericardial cyst
- Rib notching - Neurofibromatosis, Aortic Aneurysm, Taussig-Bing Operation, Aortic obstruction, Coarctation of aorta.
- **Coeur en Sabot, Flask shape heart -** TOF
- **Candle wax sign** -Melorheostosis
- **Football Sign** - Pneumoperitoneum
- **Thumb Print Sign** - Epiglotis, Ischemic Colitis
- **Double bubble sign** - Duodenal Atresia
- **Single bubble sign -** Pyloric stenosis
- **Soap bubble appearance -** Meconium ileus
- **Meniscus appearance -** CBD stone on cholangiography
- **Central dot sign -** Caroli's disease
- **Chain of lakes appearance** - Chronic pancreatitis
- **Spongy appearance with central sunburst calcification sign** - serous cyst adenoma
- **Rim sign in IVP** - Hydronephrosis
- **Cobra head deformity** - Ureterocele
- **B/L spider leg sign** - Polycystic Kidney
- **Golf hole ureter** - T.B.
- **Flower Vase pattern of pelvis in IVP** - Horse shoe kidney

374. Ans. (b) Ureterocele

Ref: Bailey & Love, 26th ed. pg. 1285

A ureterocele is a congenital saccular dilatation of terminal portion of the ureter. The most common presentation is that of urinary tract infection or uro-sepsis in children. Stasis of urine can lead to calculus formation. Some children may present with palpable mass due to hydro nephrotic kidney .Cyst may prolapse into internal urethral opening causing obstruction to bladder outflow. This condition may remain unrecognized until adult life. Ureterocele is usually discovered on radiological examination or during endoscopy.

375. Ans. (a) Leydig cells

Ref: Bailey & Love, 26th ed. pg. 1341

Rectangular, crystal-like inclusions, composed of protein, with pointed or rounded ends in the interstitial cells of the testis (Leydig cells) and hilus cells in the ovary. *Inside the Leydig cells of human males can be found Reinke's crystals.* The purpose of these crystals is uncertain, some believe that they are a by-product of a degenerative process related to aging. They appear to have no contribution to androgen or testosterone production, and they *can be used to identify Leydig cells easily when viewing testicular tissue under a microscope.*

376. Ans. (a) Seminoma

Ref: Bailey & Love, 26th ed. pg. 1385

Seminoma is the most common germ cell tumor of the testis or, more rarely, the mediastinum or other extra-gonadal locations. It is a malignant neoplasm and is one of the most treatable and curable cancers, with a survival rate above 95% if discovered in early stages.

377. Ans. (b) Para aortic

Ref: Harrison, 19th ed. pg. 589

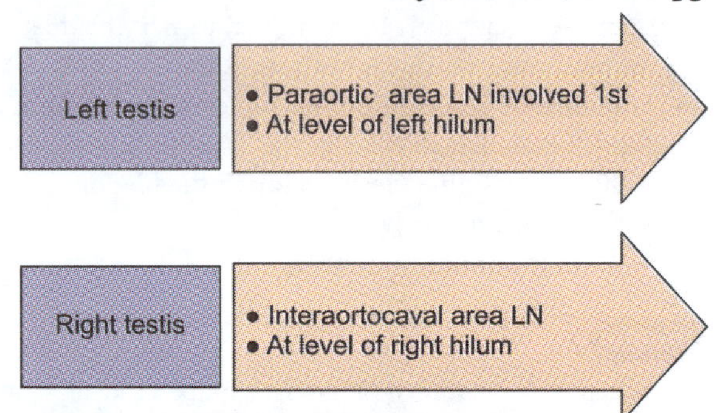

Points to Remember about testicular tumor

- **In** metastatic disease-Retroperitoneal LN is **Most commonly** involved
- **Metastasis**- Lymphatic >> Blood (m/c lung)
- **Exception is Choriocarcinoma where blood metastasis (m/c lung)** >> lymphatic metastasis.
- **Most common testicular tumor- in general** → seminoma
  - Prepubertal adults- Teratoma
  - Infant and children- Yolk sac tumor
- **Most common presentation**- nodule or painless swelling of one gonad
- Most common bilateral testicular tumor- **Malignant lymphoma**
- Most common bilateral primary testicular tumor Seminoma
- FNAC contraindicated
- **Initial IOC**- USG (hypo echoic area within tunica albuginea is suspicious)
- HPE diagnosis by-radical orchiectomy (inguinal approach)
- **Scrotal orchiectomy**- contraindicated
- **Chavesseac maneuver**- soft clamp applied to cord → biopsy from suspicious area → sent for frozen section → if + ligate cord, do orchiectomy → final HPE

378. Ans. (a) P.S.A

Ref: Bailey & Love, 26th ed. pg. 1341

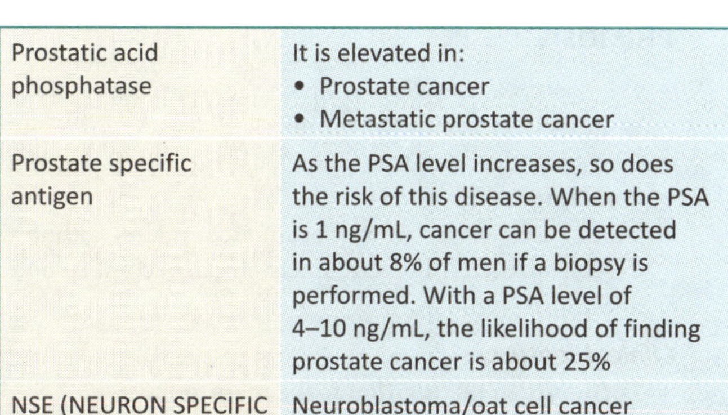

Prostatic acid phosphatase	It is elevated in: • Prostate cancer • Metastatic prostate cancer
Prostate specific antigen	As the PSA level increases, so does the risk of this disease. When the PSA is 1 ng/mL, cancer can be detected in about 8% of men if a biopsy is performed. With a PSA level of 4–10 ng/mL, the likelihood of finding prostate cancer is about 25%
NSE (NEURON SPECIFIC ENOLASE)	Neuroblastoma/oat cell cancer

379. Ans. (d) Persists in blood after prostatectomy

Ref: Bailey & Love, 26th ed. pg. 1341

- PSA is a kallikrein-related serine protease that causes liquefaction of seminal coagulum.
- It is produced by both nonmalignant and malignant epithelial cells and, as such, is prostate-specific, not prostate cancer–specific, and serum levels may also increase from prostatitis and BPH. Serum levels are not affected by DRE but the performance of a prostate biopsy can increase PSA levels up to tenfold for 8–10 weeks.
- Elimination of PSA bound to alpha 1-antichymotrypsin is slow (estimated half-life of 1-2 weeks) as it is too large to be cleared by the kidneys. Levels should be undetectable after about six weeks if the prostate has been removed.

380. Ans. (c) Prostate specific antigen only

Ref: Bailey & Love, 26th ed. pg. 1341

- The most common presentation of advanced prostate cancer is a patient with a rising PSA level in whom initial local therapy has failed. Generally, after a radical prostatectomy, the PSA level should be less than 0.2 ng/mL and, after radiation therapy, less than 0.5 ng/mL. Other important prognostic indicators include PSA velocity, time to PSA nadir, time to PSA recurrence, and pattern of PSA recurrence.
- PSA levels for all men with prostate cancer who are having radical treatment should be checked at the earliest 6 weeks following treatment, at least every 6 months for the first 2 years and then at least once a year thereafter.

381. Ans. (b) Prostatitis

Ref Bailey & Love, 27th pg. 1475

The **three-glass urine test** is valuable, if the first glass with the initial voided urine sample shows **prostatic threads**.

Prostatodynia is diagnosed by presence of perigenital pain in the absence of any objective evidence of prostate inflammation.

382. Ans. (a) Bateson plexus

Ref: Bailey & Love, 26th ed. pg. 527

- The **Bateson venous plexus** is a network of valve-less veins in the human body that connect the deep pelvic veins and thoracic veins to the internal vertebral venous plexuses.
- Because of their location and lack of valves, they are believed to provide a route for the spread of cancer metastases. These metastases commonly arise from cancer of the pelvic organs such as prostate and may spread to the vertebral column.

383. Ans. (b) Localized prostate cancer, life expectancy >10 years

Ref: Bailey & Love, 26th ed. pg. 1355

- Nerve-sparing RRP is done in patients with clinically localized prostate cancer who have at least a 10-year life expectancy and low comorbidities.
- *Patients with locally advanced disease cannot undergo nerve-sparing RRP; because of the extent of the local tumor burden (especially posteriorly), the nerve-sparing procedure can compromise the adequacy of the operation.*
- The objective of modern RP are to remove the entire cancer with negative surgical margins, minimal blood loss, no serious perioperative complications, and complete recovery of continence and potency.

384. Ans. (a) Horse shoe kidney

Ref: Bailey & Love, 26th ed. pg. 1282

- Since the contrast can be seen on both sides, absent kidney is ruled out. More over the contrast is at normal level, so undescended kidney is unlikely.
- The *horseshoe kidney* consists of two distinct functioning kidneys on each side of the midline, *connected at the lower poles by an isthmus of functioning renal parenchyma or fibrous tissue that crosses the midline of the body*
- The collecting system has a characteristic appearance on intravenous urography because of an incomplete inward rotation of the renal pelvis, which faces anterior. The axis of the collecting system is deviated inward at the lower poles because of the lower pole's connection with the isthmus.

385. Ans. (a) Renal cell cancer

- The large homogenous mass on right shows an enlarged kidney as compared to other side suggestive of malignancy. The hilum of kidney shows renal vein thrombosis.
- Due to homogenous mass present unilaterally, polycystic kidney is ruled out. Since no cystic dilatation is present, hydro-nephrosis is ruled out.

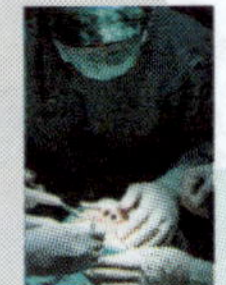

386. Ans. (b) Bladder stone

- Notice the densely radio-opaque, single large calculus.
- Fecolith is hardening of feces into lumps of varying size inside the colon, which may appear whenever chronic obstruction of transit occurs, such as in megacolon and chronic constipation but location of this radioopaque shadow in pelvis rules out fecolith.

387. Ans. (b) Carcinoma penis

Ref: Bailey & Love, 26th ed. pg. 1374

- Penile squamous cell carcinoma, the most common penile malignancy, behaves similarly to squamous cell carcinoma in other parts of the skin. This is a slow-growing cancer in its early stages, and because it seldom interferes with voiding or erectile function.
- *Bowen's disease* typically presents as a gradually enlarging, well-demarcated erythematous plaque with an irregular border and surface crusting or scaling. *About 60-85% of patients have lesions on the lower leg, usually in previously or presently sun-exposed areas of skin.*

388. Ans. (b) Inguinal lymph node metastasis operable

Ref: Bailey & Love 26th ed. pg. 1373-74

CARCINOMA PENIS

Clinical Features

- Most commonly occur in 6th decade of life
- ***Squamous cell carcinoma (80%) is the MC type,*** most commonly originates from glans> sulcus > prepuce > shaft.
- Others are transitional cell carcinoma (15%), basal cell carcinoma, malignant melanoma, sarcoma
- **MC symptom**: foul smelling discharge, with little or no pain
- More than 50% patients of CA penis presents with enlarged inguinal lymph nodes.
- **MC and earliest symptom of metastatic CA penis: Priapism**

Jackson (Extent of spread) Staging for CA Penis	
Stage I	Confined to glans or prepuce
Stage II	Extension to shaft
Stage III	Operable inguinal LN metastasis
Stage IV	Inoperable inguinal LN metastasis or local or advanced spread

389. Ans. (d) Phimosis

Ref: Bailey, 26th ed. pg. 1359

PHIMOSIS

- Phimosis is a condition in which the contracted foreskin cannot be retracted over the glans.
- Chronic infection from poor local hygiene is its most common cause.
- Most cases occur in uncircumcised males, although excessive skin left after circumcision can become stenotic and cause phimosis.

Clinical features

- **Difficulty in micturition is the main symptom.**
- Ballooning of prepuce during micturition is suggestive of phimosis.
- *Edema, erythema, and tenderness of the prepuce and the presence of purulent discharge usually cause the patient to seek medical attention.*
- Inability to retract the foreskin is a less common complaint.

HYPOSPADIAS

- Hypospadias results when fusion of urethral folds is incomplete, and urethral meatus opens on the underside of penis or perineum (ventral surface of penis).
- Because fusion of urethral folds is from posterior to anterior, Anterior forms are more common than posterior.
- **Associated pathology:** In addition to ventrally placed ectopic meatus, hypospadias has:
  - **Chordee:** Ventral curvature of penis due to contracture of fibrous cord which has replaced the distal urethra and corpus spongiosum.
  - **Hooded prepurce:** Deficient on ventral aspect and excess on dorsal aspect
  - Stenosis of ectopic meatus

EPISPADIAS

- Urethra opens on the dorsum (upper aspect) of the penis in males, in females there is a fissure in the wall of the urethra which opens above the clitoris
- **Females:** Bifid clitoris and separation of the labia. Most are incontinent because of maldevelopment of the urinary sphincters.
- **Males:** Patients with glandular epispadias seldom have urinary incontinence. However, incontinence in penopubic epispadias is 95% and penile epispadias is 75%.

POSTERIOR URETHRAL VALVE

- Exclusively an anomaly of male urethra.
- Symmetrical folds of urothelium extending distally from prostatic urethra to external urinary sphincter.
- Newborns may present with palpable abdominal masses.
- Sometimes, the valves are incomplete and the patient remains without symptoms until adolescence or adulthood.

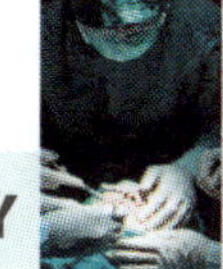

390. Ans. (b) Hypospadias

Ref: Bailey, 26th ed. pg. 1359

Refer to above explanation

391. Ans. (b) Circumcision

Ref: *Bailey & Love, 25th pg. 1371*

Balanitis xerotica obliterans (BXO)
- A condition in which the normally pliant **foreskin becomes thickened and will not retract.**
- It is difficult to keep the penis clean and there is a problem with hygiene.
- In later life there is an **increased susceptibility to carcinoma.**
- Treatment is by **circumcision**

392. Ans. (d) Infection

Ref: Campbell's Urology, 8th ed. pg. 346, 349

Principal causes of death in renal transplant patients (in decreasing order)

1. Heart disease
2. Infection
3. Stroke

HEPATOBILIARY SYSTEM

393. Ans. (d) Conservative treatment with antibiotics

Ref: Bailey and Love, 27th ed. pg. 1203

Cystic duct is the most common site of bile leak after cholecystectomy. The treatment of choice is usually conservative. Using sufficient percutaneous drainage of the biloma cavity and endoscopic retrograde cholangiography with sphincterotomy and/or stenting, the cure rate of bile leaks is greater than 90%.

394. Ans. (c) C

Ref: Bailey and Love, 27th ed. pg. 1198

Type III would have intraduodenal diverticulum and would be located at the terminal end of CBD. Option c is correct answer. Option d is ruled out to multiple intra and extra hepatic cysts seen.

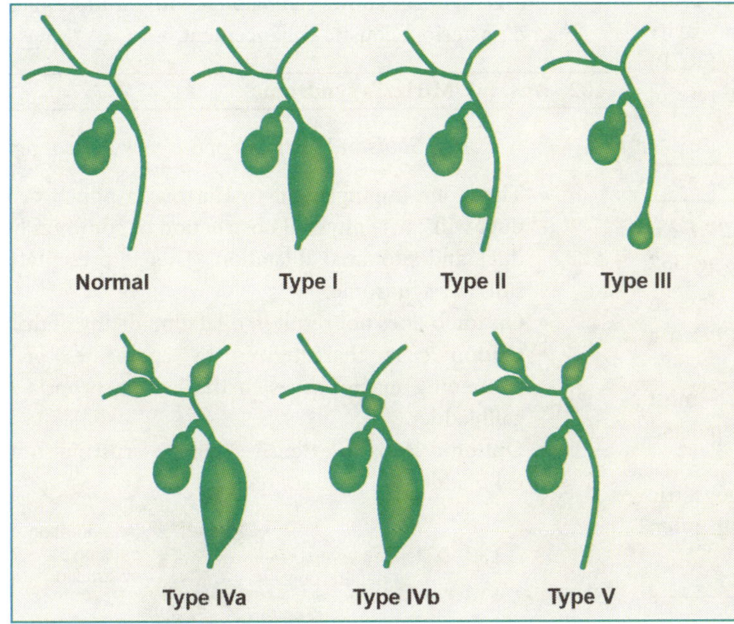

I	Cystic (Ia)/saccular (Ib)/fusiform (Ic) dilatation of the extrahepatic bile duct (accounts for 80–90% of cases)
II	Extrahepatic, supraduodenal bile duct diverticulum
III	Intraduodenal diverticulum (choledochocele)
IV	Intra and extrahepatic duct dilatation
IVa	Multiple infra and extrahepatic cysts
IVb	Multiple extrahepatic cysts only

395. Ans. (d) Reassure the patient and follow-up

Ref: Bailey and Love, Textbook of Surgery, 27th ed. pg. 1210

Polyps of the gall bladder are tumor-like lesions and polyps ≤0.5 cm are just followed up on regular basis.

All Gallbladder polyps larger than 1 cm, or symptomatic, or larger than 0.6 cm with associated risk factors for cancer are indications for cholecystectomy.

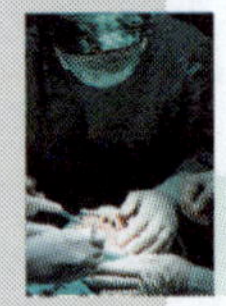

396. Ans. (b) Steatorrhea

Ref: Bailey and Love, Textbook of Surgery, 27th ed. pg. 1198

Post-cholecystectomy syndrome describes the presence of abdominal symptoms after a cholecystectomy.

- After cholecystectomy, the reduced absorption of fat results in nausea, indigestion, and steatorrhea.
- Steatorrhea occurs only when 90% of pancreatic output has been lost, due to inadequate delivery of both lipase and bicarbonate.
- The acidic environment further inactivates what lipase may be present and precipitates bile salts, worsening fat absorption.

397. Ans. (a) Bile leak at site

Ref: Bailey and Love, Textbook of Surgery, 27th ed. pg. 1202

Post op RUQ pain after laparoscopic cholecystectomy is suggestive of bile leak.

- Biliary leaks can be a severe surgical complication and are the most reported postoperative biliary injury, particularly after cholecystectomy.
- Cystic duct is the most common site of bile leak after cholecystectomy.
- The treatment of choice is usually conservative. Using sufficient percutaneous drainage of the biloma cavity and endoscopic retrograde cholangiography (ERCP) with sphincterotomy and/or stenting, the cure rate of bile leaks is greater than 90%.

398. Ans. (b) Hypovolemic shock

Ref: Bailey and Love, Textbook of Surgery, 27th ed. pg. 352

Esophageal varices are dilated sub-mucosal veins in the lower third of the esophagus. They are most often a consequence of portal hypertension.

- Bleeding from esophageal varices is the third most common cause of upper GI bleeding, after duodenal and gastric ulcers.
- In cirrhotic patients, esophageal and esophagogastric varices are the most common sites of bleeding, often responsible for hypovolemic shock.

399. Ans. (a) IV ceftriaxone

Ref: Bailey and Love, Textbook of Surgery, 27th ed. pg. 1053

The clinical diagnosis due to presence of Polymorphonuclear cell count in the ascitic fluid is spontaneous bacterial peritonitis

- It is a frequent and severe complication of decompensated cirrhosis.
- The detection of a PMN cell count >250 cells/mm^3 is highly suspicious and provides an indication to initiate empirical antibiotic treatment.
- The efficacy of cephalosporins (such as ceftriaxone and ceftazidime) administered once daily; appear to be as effective as cefotaxime.

400. Ans. (a) USG abdomen

Ref: Bailey and Love, Textbook of Surgery, 27th ed. pg. 1199

Right upper quadrant abdominal pain, arising from the GI tract or nearby organs, is the utmost recurrent and frequent cause of patients presenting in the hospital emergency and outpatient department.

- Various systems of organs are incorporated at standard RUQ USG, and an assortment of ultrasonographically diagnosable infection cycles can be recognized, including states of hepatic, pancreatic, adrenal, renal, gastrointestinal, vascular, and thoracic, all of which may bring about RUQ torment and pain.

401. Ans. (b) Multiple gallstones

Ref: Bailey and love 27th ed. pg. 1215

The USG image shows Gallbladder with multiple gallstones and posterior acoustic enhancement.

402. Ans. (a) Mirizzi's syndrome

Ref: Sabiston Textbook of Surgery 21st ed. pg. 1504

- The stone impingement in Hartmann pouch or cystic duct will cause physical obstruction of common hepatic duct and proximal dilatation. This is presentation of Mirrizi's syndrome.
- Option b does not result in dilatation of any of ducts.
- Option c is characterized by aggregates of lipid-containing macrophages in the lamina propria of the gallbladder.
- Option d leads to extensive calcium crusting in wall of gallbladder.

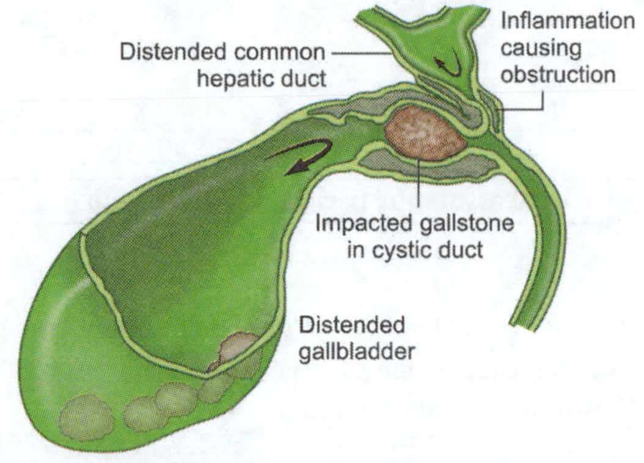

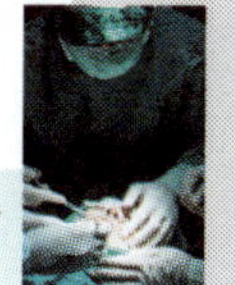

403. Ans. (a) Hydatid cyst

Ref: Bailey and Love 27th ed. pg. 68

The USG image shows water lily appearance on USG which is diagnostic of Hydatid cyst. It occurs when there is detachment of the endocyst membrane which results in floating membranes within the pericyst that mimic the appearance of a water lily.

404. Ans. (c) Arsenic

Ref: Bailey and Love 27th ed. pg. 146

A spectrum of liver lesions has also been attributed to chronic arsenic exposure.

- Angiosarcoma liver
- Cirrhosis
- Hepatocellular carcinoma
- Hepatoportal sclerosis

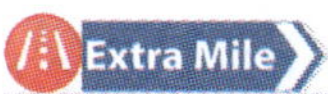

Extra Mile

Must know agents incriminated in causing cancers

Inhaled particles		Asbestos	Mesothelioma
		Wood dust	Paranasal sinus cancers
Chemicals		Environmental pollutants/ chemicals used in industry	Angiosarcoma (vinyl chloride) Bladder cancer (aniline dyes), vulcanisation of rubber) Lung, nasal cavity (nickel) Skin (arsenic) Lung (beryllium, cadmium, chromium) All sites (dioxins)
	Medical	Alkylating agents used in cytotoxic chemotherapy	Leukaemia Lymphoma Lung cancer
		Immunosuppressive treatment	Kaposi's sarcoma
		Stiboestrol	Adenocarcinoma of vagina in daughters of treated mothers
		Tamoxifen	Endometrial cancer
Fungal and plant toxins	Aflatoxins		Hepatoma
Obesity/lack of physical exercise			Breast endometrium kidney

405. Ans. (a) Carcinoma gall bladder

Ref: Bailey and Love 27th ed. pg. 1210

- Image shows a fungating mass inside the lumen of resected specimen of gall bladder which is specific for carcinoma of gall bladder.
- Option b and c would be visible as well-defined concretion or in lumen of gallbladder.
- Option d is appearance of the mucosa of GB due to multiple focal collections of triglycerides and cholesterol esters within the lamina propria of the gallbladder wall.

406. Ans. (d) Contrast CT scan

Ref: SRB 5th ed. pg. 599, 601

The clinical presentation is suggestive of liver abscess. Since the patient is anicteric, viral hepatitis is a less likely diagnosis. The initial investigation to be performed will be USG which will evaluate the echotexture of liver and give insight into altered echogenicity.

CT scan abdomen with contrast has 95% sensitivity to pick up the abscess, location, size and picks up complications as well.

407. Ans. (a) HCC

Ref: SRB 5th ed. pg. 609

Alpha-fetoprotein is raised to more than 100 IU in Hepatocellular carcinoma. It begins to rise once vascular invasion occurs by the tumor. The fibrolamellar variant of

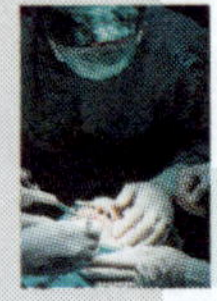

HCC does not show elevated HCC. Other tumor markers for HCC are:
- PIVKA II
- ALP-L3
- DCP (des carboxy prothrombin)

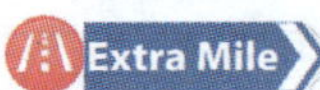

Tumor marker for fibrolamellar variant of HCC is neurotensin levels.

408. Ans. (c) E.R.C.P

Ref: SRB, 5th ed. pg. 634

The image shows presence of gastroduodenoscopy at 7'o clock position with a filling defect in CBD. The technique involves cannulation of sphincter of Oddi and dye is injected. It is done under C arm guidance and sedation like midazolam or propofol anaesthesia.

T – Tube cholangiogram	Percutaneous transhepatic cholangiography
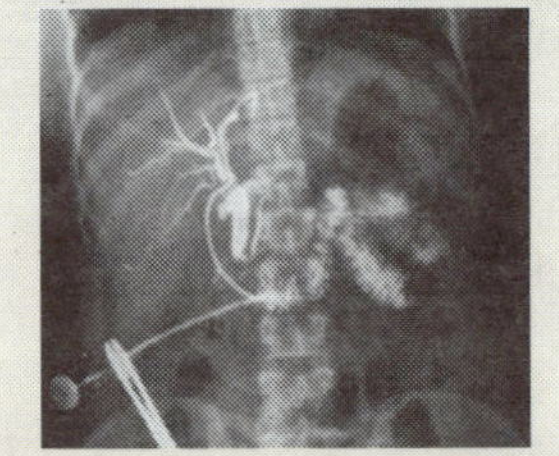	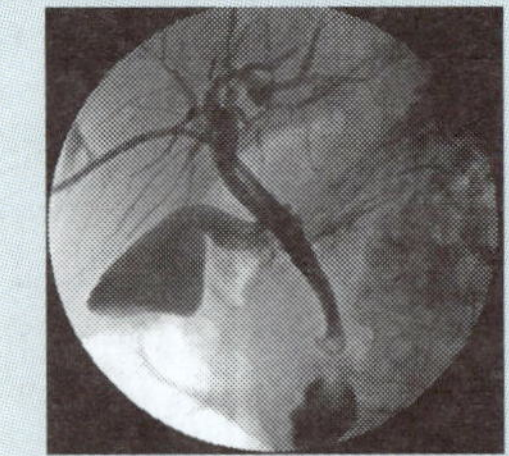
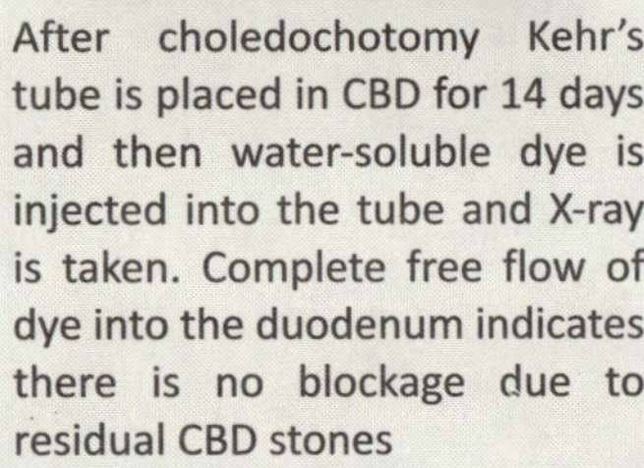 After choledochotomy Kehr's tube is placed in CBD for 14 days and then water-soluble dye is injected into the tube and X-ray is taken. Complete free flow of dye into the duodenum indicates there is no blockage due to residual CBD stones	With help of C arm fluoroscopy *Okuda needle* is passed into dilated biliary duct via the liver parenchyma. It is done to evaluate for high biliary strictures or failure of ERCP.

409. Ans. (a) Associated with MEN1

Ref: Harrison 19th ed. pg. 569

- Zollinger Ellison syndrome/Gastrinoma is the most common pancreatic tumor seen in multiple endocrine neoplasia type 1.
- The most common site is second part of duodenum and hence choice b is wrong.
- The best test for diagnosis of ZES is secretin study with measurement of fasting gastrin levels and BAO/MAO levels.
- Most common presenting symptom is epigastric pain > diarrhea.
- The most frequent metastasis is *to liver*.

410. Ans. (a) Hepatoduodenal ligament

Pringle maneuver is used to slow bleeding flow during liver surgery. *The Pringle manoeuvre is characterised by clamping of hepatoduodenal ligament.* It is effective as the liver is partially nourished by backflow from the hepatic veins. However intermittent clamping with 15 minutes of clamping and 5 minutes without clamping is less harmful.

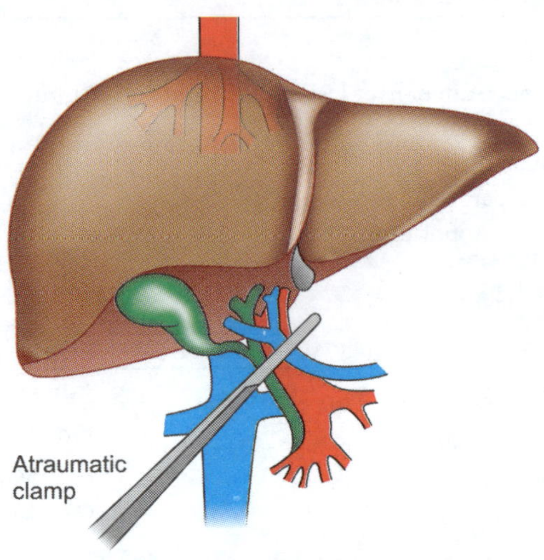

FIGURE: Pringle maneuver. Occlusion of the porta hepatis decreases blood flow to the liver to slow bleeding during liver surgery. It clamps the portal vein and hepatic artery

411. Ans. (a) Cholelithiasis

The USG image shows stones appearing as intraluminal, echogenic, mobile foci that are gravity-dependent and create a clean acoustic shadow. The gravity dependent movement of stone with change of patient position and is called as rolling stone sign.

412. Ans. (b) Aspiration + Anti amoebic drugs

Ref: Bailey, 26th ed. pg. 131

- *The presence of solitary abscess in left lobe points to amoebic liver abscess etiology and needs aspiration and anti- amoebic drugs*
- Liver involvement occurs following invasion of *E histolytica* into mesenteric venules.
- Amebae then enter the portal circulation and travel to the liver where they typically form large abscesses.
- Routine aspiration of liver abscess is not indicated.
- The aspirate is the color of chocolate/ Anchovy sauce due to mixture of blood and liver tissue.
- Choice d is performed for Hydatid cyst.

Indications of aspiration in amoebic liver abscess are:

1 Lack of clinical improvement in 24–48 hours
2. *Left lobe abscess*
3. Thin rim of liver tissue around the abscess

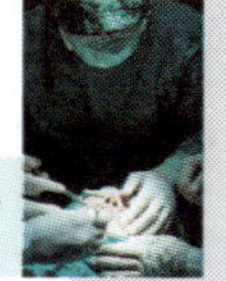

413. Ans. (a) Liver cancer

Ref: Bailey, 26th ed. pg. 131

- Aflatoxin exposure in food is a significant risk factor for Hepatocellular carcinoma.
- Aflatoxins are primarily produced by the food-borne fungi *Aspergillus flavus* and *Aspergillus parasiticus*, which colonize a variety of food commodities, including maize, oilseeds, spices, groundnuts
- Choice b is related to Smoking and aniline dye exposure
- Choice d is related to the earliest detected proto-oncogene Rb.

414. Ans. (c) Rapid transfusion of fresh blood

Ref: Bailey, 26th ed. pg. 16-17 and pg. 109

Choice a	Vasopressor or inotropic therapy is not indicated as first-line treatment of hypovolemic shock.
Choice b	Laparotomy would require General anesthesia which cannot be given in setting of decompensated shock.
Choice c	If blood is being lost, the ideal replacement fluid is blood, although crystalloid therapy may be required while awaiting blood products.
Choice d	While awaiting Blood transfusion crystalloids must be started and is a first line management.

Extra Mile

Role of vasopressors in shock

- Vasopressor agents (phenylephrine, noradrenaline) are indicated in distributive shock states (sepsis, neurogenic shock) where there is peripheral vasodilatation, and a low systemic vascular resistance, leading to hypotension despite a high cardiac output.
- Where the vasodilatation is resistant to catecholamines (e.g., absolute or relative steroid deficiency) vasopressin may be used as an alternative vasopressor.

415. Ans. (b) Amoebic liver abscess

Ref: Sabistan, 19th ed. pg. 1443

AMOEBIC LIVER ABSCESS

- Caused by Entamoeba histolytica whose cysts are acquired through the feco-oral route
- Usually Solitary and more common in **right lobe of liver**.
- It most frequently affects the cecum and ascending colon
- **In colon:** Flask-shaped ulcers (MC site: Cecum and ascending colon)

Clinical Features

- Most common symptoms is abdominal pain
- **Typical clinical picture (*as seen in the question*)**: Patient of 20–40 yrs of age, with history of travel to endemic area, presents with fever, chills, anorexia, *right upper quadrant pain*.
- Results from an obligatory colonic infection, a recent history of diarrhea are uncommon.
- USG guided aspiration: Shows anchovy sauce pus

TABLE: Difference between Amoebic liver abscess and Pyogenic liver abscess

Clinical features	Amebic liver abscess	Pyogenic liver abscess
Age (yr)	20–40	>50
Travel in endemic area	Yes	No
Diabetes mellitus	Uncommon	More common
Alcohol use	Common	Common
Jaundice	Uncommon	Common
Elevated bilirubin	Uncommon	Common
Elevated alkaline phosphatase	Common	Common

Extra Mile

- **Most common** symptom of pyogenic abscess: FEVER
- MC sign of pyogenic abscess: RUQ tenderness
- **Most common** symptom of amoebic abscess: **Abdominal pain**
- **Most common** sign of amoebic abscess: **HEPATOMEGALY**
- Hydatid cyst is mostly asymptomatic. If presents with symptom, most common presenting symptom is abdominal pain, vomiting, dyspepsia.

416. Ans. (a) Amoebic liver abcess

Ref: Bailey & Love, 26th ed. pg. 70

417. Ans. (b) Peritoneal deposits

Ref: Bailey & Love, 26th ed. pg. 1100

Advantages of ultrasound in obstructive jaundice
1. Ultrasonography (US) is the least expensive, safest, and most sensitive technique for visualizing the biliary system, particularly the gallbladder
2. Current accuracy is close to 95%. US is the procedure of choice for the initial evaluation of cholestasis and for helping differentiate extrahepatic from intrahepatic causes
3. Visualization of the pancreas, kidney, and blood vessels is also possible.

418. Ans. (a) Clonorchis sinensis

Ref: Bailey & Love, 26th ed. pg. 1115

Clonorchis sinensis is liver fluke acquired by ingestion of raw or inadequately cooked fresh water fish. In human

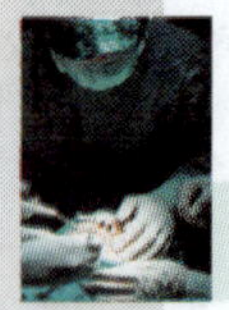

body it lives within bile ducts and causes inflammatory reaction leading to cholangitis, cholangio-hepatitis and biliary obstruction. It is well known to be a risk factor for Cholangio-carcinoma.

419. Ans. (b) Acute cholecystitis

Ref: Sabistan, 19th ed. pg. 1847

ACUTE CHOLECYSTITIS

- Acute cholecystitis is inflammation of gallbladder and is due to gallstones in 90-95% of cases.
- **Characteristic triad of cholecystits:** RUQ pain + Fever + Leucocytosis
- Obstruction of the cystic duct leading to biliary colic is the initial event in acute cholecystitis

Clinical Presentation

1. RUQ pain of much longer duration than biliary colic, is the **MC symptom**
2. **Other common symptoms:** Fever, nausea, and vomiting
3. **Upon Physical examination:** RUQ tenderness and guarding are usually present inferior to the right costal margin.
4. **Murphy's sign:** Inspiratory arrest with deep palpation in the RUQ in acute cholecystitis.
5. **Boas sign:** Hyperesthesia below right scapula in acute cholecystitis

420. Ans. (a) Acute cholangitis

Ref: Sabiston, 19th ed. pg. 1847

- Charcoat triad is seen in case of acute cholangitis.
- **It includes: Pain, Fever, Jaundice**
- Do not mix with triad of cholecystitis

421. Ans. (b) Acute Cholecystitis

Ref: Chapter 67, Bailey and Love, 26th ed. pg. 1107

- In the acute phase of Cholecystitis, the patient may have right upper quadrant tenderness that is exacerbated during inspiration by the examiner's right subcostal palpation **(Murphy's sign).**

422. Ans. (c) Cholecystitis

- Cholecystitis is inflammation of gallbladder wall. Radiological evaluation does not show elevation of right hemidiaphragm in these cases.
- Chest radiographs are abnormal in the majority of patients with amebic hepatic abscesses. Findings include **elevation of the right hemi-diaphragm**, right pleural effusion, atelectasis in the region of the base of the right lung, and a right pleural effusion.
- In case of pyogenic liver abscess and subdiaphragmatic abscess also, there is elevation of right hemi-diaphragm.

423. Ans. (c) Hemangioma

Ref: Bailey & Love, 26th ed. pg. 1083

Hemangioma being a *vascular tumor* is diagnosed by imaging techniques and liver biopsy is contraindicated. Cavernous hemangiomas arise from the endothelial cells and consist of multiple, large vascular channels lined by a single layer of endothelial cells and supported by collagenous walls. These tumors are frequently asymptomatic and incidentally discovered at imaging, surgery, or autopsy.

424. Ans. (a) Hemangioma

Ref: Bailey & Love, 26th ed. pg. 1083

- **Hemangiomas:** These are the *most common type of benign liver tumor*. Most of these tumors do not cause symptoms and do not need treatment.
- Hepatic adenomas: These are benign epithelial liver tumors that develop in the liver and are found mainly in women that using estrogens as contraceptives. Symptoms associated with hepatic adenomas are all associated with large lesions which can cause intense abdominal pain.
- Focal nodular hyperplasia (FNH) is the second most common tumor of the liver. This tumor is the result of a congenital arteriovenous malformation hepatocyte response.

425. Ans. (b) Hepatic artery

Ref: Bailey & Love, 26th ed. pg. 1073

- Pringle manoeuvre: Atraumatic clamping of the hilar vessels to control hepatic bleeding from traumatic injuries also known-as the Pringle maneuver.
- This atraumatic clamp is placed at foramen of Winslow, *across the hepatoduodenal ligament*
- It clamps the portal vein and hepatic artery, and prevents excessive blood loss during parenchymal transection.

426. Ans. (d) Pale yellow

Ref: Bailey & Love, 26th ed. pg. 1106-1107

Morphology of gall stones
Cholesterol stones:
Cholesterol stones arise exclusively in the gallbladder and are composed of cholesterol. *Pure cholesterol stones are pale yellow, round to ovoid, and have a finely granular, hard external surface.* Stones composed largely of cholesterol are radiolucent: Presence of calcium carbonate in stones makes them radiopaque
Mixed stones:
Increasing proportions of calcium carbonate, phosphates, and bilirubin, the stones exhibit discoloration and appear gray-white to black

Contd...

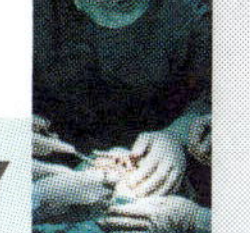

Pigment gallstones:
- Pigment stones are classified as "black" and "brown." *Black pigment stones* are found in *sterile gallbladder* bile and *brown stones* are found in *infected intrahepatic or extrahepatic ducts*.
- "Black" pigment stones contain oxidized polymers of the calcium salts of unconjugated bilirubin, small amounts of calcium carbonate, calcium phosphate, and mucin glycoprotein.
- "Brown" pigment stones contain pure calcium salts of unconjugated bilirubin, mucin glycoprotein, a substantial cholesterol fraction, and calcium salts of palmitate and stearate.

427. Ans. (a) Pigment stone

Ref: Bailey & Love, 26th ed. pg. 1106-1107

In hemolytic anemia like hereditary spherocytosis, on account of increased extravascular hemolysis, there is production of calcium bilirubinate stones (pigment stones).

428. Ans. (d) Liver cancer

Ref: Harrison, 18th ed. Ch. 91

- Aspirin suppresses cell proliferation by inhibiting prostaglandin synthesis.
- Regular aspirin use reduces the risk of colon adenomas and carcinomas as well as death from large-bowel cancer.

HEAD AND NECK

429. Ans. (b) Moderate

Ref: Harrison, 21st ed. pg. 3456

Severity	GCS*	LOC	PTA
Mild	13–15	<20 min–1 h	<24 h
Moderate	9–12	1–24 h	24 h – <7 days
Severe	3–8	>24 h	>7 days

430. Ans. (d) Squamous cell carcinoma

Ref: Bailey and Love, 27th ed. pg. 1086

Progressive Dysphagia would point to cause as esophageal cancer and SCC is the commonest one.

431. Ans. (d) Surgical excision

Ref: Bailey and Love, Textbook of Surgery, 27th ed. pg. 673

The image given above is suggestive of dermoid cyst.
- It is an abnormal growth (teratoma) containing epidermis, hair follicles, and sebaceous glands, derived from residual embryonic cells.
- Surgical removal is the only effective treatment for any type of dermoid cyst.

432. Ans. (a) Pyriform sinus

Ref: Bailey and Love, Textbook of Surgery, 27th ed. pg. 754

A branchial fistula may be unilateral or bilateral and is thought to represent a persistent second branchial cleft.
- The third branchial cleft sinus course is as follows: from the skin opening described above, the tract courses deep to platysma and course posterior to the internal carotid artery.
- It will pass between the glossopharyngeal and hypoglossal nerves and may be intimately associated with the superior laryngeal nerve.
- It then connects to the pyriform sinus in the larynx.

433. Ans. (a) Failure of fusion of maxillary and median nasal process

Ref: Bailey and Love, Textbook of Surgery, 27th ed. pg. 689

Cleft lip is a common congenital anomaly that is caused by defective fusion of the medial nasal and maxillary processes during embryologic development.
- Cleft palate is a developmental defect in the hard palate that results in a communication between the oral and nasal cavities resulting in nasal reflux during feeds. It is one of the most common congenital anomalies and has an excellent prognosis with appropriate diagnosis and surgical treatment.

434. Ans. (a) Surgical excision

Ref: Bailey and Love 27th ed. pg. 673

Angular dermoid cysts are common peri-orbital tumors in children. Characteristically benign and slow growing, they are tumors of embryonic origin that arise along bony sutures as a result of abnormal ectodermal sequestration during development. The best management is surgical excision with a well concealed scar.

435. Ans. (a) Extradural hematoma

Ref: Bailey and Love 27th ed. pg. 333

The Clinical history given is of lucid interval. The patient has regained consciousness between two periods of unconscious state. This is a characteristic feature of Extra-dural hemorrhage.

436. Ans. (d) Tracheostomy

Ref: Bailey and Love 27th ed. pg. 747

The image shows a tracheostomy tube in place.

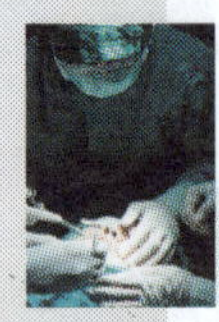

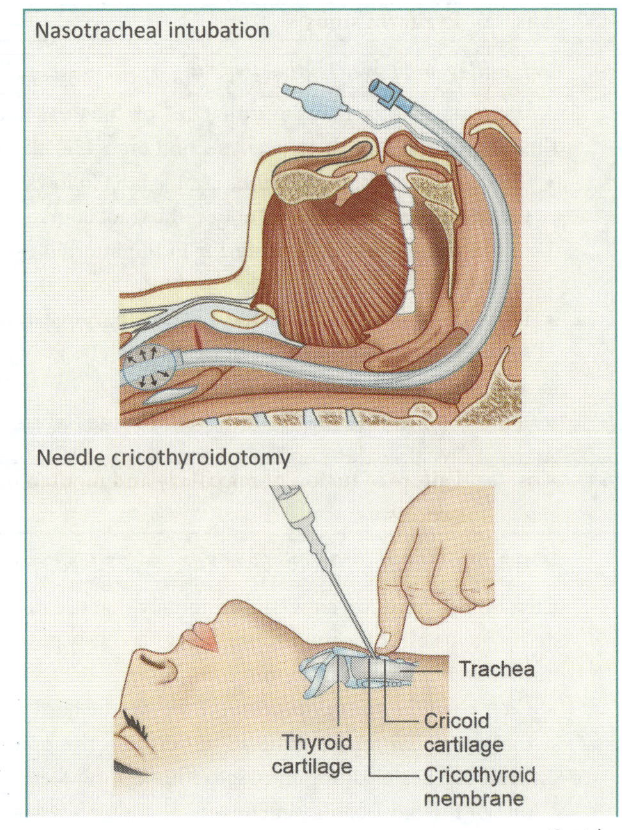

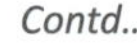

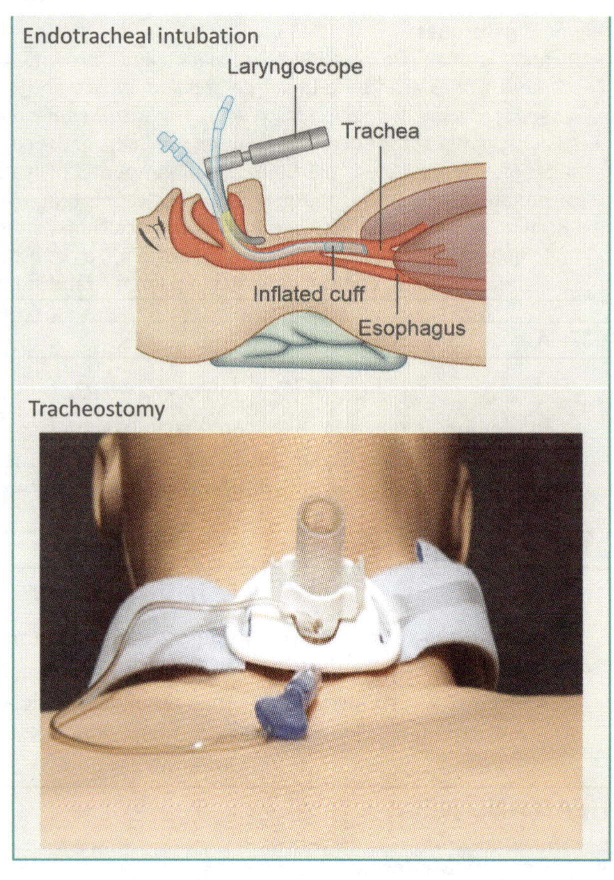

Contd...

437. Ans. (b) **Collar stud abscess**

Ref: Bailey and Love 27th ed. pg. 78

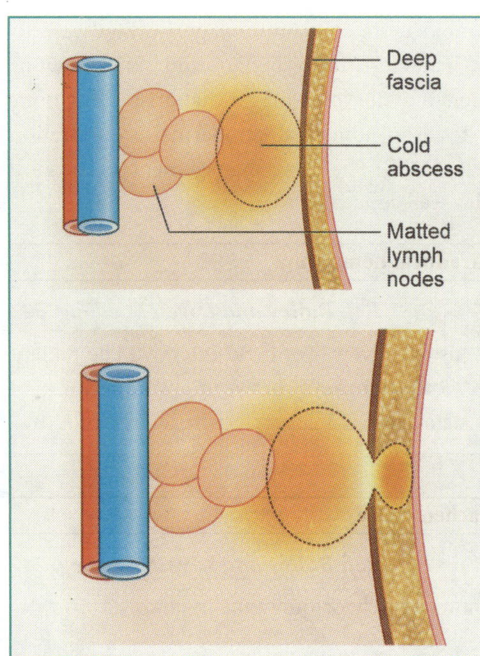

The image shows an induration at site of fistula with swelling originating from anterior triangle of neck. This is usually seen in case of Tuberculosis and is called *collar stud* abscess.

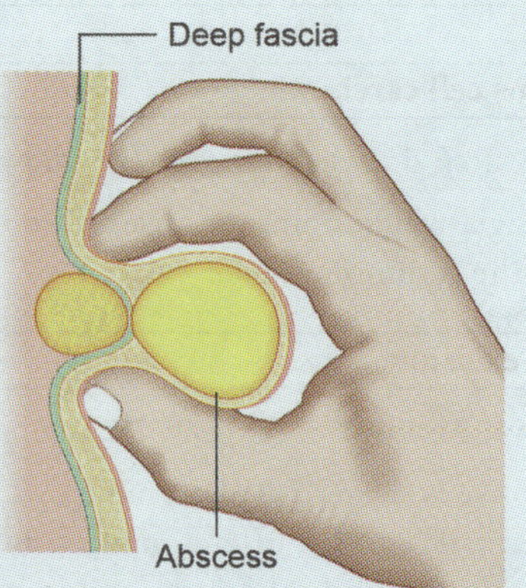

Option a is ruled out as it presents in posterior triangle of neck and does not have a fistula opening in neck.
Option c will have a watery discharge and is seen post excision of branchial cyst.
Option d is seen as midline swelling that moves with tongue protrusion.

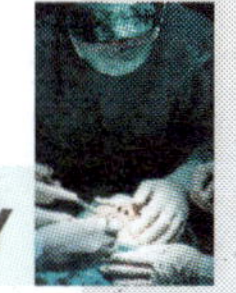

438. Ans. (c) Carotid body tumor

Ref: Bailey and Love 27th ed. pg. 757

Since the swelling is pulsatile it indicates vascular etiology. Option b and d are ruled out due to nonpulsatile nature.

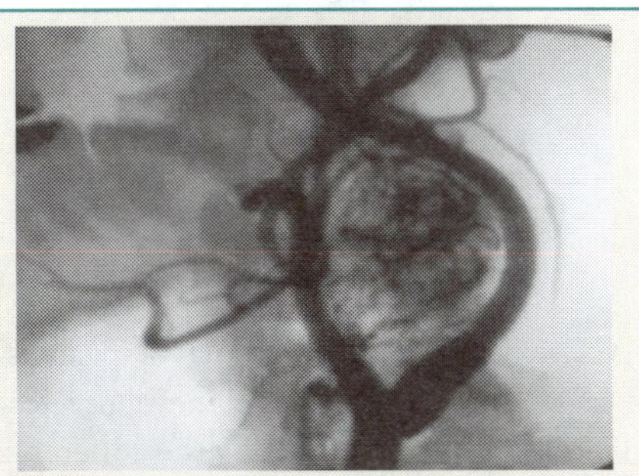

- The location of swelling at angle of jaw and producing an outward expansile impulse points to diagnosis of carotid body tumor.
- Normal carotid artery pulsations are present at lower part of neck medial to insertion of sternocleidomastoid.

439. Ans. (b) Characteristic Translucent

Ref: Bailey and Love 27th ed. pg. 779

- Ranula is a *mucous extravasation cyst* that arises from *sublingual gland* so option a and c are wrong. It is a clinical diagnosis and does not need a FNAC so option d is ruled out
- It has a characteristic translucent swelling that takes appearance of frog belly and traditional and effective way to treat it is to remove the sublingual gland.

440. Ans. (c) Oral lichen planus

Ref: SRB 5th ed. pg. 370

Conditions responsible for premalignant lesions of oral cavity

Equivocal risk lesions are:
- Oral lichen planus
- Dyskeratosis congenita
- Discoid lupus erythematosus

Medium risk lesions are:
- Oral submucosal fibrosis
- Syphilitic glossitis
- Sideropenic Glossitis/Plummer Vinson Syndrome

High risk Lesions are:
- Leukoplakia
- Erythroplakia
- Chronic hyperplastic candidiasis

441. Ans. (d) SCC of lip

Ref: SRB 5th ed. pg. 384

The image shows a fungating mass arising from mucosal part of lip. It shows everted edge with induration. The visible staining of teeth indicates that the patient may be using khaini (mixture of tobacco and lime) kept under the lip which is a common cause in Indian patients

The age of patient also favours the diagnosis. It is usually a well differentiated Squamous cell carcinoma.

Epulis	Plunging ranula	Basal cell cancer

442. Ans. (c) Nodulocystic

Ref: SRB, 5th ed. pg. 290

- The most common subtype of Basal cell cancer is rodent ulcer. It is the most common malignant skin tumor seen on face (Oghren line) and is also called tear cancer. The most common subtype is nodulocystic and noduloulcerative subtype.
- Choices a and b are subtypes of malignant melanoma. Choice d pigmented BCC mimics melanoma.

443. Ans. (c) Betel nut chewing

Ref: Harrison 19th ed. pg. 369

Causes of Submucosal Fibrosis

1. Prolonged irritation by chilies, tobacco (pan/quid), areca due to arecoline
2. Deficiency of vitamin A and B complex (riboflavin)
3. Localized collagen disorder

- It presents with soreness in mouth which increases during meals. There is trismus and difficulty in protruding the tongue. The entire area turns red and later has stiff fibrotic bands and scarring.
- Common sites are buccal mucosa, faucial pillars and soft palate.
- There is progressive nature of disease even with cessation of causative factors.

444. Ans. (d) Pain and paraesthesia in ulnar nerve distribution

- Neurologic symptoms occur in 95% of cases of thoracic outlet syndrome. The lower 2 nerve roots of the brachial plexus, C8 and T1, are most commonly (90%) involved, producing pain and paresthesias in the *ulnar nerve* distribution.

- The second most common anatomic pattern involves the upper 3 nerve roots of the brachial plexus, C5, C6, and C7, with symptoms referred to the neck, ear, upper chest, upper back, and outer arm in the radial nerve distribution.

445. Ans. (a) Frontal bone

- *Potts puffy tumor is a misnomer and is an acute osteomyelitis of frontal bone.*
- It has diffuse external swelling of scalp due to sub-periosteal pus formation and scalp oedema. It originates in frontal area.
- It presents as a boggy swelling with pitting scalp oedema. X-ray of Skull is done. It is treated with antibiotics and drainage under GA before it spreads to the CNS.
- Once it extends into the cranial cavity, it is managed by neurosurgical decompression using Dandy's Brain Cannula.

Complications
1. Osteomyelitis of frontal bone
2. Spread of infection of intracranial cavity.
3. Cortical venous thrombosis
4. Subdural empyema

446. Ans. (a) Rathke pouch

Ref: Harsh Mohan, 7th ed. pg. 787

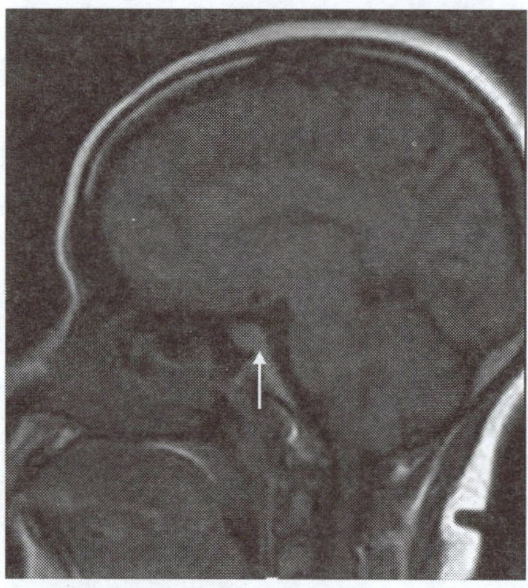

Features of Craniopharyngioma are:
- Slow-growing tumor
- Epithelial-squamous
- Calcified hence, visible even on X-ray skull
- Cystic tumor arising from remnants of the craniopharyngeal duct and/or Rathke cleft
- Occupying the (supra) sellar region.

447. Ans. (a) Extradural bleeding

Ref: Bailey, 26th ed. pg. 316

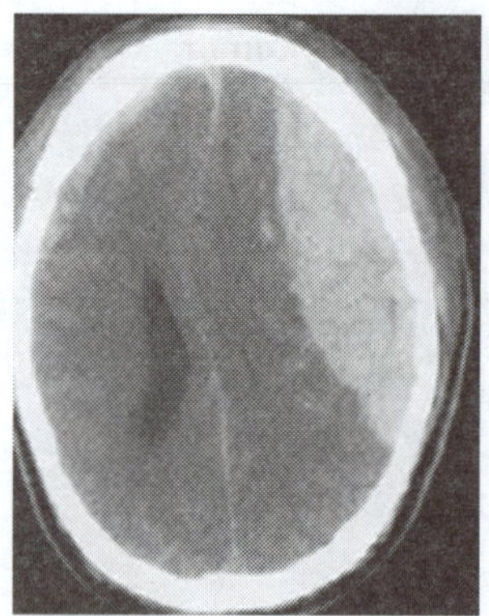

- On CT, extradural haematomas appear as a lentiform (lens shaped or biconvex) hyperdense lesion between skull and brain constrained by the adherence of the dura to the skull.
- Mass effect may be evident, with compression of surrounding brain and midline shift.
- Areas of mixed density suggest active bleeding.

448. Ans. (b) Nasopharyngeal cancer

Ref: Schwartz, 10th ed. pg. 583

Metastasis to Cervical lymph Nodes

Squamous cell carcinoma (SCC) is the most common histotype, followed by adenocarcinoma, undifferentiated carcinoma and other malignancies (for example, lymphoma and melanoma)

Common site for metastasis to neck nodes – Head and Neck (M.C.), Lungs (2nd M.C.), esophagus, stomach, ovary, pancreas. Approximately ten percent of patients with abnormal cervical nodes present without obvious primary. *Most common sites for unknown primary:*

1. Nasal Pharynx
2. Pyriform Sinus
3. Tongue Base
4. Tonsillar Crypts
5. Thyroid

The left supraclavicular node is called Virchow's node since it is on the left side of the neck where the lymphatic drainage of most of the body (from the thoracic duct) enters the venous circulation via the left subclavian vein. The metastasis blocks the thoracic duct leading to regurgitation into the surrounding nodes i.e. virchow's node.

449. Ans. (a) Astrocytoma

Ref: Harrison, 18th ed. pg. 379

- MC malignant brain tumor is astrocytoma
- Overall most common brain tumor: Metastasis (Oat cell cancer of lung)

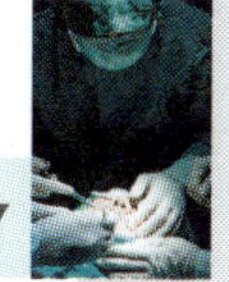

450. Ans. (a) Brain tumor

Ref: Harrison, 18th ed. pg. 379

RADIOSURGERY & STEREOTACTIC RADIOTHERAPY

- Radiosurgery refers to a single treatment with a relatively large dose of radiation by focusing many small beams of radiation from different directions onto a small tumor (up to 3 cm in diameter).
- The CyberKnife is a specially designed imaging-guided system in which a small linear accelerator is moved around the patient by a programmable robotic arm. In addition to treating tumors of the brain, the Cyberknife can be used to treat tumors of the spine and other sites such as the head and neck, prostate, liver, lung, and kidney.

There are two types of Stereotactic Radiation

- Stereotactic radiosurgery (SRS) refers to a single or several stereotactic radiation treatments of the brain or spine.
- Stereotactic body radiation therapy (SBRT) refers to one or several stereotactic radiation treatments with the body, excluding the brain or spine.
- Generally in brain the procedure is referred as stereotactic surgery if it is done in a single session or as **fractionated stereotactic radiotherapy (SRT),** if done in multiple sessions.
- If the therapy is done for other parts of the body then it is generally known as stereotactic radiotherapy

451. Ans. (d) Seminoma

Ref: Bailey & Love, 26th ed. pg. 1385

Radiosensitive tumors	Radioresistant tumors
• Neuroblastoma • Seminoma • Medulloblastoma • Wilm's tumor • Early cervical cancer and vaginal cancer • Head and neck tumors	• Renal cell cancer • Colonic cancer • Lung cancer • Melanoma • Sarcoma

452. Ans. (b) Osteosarcoma

Most common *secondary malignancy* in retinoblastoma is osteosarcoma developing in second decade of life.

453. Ans. (d) Seen with juvenile nasopharyngeal angiofibroma

Trotter's triad is seen with nasopharyngeal carcinoma

TROTTER'S TRIAD

1. Conductive deafness
2. Immobility of homolateral soft palate
3. Trigeminal neuralgia

Remember Commonly Asked Triads

Extra Mile

Triad of Alports Syndrome
- Sensorineural deafness/Progressive renal failure/Ocular anomalies

Triad of Behcet's Syndrome:
- Recurrent oral ulcers/Genital ulcers/Iridocyclitis [mnemonic: can't see, can't pee, can't eat spicy curry]

Beck's Triad
- Muffled heart sound/Distended neck veins/Hypotension

Gradenigo's Triad
- Sixth cranial n. Palsy/Persistent ear discharge/Deep seated retro orbital pain

Charcot's Triad
- Pain + fever + jaundice

Triad of Hypernephroma
- Pain + hematuria + renal mass Triad of Hypernephroma

Hutchinson's Triad
- Hutchison's teeth/Interstitial keratitis/Nerve deafness

Triad of Kwashiorkar
- Growth retardation/Mental changes/Edema

Saint's Triad
- Gall stones/Diverticulosis/Hiatus hernia

Trotter's Triad
- Conductive deafness/Immobility of homolateral soft palate/ Trigeminal neuralgia

Virchow's Triad
- Stasis/Hypercoagulabilty/Vessel injury

Fanconi Syndrome Triad
- Aminoaciduria/Proteinuria/Phosphaturia

454. Ans. (c) MC site is on Lateral margin

Ref: Bailey, & Love, 26th ed. pg. 713-14

TONGUE CANCER

- MC site is middle of lateral border or ventral aspect of the tongue.
- MC histological type is squamous cell carcinoma.
- **MC complaint:** Mid-irritation of tongue.
- MC associated risk factors are tobacco and alcohol.
- MC variety is ulcerative.
- *ONLY 30% patients present with cervical node metastasis.*
- The intrinsic tongue musculature provides little restriction to tumor growth, thus it may enlarge considerably before producing symptoms.
- Presents as painless mass or ulcer that fails to heal after minor trauma.

455. Ans. (c) Lateral margin of tongue

Ref: SRB Manual of Surgery, 4th ed. pg. 1310

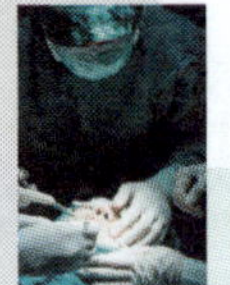

Squamous cell cancer of the tongue is the commonest cancer. The location is at the following sites:
- Lateral margin – 50%
- Posterior 1/3 rd tongue – 20%
- Dorsum – 6.5%
- Ventral surface – 6%
- Tip – 10%

456. Ans. (c) Cleft lip and palate

Ref: Bailey & Love, 26th ed. pg. 634

Orofacial clefts (ie, cleft lip [CL], cleft lip and palate [CLP], cleft palate [CP] alone, as well as median, lateral [transversal], oblique facial clefts) are among the most common congenital anomalies. *Approximately 1 case of orofacial cleft occurs in every 500-550 births.*

457. Ans. (c) Thyroglossal fistula

Ref: Dhingra's ENT, 5th ed. pg. 398

- Sublingual dermoid cyst present as midline submental swelling. This cyst is not attached to foramen cecum and hence doesn't move upon tongue protrusion or upon deglutition.
- The **thyroglossal cyst** classically moves upwards with swallowing and notably with tongue protrusion, as it is attached to foramen cecum. It merely indicates attachment to the hyoid bone.

458. Ans. (c) Cystic hygroma

Ref: Bailey & Love, 26th ed. pg. 701

CYSTIC HYGROMA/LYMPHANGIOMA

- Cystic hygromas are multiloculated cystic swelling filled with clear lymph lined by endothelial cells
- It results due to sequestration of a portion of the jugular lymph sac from the lymphatic system.
- It is associated with Turner's syndrome
- Most cystic hygromas involve the lymphatic jugular sacs
- **MC site:** Posterior neck region
- **Other common sites:** Axilla, mediastinum, inguinal and retroperitoneal regions
- Approximately 50% of them are present at birth.
- It may show spontaneous regression
- The cysts are filled with clear lymph and **lined by a single layer of endothelium epithelium.**

Clinical Features

- Usually manifests in the neonates or in early infancy (50% present at birth).
- Prone to infection and hemorrhage within the mass.
- Usually present as soft masses that distort the surrounding anatomy, can result in acute airway obstruction.
- Swelling is soft and partially compressible and invariably increases in size when the child coughs or cries.
- **Characteristic features: Brilliantly translucent**

Diagnosis: MRI plays a crucial role in preoperative planning

Treatment: Complete surgical excision is the preferred treatment.

Extra Mile

- Carotid body tumor aka potato tumor MC presents in 5th decade with firm, rubbery, mobile mass.
- Branchial cyst most commonly seen in older children or adolescents. However, all branchial remnants are present at the time of birth.

459. Ans. (d) Lined by columnar epithelium

Ref: Bailey & Love, 26th ed. pg. 700-701

VASCULAR SURGERY

460. Ans. (d) Rest pain

Ref: Bailey and Love, 27th ed. pg. 967

- Smoker with reduction in claudication distance points to Buerger's disease as the cause. Rest pain occurs in critical ischemia.
- Option a is ruled out causes severe thigh and leg tightness and pain with exercise. The pain typically takes 20-30 minutes of rest to resolve. Leg elevation can improve the time it takes to relieve the pain. In contrast, the case given dependency of legs is improving pain of the patient.
- Option b worsens on prolonged standing.
- Option c causes burning radicular pain on back of thigh and radiates down the calf and sole of foot.

461. Ans. (a) CCB

Ref: Bailey and Love, 27th ed. pg. 967

The clinical presentation is of Raynaud phenomenon and needs CCB for management of vasospasm in digital blood vessels.

462. Ans. (d) Buerger's disease

Ref: Bailey and Love, Textbook of Surgery, 27th ed. pg. 967

Buerger's disease (also known as thromboangiitis obliterans) affects blood vessels in the body, most commonly in the arms and legs.
- Arterial narrowing leads to severe ischemia and resultant pain, tissue damage, and even gangrene.
- History of smoking is the most important risk factor.

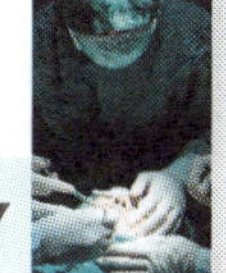

463. Ans. (a) Venous thromboembolism

Ref: Bailey and Love, Textbook of Surgery, 27th ed. pg. 986

The post-operative incidence of venous thromboembolism (VTE) is high for patients undergoing hip fracture surgery.

- Proximal femur fractures result from high velocity trauma in all age groups and could require prolonged immobilization, which is associated with increased risk of VTE.
- The diagnosis of VTE is frequently missed, however, because few signs and symptoms are recognized. It often presents as sudden breathlessness with chest pain, collapse with shock in the absence of other causes.

464. Ans. (d) CT angiography

Ref: Bailey and Love, Textbook of Surgery, 27th ed. pg. 989

A computed tomography pulmonary angiogram shows pulmonary emboli as filling defects in the pulmonary artery.

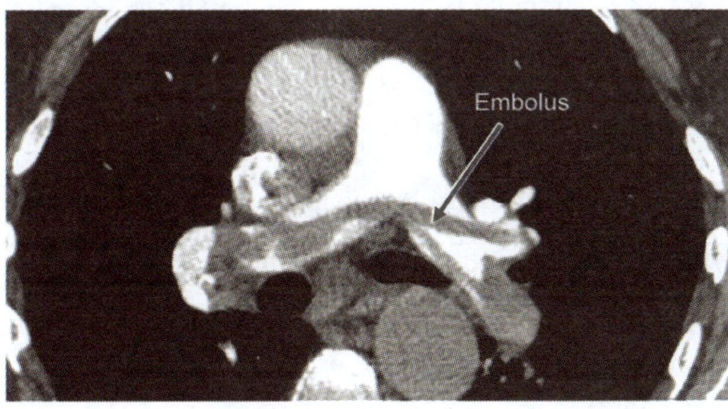

465. Ans. (a) Venous ulcer

Ref: Bailey and Love 25th ed. pg. 985

- The image shows a non-healing ulcer above medial malleolus in *skin of Gaiter region*, the area between muscles of calf and ankle. It is associated with hyperpigmentation of skin due to hemosiderin deposition. This is a feature of venous ulcer.
- This is the region where the Cockett perforators join the posterior tibial vein to surface vein called posterior arch vein.
- Choice b is seen on dorsum of foot at location of dorsalis pedis
- Optic c is seen on sole of foot at metatarsal heads or calcaneum
- Option d is seen related to sacrum.

466. Ans. (b) DVT

Ref: Bailey and Love 27th ed. pg. 986

- Prolonged immobilization is a risk factor for development of stasis of blood in calf veins/soleal veins. The development of fever and swelling in calf confirms the clinical diagnosis of Deep vein thrombosis for which a Doppler will be confirmatory.
- Option a leads to extensive redness and induration in soft tissues. Option c will cause desquamation and Option d causes prominent superficial veins in the legs.

467. Ans. (c) Deep vein thrombosis

Ref: Bailey and Love 27th ed. pg. 989

- Prolonged immobilization is a risk factor for venous stasis. The acute onset of unilateral leg swelling with tremendous increase in girth of limb with redness and shiny appearance of skin is a feature of Deep Vein thrombosis.
- Option a will produce red streak of cutaneous inflammation.
- Option b will produce painful inflamed veins especially after venous cannulation.
- Option d is a genetic condition and would be present since birth.

468. Ans. (a) Compartment syndrome

- Option d is seen post-operative and is ruled out. Option c is seen in smokers and presents with intermittent claudication. Option b is seen in immunocompromised patients or those with hematological malignancy.
- Post trauma stiffness/woody feel of muscles with pain and weak distal pulses is a feature of compartment of syndrome.

Extra Mile

6 P's of acute limb ischemia: Pain, Pallor, Paresthesias, Poikilothermia, Pulselessness, and Paralysis

Acute Compartment Syndrome

Typically presents with a rapid progression of symptoms

- Early presentation
  - Pain
    - Often not proportion to the extent of injury
    - Worse with passive stretching or extension of muscles
    - Very tight, wood -like muscles that are extremely tender to touch
  - Paresthesia (e.g., pins and needles)
  - Soft tissue swelling
  - Initially, peripheral circulation and distal pulses are maintained.
- Late presentation
  - Worsened pain and swelling
  - Muscle weakness to paralysis
  - Cold peripheries
  - Pallor or cyanosis
  - Absent (or weak) distal pulse

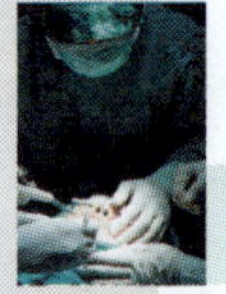

469. Ans. (c) Nonsuppurative and invasive

Ref: Bailey and Love 27th ed. pg. 48-49

Cellulitis is a non-suppurative, invasive infection of tissues related to point of injury. There is poor localization in addition to cardinal signs of spreading inflammation. It is typically caused by organisms like streptococci and C. perfringens. Tissue destruction, gangrene and ulceration may follow which cause release of proteases.

470. Ans. (c) Necrotizing fasciitis

Ref: Bailey and Love 27th ed. pg. 50

Diabetics are prone to infections. The image shows necrotizing fasciitis. It is caused by mix of organisms like coliforms, staph, Bacteroides. The aerobes destroy the tissues to allow anaerobes to thrive.

471. Ans. (a) Brodie Trendelenberg test I

Ref: SRB 5th ed. pg. 229

Clinical signs	
Brodie-trendelenberg's test I	Saphenofemoral incompetence
Brodie-trendelenberg's test II	Perforator incompetence
Perthe's test/modified perthe's	DVT
Tourniquet's test	Perforator incompetence
Schwartz test	Valvular incompetence
Fegan test	Perforator site localisation
Pratt's test	Blow outs = perforators

472. Ans. (a) Marjolin ulcer

Ref: Bailey and Love 26th ed. pg. 918

- Marjolin's ulcer is a squamous cell cancer that can develop in chronic long standing venous ulcer.
- Failure to heal an ulcer indicates it may have another coexisting cause like malignancy, Rheumatoid arthritis and arterial ulcer.
- Erythema Induratum of Bazin is a tuberculid showing lobular panniculitis. EIB is classified under cutaneous tuberculosis

473. Ans. (a) Neuralgia

Ref: Bailey and Love: 26th ed. pg. 912

COMPLICATIONS OF STANDARD VARICOSE VEIN SURGERY

- Infection
- Nerve injury. The incidence of saphenous nerve neuralgia is 7% following LSV stripping to the knee. The incidence of sural nerve neuropraxia and common peroneal nerve injury following SSV surgery is fairly high.

474. Ans. (c) Neuralgia

Ref: SRB, 5th ed. pg. 234

Two methods of Venous stripping are:
- Extraluminal collision technique using Myer's stripper
- Invagination technique using Codman stripper

COMPLICATIONS OF STRIPPING

- Saphenous neuralgia due to saphenous nerve injury/avulsion
- Numbness or tingling along femoral nerve distribution
- Hematoma
- Infections
- Ulceration
- Recurrence of disease

475. Ans. (c) Popliteal artery

Ref: SRB 5th ed. pg. 177

- About 70% of peripheral arterial aneurysms are popliteal aneurysm and 20% are iliofemoral aneurysms.
- These aneurysms frequently co-exist with abdominal aortic aneurysms.
- They usually cause limb ischemia and distal embolism.

476. Ans. (c) Relieved on standing still

Ref: Bailey 26th ed. Chapter 53, pg. 901

Intermittent claudication or vascular claudication is defined as:

- Pain that develops on walking/exercise
- Not seen with the first step (unlike osteoarthritis knees)
- Relieved by standing still (unlike neurogenic claudication)

The distance walked by the patient keeps on progressively reducing.

477. Ans. (b) Carotid angioplasty and stenting

Ref: Schwartz Principles of Surgery, 10th ed. pg. 903; Harrison 19th ed. pg. 2571-72

- Radiation induced occlusive carotid artery disease is due to Radiation given to head and neck area. It can lead to development of stroke.
- The best *screening* test is carotid Doppler and measure of carotid intimal thickness is used for diagnosis.
- The gold standard investigation is carotid angiography.
- Carotid angioplasty and stenting is the treatment of choice
- Carotid endarterectomy has higher incidence cranial nerve injury and wound infections which limits its use in these patients.

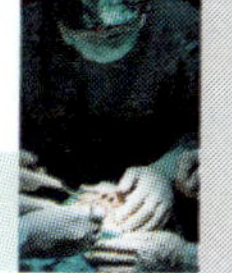

478. Ans. (d) Varicose veins

Ref: Bailey & Love, 26th ed. pg. 593/903

- Varicose veins are a cause of chronic leg edema and *not* a result of chronic leg edema.
- Edema is defined as a palpable swelling caused by an increase in interstitial fluid volume. The most likely cause of leg edema in patients over age 50 is venous insufficiency. ***Venous insufficiency affects up to 30% of the population, whereas heart failure affects only approximately 1%.***The most likely cause of leg edema in women under age 50 is ***idiopathic edema, formerly known as cyclic edema. Pulmonary hypertension and early heart failure can both cause leg edema before they become clinically obvious in other ways.***
- **Marjolin's ulcer** refers to an aggressive ulcerating squamous cell carcinoma presenting in an area of previously traumatized, chronically inflamed, or scarred skin. Histologically, the tumor is a well-differentiated squamous cell carcinoma. This carcinoma is aggressive in nature, spreads locally and is associated with a poor prognosis. Its edge is everted and not always raised. The IOC is a wedge biopsy.

479. Ans. (d) All of the above

Ref: Bailey & Love, 26th ed. pg. 899-900

- Acute-phase lesions have inflammation involving all coats of the vessel wall, especially of the veins, in association with occlusive thrombosis.
- Intermediate phase is characterized by progressive organization of the occlusive thrombus in the arteries and veins.
- Chronic phase or end-stage lesion is characterized by organization of the occlusive thrombus with extensive recanalization and prominent vascularization of the media.
- In all three phases, the normal architecture of the vessel wall subjacent to the occlusive thrombus and including the internal elastic lamina remains essentially intact.

480. Ans. (c) Small acral vessels of limb involvement causes hypohidrosis

Ref: Bailey & Love, 26th ed. pg. 899-900

- Arteries affected are plantar and digital vessels of the foot and lower leg. In advanced cases fingers and hands can be involved.
- Sympathetic overactivity can cause excessive sweating and capillary autonomic dysfunction. Raynaud's phenomenon can be a presentation with Buerger disease.
- The visceral and cerebral arteries are rarely involved.
- Phlebitis migrans and deep vein thrombosis is attributed to thrombophilia.
- Angiography shows normal proximal vasculature with cork screw collaterals.
- The most frequently affected arteries are anterior (41.4%) or posterior (40.4%) tibial arteries in the lower extremities, and the ulnar artery (11.5%) in the upper extremities.

481. Ans. (d) Saphenofemoral flush ligation with stripping

Ref: Bailey & Love, 26th ed. pg. 903-904

Sapheno-femoral flush ligation if done alone results in development of collaterals and thereby chances of recurrence. The long saphenous vein is not ligated until the T-junction has been confirmed and femoral vein has been exposed. The saphenous trunk is than retrogradely stripped to knee.

482. Ans. (d) All of these

Ref: Bailey & Love, 26th ed. pg. 899-900

- Buerger's disease is an inflammation of the arteries, veins, and nerves in the legs, principally, leading to restricted blood flow. Left untreated, Buerger's disease can lead to gangrene of the affected areas. Buerger's disease is also known as thrombo-angitis obliterans.
- Early symptoms include decrease in the blood supply (arterial ischemia) and superficial (near the skin surface) phlebitis. The main symptom is pain in the affected areas. Inflammation occurs in small and medium-sized arteries and veins near the surface of the limb. The pulse in arteries of the feet is weak or undetectable. The lack of blood flow can lead to gangrene. A cold sensitivity in the hands, similar to that seen in Raynaud's disease, can develop.

483. Ans. (b) Nerve regeneration

Ref: Bailey & Love, 26th ed. pg. 471

- **Hoffman Tinel sign** is seen in nerve regeneration and should not be confused with *Homan sign seen in deep vein thrombosis.*
- **Hoffman reflex** is elicited by a reflex test which verifies the presence or absence of lesions in the cortico-spinal tract. It is also known as the **finger flexor reflex**. The test involves tapping the nail or flicking the terminal phalanx of the middle or ring finger. A positive response is seen with flexion of the terminal phalanx of the thumb.

GENERAL SURGERY

484. Ans. (b) Epidermis and partial dermis

Ref: SRB 5th ed. pg. 136

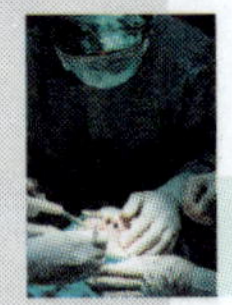

If the entire thickness of the dermis is included, the appropriate term is full-thickness skin graft (FTSG). If less than the entire thickness of the dermis is included, this graft is referred to as a split-thickness skin graft (STSG). STSGs are categorized further as thin (0.005-0.012 in), intermediate (0.012-0.018 in), or thick (0.018-0.030 in), based on the thickness of the harvested graft.

485. Ans. (d) First resuscitation then debridement and then grafting

Ref: SRB Manual of Surgery, pg. 139

- Initial step would be resuscitation to correct physiological metabolic derangements. Subsequently excise and debride the largest surface areas first, such as the anterior or posterior trunk or large areas on the extremities which will reduce the bacterial load as well.
- The delay of 24 to 48 hours before proceeding to the excision and grafting allows for the resuscitation and correction of physiologic derangements to optimize outcomes as well as providing time for the cells in the zone of stasis to become necrotic or demonstrate viability.

486. Ans. (b) Hair clippers inside the operation theater

Ref: Bailey and Love, 27th ed. pg. 52

Use of hair clippers just before surgery would cause minimal bacterial load at surgical site and reduce post operative SSI. Depilatory cream would be second best option. Shaving would create micro abrasions and increase the chances of bacterial contamination.

487. Ans. (d) Debridement and hyperbaric oxygen

Ref: SRB Manual of Surgery, pg. 65

The clinical diagnosis is necrotizing fasciitis and closure or flap closure would be contraindicated in setting of open wound for past 3 days. HBOT helps in improved wound healing.

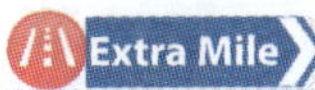

Indications for H.B.O.T
- Air embolism
- CO poisoning
- Necrotizing fasciitis
- Gas gangrene

488. Ans. (c) C

Ref: Bailey and Love, 27th ed. pg. 1309

In recent years, a transverse skin crease (Lanz) incision has become more popular, as the exposure is better and extension, when needed, is easier. The incision, appropriate in length to the size and obesity of the patient, is made approximately 2 cm below the umbilicus centred on the mid-clavicular—mid-inguinal line. When necessary, the incision may be extended medially, with retraction or suitable division of the rectus abdominis muscle.

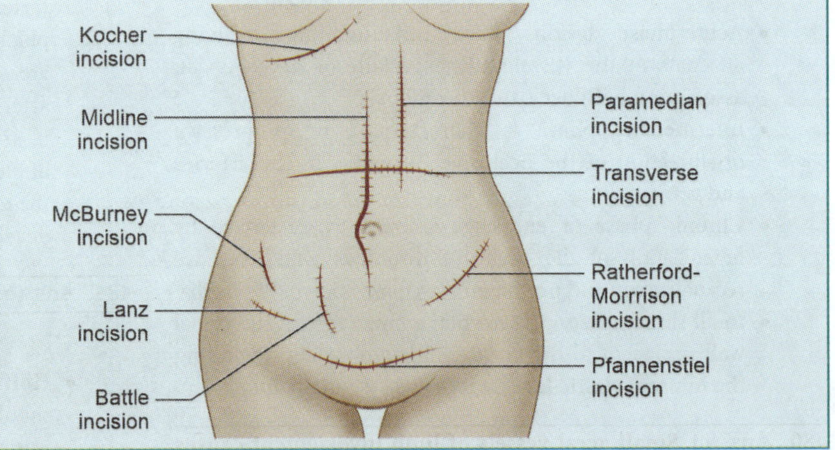

489. Ans. (d) Perforation of peptic ulcer

Ref: Bailey and Love, Textbook of Surgery, 27th ed. pg. 1116

The X-ray shows large amounts of free intraperitoneal gas, most easily appreciated under the right diaphragm and is diagnostic of perforated peptic ulcer.
- Perforated peptic ulcer is a serious complication of PUD and patients with PPU often present with acute abdomen.
- Early surgery and aggressive management of sepsis are the mainstays of therapy.

490. Ans. (c) Lung metastasis

Ref: Bailey and Love, Textbook of Surgery, 27th ed. pg. 1508, 934

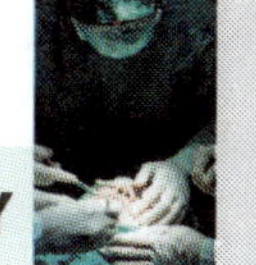

Cannon ball metastases refer to multiple large, well-circumscribed, round pulmonary metastases that appear not unsurprisingly like cannon balls.

- Cannon ball lesions in lung fields are most commonly due to hematogenous spread of a primary malignancy elsewhere; the most common primaries are as follows: Breast carcinoma, colorectal carcinoma, renal cell carcinoma.

491. Ans. (a) Pulmonary hamartoma

Ref: Bailey and Love, Textbook of Surgery, 27th ed. pg. 934

Popcorn calcification refers to amorphous calcifications often with rings and arcs that resemble popped corn kernels.

- About 30% of hamartomas show characteristic calcification on chest radiographs which often resemble popcorn.

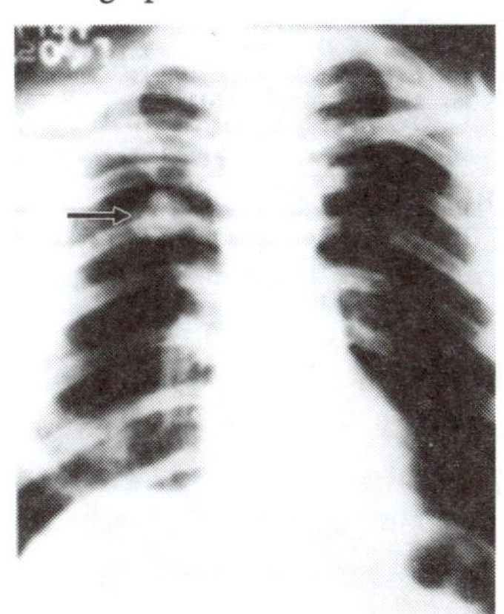

Chest radiograph showing a well-defined solitary pulmonary nodule with popcorn pattern of calcification in the right upper lobe.

492. Ans. (b) Bronchogenic carcinoma

Ref: Bailey and Love, Textbook of Surgery, 27th ed. pg. 925

Chest X-ray demonstrates an increased density in the right upper medial hemithorax with loss of volume, and shift of the trachea to the right. A mass is present at the right hilum.

- This case demonstrates the typical appearances of a reverse S sign of Golden (aka Golden S sign). This patient had a primary bronchogenic carcinoma at the hilum.

493. Ans. (a) Esophagus

Ref: Bailey and Love, Textbook of Surgery, 27th ed. pg. 1073

The esophagus is the most common site for an acute foreign body or food impaction in the gastrointestinal tract, and 80 to 90% of swallowed objects that reach the stomach will eventually pass without intervention.

- Flat objects like coins, bottle caps, or disc batteries are usually oriented in the coronal plane if they are lodged in the esophagus and appear round on the frontal (PA) view.
- However, if they are lodged in the trachea, they orient in the sagittal plane and appear round on the lateral view.

494. Ans. (d) 30 mm Hg

Ref: Bailey and Love, Textbook of Surgery, 27th ed. pg. 29

Pressure ulcers are a type of injury that breaks down the skin and underlying tissue when an area of skin is placed under constant pressure for certain period causing tissue ischemia, cessation of nutrition and oxygen supply to the tissues and eventually tissue necrosis.

- External pressure of more than 33 mm Hg occludes the blood vessel so that the underlying and surrounding tissues become anoxic and if the pressure continues for a critical duration, cell death will occur, resulting in soft tissue necrosis and eventual ulceration.

495. Ans. (a) Hypertrophic scar

Ref: Bailey and Love, Textbook of Surgery, 27th ed. pg. 31

A hypertrophic scar is a thick raised scar that's an abnormal response to wound healing and occurs *within the limits of lesion.*

- They more commonly occur in taut skin areas following skin trauma, burns or surgical incisions.
- Treatments include medication, freezing, injections, lasers and surgery.

Scar	Keloid	Hypertrophic scar
Clinical findings Extension Involution Appearance	Beyond the limits of injury Without spontaneous regression Bright, nodules, telangiectasias, thin skin, ulceration, and hyperpigmentation possible	Within the limits of the lesion Spontaneous regression Red or pinkish, rarely thicker than 4 mm
Symptom	Pain, itching	Itching
Histopathology Cellularity (fibroblasts) Collagen Type of collagen Skin appendages Stages of healing	Smaller, without myofibroblasts Thick, irregular bundles 3 Without glands or hair follicles Do not enter in the remodeling phase	Greater Arrangements in nodules, parallel to the epidermi 1 and 3 May have glands or hair follicles Can enter in the remodeling phase

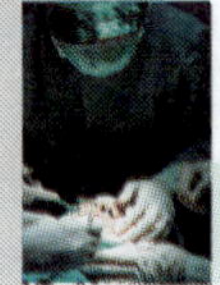

496. Ans. (d) Exploratory laparotomy

Ref: Bailey and Love, Textbook of Surgery, 27th ed. pg. 372

The following case is suggestive of hemoperitoneum in the patient following RTA.

- Hemodynamically unstable trauma patients with hemoperitoneum should undergo exploratory laparotomy without any delay.

497. Ans. (a) Cardiac tamponade

Ref: Bailey and Love, Textbook of Surgery, 27th ed. pg. 367

The image shows Hemopericardium that would cause cardiac tamponade.

- Because of the pressure the heart can't beat correctly, causing a drop in blood pressure. If not treated, it is always fatal.
- The classic signs of Beck's triad include low blood pressure, distension of the jugular veins and decreased or muffled heart sounds on cardiac auscultation.

498. Ans. (b) E2M3V3

Ref: Bailey and Love, Textbook of Surgery, 27th ed. pg. 325

TABLE: Glasgow coma scale

Behavior	Response	Score
Eye opening response	Spontaneously	4
	To speech	3
	To pain	2
	No response	1
Best verbal response	Oriented to time, place, and person	5
	Confused	4
	Inappropriate words	3
	Incomprehensible sounds	2
	No response	1
Best motor response	Obeys commands	6
	Moves to localized pain	5
	Flexion withdrawal from pain	4
	Abnormal flexion (decorticate)	3
	Abnormal extension (decerebrate)	2
	No response	1
Total score	Best response	15
	Comatose client	8 or less
	Totally unresponsive	3

499. Ans. (b) Tension pneumothorax

Ref: Bailey and Love, Textbook of Surgery, 27th ed. pg. 366

Features suggestive of Tension pneumothorax are:

- Deep Sulcus sign
- Absent vascular shadows
- Contralateral shift of the mediastinum
- Depression of the hemidiaphragm

500. Ans. (b) Perforation peritonitis

Ref: Bailey and Love, Textbook of Surgery, 27th ed. pg. 210

The imaging diagnosis of bowel perforation almost always relies on seeing pneumoperitoneum.

- Free gas under the diaphragm is a classic sign of pneumoperitoneum on the erect chest and abdomen radiographs and it is suspicious for bowel perforation.

501. Ans. (a) I 131

Ref: Bailey and Love, Textbook of Surgery, 27th ed. pg. 804

I-131 scan is an important imaging tool to aid the diagnosis and treatment of multiple thyroid disorders. Particularly pre-therapy and post-therapy scan in differentiated thyroid cancer patients allows surveillance of the disease and guide the clinician for the treatment plan.

- I-131 radiotherapy is a treatment for thyroid cancer that typically follows surgery to remove the thyroid.

502. Ans. (a) 18F

Ref: Bailey and Love, Textbook of Surgery, 27th ed. pg. 200

Positron emission tomography (PET) with 2-deoxy-2-[fluorine-18] fluoro-D-glucose (18F-FDG), an analogue of glucose, provides valuable functional information based on the increased glucose uptake and glycolysis of cancer cells and depicts metabolic abnormalities before morphological alterations occur.

- The most important current clinical applications of 18F-FDG PET/CT in breast cancer patients is for the detection and evaluation of recurrent or metastatic disease and for monitoring response to therapy.

503. Ans. (c) Chest tube insertion on right side

Ref: Bailey and love 27th ed. pg. 919

The CXR shows a hyper-translucent lung with absent vascular markings on right side. The diagnosis is right sided pneumothorax. This will require an ICD in 5th intercostal space on right side. There is also evidence of mediastinal shift.

504. Ans. (b) Keloid

Ref: Bailey and Love 27th ed. pg. 31

- The image shows a keloid over sternum. It is present at its usual site which is in area between xiphisternum and two shoulder tips.
- Atrophic scar is pale, flat and stretched which the image shows excessive tissue.
- Hypertrophic scare does not extend beyond the boundary of original incision while the image shows a scar extending outside the original incision site.

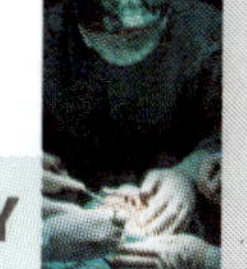

505. Ans. (d) 5% dextrose

Ref: Bailey and Love 27th ed. pg. 336

In patients with raised ICP, hypotonic fluids like 5% dextrose are contraindicated as they will cause further increase in swelling of brain and will cause deterioration. Rather we need to use hypertonic saline and mannitol.

506. Ans. (c) Hypovolemic

Ref: Bailey and Love 27th ed. pg. 14

- Since the patient is having bleeding and has CVP on lower side of normal he is having Hypovolemic shock. Normal CVP is 2-10 cm of Water.
- Option A is seen post MI. Option B is seen in spinal Shock/trauma to spinal cord. Option D is seen in anaphylaxis, septic shock and spinal cord injury.
- Spinal cord injury will reduce sympathomimetic outflow leading to it being an example of both neurogenic and distributive shock.

Cardiovascular and metabolic characteristics of shock

	Hypovolaemia	Cardiogenic	Obstructive	Distributive
Cardiac output	Low	Low	Low	High
Vascular resistance	High	High	High	Low
Venous pressure	Low	High	High	Low
Mixed venous saturation	Low	Low	Low	High

Extra Mile

Endocrine Shock

It is a combination of hypovolemic, cardiogenic or distributive shock. Important causes include hypo or hyperthyroidism and adrenal insufficiency.

Hypothyroidism causes a shock state similar to neurogenic shock due to disordered vascular and cardiac responsiveness to circulating catecholamines.

507. Ans. (c) Chest X-ray

Ref: Bailey and Love 27th ed. pg. 287

- The main advantage of a post procedure (central line insertion) CXR is to detect malposition, kinking of catheter and pneumothorax.
- Only transesophageal echocardiography can accurately detect a CVC tip in relation to superior vena cava and right atrium but its availability as a bedside tool is limited to major hospitals.
- Intraoperative monitoring of CVP is done via central line in Internal Jugular vein or subclavian vein.

508. Ans. (c) Orange

Ref: Emergencies in Anesthesia 3rd ed. pg. 483

- For resuscitation, greatest flow is through a short wide gauge cannula. Two 14G orange cannula in large forearm or antecubital fossa veins are recommended. If not available then grey 16G or white 17G cannula can be used.
- Blue cannula is used in pediatrics. Green cannula is used for routine fluid infusion or Blood transfusions in male patient.

509. Ans. (d) Carbuncle

Ref: SRB 5th ed. pg. 47

The image shows a suppurative collection with *multiple sieves* with discharging pus. This is a carbuncle and the sieves may fuse together to form a central necrotic ulcer. It is an infective gangrene of skin and subcutaneous tissue and occurs on nape of neck and back.

510. Ans. (c) Hypertonic saline

Ref: Harrison 20th ed. pg. 2077

Hypotonic fluids should not be given in case of severe head injury as they will worsen the brain swelling. It is *hypertonic fluids* like 3% saline or mannitol that will reduce the cerebral edema in cases of raised Intracranial pressure.

511. Ans. (c) Exploratory laparotomy

Ref: Bailey and Love 27th ed. pg. 1051

- The CXR shows evidence of gas under diaphragm implying perforation peritonitis. The patient will need an urgent exploratory laparotomy.
- Option a and b are done for focal fluid/pus collections while Option d would be required in sigmoid volvulus.

512. Ans. (b) Red – Yellow – Green – Black

Ref: Bailey and Love 27th ed. pg. 412

- Red = Most critically injured that need immediate treatment right now
- Yellow = Less critical need urgent treatment within hours
- Green = No limb or life-threatening injury so likely to survive if treatment is delayed by hours or days
- Black = Moribund patient, non-breathing or pulseless

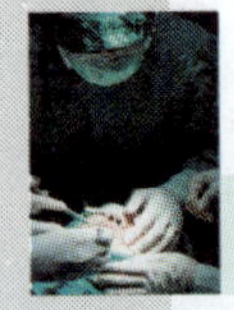

Triage categories.

Priority	Colour	Medical need	Clinical status	Examples
First (I)	Red	Immediate	Critical, but likely to survive if treatment given early	Severe facial trauma, tension pneumothorax, profuse external bleeding, haemothorax, flail chest, major intra-abdominal bleed, extradural haematomas
Second (II)	Yellow	Urgent	Critical, likely to survive if treatment given within hours	Compound fractures, degloving injuries, ruptured abdominal viscus, pelvic fractures, spinal injuries
Third (III)	Green	Non-urgent	Stable, likely to survive even if treatment is delayed for hours to days	Simple fractures, sprains, minor lacerations
Last (0)	Black	Unsalvageable	Not breathing, pulseless, so severely injured that no medical care is likely to help	Severe brain damage, very extensive burns, major disruption/loss of chest or abdominal wall structures

513. Ans. (a) 1

Ref: Sabiston E-Book pg. 1109

- Zone 1 is central retroperitoneal hemorrhage and has highest risk of vascular injury and needs exploration.
- Zone 2 is lateral and involves renal injuries. Blunt injury would require observation and follow up while renal vascular injury would require angiographic embolization.
- Zone 3 would be associated with pelvic fracture and does not require exploration as controlling bleed in pelvis would be very difficult.

514. Ans. (a) Fat embolism

Ref: Bailey and Love 27th ed. pg. 956

- Long bone fracture and subsequent development of respiratory distress favors diagnosis of Fat embolism.
- Option B is seen in post-operative state where patient is immobilized for long duration.
- Option C is seen with neurosurgery.
- Option D is seen with parasitic infestation.

515. Ans. (c) NCCT

Ref: Bailey and Love 27th ed. pg. 207

The best investigation to work out diagnosis of Extradural vs subdural vs subarachnoid vs intraparenchymal hemorrhage is Non-Contrast CT head.

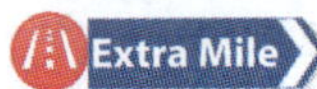

CT is the best modality to pick up Intracranial, intra-abdominal and vertebral injuries.

516. Ans. (b) Leukocytosis

Ref: Bailey and Love 27th ed. pg. 1307

Alvarado score is used for clinical diagnosis of Acute appendicitis. There are two components of Alvarado score that has value assigned as 2 points. They are tenderness in RIF and Leucocytosis. The remaining components are assigned one point each. For diagnosis of acute appendicitis score of 7 or more improves diagnostic sensitivity.

The alvarado (mantrels) score

	Score
Symptoms Migratory RIF pain	
Anorexia	1
Nausea and vomiting	1
Signs	
Tenderness (RIF)	2
Rebound tenderness	1
Elevated temperature	1
Laboratory	
Leucocytosis	2
Shift to left	1
Total	10

517. Ans. (d) Triage

Ref: Bailey and Love 27th ed. pg. 412

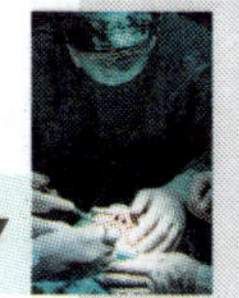

Triage categories.

Priority	Colour	Medical need	Clinical status	Examples
First (I)	Red	Immediate	Critical, but likely to survive if treatment given early	Severe facial trauma, tension pneumothorax, profuse external bleeding, haemothorax, flail chest, major intra-abdominal bleed, extradural haematomas
Second (II)	Yellow	Urgent	Critical, likely to survive if treatment given within hours	Compound fractures, degloving injuries, ruptured abdominal viscus, pelvic fractures, spinal injuries
Third (III)	Green	Non-urgent	Stable, likely to survive even if treatment is delayed for hours to days	Simple fractures, sprains, minor lacerations
Last (0)	Black	Unsalvageable	Not breathing, pulseless, so severely injured that no medical care is likely to help	Severe brain damage, very extensive burns, major disruption/loss of chest or abdominal wall structures

518. Ans. (d) Insert needle in 2nd intercostal space

Ref: Harrison 20th ed. pg. 2009

- The clinical diagnosis based on history of rib fractures, respiratory distress and hypotension is pneumothorax. There can be concomitant hemothorax but treatment of obstructive shock caused by pneumothorax is the immediate step.
- This would be done by inserting a wide bore needle in second intercostal space to reduce the impact of obstructive shock and increase systolic blood pressure.
- According to recent ATLS guidelines, wide bore needle should be inserted in 5th intercostal space.

519. Ans. (c) Sitting with neck flexed

Ref: Oxford Handbook of Clinical Medicine, pg. 773

Nasogastric tube should be inserted in a conscious patient in sitting position with slight flexion of the neck.

Procedure for inserting NG tube

- Examine the patient's nostril to check for septal deviation and identify the more patent nostril
- Instil viscous lidocaine into the patient's nostril
- Estimate the length of insertion by measuring the distance from the tip of the nose, around the ear, and down to just below the left costal margin.
- The estimated length falls in between the 2nd and 3rd pre-printed black lines on the tube
- Position the patient sitting upright with the neck partially flexed. Ask the patient to hold a cup of water in his or her hand and put a straw in his or her mouth with instructions to sip water only when asked to.

Contd...

- Gently insert the NG tube along the floor of the nose, and advance it parallel to the nasal floor (i.e. directly perpendicular to the patient's head, not angled up into the nose) until it reaches the back of the nasopharynx, where resistance will be met (10-20 cm).
- At this time, ask the patient to sip on the water through the straw and start to swallow.
- Notice the flexion in the neck of the patient while the patient is swallowing water through a straw while the NG is advanced forwards.
- Continue to advance the NG tube until the distance of the previously estimated length is reached.

520. Ans. (c) 10

Ref: Harrison 20th ed. pg. 3183

Eye opening to pain = 2

Confused= 4

Flexion on painful noxious stimuli to arm = 4

Score = 10

Eye opening (E)		Verbal response (V)	
Spontaneous	4	Oriented	5
To speech	3	Confused	4
To pressure	2	Words	3
None	1	Sounds	2
		None	1
Best motor response (M)			
Obeying commands	6		
Localizing	5		
Normal flexion	4		
Abnormal flexion	3		
Extension	2		
None	1		

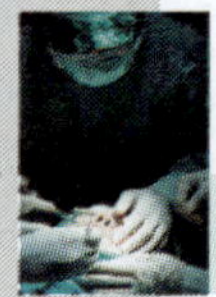

521. Ans. (b) Intramarginal excision followed by radiation

Ref: SRB, 5th ed. pg. 12

- Excisional surgery alone has been shown to yield a 45-100% recurrence rate and should very rarely be used as a solitary modality, although excision in combination with adjunct measures can be curative.
- Most studies in which excisional surgery was combined with injected steroids reported a recurrence rate of less than 50%.
- *Surgery followed by adjunctive radiotherapy has obtained recurrence rates of 0–8.6%*

522. Ans. (b) Pleural cavity

Ref: Bailey and Love: 26th ed. pg. 109

FAST looks for fluid in following *five* areas

- Perihepatic area and hepatorenal space
- Peri-splenic area
- Left and right Pericolic gutters
- Pelvis
- Pericardium

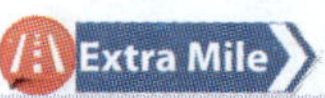

Extra Mile

Focused abdominal sonar for trauma
- It detects free fluid in the abdomen or pericardium
- It will not reliably detect less than 100 ml of free blood
- It does not identify injury to hollow viscus
- It cannot reliably exclude injury in penetrating trauma
- It may need repeating or supplementing with other investigations

523. Ans. (a) 60 minutes before skin incision

Ref: Bailey and Love 26th ed. pg. 248

- The timing of antibiotic administration may vary, but the *goal of administering preoperative systemic prophylactic antibiotics is to have the concentration in the tissues at its highest* at the start and during surgery.
- The literature supports at least 30 minutes, but no greater than 60 minutes before the skin incision is the optimal timing for the pre-operative administration of most commonly used antibiotics
- The antibiotic used most commonly is cefazolin
- The antibiotic must be stopped within 48 hours of the surgery.

524. Ans. (c) Excision

Ref: Bailey and Love: 26th ed. pg. 725

- Mucous retention cysts develop in floor of mouth either from obstructed minor salivary glans or from sublingual salivary gland.
- The term ranula applies to mucous extravasation cyst that arises from a sublingual gland producing an appearance of a frog belly.
- It can resolve spontaneously or *requires formal surgical excision of cyst and affected sublingual gland.*
- Incision and drainage results in recurrence.
- Sometimes the cyst may perforate through mylohyoid muscle diaphragm to enter the neck and is called plunging ranula.

525. Ans. (b) 24-hour urinary Fractionated Metanephrine

Ref: Bailey and Love 26th ed. pg. 784

- Catecholamines like nor-epinephrine, epinephrine and dopamine are produced in excess by chromaffin cells of pheochromocytoma.
- The end product of metabolism of these catecholamines is fractionated metanephrine levels.
- Vaniyl mandelic acid levels are used for diagnosis of neuroblastoma.

526. Ans. (a) Sebaceous cyst

Ref: SRB: 5th ed, pg. 78

The image shows a sebaceous cyst on the scalp. Other common sites apart from scalp are face and scrotum. It contains a cheesy white material with putty consistency. It is not seen in palms and soles as there are no sebaceous glands.

527. Ans. (a) Lipoma

Ref: SRB: 5th ed, pg. 72

- The image shows a solitary lipoma on dorsum of neck with probably a decubitus ulcer. They are common in males and are common in back, shoulder and upper arm.
- Choice B is seen in pediatric age group and survival up to adult age group is unlikely. Choice C is seen in posterior triangle of neck
- Choice D is unlikely at occiput.

528. Ans. (b) Gut

Ref: Bailey and Love: 26th ed. pg. 1429

Progress in small bowel transplantation has lagged behind others since intestinal transplants stimulate a strong graft rejection response *because small intestine contains large amount of lymphoid tissue.* Moreover, ischemia and rejection increase intestinal permeability and allow translocation of bacteria from the lumen of bowel.

529. Ans. (a) Kidney

Ref: Bailey and Love: 26th ed. pg.18

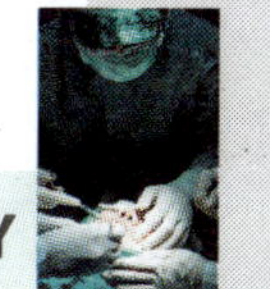

Urine out-put is a reliable indicator of end organ perfusion. The Brain and heart continue to receive blood supply at the expense of other organs. The Kidney insult in hypovolemic shock indicates decompensation process has started and resuscitative measures are not working.

530. Ans. (b) S.T.D

Ref: SRB 5th ed. pg. 36

It is a common sense question that hospital acquired infections would be surgical site infection. Urinary tract infection and pneumonia. Sexually transmitted infections would be on account of high-risk sexual behaviour prevalent amongst young adults.

531. Ans. (c) 30-40%

Ref: SRB: 5th ed. pg. 120

TABLE: Classification of Hemorrhagic shock

Shock class	Blood loss mL (%)	Heart rate beats/min	Blood pressure	Respiratory rate breaths/min	Mental status
I	<750 (15)	<100	Normal	14–20	Slightly anxious
II	750–1500 (15–30)	100–120	Normal	20–30	Mildly anxious
III	1500–2000 (30–40)	120–140	Decreased	30–40	Anxious, confused
IV	>2000 (>40)	>140	Decreased	>35	Confused, lethargic

532. Ans. (a) Wet gangrene

Ref: SRB: 5th ed, pg. 206

The image shows a gangrenous toe of left foot with a vague line of demarcation. The part is putrefied and discoloured. Notice the proximal swelling, erythema and slight ulceration. Usual causes are emboli or trauma.

Feature	Dry gangrene	Wet gangrene	Gas gangrene
Site	Commonly limbs	More common in bowel	Limbs
Mechanism	Arterial occlusion	More commonly venous obstruction	Gases produced by *Clostridium bacteria*
Macroscopy	Organ dry, shrunken, and black	Part moist, soft, swollen, rotten, and dark	Organ red, cold, pale, numb, shriveled up, and auto-amputation
Putrefaction	Limited due to very little blood supply	Marked due to congestion of organ with blood	Marked due to bacteria and infiltration of gases produced by them in tissues
Line of demarcation	Present at the junction between healthy and gangrenous parts	No clear-cut line of demarcation	No clear-cut line of demarcation
Bacteria	Bacteria fail to survive	Numerous present	Major cause
Prognosis	Generally better due to little septicemia	Generally poor due to profound toxemia	Generally poor due to quick spread to the surrounding tissues

533. Ans. (a) Subcutaneous emphysema

Ref: Bailey and Love: 26th ed. pg. 933

- The image shows puffiness of face with examination finding of crepitus the diagnosis is subcutaneous emphysema.
- Choice b is ruled out as there is history of any trauma given in the patient
- Choice c is ruled out as no history suggestive of acute kidney injury is given.
- Choice d is ruled out as no facial plethora or dilated collaterals on the chest are seen.

534. Ans. (a) 3

Ref: SRB 5th ed. pg. 1093

Eye opening = 1	Verbal response = 1	Motor response = 1

Hence the total score is 3. GCS is any way not designed to identify brain death but is used to evaluate presence of coma.

Extra Mile

- Mild head injury GCS score: 13–15
- Moderate head injury GCS score: 9–12
- Severe head injury GCS score: 3–8

535. Ans. (c) 4 L

Ref: SRB 5th ed. pg. 133

Applying the Parkland formula: 4 mL per % of burn per kg body weight

$4 \times 50 \times 40 = 8000$ mL = 8 L

Out of this total 8 L, the first 4 L is given over 8 hours and rest 4 L over the remaining 16 hours.

Extra Mile

In burns patient, Muir and Barclay formula is used to calculate the *colloid* to be given after 24 hours of admission.

536. Ans. (a) Elective intubation

Ref: SRB 5th ed. pg. 138

- Airway burns are evidenced by singeing of nasal hair and burns on face and neck.
- Hence *elective intubation is recommended with regular performance of pulmonary toilet* to remove the secretions.
- In case routine intubation is not possible, nasopharyngeal intubation should be performed.
- Tracheostomy/cricothyroidotomy can be life-saving especially in case of endotracheal intubation being not possible.
- However tracheostomy performance via burned tissue of neck has *increased complication rate and risk of sepsis as compared to elective intubation.*

537. Ans. (a) Acute limb ischemia

Ref: SRB Surgery: 5th ed. pg. 191

Treatment of Embolism and Thrombosis of Acute Limb Ischaemia

Immediate infusion of 5000-10,000 units of IV heparin and relief of pain are needed first

Surgical

- Embolectomy (surgical exploration and removal of clot) is the choice for embolus. It is done either by interventional balloon 5 French (Fogarty, 1963) embolectomy or open method. It is the standard treatment for arterial embolism. It can be repeated several times until adequate bleeding occurs
- For acute thrombosis causing acute limb ischaemica, open thrombectomy with or without bypass may be the surgical treatment: but it is not the standard treatment for acute thrombosis (standard is thrombolysis, Dotter and co, 1974)

Endovascular therapy

- Intra-arterial thrombolysis using urokinase
- *Percutaneous mechanical thrombectomy*-it is done either by suctioning clot via catheter or dissolution of thrombus by pulverisation and aspiration by high speed motors or fluid jets
- Ultrasound accelerated thrombolysis using catheter based or transdermal using acoustic cavitation to ablate thrombus

Embolectomy

- It is done as early as possible as an emergency, operation.
- Under fluoroscopic guidance. Fogarty catheter (interventional radiology) is passed beyond the embolus and the balloon is inflated. Catheter is withdrawn out gently with embolus. Procedure has to be repeated until embolectomy is completed and good back bleeding occurs. Angiogram is repeated to confirm the free flow
- Postoperatively initially heparin and later oral anticoagulants are used. Procedure is done under general anaesthesia or local anaesthesia.

538. Ans. (a) Cutting needle

- *Cutting needle* is used to suture skin, aponeurosis and tough structures.
- *Reverse cutting needle* is used to suture mucoperiosteum
- *Round body needles* are used in soft structures like peritoneum, muscle, vessel, nerves, tendons, bowel and soft tissues.

Surgical Needles

Types

Based on the edge	
• Round body needle • Cutting needle • Reverse cutting needle	• Taper cut needle • Side-to-side flat—Hagedron needle
Based on curvature	
• Straight needle • Curved needle. Half circle; 5/8 circle, etc.	

Based on Existence of the Eye

- **Atraumatic needle** is eyeless. Here suture material is attached to the needle by swaging. Size of the suture material and that of needle is same and so tissue trauma is less. Needle once used is disposed of (not reusable).
- **Traumatic needle:** It is eyed needle. Needle in the eye area is wider than the body of the needle and so tissue trauma is more. These needles are reusable.

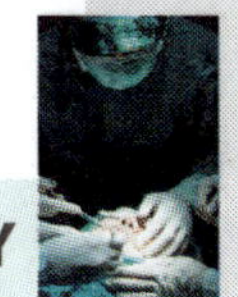

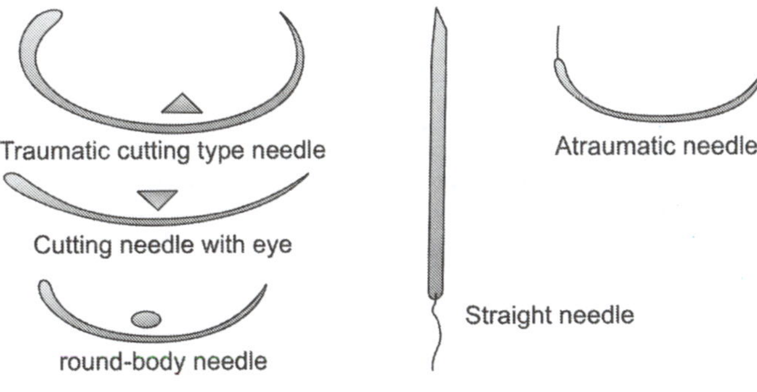

FIGURE: Needles

539. Ans. (a) Pulse rate/BP

Shock index is defined as ratio of pulse rate to blood pressure and value >1 indicates significant blood loss.

Signs of Significant Blood Loss

- Pulse >100/min
- Systolic BP <100 mm Hg
- Diastolic BP drop on sitting or standing >10 mm Hg
- Pallor/sweating
- Shock index (ratio of Pulse rate to Blood pressure >1)

Tachycardia is not reliable indicator of haemorrhage.

540. Ans. (d) All of the above

Steps to stop blood loss

- Pressure
- Packing
- Position
- Operative procedures

541. Ans. (b) Colloids

Fluids used in Burns

Fluids used are Ringer lactate, Hartmann fluid, plasma. *Ringer lactate is the fluid of choice.* Blood is transfused in later period (after 48 hours).

First 24 hours only *crystalloids* should be given (Crystalloids are one which can pass through capillary wall like saline either hypo, iso or hypertonic, dextrose saline, *Ringer lactate*).

Sodium is assessed by formula: 0.52 mmol × kg body weight × % body burns, given at a rate of 4.0 to 4.4 ml/kg hours.

After 24 hours up to 30–48 hours, *colloids* should be given to compensate plasma loss (colloids are one which are retained in intravascular compartment). Plasma haemaccel (gelatin), dextrans, hetastarch are used. Usually at a rate of 035–0.5 mL/kg/% burns is used in 24 hours.

542. Ans. (d) Urgent Angiography

- No role exists for probing or local exploration of the neck in the emergency department because this may dislodge a clot and initiate uncontrollable hemorrhage.
- Immediate surgical exploration *is only* done for patients who present with signs and symptoms of shock and continuous haemorrhage from the neck wound.
- **In our case the patient is not in shock. Hence angiography will be done to identify the presence of vascular injury. This is followed by formal neck exploration if required or conservative management is required. Read the protocol mentioned here for better understanding of the topic.**

Selective Management of Penetrating Neck Wounds

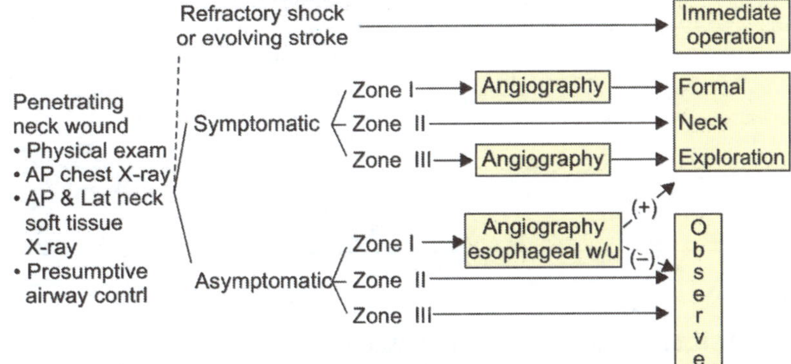

The neck may be divided into 3 zones using anatomic landmarks. Each zone has a group of vital structures that can be injured and may determine the kind of trauma management.

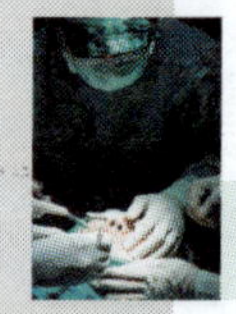

Zones of Penetrating Neck Injury

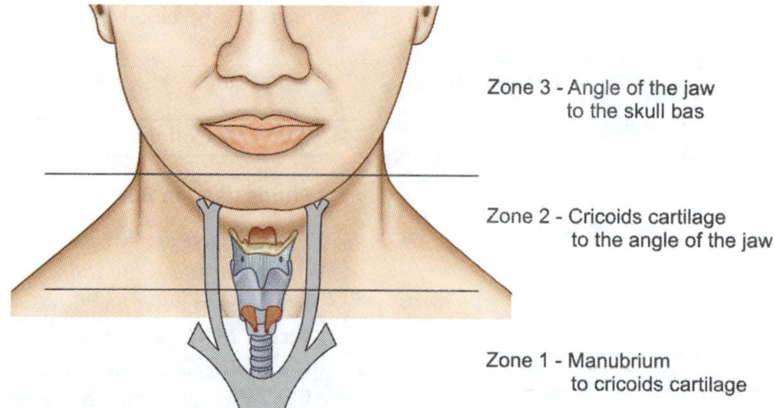

Zone 1	Horizontal area between the clavicle/suprasternal notch and the cricoid cartilage encompassing the thoracic outlet structures	The proximal common carotid, vertebral, and subclavian arteries and the trachea, oesophagus, thoracic duct, and thymus
Zone 2	Area between the cricoid cartilage and the angle of the mandible	Contains the internal and external carotid arteries, jugular veins, pharynx, larynx, esophagus, recurrent laryngeal nerve, spinal cord, trachea, thyroid, and parathyroids
Zone 3	Area that lies between the angle of the mandible and the base of the skull	Distal extracranial carotid and vertebral arteries and the uppermost segments of the jugular veins

543. Ans. (c) F.A.S.T

BAT (blunt abdominal trauma)

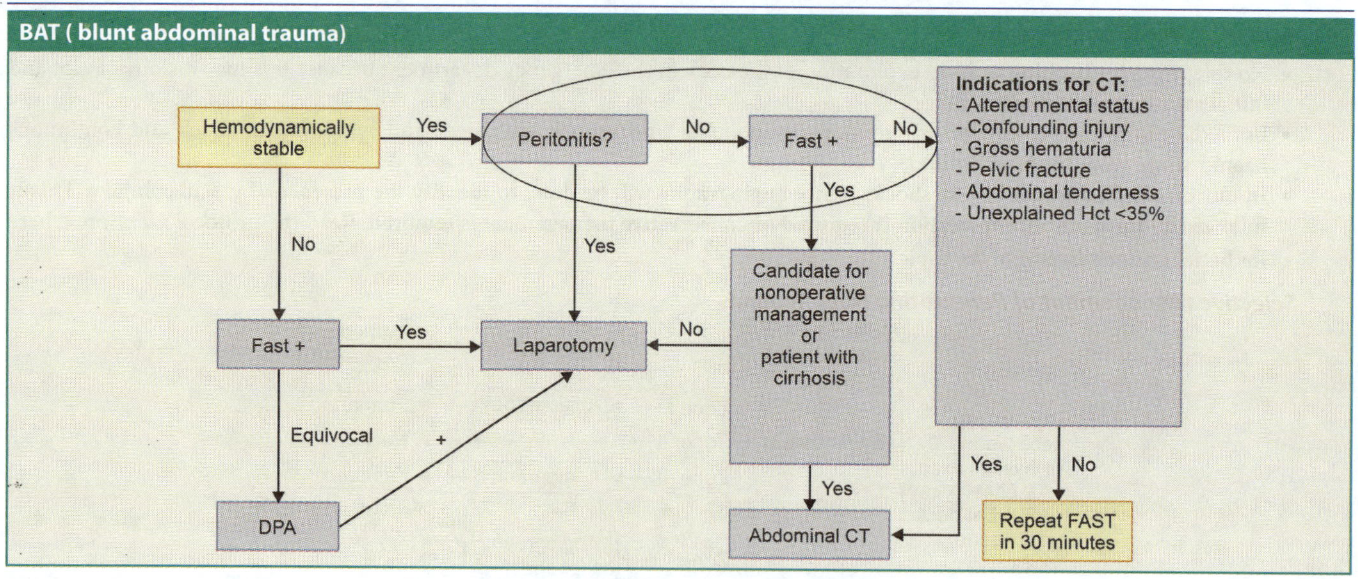

544. Ans. (a) 750

CLASSIFICATION OF HAEMORRHAGIC SHOCK (CIRCULATORY FAILURE)

Class	Blood loss	Features
I	Up to 15% (<750 mL)	Normal
II	Blood loss 15–30% (750–1500 mL)	Palor, thirsty, tachycardia
III	Blood loss 30–40% (1500–2000 mL)	Hypotension, tachycardia, oliguria, confusion
IV	Blood loss >40% (>2000 mL)	Rapid pulse, low BP, anuria, unconsciousness, MODS

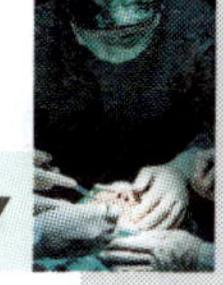

545. Ans. (a) Acute limb ischemia

Surgical Guidelines for Acute Limb Ischemia

- 5000-10,000 units of heparin
- Relief of pain
- *Embolectomy with 5Fr Fogarthy catheter. The catheter is passed beyond the embolus and balloon is inflated. Catheter is withdrawn gently with the embolus.*
- Surgical exploration and removal of clot if all else fails.

546. Ans. (b) Secondary

Ref: Bailey and Love, 26th ed. pg. 284

Primary hemorrhage	Occurs at the time of surgery or trauma.
Secondary hemorrhage	Secondary haemorrhage is defined as occurring at least 24 hours after surgery, but usually presents several days later, as it is due to postoperative infection.
Reactionary haemorrhage	• Common after first 4–6 hours after surgery. • It may be caused by ▪ Slippage of a ligature ▪ Displacement of blood clot ▪ Cessation of vasospasm, after coughing or increased mobility.

547. Ans. (c) Blood transfusion

Ref: Bailey, 26th ed. pg. 17

Choice A and B	This statement is direct quote from Bailey page 17, 26th edition • *"On balance, there is little evidence to support the administration of colloids, which are more expensive and have worse side-effect profiles."* • Most importantly, the oxygen carrying capacity of crystalloids and colloids is zero.
Choice C	*If blood is being lost, the ideal replacement fluid is blood, although crystalloid therapy may be required while awaiting blood products.*
Choice D	Fluid resuscitation must be done before General anesthesia can be given and surgeon can proceed with immediate laparoscopy.

548. Ans. (a) Urine output

Ref: Bailey, 26th ed. pg. 15

Choice A	As shock progresses, renal compensatory mechanisms fail, renal perfusion falls and urine output dips below 0.5 mL/kg/hr.
Choice C ruled out as	Hypotension is one of the last signs of shock. Children and fit young adults are able to maintain blood pressure until the final stages of shock.
Choice D ruled out	Tachycardia may not always accompany shock. Patients who are on beta-blockers or who have implanted pacemakers are unable to mount a tachycardia

The *minimum* standard for monitoring of the patient in shock is

- Continuous heart rate
- Oxygen saturation monitoring
- Frequent non-invasive blood pressure monitoring
- Hourly urine output measurement.

Since the question is asking for the best parameter, out of the given options urine output is the best answer.

Extra Mile

- Shock is the most common and therefore the most important cause of death of surgical patients.
- *Ideal way to manage shock is measure pulmonary capillary wedge pressure> urine output monitoring.*

549. Ans. (a) Detection of Pericardial fluid accumulation

Ref: Bailey, 26th ed. pg. 109

Focused assessment with sonography for trauma (FAST) looks for fluid in the

- Peri-hepatic and hepato-renal space
- Peri-splenic area
- Pelvis
- Pericardium.
  - It has a role in children but it does not detect solid organ injuries nor replace CT.
  - Bowel perforation or deep penetrating trauma requires a laparoscopy or laparotomy.
  - Isolated blunt splenic and/or liver injuries identified on a CT

550. Ans. (a) Septic shock

In Septic shock findings include:

- *Enhanced cardiac output*
- *Peripheral vasodilation*
- *Fever*
- *Leukocytosis*
- *Hyperglycemia*
- *Tachycardia*
- In septic shock, the vasodilatory effects are due in part to the upregulation of the inducible isoform of nitric oxide synthase (iNOS or NOS_2) in the vessel wall.

551. Ans. (c) Crystalloids

Ref: Bailey & Love, 26th ed. pg. 16-17

- ***Crystalloid is the first fluid of choice for resuscitation.*** Immediately administer 2 L of isotonic sodium chloride solution or lactated Ringer's solution in response to shock from blood loss. Fluid administration should continue until the patient's hemodynamics become stabilized. Because crystalloids quickly leak from the vascular space, each liter of fluid expands the blood volume by

20-30%; therefore, 3 L of fluid needs to be administered to raise the intravascular volume by 1 L.

- About the use of RL and NS in hemorrhagic shock, it has been shown that Resuscitation with NS modulates hypercoagulability after trauma and results in increased fluid requirements Administration of RL during resuscitation appears to have no effect on the hypercoagulable state induced by trauma. This hypercoagulable state may reduce bleeding and be protective initially, but may lead to thromboembolic complications later in the course of trauma admission. Due to this reason *RL may be preferred in the trauma (hemorrhagic shock) in the initial phase over NS.*
- As the RL is a little hypotonic solution large volume of RL in patients with head injury may lead to cerebral oedema therefore NS may be preferred over LR in patients of hemorrhagic shock with head injury. (Also remember that head injuries may also precipitate hyponatremia. The most common metabolic abnormality after head injury is SIADH).

552. Ans. (a) Septic shock

Plasma expanders are used to restore circulatory volume in shock, burns, sepsis, hemorrhage, surgery, and other trauma or for prophylaxis of venous thrombosis and thromboembolism.

- *Plasma expanders are most useful when there is faulty distribution* rather than real loss eg- burns, septic/endotoxic shock and trauma. They do not provide oxygen carrying capacity.
- Septic shock is associated with peripheral vasodilatation causing relative hypovolumia
- Antibiotics are the mainstay of treatment of septic shock
- Examples of plasma expanders
  - Dextran 70 & Dextran 40
  - Polyvinyl pyrrolidone
  - Gelatin polymer
  - Albumin
  - Hydroxyl ethyl starch

553. Ans. (d) Anesthesia

Ref: Bailey and Love, 26th ed. ch. 2/15

In high spinal anesthesia, Hypotension occurs due to loss of sympathetic autonomic function and unopposed parasympathetic function. Vasoconstrictor tone is lost and venous pooling occurs. Loss of cardiac accelerator fibres results in bradycardia and patients are unable to increase cardiac output by changes in heart rate.

554. Ans. (b) Normal saline

Ref: Harrison, 18th ed. pg. 270

Normal saline is the preferred fluid for volume expansion in a *crashing patient with un-recordable BP*. The main point to be noted is that if ringer lactate is infused in these patients, then lactate in the solution will never reach the liver where it is normally converted into bicarbonate. Hence the accumulated lactate will get broken into lactic acid that will worsen the status of patient of poly-trauma who is already acidotic. Dextran would not be indicated as it exhibits anti-thrombotic tendency.

555. Ans. (b) Normal saline

Ref: Harrison, 18th ed. pg. 270

Fluid of choice in Hypovolemic shock is Normal saline.

556. Ans. (b) Hypotension

Ref: Nelson, 18th ed. ch. 176

- Sepsis is defined as SIRS plus evidence of infection like positive blood culture report
- Septic shock is defined as sepsis plus evidence of hypotension for > 1 hour in spite of use of vasoactive agents.

SIRS: 2 out of 4 criteria, 1 of which must be abnormal temperature or abnormal leukocyte count

- Core temperature >38.5°C or <36°C (rectal, bladder, oral, or central catheter)
- Tachycardia: mean heart rate >2 SD above normal for age in absence of external stimuli, chronic drugs or painful stimuli; OR unexplained persistent elevation over 0.5–4 hr; OR in children <1 yr old persistent bradycardia over 0.5 hr (mean heart rate <10th percentile for age in absence of vagal stimuli, β blocker drugs, or congenital heart disease)
- Respiratory rate >2 SD above normal for age or acute need for mechanical ventilation not related to neuromuscular disease or general anesthesia
- Leukocyte count elevated or depressed for age (not secondary to chemotherapy) or >10% immature neutrophils

557. Ans. (d) Normal saline

Ref: Bailey & Love, 26th ed. pg. 482-83

The first step in the management of a newborn with myelomeningocele is a careful clinical assessment followed by **open defects which should be covered with a saline-moistened non-adherent dressing to prevent injury to and dessication of the neural placode.**

558. Ans. (a) 0.1 mEq

500 mL of 0.9% saline contains about 154 mEq of sodium and chloride per liter. Thus mathematically 1 mL contains 0.15 mEq approximately.

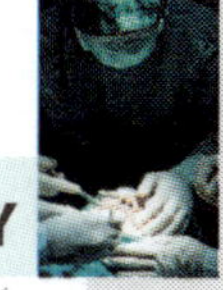

559. Ans. (a) 0.5 mEq

Since 3% NaCl has 513 mEq/L of Na and Cl in 1000 ml, mathematically the answer will be 0.5 mEq.

	Size (mL)	Composition (g/L)	Ionic concentration (mEq/L)		Osmolarity (mOsmol/L)	pH
		Sodium chloride USP (NACL)	Sodium	Chroride		
3% sodium chloride injection, USP	500	30	513	513	1027	50 (4.5 to 7.0)
5% sodium chloride injection, USP	500	50	856	856	1711	5.0 (4.5 to 7.0)
* Normal physiological osmolarity range is approximately 280 to 310 mOsmol/L. Administration of substantially hypertonic solutions (≥ 600 mOsmol/L) may cause vein damage						

560. Ans. (d) 50

Ref: Sabiston, 19th ed. pg. 138-39

TPN Formulation	
Without lipid	**With Lipid**
• Calories from amino acids: 20–25% • Calories from dextrose: 75–80%	• Calories from amino acids: 20–25% • Calories from lipids: 20% • Calories from dextrose: 55–60%

561. Ans. (a) 1%

Ref: Sabiston, 9th ed. pg. 523

- *This was a confusing question, as most students marked it as 9%, which is true for upper extremity but NOT for hand.*
- *Bailey in 26th ed. clearly mentions hand as palm and counting it as 1%*

Burn size is assessed by Wallace rule of nines (By Alfred Russel Wallace)

- Each upper extremity: 9%
- Head and neck: 9%
- Lower extremities: 18%
- Anterior and posterior aspects of the trunks: 18%
- Perineum and genitalia: 1%

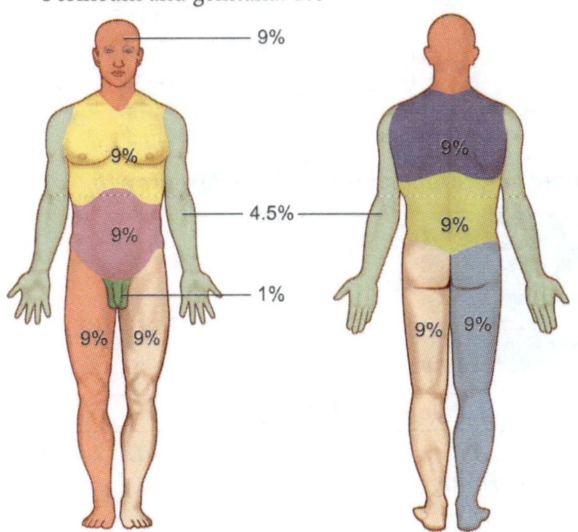

562. Ans. (a) 1%

Ref: Sabiston, 19th ed. pg. 523

Perineum involved in burns is 1% of body surface area.

563. Ans. (b) Ringer's lactate

Ref: Sabiston, 19th ed. pg. 529-30

- **IV fluid resuscitation is immediately required:** In children with burn >10% TBSA and adult with burn >15% TBSA
- Maximum fluid is given in first 8 hours (50%) rest of the fluid will be given in subsequent hours (25% + 25% in next 16 hours).
- **Most commonly used/preferred fluid: Ringer lactate** (Crystalloids). Because it is a relatively isotonic crystalloid solution that is the key component of almost all resuscitative strategies, at least for the first 24-48 hours.
- However, some centers use human albumin, FFP or hypertonic saline.
- RL is preferable to isotonic sodium chloride solution (ie, normal saline [NS]) for large-volume resuscitations because ***its lower sodium concentration (130 mEq/L vs 154 mEq/L) and higher pH concentration (6.5 vs 5.0) are closer to physiologic levels.***
- **Hypotonic fluid is not given, as it can lead to hyponatremia and water intoxication.**
- **Maintenance fluid in children:** Dextrose –saline

Extra Mile

- Hypertonic saline has been effective in treating burn shock as it produces hyperosmolarity and hypernatremia
- This reduces the shift of intracellular water to the extracellular space

564. Ans. (a) Hypotonic solutions

Ref: Sabiston, 19th ed. pg. 530-33

565. Ans. (a) Crystalloids

Ref: Bailey & Love, 26th ed. pg. 392

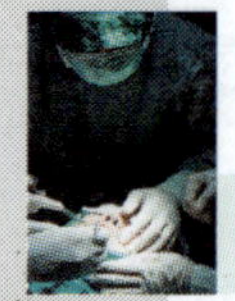

566. Ans. (a) Hematemesis is an early complication

Ref: Sabiston, 19th ed. pg. 529-32

Management of burn wound	
Exposure Method	Closed method
• Application of the agent to the wound 2-3 times a day. *No dressings are applied over wound*	• Generally closed method is preferred
• Exposure method is commonly used for face and head	• Occlusive dressing is applied over the agent and changed twice daily
• **Disadvantage:** Increased pain, heat loss Risk of cross-contamination	• **Advantage:** Less pain, less heat loss Less risk of cross -contamination
	• **Disadvantages:** If dressing is not changed twice daily, there is risk of contamination

- *Pseudomonas is the most common infection in burn patients.*
- Due to inhalation of burn particles, stridor can be present.

567. Ans. (a) Dehydration

Ref: Sabiston, 19th ed. pg. 534-35

- In this case there is 70% burn and in addition enteral feeding is not given. The most probable cause of death in this case will be dehydration/Hypovolemia.
- MCC of early death in burn patient: **HYPOVOLEMIA**
- MCC of later death in burns: **Septicemia**
- MCC of death in burns: **Septicemia**
- MC CA in burns: **Squamous cell CA**

568. Ans. (d) Hypovolemia

Ref: Sabiston, 19th ed. pg. 534-35

569. Ans. (c) Early elective intubation is safest

Ref: Bailey & Love, 26th ed. pg. 389-90

The shock Reaction after burns

- Burns produce an inflammatory reaction
- This leads to vastly increased vascular permeability
- Water, solutes and proteins move from the intra- to the extravascular space
- The volume of fluid lost is directly proportional to the area of the burn
- *Above 15 per cent of surface area, the loss of fluid produces shock*

Dangers of smoke, hot gas or steam inhalation

- *Inhaled hot gases can cause supraglottic airway burns and laryngeal oedema*
- Inhaled steam can cause subglottic burns and loss of respiratory epithelium
- Inhaled smoke particles can cause chemical alveolitis and respiratory failure
- Inhaled poisons, such as carbon monoxide, can cause metabolic poisoning
- Full-thickness burns to the chest can cause mechanical blockage to rib movement

Initial management of the burned airway

- *Early elective intubation is safest*
- Delay can make intubation very difficult because of swelling
- Be ready to perform an emergency cricothyroidotomy, if intubation is delayed

Fluids for resuscitation

- In children with burns over 10 per cent TBSA and adults with burns over 15 per cent TBSA, consider the need for intravenous fluid resuscitation
- If oral fluids are to be used, salt must be added
- Fluids needed can be calculated from a standard formula
- The key is to monitor urine output

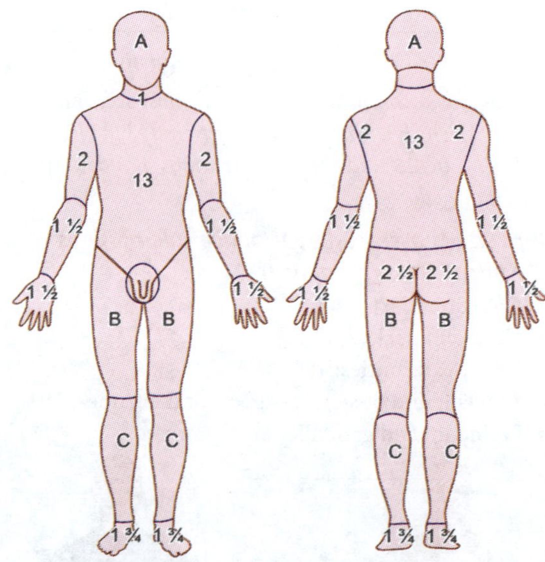

Relative percentage of area affected by growth

Relative percentage of area affected by growth

Age in years	0	1	5	10	15	Adult
A Head	9	8	6	5	4	3
B Head	2	3	4	4	4	4
C leg	2	2	3	3	3	3

570. Ans. (c) Painless and cherry red

Ref: Harrison, 18th ed. ch. 60/390

- ***Third-degree burns*** *appear white, tan, brown, black, or deep cherry red in color.*

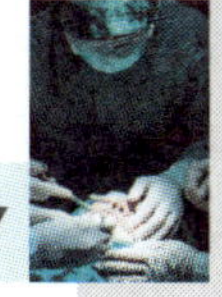

- The region of third-degree burn is usually painless because of destruction of sensory receptors.
- **Full-thickness burns** are also termed third-degree burns. The epidermis and the dermis are completely destroyed, and deeper tissue may also be involved.

571. Ans. (a) HSV

- **Viral infection in burns:** Burn patients suffer significant immunosuppression during *the first 3 or 4 weeks after hospitalization*. Herpes simplex virus (HSV) infections are commonly seen in immunosuppressed patients and may account for considerable morbidity and some mortality.
- **Bacterial infection in burns:** Burn wound *bacterial infections commonly occur in the first weeks* of hospitalization. ***S aureus* is the most common pathogen infecting burned** patients, as it is an early colonizer. *K pneumoniae* wound infections occur around the same time as infections by *S aureus* and seem to be more prevalent in the institutions that use systemic perioperative prophylaxis. As would be expected, infections by the nosocomial organisms *P aeruginosa* and *A baumannii* appear later in the course of the hospitalization (after 2 wk of admission).
- **Fungal infection in burns:** Burn wounds are also commonly infected with *fungal pathogens*. These infections are frequent after the use of broad-spectrum antibiotics. *Candida albicans* is the most common fungal infection; nonetheless, a trend towards nosocomially acquired, intrinsically resistant fungal infections (e.g., *Candida krusei*) has been reported

572. Ans. (a) Sepsis

Ref: Schwartz, 10th ed. pg. 233

Causes of Death in Burns

Cause	%
ARDS	29%
Brain injury	16%
Shock	8%
Sepsis	***47%***

573. Ans. (d) Air embolism

Ref: Schwartz, 10th ed. pg. 233

The following Complications in burns may occur

- Infections being the most common
- Pneumonia, cellulitis, urinary tract infections
- Anemia secondary to full thickness burns of greater than 10% TBSA is common.
- Electrical burns may lead to compartment syndrome or rhabdomyolysis
- Deep vein thrombosis

Long Term Morbidity with Burns

- The hypermetabolic state result in a decrease in bone density and a loss of muscle mass.
- Keloids may form subsequent to a burn
- Significant psychological trauma
- Social isolation, extreme poverty and child abandonment.

574. Ans. (a) Proptosis

Ref: Bailey & Love, 26th ed. pg. 344

Lefort I	Ecchymosis is present
Lefort II and Lefort III (common)	Gross edema of soft tissue over the middle third of the face, bilateral circumorbital ecchymosis, bilateral sub-conjunctival hemorrhage, epistaxis, CSF rhinorrhoea, dish face deformity, diplopia, enophthalmos, cracked pot sound.
Lefort II	Step deformity at infra-orbital margin, mobile mid face, anesthesia or paresthesia of cheek.
Lefort III	Tenderness and separation at fronto-zygomatic suture, lengthening of face, depression of ocular levels, Enophthalmos, hooding of eyes, tilting of occlusal plane with gagging on one side

Contd...

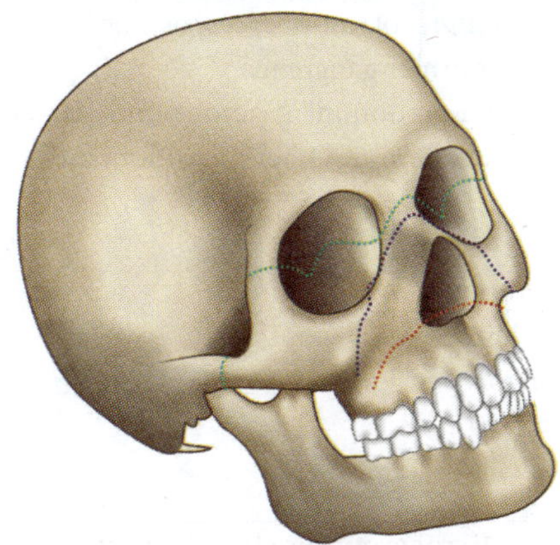

FIGURE: Le-fort fracture

575. Ans. (d) Proprioception

Ref: Harrsion, 18th ed. pg. 377

- Brown sequard consists of ipsilateral weakness (corticospinal tract) and loss of joint position and vibratory sense (posterior column), with contralateral loss of pain and temperature sense (spinothalamic tract) one or two levels below the lesion.
- Segmental signs, such as radicular pain, muscle atrophy, or loss of a deep tendon reflex, are unilateral. Partial forms are more common than the fully developed syndrome.

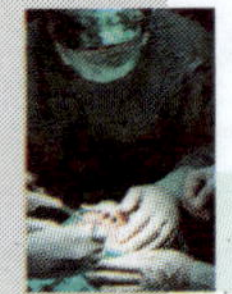

576. Ans. (b) Orbital floor

- Fracture of the orbital floor is the most common traumatic orbital fracture.
- Eyebrow Ptosis after Blowout Fracture Indicates Impairment of Trigeminal Proprioceptive Evocation That Induces Reflex Contraction of the Frontalis Muscle.
- The force of a blow to the orbit is dissipated by a fracture of the surrounding bone, usually the orbital floor and/or the medial orbital wall. Serious consequences of such injury include diplopia in upgaze where there is significant damage to the orbital floor. In blowout fractures, the medial wall is fractured indirectly.
- Fracture of the medial wall is more common than the floor, since the medial wall is slightly thinner (0.25 mm vs 0.50 mm). *However, it is known that pure blowout fractures most frequently involve the orbital floor. This is due to the honeycomb structure of the numerous bony septa of the ethmoid sinuses, thus allowing it to withstand the sudden rise in intraorbital hydraulic pressure better than the orbital floor*

577. Ans. (c) Anaerobic Streptococcus

Ref: Bailey & Love, 26th ed. pg. 1388

Current clinical studies have emphasized the *multi-organism nature* of most cases of necrotizing infection, including Fournier gangrene.

E. coli is the predominant aerobe and Bacteroides is the predominant anerobe. Other microflora include:

- Proteus
- Enterococcus
- Pseudomonas
- Clostridium
- Staphylococcus
- Streptococcus
- Klebsiella

578. Ans. (d) Microaerophilic streptococcus

Ref: Bailey & Love, 26th ed. pg. 57

- **Chronic undermining burrowing ulcer** (also known as **Meleney gangrene**, or **Meleney's ulcer**) is a cutaneous condition that is a postoperative, progressive bacterial gangrene. Synergistic gangrene is caused by micro-aerophilic streptococci acting synergistically with aerobic staphylococci, with or without Gram-negative bacilli. It occurs in debilitated patients with other disorders (e.g. diabetes, malnutrition, alcoholism. Infection spreads rapidly along fascial and subcutaneous planes without a severe inflammatory reaction.

579. Ans. (b) Insulin

Ref: Bailey & Love, 26th ed. pg. 4

- The stress response to surgery is characterized by increased secretion of pituitary hormones and activation of the sympathetic nervous system. Release of corticotrophin from the pituitary stimulates cortisol secretion from the adrenal cortex. Arginine vasopressin is secreted from the posterior pituitary and has effects on the kidney. In the pancreas, glucagon is released and insulin secretion may be diminished.
- Logic for ADH increase is that the body is trying to retain water.

Hormones increased	ACTH, GH, AVP, Cortisol, Aldostrone, Small Increase In Glucagon
Hormones decreased	Insulin, Thyroxine (T4) And T3
May increase or decrease	Tsh, Fsh, Lh

580. Ans. (c) Subsides over time

Ref: Bailey & Love, 26th ed. pg. 30

- Keloid formation is a type of scar which, depending on its maturity, is composed mainly of either type III (early) or type I (late) collagen.
- Keloids are firm, lesions or shiny, fibrous nodules, and vary from pink to flesh-colored or red to dark brown in color. A keloid scar is benign and not contagious, but sometimes accompanied by severe itchiness, pain, and changes in texture.
- **They may not improve in appearance over time and can limit mobility if located over a joint.**

581. Ans. (a) Spleen

Ref: Bailey & Love, 26th ed. pg. 1087

- The spleen is the most commonly injured viscus in blunt abdominal trauma and can result from the most trivial of traumas.
- The classical presentation is that of a hemodynamically unstable patient with a history of trauma, with severe abdominal pain and signs of peritonitis.
- The classic physical findings of splenic rupture are left shoulder pain, left upper quadrant pain and tenderness, and Kehr's sign (left shoulder pain from irritation of inferior border of left diaphragm by hematoma).
- Absence of one or more or even all of these signs does not rule out splenic injury. Diagnosis is based on a thorough physical examination and confirmed with the FAST examination

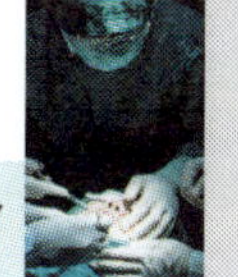

582. Ans. (c) 5–12 days

Ref: Bailey & Love, 26th ed. pg. 279

- Patients maximum at risk for wound dehiscence are those who are/have

- Obese
- Malnourished
- Abdominal distention
- Malignancy
- Multiple trauma to the abdomen
- Infected wounds are also prone to dehiscence.
- **Chronic cough are also at risk.**

Wound separation occurs especially between the fifth and eight postoperative days.

583. Ans. (a) Is a skin graft including the epidermis and part of the dermis

Ref: Bailey & Love, 26th ed. pg. 402

- Skin transplanted from one location to another on the same individual is termed an autograft. If the entire thickness of the dermis is included, the appropriate term is full-thickness skin graft (FTSG).
- *If less than the entire thickness of the dermis is included, this graft is referred to as a split-thickness skin graft (STSG).* STSGs are categorized further as thin (0.005-0.012 in), intermediate (0.012-0.018 in), or thick (0.018-0.030 in), based on the thickness of the harvested graft.

584. Ans. (d) Transplantation of living tissues/organs from one species to another

Ref: Bailey & Love, 26th ed. pg. 833

- **Xenotransplantation** is the transplantation of living cells, tissues or organs from one species to another. Such cells, tissues or organs are called **xenografts** or **xenotransplants**.
- In contrast, the term allotransplantation refers to a same-species transplant. Human xenotransplantation offers a potential treatment for end-stage organ failure, a significant health problem in parts of the industrialized world.

585. Ans. (b) Buruli ulcer

Ref: SRB Manual of Surgery, 23rd ed. pg. 23

- Buruli ulcer is an infectious disease caused by *Mycobacterium ulcerans*. The early stage of infection is characterised by a painless nodule, with non-pyogenic, necrotizing lesions developing in the skin, and occasionally in adjacent bone, as the disease progresses.
- *M. ulcerans* secretes a lipid toxin, mycolactone, which functions as an immune suppressant, necrotising agent and activator of cellular apoptosis in mammalian tissues.
- The disease is primarily an infection of subcutaneous fat, resulting in a focus of necrotic (dead) fat containing myriads of the mycobacteria in characteristic spherules formed within the dead fat cells. Skin ulceration is a secondary event.
- All other ulcers are associated with significant scarring in the tissues. Scarring in gastric ulcer/duodenal ulcer leads to gastric outlet obstruction.

586. Ans. (d) Marjolin's ulcer

Ref: Bailey & Love, 26th ed. pg. 918

- Marjolin's ulcer is a misnomer. It is a malignant degeneration arising within **a pre-existing cicatrix or scar**
- Most commonly found in the lower extremity, especially the **heel and plantar foot**.
- Causes:
  - As originally presented by Marjolin, to this day the **leading cause is old burn scars**.
- Marjolin's ulcers are 3 times more likely in **men** than in women.
- Average age of diagnosis is the **fifth decade** of life.
- As a rule, normal healing should be exhibited within the first **2 to 3 weeks**, and ulcers that repeatedly break down, do not respond to treatment and are chronic in nature, are suspicious for malignancy
- Most commonly well-differentiated **squamous cell tumors** found but can be basal cell or melanoma
- **Duration of ulceration** is directly proportional to chance of malignant transformation
- Although there is **no definitive treatment** protocol, therapy generally involves wide local excision with skin grafting or amputation proximal to the lesion depending upon size.
- **Most widely accepted treatment/most definitive option to treat the cancer, and infection/when the bone or joint is involved is amputation.**

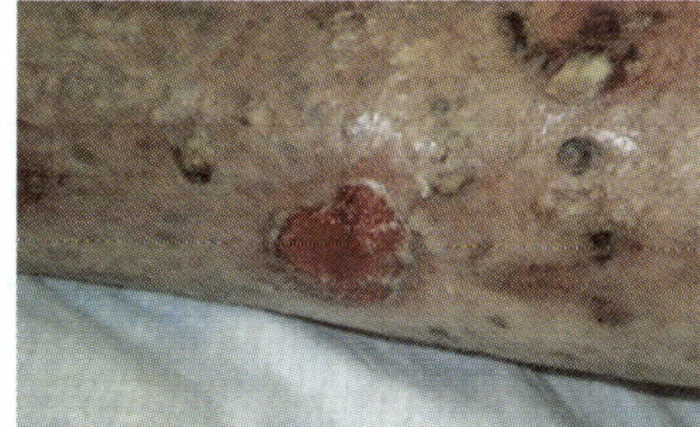

587. Ans. (a) Metaphysis

Ref: Bailey & Love, 26th ed. pg. 541

- The most common site is the rapidly growing and highly vascular metaphysis of growing bones. The apparent slowing or sludging of blood flow as the vessels make

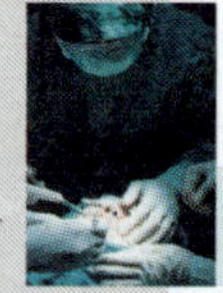

sharp angles at the distal metaphysis predisposes the vessels to thrombosis and the bone itself to localized necrosis and bacterial seeding.

- Vertebral osteomyelitis at any age is most often a secondary complication of a remote infection with hematogenous seeding.
- Direct or contiguous inoculation osteomyelitis is caused by direct contact of the tissue and bacteria during trauma or surgery.

588. Ans. (a) Primary intention

Ref: Bailey & Love, 26th ed. pg. 25

HEALING BY PRIMARY INTENTION

- It involves epidermis and dermis without total penetration of dermis healing by process of epithelialization when wound edges are brought together so that they are adjacent to each other (re-approximated).
- This minimizes scarring
- Most surgical wounds heal by primary intention healing
- Wound closure is performed with sutures (stitches), staples, or adhesive tape
- **Examples:** Well-repaired lacerations, well reduced bone fractures, healing after flap surgery

589. Ans. (a) 8–10 days

Ref: Sabiston, 18th ed. pg. 2134

Scalp suture should be removed on 6th to 8th day. Given these options, 8–10 days is the best choice.

TABLE: Day of suture removal from different body areas

Body area	Suture removal on
• Scalp	6–8 days
• Face	3–5 days
• Chest, Abdomen	8–10 days
• Ear	10–14 days
• Extremities, back	12–14 days

590. Ans. (d) Recovery time is longer

- Laparoscopy is a technique in which operations in the abdomen are performed through small incisions (usually 0.5–1.5 cm) as opposed to the larger incisions needed in laparotomy.
- Rather than a minimum 20 cm incision as in traditional (open) cholecystectomy, four incisions of 0.5–1.0 cm will be sufficient to perform a laparoscopic removal of a gallbladder.
- Since the gallbladder is similar to a small balloon that stores and releases bile, it can usually be removed from the abdomen by suctioning out the bile and then removing the deflated gallbladder through the 1 cm incision at the patient's navel.
- *Post operative stay in hospital is short.*
- The risk of Trocar injuries is increased in patients who have a low body mass index or have a history of prior abdominal surgery.
- Vascular injuries can result in hemorrhage that may be life threatening. Injuries to the bowel can cause a delayed peritonitis. It is very important that these injuries be recognized as early as possible.

591. Ans. (c) Mesentery

Ref: Bailey & Love, 26th ed. pg. 982

- Seat belt syndrome is characterized by tear of mesentery on sudden deceleration while the patient is using a seat belt.
- **In the absence of seat belt being worn by the car passenger, the chest of the victim would slam into the steering wheel resulting in hemo-pericardium and a resultant high mortality.**

592. Ans. (a) Damage to respiratory centre

Ref: Bailey & Love, 26th ed. pg. 310

The Cushing's triad is the triad of bradycardia, hypertension, and respiratory irregularity that often occupies a herniation event clinically. It is likely due to brainstem compression.

593. Ans. (a) CECT abdomen

Ref: Bailey & Love, 26th ed. pg. 208

Since the patient is in shock with history of blunt abdomen trauma, the first investigation to be done should be FAST. The main role of ultrasound includes the assessment of intraperitoneal fluid and haemopericardium In the presence of free intraperitoneal fluid and an unstable patient, the ultrasound allows the trauma surgeon to explore the abdomen as a cause of blood loss.

In the presence of fluid and a haemodynamically stable individual, further assessment by way of CT shall be performed. Occasionally, a second ultrasound scan may show free fluid in the presence of an initially negative FAST scan.

594. Ans. (a) Tetany

Ref: Harrison, 18th ed. pg. 352

- Painful lock jaw is related to inflammation of anatomical structures of jaw and surrounding structures. Tetanus is characterized by release of tetano-spasmin toxin which causes painful muscle spasm and lockjaw.
- However in the question the choice A is Tetany/ Hypocalcemia where either Chvostek sign and Carpo-pedal spasm is seen.

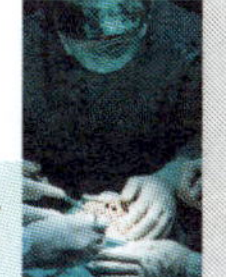

595. Ans. (c) Lower lip

Ref: Bailey & Love, 26th ed. pg. 710

- Lip cancer is the most common malignant lesion of the oral cavity, constituting 25–30% of all oral cavity cancer cases and is the second most common malignancy of the head and neck overall (after cutaneous malignancy). Unlike other sub-sites of the oral cavity, sun exposure is a well established risk factor for development of lip cancer.
- 95% of carcinoma of lip arise on lower lip and 15% rise in central one-third and commissures. The lymph nodes involved are submental and submandibular groups.

596. Ans. (a) Common peroneal nerve

- Common peroneal nerve originates from the dorsal branches of the fourth and fifth lumbar and the first and second sacral nerves. It descends obliquely along the lateral side of the popliteal fossa to the head of the fibula, close to the medial margin of the biceps femoris muscle. **Where the common peroneal nerve winds round the head of the fibula, it is palpable and vulnerable to injury.**

Remember

- Tarsal tunnel syndrome- Posterior tibial nerve
- Meralgia Parasthetica- Lateral cutaneous nerve of thigh
- Claw hand-ulnar nerve
- Mononeuritis multiplex is most commonly caused by Polyarteritis Nodosa. (If asked for India Ans. as leprosy).

597. Ans. (b) Surgical site infection

Ref: Bailey & Love, 26th ed. pg. 136/140

- Surgical site infections (SSIs) have been reported to be one of the most common causes of nosocomial infections; accounting for 20% to 25% of all nosocomial infections worldwide. SSIs have been responsible for the increasing cost; morbidity and mortality related to surgical operations and continue to be a major problem worldwide.
- Globally, surgical site infection rates have been reported to range from 2.5% to 41.9%. *Nosocomial infections can be defined as those occurring within 48 hours of hospital admission, 3 days of discharge or 30 days of an operation.*

598. Ans. (a) Right lower lobe superior basal

Ref: Complete Review of Medicine by Deepak Marwah, 1st ed.

- *In supine position and with the patient on back superior segment of RLL is the most dependent segment.*
- In right lateral decubitus position the axillary subsegments of anterior and posterior segments of RUL are the dependent site for aspiration. Abscess is located in the middle of lateral CXR corresponding to RUL bronchus take off.
- When the patient is on abdomen, aspiration does not occur, thus it is extremely unlikely for any anterior segments, middle lobe and lingula to be the site for aspiration lung abscess.
- ***The superior segments of Right Lower Lobe and axillary subsegments of anterior and posterior segments of RUL are common sites for aspiration and will account for 85% of all Lung abscesses.***

599. Ans. (d) Surgery + Imiquimod

Ref: Schwartz, 10th ed pg. 647; Bailey & Love, 26th ed. pg. 463

- Most cancers of the anus, cervix, head and neck, and vagina are epidermoid carcinomas and also called squamous cell carcinoma.
- *Treatment modalities for SCC include cautery and ablation, cryotherapy, drug therapy including imiquimod, surgical excision, Moh's microsurgery, and radiation therapy.*
- Topical fluorouracil is FDA-approved treatment for superficial Basal Cell Carcinoma.

600. Ans. (c) Number of lymph nodes involved

NEUROLOGY

601. Ans. (d) Subarachnoid hemorrhage

Ref: Bailey and Love, Textbook of Surgery, 27th ed. pg. 658

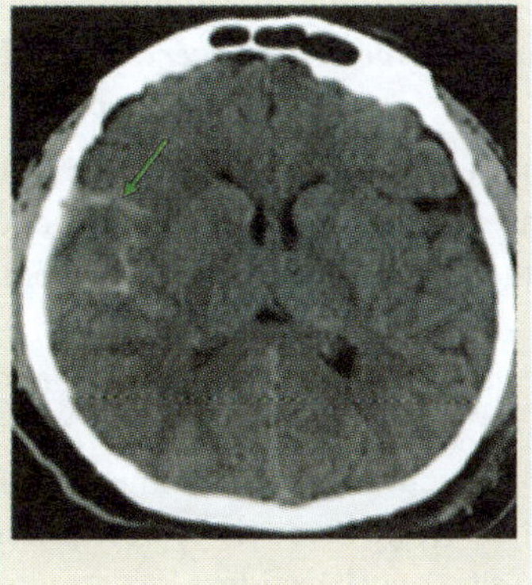

- Notice the blood in Sylvian fissure. Another keyword in the MCQ is "worst headache of my life".
- Spontaneous subarachnoid hemorrhage is usually the result of bleeding from a ruptured aneurysm (~80% of SAH) or an arteriovenous malformation.
- Most ruptured aneurysms are in the circle of Willis, at branch points in the arterial tree associated with turbulent blood flow.

602. Ans. (d) Extradural hemorrhage

Ref: Bailey and Love, Textbook of Surgery, 27th ed. pg. 333

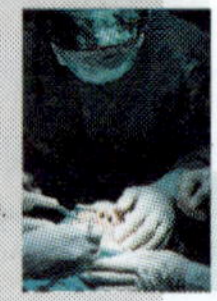

Extradural hematoma/epidural hematoma, is a collection of blood that forms between the inner surface of the skull and outer layer of the dura, which is called the endosteal layer.

- The source of bleeding is usually arterial, most commonly from a torn middle meningeal artery.
- They are usually associated with a history of head trauma and frequently associated skull fracture and history of lucid interval.

603. Ans. (b) Mannitol

Ref: Bailey and Love, Textbook of Surgery, 27th ed. pg. 336

Mannitol is the most popular osmotic agent. Osmotic therapy using mannitol reduces ICP by mechanisms that remain unclear.

- Mannitol is thought to decrease brain volume by decreasing overall water content, to reduce blood volume by vasoconstriction, to reduce CSF volume by decreasing water content.

604. Ans. (a) Bruising on mastoid

Ref: Bailey and Love, Textbook of Surgery, 27th ed. pg. 362

Battle sign is bruising over the mastoid process that is typically the result of head trauma.

- It requires significant head trauma and may indicate significant internal injury to the brain and not just the posterior cranial vault or mastoid. Basilar skull fracture is one of the leading causes.

605. Ans. (b) Extradural hematoma

Ref: Bailey and Love, Textbook of Surgery, 27th ed. pg. 333

Extradural hematomas are seen on CT scans of the brain. They are typically bi-convex (or lentiform) in shape, and most frequently beneath the squamous part of the temporal bone.

- EDHs are hyperdense, somewhat heterogeneous, and sharply demarcated.
- When acute bleeding is occurring at the time of CT scanning the non-clotted fresh blood is typically less hyperdense, and a swirl sign may be evident.

606. Ans. (c) Meningioma

Ref: Bailey and Love 27th ed. pg. 480

The image shows round lamellated calcified lesion psammoma bodies in brain biopsy specimen of a patient with intracranial space occupying lesion. It is seen in Meningioma. This lamellated concentric calcification occurs around necrotic tumor cells and is an example of dystrophic calcification.

> Psamomma bodies are seen in (Mnemonic- **PSM-A**)
> - **P**apillary thyroid carcinoma
> - **P**apillary serous carcinoma of endometrium
> - **S**erous cystadenoma of ovary
> - **M**eningioma
> - **M**esothelioma
> - **A**denocarcinoma lung

607. Ans. (d) Diffuse axonal injury

Ref: Bailey and Love 27th ed. pg. 336

- The NCCT shows punctuate hyper-densities at junction of Grey and white matter in a unconscious patient with posturing. This is a feature of Diffuse Axonal injury. In lot cases CT can be normal as well.
- Option a is ruled out as no blood is seen in Slyvian fissure.
- Option b is ruled at no concavo-convex hyper-density is seen
- Option c is ruled out as it causes weakening of wall of blood vessels and causes intraparenchymal bleeding.

MISCELLANEOUS

608. Ans. (b) Needle thoracostomy

Ref: Harrison 20th ed. pg. 2200

The CXR shows left sided pneumothorax due to absence of vascular shadows, collapsed lung border visible. The air at positive pressure will lead to mediastinal shift and compression of great veins. This leads to low BP and needs intervention in form of wide bore needle decompression followed by chest tube insertion.

609. Ans. (c) Right Empyema

Ref: Bailey and Love, 27th ed. pg. 922

The first image shows collapse of right lung due to effusion/empyema. Post Chest ICD drainage the lung has re expanded but shows underlying consolidation/re-expansion pulmonary procedure.

610. Ans. (b) Internal mammary artery

Ref: Bailey and Love, 27th ed. pg. 890

Atherosclerosis can develop in bypass grafts as well and patients may require a re-do CABG. The patency rates of 98 percent have been reported since 1980s for LIMA/internal thoracic artery to LAD.

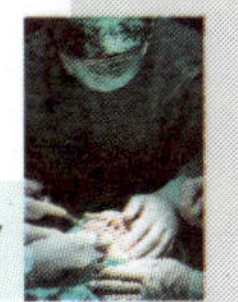

Blood vessel used as graft in CABG	Patency rate
Left internal mammary artery/Internal thoracic artery	~98%
Radial Artery	~80%
Gastroepiploic artery	~80%
Saphenous venous graft	~60%

611. Ans. (b) Isograft

Ref: Robbins Essential Pathology E-Book pg. 53

- Transplantation of organ across twins is called as isograft/syngeneic transplantation.
- Autograft is used for management of burns and hematological conditions like multiple myeloma and Hodgkins lymphoma.
- Allograft is done with HLA matched individual.
- Xenograft is done across species.

> *Interesting fact*
> Autograft in interventional cardiology
> In ross procedure the surgeon removes the abnormal aortic valve and replaces it with child's own pulmonic valve. This is an example of autograft. Then the surgeon uses a valve from cadaver to replace the pulmonic valve.

612. Ans. (d) Babcock's forceps

Ref: Bailey and Love 27th ed. pg. 1562

The image shows a forceps with atraumatic ends to cause minimal tissue damage. It is used to hold delicate tissues like appendix and fallopian tubes.

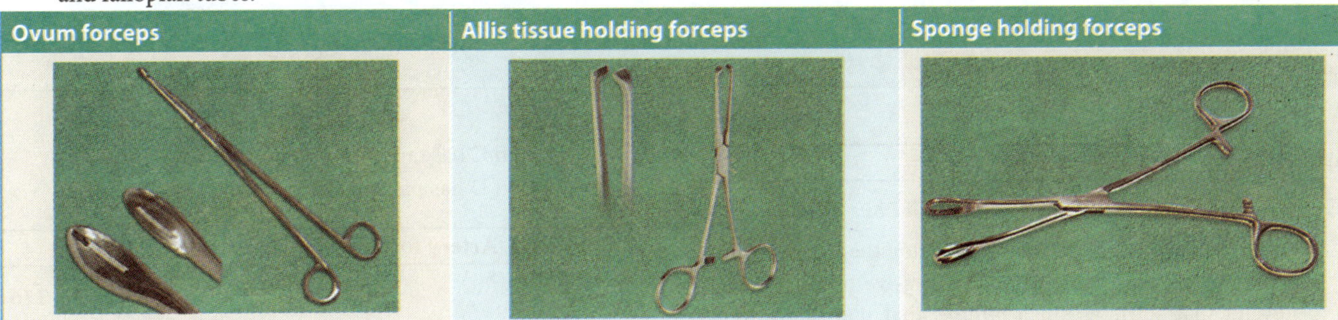

613. Ans. (c) Malignant melanoma

Ref: Bailey and Love 27th ed. pg. 610

- Option a is ruled out as Rodent ulcer is not seen. Option b is ruled out as any exophytic growth is not seen. The hyperpigmentation on malar eminences that has been increasing in size for past 6 months is strongly suggestive of Malignant melanoma.
- The incidence of this disease is more in white skinned individuals in areas of UV ray exposure.
- Option d would not show any growth.
- The leading presentation of malignant melanoma is superficial spreading melanoma that arises in pre-existent nevus after years of slow change followed by rapid growth.

614. Ans. (b) Squamous cell carcinoma

Ref: Bailey and Love 27th ed. pg. 605

- The image shows a cutaneous horn which can in future evolve into cutaneous S.C.C. Cutaneous horn is a manifestation of Actinic keratosis which occurs in area of sun exposure and shows dyskeratosis, cellular atypia and dermal inflammation.
- When the height of lesion is more than its breadth, it is called as cutaneous horn. It can evolve into SCC which is a malignant tumor of keratinizing cells of epidermis or its appendages. It arises from stratum basalis of epidermis and expresses cytokeratin 1 and 10.

615. Ans. (c) Scrofuloderma

Ref: Bailey and Love 27th ed. pg. 77

- The image shows multiple fistulous tracts with local scarring/inflammation in posterior triangle of neck

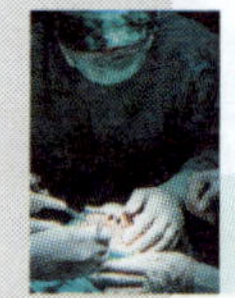

encroaching to sub occipital area. This is a feature of Tuberculous lymphadenitis which has caused direct skin infiltration and is called as Scrofuloderma.

- Castleman disease leads to benign growth of lymph nodes commonly in chest and abdomen.

616. Ans. (a) Streptococcus

Ref: Bailey and love 27th ed. pg. 597

The sharply demarcated infection of superficial lymphatics on face is erysipelas and is caused by streptococcus.

617. Ans. (d) 3rd degree burn

Ref: Bailey and Love 27th ed. pg. 622

Since the burn has involved dermis as well as subcutaneous tissue it is a full thickness/3rd degree burn.

Classification of Burns by Depth

Burn thickness	Deepest skin structure involved	Appearance	Pain	Prognosis (without surgical intervention)
Superficial (first-degree)	Epidermis	Dry, blanching erythema	Painful	Heals without scarring, 5–10 days
Superficial partial-thickness (second-degree)	Upper dermis	Blisters; wet, blanching erythema	Painful	Heals without scarring, <3 weeks
Deep partial-thickness (second-degree)	Lower dermis	Yellow or white, dry, nonblanching	Decreased sensation	Heals in 3–8 weeks; likely to scar if healing >3 weeks
Full-thickness (third-degree)	Subcutaneous structures	White or black/brown, nonblanching	Decreased sensation	Heals by contracture >8 weeks; will scar

618. Ans. (c) Basal cell cancer

Ref: Bailey and Love 27th ed. pg. 674

The leading malignant tumor involving the eyelids is Basal cell cancer. It presents as locally invasive tumor on lower eyelid that starts as small pimple, that ulcerates and has raised edges. Treatment is with complete excision while extensive lesions require Mohs micrographic surgical excision controlled by frozen section.

619. Ans. (a) Squamous cell ca

Ref: Bailey and love 27th ed. pg. 761

SCC is predominant histology for tumors originating from oral cavity. Tumors mainly arise from mucosal epithelium. This is followed by lymphomas originating around Waldeyer's Ring in oral cavity.

620. Ans. (a) Port wine stain

Ref: Bailey and Love 27th ed. pg. 613

- Port wine stain is purple stain present on head and neck often with the maxillary and mandibular dermatomes of trigeminal nerve.
- Option B is a red color capillary hemangioma seen on face and usually fade by 2 years of age.
- Option C has target lesions anywhere on the body
- Option D has painful lumps on shins

621. Ans. (a) Artery forceps

Ref: SRB: 5th ed. pg. 1164

The image shows a surgical instrument which has visible transverse serrations in distal blades with a lock in proximal part.

Use
• To catch bleeding points • To open the fascial planes in different surgeries • To pass a ligature • To hold fascial, peritoneum, aponeurosis • To hold sutures • To drain an abscess like a sinus forceps

622. Ans. (a) Tongue depressor

Ref: SRB, 5th ed, pg. 1150

The image shows a tongue depressor which can be used for posterior pharyngeal wall visualization to intubation process.

623. Ans. (a) Size of tumor

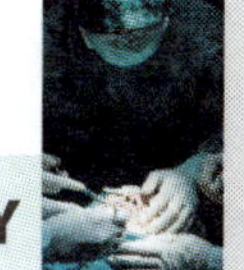

TNM is based on 3 components:

Letter	Stands for	Description
T	Tumor	Indicates the size of the primary tumor and the degree of spread into nearby tissues (local invasion)
N	Lymph nodes	Indicates whether or not the cancer has spread to nearby lymph nodes, the size of the nodes that contain cancer and how many lymph nodes contain cancer
M	Metastasis	Indicates whether or not cancer has spread (metastasized) to distant organs

Additional letters or numbers are placed after T, N and M to provide more specific details:

- X means the tumor or lymph nodes cannot be assessed or evaluated.
- T followed by a number (0–4) describes the size of tumor and how much nearby tissue it has invaded.
- N followed by a number (0–3) describes the degree of spread to the lymph nodes.
- M followed by the number 0 or 1 describes whether or not cancer has spread to other parts of the body.
- Lowercase letters (a, b or c) are used to subdivide the tumor, lymph nodes or metastasis categories to make them more specific.

624. Ans. (d) Metastasis

The X-ray spine AP shows multiple lytic lesions suggestive of malignancy metastasizing to the vertebra. The most probable origin is from the prostate which is the leading cancer is males.

Also notice the combination of osteolytic and osteosclerotic secondaries.

625. Ans. (a) Gestational age 1–7 months in abdomen

Ref: Human Embryology, 10th ed. pg. 311

- *The testes remain high in the abdomen until the 7th month of gestation, when they move from the abdomen through the inguinal canals into the two sides of the scrotum.*
- In first phase, movement across the abdomen to the entrance of the inguinal canal appears controlled by anti-müllerian hormone (AMH).
- In second phase, in which the testes move through the inguinal canal into the scrotum, is dependent on androgens (most importantly testosterone).
- In many infants with inguinal testes, further descent of the testes into the scrotum occurs in the first 6 months of life. This is attributed to the postnatal surge of gonadotropins and testosterone that normally occurs between the first and fourth months of life.

626. Ans. (d) Descending colon

Ref: High Yield Embryology, 5th ed. pg. 294

627. Ans. (d) Hepatocellular jaundice

Ref: Manipal Manual of Surgery,4th ed. pg. 520

- The anchovy sauce pus of ameobic liver abscess is sterile and is produced due to broken RBCs and damaged hepatocytes.
- Due to right branch of portal vein being more in line with portal vein the organism will have higher chances of seeding in the right lobe than the left lobe.
- Most patients will be male and alcoholic from lower socio-economic background and will present with severe right hypochondrium pain and symptoms of pleurisy and right shoulder pain.
- On examination intercostal tenderness is seen
- Bed side USG is the investigation of choice.
- Jaundice is not seen usually or if seen is of obstructive type.

628. Ans. (a) Ameobic liver abscess

Ref: Manipal Manual of Surgery, 4th ed. pg. 521

Refer to the above explanation

Hydatid cyst	Usually clinically silent *Enlarged liver with smooth surface and is non tender.*
Pyogenic liver abscess	Multiple abscess leading to spiky fever and enlarged liver.
Hepatic adenoma	Presents in young women on OCP and is solitary. Liver enlargement may or may not be seen.

629. Ans. (a) Cholesterolosis

Ref: Bailey & Love, 26th ed pg. 1108

- The submucous aggregation of cholesterol crystals in mucosa of gallbladder lends it appearance to be called strawberry gallbladder.
- Porcelain gallbladder exhibits calcification and is a risk factor for malignancy of gallbladder.

Extra Mile

Strawberry Tongue	Kawasaki Disease and scarlet fever
Strawberry nose	Rhinosporidiosis
Strawberry vagina	Trichomoniasis
Strawberry gingiva	Wegener granulomatosis

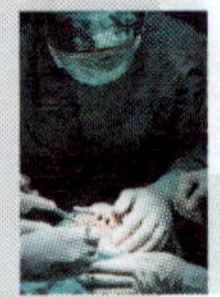

630. Ans. (d) Cholesterosis

Ref: Manipal Manual of Surgery, 4th ed. pg. 584

631. Ans. (a) Volvulus

Ref: Manipal Manual of Surgery, 4th ed. pg. 739

- In sigmoid volvulus, the X-ray abdomen erect shows hugely dilated sigmoid loop called bent inner tube sign.
- Acute sigmoid volvulus presents as intestinal obstruction and starts after straining at stool. *It occurs in anti-clockwise direction and after one and a half turns, the entire loop becomes gangrenous.*
- The percussion note on the abdomen shall be tympanitic note.

632. Ans. (b) Sigmoid volvulus

Ref: Manipal Manual of Surgery, 4th ed. pg. 738

- In sigmoid volvulus the loop of bowel twists to result in tympanitic note all over the abdomen. Hypovolemic shock develops within 6-8 hours and per rectum shows rectum to be empty.
- On performing a *contrast enema*, when the barium enters the rectum, it tapers into sigmoid colon called as *Bird Beak sign.*
- Bird beak sign on barium swallow occurs with achalasia cardia.

633. Ans. (d) Hirschsprung's disease

Ref: Manipal Manual of Surgery, 4th ed. pg. 731

Common causes of ileal obstruction	*Common causes of colonic obstruction*
• Adhesions • Obstructed hernia • Stricture • Intussusception • Ileocaecal TB • Bands	• Fecal impaction • Carcinoma colon • Hirschsprung's disease • Anorectal malformations

634. Ans. (a) Stomach

Ref: Bailey and Love 26th ed. pg. 1160

- GIST is a mesenchymal tumor with increased size and high levels of c-kit (CD117)
- *GIST tumors are found most commonly in the stomach*
- Occur most commonly in the 50-70-year age group.
- Presents with pain, nausea, hematemesis or melena.
- Surgery is the most effective way of removing GISTs, as they are radio-resistant.
- Imatinib Mesylate is the best drug

635. Ans. (a) Stomach

Ref: Advances in Oncology, Vol. 3/137

The most common extra-nodal site of lymphoma is GIT with the most common site being the stomach followed by small intestine and ileo-caecal region.

636. Ans. (a) Intussusception

Ref: Schwartz 10th ed. pg. 1237

Infants can develop in intussusception leading to intestinal obstruction. Option B, congenital bends will present in neonate age:

- Most common lead point causing intussusception in children = Meckel's Diverticulum
- Most common type of intussusception in children = Ileo-colic (Post Rota virus diarrhea)
- Most common lead point causing intussusception in Adults = Polyp (Villous Adenoma)
- Most common type of intussusception in adults = Colo-colic

637. Ans. (b) Gastroduodenal artery

Ref: Bailey and Love, 26th ed. pg. 1023

- Perforations involving the gastroduodenal artery complex occur as a sequel to transmural ulceration of the posterior duodenal wall.
- The gastroduodenal artery, is a branch of the hepatic artery, passes behind the first part of the duodenum, and is responsible for bleeding in duodenal ulcer.

638. Ans. (c) It is accurate in detecting <50 mL of free blood

Ref: Bailey and Love, 26th ed. pg. 359

- *FAST does not reliably detect less than 100 ml of free blood. Hence choice **C is False.***
- It does not identify injury to hollow viscus. It cannot reliably exclude injury in penetrating trauma.

Focused assessment with sonography for trauma (FAST) should include views of

- Hepato-renal recess (Morison pouch)
- Peri-splenic view
- Sub-xiphoid pericardial window
- Supra-pubic window (Douglas pouch).

If an extended FAST (E-FAST) examination is performed, views of

- *The bilateral hemithoraces and*
- *The upper anterior chest wall, should also be obtained.*

639. Ans. (c) Full thickness skin graft

Ref: Bailey and Love, 26th ed. pg. 404

If the entire thickness of the dermis is included, the appropriate term is full-thickness skin graft (FTSG). If less than the entire thickness of the dermis is included, this graft is referred to as a split-thickness skin graft (STSG).

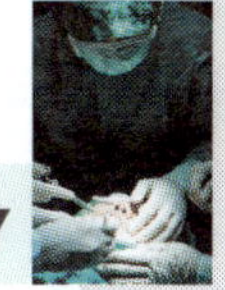

STSGs are categorized further as

- Thin (0.005–0.012 in)
- Intermediate (0.012–0.018 in)
- Thick (0.018–0.030 in)
- Split-thickness skin grafts (of varying thickness). These are sometimes called Thiersch grafts. They are used to cover all sizes of wound, are of limited durability and will contract. They may be used to provide valuable temporary wound closure before better cosmetic secondary correction after rehabilitation.
- *Full-thickness skin grafts (Wolfe grafts)*: Used for smaller areas of skin replacement where good elastic skin that will not contract is required (such as fingers, eyelids, facial parts).
- *Composite skin grafts (usually skin and fat, or skin and cartilage)*. Often taken from the ear margin and useful for rebuilding missing elements of nose, eyelids and fingertips

640. Ans. (d) Liver Laceration

Ref: Bailey and Love 26th ed. pg. 1073

- Pringle maneuver is used for control of bleeding in liver trauma
- This technique enables surgeons to *halt hemorrhage and find the source of bleeding*, allowing time for repair of the vessel. In the setting of hepatic resection of benign and malignant lesions, this maneuver *can be used to assist with control of bleeding.*
- *It involves vascular inflow occlusion by placing an atraumatic clamp across the foramen of Winslow.*

641. Ans. (b) At the induction of anaesthesia

Ref: Bailey and Love 26th ed. pg. 1109

- Prophylaxis is uniformly recommended for all clean-contaminated, contaminated and dirty procedures.
- Timing of antibiotic administration is critical to efficacy. The first dose should always be given before the procedure, preferably within 30–60 minutes *before incision.*
- Re-administration at one to two half-lives of the antibiotic is recommended for the duration of the procedure.
- In general, postoperative administration is not recommended.
- There is a delay before host defences can become mobilised after a breach in an epithelial surface, whether caused by trauma or surgery. The acute inflammatory, humoral and cellular defences take up to 4 hours to be mobilised. This is called the 'decisive period', and it is the time when the invading bacteria may become established in the tissues.
- Cefazolin provides adequate coverage for most other types of procedures.

642. Ans. (b) Polyamide polymer

Ref: Bailey and Love, 26th ed. pg. 37

TABLE: Non-absorbable suture materials

Suture	Types	Raw Material
Silk	Braided or twisted multifilament Dyed or undyed Coated (with wax or silicones) or uncoated	Natural protein Raw silk from silkworm
Linen	Twisted	Long staple flax fibres
Nylon	Monofilament or multifilament	Polyamide
Polybutester	Monofilament Dyed or undyed	Polybutylene terephthalate and polytetramethylene ether glycol
Polypropylene	Monofilament Dyed or undyed	Polybutylene terephthalate and polytetramethylene Polymer of propylene

643. Ans. (a) Anatomical abnormality is unilateral and contralateral testis should not be fixed

Ref: Bailey and Love, 26th ed. pg. 1379

Anatomical abnormality is unilateral and contralateral testis should not be fixed	*The other testis should also be fixed because the anatomical predisposition is likely to be bilateral. An infarcted testis should be removed and prosthetic device deployed.*
Prompt exploration and twisting and fixation is the only way to save the torted testis	Patient presents with sudden agonising pain in the groin and the lower abdomen. The patient feels nauseated and may vomit. If the testis is viable when the cord is untwisted it should be prevented from twisting again by fixation with non-absorbable sutures between the tunica vaginalis and the tunica albuginea.
Most common between 10 and 25 years of age	Testicular torsion is most common between 10 and 25 years of age, although a few cases occur in infancy.
Inversion of testis is the most common predisposing cause	Inversion of the testis is the most common predisposing cause. The testis is rotated so that it lies transversely or upside down.

644. Ans. (b) Pain

Ref: Handbook of Clinical Anesthesia, 3rd ed. pg. 783

Pain should be recorded as the fifth vital sign along with blood pressure, heart rate, respiratory rate and temperature.

645. Ans. (d) Squamous cell carcinoma

Ref: Devita, 9th ed. pg. 729

- Most common site oral Cancer: Carcinoma Tongue > Carcinoma Lip
- Most common histological type: Squamous Cell Cancer
- Most common site of oral Cancer in India: Cancer of Buccal Mucosa
- Max Risk of L.N. Metastasis: Carcinoma Tongue
- Min Risk of L.N Metastasis: Carcinoma lip > hard palate
- Most common age: 50-60 years

646. Ans. (b) Intestinal metaplasia

Ref: Sabiston, 19th ed. pg. 1033

- Barrett's esophagus is characterized by metaplasia of esophageal squamous epithelium into columnar in distal esophagus.
- For diagnosis of Barrett's esophagus it requires both endoscopically visible segment of columnar lining of distal esophagus and intestinal metaplasia showing goblet cells on biopsy.
- Barrett's esophagus is the single most important risk factor for adenocarcinoma of esophagus.
- Adenocarcinoma develops at the squamo-columnar junction or within 2 cm from the junction.

647. Ans. (c) Spontaneous perforation

Ref: Sabiston, 19th ed/1043, SRB manual of Surgery/1287

- Boerhaave's syndrome is spontaneous perforation of esophagus, occurring usually due to severe barotrauma when a person vomits against a closed glottis.
- Most common location of perforation is left posterolateral side of the distal esophagus.
- Tear is full thickness penetrating complete through all the layers of esophageal wall with spillage of contents into the mediastinum. (In Mallory Weiss tear it is partial thickness, extends through the mucosa and submucosa, but not through the muscular layer.)
- **Clinical finding – *Mackler's triad***
  - Vomiting
  - Thoracic pain
  - Cervical subcutaneous emphysema

648. Ans. (d) Gastric freezing

Ref: Harrison, 18th ed. pg. 2598

- Endoscopy followed by endoscopic variceal ligation should be performed.
- Balloon tamponade with Sengstaken Blakemore tube or Minnesota tube can be used in patients who cannot get endoscopic therapy immediately or who need stabilization prior to endoscopic therapy.
- Some endoscopists will use variceal injection therapy (sclerotherapy) as initial therapy, particularly when bleeding is vigorous.
- Shunt therapy (Transjugular intrahepatic portacaval shunt) has been shown to control refractory bleeding.

Pharmacologic Therapy for Variceal Hemorrhage

- Vasopressin, most potent vasoconstrictor, use is limited by side effects.
- Somatostatin and octreotide
- Octreotide is the preferred pharmacological agent

649. Ans. (c) Like toothpaste emulsion in the gallbladder

Ref: Harrison, 18th ed. pg. 2622

- It is a complication of chronic cholecystitis.
- Calcium salts in the lumen of the gallbladder in sufficient concentration may produce calcium precipitation and diffuse, hazy opacification of bile or a layering effect on plain abdominal radiography.
- This so called **limey bile or milk of calcium bile**, is usually clinically innocuous but cholecystectomy is recommended, especially when it occurs in a hydropic gallbladder.
- In the entity called porcelain gallbladder, calcium salt deposition within the wall of a chronically inflamed gallbladder may be detected on the plain abdominal film.

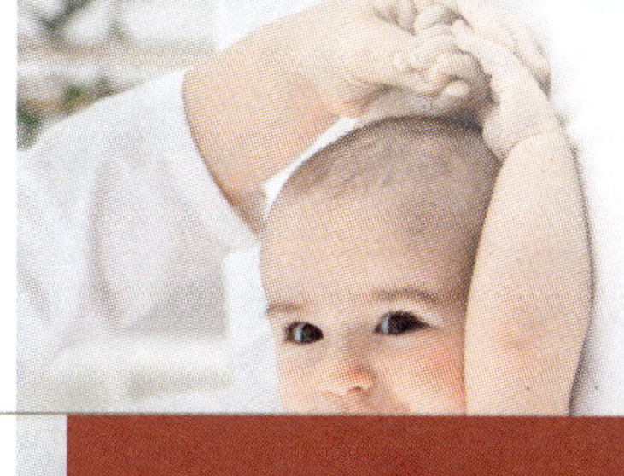

PEDIATRICS

11

MOST RECENT QUESTIONS 2023

1. What is the diagnosis of the birth defect shown in the image? ***(Most Recent Question July 2023)***

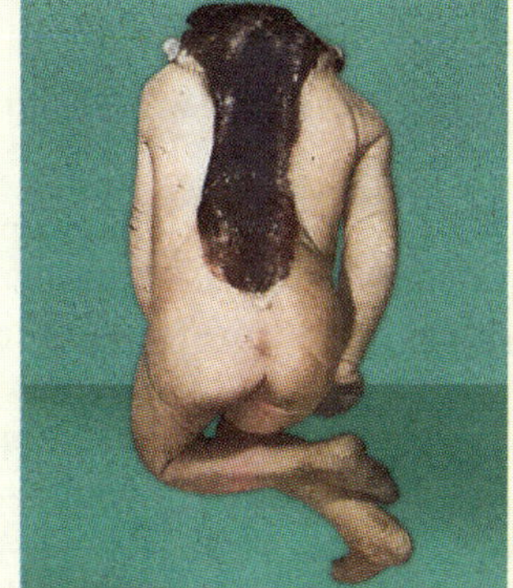

a. Craniorachischisis b. Anencephaly
c. Myelomeningocele d. Spina Bifida

2. A two-week-old infant is brought to the emergency department because of poor feeding, abdominal distention, and vomiting since he was born. Physical exam reveals bilateral cataracts and hepatomegaly. Urine has reducing substances but absence of glucose. Which of the following enzyme deficiency is responsible for this presentation? ***(Most Recent Question July 2023)***

a. GALT deficiency
b. Glucose 6 phosphatase deficiency
c. UDP Galactose 4 Epimerase
d. Galactokinase deficiency

3. What is the amount of milk given to a term baby in first 24 hours after delivery? ***(Most Recent Question July 2023)***

a. 40 mL/kg b. 50 mL/kg
c. 60 mL/kg d. 80 mL/kg

4. What is the dose of vitamin A given in a child of age 1–8 years? ***(Most Recent Question July 2023)***

a. 2 lakh IU every 6 months till 5 years
b. 2 lakh IU every 6 months till 4 years
c. 1 lakh IU every 5 months till 5 years
d. 2 lakh IU every 4 months till 4 years

5. What is the mid-arm circumference for severe acute malnutrition? ***(Most Recent Question July 2023)***

a. 12.5 cm b. 12 cm
c. 11.5 cm d. 11 cm

6. A child is brought to well-baby clinic with complaints of developing recurrent respiratory infections. Physical examination shows height for age to be less than minus 2 SD as compared to the expected. On detailed history, incorrect feeding methods were found to be used by parents. What is the appropriate term for the above-mentioned condition?

(Most Recent Question July 2023)

a. Stunting b. Wasting
c. Dwarfism d. Wasting and stunted

7. A 3-year-old child from a village is brought with complaints of developing cough, coryza and conjunctivitis for past 4 days and development of maculopapular rash which started on day 4 of illness from behind the ears and spread to rest of trunk. The clinical diagnosis is:

(Most Recent Question July 2023)

a. Measles b. Dengue
c. Rubella d. Chicken pox

8. A 2-year-old child is brought to the clinic with feeble pulses and obtundation. On examination he has severe malnutrition as deduced from anthropometric parameters. What would be the choice of resuscitation for this patient? ***(Most Recent Question July 2023)***

a. ORS
b. NS
c. RL with 5% Dextrose
d. DNS

9. In which trimester, following markers beta-HCG, Serum alpha fetoprotein, serum estriol and inhibin-A are done for antenatal screening?

(Most Recent Question July 2023)

a. 1st
b. 2nd
c. 3rd
d. 4th

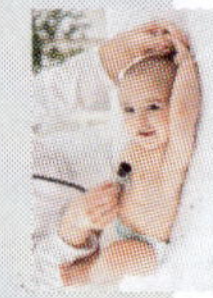

10. In a newborn child with development delay and recurrent pneumonia episodes the following appearance is noted. Comment on the diagnosis.

(Most Recent Question July 2023)

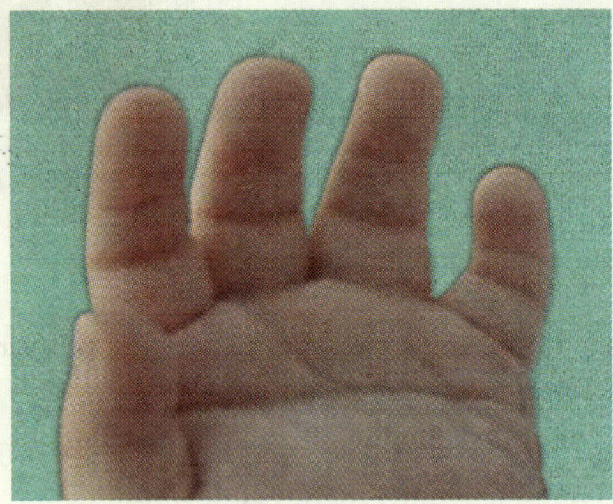

a. 47, XY (+21)
b. 45, XO
c. 47 XY (+18)
d. 47 XXY

11. A child presents with short stature. His bone age is less than the chronological age. The height of his parents is normal. What is the diagnosis?

(Most Recent Question Jan 2023)

a. Constitutional delay in growth
b. Familial short stature
c. Cretinism
d. Malnutrition

12. An 8 -month child was found to have bitot spots and nyctalopia. What is the dose of oral vitamin A required?

(Most Recent Question Jan 2023)

a. 50000 IU
b. 75000 IU
c. 100000 IU
d. 200000 IU

13. True statement regarding the image given here:

(Most Recent Question Jan 2023)

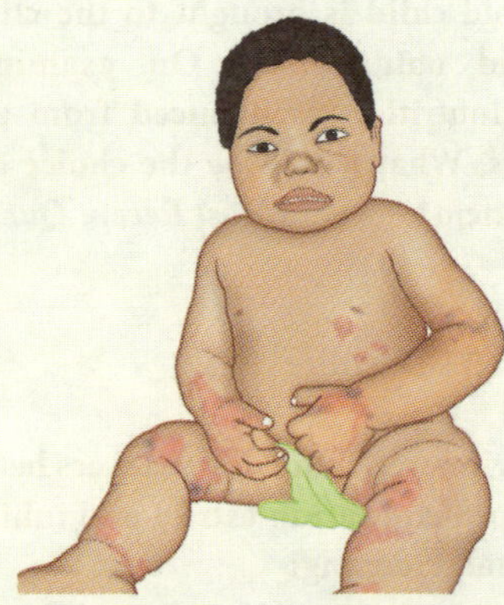

a. Kwashiorkor due to less protein intake
b. Marasmus due to less protein intake
c. Marasmus due to less calorie intake
d. Kwashiorkor due to less calorie intake

14. A 5-year-old child develops a fever with rashes. Also had cough, conjunctivitis and Coryza. The image of the child is given here. What is the diagnosis?

(Most Recent Question Jan 2023)

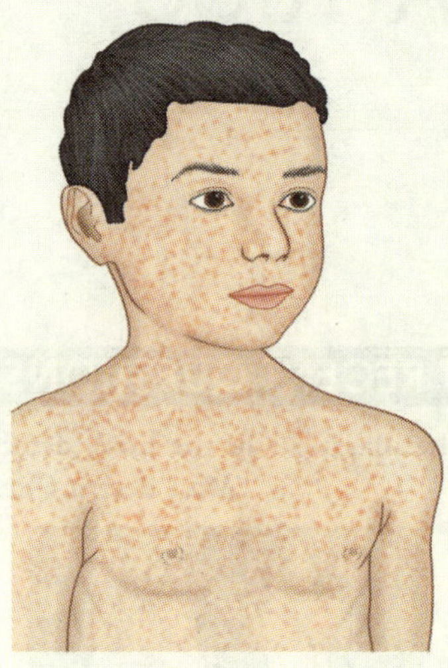

a. Measles
b. Chicken pox
c. Erythema infectiosum
d. Hand foot mouth disease

15. Within how many hours can breast feeding be initiated in a perfectly healthy child with no anatomical problems?

(Most Recent Question Jan 2023)

a. 1 hour
b. 3 hours
c. 24 hours
d. 48 hours

16. A 2-year-old child is brought to the clinic with feeble pulses and obtundation. On examination, he has severe malnutrition as deduced from anthropometric parameters. What would be the choice of resuscitation for this patient? ***(Most Recent Question Jan 2023)***

a. Ringer lactate
b. 10% Dextrose
c. Normal saline
d. Ringer lactate +5% dextrose

17. Which of the following are not correct about ABCDE in Pediatrics Advanced Life Support (PALS)?

(Most Recent Question Jan 2023)

a. A airway
b. B- breathing
c. C- circulation
d. D- dehydrate

18. According to neonatal resuscitation protocol, chest compression is initiated at heart rate of:

(Most Recent Question Jan 2023)

a. 80/min
b. 75/min
c. 70/min
d. 60/min

19. According to neonatal resuscitation protocol, how much oxygen is to be given in a term neonate with apnea and bradycardia initially? ***(Most Recent Question Jan 2023)***

a. 21%
b. 30%
c. 50%
d. 100%

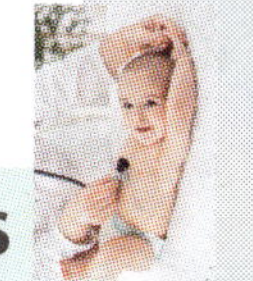

20. A neonate is unable to open the eyelid. Identify the condition given in the image here:
(Most Recent Question Jan 2023)

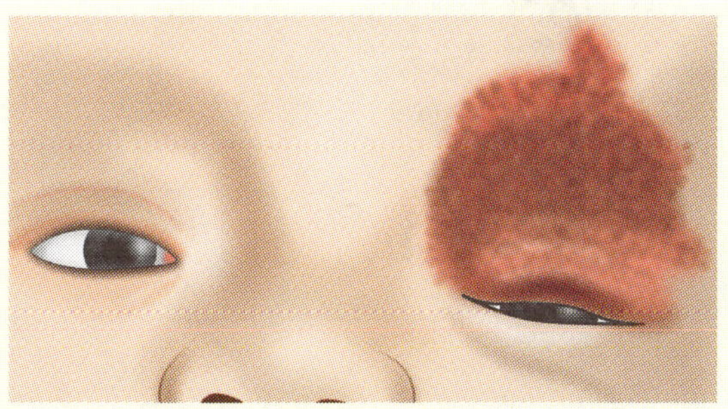

a. Capillary hemangioma
b. Mongolian spot
c. Milia
d. Erythema toxicum neonatorum

21. A neonate born to primigravida at home is brought at 12 hours of life with the history of frothiness from mouth. X-ray of the child is given here. What is the diagnosis?
(Most Recent Question Jan 2023)

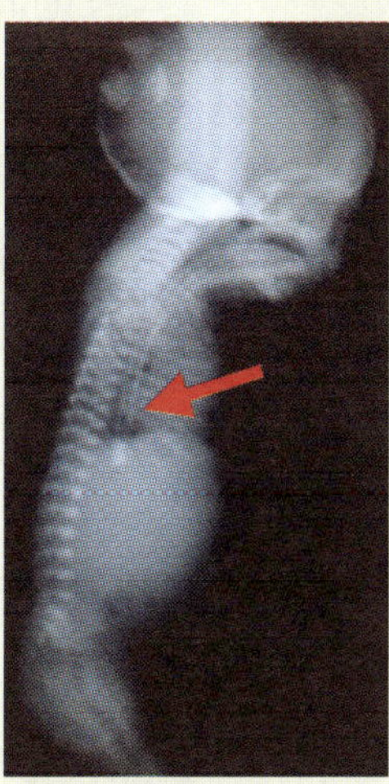

a. Transient tachypnea of newborn
b. Hyaline membrane disease
c. Esophageal atresia
d. Bochdalek hernia

22. An 8-year-old child presents with high grade fever, restlessness for last 2 days and is found to have neck rigidity. LP was done and CSF shows turbid CSF with 80% PMN cells and 20% Lymphocytes. What is the diagnosis? *(Most Recent Question Jan 2023)*

a. Bacterial meningitis
b. TB meningitis
c. Viral meningitis
d. Fungal meningitis

NEONATOLOGY

23. Vitamin K is given at birth to prevent the following?
(Most Recent Question Dec 2021)

a. Hemorrhagic disease of newborn
b. Neonatal asphyxia
c. Neonatal hypoglycemia
d. Hemolytic anemia

24. Infant of diabetic mother is at risk of development of which of the following?
(Most Recent Question Dec 2021)

a. Hypoglycemia b. Hyperglycemia
c. Anemia d. Diarrhea

25. A newborn is found to have ambiguous genitalia. Work up shows high 17 hydroxyprogesterone, progesterone and DHEAS levels. Which enzyme deficiency is responsible?
(Most Recent Question Dec 2021)

a. 21 hydroxylase
b. 17 beta hydroxylases
c. 11 hydroxylase
d. 17 alpha hydroxylase

26. Which of the following not included in Essential Newborn Care? *(Most Recent Question Dec 2021)*

a. Ear care b. Clean the baby
c. Breastfeeding d. Temperature maintenance

27. Neonate is detected to have facial abnormality, thymic hypoplasia and Tetralogy of fallot. These features would be present in which of the following syndrome?
(Most Recent Question Dec 2021)

a. DiGeorge b. Down
c. Turner d. Klinefelter

28. Which of the following reflexes is first to appear in a child? *(Most Recent Question June 2021)*

a. Palmar grasp reflex
b. Transferring object from hand to hand
c. Parachute reflex
d. Rooting reflex

29. A mother with a newborn is worried for her child as the newborn hasn't passed the meconium till after 6 hours of birth. How much maximum time should she wait for the meconium to pass out? *(Most Recent Question Dec 2020)*

a. 48 hours b. 24 hours
c. 12 hours d. 22 hours

30. A neonate who was just born, was found to have a heart rate of 120/min with weak and irregular respiratory efforts. He had a pink body with blue extremities, partially flexed and he grimaced on stimulation by catheter. What is the APGAR score for this baby?
(Most Recent Question Aug 2020)

a. 5 b. 8
c. 6 d. 7

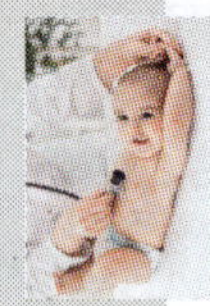

31. Neonatal jaundice becomes detectable at serum bilirubin exceeding? *(Most Recent Question 2019)*

a. 2 mg%
b. 3 mg%
c. 4 mg%
d. 5 mg%

32. Protein in Cow's milk in comparison to human milk is? *(Most Recent Question 2019)*

a. Double
b. Triple
c. Quadruple
d. Same

33. Maximum heat loss in neonate is from: *(Recent Pattern Question 2018–19)*

a. Head
b. Skin
c. Respiration
d. Trunk

34. All are features of congenital syphilis; EXCEPT: *(Recent Pattern Question 2018-19)*

a. Gumma
b. Saddle nose
c. Osteochondritis
d. Charcot joints

35. Which is the best marker for NTD? *(Recent Pattern Question 2018)*

a. αFP
b. hCG
c. Pseudocholinesterase
d. Inhibin-A

36. The pupil of a newborn is: *(Recent Pattern Question 2018)*

a. Dilated
b. Mid-dilated
c. Constricted
d. Normal

37. Gynecomastia in neonate is seen due to: *(Recent Pattern Question 2018)*

a. Transplacental transfer of estrogen
b. Transplacental transfer of progesterone
c. GnRH
d. Gonadotropins

38. A term child is brought with complaints of having jaundice on day 3 of life. How much should be the minimum level to cause jaundice? *(Recent Pattern Question 2017)*

a. 5 mg%
b. 10 mg%
c. 15 mg%
d. 20 mg%

39. A term baby is apneic and has a heart rate 90/min. Bag and mask ventilation was given for 30 seconds. Subsequently the Heart rate is still less than 100 bpm. What is the next step? *(Recent Pattern Question 2017)*

a. Reduce oxygen supply
b. Check chest movement
c. Give supplemental oxygen
d. Give chest compression

40. What is the diagnosis of the child shown in the image, whose mother is having Bronchial asthma? *(Recent Pattern Question 2016)*

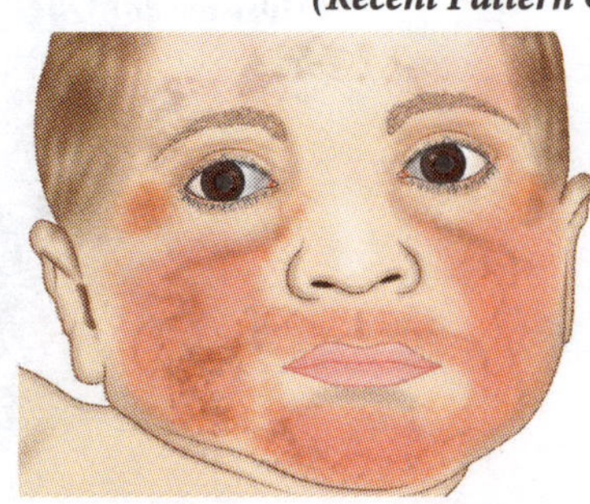

a. Atopic dermatitis
b. Contact dermatitis
c. Seborrheic dermatitis
d. Irritant dermatitis

41. Apgar score system contains all of the following criteria; EXCEPT:

a. Respiratory rate
b. Color
c. Motor activity
d. Heart rate

42. For accurate measurement of axillary temperature in newborn, thermometer is kept for:

a. 1 minute
b. 2 minutes
c. 3 minutes
d. 5 minutes

43. Anterior fontanelle corresponds to all structures; EXCEPT:

a. Frontal bones
b. Coronal suture
c. Lambdoid suture
d. Saggital suture

44. What is the most common cause of Jaundice in term newborns requiring treatment?

a. Rh incompatibility
b. ABO incompatibility
c. Physiological jaundice
d. Sepsis

45. In neonatal sepsis, acute phase reactant is:

a. WBC
b. Alpha anti trypsin
c. IL-6
d. CRP

46. True about Cephal-hematoma:

a. Jaundice is prolonged due to cephal-hematoma
b. Crosses the suture line
c. Appears on occiput in first few hours of life
d. Due to rupture of bridging arteries

47. Hutchinson teeth are seen in:

a. Early congenital spirochete infection
b. Late congenital syphilis
c. Rickets
d. Scurvy

48. Congenital Rubella Syndrome has all of the following; EXCEPT:

a. Sensorineural deafness
b. Cataract
c. Cardiac defects
d. Hydrocephalus

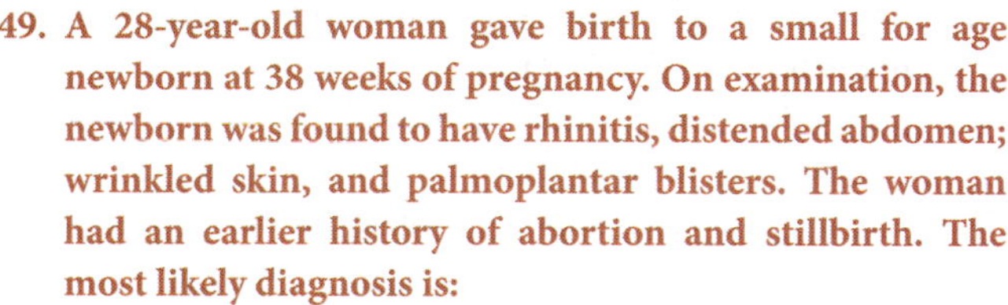

49. A 28-year-old woman gave birth to a small for age newborn at 38 weeks of pregnancy. On examination, the newborn was found to have rhinitis, distended abdomen; wrinkled skin, and palmoplantar blisters. The woman had an earlier history of abortion and stillbirth. The most likely diagnosis is:

a. Neonatal pemphigus b. Scabies
c. Congenital syphilis d. Congenital HIV infection

50. Physiological jaundice in a full term newborn usually resolves by:

a. One week b. Two weeks
c. Three weeks d. Four weeks

51. The time usually taken for air to reach the descending colon after birth in a normal infant is:

a. 1–2 hrs b. 3–4 hrs
c. 5–6 hrs d. 8–9 hrs

52. In neonatal resuscitation which is correct?

a. Put cold water on back
b. Slap on back
c. Tickle the sole
d. Suspend head down

53. Drug of choice for acute lead encephalopathy

a. Succimer b. d-penicillamine
c. EDTA d. Zinc acetate

54. Key features of kangaroo mother care are all the following; EXCEPT?

a. Skin to skin contact between mother and baby
b. Exclusive breastfeeding
c. Initiated in a facility and continued at home
d. Done for babies with cyanosis

55. Nipple confusion means?

a. Baby fed with a bottle finding it difficult and confusing to suckle at breast
b. Baby not able to suckle with bottle
c. Baby not able to feed with spoon
d. Baby not able to feed with paladi

56. Bag and mask ventilation is contraindicated in newborn resuscitation with clinical suspicion of?

a. Diaphragmatic hernia b. Intracranial hemorrhage
c. Meconium ileus d. Pneumothorax

57. A mother complains that baby is more comfortable and breathes better when held against shoulder. What important clinical problem do you suspect?

a. Nose block
b. Psychological anxiety or insecurity
c. Aerophagy with abdominal fullness
d. Orthopnea

58. The following component of human milk is not protective against GIT infections?

a. Lysozyme b. Lactoferrin
c. Bifidus factor d. β_2 transferrin

59. Increased oxygen delivery during prematurity causes all the following; EXCEPT:

a. Vasoconstriction
b. Vasodilation
c. Vaso obliteration
d. Neovascularisation

60. Expressed breast milk can be stored at room temperature for how many hours?

a. 4 b. 8
c. 16 d. 24

61. Pathological jaundice criteria includes all; EXCEPT:

a. 24 hours later but within 72 hours
b. More than 14 days persistence
c. >2 mg/dL conjugated bilirubin
d. Clay colored stool

62. Growing fetus derives energy from?

a. Amino acid b. Carbohydrate
c. Lipid d. Minerals

63. The ratio of chest compression to breathing in neonatal life support is?

a. 3:1 b. 4:1
c. 5:1 d. 6:1

64. Which type of cerebral palsy is most commonly seen as a sequel of bilirubin encephalopathy?

a. Spastic quadriparesis
b. Spastic diplegia
c. Atonic cerebral palsy
d. Extra pyramidal cerebral palsy

65. Hemorrhagic disease of the newborn is attributed to the deficiency of?

a. Vitamin A b. Vitamin E
c. Vitamin K d. Vitamin C

66. In neonate which is the indication for chest compressions?

a. Irregular breathing with heart rate 80 after 30 seconds
b. Regular breathing with heart rate 80 after 30 seconds
c. AMBU Bag ventilation for 30 seconds with heart rate of 50
d. Regular breathing with Cyanosis

MILESTONES IN CHILDREN

67. First tooth to erupt in a child is:

(Most Recent Question June 2021)

a. Lower central incisor
b. Upper central incisor
c. First molar
d. Second molar

68. What is the cut off level of imbecile?

(Recent Pattern Question 2018)

a. 0–20 b. 20–49
c. 50–69 d. >70

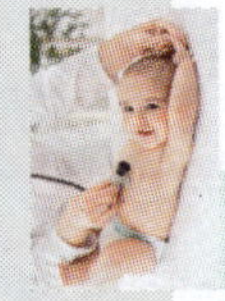

69. A baby with tripod position, bi dextrous approach, recognises strangers and can spell out mono syllable by what age:

a. 7 months b. 12 months
c. 9 months d. 10 months

70. Beyond what age, absence of social smile is regarded as abnormal:

a. 12 weeks b. 14 weeks
c. 16 weeks d. 18 weeks

71. Moro's reflex disappears by which age?

a. 3 months b. 6 months
c. 9 months d. 12 months

72. Most common cause of neonatal mortality in India?

a. Prematurity
b. Congenital malformation
c. Pneumonia
d. Metabolic (hypoglycemia)

73. A baby placed in the prone position is able to lift the head and upper chest on extended arms by?

a. 1 month b. 3 months
c. 6 months d. 9 months

BREASTFEEDING

74. Which vitamin is deficient in breast milk?
(Most Recent Question June 2022)

a. Vitamin A b. Vitamin C
c. Vitamin D d. Vitamin K

75. Absolute contraindication to breastfeeding?
(Most Recent Question Dec 2021)

a. Galactosemia in the infant
b. Maternal hepatitis C
c. Maternal CMV
d. Herpes not involving the breast

76. All are true about human colostrum; EXCEPT?
(Most Recent Question Dec 2021)

a. Thick and yellow color
b. IgA high
c. High amino acids and minerals
d. High sugar and fat

77. What should be the best initial feeding method for a baby born at 33 weeks gestation, with no perinatal complication? *(Most Recent Question Aug 2020)*

a. IV fluid b. Breastfeeding
c. Orogastric tube feed d. Paladai feeding

78. Best management for formula fed child with severe Cow milk protein allergy? *(Recent Pattern Question 2016)*

a. Soya milk
b. Hydrolysed formula feed
c. Amino acid based formula
d. Total Parenteral nutrition

79. All of the following are signs of good attachment during breastfeeding; EXCEPT:

a. Baby's mouth is wide open
b. Baby's lower lip is inverted
c. Upper areola is more visible than lower
d. Baby's chin touching the breast

80. All of the following are signs of good attachment during breastfeeding; EXCEPT:

a. Baby's mouth is wide open
b. Baby's lower lip is everted
c. Lower areola is more visible than upper
d. Baby's chin touching the breast

81. Recommendation for exclusive breastfeeding is up to:

a. 3 months b. 4 months
c. 5 months d. 6 months

82. Breast milk contains all; EXCEPT?

a. Lacta globulin b. Lactoalbumin
c. Whey protein d. Avidin

83. "Good attachment" of infant to mother's breast during breastfeeding includes all of the following; EXCEPT:

a. Chin of the infant touches mother's breast
b. Upper part of areola is visible more than the lower part
c. Lower lip of infant is inverted
d. Mouth of infant is wide open

84. Which amino acid, present in human milk in large amount helps in brain development?

a. Alanine b. Tyrosine
c. Lysine d. Taurine

GROWTH AND DEVELOPMENT

85. By WHO reference child's height for age <2 SD is called _____? *(Most Recent Question June 2022)*

a. Under weight b. Stunting
c. Wasting d. Stunting and wasting

86. A child came for regular check up in OPD. His growth chart shows that weight of the child is between 85th and 95th percentile. Comment on child status?
(Most Recent Question June 2022)

a. Obesity
b. Severe acute malnutrition
c. Overweight
d. BMI needed for interpretation

87. Chronic malnutrition in child is best evaluated by?
(Most Recent Question 2019)

a. Weight for height b. Weight for age
c. Height for age d. Ponderal index

88. Swallowing reflex appears at?
(Recent Pattern Question 2017)

a. 6 week b. 16 weeks
c. 18 weeks d. 22 weeks

89. Undescended testis is a feature of:
(Recent Pattern Question 2016)
a. Prematurity b. Post term
c. Term child d. Term small for date

90. How many teeth are present in a 3 year child?
a. 8 teeth b. 12 teeth
c. 18 teeth d. 20 teeth

91. False regarding the testicular development during fetal stage:
a. Develop in abdomen
b. Gubernaculum plays decisive role
c. 7 months into scrotum
d. Scrotum empty at 7 months

92. All of the following are common problems of pre-school children; EXCEPT:
a. Temper tantrums b. Sleep problems
c. Truancy d. Pica

93. Early sign of puberty in male is enlargement of testes. In females it is determined by:
a. Pubarche b. Menarche
c. Thelarche d. Menstruation

94. Nocturnal Enuresis is occurrence of involuntary voiding at night in a child more than:
a. 2 ½ years b. 3 ½ years
c. 4 years d. 5 years

95. An infant is considered anemic at Hemoglobin less than gm%?
a. 8 b. 9
c. 10 d. 12

96. A 3-year-old Child who has diurnal enuresis and soiling of clothes. Treatment required?
a. Urethroplasty
b. Put catheter for 7 days
c. Circumcision at 10 years
d. Behavior modification

97. Rickets in India is most commonly caused by?
a. Malnutrition b. Lack of sun exposure
c. Lactose intolerance d. Genetics

98. Age at which child can tell gender?
a. 2 years b. 3 years
c. 4 years d. 5 years

99. Concerning attention deficit hyperactivity disorder which is true?
a. Impulsive behavior is a feature
b. Higher incidence in tic disorders
c. May respond to treatment with stimulants such as amphetamine
d. All of the above

100. X-ray of choice for age detection in 6 months old child is?
a. Skull b. Hand
c. Knee d. Shoulder

101. Most common location of supernumerary teeth is?
a. Between incisors b. Between canines
c. Between molars d. Between premolars

102. Birth weight doubles by?
a. 3 months b. 5 months
c. 9 months d. 12 months

103. Birth length doubles by what age?
a. 1 year b. 2 years
c. 3 years d. 4 years

104. At what age do first permanent teeth appear?
a. 5 years b. 6 years
c. 7 years d. 8 years

105. Vocabulary of a 2 year old child is?
a. 20 words b. 50 words
c. 100 words d. 200 words

106. A child draws Triangle at what age?
a. 3 years b. 4 years
c. 5 years d. 7 years

107. A 18 month baby can do which of the following?
a. Hide & seek game
b. Write Alphabet
c. Say short sentence
d. Walk short distance

108. Which of the following is called as red flag sign in child development, if not attained?
a. Vocalization at 2 months
b. Walking at 12 months
c. Single word at 12 months
d. Social smile at 3 months

109. Which of the following-is the first sign of sexual maturity in boys?
a. Increase in height
b. Appearance of facial hair
c. Change in voice
d. Increase in testicular size

110. At what age (in years) does-a child attain a height of 100 cms?
a. 2 b. 3
c. 4 d. 5

PROTEIN ENERGY MALNUTRITION

111. A child is having growth retardation and was on exclusive breast milk until 3 years of age. Child is dull and lethargic. Pitting Edema is present on examination. Diagnosis is: *(Most Recent Question June 2022)*
a. Hypothyroidism b. Kwashiorkor
c. Marasmus d. Severe acute malnutrition

112. Sugar baby appearance is seen in:
(Most Recent Question Dec 2021)
a. Kwashiorkor b. Scurvy
c. Marasmus d. Vitamin B1 deficiency

113. Child brought to casualty has complete loss of subcutaneous fat, wrinkled skin and muscle wasting. Diagnosis is: ***(Most Recent Question Dec 2021)***

a. Carbohydrate deficiency
b. Protein deficiency
c. Lipid deficiency
d. Caloric Deficiency

114. This form of malnutrition is due to which of following? ***(Most Recent Question June 2021)***

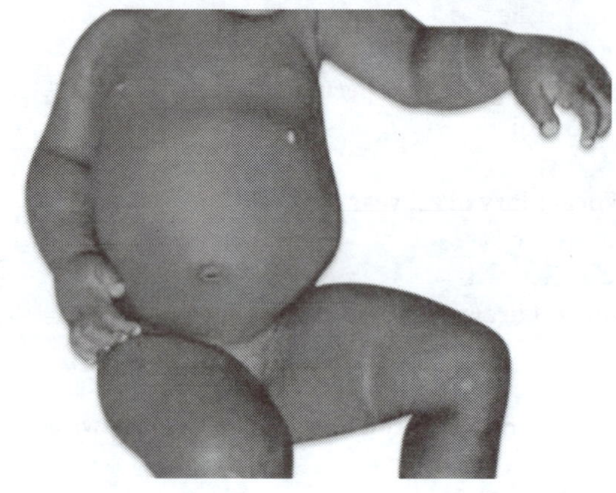

a. Less protein intake
b. Less energy intake
c. Less fat intake
d. Less iron intake

115. For severe malnutrition MAC will be less than – ***(Most Recent Question Dec 2019)***

a. 14.5
b. 13.5
c. 12.5
d. 11.5

116. Which is the most specific clinical feature for diagnosis for Kwashiorkor? ***(Recent Pattern Question 2018)***

a. Fatty liver
b. Easy pluckable hair
c. Low serum albumin
d. Edema

117. Chronic malnutrition is measured by:

a. Weight/height
b. Height/age
c. Weight/age
d. Mid arm circumference

118. Which is the best parameter for acute severe malnutrition:

a. Weight/height
b. Height/age
c. Weight/age
d. Mid arm circumference

119. BMI is measured in children by:

a. $Wt.kg/Ht.m^2$
b. $Wt.kg/Ht.cm^2$
c. $Wt.g/Ht.cm^2$
d. $Wt.g/Ht.m^2$

120. Very low birth weight child weighs:

a. 1000 g
b. <1500 g
c. <2500 g
d. <750 g

121. Extremely low birth weight baby is defined as?

a. <1000 g
b. <1500 g
c. <2500 g
d. <2800 g

122. What is the mid upper arm circumference – cut off value for malnutrition of a child:

a. 12.5 cm
b. 10.5 cm
c. 14.5 cm
d. 9.5 cm

123. Ponderal index in malnourished babies is?

a. <1
b. <2
c. <4
d. <6

124. A 4-year-old boy, with swollen bleeding gums, petechiae and dry eyes. Diagnosis:

a. Rickets
b. Marasmus
c. Scurvy
d. Dehydration

125. Flag hair sign is seen in

a. Kwashiorkor
b. Marasmus
c. Scurvy
d. Pellagra

126. All are seen in Marasmus; EXCEPT:

a. Muscle wasting
b. Hepatomegaly
c. Low insulin
d. Muscle wasting

127. All are seen in Kwashiorkor; EXCEPT:

a. Increase appetite
b. Flag sign on hair
c. Hepatomegaly
d. Apathy

128. Nutritional rickets is treated by a single dose of vitamin D of:

a. 5,000 mcg
b. 10,000 mcg
c. 15,000 mcg
d. 20,000 mcg

129. All are seen in nutritional Rickets; EXCEPT:

a. Pseudoparalysis
b. Delayed dentition
c. Widening of the wrist joint
d. Double medial malleolus

130. The metabolic defect in hereditary fructose intolerance is due to deficiency of enzyme:

a. Fructokinase
b. Aldolase-B
c. Xylitol dehydrogenase
d. Phosphofructokinase

131. Chronic malnutrition diagnosis is based upon?

a. Decreased weight for age
b. MAC <11.5 cm
c. <3.5 g% serum protein
d. Decreased height for age

132. All are seen in marasmus; EXCEPT:

a. Hunger
b. Wasting
c. Loose folds skin
d. Apathy

PEDIATRIC NEUROLOGY

133. A 8-year-old child presents with recurrent staring episodes where he stopped blinking for 20 seconds. Which of the following drug would you like to give for treatment? ***(Most Recent Question Dec 2021)***

a. Valproate
b. Phenytoin
c. Diazepam
d. Midazolam

134. A child was brought to the emergency with generalized tonic-clonic seizures. Which drug should be given first to control his symptoms? ***(Most Recent Question Aug 2020)***

a. Valproate
b. Diazepam
c. Phenytoin
d. Haloperidol

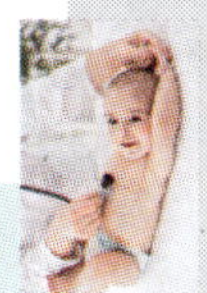

135. Medulloblastoma is: *(Recent Pattern Question 2018)*
a. Malignant tumor in adults
b. Malignant tumor in children
c. Benign brain tumor
d. Malignant cerebellar tumor in adults

136. Elevated amniotic fluid acetylcholinesterase is used for diagnosis of? *(Recent Pattern Question 2017)*
a. Neonatal myasthenia gravis
b. Spinal dysraphism
c. Hydrops fetalis
d. Neonatal heart block

137. Which of the following is a neural tube marker? *(Recent Pattern Question 2017)*
a. Pseudo-cholinesterase
b. Acetylcholinesterase
c. Transketolase
d. Beta 2 transferrin

138. NTD with maximum viability is: *(Recent Pattern Question 2017)*
a. Spina bifida occulta
b. Anencephaly
c. Myelomeningocele
d. Meningocele

139. SSPE is caused by? *(Recent Pattern Question 2017)*
a. Rubella b. Rubeola
c. Varicella d. Variola

140. A 1-year-old baby brought by the mother complaining of a cystic mass on back and inability to move both legs ever since birth. Possible diagnosis?
a. Pilonidal cyst b. Meningocoele
c. Meningomyelocoele d. Sacrococcygeal teratoma

141. All are true regarding congenital hydrocephalus; EXCEPT:
a. Stenosis of aqueduct can contribute
b. Mostly Hereditary in nature
c. Can be seen together with Spina bifida
d. Broad forehead and wide open anterior fontannel

142. In a child diagnosed with H. influenza meningitis, what investigation must be done before discharging him from the hospital?
a. BERA b. MRI
c. CT scan d. X-ray skull

143. Most common cause of meningo-encephalitis in children is?
a. HSV b. Measles
c. Adenovirus d. Enterovirus

144. All of the following are manifestations of hypervitaminosis A; EXCEPT?
a. Loss of hair
b. Generalized exfoliation
c. Decreased Intracranial pressure
d. Muscle pains

GENETICS

145. Neural tube defect shows which pattern of inheritance? *(Most Recent Question June 2022)*
a. Autosomal dominant
b. X linked recessive
c. Mitochondrial inheritance
d. Multifactorial inheritance

146. A couple is trying to have a child for past 2 years, after multiple unsuccessful trials they went for respective examination. Investigation of female came out to be absolutely normal but male shows presence of gynecomastia, small testis and scanty pubic hairs. He had a history of antisocial behavior during school days. Most probably he has: *(Most Recent Question June 2022)*
a. Williams syndrome b. Noonan syndrome
c. Klinefelter syndrome d. Marfan syndrome

147. A 7-year-old female child presents with crampy abdominal pain and rash mainly on the back of her leg, buttocks as well as on the extensor surface of his forearm. Laboratory analysis reveals proteinuria and microscopic hematuria. Diagnosis is: *(Most Recent Question June 2022)*
a. Systemic lupus erythematous
b. Hemolytic uremic syndrome
c. Post streptococcal glomerulonephritis
d. Henoch Schoenlein purpura

148. A child has a large head, large tongue and both the testicles are also large in size. The child also shows features of autism spectrum disorder. What is the probable diagnosis? *(Most Recent Question Aug 2020)*
a. Rett syndrome b. Fragile X-syndrome
c. Eisenmenger syndrome d. William syndrome

149. A child with developmental delay shows the karyotype depicted below. What is the probable diagnosis? *(Most Recent Question Aug 2020)*

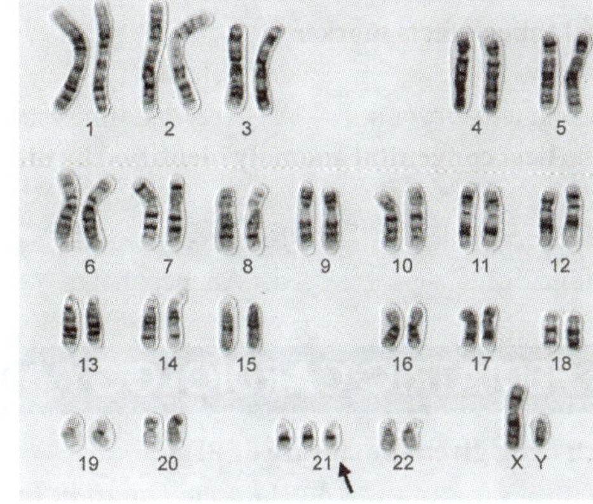

a. Turner syndrome b. Down syndrome
c. Edward syndrome d. Klinefelter syndrome

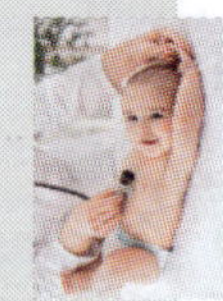

150. A 4-year-old boy is brought to the emergency unit after he is pushed down while playing. After falling on his knees, he developed swelling and bruising of his left knee. History revealed that his maternal uncle also has a similar presentation. What could be the probable mode of inheritance of this child's condition? *(Most Recent Question Aug 2020)*

a. X linked dominant b. X linked recessive
c. Autosomal dominant d. Autosomal recessive

151. Trisomy of Down's syndrome is:

a. 21 b. 22
c. 18 d. 13

152. Which is correct about estriol level in Down syndrome?

a. No change b. Low
c. Elevated d. Double-triple

153. Trisomy 18 is? *(Recent Pattern Question 2016)*

a. Down syndrome b. Edward syndrome
c. Patau syndrome d. Turner syndrome

154. Anti-mongoloid facies, Short stature, undescended testis, and pulmonic stenosis are seen in? *(Recent Pattern Question 2016)*

a. Noonan syndrome b. Down syndrome
c. Klinefelter syndrome d. Angelman syndrome

155. Which of the following marker is peculiar to quadruple test as compared to triple test used for prenatal screening of Down syndrome?

a. HCG b. Alpha feto protein
c. Inhibin d. Estriol

156. All are seen in Down's syndrome; EXCEPT:

a. Low IQ b. Brachycephaly
c. Umbilical hernia d. Hypothyroidism

157. For Prenatal diagnosis of Down's syndrome, all are true; EXCEPT?

a. Reduced femur and humerus length
b. Nuchal fold thickness >2.5 mm
c. Increased umbilical blood flow
d. Ventricular septal defect may be present

158. Neural tube defects marker

a. Estriol b. Beta hCG
c. Alpha feto-protein d. Acetylcholine esterase

159. The earliest congenital anomaly identified by ultrasound is:

a. Hydrocephalus b. Encephalocele
c. Spina bifida d. Anencephaly

PEDIATRIC CARDIOLOGY

160. Which drug given for closure of PDA? *(Most Recent Question June 2021)*

a. Indomethacin b. Mefenemaic acid
c. Paracetamol d. Ivabridine

161. All of the following are components of Tetralogy of Fallot; EXCEPT? *(Most Recent Question Aug 2020)*

a. Overriding of aorta
b. Tricuspid stenosis
c. Right ventricular hypertrophy
d. Ventricular septal defect

162. Severity of cyanosis in Fallot's physiology is best decided by: *(Most Recent Question 2019)*

a. V.S.D b. Overriding of aorta
c. Concentric RVH d. Subpulmonic stenosis

163. Most common cardiac anomaly associated with Noonan syndrome: *(Recent Pattern Question 2018–19)*

a. Pulmonic stenosis b. Coarctation of aorta
c. VSD d. TAPVR

164. Continuous murmur is heard in? *(Recent Pattern Question 2018–19)*

a. Patent ductus arteriosus b. VSD
c. ASD d. Tetralogy of Fallot

165. All of the following statements are true regarding TOF; EXCEPT: *(Recent Pattern Question 2018)*

a. Right ventricular hypertrophy
b. ASD
c. Overriding of aorta
d. Subpulmonic stenosis

166. The innocent murmur is best heard in children at: *(Recent Pattern Question 2018)*

a. Pulmonic area
b. Aortic area
c. Left lower sternal border
d. Apex

167. A 2-week-old child presents with cyanosis. Which of the following heart disease will have highest chances of 1 year survival? *(Recent Pattern Question 2017)*

a. TOF b. TGA
c. TAPVC d. Tricuspid Atresia

168. Which of the following is a feature of Tetralogy of fallot? *(Recent Pattern Question 2017)*

a. Pan-systolic murmur
b. Congestive heart failure
c. Pulmonic stenosis
d. Normal cardiothoracic ratio

169. Structure with functional closure immediately after birth? *(Recent Pattern Question 2017)*

a. Foramen Ovale b. Ductus venosus
c. Ductus arteriosus d. Umbilical artery

170. Most common heart defect in children? *(Recent Pattern Question 2016)*

a. Muscular V.S.D b. Membranous VSD
c. Ostium Secondum d. Ostium Primum

171. Which of the following is an acyanotic heart disease:

a. TOF b. TGA
c. PDA d. COA

172. All are seen in Kawasaki disease; EXCEPT:

a. Mitral regurgitation b. Ischemic heart disease
c. Myocarditis d. Pericardial tamponade

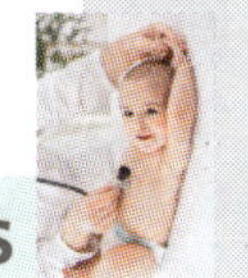

173. Which of the following is synonymous with Muco-cutaneous lymph node syndrome?
a. Scarlet fever b. Kawasaki disease
c. Behcet's syndrome d. Tuberculosis

174. In septum primum type of ASD over burden occurs in which chamber?
a. RV b. LV
c. RA d. LA

GASTROINTESTINAL TRACT

175. A 5-year-old boy presented with hematemesis and was found to have splenomegaly, on examination. There was a past history of exchange transfusion in this child for neonatal jaundice. What is the probable diagnosis? *(Most Recent Question Aug 2020)*
a. Budd-Chiari syndrome b. Portal hypertension
c. Liver cirrhosis d. Portal vein thrombosis

176. A 1-month-old baby presents with lethargy, non-bilious vomiting, excessive crying and F.T.T. The diagnosis is? *(Recent Pattern Question 2017)*
a. Ileal atresia
b. Duodenal atresia
c. Hypertrophic pyloric stenosis
d. Trachea-esophageal fistula

177. What is the dose of zinc given to 4-month-old child in diarrhoea? *(Recent Pattern Question 2016)*
a. 5 mg b. 10 mg
c. 15 mg d. 20 mg

178. In pediatrics, differential for Acute appendicitis are all; EXCEPT:
a. Gastroenteritis b. Volvulus
c. Trauma d. Torsion

179. Useful in acute diarrhea:
a. Zinc b. Magnesium
c. Calcium d. Potassium

180. IOC for congenital hypertrophic pyloric stenosis:
a. X-ray b. CT San
c. MRI d. Ultrasound

181. Which drug consumption by pregnant lady can lead to baby developing hypertrophic pyloric stenosis?
a. Vancomycin b. Nifedipine
c. Erythromycin d. Phenyl propalamine

182. Double bubble appearance is seen in?
a. Jejunal atresia b. Duodenal atresia
c. Obstructive jaundice d. Pyloric atresia

183. What is the most-likely diagnosis of a 26-day-old infant presenting with recurrent nonbilious vomiting with constipation and loss of weight?
a. Esophageal atresia b. Annular pancreas
c. Ileal atresia d. Pyloric stenosis

184. All are seen in lactose intolerance; EXCEPT?
a. Benedict test positive in urine
b. Alkaline urine
c. Acidic stool
d. Lactase enzyme deficiency

185. All are seen in lactose intolerance; EXCEPT?
a. Benedict test positive in urine
b. Non reducing sugar in urine
c. Acidic stool
d. Lactase enzyme deficiency

186. A child presents with bilious vomitting on day 2 of life and the mother gives history of polyhydramnios. The radiological imaging is shown. What's your probable diagnosis?

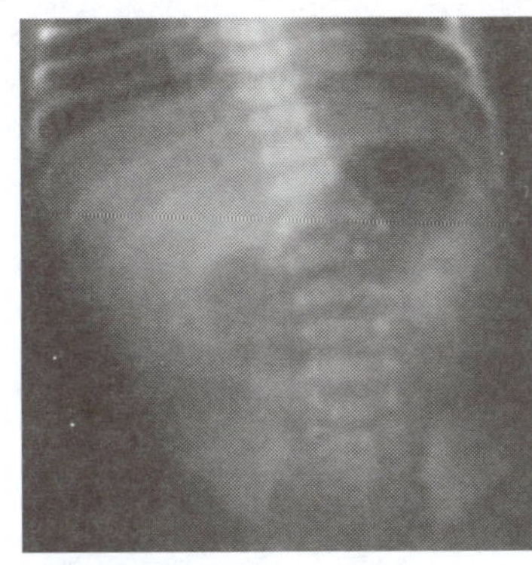

a. Duodenal atresia
b. Hypertrophic pyloric stenosis
c. Ileal atresia d. Congenital Mega-colon

187. In Hypertrophic pyloric stenosis which electrolyte should be replenished first?
a. Na^+ b. K^+
c. Ca^{++} d. HCO^{3-}

188. A 5-year-child came with dehydration. Plan A was proposed for treatment of dehydration. How much ORS should be given per loose stool?
a. 0–50 mL b. 50–100 mL
c. 100–200 mL d. 200–300 mL

FLUID & ELECTROLYTE BALANCE

189. Child presents with history of protracted vomiting, what will it cause? *(Most Recent Question June 2021)*
a. Metabolic acidosis b. Metabolic alkalosis
c. Respiratory acidosis d. Respiratory alkalosis

190. A child is admitted with iron overload. What is the antidote? *(Most Recent Question June 2021)*
a. Deferoxamine b. N-Acetylcysteine
c. Naloxone d. Ethanol

191. What is given in an irritable child with dehydration? *(Most Recent Question June 2021)*
a. ORS b. IV Ringer Lactate
c. Normal Saline d. 0.45% NS

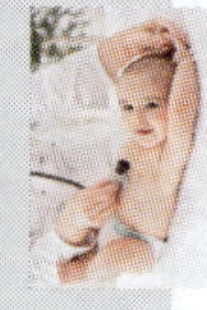

192. A 5-year-old child presents to your PHC with complaints of diarrhea and is unable to take feeds or ORS. His weight is 17 kg. What is the amount of maintenance fluid required in 24 hours? *(Most Recent Question Dec 2020)*

a. 1000 mL b. 1700 mL
c. 1350 mL d. 2000 mL

193. A 7-month-old boy was brought with a history of 18 episodes of loose stools and 2 episodes of vomiting. The child is irritable, but can drink eagerly. What is the best way to manage this child? *(Most Recent Question Aug 2020)*

a. Give IV fluids only
b. Give IV fluids for 4 hours followed by ORS
c. Give ORS only
d. Give plain water only

194. A 3-year-old child with weight of 12 kg is having loose motions. He is thirsty, drinks eagerly, tears are absent and skin pinch goes back slowly. What is the best treatment plan for this child? *(Most Recent Question 2019)*

a. 1200 mL RL over 12 hours
b. 600 mL RL over 6 hours
c. ORS 100 mL per episode of loose stool
d. ORS 50 mL per episode of loose stool

195. 24 hour normal fluid requirement for a one year old child weighing 8 kg is:

a. 700 mL b. 800 mL
c. 900 mL d. 1000 mL

196. The sodium concentration of low osmolarity ORS is:

a. 45 mmol/L b. 60 mmol/L
c. 75 mmol/L d. 90 mmol/L

197. A 2-year-old female child was brought to a PHC with a history of cough and fever for 4 days with inability to drink for last 12 hours. On examination, the child was having weight of 5 kg and respiratory rate of 45/min with fever. The child will be classified according to IMNCI as suffering from:

a. Very severe pneumonia b. Severe pneumonia
c. Pneumonia d. No pneumonia

198. Calculate the Fluid requirement for severe dehydration in a one-year-old child weighing 8 kg:

a. 600 mL b. 800 mL
c. 900 mL d. 1000 mL

199. What serum level of albumin is considered as mild degree of malnutrition:

a. 4.0 g/dL b. 3.5 g/dL
c. 3.0 g/dL d. 2.5 g/dL

200. Severe dehydration is seen in 2-year-old child. Amount of IV fluid to be given:

a. 30 mL/kg in 60 min b. 30 mL/kg in 30 min
c. 70 mL/kg in 360 min d. 70 mL/kg in 180 min

201. Intraosseous line is placed in which bone in children?

a. Femur b. Tibia
c. ASIS d. Iliac crest

202. Low Osmolar ORS composition is?

a. Na 90 mEq + 311 mOsm b. Na 75 mEq + 245 mOsm
c. Na 60 mEq + 245 mOsm d. Na 60 mEq + 240 mOsm

VACCINES

203. 1st dose of hepatitis B vaccine given at: *(Most Recent Question June 2022)*

a. Birth b. 6 weeks
c. 10 weeks d. 6 months

204. Which of the following vaccines given at birth? *(Most Recent Question June 2022)*

a. BCG, OPV, DPT b. BCG, HBV, DPT
c. BCG, OPV, HBV d. OPV, HBV, DPT

205. Oral vitamin A dosage in 2-year-old malnourished child weighing 8 kg. *(Most Recent Question Dec 2021)*

a. 50000 units b. 1 lakh units
c. 1.5 lakh units d. 2 lakh units

206. What is the upper limit of initiation of first dose of Rotavirus vaccine? *(Recent Pattern Question 2017)*

a. 6 weeks b. 10 weeks
c. 12 weeks d. 15 weeks

207. Which of the following vaccine can be given to AIDS positive child?

a. DPT b. BCG
c. Measles d. OPV

208. Which among the following is vaccine for cholera?

a. PPV 23 b. Dukoral
c. Ty 21 a vaccine d. JE-MB Nakayama

209. Osteomyelitis is side effect of which vaccine?

a. Hepatitis B vaccine b. BCG
c. Measles vaccine d. IPV

210. A child presents with redness of eyes, fever, backache and generalized rash as seen below. What is the probable diagnosis? *(Most Recent Question Aug 2020)*

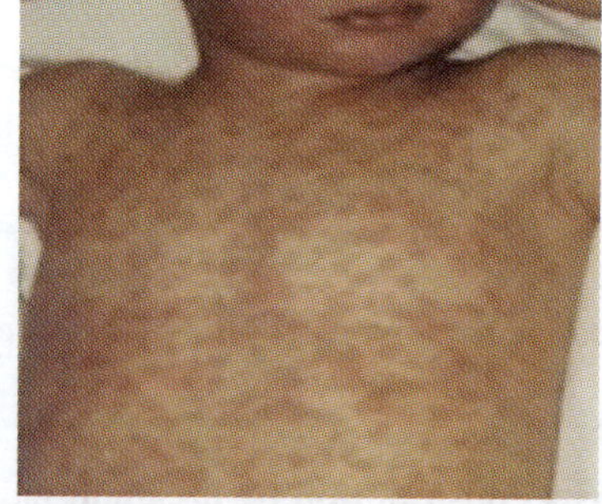

a. Measles b. Dengue
c. Chicken pox d. Herpetic rash

KIDNEY

211. A child presented with a boil on the leg 2 weeks ago and is now presenting with cola colored urine. What is the diagnosis? *(Most Recent Question Dec 2021)*

a. Minimal change disease
b. IgA nephropathy
c. Post streptococcal glomerulonephritis
d. Nodular glomerulosclerosis

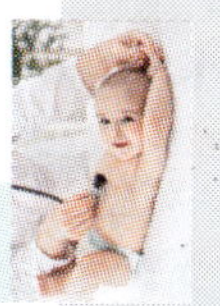

212. A child presented with palpable rash on limbs, hematuria, joint pain. There was a history of respiratory infection one week ago. What is the probable diagnosis? *(Most Recent Question Dec 2021)*

a. Henoch schonlein purpura
b. Rheumatoid arthritis
c. Hemolytic uremic syndrome
d. Reactive arthritis

213. A 6-year-old child weighing 12 kg has a urinary output of 0.4 mL/kg/hr in the last 12 hours. To which stage of KDIGO staging of Acute kidney injury does the child belong to? *(Most Recent Question Aug 2020)*

a. 1
b. 2
c. 3
d. 4

214. A male infant was brought to the emergency pediatric unit with abdominal distention. There was a history of recurrent urinary tract infections. On examination he was found to have urinary retention. Imaging showed bilateral hydronephrosis. What is the diagnosis? *(Most Recent Question Aug 2020)*

a. Renal calculi
b. PUJ obstruction
c. Posterior urethral valve
d. Urethral stricture

215. Mutation in NPHS 1 gene causes which disease?

a. Alport syndrome
b. Congenital Finnish type nephrotic syndrome
c. Focal segmental glomerulonephritis
d. Nail patella syndrome

216. Child presents with Pathological fracture, Renal stone and Psychiatric symptoms. Most probable diagnosis is?

a. Renal tubular acidosis
b. Hyperparathyroidism
c. Polycystic kidney disease
d. CRF

217. Henoch Schonlein purpura commonly involves which age group?

a. 4–8 years
b. 10–15 years
c. 15–20 years
d. >25 years

RESPIRATORY SYSTEM

218. A 2-year-old boy reported to sub center with complaint of fever and cough for 2 days with chest indrawing. His respiratory rate is 38/min. Next step is: *(Most Recent Question June 2022)*

a. Home treatment
b. Pneumonia clinical treatment
c. Severe pneumonia and referral
d. Severe pneumonia antibiotics and referral

219. A 2-year-old child who presented with fever had a RR of 36/min and chest indrawing. What is the diagnosis and treatment? *(Most Recent Question Dec 2021)*

a. Severe pneumonia; give antibiotics and refer urgently
b. Very severe disease; refer urgently
c. Pneumonia; oral antibiotics and come back after 5 days
d. Give only antipyretic and send home

220. The following line diagram represents growth of body organs with age. Which of these curves will represent lymphoid organ growth? *(Most Recent Question Dec 2021)*

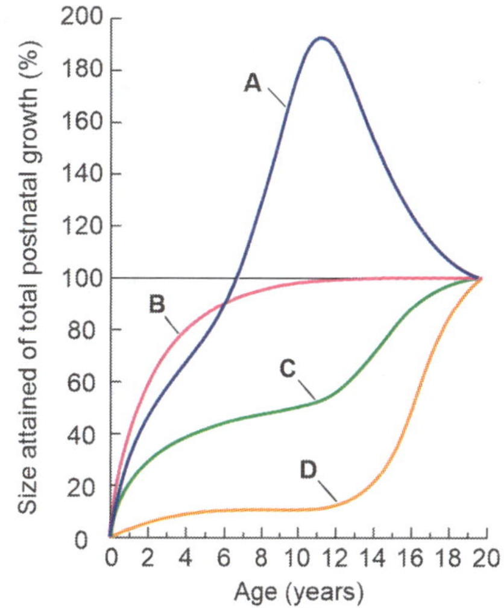

a. A
b. B
c. C
d. D

221. Comment on diagnosis based on CXR findings? *(Most Recent Question June 2021)*

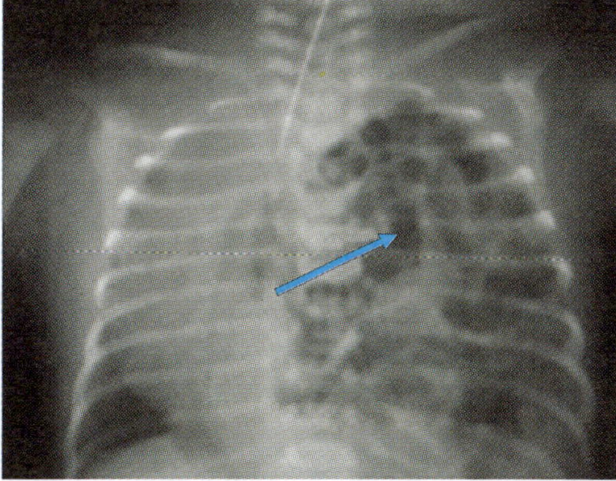

a. Congenital diaphragmatic hernia
b. ARDS
c. Pneumothorax
d. Pneumonia

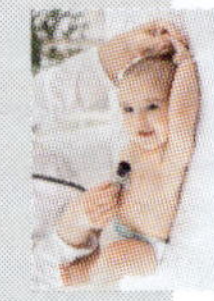

222. A 5-month-old baby has respiratory rate of 58/min and chest indrawing. The baby has not been able to feed for last 10 hours. What is the best management? *(Most Recent Question Aug 2020)*

a. Prescribe oral antibiotics and follow-up after 2 weeks
b. Give first dose ampicillin and gentamicin and refer urgently to hospital
c. Reassure mother that it is just cough and cold
d. Do nothing, refer the baby to tertiary care center

223. A one and half-year-old child presents with single episode of wheeze and breathing difficulty. CXR is done and it shows bilateral hyperinflation. Which organism is most commonly responsible? *(Most Recent Question Aug 2020)*

a. Respiratory syncytial virus
b. Streptococcus pneumoniae
c. H. influenzae
d. Coxsackie virus

224. A 3-month-old baby is brought with complaints of fever and fast breathing. On examination respiratory rate = 60/min, child is irritable but mother is able to feed the child. There is no stridor, no chest indrawing, no convulsions. Diagnosis is? *(Most Recent Question Dec 2019)*

a. Pneumonia
b. Severe pneumonia
c. Very severe pneumonia
d. No pneumonia

225. Infant is admitted with respiratory distress and prolonged expiration with Rhonchi in chest are heard. CXR shows hyperinflation. What is the diagnosis? *(Most Recent Question 2019)*

a. Pneumonia
b. Croup
c. Asthma
d. Bronchiolitis

226. Which of these is used in treatment of bronchiolitis? *(Most Recent Question 2019)*

a. Ribavarin
b. Amantadine
c. Racemic epinephrine
d. Corticosteroids

227. Which of the following clinical presentation is correct for a child with pneumonia? *(Recent Pattern Question 2018)*

a. <50/min RR, with age of 2 months
b. >40/min RR, for 2–12 months
c. >40/min RR, for 12–60 months
d. <60/min RR, for 0–2 months

228. Most common cause of common cold in children is?

a. RSV
b. Rhinovirus
c. Influenza
d. Allergic

INBORN ERRORS OF METABOLISM

229. An infant is brought to a hospital because her wet diaper turns black when they are exposed to air. Physical examination of infant is normal. This disorder is caused by a deficiency of: *(Most Recent Question June 2022)*

a. Homogentisic acid oxidase
b. Phenylalanine hydroxylase
c. Ketoacid decarboxylase
d. Tyrosinase

230. A 8-year-old child presented with hepatomegaly and hypoglycemia. He was diagnosed with glucose 6 phosphatase deficiency. The cause of hepatomegaly in this child is? *(Most Recent Question Dec 2021)*

a. Glucose accumulation in liver
b. Glycogen accumulation in liver
c. Glucose accumulation in muscles
d. Glucose 6 phosphate accumulation in liver

231. Burnt sugar smell of urine in a child; which enzyme deficiency is likely? *(Most Recent Question June 2021)*

a. Phenylalanine hydroxylase
b. Branched-chain alpha-keto acid dehydrogenase (BCKD) enzyme
c. Glucose-6-phosphate dehydrogenase
d. Lactase

232. A normal born child presents with mental retardation, blond hair and convulsions at 1 year of age. Most probable diagnosis is?

a. Albuminuria
b. Phenylketonuria
c. Gaucher's disease
d. Tyrosinemia

ENDOCRINOLOGY

233. A 7-year-old child is present with short stature. On biochemical examination, growth hormone levels are elevated with very low levels of IGF-1. Which of the following could be the possible defect in this child? *(Most Recent Question Aug 2020)*

a. GHRH Deficiency
b. GnRH receptor deficiency
c. GH deficiency
d. GH receptor deficiency

234. A 3-week-old boy was brought to the pediatric OPD with yellowish discoloration of skin and hypotonia. On examination, the baby also has large protruded tongue and umbilical hernia. Which of the following would be initial step in the evaluation of his clinical condition? *(Most Recent Question Aug 2020)*

a. Serum cortisol level
b. Serum TSH level
c. Sepsis screening
d. Serum IGF – 1 level

235. Wide open posterior fontanelle with large tongue with rough dry skin is seen in? ***(Most Recent Question 2019)***

a. Pellagra b. Down syndrome
c. Hypothyroidism d. Nutritional rickets

236. Nelson syndrome is seen in?

a. Adrenalectomy
b. Hypopituitarism
c. Deficiency of beta cells
d. Deficiency of growth hormone

MISCELLANEOUS

237. Macrocytic anemia present in: ***(Most Recent Question June 2022)***

a. Thalassemia
b. Anemia of chronic disease
c. Sideroblastic anemia
d. Liver disease

238. Menke disease is a disorder of? ***(Most Recent Question Dec 2021)***

a. Cu b. Zinc
c. Fe d. Se

239. A male child presents to you with swelling below the ear, but no systemic manifestations. There have been two other similar cases in the friends of this child is the same village. What will you do? ***(Most Recent Question Dec 2021)***

a. Immediate hospitalization
b. Incision and drainage
c. Mouthwash
d. Give antipyretics and send home

240. A 1-year-old boy presented with hemarthrosis of left knee after a history of fall. Deficiency of which factor can lead to the following condition? ***(Most Recent Question Dec 2020)***

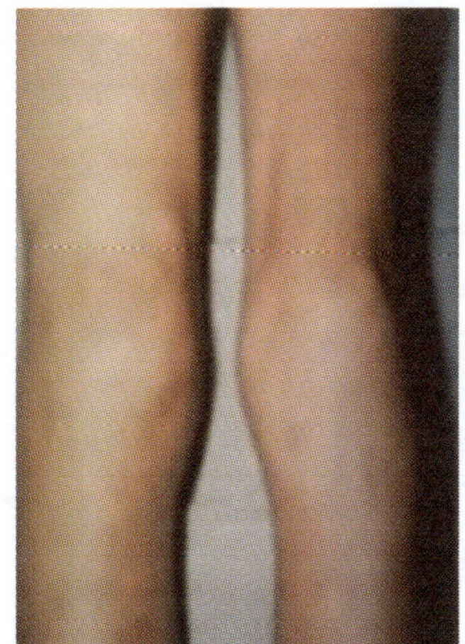

a. Von Willebrand disease b. Vitamin K deficiency
c. Thrombocytopenia d. Factor VIII deficiency

241. A boy with a history of frequent fractures presented with blue sclera. What could be the diagnosis? ***(Most Recent Question Dec 2020)***

a. Scurvy b. Rickets
c. Osteogenesis imperfecta d. Osteomalacia

242. The image given below shows a female baby with a rash on face and perineal area. What could be the underlying deficiency responsible for this rash? ***(Most Recent Question Aug 2020)***

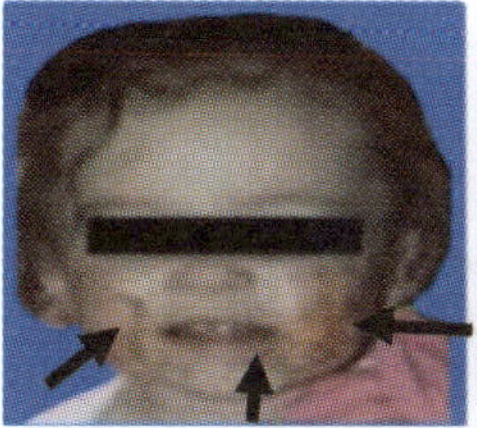
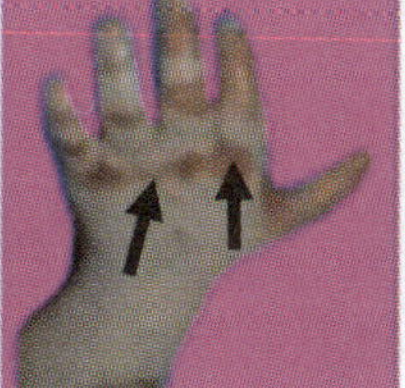
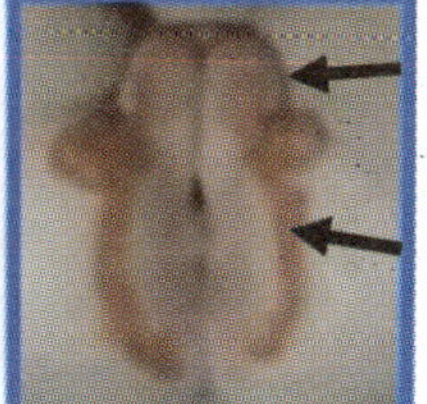

a. Copper b. Riboflavin
c. Vit C d. Zinc

243. A child presents with different types of rashes, including papules, vesicles and pustules involving the whole body and these rashes are present all at the same time and appearance of rash is associated with the onset of fever. What is the probable diagnosis? ***(Most Recent Question Aug 2020)***

a. Measles b. Chicken pox
c. Scabies d. Rubella

244. What is the organism responsible for this rash seen in an otherwise well child, who also had oral ulcers? ***(Most Recent Question Aug 2020)***

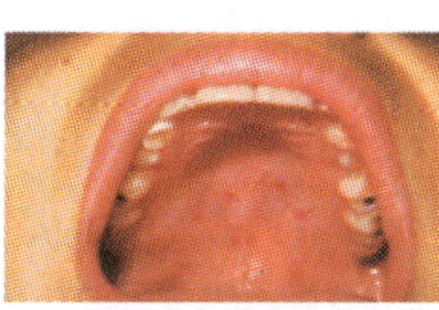
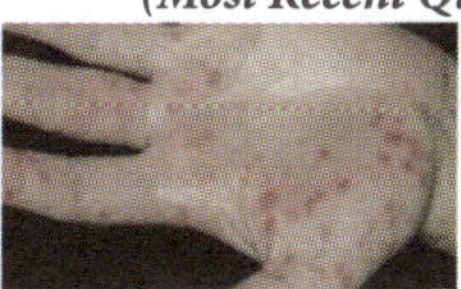
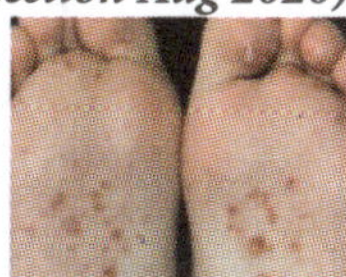

a. Pox virus b. Coxsackie virus
c. Adenovirus d. Epstein-Barr virus

245. 6th day disease is? ***(Most Recent Question 2019)***

a. Erythema Infectiosum
b. Exanthema subitum
c. Erythema marginatum
d. Erythema nodosum

246. Hand foot mouth disease is usually caused by: ***(Recent Pattern Question 2018)***

a. Coxsackie A b. Adenovirus
c. Rotavirus d. Hepatitis B virus

247. Which of the following is the cause of development of acute scrotum in a 2-year-old child? ***(Recent Pattern Question 2017)***

a. Torsion of appendix of testis
b. Epididymitis
c. Testicular trauma
d. Idiopathic swelling of scrotum

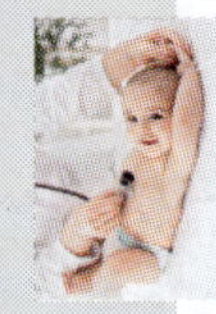

248. An 8 month baby presents with fever, cough and confluent rash on hairline, face, neck and body. Which of the following is a causative organism?

(Recent Pattern Question 2017)

a. Varicella
b. Variola
c. Rubella
d. Rubeola

249. Slapped cheeks appearance is seen in?

(Recent Pattern Question 2016)

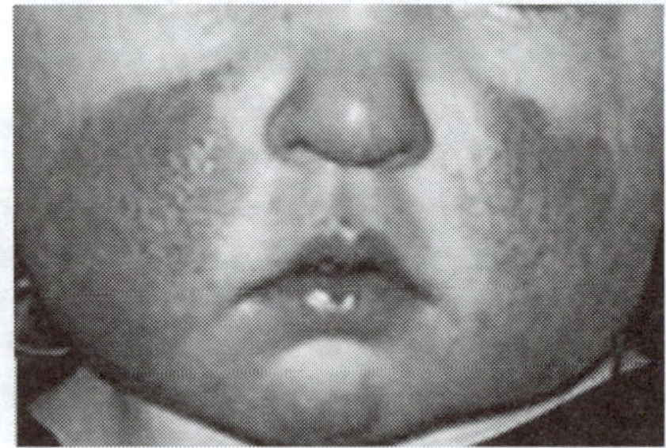

a. Erythema infectiosum
b. Measles
c. Chicken pox
d. Erythema nodosum

250. Post streptococcal glomerulonephritis in children is diagnosed by

a. Heavy proteinuria, high cholesterol, high ASO titer
b. Heavy proteinuria, hematuria, low ASO titer
c. Mild proteinuria, high hematuria, high ASO titer
d. Mild proteinuria, high cholesterol, normal ASO titer

251. Acrodermatitis enterohepatica is due to:

a. Pustular psoriasis
b. Zinc toxicity
c. Zinc deficiency
d. Collodion baby

252. What is the dose of isoniazid in infants?

a. 5 mg/kg
b. 10 mg/kg
c. 15 mg/kg
d. 20 mg/kg

253. Precocious puberty and patchy skin pigmentation is known as:

a. Albright's syndrome
b. Litter Siwe disease
c. Asherman's syndrome
d. Morquio's syndrome

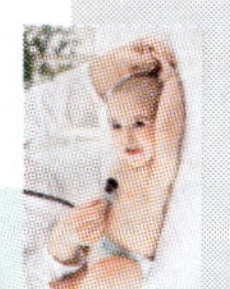

ANSWERS WITH EXPLANATIONS

MOST RECENT QUESTIONS 2023

1. Ans. (a) Craniorachischisis

Ref: Nelson, 20th ed. pg. 2805

The image shows the most severe neural tube defect where both brain and spinal cord malformation is present, this is known as Craniorachischisis.

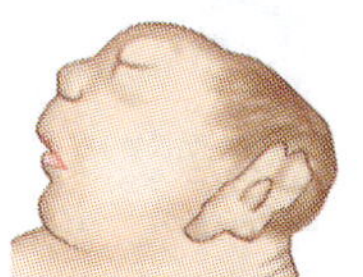

Anecephaly

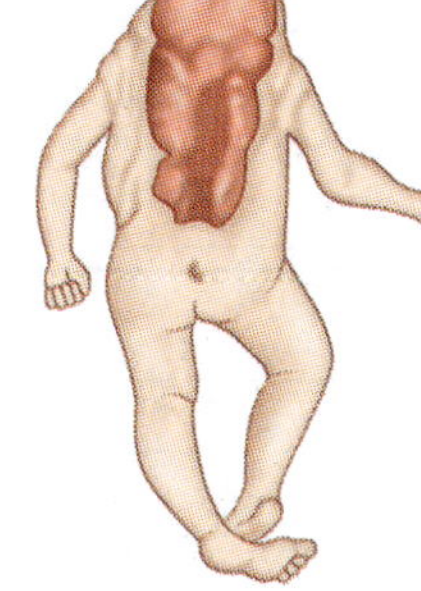

Craniorachischisis

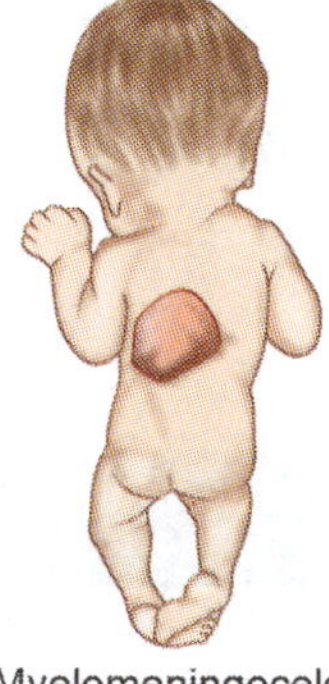

Myelomeningocele

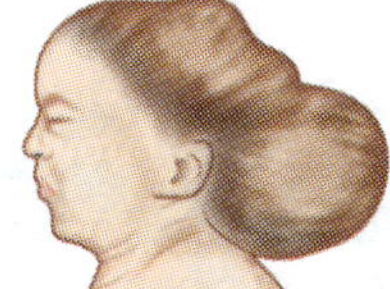

Encephalocele

2. Ans. (a) GALT deficiency

Ref: Nelson, 20th ed. pg. 717

- GALT (Galactose-1-phosphate uridylyltransferase) is responsible for hereditary galactosemia and is the most common deficiency. This enzyme catalyzes conversion of galactose-1-phosphate and UDP glucose to UDP galactose and glucose-1-phosphate. It results in failure to thrive and vomiting after feeds. Presence of bilateral cataracts points to the diagnosis of galactosemia.
- Galactokinase converts galactose to galactose-1-phosphate and is not a common deficiency.
- Uridine diphosphate (UDP) galactose-4-epimerase epimerizes UDP galactose to UDP glucose and is also uncommon.
- Option b is responsible for Von Gierke disease which does not have cataracts.

3. Ans. (c) 60 mL/kg

Ref: Nelson, 20th ed. pg. 717

Breast milk required for a baby is based on body weight and is 60 mL/kg of body weight. It should be started as soon as possible within the first hour of delivery.

4. Ans. (a) 2 lakh IU every 6 months till 5 years

Ref: who.int

Dose of vitamin A is 2 Lac IU orally every 6 months till age of 5 years. Below one year the dose is 1 Lac IU orally single dose.

5. Ans. (c) 11.5 cm

Ref: who.int

The cut-off of arm circumference for severe acute malnutrition is 11.5 cm.

DIAGNOSTIC CRITERIA FOR SAM IN CHILDREN AGED 6–60 MONTHS

Indicator	Measure	Cut-off
Severe wasting (2)	Severe wasting (2)	<-3 SD
Weight-for-height (1)	MUAC	<115 mm
Bilateral edema (3)	Clinical sign	
1 Based on WHO Standards (www.who.int/childgrowth/standards) 2, 3 Independent indicators of SAM that require urgent action		

6. Ans. (a) Stunting

Ref: who.int

Since the height for age is reduced it implies stunting in the child due to incorrect feeding by parents.

7. Ans. (a) Measles

The development of maculopapular rash that started from behind the ears and spread to trunk after few days of URT symptoms is presentation of measles. Chicken pox will have maculo-papulovesicular rash. Dengue will cause myalgia and high fever followed by hemorrhagic features like epistaxis and or circulatory failure. Rubella presents like measles but has lymphadenopathy also.

8. Ans. (c) RL with 5% Dextrose

Ref: https://www.ncbi.nlm.nih.gov/pmc/articles/PMC5590082

RL is fluid of choice for severe dehydration and 5% dextrose is required due to presence of hypoglycemia in severe acute malnutrition.

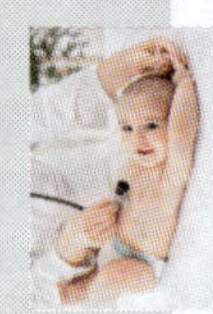

WHO RECOMMENDATIONS FOR TREATMENT OF SEVERELY MALNOURISHED CHILDREN WITH DEHYDRATION

	Shock and severe dehydration in child unable to tolerate oral fluid	No shock
Initial	15 mL/kg Ringers Lactate + 5% dextrose, over 1 hour, repeated once, if needed	ReSoMal Oral/ Nasogastric- 5 mL/kg every 30 minutes for first 2 hours.
Subsequent	Oral/Nasogastric ReSoMal alternating with F75 10 mL/kg/hr up to 10 hours, and then refeeding with F75.	Then 5–10 mL/kg/hr alternating F75 and ReSoMal for 4–10 hours

9. Ans. (b) 2nd

Ref: iapindia.org

The markers point to Quad screen test that is done in second trimester (usually 15–20 weeks) to screen for Down syndrome.

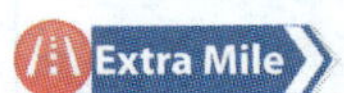

Aneuploidies	AFP	Estriol	hCG	Inhibin A
Down's syndrome	Low	Low	**High**	**High**
Turner's syndrome	Decreased	Decreased	**Very high**	**Very high**
Edward's syndrome	Unchanged	**Low**	**Very low**	Unchanged
Patau's syndrome	**Increased**	Normal	Normal	Normal

10. Ans. (a) 47, XY (+21)

Ref: Nelson, 20th ed. pg. 612

The image shows simian crease which in clinical setting of development delay and recurrent pneumonia episodes, points to Down Syndrome. Simian crease *alone is not diagnostic of Down syndrome.*

Extra Mile

Simian Crease

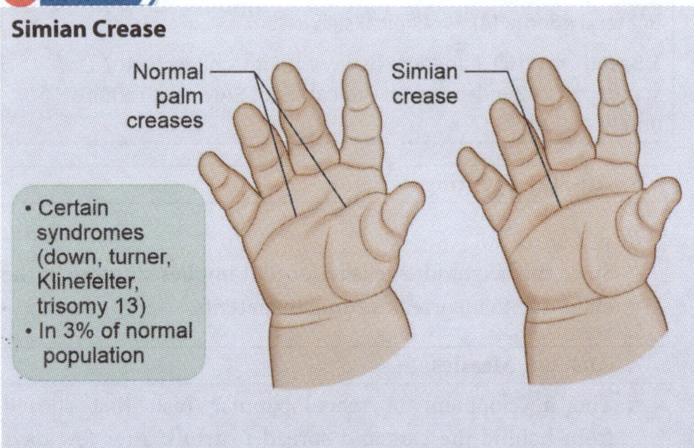

Clinical features of down syndrome in the neonatal period
Central Nervous System • Hypotonia • Developmental delay • Poor Moro reflex
Craniofacial • Brachycephaly with flat occiput • Flat face • Upward slanted palpebral fissures • Epicanthal folds • Speckled irises (Brushfield spots) • Three fontanels • Delayed fontanel closure • Frontal sinus and midfacial hypoplasia • Mild microcephaly • Short hard palate • Small nose, flat nasal bridge • Protruding tongue, open mouth • Small dysplastic ears
Cardiovascular • Endocardial cushing defects • Ventricular septal defect • Atrial septal defect • Patent ductus arteriosus • Aberrant subclavian artery • Pulmonary hypertension

Contd...

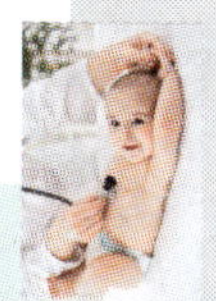

Clinical features of down syndrome in the neonatal period
Musculoskeletal • Joint hyperflexibility • Short neck, redundant skin • Short metacarpals and phalanges • Short 5th digit with clinodactyly • Single transverse palmar creases • Wide gap between 1st and 2nd toes • Pelvic dysplasia • Short sternum

11. Ans. (a) Constitutional delay in growth

Ref: Nelson, 2022 ed. pg. 673

Familial short stature	Constitutional delay in growth and puberty
Parents are short in height Bone age is equal to chronological age Normal puberty	Parents height is normal Bone age is less than chronological age Puberty is delayed

Option c will have features like obesity, myxedema and delayed milestones.
Option d is ruled out as no anthropometry parameters are given.

12. Ans. (c) 100000 IU

Ref: WHO Guidelines: Vitamin A Deficiency

For child less than 1 year of age dose of vitamin A is 1 lac IU and older than 1 year is 2 lac IU orally.

13. Ans. (a) Kwashiorkor due to less protein intake

Ref: pg. 1250: CMDT 2023

Notice the edema present in extremities and face which implies severe protein deficiency leading to Kwashiorkor.

14. Ans. (a) Measles

Ref: Nelson, 20th ed. pg. 1542

Notice the maculopapular rash on face and extremities which is seen in measles. Option b will have maculopapulovesicular rash. No vesicles are noted in the image seen. Option c will have slapped cheeks appearance. Option d will have lesion in mouth, sole of foot and in palms.

15. Ans. (a) 1 hour

Ref: WHO guidelines on breastfeeding

Breast feeding should be initiated as early as possible and preferably in first hours of birth of child.

16. Ans. (d) Ringer lactate +5% dextrose

Ref: https://www.ncbi.nlm.nih.gov/pmc/articles/PMC5590082

RL is fluid of choice for severe dehydration and dextrose is required due to presence of hypoglycemia in severe acute malnutrition.

WHO Recommendations for Treatment of Severely Malnourished Children with Dehydration

	Shock and severe dehydration in child unable to tolerate oral fluid	No shock
Initial	15 mL/Kg Ringers Lactate + 5% dextrose, over 1 hour, repeated once if needed	ReSoMal Oral/ Nasogastric- 5 mL/kg every 30 minutes for first 2 hours.
Subsequent	Oral/Nasogastric ReSoMal alternating with F75 10 mL/Kg/hr up to 10 hours, and then refeeding with F75.	Then 5–10 mL/kg/hr alternating F75 and ReSoMal for 4–10 hours

17. Ans. (d) D- dehydration

Ref: PALS

D is for disability and not for dehydration.

Airway and Breathing	Circulation	Disability	Exposure
Effort of breathing	Heart rate	Conscious level	Fever
Respiratory rate and rhythm	Pulse volume	Posture	Rash
Stridor/wheeze	Capillary refill	Pupils	Bruising
Auscultation	Skin temperature		
Skin colour			

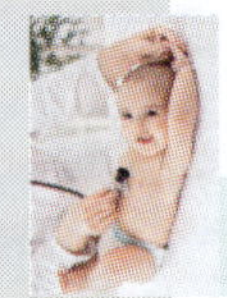

18. Ans. (d) 60/min

Ref: NRP

Check chest movement
Ventilation corrective steps if needed
ETT or laryngeal mask if needed

↓

HR below 60/min? — No (back to above)

Yes ↓

Intubate if not already done
Chest compressions
Coordinate with PPV
100% O_2
ECG monitor
Consider emergency UVC

↓

HR below 60/min?

Yes ↓

IV epinephrine
If HR persistently bellow 60/min
Consider hypovolemia
Consider pneumothorax

19. Ans. (a) 21%

Ref: NRP

At the start of bag and mask ventilation room air is used which is 21% oxygen. Later oxygen can be attached at the port behind the AMBU bag to increase the FiO_2 delivered.

20. Ans. (a) Capillary hemangioma

Ref: Nelson, 20th ed. pg. 2480

The image shows the presence of capillary hemangioma which is most common benign vascular eyelid tumor in neonates. It initially shows engorgement in the first year of life and later shows regression by 6 to 7 years of life.

Mongolian spots

Milia

Erythema Toxicum

21. Ans. (c) Esophageal atresia

Ref: Nelson, 20th ed. pg. 1783

Lateral infantogram shows a feeding tube coiled up in esophagus. There are *no gas shadows in intestine* indicating esophageal atresia. The history of frothing from mouth further confirms the diagnosis.

22. Ans. (a) Bacterial meningitis

Ref: pg. 1280, CMDT 2023

TABLE: Typical cerebrospinal fluid findings in various CNS diseases

Diagnosis	Cells/mcL	Glucose (mg/dL)	Protein (mg/dL)	Opening pressure
Normal	0–5 lymphocytes	45–85	15–45	70–180 mm H_2O
Aseptic meningitis, viral meningitis or meningoencephalitis	25–2000 (0.025–2.0 x 109/L), mostly lymphocytes[3]	Normal or low	High (>50)	Slightly elevated
Granulomatous meningitis (mycobacterial, fungal)	100–1000 (0.1–1.0 x 10^9/L), mostly lymphocytes	Low (<45)	High (>50)	Moderately elevated
Purulent meningitis (bacterial) community-acquired	200–20,000 (0.2–20 x 10^9/L) neutrophils	Low (<45)	High (>50)	Markedly elevated

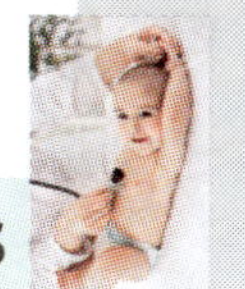

Keywords are turbid CSF with neutrophil predominance in patients with nuchal rigidity which is a key feature of bacterial meningitis. Option B will have CSF with predominant lymphocytosis and long history.

NEONATOLOGY

23. Ans. (a) Hemorrhagic disease of newborn

Ref: O.P. Ghai Essential Pediatrics, 9th ed. pg. 117

- Vitamin K is produced by gut bacteria. In neonates the gut is sterile and colonization by flora takes time.
- Hence, to counteract this vitamin K deficiency all term babies are given 1mg of vitamin K1 intramuscularly. In case this is not given like in event of home delivery the baby will develop bleeding from umbilical stump which is called hemorrhagic disease of newborn.
- In preterm babies vitamin K given is 0.5 mg

24. Ans. (a) Hypoglycemia

Ref: O.P. Ghai Essential Pediatrics, 9th ed. pg. 176

- An Infant of a Diabetic Mother is more likely to have periods of hypoglycemia shortly after birth, and during first few days of life.
- This is because the baby has been used to getting more sugar than needed from the mother.
- They have a higher insulin level than needed after birth called fetal hyperinsulinism. Insulin lowers the blood sugar.

25. Ans. (a) 21 hydroxylase

Ref: O.P. Ghai Essential Pediatrics, 9th ed. pg. 522

- The given clinical picture is suggestive of Congenital adrenal hyperplasia.
- Congenital adrenal hyperplasia due to deficiency of 21-hydroxylase or 3-hydroxysteroid dehydrogenase.
- Signs and symptoms of classic CAH may include: Insufficient cortisol, adrenal crisis, atypical genitalia, and excess androgen. Excess androgen hormones in females may result in facial hair, excessive body hair and a deepening voice.

26. Ans. (a) Ear care

Ref: https://nhm.gov.in/images/pdf/in-focus/Dakshata/Day-2/Essential_Newborn_Care.pptx

Components of ENBC includes:

Essential New-Born Care (ENBC)

1. Call out the time of birth.
2. Deliver the baby onto a warm, clean and dry towel or cloth and keep on mother's chest and abdomen (between the breasts).
3. Assess the baby's breathing while drying.
4. Immediately dry the baby with a warm clean towel or piece of cloth.
5. Clamp and cut the umbilical cord when cord pulsation stops or in 1-3 minutes (delayed cord clamping).
6. Leave the baby between the mother's breasts to start skin-to-skin care.
7. Place an identity label on the baby.
8. Cover the baby's head with a cap. Cover the mother and baby with a warm cloth.
9. Encourage the initiation of breastfeeding.
10. Administer inj. Vitamin K intramuscular to baby according to weight

27. Ans. (a) DiGeorge

Ref: O.P. Ghai Essential Pediatrics, 9th ed. pg. 633

- DiGeorge syndrome (DGS) is a congenital disorder which results from the microdeletion of chromosome 22 at a location known as 22q11.2.
- This mutation results in the failure of development of the pharyngeal pouches which are responsible for the embryologic development of the middle and external ear, maxilla, mandible, palatine tonsils, thyroid, parathyroids, thymus, aortic arch, and cardiac outflow tract.
- Features of DGS include cardiac anomalies, recurrent infections, abnormal facies, thymic hypoplasia or aplasia, cleft palate, developmental delay, and hypocalcemia.

28. Ans. (a) Palmar grasp reflex

Ref: Nelson Essentials of Pediatrics, 9th ed. pg. 17

- The palmar grasp reflex is present at 28 weeks of gestation and becomes more forceful at 32–37 weeks. It becomes less apparent and then disappears after approximately 2 months of age, when voluntary grasping becomes apparent.
- Option b comes at 5 to 6 months of age. Option c comes at 9 months, and Option d comes at birth.

29. Ans. (a) 48 hours

Ref: Nelson Textbook of Pediatrics 20th ed. pg. 797

In 99% of neonates, meconium is passed within 24 hours and the upper limit is 48 hours. If the child does not pass meconium first check the delivery notes for passage of meconium induced fetal distress.

Extra Mile

Failure to pass meconium occurs due to:
1. Intestinal obstruction
2. Imperforate anus
3. Hirschsprung's disease
4. Meconium plug

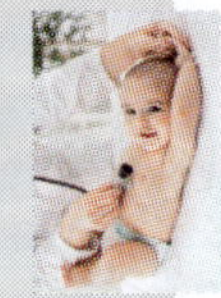

30. Ans. (c) 6

Ref: Nelson Textbook of Pediatrics 20th ed. pg. 798

Parameter given	Current assigned score
Heart rate of 120/min	2
Irregular respiration	1
Pink body with blue extremities (Acrocyanosis)	1
Partially flexed	1
Grimace on stimulation by catheter	1
Total	**6**

Score	0 point	1 point	2 points
Appearance Skin colour	Cyanotic/ pale all over	Peripheral cyanosis only	Pink
Pulse (Heart rate)	0	<100	100–140
Grimace Reflex irritability	No response to stimulation	Grimace (facial movement)/ weak cry when stimulated	Cry when stimulated
Activity Tone	Floppy	Some flexion	Well flexed and resisting extension
Respiration	Apnoeic	Slow, irregular breathing	Strong cry

APGAR - Appearance, Pulse, Grimace, Activity, Respiration.

31. Ans. (d) 5 mg%

Ref: Nelson 20th ed. pg. 871

Jaundice in neonates becomes apparent in cephalocaudal progression starting from face and progressing to abdomen and feet. Dermal pressure reveals anatomic progression. Jaundice on face starts at 5 mg/dL.

32. Ans. (b) Triple

Ref: Nelson 20th ed. pg. 417

Compositions of human colostrum, mature breast milk, and cow's milk (g/L)			
Compositions	**Human colostrum**	**Human breast milk**	**Cow's milk**
Total protein	23	11	31
Immunoglob-ulins	19	0.1	1
Fat	30	45	38
Lactose	57	71	47
Calcium	0.5	0.3	1.4
Phosphorus	0.16	0.14	0.90
Sodium	0.50	0.15	0.41

33. Ans. (a) Head

Ref: Op Ghai, 8th ed. pg. 143

Maximum heat loss in neonates occurs from the scalp.

34. Ans. (d) Charcot joints

Ref: Nelson 20th ed. pg. 2050–51

- Congenital syphilis can lead to development of rare hypersensitivity phenomenon like soft tissue gumma.
- Depression of nasal route as a result of syphilitic rhinitis destroying the adjacent bone and cartilage leads to saddle nose.
- Osteochondritis is painful and results in inability to move the involved extremity and is called pseudoparalysis of parrot.
- Seen in late congenital syphilis clutton joints are unilateral or bilateral painless joint swelling (usually involving knees) from synovitis with sterile synovial fluid. Spontaneous remission occurs after several weeks.
- *Charcot joints are seen in Tabes dorsalis in adult patient of syphilis.*

35. Ans. (a) αFP

Ref: Nelson 20th ed. pg. 2802

- Failure of closure of the neural tube allows excretion of fetal substances (*α-fetoprotein [αFP], acetylcholinesterase*) into the amniotic fluid, serving as biochemical markers for a NTD.
- Prenatal screening of maternal serum for αFP in the 16th–18th week of gestation is an effective method for identifying pregnancies at risk for fetuses with NTDs *in utero*.

Extra Mile

- Inhibin-A is a part of quadruple test for Down syndrome screening.
- Inhibin-B has negative feedback on FSH.
- It is used as tumor marker for granulosa cell tumor.

36. Ans. (c) Constricted

Ref: Advanced Pediatric Assessment, By Ellen M. Chiocca; pg. 320

- Pupil size is measured against a standardized size gauge; the normal range in infants and children is 2–6 mm
- Infants normally have miotic (constricted) pupils. Children normally have larger pupils than infants or adults.

37. Ans. (a) Transplacental transfer of estrogen

Ref: OP Ghai 8th ed. pg. 135

- Transient breast enlargement in the newborn has been reported in 20% to 30% of newborn babies. It is usually the result of the transplacental transfer of maternal and placental estrogens.

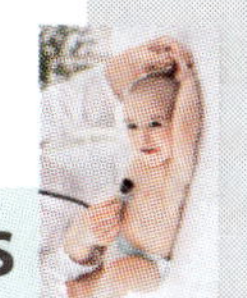

- Engorged breasts should not be squeezed or massaged as it could lead to soreness and infection.

38. Ans. (a) 5 mg%

Ref: Nelson, 20th ed. pg. 1928

Since the neonate developed Jaundice on day 3 of life it indicates physiological jaundice. It appears when total serum bilirubin exceeds 5 mg% and progresses in cephalo-caudal direction.

Dermal pressure may reveal the anatomic progression of:

1. Face = 5 mg/dL
2. Mid-abdomen = 15 mg/dL
3. Soles = 20 mg/dL

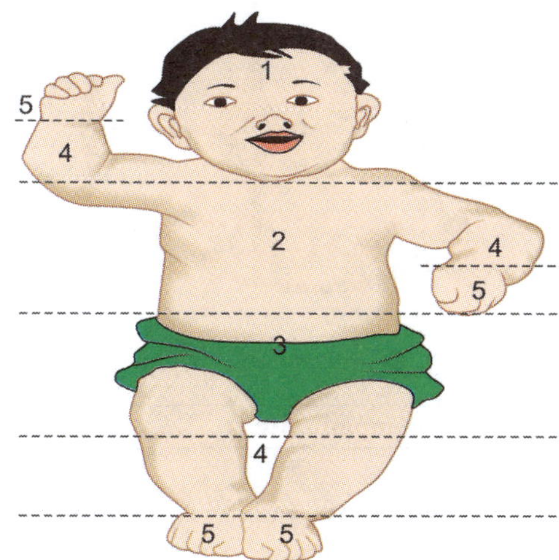

Numbers here indicate progression of Jaundice

- The yellow color usually results from the accumulation of *unconjugated, nonpolar, lipid-soluble bilirubin pigment in the skin.*
- This unconjugated bilirubin is an end product of heme-protein catabolism from a series of enzymatic reactions by heme-oxygenase and biliverdin reductase and non-enzymatic reducing agents in the reticuloendothelial cells

39. Ans. (b) Check chest movement

Ref: 2016 Update on Neonatal Resuscitation by AAP

- *Since 30 seconds of PPV has already been administered and heart rate is still less than 100/min, check chest movement to take ventilation corrective steps.*
- It could be that the face mask used is not of appropriate size or proper seal was not obtained leading to impaired ventilation.
- If the heart rate stabilizes to 100/min and spontaneous respiration is established then continue supplemental oxygen and post resuscitation care should be established.
- It is a must for you to know neonatal resuscitation. So please write down the algorithm and read it one day before the examination. For adult resuscitation protocol refer to the medicine section.

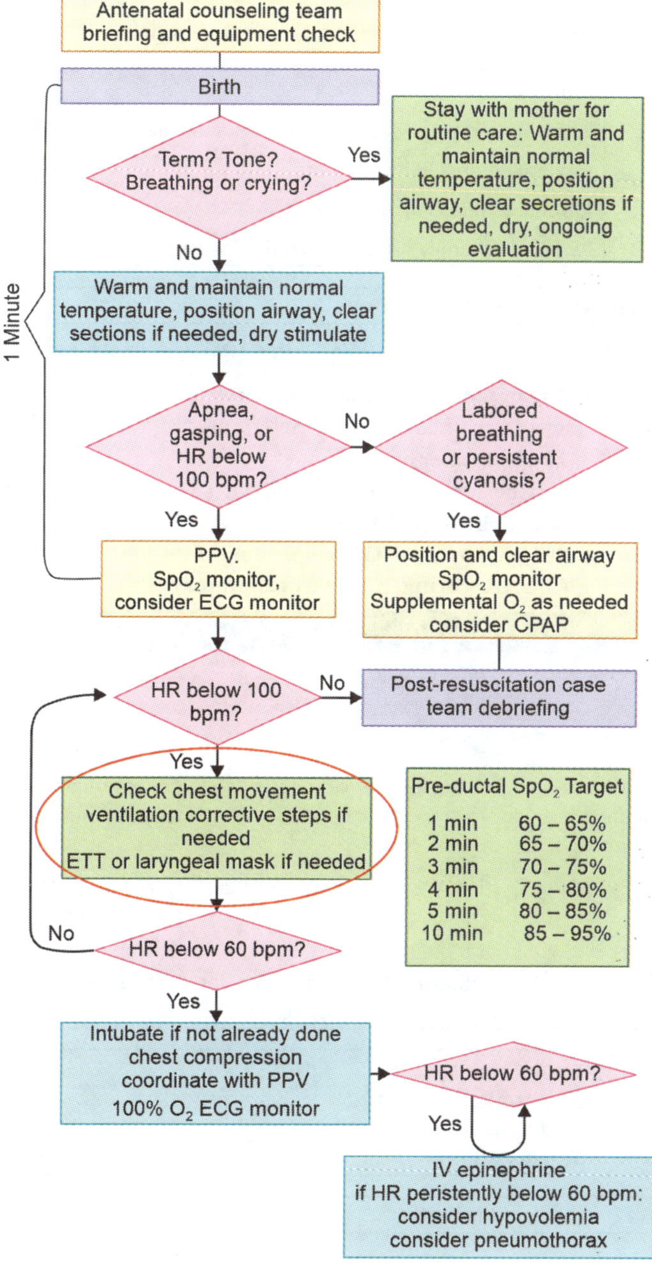

40. Ans. (a) Atopic dermatitis

Ref: Nelson, 20th ed. pg. 1096

- The most common chronic relapsing skin disease seen in infancy and childhood is atopic dermatitis.
- Affects 10–20% of children worldwide

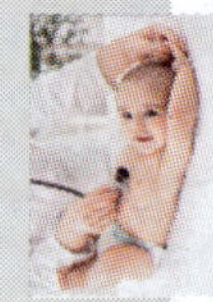

- Frequently occurs in families with asthma, allergic rhinitis, and food allergy.
- "**Atopic march**" is a term used to define infants with Atopic Dermatitis is predisposed to developing allergic rhinitis and/or asthma later in childhood.

Major Clinical Features of Atopic Dermatitis

Pruritus
Facial and extensor eczema in infants and children
Flexural eczema in adolescents
Chronic or relapsing **dermatitis**
Personal or family history of **atopic** disease

41. Ans. (a) Respiratory rate

Ref: OP Ghai, 8th ed. pg. 126

- **Apgar score:** A numerical expression of condition of new born infant, usually determined at 1 minute and 5 minutes after birth.
- **Can be remembered as APGAR (Appearance, Pulse rate, Grimace, Activity, RESPIRATORY EFFORT)**
- **Remember, its NOT respiratory rate you count in APGAR scoring, rather its respiratory effort.**

	Score 0	Score 1	Score 2
Appearance	Blue or pale all over	Blue at extremities	Pink all over
Pulse rate	Absent	<100	>100
(Grimace) Reflex irritability	No response	Grimace	Cry or pull away when stimulated
Activity	None	Some flexion	Flexed arms and legs that resist extension
Respiratory effort	Absent	Weak, irregular, gasping	Strong , lusty cry

Total score	**: 10**
No distress	: 7–10
Mild distress	: 4–6
Severe distress	: 0–3

42. Ans. (c) 3 minutes

Ref: OP Ghai, 8th ed. pg. 144

HOW TO TAKE ARMPIT (AXILLARY) TEMPERATURES in newborn

- Place the tip of the thermometer in a dry armpit.
- Close the armpit by holding the elbow against the **chest for 3 minutes**.
- Remove the thermometer after you hear the signal (usually a series of beeps) and read the temperature on the screen.
- A child has a fever if the armpit temperature is over 99°F (37.2°C). If you're not sure if it is correct, check it by taking a rectal temperature.

43. Ans. (c) Lambdoid suture

Ref: OP Ghai, 8th ed. pg. 41

- Well you can look at the diagram for the logic and memorize the diagram as it will help you in anatomy also.

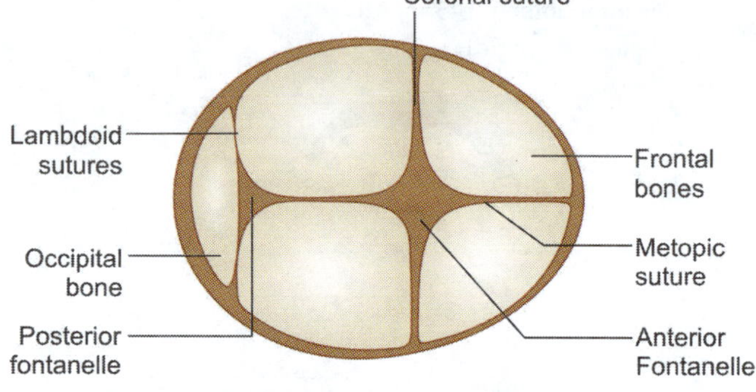

- Lambdoid suture corresponds with posterior fontanelle.

44. Ans. (a) Rh incompatibility

Ref: OP Ghai, 8th ed. pg. 175

- Most common cause of pathological jaundice in children is Rh incompatitbility.
- **Characteristics of pathological jaundice**
  - Appears within first 24 hours of birth
  - Peak values exceed >15 mg%
  - Rate of rise of Serum bilirubin >5 mg/dL/day

Management

Principles of Phototherapy

Configurational isomerization	Z isomer converted to E isomer which is excreted slowly
Structural isomerization	Bilirubin converted to lumirubin which is rapidly excreted and *responsible for phototherapy induced decline in TSB*

- **Phototherapy:** Start phototherapy if serum bilirubin >15 mg% or >12 mg% in preterm baby.
- **Exchange transfusion:** Done via the umbilical vein. O negative blood used for double volume exchange transfusion.

45. Ans. (d) CRP

Ref: Nelson, 18th ed. chapter 176

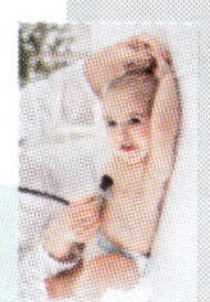

- CRP, an acute phase reactant is produced by liver and turns positive in sepsis.
- **Other abnormalities in sepsis are:**
  - Hematologic abnormalities include thrombocytopenia, prolonged prothrombin and partial thromboplastin times,
  - *Reduced serum fibrinogen levels and elevated fibrin split products, and anemia.*
  - Elevated neutrophil and *increased immature forms (bands, myelocytes, promyelocytes), vacuolation of neutrophils, toxic granulations, and Döhle bodies* can be seen with infection.
  - Neutropenia is an ominous sign of overwhelming sepsis.

46. Ans. (a) Jaundice is prolonged due to cephal-hematoma

Ref: Harrison, 18th ed. chapter 61

- Cephalhematoma is seen due to birth trauma, and represents sub-periosteal hemorrhage.
- The hematoma is limited sharply by the margins of the bone and does not cross suture lines.
- In first 2 weeks, the hematoma is of soft tissue density due to its blood contents and X skull films show the swelling as a soft tissue "mass" which is limited at its margins by the cranial sutures.

47. Ans. (b) Late congenital syphilis

Ref: OP Ghai, 8th ed. pg. 273

It is a common pattern of presentation for congenital syphilis, and consists of three phenomena *aka Hutchinson triad:*
- Interstitial keratitis
- Hutchinson incisors
- Eighth nerve deafness.

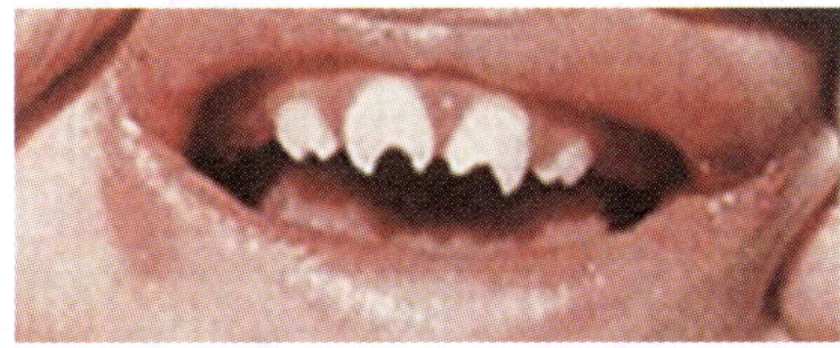

48. Ans. (d) Hydrocephalus

Ref: OP Ghai, 8th ed. pg. 272

The classic Triad for Congenital Rubella Syndrome is:

1. Sensorineural deafness (58% of patients)
2. Eye abnormalities—especially retinopathy, cataract and microphthalmia (43% of patients)
3. Congenital heart disease—especially patent ductus arteriosus (50% of patients)

*"Salt-and-pepper" retinopathy is the most common ocular manifestation of congenital rubella.

Other Manifestations of CRS may Include:

- Spleen, liver or bone marrow problems
- Mental retardation
- Microcephaly[Q]
- Eye defects
- Low birth weight
- Thrombocytopenic purpura (presents as a characteristic blueberry muffin rash)[Q]
- Hepatomegaly
- Micrognathia

49. Ans. (c) Congenital syphilis

Ref: OP Ghai, 8th ed. pg. 182, 273

Early manifestations of congenital infection vary and involve multiple organ systems.
- About 60% of infants born with congenital syphilis are asymptomatic at birth.
- Symptoms develop within the first 2 months of life. In symptomatic infants, the *most common physical finding, seen in 100% of cases, is hepatomegaly.*
- The other common findings are skeletal abnormalities, rash, and generalized lymphadenopathy.
- Radiographic abnormalities, periostitis or osteitis, involve multiple bones. Sometimes, the lesion is painful and an infant will favor an extremity (pseudopalsy).
- The rash is maculopapular and may involve palms and soles. In contrast to acquired syphilis, a vesicular rash and bullae may develop. These lesions are also highly contagious.
- Mucosal involvement may present as rhinitis ("*snuffles*"). Nasal secretions are highly contagious.
- Hematological abnormalities include anemia and thrombocytopenia.

Late-onset congenital syphilis (diagnosed >2 years)
Manifestations include neurosyphilis and involvement of the teeth, bones, eyes, and the eighth cranial nerve, as follows:

1. Bone involvement - Saber shins[Q], saddle nose
2. Teeth involvement - Notched, peg-shaped incisors (Hutchinson teeth)[Q]
3. Pigmentary involvement - Linear scars (rhagades)[Q] at the corners of the mouth
4. Interstitial keratitis - Presents in the first or second decade of life
5. Sensory-neural hearing loss (eighth cranial nerve deafness)
6. Classic Hutchinson triad[Q] - (1) defective incisors, (2) interstitial keratitis, (3) eighth cranial nerve deafness.

50. Ans. (b) Two weeks

Ref: OP Ghai, 8th ed. pg. 172

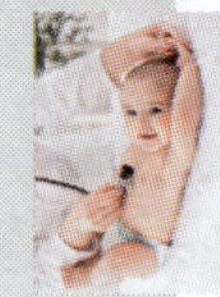

- Physiological jaundice is seen in most infants due to elevation of un-conjugated bilirubin concentration during their first week.
- **Term infants** - Jaundice lasts for about 10 days with peak of serum bilirubin up to 15 mg/dL by 3 days of age.
- **Preterm infants** - Jaundice lasts for about two weeks, with a rapid rise of serum bilirubin up to 12 mg/dL.

Mechanisms involved in physiological jaundice are mainly:

- Relatively low activity of the enzyme glucuronosyl transferase[Q]
- Shorter life span of fetal red blood cells[Q], being approximately 80–100 days in a full term infant, compared to 100–120 days in adults.
- Relatively low conversion of bilirubin to urobilinogen by the intestinal flora[Q], resulting in relatively high absorption of bilirubin back into the circulation.

51. Ans. (d) 8-9 hrs

- There is no gas in the abdomen of a new born baby. It takes 8 hours for the air to reach the descending colon and performing the X-ray shall be useful.
- Invertogram in neonates with suspected ano-rectal malformations should be done after 24 hours of life.

52. Ans. (c) Tickle the sole

Ref: Chapter 100: Delivery Room Emergencies: Nelson 18th edn.

Immediately after birth, an infant in need of resuscitation should be placed under a radiant heater and dried (to avoid hypothermia), *positioned head down and slightly extended, the airway cleared by suctioning, and gentle tactile stimulation provided (slapping the foot, rubbing the back).* Simultaneously, the infant's color, heart rate, and respiratory effort should be assessed

53. Ans. (a) Succimer

Ref: Nelson 20th edn. pg. 3433

Children with blood lead levels >45 μg/dL require 2, 3 Dimercaptosuccinic acid/succimer.

54. Ans. (d) Done for babies with cyanosis

Ref: OP Ghai, 8th ed. pg. 148

- **Kangaroo care** is a technique practiced on newborn, usually preterm, infants wherein the infant is held, skin-to-skin, with an adult.
- The kangaroo position provides ready access to nourishment.
- The parent's stable body temperature helps to regulate the neonate's temperature more smoothly than an incubator, and allows for readily accessible breastfeeding.
- Babies who are eligible for kangaroo care include pre-term infants, weighing less than 1,500 grams, and breathing independently.
- Cardiopulmonary monitoring, oximetry, supplemental oxygen or nasal (continuous positive airway pressure) ventilation, intravenous infusion, and monitor leads do not prevent kangaroo care.
- Babies who are in kangaroo care tend to be less prone to apnea and bradycardia and have stabilization of oxygen needs.

55. Ans. (a) Baby fed with a bottle finding it difficult and confusing to suckle at breast

Ref: OP Ghai, 8th ed. pg. 153

- A problem that may beset a bottlefed baby in which it forgets how to nurse on mother' nipple
- Breastfeeding requires far more vigorous mouth and tongue motions and greater muscle coordination than bottlefeeding.
- On bottle nipples or even pacifiers, a newborn can forget how to nurse properly.
- This confusion can lead to diminished or discontinued nursing. Nipple confusion is usually not a concern after the early weeks, once the baby is nursing well.

56. Ans. (a) Diaphragmatic hernia

Ref: OP Ghai, 8th ed. pg. 129

- In diaphragmatic hernia: Bag and mask will lead to over-distention of the stomach which is already lying in chest cavity. This *will worsen the mediastinal shift and compress the ipsilateral lung further leading to worsening of the patient.*
- Bag and mask ventilation is also not to be done in meconium aspiration syndrome. In choice c, it is written meconium ileus.

57. Ans. (d) Orthopnea

Ref: OP Ghai, 8th ed. pg. 397–98

- Breathing difficulty in children when lying down is a condition in which a child has trouble catching his or her breath or breathing normally when lying down.

Breathing difficulty in children when lying down (pediatric orthopnea) includes:

- Airway obstruction e.g., foreign object
- Chronic obstructive pulmonary disease
- Cystic fibrosis
- Corpulmonale
- Heart failure

Baby feels better when held against shoulders.

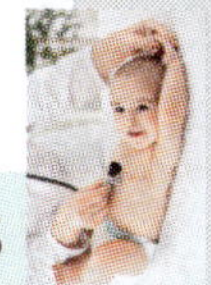

58. Ans. (d) β_2 transferrin

- Macrophages in human milk may synthesize complement, lysozyme, and lactoferrin. Breast milk contains lactoferrin, an iron-binding whey protein that is normally saturated with iron and has an inhibitory effect on the growth of *Escherichia coli* in the intestine.
- Further, the lower pH of the stool of breast-fed infants is thought to contribute to the favorable intestinal flora of these infants compared with formula fed infants (more bifidobacteria and lactobacilli; fewer *Escherichia coli*), and this helps protect against infections caused by some species of *E. coli*.

59. Ans. (b) Vasodilation

Ref: Nelson's, 18th ed. Ch: 97.2

Supplemental O_2 helps in vasoconstriction and ductal closure. Both functional and anatomical closure of ductus arteriosus is attributed to increasing O_2 levels. Increased O_2 is also responsible for neovascularization and development of retinopathy of prematurity.

Oxygen causes tissue injury through the formation of reactive oxygen intermediates and peroxidation of membrane lipids.

60. Ans. (b) 8

Ref: OP Ghai, 8th ed. pg. 155

Expressed breast milk can be stored in:

- Room temperature-for 8 hours
- Refrigerator-for 24 hours
- Deep freezer-for 3 months

61. Ans. (a) 24 hours later but within 72 hours

Ref: OP Ghai, 8th ed. pg. 172

Presence of any of the following signs denotes that the jaundice is pathological

- Clinical jaundice detected before 24 hours of age
- Rise in serum bilirubin by >5 mg/ dL/day
- Serum bilirubin >15 mg/dL
- Clinical jaundice persisting beyond 14 days of life
- Clay/white colored stool and/or dark urine staining the clothes yellow.
- Direct bilirubin >2 mg/dL at any time.

Characteristics of Physiological Jaundice

- First appears between 24 and 72 hours of age
- Maximum intensity seen on 4–5 th day in term and 7th day in preterm neonates.
- Does not exceed 15 mg/dL.
- Clinically undetectable after 14 days.
- No treatment is required but baby should be observed closely for signs of worsening jaundice.

62. Ans. (b) Carbohydrate

Ref: OP Ghai, 8th ed. pg. 8–9

- In order to supply the fetus with energy, the pregnant woman increases her hepatic glucose production by 16–30%. The transfer of glucose from the maternal circulation to the fetus takes placeby facilitated diffusion involving glucose transporter 1. (GLUT1)
- A considerable part of the trans-placentally transferred glucose is used by the fetal brain. Although enzyme systems that are necessary for glucose production (gluconeogenesis) develop early, the fetus only produces its own glucose under extreme condition such as during maternal starvation.

63. Ans. (a) 3:1

Ref: Ghai, 7th ed. pg. 691–2

- Ratio of chest compressions to rescue breaths in neonates is 3:1. In pediatric resuscitation with single rescuer, the ratio is 30:2.
- In resuscitation in adults the ratio is again 30:2 with a single/two rescuers.

Sternum should be compressed to depress approximately ***one third to one half of the anteroposterior diameter*** of the chest. Chest compression should be delivered providing ***equal time in compression and relaxation phases.***

64. Ans. (d) Extra pyramidal cerebral palsy

Ref: Ghai, 7th ed. pg. 559–560

Extrapyramidal cerebral palsy is caused by **bilirubin encephalopathy.** It is also associated with deafness.

Clinical Manifestations Include:

- Dyskinesia such as athetosis, choreiform movements, dystonia, tremors and rigidity
- ***Early indicator is inability to reach for and grasp a dangling ring by the age of 6 months.***

Types of Cerebral Palsy

Spastic cerebral Palsy: Most common type of cerebral palsy. It is of the following subtypes: Spastic Quadriparesis: More in **term babies** Spastic Diplegia: More in **preterm babies;** associated with periventricular leukomalacia Spastic Hemiplegia: recognized after 4–6 months of age
Hypotonic (atonic) cerebral palsy
Extrapyramidal cerebral palsy/athetoid cerebral palsy: Kernicterus

65. Ans. (c) Vitamin K

- Vitamin K is produced by our gut flora. The gut of a New-born baby is sterile and hence no vitamin K is being produced.

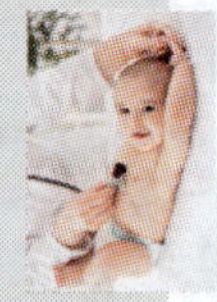

- Moreover vitamin K is negligible in breast milk. *In lieu of these factors all babies are susceptible to development of Hemorrhagic disease of New-born.*
- To prevent this from happening therefore, as standard operating procedure in all hospitals injection vitamin K_1 1 mg intramuscular is given to prevent hemorrhagic disease of new born.
- In our country where a large number of children are born via home deliveries, no vitamin K would be given to the child and therefore the *child may be brought to the hospital on day 5 with umbilical stump bleeding.*
- For management: the child should be given injection vitamin K 1mg intravenously. If bleeding is still present then FFP needs to be administered.

Extra Mile

- Type of vitamin K used for treatment of H.D.N= vitamin K_1
- Umbilical stump bleeding in child on day 1 of life= factor 13 deficiency
- Umbilical stump bleeding in child on day 5 of life= H.D.N
- Male baby with excessive circumcision bleeding= Hemophilia A
- Vaginal bleeding in a girl child on day 5 of life= No intervention required (occurs due to transplacental transfer of hormones)

66. Ans. (c) AMBU Bag Ventilation for 30 seconds with heart rate of 50

Ref: Nelson, 18th ed. Chapter 100,

Evaluate respirations, heart rate, and color
Breathing, HR>100 & Pink → Observational care
Breathing, HR>100 but cyanotic → Give supplementary oxygen
Give supplementary oxygen → Pink → Observational care
Apnea or HR < 100 → Provide positive-pressure ventilation
Give supplementary oxygen → Persistent cyanosis → Provide positive-pressure ventilation
Provide positive-pressure ventilation → Effective ventilation, HR>100 & Pink → Postresuscitation care
Provide positive-pressure ventilation → HR < 60 → • Provide positive-pressure ventilation • Administer chest compressions
• Provide positive-pressure ventilation • Administer chest compressions → HR > 60 → Provide positive-pressure ventilation
• Provide positive-pressure ventilation • Administer chest compressions → HR < 60 → Administer epinephrine and/or volume

- *If the heart rate does not improve after 30 sec with bag and mask (or endotracheal) ventilation and remains below 100/ min,* ventilation is continued and *chest compression should be initiated over the lower third of the sternum* at a rate of 120/min. The ratio of compressions to ventilation is 3:1.
- If the heart rate remains <60 despite effective compressions and ventilation, administration of epinephrine should be considered.
- AAP guidelines are given above.

MILESTONES IN CHILDREN

67. Ans. (a) Lower central incisor

Ref: O.P. Ghai Essential Pediatrics, 9th ed. pg. 39

- The first tooth to erupt is lower central incisor.
- At birth people usually have 20 primary teeth, which start to erupt at about 6 months of age.
- They fall out at various times throughout childhood. By age 21, all 32 of the permanent teeth have usually erupted.

68. Ans. (b) 20–49

Ref: Nelson 20th ed. pg. 217

IQ range	Classification
140 and over	Genius or near genius
120–140	Very superior intelligence
110–120	Superior intelligence
90–110	Normal or average intelligence
80–90	Dullness
70–80	Borderline deficiency
50–69	Moron
20–49	Imbecile
Below 20	Idiot

TABLE: Identification of cause in children with severe intellectual disability

Cause	Examples	Percent of total
Chromosomal disorder	Trisomies 21, 18, 13 Klinefelter syndrome	~20
Genetic syndrome	Fragile X syndrome Prader-Willi syndrome Rett syndrome	~20
Nonsyndromic autosomal mutations	Variations in copy number, *denovo* mutations in *SYNGAP 1, GRIK2, TUSC3*	~10

Contd...

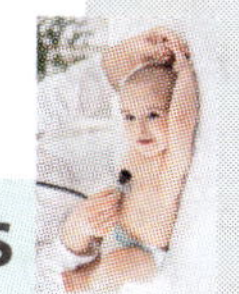

Cause	Examples	Percent of total
Developmental brain abnormality	Hydrocephalus ± meningomyelocele, lissencephaly	~8
Inborn erros of metabolism or neurodegenerative disorder	PKU, Tay-Sachs	~7
Congenital infections	HIV, toxoplasmosis, rubella, CMV, syphilis, herpes simplex	~3
Perinatal causes	HIE, meningitis, IVH, PVL, fetal alcohol syndrome	4
Postnatal causes	Trauma (abuse), meningitis, hypothyrodism	~4
Unkown	Cerebral palsy	~20

69. Ans. (a) 7 months

Ref: OP Ghai, 8th ed. pg. 49

- Lets evaluate data step wise to arrive at answer.
  1. Baby can sit in tripod position by 5th month.
  2. Bi dextrous approach by 5th month.
  3. Monosyllables by 6th month.
  4. Stranger anxiety by 7th month.

70. Ans. (a) 12 weeks

Ref: OP Ghai, 8th ed. pg. 52

There are Two Types of Smiles for Babies

- The *spontaneous* or almost reflexive smile that can occur early in the newborn period.
- The *social smile* that occurs in response to something, like when you talk or sing to baby
- The social smile is a developmental milestone that infants reach when they are one to two months old.
- *Not having a social smile by three months of age is a red flag for child to be evaluated by an expert.*

71. Ans. (b) 6 months

Ref: OP Ghai, 8th ed. pg. 142

- ***Moro reflex persists until 6 months.*** It is sometimes referred to as the startle reflex.
- The Moro reflex is present at birth, peaks in the first month of life, and *completely disappears around 6 months of age.*
- It is likely to occur if the infant's head suddenly shifts position, the temperature changes abruptly, or they are startled by a sudden noise.
- ***The legs and head extend while the arms jerk up and out with the palms up and thumbs flexed. Shortly afterward the arms are brought together and the hands clench into fists, and the infant cries loudly.***
- *Bilateral absence* of the reflex may be linked to damage to the infant's central nervous system, while a *unilateral absence* could mean an injury due to birth trauma (e.g., a fractured clavicle or injury to the brachial plexus). Erb's palsy or some other form of paralysis is also sometimes present in such cases.

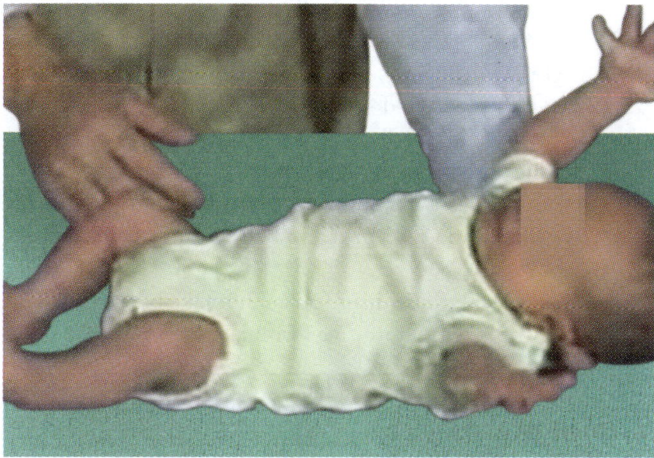

72. Ans. (a) Prematurity

Ref: OP Ghai, 8th ed. pg. 124

- Most common cause of neonatal mortality in India is prematurity (obviously lack of hospital care).
- Metabolic causes like hypoglycemia infant of diabetic mother, can be asked in questions.

73. Ans. (c) 6 months

Ref: OP Ghai, 8th ed. pg. 154

- Head lag disappears by 3 months
- Head control is achieved by 4 months
- A child in prone position at 3 months can lift chin off the bed, but it takes a while for the shoulder muscles to develop sufficient strength so as to lift the chest and head off the bed. This activity would be possible by 6 months
- Wave bye-bye by 9 months
- Stand without support at 12 months
- Run by 18 months

BREASTFEEDING

74. Ans. (d) Vitamin K

Ref: cdc.gov

Breast milk is low in vitamin K. Breast milk from mothers who are taking vitamin K supplements is also low in vitamin K.

The American Academy of Pediatrics recommends that all newborns, whether breastfed or formula fed, receive a one-time intramuscular shot of vitamin K within 6 hours after birth.

75. Ans. (a) Galactosemia in the infant

Ref: O.P. Ghai Essential Pediatrics, 9th ed. pg. 642

- Breastfeeding is contraindicated in infants with classic galactosemia. (galactose 1-phosphate uridyl-transferase [GALT] deficiency.
- The affected child will develop cataracts with delayed growth and intellectual disability, liver disease, and kidney problems.
- Galactose is a part of lactose that is found in all dairy products and also in many baby formula milk brands too.
- Babies with these disorders cannot take breast milk and may be given lactose-free formula milk.

76. Ans. (d) High sugar and fat

Ref: O.P. Ghai Essential Pediatrics, 9th ed. pg. 147

- Colostrum is high in protein and low in fat and sugar.
- It is loaded with IgA and white blood cells that give natural immunity to the child.

77. Ans. (d) Paladai feeding

Ref: Newbornwhocc.org Guidelines for Neonatal Feeding

Gestational age	Maturation of feeding skills	Initial feeding method
<28 weeks	No proper sucking efforts No propulsive motility in the gut	I.V. fluids
28–31 weeks	Sucking bursts develop No coordination b/w suck/swallow and breathing	Orogastric or nasogastric tube feeding with occasional spoon/ paladai feeding
32–34 weeks	Slightly nature sucking pattern Coordination b/w breathing and swallowing begins	Feeding by spoon/ paladai/cup
>34 weeks	Mature sucking pattern More coordination b/w breathing and swallowing	Breastfeeding

78. Ans. (c) Amino acid based formula

Ref: Nelson, 20th ed. pg. 288-89

- Most common cause associated with food intolerance during infancy: **Cow's milk proteins > Soyabean milk**
- Nearly, 50% of children affected by cow's milk protein intolerance develop soy protein intolerance as well if they are fed with soy based formulas.
- Therefore soy-based formulas should not be used for the treatment of cow's milk protein intolerance

Management of Cow Milk Protein Allergy

Exclusively breast fed child	*Formula fed child*
Maternal exclusion diet avoiding food containing Cow Milk Protein and hen's eggs is advised, since these are excreted in breast milk.	Elimination diet and avoid egg protein The elimination diet should be continued for a minimum of 2 weeks, and up to 4 weeks in cases of atopic dermatitis or allergic colitis.
If *no improvement* start Extensively hydrolyzed formula feed (eHF)	If no improvement, start *amino acid based formula*

- Use complete milk protein hydrolysates in infants who cannot be breastfed. Occasionally, children may develop intolerance toward complete hydrolysated formulas. In these cases, use amino acid–based formulas, which are now widely available and are balanced in trace elements and vitamins.

79. Ans. (b) Baby's lower lip is inverted

Correct Positioning During Breastfeeding

1. The *mother should be seated comfortably* in an upright position, so that her breasts fall naturally and she has good support for her back, arms and feet
2. The *infant should be supported* behind the shoulders and facing the mother, with his or her body flexed around the mother's body. The position must be a comfortable drinking position for the infant
3. The chin should be tucked well into the breast, and the infant's *mouth should be wide open*, with the bottom lip curled *back. More areola will be evident above* the *infant's top lip than below the bottom lip*
4. After an initial short burst of sucking, the rhythm will be slow and even, with deep jaw movements that should not cause the mother any discomfort – pauses are a normal part of the feed and they become more frequent as the feed continues

- If the cheeks are being sucked in or there is audible 'clicking', the infant is not attached correctly

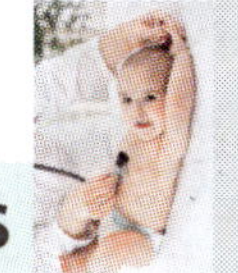

- The infant should stop feeding of his or her own accord by coming off the breast spontaneously

80. Ans. (c) Lower areola is more visible than upper

Ref: OP Ghai, 8th ed. pg. 154

Please refer to above explanation.

81. Ans. (d) 6 months

Ref: OP Ghai, 8th ed. pg. 150

- Exclusive breastfeeding is up to 6 months and should be continued uptil 2 years.
- Prelacteal feeds like water, honey, and so called health tonics are contraindicated in children <6 months of age.

82. Ans. (d) Avidin

Ref: Nelson, 18th ed. Chapter 42

- Human milk contains a variety of cells, including macrophages, T cells, stem cells, and lymphocytes.
- In early lactation, the breastfed infant may consume as many as 10^{10} maternal leukocytes per day.
- About 80% of the cells in early milk are breast milk macrophages, which originate as peripheral blood monocytes that exit the bloodstream and migrate into milk through the mammary epithelium.
- The proteins of human milk are divided into the whey and casein fractions or complexes, with each comprising of a remarkable array of specific proteins and peptides.
- *The most abundant proteins are casein, α-lactalbumin, lactoferrin, secretory immunoglobulin IgA, lysozyme, and serum albumin.*

83. Ans. (c) Lower lip of infant is inverted

Ref: OP Ghai, 8th ed. pg. 154

- The basic concept is that when the child suckles the breast the lower lip should be EVERTED.

84. Ans. (d) Taurine

Clinical studies have elucidated various mechanisms by which taurine promotes brain development, the main effect being on neurotransmitter production.

In previous year same question was asked with different choices and you need to remember that DHA- Docosa Hexanoic Acid plays an important role in brain myelination in infants. Infact studies have shown that IQ of breast fed baby is higher than that of cow milk fed baby with DHA making all the difference.

GROWTH AND DEVELOPMENT

85. Ans. (b) Stunting

Underweight	When children's weight for age is below minus two standard deviations (< –2 SD) from the WHO reference population weight.
Stunting	When children's height for age is below minus two standard deviations the WHO reference population height.
Wasting	When children's weight for height is below minus two standard deviations from the WHO

86. Ans. (c) Overweight

Ref: Nelson 20th ed. pg. 88

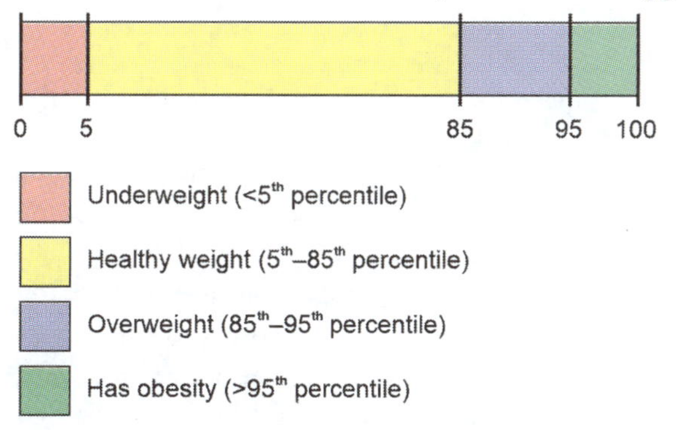

87. Ans. (c) Height for age

Ref: Nelson 20th ed. pg. 298

- Height for age is a measure of linear growth and a deficit represents cumulative effect of adverse events in first 1000 days from conception. It results in chronic malnutrition and stunting. Conversely a low weight for height or wasting indicates acute malnutrition.
- Weight for age is most commonly used index of nutritional status although is does not differentiate between wasting and stunting.

88. Ans. (b) 16 weeks

Ref: Rudolph Paediatrics, 22nd ed. pg. 183

Must know time line for fetal development

Appearance of fetal pole shadow (USG)	5–6 weeks fertilization
Heart beat (USG)	6–7 weeks
Erythropoiesis	
In liver	6 weeks
In bone marrow	16 weeks

Contd...

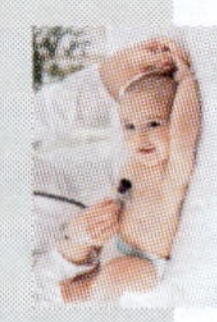

Development of lymphocytes	
In thymus	9 weeks
In lymph nodes	10 weeks
Breathing movement	11–12 weeks
Swallowing reflex	16 weeks
Appearance of meconium	20 weeks
Secretion of urine	End of first trimester

TABLE: New ballard scoring for determining prematurity

	–1	0	1	2	3	4
Skin	Sticky friable transparent	Gelatinuos red, translucent	Smooth pink, visible veins	Superficial peeling &/or rash. Few veins	Cracking pale areas rare veins	Parchment deep cracking no vessels
Plantar surface	Heel-toe 40–50 mm: –1 < 40 mm: – 2	>50 mm no crease	Faint red marks	Anterior transverse crease only	Creases ant. 2/3	Creases over entire sole
Breast	Imperceptible	Barely perceptible	Flat areola no bud	Stippled areola 1–2 mm bud	Raised areola 3–4 mm bud	Full areola 5–10 mm bud
Eye/Ear	Lids fused loosely;–1 tightly;–2	Lids open pinna flat stays folded	Slightly Curved pinna; soft; slow recoil	Well-curved pinna; soft but ready recoil	Formed & firm instant recoil	Thick cartilage ear stiff
Genitals Male	Scrotum flat, smooth	Scrotum empty faint rugae	Testes in upper canal	Testes descending few rugae	Tests down good rugae	Testes pendulous deep rugae
Genitals Female	Clitoris prominent labia flat	Prominent clitoris small labia minora	Prominent clitoris enlarging minora	Major & minora equally prominent	Majora large minora small	Majora cover clitoris & minora

89. Ans. (a) Prematurity

- Prenatal ultrasonography shows no testicular descent before 28 weeks' gestation, other than transabdominal movement to the internal inguinal ring.
- Transinguinal migration, thought to be under hormonal control, occurs at 28–40 weeks' gestation, usually resulting in a scrotal testis by the end of a full term of gestation

90. Ans. (d) 20 teeth

- All 20 teeth (10 in the upper jaw and 10 in the lower jaw) have come in by the time the child is 2½–3-year-old. The complete set of primary teeth is in the mouth from the age of 2½–3 years of age to 6–7 years of age.
  - Basic rule of thumb is that approximately 4 teeth will erupt for every 6 months of life.
  - Lower teeth erupt before upper teeth with teeth in both jaws usually erupting in pairs.
  - Primary teeth are whiter and smaller in color than the permanent teeth that will follow.
  - By the time a child is 2–3 years of age,all primary 20 teeth should have erupted.
- Shortly after age 4, the jaw and facial bones of the child begin to grow, creating spaces between the primary teeth.
- Between the ages of 6 and 12, a mixture of both primary teeth and permanent teeth reside in the mouth.

91. Ans. (c) 7 months into scrotum

Ref: OP Ghai, 8th ed. pg. 540

From the 3rd month of pregnancy and its end the testes migrate from the lumbar area to the future scrotum.

This transfer is secondary to

- Combination of growth processes and hormonal influences.
- Gubernaculum testis also plays a decisive role in this phenomenon.

Scrotum is empty at 7 months. The testis descents into inguinal canal at 7 months.

92. Ans. (c) Truancy

- ***Pre-school children are classified as children between 2 and 5 years. The usual problems seen are:***

1. **Temper tantrums** Control is a central issue. *Tantrums normally appear toward the end of the 1st year of life and peak in prevalence between 2 and 4 years of age.* ***Tantrums lasting >15 min or regularly occurring >3 times/day may reflect underlying medical, emotional, or social problems***
2. Sleep problems
3. Pica involves repeated or chronic ingestion of non-nutritive substances, which may include plaster, charcoal, clay, wool, ashes, paint, and earth.

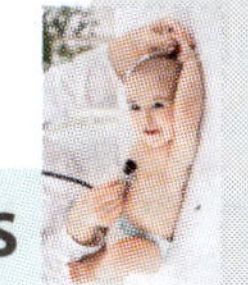

- **Truancy is seen in school going children.** Truancy **and** run-away **behavior are never** developmentally appropriate. Approximately ½ of school refusal incidents result from child and adolescent behavioral problems; the other ½ of incidents are related to mood and anxiety symptoms. ***Often, truancy represents disorganization within the home, developing personality problems, or both.***

93. Ans. (c) Thelarche

Ref: Nelson, 18th ed. Adolescence: chapter 12

IN GIRLS

- The first visible sign of puberty and the hallmark of SMR2 (Sexual maturity rating) is the **appearance of breast buds,** between 8 and 12 years of age.
- Menses typically begins 2–2½ years later, during SMR3–4 (median age, 12 years), around the peak height velocity.

IN BOYS

- ***The first visible sign of puberty and the hallmark of SMR2 is testicular enlargement, beginning as early as 9½ years.*** This is followed by penile growth during SMR3. Peak growth occurs when testis volumes reach approximately 9–10 cm^3 during SMR4.
- Under the influence of LH and testosterone, the seminiferous tubules, epididymis, seminal vesicles, and prostate enlarge. The left testis normally is lower than the right. Erections are common, and nocturnal emissions may occur. The voice deepens, and linear growth is accelerated.

Also remember: *Precocious puberty is defined as the onset of secondary sexual characteristics before 8 years of age in girls and 9 years in boys.*

94. Ans. (d) 5 years

- *OP ghai states enuresis as urinary incontinence beyond the age of 4 years for daytime and 6 years for night-time enuresis.*
- It is said to be present if it occurs twice per week for 3 consecutive months.
- *Most of children attain complete bladder control by age of 5 years*
- The prevalence of enuresis is 7% in boys and 3% in girls at age of 5 years and keeps on decreasing for every subsequent year.
- Treatment of choice for nocturnal enuresis is alarm devices with desmopressin nasal spray.

95. Ans. (d) 12

Ref: Nelson, 18th ed. Table 447–1

TABLE: Hematologic values during infancy and childhood

	Hemoglobin (G/DL)	
Age	Mean	Range
Cord blood	16.8	13.7–20.1
2 week	16.5	13.0–20.0
3 month	12.0	9.5–14.5
6 mo-6 year	12.0	10.5–14
7–12 year Adult	13.0	11.0–16.0
Female	14	12.0–16.0
Male	16	14.0–18.0

96. Ans. (d) Behavior modification

Ref: Nelson, 18th ed. Chapter 573

- In children with overactive bladder, urge incontinence, and dysfunctional voiding, voiding at predetermined times aids in retraining the child to exercise voluntary bladder control.
- *Behavioral modification has remained the mainstay of treatment for daytime wetting. These measures focus on relearning and training the normal responses from the bladder and urethra.*
- Bladder irritants such as caffeine should be eliminated from the diet.
- The child voids on waking, and subsequently at least every 2 h, during waking hours. As urgency improves, the interval between voids can be extended. In children with infrequent voiding, in whom an elevated PVR volume is encountered, double voiding will both increase functional bladder capacity and decrease the risk of infection.

97. Ans. (a) Malnutrition

Ref: Nelson, 18th ed. Chapter 45

- **Rickets,** a disease of growing bone, occurs in children due to malnutrition in India. It occurs before fusion of the epiphyses, and is due to un-mineralized matrix at the growth plates.
- Earliest presentation is craniotabes and presentation after 6 months of age is widening of Bilateral wrist joints.

98. Ans. (b) 3 years

Ref: Nelson, 18th ed. Chapter 9

Milestones at 3 years of age

1. Can tell age gender and recall story
2. Rides tricycle

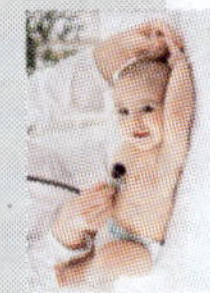

3. Stands momentarily on one foot
4. Makes tower of 10 cubes; imitates construction of "bridge" of 3 cubess
5. Copies circle
6. Imitates cross
7. Plays simple games (in "parallel" with other children)
8. Helps in dressing (unbuttons clothing and puts on shoes)
9. Washes hands

99. Ans. (d) All of the above

Ref: OP Ghai, 8th ed. pg. 59

- Attention deficit hyperactivity disorder in the (ICD-10) is a psychiatric disorder of the neurodevelopmental type in which there are significant problems of attention, hyperactivity, or acting impulsively that are not appropriate for age.
- *Symptoms must begin by age six to twelve years and persist for more than six months for a diagnosis to be made.* In school-aged individuals inattention symptoms often result in poor school performance.

Symptoms

1. Inattention
2. Hyperactivity (restlessness in adults)
3. Disruptive behavior, and
4. Impulsivity, are common in ADHD
   - Academic difficulties are frequent as are problems with relationships. Based on the presenting symptoms ADHD can be divided into three subtypes predominantly inattentive, predominantly hyperactive-impulsive, or combined.

An individual with hyperactivity may have some or all or the following symptoms:

- Fidget and squirm in their seats.
- Talk nonstop.
- Dash around, touching or playing with anything and everything in sight.
- Have trouble sitting sill during dinner, school, doing homework, and story time.
- Be constantly in motion.
- Have difficulty doing quiet tasks or activities.

100. Ans. (d) Shoulder

Ref: Ghai, 8th ed. pg. 6

Skeletal age determination	
Age	X-ray
Newborn	Knee
Infant between 3–9 months	Shoulder
1–13 years	Single film of Hand & Wrist
12–14 years	Elbow & hip

101. Ans. (a) Between incisors

Ref: Shafer's Textbook of Oral Pathology, 6th ed. pg. 46

- Supernumerary tooth or hyperdontia refers to presence of an extra tooth. It can be one or more than one.
- It develops from third tooth bud arising from the dental lamina near the permanent tooth bud or possibly by splitting of permanent tooth bud itself.
- *The most common location is anteriorly between the maxillary incisors.*

102. Ans. (b) 5 months

Ref: O.P Ghai, 8th ed. pg. 4

Birth weight doubles at 5 months, triples in an year and is four times at 2 years and becomes 5 times at 3 years.

Note: *Newborns lose 10% of body weight in first ten days due to loss of extracellular water, after which they gain 25–30 g/day for first 3 months of life.*

103. Ans. (d) 4 years

Ref: O.P Ghai, 8th ed. pg. 5

Time	Length
At birth	50 cm
3 months	60 cm
9 months	75 cm
2 years	90 cm
41/2 years	100 cm

Indian children gain 5 cm height every year until 10 years of age.

104. Ans. (b) 6 years

Ref: Nelson, 18th ed. Ch 8

105. Ans. (c) 100 words

Ref: Nelson's, 18th ed. ch: 32.2

106. Ans. (c) 5 years

Ref: Nelson's, 18th ed ch: 9

107. Ans. (d) Walk short distance

Ref: Nelson, 18th ed. chapter 10

Hide and seek game Do not confuse with peak a boo	Not mentioned but by my experience >3 years
Write alphabet	6 years
Say short sentence	2 years
Walk short distance	18 months

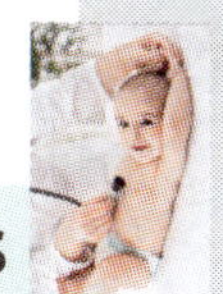

108. Ans. (d) Social smile at 3 months

109. Ans. (d) Increase in testicular size

Please refer explanation of Q. 93

110. Ans. (c) 4 years

Ref: OP Ghai 8th ed./13

- Length of Indian baby at birth = 50 cm
- Length at 1 year = 75 cm
- Length at 4½ years = 100 cm
- Subsequently 5–6 cm/year
- Pubertal growth spurt = 6–8 cm/year

PROTEIN ENERGY MALNUTRITION

111. Ans. (b) Kwashiorkor

Protein deficiency leads to Kwashiorkor and low serum albumin explains the bilateral pitting edema in these patients. Children with Kwashiorkor are dull and lethargic in contrast to marasmus where the child has a voracious appetite.

112. Ans. (a) Kwashiorkor

Ref: O.P. Ghai Essential Pediatrics, 9th ed. pg. 96

- Kwashiorkor is a type of malnutrition characterized by severe protein deficiency. They are called sugar babies due to diet that is predominantly composed up of carbohydrates as protein are relatively an expensive source of energy.
- Low serum albumin leads to pedal Edema in these patient and weight can be falsely normal.

113. Ans. (d) Caloric Deficiency

Ref: O.P. Ghai Essential Pediatrics, 9th ed. pg. 95

- Marasmus is characterized by deficiency in calorie intake and sometimes referred to as the most severe form of malnutrition.
- Children with this condition have lost a lot of muscle mass and subcutaneous fat.
- Dry skin and brittle hair are also symptoms of marasmus.

114. Ans. (a) Less protein intake

Ref: O.P. Ghai Essential Pediatrics, 9th ed. pg. 93

- Notice the bilateral extremity swelling seen due to protein deficiency in Kwashiorkor
- Edema may hide the extreme wasting of the underlying tissues.
- The skin is scaly and the hair loses its natural color/ Flag sign on hair is noticed.

115. Ans. (d) 11.5

Ref: Nelson Textbook of Pediatrics 20th ed. pg. 431

Severe acute malnutrition is defined as:

1. Severe wasting and/or
2. Bilateral edema
   - Severe wasting is extreme thinness diagnosed by a weight for length or height < - 3SD of WHO child growth standards or Mid arm circumference <115 cm using a color banded tape.
   - Bilateral edema is diagnosed by placing thumb on dorsum of foot and pressing gently and firmly for 10 seconds. A pit or dent remaining under each thumb indicates bilateral edema.

116. Ans. (d) Edema

Ref: OP Ghai 8th ed. pg. 99

- Kwashiorkor usually affects children aged 1–4 years.
- The main sign is *pitting edema*, usually starting in the legs and feet and spreading, in more advanced cases, to the hands and face.
- Because of edema, children with Kwashiorkor may look healthy because of which their parents view them as well fed.

117. Ans. (b) Height/age

Ref: Nelson's Pediatrics, 18th ed. Ch 43

The nutritional indices commonly calculated for young children are:

- **Weight for height** – an index used to measure wasting or acute malnutrition; (WHAM)
- **Height for age** – an index used to measure stunting or chronic malnutrition; (HA-CM)
- **Weight for age** – an index used to measure underweight (or wasting and stunting combined). (WASW)
- **Mid arm circumference** is a specific indicator of wasting or acute malnutrition.

Remember:

- Weight reflects only present health status of the child, whereas height indicates events in the past also
- Most sensitive measure of physical growth- WEIGHT
- Single best parameter for assessment of physical growth- WEIGHT

118. Ans. (a) Weight/height

Please refer to above explanation Q. 117

119. Ans. (a) Wt.kg/Ht.m^2

Ref: Nelson, 18th ed. chapter 44

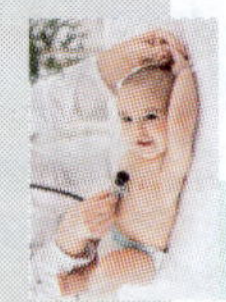

Also note that the way we diagnose obesity in children is different from adults

BMI percentile for age	Weight status
<5th percentile	Underweight
5th–84th percentile	Normal weight
85th–94th percentile	At risk for overweight
≥95th percentile	Overweight

The obesity guidelines for adults are:

BMI (kg/m²)	Weight status
<18.5	Underweight
18.5–24.9	Normal weight
25–29.9	Obesity
30–39.9	Obese
40–49.9	Morbid obesity
≥50	Super morbid obesity

120. Ans. (b) <1500 g

Ref: OP Ghai, 8th ed. pg. 125

- Normal birth weight – 2800–3000 g
- Low birth weight (LBW) – <2500 g
- Very low birth weight (VLBW) – <1500 g
- Extremely low birth weight (ELBW) – <1000 g.

121. Ans. (a) <1000 g

Ref: OP Ghai, 8th ed. pg. 125

Refer to above explanation Q. 120

122. Ans. (a) 12.5 cm

Ref: OP Ghai, 8th ed. pg. 97

- Mid arm circumference is measured by a Field instrument → Shakir's tape
- Among age group: 1–5 yrs
- <12.5 cm shows severe malnutrition

123. Ans. (b) <2

Ref: Rudolph Pediatrics, 22th ed. pg. 191

Ponderal index = Weight in grams/(Length of baby in cm)^3 multiplied by 100

- Value is <2 = Asymetrical IUGR
- Value is normal in Symmetrical IUGR

- Asymmetrical IUGR is more common. In asymmetrical IUGR, there is restriction of weight followed by length. The head continues to grow at normal or near-normal rates (head sparing). This is a protective mechanism that may have evolved to promote brain development. This type of IUGR is most commonly caused by extrinsic factors that affect the fetus at later gestational ages.
- Symmetrical IUGR is less common and is more worrisome. This type of IUGR usually begins early in gestation. Since most neurons are developed by the 18th week of gestation, the fetus with symmetrical IUGR is more likely to have permanent neurological sequelae.

124. Ans. (c) Scurvy

Ref: OP Ghai, 8th ed. pg. 120

Features of Scurvy:

- Frog leg appearance[Q]
- Bone pain
- Myalgias may occur because of reduced carnitine production.
- Skin changes with roughness, easy bruising and petechiae, gum swelling & bleeding, loosening of teeth, poor wound healing.

125. Ans. (a) Kwashiorkor

Ref: Nelson's Pedia, 19th ed. Ch 670

KWASHIORKOR

Disease occurs due to decreased protein and caloric intake.

Clinical Features are:

- **Hypoalbuminemia:** Which leads to pedal edema. This pedal oedema can mask weight loss.
- **Hepatomegaly:** Hallmark feature of kwashiorkor
- **Skin:** Sun-exposed skin is relatively spared, as are the feet and dorsal aspects of the hands;
- **Hair and Nail:** Nails are thin and soft, and hair is sparse, thin, and depigmented, sometimes displaying a **flag sign** of alternating light and dark bands that reflect alternating periods of adequate and inadequate nutrition.
- Apathy[Q]
- Lack of appetite[Q]
  - **Pellagra** presents with edema, erythema, and ***burning of sun-exposed skin on the face, neck, and dorsal aspects of the hands, forearms, and feet.***
  - **Scurvy** presents initially with follicular hyperkeratosis and ***coiling of hair.*** Perifollicular erythema and hemorrhage, swollen, erythematous gums; stomatitis; Subperiosteal hematomas lead to frog leg appearance (Pseudoparalysis)

126. Ans. (b) Hepatomegaly

Ref: OP Ghai, 8th ed. pg. 99

- **Marasmus** is characterized by failure to gain weight and irritability, followed by weight loss and listlessness until

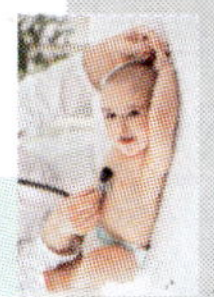

emaciation results. *The skin loses turgor and becomes wrinkled and loose as subcutaneous fat disappears. Loss of fat* from the sucking pads of the cheeks often occurs late in the course of the disease. The infant's face gives *wizened old man's look.*

- *The abdomen may be distended or flat,* with the intestinal pattern readily visible. There is muscle atrophy and resultant hypotonia.
- **Kwashiorkor** is characterized by development of pedal edema which can mask weight loss. Dietary protein deficiency leads to brain damage and apathy, and/or irritability. *When advanced, there is lack of growth, lack of stamina, loss of muscle tissue, increased susceptibility to infections, vomiting, diarrhea, anorexia, flabby subcutaneous tissues, and edema.*. It is often present in internal organs before it is recognized in the face and limbs.
- Hepatomegaly due to fatty liver is seen with flag sign on hair and skin showing flaky paint dermatosis.

127. Ans. (a) Increase appetite

Ref: OP Ghai, 8th ed. pg. 99

- Kwashiorkor is protein and calorie deficiency and hence the serum albumin of the child is very low. This causes the child to develop pedal edema and generalized anasarca later.
- Since the child is not eating proteins, essential amino acids like phenylalanine is deficient and therefore the child forms less of melanin. *This results in hair of the child being reddish in color. This color change of hair strand is seen as FLAG sign.*
- The children with kwashiorkor have a FATTY liver and thereby a hepatomegaly.
- Apathy means lack of interest in surroundings and therefore this child is not interested in playing with the mother or toys. This occurs due to brain damage secondary to chronic protein deprivation.
- Note: *Increased appetite can be seen in patients with Marasmus.*

128. Ans. (c) 15,000 mcg

Ref: OP Ghai, 8th ed. pg. 113

- 1mcg of vitamin D = 400 I.U.
- For treatment of rickets, cholecalciferol can be given in a single-day dose of 15,000 mcg (600,000 U), which is usually divided into 4 or 6 oral doses. An intramuscular injection is also available.
- An alternative regimen is to give 125–250 mcg (5000-10,000 U) daily for 2–3 months until healing is well established and the alkaline phosphatase concentration is approaching the reference range.

129. Ans. (a) Pseudoparalysis

Ref: OP Ghai, 8th ed. pg. 113

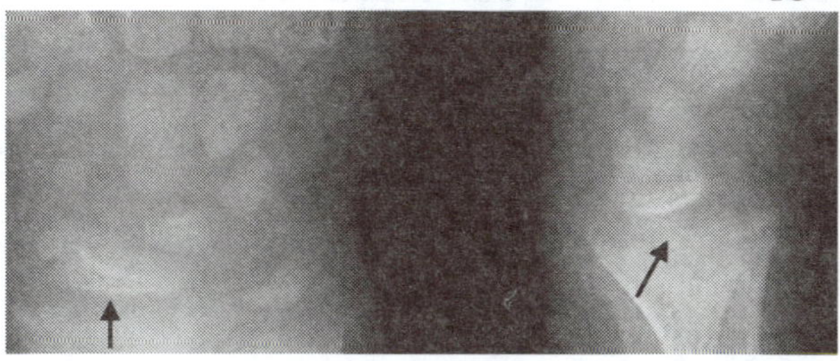

- Note the distal end of radius on the left and ulna on right. Even without experience you can notice that distal end has fraying. Mentally visualize a paint brush. The distal end of bone is widened (SPLAYED).
- ***Rickets due to deficiency of calcium and vitamin D will have delayed dentition which is defined as (ZERO TEETH AT >13 months of age.***
- The widening of wrist joint is seen usually beyond 6 months of age when the child starts crawling and creeping and weight of body fall on distal radius.
- Double medial malleolus
- Bowing of legs (GENU VARUM) and knock knees *(GENU VALGUM)* is seen.
- Pigeon chest with rachitic rosary *(non tender).*

130. Ans. (b) Aldolase-B

Ref: OP Ghai, 8th ed. pg. 696

- Hereditary fructose intolerance, or the presence of fructose in the blood (fructosemia), is caused by a deficiency of aldolase B, the second enzyme involved in the metabolism of fructose. This enzyme deficiency results in an accumulation of fructose-1-phosphate, which inhibits the production of glucose and results in diminished regeneration of adenosine triphosphate. Clinically, patients with hereditary fructose intolerance are much more severely affected than those with essential fructosuria, with elevated uric acid, growth abnormalities and can result in coma if untreated.

Remember and Don't Confuse with:

- ***Essential fructosuria*** *caused by a deficiency of the enzyme hepatic fructokinase* is a clinically benign condition characterized by the incomplete metabolism of fructose in the liver, leading to its excretion in urine.

131. Ans. (d) Decreased height for age

Ref: Nelson, 18th ed. Chapter 14

- Height for age is used for chronic malnutrition which leads to Stunting. The term "stunting" is used to describe a condition in which children fail to gain sufficient height, given their age.

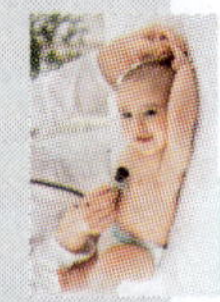

- In acute malnutrition the best parameter used is weight for height.

132. Ans. (d) Apathy

Ref: Nelson, 18th ed. Chapter 43

- **Marasmus** is characterized by weight loss and listlessness until emaciation results : MONKEY FACIES
- The skin loses turgor and becomes wrinkled and loose as subcutaneous fat disappears from buttocks leading to BAGGY PANTS appearance.
- Loss of fat from the sucking pads of the cheeks often occurs late in the course of the disease; thus, the infant's face may retain a relatively normal appearance compared with the rest of the body.
- *These children are irritable and have a voracious appetite. Apathy is a feature of kwashiorkor.*
- The abdomen has muscle wasting leading to pot belly with the intestinal pattern readily visible.

PEDIATRIC NEUROLOGY

133. Ans. (a) Valproate

Ref: O.P. Ghai Essential Pediatrics, 9th ed. pg. 556

- This is given case of absence seizure
- Typical absences are characterized by sudden loss of awareness and an EEG typically shows generalized spike wave discharges at three cycles per second.
- Valproate, Ethosuximide and lamotrigine are currently used in management of absence seizures.

134. Ans. (b) Diazepam

Ref: Nelson Textbook of Pediatrics 20th edition pg. 2875

The initial emergent therapy in management of convulsions is administration of diazepam, lorazepam and midazolam. Midazolam can be given IV, IM or Intranasal. If IV access is not possible then rectal diazepam can be given.

Extra Mile

- Management of Convulsions at home: Wait for a minute and they stop by themselves. Turn the child to left lateral position if possible, to reduce aspiration risk. Rush to hospital
- Management of febrile convulsion at home (requires training of mother in advance): Intranasal midazolam > rectal diazepam
- Leading cause of seizures in children: Febrile seizures
- Leading epilepsy in children: Benign Rolandic epilepsy

135. Ans. (b) Malignant tumor in children

Ref: OP Ghai 8th ed. pg. 571

Medulloblastoma

- These are midline cerebellar tumors and occur in infancy.
- They are fast growing and malignant.
- Craniospinal spread along neuraxis is common and death occurs early.

136. Ans. (b) Spinal dysraphism

Ref: Nelson, 20th ed. pg. 2802–2803

- Elevated amniotic fluid acetylcholinesterase is used for diagnosis of neural tube defects which are also called spinal dysraphism.
- *Tests for antenatal diagnosis of spina bifida occulta.*
  - Antenatal USG showing Frog sign
  - Amniotic fluid acetylcholinesterase

137. Ans. (b) Acetylcholinesterase

Ref: Nelson, 20th ed. pg. 2802–2803

Refer to the explanation of the question above.

138. Ans. (a) Spina bifida occulta

Ref: Nelson, 20th ed. pg. 2802–2803

- Most common neural tube defect is Spina bifida occulta.
- Most severe neural tube defect is Cranioraschisis totalis
- Best prognosis and maximum viability (survival chances) is seen with Spina bifida occulta
- If spina bifida occulta is not in choices then answer is Meningocele.

139. Ans. (b) Rubeola

Ref: Rudolph Paediatrics, pg. 2186

This disease is a complication of measles virus called rubeola. Features of SSPE

- Slowly progressive disease characterized by seizures and progressive deterioration of cognitive and motor functions, with death occurring 5–15 years after measles virus infection.
- SSPE most often develops in persons infected with measles virus at <2 years of age.
- Investigation of choice is antibody to measles virus in CSF
- EEG shows sharp wave complexes called Rademacher's complex.
- DOC is inosine prabonex.

140. Ans. (c) Meningomyelocele

Ref: Nelson's, 18th ed. Ch 592

- **Myelomeningocele** is a type of spina bifida in which the spinal canal does not close before birth.
- A **meningocele** is formed when the meninges herniate through a defect in the posterior vertebral arches.

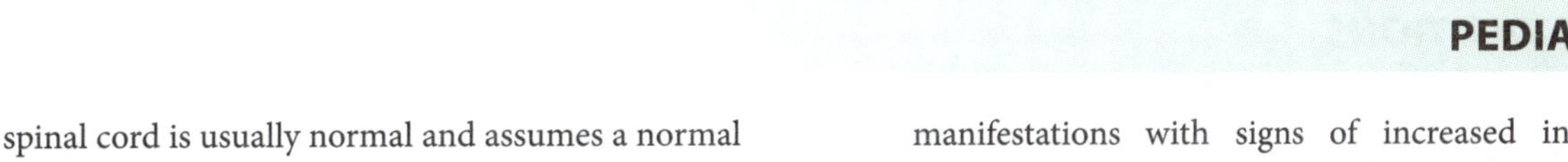

The spinal cord is usually normal and assumes a normal position in the spinal canal.

- In Meningocele, just the membranes extend through, ***while in Myelomeningocele, the spinal cord also pushes through the hole within the sac that the meninges makes by extending through the opening.***

141. Ans. (b) Mostly Hereditary in nature

Ref: Nelson's, 18th ed. Ch 592.11

- Hydrocephalus is not a specific disease; rather, it represents a diverse group of conditions that result from impaired circulation and absorption of CSF
- Congenital hydrocephalus implies hydrocephalus is present at birth. Most common cause of congenital hydrocephalus is aqueductal stenosis.

Other Causes of Congenital Hydrocephalus can be

- Dandy Walker syndrome
- Arnold chiari malformation
- Toxoplasmosis
- CMV

Clinical Manifestation

1. An accelerated rate of enlargement of the head is the most prominent sign.
2. *The anterior fontanelle is wide open and bulging, and the scalp veins are dilated.*
3. *The forehead is broad*, and the eyes may deviate downward because of impingement of the dilated supra-pineal recess on the tectum, producing the ***setting-sun eye sign.***

142. Ans. (a) BERA

Ref: OP Ghai, 8th ed. pg. 619; Oski's Pediatrics

Due to high incidence of deafness post H. influenzae meningitis, BERA should be done.

143. Ans. (d) Enterovirus

- **Meningo-encephalitis is caused by:**
  - Enterovirus (Commonest cause)
  - Coxsackie virus, echo virus – spread is mainly by mouth to mouth transmission
  - Flavi-Virus – West Nile virus, Japanese B Encephalitis
  - Herpes virus
  - Measles and mumps

144. Ans. (c) Decreased Intracranial pressure

Ref: OP Ghai, 8th ed. pg. 111–112

- Manifestations of **acute toxicity** include muscle and bone tenderness, especially over the long bones of the upper and lower extremities, as well as neurologic manifestations with signs of increased intracranial pressure (eg, children may have bulging fontanelles).
- Manifestations of **chronic toxicity** include the following: Alopecia/xeroderma with itchy skin/Skin erythema/ Skin desquamation/itching/Brittle nails/Exanthema/ Cheilitis/Petechiae/Premature epiphysial closure in children/Hepato-splenomegaly/Peripheral neuritis/ Benign intracranial hypertension.

Extra Mile

- Pseudotumor cerebri/benign intracranial hypertension = vitamin A toxicity
- Earliest sign of vitamin A deficiency = Conjunctival xerosis
- Treatment of vitamin A deficiency = Vitamin A orally 2 LAC IU on day 0,1 and day 14.

GENETICS

145. Ans. (d) Multifactorial inheritance

Ref: Nelson 20th ed. pg. 2802

- Neural tube defects (NTDs) account for the largest proportion of congenital anomalies of the CNS and result from failure of the neural tube to close spontaneously between the 3rd and 4th week of in utero development.
- Evidence suggests that many factors, including hyperthermia, drugs (valproic acid), malnutrition, low red cell folate levels, chemicals, maternal obesity or diabetes, and genetic determinants (mutations in folate-responsive or folate-dependent enzyme pathways) can adversely affect normal development of the CNS from the time of conception.

146. Ans. (c) Klinefelter syndrome

Ref: Nelson 20th ed. pg. 2650

- The key words are gynecomastia with features of hypogonadism like small testis and scanty pubic hair in a male patient showing antisocial behavior. This is seen in Klinefelter syndrome.
- Option a presents with idiopathic hypercalcemia and supravalvular aortic stenosis. Option b looks like turner syndrome and has pulmonic stenosis. Option d has tall person with arm span > height and aortic dissection.

147. Ans. (d) Henoch Schoenlein purpura

- The key word in the MCQ is extensor rash which is seen in HSP. It occurs due to IgA mediated vasculitis.
- Option a presents with butterfly rash and kidney failure. Option b leads to AKI after infection with *E. coli*

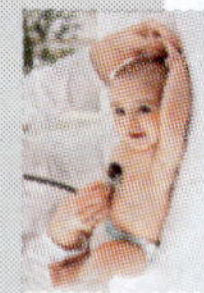

0157: H7. Option c presents with pyoderma followed by cola color urine and renal failure.

148. Ans. (b) Fragile X-syndrome

Ref: Nelson Textbook of Pediatrics 20th ed. pg. 622

Physical features of Fragile X syndrome	Neuropsychological findings of Fragile X syndrome
• Adolescent and adults have long thin face with prominent ears, prominent foreheads and facial asymmetry • Head circumference > 50th centile and prominent jaw • Large prominent ears • Hyperextensible finger joints • Single palmar crease (Also seen in Down's syndrome) • Macroorchidism in postpubertal males. In unaffected males, average testicular volume is 17 mL; in patients with fragile X syndrome, testicular volume is >25 mL • A heart murmur or click consistent with mitral valve prolapse is often auscultated and requires consultation with a cardiologist.	• Autistic behavior (most common) • ADHD • Seizures • OCD

149. Ans. (b) Down syndrome

Ref: Nelson Textbook of Pediatrics 20th ed. pg. 612

The image shows G banding (G = Giemsa) of chromosomes which in karyotype are arranged in decreasing order of size. Notice chromosome 1 is the largest chromosome. As you move down you will notice three 21 chromosomes leading to diagnosis of Down syndrome in a boy. Note the XY configuration. Age of mother >35 years is one of the important causes.

150. Ans. (b) X linked recessive

Ref: Nelson Textbook of Pediatrics 20th ed. pg. 2382

Joint bleeding is a characteristic feature of clotting factor deficiency. Since the maternal uncle also has the same problem, it implies that the males in the family are being affected. Hence the clinical diagnosis is Hemophilia A/B. The factor 8 and 9 level estimation can confirm the diagnosis. The pattern of inheritance of both is X Linked recessive.

151. Ans. (a) 21

Ref: O.P Ghai 8th ed. pg. 420

- Down syndrome is the most common chromosomal disorder, occurring with a frequency of 1:800 to 1:1000 newborns.
- Chromosome number 21 is present in triplicate, the origin of the extra chromosome 21 being maternal (due to maternal meiotic non disjunction).

152. Ans. (b) Low

Ref: Rudolph Paediatrics, 22nd ed. pg. 1415

Aneuploidies	AFP	Estriol	hCG	Inhibin A
Down's syndrome	Low	Low	High	High
Turner's syndrome	Decreased	Decreased	Very high	Very high
Edward's syndrome	Unchanged	Low	Very low	Unchanged
Patau's syndrome	Increased	Normal	Normal	Normal

153. Ans. (b) Edward syndrome

Ref: Nelson, 20th ed. pg. 611

Syndrome	Description
Down syndrome	Trisomy 21
Edward syndrome	Trisomy 18
Patau syndrome	Trisomy 13 *Patau syndrome is the least common and most severe of the viable autosomal trisomies. Median survival is fewer than 3 days.*
Turner syndrome	45 XO

154. Ans. (a) Noonan syndrome

Ref: Nelson, 20th ed. pg. 2747-48

NOONAN SYNDROME

- The term is applicable to males and females with normal karyotypes who have certain phenotypic features that occur also in females with Turner syndrome.
- Inheritance pattern is *Autosomal dominant* with variable expression.

Clinical Features:

1. Hypertelorism, epicanthus, *downward slanted palpebral fissures known as antimongoloid facies.*
2. Short stature, webbing of the neck
3. Pectus carinatum or pectus excavatum
4. Cubitus valgus
5. The cardiac defect is most often *pulmonary valvular stenosis*, hypertrophic cardiomyopathy, or atrial septal defect.

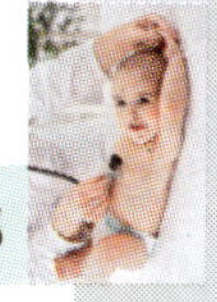

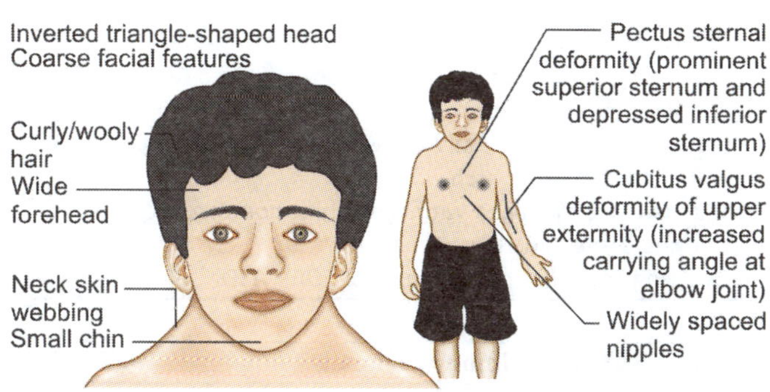

155. Ans. (c) Inhibin

***Ref:* Nelson, 18th ed. pg. Ch. 95**

- Triple test can screen trisomy 21. *(Diagnostic sensitivity 70%)*
- In addition to Down syndrome, the triple and quadruple tests screen for fetal trisomy 18 also known as Edward's syndrome, open neural tube defects, and may also detect an increased risk of Turner syndrome, trisomy 16 mosaicism, fetal death, Smith-Lemli-Opitz syndrome, and steroid sulfatase deficiency

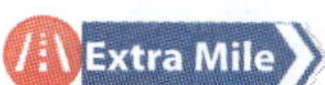
Extra Mile

Quadruple test incorporates the above parameters and Inhibin A
- High LEVELS are seen in Trisomy 21.
- Low levels are seen in Trisomy 18.
- Variable levels in Trisomy 13 (Patau syndrome)

Triple test parameters	Alpha feto protein	Unconjugated Estriol	Beta HCG
Down syndrome	*Low*	*Low*	*High*
Edward syndrome	*Low*	*Low*	*Low*
Neural tube defects Omphalocele, multiple gestation	High	Not applicable	Not applicable

156. Ans. (c) Umbilical hernia

***Ref:* OP Ghai, 8th ed. pg. 638**

- Brachycepahly implies small skull, due to premature fusion of the coronal suture. Therefore, the brain is not able to grow and results in mental retardation.
- Overall the most common cause of mental retardation is idiopathic > Down syndrome.
- Thyroid abnormalities in form of either thyroid agenesis or autoimmune thyroditis are seen in Down syndrome.
- Eye findings of down syndrome have also been asked and should be remembered as *(MEBB)*
  1. Mongoloid slant of eyes
  2. Epicanthal folds
  3. Blue dot cataract
  4. Brushfield spots in the iris

Clinical features of Down syndrome
- Flattened facies and low set ears
- Mental retardation
- Single transverse palmar crease and atypical finger prints
- Clinodactyly
- Hypotonia
- Brachycephaly
- Congenital heart disease (ASD): Endocardial cushion defect
- Macroglossia
- Epicanthix fold
- Strabismus
- Brushfield spots (Iris)

157. Ans. (c) Increased umbilical blood flow

***Ref:* OP Ghai, 8th ed. pg. 639**

- Best way for prenatal diagnosis of Down syndrome is Chorionic villus sampling. However antenatal ultrasound features are:
  - Reduced length of femur and humerus
  - Nuchal fold translucency >2.5 mm
  - Congenital heart disease like ASD, VSD.

158. Ans. (d) Acetylcholine esterase

***Ref:* OP Ghai, 8th ed. pg. 575–76**

- *NTD (anencephaly, open spina bifida or meningomyelocele, and encephalocele)* are a heterogeneous group of congenital malformations resulting from a failure of fusion of the neural tube.
- When a NTD is suspected based upon maternal serum alpha-fetoprotein (AFP) screening results or diagnosed via ultrasound, analysis of AFP and acetylcholinesterase (AChE) in amniotic fluid are useful diagnostic tools.
- AChE is primarily active in the central nervous system with small amounts of enzyme found in erythrocytes, skeletal muscle, and fetal serum.
- *Normal amniotic fluid does not contain AChE, unless contributed by the fetus as a result of an open NTD.*

159. Ans. (d) Anencephaly

***Ref:* Nelson, 18th ed. pg. Ch. 592.6**

Anencephaly is absence of cranial vault posteriorly with brain and meninges exposed. This condition can be detected by antenatal USG as early as 11–12 weeks. The USG sign is called *frog eye sign.*

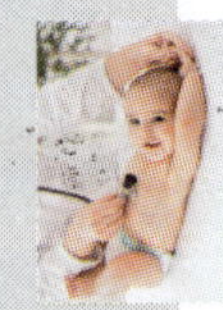

PEDIATRIC CARDIOLOGY

160. Ans. (a) Indomethacin

Ref: O.P. Ghai Essential Pediatrics, 9th ed. pg. 414-416

- Indomethacin is a non-steroidal anti-inflammatory drug that is a potent inhibitor of prostaglandin E_2 synthesis.
- After birth, the ductus arteriosus closes spontaneously within 2–4 days in term infants.
- The major factor closing the ductus arteriosus is the tension of oxygen, which increases significantly after birth.

161. Ans. (b) Tricuspid stenosis

Ref: Nelson Textbook of Pediatrics 20th ed. pg. 2216

TOF has subpulmonic stenosis and not tricuspid stenosis. Subpulmonic stenosis leads to reduction of pulmonary blood flow and is the main determinant of cyanosis. The four features of TOF are:

1. Subpulmonic stenosis
2. Concentric RV Hypertrophy
3. VSD that operates R to L (due to RV hypertrophy)
4. Overriding of Aorta

Extra Mile

Tetralogy of Fallot

1. Ductal dependent Pulmonic circulation
2. Drug of choice is Alprostadil must be started soon after birth to maintain ductal patency

Contd...

3. CXR shows three important features:
   a. Lungs appear more black than normal due to reduced pulmonary circulation
   b. Right ventricular hypertrophy leading to boot shaped heart
   c. Right sided aortic arch
4. Tet spells are managed with knee chest position, propranolol, morphine and soda bicarbonate
5. Pentalogy of Fallot has Features of TOF + ASD

162. Ans. (d) Subpulmonic stenosis

Ref: Nelson 20th ed. pg. 2212

The major determinant of cyanosis in TOF is subpulmonic stenosis which will decide the amount of blood entering into lungs.

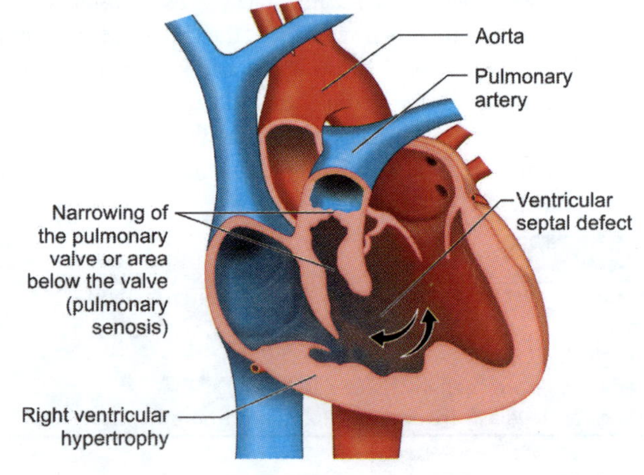

163. Ans. (a) Pulmonic stenosis

Ref: Nelson 21st ed. pg. 2995

Pulmonary stenosis, with or without dysplastic pulmonary valve and hypertrophic cardiomyopathy, are the "classic" cardiac defects reported in Noonan syndrome.

Features of Noonan Syndrome

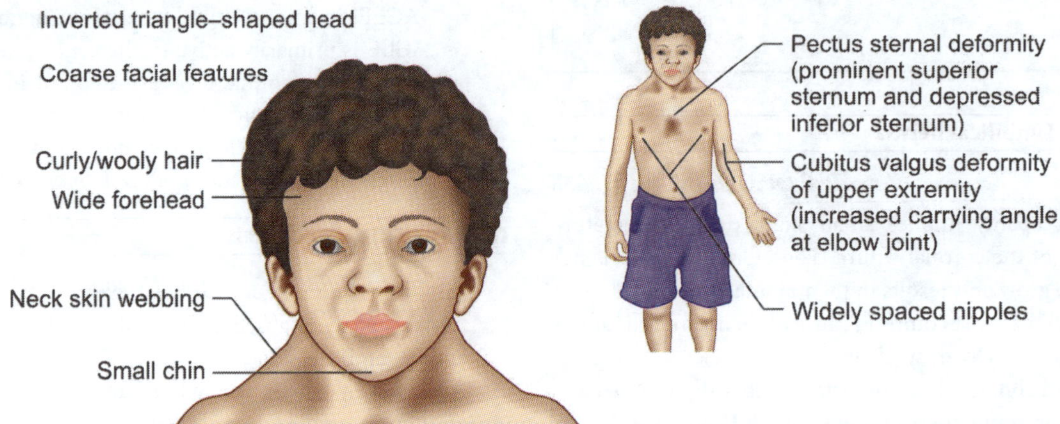

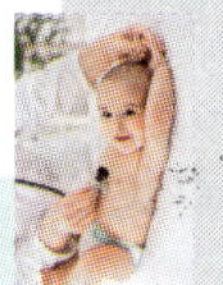

164. Ans. (a) Patent ductus arteriosus

Ref: Op Ghai 8th ed pg. 417

- Continuous murmur is heard in PDA due to huge pressure difference between aorta and pulmonary artery. It is heard both in systole and diastole and peaks at S2.

Causes of Continuous Murmurs

1. Patent ductus arteriosus
2. Coronary arteriovenous
3. Ruptured sinus of Valsalva aneurysm
4. Aortic-pulmonary window
5. Anomalous left coronary artery origin from pulmonary artery
6. Coarctation of aorta
7. Pulmonary artery atresia
8. Truncus arteriosus
9. Pulmonary artery stenosis
10. Systemic arteriovenous fistula
11. Pulmonary arteriovenous fistula
12. Mammary souffle
13. Venous hum

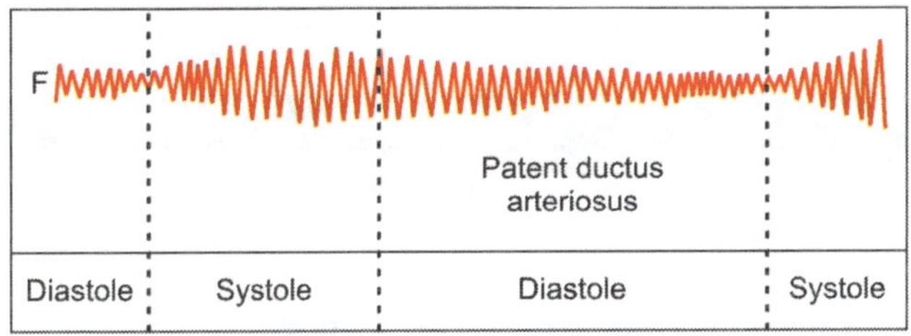

165. Ans. (b) ASD

Ref: OP Ghai 8th ed. pg. 420

Classic Tetrad of TOF

1. Severe right ventricle outflow obstruction due to sub-pulmonic stenosis
2. Large VSD
3. Over-Riding of aorta
4. Right ventricular hypertrophy.

Extra Mile

- Major determinant of central cyanosis in TOF is sub-pulmonic stenosis.
- IOC for TOF is T.T.E
- DOC for TOF is Alprostadil
- Palliative surgery for TOF is Blalock Taussig shunt.

166. Ans. (c) Left lower sternal border

Ref: Nelson 20th ed. pg. 2169

- Many murmurs in children are *not associated* with significant hemodynamic abnormalities. They are called "innocent" murmurs.
- The most common innocent murmur is a medium-pitched, vibratory or "musical," relatively short *systolic ejection murmur*, which is heard best along the left lower and midsternal border and has no significant radiation to the apex, base or back.

167. Ans. (a) TOF

Ref: Nelson 20th ed. pg. 2212–2213

- Tetralogy of Fallot is the most common cyanotic heart disease and will have the maximum viability out of the structural defects given in the choices. *After successful total correction, patients are generally asymptomatic and are able to lead unrestricted lives.*
- TGA will present with cyanosis on day 0 and will result in death due to mixing of two circulations unless atrial septostomy is done followed by switch operation. Without treatment, the prognosis is poor; most patients succumb in the 1st year of life because of heart failure, hypoxemia, and pulmonary hypertension.
- Tricuspid atresia with pulmonic atresia will lead to cyanosis on day 0 and has bad prognosis.
- TAPVC will cause overloading of right side of heart with obstructive flow in infra-cardiac variety. It again has a bad prognosis.

168. Ans. (d) Normal cardiothoracic ratio

Ref: Nelson 20th ed. pg. 2212–2213

Tetralogy of Fallot has:

1. Sub-pulmonic stenosis (Ejection Systolic murmur)
2. VSD (Right to Left Shunting)
3. Concentric right ventricular hypertrophy
4. Over- riding aorta

Due to right ventricular hypertrophy the chances of RVF is unlikely. On CXR boot shaped heart is seen with normal CT ratio.

Note: *That can concentric RVH cannot be picked up by CXR.*

Extra Mile

- Most common cause of cyanosis with normal sized heart is TOF.
- Most common cause of cyanosis with left sided enlargement of heart is tricuspid atresia.

169. Ans. (a) Foramen Ovale

Ref: Langman Embryology, pg. 47

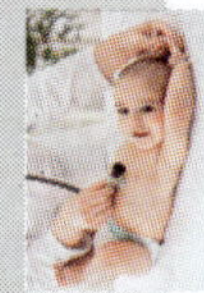

Key Functional Changes after Birth

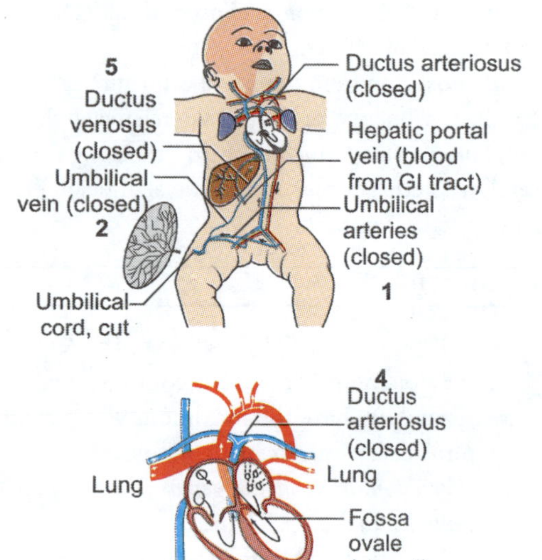

1. & 2 Umbilical cord clamped (Closure of Umbilical arteries and vein)
3. Foramen ovale closed
4. Ductus arteriosus closed
5. Ductus venosus closed

170. Ans. (b) Membranous VSD

Ref: Nelson, 20th ed. pg. 2194–95

VSD is the most common cardiac malformation and accounts for 25% of congenital heart disease. Defects may occur in any portion of the ventricular septum, but most are of the membranous type.

Types of VSD

- Membranous
- Muscular VSD or Swiss cheese type multiple defects
- Supra-cristal VSD

Types of ASD

- Ostium secondum (most common type)
- Ostium primum (associated with Down Syndrome)
- Sinus venous variety (associated with Partial anomalous venous connection)

171. Ans. (c) PDA

Ref: Nelson, 18th ed. Chapter 426

Acyanotic heart disease	Cyanotic heart disease	Obstructive heart disease
PDA VSD ASD	TOF Tricuspid atresia Transposition of great arteries	Coarctation of aorta
Presents with recurrent pneumonia and congestive heart failure	Presents with cyanosis. Tet spells and failure to thrive. On examination the child has cyanosis with single S2. CXR in TOF shows Boot shaped heart/ Coer en sabot	Presents with hypertension
Treatment PDA = Indomethacin/surgical ligation VSD = Dacron patch ASD = Occlusion device	**Treatment** Modified Blalock taussig shunt TGA= Atrial Septostomy followed by switch operation	**Treatment** Balloon dilation with stenting

172. Ans. (d) Pericardial tamponade

Ref: Nelson, 18th ed./ Ch. 165

Cardiac Manifestations of Kawasaki Disease

- Coronary artery aneurysms develop in up to 25% of untreated patients in the 2nd-3rd week of illness and are best detected by two-dimensional echocardiography.
- Myocarditis, manifested as tachycardia out of proportion to fever occurs in at least 50% of patients
- Valvular regurgitation: Mitral and Aortic regurgitation have been associated with Kawasaki disease in both early and chronic phase of the disease.
- Pericarditis with a small pericardial effusion is common during the acute illness.
- Giant coronary artery aneurysms (>8 mm internal diameter) pose greatest risk for rupture, thrombosis or stenosis, and myocardial infarction.

173. Ans. (b) Kawasaki disease

Ref: OP Ghai, 8th ed. pg. 631

174. Ans. (d) LA

Ref: OP Ghai, 8th ed. pg. 413

- Ostium primum ASDs commonly present with a cleft in the anterior leaflet of the mitral valve. This is sometimes termed a partial AV canal defect or a partial AV septal defect.

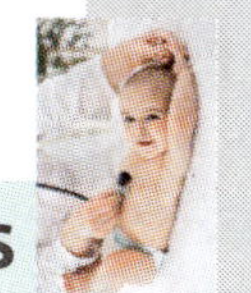

- Due to cleft in mitral valve, the LV decompresses into LA leading to overloading of left atrium. In contrast in O. Secundum ASD it is right atrium and right ventricular that develop overloading.

GASTROINTESTINAL TRACT

175. Ans. (d) Portal vein thrombosis

Ref: Nelson Textbook of Pediatrics 20th ed. pg. 1975

- The combination of clinical findings of Hematemesis and splenomegaly points to diagnosis of portal hypertension.
- Now since child underwent exchange transfusion for neonatal jaundice it implies vascular access was taken via umbilical vein. Umbilical vein catheterization carries the inherent risk of causing portal vein thrombosis.
- Once portal vein thrombosis occurs pressure in splenic vein will rise and cause congestive splenomegaly.
- Later due to rising pressure in portal vein portal systemic collaterals will develop in form esophageal varices. The rupture of esophageal varices explains the first line of the question as to why the child had hematemesis.

176. Ans. (c) Hypertrophic pyloric stenosis

Ref: Nelson, 20th ed. pg. 1787

Ileal atresia	Presents as bilious vomiting and triple bubble sign on X-ray Abdomen.
Duodenal atresia	Presents as bilious vomiting and double bubble appearance on X-Ray abdomen
Hypertrophic pyloric stenosis	The presentation is after 2 weeks of life in usually a first born boy baby. The child presents with non-bilious vomiting.
Trachea-esophageal fistula	Presents with choking after feeds with failure to thrive. Drooling of saliva in neonates indicates esophageal atresia.

177. Ans. (b) 10 mg

Ref: Nelson, 20th ed. pg. 1872-73

Zinc supplementation is given at a dose of 2RDA per day (20 mg per day for >6 months and 10 mg/day for younger than 6 months) for 14 days is effective in reducing severity of diarrhea as well as duration of episode.

178. Ans. (c) Trauma

Ref: Nelson's Pedia, 18th ed. Ch. 340

The list of illnesses that can mimic acute appendicitis includes: 1. Gastroenteritis; 2. Mesenteric adenitis; 3. Meckel diverticulitis; 4. Inflammatory bowel disease; 5. Pneumonia; 6. Cholecystitis; 7. Urinary tract infection; 8. Infectious enteritis; 9. Testicular torsion.

179. Ans. (a) Zinc

Ref: OP Ghai, 8th ed. pg. 121

- The World Health Organization (WHO) and UNICEF ***recommend daily 20 mg zinc supplements for 10–14 days for children with acute diarrhea, and 10 mg/day for infants under six-month-old, to curtail the severity of the episode and prevent further occurrences in the ensuing -two to three months, thereby decreasing the morbidity considerably.***
- One out of every five children who die of diarrhea worldwide is an Indian. Daily around 1,000 children die of diarrhea in India, which means 41 children lose their lives every hour.

180. Ans. (d) Ultrasound

Ref: Nelson, 18th ed. pg. Ch. 326.1

ULTRASONOGRAPHY

- ***The criterion standard imaging technique for diagnosing HPS***
- *Muscle wall thickness 3 mm* or greater and *pyloric channel length 14 mm* or greater *are considered abnormal* in infants younger than 30 days.

BARIUM UPPER GI STUDY

- Effective when Ultrasonography is not diagnostic.
- Should demonstrate an elongated pylorus with antral indentation from the hypertrophied muscle.
- May show the "double track" sign when thin tracks of barium are compressed between thickened pyloric mucosa or the "shoulder" sign when barium collects in the dilated pre-pyloric antrum.
- Serum electrolytes should be measured to document adequacy of fluid resuscitation and correction of electrolyte imbalances before surgical repair.
- The definitive treatment of pyloric stenosis is with surgical pyloromyotomy known as Ramstedt's procedure
- It is done by simple incision of about 3–4 cm which leads to relaxation of pyloric muscles and hence gastric outlet opens up.

The classic biochemical abnormality seen in case of HPS is hypochloremic, hypokalemic metabolic alkalosis with paradoxical aciduria.

181. Ans. (c) Erythromycin

Exposure to erythromycin between 3 and 13 days of life is associated with an eightfold risk of infantile hypertrophic pyloric stenosis (IHPS) developing shortly thereafter, according to the results of a retrospective cohort study published in the July, 2015 issue of the Archives of Pediatric and Adolescent Medicine.

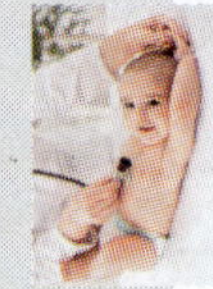

Extra Mile

Perinatal drug exposure	Teratogenic effect
Lithium	Ebstein anomaly
Vitamin D3	William syndrome (supravalvular aortic stenosis)
Thalidomide	Phocomelia
Erythromycin	Infantile hypertrophic pyloric stenosis
Carbimazole/ methimazole	Aplastic cutis congenital
Warfarin	Nasal hypoplasia and phalangeal defects
Steroids	Cleft lip and palate

182. Ans. (b) Duodenal atresia

Ref: Nelson, 18th ed. pg. Ch. 327.1

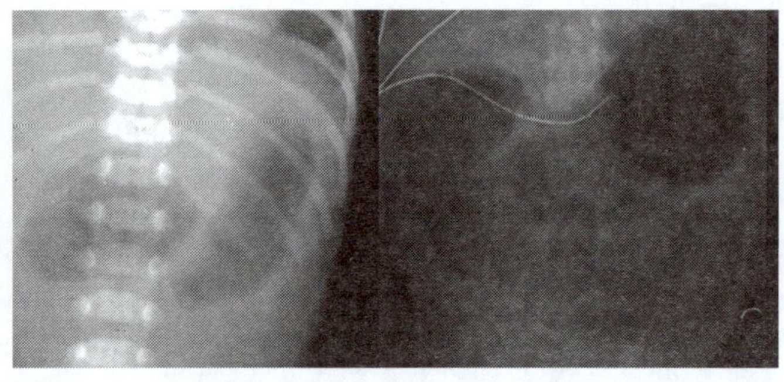

Look at the two X-rays. The left one shows double bubble appearance of duodenal atresia and the right one shows triple bubble sign of jejunoileal atresia.

183. Ans. (d) Pyloric stenosis

Ref: Nelson, 18th ed. pg. Ch. 326.1

- All babies REGURGITATE curdled milk. So the mother is instructed to always put the baby to shoulder after breastfeeding the child as this shall help the child burp and expel the swallowed air.
- However, if a male infant, first born, 2–3–weeks old is brought to your clinic with recurrent vomiting which is non-bilious and associated with failure to gain weight, then suspect-HYPERTROHPIC PYLORIC STENOSIS
- A lump may be palpable to gentle examination in the epigastrium with finding of visible peristalsis. The investigation of choice shall be USG abdomen. Surgery to be done shall be a pyloromyotomy (Ramstedt operation).

Extra Mile

- **Hypokalemic hypochloremic metabolic alkalosis** is seen in = Hypertrophic pyloric stenosis
- **Hyperkalemic hyperchloremic metabolic acidosis** is seen in = Uretero-sigmoidostomy
- MC cause of hematochezia in a preterm neonate = Necrotizing Enterocolitis
- MC cause of hematochezia in children= Rectal Prolapse> Meckel's Diverticulum
- Double bubble sign= duodenal atresia
- Inverto-gram (Special X-ray of the baby in inverted position) isused for = Anorectal malformations

184. Ans. (b) Alkaline urine

Ref: Lippincott's, 4th ed. pg. 85

LACTOSE INTOLERANCE/LACTASE DEFICIENCY

The classic example of osmotic diarrhea is lactose intolerance due to lactase enzyme deficiency. *The colonic bacteria ferment the non-absorbed lactose to short-chain organic acids, generating an osmotic load and causing water to be secreted into the lumen.*

- Lactose is by far the most commonly Mal-absorbed carbohydrate.
- Secondary lactose intolerance follows small bowel mucosal damage (celiac disease, rotavirus infection) and is usually transient, improving with mucosal healing.
- Lactase deficiency can be diagnosed by hydrogen breath test or by measurement of mucosal lactase concentration with small bowel biopsy
- *Confirmatory diagnosis is made by stool acidity test, undigested lactose creates lactic acid that can be detected in stool sample.*
- *Undigested lactose may get absorbed and eliminated in urine (Lactoseuria), hence acidic urine.*
- In lactose intolerance reducing substance will be positive by Benedict's test in urine.
- Diagnostic testing is not mandatory and often simple dietary changes that produce symptom relief. Eliminate lactose from the diet result in symptom relief
- *Treatment* of lactase deficiency *consists of a milk-free diet.*

185. Ans. (b) Non reducing sugar in urine

Ref: Lippincott's, 4th ed. pg. 85

Refer to above explanation Q. 184

186. Ans. (a) Doudenal atresia

Ref: Bailey and love 24th ed., /1199

- The hallmark of duodenal obstruction is **bilious vomiting** without abdominal distention, which is usually noted on the 1st day of life.

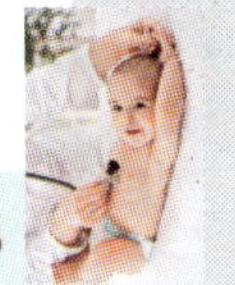

- A history of **polyhydramnios** is present in half the pregnancies and is caused by a failure of absorption of amniotic fluid in the distal intestine.
- The diagnosis is suggested by the presence of a "**double-bubble sign**" on plain abdominal radiographs. *The appearance is caused by a distended and gas-filled stomach and proximal duodenum*

187. Ans. (b) K^+

Ref: Sabiston, 18th ed./Ch .71

- Hypertrophic pyloric stenosis presents with *hypokalemic, hypochloremic metabolic alkalosis with paradoxical aciduria.*
- Treatment includes replacement of the volume deficit with isotonic saline and then potassium replacement once adequate urine output is achieved.
- For most infants, administration of fluid containing 5% dextrose and 0.45% saline with **2 to 4 mEq/kg of added potassium at a rate of approximately 150 to 175 mL/kg for 24 hours** will correct the underlying deficit. After resuscitation, a Fredet-Ramstedt pyloromyotomy is performed
- Fluid resuscitation with correction of electrolyte abnormalities and metabolic alkalosis is essential before induction of general anesthesia for operation.

188. Ans. (c) 100–200 mL

Ref: OP Ghai, 6th ed. pg. 273

PLAN A

Home Based Treatment of Dehydration

Age	Amount of ORS to give after each loose stool or other culturally appropriate ORT fluids	Amount of ORS to provide for use at home
< 2 years	50–100 mL	500 mL/day
2–10 years	100–200 mL	1000 mL/day
>10 years	As much as desired	2000 mL/day

FLUID & ELECTROLYTE BALANCE

189. Ans. (b) Metabolic alkalosis

Ref: O.P. Ghai Essential Pediatrics, 9th ed. pg. 74

- Vomiting, a common cause of hypokalemia produces volume depletion and metabolic alkalosis by the loss of gastric secretions, which are rich in hydrochloric acid (HCl). Whenever a hydrogen ion is excreted, a bicarbonate ion is gained in the extracellular space.

190. Ans. (a) Deferoxamine

Ref: O.P. Ghai Essential Pediatrics, 9th ed. pg. 712

- Deferoxamine is a chelating agent that can remove iron from tissues and free iron from plasma
- It is indicated in patients with systemic toxicity, metabolic acidosis, worsening symptoms with iron toxicity.

191. Ans. (a) ORS

Ref: O.P. Ghai Essential Pediatrics, 9th ed. pg. 766

- Irritable child with dehydration points to presence of some dehydration. This would require correction with ORS at 75 mL/kg over next 4 to 6 hours.
- Oral rehydration therapy is a type of fluid replacement used to prevent and treat dehydration, especially due to diarrhea.
- It involves drinking water with modest amounts of sugar and salts, specifically sodium and potassium.
- The glucose contained in ORS solution enables the intestine to absorb the fluid and the salts more efficiently.

192. Ans. (c) 1350 mL

Ref: Nelson Essentials of Pediatrics E-book: pg. 126

For calculation of maintenance fluid in children the following hack can be used: 100–50–20

0–10 kg body weight	100 mL/kg
10–20 kg body weight	1000 + 50 mL kg for each kg above 10 kg
>20 kg body weight	1500 + 20 mL/kg for each kg above 20 kg

0–10 kg = 100 mL /kg = 100 × 10 = 1000 mL
10–20 kg = 50 mL /kg = 50 × 7 = 350 mL
Total = 1350 mL

193. Ans. (c) Give ORS only

Ref: Nelson Textbook of Pediatrics 20th ed. pg. 388-89

- Since the child can drink orally and eagerly, it implies he is having some dehydration. Hence, he should be put on ORS @75 mL/Kg and given over next 4–6 hours.
- Drinking *eagerly* means that child will himself bring face near the cup of water as he is feeling thirsty. In contrast child with severe dehydration is listless and does not make any attempt to drink water.

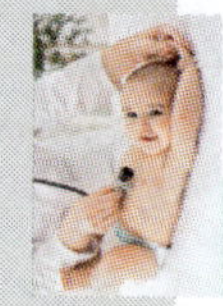

- Option a and b are for management of Severe Dehydration Option d is used for management of Hypernatremic dehydration which occurs due to administration of wrongly diluted ORS. If ORS is mixed with less than one litre of water and given to child it causes osmotic diarrhea and leads to increased concentration serum sodium due to loss of water from the body.

194. Ans. (c) ORS 100 mL per episode of loose stool

Ref: OP Ghai, 8th ed. pg. 294

- The diagnosis of this child who is thirsty and drinks eagerly with absent tears is some dehydration. Hence, ORS is to be given to this child for correction of dehydration at rate of 75 mL/Kg over the next 4–6 hours plus ongoing losses.
- For ongoing losses in children over 2 years, 100 mL per episode of loose stool should be given extra over the correction mentioned in first point.
- Choice a and b are ruled out as intravenous correction is done for severe dehydration.

Age	Amount of ORS to be given after each loose stool
<24 months	50–100 mL per episode
2–10 years	100 mL–200 mL per episode
>10 years	Ad Lib

195. Ans. (b) 800 mL

Ref: OP Ghai, 8th ed. pg. 73, 293

The fluid requirement of children less than 10 kg is *100 mL/kg of body weight.* The preffered fluid shall be N/5 in 5% dextrose with added potassium for daily requirements.

196. Ans. (c) 75 mmol/L

Ingredient	g/L	Mmol/L
Sodium chloride	2.6 g	75
Anhydrous glucose	13.6	75
Potassium chloride	1.5	20
Trisodium citrate	2.9	10

The low osmolality ORS has osmolality of 245 mOsm.

197. Ans. (a) Very severe pneumonia

Ref: OP Ghai, 8th ed. pg. 294

- The clinical presentation of severely malnourished child with fast breathing will be classified as very severe pneumonia.
- Integrated management of childhood illness encompasses a holistic approach towards a sick child where criteria based diagnosis is made and treatment initiated as per the protocol.
- The primary criteria for diagnosis of pneumonia are based on respiratory rate and the age of child.

Age of child	Pneumonia diagnosed if respiratory rate is
Less than 2 months	>60 breaths/min
2–12 months	>50 breaths/min
>1–5 yrs	>40 breaths/min

The disease is Classified as Very Severe if any of the Following is Present

- Cyanosis
- Inability to drink or breast feed
- Seizures/encephalopathy
- *PEM grade 4*

The disease is Classified as Severe Pneumonia in presence of:

- Chest in-drawing
- Sub-costal and or intercostals recessions
- Use of accessory muscles of respiration like nasal flaring/ sterno-mastoid prominent

198. Ans. (b) 800 mL

Ref: Harrison 18th ed., Chapter 54: Deficit therapy

- For correction of severe dehydration, the fluid requirement the formula = 100 mL/Kg
- The total fluid required in 8 kg child would be therefore 800 mL
- The initial fluid here would be given at a rate of 30 mL/kg = 240 mL given over 1 hour.
- The remainder fluid here would be given at a rate of 70 mL/kg = 560 mL over 5 hours.

199. Ans. (b) 3.5 g/dL

All the following criteria must be met for diagnosis of mild malnutrition

- Patient is 20% below usual weight or significant history of weight loss documented
- Serum albumin <3.4 g/dL

200. Ans. (b) 30 mL/kg in 30 min

Ref: Nelson's Pediatrics, 18th ed. Ch. 54

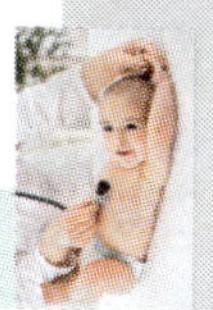

Treatment for Severe Dehydration

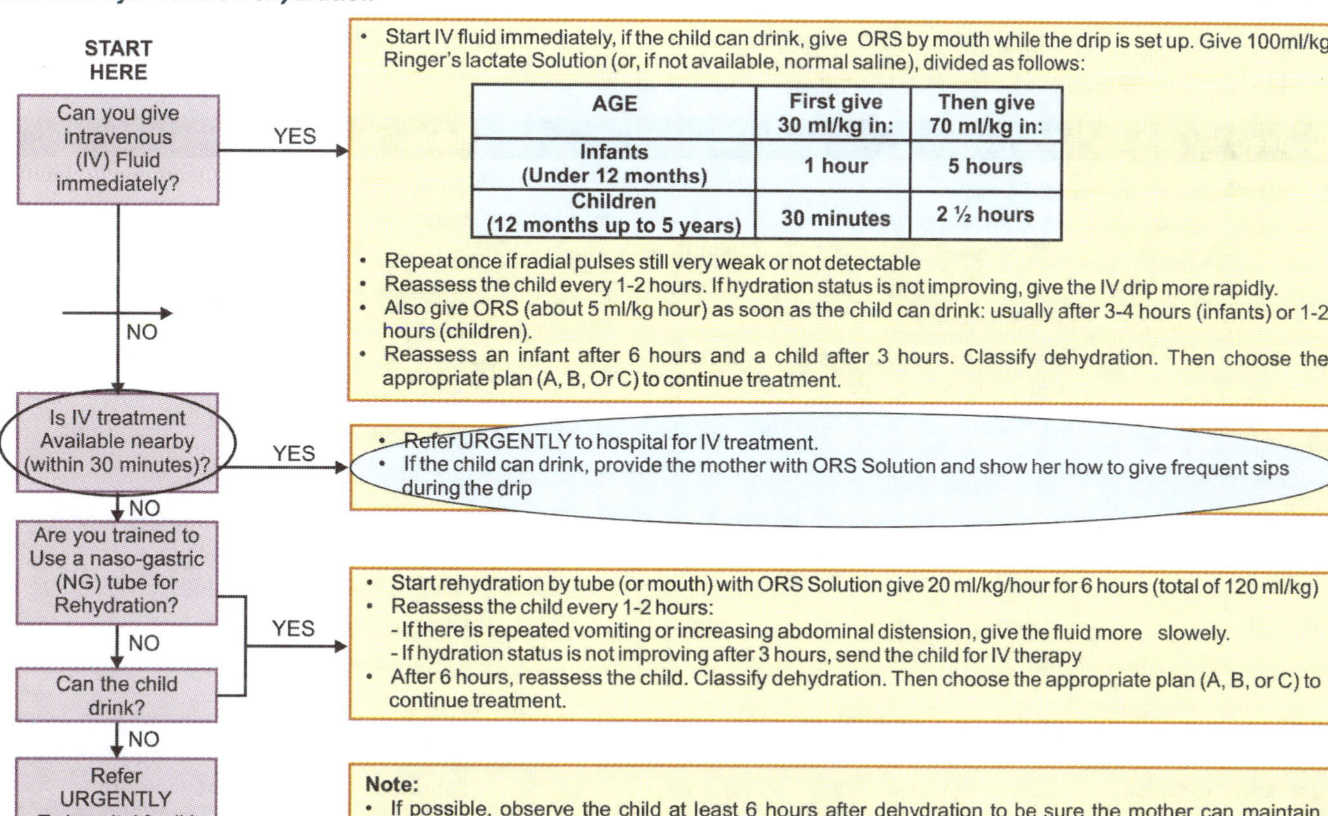

201. Ans. (b) Tibia

Ref: Nelson's, 18" ed./ ch. 66

- *If venous access is not available in an arrest situation within 1 minute, an intraosseous line should be placed in the anterior tibia (with care taken to avoid traversing the epiphyseal plate)*
- The needle should penetrate the anterior layer of compact bone, with its tip advanced into the spongy interior of the bone.
- Intraosseous needles are special rigid, large-bore needles that resemble those used for marrow aspiration. Current recommendations urge the use of intraosseous cannulation in patients for whom intravenous access proves difficult or unattainable, even in older children.
- Once the patient has received initial drug and fluid therapy through the IO line, every effort should be made to obtain more conventional central venous access and remove the I0 line as soon as possible.
- Alternative sites for intraosseous (IO) insertion include **the distal tibia, distal femur, sternum, and humerus**

202. Ans. (b) Na 75 mEq + 245 mOsm

Ref: OP Ghai, 8th ed. pg. 294

The concentration of sodium in low osmolality ORS is 75 mEq. The osmolality is 245 mOsm.

Extra Mile

*WHO recommends a special ORS formulation, known as **ReSoMal**, for management of diarrhoea in **severely malnourished children** that contains a lower amount of sodium (45mmol/L) and higher amount of potassium (40 mmol/L) than the standard WHO-ORS.*

VACCINES

203. Ans. (a) Birth

Ref: main.mohfw.gov.in

Hepatitis B subunit vaccine is given at day 0, 6 weeks and 10/14 weeks of age. The first dose of hepatitis B is given as soon as possible within 24 hours of birth.

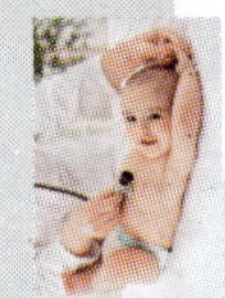

204. Ans. (c) BCG, OPV, HBV

Ref: main.mohfw.gov.in

National Immunization Schedule (NIS) for Infants

Vaccine	When to give	Dose	Route	Site
For Infants				
BCG	At birth or as early as possible till one year of age	0.1 mL (0.05 mL until 1 month age)	Intradermal	Left upper arm
Hepatitis B - Birth dose	At birth or as early as possible within 24 hours	0.5 mL	Intramuscular	Anterolateral side of mid-thigh
OPV-0	At birth or as early as possible within the first 15 days	2 drops	Oral	Oral
OPV 1, 2 and 3	At 6 weeks, 10 weeks and 14 weeks (OPV can be given till 5 years of age)	2 drops	Oral	Oral
Pentavalent 1, 2 and 3	At 6 weeks, 10 weeks and 14 weeks (can be given till one year of age)	0.5 mL	Intramuscular	Anterolateral side of mid-thigh
Rotavirus	At 6 weeks, 10 weeks and 14 weeks (can be given till one year of age)	5 drops	Oral	Oral
IPV	Two fractional dose at 6 and 14 weeks of age	0.1 mL	Intradermal two fractional dose	Intradermal: Right upper arm
Measles/MR 1st Dose	9 completed months-12 months (can be given till 5 years of age)	0.5 mL	Subcutaneous	Right upper arm
JE-1	9 completed months-12 months.	0.5 mL	Subcutaneous	Left upper arm
Vitamin A (1st dose)	At 9 completed months with measles-Rubella	1 mL (1 lakh IU)	Oral	Oral

205. Ans. (d) 2 lakh units

Ref: O.P. Ghai Essential Pediatrics, 9th ed. pg. 200

- Vitamin A reduces morbidity and mortality of measles and a single oral dose of 1,00,000 units below 1 year
- For age above the age of 1 year, 2,00,000 units is recommended.

206. (d) 15 weeks

Ref: IAP 2016 Guidelines

ROTAVIRUS (RV) VACCINES

Routine Vaccination

- Minimum age: 6 weeks for all available brands (RV-1) [Rotarix], RV-5 [RotaTeq] and RV-116E [Rotavac])
- Only two doses of RV-1 are recommended
- RV1 should preferably be employed in 10–14 week schedule.
- If any dose in series was RV-5 or RV-116E or vaccine product is unknown for any dose in the series, a total of 3 doses of RV vaccine should be administered.

Catch-up vaccination

- **The maximum age for the first dose in the series is 14 weeks, 6 days**
- Vaccination *should not be initiated for infants aged 15 weeks, 0 days or older*
- The maximum age for the final dose in the series is 8 months, 0 days

207. Ans. (a) DPT

Ref: OP Ghai, 8th ed. pg. 193

- Since all live vaccines are contraindicated in immune-compromised patients hence only DPT can be given. *Please note that the question mentions an AIDS positive patient and "not a child born to HIV positive mother".*
- If a child is born to HIV positive mother, the child may or may-not be acquire HIV infection from the mother. Hence WHO recommends BCG should be given to a baby born to HIV positive lady. ***Textbook clearly mentions that if baby has documented AIDS then live vaccines are contraindicated. In such cases IPV can be given in place of OPV***

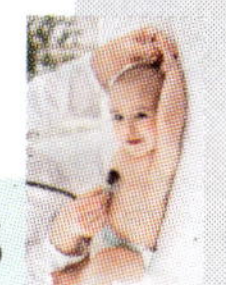

208. Ans. (b) Dukoral

Ref: Nelson, 18th ed chapter 173, http://wwwnc.cdc/gov/eid/article/17/11 11-0822 article

- Dukoral is indicated for active immunization against disease caused by *Vibrio cholerae*s ero group O1 in adults and children from 2 years of age who will be visiting endemic/epidemic areas
- The standard primary course of vaccination with Dukoral against cholera consists of 2 doses for adults and children from 6 years of age. Children 2 to below 6 years of age should receive 3 doses. Doses are to be administered at intervals of at least one week. If more than 6 weeks have elapsed between doses, the primary immunization course should be re-started.
- Immunization should be completed at least 1 week prior to potential exposure to *V. cholerae* O1.

209. Ans. (b) BCG

Ref: OP Ghai, 8th ed. pg. 191

BCG

- Although BCG vaccination often causes local reactions, serious or long-term complications are rare. *Reactions that can be expected after vaccination include moderate axillary or cervical lymphadenopathy and induration and subsequent pustule formation at the injection site*; these reactions can persist for as long as 3 months after vaccination.
- Most serious complication of BCG vaccination is disseminated BCG infection.
- The most frequent disseminated infection is BCG osteomyelitis.

210. Ans. (a) Measles

Ref: Nelson Textbook of Pediatrics 20th ed. pg. 1545

Measles	Maculopapular rash
Dengue	Petechial rash on extremities and spreading on trunk
Chicken pox	Maculo-papulo-vesicular rash
Herpetic rash	Always grouped vesicles in dermatomal distribution

Extra Mile

Measles can lead to

1. **Giant cell pneumonia:** The leading cause of death in measles is pneumonia. It can be direct viral infection or secondary bacterial infection with pneumococcus, etc.
2. **Black measles:** Hemorrhagic measles
3. **SSPE:** Occurs due to defective measles virus and presents as myoclonus with neurodegeneration

KIDNEY

211. Ans. (c) Post streptococcal glomerulonephritis

Ref: Nelson Essentials of Pediatrics, 9th ed. pg. 638

- Post-streptococcal glomerulonephritis is a disease of the kidneys which occurs after infection with nephritogenic strains of group A streptococcus.
- This results in immune complex deposition in glomerulus and resultant damage leads to dark urine referred as brown-, tea-, or cola-colored. Option a presents with nephrotic range proteinuria, option b presents with hematuria but after URTI while in this case it was after skin involvement. Option d is seen with diabetic nephropathy.

212. Ans. (a) Henoch schonlein purpura

Ref: Nelson Essentials of Pediatrics, 9th ed. pg. 361

- Henoch-Schönlein purpura (HSP) is a condition that involves inflammation of small blood vessels.
- The inflammation causes blood vessels in the skin, intestines, kidneys, and joints to start leaking.
- The main symptom is a rash with numerous small bruises, which have a raised appearance, over the legs or buttocks. Option b presents with PIP, MCP and bilateral wrist joint involvement. Option c presents with renal failure. Option d presents with urethritis, conjunctivitis, uveitis and arthritis.

213. Ans. (b) 2

Ref: KDIGO guidelines

Acute kidney injury

Stages:

Stage	Creatinine criteria	Urine output
AKI stage I	1.5–2 times baseline OR 0.3 mg/dL increase from baseline (≥26.4 mmol/L)	<0.5 mL/kg/hr for >6 hours
AKI stage II	2–3 times baseline	<0.5 mL/kg/h for >12 hours
AKI stage III	3 times baseline OR 0.5 mg/dL (44 mmol/L) increase if baseline >4 mg/dL (≥ 354 mmol/L) OR Any renal replacement therapy given	<0.3 mL/kg/h for >24 hours OR Anuria for >12 hours

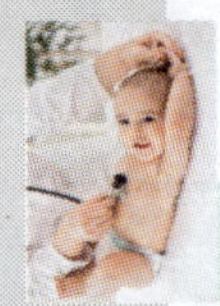

214. Ans. (c) Posterior urethral valve

Ref: Nelson Textbook of Pediatrics 20th ed. pg. 2573

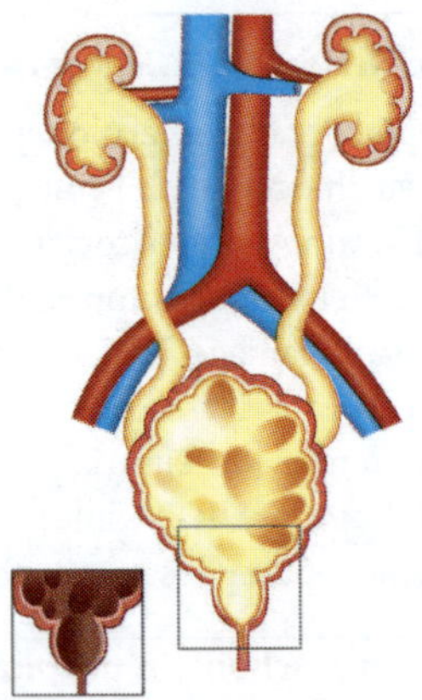

FIGURE: Posterior urethral valves (PUV)

- Bilateral hydronephrosis points to etiology present in or below the urinary bladder. A leading cause of this is posterior urethral valves which will cause a trabeculated bladder and Vesicoureteral reflux. This damages the kidney parenchyma and can lead to pyelonephritis.
- Choice a and b are usually seen unilateral and do not cause urine retention.
- Choice d is unlikely to be seen in an infant and would cause a trabeculated bladder but not a VUR.

215. Ans. (b) Congenital Finnish type nephrotic syndrome

Ref: Nelson, 18th ed./ Table 527.1

- Congenital nephrotic syndrome is one of the Finnish heritage diseases and rare form of nephrotic syndrome.
- It occurs predominantly in families of Finnish origin and manifests shortly after birth
- The condition is caused by a defect in the protein nephrin, which is found in the kidney.
- Gene responsible is NPHS 1.

216. Ans. (b) Hyperparathyroidism

Renal Tubular acidosis	RTA 1 can present with Nephrocalcinosis and renal rickets but pathological fractures and psychiatric symptoms are not seen
Hyperparathy-roidism	The increased bone resorption explains pathological fracture. Hypercalcemia leads to deposition of calcium in the kidney parenchyma. Psychiatric symptoms are seen in hyperparathyroidism.
Polycystic kidneys	Presents with CRF with cystic kidneys
CRF	Can have pathological fracture due to Osteitis Cystica Fibrosa due to secondary Hyperparathyroidism.

217. Ans. (a) 4–8 years

Henoch schonlein purpura is the most common type of vasculitis in children and presents at 4–8 years of age. IgA is incriminated in pathogenesis of HSP. The commonest presentation is extensor purpura.

RESPIRATORY SYSTEM

218. Ans. (d) Severe pneumonia antibiotics and referral

Ref: nhm.gov.in

Signs	Classify as	Identify treatment (Urgent pre-referral treatments are in bold print)
• Any general danger sign or • Chest indrawing or • Stridor in calm child	Severe pneumonia or very severe disease	• Give first dose of Cotrimoxazole • Refer urgently to hospital
• Fast breathing	Pneumonia	• Give Cotrimoxazole for 5 days • Soothe the throat and relieve the cough with a safe remedy. • Advise mother when to return immediately. • Follow-up in 2 days
• No signs of pneumonia or very severe disease.	No Pneumonia: Cough or Cold	• If coughing more than 21 days, refer for assessment. • Soothe the throat and relieve the cough with a safe remedy. • Advise mother when to return immediately. • Follow-up in 5 days, if not improving.

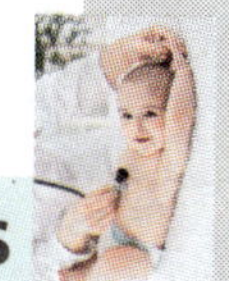

219. Ans. (c) Pneumonia; oral antibiotics and come back after 5 days

Ref: O.P. Ghai Essential Pediatrics, 9th ed. pg. 380

- If the child has rapid respiration and chest in drawing, but no hypoxia, feeding well and does not have danger signs he may be treated on ambulatory basis with oral amoxicillin twice daily for 5 days.

220. Ans. (a) A

Ref: Nelson Essentials of Pediatrics, 9th ed. pg.s 11, 12, 13

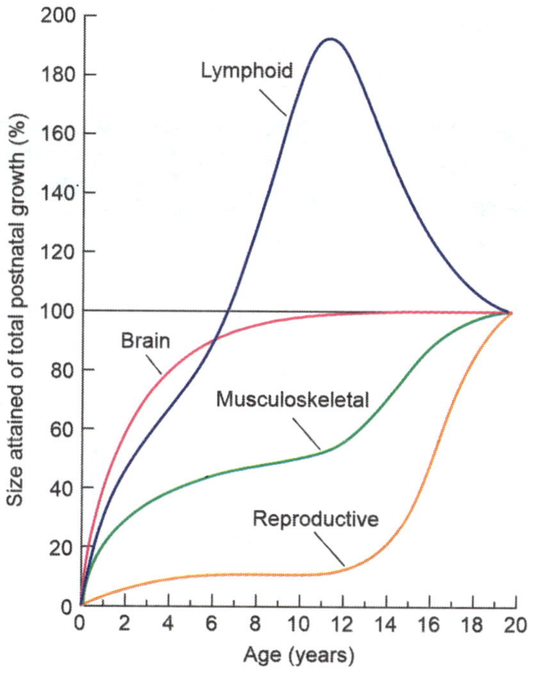

221. Ans. (a) Congenital diaphragmatic hernia

Ref: O.P. Ghai Essential Pediatrics, 9th ed. pg. 141, 172

- The X-ray suggests intestinal loops in the mediastinum which is seen in CDH.
- Congenital diaphragmatic hernia occurs when the diaphragm, the muscle that separates the chest from the abdomen, fails to close during prenatal development.
- This opening allows contents of the abdomen (stomach, intestines and/or liver) to migrate into the chest, impacting the growth and development of the lungs.
- Approximately 83% of babies with CDH have a defect on the left side of the diaphragm.

222. Ans. (b) Give first dose ampicillin and gentamicin and refer urgently to hospital

Ref: ARI control Programme, Government of India Guidelines

Signs	Classify as	Management
• General danger signs (inability to breastfeed or drink, lethargy or reduced level of consciousness, convulsions) • Chest indrawing with oxygen saturation <92% or SpO_2 facilities not available	Severe pneumonia	• Admit immediately • Administer intravenous Ampicillin (or Penicillin) Plus Gentamicin • Give oxygen if saturation <92%. • Manage airway, as appropriate.
• Fast breathing: Respiratory rates ▪ 2–11 months ≥50/min ▪ 12–59 months ≥40/min **And/or** • Chest indrawing (SpO_2≥ 92%)	Pneumonia	• Home treatment • Give Amoxycillin for 5 days • Soothe the throat and relieve cough with a safe remedy
And No signs of severe pneumonia		• Treat high fever if present • Treat wheeze if present • Assess regularly
No signs of severe pneumonia or pneumonia	No pneumonia	• Soothe the throat and relieve cough with safe remedy). • Advise the mother when to return. • Follow-up after 5 days if not improving. • If coughing for more than 14 days refer to doctor for further investigation
* If the child has wheezing, Give 3 doses of inhaled salbutamol and reassess If there is no improvement in symptoms: classify as severe pneumonia or pneumonia		

223. Ans. (a) Respiratory syncytial virus

Ref: Nelson Textbook of Pediatrics 20th ed. pg. 2045

- CXR showing bilateral hyperinflation and wheezing points to airway narrowing and obstructive airway disease. This is presentation of bronchiolitis in infants and is caused by Respiratory syncytial virus.
- Option b and c would cause auscultatory finding of bronchial breathing or crepitations.
- Option d causes Hand foot and mouth disease (Coxsackie A) and Myocarditis/fulminant diabetes (Coxsackie B)

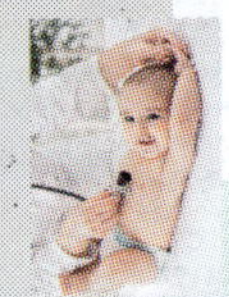

224. Ans. (a) Pneumonia

Ref: ARI control Programme, Government of India Guidelines

Signs	Classify as	Management
• General danger signs (inability to breastfeed or drink, lethargy or reduced level of consciousness, convulsions) • Chest indrawing with oxygen saturation <92% or SpO_2 facilities not available	Severe pneumonia	• Admit immediately • Administer intravenous Ampicillin (or Penicillin) Plus Gentamicin • Give oxygen if saturation <92%. • Manage airway, as appropriate.
• Fast breathing: Respiratory rates ▪ 2–11 months ≥50/min ▪ 12–59 months ≥40/min	Pneumonia	• Home treatment • Give Amoxycillin for 5 days • Soothe the throat and relieve cough with a safe remedy
And/or • Chest indrawing (SpO_2≥ 92%) **And** No signs of severe pneumonia		• Treat high fever if present • Treat wheeze if present • Assess regularly
No signs of severe pneumonia or pneumonia	No pneumonia	• Soothe the throat and relieve cough with safe remedy. • Advise the mother when to return. • Follow-up after 5 days if not improving. • If coughing for more than 14 days refer to doctor for further investigation
* If the child has wheezing, Give 3 doses of inhaled salbutamol and reassess If there is no improvement in symptoms: classify as severe pneumonia or pneumonia		

225. Ans. (d) Bronchiolitis

Ref: Nelson 20th ed. pg. 245

- The characteristic feature of bronchiolitis is prolonged expiration due to airway inflammation. It is caused by Respiratory syncytial virus.
- Choice a has presence of Bronchial breathing and crepitations and is ruled out.
- Choice b manifests as hoarseness, a seal-like barking cough, inspiratory stridor, and a variable degree of respiratory distress.
- Choice c has episodic attacks on exposure to allergens.

226. Ans. (a) Ribavarin

Ref: Nelson 20th ed. pg. 1608

Bronchiolitis caused by respiratory syncytial virus is managed with aerosol of Ribavarin. It causes only modest improvement. Hence, humified oxygen is the main stay of treatment. Latest approach is to use palivizumab for prophylaxis in high risk infants.

Virus	Clinical syndrome	Antiviral agent of choice	Alternative antiviral agents
Influenza A	Treatment	Oseltamivir (>1-year-old)	Rimantadine Amantadine
	Prophylaxis	Oseltamivir (>1-year-old)	Amantadine Rimantadine Zanamivir (>7-year-old)
Influenza B	Treatment	Oseltamivir	Zanamivir (> 7-year-old)
Respiratory syncytial virus	Bronchiolitis or pneumonia in high-risk host	Oseltamivir Ribavirin aerosol	

227. Ans. (c) >40/min RR, for 12–60 months

Ref: OP Ghai 8th ed. pg. 381

As per WHO clinical classification of acute lower respiratory infection, pneumonia is defined as:

Increased respiratory rate:	
<2-month-old	>60/min
2–12-month-old	>50/min
12–60-month-old	>40/min

228. Ans. (b) Rhinovirus

Ref: Harrison, 18th ed. chapter 186, Nelson, 18th ed. chapter 376

The most common pathogens associated with the common cold are the rhinoviruses.
In contrast bronchiolitis is caused by RSV.

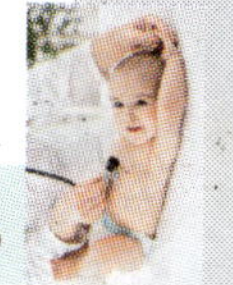

Pathogens Associated with the Common Cold

Association	Pathogen	Relative Frequency
Agents primarily associated with colds	Rhinoviruses Coronaviruses	Frequent Occasional
Agents primarily associated with other clinical syndromes that also cause common cold symptoms	Respiratory syncytial viruses *(MC cause of bronchiolitis)*	Occasional
	Influenza viruses	Occasional
	Parainfluenza viruses	Uncommon
	Adenoviruses	Uncommon
	Enteroviruses	Uncommon

INBORN ERRORS OF METABOLISM

229. Ans. (a) Homogentisic acid oxidase

Ref: Nelson Textbook of Pediatrics, pg. 642

The clinical diagnosis is Alkaptonuria. The key words are urine turning black on-air exposure. Alkaptonuria has homogentisic acid oxidase deficiency.

230. Ans. (b) Glycogen accumulation in liver

Ref: O.P. Ghai Essential Pediatrics, 9th ed. pg. 338

- Glucose-6-phosphatase deficiency (G6P deficiency), or glycogen storage disease type I, is called von Gierke disease.
- It is characterized by poor tolerance to fasting, growth retardation and hepatomegaly resulting from accumulation of glycogen and fat in the liver.

231. Ans. (b) Branched-chain alpha-keto acid dehydrogenase (BCKD) enzyme

Ref: O.P. Ghai Essential Pediatrics, 9th ed. pg. 650

- Maple syrup urine disease is characterized by deficiency of an enzyme branched-chain alpha-keto acid dehydrogenase.
- People with maple syrup urine (MSUD) disease can't break down three specific amino acids found in protein-containing foods (Leucine, Isoleucine and Valine).
- Symptoms of classic MSUD appear in newborns within 48 hours of birth. It includes Urine, sweat that smells like maple syrup or burnt sugar, poor feeding, vomiting, loss of appetite, irritability.

232. Ans. (b) Phenylketonuria

Ref: Nelson, 18th ed. chapter 85.1, Harrison's 17th ed. Ch 358

Clinical Manifestations of Classic Phenylketonuria

- The affected infant is normal at birth.
- Mental retardation may develop gradually and may not be evident for the 1st few months.
- Vomiting, sometimes severe enough to be misdiagnosed as pyloric stenosis, may be an early symptom.
- Older untreated children become hyperactive, with purposeless movements, rhythmic rocking, and Athetosis.
- Infants are lighter in their complexion than unaffected siblings with blonde hair.
- These children have an unpleasant odor of Phenyl-acetic acid, which has been described as musty or mousey.
- Most infants are hypertonic with hyperactive deep tendon reflexes.
- Microcephaly, prominent maxilla with widely spaced teeth, enamel hypoplasia, and growth retardation are other common findings in untreated children.

ENDOCRINOLOGY

233. Ans. (d) GH receptor deficiency

Ref: Harrison 20th ed. pg. 2657

- Since GH levels are elevated, hypopituitarism/GH deficiency/choice c is ruled out.
- GH receptor deficiency that leads to low production of IGF-1 levels and is called Laron syndrome.
- In choice a and b, GH levels will be low and hence are ruled out.

234. Ans. (b) Serum TSH level

Ref: Nelson Textbook of Pediatrics 20th ed. pg. 2669

- Large protruded tongue with prolongation of physiological jaundice is seen in congenital hypothyroidism. Hence, Serum TSH levels will be elevated.
- The child is not having features of sepsis or Cushingoid appearance. Hence choice a and c are ruled out.
- Hypopituitarism has normal length at birth and is diagnosed later when the child fails to gain height.

235. Ans. (c) Hypothyroidism

Ref: Nelson 20th ed. pg. 2269

- Choice a Pellagra manifests as edema, erythema, and burning of sun-exposed skin on the face, neck, and dorsal aspects of the hands, forearms, and feet.

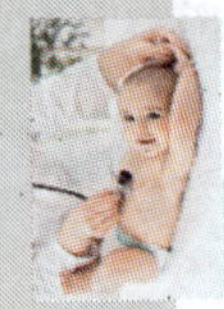

- Choice b presents as protuberant tongue with brachycephaly and early closure of fontanelles.
- Choice d presents as wide open anterior fontanelle.
- Choice c Congenital Hypothyroidism presents with patent posterior fontanelle with myxedema leading to large tongue and coarse dry skin. The leading cause of congenital hypothyroidism is thyroid dysgenesis.

236. Ans. (a) Adrenalectomy

Ref: Nelson, 18th ed./Ch. 578

Nelson syndrome is seen post adrenalectomy. The rise of ACTH post-operatively leads to hyper pigmentation of palm, sole creases.

MISCELLANEOUS

237. Ans. (d) Liver disease

Ref: Harrison 21st ed. pg. 776-777

- Option a and c presents with microcytic hypochromic anemia. Option b presents with Normocytic normochromic anemia.

The Non-megaloblastic Macrocytic Blood Picture

The most important causes here are chronic liver disease, alcoholism, and hypothyroidism.

There may be a pancytopenia with chronic liver disease, since it is often associated with protal hypertension, splenomegaly, and hypersplenism, the features of which will be added to the total picture.

238. Ans. (a) Cu

Ref: O.P. Ghai Essential Pediatrics, 9th ed. pg. 123

- Menke's disease is caused by a defect in the ATP7A gene.
- The defect makes it hard for the body to properly transport copper throughout the body.
- As a result, the brain and other parts of the body do not get enough copper, while it builds up in the small intestine and kidneys.

239. Ans. (d) Give antipyretics and send home

Ref: O.P. Ghai Essential Pediatrics, 9th ed. pg. 375

- The case presentation is of mumps. Secondary attack rate of mumps is 85%. Conservative management and home isolation is required.

240. Ans. (d) Factor VIII deficiency

Ref: Nelson Textbook of Pediatrics 20th ed. pg. 2382

Joint bleeding after minimal trauma or excessive bruisability is seen in cases of Hemophilia. The leading subtype is Hemophilia A which has factor eight deficiency and X-linked recessive pattern of inheritance. The child should be screened by coagulogram and deranged aPTT will be seen. The best investigation for diagnosis is Factor 8 level estimation and treatment is monthly factor 8 concentrates manufactured by DNA recombinant technology.

Extra Mile

- Bleeding from umbilical stump in neonate on day 0 = Glanzmann Thrombasthenia
- Bleeding from umbilical stump in neonate on day 5 = Hemorrhagic disease of newborn
- Excessive bleeding in a boy after circumcision = Factor 8 deficiency/Hemophilia A
- Bleeding in joint space in a boy after a minor fall = Factor 8 deficiency/Hemophilia A

241. Ans. (c) Osteogenesis imperfecta

Ref: Nelson Textbook of pediatrics 20th ed. pg. 3381

Blue sclera and multiple fractures are the key factors that depict a problem in connective tissue. The diagnosis in this case is Osteogenesis imperfecta. It occurs due to defect of COL1A1 or COL1A2 genes which form type 1 collagen. Therefore, all connective tissue in which type 1 collagen is found will be affected. Though large number of subtypes exist, the table below mentions the core issues to be remembered.

Classification of osteogenesis imperfect

Type	Description
I	• Most common type • Least severe type • Blue sclerae
II	• Lethal (respiratory compromise); most do not survive past early infancy
III	• Most severe form that is compatible with life • Early and numerous fractures leading to deformed limbs • Progressive in nature • Normal sclerae
IV	• Not as severe as type III • Fractures common • Bowed long bones • Normal sclerae

Extra Mile

Other important features of OI
1. Basilar invagination of skull
2. Blue sclera
3. Dentinogenesis imperfecta
4. MVP/Aortic dissection

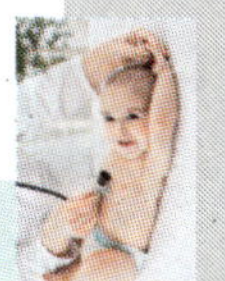

242. Ans. (d) Zinc

Ref: Nelson Textbook of Pediatrics 20th ed. pg. 3238

- The image shows perioral and acral dermatitis with key finding of perigenital dermatitis which confirms that zinc deficiency is the culprit leading to development of acrodermatitis enteropathica.
- Zinc is an essential trace nutrient that plays a role in functioning of 100 enzymes and nucleic acid metabolism. The disease can occur either due to defects in SLC39A4 gene that codes for ZIP (zinc iron transporter protein) that is expressed on enterocytes in Duodenum and Jejunum. Acquired causes can occur due to malnutrition, malabsorption or combination of both.

243. Ans. (b) Chicken pox

Ref: Nelson Textbook of Pediatrics 20th ed. pg. 1583

- In measles the rash appears on day 4 of fever while in chicken pox the rash appears on day 1. The combination of macules, papules and vesicles at the same time is characteristic of chicken pox. The lesions are called "dew drop" lesions.
- Scabies is ruled out as it would not have fever
- Rubella does not have vesicular rash

244. Ans. (b) Coxsackie virus

Ref: Nelson Textbook of pediatrics 20th ed. pg. 1564

The image shows vesicular lesion in oral cavity, palms and soles. These are classic features of hand foot and mouth disease which is caused by Coxsackie A16, A6 virus and enterovirus 71. Exclusive oral cavity involvement is called herpangina.

245. Ans. (b) Exanthema subitum

Ref: Nelson 20th ed. pg. 1594

- Human herpes-6A, Herpes-6B and HHV7 causes Roseola infantum or exanthema subitum and is called sixth disease.
- The most common cause is primary infection with human herpesvirus 6B.
- The classic presentation of roseola infantum is a 9–12-month-old infant who acutely develops a high fever and often a febrile seizure. After 3 days, a rapid defervescence occurs, and a morbilliform rash appears.

Extra Mile

Number	Other names for the disease	Etiology (ies)
First disease	Rubeola, measles, hard measles, 14-day measles, morbilli	Measles virus
Second disease	Scarlet fever, scarlatina	*Streptococcus pyogenes*
Third disease	Rubella, German measles, 3-day measles	Rubella virus
Fourth disease	Filatov-Duke's disease, staphylococcal scalded skin syndrome, Ritter's disease	Some say the disease does not exist. Other believe it is due to *Staphylococcus aureus* strains that make epidermolytic (exfoliative) toxin
Fifth disease	Erythema infectiosum	Erythrovirus (Parvovirus) B19
Sixth disease	Exanthem subitum, roseola infantum, "Sudden Rash", rose rash of infants, 3-day fever	Human herpes virus 6B or human herpes virus 7

246. Ans. (a) Coxsackie A

Ref: OP Ghai 8th ed. pg. 219

- Hand-foot-mouth disease is a common viral illness primarily affecting children below 5 years of age.
- The most common causes of hand foot mouth disease are Coxsackie virus A16 and enterovirus 71.

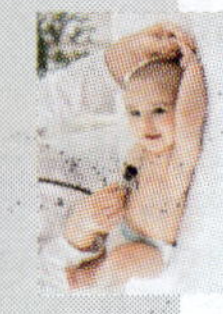

247. Ans. (a) Torsion of appendix of testis

Ref: Nelson, 20th ed. pg. 2595–96

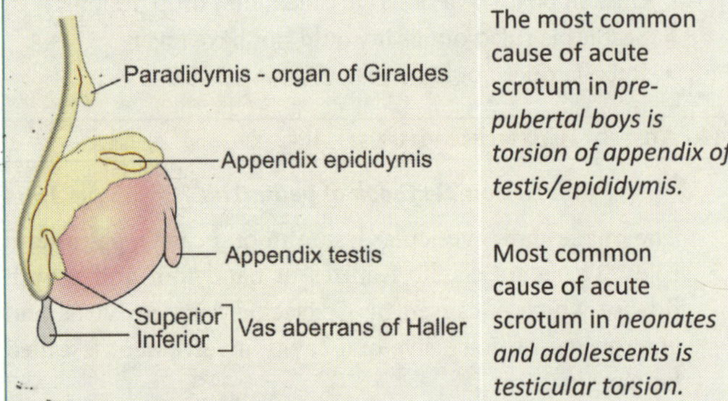

The most common cause of acute scrotum in *pre-pubertal boys is torsion of appendix of testis/epididymis.*

Most common cause of acute scrotum in *neonates and adolescents is testicular torsion.*

248. Ans. (d) Rubeola

Ref: Nelson, 20th ed. pg. 1544

- The clinical presentation given is of measles (Aka Rubeola) and is characterised by rash on face, neck and spreading to rest of the body.
- Chicken pox rash appears on extremities and is maculo-papulo-vesicular. The rash is red but has vesicles which are not given in the clinical presentation above.
- Rubella presents as measles but has posterior cervical lymphadenopathy.
- Variola is the small pox virus and the vaccine for small pox is made from a virus called *vaccinia.*

249. Ans. (a) Erythema infectiosum

- Erythema infectiosum (also known as fifth disease) is usually a benign childhood condition characterized by a *classic slapped-cheek appearance* and lacy exanthem.
- It results from infection with human parvovirus (PV) B19, an erythrovirus

250. Ans. (c) Mild proteinuria, high hematuria, high ASO titer

Ref: OP Ghai, 8th ed. pg. 474–75

- Glomerulo-nephritis is characterized by inflammation of glomerulus leading to hematuria with sub-nephrotic proteinuria. The inflammation follows a skin infection or a sore throat and therefore requires serological evidence in form of elevated ASO titer or anti DNA-ase-B.

251. Ans. (c) Zinc deficiency

Ref: Pediatric Dermatology, 3rd ed. pg. 1137

- Zinc toxicity can cause zinc shakes especially after inhalation of zinc following welding of galvanized metals.
- *Zinc deficiency is known as acrodermatitis enterohepatica*

252. Ans. (c) 15 mg/kg

Ref: OP Ghai, 8th ed. pg. Table 10.9

Drug	Pediatric dose in mg/kg	Side effect	MAX adult dose
INH	***15 mg/kg thrice weekly, under RNCTP 20–30 mg twice weekly dosages***	Peripheral neuritis	300 mg
Rifampicin	15 mg/kg	Hepatitis	600 mg
Pyrazina-mide	30–35	Gout	2000 mg
Ethambutol	20–25	Optic neuritis	1500 mg

Please note that the values for INH and rifampicin under the revised programme are equal.

253. Ans. (a) Albright's syndrome

Ref: Nelson, 18th ed. Ch. 563

McCune Albright syndrome is suspected when two of the three following features are present:

1. Endocrine hyperfunction such as precocious puberty
2. Polyostotic fibrous dysplasia
3. Unilateral Cafe-au-lait spots

OBSTETRICS AND GYNECOLOGY

12

OBSTETRICS

MOST RECENT QUESTIONS 2023

1. During delivery of a baby, which of the following maneuver is done when fetal scalp is visible at vulva?
(Most Recent Question July 2023)

a. Pinard
b. Ritgen
c. Loveset
d. Mauriceau-Smellie-Veit

2. Uterine height after delivery is at the level of:

a. 12 weeks
b. 16 weeks
c. 20 weeks
d. 28 weeks

3. What will be the most likely diagnosis if the middle swab is stained with dye in methylene blue 3 swab test?
(Most Recent Question July 2023)

a. Uterovesical fistula
b. Ureterovaginal fistula
c. Vesicovaginal fistula
d. Ureterovaginal fistula

4. Induction of labor should not be done in which of the following conditions? *(Most Recent Question July 2023)*

a. Gestational hypertension
b. Premature rupture of membranes
c. Central placenta previa
d. Abruptio placenta

5. Which of the following is required for medical termination of pregnancy at 21 weeks for fetus diagnosed with meningomyelocele?
(Most Recent Question July 2023)

a. Opinion of one doctor
b. Opinion of two doctors
c. Consent of husband
d. Her consent with opinions of two doctors

6. A 32 weeks pregnant lady presents with bleeding per-vaginum. Per abdominal examination reveals tense and tender uterus, fetal parts are not palpable. Which of the following is the most likely diagnosis?
(Most Recent Question July 2023)

a. Placenta previa
b. Polyhydramnios
c. Abruptio placentae
d. Uterine rupture

7. Which of the following hormones are secreted by Sertoli cells and Leydig cells respectively?
(Most Recent Question July 2023)

a. Testosterone and progesterone
b. Testosterone and hCG
c. Inhibin and Testosterone
d. Testosterone and Inhibin

8. A 32 weeks pregnant female presented with blood pressure 150/100 mm Hg and proteinuria on urine dip stick test is 2+. Which of the following is the most likely diagnosis? *(Most Recent Question July 2023)*

a. Abruptio placentae
b. Postpartum hemorrhage
c. Placenta previa
d. Pre-eclampsia

9. In a pregnant female, Quadruple test is done in which trimester? *(Most Recent Question July 2023)*

a. First trimester
b. Second trimester
c. Third trimester
d. Fourth trimester

10. Which of the following is not a hyperestrogenic condition? *(Most Recent Question July 2023)*

a. Low BMI
b. Use of tamoxifen
c. Nulliparity
d. Endometriosis

11. Which of the following is outlet forceps?
(Most Recent Question July 2023)

a. Kielland
b. Das
c. Piper
d. Wrigley

12. A female patient with recent history of abortion presented with amenorrhea. Serum evaluation shows the following findings: FSH: 7 IU/L, hCG: <5 IU/L. What is the most likely diagnosis?

a. PCOD
b. Uterine synechiae
c. Endometriosis
d. Adenomyosis

13. Which of the following is decreased in polycystic ovarian syndrome? *(Most Recent Question July 2023)*

a. LH
b. Testosterone
c. FSH
d. Estrogen

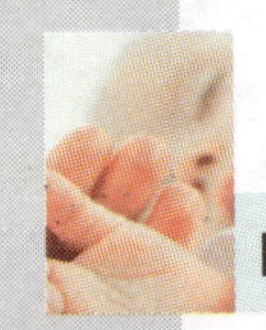

14. Which of the following investigation is performed in a patient with polycystic ovarian syndrome?
(Most Recent Question July 2023)
a. Urine culture
b. Sleep study
c. Serum testosterone
d. Thyroid profile

15. A 35-year-old female patient presented with loss of sensation over anterolateral part of thigh. There is history of vaginal delivery 2 days ago. Which of the following nerve is most likely involved?
(Most Recent Question July 2023)
a. Obturator nerve
b. Sciatic nerve
c. Lateral cutaneous nerve of thigh
d. Ilioinguinal nerve

16. Oxytocin is contraindicated in:
(Most Recent Question July 2023)
a. Postpartum hemorrhage
b. Placenta covering internal os
c. Vaginal delivery
d. Instrumental delivery

17. Which of the following statements is correct in pregnancy? ***(Most Recent Question July 2023)***
a. Decreased GFR
b. Decreased Serum creatinine
c. Decreased Plasma protein
d. Decreased plasma volume

18. McCall culdoplasty is done for:
a. Enterocele
b. Rectocele
c. Peritonitis
d. All of the above

19. Which of the following is protective factor for endometrial cancer? ***(Most Recent Question July 2023)***
a. Oral combined contraceptive
b. Obesity
c. Aspirin
d. Tamoxifen

20. A young male patient presented with history of infertility. Seminogram shows sperm count 16 million/mL, motility 40%, morphologically normal sperms < 1%. Given these findings, what is this condition called?
a. Normospermia
b. Asthenospermia
c. Teratozoospermia
d. Oligospermia

21. Galactokinesis is governed by:
a. Estrogen
b. Progesterone
c. Prolactin
d. Oxytocin

22. Identify the type of placenta previa from the given image:
(Most Recent Question Jan 2023)

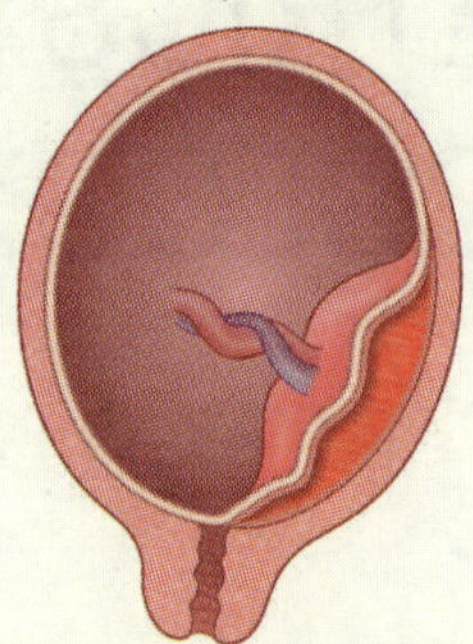

a. Marginal
b. Partial
c. Low lying
d. Complete

23. Identify the type of pelvis in the given image:
(Most Recent Question Jan 2023)

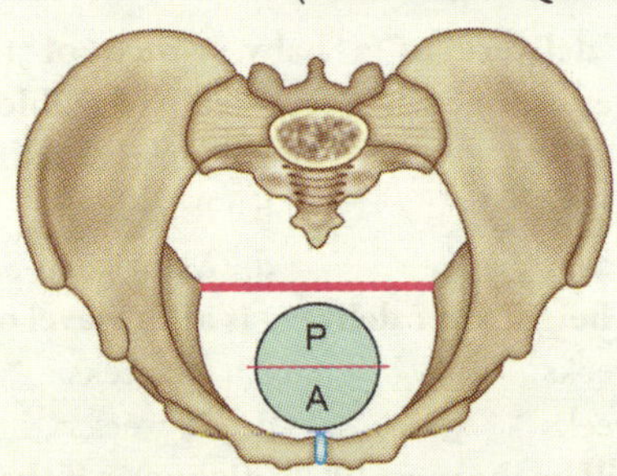

a. Gynecoid
b. Android
c. Anthropoid
d. Platypelloid

24. What will be the type of twin if division in zygote occurs between 9-12 days after fertilization?
a. Dichorionic diamniotic
b. Monochorionic diamniotic
c. Monochorionic monoamniotic
d. Siamese twins

25. Identify the forceps:
(Most Recent Question Jan 2023)

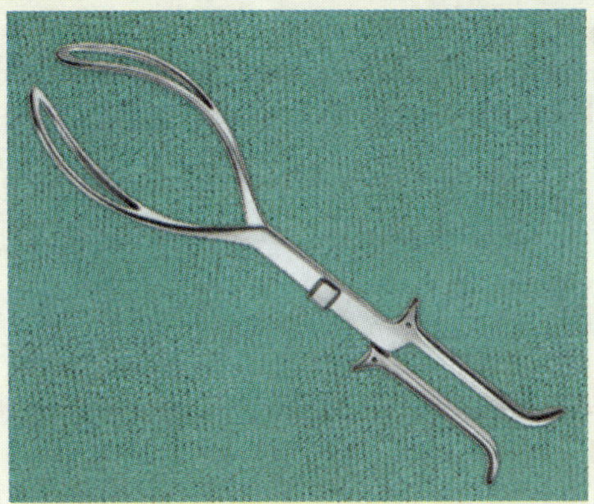

a. Kiellands
b. Outlet
c. Piper
d. Das forceps

26. Post-term pregnancy is:
a. Beyond 42 weeks
b. Beyond 41 weeks
c. Between 40 and 41 weeks
d. At 40 weeks

27. Identify the condition: ***(Most Recent Question Jan 2023)***

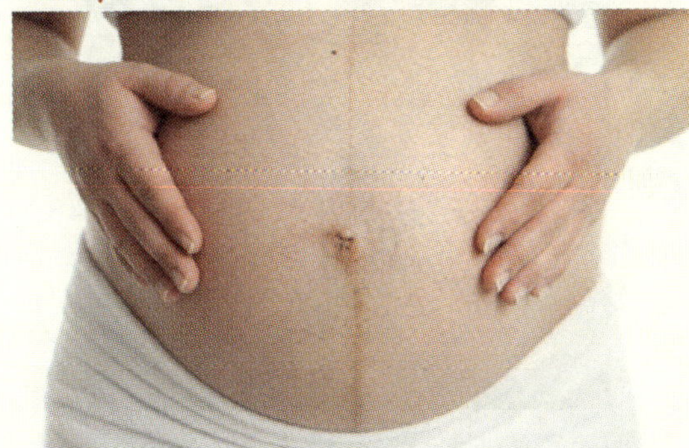

a. Linea alba
b. Linea nigra
c. Stria gravidarum
d. Cloasma

28. All of the following parameters are part of obstetric audit; except: ***(Most Recent Question Jan 2023)***
a. Fetal death
b. Injury to mother
c. Injury to fetal head
d. Preterm labor

29. Best ultrasound parameter for assessment of gestational age is: ***(Most Recent Question Jan 2023)***
a. Crown-rump length
b. Biparietal Diameter
c. Femur length
d. Sacral length

30. Order of lochia is: ***(Most Recent Question Jan 2023)***
a. Lochia rubra – lochia serosa – lochia alba
b. Lochia alba – lochia rubra – lochia serosa
c. Lochia serosa – lochia alba – lochia rubra
d. All of the above

31. A lady presents with thin frothy discharge with erythematous cervix. On saline microscopy, motility of organism is seen. What is the diagnosis?
a. Trichomonas vaginitis
b. Candida vaginitis
c. Chlamydial vaginitis
d. Bacterial vaginosis

32. All of the following are contraindications of normal vaginal delivery; except: ***(Most Recent Question Jan 2023)***
a. Previous 2 LSCS
b. Central placenta previa
c. Previous classic CS
d. Previous macrosomia

33. A lady presents with a history of lower abdominal pain and restricted movements. Laparoscopy shows pus at the fimbria ends of the fallopian tube. What is the most likely diagnosis? ***(Most Recent Question Jan 2023)***
a. Pelvic inflammatory disease
b. Endometriosis
c. Ovarian cancer
d. Cervical cancer

34. A pregnant female presented in 2nd trimester. She has a 2-year-old child. Which of the following is recommended dose of tetanus for the pregnant female? ***(Most Recent Question Jan 2023)***
a. TT dose 2 doses
b. TT dose 3 doses
c. TT booster
d. Td booster

35. A 50-year-old female presented with cervical cancer stage I-B. What is the management of this case? ***(Most Recent Question Jan 2023)***
a. Type 1 hysterectomy
b. Type 2 hysterectomy
c. Type 3 hysterectomy
d. Type 4 hysterectomy

36. Just after delivery, uterus is at the level of: ***(Most Recent Question Jan 2023)***
a. Above symphysis pubis
b. Above umbilicus
c. Below symphysis pubis
d. Below umbilicus

37. LH surge is due to: ***(Most Recent Question Jan 2023)***
a. Progesterone
b. LH
c. Estradiol
d. HCG

38. A lady presents with blood pressure 146/90 mmHg at 34 weeks gestation. What is the next step? ***(Most Recent Question Jan 2023)***
a. CBC
b. LFT
c. USG
d. Urine dipstick test

39. A patient comes with complaints of dysmenorrhea and dyspareunia. Speculum examination reveals bluish powder burn lesion on the cervix and nodularity felt on bimanual examination in the pouch of Douglas. What is the possible diagnosis? ***(Most Recent Question Jan 2023)***
a. Endometriosis
b. Adenomyosis
c. Fibroid
d. Polycystic ovarian syndrome

40. A primigravida gives birth to a male child without any complication for the mother or the neonate. After how many hours she should start the breastfeeding?
a. After 4–6 hours
b. Within 1 hour
c. Within 8–14 hours
d. After 1 day

41. The shown laparoscopic procedure is done for which condition? ***(Most Recent Question Jan 2023)***

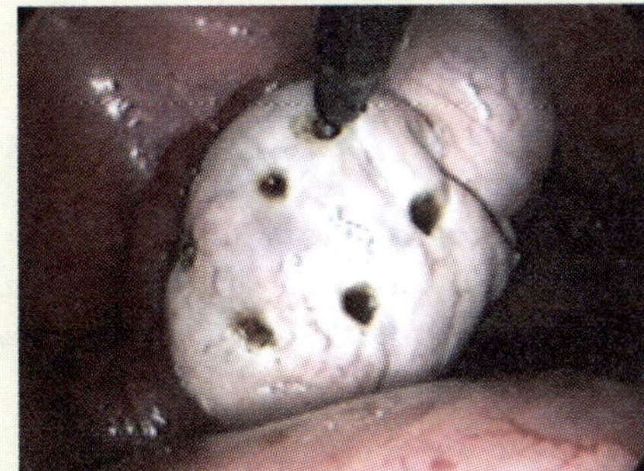

a. PCOS
b. OHSS
c. Chocolate cyst
d. Fallopian tube cyst

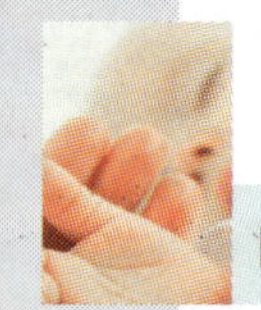

42. The shown aspirator is required for: ***(Most Recent Question Jan 2023)***

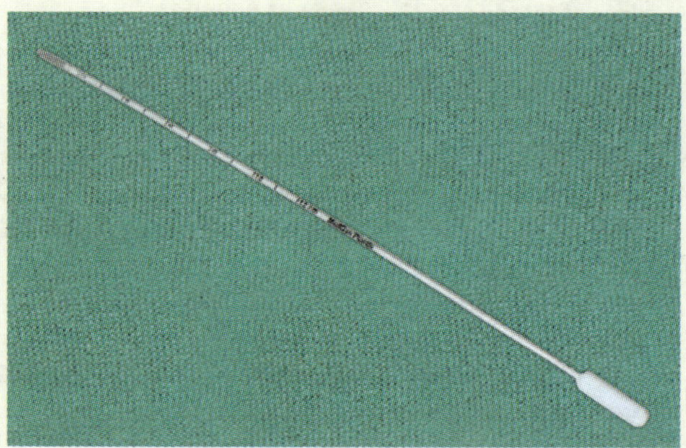

a. Endometrial biopsy
b. Cervical biopsy
c. Tubal aspiration of ectopic pregnancy
d. Termination of pregnancy

43. Fracturing clavicle to facilitate delivery of baby is: ***(Most Recent Question Jan 2023)***

a. Craniotomy
b. Symphysiotomy
c. Episiotomy
d. Cleidotomy

44. Half-life of Copper T 380A is: ***(Most Recent Question Jan 2023)***

a. 5 years b. 2 years
c. 10 years d. 1 years

45. The most common site of ectopic pregnancy is: ***(Most Recent Question Jan 2023)***

a. Ampulla b. Isthmus
c. Intramural d. Infundibular

ANATOMY AND PHYSIOLOGY

46. A couple came to clinic with complaint of infertility. On examination her husband had gynecomastia and tall stature. What is the possible diagnosis? ***(Most Recent Question June 2022)***

a. Klinefelter's syndrome
b. Turners syndrome
c. Swyer syndrome
d. Testicular feminization syndrome

47. Location of the bartholin's gland opening/Bartholin cyst: ***(Most Recent Question June/Dec 2021)***

a. Vestibule
b. Vagina
c. Sub urethral
d. Peri anal

48. A young girl with complaints of not attaining menarche presents with periodic abdominal pain to the hospital. On examination the following presentation (image) is seen. What is the likely lesion this girl is suffering from? ***(Most Recent Question June/Dec 2021)***

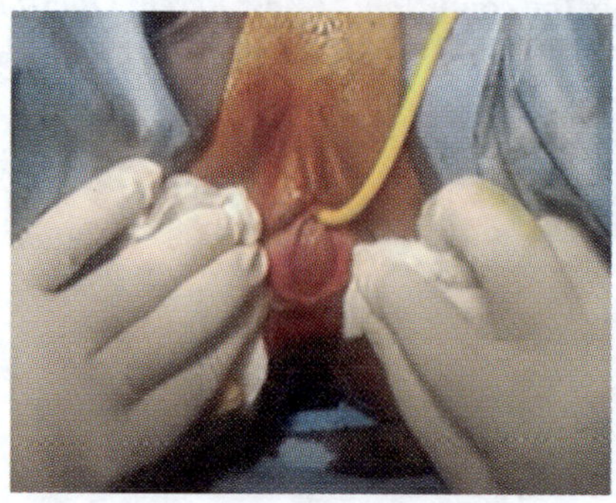

a. Imperforate hymen image b. Bartholin cyst
c. Gartners cyst d. Septate uterus

49. Epithelium of the fallopian tube; ***(Most Recent Question June/Dec 2021)***

a. Stratified squamous b. Cuboidal
c. Ciliated columnar d. Pseudo stratified columnar

50. Secondary amenorrhea after 3 months of abortion due to, serum FSH: 67 IU/L: ***(Most Recent Question June/Dec 2021)***

a. Sheehans syndrome b. Fresh pregnancy
c. Premature ovarian failure d. Asherman's syndrome

51. 16-year-old girl with primary amenorrhea. Ssc well developed. On examination there is bluish bulging hymen. What is the best management? ***(Most Recent Question June/Dec 2021)***

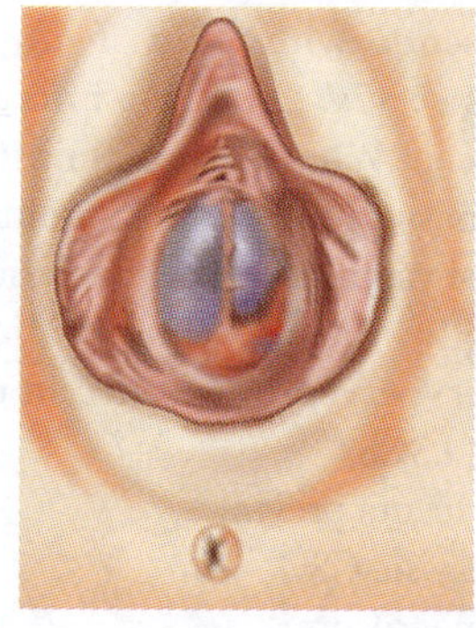

a. Cruciate incision and drainage of blood
b. Long term treatment with estrogen
c. b/l gonadectomy d. OCP

52. Which type of pelvis is associated with persistent op position? ***(Most Recent Question June/Dec 2021)***

a. Android pelvis b. Anthropoid pelvis
c. Gynecoid pelvis d. Platypelloid pelvis

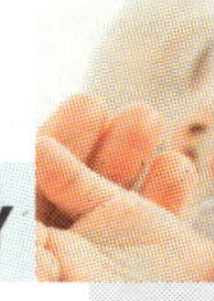

53. Identify shown HSG image:

(Most Recent Question Aug 2020)

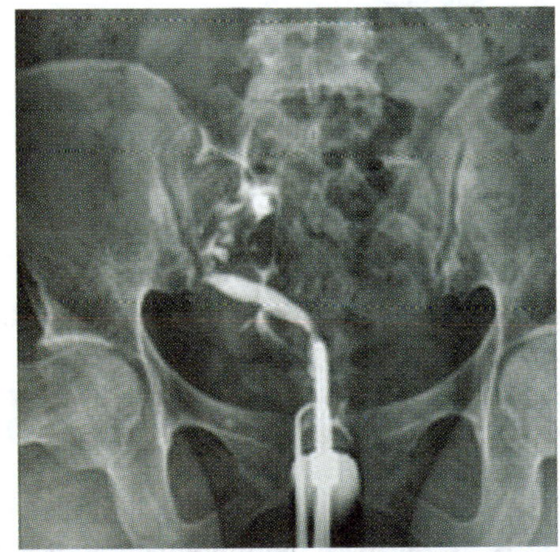

a. Unicornuate uterus b. Bicornuate uterus
c. Septate uterus d. Didelphys

54. Double decidual sign is seen in:

(Most Recent Question Dec 2019-20)

a. Uterine gestational sac b. Pseudo gestational sac
c. Threatened abortion d. None of the above

55. On the basis of given image. What is your diagnosis?

(Most Recent Question Dec 2019-20)

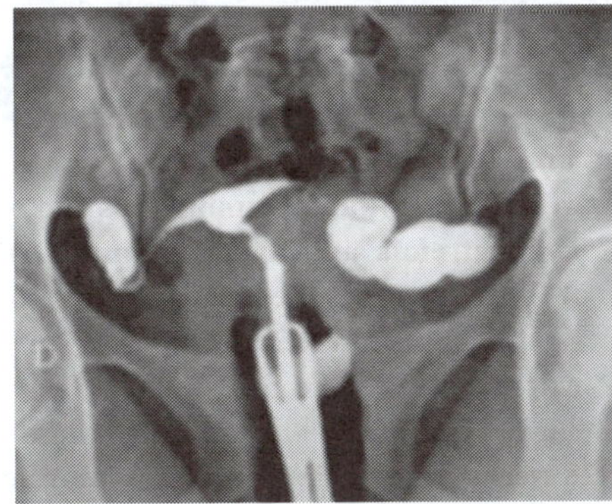

a. Hydrosalpinx b. Cornual block
c. Adnexal mass d. None of these

56. Most dependent part in a sitting female?

(Most Recent Question Dec 2019-20)

a. Pouch of Douglas b. Paracolic gutter
c. Hepatorenal pouch d. None of these

57. Testosterone secreted by:

(Most Recent Question Dec 2019-20)

a. Leydig cell b. Sertoli cell
c. Theca lutein d. Granulosa cell

58. True conjugate is? *(Most Recent Question Dec 2019-20)*

a. Lower border of pubic symphysis to sacral promontory
b. Upper border of pubic symphysis to sacral promontory
c. Posterior border of pubic symphysis to sacral promontory
d. Lower border of symphysis to ischial spine

59. In this normal menstrual cycle graph, the mark 'X' graph is due to: *(Most Recent Question 2019)*

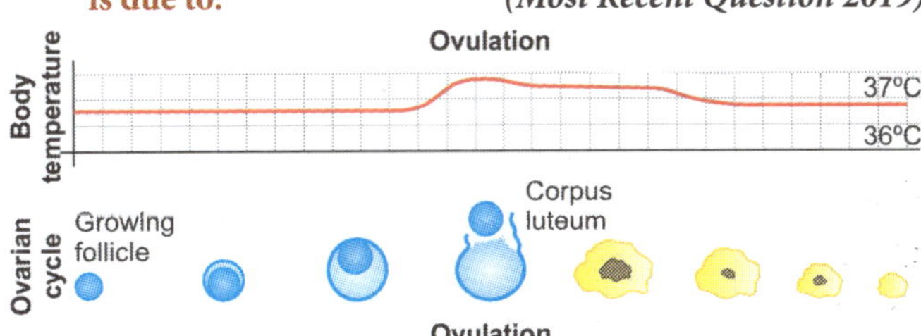

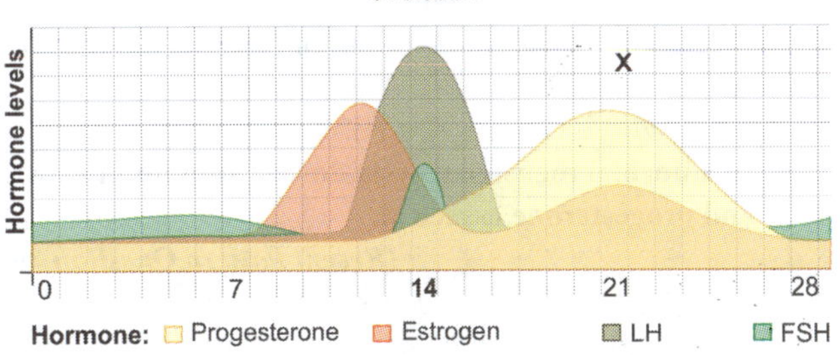

a. LH b. FSH
c. Estrogen d. Progesterone

60. Beta hCG is secreted by:

(Recent Pattern Question 2018-19)

a. Yolk sac b. Placenta
c. Syncytiotrophoblast d. Umbilical cord

61. Constipation in pregnancy is due to:

(Recent Pattern Question 2017)

a. Uterus enlargement b. Estrogen effect
c. Progesterone effect d. Excessive micturition

62. During pregnancy urine frequency increases in which trimester? *(Recent Pattern Question 2017)*

a. T1 b. T2
c. T3 d. Puerperium

63. Change in BMR(%) during pregnancy:

(Recent Pattern Question 2017)

a. Rise by 25% b. Fall by 25%
c. Rise by 50% d. Fall by 50%

64. Which is the largest diameter of fetal head?

(Recent Pattern Question 2017)

a. Mentovertical b. Occipitofrontal
c. Submentobregmatic d. Suboccipitofrontal

65. Placenta develops completely by—age of gestation:

(Recent Pattern Question 2016)

a. 3 weeks b. 4 weeks
c. 6 weeks d. 12 weeks

66. Vessel which disappears in placenta:

(Recent Pattern Question 2016)

a. Left umbilical artery b. Left umbilical vein
c. Right umbilical vein d. Right umbilical artery

67. Blood is carried from placenta to inferior vena cava through: *(Recent Pattern Question 2016)*

a. Ductus arteriosus b. Ductus venosus
c. Right umbilical vein d. Left umbilical vein

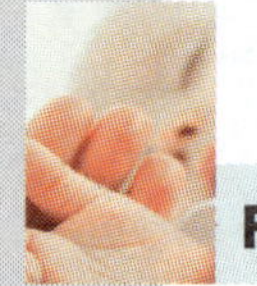

68. Which of the following decreases during pregnancy *(Recent Pattern Question 2016)*
a. Systemic venous resistance
b. CO
c. HR
d. Plasma volume

69. Normal pH of vagina *(Recent Pattern Question 2016)*
a. 2–2.5 b. 3.5–4.5
c. 4.5–5.5 d. 5.0–6.5

70. Nulliparous cervix: body uterus ratio *(Recent Pattern Question 2016)*
a. 50–50 b. 60–40
c. 30–70 d. 70–30

71. In a normal menstrual cycle, lowest amount of estrogen and progesterone is seen at: *(Recent Pattern Question 2016)*
a. Follicular phase b. Ovulation
c. At beginning of menses d. Secretory phase

72. True support of uterus:
a. Broad ligament b. Round ligament
c. Cardinal ligament d. Uterosacral ligament

73. Which gland opens on posterolateral margin of vaginal opening:
a. Skene gland b. Cooper gland
c. Bartholin's gland d. Bulbourethral gland

74. Which is the smallest transverse diameter of fetal head:
a. Biparietal b. Bitemporal
c. Bimastoid d. Super subparietal

75. Shortest diameter of pelvic outlet:
a. Anteroposterior b. Intertuberous
c. Oblique d. Interspinous

76. Largest diameter of pelvic inlet:
a. Transverse b. True conjugate
c. Oblique d. Bituberous

77. What is the least diameter of pelvic inlet? *(Recent Pattern Question 2017)*
a. Sacrococcygeal b. Pubococcygeal
c. Transverse d. Sacrocotyloid

78. Prominent iliac spine is seen in which type of pelvis:
a. Gynaecoid b. Platypelloid
c. Android d. Anthropoid

79. Which of the following is not increased during pregnancy:
a. Plasma volume b. RBC count
c. Platelet count d. Hemoglobin

80. In pregnancy which clotting factor will be decreased:
a. Factor II b. Factor V
c. Factor VII d. Factor XI

81. Most common cause of secondary amenorrhea
a. Turner syndrome b. Pregnancy
c. Mullerian agenesis d. Kallmann syndrome

82. When is the best time to do breast self-exam?
a. 3 days after menstruation
b. 3 days before menstruation
c. During menstruation
d. During ovulation

83. When is the time for ovulation:
a. 14 days after menstruation
b. Along with LH surge
c. 1 week before menstruation
d. 2 weeks before next menstruation

84. Oxygenated blood from placenta goes to fetal heart via:
a. Ductus arteriosus b. Ductus venosus
c. Foramen ovale d. Umbilical artery

85. Which of the following closes before birth:
a. Ductus arteriosus b. Ductus venosus
c. Cardinal vein d. Umbilical vein

86. Uterus is at the level of umbilicus at which age of gestation:
a. 12 weeks b. 22 weeks
c. 20 weeks d. 24 weeks

87. Oxytocin will not do the following action:
a. Milk production
b. Milk let down
c. Contraction of myo-epithelial cells
d. Vascular contraction

EMBRYOLOGY

88. Infant brought to the casualty with dehydration and tachycardia. The genitalia is ambiguous and blood work shows hyponatremia and hyperkalemia. Deficiency of which of the following is the reason for this condition ? *(Most Recent Question June/Dec 2021)*
a. 17 hydroxyprogesterone b. 3-B HSD
c. 11-B hydroxylase d. 21 hydroxylase

89. After 28 weeks AOG major amount of amniotic fluid is secreted from: *(Recent Pattern Question 2018-19)*
a. Fetal skin b. Fetal urine
c. Placental cell membrane d. Plasma

90. In a general population, the screening of Down syndrome is done by: *(Recent Pattern Question 2018)*
a. USG
b. Serum biomarkers
c. Chorionic villus sampling
d. Amniocentesis

91. Which of the following is best done for intrapartum fetal monitoring? *(Recent Pattern Question 2018)*
a. Fetal echocardiography
b. Fetal scalp pH
c. Continuous electrical fetal monitoring
d. Physical examination

92. Amniocentesis is best done by:

(Recent Pattern Question 2018)

a. 10–11 weeks b. 12–13 weeks
c. 15–18 weeks d. 20–35 weeks

93. Size of graffican follicle at the time of ovulation:

a. 10 mm b. 15 mm
c. 20 mm d. 25 mm

94. Which of the following is not related with fertilization:

a. Sperm crosses corona radiata
b. Implantation after 6 days
c. Zona pellucida facilitation by hyaluronidase
d. Zona reaction attracts the sperms

95. What is the function of zona pellucida?

(Recent Pattern Question 2017)

a. Prevent wrong implantation of embryo
b. Formation of blastocyst
c. Prevention of multiple sperm entry
d. Prevent wrong attachment of sperm

96. Which of the following is a true statement:

a. Placenta is formed at morula stage
b. Implantation starts on 10th day
c. During initial weeks corpus luteum survival is due to LH
d. Fertilization takes place in ampula

97. Implantation occurs after fertilization:

a. 5–6 days b. 7–8 days
c. 8–10 days d. 10–12 days

98. Gestational sac can be visualized via USG by:

a. 4 weeks b. 5 weeks
c. 8 weeks d. 10 weeks

99. Corpus luteum formation occurs on ________ of menstrual cycle:

a. 15th day b. 22nd day
c. 1st day d. 28th day

100. Doubling of Beta hCG levels is seen in:

a. 24 hours b. 48 hours
c. 72 hours d. 96 hours

101. Placental blood supply is established on:

(Recent Pattern Question 2016)

a. 2nd week b. 3rd week
c. 5th week d. 8th week

102. Labia minora is homologous to which organ in males?

(Recent Pattern Question 2017)

a. Glans penis b. Scrotum
c. Corpus cavernosa d. Penile urethra

103. Inferior 1/3rd of vagina is derived from:

(Recent Pattern Question 2017)

a. Metanephric bud b. Urogenital sinus
c. Mullerian duct d. Genital fold

104. When is the embryo termed as fetus?

(Recent Pattern Question 2017)

a. End of 7th week
b. After 10 weeks from LMP
c. End of 8th week after LMP
d. From end of 2nd trimester

105. Fertilization most commonly occurs at:

(Recent Pattern Question 2017)

a. Ampulla b. Interstitium
c. Isthmus d. Uterine cavity

106. When does Haematopoiesis shift to liver from yolk sac:

a. 10 weeks b. 12 weeks
c. 16 weeks d. 20 weeks

107. Maximum number of oogonia:

a. 6 million b. 4 million
c. 5 million d. 7 million

108. 1st polar body is released at the time of:

a. Birth b. Puberty
c. Menstruation d. Fertilization

109. What is released at the time of ovulation:

a. 1st polar body b. Primary oocyte
c. Female pronucleus d. 2nd polar body

110. Ovulation occurs after the extrusion of:

a. Primary oocyte b. Female pronucleus
c. 1st polar body d. 2nd polar body

111. Maternal side of placenta is derived from which layer:

a. Decidua basalis b. Zona capsularis
c. Zona parietalis d. Inner cell mass

112. True about fetal surface of placenta:

a. Derived from decidua basalis
b. It has spongy and rough surface
c. It has umbilical cord attachment site
d. It has cotyledons

LABOR AND DELIVERY

113. Ritodrine to prevent premature labor will cause all of the complications in mother; EXCEPT?

(Most Recent Question June 2022)

a. Tachycardia b. Hypotension
c. Tremor d. Pulmonary edema

114. What is the reason for abdominal pain to the mother when she is breast feeding her baby?

(Most Recent Question June/Dec 2021)

a. Prolactin b. Estrogen
c. Progesterone d. Oxytocin

115. Women with history of previous cs presented with prolonged labor. Patient is hypotensive. Fhr is not audible, fetal parts are easily palpable on pa examination, what is the diagnosis?

(Most Recent Question June/Dec 2021)

a. Abruption
b. Uterine rupture
c. Fetal intrauterine death
d. Uterine Synechiae

116. Complication associated with iv bolus oxytocin?

(Most Recent Question June/Dec 2021)

a. Hypotension b. Hypoglycemia
c. Hyperglycemia d. Hypertension

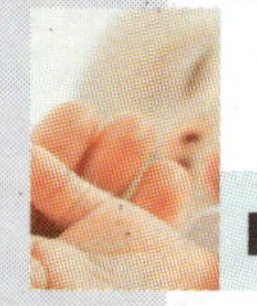

117. An intern conducting delivery observes mother developing abdominal pains breathlessness, hypotension, tachycardia and collapsing. Shock is out of proportion to bleeding. Examination reveals large boggy mass at the introitus. Possible cause:
(Most Recent Question June/Dec 2021)

a. PPH
b. Uterine inversion
c. DIC
d. Amniotic Fluid Embolism

118. A 25-year-old women visits labor room at 37 weeks. Pt. has mild labor pain for 10 hours and cervix is persistently 1 cm dilated and uneffaced. Management?
(Most Recent Question June/Dec 2021)

a. ISCS
b. Arm
c. Sedation and wait
d. Augmentation with oxytocin

119. Which of the following is used for dilation of cervix?
(Most Recent Question Aug 2020)

a. Mifepristone
b. Misoprotosol
c. Laminaria tent
d. Carboprost

120. Identify the given maneuver shown in image?
(Most Recent Question Dec 2019-20)

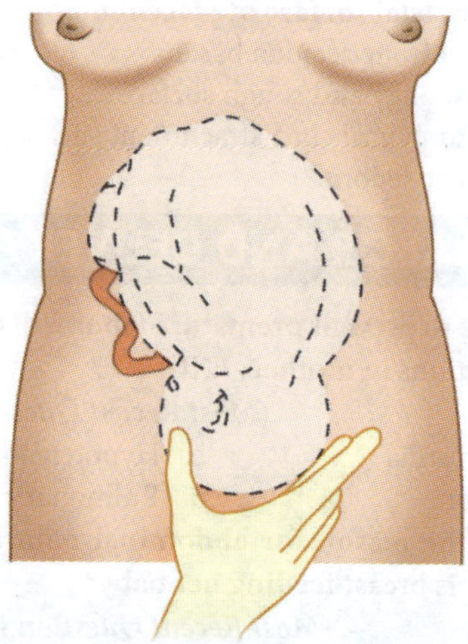

a. Leopold 1
b. Leopold 2
c. Leopold 3
d. Leopold 4

121. A patient is in labor, on per vaginal examination cervix is 5 cm dilated and fully effaced. She is in which stage of labor:
(Most Recent Question Dec 2019-20)

a. First stage
b. Second stage
c. Third stage
d. Fourth stage

122. After a normal delivery in a 27-year-old female placenta is still attached with uterus. Most common complication which can occur due to forceful traction of cord?
(Most Recent Question Dec 2019-20)

a. Haemorrhage
b. Uterine inversion
c. Uterine rupture
d. Placenta retraction

123. A lady with 36 weeks pregnancy with previous 3 C-section presented with low BP, tachycardia and on USG fluid present in peritoneum. What is diagnosis and next management: *(Most Recent Question Dec 2019-20)*

a. Uterine scar rupture and laparotomy
b. Normal labor and Laparoscopy
c. Ectopic pregnancy and abortion
d. Fetal death and abortion

124. Angle of cut in episiotomy

a. 30 degrees to the midline
b. 60 degrees to the midline
c. 90 degrees to the midline
d. 15 degrees to the midline

125. A grand multipara is a women who has given birth to births: *(Most Recent Question 2019)*

a. >2
b. >3
c. >4
d. >5

126. A 32-year-old pregnant female presented with 34-week pregnancy with complaints of pain in the abdomen, and decreased fetal movements. Upon examination, BP = 90/60, FHR = 100, upon per vaginum examination there is blood seen and cervix is closed. What is the preferred management? *(Recent Pattern Question 2018-19)*

a. Tocolytics
b. Induce labor
c. Immediate LSCS
d. Wait and watch

127. Uterus relaxation in order to delay the labor is caused by:
(Recent Pattern Question 2018)

a. Ritodrine
b. Tolterodine
c. Oxytocin
d. Labetalol

128. Which of the following the presenting part in the fetus in left occiput anterior (LOA) position:
(Recent Pattern Question 2018)

a. Suboccipito-bregmatic
b. Submentoverical
c. Brow
d. Vertex

129. Pacemaker of uterine contraction is located at:

a. Fundus
b. Anterior wall
c. Posterior wall
d. Tubal ostia

130. 1/5 head is palpable suprapubic. True statement regarding this is: *(Recent Pattern Question 2016)*

a. Brow presentation
b. 1/5 of head at pelvic brim
c. Fetal head is engaged
d. 1/5th of the head below ischial spine

131. According to the rule of 5th, when is the fetal head engagement:

a. $1/5^{th}$ of the fetal head palpable
b. $2/5^{th}$ of the fetal head palpable
c. $3/5^{th}$ of the fetal head palpable
d. $4/5^{th}$ of the fetal head palpable

132. Moulding of fetal head *(Recent Pattern Question 2016)*

a. Disappears in few weeks
b. Can damage brain
c. No alteration in shape of head
d. Complicates the delivery

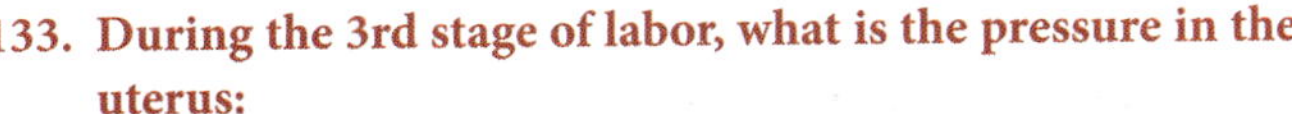

133. During the 3rd stage of labor, what is the pressure in the uterus:

a. 30–40 mm Hg b. 100–120 mm Hg
c. 80–100 mm Hg d. 40–60 mm Hg

134. Pressure inside uterus during early phase of active labor:

a. 50 mm Hg b. 100 mm Hg
c. 150 mm Hg d. 200 mm Hg

135. Duration of 2nd stage of labor in primigravida:

a. 30 minutes b. 2 hours
c. 15 minutes d. 4 hours

136. To monitor fetal heart rate in a normal delivery partogram, it should be repeated every:

a. 30 minutes b. 1 hours
c. 2 hours d. 90 minutes

137. While doing partogram, pelvic examination is done at:

a. 30 minutes b. 1 hours
c. 2 hours d. 4 hours

138. Peak of prostaglandins occurs in what stage:

a. 1st stage of labor b. 2nd stage of labor
c. 3rd stage of labor d. Before 1st stage of labor

139. Amniotic fluid at term:

a. 1000–1200 mL b. 800–1000 mL
c. 1200–1500 mL d. 700–800 mL

140. Amniotic fluid is maximum at:

a. 22–26 weeks b. 34–36 weeks
c. 38–40 weeks d. 40–42 weeks

141. Bishop score includes all; EXCEPT:

a. Cervical consistency b. Dilatation of cervix
c. Position of cervix d. Cervical shape

142. Most common fractured bone during birth is:

a. Humerus b. Scapula
c. Clavicle d. Radius

143. Cord compression leads to:

a. Late deceleration b. Early deceleration
c. Variable deceleration d. Acceleration

144. Late deceleration is due to:

a. Head compression
b. Cord compression
c. Uteroplacental insufficiency
d. All of the above

145. Identify the progress of partogram:

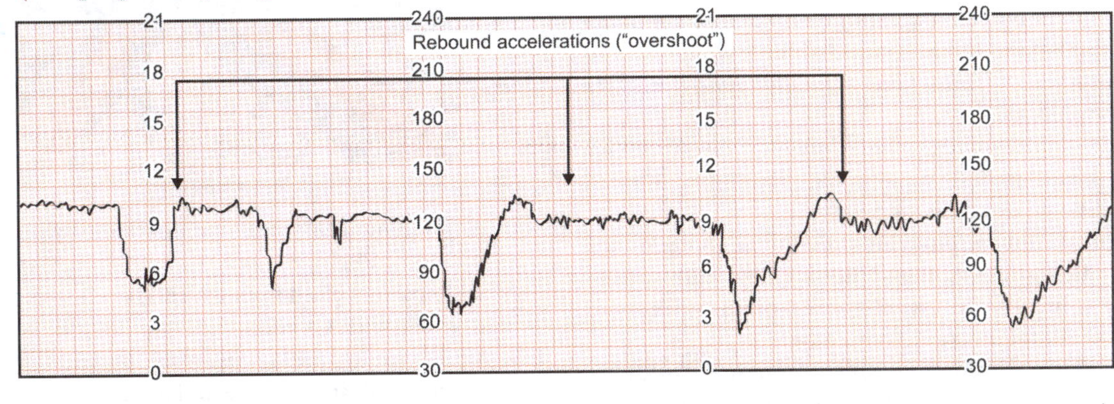

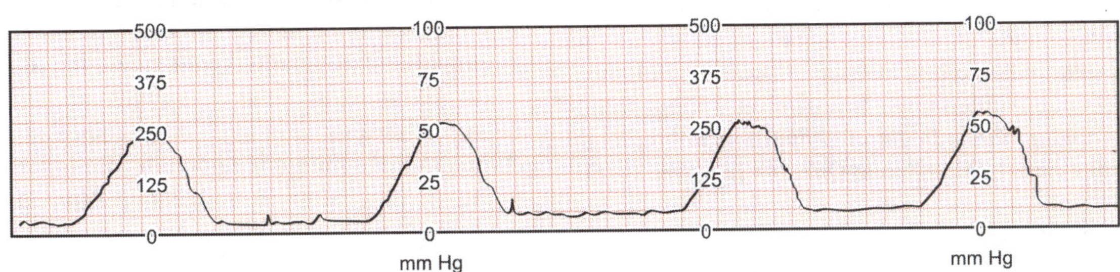

a. Early deceleration b. Variable deceleration c. Late deceleration d. Normal partogram

146. As compared to mediolateral episiotomy, median episiotomy has complications because of:

a. Poor repair b. Cosmetic problem
c. Extension to rectum d. More blood loss

147. Arrest disorder is defined as the cessation of cervical dilatation in active phase of labor of more than:

a. 1 hour b. 1.2 hours
c. 1.5 hours d. 2 hours

ANTEPARTUM AND POSTPARTUM PERIOD

148. What is the recommended dose of folic acid in a female with a history of NTD in last pregnancy ?

(Most Recent Question June/Dec 2021)

a. 4 mg b. 0.4 mg
c. 0.1 mg d. 1 mg

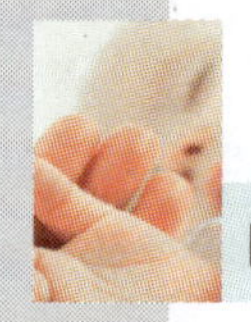

149. Maximum amniotic fluid is seen at which gestational age? *(Most Recent Question June/Dec 2021)*
a. 36 weeks
b. 40 weeks
c. 28 weeks
d. 20 weeks

150. Minimum prenatal visits *(Most Recent Question June/Dec 2021)*
a. 3
b. 4
c. 5
d. 6

151. Cardiac output comes to normal after how many days after delivery? *(Most Recent Question June/Dec 2021)*
a. 45 days
b. 21 days
c. 10 days
d. 15 days

152. Which of the following conditions require a serial determination of pregnancy test? *(Most Recent Question June/Dec 2021)*
a. Rh incompatibility
b. Molar pregnancy
c. Viability of pregnancy
d. Gender identification

153. A G2P2 postpartum presents with few weeks of spotting and history of bleeding per vaginum since 3 months now comes with heavy bleeding. She gives h/o d and c in some other hospital but still continues to bleed. What could be the reason? *(Most Recent Question June/Dec 2021)*
a. Normal lochia
b. DIC
c. Retained placenta
d. Gestational trophoblastic neoplasia

154. A pregnant women comes for check up at 18 weeks. On examination she was found uterine size corresponds to only 16 weeks. On usg, oligohydraminos was found. Which of the following is likely cause? *(Most Recent Question June/Dec 2021)*
a. Fetal anemia
b. Anencephaly
c. Renal agenesis
d. IUGR

155. An intern conducting delivery observes mother developing breathlessness, hypotension, tachycardia and collapsing. Shock is out of proportion to bleeding what is the cause? *(Most Recent Question June/Dec 2021)*
a. PPH
b. Uterine inversion
c. DIC
d. Placenta previa

156. A Lady presented 5 days after normal vaginal delivery with heaviness in breast. She complaints that her baby is unable to latch on for breastfeeding. The most likely reason amongst the following for this is? *(Most Recent Question Aug 2020)*
a. Lactation failure
b. Breast engorgement
c. Breast abscess
d. Mastitis

157. A patient presented with secondary amenorrhea, 3 months postdelivery. Before surgical intervention is considered, which of the following can be done? *(Most Recent Question Aug 2020)*
a. OCP to induce a cycle
b. Pulsatile GnRH to stimulate the ovary
c. Progesterone to give a 'withdrawal bleeding'
d. Assurance

158. Where is the common obstetric/gynaecological condition where this procedure done? *(Most Recent Question Aug 2020)*

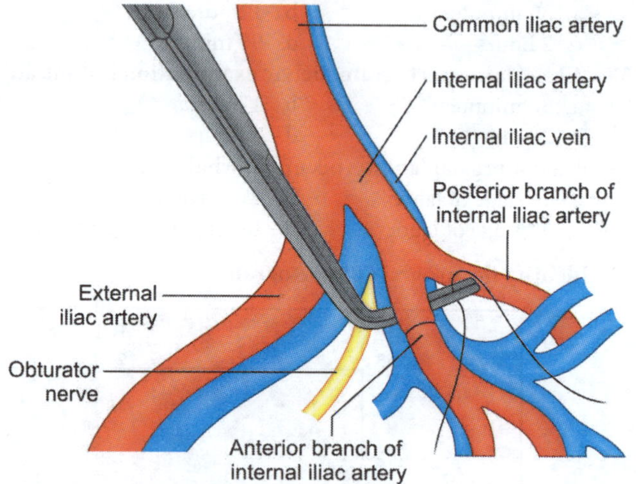

a. Dysfunctional bleed after hysterectomy
b. Atonic PPH
c. Recurrent bleed from CA cervix
d. Bleed from Ca vulva

159. A 38-year-old P3L3 woman presents with severe secondary dysmenorrhea and on USG there is a uniform enlargement of uterus up to 10 weeks. What is the provisional diagnosis? *(Most Recent Question Aug 2020)*
a. Adenomyosis
b. PID
c. Leiomyoma
d. Endometriosis

160. Which is the hormone responsible for lactation? *(Most Recent Question Aug 2020)*
a. LH
b. FSH
c. GH
d. Oxytocin

161. A 35-year-old lady with 4 children, after 5th normal vaginal delivery, had excessive bleeding after placenta removal. This is most likely due to: *(Most Recent Question Dec 2019-20)*
a. Estrogen deficiency
b. Progesterone deficiency
c. Excessive uterine contraction
d. Post-partum hemorrhage

162. EDD calculated by: *(Recent Pattern Question 2018-19)*
a. Young's rule b. Naegele's formula
c. Cardiff formula d. Hadlock formula

163. True sign of placental separation are all; EXCEPT:
(Recent Pattern Question 2018)
a. Gush of blood
b. Raised fundal height
c. Lengthening of cord
d. Discoid uterus

164. Which is correct about iron status in pregnancy?
(Recent Pattern Question 2016)
a. Serum iron is increased
b. TIBC increased
c. Serum ferritin increased
d. Serum iron: TIBC ratio increased

165. Lactiferous duct of breast contraction is due to
(Recent Pattern Question 2016)
a. Progesterone b. Estrogen
c. Oxytocin d. Prolactin

166. First investigation to be done for screening the presence of fetus:
a. TVS b. TAS
c. MRI d. Doppler

167. Placental circulation is established by:
a. 15 days b. 16 days
c. 21 days d. 25 days

168. A 35 year primigravida visited your clinic. USG given below: What is the diagnosis?

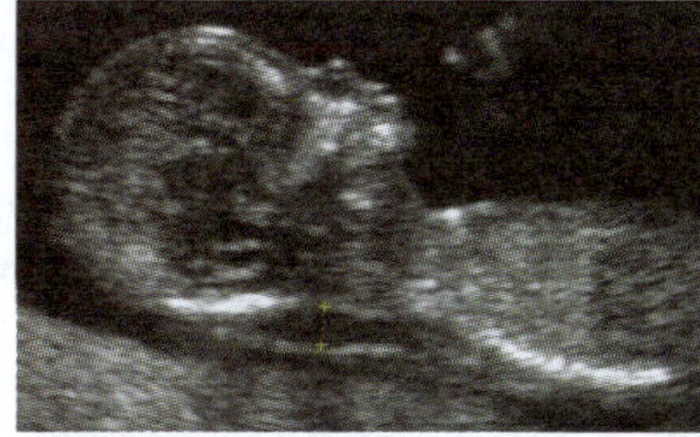

a. Anencephaly b. Holoprocencephaly
c. Nuchal translucency d. Hydrocephaly

169. Iron and folic acid supplement during pregnancy:
a. 500 mg iron + 100 mcg folic acid
b. 100 mg iron + 500 mcg folic acid
c. 100 mg iron + 100 mcg folic acid
d. 20 mg iron + 100 mcg folic acid

170. Test which identifies fetal well being by detecting fetal heart rate acceleration and fetal movement:
a. Bio-Physical profile b. Stress test
c. Non-stress test d. Contraction stress test

171. Biophysical profile scoring includes all; EXCEPT:
a. FHR deceleration b. Fetal breathing
c. Fetal movement d. Amniotic fluid

172. Length of lower uterine segment at term:
a. 5 cm b. 10–12 cm
c. 15 cm d. 20 cm

173. Hegar sign is seen earliest at:
a. 6 weeks b. 10 weeks
c. 14 weeks d. 15 weeks

174. Jacquemier's sign of pregnancy occurs in which week:
a. 6th week b. 8th week
c. 10th week d. 12th week

175. LMP of patient is 30 June 2015, EDD is__:
a. 7 March, 2016 b. 7 April, 2016
c. 30 March, 2016 d. 30 April, 2016

176. Lochia lasts for:
a. 5 days b. 2 weeks
c. 3 weeks d. 4 weeks

177. The most common site of puerperal infection is:
a. Placental site b. Cervical laceration
c. Episiotomy wound d. Vaginal laceration

178. Following are signs of placental separation; EXCEPT:
a. Uterus rises in abdomen
b. Uterus becomes discoid
c. Lengthening of cord
d. Fresh gush of blood from the vagina

179. Which of the following is a sign of placental separation in stage III of labor:
a. Gushing of blood
b. Discoid uterus
c. Filling of placenta in vagina
d. Increase in blood pressure

180. The signs and symptoms of placental separation include all of the following; EXCEPT:
a. Raised fundal height
b. Fundus of uterus below umbilicus
c. Gush of Vaginal bleeding
d. Lengthening of cord

181. Common cause of 3rd day Puerperal fever:
a. Breast Engorgement b. UTI
c. Puerperal sepsis d. Pulmonary

182. What is the most common cause of maternal mortality in India?
a. Hemorrhage b. Obstructed Labor
c. Cardiac arrest d. Anemia

183. Most common indirect cause of maternal mortality:
a. Sepsis b. Hemorrhage
c. Obstructed labor d. Anemia

184. Which of the following is the cause of amenorrhoea in a lactating mother:
a. Increased release of LH b. Increased GnRH secretion
c. Hyperestrogenic state d. Increased prolactin level

185. Weight of uterus immediately after delivery:
a. 60 g b. 500 g
c. 1000 g d. 800 g

186. Heart rate returns to normal after delivery:
a. Immediately b. 4 weeks
c. 4 hours after d. 6 weeks

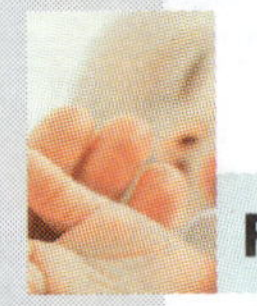

187. Cardiac output return to normal how many days after delivery:

a. 1 hour b. 4 hours
c. 2 weeks d. 4 weeks

188. The uterus becomes pelvic organ how many days after normal delivery:

a. 5–7 days b. 12–14 days
c. 16–18 days d. 20–22 days

189. Blood loss of fetal origin:

a. Placenta previa b. Vasa previa
c. Abruption Placenta d. Circumvallate placenta

190. A pregnant patient after delivery presented with hemorrhage. Immediate hysterectomy is done in:

a. Pre-eclampsia b. Rupture of uterus
c. Atonic uterus d. Inversion of uterus

191. During delivery there is a perineal tear involving the anal sphincter but anal mucosa is not involved. Which is the degree of tear?

a. I b. II
c. III d. IV

ABORTION AND THIRD TRIMESTER BLEEDING

192. Drugs for medical abortion:
(Most Recent Question June/Dec 2021)

a. Mifepristone 200 mg and methotrexate after 48 hours
b. Misoprostol 200 mg and methotrexate after 48 hours
c. Mifepristone 200 mg and misoprostol 800 microgram after 48 hours
d. Misoprostol 200 mg + mifepristone 400 microgram after 48 hours

193. Ultrasound image of the uterus show a snowstorm's appearance? ***(Most Recent Question June/Dec 2021)***

a. Hydatidiform mole b. Partial mole
c. Choriocarcinoma d. Adenomyosis

194. Most common cause of DIC?
(Most Recent Question June/Dec 2021)

a. Twin pregnancy b. Abruption
c. GDM d. Pre-eclampsia

195. A 26-year gravida 3 female with history of 3 previous mid trimester abortions present at 22 weeks of gestation with cervical length of 15/mm. What could be the possible cause of her miscarriage?
(Most Recent Question June/Dec 2021)

a. Cervical incompetence
b. Uterine anomaly
c. Hormonal disturbance
d. Chromosomal malformation

196. A 14-week-old pregnant women came to the OPD for MTP. What is the dose of misoprostol to be given with mifepristone? ***(Most Recent Question Aug 2020)***

a. 800 mcg vaginally b. 400 mcg vaginally
c. 200 mcg vaginally d. 100 mcg vaginally

197. A patient presented with bleeding per vaginum in labor and a 'tender tense' abdomen on palpation. Her BP is 150/100. Cervical dilation 5 cm and full effacement. Fetal heart rate is 144/min with adequate beat to beat variability. What is the likely diagnosis?
(Most Recent Question Aug 2020)

a. Abruptio placentae b. Placenta accreta
c. Placenta previa d. Vasa previa

198. G2P1L1 lady underwent LSCS in previous pregnancy for fetal distress. This time she had an uneventful vaginal birth after caesarean section (VBAC) but the placenta could not be removed completely. The cord snapped on traction but the placenta did not deliver. She also started to bleed more profusely now. What is the likely reason for this? ***(Most Recent Question Aug 2020)***

a. Succenturiate lobe b. Inversion of uterus
c. Placenta accreta d. Placenta previa

199. What is the dose of mifepristone in medical termination of pregnancy? ***(Most Recent Question Dec 2019-20)***

a. 600 mg b. 200 mg
c. 400 mg d. 100 mg

200. Patient presents at 11 weeks POG with mild spotting per vaginum. On USG only gestational sac is seen without fetal pole. Uterus size is normal and equal to POG and os is closed. Diagnosis? ***(Most Recent Question Dec 2019-20)***

a. Missed abortion b. Threatened abortion
c. Inevitable abortion d. Incomplete abortion

201. A 32-year-old pregnant lady in third trimester, presented with mild bleeding and pain. On examination uterus is tender and fetal heart sound is absent. What is diagnosis? ***(Most Recent Question Dec 2019-20)***

a. Abruptio placenta b. Fetal distress
c. Ectopic pregnancy d. Placenta previa

202. A lady with 12-week pregnancy with bleeding and on examination vagina is normal, internal OS is closed and live-birth sign on USG and fundal height is 13 weeks. Diagnosis? ***(Most Recent Question Dec 2019-20)***

a. Threatened abortion b. Complete abortion
c. Incomplete abortion d. Inevitable abortion

203. Couvelaire uterus is seen in: ***(Most Recent Question 2019)***

a. Placenta previa b. Vasa previa
c. Abruptio placenta d. Placenta percreta

204. A G4P2 lady presented with history of two abortions at 16 weeks and 20 weeks AOG. Which of the following could be the most suspected cause for this abortions?
(Recent Pattern Question 2018-19)

a. Chromosomal abnormality
b. Cervical incompetence
c. Placenta previa
d. Thyroid abnormality

205. Most common cause of miscarriage in 1st trimester abortions: ***(Recent Pattern Question 2018)***

a. Trisomy b. Monosomy X
c. Triploidy d. Tetraploidy

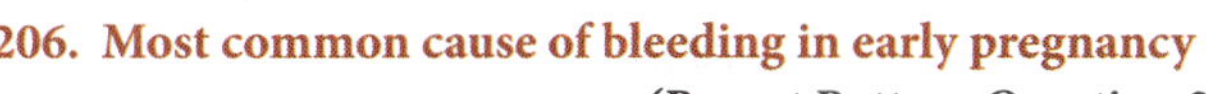

206. Most common cause of bleeding in early pregnancy ***(Recent Pattern Question 2016)***
   a. Spontaneous abortion
   b. Missed abortion
   c. Ectopic pregnancy
   d. Abruption placenta

207. Most common cause of 1st trimester abortions:
   a. Trisomy
   b. Monosomy X
   c. Triploidy
   d. Tetraploidy

208. Commonest cause of first trimester miscarriage is:
   a. Syphilis
   b. Cervical incompetence
   c. Chromosomal abnormalities
   d. Rhesus isoimmunisation

209. In Inevitable abortion:
   a. Uterus size larger than to AOG, cervix open
   b. Uterus size equal to AOG, cervix close
   c. Uterus size smaller than to AOG, cervix open
   d. Uterus size smaller than to AOG, cervix close

210. Treatment of choice of inevitable abortion less than 10 week:
   a. Dilatation and evacuation
   b. Suction and evacuation
   c. Medical management
   d. Complete hysterectomy

211. For MTP which of the following drug dosage is used:
   a. 200 mg mifepristone + 400 mg misoprostol
   b. 200 mg misoprostol + 400 mg mifepristone
   c. 200 mg mifepristone + 400 mcg misoprostol
   d. 400 mcg mifepristone + 200 mg misoprostol

212. Which one of following is the legal drug used for MTP in India?
   a. Misoprostol + Methotrexate
   b. Mitoprostane + Methotrexate
   c. Mifepristone 200 mg + Misoprostol 400 mcg oral
   d. None

213. Which of the following is not used in MTP?
   a. Misoprostol
   b. Mifepristone
   c. Misoprostol + Tamoxifen
   d. Mifepristone + Misoprostol

214. Dangerously low lying placenta is:
   a. Type I anterior
   b. Type II anterior
   c. Type I posterior
   d. Type II posterior

215. McAfee and Johnson regimen is used for:
   a. Eclampsia   b. Placenta previa
   c. Placental abruption   d. Placenta accrete

216. Patient with 37 week AOG, centrally located placenta previa presented with bleeding per vaginum. Management:
   a. Caesarean section
   b. Abortion
   c. Vaccum delivery
   d. Foreceps delivery

217. Umbilical cord attached to the margin of placenta:
   a. Circumvallate placenta
   b. Battledore placenta
   c. Velamentous insertion
   d. Vasa previa

218. Nitabuch's membrane is absent in:
   a. Placenta accreta
   b. Vasa previa
   c. Abruption placenta
   d. Placenta previa

219. Absence of Nitabuch's membrane leads to in all; EXCEPT:
   a. Placenta previa
   b. Placenta accreta
   c. Placenta increta
   d. Placenta percreta

220. Recurrence of hydatiform mole is assessed by:
   a. AFP level
   b. β-hCG level
   c. LDH level
   d. Estrogen level

221. Complete mole contains
   a. 46 YY   b. 46 XY
   c. 46 XXY   d. 69 XXX

222. In gestational trophoblastic disease, metastases most commonly occurs to:
   a. Brain   b. Liver
   c. Lungs   d. Bone

223. Theca lutein cyst are seen in
   a. Complete mole   b. Partial mole
   c. Tubal ectopic   d. Missed abortion

224. In a patient who underwent post molar evacuation by dilatation and curettage. Which of the following test used to define successful removal of H. Mole:
   a. Beta hCG   b. Per speculum
   c. Progesterone   d. USG

225. The risk of uterine rupture after previous lower transverse uterine incision at Caesarean Section is:
   a. 1%   b. 3%
   c. 5%   d. 7%

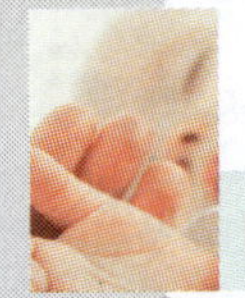

TWIN PREGNANCY

226. Identify the given image?
(Most Recent Question Dec 2019-20)

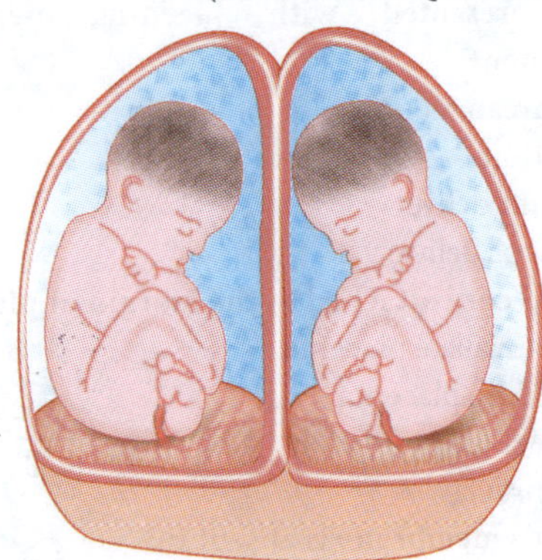

a. Dichorionic Diamniotic
b. Monochorionic Diamniotic
c. Monochorionic Monoamniotic
d. Conjoint twin

227. A 32-year-old lady with twin pregnancy dichorionic diamniotic, first baby breech presentation and second baby cephalic presentation. What is the management?
(Most Recent Question Dec 2019-20)

a. C-section
b. Assisted breech
c. Instrumental delivery
d. Normal vaginal delivery

228. If a zygote divides 2–3 days after fertilization, which of the following type of twining is seen:
(Recent Pattern Question 2018-19)

a. Monochorionic, Monoamniotic
b. Monochorionic, Diamniotic
c. Diamniotic, Dichorionic
d. Dichorionic, Monoamniotic

229. Division of zygote took place on 5th day after fertilization. What is the type of twinning?

a. Monochorionic, monoamniotic
b. Monochorionic, diamniotic
c. Dichorionic, diamniotic
d. Dichorionic, monoamniotic

230. Most common type of twin gestation is:

a. Monochorionic monoamniotic
b. Diamniotic, monochorionic
c. Conjoined twins
d. Dichorionic monoamniotic

231. Best position of twins for normal vaginal delivery:

a. A non-vertex, B vertex
b. A vertex, B non-vertex
c. A vertex, B vertex
d. A non-vertex, B non-vertex

232. Twin pregnancy is earliest detected at:

a. 10 weeks
b. 12 weeks
c. 6 weeks
d. 8 weeks

233. Twin pregnancy is least associated with:

a. Multigravida
b. Genetic
c. Young female
d. Patient receiving fertilization treatment

ECTOPIC PREGNANCY

234. Which of the following is an indication for surgery in ectopic pregnancy for a woman who is desirous of another pregnancy?
(Most Recent Question June/Dec 2021)

a. Serum beta hCG level <1000 miu/mL
b. Pt. wants to continue the pregnancy
c. Ectopic mass >4 mcs
d. Unruptured ectopic pregnancy

235. Late rupture of tubal pregnancy is seen if ectopic pregnancy occurs at this site:
(Most Recent Question Dec 2019-20)

a. Interstitium
b. Isthmus
c. Ampula
d. Fimbriae

236. In a patient with ectopic tubal pregnancy which is the earliest to rupture? ***(Recent Pattern Question 2018-19)***

a. Interstitial
b. Isthmus
c. Ampulla
d. Infundibulum

237. Most common site of ectopic pregnancy:
(Recent Pattern Question 2017)

a. Ampulla
b. Interstitium
c. Isthmus
d. Fimbrae

238. Which is the most dangerous site for Ectopic pregnancy:
(Recent Pattern Question 2017)

a. Isthmus
b. Ampulla
c. Interstitial
d. Fimbrae

239. A 29-year-old female presented with 7 weeks of pregnancy. She has complaint of vaginal spotting. USG shows empty uterus. Best treatment:
(Recent Pattern Question 2017)

a. If sac >3.5 cm do medical management
b. Laparoscopy with salpingostomy
c. Laparotomy with salpingectomy
d. Laparatomy

240. Ectopic pregnancy with adnexal mass <2.5 cm. Treatment: ***(Recent Pattern Question 2017)***

a. Medical management
b. Surgical management
c. Laparoscopy
d. Laparoscopy with salpingectomy

241. Most common complaints of ectopic pregnancy:
(Recent Pattern Question 2016)

a. Pain
b. Vaginal bleeding
c. Infection
d. Amenorrhea

242. Pain is more common than bleeding in:
(Recent Pattern Question 2016)
a. Ectopic pregnancy b. Complete mole
c. Incomplete abortion d. Missed abortion

243. Suspected ectopic pregnancy is best diagnosed by
(Recent Pattern Question 2016)
a. MRI b. TVS
c. X-ray abdomen supine d. HSG

244. Drug used for ectopic pregnancy
(Recent Pattern Question 2016)
a. Mifepristone + misoprostol
b. Misoprostol 200 mg
c. Methotrexate 50 mg IM
d. Progesterone

245. Triad of ectopic pregnancy are all; EXCEPT:
a. Vomiting b. Bleeding
c. Abdominal pain d. Amenorrhea

246. All are true about ectopic pregnancy; EXCEPT
a. Most common cause is Progestasert
b. Can be diagnosed by hCG level
c. A negative pregnancy test excludes the diagnosis
d. Methotrexate is used as medical management

247. Most sensitive diagnostic test for ectopic pregnancy:
a. Transvaginal USG
b. Serial monitoring of beta hCG
c. Culdocentesis
d. MRI

248. Criteria for medical termination of ectopic pregnancy:
a. Beta hCG < 5000 b. Mass of >3.5 cm
c. Present fetal heart beat d. 6 week pregnancy

MALPRESENTATION, DIFFICULT DELIVERY AND INSTRUMENTATION

249. This instrument is used for:
(Most Recent Question June 2022)

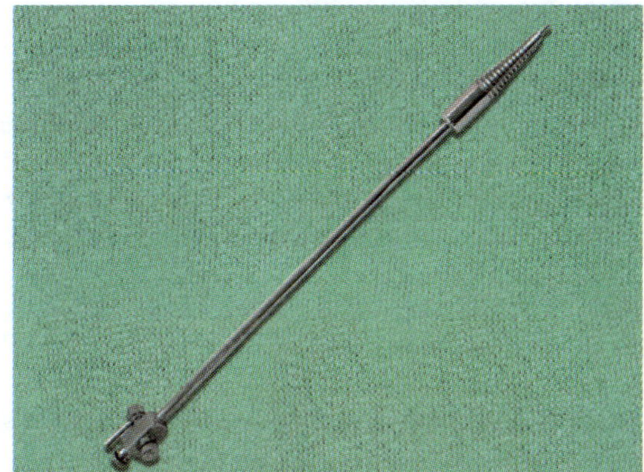

a. Hysteroscopy b. MTP
c. Sounding the uterus d. Hysterosalpingography

250. Colposcopy filter color is ?
(Most Recent Question June/Dec 2021)
a. Red b. Green
c. Orange d. Purple

251. A lady during labor presented with persistent occipito posterior position. Manual rotation was tried but it was unsuccessful. What is the pelvis type?
(Most Recent Question Aug 2020)
a. Gynaecoid b. Anthropoid
c. Osteomalatic pelvis d. Platypelloid

252. A 32 year lady with intrauterine fetal death, underwent instrumental vaginal delivery continues passing of urine from vagina. What is the most probable diagnosis?
(Most Recent Question Dec 2019-20)
a. Bladder rupture b. Vesicovaginal fistula
c. Urge incontinence d. Stress incontinence

253. The pressure used for gynecological laparoscopy:
(Recent Pattern Question 2018)
a. 10–15 mm Hg b. 15–20 mm Hg
c. 20–30 mm Hg d. 30–50 mm Hg

254. Upon hysteroscopy which of the following cannot be seen? *(Recent Pattern Question 2018)*
a. OS b. Cervix
c. Endometrium d. Uterus surface

255. True about frank breech:
(Recent Pattern Question 2018)
a. Mostly associated with congenital anomaly
b. Footling presentation
c. ECV done after 34 weeks
d. Has hip extended and knee flexed

256. Which is the most prominent part in transverse lie?
(Recent Pattern Question 2016)
a. Acromion b. Sternum
c. Buttock d. Mentum

257. In face presentation what is the presenting denominator? *(Recent Pattern Question 2016)*
a. Cheek b. Mentum
c. Forehead d. Lips

258. Breech presentation with footling. Management is:
a. Vaginal delivery b. Ceasarean section
c. Forceps delivery d. Internal podalic version

259. Which of the following is most common compound presentation:
a. Head with foot b. Head with hand
c. Hand, head and foot d. Both hand and foot

260. In Brow presentation, head of the fetus:
a. Complete hyperextension
b. Partial extension
c. Complete flexion
d. Moderate flexion

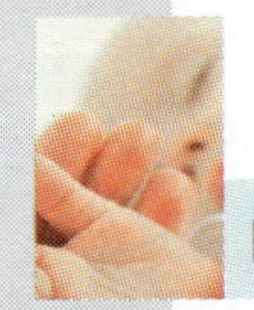

261. What is the presentation of the given image:

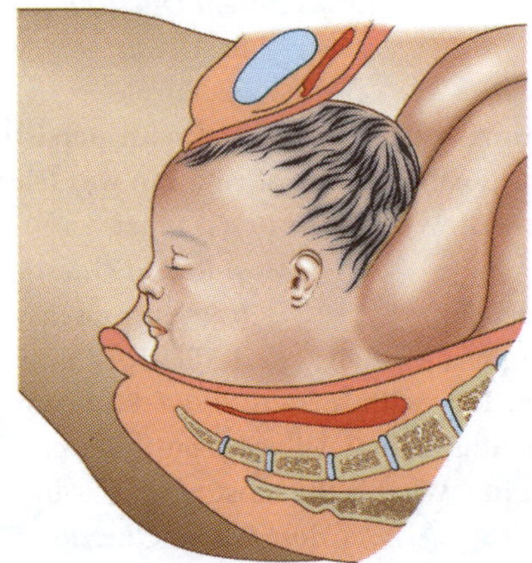

a. Face presentation b. Transverse lie
c. Brow presentation d. Vertex

262. Fetus in transverse position. Which of the following is true:

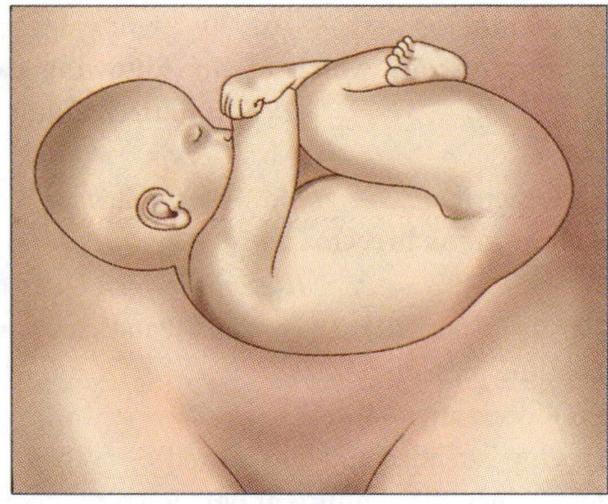

a. Polyhydramnios is a cause
b. It can be caused by abruptio placenta
c. It results to hand prolapsed in all cases
d. Shoulder dystocia is a major threat

263. Treatment of choice of acute hydramnios with fetal distress in pregnancy:

a. Amniocentesis b. Cordocentesis
c. Indomethacin d. Termination

264. Which of the following is a contraindication for trial of vaginal delivery in VBAC:

a. Breech presentation
b. Previous CS of >2
c. Presence of anesthesiologist
d. Informed consent

265. All are contraindications of Internal cephalic version; EXCEPT:

a. Shoulder presentation of first fetus
b. Face presentation
c. Transverse lie of second fetus in a twin pregnancy
d. Breech presentation of 2nd fetus in a twin

266. External cephalic version is done in all; EXCEPT:

a. Primigravida b. Flexed breech
c. Anemia d. PIH

267. Following are contraindications to External Cephalic Version; EXCEPT:

a. Contracted pelvis b. Antepartum hemorrhage
c. Multiple pregnancy d. Hydramnios

268. Low forceps are applied when:

a. Scalp is visible at the introitus
b. Fetal head is at pelvic floor
c. Fetus is at station + 2
d. Fetal head is engaged

DISEASES DURING PREGNANCY

269. A 23-year-old primigravida presents to her physician at 18 weeks with FBS >126 mg/dL Hba1c >6.5. What is the diagnosis? ***(Most Recent Question June/Dec 2021)***

a. Pregestational DM
b. GDM
c. Maturity onset diabetes mellitus
d. Impaired Glucose Tolerance

270. A 24-year-old primigravida attends anc clinic with h/o bp 160/120 mm Hg. Her lab findings shows increased liver enzymes and increased IDH. Low platelet count. Diagnosis? ***(Most Recent Question June/Dec 2021)***

a. AFLP b. HELLP
c. Hepatitis B d. Obstetric cholestasis

271. A pregnant woman with prosthetic valve on warfarin tests positive for pregnancy. What is the advice to be given? ***(Most Recent Question June/Dec 2021)***

a. Discontinue warfarin
b. To replace warfarin with heparin
c. Add vit. K with warfarin
d. To continue warfarin throughout pregnancy

272. Patient present with eclampsia. Treatment of magnesium sulphate is given what is the first sign of magnesium sulphate toxicity: ***(Most Recent Question Aug 2020)***

a. Decrease in BP b. Loss of deep tendon reflex
c. Breathing difficulty d. Asystole

273. A patient underwent OGTT at 27 weeks of gestation. Her fasting blood glucose was 130 mg/dl and at 2-hour, blood glucose was 180 mg/dL. AFI = 14. What is your next step in the management? ***(Most Recent Question Dec 2019-20)***

a. Start insulin and check at 34 weeks
b. Admit her and start insulin
c. Medical nutrition therapy and exercise
d. Start insulin and monthly checkup

274. A baby born to diabetic mother is jittery and hypoglycemic after delivery. What is the reason for hypoglycemia? ***(Most Recent Question Dec 2019-20)***

a. Due to excess insulin b. Heavy birth weight
c. Hypermotility d. Hypercalcemia

275. A patient with 37 weeks of gestation came to hospital without antenatal check-up and presented with onset of labor. On investigation the mother is hepatitis B positive, what management should be given to neonate?
(Most Recent Question Dec 2019-20)

a. Hep B vaccine only
b. Hep B vaccine + IG
c. First immunoglobulin then Hep B vaccine after 1 month
d. Only immunoglobulin

276. A 19-year-old primigravida, presents with 8 weeks amenorrhea, light bleeding and pain. USG reveals intra uterine pregnancy. What is preferred management in this case? *(Most Recent Question 2019)*

a. Estrogen plus progesterone therapy
b. D and C
c. Bed rest and progesterone
d. Beta hCG

277. A 26 weeks pregnant female presented with HTN for the first time. There is no proteinuria. Diagnosis of such condition. *(Most Recent Question 2019)*

a. Chronic hypertension
b. Eclampsia
c. Gestational hypertension
d. Preeclampsia

278. Which of the following can be a cause of Oligohydramnios? *(Most Recent Question 2019)*

a. Multiparity b. Twins
c. Renal agenesis d. Macrosomia

279. Feature of hydrops fetalis in a fetus can be due to:

a. Ebstein barr virus *(Recent Pattern Question 2018-19)*
b. Human papilloma virus
c. Parvovirus B19
d. Influenza virus

280. Cut off point for 50 gram glucose challenge test at 1 hour mg%: *(Recent Pattern Question 2018-19)*

a. 100 b. 140
c. 180 d. 200

281. Chromosome pattern in complete mole:
(Recent Pattern Question 2018-19)

a. 46 XY both maternal origin
b. 46 XX both maternal origin
c. 46 XX both paternal origin
d. 46 YY both paternal origin

282. Agent used for status eclampticus?
(Recent Pattern Question 2017)

a. Hydralazine b. Thiopentone sodium
c. Valproate d. Magnesium sulfate

283. In an eclamptic patient with raised ICT, which drug should be given: *(Recent Pattern Question 2017)*

a. Mannitol b. Furosemide
c. Labetalol d. Hydralazine

284. Maximum risk of pre-eclampsia is due to:
(Recent Pattern Question 2016)

a. CRF b. Heart disease
c. Anemia d. Liver disease

285. Antenatal mother with epilepsy on phenytoin therapy must be given:

a. Folic acid supplementation
b. Vitamin B_{12} supplementation
c. Vitamin B_6 supplementation
d. Vitamin A supplementation

286. A 42 years primigravida presents at 28 weeks period of gestation and has left upper breast mass. Choose the best investigation modality:

a. Mammography b. CT scan
c. MRI d. High Resonance ultrasound

287. Best marker in intrahepatic cholestasis of pregnant women:

a. Bile acid b. Bilirubin
c. Alkaline phosphatase d. SGPT

288. All of the following can cause DIC in women; EXCEPT:

a. Amniotic fluid embolism b. Sepsis
c. Placenta previa d. HELLP

289. All are true about HELLP syndrome; EXCEPT:

a. Increased LDH b. Low platelet
c. Increased liver enzymes d. Hyponatremia

290. DOC for candidiasis in pregnancy:

a. Metronidazole 500 mg b. Tinidazole 500 mg
c. Fluconazole 150 mg d. Metronidazole 1 g

291. A pregnant women with BP 150/100 mm Hg, proteinuria after 20 weeks. Diagnosis?

a. Pre-eclampsia
b. Pregnancy induced hypertension
c. Renal hypertension
d. Eclampsia

292. All can be done in pre-eclampsia; EXCEPT:

a. Diuretics b. Anti hypertensives
c. $MgSO_4$ d. Admission and wait

293. For controlling eclamptic patient with convulsion, which of the following will be used:

a. Mannitol b. Furosemide
c. Hydralazine d. $MgSO_4$

294. A patient presented with a pregnancy of 32 weeks with antepartum haemorrhage. Patient with hypertension. Management at this point of time:

a. Caesarean section
b. Observation on OPD basis
c. Hospitalization and observation
d. Induce labor

295. A pregnant lady with PIH is having bleeding per vagina. The decision to continue pregnancy is based on:

a. Presence of fetal cardiac activity
b. Availability of blood
c. Blood pressure
d. Adequate medical facilities

296. In a diabetic mother, most common fetal complication will be:
a. Neural tube defect
b. Congenital sacral agenesis
c. Congenital heart disease
d. Hydrocephalus

297. DOC for hyperthyroidism in pregnancy:
a. Propylthiouracil
b. Methimazole
c. I-131
d. Thyroxine

FETAL GROWTH AND DEVELOPMENT

298. Best parameter to find out age of gestation in first trimester: ***(Recent Pattern Question 2018)***
a. Dates of menstrual period
b. CRL
c. Femur length
d. Weight of the fetus

299. Breathing movement of fetus on USG is first detected at: ***(Recent Pattern Question 2017)***
a. 11 weeks
b. 20 weeks
c. 24 weeks
d. 26 weeks

300. During intrauterine life fetal waste is excreted by? ***(Recent Pattern Question 2017)***
a. Straight into mother's blood by simple diffusion
b. Diffusion into amniotic fluid
c. Ultrafiltration
d. Leakage

301. Fetal haemoglobin is maximum secreted by ***(Recent Pattern Question 2016)***
a. Liver
b. Yolk sac
c. Spleen
d. Bone marrow

302. Deoxygenated blood from the fetus to the mother is carried via:
a. Umbilical artery
b. Umbilical veins
c. Pulmonary artery
d. Pulmonary vein

303. Cardiac activity in fetus can be asessed via transabdominal scan by:
a. 6–7 weeks
b. 8–9 weeks
c. 9–11 weeks
d. 12–14 weeks

304. Crown rump length at 12 weeks:
a. 7 cm
b. 10 cm
c. 12 cm
d. 25 cm

305. At 12 weeks pregnancy "CRL" is:
a. 60 mm
b. 100 mm
c. 120 mm
d. 250 mm

306. Radiotherapy is most harmful in which week of gestation:
a. 4–16 weeks
b. 18–23 weeks
c. 28–32 weeks
d. 36–38 weeks

307. In folate + vitamin B12 combined deficiency which of the following is/are mainly seen?
a. Neural tube defects
b. Megaloblastic anemia
c. Abruptio placentae
d. Placenta previa

INTRAUTERINE FETAL DEATH

308. Intrauterine death is least likely caused by:
a. Rh-incompatibility
b. Obstructed labor
c. Low birth weight
d. Placental insufficiency

309. Which of the following sign is seen in intrauterine fetal demise:
a. Von Braun-Fernwald's sign
b. Robert's sign
c. Goodell's sign
d. Osiander sign

310. Which of the following is most likely cause of intrapartum death?
a. Cord prolapsed
b. Abruptio placentae
c. Hyaline membrane disease
d. Eclampsia

311. Methotrexate is indicated mainly in:
a. Pre-eclampsia
b. IUD
c. Prematurity
d. Ectopic pregnancy

MISCELLANEOUS

312. Identify this image: ***(Most Recent Question June 2022)***

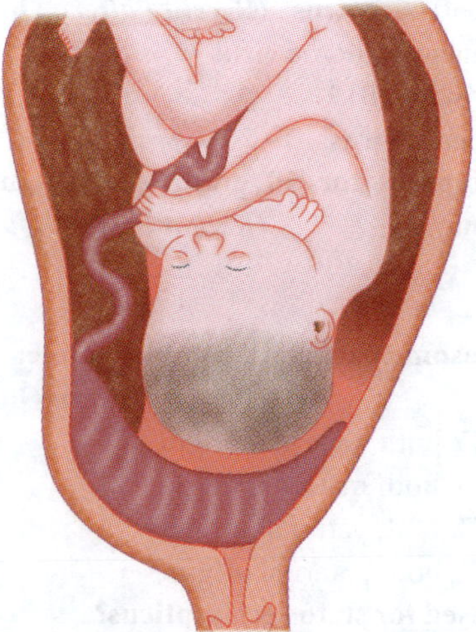

a. Vasa previa
b. Placenta accrete
c. Placenta abruption
d. Placenta previa

313. Size of Karman's cannula at 10 weeks to use for suction evacuation is? ***(Most Recent Question June/Dec 2021)***
a. 4 mm
b. 5 mm
c. 7 mm
d. 10 mm

314. Identify instrument:

(Most Recent Question June/Dec 2021)

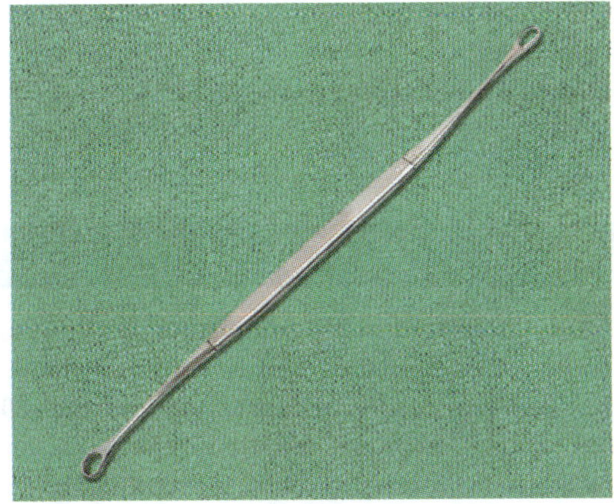

a. Dilator
b. Curette
c. Sound
d. Vaginal wall retractor

315. 46XX, presented with primary amenorrhea. Upon examination, uterus, vagina are absent with normal secondary sexual characteristics. Ovary present, FSH and LH within normal limits. Possible diagnosis?

(Most Recent Question June/Dec 2021)

a. MRKH
b. Androgen insensitivity syndrome
c. Turner Syndrome
d. Congenital Adrenal Hyperplasia

316. Which of the following peak is responsible for ovulation? *(Most Recent Question June/Dec 2021)*

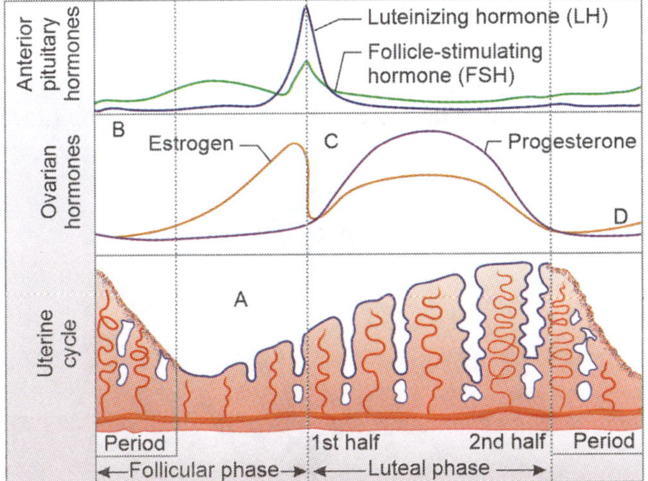

a. A
b. B
c. C
d. D

317. False statement regarding following image

(Most Recent Question June/Dec 2021)

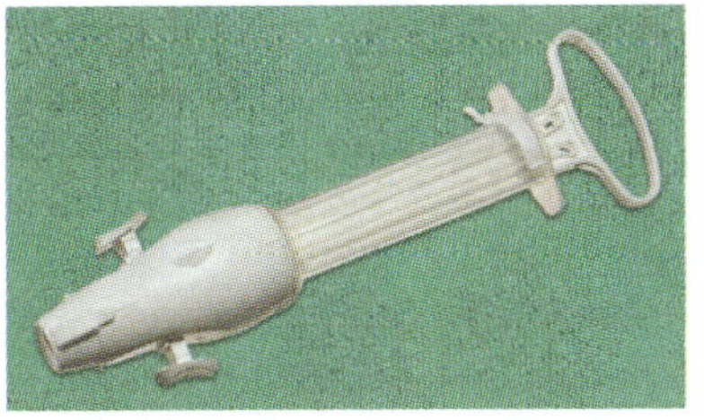

a. Do not use electricity
b. Creates a negative pressure of 60 mm Hg
c. Capacity is 60 ml
d. Can be used upto 12 weeks

318. Which of the following statement is Not true about placenta:

a. Weight of full term placenta is 508 and volume is 497 ml
b. At 17th week weight of placenta is equal to weight of fetus
c. It has 4 to 6 lobes
d. Total of lobes remain the same throughout the gestation

319. Level of which hormone are increased during post menopausal women:

a. Estrogen b. Progestron
c. FSH d. Cortison

320. Antibody to cross placenta

a. IgA b. IgG
c. IgE d. IgM

321. Earliest sex-determination is done at:

a. 1 month b. 2 months
c. 3 months d. 4 months

322. The dose of anti-D immunoglobulin to be given to non-immune Rh D negative women after delivery is:

a. 50 μg b. 150 μg
c. 300 μg d. 450 μg

GYNECOLOGY

ANATOMY, MENARCHE AND MENOPAUSE

323. In this graph of menstrual cycle – which alphabet shown is suggestive of ovulation?

(Most Recent Question Aug 2020)

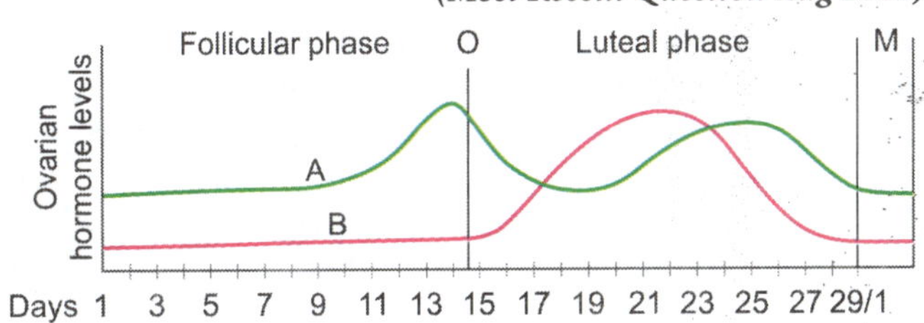

a. A b. B
c. O d. M

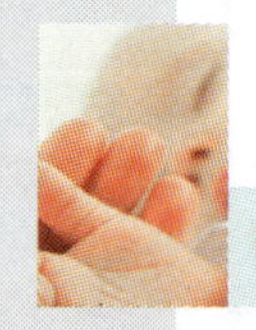

324. A 13-year-old girl presented with pain abdomen and heavy menstrual bleeding. History reveals menarche was at the age of 12 years and her menstrual cycles are irregular. What is the immediate management? *(Most Recent Question Dec 2019-20)*

a. Uterine ablation
b. Uterine artery block
c. Progesterone
d. Hysteroscopy examination

325. A 58-year-old lady with menopause and hot flushes presents to the physician. Which is correct? *(Recent Pattern Question 2018-19)*

a. Increased FSH, increased estrogen
b. Decreased FSH, decreased estrogen
c. Decreased FSH, increased estrogen
d. Increased FSH, decreased estrogen

326. A girl is said to have primary amenorrhea in absence of secondary sexual characters by what age: *(Recent Pattern Question 2018)*

a. 12
b. 13
c. 14
d. 16

327. Which of the following is the most common cause of secondary amenorrhea? *(Recent Pattern Question 2018)*

a. Pelvic irradiation
b. Diabetes
c. Kallmann syndrome
d. Imperforate hymen

328. Marker of ovarian reserve in a premenopausal female: *(Recent Pattern Question 2018)*

a. Antral follicle size
b. Raised LH/FSH ratio
c. Decreased inhibin A
d. Anti-mullerian hormone

329. According to American fertility society classification system, unicornuate uterus is classified under this class:

a. Class I
b. Class II
c. Class III
d. Class IV

330. Thelarche definition: *(Recent Pattern Question 2017)*

a. Growth of pubic and axillary hair
b. Growth of breast
c. Increase in height
d. Onset of menstruation

331. The hormone which increases on thelarche: *(Recent Pattern Question 2017)*

a. GnRH
b. Estrogen
c. Progesterone
d. GH

332. Average age of menopause: *(Recent Pattern Question 2017)*

a. 40
b. 45
c. 55
d. 60

333. Precocious puberty in females is defined as: *(Recent Pattern Question 2016)*

a. Occurrence of menarche before age of 8 years
b. Occurrence of menarche before age of 12 years
c. Appearance of secondary sexual characteristics before 8 years
d. Appearance of secondary sexual characteristics before 10 years

334. Follicles in ovary are decreasing with age, the first change is: *(Recent Pattern Question 2016)*

a. Increase FSH
b. Increase LH
c. Increase inhibin
d. Increase estradiol

335. Menstrual blood stored in vagina in:

a. Pyometra
b. Hematometra
c. Hematocolpos
d. Hematosalphinx

INFECTION

336. A lady presented with complaints of foul smelling greyish white discharge and a whiff test done on the discharge was positive. On examination clue cells were seen on microscopic examination. What is the condition and which is the drug of choice for treatment? *(Most Recent Question June/Dec 2021)*

a. Candida, fluconazole
b. Trichomonas, metronidazole
c. Gardnerella vaginalis, metronidazole
d. Gonococci, doxycycline

337. A patient presented to the OPD with symptoms of lower abdominal pain, Dyspareunia and on pelvic examination adnexal tenderness and cervical motion tenderness is observed. What could be the long-term sequelae of this condition? *(Most Recent Question Aug 2020)*

a. Recurrent pregnancy loss
b. Infertility
c. Pelvic organ prolapse
d. Amenorrhea

338. A patient presented with smelly greenish vaginal discharge 5 days after delivery (in early puerperium). What is next step in management? *(Most Recent Question Aug 2020)*

a. Antibiotics
b. USG
c. Urine analysis
d. Per vaginum examination

339. Diagnosis of the image: *(Most Recent Question 2020)*

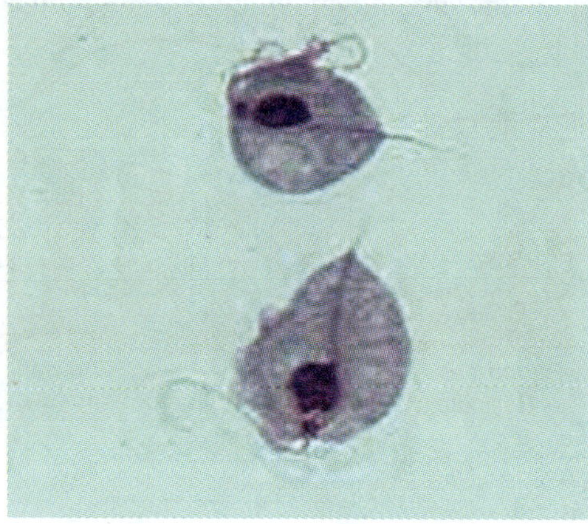

a. Trichomonas
b. Listeria
c. Pseudomonas
d. Enterobacter

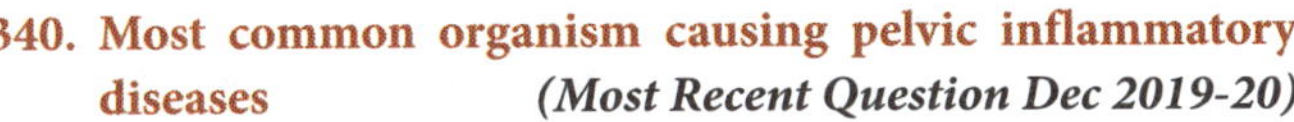

340. Most common organism causing pelvic inflammatory diseases *(Most Recent Question Dec 2019-20)*
a. E. coli
b. Gardenella vaginalis
c. Bacteroides
d. Chlamydia

341. Investigation of choice for genital TB: *(Most Recent Question Dec 2019-20)*
a. Endometrial curettage
b. Urine sample with Giemsa staining
c. Early morning urine sample
d. Incision and curettage

342. Amsel criteria is used for: *(Most Recent Question Dec 2019-20)*
a. Gardenella vaginosis
b. Candidiasis
c. Trichomoniasis
d. Chlymadia infection

343. Which is correct about presentation of C. trachomatis infection? *(Recent Pattern Question 2018-19)*
a. Pruritic vaginitis
b. Leads to infertility
c. Uveitis
d. Inclusion body pneumonitis

344. Which of the following infections can commonly lead to infertility: *(Recent Pattern Question 2018-19)*
a. Chlamydia
b. Trichomoniasis
c. Candidiasis
d. Bacterial vaginosis

345. A 32-year-old female presented with acute history of profuse mucoid vaginal discharge, abdominal pain and deep dyspareunia. Per speculum examination reveal erosion of cervix and a reddened area around cervix external os. Which of the following treatment option is preferred for this patient: *(Recent Pattern Question 2018-19)*
a. Laser therapy
b. Conization operation
c. Cryosurgery
d. Policresulen

346. Common mode of transmission in pyogenic TB salpingitis: *(Recent Pattern Question 2018)*
a. Hematogenous
b. Lymphatic
c. Direct invasion
d. Sexually transmitted

347. A 25-year-old lady who presents with curdy white discharge from vagina is likely to be suffering from: *(Recent Pattern Question 2018)*
a. Gonococcal vulvovaginitis
b. Candida vaginitis
c. Trichomoniasis
d. Chlamydia trachomatis

348. Temperature in puerperal pyrexia: *(Recent Pattern Question 2018)*
a. 98.4°F
b. 99°F
c. 100.4°F
d. 104°F

349. Which of the following organism is common cause of tubal blockage?
a. Chlamydia
b. Herpes simplex
c. Candida
d. HPV

350. A 29-year-old female presents with PID, what is the indication to hospitalize? *(Recent Pattern Question 2017)*
a. Pregnancy
b. Cervical discharge
c. TB
d. Acute mild PID

351. Most common presentation in fallopian tube TB: *(Recent Pattern Question 2017)*
a. Infertility
b. Pain
c. Abdominal cramps
d. Bleeding

352. Recurrent vulvo-vaginitis is defined as: *(Recent Pattern Question 2016)*
a. >2 infection in a year
b. >3 infection in a year
c. >4 infection in a year
d. >5 infection in a year

353. Clue cells are seen in: *(Recent Pattern Question 2016)*
a. Bacterial vaginosis
b. Cystitis
c. Candida albicans
d. Trichomoniasis

354. 10% KOH is used for diagnosing: *(Recent Pattern Question 2016)*
a. Candida
b. Trichomonas
c. Mycoplasma
d. Gardenella vaginalis

355. Fishy odor in whiff test is seen in: *(Recent Pattern Question 2016)*
a. Giardia
b. Bacterial vaginosis
c. Trichomoniasis
d. Candidiasis

356. All of the following statement are true about Bacterial vaginosis; EXCEPT:
a. Cause by gardenella vaginalis
b. Fishy odor upon whiff test
c. Infection seen when vaginal pH is <4.5
d. It is not an STD

357. Clue cells are seen in:
a. Bacterial vaginosis
b. Candidiasis
c. Trichomoniasis
d. Gonoccocal

358. Whiff test done for:
a. Gonococcal infections
b. Gardenella
c. Trichomoniasis
d. Candiasis

359. In patients with asymptomatic carrier of Chlamydia, organisms resides most commonly in:
a. Vagina
b. Urethra
c. Ectocervix
d. Endocervix

360. First symptom of fallopian tube TB:
a. Pain
b. Bleeding
c. Watery discharge
d. Uterine prolapse

361. Clubbing of fimbrial end of Fallopian tube is seen upon HSG. What could be the possible pathology:
a. Tuberculosis
b. Gonococcal
c. Hydrosalpinx
d. Mullerian anomaly

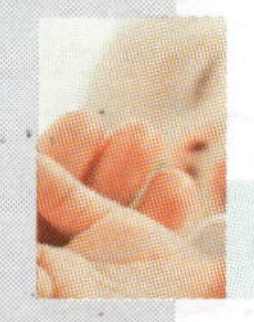

362. A young female was worked up for examined for her infertility by hysterosalpingography reveals 'Bead — like' fallopian tube and clubbing of ampulla. Which of the following is the most likely cause?

a. Gonococcus
b. Mycoplasma
c. Chlamydia
d. Mycobacterium tuberculosis

363. PID can be due to:

a. IUCD insertion b. Oral contraceptive
c. Condom d. Hypertension

364. A 40-year-old woman presents with PID. Best investigation to be done:

a. USG b. CT
c. MRI d. Laproscopy

CERVICAL CANCER

365. Causative agent for CIN 3/Ca cervix

(Most Recent Question June/Dec 2021)

a. HPV 6 b. HPV 11
c. HPV 18 d. HPV12

366. A patient underwent radiotherapy for carcinoma cervix. Which organ in the pelvis is most radiosensitive?

(Most Recent Question June/Dec 2021)

a. Uterus b. Urethra
c. Ovary d. Urinary bladder

367. A 55-year-old woman was found to have a carcinoma cervix figo stage 3b. what is the management?

(Most Recent Question June/Dec 2021)

a. Concurrent chemoradiotherapy
b. Radiotherapy + HPV vaccine
c. Schauta procedure
d. Intracavitary brachytherapy followed by EBRT

368. Which is most cost effective cheap cervical screening test? ***(Most Recent Question June/Dec 2021)***

a. VIA b. HPV-DNA testing
c. Pap smear d. Colposcopy

369. A 23-year-old lady presented with complain of post coital bleeding. On per speculum examination the following is seen, it bleeds on touch. Possible diagnosis:

(Most Recent Question Dec 2019-20)

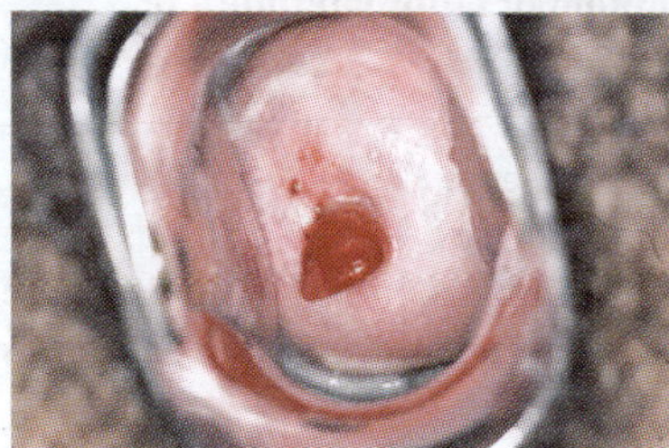

a. Cervical fibroid b. Cervical polyp
c. Cervical carcinoma d. Hemorrhagic cyst

370. Cervical cancer is mostly caused by:

(Recent Pattern Question 2018-19)

a. HPV 6 b. HPV 16
c. HPV 31 d. HPV 56

371. Most common type of cervical cancer:

a. Squamous cell CA b. Small cell CA
c. Adeno CA d. Adenoma

372. All of the following statements are true regarding etiology of cervical cancer; EXCEPT:

a. Both active and passive cigarette smoking increases the risk of cervical cancer
b. Oral contraceptives decreases the risk of cervical cancer
c. Abstinence from sexual activity and barrier protection decrease cervical cancer risk
d. Low education increases cervical cancer risk

373. Secondary level prevention of CA cervix:

a. Vaccination b. Pap smear
c. Colposcopy d. Spectroscopy

374. Screening test for cervical cancer is:

a. Biopsy b. Papaniculaou smear
c. Visual inspection d. Colposcopy

375. Cancer cervix screening according to WHO guidelines:

a. Women between the ages of 21 and 29 should have a Pap test every 3 years
b. Women between the ages of 30 and 65 should have both a Pap test and an HPV test every 5 years
c. Women over age 65 who have had regular screenings with normal results should NOT be screened for cervical cancer
d. All of the above

ENDOMETRIAL AND FALLOPIAN TUBE CANCER

376. What should be the treatment of an 8 cm endometrial cyst? ***(Most Recent Question June 2022)***

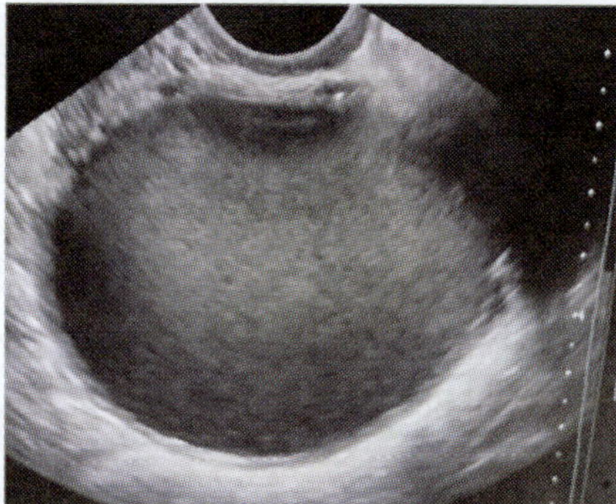

a. Needle aspiration
b. Cystectomy
c. Give GnrH agonist
d. Conservative since asymptomatic

377. A couple presented with infertility semen analysis is normal, female has menorrhagia on hsg there is distal dilation with fimbria. What is the likely cause? *(Most Recent Question June/Dec 2021)*

a. Tubal polyp b. Tubal endometriosis
c. Tubal spasm d. Tubal salphingitis

378. Investigation of choice for endometriosis: *(Most Recent Question Dec 2019-20)*

a. CT b. MRI
c. USG d. Laparoscopy

379. Risk of endometrial cancer is least in: *(Most Recent Question 2019)*

a. Nullipara b. Obesity
c. Late menopause d. Multigravida

380. Effect of tamoxifen: *(Recent Pattern Question 2018)*

a. Increased risk of endometrial carcinoma
b. Decreased risk of ovarian CA
c. Causes cardiotoxicity
d. Increased risk of osteoporosis

381. In endometriosis which of the following is not given? *(Recent Pattern Question 2018)*

a. Gonadotropin analogue b. Aromatase inhibitor
c. Mifepristone d. Estradiol

382. Radiological test for staging of endometrial carcinoma is best done with: *(Recent Pattern Question 2018)*

a. MRI b. Sonosalpingography
c. PET-CT d. Doppler USG

383. Most common presentation of adenomyosis? *(Recent Pattern Question 2017)*

a. Dyspareunia b. Infertility
c. Dysmenorrhea d. Hypomenorrhea

384. ___________% women with postmenopausal bleeding found to have endometrial cancer:

a. 20 b. 30
c. 40 d. 50

385. This type of endometrial hyperplasia leads to increased risk of endometrial cancer:

a. Simple b. Proliferative
c. Atypical d. Secretive

386. Best prognostic for endometrial pathology

a. Transvaginal ultrasound b. Biopsy
c. Hysteroscopy d. Fractional curettage

387. What would be the appropriate treatment of stage-I endometrial cancer:

a. Conservative management
b. Chemo therapy followed by radio therapy
c. Simple hysterectomy
d. Bilateral salpingo oophorectomy

388. Earliest presentation of fallopian tube cancer:

a. Painless watery discharge
b. Painless vaginal bleeding
c. Painful watery discharge
d. Painful vaginal bleeding

389. Tumor erodes serosa/adnexa of uterus in this stage of endometrial CA:

a. Ib b. II
c. IIIa d. IIIb

OVARIAN CANCER

390. Meig syndrome is? *(Most Recent Question June/Dec 2021)*

a. Benign fibroma + ascites + hydrothorax
b. Malignant fibroma + Ascites + hydrothorax
c. Ascites + hydrothorax
d. Ascites + pneumothorax

391. A 30-year female came for regular checkup found with 6 cm × 6 cm ovarian cyst. What is your next step in the management? *(Most Recent Question Dec 2019-20)*

a. CA-125 follow up
b. Laparotomy and ovariectomy
c. Laparoscopic ovariectomy
d. Combined OCP and follow up

392. Call exner bodies are seen in: *(Recent Pattern Question 2017)*

a. Granulosa cell tumor b. Yolk cell tumor
c. Teratoma d. Krukenberg tumor

393. Theca lutein cysts are common in: *(Recent Pattern Question 2016)*

a. Vagina b. Uterus
c. Ovary d. Cervix

394. All of the following are germ cell tumor; EXCEPT:

a. Dysgerminoma
b. Choriocarcinoma
c. Clear cell tumor
d. Teratoma

395. Most common germ cell ovarian tumor:

a. Dysgerminoma
b. Teratoma
c. Endodermal sinus tumor
d. Clear cell tumor

396. Most common malignant germ cell ovarian tumor:

a. Yolk sac tumors
b. Dysgerminoma
c. Dermoid cyst
d. Brenners

397. Most frequent epithelial tumors of ovary:

a. Papillary serous cystadenoma
b. Brenners
c. Endometrioid
d. Mucinous cyst adenoma

398. Most common malignant ovarian tumor?

a. Clear cell tumor
b. Serous cyst adenocarcinoma
c. Mucinous cyst adenocarcinoma
d. Granulosa cell tumor

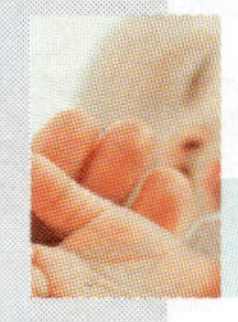

399. All of the following statements are true about choriocarcinoma; EXCEPT:
a. Can present with epigastric pain
b. Ovary is the primary site
c. Lungs are common site of metastasis
d. Snow storm appearance upon CXR

400. Syncitiotrophoblast is seen in:
a. Partial mole
b. Complete mole
c. Choriocarcinoma
d. Placental site of trophoplastoma

401. Treatment of choice in choriocarcinoma is:
a. Chemotherapy
b. External beam radiotherapy
c. Hysterectomy
d. Intracavitary brachytherapy

402. Tumor marker of CA ovary for follow up:
a. CEA
b. PSA
c. CA 125
d. BETA hCG

VULVAR AND VAGINAL CANCER

403. In a patient with Vulval ulcer. Which of the following will lead to malignancy?
a. HSV1
b. HSV2
c. STD
d. HPV

404. Vulval cancer spreads to urethra at what stage?
a. Stage I A
b. Stage I B
c. Stage II
d. Stage III A

405. Urethra is involved in which stage of Vulvar neoplasia?
a. Stage I
b. Stage II
c. Stage III
d. Stage IV

406. A Vulvar cancer of 3 cm, no lymph node involved. Treatment:
a. Simple partial vulvectomy with lymphadenectomy
b. Simple partial vulvectomy without lymphadenectomy
c. Wide local excision with lymphadenectomy
d. Radical vulvectomy

407. Treatment for vulval cancer stage 1
a. Complete radical Vulvectomy
b. Partial vulvectomy
c. Total vulvectomy and bilateral groin lymph node resection
d. CT or RT followed by resection of residual tumor

408. Infertility occurs due to carcinoma of all; EXCEPT:
a. Endometrial carcinoma
b. Ovarian carcinoma
c. Vaginal carcinoma
d. Cervix CA

DYSFUNCTIONAL UTERINE BLEEDING (DUB) AND DYSMENORRHEA

409. Which among the following is the most common cause of post-menopausal bleeding?
a. Atrophy *(Most Recent Question June 2022)*
b. CA endometrium
c. CA cervix
d. Polyps

410. Patient with breast cancer treatment with tamoxifen. She now presents with complaints of bleeding per vaginum. What is the most likely cause? *(Most Recent Question June 2022)*
a. Endometrial cancer
b. Cervical cancer
c. Endometrial polyp
d. Fibroid uterus

411. A 14-year-old girl presents with amenorrhea. On examination secondary sexual characters are seen. Uterus and ovaries were seen to be normal on USG. What is next step of management?
a. Reassurance *(Most Recent Question Aug 2020)*
b. UPT
c. Karyotyping
d. LH and FSH level and TSH

412. A 19-year-old girl presented with weight loss, secondary amenorrhea and a constant fear, that she will gain weight. Alteration in which of the following is responsible for this presentation? *(Most Recent Question Aug 2020)*
a. GnRH
b. hCG
c. Estrogen
d. Progesterone

413. A 19-year-old girl with primary amenorrhea with normal secondary sexual characteristics. On examination, uterus was absent. What is the next Best investigation to be done? *(Most Recent Question Aug 2020)*
a. USG
b. LH and FSH
c. Estimation
d. Karyotyping

414. A 52-year-old female came with 16 months of amenorrhea. The test results that you would expect would be? *(Most Recent Question Aug 2020)*
a. High LH and high FSH
b. Low FSH and low LH
c. FSH low and LH within normal limits
d. High FSH and Low LH

415. A 67-year-old female with hypertension and diabetes comes with heavy bleeding per vagina. What is the next management? *(Most Recent Question Dec 2019-20)*
a. Uterine ablation
b. Uterine artery block
c. Hysterectomy
d. Laser

416. A 30-year-old lady presented with amenorrhea and galactorrhea. Serum analysis reveals prolactin level of 150 ng/ml. Possible cause:
a. Pituitary adenoma *(Most Recent Question Dec 2019-20)*
b. Adrenal hyperplasia
c. 70 alpha hydroxylase deficiency
d. Hypoprolactinemia

417. True about endometriosis: *(Recent Pattern Question 2018-19)*
a. Presence of endometrial gland in deep myometrium
b. Presence of endometrium at ectopic locations
c. Treated with hysterectomy
d. Not associated with infertility

418. A 29-year-old female presented with infertility. There is history of abdominal pain, dyspareunia, dysmenorrhea, menorrhagia. Most likely cause: *(Recent Pattern Question 2018-19)*
a. Adenomyomatosis
b. Endometriosis
c. Myomas
d. Cervicitis

419. In a 25-year-old lady with primary dysmenorrhea, which of the following statement is true? *(Recent Pattern Question 2018)*
a. No clinical significant pelvic pathology is found
b. Menorrhagia and dyspareunia
c. More commonly seen after 3rd decade
d. Biochemical parameters are always normal

420. Most common cause of dysfunctional uterine bleeding:
a. PID
b. Endometriosis
c. Dermoid cyst
d. Anovulatory

421. Which of the following is an acyclical bleeding:
a. Menorrhagia
b. Polymenorrhoea
c. Metrorrhagia
d. Oligomenorrhoea

422. A 15-year-old girl presented with dysmenorrhea in every menstrual period. Menarche occurs at 13 years of age. Since then she experiences this very severe pain at right side associated with nausea and vomiting. She can't attend the school during menses from past year for which she consulted and started to take NSAIDs. Initially it is effective but after some time it is ineffective. What is next line of management?
a. Pelvic and abdomen USG
b. Oral contraceptive pills
c. Dilatation and curretage
d. High dose of non-specific steroid

423. Drug of choice in case of Puberty menorrhagia:
a. Progesterone
b. OCP
c. IUCD
d. Endometrial curretage

FIBROID

424. During a laparotomy of a 60-year-old woman, a mass is seen next to the uterus as shown in the picture. What is the mass likely to be? *(Most Recent Question Aug 2020)*

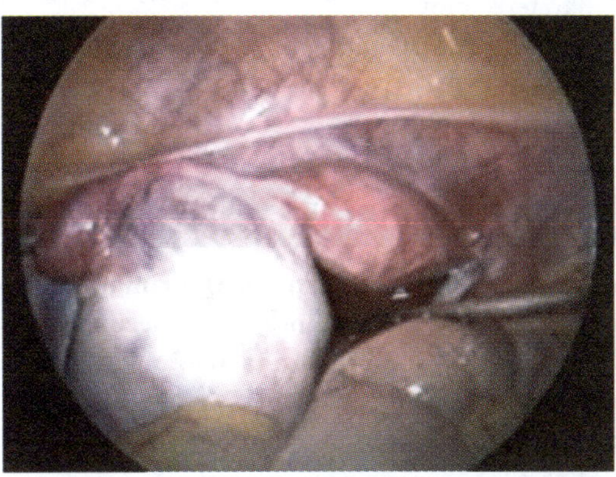

a. Ovarian CA
b. Hydrosalpinx
c. Fibroid
d. Tb adnexa

425. Patient had history of severe heart disease and now she presented with a large fibroid. Anesthesiologist classified her as a moderate risk. What procedure is NOT to be performed? *(Most Recent Question Aug 2020)*
a. Vaginal hysterectomy
b. Total abdominal hysterectomy
c. Laparoscopic hysterectomy
d. Subtotal hysterectomy

426. During caesarean section which fibroid is the easiest to remove: *(Recent Pattern Question 2018-19)*
a. Pedunculated
b. Interstitial
c. Cervical
d. Intramural

427. Which of the following is not associated with pain in submucosal fibroids? *(Recent Pattern Question 2018)*
a. Torsion
b. Large size
c. Sarcomatous change
d. Red degeneration

428. Most common type of uterine tumor is: *(Recent Pattern Question 2018)*
a. Leiomyoma
b. Endometrial cancer
c. Adenomyoma
d. Leiomyosarcoma

429. Retention of urine is caused by which type of fibroid: *(Recent Pattern Question 2017)*
a. Subserosal
b. Cervical
c. Intramural
d. Submucosal

430. Hysteroscopical excision can be done for all; EXCEPT:
a. Uterine fundus fibroid
b. Submucous fibroid
c. Subserous fibroid
d. Endometrial polyp

431. Laproscopic surgery is most applicable to which types of fibroid:
a. Subserous fibroid
b. Uterine fundus fibroid
c. Submucous fibroid
d. Endometrial polyp

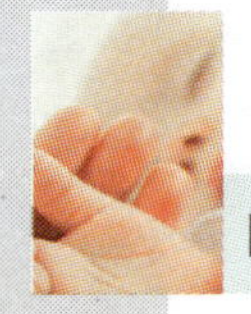

432. A pregnant female with 16 week AOG presented with bleeding. Upon USG Fibroid detected. Management:
- a. Conservative management
- b. Laparoscopic myomectomy
- c. Curettage
- d. Hysterectomy

433. Drug indicated in uterine fibroid:
- a. Danazol
- b. GnRH analogue
- c. Mifepristone
- d. All of the above

CHROMOSOMAL ANOMALIES

434. A 16-year-old girl presented with primary amenorrhea with orderly appearance of secondary sexual characteristics like breast and pubic hair. What is the next best step for this patient:
(Most Recent Question 2019)
- a. Reassure
- b. USG
- c. HSG
- d. Hormonal study

435. In Turner syndrome all are seen; EXCEPT:
- a. Webbed neck
- b. Tall stature
- c. Widening of long bones of leg
- d. XO inheritance

436. Which of the following is true about Turner syndrome?
- a. 45 X Chromosome
- b. Primary Amenorrhea
- c. Coarctation of acrta
- d. All of the above

437. Turner syndrome is
- a. 45 XO
- b. 47 XXY
- c. Trisomy 13
- d. Trisomy 18

438. Turner syndrome presents with which heart defect?
- a. PDA
- b. TOF
- c. Coaractation of aorta
- d. Mitral stenosis

439. In Down's syndrome, 2nd trimester quadruple test includes all; EXCEPT:
- a. Alpha fetoprotein
- b. hCG
- c. Inhibin A
- d. PAPP

440. Young female comes in with primary amenorrhea with normal breast, normal pubic hair. USG reveals absent uterus and cervix with short vaginal pouch and normal ovaries. Diagnosis:
- a. Klinefelter syndrome
- b. Mullerian agenesis
- c. Gonadal dysgenesis
- d. XYY

441. Female pseudohermaphroditism, all are true; EXCEPT:
- a. Mullerian inhibiting substance is not produced
- b. Karyotype 46 XX
- c. Ovaries and uterus are absent
- d. Fused posterior labia with prominent clitoral hypertrophy

TROPHOBLASTIC TUMORS

442. On the basis of given image what is your diagnosis?
(Most Recent Question Dec 2019-20)

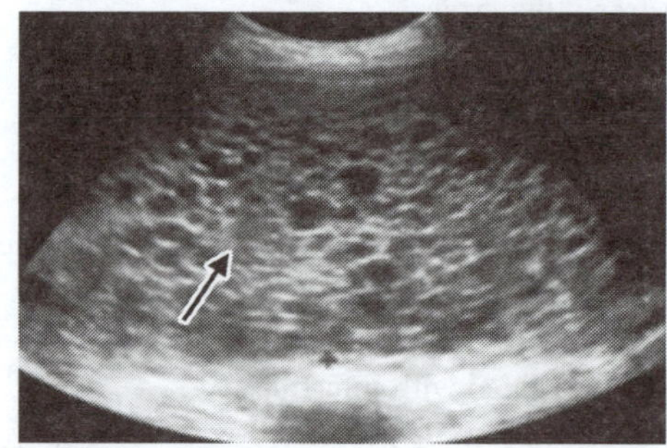

- a. Hydatiform mole
- b. Fibroid
- c. Ovarian cyst
- d. PCOS

443. Most common site of metastasis of choriocarcinoma
(Recent Pattern Question 2016)
- a. Lung
- b. Liver
- c. GIT
- d. Ovaries

444. After evacuation of molar pregnancy, monitoring is done with *(Recent Pattern Question 2016)*
- a. Serial TVS
- b. Serial serum β hCG level
- c. Speculum examination
- d. LDH level

445. Which of the following is not trophoblast related:
- a. Choriocarcinoma
- b. H. mole
- c. Placental Site tropboblast tumor
- d. Chorioangioma

INFERTILITY AND CONTRACEPTION

446. Identify the image? *(Most Recent Question June 2022)*

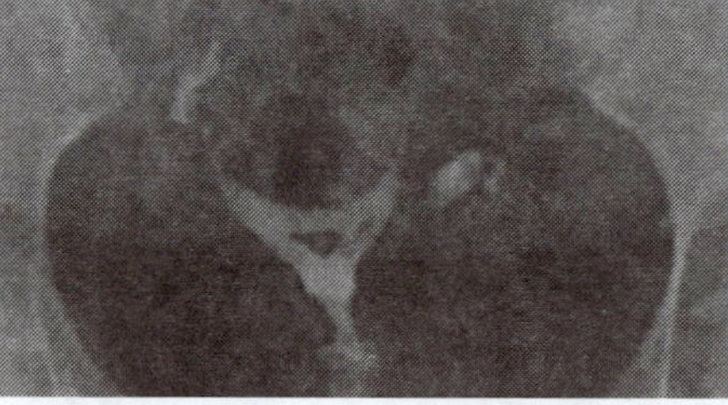

- a. Unicornuate uterus
- b. Septate
- c. Asherman syndrome
- d. Normal HSG

447. Which of the following is an absolute contraindication of IUCD insertion? *(Most Recent Question June/Dec 2021)*
- a. Unexplained vaginal bleeding
- b. History of previous PID
- c. Previous ectopic pregnancy
- d. HIV positive status

448. A female undergoing IVF was given inj. hCG for ovulation trigger now presents with nausea, vomiting and headache. The USG of pelvis done shows some ascites and the ovary looks like the image shown. What is the most probable diagnosis?

(Most Recent Question June/Dec 2021)

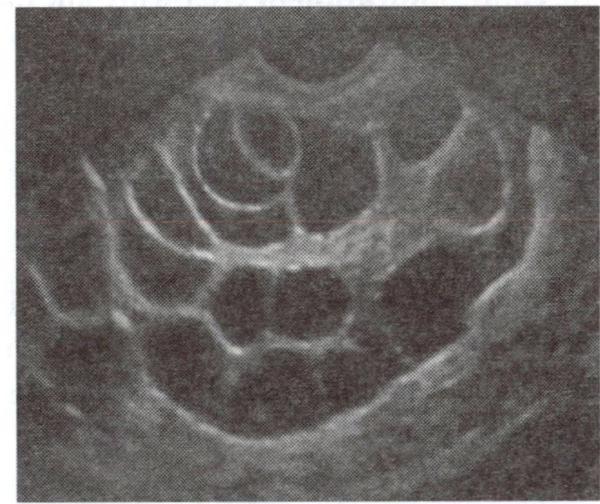

a. Serous cystadenoma
b. Theca lutein cysts
c. Ovarian hyperstimulation syndrome
d. PCOS

449. All of the following regarding 'Non scalpel vasectomy' are correct; EXCEPT?

(Most Recent Question June/Dec 2021)

a. Hematoma in up to 5% of subjects may occur
b. Sexual function following healing is rarely affected
c. Sterility immediately after vasectomy
d. Recanalization is possible

450. A lady with infertility undergoes a laparoscopy for the purpose of assessment of the pelvic anatomy for tubal patency a 'Chromotubation' involves pushing dye from a cannula in the cervix which is observed to come out from the fallopian tubes. This chromotubation is usually done using which of the following?

(Most Recent Question June/Dec 2021)

a. Saline b. Methylene blue dye
c. Carbon dioxide d. Gentian violet

451. A male had a vasectomy 1 month ago. Even after the procedure, his wife is now pregnant. What advice should have been given? *(Most Recent Question Aug 2020)*

a. Use condom for 3 months
b. Abstinence for 3 month
c. OCP for 1 month for wife
d. 1 month hormonal contraceptive

452. A patient was using IUCD as method of contraception. After 2 months of usage, she presents with repeated 'black-outs' (syncopal attacks) to the emergency room. What is the likely cause?

(Most Recent Question Aug 2020)

a. Ectopic pregnancy b. Recurrent abortion
c. Sepsis d. Coagulation abnormality

453. A 29-year-old nulliparous lady presented with endometriosis and infertility on laparoscopy there were severe pelvic adhesions and the uterus had bowel stuck to its fundus with dense adhesions. The ovaries were cystic, each around 6–8 cms in size, and were stuck to each other (kissing ovaries) what is next line of management?

a. GnRH analogues *(Most Recent Question Aug 2020)*
b. OCPs
c. Hysterectomy with oophorectomy
d. Bilateral cystectomy, adhesiolysis and prepare for IVF

454. A woman with secondary amenorrhea with history of curettage for abortion. FSH 7 miu/ml. What is your likely diagnosis? *(Most Recent Question Dec 2019-20)*

a. Pituitary failure b. Ovarian failure
c. Uterine synechiae d. Pregnancy

455. Contraindications of the device shown in image:

(Most Recent Question Dec 2019-20)

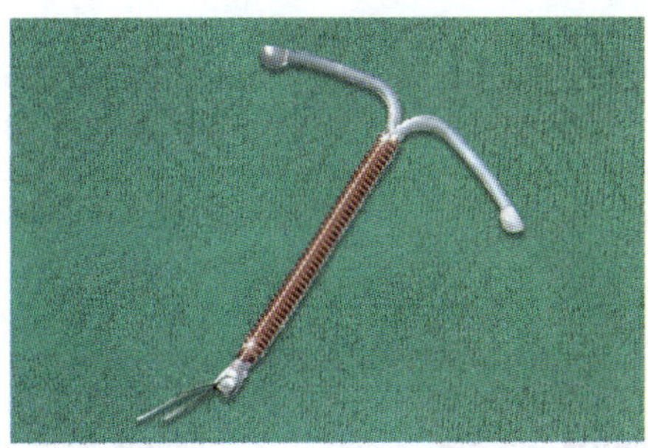

a. Breast feeding b. Monogamous
c. Hypertension d. PID

456. A 22-year-old female asking for an emergency contraception within 8 hours of sexual assault and she is on 13th day of the cycle. What is the suitable emergency contraception for her?

(Most Recent Question Dec 2019-20)

a. Levonorgestrel tablet single dose 1.5 mg
b. DMPA
c. OCP from day 1st of next cycle
d. Misoprostol

457. In a newly married couple, the woman is having irregular menstruation. What is the contraceptive of choice?

(Most Recent Question Dec 2019-20)

a. Barrier method b. OCP
c. Calendar method d. Progesterone only pills

458. The contraceptive which is contraindicated in DVT:

(Most Recent Question Dec 2019-20)

a. OCP b. Barrier method
c. Billing's method d. IUD

459. Contraceptive contraindicated during post-partum is?

(Most Recent Question Dec 2019-20)

a. Oral contraceptive pills b. Barrier method
c. Withdrawal d. IUD

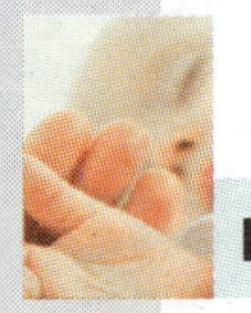

460. A woman post coitus after 96 hours, best contraceptive of choice is: *(Most Recent Question Dec 2019-20)*
a. OCP b. IUCD
c. Mifepristone d. Progesterone only pills

461. In a retroverted uterus a mass is present in lower uterine cavity. Palpated through posterior fornix. Patient is nulliparous and infertile. Tenderness is present in posterior fornix. Diagnosis? *(Most Recent Question Dec 2019-20)*
a. Adenomyosis b. Endometriosis
c. Fibroid uterus d. None

462. A young lady presents with infertility and diagnosed with bilateral cornual block on HSG. What is the next step in the management? *(Most Recent Question Dec 2019-20)*
a. IVF
b. Tuboplasty
c. Laparoscopy and hysteroscopy
d. USG

463. A 35-year-old female presented with complaints of infertility. She has previous history of PID. Preliminary investigations like USG showed normal organs and hormone levels were also normal. What is the next best investigation? *(Most Recent Question 2019)*
a. Repeat USG
b. Hysterosalpingography
c. Endometrial biopsy
d. Urine culture and sensitivity

464. Minimum sperm count for normal semen analysis according to WHO: *(Most Recent Question 2019)*
a. 2 million/mL b. 5 million/mL
c. 10 million/mL d. 20 million/mL

465. Endometrial biopsy for infertility test in women should be done at: *(Most Recent Question 2019)*
a. Ovulatory phase b. Menstrual phase
c. Anytime during cycle d. Premenstrual period

466. A patient who was using CuT for contraception, presented with a 20 weeks pregnancy. The IUCD is placed at fundus, tail visible at OS and she wants to continue the pregnancy. What is your next step in this patient: *(Most Recent Question 2019)*
a. Leave IUD in-situ, continue pregnancy
b. Do medical termination of Pregnancy
c. Remove IUCD and continue pregnancy
d. Remove IUCD and do MTP

467. A 28-year-old lady (G2P1) who does not want to conceive after abortion, which is the preferred mode of contraception: *(Recent Pattern Question 2018-19)*
a. OCP b. IUD
c. Barrier d. Implant

468. After a normal delivery OCP is to be started after___: *(Recent Pattern Question 2018-19)*
a. 2 weeks b. 6 weeks
c. 12 weeks d. 3 months

469. In a couple, initial work-up done for infertility: *(Recent Pattern Question 2018-19)*
a. Semen analysis, CXR, Montoux
b. Semen analysis, Tubal patency test, Ovulation test
c. Ovulation, tubal patency, Montoux test
d. Testicular biopsy, USG, sperm penetration test

470. Absolute contraindication of OCP's are all; EXCEPT: *(Recent Pattern Question 2018)*
a. Smoking b. Age <35 years
c. Lactation d. Breast cancer

471. OCP can lead to: *(Recent Pattern Question 2018)*
a. Hepatic adenoma b. Thyroid adenoma
c. Fibroadenoma d. Myoma

472. Which of the following is the preferred mode of contraception recommended during lactation? *(Recent Pattern Question 2018)*
a. IUCD b. DMPA
c. Progesterone only pills d. OCP

473. Which of the following is the first line drug for follicle induction in infertility? *(Recent Pattern Question 2018)*
a. Clomiphene citrate b. GnRH agonist
c. OCP d. hCG therapy

474. Which of these is true about RU_486 given for abortion? *(Recent Pattern Question 2017)*
a. Used till 11th week
b. Teratogenic effect
c. Used for emergency contraception
d. Protects from ectopic pregnancy

475. Most common complication of IUD insertion *(Recent Pattern Question 2016)*
a. Pain b. Vaginal bleeding
c. Expulsion d. Infection

476. Unexplained infertility is diagnosed in:
a. 1% of infertile couples b. 5% of infertile couples
c. 10% of infertile couples d. 2S% of infertile couples

477. Testicular biopsy is best indicated in diagnostic workup of patient with:
a. Azoospermia
b. Oligospermia
c. Necrospemnia
d. Pyospermia

478. A couple after four days of having sex, contraceptive recommended:
a. Oral contraceptive pills
b. CuT 380
c. Yuzpe method
d. Low dose POP with norgesterol

479. Failure rate of Pomeroy's technique of sterilization is:
a. 0.1% to 0.3% b. 0.3% to 1%
c. 1.0% to 1.5% d. 1.6% to 2.0%

480. Contraceptive effect of CuT-380A lasts for how many years?
a. 5 years b. 10 years
c. 15 years d. 20 years

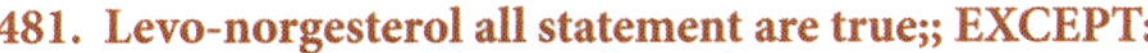

481. Levo-norgesterol all statement are true;; EXCEPT:
- a. Used in combined OCP with estrogen
- b. Composition in combined OCP is 0.15 mg
- c. Should be given for 21 days
- d. They are lipid friendly

482. All are benefits of OCPs; EXCEPT:
- a. Improve menstrual abnormality
- b. Protect against unwanted pregnancy
- c. Protect from breast cancer
- d. Protect from endometrial cancer

483. Non-contraceptive benefit of combined oral contraceptive pills include all; EXCEPT:
- a. Protection against endometrial cancer
- b. Protection against cervical cancer
- c. Relief of dysmenorrhoea
- d. Relief of menorrhagia

484. Mechanism of action of combined OCP:
- a. Prevent implantation of ovum
- b. Prevent fertilization
- c. Prevent release of ovum from ovary
- d. Reduce sperm motility

POLYCYSTIC OVARIAN SYNDROME (PCOS)/STEIN LEVANTHAL SYNDROME

485. MC cause of hirsutism: ***(Recent Pattern Question 2018-19)***
- a. Drug induced
- b. PCOS
- c. Endometriosis
- d. Adenomyosis

486. The number of ovarian follicles are increased in: ***(Recent Pattern Question 2018)***
- a. Turner syndrome
- b. Klinefelter syndrome
- c. PCOD
- d. Primary amenorrhea

487. Most common cause of hirsutism in females is:
- a. Metropathica hemorrhagica
- b. PCOD
- c. Endometriosis
- d. PID

488. Patient with history of amenorrhea and hirsutism. USG of uterus given below. Diagnosis:

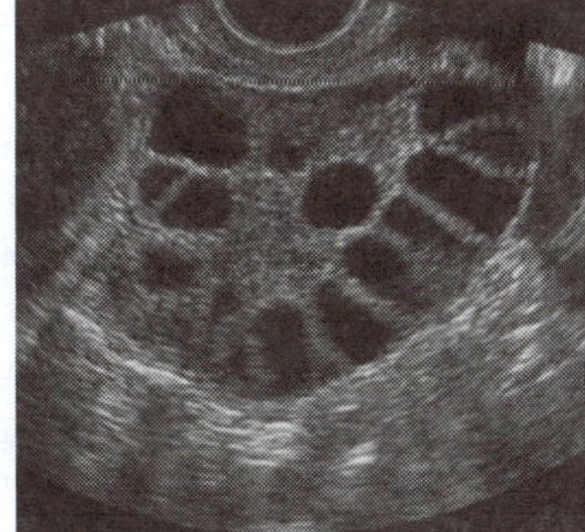

- a. PCOS
- b. Endometriosis
- c. Adenomyomatosis
- d. Choriocarcinoma

489. Primary treatment for hirsutism in PCOD:
- a. Minoxidil
- b. Progesterone
- c. GnRH analogue
- d. Combined OCP

PROLAPSE

490. 24-year-old woman presented in ER with fully outside cervix and a cystocele. What is the next step of management? ***(Most Recent Question June 2022)***
- a. Hysterectomy
- b. Le fort and posterior colporraphy
- c. Simply cystocele repair
- d. Pessary for temporary relief

491. Identify the image? ***(Most Recent Question June 2022)***

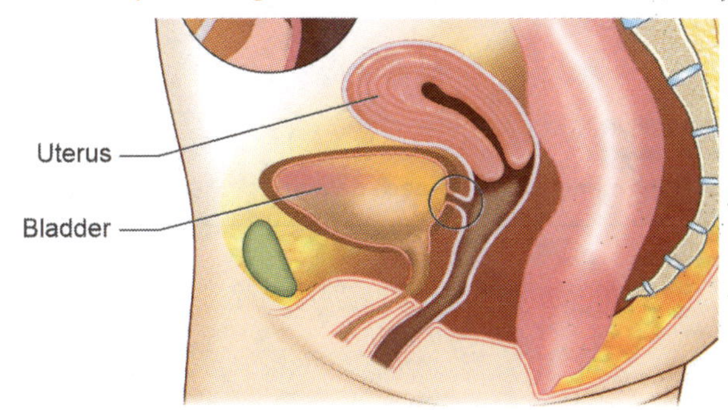

- a. Vesicovaginal fistula
- b. Uterovaginal fistula
- c. Vesico cervical fistula
- d. Uretero vaginal

492. Lady passes urine while coughing or laughing: ***(Most Recent Question June/Dec 2021)***
- a. Stress urinary incontinence
- b. Urge incontinence/OAB
- c. Urethrovaginal fistula
- d. Reflex incontinence

493. Which of the following is treatment for decubitus ulcers in uterine prolapse? ***(Most Recent Question June/Dec 2021)***
- a. Laser ablation
- b. Antibiotics
- c. Cryotherapy
- d. Packing

494. True about Pessary used in prolapse: ***(Recent Pattern Question 2018-19)***
- a. Filling type pessary used
- b. Not preferred in pregnancy
- c. Needs to be changed every 3 months
- d. Never used with Gel to insert

495. Conservative treatment for pelvic organ prolapse: ***(Recent Pattern Question 2018-19)***
- a. Perineorrhaphy
- b. Shirodkar procedure
- c. Pessary
- d. Le Fort repair

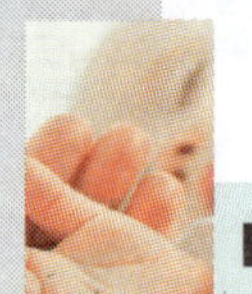

ANSWERS WITH EXPLANATIONS

OBSTETRICS

MOST RECENT QUESTIONS 2023

1. Ans. (b) Ritgen

Ref: Williams Obstetrics, 22nd ed. pg. 486

Ritgen's maneuver denotes extracting the fetal head, using one hand to pull the fetal chin from between the maternal anus and the coccyx, and the other on the fetal occiput to control speed of delivery.

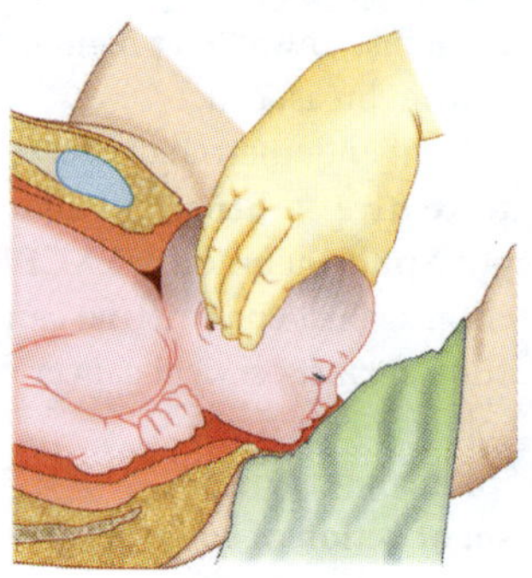

Extra Mile

Important maneuver for breech deliveries

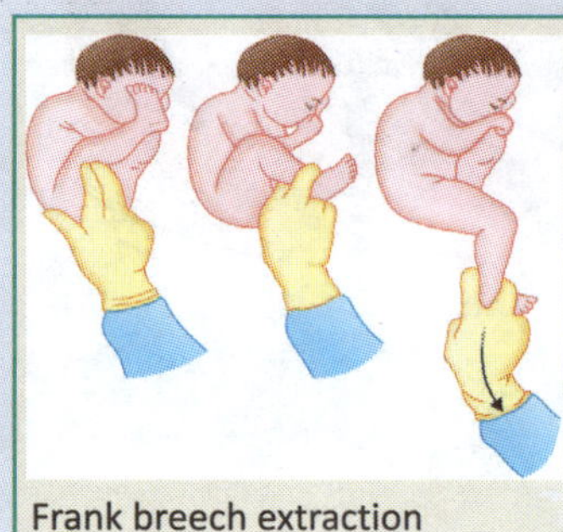

Frank breech extraction (Pinard's Maneuver)

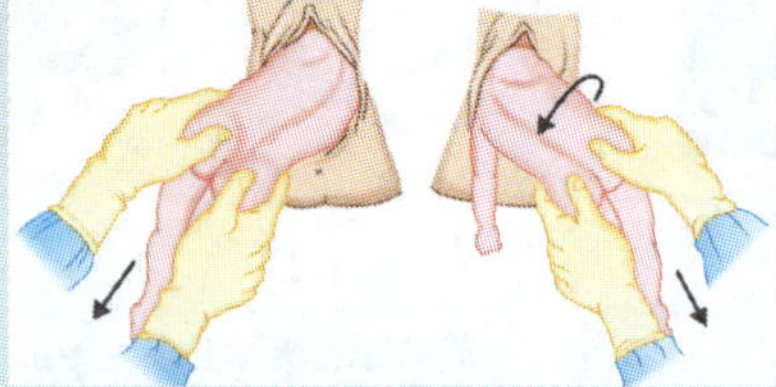

Løvset's Maneuver

It involves rotation of the trunk of the fetus during a breech birth to facilitate delivery of the extended fetal arms and the shoulders.

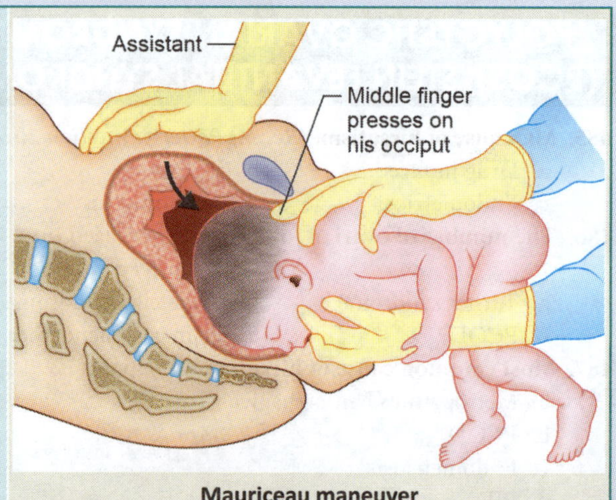

Mauriceau maneuver

2. Ans. (c) 20 weeks

Ref: Williams Obstetrics, 22nd ed. pg. 413

- Uterine height after delivery is at the lower border of umbilicus, i.e., which is same as 20 weeks age of gestation.
- Involution is ~ 1.25 cm/day and it becomes pelvic organ on day 10–11 after delivery.

Extra Mile

• Immediately after delivery	• Fundus palpable at the level of umbilicus
• 10–14 days after delivery	• At the level of pubic symphysis
• 6 weeks post-partum	• Nonpregnant size

3. Ans. (c) Vesicovaginal fistula

Ref: Williams Obstetrics, 22nd ed. pg. 1007

- A vesicovaginal fistula is an abnormal connection between the bladder and the vagina. There may be just one opening, there may be more. If fistula is present, urine will leak from the vagina.
- In methylene blue swab test, three gauze swabs are placed into the vagina using a speculum – one at the top, one in the middle, and one at the bottom. A small catheter (hollow tube) is put into the bladder and blue dye is passed through it into the bladder:
  - If uppermost swab is wet: Ureterovaginal fistula

- If middle swab is wet: Vesicovaginal fistula
- If lowermost swab is wet: Urethrovaginal fistula

4. Ans. (c) Central placenta previa

Ref: Williams Obstetrics, 22nd ed. pg. 578

- Central placenta previa is a complete contraindication to induction of labor. Therefore, expectant management includes planned cesarean section in late gestation which is done between 36 and 37 weeks.
- The primary maternal risk factor in placenta previa is massive hemorrhage, including postpartum bleeding.
- **Contraindications to Induction of Labor:**
  - Placenta previa central/major degree
  - Vasa previa
  - Umbilical cord prolapses
  - Active genital herpes infection
  - Cephalopelvic disproportion
  - Invasive cervical CA
  - Transverse lie
  - Previous history of uterine rupture
  - Hypersensitivity to cervical ripening agent

5. Ans. (d) Her consent with opinions of two doctors

- As per the recent MTP amendment Act 2021, medical termination of pregnancy can be done till 24th week age of gestation in cases of sustained fetal abnormalities (example: meningomyelocele). For this, opinions of two RMPs are required along with the consent of patient.

6. Ans. (c) Abruptio placentae

Ref: Williams Obstetrics, 22nd ed. pg. 749

- Placental abruption is when the placenta separates early from the uterus; in other words, separates before childbirth. It occurs most commonly around 25 weeks of pregnancy.
- Symptoms may include vaginal bleeding, lower abdominal pain, and dangerously low blood pressure.
- Most important risk factor for abruptio placenta: Hypertension
- In uterine rupture, fetal parts are palpable and placenta previa presents with painless vaginal bleeding.

7. Ans. (c) Inhibin and Testosterone

Ref: Williams Obstetrics, 22nd ed. pg. 228

- Sertoli cells are involved in inhibin secretion, while Leydig cells secrete testosterone.

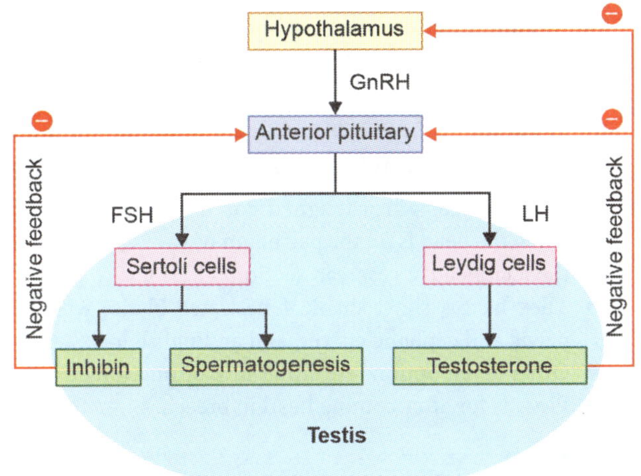

8. Ans. (d) Pre-eclampsia

Ref: Williams Obstetrics, 22nd ed. pg. 690

- Pre-eclampsia is defined as BP >140/90 on 2 occasions, 4 hours apart.
- In addition to the blood pressure criteria, proteinuria of greater than or equal to 0.3 grams in a 24-hour urine specimen, a protein (mg/dL)/creatinine (mg/dL) ratio of 0.3 or higher, or a urine dipstick protein of 1+ (if a quantitative measurement is unavailable) is required to diagnose pre-eclampsia.

9. Ans. (b) Second trimester

Ref: Williams Obstetrics, 22nd ed. pg. 144

- The quadruple screen test is a blood test done during pregnancy to determine whether the baby is at risk of certain birth defects.
- It is done in second trimester.
- The test measures levels of the following four pregnancy hormones:
  - Alpha-fetoprotein (AFP), a protein produced by the baby.
  - Human chorionic gonadotropin (hCG), a hormone produced in the placenta.
  - Unconjugated estriol (uE3), a form of the hormone estrogen produced in the fetus and the placenta.
  - Inhibin-A

10. Ans. (a) Low BMI

Ref: Williams Obstetrics, 22nd ed. pg. 103

- One form of estrogen called estradiol decreases at menopause. This hormone helps to regulate metabolism and body weight.
- Lower levels of estradiol may lead to weight gain.

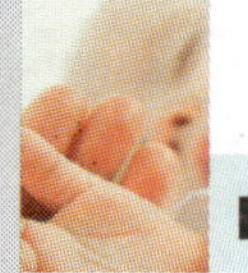

- Nulliparity endometriosis and tamoxifen use can be associated with elevated estrogen levels.

11. Ans. (d) Wrigley

Ref: Williams Obstetrics, 22nd ed. pg. 3076

- Outlet forceps are designed for use in outlet lift-out when the head is on the perineum or to assist the birth of the fetal head at cesarean section.
- They have a short shank, fenestrated blades with both pelvic and cephalic curves, and an English lock.
- Other given options are either low, or mid forceps.
- Piper is for after coming head in breech.

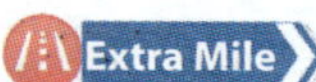

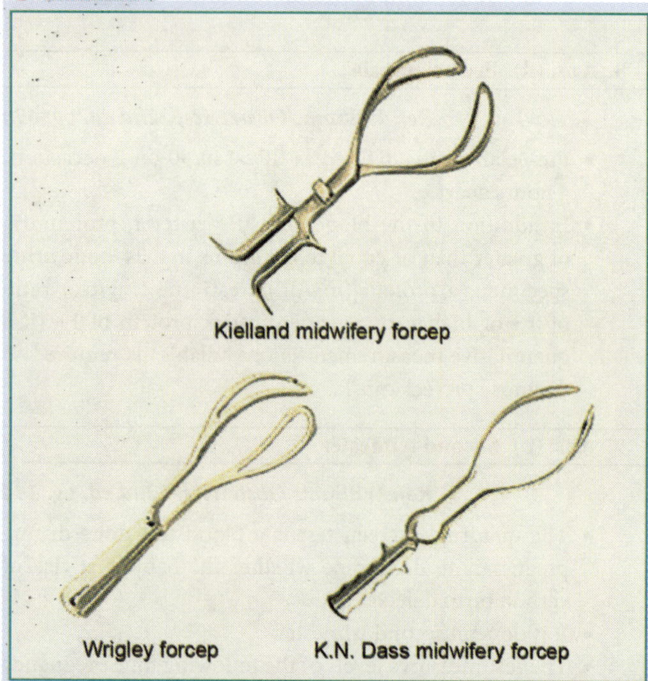

12. Ans. (b) Uterine synechiae

Ref: Williams Obstetrics, 22nd ed. pg. 204

- Asherman syndrome (intrauterine adhesions or intrauterine synechiae) occurs when scar tissue forms inside the uterus and/or the cervix.
- These adhesions occur after surgery of the uterus or after a dilatation and curettage after abortion or with tuberculosis and schistosomiasis being a less common cause.

13. Ans. (c) FSH

Ref: Williams Obstetrics, 22nd ed. pg. 300

- The normal gonadotrophin axis is disturbed in PCOS women; therefore, LH levels increase, and FSH levels decrease leading to a reversal of LH/FSH ratio.

14. Ans. (c) Serum testosterone

Ref: Williams Obstetrics, 22nd ed. pg. 302

- Polycystic ovary syndrome (PCOS) is a condition in which the ovaries produce an abnormal number of androgens.
- Women with PCOS often have an increased level of both total testosterone and free testosterone.

15. Ans. (c) Lateral cutaneous nerve of thigh

Ref: Williams Obstetrics, 22nd ed. pg. 498

- During vaginal delivery, lateral femoral cutaneous nerve injury occurs in approximately four out of 1000 parturient.
- This nerve supplies sensation to the anterolateral thigh, courses under the inguinal ligament, which makes it susceptible to compression while in lithotomy position.

16. Ans. (b) Placenta covering internal os

Ref: Williams Obstetrics, 22nd ed. pg. 412

- For vaginal delivery or for controlling postpartum hemorrhage, oxytocin is indicated. It can also be utilized while doing instrumental delivery but not in patient placenta previa.
- **Contraindications of oxytocin:**
  - Abnormal fetal position
  - Cephalopelvic disproportion
  - Cervical cancer
  - Elective induction of labor
  - Fetal distress
  - Fetal prematurity
  - Placenta previa
  - Vasa previa

17. Ans. (b) Decreased Serum creatinine

Ref: Williams Obstetrics, 22nd ed. pg. 68

- During pregnancy, blood flow to the kidneys is higher. This increases a person's GFR and the rate of creatinine excretion. Due to this, pregnant people typically have lower levels of blood creatinine.
- Pregnancy-associated plasma protein A (PAPP-A) is a key regulator of insulin-like growth factor bioavailability essential for normal fetal development. In maternal blood, this protein increases with gestational age and then rapidly decreases after delivery.

Extra Mile

Hematological changes during pregnancy

- Increased plasma volume up to 50%
- RBC volume increases ~30%
- Increased procoagulant factors

18. Ans. (a) Enterocele

Ref: Williams Obstetrics, 22nd ed. pg. 564

- McCall culdoplasty is a vaginal-approach repair of an enterocele.
- The modified McCall culdoplasty (MC) is a relatively simple procedure that is performed after the removal of the uterus and cervix from the apex of the vagina, where the angles of the vagina are attached to their respective uterosacral ligaments, and the cul-de-sac is surgically obliterated for support postoperatively.

19. Ans. (a) Oral combined contraceptive

Ref: Williams Obstetrics, 22nd ed. pg. 671

The following protective factors decrease the risk of endometrial cancer:

- Pregnancy and breastfeeding (Estrogen levels are lower during pregnancy and while breastfeeding)
- Hormonal contraceptives (COCP)
- Weight loss
- Physical activity

Note: Tamoxifen is SERM which increases the risk of endometrial cancer. Conditions like obesity, diabetes, late menopause, early menarche, nulliparity increase the risk of endometrial CA. Aspirin reduces the risk of colonic carcinoma, but does not seem to reduce endometrial carcinoma.

20. Ans. (c) Teratozoospermia

Ref: Williams Obstetrics, 22nd ed. pg. 675

- In the given seminogram, the sperm count and motility are within normal limits but morphologically they are in less number (n = at least 4%), this is a case of teratozoospermia.
- Teratozoospermia is a condition where there is a high amount of abnormal shaped sperm.

Extra Mile

Terminology	Description
Oligozoospermia	Sperm concentration ≤15 million/ml
Asthenozoospermia	Sperm progressive motility <32%
Teratozoospermia	Sperm normal morphology <4%
Oligo-astheno-teratozoospermia (OATS)	All the above three parameters
Azoospermia	No sperm detected
Normozoospermia	Normal sperm parameters

21. Ans. (d) Oxytocin

Ref: Williams Obstetrics, 22nd ed. pg. 578

- Galactokinesis is milk ejection from the breast. It is dependent on the posterior pituitary hormone, oxytocin.
- Factors that stimulate oxytocin secretion are infant suckling and other sensory inputs that mimic the infant such as cry, sight, smell, and touch.

22. Ans. (a) Marginal

Ref: DC Dutta's Textbook of Obstetrics 9th ed. pg. 228-229

Placenta previa is defined as the wrongly implanted placenta partially or completely over the lower uterine segment (over and adjacent to the internal os). The shown image is marginal type of placenta previa.

Types or degrees of placenta previa:

- **Type 1 (low lying):** The major part of the placenta is attached to the upper segment and only the lower margin encroaches onto the lower segment but not up to the os.
- **Type 2 (marginal):** The placenta reaches the margin of the internal os but does not cover it.
- **Type 3 (incomplete or partial central):** The placenta covers the internal os partially (covers the internal os when closed but does not entirely do so when fully dilated.)
- **Type 4 (central or complete):** The placenta completely covers the internal os even after it is fully dilated.

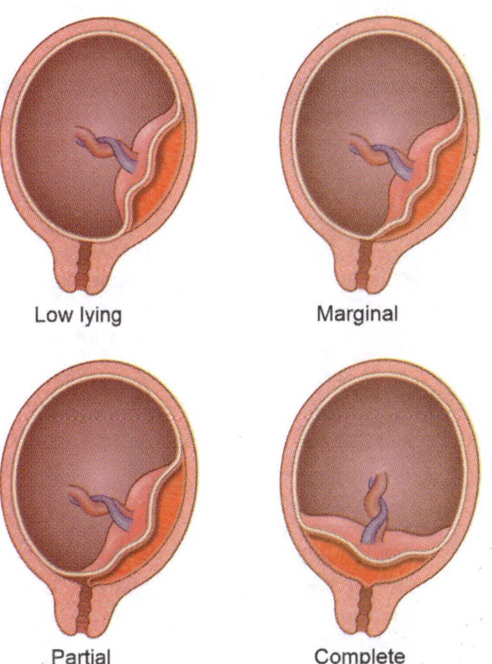

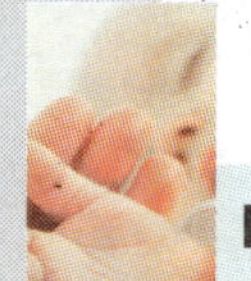

23. Ans. (a) Gynecoid

Ref: DC Dutta's Textbook of Obstetrics, 9th ed. pg. 79-85

The pelvis is anatomically divided into a false pelvis and a true pelvis. Inlet is the brim of the pelvis; the circumference of the inlet is formed by the bony landmarks. The shape of the female pelvis is usually round with the anteroposterior diameter being the shortest. This type of pelvis is known as gynecoid pelvis. Other different shapes of inlet are android, anthropoid and platypelloid.

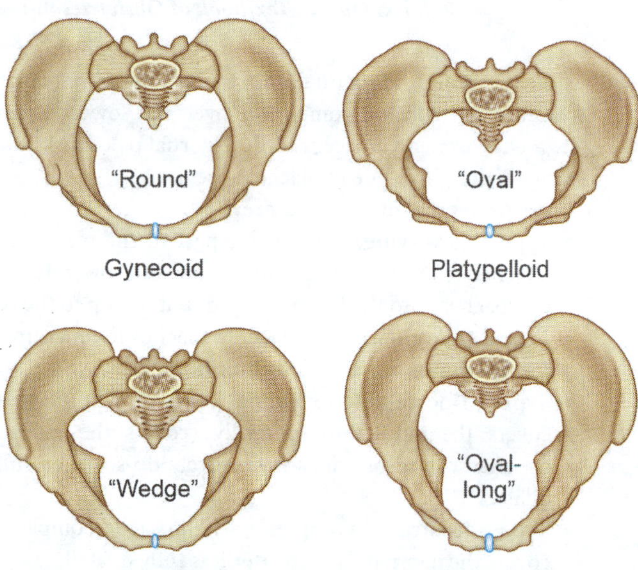

INLET

	Gynecoid	Anthropoid	Android	Platypelloid
Shape	Round	Antero-posteriorly oval	Triangular	Transversely oval
Anterior and posterior segments	Almost equal and spacious	Both increased with slight anterior narrowing	Posterior segment short & anterior segment narrow.	Both reduced- flat
Sacrum	Sacral angle >900 Inclined backwards. Well curved from above down and side to side	Sacral angle >90° Inclined posteriorly. Long and narrow	Sacral angle <90 Inclined forwards and straight.	Sacral angle >90° Inclined posteriorly.

24. Ans. (c) Monochorionic monoamniotic

Ref: DC Dutta's Textbook of Obstetrics, 9th ed. pg. 187

Determination of Chorionicity in Monozygotic Twin Pregnancy

Timing of Cleavage	Membrane status of Placenta
< 72 hours	Diamniotic-Dichorionic
4–7 days	Diamniotic-Monochorionic
8–12 days	Monoamniotic-Monochorionic
> 13 days	Conjoined (Siamese)

25. Ans. (a) Kiellands

Ref: DC Dutta's Textbook of Obstetrics 9th ed. pg. 620

- The given instrument is Kiellands forceps.
- It is usually used as rotation forceps in deep transverse arrest of occipito-posterior position of the head or in unrotated vertex or face presentation.

Other types of forceps images have been included in previous questions.

26. Ans. (a) Beyond 42 weeks

Ref: Dutta's Textbook of Obstetrics 9th ed. pg. 86-87

- Period of gestation is defined as the duration of pregnancy expressed in terms of completed weeks. A fraction of a week more than three days is considered a completed week.
- The criteria of a normal pregnancy are delivery of a single baby in good condition at term, that is between 38 and 42 weeks, with fetal weight of 2.5 kg or more and with no maternal complications. If delivery of the baby takes place before 38 weeks, it is termed preterm delivery; and if it is beyond 42 weeks, it is termed post-term delivery.

27. Ans. (b) Linea nigra

Ref: Dutta's Text Book of Obstetrics 9th ed. pg. 71

- The given image is of linea nigra. Linea nigra, often referred to as a pregnancy line, is a linear hyperpigmentation that commonly appears on the abdomen. The line runs vertically along the midline of the abdomen from the pubis to the umbilicus, but can also run from the pubis to the top of the abdomen.
- For pregnant women, Linea nigra is attributed to increased melanocyte stimulating hormone made by the placenta which also causes melasma and darkened nipples.

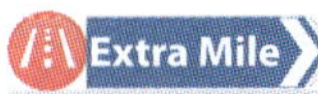

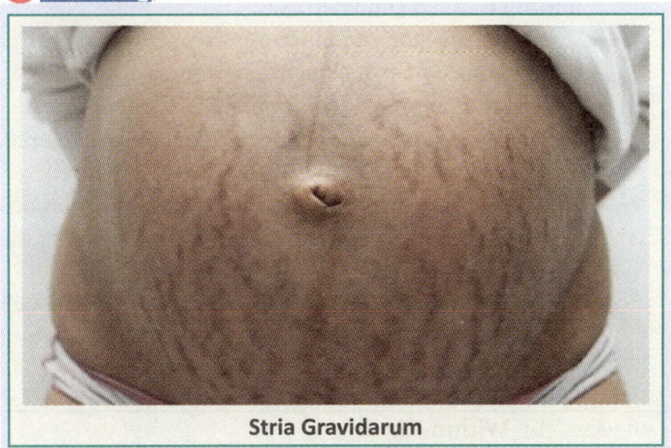

Stria Gravidarum

28. Ans. (d) Preterm labor

Ref: DC Dutta's Textbook of Obstetrics 9th ed. pg. 596

- Audit is defined as the systematic and critical analysis of the quality of medical care. Objective of carrying out an audit is to improve the quality of clinical care.
- Obstetric audit includes fetal death, injury to mother, injury to fetal head, but does not include preterm labor.

29. Ans. (a) Crown-rump length

Ref: Dutta's Textbook of Obstetrics 9th ed. pg. 63

- The best ultrasound parameter for assessment of gestational age is crown-rump length (CRL). It is usually measured using ultrasound as early as the first prenatal visit.
- Fetal gestational age is best determined by measuring the CRL between 7 and 12 weeks.
- The Doppler effect of ultrasound can pick up the fetal heart rate reliably by 10th week.

30. Ans. (a) Lochia rubra - lochia serosa – lochia alba

Ref: Dutta's Textbook of Obstetrics 9th ed. pg. 138

- Lochia is the vagina discharge for the first fortnight during puerperium. The discharge originates from the uterine body, cervix and vagina. It has got a peculiar offensive fishy smell. Depending upon the variation of the color of the discharge, it is named as: *(Mn: RSA)*
  - Lochia Rubra (red): 1–4 days
  - Lochia Serosa (yellowish): 5–9 days
  - Lochia Alba (whitish): 10–15 days

31. Ans. (a) Trichomonas vaginitis

Ref: Shaw's Textbook of Gynecology 16th ed. pg. 155

- Trichomonas vaginalis is an anaerobic flagellated, protozoan parasite, and the causative agent of a sexually transmitted disease called trichomoniasis. It is a common cause of vaginitis in women.
- 'Frothy' greenish vaginal discharge with a 'musty' malodorous smell is a characteristic feature. Only 2% of women with the infection will have a strawberry cervix. This is due to capillary hemorrhage.

32. Ans. (d) Previous macrosomia

Ref: Dutta's Textbook of Obstetrics 9th ed. pg. 546

- Previous macrosomia is not a contraindication for normal vaginal delivery. Other options are contraindications for vaginal delivery.

Indications of cesarean section

Absolute indications	Relative indications
• Central placenta previa. • Contracted pelvis or cephalopelvic disproportion • Pelvic mass causing obstruction • Advanced carcinoma cervix • Vagina obstruction (atresia, stenosis)	• Previous cesarean section. • Non-reassuring FHR • Dystocia • Antepartum hemorrhage • Malpresentation • Failed surgical induction of labor

33. Ans. (a) Pelvic inflammatory disease

Ref: Shaw's Textbook of Gynecology 16th ed. pg. 177

- Pelvic inflammatory disease (PID) is an infectious and inflammatory disorder of the upper female genital tract, including the uterus, fallopian tubes and adjacent pelvic structures. The diagnosis of acute PID is primarily based on clinical findings.
- Symptoms of PID range from fever, cervical motion tenderness over abdominal pain, new or different discharge, painful intercourse and adnexal tenderness.
- **Note:** Endometriosis, cervical cancer or ovarian cancer will not present with pus at the tubal ends.

34. Ans. (d) Td booster

Ref: DC Dutta's textbook of Obstetrics 9th ed. pg. 91

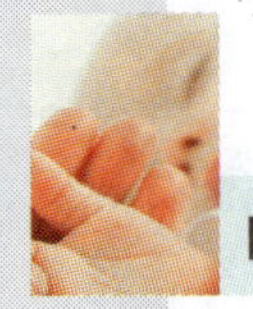

- Only Td booster dose is given to a pregnant female who has been vaccinated within three years of present pregnancy.
- Immunization against tetanus not only protects the mother but also the newborn.
- In unprotected women, 0.5 mL tetanus toxoid is given intramuscularly, 2 doses at 6 weeks interval. The first one to be given between 16 and 24 weeks.
- A booster dose of 0.5 mL is given in the last trimester to the women who have been immunized in the past.

35. Ans. (c) Type 3 hysterectomy

Ref: Shaw's Textbook of Gynecology 16th ed. pg. 485

Cervical cancer stages IA1, IA2, IB1, IB2, and IIA1 are radio sensitive and surgically operable, but surgery is preferred over radiotherapy for the stages because of the following reasons:

- Preservation of ovarian function
- Preservation of vagina for coital function
- Psychological benefit to the patient

In a 50-year-old female with carcinoma cervix, 1B, the standard management is a type 3 radical hysterectomy. Pelvic lymphadenectomy should always be included.

36. Ans. (d) Below umbilicus

Ref: DC Dutta's Textbook of Obstetrics 9th ed. pg. 137

- Just after delivery, uterus is at the lower border of umbilicus, which is around 20 weeks of gestation height.

37. Ans. (c) Estradiol

Ref: Shaw's Textbook of Gynecology 16th ed. pg. 37-47

- Peak level of estradiol is 200 pg/mL seen on D 10 to D 11. LH surge occurs after estradiol peak is sustained for 48 hours. Thus, LH surge occurs due to estrogen.

38. Ans. (d) Urine dipstick test

Ref: DC Dutta's Textbook of Obstetrics 9th ed. pg. 213

- The given clinical scenario suggests that the patient is suffering from pre-eclampsia. Among the given options, the best next step that has to be done in a patient of pre-eclampsia is urine dipstick test to check for proteinuria so as to prevent the development of eclampsia.

39. Ans. (a) Endometriosis

Ref: DC Dutta's Textbook of Gynecology, 7th ed. pg. 248-252

- Presence of endometrium in sites other than uterine mucosa is called endometriosis.
- Common sites for endometriosis can be ovaries, pelvic peritoneum, pouch of Douglas, uterosacral ligament, etc.
- Most common presenting symptom is dysmenorrhea.
- Other symptoms can be menorrhagia, dyspareunia, infertility.
- Speculum examination: Bluish powder-burn lesions may be seen on the cervix or the posterior fornix of the vagina.
- Bimanual examination: Reveal nodularity in the pouch of Douglas, nodular feel of the uterosacral ligaments and unilateral or bilateral adnexal mass (chocolate cysts).

40. Ans. (b) Within 1 hour

Ref: DC Dutta's Textbook of Obstetrics, 8th ed. pg. 172

- After normal vaginal delivery, breastfeeding should be started as soon as possible or within one hour.
- The initial secretion from the breast is called colostrum. It is a deep yellow serous fluid, alkaline in reaction. It has got a higher specific gravity; a high protein, vitamin A, sodium and chloride content but has got lower carbohydrate, fat and potassium than the breast milk (Refer to the following table).
- Colostrum contains immunologic components such as immunoglobulin A (IgA), lactoferrin.

TABLE: Percentage composition of colostrum and breast milk

	Protein	Fat	Carbohydrate	Water
Colostrum	8.6	2.3	3.2	86
Breast milk	1.2	3.2	7.5	87

41. Ans. (a) PCOS

Ref: DC Dutta's Textbook of Gynecology, 7th ed. pg. 378-382

- The given image shows the laparoscopic ovarian drilling procedure. It is done in case of polycystic ovarian syndrome (PCOS).
- This syndrome is manifested by amenorrhea, hirsutism, and obesity associated with enlarged polycystic ovaries, which is treated using the drilling procedure.

42. Ans. (a) Endometrial biopsy

Ref: DC Dutta's Textbook of Gynecology, 7th ed. pg. 462-463.

- The given image shows pipelle aspirator used for endometrial biopsy in case of abnormal postmenopausal

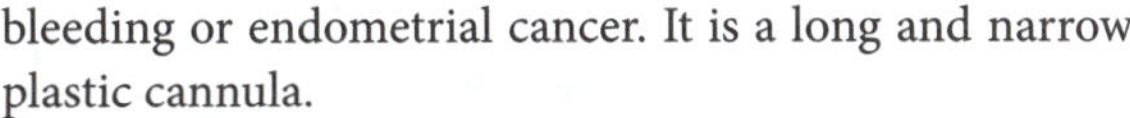

bleeding or endometrial cancer. It is a long and narrow plastic cannula.

- This is done as an outpatient department (OPD) procedure during speculum examination. Adequate sample is obtained with this procedure and the tissue is subjected to histological examination.
- It has no role in termination of pregnancy or aspiration of ectopic pregnancy.

43. Ans. (d) Cleidotomy

Ref: DC Dutta's Textbook of Obstetrics, 8th ed. pg. 469-470

- Cleidotomy is a deliberate fracture of the clavicle. One or both clavicles may be cut with scissors to reduce the shoulder girth. This is applicable to a living anencephalic baby as a first choice or in a dead fetus.
- It was earlier done in case of shoulder dystocia in gestational diabetes mellitus as a last alternative procedure but no longer recommended now.

44. Ans. (c) 10 years

Ref: DC Dutta's Textbook of Obstetrics, 8th ed. pg. 615

- Copper T 380A is a type of medicated intrauterine contraceptive device. It has a total of 380 mm square surface area of copper wire wound around the stem (314 mm^2) and each copper sleeve on the horizontal arms (33 mm^2). The frame contains barium sulfate and is radiopaque.
- Its half-life is 10 years.
- Mechanism of antifertility effects of all the IUDs is not yet clear. They act predominantly in the uterine cavity and do not inhibit ovulation.

45. Ans. (a) Ampulla

Ref: DC Dutta's Textbook of Obstetrics, 8th ed. pg. 207

- Ectopic pregnancy is defined as pregnancy in which the fertilized ovum is implanted and develops outside the normal endometrial cavity.
- Overall the most common site of ectopic pregnancy is ampulla of fallopian tube.

Various sites where ectopic pregnancy can be implanted are shown in the following chart:

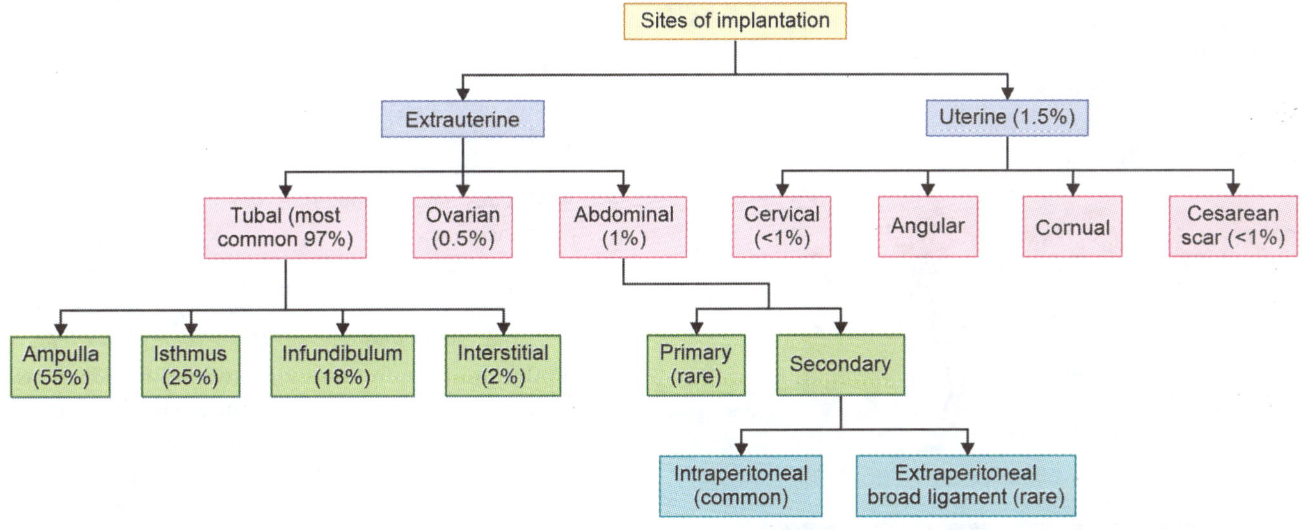

ANATOMY AND PHYSIOLOGY

46. Ans. (a) Klinefelter's syndrome

Ref: Comprehensive Gynecology 7th ed. pg. 33

- Klinefelter syndrome is a chromosomal condition in boys and men that can affect physical and intellectual development. The features of the condition are so mild that the condition is not diagnosed until puberty or adulthood.
- Children with klinefelter syndrome may have hypotonia and problems with coordination that may delay the development of motor skills, such as sitting, standing, and walking.
- Boys and men with Klinefelter syndrome typically have small testes that produce a reduced amount of testosterone.

47. Ans. (a) Vestibule

Ref: DC Dutta's 9th ed. pg. 2

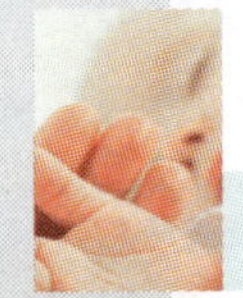

There are 4 openings into the vestibule:
1. Urethral opening
2. Vaginal orifice and hymen
3. Opening of bartholin's ducts
4. Skene's gland

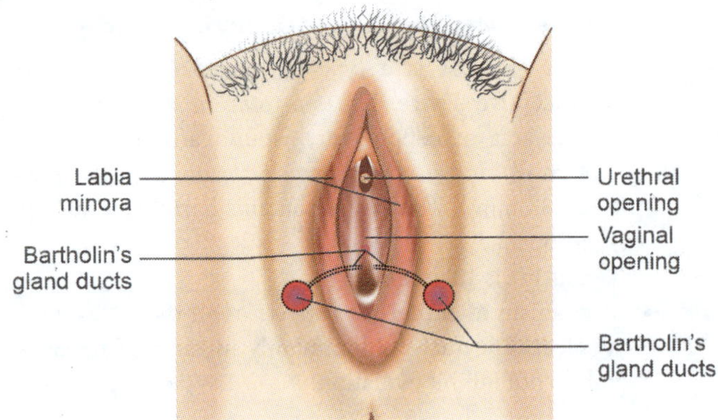

48. Ans. (a) Imperforate hymen image

Ref: DC Dutta's 9th ed. pg. 2

- An imperforate hymen is a congenital disorder where a hymen without an opening completely obstructs the vagina. It is caused by a failure of the hymen to perforate during fetal development.
- It is most often diagnosed in adolescent girls when menstrual blood accumulates in vagina and also in uterus.

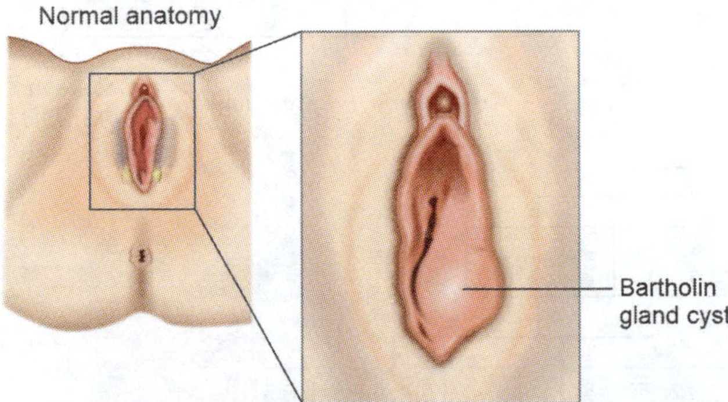

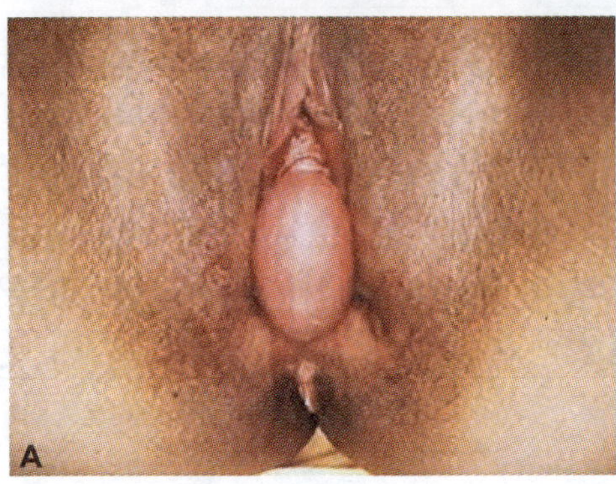

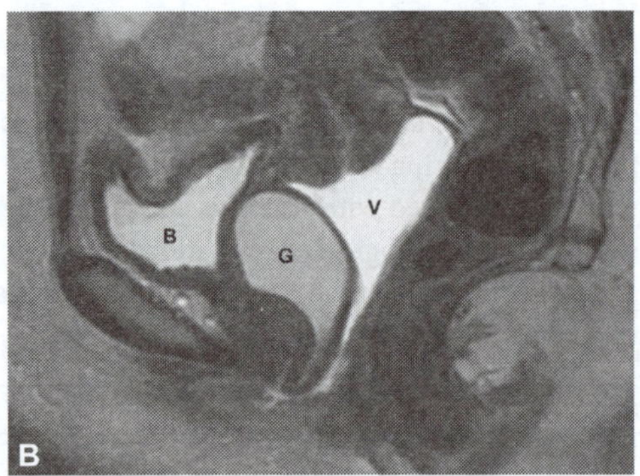

Gartner's Cyst

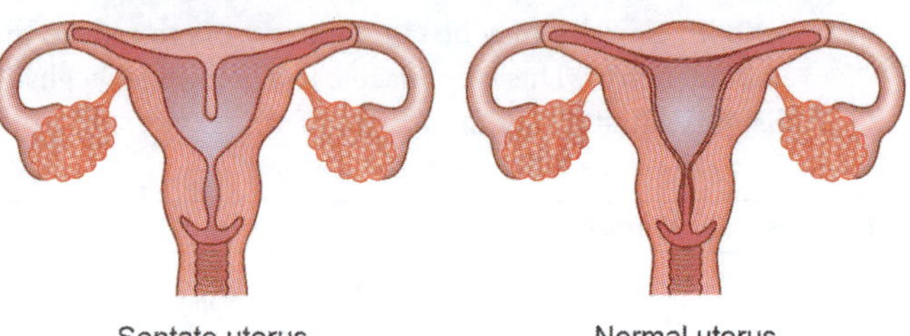

49. Ans. (c) Ciliated columnar

Ref: DC Dutta's 9th ed. pg. 7

Fallopian tube consist of layers
- **Serous:** It consist of peritoneum on all sides except along the line of attachment of mesosalpinx
- **Muscular:** Arranged in two layers- outer longitudinal and inner circular
- **Mucous membrane:** It is lined by ciliates columnar epithelium.

50. Ans. (d) Asherman's syndrome

Ref: Comprehensive Gynecology 7th ed. pg. 334

- Asherman syndrome is characterized by adhesions in the uterine cavity that can cause partial or complete obliteration of the endometrium, leading to menstrual abnormalities and amenorrhea, as well as pregnancy loss.
- In the majority cases, adhesions result from uterine curettage for pregnancy complications such as missed or incomplete abortion as well as postpartum complications such as postpartum hemorrhage or retained placental remnants.

51. Ans. (a) Cruciate incision and drainage of blood

Ref: Shaw's Textbook of Gynaecology, 7th ed. pg. 144

- Bluish bulging hymen suggests cryptomenorrhea.
- Cryptomenorrhea is a condition in which menstruation occurs but is not visible due to obstruction of outflow

tract resulting in either hematometra (blood collection within uterus) or hematocolpos (blood collection within vagina).

- A history of cyclic abdominal colicky pain, retention of urine, presence of a palpable abdominal lump and visualization of a bluish bulging membrane confirms the diagnosis.

52. Ans. (b) Anthropoid pelvis

Ref: William's Obstetrics, Chapter 2, 26th ed. pg. 89

- Persistent occipito-posterior is common in the Anthropoid type of pelvis.

The four different pelvis shapes are:

- **Gynecoid**: This is the most common type of pelvis in females and is generally considered to be the typical female pelvis. Its overall shape is round, shallow, and open.
- **Android**: This type of pelvis bears more resemblance to the male pelvis. It's narrower than the gynecoid pelvis and is shaped more like a heart or a wedge.
- **Anthropoid**: An anthropoid pelvis is narrow and deep. Its shape is similar to an upright egg or oval.
- **Platypelloid**: The platypelloid pelvis is also called a flat pelvis. This is the least common type. It's wide but shallow, and it resembles an egg or oval lying on its side.

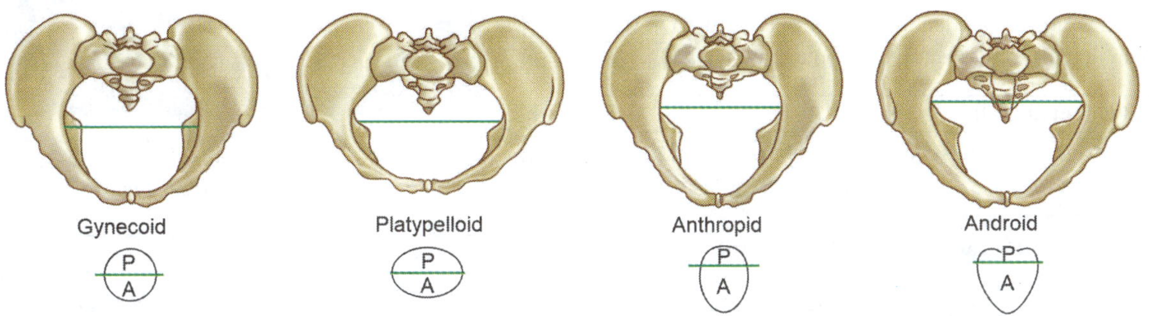

FIGURE: The four parent pelvic types of the Caldwell–Moby classification are shown by anatomic and schematic drawings. In each, the blue line passes through the widest transverse diameter and divides the pelvic inlets into posterior (P) and anterior (A) segments. Mixed types are formed by combining anterior and posterior inlet segments from different parent types.

53. Ans. (a) Unicornuate uterus

- Hysterosalpingography showing unicornuate uterus.
- It is a genetic condition in which lateral fusion defect seen i.e. two mullerian duct not able to fuse properly.
- In this uterus is smaller than normal uterus and only one fallopian tube present.

54. Ans. (a) Uterine gestational sac

Ref: William's Obstetrics, 24th ed. pg. 170

Double Decidual Sac Sign

- Seen on early pregnancy ultrasound and used to confirm an early intrauterine pregnancy
- Consists of decidua parietalis and decidua capsularis and is seen as two concentric rings surrounding an anechoic gestational sac.
- It helps in differentiating normal pregnancy from ectopic pregnancy. In ectopic pregnancy there is single decidual sac is seen.

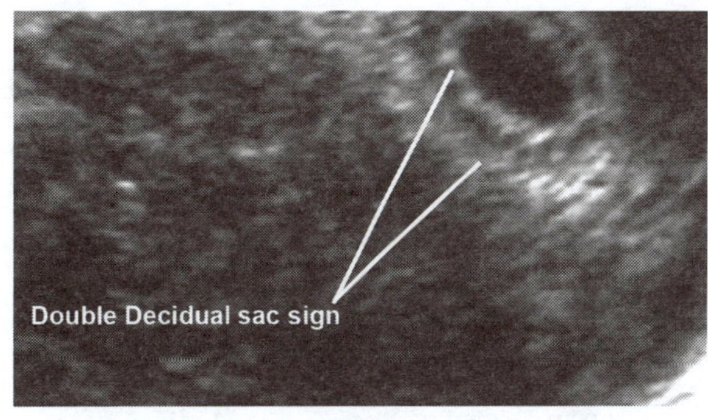

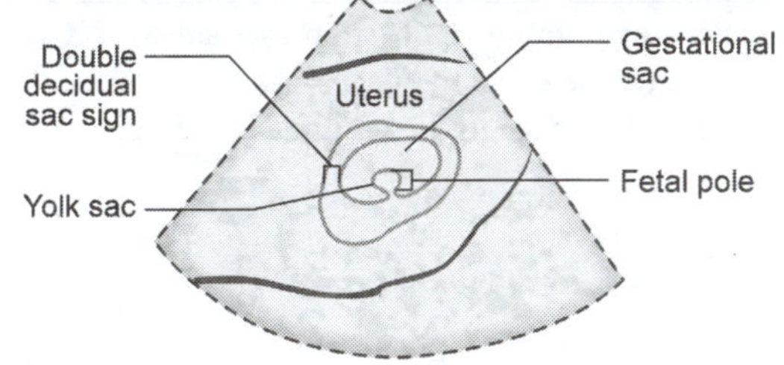

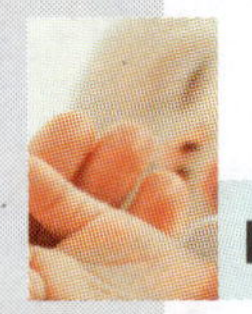

55. Ans. (a) Hydrosalpinx

Ref: Berek Novak's Gynecology 16th ed. pg. 665

- The shown image of dilatation of fallopian tube on HSG, is suggestive of hydrosalpinx.
- Hydrosalpinx is collection of mucus secretion into the fallopian tube. It is considered as end stage of pyosalpinx, when the pus is liquified.
- It is a descriptive term and refers to a fluid filled dilatation of fallopian tube.

56. Ans. (a) Pouch of Douglas

Ref: Berek and Novak's Gynecology, 16th ed. pg. 218

- The rectouterine pouch, also known as the rectovaginal pouch, cui-de-sac or pouch of Douglas, is an extension of peritoneum between the posterior wall of uterus and the rectum in females.
- It is the most dependent part of the peritoneal cavity and is analogous to the rectovesical pouch in males.

57. Ans. (a) Leydig cell

Ref: William's Obstetrics 25th ed. pg. 442

- High local levels of testosterone are integral to normal spermatogenesis.
- LH from the anterior pituitary gland stimulates production of testosterone by the Leydig cells.
- FSH increases LH receptor density on the Leydig cells, thus indirectly contributing to testosterone production.
- In addition, FSH elevates production of sex hormone-binding globulin, also called androgen-binding protein. Androgen-binding protein binds testosterone and maintains high concentrations of this hormone in the seminiferous tubules.

58. Ans. (b) Upper border of pubic symphysis to sacral promontory

Ref: Dutta's Obstetrics 8th ed. pg. 94-95

- True conjugate extends from the upper most margin of the symphysis pubis to the sacral promontory.
- Size of true conjugate: 11 cm

Other pelvic diameters have been discussed later in this book

59. Ans. (d) Progesterone

- The shown graph in question marked with X is due to progesterone effect in luteal phase.
- Follow the image for better understanding:

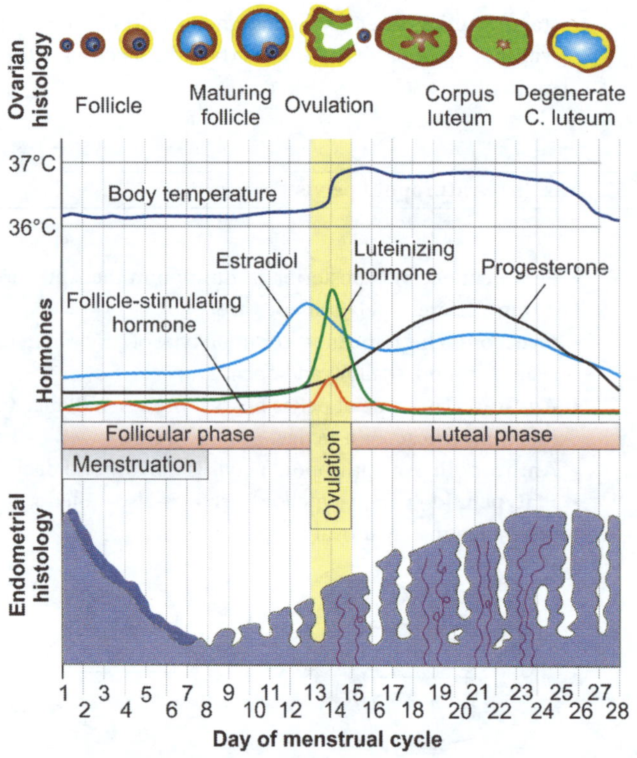

60. Ans. (c) Syncytiotrophoblast

Ref: DC Dutta 9th ed. P 53-54

- From placenta, syncytiotrophoblast is the principal site of protein and steroid hormone synthesis.
- **hCG:**
  - A glycoprotein hormone
  - MW: 36000–40,000 dalton
  - Has 2 subunits: α and β
  - α: Hormone non-specific (92 Amino acid). ***Biochemically similar to LH, FSH and TSH.***
  - **β:** Hormone specific (145 amino acid). Unique for hCG.
- **Functions:**
  - Rescue and maintenance of corpus luteum till 6 weeks of pregnancy
  - Stimulate leydig cell of male fetus (to produce testosterone)
  - Immunosuppressive activity
  - Stimulate both adrenal and placental steroidogenesis
  - Promote secretion of relaxin from the corpus luteum.

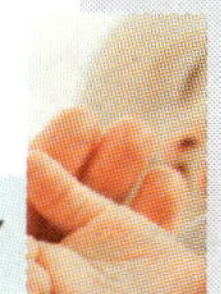

Extra Mile

- hCG disappears from circulation within 2 weeks following delivery
- **hPL (Human Placental Lactogen)** aka human chorionic somatomammotropin; Similar to GH and prolactin.
  - First detected during the 3rd week of gestation. Its plasma concentration rises proportionatally to placental mass
  - **Func:** Causes maternal lipolysis and promote transfer of glucose and amino acid to the fetus.
- **Pregnancy specific β-1 Glycoprotein (PS β-1G):** Produced by trophoblast cell. Detected in maternal serum 18–20 days after ovulation. Potent immunosuppressor → prevent rejection of conceptus.

61. Ans. (c) Progesterone effect

Ref: DC Dutta 8th ed. pg. 114

Dutta states: "*Constipation is a quite common ailment during pregnancy. Atonicity of the gut due to the* ***effect of progesterone,*** *diminished physical activity and pressure of the gravid uterus on the pelvic colon.*"

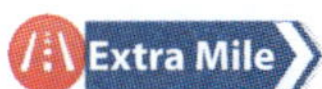

Extra Mile

Reasons of other ailments during pregnancy
- ***Leg cramps* during pregnancy** may be due to deficiency of diffusible serum calcium or elevation of serum phosphorus.
- ***Backache***: Physiological changes that contribute to backache are: joint ligament laxity (relaxin, estrogen), weight gain, hyperlordosis and anterior tilt of the pelvis. It is a common problem (50%) in pregnancy.

62. Ans. (a) T1

Ref: DC Dutta, 8th ed. pg. 53

- **Dutta states:** "*Increased frequency of micturition is noticed at 6–8 weeks of pregnancy which subsides after 12 weeks*".
- Urine frequency increases initially in first trimester. Normally, uterus is anteverted in position and is exaggerated up to 8 weeks.
- This enlarged uterus may lie on the bladder rendering it incapable of filling, clinically evident by increased frequency of micturition. Afterwards, it becomes erect, the long axis of the uterus conforms more or less to the axis of the inlet.

63. Ans. (a) Rise by 25%

Ref: DC Dutta, 8th ed. pg. 70

- During pregnancy glomerular filtration rate increases, which causes increased renal clearance of iodine.
- **Maternal serum iodine levels fall** due to increased renal loss and also due to transplacental shift to the fetus. These cause hyperplasia of the gland.
- **Therefore** iodine intake during pregnancy should be increased from 100 μg/day to 200 μg/day (as recommended by WHO).
- **There is rise in the basal metabolic rate**, which **begins at about the third month**, reaches a value of +25% **during the last trimester**.
- This increase in BMR is probably due to increase in net oxygen consumption of mother and fetus.

64. Ans. (a) Mentovertical

Ref: DC Dutta, 8th ed. pg. 96

- **Largest fetal head diameter is Mentovertical.**

TABLE: Important diameters of the skull

Diameters	Measurement in cm (inches)	Attitude of the head	Presentation
Suboccipitobregmatic—extends from the nape of the neck to the center of the bregma	9.5 cm (3¾″)	Complete flexion	Vertex
Suboccipito-frontal–extends from the nape of the neck to the anterior end of the anterior fontanel or center of the sinciput	10 cm (4″)	Incomplete flexion	Vertex
Occipitofrontal—extends from the occipital eminence to the root of the nose (Glabella)	11.5 cm (4½″)	Marked deflexion	Vertex
Mentovertical—extends from the midpoint of the chin to the highest point on the sagittal suture	14 cm (5½″)	Partial extension	Brow
Submentovertical–extends from junction of floor of the mouth and neck to the highest point on the sagittal suture	11.5 cm (4½″)	Incomplete extension	Face
Submentobregmatic—extends from junction of floor of the mouth and neck to the center of the bregma	9.5 cm (3¾″)	Complete extension	Face

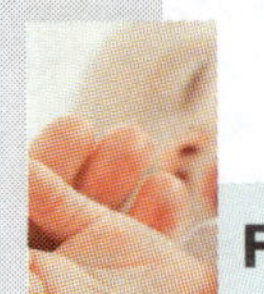

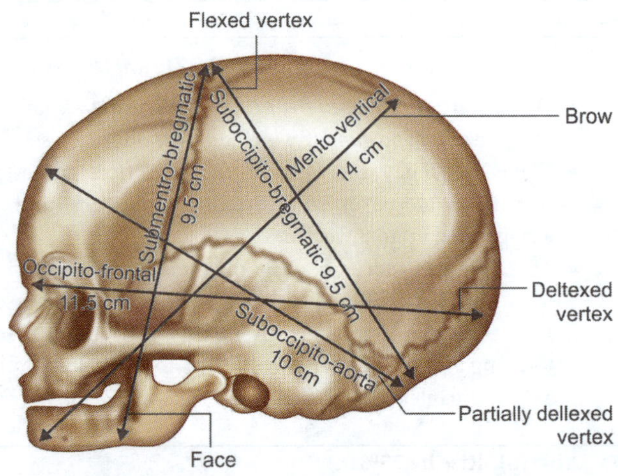

65. Ans. (d) 12 weeks

Ref: DC Dutta, 8th ed. pg. 32-33

- The placenta is developed from two sources:
  - **Fetal component:** The principal component *(which develops from the chorion frondosum)*
  - **Maternal component** consists of decidua basalis. (*Only the decidua basalis and the blood in the intervillous space are of maternal origin.*)
- **At 3rd–4th week:** Lacunar spaces become confluent with one another and form a multilocular receptacle lined by syncytium and filled with maternal blood. This space becomes the future intervillous space.
- **At 6th week:** Decidua capsularis becomes thinner and both the villi and the lacunar spaces in the embryonic area get obliterated, converting the chorion into chorion laeve.
- Because of this there is compensatory growth and proliferation of the **decidua basalis** and enormous and exuberant division and subdivision of the chorionic villi in the embryonic pole **(chorion frondosum).**
- **These two, i.e., chorion frondosum and the decidua basalis form the discrete placenta. It begins at 6th week and is completed by 12th week**

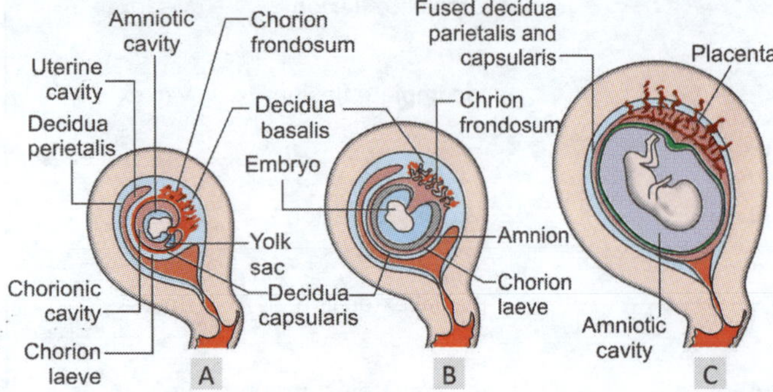

FIGURE: Relation of the aminiotic cavity, chorionic cavity and uterine cavity of successive stages; (A) End of the 8th week; (B) 10 weeks after the last period; (C) End of the 12th week

66. Ans. (c) Right umbilical vein

Ref: DC Dutta, 8th ed. pg. 37-38

- Placental circulation consists of independent circulation of blood in two systems:
  - **Uteroplacental circulation** (maternal circulation): It is the circulation of the maternal blood through the intervillous space. A mature placenta has a volume of about 500 mL of blood; **350 mL being occupied in the villi system** and **150 mL lying in the intervillous space[Q].**
  - **Fetoplacental circulation:** The **two umbilical arteries** carry the impure blood from the fetus. The fetal blood flow through the placenta is about 400 mL/min.
  - **Note:** Of the two umbilical veins, **the right one disappears by the 4th month, leaving behind left umbilical vein,** which carries oxygenated blood from the placenta to the fetus.
- Umbilical artery carry deoxygenated blood from fetus to mother

Extra Mile

TABLE: Summary of intervillous hemodynamics (V. Imp)

• Volume of blood in mature placenta	500 mL
• Volume of blood in intervillous space	150 mL
• Blood flow in intervillous space	500–600 mL/min
• Pressure in intervillous space: ▪ During uterine contraction ▪ During uterine relaxation	30–50 mm Hg
• Pressure in the supplying uterine artery	70–80 mm Hg
• Pressure in the draining uterine vein	8 mm Hg

TABLE: Summary of fetal hemodynamics (V. Imp)

• Fetal blood flow through the placenta	400 mL/min	
• Pressure in the umbilical artery	60 mm Hg	
• Pressure in the umbilical vein	10 mm Hg	
• Fetal capillary pressure in villi	20–40 mm Hg	
	Umbilical artery	**Umbilical vein**
• O_2 saturation	50–60%	70–80%
• PO_2	20–25 mm Hg	30–40 mm Hg

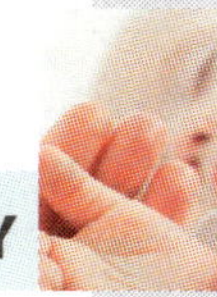

67. Ans. (b) Ductus venosus

Ref: DC Dutta, 8th ed. pg. 49

- **The umbilical vein carrying the oxygenated blood (80% saturated) from the placenta**, enters the fetus at the umbilicus and runs along the free margin of the falciform ligament of the liver. In the liver, it gives off branches to the left lobe of the liver and receives the deoxygenated blood from the portal vein.
- The greater portion of the oxygenated blood, mixed with some portal venous blood, short circuits the liver through the **ductus venosus** to enter the inferior vena cava (IVC) and thence to right atrium of the heart.

68. Ans. (a) Systemic venous resistance

Ref: DC Dutta, 8th ed. pg. 60

Changes during pregnancy:
- Increased in cardiac output
- Increase in HR
- Increase in plasma volume
- **Decrease in SVR** by (–21%) due to smooth muscle relaxing effect of progesterone, NO, prostaglandins or ANP.
- In spite of the large increase in cardiac output, the **maternal BP (BP = CO × SVR) is decreased** due to decrease in SVR. **There is overall decrease in diastolic blood pressure (BP) and mean arterial pressure (MAP) by 5–10 mm Hg**

69. Ans. (c) 4.5–5.5

pH of vagina: Normally it is acidic due to duoderlins bacilli, estrogen. Acidic pH prevents uterus from infection *(since age group is not mentioned, we will be considering the adult in reproductive age group)*
- **Normal pH throughout reproductive life is 4–4.5**
- pH during pregnancy: Less than 4 (becomes more acidic)
- pH at birth: 5.5–6.0
- pH during pre-pubertal age, menstruation and Menopause is similar: 6.5–7.5

70. Ans. (c) 30–70

Ref: DC Dutta, 8th ed. pg. 7 - 8

Cervix: Corpus ratio *(since age group is not mentioned, we will be considering the adult in reproductive age group)*
- **At birth**—1:1
- **Before puberty**—2:1
- **After puberty**—1:2
- **Reproductive life**—1:3
- **Menopause**—1:1

71. Ans. (a) Follicular phase

Ref: Shaws, 16th ed. pg. 47

- In follicular phase estradiol level is 100/200 pg/mL and progesterone level is 1 ng/mL, which is least amount together in the menstrual cycle phases.
- *Compare the levels from table*

TABLE: Hormonal levels in different phases of menstrual cycle

NORMAL				
Hormone	**Follicular phase**	**Ovulation**	**Luteal phase**	**Menstrual phase**
FSH	5–15 mIU/mL	12–30	2–9	3–15 mIU/mL
LH	6–14 mIU/mL	25–100	2–13	3–12 mIU/mL
E_2	100/200 pg/mL	300–500 pg/mL	100–200	–
Progesterone	1 ng/mL	–	15 ng/mL	–
17 ketosteroid	Normal	5–10 mg/daily	–	>25 mg in adrenal hyperplasia
Testosterone	Normal	0.2–0.8 ng/mL	–	>2 ng/mL in ovarian tumors
Androstenedione	Normal	1.3–1.5 ng/mL	–	–
DHEA	Normal	<5 mcg/mL	–	>5 mcg in adrenal hyperplasia
Cortisol	–	<5 mcg/dL	–	–
DHEAS	800 ng/mL	–	–	Adrenal hyperplasia, tumor

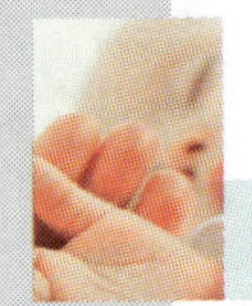

72. Ans. (c) Cardinal ligament

Ref: DC Dutta, 8th ed. pg. 7

- Cardinal ligament is also known as Mackenrodt's ligament.
- It is considered as true support of uterus.
- Normal position of uterus is: *Anteversion and Anteflexion*
- **Function of cardinal ligament:**
  - Lateral stabilization of cervix at the level of ischial spine
  - Primary vascular conduits of the uterus and vagina
- Other ligaments like round and broad ligament act as a guyrope with a steadying effect on the uterus. *They have no role in preventing descent of uterus.*

73. Ans. (c) Bartholin's gland

Ref: Gray's Basic Anatomy/248

- The orifice of urethra and vagina are associated with opening of glands.
- The ducts of para-urethral glands **(skene's gland)** opens into the vestibule, one on each side of the lateral margin of urethra.
- The ducts of greater vestibular gland **(Bartholin's gland)** open adjacent to the ***postero-lateral margin of the vaginal opening*** in the crease between the vaginal orifice and remanants of hymen.
- Bartholin gland the female homologues of the bulbourethral glands in men.

Extra Mile

- When bartholin's gland is blocked, a fluid filled cyst named bartholin's cyst develops.
- TOC for bartholin's cyst: **Marsuplization.**

74. Ans. (c) Bimastoid

Ref: DC Dutta, 8th ed. pg. 94-97

TRANVERSE DIAMETERS OF FETAL HEAD

- Biparietal: 9.5 cm
- Bitemporal: 8 cm
- *Bimastoid: 7.5 cm; smallest transverse diameter*
- Super subparietal: 8.5 cm

75. Ans. (b) Intertuberous

Ref: DC Dutta, 8th ed. pg. 94-97; William's 23rd ed. Chapter 2, Maternal Pelvic Anatomy

- *Most of the students answer interspinous for this question. Obviously interspinous is having the least diameter (10cm), but it belongs to mid pelvis.*
- The question is asking about the shortest diameter of **pelvic outlet**, which is intertuberous *(diameter between ischial tuberosity)* diameter ~**11 cm.**

PLANES AND DIAMETERS OF THE PELVIS

The pelvis is described as having four imaginary planes:

- The plane of the **pelvic inlet**—the superior strait
- The plane of the **mid pelvis**—the least pelvic dimensions
- The plane of the **pelvic outlet**—the inferior strait
- The plane of greatest pelvic dimension—of no obstetrical significance.

TABLE: Summarized data of maternal pelvis planes and diameters *(all the numerical datas are derived from standard reference i.e. William's 24th ed.)*

Plane	Diameter	Measured between	Size
Pelvic Inlet Pelvic diameters A - Anteroposterior B - Oblique C - Transverse	Transverse	Greatest distance between the linea terminalis on either side	**~13 cm**
	A-P diameter aka **true conjugate**	Extends from the uppermost margin of the symphysis pubis to the sacral promontory	**11 cm**
	Oblique diameter	Extends from one of the sacroiliac synchondroses to the iliopectineal eminence on the opposite side.	**12 cm**

Contd...

Plane	Diameter	Measured between	Size
Mid pelvis Measured at level of ischial spine	Interspinous diameter	Between the ischial spines	**10 cm**
	Anteroposterior	At the level of ischial spine	**11.5 cm**
Pelvic outlet Makes 2 traingles with common base	Antero-posterior	Coccyx to symphysis pupis	**11.5 cm**
	Transverse	Between ischial tuberosities	**11 cm**
	Posterior saggital	Sacrococcygeal angle to the midline imaginary line at base	**11.5/2 cm**
Other important pelvic diameters	**Obstetrical conjugate**	Shortest distance between the sacral promontory and the symphysis pubis	**10 cm.** Obstetrical conjugate is estimated indirectly by subtracting 1.5–2 cm from the diagonal conjugate
	Diagonal conjugate	From the lower margin of the symphysis to the sacral promontory	11.5–12 cm

76. Ans. (a) Transverse

Ref: DC Dutta, 8th ed. pg. 99-104

- If such questions are asked regardless of pelvic plain, then ***transverse diameter of pelvic inlet has largest diameter (13 cm).*** *If it is not in option, next best option is oblique diameter (12 cm)*
- Smallest diameter regardless of pelvic plain—**Bispinous (10 cm)**
- *For more details, please refer to above explanation.*

77. Ans. (d) Sacrocotyloid

Ref: DC Dutta, 8th ed. pg. 101

- **Sacrocotyloid—9.5 cm (3¾"):** It is the distance between the midpoint of the sacral promontory to iliopubic eminence (Fig.).
- It represents the space occupied by the biparietal diameter of the head while negotiating the brim in flat pelvis.

- **Other diameter of pelvic inlet:**
  - Anteroposterior: 11 cm
  - Transverse: 13 cm
  - Oblique: 12 cm

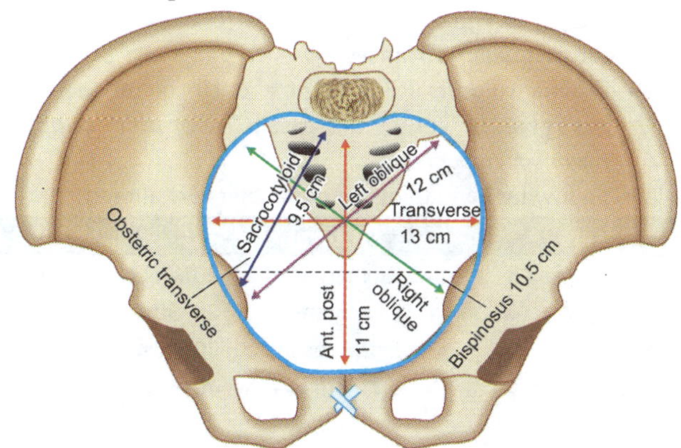

FIGURE: Different diameters of the inlet of obstetrical significance. Bispinous diameter is also demonstrated

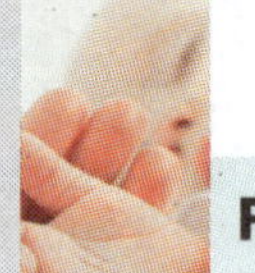

78. Ans. (c) Android

Ref: DC Dutta 8th ed. pg. 99-104

- Prominent ischial spine is seen in case of android type of pelvis.
- Pelvis type most favorable for delivery: **Gynecoid**
- MC type of pelvis in females: **Gynecoid**
- Heart shaped pelvis: **Android**
- Flat pelvis: **Platypelloid**

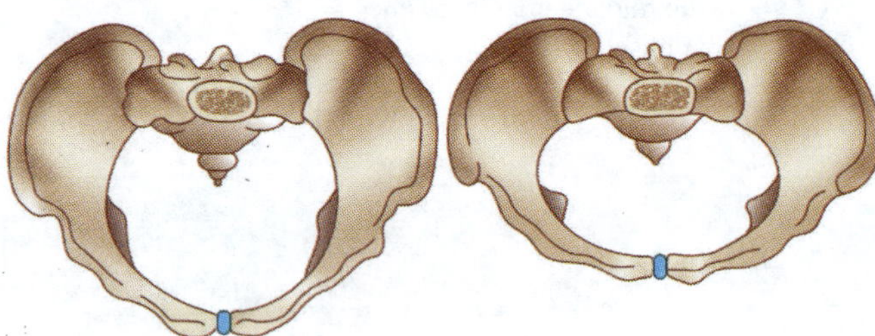

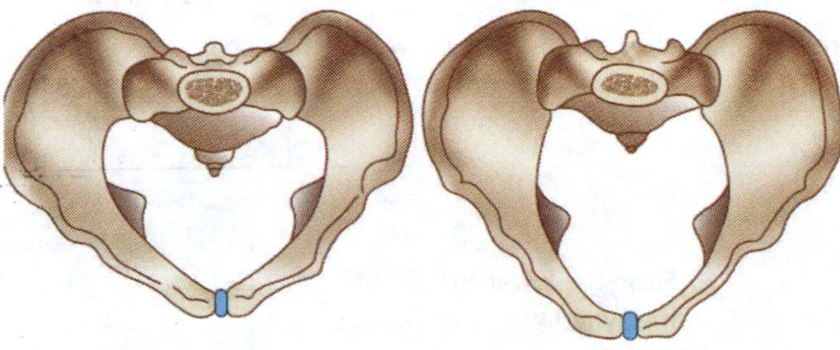

FIGURE: Types of pelvis

- **Pelvis MC associated with face and brow presentation: Platypelloid**
- **Pelvis MC associated with occipitoposterior presentation: Android**
- **Pelvis MC associated with face to pubis delivery: Anthropoid**

79. Ans. (c) Platelet count

Ref: DC Dutta, 8th ed. pg. 58-59

- During pregnancy, physiological demand increases as the pregnancy advances.
- Plasma volume, RBC count and Hb count increased, but platelet count decreased *(Idiopathic dilutional thrombocytopenia)*.
- Following hematological parameters are altered:

Parameters	Alterations
Hb	Increased by: 20%
RBC	Increased by: 20–30%
Blood volume	Increased by: 30–40%
Plasma volume	Increased by: 40–50%
Packed cell volume	Decreased
Platelet count	Decreased (dilutional thrombocytopenia)

- Maximum plasma volume is seen at **36** weeks AOG: **50%**
- Maximum cardiac output: Immediately post partum (highest cardiac output).
- BP fall post partum because of relaxation of all blood vessels.

80. Ans. (d) Factor XI

Ref: DC Dutta, 8th ed. pg. 58; William's Obstetrics 23rd ed. pg. 121-122

- Pregnancy is a hypercoagulable state. All clotting factors are increased during pregnancy except **factor XI and XIII which decreases** (11 and 13).
- **Note:** Clotting time and bleeding time remains unaffected during pregnancy.

81. Ans. (b) Pregnancy

Ref: Dutta's Obstetrics, 7th ed. pg. 431-438

- Amenorrhea is the absence of menstrual bleeding. It is a normal feature in prepubertal, pregnant, and postmenopausal females.
- **Primary amenorrhea** is defined as the absence of menses by age 16 in the presence of normal developmental and secondary sexual characteristics or by age 14 if secondary sexual characteristics have failed to develop
- **Secondary amenorrhea** refers to the absence of menses for 6 months or more in a women with previously regular menstrual cycles.

Causes

- Primary amenorrhea may result from congenital reproductive tract abnormalities or endocrine disorders that delay the onset of puberty.
  - Ex: HPA dysfunction, Kallman's syndrome, CNS tumors, turner syndrome, mullerian agenesis etc.
- *The most common cause of secondary amenorrhea is pregnancy.*
- Other causes of secondary amenorrhea can be: Tubercular Endometritis, PCOS, Cushing's disease, Sheehan's syndrome, Uterine synechiae secondary to vigorous curettage.

82. Ans. (a) 3 days after menstruation

Ref: DC Dutta, 8th ed. pg. 56, 7th ed. pg. 540

- **Breast self-examination** (BSE) is a screening method used in an attempt to detect early breast cancer. The method involves the woman herself looking at and feeling each breast for possible lumps, distortions or swelling.
- **For premenopausal women**, the most commonly recommended time is **just after the end of menstruation**, because the breasts are least likely to be swollen and tender at this time.

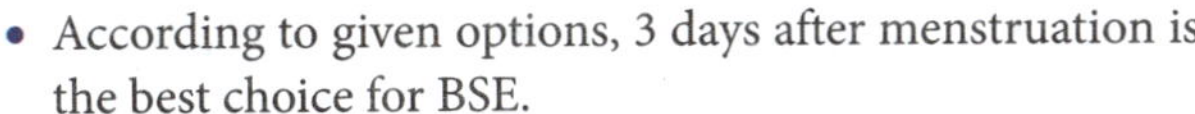

- According to given options, 3 days after menstruation is the best choice for BSE.
- For postmenopausal or have irregular cycles might do a self-exam once a month regardless of their menstrual cycle.

83. Ans. (d) 2 weeks before next menstruation

Ref: DC Dutta, 8th ed. pg. 22, 7th ed. pg. 19

- Ovulation is a process whereby a secondary oocyte is released from the ovary following rupture of a mature Graffian follicle and becomes available for conception.
- *In relation to the menstrual period, the event occurs about 14 days prior to the expected period.*

84. Ans. (b) Ductus venosus

Ref: DC Dutta, 8th ed. pg. 36; William's Obstetrics 23rd ed. Ch: 4

- Ductus venosus carries oxygenated blood from placenta and drains into IVC.
- Ductus arteriosus is a connection between aorta and pulmonary arteries, thereby bypassing lung. Persistence of ductus arteriosus leads to a congenital heart condition called Patent Ductus Arteriosus.
- Foramen ovale is connection between right atrium and left atrium.
- Umbilical artery carries deoxygenated blood from fetus to mother.

85. Ans. (c) Cardinal vein

Ref: DC Dutta, 8th ed. pg. 50

- The cardinal veins form as the basis for the intraembryonic venous part of the circulatory system. Various venous systems appear in various stages of the embryogenesis and partially disappear again. Very early in the development two paired systems appear:
  - The **superior cardinal veins** bring the blood from the head region via the left and right common cardinal vein
  - The **inferior cardinal veins** drain the blood from the lower half of the body into the two common cardinal veins
- From here, the blood is emptied into the **sinus venosus** and into the atrium via the **sinus horns**.

Rest of structures given in option closes AFTER birth, with following sequence:

U- Umbilical vein
F- Foramen ovale
A- Ductus Arteriosus
V- Ductus Venosus

86. Ans. (d) 24 weeks

Ref: DC Dutta, 8th ed. pg. 54, 78; 7th ed pg. 69

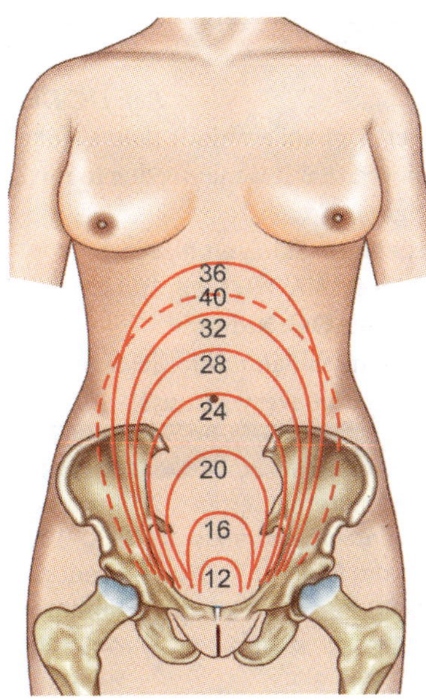

Dutta in 8th ed. States

The height of uterus is midway between symphysis pubis and umbilicus at 16th week and at the level of umbilicus at 24th week.

TABLE: Gestational age and fundal height

Gestational age	Fundal height landmark
12 weeks	Pubic Symphysis
24 weeks	Umbilicus
36 weeks	Xiphoid Process of Sternum
37–40 weeks	Regression of fundal height between 36-32 cm

87. Ans. (a) Milk production

Ref: DC Dutta, 8th ed. pg. 136, 574

Milk production is by Prolactin.

EMBRYOLOGY

88. Ans. (d) 21 hydroxylase

Ref: Shaws Textbook of Gynecology, 7th ed. pg. 78

- The most common cause of CAH is a 21-hydroxylase deficiency due to mutations or deletions of CYP21A, which accounts for >90% of CAH cases.
- The examination of the external genitalia is of primary importance and the commonest cause of ambiguous genitalia is adrenal hyperplasia.
- The prognosis is serious if not promptly recognized and treated.
- The immediate concern is to prevent rapid dehydration leading to fluid and electrolyte imbalance.

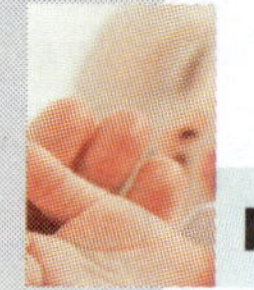

89. Ans. (b) Fetal urine

Ref: DC Dutta 9th ed. pg. 34

- The exact origin of amniotic fluid is not well understood. It is believed that it is mainly due to mixed maternal and fetal origin.
  - **Early stages:** Skin and placenta
  - **12–14 weeks AOG:** Lung and kidney
  - **20 weeks AOG:** Kidney
- The water in the amniotic fluid is completely changed and **replaced in every 3 hours**

Production	Removal
• **Transudation** of maternal serum across the placental membranes • Transudation from fetal circulation across the umbilical cord or placental membranes • **Secretion** from amniotic epithelium • **Transudation** for fetal plasma through the highly permeable **fetal skin** before it is keratinized at 20th week • **Fetal urine:** Daily output at term is about 400–1,200 mL • **Fetal lung** that enters the amniotic cavity add to its volume	• **Fetus swallows** about 500–1000 mL of liquor every day • **Intramembranous absorption** of water and solutes (200–500 mL/day) from the amniotic compartment to fetal circulation through the fetal surface of the placenta.

- Volume of amniotic fluid according to AOG:
  - At 12 weeks: 50 mL
  - At 20 weeks: 400 mL
  - At 36–38 weeks: 1 Litre (peak)
  - At **term: 600–800 mL**
  - 43 weeks: 200 mL

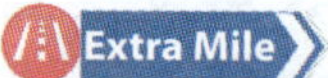

Scheme showing the source and circulation of amniotic fluid

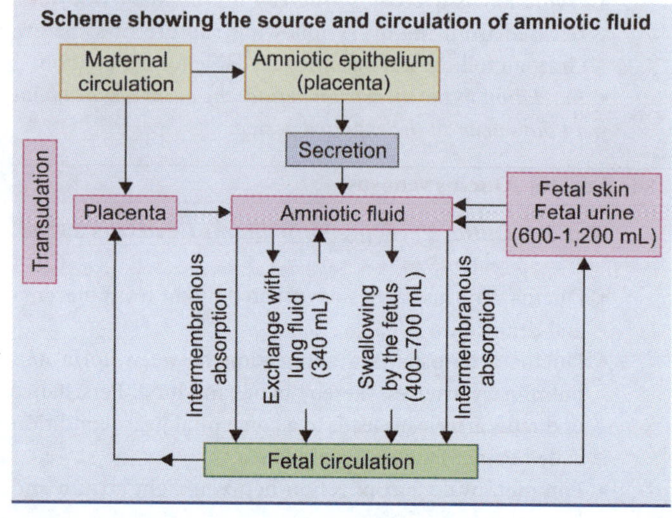

90. Ans. (a) USG

Ref: DC Dutta Obstetrics 8th ed. pg. 41

- In general population the investigation modality to screen Down syndrome is USG, which is readily available.
- **Nuchal translucency**—Increased fetal nuchal skin thickness (in the first trimester) >3 mm by TVS is a strong marker for chromosomal anomalies (trisomy 21, 18, 13, triploidy and Turner's syndrome).
- **For confirmation** fetal karyotyping is done.
- **Earliest investigation which can confirm the diagnosis is chorionic villi sampling, which can be done transcervically** between 10 weeks and 13 weeks and **transabdominally** from 10 weeks to term.

TABLE: Prenatal diagnosis: CVS, amniocentesis and cordocentesis

	Chorionic villus sampling	Amniocentesis	Cordocentesis
Time	• Transcervical 10–13 weeks • Transabdominal 10 weeks to term	After 15 weeks (early 12–14 weeks)	18–20 weeks
Materials for study	Trophoblast cells	• Fetal fibroblasts • Fluid for biochemical study	• Fetal white blood cells (others—infection and biochemical study)
Karyotype result	• **Direct preparation:** 24–48 hours • **Culture:** 10–14 days	• **Culture:** 3–4 weeks	• **Culture:** 24–48 hours
Fetal loss	0.5–1%	0.5%	1–2%
Accuracy	Accurate; may need amniocentesis for confirmation	Highly accurate	Highly accurate
Termination of pregnancy when indicated	1st trimester—safe	2nd trimester—risky	2nd trimester—risky
Maternal effects following termination of pregnancy	Very little	More traumatic; physically and psychologically	Same as amniocentesis

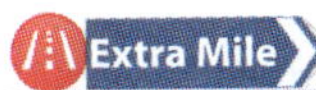

TABLE: Ultrasound markers of chromosomal abnormalities (General sonography)

Observation	Chromosomal abnormality
Head • Choroid plexus cyst • Strawberry skull • Hydrocephalus • Holoprosencephaly	Trisomy 18, 13 triploidy
Face • Cleft lip/palate • Micrognathia • Low set ears	Trisomy 13,18, Meckel-Gruber syndrome Triploidy
Nuchal translucency >3 mm	Trisomy 21, 18, 13, Turner syndrome
Cardiac defects	Trisomy 13, 18, 21
Renal anomalies • Horseshoe kidney • Bilateral dilatation of renal pelvis • Cystic dysplasia	Trisomy 13, 18, 21 Triploidy
Hands/feet • ***Flexed overlapping fingers*** • Rockerbottoms/club foot • Polydactyly • Wide gap between 1st and 2nd toes • Clinodactyly • Short femur	Trisomy 18 Trisomy 13 Trisomy 21

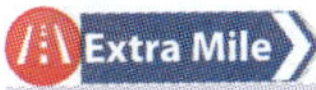

Observation	Chromosomal abnormality
GI system • Echogenic bowel • Omphalocele • Duodenal atresia	Trisomy 13, 18 Trisomy 21
General • Early IUGR • Hydrops	Trisomy 13, 18, 21 Triploidy, 45XO

91. Ans. (c) Continuous electrical fetal monitoring

Ref: DC Dutta Obstetrics 8th ed. pg. 693-94

- Continuous electronic fetal monitoring is done by using ultrasound Doppler effect. The transducers are placed on the maternal abdomen, one over the fundus and the other at a site where the fetal heart sound is best audible.
- Frequency of uterine contractions and uterine pressure are recorded simultaneously by tocodynamometer.
- **Book states:** *"**Intermittent auscultation** is an effective method. Fetuses with abnormal FHR pattern on auscultation should have EFM."*
- *"**EFM is most reliable** when FHR pattern is reassuring and when there is fetal acidosis."*

Advantages of EFM over clinical monitoring:

- Accurate monitoring of uterine contractions.
- Significant improvement of perinatal mortality.
- Can detect hypoxia early and can explain the mechanism of hypoxia and its specific treatment.
- Improvement of intrapartum fetal death by threefold.
- It is an important record for medicolegal purpose.

92. Ans. (c) 15–18 weeks

Ref: DC Dutta Obstetrics 8th ed. pg. 741

- Amniocentesis is the deliberate puncture of the amniotic fluid sac per abdomen for diagnostic and therapeutic purposes.
- ***It is best done in early months at around 15–20 weeks.*** **For diagnosis** of chromosomal and genetic disorders like:
  - Sex-linked disorders
  - Karyotyping
  - Inborn errors of metabolism
  - Neural tube defects.

93. Ans. (c) 20 mm

Ref: DC Dutta 8th ed./22; Shaw's 15th ed. /Harrison 19/e

- Preovulatory graffian follicle is **18–20 mm**

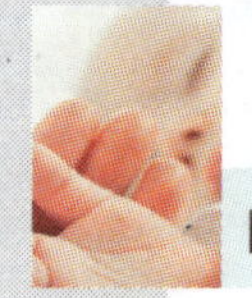

- Rate of growth of follicle **2–3 mm/day**
- Growth and size of follicle measured by **TVS,** started on 10th day of cycle (in case of infertility), done alternate day.
- Just prior to ovulation its size of follicle is **18–20 mm**, and endometrium is **trilaminar** in appearance.
- When the egg enters the fallopian tube, it is surrounded by a cumulus of granulosa cells (cumulus oophorus) and intimately surrounded by a clear zona pellucida.
- In most mammals, including humans, the egg is released from the ovary in the metaphase II stage.

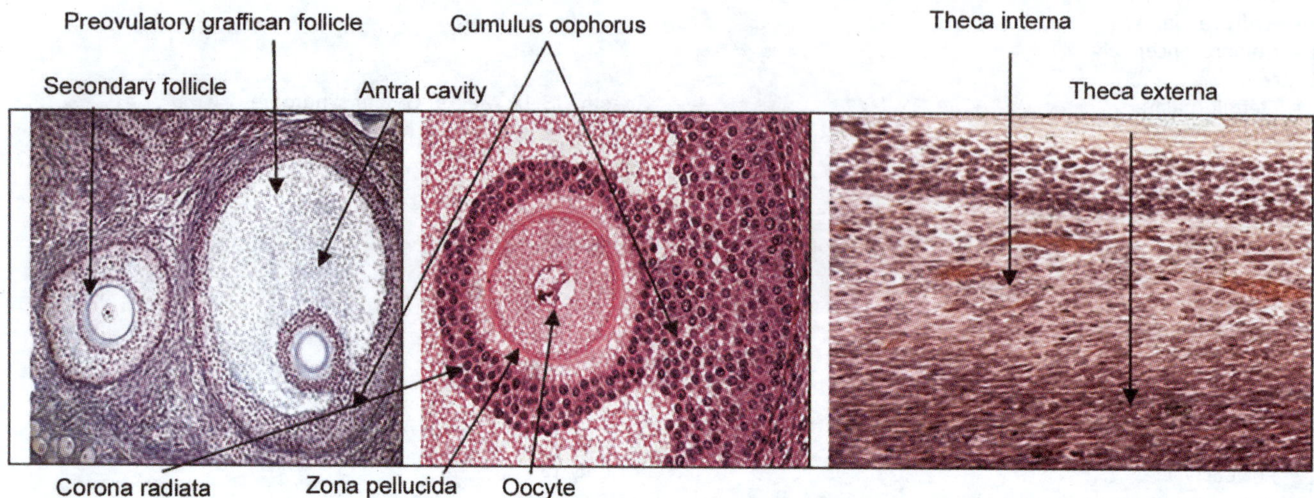

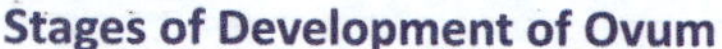

Stages of Development of Ovum

Oogonia 46XX

↓

Primary oocyte 46XX undergo meiosis I and get arrested in **PROPHASE,**which gets completed just prior to ovulation

↓

Secondary oocyte 23X+1st polar body (just prior to ovulation)
2°oocyte undergo meiosis II,which get arrested at **METAPHASE**

↓

Ova 23X + 2nd polar body (at time of fertilization)
ONLY IF FERTILIZATION OCCURS

94. Ans. (d) Zona reaction attracts the sperms

Ref: DC Dutta, 8th ed. pg. 23, 7th ed. pg. 21

Once an ovum is fertilized, zona reaction takes place.

- **Zona reaction**-Once sperm penetrates zona pellucida, the ovum become impermeable to other sperms, this prevents polyspermy. *Therefore zona reaction DOESN'T ATTRACT sperm.*
- When more than one sperm manages to enter the ovum (dispermy = 2; triploidy = 3), the fetus nearly always aborts
- 1st Cell division then occurs (20 hour) → gives rise to two-cell embryo

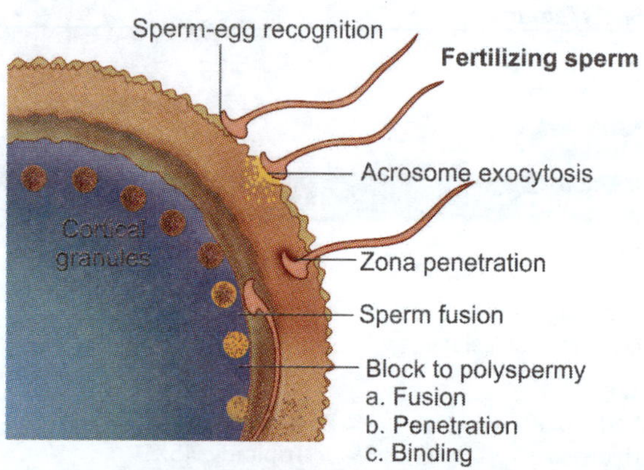

Complete Steps of Fertilization

- **Capacitation** - A period of conditioning that occurs in the **female reproductive tract.**
- **Chemotaxis** -sperm are **attracted to an egg** through the process known as chemotaxis
- Binding of **progesterone** + surface receptor on the sperm → increase in intracellular calcium ion concentration → which increases **sperm motility** (chemokinesis).
- **Acrosome reaction** *(perforations form in the acrosome)* **occurs in ampulla**
- Zonapellucida is a glycoprotein layer surrounding the membrane of oocytes (see image).

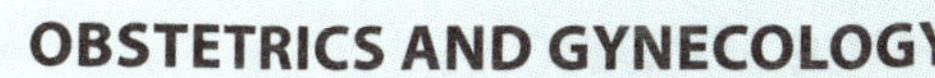

- Once sperm reaches ova, there is release of hyluronidase → **penetration of corona radiata** and cumulus cells by sperm.
- Glycoproteins on the outer surface of the sperm then bind with glycoproteins on the zonapellucida of the ovum.

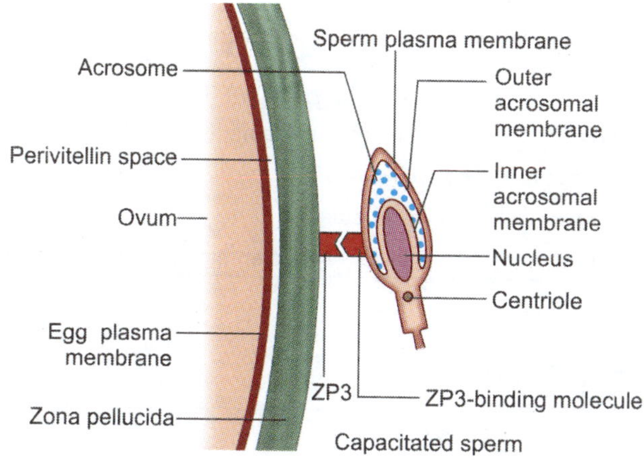

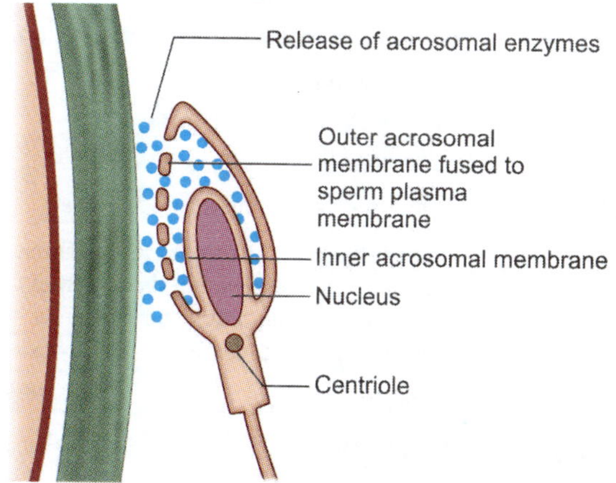

- Release of acrosin occurs → Acrosin digests the zonapellucida and membrane of the oocyte
- After this Sperm enters the cytoplasm → intracytoplasmic structures, the coronal granules, arrange themselves in an orderly fashion (around the outermost portion of the cytoplasm just beneath the cytoplasmic membrane). Swelling of sperm head then occurs, giving rise to male pronucleus.
- Doing this the egg completes its **second meiotic division,** casting off the **second polar body to a position beneath the zonapellucida.**

95. Ans. (c) Prevention of multiple sperm entry

Ref: DC Dutta, 8th ed. pg. 24

- Zona pellucida is a glycoprotein layer surrounding the membrane of oocytes.
- Once sperms reach ova, there is release of hyluronidase → **penetration of corona radiata** and cumulus cells by sperm.
- Glycoproteins on the outer surface of the sperm then bind with glycoproteins on the zona pellucida of the ovum.
- **Zona reaction: Once sperm penetrates zona pellucida, the ovum become impermeable to other sperms, this prevents polyspermy.**

96. Ans. (d) Fertilization takes place in ampula

Ref: DC Dutta, 8th ed. pg. 32-36, 7th ed. pg. 21-22

Option A-Placenta is formed by trophoblast which 1st appear at blastocyst stage, hence option A is wrong.
Option B-Implantation starts on 6th day and completes by 10th day.
Option C-During initial weeks corpus leuteum surviaval is due to hCG, not due to LH.
Option D-site of fertilization is ampulla.

97. Ans. (a) 5-6 days

Ref: DC Dutta, 8th ed. pg. 25, 8th ed. 25

- Dutta in 8th ed. states that Implantation occurs in the endometrium of the anterior or posterior wall of the body near the funduso**n 6th day**, which corresponds *to 20th day of a regular normal cycle.*
- **Implantation occurs through 4 stages:** Apposition, Adhesion, Penetration, Invasion.
- *Most students got confused here and marked the answer as 7–8 days. But if you read the question again, it is cleverly asking that implantation occurs AFTER. 5–6 days is the single best answer here.*

98. Ans. (b) 5 weeks

Ref: DC Dutta, 8th ed. pg. 734, 7th ed. pg. 68

- 1st radiological investigation for diagnosis of pregnancy is visualisation of gestational sac by TVS.
- **4½ weeks**- TVS
- **5 weeks** - by both TVS & TAS

*TVS: Transvaginal scan
*TAS: Transabdominal scan

99. Ans. (a) 15th day

Ref: DC Dutta, 8th ed. pg. 22; Williams Obstetrics 23rd ed. Ch: 3

- Following ovulation (14th day) the remaining follicular cells left by the ovulated follicle differentiate into the corpus luteum (meaning *yellow body).*
- Corpus luteum secrets progesterone, which causes secretory changes in endometrium.

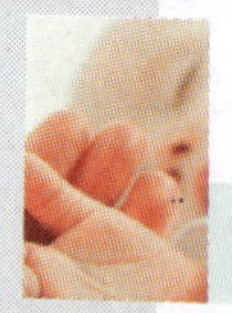

MENSTRUAL PHASES

Cycle day	1–5	6–14	15–28
Ovarian phase	Early follicle	Follicular	Luteal
Endometrial phase	Menstrual	Proliferative	Secretory
Estrogen/ Progesterone	Low levels	Estrogen	Progesterone

100. Ans. (b) 48 hours

Ref: DC Dutta, 8th ed. pg. 23, 8th ed. pg. 66, 7th ed. pg. 58-59

hCG

- hCG is a glycoprotein which is synthesized by syncytiotrophoblast of the placenta.
- The half-life of hCG is 36 hours.
- In early pregnancy the doubling time of hCG is 1.4–2 days.
- **It has 2 subunits:**
  - α-biologically similar in LH, FSH and TSH. (i.e. non-specific)
  - β-subunit-unique to hCG. (i.e. specific)
- Structurally it is similar to—FSH, LH, TSH but functionally it is similar to LH (i.e. luteotropic), i.e. helps in maintaining corpus luteum. So, the **main hormone which maintains activity of corpus luteum during pregnancy is hCG** and in **non-pregnant state is LH**.
- It can be detected in material serum as early as 8 days following fertilization/day 22 of menstrual cycle/5 days before missed period by immuno assay.°
- The level is 100 IU/L or mIU/mL around the time of the expected menses.
- The level progressively rise and reach maximum levels by about 8–10 weeks/70 days/1st trimester. It then falls until about 16 weeks and remains at low level up to term.
- hCG disappears from circulation by 2 weeks following delivery.

Action

- Sustains the corpus luteum and thereby maintains the hormonal support to the pregnancy in early weeks.
- Stimulates the leydig cells of the male fetus to produce testosterone and thereby induces development of the male external genitalia

101. Ans. (b) 3rd week

Ref: DC Dutta, 8th ed. pg. 32

- **After interstitial implantation is completed on day 11th**, the blastocyst is surrounded on all sides by lacunar spaces around cords of syncytial cells, called trabeculae.
- **On 13th day** stem villi develops from the trabeculae which connect the chorionic plate with the basal plate.
- **On 13th, 16th and 21st day** Primary, secondary and tertiary villi are successively developed respectively from the stem villi.
- **Arterio-capillary-venous system in the mesenchymal core of each villus is completed on 21st day (week 3).**

Extra Mile

TABLE: Important events following fertillization

'0' hour	Fertilization (day-15 from LMP)
30 hours	Two-cell stage (blastomeres)
40–50 hours	Four-cell stage
72 hours	Twelve-cell stage
96 hours	16 cell stage. Morula enters the urterine cavity

Extra Mile

5th day	Blastocyst
4–5th day	Zone pellucida disappears
5–6th day	Blastocyst attachment to endometrial surface
6–7th day	Differentiation of cyto and syncytiotrophoblastic layers
10th day	Synthesis of hCG by syncytiotrophoblast
9–10th day	Lacunar network forms
10–11th day	• Trophoblasts invade endometrial sinusoids establishing uteroplacental circulation • Interstitial implantation completed with entire decidual coverage
13th day	Primary villi
16th day	Secondary villi
21st day	Tertiary villi
21st–22nd day	Fetal heart. Fetoplacental circulation

102. Ans. (d) Penile urethra

Ref: Shaw, 16th ed. pg. 1

TABLE: Embroyological structure and its derivative in female and male counterparts

Embroyological structure	Female derivative	Male derivative
Genital swelling	Labia majora	Scrotum
Genital fold	Labia minora	Penile urethra
Genital ridge	Ovary	Testis
Genital tubercle	Clitoris	Penis

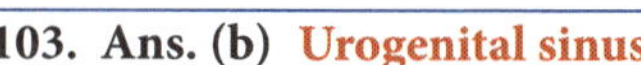

103. Ans. (b) Urogenital sinus

Ref: Shaw, 16th ed. pg. 124

- **Vagina is embroyologically derived from:**
  - **Upper 2/3rd:** Mesoderm of Mullerian duct
  - **Lower 1/3rd:** Sinovaginal bulb of endodermal sinus

104. Ans. (b) After 10 weeks from LMP

Ref: DC Dutta, 8th ed. pg. 46

The chronology in the fetal period is expressed in terms of menstrual age and not in embryonic age

Three periods are distinguished in the prenatal development of the fetus.

- **Ovular period or germinal period**—lasts for first 2 weeks following ovulation.
- **Embryonic period:** From 3rd week to 10 weeks following ovulation (8 weeks post conception).
- **Fetal period:** Begins 10 week after ovulation (after 8th week following conception) and ends in delivery.

105. Ans. (a) Ampulla

Ref: DC Dutta, 8th ed. pg. 23

- Fertilization is the process of fusion of the spermatozoon with the mature ovum.
- Almost always, fertilization occurs in the ampullary part of the fallopian tube.

106. Ans. (a) 10 weeks

Ref: DC Dutta, 8th ed. pg. 19, 7th ed. pg. 42

- **Fetal Blood:** Haematopoiesis is demonstrated in the embryonic phase first in the yolk sac by 14th day.
- By 10th week, the liver becomes the major site.
- Gradually, the red cells production sites extend to the spleen and bone marrow and near term, the bone marrow becomes the major site of red cell production.

107. Ans. (d) 7 million

Ref: DC Dutta, 8th ed. pg. 19

- The gonads begin to differentiate. During the 4th or 5th week of development.
- If there is absence of the Y chromosome, the gonads will differentiate into ovaries. As the ovaries differentiate, ingrowths called cortical cords develop where the primordial germ cells collect.
- The primordial germ cells grow and begin to differentiate into oogonia during the 6th to 8th week of female (XX) embryonic development.
- Oogonia then proliferate via mitosis during the 9th to 22nd week of embryonic development.
- By the 8th week of development, there can be up to 600,000 oogonia and **up to 7,000,000 by the 5th month of development.**

108. Ans. (b) Puberty

Ref: DC Dutta, 8th ed./19-20, 8th ed./ 21, 7th ed./17 & 19

- **Oogenesis:** The process involved in the development of a mature ovum is called Oogenesis.
- At 20th week AOG, the number of oogonia reaches at its maximum number, about 7 million.
- While the majority of the oogonia continue to divide, some enter into the prophase of the first meiotic division and are called primary oocytes.
- At birth, total number of oocyte is about 2 million.
- *The primary occytes do not finish the first meiotic division until puberty is reached.*
- ***Now, first meiotic division of primary oocyte takes place at puberty, which give rise to secondary oocyte and first polar body.***
- These two are of unequal size, the *secondary oocyte* contains nearly all the cytoplasm and haploid number of chromosomes (23, X), but the *polar body* contains scanty cytoplasm and half of the chromosomes (23, X).
- *Ovulation takes place soon after the formation of the secondary oocyte.*
- ***2nd meiotic division of secondary oocyte takes place only after fertilization of ova by the sperm.***
- This results in the formation of two unequal daughter cells, each possessing 23 chromosomes (23, X): larger one is the mature ovum and the smaller one is the second polar body containing the equal number of chromosomes.
- The first polar body may also undergo the second meiotic division.
- In the absence of fertilization, the secondary oocyte does not complete the second meiotic division and degenerates as it is.
- *Refer to the flowchart below (must remember it. There's question in almost every exam from this topic)*

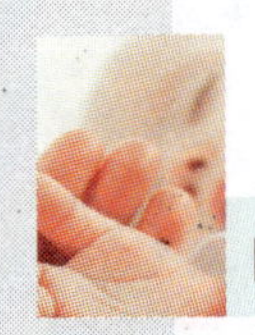

Scheme showing gametogenesis

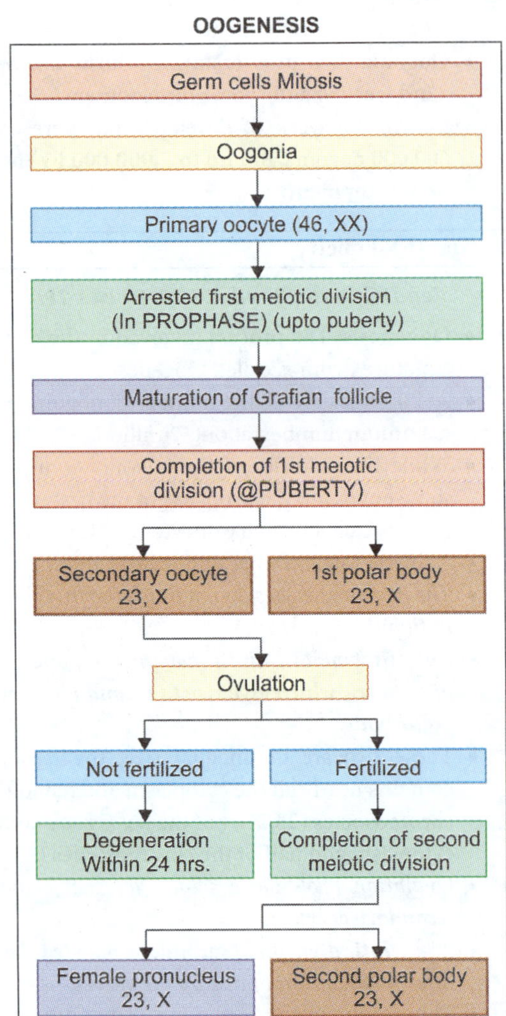

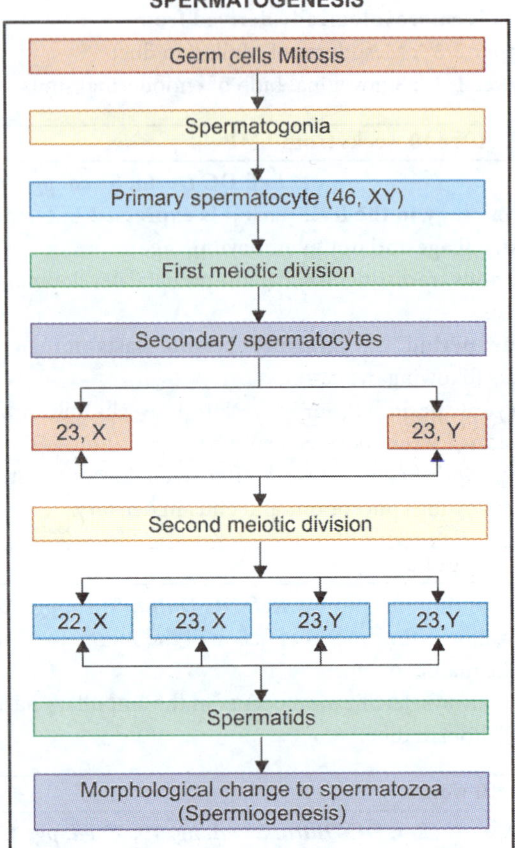

Extra Mile

- 1ST polar body released: At time of puberty/ovulation
- 2nd polar body released: At time of fertilization
- 1st site of fetal hematopoiesis: Yolk sac.

109. Ans. (a) 1st polar body

Ref: DC Dutta, 8th ed. pg. 19-20; Shaws, 15th ed. pg. 74

PROCESS OF FERTILIZATION

- Certain changes are necessary before the primary oocyte can mature for fertilization. ***Oogonia that enter the prophase of the first meiotic division are known as primary oocytes.*** Those oogonia which do not begin the first meiotic division and those not surrounded by granulosa layer atrophy.
- At puberty, under the LH surge, primary oocyte completes the first meiotic division and gives rise to secondary oocyte, containing most of the cytoplasm, 23X chromosomes, and a small polar body.
- This secondary oocyte completes its second meiotic division only after fertilization, and gives out second polar body.
- Thus, the first stage of maturation of the oocyte occurs within the Graafian follicle, but the second division occurs only after the fertilization in the fallopian tube.
- *Please refer to above explanation and flowchart also for detailed explanation.*

110. Ans. (c) 1st polar body

Ref: DC Dutta, 8th ed. pg. 21-22, 8th ed. pg. 21, 7th ed. pg. 17,19

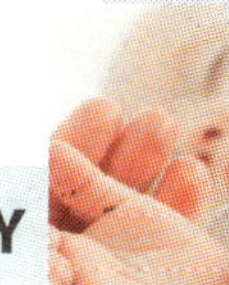

111. Ans. (a) Decidua basalis

Ref: DC Dutta, 8th ed. pg. 32

SAILENT FEATURE OF PLACENTA

- Weight 500 g
- Ratio of weight of placenta: Weight of fetus = 1: 6
- Human placenta is discoidal (disc shape) and deciduate (shed off during delivery), hemochoroidal (in contact with maternal blood)
- **Derived forms decidua basalis**
- Placental circulation established at 21-22nd day (same time heart is formed, hence fetal circulation is established.)

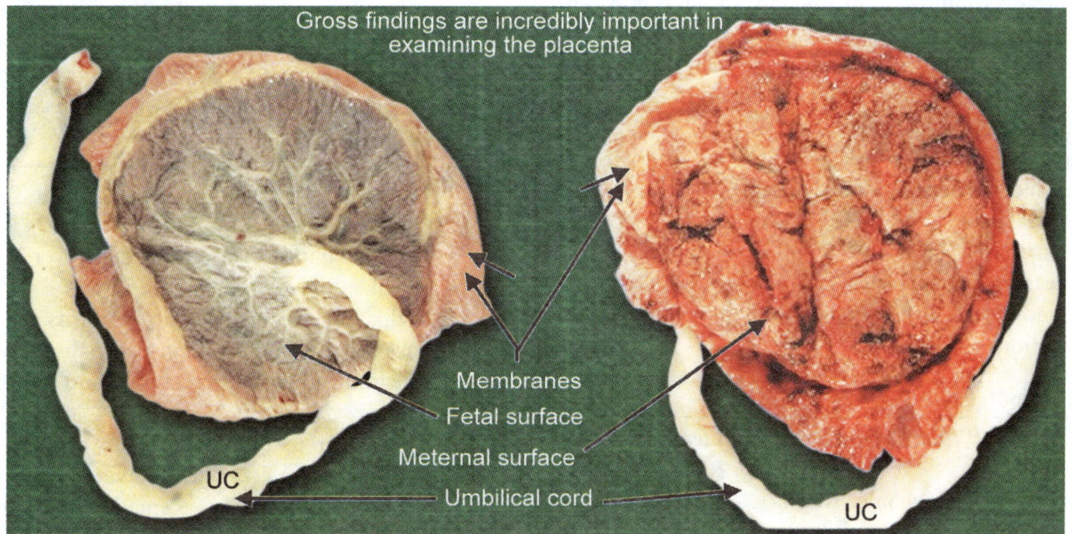

112. Ans. (c) It has umbilical cord attachment site

Ref: DC Dutta, 8th ed. pg. 34-35, 7th ed. pg. 29

Maternal surface of placenta covered by remnant of the deciduas basalis (compact and spongy layer)

Fetal surface	Maternal surface
• Smooth, glistening	• Rough, spongy
• Covered by amnion (above) and chorion (below)	• Covered by remnant of deciduas basalis
• Umbilical cord is attached	• Has 15–20 lobes/cotyledons
• 4/5 of placenta is fetal origin	• 1/5 is maternal origin
• Develops from chorionic sac (chorion frondosum)	• Derived from endometrium (functional layer - Decidua basalis).

LABOR AND DELIVERY

113. Ans. (d) Pulmonary edema

Ref: William's Obstetrics, Chapter 42, 26th ed. pg. 805, 2095

- Ritodrine is a tocolytic drug used to stop premature labor. Pulmonary Edema is not a common complication caused by Ritodrine.
- Cardiovascular side effects include tremors, tachycardia or other cardiac arrhythmias, diastolic blood pressure reduction resulting in dizziness and lightheadedness, and chest pain or tightness. Myocardial ischemia and palpitations have also been reported.

114. Ans. (d) Oxytocin

Ref: https://www.ncbi.nlm.nih.gov/books/NBK148970/

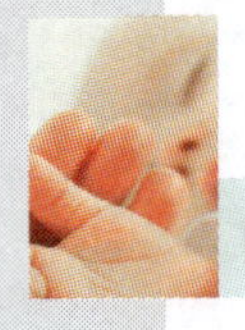

- When baby is breastfeeding, and oxytocin is released, it triggers contractions of the uterus.
- These uterine contractions are often called after pains and they feel similar to menstrual cramps.
- In the first few days after childbirth, after pains can be very strong and, as the name suggests, painful.

115. Ans. (b) Uterine rupture

Ref: William's Obstetrics, Chapter 42, 26th ed. pg. 1925

- A uterine rupture is a complete division of all three layers of the uterus.
- Most uterine ruptures occur when the uterus is gravid in the setting of a trial of labor after cesarean delivery.
- More often, rupture is secondary and associated with a preexisting incision, anomaly, or injury of the myometrium.

Symptoms:

- Vaginal bleeding and Abdominal pain
- Abdominal pain
- Hypotension
- Fetal heart rate abnormality
- Fetal body parts are palpable through per abdomen examination

116. Ans. (a) Hypotension

Ref: William's Obstetrics, Chapter 21, 26th ed. pg. 1033-1034, 1052

- Oxytocin is given to women during CS to decrease blood loss.
- When given as rapid IV bolus, it causes hypotension, tachycardia. However, the exact cause of these hemodynamic changes is lesser known.

117. Ans. (b) Uterine inversion

Ref: William's Obstetrics, Chapter 42, 26th ed. pg. 1911, 1912

- Puerperal inversion of the uterus is one of the classic hemorrhagic disasters encountered in obstetrics.
- Unless promptly recognized and managed appropriately, associated bleeding often is massive.

Clinical presentation of inversion of uterus

- Abdominal pain
- Shock out of proportion due to amount of blood loss
- Hypotension, and shock like symptoms.
- Large boggy mass appears at introitus
- MC: Hemorrhage

118. Ans. (c) Sedation and wait

Ref: William's Obstetrics, 26th ed. pg. 1022

- The presenting female is in latent phase of labor.
- During phase 1, the uterus must initiate extensive changes in its size and vascularity to accommodate fetal growth, some low intensity myometrial contractions are felt during the quiescent phase.
- These contractions do not normally cause cervical dilation, and they are common toward the end of pregnancy, especially in multiparas.
- For these patients, the most accurate management is sedation and wait for the progress of labor.

119. Ans. (c) Laminaria tent

Ref: Dutta 9th ed. pg. 618

- **Laminaria tent:** Is dehydrated, compressed, Chinese sea-weeds. It is use to dilate cervix.
- It works on hygroscopic action due to which slow dilatation of cervical canal takes place. More than one tent is to be introduced to prevent dumpling of the ends.
- It is sterilized by keeping it in absolute alcohol at least for 24 hours.

120. Ans. (c) Leopold 3

Ref: Williams Obstetrics 24th ed. pg. 437-38

- The shown image is leopold's maneuver 3, also known as Pawlik's grip.
- In this the physician will face towards patients head and does suprapubic palpation using thumb and fingers to determine the fetal presentation and station.
- **Note:**
  - In order to differentiate between head and breech presentation, leopold's manuever 1 is done
  - In order to know engagement, LM 4 is done. It is done facing the feet of patient.

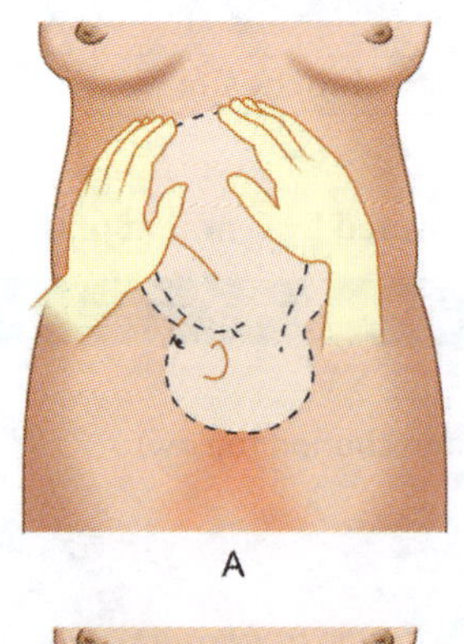

A

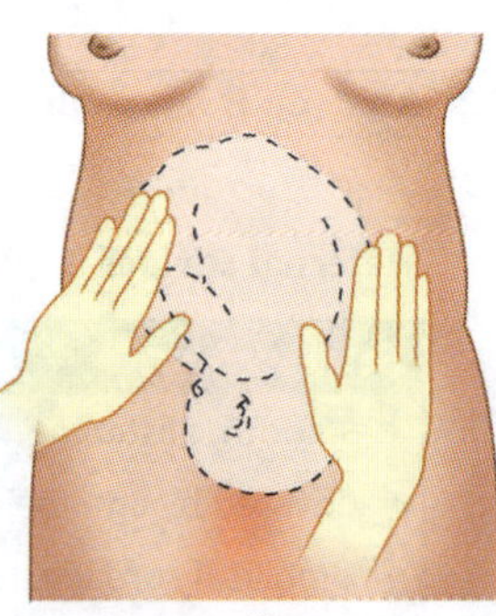

B

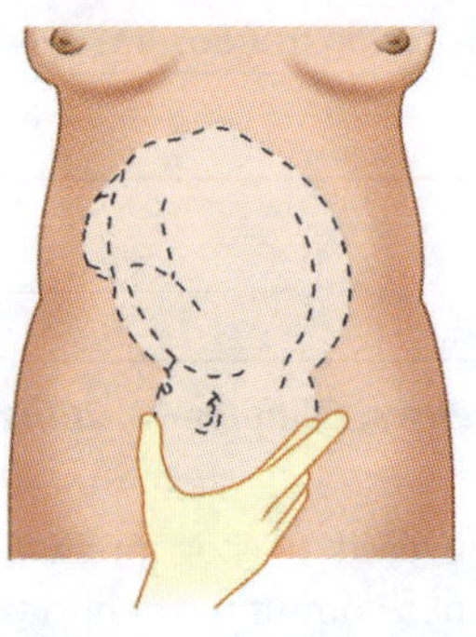

C

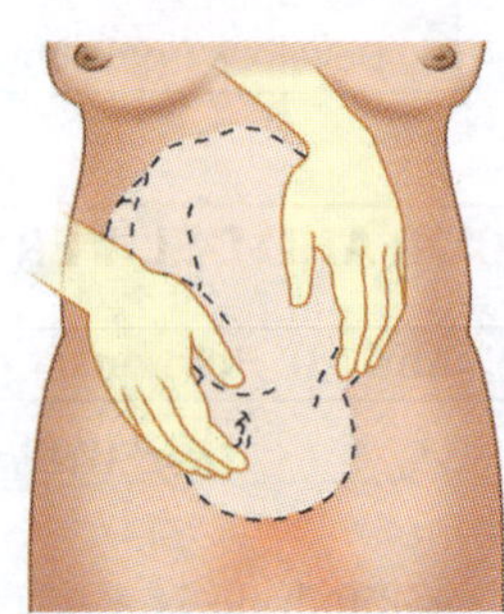

D

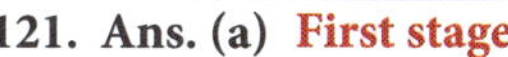

121. Ans. (a) First stage

Ref: William's Obstetrics 24th ed. pg. 409, 548

- **First stage:** Stage of contraction and cervical dilatation. Cervical dilatation is 0–10 cm
- **Second stage:** Stage of fetal descent and delivery. Full cervical dilatation to birth
- **Third stage:** Stage of placental expulsion. From birth of baby to placental expulsion
- **Fourth stage:** Stage of observation. From birth of placenta to 4 hours postpartum.

122. Ans. (b) Uterine inversion

Ref: William's Obstetrics 24th ed. pg. 787

- Uterine inversion is when the uterus turns inside out, usually following childbirth or during the forceful traction of placenta.
- Symptoms include postpartum bleeding, abdominal pain, mass in the vagina, and low blood pressure.
- Risk factors include pulling on the umbilical cord or pushing on the top of the uterus before the placenta has detached.

123. Ans. (a) Uterine scar rupture and laparotomy

Ref: William's Obstetrics 24th ed. pg. 598-99

- The most common sign of uterine rupture is a non-reassuring fetal heart rate pattern with variable decelerations that may evolve into late decelerations and bradycardia.
- Recommended step is to do immediate laparotomy.
- Few women experienced e cessation of contractions following uterine rupture. The condition usually becomes evident because of fetal distress and occasionally because of maternal hypovolemia from concealed hemorrhage.

124. Ans. (b) 60 degrees to the midline

Ref: Dutta's Obstetrics 8th ed. pg. 647

- A surgically planned incision on the perineum and the posterior vaginal wall during the second stage of labor is called episiotomy (perineotomy).
- **Objective:**
  - **To enlarge** the vaginal introitus
  - **To minimize** overstretching and rupture of the perineal muscles and fascia
- Mediolateral is the most preferred episiotomy.
  - The mediolateral episiotomy begins at the midline of the fourchette and is directed to the right or left at an angle 60 degrees of the midline.
  - This angle accounts for perineal anatomy distortion during crowning and ultimately yields an incision 45 degrees of the midline for suturing.

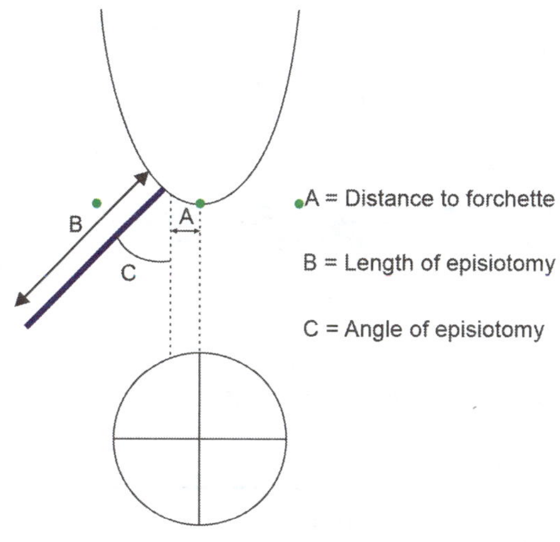

125. Ans. (c) >4

Ref: DC Dutta 9th ed. pg. 86

- A pregnant woman with a previous history of four births or more is called grand multipara.

Extra Mile

• **A nullipara** is one who has never completed a pregnancy to the stage of viability. She may or may not have aborted previously.	• **A nulligravida** is one who is not now and never has been pregnant
• **A primipara** is one who has delivered one viable child. Parity is not increased even if the fetuses are many (twins, triplets)	• **A primigravida** is one who is pregnant for the first time
• **A multigravida** is one who has previously been pregnant. She may have aborted or have delivered a viable baby	• **Multipara** is one who has completed two or more pregnancies to the stage of viability or more
• **A parturient** is a women in labor	• **A puerpera** is a woman who has just given birth

126. Ans. (c) Immediate LSCS

Ref: DC Dutta 8th ed. pg. 267

- In this case fetal distress and maternal condition does not warrant tocolytic or wait and watch policy. Therefore immediate CS should be performed.

INDICATIONS OF CESAREAN SECTION

- **When an urgent termination is indicated and the cervix is unfavorable** (unripe and closed).

- **Severe preeclampsia** with a tendency of prolonged induction—delivery interval.
- **Associated complicating factors,** such as elderly primigravidae, contracted pelvis, malpresentation, etc.

Extra Mile

Common Indications for Induction of Labor (IOL)
• Postmaturity • Pre-eclampsia/eclampsia • Intrauterine fetal death • Premature rupture of the membranes • Congenital malformation of the fetus • Antepartum hemorrhage • Chronic hydramnios

TABLE: Dangers of indication of labor

Maternal	Fetal
• Psychological upset when there is induction failure and cesarean section is done	• Iatrogenic prematurity
• Tendency of prolonged labor due to abnormal uterine action	• Hypoxia due to uterine dysfunction
• Increased need of analgesia during labor	• Prolonged labor
• Increased operative interference	• Operative interference
• Increase morbidity	

127. Ans. (a) Ritodrine

Ref: DC Dutta 8th ed. pg. 583

- **Preterm labor and delivery** can be delayed by drugs in order to improve the perinatal outcome. These agents are known as tocolytic agents.
- The commonly used drugs are:
  - **Betamimetics:** Ritodrine, Isoxuprine. Causes relaxation of uterus.
  - **Prostaglandin synthetase inhibitors/COX inhibitor:** Indomethacin, sulindac.
  - **Magnesium sulfate:** Act as **competitive inhibitor** of calcium ion.
  - **Calcium channel blockers:** Nifedipine, nicardipine.
  - **Oxytocin receptor antagonists:** Atosiban. Used as IV infusion.
  - **Nitric oxide donors:** Glyceryl trinitrate (used as patches).
  - Progesterone.

128. Ans. (d) Vertex

Ref: DC Dutta 8th ed. pg. 87

- **Anterior, posterior, right or left position is referred in relation to the maternal pelvis,** with the mother in erect position.
- **Vertex occupying the left anterior quadrant of the pelvis is the most common one** and is called left occipitoanterior (LOA). This is the first vertex position.

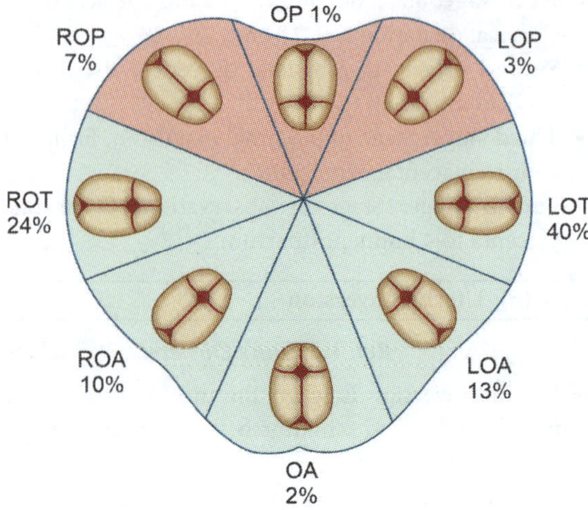

The position and relative frequency of the vertex at the onset of labor

TABLE: Pelvic diameter and presenting part

Diameters	Measurement (in cm)	Presentation
Suboccipitobregmatic	9.5 cm	Vertex
Suboccipitofrontal	10 cm	Vertex
Occipitofrontal	11.5 cm	Vertex
Mentovertical: Extend from mid-point of chin to the highest point on the sagittal suture	14 cm	Brow
Submentovertical	11.5 cm	Face
Submentobregmatic	9.5 cm	Face

129. Ans. (d) Tubal ostia

Ref: William's Obstetrics, 23rd ed. Ch: 18

- The normal contractile wave of labor originates near the uterine end of one of the fallopian tubes (tubal ostia). Thus, these areas act as "pacemakers"

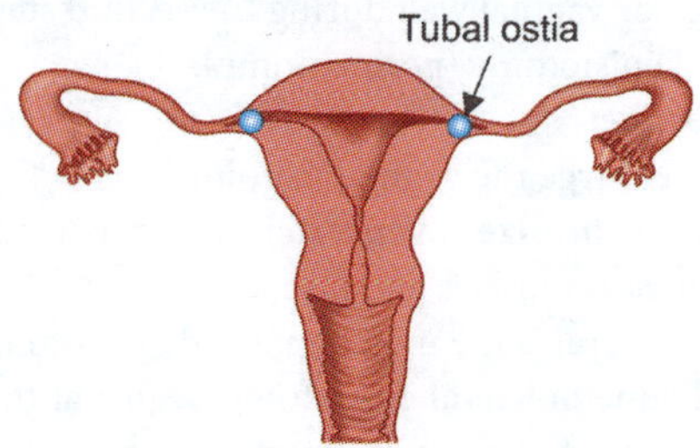

- The right pacemaker usually predominates over the left and starts most contractile waves.
- Contractions spread from the pacemaker area throughout the uterus at 2 cm/sec, depolarizing the whole organ

within 15 seconds. This depolarization wave propagates downward toward the cervix.

- Intensity is greatest in the fundus, and it diminishes in the lower uterus.

130. Ans. (c) Fetal head is engaged

Ref: DC Dutta, 8th ed. pg. 153

- Since the type of pelvis may vary from one woman to another (gynaecoid, android, anthropoid and platypelloid), the only effective measure of fetal head descent that reflects engagement is the suprapubic assessment of how much of the fetal skull remains palpable.
- The amount of fetal head felt suprapubically in finger breadth is assessed by placing the radial margin of the index finger above the symphysis pubis successively until the groove of the neck is reached.
- Progressive descent of the head can be usefully assessed abdominally by estimating the number of "fifths" of the head above the pelvic brim
- ***Dutta states:*** *"when the fetal head is* ***one-fifth above (pelvic brim***), *only the sinciput can be felt abdominally and nought-fifths represents a head entirely in the pelvis with no poles felt abdominally"*

131. Ans. (a) 1/5th of the fetal head palpable

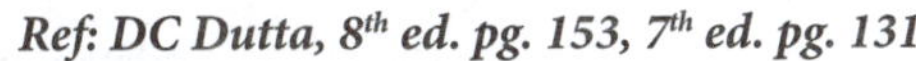

Ref: DC Dutta, 8th ed. pg. 153, 7th ed. pg. 131

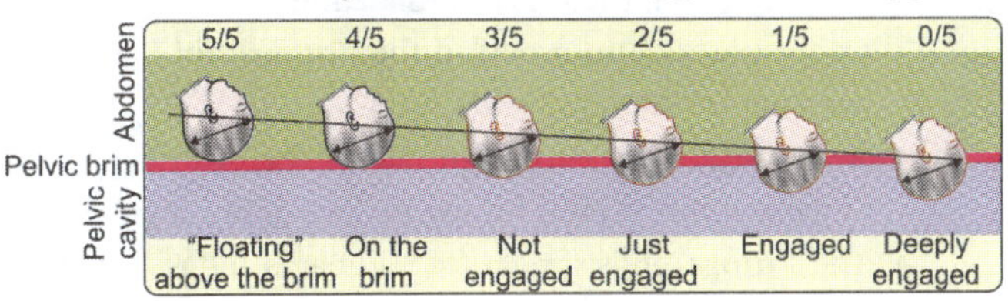

132. Ans. (b) Can damage brain

Ref: DC Dutta, 8th ed. pg. 97

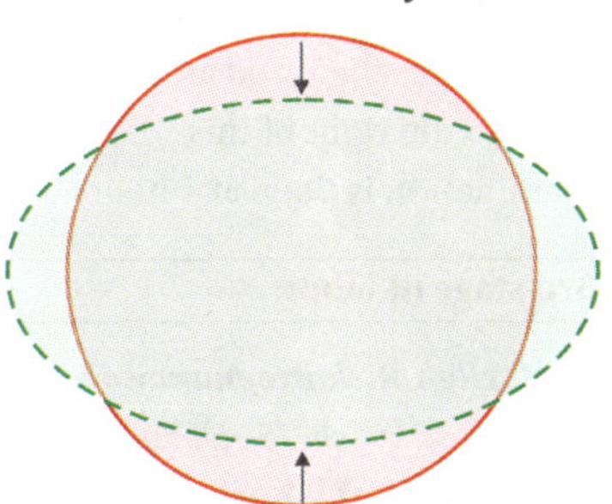

FIGURE: Diagrammatic representation showing the principle of moulding of the head

- **Moulding is alteration of the shape of the fore-coming head while passing through the resistant birth passage during labor.**
- There is very **little alteration** in size of the head.
- Normally, an alteration of **4 mm in skull diameter** commonly occurs.
- It doesn't complicate the delivery, instead it enables the head to **pass more easily,** through the birth canal.
- ***Mechanism:*** There is compression of the engaging diameter of the head with corresponding elongation of the diameter at right angle to it (Fig.)
- During the process, the parietal bones tend to overlap the adjacent bones, viz.
  - Posteriorly with occipital bone behind
  - Anteriorly, with frontal bones and the
  - At sides, with temporal bones
- **Molding disappears within few hours after birth.**

GRADING

- **Grade-1**—The bones touching but not overlapping
- **Grade-2**— Overlapping but easily separated and
- **Grade-3**—Fixed overlapping *(most severe form)*

Importance:

- **Slight molding is inevitable and beneficial.** It enables the head to **pass more easily,** through the birth canal.
- Extreme molding can result in severe intracranial disturbance in the form of **tearing of tentorium cerebelli or subdural haemorrhage.**
- Can tell the presenting part while delivery.

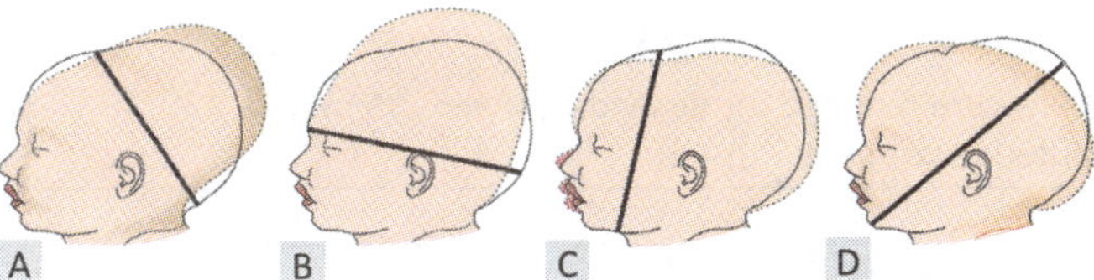

FIGURE: Types of molding in cephalic presentations (shown by dotted line): (A) Vertex presentation with well flexed head; (B) Vertex presentation with deflexed head (sugar loaf head); (C) Face presentation; (D) Brow presentation

133. Ans. (b) 100–120 mm Hg

Ref: William's Obstetrics, 23rd ed. Ch.18 intrapartum Assessment (Internal Uterine Pressure Monitoring)

- A fluid-filled plastic catheter with its distal tip located above the presenting part is used to measure amnionic fluid pressure between and during contractions.
- Clinical labor usually commences when uterine activity reaches values between *80 and 120 Montevideo units.* This translates into approximately three contractions of 40 mm Hg every 10 minutes *(40 × 3 = 120).*
- **During the first 30 weeks,** uterine activity is comparatively quiescent. Contractions are seldom greater than 20 mm Hg.
- **During first-stage labor,** uterine contractions increase progressively in intensity from approximately ***25 mm Hg at*** commencement of labor to **50 mm Hg at the end.**

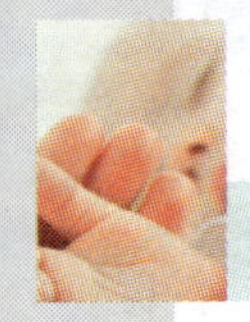

- **DC Dutta states: *"intrauterine pressure is raised to 40-50 mm Hg during 1st stage and about 100-120 mm Hg in second stage of labor during contractions. In spite of diminished pain in 3rd stage, the pressure is probably the same as that in second stage i.e. 100-120 mm Hg"***
- Uterine contractions are clinically palpable only after their intensity exceeds 10 mm Hg. Moreover, until the intensity of contractions reaches 40 mm Hg, the uterine wall can readily be depressed by the finger. At greater intensity, the uterine wall then becomes so hard that it resists easy depression.
- Uterine contractions usually are not associated with pain until their intensity *exceeds 15 mm Hg*, presumably because this is the minimum pressure required for distending the lower uterine segment and cervix.

TABLE: Uterine pressure in a nutshell

Period	Contraction pressure
During the first 30 weeks	20 mm Hg
First stage of labor	40–50 mm Hg
2nd stage of labor	100–120 mm Hg
3rd stage of labor	100–120 mm Hg
Contraction felt clinically	>10 mm Hg
Contraction associated with pain	15 mm Hg
Pressure required for distending lower uterine segment	15 mm Hg

134. Ans. (a) 50 mm Hg

***Ref:** William's Obstetrics, 23rd ed. pg. ch 18*

- According to the given options, 50 mmHg is best answer that can be chosen.
- *Please refer to above explanation.*

135. Ans. (b) 2 hours

***Ref:** DC Dutta, 8th ed. pg. 153*

Stages of Labor	Duration	
	Primipara	Multipara
Stage I: From uterine contraction to full cervical dilatation (10 cm)	12 hours	6 hours
Stage II: Full dilatation to delivery of baby	*2 hours*	30 mins
Stage III: Delivery of baby to placental delivery	15 mins	15 mins
Stage IV: 1 hour post partum to rule out PPH and vulvar hematoma.	1 hour	1 hour

136. Ans. (a) 30 minutes

***Ref:** William's 23rd ed. Chapter 17, Normal Labor and Delivery; Preadmission and Admission Electronic Fetal Heart Rate Monitoring*

- American Academy of Pediatrics and American College of Obstetricians and Gynecologists (2007) recommend that during the first stage of labor, in the absence of any abnormalities, the fetal heart rate should be checked immediately after a contraction at least every 30 minutes and then every 15 minutes during the second stage.
- ***If continuous electronic monitoring is used, the tracing is evaluated at least every 30 minutes*** during the first stage and at least every 15 minutes during second-stage labor.
- For women with pregnancies at risk, fetal heart auscultation is performed at least every 15 minutes during the first stage of labor and every 5 minutes during the second stage.
- *Given the above options, every 30 minutes monitoring is the best choice.*

137. Ans. (d) 4 hours

***Ref:** Williams, 23rd ed. Ch: 17*

- On admission, the cervical dilatation should be plotted on the partogram, provided the diagnosis of Labor has been made.
- A partogram was designed by the World Health Organization (WHO) for use in developing countries
- The partograph is similar for nulliparas and multiparas.
- Labor is divided into a latent phase (8 hrs), and an active phase. The active phase starts at 3 cm dilatation, and progress should be no slower than 1 cm/hr.
- An alert line is drawn at 1 cm/h once the active phase of Labor has been reached, and an action line is then drawn parallel and to the right of this.
- Pelvic examination is done at 4 hours.

138. Ans. (c) 3rd stage of labor

***Ref:** High Risk Pregnancy 4th ed. by James et. al, ch 75- Normal third stage of Labor*

There are four stages of labor

- **The first stage** is from the onset of true labor to complete dilation of the cervix.
- **The second stage** is from complete dilation of the cervix to the birth of the baby.
- **The third stage** is from the birth of the baby to delivery of the placenta.

- **The fourth stage** is from delivery of the placenta to stabilization of the patient's condition, usually at about 6 hours postpartum.

PROSTAGLANDINS

- Prostaglandin F (PGF), $PGF_{2\alpha}$, and oxytocin are the biochemical agents primarily involved in the third stage of labor.
- During the first and second stages of labor, only $PGF_{2\alpha}$ and oxytocin are significantly raised in maternal plasma compared with pre-labor concentrations.
- ***At 5 minutes after birth, maternal PGF and $PGF_{2\alpha}$ concentrations peak at about twice the levels found at the commencement of the second stage.*** A rapid increase in prostaglandin concentrations is also found in umbilical cord venous blood, suggesting that this postpartum prostaglandin surge originates in the placenta.
- After placental separation, the concentrations decrease but at rates slower than the metabolic clearance of prostaglandin, indicating that its production continues in the decidua and myometrium.
- Plasma oxytocin also drops to prelabor levels within 30 minutes of delivery, unless sustained by exogenous infusion.

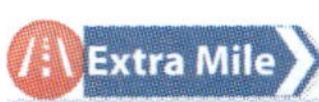
Extra Mile

Hormones	Peak level at:
Oxytocin	At birth
Prolactin	Levels decrease during labor but then rise steeply at the end of labor and **peak with birth**

139. Ans. (b) 800–1000 mL

Ref: Williams Obstetrics, 24th ed. pg. 250

NORMAL AMNIOTIC FLUID VOLUME

- Amniotic fluid volume increases as the age of gestation increases:
  - 10 weeks: 30 mL
  - 16 weeks: 200 mL
  - 3rd trimester: 800 mL
- Amniotic fluid is maximum at 28–36 week age of gestation (1000 mL).
- This fluid is approximately 98-percent water. A full-term fetus contains roughly 2800 mL of water, and the placenta another 400 mL, such that the term uterus holds nearly 4 liters of water.
- Fetal urine production begins between 8 and 11 weeks, but it does not become a major component of amniotic fluid until the second trimester.

TABLE: In order to attempt any question related to this topic we have summarized this table of the amount of amniotic fluid, fetal weight according to gestational age ***(william's OB 23rd ed. Ch 21).***

Weeks' Gestation	Fetus wt (g)	Amniotic fluid (mL)	Placenta (g)
16 weeks	100	200	100
28 weeks	1000	1000	200
36 weeks	2500	900–1000	400
40 weeks	3300	800	500

Note: *If question formed as amniotic fluid is maximum at then single best answer will be 36 weeks.*

- *This latter observation explains why fetuses with lethal renal abnormalities may not manifest severe oligohydramnios until after 18 weeks.*
- ***Fetal urination is the primary amnionic fluid source by the second half of pregnancy.***
- By term, fetal urine production may exceed 1 liter per day—such that the entire amnionic fluid volume is recirculated on a daily basis. Fetal urine osmolality is significantly hypotonic to that of maternal and fetal plasma and similar to that of amnionic fluid.

140. Ans. (b) 34–36 weeks

Ref: Williams Obstetrics, 24th ed. pg. 250

Please refer to above explanation

141. Ans. (d) Cervical shape

Ref: Dutta's Obstetrics 7th ed. pg. 523

- **Bishop score is used to predict** success rate of the induction of the labor
- **Bishop score includes:**
- Dilation of the cervix.
- Position of the cervix.
- The presenting part of the fetus
- Consistency of the cervix
- **Note:** Modified Bishop score includes cervical length by replacing the effacement.

142. Ans. (c) Clavicle

Ref: "Clavicle Fracture in Labor: Risk Factors and Associated Morbidities". J Perinatol (Dec '01)

- *Clavicle fractures are the most frequently encountered birth injury (0.5%).*
- *Brachial plexus* is also injured during child birth due to its stretch. The brachial plexus is stretched when the head is pulled in one direction and the arm in the opposite.
- *Femur fractures* also occur in as the leg is awkwardly twisted during delivery. These are rare injuries that are much less common than clavicle fractures.

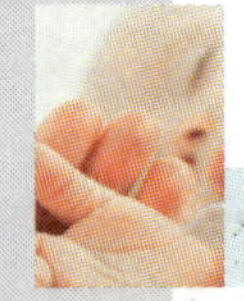

143. Ans. (c) Variable deceleration

Ref: Dutta's Obstetrics, 7th ed. pg. 612

- Deceleration is transient decrease in FHR below the baseline by 15 bpm or more and lasting for more than or equal to 15 secs.
- Three basic type of deceleration are observed:
    - **Early deceleration:** Due to head compression
    - **Late deceleration:** Uteroplacental insufficiency and fetal hypoxia
    - ***Variable deceleration:*** *Cord compression (MC type)*

144. Ans. (c) Uteroplacental insufficiency

Ref: Dutta's Obstetrics, 7th ed. pg. 612

Please refer to above explanation

145. Ans. (b) Variable deceleration

The given partogram shows variable deceleration. Now compare the different partograms

FETAL MONITOR PATTERNS

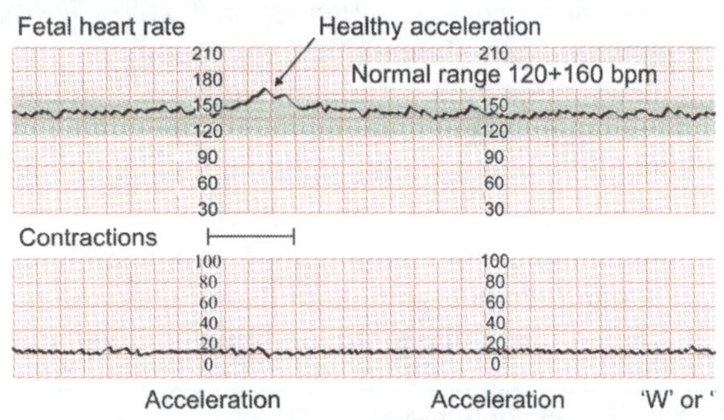

REASSURING PATTERN

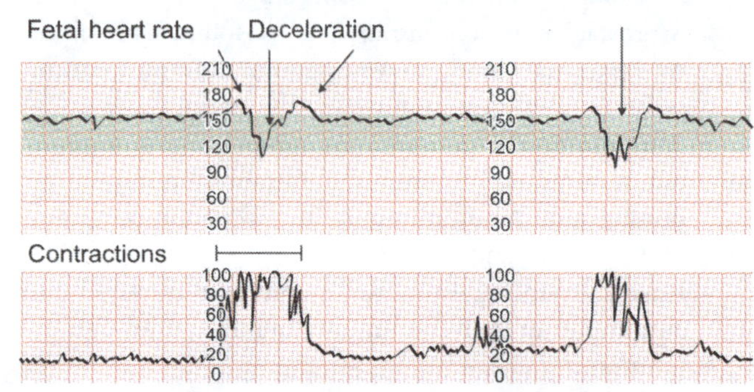

VARIABLE DECELERATIONS

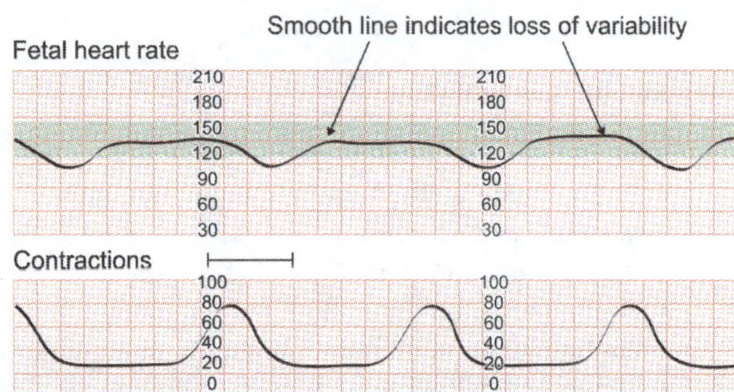

LATE DECELERATION WITH VARIABILITY LOSS

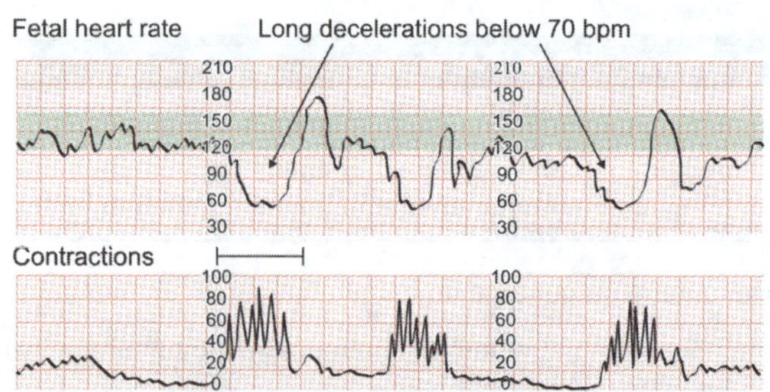

SEVERE VARIABLE DECELERATIONS

146. Ans. (c) Extension to rectum

Ref: DC Dutta, 8th ed. pg. 649-50, 5th ed. pg. 606

- **Episiotomy:** Is defined as a surgical incision of the perineum made to increase the diameter of the vulval outlet during child- birth (and not the whole birth canal).
- **Types of episiotomy:** (Only the median or mediolateral episiotomy are done commonly).
- Medio-lateral
    - Median
    - Lateral
    - 'J' shaped

Median	Mediolateral
• Muscles are not cut	• Muscles are cut
• Blood loss is less	• Blood loss is more
• Repair is easy	• Repair is difficult
• Healing is superior	• Healing is less superior
• Dyspareunia is rare	• Dyspareunia is more
• Extension, if occurs, may involve rectum	• Relative safety from rectal involvement from extension
• Incision cannot be extended	• Incision can be extended

147. Ans. (d) 2 hours

Ref: Dutta 8th ed. pg. 154-156

- **Secondary arrest** is defined when the **active phase of labor (cervical dilatation)** commences normally but stops or **slows significantly for 2 hours** or more prior to the full dilatation of the cervix.
- It is commonly **due to malposition or cephalopelvic disproportion.**

> ***'Cessation of active phase of dilatation by more than 2 hours is defined as arrest'***: Danforth.

ANTEPARTUM AND POSTPARTUM PERIOD

148. Ans. (a) 4 mg

Ref: https://www.ncbi.nlm.nih.gov/pmc/articles/PMC2329900/

The upper limit for folic acid is 1 mg/d. Women in intermediate- to high-risk categories for neural tube defects, such as a previous neural tube defect–affected pregnancy, should take 4–5 mg of folic acid daily.

149. Ans. (a) 36 weeks

Ref: William's Obstetrics, 26th ed. pg. 666

Please refer to above explanation

150. Ans. (b) 4

Ref: DC Dutta 9th ed. pg. 89

As per WHO recommendation, the visit may be curtailed to at least 4, first in the second trimester around 16 weeks, second between 24 and 28 weeks, the third visit at 32 weeks and the fourth visit at 36 weeks in developing countries.

151. Ans. (c) 10 days

Ref: DC Dutta 9th ed. pg. 48

- The cardiac output starts to increase from the 5th week of pregnancy and reaches its peak at about 30-34 weeks.
- CO is lowest in sitting and supine position and highest in the left and right lateral or knee chest position.
- CO increases further during labor and immediately following delivery over the prelabor values.
- CO comes to normal within 10 days of delivery.

152. Ans. (b) Molar pregnancy

Ref: Williams Gynaecology 3rd ed. pg. 780

- Hydatidiform mole is a benign tumor of placental origin that results from an abnormal fertilized egg and subsequent abnormal proliferation of the trophoblastic cells of the growing but ultimately non-viable 'fetus' that synthesize hCG.
- The principle use of hCG testing is the early diagnosis of pregnancy and also useful for diagnosis of some pregnancy-related disorders including hydatidiform mole (molar pregnancy).

153. Ans. (c) Retained placenta

Ref: William's Obstetrics, Chapter 36, 26th ed. pg. 1641-42

- This is a case of late postpartum hemorrhage.
- The American College of Obstetricians and Gynecologists defines secondary postpartum hemorrhage as bleeding 24 hours to 12 weeks after delivery.
- It occasionally is caused by retention of a placental fragment or by a uterine artery pseudo aneurysm.
- Rarely, retained products may undergo necrosis with fibrin deposition and neovascularization, thus forming a placental polyploid mass. Severe hemorrhage occurs in only 6% of these cases due to rupture of blood.

154. Ans. (c) Renal agenesis

Ref: William's Obstetrics, Chapter 45, 26th ed. pg. 2036,

- When the embryonic kidney cells fail to develop, the result is called renal agenesis.
- It is often detected on fetal ultrasound because there will be a lack of amniotic fluid (called oligohydramnios).
- When both kidneys are absent this condition is not compatible with life.

155. Ans. (b) Uterine inversion

Ref: William's Obstetrics, Chapter 42, 26th ed. pg. 1911, 1912

- Uterine inversion is one of the most serious complications of childbirth.
- Uterine inversion refers to the collapse of the fundus into the uterine cavity.
- Although it does not often occur, it carries a high risk of mortality due to hemorrhage and shock.

156. Ans. (b) Breast engorgement

Ref: Dutta 9th ed. pg. 410-412

- Patient present with only heaviness in breast that's why answer is Breast engorgement, this is a common breast complication in puerperium.
- It occurs due to engorgement of venous supply and lymphatics of the breast, which prevents escape of milk from lacteal system.
- This manifests after the milk secretion starts i.e. 3rd or 4th day postpartum.
- Symptoms include—pain and feeling of tenseness, heaviness in breasts, painful breastfeeding, Generalized malaise, transient rise in temperature.

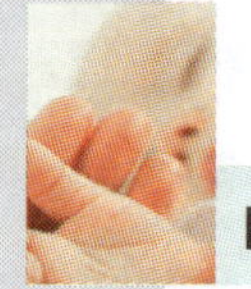

Note:

- In Mastitis patient presents with fever (102 degree or more) with chills, severe pain, tender swelling.
- In Breast abscess patient presents with brawny edema of overlying skin, marked tender with fluctuations.
- In lactation failure patient present with different causes like depression or anxiety of mother during puerperium, reluctance to nursing, infrequent suckling etc.

157. Ans. (d) Assurance

Ref: Shaw's Gynecology 16th ed. pg. 325

- **Secondary amenorrhea** is a rare condition, seen in 2–3% of the population.
- It is defined as amenorrhea of 6 months or more in a woman with previous normal menstrual patterns in the absence of pregnancy and lactation.
- In the above case, assurance is the best advise to be given to the patient, since this is a case of lactational amenorrhea and no surgical intervention is required.
- Till 6 months of postdelivery mother give exclusive breastfeeding to the baby which results in Lactational Amenorrhea.
- Due to breastfeeding disruption of pattern of pulsatile release of GnRH from hypothalamus, hence disrupts LH from pituitary, Preovulatory LH surge doesn't takes place results in either fail to rupture follicles or become atretic and cystic.
- Only after decline of lactation, preovulatory LH surge will take place which will result in normal menstruation.

158. Ans. (b) Atonic PPH

Ref: Dutta 9th ed. pg. 391-92

- This picture showing ligation of internal iliac artery — it is done in the anterior division, below the origin of posterior division. This is a method to **control PPH**.
- It reduces distal blood flow and helps stable clot (because of reduction of pulse pressure).
- No pelvic necrosis due to extensive collateral circulation.

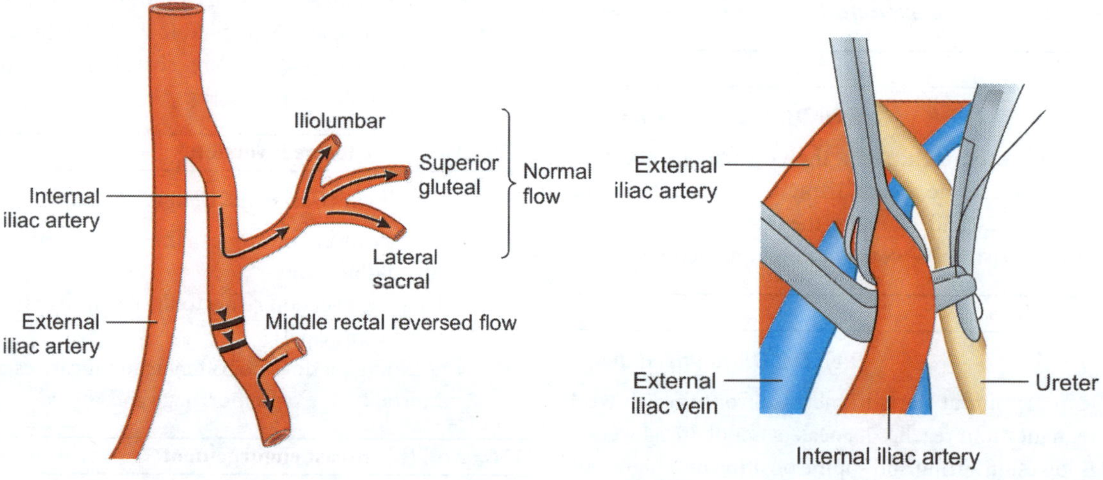

159. Ans. (a) Adenomyosis

Ref: Shaw's Gynecology 16th ed. pg. 420

- Adenomyosis is also known as uterine endometriosis, where endometrial lining is found in walls of uterus.
- Adenomyosis is mostly seen in parous females around age of 40 years, and more than 1/3rd of hysterectomy reveals adenomyosis presence.
- Gross examination reveals that uterus appears symmetrically enlarged to not more than 14 weeks size.
- Patient often remain asymptomatic and some may present with menorrhagia and progressively increasing dysmenorrhea, backache, dyspareunia.
- Here in this case uterine enlargement of up to 10 weeks and symptoms like amenorrhea, uniform enlargement (globular) of uterus, tender on touch — **direct toward Adenomyosis.**

Note:

- In leiomyoma (fibroid) – non uniform enlargement, size of it 20 weeks, non tender on touch.
- In PID, Endometriosis no engagement of uterus, as in endometriosis adnexal mass.

160. Ans. (d) Oxytocin

Ref: Dutta 8th ed. pg. 173-74

- Sucking of breast by the baby stimulates the nerves which make release of prolactin from anterior pituitary and oxytocin from the posterior pituitary.
- Prolactin is responsible for milk production i.e. detection from the tissue while Oxytocin responsible for ejection of milk so this is responsible for lactation.

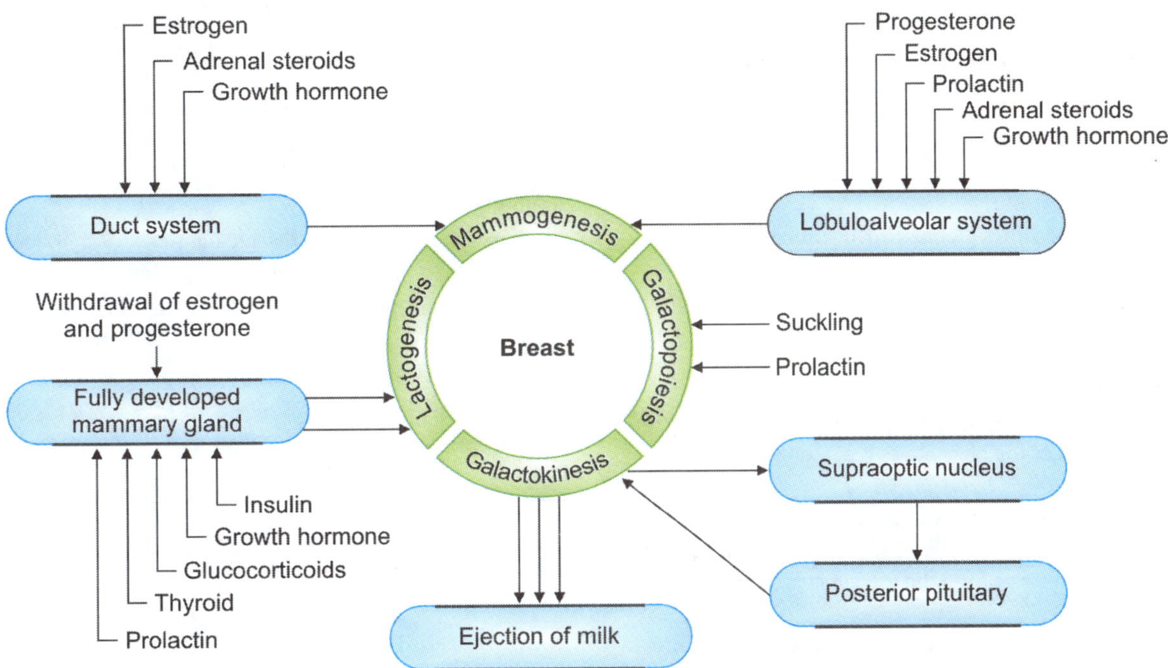

161. Ans. (d) Post-partum hemorrhage

Ref: William's Obstetrics 25th ed. pg. 777

- Following placental removal, the placenta site may bleed uncontrollably due to poorly contracted smooth muscle, which is characteristic of the lower uterine segment.
- If hemostasis at the placental implantation site cannot be obtained by adequate uterotonic administration and pressure, it can be overseen with O-chromic sutures.

162. Ans. (b) Naegele's formula

Ref: DC Dutta 9th ed. pg. 88

- Calculation of the expected date of delivery is done according to **Naegele's formula**
- 1st day of LMP + 9 months + 7 days

Extra Mile

- **Cardiff "count 10" formula:** fetal movement count. If <10 kicks in 12 hours on two successive days → Fetal compromise.
- **Hadlock formula and Shepard formula:** For fetal weight estimation according to gestational age using fetal biometric data (BPD, Head circumference, Abdominal circumference and femur length)
- **Johnsons formula:** Also for fetal weight estimation.
  - Height of uterus above symphysis pubis minus 12
- **Crichton's Fifth formula:** Assessment of progressive descent of fetal head.

- Count 3 calendar month back from 1st day of LMP +7 days
- For IVF pregnancy, date of LMP is 14 days prior to date to embryo transfer
- Based on formula labor starts on expected date in 4%. Its prediction range is about 50% with 7 days on either side of EDD.

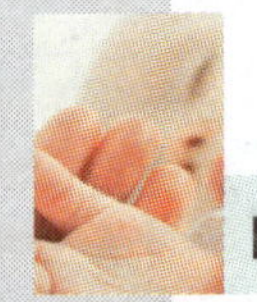

163. Ans. (d) Discoid uterus

Ref: DC Dutta Obstetrics 8th ed. pg. 143-44

- The 3rd stage of labor comprises of placental separation, its descent into lower segment and its expulsion.
- After the birth of the baby, the uterus measures about 20 cm (8″) vertically and 10 cm (4″) anteroposteriorly and the shape become discoid (before separation).

Signs Before and After Placental Separation

- **Before separation:** Uterus becomes *discoid in shape*, firm in feel and nonballottable.
  - Fundal height reaches slightly below the umbilicus
- **After separation:**
  - Uterus becomes globular firm and ballotable
  - *The fundal height is slightly raised*
  - Sudden gush of vaginal bleeding upon separation
  - Permanent lengthening of the cord.

Extra Mile

- **The separation is facilitated partly** by uterine contraction and mostly by weight of the placenta as it descends down from the active part.
- There are two types of separation of placenta:
  i. **Marginal separation:** Also known as Mathews-Duncan separation and starts from the margin. It is the most common type.
  ii. **Central separation:** Also known as **Schultze** separation. Starts at center, blood accumulates retroplacentally until whole of the placenta gets detached.

164. Ans. (b) TIBC increased

Ref: DC Dutta, 8th ed. pg. 304

- Total iron requirement during pregnancy is estimated approximately 1,000 mg
- This iron need is not squarely distributed throughout the pregnancy but mostly limited to the third trimester.
- Pregnancy is an inevitable iron deficiency state.
- There is **decreased** serum iron, serum ferritin (storage form of iron) and reduced serum iron: Serum TIBC ratio.
- TIBC is increased (as serum iron is decreased).

Extra Mile

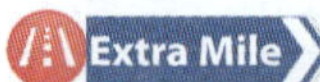

TABLE: Normal blood values in non-pregnant and pregnant state

Blood values	Non-pregnant	Second half pregnancy
Hemoglobin (Hb)	14.8 g/100 mL	11–14 g/100 mL
Red blood cells (RBC)	5 million/cu mm (mm³)	4–4.5 million/mm³
Packed cell volume (PCV) (Hematocrit)	39–42%	32–36%
Mean corpuscular hemoglobin (MCH)	27–32 micromicron (picogram-pg)	26–31 pg
Mean corpuscular volume (MCV)	75–100 cubic micron (μ³)	75–95 μ³
Mean corpuscular hemoglobin concentration (MCHC)	32–36%	30–35%
Serum iron	60–120 μg/100 mL	Slightly lowered (65–75 μg/100)
Total iron blinding capacity (TIBC)	300–350 μg/100 mL	Increaed (300–400 μg/100 mL)
Saturation percentage (Ratio-serum Iron: TIBC)	30%	Less than 16%
Serum ferritin	20–30 μg/L (mean)	15 mg/L (mean)

165. Ans. (c) Oxytocin

Ref: Textbook of Gyenecolgy by Rao, pg. 17; DC Dutta, 8th ed. pg. 17

- **Oxytocin** primarily results in stimulation of **two specific types of muscular contraction:**
  - Uterine muscular contraction during parturition
  - Breast lactiferous duct myoepithelial contraction during milk let down reflex.

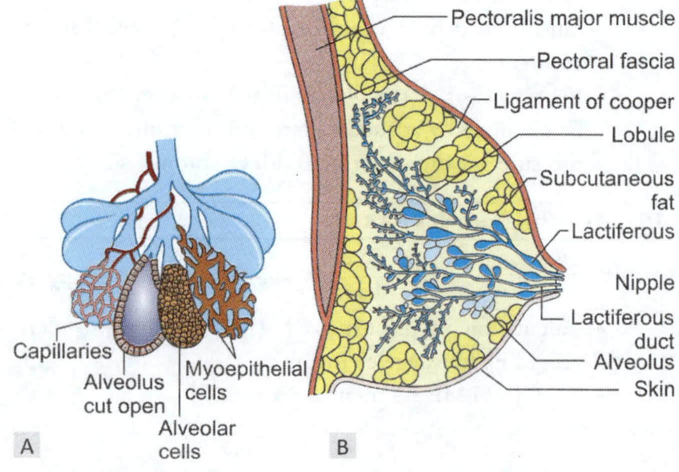

FIGURE: (A) Structure of the basic unit of the mammary gland; (B) Structure of adult female breast

A Brief on Breast Functional Anatomy

- **The areola** is central, pigmented portion of breast with a diameter of about 2.5 cm.
- Accessory glands located around the periphery of the areola are **Montgomery glands** *(they can secrete milk).*
- **The nipple** ccommodates **about 15–20 lactiferous ducts** and their openings.
- Each milk duct **(lactiferous duct)** dilates to form lactiferous sinus at about 5–10 mm away from its opening in the nipple. Lactiferous sinus acts as reservoir of milk.
- The lining epithelium of the duct near the opening is stratified squamous. Each alveolus is lined by columnar epithelium where milk secretion occurs.
- **Myoepithelial cells are the** network of branching longitudinal striated cells which surround the alveoli and the smaller ducts. There is a dense network of capillaries surrounding the alveoli. These are situated between the basement membrane and epithelial lining.
- **Contraction of these cells (in response to oxytocin) squeezes the alveoli and ejects the milk into the larger duct.**

166. Ans. (b) TAS

Ref: DC Dutta, 8th ed. pg. 733

- For screening transabdominal sonography is the best modality. However if question framed as "best investigation" or "earliest detection" then the answer will be transvaginal sonography.

167. Ans. (c) 21 days

Ref: DC Dutta, 8th ed. pg. 32

- Placental circulation is established by 21 days
- Fetal circulation is established by 21 days

Extra Mile

- Weight of placenta at term: **500 gm**
- Functional unit of placenta: **Lobule**
- Surface area of placenta at term: 12 m^2
- Placenta takes over function of corpus luteum at 8 weeks (8–10 weeks)

168. Ans. (c) Nuchal translucency

Ref: DC Dutta, 8th ed. pg. 735

- **Nuchal translucency** is a fluid behind the neck of the fetus. It is an anechoic space visible and seen in all fetuses between 11–14 weeks of age
- **The most common cause of increased nuchal translucency (>3 mm) is aneuploidy** where TURNER syndrome is the most common cause followed second by Down syndrome.
- The reason why it is seen in 11–14 weeks is because at that time fetal lymphatics are developing and peripheral resistance is high and gradually disappears.
- **Remember:** Cystic hygroma which is seen in Turner syndrome is high incidence is due to defective development of lymphatics.

169. Ans. (b) 100 mg iron + 500 mcg folic acid

Ref: DC Dutta, 8th ed. pg. 241

- **Adult** iron + folic acid tablet given in pregnancy: 1 tab/day × 100 days
- **Kids** iron + folic acid tablet given: 1 tab/day × 100 days per year- 0 to 5 years of age.

Iron and Folic Acid Tablet Content

	Iron	Folic acid
Adult tab	100 mg	500 mcg
Kids tab (1/5th)	20 mg	100 mcg

170. Ans. (c) Non-stress test

Ref: DC Dutta, 8th ed. pg. 122

NON-STRESS TEST (NST)

- In NST, continuous electronic monitoring of fetal heart rate with fetal movements are noted.
- There is an observed association of FHR acceleration with fetal movements, which when present, indicates a healthy fetus.
- It can reliably be used as a screening test.
- The FHR accelerations associated with fetal movements is basically *reflex mediated.*
- *It should be noted that the test is valuable to identify the fetal wellness rather than illness.*

Interpretation

- **Reactive (Reassuring)**–two or more accelerations of more than 15 beats per minute which lasts for 15 seconds or more in a 20 minute observation.
- **Non-reactive (Non-reassuring)**–Absence of any fetal reactivity.

Contraction stress test (CST) is based to observe the response of the fetus at risk for utero placental insufficiency in relation to uterine contractions.

171. Ans. (a) FHR deceleration

Ref: Dutta's Obstetrics, 7th ed. pg. 109

Biophysical Profile Scoring (Manning – 1992)

Observation for 30 minutes Normal score: 2 Abnormal: 0			BPP score	Interpretation
Parameters	**Minimal normal criteria**	**Score**		
Non stress Test (NST)	Reactive pattern	2	8–10	No fetal asphyxia

Contd...

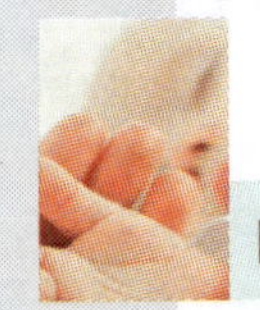

Biophysical Profile Scoring (Manning – 1992)				
Breathing movements	≥1 episode lasting >30 sec	2	6	Suspect Chronic asphyxia
Gross body movement	≥3 discrete body/ limb movements	2	4	Suspect Chronic asphyxia
Fetal muscle tone	≥1 episode of extension (limb or trunk) with return of flexion	2	0–2	Strongly suspect asphyxia
Amniotic fluid	≥1 pocket measuring 2 cm in two perpendicular planes	2		

172. Ans. (b) 10–12 cm

MATERNAL CHANGES DURING PREGNANCY

- Both ovaries are enlarged due to increased vascularity
- Uterus weight increases from 50 g in non-pregnant state to 1000 g at term.
- Capacity, shape and blood flow of uterus increases during pregnancy
- Formation of lower uterine segment: After 12 weeks, the isthmus (0.5 cm) starts to expand gradually to form the lower uterine segment **which measures 10 cm in length at term** (7.5-10 cm according to Dutta).
- The vagina becomes soft, warm, and moist with increased secretion and violet in color (Chadwick's sign) due to increased vascularity.

Difference between upper uterine segment and lower uterine segment

	Upper uterine segment	Lower uterine segment
Peritoneum	Firmly-attached	Loosely-attached
Myometrium	3 layers; outer longitudinal, middle oblique and inner circular	2 layers; outer longitudinal and inner circular
Decidua	Well-developed	Poorly-developed
Membranes	Firmly-attached	Loosely- attached
Activity	Active, contracts, retracts and becomes thicker during labor	Passive, dilates, stretches and becomes thinner during Labor

173. Ans. (a) 6 weeks

Ref: DC Dutta 8th ed. pg. 74-75

The pelvic changes during pregnancy are divers and appear different at different periods:

Signs	At AOG
Palmer's sign: Regular and rhythmic uterine contraction	4–8 weeks
Vaginal sign: Softened vaginal wall with copious mucoid discharge	6th week
Goodell's sign: Cervix feels soft and congested	6th week
Hegar's sign: Uterus is enlarged and soft; cervix empty.	6–10 weeks
Osiander sign: Increased pulsation at lateral fornices	8th week
Chadwick's sign or Jacquemier's sign: Dusky hue of the vestibule and anterior vaginal wall (due to local vascular congestion)	8th week
Piskacek's sign: Asymmetrical enlargement of the uterus if there is lateral implantation	8th week

174. Ans. (b) 8th week

Please refer to above explanation.

175. Ans. (b) 7 April, 2016

Ref: DC. Dutta's Textbook of Obstetrics, 8th ed. pg. 83-108

- Calculation of the expected date of delivery is done according to **naegele's formula**
- 1st day of LMP + 9 months + 7 days
- Count 3 calendar month back from 1st day of LMP +7 days
- Here LMP = 30th June

EDD

30th June 2015
+7 day +9 month
7th April, 2016

176. Ans. (c) 3 weeks

Ref: DC Dutta, 7th ed. pg. 146

LOCHIA

- It is the vaginal discharge for the first fortnight during puerperium.
- It has 3 phases, which may extend upto 3 weeks.
  - Lochia rubra: 1–4 days; red in color
  - Lochia serosa: 5–9 days; the color is yellowish or pink or pale brownish
  - Lochia alba: 10–15 days; pale white color
- Duration of the Lochia alba beyond 3 weeks suggests local genital lesion

177. Ans. (a) Placental site

Ref: Dutta's Obstetrics, 7th ed. pg. 433

PUERPERAL SEPSIS

- An infection of the genital tract which occurs as a complication of delivery is termed puerperal sepsis.
- Sources of infection may be endogenous where organisms are present in the genital tract before delivery.

Mode of Infection

- Puerperal sepsis is generally a wound infection.
- Placental site being a raw surface in the endometrium is the most common site for infection.
- Other causes of puerperal sepsis may be laceration of the genital tract or may be CS section wound infection by organisms like anaerobic strep, E. Coli, staph etc.
- *Anaerobic streptococcus is the most common cause of Puerperal sepsis.*
- The primary sites of infections are: Uterus, Perineum, Vagina, Cervix.

178. Ans. (b) Uterus becomes discoid

Ref: DC Dutta, 7th ed. pg. 131-312

Clinical Course of Third Stage of Labor

- Third stage includes separation, descent and expulsion of the placenta with its membrane.

Signs before and after placental separation

- **Before Separation:** Uterus becomes *discoid in shape*, firm in feel and non-ballottable.
  - Fundal height reaches slightly below the umbilicus
- **After Separation:**
  - Uterus becomes globular firm and ballotable
  - *The fundal height is slightly raised*
  - Sudden gush of vaginal bleeding upon separation.
  - Permanent lengthening of the cord.

179. Ans. (a) Gushing of blood

Ref: D.C. Dutta, 7th ed. pg. 131-312

Please refer to above explanation.

180. Ans. (b) Fundus of the uterus below umbilicus

Ref: D.C. Dutta, 7th ed. pg. 131-312

181. Ans. (c) Puerperal sepsis

Ref: D.C. Dutta, 7th ed. pg. 432, 433, 435

PUERPERAL PYREXIA (FEVER)

- A rise of temperature reaching 100.4°F (39°C) or more on 2 separate occasions at 24 hours apart (excluding first 24 hours) within first 10 days following delivery is called *puerperal pyrexia.*
- **Causes of pyrexia are:** Puerperal sepsis, Urinary tract infection, Mastitis, Infection of caesarean section wound, Pulmonary infection, Septic pelvic thrombophlebitis etc.

PUERPERAL SEPSIS

- An infection of the genital tract which occurs as a complication of delivery is termed puerperal sepsis.
- Sources of infection may be endogenous where organisms are present in the genital tract before delivery.
- *Anaerobic streptococcus is the most common cause of Puerperal sepsis.*
- The primary sites of infections are: Perineum, Vagina, Cervix, Uterus
- *Remember: A case of puerperal pyrexia is considered to be due to genital unless proved otherwise.*

182. Ans. (a) Hemorrhage

Ref: Dutta's Obstetrics, 7th ed. pg. 411

- Most common Indirect cause of maternal mortality in India: Anemia
- Most common cause of maternal mortality in India: Post partum hemorrhage (PPH)
- Most common direct cause of MMR: PPH

Direct maternal mortality	Indirect maternal mortality
It results from obstetric complication of pregnant state (pregnancy, labor and puerperium) from interventions or incorrect treatment.	It results from previous existing disease or disease that develops during pregnancy.
Ex: PPH, Obstructed labor, Sepsis	Anemia, HTN, gestational DM, Epilepsy

183. Ans. (d) Anemia

Please refer to above explanation.

184. Ans. (d) Increased prolactin level

Ref: DC Dutta, 8th ed. pg. 171, 614; 6th pg. 148

Breast feeding increases the levels of prolactin which lead to the following consequences:

- Reduced ovarian response to FSH leading to **hypo-estrogenic state**
- Suppression of LH release thereby **preventing LH surge and inhibiting ovulation**
- **Reduces GnRH secretion**

185. Ans. (c) 1000 g

Ref: Dutta's Obstetrics, 7th ed. pg. 144.

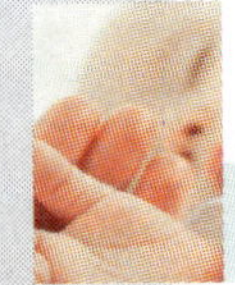

- Immediately following delivery, the uterus becomes firm and retracts with alternate hardening and softening.
- Immediately postpartum the uterus weighs about 1000 g and measures about 20 × 17 × 7.5 cm.
- ***6 weeks postpartum***, its measurement is almost similar to that of non-pregnant state and **weighs about 60 g**.

186. Ans. (b) 4 weeks

Ref: DC Dutta, 8th ed. pg. 53-54

- Heart rate returns to pre-pregnant value at around 4 weeks postpartum

187. Ans. (d) 4 weeks

Ref: Dutta's Obstetrics, 7th ed. pg. 53

- The cardiac output (CO) starts to increase from 5th week of pregnancy, reaches its peak **40-50% at about 30-40 weeks.**
- CO is lowest in the sitting or supine position and highest in the right or left lateral or knee chest position.
- It increases further during labor (+50%) and immediately following delivery (+70%) over the pre-labor values.
- Within 1–2 hours following birth, the cardiac output is estimated to be about 500 mL/min and Hr ~ 120–140/min
- **CO returns to pre labor values one hour after delivery.**
- *It returns to the prepregnancy level in 4 weeks time.*

188. Ans. (b) 12–14 days

Ref: Dutta's Obstetrics, 7th ed. pg. 144-145

- Uterus becomes pelvic organ in about 2 weeks after normal delivery.
- The rate of involution of uterus after delivery is 1.25 cm or half inch/day.
- **It regains its prepregnancy size at the end of 6 weeks.**

Extra Mile

- During pregnancy, uterus remains pelvic organ till 2 week of pregnancy. Thereon, it starts to ascend in abdomen.

189. Ans. (b) Vasa previa

Ref: Dutta's Obstetrics, 7th ed. pg. 259

VASA PREVIA

- In a vilamentous insertion of cord, the leash of blood vessels may traverse through membranes overlying the internal OS, in front of the presenting part. This condition is called Vasa previa.
- Rupture of the membranes involves the overlying vessels and leads to vaginal bleeding.
- This vaginal bleeding is, thus, entirely from fetal blood and may result in fetal exsanguination and even death.

190. Ans. (b) Rupture of uterus

Ref: William's, 23rd ed. Ch 35

- ***Postpartum hemorrhage** has been defined as the loss of 500 mL of blood or more after completion of the third stage of labor.*
- According to the given case scenario, ruptured uterus is the only indication to do immediate hysterectomy.
- Other given options like pre-eclampsia, atonic uterus or involution of uterus may present with post delivery hemorrhage, but they are not an indication for immediate hysterectomy and managed conservatively first.
- **Preeclampsia:** Because of the poorly contractile nature of the lower uterine segment, there may be uncontrollable hemorrhage following placental removal. When bleeding is not controlled by conservative means, other methods like oversewing the implantation site, bilateral internal iliac artery ligation or uninterrupted chromic sutures is the next best choice *(William's 23rd)*. If such conservative methods fail, and bleeding is brisk, then hysterectomy is necessary.
- **Uterine atony** is the most common cause of obstetrical hemorrhage. Managed initially with oxytocin, ergot derivatives, Prostaglandin analogues (PGF2α). If no effect with conservative management then hysterectomy is the choice.
- **Note:** For women whose placenta previa is implanted anteriorly in the site of a prior hysterotomy incision, there is an increased likelihood of associated placenta accreta and need for hysterectomy.
- **Inversion of the uterus** most often associated with immediate life-threatening hemorrhage. The recently inverted uterus with placenta already separated from it may often be replaced simply by pushing up on the fundus with the palm of the hand and fingers in the direction of the long axis of the vagina followed by fluid infusion and blood transfusion. If no relief then reduction via laparotomy is performed.

191. Ans. (c) III

Ref: DC Dutta, 7th ed. pg. 422-23

PERINEAL TEARS

1st degree	Is a laceration of the vaginal mucosa and the perineal skin but not the underlying fascia and muscle.
2nd degree	Involves the vaginal mucosa perineal skin and the fascia and muscles of the perineal body.
3rd degree	Involves the vaginal mucosa skin and perineal body and the anal sphincter is also disrupted
4th degree	In addition the rectal mucosa is also torn.

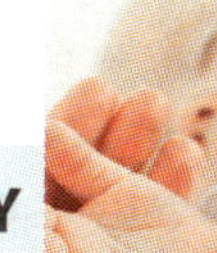

ABORTION AND THIRD TRIMESTER BLEEDING

192. Ans. (c) Mifepristone 200 mg and misoprostol 800 microgram after 48 hours

Ref: DC Dutta's 9th ed. pg. 165

	Evidence-based regimen	Original FDA-Approved regimen (as approved in 2000)
Dates in use in Ohio	Up to Jan 2011	Feb 2011 to Mar 2016
Maximum days gestation	63 d from LMP	49 d from LMP
Mifepristone dose	200 mg orally in office	600 mg orally in office
Misoprostol dose	800 mcg vaginally or buccally tablets) (4 tablets)	400 mcg orally (2 tablets)
Misoprostol timing	6–72 h after mifepristone	48 h after mifepristone
Misoprostol location	Home	Providers office
Follow-up visit	5–14 d after mifepristone	14 d after mifepristone
Cost	Lower	Higher
Minimum Number of Office Visits (Including Ohio's Required 3 Information Visit)	**3**	**4**
LMP, last menstrual period. Adapted from the American College of Obstetricians and Gynecologists [18].		
doi:10.1371/joumal.pmed.1002110.t001		

193. Ans. (a) Hydatidiform mole

Ref: Williams Gynaecology 3rd ed. pg. 782

- Transverse sonography view of a uterus with a complete hydrate form mole shows classic "snowstorm appearance" "is created by the multiple placental vesicles.
- The mole completely fills the uterine cavity, and callipers are placed on the outer uterine borders.

194. Ans. (b) Abruption

Ref: William's Obstetrics, Chapter 43, 26th ed. pg. 1946

- DIC is a leading cause of maternal mortality. It is secondary to obstetrical complications such as placental abruption, amniotic fluid embolism, HELLP syndrome, retained stillbirth and acute fatty liver of pregnancy.
- Amniotic fluid has been shown to be able to activate coagulation in vitro, and the degree of placental separation correlates with the extent of the DIC, suggesting that leakage of thromboplastin like material from the placental system is responsible for the occurrence of DIC.

195. Ans. (a) Cervical incompetence

Ref: William's Obstetrics, Chapter 11, 26th ed. pg. 537

- Incompetent cervix, this is characterized classically by painless cervical dilation in the second trimester.
- It can be followed by prolapse and ballooning of the amniotic membranes into the vagina, and ultimately, expulsion of an immature fetus.
- This sequence often repeats in future pregnancies. Of causes, prior cervical trauma is implicated.

196. Ans. (a) 800 mcg vaginally

Ref: Dutta 9th ed. pg. 165-66

- In Mid trimester termination (13–20 weeks) – Prostaglandins and their analogue are used which are very effective since it acts on cervix and uterus.
- PGEs are preferred as they have more selective action on myometrium and less side effects.
- Agent that can be used for MTP
  - **Misoprostol** (PGE1 Analogue): 400–800 ug given vaginally at interval of 3–4 hours.

    or,
  - **Mifepristone** (200 mg oral) → 36–48 hours later Misoprostol (800 ug vaginally), then misoprostol (400 ug oral) every 3 hours for 4 doses.
- Since question is asking about dose of misoprostol to be given with mifepristone, 800 ug vaginally will be the preferred answer.

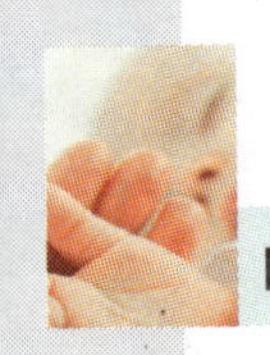

197. Ans. (a) Abruptio placentae

Ref: Dutta 9th ed. pg. 232

- **Abruptio placenta** – because painful tender abdominal with per vaginal bleed and hypertension present
- **Placenta accreta** no sign and symptoms only got to know at time of desperation of placenta—it is attached to superficial myometrium.
- **Vasa previa**—painless bleeding, in which vessel in umbilical cord get trapped between fetus and mother.
- **Placenta previa**—low lying placenta, painless bleed

TABLE: Distinguishing features of placenta previa and abruption placentae

Parameters	Placenta previa	Abruptio placentae
• **Clinical features:**		
▪ Nature of bleeding	• Painless, apparently causeless and recurrent • Bleeding is always revealed bright red	• Painful, often attributed to preeclampsia or trauma and continuous • Revealed, concealed or usually mixed
▪ Character of blood	Bright red	Dark colored
▪ General condition and anemia	Proportionate to visible blood loss	Out of proportion to the visible blood loss in concealed or mixed variety
▪ Features of preeclampsia	Not relevant	Present in one-third cases
• **Abdominal examination:**		
▪ Height of uterus	Proportionate height to gestational age	May be disproportionately enlarged in concealed type
▪ Feel of uterus	Soft and relaxed	May be tense, tender and rigid
▪ Malpresentation	Malpresentation is common. The head is high floating	Unrelated, the head may be engaged
▪ FHS	Usually present	Usually absent especially in concealed type
• **Placentography (USG)**	Placenta in lower segment	Placenta in upper segment
• **Vaginal examination**	Placenta is felt on the lower segment	Placenta is not felt on lower segment. Blood clots should not be confused with placenta

198. Ans. (c) Placenta accreta

Ref: Dutta 9th ed. pg. 235

- Placenta accreta is a rare condition in which placenta is attached to the superficial myometrium that's why not able to separate.

Note:

- **Placenta Increta:** Placenta is attached strongly with myometrium
- **Placenta percreta:** Placenta perforates/traverses the myometrium

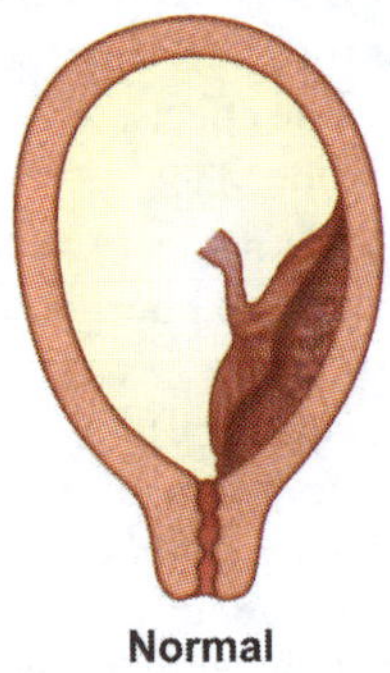

Normal

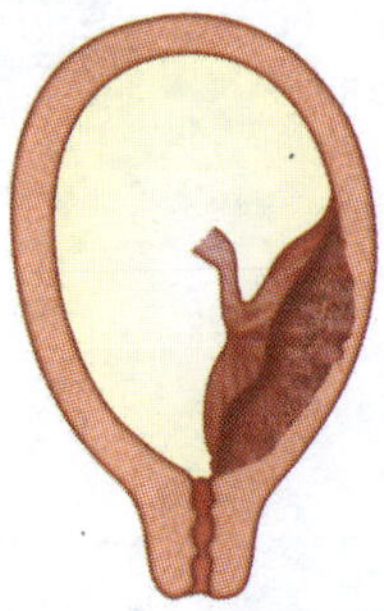

Accreta

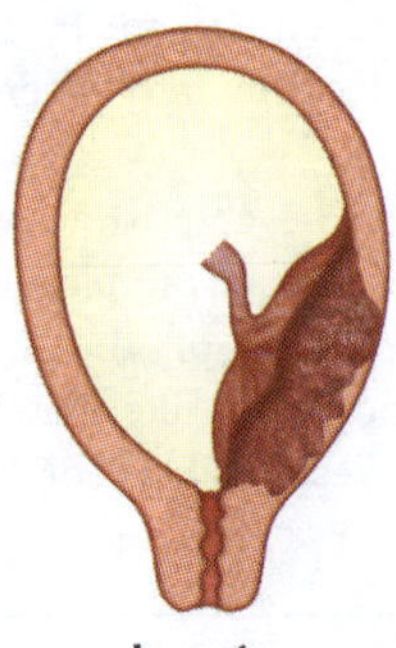

Increta

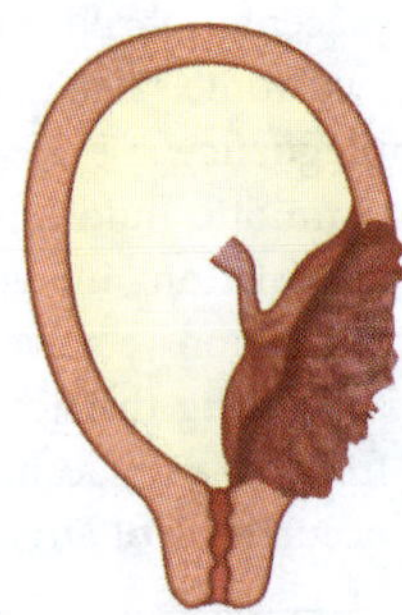

Percreta

199. Ans. (b) 200 mg

Ref: Shaw's Gynecology 16th ed. pg. 289; Berek and Novak's Gynecology, 16th ed. pg. 825

- The antiprogesterone mifepristone (RU486) is highly effective for post coital contraception.
- The usual abortifacient dose is 200mg, but a dose of 10 mg is effective for emergency contraception.
- Protocol:
  - **Day 1:** 200 mg of mifepristone given as a single dose—the woman is observed for half an hour and then allowed home.
  - **Day 3:** 400 mcg of oral misoprostol (prostaglandin) is administered (two tablets) unless abortion has occurred.
  - **Day 14:** Follow-up to confirm abortion has occurred; if not, surgical MTP is done

200. Ans. (a) Missed abortion

Ref: Williams Obstetrics 24th ed. pg. 375

- Missed abortion is also termed early pregnancy failure or loss.
- Sonogram displays anechoic sac with an anembryonic gestation.
- Upon examination, os is closed

Other types of abortion and its finding is discussed later in this book.

201. Ans. (a) Abruptio placenta

Ref: William's Obstetrics 25th ed. pg. 767

- Separation of the placenta, either partially or totally-from its implantation site before delivery is described by the term abruptio placentae.
- In the early stages of placental abruption, clinical symptoms may be absent. Even with continued bleeding and placental separation, placental abruption can still be either total or partial.
- Abruptio placenta is very common cause of bleeding in third trimester
- Most common risk factor: Hypertension

202. Ans. (a) Threatened abortion

Ref: William's Obstetrics 25th ed. pg. 348

- The diagnosis of threatened abortion is presumed when bloody vaginal discharge or bleeding appears through a closed cervical os during the first 20 weeks.

Other types of abortion have been discussed later in this book.

203. Ans. (c) Abruptio placenta

Ref: DC Dutta 9th ed. pg. 238

- Couvelaire Uterus is also known as uteroplacental apoplexy.
- It leads to severe form of concealed abruptio placentae. There is massive intravasation of blood into the uterine musculature up to the serous coat.
- The condition can only be diagnosed on laparotomy.
- Upon naked eye examination of such uterus, it is dark port wine color which may be patchy or diffuse.
- **Note:** Presence of couvelaire uterus is not an indication per se for hysterectomy.

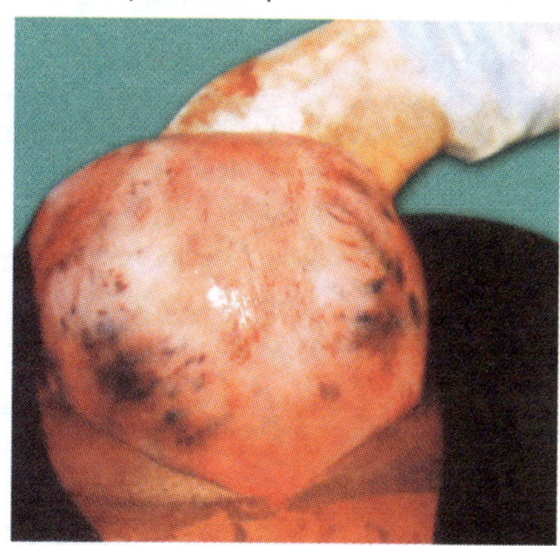

204. Ans. (b) Cervical incompetence

Ref: DC Dutta 9th ed. pg. 161

- The patient in the given case is of 2nd trimester abortion. Cervical incompetence is the most common cause that can be suspected for this patient

TABLE: Common causes of miscarriage

1st trimester	2nd trimester
• Genetic factors (50%) • Endocrine disorders like thyroid abnormalities, diabetes • Immunological disorder • Infections • Unexplained	• Anatomical abnormalities ▪ Cervical incompetence ▪ Mullerian fusion defect-bicornuate/septate uterus ▪ Uterine synechiae ▪ Uterine fibroid • Maternal medical illness • Unexplained

Cervical Incompetence/Insufficiency

- Causes of cervical incompetence can be:
  - Congenital uterine abnormalities
  - **Acquired:** More common.
    - History of D&C or D and E operation
    - Cervix amputation
    - Vaginal operative delivery through undilated cervix
    - Multiple gestations
- Patient usually present with history of mid-trimester, painless cervical dilatation and escape of liquor amnii followed by painless expulsion of the product of conceptus.

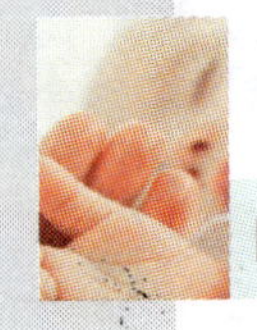

- Passage of 6–8 number hegar dilator without resistance and pain is highly suggestive

Treatment:

- ***Cerclage operation:*** Two types of operation are in current use during pregnancy
  - **Shirodkar**
  - **McDonald**
- **Principle:** It reinforces the weak cervix by a nonabsorbable tape, placed around the cervix at the level of internal os.
- **Time of operation:** Around 14 weeks of pregnancy or at least 2 weeks earlier than the previous miscarriage, as early as the 10th week.
- ***Removal of stitch*: The stitch should be removed at 37th week** or earlier if labor pain starts (preferably in OT).

Extra Mile

TABLE: Types of miscarriage and the diagnostic features

Type	Symptoms	Uterine size	Cervix (Ext. Os)	Ultrasonography
Threatened	• Vaginal bleeding present • Pelvic pain	Corresponds to gestational age	Closed	• Fetus alive • Retroplacental hemorrhage+
Inevitable	• Vaginal bleeding present • Pelvic pain	Same or smaller	Open with palpable conceptus	• Fetus often dead Retroplacental hemorrhage+
Incomplete	Vaginal bleeding (may be heavy)	Smaller	Open	Products of conception partly retained
Complete	Vaginal bleeding—trace or absent	Smaller	Closed	Uterine cavity empty
Missed	Vaginal bleeding—trace, brownish in color	Smaller	Closed	Blighted ovum or fetus without cardiac activity
Septic	Vaginal discharge: purulent, foul smelling with features of sepsis	Variable, may be larger	Open	Products of conception retained, presence of foreign body (±), free fluid in the peritoneal cavity/POD

205. Ans. (a) Trisomy

Ref: Williams 24th ed. pg. 370

- Approximately 50% of miscarriages during first trimester are anembryonic. The other 50% are embryonic miscarriages.
  - **Anembryonic:** With no identifiable embryonic elements.
  - **Embryonic:** Display a developmental abnormality of the zygote, embryo, fetus, or at times, the placenta.
- Of 50% embryonic miscarriages, 25% of all abortion are aneuploid abortions (*abnormal chromosome number*). The remaining cases are euploid (*abnormal chromosome development*) abortions.

Chromosomal aneuploidy	Incidence %
Trisomy	22–32
Monosomy X (45,X)	5–20
Triploidy	6–8
Tetraploidy	2–4
Structural anomaly	2

Note: *Most common cause of first trimester bleeding: Abortion*

206. Ans. (a) Spontaneous abortion

Ref: DC Dutta, 8th ed. pg. 185-86

- **Spontaneous abortion** is the expulsion or extraction from its mother of an embryo or fetus weighing 500 g or less when it is not capable of independent survival
- **Incidence:**
  - About 75% miscarriages occur before the 16th week and of these **about 80% occur before the 12th week of pregnancy.**

Common Causes of Miscarriage

- ***First trimester:***
  - **Genetic factors (50%)- MCC.**
  - Endocrine disorders (LPD, thyroid abnormalities, diabetes).
  - Immunological disorders (autoimmune and alloimmune).
  - Infection.
  - Unexplained.
- ***Second trimester:***
  - Anatomic abnormalities—

- Cervical incompetence (congenital or acquired).
- Mullerian fusion defects (bicornuate uterus, septate uterus).
- Uterine synechiae
- Uterine fibroid.
- Maternal medical illness
- Unexplained
- **Third trimester:** Most common cause of bleeding is: Abruptio placenta > placenta previa

207. Ans. (a) Trisomy

Ref: Williams 24th ed. pg. 370

- Approximately 50% of miscarriages during first trimester are anembryonic. The other 50% are embryonic miscarriages.
  - **Anembryonic:** With no identifiable embryonic elements.
  - **Embryonic:** Display a developmental abnormality of the zygote, embryo, fetus, or at times, the placenta.
- Of 50% embryonic miscarriages, 25% of all abortion are aneuploid abortions *(abnormal chromosome number).* The remaining cases are euploid *(abnormal chromosome development)* abortions.

Chromosomal aneuploidy	Incidence %
Trisomy	22–32
Monosomy x (45, X)	5–20
Triploidy	6–8
Tetraploidy	2–4
Structural anomaly	2

Note: *Most common cause of first trimester bleeding: Abortion*

208. Ans. (c) Chromosomal abnormalities

Ref: Dutta, 6th ed. pg. 160

With respect to first trimester abortions, 75% of the abortions take place before 16th week and out of these, about 75% occur before the 8th week of pregnancy.

- **Chromosomal abnormality in the conceptus is the commonest cause of miscarriage.**
- **Autosomal trisomy** particularly **Trisomy 16** is the commonest cause for spontaneous abortion.

209. Ans. (c) Uterus size small to AOG, cervix open

Ref: Dutta's Obstetrics, 7th ed. pg. 163

- In Inevitable abortion, condition is progressed to a stage from where continuation of pregnancy is not possible.
- Patient usually presents with bleeding per vaginum with **size of uterus smaller than age of gestation and open cervix.**
- **USG finding:** Dead fetus

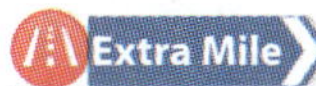

Abortion	Size of uterus	Cervix OS	USG finding
Threatened	Equal to AOG	Closed	Fetus alive
Missed	Smaller than AOG	Closed	Dead fetus
Incomplete	Smaller than AOG	Open	Retained products of conception
Complete	Smaller than AOG	Closed	Uterine Cavity empty

210. Ans. (a) Dilatation and evacuation

Ref: D.C. Dutta, 7th ed. pg. 161-162

INEVITABLE MISCARRIAGE

- It is the clinical type of abortion where the changes have progressed to a state from where continuation of pregnancy is impossible.
- **Clinical feature:**
  - Increased vaginal bleeding
  - Aggravation of pain in the lower abdomen
  - Dilated internal OS
- **Treatment**
  - Before 12 weeks
    - *Dilatation and evacuation* followed by curettage using analgesia or under general anaesthesia
    - Alternative, suction evacuation followed by curettage is also done.
  - **After 12 weeks:** Product of conception is evacuated by Oxytocin drip which increases uterine contraction.

211. Ans. (c) 200 mg mifepristone + 400 mcg misoprostol

Ref: D.C. Dutta, 7th ed. pg. 173-174

Following are the indications for termination under the MTP Act:

- **To save the life of the mother (Therapeutic or medical termination):** Ex: Grade 3–4 cardiac disease, malignant HTN, CGN, cervical or breast malignancies etc.
- **Social indications:** To prevent grave injury to the physical and mental health of the pregnant woman.
- **Humanitarian ground:** Pregnancy because of rape or incest. (MTP allowed up to 24 weeks)
- **Eugenic:** Substantial risk of the child being born with serious physical and mental abnormalities so as to be handicapped in life.

Remember

- Termination is permitted up to 20 weeks of pregnancy. When the pregnancy exceeds 20 weeks, opinion of two medical practitioners is required

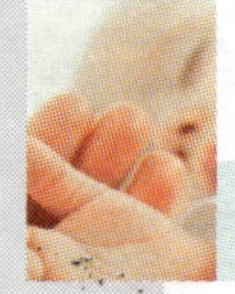

- MTP allowed up to 24 weeks in rape survivors. (MTP Amendment 2021)

Medical Methods of First Trimester Abortion

- 200 mg of mifepristone orally is given on day 1. On day 3, misoprostol (PGE_1) 400 µg orally or 800 µg vaginally is given for the MTP.
- **Note:** As per latest update on medical abortion in India till 9 weeks.
  - **Day:** Mifepristone 200 mg PO.
  - **Day:** Misoprostol 800 mg sublingual/PV/oral

212. Ans. (c) Mifepristone 200 mg + Misoprostol 400 mcg oral

Ref: Dutta's Obstetrics, 7th ed. pg. 173

Medical methods of first trimester abortion

- 200 mg of mifepristone orally is given on day 1.
- On day 3, misoprostol (PGE_1) 800 µg/L or, vaginally is given for the MTP.

213. Ans. (c) Misoprostol + Tamoxifen

Ref: Dutta's Obstetrics, 7th ed. pg. 173

- *200 mg of mifepristone orally is given on day 1. On day 3, misoprostol (PGE_1) 400 µg orally or 800 µg vaginally is given for the MTP.*
- Tamoxifen is an estrogen antagonist (SERM), which is basically used in breast cancer.

214. Ans. (d) Type II posterior

Ref: DC Dutta 8th ed./283-84; William's 23rd ed. Ch. 35.

PLACENTA PREVIA

Placenta previa is used to describe a placenta that is implanted over or very near the internal cervical os. There are several possibilities:

- **Total placenta previa**—the internal os is covered completely by placenta
- **Partial placenta previa**—the internal os is partially covered by placenta
- **Marginal placenta previa**—the edge of the placenta is at the margin of the internal os
- **Low-lying placenta**—the placenta is implanted in the lower uterine segment such that the placental edge does not reach the internal os, but is in close proximity to it.
  - ***Low lying placenta type II is posteriorly located and is considered dangerous because it*** can be compressed by the presenting part and this will cause severe fetal asphyxia and sometimes fetal death.
- **Vasa previa**—the fetal vessels course through membranes and present at the cervical os

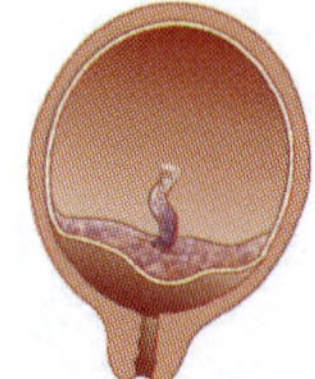
Complete

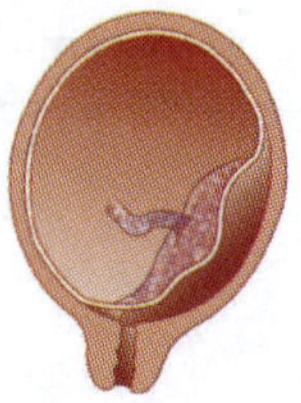
Partial

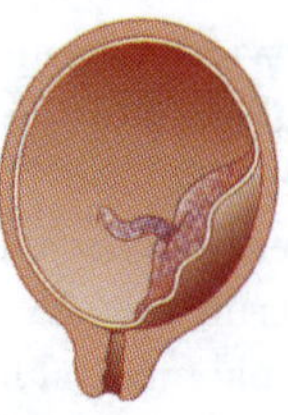
Marginal

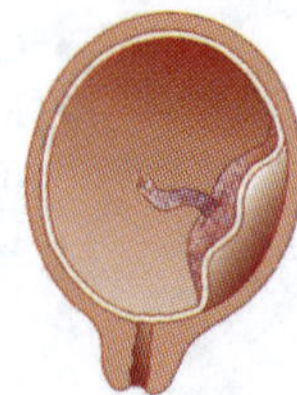
Low Lying

215. Ans. (b) Placenta previa

Ref: DC Dutta, 8th ed./290, Williams 22nd ed./ 822-823

- **MacAfee and Johnson Regimen** is a Conservative Management in Placenta Previa: This consists of complete bed rest, tocolysis, and close observation of patient.
- Steroids are generally given to enhance lung maturity.
- **To undertake this regimen (to wait and watch) all three criteria should be fulfilled:**
  - Mother should be hemodynamically stable
  - There should be no fetal distress
  - Pregnancy less than 36 weeks of gestation.
- If any of the criteria is not met then the patient should be delivered by LSCS.

Extra Mile

- Classification of abruption placentae: page/sher's/classification
- **Zuspan regimen** for the treatment of eclampsia using Magnesium sulphate (zuspan aka sibai)

Other regimens using $MgSO_4$ for treatment of eclampsia are
Pritchard's regimen (intramuscular)
Sibai regimen (intravenous)

- Most appropriate treatment of eclampsia: $MgSO_4$

216. Ans. (a) Caesarean section

Ref: DC Dutta, 8th ed. pg. 290-92; William's, 23rd ed. Chapter 35.

- Placenta previa-placenta located at LUS.
- One of the most common cause of APH.
- In case of centrally located placenta previa—mode of delivery is always CS.

Management of placenta previa depends on its type—4 types

Indication for termination(by vaginal/CS)	Indication for conservative management
• POG-37 weeks or beyond • Pt continuously bleeding • Fetal distress • Hemodynamically unstable mother • Pt is active Labor • IUD • Congenital malformation of baby which are incompatible with life	Done in patient who do not obey previous 7 rule

Contd...

Indication for termination(by vaginal/CS)	Indication for conservative management
Termination by vaginal delivery or CS (depending on type of PP) 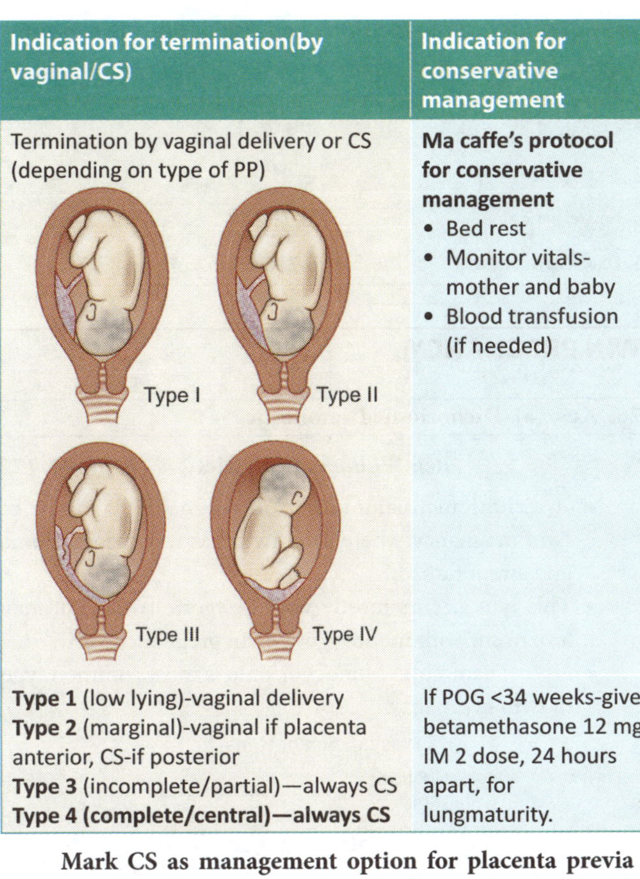 	**Ma caffe's protocol for conservative management** • Bed rest • Monitor vitals-mother and baby • Blood transfusion (if needed)
Type 1 (low lying)-vaginal delivery **Type 2** (marginal)-vaginal if placenta anterior, CS-if posterior **Type 3** (incomplete/partial)—always CS **Type 4 (complete/central)—always CS**	If POG <34 weeks-give betamethasone 12 mg IM 2 dose, 24 hours apart, for lungmaturity.

Mark CS as management option for placenta previa if any of following points give in Question

- Mother unstable
- Fetal distress
- Major degree of PP-type 3 (incomplete/partial), type 4 (complete/central)

217. Ans. (b) Battledore placenta

***Ref:* William's Obstetrics, 23rd ed. Ch: 27**

- Normally, the cord usually is inserted at or near the center of the fetal surface of the placenta.
- Cord insertion at the placental margin is sometimes referred to as a ***Battledore placenta.*** It is found in about 7% of term placentas.
- **Velamentous insertion:** This type of insertion is of considerable clinical importance. The umbilical vessels spread within the membranes at a distance from the placental margin, which they reach surrounded only by a fold of amnion. As a result, vessels are vulnerable to compression, which may lead to fetal anoxia. Incidence: 1%

218. Ans. (a) Placenta accreta

***Ref:* Williams Obstetrics, 23rd ed. Ch 35.**

- The nitabuch *layer* is a zone of fibrinoid degeneration in which invading trophoblasts meet the decidua. ***If the decidua is defective, as in placenta accreta, the Nitabuch layer is usually absent.***

Extra Mile

- **Placenta accreta** indicates that villi are attached to the myometrium.
- **Placenta increta,** villi actually invade the myometrium.
- **Placenta percreta** defines villi that penetrate through the myometrium and to or through the serosa.

219. Ans. (a) Placenta previa

***Ref:* Williams Obstetrics, 23rd ed. Ch 35.**

Absence of nitabuch membrane can lead to placenta accreta, increta or percreta.

220. Ans. (b) β-hCG level

***Ref:* DC Dutta, 8th ed. pg. 227**

Hydatiform moles are abnormal pregnancies characterized histologically by aberrant changes within the placenta. Specifically, the chorionic villi in these placentas show varying degrees of trophoblastic proliferation and edema of the villous stroma. **They are of two types: Partial and complete.**

Complete mole	Partial mole
• A molar pregnancy with some normal and some swollen villi plus fetal, cord, and/or amniotic membrane elements. • *Fetal tissue absent.* • **Karyotype:** 46, XX or 46, XY • **Villous edema:** diffuse	• A molar pregnancy with swelling of all placental villi. • *Fetal tissues are present.* • **Karyotype:** 69, XXX or 69, XXY • **Villous edema:** focal
• **Typical clinical presentation:** Molar gestation • **Postmolar malignant sequelae**- 15–20%	• **Typical clinical presentation:** Missed abortion • **Postmolar malignant sequelae**- 2–4%

Investigation

- Diagnosing in first-trimester is now common because of the routine use of serum β-hCG measurements ***(as they produce excess β-hCG due to trophoblastic proliferation)*** and transvaginal sonography.
- Although β-hCG levels are helpful, *the diagnosis of molar pregnancy more frequently is found sonographically* because of the identifiable diffuse swelling and enlargement of the chorionic villi.
- **Appearance on USG:** Snow storm appearnce

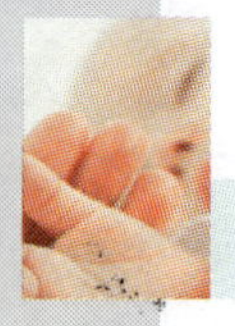

Treatment

- Suction curettage is the preferred method of evacuation regardless of uterine size in patients who wish to remain fertile.

POSTMOLAR SURVEILLANCE

- Gestational trophoblastic neoplasia (GTN) develops after approximately 15–20% of complete moles and 2-4% in partial moles.
- **Postmolar surveillance with serial quantitative serum β-hCG levels is the standard.**

Extra Mile

- GTD INCLUDES: H.Mole, Invasive mole, ChorioCA, PSTT (Placental Site Trophoblastic Tumor)
- **MC site of metastasis of GTD: Lungs**

221. Ans. (b) 46 XY

Ref: DC Dutta, 8th ed. pg. 230

Please refer to above explanation.

222. Ans. (c) Lungs

Please refer to above question.

223. Ans. (a) Complete mole

Ref: DC Dutta, 8th ed. pg. 226-30

THECA LUTEIN CYST

- **Theca lutein cysts yellow colored cyst seen in H. mole due to high circulating levels of hCG.**
- Size: Microscopic to 10 cms size.
- **Theca lutein cyst are also seen in case of:**
  - Fetal hydrops
  - Placental hypertrophy
  - Multifetal pregnancy

224. Ans. (a) Beta hCG

MONITORING

- After suction Evacuation: We send **weekly serum β-hCG.** Till they Become Normal.

Avg. time for hCG to Came Back to Normal

- After a complete Mole – 9 weeks
- After a partial Mole – 7 weeks
- After a Molar – 9 weeks
- Once hCG is Normal
- We send hCG values Monthly × 6 months

225. Ans. (a) 1%

Ref: William's Obstetrics 23/table 26-3

Types of prior uterine incisions and risk of uterine rupture

Prior incison	Rupture rate (percentage)
1. Classical	4–9%
2. T-shaped	4–9%
3. Low-vertical	1–7%
4. Low-transverse	**0.2–1.5%**

TWIN PREGNANCY

226. Ans. (a) Dichorionic Diamniotic

Ref: William's Obstetrics 24th ed. pg. 80, 127

- A dichorionic diamniotic twin pregnancy is a type of twin pregnancy where each twin has its own chorionic and amniotic sacs.
- This type occurs mostly with dizygotic twins, but may also occur with monozygotic twin pregnancies.
- Note: Diamniotic Monochorionic is most common type of twin pregnancy.

Placentation of twins

Monozygotic or dizygotic

Monozygotic

Separate placenta 1 chorions 2 amnions

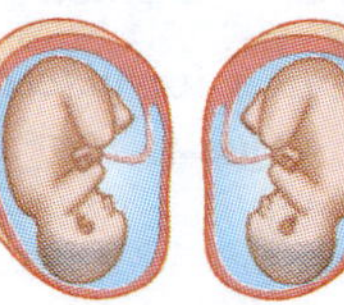

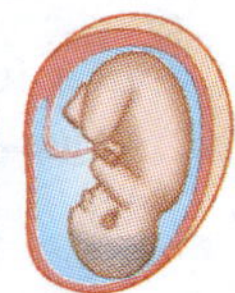

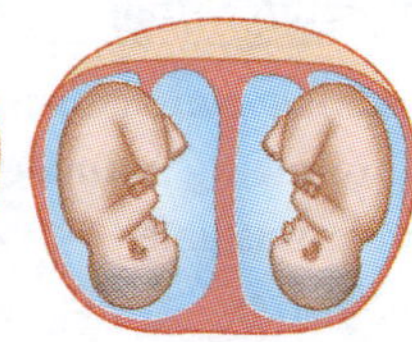

Single placenta 1 chorion 2 amnions

Fused placenta 2 chorions 2 amnions

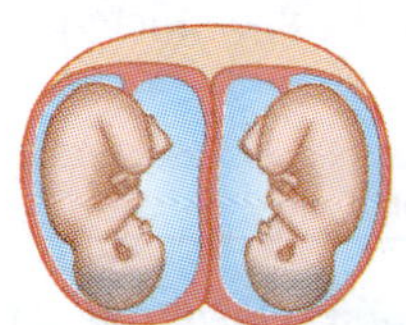

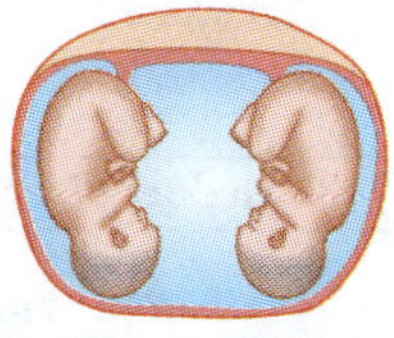

Single placenta 2 chorion 2 amnion

227. Ans. (a) C-section

Ref: William's Obstetrics 25th ed. pg. 888

- Although many possible combinations of positions may be encountered during multifetal pregnancy, those most common at admission for delivery are:
  - Cephalic-cephalic: Vaginal delivery can be done
  - Cephalic-breech
  - Cephalic-transverse.
- With the exception of cephalic-cephalic presentations, these are all unstable before and during labor and delivery.
- In twin pregnancy, if first fetus is cephalic and other is breech, then also a trial of vaginal delivery is done.
- If first twin is breech or transverse, then caesarean section is recommended.

228. Ans. (c) Diamniotic, dichorionic

Ref: DC Dutta 9th ed. P 189

TABLE: Division of zygote and types of twinning

Division of zygote on/after	Types of twining
Within 72 hours/3 days	Dichorionic, diamniotic
Between 4 and 8 days	Monochorionic, diamniotic
Between 8 and 12 days	Monochorionic, monoamniotic
>12 days	Siamese, conjoined twins

229. Ans. (b) Monochorionic, diamniotic

Ref: Dutta, 8th ed. pg. 233

Extra Mile

- Most common type of twinning is dizygotic twins: 69%
- Monozygotic twins in: 31%
- **MC type of twin gestation:** Diamniotic Monochorionic (70–75%)
- **Least common type of twin gestation:** Conjoined twins (<1%)
- **Hellin rule** is associated with multiple **pregnancy** as per which chance of twins is a1 in 80 pregnancies, triplets 1 in 80^2 and so on. It can result in complications
- **Prematurity** is the **commonest fetal complication**
- **Post partum hemorrhage** is the commonest **maternal complication.**
- **Twin to twin transfusion syndrome is seen in:** MC-DA

230. Ans. (b) Diamniotic, monochoronic

Ref: Dutta, 8th ed. pg. 233

231. Ans. (c) A vertex, B vertex

Ref: Dutta, 7th ed. pg. 202-203

- Vertex twin i.e. both baby in vertex presentation has best prognosis.

Presentations

- Both vertex (Most common) 60%
- Vertex (1st) – Breech (2nd) 20%
- Breech (1st) – Vertex (2nd) 10%
- Both Breech 8-10%

Mode of Delivery in twin presentation

- **Vertex Twin:** Mode of Delivery is Vaginal i.e. (V_x–V_x)
- **1st Breech & 2nd vertex** *C.S
    - Interlocking most commonly seen with this presentation
    - After coming head of 1st twin gets locked with forecoming Head of 2nd Twin
- 1st **Twin** Vertex and 2nd Any: Vaginal Delivery
- 1st **Twin** Transverse: C.S

232. Ans. (a) 10 weeks

Ref: D.C. Dutta, 8th ed. 237

Dutta 8th ed states: *"sonography in multifetal pregnancy is done for confirmation of diagnosis as early as **10th week AOG".*** It also helps in assessing:

- Viability of fetuses
- Chorionicity *(Lambda or twin peak sign)*
- Pregnancy dating
- Fetal growth monitoring
- Fetal anomalies
- Placental localization
- Amniotic fluid volume

Extra Mile

- Chorionicity of placenta is best diagnosed at 10–13th week AOG by USG
- **Lambda or Twin peak sign:** Indicates dichorionic placenta. In dichorionic twins there is thick septum between the two gestational sacs. It is best identified at the base of membrane where a triangular projection is seen.

233. Ans. (c) Young female

Ref: Dutta, 7th ed. pg. 202

Twin pregnancy associated with increased maternal age.

The incidence of Dizygotic twins increases with:

- Increasing maternal age
- Increasing parity
- Family history of twinning
- Ovulation induction with clomiphene citrate or gonadotrophins.

ECTOPIC PREGNANCY

234. Ans. (c) Ectopic mass > 4mcs

Ref: DC Dutta 9th ed. pg. 174

Indications for urgent surgical referral for ectopic pregnancy are:

- Hemodynamic instability
- Peritoneal signs
- Ultrasonography shows ectopic pregnancy with fetal cardiac activity
- Ultrasonography shows substantial lucid in the cul de sac
- Cases where beta hCG levels are not decreasing despite medical therapy.

235. Ans. (a) Interstitium

Ref: Dutta's Obstetrics 8th ed. pg. 207-208

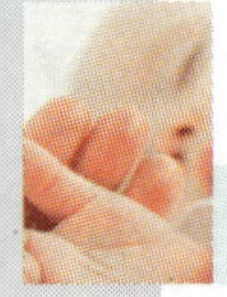

- Most common site of ectopic pregnancy: Ampula of fallopian tube
- Most common site of rupture: Ampulla
- Least common site of rupture: Interstitium (cornual)
- Least common site of tubal ectopic pregnancy: Interstitium (cornual)

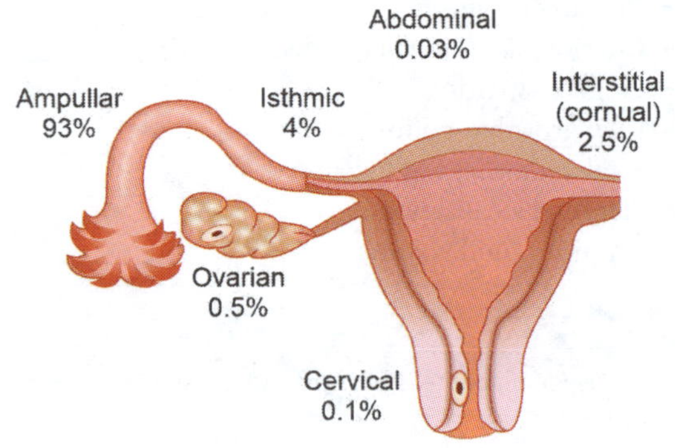

236. Ans. (b) Isthmus

Ref: DC Dutta 9th ed. P 170

- Most common site of ectopic pregnancy is Ampullary part of the fallopian tube
- **Least common variety of ectopic tubal pregnancy: Interstitial**
- MC site of tubal rupture in ectopic pregnancy: Isthmus (narrow part of tube and less distensible).
- Isthmic rupture usually occurs in:
  - **Isthmic part:** 6–8 weeks (earliest to rupture)
  - **Ampullary part:** 8–12 weeks
  - **Interstitial part:** Up to 4 months

237. Ans. (a) Ampulla

Ref: DC Dutta, 8th ed. pg. 207

- An ectopic pregnancy is one in which the fertilized ovum is implanted and develops outside the normal endometrial cavity.
- Most common site of ectopic pregnancy is fallopian tube, Ampullary part.

238. Ans. (c) Interstitial

Ref: DC Dutta 8th ed. pg. 214

- **Interstitial ectopic pregnancy is the rarest variety of tubal pregnancy**. Because of the thick and vascular musculature of the uterine wall with greater distensibility, the fetus grows dissecting the muscle fibers for a longer period **(12–14 weeks)** before termination occurs.
- The usual termination is rupture. It is **associated with massive intraperitoneal hemorrhage** due to its combined vascularization by the uterine and ovarian arteries.

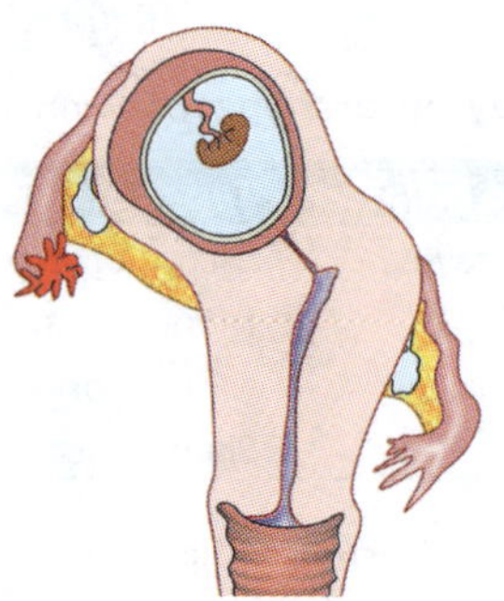

FIGURE: Interstitial pregnancy

239. Ans. (b) Laparoscopy with salpingostomy

Ref: DC Dutta, 8th ed. pg. 217-18

- The USG finding of empty uterus indicates this case as ectopic pregnancy.

Table: Management of unruptured ectopic pregnancy can be done by:

Medical management: methotrexate 50 mg/m² IM	Expectant management	Surgical management
• Serum hCG level should be <3000 IU/L • Gestational sac size <3.5 cm • Hemodynamically stable patient • Tubal diameter should be less than 4 cm without any fetal cardiac activity • There should be no intra-abdominal hemorrhage	• If sac size <3 cm • hCG < 1000 IU/L and subsequent levels are falling	• Laparoscopy is preferred over laparotomy • Salpingostomy is preferred over salpingectomy

Note: *If patient presents with unstable vitals or if laparoscopy is contraindicated, then laparotomy is advised.*

240. Ans. (a) Medical management

Ref: DC Dutta, 8th ed. pg. 217-18

241. Ans. (a) Pain

Ref: Dutta Obs, 7th ed. pg. 182; William Obs, 22nd ed. pg. 258

- An ectopic pregnancy is one in which the fertilized ovum is implanted and develops outside the normal endometrial cavity.
- **Classic Triad of Ectopic Pregnancy**
  - **Pain (100%)**

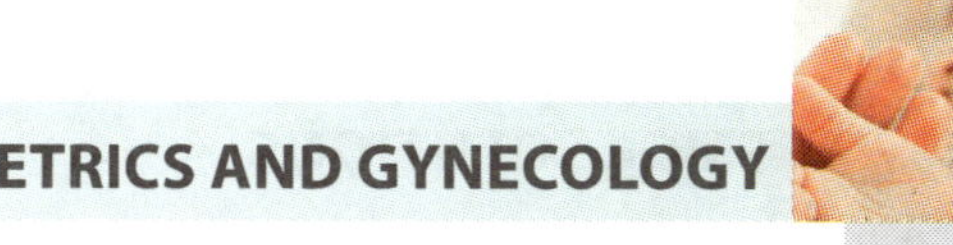

- Amenorrhea (75%)
- Bleeding per vaginum (70%)

Note: *Triad is present only in 50% case of ectopic*

- **Most common/Consistent** finding of Ectopic pregnancy: **Pain**

Symptoms

- Nausea and Vomiting
- Lower Abdominal pain/generalized Abdomen pain
- Shoulder tip pain (25%)
- Syncopal attacks (10%)

242. Ans. (a) Ectopic pregnancy

Ref: Dutta Obs, 7th ed. pg. 182; William Obs, 22nd ed. pg. 258

243. Ans. (b) TVS

Ref: DC Dutta, 8th ed. pg. 213

- Investigation of choice in a case of ectopic pregnancy/ suspected case of ectopic pregnancy is Transvaginal scan.
- Findings raising suspicion of ectopic on TVS:
  - **Empty uterine cavity: Most important**
  - Finding of complex adnexal mass
  - Fluid (echogenic) in the pouch of Douglas.
  - Adnexal mass clearly separated from the ovary.
  - Rarely cardiac motion may be seen in an unruptured tubal ectopic pregnancy.

Extra Mile

- **Estimation of B-hCG:** Urine pregnancy test—ELISA is sensitive to 10-50 mIU/mL and is positive in 95% of ectopic pregnancies. **A single estimation of B-hCG level either in the serum or in urine confirms pregnancy but cannot determine its location.**
- **Gold standard for diagnosis of ectopic pregnancy:** Laproscopy

244. Ans. (c) Methotrexate 50 mg IM

Ref: DC Dutta, 8th ed. pg. 216

Dutta states: *"For systemic therapy of ectopic pregnancy, a single dose of methotrexate (MTX) 50 mg/M² is given intramuscularly."*

245. Ans. (a) Vomiting

Ref: Dutta Obs, 7th ed. pg. 182; William Obs, 22nd ed. pg. 258

CLASSIC TRIAD OF ECTOPIC

- **Pain+ Amenorrhea+ Bleeding per vaginum**

Triad is present only in 50% case of ectopic

- **M.C/Consistent** finding of Ectopic → **pain**

Symptoms

- Nausea & Vomiting
- Lower Abdom. pain/generalized Abdom pain
- Shoulder tip pain Syncopal attacks

246. Ans. (c) A negative pregnancy test excludes the diagnosis

Ref: DC Dutta 8th ed./212, Williams Obst. 21st ed./ 892

- **Ectopic pregnancy:** Pregnancy that occurs outside the endometrial lining of uterus.
- Risk factors for ectopic pregnancy include previous ectopic pregnancies and conditions like tubal surgery, tubercular infection that disrupt the normal anatomy of the Fallopian tubes.
- Previous salpingitis/tubal disease is the most common cause of ectopic pregnancy.
- Among contraceptives, use of progestasert is the most common cause of ectopic pregnancy.
- The major health risk of ectopic pregnancy is rupture leading to internal bleeding.
- It can be diagnosed by Beta hCG level. It doesn't rise as fast as it rises in uterine pregnancy.
- ***It can also be diagnosed by pregnancy test, but a negative pregnancy test doesn't rule out the diagnosis of ectopic pregnancy.***
- On transvaginal scan presence of an adnexal mass and the absence of an intrauterine pregnancy increases the likelihood of an ectopic pregnancy.
- ***Methotrexate is considered as drug of choice for ectopic pregnancy.***

247. Ans. (a) Transvaginal USG

Ref: DC Dutta, 8th ed. pg. 212, Williams Obst, 21st ed. pg. 892

Diagnosis of Ectopic Pregnancy

- Most definite diagnosis of pregnancy is by demonstrating intrauterine sac.
- An absence of the intrauterine sac in a patient who is complaining of pain, bleeding and positive pregnancy test raise the suspicion of ectopic pregnancy.
- By doing **transvaginal USG, ectopic pregnancy can be ruled out.** If the USG demonstrates live intrauterine fetus then ectopic pregnancy is very unlikely.
- On the other hand, if the uterus is empty, an ectopic pregnancy can be diagnosed based on the visualization of an adnexal mass separate from the ovaries.
- **Beta-hCG** also helps in diagnosis of pregnancy. It is positive in virtually 100% of ectopic pregnancies.
- A positive test only confirms pregnancy and does not indicate whether it is intrauterine or extrauterine (ectopic).
- *In normal pregnancy beta-hCG should double up every 2 days but in ectopic pregnancy the rate of increase of beta hCG is slow.*

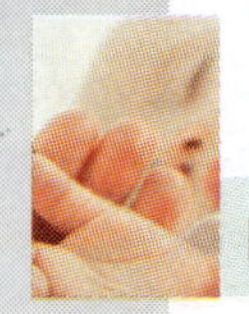

CULDOCENTESIS

- Culdocentesis is the transvaginal passage of a needle into the posterior cul-de-sac in order to determine whether free blood is present in the abdomen.
- This procedure will reveal non-clotted blood if intra-abdominal bleeding has occurred.
- Clotted bloods signify ruptured ectopic pregnancy.
- If culdocentesis is positive, laparoscopy or laparotomy should be performed immediately.

248. Ans. (a) Beta hCG <5000

Ref: DC Dutta, 8th ed. pg. 209

CRITERIA FOR MEDICAL MANAGEMENT OF ECTOPIC PREGNANCY USING METHOTREXATE

Absolute Requirements

- Hemodynamic stability
- No evidence of acute intra-abdominal bleeding
- Reliable commitment to comply with required
- Follow-up care

Preferable Requirements

- Absent or mild pain
- Serum beta hCG level <10,000 IU/L *(best results seen with hCG <2000 IU/L)*
- Absent embryonic heart activity
- Ectopic gestational mass <3.5 cm in diameter.

MALPRESENTATION, DIFFICULT DELIVERY AND INSTRUMENTATION

249. Ans. (d) Hysterosalpingography

Ref: William's Obstetrics, Chapter 42, 26th ed. pg. 121

- The given image shows HSG Cannula. It is used for the delivery of contrast media or saline into the uterine cavity during hysterosalpingography (HSG) or sonohysterography (SHG) for examination of the uterus and fallopian tubes.
- When used for HSG, the Margolin HSG Cannula can be used for evaluation of tubal patency.

250. Ans. (b) Green

Ref: Shaw's Textbook of Gynaecology, 7th ed. pg. 412

Colposcopy commonly uses a *green filter* to highlight blood vessels in the tissue. Because the green filter enables a clearer identification of disease.

251. Ans. (b) Anthropoid

Ref: Dutta 9th ed. pg. 325

TABLE: Anatomical features of parent pelvic types

		Gynecoid	Anthropoid	Android	Platypelloid
Inlet	• Shape	Round	Anteroposteriorly oval	Triangular	Transversely oval
	• Anterior and posterior segment	Almost equal and spacious	Both increased with slight anterior narrowing	Posterior segment short and anterior segment marrow	Both reduced-flat
	• Sacrum	Sacral angle (SA) more than 90°. Inclined backwards. Well curved from above down and side to side	SA more than 90°. Inclined posteriorly. Long and marrow. Usual curve	Sacral angle less than 90°. Inclined forwards and straight	SA more than 90°. Inclined posteriorly. Short and straight
Cavity	• Sacrosciatic notch	Wide and shallow	More wide and shallow	Narrow and deep	Slightly narrow and small
	• Sidewalls	Straight or slightly divergent	Straight or divergent	Convergent	Divergent
Outlet	• Ischial spines	Not prominent	Not prominent	Prominent	Not prominent
	• Pubic arch	Curved	Long and curved	Long and straight	Short and curved
	• Subpublic angle	Wide (85°)	Slightly narrow	Narrow	Very wide (more than 90°)
	• Bituberous diameter	Normal	Normal or short	Short	Wide

TABLE: Obstetric outcome in parent pelvic types

		Gynecoid	Anthropoid	Android	Platypelloid
Inlet	• Position	Occipitolateral or oblique occipito-anterior	Direct occipito-anterior or posterior	Occipitolateral or oblique occipito-posterior	Occipitolateral
	• Diameter of engagement	Transverse or oblique	Anteroposterior	Transverse or oblique	Transverse
	• Engagement	No difficulty usual mechanism	No difficulty except flexion is delayed	Delayed and difficult	Difficult by exaggerated parietal
Cavity	• Internal rotation	Easy anterior rotation	Nonrotation common	Difficult anterior rotation. Not occurs early above the ischial spines, chance of arrest	Anterior rotation usually occurs late in the perineum
Outlet	• Delivery	No difficulty	Moe incidence of face-to-pubis delivery	Difficult delivery with increased chance of perineal injuries	No difficulty

252. Ans. (b) Vesicovaginal fistula

Ref: William's Obstetrics 24th ed. pg. 536

- A vesicovaginal fistula is an opening that develops between the vagina and bladder.
- The result is that urine leaks out of the vagina.
- **Risk factors:**
  - Prolonged labor
  - Instrumental vaginal delivery
  - Caesarean section
  - Short stature

253. Ans. (a) 10–15 mm Hg

Ref: Shaw's Gyencology 16th ed. pg. 93-94

- Laparoscope is a rigid telescope varying in diameter between 4 mm and 10 mm and it is 30 cm long.
- CO_2 machine to create pneumoperitoneum is specially designed for laparoscopy. About 100 mL/min is instilled into the peritoneal cavity, maintaining intraperitoneal pressure **below 15 mm** Hg.
- About 1000 mL is required for adequate pneumoperitoneum.

254. Ans. (d) Uterus surface

Ref: Shaw's Gyenecology 16th ed. pg. 103-104

- Hysteroscopy is a diagnostic and therapeutic modality for the intrauterine pathology.
- It can visualize the OS, cervix, endometrium and their associated pathologies like fibroids, endometrial polyps, endometrial TB, adhesion of septum, *in situ* placed or misplaced IUCD.
- It cannot visualize the outer surface of uterus.
- For the procedure the uterine cavity is distended with CO_2 at the rate of 70 mL/min and pressure <100 mm Hg, or with saline, dextrose, hyskon or glycine 1.5%.
- **Types of hysteroscopes:**
  - **Microhysteroscope:** Provides magnification of 30–150 times.
  - **Contact hysteroscope:** A diagnostic tool without distending medium.

Contraindications of Hysteroscopy

- During menstruation, view is obscured and infection rate increases.
- Genital tract infection.
- Pregnancy.
- Scarred uterus and enlarged uterus more than 12 weeks size form relative contraindications.
- Cervical stenosis can cause cervical tear and uterine perforation.
- **Cardiopulmonary disorders:** Due to risk of fluid overload or anesthesia risk.

255. Ans. (c) ECV done after 34 weeks

Ref: DC Dutta 8th ed. P 435

- Breech is the most common malpresentation, with reduced incidence as the age of gestation progresses *(20% at 28th week and drops to 5% at 34th week and to 3–4% at term).*
- Thus in 3 out of 4, **spontaneous correction into vertex presentation occurs by 34th week.**
- So external cephalic version (ECV) **should not be done before 34 weeks.**
- They are **not** associated with any specific congenital anomaly.
- There are two varieties of breech presentation (*see* Fig.):
  - Complete
  - Incomplete

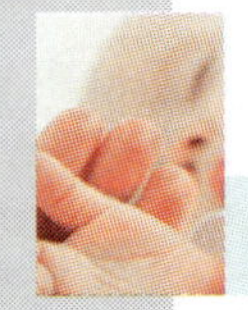

Complete (Flexed Breech)

- Thighs are flexed at hips and legs at knees.
- **Presenting part:** Two buttocks, external genitalia and two feet.
- **It is commonly present in multiparae (10%).**

Incomplete: Three varieties are possible:

- **Breech with extended legs (Frank breech):** In this condition, **thighs are flexed on the trunk and legs are extended at the knee joints** (*see* **Fig. A**). The presenting part consists of the two buttocks and external genitalia only.
  - **It is commonly present in primigravidae**, about 70% (due to tight abdominal wall and good uterine tone).

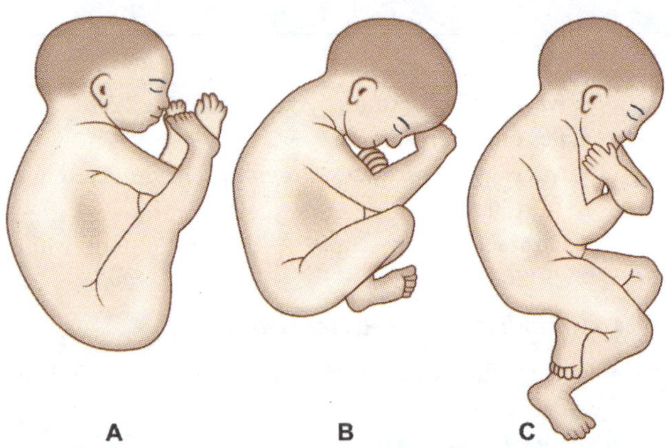

FIGURE: Varieties of breech presentation—(A) Breech with extended legs (Frank breech); (B) Flexed breech (Complete breech); (C) Footling presentation

- **Footling presentation (25%):** Both thighs and legs are partially extended bringing the legs to present at brim.
- **Knee presentation:** Thighs are extended but the knees are flexed, bringing the knees down to present at the brim. Footling and knee presentation are not so common.

256. Ans. (a) Acromion

Ref: DC Dutta, 8th ed. pg. 454

- When the long axis of the fetus lies perpendicularly to the maternal spine or centralized uterine axis, it is called transverse lie.
- In transverse lie, acromion is the presenting part/most prominent part upon vaginal examination.

Extra Mile

Presentation	Presenting part
Face	Mentum
Shoulder	Acromion
Breech	Sacrum
Cephalic	Vertex

257. Ans. (b) Mentum

Ref: DC Dutta, 8th ed. pg. 449

- Face is a rare variety of cephalic presentation where the **presenting part** is the face.
- **There is complete extension of the head** so that the occiput is in contact with the back. **The denominator is mentum.**
- Face presentation results most likely from complete extension of deflexed head of a vertex presentation.

Note: *Most common fetal cause of face presentation is anencephaly.*

258. Ans. (b) Ceasarean section

Ref: DC Dutta 8th ed./441-42, Williams 22/e/571

- **Because Breech presentation with footling has very high incidence of cord prolapse, delivery by caesarean section is recommended in these patients.**

Indication of C.S in breech are:

- Big baby (Wt >3.5 kg.)
- Hyperextension of head (stargazing fetus)
- **Footling presentation (risk of cord prolapse)**
- Suspected pelvic contraction
- Severe IUGR

259. Ans. (b) Head with hand

Ref: DC Dutta, 7th ed. pg. 397

COMPOUND PRESENTATION

When a cephalic presentation is complicated by the presence of:

- A hand or a foot or both alongside the head or
- Presence of one or both hands by the side of the breech, it is called compound presentation.
- ***The commonest one being the head with hand***
- *Rarest one being the presence of head, hand and a foot.*
- The incidence is about 1 in 600.

Causes of Compound Presentation

- Prematurity (commonest),
- Contracted pelvis
- Pelvic tumors
- Multiple pregnancy
- Macerated fetus
- High head with premature or early rupture of the membranes.

260. Ans. (b) Partial extension

Ref: William's Obstetrics, 23rd ed. Ch 17

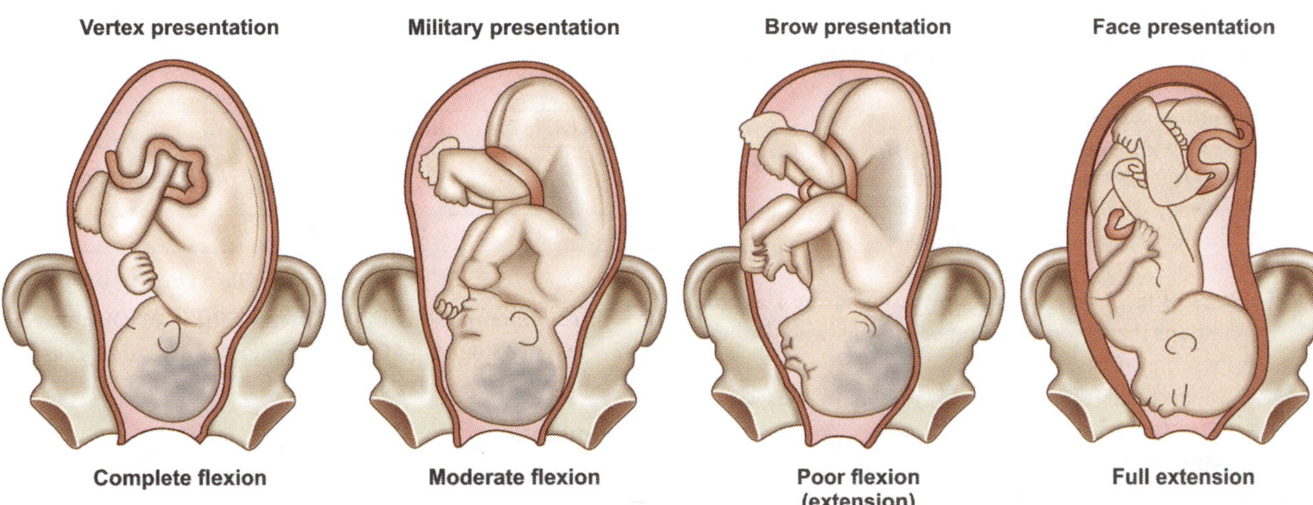

- In cephalic presentation, the fetal head may assume a position between these extremes:
  - **Vertex presentation:** Head is flexed sharply so that the chin is in contact with the thorax. The occipital fontanel is the presenting part, and this presentation is referred to as a *vertex* or *occiput presentation.*
  - **Sinciput/Military presentation:** Partially flexed head in some cases, with the anterior (large) fontanel, or bregma, as presenting.
  - **Brow presentation:** Head is partially extended (see Fig).
  - These two presentations (sinciput and brow) are usually transient. As labor progresses, sinciput and brow presentations almost always convert into vertex or face presentations by neck flexion or extension, respectively.
  - **Face presentation:** Much less commonly, the fetal neck may be sharply extended so that the occiput and back come in contact, and the face is foremost in the birth canal, giving it the *face presentation.*

261. Ans. (a) Face presentation

Ref: DC Dutta 8th ed./449, Dutta's Obstetrics pg. 392

ABNORMAL PRESENTATIONS

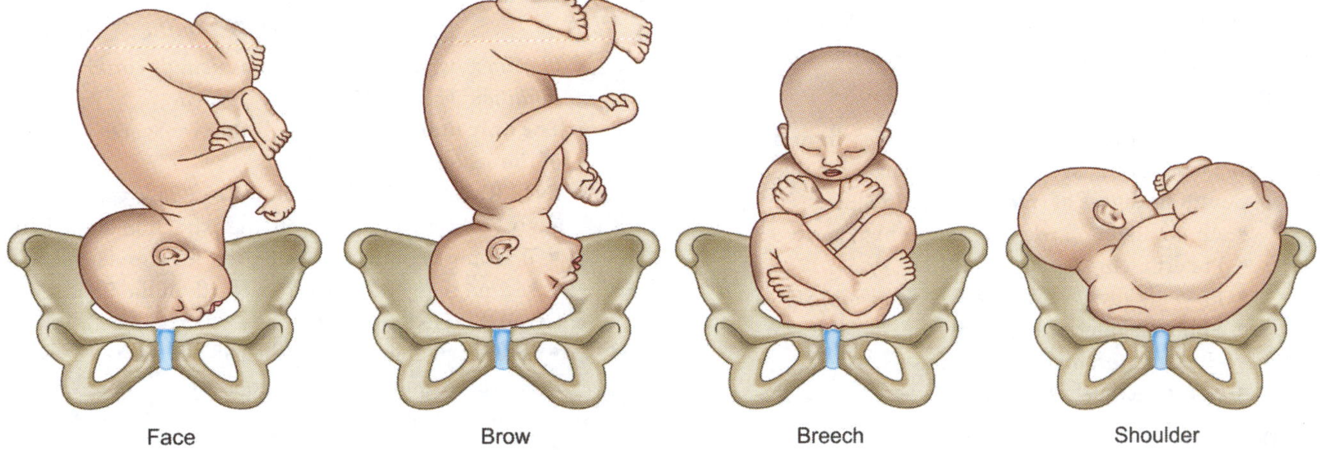

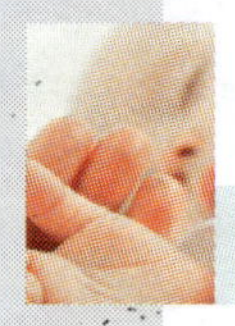

FACE PRESENTATION

- Seen in 0.5% of cases.
- With this presentation, the head is hyperextended so that the occiput is in contact with the fetal back, and the chin (mentum) is presenting.
- The fetal face may present with the chin (mentum) anteriorly or posteriorly, relative to the maternal symphysis pubis.

Etiology

- Causes of face presentations are numerous and include conditions that favor extension or prevent head flexion:
  - Preterm infants
  - Anencephalic fetuses naturally present by the face
  - In contracted pelvis or large fetuses
  - High parity is a predisposing factor to face presentation

262. Ans. (a) Polyhydramnios is a cause

Ref: William's Obstetrics 23rd ed. Ch 20, Abnormal Labor

- *For this question, most of the students usually go for 'D' shoulder dystocia is a threat for this condition. But remember one thing that shoulder dystocia usually results in longitudinal lie, where head of the baby is born and rest of the body below neck is stuck. It occurs can be secondary to contracted pelvis, macrosomic baby etc.*
- This is a clear case of transverse lie (as seen in image).

TRANSVERSE LIE

- Transverse lie is seen in 0.3% of the cases.
- In this position, the long axis of the fetus is approximately perpendicular to that of the mother.
- In a transverse lie, the shoulder is usually positioned over the pelvic inlet. The head occupies one iliac fossa, and the breech the other *(as seen in question).*
- This creates a *shoulder presentation* in which the side of the mother on which the acromion rests determines the designation of the lie as right or left acromial.

Etiology

- Women with four or more deliveries have a 10-fold incidence of transverse lie compared with nulliparas.
- **Common causes of transverse lie include:**
  - Abdominal wall relaxation from high parity
  - Preterm fetus
  - ***Placenta previa*** *(NOT abruption placentae)*
  - Abnormal uterine anatomy
  - ***Hydramnios, and***
  - Contracted pelvis.

Diagnosis

- A transverse lie is usually recognized easily, often by inspection alone.
- The abdomen is unusually wide, whereas the uterine fundus extends to only slightly above the umbilicus

Management: Active labor in a woman with a transverse lie is usually an indication for cesarean delivery.

263. Ans. (a) Amniocentesis

Ref: DC Dutta, 8th ed. pg. 248-50

264. Ans. (b) Previous CS of >2

Ref: Dutta's Obstetrics, 7th ed. pg. 330

Recommendations of American college of Obstetrician & Gynecologists (ACOG) for vaginal birth after cesarian delivery (VBAC):

Indications

- ***No more than 1 previous lower segment transverse scar***
- Availability of anesthesia and personnel for emergency cesarean delivery.
- Clinically adequate pelvis
- No history of previous uterine rupture or other uterine scars.
- Availability of physician throughout active labor.

Contraindications

- *Prior classical or T-shaped uterine incision.*
- *Previous 2 or more LSCS*
- History of uterine rupture.
- Medical or obstetrical complications that preclude vaginal birth. Ex: pre-eclampsia, placenta previa, malpresentation etc.
- Limited resources for emergency CS. Ex: lack of surgeon, anesthesia, or nursing staff.

265. Ans. (c) Transverse lie of second fetus in a twin pregnancy

Ref: DC Dutta, 7th ed. pg. 585

- *In other words, this question actually asking about condition where ICV can be performed.*
- **The only indication of ICV is the transverse lie in case of the second baby of twins.**
- **INTERNAL VERSION**: is always a podalic version and is almost always completed with the extraction of the fetus.
  - It is most commonly employed for the delivery of a second twin after the vaginal birth of the first.
- **CONDITIONS for ICV**
  - The cervix must be fully dilated
  - Amniotic fluid must be adequate for intrauterine fetal manipulation
  - Alive fetus.
- ***CONTRAINDICATIONS****: it must not be attempted in neglected obstructed labor even if the baby is living.*

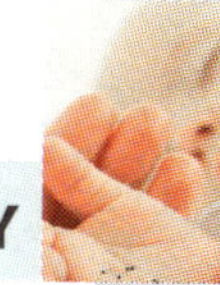

266. Ans. (d) PIH

Ref: DC Dutta, 7th ed. pg. 379-380 and 583

- External Cephalic version is done to bring the favorable cephalic pole in the lower pole of the uterus.
- **INDICATIONS of ECV:**
  - Breech presentation
  - Transverse lie
- **Benefits of ECV:**
  - Reduces maternal morbidity due to caesarean or vaginal breech delivery
  - Reduces the incidence of breech presentation at term.
  - Reduces the number of caesarean delivery
  - The success rate of external version is about 60%
- **CONTRAIDICATIONS OF ECV**
  - Multiple pregnancy
  - Previous caesarean delivery
  - Antepartum hemorrhage
  - Fetal causes like hyperextension of the head, dead or large fetus (>3.5 kg).
  - Ruptured membranes
  - Known congenital malformation of the uterus
  - Contracted pelvis
  - *Obstetric complications like Severe pre-eclampsia, obesity, Elderly primigravida, Bad obstetric History (BOH).*

Note: *Breech with extended legs is not a contraindication for external version.*

267. Ans. (d) Hydramnois

Ref: DC Dutta, 7th ed. pg. 379-380 and 583

- It's asking here about condition where ECV can be performed.
- Hydramnios always helps in bringing the favorable cephalic pole in the lower pole of the uterus.
- *Please refer to the previous Explanation.*

268. Ans. (c) Fetus is at station + 2

Ref: DC Dutta, 7th ed. pg. 573

TABLE: Classification for operative vaginal (forceps/ventouse) delivery (ACOG-2000)

Procedure	Criteria
Outlet	Scalp is visible at the introitus without separating the labia. Fetal skull at the level of the pelvic floor or on the perineum. Sagittal suture is in direct AP diameter or in the right or left occiput anterior or posterior position.
Low	Leading point of the fetal skull (station) is at +2 cm or more but has not yet reached the pelvic floor. Rotation is <45 degree Rotation is >45 degree
Mid	Fetal head is engaged. Head is 1/5 palpable per abdomen but presenting part is above +2 cm station.
High	Head is not engaged. *This type is not included in classification*

DISEASES DURING PREGNANCY

269. Ans. (a) Pregestational DM

Ref: William's Obstetrics, Chapter 40, 26th ed. pg. 2783

- Pregestational (also called preexisting) diabetes refers to type 1 or type 2 diabetes mellitus that is diagnosed before pregnancy.
- The goal of medical management of pregnant women with pregestational diabetes is to maintain blood glucose concentration at or near normoglycemic levels at the time of conception and throughout the entire pregnancy, taking into account that "normoglycemia" in pregnant women without diabetes is relatively lower than in the nonpregnant state, because good glycemic control decreases the likelihood of adverse maternal, fetal, and newborn outcomes (e.g., congenital abnormalities, preeclampsia, macrosomia, neonatal hypoglycemia).

270. Ans. (b) HELLP

Ref: William's Obstetrics, Chapter 53, 26th ed. pg. 2464

- HELLP syndrome is a pregnancy complication.
- It is a type of preeclampsia.
- It usually occurs during the third trimester of pregnancy.

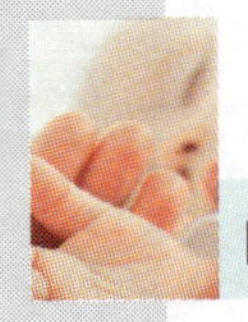

- There is no known cause of HELLP syndrome. Women who have preeclampsia or eclampsia (uncontrolled preeclampsia) have a higher risk of HELLP syndrome.

The name HELLP syndrome stands for:

H: Hemolysis

EL: Elevated liver enzymes

LP: Low platelet count

271. Ans. (b) To replace warfarin with heparin

Ref: William's Obstetrics, Chapter 52, 26th ed. pg. 2404

- With chronic heart failure, the incidence of associated thromboembolism is high, and therefore prophylactic heparin is often recommended.
- Unfortunately, warfarin is the most effective anti-coagulant for preventing maternal thromboembolism but causes harmful fetal effects.
- As a compromise, it is recommended to use heparin in early pregnancy, and then transition to warfarin in the second trimester.

272. Ans. (b) Loss of deep tendon reflex

Ref: Shaws 16th ed. pg. 221-22

$MgSO_4$ Mechanism of Action

- $MgSO_4$ acts as a membrane stabilizer and neuroprotector, also reduces motor endplate sensitivity to Ach. It also blocks neuronal calcium influx.
- It reduces cerebral vasodilation
- It dilates uterine arteries
- It increases production of prostacyclin and inhibits platelet activation

Toxicity at Levels

- At more than 7 mEq/L – loss of tendon reflex
- At more than 10 mEq/L – respiratory depression
- At more than 25 mEq/L – cardiac arrest

273. Ans. (c) Medical nutrition therapy and exercise

Ref: Williams Obstetrics 24th ed. pg. 1141

- Fasting and post prandial glucose range is in impaired glucose tolerance range. In this condition initially medical nutrition therapy and exercise is advised to the pregnant mother.
- Insulin has been considered standard therapy in women with gestational diabetes when target glucose levels cannot be consistently achieved through nutrition and exercise.

274. Ans. (a) Due to excess insulin

Ref: William's Obstetrics 24th ed. pg. 624

- **In infant of** diabetic mother, hypoglycemia in fetus is very common complication after birth, due to excessive insulin that was being produced by fetus in intrauterine life.

Conditions associated with an increased risk for neonatal hypoglycemia include

- Decreased substrate availability
- Hyperinsulinemia (infant of diabetic mother)
- Other endocrine abnormalities
- Increased glucose utilization

275. Ans. (b) Hep B vaccine + IG

Ref: William's Obstetrics 24th ed. pg. 1240

- Hepatitis B can be easily passed from a pregnant woman with hepatitis B to her baby at birth.
- Health care providers can give the baby a set of shots of hepatitis B vaccine and immunoglobulin at birth to prevent the baby from getting infected.

276. Ans. (c) Bed rest and Progesterone

Ref: DC Dutta 9th ed. pg. 153-54

- The patient is a case of threatened abortion, which can present with brisk bleeding.
- This bleeding usually stops spontaneously upon bed rest.
- **Definition of Threatened abortion:** "*a clinical entity where the process of miscarriage has started but has not progressed to a state from which recovery is impossible*"
- **Treatment:**
  - Bed rest and strenuous activity restriction
  - Treatment with progesterone induces immunomodulation to shift the Th1 (proinflammatory response) to Th2 (anti-inflammatory response)
- **Note:** Use of hCG is not preferred.

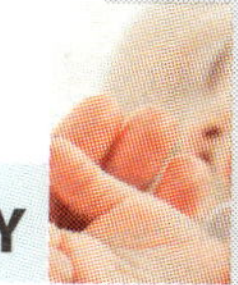

277. Ans. (c) Gestational hypertension

Ref: DC Dutta 9th ed. pg. 207

TABLE: Classification of hypertension in pregnancy (National high blood pressure education program 2000 and ACOG-2013)

<table>
<tr><th>Disorder</th><th>Definition</th><th>Disorder</th><th>Definition</th></tr>
<tr><td>Hypertension</td><td>BP $\geq$140/90 mm Hg measured two times with at least 6-hour interval</td><td rowspan="8">Chronic hypertension with superimposed pre-eclampsia and eclampsia</td><td rowspan="8">The common causes of chronic hypertension:
• Essential hypertension
• Chronic renal disease (renovascular)
• Coarctation of aorta
• Endocrine disorders (diabetes mellitus, pheochromocytoma, thyrotoxicosis
• Connective tissue diseases (Lupus erythematosus)
The criteria for diagnosis of superimposed preeclampsia:
• New onset of proteinuria >0.5 g/24 hours specimen
• Aggravation of hypertension
• Development of HELLP syndrome
• Development of headache scotoma, epigastric pain</td></tr>
<tr><td>Proteinuria</td><td>Urinary excretion of >0.3 g protein/24 hours specimen or 0.1 g/L</td></tr>
<tr><td>Gestational hypertension</td><td>BP >140/90 mm hg for the first time in pregnancy after 20 weeks, without proteinuria</td></tr>
<tr><td>Preeclampsia</td><td>Gestational hypertension with proteinuria</td></tr>
<tr><td>Eclampsia</td><td>Women with preeclampsia complicated with grand mal seizures and/or coma</td></tr>
<tr><td>HELLP syndrome</td><td>• Hemolysis (H)
• Elevated liver enzymes (EL)
• Low platelet count (LP)</td></tr>
<tr><td>Chronic hypertension</td><td>Known hypertension before pregnancy or hypertension diagnosed first time before 20 weeks of pregnancy</td></tr>
<tr><td>Superimposed preeclampsia or eclampsia</td><td>Occurrence of new onset of proteinuria in women with chronic hypertension</td></tr>
</table>

278. Ans. (c) Renal agenesis

Ref: DC Dutta 9th ed. pg. 203, 204

- Oligohydramnios is an extremely rare condition **where the liquor amnii is deficient in amount to the extent of** <200 mL at term.
- **Sonographically, it is defined** when the maximum vertical pocket of liquor is <2 cm or when amniotic fluid index (AFI) is <5 cm (<5 percentile).
- Absence of any measurable pocket of amniotic fluid is defined as Anhydramnios. AFI between 5 and 8 is termed as borderline AFI or borderline Oligohydramnios.
- Internal organ malfunction like renal agenesis can cause this problem.

Causes:

Fetal cause	Maternal cause
• Renal cause (MCC) ▪ Renal agenesis ▪ Polycystic kidney ▪ Urethral obstruction • Fetal growth restriction • Premature rupture of membranes • Post-term pregnancy • Fetal death • Drugs exposure like: PG inhibitor, ACE inhibitor	• Hypertension • Uteroplacental insufficiency • Dehydration • Idiopathic

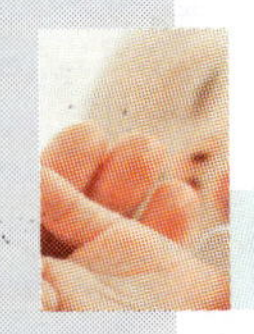

279. Ans. (c) Parvovirus B19

Ref: DC Dutta 9th ed. pg. 200, 313

- Hydrops fetalis is the most serious form of Rh hemolytic disease
- Hemolysis produces → severe anemia → Damage to liver → leading to hypoproteinemia → Causing generalized edema/Hydrops fetalis, ascites and hydrothorax.
- Hydrops fetalis is due to:
  - Rh immunization
  - Non-immune hydrops
  - Cardiothoracic anomalies
  - Fetal cirrhosis and
  - Fetal infections with TORCH and Parvovirus B19 infection.
- Incidence is 13 times higher is Rh +ve males
- **USG:** Buddha position (with halo around head due to edematous scalp)
- To counter the adversity of hypoxia due to hemolysis there is **Hyperplasia of placental tissue** as well.
- Cause of fetal death: **Cardiac failure**

280. Ans. (b) 140

Ref: DC Dutta 9th ed. pg. 263

- As a screening method for high risk pregnant patients, 50 gram oral glucose challenge test is done regardless of meal or time of the day.
- Done between 24 and 28 weeks of pregnancy
- A plasma glucose value of 140 mg% at 1 hour is considered as a cut-off point

Extra Mile

TABLE: Criteria for diagnosis of GDM with 100 gm oral glucose (O'sullivan and Mahan modified by Carpenter and Coustan) and national diabetes data group

GTT: Venous Plasma (mg/dL)		
Time	**Carpenter & Coustan**	**NDDG**
Fasting	95	105
1 hour	180	190
2 hours	155	165
3 hours	140	145
GDM is diagnosed when any two values are met or elevated		

TABLE: Criteria for diagnosis of impaired glucose tolerance and diabetes with 75 gm oral glucose (american diabetes association)

Time	Normal tolerance	Impaired glucose tolerance	Diabetes
Fasting	<100	≥100 and <126	≥126
2 hours post: Glucose	<140	≥140 and < 200	≥200

281. Ans. (c) 46 XX both paternal origin

Ref: DC Dutta 9th ed. pg. 181

- Complete mole commonly has 46XX karyotype (in 85%), the molar chromosome are derived entirely from the father.
  - Less commonly the chromosomal pattern may be 46Xy or 45X
- An empty ovum is fertilized by a haploid sperm, which duplicates its own chromosome after meiosis → Phenomenon called **Androgenesis**.
- Complete mole shows paternal: maternal ratio of 2:0, whereas partial mole shows 2:1 ratio.

TABLE: Important features of complete and partial moles

Features	Complete mole	Partial mole
Embryo/Fetus	Absent	Present
Hydropic degeneration of villi	Pronounced and diffused	Variable and focal
Trophoblast hyperplasia	Diffuse	Focal
Uterine size	More than the date (30-60%)	Less than the date
Theca lutein cysts	Common (25-50%)	Uncommon
Karyotype	46, KX (85%), Paternal in origin	Triploid (90%), diploid (10%)
β-hCG	High (>50,000)	Slight elevation (<50,000)
Classic clinical symptoms	Common	Rare
Risk of persistent GTN	20%	<5%
Immunostaining ($p57^{KF2}$)	Negative	Positive

282. Ans. (b) Thiopentone sodium

Ref: DC Dutta, 8th ed. pg. 270

- During pregnancy when fits are multiple, recurring at varying intervals **in quick succession, it is called status eclampticus.**

Treatment of status eclampticus

- **Thiopentone sodium 0.5 g** dissolved in 20 mL of 5% dextrose is given intravenously very slowly.
- **If the procedure fails,** use of complete anesthesia, muscle relaxant and assisted ventilation may be employed.
- **In unresponsive cases,** cesarean section in ideal surroundings may be a lifesaving attempt.

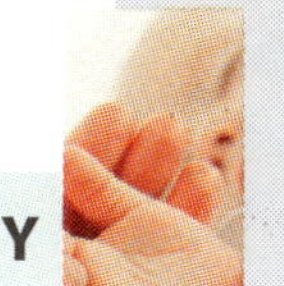

283. Ans. (a) Mannitol

Ref: DC Dutta, 8th ed. pg. 275

- A deeply unconscious patient with raised intracranial pressure needs steroid and/or diuretic therapy.
- DOC for eclampsia: $MgSO_4$.

284. Ans. (b) Heart disease

Ref: DC Dutta, 8th ed. pg. 256

- **Pre-eclampsia** is a multisystem disorder of unknown etiology characterized by development of hypertension to the extent of **140/90 mm Hg** or more with proteinuria after the 20th week in a previously normotensive and non-proteinuric woman.
- The incidence in primigravidae is about 10% and in multigravidae 5%.

Etiopathogenesis of Pre-eclampsia

- **Hypertension:** The underlying basic pathology is **endothelial dysfunction** and intense **vasospasm**, affecting almost all the vessels, particularly those of uterus, kidney, placental bed and brain. The basic underlying pathology remains as **endothelial dysfunction** and **vasospasm**.

Risk Factors for Pre-eclampsia

- Primigravida: Young or elderly (first time exposure to chorionic villi)
- Family history: Hypertension, preeclampsia
- Placental abnormalities:
  - Hyperplacentosis: Excessive exposure to chorlonic villi-(molar pregnancy twins, diabetes
  - Placental Ischemia)
- Obesity: BMI >35 kg/m², insulin resistance
- Pre-existing vascular disease
- New paternity
- Thrombophilias [antiphospholipid syndrome, protein C, S deficiency, Factor V leiden

285. Ans. (a) Folic acid supplementation

Ref: DC Dutta, 8th ed. pg. 585

- Use of anti- epileptic drugs like phenytoin, valproate and even phenobarbitone has been shown in pregnancy to contribute to acquire folic acid deficiency.
- If a lady is deficient in folic acid at the time of her pregnancy, then the baby most likely will born with neural tube defect.
- Traditionally we study that folic acid should be taken peri-conceptionally 2 months before and 3 months later to pregnant status at dose of 400 micrograms.
- However with the use of anti-epileptics drugs like phenytoin, valproate etc. the dose of folic acid needs to be supplemented at a dose of 4 mg once per day.

286. Ans. (c) MRI

Ref: William's Gyne, chapter 12- Breast Diseases; Breast CA screening

MAGNETIC RESONANCE IMAGING

- This screening option has recently been evaluated among genetically high-risk women. It is particularly attractive in this group of women, who develop breast cancer at a rate of 2 percent per year between the ages of **25 and 50,** a time during which mammography sensitivity is reduced by dense breast tissue.
- ***In general, MR imaging shows higher sensitivity and specificity than mammography.***
- *In the case given, patient is a 42 year primigravida, which in-itself is at high risk of developing congenital anomaly. By giving tests like mammography, condition can be worsened. Hence MRI is considered as the best modality of screening. Also it has higher sensitivity and specificity than other given tests.*

SCREENING MAMMOGRAPHY

- Considered as screening IOC.
- This radiographic test is currently the best available and most thoroughly validated breast cancer screening test available.
- At this time, it is generally accepted that for women aged 50–69 years, screening mammography reduces breast cancer mortality.

Screening Sonography: This modality identifies mammographically occult breast cancer in less than 1 percent of women.

287. Ans. (a) Bile acid

Ref: William's 23rd ed. Ch 50, Hepatic GB and pancreatic disorders; Intrahepatic cholestasis of Pregnancy

INTRAHEPATIC CHOLESTASIS OF PREGNANCY

- This disorder also has been referred to as recurrent jaundice of pregnancy, cholestatic hepatosis, and icterus gravidarum.
- It is characterized clinically by pruritus, icterus, or both.

Pathogenesis

- The cause of obstetrical cholestasis is unknown, but it probably occurs in genetically susceptible women.
- Whatever the inciting cause(s), bile acids are cleared incompletely and accumulate in plasma. ***Of note, total***

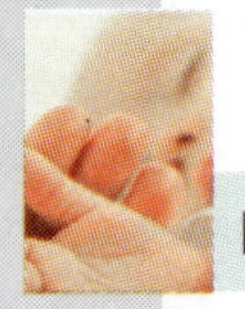

bile acid concentration may already be elevated 10- to 100-fold in normal pregnancy.

- Even *before* bile acid levels increase, associated dyslipidemia is apparent
- Total cholesterol levels are significantly higher compared with those of normal pregnancy, and ***low-density lipoprotein (LDL) cholesterol levels become elevated earliest.***
- **Hyperbilirubinemia** results from retention of conjugated pigment, but total plasma concentrations rarely exceed 4–5 mg/dL.
- **Alkaline phosphatase** is usually elevated even more so than in normal pregnancy.
- **Serum transaminase** levels are normal to moderately elevated but seldom exceed 250 U/L
- Liver biopsy shows mild cholestasis with bile plugs in the hepatocytes and canaliculi of the centrilobular regions, but without inflammation or necrosis.

Note: *These changes disappear after delivery but often recur in subsequent pregnancies or with estrogen-containing contraceptives.*

288. Ans. (c) Placenta previa

Ref: Williams, 24th ed. pg. 827

- Disseminated intravascular coagulation (DIC) aka consumptive coagulopathy is a pathologic disruption of the finely-balanced process of hemostasis.
- Massive activation of the clotting cascade results in widespread thrombosis, ***which leads to depletion of platelets and coagulation factors and excessive thrombolysis,*** *because all the clotting factors and platelets are consumed in intravascular coagulation*. The end result is multiorgan failure and hemorrhage.
- **Placental Abruption:** Is the most common cause of severe consumptive coagulopathy in obstetrics
- **Causes of DIC in pregnancy:**
  - Placental abruption (NOT placenta previa): most common cause.
  - Amnionic-fluid embolism.
  - Sepsis
  - Thrombotic microangiopathies
  - Acute kidney injury
  - Pre- eclampsia and
  - HELLP (Hemolysis, Elevated liver enzyme levels, low Platelet count) syndromes.

289. Ans. (d) Hyponatremia

Ref: DC Dutta's Textbook of Obstetrics, 7th ed. pg. 222

HELLP syndrome is rare complication of pre-eclampsia (10-15%), but can also develop without maternal hypertension.

- **H-Hemolysis (bilirubin >1.2 mg/dL)**
- **EL-Elevated Liver enzyme** (ASL and ALT >70 IU/L), **LDH >600 IU/L**, Bilirubin (>1.2 mg/dL)
- **LP-Low Platelets (1,00,000/mm^3)**

290. Ans. (c) Fluconazole 150 mg

Ref: Shaws, 15th ed. pg. 352

CANDIDAL (MONILIAL) VAGINITIS

- It is a fungal infection caused by yeast-like micro-organisms called Candida or Monilia.
- The commonest species causing human disease is Candida albicans

Clinical Features

- Vulval itching is the most common symptom, accompanied by vaginal irritation, dysuria, or both
- Thick curdy or flaky vaginal discharge.

Diagnosis

- Essentially based on clinical findings. But the diagnosis can be confirmed on microscopic examination of a smear of the vaginal discharge treated with 10% KOH solution.
- Pap smear shows **thick red-stained hyphae and dark red spores.**

Treatment

- A single dose of fluconazole 150 mg has been found to be very effective.
- Ideally, both partners should be treated and the underlying predisposing factor corrected to give long-term relief.
- Recurrent infection requires fluconazole orally 150 mg every 72 hours for 3 doses.

291. Ans. (a) Pre-eclampsia

Ref: William's Obstetrics 23rd ed. Ch 34.

GESTATIONAL HYPERTENSION CRITERIA

- Systolic BP >140 or diastolic BP >90 mm Hg for first time during pregnancy
- No proteinuria
- BP returns to normal before 12 weeks postpartum
- Final diagnosis made only postpartum
- May have other signs or symptoms of preeclampsia, for example, epigastric discomfort or thrombocytopenia.

PREECLAMPSIA

- BP >140/90 mm Hg **after 20 weeks'** gestation
- Proteinuria >300 mg/24 hours or >1+ dipstick

Eclampsia: Symptoms of pre-eclampsia + seizures *that cannot be attributed to other causes in a woman with preeclampsia.*

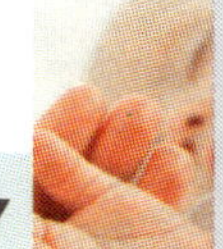

292. Ans. (a) Diuretics

Ref: KDT, 6th ed. pg. 553

- Diuretics are contraindicated in preeclampsia as they are teratogenic.

Antihypertensives in Pregnancy

Safe	Contraindicated
Labetalol-DOC	ACE inhibitors
Calcium Channel blockers	Na+ nitroprusside
Hydralazine	Diuretics
Alpha methyldopa	Reserpine
	Loratidine

293. Ans. (d) MgSO4

Ref: DC Dutta, 8th ed. pg. 271, Dutta Obs, 6th ed. pg. 235

Medical Management

- ***Seizure treatment***
  - The drug of choice for the control and prevention of convulsions is Pritchard's regimen i.e. magnesium sulphate.

Extra Mile

- DOC in eclampsia – $MgSO_4$
- 2nd DOC in eclampsia is hydralazine.

294. Ans. (c) Hospitalization and observation

Ref: DC Dutta, 8th ed. pg. 264-65

- Given these options, the best choice is hospitalization and do the observation under supervision conservatively.
- As the AOG is premature, CS or induction of labor can complicate the baby's outcome.

295. Ans. (a) Presence of fetal cardiac activity

Ref: DC Dutta, 8th ed. pg. 264

Please follow the flowchart given

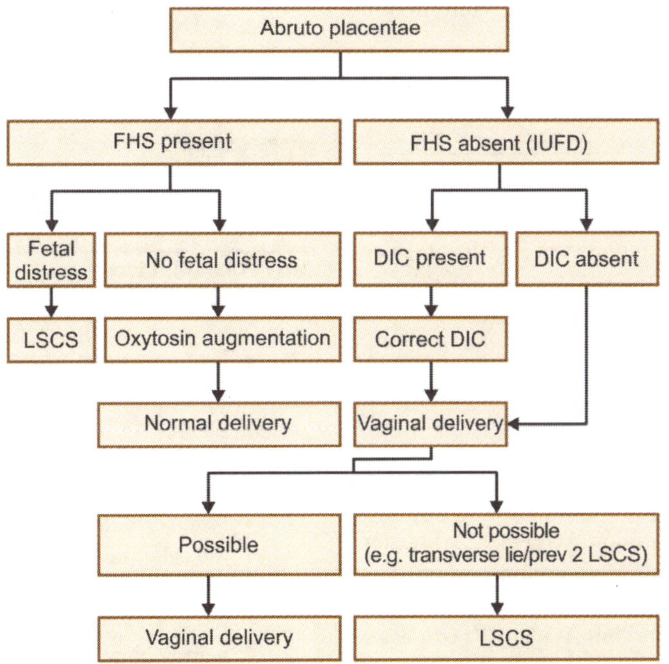

296. Ans. (c) Congenital heart disease

Ref: Danforth's Obstetrics and Gynecology, 10th ed. pg. 249-250

- In **infant of diabetic mother**, maternal hyperglycemia causes fetal hyperglycemia. In response of that, there is fetal β cell hyperplasia, which secretes enough insulin to counteract excess insulin coming from mother. This excess glucose causes glycogen and fat deposition leading to fetal macrosomia **(20-25%).**
- Soon after birth, when the cord is clamped and cut, there is cessation of glucose supply from mother while there is still higher insulin production in neonate, leading to à Hypoglycemia **(25–40%).**

- **Danforth's OBG states** "*Most frequent type of malformation involves central nervous system, cardiovascular system, gastrointestinal, genitourinary, and skeletal anomalies, with* ***cardiovascular system being the most common***"
- This ventricular wall and septal hypertrophy is thought to be due to glucose toxicity (from mother) and hyperinsulinemic state of the fetus.
- **Other fetal complications:**
  - Neonatal hyperbilirubinemia: 20–25%
  - Myocardial and septal hypertrophy: 10%
  - Congenital sacral agenesis: ~1%

297. Ans. (a) Propylthiouracil

Ref: DC Dutta 7th ed. pg. 287; Harrison's 19th ed. pg. 2297

- For the hyperthyroidism during pregnancy the mainstay of treatment in 1st trimester is PTU or methimazole.
- Methimazole is preferable avoided during first trimester of pregnancy if PTU is available.
- Methimazole and carbimazole is avoided due to fetal aplasia cutis and other defects such as choanal atresia.
- Because of its rare association with hepatotoxicity, propylthiouracil should be limited to the first trimester and then maternal therapy should be converted to methimazole (or carbimazole).

FETAL GROWTH AND DEVELOPMENT

298. Ans. (b) CRL

Ref: DC Dutta 8th ed. pg. 81, 84

- Assessment of age of gestation can also be done by first day of last menstrual period. It is greater than the postconception (fertilization) age by 2 weeks.
- The length is more reliable criterion than the weight to calculate the age of the fetus.
- In the **first trimester**, CRL (mm) + 6.5 = gestational age in weeks.
- **Best fetal parameter to find out AOG in 1st trimester:** CRL (Crown rump length). Variation ± 5 days.
- **Best fetal parameter to find out AOG in 2nd trimester:** BPD (Biparietal diameter). Most accurate when done between 12 and 20 weeks.
- **Best fetal parameter to find out AOG in 3rd trimester:** Femur length. Less reliable, variation ± 16 days.

299. Ans. (a) 11 weeks

Ref: DC Dutta, 8th ed. pg. 48

Dutta states: "***Breathing movements are identified by 11 weeks*** *but are irregular until 20th week. Their frequency varies from 30–70 per minute and is dependent on the maternal blood sugar concentration.*"

300. Ans. (a) Straight into mother's blood by simple diffusion

Ref: DC Dutta, 8th ed. pg. 41

Mechanisms involved in the transfer of substances across the placenta are:

- **Respiratory function:** Although the fetal respiratory movements are observed as early as 11 weeks, there is no gaseous exchange. Intake of oxygen and output of carbon dioxide take place by **simple diffusion** across the fetal membrane.
- **Excretory function:** Waste products from the fetus such as urea, uric acid, and creatinine are excreted in the maternal blood **by simple diffusion.**
- **Nutritive function:**
  - **Glucose,** the principal source of energy is transferred to the fetus **by facilitated diffusion.**
  - **Amino acids** are transferred by active transport
  - **Lipids, triglycerides and fatty acids** are transferred from mother and synthesized in fetus as well.
  - **Water and electrolytes** such as sodium, potassium and chloride cross through the fetal membrane by simple diffusion, whereas calcium, phosphorus and iron cross **by active transport.**
  - **Hormones:** Insulin, steroids from the adrenals, thyroid, chorionic gonadotropin or placental lactogen cross the placenta at a very slow rate.

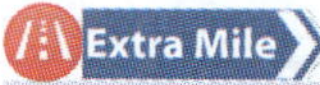

- **Neither parathormone nor calcitonin cross the placenta.**

301. Ans. (a) Liver

Ref: DC Dutta, 8th ed. pg. 47; PubMed

- Hematopoiesis is **first started in the yolk sac** by 14th day.
- **By 10th week,** the **liver becomes the major site.** The great enlargement of the early fetal liver is due to its erythropoietic function. Gradually, the red cell production sites extend to the spleen and bone marrow
- Near term, the bone marrow becomes the major site of red cell production.
- During the first half, the hemoglobin is of fetal type (α-2, γ-2) but from 24 weeks onwards, adult type of hemoglobin (α-2, β-2) **appears and at term about 75–80% of the total hemoglobin is of fetal type** (HbF).

302. Ans. (a) Umbilical artery

Ref: DC Dutta, 8th ed. pg. 36

- Deoxygenated blood from fetus to mother is carried via umbilical artery.
- Oxygenated blood is via umbilical vein.

303. Ans. (a) 6–7 weeks

Ref: DC Dutta, 8th ed. pg. 734

- Cardiac activity be assessed at the earliest by trans-vaginal scan by 5 weeks
- Cardiac activity be assessed by transabdominal scan by 6 weeks
- Fetal heart sound can be assessed by Doppler- 10 weeks
- Fetal heart sound can be assessed by stethoscope-18 weeks

304. Ans. (a) 7 cm

Ref: DC Dutta 7th ed./ 41; William's Obstetrics 22nd ed./ 91

- To determine the length of the fetus, the measurement is commonly taken from the vertex to the coccyx (crown-rump length) in earlier weeks of gestation.
  - By the end of the 12th week of pregnancy, when the uterus usually is just palpable above the symphysis pubis, the crown-rump length of the fetus is *6–7 cm.*
  - **At 16th week, CRL:** 12 cm and the weight is about 110 gm.
  - **At 28th week, CRL:** 25 cm and the weight is about 1100 gm.
  - **At 32nd week, CRL:** 28 cm and the weight is about 1800 gm.
  - **At 36th weeks, CRL:** 32 cm and the weight is about 2500 gm.
- From the end of 20th week onwards, the measurement is taken from the vertex to the heel (crown-heel length).

Extra Mile

- Best fetal parameter to find out AOG in 1st trimester: CRL (Crown Rump length)
- Best fetal parameter to find out AOG in 2nd trimester: BPD (Biparietal diameter)
- Best fetal parameter to find out AOG in 3rd trimester: Femur Length.

305. Ans. (a) 60 mm

Ref: DC Dutta 7th ed./41; William's Obstetrics 22nd ed. pg. 91

- By the end of the 12th week of pregnancy, when the uterus usually is just palpable above the symphysis pubis, the crown-rump length of the fetus is ***6 to 7 cm i.e. 60 to 70 mm.***
- *Please refer to above explanation for more details.*

306. Ans. (a) 4-16 weeks

Ref: Dutta's Obstetrics, 7th ed. pg. 647

RADIATION HAZARDS

1. **Teratogenecity:** Diagnostic range of radiation exposure (<5 Rads) is not associated with any congenital malformation.
2. **Oncogenecity:** Dividing cells particularly in **first trimester** are more sensitive to injury from radiation. Diagnostic radiation with fetal exposure is associated with an increased risk of malignancy.
3. **Genetic damage and intrauterine death**

Note: **Radiation during early stage of pregnancy can damage the embroyo. This risk can be minimized by using the "10 day rule". This rule states that:** *"No women should be exposed to X-ray for a non-urgent indication outside 10 days from her last period during reproductive period"*

307. Ans. (b) Megaloblastic anemia

Ref: Dutta's Obstetrics, 7th ed. pg. 268-69

- This is a bit confusing question though. But if we read the question carefully it is asking the outcome of combined Vitamin B_{12} and folate deficiency, which is Megaloblastic anemia according to the question.
- Neural tube defect is due to deficiency of folic acid (Vitamin B_9).
- Abruption placentae can be secondary to Vitamin B_{12} deficiency.

INTRAUTERINE FETAL DEATH

308. Ans. (b) Obstructed labor

Ref: D.C. Dutta, 7th ed. pg. 322-323

INTERAUTERINE FETAL DEATH (IUD)

- All fetal deaths weighing 500 gram or more occurring during pregnancy (antepartum death) or during labor (intrapartum).
- It is least likely caused by maternal factors like prolonged or obstructed labor, or due to uterine rupture.
- IUFD most commonly caused by fetal factors like Rh incompatibility, chromosomal abnormalities etc.

Causes of IUD

MATERNAL: 5-10%	FETAL: 25-40%
• Hypertensive disorder in pregnancy • Diabetes in pregnancy • Anti-phospholipid syndrome • Thrombophilias • *Abnormal labor: Prolonged or obstructed labor, ruptured uterus* • Post term pregnancy • Lupus Erythematosus	• Chromosomal abnormalities • *Rh-incompatibility* • Non immune hydrops • *Growth restriction*
PLACENTAL: 20-35%	**IATROGENIC**
• Antepartum haemorrhage • Cord accident • TTTS • *Placental insufficiency*	• External cephalic version • Drugs **IDIOPATHIC: 25-35%**

309. Ans. (b) Robert's sign

Ref: Dutta's Obstetrics, 7th ed. pg. 324

- **Robert's sign** refers to the presence of a gas shadow within the heart or the greater vessels, in cases of fetal death.
  - It is a rare sign caused by postmortem blood degeneration, usually seen 1–2 days after death
- **Spalding sign:** Overlapping of skull bone. *Also a sign of fetal demise.*
- **Goodell's sign:** Softening of the vaginal part of the cervix during the first trimester
- **Von Braun-Fernwald's sign:** Softening of the uterine fundus at the site of implantation at 4–5 weeks gestation.
- **Osiander sign:** Increased pulsation at lateral fornices of vagina seen at ~8th week of pregnancy.

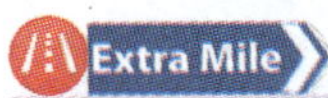

Robert Pelvis: Aka transversely contracted pelvis. Ala of both the sides are absent and sacrum is fused with innominate bones.

310. Ans. (a) Cord prolapsed

Ref: Dutta's Obstetrics, 7th ed. pg. 398

- **Most common cause of intrapartum fetal death is cord prolapsed. Overall perinatal mortality is 15-50%.**
- In other cases like abruption, Eclampsia, there are chances that we can terminate the pregnancy via emergency CS. But once there is cord prolapsed, there is sudden hypoxia to fetus leading to death.

311. Ans. (d) Ectopic pregnancy

Ref: DC Dutta, 8th ed. pg. 204, 216, 228, 486, 588

- DOC for ectopic pregnancy → Methotrexate

MISCELLANEOUS

312. Ans. (d) Placenta previa

Ref: William's Obstetrics, Chapter 42, 26th ed. pg. 1966

- In placenta previa, the placenta attaches lower in the uterus. This results in some portion of the placental tissue covering the cervix.
- It can result in bleeding during the pregnancy or during or after delivery.
- The main sign of placenta previa is bright red vaginal bleeding, usually without pain, after 20 weeks of pregnancy. Sometimes, spotting happens before an event with more blood loss.

313. Ans. (d) 10 mm

Ref: DC Dutta's 9th ed. pg. 619

- The karman cannula is a soft, flexible cannula which is used during vacuum aspiration.
- Its flexibility was claimed to reduce the risk of uterine perforation.
- Appropriate size of cannula is needed for a particular case, is same to the duration of pregnancy in weeks.
- In general, the size of the pregnant uterus and size of the cannula are:
- Uterus size 4–6 weeks: 4–7 mm of cannula
- Uterus size 7–9 weeks: 5–10 mm cannula
- Uterus size 9–12 weeks: 8–12 mm cannula.

314. Ans. (b) Curette

Ref: DC Dutta's 9th ed. pg. 617

- Uterine curette is a long metallic instrument with a small fenestrated end at each side. The shaft is there in the middle.
- It may be Sharp at both ends or sharp at one end and blunt at other end.
- It is commonly used instrument in dilatation and curettage.

315. Ans. (a) MRKH

Ref: Comprehensive Gynecology 7th ed. pg. 211; Shaw's Textbook of Gynaecology, 7th ed. pg. 145

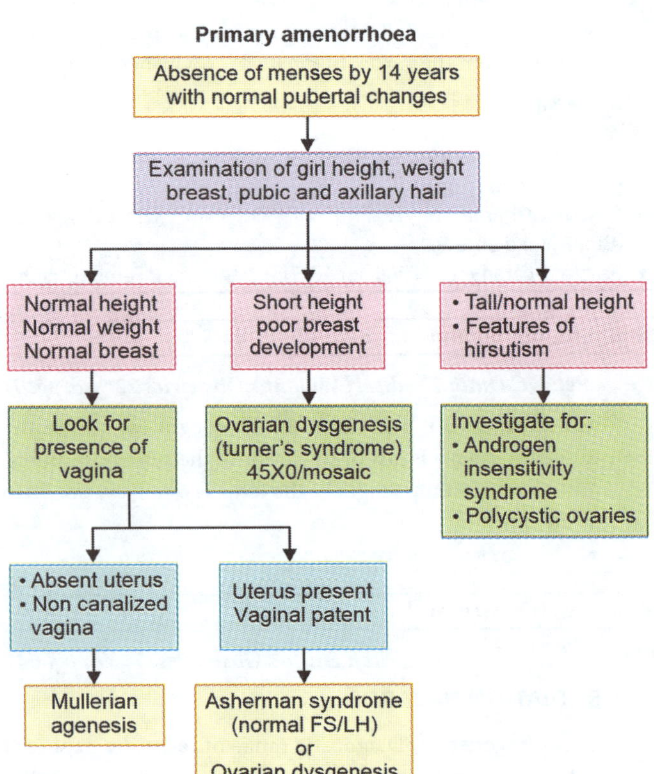

- Mayer-Rokitansky-Küster-Hauser (MRKH) syndrome is a disorder that occurs in females and mainly affects the reproductive system. This condition causes the vagina and uterus to be underdeveloped or absent, although external genitalia are normal.
- These individuals have normal pubertal development, normal ovarian function, and a 46, XX karyotype, and they commonly present with primary amenorrhea at 15 to 16 years of age.

316. Ans. (a) A

Ref: Shaw's Textbook of Gynaecology, 7th ed. pg. 49, 59

- The level of LH rises just before ovulation. LH peak is responsible for ovulation.

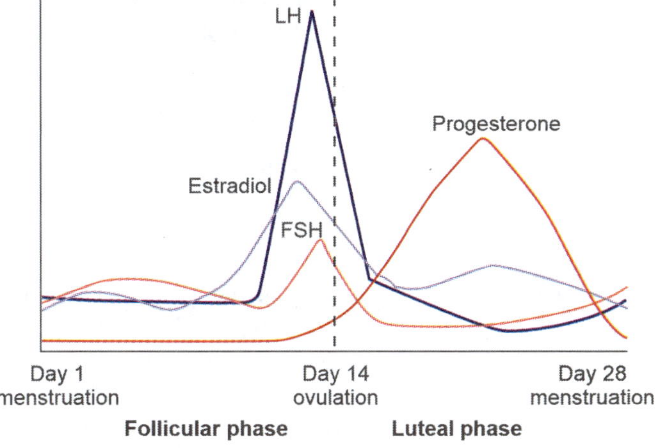

317. Ans. (b) Creates a negative pressure of 60 mm Hg

Ref: William's Obstetrics, Chapter 11, 26th ed. pg. 546; https://www.ncbi.nlm.nih.gov/pmc/articles/PMC7567277/

- Following dilation, for most first-trimester aspiration procedures, an 8–12 mm Karman cannula is appropriate.
- Small cannulas carry the risks of a longer surgery and of missed intrauterine tissue. For evacuation, the cannula is slowly moved toward the fundus until resistance is met. Suction is then activated.
- It creates a negative pressure of 660 mm Hg.
- The cannula is gradually pulled back toward the os and is simultaneously slowly turned circumferentially to cover the entire uterine cavity surface. This is repeated until no more tissue is aspirated.
- Capacity → 60 mL

318. Ans. (c) It has 4 to 6 lobes

Ref: William's obstetrics, 23rd ed. Implantation, Embroyogenesis and Placental development

PLACENTAL GROWTH

- ***In the first trimester, placental growth is more rapid than that of the fetus.***
- ***By approximately 17th weeks period of gestation, placental and fetal weights are approximately equal.***
- By term, placental weight is approximately one sixth of fetal weight.
- The average placenta at term is 185 mm in diameter and 23 mm in thickness, ***with a volume of 497 mL and a weight of 508 g.*** These measurements vary widely.
- From the maternal surface, the number of slightly elevated convex areas, ***called lobes, varies from 10 to 38.***
- Lobes are incompletely separated by grooves of variable depth that overlie *placental septa,* which arise from folding of the basal plate.
- Although grossly visible lobes are commonly referred to as cotyledons.
- ***The total number of placental lobes remains the same throughout gestation,*** and individual lobes continue to grow—although less actively in the final weeks.

319. Ans. (c) FSH

Ref: D.C. Dutta, 6th ed. pg. 56

- There is a significant fall in the level of serum estradiol from 50–300 pg/ml before menopause to 10–20 pg/ml after menopause.
- This decrease the negative feedback effect on hypothalamopituitary axis resulting in increase in FSH.
- The increase in FSH is also due to diminished inhibin.

320. Ans. (b) IgG

Ref: Robbin's, 9th ed. pg. 198-199

321. Ans. (c) 3 months

Ref: DC Dutta, 8th ed. pg. 735

322. Ans. (c) 300 μg

Ref: DC Dutta, 8th ed. pg. 387, 721

GYNECOLOGY

ANATOMY, MENARCHE AND MENOPAUSE

323. Ans. (c) O

"O" is suggestive of ovulation, for ovulation LH surge is important that occur on 14th day of mensutral cycle.

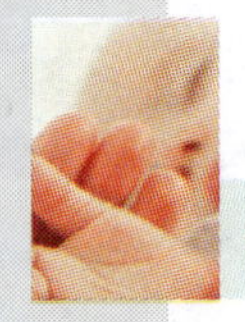

324. Ans. (c) Progesterone

Ref: William's Obstetrics 25th ed. pg. 179

- The given history reveals the case of puberty menorrhagia, where patient can present with irregular heavy menstrual bleeding.
- In these patients, therapy with progesterone with NSAIDs and reassurance is usually advised.
- Progesterone acts as an anti-inflammatory agent, and thus its deficiency raises cytokine levels in the endometrium.
- In human menstruation, progesterone plays a critical role. Two progesterone receptors (PR) are found in the endometrium, PR-A and PR-B.
- In the secretory phase, PR-B levels decline in the stromal and glandular epithelial cells of the functionalis layer.
- However, PR-A expression in this layer persists in the stromal cells, which thus remain responsive to progesterone and to its withdrawal.

325. Ans. (d) Increased FSH, decreased estrogen

Ref: Shaw, 16th ed. pg. 66–67

- Menopause is a retrospective diagnosis as it takes 12 months of amenorrhoea to confirm that menopause has set in.
- Menopause normally occurs between the ages of **45 and 50 years,** the **average age being 47 years**.
- At the time of menopause there is cessation of ovarian activity and a fall in the estrogen and inhibin levels → cause a rebound increase in the secretion of FSH and LH by the anterior pituitary gland.
- The FSH level may rise as much as 50-fold and LH 3–4 folds.
- There is 50% reduction in androgen production and 66% reduction in estrogen at menopause
  - There is a significant fall in the level of serum estradiol from 50–300 pg/ml before menopause to 10-20 pg/ml after menopause

Extra Mile

Prediction of approaching menopause:
- A fall in the level of inhibin B (not inhibin A) causes a rise in follicle-stimulating hormone (FSH) level.
- A **fall in the level of anti-müllerian hormone** suggests low ovarian reserve and low antral follicular count.
- Rise of FSH level more than normal luteinizing hormone (LH) level.

326. Ans. (c) 14

Ref: DC Dutta 7th ed. pg. 371

- The normal upper limit of menarche is 15 years.
- According to recent recommendation, primary amenorrhea is defined as:
  - Absence of menses by 14 years of age in absence of sexual characters.
  - Absence of menses by 16 years of age regardless of presence of secondary sexual characteristics.

327. Ans. (a) Pelvic irradiation

Ref: DC Dutta 7th ed. pg. 376

- Secondary amenorrhea is defined as: *"absence of menstruation for 6 months or more in a women in whom normal menstruation has been established"*
- **Book states:** *"Amenorrhea in a woman with reproductive age should be considered as pregnancy unless proved otherwise".* Therefore, pregnancy is considered as most common cause of amenorrhea in a woman of reproductive age.
- Note: Amenorrhea is physiological before puberty, during pregnancy and lactation and following menopause.
- **The most common cause of secondary amenorrhea** (pathological) is hypothalamic dysfunction. Pelvic irradiation is one of the causes of hypothalamic dysfunction.
  - Kallmann syndrome and imperforate hymen are usually associated with primary amenorrhea.
  - Diabetes and hypothyroidism is the systemic cause of secondary amenorrhea.
- **MCC of cryptomenorrhea** is imperforate hymen.
- **MCC of primary amenorrhea** is gonadal failure, abnormal chromosomal pattern, developmental defect of genital tract and disturbed action of HPO axis.

328. Ans. (d) Anti-mullerian hormone

Ref: Shaw's Gynecology 16th ed, pg. 65–66, 260

Test for ovarian reserve is indicated in:

- Women >35 years of age, smokers, presence of only one ovary and unexplained infertility.
- It involves standard day 3 FSH estimation, along with administration of 100 mg CC from day 5 to day 9, repeat FSH on day 10. FSH values must be the same as on day 3 of the cycle.

Prediction of approaching menopause:

- A fall in the level of inhibin B (not inhibin A) causes a rise in follicle-stimulating hormone (FSH) level.
- A **fall in the level of anti-müllerian hormone** suggests low ovarian reserve and low antral follicular count.
- Rise of FSH level more than normal luteinizing hormone (LH) level.

Anti-müllerian Hormone (AMH)

- AMH is a peptide secreted by the sertoli cells in the testis and granulosa cells in the ovary.
- During intrauterine life AMH inhibits the development of **müllerian** system in males. Absence of AMH results in hermaphrodite.
- In the female it helps in the follicular development and oocyte maturation.
  - Normal value is 2–6.8 ng/mL
  - **Poor ovarian reserve:** 1 ng/mL
  - **PCOD and hyperstimulation syndrome:** 0.10 ng/mL
- Estimation of serum AMH is used in the study of ovarian reserve in an infertile woman and a woman with secondary amenorrhea.
- Its level is related to precocious and delayed puberty, infertility and premature menopause.
- Its level is related and reflects the number of growing follicles.

329. Ans. (b) Class II

Ref: Shaw's 16th ed. pg. 118

American fertility society classification system classified müllerian malformations into 6 classes:

- **Class I (agenesis, hypoplasia).** Uterus is absent in total agenesis. Partial agenesis is identified as unicornuate uterus. In hypoplasia, the endometrial cavity is small with reduced intercornual distance of <2 cm.
- **Class II (unicornuate uterus)** appears **banana-shaped** without the rounded fundus and triangular-shaped uterine cavity. If present, rudimentary horn presents as a soft tissue mass with similar myometrial echogenicity. Obstruction in the rudimentary horn is recognized as haematometra on one side.
- **Class III (uterus didelphys).** The two horns are widely separated, but vaginal septum is difficult to identify.
- **Class IV (bicornuate uterus)** shows two uterine cavities, with concave fundus, with fundal cleft greater than 1 cm, and this differentiates between the bicornuate and the septate uterus. The intercornual distance is more than 4 cm.
- **Class V (septate uterus)** shows a convex or flattened fundus. The intercornual distance is normal (<4 cm) and each cavity is small.
- **Class VI (arcuate uterus)** with no fundus is of no clinical importance.

330. Ans. (b) Growth of breast

Ref: Shaw, 16th ed. pg. 56

Thelarche

- The first sign of puberty is the development of the breasts. Breast budding usually appears between the ages of 9–11 years.
- It is indicative of the competency of the hypothalamic–pituitary–ovarian axis.

331. Ans. (a) GnRH

Ref: Shaw, 16th ed. pg. 56

Endocrine mechanisms underlying puberty: These have been highlighted in the following:

- **Early in puberty**, the sensitivity of the gonadostat to the negative effects of low estradiol (E2) gradually decreases.
- **Late in puberty**, maturation of positive E2 feedback initiates the LH surge.
- Basal levels of pituitary gonadotropins **increase throughout puberty** due to enhanced hypothalamic GnRH pulse amplitude rather than frequency.

332. Ans. (b) 45

Ref: Shaw, 16th ed. pg. 66

- Menopause is defined as the time of cessation of ovarian function resulting in permanent amenorrhoea.
- Menopause is a retrospective diagnosis as it takes 12 months of amenorrhoea to confirm that menopause has set in.
- Menopause normally occurs between the ages of **45 and 50 years,** the **average age being 47 years**.

Extra Mile

- **Climacteric** is the phase of waning ovarian activity, and may begin 2–3 years before menopause and continue for 2–5 years after it. The climacteric is thus a phase of adjustment between the active and inactive ovarian function.
- Menopause setting **before the age of 40** is known as **premature menopause.**
- Menopausal age is NOT related to menarche, race, socioeconomic status, number of pregnancies and lactation, or taking of oral contraceptives.

333. Ans. (c) Appearance of secondary sexual characteristics before 8 years

Ref: Shaw's, 16th ed. pg. 59

- **Precocious puberty:** This is defined as the appearance of any of the **secondary sexual characteristics before the age of 8 years** or the **occurrence of menarche before the age of 10** years
- Precocious puberty in females is pubertal changes before the age of 8 years.
- In males it is onset of puberty before the age of 9 years

334. Ans. (a) Increase FSH

Ref: Yen and Jaffe's Reproductive Endocrinology, pg. 155

- FSH levels increase with age, before increases in LH or decrease in estradiol and a number of studies have demonstrated an inverse relationship between increase

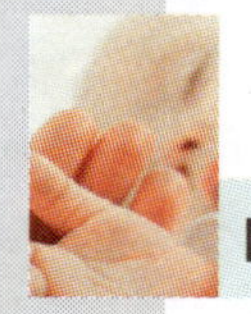

in FSH and decreasing inhibin B in association with reproductive aging."

- **Ref states:** *"Reproductive aging is associated with decline in fertility that* ***begins in third decade,*** *which accelerates after age 35. A gradual decrease in pool of ovarian follicles which first accelerates around the same age would appear to underlie this decline in fertility.* ***It is also at age 35 that an increase in FSH is first seen."***

Extra Mile

- The first evidence of primordial follicle appears at about 20 weeks of fetal life. The fetal ovary contains **7 million primordial follicles** but most degenerate, and **the newborn contains only 2 million follicles.**
- At birth, about 2 million follicles seen are reduced **to 400,000 at puberty;**
- **Only 400 follicles are available during the childbearing period for fertilization.**

335. Ans. (c) Hematocolpos

Ref: Shaws, 15th ed. pg. 96-98

- **Hematocolpos** is a medical condition in which the vagina fills with menstrual blood. It is often caused by the combination of menstruation with an imperforate hymen.
- **Hematometra:** A related disorder is, where the uterus is filled with menstrual blood.
- **Pyometra:** a type of uterine infection. Disease of the dogs, but has been also noted in humans.
- **Hematosalphinx:** Bleeding and collection of blood in fallopian tube. MCC is tubal (ectopic) pregnancy.

INFECTION

336. Ans. (c) Gardnerella vaginalis, metronidazole

Ref: Williams Gynaecology 3rd ed. pg. 51

The given clinical case is suggestive of bacterial vaginosis.

- Organisms responsible for bacterial vaginosis are *haemophilia vaginalis* and *gardnerella vaginalis.*
- It is the most common form of vaginitis overall and the most common complaint of the patient is foul smelling dirty white discharge. There is no inflammation hence no itching.
- Investigation of choice of this patient is saline microscopy, *clue cells* i.e., vaginal epithelial cells to which bacteria are adhered seen.
- Amine test/whiff test i.e., 10% KOH added to discharge is positive. Fishy odour or amine like odour obtained.
- Treatment for non-pregnant females is metronidazole or Clindamycin.
- Simultaneous treatment of male partner is not needed as it is not an STD.

337. Ans. (b) Infertility

Ref: Shaw's Gynecology 16th ed. pg. 181, 185

- Lower abdominal pain, adnexal tenderness, cervical motion tenderness – Triad is the criteria for diagnosis of PID pelvic inflammatory disease.
- **Sequelae of PID:**
  - Infertility (6–60%)
  - Ectopic pregnancy
  - Chronic pelvic pain
  - Dyspareunia
  - Fitz – Hugh Curtis Syndrome.

338. Ans. (d) Per vaginum examination

Ref: Shaw's Gynecology 16th ed. pg. 373

- Greenish yellow discharge with foul odor, most probably it is due to Trichomonas vaginitis infection.
- **Investigation of choice:** Saline microscopy done (typical motile flagellated trichomonas seen) or some motility of trichomonas seen on pap smear, if pap smear show this, a saline microscopy should be done to confirm.
- Gold standard investigation – culture.

339. Ans. (a) Trichomonas

Ref: Shaw's 16th ed. pg. 163

- These are two Trichomonas vaginalis, magnified view under a microscope (Hanging drop appearance).
- Trichomoniasis is most common STD caused by infection Trichomonas vaginalis. Discharge of green yellow color, fowl smelling, PH more than 4.5.
- On microscopy flagellated organism seen.
- Investigation of choice is Culture (Stuart's media).
- STD so partner should also be treated.
- Drug of choice – Metronidazole.

340. Ans. (a) Chlamydia

Ref: Shaw's Gynecology 16th ed. pg. 294

- Most common cause of PID include sexually transmitted infections like chlamydia trachomatis and gonorrhoea.
- Other leading causes of salpingitis are septic abortion, post-abortal sepsis and puerperal sepsis
- With reduction in the incidence of gonococcal infection, chlamydial infection predominates and causes extensive and more damage than that caused by gonococcal infection.
- **Note:** With the PID caused by chlamydial infection, risk of ectopic pregnancy increases.

341. Ans. (a) Endometrial curettage

Ref: Williams Gynecology 4th ed. pg. 56-87

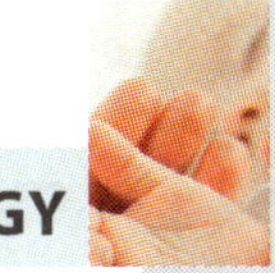

- In investigating the possibility of genital tract TB, the most accessible tissue for study with a high frequency of involvement is the endometrium.
- The histologic examination of endometrial tissues removed by biopsy or curettage, especially from the cornual area, affords a rapid method of diagnosing genital TB in at least 50% of cases.
- Endometrial biopsy is a frequent first diagnostic step, and although its sensitivity suffers from sampling errors, it can be very helpful if granulomata are found or, less commonly, if smears or cultures are positive for M. tuberculosis.

342. Ans. (a) Gardenella vaginosis

Ref: Williams Gynecology 4th ed. pg. 56-57

- Bacterial vaginosis is a common, complex, and poorly understood clinical syndrome reflects vaginal flora in which anaerobic species are over- represented.
- These include Gardnerella, Prevotella, Mobiluncus, and Bacteroides species; Atopobium vaginae, and BV-associated bacteria, provisionally named BVABI, BVAB2, and BVAB3.
- For diagnosis, clinical criteria 1st proposed by Amsel and associates (1983) include:
  - Microscopic evaluation of a vaginal secretion saline preparation
  - Release of volatile amines produced by anaerobic metabolism, and
  - Determination of the vaginal pH.

343. Ans. (b) Leads to Infertility

Ref: Harrison 20th ed. pg. 1319 - 1321

- The chlamydia species are classified mainly into 4 species:
  - *C. trachomatis*
  - *C. pneumonia*
  - *C. psittaci* (separated into 3 species: *C. psittaci*, *C. felis*, C. abortus)
  - *C. pecorum* (the last species being found in ruminants)

Infections associated with Chlamydia trachomatis

- **Trachoma:** C. trachomatis (serotype A, B, Ba and C)- can cause ocular infection trachoma and adult inclusion conjunctivitis.
- **Oculogenital infections (serotype D – K)**
  - Transmitted during sexual contact or from mother to baby during childbirth. Associated with:
    - **Female:** Cervicitis, salpingitis, acute urethral syndrome, endometritis, ectopic pregnancy, infertility, pelvic pain and PID.
      - Untreated PID and High levels of antibody to human heat-shock protein have been associated with tubal factor infertility and ectopic pregnancy.
    - **Males:** Urethritis, proctitis, and epididymitis
    - **Infants:** Conjunctivitis (inclusion body conjunctivitis) and pneumonia
- **LGV (L1, L2, L3)**
  - Characterized by acute lymphadenitis with bubo formation and/or acute hemorrhagic proctitis.

Extra Mile

- *C. pneumoniae* is a common cause of human respiratory diseases, such as pneumonia and bronchitis
- It mainly causes atypical pneumonia as seen with mycoplasma pneumonia
- The clinical spectrum of *C. pneumoniae* infection includes acute pharyngitis, sinusitis, bronchitis, and pneumonitis, primarily in young adults

344. Ans. (a) Chlamydia

Ref: Harrison 20th ed. Page 1319 - 1321

Refer to above explanation

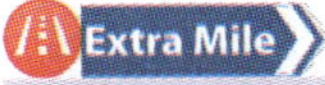

Extra Mile

TABLE: Contraindications of gastric lavage

	Symptoms signs	Examination findings	pH	Wet mount
Normal	White floccular or curdy, odorless	Discharge present in dependent portions of vagina	3.8–4.5	Normal
Bacterial vaginosis	Increased white thin discharge, increased odor	Thin whitish gray homogenous discharge sometimes frothy	>4.5 basic	Clue cells >20% shift in flora, amine odor after KOH smear
Candidiasis	Increased white thick discharge, pruritus, dysuria, burning	Thick curdy discharge, vaginal erythema	<4.5 Acidic	Hyphae or spores
Trichomonas	Increased yellow frothy discharge, increased odor, pruritus, dysuria	Yellow frothy discharge with or without vaginal or cervical erythema	>45 Basic	Motile trichomonads Increased white cells

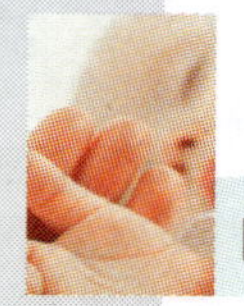

345. Ans. (c) Cryosurgery

Ref: Shaw's Gynecology 16th ed. 173-74

- The patient in this case is a case of cervicitis.
- **Acute cervicitis:** More commonly secondary to STD (chlamydia trachomatis, gonorrhoea), septic abortion and puerperal sepsis.
- **Chronic cervicitis:** More common than acute variant. Usually due to traumatic childbirth, D&C or a sequel of STD.
- **Clinical features:**
  - Profuse mucoid vaginal discharge, which can be blood stained
  - Postcoital bleeding
  - Antepartum haemorrhage
  - Low backache, abdominal pain and dyspareunia
- **Upon examination:**
  - Cervical erosion
  - Erosion takes the form of a reddened area around the external os, with its inner margin continuous with the endocervical lining and with a well-defined outer margin.
  - In chronic cases cervix is fibrosed, bulky with nabothian follicles around the area of erosion
- **Treatment:**
  - **Diathermy cauterization:** Tissues of cervix are coagulated and columnar epithelium is destroyed. It also destroys all infection lying in the depths of the racemose glands and in due course healthy epithelium grows down from the upper part of the cervical canal to cover the raw area.
    - Require opening of cervical os and anaesthesia
  - **Cryosurgery:** More preferred nowadays. Safer than cautery as it is painless and avoids accidental burn in vagina. Doesn't require anaesthesia
    - The refrigerants used in cryosurgery are carbon dioxide (–78°C), Freon (–81°C), nitrous oxide (–88°C) and nitrogen (–186°C).
    - **Disadvantage:** Extensive tissue destruction → hypokalemia
  - **Laser therapy:** Highly preferred in chronic cervicitis.
    - Fast healing and accurate/precise excision or burning of tissue
  - **Conization operation:** Preferred if above methods are ineffective or if there is extensive area involved.
  - **Policresulen:** One gram of Policresulen contains 360 mg of protein. It coagulates necrotic, pathologically altered tissue without destroying the healthy tissue.
    - Contraindicated during pregnancy.

346. Ans. (a) Hematogenous

Ref: Shaw's Gyencology 16th ed. pg. 188

- The general distribution of involvement of reproductive organs in cases of genital TB are as follows:
  - **Fallopian tube:** 90–100%
  - **Endometrium:** 50–60%
  - **Ovaries:** 20–30%
  - **Cervix:** 5–15%
  - **Vulva and vagina:** <1%
- The tubal mucosa is the most favorable nidus for **bloodborne** spread of the disease resulting in endosalpingitis—usually bilateral.
- It is the earliest lesion with a propensity for transluminal spread to the ovary and endometrium.
- Hence, fallopian tubes play the central role in the initiation and dissemination of pelvic tuberculosis.
- **Radiological appearance:** Tobacco pouch appearance.

347. Ans. (b) Candida vaginitis

Ref: Shaw's 16th ed. P 164

- Candidiasis is a fungal infection caused by yeast-like microorganisms called *Candida or Monilia.*
- The most common species causing human disease is Candida albicans. It can be sexually transmitted.

Risk Factors

- These include promiscuity, immunosuppression, HIV, pregnancy, steroid therapy, following long-term broad-spectrum antibiotic therapy, oral contraception pills, diabetes mellitus, poor personal hygiene and obesity.

Clinical Features

- **Pruritus vulva is the cardinal symptom:** It is often accompanied by vaginal irritation, dysuria, or both, and **passage of thick curdy or flaky discharge.**
- Speculum examination reveals vaginal wall congestion with **curdy discharge** often visible at the vulval mucocutaneous junction and in the posterior fornix.

Diagnosis

- Microscopic examination 10% KOH mount
- Culture on **Sabouraud agar or Nickerson's medium** helps to identify *Candida.*
- Pap smear shows thick red-stained hyphae and dark red spores.

Treatment

- **DOC:** Fluconazole 150 mg single dose. Both partners should be treated.
- Local intravaginal application of antifungal agents such as imidazole, miconazole, clotrimazole, butoconazole or terconazole vaginal pessaries or creams used for 3–6 days is very effective.

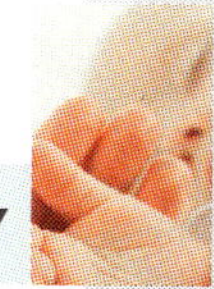

Extra Mile

- **Trichomoniasis** present with typical discharge, which is profuse, thin, creamy or slightly green in color, irritating and frothy. Itchy tender, angry looking vaginal walls and strawberry vagina.
- **Chlamydia infection** (a STD) is usually asymptomatic but may develop vaginal discharge, dysuria and **increased frequency** of micturition, and at times cervicitis. Sometimes, chlamydia may cause Reiter's syndrome with arthritis, skin lesions, conjunctivitis and genital infection.
- **Gonococcal vulvovaginitis** presents with urinary frequency and dysuria, dyspareunia, rectal discomfort, vaginal discharge. Vulvovaginal/perineal infection often results in inflammation, discharge, irritation causing pruritus and dysuria.

348. Ans. (c) 100.4°F

Ref: DC Dutta 8th ed. pg. 500

- Puerperal pyrexia is defined as a rise of temperature reaching **100.4°F (38°C)** or more (measured orally) on two separate occasions at 24 hours apart (excluding first 24 hours) within first 10 days following delivery.

Causes of Puerperal Pyrexta

- Puerperal sepsis
- **Urinary tracht infections:** Cystitis, pyelonephritis
- Mastitis, breast abscess
- **Wound infections:** CS or episiotomy
- **Pulmonary infections:** Atelectasis, pneumonia
- Septic pelvic thrombophlebitis
- A recrudescence of malaria or pulmonary tuberculosis
- **Others:** Pharyngitis, gastroenteritis

349. Ans. (a) Chlamydia

Ref: Shaw's Gynecology 16th ed. P 181

- Pelvic inflammatory disease is a leading cause of tubal obstruction and the most common associated organism is chlamydia.
- **Shaw's states:** *"Chlamydial infection causes more damage to the mucosa and the wall of the tube than gonorrhoea, leading to fibrosis and tubal blockage".*
- **Other causes** of tubal obstruction can be: Gornorrheal infeaction, tuberculosis of uterus and fallopian tube, postoperative.

350. Ans. (a) Pregnancy

Ref: Shaw, 16th ed. pg. 177-78, 183

- Pelvic inflammatory disease (PID) implies inflammation of the upper genital tract involving the fallopian tubes as well as the ovaries.
- The most common cause of PID is *sexually transmitted diseases* (STD).
- Gonococcal and chlamydial infections are most common, the incidence of the two varying in different communities. **Chlamydia being the commonest**.

Indications for hospitalization in PID

- The mild cases of acute PID are treated at home with antibiotics.
- Moderate and severe cases of PID need hospitalization.
- Those who need the diagnosis to be confirmed also require to be admitted for investigations.
- Those who need intravenous therapy need admission.

351. Ans. (a) Infertility

Ref: Shaw, 16th ed. pg. 188

- Most common site of genital TB is fallopian tube: 90–100%

Other sites:

- Endometrium: 50–60%
- Ovaries: 20–30%
- Cervix: 5–15%
- Vulva and vagina: 1%

Clinical feature:

- **Infertility:** This is an important presenting symptom. In fact, in 35–60% cases it may be the only complaint for which the patient seeks medical attention.
- **Menstrual irregularity:** This has been observed in 10–40% of cases. The menstrual disturbances reported include menorrhagia, menometrorrhagia, intermenstrual bleeding, oligomenorrhoea, hypomenorrhoea, amenorrhoea and even postmenopausal bleeding.

Chronic pelvic pain:

- Vaginal discharge
- Abdominal mass
- Fistula
- Ectopic pregnancy

352. Ans. (b) >3 infection in a year

Ref: Katz Comprehensive Gyenecology, 5th ed. Ch 22

Katz states: *"Recurrent vulvo-vaginits (bacterial vaginosis/ vulvovaginal candidiasis) is defined as three or more documented episodes in one year"*

353. Ans. (a) Bacterial vaginosis

Ref: Shaws, 15th ed. pg. 309

Gardnerella (Bacterial) Vaginosis

- **Bacterial vaginosis** is termed vaginosis rather than vaginitis, because it is associated with alteration in the normal vaginal flora rather than due to any specific infection.
- Bacterial vaginosis is a vaginal infection casued by **Gardenella vaginalis.**
- Bacterial vaginosis is diagnosed on the basis of the following findings:

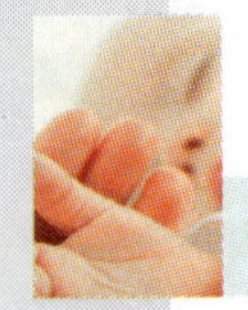

- Vaginal secretions are gray and thinly coat the vaginal walls.
- The pH of these secretions **is *higher than 4.5*** (usually 4.7 to 5.7).
- Microscopy of the vaginal secretions reveals an ***increased number of clue cells, and leukocytes are conspicuously absent.***
- The addition of **10% KOH to the vaginal secretions *(the "whiff" test)*** releases a fishy, amine-like odor.

- This infection can cause PID, chorioamnionitis, premature rupture of membrane (PROM) and preterm Labor.

Treatment: Metronidazole 500 mg BD × 1 week is effective

354. Ans. (d) Gardenella vaginalis

Ref: Shaws's, 15th ed. pg. 309

355. Ans. (b) Bacterial vaginosis

Ref: Shaws, 15th ed. pg. 309

356. Ans. (c) Infection seen when vaginal pH is <4.5

Ref: Shaws, 15th ed. pg. 308-310

- *After reading this question, usually we get this tendency to mark option D, which says bacterial vaginosis is NOT a STD, but this statement is true.*
- Bacterial vaginosis is a vaginal infection casued by Gardenella vaginalis (NOT a STD).
- ***Bacterial vaginosis is diagnosed on the basis of the following findings:***
  - Vaginal secretions are gray and thinly coat the vaginal walls.
  - The pH of these secretions **is *higher than 4.5*** (usually 4.7 to 5.7).
  - Microscopy of the vaginal secretions reveals an ***increased number of clue cells, and leukocytes are conspicuously absent.***
  - The addition of KOH to the vaginal secretions *(the "whiff" test)* releases a fishy, amine-like odor.

Extra Mile

- Most common vaginal infections during pregnancy is candidiasis
- Bacterial vaginosis (BV) is the most common vaginal infection in women of childbearing age
- Genital human papillomavirus the most common sexually transmitted infection.

357. Ans. (a) Bacterial vaginosis

Ref: Shaws, 15th ed. pg. 309

358. Ans. (b) Gardenella

Ref: Shaws, 15th ed. pg. 131-132

- Whiff test or amine test is done for gardenella (bacterial) vaginosis.
- It is performed by adding a small amount of potassium hydroxide (KOH) to a microscopic slide containing the vaginal discharge. ***A characteristic fishy odor is considered a positive whiff test*** and is suggestive of bacterial vaginosis.

359. Ans. (b) Urethra

Ref: Shaws, 15th ed. pg. 350

CHLAMYDIA

- Chlamydial infection is common in young, sexually active women. The incubation period is 6-14 days. It is sexually transmitted by vaginal and rectal intercourse.
- Chlamydia trachomatis is a small gram-negative bacteria, an obligate intracellular parasite that appears as intra cytoplasmic inclusion body, and is of two varieties, one that causes lympho granuloma venereum (LGV) and the other of non-LGV, which causes non-specific lower genital tract infection.
- Often, the infection is asymptomatic but may develop vaginal discharge, dysuria and frequency of micturition, and at times cervicitis.
- ***In asymptomatic cases, Chlamydia resides most commonly in urethra.***
- Sometimes, chlamydia may cause Reiter's syndrome with arthritis, conjunctivitis and genital infection associated with skin lesions. *(can't see, can't pee & can't walk)*

The cervix is the first site of infection. Ascending upwards causes salpingitis and infertility

Diagnosis

- The use of fluorescein-conjugated monoclonal antibody in immunofluorescence tests on smears prepared from urethral and cervical secretion allows a direct diagnosis of the infection to be made.

Note:

- Cervical ectopy with bleeding on touch and mucopurulent discharge is seen when the cervix is infected.
- Chlamydial infection and gonococcal infection often coexist and both attack the columnar epithelium of the genital tract and urethra. ***Urine can be cultured in suspected chlamydial infection.***

Treatment

- Tetracycline 500 mg and clindamycin 500 mg 6 hourly × 2 weeks is effective.

360. Ans. (a) Pain

Ref: Katz: Comprehensive Gynecology, 5th ed. Ch 23, Tuberculosis William's gynecology, ch 18

- Pelvic TB are uncommon, but when occurs, it involves **fallopian tube in most of the cases.**
- Without pasteurization of milk, bovine tuberculosis produces primary infections in the human gastrointestinal tract. This leads to Subsequent lymphatic or hematogenous dissemination results in pelvic tuberculosis.
- **The clinical presentations of this chronic infection are:**
  - ***Mild to moderate chronic abdominal and pelvic pain occur (in 35% patients)***
  - Infertility and abnormal uterine bleeding.
  - Often times, the advanced cases presents with ascites while some women may be asymptomatic.
  - The remaining patients have bilateral adnexal masses and mild adnexal tenderness, with an inability to manipulate the adnexa because of scarring and fixation.

361. Ans. (c) Hydrosalpinx

Ref: Williams Gynecology, ch. 9, Pelvic mass; Fallopian Tube pathology

HYDROSALPINX

- Results secondary to chronic PID.
- ***Grossly, the fine fimbria and tubal ostia are obliterated and replaced by a smooth, clubbed end.*** The ballooned, thin walls of the elongated tube are whitish and translucent, and the tube is typically distended with a clear serous fluid.
- Depending on the degree and location of the ipsilateral ovary, the hydrosalpinx may be adhered to it.
- Hydrosalpinx may be found in asymptomatic women during pelvic examination or incidentally during sonography or HSG done for other indications. Some women note infertility or chronic pelvic pain.

Treatment

- For women not wishing to preserve fertility, laparoscopic treatment may include lysis of adhesions and salpingectomy.
- In women who desire fertility, surgical intervention depends on the degree of tubal damage.

Extra Mile

- **HYSTEROSALPINGOGRAPHY:** To study the patency of the fallopian tubes in infertility and postoperative tuboplasty and also employed to study uterine anomalies.
- ***If in the question, clubbing of ampullary end is asked, the answer would be tuberculosis.***

362. Ans. (d) Mycobacterium tuberculosis

Ref: Shaws 15th ed. /158-159; DC Dutta 8th ed./ 158-159

TB is also an important cause of **infertility**. Other salient features about TB are as follows:

- Most common presentation of g
  enital TB is infertility.
- HSG is contraindicated in case of genital TB
- Best time to do HSG is **within 10 days** of LMP.
- Vaginal epithelium is resistant to TB.
- MC mode of spread of genital TB is **hematogenous.**
- TB salpingitis belong to stage V of PID.
- Conception rate even after treatment of genital TB is quite low.

363. Ans. (a) IUCD insertion

Ref: William's Gyenecology ch 3

- IUCD acts by causing local inflammation at endometrial site. It increases the risk of PID in female.
- Oral contraceptives decreases the risk of PID.

TABLE: Pelvic Inflammatory Disease Risk Factors

Douching
Single status
Substance abuse
Multiple sexual partners
Lower socioeconomic status
Recent new sexual partner (s)
Younger age (10 to 19 years)
Other sexually transmitted infections
Sexual partner with urethritis or gonorrhea
Previous diagnosis of pelvic inflammatory disease
Not using mechanical and/or chemical contraceptive barriers
Endocervical testing positive for *N. Gonorrhoeae* or *C. Trachomatis*

364. Ans. (d) Laproscopy

Ref: Shaws, 15th ed. pg. 451, DC Dutta, 8th ed. pg. 451

- Laproscopy is helpful in confirming the diagnosis as well as to know extent of disease.
- It is the current criterion standard for the diagnosis of PID. No single laboratory test is highly specific or sensitive for the disease.
- **Other investigations are:**
  - ESR
  - Hemogram

CERVICAL CANCER

365. Ans. (c) HPV 18

Ref: Williams Gynaecology 3rd ed. pg. 657

- The most common etiological factor associated with CA cervix is Human Papilloma Virus (HPV)
- High risk HPV include 16, 18, 31, E3, 35, 39, 45, 52, 56, 58, 59, 68
- Low risk HPV include 6 and 11, which are associated with genital warts and laryngeal papillomas.
- Most common HPV subtype associated with the CA cervix is HPV 16.
- HPV subtype most specific for the CA cervix is HPV 18.

366. Ans. (c) Ovary

Ref: Grainger & Allison's Diagnostic Radiology: A Textbook of Medical Imaging, 7th ed. pg. 882

- The most radiosensitive organ is ovary > rectum > bladder > vagina.
- Radiation tolerance dose for ovary is 2–3 Gy whereas vagina 90 Gy.
- Thus, Ovary is most radiosensitive and Vagina is most radioresistant in the pelvis.

367. Ans. (a) Concurrent chemoradiotherapy

Ref: Shaw's Textbook of Gynaecology, 7th ed. pg. 425,429

	Stagewise treatment of Cancer of the cervix
Stage Ia1	Conization or extrafascial hysterectomy (Type 1)
Stage Ia2	Modified Radical hysterectomy (Type 2)
Stage Ib1	Radical hysterectomy (Type 3)
Stage Ib2	Radical hysterectomy (Type 3) or Chemoradiation
Stage IIa	Radical hysterectomy (Type 3) or Chemoradiation
Stage II b, Stage III a, Stage III b	Chemoradiation
Stage IV	Palliative radiotherapy

368. Ans. (a) VIA

Ref: Comprehensive Gynecology 7th ed. pg. 734

- Visual inspection with acetic acid (VIA) is a simple, inexpensive test with moderate sensitivity and specificity for screening that can be combined with simple treatment procedures for early cervical lesions.

369. Ans. (b) Cervical polyp

Ref: Shaw's Gynecology 16th ed. pg. 174-75

- Cervical polyps are frequent incidental finding during speculum exams and can be a source of postcoital bleeding secondary to cervical trauma with intercourse.
- On gross examination, they appear as smooth, reddish purple lobular structures that are friable and bleed easily when touched.
- Cervical polyp arises from the mucous membrane of the cervical canal. They form a swelling about the size of a pea.

370. Ans. (b) HPV 16

Ref: Shaw's Gynecology 16th ed. pg. 485

- Women with STD, HIV infection, herpes simplex virus 2 infection, human papilloma virus (HPV) infection **(16, 18, 31, 33)** or condylomata have a high predisposition to cancer.
- Out of these HPV is now considered the most important cause.
- Most commonly caused by ***HPV 16 and 18***

Other causes/risk factors for cervical cancer:

- Coitus before the age of 18 years
- Multiple sexual partners
- Delivery of the first baby before the age of 20 years
- Multiparity
- Poor personal hygiene
- Poor socioeconomic status
- Smoking and alcohol abuse
- COC and progestogens use over 8-year periods
- Exposure to diethylstilbestrol

Extra Mile

- Average age for cervical CA: 35–45 years
- **Gardasil** is a quadrivalent vaccine against HPV 6, 11, 16, 18 to be given to adolescents at 0, 2 and 6 months intramuscularly in the deltoid muscle.
- **Cervarix** is bivalent against HPV 16, 18 to be given (0.5 mL) at 0, 1 and 6 months. Immunity is expected to last 10 years.

371. Ans. (a) Squamous cell CA

Ref: Shaws, 15th ed. pg. 964

- The two most common histologic subtypes of cervical cancer are squamous cell and adenocarcinoma.
- Of these, ***squamous cell tumors predominate, comprise 85 percent*** of all cervical cancers, and arise from the ectocervix
- Adenocarcinomas comprise **10–15%** of cervical cancers and arise from the endocervical mucus-producing glandular cells.

372. Ans. (b) Oral contraceptives decreases the risk of cervical cancer

Ref: Williams Gynecology chapter 29-30

For this question, most of the students claimed option "D" but according to william's "Lower educational attainment, older age, obesity, smoking, and neighborhood poverty are independently related to lower rates of cervical cancer screening, which contribute to increased risk of cervical cancer".

- **Use of combined oral contraceptives doesn't decrease the risk,** *but it increases the risk.* COC users and women who are within 9 years of use have a significantly higher risk of developing both squamous cell and adenocarcinoma of the cervix *(william's gyne).*
- In women who are positive for cervical HPV DNA and who use COCs, risks of cervical carcinoma increase by up to fourfold compared with women who are HPV-positive and never users of COCs.
- *Both active and passive cigarette smoking increases the risk of cervical cancer.*
- An increased number of sexual partners and early age of first intercourse have been shown to increase cervical cancer risks.
- *Abstinence from sexual activity and barrier protection during sexual intercourse have been demonstrated to decrease cervical cancer incidence.*

TABLE: Risk factors for cervical neoplasia

Behavioral risk factors	Demographic risk factors	Medical risk factors
• Infrequent or absent cancer screening Pap tests • Early coitarche • Multiple sexual partners • Male partner who has had multiple sexual partners • Tobacco smoking • Dietary deficiencies	• Ethnicity (Latin American countries, U.S. minorities) • Low socioeconomic status • Age	• Cervical high-risk human papillomavirus infection • Parity • Immuno-suppression

TABLE: Summarized staging of cervical CA

Stage I	Tumor confined to the cervix
Stage IA	Microinvasion (preclinical)
Stage IB	All other cases confined to the cervix
Stage IIA	Tumor spread to the upper two thirds of the vagina
Stage IIB	Tumor spread to paracervical tissue but not to the pelvic walls
Stage IIIA	Tumor spread to the lower third of the vagina
Stage IIIB	Tumor spread to the pelvic wall or obstruction of either ureter by tumor
Stage IV	Tumor spread to the mucosa of the bladder or rectum or outside the pelvis.

Contd...

373. Ans. (b) Pap smear

Ref: Shaws, 15th ed. pg. 957; International Journal of Obstetrics and Gynecology 2006

Cervix cancer is the second most common cause of female specific cancer after breast cancer

- **Primary prevention** of a disease requires warding it off before the pathogenic process can occur. In the case of cervical cancer, this would require that infection of the will be cervix prevented. It could be achieved either by complete abstinence from sexual activity or *with a vaccine.*
- **Secondary prevention** stops the progression of disease once it has already started. A good example of secondary prevention is cytologic screening to detect cervical cancer precursors, followed by treatment to prevent progression to cancer.

Diagnosis

- Diagnosis of cervical dysplasia is mainly based on cytological screening of the population and by signs and symptoms:
  - Many are asymptomatic.
  - Some complain of postcoital bleeding or discharge.
  - On inspection, the cervix often appears normal, or there may be cervicitis or an erosion which bleeds on touch.
  - Some present with postmenopausal bleeding.
- Routine cytological screening or Pap smear Should be done to all women above the age of 21 years who are sexually active for at least 3 years. In all women with abnormal Pap tests showing mild dysplasias, it is important to treat any accompanying inflammatory pathology and repeat the Pap test. If it persists to be abnormal, consider **colposcopic** examination and selective biopsies.

374. Ans. (b) Papaniculaou smear

Ref: Shaw's Gynae, 15th ed. pg. 403

- Pap smear is taken from cervix, with Arye spatula, rotated 360° to pick up cells from squamo-columnar junction. Vaginal smear for hormonal evaluation is taken from lateral fornix
- The objective of screening is to reduce the incidence and mortality from cervical cancer
- Pap smear test has been effective reducing the incidence of cervical cancer by 80% and the mortality by 70%.
- *Please refer to above explanation also.*

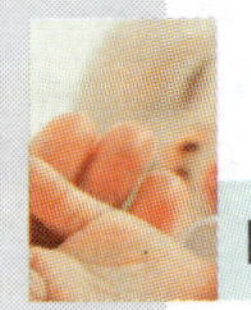

375. Ans. (d) All of the above

Ref: Shaws, 15th ed. pg. 403

The latest recommendations for cervical CA screening are:

- All women should begin cervical cancer screening at age 21 years.
- ***Women between the ages of 21 and 29 should have a Pap test every 3 years.*** They should not be tested for HPV unless it is needed after an abnormal Pap test result.
- ***Women between the ages of 30 and 65 should have both a Pap test and an HPV test every 5 years.*** This is the preferred approach, but it is also acceptable to have a Pap test alone every 3 years.
- ***Women over age 65 who have had regular screenings with normal results should not be screened for cervical cancer.*** Women who have been diagnosed with cervical pre-cancer should continue to be screened.
- Women who have had their uterus and cervix removed in a hysterectomy and have no history of cervical cancer or pre-cancer should not be screened.
- Women who have had the HPV vaccine should still follow the screening recommendations for their age group.
- Women who are at high risk for cervical cancer may need to be screened more often. Women at high risk might include those with HIV infection, organ transplant, or exposure to the drug DES. They should talk with their doctor or nurse.

ENDOMETRIAL AND FALLOPIAN TUBE CANCER

376. Ans. (b) Cystectomy

Ref: Shaw's Textbook of Gynaecology 7th ed. pg. 175, 176

- Laparoscopic cystectomy remains the first-line choice for conservative treatment of endometriotic cysts.
- Laparoscopic cystectomy when performed for endometriotic cysts with accurate surgical technique leads to no significant ovarian tissue removal and thus does not result in reduction of ovarian reserve.
- A proper blood supply is vital for the preservation of ovarian volume and antral follicular counts.

377. Ans. (d) Tubal salphingitis

Ref: Shaw's Textbook of Gynaecology, 7th ed. pg. 348-349

- Salpingitis causes inflammation of the fallopian tubes.
- Inflammation can spread easily from one tube to the other, so both tubes may become affected. It may present as distal dilation of fimbria.
- It is one of the cause of infertility in young females.

378. Ans. (d) Laparoscopy

Ref: Williams Gynecology 4th ed. Page 240

- Although imaging can add clinical information, laparoscopy is the primary method used for diagnosis of endometriosis. Endometriotic lesions can be superficial or can deeply invade the peritoneum or pelvic organs.
- Laparoscopic visualization of ovarian endometriomas has a sensitivity and specificity of 97% and 95%, respectively.

379. Ans. (d) Multigravida

Ref: Shaw's Gynecology 16th ed pg. 508

- Low parity is an increased risk factor for development of endometrial CA. Out of given choices, multigravida is at least risk of endometrial CA

Endometrial cancer: Etiology and high risk

- Unopposed estrogen or high level of estrogen
- Chronic anovulation, PCOD
- Familial predisposition
- Tamoxifen
- Obesity, hypertension, diabetes
- Feminizing ovarian tumour
- Low parity
- Late menopause

380. Ans. (a) Increased risk of endometrial carcinoma

Ref: Shaw's Gynecology 16th ed. pg. 554

- Tamoxifen is a selective estrogen receptor modulator, given for breast CA treatment.
- Tamoxifen given to women with breast cancer increases the risk of endometrial hyperplasia and cancer to two- to three-folds. It also increases the risk of ovarian CA.
- Raloxifene has no adverse effect on the endometrium.
- Tamoxifen is effective in primary and secondary prevention of breast cancer.
- It **prevents spread to the other breast and recurrence by 50% and mortality by 25%.**
- It is also bone (decrease risk of osteoporosis) and cardioprotective.
- Side effects (two-fold increase) are hot flushes, vaginal dryness (anti-E2 action), endometrial hyperplasia, polyp, endometrial carcinoma and sarcoma. Other side effects are: DVT, retinopathy, ischemic heart disease.

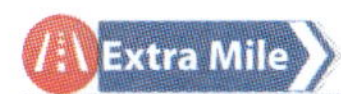

Risk Factors for Endometrial Cancer
- Endogenous estrogen dependent
- Nulliparity, low parity
- Polycystic ovary syndrome (PCOS)
- Early menarche, late menopause
- Functioning ovarian tumors
- Obesity, hypertension, diabetes, hyperlipidemia
- Exogenous estrogen
- Unopposed estrogen therapy
- Tamoxifen therapy
- Hered.ary

381. Ans. (d) Estradiol

Ref: Shaw's Gynecology 16th ed. pg. 409

- Endometriosis is ectopic benign endometrial tissues outside the cavity of the uterus, which responds to ovarian hormones.
- Usual sites of ectopic endometrial tissue is pelvic endometriosis (pelvic peritoneum, pouch of douglas, uterosacral ligament), rectovaginal endometriosis, ovary, appendix, pelvic lymph nodes, or at the scar site known as scar endometriosis.
- Symptoms can range from simple abdominal pain, dysmenorrhea, dyspareunia to infertility.

Treatment

- Endometriosis is estrogen dependent. Hormones act on the receptors in the endometriotic tissue and cause their atrophy and shrinkage.
- The purpose of administration of various hormones or drugs is to act as antiestrogens.
  - Continuous administration of gonadotropin analogue is useful in precocious puberty to down regulate and suppress pituitary gonadotropins. It causes atrophy of the endometriotic tissue in 90% cases. Drugs are: Goserelin, buserelin, nafarelin, cetrorelix, leuprolide.
  - Aromatase inhibitors available are letrozole (2.5 mg), anastrozole (1–2 mg) and rofecoxib (12.5 mg) daily for 6 months. It has antiestrogenic activity inhibiting conversion of androgen to estrogen.
  - **Combined OCP:** Intermittently or continuously, oral contraceptives may alleviate the disease. Not used much due to side effects.
  - **Oral progestogens:** They exert an antiestrogenic effect and their continuous administration causes decidualization and endometrial atrophy. Drugs commonly in use are: Norethisterone 5.0–20.0 mg daily, or dydrogesterone 10–30 mg daily. *This hormone does not prevent ovulation and is suitable for a woman trying to conceive.*
  - Mifepristone has some beneficial influence on shrinkage of fibroids and endometriosis (10–25 mg daily for 3 months).
  - Raloxifene, 60 mg daily used in endometriosis, do not cause endometrial hyperplasia.
- **Note:** Estradiol being the estrogen agonist will aggravate the symptoms. Hence should not be given.

382. Ans. (c) PET-CT

Ref: Shaw's 16th ed. 510

Radiological Tests in Endometrial CA

- **PET–CT reveals metabolic activity in the tissue and is a gold standard for staging.**
- *CT* has a predictable rate of 85% in studying the extent of spread of the lesion. Hypodensity in the myometrium suggests myometrial infiltration.
- *MRI* is superior to CT in detecting myometrial involvement and nodal enlargement with 90% detection rate and without radiation hazard.
- *Sonosalpingography* is very useful in detecting endometrial polyps which could be malignant.
- *Ultrasound* is useful in studying the endometrial thickness, irregular line, detecting polyps and associated ovarian tumor or ovarian metastasis.

383. Ans. (c) Dysmenorrhea

Ref: Shaw, 16th ed. pg. 420

Adenomyosis
- This condition is also termed as uterine endometriosis. It is observed frequently in elderly women aged more than 40.
- The disease often coexists with uterine fibromyomas, pelvic endometriosis (15%) and endometrial carcinoma.

Clinical presentation
- Some are asymptomatic, others present with **menorrhagia** and progressively increasing dysmenorrhoea.
- **Other symptoms:** Pelvic discomfort, backache and dyspareunia
- **Clinical examination** reveals a painful symmetrical enlargement of the uterus that rarely exceeds that of a 3-month pregnancy and is often mistaken for a myoma.
- A myoma is rarely painful. Therefore, a **painful, symmetrical enlargement of the uterus should suggest the diagnosis of adenomyosis.**
- **Shaw states:** *"If a patient gives a history of menorrhagia with accompanying dysmenorrhoea, one should always consider the possibility of adenomyosis"*

Investigation:
- MRI is superior to ultrasound.

Treatment
- Since most women are elderly and past the age of childbearing, **total hysterectomy** is the treatment.

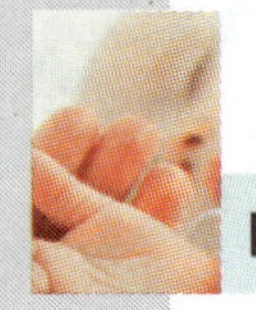

384. Ans. (c) 40

Ref: Shaws, 15th ed. pg. 151

POSTMENOPAUSAL BLEEDING

- Postmenopausal bleeding and abnormal premenopausal and perimenopausal bleeding the primary symptoms of endometrial carcinoma.
- Normally a 1-year period of amenorrhea after the age of 40 is considered as menopause. However, vaginal bleeding occurring anytime after 6 months of amenorrhoea in a menopausal age should be considered as postmenopausal bleeding and investigated.
- Even without amenorrhoea or irregular bleeding, if a woman over the age of 52 years continues to menstruate, she needs investigations to rule out endometrial hyperplasia and malignancy of the genital tract.
- ***Thirty to fifty percent of postmenopausal bleeding is attributed to malignancy of the genital tract, the most common being endometrial cancer, cervical cancer and ovarian tumors.***
- Common benign conditions are endometrial hyperplasia and polypi.

385. Ans. (c) Atypical

Ref: Shaw's Gynaecology, 15th ed. pg. 724

ENDOMETRIAL HYPERPLASIA

- This occurs in:
  - Anovulatory cycles with unopposed estrogen acting on the endometrium
  - Metropathia haemorrhagica
  - Obese women
  - Polycystic ovarian disease
  - a woman on tamoxifen
  - feminizing ovarian tumors
- Hyperplasia may be simple hyperplasia, glandular or atypical hyperplasia.
- Simple hyperplasia is at a risk of endometrial cancer in 2% and glandular hyperplasia in 4-10%. ***Atypical hyperplasia, however, has the tendency to develop carcinoma in as much as 60-70%.***

Extra Mile

- 80% cases of simple hyperplasia respond to progestogens, response of atypical hyperplasia is only 50%, but with the risk of malignancy.
- For this reason, atypical endometrial hyperplasia should be treated by hysterectomy and not merely by ablative technique.

386. Ans. (b) Biopsy

Ref: Dutta's Obstetrics, 7th ed. pg. 341 and 345

Diagnosis of Endometrial Carcinoma

- Postmenopausal bleeding is considered to be due to endometrial carcinoma unless proven otherwise.
- **Endometrial biopsy:** Histology is the definitive diagnosis
- Papanicolaou smear not a reliable test for endometrial CA. It is Positive only in 30% cases of endometrial cancer.
- **Ultrasound and color Doppler (TVS):** Findings suggestive of endometrial carcinoma are:
  - Endometrial thickness ≥ 4 mm
  - Hyperechoic endometrium with irregular outline.
  - Increased vascularity
  - Intrauterine fluid
- **Hysteroscopy:** Helps in direct visualization of endometrium and to take target biopsy.
- **Fractional curettage:** Is not only the definite method of diagnosis but can detect the extent of growth.

Prognosis

- Tumors showing poor prognosis are:
  - Poorly undifferentiated
  - Greater myometrial penetration
  - Lymphovascular space invasion
- Aneuploid tumors: worst prognosis

TABLE: Most of the prognostic factors given below in the table can be evidenced by endometrial biopsy

Prognostic factors in endometrial carcinoma

• Age at diagnosis: Older the patient poorer the prognosis.
• Stage of the disease
• **Histologic type:**
  ▪ Typical adenocarcinomas- better prognosis;
  ▪ Papillary serous, clear cell carcinoma-poor prognosis.
• Histologic differentiation.
• Histologic grade: Grade 3 tumors have 5 times more risk of recurrence and low 5 year survival rate.
• Myometrial penetration.
• Lymphovascular space invasion.
• Lymph node metastasis.

387. Ans. (c) Simple hysterectomy

Ref: William's Gyne. Ch 33

Surgical treatment options for patients with endometrial cancer:

- Simple Hysterectomy
- BSO (Bilateral salpingo oophorectomy)
- Radical hysterectomy

- Vaginal hysterectomy
- Almost three quarters of patients are stage I at diagnosis.
- ***In general, an extrafascial ("simple") hysterectomy is sufficient***, but radical hysterectomy may be preferable for women with clinically obvious cervical extension of endometrial cancer.
- **Contraindications of primary surgery include:** a desire to preserve fertility, massive obesity, high operative risk, and clinically unresectable disease.
- Vaginal hysterectomy with or without BSO is another option for those women who cannot undergo systematic surgical staging because of comorbidities.

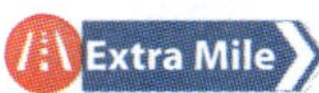

"Just so you don't miss any further question on endometrial CA staging, following table has been summarized"

TABLE: FIGO staging for endometrial CA

I A	**Tumor confined to the uterus, no or < ½ myometrial invasion**
I B	Tumor confined to the uterus, > ½ myometrial invasion
II	Cervical stromal invasion, but not beyond uterus
III A	Tumor invades serosa or adnexa
III B	Vaginal and/or parametrial involvement
III	Metastasis to pelvic and paraaortic lymph nodes
III C1	Pelvic node involvement
III C2	Para-aortic involvement
IV-A	Tumor invasion bladder and/or bowel mucosa
IV-B	Distant metastases including abdominal metastases and/or inguinal lymph nodes

Note:
- Paclitaxel (Taxol), doxorubicin (Adriamycin) and cisplatin (TAP) **chemotherapy** is the adjuvant treatment of choice for advanced endometrial cancer.
- In practice, **cytotoxic chemotherapy frequently is combined with radiotherapy** in patients with advanced endometrial cancer.
- **Primary radiation therapy** usually is considered only in rare instances when a patient is an exceptionally poor surgical candidate.

388. Ans. (a) Painless watery discharge

Ref: Shaws, 15th ed. pg. 999

FALLOPIAN TUBE CANCERS

- Primary cancer of the fallopian tubes is uncommon and account for only 0.3%.
- The tumor is often an adenocarcinoma though choriocarcinoma may develop in a tubal ectopic pregnancy or in a tubal mole.
- The tumor is highly malignant and spreads rapidly through lymphatics to the pelvic organs.

FIGO classification does not exist, Erez classification is as follows:
- **Stage I:** The tumor is limited to the mucosa and muscle.
- **Stage IIA:** The serosa is breached but the tumor has not spread to other organs.
- **Stage IIB:** The tumor invades the pelvic organs.
- **Stage III:** Metastasis outside the pelvis but within the abdominal cavity.
- **Stage IV:** Extra-abdominal metastasis is present.

Clinical Features

- The tumor occurs in menopausal women, most of them of them are nulliparous.
- ***The early symptom is painless watery discharge per vagina***, which may at times be amber-colored. Sooner or later, postmenopausal bleeding develops.
- A lump may be too small to be felt on clinical examination.
- *Pain is a late symptom.*

389. Ans. (c) IIIa

Ref: Refer to staging Shaws, 15th ed. pg. 421

OVARIAN CANCER

390. Ans. (a) Benign fibroma + ascites + hydrothorax

Ref: Williams Gynaecology 3rd ed. pg. 771

- Meigs syndrome is defined as triad of:
- Benign ovarian tumour
- Ascites
- Pleural effusion

391. Ans. (d) Combined OCP and follow up

Ref: Berek and Novak's Gynecology, 16th ed. pg. 482

- The now-routine application of ultrasound technology to gynecologic examinations led to the more frequent detection of ovarian cysts, sometimes as an incidental finding.

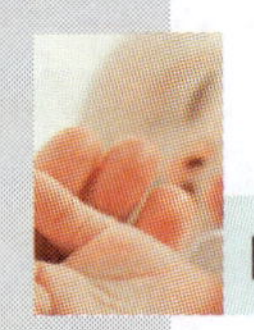

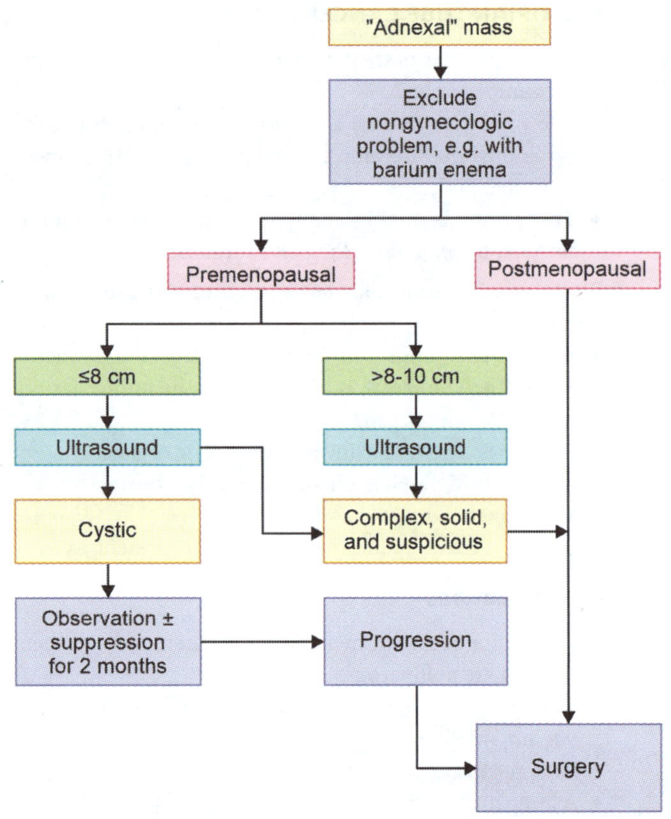

392. Ans. (a) Granulosa cell tumor

Ref: Shaw 16th ed. P 442

- Granulosa call tumor is an estrogen secreting tumor, characterized histopathologically by ***Call exner body.***

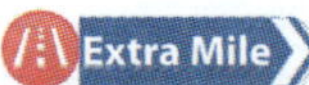
Extra Mile

Ovarian tumor	HPE characteristics
• Serous cystadenoma	Psamomma bodies
• Clear cell tumor	Hobnail cell
• Yolk sac tumor	Schiller duval bodies
• Granulosa cell tumor	Call exner bodies
• Krukenberg tumor	Signet ring cell

393. Ans. (c) Ovary

Ref: Shaws, 16th ed. pg. 430

Lutein Cysts of the Ovary

Two types of lutein cysts are recognized:
- Granulosa lutein cysts found within the corpus luteum.
- Theca lutein cysts associated with trophoblastic disease and chorionic gonadotropin therapy.

Corpus Luteum (Granulosa Lutein) Cysts

- Corpus luteum cysts are functional, non-neoplastic enlargements of the ovary.
- **Clinical presentation:** Local pain, tenderness or delayed menstruation. These cysts are often palpable clinically.
- Ultrasound reveals **spider-web-like structure** with or without a clot.

Theca Lutein Cysts

- **Theca lutein cysts** (TLC), also known as **hyperreactio luteinalis (HL)**, are a type of **functional ovarian cyst**. They are typically multiple and **seen bilaterally** and filled with straw-colored fluid.
- It is commonly associated with hydatidiform moles, choriocarcinoma and gonadotropin (hCG) or clomiphene therapy.
- The cysts spontaneously regress after elimination of the mole, therapeutic curettage, treatment of chorio-carcinoma or discontinuation of gonadotropin therapy.

394. Ans. (c) Clear cell tumor

Classification of ovarian tumor

Epithelial tumor (80%)	Germ cell tumor	Sex cord tumor
• Clear cell tumor • Brenner's tumor • Serous tumor *(MC)* • Endometrioid tumor • Mucinous tumor *Mn: CBSE-M*	• Choriocarcinoma • Dysgerminoma • Endodermal sinus tumor • Polyembroyoma • Teratoma *(MC)* *Mn: C- DEPT:*	• Theca cell tumor • Granulosa cell tumor • Androblastoma • Gynandroblas-toma • Arrhenoblastoma *Mn: The GAGA*

395. Ans. (b) Teratoma

Ref: Williams Gynae, 1st ed. Ch 36

- Germ cell tumors arise from the ovary's germinal elements and comprise a third of all ovarian neoplasms.
- The **mature cystic teratoma,** also called ***dermoid cyst,*** **is by far the most common subtype.** This accounts for 95% of all germ cell tumors and is **clinically benign**.
- In contrast, **malignant germ cell** tumors comprise fewer than 5 percent of malignant ovarian cancers in Western countries and include *dysgerminoma, yolk sac tumor, immature teratoma,* and other less common types.

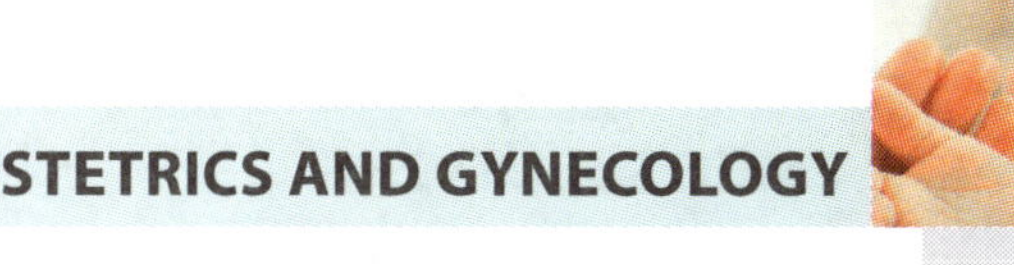

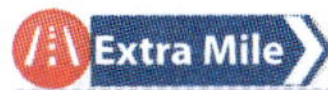

Extra Mile

- Overall, MC ovarian tumor: **Epithelial cell tumor**
- Overall, MC benign tumor of the ovary: **Dermoid cyst**
- MC benign epithelial tumor of the ovary: **Serous cystadenoma**
- MC malignant ovarian tumor: **Serous cystadenocarcinoma**
- **MC germ cell tumor: Mature Teratoma (Dermoid Cyst)**
- Most common ovarian tumor associated with pregnancy: **Dermoid Cyst**
- Most common ovarian tumor which undergo torsion: **Dermoid cyst**
- MC malignant germ cell tumor: **Dysgerminoma**
- Ovarian tumor mostly in young age: **Dysgerminoma**
- Ovarian tumor metastasized to contralateral tumor: **Granulosa cell tumor**

396. Ans. (b) Dysgerminoma

Ref: Shaws, 15th ed. pg. 933

Please refer to above explanation.

YOLK SAC TUMORS

- Yolk sac tumors account for 20% of all malignant ovarian germ cell tumors
- *Microscopically Schiller-Duval bodies* are pathognomonic when present.

397. Ans. (a) Papillary serous cystadenoma

Ref: William's Gynecology, Ch 35; Epithelial tumors of ovary

TABLE: Epithelial Ovarian Tumor Cell Types *(Katz: Comprehensive Gynecology, 5th ed.)*

Ovarian Cancers	Approximate Frequency (%)
Serous	35–40
Mucinous	6–10
Endometrioid	15–25
Clear cell (mesonephroid)	5–10
Brenner	Rare

SEROUS TUMORS

- Serous tumors are the most frequent ovarian epithelial tumors. **The malignant forms account for 40% or more of ovarian cancers.**
- During frozen section evaluation, ***psammoma bodies are essentially pathognomonic*** of an ovarian-type serous carcinoma

MUCINOUS ADENOCARCINOMAS

- About 5 to 10 percent of true epithelial ovarian cancers are mucinous adenocarcinomas
- These cells resemble cells of the endocervix or may mimic intestinal cells, which can pose a problem in the differential diagnosis of tumors that appear to originate from the ovary or intestine.

ENDOMETRIOID ADENOCARCINOMAS

- About 15–25% of epithelial ovarian cancers are endometrioid adenocarcinomas, ***the second most common histologic type.***

CLEAR CELL TUMORS

- Comprising 5–10% of epithelial ovarian cancers, *clear cell adenocarcinomas are the most frequently associated with pelvic endometriosis.*
- Microscopically **hobnail cells** are characteristic finding. These are cells with abundant glycogen and nuclei of the cells protrude into the glandular lumen.

BRENNER TUMOR

- These tumors constitute only 2–3% of all ovarian tumors.
- Brenner tumors consist of cells that resemble the transitional epithelium of the bladder and Walthard nests of the ovary.

398. Ans. (b) Serous cyst adenocarcinoma

Ref: Shaws, 15th ed. pg. 422

- Most common ovarian tumor: Serous Cystadenoma (50%)
- ***Malignant form of serous cystadenoma is serous cystadenocarcinoma.***
- Largest ovarian tumor: Mucinous cystadenoma
- Clear cell tumor is a malignant ovarian tumor of epithelial origin, characterized histopathologically by ***Hobnail Cell.***
- Granulosa call tumor is an estrogen secreting tumor, characterized histopathologically by ***Call exner body.***

Extra Mile

Ovarian tumor	HPE characteristics
Serous cystadenoma	Psamomma bodies
Clear cell tumor	Hobnail cell
Yolk sac tumor	Schiller duval bodies
Granulosa cell tumor	Call exner bodies
Krukenberg tumor	Signet ring cell

399. Ans. (b) Ovary is the primary site

Ref: Shaws, 15th ed. pg. 424

- **Choriocarcinoma** is a highly malignant tumor arising from the chorionic epithelium.

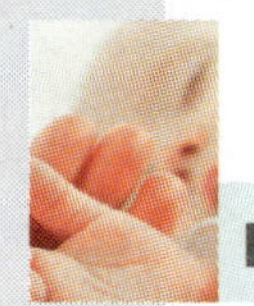

- *About 3–5% of all patients with molar pregnancies develop choriocarcinoma.*
- The primary site is usually anywhere in the uterus *(secondary involvement).*
- *Rarely, it starts in the tube or ovary.*
- The lesion is usually localized nodular type.
- **Spread:** The common sites of metastases are lungs (80%), Anterior vaginal wall (30%), brain (10%), liver (10%).

Symptoms

- Irregular vaginal bleeding, at times brisk
- Continued amenorrhoea.
- **Lung:** Cough, breathlessness, haemoptysis.
- **Cerebral:** Headache, convulsion, paralysis or coma.
- ***Liver:*** *Epigastric pain, jaundice.*
- **Chest X-ray:** Shows 'cannon ball' shadow or 'snow storm' appearance due to numerous tumor emboli.

400. Ans. (c) Choriocarcinoma

Ref: Shaws, 15th ed. pg. 424

CHORIOCARCINOMA

- Generally, choriocarcinoma is a part of a mixed germ cell tumor. Its origin as a teratoma can be confirmed in prepubertal girls, when the possibility of its gestational origin can be definitely excluded. The tumors are very vascular.
- Histologically the tumor shows adimorphic population of syncytiotrophoblasts and cyto-trophoblasts. It secretes large quantities of human chorionic gonadotropin (hCG) hormone, which forms an ideal tumor marker in the diagnosis and management of the tumor. The tumor is highly malignant, and metastasizes by bloodstream to the lungs, brain, bones and other organs.

401. Ans. (a) Chemotherapy

Ref: Shaws, 15th ed. pg. 124-125

- The treatment of choice of choriocarcinoma is mainly chemotherapy both for local and distal metastasis.
- The drug of choice for the same is **methotrexate**. It is given orally 5 mg five times a day for 5 days.
- Side effects of Methotrexate are ulcerative stomatitis, gastric hemorrhage, skin reaction, alopecia, bone marrow suppression, Liver and Kidney damage.

402. Ans. (c) CA 125

Ref: Shaws, 15th ed. pg. 422-928

- Tissue markers such as CA-125 and NB/70k are useful mainly in the follow-up of certain tumors.
- **CA-125** is a glycoprotein and surface cell antigen which is secreted by the malignant epithelial tumors.
- Level of CA-125 more than 35 U/ml suggests malignant and residual tumor, and indicates the need of chemotherapy.
- CA-125 is also raised in abdominal tuberculosis and endometriosis.
- CEA (carcinoembryonic antigen) >5 mg/L is seen in mucinous ovarian tumor.
- **Note:** CA-125 is raised in only 50% cases in Stage I and 90% in Stage II ovarian cancer.

VULVAR AND VAGINAL CANCER

403. Ans. (d) HPV

Ref: William's Gynecology Ch 31

HPV (16, 18) most comman cause of vulvar carcinoma.

- HPV infects the female → vulva, vagina, and cervix
- Male → urethra, penis, and scrotum.
- Both genders → Perianal, anal, and oropharyngeal area.

Salient Features of Vulvar Cancer

MC site- labia majora and minora	
MC symptom pruritus.	
MC type- SCC, epidermoid type (same for vaginal CA)	
MC implicated factor- HPV 16, 18.	
Premalignant lesion of vulva	
• VIN (MC) vulvar intraepithelial lesion • /ts ds • Condyloma accuminata	• Lichen sclerosis • Erythroplasia of querat • Bowen disease (type of VIN)
MC mode of spread- lymphatic 1st LN- Superficial inguinal LN 2nd LN- Deep inguinal LN	

404. Ans. (c) Stage II

Ref: Shaws 15 ed. pg. 941

Carcinoma of the Vulva (FIGO staging 2008)

Stage I	Tumor confined to the vulva
I a	Lesions ≤2 cm is size, confined to the vulva or perineum and with stromal invasion ≤1 mm, no nodal metastasis
I b	Lesions >2 cm in size or with stromal invasion >1.0 mm, confined to the vulva or perineum, with negative nodes
Stage II	**Tumor of any size with extension to adjacent perineal structures (1/3rd lower urethra, 1/3rd lower vagina, anus) with negative nodes**

Contd...

Stages III	Tumor of any size with or without extension to adjacent perineal structures (one-third lower urethra, one-third lower vagina, anus) with positive inguino-femoral lymph nodes
IIIA	• With lymph node metastasis (≥5 mm) or • 1-2 lymph node metastasis(es) (<5 mm)
IIIB	• With two or more lymph node metastases (≥5 mm) or • 3 or more lymph node metastases (<5 mm)
Stage IV A	Tumor involving any of the following: • Upper urethral and/or vaginal mucosa, bladder mucosa, rectal mucosa, or fixed to pelvic bone, or • Fixed or ulcerated inguino-femoral lymph nodes.
Stage IV	Distant metastasis including pelvic lymph nodes

Note: *According to old FIGO staging (1995) for vulvar CA (as mentioned in William's), only in stage III there is invlovement of adjacent organs like lower urethra and/or the vagina or the anus. So don't be confused, and mark answers according to latest staging as mentioned above.*

405. Ans. (b) Stage II

Ref: William's Gynecology, Ch 31

406. Ans. (b) Simple partial vulvectomy without lymphadenectomy

Ref: William's Gynecology Ch: 31

FIGO Staging of Vulvar cancer	Treatment
Stage I: Tumor confined to the vulva, Negative nodes **IA:** size <2 cm; stromal invasion <1 mm **IB:** size >2 cm; stromal invasion >1 mm	**Microinvasive surgery:** Simple/wide local excision. No Lymphadenectomy required
Stage II: Tumor of any size, with spread to lower urethra, lower vagina or anus with negative nodes **Stage III:** II + Regional lymph node metastasis (inguinal, femoral)	**Radical vulvectomy or Modified radical vulvectomy + inguinofemoral lymphadenectomy**
Stage IVA: Tumor invades upper urethra, upper vagina, bladder mucosa, rectal mucosa + Nodes	**RT + Surgery**
Stage IVB: Vulvar cancer with distant metastasis including pelvic lymph nodes	**Stage IVB: Palliative therapy**

Extra Mile

- **Radical vulvectomy:** An operation that removes the entire vulva, including subcutaneous and fatty tissue, the labia minora and majora, perineal skin, and clitoris, to treat cancer.
- **Skinning vulvectomy:** An operation that removes the skin of the vulva, including the labia majora and minora, the clitoris, and perineal skin.

407. Ans. (b) Partial vulvectomy

Ref: Shaws, 15th ed. pg. 943; William's Gynecology Ch 31, Invasive CA of Vulva

Please refer to above explanation.

408. Ans. (c) Vaginal carcinoma

- Primary vaginal carcinoma is rare and comprises only 1 to 2 percent of all gynecologic malignancies.
- The most common histologic type of primary vaginal cancer is squamous cell carcinoma, followed by adenocarcinoma.
- Vaginal carcinoma has no direct role in infertility.

Causes of Infertility

Infertitlity factors	%
Male factor	30% (most common cause)
Ovarian/anovulation factors	25%
Tubal/uterine factors	25%
Cervical factors	10%
Unexplained	10%

DYSFUNCTIONAL UTERINE BLEEDING (DUB) AND DYSMENORRHEA

409. Ans. (c) CA cervix

Ref: Comprehensive Gynecology 7th ed. pg. 669

- Postmenopausal bleeding is vaginal bleeding that occurs a year or more after the last menstrual period. It can be a symptom of vaginal dryness, polyps or other changes in reproductive system.
- Cervical cancer is as twice as common as endometrial cancer in women with postmenopausal bleeding and a thin endometrium.

410. Ans. (a) Endometrial cancer

Ref: Comprehensive Gynecology 7th ed. pg. 714

- Tamoxifen is a selective estrogen receptor modulator used for the treatment and prevention of estrogen receptor (ER)—positive breast cancer.
- However, tamoxifen increases the risk of endometrial cancer.

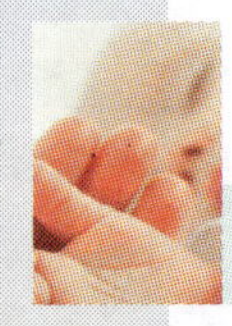

411. Ans. (a) Reassurance

Ref: Shaw's Gynecology 16th ed. pg. 322–325

- Best next step in this case is reassurance of patient, and ask her to wait for 1–2 years because –
- **Primary amenorrhea** is defined as absence of menses by 14 year of age in the absence of secondary sexual characters OR absence of menses by 16 year of age in the presence of secondary sexual characters.
- Patient's age is still 14-year-old with secondary sexual characteristics. Therefore, she doesn't need any intervention and is advised to wait for another 1–2 years.

412. Ans. (a) GnRH

Ref: Shaw's Gynecology 16th ed. pg. 325-26

CAUSES OF SECONDARY AMENORRHEA

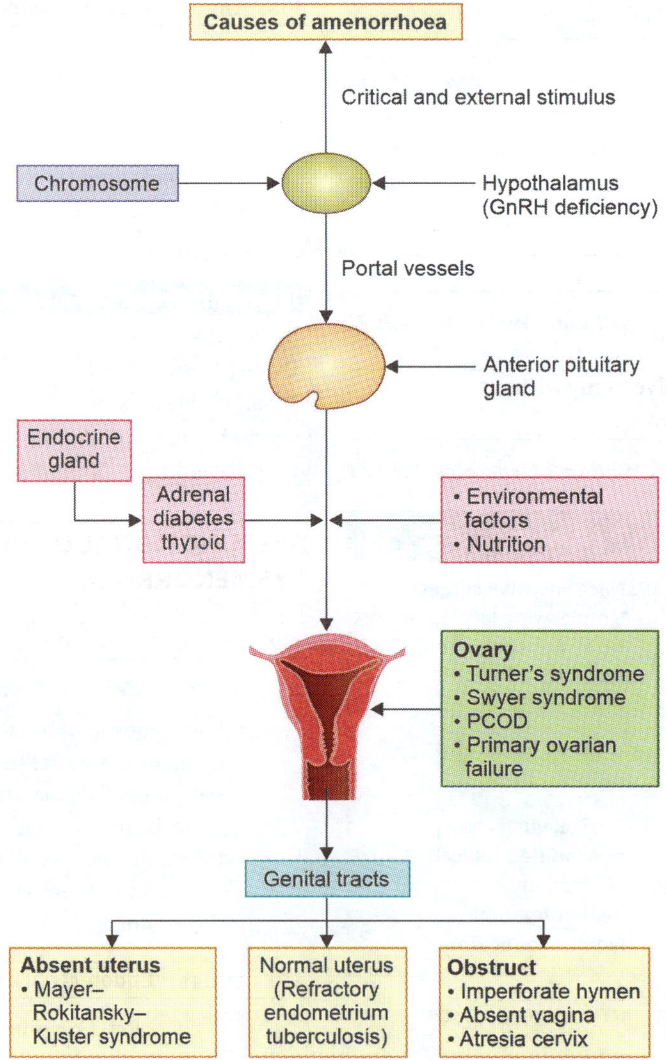

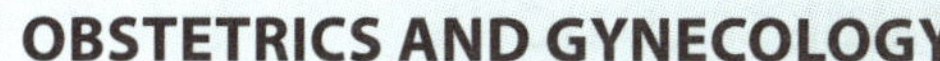
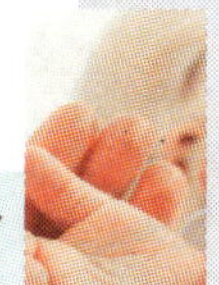

413. Ans. (d) Karyotyping

Ref: Shaw's 16th ed. pg. 327-29

- Primary amenorrhea and secondary sexual characters present so we will do examination to rule out uterus present or not. Here uterus is absent further we do karyotyping to rule out Mullerian agenesis and Androgen insensitivity syndrome.

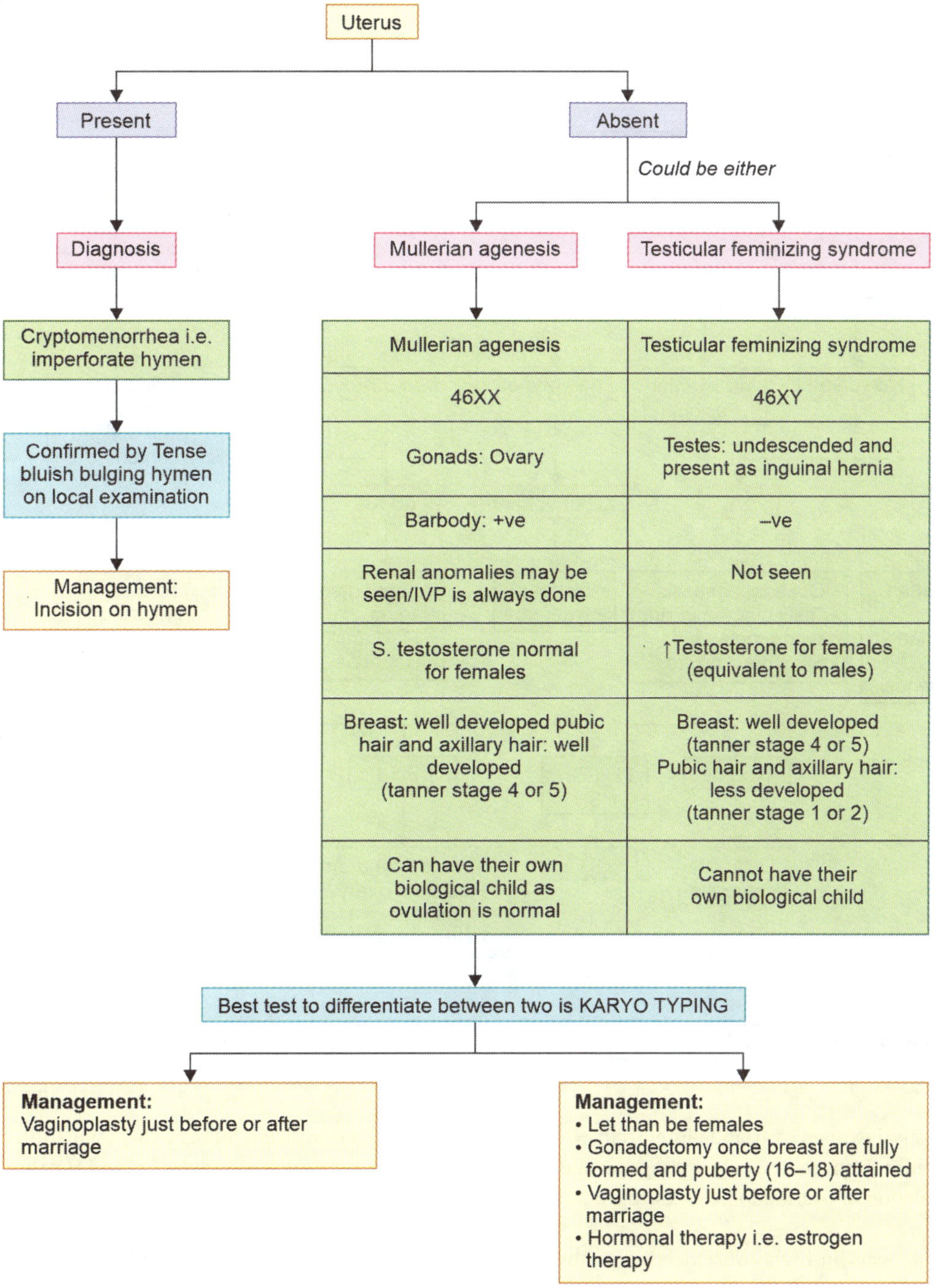

Uterus
- Present → Diagnosis → Cryptomenorrhea i.e. imperforate hymen → Confirmed by Tense bluish bulging hymen on local examination → Management: Incision on hymen
- Absent — *Could be either* → Mullerian agenesis / Testicular feminizing syndrome

Mullerian agenesis	Testicular feminizing syndrome
46XX	46XY
Gonads: Ovary	Testes: undescended and present as inguinal hernia
Barbody: +ve	–ve
Renal anomalies may be seen/IVP is always done	Not seen
S. testosterone normal for females	↑Testosterone for females (equivalent to males)
Breast: well developed pubic hair and axillary hair: well developed (tanner stage 4 or 5)	Breast: well developed (tanner stage 4 or 5) Pubic hair and axillary hair: less developed (tanner stage 1 or 2)
Can have their own biological child as ovulation is normal	Cannot have their own biological child

↓

Best test to differentiate between two is KARYO TYPING

Management:
Vaginoplasty just before or after marriage

Management:
- Let than be females
- Gonadectomy once breast are fully formed and puberty (16–18) attained
- Vaginoplasty just before or after marriage
- Hormonal therapy i.e. estrogen therapy

Investigations in Amenorrhea

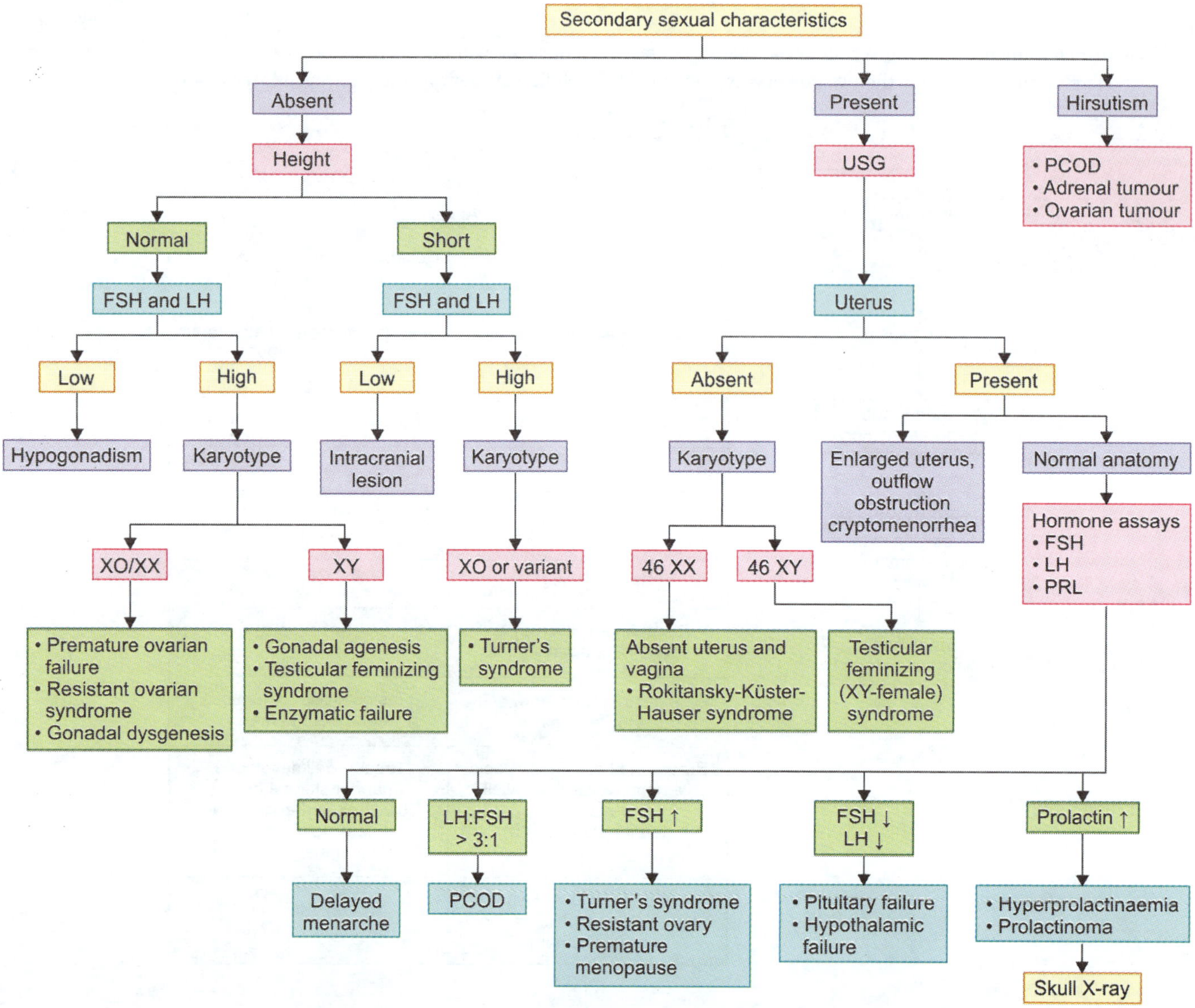

- Secondary sexual characteristics
  - Absent → Height
    - Normal → FSH and LH
      - Low → Hypogonadism
      - High → Karyotype
        - XO/XX → • Premature ovarian failure • Resistant ovarian syndrome • Gonadal dysgenesis
        - XY → • Gonadal agenesis • Testicular feminizing syndrome • Enzymatic failure
    - Short → FSH and LH
      - Low → Intracranial lesion
      - High → Karyotype
        - XO or variant → • Turner's syndrome
  - Present → USG → Uterus
    - Absent → Karyotype
      - 46 XX → Absent uterus and vagina • Rokitansky-Küster-Hauser syndrome
      - 46 XY → Testicular feminizing (XY-female) syndrome
    - Present
      - Enlarged uterus, outflow obstruction cryptomenorrhea
      - Normal anatomy → Hormone assays • FSH • LH • PRL
        - Normal → Delayed menarche
        - LH:FSH > 3:1 → PCOD
        - FSH ↑ → • Turner's syndrome • Resistant ovary • Premature menopause
        - FSH ↓ LH ↓ → • Pituitary failure • Hypothalamic failure
        - Prolactin ↑ → • Hyperprolactinaemia • Prolactinoma → Skull X-ray
  - Hirsutism → • PCOD • Adrenal tumour • Ovarian tumour

414. Ans. (a) High LH and high FSH

Ref: Shaw's 16th ed. pg. 66-67

- In Menopausal women ovarian failure occur which leads to depletion of ovarian follicles so anovulation occurs resulting no corpus luteum forms so decrease in progesterone levels so, no further negative feedback on LH so **LH value will increase**. Also due to depletion of ovarian follicles, estrogen levels will decrease so, no further negative feedback on FSH so **FSH values will increase.**
- The FSH appears in high concentration in the urine (>40 IU/L). E2/E1 ratio maintained over 1 in the premenopausal period is reduced to less than 1 in the menopausal age, causing an estrogen deficiency state.

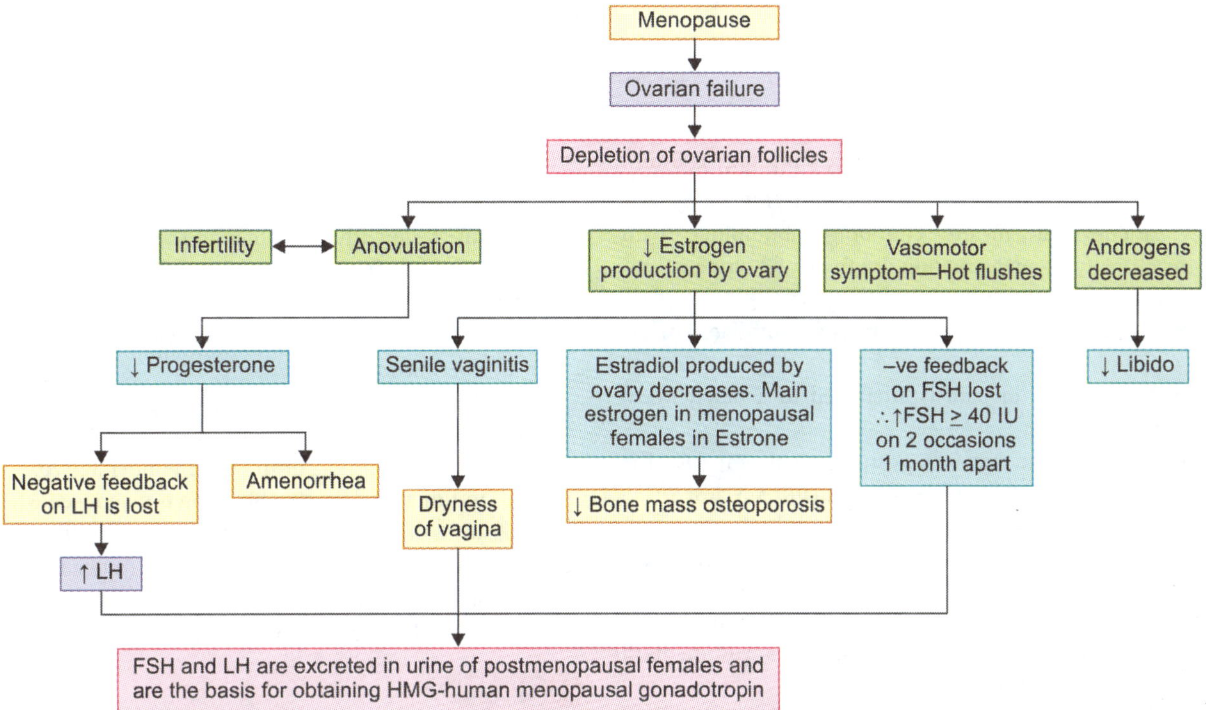

415. Ans. (c) Hysterectomy

Ref: William's Obstetrics 25th ed. pg. 47

- Some women older than 55 years may still have menstrual bleeding. However, ovulation is rare and oocytes are likely poor quality and rarely viable.
- There is also a possibility of uterine fibroids or tumors so hysterectomy is the best option for this age group.

416. Ans. (a) Pituitary adenoma

Ref: William's Obstetrics 25th ed. pg. 380

- Pituitary adenomas are the most frequent cause of acquired pituitary dysfunction.
- These most commonly secrete prolactin, but excessive secretion of any pituitary-derived hormone can result in amenorrhea. Significantly elevated serum prolactin levels (>100 ng/mL) are almost always due to a pituitary mass.
- Increased serum prolactin levels are found in as many as one-tenth of amenorrheic women, and more than half of women with both galactorrhea and amenorrhea have elevated prolactin levels (the "galactorrhea-amenorrhea syndrome").

417. Ans. (b) Presence of endometrium at ectopic locations

Ref: Shaw's Gynecology 16th ed. pg. 409-410

- Endometriosis is the occurrence of ectopic benign endometrial tissues outside the cavity of the uterus.
- The ectopic endometrial tissue responds to ovarian hormones.
- **Note:** PID closely mimics endometriosis

Endometriosis	Adenomyosis
• It is also a cause of DUB • Presence of endometrium outside uterus • **MC site:** Ovary **Rarest site:** CNS • It presents as chocolate cyst of ovary • Present with menorrhagia, pain, Infertility. • **MC symptom:** Congestive dysmenorrhea • **Gold standard Inv:** Laparoscopy (diagnostic + therapeutic)	• Also a cause of DUB • Presence of endometrial gland in myometrium • Seen in patients around 40 years • Present with menorrhagia, dysmenorrhea and pain but *no Infertility* • Uterus is tender and enlarged: 12–14 weeks size • Diagnosed with Histopathology • **Treatment of choice:** Hysterectomy

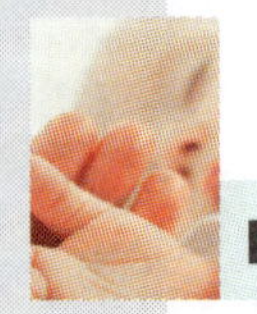

418. Ans. (b) **Endometriosis**

Ref: Shaw's Gynecology 16th ed. pg. 409-410

Refer to above explanation

419. Ans. (a) **No clinical significant pelvic pathology is found**

Ref: Shaw's Gynecology 16th ed. pg. 471

- Dysmenorrhea means cramping abdominal pain accompanying menstruation. It can be of 2 types:
- **Primary dysmenorrhea:**
  - These are not associated with any identifiable pelvic pathology.
  - Pathogenesis of pain is attributed to a biochemical derangement.
  - It affects more than 50% postpubescent women in the age group of 18–25 years with ovulatory cycles.
- **Secondary dysmenorrhea:**
  - These are associated with the presence of organic identifiable pelvic pathology, i.e. fibroids, adenomyosis, pelvic inflammatory disease (PID) and endometriosis.
  - Unilateral dysmenorrhea occurs in a rudimentary horn of a bicornuate uterus.
  - It is also seen in some women wearing intrauterine contraceptive device (IUCD) and in cases of cervical stenosis.

TABLE: Differentiating features of primary and secondary dysmenorrhea

Differentiating features	Primary	Secondary
Onset	Within 2 years of menarche	20–30 years, maybe pre- and postmenstrual
Description	Cramping–hypogastrium, back, inner things	Variable dull ache
Symptomatology	Nausea, vomiting, diarrhea, headache, fatigue	Dyspareunia, infertility, menstrual disorders
Pelvic findings	Normal	Variable, depending on cause
Etiology	Excessive myometrial contraction, ischemia, excessive prostaglandin production	Endometriosis, PID, adenomyosis, fibroids, pelvic vein congestion
Management	Reassurance, analgesics, NSAIDs, antispasmodics, OC pillls, in rare cases, surgery–Cotte's operation or laparoscopic uterosacral nerve ablation (LUNA)	Treatment directed to the cause

420. Ans. (d) **Anovulatory**

Ref: Shaws, 15th ed. pg. 301-307

- Dysfunctional uterine bleeding is irregular, abnormal uterine bleeding that is not caused by a tumor, infection or **pregnancy.**
- Dysfunctional uterine bleeding is a disorder that occurs most frequently in women at the beginning and end of their reproductive lives.
- *It is of two types:*
  1. ***Ovulatory:*** *After adolescent years and before perimenopausal years.*
  2. ***Anovulatory:*** *Postmenarcheal, premenopausal.*
- Half of the cases occur in women over 45 years of age and about one fifth occur in women under age 20.
- Dysfunctional uterine bleeding is diagnosed when other causes of uterine bleeding have been eliminated.
- Failure of the ovary to release an egg *(anovulatory)* during the menstrual cycle occurs in about 70% of women with DUB. This is probably related to a hormonal imbalance.

Extra Mile

- **Normal menstruation duration:** *28 +/–7 days, mean of 4 days duration, not >7 days*
- **Menorrhagia or hypermenorrhea:** Prolonged (>7 days) or excessive (>80 mL) bleeding at regular intervals
- **Metrorrhagia:** Bleeding in irregular but frequent intervals, variable amount
- **Menometrorrhagia:** Prolonged bleeding at irregular intervals
- **Polymenorrhea:** Bleeding in regular intervals <21 days
- **Oligomenorrhea:** Regular intervals >35 days

Endometri osis	Adenomyosis
• It is also a cause of DUB. • Presence of endometrium outside uterus. • **MC site: ovary** **Rarest site: CNS** • In ovary, it present at chocolate cyst ovary. • Present with menorrhagia, pain, Infertility. • MC symptom: Congestive Dysmenorrhea. • Gold standard Inv: Laparoscopy (diagnostic + therapeutic)	• Also a cause of DUB • Presence of endometrial gland in myometrium • Seen in patients around 40 years. • Present with menorrhagia, dysmenorrhea and pain BUT *no Infertility.* • Uterus is tender and enlarged: 12–14 weeks size. • Diagnosed with Histopathology. • Treatment of choice: Hysterectomy

421. Ans. (c) **Metrorrhagia**

Ref: Shaw, 15th pg. 283

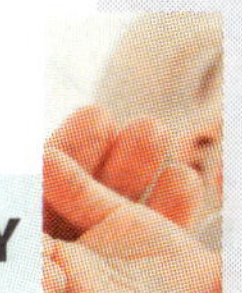

422. Ans. (a) Pelvic and abdomen USG

Ref: William's Gynecology 1st ed. Ch 11

- **Dysmenorrhea** is Cyclic pain with menstruation and accompanies most menses. This pain is classically described as cramping and is often accompanied by low backache, nausea and vomiting, headache, or diarrhea.
  - **Primary dysmenorrhea** describes cyclic menstrual pain without an identifiable associated pathology.
  - **Secondary dysmenorrhea** is cyclic menstrual pain which may frequently complicates endometriosis, leiomyomas, PID, adenomyosis, endometrial polyps, and menstrual outlet obstruction.
- The above given case is a patient of chronic pelvic pain secondary to dysmenorrhea.
- First line drug/DOC in dysmenorrhea is: NSAIDs
- If NSAIDs doesn't relieve the symptom, further work-up must be performed to rule out other pathologies.
- The next best choice for this patient is Pelvic and abdominal ultrasonography.

423. Ans. (a) Progesterone

Ref: Shaws, 15th ed. pg. 303-304

- Puberty menorrhagia is anovulatory. Therefore our first line or **DOC in puberty menorhhagia is cyclical progestin therapy.**

FIBROID

424. Ans. (a) Ovarian CA

Ref: Shaw's 16th ed. pg. 436-37

- The shown mass beside uterus is ovarian tumor.
- An ovarian tumor in adolescent and post-menopausal women is more often malignant. In the reproductive age, it is mostly benign. Most germ cell tumors occur in young girls.

TABLE: Features of benign and malignant ovarian tumours

Benign ovarian tumours	Malignant ovarian tumour
History • Not related to age or parity, though most common during childbearing period • Slow-growing tumour, no pain. No menstrual disorder unless it is a feminizing tumour or masculizing tumour	• Seen most commonly in adolescents and elderly women–mostly after 50 years of age. Low parity or infertile woman • Rapidly growing tumour, pain in advanced stage. Post-menopausal bleeding • Family history of breast, ovarian or colonic cancer
Examination • Usually unilateral, cystic, well-defined and mobile. No ascites (except in Meign syndrome). No nodules in the abdomen or pouch of Douglas	• May be bilateral and solid, fixed. Ascites may be present. Metastatic nodules may be felt per abdomen. Nodules in the pouch of Douglas
Ultrasound • Cystic well-defined with or without echoes. No ascites (except in Meigs syndrome)	• Often solid and bilateral fixed with internal echoes, ascites may be present. Metastatic nodules may be seen
Doppler ultrasound • No increased vascularity	• Increased vascularity • Pulsatile index <1 • Resistance index <0.4
MRI and CT • Similar to ultrasound findings • CA–135 normal	• Metastatic and enlarged lymph nodes may be detected • CA–125 raised more than 35 IU/mL
Operative findings • Well-defined ovarian cystic or solid tumour. No ascites or metastatic nodule. Often mobile	• Fixed solid tumour, often bilateral—with blood-stained ascites. Metastatic growth over the omentum and peritoneal cavity. Lymph nodes may be enlarged

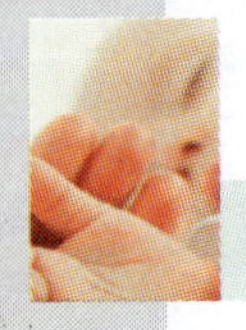

425. Ans. (c) Laparoscopic hysterectomy

Ref: Shaws 16th ed. pg. 101

Contraindications to Laparoscopy

- Extreme obesity: Its makes laparoscopic procedure and pneumoperitoneum difficult.
- Cardiac and respiratory diseases contraindicate Trendelenburg position and CO_2 pneumoperitoneum.
- Diaphragmatic hernia precludes Trendelenburg position.
- Umbilical hernia
- Previous abdominal scar (exposes the bowel to injury during trocar insertion)
- Acute pelvic infection (it can spread during laparoscopy)
- A large uterus (puerperal) and an abdominal tumor can be injured by the sharp instrument.

426. Ans. (a) Pedunculated

Ref: Shaw's Gynecology 16th ed. pg. 410-402

- Myomectomy is the most common surgical procedure done for fibroids during caesarean section
  - *Myomectomy* refers to the removal of fibroids, leaving the uterus behind
- Pedunculated myomas can easily be removed and hemostasis can be secured at the same time without endangering mother's life.
- **Vaginal myomectomy:**
  - Indicated in submucous fibroid
  - In Cervical fibroids and pedunculated fibroid polypus
  - If more than 50% submucous fibroids project into the cavity
- **Hysteroscopic myomectomy**
  - Hysteroscopic myomectomy has become possible for **submucous fibroids** not removable by the simple vaginal route.
  - The fibroid is excised either by cautery, laser or resectoscope. It is best done under laparoscopic guidance to avoid uterine perforation.

Extra Mile

- Anterior and posterior fibroids lodged in the pouch of Douglas cause increase in frequency and retention of urine
- Broad ligament fibroids can cause hydroureter and hydronephrosis

427. Ans. (b) Large size

Ref: Shaw's 16th ed. pg. 397

- In torsion very severe abdominal pain is experienced.
- **Book states:** "*Acute pain is seen when a fibroid is complicated by torsion, hemorrhage and red degeneration.*"
- Pain in a rapidly growing fibroid in an elderly woman may be due to sarcoma.
- Sarcomatous change in a myoma is extremely rare and is usually associated with intramural and submucous tumors which have a higher potential for sarcomatous change than subserous tumors.
  - It is more commonly seen in a postmenopausal woman when it is observed that the tumor grows suddenly, **causing pain** and postmenopausal bleeding.
- **A large fibroid** may be observed as an abdominal tumor which grows slowly or not at all over a long period. A rapid growth only occurs during pregnancy, due to oral contraceptive hormones and malignancy. *As many as 50% women are asymptomatic.* These fibroids are detected during gynecological check-up or ultrasound done for unrelated symptoms.

Extra Mile

TABLE: Clinical symptomatology and complications associated with uterine fibromyomas

• Menstrual disturbances—menorrhagia, polymenorrhagia, intermenstrual bleeding, continuous bleeding, postmenopausal bleeding
• Infertility
• Pain—spasmodic dysmenorrhea, backache, abdominal pain
• Lump in the abdomen or mass protruding at the introitus
• Pressure symptoms on adjacent viscera—bladder, ureters, rectum
• Pergnancy losses, postpartum hemorrhage, uterine inversion
• Vaginal discharge

428. Ans. (a) Leiomyoma

Ref: Shaw's 16th ed. pg. 507

- Most common benign tumor of uterus is leiomyoma (fibroid).
- Most common malignant tumor of uterus is endometrial carcinoma.
- **Overall most common uterine tumor:** Leiomyoma.

Endometrial CA

- Endometrial cancer is 20–25% of all genital cancers in the developed countries (*in developing countries cervical CA still predominates due to poor screening*).
- The peak incidence of endometrial cancer is 55–70 years, 20–25% occur in perimenopausal women and only 5% develop in women below the age of 45 years.
- 75% of the tumors are localized in the uterus when diagnosed and surgery is the cornerstone in its management.

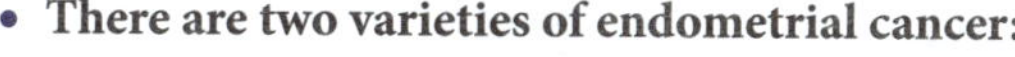

- **There are two varieties of endometrial cancer:**
  - **Type I are estrogen-dependent** and account for 90% growths. The source of estrogen may be endogenous or exogenous. They are well-differentiated with good prognosis.
  - **Type II are estrogen-independent** and develop in atrophic endometrium. They are mostly undifferentiated with poor prognosis. P_3 mutations are recognized in type II tumors.

429. Ans. (b) Cervical

Ref: Shaw's, 16th ed. pg. 392

- The distribution of myoma/Fibroid in the body of the uterus is broadly classified as follows (Figure):
- Intramural (interstitial) 75%
- Submucous 15%
- Subserous 10%
- The majority of myomas arise in the uterus. Tumors can therefore be classified as uterine and extrauterine.
- The uterine growth is further divided into those that arise from the body and those that arise from the cervix.

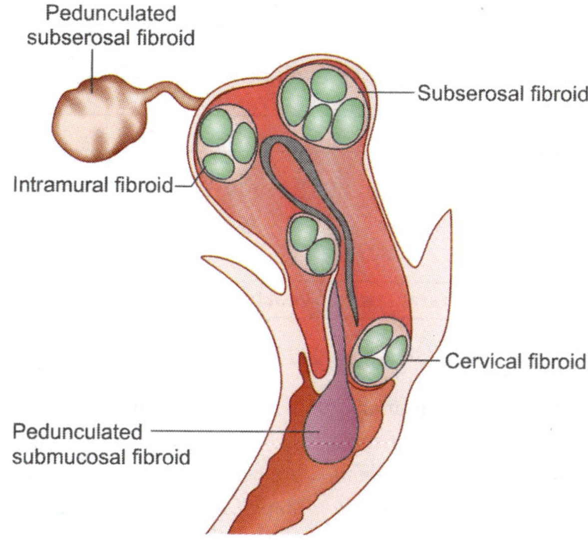

FIGURE: Varieties of submucous fibroid. Various anatomical sites of fibromyomas

Cervical Fibroid

- Cervical fibroid is a single fibroid encountered in 1% of all fibroids. It may develop as a central, anterior, posterior fibroid or grow laterally in the broad ligament.

Symptoms

- A cervical fibroid exerts pressure on the bladder, ureter and in rare cases on the rectum. A woman may feel a lump in the lower abdomen. **During pregnancy, it can cause retention of urine**. Obstructed Labor occurs if the cervical fibroid lies below the presenting part.

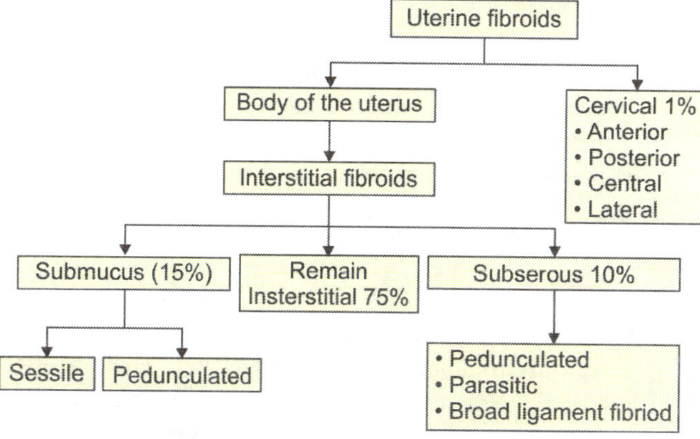

430. Ans. (c) Subserous fibroid

Ref: Shaws, 15th ed. pg. 359

- Uterine fibroids are noncancerous growths of the uterus that often appear during childbearing years. It is aka leiomyomas
- They aren't associated with an increased risk of uterine cancer and almost never develop into cancer.

Types

- **Intramural fibroids** are located within the wall of the uterus and are the **most common type.**
- **Subserosal fibroids** are located underneath the mucosal (peritoneal) surface of the uterus and can become very large. They can also grow out in a papillary manner to become pedunculated fibroids.
  - Therefore hysteroscopical excision is not possible.
  - It can be resected lapascopically or by open laparotomy.
- **Submucosal fibroids** are located in the muscle beneath the endometrium of the uterus and distort the uterine cavity; even small lesions in this location may lead to bleeding and infertility
- **Cervical fibroids** are located in the wall of the cervix (neck of the uterus)

431. Ans. (a) Subserous fibroid

Ref: Shaws, 15th ed. pg. 359

Please refer to above explanation.

432. Ans. (a) Conservative management

Ref: Shaws, 15th ed. pg. 364;
William Obstetrics 23rd ed. Ch 40

- Uterine leiomyomas (*fibroids*) are common benign smooth muscle tumors. Their incidence during

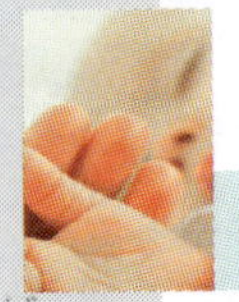

pregnancy is probably about 2% and depends on population characteristics and the frequency of routine sonography.

- **Treatment of symptomatic myomas consists of analgesia and observation.** Most often, signs and symptoms abate within a few days, but inflammation may stimulate labor.
- Surgery is **rarely** necessary during pregnancy.

433. Ans. (d) All of the above

Ref: Shaws, 15th ed. pg. 359; Williams Gynecology Ch: 9

- Leiomyomas are benign smooth muscle neoplasms that typically originate from the myometrium. They are often referred to as uterine myomas, and are incorrectly called **fibroids** because the considerable amount of collagen contained in many of them creates a fibrous consistency.
- Drugs used to decrease the size of the fibroid:
  - GnRH analogue (Buserelin, Nafarelin, Goserelin, Triptorelin, Leuprorelin acetate)
  - GnRH antagonist: Cetrirelix, Ganirelix
  - Mifepristone (anti-progesterone)
  - Danazol

CHROMOSOMAL ANOMALIES

434. Ans. (b) USG

Ref: Shaw's Gynecology 16th ed. P 329

- In a patient with primary amenorrhea and secondary sexual characteristics, we need to rule out conditions like androgen insensitivity syndrome and MRKH syndrome. But before that checking the presence or absence of uterus with help of ultrasonography decides the further steps like karyotyping or hormonal studies.

435. Ans. (b) Tall stature

Ref: Shaws, 15th ed. /110-111; Harrison 19/e 635; William's Gynecology, Ch 16

In turner syndrome

- Deletion of genetic material from an X chromosome accounts for about two thirds of gonadal dysgenesis which leads to a condition called turner syndrome (XO).
- A 45, X karyotype is found in about half of these patients, most of whom have associated somatic defects including **short stature, webbed neck,** low hairline, shield-shaped chest, widening of long bones, STREAK GONADS, renal anomalies (Horse-shoe kidney) and cardiovascular defects (COA).
- Other features of turners syndrome are summarized in the image given.

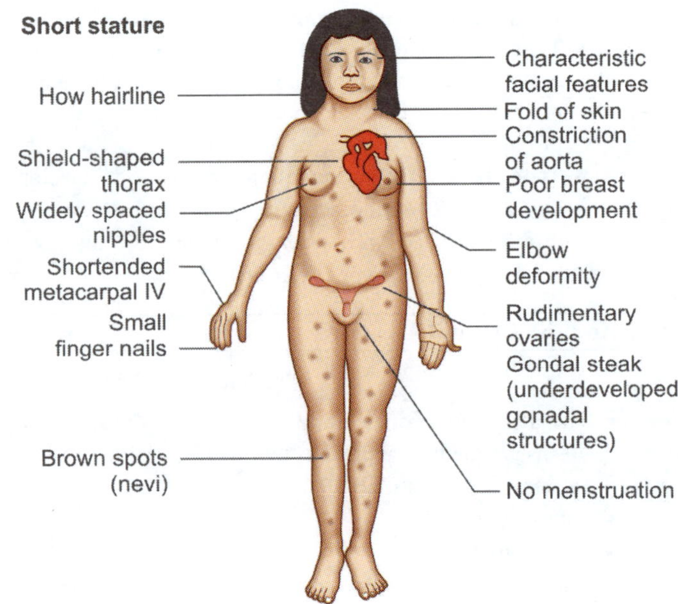

436. Ans. (d) All of the above

Ref: Shaws, 15th ed. /110-111, Harrison, 19th ed. pg. 635; DC Dutta, 6th ed. pg. 422-423

Please refer to above explanation.

437. Ans. (a) 45 XO

Ref: Shaws 15th ed. /110-111; Harrison 19/e 635; William's Gynecology Ch 16

438. Ans. (c) Coaractation of aorta

Ref: Shaws, 15th ed. pg. 111, DC Dutta, 6th ed. pg. 422-423

- Cardiac anomaly seen with turner syndrome is *coaractation of aorta.*
- *Single most common cause of increased mortality in children with Turner's syndrome:* ***Cardiovascular abnormalities (COA)***
- *Single most important cause of primary amenorrhea:* ***Turner's syndrome.***

439. Ans. (d) PAPP

- The triple test measures the following three levels in the maternal serum: *(sensitivity 71%)*
  - Alpha-fetoprotein (AFP)
  - Human chorionic gonadotropin (hCG)
  - Unconjugated estriol (UE3)
- **Quadruple test include:** Triple test + Inhibin A: *Increases sensitivity up to 80%*

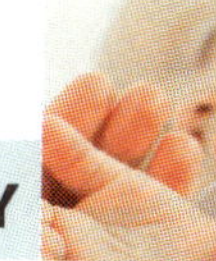

The levels may indicate increased risk for certain conditions:

AFP	UE3	hCG	Associated conditions
Low	Low	High	Down's syndrome
Low	Low	Low	Trisomy 18 (Edward's syndrome)
High	-	-	NTD, omphalocoele, gastrochisis

440. Ans. (b) Mullerian agenesis

Ref: William's Gynecology chapter 19-20

MULLERIAN AGENESIS

- Congenital absence of both uterus and vagina is referred as *müllerian aplasia*, *müllerian agenesis*, or *Mayer-Rokitansky-Küster-Hauser syndrome*.
- In classic müllerian *agenesis*, patients have a **shallow vaginal pouch**, only measuring up to 1.5 inches deep. ***In addition, the uterus, cervix, and upper part of the vagina are absent***.
- Typically, a portion of the distal fallopian tubes are present. ***In addition, normal ovaries are present***, given their separate embryonic origin.
- Most patients with müllerian *agenesis* have only small rudimentary müllerian bulbs without endometrial activity.
- Surgical excision of symptomatic rudimentary bulbs is required. With müllerian *agenesis*, traditional conception is impossible, but pregnancy may be achieved using sophisticated technology involving oocyte retrieval, fertilization, and implantation into a surrogate.

Extra Mile

- **Klinefelter syndrome, 47, XXY,** is a common sex chromosome abnormality associated with maternal age and occurs in 1/1000 live male births.
  - **Clinical features** include tall gynecoid stature, gynecomastia *(with an increased risk for breast cancer), and testicular atrophy and low IQ.*
- **Gonadal dysgenesis:** Is the most common cause of primary amenorrhea. It is most frequently due to a chromosomal disorder or deletion of all or part of an X chromosome.

In order to figure out all the MCQs based on absence or presence or breast/uterus, following table is summarized: *(Katz: Comprehensive Gynecology, 5th ed.)*

Absent breast development; uterus present
- 45, X (Turner's syndrome)
- 46, X, abnormal X (e.g., short- or long-arm deletion)
- Mosaicism (e.g., X/XX, X/XX, XXX)
- 46, XX or 46, XY pure gonadal dysgenesis
- Kallman syndrome
- 17α-hydroxylase deficiency with 46, XX
- Pituitary failure
- Hypothalamus failure

Present breast development; uterus absent
- Androgen resistance (*testicular feminization*)
- Congenital absence of uterus (*utero-vaginal agenesis*)

Absent breast development; uterus absent
- 17, 20-desmolase deficiency
- Agonadism
- 17α-hydroxylase deficiency with 46, XY karyotype

Breast development; uterus present
- Hypothalamic etiology
- Pituitary etiology
- Ovarian etiology
- Uterine etiology

441. Ans. (c) Ovaries and uterus are absent

Ref: Shaws 15th ed. /101

FEMALE PSEUDOHERMAPHRODITISM

- Results from excessive androgen exposure of an embryo or fetus
- Müllerian-inhibiting substance is not produced.
- The karyotype is 46, XX and ovaries are present.
- Because müllerian-inhibiting substance is not produced, the ovaries and female internal ductal structures such as the ***uterus, cervix, and upper vagina are present***
- Clitoral hypertrophy will be more pronounced along with fused posterior labia.
- These patients are fertile

Extra Mile

Male Pseudohermaphroditism
- Insufficient androgen exposure of a fetus destined to be a male leads to male pseudohermaphroditism.
- The karyotype is 46, XY and testes are present.
- The uterus is generally absent as a result of normal embryonic MIS production.
- These patients are most often sterile from abnormal spermatogenesis and have a smaller or inadequate phallus for sexual function.

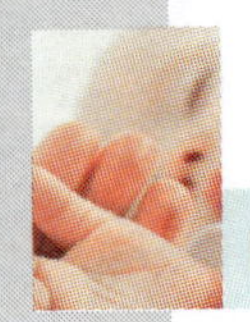

TROPHOBLASTIC TUMORS

442. Ans. (a) Hydatiform mole

Ref: Callen PW, Ultrasonography in Obstetrics and Gynaecology, 5th ed. pg. 952-963

Hyaditidiform Mole

- It is the most common benign forms of gestational trophoblastic disease
- Common complication of gestation, estimated to occur in 1 of every 1000-2000 pregnancies.

Ultrasound Features

- Enlarged uterus, Intrauterine mass with cystic spaces with or without any associated fetal parts give a **snow storm or bunch of grapes appearance.**

Note: *In PCOS, ≥20 cysts, measuring 2–9 mm diameter are arranged in peripheries and is called "string of pearl appearance".*

443. Ans. (a) Lung

Ref: Katz Comprehensive Gyenecology, 5th ed. Ch 35

- **Choriocarcinoma** is a highly malignant tumor arising from the chorionic epithelium.
- *About 3–5% of all patients with molar pregnancies develop choriocarcinoma.*
  - The primary site is usually anywhere in the uterus *(secondary involvement).*
  - *Rarely, it starts in the tube or ovary.*
  - The lesion is usually localized nodular type.
  - **Spread:** The common sites of metastases are **lungs (80%),** Anterior vaginal wall (30%), brain (10%), liver (10%)

Symptoms

- Irregular vaginal bleeding, at times brisk
- Continued amenorrhoea
- **Lung:** Cough, breathlessness, haemoptysis
- **Cerebral:** Headache, convulsion, paralysis or coma
- ***Liver:*** *Epigastric pain, jaundice*
- **Chest X-ray:** Shows **'cannon ball'** shadow or **'snow storm'** appearance due to numerous tumor emboli.

444. Ans. (b) Serial serum β-hCG level

Ref: Katz Comprehensive Gyenecology, 5th ed. Ch 35

Postmolar Surveillance

- Gestational trophoblastic neoplasia (GTN) develops after approximately 15–20% of complete moles and 2–4% in partial moles.
- **Postmolar surveillance with serial quantitative serum β-hCG levels** is the standard.

445. Ans. (d) Chorioangioma

- **Chorioangioma** *the most common tumor of the placenta*
- It is a benign vascular tumor of placental origin, and is usually found incidentally.
- They are thought to arise as a malformation of the primitive angioblastic tissue of the placenta.
- *The angiomas are perfused by the fetal circulation. Therefore when they are large, they may represent a significant impediment to fetal cardiac activity.*
- These angiomasmay also sequester platelets and can in turn give a fetal thrombocytopenia
- They can also cause increase in levels of maternal serum alpha-fetoprotein (MSAFP) and may prompt sonographic evaluation.

TABLE: Modified WHO Classification of Gestational Trophoblastic Disease

Molar lesions	Nonmolar lesions
• Hydatidiform mole ▪ Complete ▪ Partial • Invasive mole	• Choriocarcinoma • Placental site trophoblastic tumor • Epithelioid trophoblastic tumor

- **Choriocarcinoma:** A morphologic term applied to a highly malignant type of trophoblastic neoplasia in which both the cytotrophoblast and syncytiotrophoblast grow in a malignant fashion.
  - Chorionic villi are absent. These tumors tend to be hemorrhagic and necrotic
- **H. Mole:** A placental abnormality involving swollen placental villi and trophoblastic hyperplasia with loss of fetal blood vessels. There are two types: partial and complete.
  - **Partial:** A molar pregnancy with swelling of all placental villi partial. *Fetal tissues are present.*
  - **Complete:** A molar pregnancy with only villi, cord, and/or amniotic membrane elements.
- **Placental-Site Trophoblastic Tumor** A rare type of GTD arising in the uterus that secretes human placental lactogen and human chorionic gonadotrophin (hCG).
- Note: Persistent abnormal bleeding following normal pregnancy, abortion, or ectopic pregnancy should lead to a consideration of the diagnosis of GTD. ***The finding of pulmonary nodules on chest radiograph after normal pregnancy suggests GTD.***

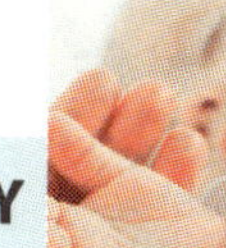

INFERTILITY AND CONTRACEPTION

446. Ans. (c) Asherman syndrome

Ref: Comprehensive Gynecology 7th ed. pg. 334-335

- Asherman's syndrome is an acquired condition where scar tissue forms inside the uterus. The scar tissue can build up, decreasing the amount of open space inside the uterus. This condition can be a complication of medical procedures.
- Hysteroscopy is the gold standard for the diagnosis of severe intrauterine adhesions.
- Intrauterine adhesions are typically seen on HSG as multiple irregular linear filling defects (may give a lacunar pattern), with the inability to appropriately distend the endometrial cavity.

447. Ans. (a) Unexplained vaginal bleeding

Ref: Williams Gynaecology 3rd ed. pg. 109

Absolute contraindications of IUCD are:

- Puerperal sepsis
- Postabortal sepsis
- Uterine distortion like fibroid
- Dysfunctional uterine bleeding/ unexplained vaginal bleeding
- Gestational trophoblastic neoplasia
- Current pelvic inflammatory disease or sexually transmitted disease within past 3 months
- Wilson disease
- Cervical cancer
- Endometrial cancer

448. Ans. (c) Ovarian hyperstimulation syndrome

Ref: Williams Gynaecology 3rd ed. pg. 453

- Ovarian hyperstimulation syndrome is an iatrogenic condition.
- It occurs due to increased capillary permeability following the administration of exogenous hormones for ovarian stimulation as a part of assisted reproduction.
- It occurs most commonly following hCG administration.
- Risk factors include: 1. Young age, 2. Low body weight, 3. PCOS, 4. High doses of exogenous hormones, 5. High or rapidly rising estrogen and 6. Prior OHSS.
- The typical imaging finding of OHSS: Bilateral symmetrical enlarged ovaries containing multiple variably enlarged cystic lesions (spoke wheel appearance) representing enlarged follicles or corpus luteum cysts in the presence of ascites.

449. Ans. (c) Sterility immediately after vasectomy

Ref: Williams Gynaecology 3rd ed. pg. 118

- No scalpel vasectomy is a unique method of gaining access to vas deferens.
- Instead of a scalpel, two specialised instruments: a ringed clamp and a dissecting forceps are used.
- Since the scrotal skin puncture made with the dissecting forceps is very small, sutures are not required.

Advantages of No-scalpel vasectomy are:

- A smaller wound than conventional method
- Earlier resumption of sexual activity after surgery
- Non time consuming
- Failure rate is very less
- Reversal is possible with microsurgery.

450. Ans. (b) Methylene blue dye

Ref: Williams Gynaecology 3rd ed. pg. 115

- *Chrome perturbation* is a method for the study of potency of Fallopian tube for suspected infertility in women caused by the obstruction of Fallopian tube.
- It is sometimes referred to as a "laparoscopy and dye" test. The dye solution used in this procedure is methylene blue or indigo Carmine.

451. Ans. (a) Use condom for 3 months

Ref: Shaw's Gynecology 16th ed. pg. 280

- Sterility doesn't occur immediately after vasectomy, it require continued contraception for about 3 months because sperms remain in semen for 15–20 ejaculations.
- So, it is advice to couple to use some form of contraception for next 3 months or 15–20 ejaculates.
- Before discontinuing any contraceptive method azoospermia should be confirmed by semen analysis at 12 weeks and 16 weeks.

452. Ans. (a) Ectopic pregnancy

Ref: Dutta 9th ed. pg. 207, 210-12

- An ectopic pregnancy is one in which the fertilized ovum is implanted and develops outside the normal endometrial cavity.
- Most common site of ectopic pregnancy: Ampulla > Isthmus > Infundibulum > Interstitium.
- Risk factors:

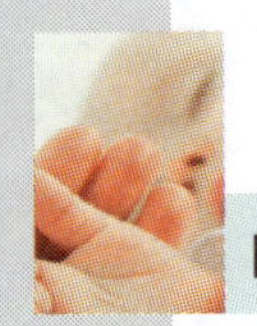

Degree of risk	Risk factors
High	Previous ectopic pregnancy
	Previous tubal surgery
	Tubal ligation
	Tubal pathology
	In utero DES exposure
	Current IUD use
Moderate	Infertility
	Previous cervicitis (gonorrhea, chlamydia)
	History of pelvic inflammatory disease
	Multiple sexual partners
	Smoking
Low	Previous pelvic/abdominal surgery
	Vaginal douching
	Early age intercourse (<18 years)

CLINICALLY IT IS PRESENTED IN THREE TYPES

Acute

- **Symptoms:** Amenorrhea, Abdominal pain, Vaginal Bleeding, vomiting fainting attack (syncopal attack).

Unruptured

- **Symptoms:** Presence of delayed period or spotting with features suggestive of pregnancy, Uneasiness on one side of the flank.

Chronic

- **Symptoms:** 6–8 weeks of amenorrhea, lower abdominal pain, vaginal bleeding (dark colored), dysuria.

453. Ans. (d) Bilateral cystectomy, adhesiolysis and prepare for IVF

- "Kissing-ovaries" are endometriotic adhesions binding down the ovaries into the pouch of Douglas 'Kissing-Ovaries'.
- Management of endometriosis in case of formation of ovarian cyst (chocolate cyst of ovary)
- Less than 5 cm – incision and drainage and destroy wall of cyst with laser
- More than 5 cm – cystectomy, adhesiolysis.
- Since this patient is young, IVF is recommended.

454. Ans. (c) Uterine synechiae

Ref: Berek and Novak's Gynecology, 15th ed. pg. 2009

- Severe trauma to the basalis layer of the endometrium with subsequent tissue bridge formation leads to intrauterine synechiae or Asherman's syndrome.
- Symptoms of severe disease include amenorrhea, menstrual irregularities, spontaneous abortion and recurrent pregnancy loss.

455. Ans. (d) PID

Ref: Berek and Novak's Gynecology, 16th ed. pg. 788

- The shown image is copper T, an IUD.
- **Contraindications to IUD use (by WHO) includes:**
  - Pregnancy
  - Puerperal sepsis
  - PID or STDs current or within the past 3 months
  - Endometrial or cervical cancer
  - Undiagnosed genital bleeding
  - Uterine anomalies
  - Fibroid tumors that distort the endometrial cavity.

456. Ans. (a) Levonorgestrel tablet single dose 1.5 mg

Ref: Berek and Novak's Gynecology,16th ed. pg. 824

- Levonorgestrel is almost as effective at 3 to 5 days after intercourse.
- WHO recommends 1.5 mg of levonorgestrel as a single dose, given up to 120 hours after intercourse.
- Levonorgestrel works only if it is administered prior to the day of ovulation.

457. Ans. (b) OCP

Ref: Berek and Novak's Gynecology, 16th ed. pg. 809

- In a newly married couple, contraception of choice is OCP, especially if the female has menstrual irregularities.

Non Contraceptive Benefits of Oral Contraceptives

Menses Related

- Increased menstrual cycle regularity
- Reduced blood loss
- Reduced iron deficiency anemia
- Reduced dysmenorrhea
- Reduced symptoms of premenstrual dysphoric disorder

458. Ans. (a) OCP

Ref: Berek and Novak's Gynecology, 16th ed. pg. 798

- Women who use estrogen containing hormonal contraceptives are at increased risk for venous thrombosis and thromboembolism.
- Normally the coagulation system maintains a dynamic balance of procoagulant and anticoagulant systems.
- Estrogens affect both systems in a dose-related fashion.

459. Ans. (a) Oral contraceptive pills

Ref: Berek and Novak's Gynecology, 16th ed. pg. 776

- Use of estrogen-progestin hormonal methods are category 2 in breastfeeding women.

- Hormonal contraceptives are not advised during lactation because of concern about reduction in the amount and quality of breast milk.
- OCP's are also contraindicated during lactation period.
- **Note:** Combined oral contraceptives are also contraindicated in a hypertensive, cardiac and diabetic women, as well as a woman with breast cancer, liver disease and previous thromboembolism. *(Remember this for future questions)*

460. Ans. (b) IUCD

Ref: Berek and Novak's Gynecology, 15th ed. pg. 442

- Reference states: *"Efficacy for emergency contraception is 100% when the device is inserted up to 5 days after intercourse, and almost 100% up to 7 days after intercourse"*

461. Ans. (b) Endometriosis

Ref: Berek and Novak's Gynecology, 16th ed. pg. 679

- There are few well-studied clinical maneuvers for use in the diagnosis of endometriosis.
- Signs may be absent or may include tender nodules in the posterior vaginal fornix, uterine motion tenderness, a fixed and retroverted uterus, or tender adnexal masses resulting from endometriomas.

462. Ans. (c) Laparoscopy and hysteroscopy

Ref: William's Obstetrics 25th ed. pg. 179

- Uterine abnormalities can he either congenital or acquired.
- Common congenital anomalies include uterine septum, bicornuate uterus, unicornuate uterus, and uterine didelphys.
- With the possible exception of a large uterine septum, the fertility effects of these anomalies have been difficult to verify.
- As a uterine septum can now be removed relatively simply and safely with hysteroscopy, most infertility specialists will proceed with laparoscopic surgery if this anomaly is identified.

463. Ans. (b) Hysterosalpingography

Ref: Shaw's Gynecology 16th ed. P 111-12

- Pelvic inflammatory disease can cause tubal blockage, which can cause infertility.
- Therefore HSG is done to rule out PID induced tubal blockage

Hysterosalpingography (HSG) is employed for the following:

- To study the patency of the fallopian tubes in infertility and postoperative tuboplasty.
- To assess the feasibility of tuboplasty by studying the location and extent of tubal pathology.
- To study uterine anomaly such as septate and cornuate uterus.
- To detect uterine synechiae.
- To detect uterine polyp.
- To study incompetence of internal OS.

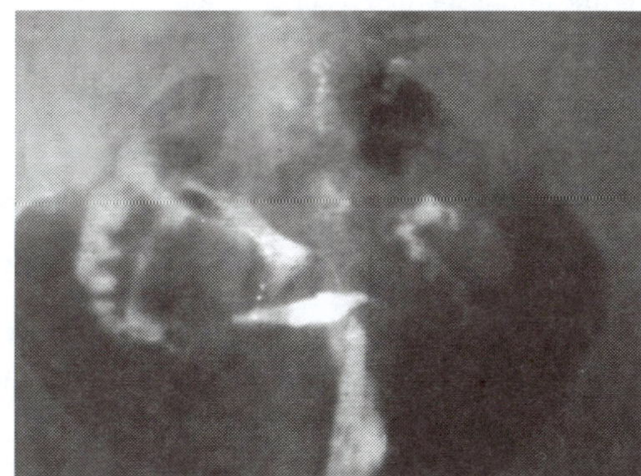

FIGURE: Genital tuberculosis—beaded blocked tubes

464. Ans. (d) 20 million/mL

Ref: Shaw's Gynecology 16th ed. pg. 243-44

TABLE: Latest WHO recommendations of normal semen analysis reference values

- Volume: 1.5–5.0 mL
- pH: >7.2
- Viscosity: <3 (scale 0–4)
- Sperm concentration: >20 million/mL
- Total sperm number: >40 million/ejaculate
- Percent motility: >50%
- Forward progression: >2 (scale 0–4)
- Normal morphology: >50% normal
- Round cells: <5 million/mL
- Sperm agglutination: <2 (scale 0–3)

Source: WHO guidelines

465. Ans. (d) Premenstrual period

Ref: Shaw Gynecology 16th ed. P 255

ENDOMETRIAL BIOPSY

- Although endometrial biopsy has been widely replaced for serial ultrasound monitoring, if ever needed, it is preferably done 1 or 2 days before the onset of menstruation.
- The material removed should be fixed immediately in formalin saline and submitted to histological scrutiny.
- Secretory changes prove that the cycle has been ovulatory.

466. Ans. (c) Remove IUCD and continue pregnancy

Ref: Shaw's Gynaecology 16th ed. pg. 271, 272

- In patients with in-situ IUCD, pregnancy occurs in 1–3 per 100 women years.

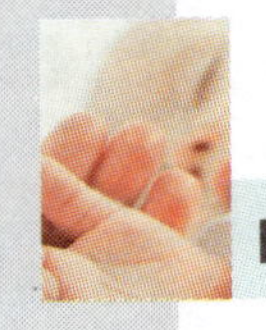

- If this happens, it is important to do ultrasound and rule out ectopic pregnancy.
- The uterine pregnancy can cause severe infection. It is therefore mandatory to remove the IUCD if the tail is visible through the os.
- While doing so, the risk of abortion should be explained to the woman. If the thread of the IUCD is not seen, termination of pregnancy is offered, not because IUCD has any teratogenic effect but because the risk of uterine infection is considerable. Alternatively, the pregnancy is continued after counseling and explaining the risk.

467. Ans. (b) IUD

Ref: DC Dutta 9th ed. pg. 498

- The best contraceptive method postplacental and postabortion is IUD
- IUD is the most effective reversible contraceptive methods.
- IUD is generally contraindicated in unmotivated persons, but since in this case the patient herself doesn't wish to conceive in near future, IUD is preferred.

Advantages of IUD:

- Ease of insertion
- Prevent uterine synechiae
- Longer action and inexpensive
- Contraceptive effect is reversible by simply removal of IUD
- Free of systemic metabolic side effects as seen with pills
- No need for continuous motivation (as seen with pills or barrier method). Only a single act of motivation is required.

Ideal IUD Candidate:

- In monogamous relationship
- Has borne at least one child
- No history of PID
- Has normal menstrual period
- Willing to check the IUD tail
- Has access to follow up and treatment

Timing of Insertion

- During menstruation or within 10 days of beginning of a menstrual period (diameter of cervical canal is greater)
- Can be done during the **first week after the delivery** before she leaves hospital *(immediate postpartum insertion).*
  - Special care required during first week as it has greater risk of perforation
- **Loop insertion:** Convenient time for loop insertion is 6–8 weeks after delivery *(postpuerperal insertion)*
- Can also be taken up immediately after first trimester abortion
  - IUD insertion after second trimester is NOT recommended → Increased risk of infection

468. Ans. (b) 6 weeks

Ref: DC Dutta 9th ed. P 623; Shaw's Gynecology 16th ed. pg. 273

- Within 6 weeks postpartum OCP's are contraindicated if the mother is lactating. In a lactating mother OCP can be started after 6 weeks (42 days) after delivery.
  - In the early phase of post-partum there is increased coagulability, which can be worsened due to estrogen containing hormonal contraceptives. Moreover lactation can also be affected.
- **The book states:** *"In a nonlactating woman, OC can be started after 3 weeks of delivery, but can be given soon after an abortion, MTP or an ectopic pregnancy"*
- **Note:** Contraceptive of choice during lactation: Mini-pill (aka Lactation pill)

Extra Mile

TABLE: Contraindications of combined oral contraceptives (WHO/FRM/FPP-2001)

Absolute			Relative
(A) Circulatory diseases (past or present) Thromboembolic disorder (current or past) • Arterial or venous thrombosis • Severe hypertension, stroke • Valvular heart disease, ischemic heart disease, angina • Diabetes with vascular complications • Focal migraine • Severe hypercholesterolemia • Smokers over age 35 years	***(B) Diseases of the liver*** • Active liver disease • Liver adenoma, carcinoma • Liver tumors	***(C) Others*** • Pregnancy • Undiagnosed genital tract bleeding • Estrogen-dependent neoplasm; e.g. breast cancer • Breast-feeding (within 6 weeks postpartum) • Major surgery or prolonged immobilization	• Age >40 years • Smoker or <35 years history of jaundice • Diabetes • Gallbladder disease • Hyperlipidemia • Postbreast cancer • Breastfeeding (postpartum 6 weeks to 6 months) • Sickle cell disease • CIN

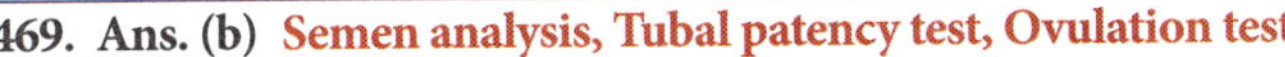

469. Ans. (b) Semen analysis, Tubal patency test, Ovulation test

Ref: Shaw's Gynecology 16th ed. pg. 240-42

- Infertility implies apparent failure of a couple to conceive, while sterility indicates absolute inability to conceive, for one or more reasons.
- If a couple fails to achieve pregnancy after 1 year of 'unprotected' and regular intercourse, it is an indication to investigate the couple.

PATHOLOGY OF INFERTILITY

- 1/3rd cases: Male is directly responsible
- 1/3rd cases: Both partners are at fault
- 1/3rd cases female is directly responsible

Faults in the Male. The factors involved include:

- Disorders of spermatogenesis—50% (Ex: Hypothalamic disorder, Kallmann syndrome, orchitis etc.)
- Obstruction of the efferent ducts—30%
- Disorders of sperm motility—15% (Kartagener syndrome)
- Sexual dysfunction- Unexplained—15% (premature ejaculation, impotence, hypospadias)

Initial work-up in an infertile couple is:

- History and physical examination
- Ovulation assessment
- Hysterosalpingogram (to check tubal patency)
- Semen analysis

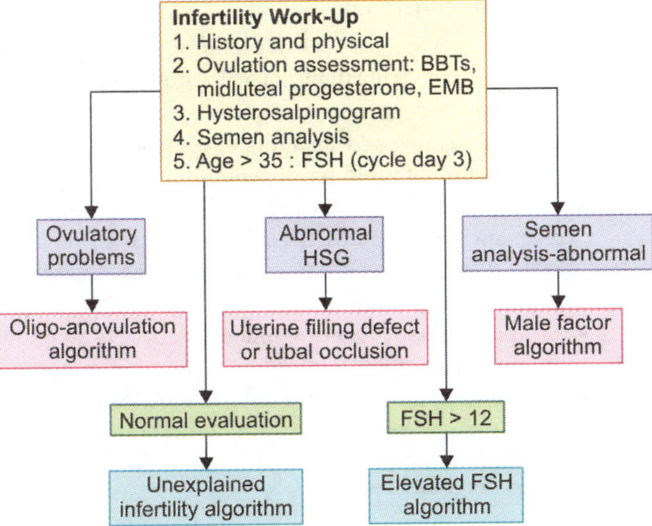

Note: *Please refer to textbook for the complete discussion of all the algorithm*

Extra Mile

Semen analysis
- It is the most important part of the male investigation.
- The best specimen is one obtained by masturbation in the vicinity of the laboratory (condom specimen is discouraged)
- Specimen best collected after a 3–5 days of abstinence.

WHO 2010 Semen Analysis

- Total volume, 2 mL (1.5 mL)
- PH—7.2–7.8
- Viscosity-3 (scale 0–4)
- Sperm concentration 20 million/mL or more (15 million/mL)
- Sperm count, >40 million/per ejaculate or more. Ten motile sperms per high field are considered normal.
- Motility >50% or more with progressive motility
- Morphology. 14% strict criteria (4%)
- Viability >75% or more (50%)
- White blood cells <1 million/mL
- Round cells <5 million/mL
- Sperm agglutination <2
- Pus cells: Absent
- **Postcoital test** (*Sims' or Huhner's test, PCT*): Postcoital (2 hs), cervical mucus collected study the sperm antibody in cervical mucus
- **Miller-Kurzrok test:** To study the penetration of sperms under the microscope.
  - Penetration less than 3 cm at 30 minutes is abnormal
- **Testicular biopsy:** Indicated in azoospermia to distinguish between testicular failure and obstruction in the vas deferens.
- **FSH level:** A high FSH level denotes primary gonadal failure

470. Ans. (b) Age <35 years

Ref: Shaw's Gyenecology 16th ed. pg. 275

OCP Pills are contraindicated in:

- Cardiac disease, hypertension, smoker >35 years.
- **Diabetes:** Because carbohydrate tolerance may be reduced
- **History of thrombosis, myocardial infarct, sickle cell anemia, severe migraine:** OCP increases the risk of thrombosis and therefore it can worsen these pathologies.
- **Chronic liver diseases such as cholestatic jaundice of pregnancy, cirrhosis of liver, adenoma, porphyrias:** Adenomas have been reported and though they are benign, rupture of a hepatoma can be fatal.
- **Breast cancer:** OCP is proved to increase the risk of breast cancer in a high-risk woman. The progestogen component of OCP has a high potential for breast cancer.
- **Gallbladder disease:** Gallbladder function may be adversely affected.
- Gross obesity.
- Patient on enzyme-inducing drugs like rifampicin, and antiepileptic except sodium valproate.
- 4–6 weeks prior to planned surgery.
- **Lactating woman:** As lactation is suppressed with combined pills.

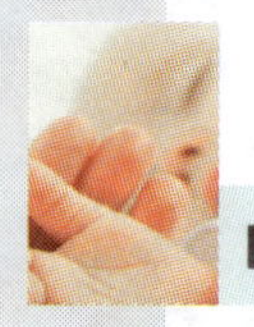

- **Monilial vaginitis:** As oral pills are associated with monilial vaginitis

Book states: *The woman can take OC for several years up to the age of 35, and thereafter until 45 years if she is healthy, slim and nonsmoker.*

471. Ans. (a) Hepatic adenoma

***Ref:** Shaw's Gynecology 16th ed. pg. 274*

Book states: *"Liver adenomas have been reported and though they are benign, rupture of a hepatoma can be fatal. Because the hormones are metabolized in the liver, chronic liver diseases and recent jaundice contraindicate the use of OCP".*

- OCP has no adverse effect on thyroid.
- It has shown to increase the risk of malignant breast CA if started in young, nulliparous females.
- No adverse effect is noted on uterine fibroids, and it is estrogen singly that increases their size.
- It has shown to increase the risk of monilial vaginitis and endocervical CA and pituitary adenoma.

472. Ans. (c) Progesterone only pills

***Ref:** Shaw's Gynecology 16th ed. pg. 275*

- **Minipill/Progestogen-only pill (POP).** The low-dose POP *(norethisterone 350 mcg, norgestrel 75 mcg or LNG 30 mcg)* have been introduced to avoid the side effects of estrogen in the combined pills.
- Given as once daily dosing, to be started within 5–7 days of menstruation and taken at the same time every day *(with a leeway of 3 hours either early or late).*
- Contraceptive agent of choice during lactation is POP.

TABLE: Advantages and disadvantages of POP

Advantages	Disadvantages
They are recommended to: • Lactating women • Women over 35 years • Those with focal migraine • Those intolerant to estrogen or estrogen contraindicated • Diabetic, hypertensive woman, sickle cell anemia • Faster return of fertility than COC users because ovulation is not suppressed in all cases (suppressed in 40%)	• Strict daily compliance • Irregular bleeding • Amenorrhea • Depression • Headache • Weight gain • More failure rate than COCP (2–3/100 women years) • Ectopic pregnancy

Contraindications of COCP

- Previous ectopic pregnancy
- Ovarian cyst, breast and genital cancers
- Abnormal vaginal bleeding
- Active liver and arterial disease
- Porphyria
- Liver tumor
  - Because of osteopenia, it is contraindicated in adolescents and young women.

473. Ans. (a) Clomiphene citrate

***Ref:** Shaw's 16th ed. pg. 258*

- Anovulation is a common problem encountered in infertility.
- **Clomiphene citrate (CC).**
  - Ovulation should be induced with CC, with a dose of 50 mg/day starting from day 2 to day 6 of the cycle for 5 days.
  - Ovulation is monitored by serial ultrasound monitoring of the follicular size, and occurrence of ovulation.
  - If the response to 50 mg CC is not satisfactory, the dose of CC should be increased to 100 mg/day from day 2 to day 6.
- If clomiphene therapy fails following 6–8 cycles, FSH and hCG therapy is recommended.
- In hypothalamic disorder, GnRH is given to stimulate the pituitary FSH and LH and the folliculogenesis monitored.

474. Ans. (c) Used for emergency contraception

***Ref:** Shaw, 16th ed. pg. 279*

RU 486 (Mifepristone)

- RU 486 is a steroid with an affinity for progesterone receptors. It does not prevent fertilization but by blocking the action of progesterone on the endometrium, it causes sloughing and shedding of decidua and prevents implantation. It is **not teratogenic.**
- A single dose of 25–50 mg is effective in preventing pregnancy in 99.1% cases (failure rate 0.9%). It causes delayed menstruation. Can be **used for emergency contraception.**
- **Ectopic pregnancy is not avoided.** The drug is expensive as compared to LNG.
- Studies have shown than it is 95% effective during the first 50 days of pregnancy.

475. Ans. (b) Vaginal bleeding

***Ref:** DC Dutta, 8th ed. pg. 618*

- **MC complication of IUD insertion:** Vaginal bleeding

Complication of IUD:

Early complication	Remote complication
• Vaginal bleed • Crampy pain • Syncopal attack • Partial or complete perforation	• Pain • Abnormal menstrual bleeding • PID • Spontaneous expulsion • Perforation

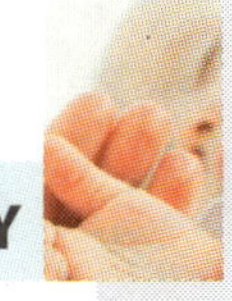

476. Ans. (c) 10% of infertile couples

Ref: Shaw, 15th pg. 202, 209

Definition of infertility: Inability to conceive even after 1 year of unprotected sexual intercourse.

Relative Prevalence of Cause of Infertility

- Male Factor 25–40%
- Female Factor 40–55 %
- Both 10%
- Unexplained 10%
  - **Disorders of the spermatogenesis** are the most common cause of **male infertility.**
  - **Ovarian causes** are the most common cause of **female infertility.**

Extra Mile

- WHO cut off limit for sperm count is 20 million/mL.
- Post coital test (Sim's or Huhner's test) is done for cervical factor of infertility
- Effective sperm count is 50 million/mL.
- Testicular biopsy can differentiate obstructive lesion at vas deferens from testicular failure.
- Most treatable form of infertility is anovulation.
- **Best investigation** for tubal patency is **laproscopic chromotubation.**
- Clomiphene citrate is the ovulation induction agent of choice
- **Ferning of cervical mucus** occurs due to **estrogen.**
- Bromocriptine is used to treat hyperprolactinemia.
- Ovarian hyperstimulation syndrome is most commonly the side effect of human menopausal gonadotropin injections used for ovulation induction.

477. Ans. (a) Azoospermia

Ref: Shaws, 15th ed. pg. 203

- Azoospermia is defined as complete absence of sperm from the ejaculate.
- It is present in about 1% of all men and in approximately 15% of infertile men.
- Azoospermia is different from aspermia, in that aspermia is the complete absence of seminal fluid emission upon ejaculation.
- In order to distinguish between obstructive and non-obstructive causes of azoospermia**, diagnostic testicular biopsy is indicated for patients with normal testicular size, at least one palpable vas deferens and a normal serum follicle-stimulating hormone level**.
- ***Testicular biopsy is indicated in azoospermic men*** with a normal-sized testis and normal findings on hormonal studies to rule out ductal obstruction.

Relative indications for testicular biopsy

- Ruling out partial obstruction in patients with severe oligospermia
- Evaluating patients with hypogonadotropism to select those likely responsive to treatment.
- Respond to gonadotropin replacement retrieving spermatozoa in azoospermic patients undergoing IVF or ICSI.

Extra Mile

- **Aspermia:** Absence of semen
- **Azoospermia:** Absence of sperm
- **Hypospermia:** Low semen volume
- **Oligozoospermia**: Low sperm count
- **Asthenozoospermia:** Poor sperm motility
- **Teratozoospermia:** Sperm carry more morphological defects than usual
- **Necrozoospermia:** All sperm in the ejaculate are dead

478. Ans. (b) CuT 380

Ref: Shaws, 15th ed. pg. 549

COPPER-T IUCD

- Can be Inserted within 5 days of intercourse
- **MOA:** Prevents implantation of a fertilized ovum.
- **Advantages:**
  - It can be inserted as late as 5 days after the unprotected intercourse.
  - cheap.
  - **Failure rate is EXCEPTIONALLY low which is 0.1%.**
  - It is long lasting, can remain as ongoing contraceptive method for 3 to 5 years.

Contraceptive	Failure rate	Method/time of administration
CuT	0.1%	Inserted within 5 days of UNPROTECTED sex
Levonorgestrel (LNG)	1.1%.	One tablet should be taken within 72 hours of unprotected sex and another 12 hours later.
Combined pill	3.2 per 100 woman years	Taken within 72 hours of intercourse followed by 2 tablets taken 12 hours later **(Yuzpe and Lancee method)**
RU 486 (mifepristone)	Failure rate 0.9%	Single dose of 10 mg
Ethinyloestra-diol	failure rate 0 to 1.5%	1 mg daily for 5 days, starting within 72 hours of unprotected sex **(Haspels and Andriesse method)**

479. Ans. (a) 0.1% to 0.3%

Ref: Shaw 15th ed. pg. 240

The most popular technique of tubal ligation is Pomeroy **technique (a type of minilaprotomy;** abdominal incision

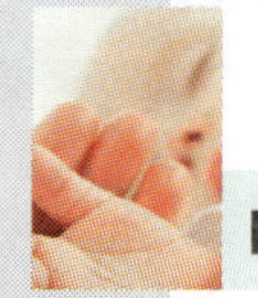

should be <5 cm). The failure rate is **only 0.4%. Catgut suture** is being used for this method of sterilization.

480. Ans. (b) 10 years

Ref: Shaw, 15th ed. pg. 227-8

Name of device	Effective period
• **CuT 380A**	**10 years**
• Nova T-Silver	5 years
• Multiload 375	5 years
• Multiload 250	3 years

481. Ans. (d) They are lipid friendly

Ref: D.C. Dutta, 7th ed. pg. 543-545

- Levonorgesterol is a progestin which is used in combined OCP with estrogen.
- The combined oral steroidal contraceptives is the most effective reversible method of contraception.
- The commonly used progestins are either levonogestrel or norethisterone or desogestrel.
- *Lipid friendly, third generation progestins are namely desogestrel, gestodene, norgestimate.*
- The oestrongens are principally confined to either ethinyl-oestradiol or menstronal.
- **Composition in OCP:** Levonorgestrel 0.15 + Ethinyl oestradiol 30
- It should normally be started on day one of the cycle.
- One tablet is to be taken daily preferably at bed time for consecutive 21 days. It is continued for 21 days and then has a seven days break.
- *Thus a simple regime of "3 weeks ON and 1 week off" is to be followed.*

482. Ans. (c) Protect from breast cancer

Ref: D.C. Dutta, 8th ed. pg. 625

BENEFITS OF COMBINED ORAL CONTRACEPTIVES (COCS)

- **Contraceptive benefits:**
  - Protection against unwanted pregnancy *(failure rate-0.1 per 100 women year)*
  - Convenient to use
  - Not intercourse related
  - Reversibility
  - Improving maternal and child health care
- **Non-contraceptive benefits:**
  - Improvement of menstrual abnormalities
  - Reduction of dysmenorrhea (40%)
  - Reduction of menorrhagia (50%)
  - Reduction of premenstrual tension syndrome (PM)
  - Prevention of malignancies like Endometrial cancer (50%), Epithelial ovarian cancer 50%, Colorectal cancer (40%).
- It increases risk of breast CA, cervical CA

483. Ans. (b) Protection against cervical cancer

Ref: D.C. Dutta, 7th ed. pg. 547

484. Ans. (c) Prevent release of ovum from ovary

Ref: DC Dutta, 8th ed. pg. 622

- Combined OCP is in combination with estrogen and progesterone. It acts by inhibiting ovulation.

POLYCYSTIC OVARIAN SYNDROME (PCOS)/STEIN LEVANTHAL SYNDROME

485. Ans. (b) PCOS

Ref: Shaw's Gynecology 16th ed. pg. 145-46

- MCC of hirsutism is: PCOS
- ***Polycystic ovarian syndrome accounts for 70 to 80% of cases of hirsutism**, with idiopathic hirsutism being the second most frequent cause.*
- In a female, hirsutism is defined as the presence of coarse, dark, terminal hairs distributed in a male pattern.
- Hirsutism in PCOS is secondary to hyperandrogenism.

Latest Definition of PCOS *(To include two out of three of the following)*

- Oligomenorrhea or anovulation
- Clinical and/or biochemical signs of **hyperandrogenism**
- Polycystic ovaries (with the exclusion of related disorders)

Signs and Symptoms/Consequences

- Patients with PCOS, complaints stem from varied endocrine effects and may include:
  - Menstrual irregularities, infertility, manifestations of androgen excess, or other endocrine dysfunction.

Short-term consequences	Long-term consequences
• Irregular menses • Hirsutism/acne androgenic alopecia • Infertility • Obesity • Metabolic disturbances • Abnormal lipid levels/glucose intolerance	• Diabetes mellitus • Cardiovascular disease • Endometrial cancer

486. Ans. (c) PCOD

Ref: Shaw's Gynecology 16th ed. pg. 145-46

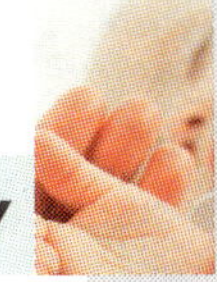

PCOD

In PCOD, upon USG:

- There are enlarged ovaries (increased size and stroma).
- Ovarian volume will be >10 mm^3.
- It shows 12 or more small follicles each of 2–9 mm in size placed peripherally.

Note: *In PCOD, there is hyperandrogenism. Androgen suppresses the growth of the dominant follicle and prevents apoptosis of smaller follicles which are normally destined to disappear in the late follicular phase. Hence there are increased numbers of follicles.*

Turner's Syndrome

- In Turner syndrome, either the short arm of X chromosome is deleted or the nucleus possesses only 45 chromosomes, i.e. 22 pairs of autosomes plus a sex chromosome XO.
- Sometimes, it is also referred as ovarian agenesis or gonadal dysgenesis because of presence of undifferentiated stromal cells with absence of sex cells, known as **streak gonads**.
- The **ovaries in Turner syndrome do not contain graafian follicles, so estrogen is not produced.**
- **In primary amenorrhea**, there is failure of HPO axis causing absence of ovarian follicles.
- In Klinefelter syndrome, there are masculine gonads.

487. Ans. (b) PCOD

Ref: Shaws, 15th ed. pg. 274; William's Gyne, Ch 17 PCOD

Please refer to above explanation for more details

Extra Mile

- **Ferriman-Gallwey Scoring System:** To quantify the degree of hirsutism
- **Most common areas affected with excess hair growth in women with PCOS include:** the upper lip, chin, sideburns, chest, and linea alba of the lower abdomen.
- Hirsutism should be distinguished from **hypertrichosis**, which is a generalized increase in lanugo, that is, the soft, lightly pigmented hair associated with some medications and malignancies.

488. Ans. (a) PCOS

Ref: Shaws, 15th ed. pg. 115-116

- **GARLAND/NECKLACE pattern on USG:** PCOS
- **Comet tail appearance:** Adenomyomatosis
- **Snowstorm appearance:** Choriocarcinoma

489. Ans. (d) Combined OCP

Ref: Williams Gynecology Ch 17

- Polycystic ovarian syndrome is also called Androgen insensitivity syndrome, where there is excess of androgen in female patient.
- Elevated androgen levels play a major role in determining the type and distribution of hair. Within a hair follicle, testosterone is converted by the enzyme 5a-reductase to dihydrotestosterone (DHT).
- Although both testosterone and DHT convert short, soft vellus hair to coarse terminal hair, **DHT is markedly more effective than testosterone.** Conversion is irreversible, and only hairs in androgen-sensitive areas are changed in this manner to terminal hairs. As a result the most common areas affected with excess hair growth in women with PCOS include the upper lip, chin, sideburns, chest, and linea alba of the lower abdomen.
- A first-line treatment for menstrual irregularities is combination oral contraceptive pills (COCs), which will induce regular menstrual cycles. In addition, COCs reduce androgen levels, Thereby, decreasing the severity of hirsutism.
- Specifically, COCs suppress gonadotropin release, which results in decreased ovarian androgen production. Moreover, the estrogen component increases SHBG levels. The progestin component antagonizes the endometrial proliferative effect of estrogen, thus reducing risks of endometrial hyperplasia due to unopposed estrogen.

PROLAPSE

490. Ans. (d) Pessary for temporary relief

Ref: William's Obstetrics, Chapter 42, 26th ed. pg. 2093

- The pessary is most commonly used in the nonsurgical management of pelvic support defects such as cystocele and rectocele.
- Multiple vaginal deliveries can weaken the musculature of the pelvic floor.
- Hysterectomy or other pelvic surgery can predispose a woman to weakness of the pelvic floor, as can conditions that involve repetitive bearing down, such as chronic constipation, chronic coughing or repetitive heavy lifting.

491. Ans. (a) Vesicovaginal fistula

Ref: Comprehensive Gynecology 7th ed. pg. 600

- Vesicovaginal fistula (VVF) is a subtype of female urogenital fistula. VVF is an abnormal fistulous tract extending between the bladder and the vagina that allows the continuous involuntary discharge of urine into the vaginal vault.

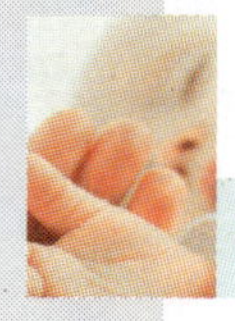

- It is the most common of all of the vaginal fistulas. Intraoperative injury to the urinary bladder is a primary risk factor for subsequent development of a postoperative VVF.
- Other risk factors for postoperative VVF formation include prior uterine surgery (cesarean section), endometriosis, infection, diabetes, arteriosclerosis, pelvic inflammatory disease, obesity, and prior radiation therapy.

492. Ans. (a) Stress urinary incontinence

Ref: DC Dutta's 9th ed. pg. 410

Stress urinary incontinence is a leakage of urine during moments of physical activity that increases abdominal pressure, such as coughing, sneezing, laughing and exercise. It is the most common type of urinary incontinence in female.

493. Ans. (d) Packing

Ref: Shaws Textbook of Gynecology, 7th ed. pg. 377

- Decubitus ulcer is seen often in a patient of utero vaginal prolapse, which occurs due to localised tissue damage and venous congestion.
- Treatment of this ulcer is done by moist vaginal packing using acriflavine and glycerine soaked gauze.

494. Ans. (c) Needs to be changed every 3 months

Ref: Shaw's Gynecology 16th ed. pg. 356; DC Dutta 9th ed. pg. 293

- Ring pessary is used for prolapse
- The ring pessary is made of soft plastic polyvinyl chloride material and is available in different sizes.
- It is inserted using gel
- Pregnant woman with prolapse needs a ring pessary in the first trimester of pregnancy
  - Uterus grows abdominally, the prolapse gets reduced, and the pessary can then be removed.
- **Current indications for use of pessary are:**
  - A young woman planning a pregnancy
  - During early pregnancy
  - Puerperium
  - Temporary use while clearing infection and decubitus ulcer
  - A woman unfit for surgery
  - In case a woman refuses for surgery

495. Ans. (c) Pessary

Ref: Shaw's Gynecology 16th ed. pg. 359-60

- Pessary is the conservative treatment for prolapse.
- All other choices are surgical repair

TABLE: Management of genital prolapse

Nulliparous	Abdominal sling operations
Pregnancy Postnatal	Ring pessary up to 16 weeks • Ring pessary and pelvic floor exercises for 3-6 months • Surgery if required thereafter
Young woman <40 years	Conservative vaginal surgery (fertility sparing surgery) • Cystocele, rectocele repair
	• Manchester repair • Sling operation
Woman beyond 40 years and multipara	Vaginal hysterectomy and pelvic floor repair

Extra Mile

Surgeries of prolapse

- **Anterior colporrhaphy:** To repair cystocoele and cystourethrocele
- **Posterior colporrhaphy:** to repair rectocoele and deficient perineum
- **Fothergill's Repair (Manchester Operation):** Anterior colporrhaphy with amputation of cervix
  - Preserves menstrual and childbearing functions
- **Shirodkar's Procedure:** Anterior colporrhaphy and attachment of Mackenrodt ligaments to the cervix on each side is exposed
  - The cervix is not amputated and subsequent pregnancy complications avoided
- **Le Fort's Repair:** reserved for the very elderly menopausal patient with an advanced prolapse.
- **Sling operation:** best for nulliparous prolapse
  - Abdominal sling operation
  - Khanna sling operation
  - Abdominal wall cervicopexy

ENT

13

MOST RECENT QUESTIONS 2023

1. **What is correct for the structure of nose?** *(Most Recent Question July 2023)*
   a. Upper ½ bone & lower ½ cartilage
   b. Upper ⅔ bone & lower ⅓ cartilage
   c. Upper ⅓ bone & lower ⅔ cartilage
   d. Upper ⅓ cartilage & lower ⅔ bone
2. **Which of the following stridor type is given in the image?** *(Most Recent Question July 2023)*

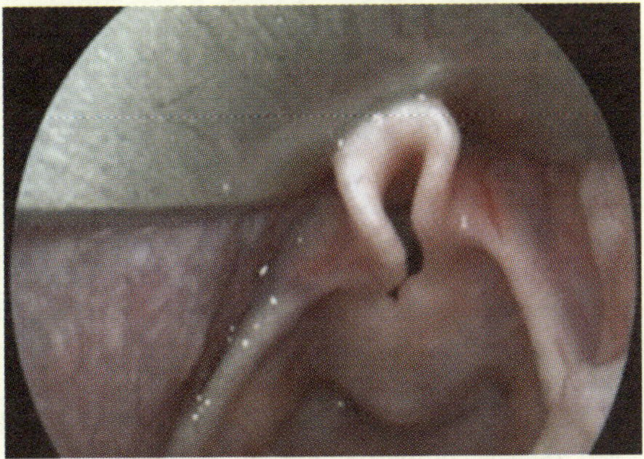

   a. Inspiratory b. Expiratory
   c. Biphasic d. None of these
3. **A neonate presented with difficulty in breathing neonate presented with difficulty in breathing. His symptoms improve with crying. In which disease, symptoms improve with crying?** *(Most Recent Question July 2023)*
   a. Atrophic rhinitis
   b. Acute rhinosinusitis
   c. Allergic rhinitis
   d. Choanal atresia
4. **Which artery is most commonly affected in cases of epistasis?** *(Most Recent Question July 2023)*
   a. Anterior ethmoidal artery
   b. Sphenopalatine artery
   c. Greater palatine artery
   d. Posterior ethmoidal artery
5. **Which of the following investigation is carried out immediately when a child has foreign body in his lungs?** *(Most Recent Question July 2023)*
   a. Ragid bronchoscopy b. Chest X-ray
   c. Direct laryngoscopy d. Flexible endoscopy
6. **A child present with swelling at the floor of mouth, below tongue and is brilliantly trans illuminant. Possible diagnosis is:**

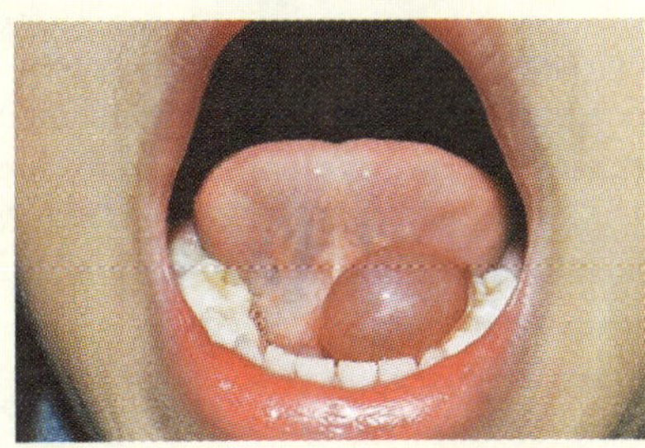

   a. Brachial cyst b. Ranula
   c. Sub lingual cyst d. Salivary gland tumor
7. **A 54-year-old male presented with nasal obstruction. On examination, there as irregular mass inside the nose. Possible cause is:** *(Most Recent Question July 2023)*
   a. Tornwaldt cyst
   b. Hypertrophic rhinitis
   c. Antrochoanal polyp
   d. Rhinolith
8. **What is the location of bulla ethmoidalis?** *(Most Recent Question July 2023)*
   a. Sphenoethmoidal recess
   b. Superior meatus
   c. Middle meatus
   d. Inferior meatus
9. **The patient with bell's palsy presented with complaints of deviation of face. The deviation is seen on which side of face?** *(Most Recent Question Jan 2023)*
   a. Same side of face
   b. Same side lower part of face
   c. Opposite side upper part
   d. Opposite side lower part

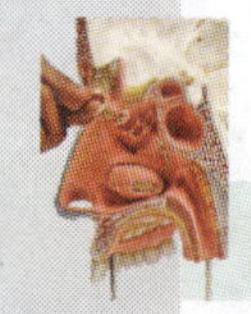

10. A 16-year-old male presented with recurrent profuse bleeding from nose. What would be the best treatment in this patient? ***(Most Recent Question Jan 2023)***

a. FNAC
b. Biopsy
c. Radiotherapy
d. Surgical excision

11. A 2-year-old male child was brought to the emergency department. The child was having difficulty in speaking and breathing. An X-ray was performed as shown here. Which among the following is the best treatment for the following condition?

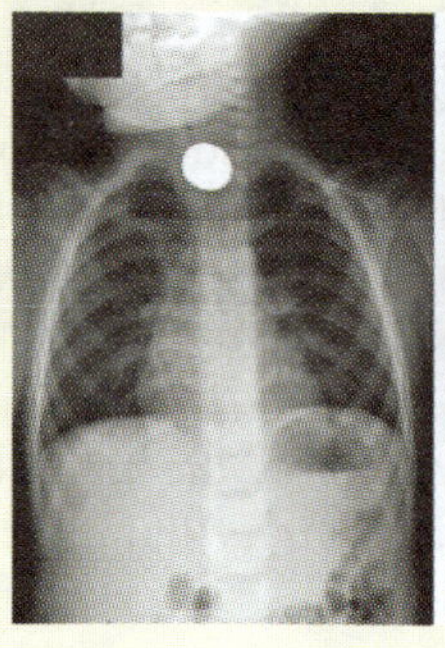

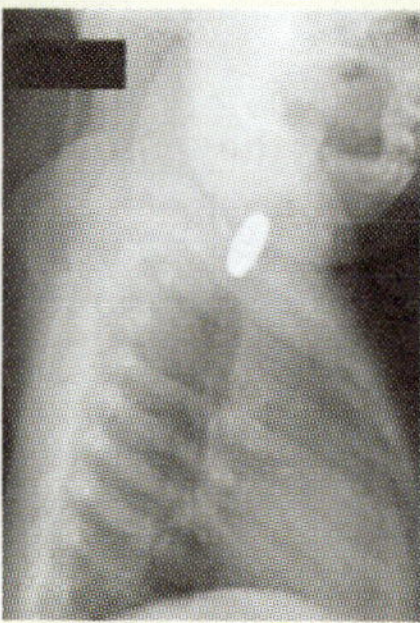

a. Bronchoscopy
b. Tracheostomy
c. Esophagoscopy
d. Heimlich maneuver

12. Which sensory nerve supplies the larynx above the vocal cord? ***(Most Recent Question Jan 2023)***

a. Internal laryngeal nerve
b. External laryngeal nerve
c. Recurrent laryngeal nerve
d. Superior laryngeal nerve

13. What is the function of utricle and saccule in inner ear? ***(Most Recent Question Jan 2023)***

a. Linear motion and angular motion
b. Linear motion
c. Helps in hearing low-frequency sound
d. Helps in hearing high-frequency sound

14. Identify the prominent sinus in the image. ***(Most Recent Question Jan 2023)***

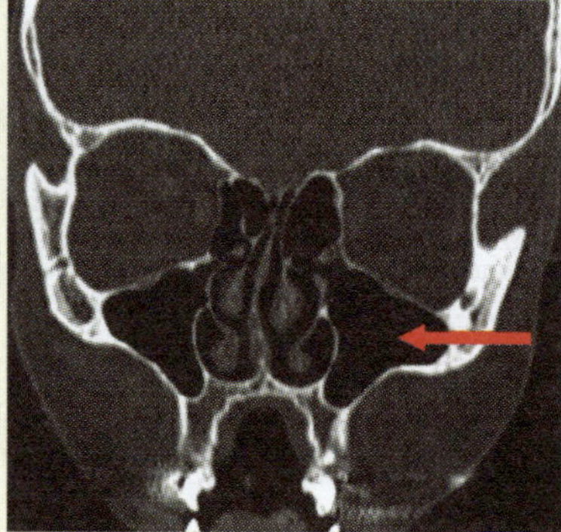

a. Sphenoid sinus
b. Ethmoid sinus
c. Maxillary sinus
d. Frontal sinus

15. A 35-year-old female took tablet of aspirin for her headache, later she presented with wheezing and breathlessness. These symptoms are most likely due to which of the following? ***(Most Recent Question Jan 2023)***

a. IgE release
b. Nasal polyp
c. Drug interaction
d. Extrinsic asthma

16. A patient who's a singer by profession presented to the clinic with complaints of hoarseness of voice. What is the possible diagnosis in this patient? ***(Most Recent Question Jan 2023)***

a. Vocal polyp
b. Vocal nodule
c. Vocal cyst
d. Reinke's edema

17. A 25-year-old female presented with complaints of decreased hearing (CHL) and pulsatile tinnitus. On examination tympanic membrane appeared red and bulging. What would be the diagnosis? ***(Most Recent Question Jan 2023)***

a. Glomus tumor
b. Serous otitis media
c. Acute otitis media
d. Chronic otitis media

18. Which type of tracheostomy tube is used in the case of an ICU patient? ***(Most Recent Question Jan 2023)***

a. Metallic tube
b. Cuffed tube
c. Uncuffed tube
d. Fenestrated cuffless tube

19. A person with Rinke's edema will have which of the following symptoms more commonly: ***(Most Recent Question Jan 2023)***

a. Dysphagia of solids more than liquids
b. Dysphagia of liquids more than solids
c. Diplophonia
d. Dysphonia

20. In a patient with Ramsay Hunt syndrome which ganglion is affected? ***(Most Recent Question Jan 2023)***

a. Geniculate ganglion
b. Otic ganglion
c. Trigeminal ganglion
d. Basal ganglion

21. The patient presents with complaints of unilateral nasal obstruction associated with watery nasal discharge or nasal bleeding. And the diagnosis of inverted papilloma is made. Which is true regarding the following condition? ***(Most Recent Question Jan 2023)***

a. Malignant
b. Benign and non-invasive
c. Benign and non-aggressive
d. Malignant and non-aggressive

ANATOMY OF AURICLE AND EXTERNAL AUDITORY CANAL & EMBRYOLOGY

22. A young woman with history of progressive moderate bilateral hearing loss came to OPD which aggravated during her pregnancy. On examination tympanic membrane was intact. What should be done to rectify this? *(Most Recent Question June 2022)*
a. Tympanoplasty
b. Conservative management
c. Tympanoplasty with stapedectomy
d. Tympanotomy with stapedectomy

23. While examining a patient's external ear syncopal attacks occurred. Which nerve is responsible for this? *(Most Recent Question June/Dec 2021)*
a. Jacobsons nerve b. Glossopharyngeal nerve
c. Arnolds nerve d. Trigeminal nerve

24. A neonate suffering from bilateral complete choanal atresia has respiratory distress since birth. What is the cause of respiratory difficulty in this neonate? *(Most Recent Question June/Dec 2021)*
a. Less lung volume
b. Associated vocal cord palsy
c. Newborns are obligatory nasal breathers
d. Insufficient lung surfactant

25. 60-year-old diabetic patient has presented with severe ear ache and blood stained ear discharge. The examination shows granulations in the external auditory canal. What is the possible diagnosis in this case? *(Most Recent Question June/Dec 2021)*
a. Malignant otitis externa
b. Diffuse otitis externa
c. Otomycosis
d. Chronic suppurative otitis media

26. Which of the following is the derivative of first pharyngeal arch: *(Recent Pattern Question 2018-19)*
a. Stapedius muscle
b. Anterior belly of digastric muscle
c. Posterior belly of digastric muscle
d. Hyoid bone

27. What is the Ossicles-lever ratio? *(Recent Pattern Question 2018)*
a. 1.3:1 b. 1.8:1
c. 21:1 d. 14:1

28. Endolymph is secreted by: *(Recent Pattern Question 2018)*
a. Basilar membrane b. Reissner's membrane
c. Stria vascularis d. Tectorial membrane

29. Surgical landmark for mastoid antrum: *(Recent Pattern Question 2017)*
a. Korner septum b. MacEwen's triangle
c. Fallopian triangle d. Antral triangle

30. Which muscle arises from 4th phyrangeal arch? *(Recent Pattern Question 2016)*
a. Cricothyroid muscle b. Cricoarytenoid
c. Posterior cricoarytenoid d. Thyroarytenoid

31. Ear lobule is made of:
a. Skin only b. Cartilage
c. Skin with fat d. Fibrous tissue

32. All of the following nerves supply auricle of ear EXCEPT?
a. Greater auricular nerve b. Lesser petrosal nerve
c. Auriculotemporal nerve d. Lesser Occipital nerve

33. All of the following nerves supply the medial aspect of auricle EXCEPT?
a. Greater auricular nerve b. Lesser occipital nerve
c. Facial nerve d. Auriculotemporal nerve

34. Major portion of auricle is supplied by:
a. Greater auricular nerve b. Lesser occipital nerve
c. Facial nerve d. Auriculotemporal nerve

35. Arnold nerve is a branch of:
a. Vagus nerve b. Hypoglossal nerve
c. Glossopharyngeal nerve d. Trigeminal nerve

36. Jacobson's nerve is a branch of:
a. Vagus nerve b. Hypoglossal nerve
c. Glossopharyngeal nerve d. Trigeminal nerve

37. Which of these is not a derivative of 3rd pharyngeal/ branchial arch?
a. Lesser cornu b. Greater cornu
c. Stylopharyngeus d. Lower hyoid

38. Greater cornu of hyoid is derived from which branchial arch:
a. I b. II
c. III d. IV

39. Which of the following intrinsic laryngeal muscles is not derived from branchial arch VI?
a. Cricoarytenoid muscle b. Interarytenoid muscle
c. Thyroarytenoid muscle d. Cricothyroid muscle

40. Thyroid cartilage is derived from which branchial arch:
a. II and III b. III and IV
c. IV and V d. IV and VI

41. Stapes is derived from which branchial arch:
a. I b. II
c. III d. IV

42. All are derived from branchial arch EXCEPT:
a. Ultimobranchial body b. Stapes
c. Laryngeal cartilage d. Mandible

43. All are true about external auditory meatus EXCEPT:
a. It extends from the bottom of concha to tympanic membrane & measures 24 mm in length
b. Fissure of santorini in cartilaginous part can transmit infection to the parotid or superficial mastoid infection.
c. Foramen of Huschke may present from Antero-inferior part of bony canal
d. Outer 1/3rd is bony and inner 2/3rd is cartilaginous

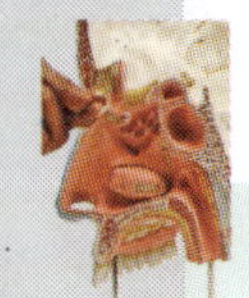

44. Length of cartilaginous part of external auditory canal:

a. 1.5 cm b. 2.4 cm
c. 8 cm d. <1 cm

45. Foramen of Huschke is a congenital pathology located between:

a. Bony part of EAC and submandibular gland
b. Cartilaginous part of EAC and submandibular gland
c. Bony part of EAC and parotid gland
d. Cartilaginous part of EAC and parotid gland

46. All are true about external ear EXCEPT:

a. Auricle is made up of frame work of single yellow elastic cartilage covered with skin
b. Area between tragus and crus of helix without cartilage is incisura terminalis
c. Cartilage from the tragus can be used in reconstructive surgery of nose
d. Composite grafts of cartilage and skin from pinna cannot be used for correction of defects of nasal ala

47. What is the length of external auditory canal?

a. 2.5 cm b. 1.5 cm
c. 1 cm d. 2 cm

48. Ceruminous glands are seen in which part of external auditory canal:

a. 2/3rd outer
b. 2/3 inner
c. 1/3rd outer
d. 1/3rd inner

49. Retromolar trigone is located at:

a. Posterior part of mandible
b. Ascending ramus of mandible
c. Submandibular area
d. Digastric muscle

ANATOMY OF MIDDLE EAR & INNER EAR

50. A boy was hit by a cricket ball while playing and next day morning he presents with headache, diplopia on looking up and enophthalmos. Which of the following is responsible for this? *(Most Recent Question June 2022)*

a. Fracture of roof of the orbit
b. Fracture of floor of the orbit
c. Subdural hematoma
d. Intracranial hemorrhage

51. A patient had mild hearing loss, along with nasal obstruction. Following is the examination finding. What is the most likely diagnosis?

(Most Recent Question June 2022)

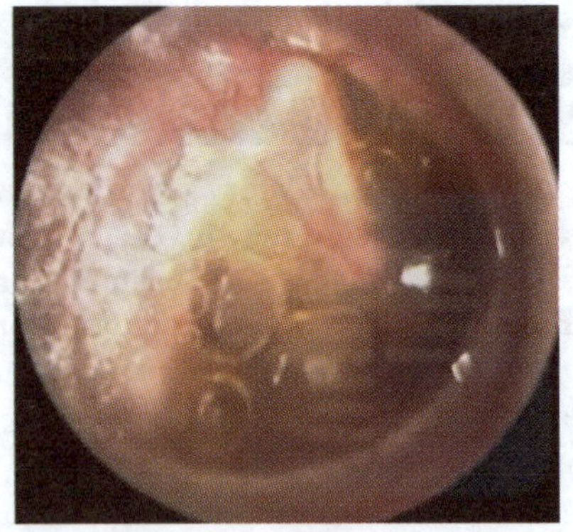

a. CSOM with central perforation
b. Serous Otitis media with effusion
c. Otomycosis
d. Otosclerosis

52. Battle's sign is due to?

(Most Recent Question June/Dec 2021)

a. Edema of mastoid
b. Bruising over the mastoid
c. Angiofibroma
d. External laryngocoele

53. A patient presented with a red mass behind tympanic membrane with pulsatile tinnitus, possible diagnosis:

(Most Recent Question June/Dec 2021)

a. Cholesteatoma b. Glomus tumour
c. Otosclerosis d. Meniere's disease

54. A 7-year-old child complaining of hearing loss and sense of fullness in the ear. The tympanometry shows type B curve. What is the diagnosis of this child?

(Most Recent Question June/Dec 2021)

a. Chronic suppurative otitis media
b. Secretory otitis media
c. Acute suppurative otitis media
d. Otitis externa

55. Which is the peripheral receptor of hearing?

(Recent Pattern Question 2017)

a. Organ of Corti b. Ampulla
c. Utricle d. Semicircular canal

56. The semi-circular canal is responsible for:

(Recent Pattern Question 2017)

a. Hearing b. Balance
c. Cough reflex d. Sneezing reflex

57. Promontory is seen in which wall of middle ear?

(Recent Pattern Question 2017)

a. Anterior b. Medial
c. Posterior d. Lateral

58. Eustachean tube opens in:

(Recent Pattern Question 2017)

a. Nasopharynx b. Oropharynx
c. Trachea d. Laryngopharynx

59. Stria vascularis is present in:

(Recent Pattern Question 2016)

a. Cochlea b. Saccule
c. Utricle d. Semi-circular canals

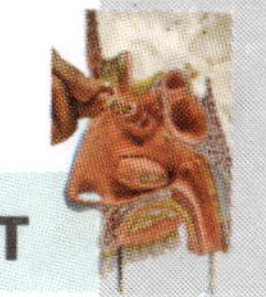

60. Autoconia is seen in: *(Recent Pattern Question 2016)*
a. Utricle
b. Superior semicircular canal
c. Lateral semicircular canal
d. Cochlea

61. Least blood supply goes to: *(Recent Pattern Question 2016)*
a. Handle of malleus b. Body of incus
c. Long process of incus d. Stapes

62. Corda tympani is seen on which wall of middle ear:
a. Anterior wall b. Medial wall
c. Posterior wall d. Lateral wall

63. Anterior wall of middle ear is also known as:
a. Outer wall b. Mastoid wall
c. Carotid wall d. Jugular wall

64. Which of the following is not a content of medial wall of middle ear?
a. Oval window
b. Round window
c. Processus cochleariformis
d. Aditus ad antrum

65. Tegmen tympani separates middle ear from:
a. Anterior cranial fossa b. Posterior cranial fossa
c. Middle cranial fossa d. Superior cranial fossa

66. Otosclerosis is seen which wall of middle ear:
a. Anterior b. Posterior
c. Lateral d. Medial

67. Tensor typmani is inserted in:
a. Tympanic membrane b. Malleus
c. Incus d. Stapes

68. Fallopian canal contains which cranial nerve?
a. 5 b. 6
c. 7 d. 8

69. Length of internal acoustic meatus:
a. 5 mm b. 1 cm
c. 2 cm d. 3 cm

70. Shortest length of middle ear:
a. 2 mm b. 4 mm
c. 6 mm d. 1 cm

71. Bill's bar divides:
a. Facial nerve and cochlear nerve
b. Facial nerve and superior vestibular cochlear nerve
c. Facial and inferior vestibule cochlear nerve
d. Superior and inferior vestibule cochlear nerve

72. Cochlea main function is:
a. Balancing b. Hearing
c. Otolith organ d. Olfaction

73. All are required for balancing EXCEPT:
a. Visual system b. Olfactory system
c. Proprioception d. Vestibule and cochlea

74. Cupula is seen in:
a. Saccule b. Utricle
c. Semicircular canal d. Cochlea

75. Stria vascularis are seen in:
a. Vestibule b. Utricle
c. Cochlea d. Middle ear

TESTS OF AUDITORY SYSTEM

76. Type B tympanogram is seen In which of the following conditions: *(Most Recent Question June/Dec 2021)*
a. Serous otitis media b. Ossicular dislocation
c. Normal ear d. Otosclerosis

77. True about BERA *(Most Recent Question Dec 2019-20)*
a. Invasive test
b. Used for SNHL
c. Used for conductive pathology
d. Is a subjective test

78. Cause of decreased bone conduction on audiogram: *(Most Recent Question Dec 2019-20)*
a. Fixation of foot plate of stapes
b. External auditory canal pathology
c. Cochlear pathology
d. Ossicular pathology

79. Why is cold water not used in syringing? *(Recent Pattern Question 2018-19)*
a. Cold water leads to wax impaction
b. Cold water leads to foreign body impaction
c. Can cause tympanic membrane rupture
d. Can cause vertigo

80. In audiometry a notch is seen at 4000 Hz. This is most likely due to: *(Recent Pattern Question 2018-19)*
a. Otosclerosis
b. Meniere's disease
c. Noise induced hearing loss
d. Age related hearing loss

81. Maximum tolerable noise according to Government of India guidelines: *(Recent Pattern Question 2018)*
a. 85 dB, 8 hrs/day for 5 days/week
b. 90 dB in 8 hrs/day for 5 days/week
c. 95 dB, 8 hrs/day for 5 days/week
d. 115 dB, 8 hrs/day for 6 days/week

82. The graph for otosclerosis in tympanometry is: *(Recent Pattern Question 2017)*
a. Ad b. As
c. A d. B

83. Which test is used for screening for neonatal deafness? *(Recent Pattern Question 2017)*
a. Tuning fork test b. ABR
c. Impedance audiometry d. Tympanometry

84. Otoacoustic emission comes from: *(Recent Pattern Question 2017)*
a. Utricle b. Cochlea
c. Saccule d. Semicircular canal

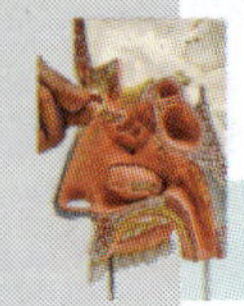

85. **Tone decay is seen in:** *(Recent Pattern Question 2017)*
    a. Otosclerosis   b. Glue ear
    c. Ossicular disruption   d. Acoustic neuroma
86. **Gelle test is done for:** *(Recent Pattern Question 2016)*
    a. Otosclerosis   b. Senile deafness
    c. Traumatic deafness   d. Congenital deafness
87. **Negative Rinne test indicates:** *(Recent Pattern Question 2016)*
    a. Meniere's disease   b. CSOM
    c. BPPV   d. Sensorineural hearing loss
88. **Pure tone audiometry symbol 'X' is used for:** *(Recent Pattern Question 2016)*
    a. Right ear, air conduction
    b. Right ear, bone conduction
    c. Left ear, air conduction
    d. Left ear, bone conduction
89. **Most common frequency of tuning fork used in ENT:**
    a. 256 Hz   b. 512 Hz
    c. 1024 Hz   d. 2048 Hz
90. **Which of the following is the best tuning fork to do Rinne's and Weber's tests?**
    a. 128 Hz   b. 256 Hz
    c. 512 Hz   d. 1024 Hz
91. **All of the following are tuning fork test EXCEPT:**
    a. Gelle test   b. Rinne test
    c. Schwabach's test   d. Pure tone audiometry
92. **Otoacoustic emissions are derived from:**
    a. Tympanic membrane   b. Ossicles
    c. Cochlea   d. Vestibule
93. **Sensorineural deafness in neonates is best diagnosed by:**
    a. ABR   b. Audiometry
    c. Tympanometry   d. Electrocochleography
94. **Caloric test is done for assessing:**
    a. Vestibular function   b. Auditory function
    c. Tactile function   d. Ocular function
95. **Calorie test with warm and cold water stimulates which of the following structures?**
    a. Saccule
    b. Lateral semicircular canal
    c. Superior semicircular canal
    d. Posterior semicircular canal
96. **Vestibular function is tested by:**
    a. Fistula test   b. Acoustic reflex
    c. Galvanic stimulation   d. Impedance Audiometry

DISEASES OF EAR, TREATMENT AND REHABILITATION

97. **Bone anchored hearing aid is used in which of the following condition?** *(Most Recent Question June 2022)*
    a. SNHL   b. Acoustic neuroma
    c. Otitis media
    d. Congenital external auditory atresia
98. **Trotters triad includes all; EXCEPT:** *(Most Recent Question June/Dec 2021)*
    a. Conductive hearing loss
    b. Retroorbital pain
    c. Palatal palsy
    d. Pain in the area of distribution of 5th nerve
99. **A patient presented with pain around mastoid, and positive reservoir sign. Most likely diagnosis:** *(Most Recent Question Aug 2020)*
    a. Mastoiditis   b. Acute otitis media
    c. Otitis media   d. CSOM
100. **All of the following is true about Meniere's disease EXCEPT:** *(Most Recent Question Dec 2019-20)*
    a. Idiopathic in origin
    b. Low frequency hearing loss
    c. Increase in endolymph
    d. Destroying the cochlear is mandatory
101. **Upon examination of oral cavity there were pulsation felt at the tonsillar area. A patient presented with of the pulsation of tonsil. The cause is:** *(Most Recent Question Dec 2019-20)*
    a. Aneurysm of the common carotid
    b. Aneurysm of the external carotid
    c. Carotid body tumor
    d. Internal carotid artery aneurysm
102. **A patient presented with profound sensorineural deafness, not responding to hearing aids, with intact auditory nerve function. Which of the following procedure is preferred in this patient?** *(Most Recent Question 2019)*
    a. BAHA   b. Cochlear implant
    c. Brainstem implant   d. Tympanoplasty
103. **Mainstay of treatment of Glue ear:** *(Recent Pattern Question 2018-19)*
    a. Antibiotics
    b. Nasal decongestants + Antibiotics
    c. Myringectomy + Gromet insertion
    d. Myringotomy + Gromet insertion
104. **The drug whose side effect is cochleotoxicity:** *(Recent Pattern Question 2018)*
    a. Kanamycin   b. Ofloxacin
    c. Imipenem   d. Minocycline
105. **Most common cause of facial nerve palsy:** *(Recent Pattern Question 2018)*
    a. Idiopathic Bell's palsy
    b. Herpes zoster oticus
    c. Mastoid surgery
    d. Chronic suppurative otitis media
106. **Flamingo pink appearance of tympanic membrane is seen in:** *(Recent Pattern Question 2018)*
    a. Glomus tumor   b. Otosclerosis
    c. Acoustic neuroma   d. Cholesteatoma

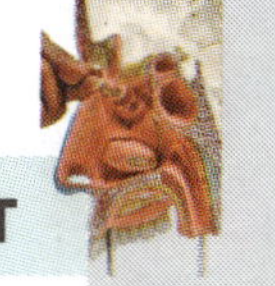

107. Ear pain, tinnitus and vertigo along with feeling of blocked ear is a feature of: ***(Recent Pattern Question 2018)***
a. Gradenigo's syndrome
b. Cantrell disease
c. Costen syndrome
d. Lermoyez syndrome

108. A patient presents with symptoms of facial nerve palsy and bulla on tympanic membrane and meatus. Possible diagnosis: ***(Recent Pattern Question 2017)***
a. Bell's palsy b. Ramsay hunt syndrome
c. Herpes oticus d. Melkersson syndrome

109. Granulomatous lesion in tympanic membrane and middle ear lateral wall is seen in: ***(Recent Pattern Question 2016)***
a. CSOM b. Bullous myringitis
c. Chronic myringitis d. Herpes zoster oticus

110. Ventilation tube is put in the ear in cases of: ***(Recent Pattern Question 2016)***
a. Otoscleorsis b. Labryinthitis
c. Serous otitis media d. CSOM

111. Impaction of wax is treated by:
a. Syringing ***(Recent Pattern Question 2016)***
b. Softening followed by syringing
c. Instrumentation
d. Suction

112. In tympanic membrane perforation, graft is taken from temporalis muscle fascia. What type of graft this? ***(Recent Pattern Question 2016)***
a. Autograft b. Allograft
c. Xenograft d. Isograft

113. Normal hearing range:
a. 20–20,000 Hz b. 30–30,000 Hz
c. 200–2000 Hz d. 300–3000 Hz

114. According to WHO moderate hearing loss is defined at:
a. 30–40 dB b. 41–60 dB
c. 56–70 dB d. 71–90 dB

115. Noise induced hearing loss is seen maximum at:
a. 1–2 khz b. 3–4 khz
c. 5–6 khz d. 7–10 khz

116. Myringitis bullosa is commonly caused by:
a. Bacteria b. Virus
c. Fungi d. Protozoa

117. Acute otitis media is most commonly caused by:
a. Streptococcus pneumoniae
b. Hemophilus influenzae
c. Staphylococcus aureus
d. Klebsiella pneumoniae

118. Which of the following is resorbed in otitis media development?
a. Pus b. Blood
c. Air d. All of these

119. According to TOS classification of chronic otitis media in which stage is the retraction pocket adherent to the handle of malleus and full extent of the retraction pocket can be clearly seen.
a. Stage 1 b. Stage 2
c. Stage 3 d. Stage 4

120. All are extracranial complications of chronic otitis media; EXCEPT:
a. Ossicular damage
b. Petrositis
c. Gradenigo syndrome
d. Lateral sinus thrombophlebitis

121. Most common intracranial manifestation of late chronic otitis media:
a. Brain abscess
b. Cerebellar abscess
c. Lateral sinus thrombophlebitis
d. Labyrinthine fistula

122. Most common extracranial complication of CSOM:
a. Meningitis b. Ossicle damage
c. Mastoiditis d. Labyrinthine fistula

123. Most common type of hearing loss in TB otitis media
a. Conductive hearing loss b. SNHL
c. Presbycusis d. Hyperacusis

124. Which one of the following is classical sign of tubercular otitis media?
a. Marginal perforation of tympanic membrane
b. Multiple perforation of pars tensa
c. Large central perforation of tympanic membrane
d. Attic perforation

125. Which of the following ear ossicle is 1st to get affected in otitis media?
a. Long process of incus b. Stapes
c. Handle of malleus d. Body of malleus

126. Gradenigo syndrome involves which cranial nerve:
a. CN IV, V b. CN V, VI
c. CN VII, VIII d. CN IX, X

127. Which is not a component of Gardenigo's syndrome?
a. Deafness b. Ear discharge
c. Retroorbital pain d. Double vision

128. Which is a causative organism for malignant otitis externa?
a. Virus b. Bacteria
c. Fungi d. Protozoa

129. Malignant otitis externa affects which cranial nerve:
a. 7th b. 8th
c. 9th d. 10th

130. Ramsay hunt syndrome is due to:
a. Herpes zoster virus
b. Herpes simplex virus
c. Varicella zoster
d. Pseudomonas

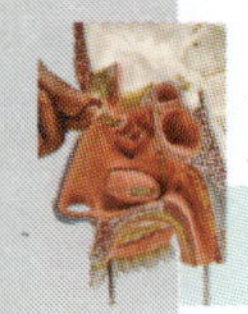

131. What will be the probable site of lesion causing slowly progressive facial palsy?
a. Skull b. Parotid
c. Geniculate ganglion d. Middle ear

132. Schwartz's sign is seen in:
a. Otosclerosis b. Meniere's disease
c. Retrocochlear lesion d. None of these

133. Carhart's notch dips at:
a. 2 Hz b. 200 Hz
c. 2000 Hz d. 2000 MHz

134. Which of the following is earliest and consistent symptom of glomus tumor?
a. Hoarseness b. Tinnitus
c. Otorrhea d. Dysphagia

135. Hennebert sign is seen in:
a. Otosclerosis b. Vestibular neuritis
c. Menier's disease d. Rotatory nystagmus

136. Hearing defect in menier's disease:
a. Hyperacusis b. Hypoacusis
c. Diplacusis d. Paracusia Willi

137. In case of BPPV, which semicircular canal is affected:
a. Lateral semicircular canal
b. Posterior semicircular canal
c. Anterior semicircular canal
d. Superior semicircular canal

138. Referred pain in the ear is commonly from:
a. Mandibular cancer b. Carcinoma of tongue
c. Laryngeal cancer d. Maxillary carcinoma

139. Trotter's triad consists of all of the following EXCEPT:
a. Palatal paralysis b. Trigeminal Neuralgia
c. Sensorineural deafness d. Conduction deafness

140. Which of the following is most prominent symptom of acoustic neuroma?
a. Ataxic gait
b. Diplopia
c. Sensorineural hearing loss
d. Parasthesia

141. Which one of the following is not a feature of adenoid hypertrophy?
a. Dull expression b. Open mouth
c. Pinched up nose d. Crowding of lower tooth

142. Adenoidectomy is contraindicated in:
a. Glue ear
b. Recurrent rhinosinusitis
c. Mouth breathing
d. Cleft palate

143. All of the following are the indications of adenoidectomy; EXCEPT:
a. Obstructive sleep apnea
b. Allergic rhinitis
c. Recurrent glue ear
d. Prior to orthodontic treatment

144. Adenoidectomy with Grommet insertion is treatment of choice for:
a. Serous otitis media in adults
b. Serous otitis media in children
c. Adenoiditis in children
d. Otitis interna in children

145. A 5-year-old child presents to your clinic with complaint of recurrent respiratory tract infection. Mother complains about this recurrent infection, mouth breathing and decreased hearing. Treatment of choice for this condition is:
a. Myringoplasty b. Adenoidectomy
c. Grommet insertion d. Myringotomy

146. Graft used for tympanoplasty:
a. Antral fascia b. Temporalis fascia
c. Preauricular fascia d. Postauricular fascia

147. Electrode of cochlear implant is passed via:
a. Round window
b. Oval window
c. Lateral semicircular canal
d. Around the auditory nerve

NOSE AND PARANASAL SINUSES

148. A 65-year-old diabetic patient with history of COVID-19 infection few months back presented in OPD with destruction of nasal portion of face. Which of the following is the drug of choice in this case? ***(Most Recent Question June 2022)***
a. Amphotericin B b. Streptomycin
c. Amikocin d. Azithromycin

149. A 35-year-old patient presented with complaints of vertigo on loud sound and blowing of nose. What is your diagnosis? ***(Most Recent Question June 2022)***
a. Labyrinthitis b. BPPV
c. Vestibular neuronitis d. Meniere's disease

150. Which fungal infection is most commonly seen in maxillary sinus? ***(Most Recent Question June 2022)***
a. Aspergilloma b. Mucormycosis
c. Candidiasis d. Rhizopus

151. A 15-year-old male presented with bleeding from nose and on examination there is a mass, probable diagnosis is: ***(Most Recent Question June/Dec 2021)***
a. Rhinosporidiosis
b. Nasopharyngeal angiofibroma
c. Nasopharyngeal ca
d. Rhinoscleroma

152. A post covid patient presented with black discharge from nasal cavity. On examination a black nasal mass extending onto orbit. Most likely cause is: ***(Most Recent Question June/Dec 2021)***
a. Tumor b. Nasal polyp
c. Acute bacterial sinusitis d. Mucormycosis

153. Which of the following X-ray views is shown in the image shown: ***(Most Recent Question June/Dec 2021)***

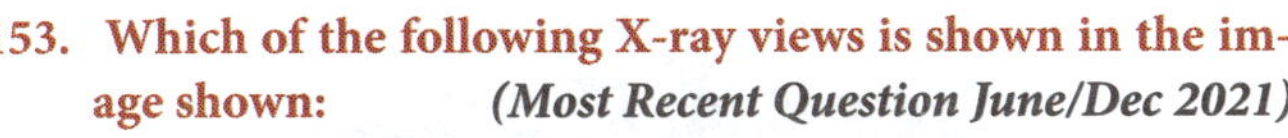

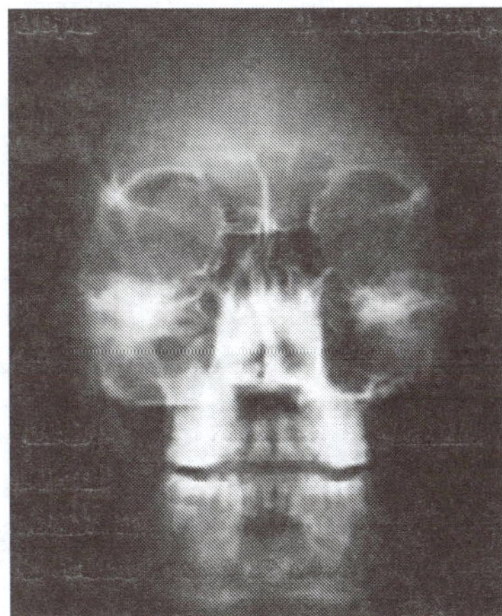

a. Caldwell's view
b. Water's views
c. Pierre's view
d. Rhese view

154. Identify the structure marked with arrow in the given X-ray image of paranasal sinuses: ***(Most Recent Question June/Dec 2021)***

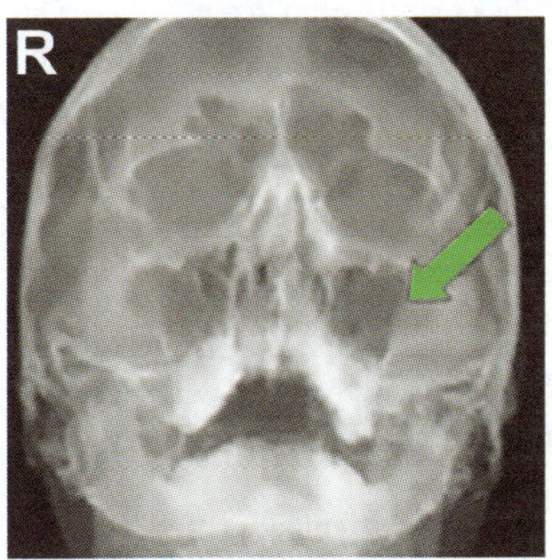

a. Sphenoid sinus
b. Frontal sinus
c. Maxillary sinus
d. Ethmoid sinus

155. A 45-year-old male presented with recurrent sinusitis. Surgical intervention is advised for this patient. Which of the following is gold standard investigation before endoscopic surgery like functional endoscopic sinus surgery (FESS): ***(Most Recent Question Aug 2020)***

a. PET scan
b. CT scan
c. MRI
d. X-ray

156. A 35-year-old male patient came to OPD in April 2020, with symptoms of cold and cough associated with loss of smell and taste. Next step in management: ***(Most Recent Question Aug 2020)***

a. Nasopharyngeal swab for SARS CoV2 testing
b. Oropharyngeal swab for rapid antigen test
c. Serum analysis for IgG
d. Serum analysis for IgM

157. A boy fell down while playing and the nose is deviated but septum was normal. Next step in management: ***(Most Recent Question Aug 2020)***

a. Lower the edema then close reduction after 7 days
b. Closed reduction and swelling automatically decreased
c. Septo-rhinoplasty
d. Open reduction

158. Syphilis affect which part of nasal septum: ***(Most Recent Question Aug 2020)***

a. Bony
b. Lateral nose
c. Vestibule
d. Floor of nose

159. Most common presentation of nasopharyngeal carcinoma; ***(Most Recent Question Dec 2019-20)***

a. Neck lymph node enlargement
b. Blockage of nose
c. Loss of smell
d. Blood tinged discharge

160. Treatment of choice is nasopharyngeal carcinoma: ***(Most Recent Question Dec 2019-20)***

a. Chemotherapy
b. Radiotherapy
c. Chemo given with radiation
d. Surgery

161. A patient with RTA presented with water nasal discharge as shown in the image below when checked upon hankerchief. The diagnosis is? ***(Most Recent Question Dec 2019-20)***

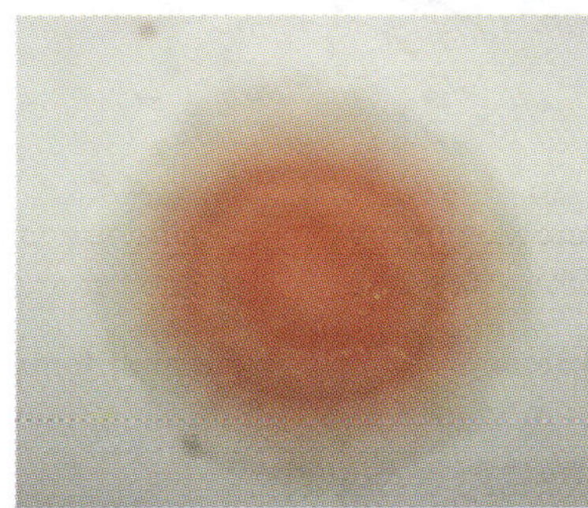

a. Schwartz sign
b. Brown sign
c. Halo sing
d. Signet ring sign

162. A lady comes to OPD after fall from scooter. Her vital are stable. She having continuous, clear watery discharge from nose after 2 days. These are most likely the feature of: ***(Most Recent Question Dec 2019-20)***

a. CSF rhinorrhoea
b. Acute respiratory infection
c. Middle cranial fossa fracture
d. Rhinitis

163. Investigation used for CSF rhinorrhoea are all except: ***(Most Recent Question Dec 2019-20)***

a. CT cisternogram
b. Skull X-ray
c. Beta 2 transferrin
d. Nasal endoscopy

164. The given image shows: *(Most Recent Question Dec 2019-20)*

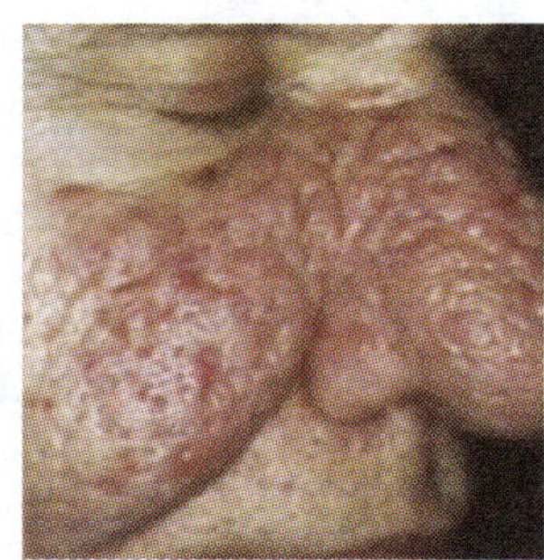

a. Rhinophyma b. Rhinosporidiosis
c. Rhinoscleroma d. Rhinolith

165. Which of the following is preferred in management of Atrophic rhinitis: *(Most Recent Question Dec 2019-20)*
a. Young's operation
b. Nasal steroid spray
c. Immunotherapy/(Or FESS)
d. NSAIDS

166. The maneuver in the image represents: *(Most Recent Question Dec 2019-20)*

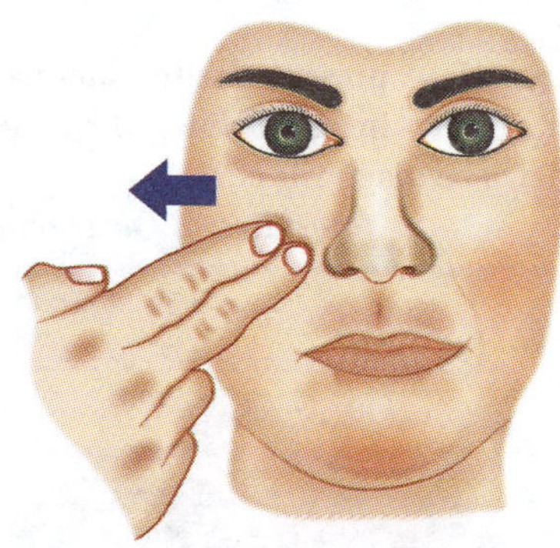

a. Cottle test b. Heimlich maneuver
c. Epley's maneuver d. Semonts maneuver

167. The sign shown in the image is: *(Most Recent Question Dec 2019-20)*

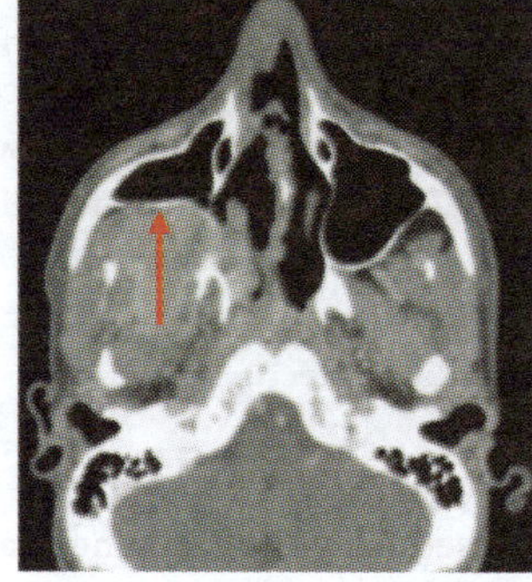

a. Hollmann miller sign b. Hondusa sign
c. Phelp sign d. Trotter sign

168. Office headache is due to inflammation of which sinus? *(Most Recent Question Dec 2019-20)*
a. Frontal b. Maxillary
c. Ethmoidal d. Sphenoid

169. The most prominent and large air cell of ethmoidal sinus? *(Most Recent Question Dec 2019-20)*
a. Agger nasi cell b. Haller cell
c. Onodi cell d. Bulla ethmoidalis

170. A 15 year boy presents with recurrent episodes of epistaxis, unilateral obstruction of nostril. Most likely cause: *(Most Recent Question 2019)*
a. Nasal polyp b. Angiofibroma
c. Nasopharyngeal CA d. Pharyngitis

171. Nasal mass with extension from maxillary sinus is most likely a case of: *(Most Recent Question 2019)*
a. Antrochoanal polyp b. Ethmoid polyp
c. Glomus tumor d. Rhinoscleroma

172. Most common symptom of Nasopharyngeal cancer: *(Recent Pattern Question 2018-19)*
a. Airway Obstruction b. Conductive hearing loss
c. Neck swelling d. Epistaxis

173. Continuous watery discharge from nose after trauma is most likely a feature of: *(Recent Pattern Question 2018-19)*
a. CSF otorrhea b. Common colds
c. CSF Rhinorrrhea d. Anterior epistaxis

174. After a head trauma a patient is unable to smell coffee and asafoetida but can smell ammonia. Which of the following statements is true about the patient? *(Recent Pattern Question 2018-19)*
a. Ammonia is used for testing olfactory nerve
b. The Olfaction system is not damaged
c. Ammonia irritates trigeminal nerve
d. All of the above

175. A male trauma patient admitted was to hospital with watery discharge from nose. On investigation it showed damage in cribriform plate. What is the possible diagnosis? *(Recent Pattern Question 2018)*
a. CSF rhinorrhea b. Vasomotor rhinitis
c. Allergic rhinitis d. Atrophic rhinitis

176. Young operation is done in: *(Recent Pattern Question 2018)*
a. Otosclerosis b. Atrophic rhinitis
c. Viral rhinitis d. Rhinitis sicca

177. Direct branch of internal carotid artery in Kiesselbach's plexus: *(Recent Pattern Question 2018)*
a. Sphenopalatine artery b. Anterior ethmoidal artery
c. Superior labial artery d. Greater palatine artery

178. Samter's triad includes: *(Recent Pattern Question 2017)*
a. Allergy, asthma, nasal polyp
b. Allergy, asthma aspirin intolerance
c. Aspirin sensitivity, asthma, nasal polyp
d. Allergy, polyp, bronchiectasis

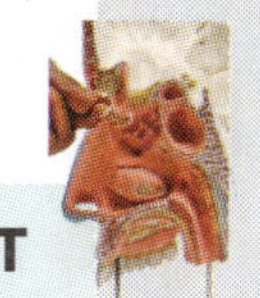

179. Which of the followng is best to prevent rhinitis medicamentosa? ***(Recent Pattern Question 2017)***
a. Give oral drug to relieve symptoms
b. Nasal drop withdrawal
c. Antihistaminic
d. Shift to nasal steroids

180. Which is the most common cancer of paranasal sinus? ***(Recent Pattern Question 2017)***
a. Squamous cell CA b. Basal cell CA
c. Adenoid cystic CA d. Melanoma

181. Sphenoid sinus opens into:
a. Superior meatus b. Middle meatus
c. Inferior meatus d. Supreme meatus

182. Location of the nasolacrimal duct:
a. Inferior meatus
b. Superior meatus
c. Sphenoethmoidal recess
d. Middle meatus

183. Nasolacrimal duct opens into:
a. Mouth opposite to 2nd molar
b. Middle meatus of the nose
c. Superior meatus of the nose
d. Inferior meatus of the nose

184. Antrochoanal polyp opens in which meatus:
a. Middle meatus b. Superior meatus
c. Inferior meatus d. Sphenoethmoidal recess

185. What is the likely source of infection for Pus from sphenoethmoidal recess?
a. Sphenoid sinus b. Ethmoidal sinus
c. Maxillary sinus d. Frontal sinus

186. Which sinus opens in inferior meatus:
a. Maxillary sinus
b. Frontal sinus
c. Anterior ethmoidal sinus
d. None of the above

187. Kiesselbach's plexus does not involve:
a. Superior labial artery b. Anterior ethmoidal artery
c. Greater palatine artery d. Posterior ethmoidal artery

188. Which of the following vessel of Little's area is not a branch of external carotid artery?
a. Sphenopalatine artery
b. Greater palatine artery
c. Anterior ethmoidal artery
d. Superior labial artery

189. Which of the following is not an etiologically derived cause for epistaxis:
a. Nose picking
b. Intra nasal tumours
c. Vascular disorders or blood dyscrasias
d. Hereditary hemorrhagic telangiectasia

190. Esthesioneuroblastoma arises from:
a. Olfactory epithelium b. Ethmoid sinus
c. Maxillary sinus d. Sphenoid sinus

191. All of the following paranasal sinuses are present at birth EXCEPT?
a. Maxillary sinus b. Ethmoid sinus
c. Sphenoid sinus d. None of these

192. Sinus absent at the birth:
a. Maxillary sinus b. Ethmoidal sinus
c. Frontal sinus d. Temporal sinus

193. Radiological evidence of frontal sinus can be seen at:
a. 2 years b. 4 years
c. 6 years d. 8 years

194. Sphenoid sinus reaches adult size at:
a. 5 years b. 10 years
c. 15 years d. 28 years

195. Ethmoid sinus reaches adult size at:
a. 5 years b. 8 years
c. 10 years d. 12 years

196. Largest sinus:
a. Frontal sinus b. Maxillary sinus
c. Ethmoidal sinus d. Aphenoid sinus

197. Caldwell luc's operation is done for:
a. Frontal sinusitis b. Maxillay sinusitis
c. Ethmoid sinusitis d. Sphenoid sinusitis

198. Young's operation is done for:
a. Atrophic rhinitis b. Vasomotor rhinitis
c. Antro-choanal polyp d. Allergic rhinitis

199. Which one of the following is a cause of nasal obstruction in Atrophic Rhinitis?
a. Secretions b. Deviated nasal septum
c. Polyp d. Crusting

200. Which of the following is the most common presentation of nasopharyngeal carcinoma?
a. Epistaxis b. Lymphadenopathy
c. Nasal obstruction d. Apnea

201. Miculicz and Russel body upon biopsy is seen in:
a. Rhinophyma b. Rhinoscleroma
c. Rhinosporidiosis d. Rhinolith

202. Rhinophyma is associated with which of the following?
a. Hypertrophy of sebaceous gland
b. Infection of hair follicles
c. Congenital deformity of the nose
d. Hypertrophy of sweat gland

203. Cause of rhinosporidiosis:
a. Bacterial b. Viral
c. Fungal d. Protozoa

204. A patient presents to you with big nasal cavity, thick crust formation and woody hard external nose. What is the probable diagnosis?
a. Vasomotor rhinitis
b. Rhinoscleroma
c. Rhinosporidiosis
d. Atrophic rhinitis

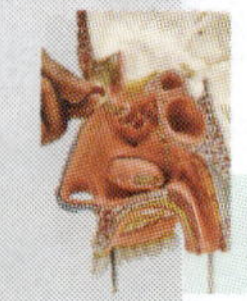

205. Woody induration of rhinoscleroma is initially seen at which stage?
a. Catarrhal stage b. Strophic stage
c. Granulomatous stage d. Cicatricial stage

206. Rhinoscleroma is caused by:
a. Virus b. Bacteria
c. Fungus d. Anaerobes

207. Most common fractured bone on face:
a. Nasoethmoid bone b. Zygomatic bone
c. Nasal bone d. Mandible

208. Chevallet fracture of nasal septum is:
a. Horizontal fracture b. Vertical fracture
c. Comminuted fracture d. Serpentine fracture

209. Impact of force in case of jarjavay septal fracture is from:
a. Above b. Below
c. Front d. Behind

210. Most common site of fracture of mandible is:
a. Neck of condyle b. Angle of mandible
c. Symphysis d. Ramus

THROAT/PHARYNX

211. In the shown X-ray, the foreign body is lodged in: *(Most Recent Question June/Dec 2021)*

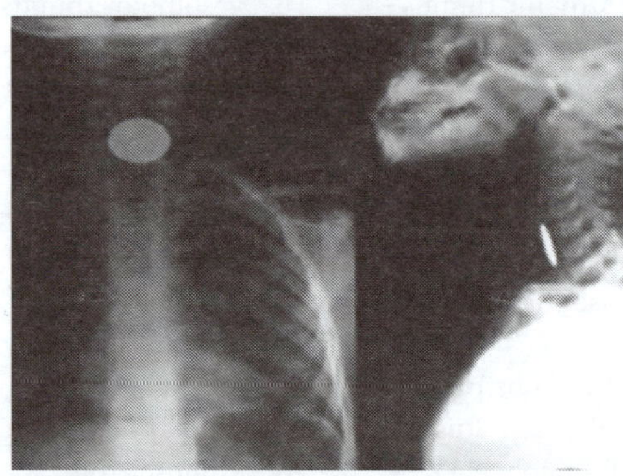

a. Trachea
b. Esophagus
c. Larynx
d. None

212. A young boy presented with mouth breathing, failure to thrive, high arched palate, and hearing loss. Management is: *(Most Recent Question June/Dec 2021)*
a. Adenoidectomy with grommet
b. Myringotomy
c. Myringotomy with grommet
d. Adenoidectomy

213. Which of the following conditions causes white membrane deposits in the throat: *(Most Recent Question June/Dec 2021)*
a. Acute tonsillitis b. Diphtheria
c. Peritonsillar abscess d. None of these

214. A 5-year-old child has fever and the neck X-ray shown has thumb sign. Most common organism in this case is: *(Most Recent Question June/Dec 2021)*

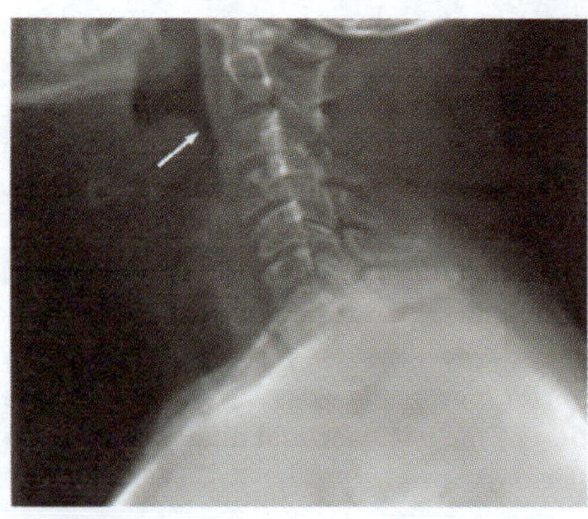

a. H. influenza b. Adenovirus
c. Parainfluenza virus d. Influenza virus

215. Which of the following is the most important artery supply of tonsils: *(Most Recent Question June/Dec 2021)*
a. Tonsillar branch of facial artery
b. Ascending pharyngeal artery
c. Ascending palatine artery
d. Dorsal lingual artery

216. Which of the following nerve is responsible for earache after tonsillectomy surgery: *(Most Recent Question June/Dec 2021)*
a. Glossopharyngeal nerve b. Vagus nerve
c. Mandibular nerve d. Maxillary nerve

217. Which of the following laryngeal cartilages does not undergo calcification: *(Most Recent Question June/Dec 2021)*
a. Epiglottis b. Cricoid
c. Arytenoid d. Thyroid

218. Which of the following muscles is an abductor of vocal cord: *(Most Recent Question June/Dec 2021)*
a. Lateral cricoarytenoid b. Posterior cricoarytenoid
c. Interarytenoid d. Cricothyroid

219. Most common cause of stridor in neonates is: *(Most Recent Question June/Dec 2021)*
a. Laryngeal papilloma b. Carcinoma
c. Polyps d. Laryngomalacia

220. Which of the following is an unpaired cartilage of larynx *(Most Recent Question June/Dec 2021)*
a. Arytenoid b. Thyroid
c. Cuneiform d. Corniculate

221. What is the exact anatomical location of Killian's dehiscence? *(Most Recent Question June/Dec 2021)*
a. Between superior and middle constrictor muscle
b. Thyropharyngeus and cricopharyngeus muscle fibers
c. Inferior constrictor muscle
d. Between middle and inferior constrictor muscles

222. A trumpet blower present with left sided neck swelling. X-ray reveals following finding. Most likely diagnosis of this patient: ***(Most Recent Question Aug 2020)***

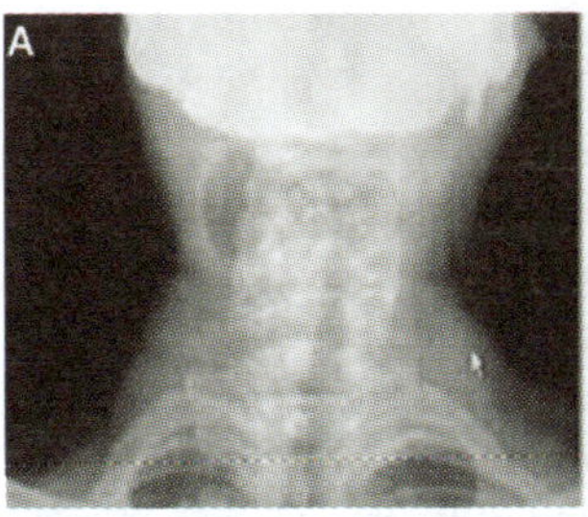

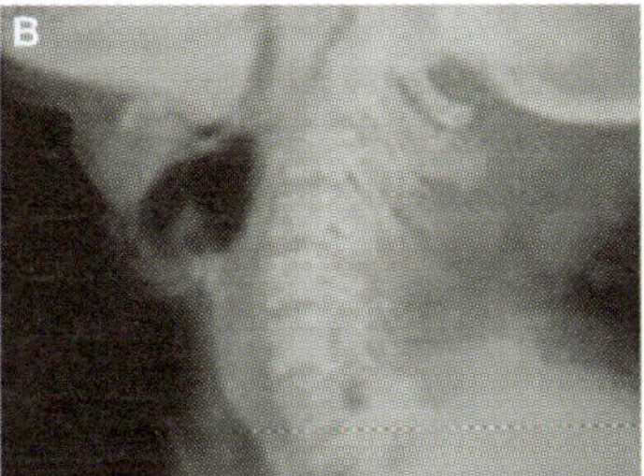

a. Laryngeal cyst
b. Thyrogossal duct cyst
c. Laryngoceoele
d. Brachial cyst

223. Pharyngeal pouch is located between: ***(Most Recent Question Aug 2020)***

a. Superior and middle constrictors
b. Middle and inferior constrictor
c. Thyropharyngeus and cricopharyngeus
d. Thyroid and cricoid

224. Upon endoscopy, the following structure is seen which is marked with arrow. Name this structure: ***(Most Recent Question Aug 2020)***

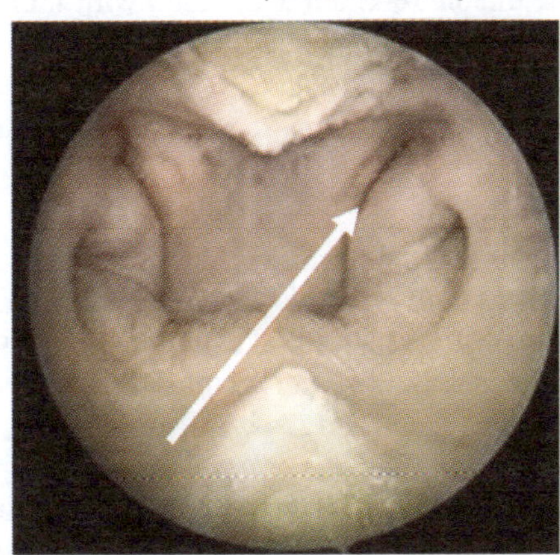

a. ET opening
b. Torus tubarius
c. Fossa of rosenmuller
d. Sphenopalatine foramen

225. In a patient with Hypopharyngeal CA, >3 cm, with the ipsilateral involvement and no extension to opposite side. Grading would be: ***(Most Recent Question Aug 2020)***

a. T1 b. T3
c. T4a d. T4b

226. The cause of nasopharyngeal carcinoma is: ***(Most Recent Question Dec 2019-20)***

a. HSV b. EBV
c. HZV d. Parainfluenza virus

227. A patient presented with bilateral neck swelling, temporoparietal neuralgia and unilateral hearing loss. The diagnosis: ***(Most Recent Question Dec 2019-20)***

a. Nasopharyngeal carcinoma
b. Juvenile nasopharyngeal angiofibroma
c. Hypopharyngeal carcinoma
d. Laryngeal carcinoma

228. Laryngeal crepitus is seen in all; EXCEPT? ***(Most Recent Question Dec 2019-20)***

a. Laryngitis
b. It is present normally in every individual
c. Post cricoid carcinoma
d. Fragment of hyoid bone and cricoid cartilage

229. A child presented with a high arched palate and mouth breathing and failure to thrive. The probable diagnosis is: ***(Most Recent Question Dec 2019-20)***

a. Tonsil hypertrophy
b. Adenoid hypertrophy
c. Lingual tonsil hypertrophy
d. Epiglottitis

230. A infant presented with inspiratory stridor, the clinical picture is shown below. The diagnosis is: ***(Most Recent Question Dec 2019-20)***

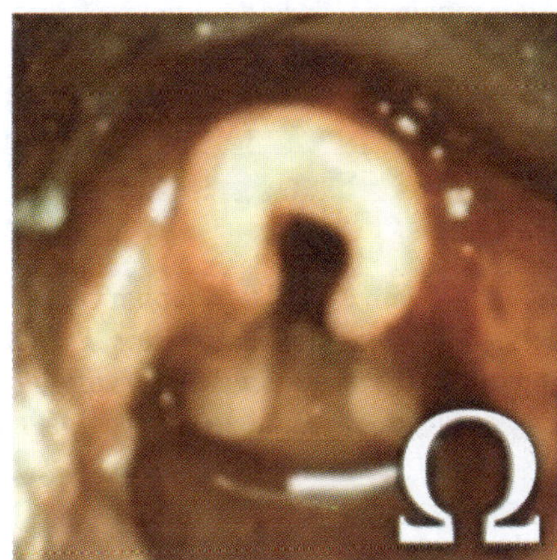

a. Acute epiglottis b. RLN palsy
c. SLN palsy d. Laryngomalacia

231. What is the causative agent croup? ***(Most Recent Question Dec 2019-20)***

a. H. influenzae
b. Parainfluenza
c. Streptococcus pneumonia
d. Rhinovirus

232. A 46-year-old boy patient came to hospital with complaints of neck swelling, sore throat and difficulty is swallowing. His pharyngeal walls were pushed medially. What will be the diagnosis: ***(Most Recent Question Dec 2019-20)***

a. Peritonsillar abscess b. Retropharyngeal abscess
c. Ludwig's angina d. Parapharyngeal abscess

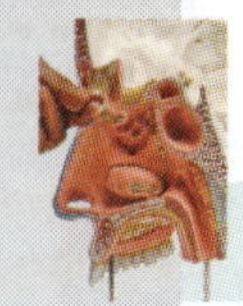

233. A young boy come to OPD with the complaints of difficulty in breathing. On examination, bilateral polyps were found. What will be the initial management? *(Most Recent Question Dec 2019-20)*

a. I and D
b. Antihistaminic
c. Conservative
d. Septoplasty

234. Adam's apple in male is due to: *(Most Recent Question Dec 2019-20)*

a. Thyroid cartilage
b. Cricoid cartilage
c. Hyoid cartilage
d. Epiglottis cartilage

235. Narrowest part of airway in infant: *(Most Recent Question 2019)*

a. Glottis
b. Subglottis
c. Supraglottis
d. Epiglottis

236. Abductor of vocal cord: *(Most Recent Question 2019)*

a. Posterior cricoarytenoid muscle
b. Interarytenoid muscle
c. Cricothyroid muscle
d. Thyroarytenoid muscle

237. In ranula management which of the following step is correct? *(Most Recent Question 2019)*

a. Excision of ranula and sublingual gland duct
b. Excision of only the cystic swelling
c. In large ranula marsuplization not preferred
d. In small ranula marsuplization is preferred

238. High tracheostomy is done in which condition? *(Most Recent Question 2019)*

a. Laryngeal carcinoma
b. Laryngeal stenosis
c. Respiratory obstruction
d. Foreign body

239. A patient presented with nasopharyngeal CA with bilateral LN, epistaxis and hearing loss. What is the most common cause of deafness in this patient: *(Most Recent Question 2019)*

a. Nerve deafness
b. Ossicular damage
c. Serous otitis media
d. Auditory canal obstruction

240. A patient presented with 3 days history of fever, throat pain, difficulty in deglutition with deviation of uvula. Most likely diagnosis: *(Recent Pattern Question 2018-19)*

a. Quinsy
b. Pre-tracheal abscess
c. Retopharyngeal abscess
d. Epiglottitis

241. Hypoglossal nerve supplies all of these muscle EXCEPT: *(Recent Pattern Question 2018-19)*

a. Palatoglossus
b. Styloglossus
c. Genioglossus
d. Hyoglossus

242. Picket fence fever is seen in: *(Recent Pattern Question 2018-19)*

a. Lateral sinus thrombophlebitis
b. Quincy
c. Laryngitis sicca
d. Croup

243. Which of the following is NOT a premalignant lesion/ condition: *(Recent Pattern Question 2018-19)*

a. Chronic hypertrophic candidiasis
b. Oral submucosal fibrosis
c. Lichen planus
d. Aphthous ulcer

244. Which of the following is preferred for treatment of nasopharyngeal carcinoma: *(Recent Pattern Question 2018)*

a. Chemoradiation
b. Surgery
c. Chemotherapy alone
d. Radiation alone

245. All of the following is seen when superior laryngeal nerve is damaged EXCEPT: *(Recent Pattern Question 2018)*

a. Aspiration
b. Stridor
c. Bowed vocal cords
d. Loss of pitch

246. Recurrent laryngeal nerve supplies all EXCEPT: *(Recent Pattern Question 2018)*

a. Cricothyroid
b. Cricoarytenoid
c. Aryepiglottic
d. Interarytenoid

247. Most common site for laryngeal web is:

a. Supraglottic
b. Subglottic
c. Glottis level
d. Epiglottis level

248. A 15-year-old boy presented with history of fever since 2 days, unable to swallow the food with muffled voice. On examination it is noted that right tonsil is shifted to midline. What is the diagnosis? *(Recent Pattern Question 2018)*

a. Quincy
b. Acute tonsillitis
c. Parapharyngeal abscess
d. Acute retropharyngeal abscess

249. Juvenile recurrent laryngeal papillomatosis is caused by: *(Recent Pattern Question 2018)*

a. EBV
b. HSV
c. HPV
d. VZV

250. A 60-year-old man presents with right sided ear pain and dysphagia. Diagnosis: *(Recent Pattern Question 2017)*

a. Achalasia cardia
b. Lower esophageal carcinoma
c. Carcinoma of pyriform sinus
d. Postcricoid carcinoma

251. Passavant's ridge is formed by: *(Recent Pattern Question 2017)*

a. Palatopharyngeus
b. Cricopharyngeus
c. Genioglossus
d. Stylopharyngeus

252. Peritonsillar abscess management: *(Recent Pattern Question 2017)*

a. Drainage
b. Analgesic plus antibiotic
c. Analgesic with antibiotic and drainage
d. Wait and watch

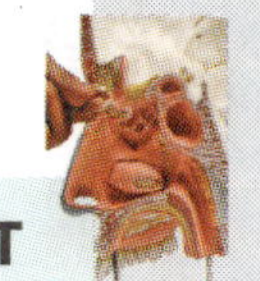

253. Elective tracheostomy is done in: *(Recent Pattern Question 2017)*
a. Deep burn of chest wall
b. Radiation burn of face
c. Burn of head and neck
d. Acid burn on ingestion

254. High tracheostomy is done in: *(Recent Pattern Question 2017)*
a. Carcinoma larynx b. Laryngomalacia
c. Thyroid surgery d. Diptheria infection

255. A singer presents with sore throat, GERD and vocal nodule. Medical treatment: *(Recent Pattern Question 2017)*
a. Direct laryngoscopy
b. PPI
c. Microscopic laryngeal surgery
d. Speech therapy plus PPI

256. Narrowest part of glottis in pediatric age group: *(Recent Pattern Question 2017)*
a. Lower part of thyroid cartilage
b. Upper part of thyroid cartilage
c. Glottis
d. Epiglottis

257. Head and neck tumour stage III according to TNM classification involves: *(Recent Pattern Question 2016)*
a. Unilateral mobile lymph nodes <3 cm
b. Unilateral mobile lymph node >3 cm
c. Bilateral mobile lymph nodes <6 cm
d. Bilateral mobile lymph nodes >6 cm

258. Abductor of vocal cords: *(Recent Pattern Question 2016)*
a. Cricothyroid b. Posterior cricothyroid
c. Posterior cricoarytenoid d. Interarytenoid

259. Mouse nibbled vocal cord is seen in: *(Recent Pattern Question 2016)*
a. Laryngeal CA b. Laryngeal TB
c. Laryngeal papilloma d. Vocal cord palsy

260. Hot potato voice is seen in *(Recent Pattern Question 2016)*
a. Acute epiglottis b. Antrochonal polyp
c. Peritonsillar abscess d. Carcinoma larynx

261. Narrowest part of airway in a child: *(Recent Pattern Question 2016)*
a. Glottis b. Supraglottis
c. Subglottis d. Epiglottis

262. Nasopharyngeal angiofibroma is most commonly seen in:
a. Elderly males b. Females
c. Young males d. Infants

263. A 13-year-old child presents with 3 year history of gradual swelling of maxilla with medial displacement of turbinates with mild proptosis. What is the most likely diagnosis:
a. Olfactory neuroblastoma b. Angiofibroma
c. Carcinoma of maxilla d. Fibrous dysplasia

264. Crypts are seen in:
a. Tonsils b. Adenoids
c. Lymph nodes d. Parotids

265. Which of the following muscle is not supplied by recurrent laryngeal nerve:
a. Cricothyroid b. Lateral cricoarytenoid
c. Thyroarytenoid d. Posterior cricoarytenoid

266. Which one of the following is an abductor of vocal cords:
a. Posterior cricoarytenoid b. Transverse arytenoids
c. Cricothyroid d. Aryepiglotticus

267. Recurrent laryngeal nerve supplies all EXCEPT:
a. Cricothyroid b. Thyroaretenoid
c. Lateral cricoaretenoid d. Posterior cricoaretenoid

268. Warthins tumor is seen in:
a. Submandibular gland b. Parotid gland
c. Sublingual gland d. All of these

269. Glossopharyngeal nerve supplies:
a. Glossopharyngeus muscle
b. Stylopharyngeus muscle
c. Anterior 2/3 of the tongue
d. All of the above

270. Omega shaped epiglottis is seen in:
a. Epiglottitis b. Laryngomalacia
c. Epiglottis CA d. Tuberculosis

271. Thumb sign is seen in:
a. Acute laryngitis
b. Acute epiglottitis
c. Acute laryngo trachea bronchitis
d. Acute tonsillitis

272. Bezold's abscess is in relation to:
a. Digastric muscle
b. Sternocleidomastoid muscle
c. Behind the mastoid
d. Submandibular region

273. All are complication of tonsillitis; EXCEPT:
a. Otitis media
b. Abscess
c. Malignant change
d. Subacute bacterial endocarditis

274. Which of the following cyst doesn't move upon deglution?
a. Ranula b. Thyroglossal cyst
c. Sublingual dermoid cyst d. Thymic cyst

275. In the early stage of which of the following carcinoma, no lymphatics involved:
a. Glottic CA b. Infraglottic CA
c. Supraglottic CA d. Hypopharyngeal CA

276. Radiation therapy is mostly useful for:
a. Glottis CA b. Epiglottis CA
c. Sub-glottis CA d. Supraglottis CA

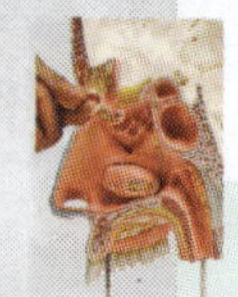

277. Hot potato voice is seen in all EXCEPT:

a. Quinsy
b. Carcinoma thyroid
c. Carcinoma tonsil
d. Streptococcus pharyngitis

278. Transillumination test is positive in:

a. Branchial cyst
b. Thymic cyst
c. Ranula
d. Thyroglossal duct cyst

279. Male patient with female like voice. This condition is called:

a. Puberphonia
b. Androphonia
c. Rhinolalia aperta
d. Rhinolalia clausa

280. Female patient with male like voice. Type of thyroplasty done:

a. I
b. II
c. III
d. IV

281. In a patient with vocal cord paralysis, the surgeon is afraid of aspiration. Thyroplasty done in order to prevent aspiration:

a. Type I
b. Type II
c. Type III
d. Type IV

282. Most common complication of tracheostomy:

a. Hemorrhage
b. Tracheal stenosis
c. Recurrent laryngeal nerve damage
d. Infection

FACE, ORAL CAVITY AND ESOPHAGUS

283. After emergency tracheostomy patient presented with surgical emphysema. What is the most likely reason?
(Most Recent Question June 2022)

a. High tracheostomy
b. Tight suture around tracheostomy site
c. Tear to posterior wall of trachea
d. Block in tracheostomy tube

284. Which of the following is the most common site of head and neck cancer in India?
(Most Recent Question June/Dec 2021)

a. Nasopharynx
b. Oropharynx
c. Oral cavity
d. Hypopharynx

285. A young child presented with lower lip swelling. Upon lip eversion, following condition is seen. Which of the following is NOT true about the given image?
(Most Recent Question Aug 2020)

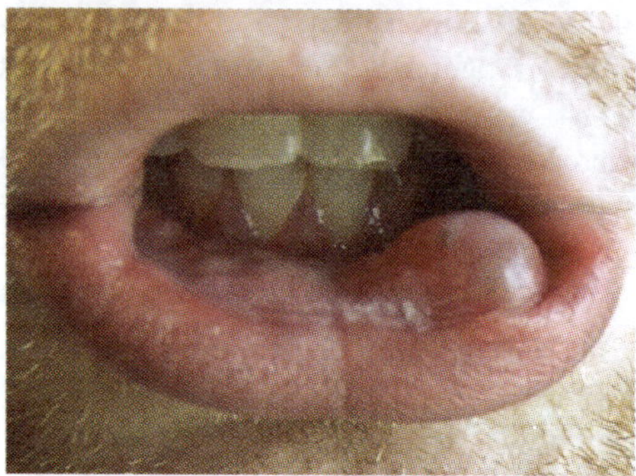

a. Its usually a retention cyst
b. Extravasation is not that common
c. It is brilliantly transilluminant
d. Mucocele of lip

286. Patient underwent removal of submandibular gland. Lingual nerve is damaged during surgery. NOT true about it:
(Most Recent Question Aug 2020)

a. Rate of sublingual secretion is decreased
b. Anterior 2/3rd taste sensation lost from tongue
c. Sensation of floor of mouth is lost
d. Tongue deviated

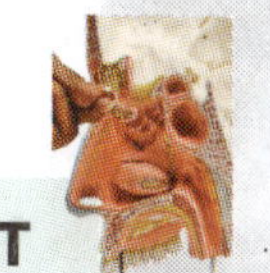

ANSWERS WITH EXPLANATIONS

MOST RECENT QUESTIONS 2023

1. Ans. (c) Upper ⅓ bone & lower ⅔ cartilage

Ref: Gray's Anatomy: The Anatomical Basis of Clinical Practice, 41st ed. pg. 515 and PL Dhingra: Diseases of Ear, Nose and Throat, 6th, ed. pg. 134

- The correct structure of the nose is that the upper one-third is composed of bone, while the lower two-thirds are made up of cartilage.
- The bony part of the nose consists of the nasal bones and the frontal processes of the maxilla, while the cartilaginous part includes the lateral nasal cartilages, septal cartilage, and alar cartilages.

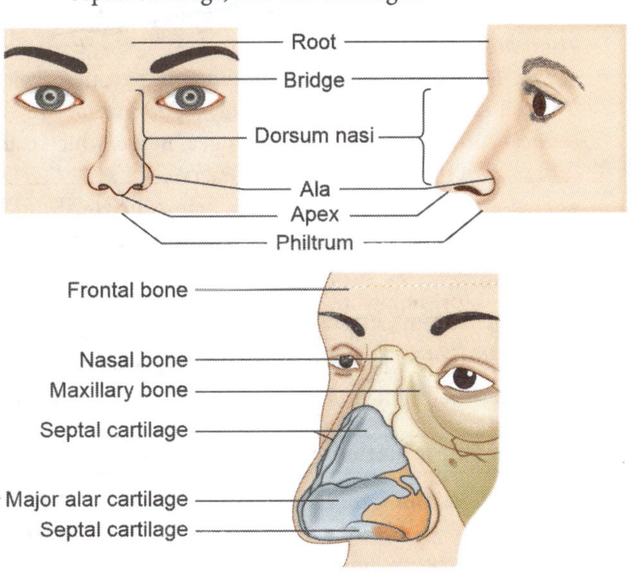

2. Ans. (a) Inspiratory

Ref: PL Dhingra: Diseases of Ear, Nose and Throat, 6th, ed. pg. 295

- The image given here is of laryngomalacia. It is self-limiting condition, that occurs due to weakness of cartilage.
- Patient in laryngomalacia presents with inspiratory stridor (noisy breathing while inhalation).

Extra Mile

- Biphasic stridor is seen in glottic or subglottic stenosis
- Expiratory stridor is seen in bronchial foreign body or tracheal stenosis

3. Ans. (d) Choanal atresia

Ref: PL Dhingra: Diseases of Ear, Nose and Throat, 6th, ed. pg. 163

- A congenital case of bilateral choanal atresia is an emergency condition, where a cyanotic neonate is brought irritability and cyanosis improves upon crying.
- In choanal atresia, there is a membrane present at the choanal area (between nose and nasopharyngeal area). Since newborns are obligate nasal breathers and nasal breathing is not easy in this case, the baby cries out of irritability and there is mouth breathing, which causes improvement of cyanosis.

4. Ans. (b) Sphenopalatine artery

Ref: PL Dhingra: Diseases of Ear, Nose and Throat, 6th, ed. pg. 177–178

- Sphenopalatine artery is major artery of septum supplying the Little's area. It is also called artery of epistaxis.
- It is the most common artery involved in anterior epistaxis.

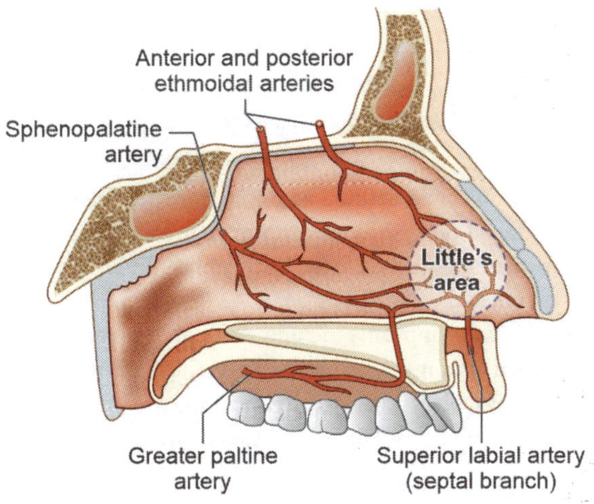

5. Ans. (b) Chest X-ray

Ref: PL Dhingra: Diseases of Ear, Nose and Throat, 6th, ed. pg. 350

- In case of foreign body aspiration, Chest X-ray should be carried out immediately.

6. Ans. (b) Ranula

Ref: PL Dhingra: Diseases of Ear, Nose and Throat, 6th, ed. pg. 224

- The given is the case of Ranula.
- Detailed discussion has been given later in this Chapter.

7. Ans. (c) Antrochoanal polyp

Ref: PL Dhingra: Diseases of Ear, Nose and Throat, 6th, ed. pg. 173–174

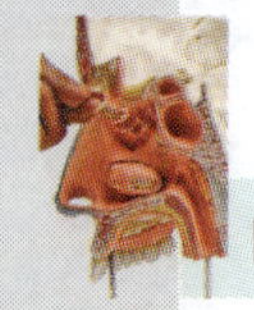

- All the nasal polyp grows anteriorly in the nose except maxillary polyp. It grows posteriorly in the choanal area due to downward sloping of nasal floor.
- Maxillary sinus is also known as antrum of Highmore and a polyp originating from here, goes toward choana, hence the name antrochoanal polyp.
- Patient will present with nasal obstruction, breathing difficulties.
- Treatment: FESS.
- Incidence of recurrence is lesser in maxillary polyp as compared to ethmoidal polyp.

8. Ans. (c) Middle meatus

Ref: PL Dhingra: Diseases of Ear, Nose and Throat, 6th, ed. pg. 137–138

- The Bulla Ethmoidalis is a bony prominence within the ethmoidal sinus, which is a part of the paranasal sinuses located in the skull.
- It is specifically found in the middle meatus of the nasal cavity.

9. Ans. (a) Same side of face

Ref: PL Dhingra: Diseases of Ear, Nose and Throat, 6th ed. pg. 95, 7th ed. pg. 103–104

- Bell's palsy is defined as idiopathic, peripheral paralysis of facial nerve of lower motor neuron type in which the ipsilateral side of face -both upper and lower part are paralyzed.
- Clinical symptoms include Bell's phenomenon, which is when attempting to close an eye, the eyeball turns up and out, unable to close the eye, drooping of angle of mouth, absence of nasolabial fold, loss of wrinkles on forehead, etc.

10. Ans. (d) Surgical excision

Ref: PL Dhingra: Diseases of Ear, Nose and Throat, 6th ed. pg. 203, 7th ed. pg. 279–281

- The above given case is suggestive of nasopharyngeal angiofibroma.
- It is a benign tumor of nasopharynx. Most commonly seen in adolescent males in the second decade. It arises from the sphenopalatine foramen.
- It is a testosterone-dependent tumor made up of highly vascular and fibrous tissue which accounts for profuse bleeding as the vessels lack muscular coat.
- The most common presentation is profuse recurrent epistaxis. At presentation, it is lobulated, smooth mass pink in color, which bleeds on touch, therefore biopsy and FNAC are contraindicated.
- Treatment of choice is surgical excision. Radiotherapy and chemotherapy can also be used.

11. Ans. (c) Esophagoscopy

Ref: PL Dhingra: Diseases of Ear, Nose and Throat, 7th ed. pg. 367

- The above shown X-rays in AP view and lateral view are suggestive of foreign body (coin) in esophagus as on lateral view coin is visible as slit-like.
- Thus, the treatment of the choice in the given scenario is removal of foreign body by esophagoscopy.
- If the coin would be in the trachea, then it would be managed by rigid bronchoscopy.
- Heimlich maneuver is used in case of foreign body lodged in the larynx, it is the sudden thrust directed upward and backward below the epigastrium.

12. Ans. (a) Internal laryngeal nerve

Ref: PL Dhingra: Diseases of Ear, Nose and Throat, 7th ed. pg. 337

- The larynx lies opposite to the 3rd to 6th cervical vertebra. The sensory supply of the larynx above the vocal cord is by the internal laryngeal nerve, which is the branch of the superior laryngeal nerve.
- The sensory supply of the larynx below the vocal cord is supplied by, recurrent laryngeal nerve, which arises from the Vagus nerve.
- The motor supply of the laryngeal muscle is by the recurrent laryngeal nerve, except the cricothyroid muscle, which is supplied by the external laryngeal nerve, which is the branch of superior laryngeal nerve.

13. Ans. (b) Linear motion

Ref: PL Dhingra: Diseases of Ear, Nose and Throat, 7th, ed. pg. 21–22

- Utricle and saccule are the part of membranous labyrinth. Utricle lies in the posterior part which receives the five openings of semicircular ducts. The sensory hair cells of the utricle and saccule is called macula which is concerned with linear acceleration and deceleration.
- Angular acceleration is detected by crista ampullaris, which is present in semicircular canals.

Note: Higher frequencies are heard at the base of cochlea while the lower frequencies are heard at the apex of the cochlea.

14. Ans. (c) Maxillary sinus

Ref: PL Dhingra: Diseases of Ear, Nose and Throat, 7th, ed. pg. 209–210

- The above given CT image is of paranasal sinuses, pointing toward the maxillary sinus, which is the largest paranasal sinus, also known as Antrum of Highmore or simply antrum.

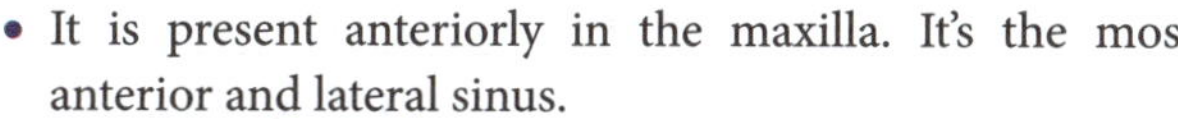

- It is present anteriorly in the maxilla. It's the most anterior and lateral sinus.
- On average, it has the capacity of 15 mL in an adult.

15. Ans. (b) Nasal polyp

Ref: PL Dhingra: Diseases of Ear, Nose and Throat, 7th, ed. pg. 193–196

- The history of the patient point toward a nasal polyp. This can be seen in an asthmatic patient with aspirin sensitivity. This is collectively known as Samter's Triad.
- **Samter's triad:** Nasal Polyp, Asthma and Aspirin sensitivity

16. Ans. (b) Vocal nodule

Ref: PL Dhingra: Diseases of Ear, Nose and Throat, 7th, ed. pg. 343

- The above clinical scenario is suggestive of vocal nodule.
- It is also known as singers or screamers nodules that occur as a result of vocal trauma when a patient screams out loud or speaks unnaturally low tone for a long time.
- It occurs at the free edge of the vocal cord at the junction of anterior 1/3rd and Posterior 2/3rd as it is subjected to the maximum vibration.
- Patient presents with hoarseness of voice, vocal fatigue and pain in the neck.

17. Ans. (a) Glomus tumor

Ref: PL Dhingra: Diseases of Ear, Nose and Throat, 7th, ed. pg. 121–123

- The above clinical scenario is suggestive of diagnosis of glomus tumor which is the most common benign tumor of the middle ear.
- It arises from Jugulotympanic paragangliomas (In association with Jacobson's and Arnold's nerves).
- It is a locally invasive and highly vascular tumor thus biopsy is contraindicated.
- It typically presents with pulsatile tinnitus, profusely bleeding polyp in EAC, conductive hearing loss.
- On examination it shows the "Rising Sun" sign as it is a red color tumor arising from the floor of the middle ear.
- Surgical excision is the treatment of choice.

18. Ans. (a) Metallic tube

Ref: PL Dhingra: Diseases of Ear, Nose and Throat, 7th, ed. pg. 359–360, 523–525.

- Tracheostomy tube used in the case of ICU patients is of metallic type.
- Tracheostomy is the procedure of making an opening in the anterior wall of trachea and converting it into a stoma on the skin surface. It simply means opening the trachea.
- It is mostly done between the second and third tracheal ring.
- Fenestrated tracheostomy tubes have holes for speech production. These are used in children for decannulation.
- Cuffed tracheostomy tube helps in the prevention of aspiration and air leak, it is used in unconscious patients.

19. Ans. (c) Diplophonia

Ref: PL Dhingra: Diseases of Ear, Nose and Throat, 7th, ed. pg. 330

- Diplophonia, also known as diphthongia, is a phenomenon in which a voice is perceived as being produced with two concurrent pitches.
- Reinke's Edema is the bilateral symmetrical swelling of the membranous part of the vocal cord that occurs due to misuse of voice, smoking, chronic sinusitis.
- Patient uses false vocal cords for voice production which results in diplophonia.

Note:

- Dysphagia of solids more than liquids is suggestive of cancer esophagus, while dysphagia of the liquid more than solids is suggestive of achalasia cardia.
- Dysphonia is the difficulty in speaking due to a physical disorder of the mouth, tongue, throat, or vocal cords.

20. Ans. (a) Geniculate ganglion

Ref: PL Dhingra: Diseases of Ear, Nose and Throat, 7th, ed. pg. 104–105

- Ramsay Hunt syndrome comprises facial nerve paralysis along with herpes zoster oticus infection.
- The geniculate ganglion is a sensory ganglion, which is situated along the course of the facial nerve, inside the bony facial canal within the petrous temporal bone. Its location is closely related to the site where the greater petrosal nerve branches off from the facial nerve at its genu.

Note:

- The otic ganglion transmits postganglionic parasympathetic secretomotor fibers to all branches of the mandibular division of the trigeminal nerve.
- Trigeminal ganglion or Gasserian ganglion is a thin, crescent-shaped structure situated in Meckel's cave within the middle cranial fossa from which trigeminal nerve arises.

21. Ans. (b) Benign and non-invasive

Ref: PL Dhingra: Diseases of Ear, Nose and Throat, 7th, ed. pg. 227

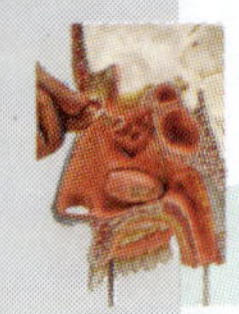

- Inverted papilloma also known as Ringertz tumor is a benign and non-invasive tumor of non-olfactory mucosa of nose and paranasal sinuses. It is the growth of hyperplastic papillomatous tissue most commonly in the middle meatus.
- It is a locally aggressive tumor.
- It most commonly presents with nasal obstruction which is mostly unilateral, nasal discharge and epistaxis.
- Treatment of choice is endoscopic medial maxillectomy.

ANATOMY OF AURICLE AND EXTERNAL AUDITORY CANAL & EMBRYOLOGY

22. Ans. (d) Tympanotomy with stapedectomy

Ref: Diseases of Ear, Nose and Throat and Head and Neck Surgery, Dhingra, 7th ed. pg. 95-98

- Otosclerosis is an abnormal bone growth in the middle ear that causes hearing loss. The stapes begins to fuse with the surrounding bone, eventually becoming fixed so it cannot move.
- Pregnancy is not a cause but may make the condition worse, so symptoms are commonly first noticed during pregnancy.
- The most common operation that is done is to replace the stapes with an artificial bone made of plastic or metal. The operation is called a stapedectomy.

23. Ans. (c) Arnolds nerve

Ref: Diseases of Ear, Nose and Throat and Head and Neck Surgery, Dhingra, 7th ed. pg. 5

- A recurrent syncopal attack provoked by light stimulation of the external auditory canal is due to auricular branch of vagus nerve stimulation. The auricular branch of the vagus nerve is often termed as Arnold's nerve.

24. Ans. (c) Newborns are obligatory nasal breathers

Ref: Diseases of Ear, Nose and Throat and Head and Neck Surgery, Dhingra, 7th ed. pg. 157

- Human infants are commonly described as obligate nasal breathers as they breathe through their nose rather than the mouth.
- Most infants, however, are able to breathe through their mouth if their nose is blocked.

25. Ans. (a) Malignant otitis externa

Ref: Diseases of Ear, Nose and Throat and Head and Neck Surgery, Dhingra, 7th ed. pg. 55

- Malignant external otitis (MEO) is an infection that affects the external auditory canal and temporal bone.
- The causative organism is usually Pseudomonas aeruginosa, and the disease commonly manifests in elderly patients with diabetes.

26. Ans. (b) Anterior belly of digastric muscle

Ref: Diseases of ENT, by Dhingra, 6th ed. pg. 285

TABLE: Derivatives of branchial/pharyngeal arches

1st Branchial arch	2nd Branchial arch	3rd Branchial arch	4th Branchial arch	6th Branchial arch
• Malleus and Incus • Maxilla • Mandible • Muscle of mastication • Anterior belly of digastric muscle • Tensor tympani muscle • Sphenomandibular ligament	• Stapes (except foot plate) • Upper half of body of hyoid • Lesser cornu of hyoid • Muscle of facial expression • Posterior belly of digastric muscle • Stylohyoid ligament	• Lower part of body of hyoid • Greater cornu of hyoid • Stylopharyngeus muscle • Common carotid artery	• Upper thyroid cartilage • Cricothyroid muscle • Extrinsic laryngeal and pharyngeal muscle	• Lower half of thyroid cartilage • Arytenoid cartilage • All intrinsic laryngeal muscle except cricothyroid
Nerve: Mandibular branch of CN 5th	**Facial Nerve**	**Glossopharyngeal nerve**	**Vagus + Superior Laryngeal nerve**	**Vagus + Recurrent laryngeal nerve**

Note: *Laryngeal cartilage like cricoid, coneiform, corniculate are formal due to fusion of Branchial arch 4 and 6.*
Epiglottic cartilage derived from hypobranchial eminence.

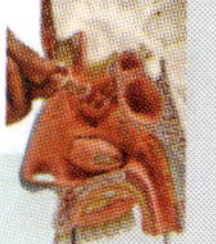

27. Ans. (a) 1.3 : 1

Ref: Dhingra's ENT 6th ed. pg. 15

- Handle of malleus is 1.3 times longer than long process of incus, providing a mechanical advantage of 1.3, giving the **ossicular-lever ratio of 1.3:1**
- **Hydraulic action of tympanic membrane:** The total area of tympanic membrane is 21 times bigger than footplate of stapes (3.2 mm), giving it a ratio of **21:1**
- As we know that only 2/3rd of tympanic membrane is effective, it gives an effective aerial ratio of 14:1
- Therefore **total transformation ratio** is: 14 × 1.3 = **18.2:1**

28. Ans. (c) Stria vascularis

Ref: Dhingrwa's ENT 6th ed. pg. 9

- **Cochlea is divided into 3 compartments:** Scala tympani, scala media and scala vestibuli by the two membranes **basilar membrane and Reissner's membrane.**
- Another membrane, i.e. stria vascularis is present on the wall of scala tympani and secretes endolymph.

29. Ans. (b) MacEwen's triangle

Ref: Dhingra's ENT, 6th ed. pg. 5

- Mastoid antrum is the largest air cell of mastoid. Its depth is ~15 mm from skin due to the thick plate of bone over it.
- Antrum is marked externally on the surface of mastoid by **Suprameatal triangle/MacEwen's triangle.**

Extra Mile

- Development of mastoid is from squamous and petrous bone. Persistence of petrosquamous suture is known as **Korner's septum.**

30. Ans. (a) Cricothyroid muscle

Ref: Diseases of ENT, by Dhingra, 6th ed. pg. 285

For explanations Please refer to above table Answer of Qs 26.

31. Ans. (c) Skin with fat

Ref: Dhingra's ENT, 6th ed. pg. 2, 5th ed. pg. 3-4

- The entire pinna is made of one yellow elastic cartilage except lobule and incisura terminalis.
  - Lobule is made of fat tissue covered with skin.
  - **Incisura terminalis:** Located between tragus and crus of helix. Can be used to gain access in external auditory meatus without cutting the cartilage.

32. Ans: (b) Lesser petrosal nerve

Ref: Dhingra's ENT, 6th ed. pg. 4

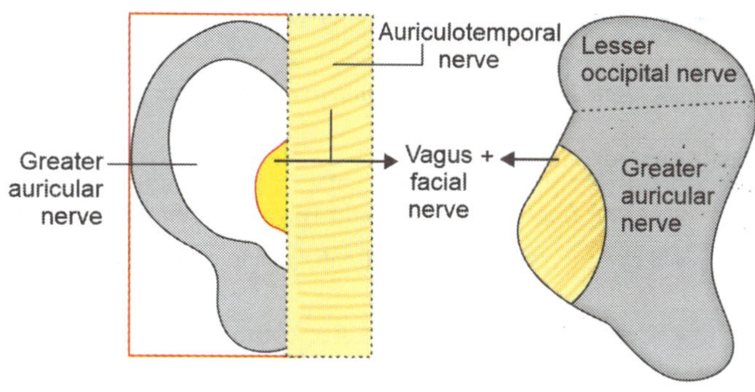

NERVE SUPPLY OF AURICLE/PINNA

Lateral Surface

- **Greater Auricular nerve**
- **Vagus (Arnold's nerve) + Facial Nerve:** Supplies concha
- **Auriculotemporal nerve**

Medial Surface

- **Lesser occipital nerve:** Supplies upper 1/3rd
- **Greater auricular nerve: Supplies lower 2/3rd**
- **Vagus (Arnold's nerve) + Facial nerve:** Supplies conchal protrusion medially (see Image)

33. Ans. (d) Auriculotemporal nerve

Ref: Dhingra's ENT, 6th ed. pg. 4

- Auriculotemporal nerve supplies only on the lateral aspect of auricle.

34. Ans. (a) Greater auricular nerve

Ref: Dhingra's ENT 6th ed. pg. 4

- Greater auricular nerve has major contribution of auricle. It supplies major portion on lateral aspect as well as on the medial aspect.

35. Ans. (a) Vagus nerve

Ref: Dhingra's ENT, 6th ed. pg. 4

- **Arnold's nerve** is the auricular branch (also known as the mastoid branch) of the vagus nerve (CN X).
- It originates from the superior ganglion of the vagus nerve
- Arnold's nerve along with facial nerve innervates concha of auricle and the external acoustic meatus *(posterior and inferior wall).*

36. Ans. (c) Glossopharyngeal nerve

Ref: Dhingra's ENT, 6th ed. pg. 4

- Jacobson's nerve is a branch of glossopharyngeal nerve (CN- IX) in middle ear.
- It supplies medial aspect of tympanic membrane.

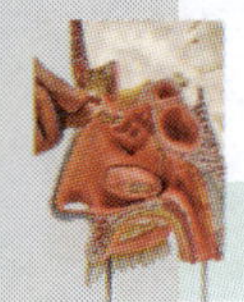

37. Ans. (a) Lesser cornu

Ref: Inderbir Singh's Embroyology, 7th ed. pg. 119-120

38. Ans. (c) III

Ref: Inderbir Singh's Embroyology, 7th ed. pg. 119-120

- Lower part of hyoid and greater cornu of hyoid is derived from branchial arch III.
- Upper part of hyoid and lesser cornu of hyoid is derived from branchial arch II

39. Ans. (d) Cricothyroid muscle

Ref: Inderbir Singh's Embroyology, 7th ed. pg. 119–120

- All intrinsic laryngeal muscles is derived from branchial arch VI EXCEPT cricothyroid muscle.
- Cricothyroid muscle is derived from branchial arch IV.

40. Ans. (d) IV and VI

Ref: Inderbir Singh's Embroyology, 7th ed. pg. 119-120

- Thyroid cartilage is derived from branchial arch IV and VI.
  - Upper part: Branchial arch IV
  - Lower part: Branchial arch VI

41. Ans. (b) II

Ref: Inderbir Singh's Embroyology, 7th ed. pg. 119-120

- Ear ossicles are derived from branchial arch I and II
- Malleus and incus: BA-I
- Stapes: BA-II

42. Ans. (a) Ultimobranchial body

Ref: Inderbir Singh's Embroyology, 7th ed. pg. 119-120

- In humans, the ultimobranchial body is an embryological structure that gives rise to the calcitonin-producing cells—**also called parafollicular cells or C cells**—of the thyroid gland.
- In humans, this body is a derivative of the ventral recess of the **fourth pharyngeal pouch.**
- **Stapes:** from 2nd Branchial arch
- **Laryngeal cartilage:** from 6th branchial arch
- **Mandible:** from 1st branchial arch

43. Ans. (d) Outer 1/3rd is bony and inner 2/3rd is cartilaginous

Ref: Dhingra's ENT, 6th ed. pg. 4-5

- In External auditory canal/meatus: **outer 1/3rd is cartilaginous, inner 2/3rd is bony**. Length is 8 mm and 16 mm respectively.
- EAC extends from bottom of concha to tympanic membrane having a total length of 24 mm.
- **Congenital pathologies associated with EAC:**
  - **Fissure of santorini:** From anterior wall of cartilaginous part of EAC to parotid gland
  - **Foramen of Huschke:** From anteroinferior wall of bony part of EAC to parotid gland
- **Note:** Any infection in parotid gland can spread to EAC or vice versa through these congenital pathologies.

44. Ans. (d) <1 cm

Ref: Dhingra's ENT, 6th ed. pg. 4-5

- **Total Length of EAC:** 24 mm (2.4 cm)
  - **Outer 1/3rd is cartilaginous: 8 mm (0.8 cm)**
  - Inner 2/3rd is bony: 16 mm (1.6 cm)

45. Ans. (c) Bony part of EAC and parotid gland

Ref: Dhingra's ENT, 6th ed. pg. 2

- **Congenital pathologies associated with EAC:**
  - **Fissure of santorini:** From anterior wall of cartilaginous part of EAC to parotid gland
  - **Foramen of Huschke:** From anteroinferior wall of bony part of EAC to parotid gland

46. Ans. (d) Composite grafts of cartilage & skin from pinna are not used for correction of defects of nasal ala

Ref: Dhingra's ENT, 6th ed. pg. 2

- **Composite grafts of cartilage and skin from pinna are used sometimes for correction of defects of nasal ala.**
- All other statements mentioned above are true.

Extra Mile

- CARTILAGE from the tragus, perichondrium from the tragus or concha and fat from lobule are frequently used for reconstructive surgery of middle ear.
- Tragal cartilage can be used to correct the depressed nasal bridge.
- Incisura terminalis is area between tragus and crus of helix. It is devoid of cartilage.

47. Ans. (a) 2.5 cm

Ref: Dhingra's ENT, 5th ed. pg. 4

- Length of external auditory canal- 24 mm (2.4 cm)
- Shape: S-shaped
- Outer 1/3rd cartilaginous part (8 mm)
- Inner 2/3rd: Bony part (16 mm)

48. Ans. (c) 1/3rd outer

Ref: Dhingra's ENT, 5th ed. / 4

- Outer 1/3rd of EAC is cartilaginous. It has hair follicles and ceruminous glands which secretes sebum.

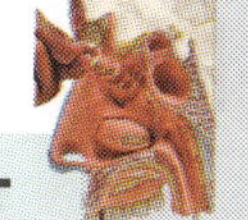

49. Ans. (b) Ascending ramus of mandible

Ref: Dhingra's ENT, 5th ed./227

- Retromolar trigone is a triangular area of mucosa covering **anterior surface of the ascending ramus of mandible.**
- Base of retromolar trigone is posterior to the last molar while its apex is adjacent to the tuberosity of maxilla.

ANATOMY OF MIDDLE EAR & INNER EAR

50. Ans. (b) Fracture of floor of the orbit

Ref: Diseases of Ear, Nose and Throat and Head and Neck Surgery, Dhingra, 7th ed. pg. 206

- Blowout fractures commonly involve the floor of orbit and may/may not be associated with fracture of medial wall or zygomatic component of lateral wall of orbit.
- Overall, physical assaults are the most common cause of orbital fractures, followed by fall from height, automobile accidents, sports related injuries, other causes in that order.

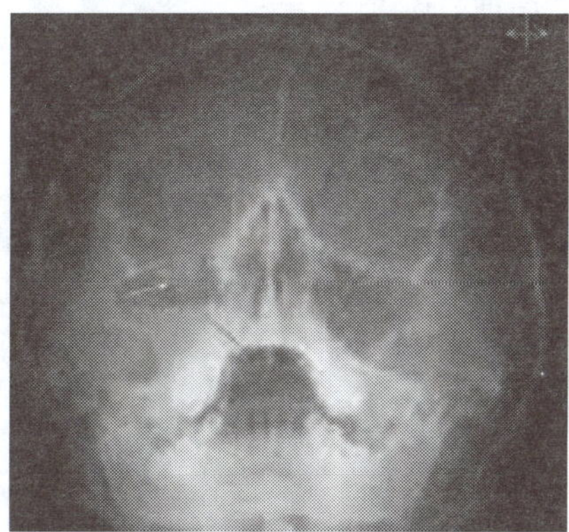

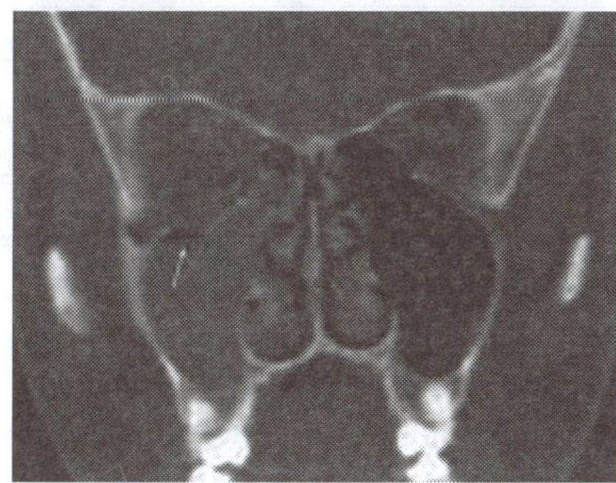

51. Ans. (b) Serous Otitis media with effusion

Ref: Diseases of Ear, Nose and Throat and Head and Neck Surgery, Dhingra, 7th ed. pg. 70

- The given image shows appearance of bubbles in the middle ear on Valsalva maneuver suggestive of Serous Otitis Media with effusion.
- Otitis media with effusion (OME) is a collection of non-infected fluid in the middle ear space. The fluid may accumulate in the middle ear as a result of a cold, sore throat or upper respiratory infection.
- Upon examination, air bubbles in middle ear is suggestive of serous otitis media/glue ear.

52. Ans. (b) Bruising over the mastoid

Ref: Bailey and Love Short Practices of Surgery, 27th ed. pg. 333

Battle sign: Bruising behind ear at mastoid region, due to petrous temporal bone fracture.

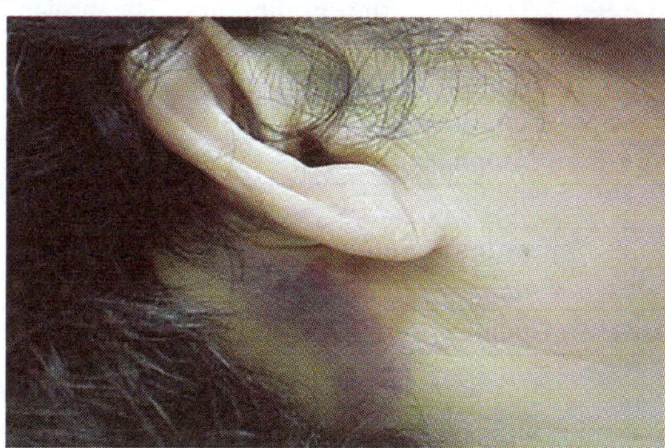

53. Ans. (b) Glomus tumor

Ref: Diseases of Ear, Nose and Throat and Head and Neck Surgery, Dhingra, 7th ed. pg. 121

- Glomus tumor is a mesenchymal tumor composed of modified smooth muscle cells that arise from the glomus body.
- The most common symptom is that of a pulsing sound as blood flows through the vessels of the tumor (pulsatile tinnitus).
- Other symptoms of a glomus tympanicum include a conductive hearing loss (caused by the tumor blocking sound transmission through the middle ear), ear pain and bleeding from the ear.

54. Ans. (b) Secretory otitis media

Ref: Diseases of Ear, Nose and Throat and Head and Neck Surgery, Dhingra, 7th ed. pg. 69

- Secretory otitis media occurs when fluid accumulates behind the eardrum and remains there after an acute middle ear infection or blockage of the eustachian tube.
- It shows type B curve of tympanometry.

55. Ans. (a) Organ of Corti

Ref: Dhingra's ENT, 6th ed. pg. 9, 10

- Organ of corti is sensory organ of hearing.

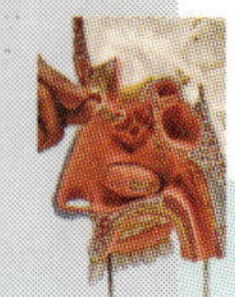

56. Ans. (b) Balance

Ref: Dhingra's ENT, 6th ed. pg. 9, 17

- There are 3 semicircular canals; the posterior, lateral and superior. They all lie in planes at right angles to each other.
- It is responsible for *balancing angular acceleration*.
- Macula, present in utricle and saccule is responsible for balancing linear acceleration.

57. Ans. (b) Medial

The most prominent portion of the medial wall of the middle ear cavity is the promontory. The projection is raised by underlying basal turn of cochlea. It has number of grooves containing tympanic plexus of nerves.

58. Ans. (a) Nasopharynx

- ET opens on lateral wall of nasopharynx.
- Bounded by ridge–Torus Tubarius

59. Ans. (a) Cochlea

Ref: Dhingra's ENT, 5th ed. pg. 12

- Upon taking the section of cochlea, we see 3 compartments and 3 membranes:
  - **Scala vestibuli:** Contains perilymph
  - **Scala media:** Contains endolymph
  - **Scala tympani:** Contains perilymph

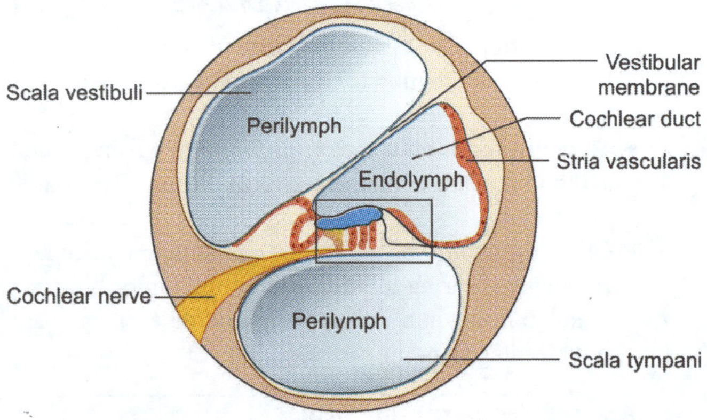

- **Three membranes are:**
  - **Reissner's membrane:** Separates scala vestibule from scala media.
  - **Basilar membrane:** Separates scala tympani from scala media. Also supports organ of corti.
  - **Stria vascularis:** On the wall of scala media. Converts perilymph into endolymph.

60. Ans. (a) Utricle

Ref: P.L. Dhingra's ENT, 6th ed. pg. 16

- Sensory organ of utricle and saccule: Macula

Structure of Macula

- Made of two parts:
  1. A **sensory neuroepithelium** made of type 1 and type 2 hair cells
  2. An **otolith membrane**. This membrane is made up of a gelatinous mass and on top, there is crystal of calcium carbonate called **otoconia or otolith.**

Extra Mile

- Sensory organ of linear motion/acceleration: Macula (In utricle and saccule)
- Sensory organ of angular motion/acceleration: Crista ampularis (in semicircular canal, ampulated portion)

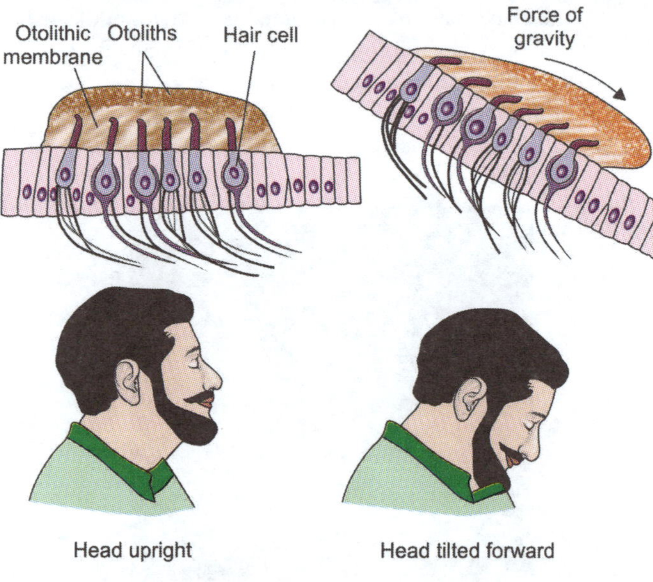

61. Ans. (c) Long process of incus

Ref: PubMed

62. Ans. (c) Posterior wall

Ref: Dhingra's ENT, 6th ed. pg. 4-5

- Chorda tympani is a branch of facial nerve which is located on posterior wall of middle ear.
- **Middle wall is box shaped cavity having 6 walls.**
- Corda tympani is a branch of facial nerve which is located on posterior wall of middle ear. It has sensory and secretomotor branches and supplies:
  - Anterior 2/3rd of tongue
  - Sublingual gland
  - Submandibular gland

Extra Mile

TABLE: Middle ear walls and their contents

Wall	Made of significance
Superior wall/roof	Made of tegmen tympani, a very thin plate of bone. **Separates middle ear from middle cranial fossa**
Inferior wall/ floor	• Aka **Jugular wall**. It is formed by tympanic plate of temporal bone. • Below the floor lies inferior jugular vein.
Lateral wall	Aka **outer wall.** Formed by tympanic membrane
Anterior wall	Aka **carotid wall**. Separates middle ear from Internal carotid artery. **Contents of anterior wall:** • Opening of eustachean tube 2 drains on lateral wall of nasopharynx • Canal of tensor tympani- Gives origin to tensor tympani muscle
Medial wall	Aka **labyrinth wall.** Separates middle ear from inner ear. **Contents:** • **Promontory:** Due to basal coil of cochlea • **Oval window:** Covered by foot plate of stapes • **Round window:** Covered by secondary tympanic membrane • **Processus cochleariformis:** Hook like structure, anterior to oval window. Tensor tympani muscle takes a turn here before inserting to neck of malleus • **Fistula ante-fenestrum: MC site for ostosclerosis** • **Fallopian canal/Facial canal:** Facial nerve runs here in horizontal direction.
Posterior wall	Aka **mastoid wall.** Separates middle ear from mastoid cavity. **Contents:** • **Pyramid:** Bony protrusion. Origin of stapedius muscle from tip of pyramid. • **Aditus ad-antrum:** Doorway to antrum of mastoid. Located on postero-superior wall. • **Facial nerve in facial canal** in vertical. direction. **Gives rise to chorda tympani.** • **Facial recess:** Landmark for intact canal wall surgery

63. Ans. (c) Carotid wall

Ref: Dhingra's ENT, 6th ed. pg. 5

Anterior wall is also known as carotid wall. Separates middle ear from Internal carotid artery. Contents of anterior wall:

- **Opening of eustachean tube:** Drains on lateral wall of nasopharynx
- **Canal of tensor tympani:** Gives origin to tensor tympani muscle.

64. Ans. (d) Aditus ad antrum

Ref: Dhingra's ENT, 6th ed. pg. 5-6

- Aditus ad antrum is located on posterior wall. It is a doorway to antrum of mastoid.
- Antrum is largest mastoid air cell.

65. Ans. (c) Middle cranial fossa

Ref: Dhingra's ENT, 6th ed. pg. 5

- Roof of middle ear is formed by tegmen tympani, a very thin plate of bone.
- It separates middle ear from middle cranial fossa.

66. Ans. (d) Medial

Ref: Dhingra's ENT, 6th ed. pg. 5

- MC site for ostosclerosis: **Fistula ante-fenestrum**
- **Location of fissula ante-fenestram:** Medial wall of middle ear

67. Ans. (b) Malleus

Ref: Dhingra's ENT, 5th ed. pg. 12

There are two important muscles of middle ear:

Muscle	Origin	Insertion	Nerve supply
Tensor tympani	Canal of tensor tympani (anterior wall)	Neck of malleus	Mandibular branch of CN - V
Stapedius	Tip of pyramid (posterior wall)	Neck of stapes	CN - VII

68. Ans. (c) 7

Ref: Dhingra's ENT, 5th ed. pg. 6

- Fallopian canal is also known as facial canal present on the walls of middle ear.
- **Direction:**
  - Entry from media wall. Facial nerve runs in horizontal direction
  - Exits on posterior wall. Facial nerve here runs in vertical direction.
  - Exits via stylomastoid foramen.

69. Ans. (b) 1 cm

Ref: Dhingra's ENT, 6th ed. pg. 9-10

- The opening to the internal acoustic meatus is located inside the cranial cavity, near the center of the posterior surface of the petrous part of the temporal bone.
- The size varies considerably; its margins are smooth and rounded. ***The canal is short (about 1 cm)*** and runs laterally into the bone.
- Length of external acoustic canal: **24 mm.**

- **Length of middle ear canal:**
  - Epitympanum – 6 mm
  - Mesotympanum – 2 mm
  - Hypotympanum – 4 mm
- **Shortest** distance between tympanic membrane to promontory: 2 mm.

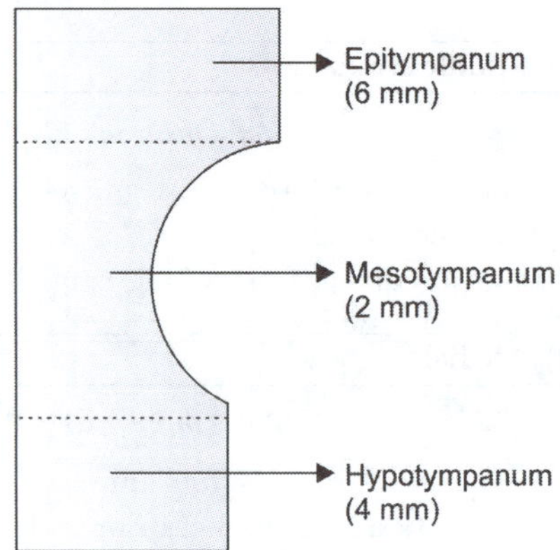

Middle ear cavity section

70. Ans. (a) 2 mm

Ref: Dhingra's ENT, 6th ed. pg. 9-10

- **Length of middle ear canal:**
  - Epitympanum – 6 mm
  - Mesotympanum – 2 mm
  - Hypotympanum – 4 mm
- **Shortest** distance between tympanic membrane to promontory: 2 mm.

71. Ans. (b) Facial nerve and superior vestibular cochlear nerve

Ref: Dhingra's ENT, 6th ed. pg. 90-91

- Bill's bar divides the superior compartment of the internal acoustic meatus into an anterior and posterior compartment.
- ***Anterior to Bill's bar, are the facial nerve*** *(in the anterior superior quadrant)* and nervus intermedius, ***and posterior to it is the superior division of the vestibular nerve*** *(in the posterosuperior quadrant).*

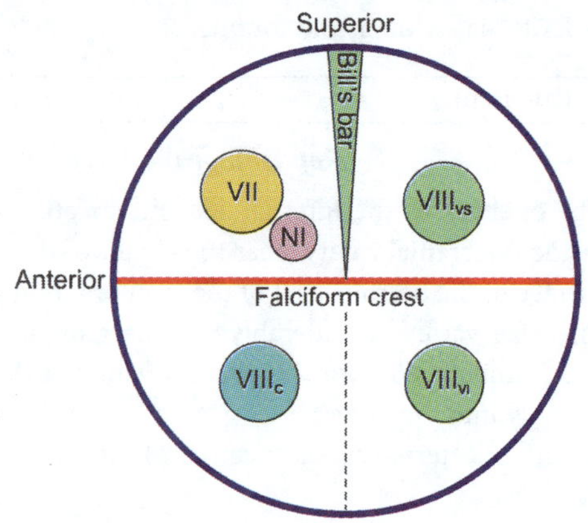

72. Ans. (b) Hearing

Ref: Dhingra's ENT, 5th ed. pg. 11

- The main function of cochlea is hearing via the hair cells present on basilar membrane
- **Sensory organ of hearing:** Organ of Corti
- **Otolith organ:** Utricle and Saccule

73. Ans. (b) Olfactory system

Ref: Dhingra's ENT, 5th ed. pg. 22

- **Requirements for balancing:**
  - Vision
  - Vestibule and cochlea
  - Proprioception
  - Cerebellum

74. Ans. (c) Semicircular canal

Ref: Dhingra's ENT, 5th ed. pg. 20

- Sensory organ of angular motion is crista ampularis which is located in semicircular canal.
- Structure of crista ampularis is a crest like mound of connective tissue on which lie the sensory epithelial cells. These sensory hair cells project into the cupula.
- **Cupula is a gelatinous mass** of polysachharides and contains canals into which project the cilia of sensory cells.

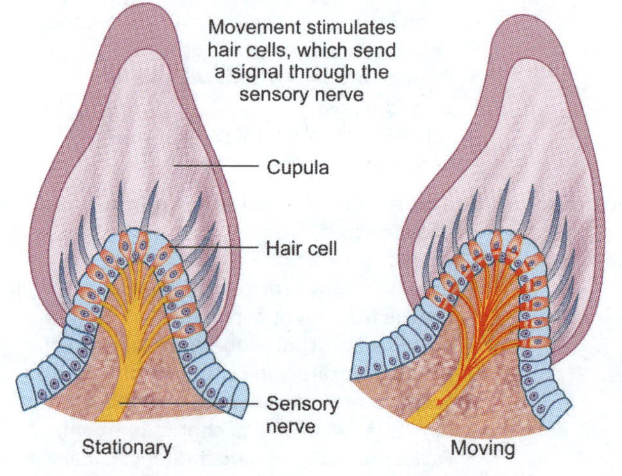

75. Ans. (c) Cochlea

Ref: Dhingra's ENT, 5th ed. pg. 12

- Upon taking the section of cochlea, we see 3 compartments and 3 membranes:
  - Scala vestibuli: Contains perilymph
  - Scala media: Contains endolymph
  - Scala tympani: Contains perilymph
- **3 membranes are:**
  - **Reissner's membrane:** Separates scala vestibule from scala media.

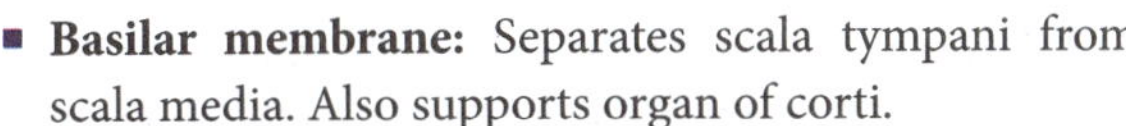

- **Basilar membrane:** Separates scala tympani from scala media. Also supports organ of corti.
- **Stria vascularis:** On the wall of scala media. Converts perilymph into endolymph.

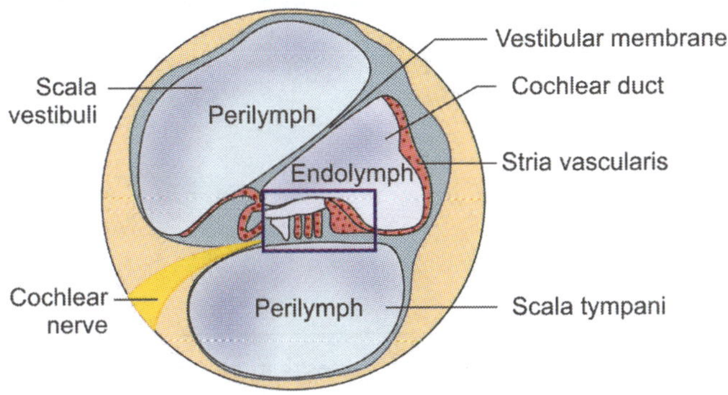

TESTS OF AUDITORY SYSTEM

76. Ans. (a) Serous otitis media

Ref: Diseases of Ear, Nose and Throat and Head and Neck Surgery, Dhingra, 7th ed. pg. 69

- **Type A tympanograms** are indicative of normal middle
- ear pressure.
- **Type A_D (deep) tympanograms** demonstrate increased compliance, as seen with ossicular chain discontinuity.
- **Type As (shallow) tympanograms** show decreased compliance, suggesting a stiff middle ear system, which can be caused by myringosclerosis or otosclerosis.
- **Type B tympanograms** with little or no mobility of the tympanic membrane are suggestive of middle ear effusion.
- **Type C tympanograms** indicate negative middle ear pressure and a retracted tympanic membrane.

77. Ans. (b) Used for SNHL

Ref: Dhingra's ENT 7th ed. pg. 29

- Brainstem Evoked Response Audiometry (BERA) aka ABR (Auditory Brainstem Response).
- It is to elicit brainstem responses to auditory stimulation by clicks or tone bursts.
- It is a **non-invasive** technique to find **the integrity of central auditory pathways** through the 8th nerve, pons and midbrain (used for SNHL assessment).
- It measures hearing sensitivity in the range of 1000–4000 Hz.
- In a normal person, 7 waves are produced in the first 10 milliseconds.
- Most stable waves: 1st, 3rd, 5th wave.

78. Ans. (c) Cochlear pathology

Ref: Dhingra's ENT 7th ed. pg. 25

- Decreased bone conduction in audiogram is seen in cochlear pathology.
- In conductive hearing loss, there is defect/abnormality associated with conducting zones like auditory canal blockage, ossicular disruption or fixation.
- Uses of audiogram (aka Pure Tone Audiometry)
  - Hearing loss present or not
  - Type and side of hearing loss
  - For prescription of hearing aid
  - To predict speech reception threshold

79. Ans. (d) Can cause Vertigo

Ref: Diseases of ENT by Dhingra 6th ed. pg. 53-54

- **External ear syringing** is done to clean/remove wax from external auditory canal.
- **Indications:**
  - Removal of wax
  - Dried fungal debris
  - Epithelial debris
  - Blunt foreign bodies
- **Direction of flow:** Postero-superior wall
- **Water** that is used is normal room temperature water (pre-boiled and cooled to room temperature)
- If too cold or too warm water used → It can stimulate labyrinth as in caloric testing and can cause vertigo.

REQUIREMENTS AND PROCEDURE OF SYRINGING

Requirements: Aural syringe 50 or 100 cc capacity, a kidney tray and warm saline at body temperature (Not to produce caloric reaction and vertigo).

Procedure: Patient sits before the operator with the ear to be syringed facing him. The nozzle of the syringe is detached and the syringe is filled with water/saline. The nozzle is then tightly reapplied and air pushed out of the syringe in vertical position. Light is thrown on to the patients ear by means of head mirror/light. The kidney tray is held below the ear. The pinna of the patient is pulled **upwards, backwards and outwards** with one hand of the operator to straighten out the meatus and by means of the syringe, the jet of the fluid is ordinarily directed towards the posterosuperior wall of the meatus. The force used should be moderate and canal washed of wax. The meatus should be inspected after each syringing to see the TM so that operator does not go on syringing unnecessarily. After syringing, the meatus should be dried with cotton wool on carrier.

Contraindications: Generalized & Localized otitis externa, Perforation of ear drum, Acute otitis media, Scarred ear drum, Recent or old fracture of base of skull, Patient suffering from heart disease for fear of vagal reflex.

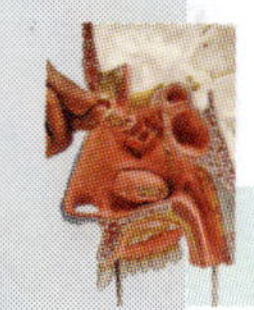

80. Ans. (c) Noise induced hearing loss

Ref: Diseases of ENT by Dhingra 6th ed. pg. 34-35

- Most common cause of acquired hearing loss: presbycusis > Noise induced hearing loss
- NIHL is usually bilateral and symmetrical
- Noise induced hearing loss (NIHL) is caused by acoustic trauma which is characterized by specific pattern of audiogram finding.
- NIHL can damage hair cells, starting in the basal turn of cochlea. Outer hair cells are affected first followed by inner hair cells.
- NIHL usually affect a person's hearing sensitivity in the higher frequencies like 3000 Hz, 4000 Hz or 6000 Hz.
- Upon audiogram a notch is seen especially at 4000 Hz.
- Tinnitus is the first symptom without any hearing impairment.

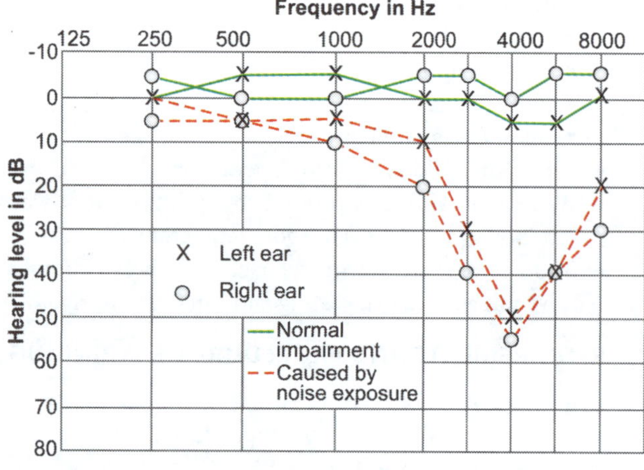

Extra Mile

- **Carhart Notch:** A sudden dip/notch at 2000 Hz. Seen in otosclerosis
- **Acoustic trauma:** Sudden, permanent, SNHL due to single exposure to an intense sound (130–140 dB) for <0.2 secd.

81. Ans. (a) 85 dB in 8 hrs/days for 5 days/week

Ref: Dhingra's ENT 6th ed. pg. 35

Book states: *"a noise of 85 dB, 8 hours a day for 5 days per week is the maximum safe limit as recommended by the ministry of labour, GOI."*

TABLE: Permissible exposure in cases of continuous noise or a number of short-term exposure (Ministry of Labor, GOI): Factory Act 1948

Noise level (dB)	Permitted daily exposure (hour)
85	8
87	6
90	4
92	3
97	1 ½
100	1
105	½
110	¼

Note: 5 dB rule of time intensity states that "any rise of 5 dB noise level will reduce the permitted noise exposure time to half".

82. Ans. (b) As

Ref: Dhingra's ENT, 6th ed. pg. 25

Types of tympanogram graphs and their interpretation:

- A: Normal
- As: Otosclerosis (reduced compliance at ambient pressure)

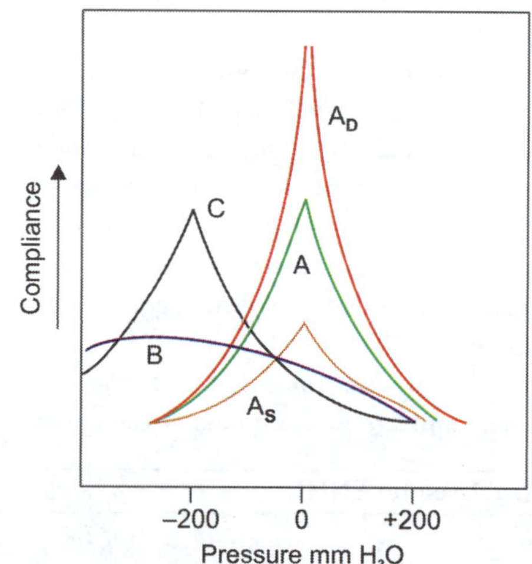

- Ad: Disruption of ossicular chain (increased compliance at ambience pressure)
- B: Glue ear/Fluid in middle ear **(Flat or dome shaped)**
- C: Eustachean tube obstruction (Maximum compliance at pressure >–200 mm H_2O; Negative pressure in middle ear)—**negative tympanogram**

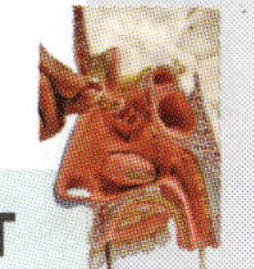

83. Ans. (b) ABR

Ref: Dhingra's ENT, 6th ed. pg. 27

ABR is auditory brainstem response. It is used for:

- Screening infants hearing
- To determine threshold of hearing in infant and in uncooperative patient.
- To diagnose brainstem pathology. E.g., multiple sclerosis.
- For intraoperative monitoring of CN.
- In acoustic neuroma surgery
- **OAE** is also used for screening of hearing in neonates.

84. Ans. (b) Cochlea

Ref: Dhingra's ENT, 6th ed. pg. 27

Otoacoustic emission test will determine cochlear, hair cell function. It is used for:

- Screening neonates exposed to aminoglycoside antibiotics.
- Differentiating sensory and neural components of sensori-hearing loss.
- Test for feign (maligned) hearing loss.
- To differentiate cochlear vs retrocochlear hearing loss

Note: *Sedation does not interfere with OAE test.*

85. Ans. (d) Acoustic neuroma

Ref: Dhingra's ENT 6th ed. pg. 450

- **Tone decay** also known as auditory fatigue, is a change in auditory threshold when a continuous tone is presented to the ear.
- It is seen in **acoustic neuroma** and other retrocochlear lesion.

86. Ans. (a) Otosclerosis

Ref: Diseases of ENT, by Dhingra, 6th ed. pg. 22-23

- Gelle's test is a Tuning fork test which can be performed using tuning fork of different frequencies such as: 128, 256, 512, 1024, 2048, 4096 Hz.
- MC used/ideal for routine clinical practice is of **512 Hz**.
- **Tests done with tuning fork:**
  - Rinne's test
  - Weber's test
  - Absolute bone conduction (ABC) test
  - Bing test
  - Gelle's test
  - Lewis test

POINTS TO KNOW ABOUT GELLE'S TEST

- Gelle's test is a bone conduction test and examines effect of increased air pressure in ear canal (*using siegel's speculum*) on hearing.
- This test is performed by placing a vibrating tuning fork on mastoid, while changes in air pressure in the ear canal are brought about by siegel's speculum.

Contd...

- In normal individuals, increased air pressure in ear canal, pushes tympanic membrane inwards which raises intralabyrynthine pressure → immobility of basilar membrane → decreased hearing **(POSITIVE TEST)**.
- In patients with fixed ossicular chain (otosclerosis) or disconnected ossicular chain, there is no change in hearing **(NEGATIVE TEST)**.

Note: *Earlier it was a popular test for otosclerosis. Now it is superceded by tympanometry.*

87. Ans. (b) CSOM

Ref: Diseases of ENT, by Dhingra, 6th ed. pg. 22

TABLE: Tests done with help of tuning fork and their interpretation

Rinne's is a tuning fork test, which is done to test the air conduction and bone conduction.
It is done by placing the tuning fork on mastoid (Bone conduction) followed by bringing it in front of ear canal (air conduction).
In normal individual and in SNHL sound is still heard when tuning fork is brought in front of ear canal (**AC > BC → Positive Rinne**)
In patients with conductive hearing loss, sound transmitted via bone conduction (mastoid) is more as compared to air conduction (**BC > AC → Negative Rinne**).
All the given conditions in options causes sensorinueral hearing loss, except the CSOM, which causes conductive hearing loss.

88. Ans. (c) Left ear, air conduction

Ref: Diseases of ENT, by Dhingra, 6th ed. pg. 30

Symbols and Lines used in Audiogram

- Broken line for bone conduction (Mn: B–B)
- Continuous line for air conduction
- Red line for right ear (Mn: R–R)
- Blue line for left ear

TABLE: Symbols used in Audiogram charting

Test modality	Right ear	Left ear
AC unmasked	○	X
AC masked	△	□
BC unmasked	<	>
BC masked	[	]

89. Ans. (b) 512 Hz

Ref: Dhingra's ENT, 5th ed. pg. 26

- Tuning fork test can be performed using tuning fork of different frequencies such as: 128, 256, 512, 1024, 2048, 4096 Hz.
- MC used/ideal for routine clinical practice is of 512 Hz.

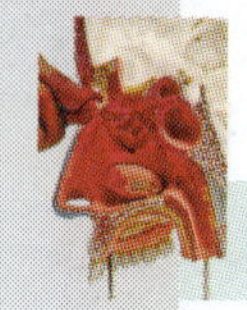

- Tuning fork of lower frequencies produce sense of bone vibration while those of higher frequencies have a shorter decay time and are thus not routinely preferred.
- Tuning fork of
- **Tests done with tuning fork:**
  - Rinne's test
  - Weber's test
  - Absolute bone conduction (ABC) test
  - Bing test
  - Gelle's test
  - Lewis test

90. Ans. (c) 512 Hz

Ref: Dhingra's ENT, 6th ed. pg. 22, 5th ed. pg. 26

91. Ans. (d) Pure tone audiometry

Tests done with help of tuning fork and their interpretation:

Test	Normal	CHL	SNHL
RINNE	AC > BC	BC > AC	AC > BC
WEBER	NO Lateralization	Lateralization deaf side	Lateralization normal side
ABC	Equal	Equal	Reduced
Schwabach's	Equal	Increased	Reduced

92. Ans. (c) Cochlea

Ref: Dhingra's ENT 5th ed. pg. 32

- Otoacoustic emission (OAE) are low intensity sounds **produced by outer hair cells of a normal cochlea.**
- These sounds produced by outer hair cells travels in a reverse direction: Outer hair cells 2 basilar membrane 2 perilymph 2 oval window 2 ossicles 2 tympanic membrane 2 ear canal.
- When outer hair cells are damaged, OAE are absent. Hence it helps to know the function of cochlea.

93. Ans. (a) ABR

Ref: Dhingra's ENT, 5th ed. pg. 31-32

- **ABR** is considered as best test for screening of hearing in neonates
- **ABR is** auditory brainstem response. Can be used as screening procedure and threshold of hearing in infants. Mainly used to diagnose retrocochlear pathology. Ex: Acoustic Neuroma.
- **Tympanometry** is considered as IOC for otosclerosis.
- **Electrocochleography:** Used to find out threshold of hearing in young infants and children. It is also the most sensitive test for Meniere's disease.

94. Ans. (a) Vestibular function

Ref: Dhingra's ENT, 5th ed. pg. 48

- Caloric test is used to assess vestibular function. The basis of this test is to induce nystagmus by thermal stimulation of the vestibular system.
- Done by taking water of 2 temperatures, cold (30°C) and hot (44°C).
- **Position of the test:** Supine then lift head at 30° forward or patient sitting with bending backwards 60°.
- **This position is used in order to make lateral/horizontal SCC in vertical position.**
- Cold water elicits nystagmus in opposite eye and warm water elicit nystagmus in same eye (Mn: COWS).
- **Interpretation:**
  - **Normal: Time** taken from start of irrigation to end point of Nystagmus is taken and it is **80 seconds –120 seconds.**
  - **Canal paresis:** Duration of Nystagmus shortened i.e. <80 secd.
- Indicates depressed function of ipsilateral labyrinth, vestibular nerve and vestibular nuclei.
- **It is seen in:**
  - Meniere's disease
  - Acoustic neuroma
  - Vestibular neuritis
  - Vestibular nerve section
  - Postural vertigo

95. Ans. (b) Lateral semicircular canal

Ref: Dhingra's ENT, 6th ed. pg. 43

96. Ans. (a) Fistula test

Ref: Dhingra's ENT, 6th ed. pg. 41

FISTULA TEST

- The aim of this test is to induce nystagmus by increasing pressure in labyrinth which is performed by applying pressure at tragus.
- **If there is fistula between middle ear and inner ear, this increased pressure leads to stimulation of labyrinth which results in nystagmus and vertigo.**
- In normal population the test is negative because the pressure changes in the external auditory canal cannot be transmitted to the labyrinth.
- **Fistula test is positive in the following cases:**
  - When there is erosion of lateral/horizontal semi-circular canal as in cholesteatoma
  - After fenestration operation- **type V tympanoplasty** *(a surgically created window in the horizontal canal)*

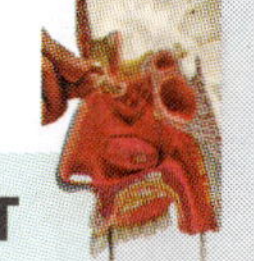

- Post stapedectomy fistula *(Abnormal opening in the oval window post-stapedectomy)*
- After rupture of round window membrane
- **A positive fistula also implies that the labyrinth is still functioning.**

- **It is absent when labyrinth is dead.**
- A false negative fistula test is also seen when cholesteatoma covers the site of fistula and doesn't allow pressure changes to be transmitted to the labyrinth.
- A false positive fistula test is seen in case of menier's disease aka endolymphatic hydrops.

Extra Mile

- **Impedance audiometry** is done in order to determine the status of the tympanic membrane and middle ear via tympanometry.
  - The other purpose of this test is to evaluate acoustic reflex pathways, which include cranial nerves VII and VIII and the auditory brainstem.
- **Galvanic vestibular stimulation** is the process of sending specific electric messages to a nerve in the ear that maintains balance.

DISEASES OF EAR, TREATMENT AND REHABILITATION

97. Ans. (d) Congenital external auditory atresia

Ref: Diseases of Ear, Nose and Throat and Head and Neck Surgery, Dhingra, 7th ed. pg. 136-137

- In the treatment of auditory canal atresia, BAHA provides superior hearing results, greater parental satisfaction and fewer complications.
- Bone-anchored hearing aid is a type of hearing aid which is based on the principle of bone conduction.
- It is primarily suited to people who have conductive hearing loss, unilateral hearing loss and those with mixed hearing loss.

98. Ans. (b) Retroorbital pain

Ref: Diseases of Ear, Nose and Throat and Head and Neck Surgery, Dhingra, 7th ed. pg. 285

- Pathognomonic features of Trotter's triad in sequential order include:
  - Ipsilateral conductive hearing loss
  - Trigeminal nerve neuralgia affecting the mandibular division and
  - Soft palate palsy
- Trotters' triad is seen in nasopharyngeal carcinoma

99. Ans. (a) Mastoiditis

Ref: Dhingra's ENT 6th ed. pg. 84-86

The given history and sign, is seen in mastoiditis.

Mastoiditis Symptoms

- Pain behind the ear seen
- Fever: Persistence of fever in otitis media → resemble development of mastoiditis
- Ear discharge - profuse

Signs

- Ear Discharge - mucopurulent profuse
- Mastoid tenderness
- Mastoid swelling
- Reservoir sign - meatus immediately fills with pus after it has been mopped out
- Sagging of posterosuperior wall
- Perforation of tympanic membrane - small perforation at para tensa
- Hearing loss - conductive type hearing loss

Treatment

- Hospitalize the patient
- Antibiotics - Amoxicillin
- Myringotomy
- Cortical Mastoidectomy in these cases

100. Ans. (d) Destroying the cochlear is mandatory

Ref: Dhingra's ENT 7th ed. pg. 111-112

- **Meniere's disease** is also known as endolymphatic hydrops. There is increased endolymphatic pressure, possibly due to increased endolymph secretion or decreased outflow.
- **Exact cause** is not known. Possibly associated with allergy, hypothyroidism, viral infection, sodium and water retention.
- **Patient present** with triad of: Sensorineural hearing loss, episodic vertigo and tinnitus.
- **Treatment:**
  - Reassurance
  - Low salt diet and avoid excess water intake
  - Cessation of smoking
  - Avoid coffee, tea, alcohol
  - **In chronic conditions** sedatives like Prochlorperazine, vasodilators like Betahistine or loop diuretics can be used
  - **Surgical options** like intratympanic gentamicin (a vestibulotoxic agent).
  - **Destructive Procedures.** They totally destroy cochlear and vestibular function and are thus used only when cochlear function is not serviceable. It is not required in every case.

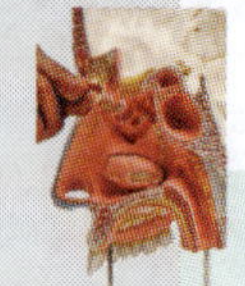

- **Labyrinthectomy:** Membranous labyrinth is completely destroyed either by opening through the lateral semicircular canal by transmastoid route or through the oval window by a transcanal approach.

101. Ans. (d) Internal carotid artery aneurysm

Ref: Dhingra's ENT 7th ed. pg. 437

- Upon examination of tonsil and tonsillar pillars, Palpation of the tonsil with a gloved finger is essential. Following findings are noted:
  - If consistency of mass is hard: Malignancy or tonsillolith
  - If there is pulsation in tonsillar area: Internal carotid artery aneurysm

102. Ans. (b) Cochlear implant

Ref: Dhingra's ENT 6th ed. pg. 125

- In the above patient of profound SNHL, cochlear implant is preferred.
- Indication of cochlear implant:
  - Bilateral Severe/profound SNHL
  - Intact auditory nerve system
- Implant has external and internal component (image). Electrode array is placed in scala tympani of cochlea.

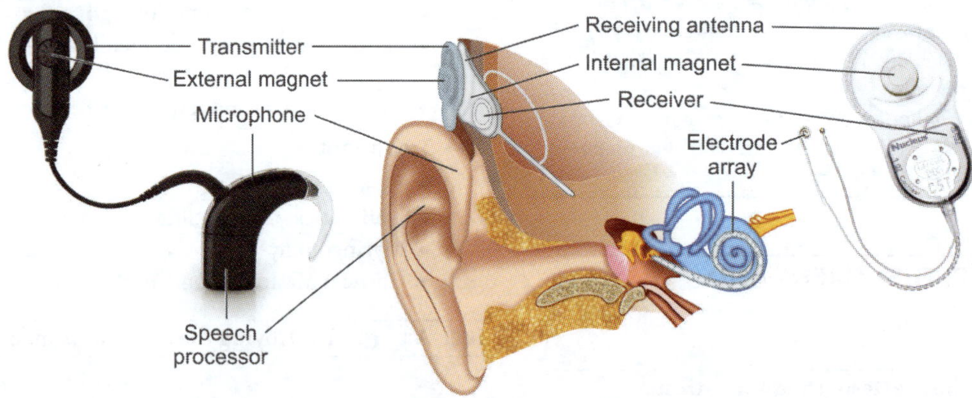

Illustration of cochlear implant components. The external parts are shown on the left, the internal components of the implant on the right. The scheme in the middle shows the position of the cochlear implant components *in situ*

103. Ans. (d) Myringotomy + Gromet insertion

Ref: Diseases of ENT by Dhingra 6th ed. pg. 65

- Main cause of otitis media is Eustachean tube obstruction/dysfunction. Can occur due to chronic rhinitis, chronic sinusitis
  - In child: MC due to adenoid hypertrophy
  - Adult: Raise suspicion of nasopharyngeal carcinoma
- **Upon examination:**
  - Severely retracted tympanic membrane
  - Dull/pale tympanic membrane
  - Presence of fluid level with air bubbles
- **Initial management:**
  - Nasal decongestant
  - Anti-allergic measures
  - Antibiotics (in cases of URTI)
  - Valsalva manuever/Politzerisation- for middle ear aeration
- Mainstay of treatment of glue ear is **myringotomy with grommet insertion** with or without adenoidectomy.

- Indications of surgery in glue ear:
  - Chronic effusion >3 months
  - CHL 40 dB
  - Suspicion of malignancy
- **Preferred site:** Postero-inferior quadrant of tympanic membrane

Extra Mile

- If aspirate is thick/glue like → two incisions are made: Antero-superior and antero-inferior quadrant known as "Beer can principle"

104. Ans. (a) Kanamycin

Ref: Goodman & Gillman 13th ed. pg. 1044-45

- All aminoglycosides have the potential to produce reversible and irreversible vestibular, cochlear, and renal toxicity and neuromuscular blockade.

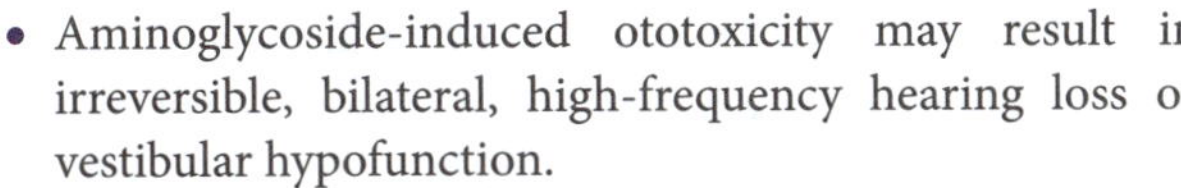

- Aminoglycoside-induced ototoxicity may result in irreversible, bilateral, high-frequency hearing loss or vestibular hypofunction.
- A high-pitched tinnitus often is **the first symptom** of cochlear toxicity.
- Drugs like amikacin, neomycin and kanamycin are specifically cochleotoxic > vestibulotoxic.
- Gentamicin, streptomycin is vestibular > cochleotoxic
- Tobramycin: Cochlear = Vestibular toxicity

105. Ans. (a) Idiopathic Bell's palsy

Ref: Dhingra's ENT 6th ed. pg. 95

- Facial nerve palsy can be central or peripheral.
- Peripheral lesion can involve nerve in its intracranial, intratemporal or extratemporal part. Peripheral lesions are more common and 2/3rd of them are idiopathic variety.
- **MCC:** 60–75% of the facial paralysis is due to **bell's palsy.** It is defined as idiopathic, peripheral facial paralysis or paresis of acute onset.
  - **Causes:** Viral infection (HSV, HZV or EBV), vascular ischemia, hereditary (~10% of patients have positive family history), autoimmune disorder.

106. Ans. (b) Otosclerosis

Ref: Dhingra's ENT 6th ed. pg. 87

- Otosclerosis is a sclerotic bone disease having two stages:
  - **Otospongiotic stage** also known as active stage
  - **Otosclerotic stage** also known as passive stage
- It is most commonly seen in females, in the age group of 20–30 years and the condition worsens during pregnancy.
- **Clinical features/symptoms:**
  - Progressive conductive hearing loss
  - Tinnitus
  - Vertigo
  - **Paracusis willis:** Patient hears better in noisy environment (as a normal person raises voice in noisy environment)
- **Signs**
  - **Schwartz sign:** Reddish hue/flamingo pink coloration seen on the promontory through tympanic membrane.
  - Pure tone audiometry shows loss of air conduction more for lower frequencies. At 2000 Hz, there is sudden dip/notch formation known as **Carhart Notch**
- **IOC: Tympanometry (finding will be "As")**
- **Treatment: Stapedectomy/Stapedotomy** with a placement of prosthesis is treatment of choice.

107. Ans. (c) Costen syndrome

Ref: Dhingra's ENT 6th ed. pg. 447

- **Costen syndrome:**
  - It is an abnormality of temporomandibular joint, and is characterized by otalgia, feeling of blocked ear, tinnitus and often vertigo as well.
  - Pain in Costen syndrome also radiates to frontal, parietal and occipital region.
- **Gradenigo's syndrome:** It is a severe form of petrositis (complication of otitis media) and involves CN V and VI. It consists of:
  - Ear discharge
  - Diplopia (due to CN VI involvement)
  - Retro-orbital pain (due to CN V involvement)

108. Ans. (b) Ramsay hunt syndrome

Ref: Dhingra's ENT, 6th ed. pg. 55, 96

- **Herpes zoster oticus** is a condition which is characterized by the appearance of vesicles on tympanic membrane, deep meatus, retroauricular sulcus and concha.
- If herpes zoster oticus involves facial nerve, this condition is called **Ramsay hunt syndrome.** Patient may present in symptoms of facial nerve paralysis along with facial anesthesia, giddiness and hearing impairment due to involvement of 5th and 8th cranial nerve.
- **Treatment:** Acyclovir + Steroids

Extra Mile

- **Bell's palsy** is usually idiopathic. However it can be infective or hereditary in origin as well. It is always diagnosis of exclusion.
- **Myringitis bullosa** is a painful condition characterized by formation of haemorrhagic blebs on the tympanic membrane. and deep meatus. Involvement of facial nerve is very less likey.
- **Melkersson syndrome** is an idiopathic condition present with triad of recurrent facial nerve paralysis, lip swelling and fissured tongue.

109. Ans. (c) Chronic myringitis

Ref: Diseases of ENT, by Dhingra, 6th ed. pg. 55

- **Myringitis granulosa**
  - It is a non-specific granulation on the outer/lateral surface of tympanic membrane.
  - It may be associated with external ear infection, impacted wax or long-standing foreign body.

110. Ans. (c) Serous otitis media

Ref: Dhingra, 5th ed. pg. 71-72

- Serous otitis media is also known as Glue ear.
- It is an insidious condition characterized by accumulation of non-purulent effusion in the middle ear cleft.
- One of common causes of serous otitis media (Glue ear) in children is blockage of Eustachian tube secondary to adenoid hyperplasia.

- Therefore, the treatment aims at removal of adenoid (adenoidectomy) and drainage of middle ear by grommet/Ventillation tube.
  - **Grommet** is a small tube inserted in tympanic membrane to drain the middle ear.
- Serous otitis media in adults should arouse suspicion of nasopharyngeal carcinoma and hence the treatment aims at removal of carcinoma.
- Adenoiditis is an acute condition and requires treatment conservatively.

111. Ans. (b) Softening followed by syringing

Ref: PL Dhingra's ENT, 6th ed. pg. 53

Dhingra states: *"If the wax is too hard and impacted to be removed by syringing or instruments, it should be softened by drops of 5% sodium bicarbonate in equal parts of glycerine and water instilled 2–3 times a day for a few days."*

Note:

- Hydrogen peroxide, liquid paraffin or olive oil may also achieve same result.
- Commercial drops like 2% paradichlorobenzene (ceruminolytic agent) can also be used to soften the wax.

Extra Mile

- If a fly or any crawling insect enters the ear canal, no attempt should be made to catch them alive. First they should be killed by instilling oil, spirit or chloroform, then suctioned out.

112. Ans. (a) Autograft

Ref: PubMed

- **Autograft:** Transplantation of tissue to the same person, from whom the tissue is harvested.
- **Isograft:** Transplantation of organ or a tissue from a donor to a genetically identical recipient like the twins
- **Allograft:** Transplant of an organ or tissue between two genetically non-identical members of same species
- **Xenograft:** Transplant of organ or tissues from one species to another.

Extra Mile

- Tympanoplasty is repairing of tympanic membrane in cases of ruptured tympanic membrane either due to infection or trauma.
- Temporalis fascia is used for tympanoplasty. It has **very low basal metabolic rate**, hence very high rate of survival.

113. Ans. (a) 20–20,000 Hz

Ref: Dhingra's ENT, 6th ed. pg. 14-15

- Normal hearing capacity is from 20 Hz to 20,000 Hz.
- Function of hearing is by cochlea, which has 2 ends broadly. Apex and Base. Apex is for low frequency sound (20 Hz) and Base is for high frequency sound (20,000 Hz).

114. Ans. (b) 41–60 dB

Ref: Dhingra's ENT, 6th ed. pg. 38

WHO classification for hearing loss:

0–25 dB	Normal hearing
26–40 dB	Mild hearing loss
41–60 dB	Moderate hearing loss
61–80 dB	**Severe hearing loss**
>80 dB	Profound hearing loss

115. Ans. (c) 5–6 khz

Ref: Noise-Induced Hearing Loss: Scientific Advances; edited by Colleen G. Le Prell, Donald Henderson, Richard R. Fay, Arthur Poppe

- When the ear is exposed to excessive sound levels or loud sounds over time, the overstimulation of the hair cells on basilar membrane leads to heavy production of reactive oxygen species, leading to oxidative cell death.
- Damage ranges from exhaustion of the "hair" (hearing) cells in the ear to loss of those cells.
- NIHL usually occurs initially at high **frequencies (3, 4, or 6 kHz),** and then spreads to the low frequencies (0.5, 1, or 2 kHz)".

116. Ans. (b) Virus

Ref: Dhingra, 5th ed. pg. 62

- **Myringitis bullosa**
  - It is a painful condition characterized by formation of haemorrhagic belbs on the tympanic membrane and deep meatus.
  - **It is most commonly caused by virus-Adenovirus**
  - However it can also be caused by mycoplasma Pneumonia
- **Another similar disease entity is:**
  - **Myringitis granulosa**
    - It is non-specific granulations on the outer surface of tympanic membrane.
    - It may be associated with external ear infection, impacted wax or long-standing foreign body.

117. Ans. (a) Streptococcus pneumoniae

Ref: Dhingra's ENT, 6th ed. pg. 62

Acute otitis media is most commonly caused by Streptococcus Pneumonia. However it can also be caused by H. influenzae and Moraxella catarrhalis.

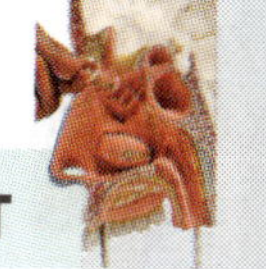

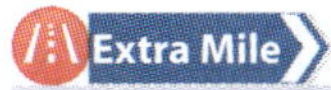

Common Infections and their most Common Causative Agents:

Infection	MC organism
Perichondritis	Pseudomonas
Malignant otitis externa	Pseudomonas
Localized otitis externa	Staphylococcus aureus
Acute suppurative otitis media	Strep pneumoniae
Chronic otitis Media	Pseudomonas

118. Ans. (c) Air

Ref: Dhingra's ENT, 5th ed. pg. 69-70

Otitis media is acute inflammation of middle ear by pyogenic organism secondary to:

- Eustachian tube blockage (MCC)
- Tympanic membrane perforation

Stages of Otitis Media Development

- **Stage of tubal occlusion:** Edema and hyperemia of nasopharyngeal end of eustachian tube blocks the tube leading to absorption of air and negative intratympanic pressure and retraction of TM with handle of malleus.
- **Stage of pre-suppuration:** Prolonged suppuration leads to growth of pyogenic organism causing appearance of inflammatory exudates, characterized by **cart-wheel appearance of TM.**
- **Stage of suppuration:** Marked formation of pus in middle ear and to some extent in mastoid air cells, characterized by red and bulging tympanic membranes with loss of landmarks. X-rays shows clouding of air cells.
- **Stage of resolution:** Rupture of TM with release of pus and subsidence of symptoms, characterized by a small perforation in antero-inferior quadrant of pars-tensa.
- **Stage of complication:** If resolution doesn't take place, disease spreads, causing mastoiditis, facial paralysis, petrositis, meningitis, etc.

119. Ans. (b) Stage 2

Ref: Dhingra's ENT, 6th ed. pg. 67-69

PARS FLACCIDA RETRACTION

- This classification described by Toss is fairly simple to apply, the only difficulty being the difficulty in making a distinction between stages 3 and 4. Hence for practical purposes these two stages are grouped together.
- Pars flaccida retractions have a vital role to play in the pathophysiology of cholesteatoma. Tos et al classified pars flaccida retraction in to four stages:
- **Stage I:** Pars flaccida is dimpled and is more retracted than normal. It is not adherent to the malleus.

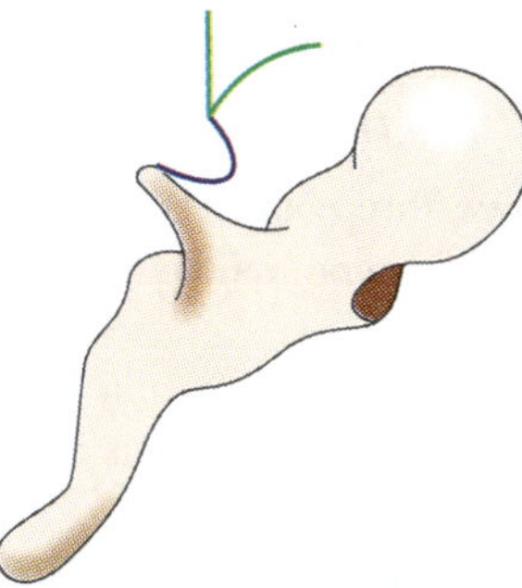

- **Stage II:** *In this stage the retraction pocket is adherent to the handle of malleus. The full extent of the retraction pocket can be clearly seen.*

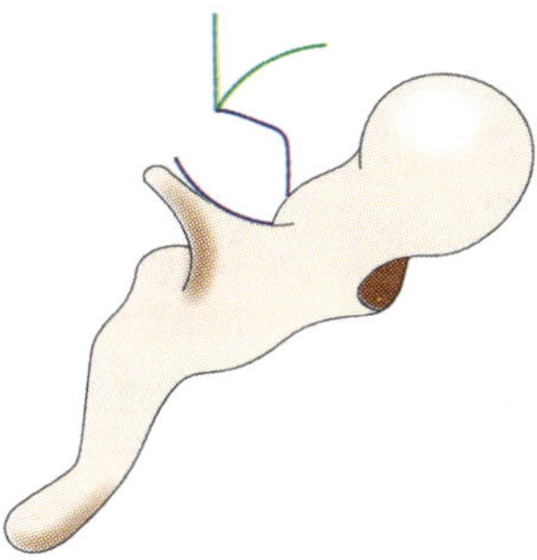

- **Stage III:** In this stage part of the retraction pocket may be hidden. There may also be associated erosion of the outer attic wall (scutum).

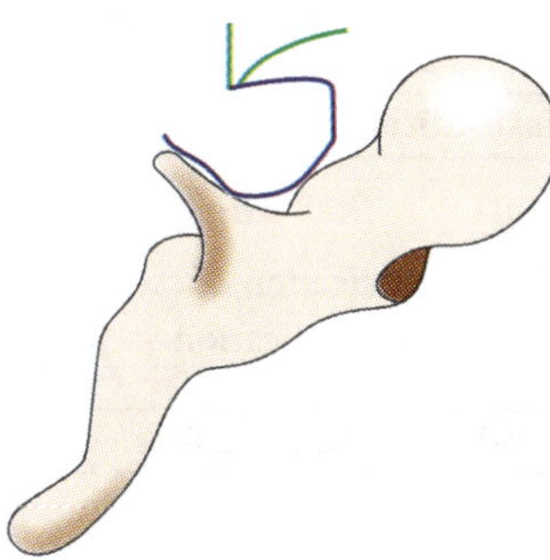

- **Stage IV:** In this stage there is definite erosion of the outer attic wall. The extent of the retraction pocket cannot be clearly seen as most of it are hidden from the view.

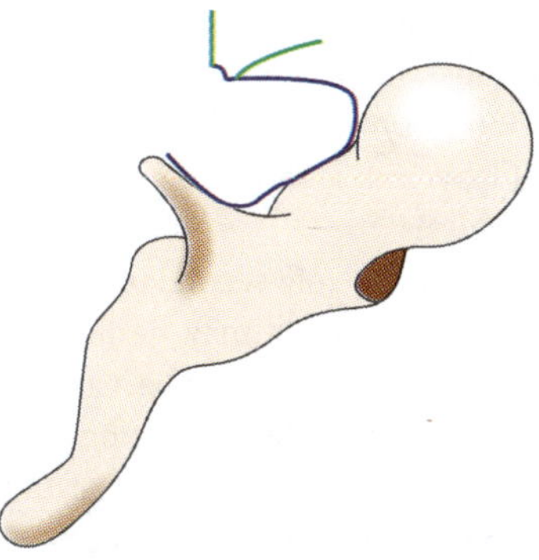

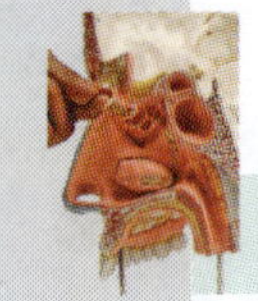

120. Ans. (d) Lateral sinus thrombophlebitis

Ref: Dhingra's ENT, 5th ed. pg. 94 and 84-86

- Lateral sinus thrombophlebitis is an inflammation of inner wall of lateral venous sinus with formation of thrombus.
- It occurs as a complication of acute coalescent mastoiditis, masked mastoiditis or chronic suppurative otitis media.

Intracranial	Extracranial
Meningitis- ***MC***	Ossicular damage
Lateral sinus thrombophlebitis	Mastoiditis ***(MC)***
Sub dural abscess	Gardenigo's syndrome
Extra dural abscess	Labyrinthine fistula/ Labyrinthitis
Otitis hydrocephalus	Petrositis
Cerebral abscess ***(2nd MC)***	Facial nerve palsy
Mn: Men Like S-Ex On Call	Mn: OMG Lady Love Peters Face

121. Ans. (a) Brain abscess

Ref: Dhingra's ENT, 5th ed. pg. 84-86, 94

MC Intracranial complication of CSOM Meningitis > Cerebral Abscess

Please refer to above explanation

122. Ans. (c) Mastoiditis

Ref: Dhingra's ENT 5th ed./ 84-86, 94

- Overall, MC complication of csom → Mastoiditis
- MC extracranial complication → Mastoiditis.

123. Ans. (a) Conductive hearing loss

Ref: Dhingra's ENT, 5th ed. pg. 83

Clinical features of Tubercular otitis media:

- **Painless foul smelling ear discharge:** Very characteristic finding.
- **Perforation:** Multiple perforations usually 2–3 on pars tensa is classical sign of disease.
- **Hearing loss:** There is a severe hearing loss, out of proportion to symptoms . **Mostly conductive**, it may be SNHL if labyrinth is involved.
- Facial paralysis
- In the presence of secondary pyogenic infection, tubercular otitis media may be indistinguishable from chronic suppurative otitis media. Culture of ear discharge for tubercle bacilli, histopathological examination of granulations and other evidence of tuberculosis in the body help to confirm the diagnosis.

Treatment

- **Systemic antitubercular therapy** as being carried for primary focus.
- **Local treatment** in the form of aural toilet and control of secondary pyogenic infection. Mastoid surgery is indicated for complications. Healing is delayed in tuberculous cases. Wound break-down and fistula formation are common.

124. Ans. (b) Multiple perforation of pars tensa

Ref: Dhingra's ENT, 5th ed. pg. 83

Please refer to above explanation

125. Ans. (a) Long process of incus

Ref: Dhingra's ENT, 5th ed. pg. 78 & 81

OSSICULAR NECROSIS IN OTITIS MEDIA

Dhingra States

- In case of tubo-tympanic CSOM *"ossicular chain is usually intact and mobile but may show some degree of necrosis,* ***particularly of the long process of incus****"*
- In case of atticoantral type CSOM *"ossicular necrosis is common in atticoantral type of CSOM.* ***Destruction may be limited to the long process of incus*** *or may also involves stapes superstructure, handle of malleus or the entire ossicular chain"*

126. Ans. (b) CN V, VI

Ref: Dhingra's ENT, 6th ed. pg. 447

- Petrositis is inflammation of petrous bone.
- Gardenigo's syndrome results due to severe petrositis, which is a complication of CSOM (Chronic Suppurative Otitis Media).
- Two cranial nerves are involved in case of Gardenigo's syndrome: CN V and CN VI.
- **It is characterized by 3 D's:**
    - Discharge
    - Diplopia
    - Deep pain/retro-orbital pain
- Remember, there is NO Deafness in case of Gardenigo's syndrome.

127. Ans. (a) Deafness

Ref: Dhingra's ENT, 6th ed. pg. 447

128. Ans. (b) Bacteria

Ref: Dhingra's ENT, 5th ed. pg. 57-58

- Malignant otitis externa is caused by pseudomonas infection in elderly, diabetics & patients on the immune-compromised drugs.

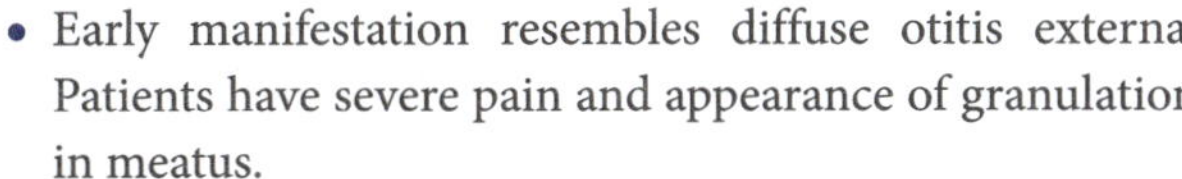

- Early manifestation resembles diffuse otitis externa. Patients have severe pain and appearance of granulation in meatus.

Infectious Etiology of Ear Canal

Bacterial	Fungal	Viral
• Localized otitis externa • Diffuse otitis externa • Malignant otitis externa	Otomycosis	• Herpes zoster oticus • Otitis externa hemorrhagica

129. Ans. (a) 7th

Ref: Dhingra's ENT, 6th ed. pg. 52-53

- Malignant otitis externa is an inflammatory condition caused by pseudomonas infection usually in elderly diabetic & those on immune-compromised drugs.
- Facial nerve paralysis is common.

130. Ans. (a) Herpes zoster virus

Ref: P.L. Dhingra, 5th ed. pg. 107

- In some cases of herpes zoster oticus, there is facial paralysis along with vesicular rash in the external auditory canal and pinna. This condition is called Ramsay Hunt Syndrome.
- **Treatment:** Acyclovir + Steroids

131. Ans. (c) Geniculate ganglion

Ref: Dhingra's ENT, 5th ed. pg. 102, 109

Course of Facial Nerve

- Motor fibers take origin from the nucleus of VIIth nerve. It leaves the brainstem at pontomedullary junction, travels through posterior cranial fossa and enters the internal acoustic meatus.
- Origin of facial nerve in inner ear is from geniculate ganglion. If there is a lesion at geniculate ganglion it can cause slow progressive facial palsy

Branches of Facial Nerve

- **Greater superficial petrosal nerve:** Arises from geniculate ganglion and carries secretomotor fibers to lacrimal gland and glands of nasal mucosa
- Nerve to stapedius
- Chorda tympani: Sensory to anterior 2/3rd of tongue and secretomotor fibers to sublingual and submandibular gland.
- Communicating branch
- Posterior auricular nerve
- Muscular branch: To stylohyoid and posterior belly of digastric
- Peripheral branches.

132. Ans. (a) Otosclerosis

Ref: Dhingra, 5th Ed. pg. 461, 98-99

- **Schwartz sign** is a pink reflex, seen through intact tympanic membrane, in the area of oval window. It indicates active otosclerosis usually during pregnancy.
- Otosclerosis is an abnormal bone growth in the middle ear that causes conductive hearing loss.

Symptoms

- Hearing loss (CHL)
- **Paracusis willi:** An otosclerotic patient hears better in noisy surrounding.
- Tinnitus
- Vertigo
- Speech

Signs

- **Schwartz's sign:** A reddish hue seen on the promontory through the tympanic membrane. This is indicative of active focus with increased vascularity.
- Pure tone audiometry shows loss of air conduction, more for lower frequencies.
- **Carhart's notch:** There is a sudden dip at 2000 Hz in bone conduction curve.

Extra Mile

- Don't get confused between schwartz sign and Schwartz surgery.
- Schwartz surgey is a simple mastoidectomy or cortical mastoidectomy in case of mastoiditis.

133. Ans. (c) 2000 Hz

- **Carhart Notch** is an audiogram finding and is an important feature in patients with Otosclerosis.
- There is a sudden dip (notch) at 2000 Hz in bone conduction curve.
- Carhart's notch disappears after stapedectomy.

134. Ans. (b) Tinnitus

Ref: Dhingra, 5th ed. pg. 120-121

- **Glomus tumor** is the most common benign neoplasm of middle ear and is so-named because of its origin from the glomus bodies.
- The tumor is often seen in the middle age (40–50 years)
- Females are affected five times more than males.
- **There are two types of glomus tumor:**
  - **Glomus jugulare** arise from the dome of jugular bulb. Invade the hypotympanum and jugular foramen.
    - They may compress jugular vein or invade its lumen
  - **Glomus tympanicum** arise from the promontory of the middle ear and cause aural symptoms and sometimes with facial paralysis.

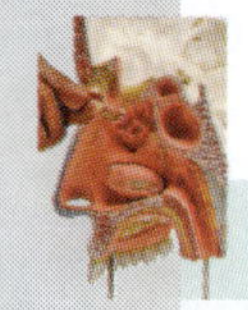

Clinical Features

- **Earliest symptoms are tinnitus** and hearing loss.
  - Tinnitus is pulsatile and of swishing character.
  - Hearing loss is conductive and slowly progressive.
- Otoscopy shows a red reflex through intact tympanic membrane.
- **"Rising sun"** appearance is seen when tumor arises from the floor of middle ear.
- In addition to hearing loss and tinnitus, there is history of profuse bleeding from the ear either spontaneously or on attempts to clean it.
- Dizzines or vertigo and facial paralysis may appear.
- Ear ache is less common.
- Otorrhea may occur due to secondary infection and the condition may simulate chronic suppurative otitis media with polyp.
- IXth–XIIth cranial nerves may be paralyzed.
- There is dysphagia and hoarseness with unilateral paralysis of the soft palate, pharynx and vocal cord with weakness of the trapezius and sternomastoid muscles.
- **Rule of 10**—Remember that 10% of the tumors are familial, 10% multicentric and up to 10% functional, i.e. they secrete catecholamines.

135. Ans. (c) Meniere's disease

Ref: Dhingra's ENT, 6th ed. pg. 448

Meniere's disease aka Endolymphatic Hydrops is a condition which is characterized by triad of:
- Episodic Vertigo
- Sensorineural Hearing loss
- Tinnitus

Meniere's disease has some special features:

- **Hennebert's sign:** False positive fistula sign
- **Tulio's phenomenon:** Vertigo in noisy environment
- Diplacusis

136. Ans. (c) Diplacusis

Ref: PL Dhingra, 5th ed. pg. 112

WHY DIPLACUSIS IN MENIERE'S DISEASE?

In the abnormal ear, neurons respond to a broader range of stimulus frequencies. But due to CNS preconditioning, the brain interprets any activity in a particular neuron as resulting from a stimulus of its normal characteristic frequency. Thus a single stimulus simultaneously processed by the normal and abnormal cochlea will be perceived as two different stimuli by the CNS, thus leading to diplacusis.

137. Ans. (b) Posterior semicircular canal

Ref: Dhingra's ENT, 6th ed. pg. 45-46

- BPPV is Benign Paroxysmal Positional Vertigo
- It occurs **due to an otolith in posterior semicircular canal,** which can result either due to head trauma, infection or drugs.
- This condition can be diagnosed by typical history and Dix-Hallpike Manoeuver.
- This condition can be treated by Epley's maneuver, where repositioning of otolith is done from posterior semicircular canal to utricle.

138. Ans. (b) Carcinoma of tongue

Ref: Dhingra, 5th ed. pg. 240

- Referred pain in the ear is most likely due to carcinoma of tongue.
- Due to common nerve supply of the tongue (lingual nerve) and ear (auriculo temporal) from the mandibular division of the trigeminal nerve, a referred pain of tongue CA presents with ipsilateral ear pain.

CARCINOMA OF TONGUE

- Carcinoma involving anterior 2/3rd of tongue is commonly seen in men in the age group of 50–70 years.
- It may also develop on a pre-existing leukoplakia, long standing dental ulcer or syphilitic glossitis
- Most common type of tongue CA: Squamous cell type
- **Site: Most common site is middle of the lateral border** or the ventral aspect of the tongue

Clinical Presentation

- A submucous nodule with induration of the surrounding tissue.
- An exophytic lesion like a papilloma.
- A non-healing ulcer with rolled edges, grayish white shaggy base and induration.

Symptomatology

- Early lesions are painless and remain asymptomatic for a long time
- Pain in the tongue locally at the site of ulcer
- **Pain in the ipsilateral ear:** Due to common nerve supply of the tongue (lingual nerve) and ear (auriculo temporal) from the mandibular division of the trigeminal nerve
- A lump in the mouth
- Enlarged lymph node mass in the neck
- Dysphagia, difficulty to protrude the tongue, slurred speech and bleeding from the mouth are late features.

139. Ans. (c) Sensorineural deafness

Ref: Dhingra's ENT, 6th ed. pg. 446-47

- Trotter's triad is seen in case of nasopharyngeal carcinoma. **It is also called Sinus of Morgagni Syndrome. Trotter's triad includes:**
  - Ipsilateral soft palate palsy (Due to CN X)

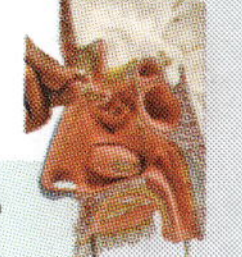

- Conductive hearing loss (Due to ET obstruction)
- Trigeminal neuralgia (Due to CN V).

140. Ans. (c) Sensorineural hearing loss

Ref: Dhingra's ENT, 5th ed. pg. 124

ACOUSTIC NEUROMA

- Acoustic neuroma is also known as vestibular schwannoma, neurilemmoma or eighth nerve tumor.
- It arises from superior division of vestibular nerve.
- The tumor arises from the Schwann cells of the vestibular, but rarely from the cochlear division of 8th nerve within the internal auditory canal.

Clinical Features

- **Age and sex:** Mostly seen in age group of 40–60 years. Both sexes are equally affected.
- **Cochleovestibular symptoms**
  - They are the earliest symptoms.
  - Most commonly manifests by Progressive unilateral sensorineural hearing loss, often accompanied by tinnitus.
  - Vestibular symptoms are imbalance or unsteadiness.
- **Cranial nerve involvement**
  - **Cranial nerve 5th is the earliest nerve to be involved** (after 8th) causing loss of corneal reflex
  - **MC clinical finding of acoustic** neuroma-loss of corneal reflex
  - **CN 7th involvement:** Although rare, it causes numbness or paraesthesia of face
  - **Hitzelberger sign:** Hypoaesthesia around posterior auricular area (due to CN 7th involvement)
  - In CN 8th sensory fibers are affected early.
  - **9th and 10th nerves:** There is dysphagia and hoarseness due to palatal, pharyngeal and laryngeal paralysis.
- **Brainstem involvement**
  - There is ataxia, weakness and numbness of the arms and legs with exaggerated tendon reflexes.
- **Cerebellar involvement**
  - Revealed by finger-nose test, knee-heel test, dysdiadochokinesia, ataxic gait, inability to walk along a straight line with tendency to fall to the affected side.
- **Raised intracranial tension**
- This is also a late feature.
- There is headache, nausea, vomiting, diplopia and papilloedema with blurring of vision.

141. Ans. (d) Crowding of lower tooth

Ref: Dhingra's ENT, 6th ed. pg. 243-44

- **Enlargement of adenoid tonsils due to infection can lead to adenoid hypertrophy.**

Clinical Features of Adenoid Hypertrophy

- Signs and symptoms of adenoid hypertrophy doesn't depend on the absolute size of the adenoid mass but are relative to the available space in the nasopharynx.
- This hypertrophy may cause nasal, aural or general symptoms.

A. Nasal Symptoms

- **Commonest symptom of adenoid hypertrophy: Nasal obstruction.**
- **Nasal discharge:** It is partly due to choanal obstruction, as the normal nasal secretions cannot drain into nasopharynx and partly due to associated chronic rhinitis. The child often has a wet bubbly nose.
- **Sinusitis:** Adenoid hypertrophy can lead to persistent nasal discharge and infection which can cause chronic maxillary sinusitis. Reverse is also true that a primary maxillary sinusitis may lead to infected and enlarged adenoids.
- **Epistaxis:** When adenoids are acutely inflamed, epistaxis can occur with nose blowing.
- **Voice change:** Decreased nasality in voice *(Rhinolalia Clausa).*

B. Aural Symptoms

- **Tubal obstruction:** Adenoid mass blocks the eustachian tube leading to retracted tympanic membrane which causes conductive hearing loss.
- Persistence can cause Chronic suppurative otitis media which may fail to resolve due to presence of infected adenoids.
- **Serous otitis media:** The waxing and waning size of adenoids causes intermittent eustachian tube obstruction with fluctuating hearing loss.

C. General Symptoms

- **Adenoid facies:** Mouth breathing and Chronic nasal obstruction can lead to characteristic facial appearance called **adenoid facies.**
  - *In adenoid facies, the child has an elongated face with dull expression, open mouth,* ***prominent crowded upper teeth****, and hitched up upper-lip,* ***pinched-in nose appearance*** *due to disuse atrophy of alae nasi.*
- **Highly arched hard palate** as the moulding action of the tongue on palate is lost. *This high arched hard palate can cause deviated nasal septum.*
- **Pulmonary hypertension:** Long-standing nasal obstruction due to adenoid hypertrophy can cause pulmonary hypertension and cor-pulmonale.

142. Ans. (d) Cleft palate

Ref: Dhingra, 5th ed. pg. 442

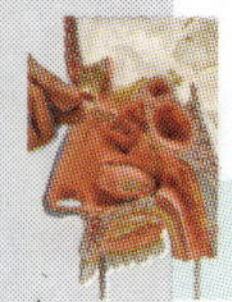

- **Adenoids**, also known as **pharyngeal tonsil**, or **nasopharyngeal tonsil**, are located at the back of the throat, above the tonsils, and are small lumps of tissue.
- They form part of the immune system of babies and young children.
- In case of their hyperplasia, there are several difficulties faced by patients like rhinousinusitis, mouth breathing, snoring etc.
- Adenoidectomy is surgical removal of adenoids to overcome those problems.

Indications and Contraindications of Adenoidectomy

Indications	Contraindications
• Adenoid hypertrophy causing snoring • Mouth breathing sleep apnea syndrome or speech abnoramlities, i.e. (rhinolalia clausa) • Recurrent rhinosinusitis • Chronic secretory otitis media associated with adenoid hyperplasia • Recurrent ear discharge in benign CSOM associated with adenoiditis/adenoid hyperplasia • Dental malocclusion	• Cleft palate or submucous palate • Removal of adenoids causes velopharyngeal insufficiency in such cases • Haemorrhagic diathesis • Acute infection of upper respiratory tract. • Bleeding disorders • Allergic rhinitis • Polio epidemic

143. Ans. (b) Allergic rhinitis

Ref: Dhingra's ENT, 6th ed. pg. 431-432

144. Ans. (b) Serous otitis media in children

Ref: Dhingra, 5th ed pg. 71-72

- Serous otitis media is also known as Glue ear.
- It is an insidious condition characterized by accumulation of non-purulent effusion in the middle ear cleft.
- One of common causes of serous otitis media (Glue ear) in children is blockage of Eustachian tube secondary to adenoid hyperplasia.
- Therefore, the treatment aims at removal of adenoid (adenoidectomy) and drainage of middle ear by grommet.
  - Grommet is a small tube inserted in tympanic membrane to drain the middle ear.
- Serous otitis media in adults should arouse suspicion of nasopharyngeal carcinoma and hence the treatment aims at removal of carcinoma.
- Adenoiditis is an acute condition and requires treatment conservatively.

145. Ans. (b) Adenoidectomy

Ref: Dhingra's ENT, 6th ed. pg. 431-32

Please refer to the previous question for explanation.

146. Ans. (b) Temporalis fascia

Ref: Dhingra's ENT, 6th ed. pg. 29-30, 400

- Tympanoplasty is repairing of tympanic membrane in cases of ruptured tympanic membrane either due to infection or trauma.
- Temporalis fascia is used for tympanoplasty. It has very low basal metabolic rate, hence very high rate of survival of graft.

147. Ans. (a) Round window

Ref: Dhinga's ENT, 5th ed. pg. 138

- Cochlear implant is an electronic device that can provide useful hearing and improved communication abilities for a person with profound sensorineural hearing loss.
- **Cochlear implant consists of two components:**
  1. **External component:** Include external speech processor and a transmitter. Speech processor may be body worn or behind the ear type.
  2. **Internal component:** It is surgically implanted and comprises the receiver/stimulator package with an electrode array. Electrode array is **passed via round window** and is ***inserted into the cochlea (scala tympani) deeper in skull.***

NOSE AND PARANASAL SINUSES

148. Ans. (a) Amphotericin B

Ref: Diseases of Ear, Nose and Throat and Head and Neck Surgery, Dhingra, 7th ed. pg. 178

- Mucormycosis is a serious fungal infection caused by a group of molds, called mucormycetes.
- Mucormycosis needs to be treated with prescription antifungal medicine, usually amphotericin B, posaconazole, or isavuconazole.

149. Ans. (d) Meniere's disease

Ref: Diseases of Ear, Nose and Throat and Head and Neck Surgery, Dhingra, 7th ed. pg. 111

- Meniere's disease is a disorder of the inner ear that can lead to vertigo and hearing loss. In most cases, Meniere's disease affects only one ear.
- Symptoms of Meniere's disease appear to be the result of an abnormal amount of endolymph in the inner ear.

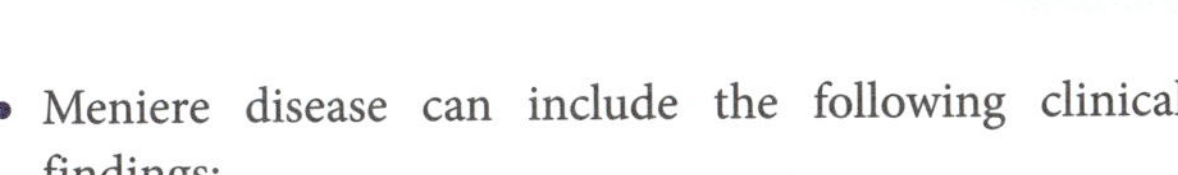

- Meniere disease can include the following clinical findings:
  - Two or more episodes of dizziness or vertigo, fluctuating aural symptoms (fullness, hearing, or tinnitus) in the affected ear, Diplacusis.
  - It can present due to multiple stimuli like loud noise. Loud noise induced vertigo is termed as **Tulio's Phenomenon.**

150. Ans. (a) Aspergilloma

Ref: Diseases of Ear, Nose and Throat and Head and Neck Surgery, Dhingra, 7th ed. pg. 220

- Aspergillomas are formed when the fungus grows in a clump in a sinus cavity or lung cavity.
- The maxillary antrum is a relatively common site for formation of an aspergilloma where it forms around a nexus of foreign body.
- In patients with aspergillus, sinusitis may report symptoms of vague chronic sinusitis, or present with no symptoms at all.

151. Ans. (b) Nasopharyngeal angiofibroma

Ref: Diseases of Ear, Nose and Throat and Head and Neck Surgery, Dhingra, 7th ed. pg. 279

- Juvenile nasopharyngeal angiofibroma is a benign tumor that tends to bleed and occurs in the nasopharynx of prepubertal and adolescent males.

152. Ans. (d) Mucormycosis

Ref: Diseases of Ear, Nose and Throat and Head and Neck Surgery, Dhingra, 7th ed. pg. 178

- Mucormycosis, also known as black fungus, is an aggressive, life-threatening infection occurs when a susceptible person comes in contact with its spores in the environment.
- Post-Covid 19 patients who are at an increased risk to develop Mucormycosis are those with a history of poorly controlled diabetes mellitus and excessive use of steroids.

153. Ans. (a) Caldwell's view

Ref: Diseases of Ear, Nose and Throat and Head and Neck Surgery, Dhingra, 7th ed. pg. 203

The Caldwell view (or Occipitofrontal view) is meant to show the frontal sinus more clearly than a standard PA skull radiograph.

154. Ans. (c) Maxillary sinus

Ref: Diseases of Ear, Nose and Throat and Head and Neck Surgery, Dhingra, 7th ed. pg. 206

- The arrow in image is pointed at maxillary sinus
- Waters' view (also known as the occipitomental view) is a radiographic view of the skull. It is commonly used to get a better view of the maxillary sinuses.

155. Ans. (b) CT scan

Ref: Dhingra's ENT 6th ed. pg. 219

- CT scan of sinuses will tell the extent of disease, predisposing structural abnormalities, amount of destruction of bony walls and any extension to orbit and cranial cavity.
- Investigation of choice for diagnosis of sinusitis is also CT scan.

156. Ans. (a) Nasopharyngeal swab for SARS COV2 testing

- During outbreak of covid, with symptoms of common colds, loss of smell and taste, raises suspicion of covid.
- RT-PCR is advised with Nasopharyngeal swab.

157. Ans. (a) Lower the edema then close reduction after 7 days

Ref: Dhingra's ENT 6th ed. pg. 203-204

- Fractures of nasal septum are the most common fracture over face. The amplitude of force can be from front or below.
- Nasal bone fracture, are also common. Traumatic forces may act from the front or side depend on amplitude.

Types

- **Depressed:** Due to frontal blow.
- **Angulated:** Due to lateral blow.

Symptoms

- Swelling within few hours of trauma
- Tenderness
- Nasal deformity
- Epistaxis
- Nasal obstruction - due to hematoma or septal injury.
- Periorbital ecchymosis

Diagnosis

- On physical examination
- X-rays should include Waters' view, right and left lateral views and occlusal view

Treatment

- Simple fractures without displacement - need no treatment
- Others - may require closed or open reduction
- Presence of edema interferes with accurate reduction by closed methods.

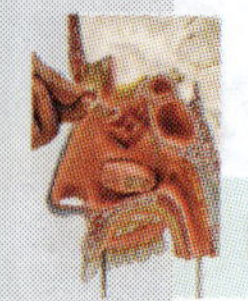

- So, best time to reduce a fracture is before the appearance of oedema, or after it has subsided, which is usually in 5–7 days.

158. Ans. (a) Bony

Ref: Dhingra's ENT 6th ed. pg. 175

- Nasal syphilis can be congenital or acquired.
- **Acquired syphilis** is the more common one and it occurs as:
  - **Primary:** Rare form. Manifest as primary chance of vestibule
  - **Secondary:** Manifest as simple rhinitis with crusting and fissuring of nasal vestibule
  - **Tertiary:** In this stage nose is commonly involved and commonly manifest as formation of gumma on nasal septum. Later this septum is destroyed also in bony and cartilaginous part both → lead to septal perforation.
    - Also has foul odor nasal discharge with crust.
    - Can lead to septal collapse and nose deformity.
- **Congenital syphilis** occurs in two forms: early and late form:
  - **Early form:** Seen in first 3 months of life and manifest as snuffles, followed by purulent discharge.
  - **Late form:** Manifest around puberty. Presents as tertiary stage of acquired syphilis.
- **Treatment:**
  - **DOC:** Benzathine penicillin 2.4 MU intramuscular weekly for 3 weeks.

159. Ans. (a) Neck lymph node enlargement

Ref: Dhingra's ENT 7th ed. pg. 283-84

Most common clinical presentation of nasopharyngeal CA: **Cervical lymphadenopathy** (neck swelling)

160. Ans. (b) Radiotherapy

Ref: Dhingra's ENT 7th ed. pg. 283-84

- Nasopharyngeal CA is the most radiosensitive tumor of head and neck
- TOC is **radiotherapy.**
  - **Stage I and II:** Radiotherapy alone
  - **Stage III and IV:** Radiation + chemotherapy
- External beam radiation of 6000–7000 cGy can be delivered by linear accelerator to the primary and both sides of neck

161. Ans. (c) Halo sing

Ref: Dhingra's ENT 7th ed. pg. 184

- The history of the given case is of CSF rhinorrhea due to cribriform plate fracture (due to history of RTA).
- CSF rhinorrhoea after head trauma is mixed with blood and shows double target sign when collected on a piece of filter paper.
- It shows central red spot (blood) and peripheral lighter halo, as seen in the image above. It is often termed as halo sign/double target sign.

162. Ans. (a) CSF rhinorrhoea

Ref: Dhingra's ENT 7th ed. pg. 184

- The shown case is a feature of CSF rhinorrhea, due to cribriform plate fracture.

Refer to above explanation

163. Ans. (d) Nasal endoscopy

Ref: Dhingra's ENT 7th ed. pg. 184

Nasal endoscopy has no role in CSF rhinorrhea.

Investigation done in CSF rhinorrhea:

- **Beta 2 transferrin level:** It is protein found in CSF and vitreous humor only and not in nasal discharge.
  - It's a sensitive and specific test
- **Beta trace protein**
- **Fracture site localization:**
  - **HRCT**
  - **MRI**
  - **Intrathecal fluorescein study**
  - **CT cisternogram:** Intrathecal injection of iohexol and a CT scan to localize the site in cases when beta-2 transferrin cannot be done

164. Ans. (a) Rhinophyma

Ref: Dhingra's ENT 7th ed. pg. 162

- The shown image is sebaceous gland hypertrophy, which is a feature of rhinophyma.
- **Rhinosporidiosis:** It is an infective condition caused by Rhinosporidiosis seeberi. It can cause polyp.
- **Rhinoscleroma:** it is a chronic granulomatous condition. Associated with infection with Klebsiella Rhinoscleromatis.

165. Ans. (a) Young's operation

Ref: Dhingra's ENT 7th ed. pg. 173

- Atrophic rhinitis is a chronic inflammation of nose characterized by nasal mucosa atrophy and turbinate atrophy.
- It is often also associated with infection with klebsiella ozaenae.
- Due to mucosal atrophy → nasal cavity becomes roomy and there is foul odor from nose.

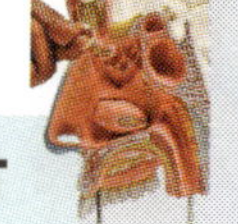

Treatment:

- Alkaline nasal douche followed by 25% glucose in glycerine topical to inhibit the growth of proteolytic organism.
- Antibiotics Streptomycin 1g/d for 10 days
- **Surgical:**
  - Young's operation
  - Modified young's operation
  - Narrowing of nasal cavities

166. Ans. (a) Cottle test

Ref: Dhingra's ENT 7th ed. pg. 167

- The shown test in the image is Cottle test.
- It is used for testing nasal obstruction due to abnormality of the nasal valve.
- In this test, cheek is drawn laterally while the patient breathes quietly. If the nasal airway improves on the test side, the test is positive and indicates abnormality of the vestibular component of nasal valve.

167. Ans. (a) Hollmann miller sign

Ref: Dhingra's ENT 7th ed. pg. 281

- CT image shown anterior pushing of maxillary sinus, causing cheek fullness.
- This sign is often termed as: **Hollman miller sign** or antral sign- Pathognomonic of angiofibroma.
- If there is pushing of eyeball, it is termed as frog eye sign.
- Hondusa sign is also the feature of angiofibroma. There is widening of gap between ramus of mandible and maxillary body.

168. Ans. (a) Frontal

Ref: Dhingra's ENT 7th ed. pg. 215

Clinical feature of acute frontal sinusitis

- Frontal headache: Usually severe and localized over affected sinus, which is periodic. It usually comes up on waking, reaches its peak and then start subsiding
- It is often termed as "**office headache**" because of its presence during office hours
- Tenderness and edema of upper eyelid
- Note: Chronic frontal sinusitis is also known as **pott's puffy tumor**

169. Ans. (d) Bulla ethmoidalis

Ref: Dhingra's ENT 7th ed. pg. 151

- **Bulla ethmoidalis** is a prominent and largest adamanterior ethmoid air cell.
- If there is failure to pneumatize, it is known as torus ethmoidalis.
- It is situated behind the uncinate process, in the middle meatus.

170. Ans. (b) Angiofibroma

Ref: Dhingra's ENT 6th ed. pg. 246–47

- Angiofibroma is a benign vascular tumor of nasopharyngeal area.
- It is the most common pharyngeal tumor of adolescent male, mostly in second decade of life.
- This tumor is thought to be testosterone dependent
- MC site: Sphenopalatine foramen

CLINICAL FEATURE

- MC clinical feature: Recurrent epistaxis
- Progressive nasal obstruction and denasal speech
- Otitis media with effusion and conductive hearing loss
- Hollman miller sign/Antral sign: Cheek swelling- Pathognomonic feature
- Frog eye sign: Proptosis

IOC: CECT

Treatment: Surgical excision

171. Ans. (a) Antrochoanal polyp

- The mentioned case is very much suggestive of antrochoanal polyp.
- These are the single polyp originated from maxillary sinus and protrudes into nasal cavity.

172. Ans. (c) Neck swelling

Ref: Diseases of ENT by Dhingra 6th ed. pg. 250-251

Nasopharyngeal cancer

- Commonly seen in chinese, elderly population (30 – 50/100,000 population)
- **MC site:** Fossa of Rosenmuller
- The tumor from fossa of Rosenmuller can grow in any direction.
  - Anterior: Can block Eustachean tube → CHL
  - Inferior: Can cause difficulty in deglutition
  - Superior: Can involve several cranial nerve if skull base is involved
    - All cranial nerves can be affected (First CN involved: CN VI)
    - Frequently involved CN are V, VI, IX and X
    - Involvement of nerve supplying ocular muscles are also seen
- **Symptoms:**
  - Neck mass: Due to cervical lymphadenopathy- most common clinical picture that patient present with

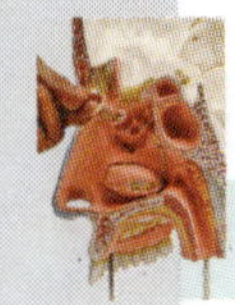

- Trotter's triad: CHL, soft palate palsy, deep facial pain
- Diplopia, nasal dysfunction, headache, etc.

- **WHO classification-on basis of histopathology**

Type I (25%)	Squamous cell carcinoma
Type II (12%)	Non-keratinising carcinoma • Without lymphoid stroma • With lymphoid stroma
Type III (63%)	Undifferentiated carcinoma • Without lymphoid stroma • With lymphoid stroma

- **Treatment:**
  - Radiotherapy is definitive treatment (it is most radiosensitive tumor of head and neck).

173. Ans. (c) CSF Rhinorrhea

Ref: Dhingra's ENT 6th ed. pg. 305

- It is a case of CSF rhinorrhea due to cribriform plate fracture.
- Cribriform plate, which is a thin plate of bone, forms the roof of nose. In patients with trauma, there is clear watery nasal discharge with or without blood tinged.
- **Causes of CSF rhinorrhea:**
  - Trauma: Most common cause
  - Surgical: During FESS, transphenoidal surgery
  - Neoplasm invading the skull base
  - Infection and mucoceole of sinuses eroding bone and dura
  - Congenital: Meningocoele, meningoencephalocoele and glioma with skull base defect
- **Symptoms:**
  - Clear watery nasal discharge which cannot be sniffed back
  - Reservoir sign: When rising in morning CSF collected in sinuses on bending head.
  - Handkerchief sign: Handkerchief stiffens if it is due to nasal discharge due to its mucus content.
- **Investigation:**
  - Beta 2 transferrin: Most sensitive and specific.
  - HRCT: IOC
  - MRI: To locate site of leak and if any associated CNS pathology.
- **Treatment:**
  - Conservative treatment along with prophylactic antibiotics.
  - Surgical repair if there is no relief from conservative management.

174. Ans. (c) Ammonia irritates trigeminal nerve

Ref: Physical Medicine and Rehabilitation, 4th ed. pg. 12

- The patient here is presenting with history of trauma, which can cause damage to olfactory nerve → leading to anosmia.
  - MC cranial nerve damaged in head trauma: Olfactory nerve
- Remember, for olfaction system two separate nerves are responsible:
  - CN I: Responsible for perception associated with quality of odour
  - CN V: Produces sensation of irritation or pungency
- Odour sensation from olfactory nerve usually do not produce physiological response. But sensation from trigeminal nerve can produce response such as runny nose, red eyes, sneezing when an irritant like ammonia/vinegar is detected.

175. Ans. (a) CSF rhinorrhea

Ref: Dhingra's ENT 6th ed. pg. 305

- It is a case of CSF rhinorrhea due to cribriform plate fracture.
- Cribriform plate, which is a thin plate of bone, forms the roof of nose. In patients with trauma, there is clear watery nasal discharge with or without blood tinged.
- **Symptom:**
  - Watery nasal discharge which cannot be sniffed back.
- **Investigation:**
  - **Beta 2 transferrin:** Most sensitive and specific.
  - **HRCT:** IOC.
  - **MRI:** To locate site of leak and if any associated CNS pathology.
- **Treatment:**
  - Conservative treatment along with prophylactic antibiotics
  - Surgical repair if there is no relief from conservative management.

176. Ans. (b) Atrophic rhinitis

Ref: Dhingra's ENT 6th ed. pg. 154

- Atrophic rhinitis is the chronic inflammation of nose characterized by atrophy of nasal mucosa and turbinate bone. This makes the nasal cavity roomy and filled with foul smelling nasal crust.
- **Pathology:** Ciliated columnar epithelium is lost and is replaced with stratified squamous type of epithelium.
- **Treatment:**
  - Alkaline nasal douching using Na^+ bicarbonate, Na^+ biborate and NaCl.
  - Followed by local application of 25% glycerin → it inhibits the growth of proteolytic organisms.
  - Antibiotics (streptomycin 1 g/day × 10 days)
  - Surgery:
    - **Young's operation:** Complete closure of both nostrils by nasal flaps.

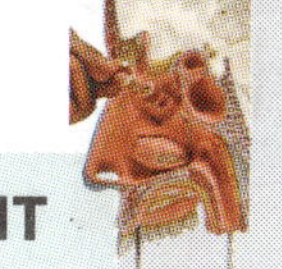

- ♦ **Modified Young's operation:** Keep the nostrils partially open ~3 mm. Its efficacy is similar to Young's operation.
- ♦ **Lautenslager operation:** Medicalization of lateral wall of nose
- ♦ **Wittmack's operation:** It is the transposition of the parotid duct into the maxillary sinus for moistening the nasal cavity.
- ♦ Submucosal Teflon paste injection.

177. Ans. (b) Anterior ethmoidal artery

Ref: Dhingra's ENT 6th ed. pg. 177

- Kiesselbach's plexus is the arterial plexus present at the anteroinferior part of septum just above the vestibule and the area is also known as Little's area.
- **Arteries of the plexus are:**
  - Sphenopalatine artery (branch of maxillary artery → Br. of external carotid artery)
  - Greater palatine artery (branch of maxillary artery → Br. of external carotid artery)
  - Superior labial artery (branch of facial artery → Br. of External carotid artery)
  - Anterior ethmoidal artery (branch of ophthalmic artery → Br. of internal carotid artery)

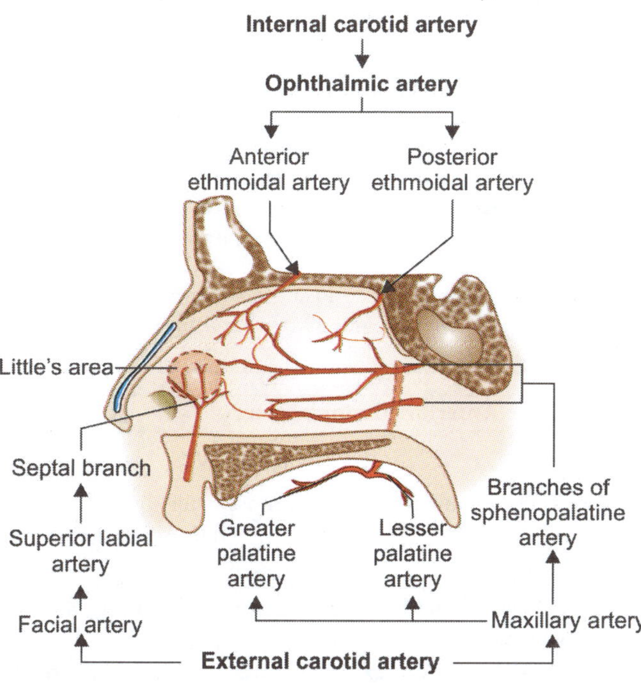

178. Ans. (c) Aspirin sensitivity, asthma, nasal polyp

Ref: Dhingra's ENT, 6th ed. pg. 240

Samter's triad consists of nasal polyp, bronchial asthma and aspirin sensitivity.

179. Ans. (b) Nasal drop withdrawal

Ref: Dhingra's ENT, 6th ed. pg. 170

- Topical nasal decongestants can sometimes cause rebound phenomenon if used for long time, the condition is known as **rhinitis medicamentosa.**
- **It is treated by:**
  - **Withdrawal of nasal drops**
  - Short course of systemic steroid therapy
  - Surgical reduction of turbinates in some cases if hypertrophied.

180. Ans. (a) Squamous cell CA

Ref: Dhingra's ENT, 6th ed. pg. 205-206

- Paranasal sinus CA most commonly affects males of age above 50 years.
- **Most common paranasal sinus CA is squamous cell CA.** Rest are adenocarcinoma, adenoid cystic CA, melanomas and various other sarcomas.
- Most common sinus associated with CA: **Maxillary sinus.**
- Most common sinus CA among workers of furniture/ wood industry: **Adenocarcinoma**

181. Ans. (d) Supreme meatus

Ref: Dhingra's ENT, 6th ed. pg. 187-88

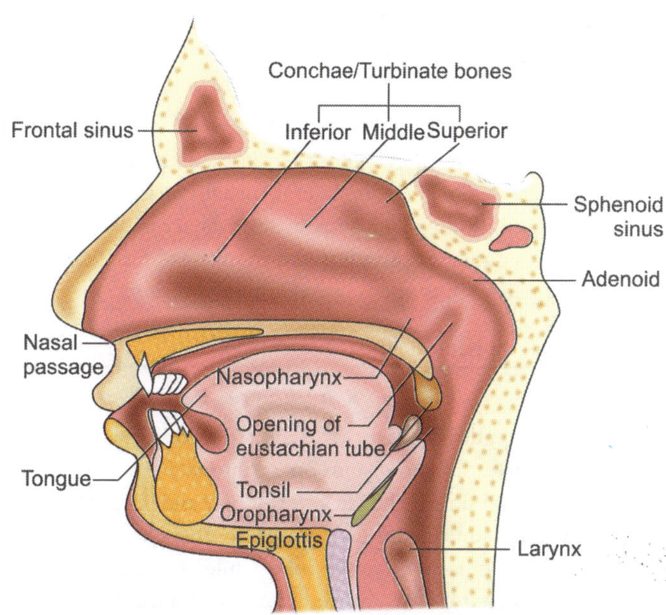

- On the lateral wall of the nose are three turbinates and four meatuses.
- **The inferior turbinate is the longest turbinate**
- The supreme meatus is also called sphenoethmoidal recess

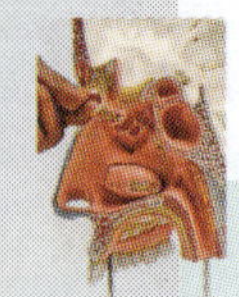

Ostia Opening in Meatuses

Meatus	Ostia
Supreme meatus/ Sphenoethmoidal recess	Sphenoid sinus ostia
Superior meatus	Posterior ethmoidal sinus ostia
Middle meatus	Has three ostias • Maxillary sinus • Frontal sinus • Anterior ethmoidal sinus
Inferior meatus	**Has no Ostia.** It has Nasolacrimal duct opening

Remember: Direction of nasolacrimal duct is ***downwards, backwards and outward.***

182. Ans. (a) Inferior meatus

Ref: Dhingra's ENT, 6th ed. pg. 187-88

- **Late**ral wall of the nose ***contains inferior meatus*** which has no ostia, ***instead it has naso-lacrimal duct***. The nasolacrimal duct (sometimes called the tear duct) carries tears from the lacrimal sac into nasal cavity.
- Inferior nasal meatus is partially covered by a mucosal fold called **valve of Hasner** or *plica lacrimalis*).

183. Ans. (d) Inferior meatus of the nose

Ref: Dhingra's ENT, 6th ed. pg. 1 87-88

Refer to above explanation

184. Ans. (a) Middle meatus

Ref: Dhingra's ENT, 6th ed. pg. 173-75

- ANTROCHOANAL POLYP most commonly seen in children. They are unilateral, usually arises from the mucosa of maxillary antrum near its accessory ostium, comes out of it & grows in the chonaa and nasal cavity.
- Maxillary sinus opens into the middle meatus.

185. Ans. (a) Sphenoid sinus

Ref: Dhingra's ENT, 6th ed. pg. 138

- Spheno ethmoidal recess is situated above the superior turbinate. Sphenoid sinus opens into it.
- Sphenoid sinus. It has an anterior part and posterior part.
  - **Anterior part:** Roof related to the olfactory tract, optic chiasma, frontal lobe while the lateral wall is related to optic nerve, internal carotid artery and maxillary nerve.
  - **Posterior part:** Roof is related to the pituitary gland in the sella turcica while each lateral wall is related to cavernous sinus, internal carotid artery and CN 3rd and all division of 5th nerve.

186. Ans. (d) None of the above

Ref: Dhingra's ENT, 6th ed. pg. 138-40

- Please read the question carefully! The question is about the sinus opening.
- In inferior meatus there is no opening of any sinuses. *It has opening for nasolacrimal duct.*

187. Ans. (d) Posterior ethmoidal artery

Ref: Dhingra's ENT, 6th ed. pg. 147,
Dhingra 4th ed. pg. 140

- Kiesselbach's area, aka Kiesselbach's plexus and Little's area, is an area on the nasal septum located on the antero-inferior part of the septum.
- In this area four arteries anastomose to form a vascular plexus called Kiesselbach's plexus.
- **The arteries are**
  1. Sphenopalatine artery (from the maxillary artery): **Main artery of plexus**
  2. Greater palatine artery (from the maxillary artery)
  3. Anterior ethmoidal artery (from the ophthalmic artery)
  4. Septal branch of the superior labial artery (from the facial artery)

Extra Mile

- Only artery of Kisselbach's plexus which is a branch of internal carotid artery: Anterior ethmoidal artery. The other three are branches of external carotid artery.
- Most common site of epistaxis: Kisselbach's area/Little's area
- **Artery of epistaxis: Sphenopalatine artery**
- **Posterior epistaxis is from:** Woodruf's plexus (very difficult to control)
- **Woodruf's Plexus:** Situated in the posterior part of meatus. Formed when sphenopalatine artery anastomosis with post-pharyngeal artery.

188. Ans. (c) Anterior ethmoidal artery

Ref: Dhingra's ENT, 6th ed. pg. 147-48

- Anterior and posterior Ethmoid artery is a branch of ophthalmic artery, which is derived from internal carotid artery.
- It is only anterior ethmoidal artery (of internal carotid) which contributes to little's area.
- **Branches from external carotid artery *(indirectly)* contributing to little's area:** Sphenopalatine artery, Greater palatine artery and superior labial artery.

189. Ans. (d) Hereditary hemorrhagic telangiectasia

Ref: Dhingra's ENT, 6th ed. pg. 176-77

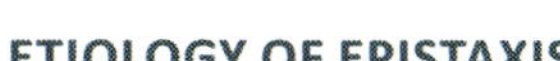

ETIOLOGY OF EPISTAXIS

- One of the most common local causes is trauma, due to nose picking or fractures.
- Some of the other local causes include nasal sprays, inflammatory reactions, anatomical deformities (i.e. septal deviation, septal spurs), foreign bodies, intranasal tumors, chemical irritants, and nasal prongs for oxygen. Systemic causes include hypertension, vascular disorders, blood dyscrasias, hematologic malignancies, allergies, malnutrition, alcohol, drugs, and infection.
- Hereditary Hemorrhagic Telangiectasia is a rare cause causing bleeding. This is also known as **Osler-Weber-Rendu disease** and an **autosomal dominant** disease.

Extra Mile

- MCC of epistaxis overall: Trauma
- MCC of epistaxis in adult: Trauma
- MCC of epistaxis in elderly: Hypertension
- MCC of epistaxis in child: Digital trauma from nose picking.

190. Ans. (a) Olfactory epithelium

Ref: Dhingra's ENT, 6th ed. pg. 204

- **Esthesioneuroblastoma** usually arise from the olfactory epthelium. It's a rare tumor of any age group.
- **Presentation of tumor:** cherry red, polypoidal spots mass in upper third of nasal cavity. It is a vascular tumor that bleeds profusely on biopsy.

191. Ans. (c) Sphenoid sinus

Ref: Dhingra, 5th ed. pg. 203

TABLE: Development and growth of paranasal sinuses

Sinuses	Status at birth	Growth	First radiologic evidence
Maxillary	Present at birth	Rapid growth from birth to 3 years and from 7–12 years. Adult size-15 yrs	4–5 months after birth
Ethmoid	Present at birth	Reach Adult size by 12 years	1 years
Frontal	Not present	Invades frontal bone at the age of 4 years. Size increases until teens	6 years
Sphenoid	Not present	Reaches sella turcica by the age of 7 years. **Reaches full size between 15 years to adult age**	4 years

192. Ans. (c) Frontal sinus

Ref: Dhingra, 5th ed. pg. 203

- *Please refer to above table*
- The first sinus that starts to develop in human embryo is maxillary sinus. It starts to develop around 10 weeks of intra-uterine life.
- ***The last sinus to develop in human embryo is frontal sinus. This sinus is absent at the time of birth & starts to develop postnatally.***
- Frontal sinus can be visualized radiologically at 6 years of age.

193. Ans. (c) 6 years

Ref: Dhingra, 5th ed. pg. 203

194. Ans. (c) 15 years

Ref: Dhingra, 5th ed. pg. 203

195. Ans. (d) 12 years

Ref: Dhingra, 5th ed. pg. 203

196. Ans. (b) Maxillary sinus

Ref: Dhingra, 5th ed. pg. 203-204

Maxillary sinus is largest sinus with volume of around 15 cc.

197. Ans. (b) Maxillay sinusitis

Ref: Dhingra's ENT, 6th ed. pg. 411-12

- **Most common sinus involved in sinusitis: Maxillary sinus** *(aka Antrum of Highmoore)*
- Treatment of acute cases is by antibiotics and symptomatic.
- Chronic cases and recurrent cases are treated by surgery. Usually performed surgeries are:
- Antral wash
- **Caldwell-Luc operation**
- FESS (Functional Endoscopic Sinus Surgery) - Most preferred currently. Best surgical option

Caldwell Luc operation Indications:	Technique
• In case of chronic maxillary sinusitis • Dental cyst or Oro-antral fistula • Fracture of maxilla or blow out fracture of orbit • Antrochoanal polyp	• Horizontal Incision below gingivolabial sulcus • Elevation of flap à Opening of Antrum à Removal of deseased antral mucosa/polyp • Making of nasoantral window • Packing the antrum à closure of wound

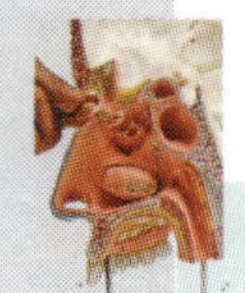

198. Ans. (a) Atrophic rhinitis

Ref: Dhingra, 5th ed. pg. 170

ATROPHIC RHINITIS (OZAENA)

- **Etiology** (Remember Mnemonic HERNIA)
  - Hereditary factors
  - Endocrinal disturbance: Disease usually starts at puberty, involves females more than males.
  - Racial factors: White and yellow races are more susceptible than equatorial African natives.
  - Nutritional deficiency. Disease may be due to deficiency of vitamin A, D or iron
  - Infective.
    - **Kelbsiella ozaenae: Most common cause**
    - Diphtheroids, P. vulgaris, E. coli, staphylococci and Streptococci

Clinical Features

- Foul smell from the nose
- **Merciful anosmia**
- **Nasal obstruction:** *Due to large crusts filing the nose*
- Epistaxis: May occur when the crusts are removed

Treatment

Medical: Nasal irrigation and removal of crusts by Alakaline Douche - **Best Treatment**

- **Alakaline nasal douche** is prepared from **(in ratio of 1:1:2):**
  - Sodium bicarbonate
  - Sodium biborate
  - Sodium chloride

Surgical

- **Young's operation:** Both the nostrils are closed completely just within the nasal vestibule by raising flaps. They are opened after 6 months.
- **Modified young operation:** To avoid the discomfort of bilateral nasal obstruction, modified Young's operation aims to partially close the nostrils.

199. Ans. (d) Crusting

Ref: Dhingra, 5th ed. pg. 170

Please refer to above explanation

200. Ans. (b) Lymphadenopathy

Ref: Dhingra's ENT, 6th ed. pg. 446-47

NASOPHARYNGEAL CARCINOMA

- Nasopharyngeal carcinoma is caused by **Ebstein Barr virus (EBV).**
- It is seen most commonly in Chinese population or South East Asian peoples.
- Most common site of nasopharyngeal carcinoma: **Fossa of Rosenmuller**.
  - This is a pyramidal shaped fossa on the lateral wall of nasopharynx.
- The most common type of nasopharyngeal carcinoma is undifferentiated carcinoma of nasopharyngeal type.

Clinical Presentation

- The most common presentation is cervical lymphadenopathy.
- **Other important presentations are**
  - Nasal obstruction
  - Nasal bleeding
  - Unilateral glue ear in adult leading to conductive hearing loss.
  - Cranial nerve palsies. *All the nerves from 3rd to 12th may be involved.*
- **Trotter's triad** seen in case of nasopharyngeal carcinoma. It is also called Sinus of Morgagni Syndrome.
  - Ipsilateral soft palate palsy
  - Conductive hearing loss
  - Trigeminal neuralgia.

201. Ans. (b) Rhinoscleroma

Ref: Dhingra's ENT, 5th ed. pg. 172

RHINOSCLEROMA

- Caused by gram negative coccobacillus- Klebsiella Rhinoscleromatis.
- **It passess through 3 stages:** Catarrhal, Granulomatous and Cicatricial.
- It causes woody infiltration of upper lip, so it is also known as Woody Nose.
- Upon biopsy characteristic cells seen are: Miculicz's cell and Russel Bodies.
- Tx: Streptomycin (1 g/day) and tetracycline (2 g/day) are given together for 4-6 weeks.

RHINOPHYMA

- It is due to hypertrophy of sebaceous glands of nasal tip.
- Associated with Acne Rosacea.
- Nose becomes big and ugly, hence also known as Potato Nose.

RHINOLITH

- It is old, calcified foreign body in nose.
- Present with foul smelling, one sided yellowish nasal discharge.

RHINOSPORIDIOSIS

- Caused by Rhinosporidiosis Seeberi
- *Present as strawberry/mulberry polyp in the nose.*

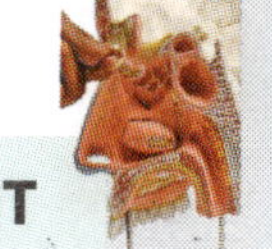

- It has very higher tendency to bleed. Hence also known as Bleeding Polyp.

202. Ans. (a) Hypertrophy of sebaceous gland

Ref: PL Dhingra, 5th ed. pg. 159, 461

RHINOPHYMA/POTATO NOSE/RUM NOSE/ COPPER'S NOSE/TOPPER'S NOSE/BRANDY NOSE

- Benign tumor due to **hypertrophy of sebaceous glands of tip of nose.**
- Seen in cases of long-standing **acne rosacea.**
- Precipitated by: Spicy food, Heat, Alcohol
- **Treatment: Laser (CO_2)** Excision with skin grafting and **Avoidance of alcohol.**

203. Ans. (d) Protozoa

Ref: Dhingra's ENT, 6th ed. pg. 158-59

- Currently rhinosporidiosis is considered as a protozoal infection caused by **RHINOSPORIDIOSIS SEEBERI.** It is most commonly seen in the coastal parts of the world, most commonly in India, Pakistan and Sri Lanka. In india most commonly reported from the coastal part Tamil Nadu.
- It most commonly infects nose and nasopharynx. Other sites: Lip, Palate, conjunctiva, brochi, skin, vulva, vagina.
- It presents as polypoid mass which bleeds easily on touch, hence also known as Bleeding polyp.
- According to very recent papers, it is classified as **aquatic protist**

Treatment

- **Medical:** Dapsone
- **Surgical:** Complete excision of mass with diathermy knife and cauterization of base

204. Ans. (b) Rhinoscleroma

Ref: Dhingra's ENT, 6th ed. pg. 156-57, 5th ed. pg. 172

RHINOSCLEROMA

- It is a chronic granulomatous disease caused by gram negative coccobacillus-**Klebsiella Rhinoscleromatis.**
- **It has 3 stages:**
  - **Catarrhal or atrophic stage:** characterized by foul smelling purulent nasal discharge and crusting *(causing obstruction). This stage resembles atrophic rhinitis.*
  - **Granulomatous stage**: In this stage there are painless and non-ulcerative granulomatous nodules in nasal mucosa. *There is also subdermal infiltration of lower part of external nose and upper lip giving a 'woody' feel.*
  - **Cicatricial stage:** The last stage which causes adverse conditions like stenosis of nares, distortion of upper lip, adhesions in the nose, nasopharynx and oropharynx. There may be subglottic stenosis with respiratory distress.
  - Rhinoscleroma causes woody infiltration of nose, so it is also known as **Woody Nose.**
  - Characteristic cells upon biopsy are: ***Miculicz's cell and Russel Bodies.***
  - **Treatment:** Streptomycin (1g/day) and tetracycline (2g/day) are given together for 4–6 weeks.

205. Ans. (c) Granulomatous stage

Ref: Dhingra's ENT, 6th ed. pg. 156-57, 5th ed. pg. 172

206. Ans. (b) Bacteria

Ref: Dhingra's ENT, 6th ed. pg. 156-57

Please refer to above explanation for more details.

207. Ans. (c) Nasal bone

Ref: Dhingra's ENT, 6th ed. pg. 147-148

- **Facial trauma**, also called **maxillofacial trauma**, is any physical trauma to the face.
- Commonly injured facial bones include the nasal bone, maxilla, and the mandible. The mandible may be fractured at its symphysis, body, angle, ramus, and condyle.
- ***Nasal fracture is the most common facial fracture, and the third most common fracture of the skeleton overall.***
- Facial fractures occur for a variety of reasons related to sports participation: Contact between players (eg, a head, fist, elbow); contact with equipment (eg, balls, pucks, handle bars); or contact with the environment, obstacles, or a playing surface (e.g., wrestling mat, gymnastic equipment, goalposts, trees).
- Facial fractures may be associated with head and cervical spine injuries and it requires a significant amount of force.

208. Ans. (b) Vertical fracture

Ref: Dhingra's ENT, 6th ed. pg. 147-48

There are two main types of fracture of septum namely: Chevallet and Jarjavay fracture

TABLE: Fracture of nasal septum

Fracture	Injury type	Impact of force
Chevallet fracture	Vertically	From below
Jarjavay fracture	Horizontally	From front

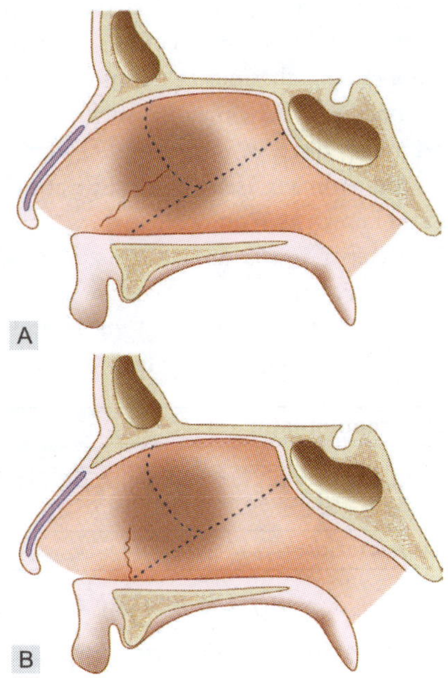

FIGURE: Fracture showing (A) Jarjaway type (B) Chevallet type

209. Ans. (c) Front

Ref: Dhingra's ENT, 6th ed. pg. 147-48

210. Ans. (a) Neck of condyle

Ref: Dhingra's ENT, 6th ed. pg. 185

- Neck of condyle is the most common site of fracture of mandible followed by angle of mandible.

THROAT/PHARYNX

211. Ans. (b) Esophagus

Ref: Diseases of Ear, Nose and Throat and Head and Neck Surgery, Dhingra, 7th ed. pg. 397

- A round metallic foreign body lies in the midline just above the aortic knob, suggestive of a coin within the esophagus.

212. Ans. (a) Adenoidectomy with grommet

Ref: Diseases of Ear, Nose and Throat and Head and Neck Surgery, Dhingra, 7th ed. pg. 69

- The given case is suggestive of Otitis media with effusion (OME).
- It is characterized by a nonpurulent effusion of the middle ear that may be either mucoid or serous.
- Surgery, in the form of grommet insertion, with or without adenoidectomy, is the most effective treatment in persistent, symptomatic cases.

213. Ans. (b) Diphtheria

Ref: Diseases of Ear, Nose and Throat and Head and Neck Surgery, Dhingra, 7th ed. pg. 328

- Pharyngeal diphtheria is characterized by the development of a pseudo membrane.
- The pseudo membrane is characterized by the formation of a dense, gray debris layer composed of a mixture of dead cells, fibrin, RBCs, WBCs, and organisms.
- The distribution of the membrane varies from local (e.g, tonsillar, pharyngeal) to widely covering the entire tracheobronchial tree.

214. Ans. (a) H. influenza

Ref: Diseases of Ear, Nose and Throat and Head and Neck Surgery, Dhingra, 7th ed. pg. 326

- The thumbprint sign seen on the X-ray suggests the diagnosis of epiglottitis.
- In children, epiglottitis is usually caused by the bacteria Hemophilus influenzae (H influenzae) type B.

215. Ans. (a) Tonsillar branch of facial artery

Ref: Diseases of Ear, Nose and Throat and Head and Neck Surgery, Dhingra, 7th ed. pg. 243

- Major artery of tonsil is tonsillar branch of facial artery.
- **Other arteries of tonsil:** Maxillary artery, Ascending pharyngeal artery, Ascending palatine artery, lingual artery

216. Ans. (a) Glossopharyngeal nerve

Ref: Diseases of Ear, Nose and Throat and Head and Neck Surgery, Dhingra, 7th ed. pg. 487

- Glossopharyngeal neuralgia (GPN) is believed to be caused by irritation of the 9th cranial nerve, called the glossopharyngeal nerve.
- This is responsible for earache after tonsillectomy surgery.

217. Ans. (a) Epiglottis

Ref: Diseases of Ear, Nose and Throat and Head and Neck Surgery, Dhingra, 7th ed. pg. 319

It is believed that the epiglottis doesn't calcify to the same extent as the laryngeal cartilages, owing to its elastic nature.

218. Ans. (b) Posterior cricoarytenoid

Ref: Diseases of Ear, Nose and Throat and Head and Neck Surgery, Dhingra, 7th ed. pg. 320

- The posterior cricoarytenoid muscles are the only muscles to open the vocal cords (Abductor). This is important in breathing.

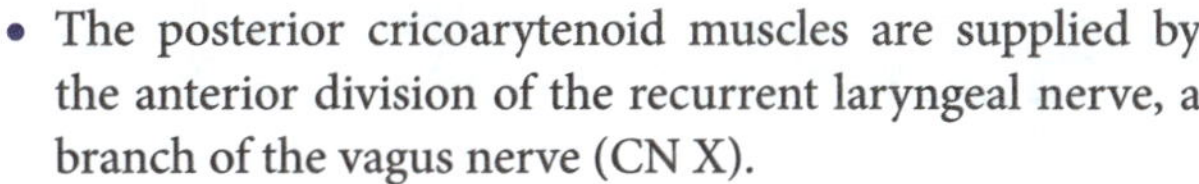

- The posterior cricoarytenoid muscles are supplied by the anterior division of the recurrent laryngeal nerve, a branch of the vagus nerve (CN X).
- Other muscles in option are adductor of vocal cord.

219. Ans. (d) Laryngomalacia

Ref: Diseases of Ear, Nose and Throat and Head and Neck Surgery, Dhingra, 7th ed. pg. 333

- Laryngomalacia is the most common cause of noisy breathing in infants.
- The most common sign of laryngomalacia is stridor (noisy breathing due to obstruction at the level of the voice box). In other words it is also said that most common cause of stridor is laryngomalacia.
- This causes the epiglottis to curl inward (become "omega-shaped").

220. Ans. (b) Thyroid

Ref: Diseases of Ear, Nose and Throat and Head and Neck Surgery, Dhingra, 7th ed. pg. 319

- There are total 9 cartilages in larynx, 3 paired and 3 unpaired.
  - **Unpaired cartilages are:** Epiglottis, Thyroid, and Cricoid.
  - **Paired cartilages are:** Arytenoids, Corniculate, and Cuneiform

221. Ans. (b) Thyropharyngeus and cricopharyngeus muscle fibers

Ref: Diseases of Ear, Nose and Throat and Head and Neck Surgery, Dhingra, 7th ed. pg. 269

- Killian's dehiscence is a triangular area in the wall of the pharynx between the cricopharyngeus and thyropharyngeus.
- It represents a potentially weak spot where a Zenker's diverticulum is more likely to occur.

222. Ans. (c) Laryngoceoele

Ref: Dhingra's ENT 6th ed. pg. 345

- Laryngocoele is a air-filled cystic swelling due to dilatation of the saccule.
- **Aquired laryngocele:** Increased pressure in the laryngeal lumen (wind instrument player).
- **Laryngopyocele:** Infected laryngocele.

It may be:

- **Internal:** Confined within the larynx and look like distension of false cord and aryepiglottic fold.
- **External:** Saccule herniates through the thyroid membrane and presents in neck.
- **Mixed** in which both internal and external components are seen.

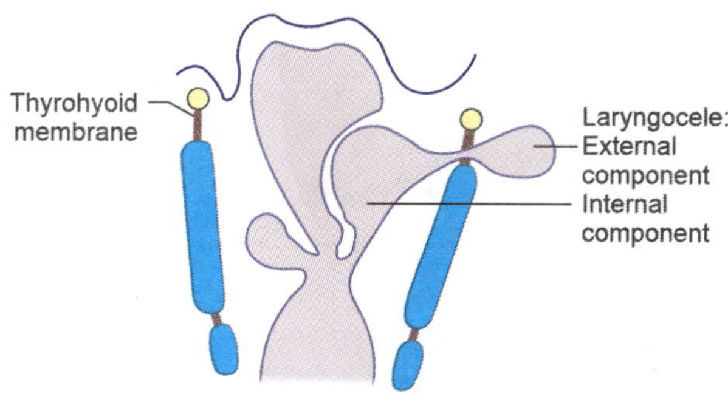

Clinical Feature

- Hoarseness, cough and if large in size then present with airway obstruction.
- It is reducible swelling in the neck which increases in size on coughing or performing Valsalva.

Diagnosis

- Made by indirect laryngoscopy, and soft tissue AP and lateral views of neck with Valsalva.

Treatment

- Internal laryngocele: treated by endoscopic laser surgery
- External laryngocele: transcervical approach

Extra Mile

Other laryngeal presentation of importance:
- Steeple sign: Croup
- Thumb sign: Acute epiglottitis

223. Ans. (c) Thyropharyngeus and cricopharyngeus

Ref: Dhingra's ENT 6th ed. pg. 310

- Pharyngeal pouch also known as hypopharyngeal diverticulum or Zenker's diverticulum.
- It is a pulsion diverticulum in which pharyngeal mucosa herniates through the Killian's dehiscence (a weak area between two parts of the inferior constrictor muscle).
- Inferior constrictor muscle has two parts—thyropharyngeus muscle with oblique fibers and cricopharyngeus muscle with transverse fibers.

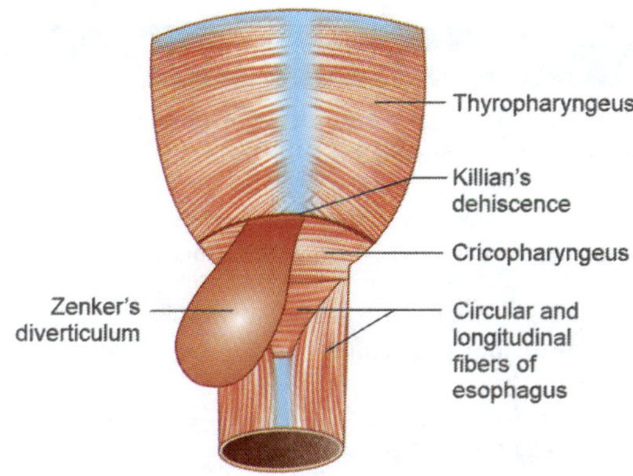

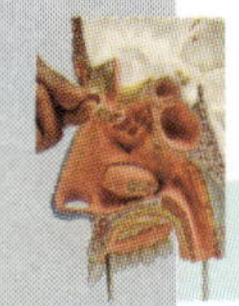

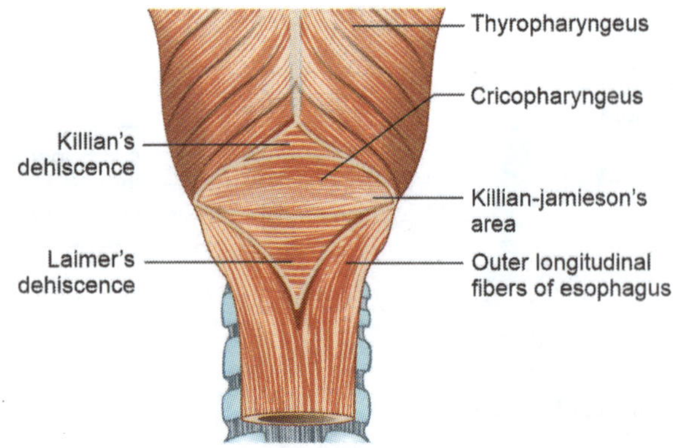

224. Ans. (c) Fossa of rosenmuller

Ref: Dhingra's ENT 6th ed. pg. 270

- Eustachian tube opening present on the lateral wall of nasopharynx, situated 1.25 cm behind the posterior end of inferior turbinate.
- An elevation known as Torus tubarius raised by the cartilage of the tube bound the tube above and behind.
- Above and behind the tubal elevation is a recess called fossa of Rosenmüller.
- Fossa of Rosenmüller is the commonest site for origin of nasopharyngeal carcinoma.
- From lower end of torus tubarius a ridge extends to the lateral pharyngeal wall and is called salpingopharyngeal fold. It is raised by corresponding muscle.

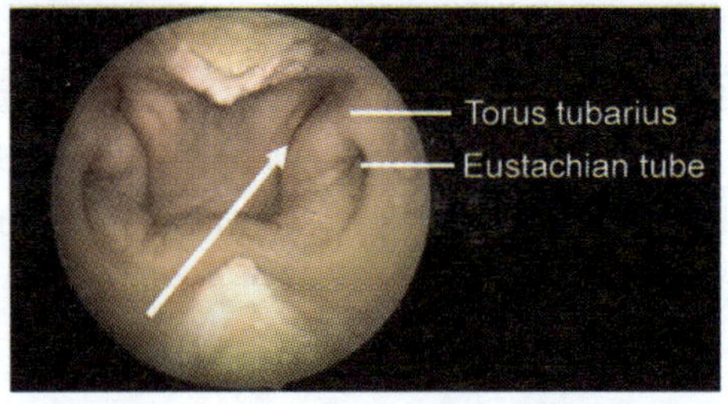

225. Ans. (b) T3 N0 M0

Ref: AJCC Cancer Staging Handbook, 7th ed. New Tork: Springer, 2010

TNM staging–AJCC 7th edition (2010)*	
T1:	Tumour limited to one subsite of hypopharynx and < 2 cm in greatest dimension.
T2:	Tumour invades more than one subsite or adjacent site or measures >2 cm but ≤ 4 cm without fixation of hemilarynx.
T3:	Tumours >4 cm or with fixation of hemilarynx or extension into esophagus.
T4a:	Tumor invades thyroid/cricoid cartilage, hyoid bone, thyroid gland, central compartment of soft tissue.

Contd...

TNM staging–AJCC 7th edition (2010)*	
T4b:	Tumor invades prevertebral fascia, encases the carotid artery or involves mediastinal structures.

*Edge SB, Byrd DR, Compton CC, et al. *AJCC Cancer Staging Handbook*, 7th ed. New York: Springer, 2010.*

T and N staging in Hypopharyngeal cancers

- N0: No regional LN
- N1: Single ipsilateral LN ≤3 cm
- N2a: Single ipsilateral LN 3–6 cm
  b: Multiple ipsilateral LNs ≤6 cm
  c: Bilateral or contralateral LNs ≤6 cm
- N3: Any LN >6 cm
- M stage:
- Mx–cannot be assessed,
- M0–no distant metastasis,
- M1–distant metastasis

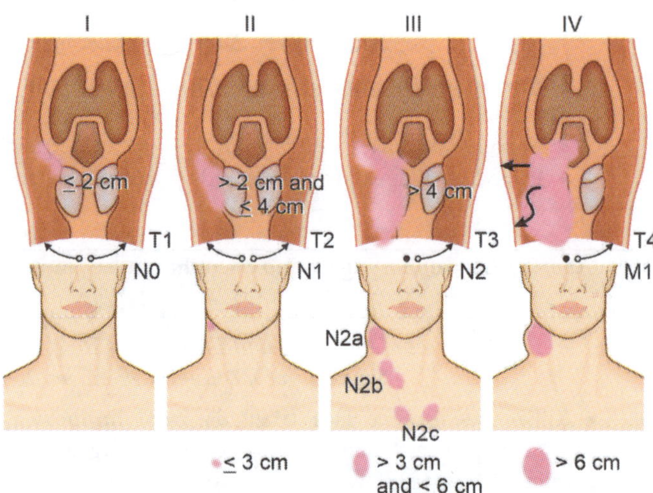

FIGURES: T and N staging in hypopharyngeal cancers

226. Ans. (b) EBV

Ref: Dhingra's ENT 7th ed. pg. 283-84

- **Causes of nasopharyngeal CA:**
  - **Genetic:** Higher incidence among Chinese
  - **Infection:** Due to EBV infection
  - **Environmental:** Air pollution, tobacco and opium smoking, dry salted fish, smoke from burning incense stick and wood.

Extra Mile

Cancers associated with EBV:
- Nasopharyngeal CA
- Burkitt's lymphoma
- Hodgkin's lymphoma
- Lymphoproliferative disease

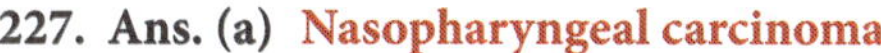

227. Ans. (a) Nasopharyngeal carcinoma

Ref: Dhingra's ENT 7th ed. pg. 283-84

- Most common clinical presentation of nasopharyngeal CA: **Cervical lymphadenopathy** (neck swelling), as seen in the case.
- **Trotter's triad** is associated with Nasopharyngeal CA. this triad includes:
  - Unilateral conductive hearing loss (due to Eustachian tube blockade)
  - Deep facial pain (due to CN V involvement)
  - Soft palate palsy (due to CN X involvement)

228. Ans. (c) Post cricoid carcinoma

Ref: Dhingra's ENT 7th ed. pg. 310

Postcricoid CA Diagnosis

- Postcricoid growths may not be visible on indirect Laryngoscopy.
- Edema and erythema of the postcricoid region and pooling of secretions in the hypopharynx are suggestive of growth.
- **Laryngeal crepitus,** felt normally while moving larynx over the cervical spine, may be lost.
- Normally, larynx moves with deglutition. It can also be moved from side to side producing a characteristic grating sound (laryngeal crepitus).
- Fixity of larynx indicates inflammation or infiltration of growth into the surrounding structures. Loss of laryngeal crepitus is due to postcricoid carcinoma.

229. Ans. (b) Adenoid hypertrophy

Ref: Dhingra's ENT 7th ed. pg. 270-72, 492

- Development of high arched palate, snoring, mouth breathing, sleep apnea and speech abnormalities is a feature of adenoid hypertrophy
- Adenoid hypertrophy can also lead to deviated nasal septum.

230. Ans. (d) Laryngomalacia

Ref: Dhingra's ENT 7th ed. pg. 333

- Omega shaped glottis is feature of laryngomalacia.
- It is the most common congenital abnormality of the larynx
- Due to extreme weakness of laryngeal cartilage, it gives an appearance of symbol omega.

Extra Mile

- Key hole epiglottis is seen in Phonesthenia
- Thumb sign on X-ray (lateral view): Acute epiglottitis
- Turban epiglottis: Laryngeal TB

231. Ans. (b) Parainfluenza

Ref: Dhingra's ENT 7th ed. pg. 327-28

- Causative agent of croup is Parainfluenza virus 1 and 2

TABLE: Differences between acute epiglottitis and acute laryngo-tracheo-bronchitis in children

	Acute epiglottitis	Acute laryngotracheo-bronchitis (or group)
Causative organism	*Haemophilus influenza type B*	Parainfluenza virus type I and II
Age	2–7 years	3 months to 3 years
Pathology	Supraglottic larynx	Subglottic area
Prodromal symptoms	Absent	Present
Onset	Sudden	Slow
Fever	High	Low grade or no fever
Patient's look	Toxic	Nontoxic
Cough	Usually absent	Present (barking seal-like)
Stridor	Present and may be marked	Present
Odynophagia	Present, with drooling of secretions	Usually absent
Radiology	Thumb sign on lateral view	Steeple sign on anteroposterior view of neck
Treatment	Humidified oxygen, third generation cephalosporin (ceftriaxone) or amoxicillin	Humidified O_2 tent, steroids

232. Ans. (d) Parapharyngeal abscess

Ref: Dhingra's ENT 7th ed. pg. 301

- Parapharyngeal space is pyramidal in shape with its base at the base of skull and its apex at the hyoid bone.
- Parapharyngeal space communicates with other spaces like retropharyngeal; submandibular, carotid and parotid space.
- **Infection to this area can occur from:**
  - Peritonsillar abscess
  - Parotid abscess
  - Submandibular gland infection
  - Masticator space abscess

Clinical Feature: Depends on Involved Compartment

- **Anterior compartment:** Produces a triad of symptoms:
  - Tonsil and tonsillar fossa prolapse
  - Trismus (due to spasm of medial pterygoid muscle)
  - Swelling at angle of jaw

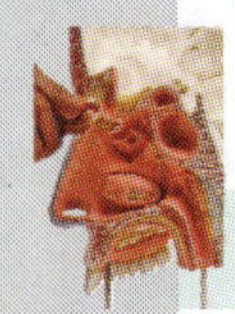

- **Posterior compartment** involvement presents with:
  - Pharyngeal bulge behind posterior pillar
  - Paralysis of CN IX, X, XI, XII and sympathetic chain
  - Swelling of parotic region.
- Fever, odynophagia, sore throat and torticollis are the other symptoms

Extra Mile

- Retropharyngeal abscess commonly seen in child <3 years. It presents with dysphagia, difficulty in breathing, stridor and torticollis.
- Ludwig angina is infection of submandibular gland
- Peritonsillar abscess (quinsy) mostly affect the adults. It rarely affects children. They present with high grade fever, chills with rigors, malaise, body ache, throat pain and muffled voice (hot potato voice).
  - Upon examination tonsil often is buried in the edematous pillars, hence doesn't appear to be enlarged.

233. Ans. (b) Antihistaminic

Ref: Dhingra's ENT 7th ed. pg. 193-94

- Nasal polyp initially is managed with antihistaminic.
- **Common cause and site of polyp:**
  - **Child:** Maxillary sinus; infective in origin
  - **Adult:** Ethmoid sinus; allergic in origin
- **TOC for this polyp:** FESS

234. Ans. (a) Thyroid cartilage

Ref: Dhingra's ENT 7th ed. pg. 319

- Adam's apple in male is due to thyroid cartilage. This cartilage is larger in male due to testosterone.
- Anatomically it is located at the level of C4.
- The two ala of thyroid cartilage meets at midline forming an angle.
  - In male: 900 (making it more prominent)
  - In female: 1200

235. Ans. (b) Subglottis

Ref: Dhingra's ENT 6th ed. pg. 285

- Book states: *"infants larynx is small and conical. The diameter of cricoid cartilage is smaller than the size of glottis, making subglottis the narrowest part."*

Note: In adults the dimensions of glottis–subglottis is same and larynx is cylindrical. However glottis is considered as the narrowest part of adult larynx

TABLE: Difference between adult and pediatric larynx

	Adult larynx	Pediatric larynx
Location	C3–C6	High in neck At rest: C3 or C4 While swallowing: C1 or C2
Cartilage	Soft	Softer
Thyroid cartilage	Elevated at thyroid angle	Flat
Shape	Cylindrical	Conical
Length of vocal cord	Female: 15–19 mm Male: 17–23 mm	Female: 6 mm Male: 8 mm

Note: *In contrary to what book says, there are recent studies that says that the narrowest portion of child larynx is same as adult i.e. glottis.*

- However many anatomist are still not agreeing to this.
- We are therefore referring here the textbook to answer this question.

236. Ans. (a) Posterior cricoarytenoid muscle

Ref: Dhingra's ENT 6th ed. pg. 283

The only abductors of vocal cord is posterior cricoarytenoid muscle

MUSCLES OF LARYNX

Intrinsic muscles of Larynx: Attaches laryngeal cartilage with each other

Muscles acting on vocal cord	Muscles acting on Laryngeal inlet
• **Abductors:** Posterior cricoarytenoid • **Adductors** ▪ Lateral cricoarytenoid ▪ Interarytenoid ▪ Thyroarytenoid (external part) • **Tensors:** ▪ Cricothyroid ▪ Vocalis muscle (internal part of thyroarytenoid)	• **Opener of laryngeal inlet** ▪ Thyroepiglottic muscle (part of thyroarytenoid) • **Closers of laryngeal inlet** ▪ Interarytenoid ▪ Aryepiglottic muscle

Extrinsic muscles of vocal cord: Connects larynx with neighbouring structure

- **Elevators of larynx:**
  - **Primary elevator:** Stylopharyngeus, Salpingopharyngeus, Palatopharyngeus and Thyrohyoid
  - **Secondary elevator:** Mylohyoid (main), Digastric muscle, Stylohyoid and Geniohyoid
- **Depressors:**
  - Sternohyoid, Sternothyroid and Omohyoid

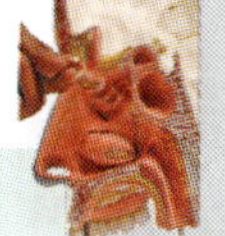

237. Ans. (a) Excision of ranula and sublingual gland duct

Ref: Dhingra's ENT 6th ed. pg. 224

- Ranula is cystic translucent lesion at the floor of mouth on one side of frenulum.
- It pushes the tongue upwards
- Arises due to obstruction of sublingual salivary gland duct.
- Sometimes when it extends into the neck → Known as plunging ranula

TREATMENT

- If small: Complete surgical excision of cyst and its duct
- If large: Marsupialization preferred

238. Ans. (a) Laryngeal carcinoma

Ref: Dhingra's ENT 6th ed. pg. 316-17

Types of Tracheostomy

- **Emergency tracheostomy:** Done in emergency/urgent setting. Vertical midline incision made in 2nd and 3rd tracheal rings
- **Elective/Routine tracheostomy/Tranquil:** Planned procedure. Transverse incision
- **Permanent tracheostomy:** May be required in bilateral abductor paralysis or laryngeal stenosis

Tracheostomy is also classified on the basis of site:

- **High tracheostomy:** Done above level of isthmus. Damages first tracheal ring
  - Complication: Perichondritis
  - Only indication: Laryngeal CA *(total laryngectomy is anyway required)*
- **Mid tracheostomy:** Preferred type. Done through 2nd or 3rd tracheal ring. Divides thyroid isthmus
- **Low tracheostomy:** Done below the level of isthmus. A difficult one, not generally recommended.

239. Ans. (c) Serous otitis media

Ref: Dhingra's ENT 6th ed. pg. 250-51

- In a patient with nasopharyngeal CA, most common clinical presentation is cervical lymphadenopathy.
- Upon superior invasion it can invade floor of skull invading several cranial nerve
- First cranial nerve to be involved: CN 6
- An anterior growth can cause eustachean tube obstruction → serous otitis media/glue ear
- **Clinical feature:** Trotter's triad
  - Soft palate palsy (due to CN 10 invasion)
  - Deep facial pain (due to CN 5 invasion)
  - Conductive hearing loss (due to eustachean tube obstruction)

Note: In adult patient with unilateral glue ear, nasopharyngeal CA should be ruled out first.

240. Ans. (a) Quinsy

Ref: Diseases of ENT by Dhingra 6th ed. pg. 265

- **Quinsy is** peritonsillar abscess where crypta magna gets infected and sealed off leading to intratonsillar abscess which then burst through tonsillar capsule leading to collection of pus in peritonsillar tissues → Peritonsillar abscess.
- **MC organism:** *Streptococcus pyogenes, Staph aureus*
- **Symptoms:** Severe throat pain, odynophagia (refusal to eat), halitosis, hot potato voice, ipsilateral earache
- **Upon examination:** Congested tonsil with edematous pillar, contralateral deviation of uvula
- **Treatment:**
  - IV antibiotics and fluid
  - Surgical drainage by incision

Extra Mile

- **Infection in pretracheal space** can lead to is dangerous and can compress major vessels, lower airways and upper digestive tract. Infection in this space is secondary to thyroiditis or perforation of anterior cervical esophagus.
- **Retropharyngeal abscess** patient can present with dysphagia, difficulty in breathing, stridor, croupy cough and torticollis (neck become stiff). Upon examination- bulge in the posterior pharyngeal wall usually seen on one side of midline.

Extra Mile

	Croup	Epiglottitis	Bacterial tracheitis	Retro-pharyngeal abscess
Peak age	1–2 years	2–7 years	1–6 years	1–5 years
Onset	Gradual (days)	Sudden (hours)	Gradual (days) with progressive worsening	Gradual (days) with progressive worsening
Prodromal URTI	Yes	Minimal, short	Yes	Yes
Fever	Low grade	High grade	Variable severity	High grade
Cough	Barking	Minimal, muffled	Barking, croup-like	Minimal
Stridor	Harsh	Soft, may become inaudible	Harsh	Variable (20–71% cases)
Discriminating features	Well child; worsens at night	Drooling: Leans forward in 'tripod' posture	Painful swallow; poor response to croup treatment	Painful swallow; neck stiffness or torticollis

URTI = Upper Respiratory Tract Infection

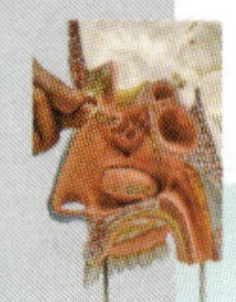

241. Ans. (a) Palatoglossus

- The hypoglossal nerve (CN XII) runs inferior to the tongue and innervates tongue muscles.
- All the intrinsic and extrinsic muscles of tongue (genioglossus, styloglossus, hyoglossus) is supplied by CN XII except palatoglossus.
- Palatoglossus is supplied by CN X

Extra Mile

Sensory supply of tongue
- **Anterior 2/3rd:**
  - General sensation: Lingual nerve
  - Special sensation: Chorda tympani (branch of CN VII)
- **Posterior 1/3rd:**
  - General and special sensation: Glossopharyngeal nerve
- **Base of tongue:**
  - General and special sensation: Internal laryngeal nerve

242. Ans. (a) Lateral sinus thrombophlebitis

Ref: Diseases of ENT by Dhingra 6th ed. pg. 84-85

- Lateral sinus thrombophlebitis is an intracranial complication of CSOM.
- The patient usually present with intermittent high grade fever termed as hectic picket fence fever associated with rigor, chills, headache.

Other clinical features:
- Anemia
- Thrombocytopenia
- Papilledema
- **Griesinger sign:** Edema over posterior part of mastoid, due to thrombosis of mastoid emissary veins.
- **Tobey-Ayer test:** If internal jugular vein compressed on healthy side, there is rise in CSF pressure.
- **Crowe-Beck test:** Pressure applied on the jugular vein of healthy side produces engorgement of retinal veins and supraorbital veins (because of thrombosed opposite side).

243. Ans. (d) Aphthous ulcer

Ref: Diseases of ENT by Dhingra 6th ed. pg. 218

- **Apthous ulcer** can be due to autoimmune process, nutritional deficiency of vitamin B12, folic acid and iron, infection, stress or food allergy.
- **Site:** mucosa of inner surface of lips and buccal mucosa, tongue, floor of mouth, soft palate
- **Spares** mucosa of hard palate and gingiva.
- **Occur in 2 forms:**
  - Minor form: 2–10 mm; multiple in number with central necrotic area and a red halo; heals without any scar in 2 weeks.
  - Major form: 2–4 cm; heals with a scar
- **Treatment:**
  - Topical application of steroids
  - Cauterization with 10% silver nitrate
  - In severe cases: 250 mg of tetracycline dissolved in 50 mL water → given as mouth rinse then to be swallowed (4 times/day)
  - Lignocaine viscous: For local pain

Extra Mile

- Erosive form of **lichen planus** can be a premalignant lesion. There is painful erosion of buccal mucosa, gigiva or lateral tongue surrounded by a keratotic periphery.
  - Malignant potential: 0.4 to 3.7%
- **Chronic hypertrophic candidiasis** aka candidial leukoplakia.
  - **MC site:** Anterior buccal mucosa just behind angle of mouth
  - It appears as white patch that cannot be wiped off
- **Oral submucal fibrosis** mostly associated with betel-nut chewing. Alcohol further increases the risk by 2 fold.
  - It is a premalignant condition. Malignant transformation is seen in 3–7.6% of cases
  - Leukoplakia and squamous cell CA is associated with submucous fibrosis, possible due to common etiological factors involved

TABLE: Some premalignant lesion and conditions

Premalignant lesions	Premalignant conditions
• Erythroplakia (aggressive) • Leukoplakia • Candidiasis • Carcinoma in situ • Leukokeratosis nicotina palatinae	• Oral submucous fibrosis • Oral lichen planus • Actinic keratosis • Syphilis • Discoid lupus erythematosus • Sideropenic dysphagia

244. Ans. (a) Chemoradiation

Ref: Dhingra's ENT 6th ed. P 252

Nasopharyngeal carcinoma is the most common malignant carcinoma (CA) of nasopharyngeal area and is most commonly seen in Chinese population.

TREATMENT OF NASOPHARYNGEAL CA:

- **Stage I and II:** Radiotherapy is the treatment of choice.
- **Stage III and IV:** Radiotherapy + chemotherapy.
- **Book states:** *"Stage III and IV CA can be cured by radiotherapy alone, but cure rate is doubled when chemotherapy is combined with radiotherapy".*
- Cisplatin or cisplatin + 5FU is used for chemotherapy.

MUST KNOW QUESTIONS ABOUT NASOPHARYNGEAL CA:

- **Most common site for nasopharyngeal CA:** Fossa of Rosenmüller
- Most common type of nasopharyngeal carcinoma is Type III (63%).

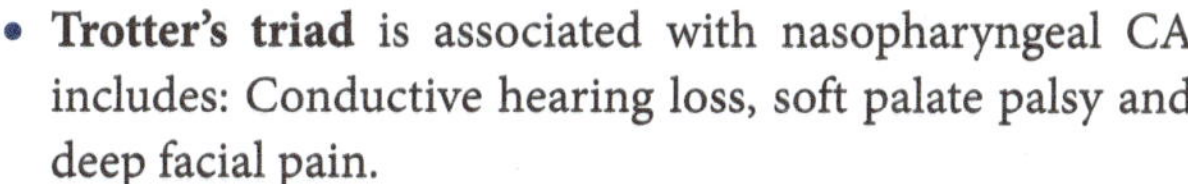

- **Trotter's triad** is associated with nasopharyngeal CA includes: Conductive hearing loss, soft palate palsy and deep facial pain.
- First cranial nerve (CN) to be affected is: CN VI (Abducens nerve).
- Nasopharyngeal CA can involve multiple cranial nerves like II, III, IV, V, VI, IX, X, XI, XII.
- Involvement of CN IX, X, XI causes *jugular foramen syndrome.*

245. Ans. (a) Aspiration

Ref: Dhingra's ENT 6th ed. pg. 326

- External branch of superior laryngeal nerve supplies cricothyroid and is mainly responsible for pitch of the voice.
- If it is injured, it causes bowing and inferior placement of vocal cord with consequent loss of pitch.

246. Ans. (a) Cricothyroid

Ref: Dhingra's ENT 6th ed. pg. 284, 298

- All the muscles of larynx are supplied by either recurrent laryngeal nerve or superior laryngeal nerve.
- External branch of **superior laryngeal nerve supplies cricothyroid muscle** and is mainly responsible for pitch of the voice. Rest all the muscles are supplied by recurrent laryngeal nerve (RLN).
- Right RLN arises from the vagus at the level of subclavian artery, hooks around it and then ascends between the trachea and esophagus.
- Left recurrent laryngeal nerve arises from vagus and hooks around arch of aorta, loose around it and then ascends into the neck in tracheoesophageal groove.
- The left RLN has much longer course and is more prone to injury and paralysis as compared to right side.

247. Ans. (c) Glottis level

Ref: Dhingra's ENT 6th ed. pg. 295

- Laryngeal web is due to incomplete recanalization of larynx.
- Most common site of this web is between the vocal cords (at the glottis level) and has a concave posterior margin.
- **Clinical features:**
  - Airway obstruction
  - Weak cry
  - Aphonia (dating from birth)
- **Treatment:**
  - **If thin webs:** Cut with a knife or CO_2 laser
  - **Thick web:** Excision via laryngofissure and placement of a silicon keel and subsequent dilatation.

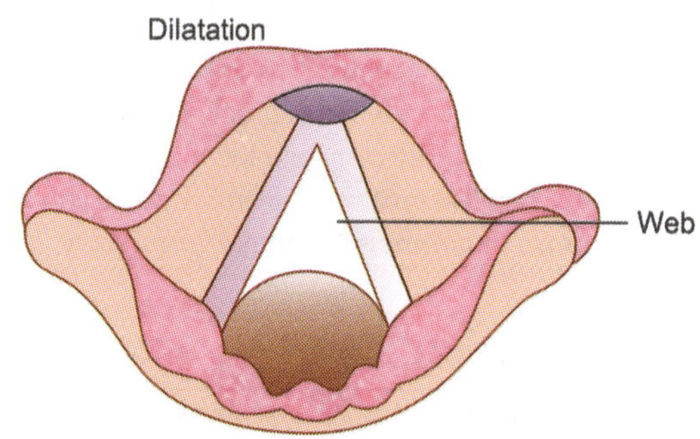

FIGURE: Laryngeal web

248. Ans. (a) Quincy

Ref: Dhingra's ENT 6th ed. pg. 265

QUINCY

- It is collection of pus in the peritonsillar space, which lies between the tonsillar capsule and superior constrictor muscle.
- It usually follows acute tonsillitis, though it may arise de novo as well.
- **MCC:** *Streptococcus pyogenes, Staphylococcus aureus.*
- **Symptoms:**
  - Acute onset high grade fever
  - Severe throat pain, usually unilateral
  - Marked odynophagia; patients are even unable to swallow their own saliva
  - **Muffled voice,** often **called hot potato voice**
  - Foul breath due to sepsis in oral cavity
  - Trismus and ipsilateral earache.
- **Signs:**
  - Swollen/enlarged tonsil
  - Swollen uvula and pushed to opposite side
  - Soft palate and anterior pillar bulging
  - Cervical lymphadenopathy.
- **Treatment:**
  - IV fluids + antibiotics + analgesics + oral hygiene
  - Surgery:
    - Incision and drainage
    - Interval tonsillectomy (I/D → then tonsillectomy after 4–6 weeks).

Extra Mile

- **Parapharyngeal and acute retropharyngeal abscess** is usually seen in children below 3 years. Symptoms can be dysphagia, stridor, bulge in posterior pharyngeal wall.

249. Ans. (c) HPV

Ref: Dhingra's ENT 6th ed. pg. 305

- Juvenile papillomatosis also known as respiratory papillomatosis is the most common benign neoplasm of larynx in the children.

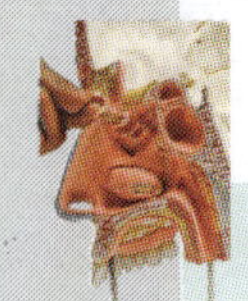

- It is most commonly caused by **HPV type 6 and 11.**
- Affected children acquire this infection at birth itself from the mothers who had vaginal HPV virus infection.
- Papilloma's mostly affects supraglottic and glottic region of larynx but can also involve subglottis, trachea and bronchi.
- **Symptoms:** Hoarseness, aphonia, respiratory difficulty, stridor.
- **Treatment:** CO_2 laser surgery.

250. Ans. (c) Carcinoma of pyriform sinus

Ref: Dhingra's ENT, 6th ed. pg. 273

Pyriform Sinus Carcinoma

- It is the most common hypopharyngeal cancer
- Mostly affect males above 40 years of age. The growth is asymptomatic for long time due to large size of the pyriform sinus.
- It can spread locally or via lymphatic spread.
- Most common and first lymph node involved: Cervical lymph node.

Clinical feature:

- Patient usually describes it as "something sticking in throat and pricking sensation" while swallowing. It is also the **earliest symptom**.
- **First sign: Mass of lymph nodes** high up in the neck
- Referred otalgia, pain on swallowing and increasing dysphagia are other symptoms which may follow.

IOC: Endoscopic biopsy

Treatment:

- **If no nodal involvement: Radiotherapy**
- **If nodal involvement: Surgery**

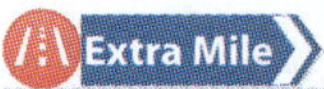

Extra Mile

Postcricoid carcinoma arises from postcricoid region and most commonly affects females in early 20's–30's. Its most common presenting symptom is progressive dysphagia.

251. Ans. (a) Palatopharyngeus

Ref: Dhingra's ENT, 6th ed. pg. 240

- **Passavant ridge** is a mucosal ridge raised by fibers of palatopharyngeus.
- It encircles the posterior and lateral walls of nasopharyngeal isthmus
- **Advantage of ridge:** Soft palate while contraction makes a firm contact with this ridge to cut off Nasopharynx from the oropharynx during speech or deglutition.

252. Ans. (c) Analgesic with antibiotic and drainage

Ref: Dhingra's ENT, 6th ed. pg. 264-65

Treatment of Peritonsillar Abscess (Quinsy)

- IV fluids to cover dehydration
- Antibiotics to cover both aerobic and anerobic organisms
- Analgesics to relieve pain
- Oral hygiene
- Incision and drainage of abscess
- Interval tonsillectomy: Tonsils are removed 4–6 weeks following attack of quinsy.

253. Ans. (c) Burn of head and neck

Ref: Dhingra's ENT, 6th ed. pg. 316

- Burn of face and neck can lead to airway edema and will require a planned tracheostomy. Elective tracheostomy can be therapeutic to relieve respiratory obstruction, remove tracheobronchial secretions. Prophylactic tracheostomy is done to guard against anticipated respiratory obstruction or aspiration of blood.
- **Elective tracheostomy** also known as routine tracheostomy is a planned, unhurried procedure. It is done when all surgical facilities are available, endotracheal tube can be put and local or general anesthesia can be given.

254. Ans. (a) Carcinoma larynx

Ref: Dhingra's ENT, 6th ed. pg. 316

- Tracheostomy can be divided into: High, Mid or Low
  - **High tracheostomy** is done above the level of thyroid isthmus. It violates the 1st ring of trachea. Only indication for high tracheostomy is CA larynx, because in such cases total larynx would ultimately be removed and in a lower down area, a fresh tracheostome is made.
  - **Mid tracheostomy** is the preferred one. Done through 2nd or 3rd ring by dividing or retracting isthmus upwards.
- **Low tracheostomy** is done below the level of isthmus. Diptheria is a common indication.

255. Ans. (d) Speech therapy plus PPI

Ref: Dhingra's ENT, 6th ed. pg. 303

- The given condition is a case of singer's nodule also known as screamer's nodule.
- It is medically treated with **speech/voice therapy** and PPI should be added to relieve GERD, which might be an aggravating factor for the patient.
- For large nodules or long standing nodules, surgery (Microscopic laryngeal surgery) may be required.

256. Ans. (a) Lower part of thyroid cartilage

Ref: Dhingra's ENT, 6th ed. pg. 285

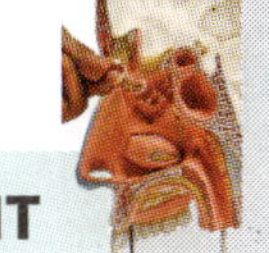

- Infants larynx is small and conical. The diameter of cricoid cartilage is smaller than size of glottis, making **subglottis the narrowest part.**
- Cricoid cartilage is located at the lower part of thyroid cartilage, hence it is the best answer of choice given these options.

257. Ans. (d) Bilateral mobile lymph nodes >6 cm

Ref: Diseases of ENT, by Dhingra, 6th ed. pg. 308

TABLE: Tumor staging

Tumor	Node	Metastasis
T1- One focal area involved **T2-** 2-3 area involved **T3-** Pre-epiglottic, Para-Glottic, Paralysis of VC, Posterior cricoid space **T4-** Trachea, Tongue base muscle, Thyroid muscle	**N0-** No LN involved **N1-** <3 cm, single, 1/L **N2a:** 3–6 cm single, 1/L **N2b:** 3–6 cm multiple, 1/L **N_2C:** 3–6, multiple, B/L **N_3:** >6 cm	**M0:** no mets **M1:** + Mets **Mx:** Can not be assessed

258. Ans. (c) Posterior cricoarytenoid

Ref: P.L. Dhingra, 6th ed. pg. 283-84

Movement	Muscles	Nerve supply
Abduction of vocal cords	Posterior cricoarytenoids only	Recurrent laryngeal nerve
Adduction of the vocal cords	• Lateral cricoarytenoids • Interarytenoids • Thyroarytenoids (external part)	Recurrent laryngeal nerve
Tensor of vocal cords	• Cricothyroid • Vocalis (internal part, part of Thyroarytenoid)	Superior laryngeal nerve
Relaxor of vocal cord	Thyroarytenoid	Recurrent laryngeal nerve
Elevation of larynx	Thyrohyoid, mylohyoid	
Depression of larynx	Sternothyroid, sternohyoid	

259. Ans. (b) Laryngeal TB

Ref: Diseases of ENT, by Dhingra, 6th ed. pg. 293

- Laryngeal TB is always secondary. It is primary most commonly from lungs.
- Most commonly involved part: Posterior wall
- First part to get affected in case of laryngeal TB: **Interarytenoid fold**
- **Important Features:**
  - **Turban epiglottis:** Due to pseudo edema
  - **Mouse nibbled appearance:** Due to ulceration of vocal cord
- **Cobble stone appearance**

260. Ans. (c) Peritonsillar abscess

Ref: Dhingra's ENT, 5th ed. pg. 279

- Hot potato voice is muffled and thick speech.
- MCC of hot potato voice is **Quincy (peritonsillar abscess),** which is an extremely painful condition.
- However it can also be seen in conditions like CA tonsil and streptococcus pharyngitis.

261. Ans. (c) Subglottis

Ref: Diseases of ENT, by Dhingra, 6th ed. pg. 285

TABLE: Difference between infant and adult larynx

Features	Infant/child	Adult
Anatomical level	C2–C3	C3–C6
Shape	Conical	Tubular
Narrowest at	Subglottis	Glottis
Important feature	Can swallow and breath at the same time	Can not swallow and breath at the same time
Cartilage	Softer	Soft

Extra Mile

TABLE: Difference between male and female larynx

Features	Male	Female
Length	44 mm	36 mm
AP diameter	43 mm	41 mm
Transverse diameter	36 mm	26 mm

262. Ans. (c) Young males

Ref: Dhingra's ENT, 5th ed. pg. 261

"Nasopharyngeal angiofibroma is seen almost exclusively in ADOLESCENT **males in the age group of 10–20 years.**"

ABOUT NASOPHARYNGEAL ANGIOFIBROMA

- It is a vascular tumor with lots of fibrous tissue without muscular coat. Hence it causes severe bleeding because of inability to contract.
- **Most common benign tumour** of nasopharynx.
- Arises from the posterior part of nasal cavity close to superior margin of **sphenopalatine foramen.**
- **Frog face deformity**—if tumor Extends to orbit and causes proptosis

- **Antral/Holman-Millar sign**—Anterior bowing of posterior wall of maxillary sinus is pathognomonic.
- Investigation of choice is **C.E.C.T.** scan
- Treatment of choice is **surgical excision.**

263. Ans. (b) Angiofibroma

Ref: Dhingra's ENT, 5th ed. pg. 261

264. Ans. (a) Tonsils

Ref: Dhingra's ENT, 6th ed. pg. 257-58

- **Crypts are inward folding of the mucosa which are found in tonsils and they increase the surface area.**
- **Crypts are also seen in small intestine.**

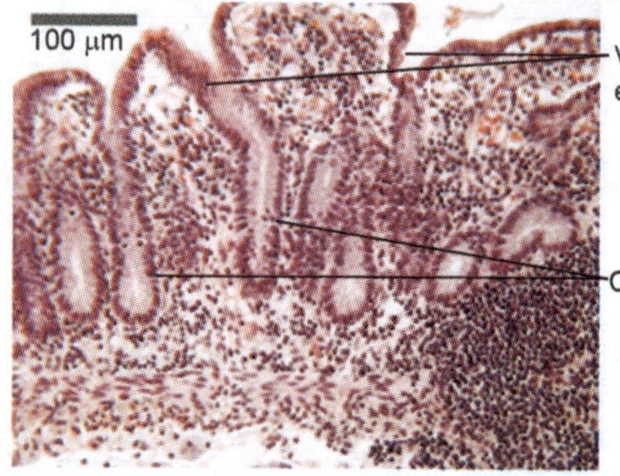

265. Ans. (a) Cricothyroid

Ref: P.L. Dhingra, 5th ed. pg. 317; BD Chaurasia Vol: 3 pg. 242, 244

- All intrinsic muscles of the larynx are supplied by the recurrent laryngeal nerve except cricothyroid which is supplied by external branch of superior laryngeal nerve.
- Recurrent laryngeal nerve supplies posterior cricoarytenoid, lateral cricoarytenoid, transverse and oblique arytenoids, aryepiglotticus, thyroarytenoid, thyroepiglotticus muscle.

266. Ans. (a) Posterior cricoarytenoid

Ref: P.L. Dhingra, 5th ed. pg. 317

Please refer to above explanation

267. Ans. (a) Cricothyroid

Ref: P.L. Dhingra, 5th ed. pg. 317

Please refer to above explanation

268. Ans. (b) Parotid gland

Ref: Dhingra's ENT, 5th ed. pg. 248

WARTHINS TUMOR

- Warthins tumor is also known as Adenolymphoma
- It is a benign, mixed type tumor of salivary gland.
- It occurs exclusively in parotid gland.
- It is the 2nd most common benign tumor of parotid gland.
- Most common benign & overall tumor of parotid gland is pleomorphic adenoma

Extra Mile

- Most common salivary gland tumors occurs in Parotid Gland (85% benign): **Pleomorphic adenoma.**
- Overall, **mucoepidermoid carcinoma** is the most common malignant tumor of the parotid gland or any salivary gland. It can be divided into low-grade and high-grade tumors.
- Second most common tumor of parotid gland is **Warthin's tumor**
- Most common malignant tumor of parotid gland is **mucoepidermoid carcinoma**
- Parotid tumor which spreads by perineural invasion is Adenoid cystic carcinoma.

269. Ans. (b) Stylopharyngeus muscle

- Cranial nerve IX (glossopharyngeal nerve) is a mixed nerve that carries afferent sensory and efferent motor information.

Functions

- **Branchial motor:** Supplies the stylopharyngeus muscle
- **Visceral motor:** Provides parasympathetic innervation to the parotid gland
- **Visceral sensory:** Carries visceral sensory information from the carotid sinus and carotid body.
- **General sensory:** Provides general sensory information from the skin of the external ear internal surface of the tympanic membrane, upper pharynx and the posterior one-third of the tongue.
- **Special sensory:** Provides taste sensation from the posterior one-third of the tongue including circumvallate papillae.

270. Ans. (b) Laryngomalacia

Ref: Dhingra's ENT, 6th ed. pg. 295

LARYNGOMALACIA

- The most common congenital disease of larynx is Laryngomalacia.
- Laryngeal cartilages are extremely soft and flabby in a child with laryngomalacia.
- **Most common clinical presentation of laryngomalacia: Stridor**
- The stridor is mainly inspiratory and increases during supine position but decreases during prone position.

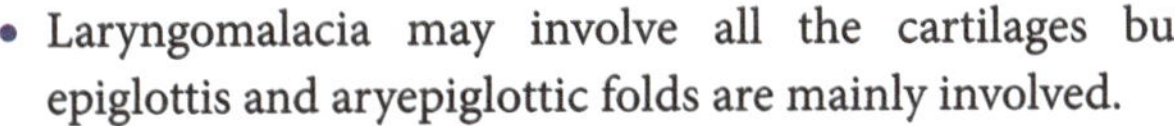

- Laryngomalacia may involve all the cartilages but epiglottis and aryepiglottic folds are mainly involved.
- **IOC:** Direct laryngoscopy.
- The finding is Omega shaped epiglottis (long and tubular epiglottis with curled up tip).

Extra Mile

TABLE: Different shape of glottis and conditions

Glottis shape	Condition
• Key hole shaped	Phonasthenia
• Omega shaped	Laryngomalacia
• Thumb sign	Acute epiglottitis
• Steeple sign	Croup/Laryngotracheobronchitis
• Turban shaped	Laryngeal TB

271. Ans. (b) Acute epiglottis

Ref: Dhingra's ENT, 6th ed. pg. 289, 4th ed. pg. 267

	Acute epiglottitis	Acute laryngo-tracheo-bronchitis (or croup)
Causative organism	• Strep. pneumoniae > Haemophilus influenza type B	Para influenza virus type I and II
Age	2–7 years	3 months to 3 years
Pathology	Supraglottic larynx	Subglottic area
Prodromal symptoms	Absent	Present
Onset	Sudden	Slow
Fever	High	Low grade or no fever
Patient's look	Toxic	Non-toxic
Cough	Usually absent	Present, (Barking seal-like)
Stridor	Present and may be marked	Present
Odynophagia	Present, with drooling of secretions	Usually absent
Radiology	***Thumb sign on lateral view***	**Steeple sign on AP view of neck**
Treatment	Humidified oxygen, third generation cephalosporin or amoxicillin	Humidified O_2 tent, steroids

Note: *According to recent papers Strep. pneumoniae is MCC of acute epiglottitis*

272. Ans. (b) Sternocleidomastoid muscle

Ref. PL Dhingra, 5th pg. 87

- **Mastoid tip is in relation to two muscles:**
  - Sternocleidomastoid muscle
  - Digastric muscle (posterior belly)
- If there is abscess from:
  - **SCM muscle**: Bezold's abscess
  - **Digastric area:** Citelli's abscess.

Extra Mile

Different MASTOID Abscess

Abscess	Location
Wild's abscess	Subperiosteal mastoid abscess
Bezold's abscess	Deep to Sternomastoid muscle
Luc's abscess	Under periosteum of the roof of bony canal
Citelli's abscess	Digastric triangle (along posterior belly of digastric muscle)

273. Ans. (c) Malignant change

Ref: Dhingra's ENT, 5th ed. pg. 272-273

- Acute tonsillitis often affects school-going children, but it can also affect adults.

Cause:

- **MCC:** Group A Beta Hemolytic streptococcus
- Acute infections of tonsil may involve these components and are thus classified as:
  - **Acute catarrhal or superficial tonsillitis:** Generalized pharyngitis and is mostly seen in viral infections.
  - **Acute follicular tonsillitis:** Infection spreads into the crypts which become filled with purulent material.
  - **Acute parenchymatous tonsillitis:** Uniformly enlarged and red tonsil.
  - **Acute membranous tonsillitis:** It is a stage ahead of acute follicular tonsillitis. In this, exudation from the crypts coalesces to form a membrane on the surface of tonsil.

Symptoms

- Sore throat, Difficulty in swallowing, Fever, Eearache, odynophagia, dysphagia
- **Constitutional symptoms**
  - Headache, general body aches, malaise and constipation.

Treatment

- Patient is put to bed and encouraged to take plenty of fluids.
- Analgesics
- Antimicrobial therapy (DOC: Penicillin)

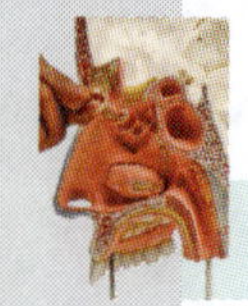

Complications

- Chronic tonsillitis with recurrent acute attacks. This due to incomplete resolution of acute infection.
- *Peritonsillar abscess.*
- *Parapharyngeal abscess.*
- Cervical abscess due to suppuration of jugulodigastric lymph nodes.
- *Acute otitis media.*
- Rheumatic fever.
- Acute glomerulonephritis.
- *Subacute bacterial endocarditis.*

Note: Malignancy is never a complication of tonsilittis.

274. Ans. (c) Sublingual dermoid cyst

Ref: Dhingra's ENT, 5th ed. pg. 398

- Sublingual dermoid cyst present as midline submental swelling. This cyst is not attached to foramen cecum and hence does not move upon tongue protrusion or upon deglutition.
- The thyroglossal cyst classically moves upwards with swallowing and notably with tongue protrusion, as it is attached to foramen cecum. It merely indicates attachment to the hyoid bone.

275. Ans. (a) Glottic CA

Ref: Dhingra's ENT, 5th ed. pg. 327

- Most common laryngeal malignancies are squamous cell CA (90–95%).
- It can be any of these three sites:

Supraglottis	2nd MC site. Nodal metastasis occur early. MC to middle jugular nodes
	Symptom: Throat pain, Dysphagia, referred pain to ear > Hoarseness
Glottis	**MC site:** Local spread present. *Nodal metastasis is always absent as glottis has no (or very few) lymphatics.*
	Symptoms: Hoarseness > Stridor > laryngeal obstruction
Subglottis	3rd MC site. Lymph nodes involved are: Prelaryngeal, Pretracheal, Paratracheal and Lower jugular nodes.
	Symptoms: Stridor > Hoarseness

276. Ans. (b) Epiglottis CA

Ref: Dhingra's ENT, 5th ed. pg. 329

- Treatment of laryngeal CA depends upon site of lesion, extent of lesion, presence or absence of nodal metastasis.
- **It consists of:**
  - Radiotherapy
  - Surgery (conservative laryngeal surgery, total laryngectomy)
  - Combined therapy
- **Radiotherapy:** Reserved for early lesions which neither impair cord mobility nor invade the cartilage or cervical nodes.
- **Superficial exophytic lesions, especially of the tip of epiglottis, and aryepiglottic folds give 70-90% cure rate.**
- RT doesn't give good results in lesions with fixed cords, subglottic extension, cartilage invasion and nodal metastasis.
- **Note:** *Early stages of all these cancers, gives good prognosis with radiotherapy. But once cord mobility is impaired, surgery is the next best choice.*

277. Ans. (b) Carcinoma thyroid

Ref: Dhingra's ENT, 5th ed. pg. 279

- Hot potato voice is muffled and thick speech.
- MCC of hot potato voice is Quincy (peritonsillar abscess), which is an extremely painful condition.
- However it can also be seen in conditions like CA tonsil and streptococcus pharyngitis.

278. Ans. (c) Ranula

Ref: Dhingra's ENT, 5th ed. pg. 237-38, 400

- **Ranula** is a cystic **transilluminant** swelling seen in the floor of mouth on one side of frenulum. It arises due to obstruction of sublingual salivary gland duct.
  - **Treatment:** Complete surgical excision if small, or marsupialization if large.
- **Thymic cyst** can be cystic or solid. Present as a neck mass anterior and deep to middle third of SCM muscle.
- **Branchial cyst** is non-transilluminant, round, fluctuant, non-tender mass present in upper part of neck anterior to SCM muscle.
- **Thyroglossal duct cyst** is cystic midline swelling in the course of thyroid duct.

279. Ans. (a) Puberphonia

Ref: Dhingra's ENT, 6th ed. pg. 314-15

- **Androphonia:** Female patient with male like voice. Cause can be psychological or organic
- **Puberphonia:** Male patient with female like voice. Cause can be psychological or organic
- **Rhinolalia aperta:** Hypernasality in voice. **Cause can be:** cleft palate, Post adenoidectomy, oroantral fistula etc.
- **Rhinolalia clausa:** Hyponasality in voice. Caused due to any pathology causing nasal obstruction.

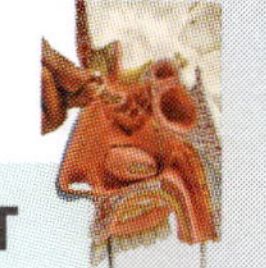

280. Ans. (d) IV

There are 4 types of thyroplasty done, depending on the pathology

- **Type I:** Medialization (Done for Abducted Vocal Cord)
- **Type II:** Lateralization (Done for Adducted Vocal Cord)
- **Type III:** Relaxation, shortening ***(in order to lower down the pitch)***
- **Type IV:** Tensioning, Lengthening ***(in order to increase the pitch)***

281. Ans. (a) Type I

- Type I thyroplasty is medialization. It is done in patient with lateralized vocal cord to prevent complications like aspiration.

282. Ans. (a) Hemorrhage

Ref: Dhingra's ENT, 6th ed. pg. 319

- Most common complication of tracheostomy: Hemorrhage > Tracheal stenosis
- MC damaged structure while tracheostomy: Isthmus of thyroid

FACE, ORAL CAVITY AND ESOPHAGUS

283. Ans. (b) Tight suture around tracheostomy site

Ref: Diseases of Ear, Nose and Throat and Head and Neck Surgery, Dhingra, 7th ed. pg. 360,361

- Subcutaneous emphysema can result from surgical, traumatic, infectious, or spontaneous etiologies.
- Subcutaneous emphysema is a condition often causing minimal symptoms, but sometimes it can be severe and even life-threatening.
- Skin incision should not be sutured or packed tightly as it may lead to development of subcutaneous emphysema.

284. Ans. (c) Oral cavity

Ref: Diseases of Ear, Nose and Throat and Head and Neck Surgery, Dhingra, 7th ed. pg. 251, 411; https://fhno.org/blog/Head-And-Neck-Cancers-in-India

- Oral cancers are the commonest of the head and neck squamous cell cancer (HNSCC) in the South-east Asian region.
- Oral cavity: Includes the lips, the front two-thirds of the tongue, the gums, the lining inside the cheeks and lips (Buccal mucosa), the floor (bottom) of the mouth under the tongue, the hard palate (bony top of the mouth), and the small area of the gum behind the wisdom teeth.

285. Ans. (b) Extravasation is not that common

Ref: Dhingra's ENT 6th ed. pg. 252

- The shown condition is mucocele of the lip
- It is retention cyst of minor salivary glands
- Most common site: Lower lip.
- Upon examination: Soft and cystic mass of bluish colour.
- It is brilliantly transilluminant
- Extravasation is very common
- Treatment is surgical excision.

286. Ans. (d) Tongue deviated

Ref: BD Chaurasia, 7th ed. volume 3, pg. 130

- Lingual nerve provide sensory (touch, pain and temperature) innervation to anterior 2/3rd of tongue.
- Lingual nerve is best considered as 2-way nerve:
  - General sensory to anterior 2/3rd of tongue
  - Taste (via chorda tympani) to anterior 2/3rd of tongue
  - Secretomotor (via chorda tympani) to sublingual and submandibular nerve.
- Lingual nerve has no motor innervation to tongue; hence tongue deviation will not be seen.

ORTHOPEDICS

14

MOST RECENT QUESTIONS 2023

1. After an injury the patient presented with a deformity as shown in the image. The X-ray showed following finding. Which nerve is most likely to be damaged?
(Most Recent Question July 2023)

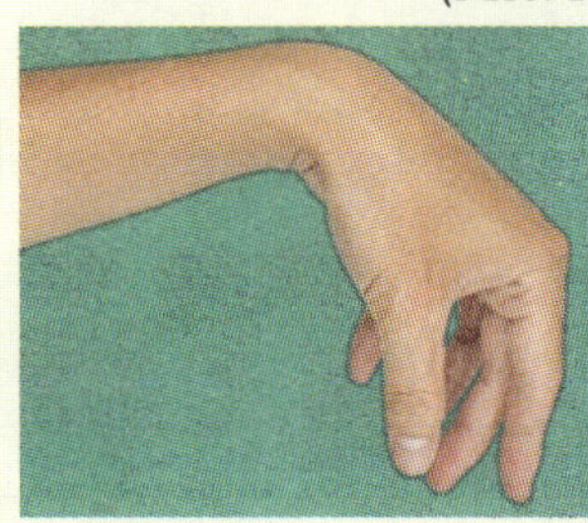
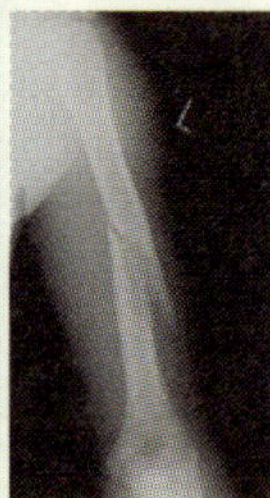

a. Median nerve
b. Radial nerve
c. Ulnar nerve
d. Axillary nerve

2. A person fell on the outstretched hand and got injured at the anatomical snuff box. Which bone is most commonly fractured at anatomical snuff box?
(Most Recent Question July 2023)

a. Lunate
b. Scaphoid
c. Trapezium
d. Pisiform

3. A person fell from the stairs while climbing upstairs and an iron nail hit on his neck. After the injury, the patient is unable to shrug/elevate his shoulder and he is having difficulty in turning his head. What structure is most likely to be damaged? ***(Most Recent Question July 2023)***

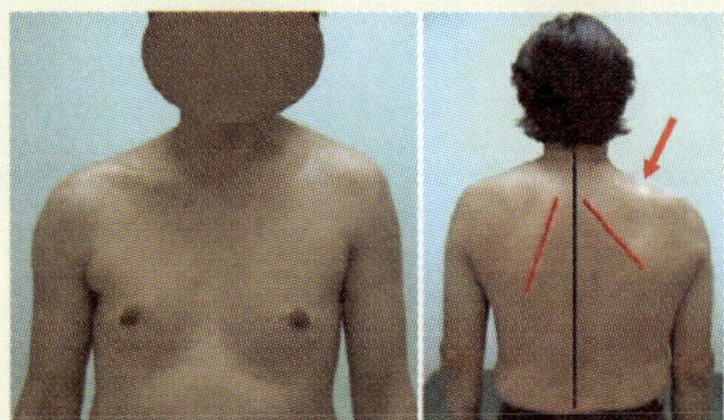

a. Vagus nerve
b. Spinal accessory nerve
c. Long thoracic nerve of bell
d. Suprascapular nerve

4. What is shown in the image?
(Most Recent Question July 2023)

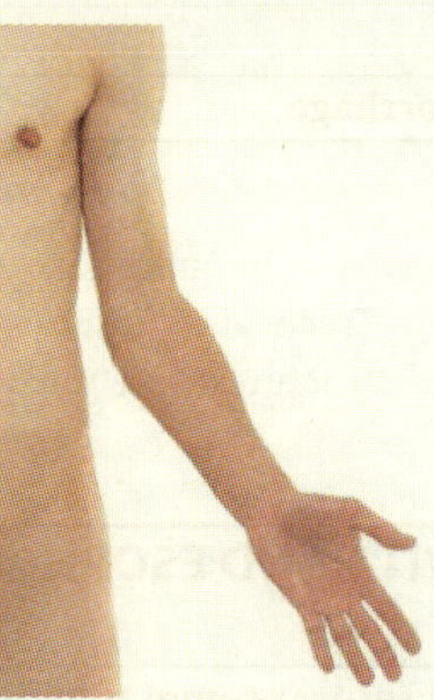

a. Cubitus varus
b. Cubitus valgus
c. Gunstock deformity
d. Dinner fork deformity

5. Identify the defect. ***(Most Recent Question Jan 2023)***

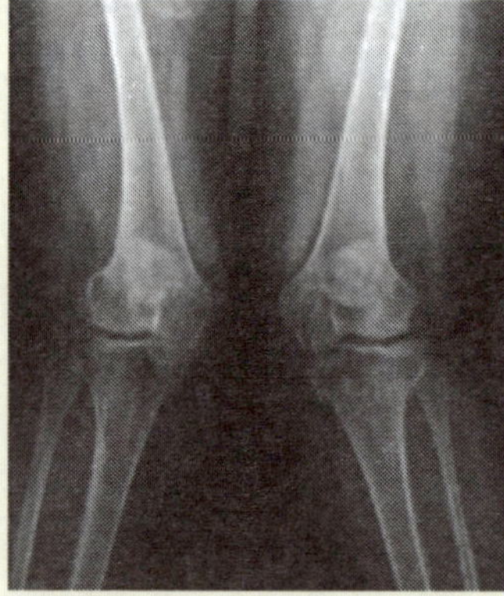

a. Genu valgum
b. Genu-varus
c. Femur fracture
d. Muscle deformity

6. A 5-year-old male child presented in your OPD with genu varum. On X-ray, osteopenia and pseudo fractures can be noticed. On blood investigations, there is decreased vitamin D and increased ALP. What is the most probable diagnosis? ***(Most Recent Question Jan 2023)***

a. Osteomalacia
b. Osteitis deformans
c. Osteopetrosis
d. Osteoporosis

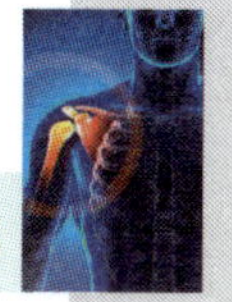

7. A 70-year-old patient presented to OPD with pain in her right knee. There is swelling on knee as well. The clinical image of the case is shown. Identify the disease.

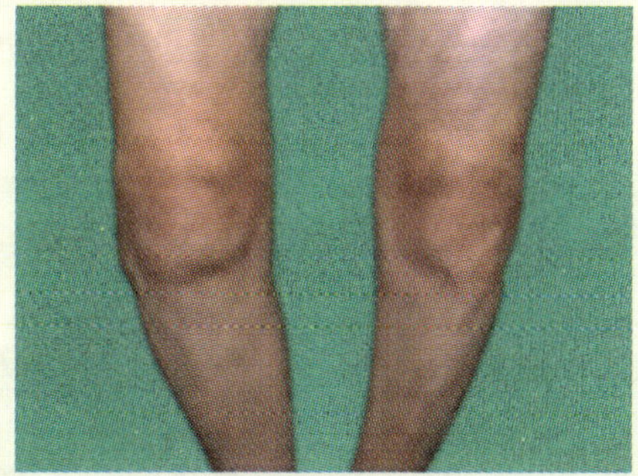

a. Paget's disease of bone b. Osteoarthritis knees
c. Rheumatoid arthritis d. Gouty arthritis

8. A 20-year-old male with pain in lateral side of his hand. X-ray shows the following finding. Identify the condition. ***(Most Recent Question Jan 2023)***

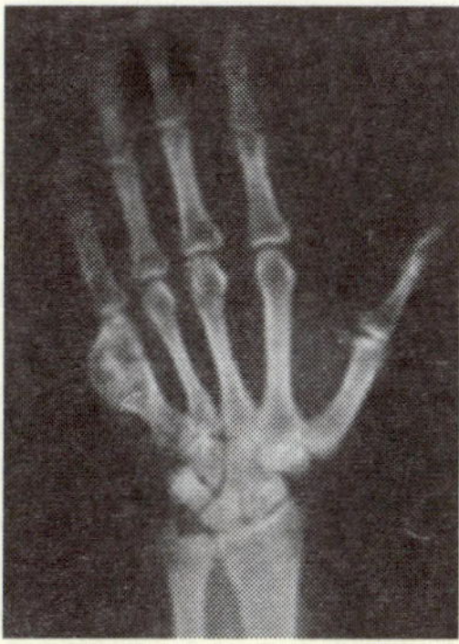

a. Giant cell tumor b. Osteoid osteoma
c. Osteoblastoma d. Enchondroma

9. A 20-year-old male presented to ortho OPD with chronic pain and swelling palpable in the knee. An X-ray shows the following finding. Identify the pathology.
(Most Recent Question Jan 2023)

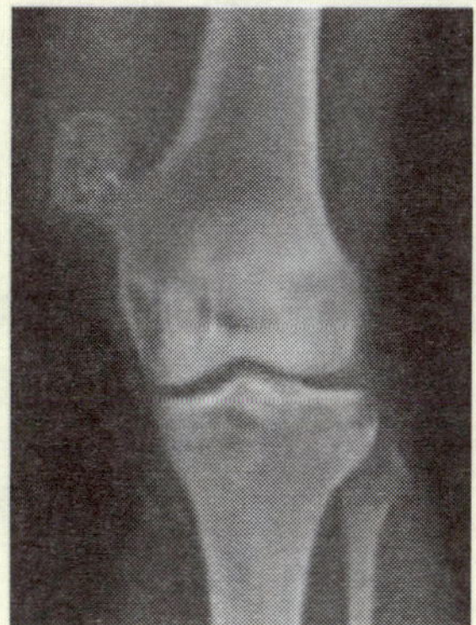

a. Osteochondroma b. Osteoblastoma
c. Osteoporosis d. Osteitis fibrosa cystica

10. A 60-year-old patient presented to the emergency department after falling on an outstretched hand. On examination, dinner fork deformity can be noticed. What can be a probable diagnosis?
(Most Recent Question Jan 2023)

a. Colles fracture b. Carpal tunnel syndrome
c. Osteoporosis d. Smith's fracture

GENERAL ORTHOPEDICS AND FRACTURES

11. Identify the condition shown below?
(Most Recent Question Dec 2019-20)

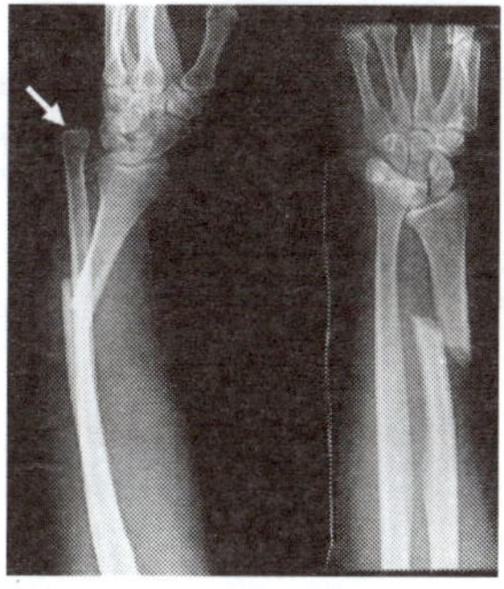

a. Galeazzi fracture b. Monteggia deformities
c. Monteggia fracture d. Green stick fracture

12. A 6-year-old child is suspected with supracondylar fracture of right hand, complaining of pain and swelling. X-ray of right elbow was not significant. What is the next best step in this case? ***(Most Recent Question 2019)***

a. Compare with X-ray of left hand
b. Closed reduction and slab
c. Closed reduction with K-wire fixation
d. Casting

13. A lady presented in emergency with history of trauma to neck region. Identify the shown fracture in image:
(Recent Pattern Question 2018-19)

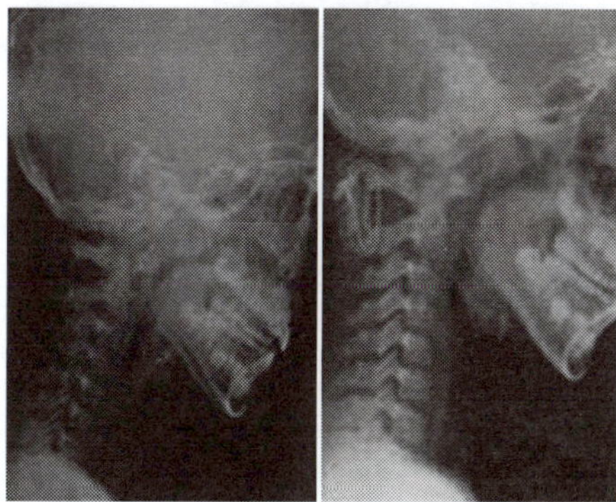

a. Atlanto-axial dislocation b. Jefferson fracture
c. Hangman fracture d. Clay-shoveler fracture

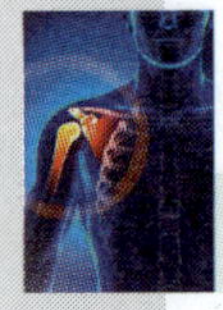

14. Jefferson fracture is: ***(Recent Pattern Question 2017)***
a. C2 fracture
b. C1 fracture
c. Fracture of talus
d. Atlanto-axial dislocation

15. Hangman fracture is: ***(Recent Pattern Question 2017)***
a. C1 ring fracture
b. C2 odontoid process fracture
c. C2 pars interarticularis fracture
d. C7 fracture

16. A male patient presents after trauma with popliteal vessel injury and fracture of 0.5 cm × 0.5 cm. What is the Anderson Gustillo classification?
(Recent Pattern Question 2017)
a. 1
b. 2
c. 3A
d. 3C

17. What is the treatment of Anderson Gustillo classification grade 3B? ***(Recent Pattern Question 2017)***
a. Intramedullary nailing
b. Intramedullary wiring
c. Close reduction
d. K-wire

18. Connection of Haversian canal are by: ***(Recent Pattern Question 2016)***
a. Canaliculi
b. Volkmann canal
c. Osteon
d. Central canal

19. Stress fracture occurs most commonly in:
a. Metatarsals
b. Metacarpals
c. Calcaneum
d. Talus

20. Runners fracture occurs in which bone:
a. Fibula
b. Metatarsals
c. Tibia
d. Calcaneum

21. Fracture and dislocation of lateral clavicle. Best treatment is:
a. Figure of 8 splint
b. Open reduction
c. Normal sling
d. Surgical repair

22. Avascular necrosis can be a possible sequelae of fracture of all of the following bones; EXCEPT:
a. Femur neck
b. Scaphoid
c. Talus
d. Calcaneum

23. Mason's classification is used for:
a. Clavicle fracture
b. Colle's fracture
c. Radial head fracture
d. Monteggia fracture

24. Which of the following fracture most likely leads to malunion:
a. Clavicle fracture
b. Femur neck fracture
c. Scaphoid fracture
d. Ulna fracture

UPPER LIMB

25. A patient falls on an out stretched hand. For management the doctor ties a cast as given in the image. Which fracture did the patient suffer from?
(Most Recent Question June 2022)

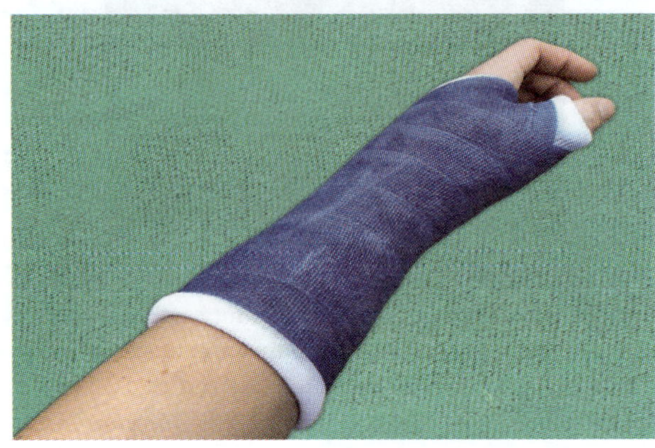

a. Colle's fracture
b. Scaphoid fracture
c. Smith's fracture
d. Galeazzi's fracture

26. A patient comes to the OPD with the chief complaint of pain and swelling in the right shoulder. A fracture of clavicle is suspected. Which is the most common site of fracture in the clavicle?
(Most Recent Question June 2022)
a. Lateral 1/3rd
b. Junction of lateral 1/3rd and medial 2/3rd
c. Junction of medial 1/3rd and lateral 2/3rd
d. Medial 1/3rd

27. A patient met with a road traffic accident and had a fracture of shaft of humerus. After injury he was unable to dorsiflex the wrist. He was advised a splint as shown in figure. Identify the splint.
(Most Recent Question June/Dec 2021)

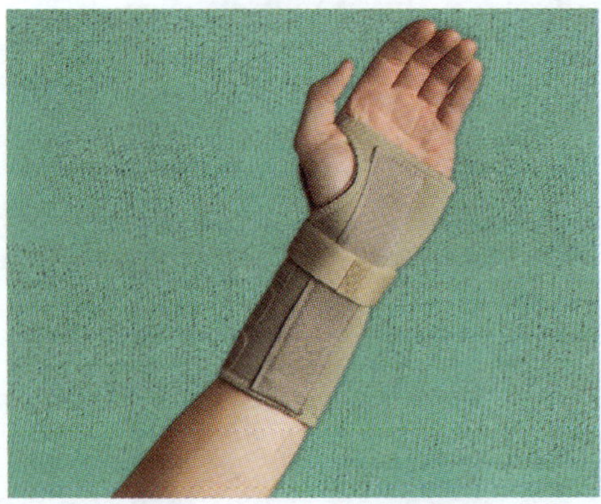

a. Aeroplane splint
b. Thomas splint
c. Cock up splint
d. Knuckle blender splint

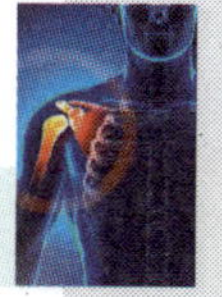

28. A patient was diagnosed as a case of supraspinatus tendinitis. What degrees and what movement of shoulder would be painful: *(Most Recent Question June/Dec 2021)*
  a. 0–15 degree of shoulder abduction
  b. 15–90 degree of shoulder abduction
  c. 0–15 degree of should adduction
  d. 15–90 degree of shoulder adduction

29. A child is unable to carry out movements of pronation supination since childhood. X-ray shown below. Possible diagnosis *(Most Recent Question Aug 2020)*

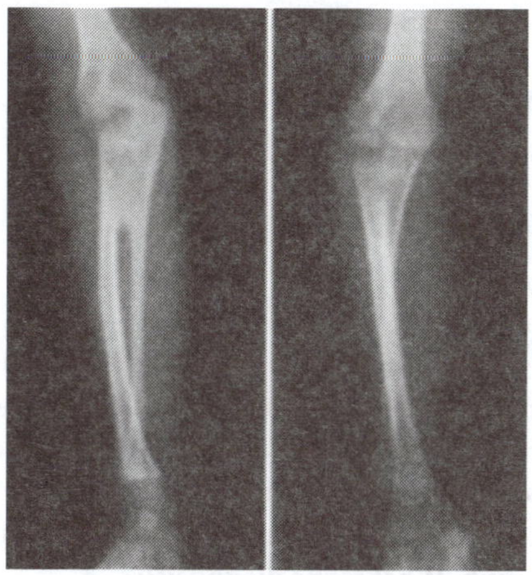

  a. Radial dislocation
  b. Congenital radial head dysplasia
  c. Radio ulnar synostosis
  d. Elbow dislocation

30. Identify the labelled structure: *(Most Recent Question Aug 2020)*

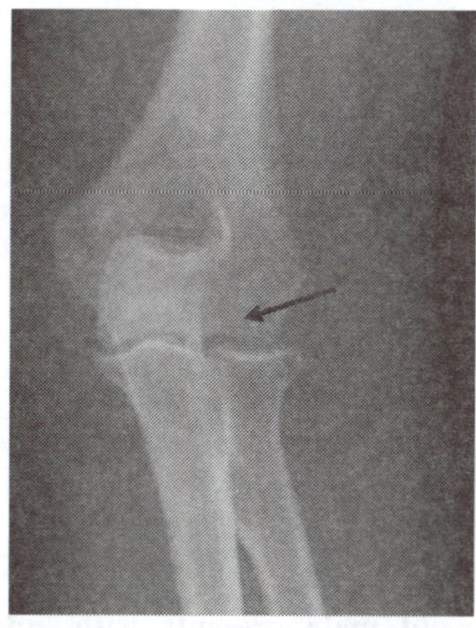

  a. Radial head b. Trochlea
  c. Capitellum d. Lateral epicondyle

31. Three point bony relationship has diagnostic value in: *(Most Recent Question 2019)*
  a. Elbow fracture b. Monteggia fracture
  c. Galeazzi fracture d. Colles' fracture

32. Management of olecranon fracture as seen in the image: *(Most Recent Question 2019)*

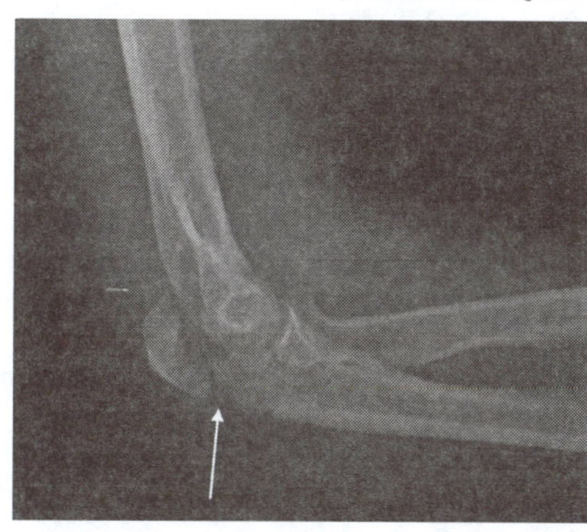

  a. Above elbow plaster slab
  b. Below elbow plaster slab
  c. Close reduction with Tension band wiring
  d. Open reduction with Tension band wiring

33. A Tennis player presents with a history of spontaneous shoulder dislocation, labrum injury. Now he states that he can himself correct the dislocation. This condition most likely is: *(Recent Pattern Question 2018-19)*
  a. Recurrent anterior shoulder dislocation
  b. Recurrent posterior shoulder dislocation
  c. Reverse hill sach's lesion
  d. Inferior shoulder dislocation

34. Herberden's arthropathy affects: *(Recent Pattern Question 2018)*
  a. Lumbar spine
  b. Sacroiliac joint
  c. Distal interphalangeal joint
  d. Knee joint

35. Muscle in 2nd compartment of wrist: *(Recent Pattern Question 2018)*
  a. Extensor pollicis brevis
  b. Extensor carpi radialis brevis and longus
  c. Abductor pollicis longus
  d. Extensor pollicis longus

36. A patient received an electric shock and fell down. He cannot do external rotation of shoulder and cannot move arm. What is the diagnosis? *(Recent Pattern Question 2018)*
  a. Anterior dislocation b. Posterior dislocation
  c. Clavicle fracture d. Luxation erecta

37. Terrible triad of elbow is: *(Recent Pattern Question 2017)*
  a. Humerus fracture with medial epicondyle fracture
  b. Shaft fracture with dislocation and ulnar fracture
  c. Elbow dislocation with shaft fracture
  d. Elbow dislocation with radial head and coronoid fracture

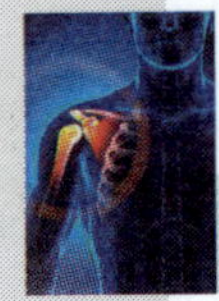

38. What is true about supracondylar fracture?
(Recent Pattern Question 2017)
a. Mostly seen in elderly population
b. Females are mostly affected
c. Most common type is extension type
d. Can cause non union

39. Nerve involved in shaft of humerus fracture
(Recent Pattern Question 2016)
a. Median b. Anterior interosseous
c. Posterior interosseus d. Radial

40. Nerve involved in carpal tunnel syndrome
(Recent Pattern Question 2016)
a. Ulnar nerve b. Radial nerve
c. Median nerve d. Medial nerve

41. Which of the following is static stabilizer of shoulder joint:
a. Supraspinatus b. Infraspinatus
c. Negative pressure in glenoid cavity
d. Subscapularis

42. Supraspinatus injury leads to which of the following:
a. Frozen shoulder b. Winging of scapula
c. Cannot abduct d. Cannot adduct

43. In Anterior dislocation of shoulder which nerve is commonly affected:
a. Axillary nerve b. Radial nerve
c. Ulnar nerve d. Median nerve

44. In a man lifting up suitcase, posterior dislocation of glenohumeral joint is prevented by:
a. Deltoid b. Latissimus dorsi
c. Coracobrachialis d. Short head of biceps

45. Which of the following test of shoulder dislocation is verified by just looking at the axillary fat folds:
a. Dugas test b. Callway test
c. Hamilton ruler test d. Bryants's test

46. Hill Sach's lesion is seen in:
a. Hip joint dislocation b. Elbow dislocation
c. Shoulder Dislocation d. Jaw dislocation

47. Colle's fracture which of the following tendons likely to rupture:
a. Flexor pollicis longus b. Flexor policis brevis
c. Extensor policis longus d. Extensor policis brevis

48. Kienbock disease is avascular necrosis of:
a. Scaphoid b. Trapezoid
c. Trapezium d. Lunate

49. Monteggia fracture is:
a. Fracture of distal radius with dislocation of head of ulna
b. Fracture of the proximal third of the ulna with dislocation of the head of the radius.
c. Fracture of distal third of ulna with dislocation of head of radius
d. Fracture of proximal one third of radius with dislocation of head of radius

50. Injury in radial groove of humerus will lead to:
a. Wrist drop b. Chauffeur's fracture
c. Skier's thumb d. Mallet finger

51. Content of anatomical snuff box
a. Radial artery b. Ulnar artery
c. Median nerve d. Superficial artery

52. Which of the following does not indicate ulnar nerve injury:
a. Clawing of medial 2 digits
b. Froment sign is present
c. Abductor Pollicis longus palsy
d. Loss of sensory supply of medial little finger and medial half of ring finger

53. First sign of volkman's ischemia is:
a. Pulselessness
b. Pallor
c. Paralysis
d. Pain

54. A pregnant woman aged 30 years, after trauma feeling tingling pain and numbness at the tips of thumb, index finger and middle finger, on examination doctor presses between the wrist joint for 30 seconds and the patient develops more pain at the tips of the middle, index finger and thumb. What is the diagnosis:
a. Carpal tunnel syndrome
b. Cubital tunnel syndrome
c. Tarsal tunnel syndrome
d. Pronator syndrome

55. Finkelstein test is done for:
a. Compound palmar ganglia
b. Carpal tunnel syndrome
c. De-quervain tenosynovitis
d. Tennis elbow

56. Dupuytren's contracture is associated with all; EXCEPT:
a. Usually not painful
b. Involves the ring and little finger
c. Table top test is negative
d. Clostridial collagenase for resolution

57. Gun stock deformity is seen in:
a. Supracondylar fracture of humerus
b. Lateral condyle fracture
c. Radial head fracture
d. Ulnar head fracture

58. A 20-year-old male presents with anterior shoulder dislocation. This injury is usually caused as a combination of which of the following?
a. Abduction and external rotation
b. Abduction and internal rotation
c. Adduction and external rotation
d. Adduction and internal rotation

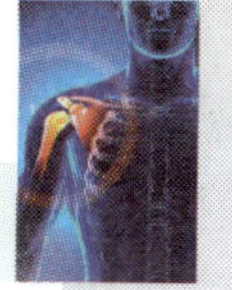

59. A 24-year-old sustained the fracture shown in the X-ray below. The nerve most likely to be injured is:

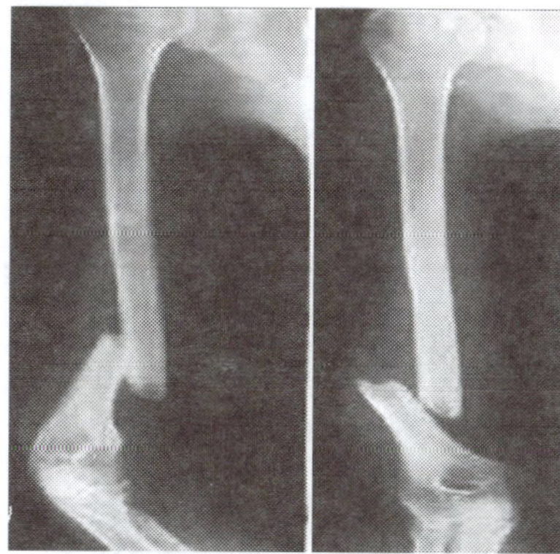

a. Ulnar nerve
b. Median nerve
c. Radial nerve
d. Musculocutaneous nerve

60. Eponym for fracture shown in below X-ray is:

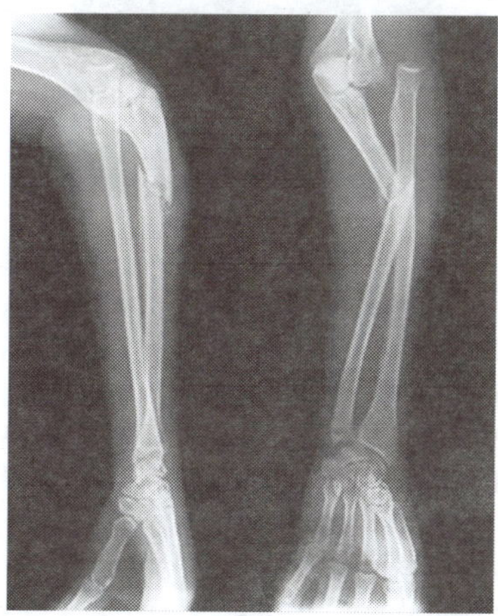

a. Monteggia fracture
b. Colles fracture
c. Galezzei fracture
d. Smith fracture

LOWER LIMB

61. What is the treatment for this fracture?

(Most Recent Question June 2022)

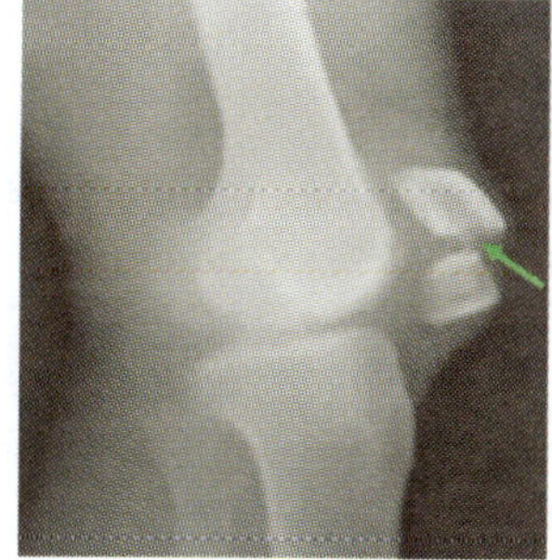

a. Total patellectomy
b. K-wire
c. Conservative treatment
d. Partial patellectomy

62. A person sitting in the front seat of car, met with a road traffic accident. Following injury his lower limb was in flexion, adduction, internal rotation (FADIR). X-ray was done as shown in figure. Most likely diagnosis:

(Most Recent Question June/Dec 2021)

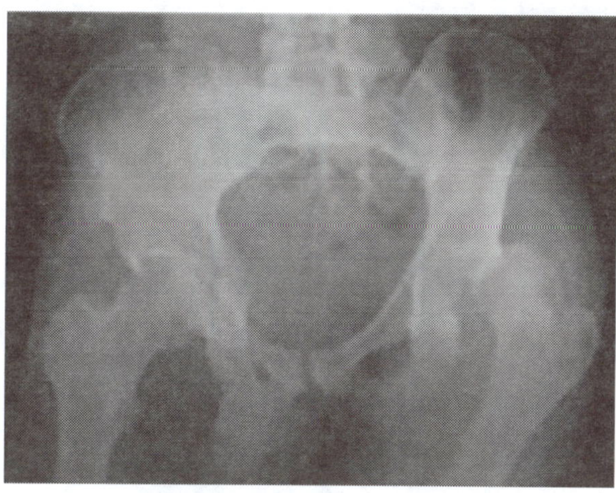

a. Anterior dislocation of hip
b. Posterior dislocation of hip
c. Fracture neck of femur
d. Fracture shaft of femur

63. Which artery is palpated behind medial malleolus

(Most Recent Question June/Dec 2021)

a. Anterior tibial
b. Posterior tibial
c. Dorsalis pedis
d. Popliteal

64. Based on the X-ray and clinical picture given below, which nerve is most commonly damaged:

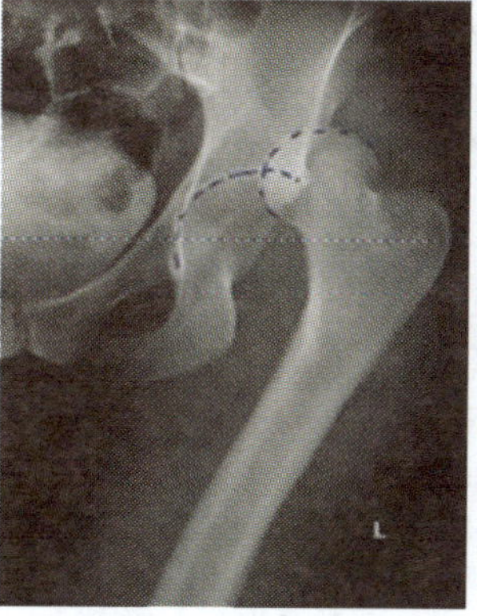

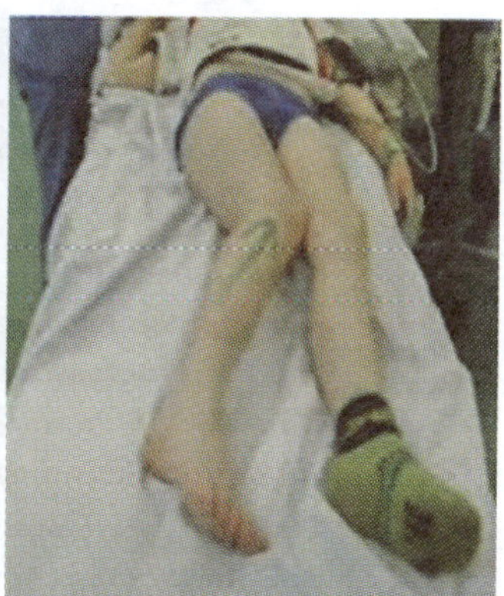

a. Pudendal nerve
b. Sciatic nerve
c. Femoral nerve
d. Obtutator nerve

65. A doctor removed the cast and found that the area was deformable but not mobile. The doctor applied the cast. What is the stage of fracture healing?

(Most Recent Question Aug 2020)

a. Callus stage
b. Modelling stage
c. Remodelling stage
d. Hematoma stage

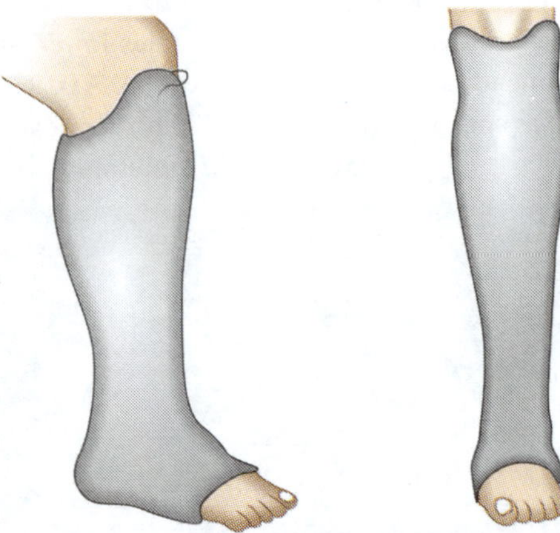

66. **A patient comes after injury. After seeing the X-ray what is the probable diagnosis?** *(Most Recent Question Dec 2019-20)*

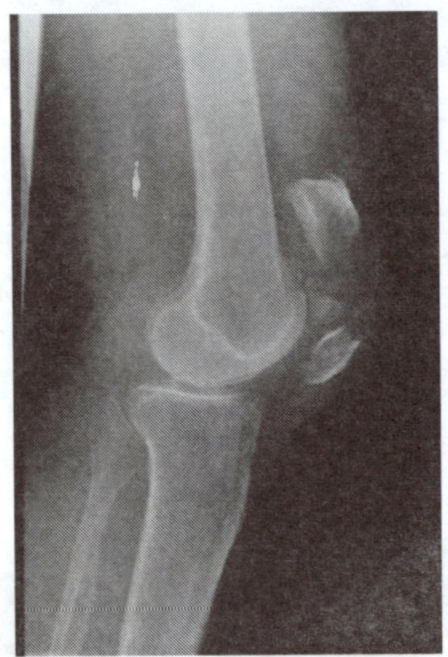

a. Tibial fracture
b. Patellar fracture
c. Knee loose body
d. Femur fracture

67. **A 60-year-old female complaints of pain in bilateral knee. The pain increases while going up and down the stairs. The X-ray shows bilateral reduced joint space what is the most likely diagnosis?** *(Most Recent Question Dec 2019-20)*
a. Osteoarthritis
b. Rheumatoid arthritis
c. Ankylosing spondylitis
d. Hemophiliac arthropathy

68. **Football player with knee injury diagnosed as medial collateral ligament injury. Which structure is most commonly associated with this type of injury?** *(Most Recent Question Dec 2019-20)*
a. Posterior collateral ligament
b. Medial meniscus
c. Posterior cruciate ligament
d. Lateral lemniscus

69. **Avascular necrosis of femur head is due to which of the following artery?** *(Most Recent Question Dec 2019-20)*
a. Medial circumflex femoral artery
b. Lateral circumflex femoral artery
c. Obturator artery
d. Profunda femoris artery

70. **The shown apparatus is:** *(Most Recent Question Dec 2019-20)*

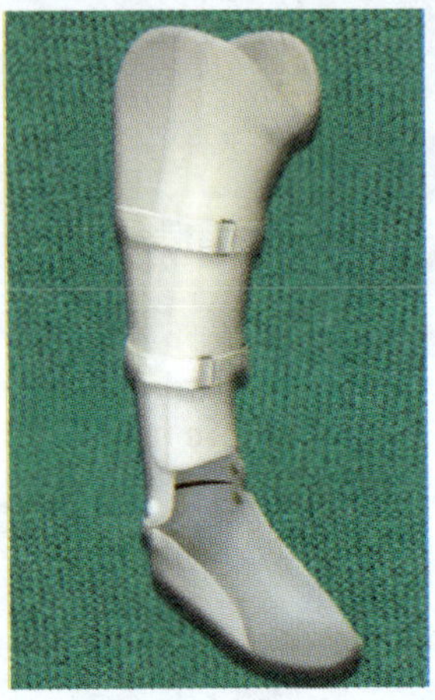

a. Ankle knee stabilizer
b. Patella tendon bearing brace
c. Thomas splint
d. Prosthetic foot

71. **Which of the following finding is noted in initial stages of TB hip:** *(Most Recent Question Dec 2019-20)*
a. Reduction of joint space
b. Increased in joint space
c. Degeneration of cartilage
d. Joint fusion

72. **The triad of triple arthrodesis includes all; EXCEPT:** *(Recent Pattern Question 2018)*
a. Calcaneocuboid joint
b. Talonavicular joint
c. Tibiotalar joint
d. Subtalar joint

73. **Lauge-Hansen classification belongs to:** *(Recent Pattern Question 2018)*
a. Femur fracture
b. Elbow fracture
c. Ankle fracture
d. Shoulder fracture

74. **Triple deformity is seen in all of the following conditions; EXCEPT:** *(Recent Pattern Question 2017)*
a. Knee TB
b. Reactive arthritis
c. Iliotibial contracture
d. Poliomyelitis

75. **Triple deformity of knee includes all; EXCEPT:**
a. Knee flexion
b. Posterior subluxation of femur
c. Lateral rotation of tibia
d. Posterior subluxation of tibia

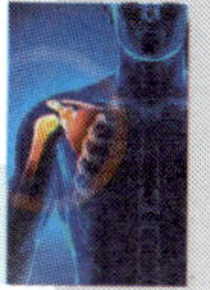

76. A patient with fracture of femur shaft develops petechiae, respiratory distress and decreased SpO_2, 5 days after injury. Possible diagnosis is:

(Recent Pattern Question 2016)

a. Hypostatic pneumonia
b. Haemolytic anemia
c. Crush syndrome
d. Fat embolism

77. Anterior cruciate ligaments prevent:

a. Anterior dislocation of ulna
b. Posterior dislocation of ulna
c. Anterior dislocation of tibia
d. Posterior dislocation of tibia

78. Which nerve is injured in fracture of fibula:

a. Posterior tibial nerve
b. Anterior tibial nerve
c. Common peroneal nerve
d. Deep peroneal nerve

79. Bumper fracture is?

a. Fracture of fibula
b. Fracture of distal tibia
c. Fracture of medial tibial plateau
d. Fracture of lateral tibial plateau

80. Main extensor of knee:

a. Gastrocnemius
b. Quadriceps femoris
c. Hamstrings
d. Peroneal muscles

81. Q angle is increased in:

a. Patellar subluxation
b. Genu varum
c. Femoral ante-flexion
d. Medial positioning tibial tuberosity

82. Gallow's traction is used for fracture of:

a. Neck of femur
b. Shaft of femur
c. Shaft of tibia
d. Tibial plafond

83. The ligaments connecting the menisci to the tibia are known as:

a. Coronary
b. Arcuate
c. Transverse
d. Oblique

84. In patient with femoral head fracture associated with femur neck fracture. What is the grading according to pipkin classification:

a. Grade I
b. Grade II
c. Grade III
d. Grade IV

85. Spot diagnosis:

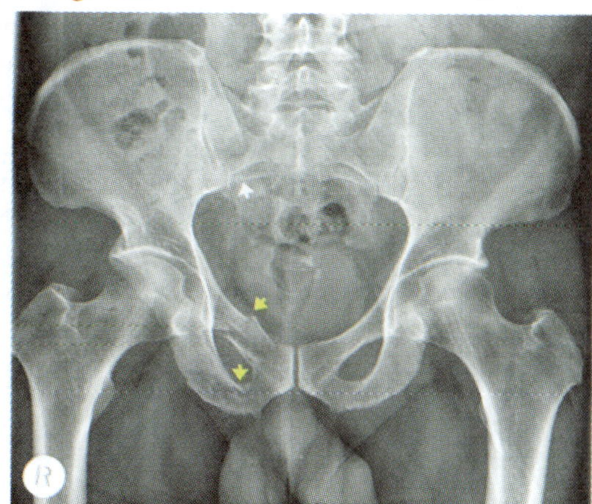

a. Malgaigne fracture
b. Straddle fracture
c. Pubic rami with penile fracture
d. Sacroiliac joint dislocation only

PELVIS AND HIP

86. In the shown X-ray of hip joint, which is the most common area affected in TB hip:

(Most Recent Question Aug 2020)

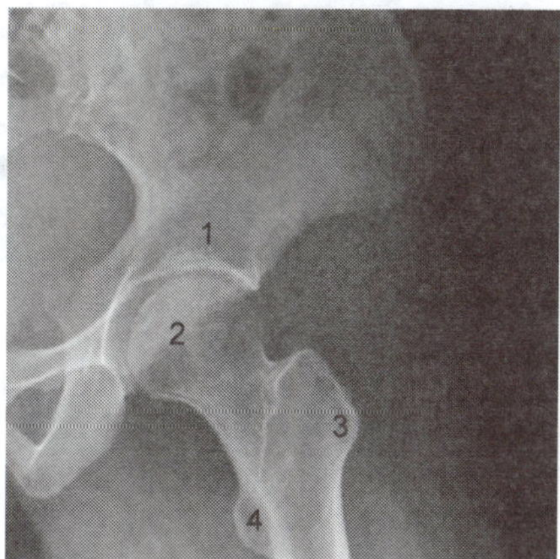

a. 1
b. 2
c. 3
d. 4

87. A 30-year-old has history of trauma and pain right hip with flexion abduction and external rotation what is the most likely diagnosis:

(Most Recent Question Dec 2019-20)

a. Hip posterior dislocation
b. Hip anterior dislocation
c. Fracture neck femur
d. Intertrochanteric fracture

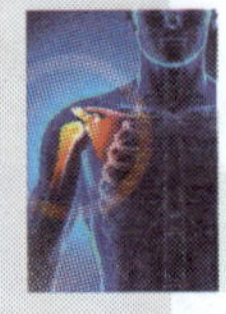

88. A 79-year-old lady presents with history of fall. There is right sided intertrochanteric fracture of hip evidenced by the given X-ray. Best management for this patient is:
(Recent Pattern Question 2018-19)

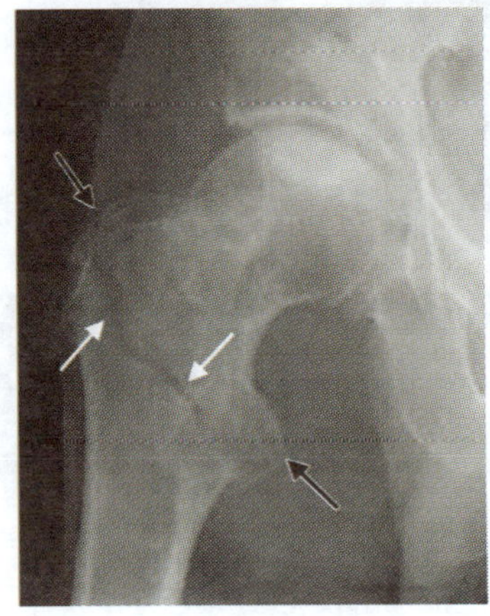

a. Bipolar Hemiarthoplasty
b. Intramedullary nail
c. Hip-Spica
d. Internal fixation

89. A 30-year-old male fell from a tree. Thereafter he complains of pain and is unable to move his legs *(image given)*. Next management *(Recent Pattern Question 2016)*

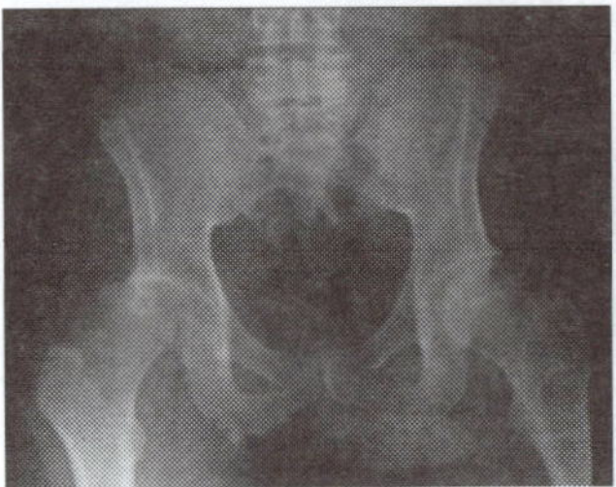

a. Open reduction
b. Urgent closed reduction
c. Traction
d. Observation

90. Patient came into emergency department with flexion, adduction and internal rotation of hip. Diagnosis?
a. Anterior dislocation of hip
b. Posterior dislocation of hip
c. Femur neck fracture
d. Femur head fracture

91. Posterior dislocation of hip results in:
a. Abduction, internal rotation, extension
b. Adduction, internal rotation, extension
c. Adduction, internal rotation, flexion
d. Abduction, external rotation, flexion

92. 82-year-old female with necrotic head of femur and bilateral osteoarthritis. What is the next step of management:
a. Uncemented total hip replacement
b. Cemented total hip replacement
c. Hemi-arthroplasty
d. Observation

93. In anterior dislocation of hip, attitude of limb is:
a. Flexion, abduction, internal rotation
b. Flexion, abduction, external rotation
c. Flexion, adduction, internal rotation
d. Flexion, adduction, external rotation

94. What is the position of leg in tubercular arthritis in synovitis stage:
a. Flexion, adduction, internal rotation
b. Flexion, abduction, internal rotation
c. Flexion, abduction, external rotation
d. Extension, abduction internal rotation

INFECTION & TUBERCULOSIS OF BONE AND JOINTS

95. What would be the probable diagnosis:
(Most Recent Question June 2022)

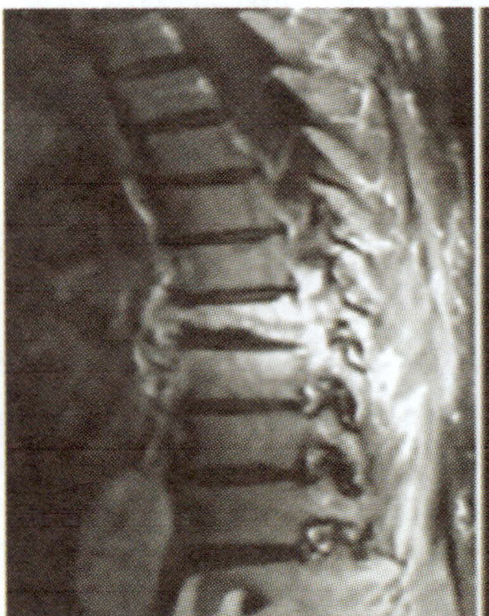
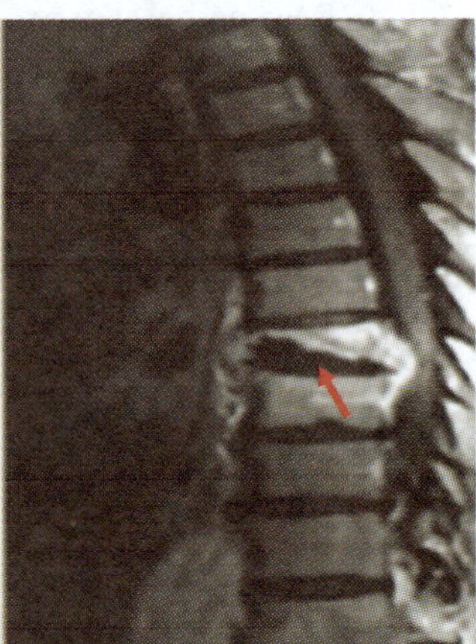

a. Pott's spine
b. Pyogenic spondylitis
c. Multiple myeloma
d. Ankylosing spondylitis

96. Person with history of hip pain from last few months and was diagnosed as a case of tuberculosis. Examination reveals true limb shortening. Which stage it is:
a. Late arthritis ***(Most Recent Question June/Dec 2021)***
b. Early arthritis
c. Early synovitis
d. Advanced arthritis

97. A young girl presented with swelling of thigh with discharging sinus from which a bony fragment came out. The parents were concerned about this bony fragment. What is the bony fragment called:
(Most Recent Question Aug 2020)

a. Involucrum
b. Cloacae
c. Sequestrum
d. Loose body

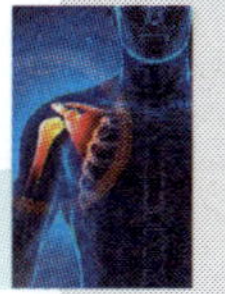

98. A patient presented with following problem (as shown in image). There is history of pin prick injury in this patient's finger. Which of the following is not true about the given image? *(Most Recent Question Aug 2020)*

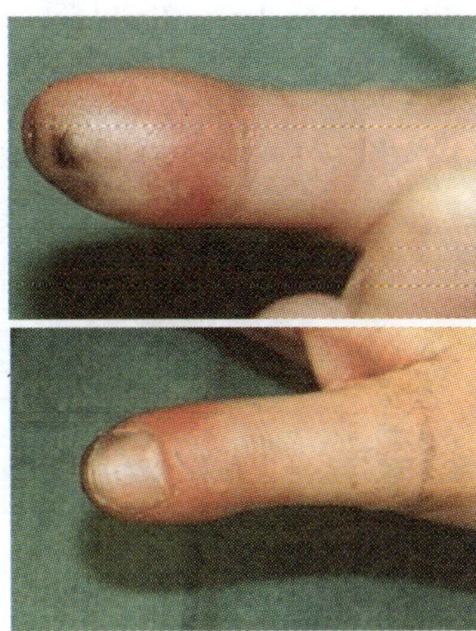

a. May cause osteomyelitis
b. May be caused due to pin prick injury
c. Causative organism is staph epidermidis
d. May be treated initially by antibiotics

99. The spina ventosa is seen in:
(Recent Pattern Question 2018)
a. Carpals
b. Phalanges
c. Dorsal spine
d. Shoulder joint

100. Most common type of lesion in Pott's spine:
(Recent Pattern Question 2018)
a. Central
b. Anterior
c. Paradiscal
d. Appendiceal

101. A 4-year-old child presented with limping and fever and has the given X-ray. Most likely diagnosis:

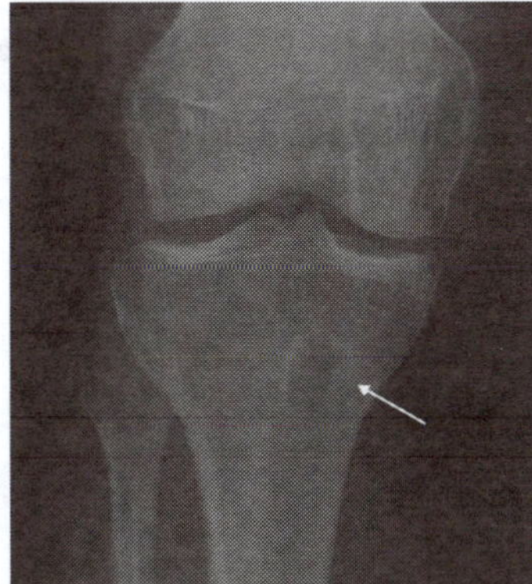

(Recent Pattern Question 2017)
a. Osteomyelitis
b. Osteosarcoma
c. Enchondroma
d. Aneurysmal bone cyst

102. Most common organism causing osteomyelitis:
a. Staph aureus
b. Strep pneumonia
c. H. Influenza
d. E. coli

103. Most common site for osteomyelitis:
a. Epiphysis
b. Metaphysis
c. Diaphysis
d. Sub-chondral growth plate

104. Earliest X-ray finding in osteomyelitis:
a. Involucrum
b. Sequestrum
c. Cloacae
d. Periosteal reaction

105. Felon means infection of:
a. Epinychium
b. Terminal pulp space
c. Deep palmar abscess
d. Subcuticular space

106. Spina ventosa is:
a. Tubercular dactylitis
b. TB of spine
c. TB of vertebral pedicles
d. Extra-axial

107. Triple deformity of knee includes all; EXCEPT:
a. Posterior subluxation of tibia
b. Medial rotation of tibia
c. Lateral rotation of tibia
d. Flexion

108. Triple deformity in tubercular arthritis of the knee is:
a. Flexion, posterior subluxation and external rotation
b. Flexion, posterior subluxation and internal rotation
c. Extension, anterior subluxation and external rotation
d. Extension, anterior subluxation and internal rotation

109. Most common area involved in tubercular spine is:
a. Paradiscal area
b. Central type
c. Anterior involvement
d. Appendicle involvement

110. True about bony ankylosis:
a. Painful condition
b. Tubercular arthritis is most common cause
c. Septic arthritis leads to bony ankylosis
d. Spine tuberculosis is the leading cause

111. The most common sequelae of tuberculous spondylitis is:
a. Fibrous ankylosis
b. Bony Ankylosis
c. Pathological dislocation
d. Chronic osteomyelitis

112. Kanavel sign includes all; EXCEPT:
a. Tenderness
b. Flexion
c. Pain upon passive flexion
d. Uniform swelling

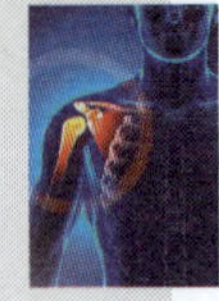

BONE ONCOLOGY AND JOINT DISORDERS

113. A 46-year-old male presents with lesion involving epiphyseal region of lower femur as shown in image. The multinucleated giant cells and mononuclear cells can be seen on histopathology. What is the most probable diagnosis? ***(Most Recent Question Aug 2020)***

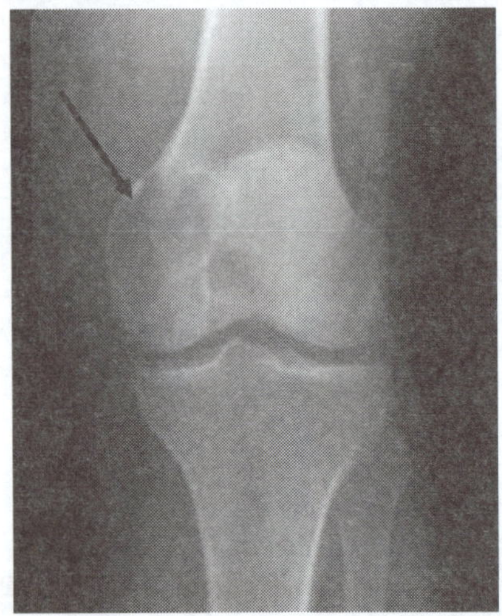

a. Unicameral bone cyst b. Aneurysmal bone cyst
c. Giant cell tumor d. Osteosarcoma

114. Which of the following is the most radiosensitive tumor? ***(Most Recent Question Dec 2019-20)***

a. Histiocytoma b. Ewing's sarcoma
c. Osteosarcoma d. Chondrosarcoma

115. A 50-year-old male patient presented with shown condition. Identify the condition shown below? ***(Most Recent Question Dec 2019-20)***

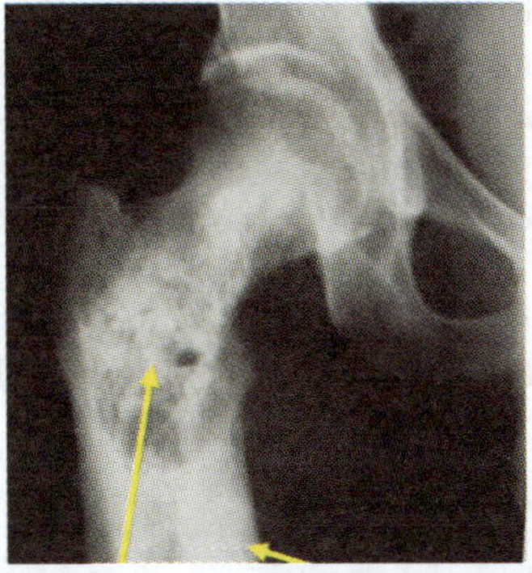

a. Osteosarcoma b. Chondrosarcoma
c. Chondroblastoma d. Ewing's sarcoma

116. Most common site of Adamantinoma: ***(Recent Pattern Question 2018-19)***

a. Radius b. Humerus
c. Tibia d. Femur

117. Sunray appearance in osteosarcoma is due to: ***(Recent Pattern Question 2018)***

a. Bone destruction b. Periosteal reaction
c. Vascular calcification d. Bone hypertrophy

118. A child with pain in lower limb presented with this X-ray. Which is the probable diagnosis? ***(Recent Pattern Question 2017)***

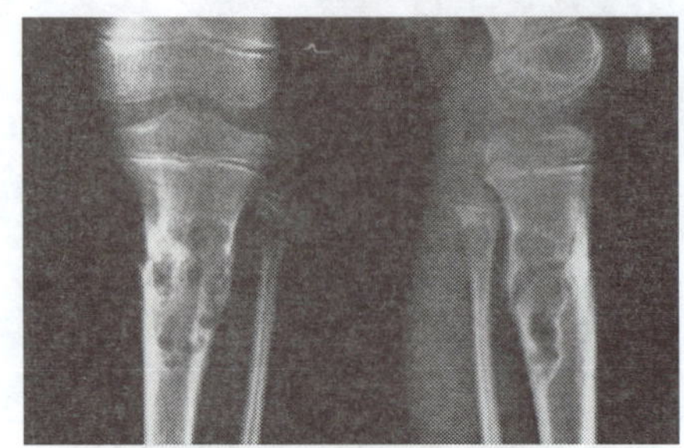

a. Osteosarcoma b. Osteoid osteoma
c. Ewing's sarcoma d. Osteofibrous dysplasia

119. Which of the following is an epiphyseal tumor? ***(Recent Pattern Question 2017)***

a. Osteoid osteoma
b. Adamantinoma
c. Osteosarcoma
d. Chrondroblastoma

120. An intramedullary tumor occurring in the lower metaphysis of the tibia in a 15-year-old male is most likely to be:

a. Ewing's sarcoma b. Giant cell tumor
c. Chondrosarcoma d. Osteosarcoma

121. Sun burst appearance usually seen in:

a. Osteosarcoma b. Osteopetrosis
c. Osteomyelitis d. Osteoradionecrosis

122. Aspirin is useful in which type of bone tumor:

a. Osteonecrosis b. Osteopetrosis
c. Osteoid osteoma d. Ewing sarcoma

123. Most common presenting age of Ewing's sarcoma is:

a. First decade b. Second decade
c. Third decade d. Fourth decade

124. X-ray wrist showing soap bubble appearance in epiphyseal region. Diagnosis:

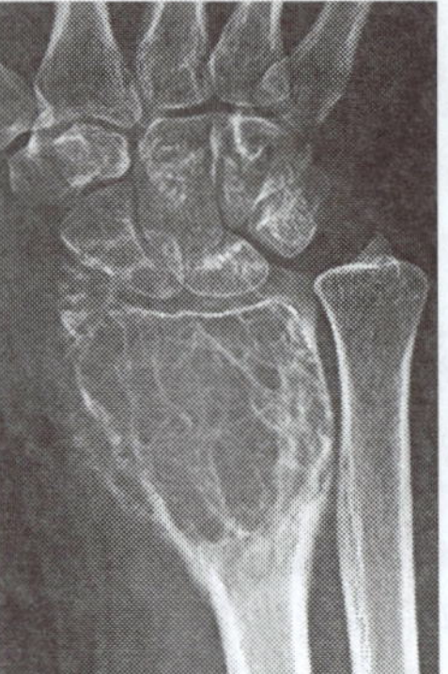

a. Giant cell tumor b. Osteosarcoma
c. Osteochondroma d. Osteoid osteoma

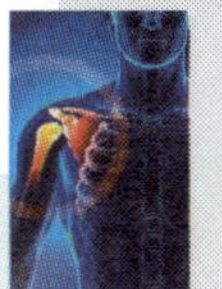

JOINT DISORDERS

125. Which is the most common joint involved in *thalassemia*? *(Recent Pattern Question 2017)*

a. Hip b. Knee
c. Shoulder d. Ankle

126. Which of the following condition present as arthritis with conjunctivitis? *(Recent Pattern Question 2017)*

a. Reiter's syndrome b. Kaplan syndrome
c. Pneumoconiosis d. Aspergillosis

127. Joint *not* involved in Rheumatoid Arthritis:

a. DIP b. PIP
c. MC d. Wrist

128. Which of the following is seen in Boutonniere's deformity:

a. Extension of PIP and DIP
b. Flexion of PIP and DIP
c. Flexion contracture of PIP and extension of DIP
d. Flexion of DIP and extension of PIP

129. All are seen in rheumatoid arthritis; EXCEPT:

a. Boutonniere's deformity b. Heberden nodes
c. Involvement of PIP d. Swan neck deformity

130. A 35-year-old female presented with MCP and PIP pain. Diagnosis:

a. Rheumatoid arthritis
b. Rheumatic fever
c. Gouty arthritis
d. Psoariatic arthritis

131. Diagnosis of the picture given:

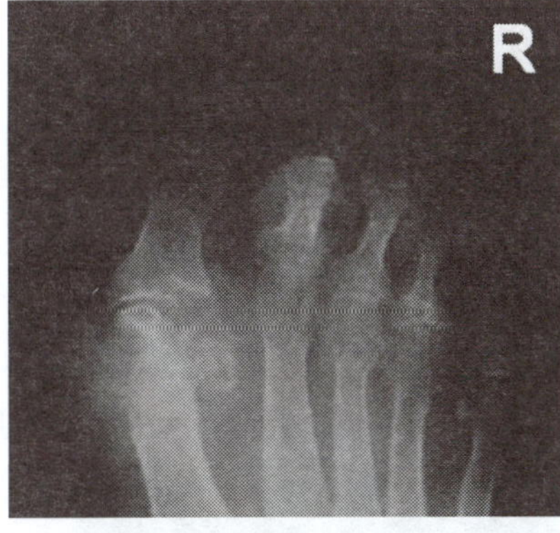

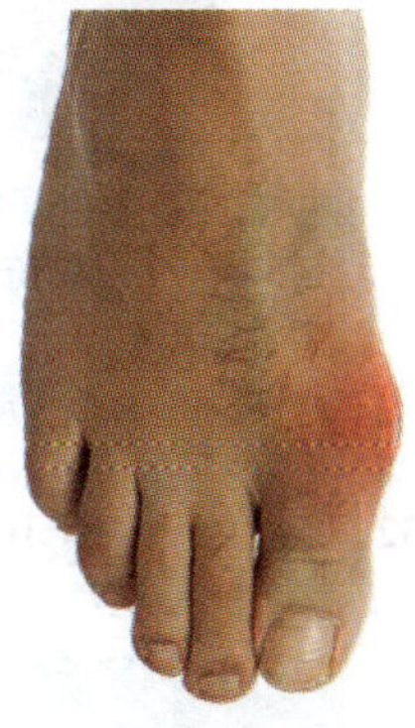

a. Osteoarthritis
b. Gouty arthritis
c. Rheumatoid arthritis
d. Pseudogout

132. Drug of choice for acute gouty arthritis:

a. Indomethacine b. Allopurinol
c. Colchicine d. Aspirin

133. Correct meaning of Poncet disease:

a. TB with Rheumatoid arthritis
b. TB of short bones
c. TB with polyarthritis
d. TB of shoulder

VERTEBRA & NEUROMUSCULAR DISEASE

134. A 30-year female has backache going to right lower limb. The following is the MRI picture. Which is the most common nerve root involved. *(Most Recent Question Aug 2020)*

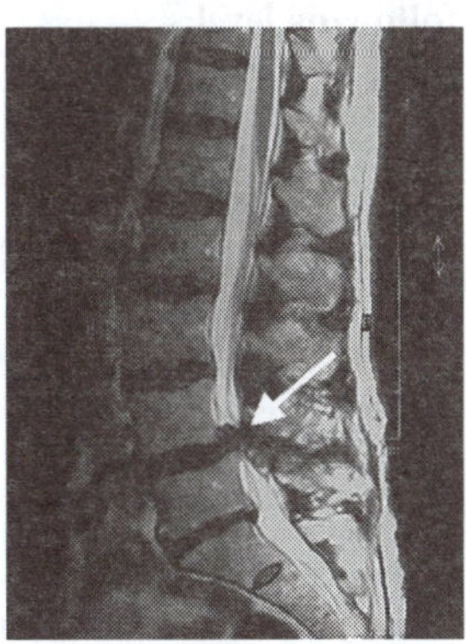

a. L3 b. L4
c. L5 d. S1

135. Identify the given image? *(Most Recent Question Dec 2019-20)*

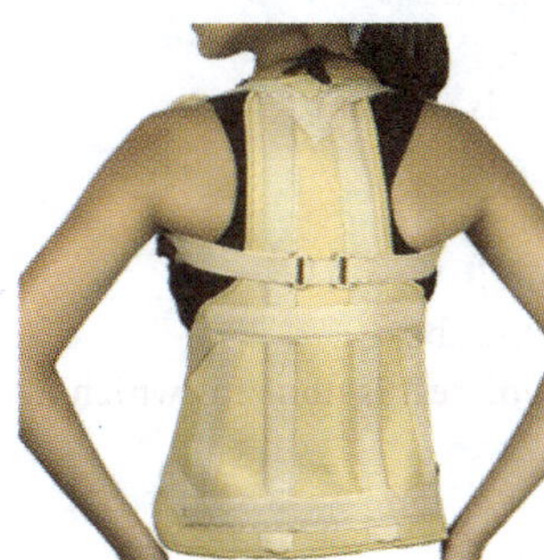

a. Taylor brace splint b. Milwaukee brace
c. Scoliosis brace d. Von rosen splint

136. The spot diagnosis of this shown image: *(Most Recent Question Dec 2019-20)*

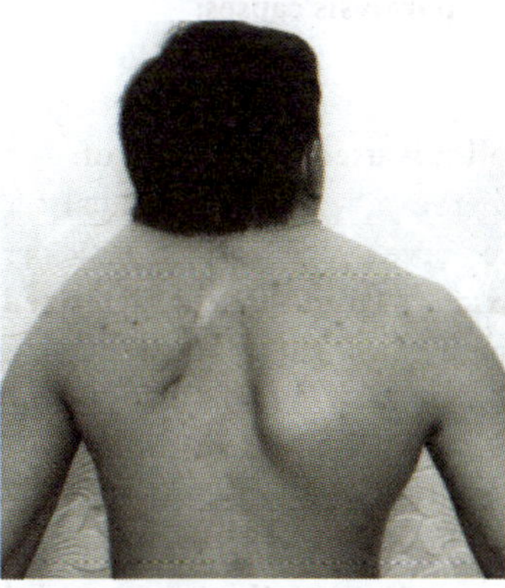

a. Scoliosis b. Disc prolapse
c. Klippel feil syndrome d. Torticollis

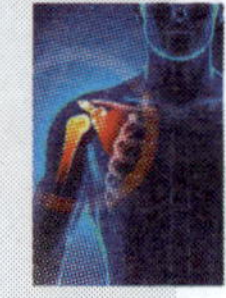

137. Cubital tunnel syndrome involves which nerve?
(Recent Pattern Question 2017)
a. Radial nerve
b. Ulnar nerve
c. Anterior interosseous nerve
d. Median nerve

138. In the lumbar spine, 90% of the disc herniations occur at which of the following level:
a. L1-L2
b. L2-L3
c. L3-L4
d. L4-L5

139. Injury to cervical nerve C5, C6 causes:
a. Erb's paralysis
b. Klumpke paralysis
c. Horner syndrome
d. Central cord syndrome

140. Sciatic nerve damage most commonly due to:
a. Degenerative
b. Iatrogenic
c. Traumatic
d. Vascular

141. Condition in which there is anterior or posterior displacement of a vertebra in relation to the vertebrae below:
a. Spondylosis
b. Spondylitis
c. Spondylolisthesis
d. Spondylolysis

142. Motor march is seen in:
a. Neurapraxia
b. Axonotmesis
c. Neurotmesis
d. None of the above

143. Card test/book test is done for which nerve injury:
a. Radial nerve
b. Ulnar nerve
c. Median nerve
d. Tibial nerve

144. Froment's sign is a feature of:
a. Radial nerve palsy
b. Ulnar nerve palsy
c. Median nerve palsy
d. Tibial nerve palsy

145. Ulnar nerve paralysis causes:
a. Ape thumb deformity
b. Wrist drop
c. Claw finger deformity
d. Meralgia perasthetica

146. Cockup splint is used in paralysis of:
a. Ulnar nerve
b. Radial nerve
c. Median nerve
d. Sciatic nerve

147. Neuropraxia is a condition characterized by:
a. Division of nerve sheath
b. Division of axons
c. Division of nerve fibres
d. Physiological block

148. Little finger of the hand corresponds to:
a. C6 dermatome
b. C7 dermatome
c. C8 dermatome
d. T1 dermatome

149. Pain due to postamputation neuroma is best treated by:
a. Infrared therapy
b. Interference therapy
c. Ultrasound therapy
d. Stump bandaging

150. The picture given below shows a hand following a nerve injury. Identify the nerve:

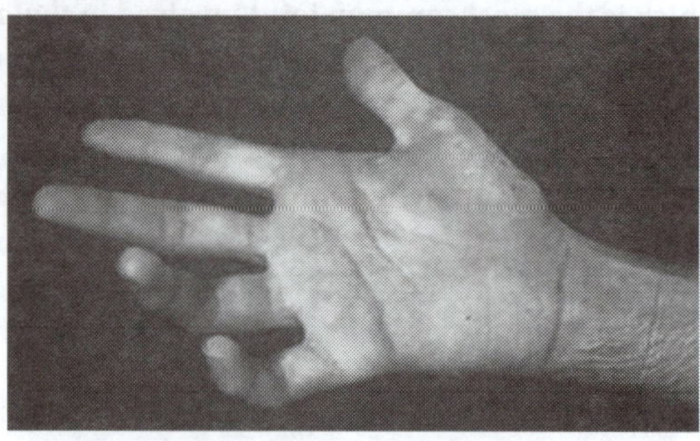

a. Median nerve
b. Ulnar nerve
c. Radial nerve
d. Musculocutaneous nerve

PEDIATRIC ORTHOPAEDICS

151. A 2-year-old baby is brought to the OPD by his worried parent with the following complaint. How would you manage the patient? *(Most Recent Question June 2022)*

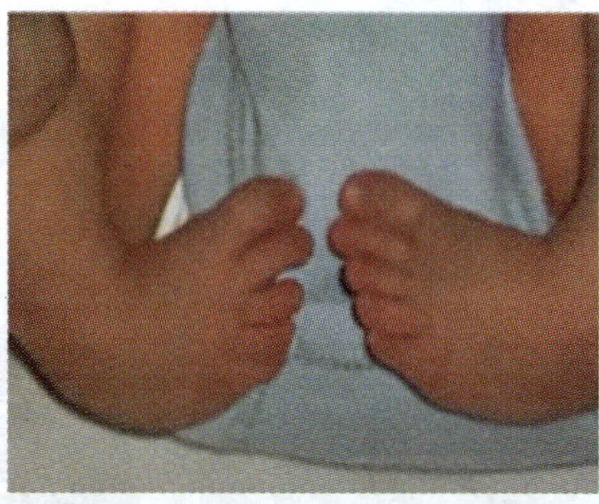

a. Manipulation and cast
b. Postero-medial soft tissue release
c. Triple arthrodesis
d. Evan's procedure

152. Identify the splint shown in the image below:
(Most Recent Question June/Dec 2021)

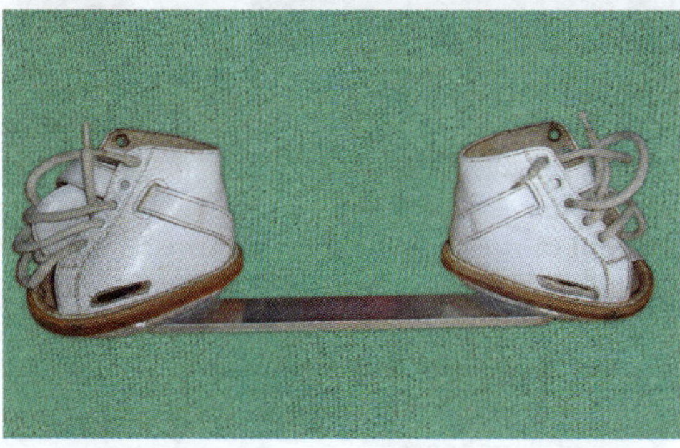

a. Aeroplane splint
b. Pavlik harness
c. Knuckle bender splint
d. Dennis brown splint

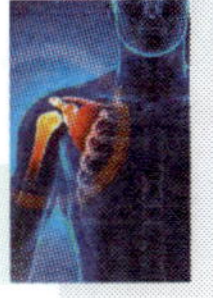

153. The following brace is used for which condition:
(Most Recent Question Aug 2020)

a. Perthes disease
b. Slipped capital femoral epiphysis
c. Congenital coxa vara
d. DDH

154. Child with widening of joint spaces presented with this X-ray. Possible diagnosis: Etiology:
(Most Recent Question Dec 2019-20)

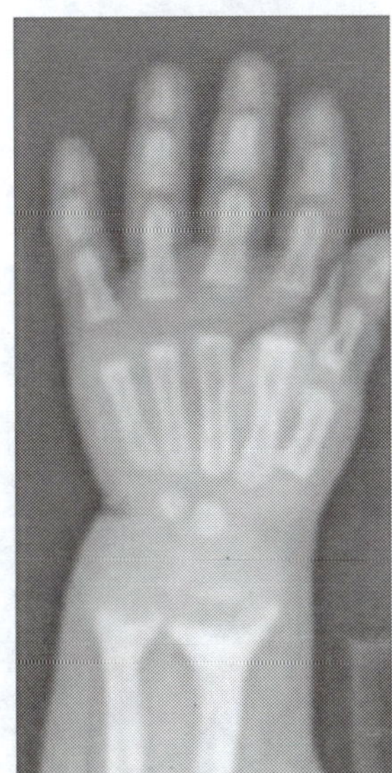

a. Scurvy
b. Rickets
c. Gout
d. Salter harris type 2 injury

155. A 5-year-old child presents with limping and limb shortening. Based on the following finding seen on X-ray, this is most likely a case of:
(Recent Pattern Question 2018-19)

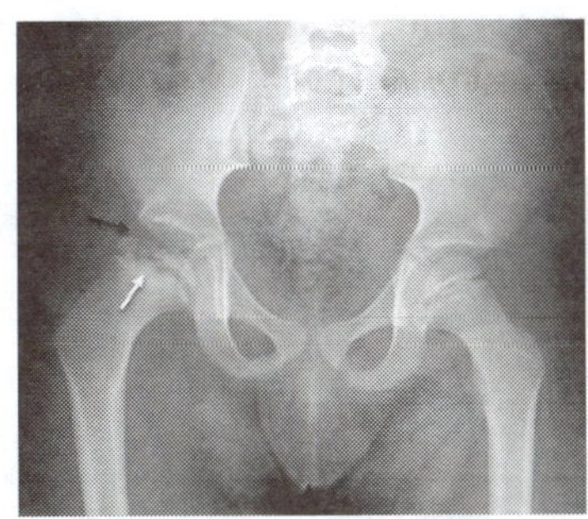

a. DDH b. Hip dislocation
c. Perthes disease d. Stage I TB hip joint

156. True about Blount disease:
(Recent Pattern Question 2018-19)

a. Dysplasia of proximal epiphysis
b. Metaplasia of distal epiphysis
c. Dysplasia of diaphysis
d. Metaplasia of diaphysis

157. Most common joint dislocation in pediatric population:
(Recent Pattern Question 2017)

a. Wrist
b. Sternoclavicular
c. Elbow
d. Hip

158. Trethovan sign is used for diagnosis of:
(Recent Pattern Question 2017)

a. Talar fracture
b. Congenital hip dysplasia
c. Clavicle fracture
d. Slipped capital femoral epiphysis

159. Investigation for screening congenital dislocation of hip in an infant is:

a. X-ray b. USG
c. CT scan d. MRI

160. Barlow test is used for testing:

a. Talar fracture
b. Slipped capital femoral epiphysis
c. Congenital dislocation of hip
d. Rickets

161. Which ligament is involved in Pes-planus:

a. Spring ligament
b. Deep transverse ligament
c. Long & short plantar ligament
d. Deltoid ligament

162. Clutton's joint is seen in:

a. Early congenital syphilis b. Late congenital syphilis
c. Tertiary syphilis d. All of these

163. Vertical talus is associated with:

a. Congenital flat foot b. Ankle dislocation
c. Talus fracture d. Pes cavus

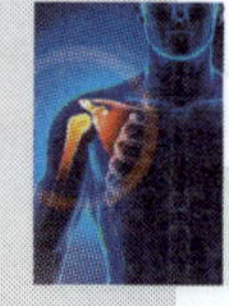

METABOLIC BONE DISORDERS

164. A 35-year-old patient from Bihar presented with generalized bone pain and had excess fluoride intake. He was diagnosed with fluorosis and presented with following condition. Fluorosis of bone is commonly associated with: ***(Most Recent Question Aug 2020)***

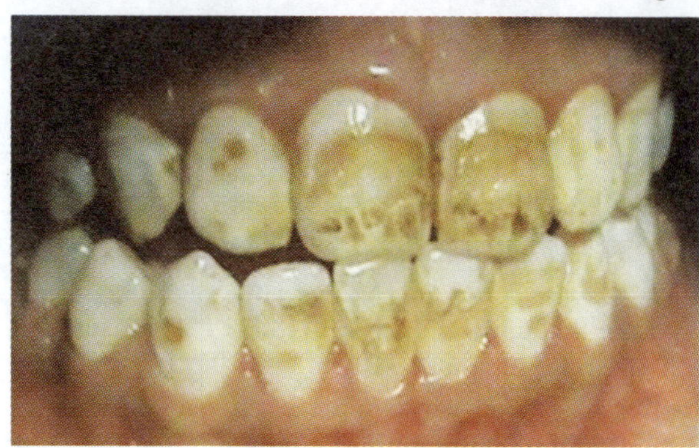

a. Osteopetrosis
b. Osteosclerosis
c. Osteoporosis
d. Osteomalacia

165. Patient has history of multiple fracture with blue sclera what is the most likely diagnosis: ***(Most Recent Question Dec 2019-20)***

a. Osteogenesis imperfecta b. Rickets
c. Scurvy d. Pagets disease

166. A patient presented with following serum parameters: Normal serum ALP, normal PTH level and increased Ca^+ and PO_4. Most likely cause: ***(Most Recent Question 2019)***

a. Vitamin D increase
b. Hyperparathyroidism
c. Osteoporosis
d. Osteomalacia

167. Marble Schonberg disease is: ***(Recent Pattern Question 2018-19)***

a. Osteomalacia
b. Osteosclerosis
c. Osteopetrosis
d. Osteoporosis

168. A patient presented finger deformity and pain in knee and fingers. In which of the following condition there is involvement of DIP, PIP, CMC (carpometacarpal joint) and sparing of wrist: ***(Recent Pattern Question 2018-19)***

a. Psoriatic arthritis b. Rheumatoid Arthritis
c. Pseudogout d. Osteoarthritis

169. Which of the following is the management for postmenopausal women with osteoporosis: ***(Recent Pattern Question 2018)***

a. Raloxifene
b. Tamoxifen
c. Bisphosphonates
d. Calcitonin

170. X-ray Wrist and hand of a child is given below. There is prominent cupping and widening of growth plate. What is the diagnosis: ***(Recent Pattern Question 2017)***

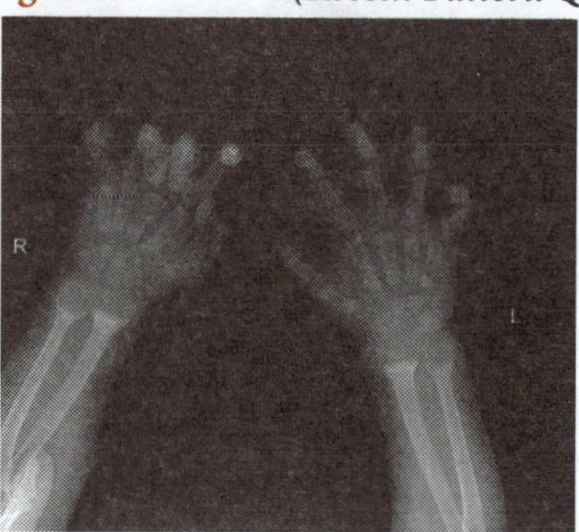

a. Fluorosis b. Plumbism
c. Vitamin C deficiency d. Vitamin D deficiency

171. A case of young patient presents to you with knee pain, irritability and gum bleeding. Upon X-ray of leg, cortex is significantly thin with a white line at the metaphysis. What could be possible cause:

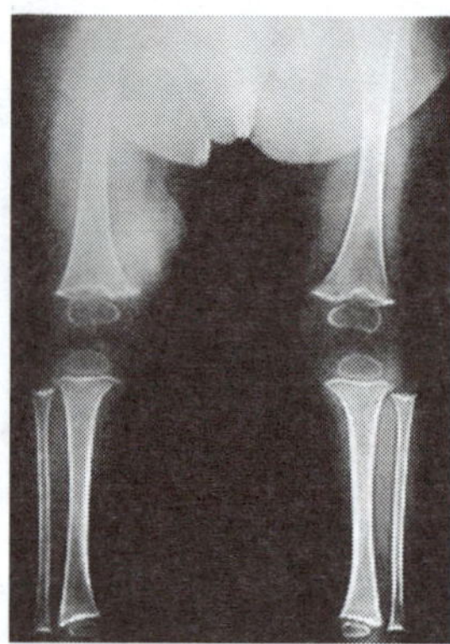

a. Fluorosis b. Rickets
c. Scurvy d. Caffey's disease

172. A 1-year-old breast fed child with excessive crying and gum bleeding and the below shown X-ray is a feature of:

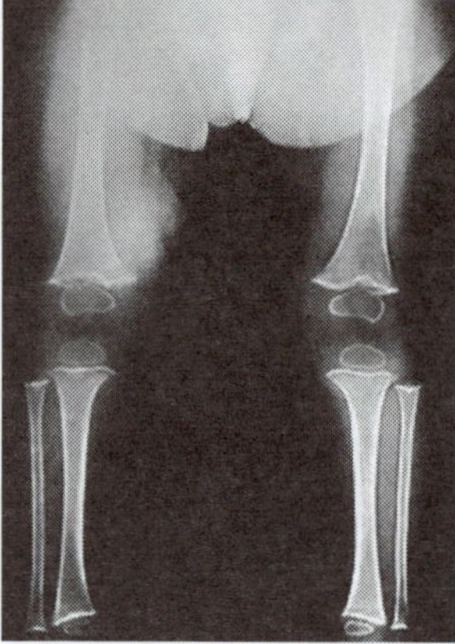

a. Rickets b. Scurvy
c. Kwashiorkor d. Marasmus

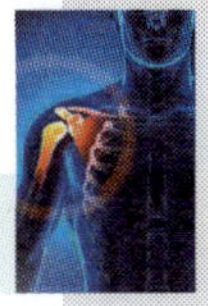

173. A 7-year-old boy presented with double medial malleolus. X-ray was performed. What is the treatment?

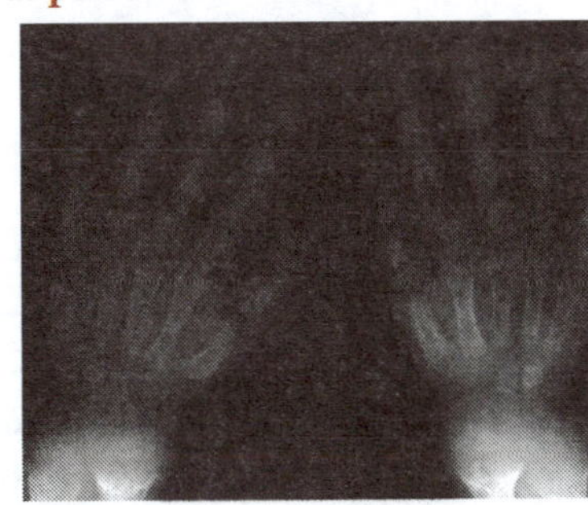

a. Vitamin B b. Vitamin C
c. Vitamin D d. Vitamin E

174. A child from a small village of Bihar has long bone pain, is weak and lethargic and on examination he has bow legs. The X-ray reports shows increase in bone density, osteophytes and dismorphic joint space. Possible diagnosis:

a. Fluorosis b. Rickets
c. Scurvy d. Caffey's disease

175. Osteopetrosis results due to defective

a. Osteoblasts b. Osteoclasts
c. Bone collagen
d. Phosphate deposition in trabecular bone

176. "Bone within bone" appearance is classically seen in

a. Osteomalacia b. Osteopetrosis
c. Renal osteodystrophy d. Vitamin C deficiency

177. Stoss therapy is used for:

a. Scurvy b. Vit D deficiency Rickets
c. Vit D Resistant rickets d. Paget's disease

178. All of the following are true about osteomalacia EXCEPT:

a. Vitamin D deficiency
b. Proximal myopathy
c. Raised serum calcium
d. Bone biopsy shows increased demineralized bone matrix

179. Looser's zones are seen in:

a. Osteoporosis b. Osteomalacia
c. Osteosarcoma d. TB spine

180. Multiple fractures in a child without healing are seen in which condition:

a. Battered baby syndrome b. Hypoparathyroidism
c. Resistant rickets d. Osteogensis Imperfecta

181. Gower's sign is seen in:

a. Gullian barre syndrome
b. Duchenne muscular dystrophy
c. Congenital myopathy
d. All of the above

182. Short 4th and 5th metacarpal is seen in:

a. Pseudohypoparathyroidism
b. Hyperparathyroidism
c. Hyperthyroidism
d. Hypothyroidism

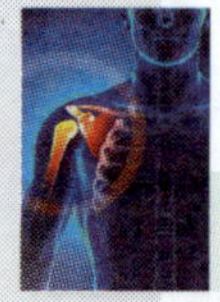

ANSWERS WITH EXPLANATIONS

MOST RECENT QUESTIONS 2023

1. Ans. (b) Radial nerve

- The image shows fracture of humerus shaft and wrist drop. On the humerus shaft, there is radial groove for radial nerve. Any fracture to shaft can lead to radial nerve injury, which presents with wrist drop.
- Radial nerve is a major nerve in the upper arm that supplies sensation to the back of the hand and the ability to extend the wrist and fingers. Damage to the nerve leads to inability extend the wrist.

2. Ans. (b) Scaphoid

- The scaphoid is the most commonly fractured carpal bone. It is located in the anatomical snuffbox, which is a depression on the thumb side of the wrist.
- The scaphoid is a small bone, and it is easily fractured by a fall on the outstretched hand.
- Scaphoid fracture risk arises from its position, between the thumb and radius.

Extra Mile

- Fall on outstretched hand in Pedia: Supracondylar humerus fracture
- Fall on outstretched hand in Elderly: Colle's fracture
- Fall on outstretched hand in adults: Scaphoid bone fracture

3. Ans. (b) Spinal accessory nerve

- The spinal accessory nerve is responsible for innervating the trapezius muscle and the sternocleidomastoid muscle.
- The trapezius muscle is responsible for shrugging the shoulder, and the sternocleidomastoid muscle is responsible for turning the head.
- If the spinal accessory nerve is damaged, the patient will be unable to shrug the shoulder or turn the head.

4. Ans. (b) Cubitus valgus

- The image represents a deformity at the elbow joint, specifically cubitus valgus.
- Cubitus valgus is characterized by an increased carrying angle at the elbow, where the forearm deviates away from the body more than usual.
- It can result from various factors, including prior fractures or developmental issues.

Other Options:

- **Cubitus varus:** Cubitus varus is the opposite deformity, where the forearm deviates toward the body.
- **Gunstock deformity:** This term is sometimes used interchangeably with cubitus varus. It can be seen due to supracondylar fracture of humerus.
- Dinner fork deformity is seen due to Colle's fracture

5. Ans. (a) Genu-Valgum

Ref: Apley's System of Orthopaedics and Fractures, 10th ed. pg. 143

- Genu valgum is a deformity where the knees are abnormally positioned in a "knock-knee" alignment, with the lower legs angling inward.
- This condition is characterized by the medial deviation of the distal femur and/or the proximal tibia.
- It can be caused by various factors, including skeletal growth abnormalities, genetic predisposition, or underlying conditions, like rickets or skeletal dysplasia.
- The treatment approach depends on the severity and underlying cause and may include observation, physical therapy, orthotic devices, or, in severe cases, surgical correction.

Extra Mile

- **Genu-Varus** is a deformity where the knees are abnormally positioned in a "bow-legged" alignment, with the lower legs angling outward.
- **Femur fracture** refers to a break in the femur bone, usually caused by trauma or injury.
- **Muscle deformity** is a general term that does not specify a particular orthopedic condition. It can refer to various muscular abnormalities or dysfunctions.

6. Ans. (a) Osteomalacia

Ref: Apley's System of Orthopaedics and Fractures, 10th ed. pg. 170

- **Osteomalacia** is a condition characterized by softening of the bones due to **vitamin D deficiency**, resulting in impaired mineralization of bone matrix.
- It typically presents with symptoms such as bone pain, muscle weakness, and skeletal deformities.
- In children, the condition is referred to as **rickets**, which can manifest as genu varum (bow legs), osteopenia (decreased bone density), and pseudo fractures (areas of bone demineralization).
- Blood investigations often reveal decreased vitamin D levels and increased alkaline phosphatase (ALP) due to compensatory bone turnover.

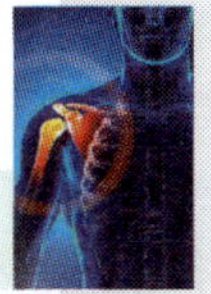

Extra Mile

- **Osteitis deformans,** also known as Paget's disease of bone, is a chronic disorder characterized by abnormal bone remodeling. It typically affects older individuals and presents with enlarged and deformed bones.
- **Osteopetrosis** is a rare genetic disorder characterized by increased bone density due to impaired bone resorption. It is typically present from birth and may lead to various complications.
- **Osteoporosis** is a condition characterized by decreased bone density and increased susceptibility to fractures. Osteoporosis may be associated with decreased vitamin D levels and is mostly seen in elderly patients.

7. Ans. (b) Osteoarthritis knees

Ref: Apley's System of Orthopaedics and Fractures, 10th ed. pg. 100

- The given clinical image shows features consistent with osteoarthritis of the knee joint.
- Osteoarthritis is a degenerative joint disease characterized by the breakdown of cartilage in the joints, leading to pain, stiffness, and swelling.
- It is commonly seen in older individuals and can be associated with factors, such as ageing, joint overuse, obesity, previous joint injuries, and genetic predisposition.
- The characteristic findings include joint space narrowing, osteophyte formation (bone spurs), and subchondral sclerosis (increased density of the bone beneath the cartilage) seen on imaging.
- Treatment options for osteoarthritis include pain management, physical therapy, lifestyle modifications, and in severe cases, surgical interventions such as joint replacement.

Note: Paget's disease is due to bone remodeling; RA presents symmetrically and involves multiple joints while gout mainly involves 1st MTP joint due to high uric acid levels.

8. Ans. (d) Enchondroma

Ref: Apley's System of Orthopaedics and Fractures, 10th ed. pg. 193

- The given X-ray shows a well-defined radiolucent lesion within the bone, which is consistent with an enchondroma.
- Enchondromas are benign cartilaginous tumors that typically arise within the medullary canal of the bone.
- They most commonly affect the small bones of the hand, causing pain and swelling in the affected area.
- Enchondromas usually have characteristic radiographic features, such as a well-defined radiolucent lesion with stippled calcifications (rings and arcs).
- Treatment depends on the size, location, and symptoms associated with the lesion, and options may include observation or surgical intervention.

9. Ans. (a) Osteochondroma

Ref: Apley's System of Orthopaedics and Fractures, 10th ed. pg. 194

- The given X-ray shows a **bony outgrowth** with a **broad base** arising from the **metaphysis** of the **distal femur,** which is characteristic of an **osteochondroma.**
- Osteochondromas are the most common benign bone tumors, typically arising during skeletal growth.
- They consist of a bony stalk covered with a cartilage cap.
- Osteochondromas are usually asymptomatic, but they can cause pain, swelling, or mechanical symptoms when they impinge on surrounding structures.
- Treatment is usually observation, but surgical excision may be considered if symptoms are significant or if complications arise.

Other options:

- **Osteoblastoma** is a benign bone tumor that can cause localized pain, but it typically presents as a larger, more expansile lesion.
- **Osteoporosis** is a condition characterized by decreased bone density, which increases the risk of fractures.
- **Osteitis fibrosa cystica,** also known as von Recklinghausen's disease, is a manifestation of hyperparathyroidism and is characterized by cystic and fibrotic changes in bone.

10. Ans. (a) Colles fracture

Ref: Apley's System of Orthopaedics and Fractures, 10th ed. pg. 797

- The presence of a **dinner fork deformity** following a fall on an outstretched hand suggests a **Colles fracture.**
- A Colles fracture is a specific type of distal radius fracture, where the distal fragment of the radius is displaced dorsally (backward) and radially (outward), resulting in a characteristic deformity resembling a dinner fork after malunion.
- This type of fracture commonly occurs due to a fall onto an outstretched hand with an extended wrist.
- Treatment typically involves closed reduction (realigning the fractured bones without surgery) followed by immobilization with a cast or splint.

Extra Mile

- **Carpal tunnel syndrome** is a condition caused by compression of the median nerve in the wrist.
- **Osteoporosis** is a condition characterized by decreased bone density and increased susceptibility to fractures
- **Smith's fracture** is a type of distal radius fracture where the distal fragment is displaced palmarly (forward) and radially (outward), resulting in a reverse deformity compared to a Colles fracture.

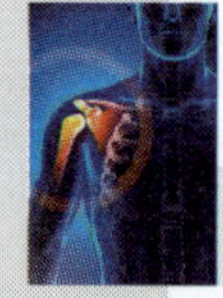

GENERAL ORTHOPEDICS AND FRACTURES

11. Ans. (a) Galeazzi fracture

Ref: Essential Orthopaedics by Maheshwari 6th ed. pg. 111

- The shown image shows Galeazzi fracture.
- It is fracture of distal 1/2 of the radius with dislocation of *distal* radioulnar joint
- **Monteggia fracture** is fracture of proximal ulna with dislocation of proximal radioulnar joint

Extra Mile

Identify these fractures:

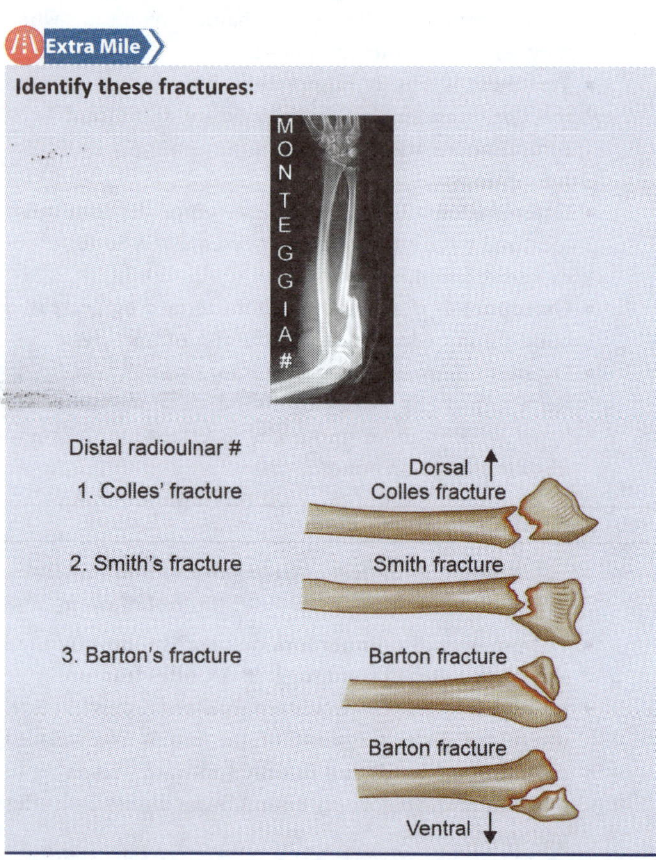

12. Ans. (a) Compare with X-ray of left hand

Ref: J. Maheshwari 6th ed. pg. 97–98

- Supracondylar fracture (SCF) is one of the most serious fracture in childhood.
- **Mechanism:** Fall on outstretched hand → as the hand strikes the ground → elbow forced into hyperextension → fracture of humerus above condyles → Known as supracondylar fracture.
- **Types of SCF:**
  - **Extension type (MC type):** Distal fragment is tilted backwards (extended) in relation to proximal fragment
  - **Flexion type:** Distal fragment is tilted forwards (flexed) in relation to proximal fragment.
- **Diagnosis:**
  - Child brought to hospital with history of fall, followed by pain, swelling, deformity and inability to move the affected elbow.
  - **Radiological investigation:** Commonly diagnosed because of wide displacement. A comparison with an X-ray of opposite shoulder might be helpful in suspected cases *(this is done in some difficult to diagnose cases of minimally displaced fracture due to presence of ossification centres around the elbow)*
- **Treatment:**
  - **Undisplaced fracture:** Require immobilisation in an above-elbow plaster slab, with elbow in 90 degree flexion.
  - **Displaced fracture:** Closed reduction and percutaneous K-wire fixation
  - **Open, displaced fracture:** Open reduction and K-wire fixation.

13. Ans. (a) Atlanto-axial dislocation

Ref: Essential Orthopaedics, Maheshwari & Mhaskar, 6th ed. pg. 3

- The shown image is a case of atlantoaxial dislocation
- Atlantoaxial dislocation commonly present with fracture, as compared to pure dislocation of C1 (Atlas) and C2 (Axis)
- Pure dislocation commonly associated with neurological deficit
- MC dislocation in atlantoaxial dislocation: Anterior
- **Treatment:**
  - Skull traction followed by immobilisation using **Minerva jacket.**

Extra Mile

- **Hangman fracture:** Fracture through pedicle and lamina of C2 vertebra, with subluxation of C2 over C3. This type of fracture seen in hanging.
- **Jefferson fracture:** Fracture of C1 vertebra
- **Clay-shoveler fracture:** Avulsion fracture of spinous process of one or more of the lower cervical or upper thoracic vertebra. Name is given as it is caused by muscular action in shovelling by labourers.

14. Ans. (b) C1 fracture

Ref: Apley's System of Orthopaedics, 9th ed. pg. 813

- **Jefferson's fracture:** Sudden severe load on the top of the head may cause a 'bursting' force which fractures the ring of the atlas.
- There is no encroachment on the neural canal and, usually, **no neurological damage.**

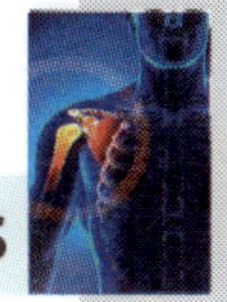

15. Ans. (c) C2 pars interarticularis fracture

Ref: Apley's System of Orthopaedics, 9th ed. pg. 814

- In the true judicial 'hangman's fracture' there are bilateral fractures of the pars interarticularis of C2 and the C2/3 disc is torn.
- The mechanism is extension with distraction.

16. Ans. (d) 3C

Ref: Apley's System of Orthopaedics, 9th ed. pg. 706

- If there is arterial injury that needs to be repaired, regardless of the amount of other soft tissue damage, it is considered as grade IIIC.

Grade	Characteristics of fracture
I	Open fracture with a wound <1 cm
II	Open fracture with a wound >1 cm without extensive soft-tissue damage
III	Open fracture with extensive soft-tissue damage
IIIa	3 with adequate soft-tissue coverage
IIIb	3 with soft tissue loss and periosteal stripping and bone exposure
IIIc	3 with arterial injury needing repair

17. Ans. (a) Intramedullary nailing

Ref: Anderson JT, Gustilo RB. Orthopedics Clinics of North America, 1980; 11:569

- For open fractures like 3B intramedullary nails are preferred over K-wires.
- With the evolution of available nails like antibiotic impregnated nails, intramedullary nailing is now performed even in 3B fractures.
- Although there was initial phobia for the use of intramedullary nails, their usage has become widespread not only in grade 1 and 2 but even in grade 3 injuries.

18. Ans. (b) Volkmann canal

Ref: Wheater's Functional Histology: A Text and Colour Atlas pg. 192

- Basic structural unit of lamellar bone is osteon. These osteons consist of concentric bone layers called lamella.
- Lamella surrounds a long passageway/central canal, known as **Haversion canal** aka longitudinal canal *(a neurovascular canal).*
- These haversian canals are joined by a transverse canal known as **Volkmann canal** *(see image)*. The neurovascular bundles connects the endosteum from periosteum via this volkmann canal.

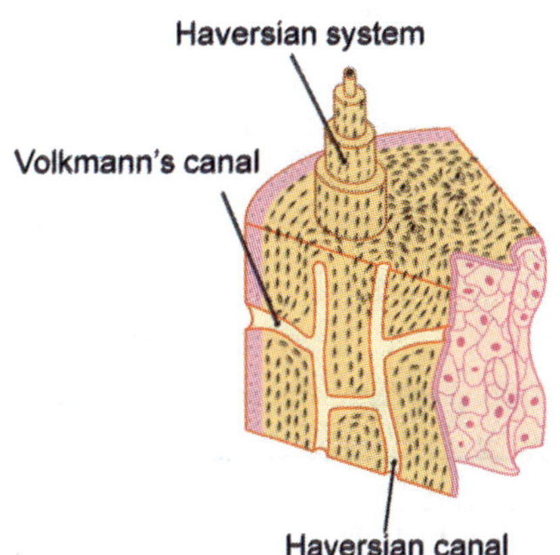

19. Ans. (a) Metatarsals

Ref: Essential Orthopedics Maheshwari, 5th ed. pg. 167

- Stress fractures often develop from overuse, such as from high-impact sports like distance running or basketball.
- Most stress fractures occur in the weight-bearing bones of the foot and lower leg. Studies show that athletes participating in tennis, track and field, gymnastics, dance, and basketball are at high risk for stress fractures.
- It most commonly occurs in metatarsals.
- It is seen due to imbalance between load and resistance on the bone.
- **Two types of stress fracture:**
  1. **FATIGUE #:** Increased load, Normal resistance of bone
  2. **INSUFFICIENCY #:** Normal load, Decreased resistance of bone
- **Examples of stress fracture:**
  - **Lower extremity:** March #- 2nd MT > 3rd MT
  - **Upper extremity:** Olecranon #
  - **Note:** MC site of stress # → lower 3rd tibia > 2nd MT

20. Ans. (a) Fibula

Ref: Apley's Orthopedics, 9th ed. pg. 724

The most common site of runner's fracture is distal shaft of fibula.

21. Ans. (d) Surgical repair

Ref: Maheshwari, 5th ed. pg. 88; Disorders of Shoulder: Diagnosis and Management, Volume 1/ 961

- Since best treatment for *lateral third fracture* and dislocation of clavicle is asked, the best choice here will surgical repair.

References State

- *"Distal third of fracture of clavicle accounts for 15% of all clavicle fracture. Non-displaced fractures of the distal*

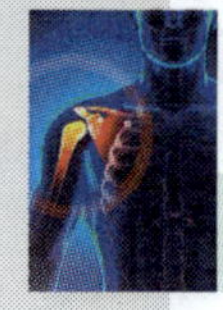

clavice are splinted and treated symptomatically with ice, analgesics and sling."

- Dislocated fractures of the distal third requires surgical intervention because of the rupture of coracoclavicular ligament.
- If displaced fracture is treated conservatively, it may cause non-union

Extra Mile

- CLASSIFICATION used for clavicular fracture → Craig's, Campbell Allman, Robinson's

22. Ans. (d) Calcaneum

Ref: Maheshwari 5th ed. pg. 50, 2nd pg. 41; Adams 9th/62

Common sites of avascular necrosis	Causes
Head of femur	• Fracture neck femur • Posterior dislocation of hip
Proximal pole of scaphoid	Fracture through waist of scaphoid
Body of Talus	Fracture through neck of talus
Lunate	Dislocation

23. Ans. (c) Radial head fracture

Fracture classification

Classification	Used for
• Mason's	• Head of radius fracture
• Campbell	• Clavicle fracture
• Neer	• Proximal humerus
• Bado	• Monteggia fracture
• Melon's	• Colle's fracture
• Garden's/Pauwels	• Neck of femur
• Pipkin	• Head of femur
• Judet	• Acetabulum #
• Tiles	• Pelvic fracture

24. Ans. (a) Clavicle fracture

- Malunion and non-union is always a worrisome complication associated with fractures.
- **Malunion** is when the fracture heals in a deformed position or with limb shortening. It can be due to improper or inadequate reduction. **It can be seen in following fractures:**
  - Intertrochantric fracture
  - Humerus supracondylar fracture
  - *Clavicle fracture*
  - Colle's fracture
- **Nonunion** is when the bone doesn't heal properly leaving the limb with pain and disability. It can be due to poor blood supply, infection.
- Femur neck #, Scaphoid #

UPPER LIMB

25. Ans. (b) Scaphoid fracture

Ref: Essential Orthopedics: Principles and Practice, Manish Kumar Varshney, 1st ed. pg. 1649

- In Scaphoid fracture, the cast is applied in a glass holding position.
- Scaphoid fractures that are closer to the thumb usually heal in a matter of weeks with proper protection and restricted activity. This part of the scaphoid bone has a good blood supply, which is necessary for healing.

26. Ans. (b) Junction of lateral 1/3rd and medial 2/3rd

Ref: Essential Orthopedics: Principles and Practice, Manish Kumar Varshney, 1st ed. pg. 1085

- The clavicle is one of the most *fractured* bones in the body. A clavicle fracture is common in children after a collision or fall onto the shoulder. These most commonly occur at the junction of lateral 1/3rd and medial 2/3rd of the bone, with the vast majority healing well without intervention beyond sling immobilization.

27. Ans. (c) Cock up splint

Ref: Essential Orthopedics: Principles and Practice, Manish Kumar Varshney, 1st ed. pg. 1746

- The shown image is of cock-up splint
- Cock-up splint helps to hold the wrists and hands "cocked-up" in a single position and immobilize the wrist during healing of wrist injuries.

28. Ans. (a) 0–15 degree of shoulder abduction

Ref: Essential Orthopedics: Principles and Practice, Manish Kumar Varshney, 1st ed. pg. 1014

- Supraspinatus tendinopathy in most cases caused by an impingement of the supraspinatus tendon on the acromion as it passes between the acromion and the humeral head.
- Pain when raising the arm forward, sideways, or above shoulder height as supraspinatus is responsible for 0–15 degrees of shoulder abduction.

29. Ans. (c) Radio ulnar synostosis

Ref: Maheshwari and Mhaskar's Essential Orthopaedics 6th ed. pg. 225

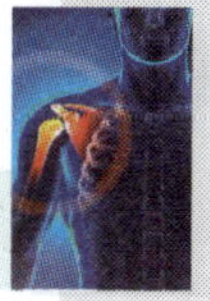

- The shown X-ray is of Radio ulnar synostosis.
- In this condition the forearm bones are joined together at the proximal end, thus preventing the forearm rotation.

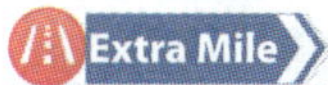

Extra Mile

- **Madelung's deformity:** Defective growth of distal radius epiphysis causing deformity of radius distal end

30. Ans. (c) Capitellum

Ref: Maheshwari and Mhaskar's Essential Orthopaedics 6th ed. pg. 107

- The shown structure in image is capitulum.
- Students are advised to know these structures in radiological image.

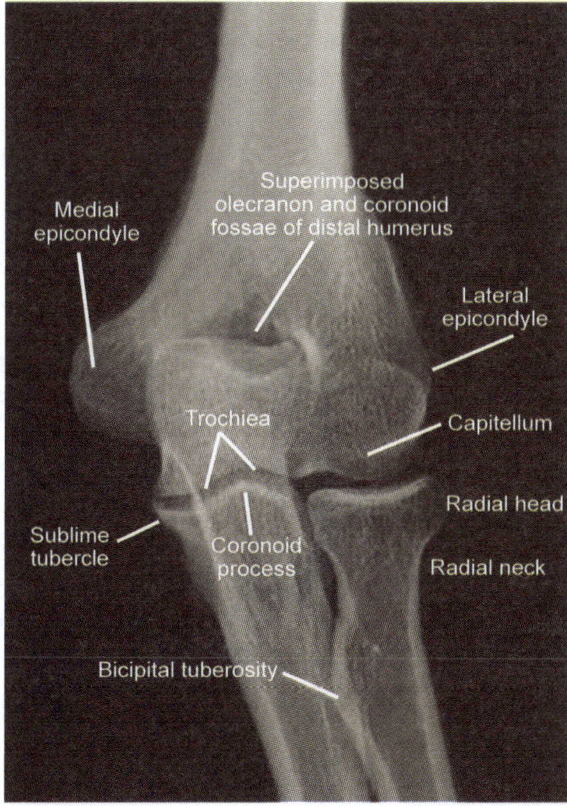

Extra Mile

- Structures around elbow and its ossification (Mn: CRITOE)

• Capitulum	2 years
• Radius head	4 years
• Internal/Medial malleolus	6 years
• Trochlea	8 years
• Olecranon	10 years
• Outer/lateral malleolus	12 years

31. Ans. (a) Elbow fracture

Ref: J. Maheshwari 6th ed. pg. 107

- Three point bony relation is made with medial malleolus, lateral malleolus and olecranon process
- This three point relationship comes in a horizontal line if elbow is extended.
- In olecranon fracture this three point bony relation is disrupted
- In supracondylar fracture, three point bony relation is maintained

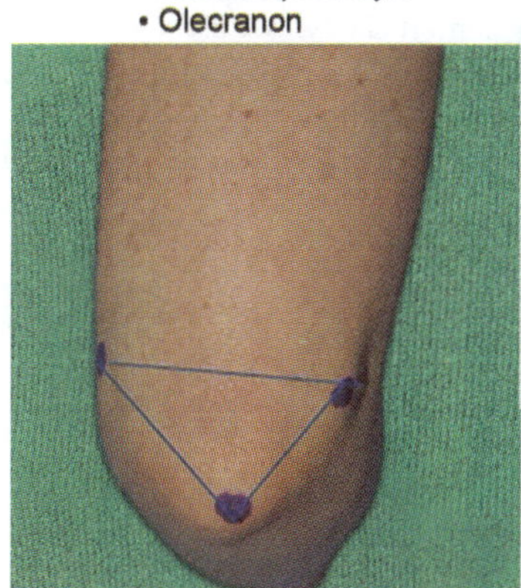

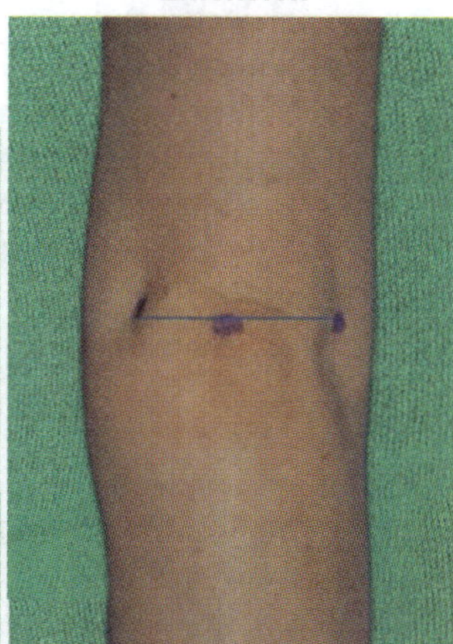

32. Ans. (d) Open reduction with Tension band wiring

Ref: J. Maheshwari 6th ed. pg. 105-106

- Olecranon fracture is commonly seen in adults due to direct injury after a fall onto the point of elbow.
- It can be of three types:

Fracture type	Treatment
Type I: Crack without displacement of fragments	Immobilize the elbow with an above elbow plaster slab in 30 degree of flexion
Type II: Clean break with separation of fragments	Open reduction and internal fixation using the technique of tension-band wiring. It is NOT possible to keep the fragments together in the plaster alone because of constant pull exerted by triceps
Type III: Comminuted fracture	**If not separated:** Treated in a plaster slab **If fragments are separated:** Tension band wiring or excision of fragments may be required.

33. Ans. (a) Recurrent anterior shoulder dislocation

Ref: Essential Orthopaedics, Maheshwari & Mhaskar, 6th ed. pg. 89-90

- **Most common joint dislocation in body:** Shoulder dislocation

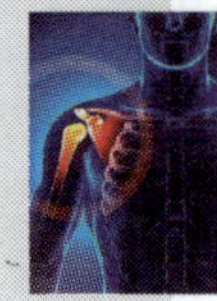

- **MC type of shoulder dislocation:** Anterior
- **Shoulder instability:** Head of the humerus is NOT stable in the glenoid. It can present with:
  - **Loose shoulder/minor shoulder instability:** Patient present with pain in shoulder upon using it. Pain occurs as a result of stretching of capsule, as the head moves out, without actual dislocation
  - **Frank dislocation:** Patient presents with abnormal movement of the head of humerus → partial movement → gets spontaneously reduced or dislocated
- **Mechanism of injury:**
  - **MC:** Fall on outstretched hand with the shoulder abducted and externally rotated.
  - Direct force (as seen in tennis player) pushing humerus head from glenoid cavity.
- **Classification of anterior shoulder dislocation:**
  - **Preglenoid:** Head of humerus lies in front of glenoid
  - **Subcoracoid: MC type;** head lies below the coracoid process
  - **Subclavicular:** Head lies below the clavicle

Extra Mile

- **Posterior shoulder dislocation** is associated with epileptiform convulsion or as a consequence of electric shock.
- **Luxatio Erecta** - inferior dislocation. Rare type of shoulder dislocation. Head comes to lie in the subglenoid position.
- **Hill–Sachs lesion**, also **Hill-Sachs fracture**, is a cortical depression in the **posterolateral** head of the humerus bone. It is seen in anterior shoulder dislocation.
- **Reverse Hill Sach's lesion** is due to posterior shoulder dislocation. Micro avulsion is seen on **antero-medial** aspect of humeral head.
- **Bankart lesion** is avulsion of anterior glenoid labrum.

34. Ans. (c) Distal interphalangeal joint

Ref: Colour Atlas of Clinical Pharmacology by N Bellamy, pg. 60

- *Heberden's arthropathy/node* is a form of joint pathology seen in osteoarthritis and involves distal interphalangeal joint.
- Another similar pathological involvement of proximal interphalangeal joint in osteoarthritis is known as *Bouchard's nodes.*

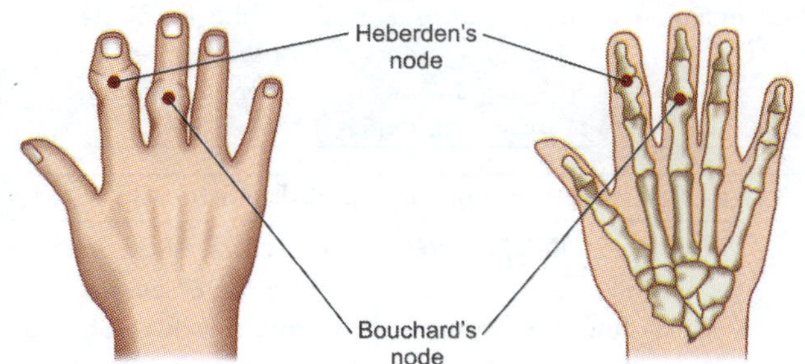

Extra Mile

TABLE: Joint involvement in several conditions

	Osteoarthritis	Rheumatoid arthritis	Psoriatic arthritis
Joint involved	PIP DIP and 1st carpometacarpal joint (1st CMC) Knee	• PIP • MCP • Wrist	• DIP • PIP and any other joints
Joint spared	MCP and wrist	DIP	Any

35. Ans. (b) Extensor carpi radialis brevis and longus

Ref: Hand and Wrist edited by James R. Doyle. pg. 94

- Second compartment of the wrist **contains two muscles namely: Extensor carpi radialis longus and extensor carpi radialis brevis.**
- On the other hand 1st dorsal compartment of hand contains muscles like abductor pollicis longus and extensor pollicis brevis.

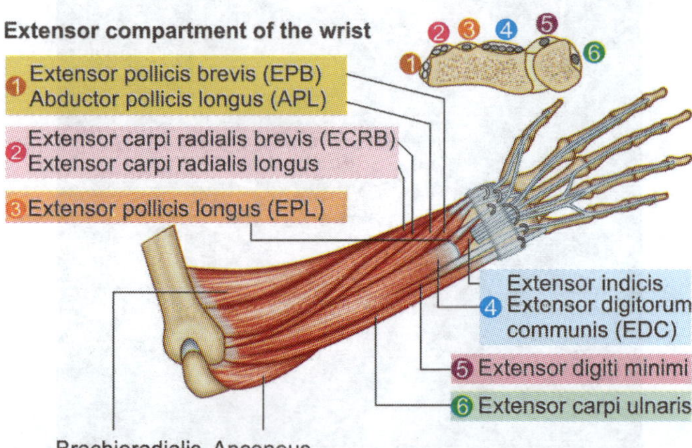

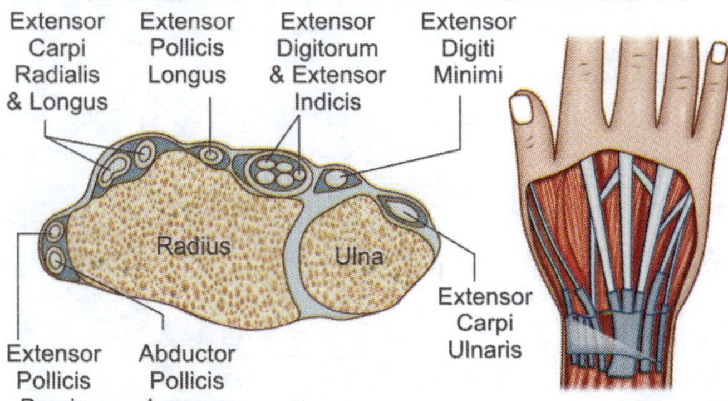

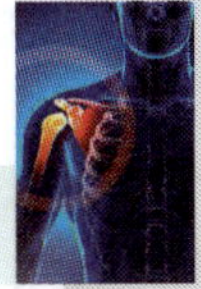

36. Ans. (b) Posterior dislocation

Ref. The Shoulder volume 1, Charles A Rockwood, pg. 151

- Electrical injury is a rare cause of posterior shoulder dislocation. Injury mechanism in electrical injury is similar to epileptic seizures, where the shoulder is forced to internal rotation, flexion and adduction.
- Posterior dislocation is seen in 2–4% patients.
- It is usually seen after electric shock, epileptic seizure, extreme trauma known as triple E syndrome.

37. Ans. (d) Elbow dislocation with radial head and coronoid fracture

Ref: Mastering Orthopedic techniques: Intra-articular Fractures by Rajesh Malhotra, pg. 149

Terrible triad of elbow includes/aka terrible triad of Hotchkiss

- Elbow dislocation
- Radial head fracture
- Coronoid fracture
  - It is called terrible because after this fracture, the joint becomes extremely unstable and fracture segments are usually quite small and hence difficult to repair.
  - In this type of injury there is recurrent instability of elbow joint.
  - This injury almost always requires surgical intervention. Non-operative treatment of this injury results in severe joint stiffness and a non-functional elbow range of motion.

38. Ans. (c) Most common type is extension type

Ref: Rockwood and Wilkins' Fractures in Children, Volume 3, pg. 489

- Supracondylar fracture is mostly seen among child age group due to fall on outstretched hand.
- Males are more commonly affected than females
- Well known complications of supracondylar fracture are:
  - Anterior interosseous nerve damage
  - Malunion of union → can cause **gun stock deformity.**
- There are two types of supracondylar fracture, based on location of its distal fragment:
  - **Extension type (MC type 75–80%):** Distal fragment displaced in posterior aspect
  - **Flexion type:** Distal fragment displaced in volar aspect.

39. Ans. (d) Radial

TABLE: Shoulders pathology and nerve involved:

Fracture	Nerve involved
• Anterior shoulder dislocation	Axillary Nerve
• Surgical neck humerus #	Axillary Nerve
• Humerus shaft #	Radial nerve
• Supracondylar #	Anterior Interosseous Nerve > Median Nerve
• Cubitus valgus	Tardy ulnar nerve palsy
• Medial condyle humerus #	Ulnar nerve

40. Ans. (c) Median nerve

TABLE: Entrapment syndromes

Entrapment syndrome	Nerve involved
Carpal tunnel syndrome aka Pronator syndrome	• Median nerve (at wrist) Median nerve (proximally compressed beneath – ligament of struthers, bicipital aponeurosis or origins of pronator teres or flexor digitorum superficialis)
Cubital tunnel syndrome/ Guyon's canal syndrome	• Ulnar nerve (between two heads of flexor carpi ulnaris or arcade of struthers) • Ulnar nerve (at wrist)
Tarsal tunnel syndrome	Posterior tibial nerve (behind & below medial malleolus)
Thoracic outlet syndrome	Lower trunk of brachial plexus, (C8 & T1) & subclavian vessels (between clavicle & first rib)
Meralgia parasthetica	Lateral cutaneous nerve of thigh
Morton's metatarsalgia	Interdigital nerve compression (usually of 3rd, 4th toe)

41. Ans. (c) Negative pressure in glenoid cavity

Ref: Maheshwari, 5th ed. pg. 87

- Shoulder joint is the most mobile joint of the body. Being the most mobile, it is also stable at its position. This can be due to following factors.

TABLE: Static stabilizer vs dynamic stabilizer of shoulder joint

Static stabilizer	Dynamic stabilizer (SITS)
• Glenoid labrum • Glenohum ligament • Negative pressure in glenoid cavity	• Supraspinatus • Infraspinatus • Teres minor • Subscapularis

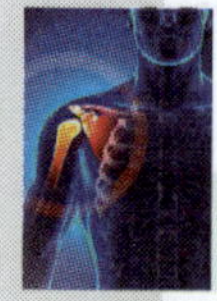

Extra Mile

- **SITS** muscle is also known as rotator cuff muscle.
- **SIT** (Supraspinatus, Infraspinatus, Teres minor) inserts on greater trochanter ***(Mn: SIT on GT)***
- **Subscapularis** inserts on lesser trochanter.
- Tendon passes in intertubercular groove-Long head of biceps brachii

42. Ans. (c) Cannot abduct

Ref: Apley's System of Orthopaedics & Fractures, 8th ed. pg. 281–82

In case of supraspinatus injury, abduction is restricted.

Function of Rotator Cuff Muscle

- **Supraspinatus:** Assists deltoid in *abduction of arm* by fixing head of humerus against the glenoid cavity.
- **Infraspinatus & Teres minor:** *Laterally (externally) rotates arm* & stabilizes the shoulder joint.
- **Subscapularis:** Internal rotation

43. Ans. (a) Axillary nerve

Ref: Maheshwari, 5th ed. pg. 91

- The shoulder is the most frequently dislocated joint. It moves almost without restriction but pays the price of stability. The shoulder's integrity is maintained by the gleno-humeral joint capsule, the cartilaginous glenoid labrum (which extends the shallow glenoid fossa), and muscles of the rotator cuff.
- ***Anterior dislocations occur in as many as 98% of cases. Anterior displacement of the humeral head is the most common dislocation seen by emergency physicians.***
- An inferior shoulder dislocation is the least common form of shoulder dislocation. The condition is also called luxatio erecta because the arm appears to be permanently held upward or behind the head, in fixed abduction. It is caused by a hyper-abduction of the arm that forces the humeral head against the acromion.

44. Ans. (c) Coracobrachialis

Ref: Maheshwari, 5th ed. pg. 88

- Glenohumeral joint is *the most important joint of shoulder complex.*
- It is a *synovial ball and socket* articulation between the head of the humerus and glenoid cavity of scapula.
- Movements at this joint includes *flexion, extension, abduction, adduction, medial rotation, lateral rotation and circumduction.*
- Posterior dislocation of glenohumeral (shoulder) joint would be prevented by the muscle which originate posteriorly and inserted anteriorly.
  - **For example: Corachobrachialis muscle** originate from **Coracoid process of scapula** and inserted at Medial aspect of shaft of humerus.
- The net vector of pull of this muscle would be anteriorly, opposing the posterior dislocation of shoulder joint.

Origin & Insertions of Muscles Around Shoulder Joint:

Muscle	Origin	Insertion
Deltoid	Ant. Fibres- Lateral 1/3rd of anterior border of clavicle Middle Fibres- Lateral border of acromion Posterior Fibres-Lower lip of crest of spine	Deltoid Tuberosity of humerus
Coracobra-chialis	Coracoid process of scapula	Medial aspect of shaft of humerus
Latissimus dorsi	Posterior 1/3rd of iliac crest, lumbar fascia, spine of lower 6 thoracic vertebrae, lower 4 ribs inferior angle of scapula	Floor of bicipital groove
Biceps	**Long head:** Supra glenoid tubercle of scapula **Short head:** Coracoids process of scapula	Tuberosity of radius

The classical clinical feature of posterior dislocation of shoulder is- ***arm is held in medial rotation and is locked in that position***, and an examiner can not externally rotate it.

45. Ans. (d) Bryant's test

Ref: Practical Orthopedics, 2th ed. pg. 479

Tests for Shoulder Dislocation can be Memorized by Simple Mnemonic: B.D.C.H.

- **Bryants test:** Look at the axillary fat fold on the dislocated side. It is displaced inferiorly if compared to normal side.
- **Dugas test:** Instruct the patient to put the hand on opposite shoulder, then bring the elbow close to chest. Inability to perform it, means positive test.
- **Callaways test:** Check for the circumference of dislocated shoulder and compare it with normal side. Circumference on dislocated side will be more than that of normal side.
- **Hamilton ruler test:** If a ruler is placed on upper arm, its two ends can easily touch the acromion and lateral condyle in a straight line. In normal person it will not be possible due to humeral head prominence.

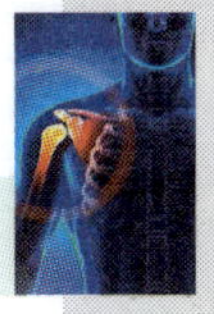

46. Ans. (c) Shoulder Dislocation

Ref: Maheshwari, 5th ed. pg. 90

- A **Hill-Sachs lesion**, also **Hill-Sachs fracture**, is a cortical depression in the **postero-lateral** head of the humerus bone.
- It is seen in anterior shoulder dislocation due to forceful impaction of the humeral head against the antero-inferior glenoid rim.

Extra Mile

- **Reverse Hill Sach's lesion** is due to posterior shoulder dislocation. Micro avulsion is seen on **antero-medial** aspect of humeral head.
- **Bankart lesion** is avulsion of anterior glenoid labrum.

47. Ans. (c) Extensor policis longus

Ref: Apley's, 9th ed. pg. 772–74

- Colle's fracture is a fracture of distal radius at corticocancellous junction with dorsal displacement of distal segment.
- **Mechanism of injury:** Fall on outstretched hand with wrist in hyperextension.

Complication of Colle's

- **Joint stiffness-most common**
- Malunion- 2nd most common
- Sudeck's osteodystrophy
- **Rupture of extensor pollicis longus tendon:** Less common complication, usually seen after 4th week of injury.

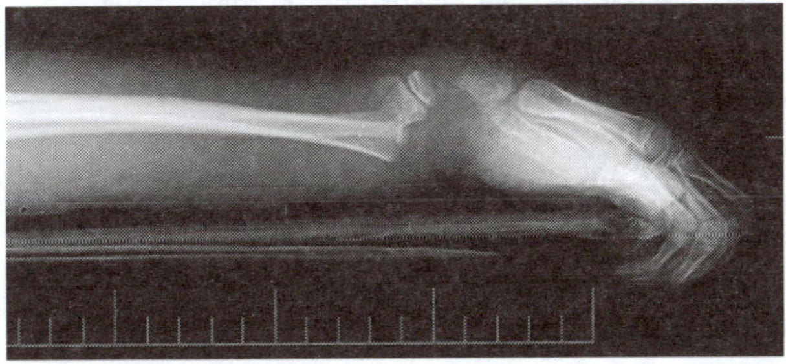

48. Ans. (d) Lunate

Ref: Maheshwari, 5th ed. pg. 318

- It is breakdown of the lunate bone, a carpal bone in the wrist that articulates with the radius in the forearm.
- ***Specifically, Kienbock's disease is another name for avascular necrosis with fragmentation and collapse of the lunate.***
- This has classically been attributed to arterial disruption, but may also occur after events that produce venous congestion with elevated inter-osseous pressure.

49. Ans. (b) Fracture of the proximal third of the ulna with dislocation of the head of the radius

Ref: Maheshwari, 5th ed. pg. 110

- **Monteggia fracture:** Fracture of the proximal third of the ulna with dislocation of proximal radio-ulnar joint.
- **Posterior interosseous nerve** is damaged in case of monteggia fracture dislocation.
- **Cause of monteggia fracture:** Fall on an outstretched hand with the forearm in excessive pronation (hyper-pronation injury).

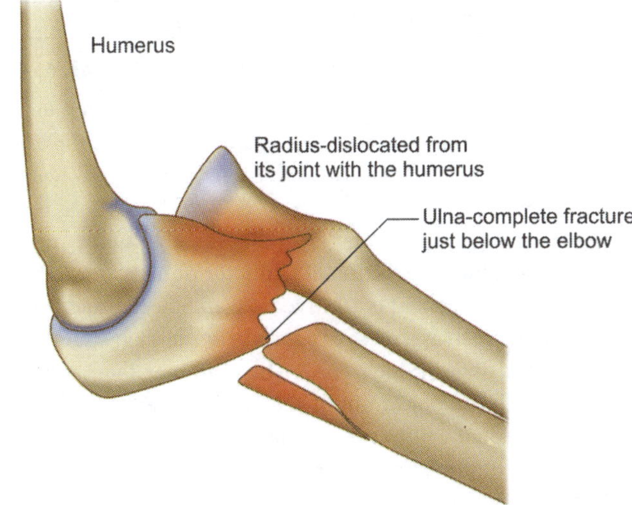

Extra Mile

- **Galeazzi Fracture:** *Fracture of the distal third of radius and dislocation of the distal radio – ulnar joint.*
- Isolated ulnar shaft fractures are most commonly seen in defence against blunt trauma (e.g. nightstick injury). Such an isolated ulnar shaft fracture is not a Monteggia fracture. It is called a **'nightstick fracture'.**

50. Ans. (a) Wrist drop

Ref: Maheshwari, 5th ed. pg. 117

- **Wrist drop:** Due to injury to radial nerve
- **Skier's thumb:** Sprain or rupture of ULNAR collateral ligament. It is due to forceful radial and palmar hyperabduction of thumb, because of snow skiing accidents.
- **Chauffeur's fracture:** Fracture of radial styloid process
- **Mallet finger:** It is flexion deformity of the **distal interphalangeal joint**, due to avulsion of extensor tendon of distal phalanx.

51. Ans. (a) Radial artery

Contents of Anatomical Snuff Box

- **Radial artery:** Only content which runs in groove *(all others are either floor or roof)*

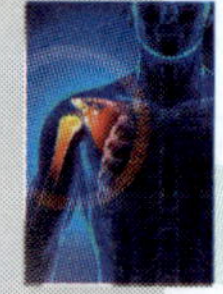

- Tendon of abductor pollicis longus
- Tendon of extensor pollicis brevis
- Scaphoid bone-Floor

Extra Mile

- **Nerve:** Superficial cutaneous branch of radial nerve
- **Partial tear of supraspinatus:** Painful arc syndrome.
- **Winging of scapula:** Long thoracic nerve palsy
- **Frozen shoulder:** Also known as *Adhesive Capsulitis*. In frozen shoulder, all range of motion is restricted. Associated with DM, hyperthyroidism, dupuytren's disease, cardiac disease etc.

52. Ans. (c) Abductor Pollicis longus palsy

Ref: Maheshwari, 5th ed. pg. 65–67

- *The abductor pollicis longus muscle is innervated by the posterior interosseous nerve, which is a continuation of the deep branch of the radial nerve after it passes through the supinator muscle.*
- ***Froment's sign*** tests for palsy of the **ulnar nerve, specifically, the action of adductor pollicis.** To perform the test, a patient is asked to hold an object, usually a flat object such as a piece of paper, between their thumb and index finger (pinch grip). The examiner then attempts to pull the object out of the subject's hands. A normal individual will be able to maintain a hold on the object without difficulty.
- However, with ulnar nerve palsy, the patient will experience difficulty maintaining a hold and will compensate by flexing the FPL (Flexor Pollicis Longus) of the thumb to maintain grip pressure causing a pinching effect.
- Injury of the ulnar nerve at different levels causes varying motor and sensory deficits.

53. Ans. (d) Pain

Ref: Maheshwari, 5th ed. pg. 102

Clinical Features of Volkman's Ischemic Contracture (VIC)

- Pain out of proportion to physical examination findings.
- ***Pain on passive stretching: 1st sign***
- Pressure increased
- Pallor/may also be pink
- Pulselessness
- Paresthesia
- Paralysis

(Pulselessness is a late sign and is unreliable for diagnosis of compartment syndrome)

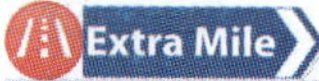

- Nerve involved in VIC: Anterior Interosseous Nerve > Median nerve

54. Ans. (a) Carpal tunnel syndrome

Ref: Maheshwari, 5th ed. pg. 303

Entrapment syndrome	Nerve involved
Carpal tunnel syndrome aka Pronator syndrome	Median nerve (at wrist) Median nerve (proximally compressed beneath–ligament of struthers, bicipital aponeurosis or origins of pronator teres or flexor digitorum superficialis
Cubital tunnel syndrome/ Guyon's canal syndrome	Ulnar nerve (between two heads of flexor carpi ulnaris or arcade of struthers) Ulnar nerve (at wrist)
Tarsal tunnel syndrome	Posterior tibial nerve (behind & below medial malleolus)
Thoracic outlet syndrome	Lower trunk of brachial plexus, (C8 & T1) & subclavian vessels (between clavicle & first rib)
Meralgia parasthetica	Lateral cutaneous nerve of thigh
Morton's metatarsalgia	Interdigital nerve compression (usually of 3rd, 4th toe)

55. Ans. (c) De-quervain tenosynovitis

Ref: Maheshwari, 5th ed. pg. 303

- Finkelstein's test is one way to determine if there is tenosynovitis in the abductor pollicis longus and extensor pollicis brevis tendons of the wrist. These two tendons belong to the first dorsal compartment.
  - **Finkelstein's test** is used to diagnose De-Quervain's tenosynovitis in people who have wrist pain.
  - To perform the test, the examining physician grasps the thumb and the hand is ulnar deviated sharply. If sharp pain occurs along the distal radius it is indicative of tenosynovitis.

56. Ans. (c) Table top test is negative

Ref: Maheshwari, 5th ed. pg. 302

- Dupuytren's contracture is a condition in which the fascia or tissue lining underneath the skin on the palm and fingers becomes thickened and scarred. As a result, the tissue lining shortens and may cause puckering of the skin or limit the ability to straighten the finger joints.
- It is usually an unpainful condition and is usually seen in northeastern European population.
- **Cause:** Idiopathic
- **Most commonly affects Ring finger > little finger. Thumb is rarely involved**

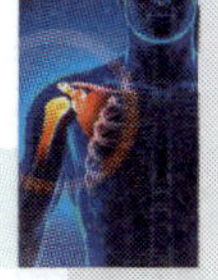

- **Most common joint involved:** Metacarpophalangeal joint > PIP joint
- Table top test involves placing palm on the table, which in presence of contracture would turn out to be impossible. ***Table top test is positive in case of Dupuytren's contracture.***
- No definite treatment but Clostridial collagenase injections have shown excellent results and are becoming the preferred method of treatment for this condition.

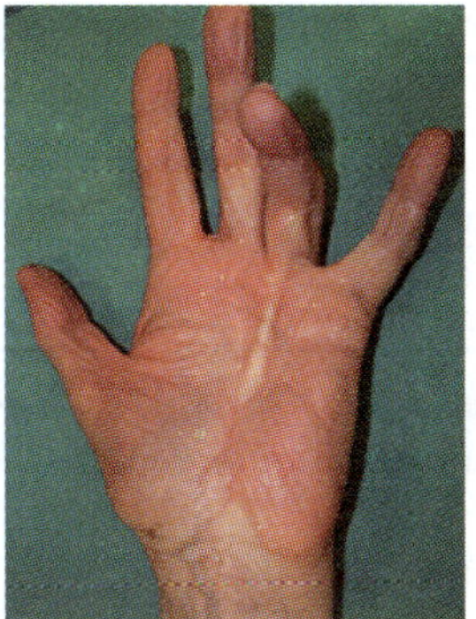

Extra Mile

- **Dupuytren disease** is another disease entity. It doesn't only affect the palms of the hands but it can also involve the back of their finger joints giving a nodule like appearance called "Garrod pads", "knuckle pads", or "dorsal Dupuytren nodules"
- Dupuytren disease can cause lumps in the arch of the feet **(Ledderhose disease)**. In severe cases, it can also involve wrist joint.

57. Ans. (a) Supracondylar fracture of humerus

Ref: Maheshwari, 5th ed. pg. 102; Essential Orthopedics by J. Maheshwari, pg. 98

- Most common complication of supracondylar fracture is malunion, which further can lead to cubitus varus deformity. This is because of the reason that fracture unites with the distal fragment tilted medially and in internal rotation.
- This cubitus varus is usually termed as gun stock deformity.
- Most common nerve damaged in supracondylar fracture: **Anterior Interosseous Nerve.**

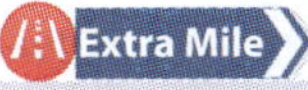
Extra Mile

A pressure >30 mm Hg → can cause compartment syndrome

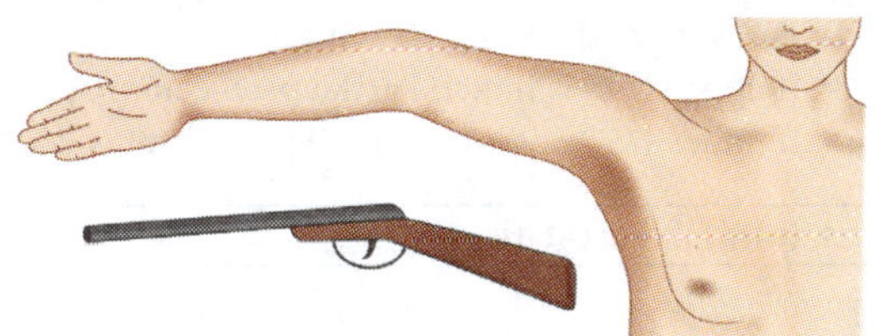

58. Ans. (a) Abduction and external rotation

Ref: Maheshwari's 'Essential Orthopaedics'; 3rd ed. pg. 74

- A fall on the outstretched hand with the shoulder abducted and externally rotated is the common mechanism of injury of anterior shoulder dislocation.
- Occasionally, it may result from a direct force pushing the humerus head out of the glenoid cavity.
- A posterior dislocation may result from a direct blow on the front of the shoulder, driving the head backwards.
- More often, however, the posterior dislocation is a consequence of an electric shock or an epileptiform convulsion.

Pathology (in recurrent cases)

- Bankart's lesion is stripping off (or an avulsion of) fibrocartilage labrum from anterior glenoid and neck of scapula.
- Hill Sachs lesion is compression fracture of postero lateral humeral head due to impression (friction) of glenoid rim which occur during repeated dislocation.

Tests for Anterior Shoulder Dislocation

- **Dugas' test:** Inability to touch the opposite shoulder.
- Hamilton ruler test:
  - Because of the flattening of the shoulder, it is possible to place a ruler on the lateral side of the arm.
  - This touches the acromion and the lateral condyle of the humerus simultaneously.
- **Callway's test:** The vertical circumference of the axilla is increased compared to the normal side.

Management:

- Commonly used reduction techniques are Stimson's gravity method, Hippocratic method and Kocher's method.
- Force direction in other dislocations of shoulder
- Posterior dislocation—Indirect force producing marked internal rotation and adduction.
- So the arm is flexed and internally rotated.

Extra Mile

Positions of leg in hip dislocation	
Dislocation of hip	Position of limb
Anterior	Flexion, Abduction, External Rotation
Posterior	Flexion, Adduction, Internal Rotation
Fracture neck of femur	Flexion, Adduction, External Rotation

59. Ans. (c) Radial nerve

Holstien Lewis Fracture

- The radiograph shows a fracture shaft of humerus.

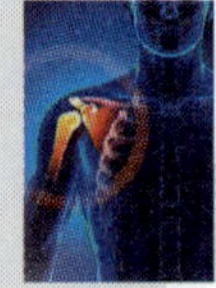

- The nerve most likely to get damaged is radial nerve, as this nerve is very close to the shaft of humerus
- **Holstein Lewis fracture:** Entrapment of radial nerve between fragments in the oblique fracture of distal third of humerus.
- Radial nerve, which is fixed to proximal fragment by lateral intermuscular septum, is trapped between fragments when closed reduction is attempted.

60. Ans. (a) Monteggia fracture

- The radiograph shows a fracture of proximal part of ulna and dislocation of head of radius (disruption of upper radioulnar joint).
- This is called Monteggia fracture dislocation.
- Treatment of Monteggia Fracture

  Acute fractures:
  - **In children:** Closed reduction and Plaster cast
  - **In adults:** ORIF with plate. Radial head reduces spontaneously.
- Old, malunited fractures: ORIF with plate for ulna fracture and radial head excision.

LOWER LIMB

61. Ans. (b) K-wire

Ref: https://radiopaedia.org/articles/patellar-fracture-2 https://www.ncbi.nlm.nih.gov/pmc/articles/PMC4127725/#:~:text=Operative%20fixation%20of%20displaced%20patella,simple%20mid%2Dpole%20patella%20fractures.

- The Modified Anterior Tension Band technique with Kirschner wires (K-wires) is one of the most common methods used for fixation of simple mid-pole patella fractures.
- The tension-band technique involves the use of two Kirschner wires placed parallel to each other and an anterior tension band of stainless-steel wire in a vertically oriented figure of eight pattern.

Extra Mile

- In comminuted fracture, If upper 1/3rd of patella is intact, partial patellectomy is done and if upper 1/3rd is not intact, total patellectomy is done

62. Ans. (b) Posterior dislocation of hip

Ref: Essential Orthopedics: Principles and Practice, Manish Kumar Varshney, 1st ed. pg. 1105

- Posterior hip dislocations are much more common than anterior hip dislocations.
- X-ray findings suggesting of Posterior hip dislocation:
  - Femoral head appears smaller than contralateral femoral head
  - Femoral head superimposes roof of acetabulum
  - Decreased visualization of lesser trochanter due to internal rotation of femur.

63. Ans. (b) Posterior tibial

Ref: Essential Orthopedics: Principles and Practice, Manish Kumar Varshney, 1st ed. pg. 1233

The posterior tibial tendon lies immediately behind the medial malleolus.

64. Ans. (b) Sciatic nerve

Ref: Essential Orthopedics: Principles and Practice, Manish Kumar Varshney, 1st ed. pg. 962, 1105

- Based on the X-ray findings, the femoral head of the thighbone is forced out of the acetabulum toward the rear (posterior dislocation).
- The sciatic nerve, usually the peroneal branch, is most often injured, and this complication can be seen after all types of posterior hip dislocation.

65. Ans. (a) Callus stage

Ref: Maheshwari and Mhaskar's Essential Orthopaedics 6th ed. pg. 10

Stages of Fracture Healing

- **Stage of hematoma:** <7 days
- **Stage of granulation tissue:** Up to 2–3 weeks
  - *Fracture is still mobile*
- **Stage of Callus:** 4–12 weeks
  - *Fracture NOT mobile in this stage*
  - ***Callus** is first sign of union visible on X-ray. Usually 3 weeks after the fracture*
- **Stage of remodelling:** 1–2 years
- **Stage of modelling:** Many years

66. Ans. (b) Patellar fracture

Ref: Essential Orthopaedics by Maheshwari 6th ed. pg. 147

- The shown image is very clearly depicting patellar fracture.
- In a transverse patella fracture, K-wire is used in management
- **In comminuted patellar fracture:**
  - If upper 1/3rd is intact: Partial patellectomy done
  - If upper 1/3rd not intact: Total patellectomy done

67. Ans. (a) Osteoarthritis

Ref: Essential Orthopaedics by Maheshwari 6th ed. pg. 295-96

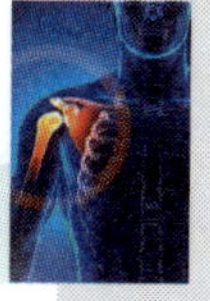

- Pain increasing on movement and bilaterally reduced joint space in elder males are suggestive of osteoarthritis.
- Osteoarthritis is a degenerative joint disease, commonly occurs due to ageing and in post-menopausal females
- **Note**: Joint stiffness in morning which improves upon movement, is feature of osteoarthritis.

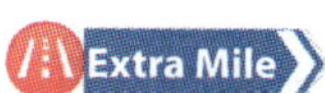
Extra Mile

Haemophilic Arthritis
- Seen mostly in males. It occurs due to a number of bleeding disorders
- Joints affected: knee, elbow and ankle
- May present as acute or chronic haemarthrosis. There are other manifestations of bleeding disorders as well
- **X-ray:** Widening of intercondylar notch in the knee

68. Ans. (b) Medial meniscus

Ref: Essential Orthopaedics by Maheshwari 6th ed. pg. 151-52

- Among the menisci, medial menisci are most commonly injured in sports injury along with medial collateral ligament.
- Overall, most common knee ligament is damaged is anterior cruciate ligament
- **Types of meniscal tear:**
  - Bucket handle tear is most common
  - Others are radial, anterior horn, posterior horn and complex tears.
- **O'Donoghue triad:** Injury to medial collateral ligament, medial meniscus and anterior cruciate ligament occur together.

69. Ans. (a) Medial circumflex femoral artery

Ref: Essential Orthopaedics by Maheshwari 6th ed. pg. 318-319

- Femoral head is mainly supplied by following branches of medial circumflex femoral artery (MCFA):
  - Lateral ascending cervical or retinacular
  - Epiphyseal branches of MCFA
- In avascular necrosis (AVN) of femoral head, following arteries are involved:
  - Medial circumflex femoral artery (most common)-due to fracture of femur neck, or due to hip dislocations
  - Lateral circumflex femoral artery

TABLE: Common sites of AVN

Site	Cause
• Head of the femur	Fracture neck of the femur. Posterior dislocation of the hip
• Proximal pole of scaphoid	Fracture through the waist of the scaphoid
• Body of the talus	Fracture though neck of the talus

70. Ans. (b) Patella tendon bearing brace

Ref: Essential Orthopaedics by Maheshwari 6th ed. pg. 18, 33

- The shown image is: Patellar tendon bearing brace.
- The brace provides adequate support to the fracture while permitting function of that limb, until the union is complete.

Uses

- Foot heel ulceration
- Tibial fractures
- Charcot's joint
- AVN of foot or ankle
- Relief of weight bearing surface in painful calcaneal fracture

71. Ans. (b) Increased in joint space

Ref: Essential Orthopaedics by Maheshwari 6th ed. pg. 194-95

- In the initial stage of TB Joint (Synovitis stage), there is effusion of the joint, causes increased joint space.
- There is apparent lengthening of limb and limb acquires flexion, abduction and external rotation position.

TABLE: Clinicoradiological classification of tuberculosis of the hip

Stages	Clinical findings	Radiologic features
Synovitis	Flexion, abduction, external rotation, apparent lengthening	Haziness of articular margins and rarefaction
Early arthritis	Flexion, adduction, internal rotation, apparent shortening	Rarefaction, osteopenia, bony erosions in femoral head, acetabulum or both. No reduction in joint space
Advanced arthritis	Flexion, adduction, internal rotation, shortening	All of the above and destruction of articular surface, reduction in joint space
Advanced arthritis with subluxation/ dislocation	Flexion, adduction, internal rotating with gross shortening	Gross destruction and reduction of joint space, wandering acetabulum

72. Ans. (c) Tibiotalar joint

Ref: Atlas Foot and Ankle Surgery, 2nd ed. pg. 272

- **Triple arthrodesis** is a surgical procedure done in order to relieve pain in the rear part of the foot, improve stability of the foot, and in some cases correct deformity of the foot, by fusing of the three main joints of the hindfoot:
  - The subtalar joint

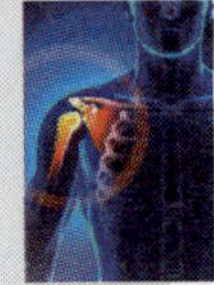

- Calcaneocuboid joint and
- Talonavicular joint.

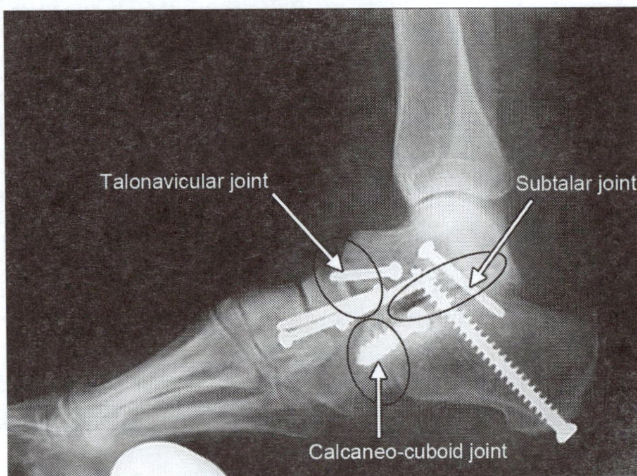

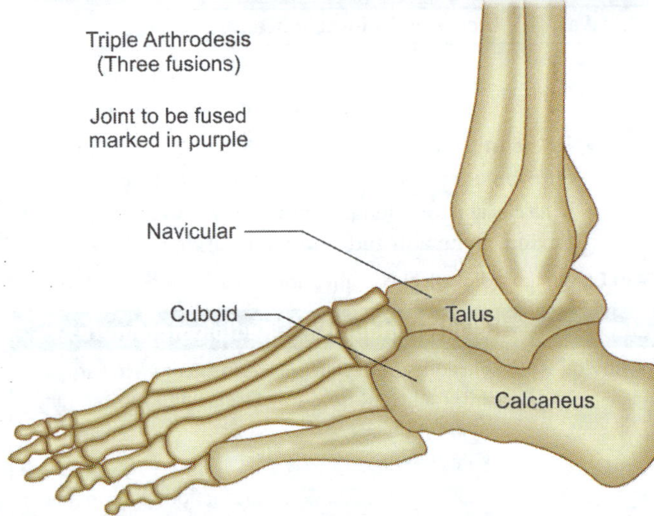

- It is commonly carried out on patients with joint degeneration resulting from arthritis or a severe flat foot deformity.

73. Ans. (c) Ankle fracture

Ref. Rockwood and Green's Fractures in Adults, Volume 1 by Charles A Rockwood, pg. 1980

- Lauge-Hansen classification is a system of categorizing ankle fractures based on the foot position and the force applied.

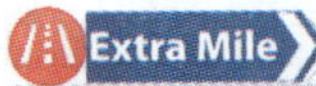
Extra Mile

Some fracture classification nomenclature

- **Femur fracture:** Winquist classification
- **Femur neck fracture:** Pauwel and Garden classification
- **Elbow fracture:** Mayo classification
- **Lateral condyle fracture:** Milch classification
- **Proximal humerus fracture:** Neer classification

74. Ans. (b) Reactive arthritis

Ref: Textbook of Orthopedics by Kotwal, pg. 98

- Triple deformity of knee can result due to spasm and contracture of biceps femoris and tensor fascia lata. It consists of:
  - Flexion at knee
  - Postero-lateral subluxation at tibia
  - Lateral rotation and abduction of the leg
- It is seen in following conditions *(remembered as TRIP)*:
  - TB knee
  - Rheumatoid arthritis
  - Iliotibial contracture
  - Polio

75. Ans. (b) Posterior subluxation of femur

- Triple deformity of knee is seen in TB knee. It includes:
  - Knee flexion
  - Posterior subluxation tibia
  - Lateral roatation
- Triple deformity seen in: (TRIP)
  - TB knee
  - RA
  - Iliotibial contracture
  - Polio

76. Ans. (d) Fat embolism

- **A fat embolism** is often caused by physical trauma such as **fracture of long bone,** soft tissue trauma and burns.

Clinical Feature

- Tachycardia, tachypnea, increased temeperature, **hypoxemia (decreased SpO_2),** hypercapnea, thrombocytopenia.
- **Pathognomonic sign: Petechial rash** on the upper anterior portion of the body, including the chest, neck, upper arm, axilla, shoulder, oral mucosa and conjunctivae.

TABLE: Factors favoring fat embolism

Traumatic	Nontraumatic
• Fracture of long bones e.g. Femur • Reaming • Mobility of fracture	• Diabetes • Fatty liver • Pancreatitis • Sickle cell anemia • Decompression sickness • Extensive burns • Inflammation of bone & soft tissue • Oil or fat introduced to body

Extra Mile

- **Crush injury** is compression of extremities or other parts of the body that causes muscle swelling and/or neurological disturbances in the affected areas of the body, while crush *syndrome* is localized crush injury with systemic manifestations. It is Characterized by major shock and renal failure after a crushing injury to skeletal muscle.

Contd...

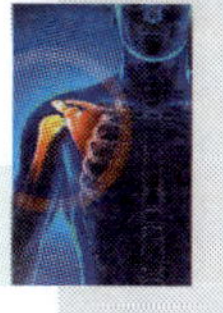

Extra Mile

- **Hypostatic pneumonia** is usually seen in elderly and debilitating patients. It results from infection developing in the dependent portions of the lungs due to decreased ventilation of those areas, with resulting failure to drain bronchial secretions.

77. Ans. (c) Anterior Dislocation of tibia

Ref: Maheshwari, 5th ed. pg. 148-149

- The anterior cruciate ligament (ACL) stretches from the lateral condyle of femur to the anterior intercondylar area.
- ***The ACL is critically important because it prevents the tibia from being pushed too far anterior relative to the femur.*** It is often torn during twisting or bending of the knee.

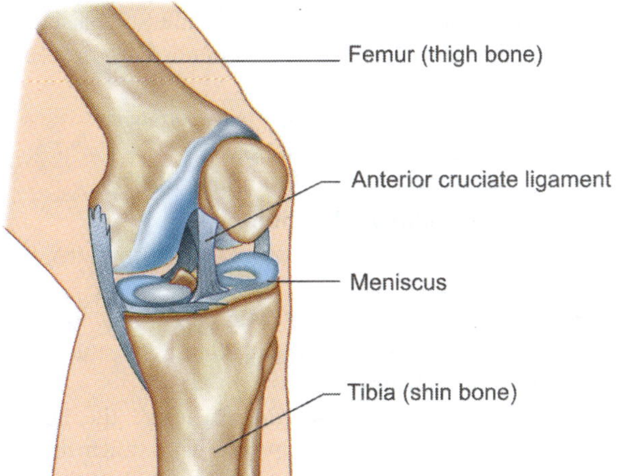

- ***ACL is considered as the major stabilizer of the knee. Therefore, ACL Tears are the most common knee injuries.***
- If there is ACL tear, reconstruction is most commonly done by autograft, meaning the tissue used for the repair is from the patient's body.
- **The two most common sources for tissue are** the patellar tendon and hamstrings tendon
- **The posterior cruciate ligament (PCL)** stretches from medial condyle of femur to the posterior intercondylar area.
- This ligament prevents posterior displacement of the tibia relative to the femur.

78. Ans. (c) Common peroneal nerve

Ref: Maheshwari, 5th ed. pg. 158

- Smaller terminal branch of sciatic nerve, the common peroneal nerve arises in the lower third of thigh. It runs downward through the popliteal fossa (lateral side) closely following the medial border of biceps femoris muscle. It leaves the fossa by crossing superficially the lateral head of the gastrocnemius muscle. It then passes behind the head of the fibula, winds laterally around the neck of the bone, pierces the peroneus longus muscle, and divides into two terminal branches superficial and deep peroneal nerve.
- ***The common peroneal nerve is extremely vulnerable to injury by direct trauma and fractures of fibula as it winds around the neck of fibula.***
- Injury to common peroneal nerve causes foot drop.

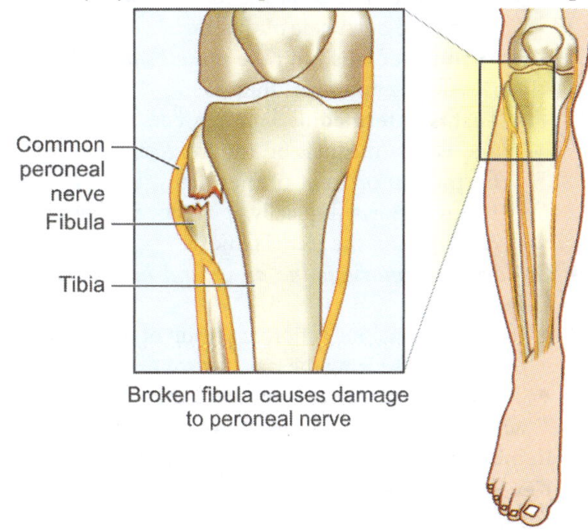

Broken fibula causes damage to peroneal nerve

79. Ans. (d) Fracture of lateral tibial plateau

Ref: BRS: Gross Anatomy, 7th ed. pg. 83

- **Bumper fracture** is a fracture of the ***lateral tibial plateau*** caused by a forced valgus applied to the knee usually by the impact bumper of a moving car on the lateral side of the knee while the foot is planted on the ground.
- This causes the lateral part of the distal femur and the lateral tibial plateau to come into contact, compressing the tibial plateau and causing the tibia to fracture.

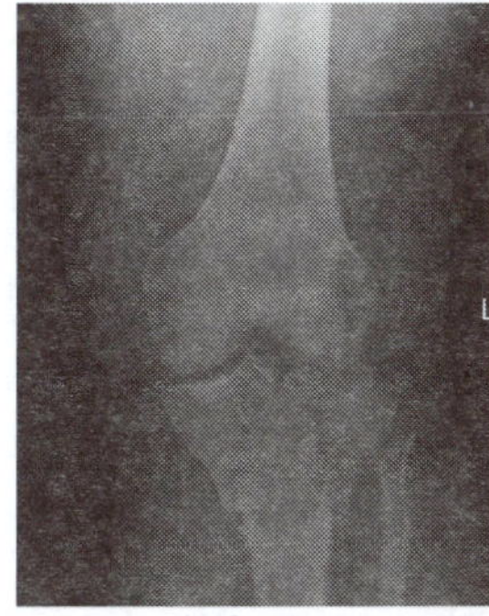

80. Ans. (b) Quadriceps femoris

Ref: Maheshwari, 5th ed. pg. 145

- Quadriceps is a large muscle group that includes the four prevailing muscles on the front of the thigh. It is the great extensor muscle of the knee. It is subdivided into four separate portions or 'heads', which have received distinctive names:

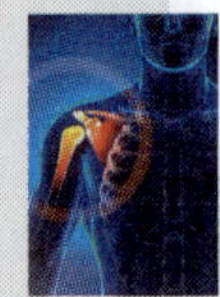

- **Rectus femoris** occupies the middle of the thigh, covering most of the other three quadriceps muscles. It originates on the ilium. It is named from its straight course.
- The other three lie deep to rectus femoris and originate from the body of the femur, which they cover from the trochanters to the condyles:
  - **Vastus lateralis** is on the *lateral side* of the femur (i.e on the outer side of the thigh).
  - **Vastus medialis** is on the *medial side* of the femur (i.e. on the inner part thigh).
  - **Vastus intermedius** lies between vastus lateralis and vastus medialis on the *front* of the femur (i.e. on the top or front of the thigh), but deep to the rectus femoris. Typically, it cannot be seen without dissection of the rectus femoris.
- ***Quadriceps femoris is the main and only extensor of knee.***
  - It produces locking action as a result of medial rotation of the femur during the last stage of extension.
  - To reverse this lock popliteus muscle comes into action and does so by the lateral rotation of femur
- **Remember: Lock is: Quadriceps femoris muscle and, Key is popliteus muscle.**

81. Ans. (a) Patellar subluxation

Ref: Practical Orthopedics, 2th ed. pg. 511

Q angle is the angle formed by a line drawn from the ASIS to central patella and a second line drawn from central patella to tibial tubercle.

- An increased Q-angle is a risk factor for patellar subluxation
- Normally Q angle is 14 degree for males and 17 degree for females

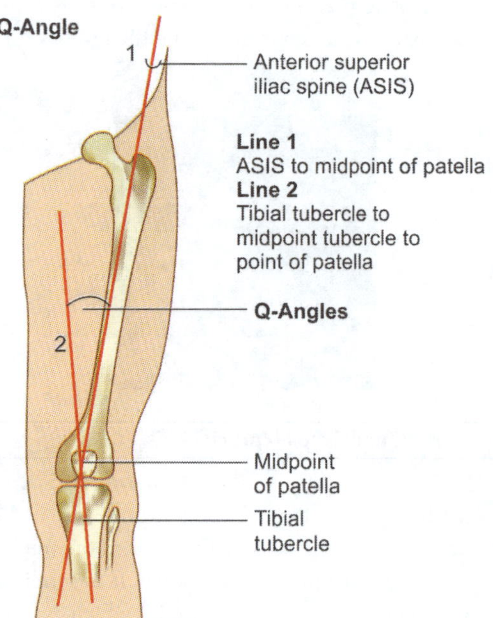

- **Q angle is increased in:**
  - Genu valgum
  - *Increased femoral anteversion*
  - External tibial torsion
  - Laterally positioned tibial tuberosity
  - Tight lateral retinaculum

82. Ans. (b) Shaft of femur

Ref: Apley's 'System of Orthopaedics and Fractures'; 9/e, p-861

Gallow's Traction

- This is used in infants and children with femoral shaft fractures.
- **Indications of Gallow's traction**
  - Child must weigh less than 12 kg
  - Femoral fractures
  - Skin must be intact
- Both the fractured and the well femur are placed in skin traction and the infant is suspended by these from a special frame.
- Vascular compromise is the biggest danger.
- Check the circulation twice daily.
- The buttocks should be just off the bed.

Bryant's or Gallow's Traction

- Do not use for children older than 18 months, best for infant under 1 year.
- Weight limit of child: 16–18 kg.
- Lie child supine with the hips flexed 90°, the legs being pulled directly upwards.
- Apply only enough weight or elevate the infant just enough to allow you to slip your hand under the nappy.
- Gallows traction has been associated with vascular problems, including severe compartment syndrome.
- This is due to the elevated position of the legs, straightness of the knees and tightness of bandages.
- Avoid complications, apply the traction carefully, use adhesive skin traction, allow some knee flexion and don't bandage too tight.

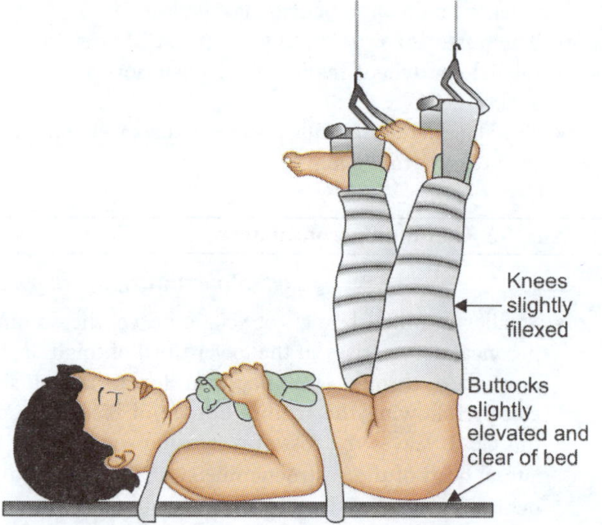

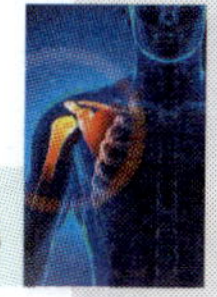

83. Ans. (a) Coronary

Ref Apley's 'System of Orthopaedics and Fractures'; 9/e, p-583

Ligaments Related to Menisci

Coronary Ligaments:

- These ligaments attach the periphery of both the menisci to the periphery of tibial condyles.
- The coronary ligaments of the knee (also known as **meniscotibial ligaments**) are portions of the joint capsule which connect the inferior edges of the fibrocartilaginous menisci to the periphery of the tibial plateaus.
- The coronary ligaments function to connect parts of the outside, inferior edges of the medial and lateral menisci to the joint capsule of the knee.

Meniscofemoral Ligaments:

- These ligaments attach the posterior part of lateral meniscus to the femur.
- These are of two types:
  - Anterior meniscofemoral ligament (Ligament of Humphrey): Runs anterior to PCL.
  - Posterior meniscofemoral ligament (Ligament of Wrisberg): Runs posterior to PCL.

Transverse Ligament:

It attaches the anterior edges of medial and lateral meniscus to each other.

- **Option 'B': Arcuate**
  Arcuate ligament is the ligament between the posterolateral femoral condyle to the fibular head.

It covers the popliteus tendon.

- **Option 'D': Oblique**
  Oblique popliteal ligament is the ligament from semi-membranous to lateral femoral condyle and it is derived from semimembranous.

84. Ans. (c) Grade III

Pipkin classification for femur head fracture (#)

- I-femoral head # caudal to fovea
- II-femoral head # cephalad to fovea
- III-femoral head # associated with femoral neck #
- IV-any of the above with acetabular #

85. Ans. (a) Malgaigne fracture

- **Straddle** #- B/L Pubic rami
- **Malgaigne#** I/L Pubis with ilium near sacroiliac joint. The image shows malgaigne's fracture
- Classification for pelvic bone fracture → Tiles classification

PELVIS AND HIP

86. Ans. (a) 1

Ref: Maheshwari and Mhaskar's Essential Orthopaedics 6th ed. pg. 195

- In the shown image, the shown number indicates:
  - 1 – Acetabulum
  - 2 – Femur head
  - 3 – greater trochanter
  - 4 – lesser trochanter
- Most common site of TB hip is acetabulum, which involves the hip joint and femur head.
- Overall, most common site of bony tuberculosis: Dorso-lumbar spine

Extra Mile

Other forms of Bony TB and their names

- **Spina ventosa:** TB of short bones (phalanges)
- **Caries sicca:** TB shoulder
- **Poncet disease:** TB with polyarthritis
- **Pott's disease:** TB spine

87. Ans. (b) Hip anterior dislocation

Ref: Essential Orthopaedics by Maheshwari 6th ed. pg. 131

- Most common hip dislocation: Posterior
- In posterior hip dislocation position of leg is: FADIR (Flexion, Adduction and Internal rotation)
- In anterior hip dislocation, position is: FABER (Flexion Abduction and External rotation).
- Anterior hip dislocation is rare. It may occur in a fall from a tree when the foot gets stuck and the hip abducts excessively, or in a road accident.
  - There can be true lengthening of limb and femur is palpable in groin.

88. Ans. (d) Internal fixation

Ref: Essential Orthopaedics, Maheshwari & Mhaskar, 6th ed. pg. 138

- In elderly population the intertrochanteric fracture is usually sustained by a sideway fall or a blow over the greater trochanter.
- In young population it occurs due to violent trauma usually due to road traffic accident.
- In the fracture the distal fragment rides up so that the femoral neck-shaft angle is reduced (coxa-vara). In most cases the fracture is comminuted and displaced.

TREATMENT:

- Most of these fractures unite by themselves if femoral neck-shaft angle is maintained. Done by conservative means like traction (require bed rest of 3–4 months).
  - **MC used traction:** Russei's traction

- In elderly population internal fixation is preferred.
  - Prolong bed rest in elderly can cause further complications like pneumonia, bed sores etc.

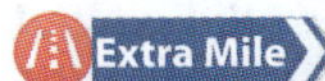

- **Hemiarthroplasty:** Used for femoral neck fracture
- **Hip spica:** Used for femoral shaft fracture (age >2 to 16 years)
- **Gallows traction:** Used for femoral shaft fracture (birth to 2 years)

TABLE: Differences between fracture neck of the femur and inter-trochanteric fracture

	Fracture neck femur	Intertrochanteric fracture
Age	After 50 years	After 60 years
Sex	F > M	M > F
Injury	Trivial	Significant
Ability to walk	May walk in impacted fracture	Not possible
Pain	Mild	Severe
Swelling	Nil	Severe
Ecchymosis	Nil	Present
Tenderness	In Scarpa's triangle	On the greater trochanter
Ext. rotation deformity	<45°	>45°
Shortening	<1 inch	>1 inch
Treatment	Int. fixation always	Can be managed in traction
Complica-tions	Nonunion	Malunion

89. Ans. (b) Urgent Closed reduction

- The shown image is case of posterior hip dislocation
- Posterior hip dislocation is usually reduced under general anesthesia as soon as possible (within the 7 day of injury).
- Most commonly this reduction is done by **closed reduction.**
- **Indication of surgical reduction:**
  - In case of failed closed reduction.
  - If associated with acetabular fracture, making hip unstable
  - Intra-articular loose fragment
- **Complications of posterior hip dislocation:**
  - Avascular necrosis of femoral head
  - Sciatic nerve injury
  - Osteoarthritis
  - Femoral head damage

90. Ans. (b) Posterior dislocation of hip

Ref: Maheshwari, 5th ed. pg. 130

POSTERIOR DISLOCATION OF HIP

- It is most common type of hip dislocation in adults and children.
- Usually this occurs in a road accident when someone seated in car is thrown forwards, striking the knee against the dashboard *(dashboard injury)*
- It is the position (direction) of hip at the time of injury that decides the pattern of injury.

Pattern of injury	Position of hip at the time of injury
Pure posterior dislocation	Flexion, adduction, internal rotation
Posterior fracture dislocation	Less flexion, less adduction (neutral or slight abduction), internal rotation
Anterior dislocation	Hyper abduction + Extension

Classification Schemes for Posterior Hip Dislocations

Thompson & Epstein	
Type I	Dislocations without or with minor fracture
Type II	Dislocation with a single large fracture of posterior acetabular rim
Type III	Dislocation with comminution of posterior acetabular rim
Type IV	Dislocation with fracture of acetabular floor
Type V	Dislocation with fracture of femoral head

Stewart and Miford	
Type I	Dislocation without fracture
Type II	Dislocation with posterior rim fracture (one or more fragments), but the hip is stable after reduction
Type III	Dislocation with fracture of rim producing gross instability
Type IV	Dislocation with fracture head or neck of femur

Type V Thompson & Epstein is Subdivided by Pipkin into Four Types (Pipkin Classification)

I. Femoral head fracture caudal to fovea centralis
II. Femoral head fracture cephalad to the fovea
III. Femoral head fracture associated with femoral neck fracture
IV. Type I, II, or III associated acetabular fracture

Note: *Thomson & Epstein, and Stewart & Milford are posterior dislocation injuries of hip and Pipkin's fracture is fracture of femoral head (& / or neck) in posterior dislocation injuries.*

91. Ans. (c) Adduction, internal rotation, flexion

Ref: Maheshwari, 5th ed. pg. 130

- Posterior dislocations comprise approximately 80–90% of hip dislocations caused by Motor Vehicle Crash.

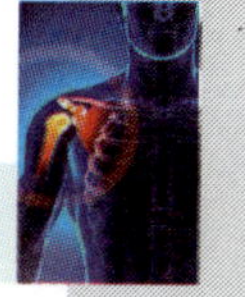

- In posterior hip dislocations, the femoral head goes posteriorly causing the femur to get adducted and internally rotated.
- ***Posterior dislocation:*** The hip is Flexed, ADducted and Internally Rotated (Mn: FADIR)
- ***Anterior dislocation:*** The hip is minimally Flexed, markedly Abducted, and Externally Rotated *(Mn: FABER).*

92. Ans. (b) Cemented total hip replacement

Ref: Maheshwari, 5th ed. pg. 138

TOTAL HIP REPLACEMENT

- Total Hip replacement may be preferrable in patients with *acetabular damage (osteoarthritis, rheumatoid arthritis, AVN), metastatic disease or Paget's disease.*
- Originally the *primary indication* for THR was the *alleviation of incapacitating* pain in patients **older than 65** years of age who could not be relieved, sufficiently by non surgical means & for whom the only surgical alternative was resection of hip joint (Girdle stone resection arthroplasty). Secondary importance is improved function of hip.
- Therefore it is mostly used for hip arthritis *(rheumatoid, ankylosing,* ***osteoarthritis****),* **avascular necrosis of femoral head,** non-union of femoral head and, or neck.

93. Ans. (b) Flexion, abduction, external rotation

Ref: Maheshwari, 5th ed. pg. 130

94. Ans. (c) Flexion abduction External rotation

Ref: Maheshwari, 5th ed. pg. 196

- The tuberculosis of hip mainly progresses through three stages.
  - **Stage of Synovitis (FABER - AL)**
  - Stage of Arthritis (FADIR - AS)
  - Stage of Erosion (FADIR - TS)
- The mnemonics indicate the orientation and appearance of the lower limb during those stages of TB
  - **FABER – AL:** stands for Flexion, ABduction, External Rotation and Apparent Lengthening.
  - **FADIR – AS:** stands for flexion, adduction, internal rotation and apparent shortening.
  - **FADIR – TS:** stands for flexion, adduction, internal rotation and true shortening.

Staging	Clinical findings	Radiologic features
Ist stage of synovitis	Flexion, abduction, external rotation, apparent lengthening	Haziness, rarefaction
IInd stage of early arthritis	Flexion, adduction, internal rotation, apparent shortening	Rarefaction, osteopenia, bony lesion in femoral head, acetabulum or both. No reduction in joint space
IIIrd stage of arthritis	Flexion, adduction, internal rotation, shorting	All of the above and destruction of articular surface, reduction in joint space
IVth stage of advanced arthritis	Flexion, adduction, internal rotation with gross shortening	Complete destruction, no joint space, wandering acetabulum

Contd...

Source: Babhulkar and Pande, Clin Ortho Rel Res 2002

INFECTION & TUBERCULOSIS OF BONE AND JOINTS

95. Ans. (a) Pott's spine

Ref: Essential Orthopedics: Principles and Practice, Manish Kumar Varshney, 1st ed. pg. 1497-1505

- Spinal tuberculosis (TB) or Pott's spine is the commonest extrapulmonary manifestation of TB.
- It spreads through hematogenous route. Clinically, it presents with constitutional symptoms, back pain, tenderness, paraplegia or paraparesis, and kyphotic or scoliotic deformities.
- Magnetic resonance imaging (MRI) is the best diagnostic modality for Pott's spine and is more sensitive than other modalities. MRI frequently demonstrates disc collapse/destruction, cold abscess, vertebral wedging/collapse, marrow edema, and spinal deformities.

96. Ans. (d) Advanced arthritis

Ref: Essential Orthopedics: Principles and Practice, Manish Kumar Varshney, 1st ed. pg. 448

- Tuberculous of the hip joint is common with a frequency of involvement next only to spinal tuberculosis.
- In Early arthritis, there is damage to bone and cartilage of the joint.
- True shortening is associated with advanced arthritis.

97. Ans. (c) Sequestrum

Ref: Maheshwari and Mhaskar's Essential Orthopaedics 6th ed. pg. 172

- Chronic infection of bone more than 3 weeks is chronic osteomyelitis.

- Hallmark feature of chronic osteomyelitis: infected dead bone within a soft tissue (sequestrum).
- **Sequestrum:** Dead necrotic bone due to osteomyelitis
- **Involucrum:** Reactive bone around sequestrum
- **Cloaca:** Draining sinus

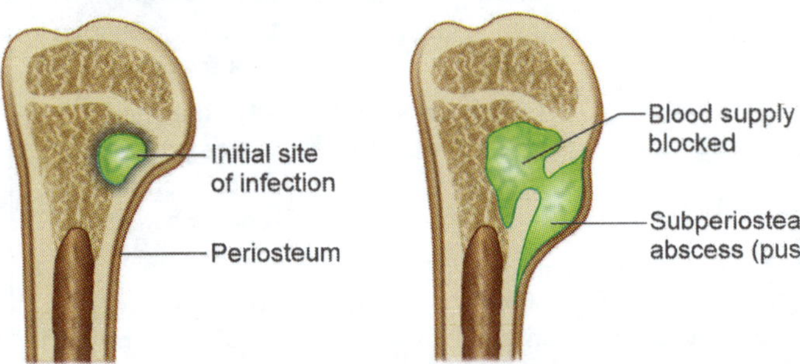

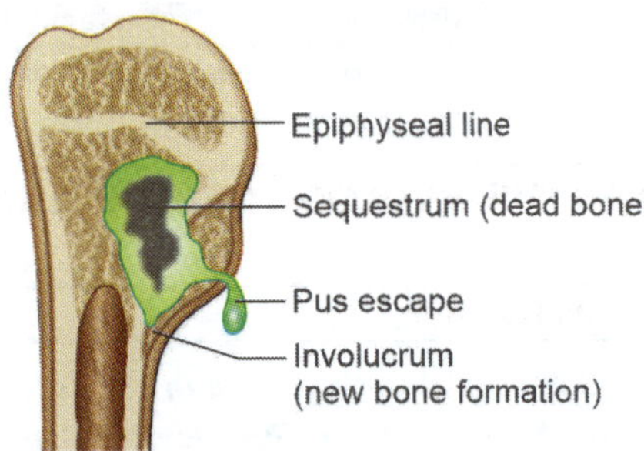

98. Ans. (c) Causative organism is staph epidermidis

Ref: Maheshwari and Mhaskar's Essential Orthopaedics 6th ed. pg. 206

- The shown condition is felon.
- Infected subcutaneous tissue of distal pulp space is called felon or whitlow.
- Most common organism associated with felon: Staph aureus
- Most common site: Thumb > Index finger
- If not treated, the subcutaneous infection can spread to bone and joints, causing osteomyelitis and tenosynovitis.
- Treatment: Vertical incision and drainage + Antibiotics.

99. Ans. (b) Phalanges

Ref: Textbook of Orthopedics by John Ebnezar, Rakesh John pg. 554

- Spina ventosa is a rare skeletal tuberculosis of short tubular bones like phalanges, metacarpals, metatarsals.
- This condition is uncommon after the age of 5 years. It is also known as tuberculosis dactylitis.
- In this condition hand is more frequently involved than foot.
- Due to abundant blood flow through the large nutrient artery, almost in the middle of the bone, the first inoculum of infection, lodged in the center of marrow cavity, leads to spindle shaped expansion of bone called *spina ventosa*.

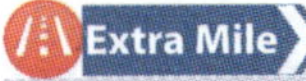

- **Caries sicca: TB** shoulder
- **Poncet disease- TB associated with polyarthritis**
- **Pott's disease**

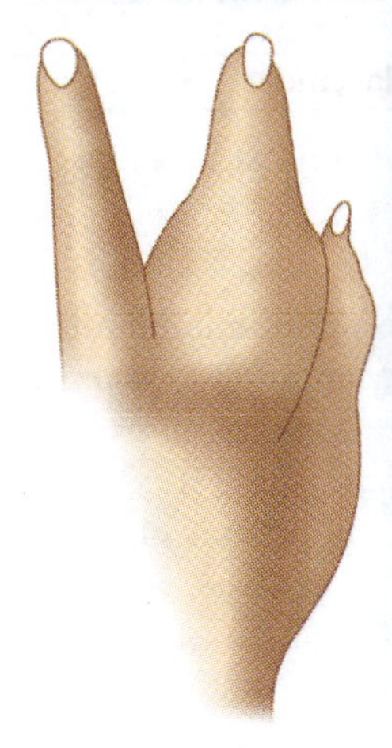

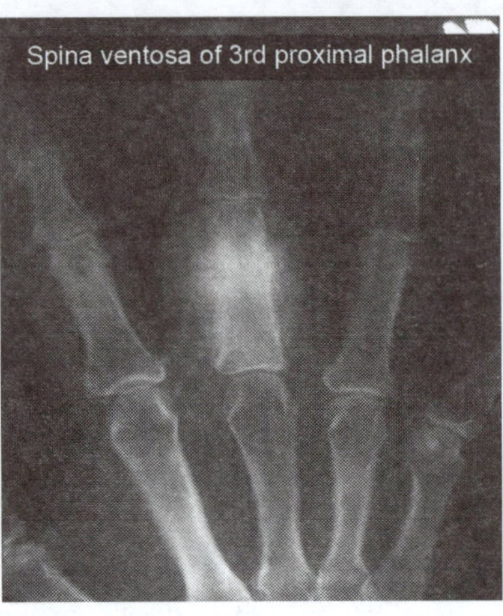

100. Ans. (c) Paradiscal

Ref. Tuberculosis of the Skeletal system, SM Tuli, P 223

- There are 4 patterns of vertebral involvement in Pott's spine:
  - I. Paradiscal (due to arterial spread)
  - II. Central (due to venous spread)
  - III. Anterior (due to subperisteal spread)
  - IV. Appendiceal and articular type (occur in isolation involving pedicles, laminae, transverse process and spinous process or in conjunction with typical paradiscal variant).

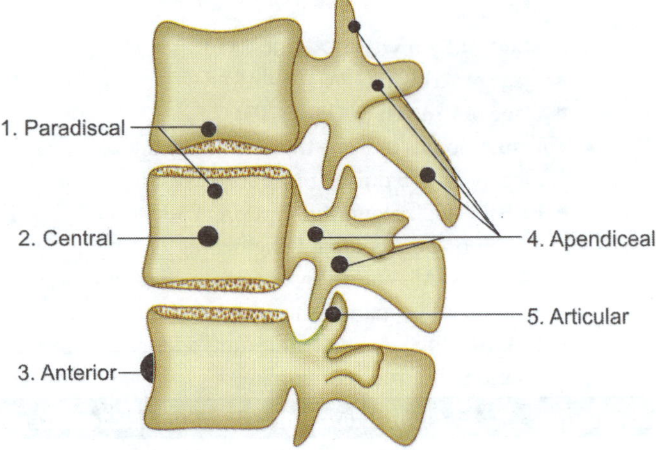

- Paradiscal is the most common type of lesion in Pott's spine.
- It spreads through arterial supply, causing reduced disc space and loss of vertebral margins.

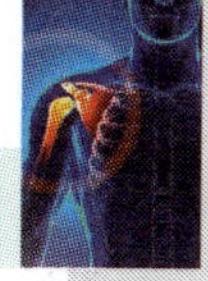

101. Ans. (a) Osteomyelitis

Ref: Apley's System of Orthopaedics, 9th ed. pg. 36

- The given image is a case of Brodie's abscess showing sclerotic margin which can be manifested sometimes in subacute osteomyelitis.

Extra Mile

- Most common bone involved in acute osteomyelitis: Lower end of femur
- Most common bone involved in subacute and chronic osteomyelitis: Upper end of tibia
- Most common organism for osteomyelitis: Staphylococcus aureus

102. Ans. (a) Staph aureus

Ref: Maheshwari, 5th ed. pg. 168

Note that responsible pathogens may be isolated in only 35-40% of infections. Bacterial causes of acute hematogenous and direct osteomyelitis include the following:

- Most common organism causing acute osteomyelitis: Staph. Aureus
- MCC of osteomyelitis in **sickle cell anemia patient: SALMONELLA**
- MCC of osteomyelitis in **IV drug abuser: PSEUDOMONAS**
- MC organism causing osteomyelitis in **open foot injury: PSEUDOMONAS**
- MC organism causing osteomyelitis in **HIV patient: Staph. Aureus**
- MC organism causing osteomyelitis in case of **animal bite: Pasteurella Multiocida**
- MC organism causing osteomyelitis in case of **human bite: Eikenella Corrodens**

103. Ans. (b) Metaphysis

Ref: Maheshwari, 5th ed. pg. 168

- Hematogenous osteomyelitis is an infection caused by bacterial seeding from the blood.
- Acute hematogenous osteomyelitis is characterized by an acute infection of the bone caused by the seeding of the bacteria within the bone from a remote source. This condition primarily occurs in children.
- The most common site is the rapidly growing and highly vascular metaphysis of growing bones. The apparent slowing or sludging of blood flow as the vessels make sharp angles at the distal metaphysis predisposes the vessels to thrombosis and the bone itself to localized necrosis and bacterial seeding.

Extra Mile

- MC site of osteomyelitis in child: Lower end of femur
- MC site of osteomyelitis in adults: Thoraco-Lumbar vertebra (Thoracic > Lumbar)
- MC site of osteomyelitis in infants: Hip

104. Ans. (d) Periosteal reaction

Ref: Maheshwari, 8th ed. pg. 169; Harrison's, 18th ed. Ch 126

- **Earliest X-ray change:** Loss of soft tissue plane which is seen after 24 hours. In case of osteomyelitis X-ray is normal during first 24 hours.
- 2nd X-ray change seen is periosteal reaction, which is usually seen 7–10 days after infection.
- **Periosteal reaction can be of 3 types:**
  - **No reaction:** seen in case of TB
  - **Narrow zone of activity:** Benign condition (Ex: in infection like osteomyelitis)
  - **Wide zone of activity:** Malignant condition (Ex: Codman's triangle in osteosarcoma)

105. Ans. (b) Terminal pulp space

Ref: Maheshwari, 5th ed. pg. 206

- Felons/Whitlow are closed-space infections of the fingertip pulp. Infection occurring within these compartments can lead to abscess formation, edema, and rapid development of increased pressure in a closed space. This increased pressure may compromise blood flow and lead to necrosis of the skin and pulp.
- **Clinical feature:** Felons are characterized by marked throbbing pain, tension, and edema of the fingertip pulp.
- **Causes:** Staphylococcus aureus, is the most common cause.
- **Management:** The felon should be incised in the area of maximum tenderness. The incision should not cross the distal interphalangeal (DIP) joint to prevent formation of a flexion contracture at the DIP flexion crease. Probing is not carried out proximally to avoid extension of infection into the flexor tendon sheath.
- **Complication of felon: Osteomyelitis > Tenosynovitis**

106. Ans (a) Tubercular dactylitis

Ref: Maheshwari, 5th ed. pg. 203

- **Spina ventosa** *("wind-filled sail")* refers to the end-stage radiographic appearance of tuberculosis dactylitis. Cystic expansion of the short tubular bones with bone destruction.
- Tuberculous dactylitis is the painless tuberculous involvement of the fingers and toes and is more common in children. It begins with fusiform soft-tissue swelling with or without periostitis.

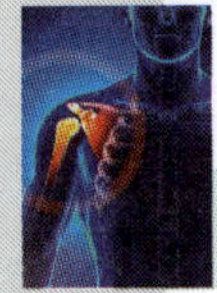

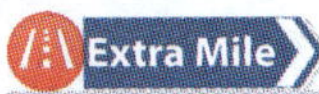

- **MC site bone TB:** Spine > Hip > Knee
- MC site in spine is *Thoracolumbar (paradiscal)*
- **Earliest symptom:** BACK PAIN
- **Triad of TB joint:** *Decreased joint space + articular damage + Juxta-articular osteoporosis*
- **Spina ventosa:** TB of short bones
- **Caries sicca:** TB shoulder
- **Poncet disease:** TB associated with polyarthritis

107. Ans. (b) Medial rotation of tibia

Ref: Practical Orthopedics, 2th ed. pg. 173

- Tuberculosis of the knee is classical cause of triple deformity. It includes:
  - Flexion
  - Lateral (external) rotation of tibia
  - Posterior subluxation of tibia
- Better treatment results are seen with ATT and arthrodesis
- This condition can also be seen in Rheumatoid arthritis.

108. Ans. (a) Flexion, posterior subluxation and external rotation

Ref: Practical Orthopedics, 2th ed. pg. 173

109. Ans. (a) Paradiscal area

Ref: Maheshwari, 8th ed. pg. 185

- **Most common site of skeletal tuberculosis:** TB Spine (50% of cases)
- **Most common site in spine**: Thoraco Lumbar vertebra followed by cervical vertebra (Thoracic vertebra > Lumbar)
- The spinal TB is always secondary to a primary lesion (ex: in lungs) and occurs due to hematogenous spread.
- **IOC for TB spine: MRI**

Clinically there are four types of Pott's Spine

- **Paradiscal lesion (most common)** *begins in the metaphysis, erodes the cartilage and destroys the disc, resulting in narrowing of the disc space.*
- **Central type** begins in the midsection of the body which further gets softened under gravity and muscle action, leading to compression, collapse and bony deformation.
- **Anterior lesions** lead to cortical bone destruction beneath the anterior longitudinal ligament. Spread of the infection is in the subperiosteal and sub ligamentous planes resulting in the loss of periosteal blood supply to the body with resultant collapse.
- **In appendicle type,** the infection settles in the pedicles, the laminae, the articular processes or the spinous processes and causes initial ballooning of the structure followed by destruction.

110. Ans. (c) Septic arthritis leads to bony ankylosis

Ref: Maheshwari, 5th ed. pg. 182

TABLE: Bony Ankylosis vs Fibrous Ankylosis

Bony	Fibrous
• Painless • MCC: Septic arthritis > TB spine	• Painful • MCC: Tubercular arthritis of hip and knee

111. Ans. (b) Bony ankylosis

Ref: Maheshwari, 5th ed. pg. 189

- Tuberculous spondylitis is most commonly localized in the thoracic portion of the spine.
- The infection coming from primary site (i.e: lungs) then spreads from two adjacent vertebrae into the adjoining intervertebral disc space. If only one vertebra is affected, the disc is normal, but if two are involved, the disc, which is avascular, cannot receive nutrients and collapses. The disc tissue dies and is broken down by caseation, leading to vertebral narrowing and eventually to vertebral collapse (Bony ankylosis) and spinal damage.
- From the choices given in the question, the most logical answer is bony ankylosis.
- Actual late complications of Tubercular spondylitis is: Vertebral collapse resulting in kyphosis, Spinal cord compression, sinus formation, paraplegia.
- **Most common cause of bony ankylosis: Septic arthritis > TB spine**

112. Ans. (c) Pain upon passive flexion

Kanavel sign is seen in tenosynovitis... infl of tendon sheath of flexor aspect of hand. It includes 4 components:

- Tenderness
- Uniform swelling
- Flexed finger
- *Pain upon passive extension*

BONE ONCOLOGY AND JOINT DISORDERS

113. Ans. (c) Giant cell tumor

Ref: Maheshwari and Mhaskar's Essential Orthopaedics 6th ed. pg. 237

- Common epiphyseal tumor are *(Mn: ECG):*
  - **Chondroblastoma:** Upper end of humerus
  - **Giant cell tumor:** MC site- Lower end femur
- Giant cell tumor is commonly seen in matured bones, lower end of femur.

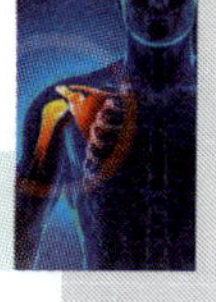

Extra Mile

Some common sites of bone tumors

Additional information: From the entrance exams point of view	
Most common sites of primary bone tumors	
Tumor	Site
Chondroblastoma	Epiphyseal (most common tumor in this region before puberty)
Osteoclastoma	Epiphyseal (most common tumor in this region after puberty)
Chondrosarcoma, osteochondroma, bone cyst, enchondroma, osteosarcoma, osteoclastoma	Metaphyseal
Ewing's tumor, lymphoma, multiple myeloma, adamantinoma, osteoma	Diaphyseal
Most common	
Tumor	Site
Solitary bone cyst	Upper end of humerus
Aneurysmal bone cyst	Lower limb metaphysis
Osteochondroma	Distal femur
Osteoid osteoma	Femur

Extra Mile

Osteoblastoma	Vertebrae
Osteoma	Skull, facial bones
Enchondroma	Short bones of hand
Chordoma	Sacrum
Adamantinoma	Tibia
Ameloblastoma	Mandible
Osteoclastoma	Lower end femur
Fibrous dysplasia	Polyostotic–craniofacial Monostotic–upper femur
Multiple myeloma	Lumbar vertebrae
Osteosarcoma	Lower end femur
Ewings's sarcoma	Femur
Chondrosarcoma	Pelvis
Secondary tumors	Dorsal vertebrae

114. Ans. (b) Ewing's sarcoma

Ref: Essential Orthopaedics by Maheshwari 6th ed. pg. 239-40

- Ewing's sarcoma is the most radiosensitive bone tumor among the given choices.
- It usually occurs in 2nd decade and commonly affects long bones like femur and tibia (diaphysis)
- Genetic defect: *Translocation*
  - t(11:22) → Most common
  - t(21:22)
  - t(7:22)
- **Symptoms:**
  - Pain and swelling of the affected bone and area
  - Systemic symptoms: Fever, anemia, weight loss, increased WBC, ESR and LDH levels.
- **X-ray:**
  - Onion peel appearance, moth eaten lesion, lytic/sclerotic lesion can also be seen
- **Treatment:**
  - It is highly radiosensitive tumor
  - Control of local tumor by radiotherapy (6000 rads), and control of metastasis by chemotherapy.
  - Chemotherapy consists of Vincristine, Cyclophosphamide, and Adriamycin in cycles, repeated every 3–4 weeks for about 12–18 cycle.

115. Ans. (b) Chondrosarcoma

Ref: Essential Orthopaedics by Maheshwari 6th ed. pg. 239, 246

- Chondrosarcoma is malignant bone tumor arising from cartilage cells.
- It can arise in normal bone: primary chondrosarcoma
- Can also arise in pre-existing cartilaginous tumor such as enchondroma: Secondary chondrosarcoma
- Commonly occurs in adult between 30–60 years
- **Symptoms:**
  - Pain and swelling
- **X-ray:**
  - Erosion of the cortex and bone destruction.
  - The tumor matrix may have mottled calcification, typical of a cartilaginous tumor
- **Treatment:**
  - Low grade tumor: Resection with wide margin
  - Amputation necessary in most tumors

116. Ans. (c) Tibia

Ref: Campbell Orthopaedics, 12th ed. P 922; Essential Orthopaedics, Maheshwari & Mhaskar, 6th ed. pg. 237

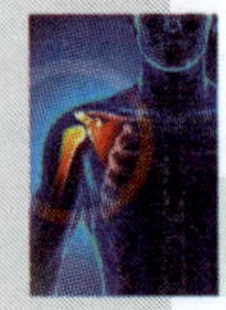

- Adamantinoma is an uncommon tumor (<1%) of long bones containing epithelial—like islands of cells
- **MC site of adamantinoma:** Tibia (85%) > Mandible
  - In mandible, it is termed as ameloblastoma
  - Can involve ipsilateral fibula
- **MC age group:** 10–35 years
- **MC symptom:** Pain
- **On X-ray:** Honey coomb like appearance/Sharply demarcated radiolucent lesions
- **Treatment:** Wide surgical resection

TABLE: Most common sites of primary bone tumors

Tumor	Site
Chondroblastoma	Epiphyseal (most common tumor in this region before puberty)
Osteoclastoma	Epiphyseal (most common tumor in this region after puberty)
Chondrosarcoma, osteochondroma, bone cyst, enchondroma, osteosarcoma, osteoclastoma	Metaphyseal
Ewing's tumor, lymphoma, multiple myeloma, adamantinoma, osteoid osteoma	Diaphyseal

TABLE: Most common sites of individual bone tumors

Tumor	Site
Solitary bone cyst	Upper end of humerus
Aneurysmal bone cyst	Lower limb metaphysis
Osteochondroma	Distal femur
Osteoid osteoma	Femur
Osteoblastoma	Vertebrae
Osteoma	Skull, facial bones
Enchondroma	Short bones of hand
Chordoma	Sacrum
Adamantinoma	Tibial
Ameloblastoma	Mandible
Osteoclastoma	Lower end femur
Fibrous dysplasia	Polyostotic–craniofacial Monostotic–upper femur
Multiple myeloma	Lumbar vertebrae
Osteosarcoma	Lower end femur
Ewing's sarcoma	Femur
Chondrosarcoma	Pelvis
Secondary tumors	Dorsal vertebrae

117. Ans. (b) Periosteal reaction

Ref: Fundamentals of Orthopedics, by Mukul Mohindra, Jitesh Kumar Jain pg. 500

- Sunray appearance in osteosarcoma is due to periosteal reaction, causing calcification along Sharpey's fiber.

IMPORTANT X-RAY SIGNS

- **Fibrous dysplasia:** Ground glass appearance, Rind sign (sclerotic margin around tumor), Shephard crook deformity (collapse of medial part of femoral neck so that proximal femur becomes hook shaped, seen in Paget's disease and Osteogenesis imperfecta also)
- **Simple bone cyst:** Fallen leaf sign (can be seen in ABC but less often).
- **Hemangiome:** Corduroy appearance (Jail house sign), Polka dot pattern.
- **Osteoid osteoma:** Nidus <1.5 cm and osteoblastoma >1.5 cm.
- **Giant cell tumor:** Soap bubble appearance.
- **Osteosarcoma:** Codman's triangle, Sunray appearance (due to calcification along sharpey's fibers).
- **Chondrosarcoma:** Popcorn like calcification.
- **Ewing's sarcoma:** Onion peel appearance (intense periosteal reaction in layers), Codman's triangle.
- **Eosinophilic granuloma:** Punched out lytic lesions in skull with double contours.
- **Multiple myeloma:** Punched out lesions without a reactive/sclerotic surrounding zone.

118. Ans. (d) Osteofibrous dysplasia

- In the given image, the lesion is in tibial shaft. Given these choices, osteofibrous dysplasia is the single best answer.
- **Apley's states:** *"tumors in the tibial shaft is fairly rare. A condition that particularly affects the tibial shaft is osteofibrous dysplasia, a tumor that almost always occurs on the tibia, predominantly in shaft area"*
- **Note:** This condition is a very close differential diagnosis of malignant adamantinoma

119. Ans. (d) Chrondroblastoma

Ref: Apley's System of Orthopaedics, 9th ed. pg. 198

CHONDROBLASTOMA

- This benign tumor of immature cartilage cells is one of the few lesions to **appear primarily in the epiphysis**, usually of the **proximal humerus, femur or tibia**.
- The presenting symptom is a constant ache in the joint; the tender spot is actually in the adjacent bone.
- X-ray shows a rounded, well-demarcated radiolucent area in the epiphysis with no hint of central calcification.

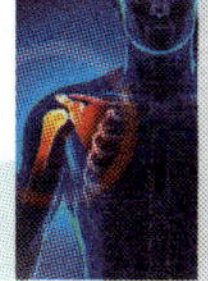

120. Ans. (d) Osteosarcoma

Ref: Maheshwari, 5th ed. pg. 239

Osteosarcoma is a malignant bone tumor, which most commonly originates from metaphyseal region and is common in second decade.

TABLE: Tumors according to their origin site in long bone

Epiphysis (Mn: ECG)	Metaphysis (Mn: ME-BOO)	Diaphysis (DEMO–A)
• **Chondroblastoma-** before physeal closure • **Giant cell tumor**-after physeal closure	• Enchondroma *(short bones)* • Bone cyst *(MC in upper humerus)* ▪ *UBC, ABC* ▪ Osteochondroma *(EXOSTOSIS)* ▪ Osteosarcoma	• Ewing's sarcoma • Multiple myeloma • Osteoid osteoma • Adamantioma

UBC = Unicameral bone cyst
ABC = Aneurysmal bone cyst

121. Ans. (a) Osteosarcoma

Ref: Maheshwari, 5th ed. pg. 239

- Osteosarcoma is an aggressive malignant neoplasm arising from primitive transformed cells of mesenchymal origin (and thus a sarcoma) that exhibit osteoblastic differentiation and produce malignant osteoid.
- Sun ray appearance: It is the most common radiological finding of primary bone cancer.
- If the lesion grows rapidly but steadily, the periosteum will not have enough time to lay down thin shell of bone, and in such cases, the tiny fibers that connect the periosteum to the bone *(Sharpey's fibers)* become stretched out perpendicular to the bone.
- ***When these fibers ossify, they produce a pattern sometimes called "sunburst" periosteal reaction.***

122. Ans. (c) Osteoid osteoma

Ref: Maheshwari, 5th ed. pg. 235

- Osteoid osteoma is a benign bone tumor characterized by pain which is relieved by non-steroidal anti-inflammatory drugs (NSAIDs), such as aspirin.
- To clarify the mechanism of the pain, five osteoid osteomas were studied immune-histochemically using polyclonal antibodies against prostaglandin E2 (PGE2), S-100 protein and protein gene product.

123. Ans. (b) Second decade

Ref: Maheshwari, 5th ed. pg. 243

"Ewing's sarcoma is generally a lesion of children and adolescents, occurring most commonly (80% to 94%) in the first 2 decades, with a peak incidence in the second decade"

EWING'S SARCOMA

- Highly malignant, undifferentiated peripheral primitive neuro ectodermal tumor (PNET)
- Most common site is diaphysis of femur
- Common in 10–20 year old male
- Histopathology shows round cells containing glycogen and reticulin; PAS positive and diastase digestible
- 80–95% tumors possess translocation; t(11, 22)
- X-ray reveals laminated periosteal new bone formation also known as *"Onion peel appearance"*

Extra Mile

TABLE Bone tumors and their Incidence age wise

Tumor	Seen at age
Unicameral bone cyst	1st decade
Aneurysmal bone cyst	2nd decade
Giant cell tumor	2nd to 4th decade

124. Ans. (a) Giant cell tumor

Ref: Maheshwari 5th ed. pg. 237; Orthopedic Pathology by Vincent J Vigorita pg. 294

- GCT is an epiphyseal tumor
- GCT usually involves subarticular region distal radius and distal femur, the proximal tibia being most common site.
- If there is a soap bubble appearance in diaphyseal region, it is adamantioma.

Extra Mile

- **Sun burst appearance:** Osteosarcoma
- **Nidu/Seed in cortex:** Osteioid osteoma
- **Onion skin appearance:** Ewing's sarcoma
- **Exostosis (cartilage cap):** Osteochondroma

JOINT DISORDERS

125. Ans. (b) Knee

- Most common joint involved in thalassemia is Knee joint.
- Most common orthopaedic symptom in thalassemia is leg pain.

Extra Mile

- Most common joint involved in haemophilia: Knee > Elbow > Ankle > Shoulder > Hip

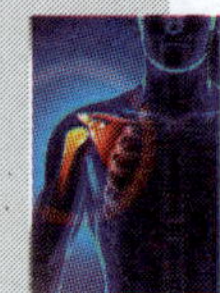

126. Ans. (a) Reiter's syndrome

Ref: Apley's System of Orthopaedics, 9th ed. pg. 70

REITER'S SYNDROME

- It is a clinical **triad** of **urethritis, arthritis and conjunctivitis** occurring some weeks after either dysentery of genitourinary infection. It is now recognized that this is one of the classic forms of reactive arthritis, i.e. an aseptic inflammatory arthritis associated with non-specific infection.

Cause

- First-degree relatives and a close association with HLA-B27 point to a genetic predisposition.
- Gut pathogens include Shigella flexneri, Salmonella, Campylobacter species and Yersinia enterocolitica. Lymphogranuloma venereum and Chlamydia trachomatis have been implicated as sexually transmitted infections.

Clinical Features

- The acute phase of the disease is marked by an asymmetrical inflammatory arthritis of the lower limb joints–usually as well. The joint may be acutely painful, hot and swollen with a tense effusion, suggesting gout or infection.
- The chronic phase is more characteristic of a spondyloarthropathy.

127. Ans. (a) DIP

Ref: Maheshwari, 5th ed. pg. 287

- Rheumatoid arthritis characteristically causes swelling of small joints in the hand like the PIP, MCP and the wrist joint bilaterally.
- Isolated DIP joint involvement is seen in psoriatic arthropathy.
- DIP joint involvement is also seen with osteoarthritis but the involvement is with pain at the base of thumb. Knee joint is the commonest large joint involved in these patients.

128. Ans. (c) Flexion contracture of PIP and extension of DIP

Ref: Maheshwari, 5th ed. pg. 288

- **Boutonniere deformity** is a deformed position of the fingers or toes, in which the joint nearest the knuckle (PIP) is permanently bent toward the palm while the farthest joint (DIP) is bent back away ***(PIP flexion with DIP hyperextension).***
- It is commonly caused by injury or by an inflammatory condition like rheumatoid arthritis.

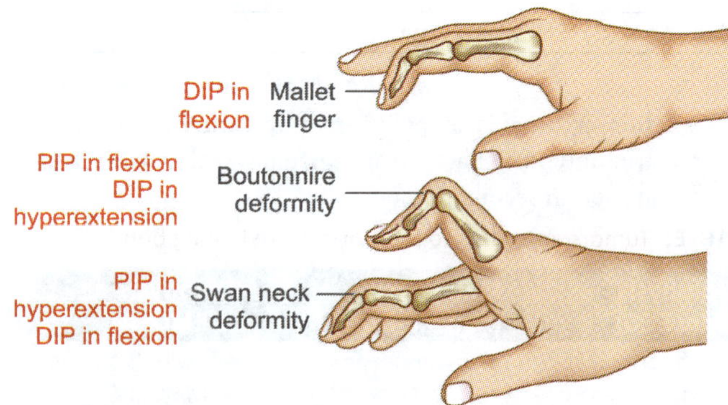

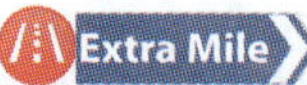

- **'Z-deformity'** i.e. radial deviation of the wrist with ulnar deviation of the digits, often with palmar subluxation of proximal phalanges.
- **'Swan – neck deformity'** i.e. hyperextension of PIP joints with compensatory flexion of the distal interphalangeal joints.
- **Wind** – sweep deformities of toes i.e. valgus deformities of toes in one foot and varus in other, *(as wind sweeps all the structure in one direction).*

129. Ans. (b) Heberdens nodes

Ref: Harrison, 18th ed./ch. 332

- ***"Heberden's nodes are hard or bony swellings that develop in the distal interphalangeal joints (DIP) in a case of osteoarthritis"***

Clinical Features of Rheumatoid Arthritis

- The presenting symptoms of RA typically result from inflammation of the joints, tendons, and bursae.
- Early morning joint stiffness lasting more than 1 hour and easing with physical activity.
- The earliest involved joints are typically the small joints of the hands and feet. The initial pattern of joint involvement may be monoarticular, oligoarticular (<4 joints), or polyarticular (>5 joints), usually in a symmetric distribution.
- ***Wrists, metacarpophalangeal (MCP) and proximal interphalangeal (PIP) joints stand out as the most frequently involved joints.***
- **Frequent hallmark of RA:** Flexor tendon tenosynovitis.

Deformities

- Ulnar deviation of the hand.
- ***Swan-neck deformity:*** Hyperextension of the PIP joint with flexion of the DIP
- ***Boutonniere deformity:*** Flexion of the PIP joint with hyperextension of the DIP joint
- ***Z deformity:*** Radial deviation of wrist with ulnar deviation of digits, often with palmar subluxation proximal phalanges.

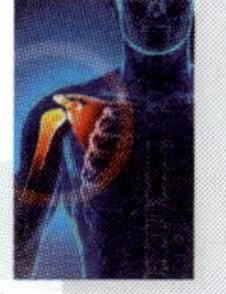

- Inflammation about the ulnar styloid and tenosynovitis of the extensor carpi ulnaris may cause subluxation of the distal ulna, resulting in a "piano-key movement" of the ulnar styloid
- **Metatarsophalangeal joint (MTP)** involvement is a feature of early disease in the feet
- **Atlantoaxial involvement of the cervical spine** can cause compressive myelopathy and neurologic dysfunction
- **Most frequent extraarticular manifestations:** Subcutaneous nodules, secondary Sjogren's syndrome, pulmonary nodules, and anemia.

130. Ans. (a) Rheumatoid Arthritis

Ref: Harrison's, 18th ed. Ch. 321

Clinical Features of RA

- Incidence of RA increases between 25 and 55 years of age.
- **Gender:** Female > Male
- Early morning joint stiffness lasting more than 1 hour and easing with physical activity.
- The earliest involved joints are typically the small joints of the hands and feet.
- The wrists, metacarpophalangeal (MCP), and proximal interphalangeal (PIP) joints stand out as the most frequently involved joints. Distal interphalangeal (DIP) joint involvement may occur in RA, but it usually is a manifestation of coexistent osteoarthritis.

131. Ans. (b) Gouty arthritis

Ref: Harrison's, 18th ed. Ch 332, 333

TABLE: Pathology and common joint involved

Pathology	Common joint involved
Gout	1st MTP; GREAT TOE
OA	DIP, PIP- sparing MCP, wrist, elbow, ankle (DIP > KNEE)
RA	Involving PIP, MCP joint
Psoriasis	DIP
Pseudogout	Knee

132. Ans. (a) Indomethacin

Ref: Harrison's, 18th ed. Ch 333

- **MC site of gout:** Meta-tarsophalangeal joint of great toe.
- In gout there is deposition of uric acid in the joint.
- **Intake of Alcohol, Diuretics and aspirin are precipitating factors of gout.**

Treatment:

- NSAIDs given in full anti-inflammatory doses are effective in ~ 90% of patients.
- The most effective drugs are NSAIDS *(except aspirin)* with a short half-life and include **indomethacin 25–50 mg TID**; naproxen, ibuprofen and diclofenac.
- **Colchicine** given orally is a traditional and effective treatment if used early in an attack. It causes GI disturbance thereby reducing the compliance.
- Ultimate control of gout requires correction of the basic underlying defect: The hyperuricemia. Uricosuric drugs like **Allopurinol and Febuxostat** both are xanthine oxidase inhibitors. *These drugs are never preferred during acute attacks and whenever given, they should always be covered by NSAIDS.*
- **DOC for chronic gout: Allopurinol.**

133. Ans. (c) TB with polyarthritis

- **Spina ventosa-TB** of short bones
- **Caries sicca-TB** shoulder
- **Poncet disease-TB with polyarthritis**
- Pott's-TB spine

VERTEBRA & NEUROMUSCULAR DISEASE

134. Ans. (c) L5

Ref: Maheshwari and Mhaskar's Essential Orthopaedics 6th ed. pg. 298-99

- The intervertebral disc between L4-L5 is shown to be affected in this MRI.
- Nerve root, passes below the level of lumbar vertebra. Example: nerve root L5 passes between L4-L5.

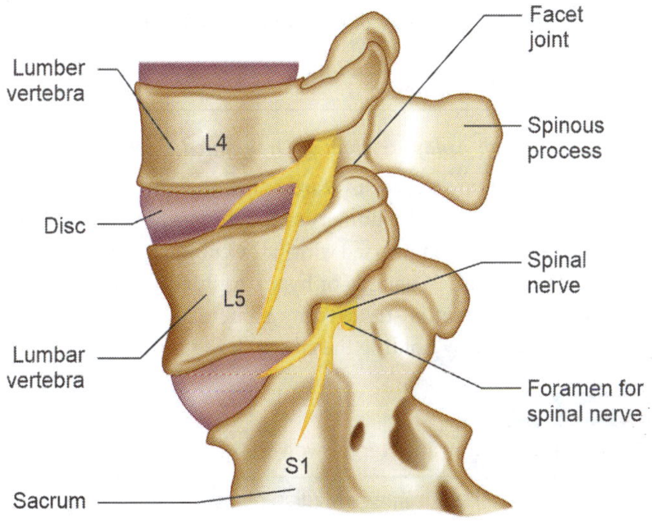

135. Ans. (a) Taylor brace splint

Ref: Essential Orthopaedics by Maheshwari 6th ed. pg. 33, 308

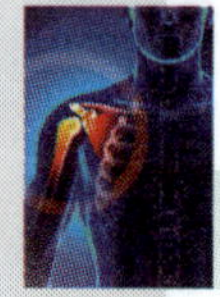

- The shown image is taylor brace splint.
- It is used in dorsolumbar immobilization and can also be used in severe osteoporotic patients to prevent pathological fracture.

Extra Mile

Uses of important braces and splint
- Biston brace and Milwaukee brace: Scoliosis
- SOMI brace: Cervical spine injury
- Toe raising splint: Foot drop
- Cock-up Splint: Radial Nerve Injury
- Knuckle bender splint: Ulnar Nerve. > Median Nerve.
- Aeroplane splint- Brachial Plexus injury
- Turn buckle splint- VIC
- Four post collar: Neck immobilization
- Aluminium splint: Immobilization of fingers

136. Ans. (c) Klippel feil syndrome

Ref: Essential Orthopaedics by Maheshwari 6th ed. pg. 224

- In Klippel feil syndrome, there is Congenital short and stiff neck due to fused or deformed cervical vertebrae.
- It occurs due to failure of normal segmentation of cervical vertebra somite between 3rd and 8th week of fetal development
- **It has 2 pattern of inheritance:**
  - AD: C2–C3 fusion
  - AR: C5–C6 fusion
- **Characterized by feil's triad:**
  - Low posterior hair line
  - Short neck
  - Limitation of head and neck movements (due to decreased range of movement of cervical spine).

137. Ans. (b) Ulnar nerve

Ref: Apley's System of Orthopaedics, 9th ed. pg. 290

- The ulnar nerve is easily felt behind the medial epicondyle of the humerus (the 'funny bone'). It can be trapped or compressed within the cubital tunnel (by bone abnormalities, ganglia or hypertrophied synovium).
- Sometimes it is stretched by a cubitus valgus deformity or simply by holding the elbow flexed for long.

Extra Mile

TABLE: Neuropathy and Nerve involved

Neuropathy	Nerve involved
• Carpal tunnel syndrome	Median nerve
• Cubital tunnel syndrome	Ulnar nerve
• Guyon canal syndrome	Ulnar nerve
• Meralgia paresthetica	Lateral cutaneous nerve of thigh
• Cheralgia paresthetica	Superficial radial nerve

138. Ans. (d) L4-L5

Ref: Maheshwari, 5th ed. pg. 253

- **Most common site of spinal disc herniation: Lumbar region (95% in L4–L5 or L5–S1).**
- **The second most common site is the cervical region (C5–C6, C6–C7).**
- Thoracic region accounts for only **0.15% to 4.0%** of cases.
- Herniations usually occur posterolaterally, where the annulus fibrosis is relatively thin and is not reinforced by the posterior or anterior longitudinal ligament.
- In the cervical spinal cord, a symptomatic posterolateral herniation between two vertebrae will impinge on the nerve which exits the spinal canal between those two vertebrae on that side. For example, a right posterolateral herniation of the disc between vertebrae C5 and C6 will impinge on the right C6 spinal nerve.

139. Ans. (a) Erb's paralysis

Ref: Apley's Orthopedics, 9th ed. pg. 279-80

Erb's paralysis	- Erb's palsy or Erb–Duchenne palsy is a paralysis of the arm caused by injury to the upper group of the arm's main nerves, specifically the severing of the upper trunk C5–C6 nerves. **Position of hand in Erb's paralysis:** Adducted, Internally rotated, and pronated
Klumpke's paralysis	Klumpke's Palsy involves the eighth cervical vertebra and the first thoracic vertebra (C8 and T1). **Position of hand:** Elbow flexed, arm supinated There may be unilateral horner syndrome
Horner syndrome	Seen with Pancoast tumor and presents with Ptosis, Miosis, enopthalmos, anhydrosis, loss of ciliospinal reflex.
Central cord syndrome	Seen most often after a hyperextension injury in an individual with long-standing cervical spondylosis. It presents with features of cortico-spinal pathway.

140. Ans. (b) Iatrogenic

Ref: Maheshwari, 5th ed. pg. 264

- The most common pathological mechanisms for sciatic nerve injury are compression, traction or direct injury by mechanical disruption as is seen in intragluteal muscle injection, or called as Sciatic neuritis.
- ***Division of the main sciatic nerve is rare except in gunshot wounds or operative (iatrogenic) accidents.***
- The sciatic nerve is the nerve most commonly injured during total hip replacement.
- Sciatic nerve is the most common nerve injured by intramuscular injections, especially in children.

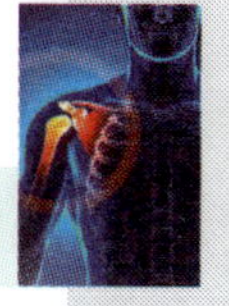

141. Ans. (c) **Spondylolisthesis**

Ref: Maheshwari, 5th ed. pg. 283-284

Spondylosis	Degenerative osteoarthritis of the joints between the center of the spinal vertebrae and/or neural foramina
Spondylitis	Spondylitis is an inflammation of the vertebra. It is a form of spondylopathy. In many cases spondylitis involves one or more vertebral joints as well, which itself is called spondylarthritis
Spondylolis-thesis	*Spondylolisthesis is the anterior or posterior displacement of a vertebra or the vertebral column in relation to the vertebrae below*
Spondylolysis	Defect of a vertebra. More specifically it is defined as a defect in the pars interarticularis of the vertebral arch

142. Ans. (b) **Axonotemesis**

Ref: Maheshwari, 5th ed. pg. 63

143. Ans. (b) **Ulnar nerve**

Ref: Clinical assessment & examination in Orthopedics pg. 67

Tests for ulnar nerve	
Card test	Palmar interossei are Adductors (PAD) tested by asking the patient to hold a card between the extended fingers and assess resistance against pulling
Egawa test	Dorsal interossei are Abductors (DAB) supplied by the ulnar nerve. It is tested by asking the patient to place the palm on table and move the middle finger both ways, i.e. towards index finger and ring finger. In Dorsal interossei palsy patient will be unable to abduct the middle finger
Book test/ Froment's sign	To test adductor pollicis ask the patient to grasp a book or card between extended thumb and index finger. An ulnar nerve palsy patient tries to grasp the book by flexing the inter-phalangeal joint of thumb.

Extra Mile

- OSCHNER CLASP TEST and PEN TEST is used to check for MEDIAN NERVE PALSY.

144. Ans. (b) **Ulnar nerve palsy**

Ref: Maheshwari, 5th ed. pg. 64

Please refer to above explanation

145. Ans. (c) **Claw finger deformity**

Ref: Maheshwari, 5th ed. pg. 64

- In ulnar nerve palsy especially in long standing cases, the hand assumes the characteristic **"claw" deformity.** It is also known as partial claw hand deformity.
- Complete claw hand deformity is due to palsy of ulnar and median nerve both.

Condition	Features
Median nerve palsy labourer nerve palsy	• Pointing index • Pen test • Ape thumb deformity • Carpal tunnel syndrome
Ulnar nerve palsy musician nerve palsy	• Book test (froment sign) • Card test • Egawa's test • Claw finger deformity
Radial nerve palsy *Lateral cutaneous nerve of thigh (entrapped)*	• Wrist drop • Thumb drop • Finger drop • Meralgia paraesthetica
Erb's palsy	**Policeman tip deformity (Porter's tip deformity)**

146. Ans. (b) **Radial nerve**

Ref: Maheshwari, 5th ed. pg. 25 Table 4.1

Cockup splint is used in cases of radial nerve injury.

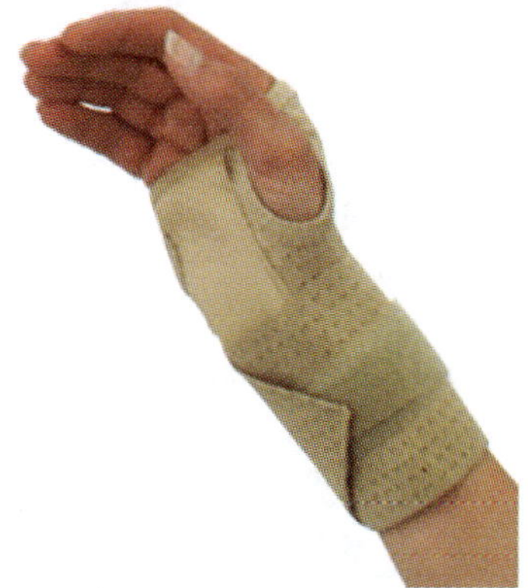

TABLE: Different splint and their Uses

Splint	Used In
Knuckle bender splint	Ulnar nerve
Aeroplane splint	Brachial plexus injury
Dennis brown splint	CTEV
Bohler Brown splint	Fracture femur (anywhere from neck to supracondylar region)
Turn buckle splint	VIC (Volkmann ischemic contracture)

147. Ans. (d) **Physiological block**

Ref: Apley's, 8th ed. pg. 231

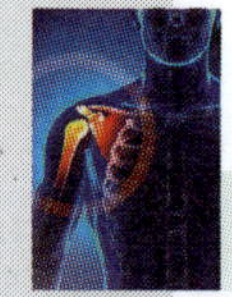

TABLE: Patterns of nerve injury

Neuropraxia	Axonotmesis	Neurotmesis
• ***Reversible physiological nerve conduction block*** • It is seen in crutch palsy, ***tourniquet palsy,*** and saturday night palsy	• There is ***loss of conduction because of axonal interruption*** but the nerve is in continuity and the neural tubes are intact • Seen in closed *fractures* and dislocations	• There is complete division of nerve with complete loss of conduction (i.e. epineurium, perineurium, endoneurium, & axon all have lost their continuity) • Seen in open *wounds*

148. Ans. (c) C8 dermatome

Ref: Apley's System of Orthopaedics & Fractures, 9th ed. pg. 229, 272

Clinically Important Dermatomes

Upper Extremity
- C6-Thumb
- C7-Middle finger
- C8-Little finger
- T1-Inner forearm
- T2-Upper inner arm

Lower Extremity
- L3-Knee
- L4-Medial malleolus
- L5-Dorsum of foot
- L5-Toes 1–3
- SI-Toes 4 and 5; lateral malleolus

Others
- C2 and C3 - Posterior head and neck
- T4-Nipple
- T10-Umbilicus

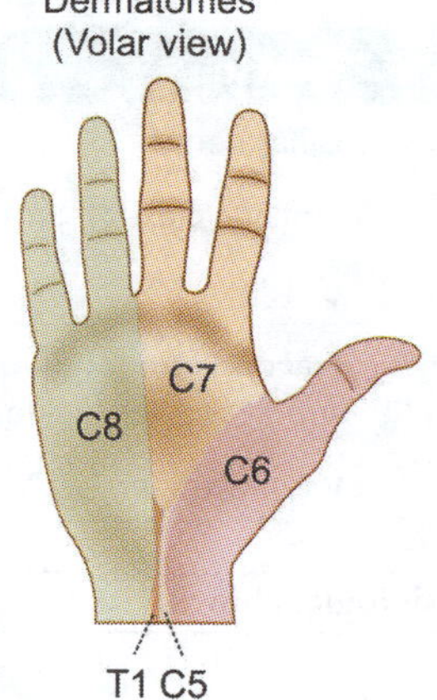

149. Ans. (c) Ultrasound therapy

Ref: De Lisa's 'Physical Medicine and Rehabilitation: Principles and Practice'; 5th ed. Vol II, pg. 1304

Treatment of Post-amputation Neuroma and Scar Pain
- Repeated injection of a local anaesthetic has proven to be an extremely useful technique.
- This should be followed by appropriate **physical therapy to the scar, usually ultrasound** followed by stretching or deep massage of the scar.
- This type of treatment has provided permanent or prolonged pain relief for longer than 6 months in many patients.
- When the local anaesthetics, with or without steroids, do not provide prolonged relief, other methods should be considered.
- Cryoanalgesia using a cryoprobe and freezing the neuroma for 1 minute at 20°C has been used with good success.
- The advantage of a cryoprobe lies in the fact that it is a physical method of blocking the nerve without further neuroma or neuritis.
- Neurolytic agents such as phenol or alcohol have been used to relieve neuroma and scar pain.
- However, incomplete block with these agents can result: In neuritis, producing severe pain.
- These neurolytic techniques should be used only after repeated injections of local anaesthetics produce consistent pain relief proportional to the duration or action of the local anaesthetic agent.
- Although surgical revision of the scar is often considered, it is not very successful when the scar cannot be stretched out and there is significant nerve entrapment.

150. Ans. (b) Ulnar nerve

Ulnar Claw Hand
- The deformity in the picture is Partial Claw Hand, i.e. Hyperextension of MCP joints and Hyperflexion of interphalangeal joints of ring and little fingers.
- Clawing of fingers is caused by Lumbrical muscle paralysis. It is also called as Intrinsic Minus Deformity or **Duchenne's sign**.
- Lumbricals of little finger and ring finger are supplied by Ulnar nerve.
- Lumbricals of Index finger and Middle finger are supplied by Median nerve.
- The ulnar nerve palsy causes partial claw hand involving little and ring fingers; **Ulnar nerve and Median Nerve combined injury causes Total claw hand involving all four fingers**
- Knuckle bender splint is used to correct the claw hand deformity.

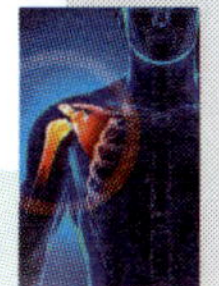

PEDIATRIC ORTHOPAEDICS

151. Ans. (c) Triple arthrodesis

Ref: Essential Orthopedics: Principles and Practice, Manish Kumar Varshney, 1st ed. pg. 800, 817

- This is a shown case of club foot.
- A triple arthrodesis is a procedure consisting of the surgical fusion of the talocalcaneal (TC), talonavicular (TN), and calcaneocuboid (CC) joints in the foot.
- The primary goals of a triple arthrodesis are to relieve pain from arthritic, deformed, or unstable joints.

152. Ans. (d) Dennis brown splint

Ref: Essential Orthopedics: Principles and Practice, Manish Kumar Varshney, 1st ed. pg. 812

- The shown image is of Dennis Brown splint
- A Dennis Brown (DB) splint is applied to CTEV children.
- Congenital talipes equinovarus (CTEV), or clubfoot, is a common foot deformity that involves a complex three-dimensional musculoskeletal abnormality.
- The deformity has 4 main components: Equinus, varus, cavus, and adduction.

153. Ans. (d) DDH

- The shown cast, is Pavlik harness cast. This is used in patients with DDH.

Other Important Casts

- **Broom stick cast:** Perthes disease
- **Minerva cast:** Cervical spine disease
- **Riser's cast:** Scoliosis
- **U-Slab/Hanging cast:** Humerus fracture
- **Hip spica:** Femur fracture (<5 years)
- **Gallows traction:** Femur fracture (<2 years)
- **Glass holding cast:** Scaphoid fracture

154. Ans. (b) Rickets

Ref: Essential Orthopaedics by Maheshwari 6th ed. pg. 310-311

- The shown image of wrist X-ray is suggestive of rickets.
- **Radiological features of rickets:**
  - Early changes observed in lower ends to radius and ulna
  - Delayed epiphysis appearance and widened epiphyseal plate
  - Cupping of the metaphysis:
  - Splaying of the metaphysis: metaphyseal end is splayed because of the pressure by the cartilage cells
  - Knock knees
- **Serum:**
  - Calcium: Normal or low
  - PO_4 is low
  - ALP is high

Types of Rickets

Type 1

- Due to vitamin D deficiency
- Due to disturbance in vitamin D metabolism (vitamin D resistant)
- It is an autosomal recessive condition

Type 2

- Defective PO_4 absorption through renal tubules (Hypophosphatemic rickets- XLD), Fanconi syndrome, RTA
- Diminished intake or absorption of PO_4

155. Ans. (c) Perthes disease

Ref: Essential Orthopaedics, Maheshwari & Mhaskar, 6th ed. pg. 318

PERTHES DISEASE

- Also known as Coxa plana or Pseudocoxalgia
- It is an osteochondritis of the epiphysis of the femoral head
- The femoral head here becomes avascular → Avascular necrosis of femoral head
- **MC age group:** 5–10 years
- **The disease progress through 3 stages:**
  - Stage of synovitis
  - Stage of trabecular necrosis
  - Stage of healing
- **Clinical picture:**
  - Pain in hip, radiating to knee
  - Limping or hip stiffness
- **Upon examination:**
  - Limb shortening
  - Limitation of abduction and internal rotation
- **X-ray:**
  - Sclerosis of femoral head epiphysis *(as seen in image of this patient)*
  - Hip joint space is increased
- **Treatment:**
  - Head containment (by plaster, splint or surgical)—Head is kept inside the acetabulum while revascularisation takes place

OTHER OPTIONS

- There is no history of trauma, so hip dislocation is unlikely
- DDH usually seen in infant, and the clinical presentation also doesn't correlate with DDH
- In Stage 1 hip there is apparent limb lengthening

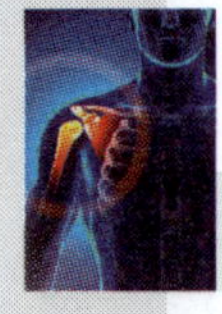

156. Ans. (a) Dysplasia of proximal epiphysis

Ref: Essential Orthopaedics, Maheshwari & Mhaskar, 6th ed. pg. 320

BLOUNT'S DISEASE

- Disease caused by abnormality of proximal posteromedial tibial epiphysis
- Classically seen in African-American obese male child (first 3 years) and in west Indies
- Presents as pathologic tibia vara (bowed legs)

TABLE: Some other developmental abnormalities of orthopaedic interest

• Olliers disease (multiple enchondromas) • Dyschondroplasia	• Not familial • Masses of cartilage in the metaphysis remain unossified • Defective ossification
Melorheostosis	• Candle bone disease
Osteopathia striata	• Striped bones disease
Osteopoikilosis	• Spotted bones disease
Morquio disease	• Familial (autosomal recessive) disease • Gives rise to dwarfism affecting both, limbs and trunk • Mental development normal • Corneal opacity sometimes present • X-ray – typical 'tonguing' of lumbar vertebrae • Keratan sulfate in urine
Hunter's disease	• Familial x-linked disease • Defect is the excretion of large amount of Keratan sulfate in urine • Dwarf with dorso lumbar kyphosis, knock knees, flat feet • Mental deficiency may occur • No corneal opacity
Hurler's disease (Gargoylism)	• Familial (autosomal recessive) disease • Give rise to dwarfism of both, limbs and trunk • Defect is an error in development of fibroblasts • There is excretion of dermatan sulfate and hepartan sulfate in urine • Typical facial appearance • Mental development abnormal • Corneal opacity present • X-ray typical 'beak ' in 2nd lumbar vertebra
Engelmann's disease	• Familial (autosomal recessive) disease • Symmetrical, fusiform enlargement and sclerosis of shafts of the long bones in children. Femur affected commonly. • Epiphysis is spared
Caffey's disease (infantile cortical hyperostosis)	• Nonfamilial disease • Starts early in life (before the 5th month) • There is a formation of sub-periosteal bone on the shafts of long bones, and on the mandible • Self-limiting course, resolves by 3 years of age • Tibia more common than ulna in familial form
Albright's syndrome	• Polyostotic fibrous dysplasia and precocious puberty
Arthrogryposis multiplex congenita (AMC)	• Defective development of muscles • Stiff, deformed joints • Multiple joint dislocations with 'shapeless extremities' • May present as clubfoot
Myositis ossificans progressiva	• Ectopic ossification, often beginning in trunk • Short big toe
Multiple epiphyseal dysplasia	• Least rare type • Affects all the epiphyses, resulting in stunted growth, deformities (varum, valgum etc.) • Epiphysis looks ill defined, irregular on X-rays
Spondylo-epiphyseal dysplasia	• Spine is also involved in addition to limb epiphyses
Metaphyseal dysplasia (Pyle's disease)	• Autosomal recessive • A modelling defect results in 'Erlenmeyer flask' deformity of the distal femur and proximal tibia
Blount's disease	• The growth of the medial-half of the proximal tibial epiphysis is retarded, resulting in severe tibia vara deformity in childhood, common in West Indies
Cleidocranil dysostosis	• Faulty development of membranous bones • Clavicles are absent • Skull sutures remain open • Coxa vara • Wide foramen magnum
Nail patella syndrome	• Familial disorder • Hypoplastic nails and absence of patella
Marfans syndrome (Arachnodactyly)	• Spider fingers • Associated atrial regurgitation • Ocular lens dislocation
Apert syndrome	• Tower shaped head

Contd...

157. Ans. (c) Elbow

- Most common joint dislocation in pediatric population: **Elbow joint**
- Most common joint dislocation in adult population: **Humerus joint**

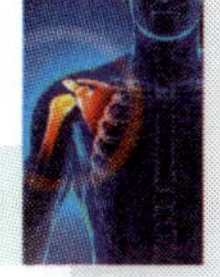

158. Ans. (d) Slipped capital femoral epiphysis

- The usual presentation of SCFE is an overweight child who has poorly localized groin, thigh or knee pain.
- Usual age of presentation is 11–14 years. M > F
- Upon examination leg is shortened and externally rotated.
- Upon radiological investigation:
  - **Trethovan's sign:** A line drawn along the superior border of the femoral neck on the AP view should pass through the femoral head. In SCFE, the line passes superior to the head rather than through the head.

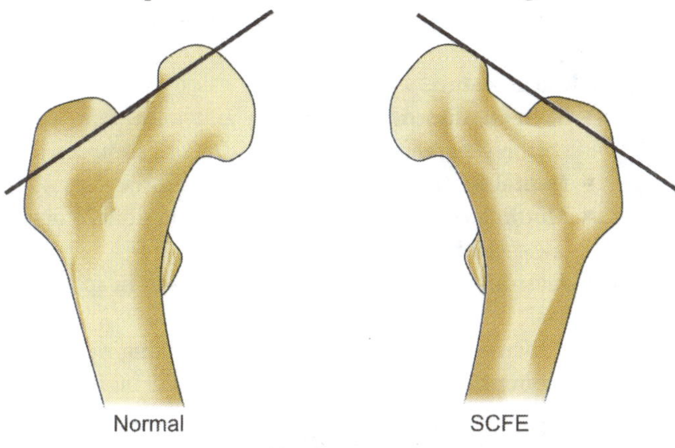

159. Ans. (b) USG

Ref: Maheshwari, 5th ed. pg. 222

TABLE: Investigations of congenital dislocation of Hip

USG	• Post natal diagnosis within the first year is best made by an ultrasound • Allows assessment even in first two months when plain radiographs can be normal • Considered as screening test of choice in case of CDH
X-Ray	Plain films may be normal in first 2–3 months, however subtle changes begin to appear at 6 weeks • Reliable depiction of DDH made after 4–6 months • Most useful in period between 2–8 months • Classical findings: (putti's triad) 1. Absent or small proximal femoral capital epiphyses 2. Lateral displacement of femur 3. Shallow acetabulum with an increased inclination of acetabular roof > 30 degrees • Disruption of shenton's line • Head lies in outer and upper quadrant
CT	Used for pre-surgical planning
MRI	Considered as IOC/Best investigation for diagnosis of CDH

160. Ans. (c) Congenital dislocation of hip

- Physical examination used for testing congenital dislocation of hip (CDH)- done together
  - **Barlow test:** Hip is dislocated by adduction
  - **Ortolani test:** relocation done by abduction

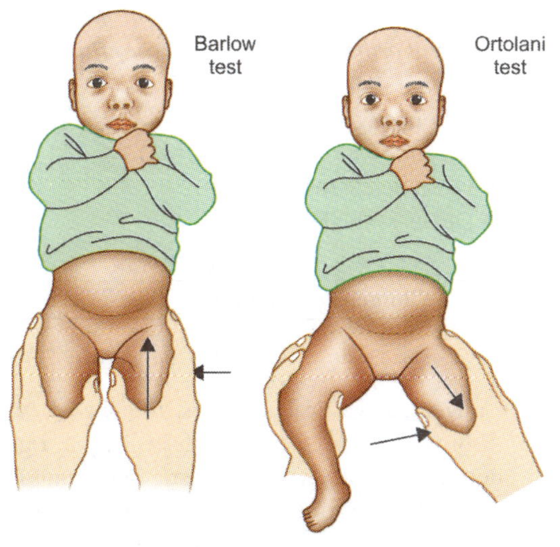

161. Ans: (a) Spring ligament

Ref: Maheshwari, 5th ed. pg. 210

- ***"Pesplanus or a flat foot is a disorder of laxity of medial longitudinal arch which is maintained by the spring ligament and plantar aponeurosis"***
- The term pesplanus denotes an excessively flat foot. There is no precise degree of flatness that defines pesplanus, but it may be either physiological or pathological.
- In physiological pesplanus, the feet are flexible and rarely problematic. In marked contrast, pathological pesplanus is often associated with stiffness and pain.
- The windlass (or 'Jack's great toe') test involves passively dorsiflexing the hallux at the metatarsophalangeal joint. This tightens the plantar aponeurosis and, in flexible pesplanus, results in accentuation of the medial longitudinal arch.
- In pathological pesplanus, no accentuation of the arch is seen. This test can also be carried out by asking the individual to stand on tiptoe and viewing the hind foot from behind. In flexible flat feet, the calcaneus swings into a varus position; in pathological pesplanus it does not.

162. Ans. (b) Late congenital syphilis

Ref: Maheshwari, 5th ed. pg. 178

- **The clinical manifestations of congenital syphilis include:**
  - **Early manifestations:** Infection appear within the first 2 years of life (often at 2–10 weeks of age)
  - **Late manifestations,** are noninfectious and appear after 2 years
- *Late congenital syphilis (untreated after 2 years of age) is subclinical in 60% of cases; the clinical spectrum in the*

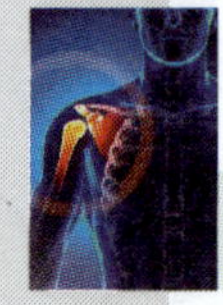

*remainder of cases may include interstitial keratitis (which occurs at 5–25 years of age), eighth-nerve deafness, and recurrent arthropathy. Bilateral knee **effusions are known as clutton's joints.***

- **Triad of congenital syphilis:**
  - Keratitis
  - Heart defect (MC: PDA)
  - Deafness (SNHL)

163. Ans. (a) Congenital flat foot

Ref: Maheshwari, 5th ed. pg. 326

- Congenital vertical talus (CVT) is an uncommon disorder of the foot, manifested as a rigid rocker-bottom flatfoot. Its characteristic radiographic feature is a dorsal dislocation of the navicular on the talus. If left untreated, CVT results in a painful and rigid flatfoot with weak push-off power. CVT has been referred to in the literature by several synonyms, including congenital convex pes valgus.
- **Presentation:**
- Presents as a rigid flatfoot with **a rocker-bottom appearance** of the foot.
- The forefoot is abducted and dorsiflexed.
- **Treatment:** Serial casting should be the initial treatment, although prior to the Dobbs article, it was usually thought to be unsuccessful. A single-stage surgical correction is another option and can be accomplished via either the **Cincinnati approach** or the dorsal approach.

METABOLIC BONE DISORDERS

164. Ans. (b) Osteosclerosis

Ref: Maheshwari and Mhaskar's Essential Orthopaedics 6th ed. pg. 314

Differential Diagnosis of Osteosclerosis

- Fluorosis
- Paget's disease
- Renal osteodystrophy
- Osteopetrosis
- Prostrate CA metastasis

Fluorosis

- An osteosclerosis disease → Excessive Ca^+ deposition in bone and soft tissue
- Due to excessive fluoride intake in drinking water (n = <1 ppm)
- **Clinical feature**
  - **Skeletal fluorosis:** Back pain and joint pain, spine stiffness, paraesthesia of limbs (d/t cord compression)
  - **Dental fluorosis:** Earliest sign of fluorosis.
  - Mottling of enamel → best seen in incisors of upper jaw → later eroded and fall off
- **X-rays:** Increased density and calcification in spine and pelvis
- **Inv:** Increased fluoride in urine and drinking water
- **Treatment:** Decrease fluoride content in drinking water

165. Ans. (a) Osteogenesis imperfecta

Ref: Essential Orthopaedics by Maheshwari 6th ed. pg. 316

- Osteogenesis imperfecta is also known as Fragilitas ossium/Vrolik's disease.
- There is defective collagen synthesis, therefore bone is usually very weak
- Characterized by frequent fracture of weak bones
- It also affects other organs like skin, sclera teeth, ligaments etc
- Note: Triad of osteogenesis imperfecta, blue sclera and otosclerosis is **Vander Hoeve syndrome**.

166. Ans. (a) Vitamin D increase

Ref: J. Maheshwari 6th ed. P 308, 313

TABLE: Actions of PTH, Vit D, and FGF23 on Gut, Bone, and Kidney

	PTH	Vitamin D	FGF23
Intestine	↑CA and P absorption (by ↑1,25 $[OH]_2$ D production)	↑Ca and phosphate absorption by 1,25 $(OH)_2D$	↓Ca and P absorption by ↓1,25 $(OH)_2$ production
Kidney	↓Ca excretion, ↑P excretion	↓Ca and P excretion by 25(OH)D and 1,25$(OH)_2D^1$	↑P excretion
Bone	↑Ca and P resorption high doses. Low doses may increase bone formation	↑Ca and P resorption by 1,25$(OH)_2D$; ↑bone formation by 1,25$(OH)_2D$ and 24,25$(OH)_2D$	↓mineralization due to hypophosphatemia
Net effect on serum levels	↑Serum Ca, ↓Serum P	↑Serum Ca and P	↓Serum P

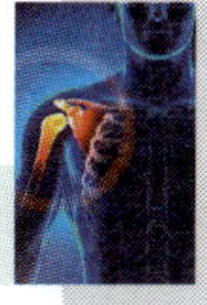

Note:
- In hyperparathyroidism serum ALP, Ca^+ is high and PO_4 is low.
- In osteoporosis all serum parameters are normal.
- Osteomalacia is due to dietary deficiency of Vitamin D causing decreased Serum Ca^+ and PO_4.

167. Ans. (c) Osteopetrosis

Ref: Essential Orthopaedics, Maheshwari & Mhaskar, 6th ed. pg. 317

OSTEOPETROSIS

- Also known as Marble bone disease or Albers-Schonberg disease
- It is characterized by dense but brittle bones also known as marble bones which occur due to reduced bone resorption and diffuse symmetrical skeletal sclerosis due to impaired formation or function of osteoclast.
- **X-ray appearances**
  - Bone within Bone appearance
  - Erlenmeyer flask deformity of long bone disease ends (flask shaped metaphysis)
  - Rugger jersey spine
  - Increased bone density

It can occur in two forms:

Autosomal dominant	Congenital Autosomal recessive
• Less severe	More severe form
• Has tendency to fracture	In child it is associated with severe anemia, jaw osteomyelitis and cranial nerve palsies
• Better survival	Poor survival

168. Ans. (d) Osteoarthritis

Ref: Harrison's 19th ed. pg. 2226

- Osteoarthritis (OA) is the most common type of arthritis.
- Commonly affected joints include the cervical and lumbosacral spine, hip, knee, and first metatarsal phalangeal joint (MTP).
- In the hands, the distal and proximal interphalangeal joints and the base of the thumb are often affected.
- Joints Spared: Wrist, elbow, and ankle
- Deformity can be due to bouchard nodes (PIP) and heberden nodes (DIP)

TABLE: Joint involvement in several conditions

	Osteoarthritis	Rheumatoid arthritis	Psoriatic arthritis
Joint involved	PIP DIP and 1st carpometacarpal joint (1st CMC)	• PIP • MCP • Wrist	• DIP • PIP and any other joints
Joint spared	MCP and wrist	DIP	Any

169. Ans. (c) Bisphosphonates

Ref. Postmenopausal Osteoporosis, Hormones & Other therapies by Andrea R Genazzari, pg. 289-90

- Bisphosphonates act by inhibiting osteoclast mediated bone resorption. Currently the 3rd generation bisphosphonate is commonly used.
- Zoledronate is the most potent and is also considered as *drug of choice for treatment and prophylaxis of osteoporosis.*
- It is also used for treatment of hypercalcemia associated with malignancy and for treatment of Paget's disease.
- Bisphosphonates have poor oral absorption. Therefore given empty stomach, around 30 minutes before meal with a glass of water. They are known to cause esophagitis, so patients are asked to remain upright after drug intake.

TABLE: Classification of bisphosphonates

1st generation	2nd generation	3rd generation
• Etidronate • Clodronate • Medronate	• Alendronate • Pamidronate	• Zoledronate (2–5 mg/year) • Risedronate (150 mg/month)

170. Ans. (d) Vitamin D deficiency

Ref: Apley's System of Orthopaedics, 9th ed. pg. 135-36

- The given image and the information on cupping and widening points towards rickets.
- Rickets and osteomalacia are different expressions of the same disease: Inadequate mineralization of bone.
- The inadequacy may be due to defects anywhere along the metabolic pathway for vitamin D: Nutritional lack, underexposure to sunlight, intestinal mal-absorption, decreased 25-hydroxylation (liver disease, anticonvulsants) and reduced 1α-hydroxylation (renal disease).

Clinical Features of Rickets

- The infant with rickets may present with **tetany** or convulsions. Later the parents may notice that there is a **failure to thrive**, listlessness and **muscular flaccidity**. Early bone changes are deformity of the skull **(craniotabes)** and thickening of the knees, ankles and wrists from physeal overgrowth. Enlargement of the costochondral junctions **('rickety rosary')** and lateral indentation of the chest **(Harrison's sulcus)** may also appear.
- Distal tibial bowing has been attributed to sitting or lying **cross-legged**.
- In active rickets there is thickening and **widening of the growth plate**, **cupping of the metaphysis** and, sometimes, bowing of the diaphysis. The metaphysis may remain abnormally wide even after healing has occurred.

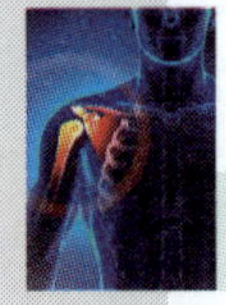

171. Ans. (c) Scurvy

Ref: Maheshwari, 5th ed. pg. 315

Scurvy causes failure of collagen synthesis and osteoid formation. It clinically presents with:
- Irritability
- Gum bleeding
- Pseudoparalysis (due to subperiosteal haemorrhage)
- Anemia and beading of costochondral junction.

Radiological features are: Frenkel's line (dense line between metaphysic and physis/epiphysis), ring sign, *thin cortex,* scurvy line (band of rarefaction on the diaphyseal side) and metaphyseal osteopenia, cleft and fractures.

Pathology: Deficiency causes failure of collagen synthesis or primitive collagen formation, throughout the body, including in blood vessels, predisposing to haemorrhage.

Extra Mile

Rickets	Scurvy
• ***Metaphysis:*** *Indistinct, frayed, splaying, and cupping of margin.* Patchy sclerosis in case of intermittent dietary deficiency • Widened epiphysis with hazed cortical margin • Generalized reduction in bone density • Looser's zone (less common) • Severe cases show Genu valgum, bow legs, thoracic kyphosis, pigeon chest, *ricketic rosary,* skull bossing, cox vera.	• **Metaphysis:** Frankel's white line, Trummerfeld, lucent zone, Pelkan spur due to fracture. • Wimberger's sign (small epiphysis surrounded by sclerotic rim) • Subperiosteal hemorrhage with periosteal elevation • Ground glass appearance of bone with pencil thin cortex.

172. Ans. (b) Scurvy

Please refer to above explanation

173. Ans. (c) Vitamin D

Ref: Maheshwari, 5th ed. pg. 311

- Double malleoli is sign of rickets which is seen due to deficiency of vitamin D.

Please refer to above explanation

174. Ans. (a) Fluorosis

Ref: Maheshwari, 5th ed. pg. 314

- Hint in the question is child from a village of Bihar with Genu varum/bow legged, long bone pain and X-Rays showing increased bone density, this characteristically focuses towards Fluorosis.

GENU VALGUM (KNOCK KNEE)

- It is *abnormal approximation of knees* with abnormally *divergent ankles.* It can be estimated by measuring the distance between the medial malleolis, when the knees are touching with the patella facing forwards; it is usually *<5 cm.* Valgus alignment of lower extremities is normal in child between *2–8 years* of age (Known as *physiological valgus* & is maximum between 2–4 years). The commonest cause of genu valgum (knock knee) is *idiopathic > rickets.*

GENU VARUM (BOW LEGS)

- Knee are abnormally divergent and ankles approximated. B/L bow legs can be estimated by measuring the distance between the medial malleoli when heels are touching; it should be *<6 cm. Normal children show maximum varus at 6 months to 1 year of age.* The *causes of genu varum are similar to genu val gum* except that the defective growth is on the medial side.

FLUOROSIS

- Fluorine in very low concentration- *1 part per million (ppm)* or less is used to reduce the incidence of dental caries. At slightly higher levels *(2–4 ppm)* it may produce *mottling of teeth.*
- In some parts of India and Africa, where fluorine concentration in the drinking water may be above *10 ppm-* chronic fluorine intoxication (flurosis) is endemic and results in skeletal anomalies.
- **Characterstic pathological feature** is *subperiosteal new bone accretion and osteosclerosis (increased bone density),* most marked in vertebrae, ribs, pelvis, forearm and leg bones, together with *hyperostosis at the bony attachments of ligaments, tendons and fascia.*
- Despite the apparent thickening and density of skeleton, tensile strength is reduced and the bones fracture more easily.
- First clinical manifestation is usually a stress fracture, ***back pain, bone pain, joint stiffness*** and neurological defects (due to hyperostosis encroaching vertebral canal).
- **Characterstic X-ray features** *are osteosclerosis, osteophytosis and ossification of ligamentous and fascial attachments.* It can be radiologically mistaken for other osteosclerotic conditions as *Paget's disease, osteopetrosis, renal osteodystrophy, idiopathic skeletal hyperostosis* etc.
- **Note:** *Fluorine stimulates osteoblastic activity; fluoroapatite crystals* are laid down in bone and these are usually *resistant to osteoclastic resorption.* This leads to *calcium retention* impaired mineralization and *secondary hyperparathyroidism.*

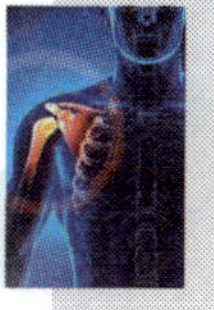

Extra Mile

- **Infantile cortical hyperostosis (Caffeys Disease)** is a *self limiting disorder* characterized by *soft tissue swelling, rapid subperiosteal new bone formation, cortical thickening of under lying bones,* fever and irritability. Classically, the onset of disease *occurs before 5th month* of life with *resolution by 3 years of age.*
- In sporadic cases, *mandible is the most common site of involvement presenting as jaw tumor* or swelling i.e. is firm, tender without heat or redness.

175. Ans. (b) Osteoclasts

Ref: Robbin's Pathology, 8th pg. 1212

"**Osteopetrosis** also known as **marble bone disease** and **Alber's Schon-berg disease** is characterized by reduced bone resorption and diffuse symmetrical skeletal sclerosis due to impaired formation or function of **osteoclasts.**"

Disease	Cause
Osteogenesis imperfecta	Deficiency in synthesis of type 1 collagen
Osteopetrosis	Osteoclasts dysfunction
Osteoporosis	Loss of bone mass
Paget disease (Osteitis Deformans)	Both osteoclast and osteoblast dysfunction
Rickets and osteomalacia	Vitamin D deficiency
Scurvy	Vitamin C deficiency

176. Ans. (b) Osteopetrosis

Ref: Sutton, 7th pg. 1339,1355, 1365

Disease	Radiological feature
Osteoporosis	• **Cod fish vertebrae** • Pencilling-in-vertebrae (loss of density of vertebral body with radiodense end plates)
Osteomalacia	• **Looser's zone/Pseudo fracture** is the Hallmark feature (B/L radiolucent band of uncalcified osteoid due to pressure of pulsating artery) • **Cod Fish** (marked biconcave) vertebrae • Pencilling in vertebrae
Osteopetrosis/ Marble Bone disease/Alberg Schowenberg disease	• **Bone within Bone appearance** • Erlenmeyer flask deformity of long bone disease ends (flask shaped metaphysis) • **Rugger jersey spine** • Increased density of bones

177. Ans. (b) Vit D deficiency Rickets

Ref: Maheshwari 5th ed. pg. 317, 311; http://www.indianpediatrics.net/july 2013/july-669-675.htm

- Different methods of treating vitamin D deficiency have been advocated, ranging from small doses for a few months to a single mega dose *(high dose)*, an approach referred to as ***stoss therapy.***
- Vitamin D deficiency rickets occurs secondary to vitamin D deficiency which can take place secondary to many factors:

Decreased vitamin D synthesis	Due to chronic liver disease
Decreased nutritional intake of vitamin	In strict vegetarian diet
Age and physiology related	Elderly, obese and institutionalized patients
Decreased maternal vitamin D stores	Exclusive breast feeding
Malabsorption	Celiac disease, pancreatic insufficiency (cystic fibrosis), biliary obstruction (biliary atresia)
Increased degradation of 25 (OH) D_3	Due to intake of drugs such as rifampicin, isoniazid, anticonvulsants, glucocorticoids

Recommended Treatment Regimen

- **Common recommendations include** vitamin D 1000-5000 units/day for several weeks or single IM injection of 6 lakh units (Stoss therapy) or 50,000 U of vitamin D_2 weekly for 8 weeks.
- Another advantage of Stoss therapy is that vitamin D is efficiently stored in adipose tissue and muscle and is continuously converted into active form.
- Stoss therapy regimens with large oral or parenteral dose of vitamin D_3 has been shown to cause increased and sustained higher levels of 25 (OH) D_3 levels, especially the regimen with **6 lakh IU.**

Note: *Vitamin D stimulates renal and GI absorption of calcium.*

PAGET'S DISEASE

- It is characterized by *excessive disorganized bone turnover,* that encompasses *excessive osteoclastic activity initially followed by disorganized excessive new bone formation.*
- **Treatment of choice for paget's disease: Calcitonin.**

178. Ans. (c) Raised serum calcium

Ref: Maheswari's, 5th pg. 310, 311

"In **osteomalacia** the **serum calcium level is low**, the phosphates are low, and alkaline phosphatase is high."

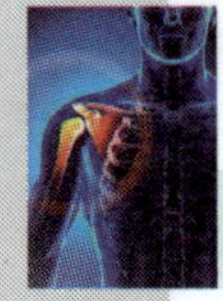

PATHOPHYSIOLOGY OF OSTEOMALACIA

Lack of sunlight exposure, nutritional deficiency of **vitamin D,** malabsorption syndrome, partial gastrectomy

↓

Failure of absorption of **calcium and phosphorous (Decreased serum calcium and phosphorous)**

↓

Decreased turnover of calcium and phosphorus in bone matrix

↓

Demineralization of bone and bony substance replaced by soft osteoid tissue

↓

Bone pains, muscular weakness (myopathy), spontaneous fractures

Note: *Osteoid matrix is secreted at normal rate but the mineralization is decreased (i.e. decrease in mineral apposition rate). This leads to increased osteoid maturation time.*

Radiological Features

- **Looser's Zone (pseudo fracture)**- Are radiolucent zones at sites of stress.
- **Triradiate pelvis** in female.

179. Ans (b) Osteomalacia

Ref: Maheshwari, 5th ed. pg. 312

- **Cortical infarctions** are wide transverse lucencies traversing bone usually at right angles to the involved cortex and are ***associated most frequently with osteomalacia*** and rickets. They are pseudo-fractures and considered a type of insufficiency fracture.
- Typically, the fractures have sclerotic irregular margins, and are often symmetrical.

Causes of Looser's Zone

- Osteomalacia
- Renal osteodystrophy
- Fibrous dysplasia
- Hyperthyroidism
- Paget's disease of bone
- X linked hypophosphataemia
- Osteogenesis Imperfecta

180. Ans. (d) Osteogenesis Imperfecta

Ref: Maheshwari, 5th ed. pg. 316

- In case of Osteogenesis Imperfecta patients are born with defective connective tissue, or without the ability to make it.
- This condition usually arises because of a **deficiency of type I collagen.**
- Deficiency of type I collagen arises from an amino acid substitution of glycine to bulkier amino acids in the collagen triple helix structure.
- The replaced larger amino acid side-chains create steric hindrance that creates a bulge in the collagen complex, which in turn influences both the molecular nano-mechanics and the interaction between molecules, which are both compromised.

Radiological Findings in Limbs in Osteogenesis Imperfecta

- Thin and under tabulated gracile bones which are normal in length or shortened
- ***Thickened or deformed bones (due to multiple fractures)***
- ***Banana fracture:*** pathological fractures tend to be oriented transversely within long bones
- Shaft fractures and metaphyseal abnormalities with florid or exuberant callus formation that can mimic an osteosarcoma.

Extra Mile

- Battered baby syndrome in this question is ruled out since fractures are seen in it in various stages of healing.
- Hypo-parathyroidism can present with short stature and features of rickets like delayed dentition.

181. Ans. (b) Duchenne muscular dystrophy

Ref: Harrison, 19th ed. pg. 462e-5

- ***Gowers' sign is classically seen in Duchenne muscular dystrophy*** but also presents itself in centro nuclear myopathy, myotonic dystrophy and various other conditions associated with proximal muscle weakness.
- This causes the patient to get up in a peculiar fashion taking support of his body or a nearby object.

182. Ans. (a) Pseudohypoparathyroidism

Ref: Harrison 19th ed. pg. 2485

Differential Diagnosis of Short 4th and 5th Metacarpal

- Post traumatic
- Ishemic diseases like sickle cell anemia
- Pseudohypoparathyroidism
- Pseudo-pseudo hypoparathyroidism
- Turner's syndrome

OPHTHALMOLOGY

15

MOST RECENT QUESTIONS 2023

1. A patient working in iron factory presents with visual disturbances and is found to have iron deposits in the eye. Which of the following conditions is most likely responsible for this ocular finding?

(Most Recent Question July 2023)

a. Chalcosis
b. Siderosis bulbi
c. Kaiser fleischer ring
d. Retinitis pigmentosa

2. A patient has a field defect where he cannot see the left side from the left eye and left side from the right eye with preserved central vision. What is the field defect?

(Most Recent Question July 2023)

a. Quadrantanopia
b. Homonymous hemianopia with macular sparing
c. Homonymous hemianopia
d. Bitemporal hemianopia

3. Which is the most common intraocular malignancy in adults? ***(Most Recent Question July 2023)***

a. Retinoblastoma
b. Choroidal metastasis
c. Uveal melanoma
d. Lymphoma

4. Oil droplet cataract is seen in:

(Most Recent Question July 2023)

a. Myotonic dystrophy
b. Galactosemia
c. Wilson's disease
d. Diabetes mellitus

5. Visual blurring in papilledema is called:

(Most Recent Question July 2023)

a. Amaurosis fugax
b. Blindness
c. Malingering
d. Amblyopia

6. In which type of cataract surgery suturing with 10–0 nylon is performed?

(Most Recent Question July 2023)

a. Phacoemulsification
b. FLACS
c. Manual small incision cataract surgery
d. Extra capsular cataract surgery

7. Which of the following dye is used in staining the anterior capsule of lens? ***(Most Recent Question July 2023)***

a. Fluorescein green
b. Trypan blue
c. Brilliant blue
d. Rose Bengal

8. In which condition is pupillary light reaction absent and accommodation reaction present?

(Most Recent Question July 2023)

a. Neurosyphilis
b. Horner's syndrome
c. Papilledema
d. Optic neuritis

9. Patient presents with vertical diplopia while walking downstairs. To correct that he tilts the head on one shoulder, which nerve palsy should be suspected?

(Most Recent Question July 2023)

a. 3 CN palsy
b. 4 CN palsy
c. 6 CN palsy
d. 7th CN palsy

10. In a patient presenting with recurrent chalazion, which cancer is suspected? ***(Most Recent Question July 2023)***

a. Sebaceous cell carcinoma
b. Squamous cell carcinoma
c. Basal cell carcinoma
d. Kaposi's sarcoma

11. On retinal examination of a hypertensive patient, multiple flame-shaped hemorrhages, cotton wool spots and disc edema were seen which grade of hypertensive retinopathy will it be classified as?

(Most Recent Question July 2023)

a. Grade 1
b. Grade 2
c. Grade 3
d. Grade 4

12. What are the yoke muscles for levo-depression?

(Most Recent Question July 2023)

a. RLR and LMR
b. RSR and LIR
c. RSO and LIR
d. RIO and LSO

13. A 60-year-old presents with chronic dacryocystitis. What should be the treatment of choice?

(Most Recent Question July 2023)

a. Lacrimal sac massage
b. Syringing
c. Dacryocystorhinostomy
d. Probing

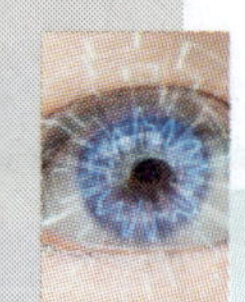

14. Diabetic male developed cataract. Which substance is deposited in cornea? ***(Most Recent Question Jan 2023)***

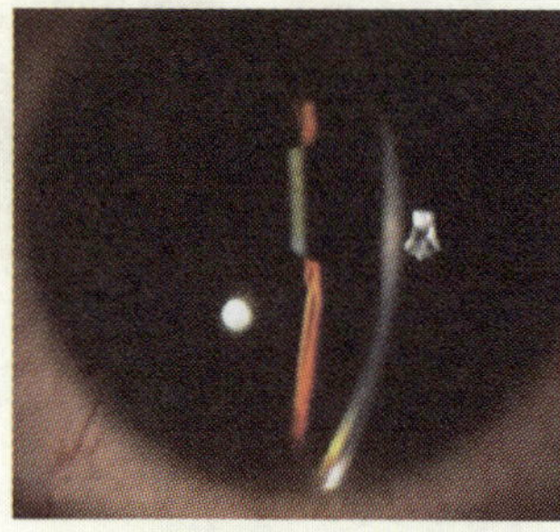

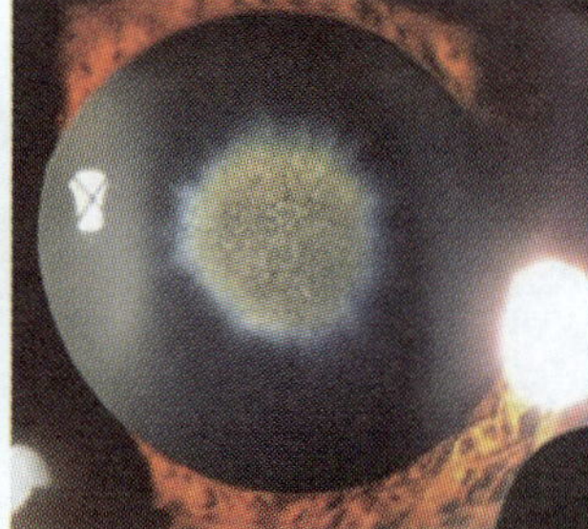

a. Copper b. Zinc
c. Iron d. Selenium

15. S in SAFE strategy of trachoma stands for: ***(Most Recent Question Jan 2023)***

a. Symptom b. Surgery
c. Spectacles d. Symbol

16. A 34-year-old male working as a Welder, came with complaint of pain, redness & watery eyes. What is the management? ***(Most Recent Question Jan 2023)***

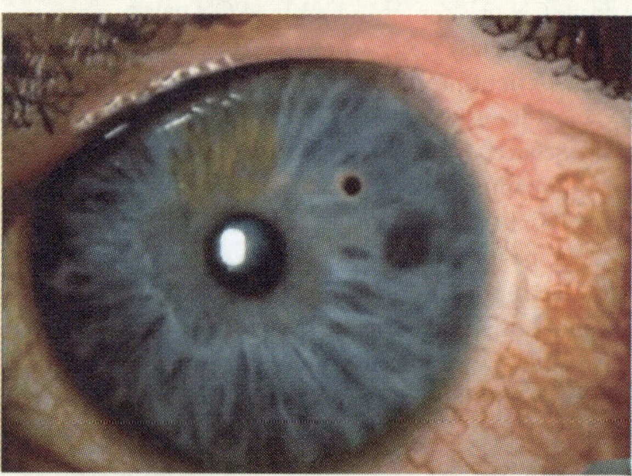

a. Syringe washing
b. Patching and antibiotics
c. Keratoplasty
d. Corneal transplant

17. What is the position of lacrimal sac in the orbit? ***(Most Recent Question Jan 2023)***

a. Medial wall
b. Lateral wall
c. Roof of the wall
d. Floor of the wall

18. Which of the following is synergistic muscle of right lateral rectus? ***(Most Recent Question Jan 2023)***

a. Lt superior oblique
b. Rt. Inferior oblique
c. Lt medial rectus
d. Lt. lateral rectus

19. Bitemporal hemianopia as shown in the image indicates that the lesion is at? ***(Most Recent Question Jan 2023)***

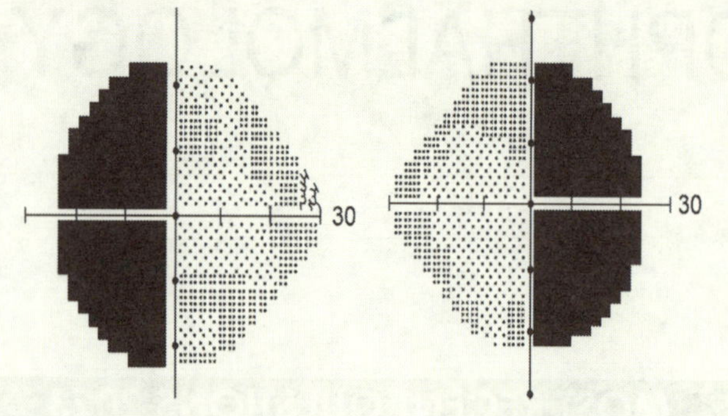

a. Optic chiasma b. Optic tract
c. Optic disc d. Optic nerve

20. Xerophthalmia causes dry eyes due to deficiency of which of the following vitamin? ***(Most Recent Question Jan 2023)***

a. Vitamin E b. Vitamin A
c. Vitamin C d. Vitamin B

21. A 70-year-old male whose cataract surgery was done a year ago, came with fibrosis of the nucleus. What is the probable diagnosis? ***(Most Recent Question Jan 2023)***

a. Index hypermetropia b. Index myopia
c. Presbyopia d. Secondary cataract

22. A 10-year-old child is diagnosed with amblyopia in one eye. What will be the best treatment? ***(Most Recent Question Jan 2023)***

a. Occlusion therapy
b. Observation
c. Refraction with near addition
d. Radial keratotomy

23. Identify the image taken from a 55-year-old diabetic patient with uncontrolled diabetes: ***(Most Recent Question Jan 2023)***

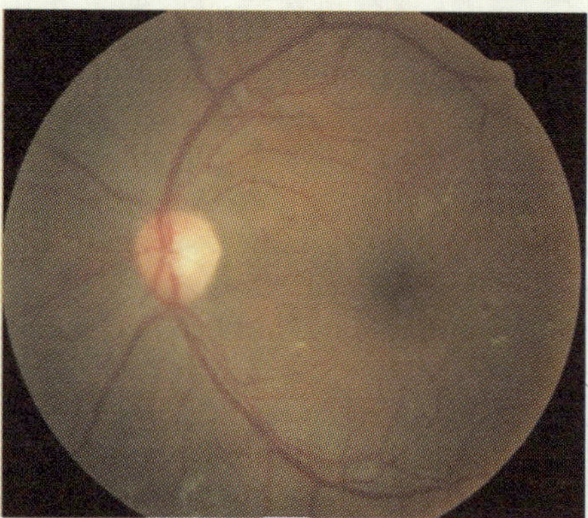

a. Primary open angle glaucoma
b. Diabetic macular edema
c. Optic nerve hypoplasia
d. Papilledema

ANATOMY, PHYSIOLOGY AND EXAMINATION OF EYE

24. In which surgery is the following instrument used?
(Most Recent Question June/Dec 2021)

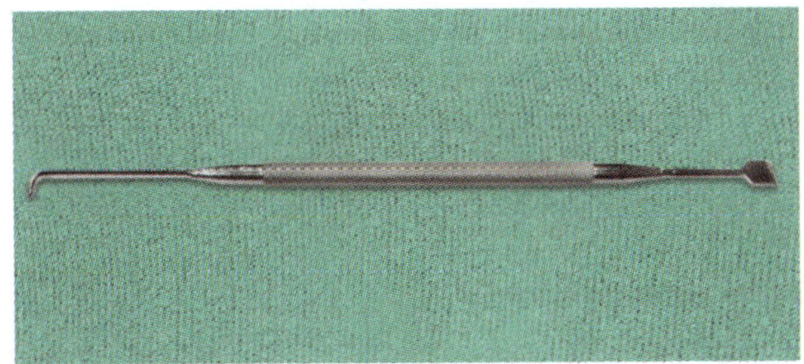

a. Enucleation
b. Dacryocystorhinostomy
c. Evisceration
d. Pterygium

25. V-Y procedure is used for correction of:
(Most Recent Question June/Dec 2021)

a. Symblepharon
b. Entropion
c. Ectropion
d. Ankylblepharon

26. A person has vision of <3/60, but >1/60 in his better eye, what is the type of blindness he has?
(Most Recent Question June/Dec 2021)

a. Social blindness
b. Economic blindness
c. Legal blindness
d. Total blindness

27. Which of the following is the gold standard for measuring intraocular pressure?
(Most Recent Question June/Dec 2021)

a. Pulse air tonometer
b. Schiotz tonometer
c. Goldmann applanation tonometer
d. None of the above

28. All of the following are true about above procedure; EXCEPT: *(Most Recent Question June/Dec 2021)*

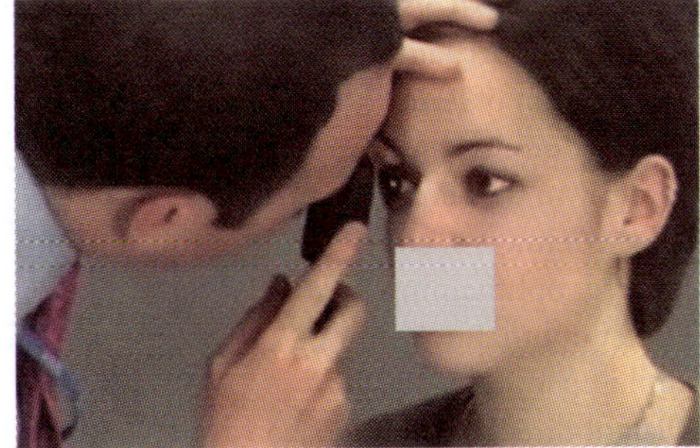

a. It can be done with the patient being in any position
b. There is no stereopsis
c. Can be used in cases of hazy ocular media
d. The retinal periphery cannot be examined

29. Which test is being demonstrated here?
(Most Recent Question Aug 2020)

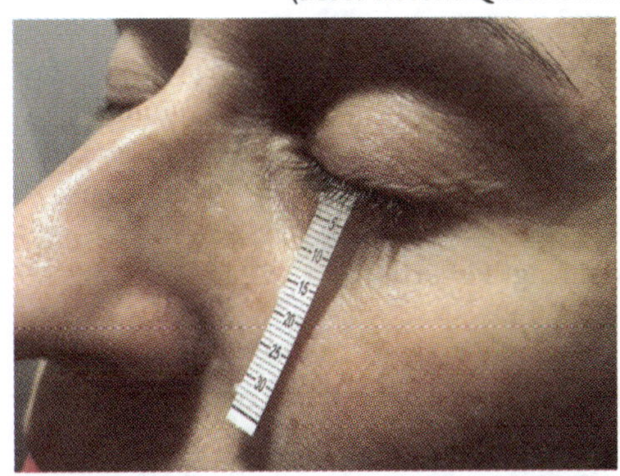

a. Jones test
b. Schirmer's test
c. Syringing and probing
d. Fluorescein staining

30. Not used for color vision testing:
(Most Recent Question 2019)

a. Holmgren wool test
b. Ishihara chart
c. FM 100 Hue test
d. Ames test

31. Corneal endothelium is derived from:
(Recent Pattern Question 2018-19)

a. Neuroectoderm
b. Neural crest
c. Mesoderm
d. Surface ectoderm

32. True about retinoscopy:
(Recent Pattern Question 2018-19)

a. In Hypermetropia the red glow moves in opposite direction
b. In high myopia, the red glow moves in same direction
c. In emmetropia the red glow moves in opposite direction
d. Done from 1 meter distance from patient

33. A child presents with night blindness, delayed dark adaptation. Which investigation to be done further to confirm the diagnosis? *(Recent Pattern Question 2018-19)*

a. Dark adaptometry
b. ERG
c. EOG
d. Retinoscopy

34. Newborn is hypermetropic by?
(Recent Pattern Question 2018)

a. +2 to +3 D
b. +1 to +2 D
c. +3 to +4 D
d. +2 to +4 D

35. Structure with highest refractive index:
(Recent Pattern Question 2018)

a. Cornea
b. Lens
c. Aqueous humor
d. Vitreous humor

36. Which is True about PHPV?
(Recent Pattern Question 2018)

a. Visual prognosis is good
b. Generally unilateral
c. Associated with microphthalmia
d. Associated with exophthalmos

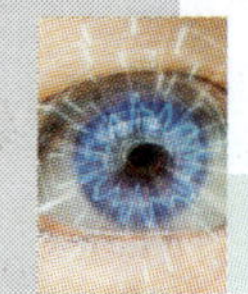

37. Maximum visual field is seen in?
(Recent Pattern Question 2016)
a. Temporal b. Nasal
c. Inferior d. Superior

38. Normal intraocular pressure ____ mm Hg?
(Recent Pattern Question 2016)
a. 5–10 b. 10–20
c. 20–25 d. 25–30

39. Axial length of orbit:
a. 2.5 mm b. 2.5 cm
c. 2 mm d. 2 cm

40. The junction between the retina and ciliary body is called:
a. Pars plana b. Pars plicata
c. Ora serrata d. Equator

41. All of the following ocular muscles are supplied by CN III; EXCEPT:
a. Superior rectus b. Superior oblique
c. Inferior rectus d. Medial rectus

42. All of the following statement are true about oculomotor nerve; EXCEPT:
a. Supplies extrinsic ocular muscles
b. Its nucleus is located in lower midbrain
c. Its nucleus is located in upper midbrain
d. Palsy may lead to ptosis

43. All are glands of eyelids; EXCEPT:
a. Glands of zeis b. Lacrimal gland
c. Meibomian gland d. Glands of moll

44. Person is not able look down. Which extra ocular muscle is affected:
a. Superior oblique b. Inferior oblique
c. Superior rectus d. Lateral rectus

45. The secondary actions of superior rectos muscle are:
a. Adduction and intorsion b. Abduction and intorsion
c. Adduction and extorsion d. Abduction and extorsion

46. Person is not able look down. Which extra ocular muscle is affected:
a. Inferior oblique b. Inferior rectus
c. Superior rectus d. Lateral rectus

47. In lateral rectus palsy of the right side, the face of the patient is turned to which of the following sides?
a. Upwards b. Downwards
c. Towards the right side d. Towards the left side

48. Synergistic muscle of right inferior oblique:
a. Right superior oblique
b. Left superior rectus
c. Left inferior rectus
d. Right superior rectus

49. The oculomotor and trochlear nerve passes through:
a. The superior orbital fissure
b. The inferior orbital fissure
c. The optic canal d. None of these

50. Maddox rod test is used for:
a. Strabismus b. Refractive error
c. Retinal hemorrhage d. Color blindness

51. By pinhole visual acuity is neutralized till:
a. 1 D b. 2 D
c. 3 D d. 4 D

52. Which component of the eye has maximum refractive index:
a. Anterior surface of the lens
b. Posterior surface of the lens
c. Centre of the lens
d. Cornea

53. Power of cornea is?
a. 41 D b. 40 D
c. 45 D d. 47 D

54. Shallow anterior chamber is seen in?
a. Myopia b. Phacomorphic glaucoma
c. Phacolytic glaucoma d. Aphakia

55. Accommodation is maximum in:
a. Children b. Young male
c. Elderly d. None

56. Surface ectoderm forms:
a. Lens of eye b. Retina
c. Iris d. Corneal stroma

57. Lens develops from.
a. Neuroectoderm b. Surface ectoderm
c. Mesoderm d. Neural crest

58. Outer epithelium of cornea is derived from?
a. Mesoderm b. Endoderm
c. Surface ectoderm d. Neural ectoderm

59. Which of the following has maximum field of vision:
a. Superior b. Inferior
c. Temporal d. Nasal

60. Neuroretinal rim is broadest in which area:
a. Temporal area b. Inferior
c. Superior d. Supero temporal

61. Which of the following is better diagnosed with distant direct ophthalmoscopy:
a. Retinal hemorrhage
b. Subluxation of lens
c. Ciliary body injury
d. Opacity in the refractive media

62. Macular edema is seen with:
a. Indirect ophthalmoscopy
b. Direct ophthalmoscopy
c. Slit lamp + 90 D
d. Distant direct ophthalmoscopy

63. Hirschberg test measures?
a. Strabismus
b. Glaucoma
c. Cataract
d. Refractive error

64. Muscle first affected in thyroid ophthalmopathy is:

a. Medial rectus b. Lateral rectus
c. Inferior rectus d. Superior rectus

65. True about Color blindness:

a. Males are more prone
b. Males and females equally affected
c. Autosomal dominant
d. Males are carrier

CORNEA, CONJUNCTIVA AND SCLERA

66. Koeppe's nodule body is seen on:

(Most Recent Question June 2022)

a. Iris b. Sclera
c. Conjunctiva d. Cornea

67. A 5-year-old child presented to the Ophthalmology Clinic with foamy lesion in eyes as shown in the image below. Which vitamin deficiency can be suspected?

(Most Recent Question June 2022)

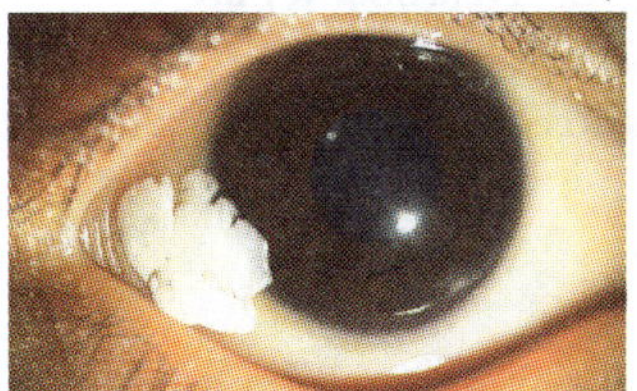
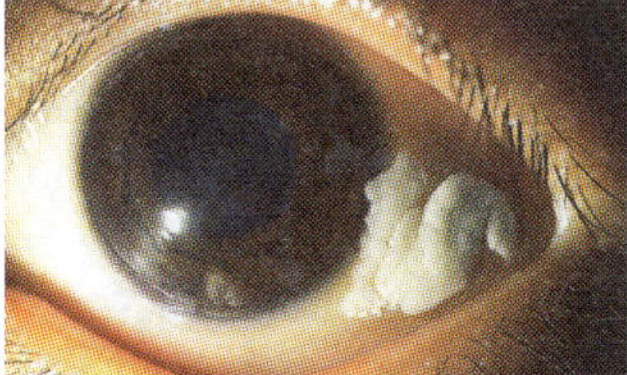

a. Vitamin A b. Vitamin D
c. Vitamin B_3 d. Vitamin B_{12}

68. A patient presents with congestion, itching, foreign body sensation in eye. He has a history of contact lens usage. What is the most probable diagnosis?

(Most Recent Question June/Dec 2021)

a. Corneal abrasion
b. Vernal keratoconjunctivitis
c. Giant papillary conjunctivitis
d. Corneal ulcer

69. A farmer presented with pain photophobia and watering from eye since last 36 hours. On examination 1 × 2 cm ulcer is seen as shown in image. Identify the lesion marked: ***(Most Recent Question June/Dec 2021)***

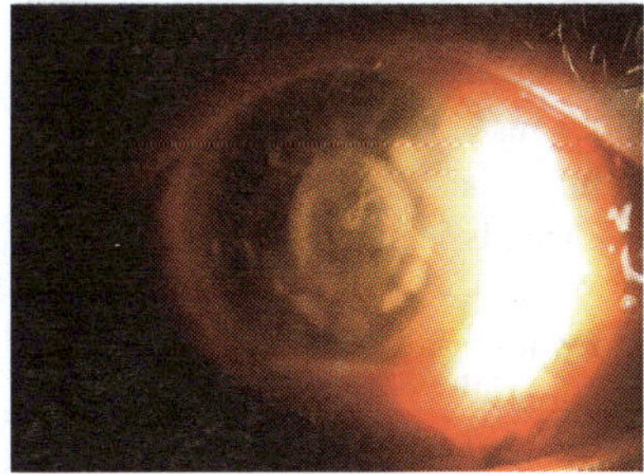

a. Hypopyon b. Satellite lesions
c. Dendritic ulcer d. Ring infiltrate

70. A young boy presents with itching, irritation and photophobia every year with onset of hot weather. What is the likely diagnosis?

(Most Recent Question June/Dec 2021)

a. Trachoma
b. Vernal keratoconjunctivitis
c. Giant papillary conjunctivitis
d. Ophthalmia neonatorum

71. A person suffers injury to eye with vegetative matter/leaf few days ago and has now developed pain and photophobia. What could be the most likely cause?

(Most Recent Question June/Dec 2021)

a. Fungal keratitis b. Acanthamoeba keratitis
c. Bacterial keratitis d. Herpes zoster

72. A child with history of malnutrition was examined and following image of the eye was seen. What is the most likely diagnosis in this case?

(Most Recent Question June/Dec 2021)

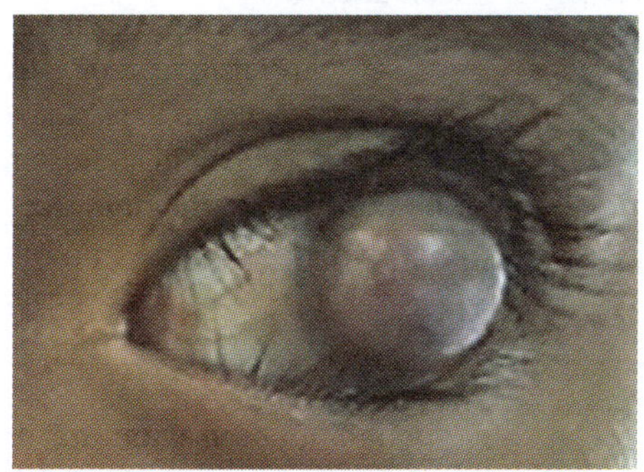

a. Anterior staphyloma b. Corneal opacity
c. Buphthalmos d. Megalocornea

73. What is the most common treatment for recurrent pterygium?

(Most Recent Question June/Dec 2021)

a. Observation b. Simple excision
c. Conjunctival autograft d. Mitomycin C

74. Spot diagnosis of the given image:

(Most Recent Question June/Dec 2021)

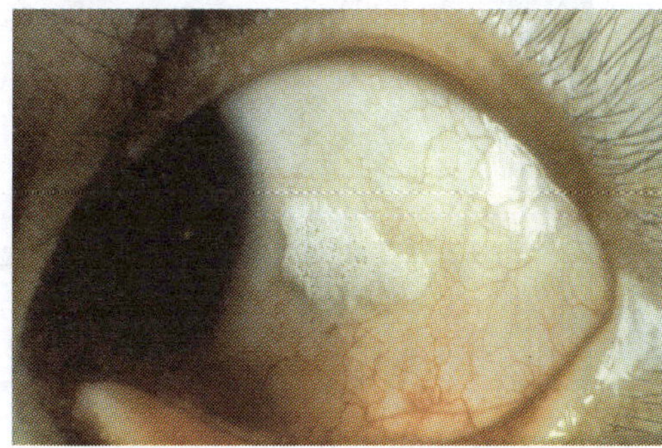

a. Pinguecula b. Pterygium
c. Bitot's spots d. Phlycten

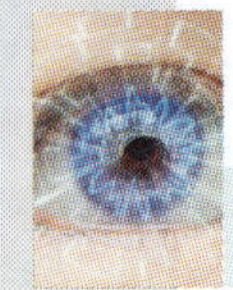

75. In which disease is corneal collagen cross-linking used?
(Most Recent Question Aug 2020)
a. Corneal ulcer   b. Corneal dystrophy
c. Keratoconus   d. Uveitis

76. What is the risk factor for acanthamoeba keratitis?
(Most Recent Question Aug 2020)
a. Extended contact lense wearing
b. Hypertension
c. Band – shaped keratopathy
d. Hyperlipidemia

77. Which part of the eye can be first involved in patients of COVID-19 patients?
(Most Recent Question Aug 2020)
a. Cornea   b. Conjunctiva
c. Retina   d. Choroid

78. Arlt's line is seen in which condition?
(Most Recent Question Aug 2020)
a. Vernal keratoconjunctivitis
b. Phlyctenular conjunctivitis
c. Ophthalmia neonatorum
d. Trachoma

79. Corneal transparency is maintained by:
(Most Recent Question Dec 2019-20)
a. Chondroitin sulphate
b. Keratan sulphate
c. Hyaluronic acid
d. Dermatan sulphate

80. A young Patient wearing lens from last 2 years started having redness and decreased vision as well. What could be the possible cause?
(Most Recent Question Dec 2019-20)
a. Bacterial corneal ulcer
b. Giant cell papillary
c. Fungal keratitis
d. HSV keratitis

81. What is NOT correct regarding the clinical condition shown in image: ***(Most Recent Question Dec 2019-20)***

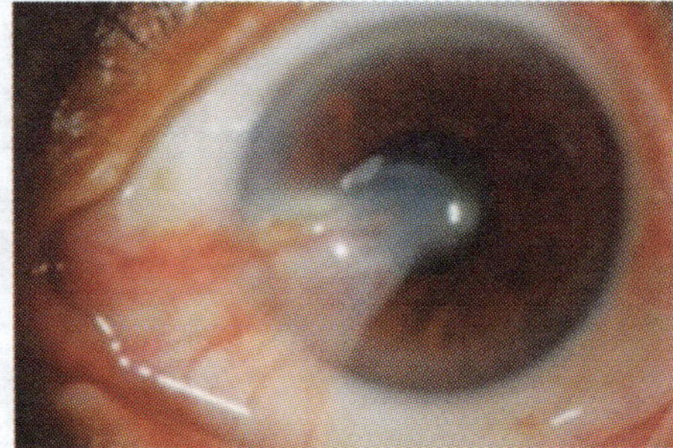

a. Occurs more commonly in warm areas
b. This structure is attached to cornea
c. It causes myopia
d. Iron deposition is found

82. A 15-year-old boy presents to clinic with difficulty in coordination of movements and abdominal pain. On further examination copper deposition in a ring form is seen in cornea. Most likely diagnosis?
(Most Recent Question Dec 2019-20)

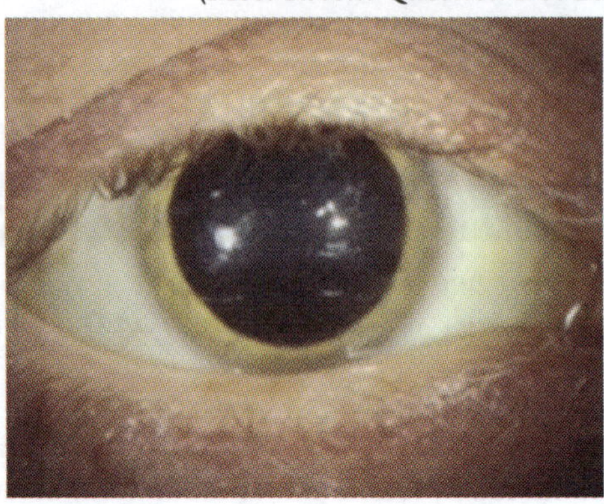

a. Keratitis   b. Munson sign
c. Wilson's disease   d. Neuroblastoma

83. Phlyctenular conjunctivitis seen due to:
(Most Recent Question Dec 2019-20)
a. Post fungal infection
b. Allergic
c. Post protozoal
d. Post tuberculoid

84. Identify the clinical condition as shown in image:
(Most Recent Question Dec 2019-20)

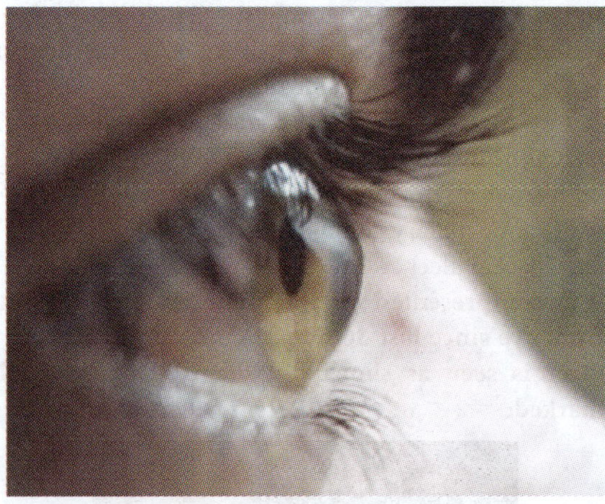

a. Keratoconus   b. Limbus
c. Keratomalacia   d. None

85. Fleischer's ring is seen in:
(Most Recent Question Dec 2019-20)
a. Keratoconus   b. Keratomalacia
c. Keratoglobus   d. Trachoma

86. Keratometer is used to assess:
(Most Recent Question Dec 2019-20)
a. Diameter of cornea   b. Thickness of cornea
c. Curvature of cornea   d. Curvature of lens

87. The following image shows: ***(Most Recent Question 2019)***

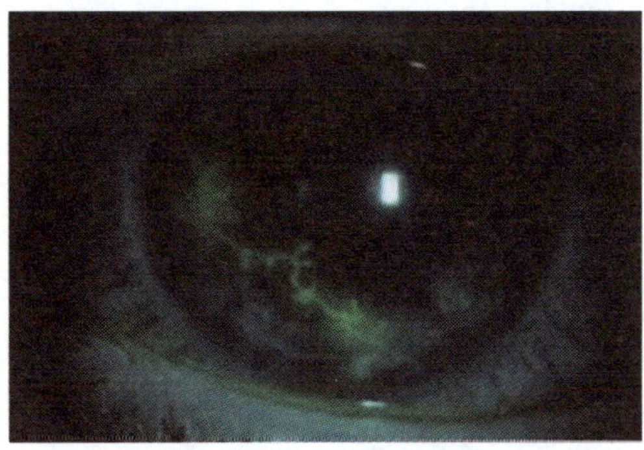

a. Bacterial keratitis b. Fungal keratitis
c. Viral keratitis d. Syphilitic keratitis

88. Drug contraindicated in keratitis: ***(Most Recent Question 2019)***

a. Tear drops b. Steroids
c. Cycloplegics d. Timolol

89. True about pterygium: ***(Recent Pattern Question 2018-19)***

a. Inflammation of cornea
b. Fatty deposition over sclera
c. Conjunctiva invasion making a flap over cornea
d. Dead epithelial debris accumulation

90. Cause of acute hemorrhagic conjunctivitis: ***(Recent Pattern Question 2018)***

a. Coronavirus b. Adenovirus
c. Enterovirus d. Herpes virus

91. Klebsiella pneumoniae causes: ***(Recent Pattern Question 2018)***

a. Stye b. Keratitis
c. Chalazion d. Entropion

92. True about dendritic ulcer: ***(Recent Pattern Question 2018)***

a. Corneal sensation decreased
b. Increased corneal thickness
c. Descemetocele
d. Hypopyon

93. Which is therapeutic indication of keratoplasty? ***(Recent Pattern Question 2018)***

a. Optic nerve atrophy b. Keratoconus
c. Myopia d. Hypermetropia

94. Swimming pool conjunctivitis is caused due to? ***(Recent Pattern Question 2017)***

a. Streptococcus b. Staph aureus
c. Chylamydia d. Hemophilus

95. To prevent disease transmission from a conjunctivitis patient, which is the most effective way: ***(Recent Pattern Question 2017)***

a. Rinse eye b. Wearing black sunglasses
c. Antibiotics d. Clean hand

96. Most common cause of bacterial corneal ulcer: ***(Recent Pattern Question 2017)***

a. Pseudomonas b. Acanthamoeba
c. Pneumococcus d. Staphylococcus

97. Salmon patch is seen in? ***(Recent Pattern Question 2017)***

a. Mooren's ulcer b. Viral keratits
c. Interstitial keratitis d. Allergic keratitis

98. Munson sign is seen in: ***(Recent Pattern Question 2017)***

a. Corneal degeneration b. Keratoconus
c. Mooren ulcer d. Pinguecula

99. Angular conjunctivitis is most commonly caused by: ***(Recent Pattern Question 2017)***

a. Moraxella b. H. influenzae
c. Strep. Pneumoniae d. Staph. Aureus

100. In case of Neurotropic keratitis which nerve is involved: ***(Recent Pattern Question 2016)***

a. Trigeminal nerve b. Oculomotor
c. Facial d. Trochlear

101. Colored halos in conjunctivitis are due to excess: ***(Recent Pattern Question 2016)***

a. Lacrimation b. Edema
c. Flakes of mucus d. Dryness

102. Angular conjunctivitis is caused by: ***(Recent Pattern Question 2016)***

a. Moraxella b. Streptococcus
c. Gonococcus d. Corynebacterium

103. Fleischer ring is seen in: ***(Recent Pattern Question 2016)***

a. Wilson's disease b. Keratoconus
c. Fungal infection d. Protozoal keratitis

104. True about bowman's membrane:

a. True elastic membrane
b. Most regenerative layer
c. Prevents infection more than descemet's membrane
d. Cellular layer

105. Keratometer is used to assess:

a. Thickness of cornea b. Refractive power
c. Astigmatism d. Curvature of cornea

106. Thickness of cornea is best detected by:

a. Keratometry b. Pachymetry
c. Placido disc d. Tonometry

107. All are seen in Keratoconus; EXCEPT:

a. Progressive vision loss due to increasing myopia and irregular astigmatism
b. Keyser Fleischer Ring
c. Scissoring reflex in retinoscopy
d. Munson sign Positive

108. Recurrent corneal erosion are seen in:

a. Corneal dystrophy b. Keratoconus
c. Keratoglobus d. Corneal degeneration

109. Recurrent corneal erosion are seen in:

a. Corneal degeneration b. Keratitis
c. Corneal dystrophy d. Keratoconus

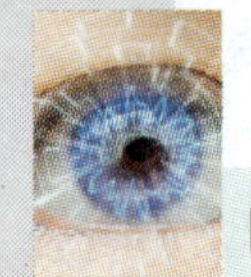

110. Which of the following drug has corneal staining property:
a. Thioridazine b. Isoniazid
c. Quinines d. Acetazolamide

111. In case of xeropthalmia secondary to Vitamin A deficiency, what does X2 indicate according to WHO:
a. Conjunctival xerosis b. Bitot's spot
c. Corneal xerosis d. Corneal ulcer

112. Which of the following does not occur due to vitamin A intoxication:
a. Xerophthalmia b. Pseudotumor cerebri
c. Dry skin d. Vomiting

113. First sign of papilledema:
a. Hyperemia of disc margin
b. Abolition of cups
c. Blurring of disc
d. Soft exudates

114. Treatment of mooren's ulcer is?
a. Topical steroids b. Corneal graft
c. Immunosuppressives d. All of the above

115. Kayer fleischer ring affects:
a. Conjunctiva b. Epithelium layer
c. Bowman's layer d. Descemets membrane

116. Giant dendritic ulceration on cornea is seen in case of:
a. Fungal infection b. Chlamydial infection
c. HSV infection d. Pneumococcal infection

117. Which one of the following drugs is contraindicated in treatment of dendritic corneal ulcer:
a. Atropine b. Cefazolin
c. Acyclovir d. Dexamethasone

118. Herpes Simplex Virus infection with disc shaped ulceration is seen in:
a. Epithelial keratitis b. Stromal keratitis
c. Syphilitic keratitis d. Interstitial keratitis

119. Nummular keratitis is seen in:
a. Bacterial keratitis
b. Herpes zoster keratitis
c. Acanthamoeba keratitis
d. Fungal keratitis

120. Interstitial keratitis is seen in:
a. Trachoma b. Bacterial conjunctivitis
c. Fungal conjunctivitis d. Syphilis

121. Which of the following is used in Acanthamoebic keratitis treatment:
a. Topical corticosteroids b. Propamidine isothionate
c. Acetazolamide d. Artificial tear

122. Acanthamoebic keratitis is associated with which of the following:
a, Lacrimal gland inflammation
b. Inturning of eyelids
c. Wearing of soft contact lenses
d. Dry eye

123. Giant Papillary Conjunctivitis is caused by:
a. Contact Lens wear
b. Ocular Prosthesis
c. Protruding corneal sutures
d. All of the above

124. Giant papillary conjunctivitis can be secondary to:
a. Trachoma
b. Contact lens
c. Phlyctenular conjunctivitis
d. Vernal kerato conjunctivitis

125. Which of the following is seen in chronic contact lens wearer:
a. Inclusion conjunctivitis
b. Giant papillary conjunctivitis
c. Vernal keratoconjunctivitis
d. Follicular conjunctivitis

126. Complication in a patient with long term use of contact lens is most commonly caused by?
a. Aspergillus b. Acanthameoba
c. Pneumococcus d. Pseudomonas

127. In which of the following corneal ulcers signs are more than symptoms:
a. Fungal corneal ulcer b. Bacterial corneal ulcer
c. Viral corneal ulcer d. Herpetic corneal ulcer

128. Satellite lesion on cornea are seen in:
a. Viral ulcer b. Bacterial ulcer
c. Fungal ulcer d. Herpetic ulcer

129. Treatment of choice of trachoma:
a. Azithromycin b. Tetracycline
c. Erythromycin d. Penicillin

130. Location of Arlt's line:
a. Sclera
b. Lens
c. Lower palpebral conjunctiva
d. Upper palpebral conjunctiva

131. Herbert pits are seen in trachoma at:
a. Limbus b. Lid margin
c. Palpebral conjunctiva d. Bulbar conjunctiva

132. Swimming pool conjunctivitis is caused by:
a. Pneumococcus b. Chlamydia
c. Pox virus d. Staph Aureus

133. Cobble stoning of conjunctiva is seen in:
a. Vernal keratoconjunctivitis
b. Simple allergic conjunctivitis
c. Gaint papillary conjunctivitis
d. Acute hemorrhagic conjunctivitis

134. Spring catarrh is treated with which of the following drugs:
a. Olopatadine drops
b. Normal saline eye drops
c. Ciprofloxacin
d. Carboxymethylcellulose (CMC) eye drops

135. Chlymadia trachomatic A-C will cause which of the following?

a. Opthalmia Neonatorum
b. Vernal Kerato conjunctivitis
c. Paratrachoma
d. Trachoma

136. Ropy discharge is seen in:

a. Conjunctival conjunctivitis
b. Bacterial conjunctivitis
c. Fungal conjunctivitis
d. Veneral conjunctivitis

137. Fat like nodules on bilateral nasal side of conjunctiva is seen in?

a. Pterygium
b. Pinguecula
c. Chalazion
d. Hordeolum

138. Intercalary staphyloma:

a. Sloughing corneal ulcer
b. Degenerative high myopia
c. Bulge in limbal area lined by root of iris
d. Penetrating injuries

139. Ciliary staphyloma is a complication of:

a. Episcleritis
b. Degenerative myopia
c. Perforated corneal ulcer
d. Scleritis

140. Posterior staphyloma is seen in:

a. High hypermetropia
b. Astigmatism
c. Emmetropia
d. Degenerative myopia

141. Scleritis is commonly seen with:

a. Reiter's syndrome
b. Rheumatoid arthritis
c. Ankylosing spondylitis
d. Wegner's syndrome

142. Keratoconjunctivitis sicca is due to:

a. Mucin deficiency
b. Lipid deficiency
c. Aqueous deficiency
d. Impaired eyelid function

RETINA AND UVEAL TRACT

143. A 67-year-old hypertensive patient presents with acute painless loss of vision. On examination his Visual Acuity is hand movement and he has relative afferent pupillary defect. Fundus image is as shown in the image below. What could be the most likely cause?

(Most Recent Question June/Dec 2021)

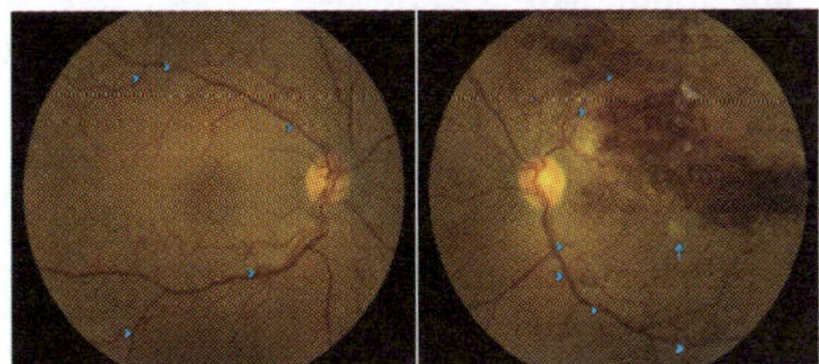

a. Central retinal vein occlusion
b. Central retinal artery occlusion
c. Branched retinal vein occlusion
d. Cystoid macular edema

144. What is the diagnosis from the given fundus image of a diabetic patient with painless loss of vision?

(Most Recent Question June/Dec 2021)

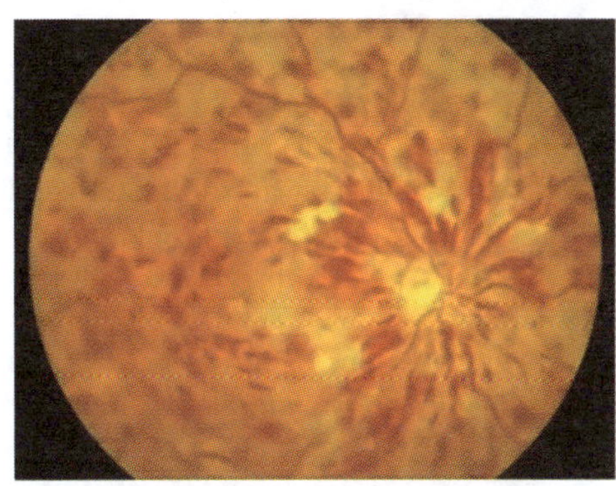

a. Proliferative diabetic retinopathy
b. Non-proliferative diabetic retinopathy
c. CRAO
d. CRVO

145. Cherry red spot is seen in:

(Most Recent Question Aug 2020)

a. Central retinal artery occlusion
b. Central retinal vein occlusion
c. Retinal detachment
d. Diabetic retinopathy

146. Microaneurysms are found in which disease?

(Most Recent Question Aug 2020)

a. Retinal detachment
b. Diabetic retinopathy
c. Uveitis
d. Cataract

147. Which of the following is used in acute anterior uveitis?

(Most Recent Question Aug 2020)

a. Pilocarpine
b. Brimonidine
c. Atropine
d. Moxifloxacin

148. Identify the investigation:

(Most Recent Question Aug 2020)

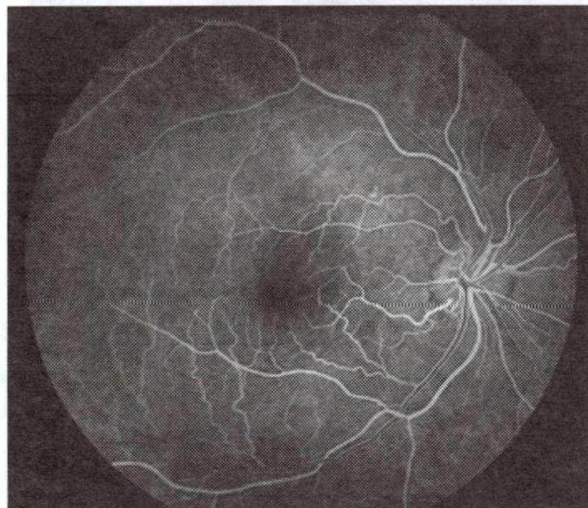

a. Fluorescein angiography
b. Optical coherence tomography
c. Ultrasound
d. Fundoscopy

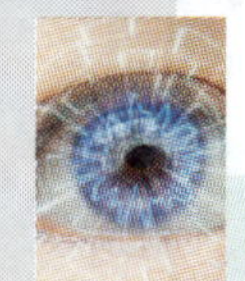

149. Which one of them is seen in iridocyclitis? *(Most Recent Question Aug 2020)*

a. Relative afferent pupillary defect
b. Keratic precipitates
c. Disc edema
d. Ectopia lentis

150. A patient presented in OPD with anterior uveitis. Which of the following can be associated with his condition? *(Most Recent Question Dec 2019-20)*

a. HLA B5 b. HLA B27
c. HLA DR3 d. HLA B53

151. A 60-year-old hypertensive and diabetic patient sudden loss of vision, 6/60 vision. Fundus picture reveals following finding. What is the diagnosis? *(Most Recent Question Dec 2019-20)*

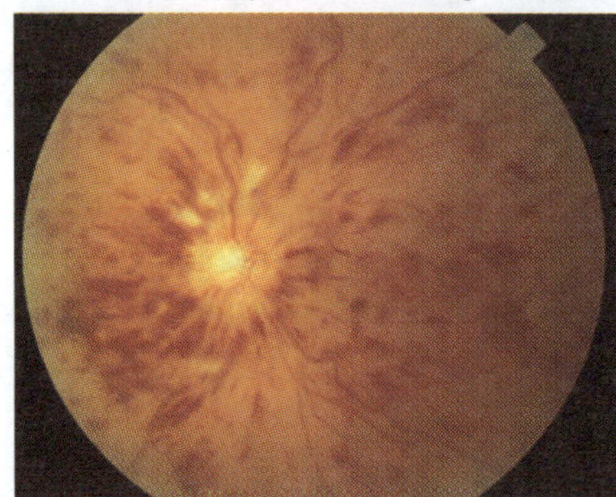

a. CRVO b. CRAO
c. Hemorrhage d. Hypertensive retinopathy

152. A young patient presented with acute onset severe pain in eye. Upon examination following finding is seen. Identify the condition: *(Most Recent Question Dec 2019-20)*

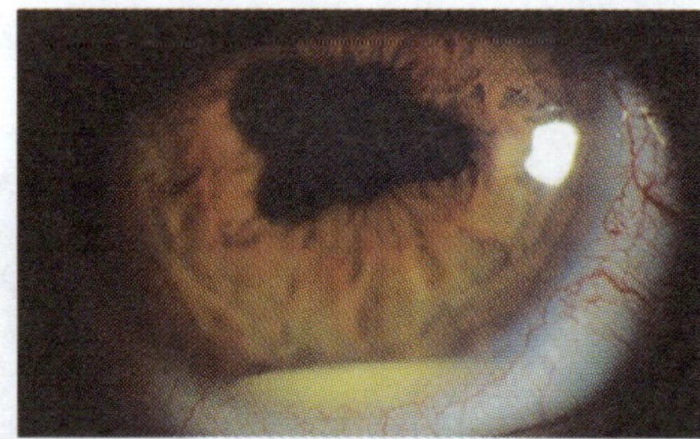

a. Anterior uveitis b. Glaucoma
c. Optic neuritis d. Keratoconus

153. Which of the following is seen retinitis pigmentosa? *(Most Recent Question 2019)*

a. Arteriolar attenuation
b. Neovascularization
c. Retinal artery thrombosis
d. Papilledema

154. Sarcoidosis is associated with: *(Recent Pattern Question 2018-19)*

a. Cataract b. Ectopia lentis
c. Anterior uveitis d. Keratitis

155. Cattle track appearance is seen in: *(Recent Pattern Question 2018)*

a. Central retinal vein occlusion
b. Central retinal artery occlusion
c. Central serous retinopathy
d. Diabetic retinopathy

156. What is the size of optic disc? *(Recent Pattern Question 2018)*

a. 0.5 mm b. 1.5 mm
c. 2 mm d. 2.5 mm

157. In uveitis, site of keratic precipitate is: *(Recent Pattern Question 2018)*

a. Corneal stroma b. Corneal endothelium
c. Lens anterior part d. Lens posterior part

158. How many years does it take to develop retinopathy in case of uncontrolled diabetes mellitus type I? *(Recent Pattern Question 2018)*

a. 1–5 b. 6–10
c. 11–15 d. 16–20

159. Which of the following is used for immediate management of acute uveitis? *(Recent Pattern Question 2017)*

a. Cycloplegics b. Steroids
c. Antimicrobials d. Eye patching

160. Granular keratic precipitates are seen in: *(Recent Pattern Question 2017)*

a. Nongranulomatous uveitis
b. Granulomatous uveitis
c. Syphilitic uveitis
d. Infective uveitis

161. Mutton fat KP is seen in: *(Recent Pattern Question 2017)*

a. Granulomatous uveitis b. Non-granulomatous uveitis
c. Traumatic uveitis d. Acute anterior uveitis

162. Which of the following condition presents with Uveitis with arthritis: *(Recent Pattern Question 2017)*

a. Kaplan syndrome b. Pneumoconiosis
c. Reiter syndrome d. Aspergillosis

163. Retinopathy of prematurity is due to? *(Recent Pattern Question 2017)*

a. Hypoxia b. Hyperoxia
c. Hypercapnea d. Apnea

164. Koeppe nodules are seen in *(Recent Pattern Question 2016)*

a. Iris stroma
b. Periphery of pupil
c. Papilla
d. Cornea

165. Retinal detachment occurs between which layers of retina?

a. Sensory and nuclear layer
b. Inner nuclear layer and outer nuclear layer
c. Sensory and pigmentary layer
d. Outer plexiform and inner plexiform layer

166. Which of the following is true about inverse Retinitis pigmentosa?
a. X linked
b. Bony spicule in fovea
c. Bony spicule in para fovea
d. Progressive Choroid degeneration

167. All of the following are features of retinitis pigmentosa; EXCEPT:
a. Bone spicule pigmentation in retina
b. Waxy pallor of disc
c. Central scotoma
d. Ring scotoma

168. A diabetic patient taking Insulin for the past 10 years complains of gradual painless loss of vision. Most likely cause of his condition is:
a. Total rhegmatogenous retinal detachment.
b. Cataract
c. Tractional retinal detachment not involving the macula
d. Vitreous hemorrhage.

169. Early stage non proliferative diabetic retinopathy is present as:
a. Microaneurysms b. Dot and Blot hemorrhages
c. Hard exudates d. Soft exudates

170. Classical sign of neovascular glaucoma is:
a. Retinal neovascularization
b. Disc neovascularization
c. Ciliary body neovascularization
d. Iris neovascularization

171. All are anti-VEGF; EXCEPT:
a. Pegaptanib b. 5FU
c. Bevacizumab d. Ranibizumab

172. Sudden painless loss of vision is due to:
a. Iridocyclitis b. Chorioretinitis
c. Vitreous hemorrhage d. Diabetic retinopathy

173. In a diabetic patient sudden severe painless loss of vision is due to?
a. Vitreous hemorrhage
b. Tractional Retinal Detachment
c. Diabetic retinopathy
d. Neovascularization

174. The most common cause of vitreous hemorrhage in a young normal male is:
a. Diabetes b. Anemia
c. Hypertensive retinopathy
d. Trauma

175. A hypertensive pregnant patient presented to you with sudden painless loss of vision what could be the possible cause?
a. Tractional retinal detachment
b. Exudative retinal detachment
c. Vitreous hemorrhage
d. Rhegmatogenous retinal detachment

176. Malignant melanoma of the choroid will produce:
a. Exudative retinal detachment
b. Traction retinal detachment
c. Retinal dialysis
d. Rhegmatogenous retinal detachment

177. All of the following are predisposing factors for rhegmatogenous retinal detachment; EXCEPT:
a. Myopia b. Diabetic retinopathy
c. Trauma d. Aphakia

178. Cherry red spot NOT seen in?
a. Trauma b. Tay Sach's
c. CRAO d. CRVO

179. The only condition amongst the following associated with cystoid macular edema is:
a. Overuse of ocular analgesics
b. Glaucoma
c. Central retinal vein occlusion
d. Topical steroid therapy

180. Candle Wax retinopathy seen in?
a. Sarcoidosis b. Amyloid
c. Diabetic retinopathy d. Hypertensive retinopathy

181. Snow banking is typically seen in:
a. Pars planitis b. Endophthalmitis
c. Coat's disease d. Eale's disease

182. Duration of cycloplegic by atropine in an adult:
a. 6 hours b. 2–3 days
c. 7–10 days d. 1–2 days

183. Drug contraindicated in uveitis is:
a. Pilocarpine b. Acetazolamide
c. Atropine d. Steroids

184. All of the following drugs are used for acute iridocyclitis; EXCEPT:
a. Atropine eye ointment b. Steroid eye drops
c. Pilocarpine eye drops d. Timolol eye drops

185. Most common complication of acute anterior uveitis:
a. Secondary glaucoma b. Cataract
c. Retinal detachment d. Macular edema

EYELID AND LACRIMAL APPARATUS

186. Identify the condition:
(Most Recent Question June/Dec 2021)

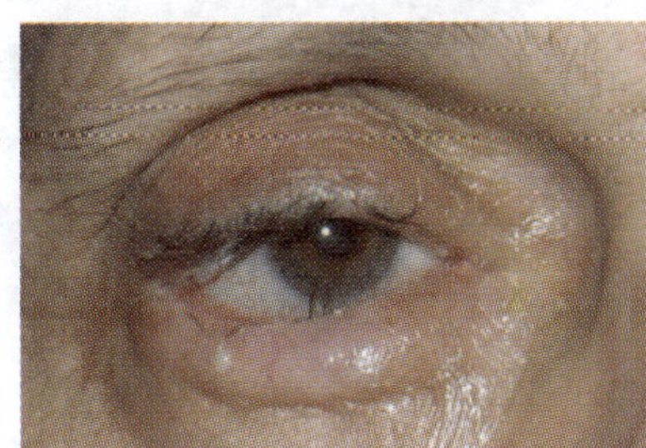

a. Ectropion b. Entropion
c. Distichiasis d. Trichiasis

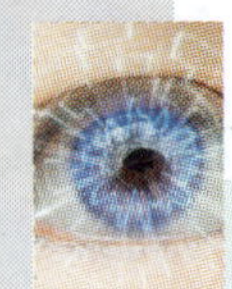

187. A patient presents with paralysis of all extraocular muscles. The most probable site of lesion is:
(Most Recent Question June/Dec 2021)

a. Upper medulla
b. Pons
c. Lower medulla
d. Midbrain

188. A young boy complains of itching, watering of eyes and rhinorrhea. On examination, the following image is seen. What is the diagnosis?
(Most Recent Question June/Dec 2021)

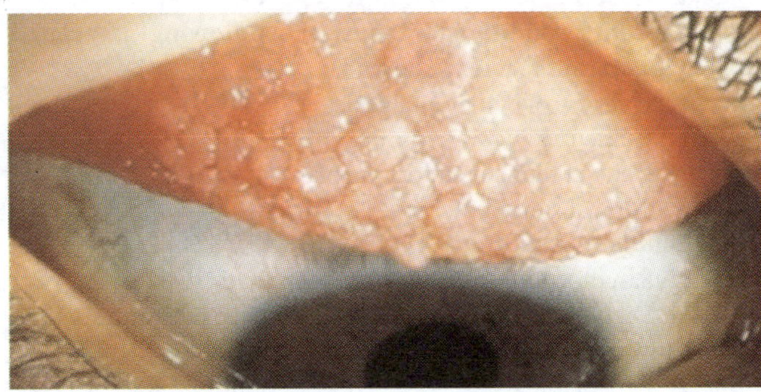

a. Trachoma
b. Vernal keratoconjunctivitis
c. Bacterial conjunctivitis
d. Acute conjunctivitis

189. A lady presents with pain, unilateral proptosis, orbital swelling and loss of vision. On examination, the given image is noted. What is the most likely diagnosis?
(Most Recent Question June/Dec 2021)

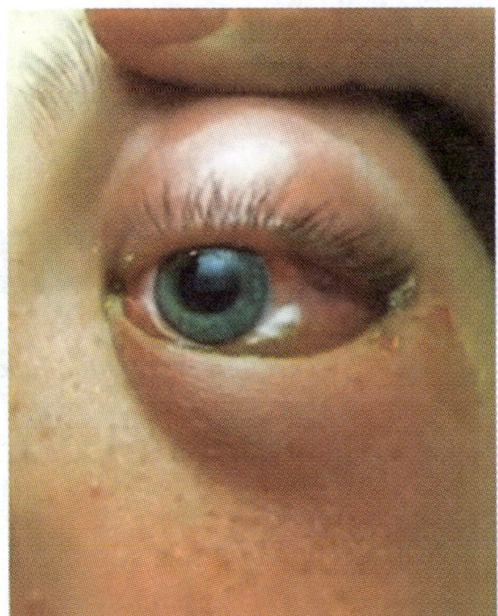

a. Preseptal cellulitis
b. Orbital cellulitis
c. Blepharitis
d. Stye

190. A person with jaundice and tremors shows following finding in the eye. What is the diagnosis?
(Most Recent Question June/Dec 2021)

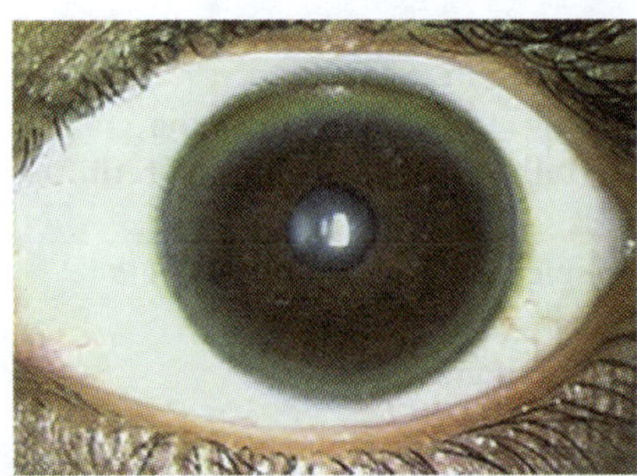

a. Wilson's disease b. Huntington's chorea
c. Heavy metal poisoning d. Sydenham chorea

191. The below pathology is associated with:
(Most Recent Question June/Dec 2021)

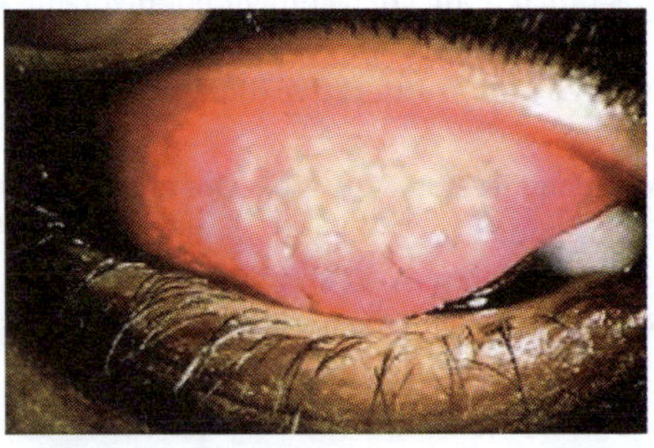

a. Chlamydia trachomatis
b. Neisseria gonorrhoeae
c. Corynebacterium diphtheria
d. Moraxella axenfeld

192. Instrument shown in the image is used for which of the following clinical condition?
(Most Recent Question Dec 2019-20)

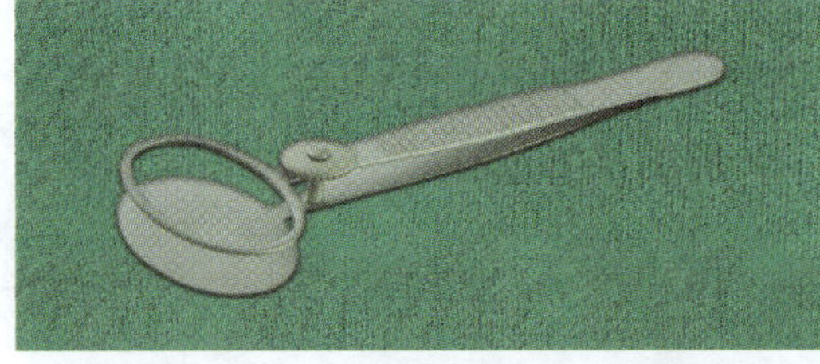

a. Instrument for ectropion b. Instrument for chalazion
c. Instrument for bitot spot d. Instrument for entropion

193. A 5-year-old suffering with chronic epiphora has appeared in the clinic. What is the next step of management? ***(Most Recent Question Dec 2019-20)***

a. Laryngeal probing and massaging
b. Dacryocystorhinostomy
c. Tarsal plate fracture
d. Lacrimal sac massage

194. Appropriate treatment for the congenital ptosis:
(Most Recent Question Dec 2019-20)
a. LPS resection
b. Antibiotics and hot compression
c. Spectacles
d. Wedge resection of conjunctiva

195. Internal hordeolum is due to inflammation of:
(Most Recent Question Dec 2019-20)
a. Zeis gland
b. Meibomian glands
c. Mohl gland
d. Lacrimal gland

196. Chronic granulomatous inflammation in upper lid with painless swelling is seen in:
(Most Recent Question Dec 2019-20)
a. Internal hordeolum
b. External hordeolum
c. Chalazion
d. Trachoma

197. In Dacryocystorhinostomy (DCR), lacrimal gland opens into: *(Recent Pattern Question 2018-19)*
a. Inferior meatus
b. Middle meatus
c. Supreme meatus
d. Superior meatus

198. Adhesion of margin of two eyelids:
a. Symblepharon
b. Lagophthalmos
c. Ankyloblepharon
d. Blepharophimosis

199. Treatment of choice for the chronic dacrocystitis?
a. Syringing
b. Dacrocystectomy
c. Conjunctivo-dacryocystorhinostomy
d. Dacrocystorhinostomy

200. In case of Ptosis which cranial nerve will be completely paralyzed?
a. 3rd CN palsy
b. 4th CN palsy
c. 5th CN palsy
d. 6th CN palsy

LENS/CATARACT

201. A child is supposed to undergo cataract surgery. Based on the guidelines, the under corrected IOL power is calculated by anticipating the expected __________
(Most Recent Question June 2022)
a. Myopic shift
b. Hypermetropic shift
c. Increase the length/size of lens capsule with the growth/age
d. Anisometropia

202. The girl patient was myopic having problem in reading and she was using her sisters contact lens. Sharing of contact lens from 1 person to another person can lead to infection by which of the following organism.
(Most Recent Question June 2022)
a. Candidiasis
b. Acanthamoeba
c. Onchocerciasis
d. Interstitial keratitis

203. A patient presents with blunt trauma to anterior part of lens. What type of cataract may develop in this patient?
(Most Recent Question June/Dec 2021)
a. Rosette cataract
b. Sunflower cataract
c. Posterior subcapsular cataract
d. Zonular cataract

204. A newborn child presents with watering and on examination, the following image is seen. What is the most probable diagnosis?
(Most Recent Question June/Dec 2021)

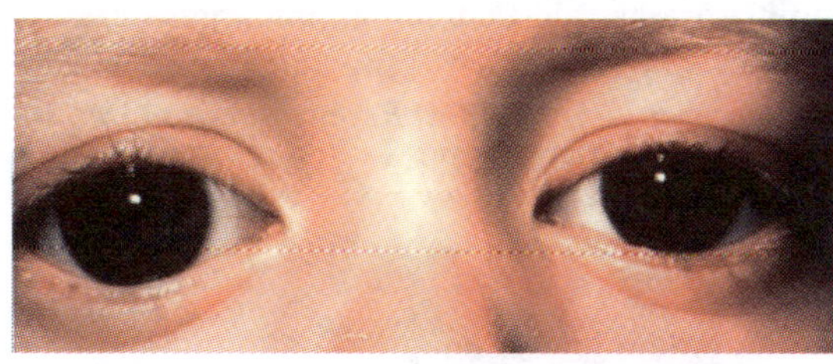

a. Megalocornea
b. Buphthalmos
c. Congenital cataract
d. Congenital Dacrocystitis

205. A patient is diagnosed with complicated cataract and on slit lamp findings are shown in the given image. What is the type of cataract seen in this case?
(Most Recent Question June/Dec 2021)

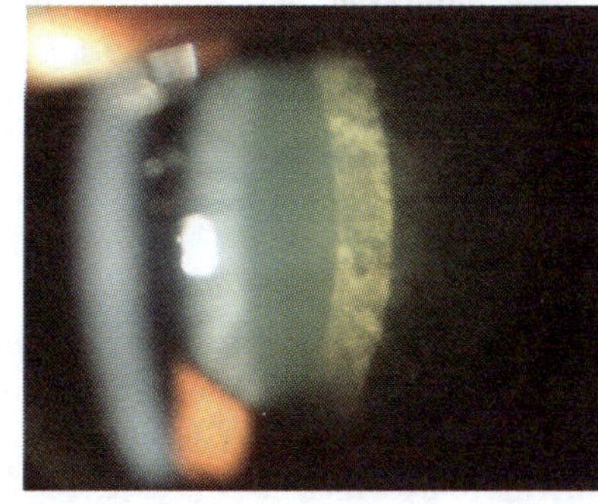

a. Anterior subcapsular cataract
b. Nuclear cataract
c. Posterior subcapsular cataract
d. Cortical cataract

206. Rosette cataract is seen due to which condition?
(Most Recent Question Aug 2020)
a. Myotonic dystrophy
b. Complicated cataract
c. Trauma
d. Diabetes

207. Shallow anterior chamber is seen in which of the following condition: *(Most Recent Question Aug 2020)*
a. Buphthalmos
b. Myopia
c. Hypermetropia
d. Total posterior synechiae

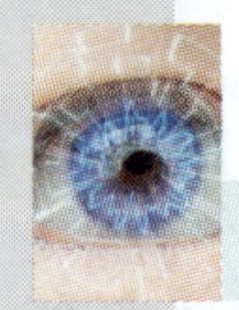

208. Which of the following is the most common ocular presentation of Marfan's syndrome?

(Most Recent Question Aug 2020)

a. Keratoconus b. Retinitis pigmentosa
c. Subluxation of lens d. Rosette cataract

209. Which laser is used in laser assisted cataract surgery?

(Most Recent Question Aug 2020)

a. Excimer b. Diode
c. Femto laser d. Nd -YAG

210. A patient comes to OPD with decreased vision in his left eye and opacification of cornea as shown in image. On history he said that he had undergone cataract surgery 6 years back. What is the next line of management in this case? *(Most Recent Question Dec 2019-20)*

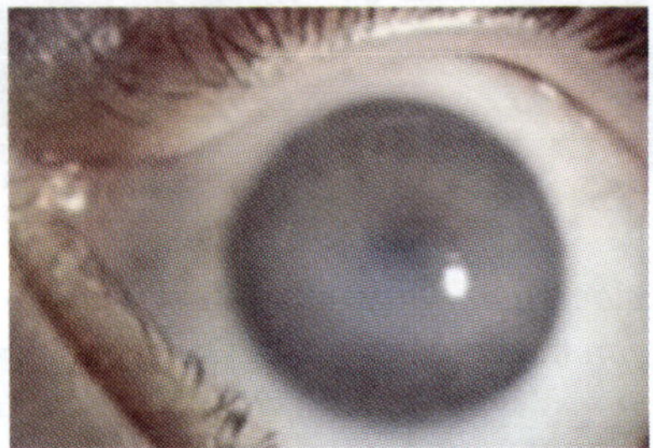

a. Keratoplasty b. Keratotomy
c. LASIK d. DCR

211. Advantage of contact lens over normal glasses:

(Most Recent Question Dec 2019-20)

a. Prismatic effect will be less
b. Prevention from UV rays
c. Decrease inflammation
d. Decrease infection

212. Most common cause of blindness in India:

(Most Recent Question 2019)

a. Cataract b. Refractive error
c. Trachoma d. Glaucoma

213. For Laser iridotomy which laser is used?

(Recent Pattern Question 2018-19)

a. Double argon laser b. ND:YAG laser
c. Excimer laser d. CO_2 laser

214. Ectopia lentis is seen in:

(Recent Pattern Question 2018-19)

a. Homocystinuria b. Refsum's disease
c. Wilson's disease d. Sarcoidosis

215. Laser used in after cataract surgery:

(Recent Pattern Question 2017)

a. Nd:YAG b. Argon
c. CO_2 d. Excimer

216. Second sight is a feature of

a. Congenital cataract *(Recent Pattern Question 2016)*
b. Cortical cataract
c. Nuclear cataract
d. Posterior subcapsular cataract

217. A 65-year-old patient presented with gradual painless reduction in vision 1 year after vitrectomy. Possible cause

a. Secondary glaucoma *(Recent Pattern Question 2016)*
b. Anterior uveitis
c. Lens protein leakage
d. Posterior-subscapular cataract due to long term use of steroids

218. Most common cause of blindness in world is:

a. Cataract b. Refractive errors
c. Trachoma d. Glaucoma

219. Which laser is used for Posterior capsular cataract:

a. Krypton b. ND:YAG
c. Argon d. Diode laser

220. Ideal site for intraocular lens implantation:

a. Behind the lens capsule
b. Anterior to the pupil
c. Behind the cornea
d. In the lens capsule

221. All of the following are Clinical features of complicated cataract; EXCEPT:

a. Polychromatic lustre
b. Axial spread of opacity
c. Opacity along sutures
d. Posterior subcapsular opacity

222. Complicated cataract caused by all; EXCEPT:

a. Subluxation of lens b. Retinal detachment
c. Vitreous movement d. Anterior Uveitis

223. Rossete cataract is seen in:

a. Trauma b. Diabetes
c. Galactosemia d. Wilson's disease

224. Vossius ring is seen at:

a. Iris
b. Cornea
c. Anterior capsule of the lens
d. Posterior capsule of the lens

225. The type of immature cataract which causes severe loss of vision is:

a. Posterior subcapsular cataract
b. Capsular cataract
c. Cortical cataract
d. Nuclear sclerosis

226. Rainbow cataract is due to:

a. Phenylketonuria b. Galactosemia
c. Diabetes mellitus d. Secondary cataract

227. All of the following systemic diseases may be associated with cataract; EXCEPT:

a. Phenylketonuria b. Galactosemia
c. Diabetes mellitus d. Wilson's disease

228. Anterior lenticonus is found in:

a. Lowe's syndrome b. William's syndrome
c. Down's syndrome d. Alport's syndrome

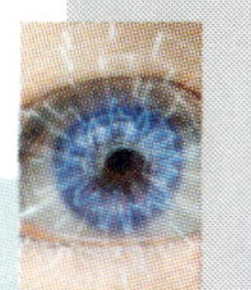

229. In Marfan's syndrome which of the following will be seen in eyes:
a. Inferonasal subluxation of lens
b. Superotemporal subluxation of lens
c. Corneal edema
d. Increased IOP

230. Location of lens in Marfan's syndrome is:
a. Inferior and nasally
b. Superior and temporally
c. Forward subluxated
d. Upward displacement

231. Jack in a box is seen in:
a. Pseudophakia
b. Aphakia
c. Squint
d. Cataract

232. Side effect of oral steroid:
a. Glàucoma
b. Cataract
c. Basement membrane thickening
d. Blepharoconjunctivitis

233. Iridodonesis is seen with:
a. Iridocyclitis
b. Subluxation of lens
c. Mature cataract
d. Intumescent cataract

GLAUCOMA

234. Which of them is not a characteristic of open angle glaucoma? ***(Most Recent Question Aug 2020)***
a. High IOP
b. Increased cup disc ratio
c. Visual field defect
d. Disc edema

235. Which is the gold standard in tonometry? ***(Most Recent Question Aug 2020)***
a. Schiotz
b. Applanation tonometer
c. Tonopen
d. Pascal dynamic contour

236. Beta blocker should be avoided in all given conditions; EXCEPT: ***(Most Recent Question Dec 2019-20)***
a. Glaucoma
b. Hypothyroidism
c. COPD
d. Diabetes

237. Phacomorphic glaucoma occurs due to: ***(Most Recent Question 2019)***
a. Intumescent cataract
b. Morgagnian cataract
c. Nuclear cataract
d. Cortical cataract

238. Which of the following is the carbonic anhydrase inhibitor used in glaucoma? ***(Recent Pattern Question 2018)***
a. Timolol
b. Mannitol
c. Latanoprost
d. Dorzolamide

239. Vertically fixed mid-dilated pupil seen in:
a. Cataract
b. Open angle glaucoma
c. Angle closure glaucoma
d. Uveitis

240. In case of Angle closure glaucoma, what is the shape of pupil:
a. Vertically dilated
b. Horizontally dilated
c. Fully constricted
d. Irregular constricted fixed

241. A 50-year-old female, presented with redness, painful, sudden loss of vision. She also claims about seeing colored haloes. Diagnosis:
a. Angular conjunctivitis
b. Retinal detachment
c. Acute congestive glaucoma
d. Keratitis

242. Primary open angle glaucoma is best treated by:
a. Peripheral Iridectomy
b. Latanoprost
c. Trabeculoplasty
d. Laser Iridotomy

243. Clinically earliest visual field defect in primary open angle glaucoma:
a. Seidel scotoma
b. Arcuate scotoma
c. Parcentral scotoma
d. Nasal spur

244. MOA of acetazolamide used in glaucoma:
a. Increase aqueous production
b. Increase uveo-scleral outflow
c. Increase trabecular outflow
d. Decrease aqueous production

245. The first line of treatment of advanced open angle glaucoma is:
a. Epinephrine
b. Latanoprost
c. Pilocarpine
d. Acetazolamide

246. Safest anti-glaucoma drug in children:
a. Acetazolamide
b. Latanoprost
c. Timolol
d. Dorzolamide

247. Which of the following drug is contraindicated in a glaucoma patient suffering from bronchial asthma:
a. Timolol maleate
b. Latanoprost
c. Betaxolol
d. Brimonidine

248. A patient of 18 year, presents with swollen, watery eyes. Examination confirms glaucoma. Which of the following is the best step that provides earliest relief:
a. Gonioscopy
b. Medical management
c. Surgical management
d. Ophthalmoscopy

249. Treatment for the given case (bilateral big blue eyes in image due to increased IOP)

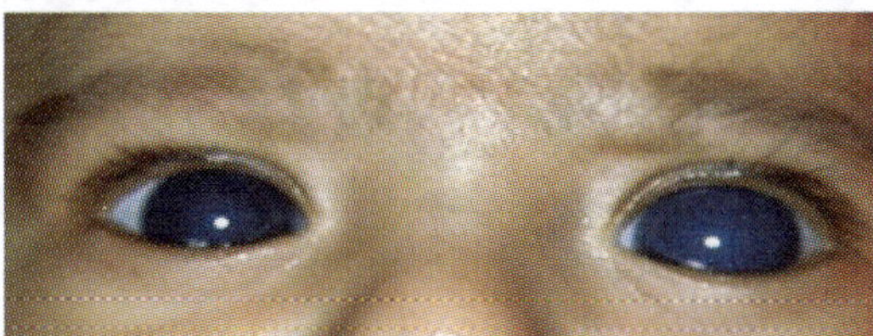

a. Goniotomy
b. Trabeculotomy
c. Trabeculectomy
d. Laser iridotomy

250. Treatment of angle closure glaucoma.
a. Peripheral Iredectomy
b. Trabeculectomy
c. Trabeculoplasty
d. Laser Iridotomy

251. Laser iridotomy is useful in:
a. Angle closure glaucoma
b. Neovascular glaucoma
c. Open angle glaucoma
d. Secondary glaucoma

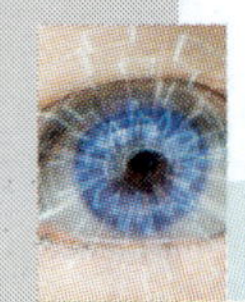

252. In acute congestive glaucoma, best prophylaxis for the other eye is:
a. Laser iridotomy
b. Topical steroids
c. Trabeculectomy
d. Surgical peripheral iridectomy

253. Treatment of choice for the other eye in open angle glaucoma is:
a. Peripheral iridectomy b. Laser trabeculoplasty
c. Laser iridotoomy d. Trabeculectomy

254. Colored haloes least seen in:
a. Cataract b. Open angle glucoma
c. Angle closure glaucoma d. Purulent conjunctivitis

255. A man present with frequent change of presbyopic lens. Diagnosis:
a. Open angle glaucoma b. Angle closure glaucoma
c. Cataract d. Astigmatism

256. Krukenberg spindles are seen at?
a. Cornea anterior surface b. Cornea posterior surface
c. Lens posterior surface d. Lens anterior surface

REFRACTIVE ERROR

257. What is the most common cause of blindness in children? ***(Most Recent Question June/Dec 2021)***
a. Cataract b. Glaucoma
c. Vitamin A deficiency d. Corneal opacity

258. On looking through a pin hole the visual acuity of a patient improves. What is the diagnosis?
(Most Recent Question June/Dec 2021)
a. Macular lesion b. Refractive error
c. Organic lesion d. Cataract

259. Biconcave lenses are used in:
(Most Recent Question June/Dec 2021)
a. Myopia b. Hypermetropia
c. Astigmatism d. Presbyopia

260. A child presents with defective vision which does not improve with glasses, but fundus is normal. Diagnosis is:
(Most Recent Question June/Dec 2021)
a. Myopia b. Hypermetropia
c. Astigmatism d. Amblyopia

261. A patient presents with a difference in visual acuity between the two eyes. What could be the most probable diagnosis?
(Most Recent Question June/Dec 2021)
a. Refractive error b. Anisometropia
c. Amblyopia d. Conjunctivitis

262. Parents of a child complain that he squeezes the eye while watching TV. What is the probable diagnosis?
(Most Recent Question June/Dec 2021)
a. Dry eyes b. Myopia
c. Hypermetropia d. Glaucoma

263. Refractive error found here is:
(Most Recent Question June/Dec 2021)

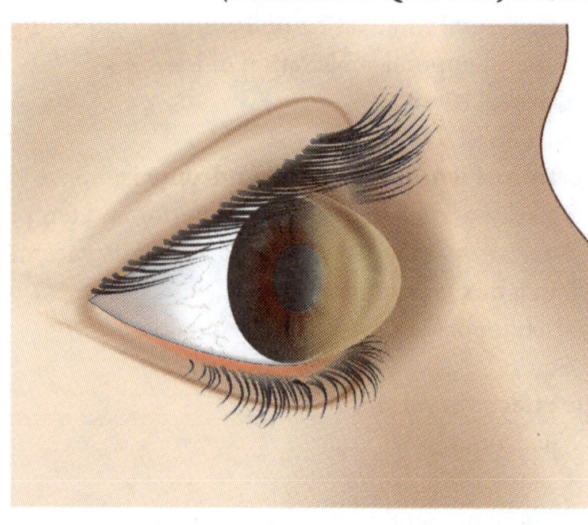

a. Myopia and astigmatism b. Hypermetropia
c. Myopia d. Astigmatism

264. In myopia image is formed at:
(Most Recent Question Dec 2019-20)
a. Anterior to retina b. Posterior to retina
c. On retina d. Uvea

265. A 20-year-old male complaints of repeatedly changes in glasses, this may possibly be due to:
(Most Recent Question Dec 2019-20)
a. Keratoconus b. Pathological myopia
c. Glaucoma d. Cataract

266. A man with convergent squint in one eye, vision is 6/60 and another eye no squint with vision 6/60. Next step in management is: ***(Most Recent Question Dec 2019-20)***
a. MRI
b. Squint surgery
c. Botulinum toxin
d. Glasses

267. In Vision 2020, which disease has been added recently for India: ***(Most Recent Question Dec 2019-20)***
a. Cataract
b. Childhood blindness
c. Glaucoma
d. Refractive errors and low vision

268. A newborn is hypermetropic by:
(Recent Pattern Question 2018-19)
a. +2.5 D b. 5 D
c. 10 D d. 1 D

269. Obstacle in manifest squint-concomitant type is:
(Recent Pattern Question 2018-19)
a. Motor obstacle b. Sensory obstacle
c. Central obstacle d. All of these

270. Crowding phenomenon is seen in:
(Recent Pattern Question 2018)
a. Hypermetropia b. Amblyopia
c. Strabismus d. Retinitis pigmentosa

271. What is the best treatment of Amblyopia? *(Recent Pattern Question 2018)*
a. Occlusion
b. Atropine penalization
c. Correction of refractive error
d. Surgery

272. Which is true statement for a patient with paralytic squint? *(Recent Pattern Question 2017)*
a. Head tilt opposite to rectus muscle paralysis
b. Head tilt towards the rectus muscle paralysis
c. Amblyopia
d. Decreased visual acuity

273. Least common cause of blindness: *(Recent Pattern Question 2016)*
a. Cataract b. Corneal opacity
c. Refractive error d. Glaucoma

274. Convex lenses are used for: *(Recent Pattern Question 2016)*
a. Myopia b. Hypermetropia
c. Astigmatism d. Myopic astigmatism

275. In convergent squint what is the angle of deviation? *(Recent Pattern Question 2016)*
a. 10° b. 15°
c. 20° d. 30°

276. In case of Myopia, the following is seen:
a. Large optic disc b. Small optic disc
c. Normal eye d. None of above

277. Excessive accommodation causes:
a. Pseudomyopia b. Pseudohypermetropia
c. Astigmatism d. Presbyopia

278. Treatment of anisometropia:
a. Glasses b. Contact lens
c. Trabeculectomy d. Trabeculoplasty

279. Lens used in Astigmatism:
a. Convex lens b. Cylindrical
c. Concave lens d. Contact lens

280. Worth 4 dot test is done for:
a. Color deficiency b. Strabismus
c. Binocular vision d. Squint

281. Different refractive power between two eyes is known as?
a. Combined astigmatism b. Aniseikonia
c. Anisometropia d. Ametropia

282. Cylindrical lens is used for:
a. Presbyopia b. High myopia
c. Hypermetropia d. Astigmatism

OCULAR INJURY AND MALIGNANCY

283. A 3-year-old boy presented to Ophthalmology clinic with a large, rapidly growing cauliflower-like mass protruding out of the left orbit and invading the surrounding soft tissues. What is the most likely diagnosis? *(Most Recent Question June 2022)*
a. Retinoblastoma b. Retinal detachment
c. Uveal melanoma d. Buphthalmos

284. 12 years old boy suffered orbit injury with a cricket ball. Next day develop diplopia with up gaze. The boy develops headache, dizziness, vomiting on looking up. Also develops bradycardia and hypotension on looking up. No congestion or proptosis of eye. Probable cause: *(Most Recent Question June 2022)*
a. Fracture floor of orbit b. Fracture roof of orbit
c. Intracranial hemorrhage d. Subdural hematoma

285. A factory worker has trauma to anterior part of eye with iron foreign body. Which of the following investigations would you do for further evaluation? *(Most Recent Question June/Dec 2021)*
a. CT scan b. MRI
c. USG B scan d. Nuclear radiology

286. A one-and-a-half-year-old child presents with a picture like the following with intraocular calcification. What is the most likely diagnosis? *(Most Recent Question June/Dec 2021)*

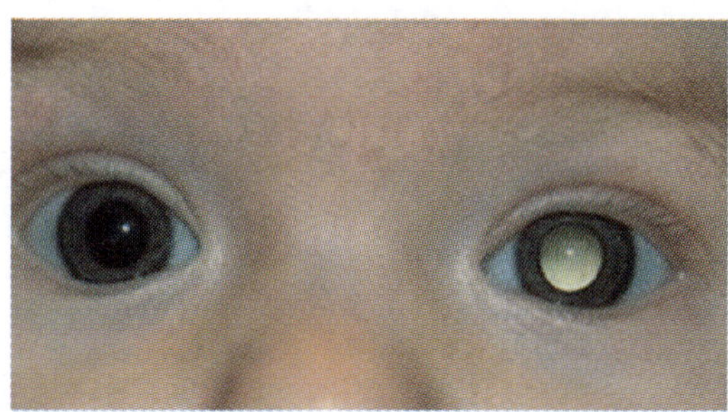

a. Congenital cataract b. Retinoblastoma
c. Eales' disease d. Toxoplasmosis

287. After a fight, patient presents with painful ocular movements and a non-reacting pupil. What is the most probable diagnosis? *(Most Recent Question June/Dec 2021)*
a. Cataract b. Glaucoma
c. Papilledema d. Option neuritis

288. A man suffered trauma to the right eye with a punch. Which of the following will be the most likely to occur in this case? *(Most Recent Question June/Dec 2021)*
a. Inferior orbital wall fracture
b. Medial wall fracture
c. Lateral wall fracture
d. Subluxation of the lens

289. If the eye has a perforating injury. Which area is most susceptible for developing sympathetic ophthalmitis? *(Most Recent Question Aug 2020)*
a. Cornea b. Sclera
c. Ciliary body d. Extraocular muscles

290. Evisceration is removal of which layer of eye ball? *(Most Recent Question 2019)*
a. Middle and inner b. Outer and middle
c. Outer and inner d. All the layers of eyeball

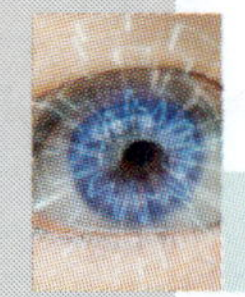

291. First sign of sympathetic Ophthalmitis is: *(Most Recent Question 2019)*
a. Circumcorneal congestion
b. Hypopyon
c. Retrolental flare
d. Iris nodule

292. A patient with a history of fall on symmetrical surface, presents with enophthalmos, diplopia on upward gaze and loss of sensitivity over cheek. True statement about this is: *(Recent Pattern Question 2018-19)*
i. Strongly suspecting orbital floor fracture
ii. It is a blow-out fracture
iii. Zygomatic bone is most likely injured
iv. Frontal bone fracture
a. Only i and ii are correct b. II, III and IV are correct
c. I, II, and III are correct d. All are correct

293. Blow out fracture can be due to:
a. Tennis ball injury *(Recent Pattern Question 2018-19)*
b. Chisel and hammer injury
c. Sudden fall
d. Punch at the chin from below

294. Most common malignant orbital tumour in children: *(Recent Pattern Question 2017)*
a. Rhabdomyosarcoma b. Retinoblastoma
c. Lipoma d. Neuroblastoma

295. Tear drop sign is seen in fracture of? *(Recent Pattern Question 2017)*
a. Orbital roof b. Orbital floor
c. Orbital lateral wall d. Orbital medial wall

296. Which gene is associated with Knudson two hit hypothesis? *(Recent Pattern Question 2017)*
a. RB gene b. PTEN
c. P16 d. P53

297. A patient presents with ocular trauma and blood in anterior chamber. Which is the best treatment? *(Recent Pattern Question 2017)*
a. Eye patch b. Hospital admission
c. Steroid d. Conservative

298. Corneal curvature is measured by: *(Recent Pattern Question 2017)*
a. Perimetry b. Gonioscopy
c. Pachymetry d. Keratometry

299. Which of the following is an etiology of axial proptosis? *(Recent Pattern Question 2017)*
a. Lacrimal gland tumour b. Optic nerve glioma
c. Orbital floor fracture d. Forehead tumour

300. Most common primary intraocular tumor in children?
a. Retinoblastoma *(Recent Pattern Question 2016)*
b. Malignant melanoma of choroid
c. Malignant melanoma of ciliary body
d. Rhabdomyosarcoma

301. Unilateral oculomotor nerve paralysis leads to? *(Recent Pattern Question 2016)*
a. Loss of accommodation b. Argyll Robertson pupil
c. Eyeball turned up and out d. Diplopia

302. Ciliary muscle damage leads to: *(Recent Pattern Question 2016)*
a. Angle closure glaucoma b. Loss of accommodation
c. ARP d. Diplopia

303. Tolosa Hunt syndrome involves:
a. Orbital floor *(Recent Pattern Question 2016)*
b. Orbital apex
c. Orbital roof
d. Orbital space

304. Which one is seen after penetrating injury in ciliary body?
a. Iridocyclitis b. Sympathetic ophthalmitis
c. Endophthalmitis d. Corneal ulceration

305. Sympathetic ophthalmitis usually results due to:
a. Glaucoma
b. Trachoma
c. Penetrating injury to Ciliary body
d. Uveitis

306. Most common foreign body to cause penetrating injury to ciliary body:
a. Ball b. Hammer and chisel
c. Gun bullet d. Vegetative material

307. Most common cause of subconjunctival hemorrhage:
a. Hypertension b. Trauma
c. Pertussis d. Diabetes

308. Pupillary reaction to light is still normal in lesion/injury to:
a. Optic nerve b. Optic disc
c. Optic tract d. Optic chiasm

309. Blow out fracture of orbit is characterized by all EXCEPT:
a. Orbital floor and medial wall involvement are common
b. Tear drop sign on X-ray
c. Diplopia
d. Exophthalmos

310. Lisch Nodules on Iris is a feature of:
a. Amyloidosis b. Neurofibromatosis
c. Tuberous Sclerosis d. None of these

311. Most common malignant eyelid tumor:
a. Squamous cell carcinoma b. Basal carcinoma
c. Sebaceous carcinoma d. Malignant melanoma

312. Most common epithelial tumor of lacrimal gland:
a. Choroid melanoma b. Pleomorphic adenoma
c. Basal cell CA d. Rhabdomyosarcoma

313. Commonest site of distant metastasis of retinoblastoma is:
a. Liver b. Brain
c. Lungs d. Long bones

314. A child with retinoblastoma will have this:

a. Esotropia b. Exotropia
c. Hypotropia d. Heterotropia

NEURO-OPHTHALMOLOGY

315. A lady suffers sudden painful loss of vision with worsening of pain on eye movements. A relative afferent papillary defect is present. On perimetry, there is a central scotoma in the involved eye. What is the most likely diagnosis in this case?

a. Optic neuritis *(Most Recent Question June/Dec 2021)*
b. Papilledema
c. Retinoblastoma
d. Central retinal vein occlusion

316. A child aged 10 years is having amblyopia in one eye. What is the best treatment in this case?

(Most Recent Question June/Dec 2021)

a. Observation b. Occlusion
c. Penalization d. None of the above

317. A 60-year-old diabetic male present with history of severe breathlessness, pyrexia, tachypnea, and generalized malaise. RT-PCR from a nasopharyngeal swab was positive for the SARS -CoV-2 virus. On day 10, patient developed bilateral orbital swelling with right eye proptosis. What could be the most common organism involved?

(Most Recent Question June/Dec 2021)

a. Aspergillus b. Pseudomonas
c. Mucormycosis d. Candida

318. A person with a brain lesion presents with macula sparing homonymous hemianopia. What could be the site of lesion? *(Most Recent Question June/Dec 2021)*

a. Optic tract b. Optic chiasma
c. Occipital cortex d. Optic nerve

319. A patient was tested for ocular motion and presented with shown ocular motion defect. The position of eyeball is shown in the image below where left eye movement was noted when the object was moved to left lower quadrant, but right eye remain static. Identify the nerve involved in following defect. *(Most Recent Question June/Dec 2021)*

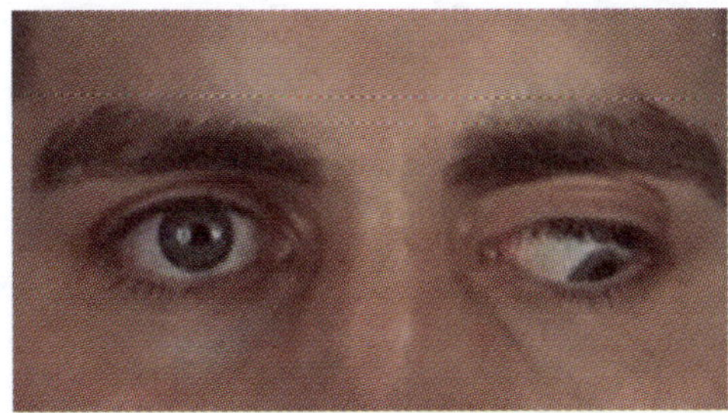

a. Oculomotor nerve b. Optic nerve
c. Trochlear nerve d. Abducent nerve

320. Identify the lesion in the image:

(Most Recent Question Aug 2020)

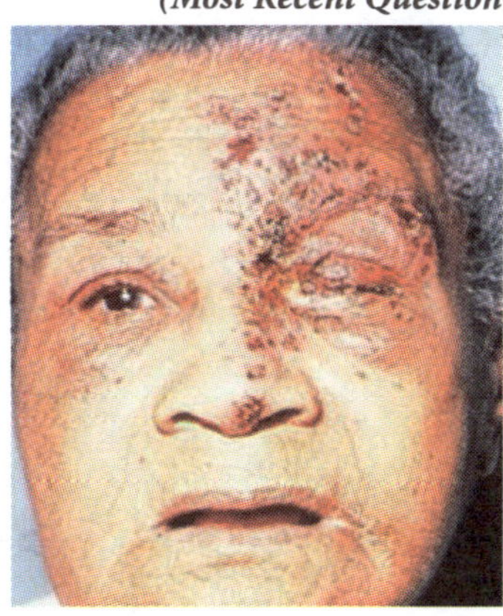

a. Falling corneal transplant
b. Anterior uveitis
c. Herpes zoster
d. Acanthamoeba keratitis

321. Identify the image and disease associated with the given image: *(Most Recent Question Dec 2019-20)*

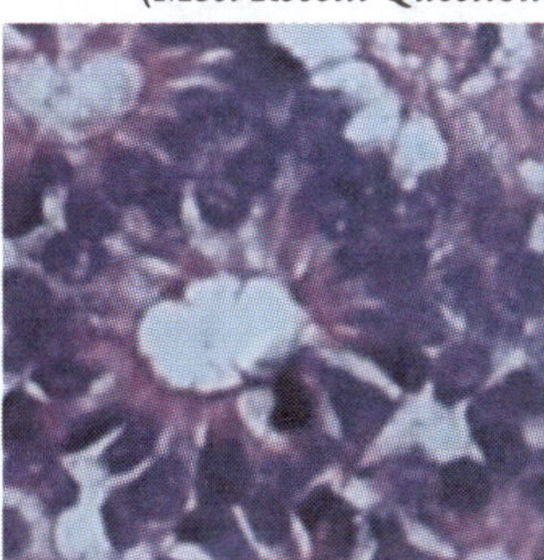

a. Retinoblastoma b. Medulloblastoma
c. Ewing's sarcoma d. Neuroblastoma

322. A patient with miosis, anhidrosis and mild drooping of eyelid as shown in the image is presented to the clinic. What is the likely diagnosis?

(Most Recent Question Dec 2019-20)

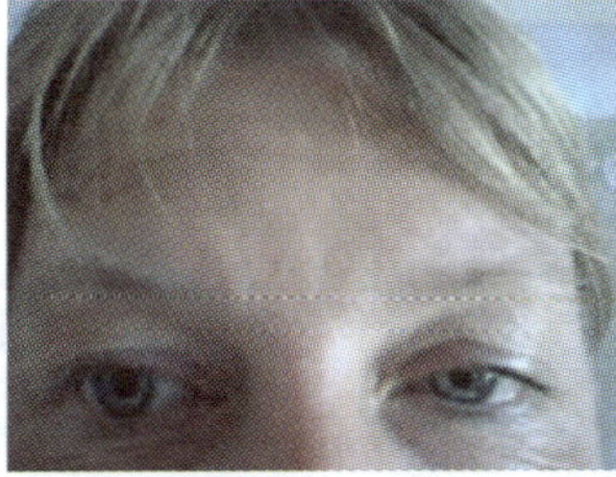

a. 3rd cranial nerve palsy b. Horner syndrome
c. 6th cranial nerve palsy d. Orbital cellulitis

323. Visual loss due to cerebral degeneration is related to which artery? *(Most Recent Question Dec 2019-20)*

a. Middle cerebral artery b. Internal carotid artery
c. Inferior cerebral artery d. Posterior cerebral artery

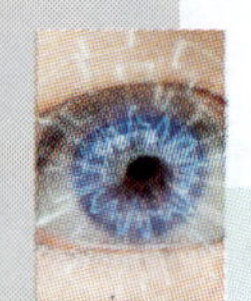

324. A tumor in the anterior pituitary causing pressure over optic chiasma will present as:
(Most Recent Question Dec 2019-20)

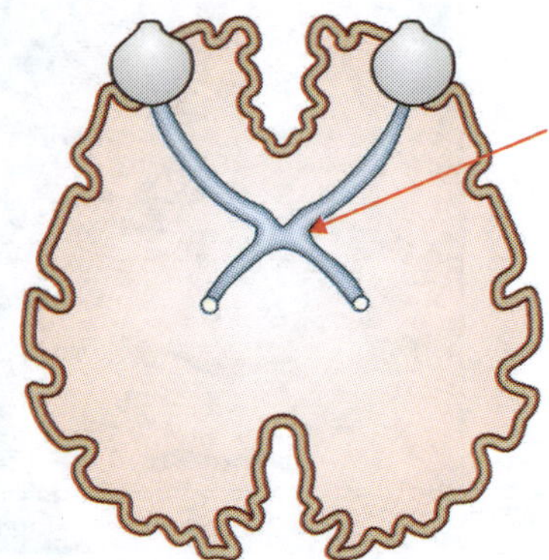

a. Homonymous hemianopia
b. Bitemporal hemianopia
c. Heteronymous hemianopia with central sparing
d. Monocular vision loss

325. In a patient of head injury, who presents with headache and increased intracranial pressure, the effect on pupil is: *(Most Recent Question 2019)*

a. Ipsilateral mydriasis
b. Contralateral mydriasis
c. Ipsilateral miosis
d. Contralateral miosis

326. All of the following conditions cause miosis; EXCEPT:
(Most Recent Question 2019)

a. Bright light
b. Horner syndrome
c. Oculomotor paralysis
d. Iridocyclitis

327. Superior quadrantic hemianopia is caused by:
(Most Recent Question 2019)

a. Craniopharyngioma
b. Meningioma
c. Pituitary adenoma
d. Temporal lobe lesion

328. Which of the following lesions occurs at optic chiasma?
(Most Recent Question 2019)

a. Bitemporal hemianopia
b. Unilateral blindness
c. Pie in floor
d. Bilateral homonymous macular defect

329. In which of the following condition there is ipsilateral 3rd nerve palsy with contralateral hemiplegia and facial palsy of upper motor neuron?
(Most Recent Question 2019)

a. Weber syndrome
b. Terson syndrome
c. Millard-Gubler syndrome
d. Foville's syndrome

330. Bilateral temporal hemianopia is due to:
(Recent Pattern Question 2016)

a. Bilateral optic nerve damage
b. Pituitary adenoma
c. Unilateral optic tract damage
d. Bilateral optic tract damage

331. Colour blindness in ethambutol toxicity:

a. Red blue
b. Red green
c. Blue
d. Red green blue

332. What will be the treatment of ptosis due to Horner syndrome:

a. Unilateral sling operation
b. Bilateral sling operation
c. Cut levator palpebrae superioris 15 mm
d. Fasanella servat operation

333. Which of the following muscle is affected in increased cranial pressure:

a. Inferior oblique
b. Lateral rectus
c. Middle rectus
d. Superior oblique

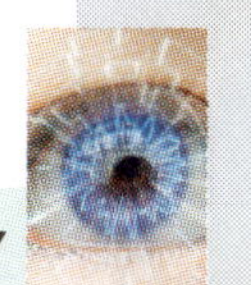

ANSWERS WITH EXPLANATIONS

MOST RECENT QUESTIONS 2023

1. Ans. (b) Siderosis bulbi

Ref: Comprehensive Ophthalmology by AK Khurana, 6th, ed. eg. 434

- Siderosis bulbi refers to the pigmentary, degenerative process of the eye following chronic retention of an iron-containing intra-ocular foreign body (IOFB). It can also occur due to iron derived from the blood.
- **Clinical feature:** Heterochromic iris, rusty posterior subcapsular opacity, cataract.

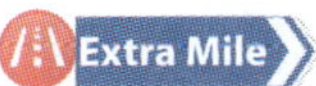

- **Chalcosis bulbi**, is a chronic reaction to a copper-containing intraocular foreign body (IOFB) with less than 85% copper content.
- **Wilson's disease** is an inborn error of copper metabolism. A commonly associated symptom is Kayser-Fleischer rings in the cornea of affected individuals.

Contd...

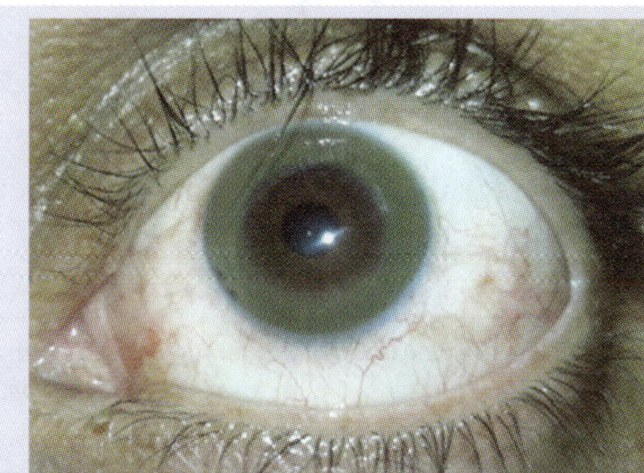

- **Retinitis pigmentosa (RP)** is a genetic disorder of the eyes that causes loss of vision. Symptoms include trouble seeing at night and decreasing peripheral vision (side and upper or lower visual field). As peripheral vision worsens, people may experience "tunnel vision".

2. Ans. (b) Homonymous hemianopia with macular sparing

Ref: Comprehensive Ophthalmology by AK Khurana, 6th ed. pg. 315

- The given case is of left side homonymous hemianopia with macular sparing, due to lesion in occipital lobe.
- Homonymous hemianopia (the inability to see in one-half of visual space in each eye) typically reflects a lesion in the contralateral optic tract, or, with sparing of macular vision, may reflect a contralateral lesion of the entire optic radiation.
- Macular sparing is seen due to dual blood supply of occipital lobe: PCA (Posterior Cerebral Artery) and MCA (Middle cerebral Artery). Occlusion of any one vessel, can be compensated by the other vessel.

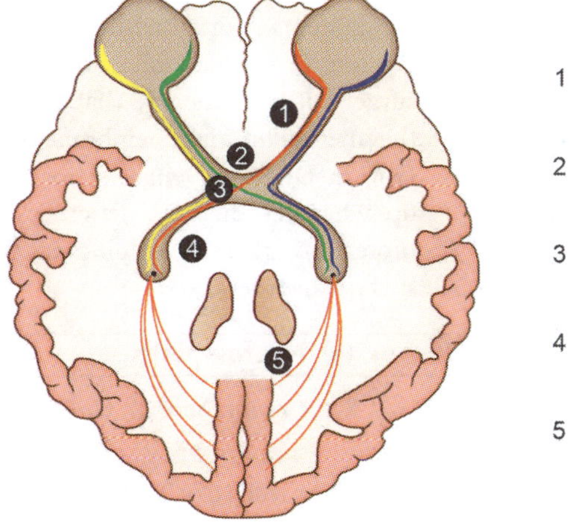

1 Total right eye visual loss
2 Bitemporal hemianopia
3 Left nasal hemianopia
4 Right homonymous hemianopia
5 Left homonymous hemianopia with macular sparing

3. Ans. (b) Choroidal metastasis

Ref: Comprehensive Ophthalmology by AK Khurana, 6th ed. pg. 460

- Choroidal metastasis is overall most common intraocular malignancy in adults.
- The choroid is the most common ocular site for metastatic disease, owing to abundant vascular supply. The primary cancers that most commonly lead to choroidal metastases include breast cancer, prostate cancer and lung cancer. Bilateral, multifocal metastases are most often secondary to breast cancer, whereas unilateral, unifocal metastasis are more commonly found with lung cancer.

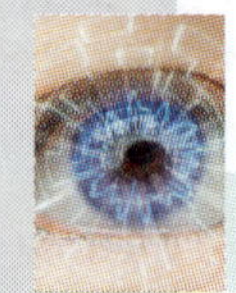

Extra Mile

- **Retinoblastoma (Rb)** is a rare form of cancer seen in pediatric age group (5-6 year). It rapidly develops from the immature cells of a retina, the light-detecting tissue of the eye.
- **Choroidal melanoma** is overall second most common intraocular tumor. It is also most common primary intraocular malignancy in adults.
- **Uveal melanoma** is primary intraocular tumor. Its incidence is lesser than choroidal metastasis.
- **Lymphoma:** MC malignant orbital tumor of adults

4. Ans. (b) Galactosemia

Ref: Comprehensive Ophthalmology by AK Khurana, 6th ed. pg. 193

- Oil Droplet Cataract is commonly seen in patients with galactosemia (a recessively inherited inborn error of carbohydrate metabolism). Patient presents with mental retardation, lethargy, refusal to feed and failure to thrive.
- Accumulation of dulcitol (galactose reduction product) within the lens cells leads to increased intracellular osmotic pressure and fluid influx into the lens.

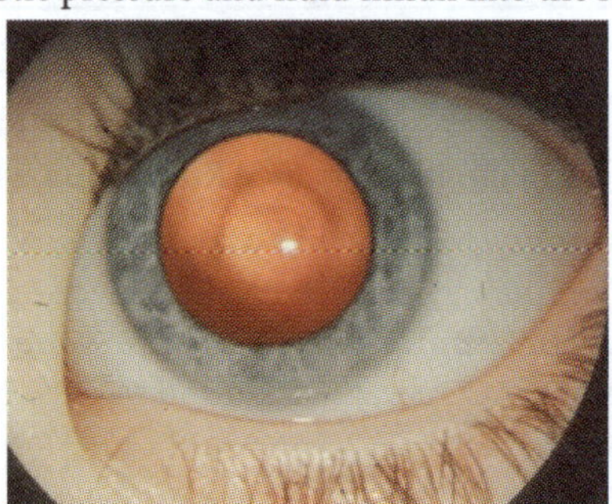

Extra Mile

Disease	Type of cataract
Myotonic dystrophy	Christmas tree cataract
Wilsons disease	Sunflower cataract
Diabetes mellitus	Snowflake cataract

5. Ans. (a) Amaurosis fugax

Ref: Comprehensive Ophthalmology by AK Khurana, 6th ed. pg. 331

- Papilledema is blurring of optic disc due to raised intracranial pressure.
- Amaurosis fugax is a temporary loss of vision in one or both eyes due to a lack of blood flow to the retina. The retina is the light-sensitive layer of tissue at the back of the eyeball.
- **Option B:** Blindness is defined as a visual acuity worse than 6/60, with the best possible correction, or a visual field of 10 degrees or less.
- **Option C:** Malingering manifest as either imitating an ophthalmic disease, or contradiction of ophthalmic disease.

6. Ans. (d) Extra capsular cataract surgery

Ref: Comprehensive Ophthalmology by AK Khurana, 6th ed. pg. 254

- In ECCE, the incision is ~ 10 mm. Suture is required here using 10-0 nylon.
- Note: Any incision beyond 6 mm requires suturing.
- Making a new incision during conversion is identical to that for a planned ECCE. The original incision is closed with a 10-0 nylon suture. The surgeon and microscope are rotated as the surgeon should sit superior.

Extra Mile

- **Phacoemulsification:** It is suture-less surgery
- **FLACS:** Femto Laser Assisted Cataract Surgery. It is surgery assisted using laser beam. No suture required.
- Manual small incision surgery doesn't require suture. This is self-sealing incision, since the 6 mm incision here is made in 3 different planes.

7. Ans. (b) Trypan blue

Ref: Comprehensive Ophthalmology by AK Khurana, 6th ed. pg. 466

- Trypan blue is used as a surgical aid during cataract eye surgery. It is a blue dye that works by staining anterior capsule of lens.

Option A: Fluorescein is a diagnostic contrast agent, particularly used in various ophthalmic procedures, such as checking for any corneal or vessel abnormalities. The application of fluorescein also extends to bioimaging whole anatomic structures and even further to cellular components in immune-histological staining.

Option C: Brilliant blue G is a surgical aid during eye surgery. It is a blue dye that works by selectively staining the internal limiting membrane of the retina.

Option D: Rose Bengal stain is for dry eye. It is taken up wherever there is deficiency of preocular tear film protection, thereby helping in the diagnosis of ocular surface disorders.

8. Ans. (a) Neurosyphilis

Ref: Comprehensive Ophthalmology by AK Khurana, 6th ed. pg. 317

- Syphilis leads to a "dorsal midbrain lesion that interrupts the pupillary light reflex pathway but spares the more ventral pupillary near the reflex pathway."
- **Argyll Robertson Pupil (ARP)** can be seen due to neurosyphilis. Students can remember easily:
  - **ARP:** Accommodation Reaction Present
  - **PRA:** Pupillary Reaction Absent
- **Option B:** The pupil on the affected side may be round and constricted (i.e., miosis). In individuals with Horner

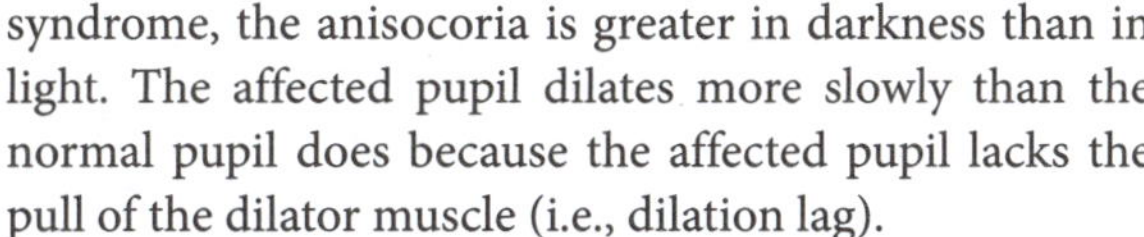

syndrome, the anisocoria is greater in darkness than in light. The affected pupil dilates more slowly than the normal pupil does because the affected pupil lacks the pull of the dilator muscle (i.e., dilation lag).

- **Option C:** In the early stages of papilledema, visual acuity and pupillary response to light are usually normal and become abnormal only after the condition is well advanced. Visual field testing may detect an enlarged blind spot.
- **Option D:** Pupillary light reflex is used to assess the brain stem function. Abnormal pupillary light reflex can be found in optic nerve injury, oculomotor nerve damage, brain stem lesions, such as tumors, and medications like barbiturates.

9. Ans. (b) 4 CN palsy

Ref: Comprehensive Ophthalmology by AK Khurana, 6th ed. pg. 336

- While walking down, downward and inward gaze is required, which is done by superior oblique muscle of the eye.
- Fourth cranial nerve palsy or trochlear nerve (CN IV) palsy causes weakness or paralysis of the superior oblique muscle that it innervates (remember mnemonic LR6-SO4).
- This condition often causes vertical or near vertical double vision as the weakened muscle prevents the eyes from moving in the same direction together.
- In right CN-IV palsy, there will be left tilt and in left CN-IV palsy, there will be right tilt due to crossing over of CN-IV.

Option A: In third Cranial Nerve Palsy the affected eye turns slightly outward and downward when the unaffected eye looks straight ahead, causing double vision. The affected eye may turn inward very slowly and may move only to the middle when looking inward. It cannot move up and down.

Option C: The abducens nerve controls the lateral rectus muscle, which abducts the eye. Abducens nerve palsy causes an esotropia due to the unopposed action of the antagonistic medial rectus muscle. The affected eye turns medially and is unable to abduct properly.

Option D: The lower motor neuron lesion of cranial nerve VII is referred to as Bell's palsy. In Bell's palsy, symptoms start acutely. Pain behind the ear may precede paralysis by 24–48 hours. There can be a transient (up to two weeks) loss of the sensation of taste.

10. Ans. (a) Sebaceous cell carcinoma

Ref: Comprehensive Ophthalmology by AK Khurana, 6th ed. pg. 365

- Chalazion is the granulomatous disease of meibomian gland.
  Note: Meibomian gland is modified sebaceous gland.
- Recurrent chalazion can increase the suspicion that it is possibly a sebaceous cell carcinoma. It most often affects the eyelids.
- **Option B:** SCC occurs usually within the exposed part of the eyeball between the lids in sun- damaged conjunctiva at the limbus. Therefore, the primary risk factor for SCC is ultraviolet B radiation.
- **Option C:** Basal cell carcinoma (BCC) is a cancer found on the skin around the body, often caused by sun exposure. It is also called a 'rodent ulcer'. It can be found on the eyelids.
- **Option D:** Kaposi sarcoma is a type of cancer that can grow from the cells lining the lymph vessels or blood vessels, usually on the face or legs and rarely on the eyelids. Kaposi sarcoma is often the result of a KSHV infection and is most common in immunocompromised people.

11. Ans. (d) Grade 4

Ref: Comprehensive Ophthalmology by AK Khurana, 6th ed. pg. 275

Hypertensive Retinopathy Grades (Modified Scheie's Classification):

- **Grade 1:** Barely detectable arterial narrowing
- **Grade 2:** Obvious arterial narrowing with focal irregularities
- **Grade 3:** Grade 2 plus retinal hemorrhages, exudates, cotton wool spots, or retinal edema
- **Grade 4:** Grade 3 plus papilledema

12. Ans. (c) RSO and LIR

Ref: Comprehensive Ophthalmology by AK Khurana, 6th ed. pg. 339

YOKE MUSCLES (CONTRALATERAL SYNERGIST)

- These are pairs of muscles, one in each eye, that produce conjugate eye movements.
- Image given here summarizes all the yoke muscles in different gazes

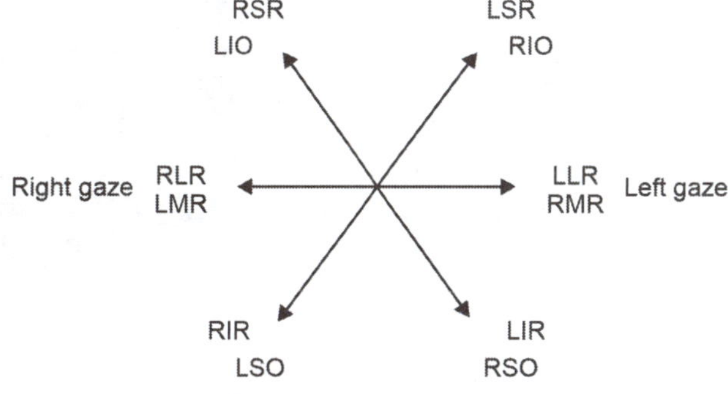

13. Ans. (c) Dacryocystorhinostomy

Ref: Comprehensive Ophthalmology by AK Khurana, 6th ed. pg. 393

- Chronic dacryocystitis is inflammation of lacrimal sac.
- Treatment depends on the age of the patient brought:

- **Age < 6 months:** Massage over the lacrimal sac area and topical antibiotics constitute the mainstay of treatment of congenital NLD block
- Lacrimal syringing (irrigation) with normal saline and antibiotic solution (up to 3 months)
- **6 months to 3 years:** Probing of NLD with Bowman's probe. It should be performed in case the condition is not cured by the age of 6 months.
- **After 3 years:** Dacryocystorhinostomy (DCR) surgery is preferred. Lacrimal sac is opened into meddle meatus, bypassing NLD
- Alternatively, balloon catheter dilation and Intubation with silicone tube can also be done.

14. Ans. (a) Copper

Ref: Comprehensive Ophthalmology by A K Khurana, 7th ed. pg. 200

- The above shown image is suggestive of sunflower cataract(right) and KF-Kayser Fleischer ring(left).
- These findings are suggestive of Wilson's disease which is an inborn error of copper metabolism.
- KF ring occurs due to the deposition of copper in the Descemet's membrane of cornea.

15. Ans. (b) Surgery

Ref: Comprehensive Ophthalmology by A K Khurana, 7th ed. pg. 67–73

- Trachoma is a type of keratoconjunctivitis that occurs due to infection by chlamydia trachomatis.
- It is characterized by, follicular and papillary response, pannus formation, cicatrisation.
- SAFE strategy is given by WHO GET 2020 program. This strategy is for prophylaxis against trachoma infection and prevention of blindness
  - S: Surgery
  - A: Antibiotic use
  - F: Facial hygiene
  - E: Environmental

16. Ans. (b) Patching and antibiotics

Ref: Comprehensive Ophthalmology by A K Khurana, 7th ed. pg. 398

The given case is of photokeratitis. Which is commonly seen among welders and persons going for skiing. It is treated with patching and antibiotics.

17. Ans. (a) Medial wall

Ref: Comprehensive Ophthalmology by A K Khurana, 7th ed. pg. 403–404

Lacrimal sac is present in the **medial wall** of the orbit.
Its function is the production of tears.

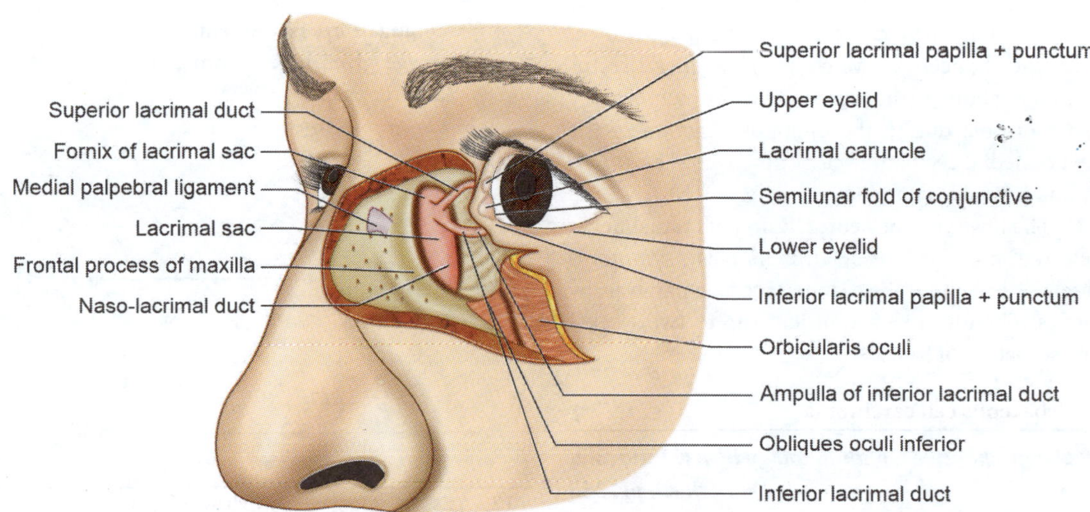

18. Ans. (b) Rt. Inferior oblique

Ref: Comprehensive Ophthalmology by A K Khurana, 7th ed. pg. 352

- Synergistic muscles are those muscles which move an eye in the same direction. Superior rectus and inferior oblique of the same eye act as synergistic muscles as both of them cause the elevation of the same eye.
- In contrary, yoke muscle is the muscle which shows synergistic action in opposite eye.

19. Ans. (a) Optic chiasma

Ref: Comprehensive Ophthalmology by A K Khurana, 7th ed. pg. 322–323

- The visual pathway starts from the retina and goes up till the visual cortex. It consists of optic nerves, optic chiasma, optic tract, lateral geniculate bodies, optic radiations and visual cortex as shown in the above flowchart.
- A lesion at optic chiasma, can cause bitemporal hemianopia.

Detailed discussion with image is given in the neuro ophthalmology section.

20. Ans. (b) Vitamin A

Ref: Comprehensive Ophthalmology by A K Khurana, 7th ed. pg. 487–488

Xerophthalmia is the collective term for all the ocular manifestations of vitamin A deficiency.

21. Ans. (b) Index myopia

Ref: Comprehensive Ophthalmology by A K Khurana, 7th ed. pg. 38–39

- In the above case scenario of the patient whose cataract surgery was done a year ago, the likely diagnosis is index myopia. Index myopia results from an increase in the refractive index of crystalline lens associated with nuclear sclerosis which is the late postoperative complication of the cataract surgery.
- In myopia, the parallel rays of light coming from infinity or focused in front of the retina when accommodation is at rest, thus the patient would be unable to look at the far objects.
- Secondary cataract is a common complication of cataract surgery, seen at the posterior subcapsular region. It doesn't cause nuclear fibrosis.

22. Ans. (a) Occlusion therapy

Ref: Comprehensive Ophthalmology by A K Khurana, 7th ed. pg. 355–356

- Amblyopia is the partial loss of sight in one or both eyes in the absence of ophthalmoscopic or other marked objective signs.
- The most sensitive period for development of amblyopia is the first six months of life.
- Treatment of amblyopia should begin at early age, and it's best when started under three years of age. Treatment of choice for a 10-year-old child is **occlusion therapy** which includes occlusion of the normal eye so that the amblyopic eye is forced to focus on objects.

23. Ans. (b) Diabetic macular edema

Ref: Comprehensive Ophthalmology by A K Khurana, 7th ed. pg. 287–289

- Diabetic macular edema is seen in patients of chronic diabetes. It can be of proliferative (PDR) or non-proliferative (NPDR) type. It occurs due to the increased permeability of the retinal capillaries.
- Diabetic macular edema is diagnosed if one of the following three criteria is present on slit lamp examination:
  - Thickening of retina at or within 500 μm of the center of fovea.
  - Hard accelerates at all within 500 μm of the center of fovea.
  - Development of a zone of retinal thickening, one disc diameter or larger in size within 1 disc diameter of the center of fovea.

ANATOMY, PHYSIOLOGY AND EXAMINATION OF EYE

24. Ans. (b) Dacryocystorhinostomy

Ref: A.K. Khurana, 7th ed. pg. 413

- The shown instrument is used for dacryocystorhinostomy (DCR).
- In DCR, nan anastomosis is created between the sac and the nasal mucosa to bypass an obstruction in the nasolacrimal duct.
- Dacryocystorhinostomy operation can be done by following techniques:
  - Conventional external approach
  - Endonasal surgical DCR
  - Endonasal laser DCR
  - Endocanalicular DCR

25. Ans. (c) Ectropion

Ref: A.K. Khurana, 7th ed. pg. 575

- The V-Y plasty technique is an island pedicle flap procedure, used for management of ectropion.

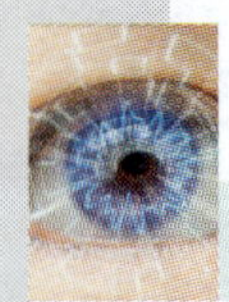

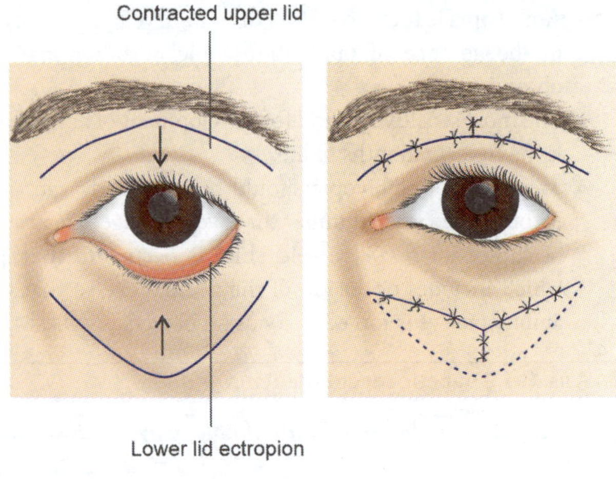

26. Ans. (a) Social blindness

Ref: A.K. Khurana, 7th ed. pg. 73

Definitions of blindness:

- **Total blindness:** Ophthalmology, Absolute (No light perception)
- **Legal blindness:** Vision in better eye <1/60 to perception light
- **Social blindness:** WHO, NPCBVI (vision in better eye <3/60 to 1/60)
- **Economic blindness:** Severe VI, work (Vision in better eye <6/60 to 3/60
- Moderate visual impairment

27. Ans. (c) Goldmann applanation tonometer

Ref: A.K. Khurana, 7th ed. pg. 530

- Goldman applanation tonometry is considered as gold standard for measuring IOP.

28. Ans. (c) Can be used in cases of hazy ocular media

Ref: A.K. Khurana, 7th ed. pg. 607

- The shown image is of direct ophthalmoscopy. It produces an Erect image (upright) and magnification 15 times.
- In hazy ocular media it cannot be used.

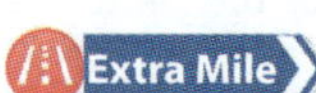
Extra Mile

Features	Direct ophthalmoscopy	indirect ophthalmoscopy
Condensing lens	Not Required	Required
Examination distance	As close to patient's eye as possible	At an arm's length
Image	Virtual, erect	Real, inverted
Illumination	Not as bright; not useful in hazy media	Bright; useful for hazy media
Area of field in focus	About 2 disc diameters	About 8 disc diameters
Stereopsis	Absent	Present
Accessible fundus view	Slightly beyond equator	Up to Oral serrata i.e. peripheral retina
Examination through hazy media	Not possible	Possible

29. Ans. (b) Schirmer's test

Ref: Khurana 7th ed. pg. 407

- Schirmer's test is used to measures total tear secretions.
- This test is used in dry eye disease.
- It is performed with the help of a 5 × 35 mm strip of Whatman-41 filter paper.

Procedure

- This paper is folded 5 mm from one end and place it in the lower fornix at the junction of lateral one-third and medial two-thirds.
- Then patient is asked to look up and not to blink or close the eyes.
- After 5 minutes wetting of the filter paper take place from the bent end then its reading is measured.
- Interpretation of Schirmer-I test -
  - More than 15 mm = Normal value
  - Value of 5-10 mm = Moderate to mild keratoconjunctivitis sicca (KCS).
  - Value less than 5 mm = severe KCS.

30. Ans. (d) Ames test

Ref: A.K. Khurana, 6th ed. pg. 330-331

- Ames test is utilized to determine the mutagenic activity of chemicals by observing they can cause mutation in test bacteria or not.
- All other test in choices are utilized in color vision testing.
- **NOTE:** FM-100 Hue test is the most sensitive test for color vision testing.

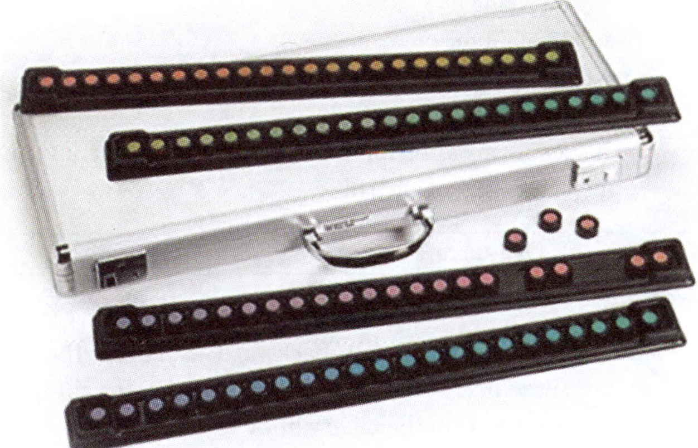

FIGURE: FM 100 Hue

31. Ans. (b) Neural crest

Ref: Comprehensive Ophthalmology by A.K. Khurana 6th ed. pg. 12–13

- Corneal epithelium is derived from surface ectoderm, while corneal endothelium is derived from neural crest.

TABLE: Embryology of eye

Surface ectoderm	Neuroectoderm	Neural crest	Mesoderm
• Tarsal plate • Epithelium of cornea & conjunctiva • Lens • Lacrimal gland	• Retina • Optic nerve • Smooth muscle of iris • Epithelium of iris and ciliary muscle, retina • Secondary vitreous	• Trabecular meshwork • Ciliary muscles • Endothelium of cornea • Stroma of cornea • **Sclera EXCEPT temporal part**	• Extraocular muscles • Primary vitreous • **Temporal sclera** • Blood Vessels
Mn: TELL	ROSES	To MESS	Extra Pulm. TB

32. Ans. (d) Done from 1 meter distance from patient

Ref: Comprehensive Ophthalmology by A.K. Khurana 6th ed. pg. 5771

- Retinoscopy aka skiascopy or shadow test is done to check the error of refraction by method of neutralization.
- Patient is made to sit at a distance of 1 meter from examiner → a light is thrown into patient's eye → through a hole in retinoscope mirror, the examiner observes the red reflex in the pupillary area of patient.
- Examiner Look for movement of red reflex/orange streak/bar of light.
  - **If NO movement:** Myopia = –1 D
  - **If opposite movement:** Myopia > –1
  - **Same side movement:** Myopia < – 1; Emmetropia = 0; Hypermetropia: +1.

33. Ans. (b) ERG

Ref: Comprehensive Ophthalmology by A.K. Khurana 6th ed. pg. 287

- Dark adaptation is ability of the eye to adapt itself to decreasing illumination. The time taken to see in dim illumination is dark adaptation time.
- Rods are more sensitive to low light (scotopic vision) while cones are for bright light.
- **Delayed dark adaptation:** Occur due to disease of rods. Ex: Deficiency of vitamin A, retinitis pigmentosa.

RETINITIS PIGMENTOSA

- Degenerative disease of the rods
- MC affects males in childhood and progress slowly
- Inherited as:
  - AR- in 25% cases; intermediate severity
  - AD- in 25% cases; least severe
  - X-linked- least common (10%); most severe
- **Clinical feature:**
  - Night blindness
  - Delayed dark adaptation
  - Tubular vision
  - **Triad:** Arterioles constriction, Bony spicule pigmentation, Waxy pallor of disc
- **IOC:** Electroretinogram (B wave affected before A wave)
- **Treatment:** Vitamin A 15000 IU orally qd, slow down progression

34. Ans. (a) +2 to +3 D

Ref: Comprehensive Ophthalmology by Khurana; 6th ed. pg. 9

EYE AT BIRTH

- AP diameter is 16.5 mm, adult size is attained by 7 to 8 years (24 mm).
- Corneal diameter 10 mm, adult size attained by 2 years.
- Lens spherical.
- Lacrimal gland underdeveloped, tears not secreted.
- Orbit is more divergent.
- Visual acuity 6/60.
- Myelination of optic nerve has reached lamina cribrosa.

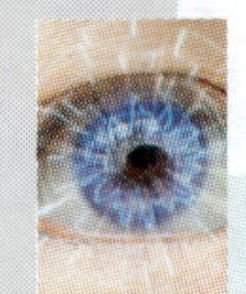

35. Ans. (b) Lens

Ref: Comprehensive Ophthalmology by Khurana 4th ed. pg. 4

- Among the given choices, lens has the highest refractive index of about 1.38 to 1.40.

Refractive index of different ocular structure

Structure	Refractive index
• Lens	1.38–1.40
• Cornea	1.376
• Aqueous humor	1.336
• Vitreous humor	1.336

36. Ans. (c) Associated with microphthalmia

Ref: Ocular Pathology; E-book, pg. 664

- The primary vitreous used information of the eye during fetal development remains in the eye upon birth and is hazy and scarred.
- The persistence of primary vitreous even after birth is said to be persistent hyperplastic primary vitreous (PHPV).
- **Symptoms are:** Leukocoria, strabismus, nystagmus and blurred vision, blindness.
- It is seen almost always unilateral (~90% of the cases)
- It is associated with:
  - Small eye (typically occurs in a microphthalmic eye)
  - Retinal detachment
  - Vitreous hemorrhage
- If diagnosed at an early stage it may be possible to aspirate the lens followed by excision of the retrolental membrane and vitrectomy.
- Visual prognosis is poor.

37. Ans. (a) Temporal

Extent of normal visual field (in degrees)

- Superior: 50°
- Inferior: 70°
- Nasal: 60°
- Temporal: 90–100°

38. Ans. (b) 10–20

Ref: A.K. Khurana's Ophthalmology, 6th ed. pg. 223

- Normal IOP refers to pressure exerted by intraocular fluids on coats of eyeball.
- Normal IOP varies **between 10 and 21 mm Hg** *(mean 16.5 +/– 2.5 mm Hg).*
- This pressure is essentially maintained by a dynamic equilibrium between the formation and outflow of aqueous humor.
- Normal aqueous production rate: 2.3 µl/L
- Normal aqueous outflow rate: 0.22/min/mm Hg

39. Ans. (b) 2.5 cm

Ref: A.K. Khurana, 6th ed. pg. 3

- Axial length of orbit is 24 mm i.e. 2.4 cm
- Volume of orbit: 6 mL
- Depth of anterior chamber: 3 mm
- Eyeball Made of 3 layers:
  - Sclera: Outer
  - Choroid: Middle *(vascular layer; a dangerous layer)*
  - Retina: Inner
- Cornea forms **anterior 1/6th** of eyeball and sclera forms **posterior 5/6th** of eyeball

40. Ans. (c) Ora serrata

Ref: A.K. Khurana, 6th ed. pg. 264

The ciliary body extends backward as far as the ora serrata, at which point the retina proper begins abruptly. The transition from the ciliary body to the choroid, on the other hand is gradual, although this line is conveniently accepted as the limit the two structures. The ora serrata thus circles the globe, but is slightly more anterior on the nasal than on the temporal side.

41. Ans. (b) Superior oblique

Ref: A.K. Khurana, 6th ed. pg. 5-6, 337

EXTRA-OCULAR MUSCLES

- The extraocular muscles control the movement of the eye.
- **Levator Palpabrae Superioris (LPS):** Muscle which elevates the palpabrae upwards resulting in opening the eye.
- When LPS gets tired, muller's muscle and frontalis muscle helps in elevation of eyelid.

- **Eyeball muscles (6):**
  - **4 Recti muscles:** Superior (SR), inferior (IR), lateral (LR) and medial rectus (MR)]
  - **2 Oblique muscles:** Superior oblique and inferior oblique
- The muscles supplied by the occulomotor nerve **(CN III)** are: superior, inferior and medial rectus and inferior oblique, sphincter papillae and ciliary muscle.
- Lateral rectus is supplied by abducens (VI)
- Trochlear nerve (CN IV) supplies superior oblique muscle.
- ***Mnemonic:*** *LR6, SO4, O3; which means lateral rectus is supplied by sixth nerve, superior oblique by fourth nerve and all other by EOM by third cranial nerve.*

42. Ans. (b) Its nucleus is located in lower midbrain

Ref: A.K. Khurana, 6th ed. pg. 7-8

- Location of **CN III** (oculomotor nerve) nucleus is **upper midbrain**
- Location of **CN IV** (trochlear nerve) nucleus is in the **lower mid-brain.**

TABLE: CN, their Respective Nucleus Location and their Function

Cranial Nerve	Nucleus Location	Function
Oculomotor III	Upper midbrain	Eyeball movements: extrinsic ocular muscles
Trochlear IV	Lower midbrain	Eyeball movements: extrinsic ocular muscles
Abducens VI	Pons	Eyeball movements: extrinsic ocular muscles
Hypoglossal XII	Medulla	Tongue muscles and movements

43. Ans. (b) Lacrimal gland

Ref: A.K. Khurana, 6th ed. pg. 386

GLANDS OF EYELIDS

- **Meibomian glands**: Also known as tarsal glands present in the stroma of tarsal plate and are arranged vertically.
  - They are modified sebaceous glands. Their ducts open at the lid margin. Their secretion constitutes the oily layer of tear film.
- **Glands of Zeis**: These are also sebaceous glands which open into the follicles of eyelashes.
- **Glands of Moll**: These are modified sweat glands situated near the hair follicle. They open into the hair follicles or into the ducts of Zeis glands.
- **Accessory lacrimal glands of Wolfring.** These are present near the upper border of the tarsal plate.

Note: *Lacrimal gland is one of the gland of lacrimal apparatus. It is NOT among the eyelid glands.*

44. Ans. (a) Superior oblique

Ref: A.K. Khurana, 6th ed. pg. 337-39

- The function of superior oblique is quite contrary to its name. Its action is depression of eyeball, which helps to see down.
- Its yoke muscle is inferior rectus, which also has the similar function as superior oblique. If superior oblique is affected patient will develop difficulty in looking down
- There are 9 Gaze:
  - Primary : Straight
  - Secondary: Up, down, left, right
  - Tertiary : Up left, Up, right, Down left, Down right
- **ACTIONS OF EOM**

Muscle	Function		
	Primary	Secondary	Tertiary
Lateral rectus	Abduction	–	–
Medial Rectus	Adduction	–	–
Inferior Rectus	Depression	Extorsion	Adduction
Superior rectus	Elevation	Intorsion	Adduction
Inferior Oblique	Extorsion	Elevation	Abduction
Superior oblique	Intorsion	Depression	Abduction

- **Mnemonics:** *SinRad (all superior muscles causes Intorsion; all rectus muscles causes Adduction EXCEPT Lateral rectus)*

45. Ans. (a) Adduction and intorsion

Ref: A.K. Khurana, 6th ed. pg. 339

46. Ans. (b) Inferior rectus

Ref: A.K. Khurana, 6th ed. pg. 337-39

- The function of inferior rectus is depression of eyeball, which helps to see down.
- Its yoke muscle is superior oblique, which also has the similar function as inferior rectus.

47. Ans. (c) Towards the right side

Ref: A.K. Khurana, 6th ed. pg. 337-39

- ***VIth nerve palsy leads to*** loss of abduction/lateral gaze leading to **abnormal head posture towards the side** of affected muscle
- ***There is*** Presence of ***convergent squint also.***

Extra Mile

IVth nerve palsy
- Diplopia on looking down
- Inability to look inferomedially

48. Ans. (d) Right superior rectus

Ref: A.K. Khurana, 6th ed. pg. 339

- **Synergistic muscle** is two muscles *functioning as same, in the same eye.* Function of superior rectus is to elevate the eye, which is same with inferior oblique.
  - Right inferior oblique and right superior rectus elevate the right eye
- Yoke muscle on the contrary, is two extraocular muscles from two eyes having same function.
  - **Ex:** Yoke muscle of right inferior oblique is left superior rectus.

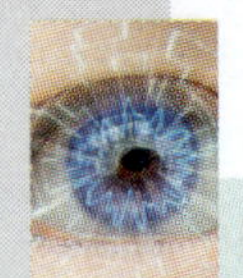

49. Ans. (a) The superior orbital fissure

Ref: A.K. Khurana, 6th ed. pg. 337, BDC, 4th ed. Vol III, pg. 25-6

TABLE: Structures passing through superior orbital fissure

Superior orbital fissure		
Medial /lower part	**Middle part (through tendinous ring)**	**Lateral/ Upper part**
• Inferior Ophthalmic vein • Sympathetic nerves around internal carotid artery ***Mn: Inferior sympathy***	• Nasociliary nerve • Occulomotor nerve • Abducent nerve ***Mnemonic –"NOA"***	• Superior Ophthalmic vein • Lacrimal nerve • Frontal nerve • Trochlear nerve ***Mn – "Superior LFT"***

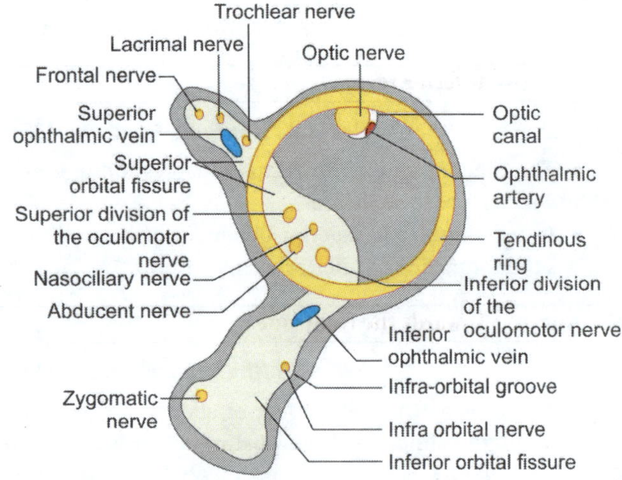

Extra Mile

Structures passing through Inferior orbital fissure
- Zygomatic branch of maxillary nerve
- Infraorbital nerve and vessels
- Rami of Pterygoid ganglion
- Communicating vein b/w inferior ophthalmic and pterygoid plexus of veins.

Mn-"ZIPC"

50. Ans. (a) Strabismus

Ref: A.K. Khurana, 6th ed. pg. 346

- **Strabismus:** A misalignment of the visual axes of the two eyes is called squint or strabismus.
- **It is classified as:**
  - Pseudostrabismus (apparent squint)
  - Heterophoria (latent squint)
  - Heterotropia (manifest squint)

HETEROPHORIA

- Heterophoria also known as 'Latent strabismus'
- It is a condition in which the tendency of the eyes to deviate is kept latent by fusion.

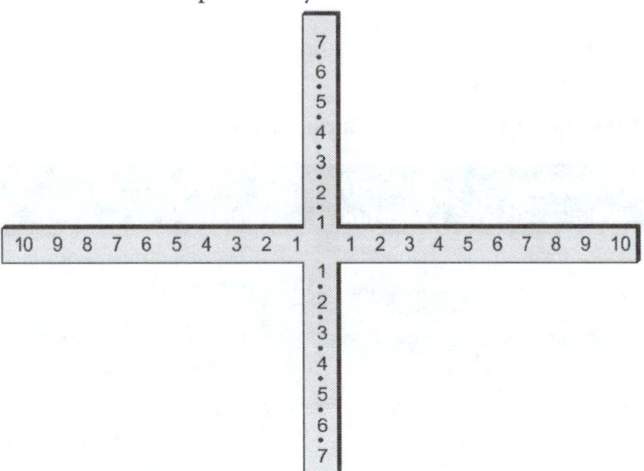

Examination of a Case of Heterophoria

- Testing for vision and refractive error.
- Cover-uncover test.
- Prism cover test
- **Maddox rod test:** Patient is asked to fix on a point light in the centre of Maddox tangent scale at a distance of 6 meters.
- A Maddox rod is placed in front of one eye with axis of the rod parallel to the axis of deviation.
- The Maddox rod converts the point light image into a line. Thus, the patient will see a point light with one eye and a red line with the other.
- Due to dissimilar images of the two eyes, fusion is broken and heterophoria becomes apparent.
- **Maddox wing test:** Also used to measure phoria of near distance.

51. Ans. (c) 3 D

Ref: A.K. Khurana, 6th ed. pg. 578

- By pinhole test visual acuity can be neutralized till 3 D. It can't accommodate more than that.
- It is a test to distinguish a refractive error from organic disease.
- A refractive error may, be corrected with glasses, whereas organic disease may signal the development of preventable blindness. If visual acuity is improved after pinhole test, the defect is refractive; if not, it is organic.
  - **Pinhole improves vision:** Refractive error, peripheral cataract
  - **Pinhole worsen vision:** Macular diseases, central lens opacities
  - **Vision static with pinhole**: Amblyopia

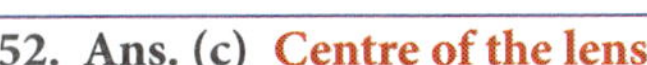

52. Ans. (c) Centre of the lens

Ref: A.K. Khurana 6th ed. /179; Parson's 20/e p-52-53

REFRACTIVE INDEX OF DIFFERENT MEDIUM

- Highest refractive index is of *center of lens* (1.406)
- Anterior and posterior lens cortex forming anterior & posterior lens surface (1.386)
- Cornea (1.376)
- Aqueous and vitreous humor (1.336)
- Air (1)

53. Ans. (c) 45 D

Ref: A.K. Khurana, 6th ed. pg. 95

POWER

- Lens= +16D
- Cornea= +44D
- Total= +60D

54. Ans. (b) Phacomorphic glaucoma

Ref: A.K. Khurana, 6th ed. pg. 3, 192-93

- **Deep anterior chamber is seen in**: Young, males and myopes
- **Shallow anterior chamber is seen in**: Women, Elderly, and Children (WEC)

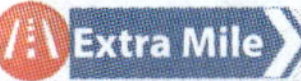

Extra Mile

Phacomorphic Glaucoma

- Phacomorphic glaucoma is angle closure glaucoma caused by mature cataract ***making the anterior chamber shallow.***

Phacolytic glaucoma

- Phacolytic glaucoma is open angle glaucoma caused by hypermature cataract in which the *anterior chamber is deep* by leaking lens material which blocks the trabecular meshwork.
- Treatment is cataract surgery

Myopia

- Myopia or 'Short sight' is a refractive error that most commonly presents as indistinct distant vision in which the light rays are focused in front of retina. As the maximum distance of clear vision is reduced the far point comes nearer. Following are types of myopia-
  - Axial Myopia
  - Curvature Myopia
  - Index Myopia
- **Axial Myopia-** eyeball larger than normal causes myopia. Every 1 mm increase in axial length has 3D increase in 1 mm = 3D
- **Curvature Myopia**- axial length normal. Cornea is curved as in keratoconus. 1 mm of curvature = 6D. So they are very high myopes.
- **Index Myopia**- corneal curvature normal. Refractive Index increases. More the difference → more the bending between two media.

Myopics are typically called short sighted, so all myopics wear concave lenses. Minification 1D = 2%

Aphakia: Aphakia means absence of crystalline lens from eye.

55. Ans. (a) Children

Ref: A.K. Khurana 6th ed. /45-49; Khurana's 4th ed. pg. 39-41

ACCOMMODATION

- Mechanism by which we can focus the diverging rays coming from a near object on the retina in an attempt to see clearly is called accommodation.
- During this there occurs increase in the power of crystalline lens due to increase in the curvature of its surface.

Mechanism of Accommodation

- When the eye is at rest (unaccommodated), the ciliary ring is large and keeps the zonules tense.
- Because of zonular tension the lens is kept compressed (flat) by the capsule.
- Ciliary muscles and zonules have inverse relation in function.
- Ciliary ring is shortened due to contraction of the ciliary muscle which releases zonular tension on the lens capsule. This allows the elastic capsule to act unrestrained to deform the lens substance. The lens then alters its shape to become more convex (conoidal).
- The lens assumes conoidal shape due to configuration of the anterior lens capsule which is thinner at the centre and thicker at the periphery
- Note: *The crystalline protein of lens and contraction of ciliary muscle is finest in child as compared to adult and elderly. Hence children have maximum accommodation.*

56. Ans. (a) Lens of eye

Ref: A.K. Khurana, 6th ed. pg. 12

Among the given options, surface ectoderm forms lens

Note:

- Iris smooth muscle is derived from Neuroectoderm
- Sclera (except temporal part) and corneal stroma is derived from Neural crest

57. Ans. (b) Surface ectoderm

Ref: A.K. Khurana, 6th ed. pg. 12

58. Ans. (c) Surface ectoderm

Ref: A.K. Khurana, 6th ed. pg. 12

Please refer to above explanation

59. Ans. (c) Temporal

Ref: A.K. Khurana, 6th ed. pg. 505, Khurana, 4th ed. pg. 481

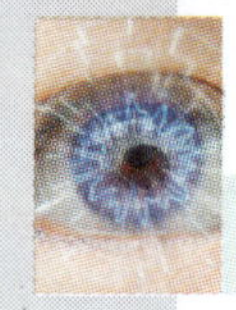

Extent of Normal Visual Field:

- Superior: 50
- Inferior: 70
- Nasal: 60
- Temporal: 90-100

60. Ans. (b) Inferior

Ref: A.K. Khurana, 6th ed. pg. 265-66

- Neuroretinal rim is the tissue outside the cup and contains the retinal nerve axons as they enter the nerve head.
- It is broadest in lower segment of the disc, then above followed by nasally and temporally.
- There is greater axonal mass and vascularity in the infero-temporal region.
- In case of primary open angle glaucoma, there is progressive loss of retinal ganglion cells, leading to enlargement of the cup, particularly in lower and upper poles of disc, leading to vertically oval cup.

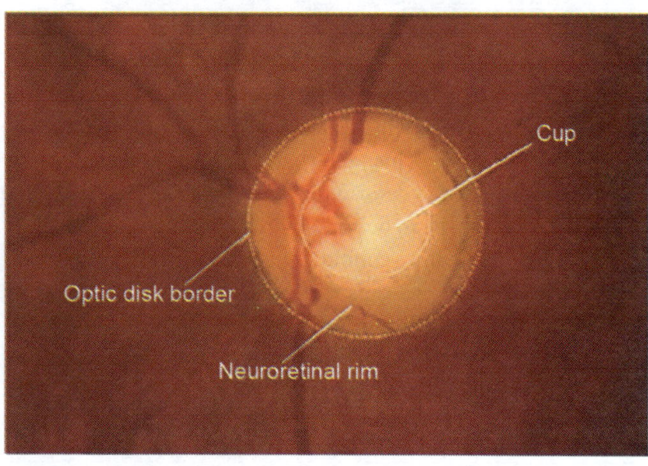

61. Ans. (d) Opacity in the refractive media

Ref: A.K. Khurana, 6th ed. pg. 586

DISTANT DIRECT OPHTHALMOSCOPY

- Used to get a preliminary idea about the status of the ocular media and fundus
- This should be done routinely before doing a direct ophthalmoscopy
- **Equipment needed:** Self-illuminated ophthalmoscope or plane mirror with a hole in centre
- **Procedure**
  - Should be performed in a semi dark room
  - The ophthalmoscope should be kept at a distance of 20–25 cm from the patient's eye
  - Normally a red reflex is seen at the pupillary area
- **Uses**
  - Opacities in the ocular media are seen as dark spots in the red glow at the pupillary area
  - The plane of the opacities can be assessed by asking the patient to move the eye from side to side while the examiner is observing the pupillary glow (based on parallax principle)
    - Opacities in front of the pupil move in the direction of eye movement
    - Opacities in the pupillary plane do not move
    - Opacities behind the pupillary plane move opposite the direction of eye movement
- To differentiate between a mole on the iris and a hole in the iris
  - In oblique illumination, both appear dark
  - In distant direct ophthalmoscopy
    - Mole–appears dark
    - Hole–red glow is seen
- To detect a retinal detachment or fundal mass
  - Both of them are visible as a grayish reflex
  - It is not possible to differentiate them in distant direct ophthalmoscopy
- The image in Indirect Ophthalmoscopy is inverted both vertically as well as laterally, which means: *What appears as right upper quadrant is actually in the left lower quadrant.*

Extra Mile

Direct ophthalmoscope	Indirect Ophthalmoscope
Virtual, Erect and Magnified 15 times: "VEM"	Real, Inverted and 4–5 times Magnified: "RIM"
Mneomonic: "DEV" i.e. Direct = Erect + Virtual	*Mnemonic: "IIR" i.e. Indirect = Inverted + Real*

62. Ans. (b) Direct ophthalmoscopy

Ref: A.K. Khurana, 6th ed. pg. 586; Khurana 4th ed. pg. 565

- **Direct ophthalmoscopy:** Disc and macula
- **Indirect ophthalmoscopy:** Whole retina, vitreous *(choice of test in retinal detachment)*
- **Distant direct ophthalmoscopy**- for any opacity, cataract, detachment
- **Retinoscopy:** For calculating refractive error

63. Ans. (a) Strabismus

Ref: A.K. Khurana, 6th ed. pg. 344-58

Classification of Squints (Strabismus)

LATENT SQUINT/HETEROPHORIA

- A condition in which the tendency of eyes to deviate is kept latent by fusion. Therefore when the influence of

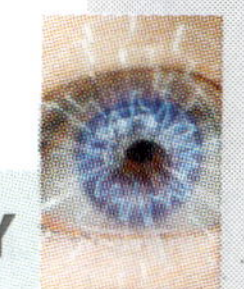

fusion is removed the visual axis of one eye axis of one eye deviates away (Orthophoria is a condition of perfect alignment of two eyes)

- **Types Esophoria is a tendency to converge**
  - Exophoria is a tendency to diverge
  - Hyperphoria is a tendency to deviate upwards
  - Hypophoria is a tendency to deviate downwards
  - Cyclophoria is a tendency to rotate around A–P axis
- **Evaluation**
  - Refraction
  - Uncover test (tells about present & type of heterophoria)
  - Maddox rod test (amount of heterophoria in degrees)
  - **Maddox wing test** (amount of phoria for near distance i.e. 33 cm)
- **Treatment:**
  - Refraction
  - Occlusion therapy (in presence of amblyopia)
  - Orthoptic exercise
  - Operative correction
  - Prism correction for remaining error.

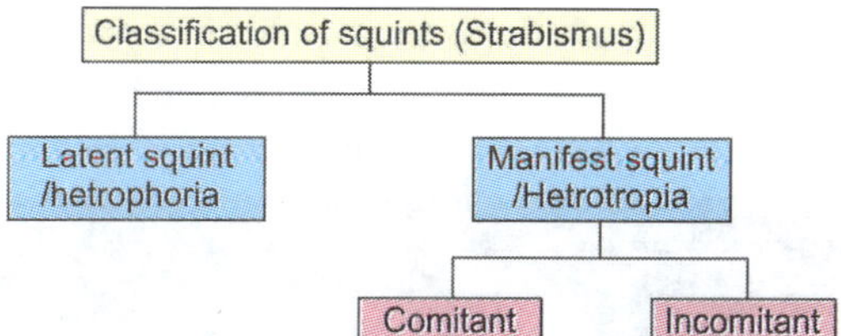

MANIFEST SQUINT (HETEROTROPIA)	
Comitant	**Incomitant**
• Amount of deviation in squinting eye remains constant (unaltered) in all directions of gaze & there is no limitation of ocular movements.	• Manifest squint in which amount of deviation varies in different directions of gaze.
• Types ▪ **Alternating squint:** when one eye fixes, the other eye deviates & either of the eyes can adopt fixation alternately & freely ▪ Esotropia (Convergent squint) ▪ Exotropia (Divergent squint) ▪ Hypertropia (Vertical squint)	• Types ▪ Paralytic squint ▪ "A" & "V" pattern hetrotrophias ▪ Special ocular motility defects ▪ **Clinical presentation:** is diplopia, confusion, nausea, vertigo & ocular deviation with restriction of eye movements, compensatory head posture & false projection & orientation, loss of stereoposis, normal visual acuity & no amblyopia.
• **Evaluation** ▪ Refraction, visual acuity, ocular motility ▪ Direct cover test (confirms the presence of manifest squint) ▪ Alternate cover test (reveal whether the squint is U/L or alternate and to differentiate concomitant squint from paralytic squint). ▪ Estimation of angle of deviation. ▪ **Hirschberg corneal reflex test:** Roughly the angle of squint is 15° and 45° when the corneal light reflex falls on the border of pupil & limbus respectively. The premise is that every millimeter of deviation from centre of pupil is equal to 7° (15Δ)	• **Evaluation** ▪ All tests of comitant squint ▪ Diplopia carting ▪ ***Hess screen test*** ▪ *Forced duction test* • Treatment of cause, diplopia (by occlusion), surgery (if no recovery in 6 months).

64. Ans. (c) Inferior rectus

Ref: A.K. Khurana, 6th ed. pg. 414

- In thyroid eye ophthalmopathy, the ocular motility defects due to restrictive myopathy *(in order of frequency)* are:
  - Elevation (due to fibrosis of inferior rectus)
  - Abduction (due to fibrosis of medial rectus)
  - Depression (due to fibrosis of superior rectus)
  - Adduction (due to fibrosis of lateral rectus).

Mnemonic - "I M Shy Lad"

65. Ans. (a) Males are more prone

Ref: A.K. Khurana, 6th ed. pg. 329

- Color blindness is an **X-Linked recessive condition**. Females are always carrier and males are always affected. Hence males are more affected than females.
- Most common type of color blindness: Deutranopia (Green color blindness)

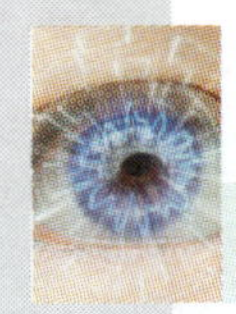

CORNEA, CONJUNCTIVA AND SCLERA

66. Ans. (a) Iris

Ref: Kanski Clinical Ophthalmology, 9th ed. pg. 427

- Koeppe nodules are inflammatory cell precipitates and could be found in non-granulomaous as well as granulomatous uveitis
- Koeppe nodules are located on the pupillary margin of iris and may be the site of posterior synechiae formation.

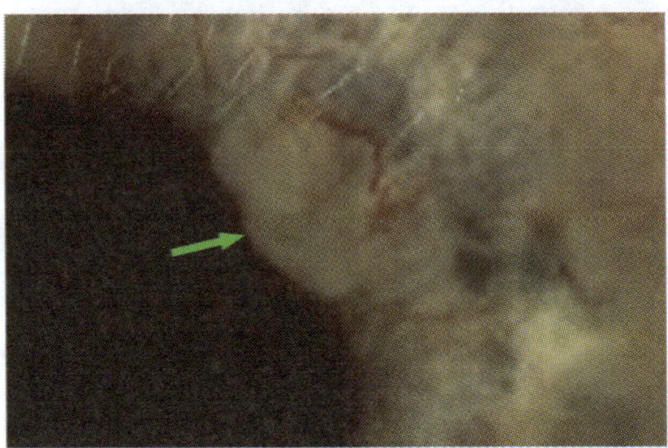

FIGURE: Koeppe nodules on pupillary margin

67. Ans. (a) Vitamin A

Ref: Kanski Clinical Ophthalmology, 9th ed. pg. 247

- Bitot's spots are typically dry-appearing triangular patches of xerosed conjunctiva with a layer of foam on the surface, usually located temporal to the cornea.
- They mainly composed of keratin admixture with gas-forming bacteria Corynebacterium xerosis, lead to foamy appearance.
- **Bitot's spots** are characteristic of Vitamin A deficiency and are not caused by any other condition.

68. Ans. (c) Giant papillary conjunctivitis

Ref: A.K. Khurana, 7th ed. pg. 84

- **Giant papillary conjunctivitis** also known as mechanically induced papillary conjunctivitis is a localized allergic response to a physically rough or deposited surface like contact lens, prosthesis, exposed nylon sutures and scleral buckle.
- It mostly presents with foreign body sensation, itching and congestion. There is associated multiple small papillae development inside of the eyelid.

69. Ans. (b) Satellite lesions

Ref: A.K. Khurana, 7th ed. pg. 117

- The given condition is of fungal keratitis. It is mostly seen among farmers.
- **MC organism:** Fusarium, Aspergillus
- Patient present with photophobia, discharge, redness, blurred vision, excessive tearing
- Upon examination: satellite lesion is seen.
- **HPE**: organism is seen as Filamentary fungi, the corneal lesions have a whitish gray infiltrate with feathery border.

70. Ans. (b) Vernal keratoconjunctivitis

Ref: A.K. Khurana, 7th ed. pg. 80

- VKC is recurrent, bilateral, chronic with exacerbations and characteristic white ROPY discharge with intense itching usually in the spring season of summer. This condition is often termed as spring catarrh.

71. Ans. (a) Fungal keratitis

Ref: A.K. Khurana, 7th ed. pg. 109

- The given case is of fungal ulcer.
- Mycotic ulcer is caused when a person gets injured by vegetative material such as crop leaf, branch of tree, straw thorn etc

Other modes of injury:

- Injury by animal tail
  - Secondary fungal ulcer

72. Ans. (a) Anterior staphyloma

Ref: A.K. Khurana, 7th ed. pg. 138

- The shown condition is anterior staphyloma
- It is a localized defect in the anterior eye wall with protrusion of uveal tissue due to alterations in scleral thickness and structure.

73. Ans. (d) Mitomycin C

Ref: A.K. Khurana, 7th ed. pg. 89

- Patients with recurrent pterygia suffer from blurred vision because of the astigmatism.
- Various surgical procedures have been proposed:
  - Conjunctival autografting
  - Conjunctival limbal autografting
  - Amniotic membrane transplantation
  - Application of mitomycin C

Extra Mile

Clinical uses of Mitomycin C in Ophthalmology

- Pterygium surgery
- Glaucoma filtering surgery
- Refractive surgeries
- Ocular surface tumors
- Squint surgeries
- Dacryocystorhinostomy (DCR)
- Allergic conjunctivitis

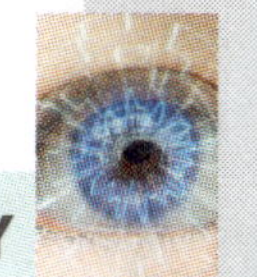

74. Ans. (c) Bitot's spots

Ref: A.K. Khurana, 7th ed. pg. 487

- The given image is of Bitot's spot, caused due to deficiency of Vit A.
- According to WHO classification of corneal diseases, it is classified under X1B.

75. Ans. (c) Keratoconus

Ref: Khurana 7th ed. pg. 137

- Keratoconus is a conical cornea
- It is progressive (slowly progress) noninflammatory bilateral ectatic condition of cornea in its axial part.
- It usually starts at puberty.
- Treatment:
  - **Spectacle correction:** Improves vision in early cases
  - **Contact lens:** Specially designes scleral contact lens (Rose-K) may be useful.
  - **Intacs**, the intracorneal ring segments. Useful due to its flattening effect.
  - **Corneal collagen cross linking** with riboflavin (CXL or C3R) and UV-A rays: It slows down the progression of disease
  - **Keratoplasty:** In advanced cases.

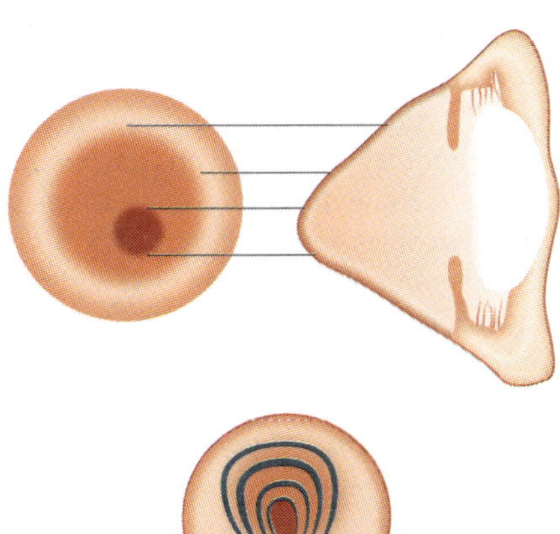

A

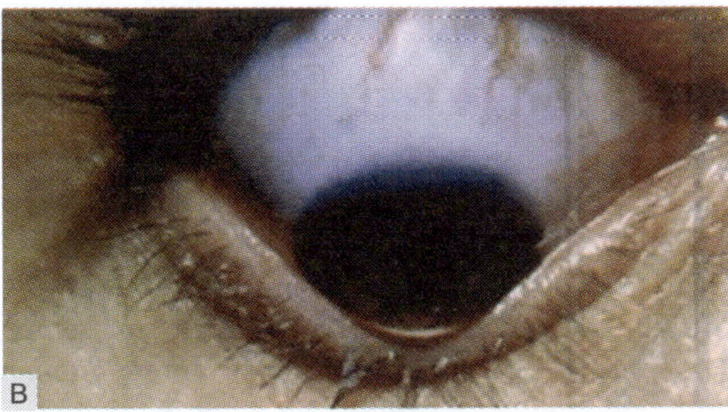

B

76. Ans. (a) Extended contact lense wearing

Ref: Khurana 7th ed. pg. 116

ACANTHAMOEBA KERATITIS

- Acanthamoeba castellanii is a Causative organism. It is a free-living genus of amoeba found in soil, fresh water, well water, sea water, sewage and air.
- In human, acanthamoeba causes:
  - Keratitis
  - Fulminant meningoencephalitis.
  - Granulomatous encephalitis
- Corneal infection with acanthamoeba occurs from direct corneal contact with any material or water contaminated

Risk factors:

- **Contact lens wearers**
- Trauma associated with contaminated matter such as vegetable matter, salt water diving.
- Occur as opportunistic infection

77. Ans. (b) Conjunctiva

Ref: American Academy of Ophthalmology

- In any viral infection including Covid-19 conjunctiva is the first part to be involved, causing conjunctivitis.

78. Ans. (d) Trachoma

Ref: Khurana 7th ed. pg. 70

- Arlt's line is a linear scar present in sulcus subtarsalis i.e. it is conjunctival scarring which may be irregular, star-shaped or linear.
- This is present in cicatricial phase of trachoma.

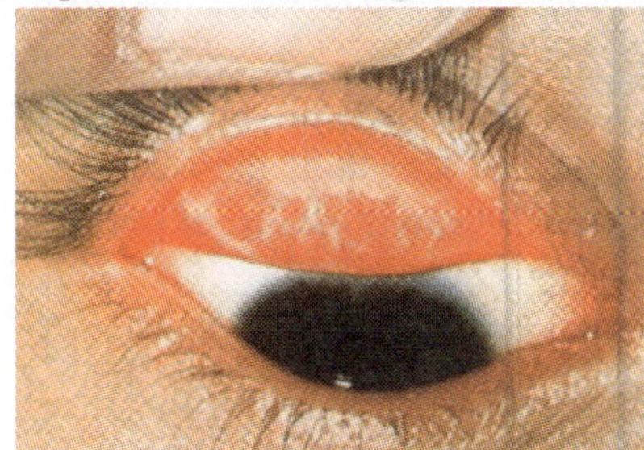

79. Ans. (b) Keratan sulphate

Ref: Comprehensive Ophthalmology by A.K. Khurana, 7th ed. pg. 100

- Keratan sulphate (KS) is the predominant glycosaminoglycan (GAG) in the cornea of the eye, where it exists in proteoglycan (PG) form.
- KS-PGs has a pivotal role in the establishment and maintenance of the array of regularly-spaced and uniformly- thin collagen fibrils which make up the corneal stroma (the thickest part of cornea).

- This characteristic arrangement of fibrils allows light to pass through the cornea.
- Mutation in the enzyme for the KS-GAG sulphation can lead to macular corneal dystrophy.

Other causes of corneal opacity:

- Avascularity
- Endothelium; which act as mechanical barrier. $Na^{+}K^{+}$ ATPase of endothelium keeps the cornea in dehydrated state.
- Failure of this pump can lead to bullous keratopathy.

80. Ans. (a) Bacterial corneal ulcer

Ref: Comprehensive Ophthalmology by A.K. Khurana, 7th ed. pg. 105, 116

- In contact lens wearers the most likely cause of redness and decreased vision is bacterial infection, which may often lead to corneal ulcer.
- The etiological organisms associated with corneal ulcer in contact lens wearers are Pseudomonas and Acanthamoeba castellanii.
- The most common source in acanthamoeba keratitis is tap water. It presents with Ring infiltrates.
- Since it is not given in the question hence the most appropriate option is bacterial corneal ulcer due to pseudomonas which produce an irregular sharp ulcer associated with hypopyon. It may perforate within 48–72 hours.

81. Ans. (c) It causes myopia

Ref: Comprehensive Ophthalmology by A.K. Khurana, 7th ed. pg. 89-90

- The shown condition in the image is pterygium.
- Pterygium is a growth of the conjunctiva or mucous membrane that covers the cornea.
- This benign or noncancerous wedge-shaped growth.
- Most common around nasal side.

Extra Mile

TABLE: Differences between pterygium and pseudopterygium

	Pterygium	Pseudopterygium
1. Etiology	Degenerative process	Inflammatory process
2. Age	Usually occurs in elder persons	Can occur at any age
3. Site	Always situated in the palpebral aperture	Can occur at any site
4. Stages	Either progressive, regressive or stationary	Always stationary
5 Probe test	Probe cannot be passed underneath	A probe can be passed under the neck

- Exact cause of pterygium is not known. One explanation is that too much exposure to ultraviolet (UV) light can lead to these growths. It occurs more often in people who live in warm climates and spend a lot of time outdoors in sunny or windy environments.

82. Ans. (c) Wilson's disease

Ref: Comprehensive Ophthalmology by A.K. Khurana, 7th ed. pg. 492

- Wilson's disease, also known as hepatolenticular degeneration, is an autosomal recessive genetic disorder of copper metabolism leading to copper accumulation in many tissues, mainly the liver, brain, cornea and kidney.
- Copper deposition leads to specific hepatic, neurological, psychiatric and ocular signs and symptoms.
- The ocular manifestations of Wilson's disease include Kayser-Fleischer ring (K-F ring) and sunflower cataract.
- K-F ring is almost always bilateral, starts superiorly first and then inferiorly, and later becomes circumferential.
- It results due to extracellular **copper deposition in the Descemet's membrane** of the cornea.

83. Ans. (b) Allergic

Ref: Comprehensive Ophthalmology by A.K. Khurana, 7th ed. pg. 100

- Phlyctenular conjunctivitis is a delayed hypersensitivity response to endogenous protein of microbes.
- It is probably a type 4 cell mediated immune response—also called as microbial allergic conjunctivitis.
- There is nodule formation on the conjunctival and corneal epithelium to endogenous allergens to which they have become sensitized.
- It is more common in girls than boys and more common in undernourished children living in overcrowded and unhygienic conditions in the peak age group of 3–15 years.
- It shows the following stages:
  - Stage of nodule formation
  - Stage of ulceration
  - Stage of granulation and
  - Stage of resolution

84. Ans. (a) Keratoconus

- The image shows V-shaped protrusion of cornea, which is termed as Munson sign. It is a feature of keratoconus.
- Other features of keratoconus:
  - Vogt's striae: Break in Descemet's membrane
  - Fleischer's ring: Iron deposition at the back of cornea
  - Upon retinoscopy: Scissoring reflex

85. Ans. (a) Keratoconus

Ref: to above Explanation for details of Keratoconus

- Fleischer ring is seen in keratoconus.
- Kayser-Fleischer ring is seen in Wilson's disease.

86. Ans. (c) Curvature of cornea

- Keratometer is used to assess curvature of cornea.
- Pachymetry is used for measurement of corneal thickness.

87. Ans. (c) Viral keratitis

Ref: A.K. Khurana, 6th ed. pg. 108-109

- The image shows dendritic ulcer, which is typical lesion for viral keratitis.
- **Signs:**
  - **Punctate epithelial keratitis:** Fine or coarse punctate lesion
  - **Dendritic ulcer:** Typical lesion for recurrent epithelial keratitis. Ulcer in irregular, zigzag, branching shape. Floor of ulcer stains with fluorescein, and the margin is stained with rose Bengal dye.
  - **Geographical ulcer:** Branches of dendritic ulcer coalesce to form geographical ulcer.

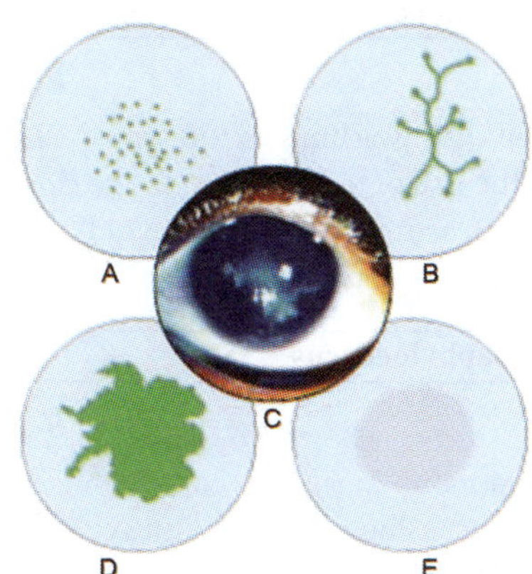

FIGURE: A. Punctate keratitis; B. Dendritic ulcer; C & D. Geographical Ulcer; E. Disciform keratitis

88. Ans. (b) Steroids

Ref: A.K. Khurana, 6th ed. pg. 64, 75

- Using steroids in active inflammation can cause flare-up of bacterial infection and corneal ulcer may develop.

89. Ans. (c) Conjunctiva invasion making a flap over cornea

Ref: Comprehensive Ophthalmology by A.K. Khurana 6th ed. pg. 87

PTERYGIUM

- It is a degenerative and hyperplastic condition of conjunctiva → elastotic degeneration and proliferation of subconjunctival tissue
- Triangular/wing shaped invasion of conjunctiva upon the cornea. It is common in dry heat, sun exposure (UV rays) and abundant dust.
- Iron deposition in the corneal epithelium at the advancing head of the pterygium is called **Stocker line.**
- It usually asymptomatic.
- **MC site:** Nasal side
  - **Primary double pterygium:** Involvement of both nasal and temporal side
- The corneal epithelium, bowman's layer and superficial stroma are destroyed
- **Treatment:** Surgical excision.
  - The commonest problem after excision is recurrence which is reduced by postoperative use of mitomycin-C/ thiotepa or by doing surgical excision with free conjunctival graft from same/other eye.

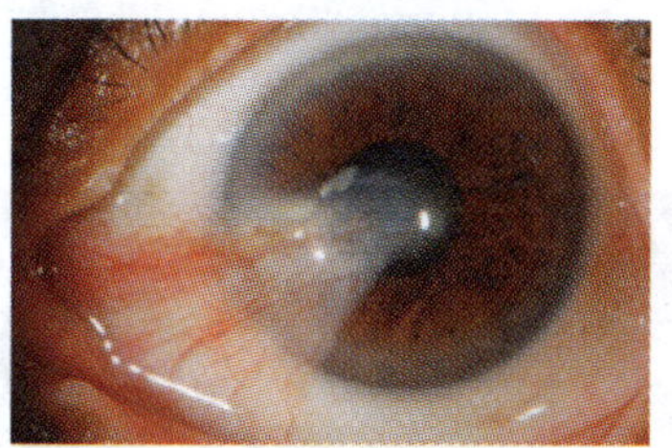

Extra Mile

TABLE: Differences between pterygium and pseudopterygium

	Pterygium	Pseudopterygium
Etiology	Degenerative process	Inflammatory process
Age	Usually occurs in elder persons	Can occur at any age
Site	Always situate in the palpebral aperture	Can occur at any site
Stages	Either progressive, regressive or stationary	Always stationary
Probe test	Probe cannot be passed underneath	A probe can be passed under the neck

90. Ans. (c) Enterovirus

Ref: Comprehensive Ophthalmology by Khurana 6th ed. pg. 23

- **Acute hemorrhagic conjunctivitis:** It is also called Apollo conjunctivitis.
- It is caused by picornavirus (enterovirus type 70).

91. Ans. (b) Keratitis

Ref: Yanoff Duker Ophthalmology; pg. 220

- Bacteria which cause purulent keratitis after epithelial injury are pseudomonas, *Staphylococcus aureus, Pneumococcus, Moraxella, Streptococcus epidermidis, E. coli, Proteus, Klebsiella.*

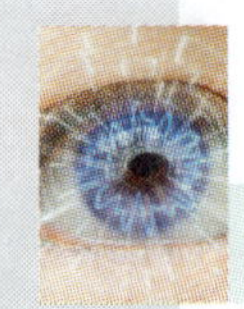

- **Clinical feature of keratitis:** Pain, lacrimation, photophobia, red eye, blurred vision.

92. Ans. (a) Corneal sensation decreased

Ref: Comprehensive Ophthalmology by Khurana 6th ed. pg. 27

- Dendritic ulcer is seen in viral keratitis which is most commonly caused by HSV. It can involve any layer of cornea but when only corneal epithelium is involved it is known as dendritic ulcer.
- Recurrent ocular herpes present as geographic ulcer, superficial punctate keratitis.
- When stroma is involved it presents as disciform keratitis and diffuse stromal necrotic keratitis.
- The characteristic hypopyon corneal ulcer is caused by pneumococcus (ulcus serpens) and pseudomonas.
- In recurrent epithelial keratitis, there is decreased corneal sensation.

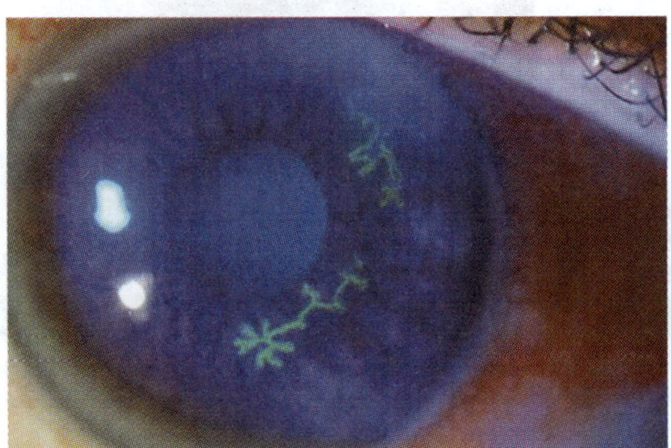

93. Ans (b) Keratoconus

Ref: Yanoff Duker; 4th ed. pg. 254

- Keratoconus is degenerative disease of cornea, where it becomes conical. It is best treated by keratoplasty.
- Keratoplasty is corneal grafting or in more simple term, corneal transplantation.
- There are two types of keratoplasty:
  - **Penetrating keratoplasty (PK)** also known as full thickness keratoplasty
  - **Lamellar keratoplasty (LK)** also known as partial thickness keratoplasty. It has highest success rate as compared to PK.
- **Indication for keratoplasty:**
  - Corneal scar
  - Non-healing ulcer
  - Chemical injuries
  - Keratoconus
  - Pseudophakic bullous keratopathy

94. Ans. (c) Chylamydia

Ref: Khurana, 6th ed. pg. 73

- **Adenovirus** is considered as the **most common** cause of swimming pool conjunctivitis. Chlorine is unable to eliminate the virus, hence it can often present as an outbreak. But it was not given in choice.
- **However, it can also be caused by chlamydia trachomatis serotypes D to K** and the condition is said to be adult inclusion conjunctivitis.

Adult inclusion conjunctivitis.

- Caused by **chlamydia trachomatis serotypes D to K.**
- **Usually** affects sexually active males and primary source of infection is urethritis in males and cervicitis in females.
- **Transmission: Either** via contaminated fingers or more commonly through contaminated water of swimming pool. Therefore it is also said to be swimming pool conjunctivitis.

95. Ans. (d) Clean hand

Ref: Khurana, 64

- Frequent handwashing is the most effective way to reduce the risk of transmission to the close contacts.
- **Other measures can be:** avoid sharing towels, handkerchief and pillows.

96. Ans. (d) Staphylococcus

Ref: Khurana, 99

- The common cause of corneal ulcer in India is Streptococcus Pneumoniae (causes central corneal ulcer) whereas the **commonest cause overall is staphylococcus aureus** (causes peripheral corneal ulcer).
- The bacterial ulcer can present with the formation of a hypopyon (sterile).
- The characteristic hypopyon corneal ulcer is due to pneumococcus and is called ulcus serpens.
- **Treatment:** Topical gentamicin/tobramycin and cephalozin with cycloplegics (atropine ointment or drops) and analgesics.

97. Ans. (c) Interstitial keratitis

Ref: Khurana, 121

- Inflammation of corneal stroma without primary involvement of epithelium or endothelium is called interstitial keratitis.
- It can have many causes like: Congenital syphilis, TB, Cogan's syndrome, acquired syphilis, malaria, sarcoidosis, leprosy.

Syphilitic interstitial keratitis

- It is associated more frequently with congenital syphilis and manifestation develops between 5 and 15 years of age.

Clinical features:

- Can present with Hutchinson triad i.e. interstitial keratitis, Hutchinson teeth and vestibular deafness.
- **Clinically it can present with three stages:**
    1. **Initial progressive stage:** Lasts for 2 weeks. Begins with edema of endothelium and deeper stroma secondary to anterior uveitis.
    2. **Florid stage:** Lasts for 2 months there is development of radial bundle of brush like vessels on cornea. Since these vessels are covered by hazy cornea, they look dull reddish pink which is called **salmon patch appearance.**
    3. **Regression stage:** May last for 1–2 years. The acute inflammation resolves with progressive appearance of vascular invasion. Resolution of the lesion leaves behind some opacities and **ghost vessels.**

Treatment:

- **Local:** Topical corticosteroid drops e.g: dexamethasone 0.1%, Atropine ointment 1% 2–3 times a day, Dark goggles or keratoplasty in case of dense corneal opacity.
- **Systemic:** Penicillin, systemic steroid.

98. Ans. (b) Keratoconus

Ref: Khurana, 131

- **Munsen's sign:** Localized bulging of lower lid when patient looks down. Seen in late stages of keratoconus.

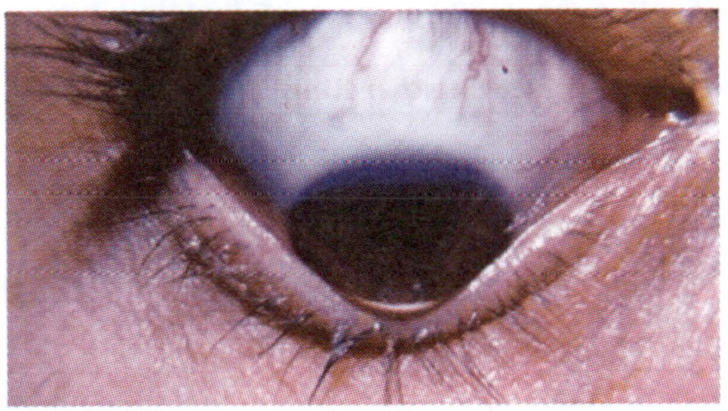

99. Ans. (a) Moraxella

Ref: A.K. Khurana's Ophthalmology, 6th ed. pg. 66

Conjunctivitis type	MC organism/comments
• **Acute mucopurulent**	• Staphylococcus • It is MC type of bacterial conjunctivitis • **(+) Halo**
• **Acute Purulent Conjunctivitis**	• Gonococcus
• **Membranous Conjunctivitis**	• C. Diphtheria • Bleeds on separation
• **Pseudomembranous Conjunctivitis**	• Adeno/Staph/Strep • Separates easily
• **Angular Conjunctivitis**	• **Moraxella Axenfeld-** MCC
• **Epidemic Keratoconjunctivitis/Madras eye**	• Adenovirus: MCC
• **Acute hemorrhagic/Apollo Conjunctivitis**	• PicoRNA virus ▪ Enterovirus 70: MCC ▪ Echovirus ▪ Coxsackie virus

Contd...

100. Ans. (a) Trigeminal nerve

Ref: A.K. Khurana's Ophthalmology, 6th ed. pg. 108–109

- Neurotropic keratitis is a corneal degenerative disease characterized by a reduction or absence of corneal sensitivity.
- In this condition, corneal innervation by **trigeminal nerve** is impaired.
- Most common ocular conditions associated with NK are herpes keratitis (zoster and simplex).
- **Other causes can be**: Topical anesthetic abuse, chemical and physical burns, contact lens abuse, topical drug toxicity, irradiation to eye or adnexa and corneal surgery.

101. Ans. (c) Flakes of mucus

Ref: A.K. Khurana's Ophthalmology, 6th ed. pg. 63

- Any condition which causes fluid accumulation on cornea, can cause colored haloes.
- **Differential diagnosis of color haloes:**
    - ACG
    - Cataract
    - Mucopurulent conjunctivitis: Due to prismatic effect of mucus present on cornea

Extra Mile

- Acute bacterial conjunctivitis is aka as acute mucopurulent conjunctivitis.
- **Causes**: Staph Aureus, Koch-weeks bacillus, Pneumococcus and streptococcus

102. Ans. (a) Moraxella

Ref: A.K. Khurana's Ophthalmology, 6th ed. pg. 66

103. Ans. (b) Keratoconus

Ref: A.K. Khurana's Ophthalmology, 6th ed. pg. 132

- **Fleischer rings** are pigmented rings in the peripheral cornea, resulting from iron deposition in basal epithelial cells, in the form of hemosiderin.
- Fleischer rings are indicative of keratoconus, a degenerative corneal condition that causes the cornea to thin and change to a conic shape.
- Signs of keratoconus:
  - **Munsen Sign:** V-Shaped protrusion of cornea on down gaze
  - **Vogt's Striae:** Break in descemet's membrane
  - **Fleischer ring:** Iron deposition at back of cornea
  - Scissoring of reflex upon retinoscopy

Extra Mile

- **Kayser-Fleischer rings** are due to copper deposition, seen in case of Wilsons disease
- **Immune ring of pessary:** In case of fungal keratitis
- Ring shaped ulcer: **Protozoal keratitis**

104. Ans. (c) Prevents infection more than descemet's membrane

Ref: A.K. Khurana 6th ed. pg. 96, Khurana, 4th ed. pg. 80.89

- Bowman's layer of cornea is acellular mass of condensed collagen fibrils
- **Thickness:** 12 μm
- It is NOT a true elastic membrane but simply a condensed superficial stroma
- Once destroyed, never regenerates
- It shows considerable resistance to *infection (descemet membrane maintains integrity of eyeball)*

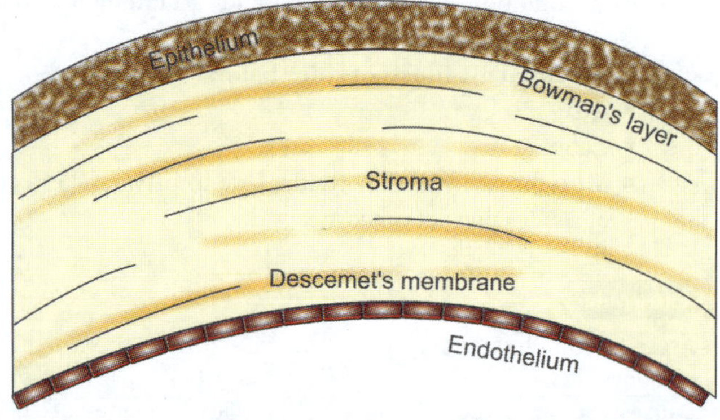

105. Ans. (d) Curvature of cornea

Ref: A.K. Khurana, 6th ed. pg. 575

Few Instruments Which are Used for Ocular Examination

Measurement parameter	Instruments/for:
• Corneal thickness	Pachymetry
• Corneal curvature	Keratometer
• Angle of anterior chamber	Gonioscope
• Corneal surface	Placido disc
• Corneal endothelium	Specular microscope
• Direct ophthalmoscope • Remembred as: "DEV"	Routine fundus examination. *"Image formed is Erect and Virtual and magnified, 15 times"*
• Indirect ophthalmoscope	For assessment of retinal detachment and other peripheral retinal lesions. *The image is real, inverted and magnified 5 times.*
• Perimetry	Optic nerve function

106. Ans. (b) Pachymetry

Ref: A.K. Khurana, 6th ed. pg. 95-96; Khurana, 4th ed. pg. 89

- Corneal thickness is measured by the method known as pachymetry. Normal corneal thickness is around (0.52–0.7 mm) 500–700 μm.

Extra Mile

- PLACIDO DISC- for corneal surface
- Keratometry- Corneal curvature
- Tonometry- for IOP

107. Ans. (b) Keyser Fleischer Ring

Ref: A.K. Khurana 6th ed. pg. 131; Khurana, 4th ed./ 141

- Fleischer's ring is seen in keratoconus and not KF rings.
- KF ring is seen in Wilsons disease (Chalcosis)

108. Ans. (a) Corneal dystrophy

Ref: A.K. Khurana, 6th ed. pg. 124-31;

Corneal dystrophies are inherited disorders in which the cells have some inborn defect due to which pathological changes may occur with time leading to hazy cornea.

- Corneal dystrophies are classified according to anatomical site involved: Anterior dystrophy, Stromal dystrophies, Posterior dystrophies.
- Among anterior dystrophies, **epithelial basement membrane dystrophy aka Cogan's microcystic dystrophy is the most common.**

- These lesions involve corneal epithelium and present as bilateral dot-like microcystic or linear finger print opacities. In 10% of cases there is recurrent corneal erosion and majority of cases remains asymptomatic.
- It is characterized by the failure of the cornea's outermost layer of epithelial cells to attach to the underlying basement membrane (Bowman's layer).
- The condition is excruciatingly painful because the loss of these cells results in the exposure of sensitive corneal nerves.
- **Cause:** There is often a history of previous corneal injury (corneal abrasion or ulcer).
- *It may also be due to corneal dystrophy or corneal disease.*
- **Treatment**- Patching with plain ointment for 1–2 days.

109. Ans. (c) Corneal dystrophy

Ref: A.K. Khurana, 6th ed. pg. 124-31

Please refer to above explanation

110. Ans. (a) Thioridazine

Ref: A.K. Khurana, 6th ed. pg. 502

- Thioridazine is an antipsychotic agent.
- Its ocular side effect (corneal staining) limits its use.
- Note: ATT drug **Ethambutol** also causes corneal staining.

111. Ans. (c) Corneal xerosis

Ref: A.K. Khurana, 6th ed. pg. 468

- **Xeropthalmia:** All the ocular manifestation of Vitamin A deficiency.
- **First clinical sign of Vitamin A deficiency:** *Conjunctival Xerosis.*
- **First clinical symptom of vitamin A deficiency:** *Night blindness.*

WHO Classification of Xeropthalmia

CLASS	SIGNS
X1A	Conjunctival xerosis
X1B	Conjunctival xerosis with bitot's spot
X2	*Corneal xerosis*
X3A	Corneal xerosis with ulceration
X3B	Keratomalacia

112. Ans. (a) Xerophthalmia

Ref: Harrison's, 19th ed. pg. 96e-6

- MC ocular manifestation of vitamin A deficiency is xerophthalmia. This condition includes milder stages of night blindness and conjunctival xerosis (dryness) with bitot's spot.

Other Features of Vitamin A Deficiency:

- Diarrhea, Dysentry, measles, malaria or respiratory. These condition can pose risk to life if associated with vitamin A deficiency.

Features of Vitamin A toxicity:

- **Acute:** Increased ICP leading to bulging fontanels, vertigo, diplopia, seizure and exfoliative dermatitis.
- **Chronic:** dry skin, Chielosis, glossitis, alopecia, bone demineralization, hyperlipidemia, hypercalcemia, amenorrhea and features of pseudotumor cerebri with increased ICP and papilledema.

113. Ans. (c) Blurring of disc

Ref: A.K. Khurana, 6th ed. pg. 323-24,
Khurana, 4th ed. pg. 299

Papilledema: Optic disc edema which is associated with the increased ICP, and is almost always bilateral.

Ophthalmoscopic Features of Early Papilledema:

- Obscuration of disc margin (nasal field involved first followed by superior > inferior > temporal).
- Blurring of peripapillary nerve fibre
- Absence of spontaneous venous pulsation at the disc
- Mild hyperemia

Features of Fully developed/Late papilledema

- Elevation of cup
- Obliteration of physiological cup
- Marked hypermia of disc
- Multiple soft exudates
- Tortuous and engorged veins
- Separation of nerve-fibre layer by edema.

114. Ans. (d) All of the above

Ref: A.K. Khurana, 6th ed. pg. 116, 4th ed. pg. 109-110

MOOREN'S ULCER

- Mooren's Ulcer/chronic serpiginous or rodent ulcer is a severe inflammatory peripheral ulcerative keratitis.
- **Treatment:**
  - Topical corticosteroids
  - Immunosuppressives with systemic steroids, e.g. cyclosporine
  - Soft contact lens
  - Lamellar or full thickness corneal grafting.

115. Ans. (d) Descemets membrane

Ref: A.K. Khurana, 6th ed. pg. 434

- **Chalcosis:** Refers to the specific changes produced by accumulation of copper in the eye.

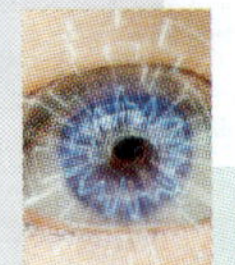

- **Clinical feature:**
  - **Kayser-fleischer ring:** It is a golden brown ring which occurs due to deposition of copper in the peripheral parts of the *Descemet's membrane of the cornea.*
  - **Sunflower cataract:** Produced by deposition of copper on the posterior capsule of the lens.
  - **Retina:** It may show deposition of golden plaques at the posterior pole which reflect the light with a metallic sheen.

116. Ans. (c) HSV infection

Ref: A.K. Khurana, 6th ed. pg. 108

- Viral keratitis causes corneal ulceration. It is caused most commonly **by Herpes simplex, Herpes Zoster and Adenoviruses.**
- Dendritic and geographical corneal ulcers are seen in herpes simplex ocular disease.
- Dendritic ulcer (branching ulcer with knobbed ends), resembles no other condition, and is *pathognomonic of herpes simplex ocular infection.*
- The use of **steroids** in dendritic ulcer hastens the formation of geographical ulcer so it is **contraindicated**.

117. Ans. (d) Dexamethasone

Ref: A.K. Khurana, 6th ed. pg. 108-109

- **Dendritic ulcer** is an irregular linear branching ulcer with knobbed ends and reduced corneal sensations seen in epithelial keratitis
- It is caused by herpes simplex infection.
- Steroids cause progression of dendritic ulcer, into **geographical ulcer** so, they are **contraindicated**.
- The treatment is done with **3% acyclovir ointment** and mechanical debridement. Other antibiotics may be required if there is a secondary infection.

118. Ans. (b) Stromal keratitis

Ref: A.K. Khurana, 6th ed. pg. 108-109

STROMAL KERATITIS

- It manifests as disciform keratitis *(**disc shape ulcer** with a surrounding Wessley immune ring formed due to delayed hypersensitivity to **HSV antigen**)* or **diffuse stromal necrotic keratitis** (due to active viral invasion and **tissue destruction**).
- **Treatment:** Steroid drops with acyclovir 3%

Extra Mile

Epithelial keratitis

- Caused by herpes simplex virus. It manifests as dendritic ulcer (irregular, linear, branching ulcer with knobbed ends and reduced corneal sensation) or geographical ulcer (large "amoeboid ulcer"). Steroids cause progression of dendritic ulcer into geographical ulcer, so, they are contraindicated.
- Treatment: 3% acyclovir ointment and mechanical debridement.

119. Ans. (b) Herpes zoster keratitis

Ref: A.K. Khurana, 6th ed. pg. 108-109

120. Ans. (d) Syphilis

Ref: A.K. Khurana, 6th ed. pg. 120-121

- Keratitis means corneal inflammation
- **Interstitial Keratitis** basically means corneal scarring due to chronic inflammation of the corneal stroma. Interstitial means space between cells i.e. corneal stroma which lies between the epithelium and the endothelium.
- It is most commonly seen in infection like syphillis

SYPHILITIC KERATITIS

- It is seen more frequently with congenital syphilis than acquired syphilis. It may present as part of Hutchinson's triad of:
  - **Interstitial keratitis**
  - Hutchinson teeth
  - Vestibular deafness

121. Ans. (b) Propomidine isothionate

Ref: A.K. Khurana, 6th ed. pg. 112

ACANTHAMOEBA KERATITIS

- Acanthamoeba is a free lying amoeba found in soil, fresh water, well water, sea water, sewage and air.
- **Mode of infection**- direct corneal contact with any material or water contaminated with the organism. **For eg:**
  - *Contact lens wearers using home-made saline from contaminated tap water is the commonest situation recognized for acanthamoeba infection.*
  - Other situations may be: mild trauma associated with contaminated vegetable matter, salt water diving, wind blown contaminant and hot tub use.
  - Opportunistic infection
- **Symptoms**. Very severe pain (out of proportion to the degree of inflammation), watering, photophobia, blepharospasm and blurred vision.
- **Treatment:** Specific medical treatment includes:
  - *0.1 % propamidine isothionate (brolene) drops;*
  - Neomycin drops
  - Polyhexamethylene biguanide (0.01–0.02% solution)
  - Chlorhexidine

122. Ans. (c) Wearing of soft contact lenses

Ref: A.K. Khurana, 6th ed. pg. 112

123. Ans. (d) All of the above

Ref: A.K. Khurana, 6th ed. pg. 82-83

GIANT PAPILLARY CONJUNCTIVITIS

- It is the inflammation of conjunctiva with formation of very large sized papillae.
- **Cause:** It is a localized allergic response to a physically rough or deposited surface *(contact lens, prosthesis, left out nylon sutures).*
- **Symptoms:** Itching, stringy discharge and reduced wearing time of contact lens or prosthetic shell.
- **Treatment:** The offending cause should be removed.
  - Disodium cromoglycate is known to relieve the symptoms and enhance the rate of resolution.

124. Ans. (b) Contact lens

Please refer to previous explanation.

125. Ans. (b) Giant papillary conjunctivitis

Ref: A.K. Khurana, 6th ed. pg. 82-83

Please refer to above explanation

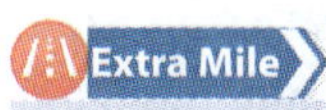

Extra Mile

Inclusion Conjunctivitis
- Caused by Chlamydia trachomatis D-K within 5–14 days of birth. Clinical features include mucoid/mucopurulent discharge, redness in conjunctiva, swollen lids and pain in eyeballs.

Follicular conjunctivitis
- It is characterized by redness in conjunctiva, formation of follicles and discharge from the eyes. It is of following types:
  - **Epidemic keratoconjunctivitis:** Adenovirus 8, 19; can cause "acute pseudomembranous conjunctivitis" in severe infection.
  - **Pharyngo-conjunctival fever:** Caused by adenovirus.
  - **Herpetic conjunctivitis:** Caused by HSV1 (more commonly) and HSV 2 (less commonly)

126. Ans. (d) Pseudomonas

Ref: A.K. Khurana, 6th ed. pg. 98

PSEUDOMONAS

- Pseudomonas is the commonest organism affecting long term use of contact lens followed by acanthameoba. SIGNS suggesting the former infection: Presence of ring shaped ulcer, lack of vascularization, pain out of proportion, pseudodendritis.

PNEUMOCOCCUS

- The commonest cause of corneal ulcer in India is Streptococcus Pneumonia (causes central corneal ulcer) whereas the commonest cause in the world is staphylococcus aureus (causes peripheral corneal ulcer).
- The bacterial ulcer can present with the formation of a hypopyon (sterile).
- The characteristic hypopyon corneal ulcer is due to pneumococcus and is called **ulcus serpens**.
- **Treatment:** Topical gentamicin/tobramycin and cephalozin with cycloplegics (atropine ointment or drops) and analgesics.

127. Ans. (a) Fungal corneal ulcer

Ref: A.K. Khurana 6th ed./106, Khurana 4th ed./100

- Fungal corneal ulcer aka fungal keratitis is most commonly caused by **Aspergillus fusarium**. Patient in this condition presents with history of trauma with vegetative matter.
- Symptoms shown by patients here are milder than signs. Signs are dry looking, greyish white corneal ulcers with feather finger like extensions (due to hyphae)

Signs of Fungal Keratitis:
- **Satellite nodule** (satellite lesion present around ulcer)
- Large organized hypopyon (non-sterile)
- **Immune ring of pessary**

Predisposing factors- topical steroids, organic matter. Worst prognosis.

Treatment: 5% natamycin or .2% fluconazole for 6-8 weeks.

128. Ans. (c) Fungal ulcer

Ref: A.K. Khurana, 6th ed. pg. 106, Khurana, 4th ed. pg. 100

Please refer to above explanation

129. Ans. (a) Azithromycin

Ref: A.K. Khurana, 6th ed. pg. 65-66

- Trachoma is caused by C. Trachomatis.
- I.P.- 5-12 days
- SAFE strategy used for control of trachoma
  - S: Surgery
  - A: Antibiotic
  - F: Face wash
  - E: Environment
- DOC for Trachoma: Azithromycin > tetracycline

130. Ans. (d) Upper palpebral conjunctiva

Ref: A.K. Khurana, 6th ed. pg. 69

- Conjunctival scarring seen in **trachoma** as irregular stellate shaped scars over sulcus subtarsalis is called Arlt's line.
- It is seen in upper palpebral conjunctiva.

131. Ans. (a) Limbus

Ref: A.K. Khurana, 6th ed. pg. 69-70; Parson's 21st ed. pg. 173

- Herbert pits are oval or circular scar which is left after healing of Herbert pit in the limbus area.

Other Signs of Trachoma:
- Conjunctival scarring *(Arlt's line)*
- **Sago grain** follicles/Bulbar follicles *(pathognomonic)*

132. Ans. (b) Chlamydia

Ref: AK Khurana, 6th ed. pg. 73-74

- Chlamydia trachomatis (D to K) is considered as most common cause of swimming pool conjunctivitis.

Disease	Causative agent
• Swimming pool conjunctivitis	Chlamydia (D to K)
• Swimming pool granuloma	*Mycobacterium marinum*
• Swimmer's itch	*Schistosoma mansoni* *S. japonicum*
• Swimmer's ear	*Pseudomonas/Staphylococcus aureus* (mixed)
• Swimming pool folliculitis	*Pseudomonas*

133. Ans. (a) Vernal keratoconjunctivitis

Ref: A.K. Khurana, 6th ed. pg. 79

CONJUNCTIVITIS

- The inflammation of the conjunctiva is characterized by redness associated with watery or mucopurulent discharge.

VERNAL KERATO-CONJUNCTIVITIS OR SPRING CATARRH

- It is a recurrent, bilateral, interstitial, self limiting, allergic inflammation of the conjunctiva seen in children usually in summer months.
- **Etiology:** It is considered a hypersensitivity reaction to some exogenous allergen such as grass pollen etc.
- **Clinical features:** Characterized by marked burning and itching sensation which is usually in tolerable.
  - Lacrimation.
  - Stringly **(ropy)** discharge.
  - Usually upper tarsal conjunctiva of both eyes are involved.
  - Lesion are characterized as **"cobble-stone"** or "pavement stone" fashion.
  - **Horner Tranta's spots:** Presence of discrete whitish raised dots along the limbus.
- **Treatment**
  - Mast Cell Stabilizers (Olopatadine)
  - Sodium Chromoglycate

Simple allergic conjunctivitis: Non specific allergic rhinitis associated with hay fever or seasonal/perennial allergic conjunctivitis.

GIANT PAPILLARY CONJUNCTIVITIS

- Conjunctivitis with formation of large sized papillae in upper tarsal conjunctiva due to localized allergy
- Against contact lens /nylon sutures/prosthesis.
- **Treatment:** Removal of offending agent
  - Mast Cell Stabilizers

- **Acute hemorrhagic conjunctivitis:** It is also called Apollo conjunctivitis. It is caused by picornavirus (enterovirus type 70).

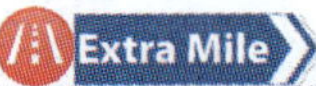
Extra Mile

Discharge	Etiological Agent
• Purulent/ mucopurulent	• Bacterial conjunctivitis
• Watery	• Viral conjunctivitis
• Ropy	• Allergic conjunctivitis
• Mucopurulent	• Chlamydial conjunctivitis

134. Ans. (a) Olopatadine drops

Ref: A.K. Khurana, 6th ed. pg. 79-80

Please refer to above explanation

135. Ans. (d) Trachoma

Ref: A.K. Khurana, 6th ed. pg. 61, 65

Trachoma: Is a chronic keratoconjunctivitis, primarily affecting the superficial epithelium of conjunctiva and cornea simultaneously.

- It is one of the leading causes of preventable blindness in the world.

Etiology

- **Causative organism:** Caused by Chlamydia trachomatis.
- The organism is epitheliotropic and produces intra-cytoplasmic inclusion bodies called H.P. bodies.
- There are 11 identified serotypes of Chlamydia: A, B, Ba, C, D, E, F, G, H, J and K
- *Serotypes A, B, Ba and C are associated with hyperendemic (blinding) trachoma*
- *Serotypes D-K are associated with paratrachoma.*

OPHTHALMIA NEONATORUM

- Bilateral inflammation of the conjunctiva occurring in an infant, <30-day-old.

Source and Mode of Infection

- **Before birth:** Very rare; through infected amniotic fluid in case of ruptured membranes.
- **During Birth:** Most common mode of infection; from infected birth canal when the child is born with face presentation or with forceps.
- **After birth:** Infection during first bath of newborn or from infected clothes or hands.

Causative Agents

- **Chemical conjunctivitis:** Silver nitrate or antibiotics used for prophylaxis.

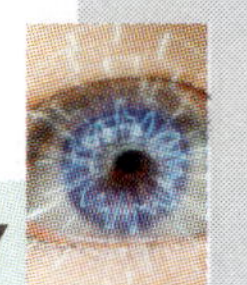

- **Gonococcal infection**
- **Neonatal inclusion conjuncitivitis** *caused by serotypes D to K of Chlamydia trachomatis* is the commonest cause of ophthalmia neonatorum.

136. Ans. (d) Veneral conjunctivitis

Ref: A.K. Khurana, 6th ed. pg. 79-80

Please refer to above explanation

137. Ans. (b) Pinguecula

Ref: A.K. Khurana, 6th ed. pg. 86

PINGUECULA

- Conjunctival fatty degeneration near limbus. It is bilateral condition, **affects more commonly nasal side** followed by involvement of the temporal side. No treatment required.
- Totally benign.

PTERYGIUM

- Triangular invasion of conjunctiva upon the cornea. It is commoner in dry heat, sun exposure and abundant dust. Iron deposition in the corneal epithelium at the advancing head of the pterygium is called STOCKER LINE. Usually asymptomatic.
- **Treatment:** Surgical excision. The commonest problem after excision is recurrence which is reduced by postoperative use of mitomycin C/thiotepa or by doing surgical excision with free conjunctival graft from same/other eye.

CHALAZION

- Chronic granulomatous inflammation of Meibomian Gland. No pain.
- **Treatment:** Incision and drainage

HORDEOLUM

- **External hordeolum/STYE:** Staphylococcus infection of Zeiss gland.
  - **Treatment**
    - Topical antibiotics.
    - Hot fomentation.
- **Internal hordeolum:** Acute Staphylococcus infection of Meibomian gland. Extremely painful.
  - **Treatment:** Incision and Drainage.

138. Ans. (c) Bulge in limbal area lined by root of iris

Ref: A.K. Khurana, 6th ed. pg. 144

- **Intercalary staphyloma** is a localized ectasia of limbal tissue lined by the root of iris.
- **Cause:** perforating injury of the peripheral cornea or perforation of marginal corneal ulcer.

Extra Mile

- **Anterior staphyloma:** Formation of pseudo cornea after perforation of a large sloughing corneal ulcer.
- **Ciliary staphyloma:** Incarceration of ciliary body and is **arises due to complication of scleritis.**
- **Equatorial staphyloma:** The ectasia of the sclera of equatorial region with incarceration of the choroid is known as equatorial staphyloma.
- **Posterior staphyloma** is an ectasia of the sclera at the posterior pole which is lined by the choroid.

139. Ans. (d) Scleritis

Ref: A.K. Khurana, 6th ed. pg. 144

140. Ans. (d) Degenerative myopia

Ref: A.K. Khurana, 6th ed. pg. 144

- Posterior staphyloma is seen in conditions like pathological myopia, posterior scleritis and perforating injuries.

Important Features Associated with Myopia

- **Simple/developmental myopia is the commonest type of myopia.**
- Foster fucks flecks is the choroidal hemorrhage in the macular region.
- Lacquer cracks are breaks in the Bruch's membrane.
- **Retinal detachment** is the **most serious complication** of myopia.

141. Ans. (b) Rheumatoid arthritis

Ref: A.K. Khurana, 6th ed. pg. 141, Khurana, 4th ed. pg. 129

- Scleritis is chronic inflammation of the sclera. Most commonly seen in elderly females (40–70 years).
- Scleritis is associated with autoimmune collagen disorders, **most commonly with rheumatoid arthritis.**
- Other causes can be PAN, SLE, ankylosis spondylitis, Wegener's granulomatosis, thyrotoxicosis, TB, syphillis.

142. Ans. (c) Aqueous deficiency

Ref: A.K. Khurana, 6th ed. pg. 389

Tear Film Consists of 3 Layers:

- **Lipid layer**-Outermost layer. Secreted by Meibomian, Zeiss and Moll gland
- **Aqueous layer**-intermediate layer. Forms bulk of tear. Secreted by lacrimal gland
- **Mucous/Mucin layer:** Innermost layer. Secreted by conjunctival goblet cells

KERATOCONJUNCTIVITIS SICCA

- It is the disease entity most commonly seen due to aqueous tear deficiency.
- Causes can be: Sjogren syndrome, hyposecretion, congenital alacrima. Decreased secretion or lack of secretion from other tear glands also contribute to this condition.
- **Symptoms of keratoconjunctivitis sicca:** Foreign body sensation, photophobia. Test is done by wetting of a filter paper (Schirmer strip test)

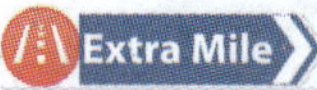

Mucin layer deficiency can lead to xerophthalmia, conjunctival scarring. Can be seen in SJS, chemical burns, trachoma.

RETINA AND UVEAL TRACT

143. Ans. (c) Branched Retinal Vein Occlusion

Ref: A.K. Khurana, 7th ed. pg. 277

- Branch Retinal Vein Occlusion is **a blockage of branches (one or more) of the central retinal vein, which runs through the optic nerve.**
- Most common site of BRVO is arterio-venous crossings and most common sector involved is supero-temporal
- **'Wedge shaped distribution of hemorrhage'** is seen on fundoscopy.

144. Ans. (d) CRVO

Ref: A.K. Khurana, 7th ed. pg. 279

- **TOMATO SPLASH/TOMATO KETCHUP APPEARANCE** due to severe hemorrhages involving periphery and posterior pole.
- It is seen in CRVO

145. Ans. (a) Central retinal artery occlusion

Ref: Khurana 7th ed. pg. 277, 546

- Cherry-red spot - present in the center of macula in contrast to the surrounding pale retina.
- It is seen due to vascular choroid shining through the thin retina in foveal region, in contrast to the surrounding pale retina

Causes of Cherry Red Spot

- Central retinal artery occlusion
- Tay-Sachs disease
- Commotio retinae (Berlin's edema)- due to trauma
- Niemann-Pick disease
- Gaucher's disease
- Sandhoff disease

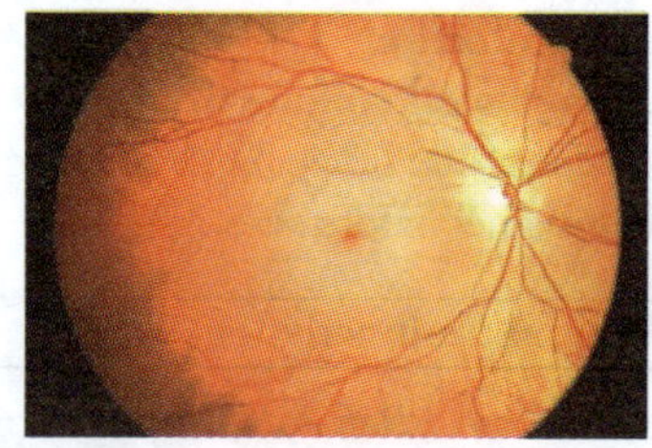

146. Ans. (b) Diabetic retinopathy

Ref: Khurana 7th ed. pg. 287, 529-30

- Microaneurysms are multiple tiny dot-like dilatations along the venous end of capillaries due to focal dilation (out pouching) of capillary wall following loss of pericyte.
- It appear as red dots and leak fluid, proteins, lipids and also fluorescein dye on FFA.
- Most commonly found in diabetic retinopathy seen in the macular area.
- Also found in:
  - Hypertensive retinopathy
  - Retinal vein occlusions
  - Eales disease
  - Sickle cell disease.

147. Ans. (c) Atropine

Ref: Khurana 7th ed. pg. 164-65

- **Acute uveitis:** Inflammation of uveal region of the eye, namely iris, choroid and ciliary body. In this sudden symptomatic onset and it lasts for about 6 weeks to 3 months.
- **Main symptoms of acute anterior uveitis:** Pain, photophobia, redness, lacrimation and decreased vision.

Treatment

- **Local therapy:**
  - **Cycloplegic drugs:** Most effective during acute phase of iridocyclitis.
  - Dose: 1% atropine sulfate eye ointment or drops instilled 2–3 times a day.
- **Mechanism of action:**
  - Gives comfort and rest to the eye by relieving spasm of muscles
  - Prevents the formation of synechiae
  - Break already formed synechiae
  - Reduces exudation
  - By relieving pressure on the anterior ciliary arteries it increases the blood supply to anterior uvea.
- **Systemic therapy:**
  - Corticosteroid (DOC)
  - NSAIDs
  - Immunosuppressive drugs

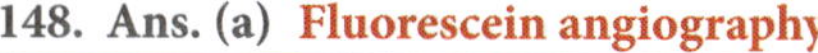

148. Ans. (a) Fluorescein angiography

- The shown investigation is fluorescein angiography.

149. Ans. (b) Keratic precipitates

Ref: Khurana 7th ed. pg. 159-60

- Keratic precipitates (KPs) are the pathognomonic sign of anterior uveitis.
- KPs are proteinaceous-cellular deposits occurring at the back of cornea, arranged in a triangular fashion present in center and inferior part of cornea due to convection currents in the aqueous humor.
- Types of KPs:
  - Mutton fat KPs—seen in chronic granulomatous diseases (Ex: Sarcoidosis, Leprosy etc)
  - Small and medium KPs (granular KPs)
  - Fine KPs, also called as 'stellate' KPs
  - Old KPs. These are sign of healed uveitis.

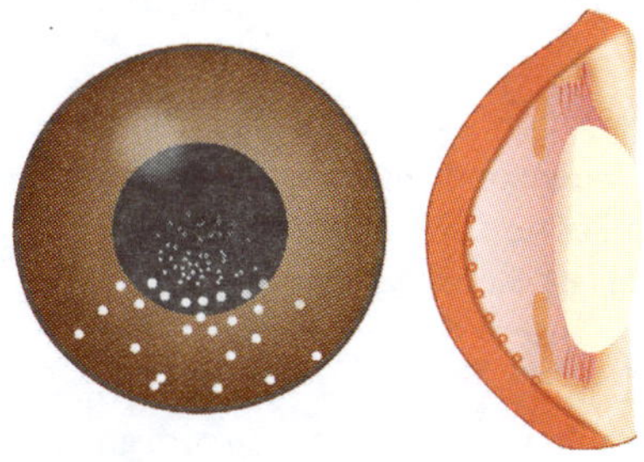

150. Ans. (b) HLA B27

Ref: Comprehensive Ophthalmology by A.K. Khurana, 7th ed. pg. 174

- Uveitis is many times associated with infectious and noninfectious systemic diseases like sarcoidosis, Behçet's disease, ankylosing spondylitis, Reiter's syndrome, juvenile idiopathic arthritis and Fuchs' heterochromic uveitis.
- In ankylosing spondylitis there is uveitis associated with an idiopathic chronic inflammatory arthritis involving the sacral iliac and posterior intervertebral joints.
- It mostly involves young people positive for HLA-B27 and the uveitis is mostly acute anterior iridocyclitis.

Conditions associated with HLA B27

- Psoriasis
- Ankylosing spondylitis
- Inflammatory bowel disease
- Reiter's syndrome

151. Ans. (a) CRVO

Ref: Comprehensive Ophthalmology by A.K. Khurana, 7th ed. pg. 278-79

- The shown image of fundus is splashed tomato fundus, which is seen in central retinal vein occlusion.
- Retinal vein occlusion (RVO) is a common cause of vision loss in older individuals.
- There are two distinct types, classified according to the site of occlusion: In central RVO (CRVO), the
  - Occlusion is at or proximal to the lamina cribrosa of the optic nerve.
  - CRVO is further divided into the categories of perfused (nonischemic) and nonperfused (ischemic).
- The pathogenesis of CRVO is believed to follow the principles of Virchow's triad for thrombogenesis, involving vessel damage, stasis and hypercoagulability.
- Age is the most important factor. Majority of patients are >55 years.
- Hyperglycemia is present in about 10% of cases over the age of 50 years but is uncommon in younger patients.
- Other risk factors include hypertension and hyperlipidemia.

152. Ans. (a) Anterior uveitis

- The irregularly dilated pupil shown in the image is festooned pupil.
- It is feature of acute anterior uveitis
- Other features of anterior uveitis: Keratic precipitate, Arlt's triangle.

153. Ans. (a) Arteriolar attenuation

Ref: A.K. Khurana 6th ed. pg. 288

Fundal changes in retinitis pigmentosa:

- Retinal pigmentary changes: Perivascular, jet black spots resembling bony corpuscles in shape
- Retinal arterioles are attenuated (narrowed), may become thread like in later stages
- Thinning and atrophy of retinal pigment epithelium
- Pale, waxy optic disc

Clinical features of RP:

- Night blindness: Characteristic earliest feature
- Delayed dark adaptation
- Tubular vision (preserved central vision, lost after many years)

RP is inherited as:

- **AR:** Most common (intermediate severity)
- **AD:** Least severe
- **X-Linked:** Least common (Most severe)

154. Ans. (c) Anterior uveitis

Ref: Comprehensive Ophthalmology by A.K. Khurana 6th ed. pg. 167

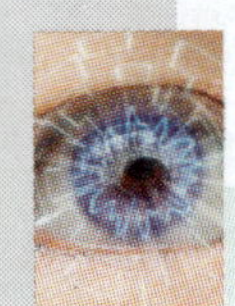

UVEITIS IN SARCOIDOSIS

- Sarcoidosis is one of the chronic granulomatous disease that can cause non-infective uveitis
- **MC age group:** 20–50 years; F > M
- **Associated feature:** Bilateral hilar lymphadenopathy, pulmonary infiltration, skin and ocular lesions
- 20–50% of sarcoidosis patients present with ocular lesions like:
- **Sarcoid uveitis:** Can cause anterior, posterior or intermediate panuveitis
  - **Anterior uveitis:** Large mutton fat KP, bussaca nodule, anterior chamber cells and flare
  - **Intermediate uveitis:** Characterized by snow balls and snow banking
  - **Posterior uveitis:** Present with cystoid macular edema, periphlebitis retinae with sheathing, appearing as candle wax dripping, peripheral multifocal chorioretinitis characterised by small, punched out atrophic spots *(it is highly suggestive of sarcoidosis).*
- **Uveoparotid fever:** Aka Heerfordt's syndrome:
  - Characterized by bilateral granulomatous panuveitis with painful enlargement of parotid gland, rash, fever and cranial nerve palsies.

DIAGNOSIS:

- Abnormal Chest X-ray (in 90% cases)
- **Kveim test:** +ve
- Serum ACE level

Treatment: Steroids

155. Ans. (b) Central retinal artery occlusion

Ref: Walsh and Hoyt; Vol. 3, pg. 3370

- **Central retinal artery occlusion (CRAO):** Presents with sudden painless loss of vision. Causes are:
  - **Artery occlusion by the Emboli:** It is most common cause.
  - **Other causes:** Giant cell arteritis, SLE, scleroderma.
  - Fundus appears milky white because of retinal edema. There is cherry red spot. Due to embolus the blood column within the retina is segmented and is known as cattle tracking.
- **Central retinal vein occlusion (CRVO):** Its incidence is more common than CRAO. Causes are:
  - Hypertension, diabetes mellitus, atherosclerosis.
  - **Upon examination:** Tortuous and engorged veins, disc edema, soft exudate and evidence of rubeosis iridis (new vessel on iris).
- **Central serous retinopathy (CSR):** It is due to accumulation of transparent fluid at the posterior pole specially macula causing a circumscribed area of retinal detachment in the macular region. Causes are:
  - Raised aldosterone level usually among type A personalities
  - Cushing syndrome, idiopathic. Fluorescein angiography shows ink blot pattern and smoke stack pattern.
- **Diabetic retinopathy:** It is of 2 types:
  - **Nonproliferative diabetic retinopathy (NPDR):** Findings/changes in NPDR are:
    - **Microaneurysm:** Earliest change
    - Retinal hemorrhage
    - Hard and soft exudates.
  - **Proliferative diabetic retinopathy (PDR):** Findings/changes in PDR are:
    - **Neovascularization:** Hallmark
    - Vitreous hemorrhage, and
    - Retinal detachment.

156. Ans. (b) 1.5 mm

Ref: Comprehensive Ophthalmology by Khurana 6th ed. pg. 6

- The average optic disc is 1500 microns (or 1.5 millimeters) in size where optic nerve enters into the back of the eye.
  - Small optic disc is said when vertical diameter of optic disc is <1.5 mm
  - Large disc is said when size of vertical diameter is >2.2 mm.
- Length of optic nerve is 47–50 mm and has 4 parts:
  - **Intraocular:** 1 mm
  - **Intraorbital:** 30 mm
  - **Intracanalicular:** 6–9 mm
  - **Intracranial:** 10 mm

157. Ans. (b) Corneal endothelium

Ref: Comprehensive Ophthalmology by Khurana 6th ed. pg. 34

- Keratic precipitate (KP) is deposition of protein on the corneal endothelium in patients with anterior uveitis.
- This KP is deposited in a triangular fashion, known as Arlt's triangle.
- In some chronic granulomatous diseases like sarcoidosis, leprosy, TB, there is deposition of special KP's known as mutton fat KP.

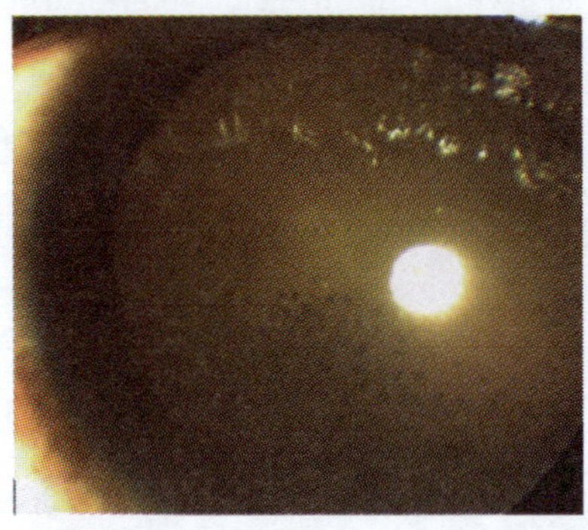

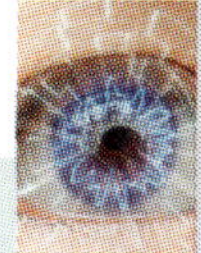

158. Ans. (a) 1–5

Ref: Harrison 19th ed. pg. 2424

- Poor sugar control (glycosylated hemoglobin > 7%) leads to development of diabetic retinopathy within 5 years in type 1 diabetes mellitus and over 15–20 years in type 2 diabetes mellitus.
- Diabetics have *25 times* higher chances of blindness as compared to nondiabetics.

Extra Mile

- Most common cause of *visual loss* in a diabetic is macular edema.
- Best method to *detect visual loss* is FFA or optical coherence tomography.
- Most common cause of blindness in diabetic is retinal detachment.
- Diabetic retinopathy and nephropathy progress over same duration and *always co-exist*.
- Best *predictor for development of retinopathy* is duration of diabetes.

159. Ans. (a) Cycloplegics

Ref: Khurana, 6th ed. pg. 159-60

- **DOC for acute anterior uveitis:** Topical glucocorticoids
- **1st line agent for immediate management of acute uveitis:** Cycloplegics
- **Khurana states:** *"Cycloplegics are very useful and most effective during acute phase of iridocyclitis"*
- Commonly used drug is 1% atropine sulphate eye ointment or drops to be instilled 2-3 times a day.
- **Mechanism of action:**
  - Relieves spasm of iris sphincter and ciliary body, which gives immediate relief and comfort from pain.
  - Prevents synechiae formation and breaks them as well.
  - Decreases hyperemia which reduces exudation.
  - Increases blood supply to anterior uvea by relieving pressure on anterior ciliary artery, which adds to more absorption of toxin.

160. Ans. (a) Nongranulomatous uveitis

Ref: Khurana, 6th ed. pg. 154

- **Granular KPs** are small and medium keratic precipitate, and are pathognomonic of non-granulomatous uveitis.
- These are small, dirty white KP arranged irregularly at the back of cornea and are usually numerous.

Extra Mile

- **Fine KP:** Aka stellate KP. They usually cover whole corneal endothelium and form endothelial dusting. They are seen in: Fuch's heterochromic iridocyclitis, Herpetic iritis and CMV retinitis.
- **Old KP:** They are irregular in shape and this is a sign of healed uveitis.

161. Ans. (a) Granulomatous uveitis

Ref: Khurana, 6th ed. pg. 154

- **Mutton fat keratic precipitates** are typically seen in granulomatous uveitis. These are composed of epithelioid cells and macrophages.
- These are large, thick, fluffy, lardaceous KP having waxy or greasy appearance. They are usually 10-15 in number

162. Ans. (c) Reiter syndrome

Ref: Khurana, 6th ed. pg. 168

- **Reiter syndrome** is characterized by triad of: Urethritis, arthritis and conjunctivitis with or without iridocyclitis.
- It mostly affects males who are positive for HLA B27.

163. Ans. (b) Hyperoxia

Ref: Khurana, 6th ed. pg. 283

- Retinopathy of prematurity (ROP), *(earlier known as retrolental fibroplasia)* is a bilateral proliferative retinopathy occurring in premature infants with low birth weight who often have been exposed to high concentration of oxygen.
- **Risk factors:**
  - Low gestation age <32 weeks
  - Low birth weight <1500 gm
  - Supplemental oxygen therapy
  - Vitamin E deficiency in mothers, respiratory distress syndrome, asphyxia, shock etc.

164. Ans. (b) Periphery of pupil

Ref: A.K. Khurana's Ophthalmology, 6th ed. pg. 153

- Granulamotous uveitis is characterized by infiltration with lymphocytes, plasma cells and mobilization and proliferation of large mononuclear cells → collectively known as iris nodule
- Iris nodule is a feature of granulomatous uveitis.
- If formed near pupillary border: **Koeppe's nodule**
- If formed near collarette: **Busaca nodule**
- If deposited at the back of cornea: Keratic precipitates

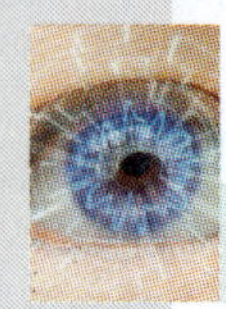

165. Ans. (c) Sensory and pigmentary layer

Ref: A.K. Khurana, 6th ed. pg. 299

- Retina has 10 layers.
- Inner 9 layers are known as neurosensory layer and outer one layer is known as pigmentary layer.
- *Retinal detachment is defined as separation of neurosensory layer of retina from pigmentary retinal layer.*

166. Ans. (a) X linked

Ref: A.K. Khurana, 6th ed. pg. 287

INVERSE RETINITIS PIGMENTOSA

- Inverse RP is a degeneration of the nerve cells in the macula, which is located in the center of the retina. Inverse or central RP is characterized by a bilateral and often symmetrical loss of cone function in the presence of a reduced rod function. Individuals with macular degeneration secondary to a central vision loss experience difficulty reading, recognizing faces, shapes and contours of objects or things.
- This is a general term for a disparate group of rod-cone dystrophies characterized by progressive **night blindness,** visual field constriction with a **ring scotoma/ tubular vision, loss of acuity, waxy pallow optic disc,** and an abnormal electroretinogram (ERG).
- It occurs sporadically or in an autosomal recessive, dominant, or **X-linked pattern.**
- **MC inheritance pattern: Autosomal Recessive**
- Irregular black **deposits of clumped pigment in the peripheral retina**, called ***bone spicules*** because of their vague resemblance to the spicules of cancellous bone, give the disease its name.
- **No definite treatment. However, Vitamin A can slow down the progression.**

167. Ans. (c) Central scotoma

Ref: A.K. Khurana, 6th ed. pg. 233, 287-88

Central scotoma is a feature of open angle glaucoma.

All other choices are considered as triad of retinitis pigmentosa (Bony spicule on retina, waxy pallor disc, Ring scotoma)

Visual field abnormalities in glaucoma are initially observed on kinetic perimetry are as follows

- **Relative paracentral scotoma:** These are areas where smaller or dimmer targets are not visualized by the patient, but larger or brighter targets are appreciated.
- **Bjerrum's Scotoma:** Extension of the blind spot in the shape of an arc in the central bjerrum's area.
- **Siedel scotoma:** One that appears to start at the poles of the blind spot and arches over the macular area, without reaching the horizontal meridian nasally.
- **Arcuate scotoma:** Also appear to start at the superior or inferior poles of the blind spot and arch over the macular area, widening as they curve down or up to end as a horizontal line nasally, which never crosses the horizontal divide of the visual field.
- **Double arcuate or ring scotoma:** Advanced glaucomatous field defects - only central and temporal islands of vision are left when two arcuate scotomas expand to involve the peripheral visual field
- **Nasal step:** The appearance of a horizontal shelf in the nasal visual field is caused by an asymmetry in the nerve fiber loss at the two poles.
- **End-stage or near-total field defect** with only a residual temporal island of vision, occurs at the last stage, sparing of blind spot.

168. Ans. (c) Tractional retinal detachment not involving the macula

Ref: A.K. Khurana, 6th ed. pg. 276-77

- Diabetic retinopathy leads to tractional retinal detachment, which presents with slowly progressive loss of vision.
- There is no photopsia or floaters unless macula is involved because the vitreo-retinal traction develops very slowly.

169. Ans. (a) Microaneurysms

Ref: A.K. Khurana, 6th ed. pg. 276-77

DIABETIC RETINOPATHY

- The retinal change seen in diabetes are called as diabetic retinopathy. In diabetes, there is pericytes necrosis. Normally ratio 1 pericytes: 1 endothelial cell. But in diabetic retinopathy 1 pericyte: 3 endothelial cell. The vessels wall is weakened and leakage occurs. Classification–
  - Non proliferative diabetic retinopathy
  - Proliferative diabetic retinopathy

Non proliferative diabetic retinopathy (NPDR)	Proliferative diabetic retinopathy (POR)
• **Microaneurysms-** early manifestation • Dot and Blot hemorrhages • Hard exudates • Soft exudates	• Neovascularization of the disc • Neovascularization of anywhere else from the disc • Neovascularization of iris-RUBIOSSIS IRIDIS

170. Ans. (d) Iris neovascularization

Ref: A.K. Khurana, 6th ed. pg. 250-51

- Neovascular glaucoma results from the formation of a neovacular membane involving the anterior chamber secondary to diffuse retinal hypoxia. There is release of factors like vascular endothelial growth factor (VEGF) from the vitreous which causes formation of abnormal

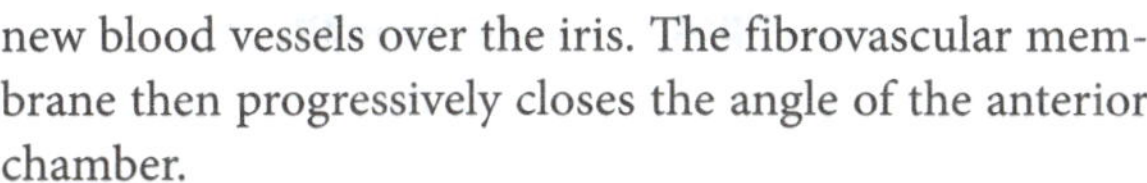

new blood vessels over the iris. The fibrovascular membrane then progressively closes the angle of the anterior chamber.

- It is usually associated with **neovascularisation of the iris (rubeosis iridis).**

171. Ans. (b) 5FU

Ref: A.K. Khurana, 6th ed. pg. 251-52

- Anti-VEGF are class of drugs which are used for treatment of diabetic retinopathy with neovascularization (proliferative diabetic retinopathy-PDR).
- Available anti-VEGF are: Ranibizumab, Bevacizumab, Pegaptanib.

Note: *TOC for PDR- Laser photocoagulation*

172. Ans. (c) Vitreous hemorrhage

Ref: A.K. Khurana, 6th ed. pg. 260-61

- Vitreous hemorrhage usually occurs from the retinal vessels and may present as pre-retinal or an intragel hemorrhage.

CAUSES

Causes of Vitreous Hemorrhage are as Follows:

- **Spontaneous** vitreous hemorrhage from retinal breaks especially those associated with PVD.
- **Trauma to eye:** Blunt or perforating
- **Inflammatory diseases** such as chorioretinitis and periphlebitis
- **Vascular disorders** e.g., hypertensive retinopathy, and centreal retinal vein occlusion.
- **Metabolic diseases** as diabetic retinopathy.
- **Blood dyscrasias** e.g.: Retinopathy of anaemia, leukaemias, polycythemias sickle-cell
- **Neoplasms**

Clinical Features

- **Symptoms:** Sudden development of floaters occurs when the vitreous hemorrhage is small.
  - In massive vitreous hemorrhage, sudden painless loss of vision.
- **Signs**
  - Distant direct ophthalmoscopy reveals black shadows against the red glow in small hemorrhages and no red glow in a large hemorrhage.
  - Direct and indirect ophthalmoscopy may show presence of blood in the vitreious cavity.
  - Ultrasonography with b-scan is particularly helpful in diagnosing vitreous hemorrhage.

173. Ans. (a) Vitreous hemorrhage

Ref: A.K. Khurana, 6th ed. pg. 260-61

Causes of Painless and Painful Loss of Vision

Sudden painless loss of vision	Sudden painful loss of vision
• Vascular occlusion (CRAO, CRVO) • *Retinal detachment* • ***Vitreous hemorrhage*** • Ischemic optic neuropathy	• Acute iridocyclitis • Chemical injuries • Mechanical injuries • Acute congestive glaucoma • Optic neuritis
Gradual painless loss of vision	**Gradual painful loss of vision**
• Progressive pterygeum involving the pupil • Corneal degeneration • Corneal dystrophy • Developmental cataracts • Senile cataracts • Optic atrophy • Chorioretinal degeneration • Age- related macular degeneration • *Diabetic retinopathy* • Refractive errors • Papilledema and Papillitis	• Chronic iridocyclitis • Corneal ulceration • Chronic simple glaucoma

174. Ans. (d) Trauma

Ref: A.K. Khurana, 6th ed. pg. 260-61

- Vitreous hemorrhage is defined as the presence of extravasated blood within the space outlined by the zonular fibers and posterior lens capsule anteriorly, the nonpigmented epithelium of the ciliary body laterally, and the internal limiting membrane of the retina (lamina limitans interna) posteriorly and posterolaterally.
  The 3 most common causes of vitreous hemorrhage are proliferative diabetic retinopathy, posterior vitreous detachment (PVD) with or without retinal tears, and ocular trauma (e.g., shaken baby syndrome).
  - Any cause of peripheral neovascularization may result in vitreous hemorrhage, **but trauma is the leading cause of vitreous hemorrhage in young people.**

The most common cause found in adults is diabetic retinopathy

MCC of recurrent vitrous hemorrhage in young adult: Eale's disease

175. Ans. (b) Exudative retinal detachment

Ref: A.K. Khurana, 6th ed. pg. 273

Please refer to above table.

RETINAL DETACHMENT

- Retinal detachment is the separation of neurosensory retina from the retinal pigmentary epithelium by subretinal fluid. Depending on the mechanism of

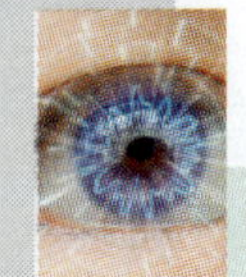

subretinal fluid accumulation retinal detachment are of following types:

- Exudative retinal detachment
- Tractional retinal detachment
- Rhegmatogenous retinal detachment

Exudative retinal detachment: Lesions of retinal pigment epithelium. **Commonest causes are:**

- **Malignant melanoma of choroid**
- ***Followed by pregnancy induce hypertension, 140/90 after 20th week of gestation.***
- Malignant hypertension 200/120 end stage hypertension.

TRACTIONAL RETINAL DETACHMENT

- Caused by mechanical traction (progressive contraction) of fibrovascular membrenes over large areas of vitreoretinal adhesion. *Characterized by slow painless loss of vision* (only retinal detachment that is slow). Causes are:
  - *Most common cause is diabetes mellitus*
  - Retinopathy of pregnancy
  - Sickle cell anemia

RHEGMATOGENOUS RETINAL DETACHMENT

- Characterized by the presence of retinal break held open by vitreo retinal traction that allows accumulation of liquefied vitreous (syneresis) under neurosensory retina, separating it from retinal pigment epithelium.
- The predisposing conditions of **rhegmatogenous retinal detachment** are **Myopia**, previous intraocular surgery such as **aphakia** or pseudophakia, a family history of retinal detachment, **trauma** and inflammation.

VITREOUS HEMORRHAGE

- Vitreous hemorrhage is not a (clinical) feature of retinal detachment. *Characterised by sudden painless loss of vision; floaters, no flashing of light.* **Causes are:**
  - **Diabetic retinopathy: Most common cause**
  - In young patient most common cause is Trauma and Eale's disease.

176. Ans. (a) Exudative retinal detachment

Ref: A.K. Khurana, 6th ed. pg. 273, 299

177. Ans. (b) Diabetic retinopathy

Ref: A.K. Khurana, 6th ed. pg. 273, 299; Parson's Ophthalmology 20/312

178. Ans. (d) CRVO

Ref: A.K. Khurana, 6th ed. pg. 269, 431

Cherry Red Spot of Retina is seen in—

- CRAO
- Trauma (Blunt trauma, Berlin's edema)
- Neimann pick disease
- Gaucher's disease
- Tay – Sach's disease
- Sand hoff's disease

Mnemonic: Cherry Tree Never Grow Tall in Sand.

179. Ans. (c) Central retinal vein occlusion

Ref: A.K. Khurana, 6th ed. pg. 214, 271, 294

CYSTOID MACULAR EDEMA (CME)

- Collection of fluid in the **outer plexiform (Henle's layer) a nuclear layer** of the retina is called CME.
- It is associated with Central Retinal Vein Occlusion/ post operative complication of cataract extraction and penetrating keratoplasty/diabetic retinopathy/Retinitis pigmentosa
- Minimal to moderate loss of vision is seen.
- It is **best examined with slit lamp/+90D** lens
- Ophthalmoscopy shows **"honeycomb appearance" of macula.**
- Fundus flurorescein angiography shows **"flowerpetal appearance".**
- Treatment of underlying primary cause and drugs (topical steroids triamcinofone/topical NSAIDs like flurbiprofen) is beneficial.

Extra Mile

- **100 day glaucoma'** is seen with CRVO
- **CATTLE TRUCK** appearance seen with CRAO
- IRVIN GASS SYNDROME is seen with post cataract CME

180. Ans. (a) Sarcoidosis

SARCOIDOSIS

- Sarcoidosis is a granulomatous disease of unknown etiology.
- It occurs most frequently in young adults (20 to 40 years), has a predilection for women.
- Around 20% patients with sarcoidosis has ocular involvement.
- **The most prevalent ocular sign** is unilateral, anterior, granulomatous uveitis.
- The common clinical ocular findings associated with sarcoid uveitis include:
  - Decreased or hazy vision, pain, photophobia, lacrimation, conjunctival injection, cells and flare in the anterior chamber, granulomatous iritis with large *"mutton fat"* keratic precipitates scattered over

the back surface of the corneal endothelium, iritis spill over leading to anterior vitritis, true vitritis with white exudative debris in the region of the ora serrata (snowball or snowbank retinopathy) with retinal vasculitis ***(candle wax drippings)*** and phlebitis (venous sheathing).

AMYLOIDOSIS

- **Orbit/adnexal:** Include ptosis, keratoconjunctivitis sicca, proptosis, ocular motility disturbances, palpable mass lesions and pupillary abnormalities. Pain uncommonly accompanies orbital amyloidosis, and its presence should prompt the examiner to consider alternative diagnosis.
- **Conjunctiva:** Ptosis, a visible or palpable mass, and recurrent subconjunctival hemorrhage are commonly reported symptoms.
- **Anterior chamber/iris:** A "scalloped" configuration of the iris margin may signify amyloid deposition in the iris stroma or, alternatively, disruption of the parasympathetic innervation of the iris sphincter. Anterior chamber involvement appears as whitish, flocculent debris in the aqueous, on the lens capsule or on the iris surface.
- **Lens:** Pseudopodia lentis, punctate dots on the posterior capsule resembling ameboid foot processes, are considered pathognomonic of vitreoretinal amyloidosis in patients with heredofamilial disease.
- **Vitreous/retina:** Vitreoretinal amyloidosis manifests as **"lacy," "cobweb-like," "sheet-like" or "stringy"** veils of gray or yellowish-white material in the vitreous. Symptoms include floaters, blurry vision or glare, or patients may be asymptomatic.
- **Diagnosis:** Congo red staining demonstrating apple-green birefringence when viewed through crossed polarimetric filters remains the gold standard for establishing the diagnosis of amyloidosis.
- **Treatment:** Surgical excision or debulking remains the treatment of choice.

181. Ans. (a) Pars planitis

Ref: A.K. Khurana, 6th ed. pg. 150-51

INTERMEDIATE UVEITIS (PARS PLANITIS)

- It denotes inflammation of pars plana part of ciliary body and most peripheral part of the retina.
- **Etiology:** It is an idiopathic disease usually affecting both eyes (80 percent) of children and young adults.

Clinical Features

- **Symptoms:** Most of the patients present with history of floaters.
- **Signs:** The eye is usually quiet.
  - Slit-lamp examination may show: Mild aqueous flare, and fine KPs at the back of cornea.
  - Fundus examination with indirect ophthalmoscope reveals the whitish exudates in the inferior quadrant present near the ora serrata.
  - These typical exudates are referred as *snow ball opacities*. These may coalesce to form a grey white plaque called *snow banking*.

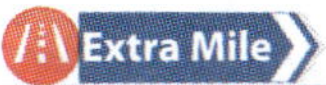

TABLE: Comparison of Anterior, Intermediate and Posterior Uveitis

	Anterior	Intermediate	Posterior
Aka	Iridocyclitis	Pars Planitis	Chorioretinitis
Cause	Idiopathic	Idiopathic	Toxoplasmosis
Clin. Feature	Sudden painless loss of vision	Floaters	Sudden painless loss of vision
Cells	WBC's **Keratic precipitate**	**Snowballs/ snowbanks**	**Headlight in fog appearance**
Treatment	Topical steroids-DOC Cycloplegics	Inj: Triamcinilone	Antimicrobials Systemic steroids

182. Ans. (c) 7–10 days

Ref: A.K. Khurana, 6th ed. pg. 573, Khurana, 4th ed. pg. 146

TABLE: Cycloplegics and its duration of action

Drug	Duration of Effect (days)
Atropine	7–10
Scopolamine	3–7
Homatropine	1–3
Cyclopentolate	1
Tropicamide	days (6 hrs)

183. Ans. (a) Pilocarpine

Ref: A.K. Khurana, 6th ed. pg. 159-50, Khurana's, 4th ed. pg. 146, 47

- **DOC for acute anterior uveitis:** Topical glucocorticoids
- **1st line agent:** Cycloplegics
- In case of uveitis, there is spasm of ciliary muscle and constriction of pupil (miosis). Pilocarpine is a parasympathomimetic agent, which causes further spasm of ciliary muscles and miosis.
- **Note:** *In case of anterior uveitis, there is irregular constriction of pupil called, festooned pupil.*

184. Ans. (c) Pilocarpine eye drops

Ref: A.K. Khurana, 6th ed. pg. 159-60

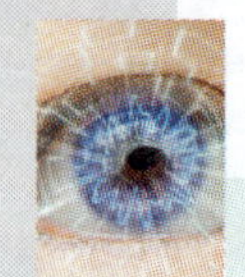

185. Ans. (a) Secondary glaucoma

Ref: A.K. Khurana, 6th ed. pg. 157

Complications of Anterior Uveitis:

- *Secondary glaucoma (most common)*
- Band shaped keratopathy: More common in children with JRA
- Anterior & posterior synechiae
- Seclusio occlusio pupillae
- *Complicated cataract*
- Pseudoglioma due to vitreous exudation
- *Cystoid macular edema* is common cause of visual impairment
- Pthisis & atrophic bulbi
- Tractional retinal detachment

Extra Mile

- Retinal detachment is a rare and late complication of anterior uveitis
- It is more common in pars-planitis and posterior uveitis).

EYELID AND LACRIMAL APPARATUS

186. Ans. (b) Entropion

Ref: A.K. Khurana, 7th ed. pg. 387

- The shown image is of entropion.
- Entropion refers to inward rolling and rotation of the lid margin toward globe.
- Ectropion: Outward rotation of lower eyelid.

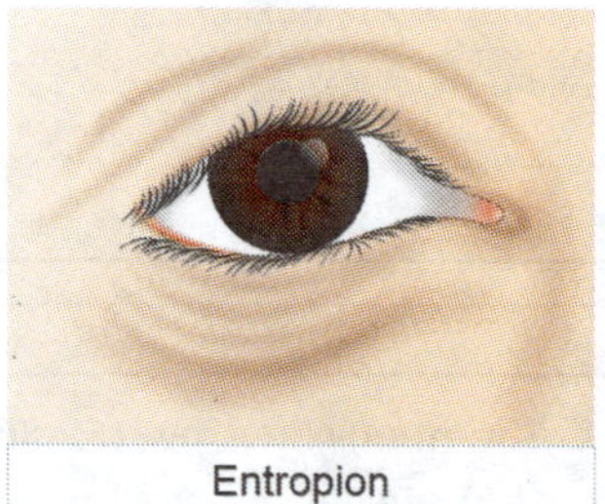

Entropion

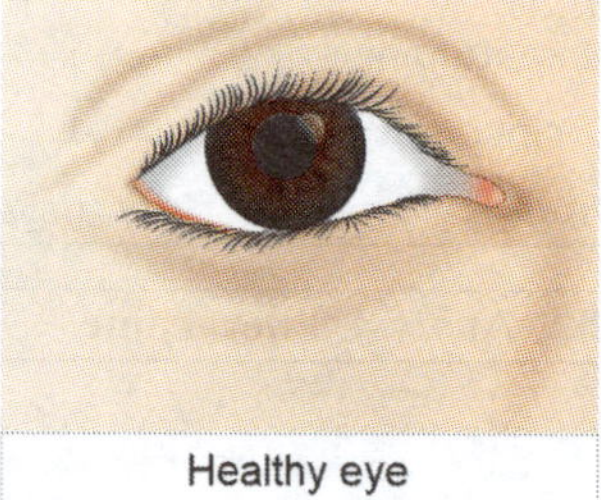

Healthy eye

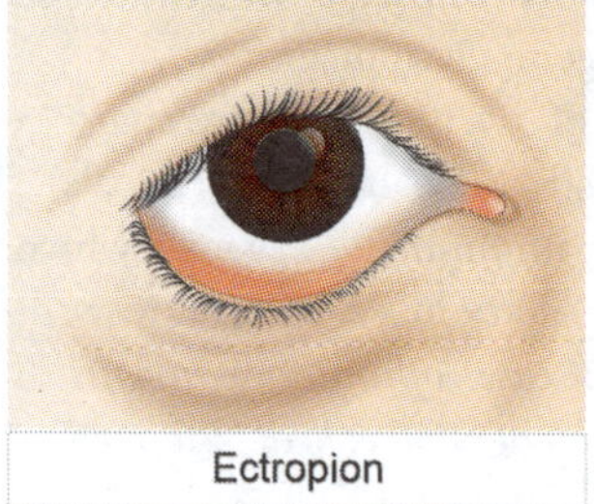

Ectropion

187. Ans. (d) Midbrain

Ref: A.K. Khurana, 7th ed. pg. 349

- The extraocular muscles are supplied by 3, 4 and 6th cranial nerve.
- All the nerves are present in midbrain. Therefore, injury to midbrain can lead to damage of nerves supplying extraocular muscles.
- CN 3 supplies superior medial and inferior recti and inferior oblique muscles. CN 4 supplies the superior oblique. CN 6 supplies lateral rectus muscle. *(Mn: LR6-SO4)*

188. Ans. (b) Vernal keratoconjunctivitis

Ref: A.K. Khurana, 7th ed. pg. 80

- The given image is of palpebral form of VKC.
- Upon examination: **Cobblestone** or '**Pavement Stone**' appearance with conjunctival hyperemia.

189. Ans. (b) Orbital cellulitis

Ref: A.K. Khurana, 7th ed. pg. 426

- **Orbital cellulitis** is an infection of the fat and muscles around the eye.

Causes:

- Streptococcus species
- Staphylococcus species
- Extension of infection from neighboring structures

Extra Mile

Causes of Proptosis

Unilateral	Bilateral
1. Congenital – Dermoid/ Teratoma	Developmental Anomalies – Oxycephaly
2. Traumatic – Orbital Hrage/ Emphysema/IOFB	Osteopathies – Rickets/ Acromegaly
3. Inflammation – Orbital Cellulitis/Abscess/Cavernous Sinus Thrombosis/ Pseudotumor/Tuberculosis GUMMA/Sarcoidosis	Tumors-Lymphoma/ Leukemia/Ewings Sarcoma/ Neuroblastoma
4. Vascular-Orbital Varix	Endocrinal – Thyroid Eye Disease
5. Cysts parasitic	Inflammatory – Wegener's/ Histiocytosis /Sjogren's/ Fungal Granuloma
6. Tumor – Primary or Secondary	
7. Mucocoele of Paranasal Sinuses	

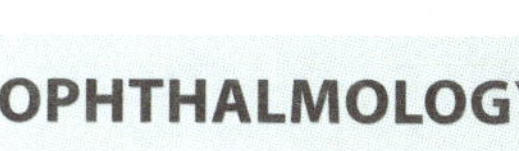

190. Ans. (a) Wilson's disease

Ref: A.K. Khurana, 7th ed. pg. 492

- The shown image along with clinical findings are suggestive of sunflower cataract, which is seen in Wilson's disease
- Copper deposited starts at limbus in ring form over Descemet membrane of cornea, often termed as KF ring.

191. Ans. (a) Chlamydia trachomatis

Ref: A.K. Khurana, 7th ed. pg. 67

- The shown image is **SAGO GRAIN FOLLICLES** in upper palpebral conjunctiva.
- It is suggestive of trachoma infection which is caused by chlamydia trachomatis.

192. Ans. (b) Instrument for chalazion

Ref: Comprehensive Ophthalmology by A.K. Khurana, 7th ed. pg. 621

- Chalazion clamp is applied to the everted lower lid. The clamp is tightened and used to evert and expose the conjunctival aspect of the eyelid.
- The clamp aid controls bleeding during the procedure and helps in fair localization of the lesion.
- Chalazion clamp consists of two limbs like a forceps which can be clamped with the help of a screw.
- One of the limbs that are placed on the skin side is in the form of a disc while the one that is placed on the conjunctival side is a circular ring.

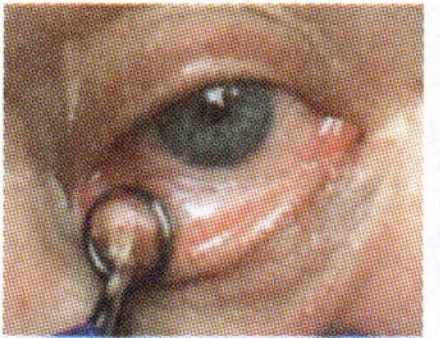
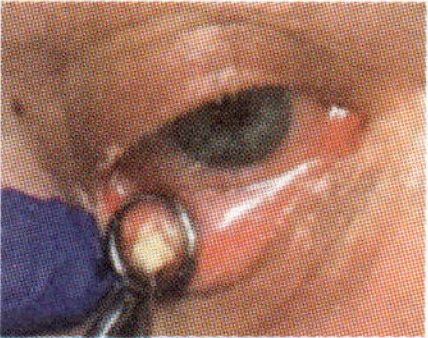
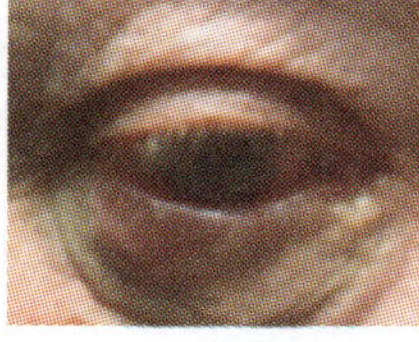

193. Ans. (b) Dacryocystorhinostomy

Ref: Comprehensive Ophthalmology by A.K. Khurana, 7th ed. pg. 413

- Dacryocystorhinostomy (DCR) is a surgical procedure to restore the flow of tears into the nose from the lacrimal sac when the nasolacrimal duct does not function.
- Reference states: The operation can be performed by following techniques
  - Conventional external approach
  - Endonasal surgical DCR
  - Endonasal laser DCR
  - Endocanalicular laser DCR
- NOTE: Atrophic rhinitis is an absolute contraindication of DCR.
- In case of acute dacryocystitis, this operation cannot be done immediately, rather it is done after a period of time.
- In case of elderly patients (above 70 years of age), dacryocystectomy is more preferred than dacryocystorhinostomy as old age naturally causes atrophy in nasal mucosa.

194. Ans. (a) LPS resection

Ref: Comprehensive Ophthalmology by A.K. Khurana, 7th ed. pg. 396-97

- For congenital ptosis surgery is the treatment of choice.
- Ptosis is drooping of eyelids and its severity is graded by: (Amount of cornea covered by eyelid – 2)
  - **Mild ptosis:** 2 mm
  - **Moderate ptosis:** 3 mm
  - **Severe ptosis:** 4 mm
- In severe cases surgery should be performed as soon as possible in order to avoid amblyopia.
- In mild and moderate cases surgery can be delayed until the age of 3 to 4 years.
- **There are many surgeries for ptosis like**
  - Fasanella Servat Operation for mild ptosis
  - Blaskovics operation, LPS Resection for moderate-severe ptosis
  - Frontalis Sling Surgery for completely paralyzed levator muscle

Note:

- Tarsal fracture and Wedge resection are the surgeries for entropion.

195. Ans. (b) Meibomian glands

GLANDS OF EYE AND ITS ASSOCIATED PATHOLOGY

Gland	Associated pathology
Meibomian gland	**Internal hordeolum:** Staphylococcal infection of meibomian gland. Painful condition. Treated with I/D and antibiotics support **Chalazion:** Chronic granulomatous disease occurred due to blocked meibomian gland. Nonpainful condition. Treated with incision and curettage.
Zeis gland	**External hordeolum/Stye:** Staphylococcal infection of Zeis gland. Treated with topical antibiotics.

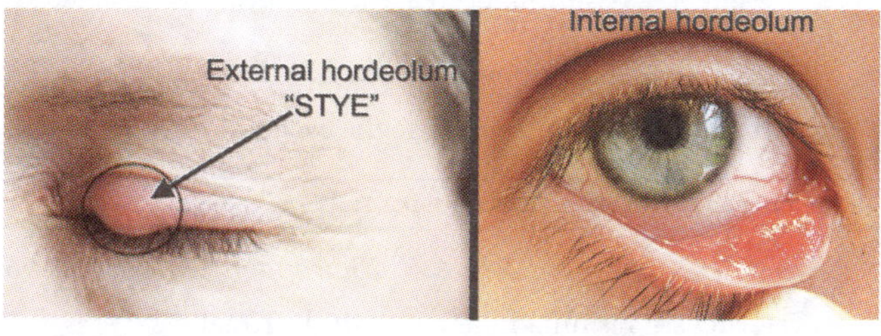

196. Ans. (c) Chalazion

- Chalazion is Chronic granulomatous painless inflammation of Meibomian Gland.
- Treatment: Incision and drainage

Note:

- Internal and external hordeolum is a staphylococcal infection and painful in nature.

197. Ans. (b) Middle meatus

Ref: Comprehensive Ophthalmology by A.K Khurana 6th ed. pg. 396

- **Dacryocystorhinostomy** (DCR) is a surgical procedure of choice in patients with dacryocystitis (inflammation of lacrimal sac)
- It is done by creating a new drainage of tear into nose, which opens in middle meatus.
  - **Remember:** Normally nasolacrimal duct opens into inferior meatus.
- The medial wall of lacrimal sac is anastomosed with middle meatus of nose → overcoming the obstruction at the junction of lacrimal sac and nasolacrimal duct.
- Performed in patients below 60 years.

Extra Mile

- **Dacryocystectomy (DCT):** used only when DCR is contraindicated or when the patient is too young (<4 years) or too old (>60 years) or in cases of chronic granulomatous disease induced obstruction like syphilis, TB, leprosy.
- **Conjunctivodacryocystorhinostomy (CDCR):** Done in presence of blocked canaliculi

198. Ans. (c) Ankyloblepharon

Ref: A.K. Khurana, 6th ed. pg. 377

- **Symblepharon:** Lids become adherent with the eyeball as a result of adhesions between the palpebral and bulbar conjunctiva.
- ***Ankyloblepharon:*** *Adhesions between margins of the upper and lower lids.*
  - It may occur as a congenital anomaly or may result after healing of chemical burns, thermal burns, ulcers and traumatic wounds of the lid margins.
- **Blepharophimosis:** In this condition the extent of the palpebral fissure is decreased. It appears contracted at the outer canthus.
- **Lagophthalmos:** This condition is characterized by inability to voluntarily close the eyelids.

199. Ans. (d) Dacrocystorhinostomy

Ref: A.K. Khurana, 6th ed. pg. 395-96

Dacrocystits is inflammation of the lacrimal sac

CHRONIC DACROCYSTITIS

- Chronic dacryocystitis is more common than the acute dacrocystitis.
- **Cause:** Vicious cycle of stasis and mild infection of long duration.
- **Factors responsible for stasis of tears in lacrimal sac:**
  - Anatomical factors: Narrow bony canal
  - **Foreign bodies** in the sac may block opening of NLD.
  - **Excessive lacrimation**
  - **Mild grade inflammation:** May block the NLD
  - **Obstruction of lower end of the NLD** by nasal diseses such as polyps, hypertrophied inferior concha, severe deviated nasal septum.
- **Source of infection:** It may get infected from the conjunctiva, nasal cavity (retrograde spread), or paranasal sinuses by: Staphylococci, pneumococci, streptococci and pseudomonas pyocyanea.
- **Clinical Feature**
  - **Stage of chronic catarrhal dacryocystitis:** Characterised by mild inflammation of the lacrimal sac associated with blockage of NLD.
  - **Stage of lacrimal mucocoele:** Characterized by constant epiphora associated with a swelling just below the inner canthus.
  - **Stage of chronic suppurative dacryocystitis:** Characterized by epiphora, associated recurrent conjunctivitis and swelling at the inner canthus with mild erythema.
  - **Stage of chronic fibrotic sac:** Repeated infections may result in a small fibrotic sac due to thickening of mucosa, which is associated with epiphora and discharge.
- **Treatment**
  - **Conservative treatment** by repeated lacrimal syringing.
  - ***Dacryocystorhinostomy (DCR).*** *It is considered as surgery of choice as it re-establishes the lacrimal drainage.*
  - **Dacryocystectomy (DCT).** It should be performed only when DCR is contraindicated.
  - **Conjunctivodacryocystorhinostomy (CDCR).** It is performed in the presence of blocked canaliculi.

200. Ans. (a) 3rd CN palsy

Ref: A.K. Khurana, 6th ed. pg. 379

- Ptosis is drooping of eyelid.
- Eyelid is comprised of 4 muscles:

TABLE: Muscles, their innervation and function

Muscle	CN innervation	Function
LPS	III	Opens the eyelid
Muller's muscle	III	Opens eyelid when LPS tired
Frontalis	VII	Closes the eyelid
Orbicularis oculi	VII	Closes the eyelid

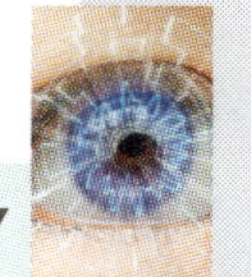

- CN III palsy leads to drooping of eyelid (Ptosis).
- CN VII palsy may also cause ptosis.

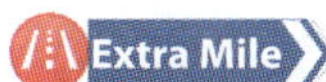

Extra Mile

- All the extraocular muscles are supplied by CN III except lateral rectus and superior oblique.
- Lateral rectus supplied by—CN VI
- Superior oblique supplied by—CN IV

Remember: LR6, SO4; all other by CN III

LENS/CATARACT

201. Ans. (a) Myopic shift

Ref: Kanski Clinical Ophthalmology, 9th ed. pg. 319

https://www.ncbi.nlm.nih.gov/pmc/articles/PMC6174295/

- The major postoperative refractive error at the follow-up is myopia. Thus, it is important to adjust the IOL calculation formula to specify more undercorrection, with the aim of achieving more optimal refractive outcomes in adulthood.
- Based on guidelines, the under corrected IOL power was calculated by anticipating the expected myopic shift.

Under correction:

- By 20% if the age is <2 years
- By 10% if the age is <8 years
- Full correction after 8 years, because of emmetropia

202. Ans. (b) Acanthamoeba

Ref: Kanski Clinical Ophthalmology, 9th ed. pg. 232

- Acanthamoeba keratitis is a serious corneal infection that can lead to visual loss or a need for corneal transplant.
- Acanthamoeba keratitis is most frequently associated with contact lens wear, especially if tap water is used for rinsing.
- Symptoms of an infection include redness, pain, tearing, increased light sensitivity, blurry vision, foreign body sensation, discharge or swelling.

203. Ans. (a) Rosette cataract

Ref: A.K. Khurana, 7th ed. pg. 448

- **Rossette Shaped Cataract** is a posterior subcapsular developed due to minute ruptures in lens capsule with influx of aqueous leading to opacification.
- It is caused due to blunt trauma

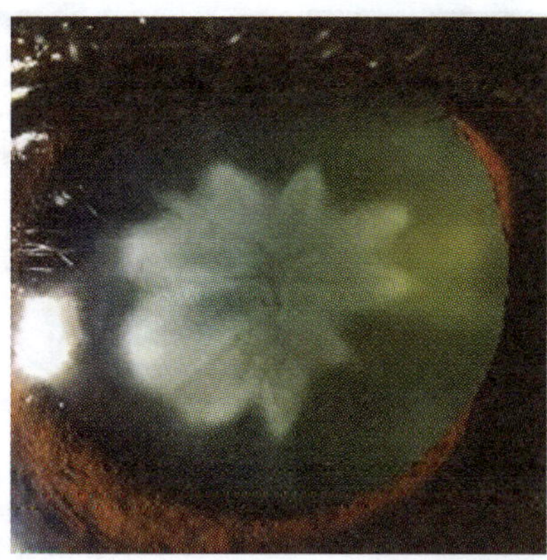

204. Ans. (b) Buphthalmos

At present, the term "buphthalmos" is used to describe the visible enlargement of the eyeball detected at birth or soon after, due to any uncontrolled glaucoma in early childhood.

Clinical features of Buphthalmos:

- Tearing
- Sensitivity to light
- Eye irritation
- Haziness in the eye

205. Ans. (c) Posterior subcapsular cataract

Ref: A.K. Khurana, 7th ed. pg. 189

- The shown image is of Posterior Subcapsular Cataract (PSC). There is formation of granular or plaque like opacity in the posterior subcapsular cortex.
- PSC causes maximum visual disability due to its location at/near the NODAL POINT of the eye.
- **Clinical feature:**
  - Loss of near vision more than far vision
  - Vision improves in dim illumination
  - Glare

206. Ans. (c) Trauma

Ref: Khurana 7th ed. pg. 527, 448

- Rosette-shaped cataract, early as well as late, is typical of concussion injury of lens.
- Rosette cataract is a complication of blunt trauma.
- **Early rosette:** Feathery lines of opacities along the star-shaped suture lines, usually in the posterior cortex.
- **Late rosette:** Develops in the posterior cortex 1 to 2 years after the injury.
- Sutural extensions are shorter and more compact than the early rosette cataract.

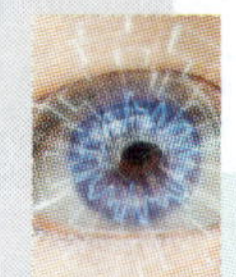

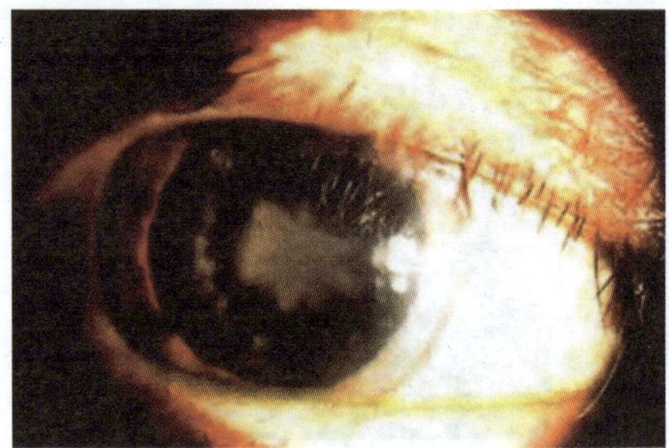

FIGURE: Rosette shaped cataract following blunt trauma

207. Ans. (c) **Hypermetropia**

Ref: Khurana 7th ed. pg. 296-97

- Anterior chamber is the space between posterior surface of cornea to anterior surface of lens.
- Normal depth: 2.5 mm and contains 0.25 mL of aqueous humor
- NOTE: Chamber depth decreases by 0.01 mm/year of life
- **Anterior chamber is shallow in:**
  - **Physiological:** Young age and in Elderly persons
  - **Diseases:** ACG, Hypermetropia, perforated cornea, iris bombe, adherent leucoma can cause shallow anterior chamber
- **Anterior chamber is deep in:**
  - Aphakia, Myopia, Keratoconus, Keratoglobus, Buphthalmos, total posterior synechiae can cause deep anterior chamber.

208. Ans. (c) **Subluxation of lens**

Ref: Khurana 7th ed. pg. 222

- Marfan's syndrome is an autosomal dominant mesodermal dysplasia.
- In this lens is displaced upwards and temporally bilaterally symmetrical.

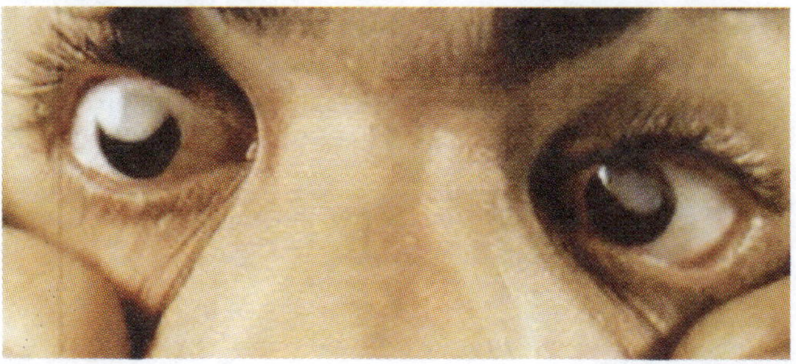

209. Ans. (c) **Femto laser**

Ref: Khurana 7th ed. pg. 212

- **Femto second laser assisted cataract surgery (FLACS)** - It is the best available procedure presently for doing cataract surgery.
- FLACS is basically a microincision cataract surgery (MICS) in which femtosecond laser (FSL) is used.

Note:

- Laser iridotomy for ACG (uses ND:YAG laser)

Argon laser trabeculoplasty for OAG

210. Ans. (a) **Keratoplasty**

Ref: Comprehensive Ophthalmology by A.K. Khurana, 7th ed. pg. 142-43

- Corneal transplantation, also known as corneal grafting, is a surgical procedure where a damaged or diseased cornea is replaced by donated corneal tissue (the graft).
- Keratoplasty simply means surgery to the cornea. The graft is taken from a recently deceased individual with no known diseases or other factors that may affect the chance of survival of the donated tissue or the health of the recipient.
- Types of keratoplasty:
  - **Penetrating keratoplasty:** Entire cornea is replaced
  - **Lamellar keratoplasty:** Only part of the cornea is replaced

211. Ans. (a) **Prismatic effect will less**

Ref: Comprehensive Ophthalmology by A.K. Khurana, 7th ed. pg. 51

Contact lens have the following advantages over spectacles:

- Irregular corneal astigmatism can be corrected
- They provide normal field of vision
- Prismatic distortions can be corrected
- Binocular vision can be retained in high anisometropia
- Cosmetically better

212. Ans. (a) **Cataract**

Ref: A.K. Khurana 6th ed. pg. 477

- Globally, MCC of blindness is cataract, affecting 17.6 million (39%), followed by glaucoma which affects 4.5 million (10%) population.
- MCC of blindness in India: Cataract
- MCC of blindness in developed countries: Age Related Macular Degeneration (50% of all blindness in developed countries)

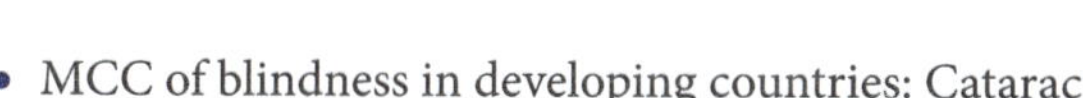

- MCC of blindness in developing countries: Cataract
- MC preventable cause of blindness worldwide: Trachoma

213. Ans. (b) ND:YAG laser

Ref: Comprehensive Ophthalmology by A.K. Khurana 6th ed. pg. 462

- Lasers for glaucoma:
  - Laser iridotomy for ACG (uses ND:YAG laser)
  - Argon laser trabeculoplasty for OAG
  - Laser goniopunctures for developmental glaucoma
  - Pan retinal photocoagulation: For prophylactic/ treatment of neovascular glaucoma
  - **Cyclophotocoagulation:** For absolute glaucoma or near absolute glaucoma
- Nd:YAG laser typically emits light with wavelength of **1064 nm** in the infrared
- **Uses of Nd:YAG laser:**
  - Correct posterior capsular opacification
  - Peripheral laser iridotomy in ACG
  - Double frequency ND:YAG (wavelength: 532 nm) used for pan-retinal photocoagulation.

Extra Mile

- **Excimer lasers** are used for photoablation—these lasers act by tissue remodelling. Used for:
  - Photorefractive keratectomy (PRK)
  - LASIK surgery
  - Phototherapeutic keratectomy (PTK) for corneal diseases such as band shaped keratopathy.

TABLE: Lasers used in ophthalmology

Type of laser	Wave length (nm)	Atomic environment used	Effects produced
• Argon	514	Argon gas	Photocoagulation
• Krypton	647	Krypton gas	Photocoagulation
• Diode	840	Diode crystal	Photocoagulation
• Diode Pumped frequency doubled Nd:YAG	532	Diode and Nd:YAG crystals	Photocoagulation
• Nd: YAG	1064	A liquid dry or a solid compound of yttrium-aluminium garnet and neodymium	Photodisruption
• Excimer	193	Helium and fluorine gas	Photoablation
• Femto-second	1053	Neodymium-glass	Photodisruption

214. Ans. (a) Homocystinuria

Ref: Comprehensive Ophthalmology by A.K. Khurana 6th ed. pg. 216

Systemic conditions associated with ectopia lentis:

- **Marfan syndrome:** MCC of hereditary ectopia lentis. AD condition. Lens displaced supero-temporally (bilaterally symmetrical)
- **Homocystinuria:** 2nd MCC of of hereditary ectopia lentis. AR condition. Lens subluxated inferior and nasally.
- **Weil Marchesani syndrome:** AR condition. Associated with mental retardation, short stature and stubby fingers. Lens subluxated anteriorly.
- **Sulphite oxidase deficiency:** AR condition. Ectopia lentis is universal ocular feature
- Hyperlysinnemia

Extra Mile

- **Simple ectopia lentis:** Superior displacement of lens
- **Sunset syndrome:** Inferior subluxation of IOL
- **Sunrise syndrome:** Superior subluxation of IOL
- **Lost lens syndrome:** Complete dislocation of IOL into vitreous cavity.

215. Ans. (a) Nd:YAG

- ND-YAG (Neodymium- Yttrium-Aluminium-Garnet) laser is used for posterior capsulotomy in after cataract surgery.

216. Ans. (c) Nuclear cataract

Ref: A.K. Khurana's Ophthalmology, 6th ed. pg. 191

- Nuclear cataract can cause nuclear sclerosis, which causes deterioration of distant vision (due to progressive index myopia). These patients may be able to read without presbyopic glasses. This improvement in near vision is referred to as ***"second sight"***

217. Ans. (d) Posterior-subscapular cataract due to long term use of steroids

Ref: A.K. Khurana's Ophthalmology, 6th ed. pg. 194-95

218. Ans. (a) Cataract

Ref: A.K. Khurana, 6th ed. pg. 180-81, Khurana 4th ed. pg. 171, 175

- **MCC of blindness in world & India:** Cataract
- Cataract most commonly seen in females

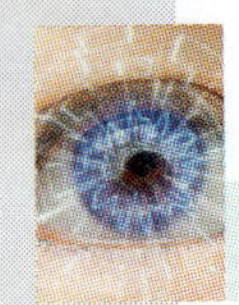

- **2nd MCC of blindness:** Glaucoma
- **MC infective cause of blindness:** Trachoma
- **MCC of ocular morbidity:** Refractive error

219. Ans. (b) ND-YAG

Ref: A.K. Khurana, 6th ed. pg. 187-89

- ND-YAG (Neodymium- Yttrium-Aluminium-Garnet) laser is used for posterior capsulotomy in after cataract.
- Diode, Argon and Krypton laser is used for retinal photocoagulation.

220. Ans. (d) In the lens capsule

Ref: A.K. Khurana, 6th ed. pg. 186, 195-96

INTRAOCULAR LENS IMPLANTATION

- Presently, intraocular lens (IOL) implantation is the method of choice for correcting aphakia.

Types of Intraocular Lenses

- **Anterior chamber IOL**: These lenses lie in front of the iris and are supported in the angle of anterior chamber.
- ACIOL can be inserted after ICCE or ECCE *(Intra/Extra Capsular Ccataract Extraction).*
- **Iris –supported lenses:** These lenses are fixed on the iris with the help of sutures or claws.
- **Posterior Chamber lenses:** PCIOL implanted behind the iris. They may be supported by the ciliary sulcus or capsular bag.
- **At present** the trend is *"In the Bag"* fixation.

Extra Mile

Cataract Surgeries and their Main Indications

Cataract	Surgery
Immature cataract	Phacoemulsification
Mature/hyper mature cataract	ECCE
Subluxated	ICCE

221. Ans: (c) Opacity along sutures

Ref: A.K. Khurana, 6th ed. pg. 194-95

- **Complicated cataract**: Cataract secondary to some intraocular disease which may be:
  - **Anterior *cortical*** in anterior segmental lesion as glaucoma, acute iritis, or,
  - **Posterior cortical** in posterior segmental lesion as uveitis, RD, pigmentary retinal dystrophy.
- The second type of complicated cataract presents with posterior cortical bread crumb appearance/ polychromatic lusture or rainbow cataract.
- *Bread crumbs appearance* is Pathognomonic of posterior cataract.
- *Opacity usually commence in posterior cortex and spread axially and NOT along sutures.*
- Vision is much impaired even in early stage, owing to the position of the opacity near the nodal point of the eye.

222. Ans. (c) Vitreous movement

Ref: A.K. Khurana, 6th ed. pg. 194-95

- **Complicated cataract occurs secondary intraocular disease e.g.**
  - Inflammatory conditions as uveitis.
  - Degenerative conditions as retinitis pigmentosa, high myopia etc.
  - Intraocular tumors
  - Retinal detachment, Glaucoma etc.

Extra Mile

TABLE: Types of cataract and their causes

Type of cataract	Cause
Snow flake/snow storm cataract	Diabetes mellitus/Down's syndrome
Sunflower/Petals of flower cataract	Wilson's disease Chalcosis (mild reaction to copper) Penetrating trauma (with retention to copper)
Blue dot cortical cataract	Atopic dermatitis Myotonic dystrophy
Vossius ring/Rosette shaped cataract	Blunt trauma
Christmas tree cataract	Myotonic dystrophy
Oil drop cataract Dust like lenticular opacity	Galactosemia
Breadcrumb appearance Polychromatic lusture Rainbow cataract	Complicated cataract/Secondary cataract
Morgagnian cataract	Hypermature senile cataract

223. Ans. (a) Trauma

Ref: A.K. Khurana, 6th ed. pg. 429, Khurana, 4th ed. pg. 405

224. Ans. (c) Anterior capsule of the lens

Ref: A.K. Khurana, 6th ed. pg. 429, Parsons' Diseases of the Eye, 20th ed. pg. 367

- **Blunt trauma** to eye leads to formation of ***vossius ring on anterior surface of lens***
- It is a faint or stippled opacity seen on the anterior capsule of the lens due to multitudes of brown amorphous granules of pigment lying on the capsule

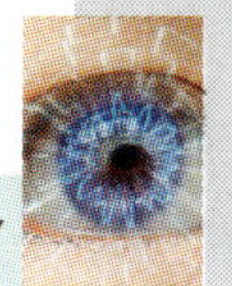

- Produced by the impress of the iris on the lens as a result of a force that drives cornea and iris backwards.
- It is about the same diameter as the *contracted pupil.*

225. Ans. (a) Posterior subcapsular cataract

Ref: Levin's Ophthalmology, 232

"**Posterior sub capsular cataracts** typically account for less than 10% of age related cataracts. They arise from epithelial cells that fail to differentiate properly into fiber cells. These cells migrate or are carried by their neighbors to the posterior pole of lens where they swell and form a plaque that scatters light. Because these plaques are in the **optic axis** they **significantly degrade vision** even when quite small.

226. Ans. (d) Secondary cataract

Ref: A.K. Khurana, 6th ed. pg. 214

227. Ans. (a) Phenylketonuria

Ref: A.K. Khurana, 6th ed. pg. 181-215

228. Ans. (d) Alport's syndrome

Ref: A.K. Khurana, 6th ed. pg. 218-219

- Anterior lenticonus is seen *in Alport's syndrome* (90%)
- It is a disorder of basement membrane and is characterized by:
  - *Familial haemorrhagic nephritis*
  - *Sensory-neural deafness* and
  - *Ocular features like anterior lenticonus,* cataract, retinal flecks and posterior polymorphous corneal dystrophy.

229. Ans. (b) Superotemporal subluxation of lens

Ref: Khurana, 4th ed. pg. 202

- Marfan's syndrome is an **autosomal dominant** condition.
- Subluxation of lens is a common finding, which is seen in upward and temporal area, bilaterally symmetrical.
- Other abnormalities includes: Spider finger, long extremities, high arched palate and dissecting aortic aneurysm with normal IQ.

Extra Mile

Suluxation of lens also seen in:
- **Homocystinuria:** Autosomal Recessive condition; Downward and nasally displaced lens.
- **Weil marchesani syndrome:** Forward subluxation and spheroaphakia
- **Sulphite oxidase deficiency:** Ectopia lentis is universal ocular feature
- **Ehler's danlos syndrome**
- Hyperlysinemia
- Stickler syndrome

230. Ans. (b) Superior and temporally

Ref: A.K. Khurana, 6th ed. pg. 215

Please refer to above condition

231. Ans. (b) Aphakia

Ref: A.K. Khurana, 6th ed. pg. 37, 187

- Jack in a box phenomenon is seen after cataract surgery where the lens of the patient is removed. This causes disproportion in power of the eye. To correct aphakia, patients are prescribed with glasses.
- To correct the refractive error in aphakia about 10 dioptre of convex lenses are required for distance vision and about 13 dioptre for near vision. Such high power lenses are associated with numerous physical and optical problems. The most important of these problems are:
  - Magnification
  - Roving Ring Scotoma
  - **Jack-in-the-box Phenomenon**

232. Ans. (b) Cataract

- Side of oral/systemic steroid: **Cataract**
- Side effect of topical steroid: **Glaucoma**
  - *Mn: GTCS (Glaucoma-topical; Cataract- Systemic)*
- Blepharoconjuncivitis is Side effect of **Timolol**

233. Ans. (b) Subluxation of lens

Ref: A.K. Khurana, 6th ed. pg. 215, 500;
Khurana, 4th ed. pg. 203-204, 473

- Iridodonesis is tremulousness of iris.
- It is observed when its posterior support is lost as in aphakia and subluxation of lens.

GLAUCOMA

234. Ans. (d) Disc edema

Ref: Khurana 7th ed. pg. 236

- Primary open-angle glaucoma also known as chronic simple glaucoma of adult onset.
- Characterized by:
  - Slowly progressive raised intraocular pressure (>21 mm Hg at least on few occasions)
  - Open normal appearing anterior chamber angle
  - Characteristic optic disc cupping
  - Specific visual field defects.

235. Ans. (b) Applanation tonometer

Ref: Khurana 7th ed. pg. 531

- Applanation tonometry based on Imbert-Fick law (pressure inside a sphere (P) is equal to the force (W) required to flatten its surface divided by the area of flattening (A).

- The commonly used applanation tonometer are:
  - Goldmann tonometer—it is the most popular and accurate tonometer, consists of a double prism mounted on a standard slit-lamp. The prism applanates the cornea in an area of 3.06 mm diameter.

236. Ans. (a) Glaucoma

Ref: Comprehensive Ophthalmology by A.K. Khurana, 7th ed. pg. 470

- Topical beta-blockers have long been the mainstay of open-angle glaucoma therapy.
- When an individual is already using systemic beta-blockers, the response to topical beta-blockers is often not optimal.
- Preferred beta blocker in OAG: Timolol
- Preferred beta blocker in patients with history of bronchial asthma: Betaxolol.

237. Ans. (a) Intumescent cataract

Ref: A.K. Khurana, 6th ed. pg. 193, 248

- Phacomorphic glaucoma is most common lens induced glaucoma (secondary ACG).
- It is caused due to intumescent/swollen, cataractous lens.
- The swollen lens pushes the iris forward resulting in secondary ACG.

238. Ans. (d) Dorzolamide

Ref: Katzung Pharmacology; 11/ed. pg. 89

- **Timolol:** Beta blocker. Decreases aqueous secretion from ciliary epithelium. DOC for POAG in India.
  - Overall, DOC for OAG is latanoprost.
- **Mannitol:** A hyperosmotic agent. Reduces vitreous volume and deepens anterior chamber.
- **Prostaglandin analogue: Latanoprost, Bimatoprost:** Increases uveoscleral aqueous outflow. Considered as DOC for OAG.
- **Carbonic anhydrase inhibitor: Acetazolamide, dorzolamide, brinzolamide.** Acts by decreasing aqueous secretion.

239. Ans. (c) Angle closure glaucoma

Ref: A.K. Khurana, 6th ed. pg. 239-40

- In case of angle closure glaucoma, pupil is mid-dilated, vertically fixed. At this position of pupil, iris and lens are at maximum approximation which precipitate the condition and patient presents with sudden painful loss of vision.
- Open angle glaucoma is due to blockage of trabecular meshwork. Patient gives a history of slow painless loss of vision.
- Uveitis is inflammation of uveal component. Pupil here called festooned pupil *(anterior uveitis)*.

240. Ans. (a) Vertically dilated

Ref: A.K. Khurana, 6th ed. / 239-40, Khurana 4th ed./ 225

- In case of angle closure glaucoma, pupil is mid dilated, vertically fixed.
- Irregularly constricted fixed pupil is seen in anterior uveitis *(known as festooned pupil)*.

241. Ans. (c) Acute congestive glaucoma

Ref: A.K. Khurana, 6th ed. pg. 239-41

- Acute congestive glaucoma usually presents with sudden painful loss of vision associated with colored haloes. ACG more commonly seen in middle to elderly females.
- **D/dx of color haloes:**
  - ACG
  - Cataract
  - Mucopurulent conjunctivitis (Not in angular)
- RD presents with sudden painless loss of vision associated with flashes of light.

242. Ans. (b) Latanoprost

Ref: A.K. Khurana, 6th ed. pg. 228-30

GLAUCOMA

- It is a group of conditions characterized by progressive optic neuropathy with characterstic optic disc appearance and irreversible visual field defects.
- It is caused due to retinal ganglion cell death by increase in intraocular pressure (IOP) (usually) or other factors (excitotoxicity/optic nerve spasm)

Classical Triad

- Increase IOP (>21)
- Visual Field decrease
- Optic disk/Nerve changes (damage)

Atleast 2 conditions is required for diagnosis

PRIMARY OPEN ANGLE GLAUCOMA

- It is also known as chronic simple glaucoma of adult onset and is characterized by the:
  - Slowly progressive raised IOP
  - Optic disc cupping
  - Specific visual field defects

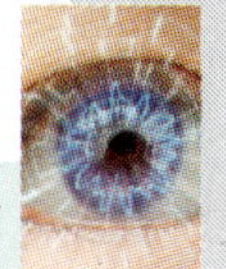

Clinical Features and Risk Factors for OAG

Clinical features	Risk factors
• Frequent change in presbyopic glasses. • Delayed dark adaption. • Painless • No corneal edema • No loss of vision • No coloured halos	• Age • Race- Indians, Japanese. • Myopes • Diabetes, hypertension, hyperthyroidism • Mustard oil intake

Treatment: POAG is best treated by PG analogue Latanoprost (DOC)

Surgery: Trabeculectomy

- Surgical–Argon/diode laser trabeculoplasty can also be done.

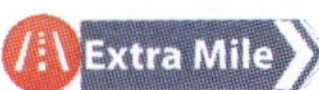

Extra Mile

- **Peripheral Iridectomy:** Surgical treatment done in primary angle closure glaucoma. *Treatment of choice for acute congestive glaucoma.*
- **Laser Iridotomy:** Treatment of choice for angle closure glaucoma.

243. Ans. (c) Parcentral scotoma

Ref: A.K. Khurana, 6th ed. pg. 233, 238

Visual field defects in glaucoma

1. Isopter contraction: *Earliest*
2. Baring of blind spot
3. Isolated paracentral scotoma (earliest chinically significant)
4. Seidel scotoma
5. Bjerrum or arcuate scotoma
6. Roenne's central nasal step
7. Double arcuate scotoma leads to tubular vision
8. Temporal island of vision is also lost with no light perception

244. Ans. (d) Decrease aqueous production

Ref: A.K. Khurana, 6th ed. pg. 451-52

- **ACETAZOLAMIDE** is a carbonic anhydrase inhibitor which acts in OAG by decreasing aqueous production.
- **Carbonic anhydrase derivatives are:** Acetazolamide, **Dorzolamide,** Brinzolamide
- Dorzolamide is mildest carbonic anhydrase inhibitor, hence considered as DOC for glaucoma in children.
- Alpha-2 agonist (Brimonidine, Apraclonidine) also act by decreasing aqueous production.
- **Class of drugs which act by increasing outflow:**
  - ↑ **Trabecular outflow:** Pilocarpine, Epinephrine
  - ↑ **Uveoscleral outflow:** PG Analogue (Latanoprost)

Extra Mile

TREATMENT OF Glaucoma

- **First line DOC for ACG:** Mannitol
- **TOC for ACG:** Laser iridotomy
- **DOC for OAG:** PG analogue (Latanoprost)
- **Most powerful anti glaucoma drug:** Latanoprost
- **DOC for OAG in India-** Timolol
- **Safest anti-glaucoma for children-** Dorzolamide

245. Ans. (b Latanoprost

Ref: A.K. Khurana, 6th ed. pg. 453

246. Ans. (d) Dorzolamide

Ref: A.K. Khurana, 6th ed. pg. 452-454

247. Ans. (a) Timolol maleate

Ref: A.K. Khurana, 6th ed. pg. 236-37

- Although timolol is considered as DOC for OAG in India, it is contraindicated in glaucoma patients suffering from bronchial asthma.
- Timolol is a non selective Beta blocker which might aggravate the asthma of the patient.
- For such patient Betaxolol is next best choice.

248. Ans. (c) Surgical management

Ref: A.K. Khurana, 6th ed. pg. 225-227

- Once the patient presents with symptoms of primary developmental glaucoma like photophobia, blepharospasm, lacrimation, eye rubbing, the next procedure is to do careful examination in which following things done: IOP measurement, ophthalmoscopy and gonioscopic examination of the angle of anterior chamber.
- The next best step once examination confirms glaucoma is to undergo surgical management (goniotomy) in order to decrease the IOP.

249. Ans. (b) Trabeculotomy

Ref: A.K. Khurana, 6th ed. pg. 225-227,

- Manifestation of congenital glaucoma below age of 3 years is termed as buphthalmos *(as given in case).* This condition occur due to developmental anomaly of the angle of anterior chamber.
- **Treatment:**
  - **Goniotomy** is preferred treatment, where barkaan's goniotomy knife is used to make an incision in the angle under gonioscopic control.
  - **Trabeculotomy** is preferred when corneal clouding prevents visualization by gonioscopy. *(as seen in given case)*

- **Combined trabeculotomy and trabeculectomy** is preferred treatment nowadays with better result.

250. Ans. (d) Laser iridotomy

Ref: A.K. Khurana, 6th ed. pg. 247

- **Laser Iridotomy:** Treatment of choice for angle closure glaucoma.
- **Peripheral Iredectomy:** Surgical treatment done in primary angle closure glaucoma. Treatment of choice for acute congestive glaucoma.
- **Trabeculectomy:** It is a filtration surgery done in primary open angle glaucoma.
- **Trabeculoplasty:** Primary open angle glaucoma is also treated by Trabeculoplasty.

251. Ans. (a) Angle closure glaucoma

Ref: A.K. Khurana, 6th ed. pg. 247

252. Ans. (a) Laser iridotomy

Ref: A.K. Khurana, 6th ed. pg. 247-48

- Please refer to above explanation
- Treatment of choice for primary angle closure glucoma *(fellow eye,* latent stage, *subacute or intermittent stage,* chronic stage) is *laser iridotomy*
- Peripheral surgical iridectomy can also be used.
- In acute congestive stage of PACG *drug of choice is Pilocarpine, till the time laser iridotomy can be performed.*

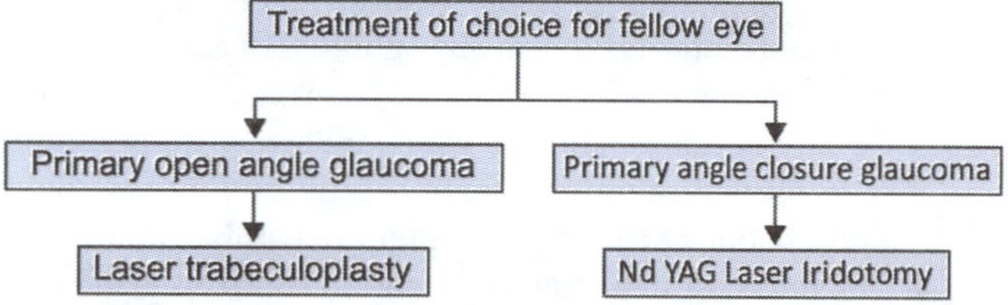

253. Ans. (b) Laser trabeculoplasty

Please refer to above explanation

254. Ans. (b) Open angle glucoma

- In case of OAG colored haloes are very late feature.
- Coloured halos are most commonly seen in ***primary angle closure glaucoma, cataract & acute purulent conjunctivitis.*** These are differentiated by:
  - **Emsley-Fincham's test:** a stenopaeic slit is passed across the pupil.
    - In case of Primary angle closure glaucoma: Haloes remain intact
    - In case of Immature cataract: Haloes broken into segments.
  - **Conjunctivitis:** Haloes eliminated after irrigating the discharge.
- Therefore given these options, our best choice will be OAG.

255. Ans. (a) Open angle glaucoma

Ref: A.K. Khurana, 6th ed. pg. 229

Frequent change of presbyopic lens is a typical characteristic feature of open angle glaucoma.

Extra Mile

FREQUENT CHANGE OF GLASSES in young:
- If power also increases → PATHOLOGICAL Ex: OAG
- If NO increment in power → KERATOCONUS

256. Ans. (b) Cornea posterior surface

Ref: A.K. Khurana, 6th ed. pg. 250; Khurana, 4th ed. pg. 234

- Krukenberg spindles are pigmentary granules which are seen on posterior surface of cornea in shape of spindles in **cases of secondary open angle glaucoma** (pigmentory glaucoma). It can be seen on iris.
- This condition is most commonly seen in young males and myopics.

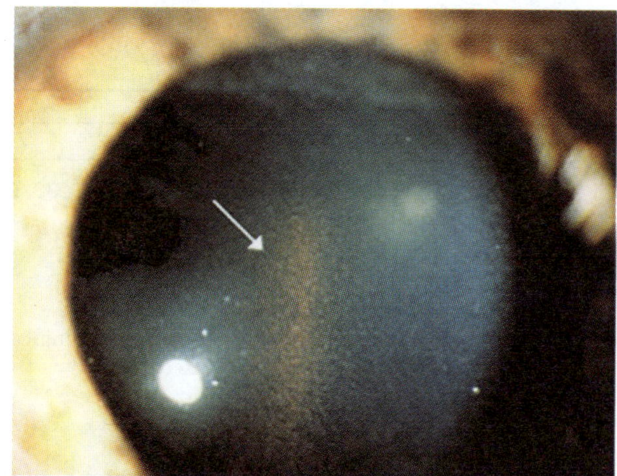

REFRACTIVE ERROR

257. Ans. (d) Corneal opacity

Ref: A.K. Khurana, 7th ed. pg. 138

- In developing countries like India vit A deficiency is the most common cause of blindness in children but corneal opacity causes loss of vision in children throughout world.
- MCC of vision loss in adults: Cataract

258. Ans. (b) Refractive error

Ref: A.K. Khurana, 7th ed. pg. 599

- Pin hole helps in confirming whether the optical correction in trial frame is correct or not.

- An improvement in visual acuity while looking through a pin hole indicates that optical correction in the trial frame is incorrect, and the possible cause of low vision is refractive error.

259. Ans. (a) Myopia

Ref: A.K. Khurana, 7th ed. pg. 41

- Biconcave lens is used for correction of myopia.

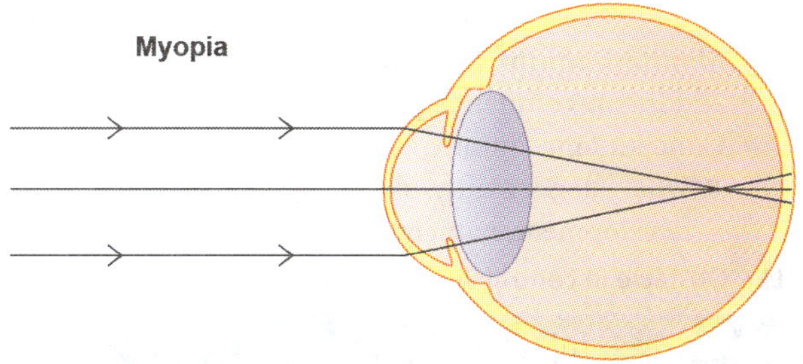

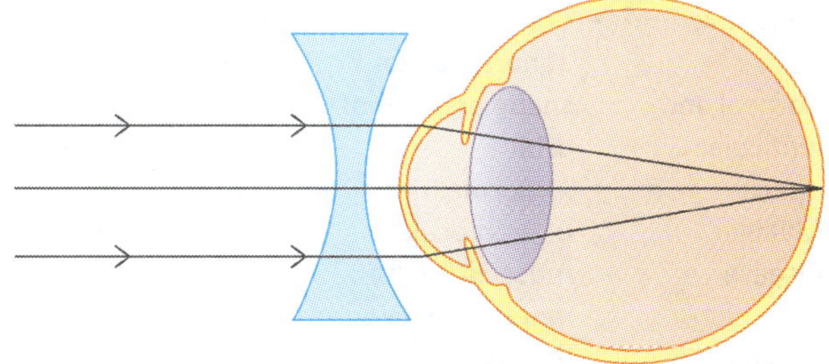

260. Ans. (d) Amblyopia

Ref: A.K. Khurana, 7th ed. pg. 344

Amblyopia implies a partial loss of sight in one or both the eyes, in the absence of ophthalmoscopic or other marked objective signs.

261. Ans. (b) Anisometropia

Ref: A.K. Khurana, 7th ed. pg. 44

- **Anisometropia** is the difference in vision between the two eyes and it interferes with normal binocular vision.

262. Ans. (b) Myopia

Ref: A.K. Khurana, 7th ed. pg. 34

- Myopia or shortsightedness is a type of refractive error in which parallel rays of light coming from infinity are focused in front of the retina where accommodation is at rest.
- A myopic child often presents with symptoms like:
  - Moving closer to TV
  - Squeezing eye while watching TV
  - Decreased performance at school
  - Headache or tired looking eyes
  - Blurred vision

263. Ans. (d) Astigmatism

Ref: A.K. Khurana, 7th ed. pg. 42

- The shown image is keratoconus (conical cornea), which is seen in patients with astigmatism.
- Astigmatism occurs when the cornea or lens is curved more steeply in one direction than in another.

264. Ans. (a) Anterior to retina

Ref: Comprehensive Ophthalmology by A.K. Khurana, 7th ed. pg. 38-39

- Near-sightedness, also known as short-sightedness and **myopia**, is an eye disorder where light focuses in front of, instead of on, the retina.
- This causes distant objects to be blurry while close objects appear normal.
- Other symptoms may include headaches and eye strain. Severe near-sightedness is associated with an increased risk of retinal detachment, cataracts, and glaucoma.

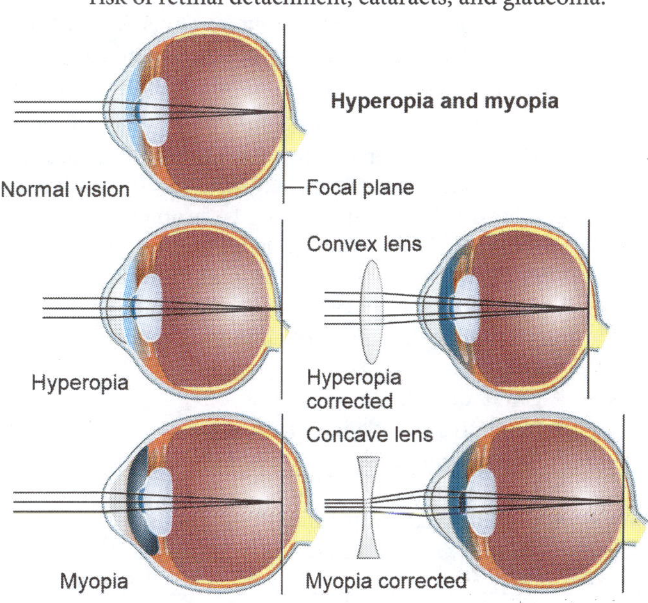

265. Ans. (a) Keratoconus

Ref: Comprehensive Ophthalmology by A.K. Khurana, 7th ed. pg. 136-37

- In keratoconus the patient presents with progressive myopia and irregular astigmatism due to change in the curvature of the cornea. The vision becomes more blurred and distorted which can be associated with colored halos glare and photo phobia.
- The patient presents with frequent change of glasses because of this progressive change.

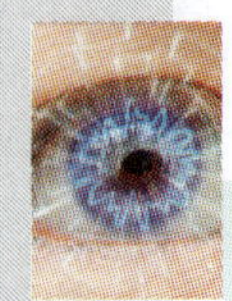

- Glaucoma also presents with frequent change of glasses but it is mostly a frequent change of presbyopic glasses in an elderly person.

266. Ans. (b) Squint surgery

Ref: Comprehensive Ophthalmology by A.K. Khurana, 7th ed. pg. 372

- Squint surgery usually involves tightening or moving one or more of the outside ocular muscles which move the eye to change the eye position.
- These muscles are attached quite close to the front of the eye under the conjunctiva, the clear surface layer. The eye is never taken out of the socket during surgery. Stitches are used to attach the muscles in their new positions.
- Muscle recession surgery means weakening the muscle and muscle resection surgery means strengthening the muscle.
- The **recession surgery** is done in **restrictive squint** whereas the **resection surgery** is done in the **paralytic squint**.

267. Ans. (c) Glaucoma

Ref: Comprehensive Ophthalmology by A.K. Khurana, 7th ed. pg. 500; https://www.ncbi.nlm.nih.gov/pmc/articles

- Vision 2020 "Right to Sight" was launched as a collaborative movement by World Health Organization (WHO) and International Agency for Prevention of Blindness (IAPB) [representing governments and non-governmental organizations] in Geneva on February 18, 1999.
- Vision 2020 has identified certain conditions which require immediate attention in India. These are:
  - Cataract
  - Childhood blindness
  - Refractive errors and low vision
  - Corneal blindness
  - Diabetic retinopathy and
  - Glaucoma (recently added)

268. Ans. (a) +2.5 D

Ref: Comprehensive Ophthalmology by A.K. Khurana 6th ed. pg. 13

- A newborn is hypermetropic by +2 to +3 D (average: 2.5 D)

EYE AT BIRTH

- **AP diameter:** 16.5 mm (adult size 24 mm by 7–8 years)
- **Corneal diameter:** 10 mm (adult size 11.7 mm 2 years)
- NB hypermetropic by 2–3 D
- Fixation starts at 1 month. Completed by 6 months
- **Retina:** Fully developed except macular area
  - Macula fully developed by 4–6 months
  - Fusional reflex and accommodation well developed by 4–6 months
  - 3D depth perception/stereopsis - 6 years
- **Lacrimal gland:** Underdeveloped (tears not secreted)
- **Anterior chamber:** Shallow and angle is narrow
- Orbit is more divergent (50°) as compared to adults (45°)

269. Ans. (d) All of the above

Ref: Comprehensive Ophthalmology by A.K. Khurana 6th ed. pg. 347-348

- **Manifest squint is of two types:** Concomitant squint and Incon-comitant squint.
- Concomitant squint:
  - Due abnormality/obstacle in binocular vision development, namely sensory, motor and central

TABLE: Obstacle in central vision development

Sensory obstacle	Motor obstacle	Central obstacle
• Refractive error • Corneal and lenticular opacity • Macular disease • Incorrect spectacle use • Optic atrophy	• Congenital abnormality of shape and size of orbit • Abnormalities of extraocular muscles (faulty innervation & insertion) • Abnormalities of accommodation and convergence	• Deficient development of fusion • Abnormality of cortical control of ocular movement (as seen in mental trauma, hyperexcitability of CNS)

270. Ans. (b) Amblyopia

Ref: Handbook of Pediatric Strabismus and Amblyopia edited by Kenneth W. Wright, Peter H. Spiegel, pg. 116

The visual deficit associated with amblyopia has certain unique characteristics, including the crowding phenomenon, the neutral density filter effect, and eccentric fixation. The crowding phenomenon relates to the fact that patients with amblyopia have better visual acuity reading single optotype than reading multiple optotypes in a row (linear optotypes). Often, patients with amblyopia will perform 1 or 2 Snellen lines better when presented with single optotypes versus linear optotypes. This crowding phenomenon may have something to do with the relatively large receptive field associated with amblyopia. Crowding bars are often used around a single optotype to provide a more sensitive test for amblyopia.

271. Ans. (a) Occlusion

Ref: Comprehensive Ophthalmology by Khurana; 6/ed. pg 63

- Amblyopia refers to a reversible decrease of vision, and is also referred as to lazy eye.
- Treatment of amblyopia should be started as early as possible, younger the child better is the prognosis.
- Occlusion therapy is the mainstay of therapy in which healthy eye is occluded to force the fixation of amblyopic eye.
- Before occlusion any opacity in the media should be removed and any refractive error should be corrected.
- However atropine penalization can also be done in better eye. Atropine causes cycloplegia and hence blurring of vision, which also forces the fixation of amblyopic eye.

272. Ans. (b) Head tilt towards the rectus muscle paralysis

Ref: Khurana, 6th ed. pg. 354

Paralytic squint

- Refers to ocular deviation resulting from complete or incomplete paralysis of one or more extraocular muscles.
- **Causes may be:** Neurogenic, myogenic or at the level of neuromuscular junction.

Clinical features:

Symptoms	Signs
• Diplopia: It is the main symptom and is more marked in the field of action of paralyzed muscle • Confusion • Nausea and vertigo • Ocular deviation	• **Primary deviation:** Deviation of the affected eye and is away from the action of paralyzed muscle. Eg: if medial rectus palsy, the eye is diverged. • **Secondary deviation:** Deviation of normal eye • **Ocular movement restriction:** Occurs in direction of action of paralyzed muscle • **Compensatory head posture:** In the direction of action of paralyzed muscle. It is adopted to avoid diplopia and confusion.

Note: *In case of paralytic squint, visual acuity is normal and there is no amblyopia as in most cases paralytic squint develops in adults when visual acuity has already developed.*

273. Ans (c) Refractive error

Ref: A.K. Khurana's Ophthalmology, 6th ed. pg. 34-36; Harrison's, 19th ed. pg. 195

- Most common cause of blindness in the world: Cataract
- Second Most common cause of blindness in world: Glaucoma> ARMD
- Most common infective cause of blindness: Trachoma
- Most common cause of ocular morbidity: Refractive error
- Given these choices, refractive error is the least common cause of blindness. **Harrison states:** *"Refractive errors usually develop slowly and* ***remain stable*** *after adolescence, except in unusual circumstances. For example, the acute onset of diabetes mellitus can produce sudden myopia because of lens edema induced by hyperglycemia."*
- Corneal opacities like Nebula, Macula and Leucoma also contribute significantly to blindness.

274. Ans. (b) Hypermetropia

Ref: A.K. Khurana's Ophthalmology, 6th ed. pg. 36

- Convex lens (plus lens) is used for treatment of hypermetropia.

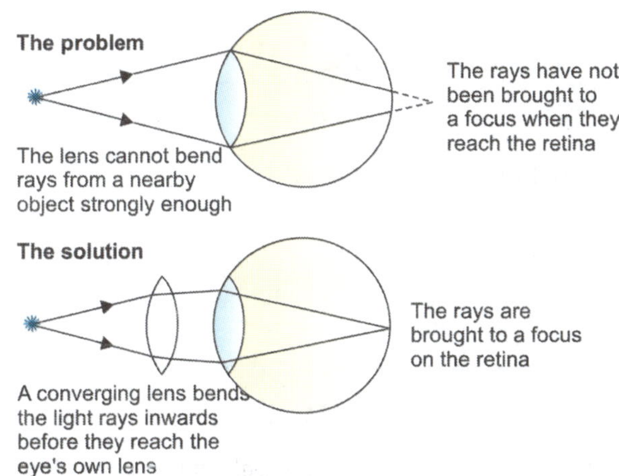

Extra Mile

- Lens used in myopia: Concave lens (Minus lens)
- Lens used in presbyopia: Convex lens

275. Ans. (d) 30°

Ref: A.K. Khurana's Ophthalmology, 6th ed. pg. 348

Concomitant squint is of three types:

- Convergent squint (esotropia)
- Divergent squint (exotropia)
- Vertical squint (hypertropia)

CONVERGENT SQUINT (ESOTROPIA)

- It denotes inward deviation of one eye. It is the most common type of squint in children

TYPES

- **Infantile esotropia**
  - **Clinical features:**
    - Age: Onset at 1–2 month, but can occur at any time in first 6 months of life
    - **Angle of deviation:** Usually constant and fairly large (>30°)

- Amblyopia in 25–40% of cases
- Fixation pattern: Binocular vision does not develop and there is alternate fixation in primary gaze and cross fixation in lateral gaze.

- TOC: Surgery
- Time for surgery: Between first 6 months to 2 years (preferable before 1 year of age).

- **Accommodative esotropia:** Develops at around 2–3 years of age. Associated with high hypermetropia (+4 to +7 D)
- **Acquired non-accomodative esotropia**
- **Sensory esotropia**
- **Consecutive esotropia**

276. Ans. (a) Large optic disc

Ref: A.K. Khurana, 6th ed. pg. 38

MYOPIA

- Also known as short sightedness.
- It is a type of refractive error in which parallel rays of light coming from infinity are focused in front of retina when accommodation is at rest.
- Myopic patients have short eyeballs.

Fundus Examination of Myopia

- *Optic disc appears large and pale* and at its temporal edge a characteristic myopic crescent is present
- Degenerative changes in retina and choroid are common in progressive myopia
- Posterior staphyloma at posterior pole may be apparent due to ectasia of sclera.
- Degenerative changes in vitreous include: liquefaction, vitreous opacities, and posterior vitreous detachment (PVD).

277. Ans. (a) Pseudomyopia

Ref: A.K. Khurana, 6th ed. pg. 47

"Accommodation refers to a process whereby a change in position as well **as increased curvature of the crystalline lens** increases the conjugation power of the eye i.e. its ability to **converge an image to focus on retina.**

From the above paragraph it can be concluded that more is the accommodation, more is the curvature of lens and the ray will converge more and hence image will be formed in front of retina i.e. pseudomyopia.

278. Ans. (b) Contact lens

Ref: A.K. Khurana, 6th ed.

- Anisometropic patients cannot wear glasses as it causes diplopic vision so contact lens are prescribed.
- Glasses can only tolerate and correct upto 4D.
- **Trabeculectomy:** It is a filtration surgery done in primary angle closure glaucoma.
- **Trabeculoplasty:** Primary open angle glaucoma is treated by Trabeculoplasty.

279. Ans. (b) Cylindrical

Ref: A.K. Khurana, 6th ed. pg. 42-423

- Astigmatism is a common eye condition that's easily corrected by eyeglasses, contact lenses, or surgery.
- It is caused by an eye that is not completely round. It is a type of refractive error.
- **Cause:** Astigmatism is a natural and commonly occurring cause of blurred or distorted vision. The exact cause in not known.
- **Symptom:** Blurring of vision which can be associated with fatigue and eyestrain.
- **Cylindrical lens** is used for the management of astigmatism.

Extra Mile

- Myopics are said to be short sighted. Concave lenses are used in myopics
- Convex lens are used in hypermetropics.

280. Ans. (c) Binocular vision

Ref: A.K. Khurana, 6th ed. pg. 342

- **Worth four dot test (WFDT)** is a test for binocular vision using red-green color dissociation.
- It is a dissociation test which can be used with both distance and near fixation and differentiate between binocular single vision, abnormal retinal correspondence and suppression.
- **Note:** Result of WFDT can only be interpreted if the presence or absence of manifest squint is known at the time of testing.

281. Ans. (c) Anisometropia

Ref: A.K. Khurana, 6th ed. pg. 44-45,
Khurana, 4th ed. pg. 38

- **Isometropia:** Two eye with equal refraction
- **Anisometropia:** Two eye with unequal refraction of power >2.5D
- **Aniseikoinia:** Difference in size/shape of image of >5% on visual cortex by retina.

282. Ans. (d) Astigmatism

Ref: A.K. Khurana, 6th ed. /42-43, Harrison's 19th ed./ 195

- Astigmatism is a type of refractive error which arises due to irregular curvature of cornea.
- Correction of astigmatism is done by using cylindrical lens.

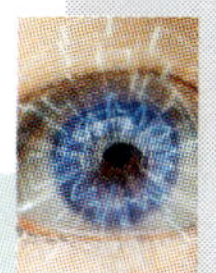

OCULAR INJURY AND MALIGNANCY

283. Ans. (a) Retinoblastoma

Ref: Kanski Clinical Ophthalmology, 9th ed. pg. 860

- Retinoblastoma is the most common primary intraocular malignancy of childhood
- Leukocoria (white pupillary reflex) is the commonest presentation
- Tumors are composed of small basophilic cells (retinoblasts) with large hyperchromatic nuclei and scanty cytoplasm
- Well-differentiated tumour shows abundant Flexner–Wintersteiner rosettes

284. Ans. (a) Fracture floor of orbit

Ref: Kanski Clinical Ophthalmology, 9th ed. pg. 894

- A blow-out fracture of the orbital floor is typically caused by a sudden increase in the orbital pressure from an impacting object that is greater in diameter than the orbital aperture.
- The common mechanisms are falls, high-velocity ball-related sports, traffic accidents, and interpersonal violence.
- The trauma mechanism is a blunt, directed force that may be aimed at the eye without a pressure component toward the eye rim, leading to an increase of pressure inside the orbit with a fracture of the bony structures.

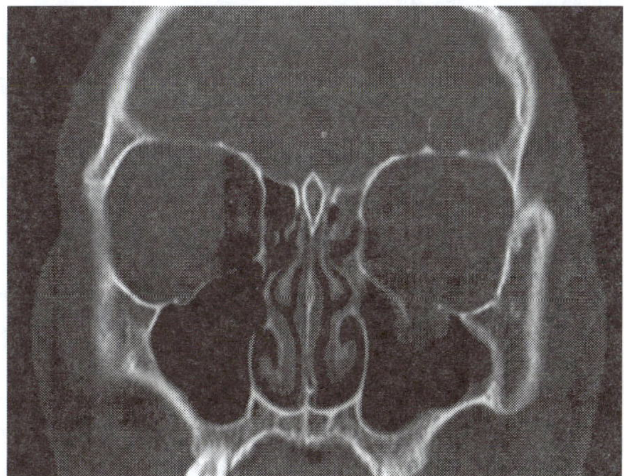

FIGURE: Tear drop sign on CT scan is characteristic finding of orbital floor fracture

285. Ans. (a) CT scan

Ref: A.K. Khurana, 7th ed. pg. 450

- CT scan is the investigation of choice for metallic FB.
- MRI is contraindicated for metallic FB.
- There is no significance of nuclear imaging here
- USG B scan is mainly done for the posterior segment of eyeball.

286. Ans. (b) Retinoblastoma

Ref: A.K. Khurana, 7th ed. pg. 314

- **Leucocoria** or yellowish white pupillary reflex is seen in the shown image. This also known as amaurotic cat's eye appearance.
- It is seen in retinoblastoma, a most common intraocular tumor among pediatric population.

287. Ans. (d) Optic neuritis

Ref: A.K. Khurana, 7th ed. pg. 335

- The given clinical feature suggests traumatic optic neuropathy.
- **Traumatic optic neuropathy** is of two types –direct and indirect.
- Characteristic features include:
  - Loss of vision
  - Dilatation of pupil
  - Loss of direct light reflex on affected side
  - RAPD

288. Ans. (a) Inferior orbital wall fracture

Ref: A.K. Khurana, 7th ed. pg. 455

- Punch/ball injury to eye commonly leads to orbital floor fracture
- Blow out fracture usually involves the floor of orbit.

Signs include:

- Periocular ecchymosis, edema
- Infraorbital nerve anesthesia
- Double diplopia

289. Ans. (c) Ciliary body

Ref: Khurana 7th ed. pg. 455

- Sympathetic ophthalmitis is Bilateral granulomatous panuveitis which follows a penetrating ocular trauma.
- In penetrating injury ciliary body injury is more common. Ciliary region the so-called dangerous zone is more prone to injury due to penetrating trauma.
- Wounds with incarceration of the iris, ciliary body or lens capsule are more vulnerable.
- Injured eye is exciting eye and the fellow eye also develops uveitis is called sympathizing eye.

Pathology

- Allergic theory is the most accepted theory which postulates that the uveal pigment acts as an allergen and excites plastic uveitis in the sound eye (normal eye).

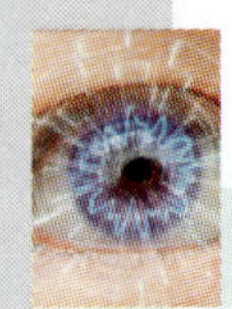

290. Ans. (a) Middle and inner

Ref: A.K. Khurana, 6th ed. pg. 173

- Eyeball has 3 layers: Sclera, Choroid and Retina
- Evisceration is removal of content of eyeball leaving behind the sclera (the outer layer).
- Frill evisceration is preferred over simple evisceration, where about 3 mm frill of the sclera is left round the optic nerve.

Indications:
- Panophthalmitis
- Expulsive choroidal hemorrhage
- Bleeding anterior staphyloma

Extra Mile

- **Enucleation** is excision of eyeball.
- In adults performed under local anaesthetics and in children under general anaesthetics
- **Indications:**
  - Retinoblastoma and Malignant melanoma
  - Painful blind eye
  - MC indication for enucleation: Eye donation from cadaver

291. Ans. (c) Retrolental flare

Ref: A.K. Khurana, 6th ed. pg. 437

- Sympathetic ophthalmitis is bilateral granulomatous panuveitis. It occurs as a result of penetrating ocular trauma (exciting eye), which can involve the contralateral eye (sympathizing eye) due to uveal pigment allergen released from the injured eye.
- **Symptom:**
  - Photophobia and transient indistinctness of near object
- **Signs:**
  - **First sign:** Presence of retrolental flare and cells or the presence of few keratic precipitates at the back of cornea.
  - Mild ciliary congestion
  - Edematous disc
- **Treatment:**
  - **Best prophylactic therapy:** Early excision of injured eye
  - **If there is hope of saving injured eye:** Repair the wound + topical and systemic steroid and antibiotics along with atropine
  - If no relief or photophobia, KP and lacrimation persist after 2 weeks of treatment → excise the injured eye immediately

292. Ans. (a) Only i and ii are correct

Ref: Comprehensive Ophthalmology by A.K. Khurana 6th ed. pg. 422-23

- Blow out fracture is comminuted fracture of orbital floor >> and medial wall.
- It result from trauma to orbit by relatively large, round object like tennis ball, cricket ball, human fist or a part of automobile.
- Orbit is made of 7 bones:
  - **Orbital floor**: Maxillary and palatine bone
  - **Medial wall:** Ethmoid and Lacrimal bone
  - **Lateral wall:** Zygomatic and Greater wing of sphenoid
  - **Roof:** Frontal bone
- **Clinical picture:**
  - Periorbital edema
  - **Paraesthesia and anaesthesia:** Over cheek, side of nose, lower eye-lid, upper lip due to involvement of infraorbital nerve.
  - **Enophthalmos:** Due to protrusion of orbital fat into maxillary *sinus (X-ray: Tear drop sign).*
  - **Diplopia:** Due to extraocular nerve entrapment
- **Treatment:**
  - Avoid nose blowing
  - Systemic antibiotics (as prophylaxis) and analgesics
  - Cold compress (decreases swelling by vasoconstriction)
  - Surgical repair of plate (10–14 days after injury)

293. Ans. (a) Tennis ball injury

Ref: Comprehensive Ophthalmology by A.K. Khurana 6th ed. pg. 422-23

Refer to above explanation

294. Ans. (a) Rhabdomyosarcoma

Common Malignancies of Eye
- ***Retinoblastoma is most common secondary intraorbital tumor of children***
- *Squamous cell CA is most common secondary orbital tumor of adult*
- ***Rhabdomyosarcoma** is most common primary malignant orbital tumor of children* and most common soft tissue malignancy of childhood.
- Lymphoma is the most common primary malignant orbital tumor of adult
- ***Choroid melanoma** is most common intraocular malignancy in adult*
- **Capillary hemangioma** is most common tumor of orbital & periorbital areas in children.
- **Cavernous hemangioma** is most common benign orbital tumor in adults.
- **Pleomorphic adenoma** (benign mixed tumor) is most common epithelial tumor of lacrimal gland.
- **Neuroblastoma** is *most common cause of orbital metastasis in children*

- **Breast** (> Bronchus > Prostate > Skin melanoma) is the most common cause of orbital metastasis in adult.
  - CA Breast (Female)
  - CA Breast (Male)
- **Choroid** is the most common site for metastasis (90%) followed by iris & ciliary body. *Metastatic tumors to choroid are more common than primary malignancies.*

295. Ans. (b) Orbital floor

- Orbital floor is made of maxillary and palatine bone. In case of orbital floor fracture, content of orbit protrudes into maxillary sinus which on radiological image is seen as tear drop.

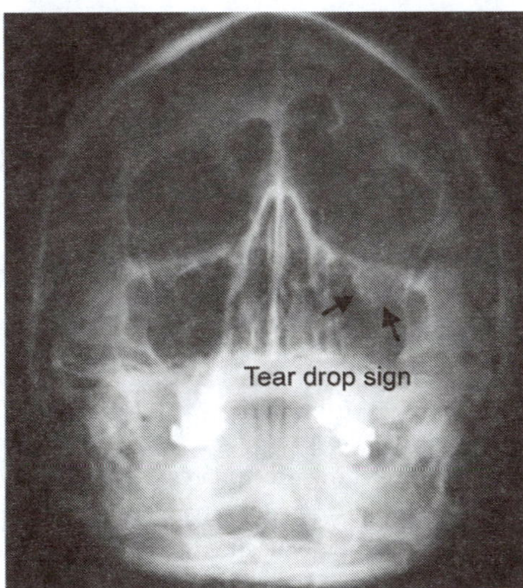

296. Ans. (a) RB gene

Ref: Khurana, 6th ed. pg. 303

- Retinoblastoma (RB) gene has been identified as 14 band on long arm of chromosome 13 (13q14) and is a cancer suppressor or antioncogenic gene. Deletion or inactivation of both the normal alleles of this protective gene by two mutation **(Knudson two hit hypothesis)** results in occurrence of retinoblastoma.

297. Ans. (d) Conservative

Ref: Khurana, 6th ed. pg. 429

- It is a case of traumatic hyphema (blood in anterior chamber).
- **Khurana states:** *"Conservative treatment is aimed at prevention of rise in IOP and occurrence of secondary haemorrhage. A small hyphaema usually clears up with conservative treatment, however a large non resolving hyphaema should be drained to avoid blood staining of cornea"*
- If hyphema is associated with rise in IOP, it can be lowered by acetazolamide and hyperosmotic agents.

298. Ans. (d) Keratometry

INSTRUMENTS USED FOR OCULAR EXAMINATION

Measurement parameter	Instruments for:
• Corneal thickness	Pachymeter
• Corneal curvature	Keratometer
• Angle of anterior chamber	Gonioscope
• Corneal surface	Placido disc
• Corneal endothelium	Specular microscope
• Direct ophthalmoscope **(Remembered as: "DEV")**	Routine fundus examination. *"Image formed is **Erect** and **Virtual** and magnified, 15 times"*
• Indirect ophthalmoscope	For assessment of retinal detachment and other peripheral retinal lesions. *The image is real, inverted and magnified 5 times.*
• Perimetry	Optic nerve function

299. Ans. (b) Optic nerve glioma

Ref: Khurana, 6th ed. pg. 419

Optic nerve glioma

- It is a slow growing tumor arising from the astrocytes, usually occurs in 1st decade of life in a child between 4-8 years of age.
- It may present either as a solitary tumor or as a part of von Recklinghausen neurofibromatosis.

Clinical features:

- It is characterized by gradual vision loss associated with a gradual, **painless unilateral axial proptosis.**
- **Fundus exam shows:** Optic atrophy or papilledema and venous engorgement.

Treatment: Observation, followed by surgical excision.

300. Ans. (a) Retinoblastoma

Ref: A.K. Khurana's Ophthalmology, 6th ed. pg. 303

COMMON MALIGNANCIES OF EYE

- ***Retinoblastoma** is most common intraocular (not orbital) malignancy in children (1 in 15000 to 20,000 live births)*
- *Retinoblastoma is confined to infancy and very young children usually seen between 1 and 2 years of age.*
- *Occurs bilaterally in 25–30% cases*

301. Ans. (a) Loss of accommodation

Ref: A.K. Khurana's Ophthalmology, 6th ed. pg. 355

FUNCTION OF OCULOMOTOR NERVE (CN.III)

- The third cranial nerve controls the movement of four of the six eye muscles. These muscles move the eye inward, up and down, and they rotate the eye. The third cranial nerve also controls constriction of the pupil, the positioning of the upper eyelid, and the ability of the eye to focus.
- *With unilateral third nerve palsy, diplopia is masked due to development of ptosis.*
- **Other findings:**
  1. Ptosis: Due to paralysis of LPS muscle
  2. Deviation: Eyeball is turned *downward and outward*
  3. Restricted ocular movements in all direction except outward.
  4. Fixed and dilated pupil: Due to paralysis of sphincter pupillae muscles.
  5. **Accommodation is completely lost** due to paralysis of ciliary muscle.

302. Ans. (b) Loss of accommodation

Ref: A.K. Khurana's Ophthalmology, 6th ed. pg. 147-48

FUNCTION OF CILIARY BODY

- Formation of aqueous humor (*by pars plicata*)
- Ciliary muscles helps in accommodation (*its damage leads to loss of accommodation*)

303. Ans. (b) Orbital apex

Ref: A.K. Khurana's Ophthalmology, 6th ed. pg. 413

- Tolosa hunt syndrome refers to idiopathic non-specific granulomatous inflammation involving the superior orbital fissure and/or orbital apex and/or cavernous sinus
- **Clinical presentation:**
  - Depending on the involvement of orbital, it can present as either orbital apex syndrome or as superior orbital fissure syndrome.
    - **Superior orbital fissure syndrome:** Symptoms depend on involvement of structure passing through the superior orbital fissure.
      - **CN V #:** Retroorbital pain, loss of sensation in ophthalmic division of CN V.
      - **CN III, IV, VI #:** Ipsilateral ophthalmoplegia
      - **CN III #:** Ptosis
  - **Orbital apex syndrome:** Symptoms are due to involvement of structure present at orbital apex. Optic nerve involvement causing early vision loss and afferent pupil defect plus symptoms of superior orbital fissure syndrome.

304. Ans. (b) Sympathetic ophthalmitis

Ref: A.K. Khurana, 6th ed. pg. 163, 437

- Sympathetic ophthalmitis is a serious bilateral granulomatous panuveitis which usually occurs due to penetrating trauma to ciliary body.
- The injured eye is called exciting eye.
- Fellow eye which also develops uvieitis is called sympathizing eye.

Features

- Always follows a penetrating wound.
- More common in children than in adults.
- It doesn't occur when actual suppuration develops in the injured eye

Pathologies

- Uveal pigment acts as allergen and excites plastic uveitis in the sound eye.
- Dalen-Fuchs' nodules are formed due to proliferation of the pigment epithelium (of the iris, ciliary body and choroid) associated with invasion by the lymphocytes and epithelioid cells.

Clinical Picture

- **Prodromal stage:** Sensitivity to light (photophobia) transient indistinctness of near objects is *the earliest symptoms.*
- *First sign* may be presence of retrolental flare or the presence of a keratic precipitates (KPs) at back of cornea.
- **Fully-developed stage**: Has typical signs and symptoms consistent with acute plastic iridocyclitis.
- **Dalen Fuch's Nodules** are characteristic of SO.
- **Exciting (injured) eye:** Keratic precipitates may be present at the back of cornea
- **Sympathizing (sound) eye:** Usually involved after 4-8 weeks of injury in the other eye.
- **Treatment** – Early excision of the injured eye.
  - Topical cycloplegics + IV/oral steroids are also used for treatment.

305. Ans. (c) Penetrating injury to Ciliary body

Ref: A.K. Khurana, 6th ed. pg. 163, 437

Please refer to above explanation.

306. Ans. (b) Hammer and chisel

Ref: A.K. Khurana, 6th ed. pg. 163, 437

307. Ans. (b) Trauma

Ref: A.K. Khurana, 6th ed. pg. 91, 335

SUBCONJUNCTIVAL HEMORRHAGE

- A subconjunctival hemorrhage is blood that is located between the conjunctiva and the underlying sclera.

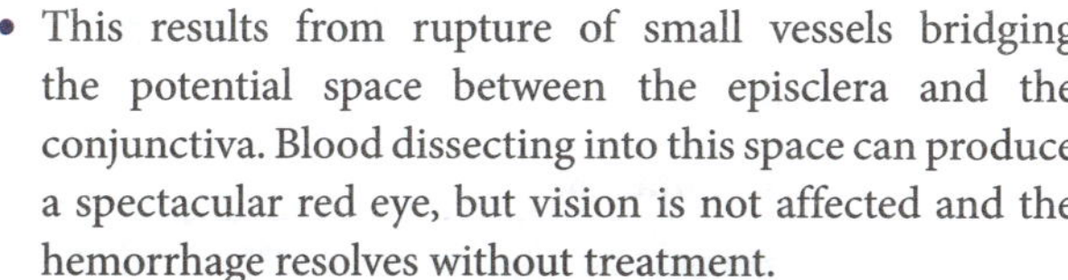

- This results from rupture of small vessels bridging the potential space between the episclera and the conjunctiva. Blood dissecting into this space can produce a spectacular red eye, but vision is not affected and the hemorrhage resolves without treatment.

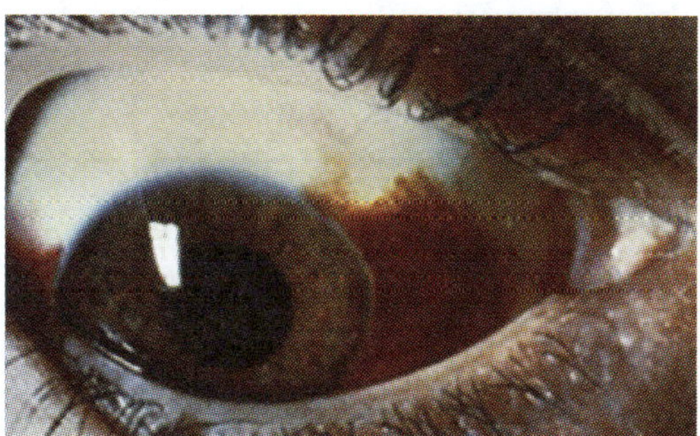

- Subconjunctival hemorrhage is usually spontaneous **but can result from blunt trauma**, eye rubbing, or vigorous coughing. Occasionally it is a clue to an underlying bleeding disorder.
- **Sx:** The most obvious sign of a subconjunctival hemorrhage is a bright red patch on the white (sclera) of your eye.
- Despite its bloody appearance, a subconjunctival hemorrhage should **cause no change in vision**, no discharge from eye and no pain.
- **Note:** *If trauma is not is option, the next best option you can choose is pertusis or chronic cough.*

308. Ans. (b) Optic disc

- Optic disc is not involved in papillary light reflex.
- Pathway of papillary light reflex:

> Retina → Optic Nerve → Optic Chiasma → Optic Tract → Prerectal Nucleus → Edinger Westphal Nucleus → Inferior Division of 3rd Nerve → Ciliary Ganglion → Short Ciliary Nerves → Sphincter Pupillae

309. Ans. (d) Exophthalmos

***Ref:* A.K. Khurana, 6th ed. pg. 422-23, Khurana's, 4th ed. pg. 397-398**

- *Blowout fractures mainly involve orbital floor and medial wall.*
- It usually result from trauma to the oribit by a relatively large, often rounded object, such as tennis ball, cricket ball etc.
- With a resultant fracture of the weakest point of the orbital wall.

Classification

- **Pure blow-out fractures:** Not associated with involvement of the orbital rim.
- **Impure blow-out fractures:** Associated with other fractures about the middle third of the facial skeleton.

Clinical Feature

- Periorbital edema and blood extravasation in and around the orbit
- Emphysema of the eyelids occurs more frequently with medial wall than floor fractures.
- Paraesthesia and anaesthesia
- Ipsilateral epistaxis
- Proptosis and Ptosis
- Enophthalmos; NOT Exophthalmos
- Diplopia

- **Plain X-rays** (Water's view): Fragmentation and irregularity of the orbital floor; depression of bony fragments and *'hanging drop/tear drop'* opacity of the superior maxillary antrum from orbital contents herniating through the floor.

310. Ans. (b) Neurofibromatosis

***Ref:* A.K. Khurana, 6th ed. pg. 309-10**

- In some patients who have neurofibromatosis type 1, multiple uveal nevi develop in both eyes. These lesions must be differentiated from the small, tan, melanocytic iris lesions **(Lisch nodules)** that arise multifocally from the anterior surface of the iris.
- Lisch nodules appear to be nodular aggregates of dendritic melanocytes and not true nevi.
- They usually become evident by the age of 10–15 years and are *highly characteristic of NF-1.*

311. Ans. (b) Basal carcinoma

***Ref:* A.K. Khurana, 6th ed. pg. 384**

BASAL CELL CANCER OR RODENT ULCER

- *It is the most common malignant tumor of the eyelid.*
- Most common site of origin of BCC: Lower eyelid followed by medial canthus.
- Noduloulcerative basal cell cancer is the most common presentation
- The treatment is done by surgical excision with primary repair.

312. Ans. (b) Pleomorphic adenoma

***Ref:* A.K. Khurana, 6th ed. pg. 399-400**

- Most common Epethilial tumor of lacrimal gland: Pleomorphic Adenoma (MC benign lacrimal gland tumor)
- Most common malignant eyelid tumor: Basal cell CA > Squamous cell CA
- Most common benign eyelid tumor: Papilloma

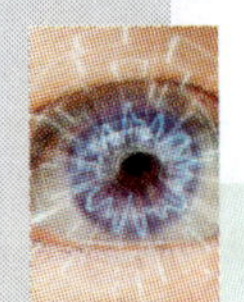

313. Ans. (b) Brain

Ref: A.K. Khurana, 6th ed. pg. 303-304

- The child is usually brought to the surgeon on account of a peculiar white reflex from the pupil, sometimes called leucocoria 'amaurotic cat's eye'.
- Other modes of presentation include a convergent or divergent squint, cataract, buphthalmos, a hypopyon or proptosis.
- If left untreated retinoblastoma runs through the same stages as melanoma of the choroid:
  - Quiescent stage, lasting from six months to a year
  - Glaucomatous stage
  - Stage of extraocular extension
  - Stage of metastasis
- Metastasis first occurs in the pre-auricular and neighbouring lymph nodes, later in the cranial and other bones.
- **Direct extension by-continuity to the optic nerve [which is affected early) and Brain is more common, while metastases in other organs, usually the liver are relatively rare.**
- Clinically cauliflower-like mass-arising from the retina is seen extending into the vitreous. There is neovascularization on the surface with white areas of calcification. Vitreous or anterior chamber seedings are seen as fluffy whitish-grey deposits. The endophytic type of retinoblastoma presents as an exudative retinal detachment.

314. Ans. (a) Esotropia

Ref: A.K. Khurana, 6th ed. pg. 303-304

NEURO-OPHTHALMOLOGY

315. Ans. (a) Optic neuritis

Ref: A.K. Khurana, 7th ed. pg. 329

Optic neuritis has 3 anatomical types:

- Papillitis
- Neuroretinitis
- Retrobulbar neuritis

316. Ans. (b) Occlusion

Ref: A.K. Khurana, 7th ed. pg. 344

Occlusion therapy using an eye patch to cover the non-amblyopic eye for a couple of hours each day.

317. Ans. (c) Mucormycosis

- Clinical features and positive RT-PCR is suggestive of infection by mucormycosis is a fungal infection caused by zygomycetes.
- Symptoms include: Fever, headache, shortness of breath etc.
- Complications include blindness, organ dysfunction, or death.

318. Ans. (c) Occipital cortex

- Homonymous hemianopia is seen if there is lesion at the site of optic tract
- Homonymous hemianopia sparing macula is seen if there is lesion in occipital cortex.

319. Ans. (c) Trochlear nerve

Ref: A.K. Khurana, 7th ed. pg. 349

- In the shown image right eye remain fixed upon moving the object to left lower quadrant. The muscle involved in such movement is superior oblique muscle. Nerve supplying superior oblique muscle is CN-IV (Trochlear nerve).
- Function of superior oblique: Inferior and Abduction
- The given image is of TROCHLEAR NERVE PALSY.
- Trochlear nerve supplies superior oblique muscle.

320. Ans. (c) Herpes zoster

Ref: Khurana 7th ed. pg. 113-14

- This is looking like herpes zoster infection.
- **Hutchinson's rule:** It implies that ocular involvement is frequent if the side or tip of nose presents vesicles, this is due to cutaneous involvement of nasociliary nerve.

321. Ans. (a) Retinoblastoma

Ref: Comprehensive Ophthalmology by A.K. Khurana, 7th ed. pg. 314-15

- The shown histopathological image is Flexner-Wintersteiner rosettes, which is a characteristic finding of retinoblastoma.
- Retinoblastoma (Rb) is a rare form of cancer that rapidly develops from the immature cells of a retina, the light-detecting tissue of the eye.
- It is the most common primary malignant intraocular cancer in children, and it is almost exclusively found in young children.
- Almost half of children with retinoblastoma have a hereditary genetic defect associated with retinoblastoma.
- In other cases, it is caused by a congenital mutation in the chromosome 13 gene 13q14 (retinoblastoma protein).

322. Ans. (b) Horner syndrome

Ref: Comprehensive Ophthalmology by A.K. Khurana, 7th ed. pg. 395

- Horner's syndrome, also known as oculosympathetic paresis, is a combination of symptoms that arises when a group of nerves known as the sympathetic trunk is damaged.

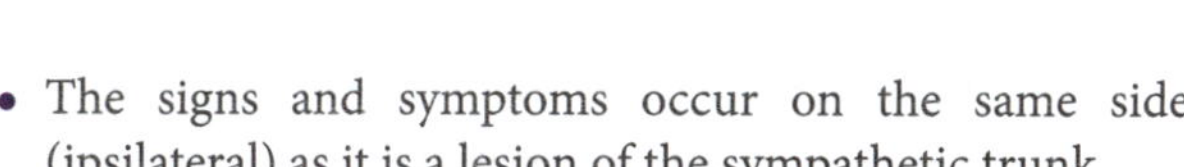

- The signs and symptoms occur on the same side (ipsilateral) as it is a lesion of the sympathetic trunk.
- It is characterized by miosis (a constricted pupil), partial ptosis (a weak, droopy eyelid), apparent anhidrosis (decreased sweating), with apparent enophthalmos (inset eyeball).

323. Ans. (d) Posterior cerebral artery

Ref: Comprehensive Ophthalmology by A.K. Khurana, 7th ed. pg. 326-27

- The medial face of the visual cortex receives branches from the posterior cerebral artery (throughout its collaterals: calcarine artery, parieto-occipital artery and posterior temporal artery.
- Its lateral surface receives cortical branches from the middle cerebral artery and its inferior surface is irrigated from collaterals of the posterior temporal and temporo-occipital arteries.
- Some of the branches penetrate directly the visual cortex perpendicularly and others form at first, a superficial, pial network.

324. Ans. (b) Bitemporal hemianopia

- Any optic chiasmal lesion like pituitary adenoma, will cause bitemporal hemianopia.
- Detailed image and description of this is discussed in neuro-ophthalmology section of this book.

325. Ans. (a) Ipsilateral mydriasis

Ref: A.K. Khurana, 6th ed. pg. 335

Ocular signs in head injury can be seen due to concussion injury or base of skull bone fracture.

Concussion Injury: Associated with subdural hemorrhage and unconsciousness, and produces following ocular signs:	**Fractured skull base** • **Cranial nerve palsies:** Commonly associated with fractured base of skull. MC being ipsilateral facial paralysis of lower motor neuron type.
• **Hutchinson pupil:** Characterized by ipsilateral miosis followed by mydriasis, with no light reflex due to raised ICP. • **Papilledema:** If occurs within 48 hours of trauma → indicates extra or intracerebral hemorrhage. If occurs after a week of head injury, it is usually due to cerebral edema	• **Optic nerve injury:** Can cause optic nerve atrophy 2-4 weeks after injury • Subconjunctival Hemorrhage • **Pupillary signs:** Inconsistent sign. Pupil size is usually dilated on the affected side.

326. Ans. (c) Oculomotor paralysis

Ref: A.K. Khurana, 6th ed. pg. 504

TABLE: Condition causing miosis and mydriasis

Causes of miosis	Causes of mydriasis
• Parasympathomimetic drugs	• Topical sympathomimetic drug (phenylephrine)
• Systemic morphine	• Topical parasympatholytics (atropine)
• Iridocyclitis (irregular, non-reactive pupil)	• Acute congestive glaucoma; Absolute glaucoma
• Horner's syndrome	• Optic atrophy
• Head injury (pontine hemorrhage)	• Retinal detachment
• As an effect of strong light	• CN 3 (oculomotor nerve) palsy
• During sleep	• Belladonna poisoning

327. Ans. (d) Temporal lobe lesion

Ref: A.K. Khurana, 6th edit pg 314

- Superior quadrantic hemianopia is also termed as *"pie in the sky"*.
- It is produced when inferior fibres are involved in temporal lobe lesions. Inferior most fibres of optic radiation form the so called Meyer's loop.
- Remember, inferior fibres of optic radiations contain fibres from ipsilateral lower temporal retina and contralateral lower nasal retina.
- Inferior quadrantic hemianopia is *"pie on the floor"*. It is produced when superior fibres are involved in parietal lobe lesions
- Other choices like pituitary adenoma (MCC), craniopharyngioma and meningioma are the causes of chiasmal lesions, which causes bitemporal hemianopia.

Lesion of parietal lobe (Pie on floor)

Inferior quadrantic hemianopia

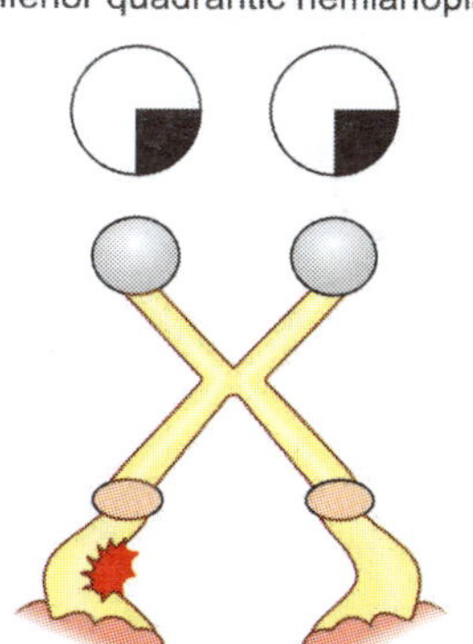

Lesion of temporal lobe (Pie on sky)

Superior quadrantic hemianopia

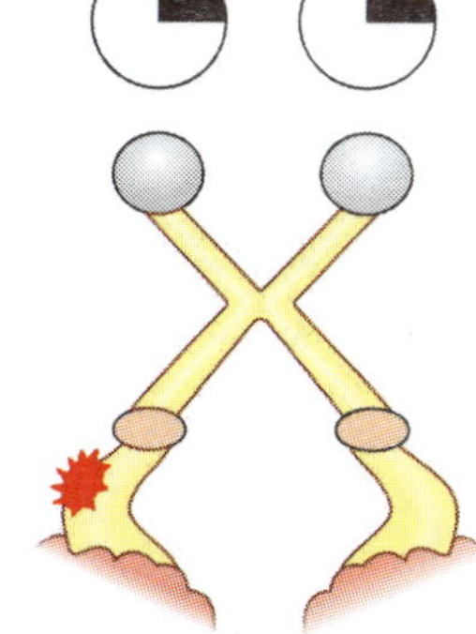

328. Ans. (a) Bitemporal hemianopia

Ref: A.K. Khurana, 6th ed. pg. 312

- An optic chiasmal lesion can cause bitemporal hemianopia.

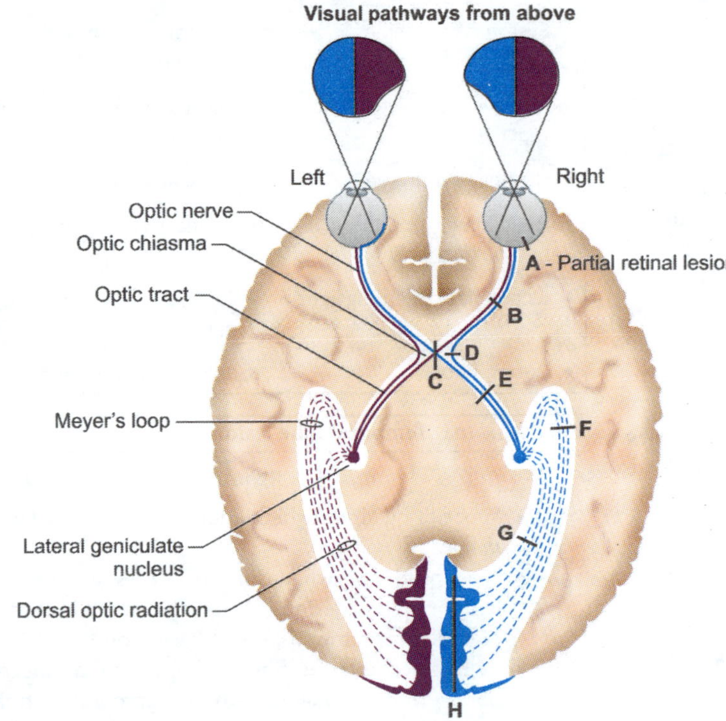

A. Monocular scotoma
B. Right anopia
C. Bitemporal hemianopia
D. Right nasal hemianopia
E. Left homonymous hemianopia
F. Left homonymous superior quadrantanopia ("Pie in the sky")
G. Left homonymous inferior quadrantanopia ("Pie on the floor")
H. Left homonymous hemianopia with macular sparing

329. Ans. (a) Weber syndrome

Ref: A.K. Khurana, 6th ed. pg. 334

- **Weber syndrome:** Characterized by ipsilateral CN 3 palsy, contralateral hemiplegia and facial palsy of upper motor neuron type.
- **Benedict's syndrome:** Characterized by ipsilateral CN 3 palsy associated with tremors and jerky movements of the contralateral side due to involvement of the red nucleus.
- **Millard-Gubler syndrome:** Consist of ipsilateral CN 6 palsy, contralateral hemiplegia and ipsilateral facial palsy.
- **Foville's syndrome:** CN 6th paralysis is replaced by a loss of conjugate movement on the same side.
- **Terson syndrome:** Combination of bilateral intraocular hemorrhages and subarachnoid hemorrhage due to aneurysmal rupture.

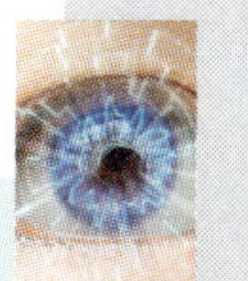

330. Ans. (b) Pituitary adenoma

Ref: A.K. Khurana's Ophthalmology, 6th ed. pg. 313-14

Type of visual field defect

1. **Unilateral blindness:** U/L optic nerve lesion
2. **Bitemporal hemianopia**: Optic chiasmal lesion *(ex: Pituitary adenoma).*
   - **Binasal hemianopia:** 2 separate lesion at chiasma laterally
4. **Homonymous hemianopia:** Lesion at U/L optic tract.
5. **Superior quadrantopia**: Temporal lobe lesion *(pie on the sky).*
6. **Inferior quadrantopia**: Parietal Lobe lesion *(pie on the floor)*
7. **Homonymous hemianopia with macular sparing**: Occipital lobe lesion

Site of lesion

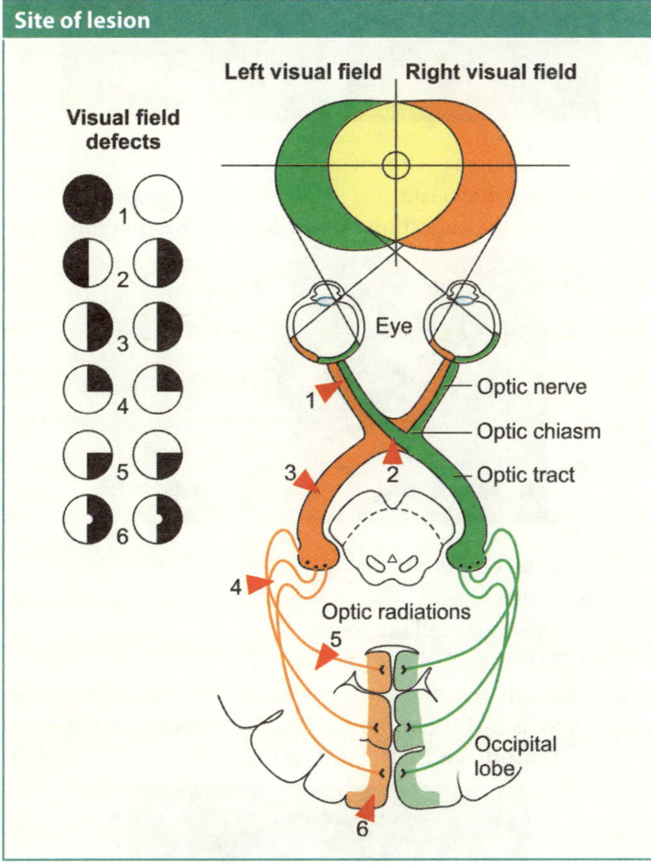

331. Ans. (b) Red green

Ref: A.K. Khurana, 6th ed. pg. 329

- Optic neuritis, the most serious adverse effect reported due to ethambutol toxicity, typically presents as reduced visual acuity, central scotoma, and loss of the ability to see green (or, less commonly, red).
- *Please refer to pharmacology section for detailed discussion on ATT and their side effect.*

332. Ans. (d) Fasanella servat operation

Ref: A.K. Khurana, 6th ed. pg. 381

- **Fasanella-servat operation** or Tarso-conjunctivo-mullerectomy is the surgery of choice for ptosis due to Horner syndrome: as the ptosis in Horner syndrome is mild (2 mm) and is due to Muller's muscle dysfunction (sympathetic supply)
- **Sling surgery** is done in severe ptosis with poor Levator action. Here the ptosis is mild so sling is not advised
- Levator resection upto 15 mm strengthens levator muscle and is done to correct mild degree of ptosis. If fasanella Servat operation is not provided, that it is the best correct option.

333. Ans. (b) Lateral rectus

- In raised intracranial tension, the nerves affected are the ones which have long intracranial course leading to false localizing signs. Since the CN VI emerges straight from the brainstem (while others originate obliquely), this nerve is more liable to get affected in increased intracranial pressure.
- CN VI supplies, lateral rectus muscle. Hence lateral rectus muscle is the first one to be affected in increased ICP.

DERMATOLOGY

16

MOST RECENT QUESTIONS 2023

1. A 50-year-old man came with the lesions as shown in the image. On examination, painful and swollen fingers noted along with inflamed wrist joint. What is the most likely diagnosis? ***(Most Recent Question July 2023)***

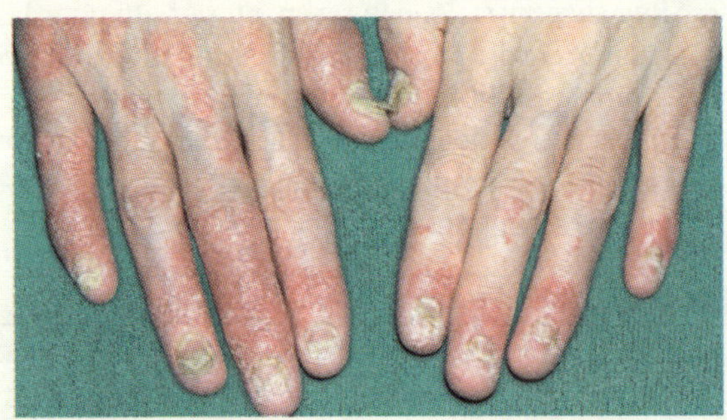

a. Reactive arthritis
b. Psoriatic arthritis
c. Osteoarthritis
d. Pseudogout

2. A patient presented with shown lesions to a physician and he is treated with topical steroids. What is this condition called? ***(Most Recent Question July 2023)***

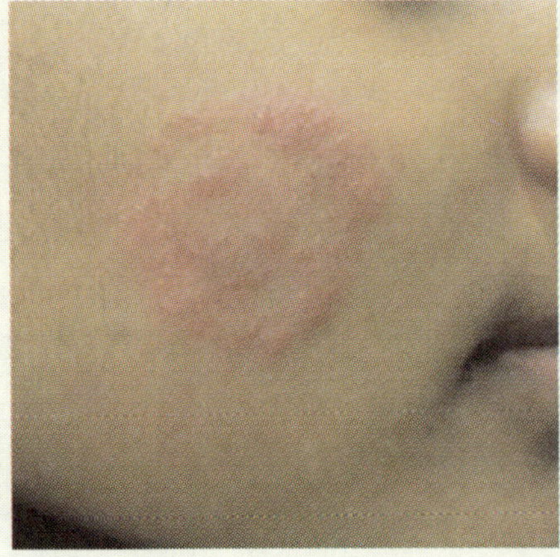

a. Tinea corporis b. Tinea cruris
c. Tinea incognito d. None of the above

3. Identify the condition: ***(Most Recent Question July 2023)***

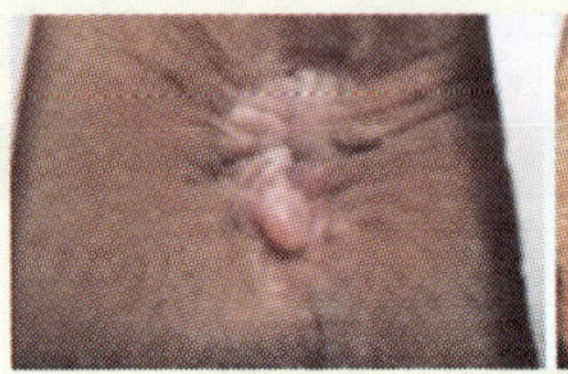
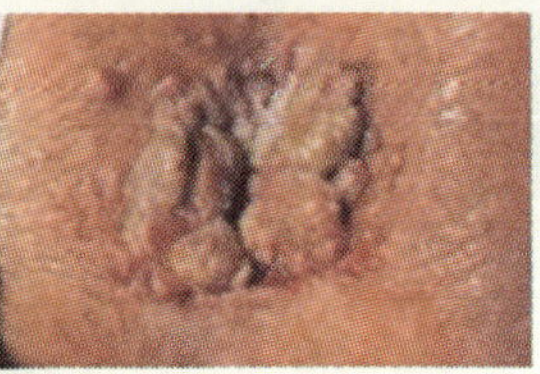

a. Condyloma acuminata b. Herpes genitalis
c. Condyloma lata d. Hemorrhoids

4. Identify the condition: ***(Most Recent Question July 2023)***

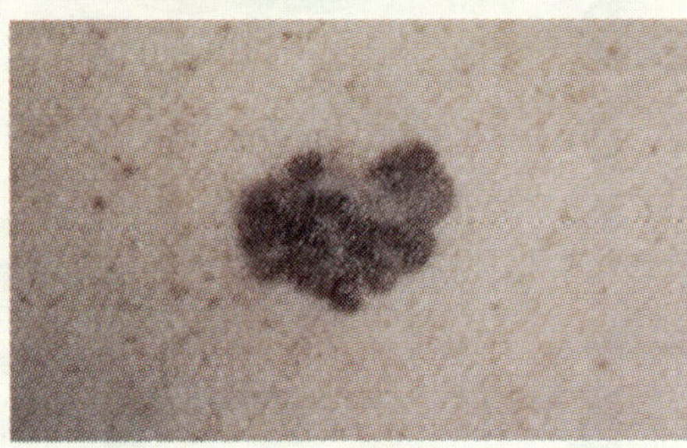

a. Basal cell carcinoma
b. Melanoma
c. Squamous cell carcinoma
d. Malignant nevus

5. A patient presents with the shown condition as in image. There is history of burn around 3 years ago, what is the probable diagnosis? ***(Most Recent Question July 2023)***

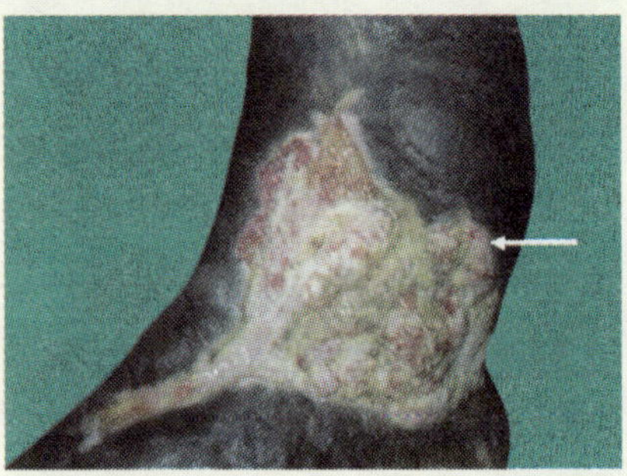

a. Marjolin's ulcer b. Diabetic ulcer
c. Chronic burn lesion d. Buerger's disease

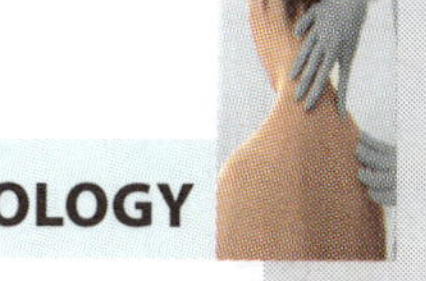

6. A patient presents with multiple blisters on an erythematous base. Along a dermatome on the trunk as shown in the image. Diagnosis is: ***(Most Recent Question Jan 2023)***

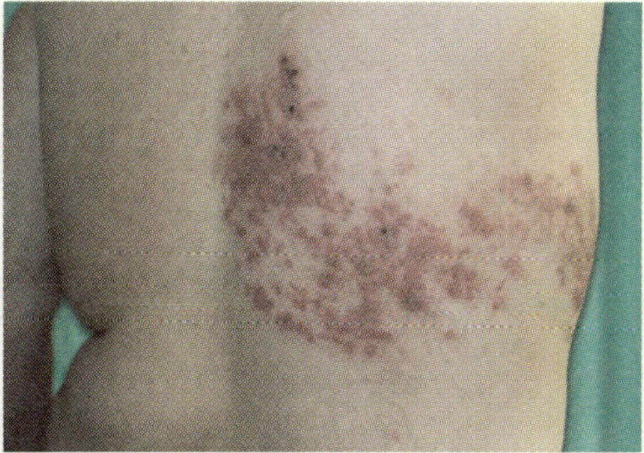

a. Herpes simplex
b. Herpes zoster
c. Molluscum contagiosum
d. Chicken pox

7. A 3-month child is presented to the hospital with the bright red birth mark as shown in the image, what will be the diagnosis? ***(Most Recent Question Jan 2023)***

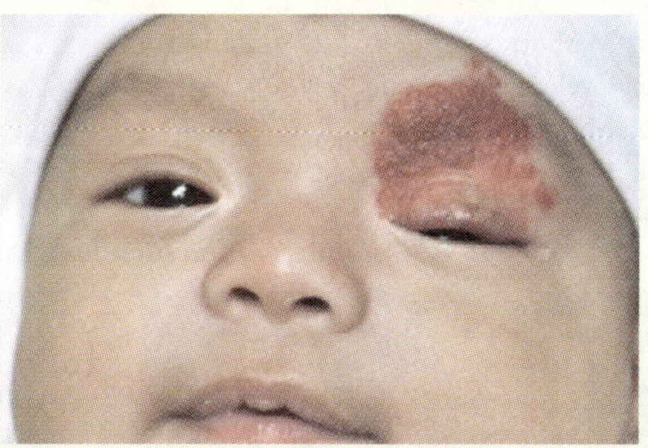

a. Capillary hemangioma
b. Molluscum contagiosum
c. Chicken pox
d. Herpes zoster

8. A 29-year-old female presents to the dermatological OPD as shown here, what is the finding? ***(Most Recent Question Jan 2023)***

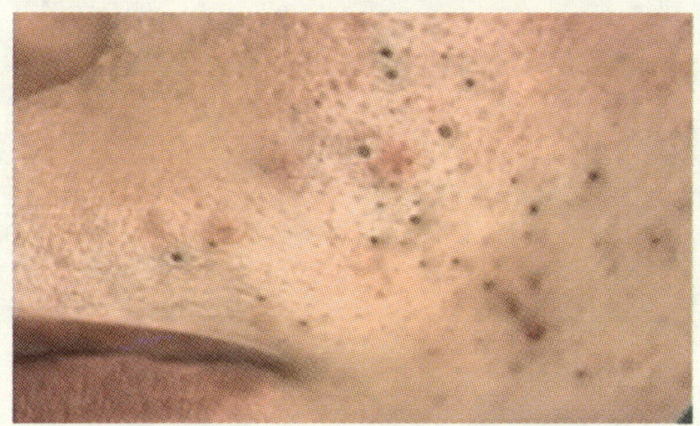

a. Comedones
b. Papules
c. Pustules
d. Abscess

9. A 50-year-old presents to the dermatology OPD with the white patchy lesions as shown in the image here, what is the diagnosis? ***(Most Recent Question Jan 2023)***

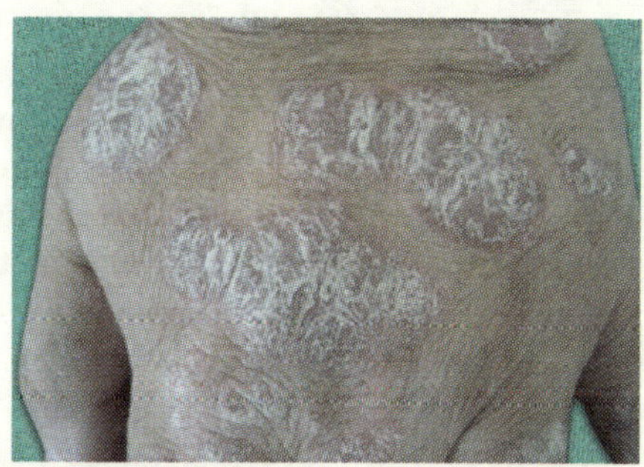

a. Psoriasis
b. Fungal infection
c. Secondary syphilis
d. Maculopapular drug eruptions

10. Koebner's phenomenon is seen in all; EXCEPT: ***(Most Recent Question June 2022)***

a. Vitiligo
b. Psoriasis
c. Lichen planus
d. Herpes

11. Identify the variant of psoriasis in the image below: ***(Most Recent Question June 2022)***

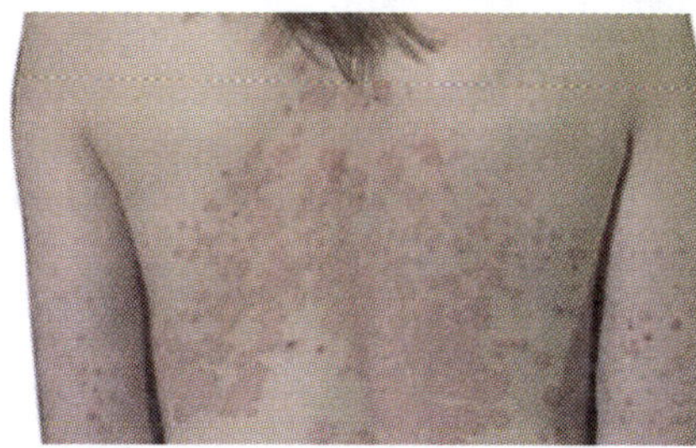

a. Guttate
b. Erythrodermic
c. Pustular
d. Inverse

12. Identify the given condition? ***(Most Recent Question June 2022)***

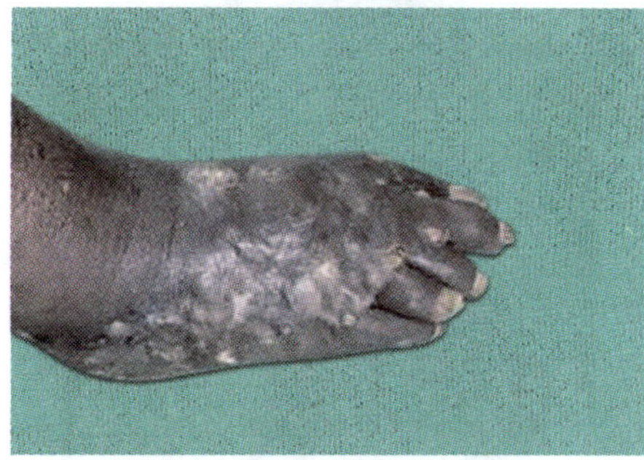

a. Madura foot
b. Chromoblastomycosis
c. Tuberculosis verrucosa cutis
d. Cellulitis

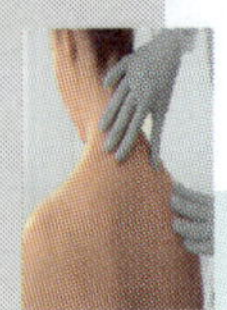

13. Neurofibromatosis type 1 (NF1) is a hereditary condition commonly associated with multiple café-au-lait spots on the skin. Which pattern of inheritance seen in this?

(Most Recent Question June 2022)

a. Autosomal dominant
b. Autosomal recessive
c. X linked dominant
d. X linked recessive

14. A 25-year-old female came with chief complaint of vaginal discharge with lower abdominal pain and tenderness, which color kit will you prescribe to her?

(Most Recent Question June/Dec 2021)

a. Grey kit (Kit 1)
b. Red Kit (Kit 5)
c. Yellow kit (kit 6)
d. Black kit (kit 7)

15. A patient came to OPD with complaints of diarrhea, dermatitis and mental retardation. It was also found that he was maize eater. Which of the following could be most probable diagnosis?

(Most Recent Question June/Dec 2021)

a. Beri Beri
b. Night blindness
c. Pellagra
d. Kwashiorkor

16. All are seen in lichen planus; EXCEPT?

(Most Recent Question June/Dec 2021)

a. Munro microabscess/kogoj
b. Gestational diabetes mellitus
c. Saw tooth acanthosis
d. Civatte bodies/shiny plaques

17. Patient on treatment with 13-cis-retinoic Acid. Which of the following is a known side effect on the drug?

(Most Recent Question June/Dec 2021)

a. Teratogenic
b. Neural tube defect
c. Follicular hyperkeratosis
d. Photo onycholysis

18. A patient presented with hypopigmented macules over back and upper trunk. KOH mount shows spaghetti and meat ball appearance. What can be the causative agent?

(Most Recent Question June/Dec 2021)

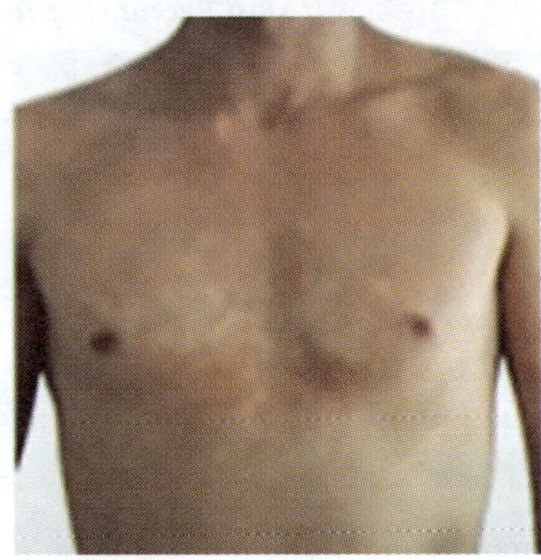

a. Malassezia furfur
b. Tinea Nigra
c. Trichosporon
d. Candida

19. Patient presented with lesion as shown in the image below, later patient also developed arthritis. What is the treatment? ***(Most Recent Question June/Dec 2021)***

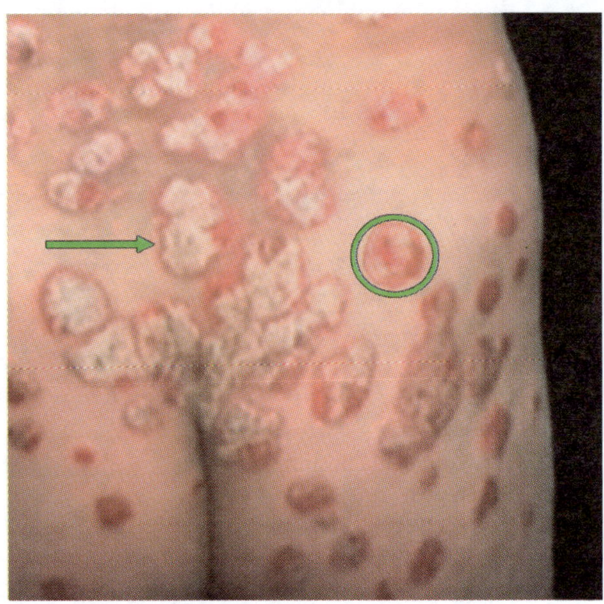

a. Methotrexate
b. Cyclophosphamide
c. Mycophenolate mofetil
d. Rituximab

20. Identify the condition:

(Most Recent Question June/Dec 2021)

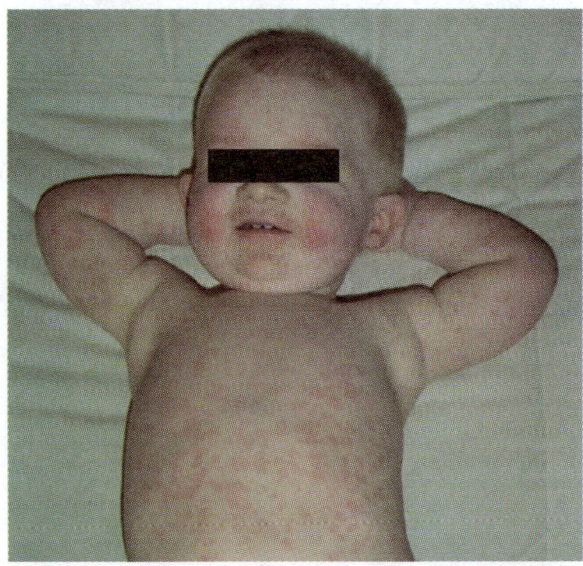

a. 1st disease
b. 5th disease
c. 6th disease
d. 3rd disease

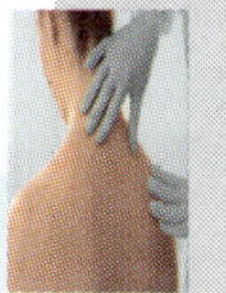

21. A patient presented with the following lesion. What is the most likely diagnosis?

(Most Recent Question June/Dec 2021)

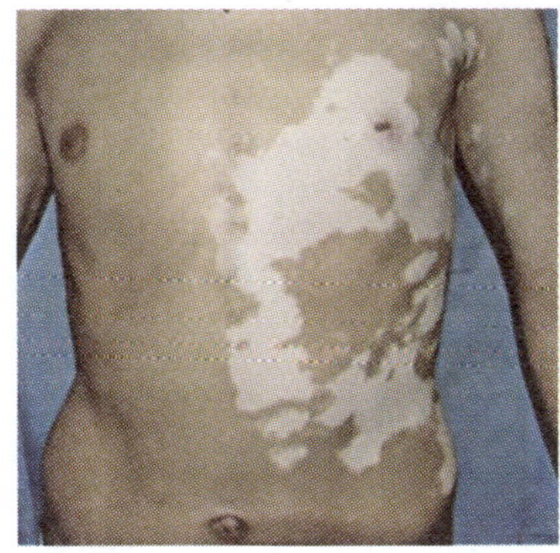

a. Nevus of ITO
b. Becker's nevus
c. Hypomelanosis of Ito
d. Segmental vitiligo

22. What could be the diagnosis for this image where exclamation mark is seen in Trichoscopy?

(Most Recent Question June/Dec 2021)

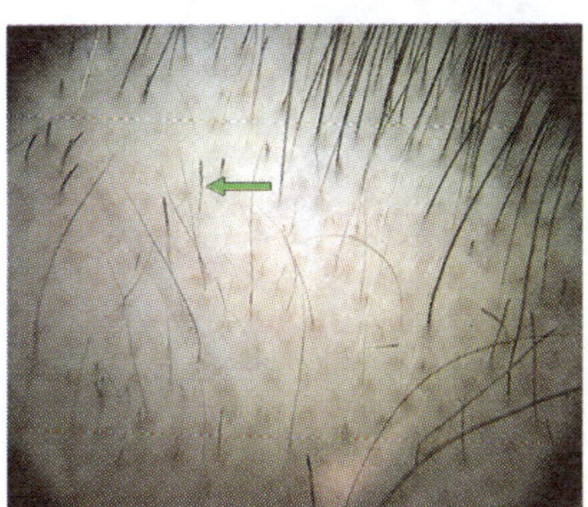

a. Telogen effluvium
b. Trichotillomania
c. Anagen effluvium
d. Alopecia areata

23. A 70-year-old patient develop the following lesion over face for 2 years. What is the possible diagnosis?

(Most Recent Question June/Dec 2021)

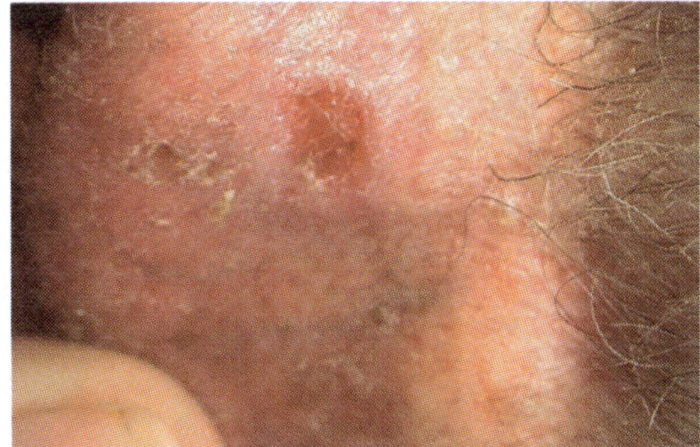

a. Malignant melanoma
b. Keratoacanthoma
c. Basal cell carcinoma
d. Squamous cell carcinoma

24. A young lady presents with following lesion in the oral cavity. What is the diagnosis?

(Most Recent Question June/Dec 2021)

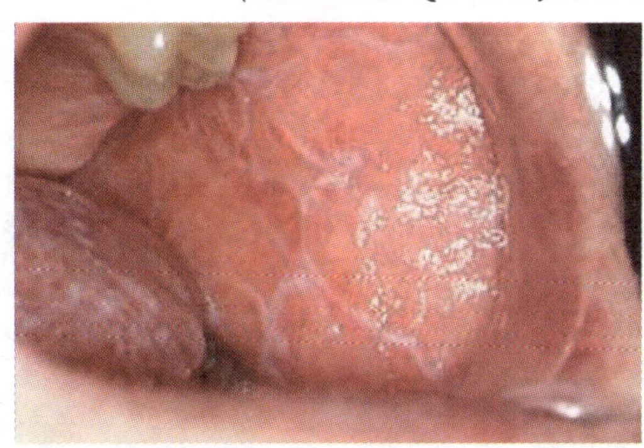

a. Lichen planus
b. Oral leukoplakia
c. Candidiasis
d. Psoriasis

25. Auspitz sign is seen in?

(Most Recent Question Aug 2020)

a. Pemphigus vulgaris
b. Psoriasis vulgaris
c. Pustular psoriasis
d. DLE

26. Ulcer "with overhanging/undermined edges" in the neck region as shown in the image given below. Diagnosis?

(Most Recent Question Aug 2020)

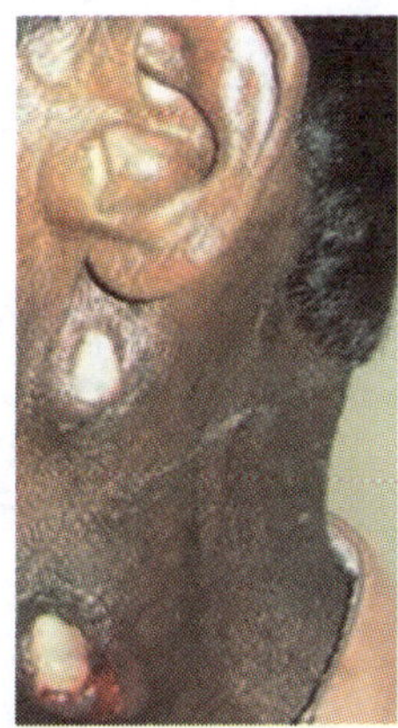

a. Tubercular lymph node
b. Malignant Cervical lymphadenopathy
c. Syphilis
d. Reactive lymphadenopathy

27. Which mineral deficiency can lead to following condition? ***(Most Recent Question Aug 2020)***

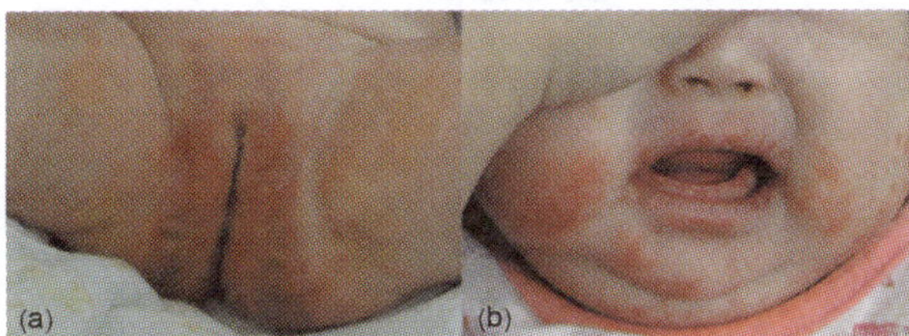

a. Zinc
b. Iron
c. Calcium
d. Vitamin

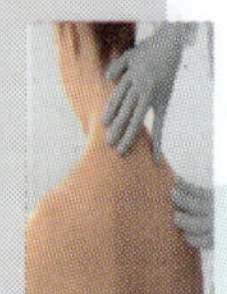

28. **First line treatment for acne comedones as shown in image:** ***(Recent Pattern Question Aug 2020)***

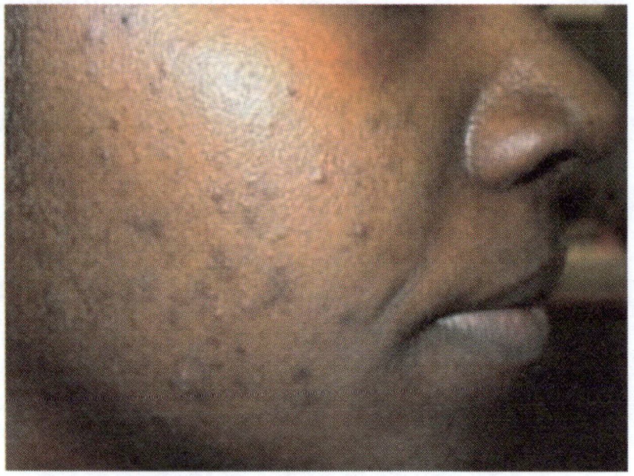

a. Topical steroid b. Topical antibiotics
c. Benzyl peroxide d. Topical retinoids

29. **A 20 year patient presented with the shown condition. The lesion increased in size and shape in last few weeks. Identify the condition shown in the image?** ***(Most Recent Question Aug 2020)***

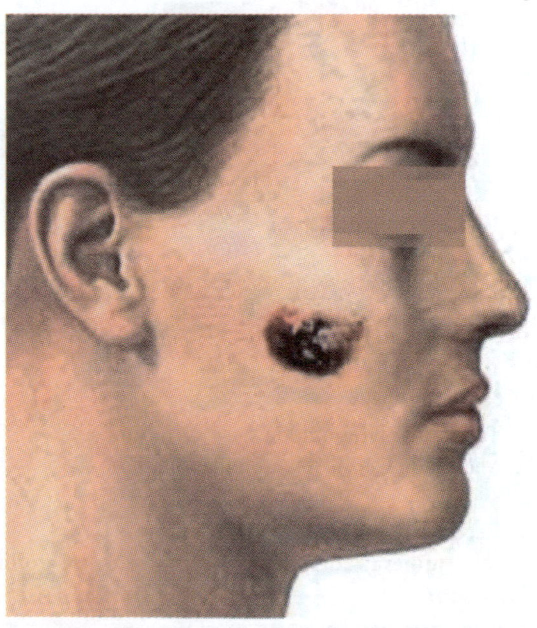

a. Malignant melanoma
b. BCC
c. Squamous cell carcinoma
d. Nevus pilus

30. **Organism responsible for causing erysipelas:** ***(Most Recent Question Aug 2020)***

a. Streptococcus b. Staphylococcus
c. Bacteroides d. Fungus

31. **Cutaneous horn as shown in the image is associated with which of the following skin cancer?** ***(Most Recent Question Aug 2020)***

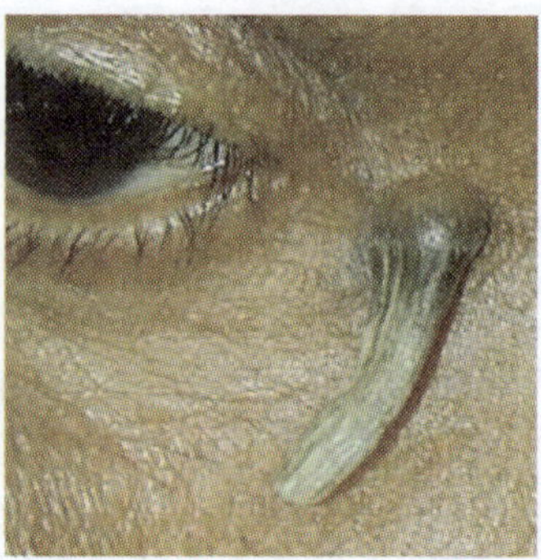

a. Squamous cell carcinoma
b. Melanoma
c. BCC
d. Actinic keratosis

32. **Identify the condition shown in the image?** ***(Most Recent Question Aug 2020)***

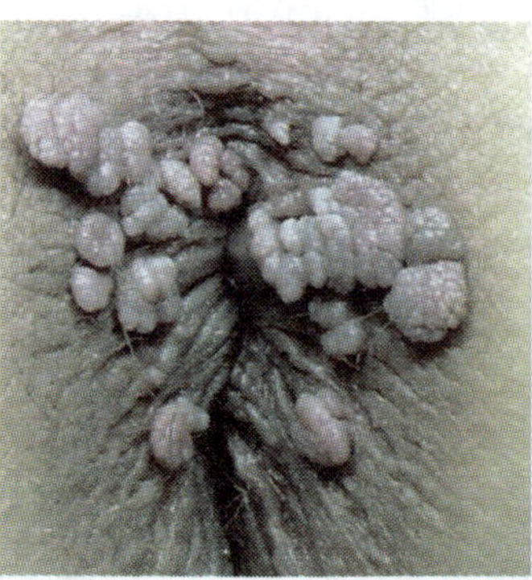

a. Condyloma acuminata b. Bowen disease
c. Condyloma lata d. Hemorrhoids

33. **Patient suffering from ulcerative colitis presents with ulcer on anterior leg as shown in the image. Diagnosis:** ***(Most Recent Question Aug 2020)***

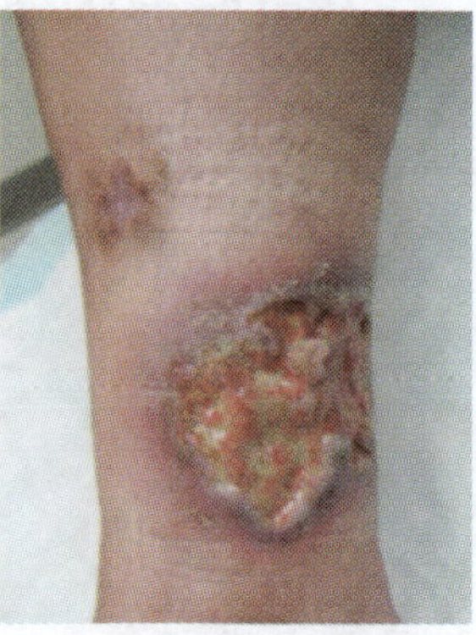

a. Pyoderma gangrenosum b. Venous ulcer
c. Tubercular ulcer d. Chancroid

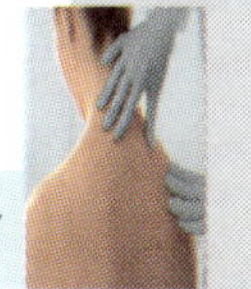

34. Common complication associated with the following condition: ***(Most Recent Question Aug 2020)***

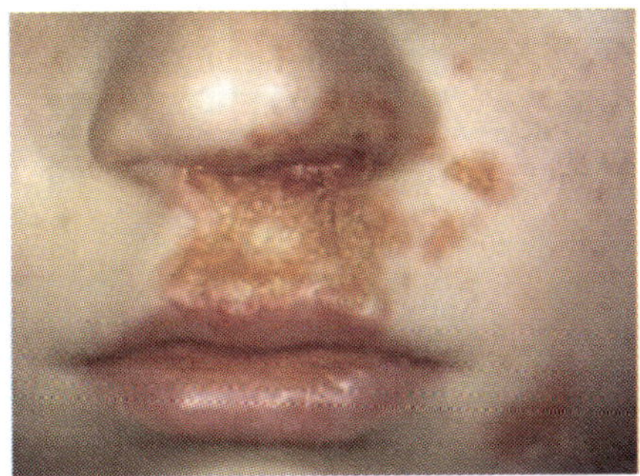

a. Post streptococcal glomerulonephritis
b. SSSS
c. Encephalitis
d. Pneumonitis

35. A tourist guide in Mt. Everest, after one of his trips developed blisters on the feet as shown in the image. Which is not useful for his treatment? ***(Recent Pattern Question Aug 2020)***

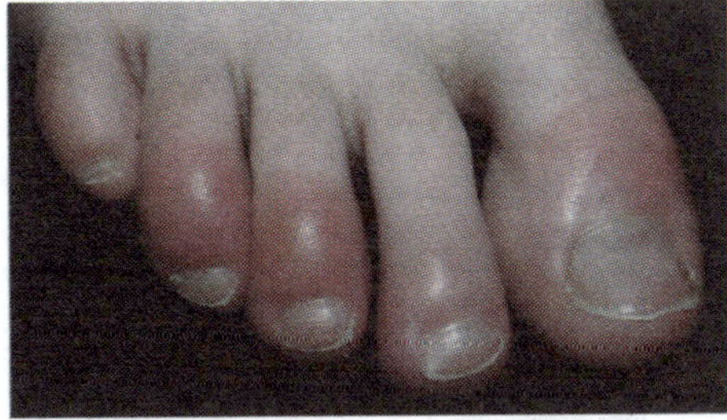

a. Hyperbaric Oxygen
b. Aspirin
c. Phenylephrine
d. Pentoxifylline

36. Patient presents with history of severe sunburn after only a few minutes in the sun, freckling in sun exposed areas, dry skin and changes in skin pigmentation. Diagnosis? ***(Most Recent Question Aug 2020)***

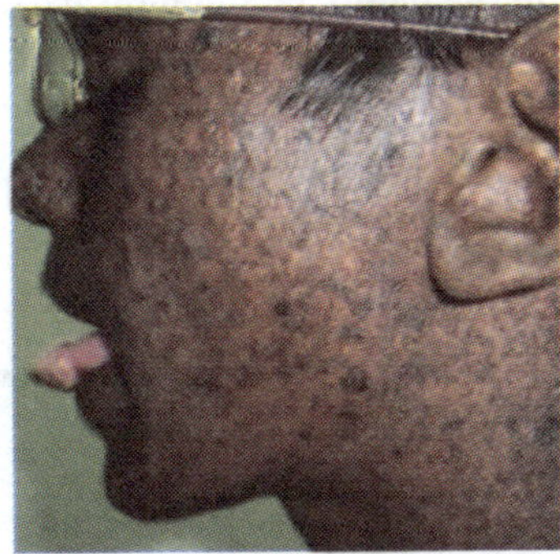

a. Xeroderma pigmentosum
b. Bloom syndrome
c. Warts
d. Melanocytes nevus

37. Child presents with sores in the mouth and a rash on the hands and feet as shown in the image below. What is the causative organism for it? ***(Most Recent Question Aug 2020)***

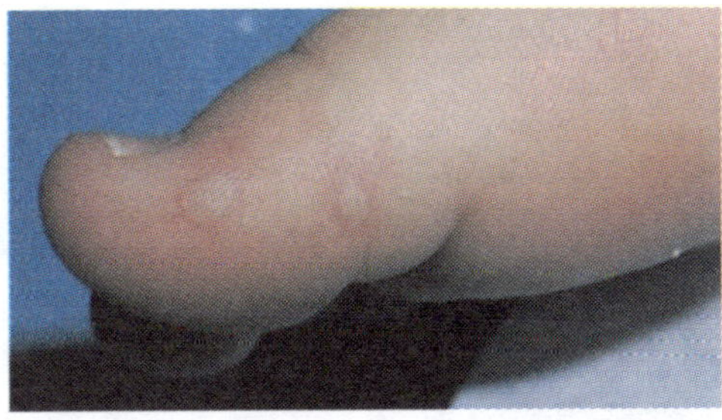

a. Pox virus
b. Herpes virus
c. Human papilloma virus
d. Coxsackievirus A16

38. Child presents with fever and pleomorphic rash as shown in the image. Diagnosis? ***(Most Recent Question Aug 2020)***

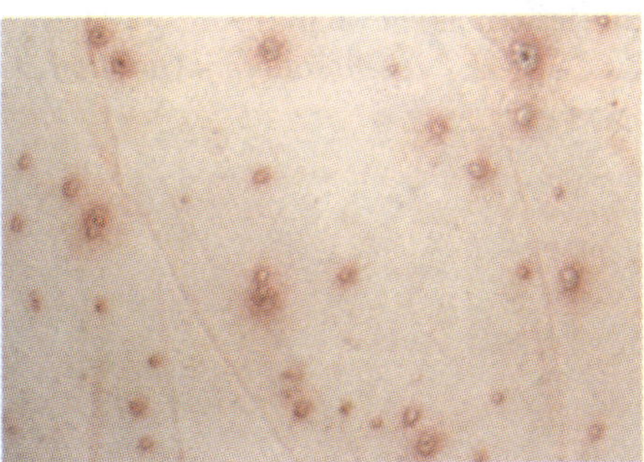

a. Chicken pox
b. Small pox
c. Measles
d. Rubella

39. A 40-year-old female comes with complaint of pain in her finger nail. On examination red nail fold with pus discharge are noted. The most likely diagnosis is: ***(Most Recent Question Aug 2020)***

a. Paronychia
b. Yellow nail syndrome
c. Psoriasis
d. Alopecia areata

40. Which sign is shown in the given picture? ***(Most Recent Question Dec 2019-20)***

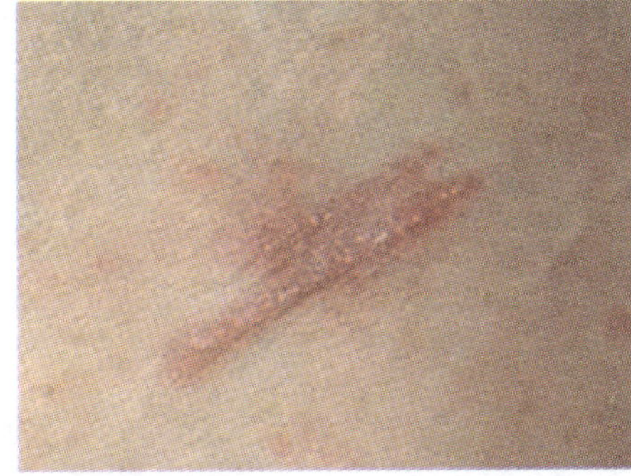

a. Auspitz sign
b. Dermographism
c. Koebner's phenomenon
d. Nikolsky's sign

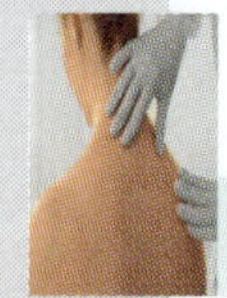

41. A patient who was on anti-convulsant medication, presented with lesion as shown in the given image. What could be the diagnosis?

(Most Recent Question Dec 2019-20)

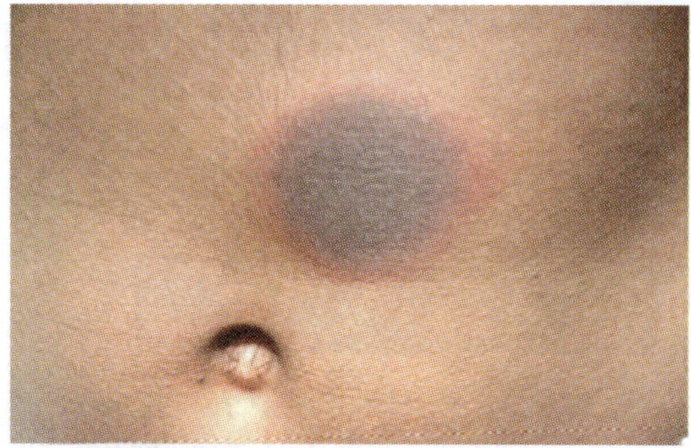

a. Urticaria b. Fixed drug eruption
c. Angioedema d. Cellulitis

42. A patient presented with hypopigmented rash with satellite lesions as shown in the image. Diagnosis?

(Most Recent Question Dec 2019-20)

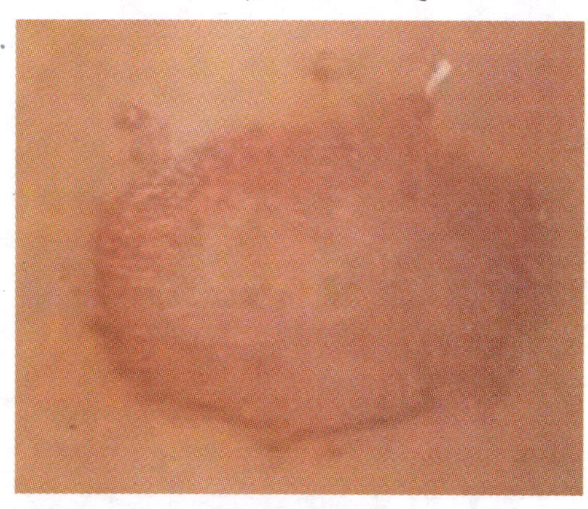

a. BT b. BL
c. LL d. TT

43. Identify the condition in this image?

(Most Recent Question Dec 2019-20)

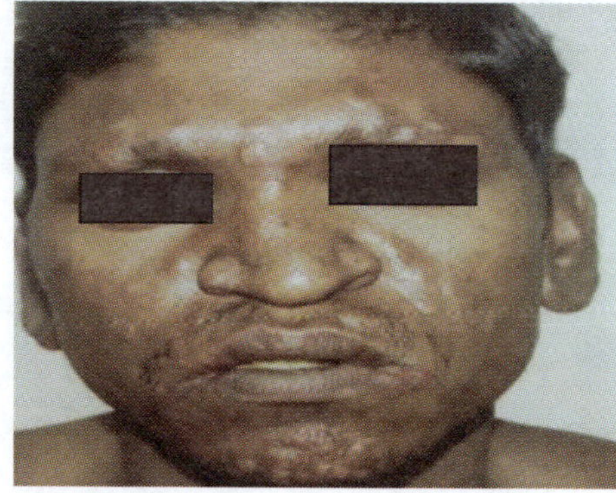

a. Leishmania cutanea b. Lepromatous leprosy
c. Post kala azar dermatitis d. Tuberculoid leprosy

44. A truck driver with history of painless lesion on penis undergoing treatment present with rashes as shown in the image. What is the diagnosis?

(Most Recent Question Dec 2019-20)

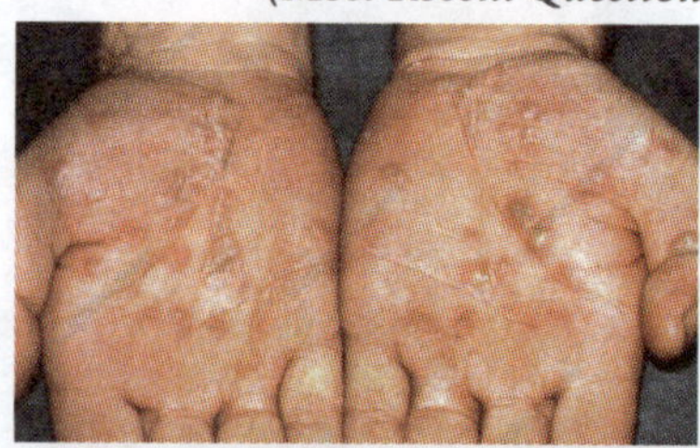

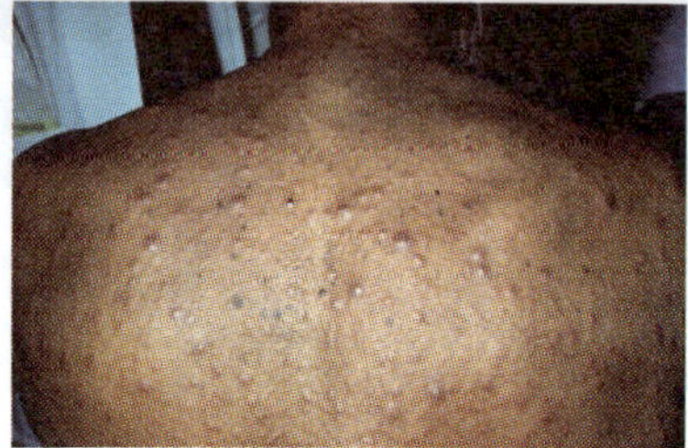

a. Secondary syphilis b. Drug eruption
c. TEN d. Steven Johnson syndrome

45. Identify the image shown below?

(Most Recent Question Dec 2019-20)

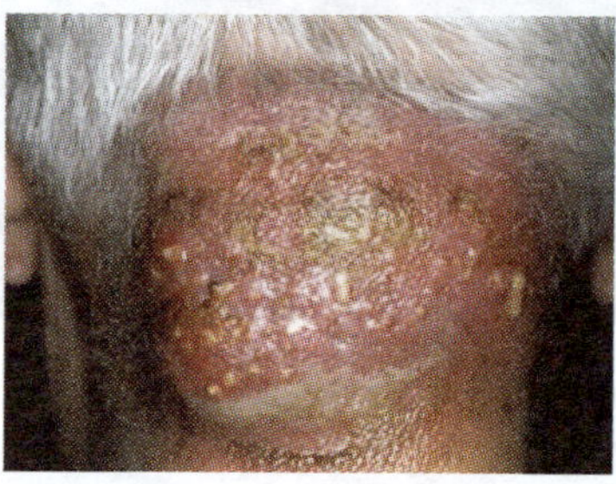

a. Carbuncle b. Follicular abscess
c. Cellulitis d. Erysipelas

46. A farmer presented to OPD with a swelling over his palm as shown in the photo. Few months back he got injured with a thorn. What is the most likely condition given below? ***(Most Recent Question Dec 2019-20)***

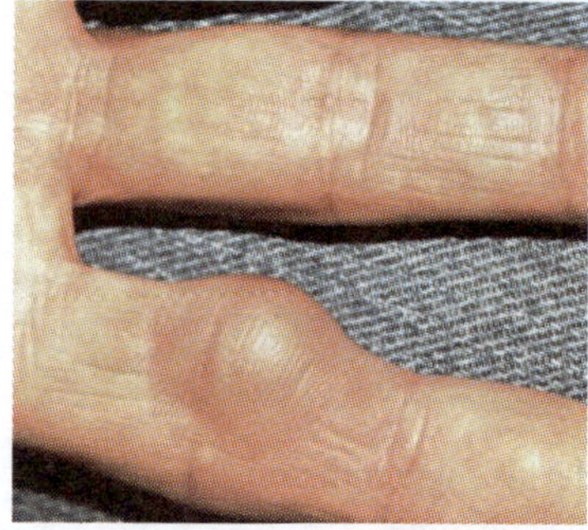

a. Sequestration dermoid b. Implantation dermoid
c. Teratomatoid dermoid d. Ameloblastoma

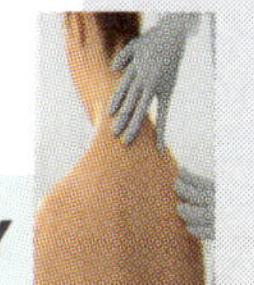

47. Which nail finding is characteristic for psoriasis vulgaris as shown in the image?
(Most Recent Question Dec 2019-20)

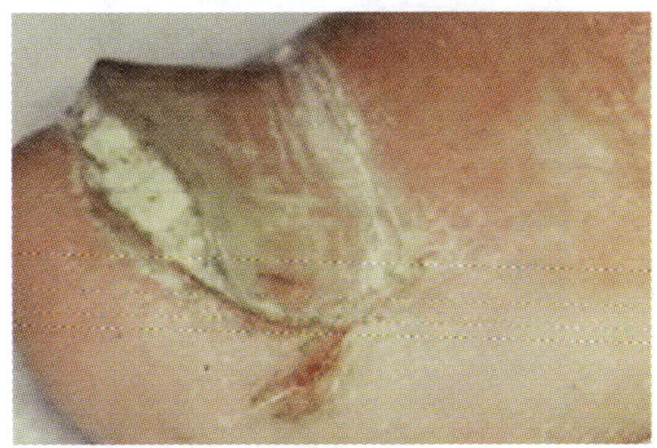

a. Subungual hyperkeratosis
b. Auspitz sign
c. Oil drop sign
d. Onycholysis

48. Identify the shown condition in the image?
(Most Recent Question Dec 2019-20)

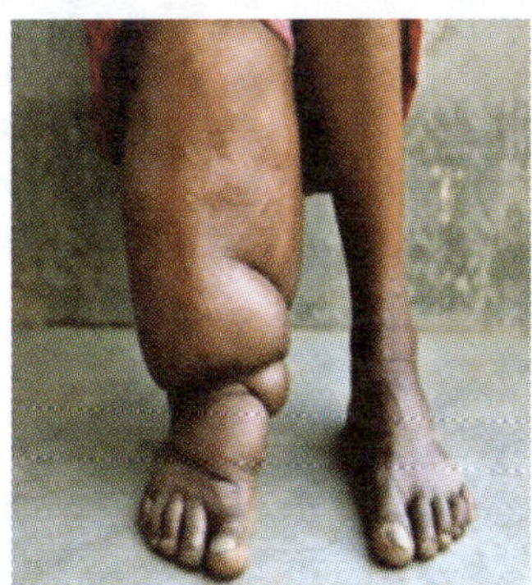

a. Verrucous vulgaris
b. Elephantiasis
c. Leprosy
d. Leishmaniasis

49. Identify condition in the shown image?
(Most Recent Question Dec 2019-20)

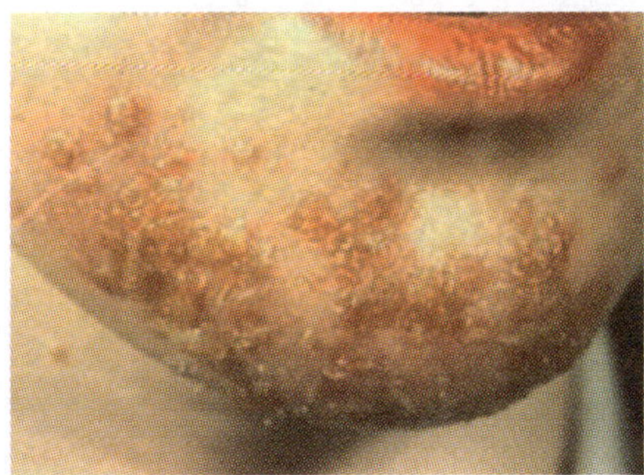

a. Impetigo contagiosa
b. Contact dermatitis
c. Molluscum contagiosum
d. HSV

50. Exclamation mark hair is seen in?
(Most Recent Question Dec 2019-20)

a. Alopecia areata
b. Androgenic alopecia
c. Anagen effluvium
d. Hirsutism

51. What is the name of this appearance which is seen in pellagra? *(Most Recent Question Dec 2019-20)*

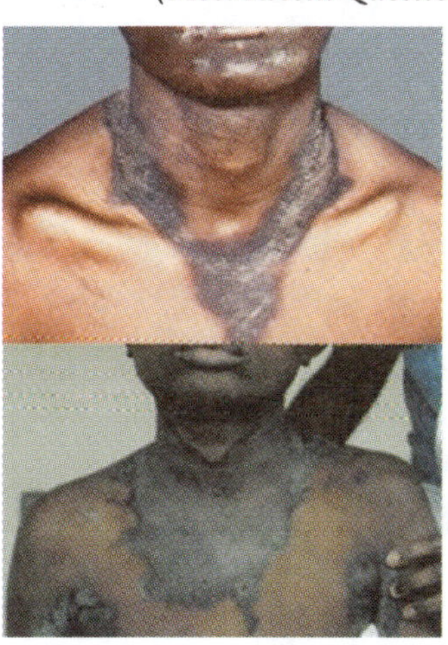

a. Burn
b. Castle necklace appearance
c. Shawl sign
d. Gottron's papule

52. A 25-year-old female presents with history of fever and oral ulcers and has developed erythematous lesions on her face. Comment on the diagnosis.

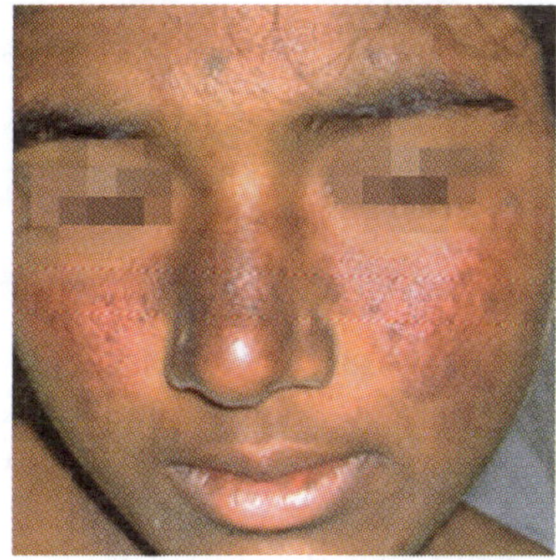

a. SLE
b. Dermatomyositis
c. Melasma
d. Rosacea

53. The following lesion was noticed in a patient with history of involuntary weight loss. What is the diagnosis?

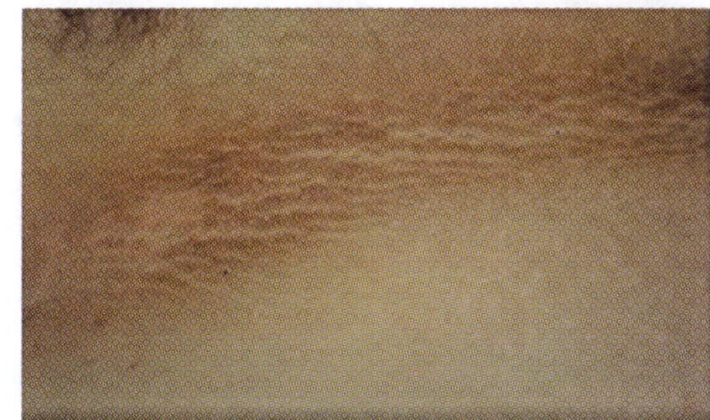

a. Acanthosis nigricans
b. Leser-Trélat sign
c. Actinic keratosis
d. Intertriginous Candida

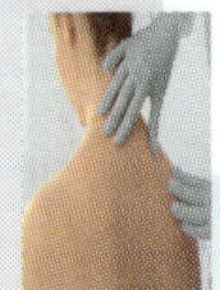

54. Which is not correct about the lesion shown?

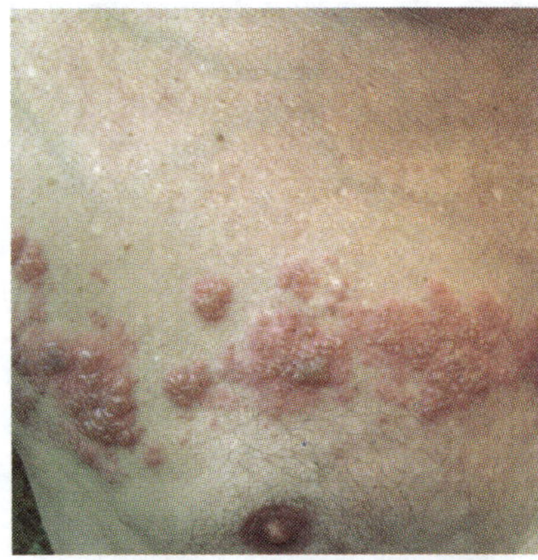

a. The lesions are infectious to seronegative individuals
b. Can be associated with meningoencephalitis
c. Bilaterally symmetrical dermatomal vesicular eruption
d. Geniculate ganglion is involved in Ramsay Hunt syndrome

55. The shown instrument is:

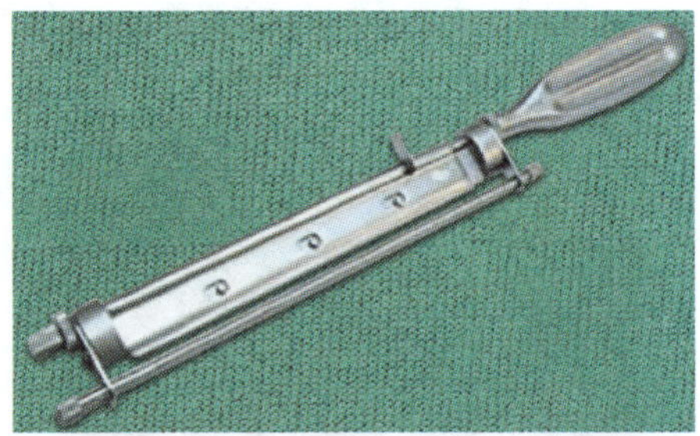

a. Single cutting razor b. Double cutting razor
c. Humby's knife d. Finochietto knife

56. Most appropriate Management to reduce recurrence of keloid:

a. Intralesional steroids b. Surgery
c. Cryotherapy d. Electrocoagulation

57. An infant presents with the condition as shown below after a pharyngeal infection. The shown condition is:

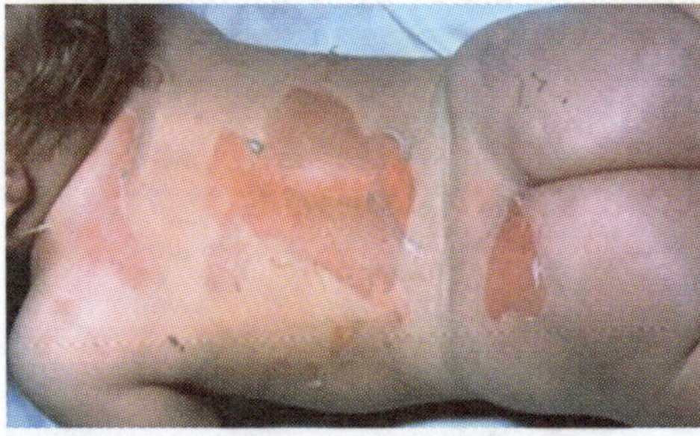

a. Staphylococcal scalded skin syndrome
b. Epidermolysis bullosa simplex
c. Impetigo contagiosa
d. Pemphigus foliaceus

58. The shown penile lesion is:

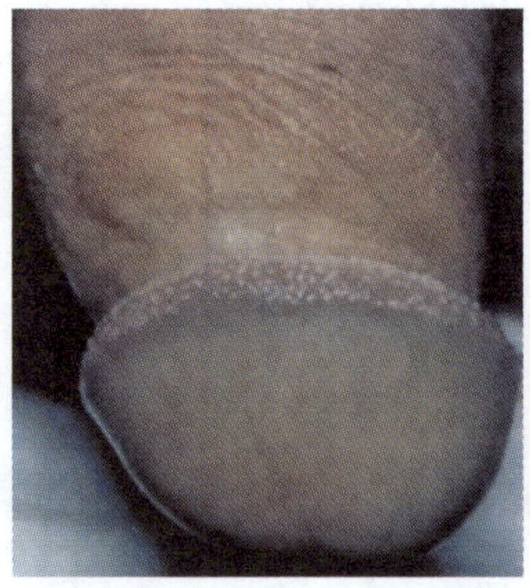

a. Genital wart
b. Pearly penile papule
c. Balanitis
d. Sebaceous gland prominence

59. The shown lesions are:

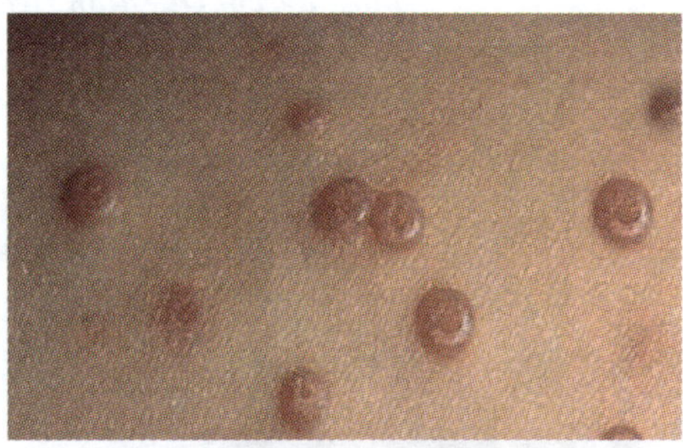

a. Molluscum contagiosum b. Chicken pox
c. Pemphigus d. Common warts

60. Identify condition in the shown image:
(Recent Pattern Question 2018-19)

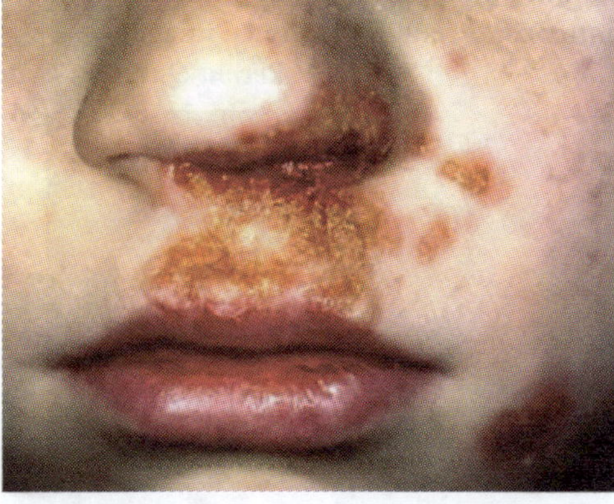

a. Impetigo b. Chickenpox
c. Pemphigus d. Traumatic crust

61. Common neurological tumour associated with NF-2:
(Recent Pattern Question 2018-19)

a. Acoustic neuroma b. Optic glioma
c. Café-Au-Lait macules d. Meningioma

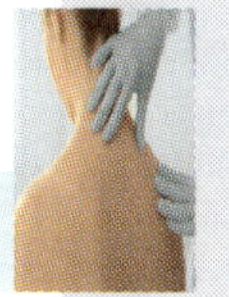

62. What are these colored divisions on body called:
(Recent Pattern Question 2018-19)

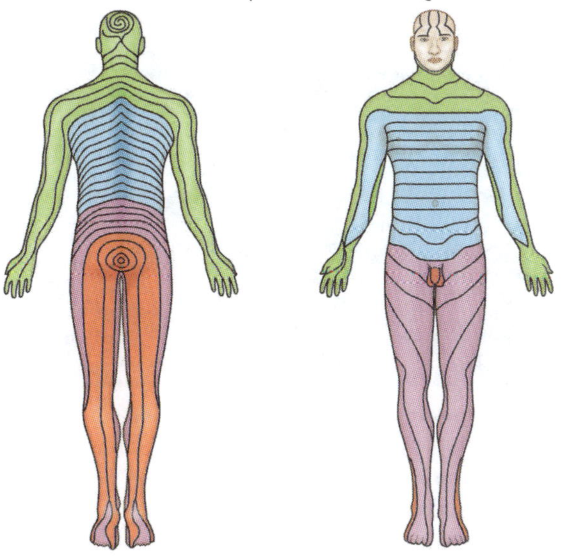

a. Lymphatic development b. Dermatomes
c. Blaschko Lines d. Vascular development

63. Which of the following is NOT seen in congenital syphilis: ***(Recent Pattern Question 2018-19)***

a. Maculopapular skin lesion
b. Hutchison teeth
c. Bow legs
d. Gumma ulcers

64. Which of the following is used for treatment of Vitiligo?
(Recent Pattern Question 2018-19)

a. Retinoids b. Systemic steroids
c. Psoralen PUVA d. Nd-YAG laser

65. Tzanck smear as shown in the image shows:

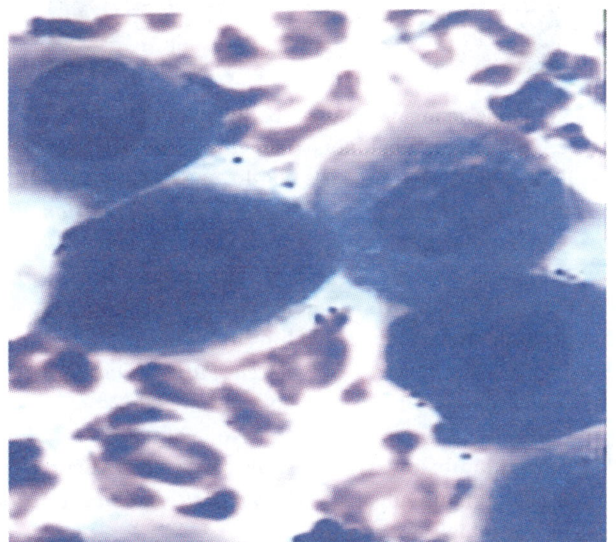

a. Acanthosis b. Acantholytic cells
c. Smudge cells d. Anaplasia

66. Name the horizontal lines shown in the image:
(Recent Pattern Question 2018-19)

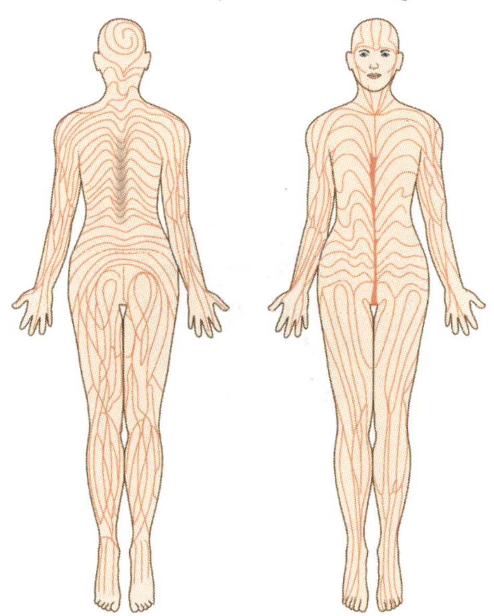

a. Langer lines b. Blaschko lines
c. Kraissl lines d. Borges lines

67. In which condition is Nikolsky's sign positive and bulla spread sign seen? ***(Recent Pattern Question 2018)***

a. Dermatitis herpetiformis
b. Pemphigus vulgaris
c. Bullous pemphigoid
d. Erythema multiforme

68. Identify the given image: ***(Recent Pattern Question 2018)***

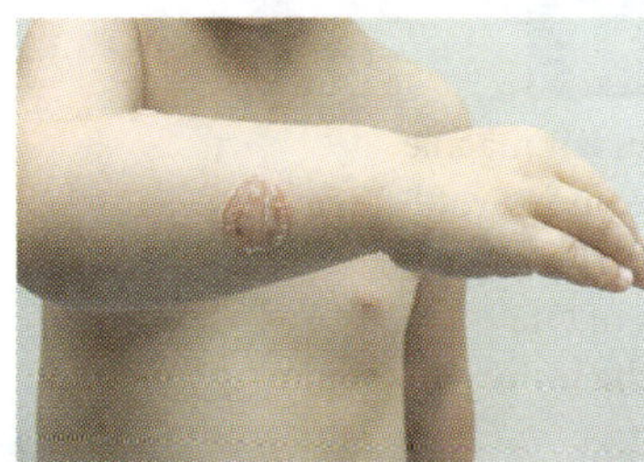

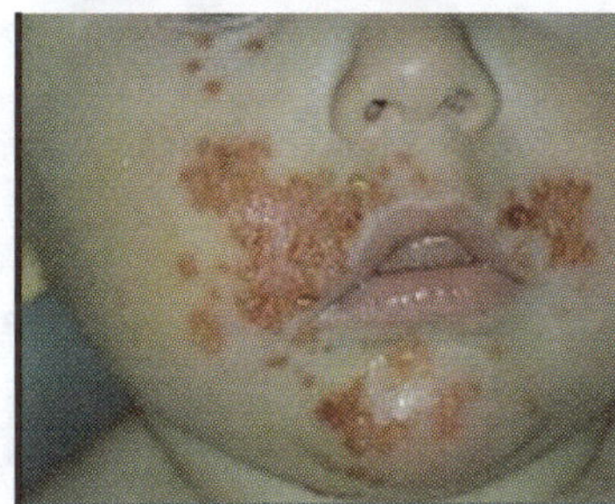

a. Chicken pox
b. Eczema
c. Molluscum contagiosum
d. Impetigo

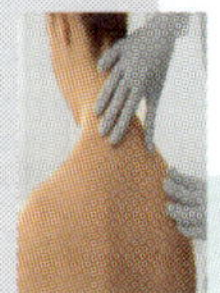

69. **Fordyce's spots involves:** ***(Recent Pattern Question 2018)***
    a. Sweat gland b. Mucus gland
    c. Sebaceous gland d. Moll glands

70. **The shown image is the causative agent for:** ***(Recent Pattern Question 2018)***

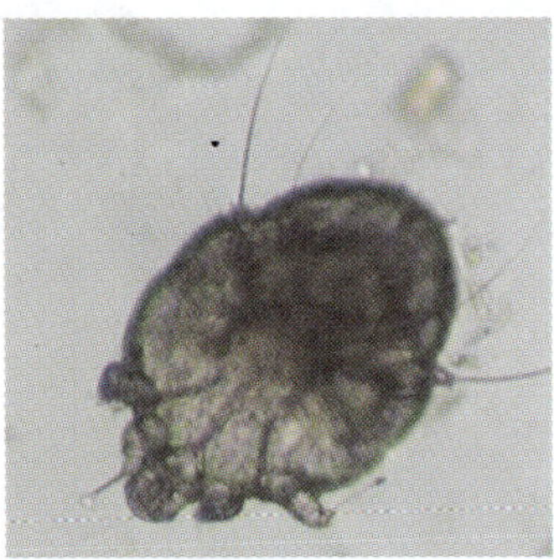

    a. Scabies b. Pediculosis
    c. Molluscum contagiosum d. Pthirus pubis

71. **Identify the type of nevus:** ***(Recent Pattern Question 2018)***

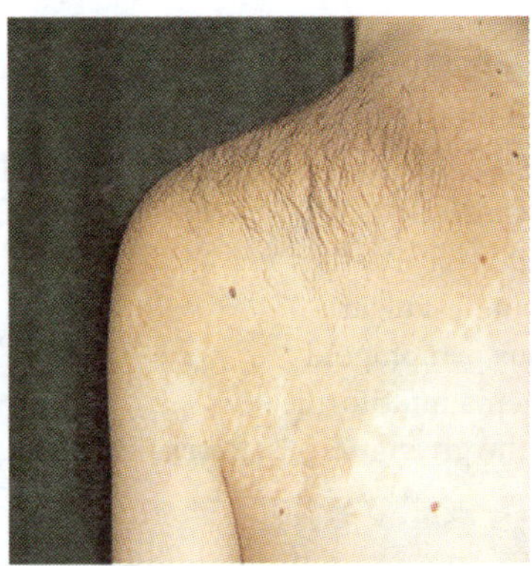

    a. Café au lait macule
    b. Plexiform neurofibroma
    c. Becker nevus
    d. Nevus of Ota

72. **Identify the lesion on trunk:** ***(Recent Pattern Question 2018)***

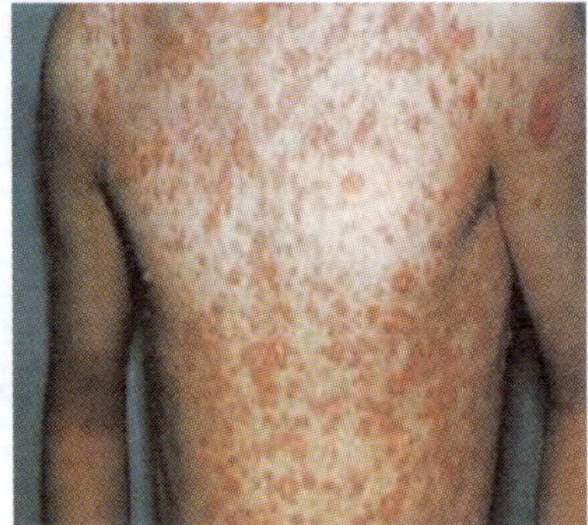

    a. Pityriasis alba b. Pityriasis rosea
    c. Pityriasis versicolor d. Chicken pox

73. **Possible diagnosis based on wood lamp examination?** ***(Recent Pattern Question 2017)***

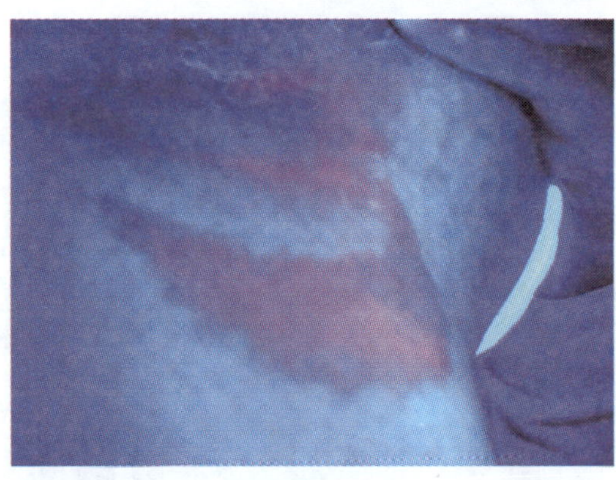

    a. Psoriasis
    b. Erythrasma
    c. Pityriasis versicolor
    d. Tinea versicolor

74. **A middle age patient presented to you with the shown type of baldness. Diagnosis:** ***(Recent Pattern Question 2017)***

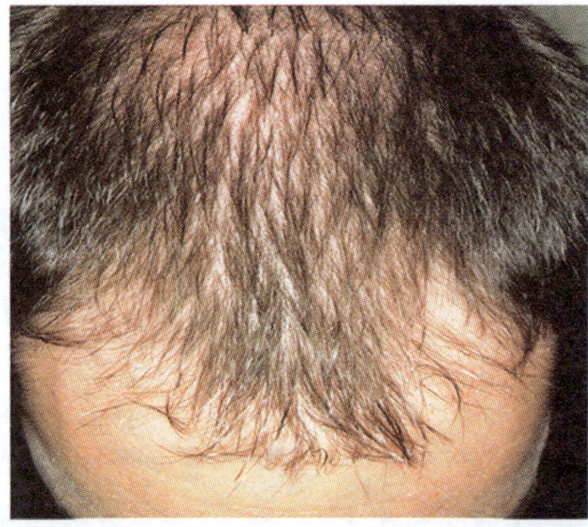

    a. Alopecia areata b. Telogen effluvium
    c. Male pattern baldness d. Cicatricial hair loss

75. **Pemphigus foliaceous is a condition which is seen due to antibody against:** ***(Recent Pattern Question 2017)***
    a. Desmoglein 1 b. Desmoglein 2
    c. Desmoglein 3 d. Desmoglein 4

76. **Pemphigus vulgaris can be seen due to antibodies against desmosomal cadherin cell binding protein:** ***(Recent Pattern Question 2017)***
    a. Desmoglein 1 b. Desmoglein 3
    c. Both d. None of these

77. **Row of tombstone is seen in which skin disorder:** ***(Recent Pattern Question 2017)***
    a. Pemphigus vulgaris
    b. Pemphigus foliaceous
    c. Paraneoplastic pemphigus
    d. Bullous pemphigoid

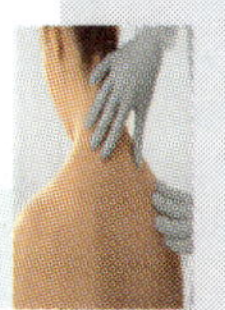

78. The shown immunofluroscence pattern in skin biopsy is suggestive of: *(Recent Pattern Question 2017)*

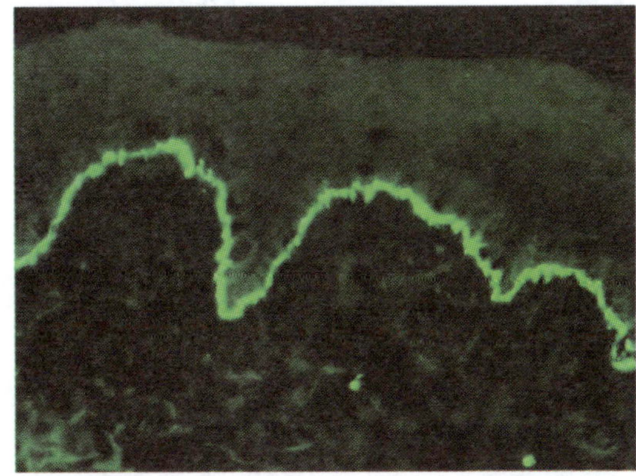

a. Pemphigus vulgaris
b. Pemphigus foliaceous
c. Paraneoplastic pemphigus
d. Bullous pemphigoid

79. Identify the lesion: *(Recent Pattern Question 2017)*

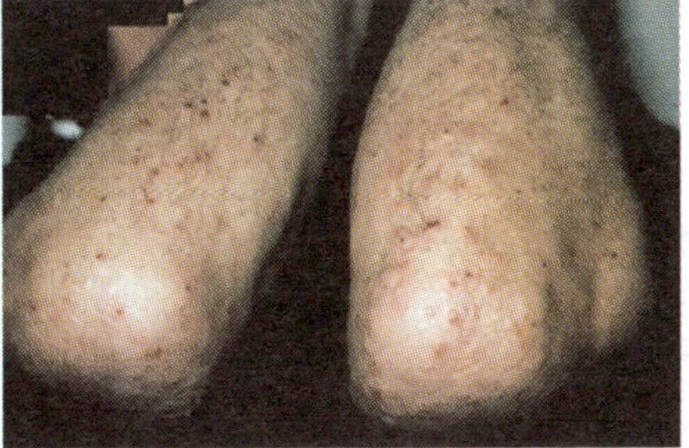

a. Erythema marginatum
b. Dermatitis herpetiformis
c. Psoriasis
d. Dermatomyositis

80. Hertoghie's sign is seen in: *(Recent Pattern Question 2017)*

a. Contact dermatitis
b. Atopic dermatitis
c. Seborrheic dermatitis
d. Neurodermatitis

81. A young girl having low intelligence presented as shown below. There is history of epilepsy. Diagnosis: *(Recent Pattern Question 2017)*

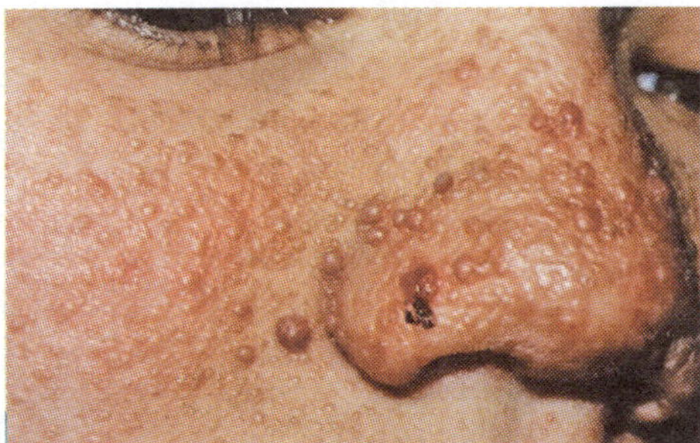

a. Neurofibromatosis
b. Tuberous sclerosis
c. Systemic lupus eythematous
d. Systemic sclerosis

82. A patient presented with blue marks on face as shown in image. Most likely diagnosis: *(Recent Pattern Question 2017)*

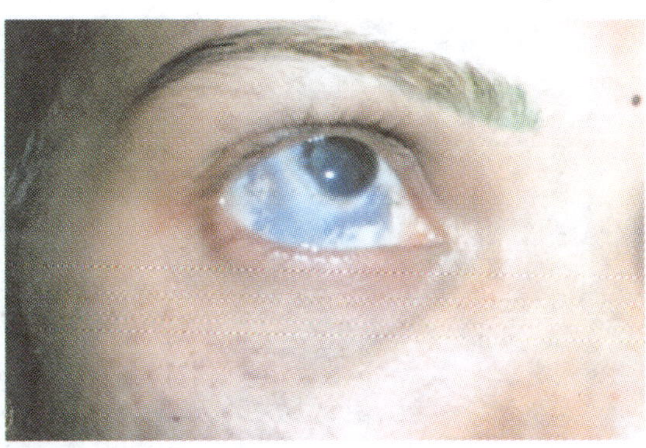

a. Nevus Ito
b. Nevus ota
c. Blue nevus
d. Tuberous sclerosis

83. A patient presented with lesions in interdigital clefts. The oral drug used is: *(Recent Pattern Question 2017)*

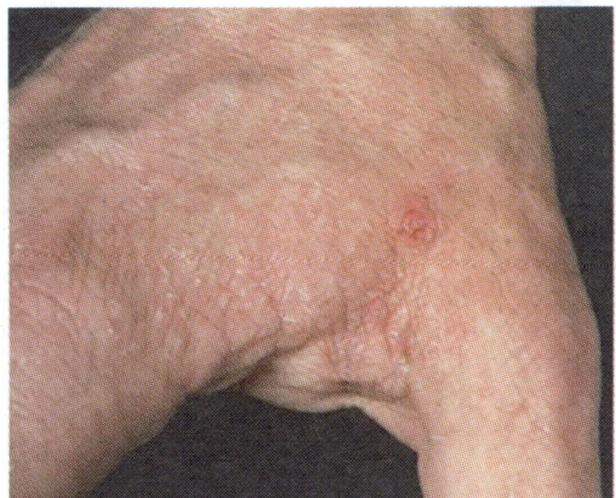

a. Permethrin
b. Ivermectin
c. Benzyl benzoate
d. Sulphur

84. A baby presents with fever, erythema around face and rash all over body. Treatment to be initiated: *(Recent Pattern Question 2017)*

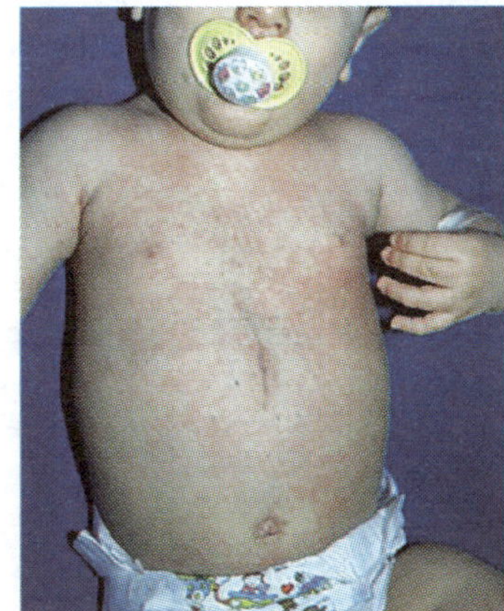

a. Acyclovir
b. Valcyclovir
c. Raltegravir
d. Antipyretics

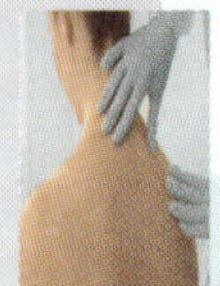

85. A patient presents with lesion on occipitotemporal region of head as shown in image. Possible diagnosis:
(Recent Pattern Question 2017)

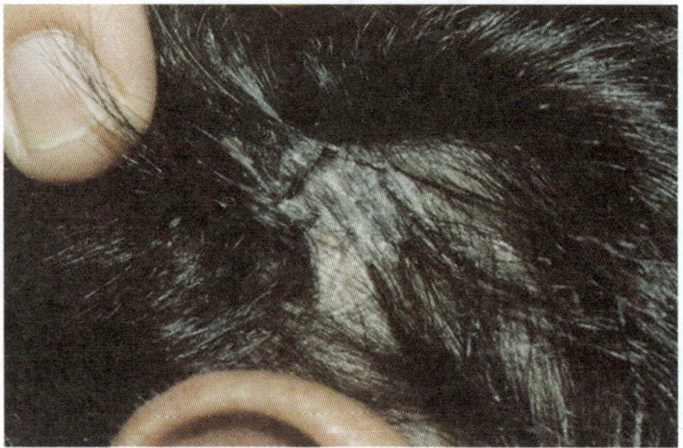

a. Dermatitis herpeteformis b. Lichen planus
c. Tinea captitis d. Traumatic alopecia

86. Patient presented with patchy rash involving trunk and back as shown in image. Diagnosis is?
(Recent Pattern Question 2017)

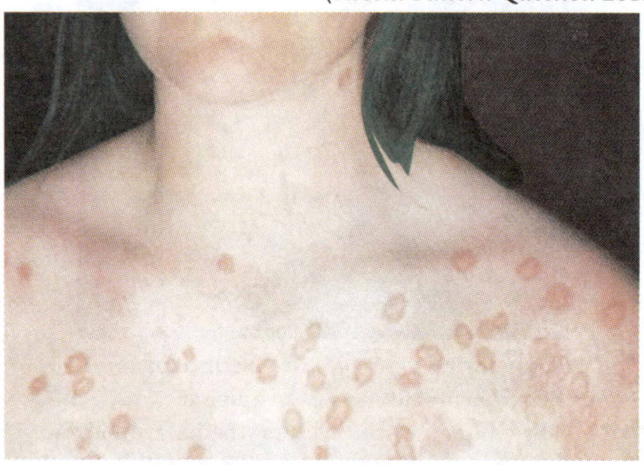

a. Candida b. Tinea corporis
c. Tinea versicolor d. Tinea capitis

87. Possible diagnosis is: ***(Recent Pattern Question 2017)***

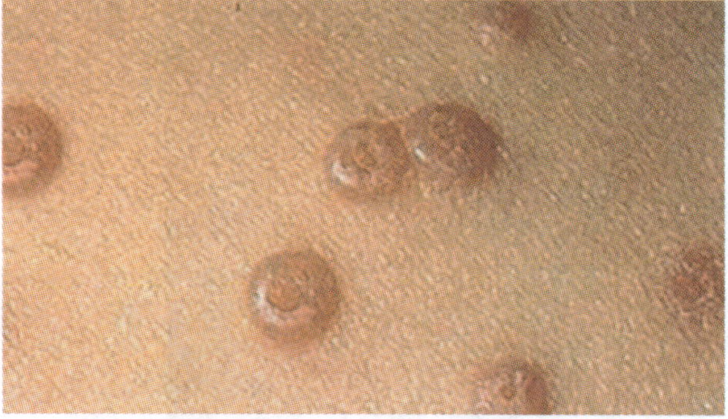

a. Molluscum contagiosum b. Pityriasis versicolor
c. Pityriasis rosea d. Tinea corporis

88. A 60-year-old lady presents with lesion on upper eyelid as shown in image. Diagnosis is:
(Recent Pattern Question 2017)

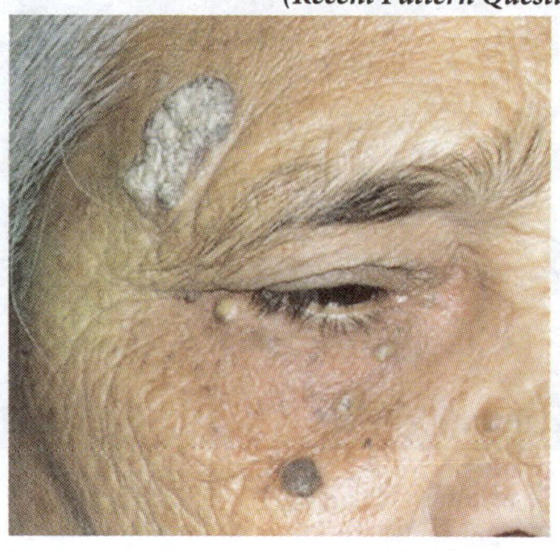

a. Kerato-acanthoma b. Basal cell cancer
c. Bowen' disease d. Psoriasis

89. A hypothyroid female patient presents with alopecia. Diagnosis is: ***(Recent Pattern Question 2017)***

a. Alopecia areata b. Androgenic alopecia
c. Telogen effluvium d. Traumatic alopecia

90. Acrodermatitis enterohepatica occurs due to?
(Recent Pattern Question 2017)

a. Copper deficiency
b. Zinc deficiency
c. Iron deficiency
d. Folic acid deficiency

91. Malassezia furfur is a causative organism for:
(Recent Pattern Question 2017)

a. Tinea versicolor
b. Tenia coli
c. Tinea capitis
d. Tinea corporis

92. In the shown lesion scratching leads to bleeding followed by further formation of similar lesion is suggestive of?
(Recent Pattern Question 2017)

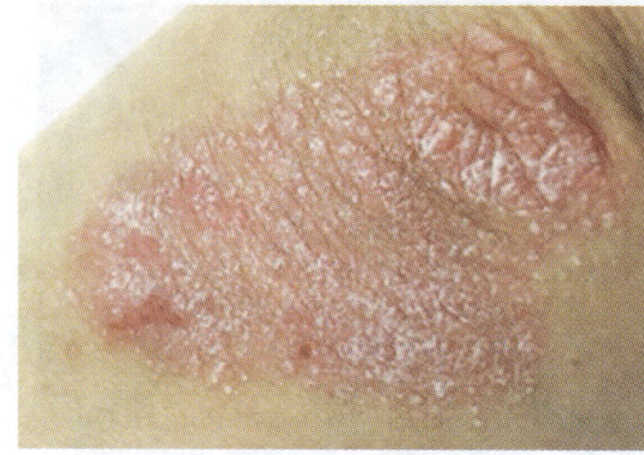

a. Pityriasis versicolor b. Psoriasis
c. Lichen vulgaris d. Psoriasis

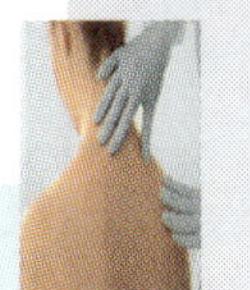

93. 25-year-old Truck driver with repeated Herpes infection presents with following skin lesions. Diagnosis is: ***(Recent Pattern Question 2017)***

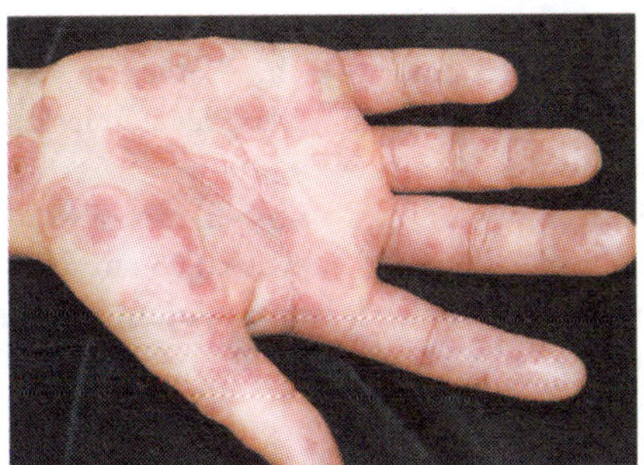

a. Hand foot mouth disease
b. Steven Johnson syndrome
c. Erythema multiforme
d. Dermatitis herpetiformis

94. True about chickenpox rash are all; EXCEPT: ***(Recent Pattern Question 2016)***

a. Superficial
b. Pleomorphic
c. Centripetal
d. Palms and soles involved

95. A 25-year-old patient present with violaceous lesion on arms. What is the likely diagnosis: ***(Recent Pattern Question 2016)***

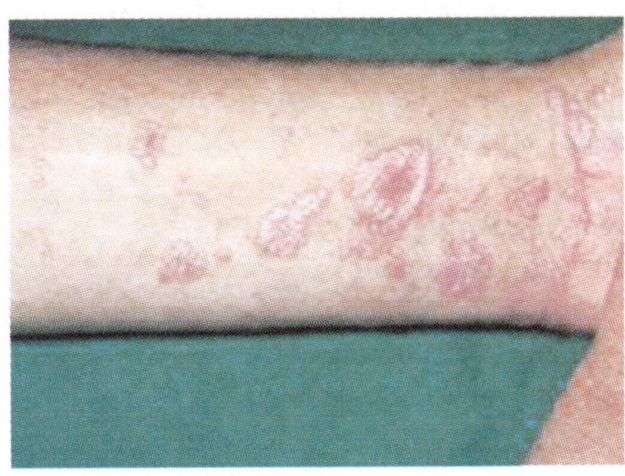

a. Psoriasis
b. Pityriasis rosea
c. Lichen planus
d. Dermatophytosis

96. What is the diagnosis of the given image? ***(Recent Pattern Question 2016)***

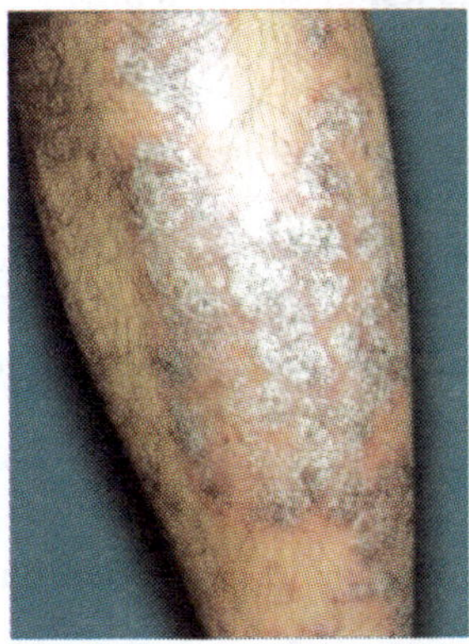

a. Lichen planus
b. Lichenoid dermatitis
c. Psoriasis
d. Pityriasis rosea

97. Best treatment of 24-year-old female with the following lesions? ***(Recent Pattern Question 2016)***

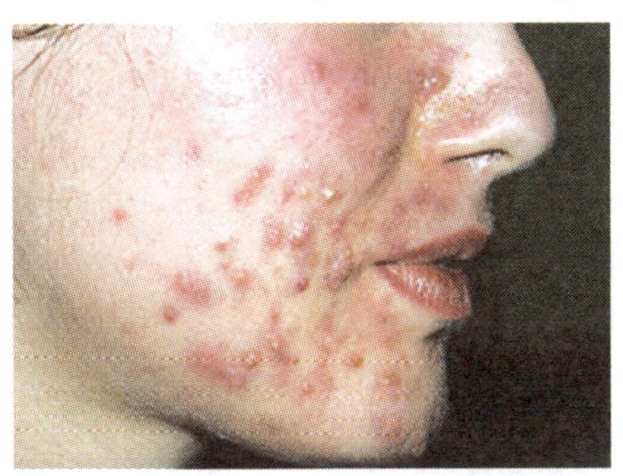

a. Steroids
b. Isotretinoin
c. Tetracycline
d. Erythromycin

98. Patient present with axillary frecking (as shown in image). Diagnosis: ***(Recent Pattern Question 2016)***

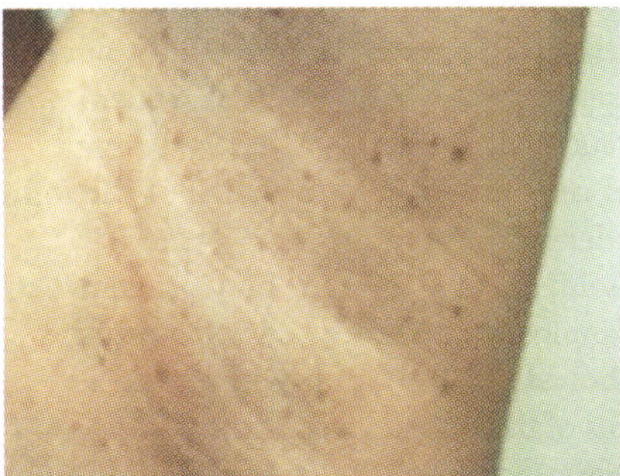

a. Neurofibromatosis
b. Tuberous sclerosis
c. Ichthyosis vulgaris
d. Von Hippel–Landau

99. What is the likely diagnosis? ***(Recent Pattern Question 2016)***

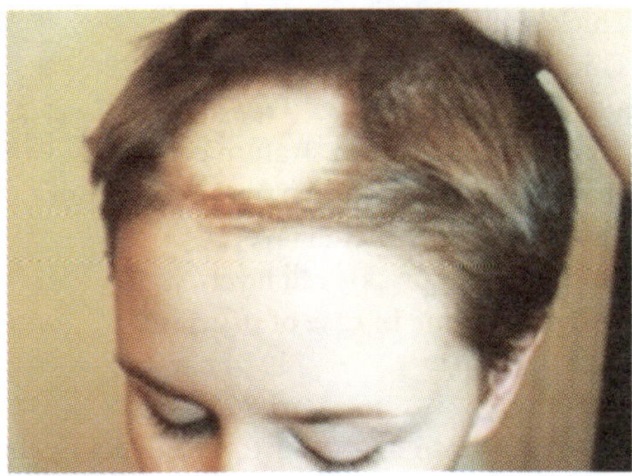

a. Alopecia areata
b. Androgenic alopecia
c. Telogen effluvium
d. Tinea capitis

100. Sunscreen lotion contains: ***(Recent Pattern Question 2016)***

a. Mercury
b. Selenium
c. Sulfide
d. Zinc oxide

101. Average weight of skin:

a. 5 kg
b. 10 kg
c. 15 kg
d. 18 kg

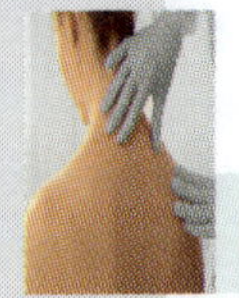

102. Deepest layer of epidermis:
a. Stratum corneum b. Stratum spinosum
c. Stratum granulosum d. Stratum germinatum

103. Synthesis of keratin mainly takes place in this layer of epidermis:
a. Stratum basale b. Stratum cornuem
c. Stratum cranulosum d. Stratum spinosum

104. Hyperkeratosis is:
a. Thinning of stratum corneum
b. Thickening of stratum corneum
c. Thinning of stratum basale
d. Thickening of stratum basale

105. Odland bodies are seen in this layer of epidermis:
a. Stratum cornuem b. Stratum granulosum
c. Stratum spinosum d. Stratum basale

106. Principal cell of epidermis:
a. Melanocytes b. Langerhans cell
c. Keratinocytes d. Merkel cell

107. Langerhan cell present in which layer of epidermis:
a. Basale b. Cornuem
c. Granulosum d. Spinosum

108. Merkel cells are present in which of the following layers on epidermis:
a. Basale b. Cornuem
c. Granulosum d. Spinosum

109. Acantholysis is:
a. Lysis of basale cell layer
b. Separation of keratinocytes
c. Thickening of granular layer
d. Thickening of corneum layer

110. Acanthosis is:
a. Separation of keratinocytes
b. Thickening of granular layer
c. Thickening of corneum layer
d. Thickening of prickle cell layer

111. Parakeratosis is:
a. Absence of nucleus in stratum corneum
b. Persistence of nucleus in stratum corneum
c. Thickening of corneum layer
d. Thickening of prickle cell layer

112. Skin turnover time in case of psoriasis:
a. 2 days b. 4 days
c. 8 days d. 10 days

113. A person starts to sweat on forehead and gets a runny watery nose whenever he eats hot and spicy meals. This kind of sweating is:
a. Mental sweating b. Physical sweating
c. Thermogenic sweating d. Gustatory sweating

114. True about fordyce spot:
a. Axilla is most common site
b. Lips are most common site
c. Blockage of eccrine gland ducts
d. Blockage of apocrine gland ducts

115. Most common site of fordyces spot:
a. Lips b. Below tongue
c. Axilla d. Groin

116. True about macule:
a. Flat lesion >2 cm b. Flat lesion <2 cm
c. Elevated lesion >2 cm d. Elevated lesion <2 cm

117. Size of papule:
a. <5 cm b. <5 mm
c. <0.5 mm d. <0.05 cm

118. A papule that is raised, non-purulent is most probably due to:
a. Insect bite b. Urticaria
c. Angioedema d. Erythema nodosum

119. Green color at bruise site is due to:
a. Hemotidin b. Bilirubin
c. Hemosiderin d. Biliverdin

120. All of the following statements are true about Propniobacterium acnes; EXCEPT:
a. Normal flora of skin
b. Causes acne vulgaris
c. Sulfur granules in the purulent sinuses are characteristic
d. Can be found in GI tract also

121. Deposition of IgA in dermoepidermal junction. What could be probable diagnosis:
a. Nummular eczema b. Pemphigus vulgaris
c. Bullous pemphigoid d. Dermatitis herpetiformis

122. Acantholytic cells are seen in?
a. Pemphigus vulgaris
b. Bullous pemphigoid
c. Cicatricial pemphigoid
d. Dermatitis herpetiformis

123. Pemphigus vulgaris is caused by:
a. Bacteria b. Virus
c. Autoimmune d. Fungal

124. Pemphigus bullae are located at:
a. Subepidermal b. Intraepidermal
c. Subdermal d. All of these

125. Subepidermal lesions are seen in?
a. Pemphigus vulgaris b. Pemphigoid bullae
c. Burns d. Bullous impetigo

126. Intraepidermal bulla is seen in:
a. Bullous pemphigoid b. Pemphigus vulgaris
c. Bullous impetigo d. Dermatitis herpetiformis

127. All are true about pemphigus bullae; EXCEPT:
a. Flaccid bullae located intradermal area
b. Nikolsky sign absent
c. Usually involves mucosa
d. Acantholysis present

128. Intercellular antibodies deposition on immunofluorescence is seen in:
a. Psoriasis b. Pemphigus
c. Pemphigoid d. Porphyria

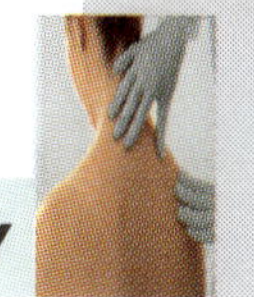

129. Drug of choice for dermatitis herpetiformis:
a. Dapsone b. Rifampicin
c. Ketokonazole d. Azithromycin

130. Darrier sign is seen in:
a. Atopic dermatitis b. Pemphigus vulgaris
c. Urticaria pigmentosa d. Bullous pemphigoid

131. Most common site of angioedema:
a. Hands b. Lips
c. Skin d. Eyelid

132. Angioedema is characterized by swelling of the
a. Subcutaneous tissue b. Epidermis
c. Dermis d. Blood vessels

133. All are true about Xeroderma Pigmentosa; EXCEPT:
a. Due to deficiency of IgA
b. Has marked sensitivity to UV light
c. Due to defective DNA repair
d. Autosomal recessive

134. Acrodermatitis enteropathica is due to deficiency of:
a. Iron b. Copper
c. Zinc d. Magnesium

135. All are true about Keloid; EXCEPT:
a. May be familial
b. Appears mostly on sternum
c. Subsides over time
d. Hyperkeratotic

136. Which of the following presents with hypopigmented patches:
a. Blue nevus b. Nevus ito
c. Nevus becker d. Nevus anemicus

137. Dermatophytes are:
a. Tinea versicolor b. Trichophyton rubrum
c. Sporothrix d. All of these

138. Which of the following structure is affected by dermatophytes:
a. Skin b. Hair
c. Nail d. All of these

139. Trichophyton infects:
a. Skin + nail b. Skin + hair
c. Hair + nail d. Skin + hair + nail

140. Which of the following infects skin and hair:
a. T. verrucosum b. M. Gypseum
c. Both d. None of these

141. A case of 12-years-old boy presents to you with boggy swelling and easily pluckable hair. What would be the probable diagnosis:
a. Lichen planus b. Tinea capitis
c. Epidermophytosis d. Alopecia areata

142. An adult male presented 4 weeks after intercourse with fever, rubbery consistency ulcer, inguinal lymphadenopathy. Causative organism:
a. LGV b. Syphillis
c. Chancroid d. HIV

143. Painful ulcer on glans penis is seen in:
a. Syphilis
b. Lymphogranuloma venerum
c. Chancroid
d. Chancre

144. School of fish appearance is seen in?
a. Bacterial vaginosis b. Hemophilus ducreyi
c. Gonococcus d. Chlamydia

145. Moth eaten alopecia is caused by:
a. Secondary syphilis b. Primary syphilis
c. Tertiary syphilis d. Early relapsing syphilis

146. All cause genital ulcer; EXCEPT:
a. Gonorrhoea b. Chancroid
c. HSV d. LGV

147. Child with recurrent mouth ulcer which usually begins as a round yellowish elevated spot surrounded by a red halo and heals within 7–10 days:
a. Gingivitis b. Aphthous ulcers
c. Malignancy d. Herpetic ulcer

148. Alopecia areata is due to defect of this stage of hair growth:
a. Anagen effluvium b. Telogen effluvium
c. Catagen d. None of these

149. Infection caused by human papilloma virus is called as?
a. Condylama lata b. Condyloma acuminata
c. Verrucous wart d. Plantar wart

150. Which of the following is the causative organism of Verruca vulgaris:
a. CMV
b. Human immunodeficiency virus
c. Human papilloma virus
d. Ebstein barr virus

151. All of the following tests are used for diagnosis of leprosy; EXCEPT:
a. Clinical examination b. Lepromin test
c. Slit skin smear d. Skin biopsy

152. Thalidomide is mostly effective in:
a. Nerve Abscess
b. Type I Lepra reaction
c. Type II Lepra reaction
d. Both type I and II leprae reaction

153. TB presents with all of the following skin conditions; EXCEPT:
a. Lupus vulgaris b. Scrofuloderma
c. Erythema nodosum d. Lichen scrofulosorum

154. Lichen planus is associated with:
a. Koilonychia b. Tinea versicolor
c. Psoriasis d. Pterygium of nail

155. Bandlike infiltrate of lymphocytes at the dermoepidermal junction, and "saw-tooth" rete ridges are diagnostic histological features of:
a. Lichen planus b. Lupus erythematosus
c. Psoriasis vulgaris d. Seborrhoeic dermatitis

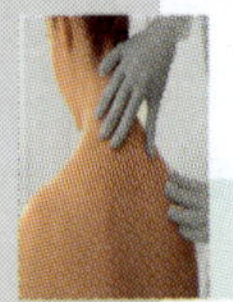

ANSWERS WITH EXPLANATIONS

MOST RECENT QUESTIONS 2023

1. Ans. (b) Psoriatic arthritis

- Psoriatic arthritis is commonly associated with psoriasis and can cause joint pain, swelling, and inflammation, particularly involving the fingers.
- The characteristic "sausage-like" swelling of the fingers, known as dactylitis, is a hallmark feature of psoriatic arthritis.
- It commonly involves proximal and distal interphalangeal joints (PIP, DIP) and metacarpophalangeal joints (MCP).

Other deformities in psoriatic arthritis:

- Marginal erosions with the adjacent bony proliferation.
- Small joint ankylosis and osteolysis of phalangeal and metacarpal bones.
- Telescoping of digits, periostitis, and proliferative new bone.
- Axial changes, like asymmetric sacroiliitis.

2. Ans. (c) Tinea incognito

- Tinea incognito refers to fungal infections, typically tinea, that have been altered by the inappropriate use of topical steroids.
- The use of steroids can modify the appearance of the infection, leading to a less typical clinical presentation.
- In this case, the patient has a fungal infection (tinea cruris) in the groin area and was treated with topical steroids.

Extra Mile

- **Tinea corporis** is a fungal infection affecting the body's skin.
- **Tinea cruris** is a fungal infection affecting the groin area.

3. Ans. (a) Condyloma acuminata

- Condyloma acuminata, also known as genital warts, is a sexually-transmitted infection caused by human papillomavirus (HPV) 6 and 11.
- The images depict raised, cauliflower-like growth on the genital area, which is the characteristic of condyloma acuminata.

Extra Mile

- **Herpes genitalis** presents with painful vesicles that can ulcerate.
- **Condyloma lata** are flat, broad-based lesions associated with secondary syphilis.
- **Hemorrhoids** are swollen blood vessels around the rectum or anus.

4. Ans. (b) Melanoma

- The image shows an asymmetric, irregularly pigmented lesion with uneven borders, which are concerning features for melanoma.
- Melanoma is a malignant tumor arising from melanocytes, the pigment-producing cells.
- The ABCDE rule (Asymmetry, Border irregularity, Color variation, Diameter >6 mm, Evolution) helps in assessing melanoma risk.

Extra Mile

- **Basal cell carcinoma** is common but typically appears as a raised, pearly nodule.
- **Squamous cell carcinoma** can appear irregular and crusted.
- A **malignant nevus**, or dysplastic nevus, may have atypical features but is less aggressive than melanoma.

5. Ans. (a) Marjolin's ulcer

- The image shows an ulcerated and irregularly-shaped lesion with raised edges and surrounding erythema and inflammation. This is characteristic of Marjolin's ulcer.
- Marjolin's ulcer is a malignant transformation that can occur in long-standing scars or chronic wounds, such as those resulting from burns.
- Chronic inflammation and tissue damage can lead to cellular changes and the development of a squamous cell carcinoma.
- No history of diabetes and smoking rules out diabetic ulcer and Buerger's disease.

6. Ans. (b) Herpes zoster

Ref: Rook's Textbook of Dermatology, 9th ed. pg. 25.27-30

The clinical scenario/image is suggestive of diagnosis of **herpes zoster**, also known as shingles.

- It is the collection of vesicles which are unilateral, painful and along the single dermatome.
- It occurs due to the reactivation of latent herpes zoster virus from dorsal root ganglia for which an earlier infection with varicella is essential.
- The most commonly involved dermatome is thoracic dermatome.
- It is a self-limiting infection with drug of choice. Acyclovir is given in case of painful zoster infection or facial zoster.

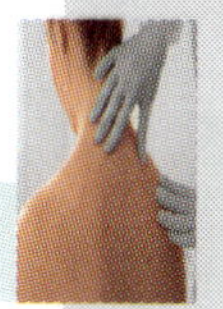

Extra Mile

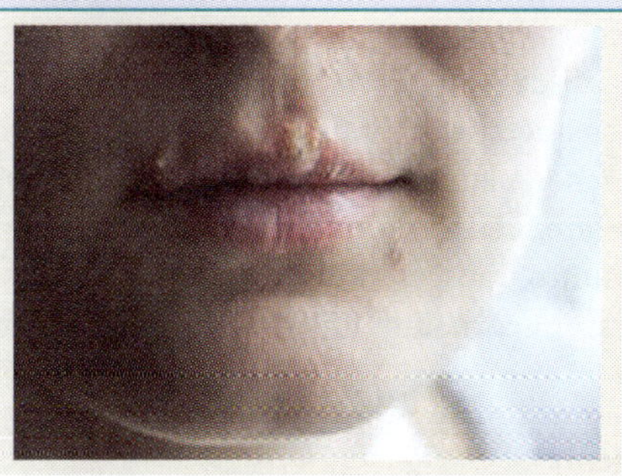
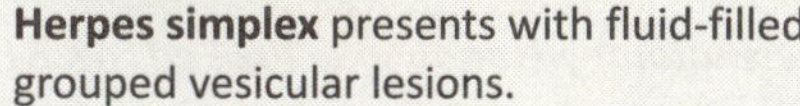

Herpes simplex presents with fluid-filled grouped vesicular lesions.

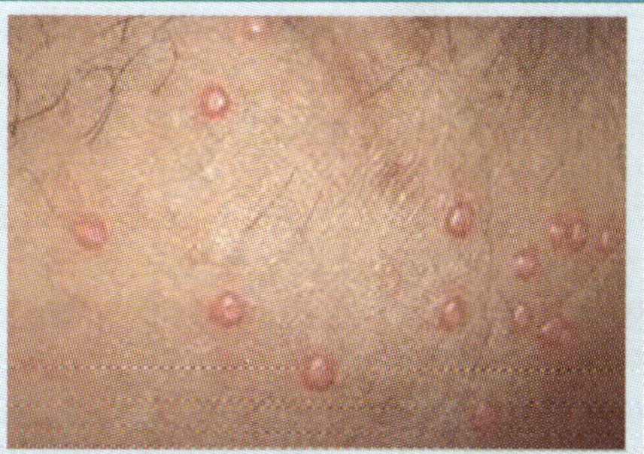

Molluscum contagiosum is characterized by the pearly umbilicated raised papules.

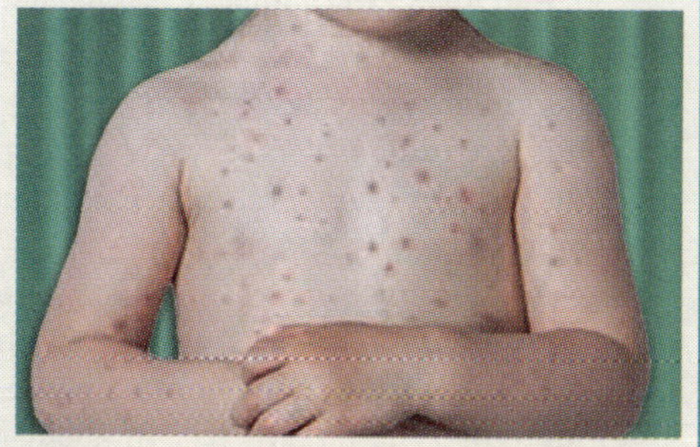

Chicken pox presents with fever, centripetal rash which are dew drops on rose petal type.

7. Ans. (a) Capillary hemangioma

Ref: Rook's Textbook of Dermatology, 9th ed. pg. 137.26-28

The above clinical scenario/an image is suggestive of capillary hemangioma.

- These are the most common benign orbital tumors of childhood.
- These are superficial red raised lesions which are commonly seen under the age of 1 year.
- Involving the upper eyelid, can cause astigmatism or amblyopia leading to severe vision loss if left untreated.
- First-line treatment is beta-blockers (Propranolol).

8. Ans. (a) Comedones

Ref: Rook's Textbook of Dermatology, 9th ed. pg. 90.1-5

Comedones are a special type of lesions seen in Acne vulgaris.

- These are noninflammatory types of lesions which are of two types—open and closed. These are also known as whiteheads and blackheads, respectively.
- They can be present on the face, back or chest as these are the most frequently affected sites.
- Papules are raised solid lesions of <0.5 cm.
- Pustules are pus-filled lesions.

9. Ans. (a) Psoriasis

Ref: Rook's Textbook of Dermatology, 9th ed. pg. 123.2

This image shows white silvery or mica-like scales on the dorsal aspect of the palm which are suggestive of psoriasis.

- These scales are characteristic of parakeratosis.
- Psoriasis is typically seen on extensor areas.
- Psoriasis shows true Koebner's phenomenon, i.e., the lesions start developing along the lines of trauma.
- In secondary syphilis, all types of lesions can be seen except vesiculobullous lesions.
- Fungal infection is characterized by an annular lesion with central clearing.
- Maculopapular drug eruptions are allergic drug reactions due to a particular drug intake, most commonly seen on lips and genitalia.

10. Ans. (d) Herpes

Ref: Rook's Dermatology Handbook, 2022 ed. pg. 157, 255

- The Koebner phenomenon or isomorphic response refers to the appearance of lesions along a site of injury.
- Causes of the Koebner phenomenon that are secondary to scratching rather than an infective or chemical cause include vitiligo, psoriasis, lichen planus, lichen nitidus, pityriasis rubra pilaris, and Darier disease.

11. Ans. (b) Erythrodermic

Ref: Rook's Dermatology Handbook, 2022 ed. pg. 163

- Psoriatic erythroderma represents a form of psoriasis that affects all body sites, including the face, hands, feet, nails, trunk, and extremities.
- Patients with this psoriasis subtype typically present with erythema involving more than 75 percent of the body surface area and associated scale, pustules, or exfoliation of the skin.

12. Ans. (a) Madura foot

Ref: Rook's Dermatology Handbook, 2022 ed. pg.118, 119

- The shown image is of Madura foot.
- Madura foot is a chronic granulomatous infection of the bones and soft tissues of the foot resulting in mycetoma formation and gross deformity.
- The infection can be caused by true fungi (eumycetoma) in 40%, or filamentous bacteria (actinomycetoma) in 60%.
- Actinomycetoma may be due to Actinomadura madurae, Actinomadura pelletieri, Streptomyces somaliensis, Nocardia spp.

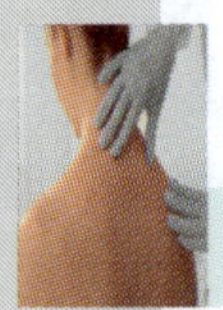

13. Ans. (a) **Autosomal dominant**

Ref: Rook's Dermatology Handbook, 2022 ed. pg. 464

- Neurofibromatosis 1 (NF1), also known as von Recklinghausen's disease.
- It is a condition characterized by skin pigmentation and the growth of tumors along nerves in the skin, brain, and other parts of the body.
- Neurofibromatosis type 1 is considered to have an **autosomal dominant** pattern of inheritance. People with this condition are born with one mutated copy of the NF1 gene in each cell. In about half of cases, the altered gene is inherited from an affected parent.

14. Ans. (c) **Yellow kit (kit 6)**

Ref: Park Textbook of Preventive and Social Medicine, 25th ed. pg. 472

- For syndromic management of sexually transmitted infections, different kits are given at Suraksha Clinic.
- Kit 6 is yellow in color and is used for lower abdominal pain

Colour coded STI/RTI drugs kits according to syndrome available at Suraksha Clinics

Kit	Colour
Kit 1	Grey: Urethral discharge, cervicitis
Kit 2	Green: Vaginitis
Kit 3	White: Genital ulcers
Kit 4	Blue: Genital ulcers
Kit 5	Red: Genital ulcers
Kit 6	Yellow: Lower abdominal pain
Kit 7	Black: Scrotal swelling

15. Ans. (c) **Pellagra**

Ref: Rook's Dermatology Handbook, 2022 ed. pg. 368

- Pellagra is a disease that occurs when a person does not get enough Niacin (one of the B complex vitamins) or tryptophan (an amino acid).
- It's marked by dementia, diarrhea, and dermatitis. Maize lacks nicotinic acid as well as tryptophan, a precursor that can be converted in the body to nicotinic acid.

16. Ans. (a) **Munro microabscess/kogoj**

Ref: Rook's Dermatology Handbook, 2022 ed. pg. 168

- Lichen planus (LP) is an inflammatory disorder of the skin and mucous membranes with no known cause.
- It appears as pruritic, violaceous papules and plaques most commonly found on the wrists, lower back, and ankles.
- A lattice-like network of white lines called **Wickham striae** overlies the lesions but is most easily observed on the buccal mucosa.
- The presence of numerous **civatte bodies (CBs)** in biopsies is a characteristic finding in skin lesions of patients with Lichen planus.
- **Kogoj pustules** are seen in pustular psoriasis.

Note: Micro Munro abscess/Kogoj is collection of neutrophils in stratum corneum. It is seen in patients with psoriasis.

17. Ans. (a) **Teratogenic**

Ref: Rook's Dermatology Handbook, 2022 ed. pg. 513

- Evidence suggests that 13-cis-retinoic acid is involved in teratogenicity.
- Malformations from exposure to 13-cis-retinoic acid causes defects, in developing fetuses, in the central nervous system, such as fluid buildup inside the brain, underdevelopment of the cerebellum, and structural malformation of the cerebral cortex.
- Other features like NTD, follicular hyperkeratosis and photo oncholysis is not associated with 13 Cis-Retinoic Acid exposure

18. Ans. (a) **Malassezia furfur**

Ref: Rook's Dermatology Handbook, 2022 ed. pg. 107

- Pityriasis versicolor is an infection of the stratum corneum caused by the yeast Malassezia furfur.
- Infection is characterized by brown, scaly macules on the trunk or upper arms.
- Malassezia (Pityrosporum) is present as a combination of both short pseudohyphae and spores, the light microscopic appearance of which is referred to as "spaghetti and meatballs" pattern.

19. Ans. (a) **Methotrexate**

Ref: Rook's Dermatology Handbook, 2022 ed. pg. 166

- The shown condition seems to be severe plaque psoriasis
- Methotrexate is used to treat moderate to severe plaque psoriasis, psoriatic erythroderma, generalized pustular psoriasis, nail psoriasis, palmoplantar psoriasis, and psoriatic arthritis.

20. Ans. (b) **5th disease**

Ref: Rook's Dermatology Handbook, 2022 ed. pg. 733

- Fifth disease is a viral disease that often results in a red rash on the arms, legs, and cheeks.
- It's sometimes called slapped-cheek disease because of the distinctive face rash that develops. It is caused by parvovirus B19.

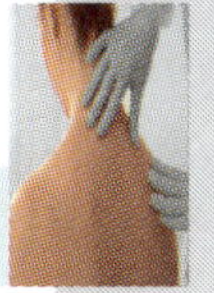

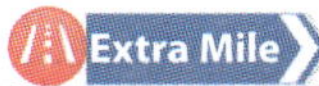

Extra Mile

The six classic childhood exanthems

Numbered disease	Names	Etiologic agent
First disease	Measles, rubeola	Measles virus
Second disease	Scarlet fever	*Streptococcus pyogenes*
Third disease	Rubella, German measles	Rubella virus
Fourth disease	Filatov-Duke's disease	Obsolete classification
Fifth disease	Erythema infectiosum	Human parvovirus B19
Sixth disease	Roseola, exanthema subitum	Human herpes virus 6

21. Ans. (d) Segmental vitiligo

Ref: Rook's Dermatology Handbook, 2022 ed. pg. 418

- Segmental vitiligo is an uncommon form of localized vitiligo, characterized by dermatomal distribution.
- It is often unilateral and asymmetrical that never crosses the midline of body. In segmental vitiligo, a CD8-dominant infiltrate around melanocytes is observed ultimately leading to melanocyte destruction.

22. Ans. (d) Alopecia areata

Ref: Rook's Dermatology Handbook, 2022 ed. pg. 394,395

- Alopecia areata is an autoimmune disorder that usually results in unpredictable, patchy hair loss.
- Alopecia areata occurs when the immune system attacks hair follicles and may be brought on by severe stress. The arrow points to an exclamation point hair on the scalp in a patient with alopecia areata.
- Exclamation point hairs are short, broken hairs that can be extracted with minimal traction and where the proximal end of the hair is narrower than the distal end.

23. Ans. (c) Basal cell carcinoma

Ref: Rook's Dermatology Handbook, 2022 ed. pg. 691

- The shown condition seems to be basal cell carcinoma.
- Basal cell carcinoma is a type of skin cancer that most often develops on areas of skin exposed to the sun, such as the face.
- BCC typically presents as a shiny, pink- or flesh-colored papule or nodule with surface telangiectasia. The tumor may enlarge and ulcerate. The most common cause is UV radiation from the sun.

Extra Mile

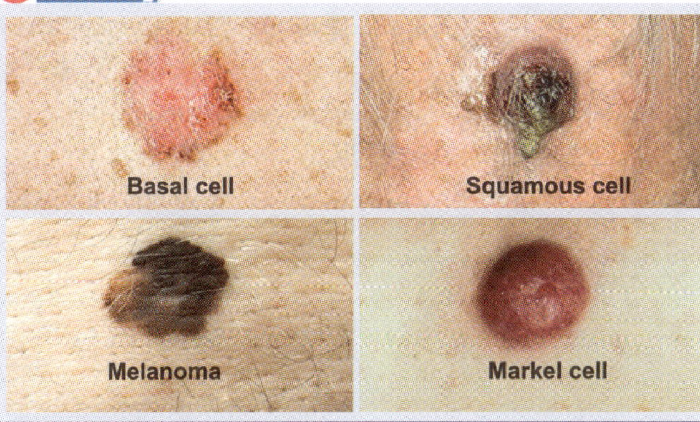

24. Ans. (a) Lichen planus

Ref: Rook's Dermatology Handbook, 2022 ed. pg. 679

- The shown condition is possibly lichen planus.
- When Lichen planus affects the mouth, it is called oral lichen planus.
- Lesions can appear as either white, lacy, raised patches of tissue that resemble spiderwebs or tender, swollen patches that are bright red.

25. Ans. (c) Psoriasis vulgaris

Ref: Rooks Textbook of Dermatology 9th ed. pg. 35.10 / 1142

- Auspitz's sign: Appearance of punctate bleeding spots when psoriatic scales are scraped off. This occur because of thinning of epidermal layer over papillae and due to dilatation of blood vessels these get bleed readily when scale is removed
- Auspitz's sign present in psoriasis. It is not seen in Guttate psoriasis, Pustular psoriasis, Erythrodermic psoriasis. It can also be seen in conditions like Darier's disease and actinic keratosis.

Steps

- First Gently scrape lesion with a glass slide. This accentuates the silvery scales will accentuates (Grattage test positive). Scrape off all the scales.
- Turn glistening white adherent membrane (Bulkley's membrane) appears
- On removing the membrane, punctate bleeding points become visible.

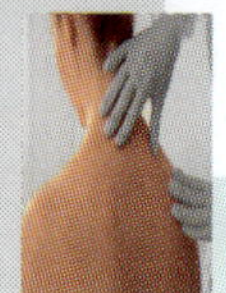

26. Ans. (a) Tubercular lymph node

Ref: Rooks Textbook of Dermatology 9th ed. pg. 767 / 27.13

Ulcers with undermined edges are seen in:
- Pyoderma gangrenosum
- Chancroid
- Cutaneous Tuberculosis/Scrofuloderma

27. Ans. (a) Zinc

Ref: Rooks Textbook of Dermatology 9th ed. pg. 1677/ 63.25

Features of Zinc Deficiency

- Scaly eczematous plaques in the - Periorificial region (around mouth, nose, genitals, and anus), acral areas, and bony prominences (like occiput)
- Diarrhoea.
- Nonscarring alopecia

Etiology

- **Acrodermatitis enteropathica** is an autosomal recessive trait, is the prototype zinc deficiency syndrome.
- Can also occur during parenteral hyperalimentation e.g. after intestinal surgery.
  - This is seen in infants being weaned off mother's milk and characterised by above cutaneous lesions. Systemic manifestation can also occur like irritability, diarrhea, growth retardation.

28. Ans. (d) Topical retinoids

Ref: Rooks Textbook of Dermatology 9th ed. pg. 90.38/2380

COMEDONES ARE THE MOST CHARACTERISTIC LESIONS IN ACNE VULGARIS

Grades of Acne

- **Grade 1** Predominantly Comedones
- **Grade 2** Predominantly Papules
- **Grade 3** Predominantly Pustules
- **Grade 4** Predominantly Nodules and Cysts

Topical Retinoids are preferred in management of comedones, preferably adapalene.

Mechanism of Action

- Effective against comedones by normalizing follicular keratinization as it Increases epidermal cell turnover and also increases dehiscence of stratum corneum.
- Also effective against inflammatory lesions, especially adapalene.

E.g. of retinoids are—adapalene, isotretinoin, and tazarotene.

Used in:
- In active disease: Effective for both comedones and inflammatory acne.
- For maintenance: Reduces formation of microcomedo.

29. Ans. (a) Malignant melanoma

Ref: Rooks Textbook of Dermatology 9th ed. pg. 143.2/3974

- It is malignant melanoma
- **Clinical feature:** It is a mole that has- (Mn: ABCDE)
  - **A**symmetrical lesion
  - **B**lurry anterior edge
  - **C**olour is multiple
  - **D**iameter is bigger (6 mm or 14 inch)
  - **E**volution (change in sudden size, shape and colour)

Extra Mile

- Classification best used for malignant melanoma: Breslow's
- Best prognostic indicator: Depth of lesion

SCC	BCC
Pre-existing disease: Occurs on damaged skin (scars, radiodermatitis, photodamaged skin). Can also develop in mucosa (leucoplakia)	Occurs on photodamaged skin. Mucosal lesions not seen.
Morphology: Fungating, indurated lesion with everted margin	Well-defined, firm lesion with waxy beaded margin
Growth: Rapid/slow gorwing	Slow growing
Sites: Anywhere on body including mucosae	Upper part of face. Superficial variant on trunk.
Metastases: Lymphadenopathy frequent. Visceral metastasis infrequent	Only local invasion

- Melanocytic nevus (MN)

SCC	BCC
Morphology: Pigmented or skin colored papule with smooth or hyperkeratotic surface; does not ulcerate	Noduloulcerative lesion with a pearly, beaded edge
Growth: Not destructive	Locally invasive, so called rodent ulcer

30. Ans. (a) Streptococcus

Ref: Rooks Textbook of Dermatology 9th ed. pg. 684/26.18

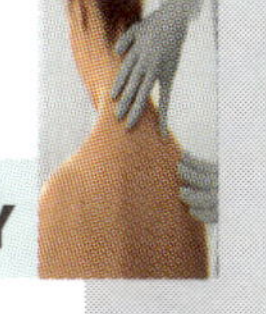

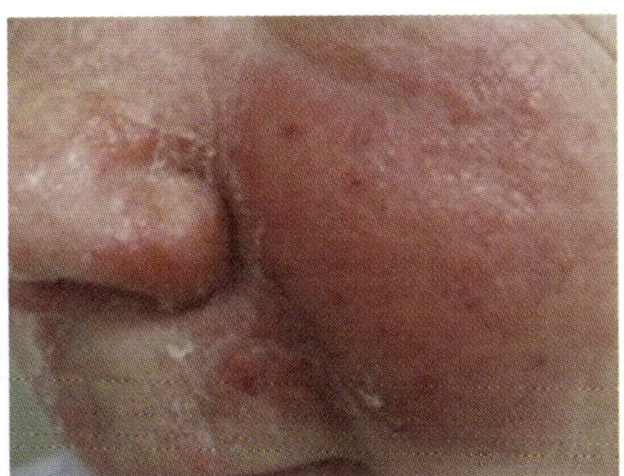

- Erysipelas is a superficial spreading pyoderma caused by Group A Beta Haemolytic Streptococcus (Streptococcus pyogenes, less frequently Streptococcus aureus)
- Acute erythematous, warm, indurated (firm to hard), rapidly spreading plaques, margin is sharply defined and superficial vesiculation may occur on the plaque.
- Note: Milian Ear sign is positive in Erysipelas that is ear is involved in Erysipelas , but spared in Cellulitis.

31. Ans. (a) Squamous cell carcinoma

Ref: Rooks Textbook of Dermatology 9th ed. pg. 108.25 2961

- Cutaneous Horn can occur secondary to underlying
  - Squamous cell carcinoma
  - Actinic keratosis (Pre Malignant condition)
  - Epidermal nevus
  - Verruca vulgaris
  - Seborrheic keratosis

Features of SCC

- Plaque or ulcer with indurated base and everted edges.
- Fixity to underlying tissue.
- Occur near damaged skin.
- Lymph node metastasis frequent in SCC arising in scarred skin.

Treatment: Excisional Biopsy

32. Ans. (a) Condyloma acuminata

Ref: Rooks Textbook of Dermatology 9th ed. pg. 3251/ 115.3

- Condyloma acuminata is a typical variant of Anogenital warts cause by Human papilloma virus type 6 > 11, 16, 18, (more frequently) 31, 33, 35, 39, 51–59 (less frequently).
- **Condyloma acuminata presents as:**
  - Soft, fleshy, sessile or pedunculated, pinkish or skin colored papules.
  - Initially small after sometime may enlarge to form cauliflower tumors.
- **Treatment:** Imiquimod > Podophyllotoxin (Teratogenic)

33. Ans. (a) Pyoderma gangrenosum

Ref: Rooks Textbook of Dermatology 9th ed. pg. 1377/49.1

Pyoderma Gangrenosum

- It is a noninfectious neutrophilic dermatosis associated with underlying systemic diseases including inflammatory bowel disease (Ulcerative colitis > **Crohn's disease**), arthritis, hematological malignancies, and monoclonal gammopathies.
- A papule, pustule or bulla which evolves into a rapidly progressive, painful, necrolytic ulcer.
- Ulcer is irregular in shape, undermined, violaceous border.
- Heals with cribriform scarring.
- Rapid response to oral steroids.

34. Ans. (a) Post streptococcal glomerulonephritis

Ref: Rooks Textbook of Dermatology 9th ed. pg. 679/26.13

- This picture showing is Non Bullous Impetigo/Impetigo contagiosa showing Golden yellow/Honey coloured Crusting
- Caused by - S. aureus, S. pyogenes (gp A) Or by both.
- Complication of this results - post streptococcal glomerulonephritis

Lesion Feature:

- Plaque covered with honey-colored crusts. Several lesions coalesce to form polycyclic plaque.
- The lesion spreads peripherally without central healing.
- Removal of the crust reveals an erosion.
- On drying, the crust falls leaving erythema which fades without scarring.

35. Ans. (c) Phenylephrine

- In the shown history and image, which is a case of frost bite, alpha receptor agonist like phenylephrine will NOT be used.
- In frost bite management, vasodilators will be used and vasoconstrictors are contraindicated.

36. Ans. (a) Xeroderma pigmentosum

Ref: Rooks Textbook of Dermatology 9th ed. pg. 2011/78.1

Xeroderma Pigmentosa

- Hallmark feature: Photosensitivity
- DNA repair defect
- On photo exposed parts multiple freckles develop and hypopigmented macules develops on dry rough skin (xeroderma).
- Patients eventually develop:

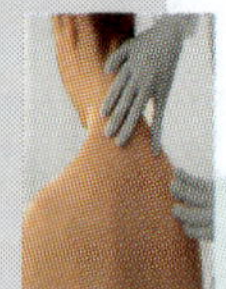

- Actinic keratosis
- keratoacanthoma
- Basal cell carcinoma
- Squamous cell carcinoma
- Malignant melanoma

37. Ans. (d) Coxsackievirus A16

Ref: Rooks Textbook of Dermatology 9th ed. pg. 651/25.81

- Coxsackievirus is an enterovirus that belongs to picornavirus family.
- Hand, Foot, and Mouth Disease (HFMD) Is caused by picorna virus (Coxsackievirus A16 and Enterovirus 71).
- It is present in both adults and children but more severe in infants and children.
- Present with Mucocutaneous lesions which is painful vesicles in oral mucosa, and occasionally on palms, soles and interdigital skin.

38. Ans. (a) Chicken pox

Ref: Rooks Textbook of Dermatology 9th ed. pg. 594/25.24

- Chicken pox is caused by Varicella-zoster virus.
- Patient presents with low grade fever and malaise.

Morphology

- Crops of papules with erythematous halo become vesicular then pustular.
- Vesicle of varicella is superficial and thin walled look like dew drops on rose petal appearance.
- Over it Crust become in few days and heal without scarring.
- Adults usually have a more severe eruption.
- Site: Profused on trunk least on face and limbs.
- Treatment: Acyclovir

39. Ans. (a) Paronychia

Ref: Rooks Textbook of Dermatology 9th ed. pg. 95.35/2509

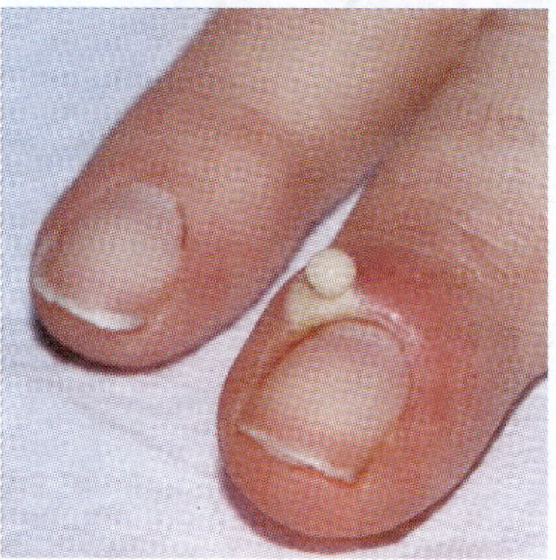

Paronychia (Infection of nail fold).

There are 2 types

- Acute paronychia (Staphylococcus aureus)
- Chronic paronychia (Candidial infection)

40. Ans. (c) Koebner's phenomenon

Ref: Rook's Textbook of Dermatology 9th ed. pg. 123.2-3

- **True koebner phenomenon** is seen in conditions like: Psoriasis, Vitiligo, Lichen planus, Kaposi sarcoma, Darrier disease.
- **Pseudo koebner's phenomenon** is seen in: Molluscum contagiosum, viral warts.

41. Ans. (b) Fixed drug eruption

Ref: Rook's Textbook of Dermatology 9th ed. pg. 118.11-12

- The shown condition after an anti-epileptic drug intake, is very characteristic of fixed drug eruption.
- Fixed drug eruption (FDE) is a cutaneous adverse drug reaction characterized by recurrent well-defined lesions occurring in the same sites each time the offending drug is taken
- It usually occurs 30 minutes to 8 hours after the drug exposure
- Most commonly associated with NSAIDs
- Drugs associated with fixed drug eruption commonly are:
    - NSAIDs, paracetamol, cotrimoxazole, tetracyclines, barbiturates, penicillin, antiepileptics.
- Lesions typically present are sharply defined, round or oval erythematous plaque, which are usually solitary or few in number.
- Commonly affected sites include the lips, genitals, palms and soles.

42. Ans. (a) BT

Ref: Rook's Textbook of Dermatology 9th ed. pg. 28.8-9

- **Satellite lesion** is a cluster of lesions around a larger central lesion.
- In BT type of leprosy, the immunity is not able contain the infection, so new lesions appear surrounding the older one.
- In borderline tuberculoid leprosy, there are four or more lesions asymmetrically distributed.
- Macules or plaques of variable sizes with well- or ill-defined margins and associated with satellite lesions.

43. Ans. (b) Lepromatous leprosy

Ref: Rook's Textbook of Dermatology 9th ed. pg. 28.8

- The shown image is of lepromatous facies, where the patient develops leonine facies and madarosis (loss of lateral 1/3rd of eyebrows).

- The first clinical manifestations of lepromatous leprosy are usually dermal (because early nerve involvement is usually asymptomatic).
- Dermal signs comprise macules, diffuse papules, infiltration or nodules, or all four.
- Macules are small, multiple, erythematous or faintly hypopigmented, with vague edges and shiny surface.

TABLE: Characteristics of lesions of polar leprosy

	Tuberculoid	Lepromatous
Number of lesions	1–10	Hundreds, confluent
Distribution	Asymmetrical, anywhere	Symmetrical, avoiding 'spared' areas
Definition and charity	Defined edge, markedly hypopigmented	Vague edge, slight hypopigmentation
Anaesthesia	Early, marked, defined, localized to skin lesions or major peripheral nerve	Late, initially slight, ill-defined, but extensive, over 'cool' areas of body
Autonomic loss	Early in skin and nerve lesions	Late, extensive as for anaesthesia
Nerve enlargement	Marked, in a few nerves	Slight but widespread
Mucosal and systemic	Absent	Common, severe during type 2 reactions
Number of *Mycobacterium leprae*	Not detectable	Numerous in all affected tissues

44. Ans. (a) Secondary syphilis

Ref: Rook's Textbook of Dermatology 9th ed. pg. 29.10

- The history is consistent with secondary syphilis.
- The palmar as shown in image is palmar syphilids.
- Upon pressing the lesion with blunt end of pin, patient experiences tenderness. This sign is known as Buschke olendroff sign.

Features of Secondary Syphilis

- 2–12 weeks of development of primary syphilis–patient manifests with symptoms of secondary syphilis
- Characterized by low-grade fever, malaise, sore throat, headache, adenopathy and cutaneous or mucosal rash.
- Manifest as–Evanescent copper-colored macular rash
- A few days later, symmetric papular eruption appears, involving entire trunk and the extremities, palm and soles
- Papules–reddish brown, scaly, discrete, 0.5–2 cm in diameter.

45. Ans. (a) Carbuncle

Ref: Rook's Textbook of Dermatology 9th ed. pg. 26.25-26

- Carbuncle is a cluster of furuncles that have multiple pus heads. It is usually caused by staphylococcal infection. It involves the adjacent follicles as well.
- They are connected subcutaneously and are more superficial than subcutaneous abscesses.

Extra Mile

Description of Bacterial Skin Infection

Disease	Description
Carbuncle	A network of furuncles connected by sinus tracts
Cellulitis	Painful, erythematous infection of deep skin with poorly demarcated borders
Erysipelas	Fiery red, painful infection of superficial skin with sharply demarcated borders
Folliculitis	Papular or pustular inflammation of hair follicles
Furuncle	Painful, firm or fluctuant abscess originating from a hair follicle
Impetigo	Large vesicles and/or honey-crusted sores

46. Ans. (b) Implantation dermoid

Ref: Rook's textbook of Dermatology 9th ed. pg. 110.10

- The given history and image are suggestive of implantation dermoid.
- It is more commonly seen in women, tailors, farmers who are prone to repeated injuries
- After a sharp injury epidermal cells are implanted in subcutaneous plane → forming dermoid cyst which is hard in consistency.
- **Common sites:** Fingers, palm, sole of foot

Extra Mile

Know the 4 types of Dermoid
- **Sequestration:** Inclusion of epithelium burried at line of embryonic fusion e.g., near head and neck
- **Implantation dermoid:** Indriven epithelium beneath skin due to puncture injury e.g. exposed part of body
- **Tubulodermoid:** Cyst from unobliterated portion of congenital ectodermal duct or tuber e.g., thyrolossal cyst, post and cyst, ependymal cyst in brain
- **Teratomatoid dermoid:** From totipotent cells e.g., ovary testis

47. Ans. (a) Subungual hyperkeratosis

Ref: Rook's Textbook of Dermatology 9th ed. pg. 95.40

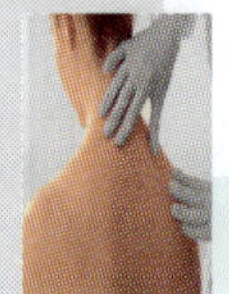

- Psoriasis is the most common disorder affecting the nails in almost 50% patients.
- **Nail changes are as follows:**
  - **Pitting:** Punctate depressions over nail
  - **Subungual hyperkeratosis:** It is seen mostly distally and extends proximally
  - **Splinter hemorrhage:** Due to increased capillary prominence in nail bed
  - **Onycholysis:** Separation of nail from the nailbed

48. Ans. (b) Elephantiasis

***Ref:** Rook's Textbook of Dermatology 9th ed. pg. 105.6-7*

- The shown image is of elephantiasis
- In this condition, there is abnormal accumulation of watery fluid in the tissues causing swelling, which is severe.
- **Causative organism:** W. bancrofti and Brugia malayi
- Note: Humans are definitive host for these parasites
- Spread by species of night feeding mosquitos, causing lymphatic filariasis, often termed as elephantiasis.
- **Affected system:** Lymphatics

49. Ans. (a) Impetigo contagiosa

***Ref:** Rook's Textbook of Dermatology 9th ed. pg. 26.13-14*

- The shown image the patient with honey colored crust is of impetigo.
- Impetigo is a superficial skin infection that is mostly seen in children and highly contagious condition.
- **It is caused by:**
  - **Bullous impetigo:** Staph aureus
  - **Non-bullous impetigo:** S. aureus, Group A streptococcus
- **Treatment:**
  - Clindamycin
  - Mupirocin and Bacitracin ointment

50. Ans. (a) Alopecia areata

***Ref:** Rook's Textbook of Dermatology 9th ed. pg. 89.31*

- Exclamation mark in the hair is a feature of alopecia areata
- **Exclamation mark hairs means:**
  - Broken hairs of 3–4 mm long which taper off towards scalp
  - Broad distal and thin proximal end

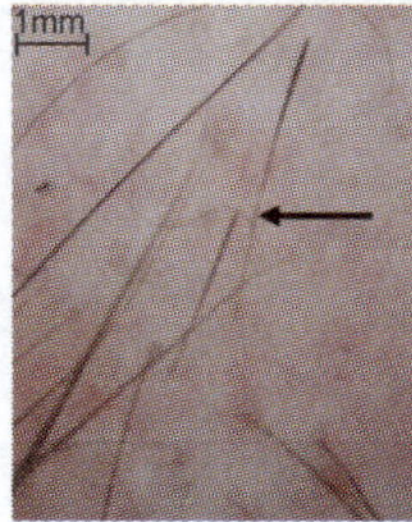

51. Ans. (b) Castle necklace appearance

***Ref:** Rook's Textbook of Dermatology 9th ed. pg. 63.16-17*

- Castle necklace appearance is a dermal manifestation of pellagra.
- Pellagra usually occurs due to dietary deficiency of Niacin (vitamin B3, Nicotinic acid) and tryptophan.
- **Other symptoms of pellagra:** Gingivitis with wedge shaped, punched out ulcers.
- **Often defined with 3 D's:** Dermatitis, dementia and diarrhea. It left untreated, it can lead to death (4th D).

52. Ans. (a) SLE

***Ref:** Harrison 20th ed. pg. 2518-2519*

- The image shows an erythematous rash sparing the nasolabial folds which coupled with clinical history points to diagnosis of SLE.
- Choice B leads to heliotrope rash involving the upper eye lid and proximal muscle weakness.
- Choice C presents as grey-brown patches, usually on the face on the cheeks, bridge of the nose, forehead, chin, and above the upper lip. It can also appear on sun-exposed parts of body, such as the forearms and neck.
- Choice D presents as redness, and can slowly spread beyond the nose and cheeks to the forehead and chin. There will be flushing, visible blood vessels and acne like breakouts.

53. Ans. (a) Acanthosis nigricans

***Ref:** Fitzpatrick Colour Atlas and Synopsis of Clinical Dermatology pg. 88*

- The image shows presence of *asymmetric, velvety hyperpigmentation* at the back of the neck of the patient suggestive of diagnosis of acanthosis nigricans. It is seen in patients with impaired glucose tolerance and internal malignancy.
- Choice B is seen in patients with internal malignancy but has multiple pigmented skin lesions.
- Choice C is a crusty, scaly growth caused by damage from exposure to ultraviolet (UV) radiation.
- Choice D has red inflamed lesions and is hence ruled out.

54. Ans. (c) Bilaterally symmetrical dermatomal vesicular eruption

***Ref:** Harrison 20th ed. pg. 1355*

- The image shows lesions of Herpes Zoster that develop unilaterally in a single dermatome.
- Choice A is correct since seronegative individuals on contact with these patients can develop chicken pox.

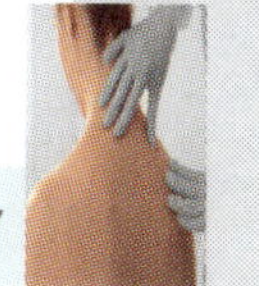

- Choice B is correct since neurological complication can develop in the form of meningoencephalitis.
- Choice D is correct since Ramsay Hunt syndrome leads to eruption in external auditory canal and the geniculate ganglion of sensory division of facial nerve is involved.

55. Ans. (c) Humby's knife

- The shown instrument is used in plastic surgery for skin feeling during grafting procedure. The instrument is Humby's knife.

56. Ans. (a) Intralesional steroids

- In patients with recurrent keloids, intralesional steroids are often very effective.
- Uniform protocol of corticosteroid injections and ointment application reduces recurrence rate of keloid drastically.
- Book says: "Intralesional steroids have been the mainstay of treatment of keloids"
- MC used steroid: Triamcinolone acetonide in concentration 10–40 mg/mL, administered intra-lesionally with 25–27 G needle at 4–6 weeks interval.
- Other modalities that can be used (less effective)
  - Silicon gel sheets and silicone occlusive dressing
  - Topical corticosteroid impregnated tape
  - Cryotherapy
  - Radiation therapy

57. Ans. (a) Staphylococcal scalded skin syndrome

- Staphylococcal Scalded Skin Syndrome aka Dermatitis Exfoliativa Neonatorum
- **Cause:** Toxin producing Staph aureus (exfoliative toxins A and B)
- **Characterized** by erythema and widespread loss of superficial epidermal layers, resembling burn
- **Symptoms:**
  - After staphylococcal infection like otitis, pharyngitis or conjunctivitis → fever with erythema resembling scarlet fever
  - It later becomes small unstable blisters → erodes quickly and leads to widespread skin loss (generalized).
  - Blister contains stratum corneum (in TEN, full thickness epidermal damage), subcorneal blisters and acantholysis.
- **Treatment:** Fluid replacement + Antibiotics

58. Ans. (b) Pearly penile papule

Ref: Dermatology Essentials E-Book, pg. 936

- The shown condition is pearly penile papule (PPP)
- Patients with pearly penile papule usually present with concern that they might have genital warts.
- PPP are benign, 1–2 mm dome shaped spots, asymptomatic angiofibromas that occur in rows, circumferentially around the coronal sulcus of penis.
  - **Incidence:** 8–30%; MC in 3rd decade
  - Mostly seen in circumcised males. It is not related to HPV
  - **Note:** Warts are not as linear or as clearly defined as PPP.
  - **Treatment:**
    - Usually not required; Reassurance
    - For lesion removal: Podophyllin application, cryotherapy, Electrodessication and curettage and CO_2 laser.

Extra Mile

- **Balanitis:** It is inflammation of glans of penis or prepuce due to poor personal hygiene by Candida species, streptococci, HPV, HSV, Gardnerella, etc.

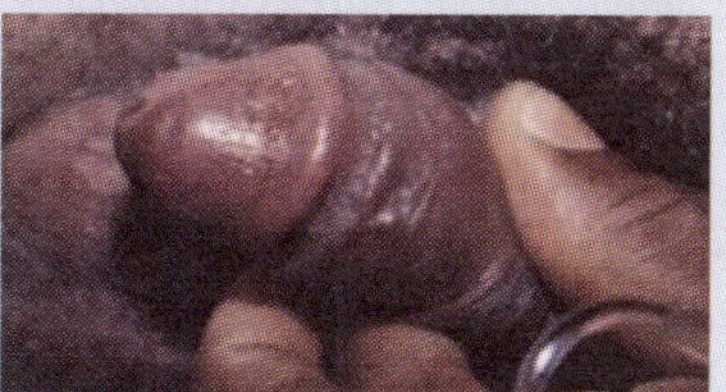

BALANITIS

- Sebaceous gland prominence

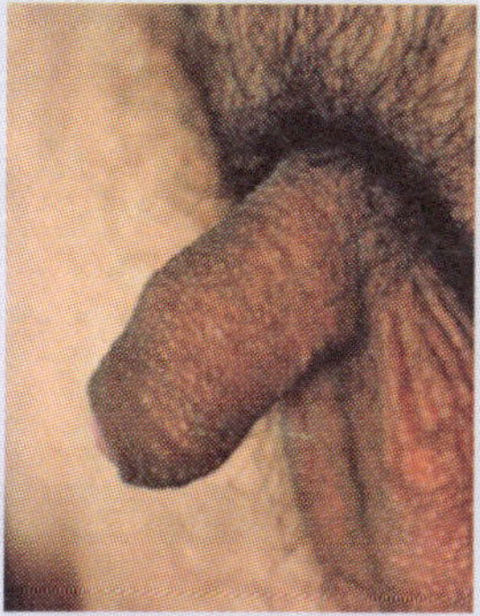

- Psoriasis of glans and shaft of penis

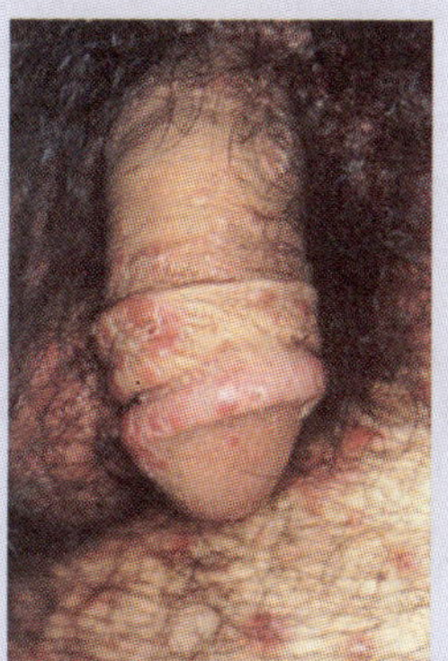

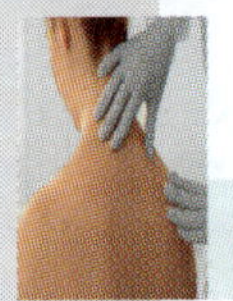

59. Ans. (a) Molluscum contagiosum

- Molluscum contagiosum caused by large DNA virus of pox group.
- Characterized by multiple, umbilicated pearly lesion
- More common in childhood and on face
- It tends to resolve spontaneously
- Lesion occurring on genitalia or lower abdomen in adult are almost always sexually transmitted.
- **HPE:** Molluscum bodies—multinucleated giant cell in the central keratinous core of lesion of giemsa stain.
- **Treatment:** Cryotherapy or KOH or Phenol application

60. Ans. (a) Impetigo

Ref: Pediatric Dermatology E book by Lawrence Schachner pg. 1338

- Impetigo is a highly contagious bacterial infection of superficial layer of epidermis.
- MCC: *Staphylococcus aureus* and *Streptococcus*.
- **It occurs in two forms:**
  1. **Non-bullous impetigo:** Caused by *Staphylococcus aureus*. Most commonly affects child age group and characterized by honey colored crust (*as seen in this patient*).
  2. **Bullous impetigo:** Can be caused by *Staphylococcus aureus* or *Streptococcus*. Common in all age groups.

61. Ans. (a) Acoustic neuroma

Ref: Neurofibromatoses in Clinical Practice, pg. 47-48

- Neurofibromatosis is a type of autoimmune skin disorder, and is associated with several other systemic conditions/tumors.
- Acoustic neuroma is the most common neural tumor associated with NF-2

TABLE: Differences between NF1 and NF2

NF1	NF2
• Common (90% of all NF cases)	• Much less common (10% of all NF cases)
• Chromosome 17 mutations	• Chromosome 22 mutations
• Almost always diagnosed by age 10	• Usually diagnosed in second to fourth decades
• Cutaneous lesions common (>95%) ▪ Cafe au lait spots ▪ Lisch nodules ▪ Cutaneous NFs (often multiple) ▪ Plexiform NFs (pathognomonic)	• Cutaneous, eye lesions less prominent • Mild/few cafe au lait spots Juvenile subcapsular opacities
• CNS lesions less common (15-20%) ▪ 72/FLAIR hyperintensities (myelin vacuolization; lesions wax, then wane) ▪ Astrocytomas (optic pathway gliomas—usually pilocytic—other gliomas) ▪ Sphenoid wing, dural dysplasias ▪ Moyamoya ▪ Neurofibromas of spinal nerve roots	• CNS lesions in 100% ▪ Bilateral vestibular schwannomas (almost all) ▪ Nonvestibular schwannomas (50%) ▪ Meningiomas (50%) ▪ Cord ependymomas (often multiple) ▪ Schwannomas of spinal nerve roots

Extra Mile

Diagnostic criteria of NF1
Two or more of the following:
• At least six café-au-lait macules (>5 mm diameter in prepubertal individuals and >15 mm in postpubertal individuals)
• Freckling in axillary or inguinal regions
• Optic glioma
• At least two Lisch nodules (iris hamartomas)
• At least two neurofibromas of any type, or one plexiform neurofibroma
• A distinctive osseous lesion (sphenoid dysplasia or tibial pseudarthrosis)
• A first degree relative with NF1

TABLE: Diagnostic criteria for NF-2

Main criteria
Bilateral vestibular schwannomas or
First-degree relative with neurofibromatosis type 2 plus 1. Unilateral vestibular schwannomas or 2. Any two of the following: Meningioma, glioma, schwannoma, or juvenile posterior lenticular opacities

62. Ans. (b) Dermatome

Ref: PubMed

- The shown division is dermatomal division
- Dermatome is the area of the skin of the human anatomy that is mainly supplied by branches of a single spinal sensory root.

> - Blaschko lines or the lines of Blaschko are thought to represent pathways of epidermal cell migration and proliferation during the development of the fetus.
> - These lines are invisible but many inherited and acquired diseases of skin manifest themselves according to these patterns creating the visual appearance of these lines.

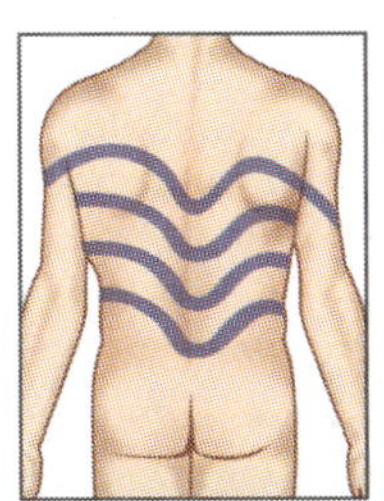

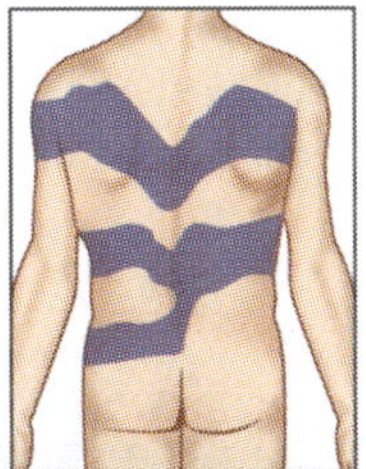

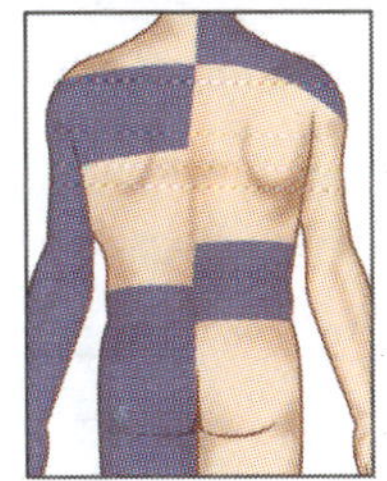

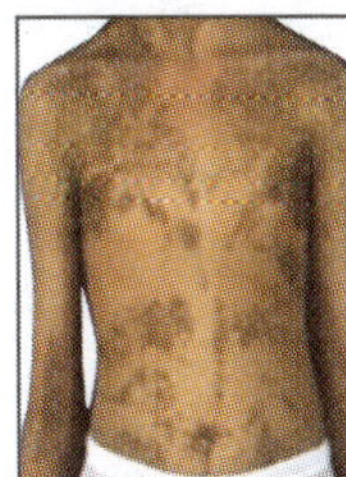

63. Ans. (c) Bow legs

Ref: Avery's Neonatology: Pathophysiology & Management of the New born, pg. 1040-41

FEATURES OF CONGENITAL SYPHILIS:

- Skin lesion: Maculopapular rash
- Hepatosplenomegaly and lymphadenopathy
- Failure to thrive
- Anaemia, jaundice
- Gummatous ulcer
- Saddle nose, prominent forehead
- Interstitial keratitis
- CN-VIII involvement: SNHL
- Syphilitic rhinitis- purulent nasal discharge
- Dental deformities: Hutchinson's teeth

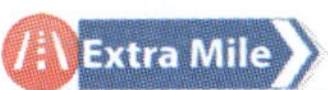
Extra Mile

Hutchinson triad:
- Interstitial keratitis
- SNHL
- Hutchinson teeth

64. Ans. (c) Psoralen PUVA

Ref: Bhutani Atlas of Dermatology, 6th ed. pg. 209-210

- Vitiligo is an acquired autoimmune condition targeting melanocytes and presents with localized or widespread white depigmented patches.
- Thyroid dysfunction is the most common association.

TREATMENT OF VITILIGO

- Mainstay of therapy: Psoralen with UVA (PUVA)
- No therapy is effective alone
  - Topicals
    - Corticosteroids
    - Immunomodulators
  - Light Therapy:
    - UVA or UVB 2
    - UVA + Psoralen = PUVA (Topical and Systemic)
    - UVB = Laser
  - Systemic Treatment: NOT USED
  - Surgical Rx:
    - Melanocyte Transplant
    - Skin Grafts Transplant
  - Bleaching Agents: Depigment all skin

65. Ans. (b) Acantholytic cells

Ref: Fitzpatrick Colour Atlas, 8th ed. pg. 681

- The image shows Acantholytic cells with ground glass nuclei consistent with tzanck cells.
- *Acantholysis is defined as the loss of coherence between epidermal cells due to the breakdown of their intercellular bridges.* In contrast Acanthosis implies thickening of skin due to diffuse epidermal hyperplasia.

Extra Mile

- **Hyperkeratosis:** Hyperplasia of the stratum corneum with abnormal keratin.
- **Papillomatosis:** Surface elevation caused by hyperplasia and enlargement of dermal papillae.
- **Parakeratosis:** Keratinization characterized by retention of the nuclei in the stratum corneum. On squamous mucosal membranes, such as buccal mucosa parakeratosis is normal.
- **Spongiosis:** Intercellular edema of the epidermis

66. Ans. (b) Blaschko lines

Ref: Fitzpatrick Dermatology, 9th ed. pg. 302

- The image shows lines of Blaschko which represent a pattern assumed by many different nevoid and acquired skin diseases on the human skin and mucosae.
- They represent *normal developmental growth pattern of skin*
- These lines do not correspond to any known nervous, vascular or lymphatic structures.
- *Langer's lines* correspond to alignment of *collagen fibers* in the dermis. They are used to determine direction with the human skin along which the skin has the least flexibility.
- *Kraissl lines* differ from Langer's lines in that unlike Langer's lines, which are defined in term of collagen orientation, Kraissl's lines are oriented *perpendicular to the action of the underlying muscles.*
- *Borges lines are relaxed skin tension lines.* The relaxation is achieved by joint mobilization, muscle contraction, or pinching.

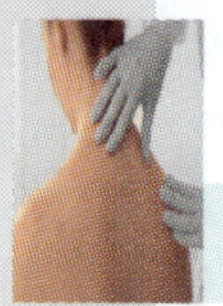

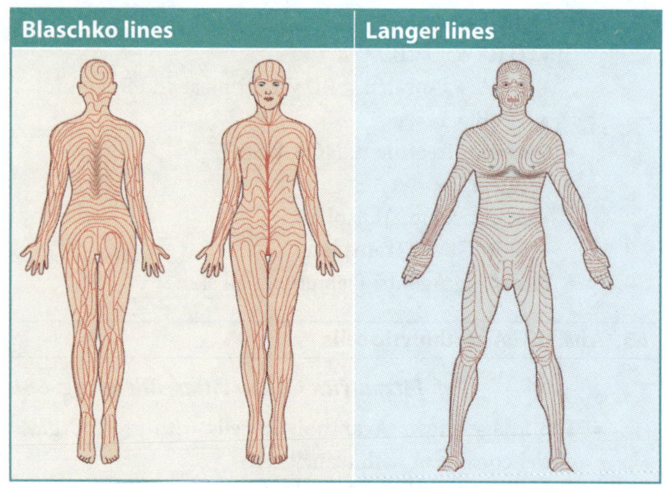

67. Ans. (b) Pemphigus vulgaris

Ref: TB of Dermatology, leprology & Venereology Devinder Mohan Thappa E book Chapter 4

- **Pemphigus vulgaris:** The antibodies are directed against Desmoglein 3 (*which binds the epidermal cells together*), causing loss of cell to cell adhesion.
  - **In mucosal *Proteus vulgaris*:** Antibody against only DSG3
  - **In mucocutaneous *P. vulgaris*:** Antibody against DSG 1 and 3
- **Upon examination and HPE following findings are seen:**
  - Bulla spread sign, Nikolsky's sign, acantholytic cells.
  - HPE shows suprabasal blister with row of tomb stone appearance.
  - Direct immunofluorescence shows intraepidermal IgG deposits in fishnet pattern.

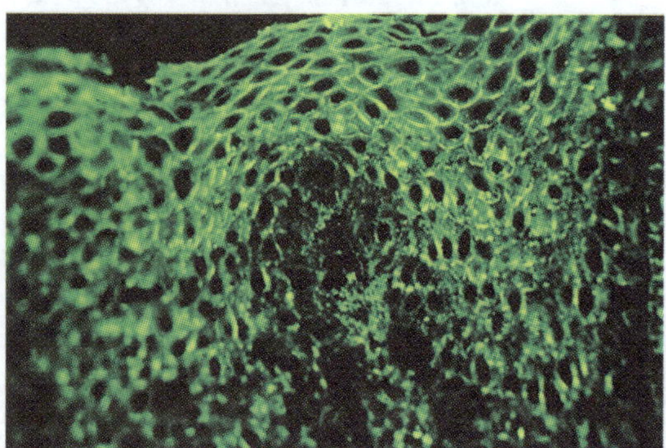

- **Bullous pemphigoid:** Most common autoimmune bullous disease. Presence of large, tense bullae. Common in elderly.
- **Dermatitis herpetiformis:** Gluten sensitive enteropathy. Very commonly (70–100%) have coeliac disease. Its dermal manifestation is severe itching. HPES shows IgA deposited in dermal papilla.
  - **Rx:** Gluten free diet and dapsone (DOC) is used for treatment.
- **Erythema multiforme:** Most commonly caused by HSV virus. Others causes can be malignancy, drug, mycoplasma, idiopathic. Has a characteristic target lesion.

Extra Mile

TABLE: Autoimmune bullous diseases—target antigens

Disease	Target antigens
Pemphigus foliaceus	Desmoglein 1
Herpetiform pemphigus	Desmoglein 1
IgA pemphigus (SPD type)	Desmocollin 1
IgA pemphigus (IEN type)	Desmoglein 1 or 3
Pemphigus vulgaris	Desmoglein 3
Epidermolysis bullosa acquisita	Type VII collagen

68. Ans. (d) Impetigo

Ref: Pediatric Dermatology E book by Lawrence Schachner pg. 1338

- Impetigo is a highly contagious bacterial infection of superficial layer of epidermis. It is caused most commonly by *Staphylococcus aureus* and *Streptococcus*.
- **It occurs in 2 forms:**
  - **Non-bullous impetigo:** Caused by *Staphylococcus aureus*. Most commonly affects child age group and characterized by honey colored crust (*as seen in this patient*).
  - **Bullous impetigo:** Can be caused by *Staphylococcus aureus* or *Streptococcus*. Common in all age groups.

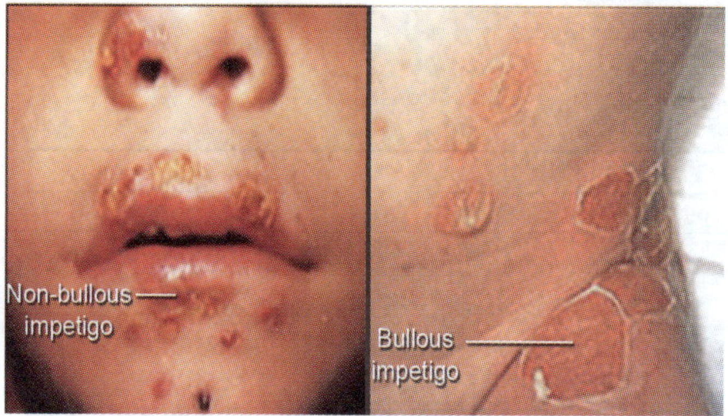

69. Ans. (c) Sebaceous gland

Ref: Illustrated Synopsis of Dermatology & Sexually transmitted diseases E book by Neena Khanna pg. 123

- Fordyce spot is ectopic sebaceous gland.
- **Most common site:** Upper lip and buccal mucosa.
- Usually asymptomatic condition. No treatment required.

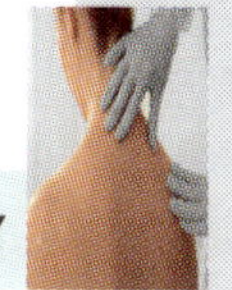

Extra Mile

- **Fox Fordyce disease:** Keratin obstruction of apocrine ducts
- **Hidradenitis suppurativa:** Keratin obstruction of apocrine ducts extending into hair follicles. Also known as inverse acne.
  - Most common site axilla.
- **Acne vulgaris:** Obstruction of pilosebaceous gland.
- **Miliaria:** Occlusion of eccrine gland due to *Staphylococcus epidermidis*.

70. Ans. (a) Scabies

Ref: Illustrated Synopsis of Dermatology & Sexually transmitted diseases E book by Neena Khanna pg. 14-15

- Scabies is a contagious skin infestation caused commonly by female mite Sarcoptes scabiei *(the shown image)*.
- Incubation period 3–4 weeks.
- **In infant scabies:** Face, palms and soles involved.
- S shaped burrow is pathognomonic of scabies infestation.
- Adult scabies spares face.
- Scabies is one of the water washed disease, involves axillae, elbow, flexures, wrist, finger, webs, umbilicus, lower abdomen and genitalia. These involved areas if joined with an intersecting lines is known as circle of hebra.
- **DOC:** 5% permethrin.
- **Oral DOC for scabies:** Ivermectin.

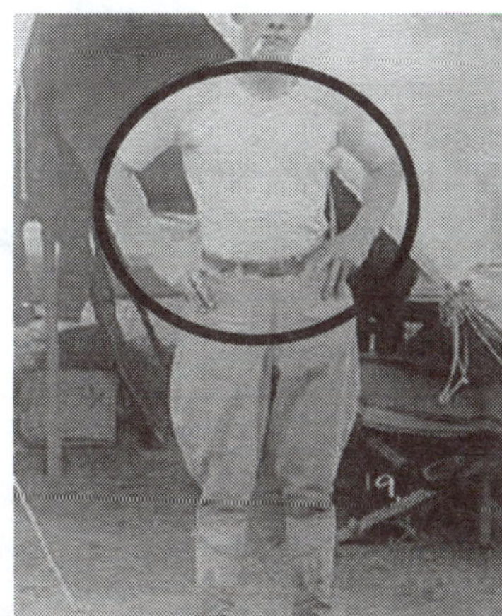

Circle of hebra

Extra Mile

- **Pediculosis (vagabond disease)**
  1. Head louse: *P. capitis*
  2. Body louse: *P. corporis*
  3. Pubic/crab louse: Pthirus pubis DOC is 1% permethrin.
- **Molluscum contagiosum**
  - Caused by Pox virus. Pearly white papules with umbilication. Common in children on face. Inclusion body known as molluscum body or *Henderson Peterson body*.

71. Ans. (c) Becker nevus

Ref: Illustrated Synopsis of Dermatology & Sexually transmitted diseases E book by Neena Khanna pg. 35

- Becker's nevus, also called pigmented hairy epidermal nevus, is a cutaneous hamartoma that can have increased epidermal (melanocyte), dermal (smooth muscle), and appendageal (hair follicle) components.
- Classically, Becker's nevus is first noticed around puberty on the shoulders and chest in males. The prevalence in postpubertal males is approximated to be 0.5%, or 1 in 200.
- It may involve only surface of body in women.

Note:

- **Nevus of Ota:** Seen usually around eyes.
- Café au lait macule is light brown macule commonly seen on trunk and has smooth edges.

72. Ans. (b) Pityriasis rosea

Ref: Illustrated Synopsis of Dermatology & Sexually transmitted diseases E book by Neena Khanna pg. 39

- Pityriasis rosea is a noncontagious, erythematous skin lesion, caused by human herpesvirus 6 and 7.
- Classically it begins with typical **Herald patch** (single red and scaly), and then becomes generalized patch.
- Sometimes, these patches are also referred to as Cigarette paper scales.
- Herald/mother's patch is the first sign of Pityriasis rosea.
- *Fir-tree or Christmas-tree appearance* due to distribution of lesion along the line of cleavage on trunk.
- Mainly involves trunk. Spares palm and soles (*this feature differentiates it from secondary syphilis*)

73. Ans. (b) Erythrasma

Ref: Dermatology by Jean L. Bolognia, Joseph L. Jorizzo, Ronald

- *Erythrasma* is a superficial, localized, mild and often chronic skin infection caused by *Corynebacterium minutissimum*.
- The growth of the organism is favoured by moist, occluded intertriginous areas, including groin, axilla, intergluteal fold and inframammary and periumbilical areas.
- These lesions are irregular in shape and size, red, well defined patches covered with fine scales and wrinkling.
- The infection begins as a proliferation of C. minutissimum within the stratum corneum.
- **Under wood's lamp examination:** Bright coral red fluorescence.
- This *bright coral red fluorescence under wood's lamp* is as a *result of porphyrin production* by the bacteria. It is considered as the best way to make diagnosis.

Extra Mile

- Tinea versicolor may resemble erythrasma, but does not tend to localize to body folds.

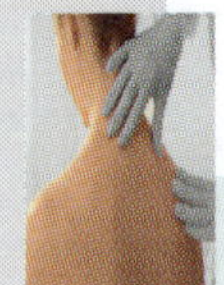

74. Ans. (c) Male pattern baldness

- The shown image is a case of *male pattern baldness.*
- Male pattern hair loss is an androgen dependent process.
- In majority of cases, this balding is patterned. The two major components being *frontotemporal recession* and *loss of hair over the vertex.*

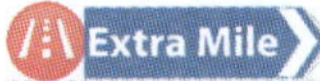

Alopecia areata: Autoimmune disease characterized by patchy hair loss with no visible signs of inflammation, exclamation mark hair and geometric pitting of the nails

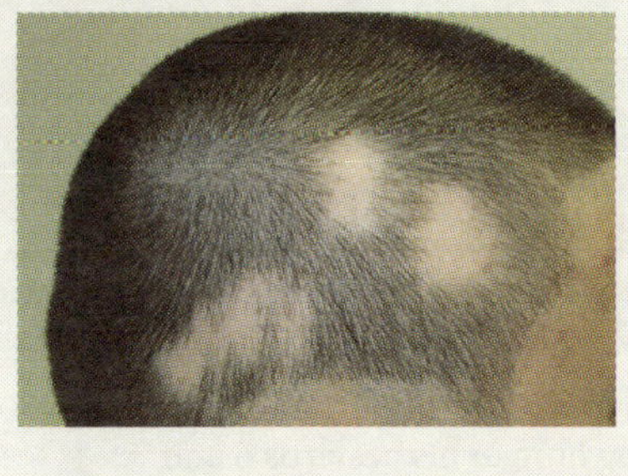

Telogen effluvium: This type of hair loss happens when hair follicles are fluctuated into the telogen or resting phase prematurely. There are large amount of hair that begin to fall prematurely at the same time secondary to certain stress like chronic illness, pregnancy, depression, etc.
Mostly seen in female.

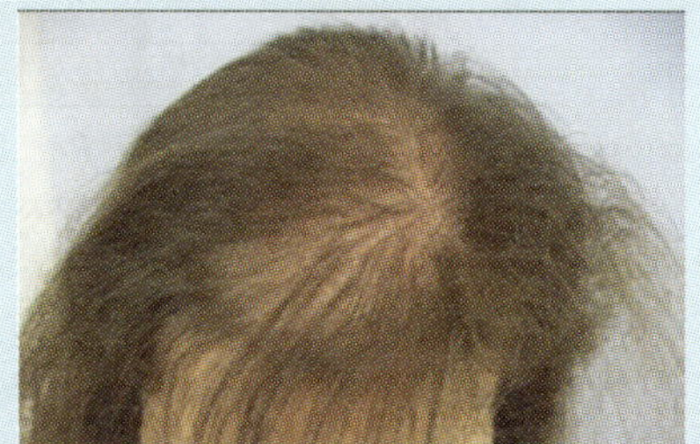

Cicatricial alopecia
Occurs due to inflammatory disorders that cause permanent destruction of pilosebaceous unit and irreversible hair loss

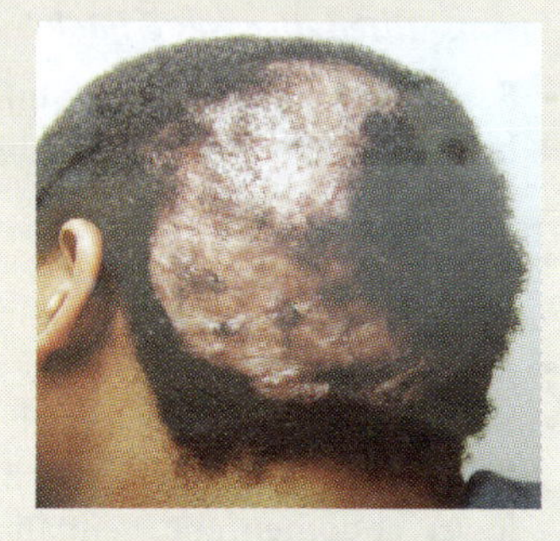

75. Ans. (a) Desmoglein 1

Ref: Inflammatory Dermatopathology: A Pathologist's Survival Guide, pg. 159

- Pemphigus foliaceous is a condition which arises due to antibody against desmoglein 1 (*remember F = First*)
- *Desmogleins* along with *desmocollins* connect two cells of epidermis. It is expressed in different layers of skin and mucosa.
- Desmogleins have several isoforms and if antibody forms against them, it will lead to different disease entity.

Desmogleins	DSG 1	DSG 3
Location	Epidermis, *subcorneal layer* It is not expressed in mucosal layer	Epidermis, *stratum basale* It is expressed in mucosal layer as well
Associated disease if antibody formed (IgG antibody)	Pemphigus foliaceous (subcorneal blister)	Pemphigus vulgaris (can involve DSG 1 as well)

76. Ans. (c) Both

Ref: Inflammatory Dermatopathology: A Pathologist's Survival Guide pg. 159

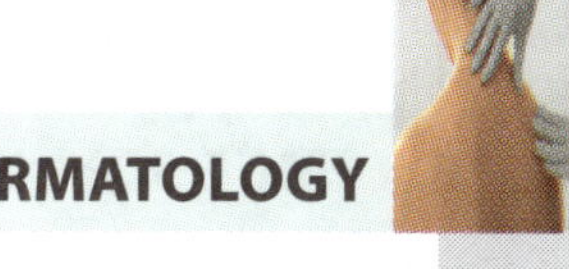

The antibodies in *pemphigus vulgaris* are directed against *desmoglein* 3, a desmosomal cadherin that mediates cell binding. Desmoglein 3 is expressed in greater concentration in the lower epidermis, the location of the suprabasal acantholytic blister of pemphigus vulgaris.

- More than half of sera from patients with pemphigus vulgaris also have circulating antibodies against desmoglein 1.
- Established lesions of pemphigus vulgaris demonstrate suprabasilar acantholysis with frequent involvement of follicular external root sheaths
- The basal keratinocytes separate from one another but remain attached to the dermis, reminiscent of a "row of tombstones"

77. Ans. (a) Pemphigus vulgaris

Please refer to above explanation

- Pemphigus vulgaris is characterized by following signs:
  1. Bulla spread sign
  2. Perilesional and distant nikolsky sign
  3. Tzanck smear: Acantholytic cell
- Histopathology shows suprabasal blister with row of tomb stone appearance of basal cells.
- Direct immunofluorescence from perilesional skin demonstrated intraepidermal IgG deposites in a *fishnet pattern.*

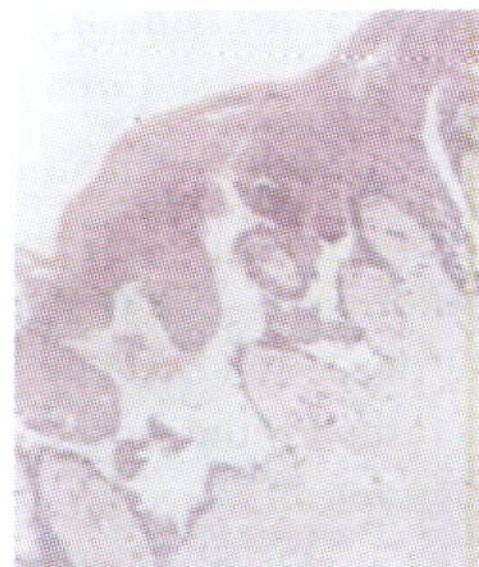

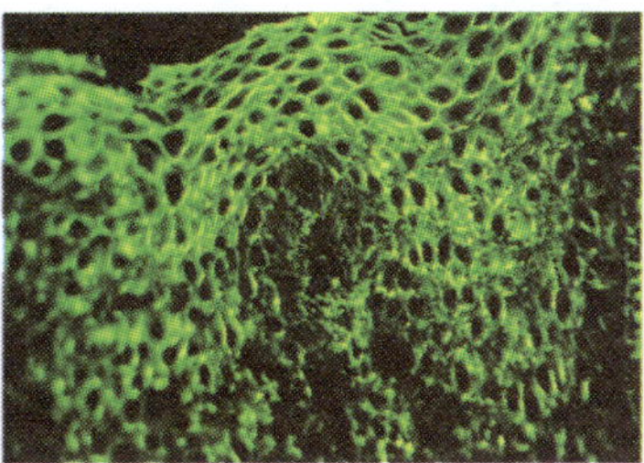

FIGURE: Pemphigus vulgaris, shows suprabasal cleavage with acantholysis. "Row of tomb stones appearance" can be seen in the floor of bulla

78. Ans. (d) Bullous pemphigoid

Ref: Mayo Clinic Internal Medicine Board Review, pg. 162

- Bullous pemphigoid is the *most common autoimmune bullous disease.*
- It occurs predominantly in elderly population.
- It presents as *large, tense bullae* with a predilection for flexural areas.
- Immunofluroscence testing is important for its diagnosis.
- Almost all cases have deposition of C3 and IgG in a *linear pattern at the basement membrane zone* (*as shown in the image of question*).

79. Ans. (b) Dermatitis herpetiformis

Ref: Bhutani Atlas of Dermatology, 6th ed. pg. 179

- Dermatitis herpetiformis is a condition seen in middle aged patients with male predilection.

Clinical Features

Dermatitis herpetiformis is an immunopathologic vesiculobullous disease of skin rarely showing oral manifestations. The condition represents the *cutaneous expression of gluten enteropathy* (gliadin sensitivity). The skin lesions are *pruritic* and are located primarily on the extremities and buttocks. They are *vesicular with a tendency to rupture and desquamate.* Oral bullae may be encountered and many patients present with aphthous like ulcers. The disease is chronic, lasting for many years, yet is not life threatening.

HPE: Neutrophilic microabscess in dermal papillary tip is **characteristic.**

Direct immunofluorescence: Shows granular IgA deposition in dermal papillary area.

80. Ans. (b) Atopic dermatitis

- **Hertoghe's sign** is lateral thinning of the eyebrows. It is seen in condition like atopic dermatitis.

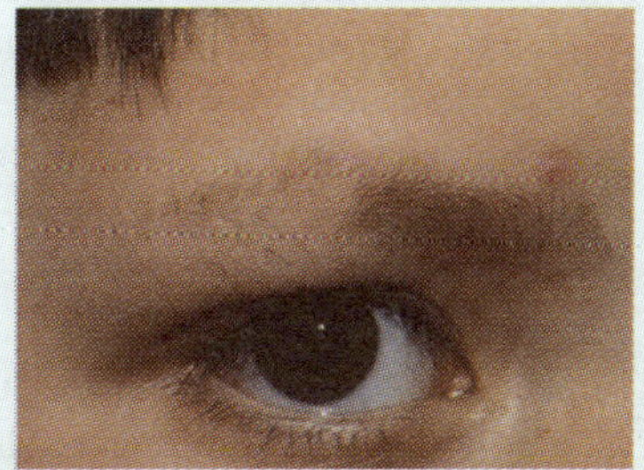

- **Dennie morgan fold:** A deep fold that can be found under the lower lid. Also seen in atopic dermatitis.

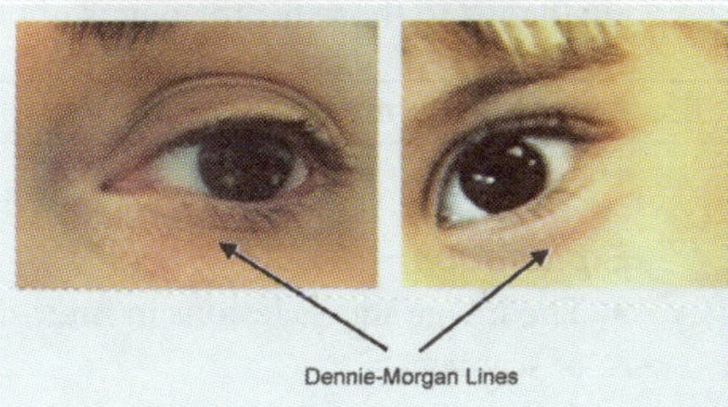

81. Ans. (b) Tuberous sclerosis

Ref: Harrison's, 19th ed. pg. 359

- **Triad of tuberous sclerosis** is remembered with simple mnemonic **EpiLoA**: **Epi**lepsy, **Lo**w IQ, and **a**denoma sebaceum.
- The patient in image presented with adenoma sebaceum and other triad of tuberous sclerosis.
- The **earliest cutaneous sign** tuberous sclerosis, is macular hypomelanosis, referred to as an *ash leaf spot.*

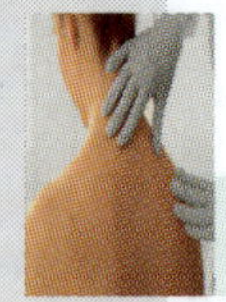

- Examination of the patient for additional cutaneous signs such as multiple angiofibromas of the face *(adenoma sebaceum)*, ungual and gingival fibromas, fibrous plaques of the forehead, and connective tissue nevi *(shagreen patches)* is recommended.
- Internal manifestations include seizures, mental retardation, central nervous system (CNS) and retinal hamartomas, pulmonary lymphangioleiomyomatosis (women), renal angiomyolipomas, and cardiac rhabdomyomas.

82. Ans. (b) Nevus ota

Ref: Oski's Pediatrics, Principle and Practice, pg. 829

- *Nevus of Ota*, is a hamartoma of dermal melanocytes.
- It is a bluish or gray-brown patch of pigmentation that occurs on the skin of the face, usually in the distribution of the first and second branches of the trigeminal nerve. Perhaps two-thirds of affected infants have an *associated ipsilateral bluish discoloration of the sclera*.
- Histologically, a nevus of Ota is *identical to a Mongolian spot* and likely results from errors in migration spot, however, the nevus of Ota does not undergo spontaneous regression. If scleral pigmentation is present, glaucoma may occur.
- Malignant degeneration occurring within a nevus of Ota is rare. Management options for the nevus include the use of a covering cosmetic or treatment with a pigmented lesion laser.

Nevus of Ito: A patch of hyperpigmentation similar to the nevus of Ota but *occurring over the shoulders*, in the supraclavicular areas, and on the sides of the neck, the upper arms, and the scapulae is known as the *nevus of Ito*. These lesions persist throughout life. Treatment options are analogous to those for the nevus of Ota.

83. Ans. (b) Ivermectin

Ref: KDT, 6th ed. pg. 864

Explanation:

- The image shows lesions in inter-digital clefts suggestive of scabies.
- Scabies is caused by an ectoparasite Sarcoptes scabiei. It is highly contagious. The mite burrows through the epidermis, laying eggs which form papules that itch intensely.
- Most common site of entry—finger webs.
- Drugs used are:
  - **Permethrin:** Broad spectrum and potent insecticide, currently most efficacious.
    - It is preferred topical drug for scabies.
    - **MOA:** It causes neurological paralysis in insects by delaying depolarization.
    - Single application needed in most cases.
    - Very less toxicity; 100% cure rate.
  - **Lindane:** Another broad spectrum insecticide. Efficacy lower than permethrin.
    - **MOA:** Kills lice and mites by penetrating through their chitinous cover and affecting the nervous system.
  - **Benzyl benzoate:** Oily liquid with a faint aromatic smell.
    - It is applied over face and neck after a bath. A second coat is applied next day which is washed after 24 hours.
  - Crotamiton
  - Sulfur

Extra Mile

- **Ivermectin:** Highly effective in scabies pediculosis and Norwegian scabies
  - It is the only orally administered drug which is used for scabies (ectoparasitosis). Oral DOC for scabies.
  - A single dose of 0.2 mg/kg has cured almost 90–100% of population.
  - *It is contraindicated in children <5 years, pregnant and lactating women.*

84. Ans. (d) Antipyretics

Ref: Primary Care Dermatology, An Issue of Primary Care, pg. 526

- The shown image is a case of roseola infantum also known as 6th day disease.
- Roseola infantum, also known as 3-day fever, is characterized by high-grade fever followed by abrupt defervescence and onset of a rash. It is the most common exanthem before age 2. It is typically seen in children between the ages of 6 months and 4 years, with a peak age of acquisition between 9 and 21 months.
- *It is most commonly caused by human herpes virus (HHV) -6 and less commonly by HHV-7, enterovirus, adenovirus, and parainfluenza virus.*
- The modes of transmission and incubation periods vary depending on the etiologic agent. In most patients with roseola caused by HHV-6 the average incubation period is 9–10 days. Usually by the time the rash appears, viremia has already resolved.

85. Ans. (c) Tinea captitis

Ref: Harrison's, 19th ed. pg. 355

- The image shows a boggy scalp of Tinea capitis

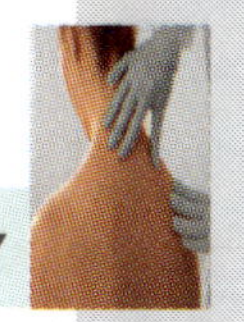

Tinea capitis	Varies from scaling with minimal hair loss to discrete patches with "black dots" (broken infected hairs) to boggy plaque with pustules (kerion)	Invasion of hairs by dermatophytes, most commonly *Trichophyton tonsurans*	Oral griseofulvin or terbinafine plus 2.5% selenium sulfide or ketoconazole shampoo; examine family members
Traumatic alopecia	Broken hair, often of varying lengths irregular outline	Traction with curlers, chemicals (e.g., hair straighteners) Mechanical pulling (trichotilloma-nia)	Discontinuation of offending hair style of chemical treatments; require observation of shaved hairs (for growth) or biopsy, possibly followed by psychotherapy

86. Ans. (b) Tinea corporis

Ref: Oski's Essential Pediatrics, pg. 155

- The annular lesion with central clearing, is most likely indicative of tinea corporis.
- The infection of nonhairy areas of the skin by dermatophytes is limited to the epidermis, only the most superficial layers of the skin are involved. The rings are generally erythematous. As the inflammation spreads, the active infection in the center of the lesions is destroyed, and this area clears, frequently resulting in the picture of an advancing border with central clearing.
- The organism responsible for most cases of tinea corporis is *Trichophytom tonsurans. Microsporum canis, Microsporum audouinii,* and *Trichophyton mentagrophytes* infections are also seen.

87. Ans. (a) Molluscum contagiosum

Ref: Harrison's, 19th ed. pg. 220e-1

- Vesicle with central umbilication is most likely suggestive of molluscum contagiosum.
- Molluscum contagiosum is a cutaneous poxvirus infection characterized by multiple umbilicated flesh-colored or hypo-pigmented papules.
- Molluscum contagiosum is highly prevalent among children and is the most common human disease resulting from poxvirus infection.
- Swimming pools are a common vector for transmission.

88. Ans. (b) Basal cell cancer

Ref: Harrison's, 19th ed. pg. 501

The image shows a lesion on face showing *raised and beaded appearance*. It is suggestive of diagnosis of BCC. The *most common site* is the face with a line drawn between angle of mouth and ear Lobule–*Onghren's line.*

89. Ans. (a) Alopecia areata

Ref: Harrison's, 19th ed. pg. 355

	Clinical	Pathogenesis	Treatment
Telogen effluvium (choice C)	• Diffuse shedding of normal hairs • Follows major stress (high fever, severe infection) or change in hormone levels (postpartum) • Reversible without treatment	Stress causes more of the asynchronous growth cycles of individual hairs to become synchronous; therefore, larger numbers of growing (anagen) hairs simultaneously enter the dying (telogen) phase	Observation, discontinue any drugs that have alopecia as a side effect, must exclude underlying metabolic causes, e.g. hypothyroidism, hyperthyroidism
Androgenetic alopecia (male pattern; female pattern) (choice B)	• Miniaturization of hairs along the midline of the scalp • Recession of the anterior scalp line in men and some women	• Increased sensitivity of affected hairs to the effects of androgens • Increased levels of circulating androgens (ovarian or adrenal source in women)	If no evidence of hyperandro-genemia, then topical minoxidil finastheride[Q] spironolactone (women); hair transplant
Alopecia areata (choice A)	• Well-circumscribed, circular areas of hair loss, 2–5 cm in diameter • In extensive cases, coalescence of lesions and/or involvement of other hair-bearing surfaces of the body • Pitting or sandpapered appearance of the nails	The germinative zones of the hair follicles are surrounded by T lymphocytes **Occasional associated disease: hyperthyroidism, hypothyrodidism, vitiligo. Down syndrome**	Topical anthralin or tazarotene; intralesional glucocorticoids; topical contact sensitizers

Contd...

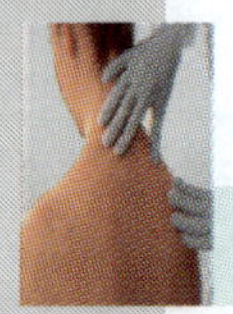

	Clinical	Pathogenesis	Treatment
Traumatic alopecia (choice D)	Broken hairs, often of varying lengths irregular outline	• Traction with curlers, rubber bands braiding • Exposure to heat or chemical (e.g. hair straighteners) • Mechanical pulling (trichotillomania)	Discontinuation of offending hair style or chemical treatments; diagnosis of trichotillomania may require observation of shaved hairs (for growth) or biopsy, possibly followed by psychotherapy

90. Ans. (d) Zinc deficiency

Ref: Harrison's, 19th ed. pg. 96e-9

Acrodermatitis Enteropathica (AE)

- *AE is characterized by abnormalities in zinc absorption* due to defect in intestinal zinc transporter *which leads to zinc deficiency.*
- It is a rare autosomal recessive (AR) disorder which classically present during infancy on weaning from breast milk to formula or cereal which have lower zinc bioavailability than breast milk.
- **Classical features of AE include:** ***(Mnemonic-"DEAL")***
  - **D**iarrhea, Depression
  - **E**czematous erosive dermatitis
  - **A**lopecia (non scarring), **A**pathetic look
  - **L**ethargy, irritability, whining and crying.

91. Ans. (a) Tinea versicolor

Ref: Harrison's, 19th ed. pg. 350

- *Malassezia furfur*, a normal inhabitant of the skin is a nondermatophytic, dimorphic fungus is a causative organism for *Tinea versicolor*.
- The expression of infection is promoted by heat and humidity. The typical lesions consist of oval scaly macules, papules, and patches concentrated on the chest, shoulders, and back.
- On dark skin the lesions often appear as hypopigmented areas, while on light skin they are slightly erythematous or hyperpigmented.
- A KOH preparation from scaling lesions will demonstrate a confluence of short hyphae and round spores *("spaghetti and meatballs")*.

92. Ans. (d) Psoriasis

Ref: Harrisons, 19th ed. pg. 347

- The silver scaly lesion as shown in the patient in the given image is more likely a case of psoriasis.

PSORIASIS

- Psoriasis is one of the most common dermatologic diseases, affecting up to 2% of the world's population.
- **Clinical feature:** Characterized by—
  - Erythematous, sharply demarcated papules and rounded plaques covered by silvery micaceous scale. The skin lesions of psoriasis are variably pruritic.
  - *Koebner* or isomorphic phenomenon: Traumatized areas often develop lesions of psoriasis.

93. Ans. (c) Erythema multiforme

Ref: Harrison's, 19th ed. pg. 134

- The shown target lesions on palm are diagnostic of erythema multiforme.
- The classic target lesions of *erythema multiforme* appear symmetrically on the elbows, knees, palms, soles, and face.
- In severe cases, these lesions spread diffusely and involve mucosal surface.
- Choice B, Steven Johnson syndrome is ruled out due to presentation of vesico-bullous lesions

Disease	Etiology	Description	Group affected/epidemiologic factor	Clinical syndrome
Hand-foot-and-mouth disease (Choice A)	Coxsackievirus A16 most common cause	Tender vesicles, erosions in mouth; 0.25 cm papules on hands and feet with rim of erythema	Summer and fall; primarily children <10 years old; multiple family members	Transient fever
Erythema multiforme (EM) (Choice C)	• Infection • Drugs • Idiopathic	• Target lesions (central erythema surrounded by area of clearing and another rim of erythema) up to 2 cm, symmetric on knees, elbows, palms, soles. • When extensive and involving mucous membranes, it is termed as EM major	Herpes simplex virus or *Mycoplasma pneumoniae* infection; drug intake (i.e., sulfa, phenytoin, Penicillin)	50% of patients <20 years old; EM major, which can be confused with Stevens-Johnson syndrome (but EM major lacks prominent skin sloughing)

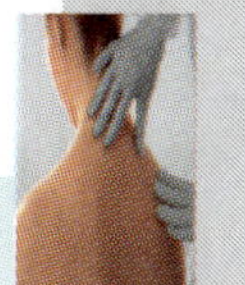

94. Ans. (d) Palms and soles involved

Ref: Robbins, 9th ed. pg. 358

- IP of chickenpox-**10–21 days**
- Infectious period is **2 days before to 5 days after** the onset of rash
- **Chickenpox** is caused by VZV and reactivation of latent VZV causes shingles (also called *herpes zoster*).
- Like HSV, VZV infects mucous membranes, skin, and neurons and causes a self-limited primary infection in immunocompetent individuals.

Small pox	Chicken pox
• Face involved	• Involves trunk mainly
• Centrifugal; involves palms and soles	• Centripetal; palm and soles not involved
• Umbilicated, deep lesion	• Superficial lesion
• Same stage at one point of time	• Pleomorphic rash
• Extensor aspect involved/ axilla, mucous not involved	• Axilla, mucosa involved
• Heals slowly	• Rapid healing
• Scab formation 10–14 days	• Scab formation 4–7 days

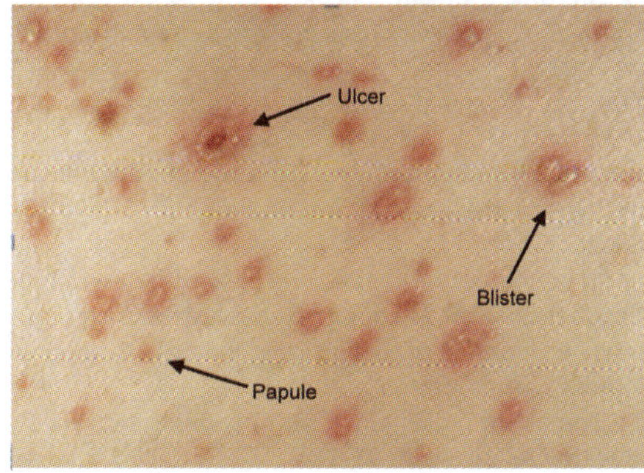

95. Ans. (c) Lichen planus

Ref: Harrisons, 19th ed. pg. 349

LICHEN PLANUS

- Lichen planus (LP) is a *papulosquamous disorder* that may affect the skin, scalp, nails, and mucous membranes.
- The primary cutaneous lesions of LP are pruritic, **polygonal, flat-topped, violaceous papules**.
- **Most common site** can occur anywhere but have a predilection for the **wrists, shins,** lower back, and genitalia.

Characteristic Feature

1. **Wickham's striae:** A network of gray lines on the surface of papules.
2. **Lichen planopilaris:** Involvement of the **scalp may lead to scarring alopecia**, and nail involvement may lead to permanent deformity or loss of finger nails and toe nails.
3. Lichen planus commonly involves mucous membranes, particularly the buccal mucosa (Erosive stomatitis) which may persist for years and linked to an *increased risk of oral squamous cell carcinoma.*
4. **LP may be associated with hepatitis C infection.** The course of LP is variable, but most patients have **spontaneous remissions 6 months to 2 years** after the onset of disease.

Treatment of choice: Topical glucocorticoids.

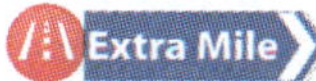

TABLE: Papulosquamous disorders

	Clinical features	Other notable features	Histologic features
Psoriasis	Sharply demarcated, erythematous plaques with *mica-like scale;* predominantly on elbows, knees, and scalp; atypical forms may localize to intertriginous areas; eruptive forms may be associated with infection	May be aggravated by certain drugs, infection; severe forms seen in association with HIV	Acanthosis, vascular proliferation
Lichen planus	*Purple polygonal papules marked by severe pruritus;* lacy white markings, especially associated with mucous membrane lesions	Certain drugs may induce; thiazides antimalarial drugs	Interface dermatitis

96. Ans. (c) Psoriasis

Ref: Harrisons, 19th ed. pg. 347

- The silver scaly lesion on the skin of the patient in the given image is more likely a case of psoriasis.

PSORIASIS

- Psoriasis is one of the most common dermatologic diseases, affecting up to 2% of the world's population.
- **Clinical feature:** Characterized by—
  - Erythematous, sharply demarcated papules and rounded plaques covered by silvery micaceous scale. The skin lesions of psoriasis are variably pruritic.
  - *Koebner* or isomorphic phenomenon: Traumatized areas often develop lesions of psoriasis.

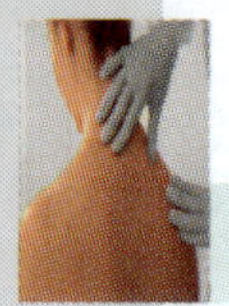

Types of Psoriasis

1. **Plaque-type:** It is the **most common variety** of psoriasis.
   - Patients present with stable, slowly enlarging plaques, which remains unchanged for long periods of time.
   - The **most commonly involved areas are** the elbows, knees, gluteal cleft, and scalp. Involvement tends to be **symmetric**.
2. **Inverse psoriasis** affects the intertriginous regions, including the axilla, groin, submammary region, and navel.
3. **Guttate psoriasis (eruptive psoriasis):** This is **most common in children** and young adults.
   - Patients present with many small erythematous, scaling papules**, frequently after upper respiratory tract** infection with β-hemolytic streptococci.
4. **Pustular psoriasis:** Usually localized to the **palms and soles**, or may be generalized. Can present with fever and or pustular eruptions.

Treatment

- **Limited psoriasis:** Topical glucocorticoids, Calcipotriene (topical vitamin D analogue), retinoid (tazarotene).
- Widespread psoriasis:
  - **UV light:** Ultraviolet B (UVB), narrow band UVB, and ultraviolet A (UV A) light with either oral or topical **psoralens (PUVA)** is used.
  - **Methotrexate** is an effective agent, especially in patients with psoriatic arthritis.

Note: ***Oral glucocorticoids should not be used*** for the treatment of psoriasis due to the potential for development of life-threatening pustular psoriasis when therapy is discontinued.

97. Ans. (c) Tetracycline

Ref: Harrisons, 19th ed. pg. 352

ACNE VULGARIS

- It is a self-limited disorder primarily of teenagers and young adults.
- Increase in sebum production by sebaceous glands after puberty is a the permissive factor for the disease expression.
- **Clinical hallmark of acne vulgaris:** Comedone, which may be closed (*whitehead*) or open (*blackhead*).
- **The earliest lesions seen in adolescence** are generally mildly inflamed or noninflammatory comedones on the forehead.
- **Most common location for acne** is the face, but involvement of the chest and back is common.

Treatment of Acne

- **Minimal to moderate pauci-inflammatory disease** respond adequately to local therapy alone: Topical agents such as retinoic acid, benzoyl peroxide, or salicylic acid.
- *Given the image, it is obvious that the case is not a minimal to moderate case of acne vulgaris. It is more likely moderate to acne vulgaris with inflammatory papules, pustules and comedones.*
- **Harrisons states:** *"Patients with moderate to* ***severe acne with a prominent inflammatory component*** *will benefit from the addition of systemic therapy, such as* ***tetracycline*** *in doses of 250–500 mg BD or doxycycline in doses of 100 mg BD"*
- **If patients with** severe nodulocystic acne are unresponsive to the therapies discussed above: Treatment with the synthetic retinoid isotretinoin is the choice. Its dose is based on the patient's weight, and it is given once daily for 5 months.
- Isotretinoin gives excellent result, but its teratogenic side effects limits its use in reproductive age group females.

98. Ans. (a) Neurofibromatosis

Ref: Harrisons, 19th ed. pg. 2331

NF-1 is diagnosed when *any two of the following seven signs* are present:

1. Six or more café au-lait macules. *Café au-lait spots are the* ***hallmark of*** *neurofibromatosis and are present in almost 100% of patients.*
2. Axillary or inguinal freckling consisting of multiple hyperpigmented areas 2–3 mm in diameter.
3. Two or more iris Lisch nodules. Lisch nodules are hamartomas located within the iris and are best identified by a slit-lamp examination.
4. Two or more neurofibromas or one plexiform neurofibroma.
5. Osseous lesion such as sphenoid dysplasia (which may cause pulsating exophthalmos) or cortical thinning of long bones with or without pseudoarthrosis.
6. Optic gliomas are present in ≈15% of patients with NF-1.
7. First Degree relative with NF-1

99. Ans. (a) Alopecia areata

Ref: Harrisons, 19th ed. pg. 354-55

- **Alopecia is of two types:** Scarring and Nonscarring.

Scarring alopecia	Nonscarring alopecia
• It is associated **with fibrosis, inflammation,** and loss of hair follicles.	• In this type **the hair shafts are absent** or miniaturized, but the **hair follicles are preserved** *(reversible condition)*
• **Most common causes** of scarring alopecia are primary cutaneous disorder such as *lichen planus, folliculitis decalvans, chronic cutaneous (discoid) lupus,* or *linear scleroderma (morphea).*	• **The most common causes** of nonscarring alopecia include 1. *Androgenetic alopecia* 2. *Telogen effluvium* 3. *Alopecia areata* 4. *Tinea capitis,* and the early 5. Phase of *traumatic alopecia.* 6. SLE

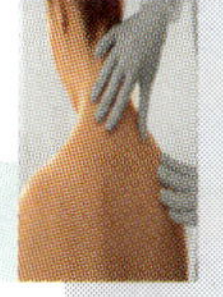

Extra Mile

- SLE has non-scarring alopecia
- This non-scarring alopecia coincides with flare up of systemic disease and presents as lupus hairs.
  - Discoid lupus erythematosus has scarring alopecia
  - Linear scleroderme [Morphea] has scarring alopecia

100. Ans. (d) Zinc oxide

Ref: Robbins, 9th ed. pg. 391

- Sunscreens are rated for their photoprotective effect by their sun protection factor (SPF).
- The SPF is simply **a ratio of the time required to produce sunburn erythema with and without sunscreen application.**
- The SPF of most sunscreens reflects protection from UV-B but not from UV-A.
- US. Food and Drug Administration (FDA) has recognized category-I ingredients as safe and effective. Those ingredients are listed in the table below:

FDA Category I Monographed Sunscreen Ingredients

Ingredients	Maximum concentration, %
p-Aminobenzoic acid (PABA)	15
Avobenzone	3
Cinoxate	3
Dioxybenzone (benzophenone-8)	3
Ecamsule	15
Homosalate	15
Methyl anthranilate	5
Octocrylene	10
Octyl methoxycinnamate	7.5
Octyl salicylate	5
Oxybenzone (benzophenone-3)	6
Padimate O (octyl dimethyl PABA)	8
Phenylbenzimidazole sulfonic acid	4
Sulisobenzone (benzophenone-4)	10
Titanium dioxide	25
Trolamine salicylate	12
Zinc oxide	25

101. Ans. (a) 5 kg

- Average weight of skin is ~4 kg. Skin is considered to be the largest organ of the body.
- It is 12-15% of the total body weight.
- *Given these options, 5 kg is closest and best choice.*

102. Ans. (d) Stratum germinatum

Ref: Fitzpatrick, 7th ed. pg. 384

- **Epidermis of the skin has 4 layers:**
  1. **Stratum basale/Germinatum:** Deepest most layers having single row **columnar** epithelial cells. It is actively dividing layer.
  2. **Stratum spinosum:** Also known as prickle cell layer. Polygonal in shape. ***Synthesis of keratin mainly takes place here.***
  3. **Stratum granulosum:** Diamond shaped. *Microscopically there is presence of* ***keratohyaline granules and Odland bodies*** *(membrane coating granules)*
  4. **Stratum corneum:** Also known as horny cell layer. Most superficial layer of skin. This layer is a nuclear dead cell layer.
- **Note:** *Stratum lucidum is the 5th layer of skin found on palm and soles. It is located between stratum granulosum and corneum.*

Extra Mile

- **Stratum corneum** develops last. Therefore this layer is absent in premature babies
- **Stratum corneum is dead layer of epidermis**
- **Hyperkeratosis: Thickening of stratum corneum.**

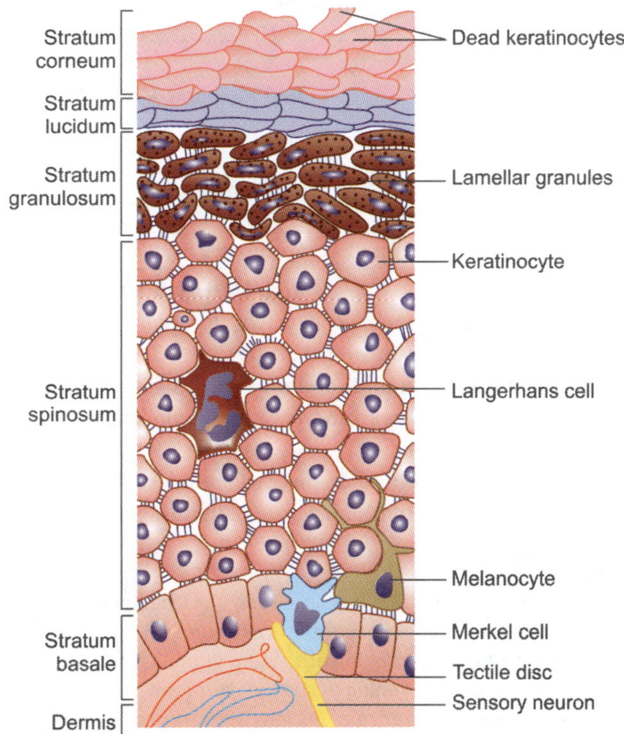

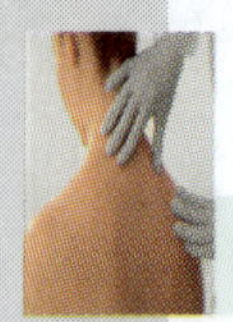

103. Ans. (d) Stratum spinosum

Ref: Fitzpatrick, 7th ed. pg. 384

104. Ans. (b) Thickening of stratum corneum

Ref: Fitzpatrick, 7th ed. pg. 384

105. Ans. (b) Stratum granulosum

Ref: McGraw Hill Speciality Board Review Dermatology 2nd ed. pg. 561

106. Ans. (c) Keratinocytes

Ref: Fitzpatrick, 7th ed. pg. 100

CELLS OF EPIDERMIS

- **Keratinocytes:** These are considered as the principal cells of epidermis. They proliferate in basal layer and differentiation occurs in spinosum and granulosum layer which further matures fully and dies in corneum. *(keratinocytes are present in all 4 layers of epidermis)*
- **Melanocytes and Merkel cell:** Present in stratum basale.
  - **Melanocytes** synthesize melanin pigment and transfer to keratinocytes
  - **Merkel cells** for touch sensation. Also known as touch cells
- **Langerhan cell** found in stratum spinosum and act as **antigen presenting cells** (macrophages).
  - They contain **tennis racquet shaped granules** also known as **Bierbeck granules.**

107. Ans. (d) Spinosum

Ref: Fitzpatrick, 7th ed. pg. 384

108. Ans. (a) Basale

Ref: Fitzpatrick, 7th ed. pg. 62

109. Ans. (b) Separation of keratinocytes

Ref: Harrison, 19th ed. pg. 370

- Keratinocytes are connected to one another by intracellular desmosomal bridges.
- If there is loss of these desmosomal bridges, it will lead to **separation of keratinocytes** and the condition is known as **acantholysis.**
- If separation continues, there will be intracellular edema, and the condition is known as **Ballooning**.

Extra Mile

- Degeneration of stratum basale is seen in: Lichen planus
- **Acanthosis:** Thickening of stratum spinosum
- **Hypergranulosis:** Thickening of stratum granulosum
- **Hyperkeratosis:** Thickening of stratum corneum
- **Parakeratosis:** Persistence of nucleus in stratum corneum layer

110. Ans. (d) Thickening of prickle cell layer

Ref: Harrison, 19th ed. pg. 370

- **Acanthosis:** Thickening of stratum spinosum aka prickle cell layer.

111. Ans. (b) Persistence of nucleus in stratum corneum

- Stratum corneum is the most superficial layer of the skin and is devoid of nucleus.
- Parakeratosis is retention of nucleus in stratum corneum
- If there is presence of nucleus in this layer it can be a normal case or can be associated with some pathology.
- **Normally** nucleus in cornuem persists in vagina and in mucous membrane of mouth.
- **Pathologies having nucleus in stratum corneum:** seborrheic dermatitis, squamous cell CA, Actinic keratosis, psoriasis, etc.

112. Ans. (b) 4 days

Ref: Neena Khanna: Synopses of Dermatology 4th ed. pg. 52

- Normal skin turnover from basal cell layer to corneum layer takes around **4–5 weeks.**
- **In conditions like psoriasis**, the mitotic activity is increased and the turnover time is highly reduced to 3–7 days with an **average of 4 days**.

113. Ans. (d) Gustatory sweating

Types of Sweating

- **Gustatory sweating:** Sweating on scalp, forehead and nose in response to hot and spicy meals.
- **Mental sweating:** Occurs in response to emotional stimuli like. For example, mental stress, emotional stress. Sweating usually noticed on palms, soles and axilla.
- **Thermogenic sweating:** Sweating in response to pre-optic stimulation of hypothalamus in order to maintain the body temperature.

114. Ans. (b) Lips are most common site

Ref: Harrison, 19th ed. pg. 127

- **Fordyce's spots** are ectopic sebaceous glands.
  - **MC site: Lips > oral mucosa > Vulva and Penis (Tysons gland)**
  - **MC age group:** Puberty
  - M > F
  - **Characterized as** discrete pin headed size, yellowish maculo-papular lesions in mucus membrane of lips and oral cavity.
  - **Mimicks** or are very often confused as **koplik's spot of measles.**

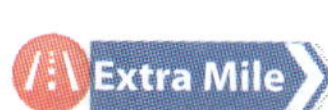

- **Obstruction of eccrine sweat gland ducts:** Miliaria
- **Obstruction of apocrine sweat gland ducts:** Fox fordyces spot/disease aka Apocrine Miliaria
- **MC site of fox fordyces disease:** Axilla
- **MC age group of fox fordyces spot:** 13–35 years ***(Females are MC affected).***

115. Ans. (a) Lips

Ref: Harrison, 19th ed. pg. 240 table 45.2/

116. Ans. (b) Flat lesion <2 cm

Ref: Harrison's, 19th ed. pg. 319

DESCRIPTION OF PRIMARY SKIN LESIONS

Macule

- A flat, colored lesion, <2 cm in diameter, not raised above the surface of the surrounding skin. A "freckle" or ephelide, is a prototypical pigmented macule.

Patch

- A large (>2 cm) flat lesion with a color different from the surrounding skin. This differs from a macule only in size.

Papule

- A small, solid lesion, <0.5 cm in diameter, raised above the surface of the surrounding skin and thus palpable (e.g. a closed comedone, or white-head in acne).

Nodule

- A larger **(0.5–5.0 cm)**, firm lesion raised above the surface of the surrounding skin. This differs from a papule only in size (e.g. a large dermal nevomelanocytic nevus).

Tumor

- A solid, raised growth **>5 cm** in diameter.

Plaque

- A large **(>1 cm)**, flat-topped, raised lesion; edges may either be distinct (e.g,. psoriasis) or gradually blend with skin (e.g. in eczematous dermatitis).

Vesicle

- A small, fluid lesion, **<0.5 cm** in diameter, raised above the pane of surrounding skin. Fluid is often visible, and the lesions are translucent (e.g. vesicles in allergic contact dermatitis caused by Toxicodendron [poison ivy]).

Pustule

- A vesicle filled with leukocytes. Note: The presence of pustules does not necessarily signify the existence of an infection.

Bulla

- A fluid-filled raised often translucent lesion **>0.5 cm** in diameter.

Wheal

- A raised erythematous, edematous papule of plaque, usually representing short-lived vasodilatation and vasopermeability.

Telanglectasia

- A dilated, superficial blood vessel.

117. Ans. (b) <5 mm

Ref: Harrison's 19th ed. pg. 319

Please refer to above explanation

118. Ans. (a) Insect bite

- **Insect bite:** Presents as papule. It can be painful or painless
- **Angioedema:** Edema of subcutaneous and submucosal tissue can be due to allergic reaction.
- **Urticaria** is an autoinflammatory condition. MC symptom is itching.
- **Erythema nodosum:** Inflammation of submucosal fatty cells.

119. Ans. (d) Biliverdin

- Bruise is a skin contusion which is also known as hematoma of skin
- Capillaries and sometimes venules are damaged by trauma, allowing blood to seep, hemorrhage, or extravasate into the surrounding interstitial tissues.
- Larger bruises may change color due to the breakdown of hemoglobin from within escaped RBC in the extracellular space.
- The striking colors of a bruise are caused by the Phagocytosis and sequential degradation of hemoglobin to biliverdin to bilirubin to hemosiderin.
- The color changes noted at the site of bruise is secondary to:
  - **Hemoglobin** itself producing a red-blue color
  - **Biliverdin producing a green color**
  - **Bilirubin** producing a yellow color
  - **Hemosiderin** producing a golden-brown color

120. Ans. (c) Sulfur granules in the purulent sinuses are characteristic

Ref: Harrison, 19th ed. pg. 1090

- **Propionibacterium acne** is a Gram-positive bacterium, which is a normal flora of the skin.
- It can also cause chronic blepharitis and endophthalmitis.
- It is basically linked to the skin condition acne.
- Aside from skin it lives primarily on fatty acids in sebum secreted by sebaceous glands in the follicles.

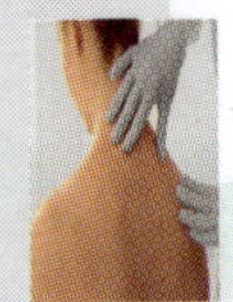

- It may also be found throughout the gastrointestinal tract in humans.
- The antibiotics most frequently used to treat acne vulgaris are: Erythromycin, clindamycin, doxycycline and minocycline.
- *Actinomyces israelii is an opportunistic pathogen which causes actinomycosis.*
- Its lesions are often characterized as "wooden". Sulfur granules form in a central purulence surrounded by neutrophils is very characteristic of actinomycosis.

121. Ans. (d) Dermatitis herpetiformis

Ref: Harrison, 19th ed. pg. 373

Diagnosis of Dermatitis Herpetiformis is confirmed by a simple blood test for IgA antibodies, and by a skin biopsy in which the *pattern of IgA deposits in the dermo-epidermal junction*, revealed by direct immunofluorescence.

Extra Mile

TABLE: Differentiating dermatitis herpetiformis, pemphigus and pemphigoid vulgaris

Feature	Dermatitis herpetiformis	Pemphigus vulgaris	Pemphigoid
Lesion	Intensely itchy vesicles, papulovesicles	Thin walled, delicate, flaccid bullae/ blister that rapidly rupture & erode	Large, tense often blood stained blisters
Area of predilection	Knees, elbows, scalp, buttock, & around axilla	Upper part of body Buccal mucosa is commonly involved	Lower part of body Mucosa not involved
Associated with	G.I. absorptive defect due to gluten enteropathy	• Acantholysis • Nikolsky sign	–
Lab finding	• Small intestine biopsy: partial villous atrophy • Lesion biopsy: Subepidermal blisters • IgA & neutrophils in papillary tips	• Lesion biopsy: ▪ **Acantholysis** ▪ ***Intraepidermal blisters*** ▪ Row of tomb stone ▪ IgG, C_3 complement deposition between epidermal cells.	• Lesion biopsy: ▪ **Subepidermal blisters** ▪ Subepidermal collection of IgG, C_3-complement, eosinophils, polymorphs.
Treatment	• Gluten free diet • *Dapsone (DOC)*	• Systemic steroid • Immunosuppresant	• Systemic steroid • Immunosuppresant

122. Ans. (a) Pemphigus vulgaris

Ref: Harrison, 19th ed. pg. 370

- The rounded keratinocytes with hyperchromatic nuclei and perinuclear halo (due to condensing of cytoplasm in periphery) are called **acantholytic cells.**
- It is seen in case of pemphigus vulgaris
- **Acantholytic cells** can be demonstrated in bed side by **Tzanck test.**

123. Ans. (c) Autoimmune

Ref: Harrison, 19th ed. pg. 370

PEMPHIGUS

- *Pemphigus is an autoimmune blistering disorder*
- It results from the loss of integrity of normal intercellular attachments with the epidermis.
- Commonly affects individuals of age between 40 and 60.
- Equal prevalence among males and females.
- There are five variants of pemphigus:
  - ***Pemphigus Vulgaris:*** *Most common type*
  - **Pemphigus Foliaceous:** Superficial pemphigus
  - **Pemphigus Vegetans.** Least common type
  - **Pemphigus Erythematous**
  - **Fogo Selvagem:** An endemic form of pemphigus foliaceus.
- ***Refer to above table***

124. Ans. (b) Intraepidermal

Ref: Harrison, 19th ed. pg. 371-72

- ***Pemphigus has intraepidermal bullae and Pemphigoid has subepidermal bullae***

TABLE: Difference between pemphigus and pemphigoid bullae

Features	Pemphigus	Pemphigoid
Row of Tomb stone	Present	Absent
Nikolsky Sign	Present	Absent
Bullae location	**Intraepidermal – flaccid Bullae**	**Subepidermal & tense Bullae**
Mucosa involvement	Present (common)	Absent or less common
Acantholysis	Present	Absent
Prognosis	Poor	Good

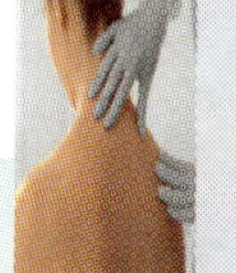

125. Ans. (b) **Pemphigoid bullae**

Ref: Harrison, 19th ed. pg. 371-72

- Pemphigus has intraepidermal bullae
- Pemphigoid has subepidermal bullae
- *Refer to the previous answer for detailed explanation.*

126. Ans. (b) **Pemphigus vulgaris**

Please refer to above explanation.

127. Ans. (b) **Nikolsky sign absent**

Ref: Harrison, 19th ed. pg. 370

Nikolsky sign is present in pemphigus bullae. It is absent in pemphigoid bullae.

128. Ans. (b) **Pemphigus**

Ref: Neena Khanna, 3rd pg. 61-6

- In Pemphigus, there is production of **IgG auto antibodes** against polypeptide complexes present in the **intercellular substance of epidermis.**
- Lesional sites show a characteristic **Fish net like pattern of intercellular IgG** deposits in the intercellular area.

129. Ans. (a) **Dapsone**

Ref: Katzung, pg. 1468

- **Dermatitis herpetiformis** is a chronic blistering skin condition, characterized by blisters filled with a watery fluid.
- DH is neither related to nor caused by herpes virus: the name means that it is a skin inflammation having an appearance similar to herpes.
- It characterized by intensely itchy, chronic papulovesicular eruptions, usually distributed symmetrically on extensor surfaces (buttocks, back of neck, scalp, elbows, knees, back, hairline, groin, or face).
- **Diagnosis** is confirmed by a simple blood test for IgA antibodies, and by a skin biopsy in which the pattern of IgA deposits in the dermo-epidermal junction, revealed by direct immunofluorescence.
- **Treatment:** Dapsone is considered as drug of choice for DH.
- In case of intolerance to dapsone, other drugs which can be used are: Colchicine, Tetracycline, Sulfapyridine.

130. Ans. (c) **Urticaria pigmentosa**

Ref: Harrison, 19th ed. pg. 367

- **Urticaria pigmentosa:** Excess of mast cells in many tissues lead to numerous red-brown/pink papules over trunk & limbs. Present as red/pink nodules in infants & young children but disappear later in childhood.
- **Atopic dermatitis:** WHITE DERMATOGRAPHISM: running a blunt object as key on affected skin produces a white line.
- **Pemphigus vulgaris:** Manual pressure on the skin elicits the separation of epidermis called NIKOLSKY SIGN.
- **Bullous pemphigoid:** Urticarial/eczematous prodrome with faint dusky erythema in a figurative pattern.

131. Ans. (b) **Lips**

Ref: Harrison, 19th ed. pg. 363; Harwood Clinical Practice pg. 855

- Angioedema is the swelling of deep dermis, subcutaneous, or submucosal tissue due to vascular leakage.
- Acute episodes often involve the eyelids, lips, tongue, larynx, GI tract and face; however, angioedema may affect other parts of body, including respiratory and gastrointestinal (GI) mucosa.
- Most common site of angioedema lips.
- Laryngeal swelling can be life-threatening.

Extra Mile

- **Angioneurotic edema (swelling of face & lips) in presence of intense pruritis and evidence of vascular collapse (hypotension)** suggest a diagnosis of **anaphylaxis.**

132. Ans. (a) **Subcutaneous tissue**

Ref: Harrison, 18th ed. pg. 2711

133. Ans. (a) **Due to deficiency of IgA**

Ref: Harrison, 19th ed. pg. 386

- Disease entity which is caused due to deficiency to zinc is Acrodermatitis enteropathica

XERODERMA PIGMENTOSA

- It is an *autosomal recessive skin disorder* with cellular hypersensitivity to ultraviolet radiation & certain chemical agents and cancer chemotherapeutic agents like cisplatin, carmustine, etc.
- Covalent linkage between adjacent pyrimidines in DNA is damaged by UV rays & chemicals.
- In normal circumstances, damaged DNA is repaired by nucleotide excision & repair pathway (NER) but in case of Xeroderma Pigmentosa, *NER is defective* leading to clinical signs and symptoms.

Clinical Presentation of XP Includes

1. **Skin involvement**
   - Hallmark of XP is *Photosensitivity* which causes acute sunburn reaction on minimal UV exposure.
   - Skin is like dry parchment and pigmented, which gives the name Xeroderma pigmentosa.
2. **Ocular involvement**
   - Loss of lashes
   - Conjunctival infection
   - Keratitis
3. **Neurological involvement**
   - Mild case: Hyporeflexia
   - Severe cases: Mental retardation, sensorineural deafness, spasticity & seizures.

134. Ans. (c) Zinc

Ref: O.P. Ghai, 8th ed. pg. 121

ACRODERMATITIS ENTEROPATHICA (AE)

- *AE is characterized by abnormalities in zinc absorption* due to defect in intestinal zinc transporter *which leads to zinc deficiency.*
- It is a rare autosomal recessive (AR) disorder which classically present during infancy on weaning from breast milk to formula or cereal which have lower zinc bioavailability than breast milk.
- **Classical features of AE include: *(Mnemonic-"DEAL")***
  - **D**iarrhea, Depression
  - **E**czematous erosive dermatitis
  - **A**lopecia (non scarring), **A**pathetic look
  - **L**ethargy, irritability, whining & crying.

135. Ans. (c) Subsides over time

Ref: Manipal Manual of Surgery, 4th ed. pg. 9

- Keloids can be remembered as *"scars that don't know when to stop."*
- A keloid, sometimes referred to as a keloid scar, is a tough heaped-up scar that rises quite abruptly above the rest of the skin.
- It can appear few day to few weeks after surgery.
- It usually has a smooth top and a pink or purple color. Keloids are irregularly shaped and tend to enlarge progressively.
- *Unlike scars, keloids do not subside over time.* Instead it spreads and includes normal skin also.
- Keloid scars are made of dense collagen fibres.
- Recurrence is possible after local excision.
- It can be familial.
- *Most common site of keloid: Sternum.*
- It can be treated by intrakeloid injection of Triamcinolone.
- Best cure of keloid is achieved by excision and radiotherapy.

136. Ans. (d) Nevus Anemicus

Ref: Neena Khanna Synopsis of Dermatology, 4th ed. pg. 147

NEVUS ANAEMICUS

- Nevus is circumscribed malformation of skin.
- Nevus anemicus is a congenital anomaly that presents clinically as a hypopigmented macule or patch.
- It usually presents at birth and is unilateral.
- It does not increase in size
- Pressure with glass slide makes the lesion disappear & indistinct from surrounding skin.

Extra Mile

Nevus anemicus	Functional development defect in vascular filling, characterized by pale round flat lesions.
Becker nevus	Irregular pigmentation of shoulder, upper chest or scapular area.
Ito nevus	Pigmentation of skin innervated by lateral branches of the supraclavicular nerve.
Ota nevus	Occulodermal melanosis
Freckles	Yellowish or brownish macules of hyperpigmentation, seen on the exposed parts of the skin.

137. Ans. (b) Trichophyton rubrum

Ref: Harrison, 17th ed. pg. 1309

DERMATOPHYTOSIS OR RING WORM (TINEA) INFECTION

- Dermatophytes include a group of fungi (ring worm) that under most conditions have the ability to infect & survive only on dead keratin; that is the superficial topmost layer of skin (stratum corneum or keratin layer), hair and nails.
- They cannot survive on mucosal surfaces (e.g. mouth or vagina) where the keratin layer does not form.
- The ring worm fungi belongs to 3 genera:

Trichophyton	Microsporum	Epidermophyton
• Infects skin, hair & nail • Infecting species include: ▪ Trichophyton rubrum ▪ Mentagrophyte ▪ Violaceum ▪ Verrucosum ▪ Schoenleinii	• *Infects skin and hair* but does not involve nails • Several infecting species include: Microsporum audounii, M. gypseum and M. canis	*Infect skin & nails* but does not involve hair Only infecting species is Epidermophyton floccosum.

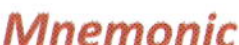

Mnemonic

- ***TSH-N*** *(Trichophyton infects Skin, Hair and Nail)*
- ***MSH*** *(Microsporum infects Skin and Hair)*
- ***ESN*** *(Epidermophyton infects Skin and Nail)*

138. Ans. (d) All of the above

Please refer to above explanation

139. Ans. (d) Skin + Hair + Nail

Ref: Roxburg, 17th ed. pg. 39

- Trichophyton Infects skin, hair & nail.
- Infecting species include:
  - Trichophyton rubrum, mentagrophytes, violaceum, verrucosum and Schoenleinii.

140. Ans. (c) Both

- In the given choices, T. verrucosum and M. gypseum both infect skin and hair.

Please refer to above explanation

141. Ans. (b) Tinea capitis

Ref: Roxburg, 17th ed. pg. 41

- **Tinea capitis** is most commonly caused by Microsporum canis.
- Second MCC of Tenia capitis is Trichophyton tonsurans.
- It is never caused by epidermophyton as it does not involve hair.
- It presents with localized non-cicatricial alopecia, itching, scaling with or without boggy swelling of scalp & *easily pluckable hair.*
- Tenia capitis is diagnosed by potassium hydroxide (KOH) wet mounts of hair & scale.
- **Treatment:** Griseofulvin is DOC

142. Ans. (a) LGV (b) Syphillis

Ref: Neena Khanna Synopsis of Dermatology, 4th ed. pg. 322

- LGV is a STD, caused by chlamydia presents classically with painless lymphadenopathy.
- Mnemonic to remember LGV:
  - **ABCDEFG:** Asymptomatic, Bubo, Chlamydia, Doxy, Esthiomine, Fries test, Groove sign
- Syphilis: Genital ulcer (Hard Chancre: Single, clean based, indurated, non tender, does not bleed on touch)

Disease	Ulcer	Lymph node
Syphilis	Painless	Painless
Chancroid	Painful	Painful
LGV	Painless	Painful (Bubo)

143. Ans. (c) Chancroid

Ref: Harrison, 19th ed. pg. 881, 1134

- **Chancroid** is a bacterial STD caused by H.Ducreyi. It is characterized by **painful sores** on the genitalia. Chancroid is known to spread from one individual to another solely through sexual contact.

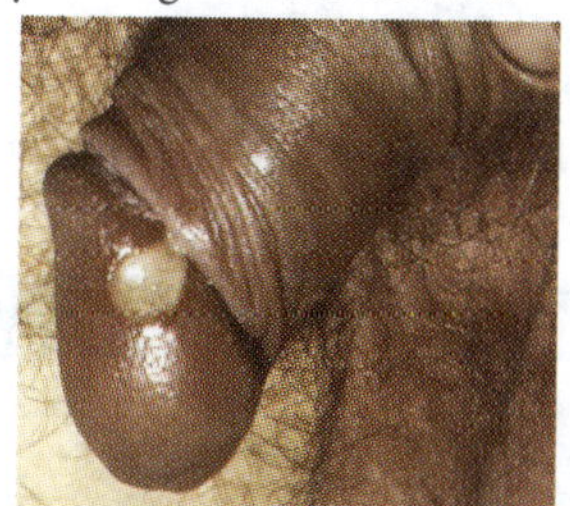

- A **chancre** on the other hand is a painless ulceration/ sore most commonly formed during the primary stage of syphilis.

144. Ans. (b) Hemophilus Ducreyi

Ref: Harrison, 19th ed. pg. 1012

- **School of fish appearance** stained smear from genital lesions in cases of chancroid. Causative agent of chancroid is Hemophilus ducreyi.
- H. Ducreyi a major cause of genital ulceration in developing countries characterized by painful sores on the genitalia. Another early symptom is dark or light-green shears in excrement.
- Chancroid starts as an erythematous papular lesion that breaks down into a painful bleeding ulcer with a necrotic base and ragged edge.
- ***H. ducreyi*** **can be cultured on chocolate agar.**

145. Ans. (a) Secondary syphilis

Ref: Harrison, 19th ed. pg. 1132

- **Hallmark features of SECONDARY SYPHILIS:** asymptomatic, bilateral symmetrical pleomorphic maculo-papular rash on palms and soles, non-tender lymphadenopathy.
- **Other findings:** Condyloma Lata, ***Moth Eaten Alopecia*** arthritis, proteinuria.
- **Features that are never seen:** Vesico-bullous lesions, intense pruritus, Interstitial Keratitis.

146. Ans. (a) Gonorrhoea

Ref: Harrison, 19th ed. pg. 1107-08

- Gonorrhea is STD caused by Neisseriae gonorrhea. It doesn't present with genital ulcer.
- Patient presents with *greenish yellow or whitish discharge from the vagina*, lower abdominal or, pelvic pain, burning when urinating, conjunctivitis, swelling of the vulva (vulvitis), burning in the throat (due to oral sex), swollen glands in the throat (due to oral sex)

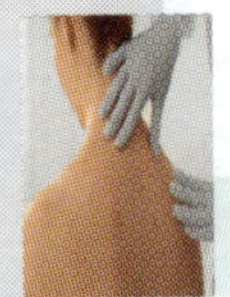

- A **genital ulcer** is located on the genital area, usually caused by a sexually transmitted disease such as genital herpes, syphilis, chancroid, or chlamydia trachomatis.
- Genital ulcers are not strictly a sign of an STD. They can occur in patients with Behçet's syndrome, lupus, and some forms of rheumatoid arthritis (all non-communicable diseases).
- Genital tuberculosis, often caused by direct genital contact with infected sputum, can also present as genital ulcer.

TABLE: Causes of genital ulcer

Bacterial	Viral	Parasitic	Non-infectious
• Hemophilus ducreyi • Treponema pallidum • Chlamydia trachomatis • Donovanosis • Balanitis	• Herpes simplex • Varicella zoster • EBV • Cytomegalovirus	• Sarcoptes scabiei • Phthirus pubis • Entamoeba histolytica • Trichomonas vaginalis	• Trauma • Pyoderma gangrenosum • Reiter's syndrome • Wegener granulomatosis • Neoplasms

147. Ans. (b) Aphthous ulcers

Ref: Harrison's, 19th ed. pg. 239

- Apthous ulcers are also called as canker sores/apthous stomatitis and present as round ulcer with yellowish base and surrounded by a red halo.
  - The usual sites are oral mucosa on the insides of lips, cheeks or below the tongue.
  - Most of apthous ulcers are <5 mm in size and heal within 1–2 weeks.
  - *Painless* recurrent apthous ulcers are seen in SLE
  - *Painful* recurrent apthous ulcers in oral cavity and genitalia is seen are in Behcet disease

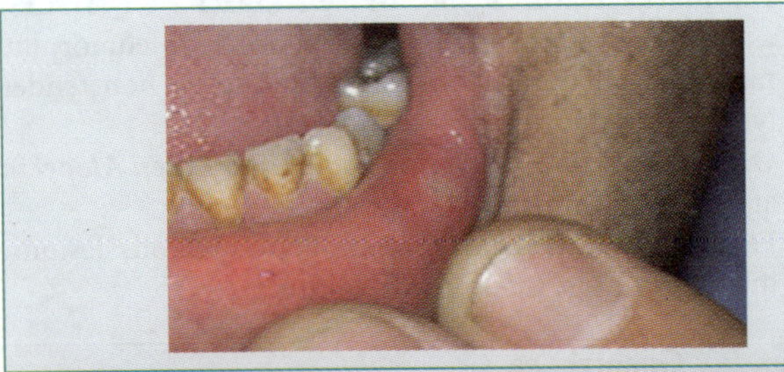

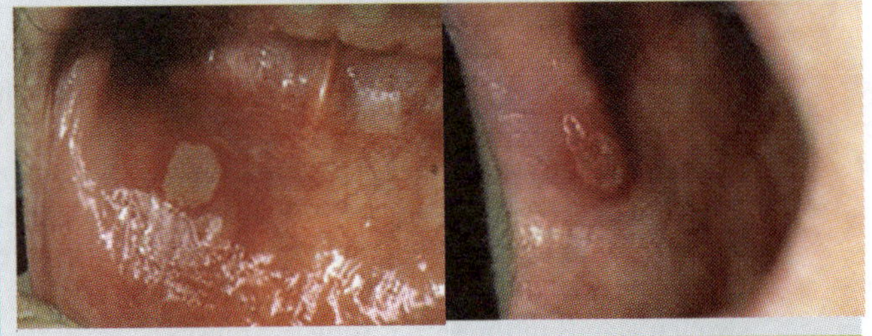

148. Ans. (a) Anagen effluvium

Ref: Fitzpatrick Dermatology, 7th ed. pg. 763

- **Alopecia areata is an autoimmune disorder, in which anagen is prematurely arrested**. It presents as non-inflamed bald patches on scalp.
  - **Pathognomonic feature:** *Exclamation mark hairs*, which taper as they approach scalp.
  - **Treatment:** Depends on extent of disease. Localized condition: Intra lesional steroids. In extensive condition application of diphencyprone is effective.
- **Telogen Effluvium:** Hair follicles are usually not involved in this phase , if synchronised into telogen resting mode, they will be shed in about 3 months later. It might be seen in severe stress, high fever, child birth, surgery.
- **Catagen:** It is a resting phase of hair follicle development and lasts for 3–4 weeks. Hair protein synthesis stops and follicle retreats towards the surface. 10–20% Scalp hair are in this phase.

149. Ans. (b) Condyloma acuminata

Ref: Fitzpatrick Dermatology, 8th ed. pg. 862

WARTS

- Caused by Human Papilloma virus (HPV). It is the most common virus induced tumor and shows Koebner's phenomenon.
- Condyloma acuminata are genital warts caused most commonly by human papilloma virus type 6 and 11.
- **DOC:** 20% podophyllin or glutaraldehyde.
- **Treatment of choice in pregnancy:** Cryotherapy. If not available: Trichloroacetic acid
- ***Most common cutaneous wart:*** *Verruca Vulgaris*

Extra Mile

Warts	Seen in
Plane wart	*Verruca plana*
Filiform wart	*Verruca filiformis*
Plantar wart	*Verruca plantaris or myrmecia wart*
Veneral wart	Condylomata accuminata
Massive wart	Buschke lowen stein tumor
Condyloma lata	Treponema pallidum

150. Ans. (c) Human papilloma virus

Ref: Fitzpatrick Colour Atlas, 7th ed. pg. 639

- Causative organism of Verruca vulgaris is human papilloma virus.
- Most common types of HPV associated with warts

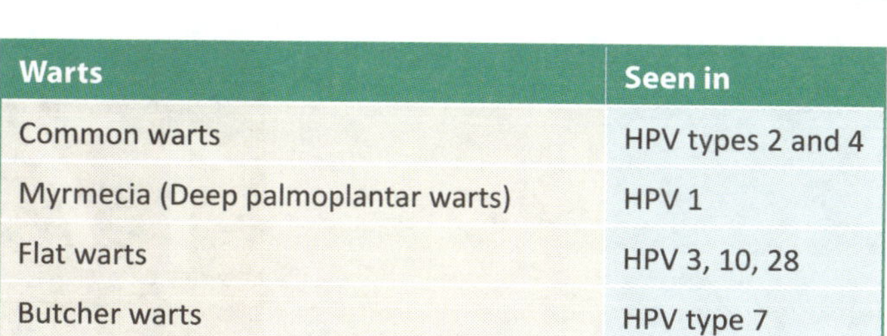

Warts	Seen in
Common warts	HPV types 2 and 4
Myrmecia (Deep palmoplantar warts)	HPV 1
Flat warts	HPV 3, 10, 28
Butcher warts	HPV type 7
Focal epithelial hyperplasia (Heck disease)	HPV type 13, 32

151. Ans. (b) Lepromin test

Ref: Harrison, 19th ed. pg. 1126

- **Lepromin test** has only prognostic significance because it tells about cell mediated immunity & classifies the type of disease.
- It has no diagnostic value.

Diagnosis of Leprosy

- **Clinical examination**
  - Sensory testing
  - Peripheral nerve examination
- **Demonstration of acid fast bacilli**
  - In skin smear prepared by slit & scrape method
  - Nasal swabs by modified ziehl–nelson method
- Nerve biopsy
- Foot pad culture (in mouse)
- **Skin biopsy**
  - Periappendiceal lymphocytosis
  - Virchow (lepra/foam) cells are diagnostic

152. Ans. (c) Type II Lepra

Ref: Harrison, 19th ed. pg. 1127-28

Type I Leprae Reaction: Reversal Reaction	Type II Leprae Reaction: Erythema nodosum Leprosum
• Type IV delayed Hypersensitivity reaction	• Type III Hypersensitivity (Jarisch- Herxheimer) reaction
• Found in TT (tuberculoid type)	• Found in LL (Lepromatous Leprosy)
• Thalidomide has no role	• *Thalidomide is most effective drug*
• *DOC is corticosteroid*	• *DOC is corticosteroid*

- ***Remember:*** *Thalidomide is absolutely contraindicated in women of child bearing age due to chances of phocomelia (seal limb deformity)*

153. Ans. (c) Erythema nodosum

Ref: Harrison, 19th ed. pg. 132

Lupus vulgaris: Can be endogenous & exogenous. Presents with non itchy annular plaque or long standing duration with atrophy. Apple jelly nodules are present in 10% of cases

Scrofuloderma: Contagious spread of TB may be from underlying lymph nodes, fascia or bone.

Most common site is cervical *lymph nodes.*

Ulcer with bluish edges with undermined edges. After healing puckered scarring marks will develop.

Lichen Scrufulosorum: Seen in children. Multiple grouped white papules all over the body, most commonly trunk. It is a source of TB lymphadenitis.

Erythema nodosum: It is a panniculitis that presents as a painful red nodule on lower limbs. It is due to C1 deposition in vessels of subcutis.

Causes: Idiopathic, Bacterial, fungal, viral infection, drugs (sulphonamides, contraceptives), IBD, Sarcoidosis, Behcet's disease.

154. Ans. (d) Pterygium of nail

Ref: Fitzpatrick Color Atlas, 7th ed. pg. 1008-09

- **Lichen planus** (LP) is a disease of the skin and/or mucous membranes that resembles lichen.
- It is an autoimmune disorder.
- Lichen planus may be categorized as affecting mucosal or cutaneous surfaces.
- **Cutaneous forms** are those affecting the skin, scalp, and Nails
- *Pterygium of nail is characteristically seen in lichen planus.*
- Koilonychia is found in Iron deficiency anemia (not megaloblastic anemia).

Extra Mile

TABLE: Patterns of Nail Involvement in different Conditions

Condition	Nail involvement
• Iron deficiency anemia	• Koilonychia
• Arsenic poisoning	Mee's Line
• Lichen planus	Pterygium, Onychia, Onychorrhexis, Pitting
• Psoriasis	Pitting of nail (thimble nail) Oil drop nails Onycholysis: Detachment of nail plate

155. Ans. (a) Lichen planus

Ref: Harrison, 19th ed. pg. 349

The Characteristic Features of Lichen Planus are:

- Hyperkeratosis with absence of parakeratosis (which is a mode of keratinization characterized by the retention of nuclei in the stratum corneum)
- Hypergranulosis (which is thickening of the granular layer) with Basal cell degeneration
- *Presence of irregular acanthosis with saw-tooth appearance of the rete-ridges.*
- Presence of upper *dermal band-like lympho-histiocytic infiltrate* that impinges on the epidermis, leading to obliteration of the dermo-epidermal interface
- Presence of *Civatte bodies* (also known as colloid bodies and hyaline bodies), representing degenerated, apoptotic keratinocytes.

ANESTHESIA

17

MOST RECENT QUESTIONS 2023

1. Identify this classification.

(Most Recent Question July 2023)

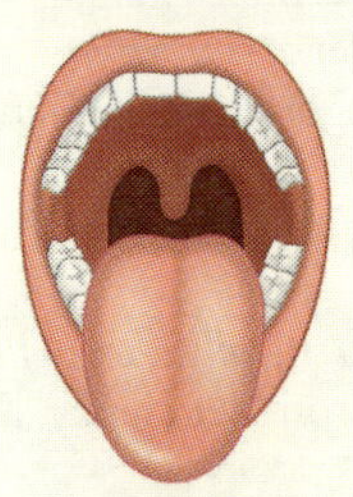

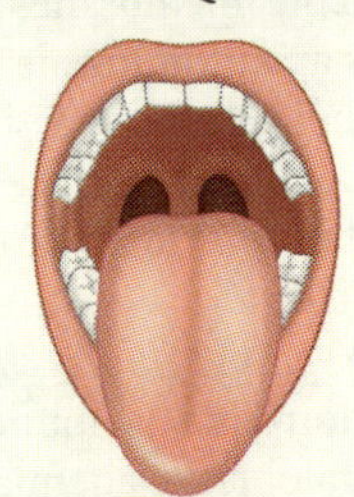

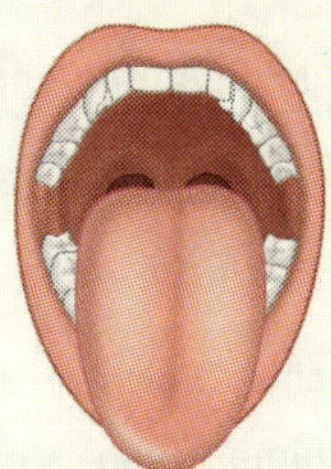

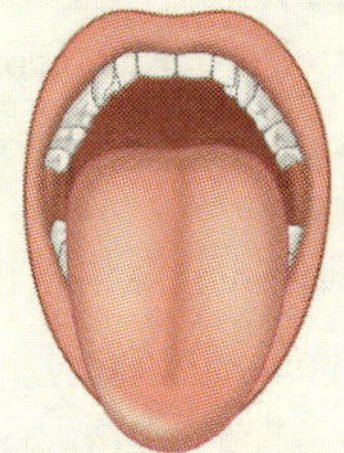

a. Mallampati classification
b. Brodsky classification
c. Friedman classification
d. Cormack–Lehane classification

2. What is the fluid of choice for surgery?

(Most Recent Question July 2023)

a. Blood
b. Colloid
c. Crystalloid
d. FFP

3. Which of the following is not used in ACLS?

(Most Recent Question July 2023)

a. Adrenaline
b. Amiodarone
c. $NaHCO_3$
d. High voltage defibrillator

4. What is this device used for?

(Most Recent Question July 2023)

a. In spinal anesthesia
b. In epidural anesthesia
c. To create pneumoperitoneum
d. In lumbar puncture

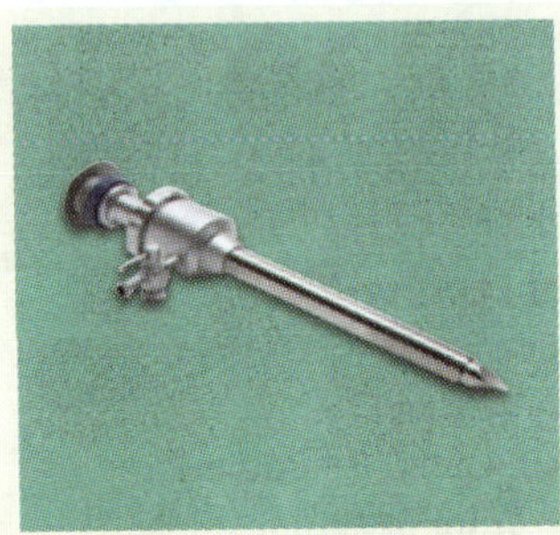

5. What is true about nasal cannula shown in the image?

(Most Recent Question Jan 2023)

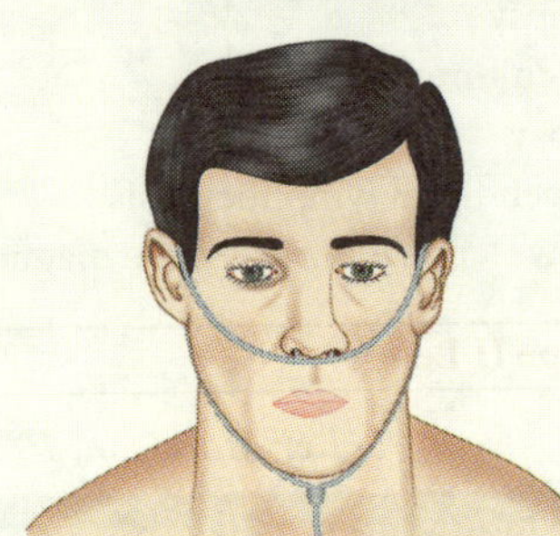

a. FiO_2 is 0.24 to 0.45
b. FiO_2 is 1.25 to 1.55
c. FiO_2 is 0.844 to 0.490
d. FiO_2 is 1.26 to 1.55

6. A 30-year-old male met with a roadside accident. He presented to hospital and underwent the procedure known as tracheostomy subsequently an endotracheal tube was inserted. Which of the following factor mainly affects the air resistance in the endotracheal tube?

(Most Recent Question Jan 2023)

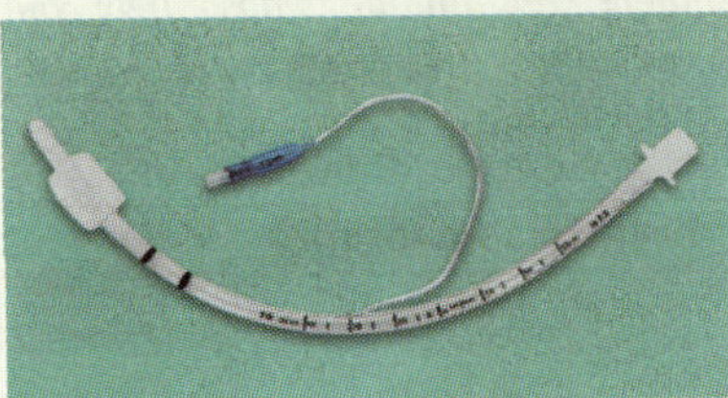

a. Balloon size
b. Width
c. Length
d. Radius

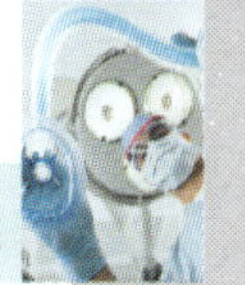

7. **Which of the following is the choice of inhalational anesthesia agent in children?** *(Most Recent Question Jan 2023)*
   a. Propofol b. Sevoflurane
   c. Desflurane d. Halothane

LOCAL ANESTHETICS AND INSTRUMENTS

8. **A patient of COVID-19 requires oxygen therapy. Which of the following cylinders should be used to provide oxygen to this patient?**
   (Most Recent Question June/Dec 2021)

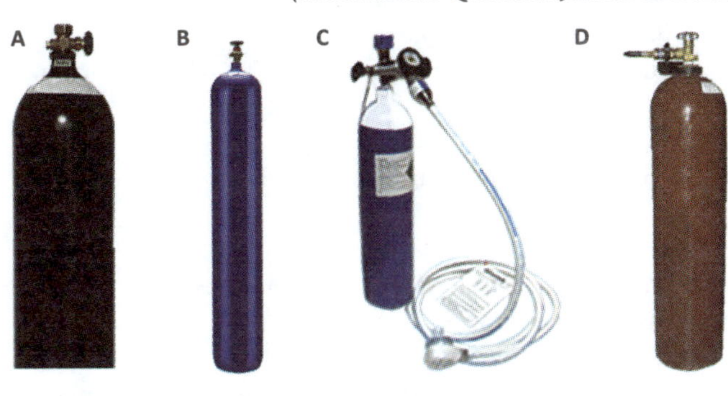

   a. A b. B
   c. C d. D
9. **Action of local anesthetic agent is by blocking which of the following ion channel?**
   (Most Recent Question Dec 2019-20)
   a. Sodium channel b. Potassium channel
   c. Calcium channel d. Chloride channel
10. **A patient has had a gunshot injury with hypotension. By which of the following cannula size maximum fluid can be given rapidly?** *(Most Recent Question Dec 2019-20)*
    a. 14 b. 16
    c. 18 d. 20
11. **What type of anesthesia is required for dental surgery?**
    (Most Recent Question Dec 2019-20)
    a. Field block b. Nerve block
    c. Infiltration d. All of these
12. **Identify the shown instrument:**
    (Most Recent Question Dec 2019-20)

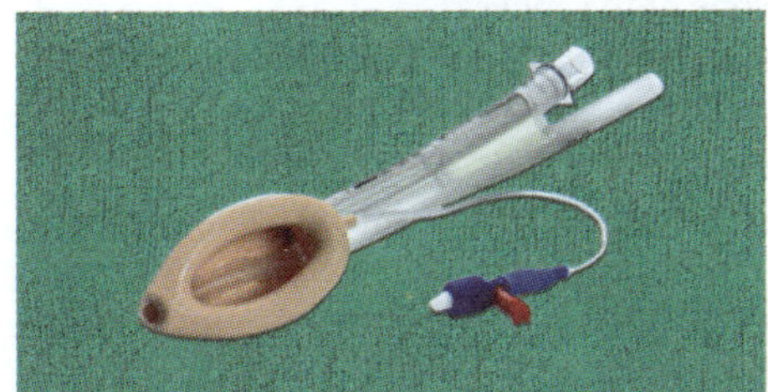

    a. Classic LMA
    b. I- gel
    c. Proseal laryngeal mask airway
    d. Laryngeal mask airway supreme
13. **Identify the shown image:**
    (Most Recent Question Dec 2019-20)

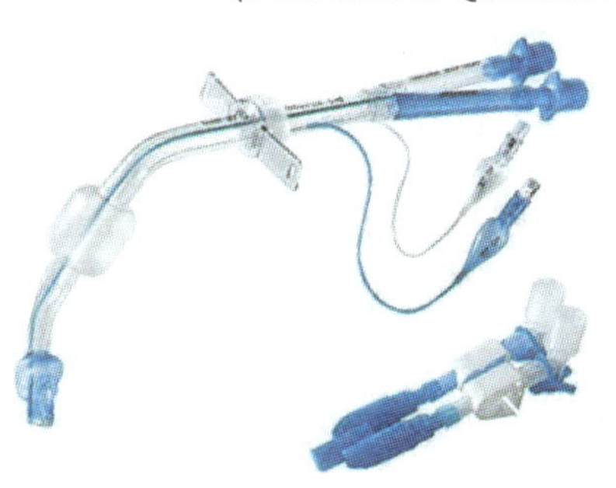

    a. Endotracheal tube
    b. Laryngeal mask airway
    c. Double lumen tube
    d. Tracheostomy tube
14. **Identify the shown needle:**
    (Most Recent Question Dec 2019-20)

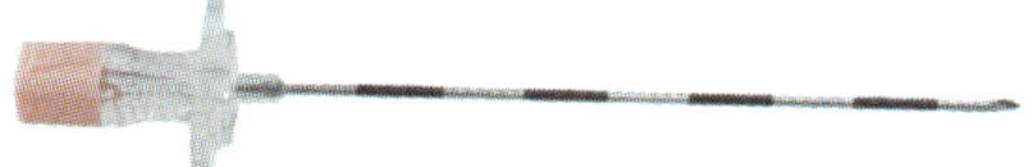

    a. Sprotte b. Whitacre
    c. Quincke d. Tuohys
15. **Colour of nitrous oxide cylinder is:**
    (Most Recent Question 2019)
    a. Blue
    b. Blue body with white shoulder
    c. White
    d. Black
16. **Drug used for Hypotensive episode during spinal anesthesia:** *(Recent Pattern Question 2018-19)*
    a. Nor adrenaline b. Phenelzine
    c. Ephedrine d. Na^+ Nitroprusside
17. **Shortest acting local anesthetics agent:**
    (Recent Pattern Question 2018-19)
    a. Bupivacaine b. Lidocaine
    c. Tetracaine d. Prilocaine
18. **True about nasal cannula:**
    (Recent Pattern Question 2018-19)
    a. 10 L oxygen flow, variable performance device
    b. Low flow, fixed performance device
    c. Low flow, variable performance device
    d. High flow fixed performance device
19. **Which of the following ligament is pierced during lumbar puncture right before entering dura mater?**
    (Recent Pattern Question 2018)
    a. Supraspinous ligament b. Interspinous ligament
    c. Infraspinous ligament d. Ligamentum flavum
20. **Which of the following local anesthetics causes methemoglobinemia?** *(Recent Pattern Question 2018)*
    a. Lignocaine b. Benzocaine
    c. Chloroprocaine d. Dibucaine

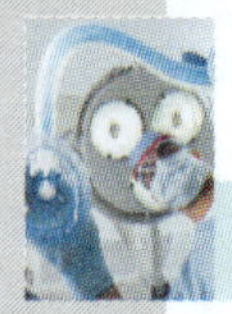

21. Correct sequence of resuscitation is: ***(Recent Pattern Question 2018)***
a. Early assessment, CPR, defibrillator, advance life saving
b. CPR, early assessment, defibrillator, advance life saving
c. CPR, defibrillator, early assessment, advance life saving
d. Early assessment, defibrillator, CPR, advance life saving

22. Which peripheral nerve fibers are mainly affected by Local anesthesia? ***(Recent Pattern Question 2017)***
a. A beta
b. A delta
c. B fibers
d. C fibers

23. Tourniquet applied in Bier's block can provide anesthesia for? ***(Recent Pattern Question 2017)***
a. ½ hour
b. 1 hour
c. 2 hours
d. 3 hours

24. Which is true about Cracking of cylinder valve? ***(Recent Pattern Question 2017)***
a. Should be performed rapidly and for prolonged duration
b. Momentarily opening it to blow away foreign matter from the outlet
c. It increases the likelihood of flash fire
d. It refers to a fracture of stem of the valve

25. What is the use of soda lime in anesthesia machine? ***(Recent Pattern Question 2017)***
a. In vaporizers
b. In oxygen concentrators
c. In breathing circuits to absorb CO_2
d. To treat metabolic abnormality

26. The purpose of cuff in endotracheal tube is? ***(Recent Pattern Question 2017)***
a. To reduce incidence of pressure necrosis
b. To prevent pneumothorax
c. To prevent the tube from slipping out
d. To prevent regurgitation of gastric contents

27. Capnography monitors: ***(Recent Pattern Question 2017)***
a. Concentration of inhaled O_2
b. Concentration of exhaled CO_2
c. Concentration of electrolyte
d. Blood pressure blood flow to the peripheral organs

28. What is this instrument used for:

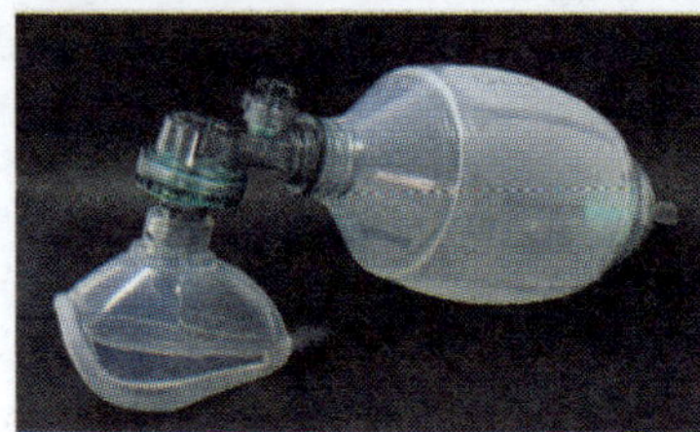

a. Ventilation
b. Feeding
c. TURP
d. Cholestomy

29. Laryngeal Mask Airway (LMA) is used for:
a. Maintenance of the airway
b. Facilitating laryngeal surgery
c. Prevention of aspiration
d. Removing oral secretions

30. A patient is on mechanical ventilation in Intensive Care unit (ICU), ventilator show alarms for increase in both peak and plateau pressure during inspiration. This indicates:
a. Obstruction of tracheal tube
b. Decrease in distensibility of lungs and chest wall
c. Acute bronchospasm
d. Increase compliance of lungs

31. Oxygen cylinder color:
a. Black body white shoulder
b. White body black shoulder
c. Brown body and shoulder
d. Blue body and shoulder

32. Pin index system for oxygen?
a. 1,5
b. 2,5
c. 4,5
d. 3,5

33. Pin index system for nitrous oxide?
a. 1,6
b. 2,5
c. 3,5
d. 1,5

34. Pin index safety mechanism in anesthesia machines are basically used to:
a. Prevent wrong attachment of cylinder
b. Prevent incorrect attachment of anesthesia machines
c. Prevent wrong inhalational drug delivery
d. Prevent incorrect anesthesia face mask attachment

35. ETT is not useful for:
a. Pneumothorax
b. Pulmonary toilet
c. Obstruction
d. Decreased level of consciousness

36. American society of anesthesiologist scoring is used to assess?
a. Oral cavity for intubation
b. Overall health status of patient
c. Risk actor
d. Pain scale

37. Local anesthesia acts by blocking
a. Calcium channel
b. Sodium channel
c. By blocking both sodium and calcium
d. None of the above

38. Local anesthetics block which ion channel:
a. K^+
b. Ca^+
c. Na^+
d. Cl^-

39. Anesthetic agent with vasoconstrictor is contraindicated in:
a. Spinal block
b. Regional block
c. Epidural block
d. Ring block

40. Which of the following doesn't belong to ester group of local Anesthetics:
a. Chlorprocaine
b. Tetracaine
c. Benzocaine
d. Dibucaine

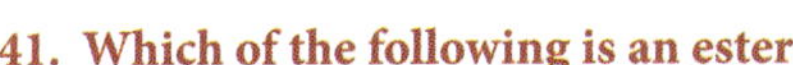

41. Which of the following is an ester:
a. Chlorprocaine b. Bupivacaine
c. Dibucaine d. Prilocaine

42. Which of the following is an ester:
a. Prilocaine b. Bupivacaine
c. Lignocaine d. Procaine

43. All are esters; EXCEPT:
a. Prilocaine b. Cocaine
c. Tetracaine d. Chlorprocaine

44. Which of the following statement is true about ether as an anesthetic agent?
a. Used with muscle relaxant
b. Slow induction
c. High risk of cardiac arrhythmia
d. Recovery faster

45. Most cardiotoxic local Anesthetic:
a. Dibucaine b. Bupivacaine
c. Lignocaine d. Chlorprocaine

MUSCLE RELAXANTS AND ANALGESICS

46. The shortest acting opioid is:
(Recent Pattern Question 2018)
a. Fentanyl b. Sulfentanil
c. Remifentanil d. Alfentanyl

47. The drug shown can be given by all of the following routes; EXCEPT: ***(Recent Pattern Question 2018)***

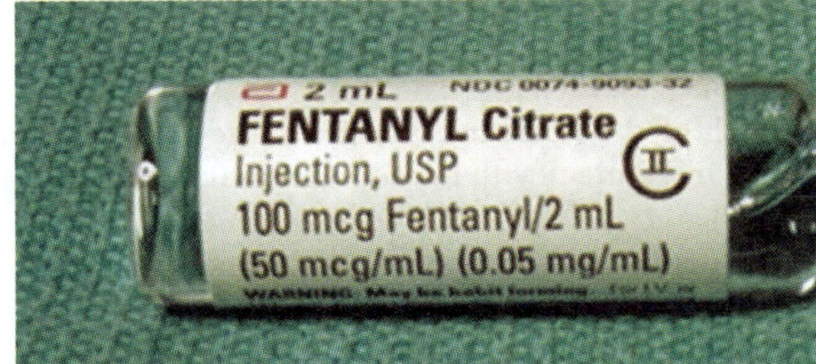

a. Epidural b. Intravenous
c. Intrathecal d. Intradermal

48. Hoffman degradation is seen in metabolism of?
(Recent Pattern Question 2017)
a. Atracurium b. Pancuronium
c. Vecuronium d. Nitrous oxide

49. A 60-year-old patient undergoing surgery has serum bilirubin = 8.9 mg% and serum creatinine = 1.9 mg%. Which anesthetic drug is preferred?
(Recent Pattern Question 2017)
a. Atracurium b. Nitrous oxide
c. Vacuronium d. Mivacurium

50. Malignant hyperthermia is due to defect in which receptor? ***(Recent Pattern Question 2017)***
a. Succinylcholine receptor b. Ryanodine receptor
c. Kainate receptor d. AMPA receptor

51. Which is the fastest non depolarising muscle relaxant?
(Recent Pattern Question 2017)
a. Mivacurium b. Rocuronium
c. Succinylcholine d. Atracurium

52. Side effect of alfentanil:
a. Chest wall rigidity b. Hypotension
c. Convulsion d. Hallucination

53. Muscle rigidity by fentanyl is due to which receptor:
a. Mu (μ) b. Kappa (k)
c. Delta (δ) d. Sigma (σ)

54. Which of the following drug causes malignant hyperthermia:
a. Mivacurium b. Pancronium
c. Succinylcholine d. Atracurium

55. Malignant hyperthermia is caused by:
a. Ryanodine receptor b. Nicotinic receptor
c. Muscarinic receptor d. NMDA receptor

56. All are true about Succinylcholine; EXCEPT:
a. Shortest acting muscle relaxant
b. Neostigmine antagonizes its action
c. Responsible for post-op muscle pain
d. Depolarizing agent

57. Which of the following is shortest acting non depolarizing muscle relaxant?
a. Vecuronium b. Mivacurium
c. Succinylcholine d. Atracrium

58. Which of the following agent is most commonly associated with malignant hyperthermia is a patient:
a. Dantrolene
b. Chloroprocaine
c. Succinylcholine
d. Mivacurium

59. Longest acting neuromuscular blocking agent is
a. Atracuronium b. Vecuronium
c. Doxacuronium d. Pancuronium

GENERAL ANESTHETIC, IV/INHALATION AGENTS

60. Which of the inhalational anesthetic uses special vaporizer? ***(Most Recent Question June 2022)***
a. Desflurane b. Sevoflurane
c. Isoflurane d. Halothane

61. A young patient underwent surgery under GA with O_2, N_2O and Desflurane. Just after extubation, the patient started to desaturate. On auscultation, there are crepitation. What could be the most common cause?
(Most Recent Question June/Dec 2021)
a. Pleural effusion
b. ARDS
c. Negative pressure pulmonary edema
d. Atelectasis

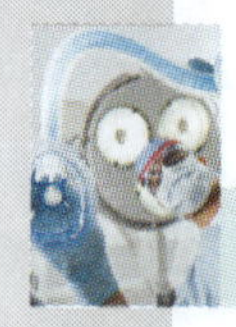

62. Which of the following anesthetic agent is best for cardiac patient? *(Most Recent Question June/Dec 2021)*
a. Halothane
b. Isoflurane
c. Nitrous oxide
d. Sevoflurane

63. Which of the following options contains all intravenous hypnotic agents? *(Most Recent Question June/Dec 2021)*
a. Propofol, Sodium thiopentone, Etomidate
b. Halothane, Sevoflurane, Desflurane
c. Sugammadex, Sufentanil,Tramadol
d. Vecuronium, Rocuronium, Atracurium

64. Which of these agents is preferred for day care anesthesia? *(Most Recent Question Dec 2019-20)*
a. Propofol b. Ketamine
c. Thiopentone d. Etomidate

65. Which anesthetic agent is contraindicated in acute intermittent porphyria? *(Most Recent Question Dec 2019-20)*
a. Propofol b. Thiopentone
c. Ketamine d. Etomidate

66. Spinal anesthesia in an adult is given at this level: *(Most Recent Question 2019)*
a. T12–L1 b. L1–L2
c. L3–L4 d. L5–S1

67. The duration of spinal anesthesia is based directly on: *(Most Recent Question 2019)*
a. Dose b. Height
c. Age d. Total body fat

68. On repeated use, which of the following inhalational anesthetic agent can cause hepatitis: *(Most Recent Question 2019)*
a. Isoflurane b. Halothane
c. Sevoflurane d. Ether

69. Which of the following is used for day care surgery? *(Most Recent Question 2019)*
a. Ketamine b. Thiopentone
c. Propofol d. Etomidate

70. An anesthetic agent causing Hepatitis: *(Recent Pattern Question 2018-19)*
a. Halothane b. Etomidate
c. Prilocaine d. Bupivacaine

71. MC gas used for pneumoperitoneum? *(Recent Pattern Question 2018-19)*
a. Carbon dioxide b. Oxygen
c. Air d. Nitrogen

72. Drug used to control secretions in general anesthesia?
a. Hyoscine b. Glycopyrrolate
c. Pethidine d. Lorazepam

73. Anesthetic agent of choice in pediatric patients:
a. Ketamine b. Desflurane
c. Sevoflurane d. Propofol

74. Best Anesthetic drug to be given in day care surgery:
a. Ketamine b. Sevoflurane
c. Desflurane d. Propofol

75. Regarding propofol, which one of the following is false:
a. It is used as an induction agent
b. It possess anti-pruritic action
c. It is painful on injecting intravenously
d. It has strong tendency to cause vomiting

76. Postanesthetic nausea and vomiting is uncommon with:
a. Propofol b. Halothane
c. Fentanyl d. Sufentanil

77. Which one of the following is the fastest acting inhalational agent?
a. Halothane b. Ether
c. Isoflurane d. Sevoflurane

78. In renal failure, IV anesthetic used is?
a. Atracurium b. Vivacurium
c. Pancuronium d. Cisatracurium

79. All of the following drugs will cause malignant hyperthermia; EXCEPT:
a. Nitrous oxide b. Desflurane
c. Isoflurane d. Sevoflurane

80. Drug producing dissociative anesthesia:
a. Propofol b. Enflurane
c. Ketamine d. Sevoflurane

81. All of the following are pharmacological effects of ketamine; EXCEPT:
a. It causes profound analgesia
b. It causes severe fall in blood pressure
c. It causes amnesia
d. It increases cerebral blood flow

82. Which of the following anesthetic agent is contraindicated in a patient with raised intracranial pressure:
a. Etomidate b. Thiopentone
c. Propofol d. Ketamine

83. Ketamine not used in:
a. Full stomach b. Increased ICT
c. Pediatric patient d. Asthma patient

84. Which anesthetic agent is contraindicated in porphyria:
a. Propofol b. Ketamine
c. Thiopentone d. Etomidate

85. Absolute contraindication to thiopentone:
a. Cardiotoxicity
b. Acute intermittent phorphyria
c. Malignant hyperthermia
d. Methemoglobinemia

86. Chloroform is:
a. Hepatotoxic b. Cardiotoxic
c. Both d. None of these

87. High spinal anesthesia is characterized by?
a. Hypertension, tachycardia
b. Hypertension, bradycardia
c. Hypotension, tachycardia
d. Hypotension, bradycardia

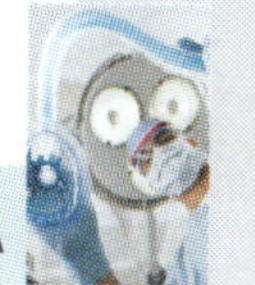

PRE-OP ANESTHETIC PREPARATION

88. At a random place you and saw a guy collapse. You started CPR after checking vitals and soon advance cardiac support arrived at the scene. What should be the next step of management? *(Most Recent Question June 2022)*
a. Handover patient to them and leave
b. Ask them to apply the paddles while you continue CPR
c. Stop CPR and left them apply the paddles
d. Continue 1 round of CPR and then use defibrillator

89. Before laparoscopic surgery, what advise should be given to the patient by surgeon? *(Most Recent Question June/Dec 2021)*
a. NPO 8–12 hours before OT
b. NPO 24 hours before OT
c. On the table hair removal by razor
d. None of the above

90. Patient underwent surgery and during recovery he was shouting and having hallucinations. Which anesthetic agent was used? *(Most Recent Question Dec 2019-20)*
a. Ketamine
b. Halothane
c. Etomidate
d. Midazolam

91. A patient with uterine fibroid & suffering from moderate to severe cardiac ailment. Which of the following should be avoided? *(Most Recent Question Dec 2019-20)*
a. Subtotal hysterectomy
b. Total hysterectomy
c. Laparoscopic hysterectomy
d. Vaginal hysterectomy

92. Preanesthetic evaluation of airway intubation in an elderly lady is done by:
a. ASA scoring *(Recent Pattern Question 2018-19)*
b. Mallampati scoring
c. Aldrete scoring system
d. Wilson scoring system

93. Thiopentone is preferred as an induction agent because of? *(Recent Pattern Question 2017)*
a. Smoothness of induction
b. Rapid recovery
c. Both
d. None of the above

94. Which is not a complication of giving anesthesia to a chronic smoker?
a. Intra-operative bronchospasm
b. Increased mucosal clearance
c. Atelectasis
d. Post-operative pneumonia

INTRA-OP AND POST-OP PATIENT CARE

95. A sick patient in ward needs supplement oxygen. It will be given from which of the following cylinder? *(Most Recent Question June/Dec 2021)*

a. 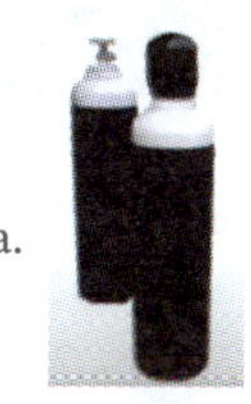

b. 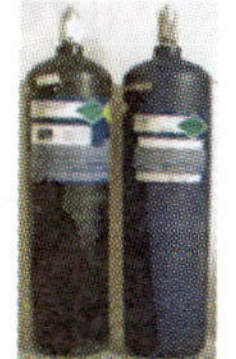

c. 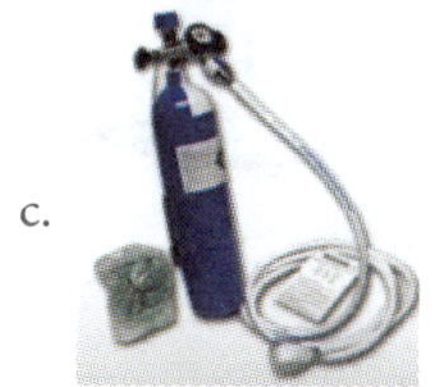

d. 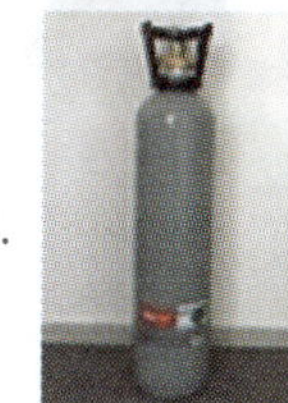

96. A COPD patient admitted in ICU was on oxygen therapy with mask with 2 liter of oxygen. He was found to be hypo-ventilating. His pCO_2 on blood gas analysis was 64 mm Hg. Which of the following should be done? *(Most Recent Question June/Dec 2021)*
a. Increase the FiO_2
b. Decrease the FiO_2
c. Start BIPAP
d. Intubate and start on ventilator

97. Which of the following structure is not encountered during epidural anesthesia? *(Most Recent Question June/Dec 2021)*
a. Supraspinous ligament
b. Interspinous ligament
c. Ligament flavum
d. Dura

98. Endotracheal tube in the esophagus is best assessed by: *(Most Recent Question Dec 2019-20)*
a. CO_2 exhalation
b. Chest wall movement
c. Auscultation
d. Chest tube passes through vocal cords

99. The proper ET tube position is best confirmed by: *(Recent Pattern Question 2018-19)*
a. Mapleson circuit
b. Capnography
c. Laryngeal mask airway
d. Bag mask ventilation

100. Instructions for routine intubation are all; EXCEPT:
a. Head tilt
b. Chin lift
c. Cricoid pressure
d. Jaw thrust

101. According to ASA what is the initial management for cardiac arrest:
a. Secure airway
b. Carotid pulse palpation
c. IV adrenaline
d. Cardiac compression

102. Sellick' s maneuver is used for?
a. To prevent alveolar collapse
b. To prevent gastric aspiration
c. To facilitate Respiration
d. To reduce dead space

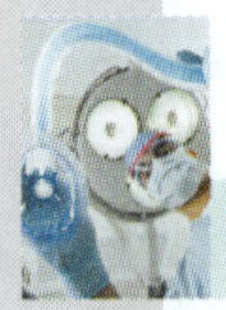

103. Factors favoring fat embolism in a patient with major trauma?
a. Hypovolemic shock b. Respiratory failure
c. Diabetes d. Mobility of fracture

MISCELLANEOUS

104. Identify the instrument given in image below. ***(Most Recent Question June/Dec 2021)***

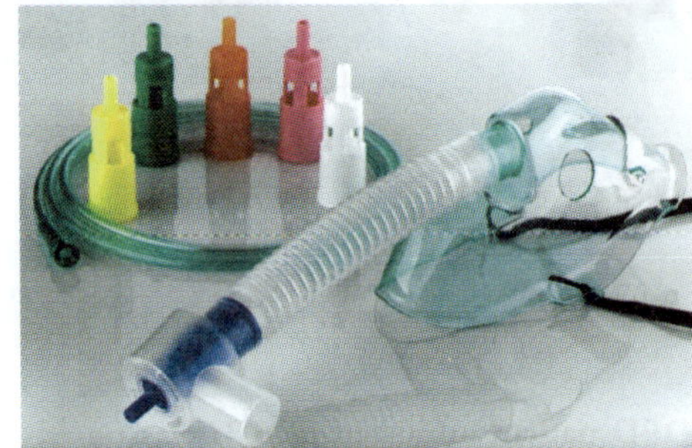

a. Anesthesia face mask b. Nebulizer
c. High flow nasal cannula d. Venturi mask

105. In CPR, number of chest compression per minute in an adult: ***(Most Recent Question 2019)***
a. 30–50 per minute b. 50–72 per minute
c. 100–120 per minute d. 120–200 per minute

106. Heimlich maneuver is performed to dislodge foreign body located in: ***(Recent Pattern Question 2017)***
a. Esophagus b. Bronchus
c. Trachea d. Upper stomach

107. Hallucinations are seen with:
a. Propofol b. Sevoflurane
c. Ketamine d. Isoflurane

108. Succinylcholine causes:
a. Severe hyperkalemia b. Paraplegia
c. Liver failure d. Renal failure

109. Mendelson's syndrome is due to:
a. Hypersensitivity reaction to anesthetic agent
b. Gastric contents aspiration
c. Faulty intubation
d. Asphyxia due to tracheal stenosis

110. Anesthetic agent not metabolized by body is:
a. N20 b. Gallamine
c. Sevofluorane d. Halothane

111. Compression depth in CPR in adults is:
a. 1 inch b. 2 inch
c. 3 inch d. 4 inch

112. What is true about laryngeal mask airway?
a. Prevents aspiration
b. Used in oral surgeries
c. Used in laryngeal surgeries
d. Maintains airway

113. Lignocaine is used as:
a. 0.5% jelly, 1 % injection b. 1% jelly, 2 % injection
c. 2% jelly, 4% injection d. 4% jelly, 5% injection

114. PIN index of nitrous oxide is:
a. 1-5 b. 2-5
c. 3-5 d. 1-6

115. The muscle relaxant that can be given in renal disease is:
a. Doxacurium b. Pancuronium
c. Vecuronium d. Gallium

116. Fastest onset skeletal muscle relaxant is:
a. Vecuronium b. Rocuronium
c. Mivacurium d. Atracurium

117. Hoffman elimination is seen in:
a. Cisatracurium b. Mivacurium
c. Pipecuronium d. Vecuronium

118. All are true about halothane; EXCEPT?
a. Amber coloured bottles
b. Arrythmogenic
c. Hepatitis
d. Bronchospasm

119. Mallampati classification in which tonsillar pillars, uvula is not seen?
a. Class I b. Class II
c. Class III d. Class IV

120. Most efficient Mapelson circuit for spontaneous ventilation?
a. Mapelson A b. Mapelson B
c. Mapelson C d. Mapelson D

121. Shortest acting spinal Anesthetic agent?
a. Lidocaine b. Bupivacaine
c. Tetracaine d. Ropivacaine

122. High spinal anesthesia leads to:
a. Bradycardia and Hypotension
b. Bradycardia and increased BP
c. Tachycardia and increased BP
d. Tachycardia and decreased BP

123. Meyer Overton rule is for?
a. Inhalational Anesthetics
b. Local Anesthetics
c. Depolarising neuromuscular blockade
d. Non depolarising neuromuscular blockade

124. Celiac block is given for?
a. Abdominal malignant growth
b. Chest pain
c. Sciatica
d. Perineal pain

125. Side effect of alfentanil:
a. Chest wall rigidity b. Hypertension
c. Convulsion d. Hallucination

126. Muscle rigidity by fentanyl is due to which receptor
a. Mu (μ) b. Kappa (k)
c. Delta (δ) d. Sigma (σ)

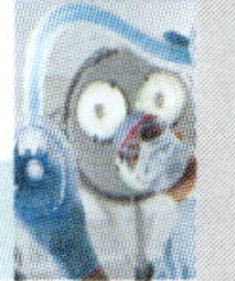

127. Anesthesia of choice in pediatric patients:
a. Ketamine
b. Desflurane
c. Sevoflurane
d. Propofol

128. Which one of the following is the fastest acting inhalational agent?
a. Halothane
b. Ether
c. Isoflurane
d. Sevoflurane

129. In renal failure, IV anesthetic used:
a. Atracurium
b. Vivacurium
c. Pancuronium
d. Cisatracurium

130. Which anesthetic agent is contraindicated in porphyria:
a. Propofol
b. Ketamine
c. Thiopentone
d. Etomidate

131. Absolute contraindication for thiopentone:
a. Cardiotoxicity
b. Acute intermittent phorphyria
c. Malignant hyperthermia
d. Methemoglobinemia

132. According to ASA what is the initial management for cardiac arrest:
a. Breathing
b. Carotid pulse palpation
c. IV adrenaline
d. Chest compressions

133. First sensation to be lost in local anesthetic use is:
a. Touch
b. Pain
c. Temperature
d. Pressure

134. Longest acting local Anesthetic drug is:
a. Procaine
b. Prilocaine
c. Lignocaine
d. Bupivacaine

135. Hoffmann elimination is seen with:
a. Gallamine
b. Thiopentone
c. Atracurium
d. Lignocaine

136. Which day is considered as "World anesthesia day"?
a. 16th September
b. 16th October
c. 16th November
d. 16th December

137. Agent causing malignant hyperthermia is:
a. Succinylcholine
b. N_2O
c. Dantrolene sodium
d. Gallamine

138. Ketamine is not given in?
a. Hypertensive patients
b. Hypovolemic patients
c. Septic
d. Asthmatic patients

ANSWERS WITH EXPLANATIONS

MOST RECENT QUESTIONS 2023

1. Ans. (a) Mallampati classification

Ref: Miller's Anesthesia 9th ed, pg. 1379

- The Mallampati classification is a valuable tool used in anesthesia and airway management. It assesses the view of the oropharynx to **predict the ease of intubation.**
- It involves a patient who is sitting upright, with open mouth, and maximum extended tongue while the clinician observes the visibility of the tonsillar pillars, the uvula, and the soft palate.
- This classification helps anesthetists determine the potential difficulty of intubation and make informed decisions about airway management techniques.

Extra Mile

- **Brodsky classification:** Brodsky classification assesses the severity of tonsillar hypertrophy, primarily for evaluating obstructive sleep apnea.
- **Friedman classification:** Friedman classification is used to assess the degree of obstructive sleep apnea by considering the factors, like tonsil size and lateral pharyngeal wall collapse.
- **Cormack–Lehane classification:** Cormack–Lehane classification is employed to grade laryngeal views during direct laryngoscopy, assisting in predicting the ease of intubation.

2. Ans. (c) Crystalloid

Ref: Sabiston's Surgery 21st ed, pg. 1538–1540

- Crystalloid solutions are the preferred intravenous fluids for surgical procedures. They consist of water, electrolytes, and sometimes glucose.
- These solutions are versatile and commonly used to maintain intravascular volume, they replace fluid losses, and correct electrolyte imbalances.
- Examples of crystalloid solutions include normal saline and Ringer's lactate. Their balanced electrolyte composition makes them suitable for various surgical scenarios.

Extra Mile

- Blood transfusion is administered when there is significant blood loss or specific clinical indications.
- Colloid solutions contain larger molecules and are used when there's a need to maintain colloid osmotic pressure or intravascular volume.
- Fresh Frozen Plasma (FFP) is used to correct coagulopathies and provide clotting factors.

3. Ans. (c) $NaHCO_3$

Ref: Sabiston's Surgery 21st ed, pg. 2717–2718

- Sodium bicarbonate (NaHCO3) was traditionally used in Advanced Cardiac Life Support (ACLS) to treat metabolic acidosis and certain arrhythmias. However, recent guidelines have shifted away from routine use of $NaHCO_3$ during ACLS. The focus is now on optimizing perfusion, early defibrillation, and appropriate administration of medications.
- ACLS drugs, like adrenaline (epinephrine) are administered to increase blood flow and perfusion during cardiac arrest. Amiodarone is used to manage certain shock-resistant ventricular arrhythmias.
- High voltage defibrillators are used to deliver synchronized shocks during ACLS to restore normal heart rhythms when appropriate.

4. Ans. (c) To create pneumoperitoneum

Ref: Schwartz Surgery 11th ed, pg. 459–460

- The shown device is a Veress needle, commonly used in laparoscopic surgery to create pneumoperitoneum. Pneumoperitoneum involves introducing carbon dioxide (CO_2) gas into the abdominal cavity, which lifts the abdominal wall away from internal organs and creates a space for laparoscopic instruments.
- Pneumoperitoneum provides a clear visual field and allows for safe insertion of laparoscopic instruments during minimally invasive procedures.

5. Ans. (a) FiO_2 is 0.24 to 0.45

Ref: Morgan and Mikhail, Clinical Anesthesia 7th ed, pg. 2147

The image shown here is of nasal cannula.

- It is a soft single-ended plastic tube with nasal prongs for the nose connected overhead.
- FiO_2 of the nasal cannula is between 0.24 and 0.45
- FiO_2 is the concentration of oxygen that a person inhales during inspiration.
- The actual FiO_2 delivered to adults with nasal cannula is determined by:
  - Oxygen flow-major factor
  - Nasopharyngeal volume
  - Patient's inspiratory flow

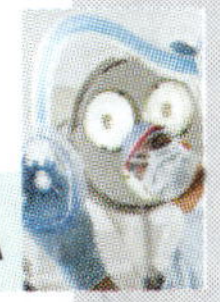

Extra Mile

Device/system	Oxygen flow rate (L/min)	FiO2 range	Images
Nasal cannula	1 2 3 4 5-6	0.21-0.24 0.23_0.28 0.27-0.34 0.31-0.38 0.32-0.44	
Simple mask	5-6 7-8	0.30-0.45 0.40-0.60	
Mask with reservoir	5	0.35-0.50	
Partial rebreathing mask-bag	7 15	0.35-0.75 0.65-1.00	
Nonrebreathing mask-bag	7-15	0.40-1.00	
Venturi mask and jet nebulizer	4-6 (total flow = 15) 4-6 (total flow = 45) 8-10 (total flow = 45) 8-10 (total flow = 33) 8-12 (total flow = 33)	0.24 0.28 0.35 0.40 0.50	

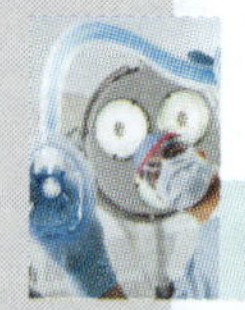

6. Ans. (d) Radius

Ref: Morgan and Mikhail, Clinical Anesthesia 7th ed. pg. 495

The image shown here is of the endotracheal tube.

- Endotracheal tube is employed for the conduct of general anesthesia and to facilitate the ventilator management of the critically ill patients both.
- Resistance to airflow depends primarily on the diameter of the tube.
- The choice of tube diameter is always a compromise between maximizing flow with a larger size and minimizing airway trauma with a smaller size.
- **Note:** Balloon in tube is used for stabilizing the tube after insertion.

7. Ans. (b) Sevoflurane

Ref: Morgan and Mikhail, Clinical Anesthesia 7th ed. pg. 287

- Sevoflurane is the choice of inhalational anesthetic agent in children.
- Its sweet smell and rapid increase in alveolar anesthetic concentration, make Sevoflurane an excellent choice for smooth and rapid inhalation inductions in pediatric and adult patients.
- Desflurane and isoflurane have a pungent smell and cause irritation thus they are not the agent of choice in the children.

LOCAL ANESTHETICS AND INSTRUMENTS

8. Ans. (a) A

- Fig. A is Oxygen Cylinder with black body and white shoulder.
- Fig. B is N_2O Cylinder which is blue colored.
- Fig. C is Entonox Cylinder with blue body and white shoulder.
- Fig. D is Helium Cylinder which is brown in colored.

	Body color	Shoulder color	Pressure, kPa (room T)
Oxygen	Black	White	13700
Nitrous oxide	Blue	Blue	4400
Carbon dioxide	Grey	Grey	5000
Air	Grey	White/Black quarters	13700
Entonox	Blue	White/Blue quarters	13700
Oxygen/helium	Black	White/Brown quarters	13700

9. Ans. (a) Sodium channel

- Local anesthetics like lidocaine act by Na^+ channel blockade → prevent generation and conduction of nerve impulse.

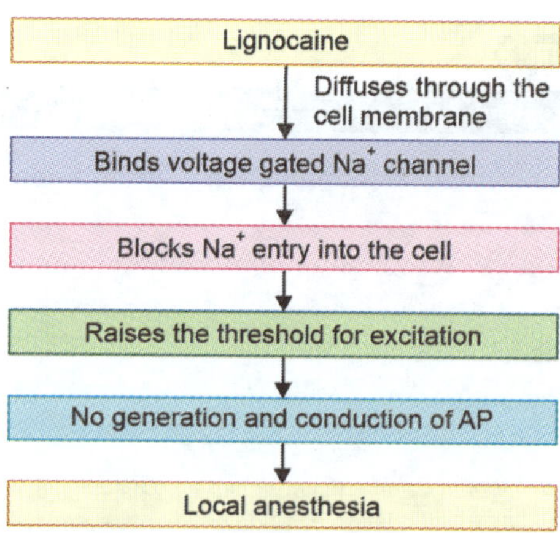

10. Ans. (a) 14

- Among the given choices, maximum fluid will be given by cannula size 14 G (orange color cannula).
- Flow rate with 14 G cannula is 270 mL/min

Compare the flow rate with other cannulas:

Color-coding of IV cannulas

Color	Gauge	Maximal flow rate (ml/min)
Yellow	24G	13
Blue	22G	31
Pink	20G	67
Green	18G	103
Grey	18G	236
Orange	14G	270

11. Ans. (d) All of the above

Definitions of dental local anesthetic injections

Infiltration	Injection of local anesthetic directly into an area of terminal nerve endings. (Superficial and infiltration anesthesia are collectively referred to as topical anesthesia)
Field block	Submucosal injection of a local anesthetic affecting the nerve branches in an area bordering the field to be anesthetized, typically providing pulpal anesthesia of one or two teeth. Field blocks are commonly referred to as "infiltrations".
Peripheral nerve block	Injection of local anesthetic in the vicinity of a peripheral nerve to anesthetize that nerve's entire area of innervation, which is also referred to as a "nerve block" "mandibular block," "division 2 block," or "block"
Regional anesthesia	Rendering a specific area of the body unresponsive to stimuli; all types may be used to accomplish regional anesthesia including topical and infiltration anesthesia. Generally refers to the anesthesia provided by field and peripheral nerve block techniques

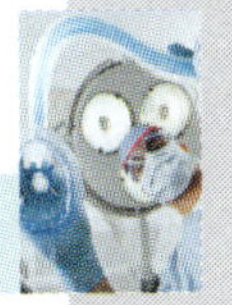

12. Ans. (c) Proseal laryngeal mask airway

- The shown image is proseal laryngeal mask airway (LMA). It has multiple advantages over classical LMA.

Classic LMA

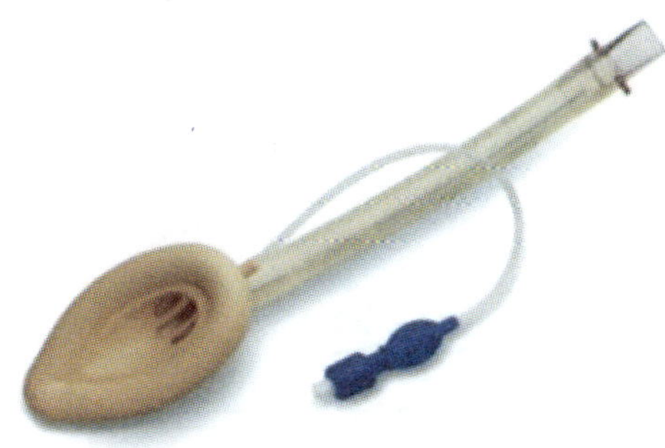

Proseal LMA

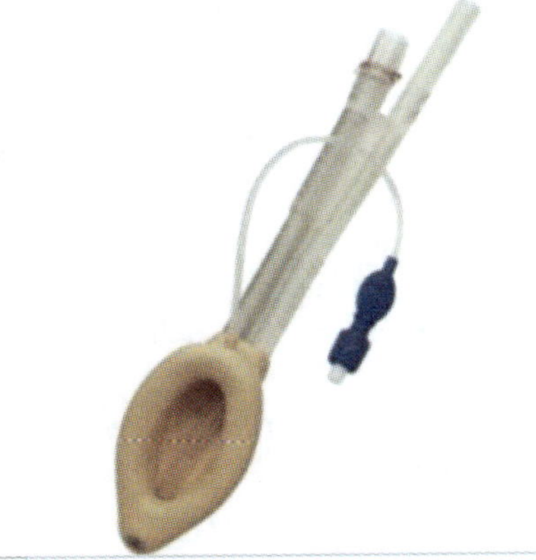

Modifications over classic LMA

- Larger and deeper bowl with no grille
- Gastric drainage tube running parallel to airway
- Larger deeper bowl and dorsal extension of cuff
- Bite block

Identify these images:

LMA Supreme

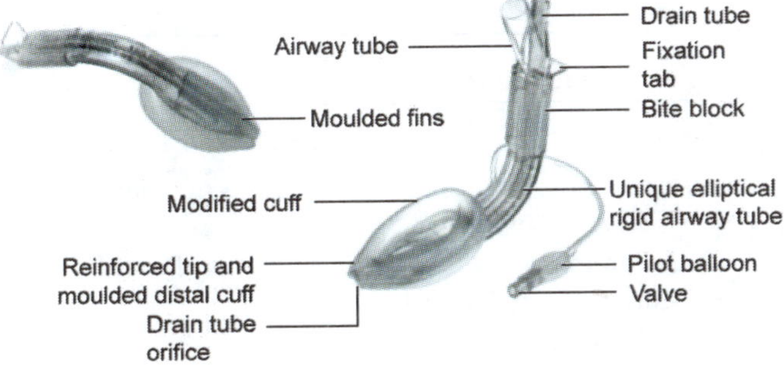

LMA Fastrach

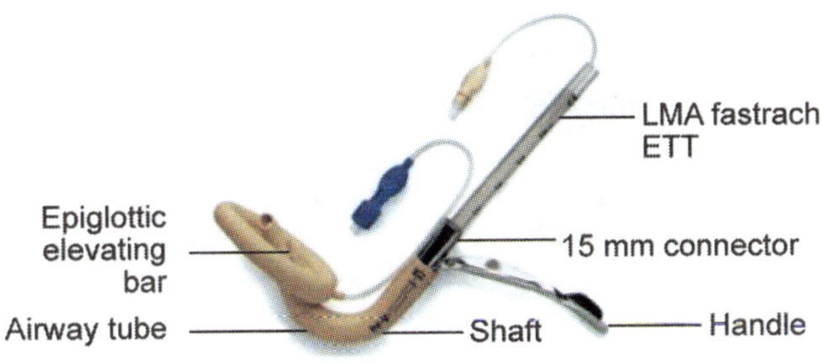

LMA Unique

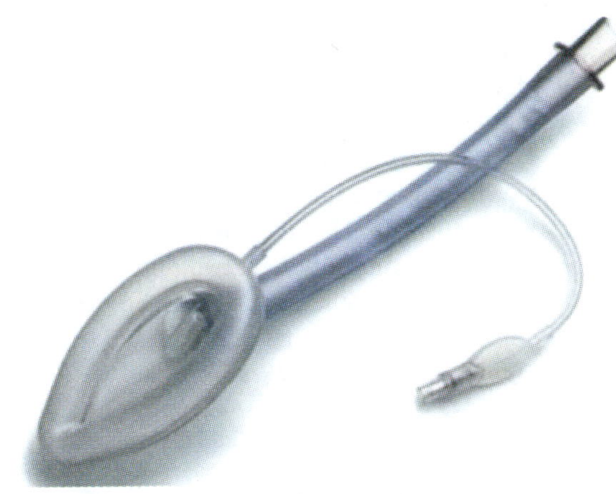

LMA Flexible

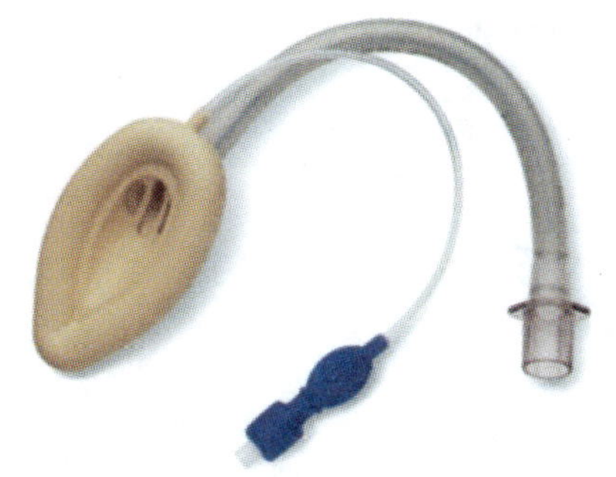

i-GEL

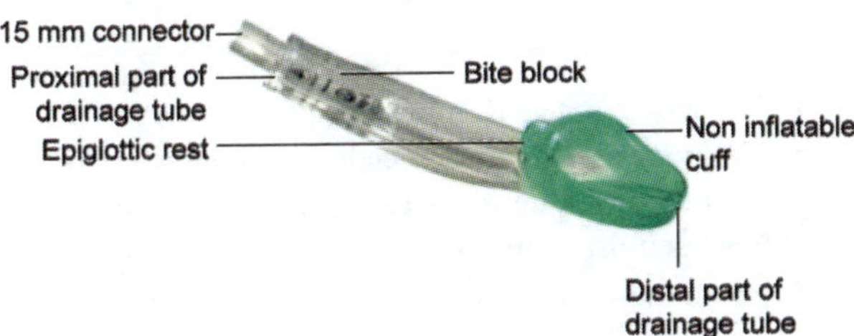

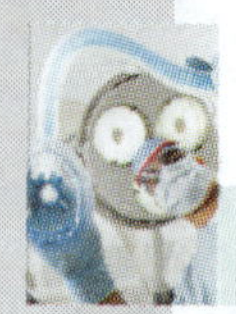

Endotracheal Tube

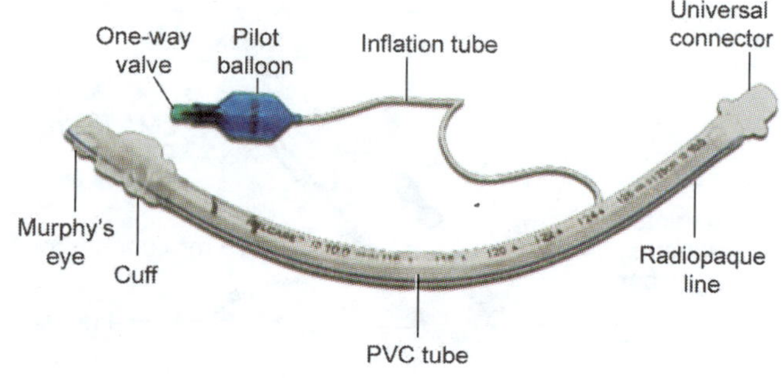

13. Ans. (c) Double lumen tube

- The shown image is double lumen tube
- Multiple types of double lumen tube are available like:
  - **Robertshaw:** Most widely used double lumen tube
  - **Carlens:** A left sided + carinal hook
  - **White**, a right sided carlens tube
  - **Bryce-smith:** Has no hook but a slotted cuff on right
- All double lumen tube have two cuffs, one terminating in trachea and the other in mainstem bronchus
- This tube is available in right sided and left sided
- Available sizes are: 41, 39, 37, 35, 28

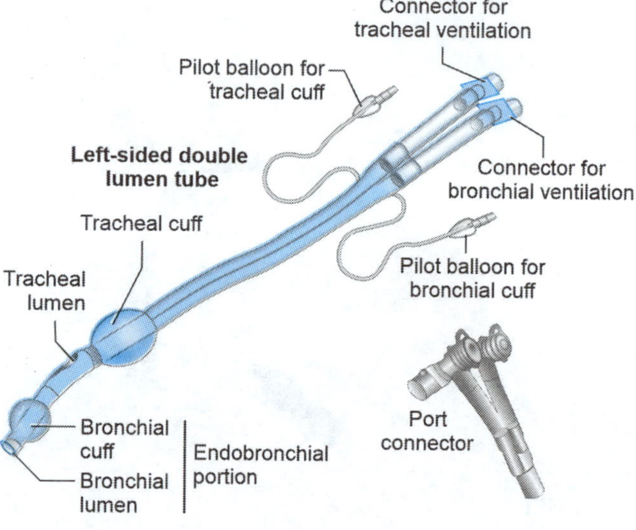

14. Ans. (d) Tuohys

- The shown image is Tuhoy's needle
- **Tuohy needle**/Epidural needle is a hollow hypodermic needle which is designed to be placed into epidural space.
- It is the most commonly used epidural needle
- It has a curved tip, which helps to prevent puncture of dural membrane.

15. Ans. (a) Blue

TABLE: Color coding of different gas cylinders

Gas	Shoulder	Body
Oxygen	White	Black
Nitrous oxide	Blue	Blue
Cyclopropane	Orange	Orange
Carbon dioxide	Grey	Grey
Air	White	Grey
Nitrogen	Black	Black
Entonox	White	Blue

16. Ans. (c) Ephedrine

Ref: Goodman & Gillman 13th ed. pg. 415

- Hypotension is commonly associated with spinal anesthesia.
- Treatment of hypotension is usually warranted when the BP decrease to about 30% of resting values.
- Aim of therapy: To maintain brain and cardiac perfusion and oxygenation

Treatment of hypotensive episode:

- Prior to spinal anesthesia a bolus of fluid (500-1000 ml) is administered
- Usual cause of hypotension is decreased venous return, possibly complicated by decreased heart rate, drugs with preferential vasoconstrictive and chronotropic properties are preferred.
- **Drug of choice:** Ephedrine, 5–10 mg intravenously.
- **Other treatment options:** Phenylephrine, Oxygen, fluid infusion, administration of vasoactive drugs.

Extra Mile

- Noradrenaline, a sympathomimetic agent, itself causes reflex bradycardia.
- Phenelzine is one of the MAO inhibitor, has no role
- Na+ Nitroprusside: Strong vasodilator. It can precipitate hypotension

17. Ans. (b) Lidocaine

Ref: Goodman & Gillman 13th ed. pg. 418

- Among the given choices, lidocaine is the shortest acting local anesthetic agent.
- Lidocaine can be used as several forms of anesthesia and duration of action varies:
  - Local anesthesia: ~ 30 min
  - Nerve block: 60–90 min
  - Spinal/Epidural anesthesia: 60–90 min

EPIDURAL ANESTHESIA • Use with epinephrine- containing test done • Risk of intravenous injection • Spread of block dependent on dose and volume injected • Epidural catheter allows repeated dosing • Consider coagulation status of patient		
Chloroprocaine	• Short duration • Epinephrine prolongs action	• 2–3% solution • Possible increased incidence of post procedure back pain
Lidocaine	• Intermediate duration • Epinephrine prolongs action	• 2% solution • Maximal healthy adult dose, ~4 mg/kg
Bupivacaine	• Long duration	• 0.5% solution • Maximal healthy adult dose, ~2–3 mg/kg
Ropivacaine	• Long duration	• 0.5–1.0% solution • Maximal healthy adult dose, ~2–3 mg/kg • May have less toxicity than equi- efficacious dose of bupivacaine
SPINAL ANESTHESIA • Dose and baricity of anesthetic strongly influences spread • Addition of opioids can prolong analgesia • Consider coagulation status of patient		
Lidocaine	• Short duration (60–90 min)	• ~25–50 mg for perineal and lower extremity surgery • Association of spinal lidocaine with transient neurological symptoms
Tetracaine	• Long duration (210–240 min)	• Duration increased by epinephrine • ~5 mg for perineal surgery • ~10 mg for lower extremity surgery
Bupivacaine	• Long duration (210–240 min)	• ~10 mg for perianal and lower extremity surgery • 15–20 mg for abdominal surgery

Note: *The shortest acting local anesthetic is chloroprocaine. Book states: "The onset and duration of action of spinal chloroprocaine are even shorter than those of lidocaine"*

- Tetracaine is a long-acting amino ester.
- Prilocaine is an intermediate-acting amino amide. (Goodman & Gillman 13 edition page 412)
- Bupivacaine is also a long acting local anesthetic.

18. Ans. (c) Low flow, variable performance device

Ref: Airway Management pg. 88; Emergency Care and Transportation of Sick and Injured, pg. 208

- Nasal cannula is an oxygen delivery system
- It is used for low-medium concentration of oxygen for the patients with mild to moderate respiratory distress (used when patient cannot tolerate mask)
- Can be used continuously with meals and activity
- **Flow rate:**
  - **Adult:** 4–6 L/m (delivers up to 40% FiO_2)
  - **Child:** < 3 L/m
  - **Infant/toddler:** <2 L/m
  - Flow rate >4L can cause irritation and dryness
- Depth and rate of breathing affect amount of oxygen reaching the lungs
- **Formula for FiO_2 calculation:**
  - 20% + (4 × oxygen liter flow)

OXYGEN DELIVERY DEVICES

Low flow (variable performance devices)	Reservoir system (variable performance devices)	High flow (fixed performance devices)
• Nasal cannula • Nasal catheter • Transtracheal catheter	• Reservoir cannula • Simple face mask • Partial rebreathing mask • Non rebreathing mask • Tracheostomy mask	• Venturi mask • Aerosol mask • T-piece with nebulisers

Extra Mile

OXYGEN DEVICES AND THEIR FLOW RATES

- **Masks:**
  - Simple mask: Flow rate 5–10 L/m. Delivers 35–40% FIO_2
  - Partial rebreathing mask: Flow rate 10–12 L/m. Delivers 50 – 60% FiO_2
  - Non breathing mask: Flow rate 10–15 L/m. Delivers up to 90% FiO_2
- **Enclosure systems:**
  - **Hoods:** Flow rate 10–15 L/m. Delivers 80–90% FiO_2
  - **Tents:** using high flow rate can deliver up to 50% FiO_2

19. Ans. (d) Ligamentum flavum

Ref: Clinical Neuroanatomy by Richard; S Snell, pg. 29

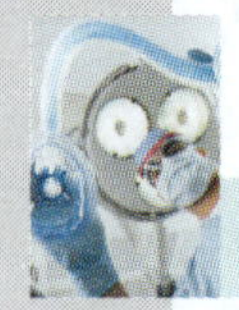

Structures which are pierced while doing lumbar puncture:

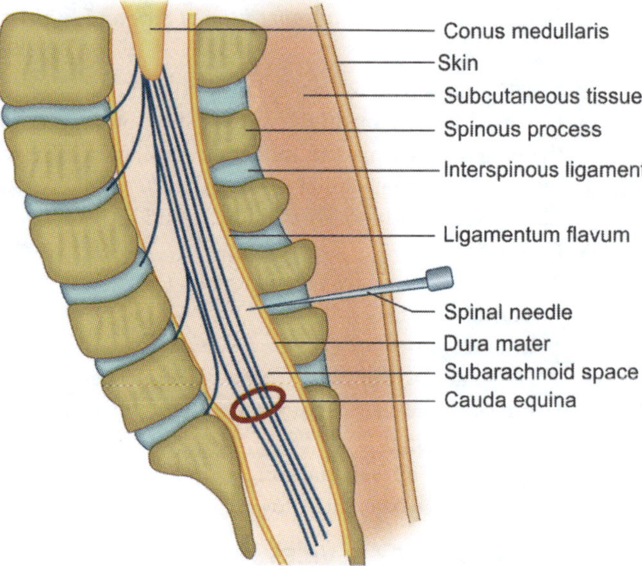

Lumbar puncture

- Skin → Subcutaneous tissue → Supraspinous ligament → Interspinous ligament → Ligamentum flavum → Dura mater → Arachnoid membrane

Needle Used

- **Dura cutting needle/Quincke's needle:** More traumatic
- **Dura separating needle/Whitacre needle:** Atraumatic. Less incidence of postpuncture headache
- **Size:** 25G (Preferred)

20. Ans. (b) Benzocaine

Ref: Handbook of Local Anesthetics, By Stanley F. Malamed; E-book, P 153

- Local anesthetics causing methemoglobinemia are: Benzocaine and prilocaine (prilocaine mainly in neonates).
- **Dibucaine:** Longest acting, most potent and most toxic LA.
- **Chloroprocaine:** Shortest acting LA.
- **LA highest incidence of malignant hyperthermia:** Lignocaine
- **Inhalational agent having highest incidence of malignant hyperthermia:** Halothane

21. Ans. (a) Early assessment, CPR, defibrillator, advance life saving

Ref: ABC of Resuscitation by Jasmeet Soar, Gavin D Perkins; Jerry Nolan, Ch 9

In an unresponsive patient:

- **Assess** pulse and breathing, on carotid artery for less than 10 seconds, if there is absent pulse, **start CPR.**
  - **Site of chest compression:** At the center of chest, lower half of sternum
  - **Depth of compression:** 2 inches or 5 cm
  - Rate 100/min
  - **Number of chest compression given per cycle of CPR:** 30
  - Maintain patent airway by head tilt, chin lift, jaw thrust
- Defibrillator is used next
- Call for advance life support help.

22. Ans. (b) A delta

Ref: Miller's Anesthesia, E-book pg. 922

Susceptibility order of nerve fibers are as follows:

- **Pressure:** $A\alpha > A\beta > A\gamma > A\delta > B > C$
- **Local anesthetic:** $A\gamma$ & $A\delta >> A\alpha$ & $A\beta >> B >> C$
- **Hypoxia:** B > A > C
- **Paresthesias** (inappropriate sensations such as burning or prickling) usually seen when A-delta is involved.

Book States

Small myelinated axons (A Gamma motor and A. delta sensory fibers) are most susceptible to impulse annihilation. Next in order of block are large myelinated fibers ($A\alpha$ and $A\beta$) and least susceptible are small non-myelinated C-fibers.

Book Further Adds

Nerve fiber with slowest conduction velocity (0.5–0.8 m/sec) are most resistant to local anesthetic.

23. Ans. (b) 1 hour

Ref: Morgan Clinical Anesthesia, 4th ed. pg. 341

- Bier's block can provide intense regional anesthesia for 45-60 minutes and short surgical procedures can be done on forearm, hand and leg.
- The procedure is usually done for *carpal tunnel release.*

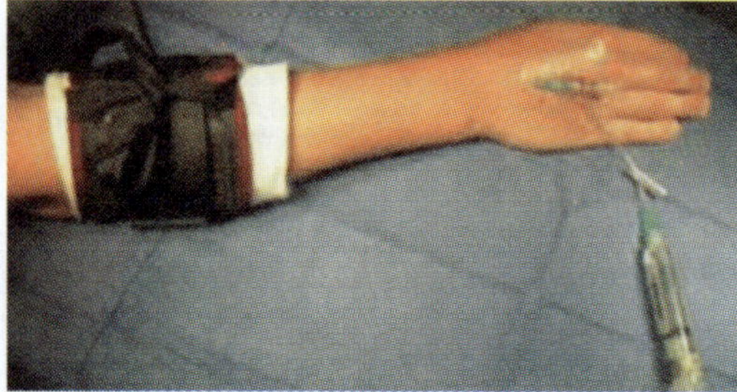

- An intravenous Catheter is inserted on the dorsum of the hand and *double pneumatic tourniquet* is placed on the arm.

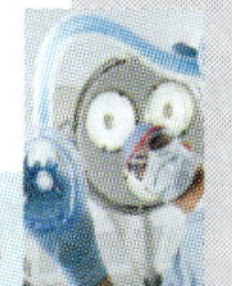

- The extremity is elevated and exsanguinated by wrapping an *esmarch elastic bandage* from a distal to proximal direction.

24. Ans. (b) Momentarily opening it to blow away foreign matter from the outlet

Ref: Objective Anesthesia Review: A Comprehensive Textbook for Examinees, pg. 358

Before connecting the cylinder to the anesthesia machine the protective cap should be removed and the valve should be opened slowly and briefly. While opening the valve the port should point away from the user or other personnel. This is known as cracking the valve. *It helps to clear dust and other foreign materials from the valve outlet before it is connected to the machine.* It reduces the possibility of fires and explosions when the valve is opened after connecting it to the machine. It also prevents the dust from being blown into the machine and clogging the filters.

25. Ans. (c) In breathing circuits to absorb CO_2

Ref: Ajay Yadav's Textbook of Anesthesia, pg. 29-30

- Soda lime is mixture of
  1. Calcium hydroxide 94%
  2. Sodium hydroxide 5%
  3. Potassium hydroxide 1%.
- They react with CO_2 to form calcium carbonate.
- Soda lime also contains small amounts of silica to make the granules less likely to disintegrate into powder and a chemical dye which changes color with change in pH.
- As more CO_2 is absorbed the pH decreases and the *color of the dye changes from pink to yellow/white* (Clayton yellow-pH indicator).

26. Ans. (d) To prevent regurgitation of gastric contents

- Cuffs prevent leakage between the endotracheal tube and the trachea-both leakage of gas outwards during IPPV and of gastric contents, blood and mucus into the lungs.

27. Ans. (b) Concentration of exhaled CO_2

- Capnography–Measures end tidal CO_2 in inspired and expired gases.
- End tidal CO_2 is a reliable estimate of $PaCO_2$ in most settings.

28. Ans. (a) Ventilation

Ref: Miller's Anesthesia, 7th ed. pg. 2139

- AMBU Bag stands for *Ambulatory Breathing Unit.*
- It is a self-refilling bag-valve-mask unit with 1-1.5L capacity, used for ventilating and oxygenating intubated patients, allowing both spontaneous and artificial respiration.

29. Ans. (a) Maintenance of the airway

Ref: Miller's Anesthesia, 7th ed. pg. 1683

It is placed blindly in oropharnyx and the cuff is inflated with large volume of air (**30 to 40 ml** for adult size). Inflated cuff seals the lateral and posterior pharyngeal walls and patient can be ventilated through ventilation ports.

Indications

1. As an alternative to intubation where difficult intubation is anticipated
2. Securing airway in emergency where intubation and mask ventilation is not possible.
3. As an elective method for minor surgeries where anesthetist wants to avoid intubation.
4. As a conduit for bronchoscopes, small size tubes, gum elastic bougies.

Advantages

- Easy to insert (even paramedical staff can insert].
- Does not require any laryngospasm and muscle relaxants.
- Does not require any specific position of cervical spine so can be used in cervical injuries.

Disadvantages

- It does not prevent aspiration so should not be used for full stomach patients.
- High incidence of laryngsospasm and bronchospasm.

Contraindications

- Full stomach patients.
- Hiatus hernia, pregnancy (where chances of aspiration are high)
- Oropharyngeal abscess or mass.
- Patients who are vulnerable to go in bronchospasm.

30. Ans. (a) Obstruction of tracheal tube

Ref: Handbook of Mechanical Ventilation, 2nd ed.

Setting-off of an alarm for peak inspiratory pressure during ventilation indicates an endotracheal tube kinking/ obstruction

Complications of Intubation

Perioperative

1. Esophageal intubation: This is a hazardous complication. If not detected in time, can cause severe hypoxia and even death.
2. Ischemia, edema and necrosis at local site (especially with red rubber tubes).
3. Aspiration (if cuff is not properly inflated).
4. Bronchial intubation and collapse of other lung.
5. **Tracheal tube obstruction by secretions, kinking.**
6. Accidental extubation

7. Trauma to gums, lip, epiglottis, pharynx, larynx and nasal cavity (in nasal intubation).
8. Reflex disturbances like laryngospasm, bronchospasm, breath holding.
9. Cardiac arrhythmias, hypertension or even cardiac arrest.

31. Ans. (a) Black body white shoulder

Ref: Miller's Anesthesia, 7th ed. pg. 675

Gas	Color Code		Pin index position
	Body	Shoulder	
Oxygen	*Black*	*White*	*2, 5*
Nitrous oxide	Blue	Blue	3, 5
CO_2	Grey	Grey	1, 6
Helium	Brown	Brown	2, 5
Air	Grey	White/black quartered	1, 5

32. Ans. (b) 2, 5

Ref: Miller's Anesthesia, 7th ed. pg. 675

- Pin index for oxygen is 2, 5.
- Cylinder of oxygen is black body with white shoulder.
- *Please refer to previous answer for explanation.*

33. Ans. (c) 3, 5

Ref: Miller's Anesthesia, 7th ed. pg. 675

Please refer to above table

34. Ans. (a) Prevent wrong attachment of cylinder

Ref: Miller's Anesthesia, 7th ed. pg. 675

- Each gas cylinder has two holes in its cylinder valve that mate with corresponding pins in the yoke of anesthesia machine.
- Each cylinder has a particular pin code and unless the correct cylinder valve is attached, the pins & holes will not coincide.
- Thus it is practically impossible to fit any cylinder to wrong yoke.
- To discourage incorrect cylinder attachment a pin index safety system has been adopted
- To prevent misconnection, gas cylinder valve blocks have holes drilled in 2 of 6 positions (a single hole in entonox)
- The pin index safety system is also ineffective if yoke pins are damaged or cylinder is filled with wrong gas or using extra sealing washers.

35. Ans. (a) Pneumothorax

Ref: Miller's Anesthesia, 7th ed. pg. 288

ETT is Endotracheal Tube Toilet

- It involves clearance of airway secretions, and is a normal process needed for the preservation of airway patency and the prevention of respiratory tract infection.
- Impaired clearance of airway secretions like in patients with depressed level of consciousness can result in atelectasis and pneumonia, and may contribute to respiratory failure.
- The primary indications for tracheal suctioning is to remove secretions in order to enhance oxygenation or to obtain samples of lower respiratory tract secretions for diagnostic tests. In the end, perform tracheal suctioning after endotracheal intubation to clear the airway of aspirated material or secretions or to enhance oxygenation in a tracheostomy patient with respiratory insufficiency.
- Perform bronchopulmonary toilet when secretions are visible in the endotracheal tube or at the orifice of the tracheostomy tube. Perform tracheal suctioning when the patient has coarse rales, rhonchi, or tubular breath sounds; acute or worsening dyspnea; or arterial oxygen desaturation.

36. Ans. (b) Overall health status of patient

Ref: Fundamentals of Anesthesia, 3rd ed. pg. 4

ASA Physical Status Scale

Class	Physical status
1	Healthy patient with no organic or psychological disease process.
2	Mild disease/mild systemic illness but no functional limitation
3	Systemic illness with functional limitation
4	A patient with severe systemic disease which is a constant threat to life (e.g. unstable angina)
5	A moribund patient unlikely to survive with or without surgery.
6	Brain dead patient (for organ transplant)

37. Ans. (b) Sodium channel

Ref: Miller's Anesthesia, 7th ed. pg. 353

- The local anesthesia (LA) acts by blocking sodium channel. With this blockage, there is decrease in entry of Na+ ions during action potential (AP). As the LA concentration is increased, the rate of rise of AP and maximum depolarization decreases, causing slowing of conduction.
- A time comes when local depolarization fails to reach the threshold potential and conduction block ensues.

- Exposure to higher concentration of calcium reduces the inactivation of Na^+ channels and lessens the degree of block.

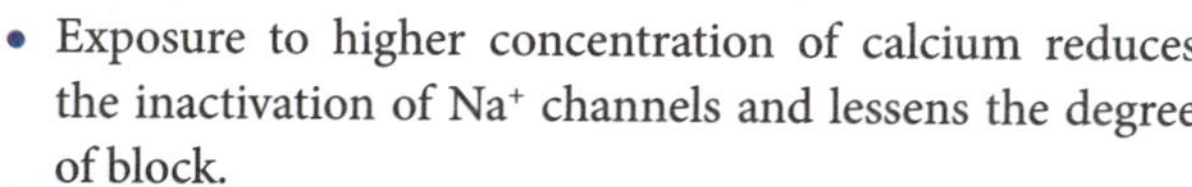

Extra Mile

- Lignocaine is most commonly used local Anesthetic.
- It is **drug of choice** for treatment of **ventricular arrhythmias** but due to digitalis toxicity but it is ineffective ***in atrial arrhythmias.***

38. Ans. (c) Na^+

Ref: KDT, 6th ed. pg. 353

39. Ans. (d) Ring block

Ref: Morgan, Clinical Anesthesiology, 4th ed. pg. 34

- Vasoconstrictor should not be added for ring block of hand, finger, toes, penis, pinna as all these organs are supplied by end arteries and ischemic damage may occur
- Adrenaline is most commonly used vasoconstrictor.
- Felypressin is preferred in cardiovascular disease patient.

40. Ans. (d) Dibucaine

Ref: KDT, 6th ed. pg. 352

- Dibucaine is amide group of local anesthetics.

TABLE: Ester and amides

Ester *(one 'I' in name)*	**Amides** *(2 'I' in name)*
• Cocaine • Benzocaine • Chlorprocaine • Tetracaine	• Lignocaine • Bupivacaine • Prilocaine • Dibucaine • Etidocaine

- All LA causes vasodilation and hypotension, except Cocaine. It causes vasoconstriction and significant rise in BP.

41. Ans. (a) Chlorprocaine

Please refer to previous question for explanation.

42. Ans. (d) Procaine

Ref: KDT, 6th ed. pg. 352

Please refer to above explanation

43. Ans. (a) Prilocaine

Ref: KDT, 6th ed. pg. 352

44. Ans. (b) Slow induction

Ref: KDT, 6th ed. pg. 371

- Blood gas coefficient of ether is 12 which means ether has **slow induction & slow recovery**.
- Irritant vapour, which can readily induce laryngeal spasm and make induction even slower and stimulates salivary and bronchial secretions, *So atropine as pre medication is required.*
- Ether is highly inflammable and causes explosion with cautery. It should not be used when diathermy is needed in the airways because of risk of fire or explosion. *Muscle relaxants need not be used as ether itself produces excellent relaxation.*
- Ether liberates catecholamines and tends to maintain blood pressure. *Cardiac arrhythmia occur rarely* with ether and there is no sensitization of myocardium to circulating catecholamines.
- Adrenaline is relatively safe with ether. Bronchial smooth muscle is relaxed.

45. Ans. (b) Bupivacaine

Ref: KDT, 6th ed. pg. 357

- Bupivacaine is a local anesthetic agent from Amide group.
- It is most cardiotoxic LA.
- Shortest acting LA: Chlorprocaine
- Longest acting LA: Dibucaine
- Most commonly used LA: Lignocaine
- Local anesthetic which causes methemoglobinemia: Prilocaine

MUSCLE RELAXANTS AND ANALGESICS

46. Ans. (c) Remifentanil

Ref: Smith and Aitken's Textbook of Anesthesia; E-book, pg. 460

- Remifentanil is shortest acting opioid due to its metabolism by plasma esterase. Dose reduction is not necessary in hepatic or renal disease.
- **Most potent opioid:** Sulfentanil.
- Alfentanyl is opioid of choice for day care surgery.
- **Opioid causing neuroleptic analgesia:** Fentanyl + Droperidol
- **Opioid causing neuroleptic anesthesia:** Fentanyl + Droperidol + N_2O.

47. Ans. (d) Intradermal

Ref: Pain Assessment and Pharmacological Management; E-book, pg. 369

- Fentanyl can be given by intravenous, intrathecal, epidural and transdermal patch.
- Side effects of fentanyl are muscle rigidity, respiratory depression and bradycardia.

48. Ans. (a) Atracurium

Ref: Essentials of Clinical Anesthesia, pg. 139

- *Hoffman degradation is simply spontaneous breakdown of the molecule at physiologic pH and temperature.* This process occurs despite renal or hepatic failure, and therefore the duration of action of atracurium and cisatracurium is essentially unchanged inpatient with renal or hepatic impairment.
- Therefore, Atracurium and Cisatracurium can be given in renal failure and hepatic failure.

49. Ans. (a) Atracurium

Ref: Broody's Human Pharmacology, pg. 144

- Since in this case, there is both renal and hepatic impairment, the anesthetic agents have to be given very carefully. Agent of choice in such cases is atracurium, because of its unique degradation that is unaffected by renal or hepatic dysfunction.

50. Ans. (b) Ryanodine receptor

Ref: Miller's Anesthesia, 2015 ed. pg. 1314

- Malignant hyperthermia is a condition that is usually triggered by exposure to certain drugs used for general anesthesia, specifically the volatile anesthetic agents and the neuromuscular blocking agent succinylcholine.
- **Succinylcholine** is depolarizing/noncompetitive M.R. with shortest duration of action (3-5 minutes) due to rapid hydrolysis by pseudo cholinesterase.
- It causes dual/biphasic block. It causes hyperkalemia, increased intraocular & intragastric pressure and temperature which leads to ***malignant Hyperthermia.***
- Susceptibility to MH is often inherited as an *autosomal dominant disorder*, for which there are at least 6 genetic loci of interest, most prominently the **Ryanodine receptor gene (*RYR1*).**
- **DOC for malignant hyperthermia:** Dantrolene
- Propofol is the intravenous Anesthetic of choice in the patients with **malignant hyperthermia.**

Extra Mile

- Glutamate-activated ion channels have been classified, based on selective agonists, into three categories: AMPA receptors, Kainate receptors, and NMDA receptors. AMPA and Kainate receptors are relatively nonselective monovalent cation channels involved in fast excitatory synaptic transmission, whereas NMDA channels conduct not only Na+ and K+ but also Ca++ and are involved in long-term modulation of synaptic responses (long-term potentiation).

51. Ans. (b) Rocuronium

- Fastest acting NDMR- **Rocuronium**
- Longest acting NDMR- **DOXACURIUM > PANCURONIUM**
- Shortest acting NDMR *(Non-depolarizing muscle relaxant)*-GANTACURIUM > MIVACURIUM
- Shortest acting depolarizing muscle relaxant: Sch

52. Ans. (a) Chest wall rigidity

Ref: Miller's Anesthesia, 7th ed. pg. 806

- **Alfentanil** is a short-acting synthetic opioid analgesic drug, used for anesthesia in surgery. It is an analogue of fentanyl, with lower potency.
- **Adverse side effect of alfentanil:** Chest wall rigidity, followed by others like respiratory depression, arrhythmia, Bradycardia, hypertension, blurred vision etc.

Extra Mile

- *Remifentanyl, Alfentanyl & Sufentanil* have short duration of action so can be used as outpatient anesthetic agents
- *Best anesthetic agent for OPD patients: Alfentanyl*

53. Ans. (a) Mu (μ)

Ref: Miller's Anesthesia, 7th ed. pg. 914

Opioid receptors are – mu (μ), Kappa (k), delta (δ)

Receptor	Location	Function
Mu(μ) receptors	Brain, cortex (laminae 3 and 4)	Respiratory depression, Miosis, Euphoria, Muscular rigidity, sadation, Physical dependence
Kappa (κ) receptors	Brain	Analgesia, diuresis, dysphoria, miosis
Delta (δ) receptors	Brain	Analgesia, antidepressant effect,
Nociception/ Orphan receptor	Brain, cortex, spinal cord, amygdala, hypothalamus	Anxiety, Depression

54. Ans. (c) Succinylcholine

Ref: Miller's Anesthesia, 7th ed. pg. 866

- Malignant hyperthermia is a condition that is usually triggered by exposure to certain drugs used for general anesthesia, specifically the volatile anesthetic agents and the neuromuscular blocking agent succinylcholine.
- **Succinylcholine** is depolarizing/noncompetitive M.R. with shortest duration of action (3-5 minutes) due to rapid hydrolysis by pseudo cholinesterase.

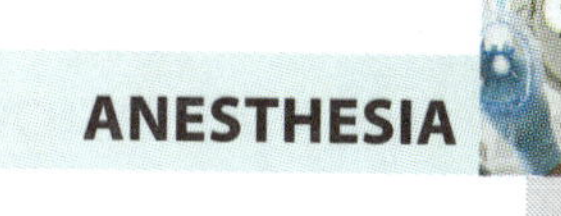

- It causes dual/biphasic block. It causes hyperkalemia, increased intraocular & intragastric pressure and temperature which leads to ***malignant Hyperthermia.***
- Susceptibility to MH is often inherited as an autosomal dominant disorder, for which there are at least 6 genetic loci of interest, most prominently the **Ryanodine receptor gene (*RYR1*).**
- **DOC for malignant hyperthermia:** Dantrolene

55. Ans. (a) Ryanodine receptor

Please refer to above explanation

56. Ans. (b) Neostigmine antagonizes its action

Ref: KDT, 6th ed. pg. 344

Reversal of Muscle Relaxation

- Depolarizing (Noncompetitive) muscle relaxants are not antagonized.
- Nondepolarizing (competitive) muscle relaxants are antagonized by Acetyl choline or Anticholinesterase: Neostigmine, Pyridostigmine, Edrophonium
- In order to prevent muscarinic effects atropine is given in combination.

57. Ans. (b) Mivacurium

Ref: KDT, 6th ed. pg. 343

- Shortest acting non-depolarizing muscle relaxant: Gantacurium > (5–10 min) Mivacurium (15–20 min).
- Shortest acting depolarizing muscle relaxant: Sch (6–11 minutes)
- Overall shortest acting muscle relaxant: Gantacurium (5–10 minutes)
- Shortest acting local Anesthetic: chlorprocaine
- Sch duration of action 6–11 minutes

Classification of Muscle Relaxants

Neuro Muscular Blocking agent	
Depolarizing (Non-competitive) muscle relaxant	**Non-depolarizing (Competitive) muscle relaxant**
1. Suxamethonium 2. Succinyl choline 3. Scoline Decamethonium	• Gantacurium • Gallamine, • D-tubocurarine, Atracurium, • Mevacurium • Vecuronium • Pancuronium • Rocuronium • Doxacurium

58. Ans. (c) Succinylcholine

Ref: KDT, 6th ed. pg. 342

- Malignant hyperthemia is a genetic condition seen due to mutation in ryanodine receptor
- Overall MC drug causing it is – SCH
- MC local anesthetic causing – LIDOCAINE
- MC inhalational agent causing malignant hyperthermia – HALOTHANE
- DOC – DANTROLENE

59. Ans. (c) Doxacuronium

Ref: KDT, 6th ed. pg. 343

- Doxacuronium is the longest acting neuromuscular blocking agent. Duration of action of doxacuronium is 120 minutes.
- Atracuronium duration of action- 45 minutes
- Vecuronium duration of action- 25–40 minutes
- Pancuronium duration of action 85–100 minutes

Extra Mile

- Most potent skeletal muscle relaxant: **Doxacuronium**
- Least potent skeletal muscle relaxant: **Succinylcholine**
- Least potent non-depolarizing muscle relaxant: **Rocuronium**
- Most commonly used muscle relaxant for routine surgery: **Vecuronium**

GENERAL ANESTHETIC, IV/INHALATION AGENTS

60. Ans. (a) Desflurane

Ref: Morgan and Mikhail's Clinical Anesthesiology, 5th ed. pg. 12-13

- Desflurane uses a specialized vaporizer Tec 6. The Tec 6 vaporizer is an electrically heated, thermostatically controlled, constant temperature, pressurized, electromechanically coupled dual circuit, gas/vapor blender.
- The pressure in the vapor circuit is electronically regulated to equal the pressure in the fresh gas circuit.

61. Ans. (c) Negative pressure pulmonary edema

Ref: Miller's Anesthesia 9th ed. pg. 286

- Negative-pressure pulmonary edema (NPPE) or post-obstructive pulmonary edema is a well-described cause of acute respiratory failure that occurs after intense inspiratory effort against an obstructed airway, usually from upper airway infection, tumor, or laryngospasm.

62. Ans. (b) Isoflurane

Ref: https://clinicaltrials.gov/ct2/show/NCT01477151

- With Isoflurane cardiac output is maintained and it produces controlled hypotension. Therefore, it is inhalational anesthetic agent preferred in cardiac surgery.

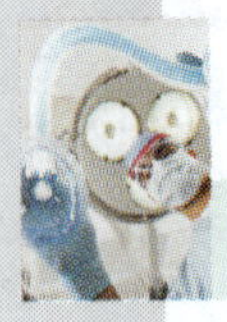

- Current evidence supports the superiority of sevoflurane for myocardial protection during cardiac surgery when compared to total intravenous anesthesia with propofol.

Extra Mile

- Isoflurane causes least increase in ICP, hence preferred in neurosurgery
- It is also safe in pheochromocytoma patients.

63. Ans. (a) Propofol, Sodium thiopentone, Etomidate

- Among the given choices only option A contains all the IV hypnotic drugs, namely Propofol, Thiopentone and Etomidate
- **Option B:** Halothane is inhalational anaesthetic agent
- **Option C:** Sugammadex is an antidote of NDMR overdose (like Rocuronium)
- **Option D:** These agents are Non depolarizing muscle relaxant.

64. Ans. (a) Propofol

Propofol:

- It is most commonly used IV anesthetic agent for day care surgery
- It has less residual impairment
- Onset of action: 45 seconds
- Duration of action: ~ 15 minutes
- Non irritant to airways and has antiemetic property

Extra Mile

- Anesthetic agent of choice for day care surgery: **Propofol**
- IV anesthetic agent of choice in patients with malignant hyperthermia: **Propofol**
- Agent of choice for induction in children: **Sevoflurane**
- Anesthetic agent preferred in neurosurgery: **Isoflurane**
- Anesthetic agent safest in unskilled hand and is highly inflammable: **Ether**
- Preferred anesthetic agent in bronchial asthma: **Halothane**
- Agent with high MAC, and has second gas effect: **Nitrous oxide**
- Agent preferred in aneurysm surgery and cardiac disease: **Etomidate**

65. Ans. (b) Thiopentone

- Barbiturates increases heme synthesis by inducing mitochondrial enzyme ALA synthetase, which can precipitate acute intermittent porphyria. Therefore, barbiturates are contraindicated in patients with AIP.
- Example of drugs that can precipitate AIP: Phenytoin, Rifampicin, OCP, Barbiturates, Sulfonamides.

Extra Mile

CONTRAINDICATION OF BARBITURATES

- Impaired hepatic and renal function
- Emphysema and pulmonary insufficiency
- Acute intermittent porphyria
- CHF and Hypovolemic shock
- Idiosyncratic patients

66. Ans. (c) L 3–L4

Ref: Basic Clinical Anesthesia by Paul K pg. 217

- Spinal anesthesia is required mainly in lower abdominal surgery such as inguinal herniorrhaphy, appendectomy, abdominal hysterectomy or caesarean delivery.
- It is preferably given at L3–L4
- Above L3 there is a risk of traumatic damage to spinal cord

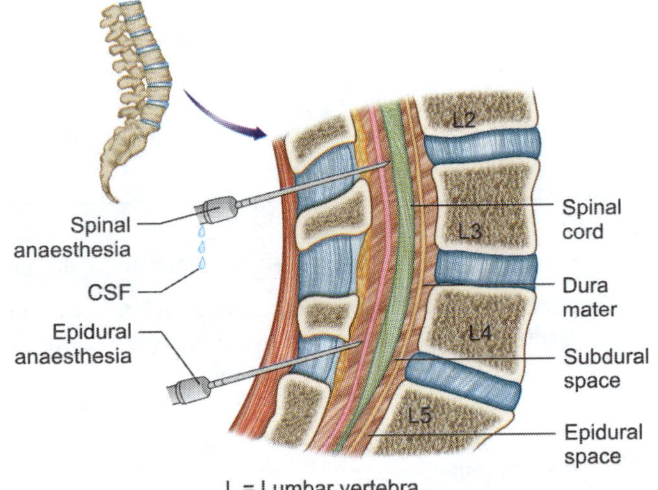

67. Ans. (a) Dose

Ref: https://www.ncbi.nlm.nih.gov/pmc/articles/PMC4823409

- The duration of spinal anesthesia is based directly on dose or concentration of anesthetic agent.
- One study also states that final level of block can be predicted by patient height and weight.
- The data shows that the time to attain a suitable sensory level for surgery and duration of action correlates incrementally with height and inversely related to weight.

68. Ans. (b) Halothane

Ref: Katzung 14th ed. pg. 449

- Halothane is known anesthetic agent to produce hepatotoxicity (Halothane hepatitis).
- **Incidence:** 1 in 20,000 to 35,000. Seen on repeated exposure with halothane and NOT with other

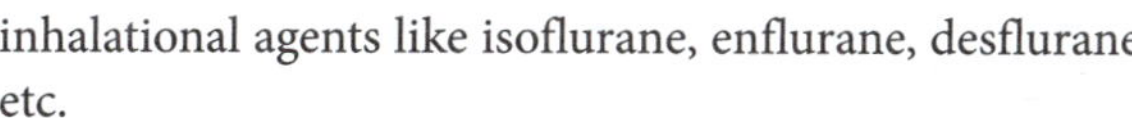

inhalational agents like isoflurane, enflurane, desflurane etc.

- **Proposed MOA for hepatotoxicity:** Formation of reactive metabolites that either cause direct hepatocellular damage (e.g., free radicals) or initiate immune mediated responses.

Extra Mile

- Inhalational agents like halothane, enflurane, desflurane, sevoflurane are known to depress cardiac contractility → decrease MAP (mean arterial pressure)
- They also known to increase myocardial sensitivity to epinephrine

69. Ans. (c) Propofol

Ref: Katzung 14th ed. pg. 450

- Propofol is a preferred alternative to inhaled anesthetics. Given by continuous infusion
- It is preferred anesthetic agent in day care surgery
- **Preferred day care anesthetic agents:** Propofol, Alfentanil, Isoflurane and congener, Mivacurium *(Mn: PAIM)*
- IV anesthetic agent of choice in malignant hyperthermia: **Propofol**
- Agent of choice in induction in children: **Sevoflurane**
- Agent of choice in CHF and shock patients: **Ketamine**
- Agent of choice in aneurysm surgery and cardiac disease: **Etomidate**

70. Ans. (a) Halothane

Ref: Goodman & Gillman 13th ed. pg. 395

- Halothane is one of the light sensitive anesthetic agent, marketed in amber color bottles
- **Side effect:** Fulminant hepatic necrosis (halothane hepatitis).
- **Incidence:** ~1 in 10,000 patients receiving halothane
- **Fatality:** 50%
- Halothane hepatitis is a syndrome which is characterized by fever, anorexia, nausea, vomiting and can be accompanied by a rash and peripheral eosinophilia.
- Halothane hepatitis may be the result of an immune response to hepatic proteins that become trifluoroacetylated as a consequence of halothane metabolism.

Extra Mile

Important side effects

- **Lidocaine:** Methemoglobinemia, cauda equine syndrome
- **Prilocaine:** Methemoglobinemia
- **Etomidate:** Adrenal suppression
- **Bupivacaine:** Most cardiotoxic LA, ventricular arrhythmia
- **Ketamine:** Dissociative anesthesia, hypertension and tachycardia
- **Nitrous oxide:** Bone marrow depression, diffusion hypoxia

71. Ans. (a) Carbon dioxide

Ref: Morgan Clinical Anesthesia, pg. 582:

Laparoscopic surgery involves insufflation of carbon dioxide into the peritoneal cavity producing a pneumoperitoneum. This causes an increase in intra-abdominal pressure (IAP).

- Carbon dioxide is insufflated into the peritoneal cavity at a rate of 4–6 L/min^{-1} to a pressure of 10–20 mm Hg. The pneumoperitoneum is maintained by a constant gas flow of 200–400 mL/min^{-1}.

72. Ans. (b) Glycopyrrolate

Ref: Ajay Yadav's Anesthesia, 4th ed. pg. 48

- **To control secretions, anti-cholinergics are used:** Glycopyrrolate, Atropine and Scopolamine.
- Glycopyrrolate is preferred over atropine and scopolamine because it doesn't cross blood brain barrier. *Therefore it is devoid of central side effects.*

Drugs Used for Premedication:

- **Sedative/Anti-anxiety:**
  - Lorazepam MC used
  - Midazolam in day care surgery
- **Anti-emetics:** Hyoscine *(Most potent),* Ondensatron, Metoclopramide
- **To decrease pain:** Morphine and Pethidine

73. Ans. (c) Sevoflurane

Ref: KDT, 6th ed. pg. 373-374

SEVOFLURANE

- Induction and emergence of anesthesia is rapid with sevoflurane.
- Absence of pungent smell makes it pleasant and administrable through face mask and is ***considered as anesthesia of choice in pediatric patient.***
- Side effect: Respiratory depression and Arrhythmia.

DESFLURANE

- Desflurane is one of the inhalation (volatile liquid) anesthetic agents.
- It is fastest acting but less soluble than isoflurane.
- It has the most pungent odor, which make it unsuitable for induction.
- It irritates air passage, which may induce coughing, laryngeal spasm.

PROPOFOL

- Anesthesia of choice for **day care surgery.**
- Short acting, action diminishes the same day.
- **Advantage:** Has anti emetic property. It is safe in porphyria.

- **Disadvantages:** Causes myocardial depression and hypotension.

KETAMINE

- Has maximum analgesic property.
- Produces **dissociative anesthesia.**
- Induction agent of choice in asthma patient.

74. Ans. (d) Propofol

Ref: KDT, 6th ed. pg. 373-374

PROPOFOL

- Anesthesia of choice for **day care surgery.**
- Short acting, action diminishes the same day.
- **Advantage:** Has anti emetic property. *It is safe in porphyria.*
- **Disadvantages:** Causes myocardial depression and hypotension.

75. Ans. (d) It has strong tendency to cause vomiting

Ref: KDT, 6th ed. pg. 375

Salient Features of Propofol

- It is a **milky white powder** that is **preservative free.** Therefore, it must be used within 6 hours.
- It is an **oil based preparation**, therefore injection is *painful.*
- Onset of action: 15 seconds
- Duration of action: 5-10 min. (due to redistribution)
- Due to rapid action, post anesthetic nausea and vomiting is uncommon with propofol
- It possesses very **strong antiemetic and antipruritic action.**
- It *decreases blood pressure* and impairs baroreceptor reflexes.
- It produces more severe and prolonged *respiratory depression* than thiopentone.
- It has no *muscle relaxant property.*
- It has cerebroprotective activity but does not possess anticonvulsant activity. Rather, **myoclonic jerking and muscle twitching** can be seen with the use of propofol.
- It is the intravenous Anesthetic of choice for **day care surgery.**
- It is also the intravenous Anesthetic of *choice for sedation in ICU.*
- Propofol is the intravenous Anesthetic of choice in the patients with **malignant hyperthermia.**
- Along with opioids (alfentanil or fentanyl) *propofol is the agent of choice for total intravenous anesthesia (TIVA).*
- Propofol infusion syndrome (on long term use as a continuous infusion >48 hours) leads to acute cardiac failure, hepatomegaly, lipemia, rhabdomyolysis.

76. Ans. (a) Propofol

Please refer to above explanation

77. Ans. (d) Sevoflurane

Ref: KDT, 6th ed. pg. 373-74

- Non pungency & rapid increase in alveolar anesthetic concentration, makes sevoflurane an excellent choice for smooth & rapid inhalational induction in pediatrics & adult population.
- *Induction and recovery are very fast in desflurane.* Due to its short action it is commonly used as *anesthesia for OPD.*
- Blood gas partition coefficient of sevoflurane is lesser than halothane and isoflurane *(halothane-2.3, isoflurane-1.4, sevoflurane-0.69, desflurane 0.42)*, which makes it *fastest acting inhalational agent among the choices.*

78. Ans. (a) Atracurium

Ref: KDT, 6th ed. pg. 345

- Atracurium and Cisatracurium undergoes spontaneous degradation by Hoffmann elimination. *So its pharmacokinetics are independent of renal and hepatic functions.* Therefore, it can be given in renal failure.
- Muscle relaxant of choice in renal failure: **Atracurium**
- Muscle relaxant of choice in renal and, or hepatic failure: **Cis-atracurium**
- Muscle relaxant in which Hoffman elimination is seen: **Atracurium, Cis-atracurium**

79. Ans. (a) Nitrous oxide

Ref: KDT, 6th ed. pg. 370-71

- Malignant hyperthermia (MH) is a life-threatening clinical syndrome of hypermetabolism involving the skeletal muscle.
- It is triggered in susceptible individuals primarily by the volatile inhalational anesthetic agents and the muscle relaxant succinylcholine.
- The most common triggering agents are volatile anesthetic agents such as: Halothane, Sevoflurane, Desflurane, Isoflurane, Enflurane or the depolarizing muscle relaxants suxamethonium and dexamethonium.
- *Anesthetic agents which are considered safe* include local anesthetics:
  - Lidocaine, bupivicaine, mepivacaine, opiates (morphine, fentanyl), ketamine, barbiturates, *nitrous oxide*, propofol, etomidate and benzodiazepines.
- Non-depolarizing muscle relaxants which are safe:
  - Pancuronium, cisatracurium, atracurium, mivacurium, vecuronium and rocuronium also do not cause malignant hyperthermia.

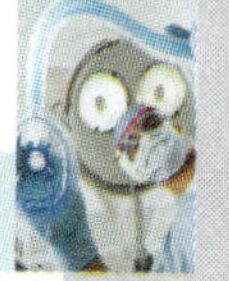

80. Ans. (c) Ketamine

Ref: Katzung, 9th ed. pg. 1604; KDT, 6th ed. pg. 376

- Ketamine is the only intravenous anesthetic that possesses analgesic properties and produces cardiovascular stimulation.
- It causes ***"dissociative anesthesia"*** which is characterized by profound analgesia, immobility, amnesia and feeling of dissociation from one's own body and the surrounding.
- **In addition it also causes:**
  - Hallucination
  - Delusion and illusion.
  - Profound analgesia
- **Ketamine increases all pressures like:**
  - BP (hypertension)
  - Intracranial tension (ICT)
  - Intraocular pressure (IOP)
- It is **contraindicated** in intracerebral mass/hemorrhage.

Extra Mile

About Ketamine: (Remembered as:)

K	Kids: Can be given to kids
E	Emergence reaction: s/e occurring during recovery
T	Thalamo-cortical junction affected: Dissociative Anesthesia
A	Analgesia strongest
M	**Meal:** Can be given with full stomach
I	**Increase: BP/IOP/ICT**
N	NMDA receptor blocker
E	Excellent bronchodilator: inducing agent of choice in asthma patient.

Extra Mile

- **PROPOFOL** causes myocardial depression and fall in BP.

81. Ans. (b) It causes severe fall in blood pressure

Ref: KDT, 6th ed. pg. 376

Ketamine causes increase in blood pressure.

Please refer to above explanation

82. Ans. (d) Ketamine

Ref: KDT, 6th ed. pg. 376

- *Please refer to above explanation.*
- Ketamine causes increase in all pressure i.e. intracranial, intraocular, intragastric and intravascular pressure.
- Therefore, it is not used in raised ICT/IOT & hypertension as it may increase the pressure to morbid levels.
- Anesthetic agents of choice in head injury/increased ICP are:
  - Thiopentone *(cerebro protective)*
  - Propofol
  - Etomidate *(protection against circulatory depression)*
  - Isoflurane

83. Ans. (b) Increased ICT

Ref: Katzung, 9th ed. 1604; KDT, 6th ed. pg. 376

84. Ans. (c) Thiopentone

Ref: KDT, 6th ed. pg. 374

- Thiopentone is an ultrashort acting thiobarbiturate because of rapid redistribution.
- It has poor analgesic property.
- I/v injection is very painful. Therefore it is contraindicated unless opioids or N_2O has been given.
- Contraindicated in porphyria patients

Extra Mile

- Etomidate is contraindicated in adrenal insufficiency.
- *Anesthetic drug safe in patients with porphyria: Propofol*

85. Ans. (b) Acute intermittent phorphyria

Extra Mile

- Thiopentone is C/I in acute intermittent porphyria.
- Etomidate is C/I in adrenal insufficiency.
- LA which causes methemoglobinemia: Prilocaine
- Malignant hyperthermia is caused by: Succinylcholine
- DOC for malignant hyperthermia: Dantrolene

86. Ans. (c) Both

Ref: Principles of Anesthesia, 4th ed. pg. 73

Chloroform is both hepatotoxic and cardiotoxic.

87. Ans. (d) Hypotension, bradycardia

Ref: KDT, 6th ed. pg. 360

Systemic Effects (Physiological Alterations) of Central Neuraxial Blocks

CARDIOVASCULAR SYSTEM

The most prominent effect is hypotension which is because of the following factors:

- Venodilatation which is because of sympathetic block which maintains the venous tone.
- Dilatation of post arteriolar capillaries which is again because of loss of sympathetic tone.
- **Decreased cardiac output which is because of:**
  - **Decreased venous return:** Due to blood pooling in veins of lower limb and lower abdomen.
  - **Bradycardia:** Bradycardia can occur as a result of:

- Decreased atrial pressure because of decrease venous return (Bainbridge reflex) and
- Direct inhibition of cardioaccelerator fibers (T1 to T4).

- Paralysis of nerve supply to adrenal glands with consequently decreased catecholamine release.
- Direct absorption of drug into systemic circulation.
- Compression of inferior vena cava and aorta by pregnant uterus, abdominal tumors (supine hypotension syndrome).

NERVOUS SYSTEM

- Autonomic fibers (mediated by C fibers) are most sensitive and they are blocked earliest followed by sensory and then motor fibers. So, sequence of block is Autonomic - Sensory - Motor. The recovery occurs in reverse order although number of studies have suggested return of autonomic activity before sensory.

PRE-OP ANESTHETIC PREPARATION

88. Ans. (b) Ask them to apply the paddles while you continue CPR

Ref: https://www.acls-pals-bls.com/algorithms/acls/

- CPR should be started before the rhythm is identified and should be continued while the defibrillator is being applied and charged.
- Apply the AED electrode pads to the bare chest of the victim and follow the prompts as instructed. Uninterrupted CPR is an important factor in increasing the recovery rate of cardiac arrest patients.

89. Ans. (a) NPO 8-12 hours before OT

Ref: https://www.ncbi.nlm.nih.gov/pmc/articles/PMC8661208/

- Preoperative fasting is mandatory before anesthesia to reduce the risk of aspiration.
- Therefore, patients are generally not allowed to eat for 8–12 hours or to drink for 4–6 hours prior to surgery.

90. Ans. (a) Ketamine

Ref: Katzung 14th ed. pg. 456

- Ketamine is one of the general anesthetics, act by NMDA receptor blockade.
- It produces a state known as "dissociative anesthesia" where the patients eye remains open with a slow nystagmus gaze (cataleptic state).
- **CNS effects:**
  - It causes cerebral vasodilation → increases ICP
  - Unpleasant reactions like vivid colorful dreams, hallucination, tactile and auditory hallucination.
- **CVS effects:**
  - Causes sympathetic stimulation which Increases HR, BP, cardiac output.

91. Ans. (c) Laparoscopic hysterectomy

- Laparoscopic procedure is contraindicated in cardiac patients due to CO_2 used in laparoscopic procedures.
- Other contraindications of laparoscopy:
  - Morbid obese patients
  - Severe cardiac disease
  - Multiple previous abdominal procedures
  - In pregnancy with uterine sixe >12 weeks
  - Hb level less than 7 g/dL
  - Hypovolemic shock
  - Generalized peritonitis

92. Ans. (b) Mallampati scoring

Ref: Airway management, An Issue in Anaesthesiology clinic, pg. 284

- Mallampati scoring is used to predict the ease of endotracheal intubation

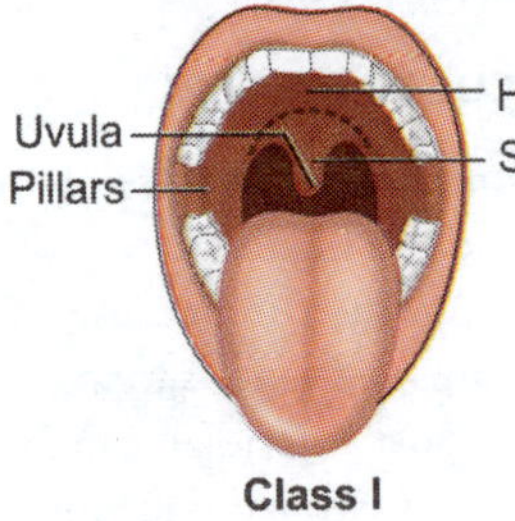

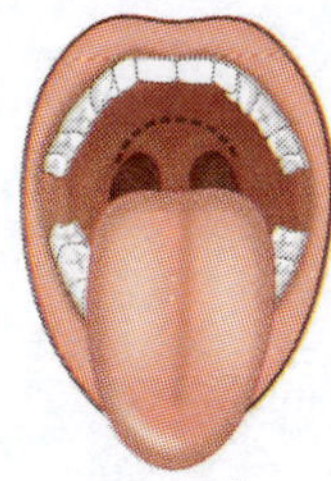

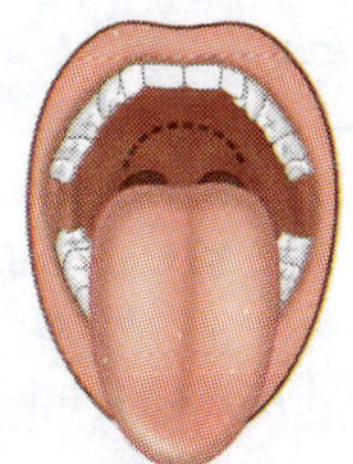

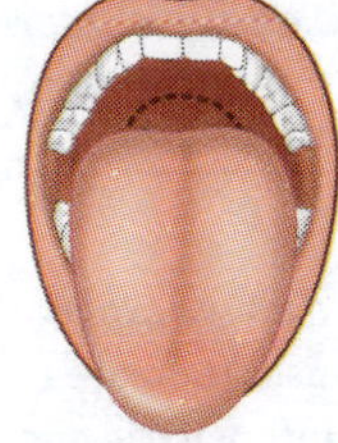

- Class I : Uvula, fauces, soft palate, pillars visible
- Class II : Uvula, soft palate, fauces visible
- Class III : Base of uvula visible, soft palate
- Class IV : Only hard palate visible

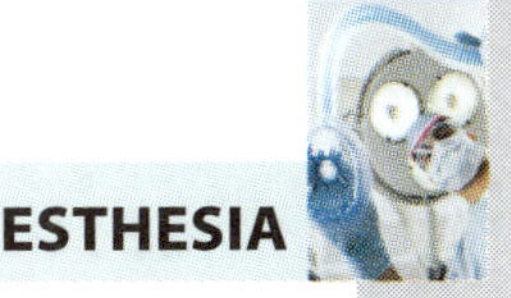

ASA SCORING

- **American Society of Anesthesiologist** classification system developed to categorize patient's physiological status that helps in predicting the operative risk.

ASA classification	Description	Example	Perioperative mortality risk
1	A normal healthy patient		0.1%
2	Patient with mild systemic disease	Controlled epileptic patient	0.2%
3	Patient with severe systemic disease	Poorly controlled diabetes mellitus	1.8%
4	Patient with severe systemic disease that is constant threat to life	Dyspneic patient	7.8%
5	A moribund patient who is not expected to survive without operation	Hypovolemic shock	9.4%
6	Declared brain dead, whose organs are being removed for donation		

Extra Mile

- **Aldrete/Modified aldrete scoring system:** For determination of discharge of patient from anesthesia care unit
- **Wilson scoring system:** For ease of laryngoscopy *(score < 5 = easy laryngoscopy; Score > 7 = Severe difficulty in laryngoscopy)*
- **P-POSSUM scoring system:** For predicting the mortality of neurosurgical patients

93. Ans. (c) Both

Thiopentone is preferred as an induction agent because of:

- Ease and rapidity of induction
- Absence of stage of delirium
- Rapid recovery
- Ability to increase depth rapidly

94. Ans. (b) Increased mucosal clearance

Ref: Handbook of Clinical Anesthesiology 3rd ed. by Brian Pollard 120

- *From an anesthesiologist's perspective, smoking increases the relative risk of postoperative pulmonary complications by up to six times.*
- A common concern is the increased risk of laryngospasm and bronchospasm.
- *Smoking increases airway mucous production and impairs ciliary function resulting in poor sputum clearance. This in combination with smoke-induced impairment of immune function, increases the likelihood of developing postoperative pneumonia.*
- **The pre-operative effect of smoking on respiratory system are:**
  - Hyper-reactive airways especially small airways
  - Reduced muco-ciliary clearance
  - Increased mucus secretion
  - Altered surfactant and permeability
  - V/Q mismatch

INTRA-OP AND POST-OP PATIENT CARE

95. Ans (a) A

Ref: Morgan and Mikhali's Clinical Anesthesia 5th ed. pg. 10-12 https://www.ncbi.nlm.nih.gov/pmc/articles/PMC3821267/

- The oxygen cylinder color code in India is a black body and white shoulder-coloured cylinder. Therefore, oxygen cylinder marked at A will be given to this patient
- Note: *Detailed data about color coding of cylinder and pin index is given later in this book*

96. Ans. (b) Decrease the FiO_2

Ref: Morgan and Mikhali's Clinical Anesthesia 5th ed. pg. 1297

- The highest priority at the start of oxygen therapy is providing effective oxygenation.
- In this case, the patient is hypoventilating which is causing CO_2 retention.
- To overcome this, we have to decrease the FiO_2 in order to maintain adequate ventilation and to wash off excess CO_2.

97. Ans. (d) Dura

Ref: Grey's Anatomy 41st ed. pg. 762

- For Epidural anesthesia the needle must pass through five distinct tissue layers: Skin, subcutaneous fat,

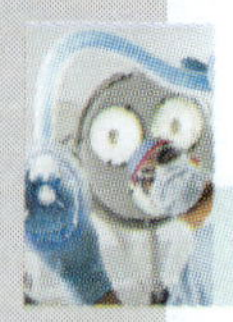

supraspinous ligament, interspinous ligament, and ligamentum flavum.
- It does not encounter the dura layer.

98. Ans. (a) CO_2 exhalation

- Endotracheal tube in esophagus is best assessed by capnography (measurement of CO_2 exhalation).
- Endotracheal intubation is the most preferred method of airway control. Following are the different ways of confirmation of proper and right placement of tube:
  - Symmetrical chest wall movement
  - Bilateral breath sounds and absence of epigastric auscultation during ventilation
  - By direct visualization
  - Humidity fogging the endotracheal tube
  - End tidal CO_2 is maintained after 5 breaths
  - Maintaining of oxygenation by pulse oximetry

99. Ans. (b) Capnography

Ref: www.capnography.com

CAPNOGRAPHY

- Best/confirmatory sign of endotracheal intubation
- Measures end tidal CO_2 in inspired and expired gases
- It is the most reliable tool to confirm placement of an advanced airway, both for endotracheal (ET) tubes and supraglottic-airway devices.
- When a device is placed correctly, a waveform and end-tidal CO_2 ($ETCO_2$) reading appear within seconds after the first ventilation is delivered to the patient.
- **Characteristics of normal capnogram:**
  - Rapid increase from B to C
  - Horizontal (rising) plateau from C to D
  - Rapid decrease from D to E

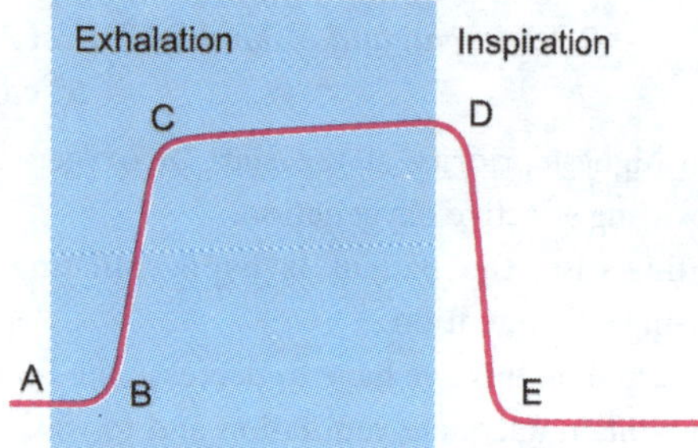

- **Phases of capnograph:**
  - **Phase I:** Inspiratory baseline (beginning of expiration)
  - **Phase II:** Expiratory upstroke (mixing of alveolar gas with dead space)
  - **Phase III:** Alveolar plateau
  - **Phase IV:** Inspiratory down stroke

TYPES OF CAPNOGRAM

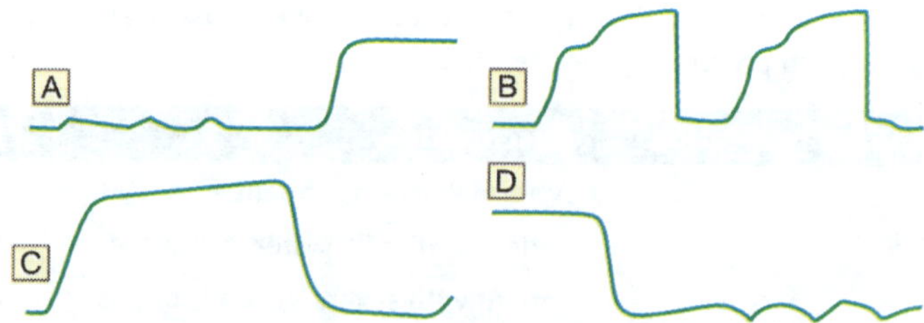

A Near flat-line of apnea to normal rounded rectangle
B Irregular top indicating problem with airway placement
C Near-normal shape indicates successful airway placement
D Sudden drop indicating displacement of airway or cardiac arrest

Extra Mile

Some typical capnograph appearances
- **Shark fin appearance:** Bronchospasm/COPD
- **Biphasic/Dual waveform aka curare cleft:** Endobronchial intubation
- **Tooth like hump at the end of expiratory phase aka cardiogenic oscillation:** Heart beating against lungs
- **Steeple sign capnogram:** Due to loose connection between sampling tube and monitor
- **Tail/Pig tail capnogram:** Slit in sampling tube

100. Ans. (c) Cricoids pressure

Ref: Miller's Anesthesia, 7th ed. pg. 2430

- Cricoid pressure is called Sellick's manuever
- It is a method of preventing regurgitation in an anesthesized patient during rapid endotracheal intubation by applying pressure to the cricoid cartilage.
- It is indicated only for *high risk cases* where patient is not fasting example: Upper GI surgery, obstetric anesthesia.
- Studies have not shown any mortality reduction.

101. Ans. (d) Cardiac compression

Ref: Harrison, 19th ed. pg. 1768

- Since cardiac arrest is already, mentioned in the question, initiate chest compressions.
- If a clinical question of a patient collapsing suddenly is given, then check carotid A pulsation and respiratory efforts in 6 second interval. If both are absent it implies cardio-respiratory arrest. Then perform CPR.

102. Ans. (b) To prevent gastric aspiration

Ref: Miller's Anesthesia, 7th ed. pg. 2430

- Sellick's manuever is a method of preventing regurgitation of an anesthesized patient during endotracheal intubation by applying pressure to the cricoid cartilage.
- Or in other words, Sellick's maneuver is application of *backward pressure on cricoid cartilage to prevent gastric aspiration (Mendelson's syndrome).*

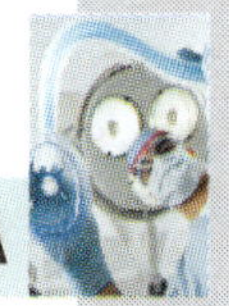

103. Ans. (d) Mobility of fracture

Ref: Textbook of Neurosurgery, 3th ed. pg. 2713

Factors Favoring Fat Embolism

Traumatic	Non- traumatic
• Fracture of long bones e.g. Femur • Reaming • Mobility of fracture	• Diabetes • Fatty liver • Pancreatitis • Sickle cell anemia • Decompression sickness • Extensive burns • Inflammation of bone & soft tissue • Oil or fat introduced to body

MISCELLANEOUS

104. Ans. (d) Venturi mask

Ref: Miller's Anesthesiology 8th ed. pg. 756-758

- The shown instrument is Venturi mask
- Venturi masks are low-flow masks that use the Bernoulli principle to entrain room air when pure oxygen is delivered through a small orifice, resulting in a large total flow at predictable FiO_2.
- While the Venturi mask is effective at delivering accurate oxygen concentrations (FiO_2), it requires relatively high oxygen flow rates to achieve this.

105. Ans. (c) 100–120 per minute

Ref: American Red Cross CPR Guidelines 2018-19

- CPR is cardiopulmonary resuscitation. According to latest 2018-19 CPR guidelines, the number of chest compression per minute in adult or infant is same i.e. 100 per minute.

TABLE: American Red Cross- New CPR Guidelines 2019

	Adult	Infant
Depth of compression	At least 2"	1 ½"
Breathing	Look for chest rise Deliver breaths over 1 second	Look for chest rise Deliver breaths over 1 second
Compression to breath ratio	30 : 2	30 : 2
Compression rate	100-120/minute (until help/paramedics arrive)	100/min
Site of chest compression	One hand should be placed on the breast bone in the center of the chest, second hand should be placed on first while keeping fingers off the chest (Image)	Use 2–3 fingers in the center of the chest on the lower half of the breast bone to compress the chest about 1 ½" (Image)

106. Ans. (c) Trachea

Ref: Emergency Procedure and Techniques, pg. 48

HEIMLICH MANEUVER

The primary indication for use of the Heimlich maneuver is *upper airway obstruction due to a bolus of food* or any aspirated foreign material unrelieved by coughing and traditional means that now is causing complete airway obstruction and threatening asphyxiation.

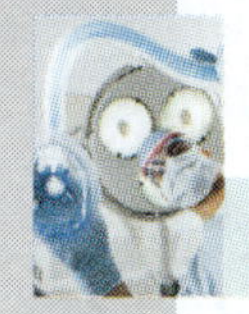

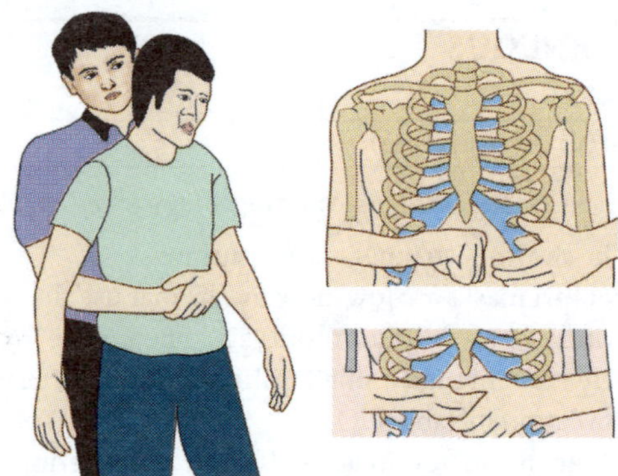

107. Ans. (c) Ketamine

Ref: Anesthesia for Medical Students by Sullivan 1999 ed. pg. 83

108. Ans. (a) Severe hyperkalemia

Ref: Miller 4th ed. Ch: 9

109. Ans. (b) Gastric aspiration

Ref: Fundamentals of Anesthesia by Tim Smith 3rd edn. pg. 5

110. Ans. (a) N20

Ref: Miller's 7th ed. ch: 24

111. Ans. (b) 2 inch

Ref: 2015 AHA Guidelines

112. Ans. (d) Maintains airway

Ref: Ajay Yadav, 2nd ed. p-36

113. Ans. (c) 2% jelly, 4% injection

Ref: Morgan's 4th ed. p-270, KDT 6th ed. p-357

114. Ans. (c) 3-5

Ref: Morgan 4th ed. p-2

115. Ans. (c) Vecuronium

Ref: Fundamentals of anesthesia by Tim Smith p-618

Vecuronium is primarily eliminated by hepatic mechanisms. Since 30% of dose is excreted unchanged in urine, the elimination half-life of drug is increased.

116. Ans. (b) Rocuronium

Ref: Lee 13th ed. p-188, Miller's 6th ed. p-492-535

117. Ans. (a) Cisatracurium

118. Ans. (d) Bronchospasm

119. Ans. (c) Class III

120. Ans. (a) Mapleson A

121. Ans. (a) Lidocaine

122. Ans. (a) Bradycardia and hypotension

123. Ans. (a) Inhalational Anesthetics

124. Ans. (a) Abdominal malignant growth

125. Ans. (a) Chest wall rigidity

126. Ans. (a) Mu (μ)

127. Ans. (c) Sevoflurane

128. Ans. (d) Sevoflurane

129. Ans. (a) Atracurium

130. Ans. (c) Thiopentone

131. Ans. (b) Acute intermittent phorphyria

132. Ans. (d) Cardiac compression

133. Ans. (b) Pain

Ref: Oral and Maxillofacial Surgery, 3rd ed. Elsevier pg. 77

The classical order of sensation loss during local anesthesia is:

1. Pain
2. Temperature
3. Touch
4. Deep pressure
5. Motor (Recovery is in reverse order)

The order of sensation loss in spinal anesthesia is cold/warm followed by pin-pnick, pain.

134. Ans. (d) Bupivacaine

Ref: Morgan's Anaesthesiology 4/e, p 269

135. Ans. (c) Atracurium

Ref: Lee Synopsis of Anesthesia 12/e, p 215

136. Ans. (b) 16th October

Ref: Miller's 7/e, ch-1

137. Ans. (a) Succinylcholine

Ref: Goodman and Gillman p 152, 11/e, 352-54

138. Ans. (a) Hypertensive patients

Ref: Miller's 7/e, Ch 26

PSYCHIATRY

18

MOST RECENT QUESTIONS 2023

1. Which of the following is considered as key symptoms of depression? ***(Most Recent Question July 2023)***

a. Low mood b. Suicidal ideations
c. Loss of energy d. Loss of appetite

2. Capgras syndrome is mostly seen in which type of dementia? ***(Most Recent Question July 2023)***

a. Alzheimer's b. Dementia with Lewy body
c. Vascular dementia d. Frontotemporal dementia

3. The following are features of pseudo hallucinations, EXCEPT: ***(Most Recent Question July 2023)***

a. They occur without stimulus
b. They are perceived in the objective space
c. They are vivid
d. They are not under the control of the patient

4. A female patient presents five days after delivery with symptoms like sadness of mood, irritability, restlessness and reduced sleep. Diagnosis is: ***(Most Recent Question July 2023)***

a. Postpartum blues b. Postpartum depression
c. Postpartum psychosis d. Postpartum anxiety

5. A patient is showing stubbornness and frugality. As per psychosexual stages of development, the fixation is in which stage? ***(Most Recent Question July 2023)***

a. Anal b. Oral
c. Phallic d. Genital

6. Identify the image and make the diagnosis: ***(Most Recent Question July 2023)***

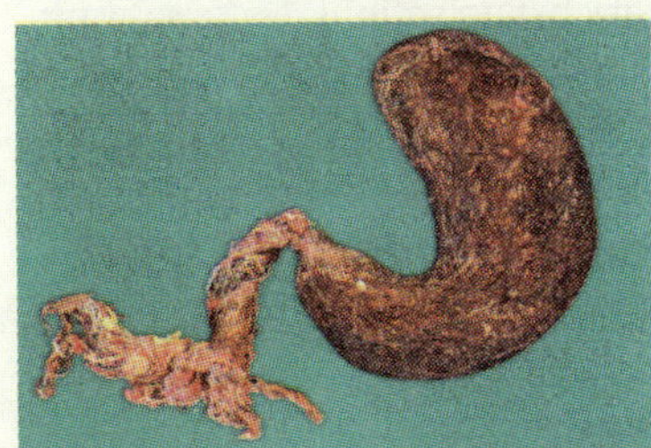

a. Trichobezoar b. Splenic rupture
c. Pancreatic necrosis d. Phytobezoar

7. A 27-year-old patient is presented with complaint that aliens are communicating with him and they are sending an electromagnetic radiation to his brain and are asking him to kill distant relatives. His relative said he has been suffering from this disease for the last 20 years, The patient does not work on farm and stopped going in social functions, patient is aware of time, place and person. What is the most likely diagnosis? ***(Most Recent Question Jan 2023)***

a. Depression b. Mania
c. Delusional disorder d. Schizophrenia

8. On MME patient is asked to subtract 7 from 100. What does it assess? ***(Most Recent Question Jan 2023)***

a. Orientation
b. Memory
c. Confusion
d. Concentration

9. What is the common effect of cannabis/marijuana intake? ***(Most Recent Question Jan 2023)***

a. Anxiety
b. Depression
c. Physical dependance
d. A state of dreaminess with altered consciousness

10. A patient present with sudden and irresistible urges to take an action, this is characteristic of which symptoms? ***(Most Recent Question Jan 2023)***

a. Impulse b. Hallucination
c. Delusion d. Pseudo hallucinations

SCHIZOPHRENIA AND PSYCHOSIS

11. A 21-year-old girl suspects that the college principal is making a conspiracy against her and is planning to fails her in the upcoming exam. She feels that other teachers have also joined the conspiracy and students are helping them too? What is the diagnosis: ***(Most Recent Question Aug 2020)***

a. Delusion of persecution b. Delusion of reference
c. Delusion of infidelity d. Othello syndrome

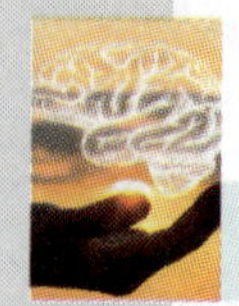

12. A 37-year-old man reports that after suffering from sudden financial loss, he developed certain symptoms. He started feeling fearful that someone is about to harm him, he could not sleep or eat properly. He also began to hear voices of a female and that voice would abuse him and say that he was useless and should kill himself. His symptoms stopped after approximately one week. There was no relevant past history of, drug abuse. What is the likely diagnosis? ***(Most Recent Question Aug 2020)***

a. Schizophreniform disorder
b. Brief psychotic disorder
c. Schizoaffective disorder
d. Schizophrenia

13. Delusion is:

a. Disorder of thinking
b. Disorder of memory
c. Disorder of perception
d. Disorder of affect

14. A female was brought to psychiatry after 3 weeks of delivery. She has fearfulness, irritability and getting suicidal thoughts. Diagnosis is: ***(Most Recent Question Dec 2019-20)***

a. Postpartum blues
b. Postpartum depression
c. Postpartum psychosis
d. Schizophrenia

15. A 24-year-old lady presented with sudden onset chest pain like heart attack, palpitations lasting for about 20 minutes. There has been previous recurrent episode of same. She says there were 3 similar episodes last month: ***(Most Recent Question 2019)***

a. Acute psychosis
b. Panic attack
c. Post-traumatic stress disorder
d. Mania

16. Management of violent patient in psychiatry is treated with all; EXCEPT: ***(Recent Pattern Question 2018-19)***

a. Benzodiazepines
b. Cognitive behavioral therapy (CBT)
c. Electroconvulsive therapy
d. Haloperidol

17. Negative symptoms of schizophrenia are all; EXCEPT: ***(Recent Pattern Question 2018-19)***

a. Overactivity
b. Anhedonia
c. Alogia
d. Apathy

18. Capgras syndrome is? ***(Recent Pattern Question 2017)***

a. Familiar person replaced by impostor
b. Nonfamiliar person appears to be familiar
c. Wife cheating with another man
d. Famous person is in love with patient

19. Fregoli syndrome is: ***(Recent Pattern Question 2017)***

a. Familiar person replaced by impostor
b. Nonfamiliar person appears to be familiar
c. Wife cheating with another man
d. Famous person is in love with patient

20. Which of the following atypical antipsychotic agents is associated with the most weight gain? ***(Recent Pattern Question 2017)***

a. Olanzapine
b. Ziprasidone
c. Aripiprazole
d. Quetiapine

21. Which of the following is seen in Catatonia ***(Recent Pattern Question 2016)***

a. Cataplexy
b. Echolalia
c. Positivism
d. Disobedience

22. An old patient was brought to the hospital with the history of auditory hallucinations. He states that, some unknown peoples are conspiring against him. He hears them talking on his every actions continuously. What could be the most likely diagnosis?

a. Dementia
b. Delusional disorders
c. Schizophrenia
d. Acute psychosis

23. A patient is brought to your clinic with complaint of unrealistic behavior from last 5–6 months. Family members mentioned about loss of his wife few years back. They also mentioned about his talking behavior in absence of everyone and sometimes muttering to himself loudly inside his room. The most likely diagnosis is:

a. Major depression
b. Schizophrenia
c. Conversion disorder
d. Delusion

24. A schizophrenia patient refuses to take drugs, because he complains that he is persistently hearing people talking in spite of taking the medications. Which drug will be most suitable for his condition?

a. Chlorpromazine
b. Clozapine
c. Resperidone
d. Fluphenazine

25. A 43-year-old male is diagnosed with Schizophrenia but he refused to take treatment. Which of the following antipsychotic drug is the treatment of choice for this patient?

a. Clozapine
b. Risperidone
c. Olanzapine
d. Fluphenazine

26. Clinical manifestation of Schizophrenia are all of the following; EXCEPT:

a. Delusion
b. Altered sensorium
c. Auditory hallucinations
d. Catatonia

27. Which of the following is not a characteristic symptom/ sign of schizophrenia:

a. Inappropriate affect
b. Disturbance of thought process
c. Visual hallucinations
d. Auditory hallucinations

28. Prognosis in Schizophrenia is less favorable if:

a. Occurs in women
b. History of depression
c. Gradual onset
d. Acute onset

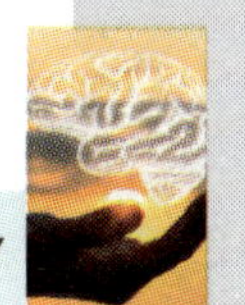

29. Schizophrenia with best prognosis:

a. Paranoid b. Catatonic
c. Hebephrenic d. Simple

30. A college student was caught by police for fighting with classmates because he thought they were planning to kill him. He states that his dead grandfather talks to him every now and then for last one month. He is delusional from past few weeks also. What will be the most likely diagnosis:

a. Delusional disorder
b. Post traumatic stress disorder
c. Mania
d. Schizophrenia

31. A 13-year-old young boy is brought by his parents with history of frequent fighting at school, disciplinary problems, stealing money, assaulting his batch mates and being weak in studies. What is the most appropriate diagnosis for this child.

a. Attention deficit hyperactivity disorder
b. Conduct disorder
c. Autism
d. Nothing abnormal (teenage phenomenon)

32. Which of the following is *not* Bleuler's 4 A's of Schizophrenia?

a. Association b. Inappropriate Affect
c. Automatism d. Ambivalence

33. All of the following are Schneider's first rank symptoms; EXCEPT:

a. Running commentary b. Primary delusion
c. Thought insertion d. Delusion of guilt

34. Antipsychotic drugs relieve positive symptoms of schizophrenia by targeting which of the following neurotransmitters:

a. Acetylcholine b. GABA
c. Dopamine d. Serotonin

35. All are first rank symptoms of schizophrenia; EXCEPT?

a. Voices commenting b. Thought broadcasting
c. Delusion of persecution d. Somatic passivity

36. Which of the following is not a component of 4A's of schizophrenia?

a. Autism b. Affect
c. Auditory hallucination d. Ambivalence

37. Not a negative symptom in schizophrenia

a. Anhedonia
b. Decreased emotional expression
c. Diminished social engagement
d. Delusions

38. Prognosis in Schizophrenia is less favorable if:

a. Occurs in women
b. History of depression
c. Gradual onset
d. Acute onset

39. Ganser syndrome is related to?

a. Approximate answer
b. Ataxia
c. Confusion
d. Repeated answers

40. Delusion is a disorder of?

a. Thought b. Personality
c. Memory d. Cognition

41. A child with schizophrenia was on medications. Suddenly he developed neck stiffness and spasm. Best treatment of such a case is?

a. Benztropine b. Lorazepam
c. Diphenhydramine d. Propranolol

42. Delusion that an identical looking individual has been replaced by imposter is?

a. De clerambault's syndrome
b. Capgras syndrome
c. Cotard's syndrome
d. Ekbom's syndrome

43. Squeeze technique is used for: ***(2018)***

a. Premature ejaculation
b. Azoospermia
c. Depression
d. Anxiety

DEPRESSION, SUICIDE AND ADJUSTMENT DISORDER

44. A patient had covid infection around 3 months back. Now he presents with the complaints of excessive sweating, palpitations, and fear the he is about to die. The physical examination and investigations didn't reveal any abnormality. What is the likely diagnosis? ***(Most Recent Question June/Dec 2021)***

a. Post-traumatic stress disorder
b. Depression
c. Mania
d. Panic attack

45. Which of the following is NOT a symptoms of panic attack: ***(Most Recent Question June/Dec 2021)***

a. Suicide attempt
b. Sudden anxiety
c. Episodic anxiety
d. Feeling of impending doom

46. A 32-year-old female presented with symptoms of mild depression for first time, what should be the initial treatment: ***(Most Recent Question June/Dec 2021)***

a. Cognitive behavior therapy
b. Antidepressant
c. CBT+ antidepressant
d. Electro convulsive therapy

47. **A 31-year-old female with history of recent divorce presents to emergency with complaints of palpitations sweating, heaviness and pain in chest. She has multiple similar episodes in last few weeks and is not able to sleep properly from past few days. The blood investigations, and ECG are normal. In the past too, investigations revealed no abnormality what is the next best step?** ***(Most Recent Question Aug 2020)***
    a. Admit for detailed investigation
    b. Start counselling sessions
    c. Use benzodiazepines for symptoms relief
    d. Use beta blockers
48. **A 25-year-old male had RTA after that he is fearful of driving vehicle and going to that place since 6 weeks and he is having flashbacks of Incidents and he is not going to his office also. What is diagnosis?** ***(Most Recent Question Dec 2019-20)***
    a. Post-traumatic stress disorder
    b. Acute stress
    c. Depression
    d. Acute panic disorder
49. **A person is unable to find pleasure in doing old activities which he used to enjoy earlier. Mostly he is suffering from:** ***(Most Recent Question Dec 2019-20)***
    a. Alexithemia b. Depression
    c. Anhedonia d. Derailment
50. **A clinician asked the patient how is your mood', patient replied 'up and down', what could be the diagnosis?** ***(Most Recent Question Dec 2019-20)***
    a. Neologism b. Tangentiality
    c. Clanging d. Derailment
51. **Double depression is:** ***(Recent Pattern Question 2018-19)***
    a. Major depressive disorder from 2 years
    b. Major depression with OCD
    c. Depression with dysthymia
    d. Depression with anxiety attack
52. **Indoor management of anorexia nervosa is done on priority in patients with:** ***(Recent Pattern Question 2018)***
    a. Forced eating symptoms
    b. Weight loss >75%
    c. Amenorrhea
    d. Depression
53. **Copycat suicide is seen at age of:** ***(Recent Pattern Question 2018)***
    a. Adolescence b. Pre-school age
    c. Adult age d. Old age
54. **What would be the choice of initial treatment when a 65-year-old man with carotid artery stenosis develops severe depression and hypersomnia:** ***(Recent Pattern Question 2017)***
    a. Amitriptyline b. Milnacipran
    c. Nortriptyline d. Phenelzine
55. **The most common psychiatric disorder associated with stroke is:** ***(Recent Pattern Question 2017)***
    a. Psychosis b. Bipolar disorder
    c. Depression d. Mania
56. **Dysthymia is seen in** ***(Recent Pattern Question 2016)***
    a. Bipolar Mood disorder
    b. Major depressive disorder
    c. Minor depressive disorder
    d. Persistent depressive disorder
57. **Which of the following is true about depression:**
    a. Increased Serotonin and Norepinephrine
    b. Increased serotonin decreased Norepinephrine
    c. Decreased serotonin and Norepinephrine
    d. Decreased serotonin increased Norepinephrine
58. **Neurotransmitters mainly involved in depression are:**
    a. Serotonin and Dopamine
    b. Serotonin and GABA
    c. Dopamine and GABA
    d. Serotonin and Norepinephrine
59. **All of the following are the feature of masked depression; EXCEPT:**
    a. Body aches and pains
    b. Gastrointestinal symptoms
    c. Functional impairment
    d. Depressed mood
60. **What is the most common cause of DALY'S in world?**
    a. Schizophrenic b. Mania
    c. Depressive disorder d. Alzheimer's
61. **In clinical practice, most common psychiatric illness seen is:**
    a. Maniac disorder
    b. Schizophrenia
    c. Depressive disorder
    d. Bipolar disorder
62. **A 40-year-old man is diagnosed with terminally ill cancer. He is not able to digest the fact. He previously indulged with his children like playing with his daughter, dropping her at school, but now he is not pleasurable in such events. He even stopped meeting friends and has difficulty in sleeping also. What could be the possible diagnosis:**
    a. Post traumatic stress disorder
    b. Adjustment disorder
    c. Major depression
    d. Sleep disorder
63. **A patient who after getting fired from her job prefers to stay isolated, has anhedonia and also lost weight. She thinks that because of her worthlessness she got fired. What could be the possible diagnosis:**
    a. Adjustment disorder
    b. Major depressive disorder
    c. Post traumatic stress disorder
    d. Sleep disorder

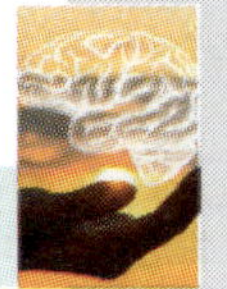

64. The son of a construction worker died at his work place. After that he is neither going out, nor eating food properly. His wife consulted a physician and stated that he has been doing this for over 2 months. What is the most likely diagnosis:
   a. Adjustment disorder
   b. PTSD
   c. Severe depression
   d. Bipolar

65. Suicide is least commonly seen in:
   a. Early depression
   b. After recovery from depression
   c. Living alone
   d. Severe depression

66. Most common cause of impotency in male:
   a. Generalized disorder
   b. Local disorder
   c. Psychogenic
   d. Somatic disorder

67. Outside environment seems strange in?
   a. Déjà vu phenomenon
   b. Derealisation
   c. Jamais vu phenomenon
   d. Mania

68. Most common symptom of psychiatric illness?
   a. Anxiety
   b. Depression
   c. Schizophrenia
   d. Somatoform illness

69. Son of a construction worker died at his work place. After that he is not going out, not eating food properly. His wife consulted physician and states that he has been doing this over 2 months. What is the most likely diagnosis?
   a. Adjustment disorder
   b. PTSD
   c. Severe depression
   d. Bipolar

70. Bright light therapy is used for?
   a. Seasonal affective disorder
   b. Schizophrenia
   c. Adjustment disorder
   d. Anxiety

71. Treatment of depression with suicidal tendencies is?
   a. Clozapine
   b. Mitrazapine
   c. ECT
   d. Olenzapine

72. Minimum time period to diagnose depression with daily manifestation is?
   a. 1 weeks   b. 2 weeks
   c. 4 weeks   d. 8 weeks

PERSONALITY DISORDER/OCD

73. A person repeatedly washes hands as shown in the image, diagnosis is: ***(Most Recent Question June 2022)***

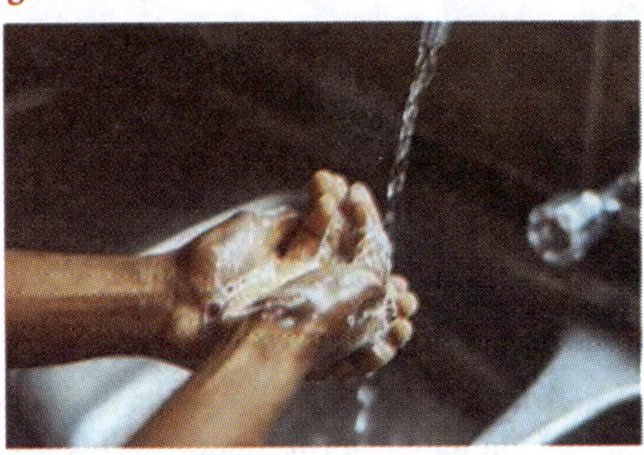

   a. OCD
   b. Panic Attack
   c. Body dysmorphic disorder
   d. Acute psychosis

74. A patient in ward is asked what is your name? Patient repeat the same sentence 'What is your name?' This phenomenon is: ***(Most Recent Question June 2022)***
   a. Echolalia   b. Echoprexia
   c. Perseveration   d. Circumstantiality

75. Hair inside stomach found during surgery as shown in the image. Which doctor is required to diagnose this condition? ***(Most Recent Question June 2022)***

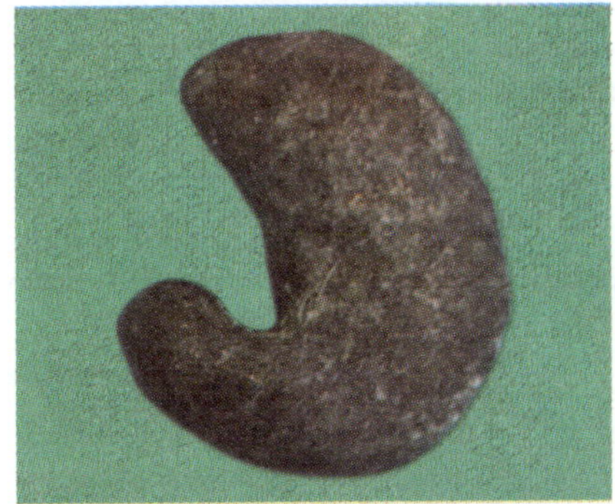

   a. Cardiologist   b. Psychiatrist
   c. Neurologist   d. Intensivist

76. Uncontrolled and excessive sexual desire in men is called as? ***(Most Recent Question June/Dec 2021)***
   a. Voyeurism   b. Sadism
   c. Nymphomania   d. Satyriasis

77. Excessive fear of getting contaminated, repeated washing, repetitive checking behaviour and excessive doubts are features of: ***(Most Recent Question Aug 2020)***
   a. Panic attacks
   b. Agoraphobia
   c. Obsessive compulsive disorder
   d. Generalized anxiety disorder

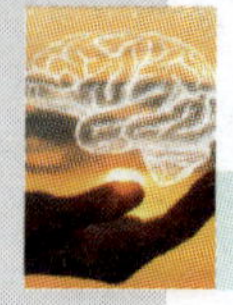

78. A patient has a long-term history about waking up in night and thinking that his family going to meet with an accident. Probable diagnosis? *(Most Recent Question Dec 2019-20)*
   a. Adjustment disorder
   b. Generalised anxiety disorder
   c. OCD
   d. Panic disorder

79. A 20-year-old female scared of elevator since birth. She prefers stairs instead elevator. Diagnosis: *(Most Recent Question Dec 2019-20)*
   a. Agoraphobia   b. Specific phobia
   c. Social phobia   d. Acrophobia

80. In nondiabetic nonhypertensive patient having some extra beats in pulse. Doctor informed it is benign. But patient is still going for investigations from doctor to doctor. This is a type of: *(Recent Pattern Question 2018)*
   a. Conversion disorder   b. Hypochondriac disorder
   c. Somatoform pain   d. Depression

81. A 6-year-old child with no interest in daily activity and not engaging with other children of his age group is likely to be suffering from: *(Recent Pattern Question 2018)*
   a. Autism   b. ADHD
   c. Depression   d. Bipolar disorder

82. What is the drug of choice for OCD? *(Recent Pattern Question 2017)*
   a. Buspirone   b. Risperidone
   c. Fluoxetine   d. Chlorpromazine

83. Goal directed repetitive behaviour is seen in: *(Recent Pattern Question 2017)*
   a. Depression   b. OCD
   c. Mania   d. Schizophrenia

84. Psychological separation of a mental function from the rest of the personality is called as? *(Recent Pattern Question 2017)*
   a. Isolation   b. Dissociation
   c. Acting out   d. Paranoia

85. Skinnerian conditioning is: *(Recent Pattern Question 2016)*
   a. Pavlov method   b. Classical conditioning
   c. Operant conditioning   d. Stimulus response

86. A 25-year-old man has presented to you with sexual indulgence and increased alcohol consumption, irritability and decreased sleep, from last 10 days. The family members stated that he was career oriented remained wide awake and had prolonged periods of activity without getting fatigued. What would be the most likely diagnosis:
   a. Schizophrenia
   b. Mania
   c. Impulsive control disorder
   d. Alcohol dependence

87. Which one of the following is not a characteristic feature of mania?
   a. Elated mood
   b. Increased energy
   c. Heightened concentration
   d. Impaired judgment

88. True about obsession:
   a. Ego dystonic
   b. Ego syntonic
   c. Feel pleasure and enjoy
   d. Must be followed by compulsion

89. Which of the following is part of the treatment for OCD:
   a. MAO inhibitor
   b. Exposure and response prevention
   c. Diazepam
   d. Neurosurgery

90. Treatment of choice for phobia:
   a. Behavior therapy   b. Psychotherapy
   c. Relaxation therapy   d. Covert sensitization

91. Which of the following best explains behavioral therapy in phobia?
   a. Exposure and response prevention followed by flooding
   b. Systemic desensitization followed by exposure and response prevention
   c. Exposure and response prevention followed by systemic desensitization
   d. Flooding followed by systemic desensitization

92. All of the following is good prognostic factor for bipolar disorder; EXCEPT:
   a. Acute onset
   b. Early age of onset
   c. Early responsive treatment
   d. Associated with depression

93. Lithium most commonly used in:
   a. Bipolar disorder   b. Depressive disorder
   c. Personality disorder   d. Headache

94. Which one of the following is *not* used in therapy of bipolar affective disorders:
   a. Lithium carbonate   b. Sodium valproate
   c. Phenytoin sodium   d. Topiramate

95. A sensitive person, gets affected easily and has difficulty in controlling anger and doesn't meet people. What is the personality defect:
   a. Maniac   b. Schizoid personality
   c. Borderline   d. Paranoid personality

96. Anorexia nervosa is an eating disorder characterized by all; EXCEPT:
   a. Menorrhagia
   b. Salivary gland enlargement
   c. Acrocyanosis
   d. Bradycardia

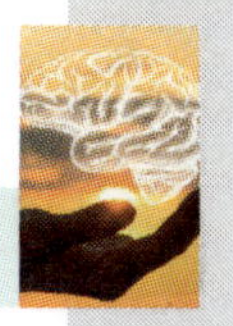

97. A 20-year-old man was found in a city far away from his home town, working in a factory. He was unable to tell about his previous life. Which of the following is the likely diagnosis:
a. Post traumatic stress disorder
b. Body dysmorphic disorder
c. Dissociative fugue
d. Dissociative identity disorder

98. A 21-year-old girl is disturbed that her nose is too big. She is convinced that it is disfiguring though no one else can see that way. What is the likely diagnosis:
a. Delusional disorder
b. Obsessive compulsive disorder
c. Body dysmorphic disorder
d. Specific phobia

99. A lady washes her hands 40 times per day for no apparent reason. Cognitive behavior therapy for her treatment should include?
a. Response prevention b. Aversion
c. Thought stopping d. Desensitization

100. Kleptomania is?
a. Fear of heights
b. Impulse control disorder
c. Compulsive eating disorder
d. None of the above

101. Dialectical behaviour therapy is used for?
a. Personality disorder
b. Somatoform disorder
c. Schizophreniform disorder
d. Schizophrenia

102. Fear of being alone in a crowd or fear of travelling alone in a bus?
a. Agoraphobia
b. Generalised anxiety disorder
c. Dissociative fugue
d. Obsessive compulsive disorder

103. True about obsession
a. Ego dystonic b. Ego syntonic
c. Feel pleasure and enjoy
d. Must be followed by compulsion

DELIRIUM, DEMENTIA AND ALZHEIMER'S DISEASE

104. A patient after getting operated for appendicitis developed confusion and hallucinations. His wife informed that he takes alcohol occasionally. What could be the most probable cause for his condition:
a. Delirium *(Most Recent Question Dec 2019-20)*
b. Alcohol hallucinosis
c. Acute transient psychotic disorder
d. Mania

105. Most commonly psychiatric illness seen in medico-surgical patient: *(Recent Pattern Question 2018-19)*
a. Depression b. Schizophrenia
c. Delirium d. Dementia

106. Most common acute organic mental disorder:
(Recent Pattern Question 2018-19)
a. Delirium b. Dementia
c. Amnesia d. Anxiety disorder

107. Clouding of consciousness is seen in:
a. Dementia b. Delirium
c. Schizophrenia a. Depression

108. Which of the following present with loss of consciousness:
a. Schizophrenia b. Dementia
c. Mania d. Organic brain syndrome

109. All are true about Dementia; EXCEPT:
a. Impaired memory
b. Loss of consciousness
c. Normal wake-sleep cycle
d. Deterioration of personality

110. Dementia pugilistica occurs due to:
a. Old age b. Trauma
c. Antiepileptic drugs d. Hydrocephalus

111. Drug used in alzheimer's disease are all; EXCEPT:
a. Biperidin b. Donepezil
c. Rivastigmine d. Memantine

112. Reversible dementia is seen in all; EXCEPT:
a. Wernicke's encephalopathy
b. Alzheimer's
c. Hypothyroidism d. Head trauma

113. Term "Dementia precox" was coined by:
a. Sigmund freud b. Bleuler
c. Kraepelin d. Schneider

114. Which of the following presents with loss of conciousness?
a. Schizophrenia b. Dementia
c. Mania d. Organic brain syndrome

115. In case of Alzheimer's disease Dementia pugilistica occurs due to:
a. Old age b. Trauma
c. Antiepileptic drugs d. Hydrocephalus

116. Pseudodementia is seen in:
a. Depression b. Schizophrenia
c. Parkinson's disease d. Dissociative disorder

SUBSTANCE ABUSE

117. After 72 hours of cessation of alcohol use, which of the following is seen in patients with alcohol dependence syndrome? *(Most Recent Question June/Dec 2021)*
a. Sweating
b. Alcoholic hallucinosis
c. Alcoholic withdrawal seizures
d. Delirium tremens

118. Earliest symptom of alcohol withdrawal is: *(Most Recent Question June/Dec 2021)*
a. Tremors b. Hallucinations
c. Seizures d. Delirium

119. A chronic alcoholic patient develops delirium tremens after stopping alcohol. Patient should be treated with: *(Most Recent Question June/Dec 2021)*
a. I/V Methylcobalamine
b. I/V Thiamine
c. I/V Thiamine + Lorazepam
d. I/V Methylcobalamine + Lorazepam

120. A patient admitted with tachycardia, arrythmia and scratch marks on skin. The most probable substance causing such presentation is: *(Most Recent Question June/Dec 2021)*
a. Cocaine b. Heroin
c. Cannabis d. Alcohol

121. A patient presented with history of visual hallucinations and disorientation. He was a chronic alcoholic and last intake was 2 days back? What is the likely diagnosis? *(Most Recent Question Aug 2020)*
a. Alcohol withdrawal seizures
b. Alcohol withdrawal delirium
c. Alcoholic hallucination
d. Schizophrenia

122. Antidote of choice for methyl alcohol poisoning: *(Recent Pattern Question 2018)*
a. Disulfiram b. Methycobalamin
c. Fomepizole d. Benzodiazepine

123. Disulfiram is a type of: *(Recent Pattern Question 2018)*
a. Aversion therapy b. Anticraving therapy
c. Maintenance therapy d. Alcohol withdrawal therapy

124. Date rape drug *(Recent Pattern Question 2016)*
a. Diazepam b. Lorazepam
c. Temazepam d. Flunitrazepam

125. Grass/Weed/pot slang is used for *(Recent Pattern Question 2016)*
a. Cocaine b. Cannabis
c. LSD d. Opioid

126. Trip word in LSD is defined as *(Recent Pattern Question 2016)*
a. Occasional use with long absistence
b. Frequent use with short absistence
c. Single use for lifetime
d. Occasional use with short abstinence

127. Alcohol withdrawal presents with all; EXCEPT:
a. Hallucinations b. Tremors
c. Bradycardia d. Sweating

128. After cessation of drinking in a person dependent on alcohol, when does the risk of alcoholic seizures peak:
a. 6-8 hours after cessation of alcohol
b. 8-12 hours after cessation of alcohol
c. 12-24 hours after cessation of alcohol
d. 24-48 hours after cessation of alcohol

129. The treatment of acute alcohol intoxication is based on which of the following?
a. Severity of respiratory and CNS depression
b. Age and sex of the patient
c. Medical fitness of the patient
d. Amount of breath odor

130. Which of the following is *not* a form of cannabis?
a. Bhang b. Charas
c. Cocaine d. Ganja

131. Early and rapid addiction is seen with:
a. Smoking b. Chewing betal seeds
c. Alcohol d. Narcotics

132. "Bad-trip" is associated with:
a. Bhang b. Ganja
c. Cocaine d. LSD

133. IQ range of Severe Mental Retardation:
a. Below 20 b. 21–34
c. 21–40 d. 35–49

134. CAGE questionnaire is used for?
a. Sex addiction b. Alzheimer's disease
c. Alcohol addiction d. Opioid addiction

135. "Bad-trip" is associated with:
a. Bhang b. Ganja
c. Cocaine d. LSD

136. Which of the following is a symptom of opioid withdrawal?
a. Pupillary constriction b. Piloerection
c. Hypotension d. Constipation

CHILD PSYCHIATRY

137. A 13-year-old boy was brought to the child psychiatrist for misbehaving frequently at home and in school with the teacher, often bullies the younger kids and has been caught stealing money on multiple occasions. What is the likely diagnosis? *(Most Recent Question Aug 2020)*
a. Antisocial personality disorder
b. Attention – deficit hyperactivity disorder
c. Conduct disorder
d. Oppositional defiant disorder

138. A child with IQ appropriate to his age and normal learning skills is poor in mathematics and getting poor marks in it. The appropriate diagnosis is? *(Most Recent Question Dec 2019-20)*
a. Autism
b. ADH
c. Specific learning disorder
d. Exam phobia

139. IQ range of moderate mental retardation:
a. Below 20 b. 21-34
c. 21-40 d. 35-49

140. Cause of death in retts syndrome is?
a. Hypoglycemia b. Cardiac arrythmia
c. Seizures d. Respiratory failure

141. An IQ of 50-60 is which type of mental retardation?
a. Mild b. Moderate
c. Severe d. Very severe

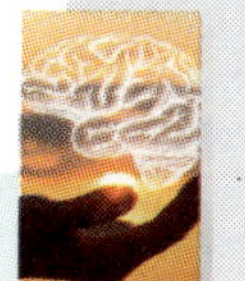

ANSWERS WITH EXPLANATIONS

MOST RECENT QUESTIONS 2023

1. Ans. (a) Low mood

Ref: Kaplan and Sadock's Synopsis of Psychiatry 11th ed. pg. 357

- Depression is a mental health disorder characterized by a persistent and pervasive **low mood** or sadness. It is often accompanied by a range of emotional, cognitive, and physical symptoms.
- The key feature of depression is the presence of a low mood that persists for most of the day, nearly every day, for at least two weeks.
- **Synopsis of Psychiatry states:** "*A depressed mood and a loss of interest or pleasure are the key symptoms of depression. In a patient with depression, the depressed often has a distinct quality that differentiate it from a normal emotion of sadness or grief*"

The diagnostic criteria for major depressive disorder are as follows:

Five or more of the following symptoms are present during the same 2-week period. At least one of the symptoms is either depressed mood or loss of interest or pleasure.

- Depressed mood most of the day
- Markedly diminished interest or pleasure in activities (anhedonia)
- Significant weight loss when not dieting or weight gain, decrease or increase in appetite
- Insomnia or hypersomnia
- Psychomotor agitation or retardation
- Fatigue or loss of energy
- Feelings of worthlessness or excessive or inappropriate guilt
- Diminished ability to think or concentrate, or indecisiveness
- Recurrent thoughts of death, recurrent suicidal ideation

2. Ans. (b) Dementia with Lewy body

Ref: Kaplan and Sadock's Synopsis of Psychiatry 11th ed. pg. 332-333

- Capgras syndrome is a neuropsychiatric disorder characterized by a delusional belief that a close family member or friend has been replaced by an identical imposter.
- This syndrome is most commonly associated with Dementia with Lewy bodies, a type of neurodegenerative dementia that shares features of both Alzheimer's and Parkinson's diseases.

3. Ans. (b) They are perceived in the objective space

Ref: Kaplan and Sadock's Synopsis of Psychiatry 11th ed. pg. 1407-18

- Pseudo-hallucinations are sensory experiences that are vivid, detailed, and intense, similar to true hallucinations. It occurs in subjective space, not objective space.
- However, they are distinct in the sense that they are experienced in the mind's eye, rather than being projected into the external world.
- Pseudo-hallucinations occur without an external stimulus and are often more dream-like and surreal and not under control of the patient.

4. Ans. (a) Postpartum blues

Ref: Kaplan and Sadock's Synopsis of Psychiatry 11th ed. pg. 839-40

- Postpartum blues, also known as "baby blues," is a common and mild mood disturbance that occurs in the days following childbirth.
- It is characterized by symptoms, such as sadness, irritability, mood swings, restlessness, and fatigue.
- It is a self-limiting condition that usually resolves within a few days to a couple of weeks and does not require specific treatment.

Note: Postpartum depression develops within weeks to months after childbirth.

5. Ans. (a) Anal

Ref: Kaplan and Sadock's Synopsis of Psychiatry 11th ed. pg. 167-68

- According to Sigmund Freud's theory of psychosexual development, the anal stage occurs from around 18 months to 3 years of age.
- During this stage, a child's pleasure centers around the elimination and retention of feces.
- Fixation at the anal stage can result from inconsistent or overly strict toilet training, leading to personality traits such as stubbornness, frugality, and an excessive need for orderliness.

Extra Mile

- **Fixation at the oral stage** can lead to dependency, passivity, and an excessive need for nurturance.
- **The phallic stage** involves the Oedipus and Electra complexes, leading to development of sexual identity and potential conflicts.
- **The genital stage** represents the mature stage of psychosexual development, where individuals focus on adult sexual relationships.

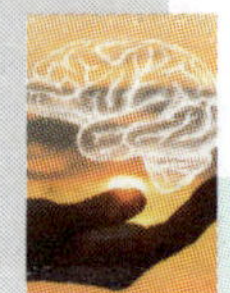

6. Ans. (a) Trichobezoar

Ref: Kaplan and Sadock's Synopsis of Psychiatry 11th ed. pg. 433

- A trichobezoar is a mass of hair that forms in the stomach or intestines due to a condition known as trichophagia, where individuals compulsively ingest their own hair.
- Trichobezoars are most commonly associated with trichotillomania (hair-pulling disorder) and often require surgical removal.
- These patients should immediately be sent for psychiatry referral.

Note: Phytobezoars are concentration of indigested food and vegetative matters in GIT

Extra Mile

Phytobezoar

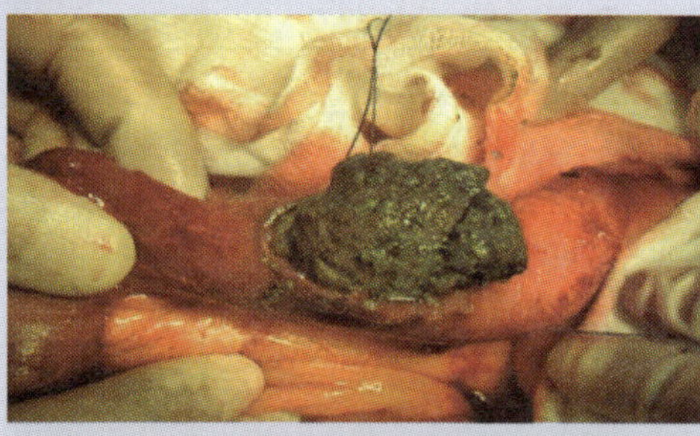

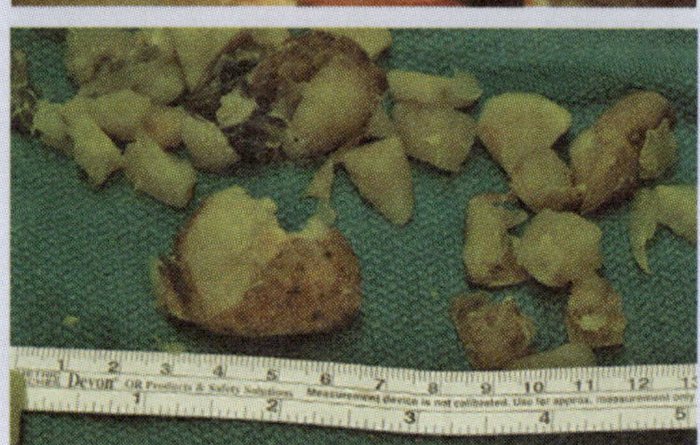

7. Ans. (d) Schizophrenia

Ref: Kaplan and Sadock's Concise Textbook of Clinical Psychiatry 11th ed. pg. 307

- The most likely diagnosis in the given case is **schizophrenia**.
- The presence of **delusions**, third person auditory hallucinations, specifically the belief in **alien communication** and **harmful commands**, is a characteristic symptom of schizophrenia.
- The absence of mood disturbance (depression or mania) makes depression and mania less likely diagnoses.

8. Ans. (d) Concentration

Ref: Kaplan and Sadock's Concise Textbook of Clinical Psychiatry 11th ed. pg. 233

- The specific task of subtracting **7 from 100 on the MMSE** primarily assesses concentration.
- The **subtraction task** on the MMSE assesses concentration by requiring the individual to concentrate, perform mental calculations, and maintain accuracy while subtracting a specific number.
- Other components of the MMSE assess various cognitive domains, such as orientation, memory, language, and visuospatial skills.

Extra Mile

- **Orientation** refers to awareness of time, place, and person.
- **Confusion** is a general term used to describe a state of disorientation, impaired thinking, and cognitive difficulties.
- **Memory** involves recalling recent or remote memory, like what you had in breakfast this morning or when is your marriage anniversary.

9. Ans. (d) A state of dreaminess with altered consciousness

Ref: Kaplan and Sadock's Concise Textbook of Clinical Psychiatry 11th ed. pg. 288

- The common effect of **cannabis/marijuana** intake is a state of **dreaminess with altered consciousness**.
- Cannabis/marijuana use can induce relaxation, euphoria, and alterations in perception, including distortions of time, space, and sensory experiences.
- The specific psychoactive compound in cannabis, delta-9-tetrahydrocannabinol (THC), is responsible for these effects.
- It is important to note that the effects of cannabis can vary from individual to individual and depend on factors such as dosage, method of consumption, and individual sensitivity.

10. Ans. (a) Impulse

Ref: Kaplan and Sadock's Synopsis of Psychiatry 11th ed. pg. 613

- **Impulses** are strong and often irresistible urges to perform certain actions without much consideration of the potential consequences.
- Impulsive behaviors are driven by immediate desires or emotions and can lead to risky or unwise decisions.

Other options:

- **Hallucinations** are false sensory perceptions, such as hearing voices or seeing things that are not present in reality.
- **Delusions** are false beliefs that persist despite evidence to the contrary.
- **Pseudo hallucinations** involve sensory experiences that occur within the mind's eye, rather than being projected externally.

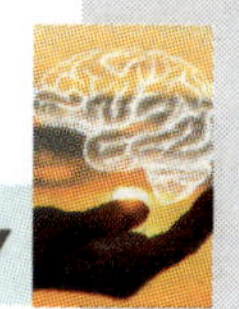

SCHIZOPHRENIA AND PSYCHOSIS

11. Ans. (a) Delusion of persecution

Ref: Neeraj Ahuja, pg. 56

- **Delusion:** A belief or altered reality that is persistently held despite evidence or agreement to the contrary, generally in reference to a mental disorder.
- Delusion of being persecuted against e.g. people are against me.

12. Ans. (b) Brief psychotic disorder

Ref: Neeraj Ahuja 20th ed. pg. 85-86

Acute and Transient Psychotic Disorder

- According to ICD 10 these have abrupt (less than 48 hrs) or acute (<2 weeks), associated with identifiable acute stress (not compulsorily) regarded as stressful condition to most of the people.
- Acute onset has better outcome, recovery occur within 2–3 months or even earlier.
- These should not satisfy the criteria of Organic mental disorder, mood disorder, psychoactive substance use disorder, schizophrenia.

Subtypes

- **Acute polymorphic psychotic disorder without symptoms of schizophrenia** - from nonpsychotic to psychotic, unstable and variable clinical picture, different type of hallucinations or/and delusions changing from day-to-day or within same day.
- **Acute polymorphic psychotic disorder with symptoms of schizophrenia**—along with above description here schizophrenic symptoms present if these symptoms present more than 1 month it is diagnosed as schizophrenia.
- **Acute schizophrenia like psychotic disorder**- psychotic symptoms are stable and not polymorphic and schizophrenic symptoms presents for less than 1 month.
- Other acute predominantly delusional psychotic disorder—main symptoms are delusion or hallucination but not fulfill the criteria of schizophrenia.

13. Ans. (a) Disorder of thinking

Reference: https://www.ncbi.nlm.nih.gov/pmc/articles/PMC3016695/

- A delusion is a belief that is clearly false and that Indicates an abnormality in the affected person's content of thought.
- The false belief is not accounted for by the person's cultural or religious background or his or her level of Intelligence.

14. Ans. (b) Postpartum depression

Ref: https://www.webmd.com/depression/gulde/postpartum-depression

- Postpartum depression (PPD) is a complex mix of physical, emotional, and behavioural changes that happen in some women after giving birth.
- According to the DSM-5, a manual used to diagnose mental disorders, PPD is a form of major depression that begins within 4 weeks after delivery.
- The diagnosis of postpartum depression is based not only on the length of time between delivery and onset, but also on the severity of the depression.

15. Ans. (b) Panic attack

Ref: Harrison's 19th ed. pg. 3262

- Panic disorder is defined by the presence of recurrent and unpredictable panic attacks, which are distinct episodes of intense fear and discomfort associated with a variety of physical symptoms like chest pain, fear of impending doom, palpitation, sweating, trembling, paresthesias, GI distress etc.
- **Diagnostic criteria:** 1 month of concern or worry about the attack or behavioural change related to them
- Lifetime prevalence of panic disorder is 2–3%
- Symptoms are always sudden onset, in an unexpected fashion, developing within 10 minutes and usually resolving within an hour.
- Frequency of panic attack varies: ranging from once a week to clusters to attacks separated by months of well being

16. Ans. (b) Cognitive behavioral therapy (CBT)

Ref: Kaplan's Textbook of Psychiatry Ch 29.2

- Violence is one of the common psychiatric emergencies. It is characterized by physical aggression of one person on another.
- It is most commonly associated with psychotic disorder and personality disorders.

Management

- Physical restraint *(only if necessary).*
- Give injection of Haloperidol (5 mg IM/IV) with or without lorazepam (2 mg IV). Repeat every 2 hours if necessary.
- Hospitalization → Referral to psychiatric services for further management
- In acute cases ECT can also be used.
- **Note:** CBT is not done in any of the acute psychiatric illness including depression.

17. Ans. (a) Overactivity

Ref: Kaplan's Textbook of Psychiatry Ch 12.8

NEGATIVE SYMPTOMS OF SCHIZOPHRENIA

- Affect flattening/blunting
- Alogia (poverty of speech/content)
- Avolition/apathy (lack of interest/motivation)
- Anhedonia (a sociality)
- Lack of attention

Note

- Over activity is NOT a negative symptom of schizophrenia.
- Example of positive symptoms: Conceptual disorganization, delusions, auditory hallucination or hallucinations
- Negative symptoms are associated with poor prognosis, while positive symptoms are associated with good prognosis.

18. Ans. (a) Familiar person replaced by impostor

Ref: Patient based approach to cognitive neurosciences pg. 155

Capgras syndrome: Chronic paranoid psychosis who is convinced that multiple persons, including members of family, had been replaced by imposters.

19. Ans. (b) Nonfamiliar person appears to be familiar

Ref: Patient based approach to cognitive neurosciences pg. 155

- **Fregoli syndrome** involves the belief that a person who appears to be well known to the patient is really impersonating.
- Christodoulou suggested that capgras syndrome is characterized by a "hypoidentification" of a person known by the patient, who is felt to be an imposter, while Fregoli syndrome was the manifestation of "hyperidentification" in which a known person could be seen in the disguise of others.

20. Ans. (a) Olanzapine

- Most common atypical antipsychotics associated with weight gain is: **Clozapine, Olanzapine**
- Other drugs associated with weight gain are Quetiapine, Risperidone and Asenapine, sertindole.

21. Ans. (b) Echolalia

Ref: Harrison's, 19th ed.

- Catatonia is a syndrome. It is a state of neurogenic motor immobility and behavioral abnormality manifested by stupor.
- It can be a part of medical illness or a psychiatric illness.
- **Signs and symptoms:**
  - **Echolalia:** Repetition of words or sentences heard by patient. Ex: what is this color? Patient replies: what is this color.
  - **Echopraxia:** Repetition of action
  - **Rigidity**
  - **Negativism:** Opposition or no response to instructions or external stimuli
  - **Automative obedience:** Excessive obeying of command without thinking of its consequence
  - **Catalepsy:** Waxy flexibility
  - **Posturing:** Spontaneous and active maintenance of a posture against gravity
  - **Mitgehen:** Excessive movement with slight pressure
  - **Gegenhalten:** Resistance of movement with proportional force
  - **Staring:** Persistent glaring/staring at one place

DIAGNOSIS

- **According to ICD 10:** Any one symptom if present is diagnostic
- **DSM 5 says:** Any 3 symptoms present is diagnostic

Treatment: IV Lorazepam

Note: *Cataplexy is symptom of narcolepsy, while catalepsy is a feature of catatonia.*

22. Ans. (c) Schizophrenia

Ref: Harrison, 19th ed. pg. 2720

- Hallucinatory voice commenting (keeping up a running commentary) on one's behavior, thought or action in the third person *(third person hallucination)* is a classical presentation of schizophrenia.
- The patient presented here presents with 3rd party auditory hallucination, which is a very characteristic finding of Schizophrenia.

TABLE: Diagnostic criteria for schizophrenia according to ICD 10 and DSM-V

ICD-10	A. At least one of the following: echoing/insertion/ withdrawal/ broadcasting of thought, delusional perceptions, hallucinatory voices, impossible delusions of some kind or B. At least two of the following: persistent hallucinations in any modality, incoherence or irrelevant speech, catatonic behaviour, negative symptoms C. Present for most of the time for at least 1 month D. Disorder is not caused by substance use or organic brain disease

Contd...

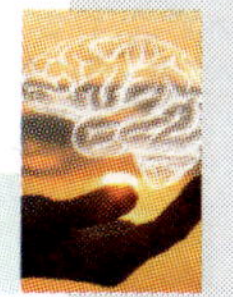

DSM-5	
	A. At least two of the following (at least one must be 1, 2 or 3) for at least 1 month: 1.Delusions, 2. Hallucinations, 3. Disorganized speech, 4. Grossly disorganized or catatonic behaviour, 5. Negative symptoms B. Level of functioning has to be significantly and long term lowered compared to the previously achieved level C. Continuous signs of the disturbance persist for at least 6 months, must include criterion A symptoms for at least 1 month D. Schizoaffective disorder and depressive or bipolar disorder with psychotic symptoms ruled out E. The disturbance is not caused by substance use or medical conditions F. If a patient has a history of autism spectrum or communication disorders from childhood, schizophrenia diagnosis can be made in case of prominent delusions/ hallucinations and other required symptoms of schizophrenia are present for at least 1 month

ICD-10, The International Statistical Classification of Diseases and Related Health Problems, 10th revision

DSM-5, The Diagnostic and Statistical Manual of Mental Disorders, 5th Edition

- Negative symptoms respond poor to treatment *(poor prognosis)* while positive symptoms are well responsive to treatment *(better prognosis).*

Positive Symptoms	Negative Symptoms
• Hallucination • Delusion • Illusion • Thought disorder • Aggressive behavior • Irrational conclusion	• Anhedonia: loss of interest in things which were interesting before. • Avolition: lack of desire to achieve goal • Alogia: poverty of speech • Attention deficit and cognition deficit • Social withdrawal/poor socialization skill • Emotional blunting

23. Ans. (b) Schizophrenia

Please refer to above explanation

24. Ans. (b) Clozapine

Ref: Harrison, 19th ed. pg. 2271, 2617

- The patient here is a case of resistant schizophrenia as the auditory hallucination is not responding to treatment. As we know that:
  - *Auditory hallucinations are first symptom to go with treatment and also 1st symptoms to reappear after drug resistance.*
- **Clozapine is:**
  - A reserve drug for resistant schizophrenia
  - Drug with least extra pyramidal side effects (ex-tardive dyskinesia)
  - Major side effect of clozapine is agranulocytosis, sedation, sialorrhea, weight gain and metabolic syndrome.

Extra Mile

Antipsychotic	
Longest acting	Paliperidone (Inj)
With antidepressant action	Flupenthixol
Least extrapyramldal side effect	Clozapine
Least potent	Thioridazine
Least Hypotensive & Least Antiemetic	Molindone

25. Ans. (d) Fluphenazine

Ref: Harrison, 19th ed. pg. 2722

Fluphenazine can be given as monthly intramuscular depot preparation. Thus it is preferred in non-compliant patients.

Important Points Regarding Anti-Psychotic Agents

- Fluphenazine (enanthate and decanoate) and haloperidol (decanoate) are long-acting injectable (s.c. or i.m) forms of typical antipsychotics.
- **Risperidone** is the first atypical antipsychotic available in *long-acting injectable form.*
- Most commonly used antipsychotic by *intravenous* route is **haloperidol**
- **Ziprasidone, aripiprazole, asenapine and iloperidone** has *negligible risk to cause metabalic adverse effects* (weight gain, hyperlipidemia and new onset diabetes mellitus)
- **Asenapine, paliperidone and ziprasidone** has greatest potential to *prolong QT interval.*
- Asenapine → available as sublingual

26. Ans. (b) Altered sensorium

Ref: Harrison, 19th ed. pg. 2270-71

- Schizophrenia is a formal thought disorder, characterized by third person hallucination & inappropriate emotion (affect)
- Altered consciousness (sensorium) is a characteristic feature seen in delirium *(not in szchizophrenia)*

Characteristics

- Only 3rd person auditory hallucinations are characteristic of schizophrenia.
- Third person hallucination means: Two or more voices talking to one another, discussing about the patient; and giving a running commentary on his actions or thoughts.
- *Auditory hallucination is most characteristic of Schizophrenia.*

27. Ans. (c) Visual hallucinations

Ref: Harrison, 19th ed. pg. 2270-71

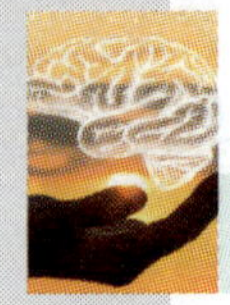

28. Ans. (c) Gradual onset

Ref: Harrison, 19th ed. pg. 2271

Prognostic Factor of Schizophrenia

Good prognostic factor	Bad prognostic factor
• *Female sex* • Acute onset (late onset) • No family history of schizophrenia • History of depressive order • Premorbid personality • Positive symptoms	• Male sex • Gradual onset (early onset) • Family history of schizophrenia • Emotional blunting • Negative symptoms

29. Ans. (b) Catatonic

Ref: Harrison, 19th ed. pg. 2271

- Catatonic schizophrenia has best prognosis

TABLE: Types of Schizophrenia

Paranoid	Hebephrenic	Simple
• Most common type. • Late onset. • It has more positive and less negative symptom • Has better prognosis	• Early onset • Personality and emotions get affected • Poor prognosis	• No positive symptom at all • Only negative symptoms • **Worst prognosis**
	Catatonic Due to imbalance of NT, there is hyperactivity and hypoactivity. BEST prognosis	**Undifferentiated** • Can't be categorized in one particular category. • Has >1 category.

30. Ans. (d) Schizophrenia

Ref: Harrison, 19th ed. pg. 2270-71

- Patient in the given case is delusional and has disorganized behavior with his classmates.
- He even hears his dead grandfather talking to him (auditory hallucination), which is a very characteristic finding of schizophrenia.
- In case of delusional disorder, hallucinations are rare, and in case they are present, they are usually tactile or olfactory

TABLE: Differentiating delusions of different causes

Delusion due to delusional disorder	Delusion due to schizophrenia
• Delusions are non bizarre (i.e. involving situations that occur in life as being followed, deceived, infected, loved etc.)	• Bizarre delusions
• Behaviour & personality is normal except in the delusional area	• Behaviour & personality is deteriorated in almost all areas
• Hallucinations are very rare & if occur are of tactile or olfactory variety	• Hallucinations are very common • Auditory variety is most common • *3rd person hallucination* is characteristic

Contd...

31. Ans (b) Conduct disorder

Ref: Ahuja 5th ed. pg. 173, Kaplan, 9th ed. pg. 1234-6

The child is not normal and suffers from conduct disorder.

TABLE: Differentiation between different disorders mentioned in the question

Autism	Attention deficit disorder	Conduct disorder
There is marked impairment of reciprocal social and interpersonal interaction: ***Absence of social smile*** • ***Absence of fear*** • Lack of attachment to parents and absence of separation anxiety • ***Lack of friends***	More common in males, the onset occurs before the age of 7 years, characterized, by: • *Poor attention span with distractibility* • *Hyperactivity* • *Impulsivity* • *Moving about here and there*	There is violation of rights and rules like: • **Frequent lying** • **Stealing** or robbery Running away from home & school • **Physical violence** • Cruelty • Poor at studies

32. Ans. (c) Automatism

Ref: Kaplan & Saddock, 10th ed. pg. 468

- Autism, NOT automatism is part of Bleuler's four A's
- Eugene Bleuler's Fundamental symptoms of schizophrenia *(4 A's of Blueler)*:
  - **Ambivalence**—Inability to decide for or against (confusion)
  - **Autism**—Withdrawal into self
  - **Association disturbance**—Loosening of association, thought disorder
  - **Affect disturbance**—Inappropriate affect

33. Ans. (d) Delusion of guilt

Ref: Harrison, 19th ed. pg. 2271

- **Schneider's first rank symptoms of schizophrenia include**: Hallucination, Delusion *(primary delusion, NOT delusion of guilt)*, Passivity (made) phenomenon, and thought alienation phenomenon.

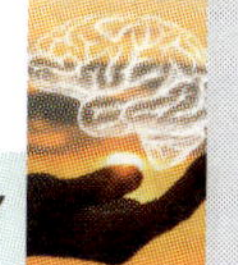

- *Presence of one symptom is diagnostic of schizophrenia.*

Hallucination

- Hearing Audible thought
- Voice heard arguing or discussing or both
- Voice commenting on one's action
- Hallucinations in form of commentary
- 3rd person hallucination
- Somatic hallucination

Thought Alienation Phenomenon

- Thought withdrawal
- Thought insertion
- Thought broadcasting

Passivity

- Made feeling (affect)
- Made impulse
- Made volition
- Somatic passivity

Delusional Perception

- Primary delusion

34. Ans. (c) Dopamine

Ref: Harrison, 19th ed. pg. 215

- Antipsychotics targeting positive symptoms probably act by *blocking the postsynaptic dopamine (D_2) receptors in the mesolimbic system*. Other receptors such as 5-HT, muscarinic receptors and GABA are also probably important. Atypical antipsychotics are also called as Serotonin Dopamine Antagonists (SDAs) due of their action on both dopamine and 5-HT.
- Overactivity of DA receptor causes positive symptoms
- Their blockage of D2 antagonist relieves from positive symptoms
- Underactivity of NMDA receptor is responsible for negative symptoms.

35. Ans. (c) Delusion of persecution

Ref: Kaplan 10th ed. pg. 468

36. Ans. (c) Auditory hallucination

Ref: Kaplan and Sadocks Synopsis of Psychiatry, 10th ed. ch-13

37. Ans. (d) Delusions

38. Ans. (c) Gradual onset

39. Ans. (a) Approximate answer

Ref: Kaplan and Sadocks Concise Textbook of clinical psychiatry 3rd ed. pg. 302

40. Ans. (a) Thought

Ref: Kaplan 9th ed. /281

41. Ans. (a) Benztropine

Ref: Handbook of Psychiatric Drug Therapy by Lawrence 3th ed. pg. 869)

42. Ans. (b) Capgras syndrome

Ref: Kaplan and sadock's 10th ed. /508-510

43. Ans. (a) Premature ejaculation

Squeeze technique is used in premature ejaculation

DEPRESSION, SUICIDE AND ADJUSTMENT DISORDER

44. Ans. (d) Panic attack

Ref: Kaplan and Sadock's, Comprehensive Textbook of Psychiatry, 10th ed. pg. 6648

- A panic attack is a sudden episode of intense fear that triggers severe physical reactions when there is no real danger or apparent cause.
- Panic attacks often happen at random and can leave you shaken. Some people become so fearful of these attacks that they develop panic disorder, a type of anxiety disorder.

45. Ans. (a) Suicide attempt

Ref: Kaplan and Sadock's, Comprehensive Textbook of Psychiatry, 10th ed. pg. 8216

- A suicide attempt is when people harm themselves with the goal of ending their life, but they do not die.
- It is not a part of symptoms associated with panic attack.

46. Ans. (a) Cognitive behavior therapy

Ref: Kaplan and Sadock's, Comprehensive Textbook of Psychiatry, 10th ed. pg. 8302

- Cognitive Behavior Therapy (CBT) for depression is a type of psychotherapy that modifies thought patterns to change moods and behaviors.
- CBT has been proven to be effective in treating mild to moderate levels of depression.

47. Ans. (c) Use benzodiazepines for symptoms relief

Ref: Neeraj Ahuja 20th ed. pg. 194-96

- Patient's history and symptoms are suggestive of panic attack, anxiety and insomnia.
- Benzodiazepines are the preferred agent in this patient with anxiety and insomnia.

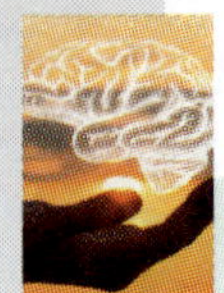

Mechanism of action: Opens GABA mediated Chloride channel.

Drugs: Mainly short acting drugs are used:

- Midazolam, Alprazolam, Lorazepam, Estazolam, Triazolam, Temazepam, Oxazepam

Indications

- Generalized anxiety disorder
- Panic disorder, agoraphobia
- Agitated depression
- For Nightmares
- Short-term treatment of insomnia.
- For treatment of alcohol withdrawal.
- For stage 4 NREM sleep disorders.

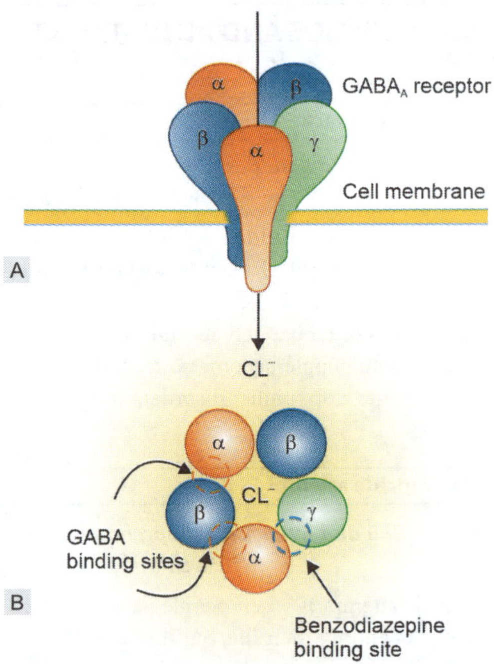

48. Ans. (a) Post-traumatic stress disorder

- Post-traumatic stress disorder (PTSD) is a mental health condition that's triggered by a terrifying event - either experiencing It or witnessing it.
- Symptoms may include flashbacks, nightmares and severe anxiety, as well as uncontrollable thoughts about the event.

49. Ans. (c) Anhedonia

Ref: https://www.ncbi.nlm.nih.gov/pmc/articles/PMC3181880/

- Anhedonia refers to the reduced ability to experience pleasure, and has been studied in different neuropsychiatric disorders.
- Anhedonia is considered as a core feature of major depressive disorder, according to DSM 5 criteria for major depression.

50. Ans. (b) Tangentiality

Ref: Brain Calipers: Descriptive Psychopathology and the Psychiatric Mental Status

- Tangentiality is one of the thought disorders.
- Tangential speech can be followed remains logical, and stays within the "ballpark of the topic at hand. Proper words and grammar are used."
- The distinctive factor here is that the person does not arrive at the main substance/conclusion.
- It may also be described as replying to a question in an oblique, tangential or in irrelevant manner. The reply is usually related to the question in some distant way. Like in question the patient replied 'up and down'

Extra Mile

Terms	Example
Derailment (loosening of associations)	When asked about a symptom of breathlessness: 'I felt breathless, like running a marathon. Marathon, the ancient Greek town. Democracy today has gone wild, hasn't it?'
Tangentiality (giving answers in an oblique fashion)	When asked how they hurt their arm: 'Well, I was riding my horse, and it was so sunny, but I suppose that is normal for this time of year. I prefer the summer months.'
Incoherence ('word salad', schizophasia)	'Glasses without a square battery mouse nor lacking table is the bottle and yes dancer'
Illogicality (drawing conclusion that do not follow basic logic)	'I was born on a Wednesday and today is a Wednesday so it will not rain today.'
Circumstantiality	Excessive long-windedness in reaching a conclusion in answer to a question
Pressure of speech	Increased production of spontaneous speech
Distractibility of speech	The subject of conversation is changed in response to a stimulus. 'I was walking to the shops when. What is your favourite song?'
Clanging	The sounds of words (such as their rhyming) dictates word choice: 'I still live on the hill, and that's quite a thrill, if you will.'

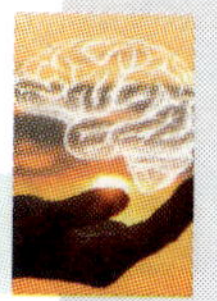

51. Ans. (c) Depression with dysthymia

Ref: Harrison's 20th ed. pg. 3269

- Prolong/persistent disorder is known as dysthymia. Therefore dysthymia is also known as persistent depressive disorder.
- It consist of a pattern of chronic (at least 2 years), ongoing depressive symptoms that are usually less severe than we seen in major depression.
- Often times the conditions like depression and dysthymia occur together and is difficult to separate.
- This persistence of depression with dysthymia is known as double depression.

52. Ans. (b) Weight loss >75%

Ref: Treatment manual for anorexia nervosa; 2/ed. pg. 277-278

- Anorexia nervosa (AN) is a type of eating disorder marked by an inability to maintain a normal healthy body weight, often dropping below 85% of ideal body weight (IBW).
- Bulimia nervosa (BN) is characterized by recurrent episodes of binge eating in combination with some form of inappropriate compensatory behavior.
- Indian patients chiefly present with refusal to eat, persistent vomiting, marked weight loss, amenorrhea and other somatic symptoms, but do not show over activity or disturbances in body image seen characteristically in anorexia nervosa.
- Nutritional rehabilitation along with some form of re-educative psychotherapy remains the mainstay of management of anorexia nervosa.
- In bulimia nervosa, both fluoxetine and cognitive behavior therapy have been found to be effective.

53. Ans. (a) Adolescence

Ref: Dying, Death and Bereavement; pg. 323

- Copycat suicide also known as Werther effect, is an imitative suicidal behaviour that occurs after exposure to another suicide
- This is more common after exposure to media reports of a celebrity's suicide and exert considerable copycat effect on at-risk individuals.
- It is commonly seen among teenagers and adolescents.

54. Ans. (b) Milnacipran

- Elderly patients are often sensitive to the hypotensive, sedative and anticholinergic effects of TCA, and this patient is at special risk for hypotension because of his carotid artery stenosis. Milnacipran is *least likely* to cause these side effects.
- It is a SNRI

55. Ans. (c) Depression

Ref: Comprehensive Clinical Psychiatry, Theodore, 2nd ed. pg. 221

- Depression is more commonly associated with frontal lobe lesions
- Left frontal lobe lesions are more commonly associated than the right frontal lobe.
- Depression occurs in 30 to 50% of stroke patients within two years of the event.
- Mania is less common and it occurs almost exclusively with right hemisphere lesions. Many of the patients who develop mania have a family history of affective disorders.

56. Ans. (d) Persistent depressive disorder

Ref: Harrison's, 19th ed. pg. 2706

- Persistent depressive disorder, also called dysthymia is a continuous long-term (chronic) form of depression.
- **Dysthymia** is, sometimes called **neurotic depression**, **dysthymic disorder**, or **chronic depression**, is a mood disorder consisting of the same cognitive and physical problems as in depression, with **less severe but longer-lasting symptoms.**

57. Ans. (c) Decreased serotonin and norepinephrine

Ref: Harrison 19th ed./2714-2715

- Depression is one of the mood disorders
- It is considered as second most common psychiatric disorder.
- Most commonly seen in middle age females. M:F ratio= 1:2
- ***Neurotransmitters involved are serotonin a NE and DA. All 3 are decreased. (Monoamine Hypothesis)***

Diagnostic Criteria of Depression

Major criteria	Minor criteria
Persistent sadness of mood	Loss of appetite
Loss of pleasure in activities	Sleep disturbance
Easy fatiguability	Decreased libido
	Decreased concentration
	Ideas of guilt, worthlessness, hopelessness
	Suicidal ideas

Depression Category on Basis of Severity

- Mild Depression : 2 major + 2 minor
- Moderate Depression : 2 major + 3 minor
- Severe Depression : 2 major + 4 minor

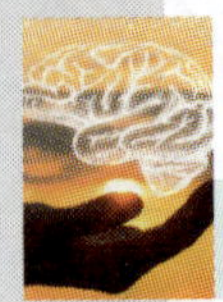

Extra Mile

Disease	Related Neurotransmitter
Alzheimer's disease	Acetyl choline decreased
Depression	Norepinephrine, Serotonin (5-HT) & dopamine are DECREASED
OCD	Serotonin (5 HT) decreased
Schizophrenia	Dopamine, Serotonin increased Glutamate decreased

58. Ans. (d) Serotonin and norepinephrine

Please refer to the previous answer for explanation.

59. Ans. (d) Depressed mood

Ref: Ahuja, 5th ed. pg. 81,109-110

- Masked depression means hidden depression which practically means that the patient is having a depression which manifests in somatic symptoms like vague body aches, bowel complaints and inability to carry out normal activities. However, the mood is not seems to be depressed.

60. Ans. (c) Depressive disorder

- DALY's is Disability Adjusted Life years.
- It is a measure of the burden of disease in a population and the effectiveness of the intervention.
- DALYs express years of life lost to premature death and years lives with disability adjusted for the severity of the disability.
- One DALY is "one lost year of healthy life"
- *According to Park 23rd ed. Most common cause of DALY's is depressive disorder.*

61. Ans. (c) Depressive disorder

Ref: Kaplan Synopsis 10th ed. pg. 528-30

- Most common psychiatric disorder and worldwide: **Anxiety disorders > depression**
- Female is most commonly affected as compared to males
- Depression is the most common psychiatric disorder associated with severe medical illness like hypothyroidism, cancer, AIDS, post MI, stroke, etc.

62. Ans. (c) Major depression

Ref: Harrison, 19th ed. pg. 2714

- Major depression is the second most common psychiatric disorder world wide & in India with highest life time prevelance (17%), ***most commonly involving middle (old) age females.*** Independent of culture or country, is *two fold greater prevalent in females than in males.*
- It is the most common psychiatric disorder associated with severe medical illness as myxedema (hypothyroidism, cancer, AIDS, post partum, post MI and post surgery etc.)
- In depression monoamine neurotransmitters (monoaminergic NTs) NE and serotonin (and dopamine also) are reduced.
- **For diagnosing major depression**
  - **>1 essential criteria**
    - Depressed/low mood
    - Loss of interest or pleasure
  - **>4 of the following for > same 2 weeks**
    - Appetite or weight loss
    - Sleep loss
    - Psychomotor activity (not meeting friends)
    - Concentration loss
    - Low energy (feeling of fatigue, weekness)
    - Feeling of worthlessness or guilt
    - Suicidal thoughts
- Patient given in the question fits in the critera:
- **1st criteria:** He has depressed mood and loss of interest or pleasure in dropping his daughter at school
- **In 2nd criteria**: Difficulty in sleeping, Not meeting with friends, decrease in energy.

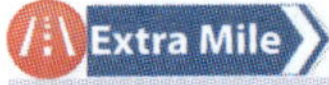

Extra Mile

MC psychiatric disorder is Anxiety spectrum disorders > depression

Ref: Harrison 19th ed. pg. 2708

63. Ans. (b) Major depressive disorder

Ref: Harrison, 19th ed. pg. 2714-15

Please refer to above explanation.

64. Ans. (a) Adjustment disorder

Ref: Kaplan & Sadock, 10th ed. pg. 790

- Adjustment disorder is a short-term condition that occurs when a person is *unable to cope with, or adjust to, a particular source of stress*, such as a major life change, loss, or event.

Diagnostic Criteria

- Development of emotional or behavior symptoms *in response to identifiable stressor (not of an unusual or catastrophic type),* ***occurring within 3 months of onset of stressor*** & does not persist for >6 months if stressor is terminated.
  - Marked distress that is in excess of what would be expected
  - Significant impairment in social or occupational life

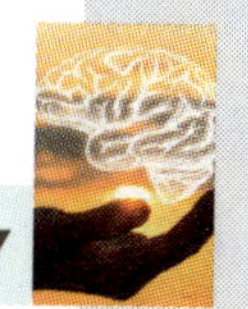

- *In this question, the examiner wanted us to mis-diagnose as severe depression, but the arousal of symptoms, i.e. within 3 months of stressor favours diagnosis of adjustment.*
- The type of stress that can trigger adjustment disorder varies depending on the person, but can include:
  - Ending of a relationship or marriage
  - Losing or changing job
  - **Death of a loved one** *(as seen in this case)*
  - Developing a serious illness (yourself or a loved one)
  - Being a victim of a crime
  - Having an accident
  - Undergoing a major life change *(such as getting married, having a baby, or retiring from a job)*
  - Living through a disaster, such as a fire, flood, or hurricane.
- A person with adjustment disorder develops emotional and/or behavioral symptoms as a reaction to a stressful event. ***These symptoms generally begin within three months of the event and rarely last for longer than six months after the event or situation.***
- Adjustment disorder is not the same as post-traumatic stress disorder (PTSD). *PTSD generally occurs as a reaction to a life-threatening event and tends to last longer.* Adjustment disorder, on the other hand, is *short-term*, rarely lasting longer than six months.

65. Ans. (d) Severe depression

Ref: Kaplan & Sadock, 10th ed. pg. 428

- Mood disorders (major depression) and alcohol dependence are two most common causes of suicide.
- Men **COMMIT** suicide four times as often as women. Women **ATTEMPT** suicide four times as often as men. Women usually take psychoactive substance while men use firearms.
- **Suicidal risk is much more in presence of following risk factors:**
  - *Early in illness* (than later), ***more commonly in men (than women) of middle or old age (>40 years).***
  - Single, separated, divorced, widowed, or recently bereaved, social isolation, unemployed.
  - *At the onset or end of depressive episode (i.e. depression in involution). Early* treatment particularly with SSRIs may increase suicidal feelings & attempts. As with other psychiatric patients, the months after discharge from a hospital are time of high risk. Subtherapeutic doses may increase risk.
- Presence of *marked haplessness.*
- At the peak of depression, the patient is either too retarded or depressed to commit suicide. *So, early stages of depression, during recovery (involution) from depression and 3 months period from recovery is high risk period for suicide.*

Suicide	
Biological factors • Decreased *central serotonin (5 HT)* plays an important role in suicide • Decreased concentrations of serotonin metabolite *5-HIAA in CSF*	Most important risk factors • Psychosis • Substance abuse • Personality disorder • Hypochondriac
Most important causes: • *Major depression* • *Substance abuse* • *Schizophrenia*	

66. Ans. (c) Psychogenic

Ref: Kaplan & Sadock 10th ed. pg. 693

- Most common cause of impotency in male is psychogenic.

67. Ans. (b) Derealisation

Ref: Kaplan and Sadocks 10th ed ch-20, Oxford Handbook of Psychiatry by davidSemple, Roger Smyth, Jonathan Burns pg. 372

68. Ans. (a) Anxiety

69. Ans. (a) Adjustment disorder

70. Ans. (a) Seasonal affective disorder

Ref: Principles and Practice of Psychopharmacotherapy by Pavuluri pg. 244

71. Ans. (c) ECT

Ref Kaplan Synopsis 10th ed. pg. 557

72. Ans. (b) 2 weeks

Ref: American Psychiatric Association, Diagnostic and Statistical Menual of Mental Disorders, 4/e

PERSONALITY DISORDER/OCD

73. Ans. (a) OCD

Ref: Kaplan and Sadock's, Comprehensive Textbook of Psychiatry, 10th ed. pg. 4576

- Many people with OCD engage in repetitive hand washing. This habit can become excessive, at times resulting in raw and broken skin.
- Specific to contamination-based OCD, signs include increased hand washing, soap being used up more, and frequent, long showers.

74. Ans. (a) Echolalia

Ref: Kaplan and Sadock's, Comprehensive Textbook of Psychiatry, 10th ed. pg. 3716

- **Echolalia** is the repetition or echoing of words or sounds that you hear someone else say.
- **Echolalia** is a feature of schizophrenia (especially the catatonic form).
- **Echopraxia:** The involuntary imitation of the movements of another person.
- Perseveration is the act of repeating something, such as words or actions, over and over again
- **Circumstantiality** is non-direct thinking or speech that digresses from the main point of a conversation.

75. Ans. (b) Psychiatrist

Ref: Kaplan and Sadock's, Comprehensive Textbook of Psychiatry, 10th ed. pg. 4600

- A trichobezoar is a mass of undigested hair within the gastrointestinal tract. Trichobezoars are often associated with trichotillomania (hair pulling), and trichophagia (hair swallowing).
- A psychiatrist can help in evaluating the exact cause of this disorder.

76. Ans. (d) Satyriasis

Ref: Kaplan and Sadock's, Comprehensive Textbook of Psychiatry, 10th ed. pg. 5047

- In men, hypersexuality is termed as satyriasis, while similar behavior in women was described as nymphomania.

77. Ans. (c) Obsessive compulsive disorder

Ref: Neeraj Ahuja 20th ed. pg. 95

- **Obsession:** An idea, impulse, image which intrudes into conscious awareness repeatedly.
  - Insight present, patient tried to resist but unable to which leads to distress.
- **Compulsion:** Form of behavior usually follows obsession, aim at preventing or neutralizing distress arising from obsession, insight present so patient realizes irrationality of compulsion.

ICD 10 Classifies OCD

- Predominantly obsession thoughts
- Predominantly compulsion acts
- Mixed obsessional thoughts and acts

Examples

- **Washers:** Commonest type e.g., obsession of contamination and compulsion is washing it.
- **Checkers:** Person have multiple doubts e.g. door has not been locked and compulsion is checking repeatedly to remove doubts.

78. Ans. (b) Generalised anxiety disorder

Ref: https://www.nhs.uk/conditions/generalised-anxiety-disorder/

Anxiety is a feeling of unease, such as worry or fear, that can be mild or severe.

Anxiety is the main symptom of several conditions, Including:
- Panic disorder
- Phobias, such as agoraphobia or claustrophobia
- Post-traumatic stress disorder (PTSD)
- Social anxiety disorder (social phobia)

79. Ans. (a) Agoraphobia

- Agoraphobia is a fear of being in situations where escape might be difficult or that help wouldn't be available if things go wrong.
- Someone with agoraphobia may be scared of: travelling on public transport, visiting a shopping centre, leaving home.

80. Ans. (b) Hypochondriac disorder

Ref: Handbook of outpatient treatment of adults: Non psychotic mental disorder; pg. 300

- **Hypochondriasis** is a condition in which a person is inordinately worried about having a serious illness. The person is preoccupied with thoughts of a serious life threatening diagnosis or medical illness.
- **Somatoform pain:** Only pain of one location of long standing duration.
- **Conversion disorder:** Anxiety due to conflict.

81. Ans. (a) Autism

Ref: Textbook of Autism Spectrum Disorders, edited by Eric Hollander e.g. al; pg. 99-102

- **Autism:** Impairment in social communication and interaction, language development delay, restrictive repetitive stereotyped behavior.
- **ADHD:** Child is hyperactive, impulsive, attention deficit.

82. Ans. (c) Fluoxetine

- The drugs of choice for OCD are SSRI
  - **SSRIs:** *Fluoxetine, Fluvoxamine, Paroxetine, Sertraline, Citalopram, Escitalopram*
- Exposure and Response Prevention is a part of cognitive and behavior therapy for OCD.

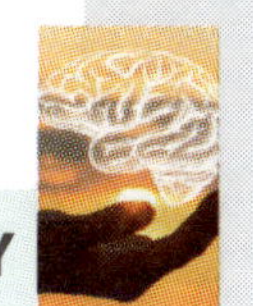

- Combination of behavior therapy & drug therapy gives best results for treatment of OCD.

83. Ans. (b) OCD

- O.C.D does not arise from any cognition bias but a goal directed dysfunction that interacts with anxiety and irrational belief. They cannot exert necessary control over their actions to realize this goal.

84. Ans. (b) Dissociation

Ref: Ahuja 5th ed. pg. 213

- Dissociation is a neurotic/immature defence mechanism characterized by involuntary splitting or suppression of a mental function or a group of mental function from rest of the personality in a manner that allows expression of forbidden unconscious impulses without having any sense of responsibility for actions.

85. Ans. (c) Operant conditioning

Ref: PubMed

- B.F. Skinner (1904–1990) is often referred to as the **father of operant conditioning.** This conditioning is based on behavioural change with reinforcement or punishment.

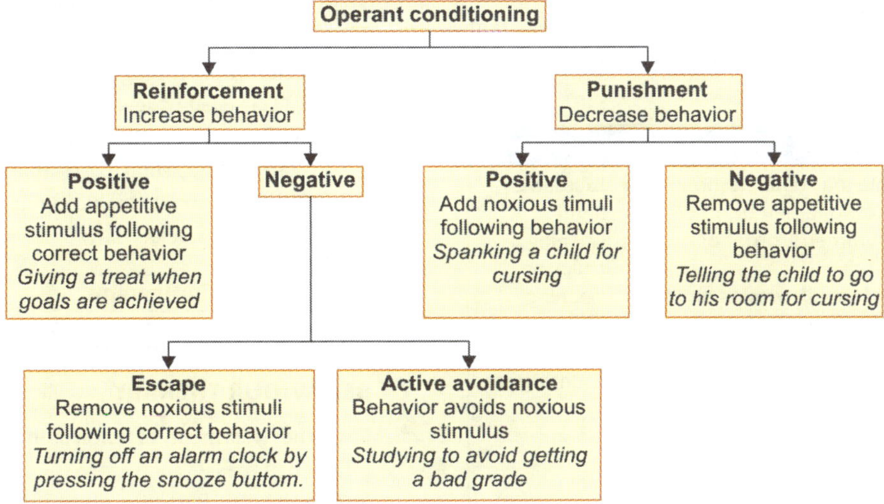

Note: *Classical conditioning differs from operant or instrumental conditioning: in classical conditioning, behavioral responses are elicited by antecedent stimuli (e.g: chocolate wrapper stimulate salivation), whereas in operant conditioning behaviors are strengthened or weakened by their consequences (i.e., reward or punishment).*

86. Ans. (b) Mania

Ref: Kaplan & Sadock, 10th ed. pg. 2717

DSM- IV Diagnostic Criteria of Mania

- Abnormally & persistently elevated, expansive, or irritable mood lasting for at least 1 week or any duration, if requires hospitalization.
- **> 3 are needed**
  - Inflated self esteem or grandiosity
  - Decreased need for sleep ($\leq$ 3 hours)
  - More talkative or pressure to keep talking
  - Flight of ideas or subjective experience that thoughts are racing
  - Distractibility (i.e. attention to easily drawn to unimportant or irrelevant external stimuli)
  - Increase in goal-directed activity (social spiritual religious, sexual) or psychomotor agitation
  - Excessive involvement in pleasurable activities *(eg. unrestrained buying sprees, foolish business investments, donations or sexual indiscretions)* that have a high potential for painful consequences.

Why Mania: This patients satisfies the criteria and his conditions fits into it.

- The patient is irritable for 10 days (i.e. criteria A-abnormally & persistently elevated mood for atleast 1 week). There are $\geq$ 3 criteria B features: increased sexual indulgence & alcohol consumption *(excessive involvement*

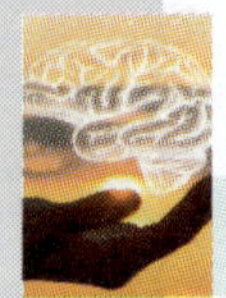

in pleasureable activity), decreased need for sleep and career oriented prolonged work without getting tired.

87. Ans. (c) Heightened concentration

Please refer to above explanation

88. Ans. (a) Ego dystonic

Ref: Kaplan & Sadock 10th ed. pg. 279

- The idea in OCD is Egodystonic or ego-alien (foreign to one's own personality), NOT ego syntonic.
- Persons with OCD are stubborn, rigid, overconscious, scrupulous & inflexible about matters of morality & ethics (not indecisive).
- ***Shows perfection that interferes with task completion***
- Is excessively devoted to work and productivity to the exclusion of leisure activities & friendships. Is reluctant to delegated task or work to others. Adopts a miserly spending style.

Obsession	Compulsion
• Fear something terrible may happen (fire, death, or illness of loved one, self or others • Concern or need for symmetry, order or exactness • Concern or disgust with bodily wastes or secretion (urine, stool, saliva), dirt, germs, environmental toxins • Scrupulosity (excessive praying or religious concerns out of keeping with patients background) • Forbidden or perverse sexual thoughts, images or impulses • Believes in Luck & unlucky numbers. • Intrusive nonsense sounds, words or music	• Excessive hand washing, checking, cleaning, ordering, arranging, counting etc.

89. Ans. (b) Exposure and response prevention

Ref: Harrison, 19th ed. pg. 2713

Exposure and Response Prevention is a part of cognitive and behavior therapy for OCD.

MANAGEMENT OF OBSESSIVE COMPULSIVE DISORDER

Behaviour Therapy (BT)

- ***It is treatment of choice for OCD***
- Exposure & response prevention is the preferred & principal approach. It is most effective in obsessional rituals (i.e. compulsions)
- In this form of therapy, the patient is asked to endure, in a graduated manner, the anxiety that a specific obsessional fear provokes while refraining from compulsions that allay (reduce) that anxiety. The principle behind success of treatment are based on habituation based on response prevention.

Pharmacotherapy

- The drug of choice for OCD are SSRI or clomipramine (2nd drug of choice)
  - **SSRI's**
    - ***FLUXOETINE, FLUVOXAMINE, PAROXETINE, SERTRALINE, CITALOPRAM, ESCITALOPRAM***
- Combination of behavior therapy & drug therapy gives best results for treatment of OCD.
- **Clomipramine:** It is the most selective for serotonin reuptake versus norepinephrine re-uptake & exceeds in the respect only by SSRI's.
- **2nd line drugs:** If treatment with SSRIs or clomipramine is unsuccessful, valproate lithium or carbamazepine are used.

Psychotherapy

- To treat OCD, Psychoanalytic prolonged insight oriented or exploratory & interpretative psychotherapy is used in educated & psychologically oriented patients.
  - **ECT:** is used in severe depression with OCD
  - **Psychosurgery:** It is indicated only for most chronic, treatment resistant cases that have resisted (IPD or OPD) treatment (including drug of behavior therapy) for at least a year.

90. Ans. (a) Behavior therapy

Ref: Kaplan & Sadock, 10th ed. pg. 605

BEHAVIOUR THERAPY

It is the treatment of choice in phobia, which may of following types

- *Exposure & Response prevention is 1st line of behavior therapy*
- Flooding (implosion or intensive exposure)
- Systemic desensitization: Progressive exposure to anxiety evoking stimulus .
- Relaxation techniques

Medications

- Anxiolytic drugs
- Tricyclic antidepressant
- SSRI
- MAO inhibitors

COVERT SENSITIZATION

- It is an aversion therapy, used for the treatment of conditions which are pleasant but undersirable. Eg. Alcohol dependence, and sexual deviations like homosexuality & transvestism etc.
- The main aim of aversion therapy is pairing of pleasant stimulus with an unpleasant response so that pleasant stimulus becomes unpleasant by association.

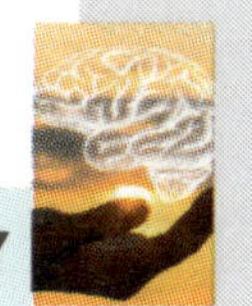

91. Ans. (c) Exposure and response prevention followed by systemic desensitization

Ref: Harrison, 19th ed. pg. 2712-13

BEHAVIOR THERAPY

- It is the treatment of choice in phobic disorders and several other psychiatric illness. Exposure and response prevention followed by systemic desensitization behavior therapy is the treatment of choice in phobia. It can be of following types:
- Exposure & Response prevention is **1st line of behavior therapy**
- Systemic desensitization: progressive exposure to anxiety evoking stimulus *(2nd line)*
- Flooding (implosion or intensive exposure)
- Relaxation techniques

92. Ans. (b) Early age of onset

Good prognostic factors	Poor prognostic factors
• Acute or abrupt onset • Typical clinical features • Severe depression • Well-adjusted premorbid personality • Good response to treatment	• Co-morbid medical disorder, personality disorder or alcohol dependence • Double depression (acute depressive episode superimposed on chronic depression or dysthymia) • Catastrophic stress or chronic ongoing stress • Unfavourable early environment and *early age of onset* • Marked hypochondriacal features, or mood incongruent psychotic features • Poor drug compliance

93. Ans. (a) Bipolar disorder

Ref: Harrison, 19th ed. pg. 2717

- **DOC for prophylaxis of bipolar disorder- Lithium**
- DOC for acute mania: Benzodiazepines atypical antipsychotic + Lithium
- Lithium can also be used in treatment of neutropenia, Cluster headache and major depression episodes.
- **Therapeutic level of lithium: 0.6–1.5 mEq/L**
- **Toxicity seen after >1.5 mEq/L**
- Most common side effect of lithium: Coarse tremor
- **Side effects of lithium (Mn: LITTH)**
  - Leukocytosis
  - Insipidus (DI)
  - Tremor, teratogenic (MC-Ebstein anomaly)
  - Hypothyroidism
- Lithium is contraindicated in pregnancy. It can cause congenital heart defect- **Ebstein anomaly.**

94. Ans. (c) Phenytoin sodium

Ref: Harrison, 19th ed. pg. 2718, 4665e-2

- Lithium has traditionally been the drug of choice for the treatment of manic episode (acute phase) as well as for prevention of further episodes in bipolar mood disorder. It has also been used in treatment of depression with less success.
- Antipsychotics are an important adjunct in the treatment of mood disorder. The commonly used drugs include risperidone, obnzapine, quetiapine, haloperidol, and aripiprazole.

The other mood stabilizers which are used in the treatment of bipolar mood disorders include

- Sodium valproate
- Carbamazepine and Oxacarbazepine
- Benzodiazepines Lorazepm (IV and orally) and clonazepam
- Lamotrigine
- Topiramate

95. Ans. (c) Borderline

Ref: Harrison, 19th ed. pg. 2720

Personality disorders and their clinical manifestation:

- **Borderline:** Pervasive pattern of unstable and intense interpersonal relationship, difficulty in controlling anger hence avoids meeting people.
- **Paranoid:** Generalized mistrust and suspiciousness
- **Schizoid:** Markedly detached from others. Excessive preoccupation with fantasy and introspection and emotional coldness.

96. Ans. (a) Menorrhagia

Ref: Harrison, 17th ed. pg. 471-7

Amenorrhea ***(and not menorrhagia)*** **is seen in 100% patients** of anorexia nervosa. It is a mandatory finding diagnostic criterion to be fulfilled for anorexia nervosa.

	Anorexia nervosa	Bulimia nervosa
Feature	Refusal to maintain body weight above a minimal normal	Irresistible craving for food with episodes of over eating in less time (Binge eating)
Method of weight control		Attempts to counter act the effects of over eating by self-induced vomiting: • Purgative abuse, • Periods of starvations • Appetite suppressants

Contd...

	Anorexia nervosa	Bulimia nervosa
Ritualised excercise	Common	Rare
Amenorrhea	**100%**	50%
Decreased Vitals ↓ BP, ↓ Pulse	**Common**	Uncommon
Hypothermia	**Common**	Rare
Skin changes (Hirsutism)	**Common**	Rare
Medical Complications	Hypokalemia Cardiac arrythmias	Hypokalemia Cardiac arrythmias

97. Ans. (c) Dissociative fugue

DISSOCIATIVE FUGUE

- Dissociative fugue is characterized by *episodes of wandering away (usually away from home)*. During the episode, the person usually *adopts a new identity* with *complete amnesia for the earlier life*. The onset is usually sudden, often in the presence of severe stress. The termination too is abrupt and is followed by amnesia for the episode, but with recovery of memories of earlier life.

MULTIPLE PERSONALITY (DISSOCIATIVE IDENTITY) DISORDER

- In this dissociative disorder, the person is dominated by two or more personalities, of which only one is being manifest at a time. These personalities are usually different, at times even opposing.

POST-TRAUMATIC STRESS DISORDER

- Arises as a delayed and/protracted response to an exceptionally stressful or catastrophic life event or situation, which is likely to cause pervasive distress in 'almost any person' (e.g. disasters, war, rape or torture, serious accident). The symptoms of PTSD may develop, after a period of latency, within six months after the stress or maybe delayed beyond this period
- PTSD is characterized be recurrent and intrusive recollections of the stressful event either in flashbacks or in dreams.

98. Ans. (c) Body dysmorphic disorder

- Body dysmorphic disorder is a somatoform disorder, wherein the affected person is concerned with body image
- It manifests as excessive concern about and preoccupation with a perceived defect of their physical features.
- The person is under an impression that they have a defect in either one feature or several features of their body, which causes psychological distress that causes clinically significant distress or impairs occupational or social functioning.
- *This condition co-exists with emotional depression and anxiety, social withdrawal or social isolation.*

99. Ans. (a) Response prevention

Ref: Kaplan and Sadocks 10th ed. pg. 953

100. Ans. (b) Impulse control disorder

Ref: Kaplan and Sadocks 10th ed. pg. 25

101. Ans. (a) Personality disorder

102. Ans. (a) Agoraphobia

103. Ans. (a) Ego dystonic

- *Ego-syntonic* refer to instincts or ideas that are *acceptable* to self and compatible with one's values and ways of thinking. Example for a thief, stealing would be considered ego-syntonic. Another such example is anorexia nervosa.
- *Ego-dystonic* refers to behaviour, ideas which are distressing, *unacceptable* or to one's self concept. Example millionaire thinking of begging for food or obsessive compulsive disorder.

DELIRIUM, DEMENTIA AND ALZHEIMER'S DISEASE

104. Ans. (a) Delirium

Ref: Delirium: Acute Confusional State, pg. 85

- Hallucinations in any sensory modality may occur in delirium, but the visual ones are the most common.
- Commonly seen in post op patients.

105. Ans. (c) Delirium

Ref: Kaplan's Textbook of Psychiatry Ch 10.2

- Delirium is the most common psychiatric condition seen in medico-surgical patient.

TABLE: Delirium incidence and prevalence in different scenarios

Population	Prevalence Range (%)	Incidence Range (%)
General medical inpatients	10–30	3–16
Medical and surgical inpatients	5–15	10–55
General surgical inpatients	N/A	9–15 postoperatively
Critical care unit patients	16	16–83
Cardiac surgery inpatients	16–34	7–34

Contd...

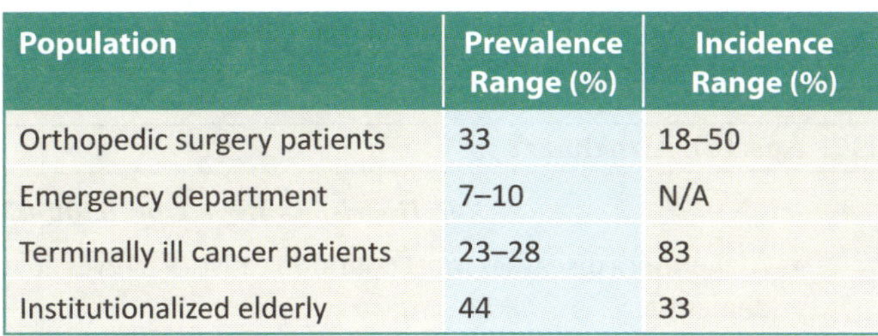

Population	Prevalence Range (%)	Incidence Range (%)
Orthopedic surgery patients	33	18–50
Emergency department	7–10	N/A
Terminally ill cancer patients	23–28	83
Institutionalized elderly	44	33

106. Ans. (a) Delirium

Ref: Kaplan's Textbook of Psychiatry Ch 12.2

- Delirium is also known as organic brain syndrome/acute brain failure/cerebral insufficiency.
- Delirium is occasionally termed to denote the acute form organic mental syndrome. It is most common organic mental disorder seen in clinical practice.

107. Ans. (b) Delirium

Ref: Harrison, 19th ed. pg. 166

DELIRIUM

- It is characterized by global impairment of consciousness *(clouding of consciousness)*, resulting in reduced levels of alertness, attention & perception of environment along with acute onset of fluctuating cognitive impairment.
- It is the commonest organic mental disorder

Clinical Features & Diagnosis

- Global impairment of consciousness & attention is the hallmark/cardinal feature of Delirium. It manifests as:
  - Diminished ability to focus, sustain or shift attention.
  - Reduced levels of alertness, attention, and perception of environment.
  - Drowsiness (mental slowness), distractibility & disorientation.
- Global impairment of cognition is manifested as:
  - Disorientation (in time, place and person)
  - *Disturbance of immediate & recent memory*
  - *Remote memory is intact.*

108. Ans. (d) Organic brain syndrome

ORGANIC BRAIN SYNDROME

- It is also known as organic brain disease which is decreased mental function due to a medical disease, other than a psychiatric illness.
- Cognitive or higher mental functions *(i.e. consciousness, orientation & abstract thinking)* are impaired in organic brain syndrome.

109. Ans. (b) Loss of consciousness

Ref: Harrison, 19th ed. pg. 170, 173

- Impairment of higher mental function is noted in case of dementia, but there is NO impairment of consciousness.
- Impairments in dementia *(Mn: A Thinking Memorable Intelligent Judge Can't be Impulsive)*
  - Abstract thinking
  - Memory *(recent > remote)*
  - Intellectual function
  - Judgment
  - Continence (fecal & urinary)
  - Impulse control (catastrophic reaction)
  - Personality & personal care
- Memory impairment (ex. Forgetfulness) is typically an early & prominent feature in dementia
- No matter how severe the dementia, patients show no impairment in their level of consciousness.
- Hallucinations & Delusion can occur in 20–40% of patients with dementia.

Feature of Cortical & Subcortical Dementia

Features	Cortical Dementia	Subcortical Dementia
Site	Cortex (frontal, parietal, temporal, occipital, hippocampus)	Subcortical grey matter
Memory impairment	• Severe, early • Recall helped very little by cues	• Mild to moderate • Recall helped partially by cues & recognization tasks
Mathematical skills	• Impaired early (Acalculia)	• Preserved
Language	• Early, Dysphasia (Aphasia)	• Normal & Anomia (in severe cases)
Speech	• Articulate until late	• Dysarthria
Personality	• Indifferent	• Apathetic, inert

Etiology of Dementia

1. Decreased level of NE in locus cereuleus
2. Decreased level of Acetylcholine in Nucleus basalis of meynert
3. In moderate to severe dementia: *Increased* level of Glutamate.

110. Ans. (b) Trauma

Ref: Harrison, 19th ed. pg. 173

- Dementia Pugilistica is also known as punch drunk syndrome. It is a form of dementia usually secondary to some trauma to head.

ALZHEIMER'S DISEASE

- Alzheimer's disease, the most common cause of dementia.

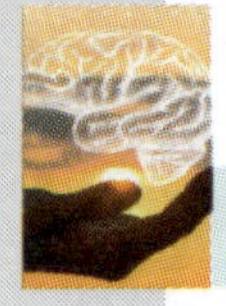

- It initially presents with minor forgetfulness & gradually progressive short term memory loss
- The memory is lost for recent events first with a delayed loss of long term memory mainly affecting episodic memory.
- **Feature of Alzheimer dementia are**
  - *Memory impairment without impairment of consciousness*
  - Aphasia: Language disturbace
  - Apraxia: Impaired ability to carry out motor activities despite intact motor function
  - Agnosia: Failure to recognize or identify objects despite intact sensory function
  - Agnosia: Failure to recognize or identify objects despite intact sensory function
  - Anosognosia *(Unware of his problem)*, Prosopognosia *(difficulty in identifying known faces)*
  - Disturbance in executive functioning (i.e planning organizing, sequencing, abstracting)
  - Focal neurological signs (ex asymmetrical hyper-reflexia or weakness)

Extra Mile

Neuropathological findings of Alzheimer's disease

Gross	Microscopic
• Diffuse atrophy with flattened cortical sulci & enlarged cerebral ventricles	• Senile (Amyloid) plaques • *Neurofibrilary tangles* • Neuronal – loss (especially in cortex & hippocampus) • Synaptic loss • Granulovascular degeneration of the neurons

Remember

Neurofibrillary tangles are not unique to Alzheimer's disease but also occur in Down's syndrome, Dementia pugilistica (punch-drunk syndrome), Parkinson dementia complex.

111. Ans. (a) Biperidin

Ref: Harrison, 19th ed. pg. 2601-02

- Alzheimer's disease is most common cause of dementia.
- Cause → Decreased level of Ach in nucleus basalis of meynert

Drugs Used in the Treatment of Alzheimer's are:

- Acetycholine esterase inhiitors: (It increases Ach level)
  - Donepezil
  - Tacrine (Hepatotoxic; not used)
  - Galantamine
- **Rivastigmine:** Carbamate derivative of physostigmine
- **Memantine:** NMDA glutaminergic antagonist
- Biperidin is an anti cholinergic drug used to treat parkinsonism.

112. Ans. (b) Alzheimer's

Ref: Harrison's 18th ed. pg. 3300-07

- Alzheimer's disease is most common cause of irreversible dementia.

TABLE: Reversible vs irreversible dementia

Reversible	Irreversible
• Vitamin deficiency ▪ B1- Wernicke's ▪ B12- SCID ▪ Nicotinic acid- Pellagra	Alzheimer's
Endocrine ***(Hypothyroidism,*** *adrenal insufficiency, cushing's)*	Vascular dementia (Multi-infarct)
• Head trauma and diffuse brain damage • Haemorrhage-*subdural, epidural, normal pressure hydrocephalus*	Leucoencephalopathy
Primary metastatic brain tumor	Metabolic disorder *(Wilson's disease, Leigh disease, Leucodystrophy)*
• Toxic dementia ***(MCC of reversible dementia)***	Degenerative disorder 1. *Parkinsonism* 2. *Pick's disease* 3. *Prion's disease,* 4. *Multiple sclerosis* 5. *Huntington's disease* 6. *Diffuse lewy body dementia*

113. Ans. (c) Kraepelin

Ref: Kaplan 10th ed. pg. 467

114. Ans. (d) Organic brain syndrome

115. Ans. (b) Trauma

116. Ans. (a) Depression

Ref: Kaplan and Sadock's Synopsis of Psychiatry: Behavioral Sciences Clinical Psychiatry 10th ed. /339, Table 10.3-11

SUBSTANCE ABUSE

117. Ans. (d) Delirium tremens

Ref: Kaplan and Sadock's, Comprehensive Textbook of Psychiatry, 10th ed. pg. 6721

- Delirium tremens is a severe form of alcohol withdrawal. It involves sudden and severe mental or nervous system changes manifested by altered mental status,

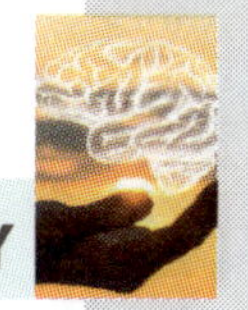

global confusion and sympathetic overdrive, which can progress to cardiovascular collapse.

118. Ans. (a) Tremors

Ref: Kaplan and Sadock's, Comprehensive Textbook of Psychiatry, 10th ed. pg. 6721

- Alcohol withdrawal symptoms occur when patients stop drinking or significantly decrease their alcohol intake after long-term dependence.
- Earliest symptom of alcohol withdrawal is tremors.
- Withdrawal has a broad range of symptoms from mild tremors to a condition called delirium tremens, which results in seizures and could progress to death if not recognized and treated promptly.

119. Ans. (c) I/V Thiamine + Lorazepam

Ref: Kaplan and Sadock's, Comprehensive Textbook of Psychiatry, 10th ed. pg. 7634

- The hallmark of management for severe symptoms is the administration of benzodiazepines.
- The most commonly used benzodiazepines are intravenous diazepam or intravenous lorazepam for management.
- Due to the risk of a comorbid condition called Wernicke-Korsakoff syndrome, thiamine is also given to the patients.

120. Ans. (a) Cocaine

Ref: Kaplan and Sadock's, Comprehensive Textbook of Psychiatry, 10th ed. pg. 3252

- Cocaine is an addictive stimulant drug. It can be snorted, injected, or smoked.
- Some other names for cocaine include: coke, blow, powder, crack
- Cocaine has NET inhibitory property, due to which there is increased level of noradrenaline which causes symptoms like tachycardia or arrhythmia. It also produces a tactile hallucination where patient feels like a bug crawling under the skin (cocaine bug), which prompts the patient to scratch the skin.

121. Ans. (b) Alcohol withdrawal delirium

Ref: Neeraj Ahuja 20th ed. pg. 38

Delirium Tremens

- It is a most severe alcohol withdrawal syndrome.
- It is usually seen 2–4 days after complete abstinence of alcohol.

Characterized by

- Disorientation of time, place
- Insomnia
- Visual hallucination, illusion, Tactile hallucination of insects.
- Dehydration with electrolyte imbalance.
- Psychomotor ataxia, agitation
- Marked autonomic disturbance.

Alcoholic Seizures

- Generalized tonic-clonic seizure seen in some alcoholic dependent patient.
- It occurs 12–48 hours after a heavy bout of drinking.

Alcoholic Hallucination

- Occurs during partial or complete abstinence of alcohol and it persist even after alcohol withdrawal syndrome is over.

122. Ans. (c) Fomepizole

Ref: Safe and Effective Medication use in Emergency Department, By Victor Cohen; pg. 120

- The primary antidotal treatment of methanol or ethylene glycol involves blocking alcohol dehydrogenase, this enzyme is inhibited by fomepizole or ethanol.

123. Ans. (a) Aversion therapy

Ref: Principles of Addiction Medicine; pg. 843

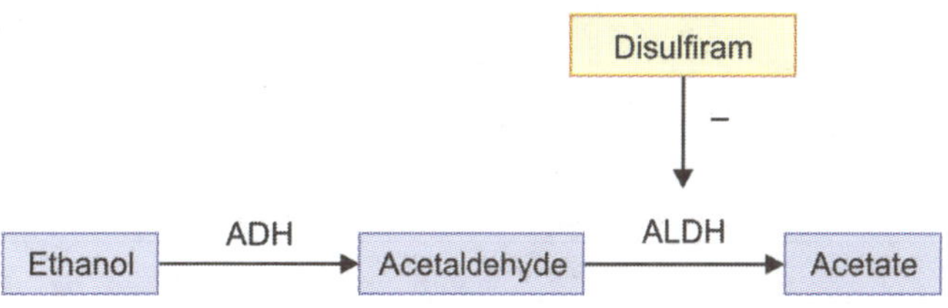

- Disulfiram acts by inhibiting aldehyde dehydrogenase, which causes accumulation of acetaldehyde.
- This accumulation of acetaldehyde leading to distressing symptoms like hot flushes, pulsatile headache, respiratory difficulty, nausea, vomiting, sweating, orthostatic syncope, chest pain, hypotension, confusion and blurred vision.
- This particular reaction produces aversion from intake of alcohol.

Anticraving medication: Naltrexone, acamprosate, baclofen, fluoxetine, topiramate.

124. Ans. (d) Flunitrazepam

Ref: Harrisons, 19th ed. pg. 469e1; PubMed

- **Flunitrazepam (Rohypnol)** is a tasteless, odorless benzodiazepine derivative primarily used to treat insomnia, but it has significant abuse potential because of its strong hypnotic, anxiolytic, and amnesia-producing effects. It is a club drug commonly referred to as a **"date-rape drug" or "roofies."**

- Earlier, it was used in some countries to treat severe insomnia and in fewer, early in anesthesia.
- **Mechanism of action:** The drug enhances GABAA receptor activity.
- **Toxicity/overdose:** Treated with **flumazenil**, a benzodiazepine receptor antagonist.

Extra Mile

- Commonly abused club drugs include flunitrazepam, GHB (Gamma Hydroxybutyrate), and ketamine
- GHB and ketamine can be identified in blood.
- Flunitrazepam can be identified in urine and hair samples.

125. Ans. (b) Cannabis

Ref: Pub Med

TABLE: Common abused substances and their slang names

Abused substance	Slang names
Cannabis/Marijuana	Aunt mary/Dope/Ganja/Grass/Green/ Joint/Pot/weed
Cocaine	Coke/snow/toot/coca
Heroin	Brown sugar/china white/Dope/Junk/Hell dust/Smack
LSD	Acid/Blotters/Blue heaven/micro dots/ yellow sunshine
Hashish	Boom/Gangster/Hash/hemp
Phencyclidine (PCP)	Angel dust/Boat/Peace pill/Sherm

126. Ans. (a) Occasional use with long absistence

Ref: Neeraj Ahuja, 7th ed. pg. 49

- The textbook quotes: *"Although tolerance as well as psychological dependence can occur with LSD use, no physical dependence or withdrawal syndrome is reported. A common pattern of LSD use is a trip **(occasional use followed by a long term period of abstinence)**".*

127. Ans. (c) Bradycardia

Ref: Harrison, 19th ed. pg. 2727

- The symptoms which arises when an alcoholic reduces or stops alcohol consumption after prolonged periods of excessive alcohol intake.
- *In case of alcohol withdrawal there is hallucinations,, tremors, sweating and tachycardia, NOT bradycardia.*
- **Clinical presentation**
  - Hangover next morning: *Most common withdrawal syndrome*
  - Mild tremors *(Most Common symptom)*
  - Nausea, vomiting
  - Weakness, insomnia, anxiety
  - Delirium tremens: Most severe withdrawal syndrome
  - Alcoholic seizures (Rum fits)
  - Alcoholic hallucinosis

TABLE: Appearance of Alcohol withdrawal symptoms

Time	Symptoms
6–12 hours	Minor withdrawal symptoms: Insomnia, tremulousness, anxiety, GIT upset, headache, diaphoresis, palpitations, anorexia
12–24 hours	Alcoholic hallucinosis; visual, auditory, or tactile hallucination
24–48 hours	*Withdrawal seizures:* Generalized tonic-clonic seizures
48–72 hours	Derlirium tremens; visual hallucinations, disorientation, *tachycardia*, hypertension, low-grade fever, agitation, diaphoresis

128. Ans. (d) 24–48 hours after cessation of alcohol

Ref: Harrison, 19th ed. pg. 2727

129. Ans. (a) Severity of respiratory and CNS depression

Ref: Harrison, 19th ed. pg. 2727

- CNS depression predisposes to chances of aspiration due to suppression of airway defence mechanisms. Hence it is the most important parameter determining hospitalization in acute intoxication of any etiology.

Acute Alcohol intoxication:

- After a brief period excitation, there is a generalized central nervous system depression with alcohol use.
- With increasing intoxication, there is increased reaction time, slowed thinking, distractibility and poor motor control.
- Later, dysarthria, ataxia and incoordination can occur. There is progressive loss of self control with frank disinhibited behavior.
- The duration of intoxication depends on the amount and the rapidity of ingestion of alcohol. Usually the signs of intoxication are obvious with blood levels of 150–200 mg %. With blood alcohol levels of 300–450 mg % increasing drowsiness followed by coma and respiratory depression develop.

130. Ans. (c) Cocaine

Ref: Harrison, 19th ed. pg. 469e-1

- Cannabis and its products contain (-) D-9 TetraHydro Coannabinol (Δ9-THC).
- It is obtained from Indian hemp plant known as cannabis Sativa.
- Different parts of plants have different product:
  - Dried leaves: *Bhang*

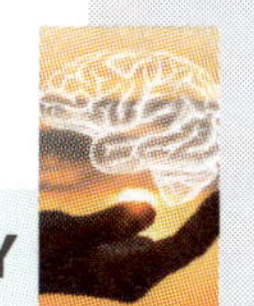

- Dried female inflorescence: *Ganja*
- Resinous extract from flowering tops: *Charas /Hashish*
- *Marijuana/Marihuana: Other name for cannabis*

- In case of cannabis abuse there is an episode of acute violent behavior for which the person claims amnesia. This is known as ***Run Amok.***

Extra Mile

Substance	Characteristic clinical feature
• Cocaine	Magnus symptoms (cocaine bugs or Tactile hallucination)
• Cannabis	• Run Amok • Amotivation syndrome • Flashbacks
• Alcohol	• Mc-Evan's sign Morbid jealousy
• LSD	• Bad Trips • Flash backs
• Amphetamine	Paranoid Halucinatory syndrome (like paranoid schizophrenia)
• Phencyclidine (Angel dust)	Dissociative anesthesia

131. Ans. (a) Smoking

Ref: Harrison, 19th ed. pg. 17, 266e-4

- **Alcohol is the most common substance abused in India and worldwide.**
- **Early and rapid addiction has been seen with SMOKING**
- **Most common illicit drug/substance abused: Cannabis > Amphetamine (2nd MC).**
- **Nicotine (tobacco/smoking):** Highly addictive and heavily used drug/substance

132. Ans. (d) LSD

Ref: Harrison, 19th ed. pg. 469e-4

- LSD intoxication causes *bad trips*, which is acute panic reaction in which the individual experience a loss of control over his self.
- Spontaneous recurrence of LSD, or sometimes cannabis use experience even during a withdrawal state is known as *Flash back.*

133. Ans. (b) 21–34

Ref: O.P. Ghai 8th ed./584-85

Categories of mental retardation based on IQ levels

Mental retardation	IQ range
Mild MR	50-69
Moderate MR	35-49
Severe MR	21-34
Profound MR	20 or below

Contd...

134. Ans. (c) Alcohol addiction

135. Ans. (d) LSD

136. Ans. (b) Piloerection

Ref: Kaplan and Sadock's Synopsis of Psychiatry 10/e, chapter 12.10

CHILD PSYCHIATRY

137. Ans. (c) Conduct disorder

Ref: Neeraj Ahuja 20th ed. pg. 167

- **Conduct disorder (CD)** in which basic rules of others are violated and rules of the society not followed.
- Diagnosis only when Conduct is far in excess of the routine mischief of children and adolescents.
- Age of onset before 18 year of age.

Symptoms

- Frequent lying
- Robbery
- Running away from home and school
- Cruel towards others and animals
- Physical violence like rape, assault, use of weapons etc.

Subtypes

- Conduct Disorder Confined to family context
- Unsocialized CD
- Socialized CD
- Oppositional defiant disorder.

138. Ans. (c) Specific learning disorder

Ref: https://www.churchillstl.org/learning-disabili tv-resources/specific-learning-disabilities/

- A specific learning disability is a disorder that interferes with a student's ability to listen, think, speak, write, spell, or do mathematical calculations.
- Students with a specific learning disability may struggle with reading, writing, or math.

139. Ans. (d) 35–49

140. Ans. (d) Respiratory failure

Ref: Nelson's 18/e, chapter 599

141. Ans. (a) Mild

Ref: Current Diagnosis and Treatment in Osychiatry pg. 543

RADIOLOGY

19

MOST RECENT QUESTIONS 2023

1. Which investigation is best for diagnosis of the following presentation? ***(Most Recent Question July 2023)***

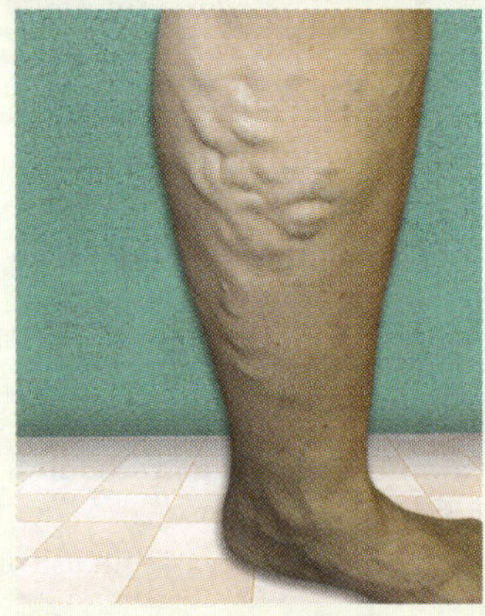

a. Plethysmography
b. MRI
c. CT
d. Duplex imaging

2. The following instrument is used to evaluate: ***(Most Recent Question July 2023)***

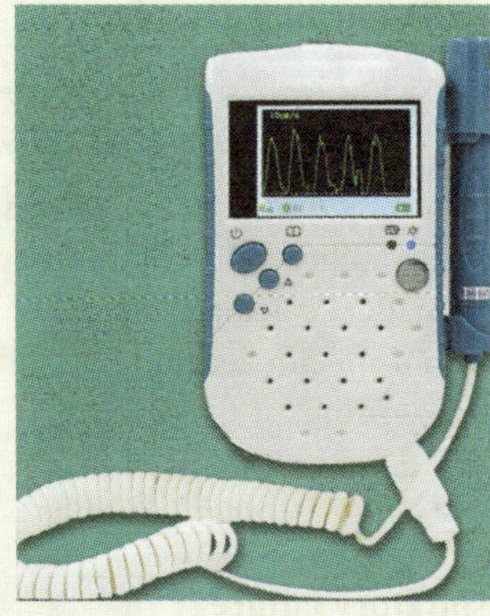

a. Regional Lymphatic flow
b. Nerve conduction velocity
c. Blood flow velocity
d. Thickness of artery

3. A 30-year-old female patient presents with chills and rigors. She has severe pain in right flank region with tenderness noted at costovertebral angle. X-ray abdomen was done in emergency department. What is the diagnosis? ***(Most Recent Question July 2023)***

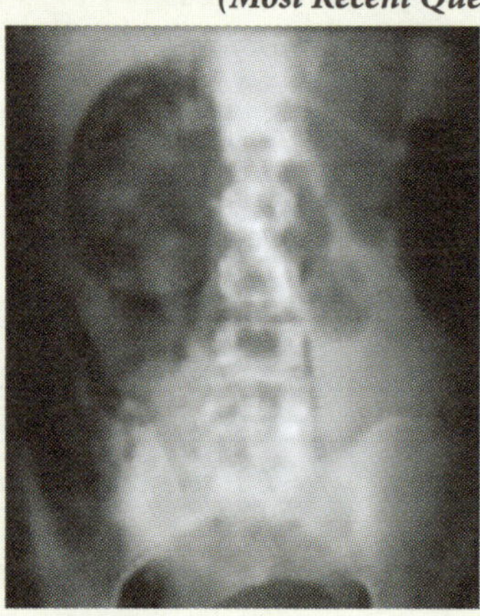

a. Papillary necrosis
b. Renal Tuberculosis
c. Acute tubular necrosis
d. Emphysematous pyelonephritis

4. Comment on the diagnosis from the following radiograph: ***(Most Recent Question July 2023)***

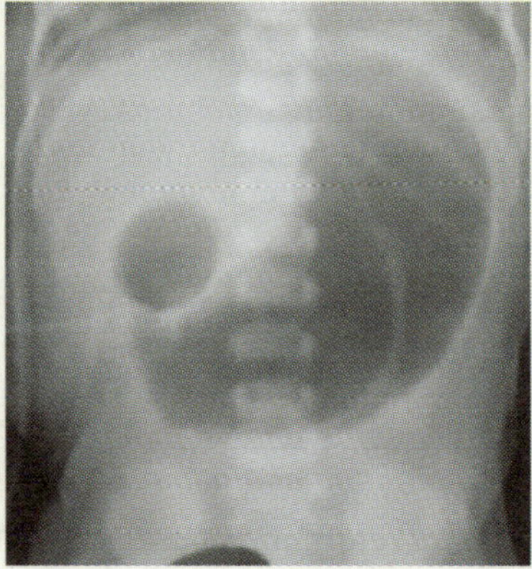

a. Volvulus
b. Duodenal atresia
c. IHPS
d. Ileal atresia

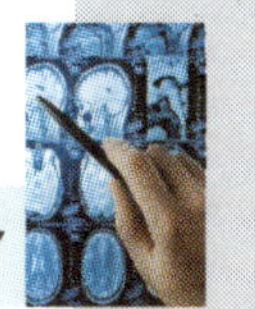

5. A construction worker fell from a bamboo ladder after being accidentally hit on the head by the hammer of his colleague. CT head is shown below, what is likely the diagnosis? ***(Most Recent Question July 2023)***

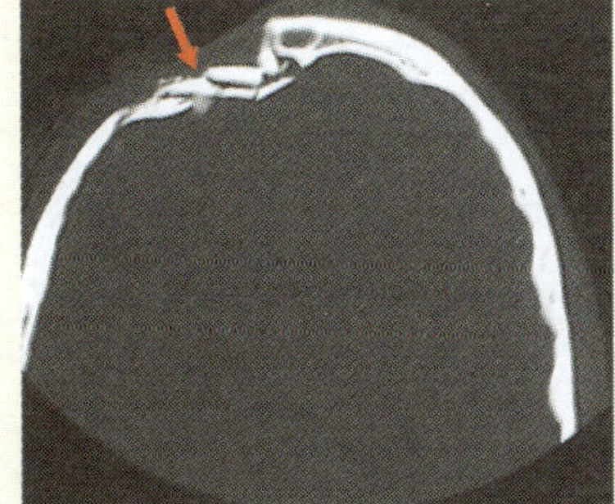

a. Concussion
b. Epidural hematoma
c. Depressed skull fracture
d. Sub-arachnoid hemorrhage

6. LINAC is used for ___________ ***(Most Recent Question July 2023)***

a. Brachytherapy
b. External beam radiotherapy
c. Radioisotope seed implants
d. Systemic radiotherapy

7. Most common long term chronic effect of head and neck radiotherapy is: ***(Most Recent Question July 2023)***

a. Xerostomia b. Mucositis
c. Alopecia d. Enteritis

8. Intensity of X-rays incident on the image receptor is _______________to the source to the image distance _________? ***(Most Recent Question July 2023)***

a. Inversely proportional, squared
b. Directly proportional, squared
c. Inversely proportional, tripled
d. Directly proportional, tripled

9. Identify the marked structure in the given chest X-ray: ***(Most Recent Question Jan 2023)***

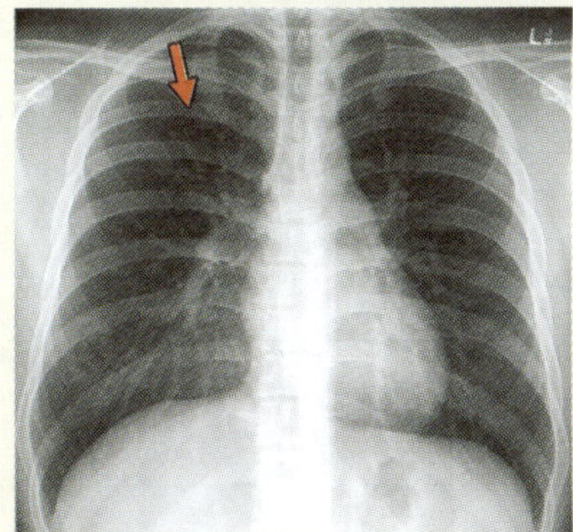

a. 3rd rib anterior part b. 3rd rib posterior part
c. 4th rib anterior part d. 4th rib posterior part

10. A patient presented to OPD with complaints of bone pain, and recurrent episodes of abdominal pain due to constipation. He has had renal colic causing hospitalization in 2021 and 2022 and also had to visit psychiatrist for consultation. You suspect it to be a case of hyperparathyroidism. Which of the following investigation can be useful in this condition? ***(Most Recent Question Jan 2023)***

a. Sestamibi scan b. USG neck
c. CT neck d. PET scan

11. Gold standard investigation for fistula-in-ano is: ***(Most Recent Question Jan 2023)***

a. CT scan b. X- ray
c. MRI d. USG

12. A patient with chronic knee pain is presented to your OPD. An X-ray was performed which is shown here. Identify the disease. ***(Most Recent Question Jan 2023)***

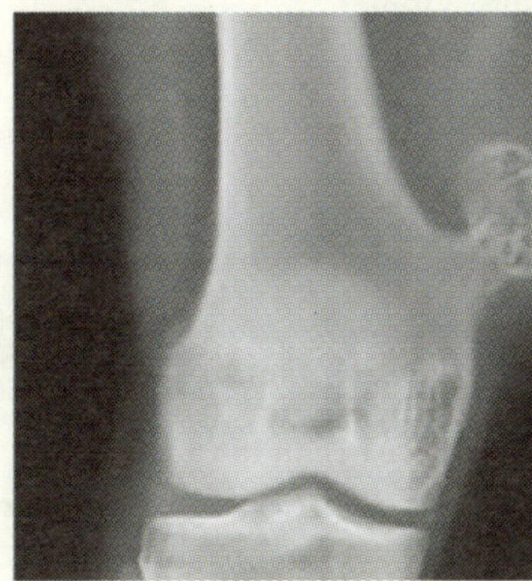

a. Ostechondroma b. Giant cell tumor
c. Osteosarcoma d. Ewings sarcoma

13. A 50-year-old patient presented to your OPD with severe pain in flanks radiating to umbilicus and penis. He says he urinates more often than usual and has burning sensation during urination, and passes small amount of urine which is red in color and foul smelling. An abdominal X-ray was performed. Which is the best for management of this case? ***(Most Recent Question Jan 2023)***

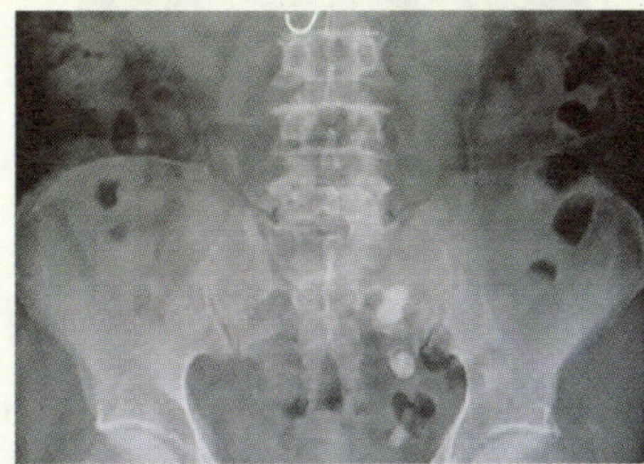

a. Ureteroscopy b. Shock wave lithotripsy
c. Pyelolithotomy d. Cystolitholapaxy

14. Identify the condition from abdominal CT scan of 25-year-old presenting with recurrent abdominal pain episodes.
(Most Recent Question Jan 2023)

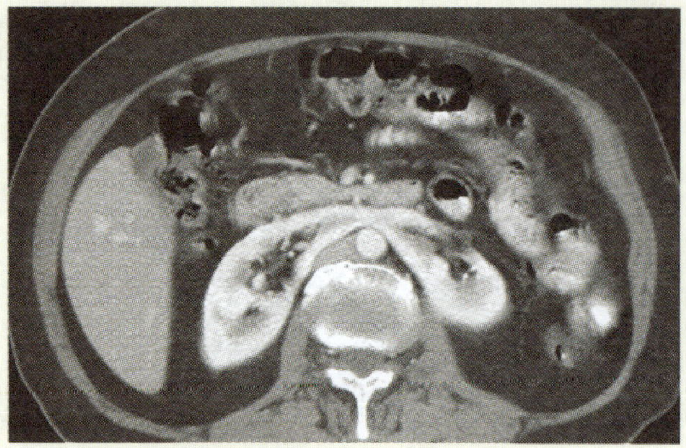

a. Horse-shoe kidney
b. Pancake kidney
c. Polycystic kidney
d. Putty kidney

BASIC RADIOLOGY PRINCIPLES AND RADIOTHERAPY

15. Most radiosensitive organ in the body is:
(Most Recent Question Dec 2021)
a. Ovaries b. Brain
c. Lungs d. GIT

16. What is the imaging modality shown below?
(Most Recent Question Dec 2021)

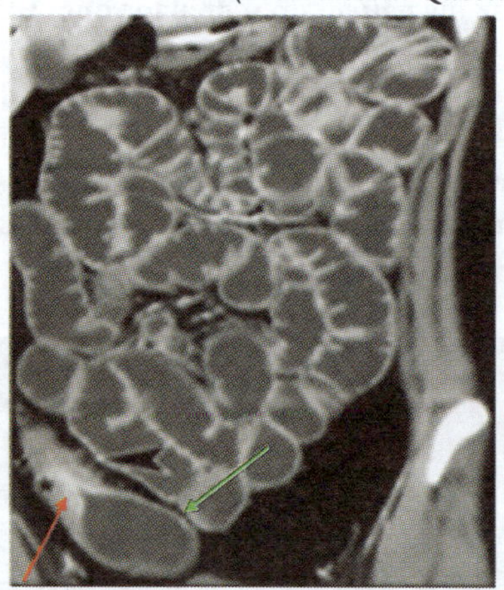

a. MRI b. Barium enema
c. X-ray d. CT Enteroclysis

17. Identify the key radioisotope used in PET imaging.
(Most Recent Question June 2021)
a. F-18 b. P-32
c. Co-60 d. I-31

18. Time for manifestation of gross biological effects of ionizing radiation is? *(Most Recent Question June 2021)*
a. Milli sec b. Seconds
c. Minutes d. Hours to days

19. What is the thickness of lead apron used in radiation protection? *(Most Recent Question Dec 2020)*
a. 0.1 mm b. 0.2 mm
c. 0.3 mm d. 0.5 mm

20. A patient with prostate cancer receives sequential radiotherapy at a dose of 1.8-2.4 Gy for 5 days every week, for 5-7 weeks. This is known as:
(Most Recent Question Aug 2020)
a. Regular fractionated radiotherapy
b. Hypofractionated radiotherapy
c. Hyperfractionated radiotherapy
d. Accelerated radiotherapy

21. Gold standard investigation for FESS is:
(Most Recent Question Aug 2020)
a. X-ray b. MRI
c. CT scan d. PET scan

22. Maximum radiation exposure is seen with:
(Most Recent Question 2019)
a. X-ray abdomen b. HSG
c. IV Angiography d. Barium enema

23. Which of the following investigations work on the same principle? *(Recent Pattern Question 2018-19)*
a. CT and MRI b. CT and X-ray
c. USG and HIDA scan d. MRI and PET scan

24. Which of the following investigation must be performed before giving contrast to the patient?
(Recent Pattern Question 2018)
a. KFT b. LFT
c. Urine specific gravity d. Serum electrolytes

25. What is the gold standard investigation of choice for deep vein thrombosis? *(Recent Pattern Question 2017)*
a. Double contrast duplex b. Venography
c. CT scan d. MRI

26. The shown image modality is:
(Recent Pattern Question 2017)

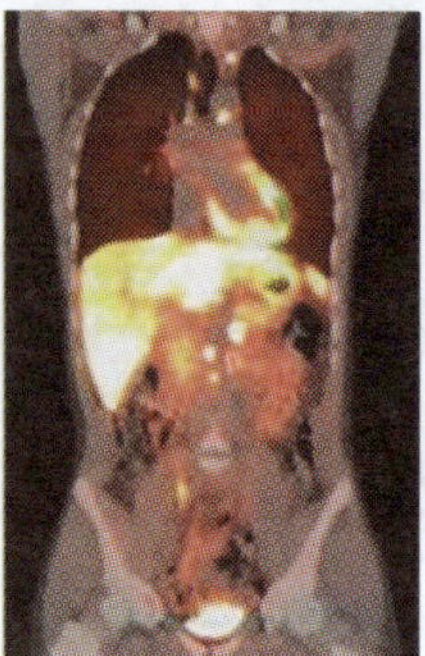

a. PET- CT scan b. PET–MRI
c. CECT d. X-ray

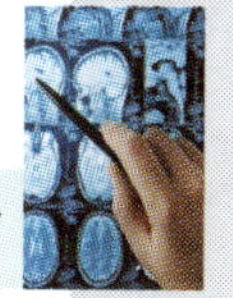

27. What is this image called?

(Recent Pattern Question 2016)

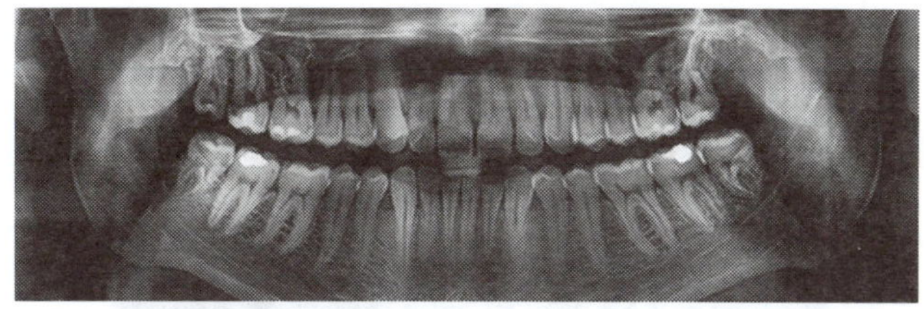

a. Orthopantogram b. Lateral cephalogram
c. Towns view d. Stenver view

28. Loss of proton and electron both when rays travel through the body:

a. Compton effect b. Loss of linear energy
c. Loss of biological dose d. Photoelectric effect

29. Maximum penetrating rays:

a. Alpha b. Beta
c. Gamma d. Delta

30. Unit of radiation exposure:

a. Rad b. Gray
c. Sievert d. Roentgen

31. Iridium 192 half life is:

a. 2.7 days b. 8 days
c. 74 days d. 16 hours

32. Radioiodine 131 half life is:

a. 8 days b. 15.7 days
c. 74.3 days d. 13 hours

33. Half- life of cobalt-60 is:

a. 53 years b. 5.3 years
c. 0.53 years d. 7.8 years

34. Half- life of radium 226 is?

a. 15.9 years b. 159 years
c. 1620 years d. 15900 years

35. Radioisotope used for thyroid treatment of metastasis/ ablation

a. I-123 b. I-31
c. I-83 d. I-90

36. The radioisotope used for ablation of thyroid gland is:

a. Iodine 123
b. Iodine 125
c. Iodine 131
d. Technetium 99 pertechnate

37. Which of the following is not used as a Radioisotope:

a. Iodine-131
b. Caesium-137
c. Iridium-192
d. Iodine-135

38. Who discovered gamma knife?

a. Rutherford
b. Roentgen
c. Leksell
d. John R Adler

39. PET scan isotope is:

a. Phosphorus-32 b. 18-fluoro-deoxyglucose
c. Iridium-77 d. Radium-226

40. Ionizing radiation with maximum penetration is:

a. Alpha particles b. Beta particles
c. Gamma rays d. Microwaves

41. Purely beta emission comes from:

a. P 32 b. I 131
c. Cobalt 60 d. Ra 226

42. Occupational radiation exposure allowed per year to Indian population:

a. 2 mSv b. 5 mSv
c. 10 mSv d. 20 mSv

43. Which of the following is a functional investigation?

a. CT scan b. MRI
c. USG d. PET scan

44. Gadolinium is a contrast agent used for:

a. CT - angiography b. Bronchography
c. MRI - Imaging d. Contrast Sonography

45. Absolute contraindication for MRI:

a. Pacemaker b. Claustrophobia
c. Penile prosthesis d. Joint replacement

46. Correct regarding B-scan on ultrasound is

a. 2D image b. 3D image
c. Visualizing blood flow d. All of these

47. Which phase of the cell cycle is most sensitive to radiotherapy?

a. G2M phase
b. S phase
c. M phase
d. G_2 phase

48. Most common complication of radiotherapy of head and neck cancer

a. Dryness of mouth b. Jawbone necrosis
c. Odynophagia d. Bleeding

49. The most radio sensitive tumor amongst the following is:

a. Small cell lung cancer b. Seminoma
c. Soft tissue sarcoma d. Osteosarcoma

50. Maximum radiation exposure occurs in:

a. Bone scan b. MRI
c. CT scan d. X-ray

51. Which of the following is a non-iodinated contrast?

a. Gadolinium
b. Visipaque
c. Iopamidol
d. Ditriazoate

52. All of the following about MRI are correct; EXCEPT:

a. MRI is useful for localizing small lesions in the brain
b. MRI is useful for evaluating bone marrow
c. MRI is better for calcified lesions
d. MRI is contraindicated in patients with pacemakers

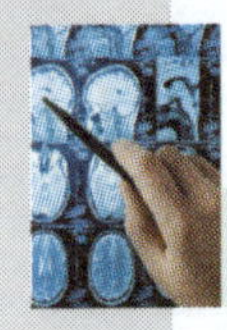

UROLOGY AND BONE IMAGING

53. A 34-year-old male complaints of lower back pain for six months. He is previously diagnosed as a case of ulcerative colitis. X-ray picture of lumbar spine given below. What is the likely diagnosis?

(Most Recent Question June 2022)

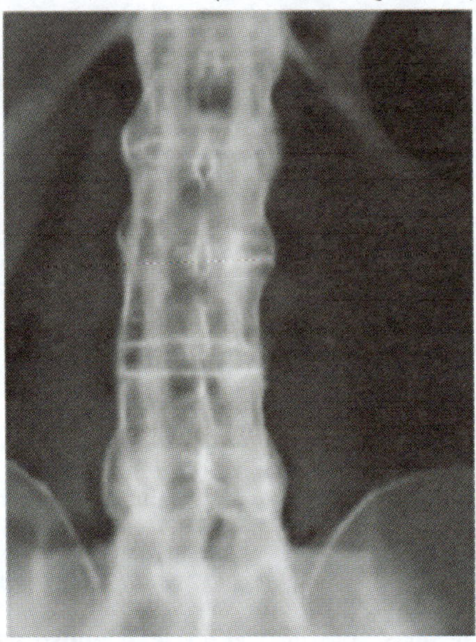

a. Pott's spine
b. Ankylosing spondylitis
c. Psoriatic arthritis
d. Rheumatoid arthritis

54. Identify the bone marked in the X-ray of the foot.

(Most Recent Question Dec 2021)

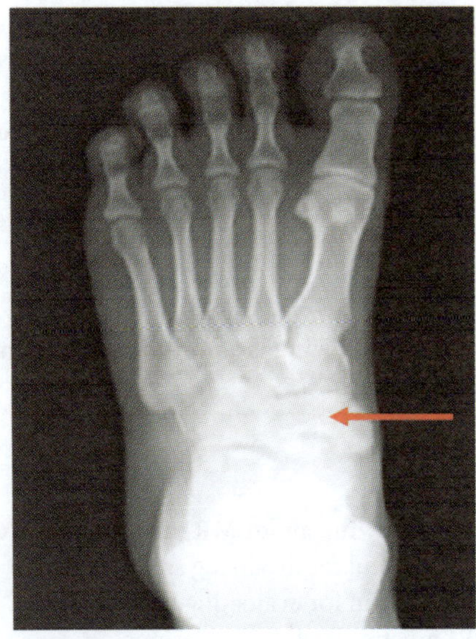

a. Cuneiform
b. Navicular
c. Cuboid
d. Talus

55. A 35-year-old male presented with pain and swelling around the wrist joint. There is no history of injury. Comment based on the X-ray shown below.

(Most Recent Question Dec 2021)

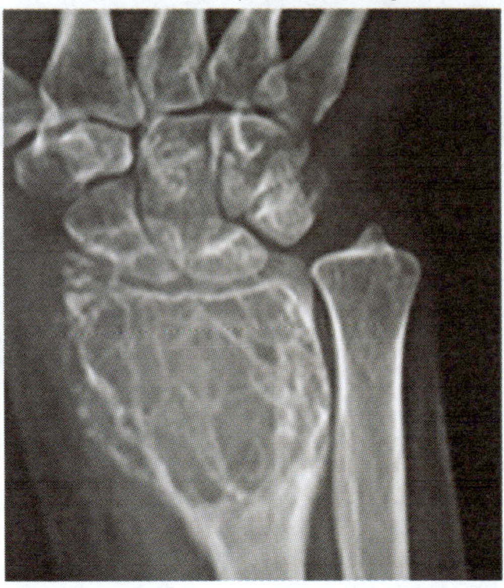

a. Osteosarcoma
b. Rickets
c. Colle's fracture
d. Giant cell tumor

56. A 70-year-old male presented with multiple areas of bone pain, anemia, renal failure, proteinuria and hypercalcemia. X-ray skull is shown in the image. What is the most likely diagnosis? ***(Most Recent Question Dec 2021)***

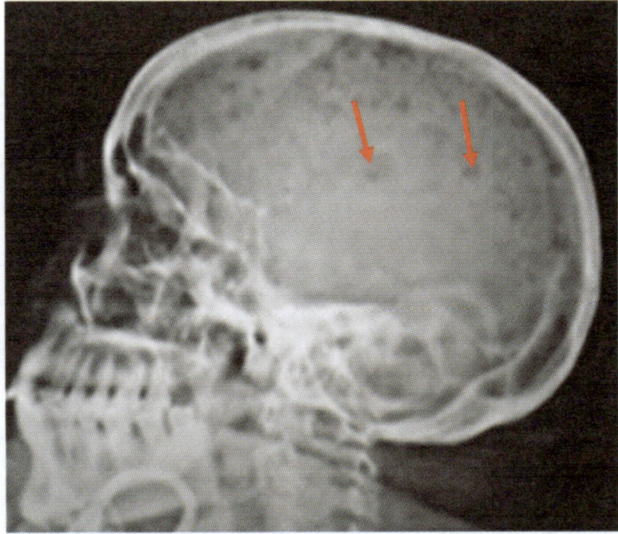

a. Carcinoma prostate
b. Multiple myeloma
c. Primary hyperparathyroidism
d. Secondary hyperparathyroidism

57. What is the likely diagnosis?

(Most Recent Question Dec 2021)

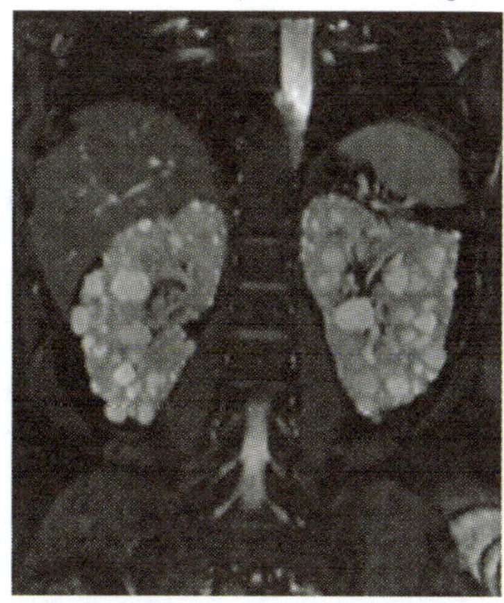

a. CT AD PCKD
b. MR-AD PCKD
c. CT-AR PCKD
d. MR-AR PCKD

58. Identify the X-ray view shown.

(Most Recent Question June 2021)

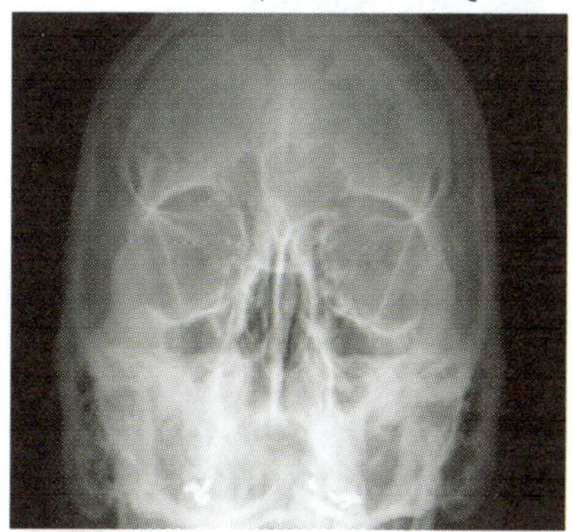

a. Caldwell
b. Water's
c. Schuller
d. Towne

59. What can be the diagnosis for the given image?

(Most Recent Question Dec 2020)

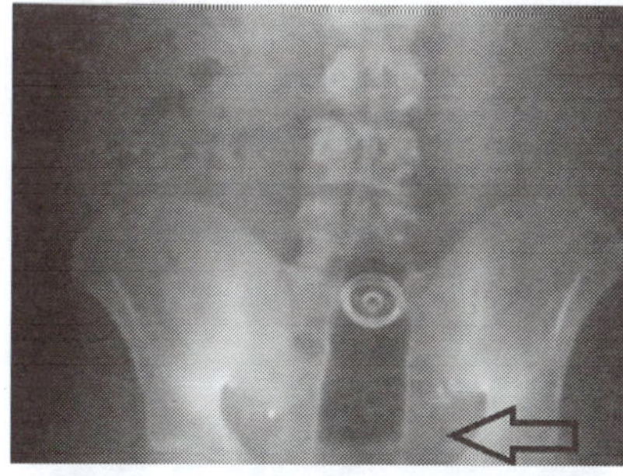

a. Iliac crest fracture
b. Foreign body
c. Ureterocele
d. Bladder stone

60. Which of the following is the most radiosensitive bone tumor? *(Most Recent Question Dec 2020)*

a. Enchondroma
b. Osteosarcoma
c. Ewing's sarcoma
d. Osteochondroma

61. Identify the fracture shown in given radiograph

(Most Recent Question Dec 2020)

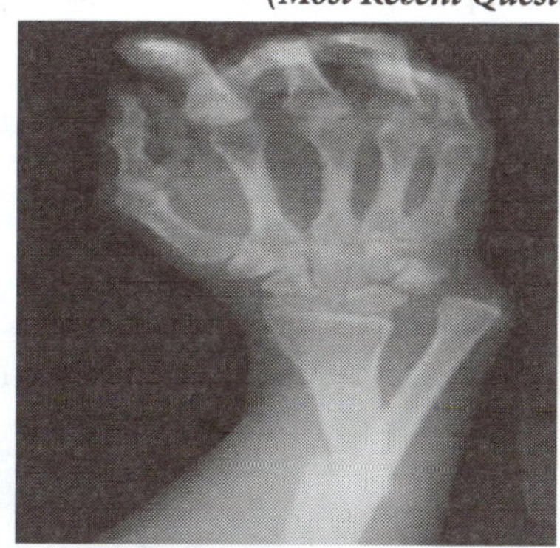

a. Monteggia fracture
b. Galeazzi fracture
c. Clayshoveler fracture
d. Jefferson fracture

62. A patient presents with fever for last 2 weeks with antalgic gait and low back pain. He has past medical history of taking incomplete treatment for tuberculosis. Diagnosis is: *(Most Recent Question Dec 2020)*

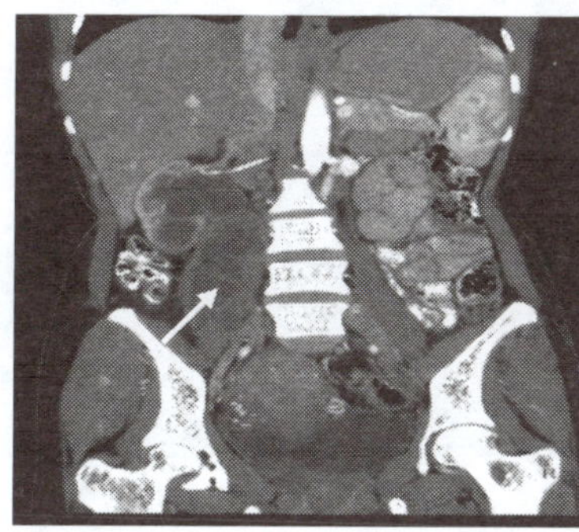

a. Perthes disease
b. Psoas abscess
c. Annular pancreas
d. Nephroblastoma

63. Identify the condition based on the given radiograph.

(Most Recent Question Dec 2020)

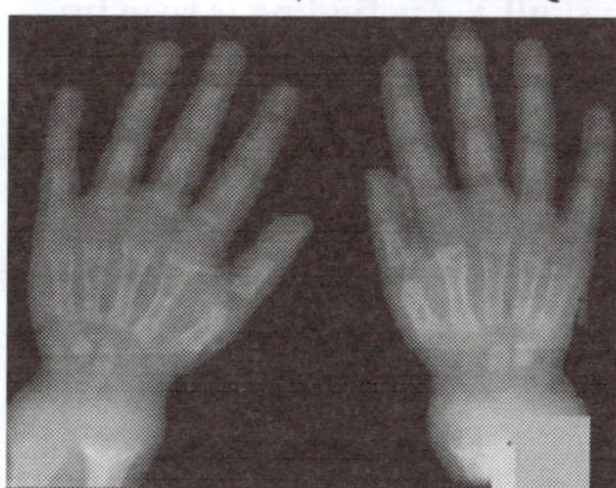

a. Scurvy
b. Rickets
c. Achondroplasia
d. Osteogenesis imperfecta

64. **A patient presents with 4 months history of fall, with swelling and pain around the knee. The following X-ray is obtained from the patient, what is the most likely diagnosis?** ***(Most Recent Question Dec 2020)***

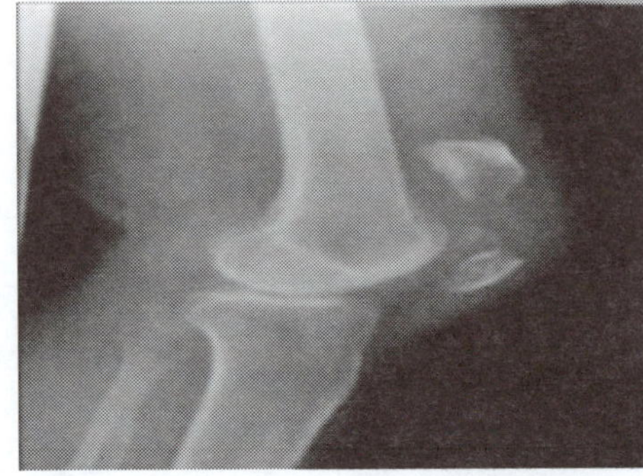

a. Fracture patella b. Tibia fracture
c. Osseous metaplasia d. Myositis ossifications

65. **Which muscle attaches to the area pointed by the arrow?** ***(Most Recent Question Dec 2020)***

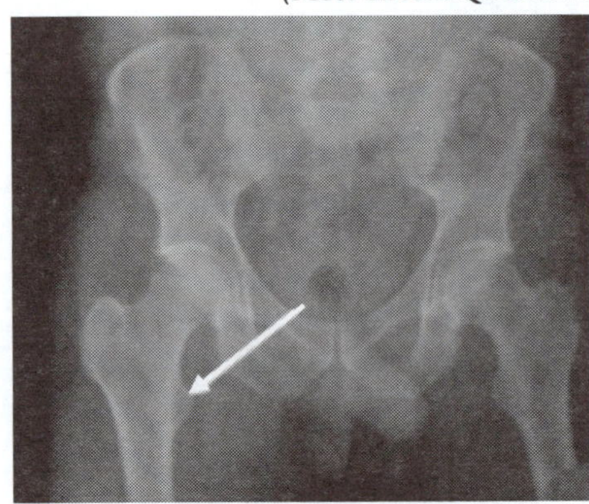

a. Iliopsoas muscle b. Pectineus
c. Gluteus maximus d. Sartorius

66. **A 5-year-old boy is unable to pronate and supinate since childhood. What is the diagnosis?** ***(Most Recent Question Aug 2020)***

a. Radioulnar synostosis b. Radial head dislocation
c. Monteggia fracture d. Myositis ossification

67. **The given skull X-ray finding is seen in:** ***(Most Recent Question Aug 2020)***

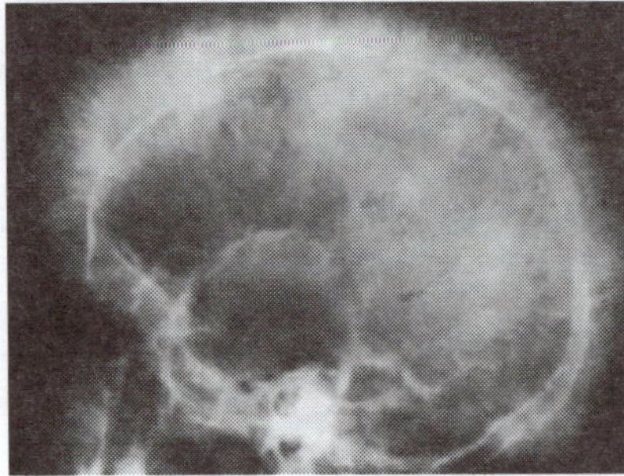

a. Hemolytic anemia b. Multiple myeloma
c. Increased ICT d. Osteopetrosis

68. **Identify the given IVP image:** ***(Most Recent Question Aug 2020)***

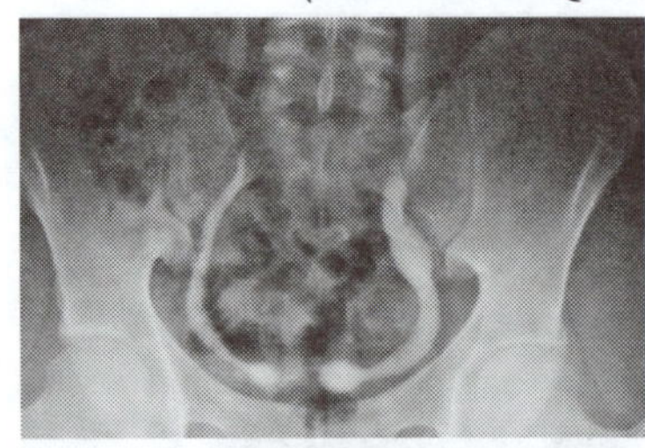

a. Ureterocele b. Hydronephrosis
c. Staghorn calculi d. Bladder calculi

69. **Thimble bladder is seen in:** ***(Most Recent Question Dec 2019)***

a. TB b. Ureterocele
c. Stage 1 Bladder cancer d. Interstitial cystitis

70. **Which of the following is a gold standard investigation for diagnosis of renal stone?** ***(Recent Pattern Question 2018)***

a. USG
b. Helical CT with Non-contrast
c. Helical CT with Contrast
d. MRI

71. **Identify the bone marked with arrow:** ***(Recent Pattern Question 2017)***

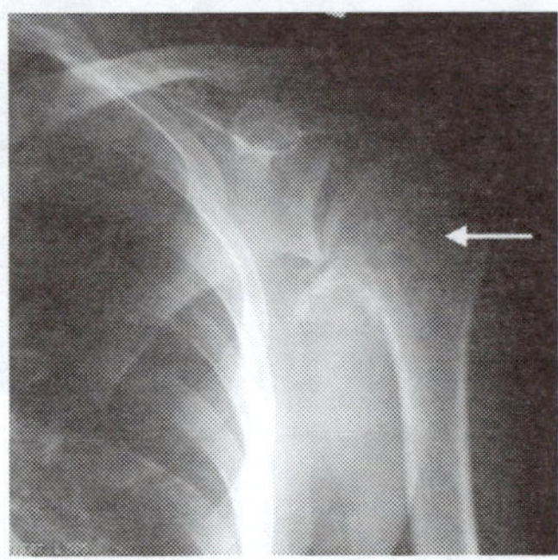

a. Radius b. Ulna
c. Humerus d. Clavicle

72. **On IVP this image was obtained. What is the diagnosis?** ***(Recent Pattern Question 2017)***

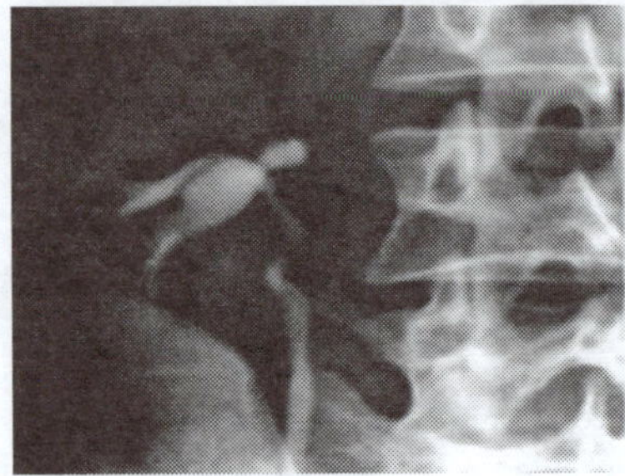

a. Horse shoe kidney
b. Duplex collecting system
c. Cross fused ectopic kidney
d. Polycystic kidney

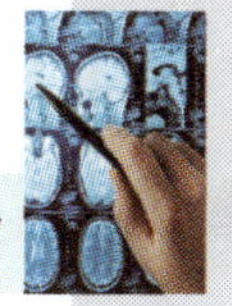

73. MRI spine shows following finding. What is the diagnosis? ***(Recent Pattern Question 2017)***

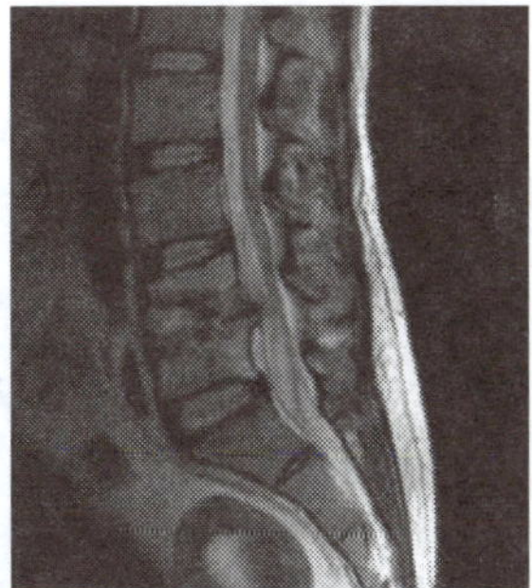

a. Osteoporosis
b. Metastasis
c. TB spine
d. Osteopetrosis

74. X-ray pelvis image is shown. What is the structure marked with arrow? ***(Recent Pattern Question 2017)***

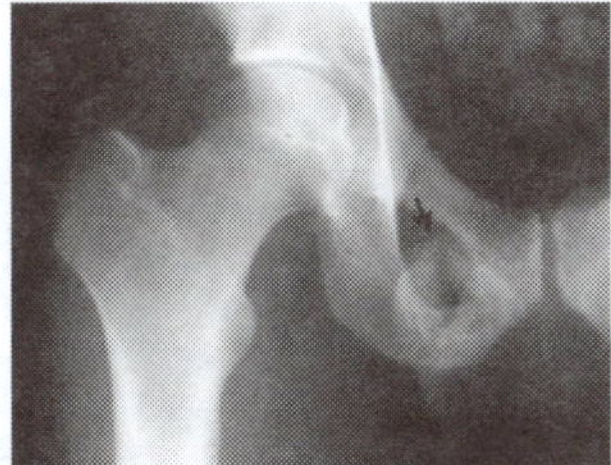

a. Acetabulum
b. Obturator foramen
c. Ischial foramen
d. Symphysis pubis

75. Ring sign is seen on urography. What is the diagnosis of the patient is: ***(Recent Pattern Question 2017)***

a. Hydronephrosis
b. Polycystic kidney
c. Papillary necrosis
d. Renal cell carcinoma

76. Which of the following condition is most predisposed for contrast nephropathy?

a. Diabetes
b. Hypertension
c. Malignant hypertension
d. Hypertensive glomerulosclerosis

77. Which of the following cancer is LEAST LIKELY to occur secondary to radiation exposure:

a. Hepatocellular CA
b. Renal cell CA
c. Stomach CA
d. Colon CA

78. Ring sign is seen on Urography film in a diabetic is due to?

a. Hydronephrosis
b. Polycystic kidney
c. Papillary necrosis
d. Emphysematous pyelonephritis

79. Spider leg sign on IVP suggests:

a. Renal stone
b. Polycystic kidney
c. Hypernephroma
d. Hydronephrosis

80. Spider-leg deformity of pelvicalyceal system on intravenous urography (IVU) is a constant feature of:

a. Tuberculosis
b. Renal cell carcinoma
c. Polycystic disease
d. Wilm's tumor

81. Adder head on I.V.P. is seen in:

a. Ureterocoele
b. Cystocele
c. Enterocele
d. Omentocele

82. Which of the following investigation is preferred for diagnosis of vesicoureteric reflux:

a. Intravenous urography
b. Micturating cystourethrogram
c. Retrograde pyelography
d. Ultrasonography

83. Crew cut appearance on X ray skull is seen in:

a. Thalassemia
b. Megaloblastic anemia
c. Autoimmune hemolytic anemia
d. Dimorphic anemia

84. Bone within a Bone appearance is seen in:

a. Osteonecrosis
b. Osteoporosis
c. Osteopetrosis
d. Osteomyelitis

85. 'Hair on end' appearance in skull X-ray is characteristic of:

a. G6PD deficiency
b. Sickle cell anemia
c. Rickets
d. Scurvy

86. Martel sign is seen in

a. Gout
b. Ankylosing spondylitis
c. Osteoarthritis
d. Rheumatoid arthritis

87. Nuchal thickness is evaluated in:

a. Ante natal USG first trimester
b. Prenatal USG screening
c. Antenatal USG second trimester
d. Antenatal USG third trimester

ABDOMEN IMAGING

88. A 50-year-old female came to the OPD with complaints of dysphagia and recurrent episodes of chest pain. The patient was further evaluated with barium swallow which is shown below. What is the most probable diagnosis? ***(Most Recent Question Dec 2021)***

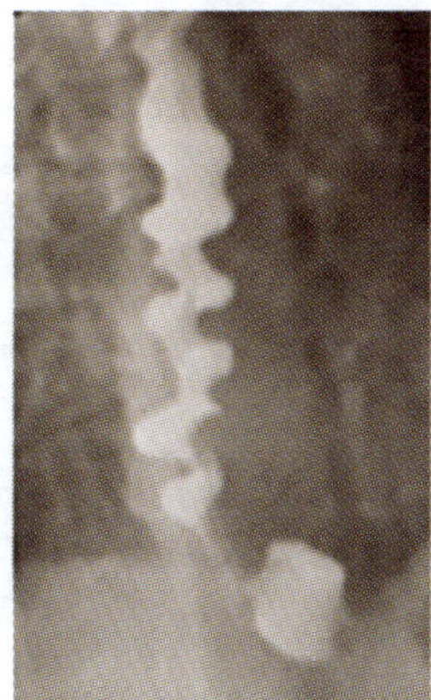

a. Carcinoma esophagus
b. Diffuse esophageal spasm
c. Achalasia cardia
d. Esophageal web

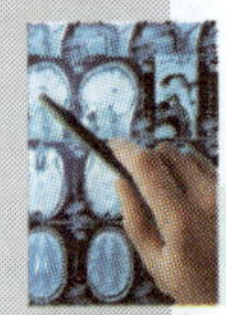

89. Identify the pattern seen in Barium enema shown here.

(Most Recent Question June 2021)

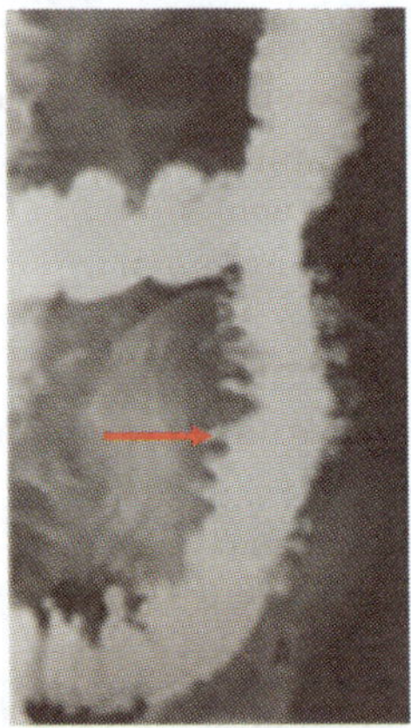

a. Saw tooth sign
b. Apple core sign
c. Corkscrew appearance
d. String sign

90. A 35-year-old female presents with dysphagia, regurgitation and weight loss. What is the likely diagnosis?

(Most Recent Question June 2021)

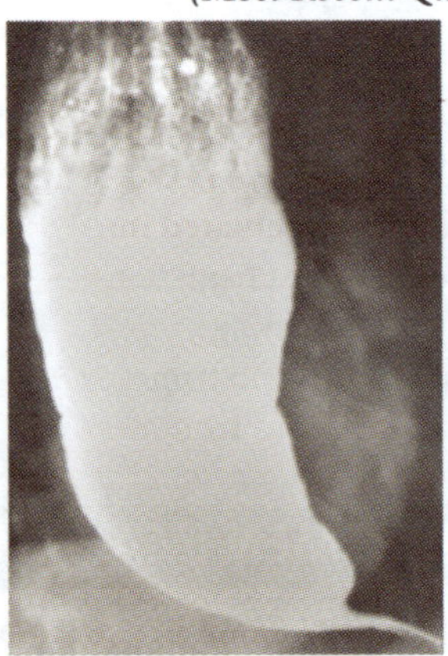

a. Diffuse esophageal spasm
b. Achalasia cardia
c. Malignancy
d. Leiomyoma

91. Identify the pathology in the given Ultrasound image.

(Most Recent Question Dec 2020)

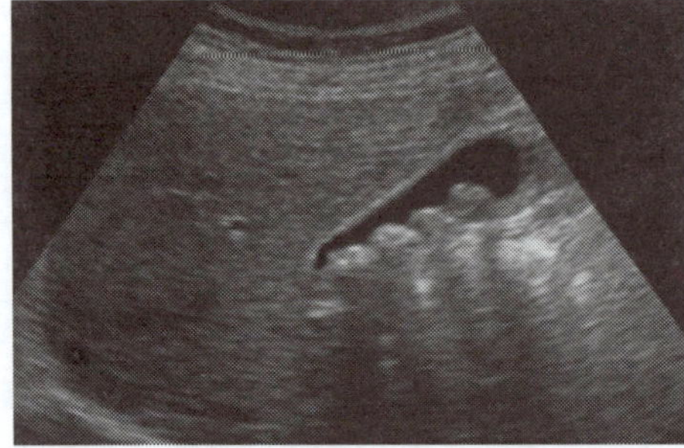

a. Multiple gallstones
b. Choledocholithiasis
c. Hydatid cyst
d. Gallbladder cancer

92. A 30-year-old patient comes to the emergency room with multiple episodes of vomiting and severe abdominal pain. On investigation the following image is obtained. What is the likely diagnosis?

(Most Recent Question Dec 2020)

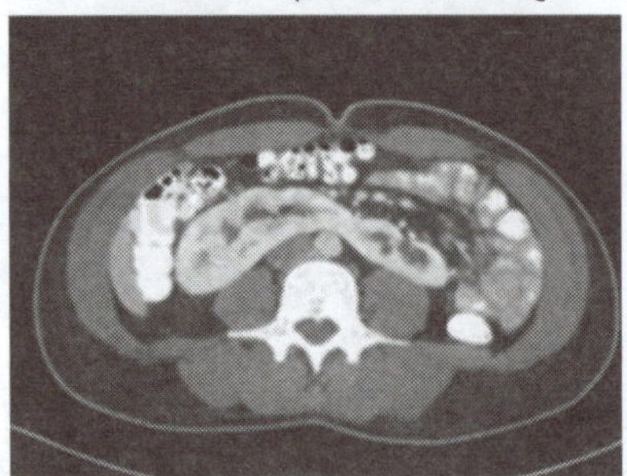

a. Pancake kidney
b. Ectopic kidney
c. Horseshoe kidney
d. Cross fused kidney

93. Identify the given image below.

(Most Recent Question Dec 2020)

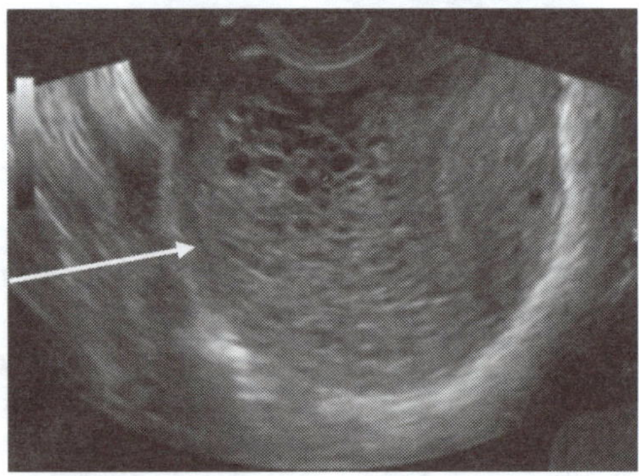

a. Complete mole
b. Incomplete mole
c. Retained products of conception
d. Polycystic Ovarian Disease

94. Identify the given HSG image.

(Most Recent Question Dec 2020)

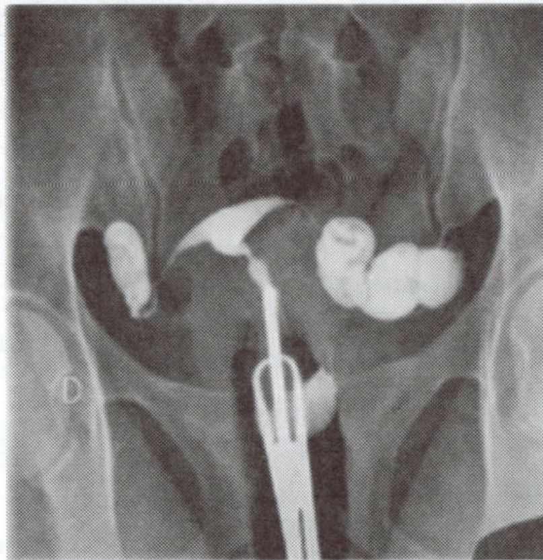

a. Para-ovarian cyst
b. Ovarian cancer
c. Bilateral Hydrosalpinx
d. Fibroid

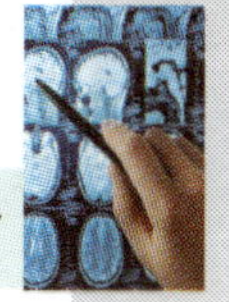

95. Diagnose based on the given image below. *(Most Recent Question Dec 2020)*

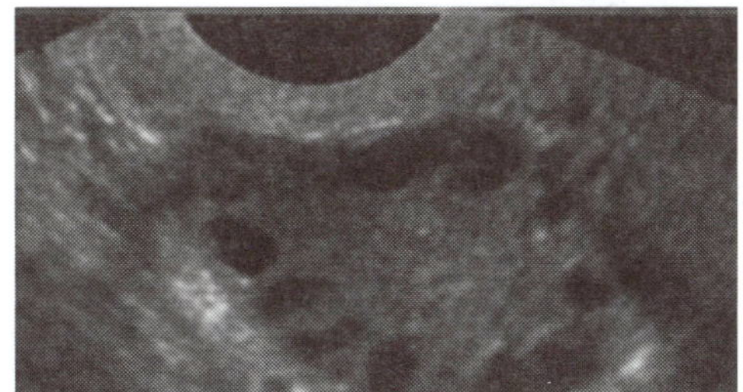

a. Ovarian hyperstimulation syndrome
b. PCOD
c. Ovarian cyst
d. Endometriosis

96. A female visits the OPD with her 2-day-old child presenting with inability to breast feed, bilious vomiting and abdominal distention. The X-ray of the neonate shows. *(Most Recent Question Dec 2020)*

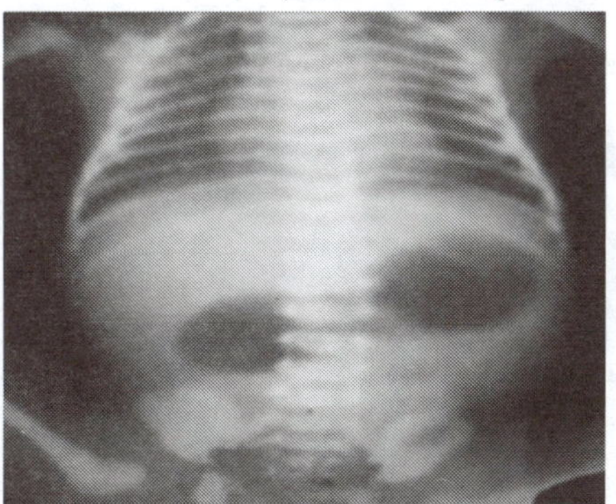

a. Congenital hypertrophic pyloric stenosis
b. Duodenal atresia
c. Jejunal obstruction
d. Hirschsprung disease

97. A 2-week-old child is brought to the emergency room by her mother with symptoms of nonbilious vomiting and lump in the epigastric area. What is most appropriate diagnosis? *(Most Recent Question Dec 2020)*

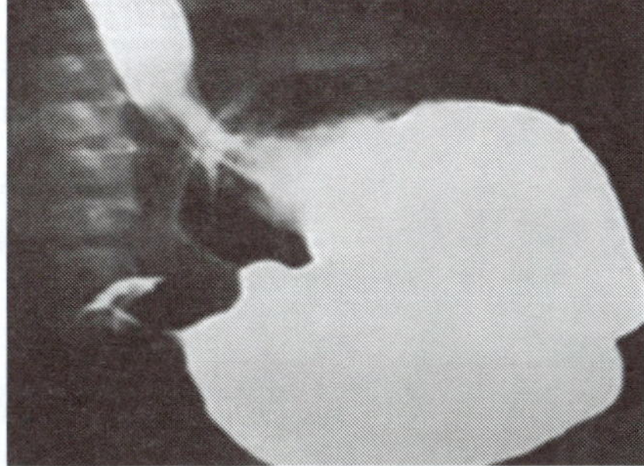

a. Congenital hypertrophic pyloric stenosis
b. Esophageal atresia
c. Jejunal atresia
d. Duodenal atresia

98. X-ray of 2-year-old child is given, what is the possible diagnosis? *(Most Recent Question Aug 2020)*

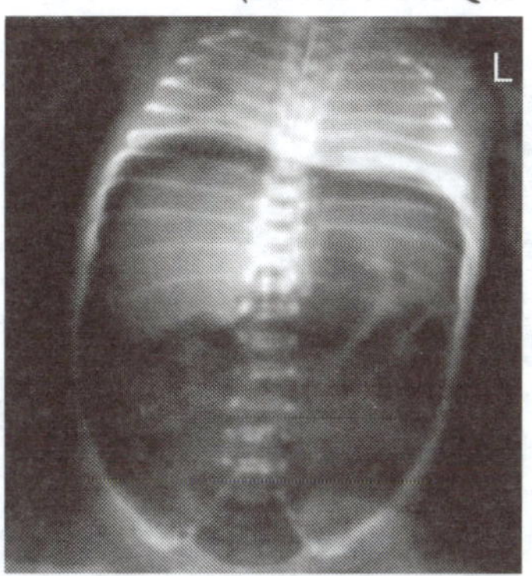

a. Pneumatosis intestinalis
b. Pneumoperitoneum
c. Subcutaneous emphysema
d. Duodenal atresia

99. Identify the given barium enema image. *(Most Recent Question Aug 2020)*

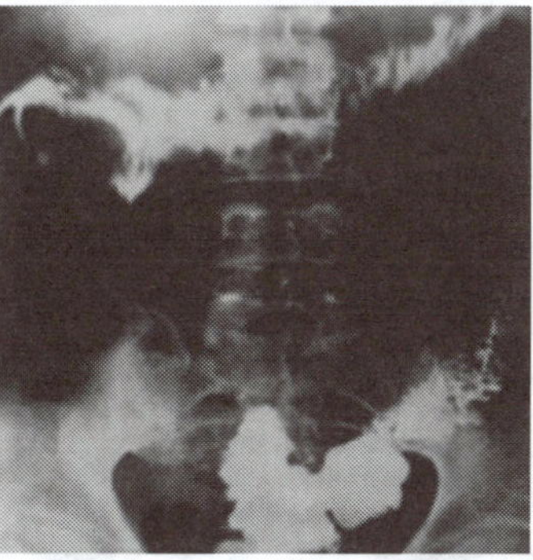

a. Intussusception
b. Ulcerative colitis
c. Cecal cancer
d. Ileocecal TB

100. A 25-year-old female patient presents with progressive dysphagia. Barium swallow image is shown. What is the likely diagnosis? *(Most Recent Question Aug 2020)*

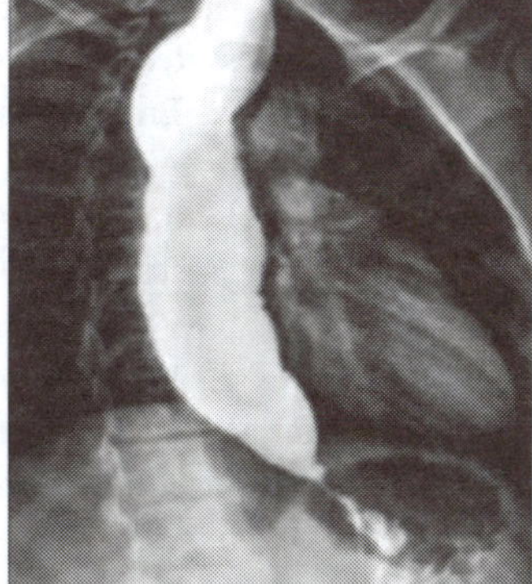

a. Achalasia cardia
b. Esophageal cancer
c. Diffuse esophageal spasm
d. Esophagitis

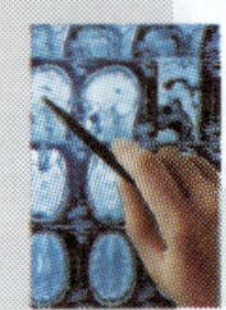

101. Identify the given HSG image.
(Most Recent Question Aug 2020)

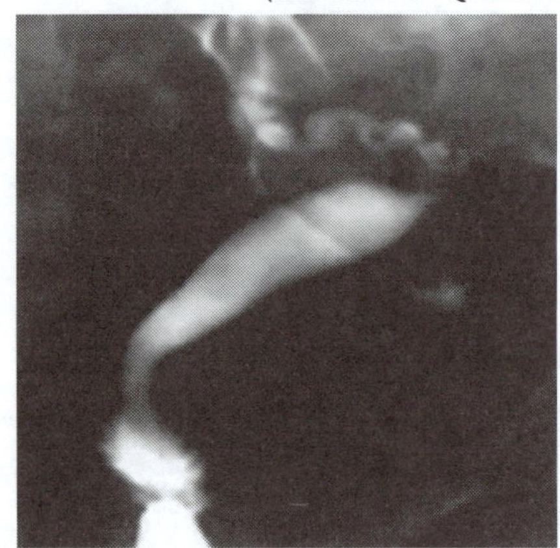

a. Bicornuate b. Unicornuate
c. Septate d. Didelphys

102. Identify the structure being pointed by the arrows.
(Most Recent Question Aug 2020)

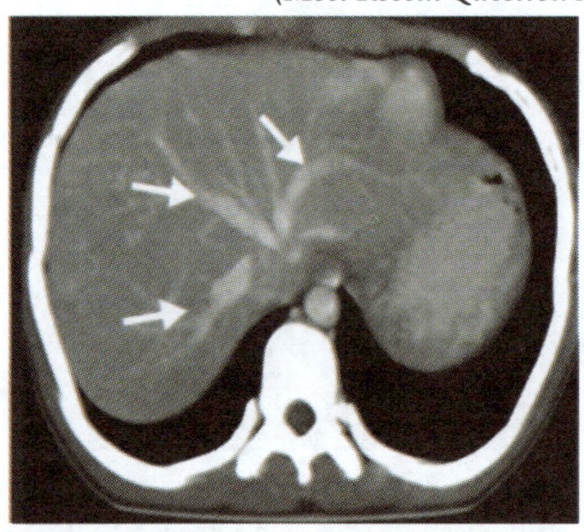

a. Hepatic artery b. Portal vein
c. Hepatic vein d. Inferior Vena Cava

103. Patient with right hypochondrial pain, has a water lily sign in ultrasound. What is the diagnosis?
(Most Recent Question Aug 2020)

a. Hydatid cyst b. Entamoeba
c. Schistosoma d. Ascariasis

104. All of the following areas are scanned in FAST; EXCEPT:
(Most Recent Question 2019)

a. Pericardium b. Pleural cavity
c. Spleen d. Liver

105. Investigation of choice for acute cholecystitis is:
(Recent Pattern Question 2018-19)

a. H.I.D.A scan b. USG
c. CT scan d. Biopsy

106. Investigation of choice for GERD:
(Recent Pattern Question 2018-19)

a. USG b. HIDA
c. Manometry d. 24-hour pH monitoring

107. Comment on the diagnosis of the image shown below:
(Recent Pattern Question 2018)

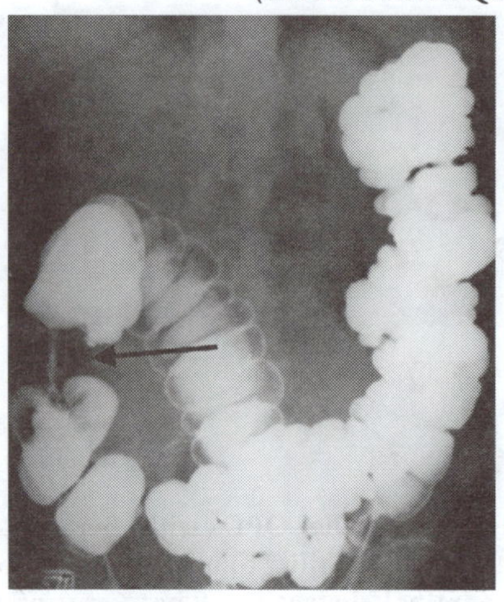

a. Apple core appearance b. Claw sign
c. Coffee bean appearance d. String sign of kantor

108. Name the structure marked with arrow:
(Recent Pattern Question 2017)

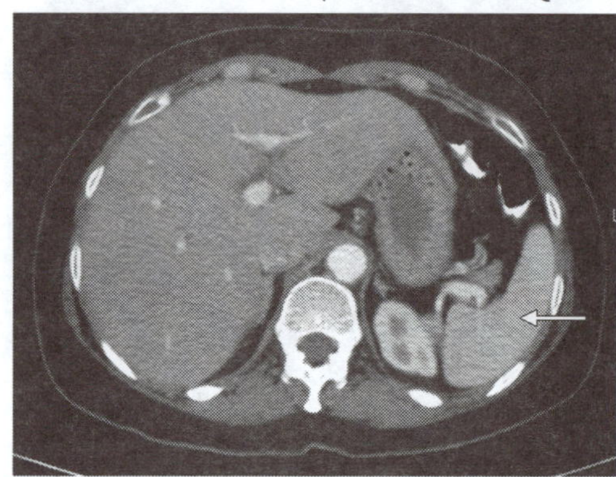

a. Right kidney b. Left kidney
c. Spleen d. Stomach

109. A 7-year-old child presented with abdominal pain, fever and jaundice. CT abdomen is given below. What is the most likely diagnosis? *(Recent Pattern Question 2017)*

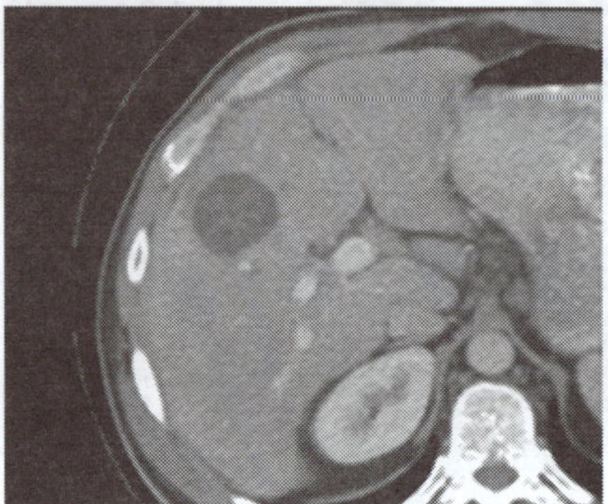

a. Amebiasis b. Hemangioma
c. Hepatoma d. Hydatid cyst

110. Identify the organ shown with an arrow:
(Recent Pattern Question 2016)

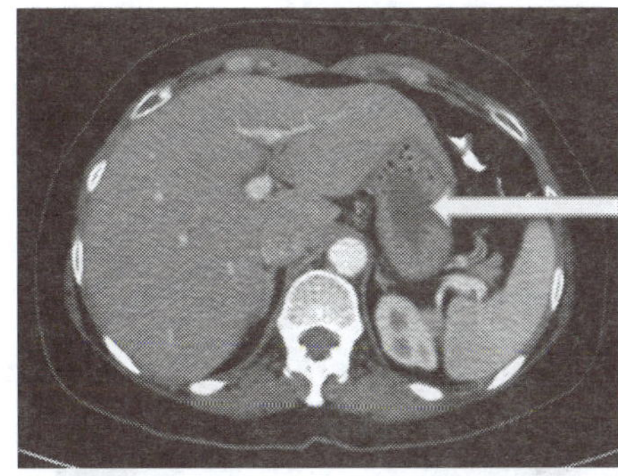

a. Spleen b. Kidney
c. Stomach d. Liver

111. Most useful investigation of choice for liver abscess is:

a. Exploratory laparotomy b. Ultrasound
c. Liver enzymes d. Parasite in the stool

112. Normal thickness of gallbladder wall:

a. 1 mm b. 1 cm
c. 3 mm d. 5 cm

113. Thumb print on barium is seen in:

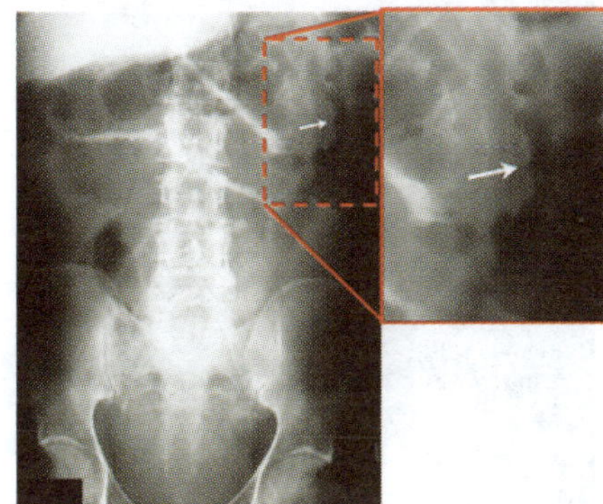

a. Volvulus b. Ischemic colitis
c. Crohn's disease d. Intussusception

114. Diagnosis of the given X-ray of abdomen:

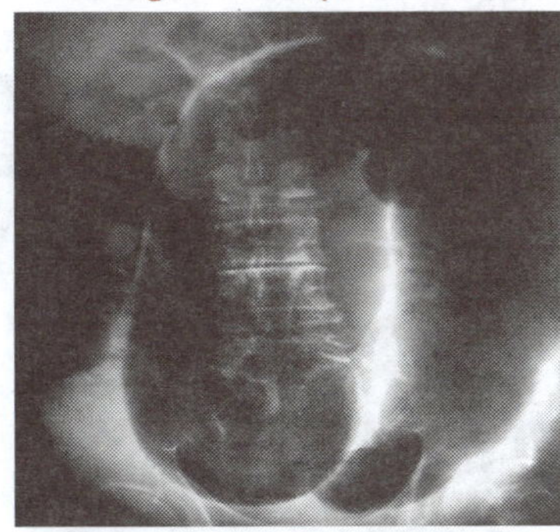

a. Small intestine obstruction
b. Pneumointestinalis
c. Sigmoid volvulus
d. Intussusception

115. Double bubble sign is seen in:

a. Duodenal atresia
b. Jejunal atresia
c. Ileal atresia
d. Hypertrophic pyloric stenosis

116. Double barrel sign is seen in?

a. Primary Sclerosing cholangitis
b. Primary Biliary cirrhosis
c. Obstructive jaundice
d. Duodenal atresia

117. Cobble stoning of intestine with string sign of kantor is seen in:

a. Crohn's disease
b. Ulcerative colitis
c. Ischemic colitis
d. Amoebic colitis

118. Pipe stem colon on barium enema is seen with:

a. Crohn's disease b. Ulcerative colitis
c. Ischemic colitis d. Irritable bowel syndrome

119. Target sign is seen in:

a. Ischemic colitis b. Meckel's Diverticulum
c. Intussuception d. Volvulus

120. Cork screw appearance on barium swallow is seen in:

a. Achalasia cardia b. Diffuse esophageal spasm
c. Zenker's diverticulum d. Scleroderma

121. IOC for neonatal hypertrophic pyloric stenosis:

a. X-ray b. CT scan
c. MRI d. Ultrasound

122. Saw tooth appearance is seen in:

a. Diverticulosis b. Cholecystitis
c. Appendicitis d. Hiatus hernia

123. Apple core appearance on barium enema is seen in?

a. Carcinoma colon b. TB caecum
c. Crohns disease d. Ulcerative colitis

124. IOC acute pancreatitis:

a. Contrast CT b. USG
c. Serum lipase d. Serum amylase

125. Sentinel loop on X-ray:

a. Meckel's diverticulum
b. Acute cholecystitis
c. Acute mesenteric adenitis
d. Acute pancreatitis

126. A patient presents with right hypochondrium pain. Which of the following investigations should be done:

a. CT b. MRI
c. USG d. Cholecystogram

127. RTA brought in casualty. On examination liver rupture is suspected. Which of the following investigation is to be done first?

a. CT b. MRI
c. USG d. Peritoneal lavage

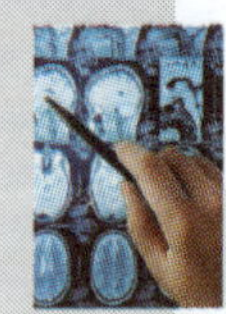

128. Identify the image:

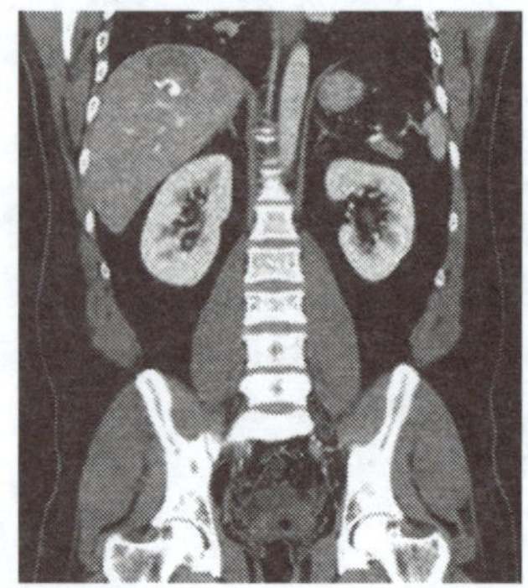

a. Digital X-ray   b. CT
c. PET scan   d. USG

THORAX IMAGING

129. A patient comes to the OPD with complaints of daily purulent sputum production. Identify the condition given in this image? ***(Most Recent Question June 2022)***

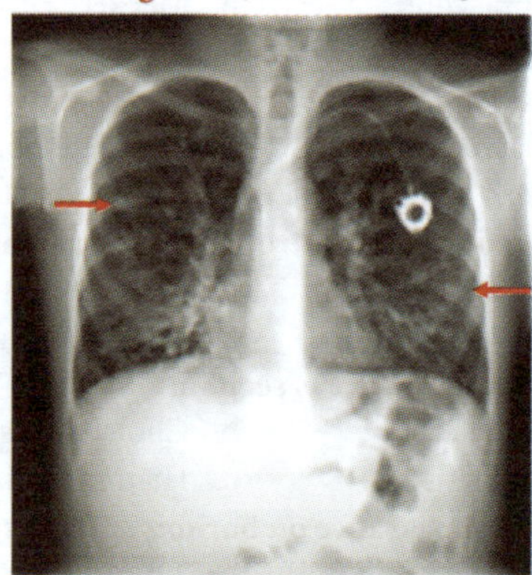

a. Chronic bronchitis   b. Bronchiectasis
c. Emphysema   d. Pneumonia

130. What does the following X-ray depict? ***(Most Recent Question June 2022)***

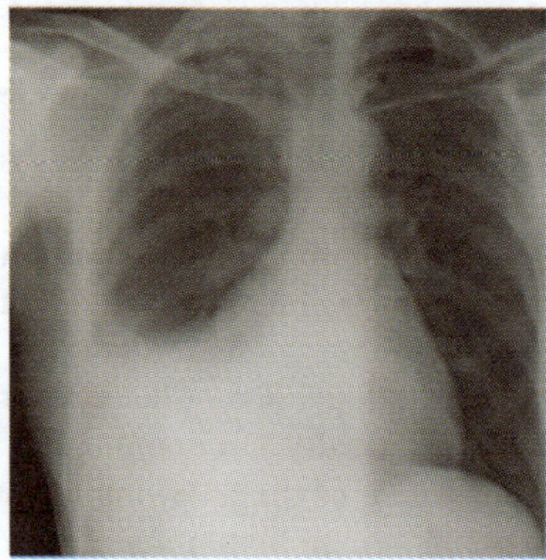

a. Pleural effusion   b. Tension pneumothorax
c. Emphysema   d. Bronchiectasis

131. A patient came to the emergency with sharp, stabbing pain in the chest. An X-ray was taken. Identify the condition. ***(Most Recent Question June 2022)***

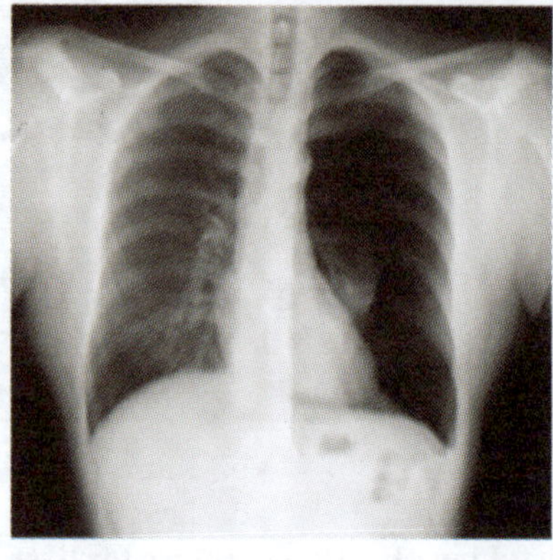

a. Pneumothorax   b. Pneumonitis
c. Emphysema   d. Bronchiectasis

132. A 60-year-old woman presented in a state of shock and abdominal distension with history of peptic ulcers. X-ray of chest is given below. Identify the condition? ***(Most Recent Question Dec 2021)***

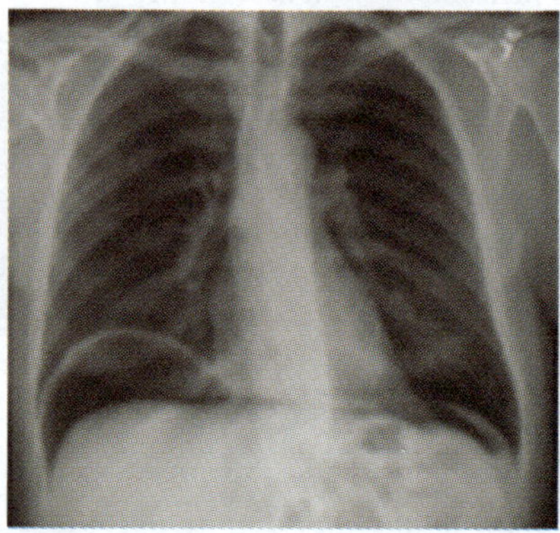

a. Perforation peritonitis   b. Pneumothorax
c. Pleural effusion   d. Hydropneumothorax

133. The following appearance is present in: ***(Most Recent Question Dec 2021)***

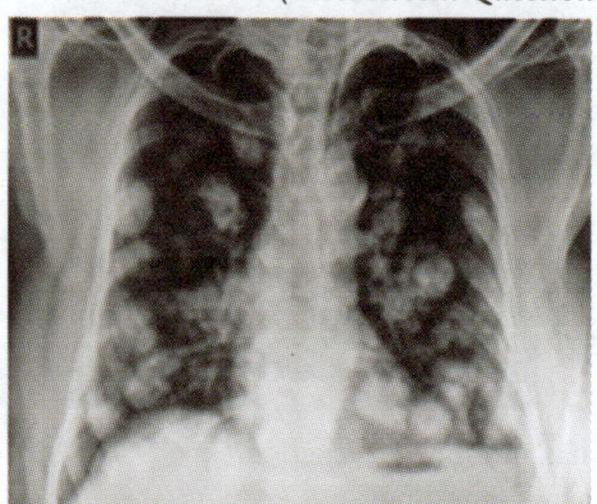

a. TB   b. Bronchogenic Ca
c. Metastasis   d. Hamartoma

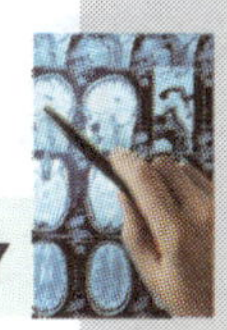

134. What is the likely diagnosis?

(Most Recent Question Dec 2021)

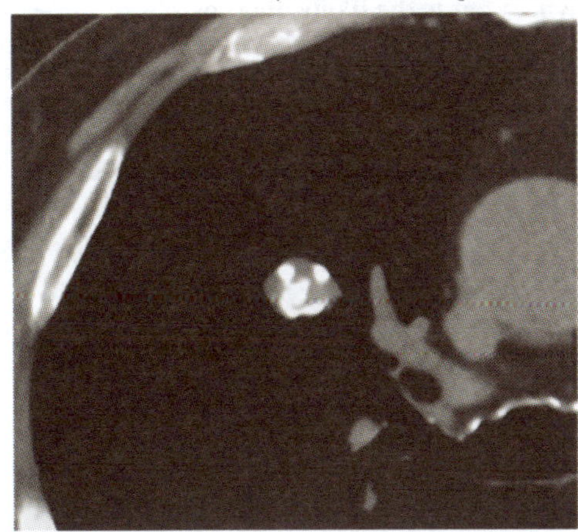

a. Hamartoma
b. Carcinoid
c. Ca lung
d. TB

135. Identify the location of the lead of device shown.

(Most Recent Question June 2021)

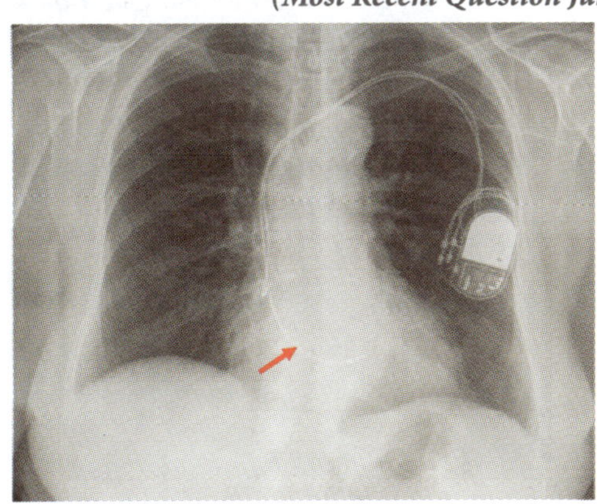

a. RA
b. RV
c. LA
d. LV

136. A 30-year-old patient presents with high grade fever and productive cough. Comment on the CXR finding shown. *(Most Recent Question June 2021)*

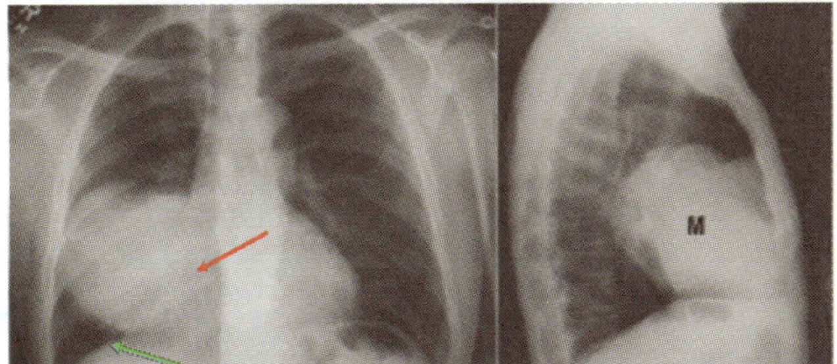

a. Right lower lobe consolidation
b. Right hydatid cyst
c. Right sided eventration of diaphragm
d. Right middle lobe consolidation

137. A 40-year-old man had a RTA. He is having shortness of breath and chest pain. CXR done shows?

(Most Recent Question June 2021)

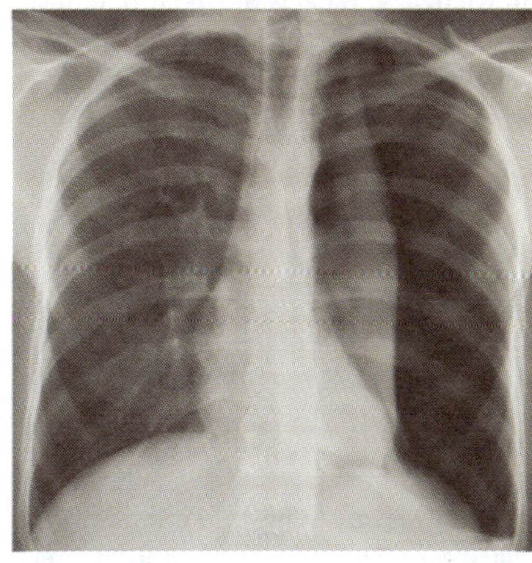

a. Hemothorax
b. Pneumothorax
c. Lung contusion
d. Diaphragmatic tear

138. A patient presents after 10 weeks of acute pancreatitis. Diagnosis is: *(Most Recent Question June 2021)*

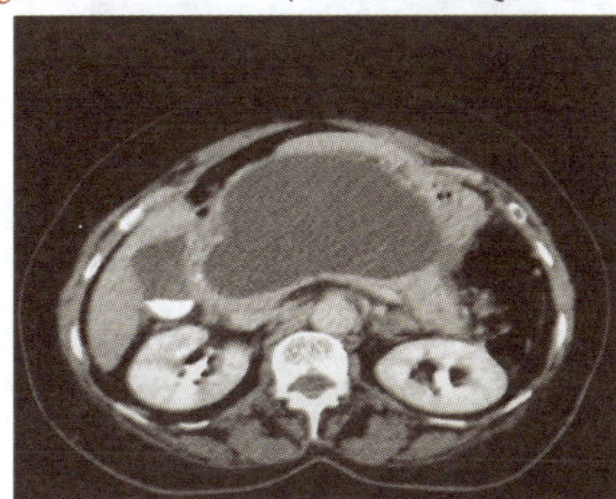

a. Liver abscess
b. Gastric outlet obstruction
c. Pancreatic pseudocyst
d. Acute pancreatitis

139. Which of the following is the likely finding?

(Most Recent Question Dec 2021)

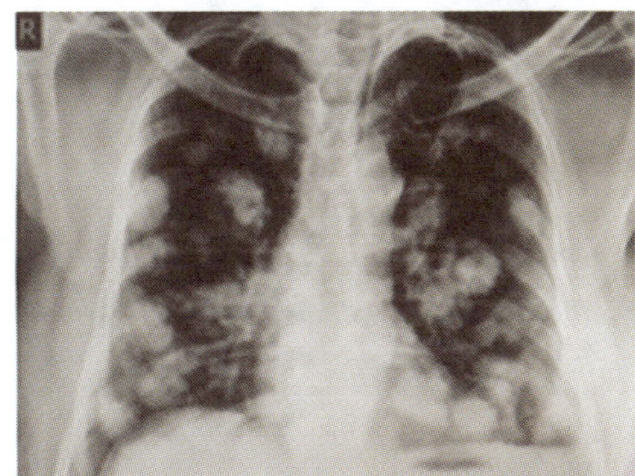

a. Cannon ball metastasis
b. Aspergillosis
c. Mesothelioma
d. Tuberculosis

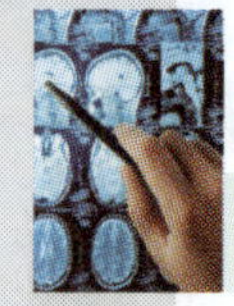

140. A 50-year-old patient presents with breathlessness and pedal edema for last 3 months. Past medical history is significant for tuberculosis. A chest radiograph is taken and shown below. What is the likely diagnosis?
(Most Recent Question Dec 2020)

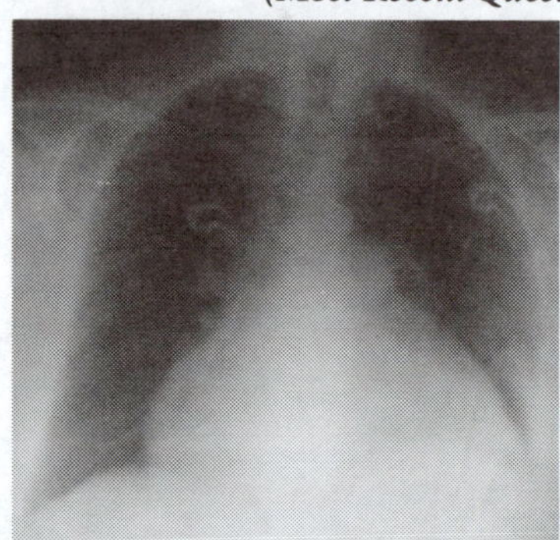

a. Constrictive pericarditis b. Pericardial effusion
c. Dilated cardiomyopathy d. Cardiac tamponade

141. A cattle handler from a village with cough, hemoptysis and chest pain underwent a chest radiograph and is shown below. What is the probable diagnosis?
(Most Recent Question Dec 2020)

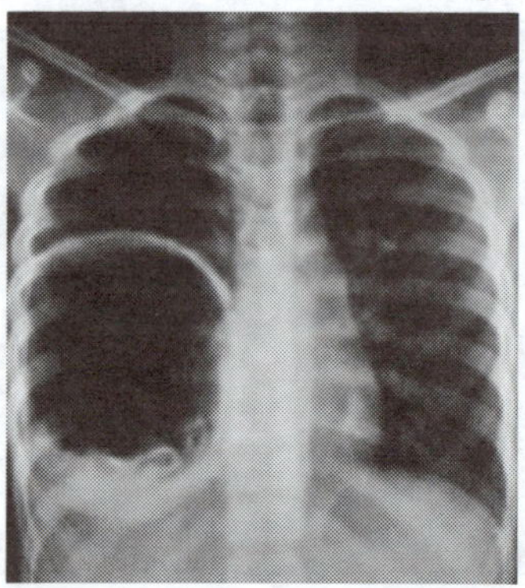

a. Hydatid cyst b. Anthrax
c. Byssinosis d. Lung abscess

142. A 6-day-old neonate with respiratory distress showed the following findings on chest X-ray?
(Most Recent Question Dec 2020)

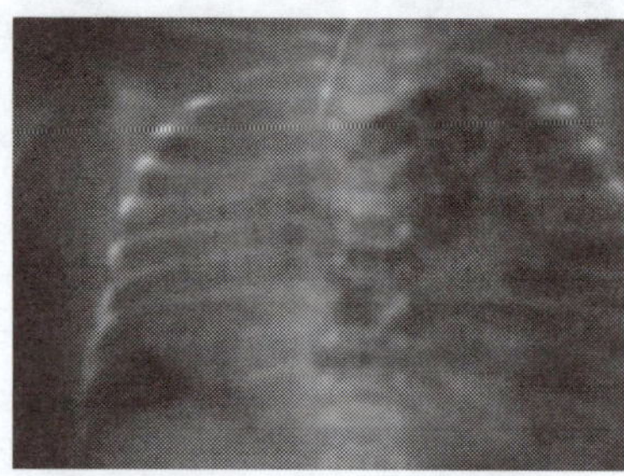

a. Cystic adenomatoid malformation
b. Bronchogenic cyst
c. Hyaline membrane disease
d. Congenital diaphragmatic hernia

143. A 30-year-old patient presents with high-grade fever, chills and cough with sputum, radiograph taken is shown. What is the likely diagnosis?
(Most Recent Question Aug 2020)

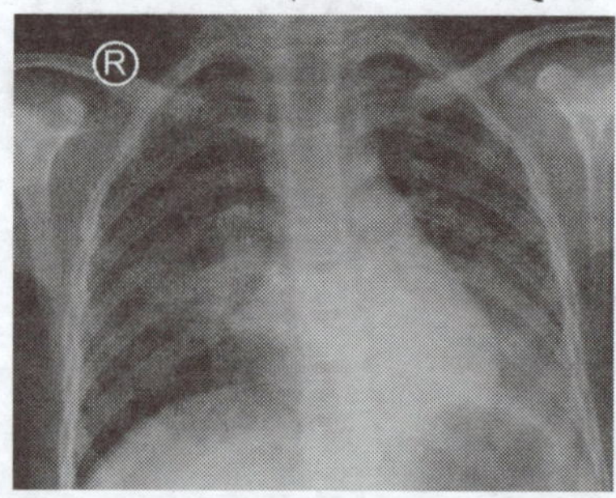

a. Rt middle lobe consolidation
b. Rt lower lobe consolidation
c. Atelectasis
d. Pneumothorax

144. A 45-year-old female came for post-surgery follow up, a CXR was taken. What is the most likely diagnosis?
(Most Recent Question Aug 2020)

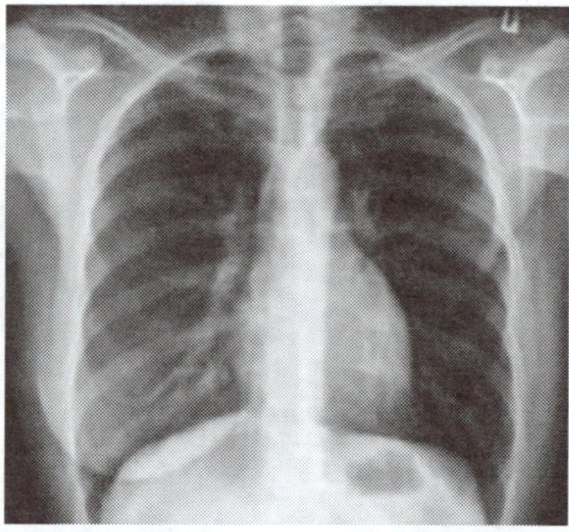

a. Left sided mastectomy b. Malignancy
c. Fibroadenoma d. Emphysema

145. Identify the diagnosis in the given chest radiograph.
(Most Recent Question Aug 2020)

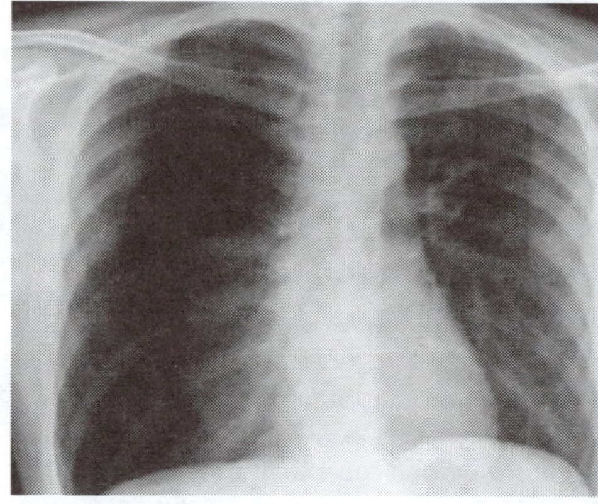

a. Pneumothorax b. Hydropneumothorax
c. Pericardial effusion d. Emphysema

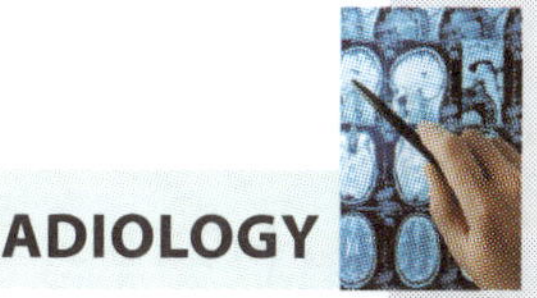

146. A 33-year-old female with fever, weight loss, elevated levels of ACE levels with hilar lymphadenopathy on X-ray. What is the probable diagnosis?
(Most Recent Question Aug 2020)

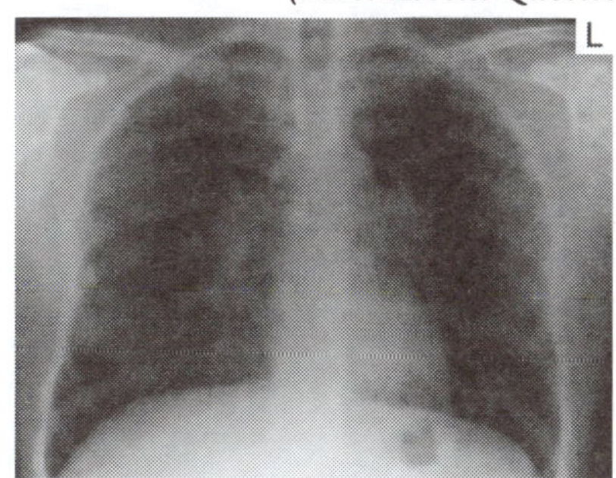

a. TB b. Sarcoidosis
c. Silicosis d. Small cell cancer

147. A 2-year-old child presents with sudden onset of breathlessness, wheezing and decreased breath sounds in right lung. Chest radiograph shows diffuse opacity in right hemithorax. What is probable diagnosis?
(Most Recent Question Aug 2020)

a. Bronchial asthma b. Pneumonia
c. Foreign body aspiration d. Pneumothorax

148. Identify the findings given in the X-ray.
(Most Recent Question Aug 2020)

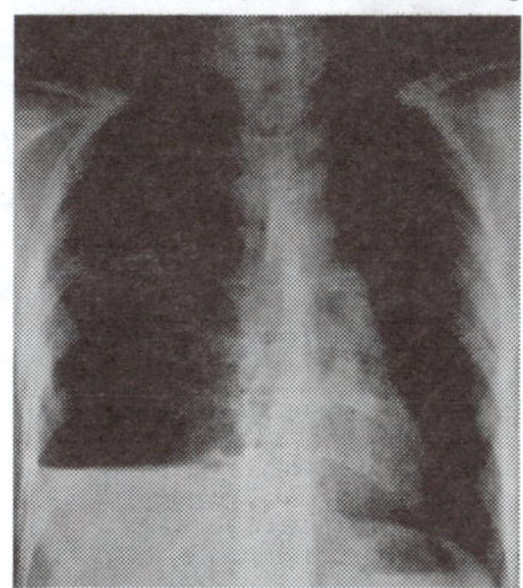

a. Hydropneumothorax b. Pneumothorax
c. Cardiac tamponade d. Lower lobe pneumonia

149. A 35-year-old female who is a known case of HIV, with CD4 <500, presents with fever, dyspnea, cough. Chest X-ray has been taken, what is the most likely diagnosis?
(Most Recent Question Aug 2020)

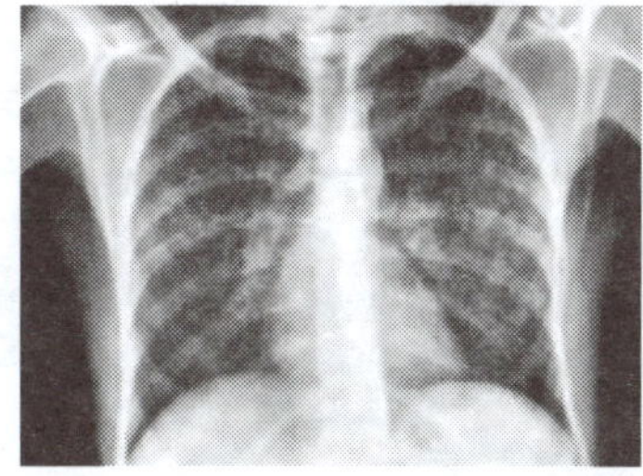

a. Staphylococcus b. Streptococcus
c. Histoplasmosis d. Military TB

150. Comment on the diagnosis of CT chest shown below.
(Most Recent Question 2019)

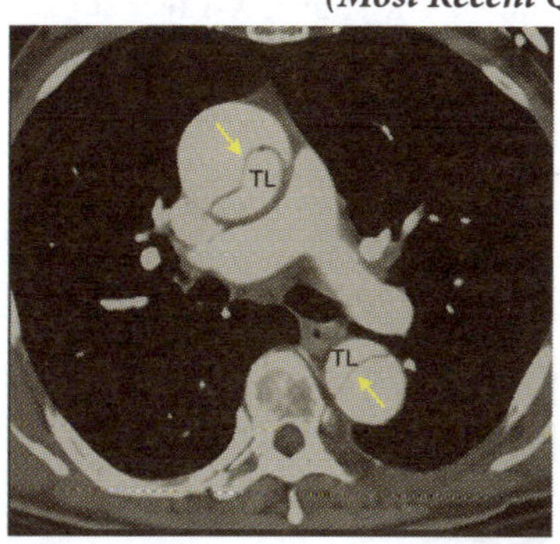

a. Aortic dissection b. Pulmonary embolism
c. Cardiac myxoma d. Aortic aneurysm

151. Which is used for calculation of ejection fraction?
(Most Recent Question 2019)

a. MUGA
b. SPECT using thallium 201
c. PET myocardial perfusion imaging
d. Sestamibi scan with pharmacological stress

152. The shown radiograph is a case of:
(Most Recent Question 2019)

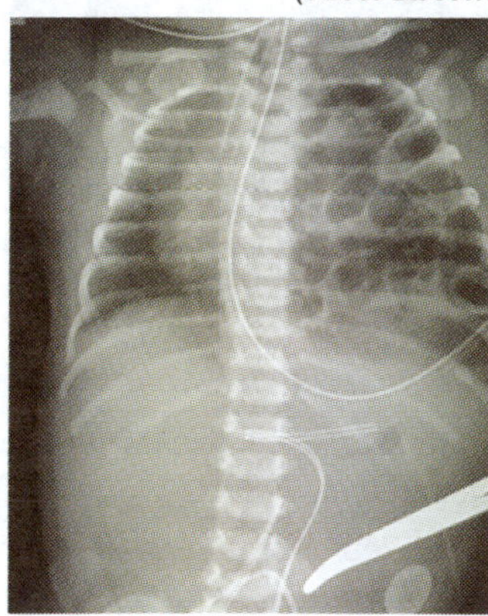

a. Diaphragmatic hernia b. Intestinal obstruction
c. Pleural effusion d. Pneumonia

153. In the shown lateral view of chest X-ray, what is the structure marked with X or white arrow head?
(Most Recent Question 2019)

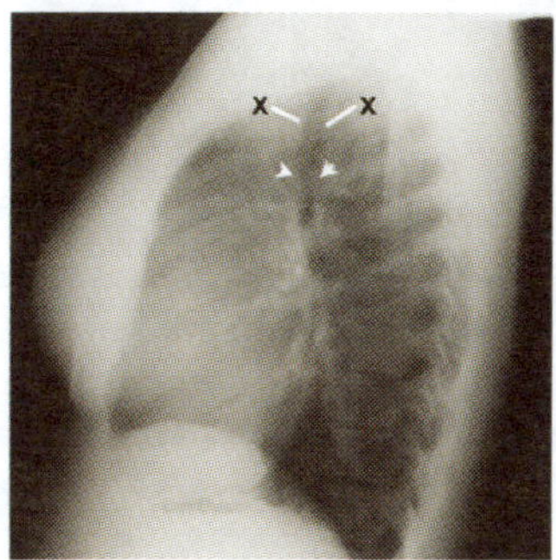

a. Esophagus b. Pulmonary artery
c. Trachea d. Left atrium

154. A patient presented with complaints of low grade fever with dyspnoea. The shown X-ray is suggestive of:
(Most Recent Question 2019)

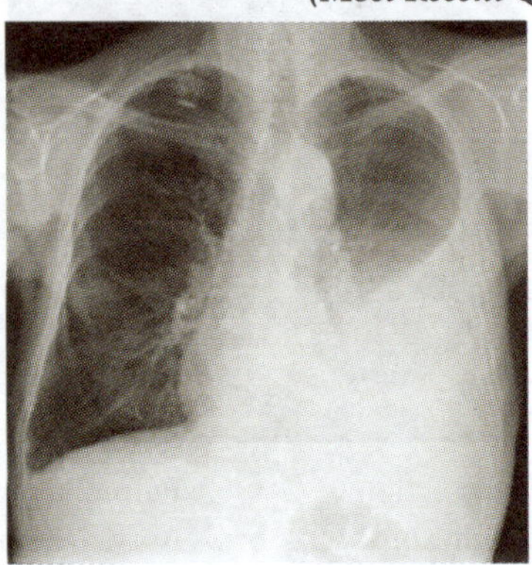

a. Consolidation
b. Exudative pleural effusion
c. Pneumothorax
d. Hydropneumothorax

155. Identify the pathology in the given X-ray:
(Recent Pattern Question 2018-19)

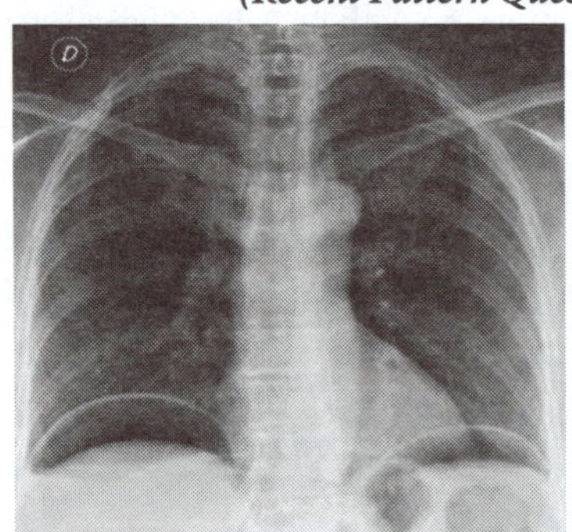

a. Pneumothorax
b. Pneumoperitoneum
c. Hydrothorax
d. Normal X-ray

156. The following image shows:
(Recent Pattern Question 2018-19)

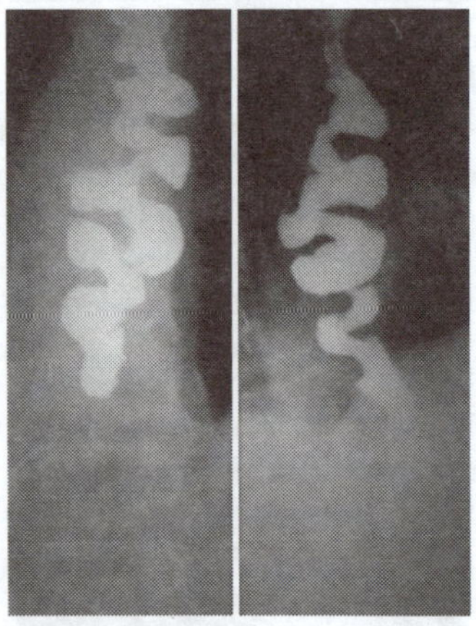

a. Achalasia cardia
b. Diffuse esophageal spasm
c. Carcinoma esophagus
d. Schatzki's ring

157. The Lateral view X-ray lung shows:
(Recent Pattern Question 2018)

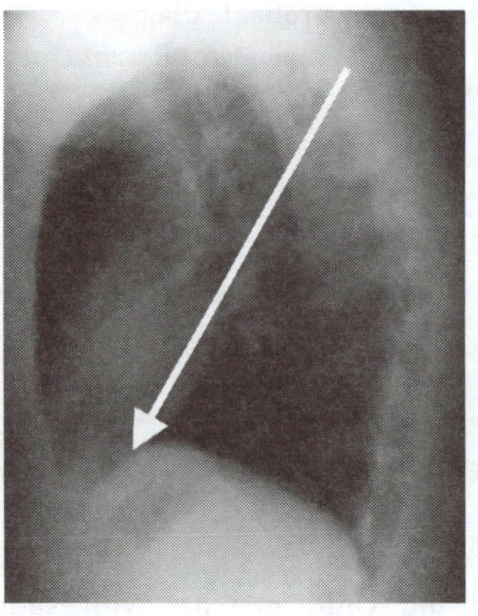

a. Major fissure
b. Minor fissure
c. Azygos fissure
d. Transverse fissure

158. Comment on the diagnosis:
(Recent Pattern Question 2017)

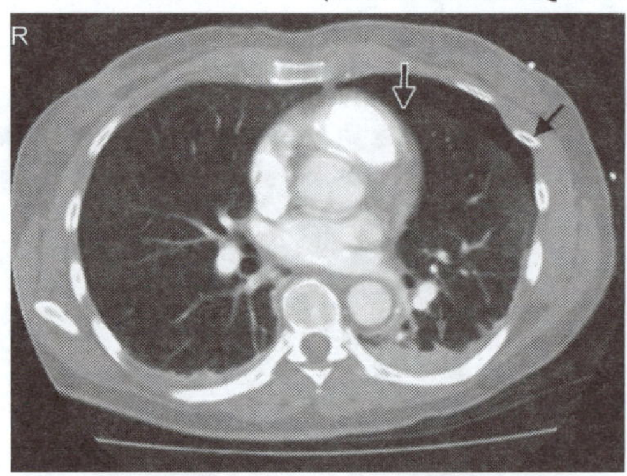

a. Hydrothorax
b. Pneumothorax
c. Pleural effusion
d. Hydropneumothorax

159. CT chest is as shown below. What is the diagnosis?
(Recent Pattern Question 2017)

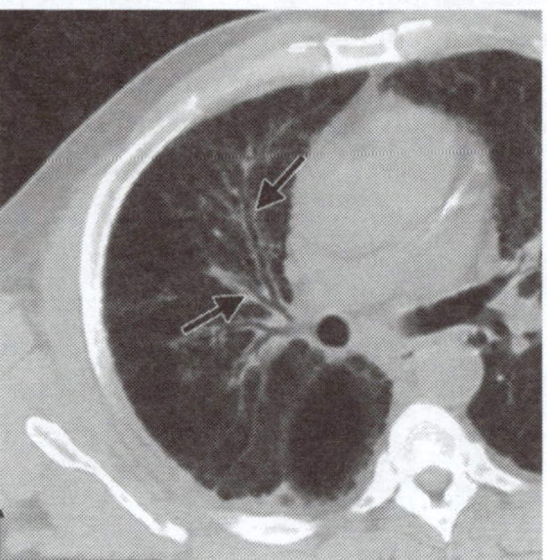

a. Bronchiectasis
b. Pneumonia
c. Pulmonary TB
d. COPD

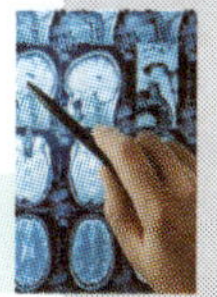

160. The shown investigation is:

(Recent Pattern Question 2017)

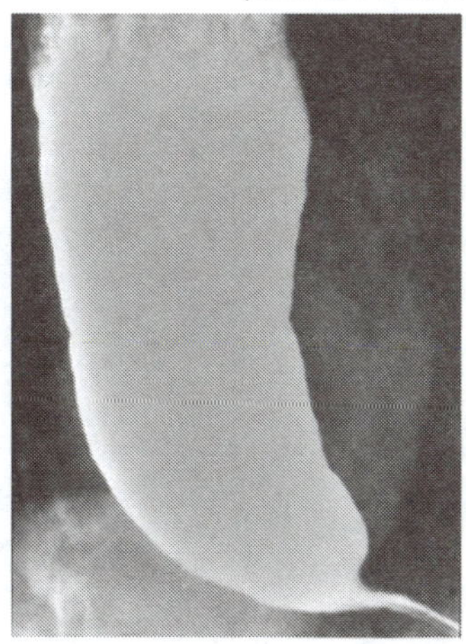

a. Barium enema
b. Barium swallow
c. Plain X-ray
d. Fluoroscopy

161. Identify the pathology in the given chest X-ray:

(Recent Pattern Question 2017)

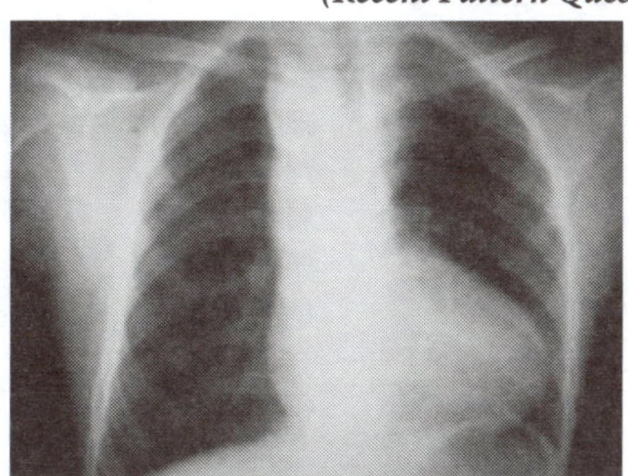

a. Tetralogy of Fallot
b. Transposition of great arteries
c. Pericardial effusion
d. Total anomalous pulmonary veinous return

162. In the CECT shown below what is the structure marked with arrow? *(Recent Pattern Question 2017)*

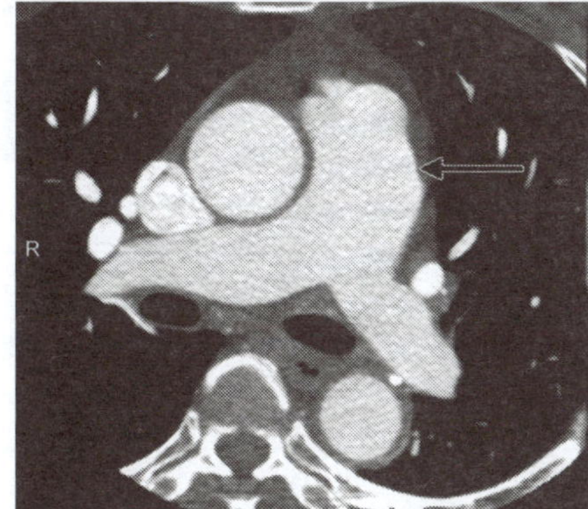

a. Aorta
b. Trachea
c. Descending aorta
d. Main pulmonary artery

163. The arrow at CXR points to:

(Recent Pattern Question 2017)

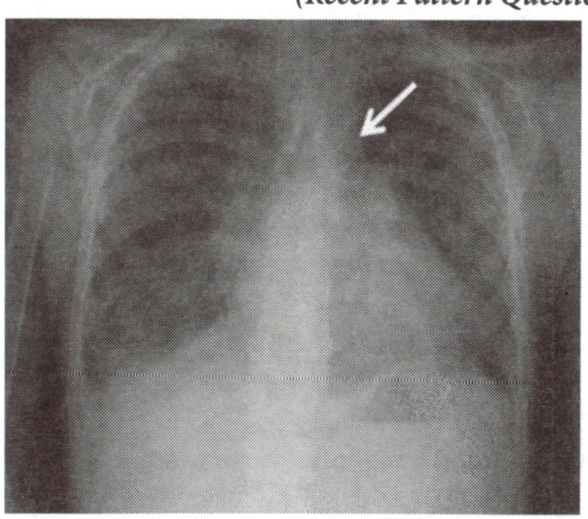

a. Left atrium
b. Left atrial appendage
c. Lingular lobe lung
d. Aortic knuckle

164. The following image shows

(Recent Pattern Question 2016)

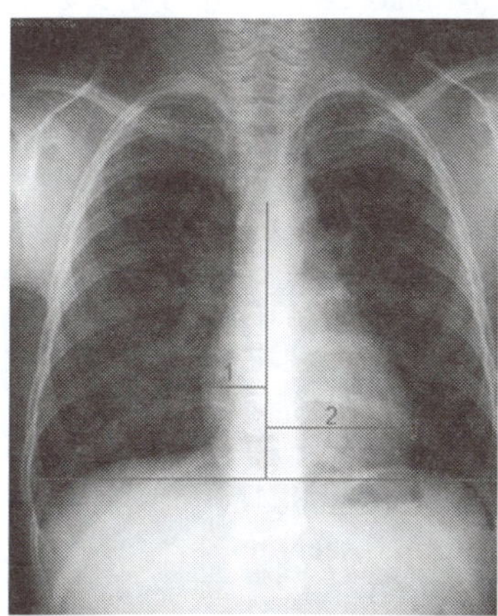

a. Pulmonary edema
b. CT ratio being measured
c. Atelectasis
d. Bronchiectasis

165. In a patient with bronchopneumonia lung, finding on CXR: *(Recent Pattern Question 2016)*

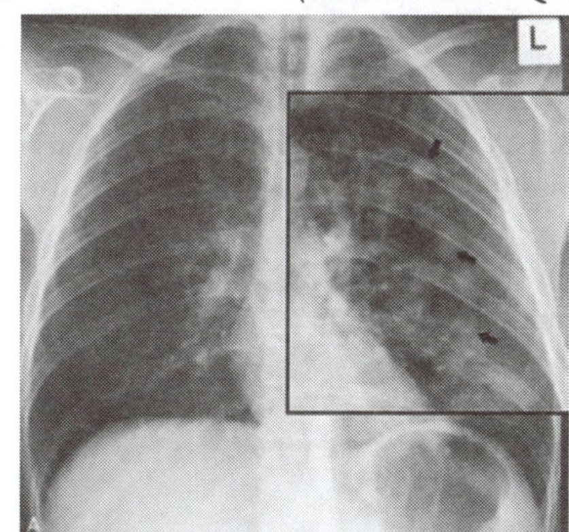

a. Patchy consolidation
b. Diffuse consolidation
c. Mediastinal shift
d. Massive pleural effusion

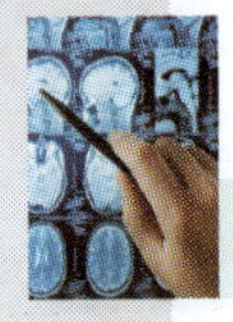

166. All of the following are true in chest X-ray PA view; EXCEPT:
a. Right ventricle forms the right heart border
b. Left ventricle forms the left heart border
c. Cardiothoracic ratio in adults is normally 50% or less than that
d. Right atrium forms the right heart border

167. Transesophageal echocardiography is better than transthoracic Echocardiography because of better evaluation of?
a. Diastolic dysfunction
b. Left ventricular hypertrophy
c. Systolic function
d. Left atrial appendage clots

168. Most common congenital cardiac anomaly diagnosed in adulthood:
a. ASD
b. VSD
c. PDA
d. TAPVR

169. Box shaped heart is seen in which of the following condition:
a. Coaractation of aorta
b. Pericardial effusion
c. Tetralogy of fallot
d. Ebstein anomaly

170. Curschmann spirals and flattening of diaphragm is seen in:
a. Asthma
b. COPD
c. Silicosis
d. Pulmonary embolism

171. Flexible Bronchoscope contains holes for all of these functions; EXCEPT:
a. Ventilation
b. Drainage of secretion
c. For biopsy
d. To remove foreign body

172. Hampton hump is seen in:
a. Pulmonary TB
b. Bronchogenic carcinoma
c. Pulmonary embolism
d. Pulmonary hemorrhage

173. Westermark's sign is seen in:
a. Pulmonary embolism
b. Pulmonary sequestration
c. Pulmonary alveolar proteinosis
d. A.B.P.A (Allergic Broncho-pulmonary Aspergillosis)

174. Continuous diaphragm sign is seen on X-ray. Diagnosis is?
a. Pneumopericardium
b. Pneumomediastinum
c. Pneumothorax
d. Pericardial abscess

175. Air Bronchogram is seen in:
a. Pneumonia
b. Pleural effusion
c. Pneumothorax
d. Pneumo-peritoneum

176. IDENTIFY: *(X-ray chest showing big mass on left upper lobe, touching sternum)*

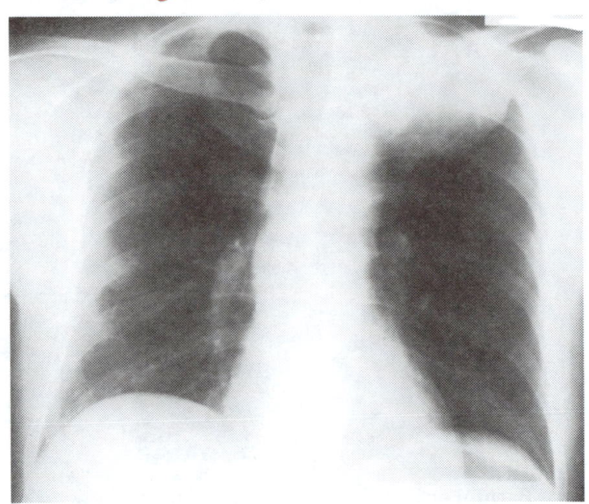

a. Lung carcinoma
b. Hydatid cyst
c. Lung Abscess
d. Aspergilloma

177. Golden S sign is seen in:

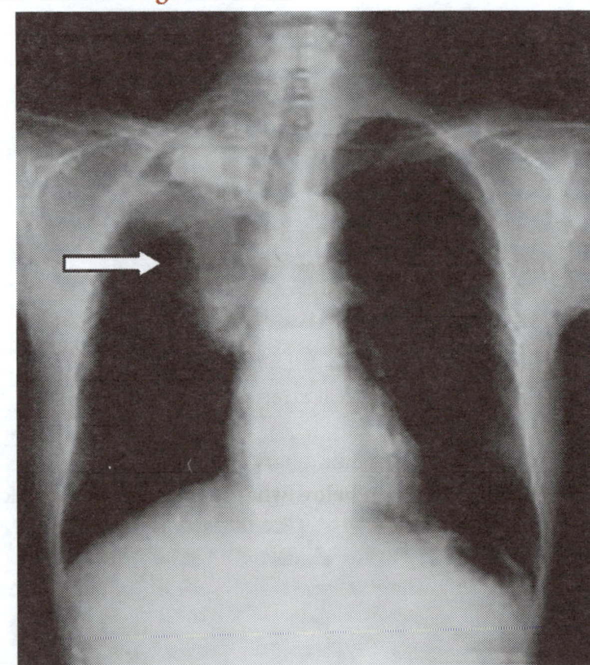

a. Bronchogenic carcinoma with collapse of lung
b. Traction Bronchiectasis with apical scarring
c. Emphysema with increased lucency and flattened diagphragm
d. Pulmonary edema

178. Pop-corn calcification is seen with?
a. Pulmonary tuberculosis
b. Pulmonary hamartoma
c. Klebsiella infection
d. Foreign body

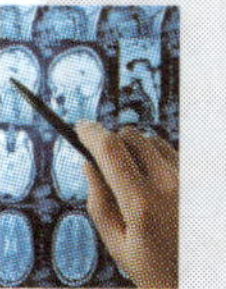

NEUROLOGY IMAGING

179. A newborn is seen to have an abnormal lump in the lower back. Identify the condition given in below MRI?
(Most Recent Question June 2022)

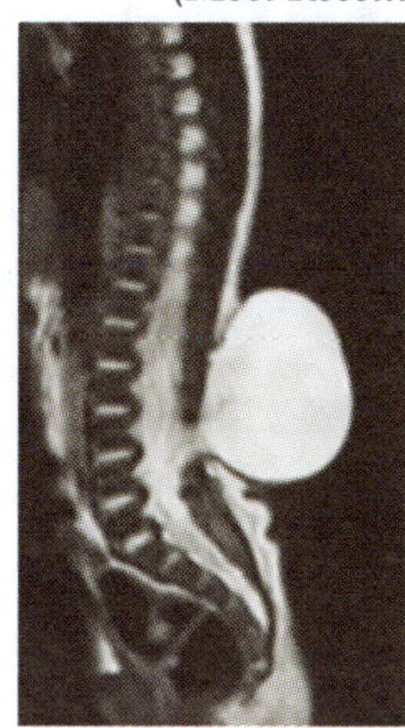

a. Meningocele
b. Spina bifida occulta
c. Myelomeningocele
d. Bone cyst

180. A 35-year-old female presents with thunderclap headache. What is the likely diagnosis based on image?
(Most Recent Question Dec 2021)

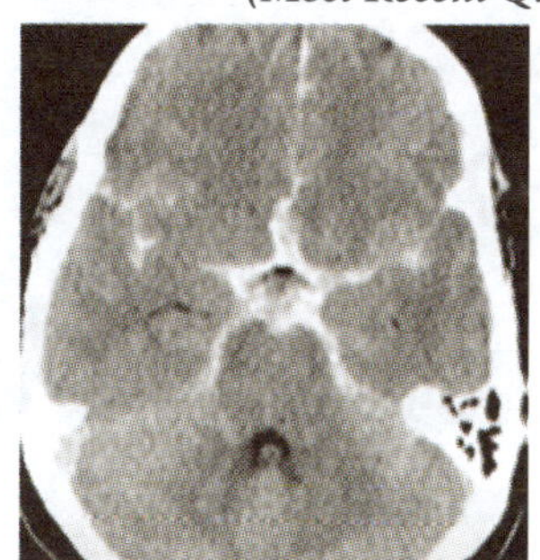

a. SDH
b. SAH
c. EDH
d. IVH

181. A 40-year-old male meets with a RTA after rash driving his bike without the helmet on. NCCT head shows:
(Most Recent Question June 2021)

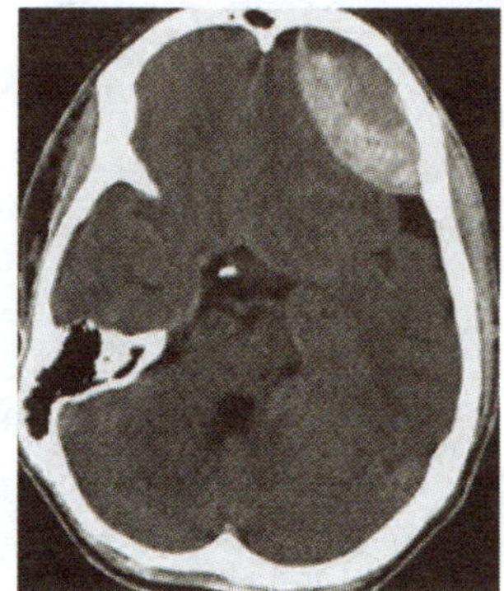

a. SDH
b. SAH
c. EDH
d. Cerebral contusion

182. Comment on the marked structure in the NCCT head.
(Most Recent Question June 2021)

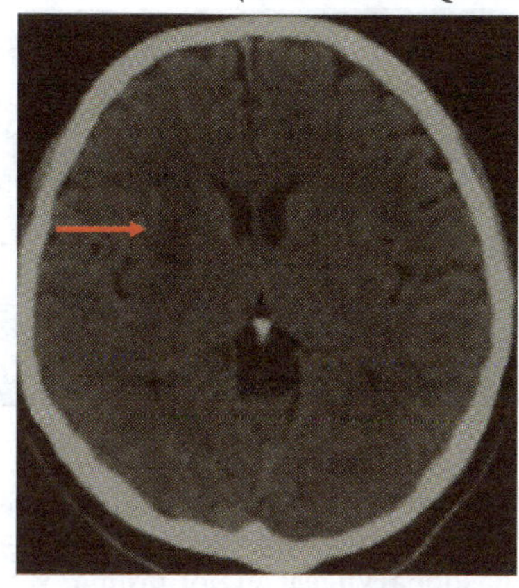

a. Caudate nucleus
b. Lenticular nucleus
c. Substantia nigra
d. Superior colliculus

183. A 30-year-old man had an RTA. On examination limb shortening was noted. Which of the following nerve is likely to be injured in this case?
(Most Recent Question June 2021)

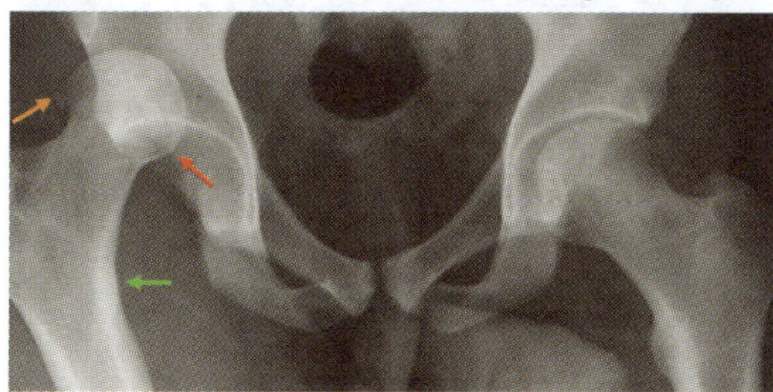

a. Femoral nerve
b. Obturator nerve
c. Sciatic nerve
d. Lumbar plexus

184. Which arterial territory is involved on this CT scan image of a patient with brain infarction?
(Most Recent Question Dec 2020)

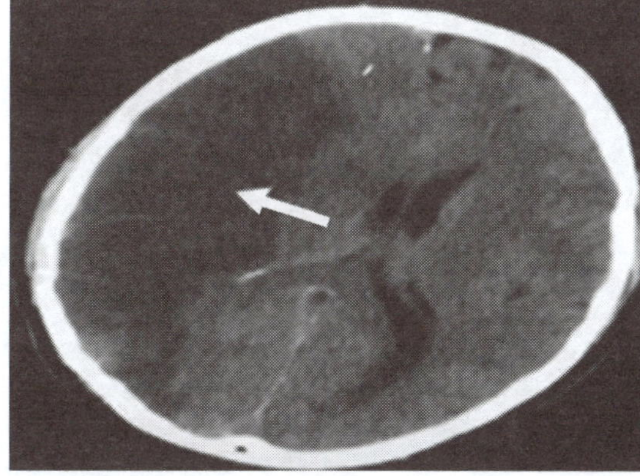

a. Anterior cerebral artery
b. Middle cerebral artery
c. Posterior cerebral artery
d. Posterior communicating artery

185. Identify the structure marked in the given image.
(Most Recent Question Dec 2020)

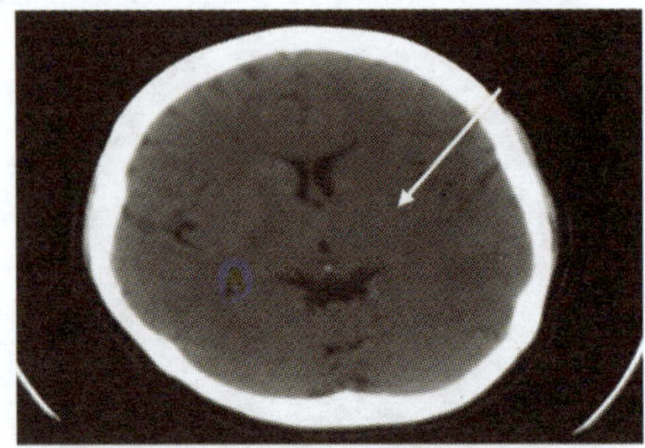

a. Caudate nucleus
b. Thalamus
c. Lentiform nucleus
d. Internal capsule

186. A patient presenting with epistaxis was diagnosed with juvenile nasopharyngeal angiofibroma. What is the sign demonstrated in the given image?
(Most Recent Question Dec 2020)

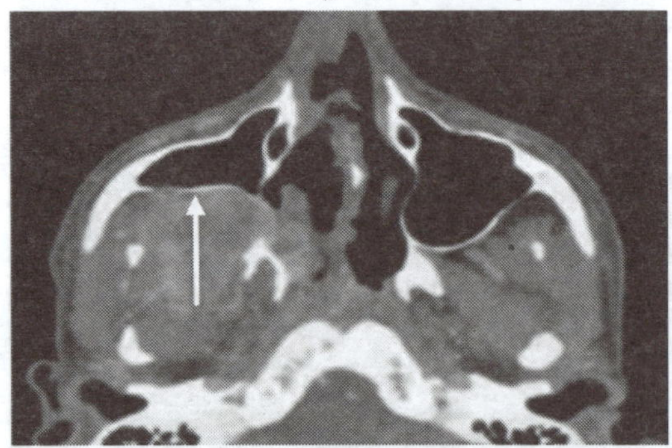

a. Holman Miller sign
b. Phelp sign
c. Griesinger sign
d. DODD sign

187. A 65-year-old hypertensive patient on irregular medication has headache and a BP 220/110. CT head is shown below. Comment on the diagnosis.
(Most Recent Question Aug 2020)

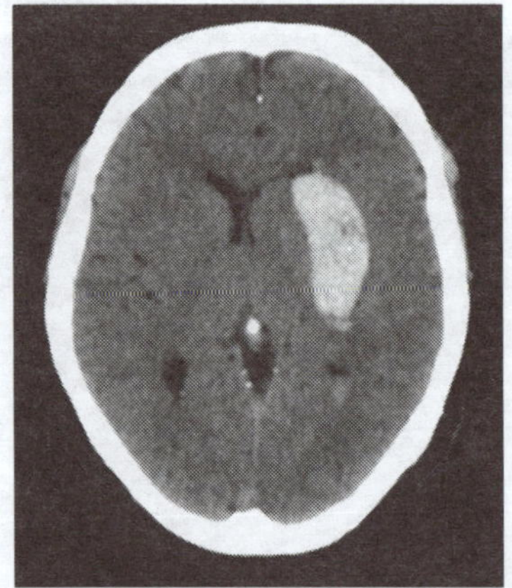

a. Intraventricular bleed
b. Putaminal bleed
c. Subarachnoid hemorrhage
d. Pontine hemorrhage

188. Identify the marked structure on CT head:
(Most Recent Question Aug 2020)

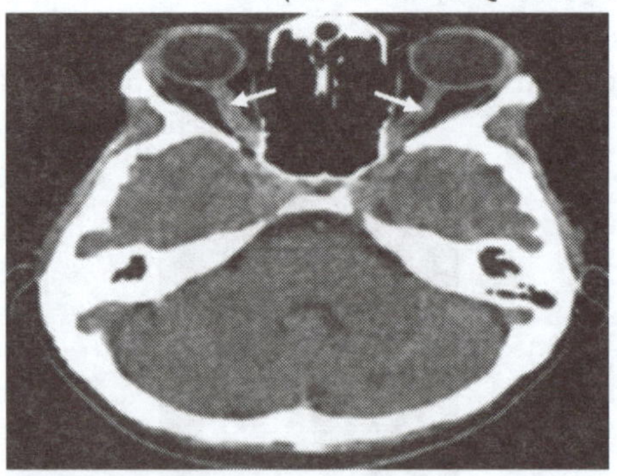

a. Optic nerve
b. Optic chiasma
c. Optic tract
d. Superior ophthalmic artery

189. Identify the marked structure shown by the arrow:
(Most Recent Question Aug 2020)

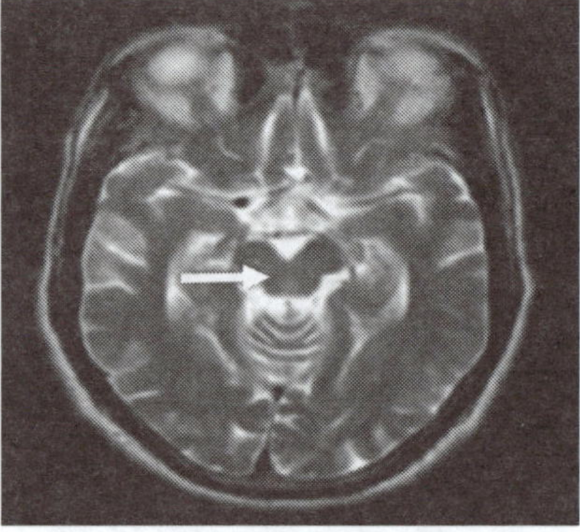

a. Medulla
b. Pons
c. Midbrain
d. Spinal cord

190. A 65-year-old female fell down in the bathroom & sustained head injury, CT scan head was performed. What is the diagnosis? ***(Most Recent Question Aug 2020)***

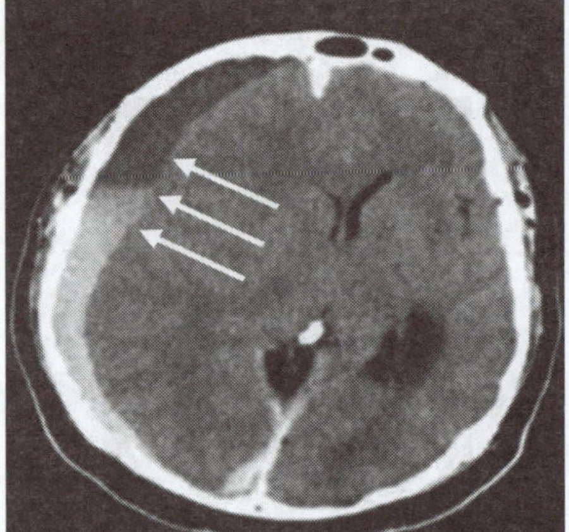

a. Extradural hematoma
b. Intracranial bleed
c. Thrombosis
d. Subdural hematoma

191. A patient met with a RTA, is unconscious and the CT scan does not show any findings except for few petechial hemorrhages. What is the probable diagnosis?

(Most Recent Question Aug 2020)

a. Diffuse axonal injury b. Concussion
c. Contusion d. Subarachnoid hemorrhage

192. A patient with brain metastasis had to undergo head and neck irradiation, what is the most common delayed symptom with head and neck irradiation?

(Most Recent Question Aug 2020)

a. Xerostomia b. Dysphagia
c. Dysgeusia d. Anhidrosis

193. Identify the arrow marked structure in the given image:

(Most Recent Question Dec 2019)

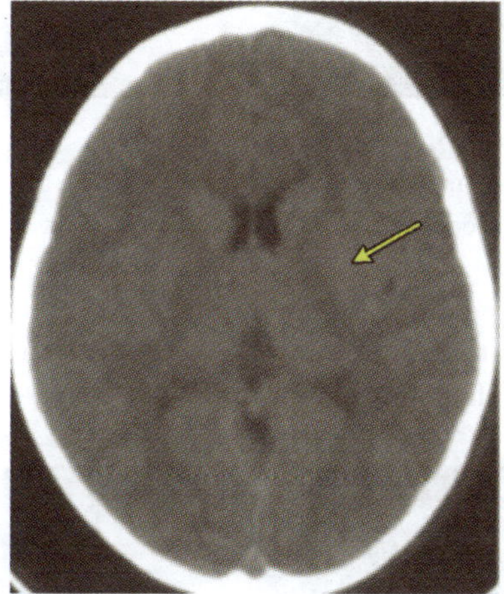

a. Thalamus b. Caudate nucleus
c. Lentiform nucleus d. Claustrum

194. Identify the pathology in the shown CT:

(Recent Pattern Question 2018-19)

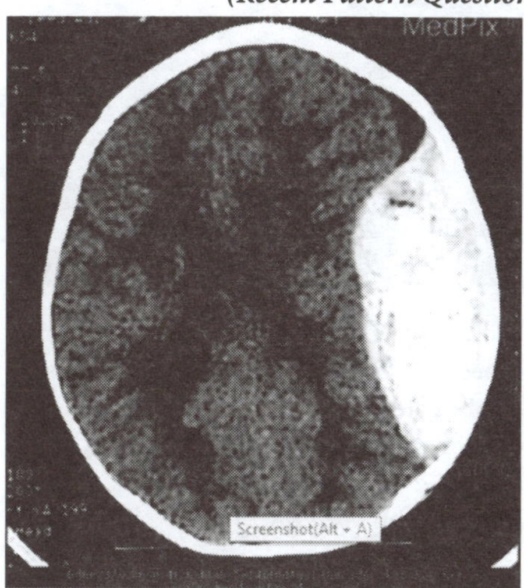

a. Intraventricular bleed
b. Massive Epidural hemorrhage
c. Subdural hemorrhage
d. Subarachnoid haemorrhage

195. Identify the image given below:

(Recent Pattern Question 2018)

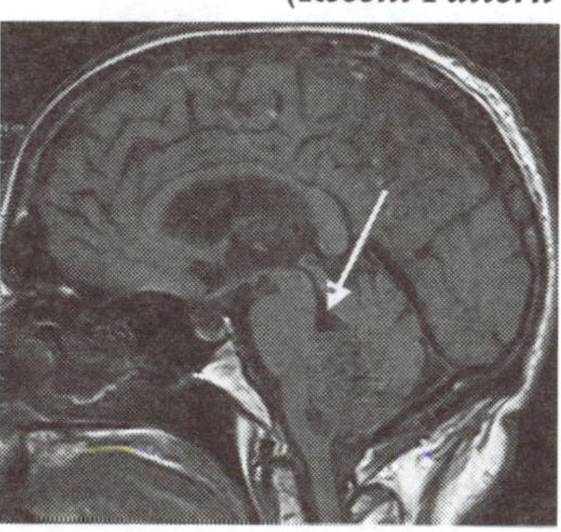

a. Lateral ventricle b. Corpus callosum
c. 3rd ventricle d. 4th ventricle

196. Angiography of brain blood vessels of brain as is shown in image. Identify the artery marked with arrow?

(Recent Pattern Question 2017)

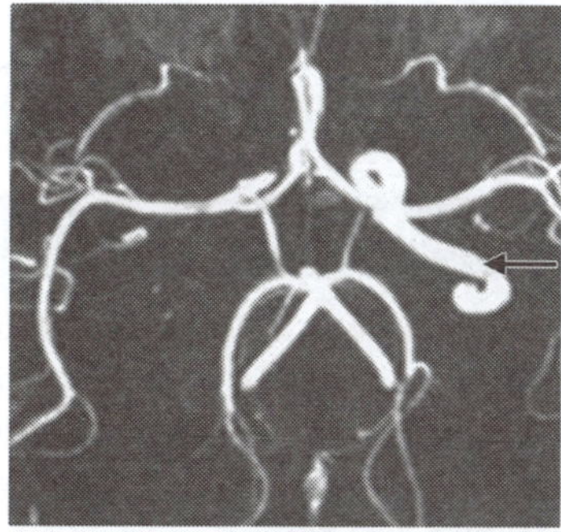

a. Anterior communicating artery
b. Posterior cerebral artery
c. Middle cerebral artery
d. Internal carotid artery

197. In the given imaging, what is the structure marked with arrow? ***(Recent Pattern Question 2017)***

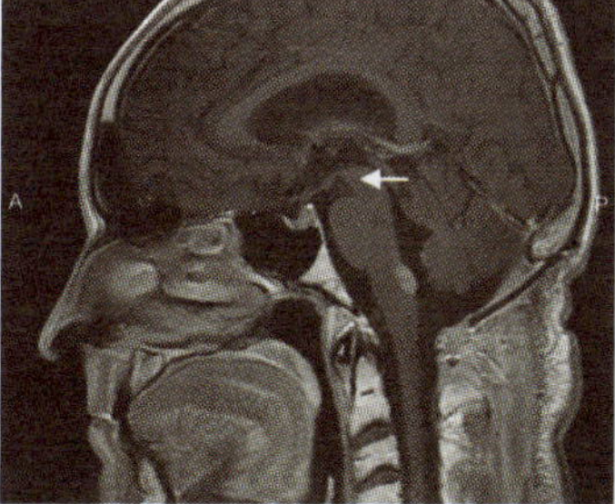

a. Midbrain b. Pons
c. Medulla d. Cerebellum

198. Most common investigation done in brain tumor:

(Recent Pattern Question 2016)

a. CT b. MRI
c. Digital X-ray d. USG

199. IOC for sub-arachnoid hemorrhage:

a. CT scan b. MRI
c. Lumbar puncture d. MRA

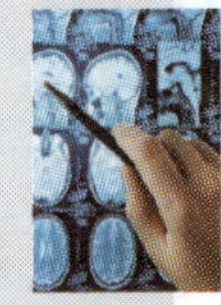

200. Extradural hemorrhage is seen as:

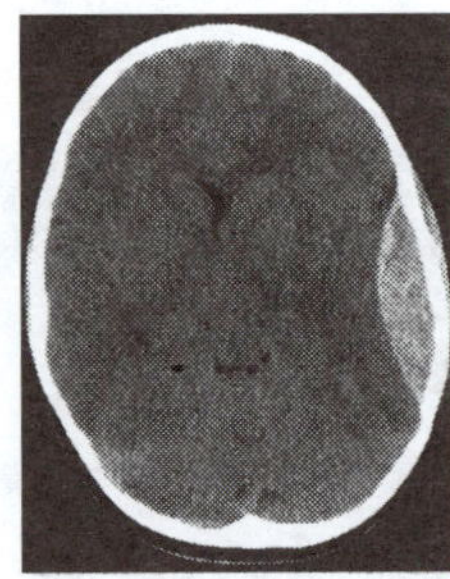

a. Hypodense bi concave b. Hypodense bi convex
c. Hyperdense bi concave d. Hyperdense bi convex

201. Intracranial calcification is best diagnosed by:

a. Plain X-ray skull b. CT scan
c. FDG-PFT scan d. MRI

202. The investigation of choice for meningeal carcinomatosis in CNS is:

a. Enhanced MRI b. SPECT
c. PET d. NCCT

MAMMOGRAPHY

203. The most appropriate technique for mammography is:

a. Spot Compression view b. Medial lateral oblique view
c. Lateral view d. Bird's eye view

204. Which one of the following statements regarding mammography is FALSE:

a. It can detect 95% of early breast cancers
b. Normal mammogram rules out breast cancer
c. The sensitivity of this investigation increases with age as the breast becomes less dense
d. Mammography is a safe investigation even after radiation exposure

OBSTETRICAL IMAGING

205. A 35-year-old female presents with a history of nausea and vomiting. She is undergoing IVF treatment. What is the likely diagnosis? ***(Most Recent Question Dec 2021)***

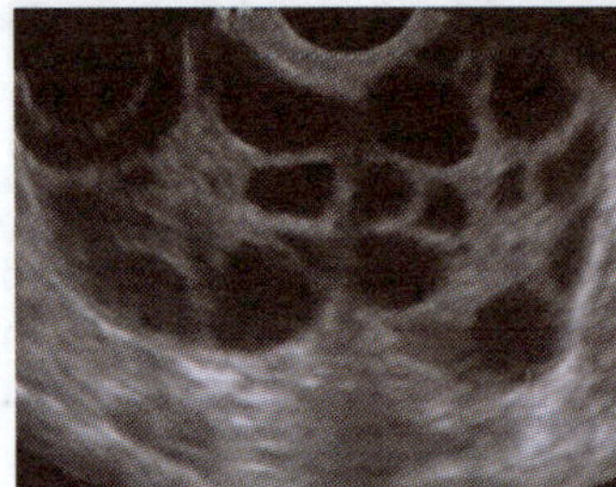

a. PCOD
b. Ovarian Hyperstimulation syndrome
c. Theca – Lutein cyst
d. Mucinous cystadenoma

206. What is the likely diagnosis based on the image below? ***(Most Recent Question Dec 2021)***

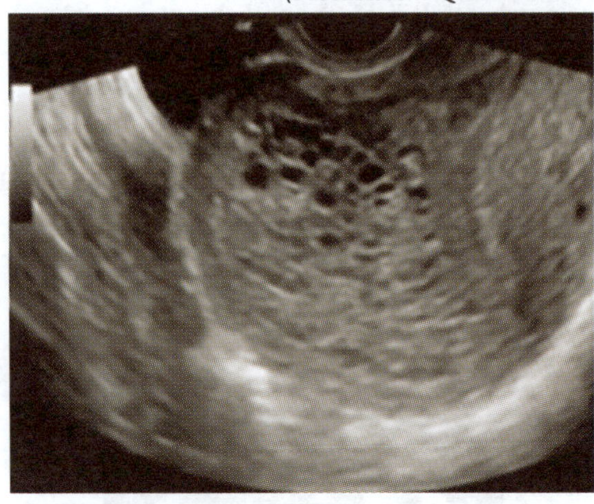

a. Ectopic pregnancy
b. Molar pregnancy
c. Retained products of conception
d. PCOD

207. A post-menopausal female with intermittent pelvic pain presents to the OPD and X-ray abdomen was performed. What is the likely diagnosis? ***(Most Recent Question June 2021)***

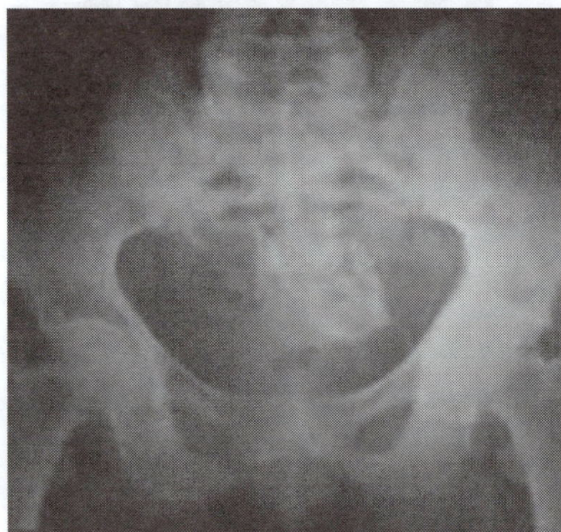

a. Bladder stone b. Calcified fibroid
c. Chocolate cyst d. Ovarian mass

208. Father of obstetrical ultrasound:

a. Ion Donald
b. John Wild
c. Doppler John
d. Hounsfield

209. By ultrasonography, the earliest sign of conception is:

a. Small white gestational ring
b. Presence of foetal pole
c. Presence of yolk sac
d. Presence of cardiac pulsations

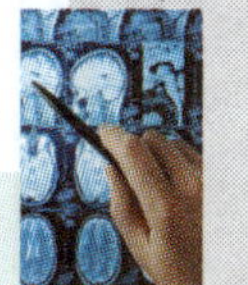

ANSWERS WITH EXPLANATIONS

MOST RECENT QUESTIONS 2023

1. Ans. (d) Duplex imaging

Ref: Bailey and Love 27th ed. pg. 975

The image shows varicose veins and the best investigation to confirm the diagnosis is Duplex imaging/ Doppler scan.

2. Ans. (c) Blood flow velocity

Ref: Bailey and Love 27th ed. pg. 976

The image shows a portable Doppler device that displays blood flow velocity waveform. Hampering blood flow will lead to thrombus formation.

3. Ans. (d) Emphysematous pyelonephritis

Tenderness in costovertebral angle indicates renal pathology with infective origin. X-ray abdomen shows gas shadow along the contour of kidney indicating infection with gas forming organism. The diagnosis is Emphysematous pyelonephritis.

- Option a is diagnosed on CT scan or IVP.
- Option b will have calcified kidney.
- Option c is a pathological diagnosis.

4. Ans. (b) Duodenal atresia

The image shows double bubble sign with dilated end of proximal duodenum and stomach seen in case of Duodenal atresia.

Extra Mile

Polyhydramnios in antenatal ultrasound and bilious vomiting in the first 2 days of life point to its presence.

5. Ans. (c) Depressed skull fracture

6. Ans. (b) External beam radiotherapy

LINAC/Linear accelerators are used to provide patients with external beam radiation therapy. External beam therapy is a common technique used to treat malignant tumors or benign lesions through the delivery of high doses of X-rays or electrons reducing the dose to the surrounding normal tissues.

7. Ans. (a) Xerostomia

- Option d is ruled out as it is too far away from the area being subjected to radiotherapy. Option b is ruled out as is an acute effect of RT.
- The acute effects of RT include mucositis, thickened secretions, mucosal infections, pain, and sensory disruptions.
- The long-term chronic effects of head and neck RT comprise tissue fibrosis, salivary gland dysfunction, increased susceptibility to mucosal infections, neuropathic pain, sensory disorders and an increased susceptibility to dental caries and periodontal disease.

8. Ans. (a) Inversely proportional, squared

Ref: Diagnostic Radiology pg. 13

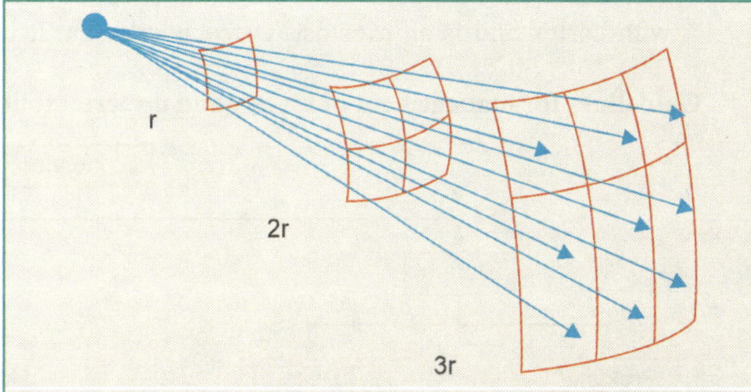

As we move further away from the X-ray source within the cone that the X-rays fluency, or the number of X-rays passing through a given area reduces as 1/R^2 where R is the distance from the X-ray source to the image receptor. This is why this effect is termed the **inverse square law** and is also written as 1/(SID)^2.

9. Ans. (c) 4th rib anterior part

The hack to solve this question is that just below the clavicle shadow, aligned *horizontally* is the 4th rib. The confusion between 3rd and 4th ribs can be resolved by looking at the adjacent image.

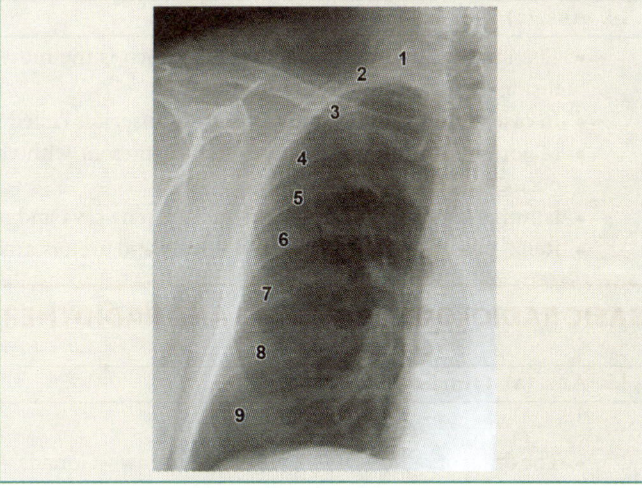

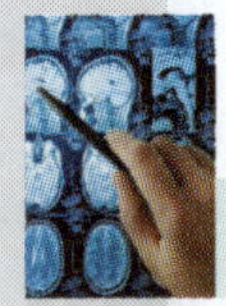

10. Ans. (a) Sestamibi scan

The clinical presentation is of psychic moans, bone pains and groans of hyperparathyroidism. To locate parathyroid tumor, the nuclear scan ordered is Tc-99 sestamibi scan.

11. Ans. (c) MRI

MR imaging allows precise definition of the fistulous track and identification of secondary fistulas or abscesses. It provides accurate information for appropriate surgical treatment, decreasing the incidence of recurrence and allowing the side effects such as fecal incontinence to be avoided.

12. Ans. (a) Ostechondroma

- The image shows a bony outgrowth that is continuous with cortex and is an exostosis/Osteochondroma. It is made up of both bone and cartilage. Since tumor can be present below the tendon it can damage the bone as well as tendon causing pain as mentioned in the question. As a child grows, an osteochondroma may grow larger as well. Once a child has reached skeletal maturity, the osteochondroma typically stops growing too.
- Option b produces soap bubble appearance in distal part of radius.
- Option c has sunburst appearance.
- Option d has onion peel appearance.

13. Ans. (a) Ureteroscopy

Considering multiple ureteric calculi in both proximal and distal part of ureter, ureteroscopy would be done. SWL can also be done, but risk of Steinstrasse: which is the German term for stone street, would be higher.

Guidelines for management of kidney and ureteric stones

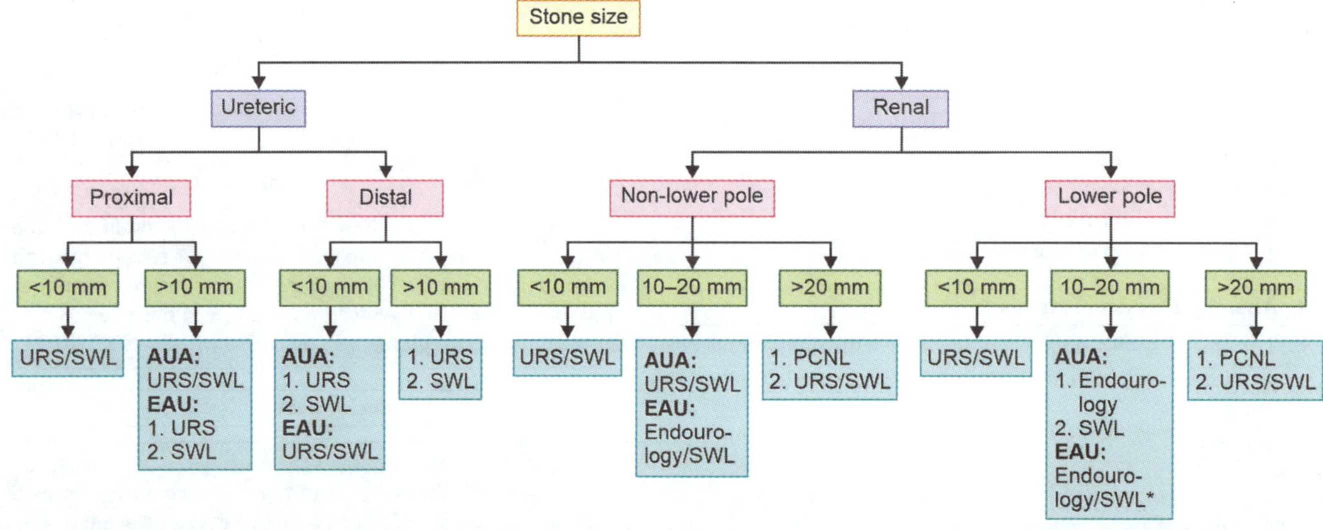

14. Ans. (a) Horse-shoe kidney

- The image shows horse-shoe kidney which is the most common fusion abnormality of the kidney with 90% cases showing fusion at the lower pole.
- In case, both the upper and lower poles fuse, it is called pancake or doughnut kidney.
- Majority are asymptomatic and rest are present with vague abdominal pain. Hydronephrosis, stones and infection can also occur.
- Isthmus is anterior to aorta and inferior vena cava and posterior to inferior mesenteric artery.
- Renal pelvis is usually rotated anteriorly and ureters arise anteriorly or laterally.

BASIC RADIOLOGY PRINCIPLES AND RADIOTHERAPY

15. Ans. (a) Ovaries

Ref: Principles of Radiation Oncology Perez, pg. 323

- The order of radiosensitivity is Bone marrow > Gonads > GIT. The concept is that the faster a tissue divides, more radiosensitive it will be.

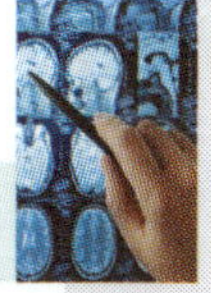

Radiosensitivity of organs and tissues

Mechanism of causing effects on human body

Active cell division — **High sensitivity**

- **Hematopoietic system**: Bone marrow and lymphatic tissues (spleen, thymus gland, lymph node)
- **Reproductive system**: Testis and ovary
- **Gastrointestinal system**: Mucus membrane and small-intestinal villus
- **Epidermis and eyes**: Hair follicle, sweat gland, skin and lens
- **Other**: Lung, kidney, liver and thyroid gland
- **Support system**: Blood vessel, muscle and bone
- **Transmission system**: Nerve

No cell division — **Low sensitivity**

16. Ans. (d) CT Enteroclysis

Ref: SRB Manual of Surgery pg. 936

- The image shows Bowel loops highlighted with contrast. Also visualized is Bone which is hyperdense. This is a hybrid technique known as CT-Enteroclysis.
- Procedure entails introduction of 12 to 14F Enteroclysis tubes under fluoroscopy or through duodenoscope. The tip of the tube is placed distal to Ligament of Treitz.

17. Ans. (a) F-18

Rf: Harrison 20th ed. pg. 2732

- The radioactive F-18 is a positron emitter and deoxyglucose is the ligand that will be picked up by cancer cells. The gamma camera will pick up the Gamma rays generated in the process.
- Option B, C and D are used in radiotherapy.

18. Ans. (d) Hours to days

Ref: ncbi.nlm.gov.in

Gross biological effect would mean development of cell death which can take few minutes to weeks depending on magnitude of radiation exposure.

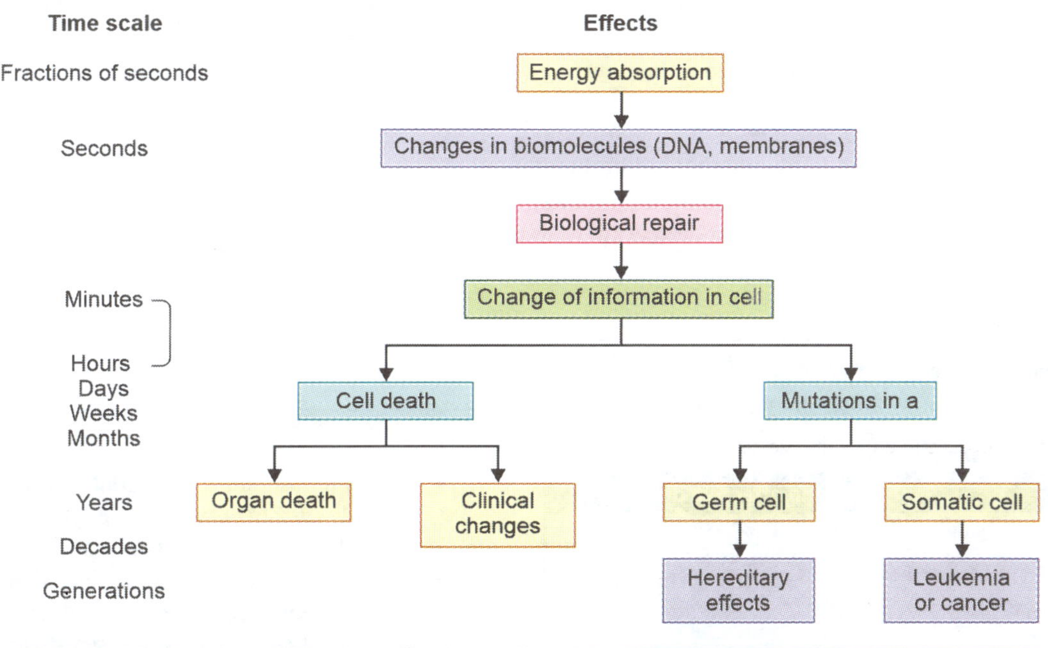

Skin erythema	Gy
Irreversible skin damage	20 Gy
Hair loss	Gy
Sterility	Gy
Cataracts	0.5 Gy
Lethality (Whole body)	3–5 Gy
Fetal abnormality	0.1–0.5 Gy

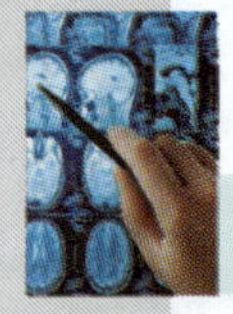

19. Ans. (d) 0.5 mm

Shielding is mainly achieved by wearing protective lead aprons of **0.5 mm** thickness, which have been cited to attenuate over 90%–99% of the radiation dose.

20. Ans. (a) Regular fractionated radiotherapy

- In the case given equal amount of radiation (2 Gy) is delivered at regular intervals for 5 days per week. The objective is to maximize destruction while minimizing damage to healthy tissues.
- Option B delivery is done for max 15 days and will deliver higher dose of radiation in later weeks while in the case given equal amounts are being given. The reason for increasing dose is to neutralize the accelerated tumor growth in later stage of radiotherapy.
- Option C involves treatment given more than once per day of lesser dose 1 Gy
- Option D involves two or more deliveries per day as well on weekends

21. Ans. (c) CT scan

- Functional endoscopic sinus surgery is a minimally invasive technique used to restore sinus ventilation and normal function.
- Fiberoptic telescopes are used for diagnosis and during the procedure, and *computed tomography is used to assess the anatomy and identify diseased areas.*
- The most suitable candidates for this procedure have recurrent acute or chronic infective sinusitis, and an improvement in symptoms of up to 90 percent may be expected following the procedure.

22. Ans. (d) Barium enema

Ref: Radiation dose in X-ray and CT exams; https://www.radiologyinfo.org/en/pdf/safety-xray

TABLE: Radiation exposure in different investigations

Procedure	Mean effective dose (mSv)
• Chest X-ray (PA View)	0.02
• Chest X-ray (PA + Lateral view)	0.1
• Mammogram	0.4
• Abdomen X-ray	0.7
• HSG	0.9 – 1.3
• CT Brain	2.2
• IVP	3
• ERCP	4
• Coronary angiography	7 (2–16)
• Barium enema	8 (2–18)
• CT Colonography	6
• CT Abdomen and Pelvis	10
• Thallium scan	16.9

Contd...

23. Ans. (b) CT and X-ray

- Out of given choices, CT and X-ray work on the same principle.
  - X-rays passed through the body are either absorbed or attenuated (weakened) at different levels
  - The image contains shadow of the dense tissues of body
  - If 3D image required, as in CT, a detector is placed opposite to radiation source. The software takes pictures from different angles and performs reconstruction of image by computer.

Extra Mile

- **Working principle of other radiological procedures:**
  - **Ultrasound:** Uses sound waves (Piezoelectric effect)
  - **MRI:** Uses magnetic fields/radio-frequency waves
  - **Nuclear medicine:** Uses gamma rays
  - **PET scan:** Uses short-lived positron emitting isotopes (each positron gives two gamma rays)

24. Ans. (a) KFT

Ref: Harrison: 19th ed, pg. 1803

The contrast can lead to development of renal shutdown due to contrast nephropathy. Serum creatinine should be checked before any contrast study is performed. Adequate hydration of the patient can prevent such a mishap. Drug of choice for management of contrast nephropathy is N-acetyl Cysteine.

25. Ans. (b) Venography

- Duplex ultrasound is the **initial investigation of choice** in nearly all patients with suspected DVT.
- Its reliability is dependent upon the skill of the user.
- Major axial veins of the lower limb are well displayed.
- It has a sensitivity of 98.7% and specificity of 100% for above-knee DVT and a sensitivity of 85.2% and specificity of 98.2% for below-knee DVT.
- **Gold standard/Best test** for venous occlusion is **invasive venography.**

26. Ans. (a) PET-CT scan

- The shown image is of PET-CT.

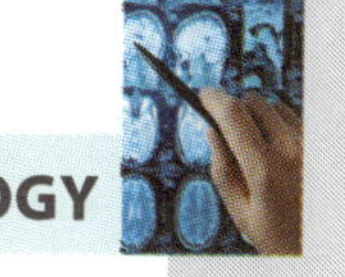

- Shown below are three images. First image is of CT scan, second image PET scan. When these two images are superimposed, the image is said to be PET-CT.

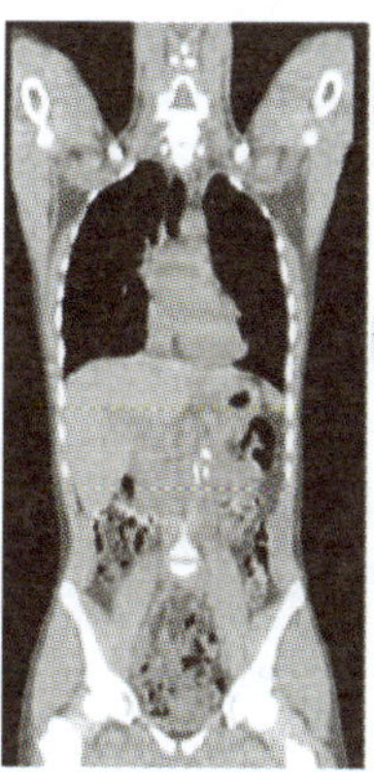
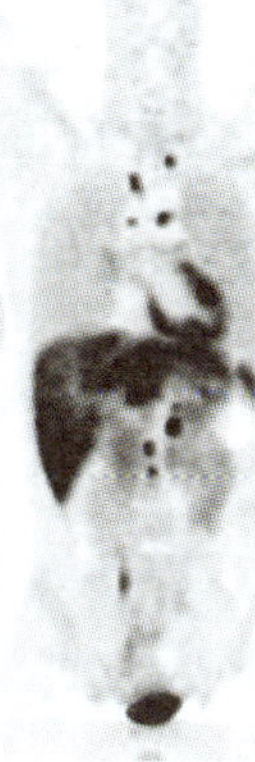
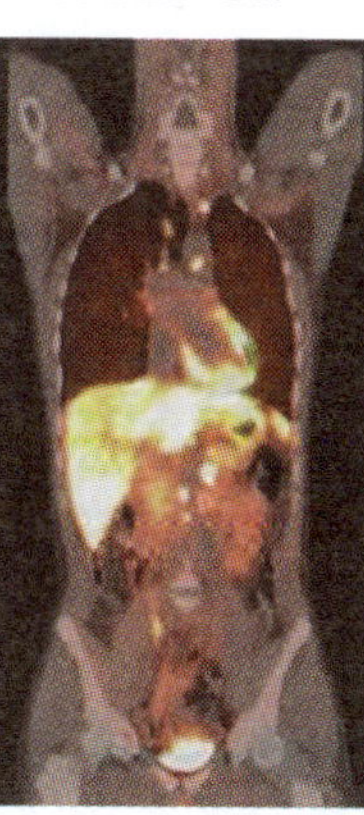

27. Ans. (a) Orthopantogram

- **An orthopantogram is a panoramic or wide view X-ray of the lower face,** which displays all the teeth of the upper and lower jaw on a single film. It demonstrates the number, position and growth of all the teeth including those that have not yet surfaced or erupted.
- **A lateral cephalogram is a lateral or side view X-ray of the face,** which demonstrates the bones and facial contours in profile on a single film (*image*).

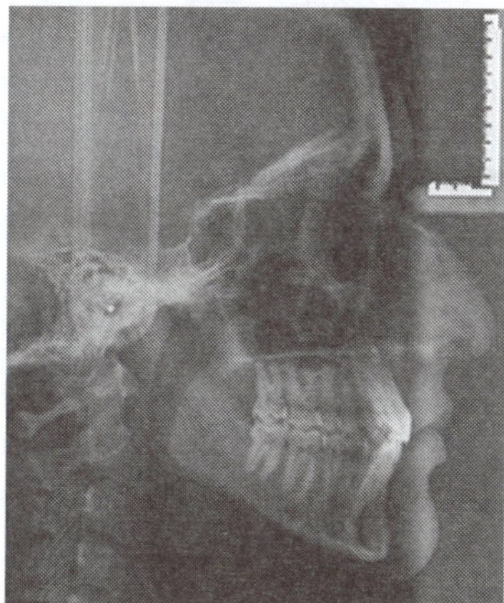

FIGURE: Lateral cephalogram

- **Towns view and stenver view** is used to visualize the petrous part of the pyramids, the dorsum sellae and the posterior clinoid processes, which are visible in the shadow of the foramen magnum.

28. Ans. (a) Compton effect

Ref: Comprehensive Biophysics, 2014 ed. pg. 1

When X-rays travel through the body it can cause two effects:
Photoelectric effect and Compton effect.

The *photoelectric effect* is the observation that many metals emit electrons when light shines upon them.

Compton Effect

- *Compton scattering* is the inelastic *scattering* of a photon by a charged particle, usually an electron. It results in a decrease in energy (increase in wavelength) of the photon (which may be an X-ray or gamma ray photon), called the *Compton effect.*
- This is the reason, it is advised to wear lead apron ***(thickness—0.5 mm)*** in the procedure room.

29. Ans. (c) Gamma

Ref: Essentials of Radiological Science, 2nd ed. pg. 10

- *Maximum penetrating is gamma rays, therefore least dangerous. Hence gamma camera is used therapeutically for myocardial perfusion imaging.*
- *Least penetrating is alpha rays, therefore most dangerous*

30. Ans. (d) Roentgen

Ref: Essentials of Radiological Science, 2nd ed. pg. 3

- Unit of radiation exposure- **Roentgen** (SI = Coloumb/kg)
- Unit of absorbed radiation **RAD** (SI = GRAY)
- Unit of biologic effect of radiaiton **Rem** (SI = Sievert)

31. Ans. (c) 74 days

Ref: Basic Radiological Physics, 2nd ed. pg. 180

- Iridium-192, emits gamma rays. It has energy of 0.4 MeV.
- T1/2 of iridium 192: 74 days

Important Half Life of Radionuclides

- **Gold-198:** 2.7 days
- **Iodine-123:** 13.3 hours
- **Iodine-131:** 8 days
- **Phosphorus-32:** 14.3 days
- **Yttrium 90:** 64 hours
- **Cobalt-60:** 5.26 years
- **Caesium-137:** 30 years
- **Radium-226:** 1620 years

32. Ans. (a) 8 days

Ref: Basics Radiological Physics, 2nd ed. pg. 180

Please refer to above explanation

33. Ans. (b) 5.3 years

Ref: Basics Radiological Physics, 2nd ed. pg. 180

Please refer to above explanation

34. Ans. (c) **1620 years**

Ref: Basics Radiological Physics, 2nd ed. pg. 180

Please refer to above explanation

35. Ans. (b) **I-31**

Ref: Sutton, 7th ed. pg. 1504

- **Iodine-131** has a radioactive decay half-life of about eight days.
- Iodine-131 exhibits a beta mode of decay, and leads to death in cells that it penetrates up to several millimeters and hence is useful for thyroid ablation.
- **I-123** has a half-life of 13.22 hours and is a radioactive isotope of iodine used in nuclear medicine imaging, including single photon emission computed tomography.

36. Ans. (c) **Iodine 131**

Ref: Sutton, 7th ed. pg. 1504

37. Ans. (d) **Iodine-135**

Ref: Essentials of Radiological Science, 2nd ed. pg. 15

- **Iodine-131** is used to treat the thyroid for cancers and other abnormal conditions such as hyperthyroidism
- **Iridium-192** can be implanted into cancers of the tongue.
- **Iodine-135** is an isotope of iodine which is an important isotope from the viewpoint of nuclear reactor physics. It is produced in relatively large amounts as a fission product, and decays to xenon-135, *which is a nuclear poison.*
- **Caesium-137** is another example of an implantable radioactive isotope used in the treatment of uterine or vaginal cancers.
- **Radium-223:** This is a new radioisotope used in treatment for secondary cancer in the bones.
- **Strontium-89 and samarium-153:** Used for treatment of secondary bone CA.

38. Ans. (c) **Leksell**

- The *Gamma Knife* is an advanced radiation treatment for adults and children with small to medium brain tumors. This surgery sometimes referred to as **stereotactic radio surgery** (SRS), is a non-invasive method for treating brain disorders. It is the delivery of a single, high dose of irradiation to a small and critically located intracranial volume through the intact skull.
- **Prof Rutherford**- Father of nuclear physics
- John R. Adler- Cyberknife therapy
- Wilhelm Röentgen- discovered X-rays.

39. Ans. (b) **18-fluoro-deoxyglucose**

Ref: Harrison, 19th ed. pg. 102e-12

- Radionuclides used in PET scanning are typically isotopes with short half-lives such as carbon-11 (~20 min), nitrogen-13 (~10 min), oxygen-15 (~2 min), fluorine-18 (~110 min), or rubidium-82 (~1.27 min).
- These radionuclides are incorporated either into compounds normally used by the body such as glucose (or glucose analogues), water, or ammonia, or into molecules that bind to receptors or other sites of drug action. Such labelled compounds are known as radiotracer.
- ***At present, however, by far the most commonly used radiotracer in clinical PET scanning is fluorodeoxy-glucose (also called FDG or fludeoxy-glucose),*** an analogue of glucose that is labeled with fluorine-18.
- This radiotracer is used in essentially all scans for oncology and most scans in neurology, and thus makes up the large majority of all of the radiotracer (>95%) used in PET and PET/CT scanning.

40. Ans. (c) **Gamma rays**

Ref: Essentials of Radiological Science, 2nd ed. pg. 10

- **Alpha** particles are emitted from the nuclei of radioactive atoms and have high speeds and high energy and are the least penetrating. Their maximum range in air is about 10 cm and can be stopped by the outer layer of skin. If they enter the body, alpha emitters are hazardous to human health. As they disintegrate, they can damage tissue. The normal route of entry by alpha particles are inhalation, digestion and through wounds.
- **Beta** particles are also emitted from the nuclei of radioactive atoms, but they are much smaller in mass than alpha particles and have considerably more penetrating power. Beta emitters are capable of penetrating wood to 4 cm and the human body to 1 cm. Like alpha emitters, they are internal radiation hazards and have the same routes of body entry. They can be stopped by ordinary wall or a 1.3-cm thick sheet of aluminum.
- ***Gamma** radiation originates in the nucleus of an atom. It can penetrate deeply into tissue, and may produce burns similar to deep sunburn, alter genes to cause mutations, and reduce the white blood cell count and encourage infections.*
- **X-rays** cause cancer by inducing mutations. X-rays are a form of electromagnetic radiation that is produced when high-speed electrons strike the target material inside the X-ray tube. The quality of the X-ray, which is the power to penetrate through matter, depends upon the wavelength and the material being irradiated. Hard X-rays with short wavelengths will penetrate thick steel plate. Soft X-rays with long wavelengths are less penetrating.
- **Neutrons** are particles released upon the disintegration of radioactive isotopes. Neutron particles are highly penetrating and require heavy shielding. They are

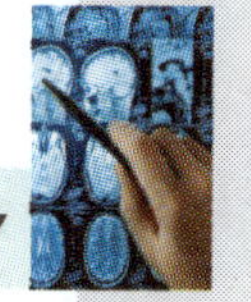

capable of penetrating the human body to several centimeters. Within the body the neutrons release excess energy which can cause tissue damage. Secondary releases of energy may also occur from alpha, beta, and gamma emitters released from the neutrons.

41. Ans. (a) P 32

- **Radioactive phosphorus:** Pure beta emission
  - Used in Bone tumor and polycythemia
- **Cobalt 60**- emits gamma rays
- **Radium-226**- Emits α, β, γ

42. Ans. (d) 20 mSv

Natural Radiation exposure	2.5 mSv
Yearly dose limit for public	1.0 mSv
Yearly dose limit for occupational workers	**20 mSv**
Dose level at which chromosomal aberrations can be measured	100 mSv
Dose at which nausea, vomiting may start	Approx 1000 mSv (1 Sv)
Dose level for 50% death of exposed population in 60 days	Approx 4,000 mSv (4Sv)

- The US Nuclear Regulatory Commission (NRC) guidelines mandate:
  - To limit human-made radiation exposure for individual members of the public to 100 mrem (1 mSv) per year
  - To limit occupational radiation exposure to adults working with radioactive material to 5,000 mrem (50 mSv) per year
- The radiation exposure of occupationally exposed individuals is carefully monitored with the use of pocket-pen-sized instruments called dosimeters.

43. Ans. (d) PET scan

- Positron emission tomography (PET) is a nuclear medical imaging modality that produces a three-dimensional image of functional processes in the body.
- The most common indication for a PET scan is to detect *cancer metastasis.*
- The technique operates on the principle of detecting gamma rays emitted indirectly by a positron-emitting radionuclide (tracer).
- Three dimensional imaging is done with the aid of a CT X-ray scan performed on the patient during the same session.
- The biologically active molecule chosen for PET is FDG (*18-Fluoro deoxy glucose*), an analogue of glucose, the concentrations of tracer imaged will indicate tissue metabolic activity by virtue of the regional glucose uptake.
- **Also remember:** Functional magnetic resonance imaging or functional MRI (fMRI) is an imaging procedure that measures brain activity by detecting associated changes in blood flow. This technique relies on the fact that cerebral blood flow and neuronal activation are coupled. It is used for diagnosis of alzeihmer's disease.

44. Ans. (c) MRI-Imaging

Ref: Harrison, 19th ed. pg. 440

- **The most commonly used compounds for contrast enhancement are gadolinium-based** and they improve the visibility of internal body structures in magnetic resonance imaging.
- *MRI contrast agents alter the relaxation times of atoms within body tissues where they are present after oral or intravenous administration.*
- This relaxation emits energy which is detected by the scanner and is mathematically converted into an image.
- *Gadolinium containing MRI* contrast agents are used for enhancement of vessels in MR angiography or for brain tumor diagnosis which is associated with the degradation of the blood-brain barrier.

45. Ans. (a) Pacemaker

Ref: Harrison, 19th ed. pg. 440e-t

Contraindications of MRI

Absolute contraindication	Relative contraindication
• Pacemaker • Metallic foreign body in the eye • Deep brain stimulator • Swan-Ganz catheter • Bullets or gunshot pellets • Cerebral aneurysm clips • Cochlear implant • Magnetic dental implants	• AAA stent • Stapes implant • Implanted drug infusion device • Neuro or bone growth stimulator • Surgical clips, wire sutures, screws or mesh • Ocular prosthesis • Penile prosthesis • Joint replacement or prosthesis • Other implants, in particular mechanical devices

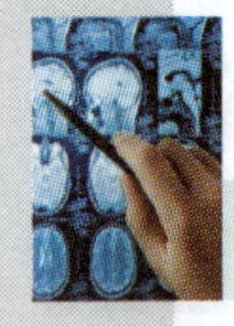

46. Ans. (a) 2D image

Modes of Ultrasound used in Medical Imaging

Mode	Principle	Application in practice
A-mode: (amplitude mode)	Simplest type of ultrasound. Single transducer scans a line through the body with the echoes plotted on screen as a function of depth	Therapeutic ultrasound aimed at a specific tumor or calculus to allow for pinpoint accurate focus of the destructive wave energy
B-mode (brightness mode)	Horizontal array of transducers scan a plane through the body that can be viewed as a two-dimensional image on screen.	Commonly known as 2D mode now
C-mode	C-mode image is formed in a plane normal to a B-mode image	Selects data from a specific depth from an A-mode line is used; then the transducer is moved in the 2D plane to sample the entire region at this fixed depth.
M-mode (motion mode) ultrasound	Pulses are emitted in quick succession and either an A-mode or B-mode image is taken.	Used to determine the velocity of specific organ structures like in valvular heart disease.
Doppler mode	Makes use of the Doppler effect in measuring and visualizing blood flow	Used in evaluation of buergers disease and valvular heart disease.

Also Remember

Types of Doppler

- **Color Doppler:** Velocity information is presented as a color-coded overlay B-mode image
- **Pulsed wave (PW) Doppler:** Doppler information is sampled from only a small sample volume (defined in 2D image), and presented on a timeline.
- **Duplex:** A common name for the simultaneous presentation of 2D and (usually) PW Doppler information.

47. Ans. (a) G2M phase

- Dividing cells are most sensitive to radiotherapy. The phase that is most sensitive to radiation is G2M.

Remember the Sensitivity in this Order

G2M > G2 > M > G1 > early S > Late S

48. Ans. (a) Dryness of mouth

DRYNESS OF MOUTH is the most common complication noted in patients undergoing radiotherapy of head and neck CA.

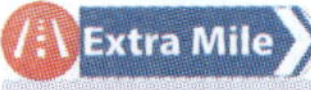

- Most radiosensitive tissue: **Bone Marrow**
- Least radiosensitive: **Nervous tissue**
- Most radiosensitive cell: **Lymphocyte**
- Least radiosensitive cell: **Platelets**
- Most sensitive phase of cell cycle: **G2-M phase**
- Least radiosensitive: **Late S2**
- Most radiosensitive cancer of head and neck: **Nasopharyngeal carcinoma**

49. Ans. (b) Seminoma

Ref: Devita, 7th ed. p-1907

- **Most radiosensitive tumor:** HL > Ewing's
- **Most radiosensitive tumor of head and Neck:** Nasopharyngeal CA > Glottic CA

Radiosensitivity of tumors

Highly sensitive	Moderate sensitive	Relatively resistant	Highly resistant
• **Ewlng's sarcoma** • **Lymphoma** • Wilms tumor • Multiple myeloma • **Seminoma**	• **Nasopharyngeal CA** • **Dysgerminoma** • **Medulloblastoma** • **Small cell cancer lung** • Breast cancer • Ovarian cancer • Basal cell cancer • **Nasopharyngeal cancer** • **Dysgerminoma** • **Small cell cancer lung** • Breast cancer • Ovarian cancer • Basal cell cancer	• Renal cell CA • Rectal/colon cancer • Bladder carcinoma • **Soft tissue sarcoma squamous cell carcinoma of lung** • Cervix cancer	• Hepatoma • Melanoma • Pancreatic cancer • **Osteosarcoma**

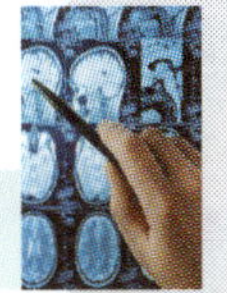

50. Ans. (a) Bone scan

Ref: Review of Radiology by Sumer Sethi, 5th ed. pg. 23.

- Radiation exposure for **CT Head** is equivalent to **115 CXR.**
- CT whole Body **is around** 400 CXRs.
- Radiation exposure of **Bone Scan** is equivalent to **200 CXR**.

51. Ans. (a) Gadolinium

- Gadolinium is a lanthanide.
- Gd-DTPA is classed as an acyclic, ionic gadolinium contrast medium.
- Its paramagnetic property reduces the T1 relaxation time.
- *Gadolinium* based agents *may cause* a toxic reaction known as *nephrogenic systemic fibrosis (NSF)* in patients with severe kidney problems.
- Rest all are iodinated contrast agents.

52. Ans. (c) MRI is better for calcified lesions

MRI Versus CT

- CT is superior to MRI for calcification **and acute intracranial haemorrhage.**
- Cortical bone is better evaluated by CT.
- **MRI is better for brain,** spine pathologies other than head injury, stroke, calcification, brain haemorrhage.
- MRI is better for bone marrow.
- **MRI is contraindicated in pacemakers,** cochlear implants, and metallic foreign bodies in sensitive locations.

UROLOGY AND BONE IMAGING

53. Ans. (b) Ankylosing spondylitis

Ref: Grainger and Allison's Diagnostic Radiology: A Textbook of Medical Imaging, 7th ed. pg. 1344, 1345

- Ankylosing spondylitis is a seronegative spondyloarthropathy, which results in fusion of the spine and sacroiliac (SI) joints, although involvement is also seen in large and small joints.
- In the given radiograph, interspinous ligament ossification giving a "dagger spine" appearance is seen.
- Features of arthritis are seen in patients with UC.

54. Ans. (b) Navicular

Ref: Netter clinical anatomy E-Book pg. 312

The arrow points at Navicular bone, posterior to which is a more dense area which is due to overlapping shadow of Talus and Calcaneus. An easy hack is to identify the three cuneiforms anterior to the marking.

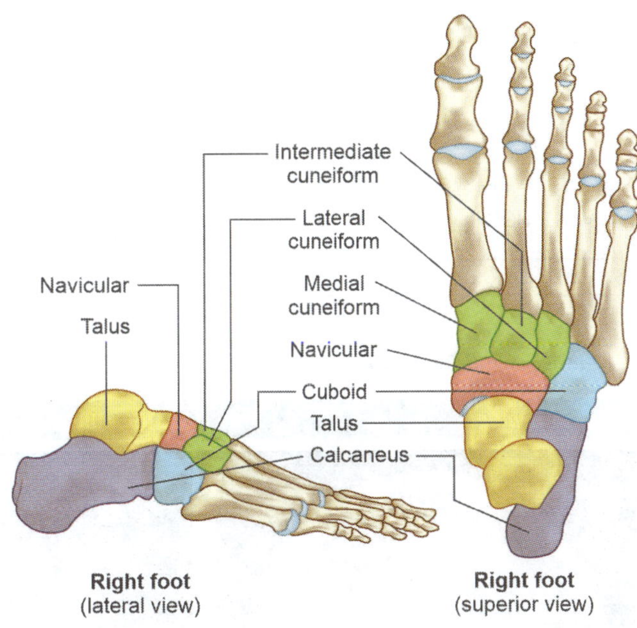

55. Ans. (d) Giant cell tumor

Ref: Maheshwari Orthopedics, 5th ed. pg. 254

The X-ray of distal end of radius shows multiloculated lesions starting from epiphysis and producing a classical soap bubble appearance of Giant cell tumor. Options A will produce a sunburst appearance in Lower extremity bones and arises from metaphysis. Option B produces Cupping, splaying and fraying at distal end of radius. Option C is due to trauma which is not mentioned in the case given.

56. Ans. (b) Multiple myeloma

Ref: Harrison 20th ed. pg. 797

The X-ray-Skull shows lytic punched out lesions in rain drop configuration in the skull. Myeloma like events like hypercalcemia, renal insufficiency and anemia are also given.

Triad of multiple Myeloma

- BM picture shows >10% Myeloma cells
- Serum protein electrophoresis shows a M-Spike >30 g/L
- Myeloma defining events: CRAB: Hyper**C**alcemia, **R**enal failure, **A**nemia and **B**ony lytic lesions

- Option A produces osteosclerotic lesions in lumbosacral spine.
- Option C will not present with anemia and renal failure. Option D will not have anemia and will have low calcium due to less synthesis of vitamin D3.
- Option D Secondary hyperparathyroidism occurs due to chronic renal insufficiency.

57. Ans. (b) MR-AD PCKD

Ref: Harrison 20th ed. pg. 2153

- The image shows MRI abdomen since the vertebra appear black. The presence of large cortical and medullary cysts with loss of corticomedullary differentiation refers to AD PCKD. Also notice that the shape of the kidney is complete distorted, which is seen in AD PCKD.
- AR PCKD would have bilateral nephromegaly with reniform shaped kidneys and homogenous parenchymal signal pattern.

58. Ans. (a) Caldwell

Ref: Dhingra 7th ed. pg. 493

Notice that only the frontal sinus and anterior ethmoidal sinuses are visible and this is seen in Caldwell view.

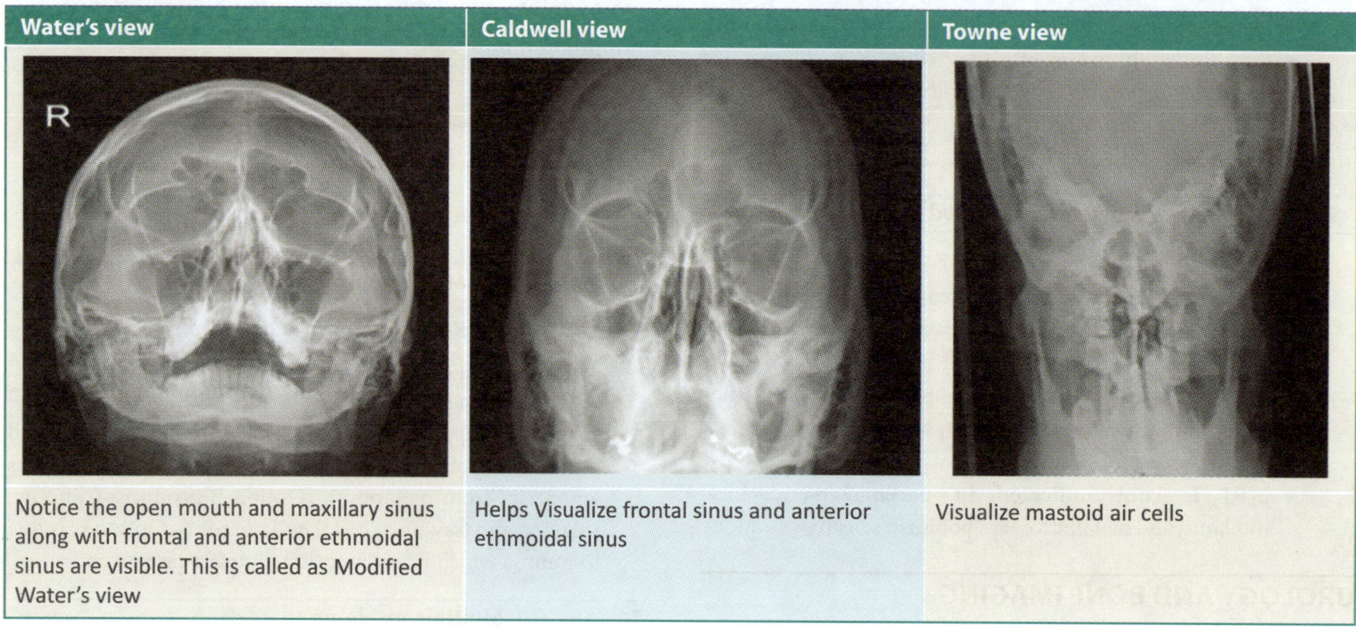

Water's view	Caldwell view	Towne view
Notice the open mouth and maxillary sinus along with frontal and anterior ethmoidal sinus are visible. This is called as Modified Water's view	Helps Visualize frontal sinus and anterior ethmoidal sinus	Visualize mastoid air cells

59. Ans. (b) Foreign body

The image shows an X-ray pelvis with a radioopaque shadow of foreign body that would have been inserted per anus. Option C is seen with IVP and Option D with CT pelvis and are ruled out.

60. Ans. (c) Ewing's sarcoma

- Ewing Sarcoma is a highly radiosensitive bone tumor.
- It is the second most common malignant primary bone tumor of childhood after osteosarcoma
- It typically arises from the medullary cavity with the invasion of the Haversian system.
- It usually presents as moth-eaten destructive permeative lucent lesions in the shaft of long bones with large soft tissue component without osteoid matrix and typical *onion skin periostitis.*

61. Ans. (b) Galeazzi fracture

- The X-ray shows fracture of distal part of radius with dislocation of distal radioulnar joint and intact ulna. This is characteristic of Galeazzi fracture
- In contrast Monteggia fracture has proximal 1/3 ulnar fracture with associated radial head dislocation.
- Jefferson fracture is a bone fracture of the vertebra C1
- Clay-shoveler fractures are fractures of the spinous process of a lower cervical vertebra.

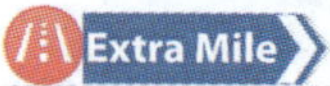

Mnemonic
MUGGER
MU = **M**onteggia: **U**lnar fracture
GR = **G**aleazzi: **R**adius Fracture

62. Ans. (b) Psoas abscess

- The CT abdomen shows right sided iliopsoas abscess. Compare with outline of psoas muscle on opposite side seen paravertebrally. Section of pelvic bones, kidney and

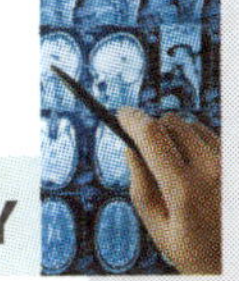

some air containing bowel loops is seen. The bowel loops appear thickened. It is possible that this patient had GI TB that spread locally to cause this abscess.

- The question can also be solved by classic triad of Antalgic gait, low back pain and fever which is seen in 30% cases of psoas abscess. Other non-specific symptoms seen would be low abdominal pain, malaise and weight loss.
- The hip lies in flexion and external rotation at test and passive extension or internal rotation of affected hip will elicit pain.

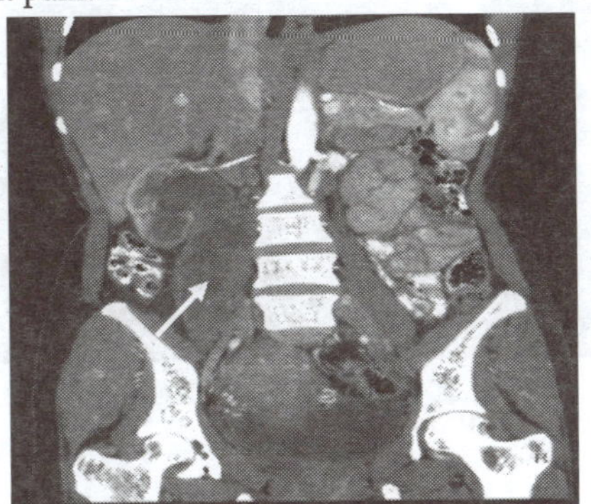

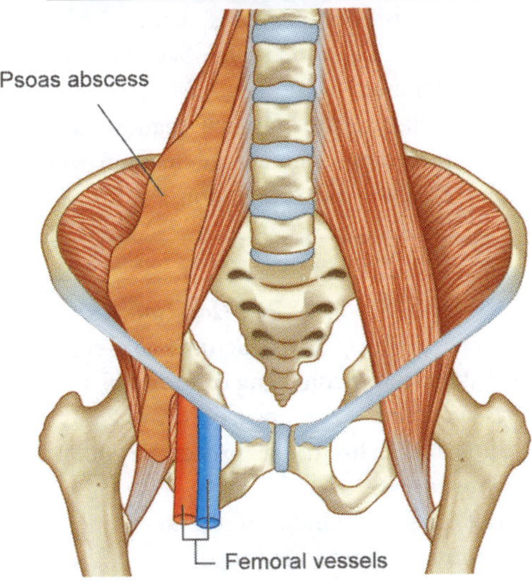

63. Ans. (b) Rickets

The image shows cupping of distal end of radius in left hand (marked with arrow) and is classical feature of nutritional rickets.

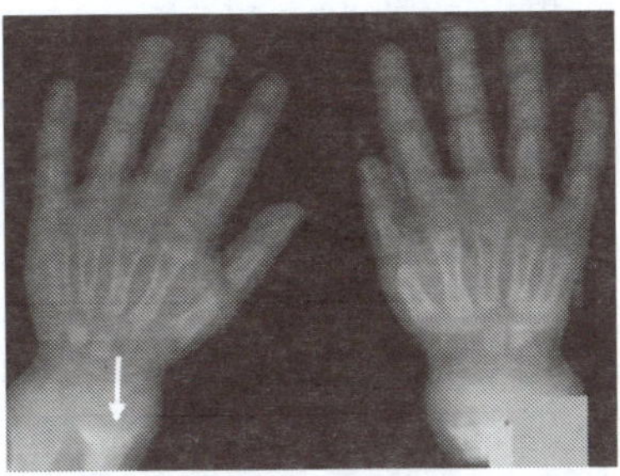

64. Ans. (a) Fracture patella

The X-ray lateral view of knee joint shows comminuted fracture of patella.

Option C and D are same and are ruled out. Tibia head has a normal outline.

65. Ans. (a) Iliopsoas muscle

The marking shown is of lesser trochanter of femur. The muscle inserted is iliopsoas.

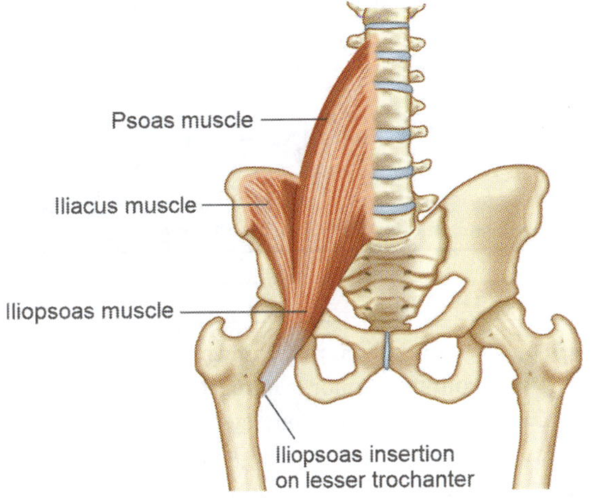

66. Ans. (a) Radioulnar synostosis

- Option B is seen in infants and children when child is pulled by or lifted by the hand or wrist while his or her arm is held straight.
- Option C and D are seen post-trauma while the clinical description in question says that problem is present since birth.
- The answer by exclusion is Radioulnar synostosis. The average age of diagnosis is 6 years and the condition will cause difficulty in following tasks:
  - Keyboard and table top activities: Deficient pronation
  - Eating, washing face and catching a ball: Defective supination

67. Ans. (a) Hemolytic anemia

X-ray of this child shows expansion of outer and inner table of skull. The bone trabeculations are appearing more prominent and shows classical hair on end appearance. Hence the diagnosis is Hemolytic anemia.

68. Ans. (a) Ureterocele

The given IVP shows bilateral cobra head appearance of distal ureter diagnostic of ureterocele.

69. Ans. (a) TB

Thimble bladder implies extreme fibrosis and contracture of the bladder walls, resulting in a tiny bladder.

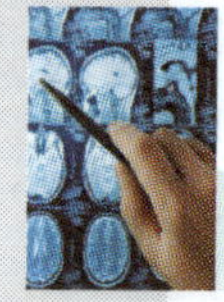

The term is usually used to describe changes from advanced genitourinary tuberculosis.

70. Ans. (b) Helical CT with noncontrast

Ref: SRB Manual of Surgery, 5th ed. P 1190, 1107

- The best investigation for kidney stone and ureteric stone is non-contrast helical CT abdomen.
- The limitation of USG is that it is less sensitive and can scan only the kidney and proximal ureter.
- Helical CT can detect stones as small as 1 mm which can be missed by other modalities.

Extra Mile

IOC for Ureteric Stones is helical Non-contrast CT abdomen
IOC for Polycystic kidneys is non-contrast CT/MRI. Contrast may be used depending on level of renal function.
Always check serum creatinine before giving contrast

71. Ans. (c) Humerus

- The structure shown in the image is humerus
- A very common tumor of humerus upper end is unicameral bone cyst/simple bone cyst, which is characterized radiologically by *trap door sign or falling leaf sign*

72. Ans. (b) Duplex collecting system

- The shown IVP finding in image is known as drooping lily sign, which is a characteristic finding of duplex ureter.

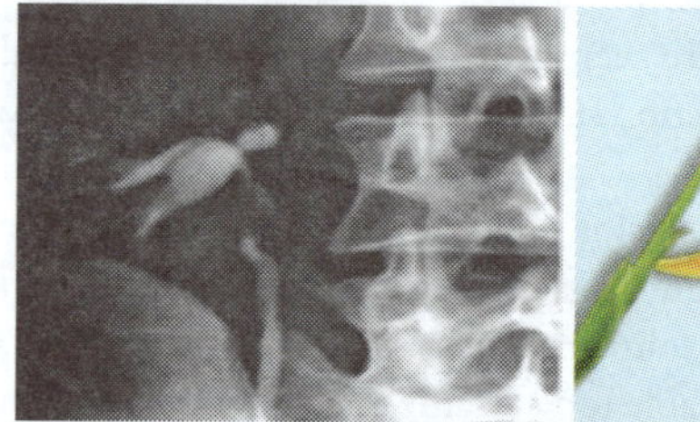

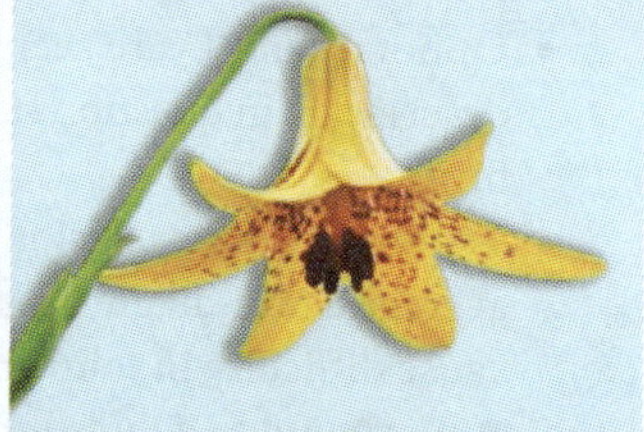

- The **drooping lily sign** is a radiological sign in patients with a duplicated collecting system. It refers to the inferolateral displacement of the opacified lower pole. The size of calyces in kidney is also smaller.

73. Ans. (c) TB spine

- Notice the vertebral body collapse, which is diagnostic of pott spine.
- IOC for Pott's spine: MRI
- The **earliest sign** of infection are local **osteoporosis of two adjacent vertebra and narrowing of intervertebral disc space**, with fizziness of end plates.
- Progressive disease is associated with signs of bone destruction and collapse of adjacent vertebral bodies into each other.

74. Ans. (b) Obturator foramen

(Revise the pelvic anatomy as shown on X-ray from this image given below)

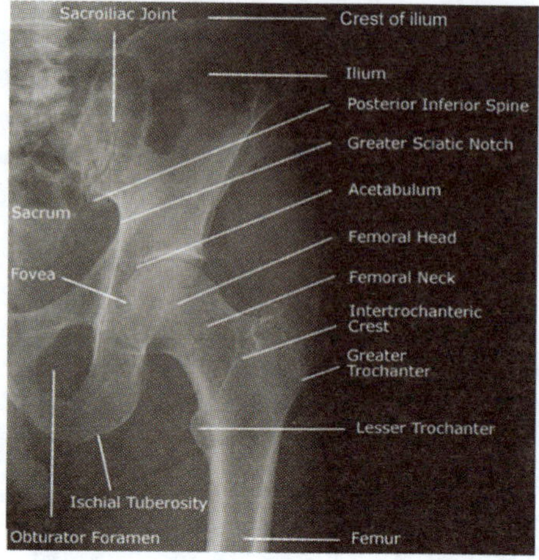

75. Ans. (c) Papillary necrosis

- *Ring sign appearance by CT urography* or IVP shows radio-contrast outlines of sloughed renal papillae in *papillary necrosis*, which often have a triangular shape.
  Also remember:
- **Cortical ring sign:** A circular shadow cast by a rotated scaphoid in scapho-lunate subluxation which is due to scaphoid's abnormal orientation.

76. Ans. (a) Diabetes

Ref: Harrison, 19th ed. pg. 270e-9

- Contrast nephropathy is defined as a condition arising after an investigation using contrast agent.
- *A rise in serum creatinine level above 25%* from baseline within 48-72 hours of procedure *indicates contrast nephropathy.*
- Out of the given condition diabetes is most predisposed for contrast induced nephropathy.

77. Ans. (b) Renal cell CA

Ref: Harrison, 19th ed. pg. 263e-7

Cancers associated with high dose exposure include leukemia, breast, bladder, colon, liver, lung, esophagus, ovarian, multiple myeloma, and stomach cancers.

78. Ans. (c) Papillary necrosis

Ref: Harrison, 19th ed. pg. 1860

Refer to above explanation

79. Ans. (b) Polycystic kidney

Ref: Radiological and Imaging Secrets, 2nd ed. pg. 79

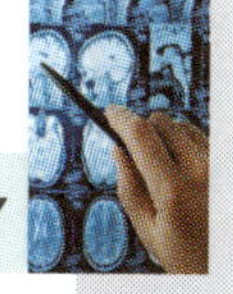

- Polycystic kidney autosomal dominant and recessive forms multiple cysts that deform the pelvi-calyceal system resulting in spider leg sign.
- MC extra-renal malformation in polycystic kidney disease = Hepatic cysts
- MC Cardiac malformation in polycystic kidney disease = Mitral valve prolapse
- MC GIT malformation in polycystic kidney disease = colonic diverticulosis

Extra Mile

Remember these Important Radiological Signs in Urology
- Spider leg appearance—polycystic kidney
- Cobra head appearance—ureterocele
- Flower vase appearance of ureters—horse shoe kidney
- Sandy patches—schistosomiasis of bladder
- Soap bubble appearance—hydronephrosis

80. Ans. (c) Polycystic disease

81. Ans. (a) Ureterocoele

Ref: SRB Manual of Surgery, 4th ed. pg. 1279

The ***adder head/cobra head sign*** refers to dilatation of the distal ureter, surrounded by a thin lucent line, which is seen in patients with an adult-type ***ureterocoele.*** The presence of this cobra head appearance is an indicator of ureterocele.

A ureterocele is a submucosal cystic dilation of the terminal segment of the ureter.

82. Ans. (b) Micturating cystourethrogram

Ref: SRB Manual of Surgery, 4th ed. pg. 1118

Steps in MCU

- Catheterization to fill the bladder with a radio-contrast agent, typically cystografin.
- Under fluoroscopy, we can see the contrast entering the bladder.
- If the contrast moves into the ureters and back into the kidneys, the radiologist makes the diagnosis of vesicoureteral reflux.

Indication of MCU

1. All males with recurrent UTIs, or abnormality on ultrasound if first UTI urinary tract infection
2. First episode UTI in females <3 years of age
3. Febrile UTIs in females <5 years of age
4. Older females with pyelonephritis or recurrent UTIs
5. Suspected obstruction (e.g. Bilateral hydronephrosis)
6. Suspected bladder trauma or rupture
7. Stress incontinence (urine)

83. Ans. (a) Thalassemia

Ref: Harrison, 19th ed. pg. 637

- Crew cut appearance in thalassemia occurs due to expansion of the marrow on account of extra-medullary hematopoiesis.
- ***The widened diploic spaces on X-ray skull lateral view appears as Crew cut or hair on end appearance.***

84. Ans. (c) Osteopetrosis

Ref: Harrison, 19th ed. pg. 426e-4

- **Bone within a bone** describes the bones that appear to have another bone within them.

Causes: P.O.S.T-C.G.D
- **P**aget's disease of bone
- **O**steopetrosis
- **S**ickle cell disease
- **T**halassemia
- **C**affey's disease
- **G**aucher's disease
- **G**rowth recovery lines (after infancy)
- Hypervitaminosis **D**

85. Ans. (b) Sickle cell anemia

- Hair on end appearance of the skull is a characteristic feature of chronic haemolysis usually seen in patients with thalassemia and sickle cell anaemia. It results from accentuated vertical trabeculae between the inner and outer tables of the skull because of excessive bone marrow hyperplasia.

Conditions where 'Hair on End Appearance' is seen:
Mnemonic: HI NEST
- Hereditary spherocytosis
- Neuroblastoma
- Enzyme deficiency (e.g. G-6-P deficiency causing haemolytic anaemia)
- Sickle cell disease
- Thalassemia major

86. Ans. (a) Gout

Ref: Harrison Rheumatology, 2006 ed. pg. 261

- **Martel sign or rat bite sign-** Sharply marginated, bony erosions from a long-standing soft-tissue tophus, seen in X-ray in a patients with gout.

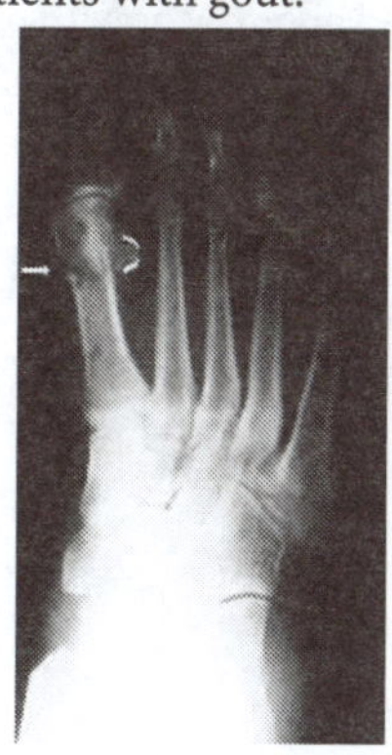

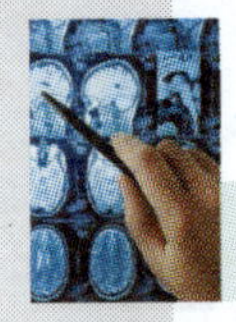

87. Ans. (c) Ante-natal USG second trimester

- The **nuchal thickness** is a parameter that is measured in a second trimester scan (18–22 weeks) *and it is not to be mixed with nuchal translucency (which is measured in the first trimester at 11-14 weeks).*
- The **nuchal thickness** is measured in a second trimester scan.
- Nuchal translucency scan is performed between 11 and 14 weeks of gestation, because the accuracy is best in this period.
- The scan is obtained with the fetus in sagittal section and a neutral position of the fetal head
- The head of the fetus should neither be hyper-flexed nor extended, either of which can influence the nuchal translucency thickness.
- Both are used for diagnosis of Trisomy 21 prenatally.

ABDOMEN IMAGING

88. Ans. (b) Diffuse esophageal spasm

Ref: Harrison 20th ed. pg. 2214

- The barium swallow shows corkscrew appearance/ multiple indentations in esophagus due to motility defect known as diffuse esophageal spasm.
- Option A is ruled since it shows a shouldering sign/ irregular filling defect. Option C will show abrupt tapering near LES.
- Option D will require endoscopy for diagnosis and is likely to be missed as it produces a shelf like defect which may be misinterpreted as an artifact.

89. Ans. (a) Saw tooth sign

Ref: Final Edge, 3rd ed. pg. 142

The image depicts a barium enema showing serrated edges known as saw tooth pattern. This occurs in diverticulosis. This condition mainly affects the sigmoid colon which happens to be the narrowest part of colon.

Extra Mile

- Saw tooth pattern in EEG: REM Sleep
- Saw tooth pattern in ECG: Atrial flutter

90. Ans. (b) Achalasia cardia

Ref: Final Edge, 3rd ed. pg. 358

- Notice the abrupt tapering at the distal end of esophagus. The esophagus also looks grossly dilated just proximal to tapering. This is seen in Diffuse esophageal spasm.
- Option A would have corkscrew appearance
- Option C will have irregular filling defect in lower or middle part of esophagus
- Option D will produce a local filling defect with relatively smooth margins in any part of esophagus

91. Ans. (a) Multiple gallstones

- The image shows multiple acoustic shadows in gallbladder indicative of cholelithiasis
- Option B may be missed on USG if stones are in distal CBD
- Option C is seen in liver parenchyma
- Option D will be a fungating mass that would be better evaluated with MRCP

92. Ans. (c) Horseshoe kidney

The image shows CT abdomen with both kidneys fused together on Hilar side and is called Horseshoe kidney.

- Fusion is at lower pole in 90% of cases
- The majority of each kidney lies on its own side of the spine
  - In crossed fused ectopia, both fused kidneys lie on the same side of the spine
- May occur as isolated anomaly or with other anomalies (1/3), such as
  - Reflux, hypospadias, retrocaval ureter, imperforate anus, Meckel diverticulum

Clinical Findings

- About 1/3 are asymptomatic
- When present, symptoms stem from hydronephrosis, stones, infection
- Vague abdominal pain may be most common presenting symptom

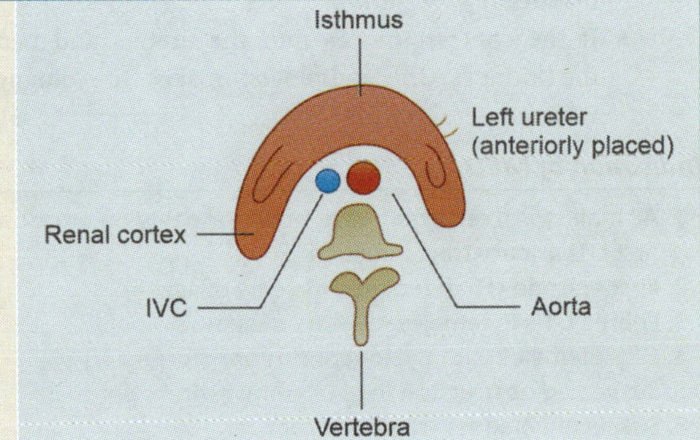

Contd...

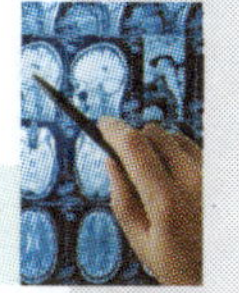

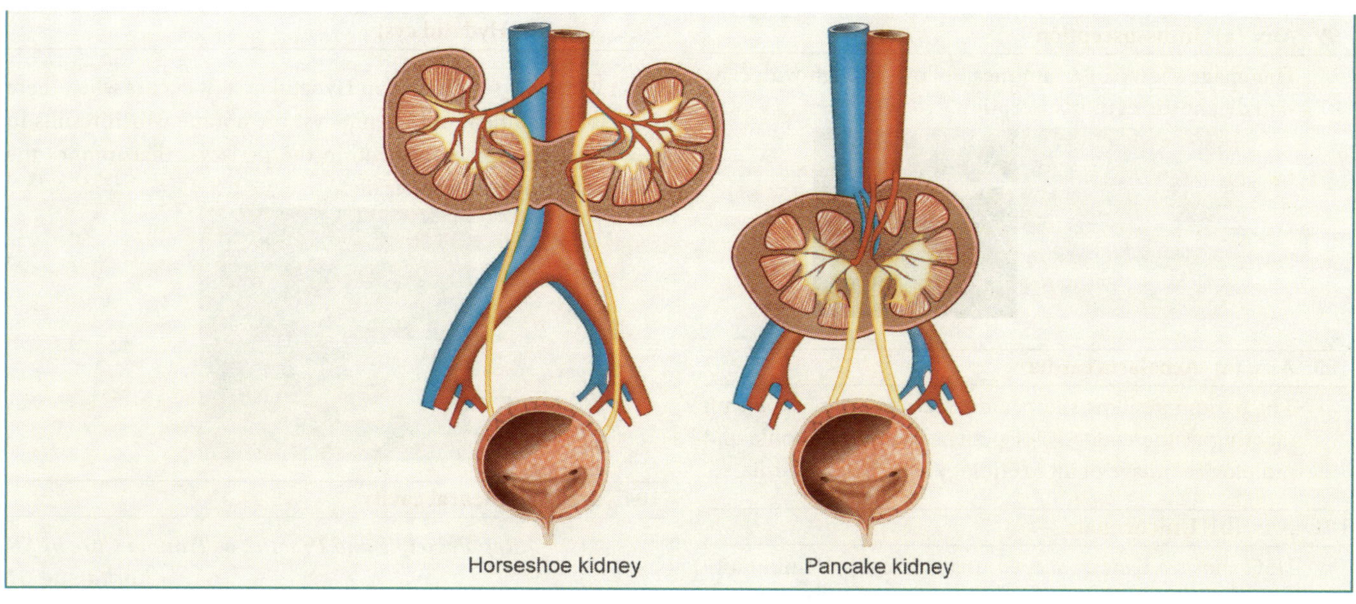

93. Ans. (a) Complete mole

The USG image shows Snow storm appearance diagnostic of complete Mole. Option B is ruled out as baby parts are not visualized.

94. Ans. (c) Bilateral hydrosalpinx

- The image shows HSG with bilateral malformed tubes due to chronic PID.
- Option A needs USG for evaluation.
- Option B needs MRI/CT abdomen for diagnosis and staging
- Option C needs USG for diagnosis.

95. Ans. (b) PCOD

The TVS image shows multiple follicles in ovary which is suggestive of diagnosis of PCOD.
USG Criteria for PCOD
Transvaginal ultrasound is considered the gold standard in the diagnosis of polycystic ovaries. Features can affect either one (unilateral polycystic ovary) or both ovaries.
Features include:

- Increased follicle number per ovary (FNPO) – usually 20 or greater
- Individual follicles are generally similar in size and measure 2–9 mm in diameter
- Peripheral distribution of follicles; this can give a "string of pearls" appearance
- Background ovarian enlargement (volume greater than 10 mL)
- Central stromal brightness +/– prominence

Only one ovary fitting these criteria is sufficient to define PCO. If there is evidence of a dominant follicle (>10 mm) or a corpus luteum, the scan should be repeated during the next cycle.

Extra Mile

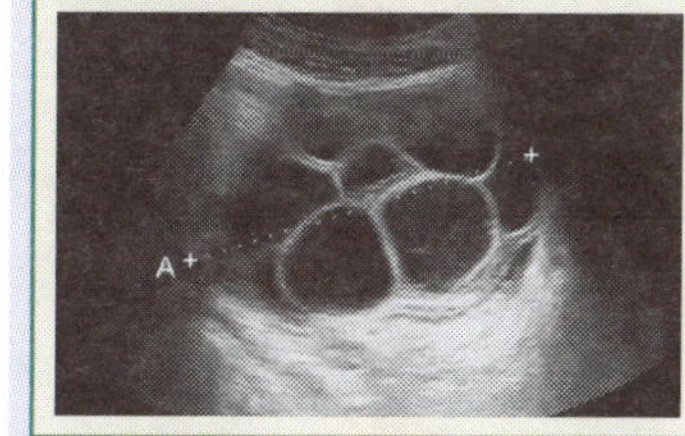

Ovarian Hyperstimulation syndrome should have history of usage ovarian induction therapy. The cysts are larger and are present juxtaposing each other.

96. Ans. (b) Duodenal atresia

The X-ray abdomen shows double bubble appearance in a neonate with bilious vomiting that points to diagnosis of Duodenal atresia.

97. Ans. (a) Congenital hypertrophic pyloric stenosis

A neonate at second week of life with non-bilious vomiting and barium study showing minimal contrast passage via pylorus is diagnostic of CHPS.

98. Ans. (b) Pneumoperitoneum

- The Abdominal X-ray shows football sign diagnostic of pneumoperitoneum in this 2-year-old child.
- Option A is seen in neonates
- Option C will have air dissection into anterior abdominal wall while in this case air is present in entire peritoneal cavity.
- Option D will have double bubble appearance

99. Ans. (a) Intussusception

The image shows a Barium meal follow through with claw sign diagnostic of intussusception.

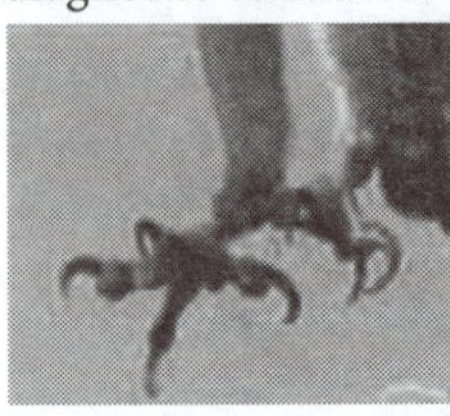
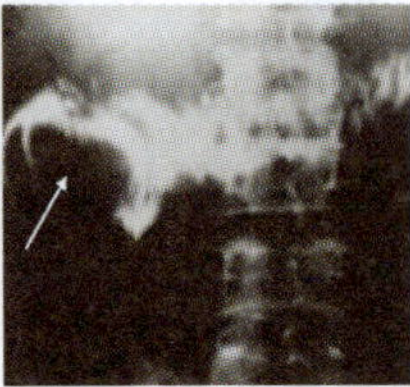

100. Ans. (a) Achalasia cardia

The barium swallow shows a dilated megaesophagus with tapering at the end. Age of patient, symptom profile and radiological image point to etiology as Achalasia cardia.

101. Ans. (b) Unicornuate

HSG shows a banana-shaped uterus usually draining into a single Fallopian tube. This pattern is seen in unicornuate uterus.

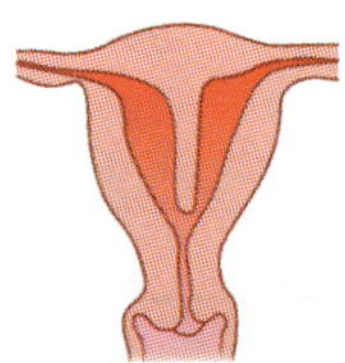
Uterine septum

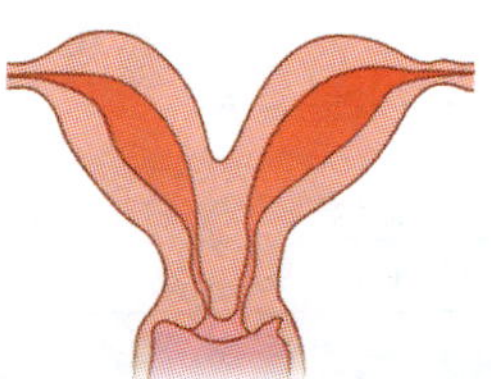
Bicornuate uterus

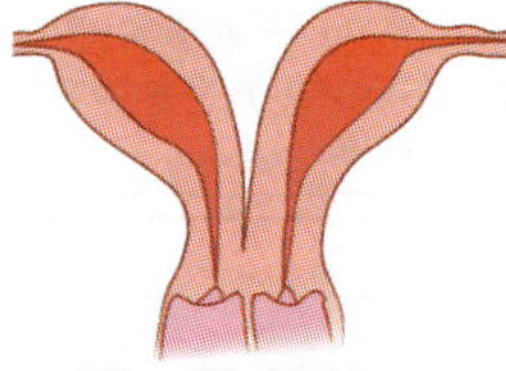
Uterus didelphys

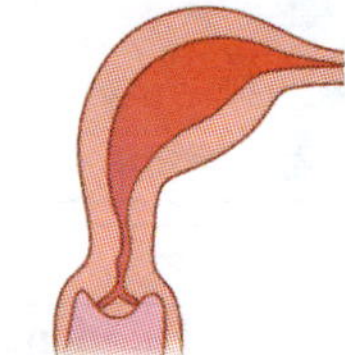
Unicornuate uterus

102. Ans. (b) Portal vein

The marked blood vessels shown are tributaries of portal vein entering into liver and bifurcating into right, left and middle hepatic veins respectively.

How would hepatic artery entering into liver look like?

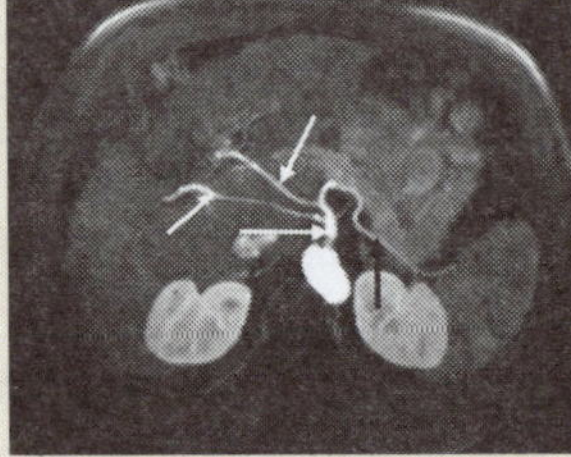

Notice the celiac trunk and **two** bifurcations of right and left hepatic arteries. In the image given in the question three branches can be seen originating from a focal point.

103. Ans. (a) Hydatid cyst

Water lily sign is seen in Hydatid cyst. It occurs when there is detachment of the endocyst membrane which results in floating membranes within the peri-cyst that mimics the appearance of a water lily.

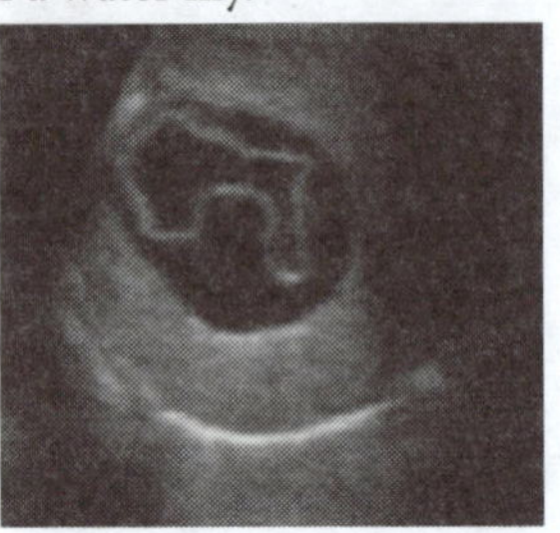

104. Ans. (b) Pleural cavity

Ref: Principle and Practice of Trauma Care by SK Kochar, pg. 51

- FAST scan is Focused Assessment with Sonography for Trauma
- It is a rapid, decision making scan done on the patients immediately at the time of trauma. It has sensitivity of ~90% and specificity of ~95%.
- Aim of this scan is to identify intraperitoneal free fluid (to rule out hemoperitoneum), which helps in precise decision making on immediate transfer of patient to operation theatre.
- Four regions that are mainly assessed by FAST scan are:
  1. **Pericardial/Subxiphoid view:** To rule our pericardial effusion
  2. **Right upper quadrant view/Perihepatic view/Morison pouch view:** To rule out fluid in the hepatorenal interface (morison pouch) due to hepatorenal trauma
  3. **Left upper quadrant/Perisplenic view:** To rule out fluid in perisplenic space due to spleen trauma
  4. **Pelvic/Suprapubic view:** This space (pouch of Douglas) is most dependent peritoneal space. It rules out bladder or other pelvic organ damage.
- Extension of FAST is eFAST, which includes scanning of pleural space also, to rule out any injury to lungs or pleural effusion.

105. Ans. (b) USG

- **USG is IOC for:**
  - Acute cholecystitis
  - Cholelithiasis, Renal stone
  - Intrauterine pathology
  - Intrauterine assessment of foetus
  - To see minimal pleural fluid/ascitic fluid
  - Hydrocephalus in infants
  - Congenital hypertrophic pyloric stenosis (CHOPS)
- Most sensitive and specific test for cholecystitis: HIDA scan

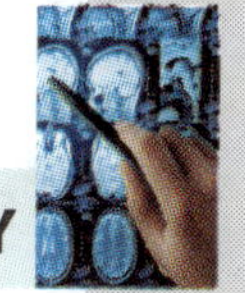

106. (d) 24-hour pH monitoring

- **IOC for GERD:** 24-hour pH monitoring
- It is the **most accurate/most sensitive/Gold standard** test for measuring pattern, frequency and duration of reflux episodes.
- It quantifies the actual time the esophageal mucosa is exposed to gastric juice

Extra Mile

- **Manometry:** IOC for motility disorders of esophagus (Ex: Achalasia cardia, diffuse esophageal spasm, corkscrew esophagus).
- **Uses of HIDA scan:**
  - Biliary atresia
  - Neonatal hepatitis (parenchymal liver disease)
  - Abnormal biliary leakage
  - Acute/Chronic cholecystitis

107. Ans. (a) Apple core appearance

Ref: SRB Manual of Surgery: 5th ed. pg. 905

- The image shows an appearance of an annular *constricting* carcinoma of the bowel, usually the colon form the circumferential involvement of lumen.
- The string sign of Kantor is seen in Crohn's disease at the junction of ileum entering into the caecum. In this image small intestine is not visualized.
- Claw sign is seen on barium enema in intussusception.
- Coffee bean sign is seen on X-ray abdomen in case of sigmoid volvulus.

108. Ans. (c) Spleen

Check out the structures on CT scan and their names in given image.

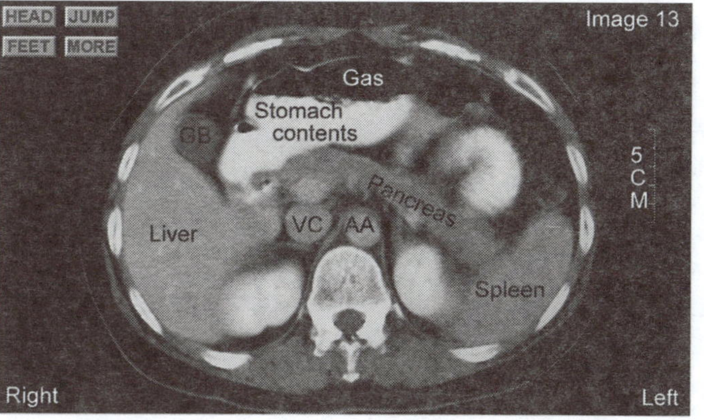

109. Ans. (d) Hydatid cyst

- **Hepatic hydatid disease** is a parasitic zoonosis caused by the *Echinococcus* tape worm. In the liver, two agents are recognised as causing disease in the human:
  - *Echinococcus granulosus*
  - *Echinococcus multilocularis*
- In the human manifestation the disease caused by echinococcus is most commonly localized to liver (in 75% of cases), followed by lungs (in 5–15% of cases) and other organs in the body such as the spleen, brain, heart, and kidneys (in 10–20% of cases).
- If the patient has cysts in the liver, symptoms abdominal discomfort, hepatomegaly with an abdominal mass, jaundice, fever and/or anaphylactic reaction.

Radiographic features:

- **Plain radiograph:** Shows a curvilinear or ring calcific shadow overlying the liver due to calcification of the pericyst.
- **Ultrasound:** Multiseptate cyst with "daughter" cysts and echogenic material between cysts.
- **CT scan:** Septation and daughter cysts may be visualised. The **water-lily sign** indicates a cyst with floating, undulating membrane, caused by a detached endocyst. It may also show hyperdense internal septa representing a **spoke wheel pattern** within a cyst.

Extra Mile

- Definitive host of echinococcus granulosus: Dog
- Intermediate host of echinococcus granulosus: Sheep
- **Accidental host for echinococcus granulosus is Man.**
- MCC of amoebic liver abscess is **Entamoeba histolytica.** This condition is mostly associated with alcoholic liver diseases (in ~ 80% of cases). M:F = 10:1
- MCC of pyogenic liver abscess in E. coli. associated with alcoholic liver disease in 20–30% cases. M:F = 1.5:1

110. Ans. (c) Stomach

For explanation, read the CT image

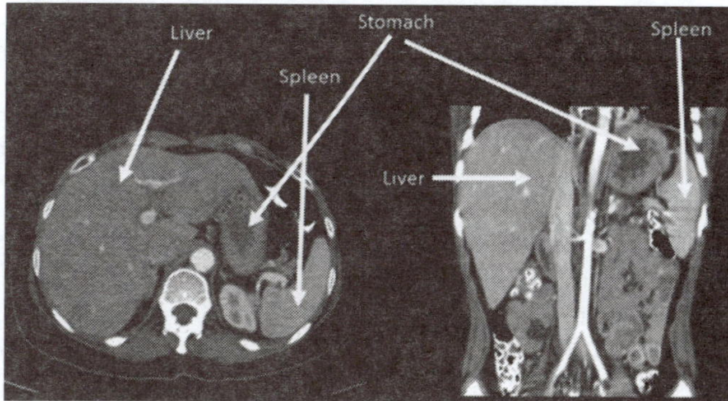

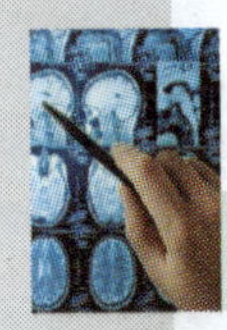

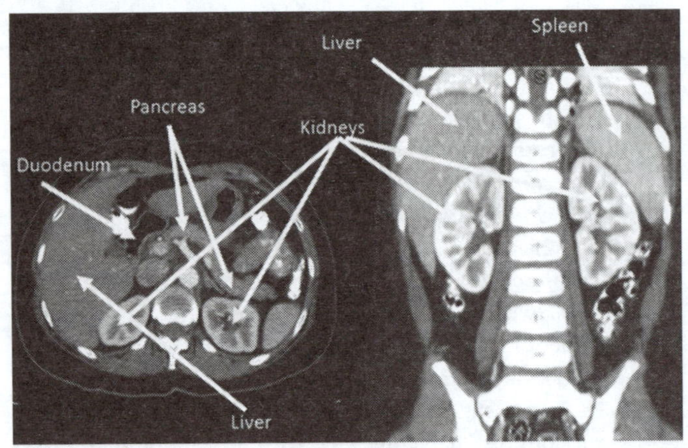

- *Multiple questions have been framed on this image in last many exams.*

111. Ans. (b) Ultrasound

Ref: Bailey & Love, 25th ed. pg. 69

- On ultrasound, an abscess cavity in the liver is seen as a hypoechoic or anechoic lesion with ill-defined borders; internal echoes suggest necrotic material or debris. **The investigation is very accurate and is used for aspiration, both diagnostic and therapeutic.**
- Where there is doubt about the diagnosis, a computerized tomography (CT) scan may be helpful.

Extra Mile

- Bloody mucoid diarrhoea in a patient from an endemic area or following a recent visit to such a place
- Upper abdominal pain, fever, cough, malaise
- In chronic cases, a mass in the right iliac fossa = ***amoeboma***
- Sigmoidoscopy shows typical ulcers—biopsy and scrapings may be diagnostic
- Serological tests are highly sensitive and specific outside endemic areas
- **Ultrasound and CT scans are the imaging methods of choice.**

112. Ans. (c) 3 mm

Ref: Clinical Sonography, 4th ed. pg. 88

- GB wall thickness Measured in the side in contact with the liver with the help of ultrasonography.
- *Normally it is up to 3 mm.*
- *From 3–5 mm: suspicion of wall thickness*
- *More than 5 mm >>> It is a thick wall gallbladder which is seen in:*

1. Cholecystitis (acute-chronic)
2. Ascites
3 Hepatitis (viral)
4. Schistosomiasis

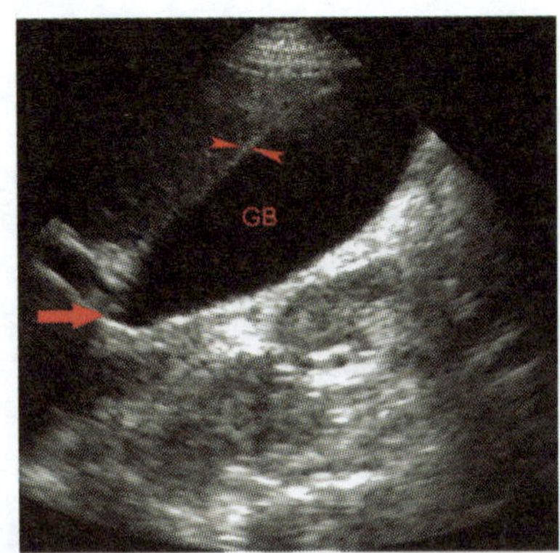

Extra Mile

Size of GB

- Long axis 6–12 cm, short axis 3–5 cm
- Contracted <5 cm
- Distended >12 cm

113. Ans. (b) Ischemic colitis

Ref: Harrison, 19th ed. pg. 267, 1857

- **Ischemic colitis** occurs due to inflammation of the colon secondary to vascular insufficiency and ischemia. Abdominal radiographic findings are include:
  - **'Thumb-printing' sign is due to mucosal edema and hemorrhage**
  - Ileal Distention
  - Localized intramural gas

TABLE: Radiological findings and their respective pathology

Barium enema findings	Associated pathology
Apple core deformity **Irregular filling defect**	Colon CA
Bird beak sign, Ace of spades	Volvulus
Bird beak appearance	Achalasia cardia
Claw sign **Coiled spring sign**	Intussusception
Coffee bean sign	Sigmoid volvulus
Corkscrew appearance **Nut cracker esophagus** **Curling esophagus**	Diffuse esophageal spasm
Dilated proximal zone with narrow distal zone of coning	Hirschsprung disease
Inverted 3 sign of Frosberg **Widening of C loop of duodenum/** **Antral pad sign.**	Pancreas head CA
Lead pipe appearance **Loss of haustrations**	Ulcerative colitis
Rat tail appearance	Esophageal CA

Contd...

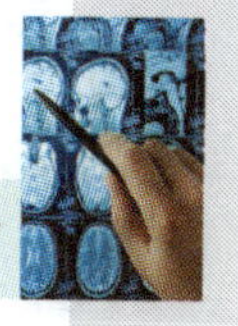

Barium enema findings	Associated pathology
String sign of kantor Raspberry thorn ulcers	Crohn's disease
Smooth irregular filling defects	Colonic polyps
Saw tooth appearance Champagne glass sign	Diverticulosis of colon
String sign	Congenital hypertrophic pyloric stenosis
Thumb print sign	Ischemic colitis

114. Ans. (c) Sigmoid volvulus

Ref: SRB Manual of Surgery, 4th ed. pg. 1329

- The given image shows coffee bean sign, which is seen in sigmoid volvulus.
- It is a cause of large bowel obstruction and occurs when the sigmoid colon twists on the sigmoid mesocolon.

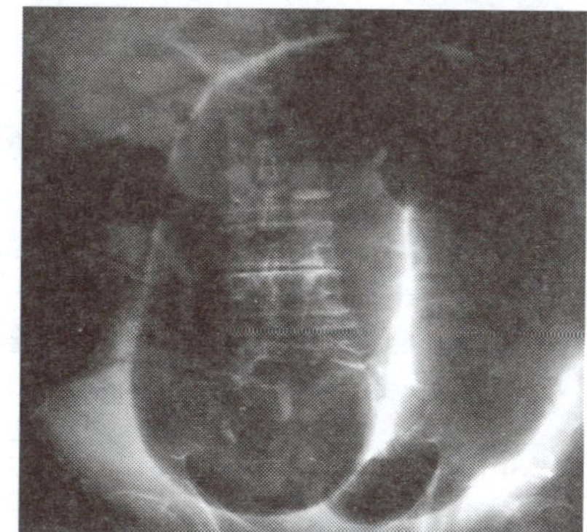

Clinical Presentation

- Constipation
- Abdominal bloating
- Nausea and/or vomiting

Causes

- Chronic constipation and/or laxative abuse
- Fibre-rich diet (especially in Africa)
- Chagas disease (especially in South America)

Treatment

- Rectal tube insertion is successful in treating 90% of cases.
- The most serious complication is bowel ischaemia.

115. Ans. (a) Duodenal atresia

Ref: SRB manual of Surgery, 4th ed. pg. 1280

- The diagnosis of duodenal atresia on X ray abdomen shows two large air filled spaces, called "**double bubble**" **sign.**
- The air is trapped in the stomach and proximal duodenum, which are separated by the pyloric sphincter, creating the appearance of two bubbles visible on X-ray.
- Since the closure of the duodenum is complete in duodenal atresia, no air is seen in the distal duodenum.

116. Ans. (c) Obstructive jaundice

Ref: Abdominal Ultrasound, 3rd ed. pg. 82

- Biliary dilatation is also easily seen on ultrasound, appearing as an extra tube running alongside the intrahepatic portal veins and hence gives an appearance of a double barrel gun aka ***double-barrel sign.***

Extra Mile

Some important radiological signs

- **Double bubble sign** is seen in (LAD): Ladd band/malrotation, Annular pancreas, Duodenal atresia
- **Single bubble appearance**: pyloric stenosis
- **Thumb print sign**: ischemic colitis
- **Multiple air fluid level:** Ileal/Jejunal obstruction

117. Ans. (a) Crohn's disease

- **Cobble stone mucosa** is appearance of the intestinal mucosa in Crohn's disease ***to the endoscopist,. Cobblestoning refers to the uniform nodules–due to the sub-mucosal fibrosis.***
- **String sign of Kantor is due to involvement of** the terminal ileum in Crohn's disease.
- It is caused by severe spasm due to irritability of the loop producing the appearance of a frayed cotton string.
- Subsequently the wall of the ileum may become fibrotic and the lumen fixed in diameter.

118. Ans. (b) Ulcerative colitis

Barium Enema Findings in Ulcerative Colitis

- *Earliest finding on air-contrast Barium enema is loss of and fine mucosal granularity.*
- *Pseudo-polyps which are scattered islands of edematous mucosa in vast expanse of ulcerated mucosa*
- Double-tracking- long, longitudinal ulcers in submucosa
- Bowel margins appear spicule like from tiny, multiple ulcerations
- Collar button ulcers-from undermining
- Shortening of the colon-may be from spasm of longitudinal muscles or from irreversible fibrosis (lead-pipe colon/pipe stem colon)
- Loss of haustrations on left side of colon.

119. Ans. (c) Intussusception

Ref: SRB Manual of Surgery, 4th ed. pg. 996

- Target sing is seen in intussusception.

- Other signs which is seen in case of Intussusception are: Coiled spring appearance, claw sign.
- The appearance is generated by concentric alternating echogenic and hypo-echogenic bands. The echogenic bands are formed by mucosa and muscularis whereas the submucosa is responsible for the hypo-echoic bands.

Also Remember

- The **pseudo kidney** of intussusception refers to the longitudinal ultrasound appearance of the intussuscepted segment of bowel.
- **Coffee bean sign:** Sigmoid volvulus
- **Whirlpool sign on USG:** Midgut volvulus
- **Thumb print sign:** Ischemic colitis
- **Saw tooth appearance on barium enema:** Diverticula of colon
- **Seagull/Mercedez Benz/Crow Feet Sign:** Radiolucent gall stone with gas
- **Bird's beak appearance on barium swallow:** Achalasia cardia
- **Bird's beak appearance on barium enema:** Volvulus
- **Corkscrew appearance on barium swallow:** Diffuse esophageal spasm.
- **Beak sign; Double track or Tram track sign; Shoulder sign; String sign:** Hypertrophic pyloric stenosis.

120. Ans. (b) Diffuse esophageal spasm

Ref: SRB Manual of Surgery, 4th ed. pg. 1323

- **Cork screw appearance** on barium swallow is seen with diffuse esophageal spasm.
- **Bird beak appearance** is seen with achalasia cardia.
- **Rat tail appearance** as per bailey and love is seen with carcinoma esophagus.

121. Ans. (d) Ultrasound

Ref: SRB Manual of Surgery, 4th ed. pg. 877

- Ultrasound abdomen is the investigation of choice for diagnosing hypertrophic pyloric stenosis.
- It is reliable, highly sensitive, highly specific, and easily performed.
- The mandatory measurements include pyloric muscle thickness and pyloric channel length.
- *Muscle wall thickness 3 mm or greater and pyloric channel length 14 mm or greater are considered abnormal in infants younger than 30 days.*

122. Ans. (a) Diverticulosis

Ref: SRB Manual of Surgery, 4th ed. pg. 952

- *Most common site of diverticulosis is the sigmoid colon in as many as 95% of patients with cecum being involved in 5% of patients.*
- *Reasons for sigmoid colon being the main site of diverticulosis and leading to saw tooth appearance:*
  - Sigmoid colon is the narrowest portion of the colon, and generates the highest intra-segmental pressures
  - Combination of numerous haustra and dehydrated stool in the sigmoid colon leads to segmentation, in which the sigmoid colon functions as multiple small compartments.

Also Remember

TABLE: Pathologies and their radiological findings

Diverticulosis	Saw tooth appearance on barium enema
Intussception	Claw sign on barium sign
Volvulus	Coffee bean sign/bird of prey sign
Ischemic colitis	Thumb printing sign

123. Ans. (a) Carcinoma colon

Ref: Bailey, 26th ed. pg. 70

- On double contrast barium enema of the rectum and distal sigmoid colon demonstrates a typical annular constricting carcinoma of the colon with overhanging edges on both the proximal and distal margins forming a so called "apple-core" lesion.

124. Ans. (a) Contrast CT

Ref: Bailey, 26th ed. pg. 192, 1121

- CECT can be used to assess the severity of acute pancreatitis and to estimate the prognosis. Balthazar et al developed a grading system in which patients with acute pancreatitis are classified into one of the following 5 grades:
  - **Grade A** - Normal-appearing pancreas
  - **Grade B** - Focal or diffuse enlargement of the pancreas
  - **Grade C** - Pancreatic gland abnormalities associated with peri-pancreatic fat infiltration
  - **Grade D** - A single fluid collection
  - **Grade E** - Two or more fluid collections

125. Ans. (d) Acute pancreatitis

Ref: Bailey, 26th ed. pg. 1128-29

- The most commonly recognized radiologic signs associated with acute pancreatitis include the following:
  - Air in the duodenal C-loop
  - ***The sentinel loop sign,*** which represents a focal dilated proximal jejunal loop in the left upper quadrant.
  - ***The colon cut-off sign,*** which represents distention of the colon to the transverse colon with a paucity of gas distal to the splenic flexure.

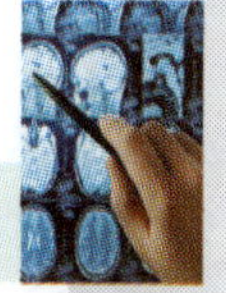

126. Ans. (c) USG

Ref: Bailey, 26th ed. pg. 1100

127. Ans. (c) USG

Ref: Bailey, 26th ed. pg. 109

- In any case of bunt abdominal trauma, first investigation to be performed is ultrasonography.
- In emergency situation, USG technique used is FAST (Focussed Assessment with Sonography for Trauma).
- In FAST, the radiologist, immediately performs the USG abdomen keeping in mind to assess the four major areas to see any collection of fluid due to abdominal organ rupture.
- **Four areas assessed in FAST:** Perihepatic area, Perisplenic area, Pericardial area, Pelvis
- **Updated modality of FAST is eFAST (Extended FAST): Pleural areas are also assessed along with superior mediastinal area.**

128. Ans. (b) CT

THORAX IMAGING

129. Ans. (b) Bronchiectasis

Ref: Grainger and Allison's Diagnostic Radiology: A Textbook of Medical Imaging, 7th ed. pg. 136

- Bronchiectasis is defined as irreversible dilatation of a portion of the bronchial tree. The three most important mechanisms that contribute to the pathogenesis of bronchiectasis are infection, airway obstruction and peribronchial fibrosis.
- In the given CXR, the arrows demonstrate mucous plugging of dilated airways.

CXR findings:

Direct Signs

- Parallel line opacities (tram track appearance)
- Tubular opacities (mucous filled bronchi)
- Ring opacities (dilated end-on bronchi)

Indirect Signs

- Lobar atelectasis (secondary to mucous plugging)
- Compensatory overinflation of the less affected lobe/ lung

130. Ans. (a) Pleural effusion

Ref: Grainger and Allison's Diagnostic Radiology: A Textbook of Medical Imaging, 7th ed. pg. 43

- Chest radiographs are the most commonly used examination to assess for the presence of pleural effusion. Upright chest radiography is highly sensitive in detecting pleural effusion.
- Most common radiographic sign is pleural meniscus as evident in the CXR.
- The diaphragmatic contour is partially or completely obliterated, depending on the amount of the fluid (silhouette sign).

131. Ans. (a) Pneumothorax

Ref: Grainger and Allison's Diagnostic Radiology: A Textbook of Medical Imaging, 7th ed. pg. 50

Pneumothorax refers to the presence of gas in the pleural space. When this collection of gas is constantly enlarging with resulting compression of mediastinal structures, it can be life-threatening and is known as a tension pneumothorax (if no tension is present, it is a simple pneumothorax).

Features of Pneumothorax on CXR:

- Visible visceral pleural edge is seen as a very thin, sharp white line
- No lung markings are seen peripheral to this line
- Peripheral space is radiolucent compared to the adjacent lung
- Lung may completely collapse
- Mediastinum should not shift away from the pneumothorax unless a tension pneumothorax is present
- Subcutaneous emphysema

132. Ans. (a) Perforation peritonitis

Ref: SRB Manual of Surgery, 2019 ed. pg. 822

- The X-ray abdomen taken in erect position shows gas under diaphragm. This is seen in pneumoperitoneum due to viscus perforation. Most of the time this is due to Peptic ulcer disease.
- Option B has deep sulcus sign and absent vascular markings. Option C and D will have blunting of CP angle.

133. Ans. (c) Metastasis

Ref: Crofton's Respiratory Diseases pg. 1145

- The CXR shows multiple rounded opacities in the bilateral lung fields which is classical for canon ball metastasis. This is seen with choriocarcinoma, RCC and breast Cancer.
- Option B will produce a cavity or consolidation in upper lobe on one side
- Option C will produce a solitary mass lesion. Option D will produce a solitary popcorn calcification.

134. Ans. (a) Hamartoma

Ref: ncbi.nlm.nih.gov

The CT chest shows a well-defined round lesion with irregular calcification in the middle of lung window. This is known as "popcorn appearance" which is seen with pulmonary hamartoma. It happens to be the most common benign tumor of lungs.

135. Ans. (b) RV

Ref: Brunner and Suddarth pg. 743

The image shows a dual chamber pacemaker with two leads one in RA and other one in RV. The marked lead is delivering timed electrical impulses to endocardium of right ventricle. There is a possibility that image was of single chamber (lead) pacemaker. The Explanation will not change as a single lead pacemaker also controls the right ventricle.

136. Ans. (d) Right middle lobe consolidation

Ref: ncbi.nlm.gov.in

The CXR PA view shows silhouette sign suggestive of right middle lobe pneumonia.

Right middle zone pneumonia	Right lower zone pneumonia
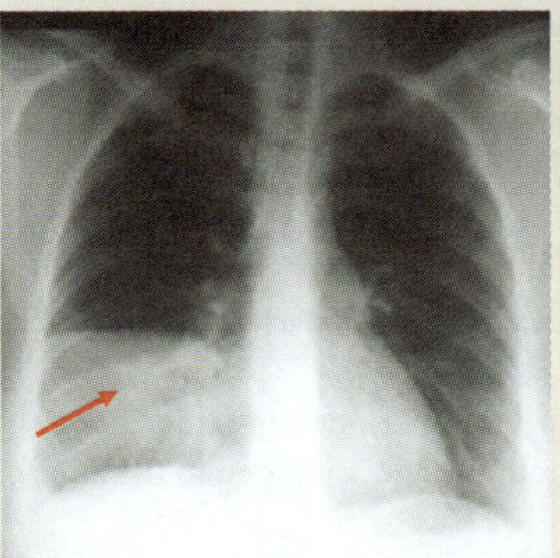 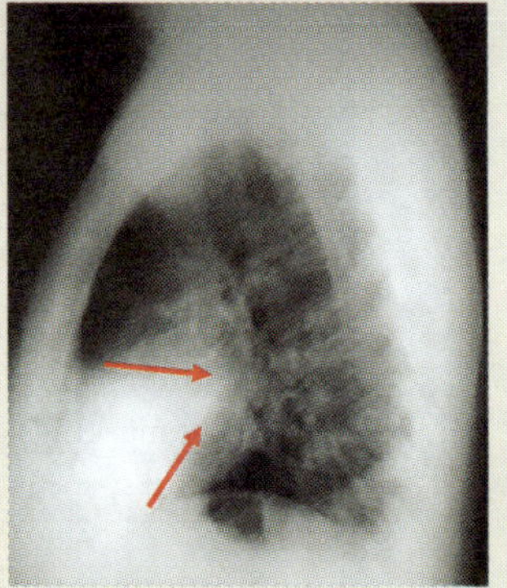	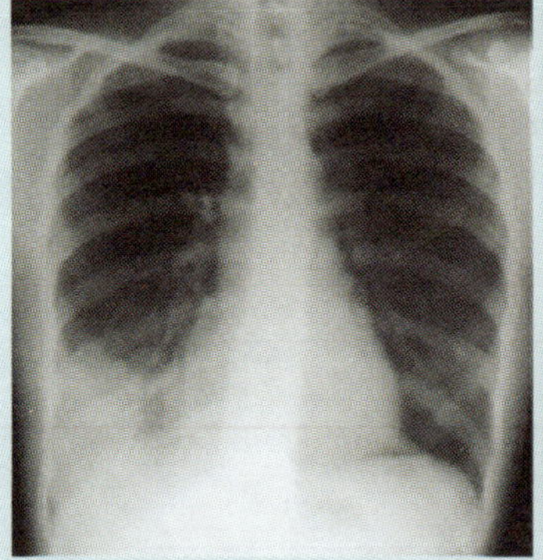 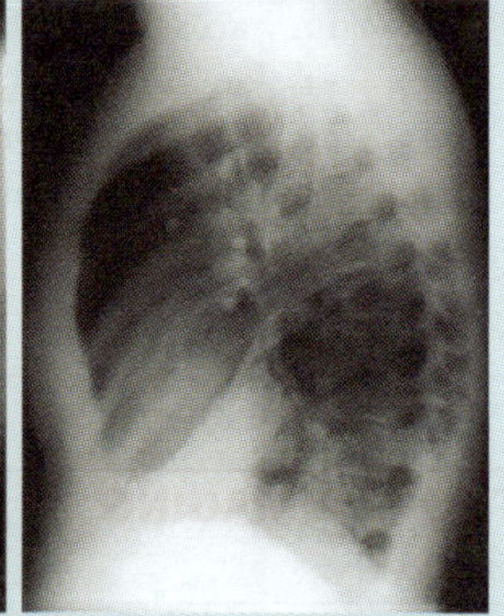
Notice the two red lines in lateral view that are representing the middle lobe which is present anteriorly	Notice that the lower lobe in lateral view is present more posteriorly Also notice that lower lobe consolidation in PA view will not cause significant obliteration of right heart border

137. Ans. (b) Pneumothorax

Ref: Final Edge, 3rd ed. pg. 110

- CXR shows deep sulcus sign on the left side with lung collapse. The area which is appearing blacker on left side is devoid of any vascular markings. The trachea also shows right sided shift. All these features point to left sided pneumothorax.
- Option A will produce Blunting of CP angle
- Option C will produce segmental defect in one lung
- Option D will cause herniation of bowel contents into the chest wall

138. Ans. (c) Pancreatic pseudocyst

Ref: SRB, 5th ed. pg. 659

- CT Abdomen shows a hypodense shadow of fluid collection in the parenchyma of pancreas. Seen posterior to it are the abdominal aorta, part of liver and both the kidneys. Based on past-history of acute pancreatitis and fluid collection in pancreatic tissue on CT abdomen the diagnosis pseudo-pancreatic cyst.
- It is called pseudo because the wall is made up of fibrotic tissue rather than plain epithelial lining.

139. Ans. (a) Canon ball metastasis

Ref: Chest Radiology Essentials by Wolter Kluwer pg. 707

CXR shows bilateral multiple opacities due to canon Ball metastasis.

Causes of Canon ball metastasis
1. Renal cell carcinoma
2. Breast cancer
3. Choriocarcinoma
4. Germ cell tumors

140. Ans. (b) Pericardial effusion

- The Chest X-ray shows increased CT ratio. In setting of TB this can be due to pericardial effusion. Notice the

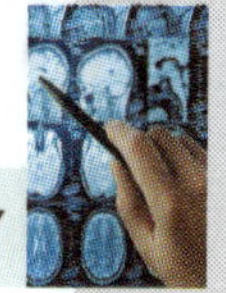

narrow vascular pedicle from top giving it a water bottle appearance.

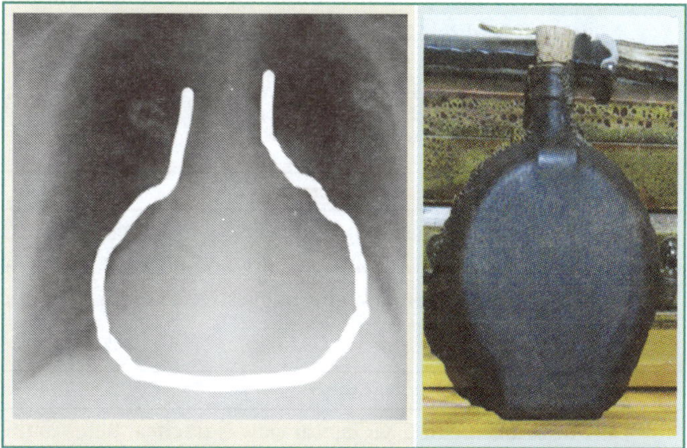

- Option A will show normal CT ratio with pericardial calcification.
- Option C is a close choice due to increased CT ration but not seen with TB. DCM should show evidence of pulmonary edema but the current CXR shows normal vascular shadows
- Option D is diagnosed only on basis of Becks triad or presence of pulsus paradoxus and echocardiography findings.

141. Ans. (a) Hydatid cyst

- The CXR shows a Boundary of a cystic lesion in right middle and lower lobe.
- Option B will cause Bilateral pneumonia with hemorrhagic mediastinitis.
- Option C will show pulmonary fibrosis and shrunken lungs.
- Option D will show circumscribed shadow with an air fluid level due to pus settling at dependent part of abscess.

142. Ans. (d) Congenital diaphragmatic hernia

- The CXR shows shadow of Bowel loops in left chest cavity which is diagnostic of Congenital Diaphragmatic hernia.
- Option A shows some cystic areas with adenomatous overgrowth of the terminal bronchioles and normal lung tissue. In the given CXR normal lung tissue is not seen.
- Option B is usually a single lesion.
- Option C is ruled out as it is seen in preterm babies and presents immediately after birth.

143. Ans. (a) Rt middle lobe consolidation

The CXR shows consolidation in right paracardiac area extending in to involve right middle zone.

Extra Mile

How to differentiate between consolidation and atelectasis?

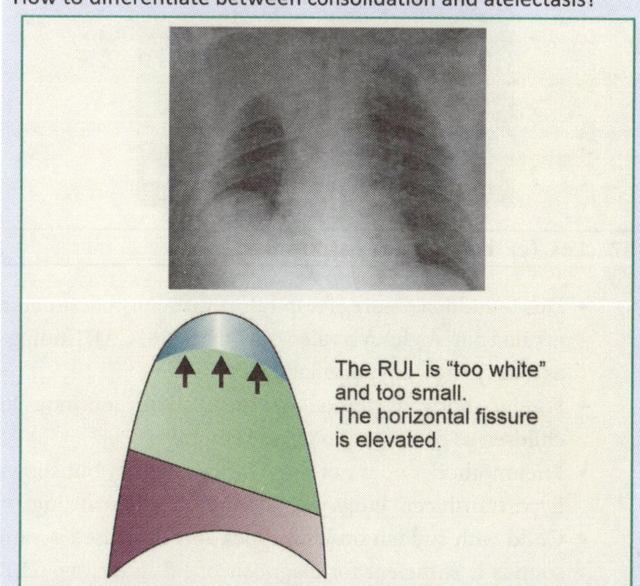

Atelectasis is also white but always shows curvature in lung fissures

144. Ans. (a) Left sided mastectomy

- The CXR shows absent breast shadow on left side.
- Trachea is central. Lung parenchyma and broncho-vascular markings are normal. CP angle is normal. CT Ratio is normal.
- Diagnosis of this post op patient is left sided mastectomy.

145. Ans. (a) Pneumothorax

The CXR shows hypertranslucent lung with absent vascular markings. The pleural reflection of collapsed lung (white arrow) can be seen. Diagnosis is left sided pneumothorax.

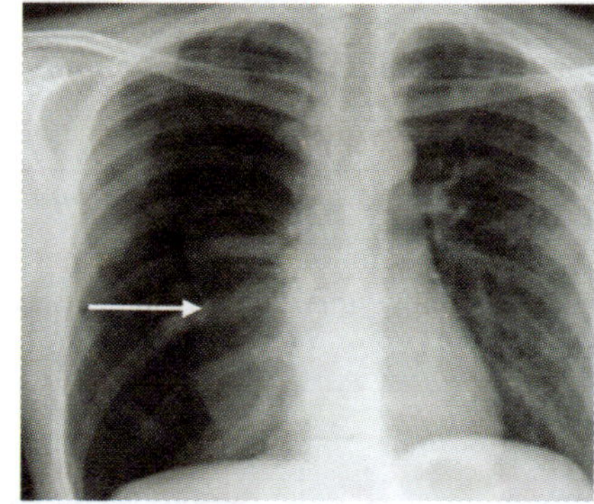

146. Ans. (b) Sarcoidosis

Elevated ACE levels with Bilateral hilar lymphadenopathy is characteristic feature of Sarcoidosis. CXR shows increased bronchovascular markings with enlarged lymph nodes (red markings) visible above aortic knuckle.

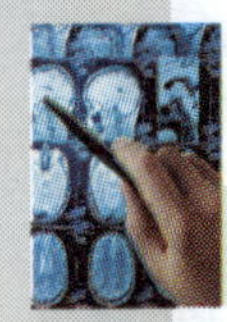

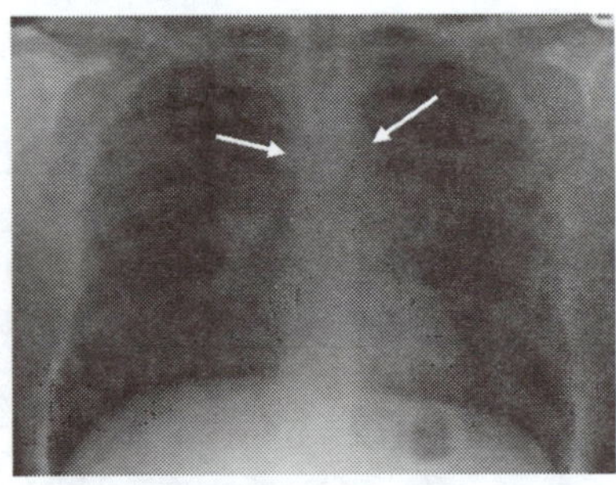

147. Ans. (c) Foreign body aspiration

- Due to sudden nature of respiratory difficulty pneumonia is ruled out. Asthma is ruled out on basis of CXR findings as it only shows hyperinflation.
- Foreign body aspiration is much more common in children as compared to pneumothorax.
- Pneumothorax does not show diffuse opacity but shows hypertranslucent lungs with absent vascular markings.
- Child with sudden onset dyspnea and decreased breath sounds is sufficient for diagnosis of FB in airway. CXR findings take some time to develop.

148. Ans. (a) Hydropneumothorax

- The CXR shows a straight-line indicating demarcation of fluid and air and is seen in hydropneumothorax. Option B is ruled out as white in right lung field indicates fluid in pleural space
- Option C is ruled out as it has increased CT ratio
- Option D will not have straight well-defined margins as seen in the image

149. Ans. (d) Military TB

CXR shows multiple millet like seeding of TB bacilli in the lung in an AIDS Positive patient with symptoms of LRTI. The leading opportunistic infection in AIDS Positive patient is TB. Low immunity favors dissemination.

150. Ans. (a) Aortic dissection

Ref: Harrison 20th ed. pg. 1921

The given image is of a CT chest showing intimal flap of aortic dissection and involves both ascending and descending aorta.

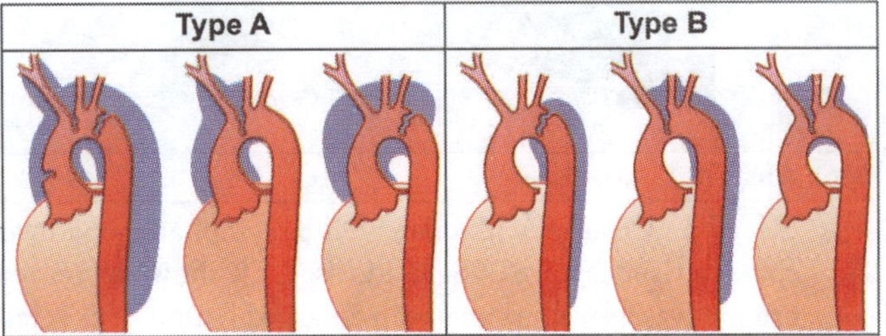

151. Ans. (a) MUGA

Ref: Harrison 20th ed. pg. 675

MUGA or Multiple Uptake Gated Acquisition Angiography and is used to asses LV function and Volume. Choices B, C and D are used for angiographically significant Coronary artery disease.

152. Ans. (a) Diaphragmatic hernia

- The shown image is suggestive of diaphragmatic hernia.
- Intestinal loop in thoracic cavity and absence of bowel loops in abdomen is highly suggestive of diaphragmatic hernia.

153. Ans. (c) Trachea

- The structure in CXR lateral view is trachea. Refer to the image below

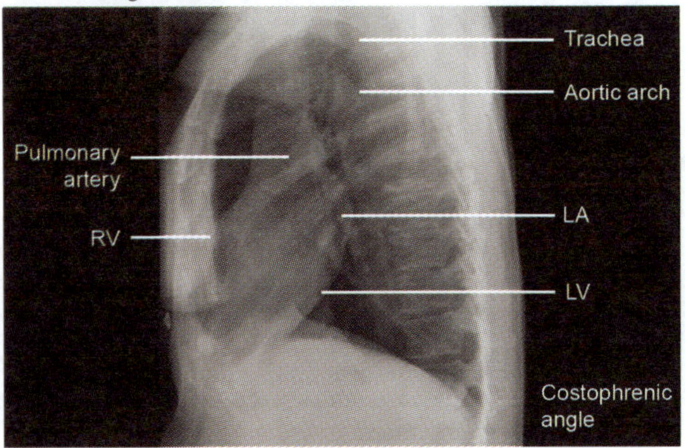

154. Ans. (b) Exudative pleural effusion

- The given X-ray shows massive pleural effusion. Since there is history of low grade fever and dyspnea, this can be secondary to some underlying pathology, producing exudative effusion.

155. Ans. (b) Pneumoperitoneum

- **IOC for pneumoperitoneum:** Chest X-ray PA view in erect position (including diaphragm)

RADIOLOGICAL SIGNS OF PNEUMOPERITONEUM

- **Gas under diaphragm sign:** Accumulation of gas under right side hemidiaphragm
- **Mustache sign**/Cupola sign/Saddle bag sign
- **Rigler sign:** Air outlining both internal and external intestinal wall
- **Urachus sign:** Air outlining middle umbilical ligament
- **Inverted V sign:** Air outlining both umbilical ligaments
- **Falciform ligament sign:** Air surrounding falciform ligament (becomes prominent).

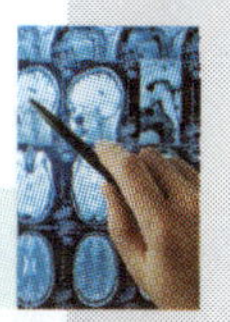

156. Ans. (b) Diffuse oesophageal spasm

- The finding shown in image is corkscrew esophagus, which is seen in patients with diffuse esophageal spasm (due to uncoordinated activity of esophageal smooth muscles).
  - This is possible due to fragmental degeneration of vagal nerve fibres
  - Simultaneous and repetitive contraction in esophagus body with normal lower esophageal sphincter.
- **Clinical feature:**
  - Chest pain, Nonprogressive dysphagia with solids and liquids and non exertional chest pain, which responds to nitroglycerin.
- **IOC for DES:** Manometry
- **Upon barium swallow:** Corkscrew appearance
- Similar to DES, there is **nutcracker esophagus** where there is high-amplitude peristalsis (>80 mm Hg) for increased duration.

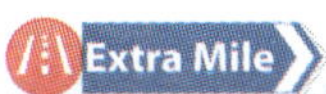

Other radiological findings of esophageal pathology
- **Barium swallow:** Bird beak/Pencil tip: Achalasia cardia
- **Barium swallow-rat tail appearance (with filling defect):** Achalasia cardia
- **Barium swallow:** Worm eaten appearance: Esophageal varices

157. Ans. (a) Major fissure

Ref: Fundamentals of Radiology by Squire, pg. 136

The image shows left lung with *major* fissure separating the left upper lobe from the lower lobe.

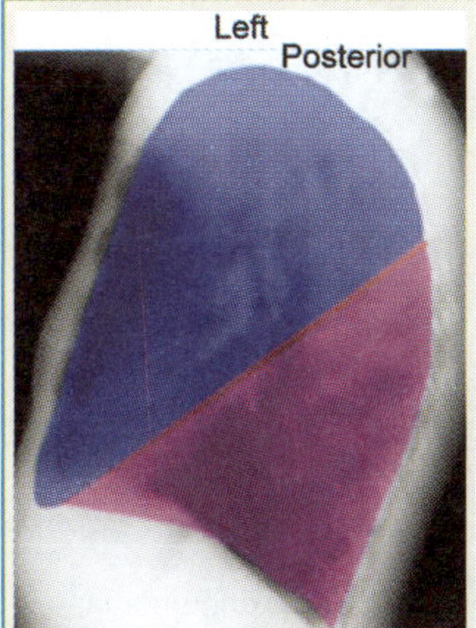

Notice the major fissure in left lung segregating the upper and lower lobes. Compare with the image given below.

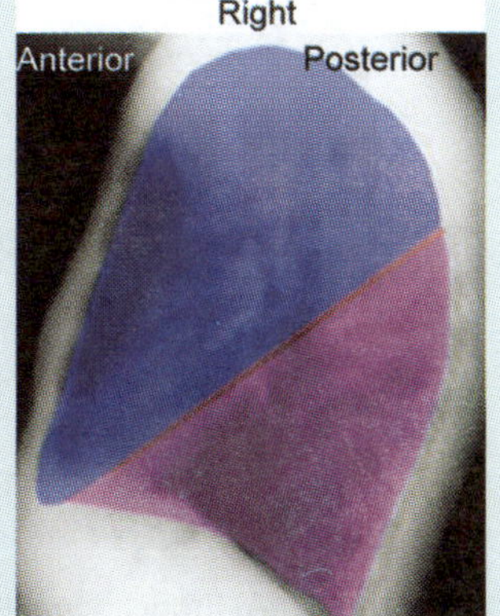

Notice the major fissure and minor fissures in right lung. Compare with the image given below.

Contd...

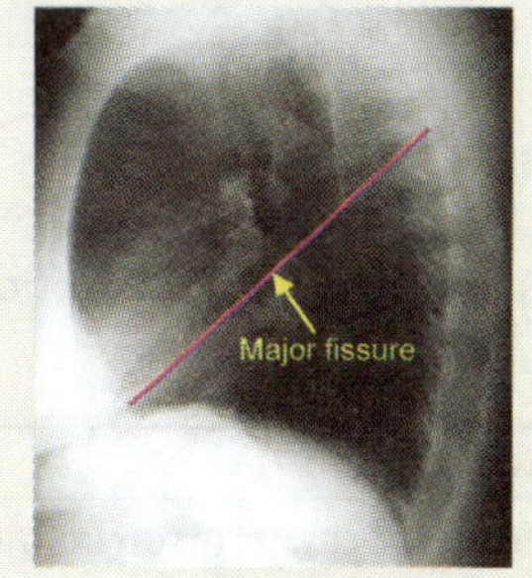

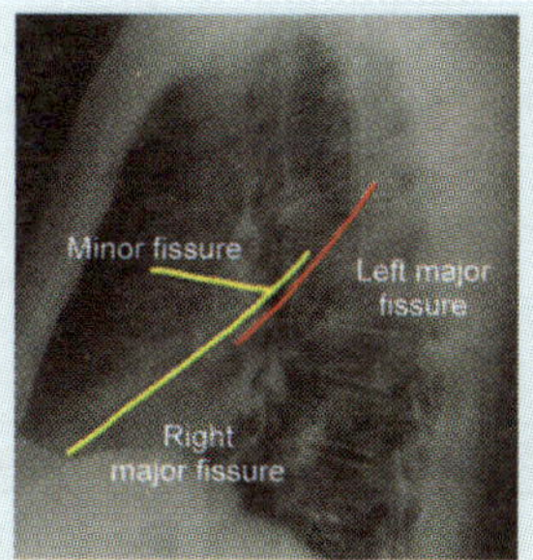

Azygos fissure is seen as a curvilinear density in upper right lung, convex towards the chest wall. Azygos lobe is found as an anatomic variant in 1% of population.

Extra Mile

- Shift in the position of fissures is seen in segmental atelectasis
- **Comet tail sign:** Rounded atelectasis
- **S sign of golden:** Upper lobe atelectasis

158. Ans. (b) Pneumothorax

- The shown CT scan clearly shows air in the pleural cavity (arrow) around left lung. This condition is pneumothorax.
- In case of pleural effusion, the water will appear relatively white and at lower aspect on CT (*due to gravity*).

159. Ans. (a) Bronchiectasis

- The shown image of CT, is suggestive of bronchiectasis, characterized by tram *track sign of airways*.
- Bronchiectasis is an abnormal dilatation of airway.
- **Radiological findings:**
  - Tram track sign
  - Cluster of grape appearance
  - Signet ring sign

160. Ans. (b) Barium swallow

- The given imaging here is barium swallow, showing achalasia cardia.
- Barium swallow is done for esophageal pathology.
- Barium meal is for stomach and first part of duodenum.
- Barium meal follow through is for small intestine.
- Barium enema is for colon.

161. Ans. (a) Tetralogy of Fallot

- The given image shows boot shaped heart, which is a characteristic finding seen in Tetralogy of Fallot.

Also Remember

Radiological findings of congenital heart disease:

- Figure of '8' appearance or Snowman appearance: **TAPVR (type I)**

- "Egg on its side" or "Apple on a stem" appearance: TGA (transposition of great arteries)
- **"Boot-shaped Heart"** /Classic coeur en sabot: TOF
- Box/Balloon shaped heart: Ebstein Anomaly
- '3 sign' and inferior rib notching on CXR: Coarctation of Aorta

162. Ans. (d) Main pulmonary artery

(Revise the chest CT anatomy from the image given below)

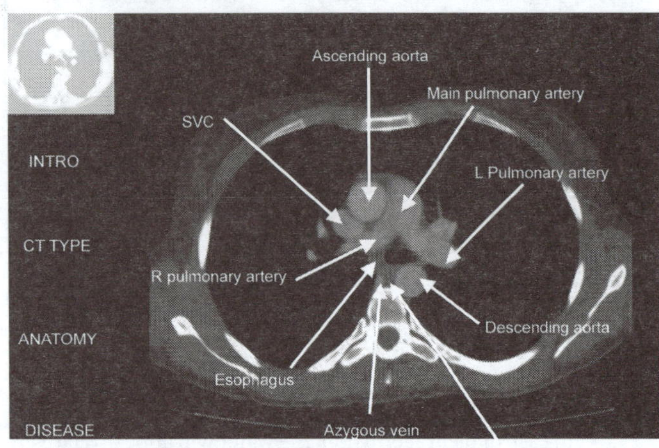

163. Ans. (d) Aortic knuckle

- Right border of heart is formed by:
  - Superior vena cava
  - The right atrium
  - Small part of inferior vena cava
- Left heart border is formed by:
  - Aortic nuckle
  - The pulmonary bay
  - The auricle of left atrium
  - The left ventricle.

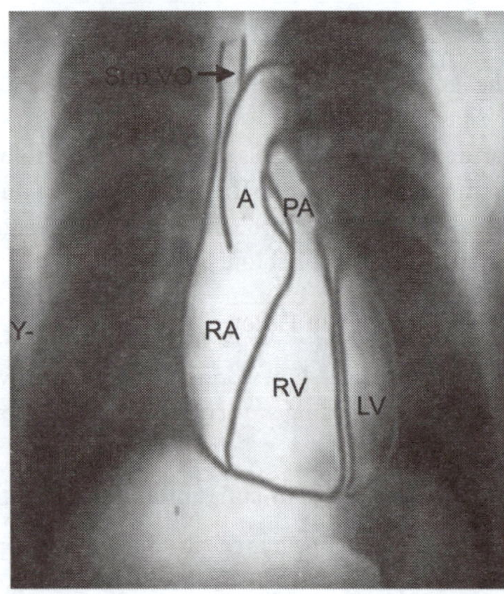

164. Ans. (b) CT ratio being measured

Cardiothoracic ratio

- It is a estimation of cardiac size
- Vertical line is drawn through the midsternal line
- Maximal distances of the right and left heart borders from the midsternal line are added
- Greatest transverse diameter of thorax is obtained
- Normal value = $\leq 50\%$

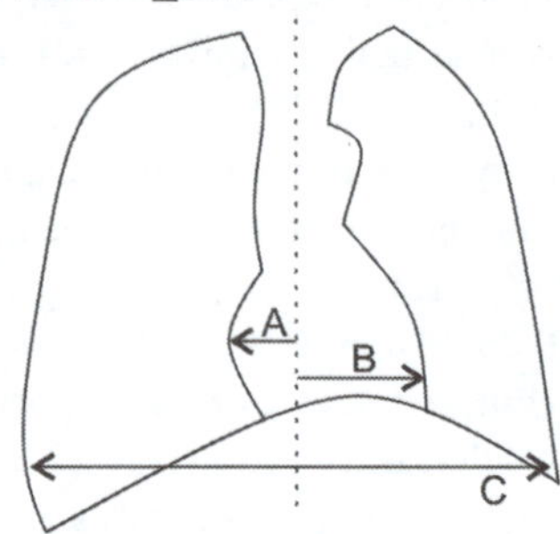

FIGURE: Cardiothoracic ratio

165. Ans. (a) Patchy consolidation

- In **bronchopneumonia there is patchy consolidation**, no mediastinal shift.
- In **lobar pneumonia there is diffuse consolidation.**
- In collapse, there is mediastinal shift on the same side.
- In pleural effusion, there is contralateral mediastinal shift.

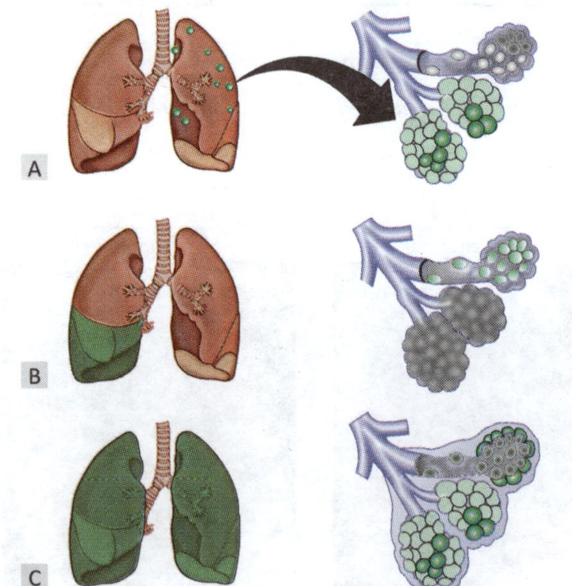

FIGURES: (A) Bronchopneumonia; (B) Lobar pneumonia; (C) Interstitial pneumonia

166. Ans. (a) Right ventricle forms the right heart border

Ref: Essential Radiology, 2nd ed. pg. 22

- **Right ventricle is not a border forming structure in PA view.** However, it forms anterior border in lateral view of Chest X-ray.

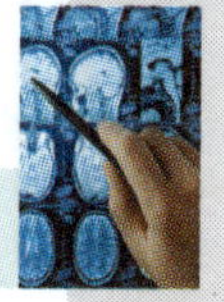

Right Heart Border

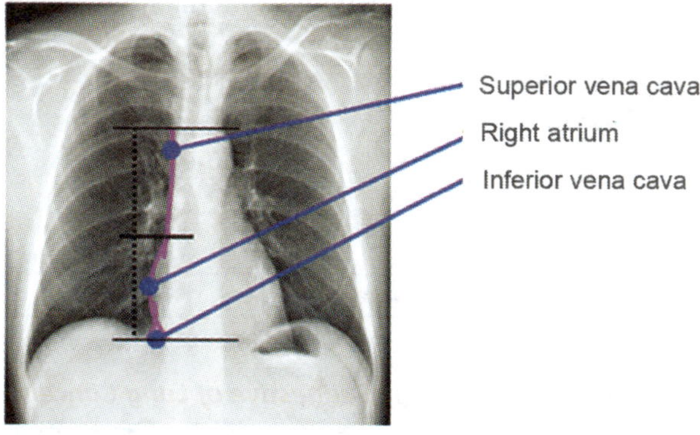

Left Heart Border

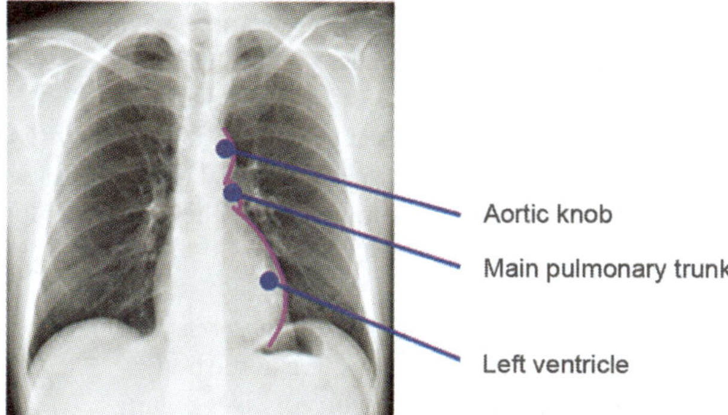

FIGURE: Heart border forming structures

167. Ans. (d) Left atrial appendage clots

Ref: Harrison, 19th ed. pg. 270e-2

T.E.E. is preferred over the routine Transthoracic echocardiography for the following situations:

1. Internal heart structures and path of blood flow in congenital heart disease is better evaluated.
2. To evaluate the effects of surgical intervention to the heart, such as repair of congenital heart defects.
3. When T.T.E is indicated, but circumstances (i.e., pulmonary disease like emphysema) that may interfere with the ability to obtain adequate images.
4. Mitral valve disease
5. Blood clots or masses inside the heart
6. Aortic Dissection
7. Implanted prosthetic heart valves
8. To evaluate for blood clots in the heart prior to cardioversion or ablation procedures.

168. Ans. (a) ASD

Ref: Harrison, 19th ed. pg. 1520

ATRIAL SEPTAL DEFECT (ASD)

- In atrial septal defect there is congenital defect in the interatrial septum.
- *It is Most common CHD diagnosed in adulthood*

TYPES Based on Defects with Different Locations Functionally the same

- *Primum*- lower part of the septum
- *Secundum*- located near the foramen ovale or fossa ovalis
- *Sinus venosus*- caval location
- *Coronary sinus- least common* → near SVC entry

Also Remember

- Most common CHD **diagnosed in infancy- VSD**
- 2nd OVERALL MOST COMMON CONGENITAL CARDIAC ANOMALY- **VSD**
- In VSD all chambers are enlarged EXCEPT: **Right Atrium**
- MC cyanotic congenital heart disease: **Tetralogy of Fallot (TOF)**
- **2nd most common cyanotic CHD after TOF- TGA**
- **Most common cause of cyanosis in neonate: Transposition of Great arteries**
- Most common cause of congenital heart disease beyond the neonatal period: **Tetralogy of Fallot**

Radiological Features:

- All chambers are enlarged in ASD EXCEPT Left ventricle.
- **Increased vascularity:** Pulmonary artery over loading.
- Enlarged main (dilated MPA) and central pulmonary arteries

169. Ans. (d) Ebstein anomaly

Ref: Pediatric Radiology, 1st ed. 57

- **Ebstein anomaly** is a congenital heart defect in which the septal and posterior leaflets of the tricuspid valve are displaced towards the apex of the right ventricle of the heart.
- **It causes atrialization of right ventricle.**

Radiographic Features In Different Congenital Heart Diseases:

- Figure of '8' appearance or Snowman appearance: **TAPVR (type I)**
- Egg on its side" or "Apple on a stem" appearance: TGA
- **Boot-shaped Heart"** /Classic coer en sabot: TOF
- **Box/Balloon shaped heart: Ebstein Anomaly**
- **'3 sign' on CXR: Coaractation of Aorta**

170. Ans. (a) Asthma

Ref: Harrison, 19th ed. pg. 1675

- Flattening of diaphragm is seen with obstructive airway diseases due to the process of air trapping.
- The point that clinches the diagnosis in favor of asthma is the curschmann spirals which represent the cast of the airways formed by mucus plugs in small airways in these patients.

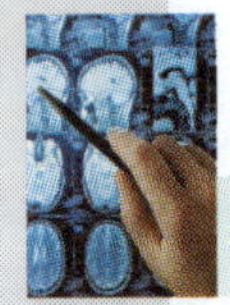

171. Ans. (d) To remove foreign body

Ref: Harrison, 19th ed. pg. 1667

Foreign body is removed by rigid bronchoscopy.

Indications for Rigid Bronchoscopy

- Bleeding or hemorrhage
- Foreign body extraction
- Deeper biopsy specimen when fiber-optic specimen is inadequate
- Dilation of tracheal or bronchial strictures, relief of airway obstruction, insertion of stents, and pediatric bronchoscopy.
- It is also used for tracheobronchial laser therapy or other mechanical tumor ablation.

172. Ans. (c) Pulmonary embolism

Ref: Harrison, 19th ed. pg. 1633

HAMPTON HUMP is a radiologic sign which consists of a shallow wedge-shaped opacity in the periphery of the lung with its base against the pleural surface.

173. Ans. (a) Pulmonary embolism

Ref: Harrison, 19th ed. pg. 1633

Westermark sign is due to focus of oligemia in pulmonary embolism (PE). The sign develops due to following reasons:

- Dilation of the pulmonary arteries proximal to the embolus
- Collapse of the distal vasculature creating the appearance of a sharp cut off on chest X-ray

The chest X-ray is normal in the majority of PE cases, the Westermark sign is seen in 2% of patients

174. Ans. (b) Pneumomediastinum

Ref: Harrison, 19th ed. pg. 1720

- Normally the central portion of the diaphragm is not discretely visualised on chest X-ray as it merges with the cardiac borders.
- However if the diaphragm can be seen continuously across the midline then this is diagnostic of free gas within the mediastinum, pericardium or peritoneal cavity.
- **Continuous diaphragm sign** is seen in pneumomediastinum.

175. Ans. (a) Pneumonia

Ref: Harrison, 19th ed. pg. 806

- **Air bronchogram** refers to the phenomenon of air-filled bronchi (*dark*) being made visible by the opacification of surrounding alveoli (*grey - white*).
- It is almost always caused by a pathologic airspace (alveolar) process, in which something other than air fills the alveoli.
- Air bronchograms will not be visible if the bronchi themselves are opacified (e.g. by fluid).
- Air bronchograms can be seen with several processes, including the following:
  - *Pulmonary consolidation* (pneumonia)
  - Pulmonary oedema
  - Non-obstructive atelectasis
  - Severe interstitial lung disease

176. Ans. (a) Lung carcinoma

Ref: Harrison, 19th ed. pg. 511

Findings in Chest X-ray Suggestive of Lung Cancer

- Central lesions appear as a bulky hilum, representing the tumor and local nodal involvement.
- In contrast a more peripheral location may appear as a rounded or spiculated mass.
- Cavitation may be seen as an air-fluid level.
- Destruction of the adjacent rib or evidence of soft tissue growing into the soft tissues superficial to the ribs as seen in the above case where lung CA is in the right upper lobe.

HYDATID CYSTS

It result from infection by the *Echinococcus* worm, and can result in cyst formation anywhere in the body.

- **Most common organ involved**: Liver > Lung

There are several clinical signs in hydatid disease:

- **Cumbo sign:** Air is seen between the pericyst and the laminated membrane of the cyst.
- **Serpent sign:** Internal rupture of the cyst with collapse of membranes of parasite into the cyst.
- **Spin sign/whirl sign:** Detached membranes with small pleural reaction seen in hydatid cyst of lung.
- **Empty cyst sign:** May be seen after complete evacuation of parasitic membranes.

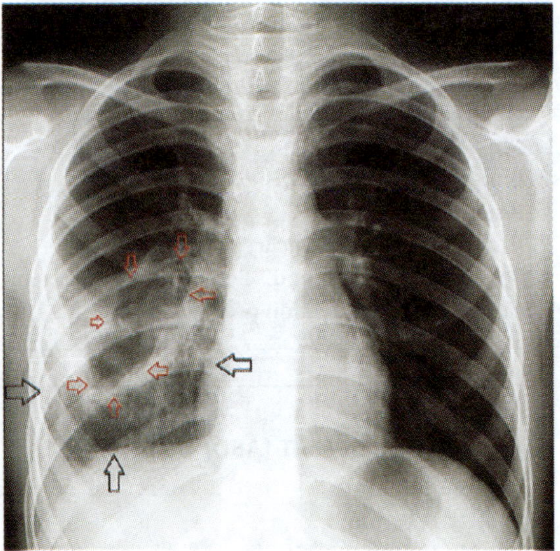

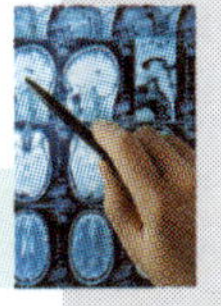

LUNG ABSCESS

- A **lung abscess** is a circumscribed collection of pus within the lung.
- Most commonly seen in superior segment of lower lobes or posterior segments of lower lobes.
- **X-ray:** The classical appearance of a pulmonary abscess is a cavity containing an air-fluid level.
- **IOC for abcess:** Contrast CT.

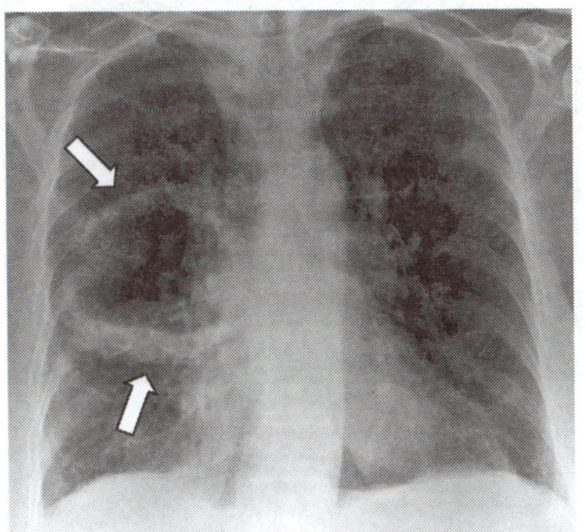

ASPERGILLOMA

- **Aspergillomas** are mass-like fungus balls that are typically composed of *Aspergillus fumigatus* and is a non-invasive form of pulmonary aspergillosis
- **CXR:** Aspergillomas typically appear as rounded or ovoid soft tissue attenuating masses located in a surrounding cavity and outlined by a crescent of air.
- **CT**: Appearances are those of a well formed cavity with a central soft tissue attenuating rounded mass surrounded by an *air crescent sign or a Monad sign.*

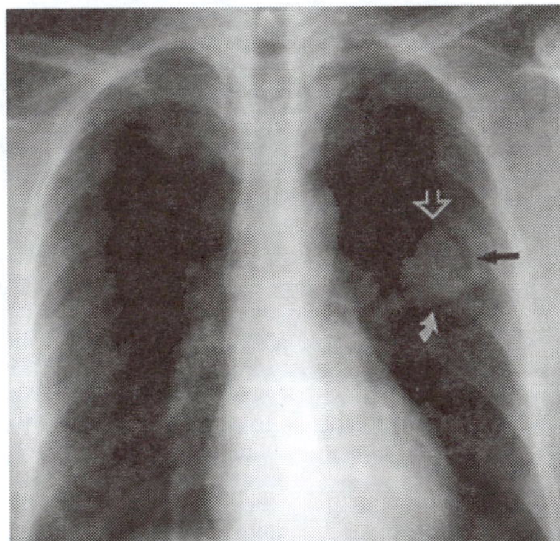

177. Ans. (a) Bronchogenic carcinoma with collapse of lung

- The Golden S sign (reverse S sign of Golden) is seen in PA chest radiographs with right upper lobe collapse.
- It is caused by a central mass obstructing the upper lobe bronchus and should raise suspicion of a primary bronchogenic carcinoma.
- The right upper lobe appears dense and shifts medially and upwards with a central mass expanding the hilum. The combination of two changes together form a reverse S shape.

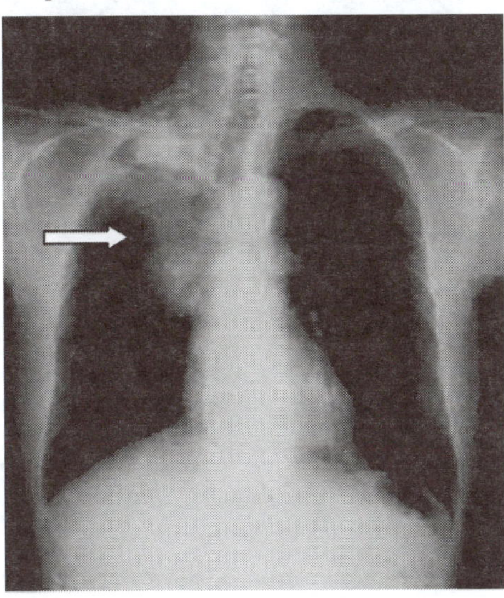

178. Ans. (b) Pulmonary hamartoma

Ref Robbins, 8th ed. pg. 1433

- Lung hamartoma is a lesion seen as rounded focus of radio-opacity called as coin lesion or as popcorn lesion on X-ray.
- It is a benign neoplasm rather than a lung malformation and the finding of chromosomal aberration **6p21 or 12q14,** indicates a **clonal origin.**
- **Note:** Popcorn calcification on mammography: FIBROADENOMA

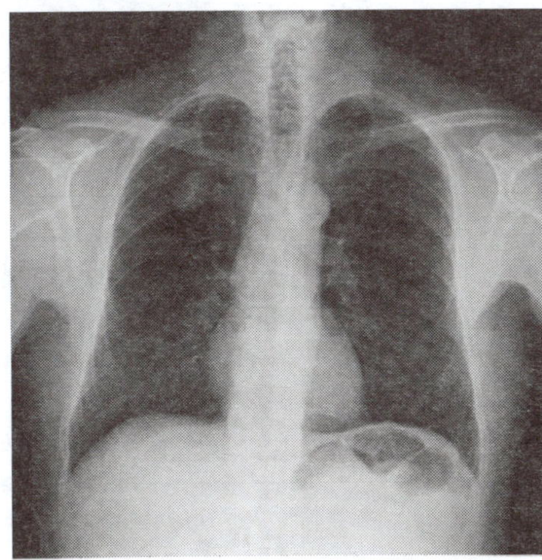

FIGURE: Popcorn calcification in lung-pulmonary hamartoma

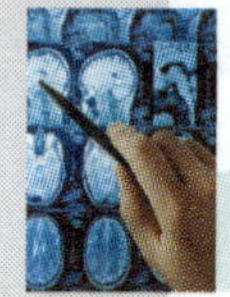

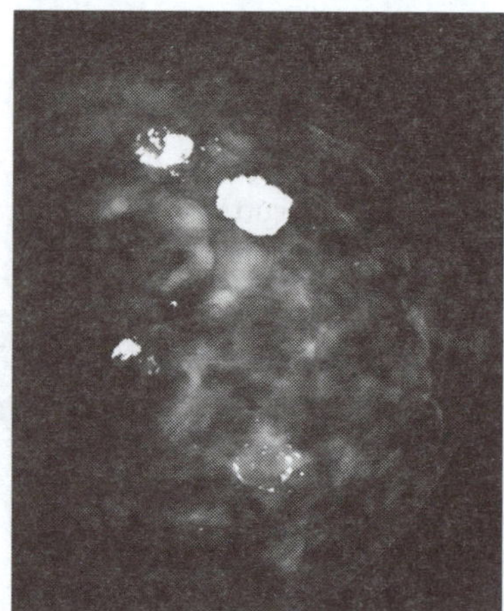

FIGURE: Popcorn calcification in breast-fibroadenoma

NEUROLOGY IMAGING

179. Ans. (a) Meningocele

Ref: Grainger and Allison's Diagnostic Radiology: A Textbook of Medical Imaging, 7th ed. pg. 1313

- Meningocele results from a failure to develop the caudal end of the neural tube resulting in a protrusion that contains cerebrospinal fluid, meninges, overlying skin, and does not have the spinal cord as its content.
- Open NTDs are the result of defects in primary neurulation and involve any area of the central nervous system (CNS).
- Closed NTDs are due to defects in secondary neurulation and present in the spine.

180. Ans. (b) SAH

Ref: Harrison 20th ed. pg. 2084

CT head shows blood in Sylvian fissure and Basal cisterns which is classical presentation of subarachnoid hemorrhage. Another key word to be picked up is "Thunderclap headache" or "Worst headache of my life".

181. Ans. (c) EDH

Ref: Final Edge, 3rd ed. pg. 365

The NCCT head shows a biconvex hyper-density in right frontal area suggestive of extradural hemorrhage. Also visible is subperiosteal hemorrhage on right side.

182. Ans. (b) Lenticular nucleus

Ref: Final Edge, 3rd ed. pg. 743

The arrow marking is at lenticular nucleus. This happens to be a common site of intraparenchymal bleeding and is the reason that it is so commonly asked in the exam. The marking given in the CT head are a must know and are regularly asked in the exam.

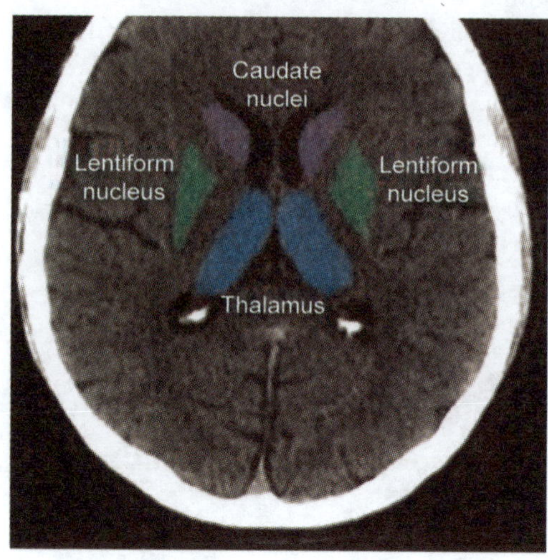

183. Ans. (c) Sciatic nerve

Ref: ncbi.nlm.gov.in

- Step 1 Compare the size of femoral head on right side. It looks smaller and is marked in red and orange arrows.
- Step 2 Look at the lesser trochanter (yellow arrow). It appears missing.
- Both are features of posterior dislocation of hip. The sciatic nerve, usually the peroneal branch, is most often injured, and this complication can be seen after all types of posterior fracture-dislocations and simple posterior dislocations. The sciatic nerve can be acutely lacerated, stretched, or compressed, or later encased in heterotopic ossification.

Anterior hip dislocation	Posterior hip dislocation
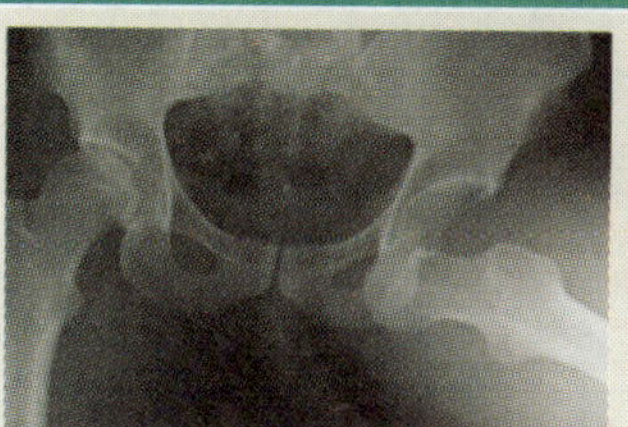 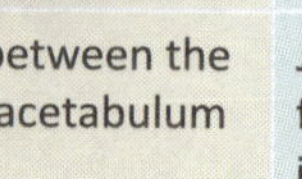	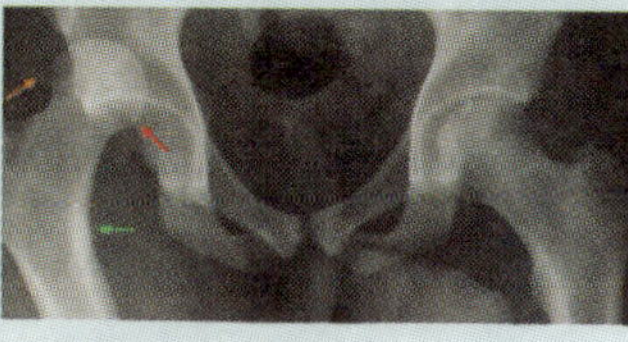
Joint congruency between the femoral head and acetabulum is affected. Notice that the head looks *bigger* It is displaced *infero medially* Lesser trochanter is *visible* and prominent.	Joint congruency between the femoral head and acetabulum is affected. Notice the head looks *smaller* It is displaced *supero-laterally* Lesser trochanter is *not visible*

184. Ans. (b) Middle cerebral artery

- The image shows large hypodensity on right hemisphere indicating occlusion of main trunk of middle cerebral artery. The patient has developed acute ischemic stroke.
- Option A will only cause frontal lobe damage
- Option C will cause mid brain stroke
- Option D will cause 3rd nerve palsy

185. Ans. (c) Lentiform nucleus

The image shows NCCT head with the marking shown to be of lenticular nucleus.

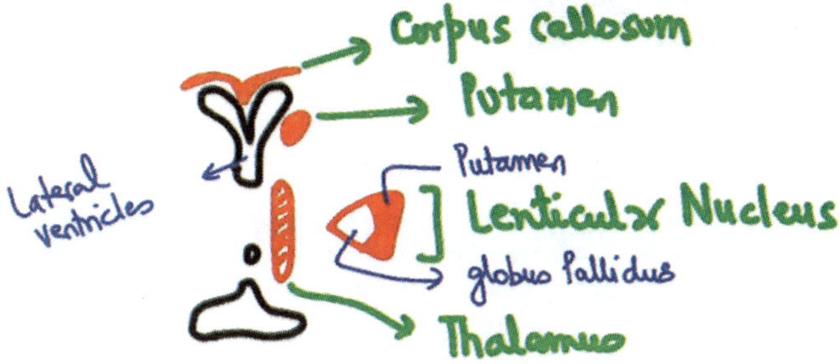

186. Ans. (a) Holman Miller sign

- The image shows a cross section CT of paranasal sinuses showing anterior bowing of posterior wall of maxillary antrum.
- It can be produced by any slowly-growing mass leading to erosion of the pterygoid lamina and is pathognomonic for juvenile nasopharyngeal angiofibroma.
- Dodd sign has X-ray finding of crescent of air between the antrochoanal polyp and posterior pharyngeal wall.
- Phlep sign is seen in Glomus jugulare paraganglioma that leads to erosion of the caroticojugular spine between the carotid canal and jugular fossa may be present
- Griesinger sign refers to edema of the postauricular soft tissues overlying the mastoid process as a result of thrombosis of the mastoid emissary vein. It is a complication of acute otomastoiditis and may be associated with dural sinus occlusive disease

187. Ans. (b) Putaminal bleed

The NCCT head shows a left sided hyperdensity encroaching on internal capsule and lenticular nucleus (Putamen + Globus Pallidus). In setting of uncontrolled hypertension, the diagnosis is left sided Hemorrhagic stroke.

188. Ans. (a) Optic nerve

- NCCT head shows marking at retro-orbital area where optic nerve is present.
- Option B and C are posteriorly located as compared to optic nerve.
- Option D would require a contrast enhanced CT to be visualized.

189. Ans. (c) Midbrain

MRI head shows midbrain and distinct shape of cerebral peduncles can be seen anteriorly.

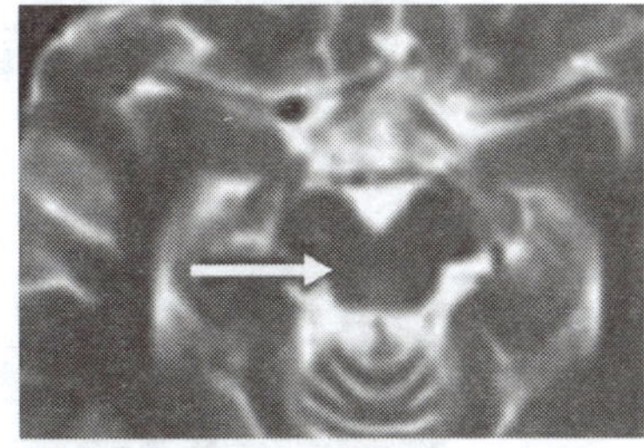

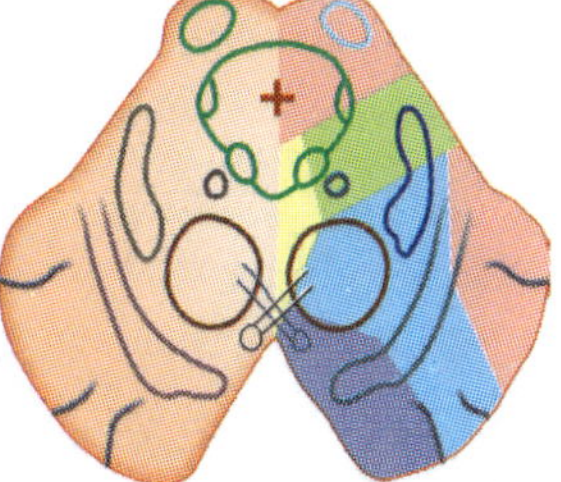

190. Ans. (d) Subdural hematoma

NCCT head show a concavo-convex hematoma diagnostic of Subdural hemorrhage with a mass effect of bleed leading to midline shift. This mid line shift is also called subfalcine herniation.

191. Ans. (a) Diffuse axonal injury

- Normal CT scan after RTA rules out Contusion and SAH.
- Concussion is common after contact or body contact sports. There is an alteration of mental status with or without associated loss of consciousness.
- Diffuse axonal injury is predominant TBI requiring hospital admission after motor vehicle crashes. There is widespread axonal damage.
- The main mechanical force causing DAI is rotational acceleration of brain which produces shearing and tensile forces due to which axons can be pulled apart at microscopic level
- NCCT head may show multiple petechial hemorrhages characteristically located at the gray-white matter interface.

192. Ans. (a) Xerostomia

- Head and neck radiation will affect salivary glands which may undergo fibrosis. This will reduce saliva production and causes xerostomia.
- Option B will be seen with Chest radiation.
- Option C is alternation of taste, while people with dry tongue due to saliva reduction will develop ageusia.
- Option D is seen with damage to sympathetic ganglia in Horner syndrome and is usually a mass effect of tumor.

193. Ans. (c) Lentiform nucleus

- The marked structure in the CT brain image is lentiform nucleus.
- Learn to identify the other important structure in the image given below

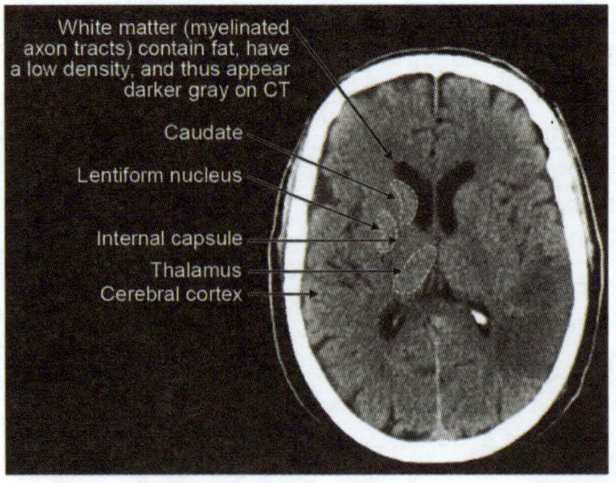

194. Ans. (b) Massive epidural hemorrhage

TABLE: Difference between different kinds of intracranial bleed

	Epidural hemorrhage	Subdural hemorrhage	Subarachnoid hemorrhage
Site	Above dura (between brain and skull)	Below dura (between dura and arachnoid mater)	Below arachnoid (between arachnoid and Pia mater)
Source of bleed	Middle meningeal artery	Cortical bridging vein tear	Circle of Willis
CT appearance	Biconvex white/Lenticular	Concavo-convex/Moon crescent	Star shaped opacity
Image			

195. Ans. (d) 4th ventricle

Ref:* *Fundamentals of Radiology by Squire, P 532

- The image shows the arrow pointed at fourth ventricle just posterior to brainstem and anterior to cerebellum.
- CSF flows via cerebral aqueduct (between third and fourth ventricles) into the fourth ventricle.
- It then leaves the ventricular system via two foramina of *luschka* at sides of inferior aspect of cerebellum and foramen of *magendie* at the back of inferior cerebellum.
- CSF then flows above the cerebral hemispheres within the subarachnoid space and is *absorbed by arachnoid granulations* at superior sagittal sinus.

196. Ans. (d) Internal carotid artery

- The shown image is angiographic image of Circle of Willis.
- The artery marked with arrow is internal carotid artery.

*(**Keywords in image:** PCA, posterior cerebral artery; PCoA, posterior communicating artery; ACA, anterior cerebral artery; ACoA, anterior communicating artery; MCA, middle cerebral artery; ICA, internal carotid artery).*

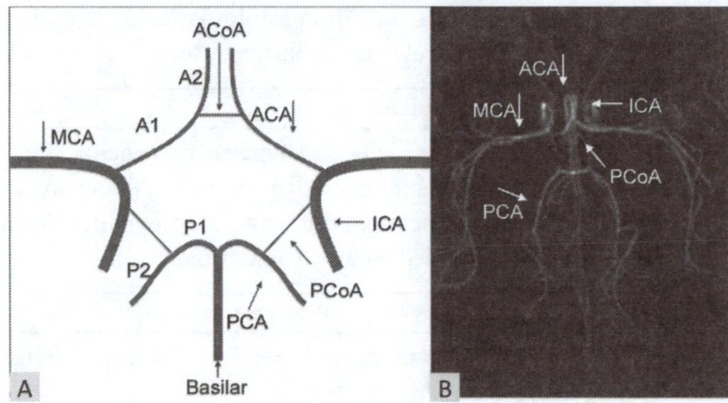

197. Ans. (a) Midbrain

(Revise the brainstem anatomy as shown in the given figure.)

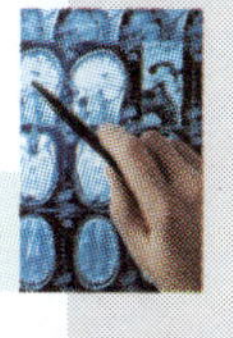

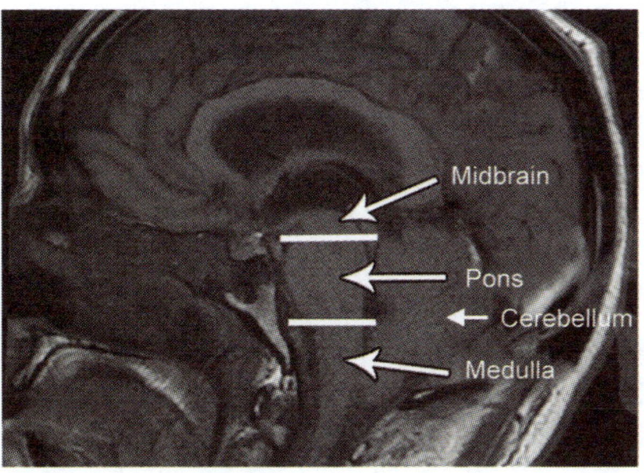

198. Ans. (b) MRI

IOC for certain conditions:

Conditions	Investigation of choice
Interstitial lung disease, bronchiectasis, fibrosis	HRCT
Gall stone, pleural effusion	USG
Spinal cord Neural tissue Chronic subarachnoid haemorrhage Stress fracture Femur neck fracture Bone marrow study	MRI
Cortical bone Calcification Acute head Injury Skull fracture Pelvic fracture	CT scan
Characterization of renal stone calculi	Dual source CT
Chronic pancreatitis	MRCP

199. Ans. (a) CT scan

Ref: Harrison, 19th ed. pg. 1786

- The diagnosis of subarachnoid hemorrhage (SAH) usually depends on a high index of clinical suspicion combined with radiologic confirmation via urgent computed tomography (CT) scan without contrast.
- Traditionally, a negative CT scan is followed with lumbar puncture (LP). However, non-contrast CT followed by CT angiography (CTA) of the brain can rule out SAH with greater than 99% sensitivity.

200. Ans. (d) Hyperdense bi convex

Ref: Harrison, 19th ed. pg. 457e-2

- In extradural hematoma or epidural hematoma, the tightly attached dura is stripped from the inner table of the skull, producing a characteristic ***lenticular shaped hemorrhage*** on noncontrast CT scan.
- ***Epidural hematomas are usually caused by tearing of the middle meningeal artery*** following fracture of the temporal bone.
- And the acute hematomas are hyperdense on NCCT and are hypodense only when they are chronic and becomes difficult to differentiate the chronic epidural hematoma (B/L and U/L) from hygromas which are collection of CSF from the rent of sub arachnoid space.

201. Ans. (b) CT scan

Ref: Harrison, 19th ed. pg. 426e-7

- When the Hounsfield units (Hu) exceed an established threshold (100 Hu), the source is believed to be calcification. **CT imaging is the gold standard in detecting calcification.**
- Calcifications of the pineal gland, choroid plexus, basal ganglia anal dura mater are commonly seen with aging and are usually not associated with pathological clinical phenomena. However calcium deposits can be associated with several intracranial pathologies including tumors, cerebrovascular diseases, congenital conditions, trauma and endocrine/metabolic disorders.

202. Ans. (a) Enhanced MRI

Ref: Multiple Journals

- Leptomeningeal carcinomatosis (LC) refers to *diffuse seeding of the leptomeninges by tumor metastases.*
- LC occurs in an estimated 20% of patients diagnosed with cancer and is most commonly found in breast carcinoma, lung carcinoma, and melanoma in adults and hematogenous malignancies and primitive neuroectodermal tumor (PNET) in children.
- *Contrast-enhanced MRI of the brain and spine is the imaging modality of choice* because of its safety, excellent contrast resolution, and multiplanar abilities.

MAMMOGRAPHY

203. Ans. (b) Medial lateral oblique view

Ref: Harrison, 19th ed. pg. 525

There are numerous mammography views that can broadly be split into two groups

- **Standard views:** Medio-Lateral, Medio-lateral oblique, Craniocaudal
- **Supplementary views:** Additional information or problem solving
  - The **mediolateral oblique (MLO) view** is one of standard mammographic views. It is the most important projection as it allows to depict most breast tissue.

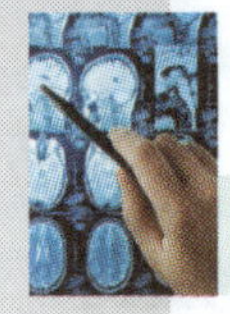

- **The Mediolateral view** loses significant tissue volume in the upper outer quadrant of the breast where statistically the most breast cancers are found. By doing an MLO view you get extra tissue without extra exposure.

204. Ans. (b) Normal mammogram rules out breast cancer

Ref: Bailey & Love, 25th ed. pg. 828

- Soft tissue radiographs are taken by placing the breast in direct contact with ultrasensitive film and exposing it to low-voltage, high amperage X-rays.
- ***The dose of radiation is approximately 0.1 cGy and, therefore, mammography is a very safe investigation.***
- ***The sensitivity of this investigation increases with age as the breast becomes less dense.***
- In total, 5% of breast cancers are missed by population-based mammographic screening programmes; even in retrospect, such carcinomas are not apparent. Thus, a **normal mammogram DOES NOT exclude the presence of carcinoma.**
- Digital mammography allows manipulation of the images and computer aided diagnosis.
- **Tomo-mammography** is also being assessed as a **more sensitive** diagnostic modality

OBSTETRICAL IMAGING

205. Ans. (b) Ovarian hyperstimulation syndrome

Ref: DC Dutta Textbook of Gynecology pg. 437

- Since the history of IVF treatment is given, the patient must be on Clomiphene which is an ovulation inductor. USG shows bulky ovaries with multiple large cysts. The Explanation is ovarian hyperstimulation syndrome.
- Option B is ruled as it is seen with H. Mole where the USG shows snow-storm appearance.
- Option D would have single large mass instead of multiple cystic lesions
- PCOD would have been considered if USG showed a string of pearl appearance as given in the image below.

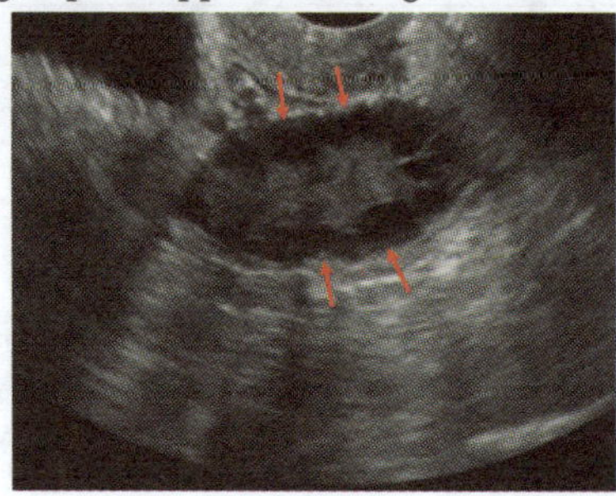

206. Ans. (b) Molar pregnancy

Ref: DC Dutta, Textbook of Obstetrics pg. 225

- The USG shows classical snowstorm appearance seen with molar pregnancy.
- Option A will show lesion in fallopian tumor and not in uterine wall
- Option C will show some fetal parts and is unlikely to be asked at undergraduate level
- Option D will show string of pearl appearance

207. Ans. (b) Calcified fibroid

Ref: SRB, 5th ed. pg. 1030

The X-ray shows a radiopaque shadow in the pelvis. It is unlikely to be a bladder stone since a stone of this size would have caused local trauma to bladder causing hematuria. The supra-pubic pain will be much more than what is described in the stem of the question. Option C can be picked up only on Laparoscopy and option D on CT abdomen and both are not radiopaque. The patient has a womb stone/calcified fibroid.

208. Ans. (a) Ion Donald

- Father of USG: **JOHN WILD**
- Father of Obstetrical USG: **ION DONALD**
- Father of Doppler: **Doppler John**
- Father of CT Scan: Godfrey Hounsefield
- Father of X-Ray: Roentgen
- Father of MRI: **Laterbuer and Mansfield**

209. Ans. (a) Small white gestational ring

Ref: Rosen's Emergency Medicine, 7th ed. pg. 175

- Although the blastocyst begins to implant in the endometrium at 3 weeks menstrual age (1 week after conception), **the first definitive ultrasound sign of pregnancy is the "gestational sac."** This is a sonographic not an anatomic term.
- Before the appearance of the gestational sac, the endometrium is markedly echogenic and the arcuate vessels are somewhat prominent. This, however, is nondiagnostic and can often be seen in the normal late secretory phase. In ultrasound images, the gestational sac appears as a thick echogenic ring surrounding a sonolucent center.
- Sonographically, the chorionic sac (gestational sac) is embedded in the depth of the thick endometrium (decidua) and appears on one side of the cavity line, not in the middle of it. This sonolucent center is actually the fluid-filled chorionic sac.
- **The sac grows @1 mm/day in mean diameter during early pregnancy.** With further growth, first the yolk sac and later the embryo become visible sonographically inside the chorionic cavity. The yolk sac has a very bright echogenic rim around a sonolucent center. When it first appears at <5 weeks, it may only be **1–3 mm** in diameter
- Discriminatory size of the gestational sac for trans-vaginal visualization of the yolk sac is reported from 5 to 13 mm in mean sac diameter.

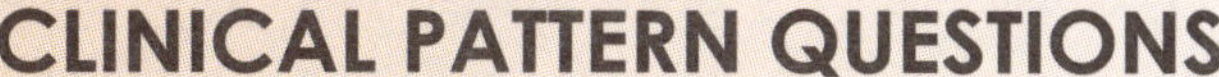

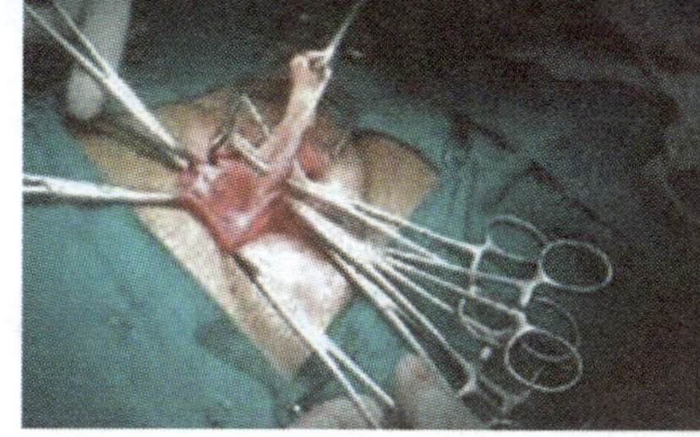

CLINICAL PATTERN QUESTIONS

Important Points

- These are integrated questions covering more than one subject and hence are not segregated subject wise
- These questions comprise 30%–40% of paper. Do not get distracted by their length but focus to identify pick up points in each of these questions. The explanations of these questions will help you pick up those subtle hints given by the examiner.
- Ideally attempt these questions when you are done with first read of all 19 subjects to increase the strike rate.

CASE 1

A 30-year-old AIDS positive truck driver is suffering from fever and breathlessness for last 5 days. On auscultation occasional crepitations are heard in bilateral lung fields and sp02= 80%. CXR was done along with Bronchoalveolar lavage. What drug treatment will be started for this patient?

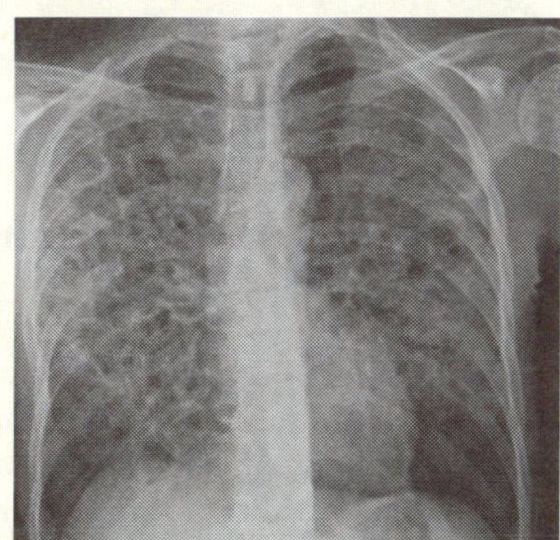

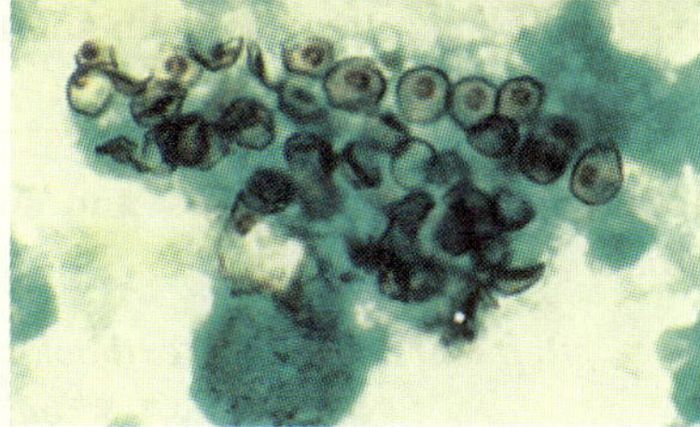

a. Azithromycin b. Cotrimoxazole
c. Anti-Tubercular drugs d. Fluconazole

Ans. (b) Cotrimoxazole

Ref: Harrison 20th ed. pg. pg. 1547

- AIDS Positive status points to opportunistic infections being present. CXR shows bilateral infiltrates.
- Bronchoalveolar lavage shows a green background with black cysts of Pneumocystis jirovecii. The stain used is Gomori methenamine stain
- Cotrimoxazole is used for treatment of P. jirovecii. The question integrates microbiology with pharmacology.

CASE 2

A 35-year-old woman presents with weakness in both legs for past 2 days leading to inability to stand. On examination bilateral knee jerk and ankle jerk are absent with power of 1/5 in both legs for all muscle groups. There is no sensory deficit and bladder bowel control is present. Skirrow media was used in the patient for identification of aetiology of presentation. Which of the following organism is incriminated?

a. Brucella Abortus b. Bordetella
c. Listeria Monocytogenes d. Campylobacter jejuni

Ans. (d) Campylobacter jejuni

Ref: Jawetz Microbiology 25th ed. pg. 240 and Harrison 20th ed. pg. 3227

- Patient has developed paraplegia with areflexia indicating lower motor neuron lesion involving the spinal cord. This is a presentation of Guillain Barre syndrome. The mention of Skirrows media in the question itself points to the incriminated agent which is Camplyobacter jejuni.
- GBS is an example of type 4 hypersensitivity which presents with ascending symmetrical flaccid paralysis with Lumbar puncture findings of Albumino cytological dissociation. The incriminated agents are Campylobacter jejuni and more recently COVID -19 and zika virus.

CASE 3

An 80-year-old man is having severe low backache leading to difficulty in daily activity. He takes pain killers daily but no relief is noted. Recently he has also started developing swelling around eyes in the morning which resolves as the day progresses and comes back next morning. MRI spine shows lytic lesions in L4 and L5 vertebra. On blood work: Hb =8 gm%, Normocytic normochromic anemia, TLC = 15,000, ESR= 100 mm fall in 1st hour, Serum creatinine = 3 mg%, Blood urea nitrogen= 80 mg, urine routine examination by dipstick is normal. Which is next best step for management of this patient?

a. Start hemo-dialysis
b. Check urine for paraproteins
c. Schedule a kidney biopsy
d. Start prednisolone for next 8 weeks

Ans. (b) Check urine for paraproteins

Ref: Harrison 20th ed. pg. 797

Lower backache in an old man with lytic lesion in lumbar vertebra points to two possible aetiologies-

- Metastasis from solid organ tumor like carcinoma prostate
- Lesions of multiple myeloma

Points in favour of multiple myeloma, using **CRAB** mnemonic (Hyper**c**alcemia, **R**enal failure, **A**nemia and **B**ony lytic lesions)

- Old age
- ESR of 100 mm fall in 1st hour
- Elevated creatinine indicative of renal failure
- Anemia due to Hb of 8 mg%
- Bony lytic lesions confirmed by MRI spine

Hence the urine of patient should be checked for Bence Jones proteins which are also called paraproteins.

CASE 4

A 65-year-old man experiences difficulty in changing channels in a television remote and buttoning up his shirt. He takes longer than usual for his morning walk and feels that he may fall. On examination, rigidity and bradykinesia are noted in all the limbs with normal plantar reflexes and deep tendon reflexes. Cranial nerve examination is within normal limits. Which of the following drugs shall not be used in management of this patient?

a. Entacapone
b. Cabergoline
c. Apomorphine
d. Tetrabenazine

Ans. (d) Tetrabenazine

Ref: Harrison 20th ed. pg. 3126-27

- Bradykinesia (slowness in doing activity) with rigidity points to clinical diagnosis of Parkinsonism. The question integrates medicine with pharmacology.
- Option A is a COMT inhibitor that is used to reduce off time with Levodopa carbidopa.
- Option B is a Dopamine agonist that reduces symptoms in PD while option C is an injectable drug used for severe off time seen in PD patients.
- Option D is a Dopamine depleter and will worsen a patient of PD who already has dopamine depletion in substantia nigra.

Extra Mile

- Tetrabenazine is used in management of Huntington's chorea
- Bradykinesia with any of following: resting tremors, rigidity and postural instability is used for diagnosis of PD
- Off and on phenomenon is seen with effects of levodopa in patients of PD

CASE 5

A 25-year-old burn victim is admitted in the hospital for last one week for management of extensive burns on legs due to blast in the cooking stove. On day eight of admission, she is having high grade fever with chills and rigors, Pulse rate = 120/min with BP = 100/60 mm Hg on dobutamine. Blood culture of the patient is likely to reveal characteristics of which organism?

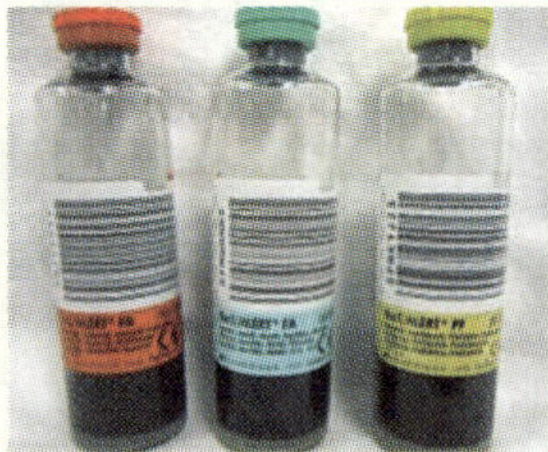

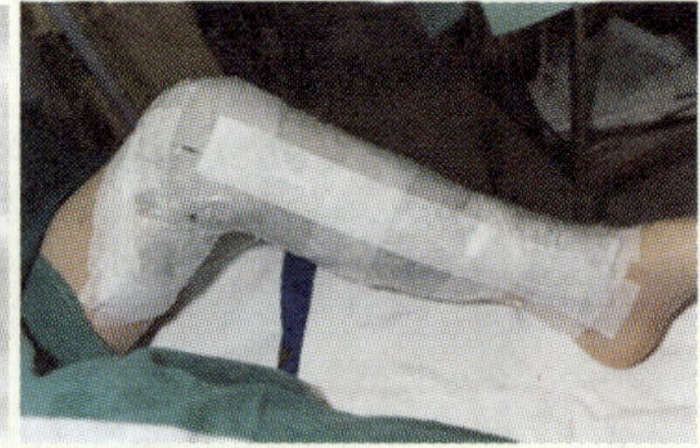

a. Gram positive cocci in grape like clusters
b. Gram positive cocci in chains
c. Gram negative rod, motile with multiple flagella
d. Gram negative rod, motile with single polar flagellum

Ans. (d) Gram negative rod, motile with single polar flagellum

Ref: Jawetz Microbiology, 25th ed. pg. 30

- Post burns sepsis is a common complication and occurs due to pseudomonas colonization of burnt surface and subsequent bacteremia.
- The low BP and use of dobutamine points to development of septic shock in the patient.
- Pseudomonas aeruginosa is a gram-negative rod which is motile with single polar flagellum.

CASE 6

A 50-year-old man has been diagnosed with liver cancer. He used to do needle sharing in college days to take IV drugs and had tested positive for hepatitis C. Which is correct about the primary malignant liver tumor that he has developed?

a. Depletion of CD95 receptors and inhibition of apoptosis
b. Activation of CD95 receptors and inhibition of apoptosis
c. Overexpression of beta catenin protein and inhibition of apoptosis
d. Under expression of beta catenin protein and inhibition of apoptosis

Ans. (a) Depletion of CD95 receptors and inhibition of apoptosis

Ref: Harsh Mohan Textbook of Pathology, 7th ed. pg. 207-208

- Hepatocellular carcinoma develops in patients who had hepatitis B or C infection in the past. The reason for development of cancer is inhibition of apoptosis via depletion of CD95 receptor.
- Beta catenin protein is related to APC gene and development of Familial adenomatous polyposis. APC gene is inhibitory to mitosis and acts via cytoplasmic protein Beta catenin. Hence Option C and D are ruled out.

CASE 7

A 20-year-old man visited a red-light area and had unprotected sexual exposure. He developed a lesion on his penis and visited the STD clinic of your hospital. You prescribed benzathine penicillin single dose. After 10 days he comes back with development of urticaria and morbilliform rash on his extremities as shown. Vitals are stable. Which of the following hypersensitivity reaction is responsible for this presentation?

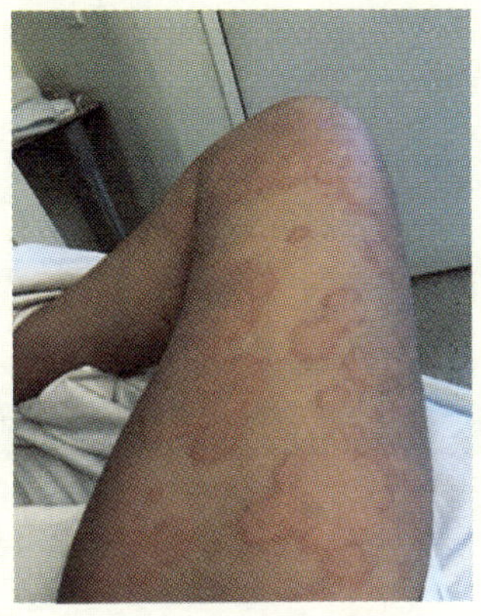

a. Type 1
b. Type 2
c. Type 3
d. Type 4

Ans. (c) Type 3

Ref: Katzung Pharmacology: 11th ed. pg. 459

- The presence of rash and urticaria 10 days after administration of antibiotic points to immune complex mediated type 3 hypersensitivity.
- Type 1 hypersensitivity occurs immediately after administration of drug or vaccine and leads to hemodynamic compromise. In this case patient has come after 10 days and vitals are stable.
- Type 2 Hypersensitivity is seen with mismatched BT and Rh incompatibility
- Type 4 is delayed hypersensitivity as is seen with Mantoux test, Lepromin test and disorders like contact dermatitis.

CASE 8

A 50-year-old obese smoker who is a lawyer by profession started having chest pain during a court hearing. He was rushed to the nearest hospital where ECG showed ST segment depression with T wave inversion. His cardiac biomarkers were grossly elevated. Which of the following is a late complication of the medical condition he has acutely developed?

a. Heart failure
b. Arrhythmia
c. Dressler syndrome
d. Cardiac rupture

Ans. (c) Dressler syndrome

Ref: Robbins 10th ed. pg. 557

- Cardiac biomarker elevation with ECG finding of ST depression and T wave inversion in setting of chest pain at rest point to diagnosis as NSTEMI.
- Option A and B are early complications that occur due to myocardial ischemia and occur on first day of MI.
- Option D is present in transmural infarction seen with main left coronary artery thrombosis. The necrosis of entire thickness of cardiac chamber can lead to a blow out and cardiac rupture. This complication is rare but occurs within few days.
- Dressler syndrome is a late complication of MI that occurs after 5–7 days.

CASE 9

A 15-year-old boy has a valvular heart disease leading to poor performance in sports in school. He has a past medical history of developing fever with recurrent sore throat. On cardiac auscultation Loud S1 and diastolic rumble could be heard. Work up shows CRP was positive, ESR = 80 mm fall in first hour and ASO titer was 200 IU. Which of the following is correct about this case?

a. Erythema Nodosum on lower extremities
b. Development of intentional tremors in upper extremities
c. Chronic adhesive pericarditis
d. Type III hypersensitivity reaction

Ans. (c) Chronic adhesive pericarditis

Ref: Robbins 10th ed. pg. 566

- Loud S1 and diastolic rumble (implies murmur) is a feature of Mitral stenosis. Elevated ASO titer indicates Rheumatic fever being the aetiology responsible for mitral stenosis.
- Option A is ruled out as it is seen in Sarcoidosis. In RF, erythema marginatum is seen.
- Option B is ruled out as it is seen in Cerebellar disease. In RF, chorea is seen
- Option D is ruled out as RF is an example of type II hypersensitivity reaction.

CASE 10

A 35-year-old smoker has an ulcer in the buccal cavity that is not healing for the last 3 months and he has visited various doctors. At your district hospital you have advised a biopsy from the lesion. Which of the following features will confirm that the lesion is malignant?

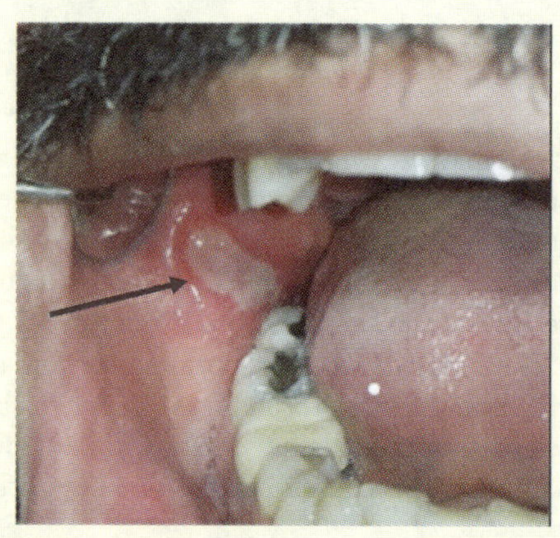

a. Basal polarity is retained
b. Pleomorphism is not present
c. N:C ratio is normal
d. Anisonucleosis is present

Ans. (d) Anisonucleosis is present

Ref: Harsh Mohan Textbook of Pathology, 7th ed. pg. 486

Biopsy Findings in Malignancy

- Loss of polarity
- Pleomorphism
- Change in Nuclear cytoplasmic ratio with variation in size of nuclei of cancer cells which stain intense basophilic
- Poor resemblance to tissues of origin
- Hyperchromatism with increased mitotic figures
- Local infiltration

(a) Normal Epithelium

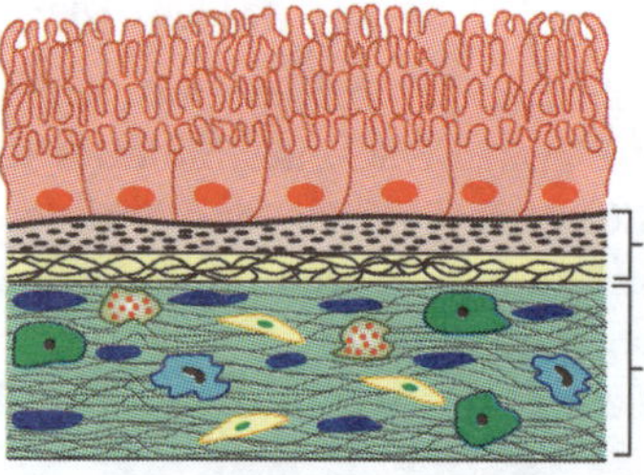

(b) Tumor Epithelium

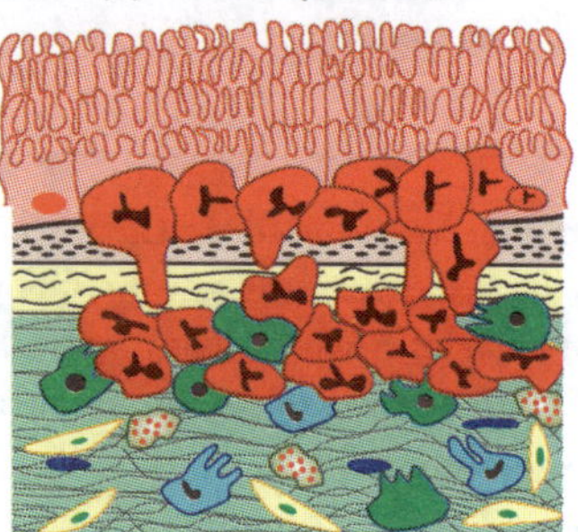

CASE 11

Which is not a feature of Gray matter disease?
a. Dementia
b. Psychological symptoms
c. Abnormal brain stem evoked response
d. Basal ganglia symptoms

Ans. (c) Abnormal brain stem evoked response

Ref: IAP Textbook of Pediatrics 2019 ed. pg. pg. 440

- BERA checks for VIII cranial nerve function which is made up of white matter.
- Cortical atrophy leading to dementia with behavioral changes are early features of Gray matter disease. Basal ganglia also are included in gray matter and damage can lead to dystonia or involuntary movements like chorea.

TABLE: Clinical features of gray- and white-matter diseases

Features	Gray matter	White matter
Dementia	Early	Late
Seizures	Early and prominent	Late
Psychological symptoms	May be present	Uncommon
Basal ganglia signs and symptoms	Often present	Absent
Retinitis pigmentosa	May be present	Absent
Primary optic atrophy	Rare	May be seen
Primary neuropathy	Rare	May be seen
MRI	Cortical atrophy, abnormalities in basal ganglia, cerebellum	Clearly identifies abnormalities in white matter
ERG	May be abnormal	Normal
Visual-evoked response	May be abnormal	Normal
Brainstem auditory-evoked responses	Usually normal	Abnormal

CASE 12

A biker had an accident and was brought to the ER. Pulse rate is 120/min with thready pulse, BP is 70/50 mm Hg and GCS is 12/15. He was subject to FAST USG and urgent laparotomy was done for emergent splenectomy. His blood group is B positive and he was given 6 units of packed RBC post-surgery to compensate for blood loss. However, he developed a rash and urticaria on the arm in which packed RBC were being given with flank pain and low BP. Which of the following is responsible for this complication?

a. IgM
b. Ig G
c. Ig A
d. Ig E

Ans. (a) IgM

Ref: Harrison 20th ed. pg. 812

The patient is having an allergic reaction to administration of blood products. Considering hemodynamic instability, he is having IgM mediated hemolysis/Type 2 hypersensitivity reaction. The transfusion must be stopped and evaluation for mismatched blood transfusion should be done. Hydrocortisone and chlorpheniramine must be given with BP monitoring.

CASE 13

A patient presents with Limb ataxia. Which part of cerebellum is involved?

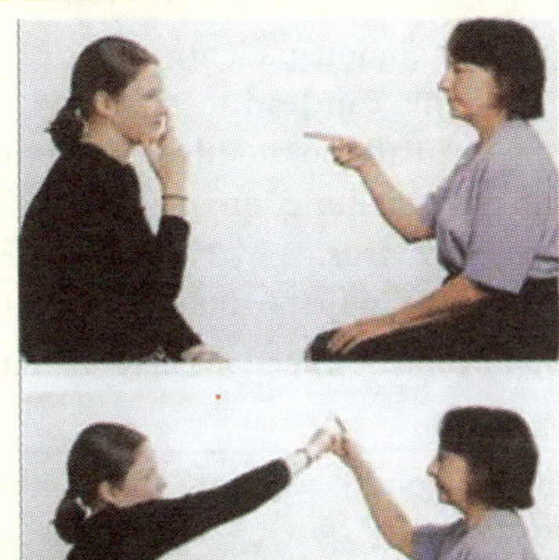

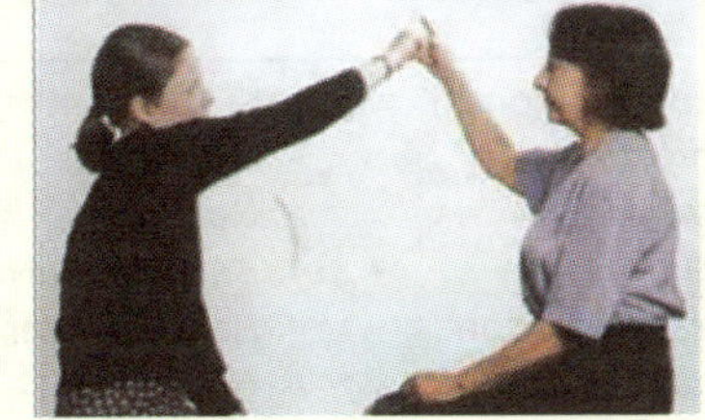

a. Paleocerebellum
b. Neocerebellum
c. Archicerebellum
d. Superior cerebellar peduncle

Ans. (b) Neocerebellum

Ref: Ganong 25th ed. pg. 252

The image shows finger nose test being done in the patient for evaluation of limb ataxia seen in cerebellar lesions. This is a feature of damage to neocerebellum.

Functional parts of cerebellum	Manifestations in case of damage
Neocerebellum	Limb ataxia (Tested by finger nose test)
Archicerebellum	Truncal ataxia
Paleocerebellum	Gait ataxia (Tested by Tandem Gait on straight line)

CASE 14

A 50-year-old post-menopausal woman started having abdominal distension with development of cachexia. On examination abdomen is bloated, fluid thrill is present with reduced intensity of bowel sounds. MRI abdomen showed presence of 10 X 12 cm tumor originating in her left ovary and free fluid in the abdomen. Which of the following is the method of spread of this tumor?

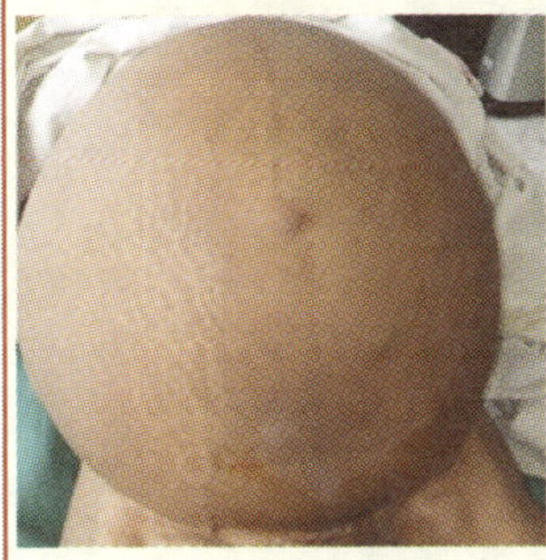

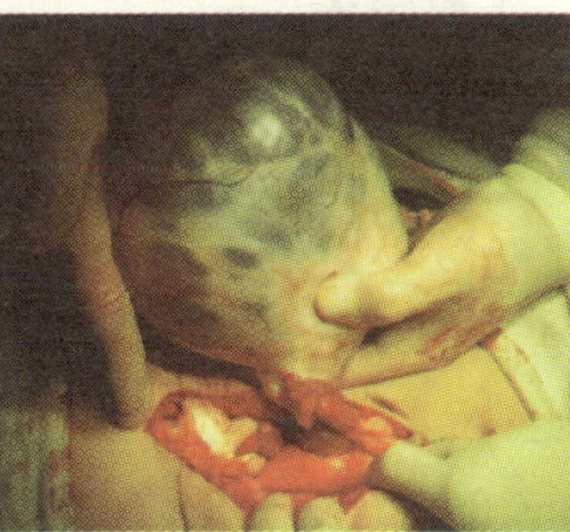

a. Direct implantation
b. Transcoelomic spread
c. Lymphatic dissemination
d. Hematogenous dissemination

Ans. (b) Transcoelomic spread

Ref: DC Dutta Textbook of Gynaecology pg. 305

- Fluid thrill and gross abdominal distension points to presentation of ascites. Since MRI showed an ovarian tumor the patient had developed a malignant ascites.
- The main route of spread of ovarian tumor is transcoelomic spread which means via exfoliation of cells. These exfoliated cells then spread along the peritoneal surfaces as well on under-surface of diaphragm.

CASE 15

A 60-year-old smoker developed multiple episodes of blood in sputum in last 2 months associated with significant weight loss. HRCT Chest shows a 3 X 3 cm endobronchial mass which was biopsied and diagnosed as small cell cancer. Genome scan showed L-myc proto-oncogene. Which is correct about mechanism of development of this cancer?

a. Translocation
b. Amplification
c. Point mutation
d. Point Deletion

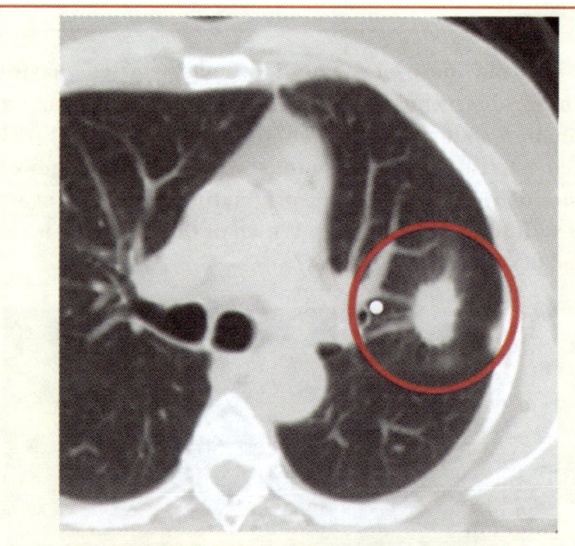

Ans. (b) **Amplification**

Ref: Harsh Mohan Textbook of Pathology, 7th ed. pg. 203

HRCT shows a lung mass with ill-defined margins suggestive of malignancy. Biopsy has confirmed it to be the most aggressive lung cancer. Cytogenetic studies show L – myc proto-oncogene which works *via amplification* and causes uncontrolled mitosis of cells.

Nuclear transcription factors		
Proto-oncogene	Mechanism	Associated human tumors
L-MYC	Amplification	Small cell ca lung
N-MYC	Amplification	Neuroblastoma and small cell ca lung
C-MYC	Translocation	Burkitt lymphoma

CASE 16

A 65-year-old man has had multiple episodes of painless hematuria over the last 4 months. Now he has developed urinary retention and urosepsis. Which of these will be the most relevant question to be asked to the patient?

a. Use of hair dye
b. Previous occupation of patient
c. History of surgical removal of large size kidney stones in past
d. Exposure to vinyl chloride

Ans. (b) **Previous occupation of patient**

Ref: Harrison 20th ed. pg. 619

Recurrent episodes of painless haematuria are seen with bladder cancer. Aniline dye exposure is incriminated in causing bladder cancer and hence occupational history would matter in this case.

CASE 17

A 65-year-old type 2 Diabetes Mellitus patient had undergone kidney transplantation at your tertiary care hospital in month of January 2020. Now he has a graft failure in the month of October 2020. Which of the following is the leading cause of this presentation?

a. EBV
b. Polyoma (BK) virus
c. E. Coli
d. Pneumocystis jiroveci

Ans. (b) **Polyoma (BK) virus**

Ref: Harrison 20th ed. pg. 2130

- Post kidney transplantation, patients are put on immunosuppressive therapy. This can lead to opportunistic infections and leading one seen after 6 months (patient had transplant in Jan 2020 and graft malfunction occurred in October 2020) is polyoma virus/ BK virus.
- CMV infection is seen in first 6 months post transplantation.

Most common opportunistic infections in renal transplant recipients

- Peritransplant (<1 month)
  - Wound infections
  - Herpesviws
  - Oral candidiasis
  - Urinary tract infection
- Early (1-6 months)
  - *Pneumocystis carinii*
  - Cytomegalovirus
  - *Legionefla*
  - *Listeria*
  - Hepatitis B
  - Hepatitis C
- Late (>6 months)
  - Aspergillus
  - Nocardia
  - BK virus (polyoma)
  - Herpes zoster
  - Hepatitis B
  - Hepatitis C

CASE 18

A 35-year-old female came to gynae OPD with complaints of developing post coital bleeding and poor genital hygiene. Per Speculum examination showed a lesion on ectocervix. A biopsy of lesion was performed which showed Koilocytes and dysplasia of cervical epithelium. Which is correct about the condition developing in this patient?

a. Over expression of viral proteins E6 and E7 and loss of p53 and pRB
b. Under expression of viral proteins E6 and E7 and loss of p53 and pRB
c. Over expression of viral proteins E6 and E7 and gain of function of p53 and pRB
d. Under expression of viral proteins E6 and E7 and gain of function of p53 and pRB

Ans. (a) Over expression of viral proteins E6 and E7 and loss of p53 and pRB

Ref: Harsh Mohan Textbook of Pathology, 7th ed. pg. 218

- Koilocytes are HPV infected cervical epithelial cells.
- HPV integrates into host cell DNA which results in overexpression of viral proteins E6 and E7. These two then cause loss of p53 and pRB activity which are the most important tumor suppressor genes.
- These viral proteins now activate cyclin A and E and inactivate CDK1 permitting further cell proliferation.

CASE 19

A 15-year-old boy has liver cirrhosis leading to portal hypertension. He has developed behavioural problems, dystonia, rigidity. Liver biopsy was performed for finding the aetiology. Which of the following stains will be useful for diagnosis?

a. Hemosiderin
b. Sudan Black
c. Von Kossa
d. Rubeanic acid

Ans. (d) Rubeanic acid

Ref: Practical Hepatic Pathology E-Book pg. 162

- The combination of liver cirrhosis and neurological findings point to probable diagnosis of Wilson disease/ Hepatolenticular degeneration.
- For confirmation of Wilson disease liver biopsy is done with estimation of hepatic copper content. The stain used is Rubeanic acid.
- Option A is used for Iron, option B for fat and Option C for calcium

CASE 20

A 50-year-old obese smoker has developed atherosclerosis of abdominal aorta. Which of the following will occur on fissure of atherosclerotic plaque in aorta?

a. Aortic dissection
b. Cholesterol Embolism
c. Fat Embolism
d. Aortic aneurysm

Ans. (b) Cholesterol Embolism

Ref: Robbins and Cotran Atlas of Pathology pg. 290

- Fissure of atherosclerotic plaque will expose the core that contains foam cells and collagen. The cholesterol fragments will embolize to systemic circulation and can lead to Hollenhorst plaques seen on fundus examination. Exposure of collagen can result in thrombus formation.
- Option A is seen with HTN and leads to an extensive tear extending deep into tunica media.
- Option C is seen with fracture of long bones
- Option D is seen due to atherosclerotic damage to abdominal aorta. But in this question, he is asking manifestation of atherosclerotic plaque fissure and not about cause of aortic aneurysm.

CASE 21

A 40-year-old alcoholic patient is having hematemesis. On examination HR = 100/min, BP = 110/70 mm Hg, normothermic and GCS of 15/15. Per abdomen examination of patient was done. The image shows elicitation of:

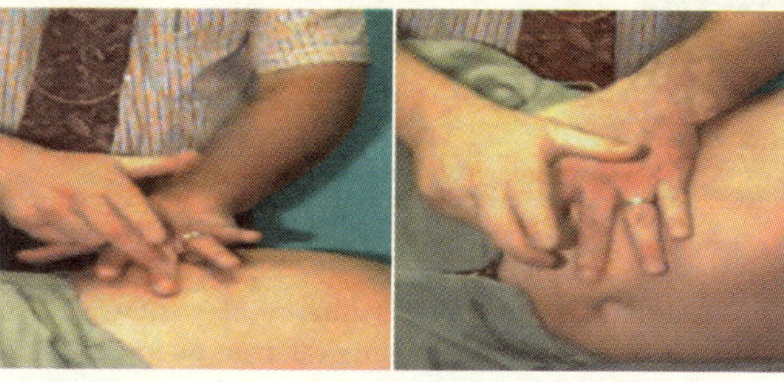

a. Fluid thrill
b. Shifting dullness
c. Puddle sign
d. Succussion splash

Ans. (b) Shifting dullness

Ref: Harrison 20th ed. pg. 2412

Alcoholic patient with hematemesis points to diagnosis of portal hypertension. One of important findings in portal hypertension is development of ascites which the physician is evaluating in this case.

The image shows physician performing percussion over anterior abdominal wall with patient in a supine position. In second image notice the patient is lying in lateral decubitus position as umbilicus can be seen. The physician is looking for shifting dullness.

Option A

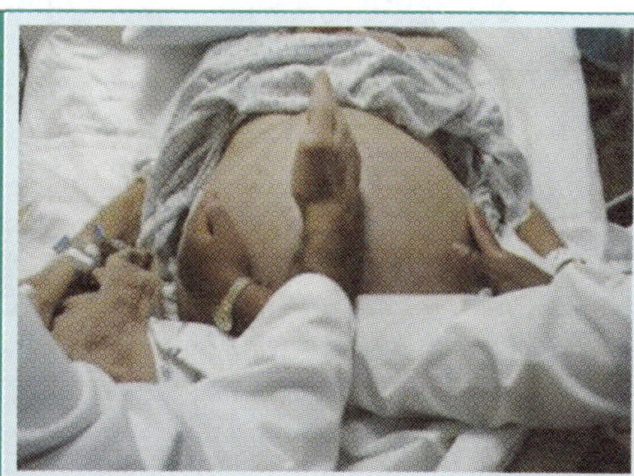

Notice the doctor flicking over anterior abdominal wall to check for fluid thrill. His assistant is keeping his hand in midline to reduce transmission of impulse via subcutaneous soft tissue

CLINICAL PATTERN QUESTIONS

Option C	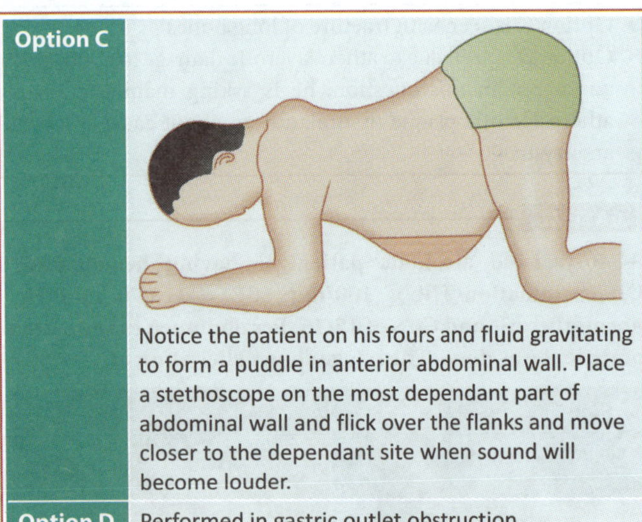 Notice the patient on his fours and fluid gravitating to form a puddle in anterior abdominal wall. Place a stethoscope on the most dependant part of abdominal wall and flick over the flanks and move closer to the dependant site when sound will become louder.
Option D	Performed in gastric outlet obstruction

CASE 22

Coronaviridae are capable of trans species transmission. Which is correct about the physical type of nucleic acid present in this RNA virion?

a. SS Positive sense, enveloped
b. SS segmented, enveloped
c. DS circular, enveloped
d. SS/DS circular, enveloped

Ans. (a) SS Positive sense, enveloped

Ref: www.cdc.gov.in *and Lancet*

Corona-viruses

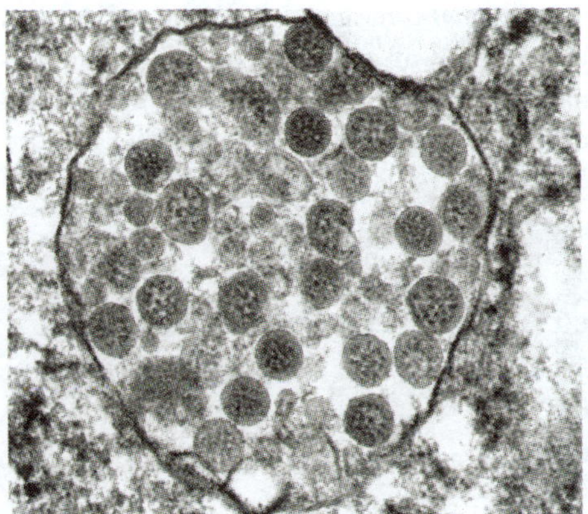

Image courtesy lancet: Virus isolate in cell culture

Capsid symmetry	Helical
Enveloped or naked	Enveloped
Physical type of nucleic acid	Positive sense Single stranded RNA
Virus family	Coronaviridae

CASE 23

Which is correct about the device shown in the given image?

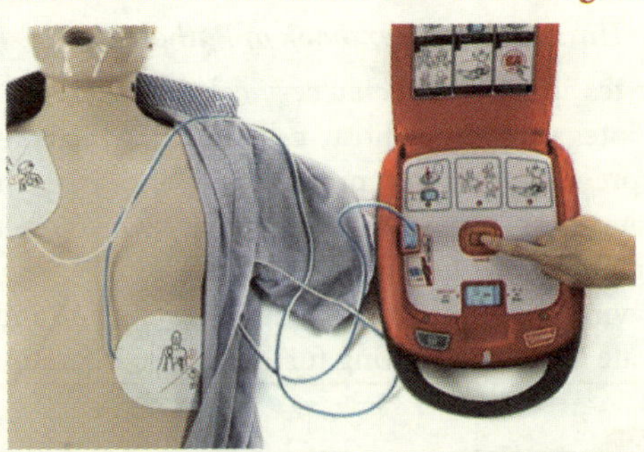

a. Deliver a DC shock of 200 J biphasic in Flat line ECG
b. Delivers a DC shock of 200 J biphasic in Agonal rhythm
c. Delivers a DC shock of 200 J biphasic in pulseless electrical activity
d. Deliver a DC shock of 200 J biphasic in pulseless ventricular tachycardia

Ans. (d) Deliver a DC shock of 200 J biphasic in pulseless ventricular tachycardia

Ref: AHA 2020 Guidelines

The image shows an automated external defibrillator and it is used in basic life support to manage shockable rhythm.

The paddles are placed on the chest as show in the image and the device can analyse the rhythm as Ventricular fibrillation or ventricular tachycardia and will give a warning beep. This means nobody should be touching the patient and then it will deliver a DC shock of 200 J biphasic.

Option A, B and C are non-shockable rhythms and require Adrenaline along with CPR.

Extra Mile

Shockable Rhythms	Non shockable rhythms
• Ventricular fibrillation • Ventricular tachycardia	• Asystole • Electromechanical dissociation • Pulseless electrical activity due to cardiac tamponade or tension pneumothorax

CASE 24

A marathon runner develops severe muscle cramps and collapses before the finish line. He is rushed in an ambulance to your hospital. On examination he is disoriented in time space and person, Heart rate = 60/ min, BP = 100/80 mm Hg, normothermic to touch with dry oral mucosa, lips. Blood work was done and shows sodium = 125mEq, potassium = 3.5 mEq and Chloride = 100 mEq. Which of the following is best for management of this patient?

a. Start 3% hypertonic saline
b. Start N/2 in 5% dextrose
c. Start normal saline
d. Start Ringer lactate

Ans. (c) Start normal saline

Ref: Harrison 20th ed. pg. 301

- A marathon runner has developed muscle cramps and disorientation due to electrolyte imbalance and dehydration. Especially running long distance in warm weather will lead to excessive sweating and loss of salt and water. Since patient is having hypovolemic hyponatremia, fluid replacement with normal saline will be started.
- Option A is used in raised ICP
- Option B is used in symptomatic hypernatremia
- Option D is used in metabolic acidosis like in diarrhea, burns

CASE 25

An 85-year-old man presents with a sudden onset of severe occipital headache and has vomited on two occasions since the headache began. He also complains of double vision.

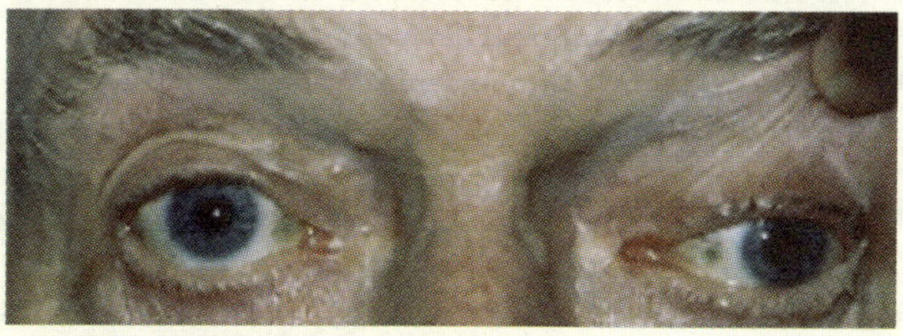

His examination findings are as follows:
Glasgow Coma Scale 15/15
Neck stiffness +++
Comment on where is the likely site of pathology?

a. Anterior communicating artery
b. Posterior communicating artery
c. Lenticulostriate artery
d. Posterior cerebral artery

Ans. (d) Posterior communicating artery

Ref: Harrison 20th ed. pg. 2085

- Vomiting and headache of sudden origin points to CNS event and possible raised ICP
- Neck stiffness of sudden onset in absence of fever is suggestive of subarachnoid haemorrhage
- Double vision is due to cranial nerve palsy and notice the left eye deviated outwards and downwards implying oculomotor nerve paralysis of left side
- This can be explained by Aneurysm in left posterior communicating artery which runs adjacent to oculomotor nerve and its rupture has caused both cranial nerve palsy apart from blood in meninges leading to neck stiffness.

Extra Mile

Most common cranial nerve involved in ruptured/ unruptured berry aneurysm= Oculomotor
Most common cranial nerve involved in raised ICP = Abducens
Most common cranial nerve involved in middle cranial fossa fracture= Seventh
Most common cranial nerve involved in GBS= Seventh
Most common cranial nerve involved in sarcoidosis = Seventh

CASE 26

An elderly man collapses at Delhi Metro gate and you are first responder on the scene. Which is the first step you shall perform?

a. Check for breathing efforts
b. Check for carotid pulse
c. Apply AED and do rhythm check
d. Start chest compressions

Ans. (a) Check for breathing efforts

Ref: AHA 2020 Guidelines

BLS steps to be followed are:

- Verify scene safety
- Check responsiveness
- Shout for help
- Activate emergency response via app (if available)
- Get AED or send someone to procure it
- Look for no breathing and check pulse

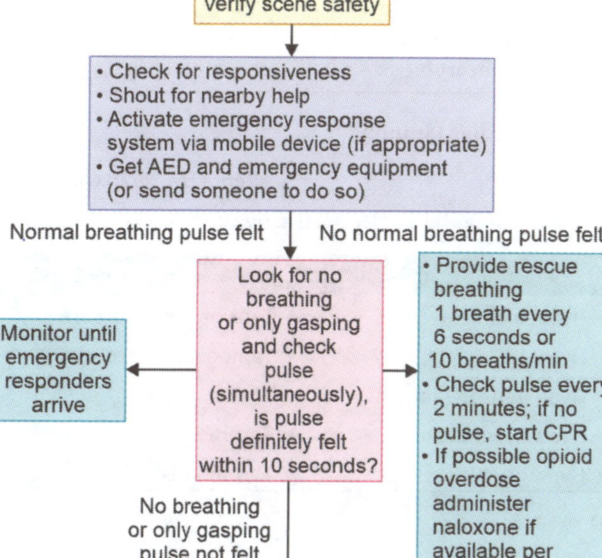

CASE 27

A previously healthy 45-year-old woman has been unable to open her left eye since awakening that morning. Which of the following cranial nerves is most likely to be affected?

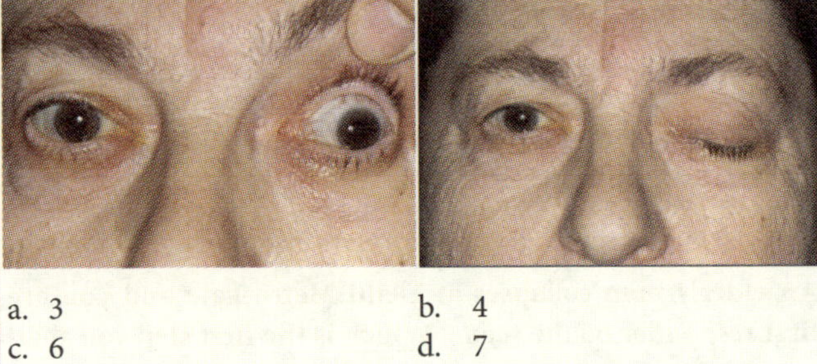

a. 3 b. 4
c. 6 d. 7

Ans. (a) 3

Ref: Netters Cranial Nerve E-Book pg. 16

- In the first image the patient is having outward deviation of left eye that has been forcibly opened. In second image the patient is having ptosis of left eye
- This would be seen in oculomotor nerve palsy leading to unopposed action of 6th nerve and resultant divergent squint along with paralysis of LPS resulting in ptosis.
- In seventh nerve palsy there is no squint or ptosis but rather inability to close eyes.

CASE 28

Which of the following leads to pulseless electrical activity?

a. Asystole
b. Ventricular fibrillation
c. Cardiac tamponade
d. Complete heart block

Ans. (c) Cardiac tamponade

Ref: AHA 2020 Guidelines

5H and 5T of pulseless electrical activity

5H	5T
• Hypovolemia	• Tension pneumothorax
• Hypoxia	• Tamponade, cardiac
• Hydrogen ion (acidosis)	• Toxins
• Hypo-hyperkalemia	• Thrombosis, pulmonary
• Hypothermia	• Thrombosis, coronary

CASE 29

Which of the given steps is not useful in management of pulseless Ventricular tachycardia?

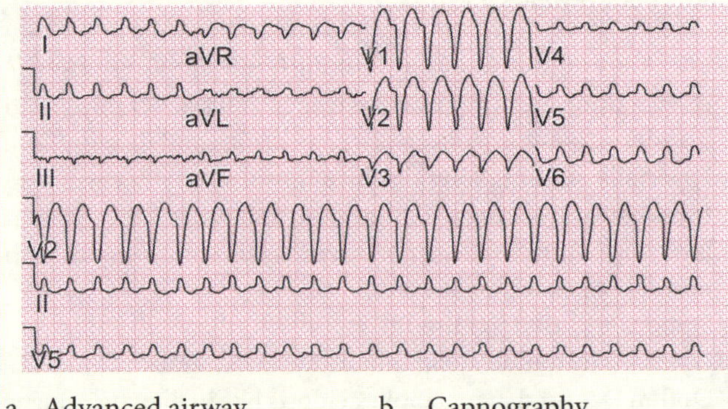

a. Advanced airway b. Capnography
c. Chest compressions d. Ibutilide

Ans. (d) Ibutilide

Ref: Harrison 20th ed. pg. 1758

- The ECG shows broad qRS complex tachycardia with HR of 200/min with extreme axis deviation.
- This is a feature of Monomorphic Ventricular Tachycardia. Since most patients will have hemodynamic collapse the patient will become pulseless and cerebral ischemia can damage respiratory centre in brain stem. Hence breathing may also stop
- To secure airway of this unconscious patient, intubation will be done which is called as advanced airway. Hence Choice A is correct
- Capnography is recommended to confirm presence of endotracheal tube and proper ventilation. Hence Choice B is correct
- Chest compressions would be required before we use defibrillator to deliver a non-synchronized DC shock. Hence Choice C is correct
- Ibutilide is used in supraventricular arrhythmias like atrial fibrillation and atrial flutter for rhythm control.

CASE 30

A 30-year-old alcoholic male has come with complaints of multiple episodes of right upper quadrant pain. LFT shows Serum Bilirubin= 0.8 mg%, SGOT = 150 U/L and SGPT = 40 U/L and PT = 20/15 seconds. USG shows mild hepatomegaly with preserved echogenicity. Which of the following drugs will be useful for management of this patient?

a. Thiamine b. Disulfiram
c. Steroids d. Ursodeoxycholic acid

Ans. (c) Steroids

Ref: Harrison 20th ed. pg. 2400

- Alcoholic with hepatomegaly rules out cirrhosis as diagnosis. SGOT elevation favours diagnosis of Alcoholic hepatitis and treatment is steroids
- Thiamine is used in Wernicke encephalopathy and wet beri beri that presents with CHF
- Disulfiram is used to control alcohol craving
- Ursodeoxycholic acid is used for management of pruritus in cholelithiasis/obstructive jaundice

CASE 31

A 60-year-old man is having multiple episodes of painless hematochezia for last one year. Work up involved colonoscopy which was normal. But since the episodes persisted a second colonoscopy was done 1 year later and was again normal. His bowel habits are normal and weight is same as last year. He occasionally consumes chicken and meat and rest of his meals are vegetarian. Which of the following is the possible etiology of his presentation?

a. Inflammatory bowel syndrome
b. Irritable bowel syndrome
c. Cancer Rectum
d. Angiodysplasia of colon

Ans. (d) Angiodysplasia of colon

Ref: Harrison 20th ed. pg. 2198

- The lesions of proctitis in option A, IBD and fungating mass in option C, cancer rectum is unlikely to be missed on repeated colonoscopy.
- Option B is ruled out as it does not cause bleeding but presents with abdominal pain relieved by defecation.
- The lesion missed on repeated colonoscopies is a vascular lesion that causes pin point bleeds and may not be bleeding on the day the colonoscopy was done.

CASE 32

A 50-year-old rickshaw puller presents with complaints of early satiety, recurrent vomiting episodes and significant weight loss. On examination a lump in epigastrium is felt which is hard in consistency. Which of the following should be the first differential diagnosis of this patient?

a. Peptic ulcer disease
b. Carcinoma stomach
c. Carcinoma pancreas
d. Abdominal tuberculosis

Ans. (b) Carcinoma stomach

Ref: Bailey and Love 27th ed. pg. 1133

- Option A, PUD does not present with lump in epigastrium
- Option C, Ca pancreas presents with obstructive jaundice
- Option D produces lump in Right iliac fossa while in this patient of cachexia, the lump is in the epigastrium, favouring diagnosis as carcinoma stomach.

CASE 33

A 35-year-old alcoholic has multiple episodes of vomiting after binge drinking. The last episode of vomiting had blood in it and he got alarmed on seeing it. On examination he is anxious, diaphoretic, vitals are stable. Per abdomen examination reveals presence of enlarged spleen with free fluid in abdomen. What is the source of bleeding in this patient?

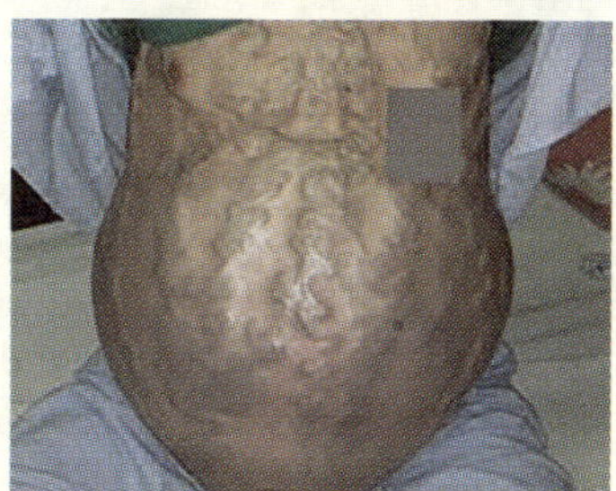

a. Gastroduodenal artery
b. Portosystemic collaterals
c. Left gastric artery
d. Azygos and hemi-azygos veins

Ans. (b) Portosystemic collaterals

Ref: Bailey and Love 27th ed. pg. 1129

- Alcoholic with hematemesis and splenomegaly implies development of portal HTN.
- The dilated veins over anterior abdominal wall are caput medusae and the reason he bled is because of rupture of esophageal varices. Both of these are due to formation of portosystemic collaterals. The ones in lower esophageal are thin walled and are prone to rupture leading to hematemesis

CASE 34

A 50-year-old alcoholic patient is having repeated episodes of epigastric pain radiating to back. He has vomited thrice in last one hour and presented in the ER. GPE shows pulse rate of 110/min, BP = 130/80 mm Hg, circumoral pallor and dry tongue. Per abdomen reveals extreme tenderness in epigastric area, rebound tenderness is absent and reduced bowel sounds. There is no evidence of free fluid in abdomen and spleen is not palpable. What is the clinical diagnosis?

a. Acute cholecystitis
b. Portal Hypertension
c. Acute pancreatitis
d. Mallory Weiss Syndrome

Ans. (c) Acute pancreatitis

Ref: Bailey and Love 27th ed. pg. 1222

- Alcoholic patient with severe epigastric pain radiating to the back, points to diagnosis of acute pancreatitis.
- Option A acute cholecystitis is ruled out as it leads to Right upper quadrant pain
- Option B Portal Hypertension presents with ascites, splenomegaly and oesophageal varices.
- Option D Mallory Weiss can have same presentation but there are two points against this diagnosis.
  1. Repeated episodes are seen in pancreatitis and not Mallory Weiss
  2. It will mainly cause chest pain and not epigastric pain radiating to back
- To resolve it a CT abdomen will help in picking up acute pancreatitis with Serum lipase levels.

CASE 35

A 65-year-old retired banker has developed sudden onset right arm weakness with aphasia for last 3 hours. Neurological examination reveals upgoing plantars with power of 1/5 at all joints in right arm. NCCT head was done and was normal. Which of the following is the best management of this patient?

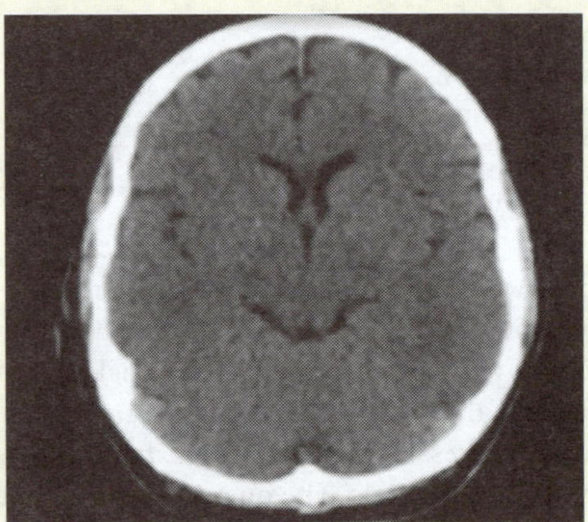

a. Reassure the patient that weakness will self-resolve and start aspirin and statins
b. Admit the patient and start thrombolysis
c. Admit the patient and schedule for mechanical thrombectomy
d. Admit the patient and start mannitol

Ans. (d) Admit the patient and start thrombolysis

Ref: Harrison 20th ed. pg. 3080

- Sudden onset focal neurological deficit in form of arm weakness and aphasia persisting for 3 hours points to diagnosis of stroke despite a normal CT head. This is because CT findings of Ischemic stroke take 6 hours or more to appear. We cannot wait for findings to appear but will start thrombolysis with reteplase to destroy the thrombus occluding left middle cerebral artery of this patient.
- Option A is ruled out as neurological deficit resolves in transient ischemic attack
- Option C is ruled out as it is done in ischemic stroke presenting after 6 hours
- Option D is ruled out as it is used for management of raised ICP in hemorrhagic stroke.

CASE 36

A 20-year-old patient went to a camping trip and developed acute gastroenteritis. He has had 15 episodes of loose motions in last 3 hours and is having prostration and extreme fatigue with cramps in legs. Which is correct about the electrolyte imbalances expected in this patient?

a. Hypovolemic hyponatremia with hypokalemia
b. Euvolemic hyponatremia with hypokalemia
c. Hypervolemic hyponatremia with hypokalemia
d. Pseudo hyponatremia

Ans. (a) Hypovolemic hyponatremia with hypokalemia

Ref: Harrison 20th ed. pg. 298

- Acute gastroenteritis leads to loss of water and salt and hence Hypovolemic hyponatremia is present. The muscle cramps are due to loss of potassium in liquid stools.
- Choice B, Euvolemic Hyponatremia is seen in SIADH.
- Choice C, Hypervolemic hyponatremia is seen in CHF and Ascites
- Choice D is seen in Multiple Myeloma and Hyperlipidemia

CASE 37

A 20-year-old patient went to a camping trip and developed acute gastroenteritis. He has had 15 episodes of loose motions in last 3 hours and is having prostration and extreme fatigue with cramps in legs. Which is correct about this patient?

a. Increased anion gap metabolic acidosis
b. Decreased anion gap metabolic acidosis
c. Mixed metabolic and respiratory acidosis
d. Normal anion gap metabolic acidosis

Ans. (d) Normal anion gap metabolic acidosis

Ref: Harrison 20th ed. pg. 317

- Diarrhea leads to under-perfusion of tissues due to depletion of fluids from body.
- Shock leads to metabolic acidosis. Anion gap value remains equal in diarrheal stool because both positive and negative charges are lost in equal amount.

High anion gap metabolic acidosis	Normal anion gap metabolic acidosis
KULT Ketoacidosis Uremia Lactic acidosis Toxins (ethylene glycol)	DR FUSE Diarrhea Renal tubular acidosis Fistula Ureterosigmoidostomy

CASE 38

A 35-year-old banker was recently diagnosed with hypertension and was started on ACEI. He is currently having severe flank pain. USG done in ER shows enlarged kidneys with multiple cysts. Which of the following finding is next expected in this patient?

a. Lung cysts
b. Liver cysts
c. Renal vein thrombosis
d. Renal artery stenosis

Ans. (b) Liver cysts

The clinical diagnosis of patient is ADPKD based on bilateral enlarged cystic kidneys along with complaints of flank pain. The leading extra renal complication in ADPKD is liver cysts.

CASE 39

A 15-year-old child has developed dystonia and poor school grades. Slit examination is shown below. Which is the initial investigation recommended for the patient?

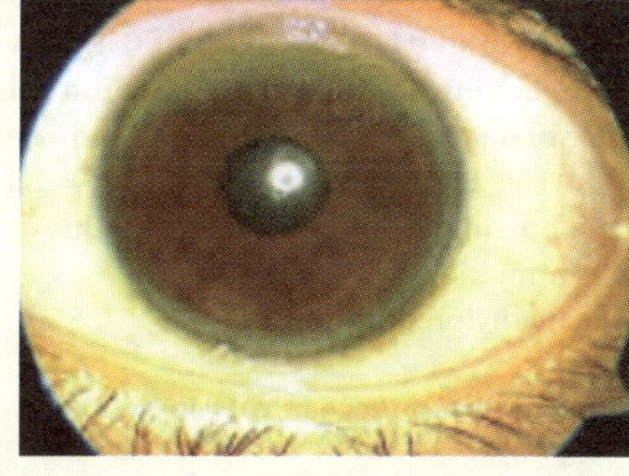

a. Serum ceruloplasmin
b. Serum copper
c. 24 hr urinary copper
d. Liver biopsy

Ans. (c) 24 hr urinary copper

Ref: Harrison 20th ed. pg. 2982

- The image shows KF ring in a child with neurological features suggestive of basal ganglia damage and neurodegeneration leading to poor school grades. Clinical diagnosis is Wilson Disease.
- The best screening test for diagnosis is 24-hour urinary copper values.

CASE 40

A 40-year-old man has experienced weight loss and recurrent episodes of colicky pain for last one year and has consulted many physicians but has not got any relief. Your work shows positive A.S.C.A and CT abdomen with contrast shows multiple strictures in small and large bowel. A diagnosis of Crohn disease is made. The Initial treatment for management of mild to moderate Crohn's disease is?

a. Mesalamine
b. Infliximab
c. Budesonide
d. Sulfasalazine

Ans. (c) Budesonide

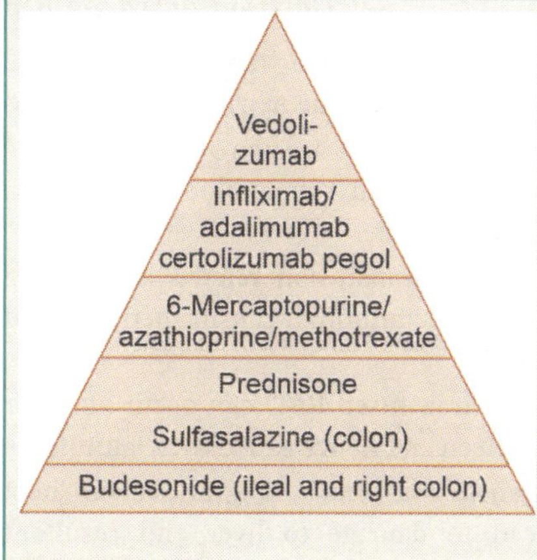

For management of mild to moderate Crohn's disease Budesonide is used along with sulfasalazine that helps in healing of lesions in colon. Subsequently if the disease worsens as a part of step-up treatment biologicals like Certolizumab and Vedolizumab are used.

CASE 41

A 40-year-old alcoholic is admitted with symptoms of confusion and repeated falls with gait ataxia. Cranial nerve examination shows nystagmus with bilateral lateral rectus palsy. Rest of CNS examination could not be completed due to non-cooperation of patient. Which of the following is the best management of this patient?

a. IV thiamine plus 10 percent dextrose
b. IV N/2 in 5% dextrose plus thiamine
c. CT scan to rule out CNS bleed due to falls
d. IV diazepam

Ans. (a) IV thiamine plus 10 percent dextrose

Ref: Harrison 20th ed. pg. 3113

The combination of gait abnormalities leading to Ataxia, confusion and ophthalmoplegia (6th nerve palsy) in an alcoholic point to diagnosis of Wernicke's Encephalopathy. For management IV thiamine is required. Dextrose infusion is given since there is concomitant hypoglycemia as well in these patients.

CASE 42

A child of thalassemia intermedia has a 20 percent increase in transfusion requirement in 2021 as compared to last year. Which of the following is not a complication of recurrent packed RBC transfusion?

a. Circulatory overload
b. Acute lung injury
c. Jaundice
d. Diarrhea

Ans. (a) Circulatory overload

Ref: Harrison 20th ed. pg. 813

- Patients of Thalassemia intermedia have packed RBC transfusion dependency as their bone marrow is not able to produce normal RBC.
- Circulatory overload is seen with Whole blood transfusion and not packed Red blood cells.
- Packed RBCs can lead to transfusion related Acute lung injury due to donor derived antibodies causing activation of recipient neutrophils.
- The hemolysis of these transfused RBC can occur at faster rate due to enlarged spleen and hence can lead to jaundice
- Recurrent PRBC transfusions leads to graft versus host disease that can lead to damage to liver and resultant jaundice.

CASE 43

A 40-year-old patient of chronic hepatitis B was non-compliant to medication. He has now developed features of hepatic encephalopathy due to decompensated cirrhosis. Which of the following shall be noted in this patient?

a. Motor aphasia
b. Sensory aphasia
c. Conduction aphasia
d. Anomic aphasia

Ans. (d) Anomic aphasia

Ref: Harrison 20th ed. pg. 160

- Metabolic encephalopathy due to ammonia intoxication leads to difficulty in naming objects and is called anomic aphasia
- Option A is seen in damage to Broca's area
- Option B is seen in damage to Wernicke's area
- Option C is seen in damage to Arcus Fasiculus

CASE 44

Which cranial nerve is involved in this case?

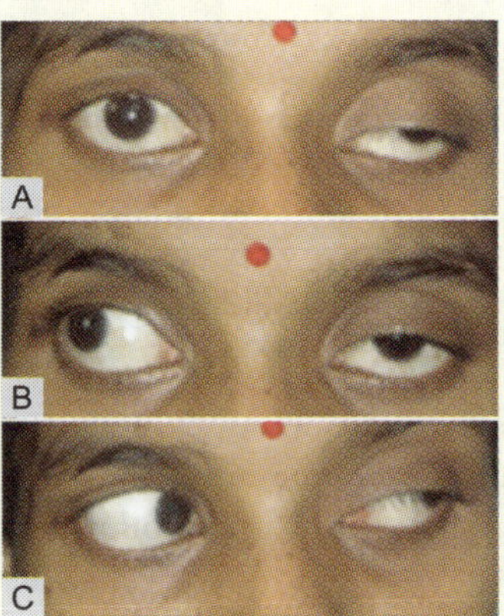

a. Left 3rd nerve palsy
b. Left 6th nerve palsy
c. Right 3rd nerve palsy
d. Right 6th nerve palsy

Ans. (a) Left 3rd nerve palsy

Ref: Harrison 20th ed. 3027

The image shows left sided ptosis with outward deviation of left eye due to unopposed activity of lateral rectus muscle. The patient has developed Left oculomotor nerve palsy. Right side abduction and adduction movements are normal.

CASE 45

A 20-year-old patient has developed flaccid paraplegia with ascending symmetrical paralysis. LP shows albumin cytological dissociation and Nerve Conduction velocity test shows evidence of demyelination. The ABG shows pH = 7.30, pCO_2 = 50 mm Hg, HCO_3 = 26 mEq and pO_2 = 70 mm Hg. Which of the following will not be useful for this patient?

a. Intravenous immunoglobulins
b. Intravenous methylprednisolone
c. Plasmapheresis
d. Elective intubation and mechanical ventilation

Ans. (b) Intravenous methylprednisolone

Ref: Harrison 20th ed. pg. 3228-9

- The clinical diagnosis based on ascending symmetrical paralysis with albumin-cytological dissociation is Guillain barre syndrome.
- Drug of choice for GBS is IVIG
- In some cases, plasmapheresis helps in removing the circulating antibodies that cause demyelination of spinal cord and peripheral nerves
- In setting of diaphragmatic paralysis in GBS, elective intubation is required with mechanical ventilation.

CASE 46

A 20-year-old student has complaints of daily episodes of loose motions leading to disturbed academics. On follow up significant weight loss is noted with features of vitamin deficiencies. Which of the following test is not useful for diagnosis of this patient?

a. D-Xylose absorption test
b. Fecal fat estimation
c. Urine aminoaciduria
d. Breath Hydrogen test

Ans. (c) Urine aminoaciduria

Ref: Harrison 20th ed. pg. 2249

- The clinical diagnosis is malabsorption syndrome based on diarrhoea, weight loss and nutritional vitamin deficiencies.
- Option A and Option D is used for carbohydrate malabsorption
- Option B is used for fat malabsorption

CASE 47

A 70-year-old man suffered a massive anterior wall myocardial infarction and is admitted in your coronary care unit. His urine output is zero since admission and Serum creatinine is 6mg%. Which of the following imbalance is likely to be present in this patient?

a. Hyperkalemic alkalosis
b. Hypokalemic alkalosis
c. Hyperkalemic acidosis
d. Hypokalemic acidosis

Ans. (c) Hyperkalemic acidosis

Ref: Harrison 20th ed. pg. 309

- Anterior wall MI will result in Left ventricular failure and fall in Systolic Blood pressure. This will reduce renal blood flow and lead to Acute kidney injury. Hence his urine output is reduced to zero and serum creatinine is highly elevated.
- The failure of kidney leads to inability to excrete potassium and hydrogen and results in hyperkalemic acidosis.

CASE 48

A 20-year-old medical student came to you with complaints of hair loss mainly from lower back of scalp and is worried about his appearance. Comment on the diagnosis?

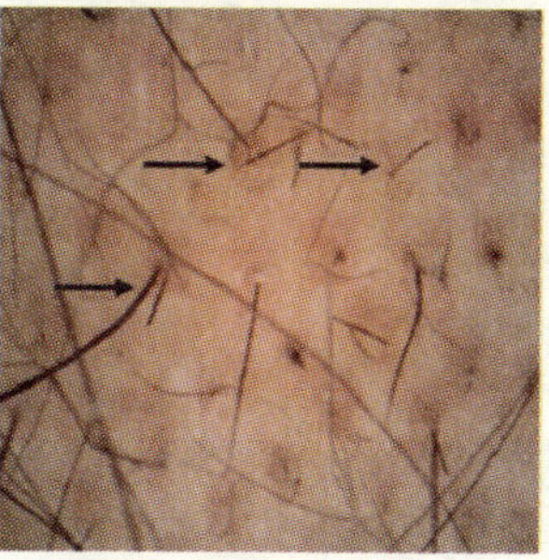

a. Androgenetic alopecia
b. Trichotillomania
c. Telogen effluvium
d. Alopecia areata

Ans. (d) Alopecia areata

Ref: Fitzpatrick Dermatology Atlas 8th ed. pg. 792

- The image shows exclamation mark hair (white arrows) on lower back of scalp which is seen in alopecia areata.
- Option A is ruled out as it shows crown involvement with bitemporal recession
- Option B will be ruled out as it involves central areas and has varying lengths of hair inside area of hair loss.
- Option D is ruled out as it associated with high fever, malignancy, severe infection, crash dieting or postpartum.

CASE 49

A 25-year-old woman who was married recently is having severe acne and weight gain for last 8 months which is not responding to topical agents. She is also concerned about darkening of skin of under arms. Which of the following will be useful for this patient?

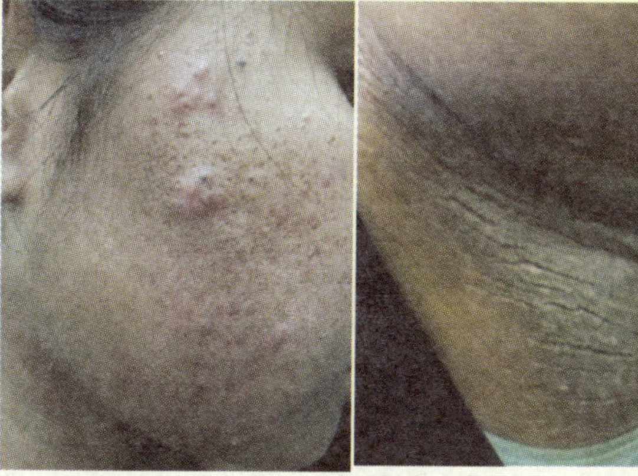

a. Adapalene
b. Azelaic acid
c. Minocycline
d. Cyproterone

Ans. (d) Cyproterone

Ref: Fitzpatrick Dermatology Atlas 8th ed. pg. 4

The image shows nodulocystic acne with black comedones that are non-responsive to topical agents. She is also having features of acanthosis nigricans with weight gain that implies development of PCOD and hormonal cause of acne. The DOC for PCOD associated acne is cyproterone acetate.

CASE 50

A 35-year-old female came with complaints of rash on convexities of face. The lesions worsen on consumption of hot drinks, exposure to sunlight and emotions. Comment on the diagnosis of this patient.

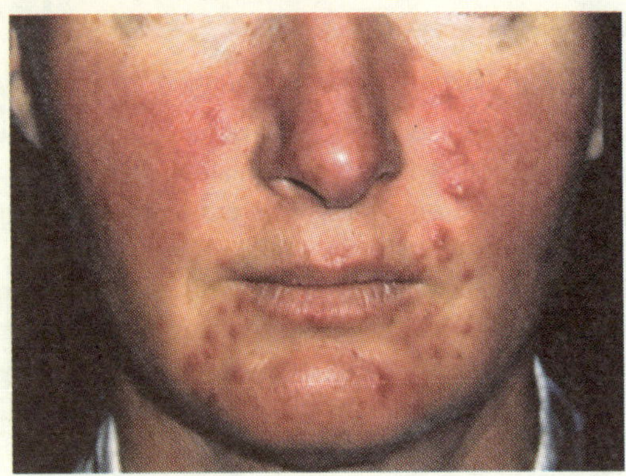

a. Drug induced lupus
b. Systemic lupus erythematosus
c. Acne rosacea
d. Nodulocystic acne

Ans. (c) Acne rosacea

Ref: Harrison 20th ed. pg. 337

- The image shows erythema involving central face (cheeks, chin and nose) with periocular and perioral sparing.
- This is not a butterfly rash of SLE. Notice some papular acneiform lesions on left cheek extending up to chin. This along with red rash on convexities of face is a feature seen with Acne rosacea.

CASE 51

A 40-year-old woman has developed progressive breathlessness since last one year. Initially it used to develop on climbing stairs but now it is present on even going to the bathroom. The work up of the patient showed bilateral enlarged lymph nodes. Since last one month painful palpable dusky blue nodules have developed on anterior shins of the patient. Comment on the diagnosis.

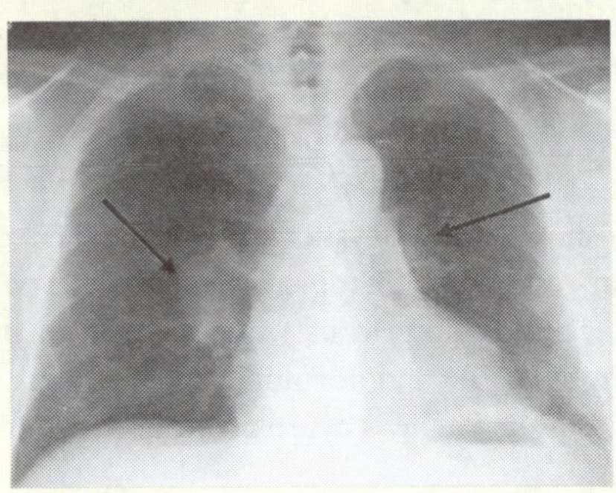

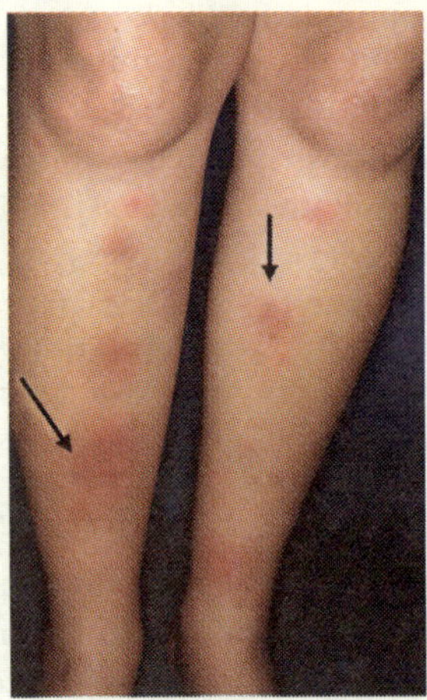

a. Erythema marginatum
b. Erythema migrans
c. Erythema multiforme
d. Erythema nodosum

Ans. (d) Erythema nodosum

Ref: Harrison 20th ed. pg. 112

- The Chest X-ray shows bilateral enlarged lymph nodes with progressive dyspnea (Grade III to Grade IV). Gender of patient is female. This favours diagnosis as Sarcoidosis. The cutaneous manifestation of sarcoidosis that can be visualized is Erythema nodosum.
- Option A is seen in Rheumatic fever
- Option B is seen in Lyme's disease
- Option C is seen in with various infections and drugs

CASE 52

A 40-year-old patient of inflammatory bowel disease is on sulfasalazine and steroid enemas. He has developed an ulcer on the shin which is not healing. What is the diagnosis?

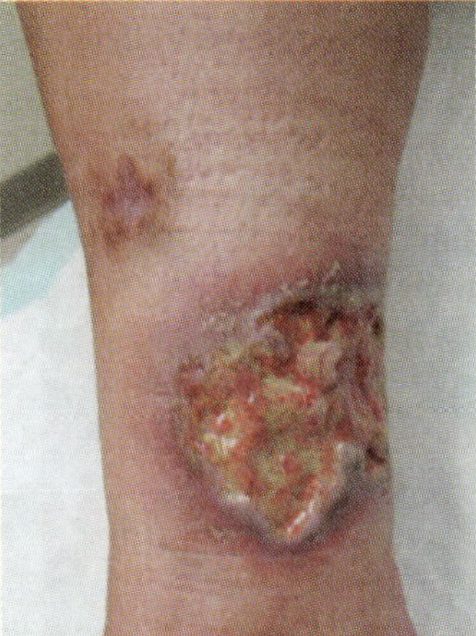

a. Venous ulcer
b. Hunner ulcer
c. Pyoderma Gangrenosum
d. Erythema pernio

Ans. (c) Pyoderma Gangrenosum

Ref: Harrison 20th ed. pg. 265

- The image shows an ulcer on the shin with purple margins in a patient of inflammatory bowel disease. This is a cutaneous manifestation of IBD called Pyoderma gangrenosum.
- Option A is seen on medial malleolus with hyperpigmentation
- Option B is seen inside urinary bladder in case of interstitial cystitis.
- Option D is seen after exposure to extreme cold environment on acral parts like finger tips and toes

CASE 53

A 70-year-old male with type 2 diabetes mellitus comes and offers you namaste (greetings). He then tells you that he has weakness of grip, clumsiness, and decreased dexterity due to reduced ability to perform fine movements. What is correct about this patient?

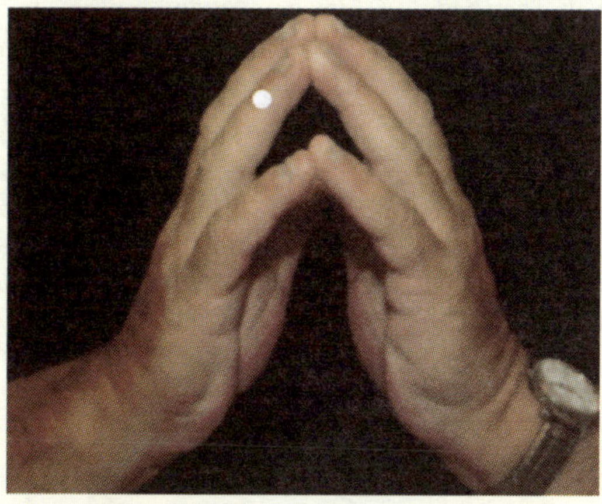

a. Patient has diabetic Cheiroarthropathy
b. Work up rheumatoid arthritis
c. Work up for Osteoarthritis
d. Reassure the patient as this is normal in old age

Ans. (a) Patient has diabetic Cheiroarthropathy

Ref: Harrison 20th ed. pg. 2875

- The image shows prayer sign which a patient of Diabetes mellitus will describe as stiff hand syndrome. It leads to skin thickening of hands leading to inability to extend the MCP joints fully. Elevated blood sugar leads to increased glycation of connective tissues and resultant deformity.
- Option B leads to swan neck deformity or boutonniere deformity with involvement of both PIP and MCP
- Option C leads to DIP involvement with formation of Heberden nodes and/or Bouchard nodes.

CASE 54

A 6-year-old child is having fever with pharyngitis for last 5 days with rash shown below that has sand paper consistency. The clinical diagnosis is?

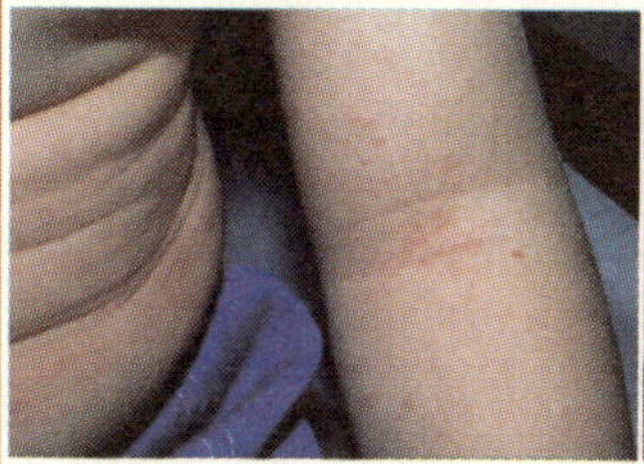

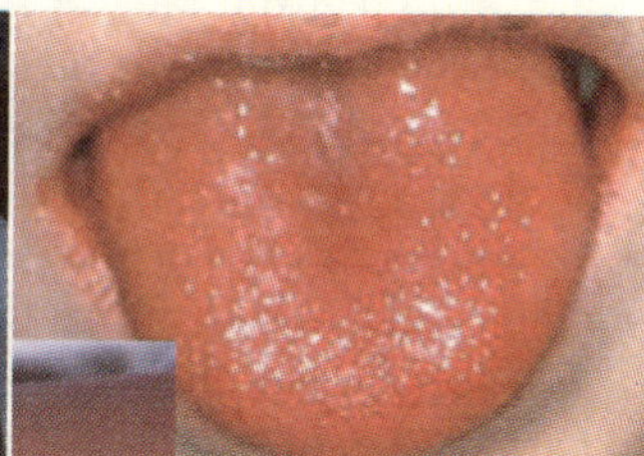

a. Erysipelas
b. Kawasaki disease
c. Scarlet fever
d. Erythrasma

Ans. (c) Scarlet fever

Ref: Harrison 20th ed. pg. 110

- The key word in MCQ is sand paper consistency of rash which is seen in first image at flexural creases of cubital fossa. The last image shows strawberry tongue. The diagnosis is Scarlet fever.
- Kawasaki disease has same features but sand paper consistency of rash is absent with presence of unilateral cervical lymphadenopathy, non-purulent bulbar congestion and desquamation of periungual skin with oedema of hands and feet.

CASE 55

A 60-year-old patient woke up in the morning with this rash on the face which was associated with severe pain in the eye. What is correct about the lesion shown below?

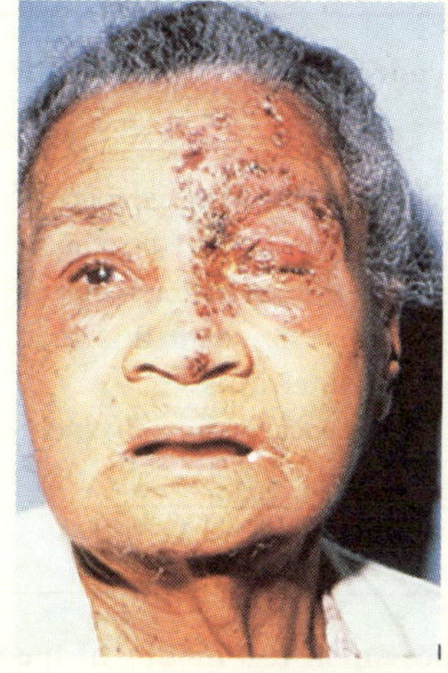

a. Neuro syphilis
b. Herpes zoster opthalmicus
c. Sarcoidosis
d. Reiter syndrome

Ans. (b) Herpes zoster opthalmicus

Ref: Harrison 20th ed. pg. 1356

- The image shows grouped vesicular eruption in dermatomal distribution involving distribution of ophthalmic division of trigeminal nerve. The tip of nose involvement is called Hutchison sign. This is a feature of Herpes zoster Opthalmicus.
- Option A leads to Argyl-Robertson pupil and Tabes dorsalis.
- Option C leads to bilateral hilar lymphadenopathy with dyspnea on exertion.
- Option D leads to arthritis, uveitis, conjunctivitis, urethritis and keratoderma blenorrhagicum.

CASE 56

A 4-day-old neonate is having extensive redness of skin with desquamation. Comment on the diagnosis.

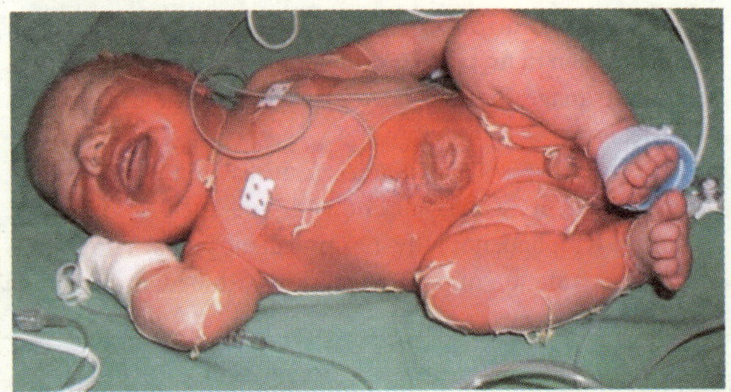

a. Acrodermatitis enteropathica
b. Ritter syndrome
c. Erysipelas
d. Non bullous impetigo

Ans. (b) Ritter syndrome

Ref: IAP Color Atlas pg. 68

- The image shows neonate with extensive desquamation of skin and erythema. This is seen in Staphylococcal scalded skin syndrome also called as Ritter syndrome.
- Option A does not have desquamation and rash is present in peri-oral and peri-genital areas.
- Option C and D have localised involvement only and do not cause peeling of skin.

CASE 57

A 25-year-old sportsman has lesions in the sole of foot as shown below. Which of the following is causative of these lesions in sole of foot?

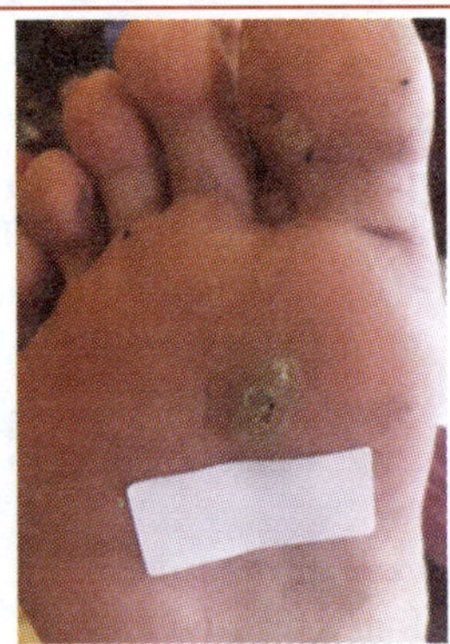

a. HPV 1
b. HPV 2
c. HSV 1
d. HSV 2

Ans. (a) HPV 1

Ref: Fitzpatrick 8th ed. pg. 2423

The image shows plantar warts/myrmecia which are causes by HPV 1. They begin as shiny papules and progress to round lesions with keratotic surface. Commonly seen on weight bearing areas like metatarsal heads and heel.

CASE 58

A patient of airway burns is having respiratory difficulty and spO_2 of 78%. Since he cannot be intubated or ventilated the resident has decided to do the following procedure in the patient. Name the procedure.

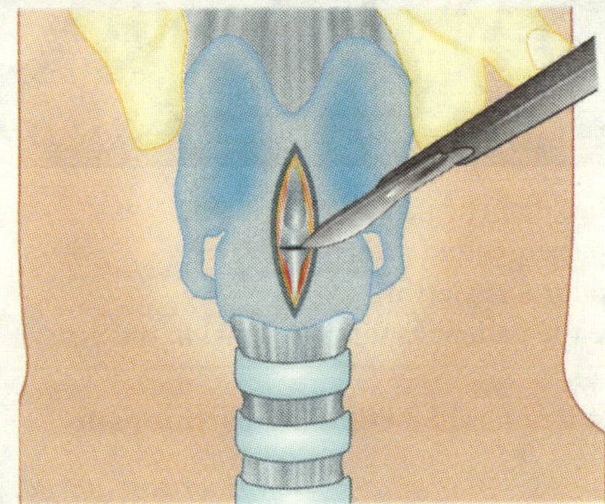

a. Tracheostomy
b. Cricothyrotomy
c. Thyroplasty
d. Laryngoplasty

Ans. (b) Cricothyrotomy

Ref: Lee Synopsis of Anesthesia, E-Book, page 233

- The image shows cricothyroid membrane being incised to get airway access in a patient with obstructed airway due to airway swelling post burns.

- This is an option when all other means of opening the airway have been unsuccessful. When skilled doctor is available and both intubation and LMA insertion has failed, then formal surgical cricothyroidotomy has higher success rate and is intervention of choice.
- Following the skin incision, a 12-14 gauze cannula pierces the cricothyroid membrane and jet insufflation is done.

CASE 59

A biker falls on the road on outstretched hand. Which of the following is likely to develop in this patient?

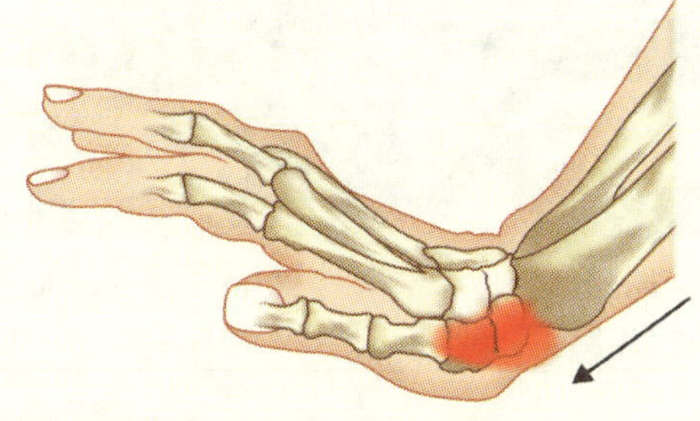

a. Dislocation of distal radioulnar joint
b. Fracture of lister's tubercle
c. Fracture of scaphoid and avascular necrosis of distal part
d. Fracture of Scaphoid and Avascular necrosis of proximal part

Ans. (d) Fracture of Scaphoid and Avascular necrosis of proximal part

Ref: Netters Clinical Anatomy E-book pg. 410

- Scaphoid bone is the most commonly fractured carpal bone in case of fall sustained on outstretched hand. The characteristic feature is pain and tenderness in anatomical snuff box.
- The scaphoid is at a risk of developing AVN due to Retrograde blood supply which enters the distal end. So, the fracture of waist or middle part will interrupt supply to proximal part leading to its necrosis. In cases the fracture is minimal these patients will develop osteoarthritis of wrist in later life.
- Lister's tubercle is a bony prominence on distal end of radius and serves as pulley for tendon for extensor pollicis longus. Hyperextension of wrist can lead to damage to lister tubercle.

CASE 60

A 25-year-old male has presented with complaints of blood in the stool for last 4 weeks. Proctoscopy of patient was performed. Which of the following is the source of bleeding in this patient?

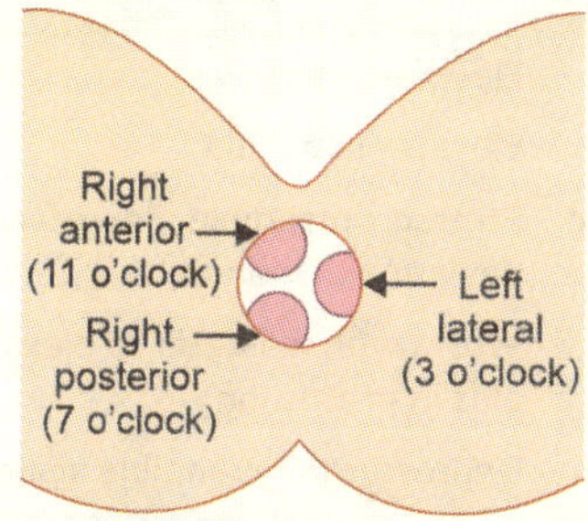

a. Superior rectal vein
b. Inferior rectal vein
c. Superior rectal artery
d. Inferior rectal artery

Ans. (a) Superior rectal vein

Ref: Volume III Vishram Singh Anatomy: 2020 ed. pg. 280

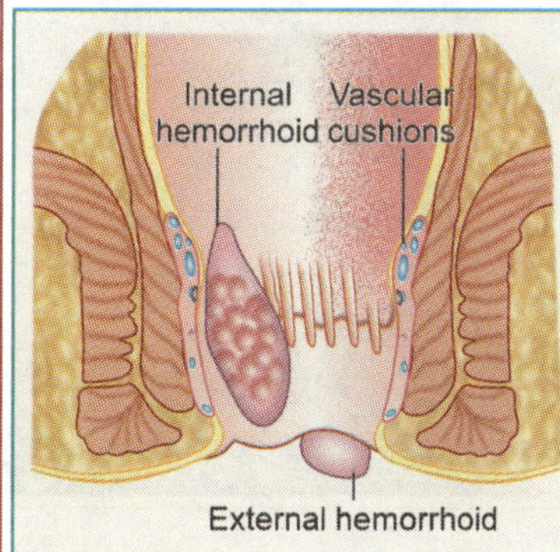

The internal hemorrhoidal plexus is placed submucosally *above the dentate line* and below the anorectal ring.
The superior (SRV) and middle (MRV) rectal veins are commonly the predominant venous branches of the internal haemorrhoid cushions.
Internal hemorrhoids drain through the superior rectal vein into the portal system.
External hemorrhoids drain through the inferior rectal vein into the inferior vena cava.

CASE 61

A 24-year-old medical student is watching Live anatomy video lectures and feeling bored. He is yawning again and again. The anatomy teacher asks him which muscle is involved in yawning?

a. Medial pterygoid
b. Lateral pterygoid
c. Temporalis
d. Masseter

Ans. (b) Lateral pterygoid

Ref: Netter Clinical Anatomy E-book pg. 457

The prolonged and forcible contraction of the lateral pterygoid muscles help to open the mouth in yawning.

Muscles	Actions
Temporalis	Elevates mandible
Masseter	Elevates mandible
Lateral pterygoid	Protracts mandible, depresses chin, lateral deviation of mandible
Medial pterygoid	Works with masseter to elevate mandible, aids in protrusion
Digastric Stylohyoid Mylohyoid Geniohyoid	Depresses the mandible against resistance when infrahyoid muscles stabilize or depress hyoid bone
Platysma	Depresses mandible against resistance

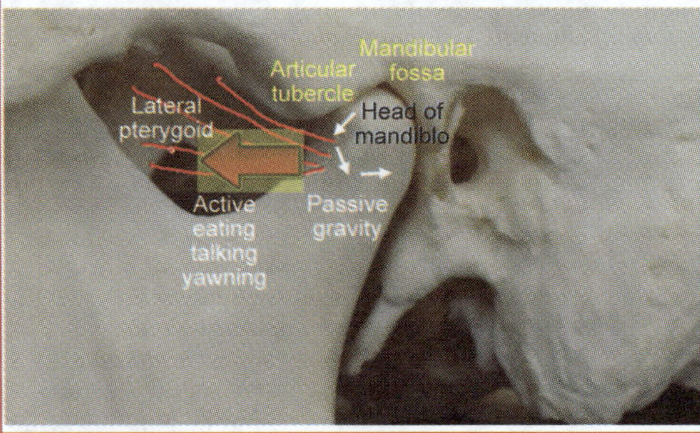

CASE 62

A young intern has his final year exams. He has to demonstrate vagus nerve testing. Which of the following is correct about this examination?

a. Check heart rate
b. Check uvula position
c. Check tongue deviation on protrusion
d. Nasal intonation of voice

Ans. (b) Check uvula position

Ref: Netter's Cranial Nerve Collection E-book pg. E-44

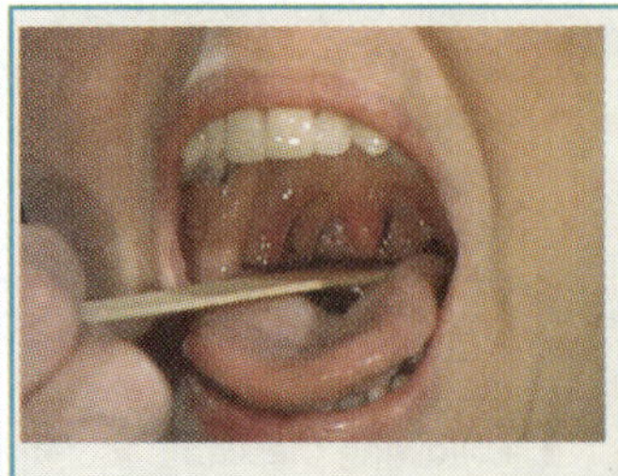

The image shows gag reflex being tested. While testing the gag reflex note the position of uvula and look for symmetric *elevation* of soft palate and look for uvular deviation *away* from side of lesion

Also notice patient's voice. Isolated RLN palsy results in hoarse voice. When patient is asked to cough, the failure of vocal cord closure produces a bovine sound.

CASE 63

Which position is shown below?

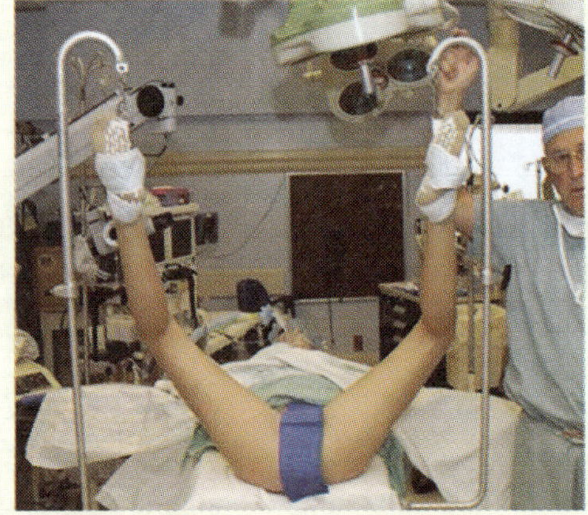

a. Fowler position
b. Lithotomy position
c. Trendelenburg
d. Reverse Trendelenburg

Ans. (b) Lithotomy position

Ref: DC Dutta Textbook of Obstetrics pg. 498

The image shows a patient placed in lithotomy position

Fowler posiiton	Lithotomy position
60°	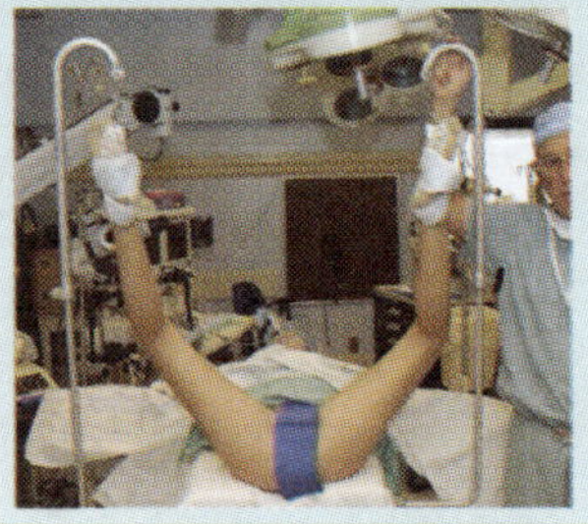

Trendelenburg position	Reverse Trendelenburg position

CASE 64

The following catheter is used for?

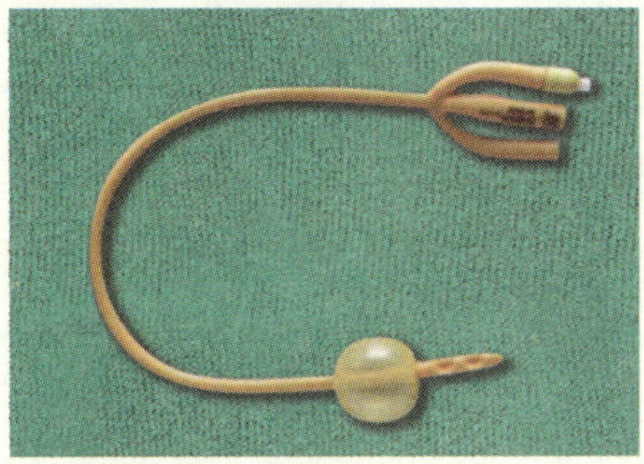

a. Suprapubic aspiration of urine
b. Bladder irrigation post-prostatectomy
c. Bladder drainage in urine retention
d. Producing tamponade effect in urethral trauma

Ans. (b) Bladder irrigation post-prostatectomy

Ref: SRB Clinical Methods in Surgery pg. 734

- The image shows a three-way foley's catheter that is used for giving bladder irrigation following TURP.
- Option A is used for diagnosis of UTI in children.
- Option C, Standard 2-way foleys catheter is used

CASE 65

Which structure marked as 3 in the CT image shown below?

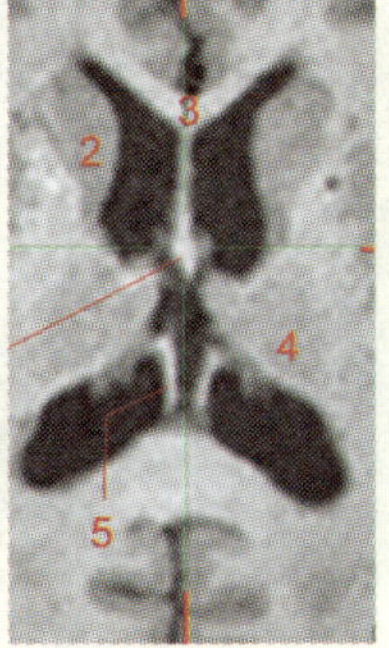

a. Corpus callosum
b. Fornix
c. Vein of galen
d. Caudate nucleus

Ans. (a) Corpus callosum

Ref: Netters Atlas of Neurosciences, E-Book pg. 66

Corpus callosum is a C-shaped nerve fiber bundle found beneath the cerebral cortex. It stretches across the midline of the brain, connecting the left and right cerebral hemispheres.

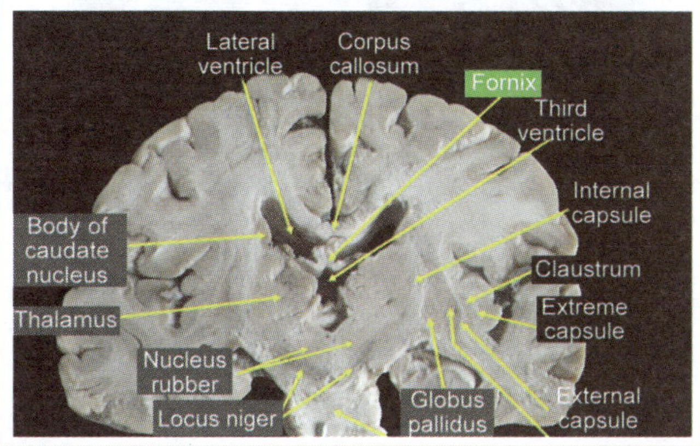

CASE 66

Which of the following structures is marked in the MRI head shown here?

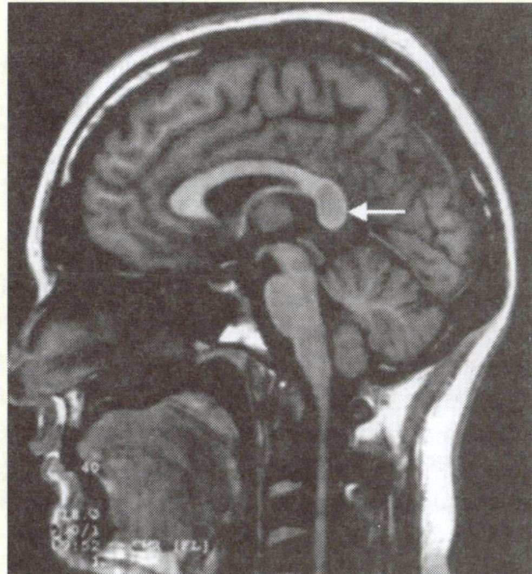

a. Pineal Gland
b. Tectum
c. Tegmentum
d. Splenium

Ans. (d) Splenium

Ref: Netters Atlas of Neurosciences, E-book pg. 66

The marking in the image is splenium which is posterior part of corpus callous in MRI head lateral view.

CASE 67

What is the name of the structure marked as 14 in the MRI head shown?

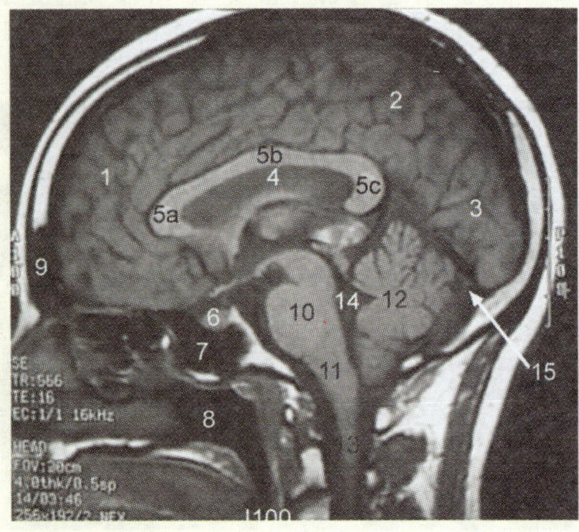

a. Neocerebellum
b. Midbrain
c. Fourth ventricle
d. Medulla oblongata

Ans. (c) Fourth ventricle

Ref: Netters Atlas of Neurosciences, E-book pg. 89

The structure marked is fourth ventricle. It is posterior to brain stem and anterior to cerebellum.

CASE 68

A 30-year-old body builder presents with complaints of dragging sensation in left testis. On examination "bag of worms" sensation in felt while examining the left scrotal sac. What is the diagnosis and which of the following is correct?

a. Varicocele and Left testicular vein drains into Right testicular vein
b. Varicocele and left testicular vein drains into left renal vein
c. Varicocele and Left testicular vein drains into IVC
d. Varicocele and Left testicular vein drains into Pampiniform plexus of right side

Ans. (b) Varicocele and left testicular vein drains into left renal vein

Ref: Textbook of Anatomy Vishram Singh 3rd ed. pg. 65

The left testicular vein drains into left renal vein. The right testicular vein drains into right renal vein. In case of left sided varicocele, it is important to always rule out renal cell cancer.

In case of Renal cell cancer of left side, the left testicular vein draining into left renal vein will be compressed. This will cause a left sided varicocele. Hence in a young male with left sided varicocele, USG abdomen must be done.

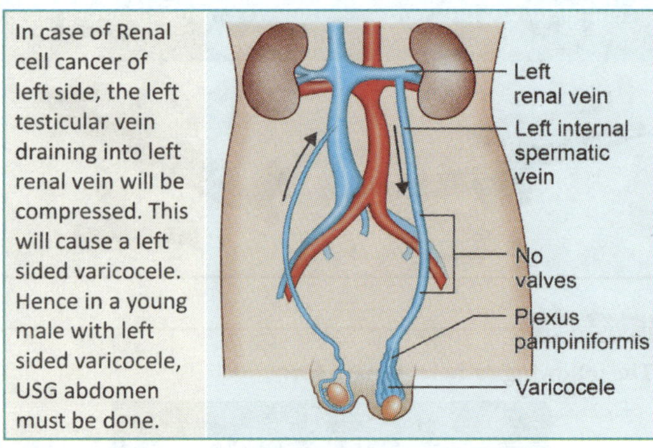

CASE 69

In which of the following body organ will an anatomist demonstrate Reidel's lobe?

a. Liver
b. Lung
c. Kidney
d. Prostate

Ans. (a) Liver

Ref: Text book of Anatomy, Vishram Singh 3rd ed. pg. 120

Riedel's lobe of the liver

- It was originally defined as a tongue-like projection of the right hepatic lobe to or beyond the level of the umbilicus
- But in recent years the definition has been refined to a caudal extension of the liver beyond the most inferior costal cartilage on cross-sectional imaging.

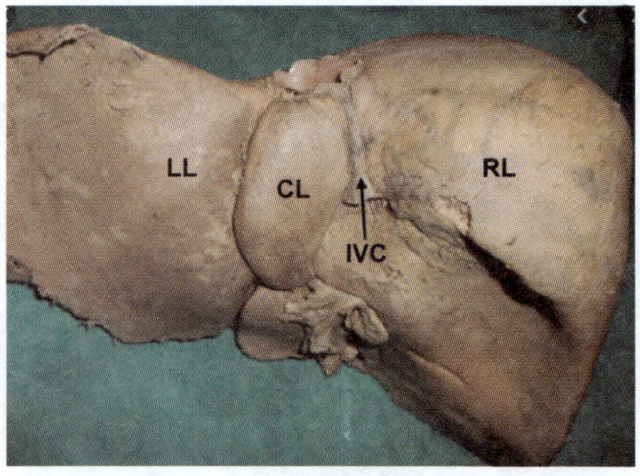

Extra Mile

• Largest gland in the body	Liver
• Gateway of the liver	Porta hepatis
• Cantlie line/plane	Line/plane of demarcation between right and left true (physiological lobes of the liver)
• Obvious feature on the visceral surface of the liver	Porta hepatis
• Fibrous appendix of the liver	Fibrous band at the left extremity of the liver representing the degenerated part of the left lobe
• Riedel's lobe	Tongue-like process projecting from the inferior border of the liver just to the right of the gallbladder

CASE 70

The following structure marked with a red arrow is derived from ___ branchial pouch.

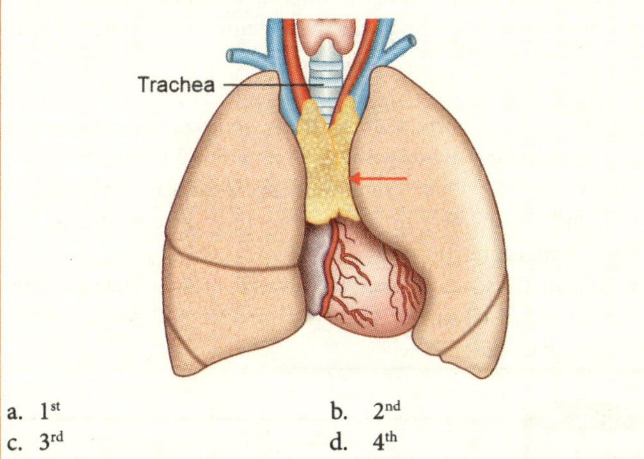

a. 1st b. 2nd
c. 3rd d. 4th

Ans. (c) 3rd

Ref: Textbook of Embryology, Vishram Singh 2020 ed. pg. 129

The image shows marking at thymus which is derived from third branchial pouch.

Derivatives of pharyngeal pouches

Pouch	Derivatives
First pouch	Pharyngotympanic tube Tympanic (middle ear) cavity
Second pouch	Palatine tonsil Intratonsillar cleft
Third pouch	Inferior parathyroid gland Thymus
Fourth pouch	Superior parathyroid gland Caudal pharyngeal complex* (ultimopharyngeal body)

Contd...

* The neural crest cells that migrate into caudal pharyngeal complex (ultimobranchial body) form parafollicular/C cells of the thyroid gland.

CASE 71

The muscles which stabilize the medial knee joint to Valgus forces and are known as Pes Anserine muscles. Which of the following combinations correctly describe these muscles?

a. Sartorius, Gracilis and semitendinosus
b. Sartorius, semi-membranous and semitendinosus
c. Sartorius, semi-membranous and peroneus longus
d. Sartorius, semi-membranous and peroneus brevis

Ans (a) Sartorius, Gracilis and semitendinosus

Ref: Grays Anatomical Basis of Clinical Practise, 2020 ed. pg. 1382

The distal tendon of Sartorius along with gracilis and semitendinosus muscle are called Pes Anserine muscles. They stabilize the medial knee joint to valgus forces that would buckle the knee joint medially.

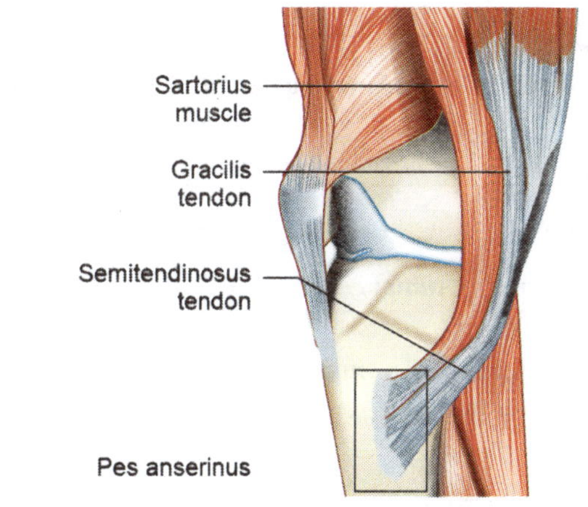

CASE 72

A 14-day-old male neonate is brought to your OPD with mother noticing that when the child urinates some fluid that smells like urine also escapes from the umbilicus of the baby and causes soiling of clothes. You make a provisional diagnosis of urinary fistula. Which of the following is responsible for this presentation?

a. Persistent urachus
b. Persistent vitello-intestinal duct
c. Urogenital sinus Remnant
d. Gubernaculum Remnant

Ans. (a) Persistent urachus

Ref: Textbook of Anatomy, Vishram Singh, 2020 ed. pg. 230

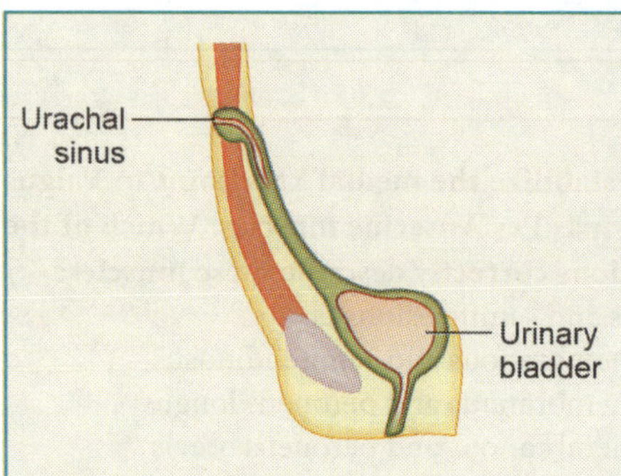

Urachus is a remnant of a channel between the bladder and the umbilicus where urine initially drains in the fetus during the 1st trimester of pregnancy. The channel of the urachus usually seals off and obliterates around the 12th week of gestation and all that is left is a small fibrous cord between the bladder and umbilicus called the median umbilical ligament.

Patent urachus will cause urine to leak from the umbilicus
Option B will cause fecal discharge from umbilicus
Option C forms Cowper glands in males and Bartholin glands in females.
Option D forms Gubernaculum in males and ovarian and round ligaments in females.

CASE 73

Scalene tubercle is located on which of the following bones?

a. Talus
b. Navicular
c. Hamate
d. Rib

Ans. (d) Rib

Ref: Textbook of Anatomy Volume-1, Vishram Singh, 2020 ed. pg. 209

The Scalene tubercle on first rib provides attachment to Scalenus anterior muscle.

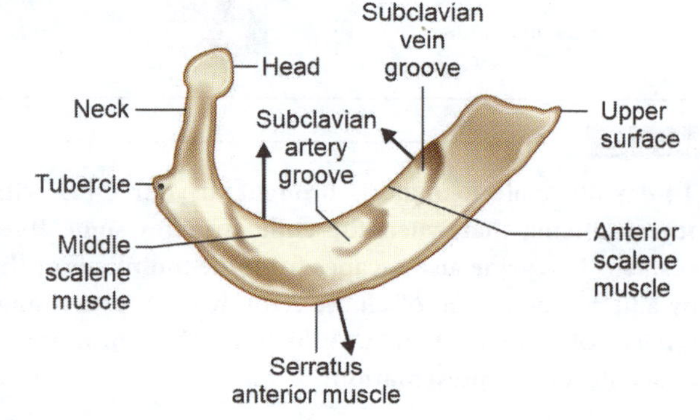

CASE 74

An 18-month-old child has failure to thrive, pallor and increased bruising around the shin. On per abdomen examination spleen is found to be enlarged up to the pelvis. Elder sibling of the child had expired at 3 years of age. Work up shows less than 15% Glucocerebrosidase activity in peripheral blood leucocytes. Which is Not correct about this condition?

a. Crumpled tissue paper appearance of Macrophages
b. Lysosomal storage disorder
c. Enzyme replacement therapy reverses Visceral and haematological manifestations
d. Increased plasma lactate values

Ans. (d) Increased plasma lactate values

Ref: Nelson 20th ed. pg. 301

- Reduced glucocerebrosidase activity in a child with failure to thrive and massive splenomegaly points to diagnosis of Gaucher disease.
- Option A and B is correct as Gaucher disease is a lysosomal storage of Glucocerebroside in cells of monocyte macrophage system which leads to formation of Gaucher cells in which the cytoplasm appears to have a crumpled tissue paper appearance. The child will show neurodegeneration due to neuronal loss in this condition and hence milestones will regress.
- Option C is correct as Enzyme replacement **therapy** is indicated for patients with type 1 and type 3 **Gaucher** disease who exhibit clinical signs and **symptoms** of the disease, including anemia, thrombocytopenia, skeletal disease, or visceromegaly.
- Option D is not correct as elevated plasma lactate values are seen in Glycogen storage disorders and not lysosomal storage disorders.

CASE 75

A politician on a hunger strike was brought in an unconscious state. ABG shows acidosis. Which of the following urine test should be done for further evaluation?

a. Heat test
b. Rothera's test
c. Hay's test
d. Fouchet test

Ans. (b) Rothera's test

Ref: Harper Biochemistry, 30th ed. pg. 321

- Prolonged starvation leads to ketoacidosis. Low pH damages the blood brain barrier and causes cerebral edema which explains the loss of consciousness of patient. For detection of ketones plasma beta hydroxybutyrate levels are preferred. However a cost-effective method is to test the urine of these patients using Rothera' test to detect ketonuria.

- Option A is used for detection of proteins in urine sample.
- Option C is used for detection of bile salts in urine sample.
- Option D is used for detection of bilirubin in urine sample.

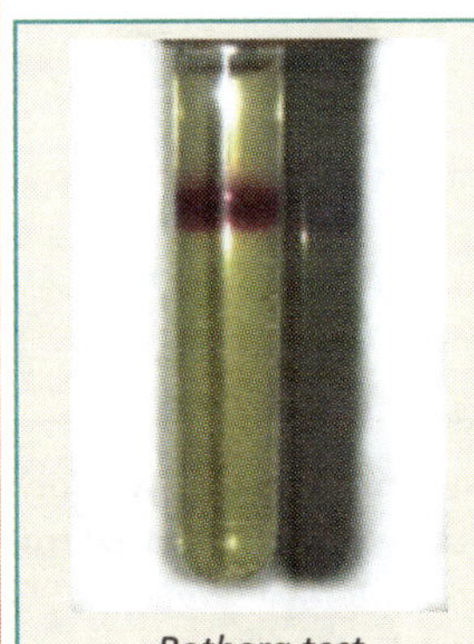
Rothera test

Principle: Nitroprusside in alkaline medium reacts with a ketone group to form a purple ring. It is given by acetone and acetoacetate, but not by Beta hydroxy butyric acid.

CASE 76

A 6-year-old boy has been diagnosed with Hunter disease. Which of the following features is not seen in this condition?

a. Coarse facies
b. Enlarged tongue
c. Corneal opacity
d. Mental retardation

Ans. (c) Corneal opacity

Ref: IAP Textbook of Pediatrics, 2019 ed. pg. 438

Hunter's disease is a subtype of Mucopolysaccharidosis. The way to remember this is that a hunter should have a good eye sight to focus on a target. So visual problems are not seen in Hunter disease in contrast to Hurler syndrome which is also a subtype of Mucopolysaccharidosis.

Disorder	Deficient Enzyme	Inheritance Pattern	High-Yield Associations
Hurler syndrome (mucopolysaccharidosis type I H)	α-L-Iduronidase	Autosomal recessive	Coarse facial features (gargoylism), hepatosplenomegaly, mental retardation, joint and skeletal abnormalities, cardiac disease, corneal clouding
Hunter syndrome (mucopolysaccharidosis type II)	Iduronate sulfatase	X-linked recessive	Same features but with milder mental retardation with aggressive behavior and no corneal clouding

CASE 77

A 9 month old child born to a consanguineous marriage is brought your OPD with complaints of hoarse cry since birth, failure to thrive and delayed milestones. You notice child has enlarged liver and periarticular subcutaneous nodules. You have referred the child to genetics unit which has demonstrated defect of ASAH1 gene and made a diagnosis of Farber disease. Which of the following is correct about Farber disease?

a. Deficiency of acid ceramidase
b. Deficiency of alpha galactosidase
c. Deficiency of beta galactosidase
d. Deficiency of arylsulfatase

Ans. (a) Deficiency of acid ceramidase

Ref: Harper Biochemistry, 30th ed. pg. 251

- Farber disease occurs due to deficiency of acid ceramidase. It is an autosomal recessive, lysosomal storage disorder. Consanguineous marriages are a important reason for presentation of such genetic defect.
- Option B, Alpha Galactosidase deficiency leads to Fabry's disease
- Option C, Beta-galactosidase deficiency is associated with three distinct autosomal recessive lysosomal storage disorders: GM1 gangliosidosis (GM1), mucopolysaccharidosis type IVB (MPS IVB), and galactosialidosis.
- Option D, arylsulfatase deficiency leads to Metachromatic leukodystrophy.

CASE 78

A 15-day-old neonate has multiple episodes of subtle seizures. On examination blond hair and blue iris are noted while the parents have black hair and brown eyes. Which disease is suspected?

a. Albinism
b. Tyrosinemia
c. PKU
d. MSUD

Ans. (c) PKU

Ref: Harper Biochemistry, 30th ed. pg. 304

- Subtle seizures are the commonest type of seizures in neonates. Since they are occurring in 2nd week of life, inborn errors of metabolism should be considered. The presence of blond hair and blue iris implies deficiency of melanin. The clinical diagnosis is phenylketonuria.
- This can occur due to defect in metabolism of phenylalanine. The defective metabolism leads to production of phenylpyruvate which leads to seizures and impaired production of tyrosine leads to melanin production being reduced.

CASE 79

Which of the following products is known as Vitamin H?

a. Biotin
b. Pantothenic acid
c. Pyridoxal
d. Nicotinic acid

Ans. (a) Biotin

Ref: Harper Biochemistry 30th ed. pg. 561

- Vitamin H/B7 is biotin. It is an important cofactor for carboxylation reactions like acetyl CoA to Malonyl CoA. It is seen with excess ingestion of egg whites which contain avidin, a protein that binds biotin and prevents in absorption.
- Deficiency leads to Dermatitis, alopecia, paraesthesia and enteritis.

CASE 80

A 24-year-old clerk recruited into Central government service was undergoing routine medical check-up. The technician has given a report of positive benedict test on his urine sample. You checked his random blood sugar which is normal and HbA1C which is 5.4%. Which of the following substances could have contributed to this report?

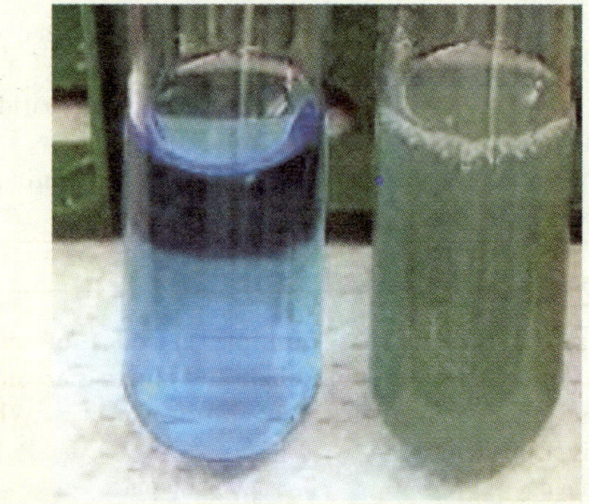

a. Ascorbic acid
b. Pantothenic acid
c. BUN
d. Triacylglycerol

Ans. (a) Ascorbic acid

Ref: Harper Biochemistry, 30th ed. pg. 7

Benedict test is used to test for presence of sugar in urine. In normal person there is no sugar in urine but a false positive Benedict's can occur due to excess intake of vitamin C.

Non-Carbohydrates giving positive Benedict's test

- High concentration of uric acid and ketones
- Homogentisic acid (solution turns black due to black colored oxidized homogentisic acid)
- Vitamin C (even without boiling)
- Certain drugs like aspirin, cephalosporins

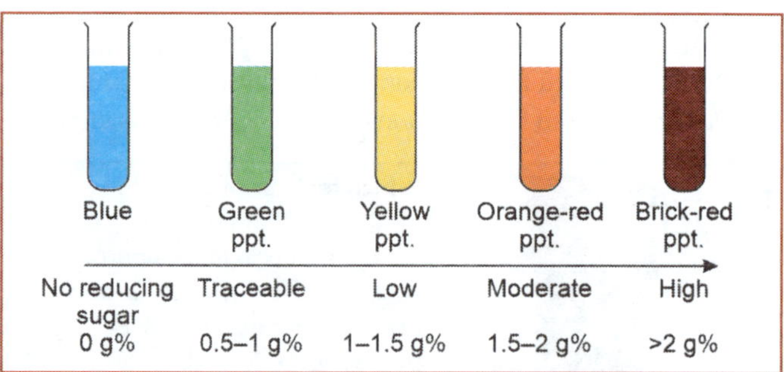

CASE 81

A 6-year-old presented with fatigue on outdoor activity. Work up shows elevated Serum lactate, triglycerides, cholesterol and blood sugar is 60mg%. Uric acid is highly elevated. USG shows enlarged liver and kidneys. The diagnosis is?

a. Von Gierke disease
b. Cori's disease
c. Pompe's disease
d. McArdle Syndrome

Ans. (a) Von Gierke disease

Ref: Harrison 20th ed. pg. 3010

- Enlargement of liver and kidney with lab findings of hypoglycemia and hyperlipidemia points to diagnosis of Von Gierke disease. Infact we don't read about *renomegaly* in any other storage disorder.
- Cori's disease also shows hepatomegaly with hyperlipidemia and muscle weakness but renal enlargement is not seen.
- Pompe disease presents with hypotonia, muscle weakness and cardiac enlargement
- McArdle syndrome presents with muscle cramps after minimal exercise and myoglobinuria leading to burgundy red urine.

CASE 82

A 25-year-old sex worker presents with following lesions after unprotected sexual exposure. Which of the following is the causative agent?

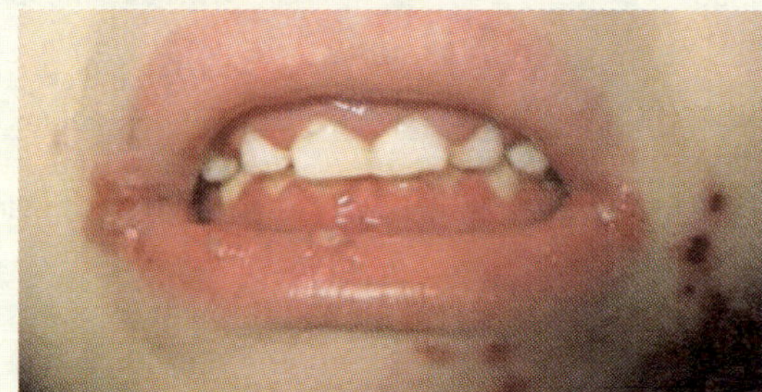

a. HPV 1
b. HPV 2
c. HSV 1
d. HSV 2

Ans. (c) HSV 1

Ref: Harrison 20th ed. pg. 1348

- Gingivostomatitis and pharyngitis are most common clinical manifestations of first episode of HSV-1 infection while recurrent herpes labialis is leading manifestation of reactivation of HSV-1 infection.
- HSV-2 infections of pharynx results in exudative or ulcerative lesions of posterior pharynx and tonsillar pillars.

CASE 83

Sago grain/tapioca like pruritic lesions in palms are seen in?

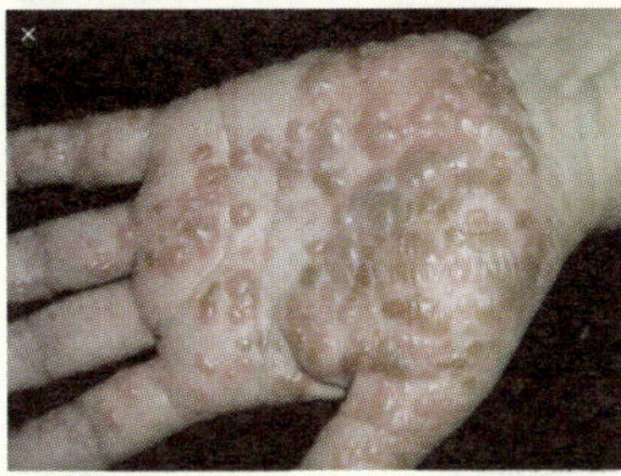

a. Atopic dermatitis
b. Pompholyx
c. Xerotic eczema
d. Asteatotic eczema

Ans. (b) Pompholyx

Ref: Fitzpatrick Color Atlas and Synopsis pg. 45

- The image shows vesicles and blisters developing in hands of patient. This is called as vesicular hand dermatitis or pompholyx.
- Option B, Atopic dermatitis will present in flexural areas like elbows, behind knees and neck creases.
- Option C, Xerotic eczema affects legs and occurs in winter and dry months. The skin becomes dry, red, itchy and cracked.
- Option D, Asteatotic eczema leads to pruritic, dry, cracked, and polygonally fissured skin with irregular scaling.

CASE 84

Comment on the condition where the following nail changes are seen?

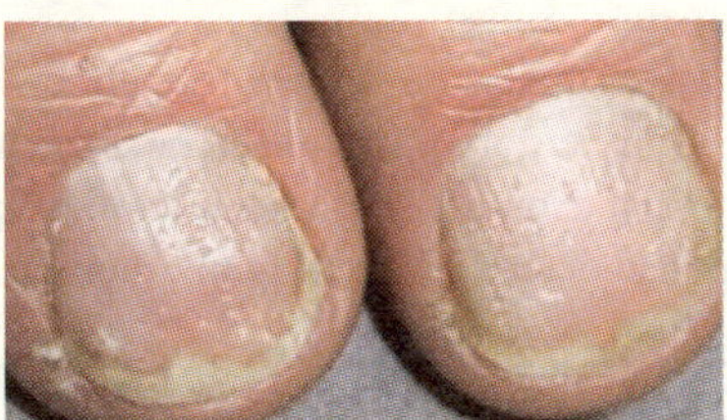

a. Psoriasis
b. Alopecia areata
c. Onchomycosis
d. Lichen planus

Ans. (a) Psoriasis

Ref: Macloed's Clinical Examination pg. 81

The image shows thimble pitting of nails which is seen in psoriasis. The pitting spots are irregular in arrangement. In contrast in alopecia areata the pitting is organised in transverse rows giving nails a hammered brass appearance.

Extra Mile

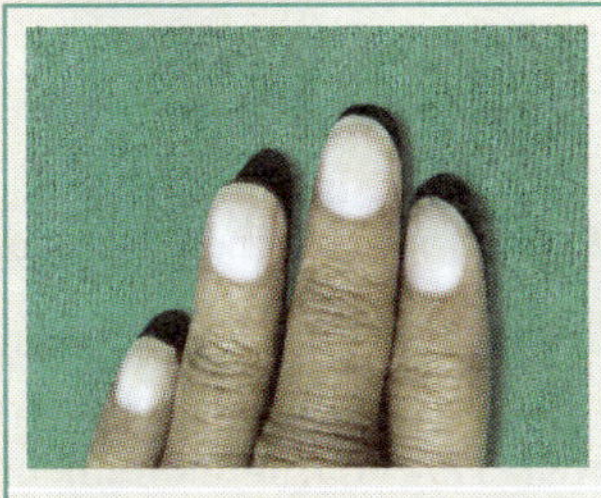

Leukonychia: Notice absence of lunula and uniformity white nail seen in Chronic liver disease.

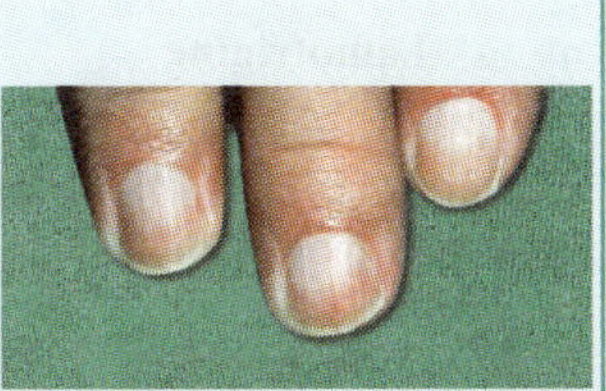

Nail and half nail sign seen in Chronic renal failure.

CASE 85

A 21-year-old female medical student comes to casualty with complaints of tachycardia, sweating, dyspnea and tremors. She says she is having a heart attack. The symptoms started suddenly when she was in a shopping mall and have occurred last month also. Her CVS examination is normal except presence of tachycardia. Diagnosis is?

a. Arrhythmia
b. Panic disorder
c. Generalized anxiety disorder
d. Dissociative disorder

Ans. (b) Panic disorder

Ref: Harrison 20th ed. pg. 3263

- The sympathomimetic symptoms are suggestive of panic disorder.
- Option A will require ECG and cannot be made from clinical history provided
- Option C, GAD is ruled out as diagnostic criteria mandate at least 6 months of symptom duration to be present. Patients with GAD worry over trivial matters and symptoms like those given in question like tachycardia and shortness of breath are relatively rare. Moreover, in the given case given only two episodes are described. One is current episode and second one occurred one month back.
- Option D, symptoms of a dissociative disorder usually first develop as a response to a traumatic event, such as abuse or military combat, to keep those memories under control.

CASE 86

What anticonvulsive agent would be MOST appropriate as first-line therapy for a 21-year-old woman recently diagnosed with focal seizures without dyscognitive features?

a. Lamotrigine
b. Carbamazepine
c. Topiramate
d. Phenytoin

Ans. (a) Lamotrigine

Ref: Harrison 20th ed. pg. 3061

For management of focal seizures in a young female patient Lamotrigine is recommended as it would be safe in future reproductive life of patient as well. However, if she remains asymptomatic for 2 years then dose can be tapered.

TABLE: Selection of antiepileptic drugs

Generalized onset tonic-clonic	Focal	Typical absence	Atypical absence, myoclonic, atonic
First-line			
Lamotrigine Valproic acid	Lamotrigine Carbamazepine Oxcarbazepine Phenytoin Levetiracetam	Valproic acid Ethosuximide Lamotrigine	Valproic acid Lamotrigine Topiramate

CASE 87

A 20-year-old male patient has deep seated retro-orbital pain with epiphora and nasal stuffiness. Such episodes have occurred earlier also and show poor response to pain killers. Neurologist has diagnosed this patient as suffering from cluster headache. What will be the first line drug for management of future such episodes?

a. Sumatriptan
b. Rizatriptan
c. Steroids
d. High flow oxygen

Ans. (d) High flow oxygen

Ref: Harrison 20th ed. pg. 3104

Features of cluster headache		Management of cluster headache
Gender	**M > F**	*Acute episode* High flow oxygen Sumatriptan injection or nasal spray Vagal nerve stimulation to prevent future episodes *Prophylaxis* Verapamil/Topiramate/Melatonin/Lithium
Pain Type Severity Site	 Stabbing, boring Excruciating Orbit, temple	
Attack frequency	1/alternate day-8/d	
Duration of attack	15-180 min	
Autonomic features	Yes	
Migrainous features	Yes	
Alcohol trigger	Yes	
Cutaneous triggers	No	
Indomethacln effect	—	

CASE 88

A 26-year-old man is being treated with chemotherapy for Hodgkin's lymphoma. During his treatment, he has severe vomiting. Which of the following areas of the brain is responsible for multiple episodes of vomiting?

a. Dorsal midbrain
b. Area postrema
c. Ventral pons
d. Thalamus

Ans. (b) Area postrema

Ref: Ganong 26th ed. pg. 491

- Area postrema is known as chemoreceptor trigger zone and leads to severe vomiting episodes. It is a V shaped band of tissue on lateral walls of fourth ventricle near the obex. It lies outside the blood brain barrier and hence can be irritated by chemotherapeutic drugs.
- Lesions of area postrema have little effect on vomiting response to GI irritation or motion sickness. But they abolish the vomiting that occurs following injection of apomorphine. Such lesions also decrease vomiting in uraemia and radiation sickness.

CASE 89

A 70-year-old woman has a progressive neurological disorder resulting in degeneration of the anterior horn cells throughout her spinal cord and brainstem. Which of the following abnormal movements is she most likely to exhibit?

a. Asterixis
b. Chorea
c. Fasciculations
d. Gait Apraxia

Ans. (c) Fasciculations

Ref: Ganong 26th ed. pg. page 235

- Anterior horn cells in spinal cord are part of lower motor neuron circuit. Axons that start from these cells terminate on skeletal muscles.
- Damage to these neurons is associated with flaccid paralysis, muscular atrophy and fasciculations.
- Fasciculations are visible muscle twitches that appear as flickers under the skin.
- Muscle tone is reduced in these patients leading to flaccid paralysis.

CASE 90

Which of the following is true of Bell's palsy?

a. The onset is typically over a period of days/weeks
b. It is a palsy of the 8th cranial nerve
c. It is associated with contralateral peri-aural numbness or pain
d. Decreased taste is a typical symptom

Ans. (d) Decreased taste is a typical symptom

Ref: Harrison 20th ed. pg. 3169

- Option A is false as onset of Bell's palsy is abrupt with maximal weakness developing over 48 hours
- Option B is wrong as Seventh nerve palsy is seen.
- Option C is wrong as pain behind the ear may be present on same side of development of paralysis for few days before onset.
- Option D is correct due to involvement of chorda tympani branch of facial nerve.

CASE 91

A 70-year-old male presents with a one-year history of progressive ataxia, urinary incontinence and memory loss. What is the *most likely* diagnosis?

a. Normal pressure hydrocephalus
b. Cerebellar astrocytoma
c. Lewy body dementia
d. Multiple sclerosis

Ans. (a) Normal pressure hydrocephalus

Ref: Harrison 20th ed. pg. 144

- The triad of DAI (**D**ementia, **A**taxia and **I**ncontinence of urine) is seen in normal pressure hydrocephalus
- Option B, cerebellar lesions do not cause dementia
- Option C, does not have ataxia
- Option D, presents with pure white matter involvement and does not have dementia.

CASE 92

All are correct about Lumbar puncture procedure except?

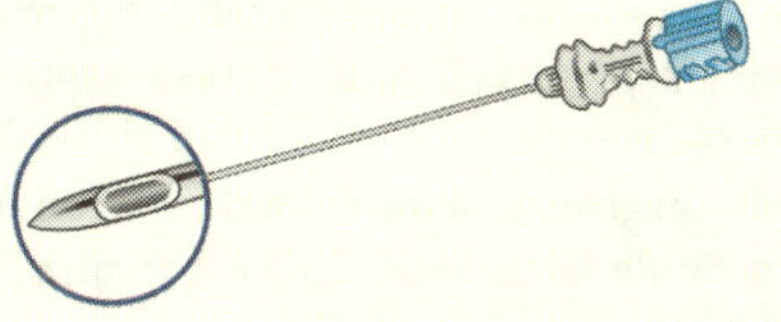

a. Done with patient in lateral decubitus position
b. Aspirate CSF once the dura mater is breached with a pop sound
c. Maximum CSF that can be removed safely is about 20 ml
d. Contraindicated in raised ICP

Ans. (b) Aspirate CSF once the dura matter is breached with a pop sound

Ref: Harrison 20th ed. pg. 992

- Lumbar puncture is done with patient in lateral decubitus position. The CSF flows out by itself and does not need to be aspirated.
- CSF that can be removed is 20-30 ml for diagnostic and therapeutic reasons. If LP is done in case of raised ICP, then chances of brain herniation leading to cardio respiratory arrest is increased.

CASE 93

A known epileptic patient who is non-compliant is having seizures for past 10 minutes. IV access could not be obtained. Which medication would be most suitable to administer at this stage to treat the patient's seizure?

a. Sodium Valproate
b. Levetiracetam
c. Diazepam
d. Lorazepam

Ans. (c) Diazepam

Ref: Harrison 20th ed. pg. 3067

In case of failure to obtain Intravenous access if the patient is having convulsions, either rectal diazepam or intranasal midazolam can be used depending on the resources available.

CASE 94

Mr X was injured in a car accident several months ago. Now when he speaks, though fluent, the sentences seem muddled and don't make sense. He also sometimes makes up words, although he seems unaware of his speech difficulties. Which area of the brain was most likely damaged in the patient's car accident?

a. Broca's area
b. Wernicke's area
c. Arcus fasciculus
d. Pre-frontal cortex

Ans. (b) Wernicke's area

Ref: Harrison 20th ed. pg. 159

- Since fluency is preserved in this patient, Option A is ruled out.
- The description given is of word salad or jargon speech where patient is creating new words. This is a feature of Wernicke's area being damaged.
- Option C is ruled out as there is no mention of repetition being impaired.
- Option D is ruled out as adults who suffer damage to the prefrontal cortex develop problems with making decisions and with behaving appropriately in social situations.

Extra Mile

TABLE: Clinical features of aphasias and related conditions commonly seen in cerebrovascular accidents

	Comprehension	Repetition of spoken language	Naming	Fluency
Wernicke's	Impaired	Impaired	Impaired	Preserved or increased
Broca's	Preserved (except grammar)	Impaired	Impaired	Decreased
Global	Impaired	Impaired	Impaired	Decreased
Conduction	Preserved	Impaired	Impaired	Preserved

CASE 95

Whilst working on the gastroenterology ward, you notice that a 47-year-old man with known liver cirrhosis has become unresponsive. You decide to calculate this man's GCS. You note that he flexes his elbows and wrists and only opens his eyes when you rub his sternum. He groans but does not say any words.

What is this man's GCS?

a. 6
b. 7
c. 8
d. 9

Ans. (b) 7

Ref: Harrison 20th ed. pg. 3183

Normal Flexion = 3
Open his eye on pain stimulus = 2
Groans/moans = 2
Hence GCS score = 7

CASE 96

Which of the following investigation is likely to be least helpful in determining the cause of the stroke?

a. Lipid profile
b. Carotid artery doppler
c. EEG
d. Autoimmune panel

Ans. (c) EEG

Ref: Harrison 20th ed. pg. 3069

- Option A will help to determine aetiology of ischemic stoke
- Option B will help to determine carotid artery atherosclerosis. The fragments from atherosclerotic plaque will cause ischemic stoke
- Option C does not help in determining ethology of stroke but helps in confirming subtypes of epilepsy.
- Option D will help in determining aetiology of ischemic stroke as autoimmune diseases lead to accelerated atherosclerosis.

CASE 97

Which type of brain herniation is called as subfalcine herniation?

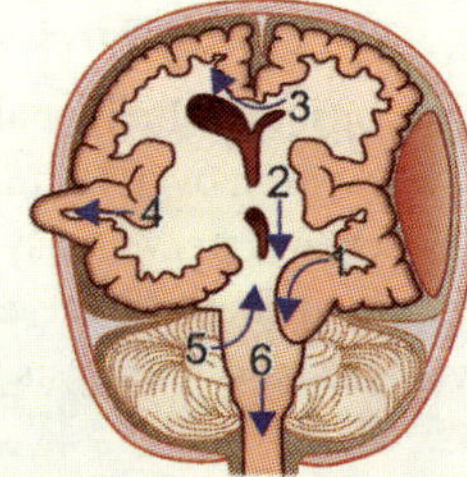

a. 1
b. 2
c. 3
d. 4

Ans. (c) 3

The image shows different types of brain herniation possible with CNS hemorrhage. Marking at point no. 3 shows subfalcine herniation where due to mass effect of bleed, one part of cerebral cortex is pushed into and below the contralateral cerebral cortex. It is also called as midline shift.

1 = Midbrain /Uncal herniation
2 = Trans-tentorial herniation
3 = Subfalcine/cingulate herniation

4 = Transcalvarial herniation
5 = Upward cerebellar transtentorial
6 = Downward cerebellar tonsillar

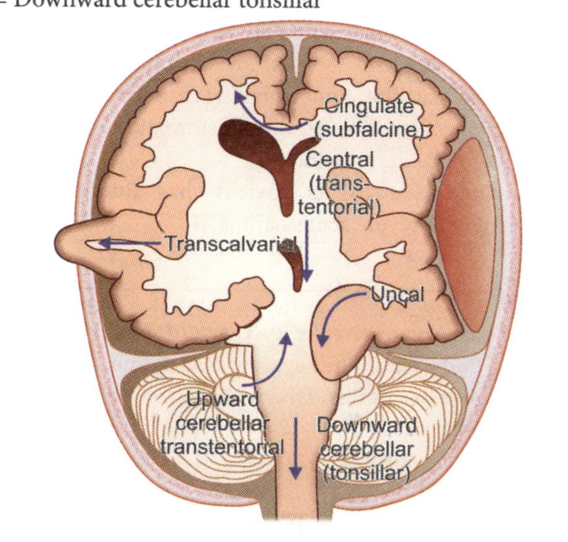

CASE 98

A 6-year-old boy has toe walking and lordotic posture. The following clinical sign was elicited. The diagnosis is?

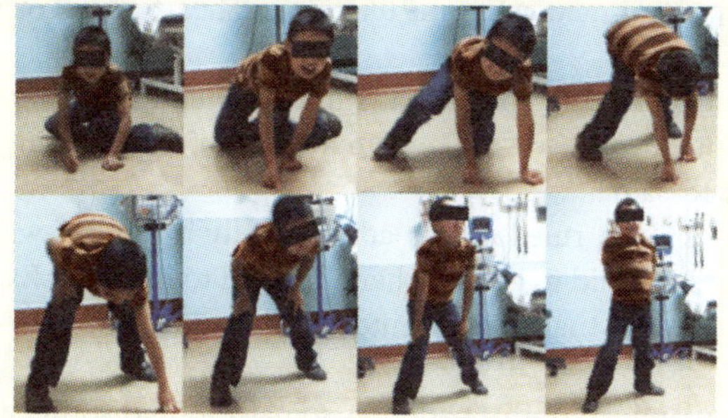

a. Dystrophinopathy
b. Neuropathy
c. Motor neuron disease
d. Myopathy

Ans. (a) Dystrophinopathy

Ref: Harrison 20th ed. pg. 3240

The image shows a child trying to get up from the floor. Notice that he uses his arms to propel himself to stand gradually. The hand of child is on the knee joint to generate traction to compensate for weakness in muscles of hip joint. This is called as Gower sign and is seen in Duchenne muscular dystrophy which is characterized by defect in dystrophin gene.

CASE 99

Glove and stocking anaesthesia are a feature of?

a. Neuropathy
b. Myopathy
c. Extrapyramidal lesion
d. Cerebellar lesion

Ans. (a) Neuropathy

Ref: Harrison 20th ed. pg. 142

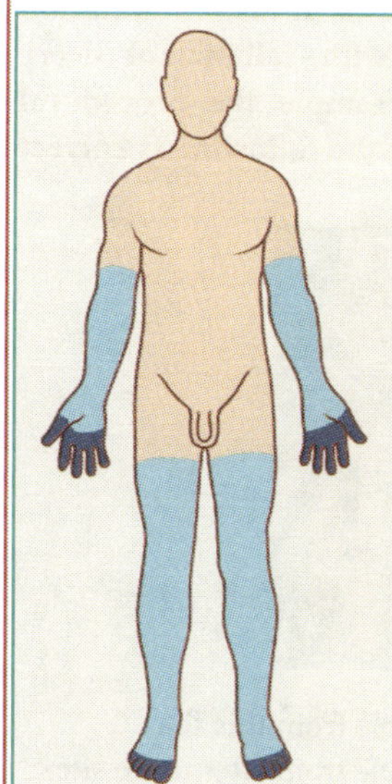

Neuropathies mostly affect the long fibres first, starting in the feet and progressing upward. Once they have progressed to the calf, symptoms may appear in the hands.

Important causes of neuropathies

- Alcohol
- Thiamine deficiency
- Niacin deficiency
- Pyridoxine deficiency
- B12 deficiency
- Pantothenic acid deficiency
- Folate deficiency
- Hypophosphatemia following TPN
- Bariatric surgery

CASE 100

A 70-year-old man is having complaints of dizzy spells and fell down in the bathroom in the night. He was brought to ER next day and subperiosteal bleed can be felt on left side of frontal bone. GCS is 15/15, higher mental functions are normal and cranial nerve examination is normal. CVS examination shows irregular pulse rhythm so ECG was done. Which is the best intervention for this patient?

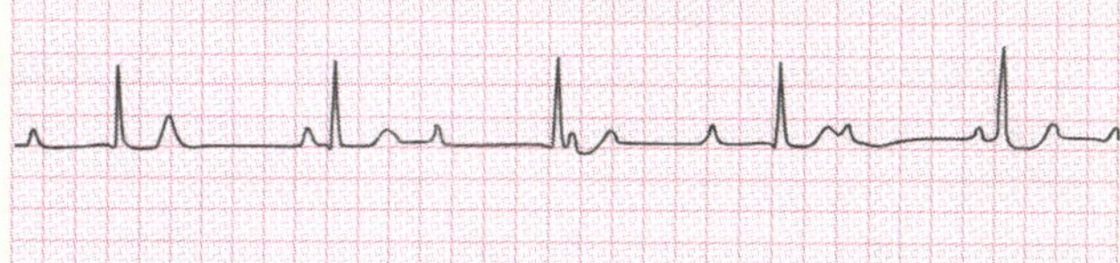

a. Adrenaline
b. Amiodarone
c. DC Shock
d. Pacemaker

Ans. (d) Pacemaker

Ref: Harrison 20th ed. pg. 1730

- The heart rate of the patient is 300/ RR interval = 300/7 = 40/ min. P-P interval and RR interval are not matching indicating AV dissociation. The patient is having complete heart block for which Permanent pacemaker is warranted.
- Option A is ruled out as it is used in case of cardiac arrest
- Option B is ruled out as it is used in Ventricular tachycardia
- Option C is ruled out as it is used in tachyarrhythmias while the given patient has bradycardia.

CASE 101

A 60-year-old smoker is admitted with acute exacerbation of Chronic bronchitis. He is started on Non-invasive ventilation with nebulization intermittently with salbutamol every 20 minutes. Before taking ABG sample the procedural guidelines were followed. Which of the following is correct about the test being performed?

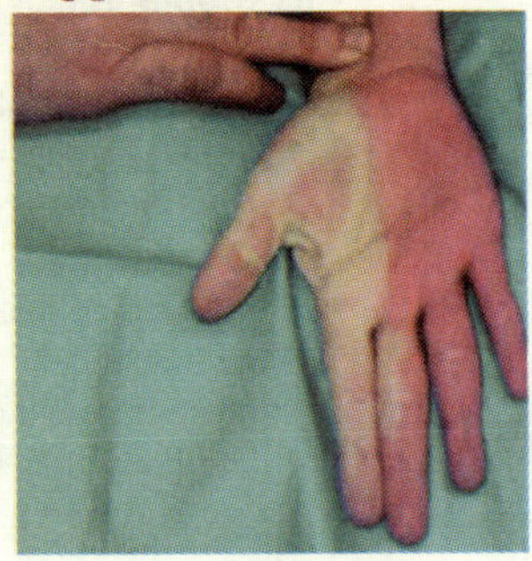

a. Positive allen test, Take ABG sample from this site
b. Positive allen test, Take ABG sample from alternative site
c. Negative allen test, take ABG sample from this site
d. Negative allen test, Take ABG sample from alternative site

Ans. (b) Positive allen test, Take ABG sample from alternative site

Ref: ABG Made Easy pg. 49

- The image shows doctor obliterating the radial artery leading to blanching of entire thumb and index finger since the collateral circulation from ulnar artery is not sufficient. The interpretation is positive Allen test and ABG sample should not be taken from this side.
- If the doctor neglects this and takes sample from the radial artery, the spasm of radial artery due to hypodermic needle and insufficient radio-ulnar collateral circulation can even lead to potential gangrene of digits.

CASE 102

A 25-year-old asthmatic patient is having an exacerbation of asthma after Diwali festival. He is feeling breathless and his respiratory rate is 30/min with use of accessory muscles of respiration. On Lung field auscultation silent chest is noted. CVS examination shows pulsus paradoxus with heart rate of 120/min. Which of the following interventions would be least useful for this patient?

a. Hydrocortisone
b. Albuterol
c. Theophylline
d. Magnesium sulphate

Ans. (c) Theophylline

Ref: Harrison 20th ed. pg. 1968

- Asthmatic patient developing severe respiratory distress and pulsus paradoxus points to clinical diagnosis of status asthmaticus/severe acute asthma.
- Steroids/Hydrocortisone is useful to reduce leukotrienes production by inhibition of phospholipase A2.
- Albuterol nebulization will help in reducing the hypoxia on immediate basis by increasing FEV1
- Magnesium sulphate works by inhibiting action of intracellular calcium and reducing bronchospasm. It is used in acute deterioration of an asthmatic progressing to impending respiratory failure.
- Theophylline due to its toxicity has limited use in management of severe acute asthma.

CASE 103

A 50-year-old woman has a 20-year-old history of vague fatigue and body pain. She says she is sick and no doctor is able to diagnose her illness. Diagnosis is?

a. Hypochondriasis
b. Munchausen syndrome
c. Somatization disorder
d. Munchausen syndrome by proxy

Ans. (c) Somatization disorder

Ref: Harrison 20th ed. pg. 3273

- Option A is ruled out as patient will make self-diagnosis with use of medical terms like cancer, heart attack or ulcers in intestine.
- Option B is ruled out as patient fakes medical history to get admitted to hospital like complaining of excruciating right iliac fossa pain.
- Option D is ruled out as adult usually a mother will fake illness of child to get him/her admitted to hospital. Example she may say that child vomited blood or was bitten by snake etc.
- The diagnosis of this patient is somatization disorder.

CASE 104

A 65-year-old smoker with 40-year history of smoking 2 packs of bidi (cigarette) every day is admitted with complaints of shortness of breath. Since he is very drowsy and Sp02 on high flow oxygen is 85%, ABG sample was drawn. pH= 7.3, $p0_2$= 78 mm Hg, PCO_2= 50, HCO_3 = 27 mEq. Comment on his blood gas analysis report.

a. Partially compensated respiratory acidosis
b. Fully compensated respiratory acidosis
c. Uncompensated respiratory acidosis
d. Mixed respiratory and metabolic acidosis

Ans. (a) Partially compensated respiratory acidosis

Ref: Harrison 20th ed. pg. 315

- pH is low which implies acidosis

- CO_2 is elevated (Normal pCO_2 = 35 -45 mm Hg) which implies respiratory etiology
- Bicarbonate is elevated (Normal HCO3 = 22-26 mEq) to neutralise the excess protons produced by respiratory acidosis.
- Therefore, the patient has partially compensated respiratory acidosis.

CASE 105

A 60-year-old Diabetes mellitus patient with constant headache for past couple of weeks is found having persistent high BP in spite of regular intake of Ramipril 5 mg. His work up shows HbA1c= 8 %, urine examination with dipstick shows absence of ketones with 4+ sugar and 4+ protein, Serum sodium= 135 mEq and Serum potassium= 6 mEq. Comment on the possible diagnosis.

a. Hyperglycemic hyperosmolar coma
b. Diabetic ketoacidosis
c. Diabetic nephropathy
d. Subarachnoid haemorrhage

Ans. (c) Diabetic nephropathy

Ref: Harrison 20th ed. pg. 2878

- HbA1c of 8% indicates poorly controlled diabetes mellitus. Urine examination shows proteinuria with elevated potassium. Both of these point to development of diabetic nephropathy. Less GFR will cause Increased RAAS activity and resultant hyperaldosteronism explains poor control of Blood pressure.
- Option A is ruled out as it presents with loss of consciousness
- Option B is ruled out as ketones by dipstick are absent and patient is well oriented
- Option D is ruled out as no features suggestive of raised ICP are present.

CASE 106

A 60-year-old man with hypertension has a deranged lipid profile. He has presented with weakness and pain in thigh and calf muscles. Which of the following drugs is responsible?

a. Aspirin
b. Atorvastatin
c. Atenolol
d. Apixaban

Ans. (b) Atorvastatin

Ref: Braunwald Cardiology pg. 1803

- The patient has statin associated myopathy. CPK MM levels will confirm the diagnosis.
- Aspirin can lead to GI bleeding. Metoprolol can lead to dizziness and hypotension. Apixaban toxicity can lead to bleeding.

CASE 107

A 24-year-old lady has complaints of oligomenorrhea, diarrhea and weight loss. On examination pulse rate is 120/min with BP = 140/100 mm Hg and fine tremors in hand. The following finding is noted in the legs of the patient. Comment on the diagnosis.

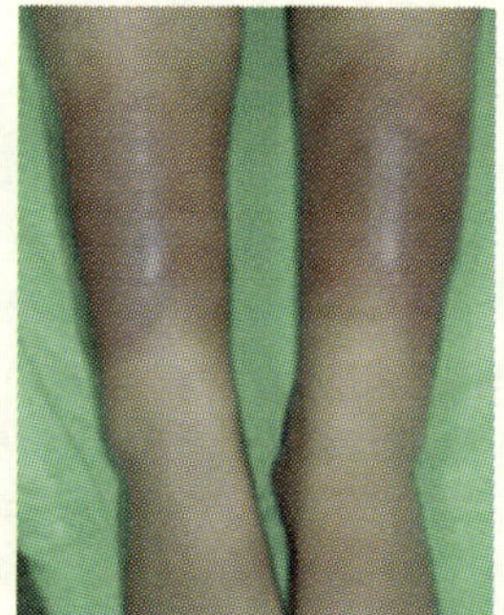

a. Pretibial myxedema
b. Necrobiosis lipidoica
c. Asteatotic eczema
d. Filariasis

Ans. (a) Pretibial myxedema

Ref: Harrison 20th ed. pg. 2704

- Features of sympathomimetic stimulation like fine tremors, tachycardia with weight loss in female patient points to diagnosis of hyperthyroidism. The image shows pretibial myxedema that is seen with Grave's disease.
- Option B leads to diabetes mellitus
- Option C leads to dry skin on shins but none of the symptoms and examination findings given in the case would be present
- Option D is ruled out due to symptom profile of the patient

CASE 108

A 60-year-old female is having cough for last 3 months and chest pain episodes that worsen with deep inspiration. On examination the finding shown in hands is noted. Further work up showed a pleural effusion showing low sugar with elevated protein and malignant cells. Which of the following is unlikely to be a cause of this presentation?

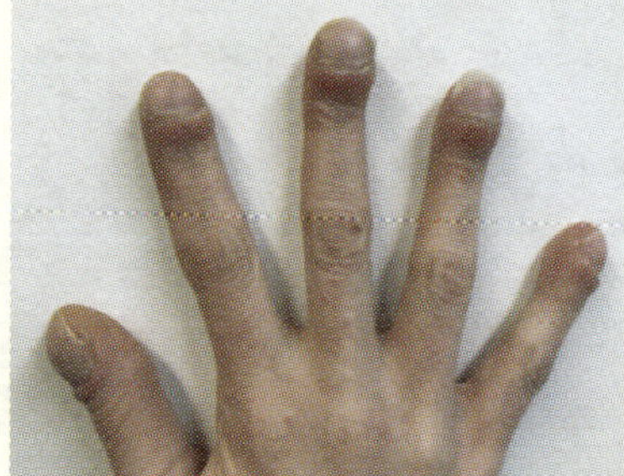

a. Adenocarcinoma lung
b. Squamous cell cancer lung
c. Large cell cancer lung
d. Small cell cancer lung

Ans. (d) Small cell cancer lung

Ref: Harrison 20th ed. pg. 541

The image shows presence of clubbing in patient with cough for last 3 months. The patient went on to develop malignant pleural effusion. The patient has developed lung cancer and subtype will be confirmed by examination of biopsy specimen. However, clubbing is less likely to be seen with small cell cancer.

Extra Mile

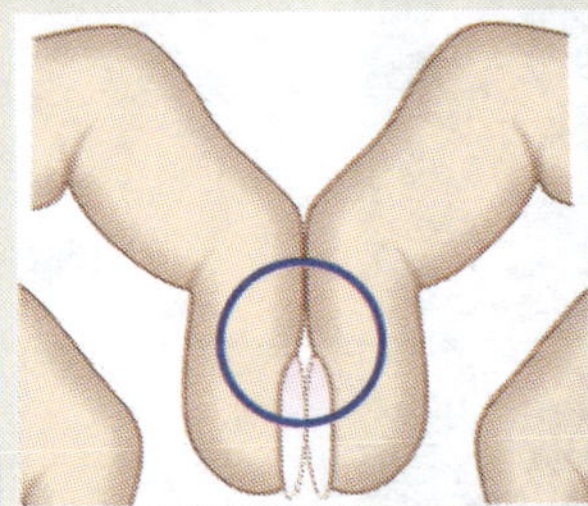

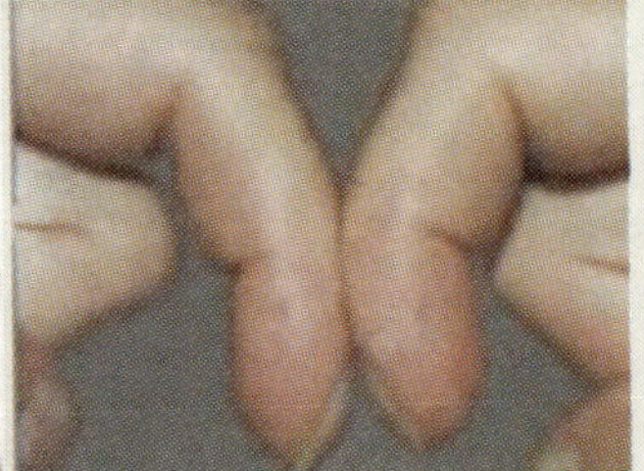

Notice diamond shaped space in between opposed fingers of normal person.

Schamroth window test can be used to identify or confirm clubbing.
If two opposing fingers are held back-to-back against each other, a diamond-shaped space should normally appear between the nail beds and the nails of the 2 fingers.
In clubbing, this space (or window) is missing.

CASE 109

An 18-year-old boy with documented valvular heart disease is having high grade fever with chills and rigors for past 2 weeks. On examination findings shown below are noted in palms and fundus examination of the patient. Which of the following is a major criterion for diagnosis of this condition?

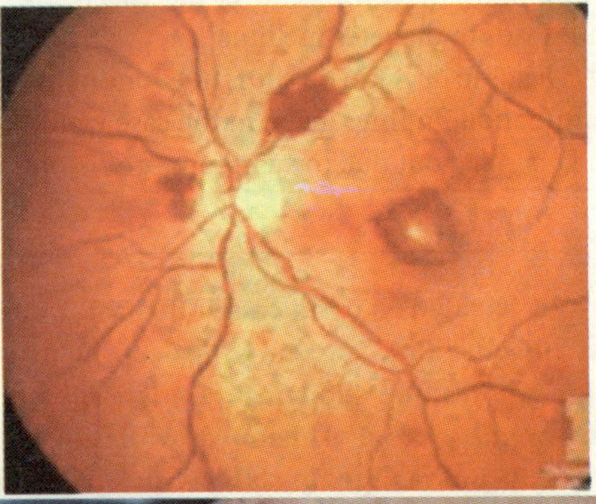

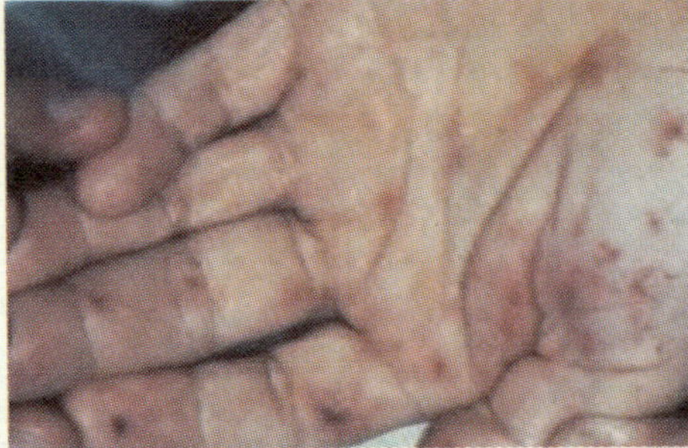

a. Prolonged PR interval
b. ASO titer elevation
c. Commissural fusion of leaflets due to Aschoff nodules
d. Positive Blood culture

Ans. (d) Positive Blood culture

Ref: Harrison 20th ed. pg. 925

- The fundus examination shows Roth spots and palms show Janeway lesions in a known case of valvular heart disease. The clinical diagnosis is infective endocarditis.
- Option A is a minor criterion for diagnosis of Rheumatic fever and not infective endocarditis.
- Option B is a lab feature seen during evaluation of patient of Rheumatic fever
- Option C is a manifestation of Rheumatic endocarditis
- Option D is major modified duke criterion for diagnosis of infective endocarditis

Extra Mile

TABLE: The modified duke criteria for the clinical diagnosis infective endocarditis

Major Criteria
1. Positive blood culture Typical microorganism for infective endocarditis from two separate blood cultures Viridans streptococci, *Streptococcus gallolyticus*. HACEK group organisms, *Staphylococcus aureus*, *or* Community-acquired enterococci in the absence of a primary focus *or* Persistently positive blood culture. defined as recovery of a microorganism consistent with infective endocarditis from: Blood cultures drawn >12 h apart: *or* All of 3 or a majority of ≥4 separate blood cultures, with first and last drawn at least 1 h apart

Contd...

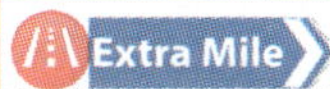

Extra Mile

Major Criteria

or

Single positive blood culture for *Coxiella burnetii* or phase I IgG antibody titer of >1:800

2. Evidence of endocardial involvement

Positive echocardiogram[b]

Oscillating intracardiac mass on valve or supporting structures or in the path of regurgitant jets or in implanted material, in the absence of an alternative anatomic explanation, *or*

Abscess, *or*

New partial dehiscence of prosthetic valve,

or

New valvular regurgitation (increase or change in preexisting murmur not sufficient)

Minor Criteria

1. Predisposition: predisposing heart conditions or injection drug use
2. Fever ≥38.0°C (≥100.4°F)
3. Vascular phenomena: Major arterial emboli, septic pulmonary infarcts, mycotic aneurysm, intracranial hemorrhage, conjunctival hemorrhages, Janeway lesions
4. Immunologic phenomena: Glomerulonephritis, Osler's nodes, Roth's spots, rheumatoid factor
5. Microbiologic evidence: Positive blood culture but not meeting major criterion, as noted previously, or serologic evidence of active infection with an organism consistent with infective endocarditis

CASE 110

A 90-year-old patient complains of recurrent episodes of dizziness and syncopal episodes. His ECG and CXR is shown below. Which of the following devices is visible in Chest X-ray?

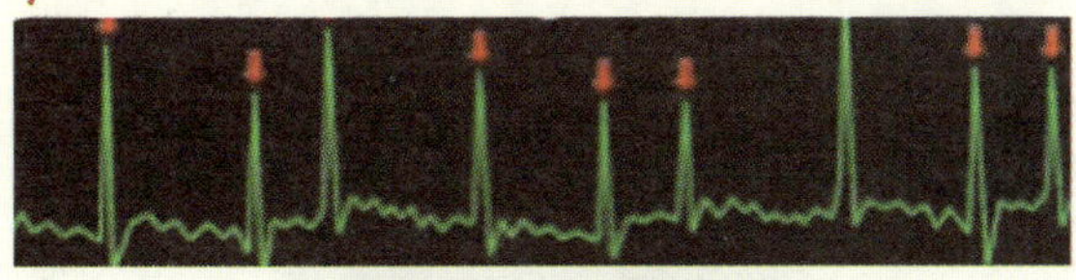

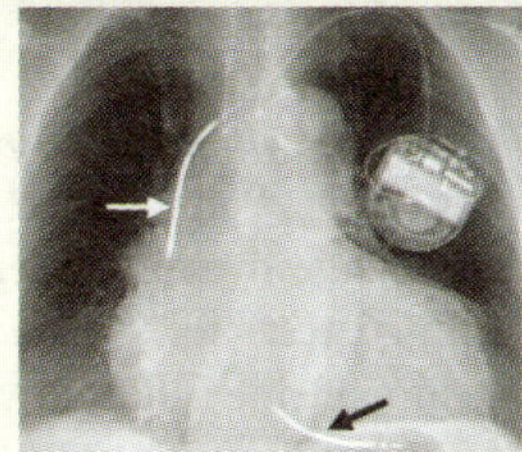

a. Implantable cardioverter defibrillator
b. Pacing Device
c. Vagal nerve stimulator
d. Chemo-port

Ans. (a) Implantable cardioverter defibrillator

Ref: Harrison 20th ed. pg. 1755

- The ECG shows irregular RR interval with absent P waves. The diagnosis is atrial fibrillation which a tachyarrhythmia. For termination of tachyarrhythmias, implantable cardioverter defibrillator is used.
- Option B is used for management of Brady arrhythmias.
- Option C is used for medically refractory epilepsy.
- Option D is used for delivery of chemotherapy directly into central veins

CASE 111

A 45-year-old man has weight gain and centripetal obesity. His BP = 150/100 mm Hg and lipid profile shows elevated triglycerides with low HDL. Fasting blood sugar is 120 mg % and 2-hour sugar value is 186 mg%. Comment on the diagnosis.

a. Syndrome X
b. Metabolic syndrome
c. Hypothyroidism
d. Maturity onset diabetes in young

Ans (b) Metabolic syndrome

Ref: Harrison 20th ed. pg. 2903

- Combination of features of centripetal obesity with hypertension, impaired glucose tolerance and hypertriglyceridemia with low HDL points to diagnosis of metabolic syndrome.
- Option A leads to narrowing of perforator branches of coronary arteries and development of chest pain on exertion.
- Option C does not have impaired glucose tolerance
- Option D does not have features of hypertension and weight gain

CASE 112

A 40-year-old female has constipation with alopecia. She tends to forget things easily and is also having menstrual abnormalities for which she has visited her gynecologist multiple times. For her dry skin she has tried all brands of moisturizers but there is no relief. The physician has ordered a thyroid function test. Which of the following is the likely report of this patient?

a. Elevated TSH and low Free T4
b. Elevated TSH and elevated Free T4
c. Low TSH and elevated T4
d. Low TSH and low Free T4

Ans. (a) Elevated TSH and low Free T4

Ref: Harrison 20th ed. pg. 2698

Dry skin, constipation and alopecia in a female with irregular menses should be worked up for primary hypothyroidism. Since the production of T4 from the gland is reduced, TSH will become elevated by feedback mechanism.

CASE 113

You have started blood transfusion in a 25-year-old primigravida, B positive patient for severe anemia before her scheduled induction of labour the next morning. Post transfusion she complains of fever, chills, rash in the arm where transfusion is being given. The nurse injects 2 ml Injection Avil and 100 mg Hydrocortisone but the symptoms are worsening and she is also having breathing difficulty with low oxygen saturation. Chest auscultation shows bilateral normal air entry. What is the diagnosis?

a. Febrile non hemolytic transfusion reaction
b. Transfusion related acute lung injury
c. Transfusion related circulatory overload
d. Tetany

Ans. (b) Transfusion related acute lung injury

Ref: Harrison 20th ed. pg. 813

- Allergic reactions can be seen post blood transfusion even if blood group is same as there are multiple antigens on RBC which differ amongst different people.
- However, breathing issues with drop of oxygen saturation points to transfusion associated acute lung injury. This usually develops in first 6 hours of transfusion and can even lead to death due to non -cardiogenic pulmonary edema.
- Option A will only cause fever and chills but BP and spO2 remain normal
- Option C will cause Congestive heart failure with bilateral crepitations. The lungs fields are clear in the case given.
- Option D leads to carpopedal spasm and Chvostek sign.

Extra Mile

TRALI

Occurs in first 6 hours of transfusion

Caused by activation of recipient neutrophils by donor-derived antibodies targeting human leukocyte antigen or human neutrophil antigen, in most cases.

CASE 114

A 50-year-old woman on day 3 post-operative total thyroidectomy complains of breathlessness and difficulty in speaking. The following test was performed in the patient. What will be the best management of this patient?

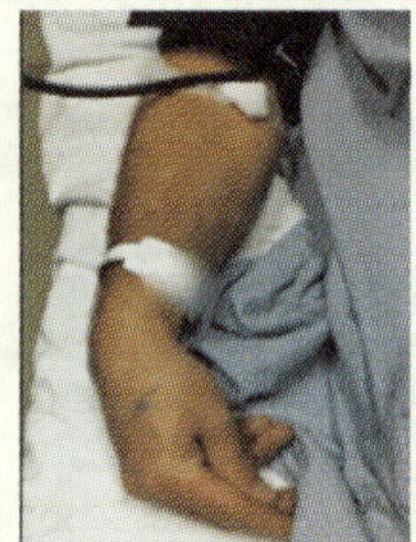

a. Reassure the patient
b. Intubate and transfer to OT for management of tension hematoma
c. Put ECG monitor and give calcium gluconate
d. Start Sodium nitroprusside drip titrated to blood pressure values

Ans. (c) Put ECG monitor and give calcium gluconate

Ref: Harrison 20th ed. pg. 314

- The image shows carpopedal spasm on inflation of BP cuff above Systolic BP. This occurs due to tetany which is commonly seen day 3 onwards in post total thyroidectomy patients.
- Urgent ECG will show QT prolongation. Samples should be drawn for serum calcium, ionised calcium and serum albumin.
- Then initiate 10% calcium gluconate slow infusion
- Option B is done for relief of tension hematoma which presents in post op patients of total thyroidectomy on day 1 with respiratory distress.
- Option D will be used for HTN crisis.

CASE 115

A 30-year-old woman has features of palpitations, headache and excessive sweating. BP charting was advised for next one week which shows intermittent paroxysmal hypertension. Which screening test will be advised for this patient?

a. 24-hour urinary Metanephrine levels
b. 24-hour urinary Vanillylmandelic acid levels
c. 24-hours urinary Homovanillic acid levels
d. 24-hours urinary 5- Hydroxyindole acetic acid levels

Ans. (a) 24-hour urinary Metanephrine levels

Ref: Harrison 20th ed. pg. 2741

- The symptoms of PHD: **P**alpitations, **h**eadache /HTN and **d**iaphoresis are suggestive of presence of pheochromocytoma. Screening test for pheochromocytoma is 24-hour urinary metanephrine values.
- Option B is used for screening for neuroblastoma
- Option C is used for evaluating end products of dopamine metabolism.
- Option D is used for evaluating possibility of carcinoid syndrome

CASE 116

A 45-year-old woman has diarrhea for last 6 months that is non-responsive to fasting. Her urine output is normal but she is having muscle weakness and cramps. Serum potassium was tested and was found to be 3 mEq/L. Which is correct about next step in management of this patient?

a. Start ORS 2 packets daily and give IV Amikacin for 7 days
b. Start Ringer lactate 5 L over next 24 hours and give IV Metronidazole for 7 days
c. Perform stool osmotic gap
d. Start oral potassium replacement and give IV flu ids based on severity of dehydration

Ans. (c) Perform stool osmotic gap

Ref: Harrison 20th ed. pg. 2244

- Diarrhea which is non-responsive to fasting is secretory diarrhea. Muscle cramps are explained by hypokalemia seen with fluid losses.
- Stool osmotic gap is used to confirm this finding. SOG > 50 is compatible with osmotic diarrhea.
- Option A and B is used in infective diarrhea and correction of dehydration.
- Option D is ruled out as IV fluids will correct dehydration currently but the problem will re-occur.
- The patient needs a subsequent work for neuroendocrine tumors like gastrinoma, insulinoma or villous adenoma that can lead to secretory diarrhea.

CASE 117

A 30-year-old marketing professional complains of episodic chest pain both at rest and sometimes on walking. His CVS examination is normal and ECG is within normal limits. There is no tenderness at any costochondral junction. Which of the following is the most likely etiology of his illness?

a. Unstable Angina
b. Prinzmetal angina
c. Tietze syndrome
d. Gastroesophageal reflux

Ans. (d) Gastroesophageal reflux

Ref: Harrison 20th ed. pg. 2215

- Option A presents with chest pain at rest and ECG findings of T wave inversion and ST depression
- Option B presents with chest pain at rest with ST segment elevation
- Option C presents with tenderness at costochondral junction
- Option D presents with retrosternal chest pain and is the first differential to be ruled out.

CASE 118

A soldier posted at Siachen glacier is having muscle cramps and weakness. Pulse oximeter reading shows saturation of 95% in room air. ABG shows pH = 7.5, PO_2 = 90 mm Hg, PCO_2 = 30 mm Hg and HCO_3 = 24 mEq/L. Comment on the diagnosis.

a. Partially compensated Respiratory alkalosis
b. Fully compensated respiratory alkalosis
c. Mixed respiratory and metabolic alkalosis
d. Uncompensated respiratory alkalosis

Ans. (d) Uncompensated respiratory alkalosis

Ref: Harrison 20th ed. pg. 315

- pH = 7.5 is diagnostic of alkalosis
- Low PCO_2 indicates hyperventilation and presence of respiratory alkalosis.
- In respiratory alkalosis, bicarbonate should be lost in urine. But in this patient bicarbonate is normal indicating uncompensated respiratory alkalosis.

CASE 119

A COVID-19 pneumonia patient is having severe respiratory distress. He has been given remdesivir with dexamethasone and following method of oxygen delivery. This is known as?

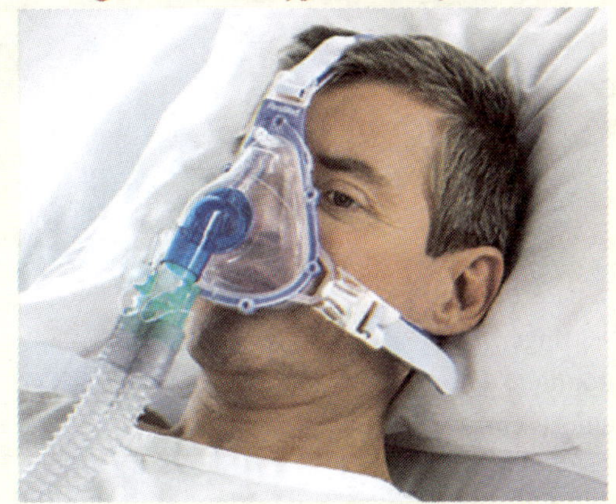

a. Venti mask
b. Non rebreather mask
c. (HFON) High flow oxygen with nasal cannula
d. Non-invasive ventilation

Ans. (d) Non-invasive ventilation

Ref: https://www.mohfw.gov.in/pdf/Updated Clinical Managementprotocol

The image shows a tight-fitting face mask used for non-invasive ventilation in cases of severe COVID-19 for maintaining oxygen saturation.

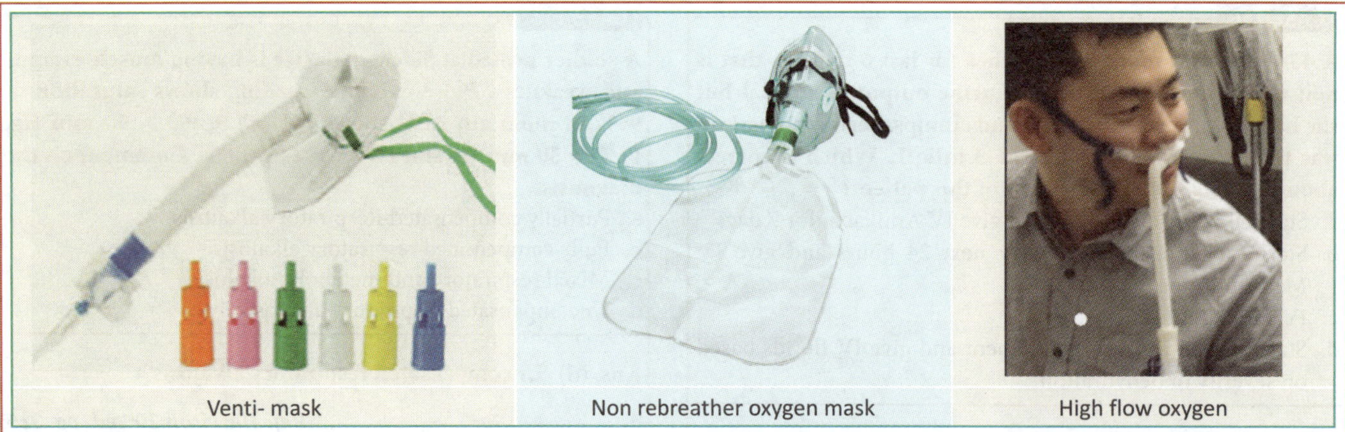
Venti- mask | Non rebreather oxygen mask | High flow oxygen

CASE 120

A 30-year-old female presents with this deformity. Comment on the diagnosis based on the image shown below.

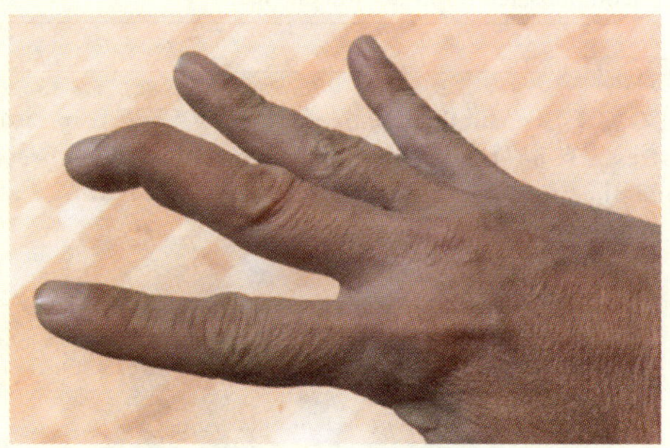

a. Swan neck deformity
b. Mallet finger
c. Boutonniere deformity
d. Calcinosis cutis

Ans. (b) Mallet finger

Ref: Essential Orthopaedics by J. Maheswari pg. 76

- The image shows flexion at DIP which is seen due to avulsion of extensor tendon which is inserted into distal phalanx. It is commonly seen in sports like cricket or football.
- Option A is ruled out as it shows flexion at DIP but extension at PIP
- Option C is ruled out it shows extension at DIP but flexion at PIP
- Option D presents as calcified plaques in skin in patients with hypercalcemia.

CASE 121

A 30-year-old woman complains of the following changes in her finger tips on cold exposure. There are no other complaints and lab work up is normal. What is the diagnosis?

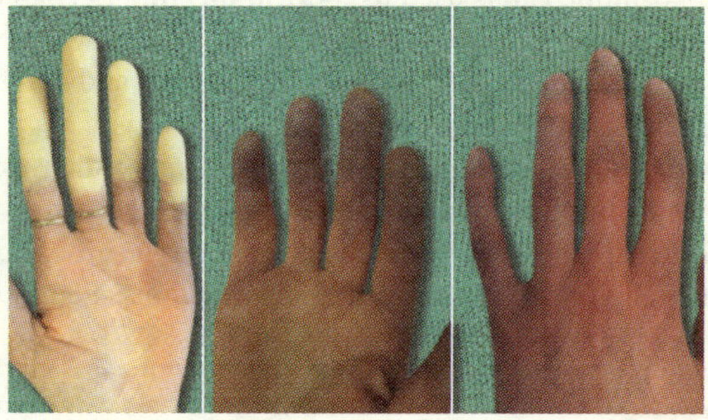

a. Raynaud's disease
b. Secondary Raynaud phenomenon
c. Hammer hand
d. Mechanic's hand

Ans. (a) Raynaud's disease

Ref: Harrison 20th ed. pg. 362

- The image shows colour change in finger tips from white—blue—red and is known as Raynaud's phenomenon. When it occurs idiopathically it is called Raynaud disease.
- When the same complaint occurs in a patient with concomitant disorders like SLE, Rheumatoid arthritis, Sjogren's syndrome, Antiphospholipid antibody syndrome then it is called as secondary Raynaud phenomenon.
- Drugs, such as antimigraine medications, interferon alpha and beta, cyclosporine, and nonselective beta blockers, can also cause secondary Raynaud phenomenon.
- Option C is Raynaud's phenomenon seen in construction workers.
- Option D is seen in patients of Scleroderma and presents as cracks and abrasion in tip of fingers as seen in car mechanic whose hands come in contact with abrasives and engine oil.

CASE 122

Comment on the diagnosis based on physical findings of this 35-year-old female with difficulty in climbing stairs.

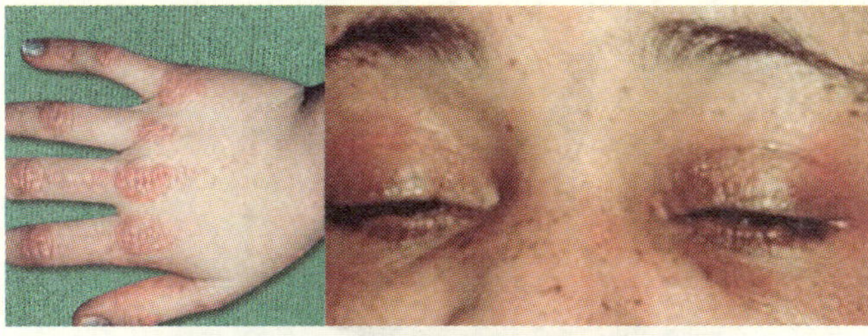

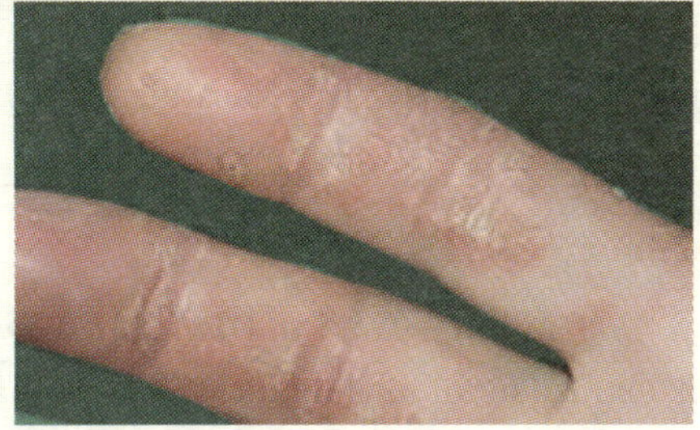

a. Dermatomyositis
b. CREST syndrome
c. Scleroderma
d. Mixed connective tissue disorder

Ans. (a) Dermatomyositis

Ref: Harrison 20th ed. pg. 2591

The image shows Gottron papules on knuckles of the patient, Heliotrope/purplish discoloration around upper and lower eyelids and dry cracked skin at finger tips called as mechanic hands. These are cutaneous manifestations of Dermatomyositis. The myositis part is given in the question in form of proximal muscle involvement leading to difficulty in climbing stairs.

CASE 123

Otto Veraguth fold is seen in?

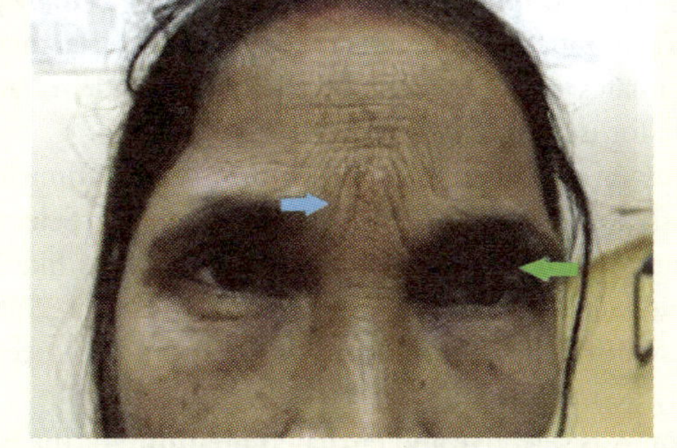

a. Depression b. Mania
c. Anxiety d. Psychosis

Ans. (a) Depression

Ref: Kaplan and Saddock Synopsis of Psychiatry pg. 548

- Otto Veraguth fold is seen in depression. Notice the black arrow in the image. It appears as triangular palpebral folds running diagonally from the lateral corners of the eyes, medially upward to the medial end of the eyebrows
- The white arrow in the figure is called omega sign. It occurs due to excessive use of muscle of grief, corrugator cili.

CASE 124

A 65-year-old man presents with fever with chills for last one week. Work up is negative for COVID-19, Typhoid, malaria and dengue. His past medical history reveals that he had developed calcification of aortic valve leading to severe aortic stenosis and had undergone aortic valve replacement in January 2020. Which of the following is the possible organism responsible for current presentation?

a. Staph aureus b. C. O.N. S
c. Strep viridans d. Enterococcus

Ans. (c) Strep viridans

Ref: Harrison 20th ed. pg. 922

Development of fever in a known case of prosthetic heart valve disease and negative reports for common infections is suggestive of first differential diagnosis as Infective endocarditis. Since the infection is developing after one year of actual valve replacement the leading organism responsible is Streptococcus viridans.

CASE 125

A 10-year-old unimmunised child from a village is brought with fever, sore throat and difficulty in breathing for last 5 days. On examination a membrane is noted in pharyngeal wall. Throat swab was taken to the microbiology lab. It should be plated on which culture media?

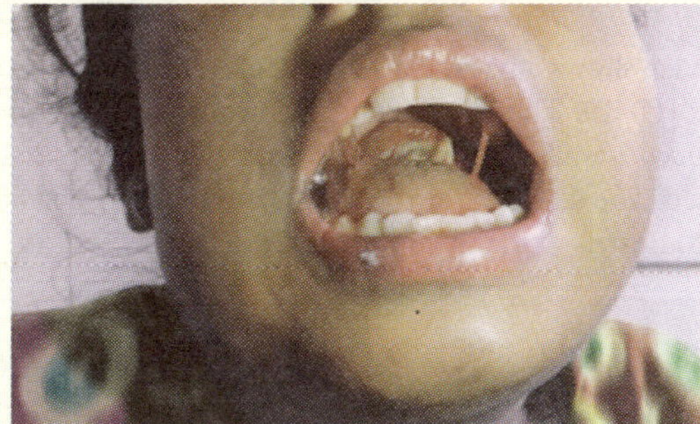

a. Pike media
b. Ludlam media
c. Potassium tellurite
d. Robertson cooked meat broth

Ans. (c) Potassium tellurite

Ref: Manson Tropical disease, E-Book pg. 1134

- The image shows a whitish membrane in posterior pharyngeal wall of an unimmunized child. First differential diagnosis is faucial diphtheria. The culture media for diphtheria is potassium tellurite. Faucial diphtheria is the most common form of diphtheria.
- At the beginning of illness, diphtheria can look like any type of tonsillitis. The membrane may extend to uvula, soft palate, oro-pharynx or larynx. The lymph nodes in neck are enlarged and painful and neck is swollen.

CASE 126

Mr Gupta is a businessman who has come to your hospital for testing for COVID-19 as he has to fly to Dubai on a business trip and has to produce the COVID -19 testing certificate at the immigration. Which is correct about the nasopharyngeal swab testing?

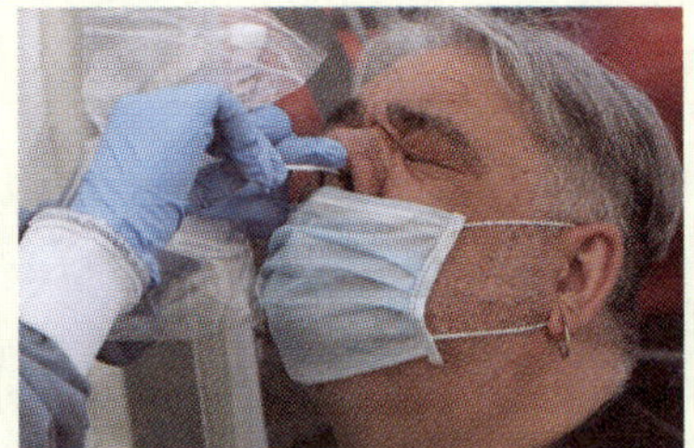

a. Insert minitip swab upwards to palate to distance equal to ear to nostril
b. Insert minitip swab parallel to palate to distance equal to ear to nostril
c. Use a different swab in case of deviated nasal septum or difficulty in obtaining specimen
d. All of the above

Ans. (b) Insert minitip swab parallel to palate to distance equal to ear to nostril

Ref: https://www.mohfw.gov.in/pdf/Updated Clinical Management Protocol

The image shows a nasal swab being taken for RT-PCR testing for COVID-19. The CDC guidelines mention the swab to be introduced parallel to hard palate with patient's neck slightly extended. The distance for the tip of swab to be pushed is equal to ear to nostril so that it can reach nasopharynx.

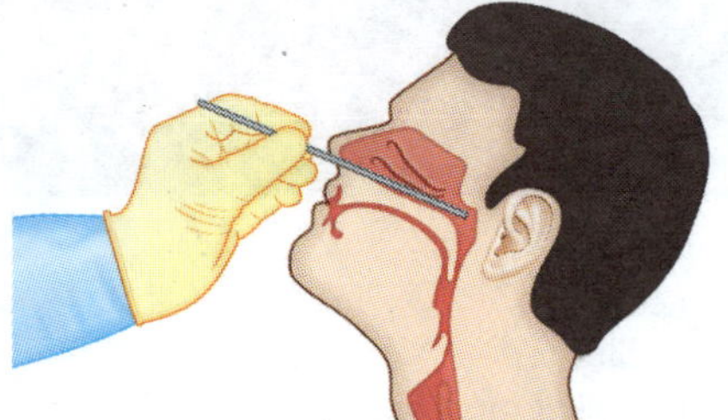

CASE 127

A patient has developed a jaw abscess followed by a draining sinus post dental extraction from a quack. Which organism is incriminated in this lesion?

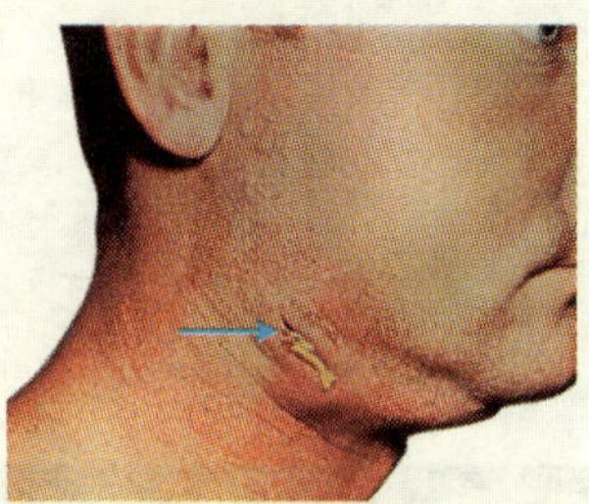

a. Actinomycetes
b. Nocardia
c. Madurella
d. Actinomyces

Ans. (d) Actinomyces

Ref: Manson Tropical Disease, E-Book pg. 1086

Post dental extraction of mandibular molar a patient can develop cervicofacial actinomycosis due to use of non-sterile instruments and poor dental hygiene.

If an abscess occurs, the infection drains mostly through the skin and generates a sinus tract. Common accompanying symptoms are fever, mild or no pain, swelling or a hard, red to reddish-purple lump on the affected site.

CASE 128

A neonate has developed meningitis and neonatologist is suspecting causative organism to be Listeria monocytogenes. Which of the following culture media is useful for isolating this organism?

a. Thayer martin
b. Castaneda method
c. Robertson cooked meat broth
d. PALCAM media

Ans. (d) PALCAM media

Ref: Manual of Applied Microbiology E-Book pg. 213

- Listeria monocytogenes is a rare cause of bacterial meningitis in neonates and CSF sample must be plated in PALCAM media for isolation of this bacteria.
- Polymyxin acriflavine lithium chloride ceftazidime aesculin mannitol (PALCAM) is a selective medium. Selectivity is attained mainly by the inhibitory components like lithium chloride, acriflavine, polymyxin and ceftazidime. This aids in easy differentiation of *Listeria* spp. from enterococci and staphylococci.
- Option A is selective and enriched **medium** for the isolation and cultivation of Neisseria species
- Option B is used for isolation of brucella and Option C is used for isolation of anaerobes.

CASE 129

The culture plate shown below is used for isolation of which organism?

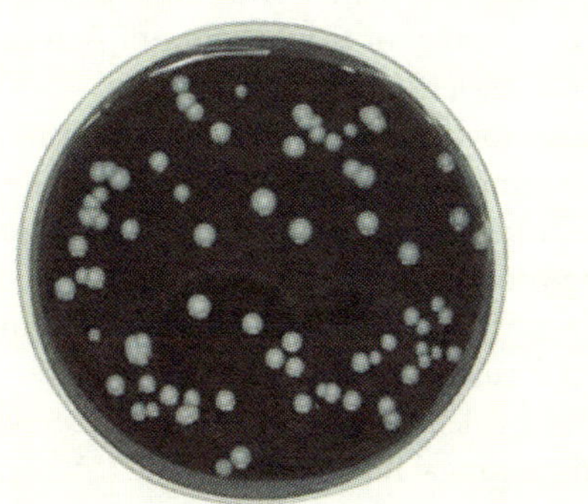

a. Haemophilus influenzae
b. Haemophilus parainfluenzae
c. Legionella pneumophila
d. E. Coli

Ans. (c) Legionella pneumophila

Ref: Manual of Applied Microbiology E-Book pg. 345

The image depicts a black color culture plate showing bacterial colonies. The black color is due to presence of charcoal. The culture media is BYCE: Buffered Yeast Charcoal Extract.

It is used to pick up organism responsible for atypical pneumonia from clinical or water specimens: Legionella pneumophila

CASE 130

The new malaria vaccine is based on which strain?

a. Jeryl Lynn strain
b. SA- 14-14-2
c. G1P
d. $RTS_1S/AS01$

Ans. (d) $RTS_1S/AS01$

Ref: WHO

- Option A is used for mumps vaccine. Option B is live JE vaccine. Option C is for Rota virus vaccine.
- Option D is the world's first malaria vaccine shown to provide partial protection to children against Plasmodium Falciparum malaria and has been launched in Africa.

CASE 131

Which is true about Nipah virus infection?

a. Transmitted by bite to person by Fruit bats
b. No human-to-human transmission
c. Leads to development of Encephalitis
d. Live vaccine single dose provides life-long immunity

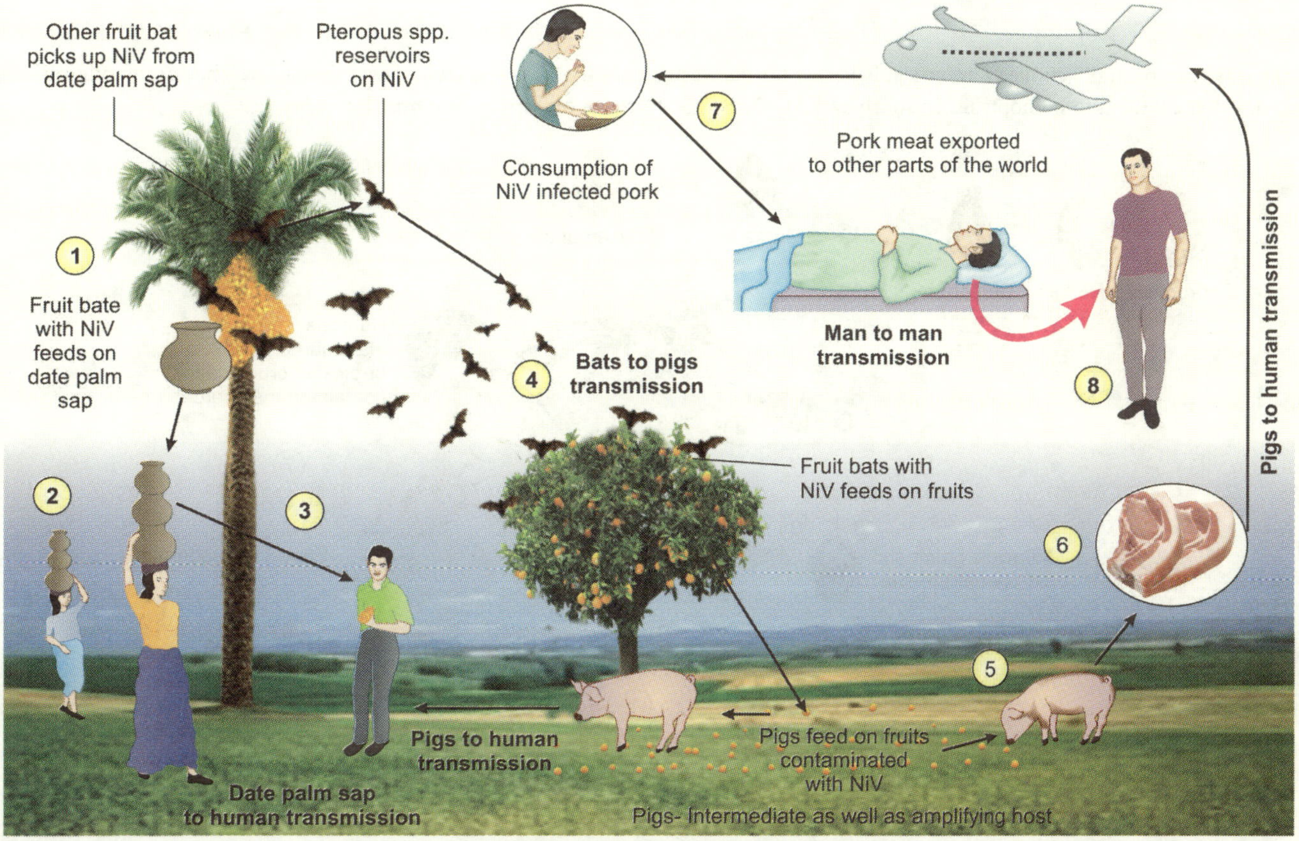

Ans. (c) Leads to development of Encephalitis

Ref: CDC

- Option A is wrong as it is transmitted by eating fruits contaminated by saliva or feces of fruit bats.
- Option B is wrong as Human to human transmission occurs
- Option D is wrong as no vaccine has been documented to prevent Nipah virus infection.
- Nipah virus leads to encephalitis.

CASE 132

A 20-year-old patient has developed fever, headache and features suggestive of meningoencephalitis after swimming in stagnant water in village pond. The causative organism is?

a. Pneumococcus
b. Group B streptococcus
c. Naegleria Fowleri
d. Cryptococcus

Ans. (c) Naegleria Fowleri

Ref: Harrison 20th ed. pg. 1574

- Meningoencephalitis after swimming in stagnant water can occur due to entry of trophozoites of Brain eating amoeba "Naegleria Fowleri".
- It is a heat-loving (thermophilic) organism. It grows best at higher temperatures up to 46°C especially in hot Indian summers when people in villages might go for swimming in the village pond.
- Option A is ruled out as it leads to bacterial meningitis
- Option B is ruled out as it is seen in neonates
- Option D is ruled out as it is seen in AIDS positive patients and leads to fungal meningitis.

CASE 133

In a village in Goa multiple people are having complaints of chest tightness, cough and haemoptysis. Epidemiological investigation revealed that all of them had attended a wedding one month back where crab meat and other sea food items were served. Which of the following is the possible incriminating agent?

a. Clonorchis sinesis
b. Schistosomiasis
c. Paragonimus westermani
d. Toxoplasma gondii

Ans. (c) Paragonimus westermani

Ref: Harrison 20th ed. pg. 1636

The parasite in partially cooked Crab meat is Paragonimus westermani which is ingested as metacercariae. The adults cause cavities in lungs that can lead to hemoptysis. In south east Asia this infection can present as Endemic hemoptysis.

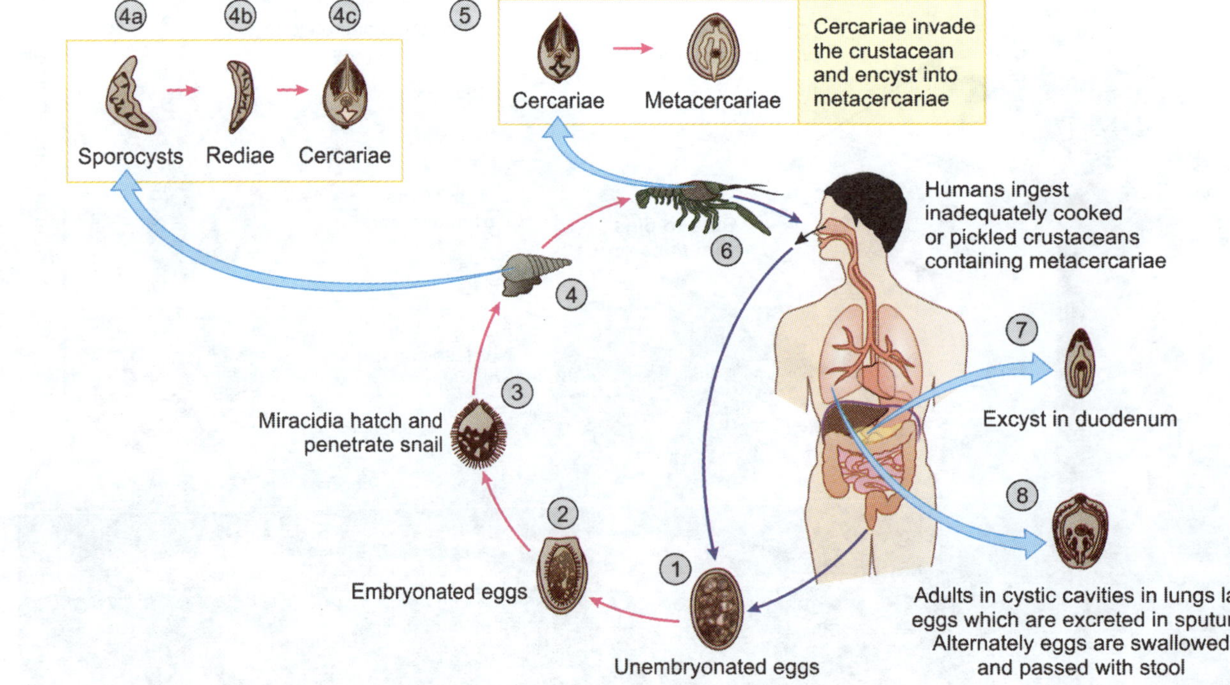

CASE 134

A 6-year-old child cries a lot at night and scratches his perianal area. The doctor has decided to perform a scotch tape test. This test is used for diagnosis of?

a. Pin worm
b. Round worm
c. Hook worm
d. Loa Loa

Ans. (a) Pin worm

Ref: Harrison 20th ed. pg. 1555

Diagnosis of *Enterobius vermicularis*

Diagnosis is commonly used.

Use of double-stick tape on a tongue depresser

This is pressed against the perianal folds where eggs will stick to the tape

Tape is then stuck onto a microscope slide and examined for eggs

CASE 135

Which of the following schistosome eggs has a terminal spine?

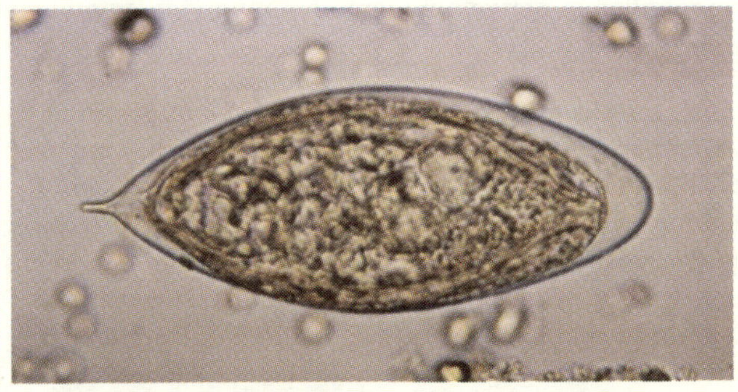

a. Schistosoma haematobium
b. Schistosoma mansoni
c. Schistosoma japonicum
d. All of the above

Ans. (a) Schistosoma haematobium

Ref: Harrison 20th ed. pg. 1552

TSH: Egg with **T**erminal spine is **S**chistosoma **H**ematobium.

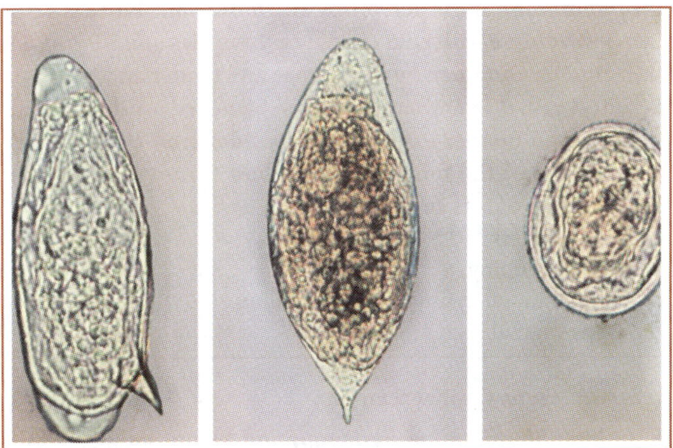

CASE 136

A 30-year-old AIDS positive truck driver is having loose motions since last 2 days. He feels tired and weak. On examination his pulse rate = 100/min with BP= 110/70 mm Hg. Tongue and oral mucosa appear dry. Stool of patient was subjected to modified cold Kinyoun acid-fast staining technique, and examined under an oil immersion lens. Which of the following is the causative organism?

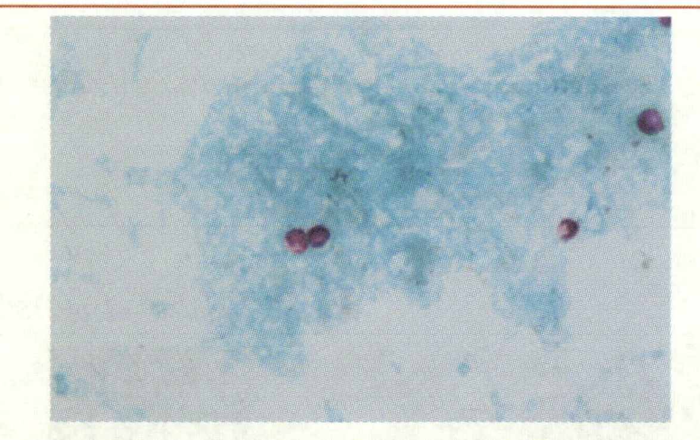

a. Balantidium coli
b. Cryptosporidium
c. Cryptococcus
d. Entamoeba histolytica

Ans. (b) Cryptosporidium

Ref: Harrison 20th ed. pg. 1553-54

The leading cause of diarrhea in an AIDS positive patient is Cryptosporidium parvum. The Kinyoun stain shows oocysts of cryptosporidium. The drug that should be started in this case is nitazoxanide.

CASE 137

A 25-year-old primigravida presents with 6 weeks amenorrhea with severe pain in lower abdomen since morning followed by two episodes of vomiting and prostration. In ER she tells about occasional spotting noticed for last one day, she is perspiring and looks pale. Pulse is 120/min low volume with cold clammy extremities and BP=80/60 mm Hg. Per abdomen bowel is tense and tender and no mass is felt. Vaginal examinations show blanched white vaginal mucosa and further examination was deferred as patient is sick. Which of the following is the best test to confirm the presentation of this case?

a. Culdocentesis
b. Blood grouping
c. Estimation of serum Beta HCG values
d. Trans vaginal scan

Ans. (d) Trans vaginal scan

Ref: DC Dutta Obstetrics, 8th ed. pg. 213

- The clinical scenario is suggestive of ruptured ectopic pregnancy. Due to internal bleeding, patient has gone into hypovolemic shock. A bedside transvaginal scan will reveal blood in cul-de-sac.
- Option A is invasive and less preferred.
- Option B will not confirm the diagnosis. It would however be required for giving blood transfusion to the patient.
- Option C will confirm pregnancy but ectopic nature will not be confirmed.

CASE 138

A 35-year-old G4P3A0L3 female with 12 weeks of amenorrhea presents with vaginal bleeding and has noticed some grape like vesicles expelled per vaginum with lower abdominal discomfort. On pelvic examination uterus is enlarged more than period of gestation and feels doughy. Cervix is favourable and FHS is not heard. Sonography report is shown below. Which is best management of this case?

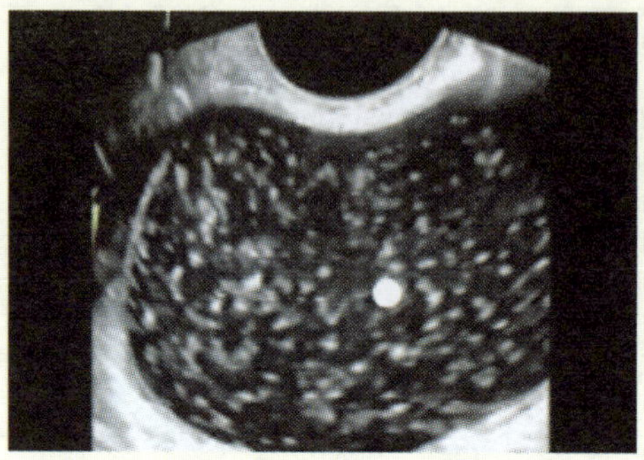

a. Suction evacuation
b. Hysterectomy
c. Hysterotomy
d. Methotrexate

Ans. (a) Suction evacuation

Ref: DC Dutta Obstetrics, 8th ed. pg. 226

- Expulsion of grape like vesicles in a lady with amenorrhea for past few weeks and USG showing snow storm appearance is diagnostic of complete mole.
- The preferred treatment is Suction evacuation. It is rapid, safe and effective in almost all cases and can be even done when the uterus is of 28 weeks gestation.

CASE 139

A 24-year-old primigravida with 26 weeks of gestation by USG report is having complaints of daily headaches and some swelling in her feet. Her BP is measured to be 150/90 mm Hg. She is previously normotensive as per her medical records. Work up shows 2 random clean catch urine specimens having no proteinuria. Fundus examination is normal. KFT and serum uric acid are normal. Which is correct about her diagnosis?

a. Eclampsia
b. Gestational Hypertension
c. Pre-eclampsia
d. Chronic Kidney disease

Ans. (b) Gestational Hypertension

Ref: DC Dutta Obstetrics 8th ed. pg. 255

- The patient has developed hypertension in second trimester of pregnancy but does not have proteinuria or elevated uric acid levels. Pre-eclampsia cannot be diagnosed without presence of proteinuria.

- The clinical diagnosis is gestational hypertension.
- Option A is ruled out as it presents at time of labour. Option D is ruled out KFT is normal.

Features	Gestational HTN	Pre-eclampsia
Hypertension	+	+
Primiparity	+	10%
Recurrence	25–45 %	5%
Proteinurio	Negative	Positive
Gestational age	Usually late (>20 weeks)	Usually early (<20 weeks)
Complications	Rarely	Increase risk
Post partum	Resolve <12 weeks	Resolve <6 weeks

CASE 140

A 30-year-old female was diagnosed as having severe pre-eclampsia and was started on Pritchard regimen. Which of the following is not useful for monitoring of this patient while on Pritchard regimen?

a. Loss of Ankle and knee jerks bilaterally
b. Severe respiratory depression with elevated pCO_2
c. ECG showing Bradycardia
d. Urine output charting showing output less than 60 ml per hour

Ans. (d) Urine output charting showing output less than 60 ml per hour

Ref: Dutta Textbook of Obstetrics: 8th ed. pg. 273

- Pritchard regimen entails administration of magnesium sulphate intramuscularly to a patient of eclampsia. Magnesium reduces release of calcium at neuromuscular junction that regulates Ach release.
- Option A is correct as Ach release at NMJ will reduce with Magnesium administration
- Option B is correct as less Ach at level of diaphragmatic innervation will reduce diaphragm function. This will cause hypoventilation leading to CO_2 retention
- Option C is correct as reduce functioning of Pacemaker of heart will cause drop-in heart rate.
- Urine output can be affected by multiple factors like blood loss during delivery, presence of sepsis and excess drip rate of oxytocin. Hence it would not be a reliable method of determining magnesium toxicity.

CASE 141

Which of the following conditions in a pregnant woman/will have least risk of maternal mortality?

a. Coarctation of aorta
b. Mitral stenosis with Dyspnea grade IV
c. Uncorrected Fallot's tetralogy
d. Bioprosthetic valve

Ans. (d) Bioprosthetic valve

Ref: Dutta Textbook of Obstetrics 8th ed. pg. 321

Risk of Maternal Mortality with Heart Disease (NYHA, 1992)	
Cardiac Disease	Mortality (%)
Group 1 (minimal risk): ASD, VSD, PDA, Fallot tetralogy (corrected), Mitral stenosis (NYHA) — Grade I and II), Bioprosthetic valve	0-1
Group 2 (moderate risk): MS (NYHA—III and IV) AS, Marfan Syndrome (normal aorta) Fallot tetralogy (uncorrected), M S with atrial fibrillation, artificial valve	5-15
Group 3 (major risk): Pulmonary hypertension, Marfan syndrome (aortic involvement) aortic coarctation with valvular involvement	25-50

CASE 142

A 30-year-old know case of GTCS on Sodium valproate for last 5 years has presented with 32 weeks of pregnancy completed at your tertiary care hospital. Which of the following is unlikely to be seen in the fetus?

a. Cleft lip/Palate
b. Anencephaly
c. Neonatal haemorrhage
d. Neonatal Seizures

Ans. (d) Neonatal Seizures

Ref: Dutta Textbook of Obstetrics 8th ed. pg. 338

- Use of anti-epilepsy drug like Sodium Valproate in a female in the first trimester of pregnancy will lead to neural tube defects like anencephaly and cranio-facial malformations.
- Valproate leads to vitamin K deficiency and increased incidence of haemorrhagic disease of newborn. This can present as intracranial haemorrhage.

CASE 143

A 28-year-old G2P1A0L1 female presents in labour pain at 34 weeks of gestation for past 6 hours. On examination she looks tired, anxious and HR = 110/min with BP of 140/90 mm Hg. Pelvic examination shows periodic uterine contraction with fetal heart rate of 80/min. CTG was done and shows FHR of persistently < 100/min. Which of the following is not to be done in this case?

a. Give Betamethasone to mother
b. Left lateral position
c. Tocolysis with Atosiban
d. Requisition for Blood transfusion and Plan for urgent LSCS

Ans. (c) Tocolysis with Atosiban

Ref: DC Dutta Obstetrics, 8th ed. pg. 367-68

- The patient is in preterm labour with regular contractions with evidence of fetal distress. Hence, steroids should be administered to mother to accelerate fetal lung maturation. She should be placed in left lateral position to improve venous return to her heart. OT needs to be prepped up as she will need an urgent LSCS in lieu of fetal distress.
- There is no role of tocolysis in scenario of preterm labour with fetal distress.

CASE 144

A primigravida 30-year-old female has developed Leakage per vaginum for last 36 hours at 32 weeks of gestation. Which complication can develop in the mother?

a. Amniotic fluid embolism
b. Complete abortion
c. Chorioamnionitis
d. Respiratory distress syndrome

Ans. (c) Chorioamnionitis

Ref: Dutta Textbook of Obstetrics 8th ed. pg. 371

The patient has gone into preterm labour with premature rupture of membranes for > 24 hours. She is at risk of developing ascending infection from vagina leading to chorioamnionitis.

CASE 145

A 34-year-old nulliparous woman is having anemia. Menstrual history has irregular cycles with heavy bleeding. TVS and Color Doppler shows multiple fibroids in an enlarged uterus. All are true about this condition except?

a. Centre of fibroid is least vascular and is likely to degenerate
b. Cervical fibroids can kink the ureter
c. Mifepristone is effective to reduce fibroid size and menorrhagia
d. Subserous pedunculated fibroid is best diagnosed with Saline infusion sonography

Ans. (d) Subserous pedunculated fibroid is best diagnosed with Saline infusion sonography

Ref: Dutta Textbook of Obstetrics 8th ed. pg. 225

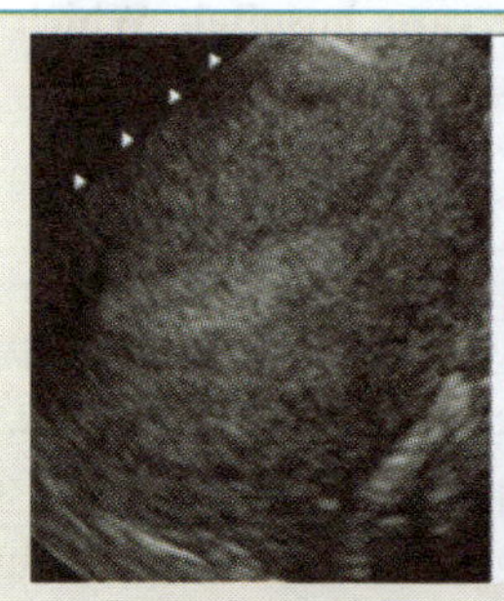

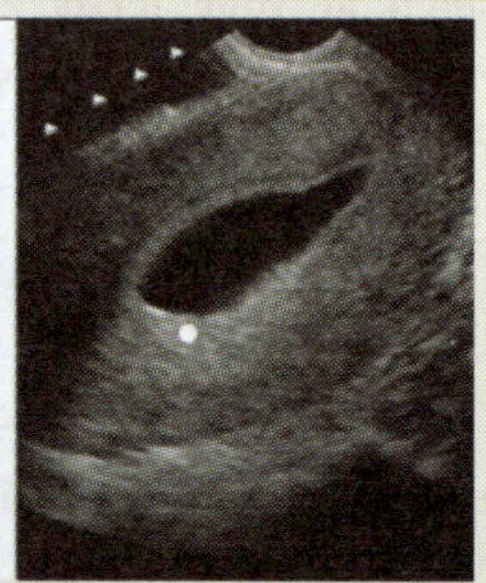

Notice that uterine walls are opposed. Infusion of saline will separate the walls and ensure evaluation of endometrium as well as submucosal fibroids

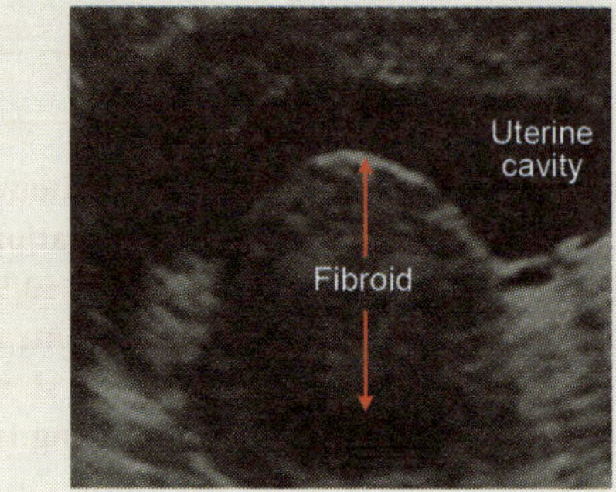

Sub serous fibroids *cannot* be diagnosed by transvaginal scan.
Option A is correct as its blood supply tapers towards the middle of growth
Option B is correct as ureter is 1.25 cm lateral to internal os and hence a cervical fibroid can easily kink the ureter as it grows.
Option C is Correct as Mifepristone (RU-486) competitively binds and inhibits progesterone receptors. Studies have suggested that fibroid growth depends on the sexual steroids. Mifepristone has been shown to decrease fibroid size and reduce the associated bleeding.

CASE 146

Cervical cancer that extends into ureter leading to hydroureter and hydronephrotic changes in the kidney belong to stage _____ as per FIGO staging.

a. I
b. II
c. III
d. IV

Ans. (c) III

Ref: Dutta Textbook of Gynecology, 7th ed. pg. 283

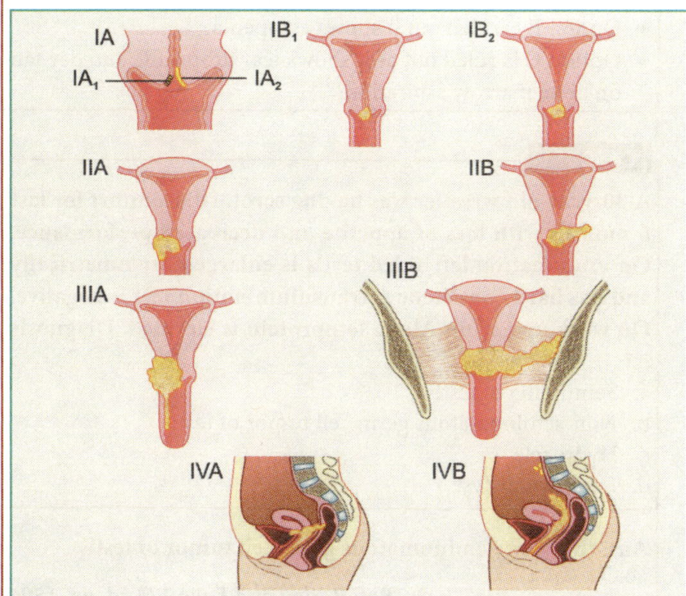

Spread of cervical cancer to ureter and development of hydronephrosis is seen in stage III. The resultant uraemia is the leading cause of death in undiagnosed cervical cancer.
Infiltration of cancer directly to bladder and rectum constitutes stage IV.
The leading route of spread of cervical cancer is via direct spread.

CASE 147

A 55-year-old woman developed sudden onset excruciating eye pain and blurring of vision while watching a movie in cinema hall. She has to leave the movie hall use washroom as she had 2 episodes of vomiting and eye pain has worsened. On examination her left cornea appears hazy and left pupil mid dilated, vertically oval pupil which is fixed and does not react to light. What is the diagnosis?

a. Cluster headache
b. Acute angle closure glaucoma
c. Acute iridocyclitis
d. Sub arachnoid haemorrhage

Ans. (b) Acute angle closure glaucoma

Ref: Harrison 20th ed. pg. 87

- The key word in this patient presenting with acute red eye and retroorbital pain is vertically oval pupil which is seen with acute angle closure glaucoma. The trigger in this case is pupillary dilatation due to watching movie in dark.
- Option A is ruled out as it does not have hazy cornea or pupillary findings
- Option C is ruled out as it presents with circumcorneal flush and aqueous flare
- Option D is ruled out as it presents with headache and features of raised ICP.

CASE 148

A 4-year-old child from low socioeconomic strata is brought by his mother for complaints of excessive crying at night. You are the intern posted at PHC and identify the cheesy lesions on temporal side of cornea bilaterally. Which of the following is responsible for development of this lesion?

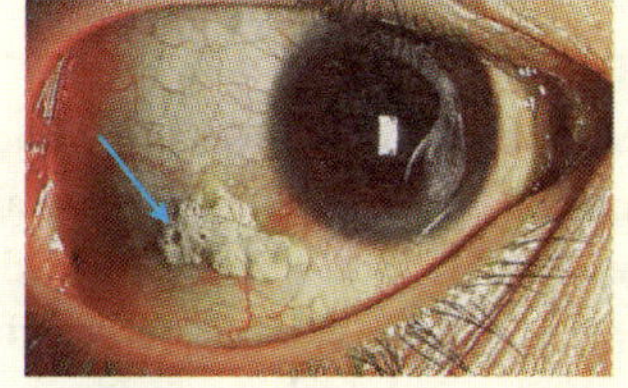

a. Moraxella catarrhalis
b. Corynebacterium Xerosis
c. Riboflavin deficiency
d. Niacin deficiency

Ans. (b) Corynebacterium Xerosis

Ref: Parson Diseases of Eye: 23rd ed. pg. 163

- The child is having features of Vitamin A deficiency that leads to xerophthalmia. Since the child is not able to see the mother at night, he/she will be afraid and cries himself to sleep. The image shows bitot spots that are seen bilaterally on temporal side of cornea.

- The chief changes are in the epithelium of conjunctiva which stops to secrete mucus and becomes epidermoid like that of skin with granular and horny layers. It has been documented that Corynebacterium xerosis grows profusely in these lesions.

CASE 149

A 30-year-old female is complaining of dyspnea at rest for last 4 months with noisy breathing. CXR of patient was done and showed Hilar lymphadenopathy. CT guided biopsy of lung tissue showed presence of Asteroid bodies. Diagnosis is?

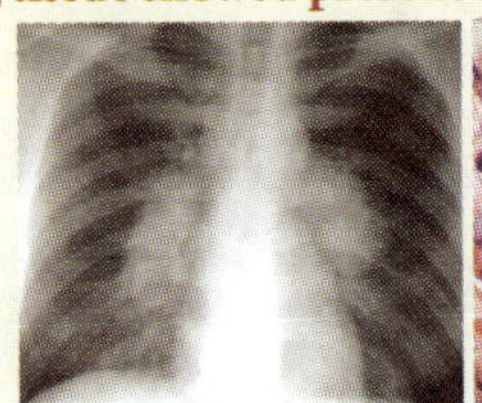

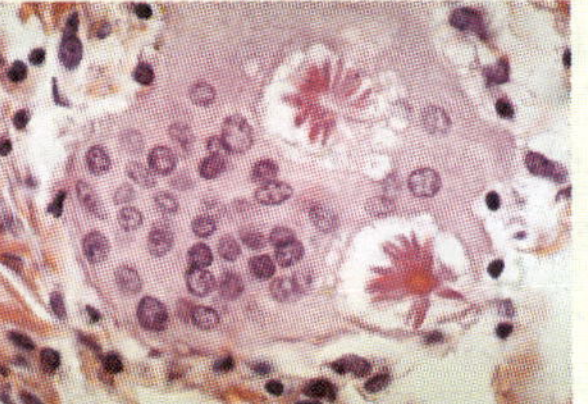

a. Silicosis
b. Anthracosis
c. Sarcoidosis
d. Coal workers' pneumoconiosis

Ans. (c) Sarcoidosis

Ref: Harrison 20th ed. pg. 2601

- The CXR shows bilateral hilar lymphadenopathy with some reticular opacities seen in right lower lung field. CT guided biopsy shows asteroid bodies. These features are diagnostic of sarcoidosis.
- Option A can have bilateral hilar lymphadenopathy but occupational history of working in glass industry should be present. Asteroid bodies are seen in sarcoidosis while silicosis patients have higher incidence of tuberculosis.
- Option B and D are ruled out in absence of any occupational exposure.

CASE 150

A 70-year-old man developed severe low backache and had difficulty in ambulation. MRI Lumbo-sacral spine showed multiple lytic lesions. Hence work up was done and shows Hb = 9 gm%, Increased TLC, ESR of 100 mm fall in first hour, normal serum alkaline phosphatase. Bone marrow biopsy showed the following cells. What is the diagnosis?

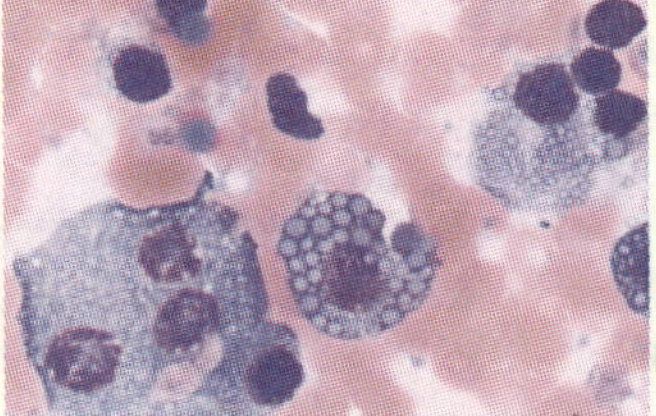

a. Osteoporosis
b. Myelodysplasia
c. Myelofibrosis
d. Plasmacytoma

Ans. (d) Plasmacytoma

Ref: Harrison 20th ed. pg. 793

- Multiple lytic lesions in spine with normal SAP and Bone marrow biopsy showing mott cells is diagnostic of plasmacytoma/multiple myeloma.
- Option A is ruled out as it does not anemia, elevated ESR and any abnormal cells in blood or bone marrow.
- Option B is ruled out it shows cytopenia.
- Option C is ruled out as it shows tear drop RBC and dry tap on bone marrow aspiration.

CASE 151

A 30-year-old wrestler was having scrotal discomfort for last 6 months with loss of appetite and decreased performance. On examination left sided testis is enlarged asymmetrically and has hard consistency. Transillumination test is negative. On work up Serum Alpha fetoprotein is elevated. Diagnosis is?

a. Seminoma of testis
b. Non-seminomatous germ cell tumor of testis
c. Hydrocele
d. Epididymal cyst

Ans. (b) Non-seminomatous germ cell tumor of testis

Ref: Bailey and Love 27th ed. pg. 1506

- Testicular mass that distorts the shape of testis with elevated alpha feto protein values is suggestive of non-seminomatous testis tumor.
- Transillumination test is positive in cystic lesions like hydrocele. It is negative in this case as it a solid tumor.

	Seminoma	Nonseminomatous
	Localized to the testis	Extension to the epididymis, spermatic cord, or scrotal sac
Stage	I or II	II or III
Metastasis	Lymphatic	Lymphatic hematogenous to lung or liver
Treatment	Radiotherapy	Chemotherapy
Prognosis	Good	Depend on the tumor type

CASE 152

A 30-year-old patient from rural India is admitted with symptoms of abdominal pain and fever for last 2 weeks. His blood culture is drawn with complete blood count and intravenous ceftriaxone with ofloxacin was started in the patient. Immediately the patient turned blue and had difficulty in breathing. Which of the following cells is responsible for the following presentation?

a. Eosinophil
b. Basophil
c. Monocyte
d. Macrophage

Ans. (b) **Basophil**

Ref: Robbins 10th ed. pg. 208

- On administration of third generation cephalosporin the patient developed features of anaphylaxis.
- Basophils play the major role in IgG-mediated systemic anaphylaxis. Upon capture of IgG-allergen complexes, basophils release platelet-activating factor that increases vascular permeability, leading to anaphylactic shock.

CASE 153

A 30-year-old man is having recurrent episodes of purulent bronchorrhea for last 2 years. He has presented at night in ER with one episode of hemoptysis. On examinations vitals are stable, gag reflex is intact and changes in nails of patient were noted. An urgent HRCT was done in the case and image is attached. Which is the most common histopathological subtype of the clinical diagnosis of patient?

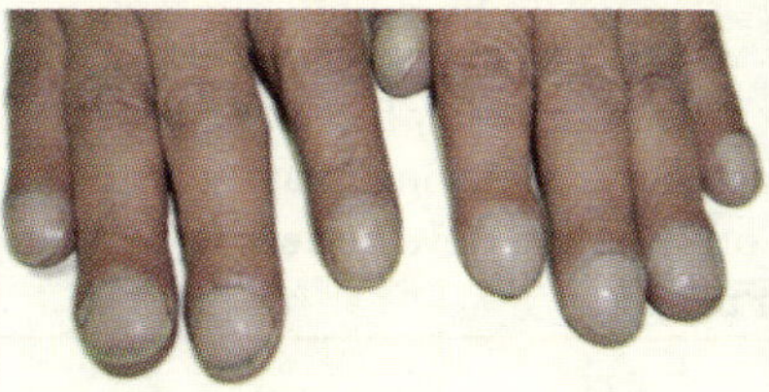

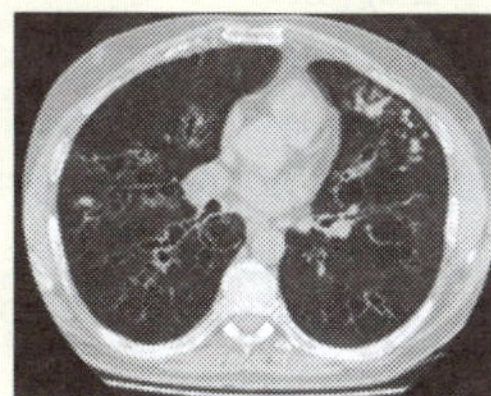

a. Cylindrical subtype
b. Fusiform subtype
c. Centroacinar subtype
d. Panacinar subtype

Ans. (a) **Cylindrical subtype**

Ref: Robbins 10th ed. pg. 691

Presence of purulent bronchorrhea with haemoptysis can be seen in chronic bronchitis as well as bronchiectasis.

The image shows digital clubbing with HRCT showing dilated airways with distorted morphology. This implies patient is having bronchiectasis.

Leading histopathological subtype of bronchiectasis is cylindrical one.

CASE 154

A 60-year-old smoker is having flank pain and haematuria episodes for last 3 months. On examination a lump was felt in right paraumbilical area which was bimanually palpable and ballotable. CT abdomen shows a mass originating from the left kidney and invading the inferior vena cava. Which of the following is the rarest variety of RCC?

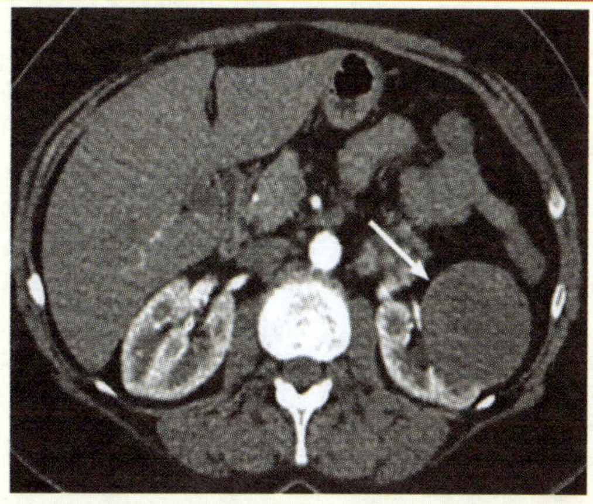

a. Clear cell type
b. Collecting duct type
c. Papillary type
d. Chromophobe type

Ans. (b) **Collecting duct type**

Ref: Robbins 10th ed. pg. 950

The image shows an exophytic mass growing and distorting the left kidney parenchyma. The same mass is bimanually palpable and ballotable on per abdomen examination. The diagnosis is renal cell cancer. The least common subtype of RCC is collecting duct type.

It is also called as Bellini duct carcinoma and arises from collecting duct cells in the medulla.

CASE 155

A 30-year-old female is having severe epigastric pain since last evening. She has been given Pantoprazole oral as well as intravenously but the pain is persisting. She feels nauseous but says she is not able to vomit. NG tube was introduced in high fowler position but the NG tube is getting stuck. Hence, oral contrast was given and an X-ray was done. There is no past history of such episodes. Which of the following is the probable diagnosis of this patient?

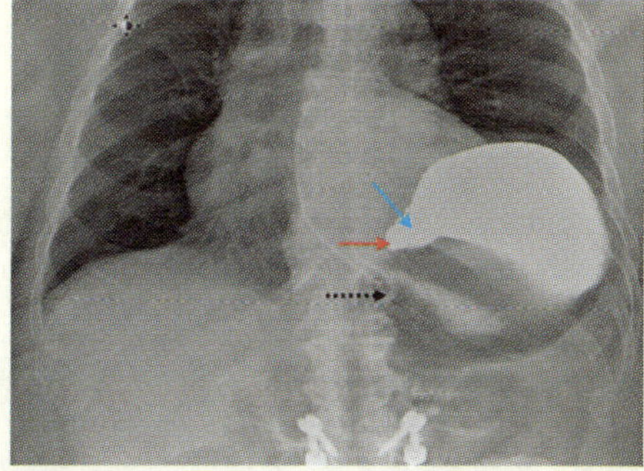

a. Empyema Gall Bladder
b. Stomach Volvulus
c. Schatzki ring of Esophagus
d. Stricture of Esophagus

Ans. (b) Stomach Volvulus

Ref: Sabiston 19th ed. pg. 1223

- The main catchword is inability to pass NG tube in a patient with epigastric pain and retching without vomiting. This is feature of Borchardt triad used to diagnose stomach Volvulus.
- Option A is ruled out as it will present with fever, chills and RUQ pain
- Option B leads to non-progressive dysphagia mainly to non-vegetarian food items.
- Option C will have history of corrosive ingestion

CASE 156

A 30-year-old female has multinodular goiter and is having extensive weight loss in spite of medication. One of the nodules has grown rapidly in last 6 months and is currently 4 X 4 cm. It is stony hard in consistency and berry sign is positive. Bone scan shows metastasis to skull. Total Thyroidectomy with central node compartment dissection was done. Which is not correct about this condition?

a. Thyroglobulin estimation is done for follow up
b. FNAC is inconclusive and on table frozen section biopsy is useful to confirm diagnosis
c. Post-operative radioactive iodine is used and patient is kept in isolation
d. Paraffin section of formalin tissue will reveal orphan Annie eye nucleus appearance

Ans. (c) Post-operative radioactive iodine is used and patient is kept in isolation

Ref: Bailey and Love 27th ed. pg. 818-19

- Rapid growth of thyroid nodule with weight loss points to thyroid malignancy.
- Bony metastasis is seen with follicular cancer of thyroid. Berry sign implies infiltration of thyroid cancer around carotid artery leading to difficulty to palpate the carotid artery of the patient.
- Option A is correct as thyroglobulin levels are used to identify recurrence of follicular cancer of thyroid
- Option B is correct as follicular nature will be distorted on FNAC and hence intra-op frozen section will confirm diagnosis
- Option C is correct as Radioactive iodine ablation is used to treat the metastasis that have occurred by hematogenous route but are not being diagnosed by conventional imaging methods.
- Option D is wrong as orphan Annie eye nucleus is found in papillary carcinoma of thyroid.

CASE 157

A 45-year-old post-menopausal woman presents with a soft swelling close to lateral canthus which has been present since childhood. It is painless, with smooth surface, and indents the adjacent bone. The overlying skin is normal and freely mobile over the swelling. Comment on the diagnosis.

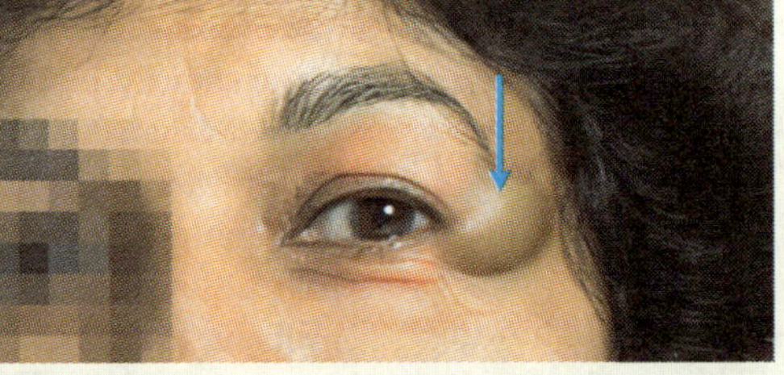

a. Lipoma
b. Dermoid
c. Sebaceous cyst
d. Glomus tumor

Ans. (d) Dermoid

Ref: Bailey and Love 27th ed. pg. 673

Angular dermoid cysts are common peri-orbital tumors in children and if neglected can become disfiguring in adult life. Characteristically benign and slow growing, they are tumors of embryonic origin that arise along bony sutures as a result of abnormal ectodermal sequestration during development. The best management is surgical excision with a well concealed scar.

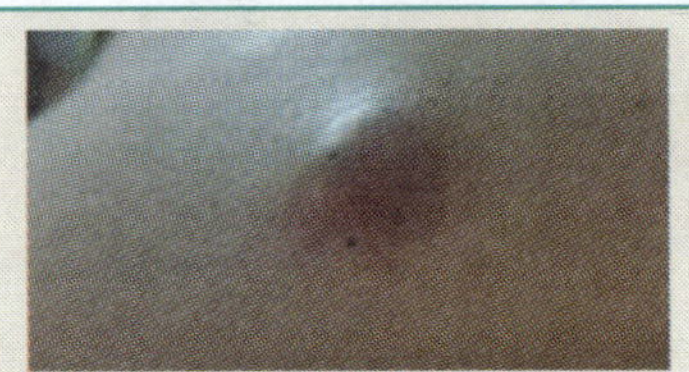

Sebaceous cyst

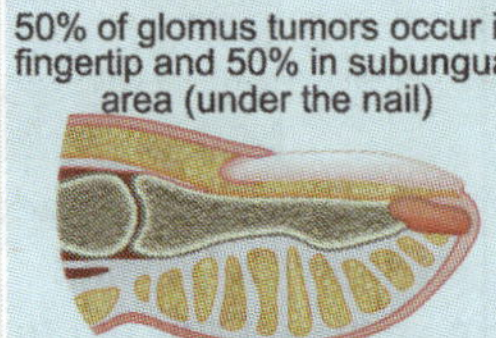

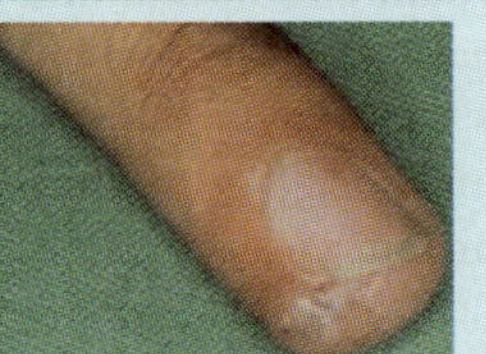

Glomus tumor in finger tip

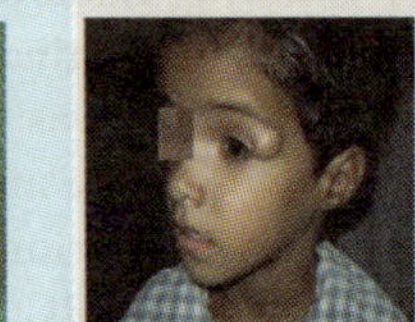

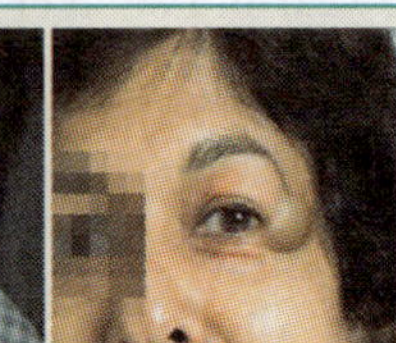

Angular dermoid

CASE 158

A 60 Kg patient is admitted with dehydration due to multiple vomiting episodes. You order one vac of isotonic 0.9% saline using the cannula shown in the image. The nurse has set up the drip. Which is correct about the images shown?

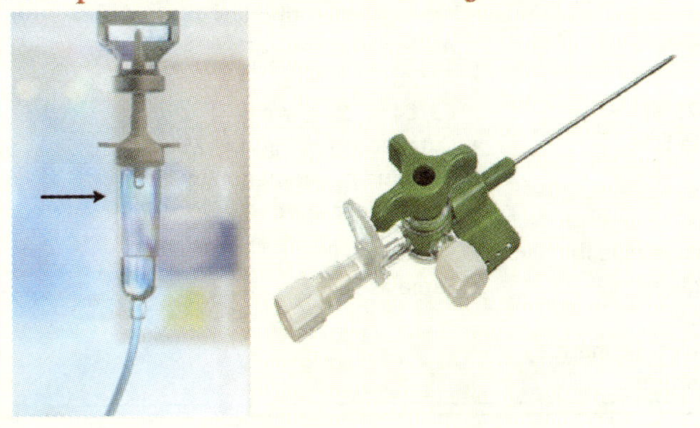

a. 1 ml = 16 drops per minute, 18 G cannula
b. 1 ml = 60 drops per minute, 20 G cannula
c. 1 ml = 16 drops per minute, 20 G cannula
d. 1 ml = 60 drops per minute, 18 G cannula

Ans. (a) 1 ml = 16 drops per minute, 18 G cannula

Ref: Oxford Surgical Handbook E-Book pg. 65

The image shows a 18G green cannula use to transfuse blood or IV fluids. The drip rate of 16 drops per minute implies 1ml has been infused. In pediatric drip set 60 micro drops constitute 1 ml. The calibration is important as fluids or drugs may be given as infusion per minute or hour.

CASE 159

Which of the following is not present in Ringer lactate?

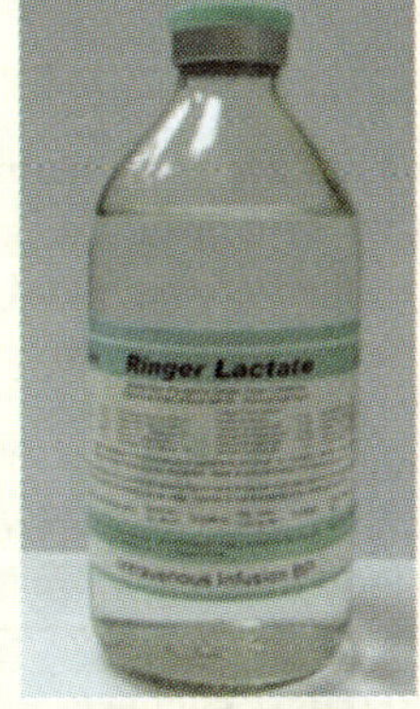

a. Sodium
b. Glucose
c. Calcium
d. Bicarbonate

Ans. (b) Glucose

Ref: Bailey and Love 27th ed. pg. 323, 624

Ringer Lactate

- Most physiological solution
- Electrolyte composition similar to ECF
- One litre of lactated Ringer's solution contains:
  - Sodium ion = 130 mmol/L.
  - Chloride ion = 109 mmol/L.
  - Lactate = 28 mmol/L.
  - Potassium ion = 4 mmol/L.
  - Calcium ion = 1.5 mmol/L
  - Osmolarity of 273, pH of 6.5

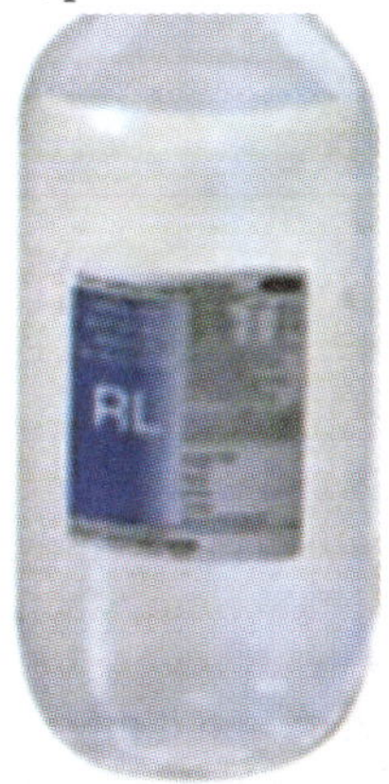

CASE 160

A 65-year-old lady was having facial skin lesions. Her dermatologist tested her for anti-histone antibodies which are positive. All of the following can cause drug induced lupus except?

a. Hydralazine
b. Isoniazid
c. Sulfonylurea
d. Penicillamine

Ans. (c) Sulfonylurea

Ref: Harrison 20th ed. pg. 2517

The causes of Drug induced lupus is SHIP2
S: Sulpha drugs like Sulfonamides
H: Hydralazine
I: INH
P: Procainamide, d-Pencillamine

Findings	SLE	DILE
• Clinical	• Average age of onset of 20-30 y • Affects blacks more than whites • Female-to-male ratio of 9:1	• Average age of onset of 50-70 y • Affects whites more than blacks • Female-to-male ratio of 1:1
• Laboratory	• Antihistone antibodies in 50% • Anti-dsDNA present in 80% • C3/C4 levels decrease • Cutaneous findings in >75% • Raynaud phenomenon in 50% • Antinuclear antibodies in >95%	• Antihistone antibodies in >95% • Anti-ssDNA present • Anti-dsDNA rare • C3/C4 levels normal • Cutaneous findings in ~25% • Raynaud phenomenon in 25% • Antinuclear antibodies in >95%
• Immunofluorescence Histopathology	• Direct immunofluorescence reveals granular deposition of IgG at dermoepidermal junction • Lymphohistiocytic interface dermatitis • Apoptosis basal vacuolization	• Same as SLE • Same as SLE

CASE 161

A 25-year-old tall thin man comes to your OPD with complaints of dragging sensation in groin and scrotum on left side. On examination in standing position impulse of coughing is present. His scrotum feels like a bag of worms and supine position leads to reduction of the tortuous swelling. Which is correct about this condition?

a. USG abdomen to look for tumor of Adrenals
b. Unilocular acquired retention cyst
c. Urgent aspiration
d. Excision via scrotal approach

Ans. (d) Excision via scrotal approach

Ref: SRB: 5th ed. pg. 1076

- The clinical finding of bag of worms feeling in scrotum points to Varicocele. It leads to dilatation and tortuosity of pampiniform plexus of veins and testicular veins. It is more common on left side.
- The leading cause is idiopathic but can occur due to left sided renal cell cancer with tumor thrombus in left renal vein leading to obstruction to venous flow of left testicular vein.
- *Venous doppler should be done for scrotum and groin and since it is mentioned as a tortuous swelling, excision of veins should be done.*

CASE 162

Middle aged male presents with a scrotal swelling which has been present for previous 6 months. It shows positive fluctuation and the surgeon can get above the swelling. Which of the following is not to be done in the patient?

a. Lord's plication
b. Jaboulay's procedure
c. Aspiration
d. Evacuation and Eversion

Ans. (c) Aspiration

Ref: SRB: 5th ed. pg. 1072

The clinical presentation is of a hydrocele. The key word is that surgeon can get above the swelling. The surgeries for hydrocele are:

- Subtotal excision of sac
- Jaboulay's Operation
- Evacuation and Eversion
- Lord's plication
- Sharma and Jhawers Technique (After excision, the sac with the testis is placed in newly created pocket between the fascial layers of the scrotum).

CASE 163

A 25-year-old male presents with inability to place back the retracted preputial skin over the glans. The glans is edematous, swollen with severe pain and tenderness. Which is initial management of this condition?

a. Dorsal slit to relieve edema
b. Urgent circumcision
c. Injection of lignocaine in swollen part to reduce pain
d. Part elevation and local dressing

Ans. (a) Dorsal slit to relieve edema

Ref: SRB: 5th ed. pg. 1061

The key word in the question in inability to push back the preputial skin over the glans penis post intercourse indicating development of Paraphimosis.

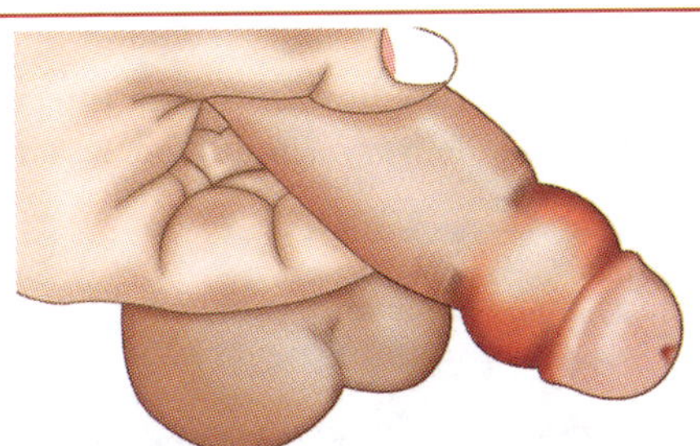

Manual reduction should be tried. If it fails, initial dorsal slit is made to reduce edema and compression. Antibiotics and analgesics are given. Circumcision is done after 3 weeks.

CASE 164

A 35-year-old alcoholic has presented with 2 episodes of hematemesis. On examination his pulse rate is 100/min with BP of 90/60 mm Hg. Per abdomen examination shows spleen palpable 3 cm below costal margin. Which is true about this patient?

a. Elevated CRP and Low C3
b. Most common site of bleeding is First part of duodenum
c. Urgent Elective intubation of patient
d. The increased portal vein pressure should be lowered with octreotide

Ans. (d) The increased pressure of portal vein pressure should be lowered with octreotide

Ref: CMDT 2019 pg. 627

- The presence of splenomegaly with hematemesis points to etiology of portal hypertension. Hence after stabilization of patients with fluids, octreotide should be started to lower the pressure in portal vein.
- The leading cause of hematemesis is peptic ulcer disease *but* this patient is having portal hypertension leading to vomiting of blood.

CASE 165

A pregnant lady was admitted with diagnosis of PIH for monitoring and bed rest. In supine position which of the following is a complication of the below representation?

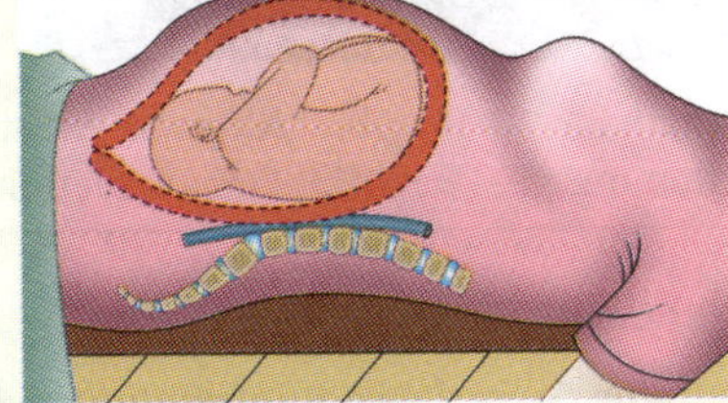

a. Abdominal aorta syndrome
b. Supine vena cava syndrome
c. Ascending aorta syndrome
d. Superior vena cava syndrome

Ans. (b) Supine vena cava syndrome

Ref: William Obstetrics pg. 1369

The image shows the developing baby compressing the IVC of the mother. This will lead to reduced venous return and development of dizziness and hypotension in the mother. This is called supine hypotension syndrome or supine vena cava syndrome.

CASE 166

A 25-year-old primigravida has presented in obstructed labor. On examination she is exhausted and has a tender uterus with a groove felt per abdomen as shown in the image. Fetal parts are not felt. What is the diagnosis?

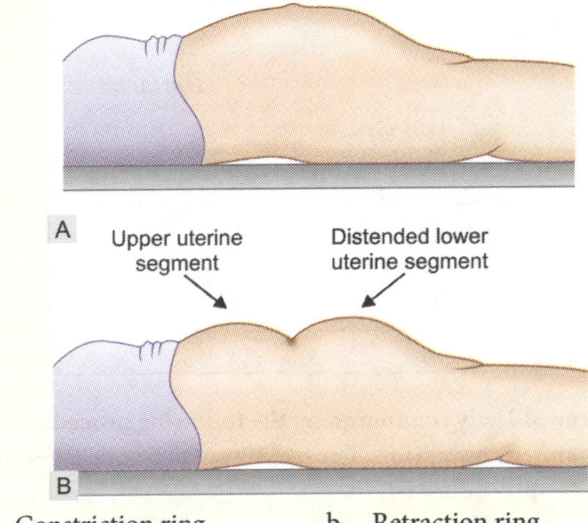

a. Constriction ring
b. Retraction ring
c. Abruptio placentae
d. Cervical dystocia

Ans. (b) Retraction ring

Ref: Dutta 8th ed. pg. 421

The presence of an exhausted patient with a tender uterus favours diagnosis of retraction ring. Please note that constriction ring is *only revealed during CS in first stage, forceps application during second stage and during manual removal in 3rd stage.*

Pathological retraction ring	Constriction ring
Occurs in prolonged 2nd stage	Occurs in the 1st, 2nd or 3rd stage
Always between upper and lower uterine segments	At any level of the uterus
Rises up	Does not change its position
Felt and seen abdominally	Felt only vaginally
The uterus is tonically retracted, tender and the fetal parts cannot be felt	The uterus is not tonically retracted and the fetal parts can be felt
Maternal distress and fetal distress or death	Maternal and fetal distress may not be present
Relieved only by delivery of the fetus	May be relieved by anesthetics or antispasmodics

CASE 167

The following instrument is used for performing aspiration of uterine cavity within ________ days of a missed period in a woman with previously normal cycle

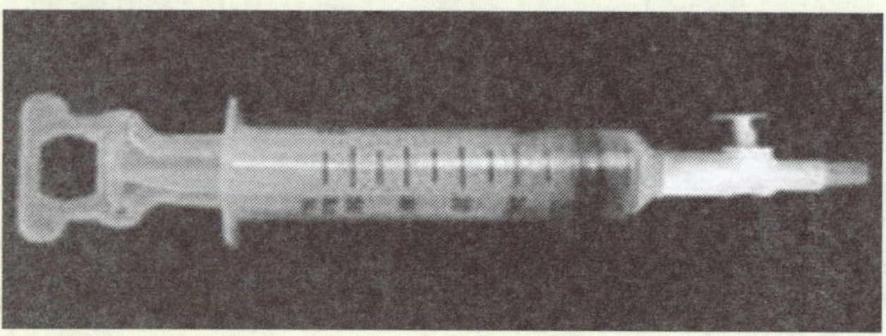

a. 14 days
b. 28 days
c. 42 days
d. 72 days

Ans. (a) 14 days

Ref: Datta: 8th ed. pg. 646

The image shows 50 ml syringe used for performing menstrual regulation. After cervical dilatation, Karman cannula is inserted and attached to the syringe for aspiration. The cannula is rotated, pushed in and out with gentle strokes. This method is used within 14 days of a missed period in a woman with a previous normal cycle.

CASE 168

A 25-year-old lady is undergoing the following procedure for an unplanned conception. The maximum pressure generated during the procedure is?

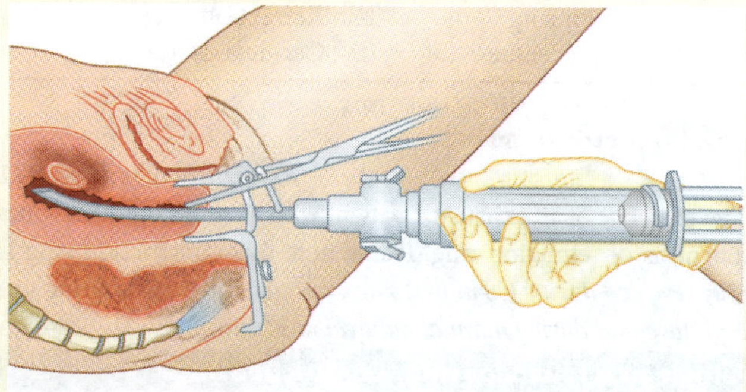

a. 100–200 mm Hg
b. 200–400 mm Hg
c. 400–600 mm Hg
d. 600–800 mm Hg

Ans. (c) 400–600 mm Hg

Ref: Datta 8th ed. pg. 646

The image shows suction evacuation being performed. The pressure of suction is raised to 400–600 mm Hg. The end-point of the suction evacuation procedure is when the cannula is gripped by a contracted uterus with a grating sensation.

CASE 169

During the following procedure, optimum interval between uterine incision and delivery should be less than _____ seconds.

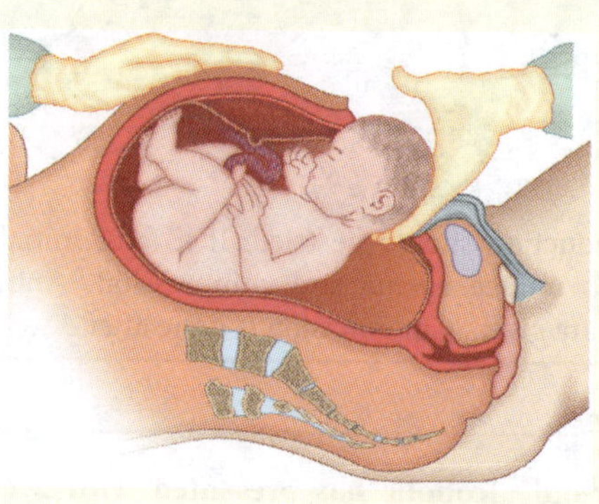

a. 30 seconds
b. 45 seconds
c. 60 seconds
d. 90 seconds

Ans. (d) 90 seconds

Ref: Datta, 8th ed. pg. 673

The image shows LSCS being performed, with the head being delivered by hooking fingers carefully between the lower uterine flap. The head is delivered by elevation and flexion using the palm as fulcrum and the *optimum time between the uterine incision and delivery should be less than 90 seconds.*

CASE 170

The following patient presented to the OPD with history of hair loss. There was no erythema, scarring or scratching. Diagnosis is?

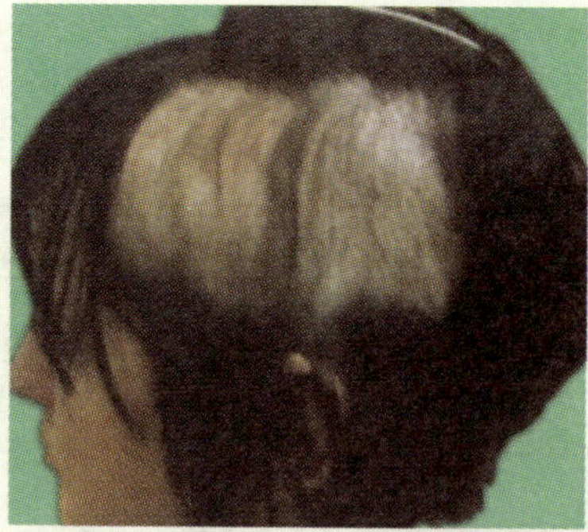

a. Trichotillomania
b. Alopecia Areata
c. Telogen Effluvium
d. Tinea infection

Ans. (a) Trichotillomania

Ref: Rook's Textbook of Dermatology, 9th ed. pg. 86

- In Trichotillomania, the hairs are plucked from fronto-parietal region and a *bizarre angular pattern of hair loss* is produced.

- Telogen effluvium develops when hair follicles go into telogen or resting face prematurely. It is related to stress like chronic illness, depression and pregnancy. It is more common in women
- Alopecia areata has a *clear demarcation* without any signs of inflammation or exclamation mark hair.

CASE 171

A child has been brought with the following scalp lesion with history of itching in scalp and hair loss for past 2 months. Which of the following is useful for diagnosis of this patient?

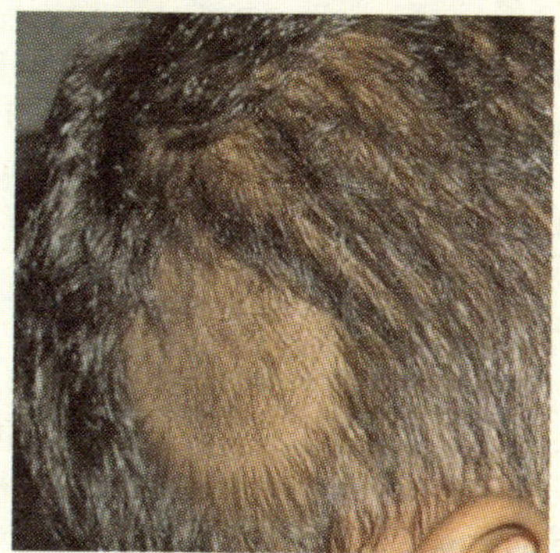

a. Gram stain
b. KOH mount
c. Slit Skin smear
d. Tzanck smear

Ans. (b) KOH mount

Ref: Fitzpatrick's Dermatology, 8th ed. pg. 2284-85

The image shows *black dot sign* classical of tinea capitis. The hairs are damaged due to endothrix infection and break easily.

CASE 172

The following image shows?

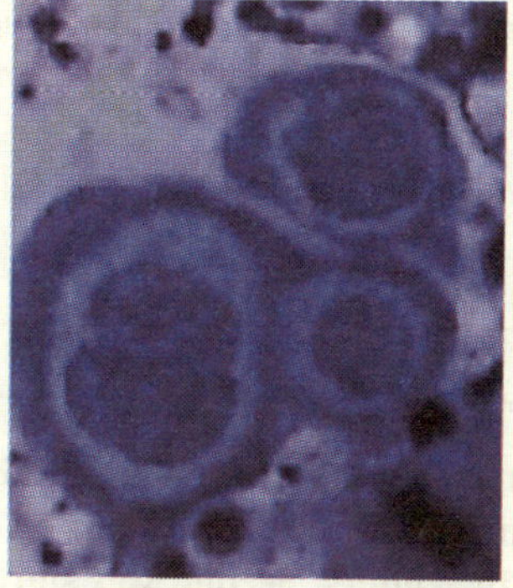

a. Acanthocyte
b. Acantholytic cell
c. Sezary cells
d. Clue cells

Ans. (b) Acantholytic cell

Ref: IAVDL Colour Atlas of Dermatology pg. 565

The image shows multinucleate giant cell with peripheral rim of cytoplasm. This is an acantholytic cell (Tzanck cell) which is a large rounded keratinocyte.

Primary acantholysis	Secondary acantholysis
• Pemphigus • Staphylococcal scalded skin syndrome • Darier disease • Hailey-Hailey disease	Seen in viral infection like herpes

CASE 173

A 10-year-old child presents with fever and wound with discharging pus from right thigh for 4 months. Given below is the X-ray of the patient. Identify the marked area.

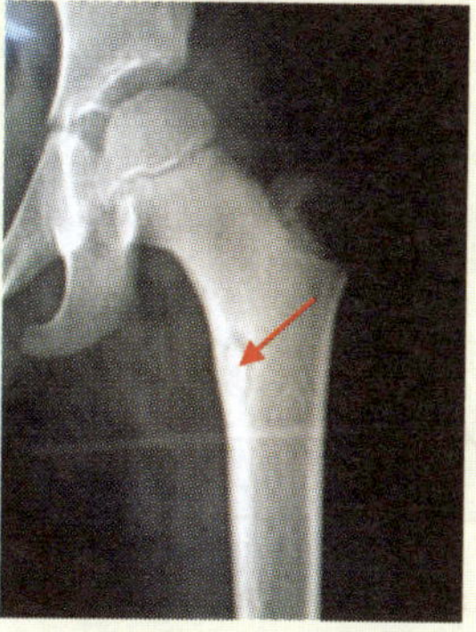

a. Sequestrum
b. Cloacae
c. Involucrum
d. Woven bone

Ans. (a) Sequestrum

Ref: Essential Orthopaedics, Maheshwari 5th ed. pg. 172

- The image shows a radio-dense area (marked by blue arrow) than the surrounding bone. Between the marked devitalized irregular bone fragment and normal bone is a radiolucent rim of granulation tissue.
- Involucrum is the *subperiosteal* reactive bone and hence, is ruled out due to location.

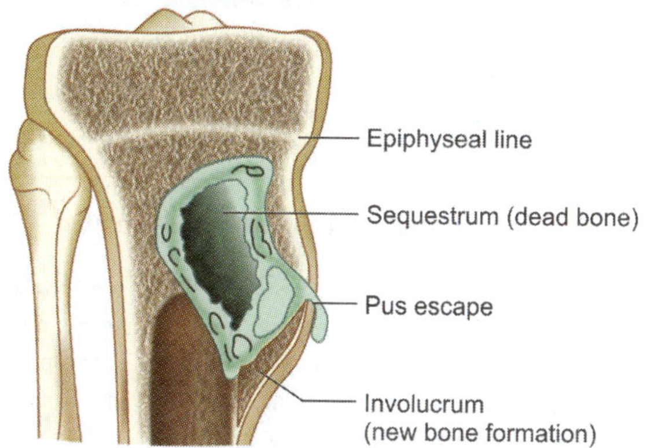

CASE 174

A 4-year-old boy fell on outstretched hand. X-ray is shown below. Which blood vessel is most commonly affected?

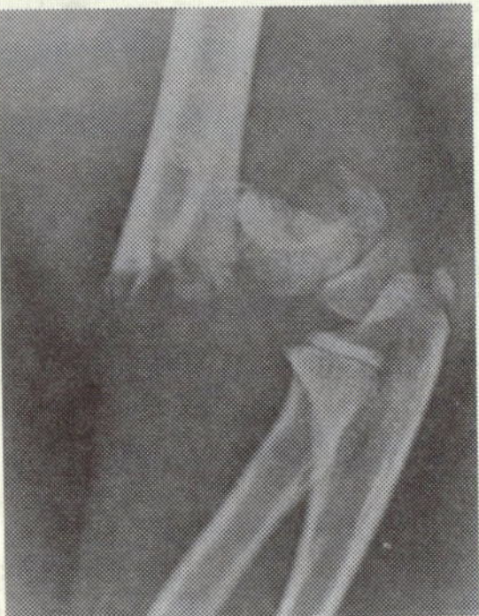

a. Ulnar artery
b. Radial artery
c. Brachial artery
d. Cubital vein

Ans. (c) **Brachial artery**

Ref: Essential Orthopaedics, Maheshwari 5th ed. pg. 97

The image shows displaced supracondylar fracture of humerus and the spike of proximal segment can easily traumatize the brachial artery.

CASE 175

An elderly patient slipped in the bathroom and sustained injury over the hip joint. X-ray is shown below. Her attitude of leg will be?

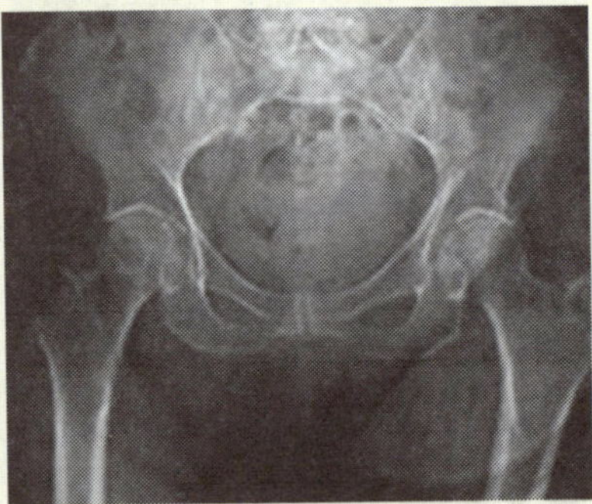

a. Shortened, abducted and externally rotated
b. Shortened and abducted
c. Lengthened and internally rotated
d. Flexed and adducted and internally rotated

Ans. (a) **Shortened, abducted and externally rotated**

Ref: Essential Orthopaedics, Maheshwari 5th ed. pg. 134

The image shows fracture of neck of femur on right side. This is commonly seen due to trivial trauma in older patients. Minimal limb shortening can be seen with limb showing flexion, abduction and external rotation.

CASE 176

A 40-year-old male complains of hot flushes each time he bathes. Hb: 20%gm, Platelet: 1,89,000/mm^3, WBC: 30,000/mm^3, Investigation revealed JAK2 mutation. What is the most likely diagnosis?

a. Progressive massive fibrosis
b. Chronic myeloid leukaemia
c. Polycythemia vera
d. Essential thrombocytosis

Ans. (c) **Polycythemia vera**

Ref: Harrison 20th ed. pg. 734

The clinical diagnosis of polycythemia is based on presence of JAK 2 mutation with elevated cell counts and *characteristic aquagenic pruritus*. The elevated basophils produce histamine which leads to intense pruritus, after exposure to water.

CASE 177

A patient with thalassemia with a need of recurrent transfusion, develops transfusion reaction like fever and chills. What can be done to the blood to decrease the rate transfusion reactions?

a. Leucocyte depletion
b. Antibiotics
c. Deglycerolization
d. Washed RBCs

Ans. (a) **Leucocyte depletion**

Ref: Wintrobe' Clinical Hematology: 13th ed. pg. 554

- In setting of recurrent transfusions, the donor leucocytes increase the risk of development of febrile nonhemolytic transfusions as well as graft versus host disease.
- Of the methods available to reduce the number of WBC in blood products, washing of red cells, freezing and deglycerolization are effective and yield a product with short shelf life. Modern generation of leukoreduction filters and apheresis machines can provide greater than 4 log reduction of WBC.
- *Leukoreduction of blood products should produce blood products with residual WBC <5 X 10^6 per unit (99.9 percent or log 3 reduction.*

CASE 178

A CKD patient had to undergo dialysis. His Hb was 5.2 gm% so two blood transfusions were to be given. First bag was completed in 2 hours. Second was started and midway he developed shortness of breath, hypertension. Vitals: BP 180/120 mm Hg and pulse rate 110/min. What is the cause?

a. Allergy
b. Transfusion related circulatory overload
c. TRALI
d. FNHTR

Ans. (b) **Transfusion related circulatory overload**

Ref: Harrison 20th ed. pg. 814

- This CKD patient has developed severe anemia which is a compensated heart failure state. *The patient was given first unit of blood in two hours instead of standard four hours and he is already in compensated heart failure.*
- The acute decompensation due to volume overloading that has subsequently occurred will result in pulmonary edema and shortness of breath. This presentation is called as transfusion associated circulatory overload.
- Ideally patients of CKD should be given erythropoietin injections to reduce the incidence of having severe anemia.

CASE 179

A 57-year-old man presents with sudden onset of severe and central chest pain radiating to the back. ECG shows ST segment elevation in lead V1-V6, I, aVL. The chest X-ray shows a widened mediastinum. The diagnosis is:

a. Aortic dissection
b. Acute cor pulmonale
c. Acute myocardial infarction
d. Acute Pericarditis

Ans. (a) **Aortic dissection**

Ref: CMDT 2019 pg. 496

The ECG finding of ST Elevation prompts diagnosis of Myocardial infarction. But the CXR showing mediastinal widening is the key word which favors diagnosis as tear in the aorta.

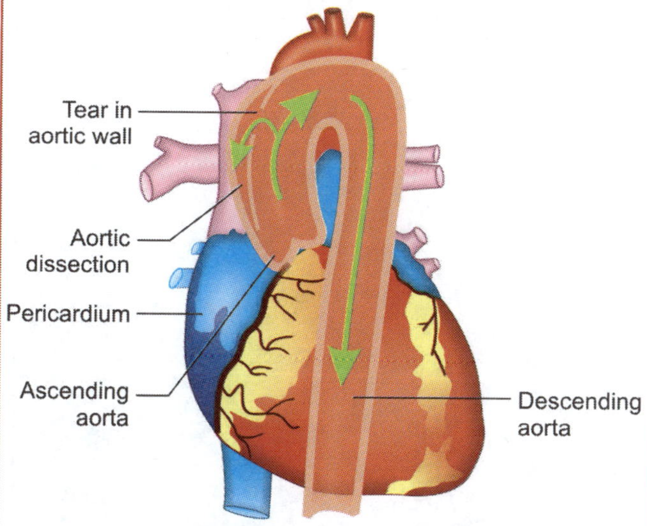

The answer is aortic dissection which exhibits a retrograde extension that can affect the coronary artery and can explain the resultant MI in this patient.

CASE 180

A 43-year-old 190 cm man post a flight to Chennai presents with left-sided chest discomfort and dyspnea. On chest X-ray, there is a small area devoid of lung markings in the apex of the left lung. Diagnosis is?

a. Spontaneous pneumothorax
b. Myocardial infarction
c. Acute cor pulmonale
d. Aortic dissection

Ans. (a) **Spontaneous pneumothorax**

Ref: CMDT 2019 pg. 325

Spontaneous pneumothorax occurs from a rupture of an apical pleural bleb and is associated with tall, young males and is also seen with *aeroplane ascent.*

CASE 181

A 52-year-old businessman with nephrotic syndrome after a non-stop flight from New York to New Delhi presents with sudden onset of breathlessness, hemoptysis, and chest pain. He is brought into Casualty in shock. His chest X-ray is normal. The ECG shows sinus tachycardia. The diagnosis is:

a. Pneumothorax
b. Myocardial infarction
c. Pulmonary embolism
d. Aortic dissection

Ans. (c) **Pulmonary embolism**

Ref: CMDT 2019 pg. 312

- Long distance air travel is contraindicated in patients with hypercoagulable state. Patients of nephrotic syndrome have a hypercoagulable state. This patient has developed pulmonary embolism. *Pulmonary embolism leads to Sinus tachycardia. The small clots obstructing the small blood vessels of lungs cannot be seen in CXR. Hence the CXR is normal.*
- Choice A on CXR will show Deep sulcus sign and absent vascular shadows. Choice C will show bat wing pulmonary edema. Choice D will show pulmonary edema and widened mediastinum.

CASE 182

A 42-year-old man presents with central, crushing chest pain that radiates to the jaw. The pain occurred while jogging around the local park. The pain was alleviated with rest. The ECG is normal. Diagnosis is?

a. Angina pectoris
b. Acute Pericarditis
c. STEMI
d. NSTEMI

Ans. (a) Angina pectoris

Ref: CMDT 2019 pg. 369

The patient is having chest pain on jogging which is a presentation of chronic stable Angina. It is aggravated by cold, by anxiety, and by exercise. In the case of a normal resting ECG, an exercise ECG should be obtained. All other choices present with chest pain on rest.

CASE 183

A 53-year-old woman with ovarian tumor presents with breathlessness and right-sided chest pain. The chest X-ray shows obliteration of the right costophrenic angle. Diagnosis?

a. Pleurisy
b. Pericarditis
c. Myocardial infarction
d. Parapneumonic effusion

Ans. (a) Pleurisy

Ref: CMDT 2019 pg. 323

Ovarian tumor (Fibroma and thecoma) can be associated with a right-sided pleural effusion (Meigs syndrome). The obliteration of CP angle on X-ray is another pointer for pleural involvement of this patient.

CASE 184

A 32-year-old man involved in a high-speed Road traffic accident is found unconscious at the scene. He is breathing spontaneously. In Accident and emergency, the ECG monitor now shows an irregular rhythm and no P, QRS, ST, or T waves. The rate is rapid. Which is the best management of this patient?

a. CPR until a defibrillator is present
b. IV adrenaline
c. Urgent Echo guided pericardiocentesis
d. IV amiodarone

Ans. (a) CPR until a defibrillator is present

Ref: CMDT 2019 pg. 411

The patient is in ventricular fibrillation and needs an urgent CPR to maintain blood flow to the brain in ratio of 30:2.

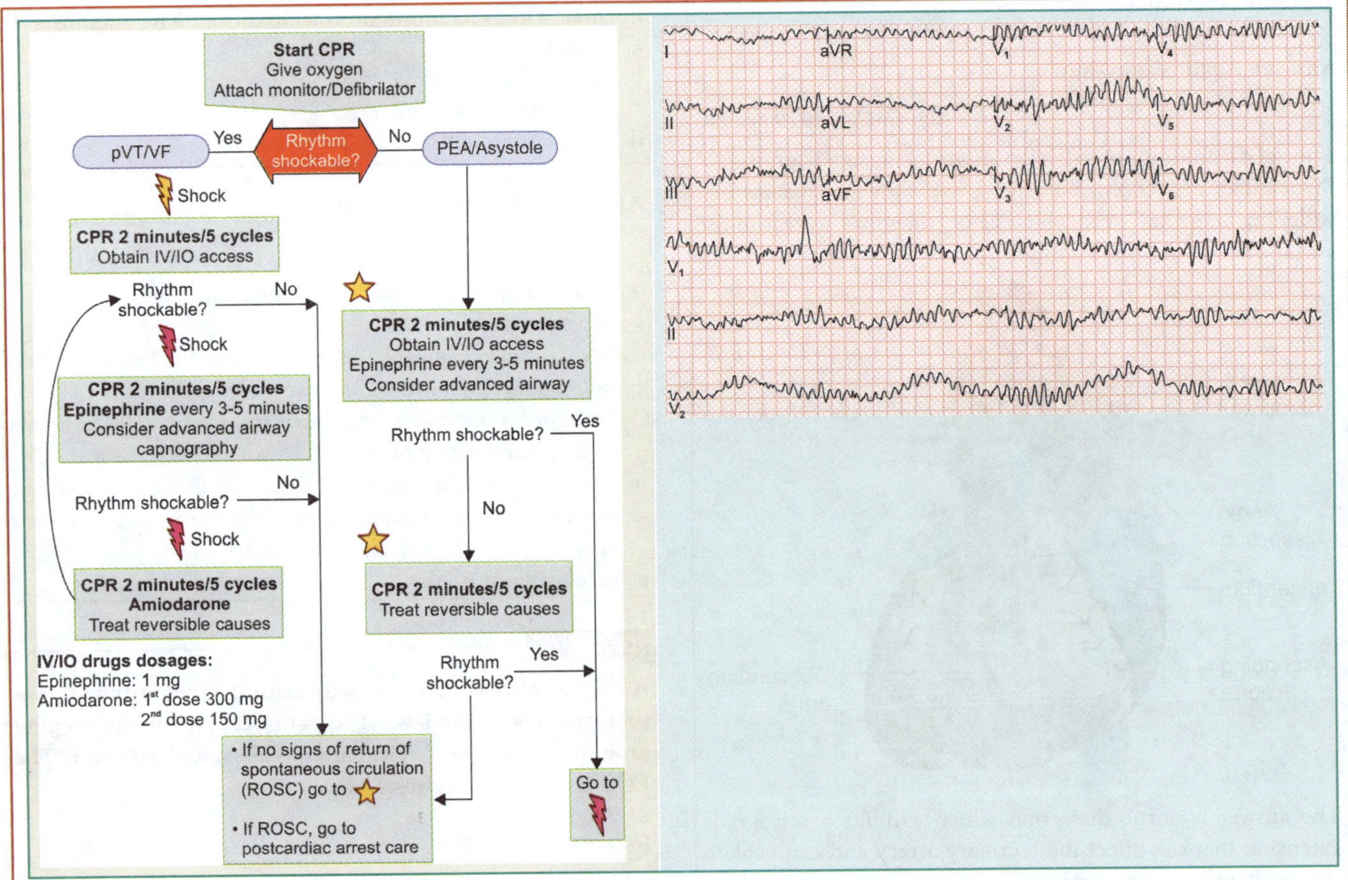

FIGURE: AHA ACLS cardiac arrest algorithm

CASE 185

A 53-year-old man presents to Casualty with severe chest pain. He has a history of angina. ECG shows ST elevation of 4 mm in leads V_1 and V_4. Thrombolysis has been done but pain and ECG findings are persisting 90 minutes after start of thrombolysis. What is the best management of this patient?

a. Rescue PCI
b. Primary PCI
c. Delayed PCI
d. IV Abciximab

Ans. (a) **Rescue PCI**

Ref: CMDT 2019 pg. 386

The patient is having failure of thrombolysis. In case of failure of thrombolysis, rescue PCI is performed. Primary PCI is done for STEMI. Delayed PCI is done for NSTEMI and hence are ruled out.

CASE 186

A 42-year-old pedestrian has been struck by a speeding car driven by a juvenile. She is brought into emergency wearing a pneumatic anti-shock garment for an extensive injury to her pelvis which is distorted. She is intubated with fluids running via two grey color cannulas. Her current blood pressure is 100/60 mm Hg. Which is the next step in management of this patient?

a. Transfuse O negative blood and apply external fixator
b. Start Packed RBC and perform exploratory laparotomy
c. Start Packed RBC and perform decompressive hemicraniectomy
d. Start vasopressors and perform pelvic drainage of blood

Ans. (a) **Transfuse O negative blood and apply external fixator**

Ref: CMDT 2019 pg. 507-8

This patient's chief concern will be massive blood loss. No delay should be taken to crossmatch blood. Ideally O negative Blood should be transfused immediately. The blood pressure may be misleading, as she is wearing an anti-shock garment. An external fixator applied by the surgeons will aid in pelvic fracture stabilisation and stem blood loss.

CASE 187

A 10-year-old boy with smoke inhalation is brought into Casualty with worsening stridor. A face mask with 100% oxygen is covering his face, but his oxygen saturation continues to fall. What is next step in management of this patient?

a. Emergency tracheostomy
b. Hyperbaric oxygen therapy
c. Urgent intubation with positive pressure ventilation
d. Extracorporeal membrane oxygenation

Ans. (a) **Emergency tracheostomy**

Ref: CMDT 2019 pg. 316

Due to hot smoke probably both the nasopharynx and oropharynx are compromised, and a tracheostomy to achieve an airway is essential. Choice B is used for management of carbon monoxide poisoning which may be considered in this patient but would be performed after tracheostomy has failed to relieve symptoms of this patient.

CASE 188

A 4-year-old asthmatic child is brought to casualty. She is not speaking and has fast shallow breathing with pulsus paradoxus. ABG shows respiratory acidosis. What is the next best step in management of this patient?

a. Urgent endotracheal intubation
b. Hyperbaric oxygen therapy
c. MDI with salbutamol and corticosteroids
d. Terbutaline subcutaneous with aminophylline drip

Ans. (a) **Urgent endotracheal intubation**

Ref: CMDT 2019 pg. 256

The child is having impending respiratory arrest due to severe exacerbation of asthma. Carbon dioxide narcosis will necessitate elective intubation and ventilation.

	Mild	Moderate	Severe	Respiratory arrest imminent
Symptoms				
Breathlessness	While walking	At rest, limits activity	At rest, interferes with conversation	While at rest, mute
Talks in	Sentences	Phrases	Words	Silent
Alertness	May be agitated	Usually agitated	Usually agitated	Drowsy confused
Sings				
Respiratory rate	Increased	Increased	Often >30/minute	>30/minute

Contd...

	Mild	Moderate	Severe	Respiratory arrest imminent
Body position	Can lie down	Prefers sitting	Sits upright	Unable to recline
Use of accessory muscles; suprasternal retraction	Usually not	Commonly	Usually	Paradoxical thoracoabdominal movement
Wheeze	Moderate, often only end expiratory	Loud; throughout exhalation	Usually loud; throughout inhalation and exhalation	Absent
Pulse/minute	<100	100–120	>120	Bradycardia
Pulsus paradoxus	Absent <10 mm Hg	May be present 10–25 mm Hg	Often present >25 mm Hg	Absence suggests respiratory muscle fatigue

CASE 189

A 13-year-old known asthmatic presents with severe wheezing and a respiratory rate of 40. Her pulse rate is 120. What is the next best step in management of this patient?

a. Oxygen and nebulized salbutamol
b. Oxygen and Metered dose inhaler of salmeterol
c. Oxygen and intravenous Aminophylline
d. Oxygen and Intravenous magnesium sulphate

Ans. (a) **Oxygen and nebulised salbutamol**

Ref: CMDT 2019 pg. 256

An acute asthmatic attack is treated initially with oxygen and salbutamol. If necessary IV hydrocortisone is added.

CASE 190

A 33-year-old cyclist is struck by a car in a head-on collision and arrives intubated to emergency department. Upon arrival, his Glasgow Coma Scale is 3. He has fixed and dilated pupils with absent gag reflex and with absence of spontaneous breathing efforts. EEG shows isolated bursts along a flat line. What is the next step in management of this patient?

a. Pronounce the patient as brain dead
b. Do urgent craniotomy
c. Do urgent ventriculostomy
d. Do urgent Burr hole surgery

Ans. (a) **Pronounce the patient as brain dead**

Ref: Bailey and Love, 26th ed. pg. 1418

A Glasgow Coma Scale of 3 is the lowest score possible with absent gag reflex and light reflex, no breathing efforts. If indicate brain-stem death. This is further confirmed by flat line on EEG.

American Academy of Neurology (AAN) guidelines for brain death in adults require one neurologic examination and one apnea test. Pediatric brain death guidelines from the American Academy of Pediatrics, Child Neurology Society, and Society of Critical Care medicine require two different physicians to conduct two neurologic examinations and two apnea tests, separated by an observation period.

AAN Guidelines for Brain Death in Adults

Clinical evaluation (prerequisites)	Clinical evaluation (neurologic assessment)	Ancillary tests	Documentation
Establish irreversible and proximate cause of come	The following must be assessed	Ordered only if	Time of death is documented
Achieve normal core temperature	Coma	Clinical examination cannot be performed	A checklist is filled out, signed, and dated
Achieve normal systolic blood pressure	Absence of brainstem reflexes	Apnea testing is inconclusive or aborted	
Perform one neurologic examination	Apnea		

CASE 191

A 62-year-old man is brought to Accident and emergency following assault to the head. He has a face mask and reservoir bag delivering 15L/min of oxygen, a stiff cervical collar and is attached to an intravenous drip. He has no spontaneous eye opening except to pain, makes incomprehensible sounds, and does not obey commands. He demonstrates flexion withdrawal to painful stimuli. On suction, he has no gag reflex. What is the next best step in management of this patient?

a. Intubate the patient
b. Urgent decompressive hemicraniectomy
c. Urgent NCCT head
d. Give mannitol and perform burr hole surgery

Ans. (a) Intubate the patient

Ref: AHA 2015 Guidelines

A GCS of 8 or less or absence of a gag reflex are both indications for urgent intubation. The patient has sustained head injury and after securing his airway, imaging would be performed to asses nature of CNS injury.

CASE 192

A 17-year-old girl presents with fever, odd behaviour, purpura, and conjunctival petechiae. Her lumbar puncture reveals Gram-negative cocci. Best treatment of this patient is?

a. Ceftriaxone with vancomycin
b. Ampicillin with gentamycin
c. Ceftriaxone with dexamethasone
d. Piperacillin with tazobactam

Ans. (a) Ceftriaxone with vancomycin

Ref: CMDT 2019 pg. 1305

The clinical diagnosis is Meningococcal meningitis and empirical ceftriaxone is started with vancomycin.

Indication	Antibiotic
Preterm infants to infants <1 month	Ampicillin + cefotaxime
Infants 1–3 months	Ampicillin + cefotaxime or ceftriaxone
Immunocompetent children >3 months and adults <55	Cefotaxime, ceftriaxone, or cefeprime + vancomycin
Adults >55 and adults or any age with alcoholism or other debilitating illnesses	Ampicillin + cefotaxime, ceftriaxone or cefepime + vancomycin
Hospital-acquired meningitis, post-traumatic or postneurosurgery meningitis, neutropenic patients, or patients with impaired cell-mediated immunity	Ampicillin + ceftazidime or meropenem + vancomycin

CASE 193

A 22-year-old woman presents with a plethora of signs and symptoms. She complains of arthralgia, depression, alopecia, fits, oral ulceration, and facial rash. She is found to have proteinuria and a normocytic normochromic anaemia. What is the best test for her diagnosis?

a. Anti-Nuclear antibody
b. Anti-Smith antibody
c. Anti-Ribosomal P antibody
d. Anti-Topoisomerase Antibody

Ans. (a) Anti-Nuclear antibody

Ref: CMDT 2019 pg. 855

The clinical diagnosis of patient is Systemic lupus erythematosus and diagnosis is based on positive ANA.

CASE 194

A 67-year-old hypertensive man presents with lower abdominal pain and back pain. An expansive abdominal mass is palpated lateral and superior to the umbilicus. What is the best investigation for this patient?

a. X-ray KUB
b. Ultrasound abdomen
c. Coronary angiography
d. Intravenous Pyelography

Ans. (b) Ultrasound abdomen

Ref: CMDT 2019 pg. 492

The presentation is suggestive of abdominal aortic aneurysm. The size should be evaluated by ultrasound and surgical repair is advisable if the aneurysm is greater than 5.5 cm in diameter as it can exhibit spontaneous rupture.

CASE 195

An 83-year-old woman suffering from rheumatoid arthritis presents with severe epigastric pain and vomiting. She also complains of shoulder tip pain. What investigation should be done in the emergency room?

a. USG chest
b. Serum electrolytes
c. Upper GI endoscopy
d. Erect chest X-ray

Ans. (d) Erect chest X-ray

Ref: CMDT 2019 pg. 640

Steroid usage for rheumatoid arthritis puts this woman at risk for a perforated peptic ulcer. Hence an urgent Erect CXR should be done to look for gas under diaphragm.

CASE 196

A 42-year-old woman with benign ovarian tumor presents with ascites and breathlessness. CXR is performed. The clinical diagnosis is?

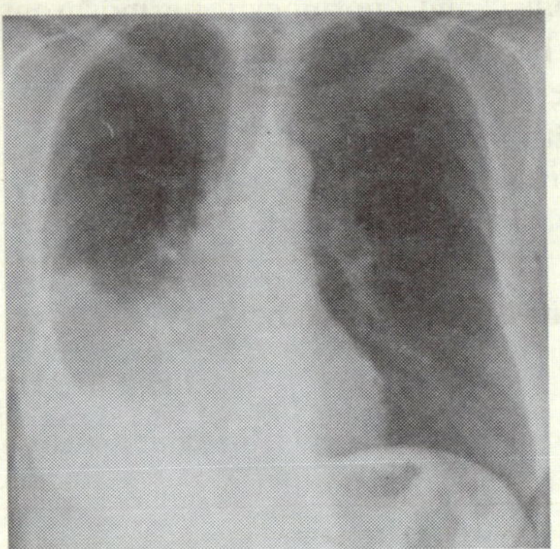

a. Meigs syndrome
b. Dressler syndrome
c. Budd-Chiari syndrome
d. Cholangiocarcinoma

Ans. (a) Meigs syndrome

Ref: CMDT 2019 pg. 323

- The CXR shows presence of right sided pleural effusion along with history of ascites and a benign ovarian tumor. This a triad seen in Meigs syndrome.
- Choice B is seen in post MI patients
- Choice C leads to acute onset ascites and right upper quadrant pain
- Choice D leads to obstructive jaundice and cachexia.

CASE 197

A 25-year-old woman develops nausea, vomiting, and abdominal pain. On examination, she has tender hepatomegaly and ascites. She was recently started on oral contraceptives. The clinical diagnosis is?

a. Budd-Chiari syndrome
b. Acute viral hepatitis
c. Portal hypertension
d. Acute cholecystitis

Ans. (a) Budd–Chiari syndrome

Ref: CMDT 2019 page 726

Budd-Chiari syndrome occurs from thrombosis of the major hepatic veins and has been associated with oral contraceptives. The main diagnostic features are

- Right upper quadrant pain and tenderness
- Ascites
- Imaging studies show occlusion/absence of flow in the hepatic vein(s) or inferior vena cava
- Clinical picture is similar in sinusoidal obstruction syndrome but major hepatic veins are patent.

CASE 198

A 42-year-old woman presents with ascites. On examination, she has large 'a' wave in JVP and a low volume pulse. She has history of rheumatic fever. Clinical diagnosis is?

a. Right ventricular hypertrophy due to pulmonary artery hypertension
b. Right ventricular failure due to tricuspid regurgitation
c. Left heart failure due to mitral stenosis
d. Left heart failure due to aortic regurgitation

Ans. (a) Right ventricular hypertrophy due to pulmonary artery hypertension

Ref: CMDT 2019 pg. 347

- The most common valvular lesion in rheumatic etiology is mitral stenosis. Long standing mitral stenosis leads to pulmonary edema and resultant Pulmonary artery hypertension. This will lead to compensatory right ventricular hypertrophy.
- Choice B is ruled out as it leads to large V wave in JVP.
- Choice C is ruled as mitral stenosis does not lead to left heart but right heart enlargement
- Choice D does not lead to ascites, and instead leads to collapsing pulse.

CASE 199

A 52-year-old woman presents with exertional fatigue and ascites. She is noted to have a rapid, irregular pulse rate. The chest X-ray reveals a small heart with calcification seen on the lateral view. The 12-lead ECG demonstrates low QRS voltage. Clinical diagnosis is?

a. Rheumatic pancarditis
b. Constrictive pericarditis
c. Restrictive cardiomyopathy
d. Acute cor pulmonale

Ans. (b) Constrictive pericarditis

Ref: CMDT 2019 pg. 441

The presence of rapid irregular pulse points to presence of atrial fibrillation. The CXR finding of calcification narrows down the diagnosis to constrictive pericarditis. The impaired filling of ventricles explains the ascites. Since the left side of heart also receives less blood it can explain presence of exertional fatigue. Low voltage ECG occurs due to calcification impairing the flow of current to recording electrodes.

CASE 200

A 34-year-old female presents with hypertension, pinched facies and progressive dysphagia with decreased tone of lower esophageal sphincter (LES) The clinical diagnosis is?

a. Scleroderma
b. Hiatus hernia
c. Rolling hernia
d. Diffuse esophageal spasm

Ans. (a) Scleroderma

Ref: CMDT 2019 pg. 323

- Pinched facies with hypertension points to presence of scleroderma. The tone of LES is reduced in scleroderma due to fibrosis.
- Choice B and C can lead to GERD but it does not have other features like systemic hypertension.
- Choice D presents with chest pain and dysphagia and is hence ruled out.

CASE 201

A 70-year-old man presents with a 16-week history of progressive dysphagia, and recurrent pneumonia episodes. He also has palpable stony hard neck nodes on examination. Diagnosis is?

a. Carcinoma of the esophagus
b. Achalasia Cardia
c. Diffuse esophageal spasm
d. Zenker's diverticulum

Ans. (a) Carcinoma of the esophagus

Ref: Bailey and Love, 26th ed. pg. 1004

Esophageal cancer presents with mechanical symptoms, principally dysphagia, but sometimes also regurgitation. The main feature for malignancy in this case is stony hard consistency of neck Lymph nodes.

CASE 202

A 70-year-old man presents with regurgitation of food, dysphagia, halitosis, and a sensation of 'lump in the throat'.

a. Pharyngeal pouch
b. Carcinoma esophagus
c. Diffuse esophageal spasm
d. Esophageal Dysmotility

Ans. (a) Pharyngeal pouch

Ref: Bailey and Love, 26th ed. pg. 1018

The key word is regurgitation of food with dysphagia which is seen with Pharyngeal pouch. When it is small, symptoms largely reflect only in-coordination with predominantly pharyngeal dysphagia. As the pouch enlarges, it tends to fill with food on eating, and the fundus descends into the mediastinum. This leads to halitosis and esophageal dysphagia.

CASE 203

A 63-year-old man recently treated for renal tuberculosis presents with weight loss, diarrhea, hypoglycemia, hypotension, and is noted to have hyperpigmented buccal mucosa, palmar and hand creases. Which investigation is most suitable for this clinical presentation?

a. Serum iron and ferritin
b. Serum copper and ceruloplasmin
c. Plasma ACTH and cortisol
d. Gene XPERT and Intravenous pyelography

Ans. (c) Plasma ACTH and cortisol

Ref: CMDT 2019 pg. 323

- The key finding of hyperpigmentation of buccal mucosa, palmar and sole creases point to etiology of Addison disease. The leading cause of Addison's disease in India is tuberculosis.
- The presence of hypotension indicates hypoaldosteronism in Addison's disease. Simultaneous mention of hypoglycemia indicates cortisol deficiency.
- Choice B is done in case of hemochromatosis and bronze diabetes
- Choice C is done in case of Wilson disease
- Choice D is done in for diagnosis of tuberculosis

CASE 204

A 66-year-old man presents with a sudden onset of diabetes, anorexia, weight loss, epigastric pain with radiation to back. Next best investigation for this patient is?

a. Ultrasound of abdomen
b. CT abdomen
c. Enteroclysis
d. Triple contrast barium enema

Ans. (b) CT abdomen

Ref: Bailey and Love: 26th ed. pg. 1137

- The clinical history of epigastric pain radiating to back points to pancreatic etiology. This patient may have developed pancreatic cancer. Sudden onset of diabetes in the elderly is also suggestive. *The best imaging modality to image chronic pancreatitis or pancreatic malignancy is CT abdomen.*
- Choice A is ruled out as gas shadows of stomach obscure ultrasound view of pancreas.
- Choice C is fluoroscopic intubation-infusion small-bowel examination which is used to evaluate for small bowel pathology while this patient has pancreatic lesion
- Choice D is ruled out as it used for large bowel evaluation.

CASE 205

A 53-year-old woman presents with weight loss, increased appetite, sweating, palpitations, and preference for cold weather, hot, moist palms, and tremors. What is the best investigation for the clinical diagnosis of this patient?

a. TSH levels
b. Autoimmune panel
c. Plasma catecholamines
d. Plasma Cortisol

Ans. (a) TSH levels

Ref: CMDT 2019 pg. 1139

This patient presents with classic signs and symptoms of hyperthyroidism. The increased Basal metabolic rate and calorigenesis explain the symptoms of the patient. These patients have highly suppressed TSH levels. The highlights of hyperthyroidism are:

- Sweating, weight loss or gain, anxiety, palpitations, loose stools, heat intolerance, fatigue, menstrual irregularity.
- Tachycardia; warm, moist skin; stare; tremor.
- **Graves disease:** Majority have a palpable goiter (sometimes with bruit); ophthalmopathy.
- Suppressed TSH in primary hyperthyroidsim; usually increased T_4, FT_4, T_3, FT_3.

CASE 206

A 69-year-old man is noted to have a glucose level of 600 mg% and a Na of 163 mmol/L. pH of blood is normal. There is no previous history of Diabetes mellitus. What is best management for this patient?

a. Insulin sliding scale and 5% dextrose
b. Insulin sliding scale and 0.9% normal saline
c. Insulin sliding scale and 3% saline
d. Insulin sliding scale and 0.45% saline

Ans. (b) Insulin sliding scale and 0.9% normal saline

Ref: CMDT 2019, pg. 323

- The blood sugar of 600 mg% leads to increased plasma osmolality and resultant fluid shift across the brain leading to loss of consciousness.
- The clinical diagnosis is nonketotic hyperosmolar coma.
- It occurs in patients with mild or occult diabetes, and most patients are typically middle-aged to elderly.
- It is characterized by severe hyperglycemia in the absence of significant ketosis, with hyperosmolality and dehydration.

CASE 207

A patient tested positive for MTB on sputum CBNAAT. He did not come again to the hospital despite multiple reminders. Today he presents with massive hemoptysis and is alarmed. What is the next best step for this patient?

a. Urgent coagulation studies
b. Perform multi slice CT scan chest
c. Schedule a flexible fibre optic biopsy
d. Urgent rigid bronchoscopy and prophylactic balloon tamponade

Ans. (b) Perform multi slice CT scan chest

Ref: CMDT 2019, pg. 26-27

Multislice computed tomography is the diagnostic imaging modality that yields most information on the cause and site of hemoptysis.

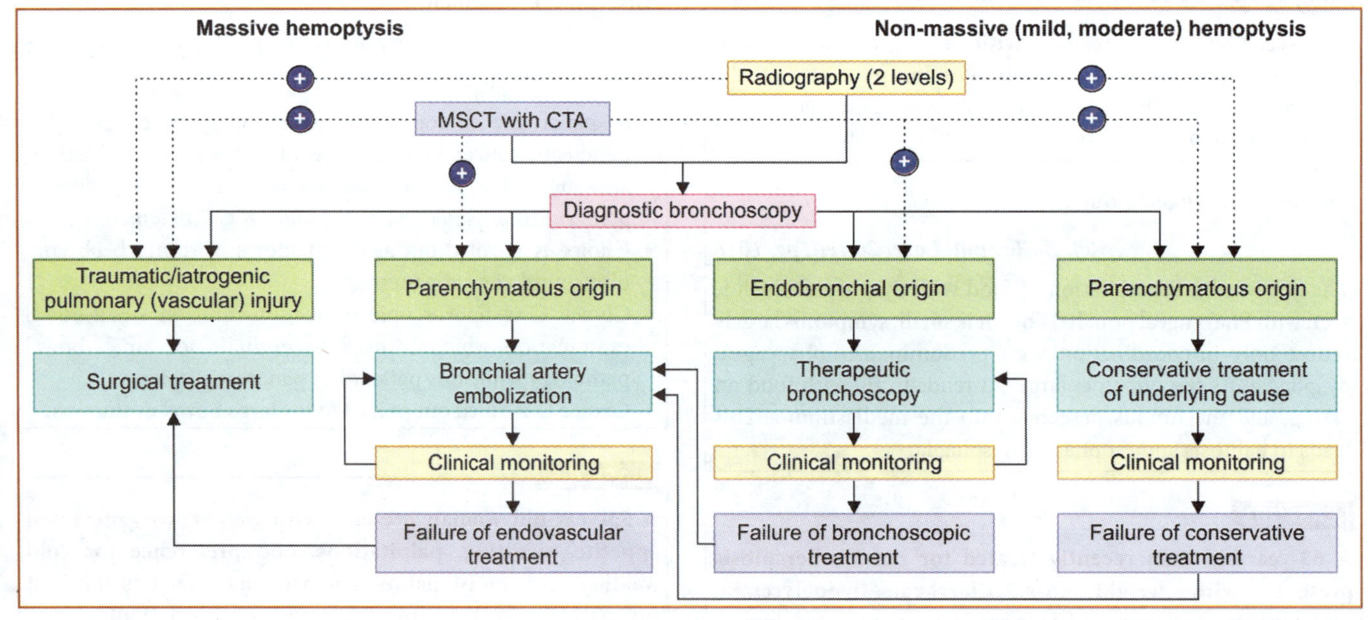

CASE 208

A 45-year-old smoker presents with sudden onset unrelenting chest pain with loss of peripheral pulses. BP measured in both arms is different. First differential diagnosis is?

a. Mirizzi syndrome
b. Aortic dissection
c. Viral pericarditis
d. Spontaneous pneumothorax

Ans. (b) Aortic dissection

Ref: CMDT 2019, pg. 28

The clinical presentation of chest pain with loss of peripheral pulses points to diagnosis of aortic dissection. The antegrade progression of tear leads to unequal BP between left and right arms.

CASE 209

A patient develops chest pain after bout of vomiting with subcutaneous emphysema. Comment on the diagnosis.

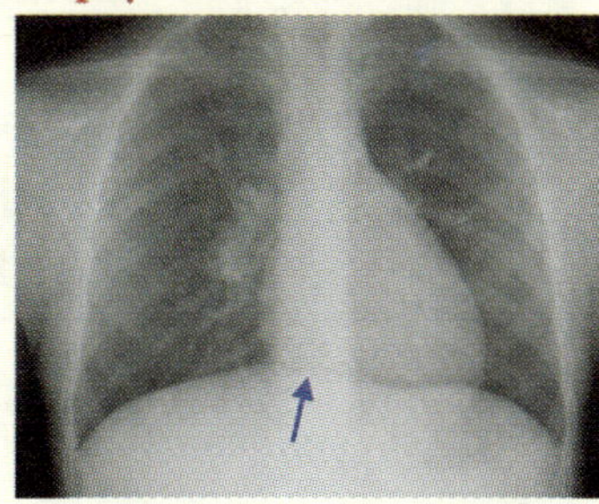

a. Eventration of diaphragm
b. Hampton hump
c. Pneumomediastinum
d. Water bottle heart

Ans. (c) Pneumomediastinum

Ref: Bailey and Love, 26th ed. pg. 992

The CXR shows continuous diaphragm sign. The presence of vomiting, chest pain and subcutaneous emphysema points to Mackler's triad of Boerhaave's syndrome. The rupture of esophagus due to vomiting against a closed glottis leads to contents of esophagus to spill over into mediastinum. This leads to chemical mediastinitis and pneumomediastinum.

CASE 210

A 70-year-old woman has a progressive neurological disorder resulting in degeneration of the anterior horn cells throughout her spinal cord and brainstem. Which of the following abnormal movements is she most likely to exhibit?

a. Asterixis
b. Chorea
c. Fasciculations
d. Gait Apraxia

Ans. (c) Fasciculations

Ref: Ganong 25th ed. pg. 240

- The lesion at anterior horn cells of spinal cord leads to lower motor neuron lesion of spinal cord. It causes twitching of muscles leading to fasciculations.
- Choice A is seen in hepatic and uremic encephalopathy
- Choice B is seen in basal ganglia damage
- Choice D is seen in frontal lobe damage.

IMAGE-BASED QUESTIONS

ANATOMY

1. Which part of brain is present in Turkish saddle-shaped space in cranium?

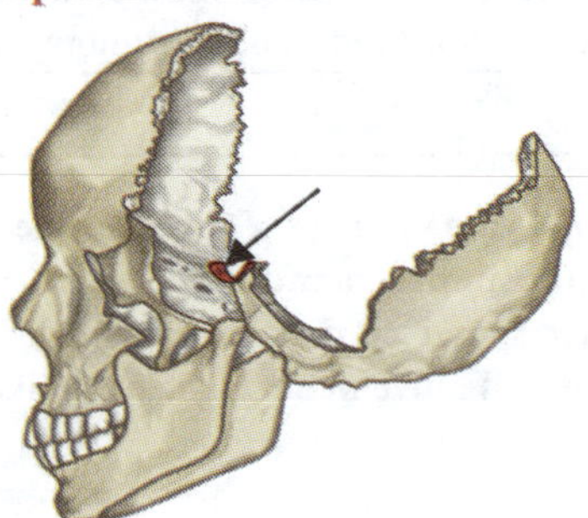

a. Pituitary gland　b. Frontal lobe
c. Hypothalamus　d. Basal ganglia

4. Which nerve is marked by an arrow in the vicinity of popliteal fossa?

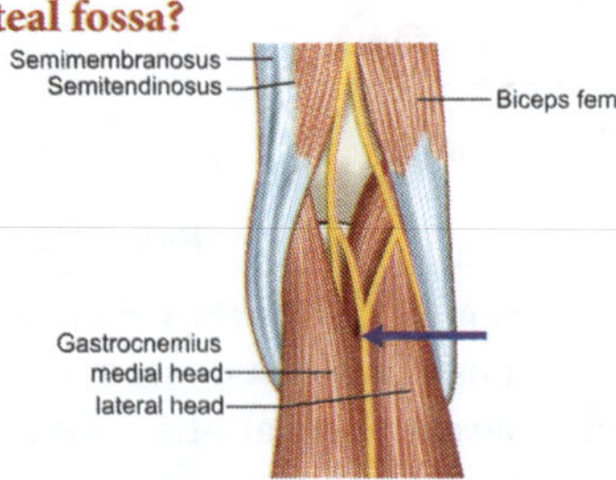

a. Common peroneal nerve
b. Deep peroneal nerve
c. Sural nerve
d. Sciatic nerve

2. Which nerve is involved in this presentation?

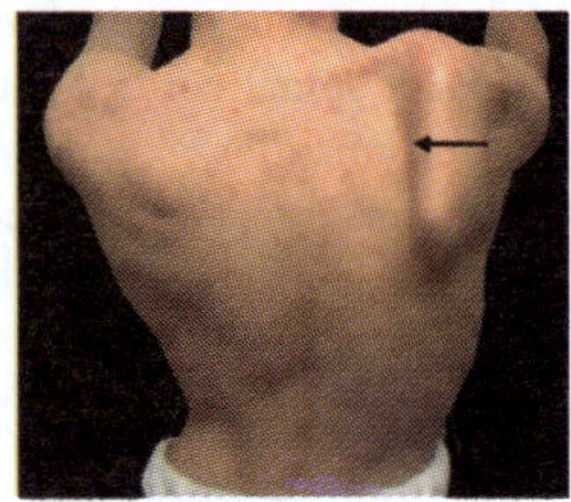

a. Long thoracic nerve
b. Musculocutaneous nerve
c. Lateral anterior thoracic nerve
d. Thoracodorsal nerve

5. A patient complains of pain in the distribution shown below. All are true about the condition except:

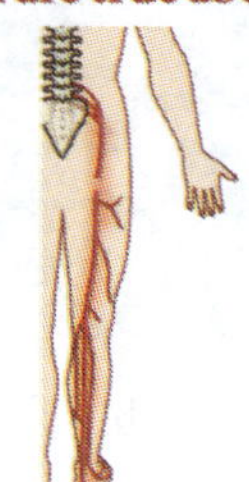

a. Sciatic nerve is involved b. Pain worse on standing
c. Straight leg raising leads to pain in opposite leg indicating disc herniation
d. Nerve originates from nerve roots L5-S2

3. Name the ligament:

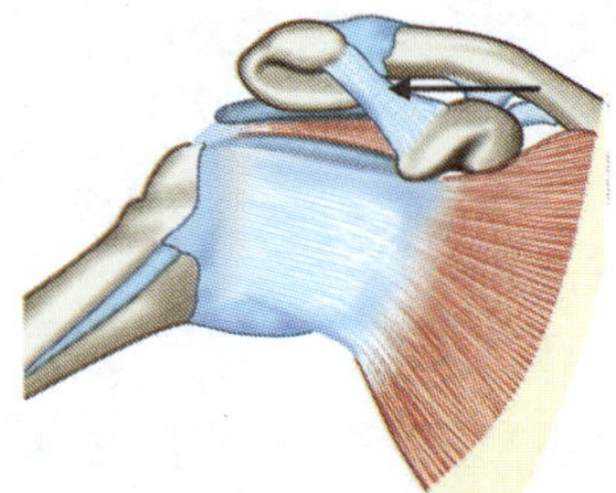

a. Coracoacromial ligament
b. Acromio-clavicular ligament
c. Coraco-humeral ligament
d. Sterno-clavicular ligament

6. Which of the following is branch of external carotid Artery?

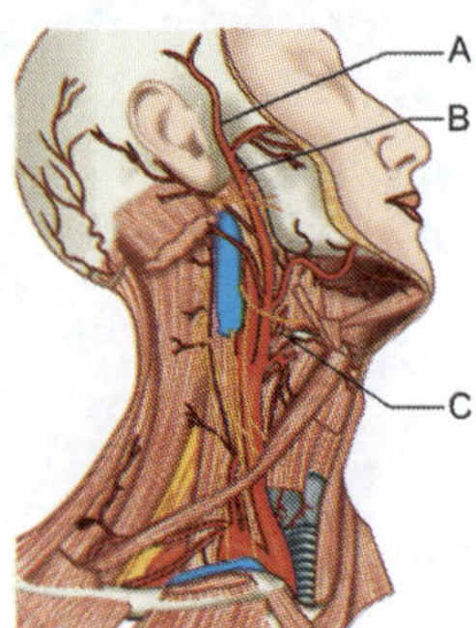

a. A　b. B
c. C　d. All of these

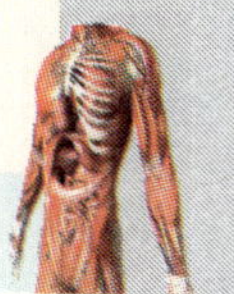

7. The blockage of which of the following blood vessels will lead to medial medullary syndrome?

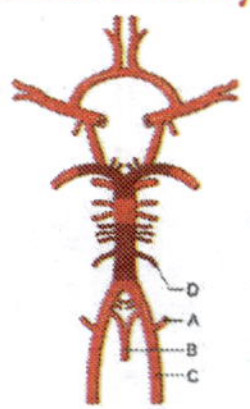

a. A b. B
c. C d. D

8. What is the insertion of shown muscle? ***(2018)***

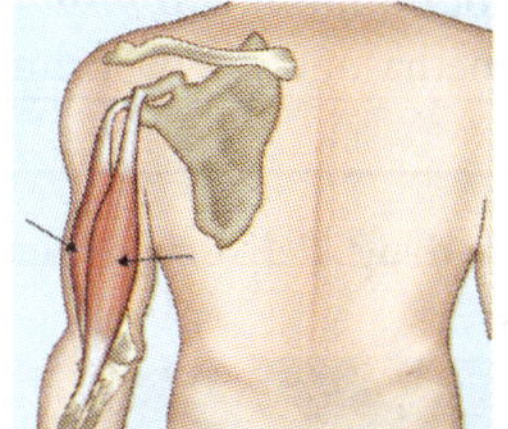

a. Supraglenoid tubercle of scapula
b. Tip of coracoid process of scapula
c. Radial tuberosity d. Ulnar tuberosity

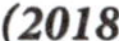

9. The marked area in skull represents: ***(2018)***

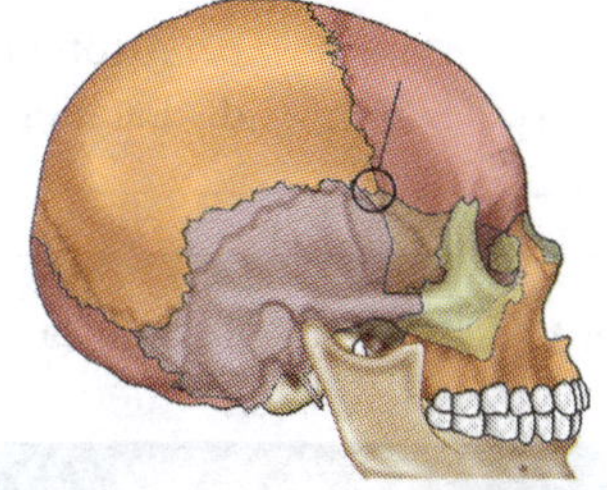

a. Asterion b. Pterion
c. Bregma d. Lambda

10. The arrow in the image denotes which of the following muscles?

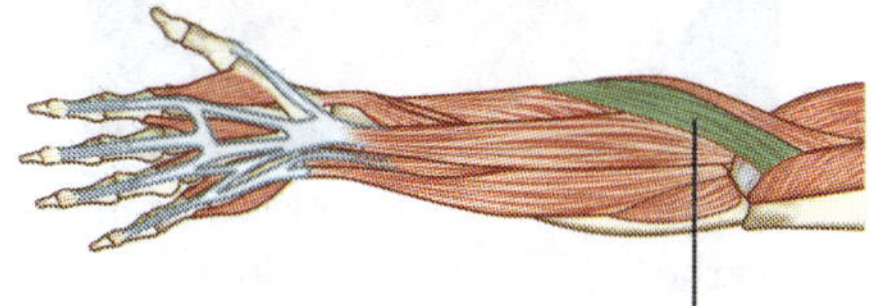

a. Brachioradialis b. Supinator
c. Extensor carpi radialis longus
d. Flexor carpi radialis brevis

11. What is the nerve supply of the structure marked in the image below?

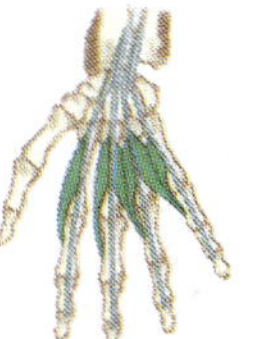

a. Median nerve b. Radial nerve
c. Posterior interosseus nerve
d. Ulnar nerve

12. The shown muscle in the image is innervated by:

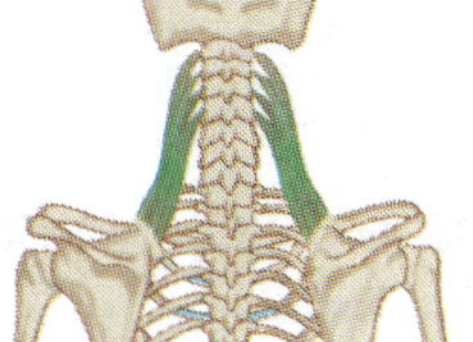

a. Dorsal scapular nerve
b. Suprascapular nerve
c. From the dorsal rami of C1
d. Subscapular nerve

13. Identify the sign shown in the image below:

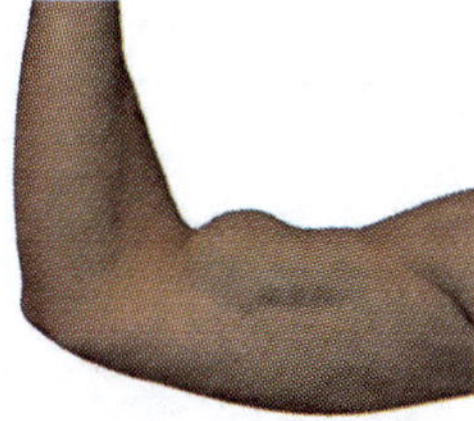

a. Popeye sign b. Hill-Sachs sign
c. Griesinger sign d. Rising sun sign

14. Identify the green marked structure in the image:

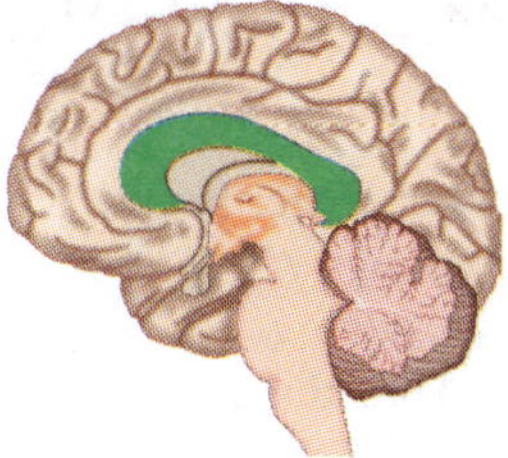

a. Corpus callosum b. Orbital cortex
c. Striate cortex d. Optic chiasma

15. Test shown is:

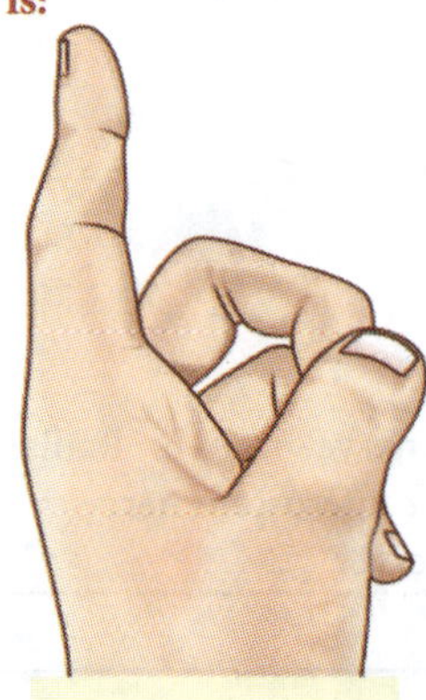

a. Card test
b. Froment's sign
c. Pointing index
d. Pen test

PHYSIOLOGY

16. Which of the following is QT interval?

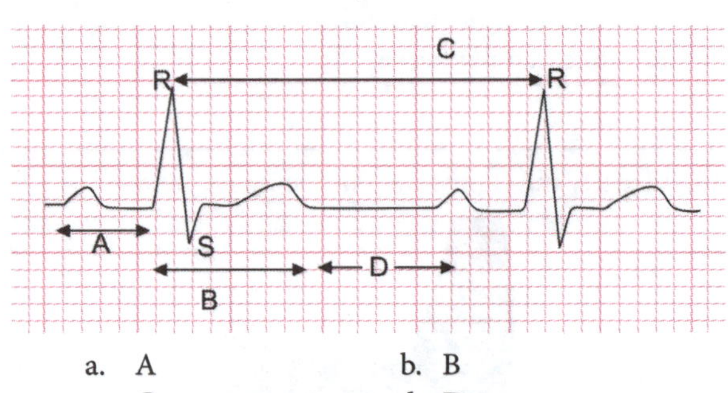

a. A
b. B
c. C
d. D

17. Which type of breathing is shown in below image?

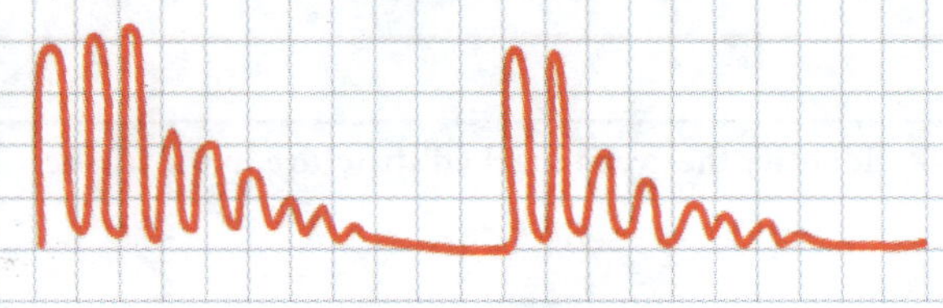

a. Cheyne stokes breathing
b. Biot breathing
c. Normal breathing
d. Kussmaul breathing

PHARMACOLOGY

18. Which of the following drugs is likely to be associated with these findings?

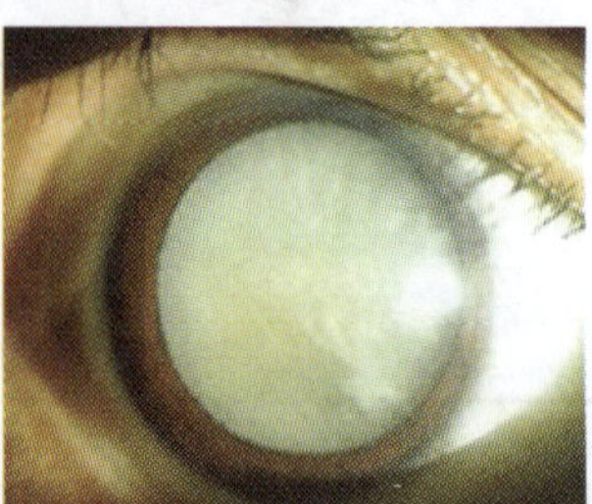

a. Timolol
b. Apraclonidine
c. Dexamethasone
d. Brimonidine

19. The shown drug delivery device is used for the delivery of:

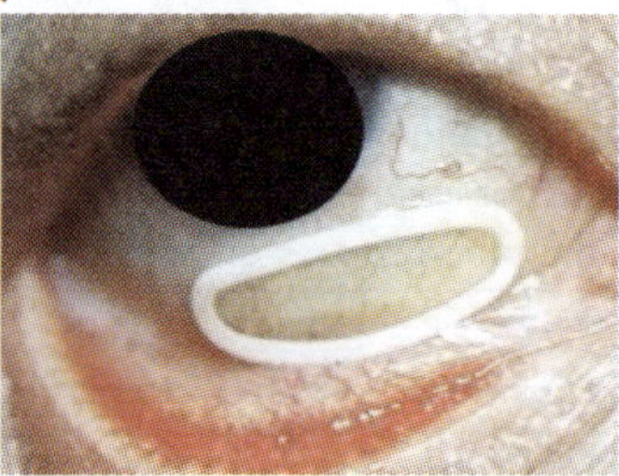

a. Clinidipine
b. Atropine
c. Pilocarpine
d. Latanoprost

20. Which anti-diabetic agent can cause the adverse effect a show in the image?

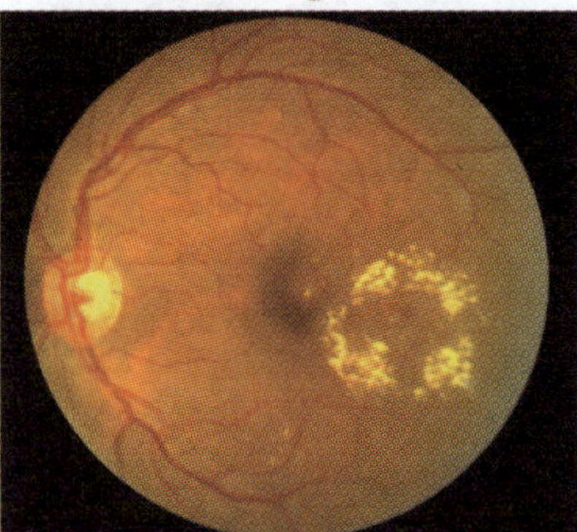

a. Glipizide
b. Metformin
c. Acarbose
d. Pioglitazone

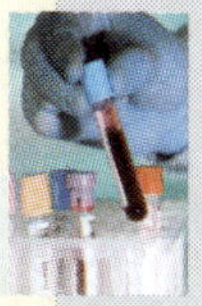

21. A 30-year-old patient presented with following condition. All of the following agents can lead to this presentation, except:

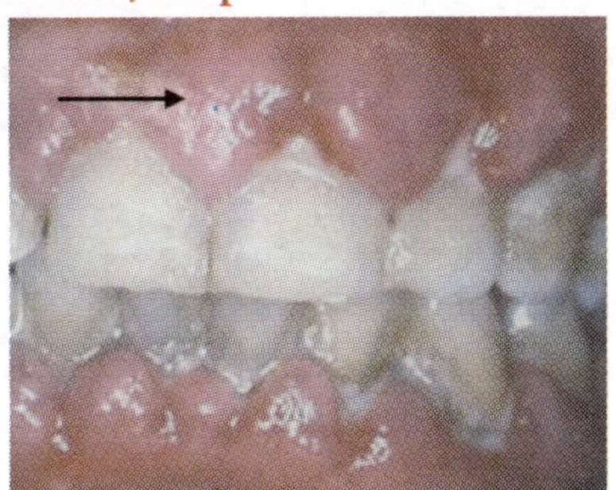

a. Phenytoin b. Labetalol
c. Nifedipine d. Tacrolimus

22. A patient, on an anticancer drug for his testicular carcinoma, presents with the shown condition. Which of the following anti-cancer drugs is associated with this presentation?

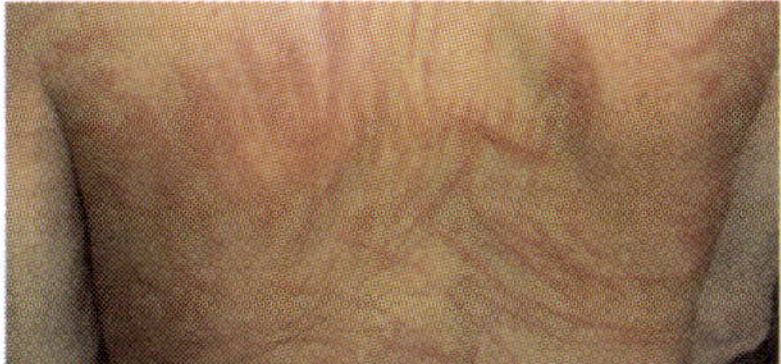

a. Busulfan b. Bleomycin
c. Doxorubicin d. Dactinomycin

23. The image shows presence of:

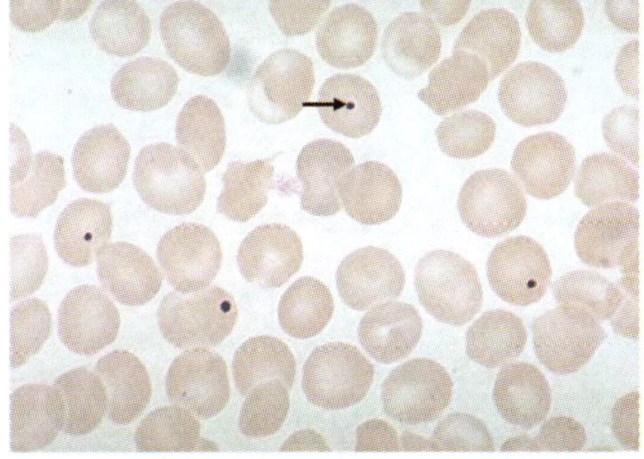

a. Howell-Jolly bodies b. Heinz bodies
c. Cabot rings d. Pappenheimer's bodies

24. Identify the cell marked:

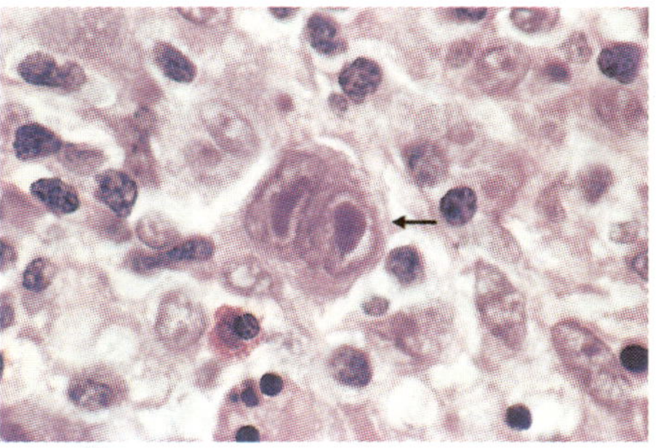

a. Orphan Annie-eye nucleus
b. Reed-sternberg cell
c. Owl eye inclusions
d. Russel bodies

25. What is the diagnosis?

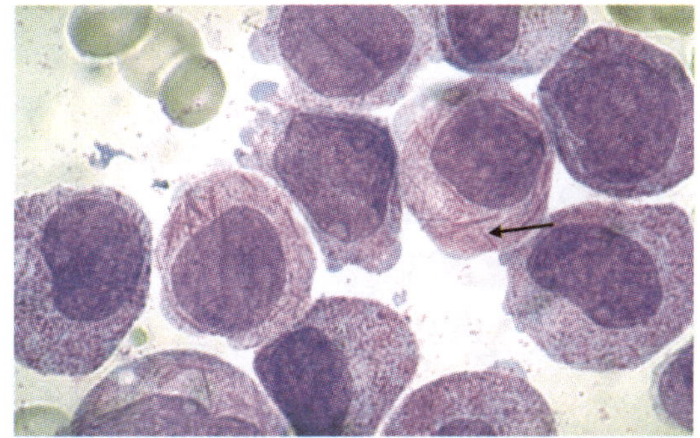

a. Lymphoblast b. Myeloblast
c. Megakaryoblast d. Normoblast

26. Identify the cell:

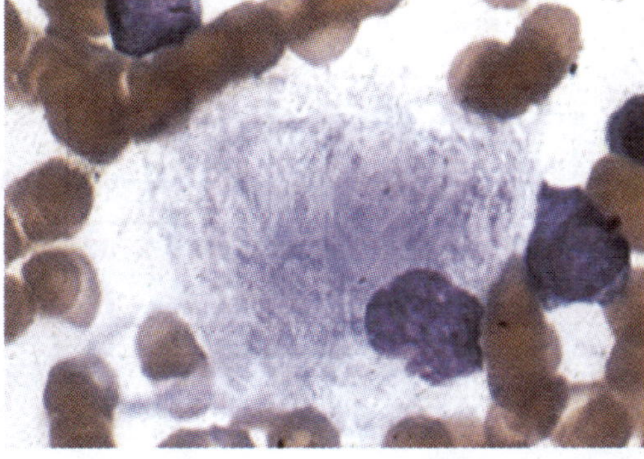

a. Gaucher cell b. Reed-sternberg cell
c. Anitschkow cell d. Pop corn cell

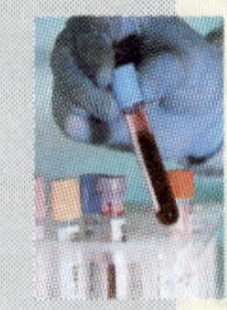

27. Spot the diagnosis:

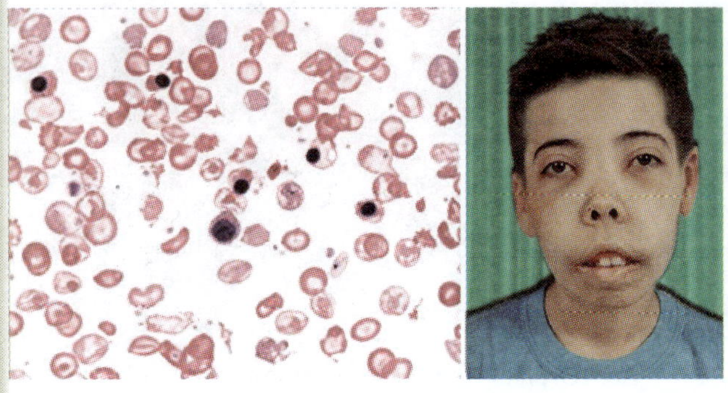

a. Iron deficiency anemia
b. Thalassemia
c. Acute leukemia
d. Hodgkin lymphoma

28. The following image shows:

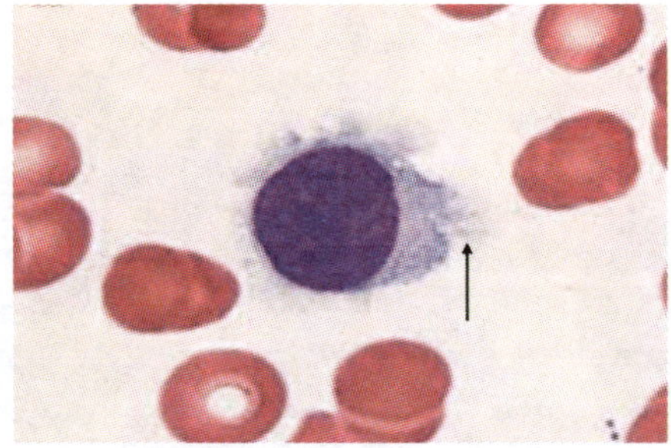

a. Hairy cell leukemia
b. Target cell
c. Acanthocyte
d. Pseudo-Pelger-Huet anomaly

29. The following image shows presence of:

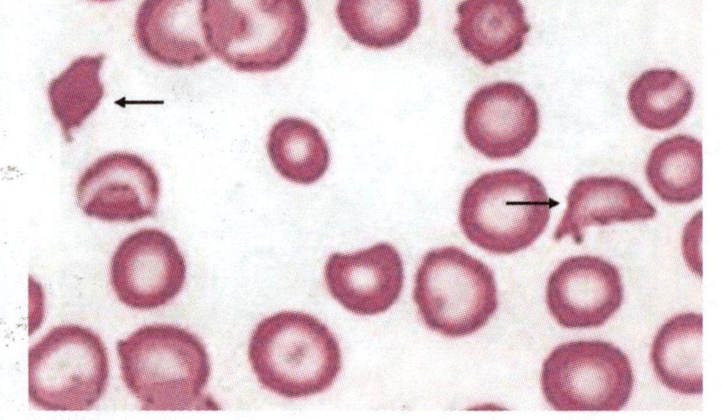

a. Target cell
b. Schistocyte
c. Sickle cell
d. Spherocyte

30. What is correct about the histopathological slide?

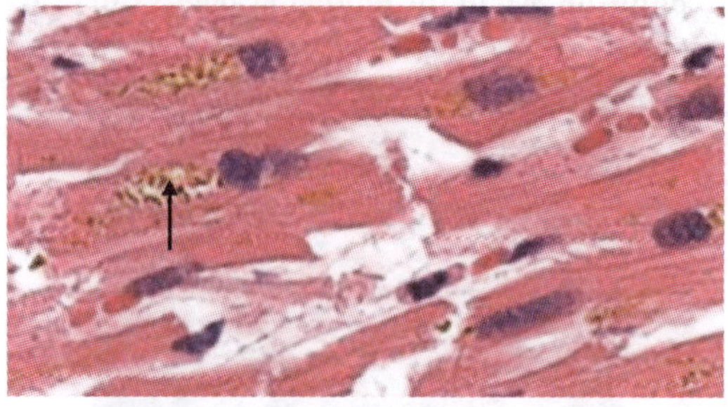

a. Lipofuscin in cardiac tissue
b. Melanin in cardiac tissue
c. Hemosiderin in kidney tubules
d. Hemopexin in hepatocytes

31. Which is true about the image shown?

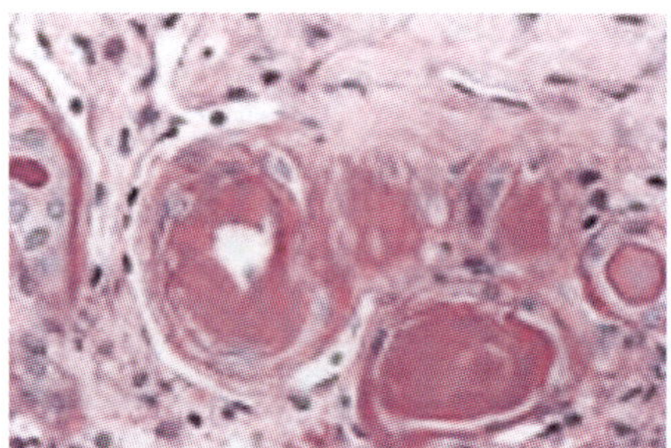

a. Monckeberg's arteriosclerosis
b. Hyaline arteriosclerosis
c. Hyperplastic arteriosclerosis
d. Fibrinoid necrosis

32. Which is true about the image shown?

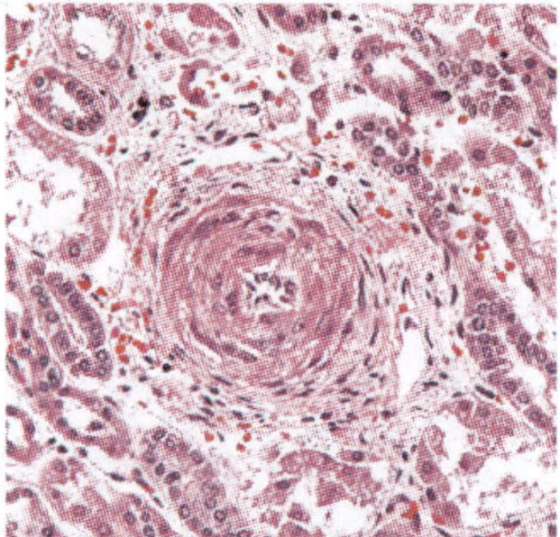

a. Hyaline arteriosclerosis
b. Hyperplastic arteriosclerosis
c. Monckeberg's arteriosclerosis
d. Fibrinoid necrosis

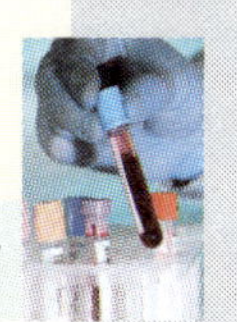
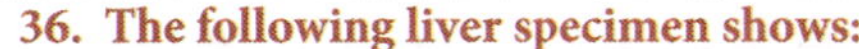

33. **The histopathological slide shows:**

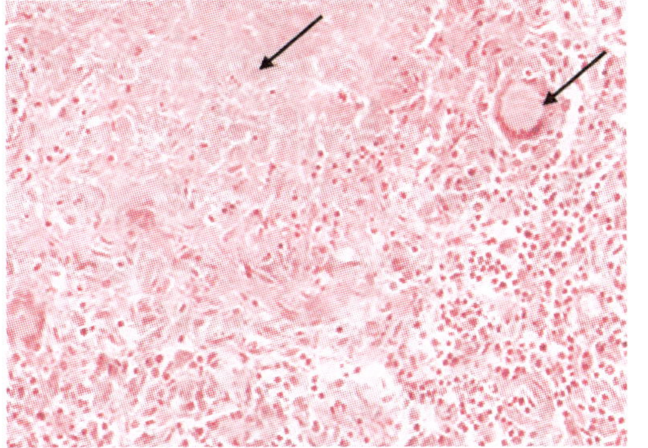

a. Coagulative necrosis b. Liquefactive necrosis
c. Caseous necrosis d. Fat necrosis

34. **Postmortem lung specimen of a patient who developed severe respiratory distress and petechiae after fracture of shaft of femur is given below. All are true about the condition given below, except:**

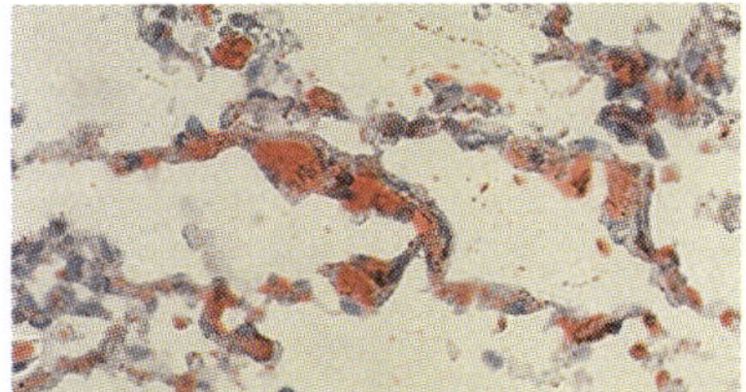

a. Oil Red O stain for fat
b. Noncardiogenic pulmonary edema
c. Gurd criteria
d. Diffuse white matter petechial hemorrhage

35. **Kidney biopsy depicted in the image shows:**

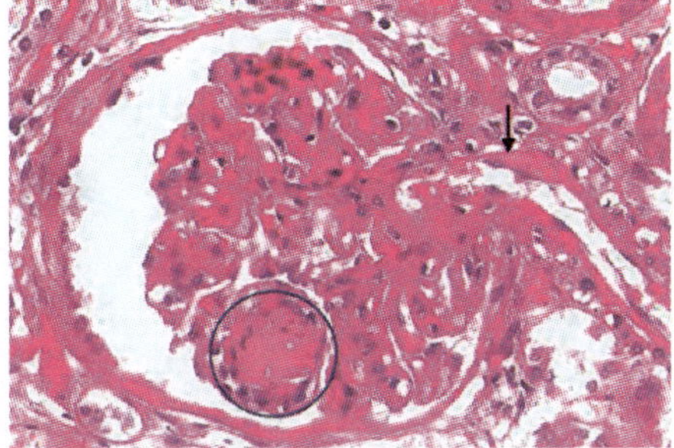

a. Focal segmental glomerulosclerosis
b. Nodular glomerulosclerosis
c. Armanni-Ebstein changes
d. Membranoproliferative glomerulonephritis

36. **The following liver specimen shows:**

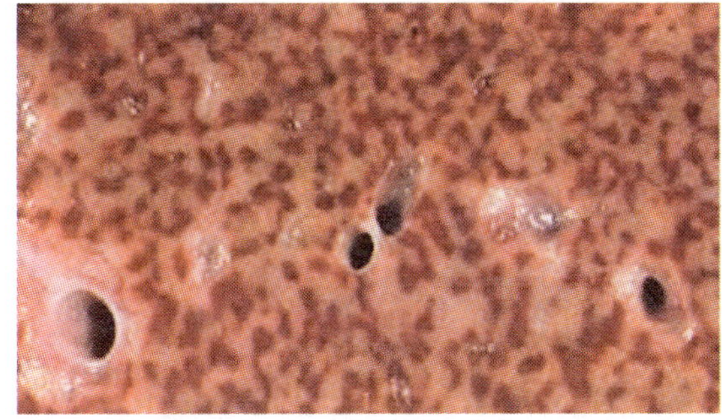

a. Postnecrotic cirrhosis
b. Dubin-Johnson syndrome
c. Miliary tuberculosis (TB)
d. Nutmeg liver

37. **All are true about the marking X in histopathological specimen from a patient of fatty liver, except:**

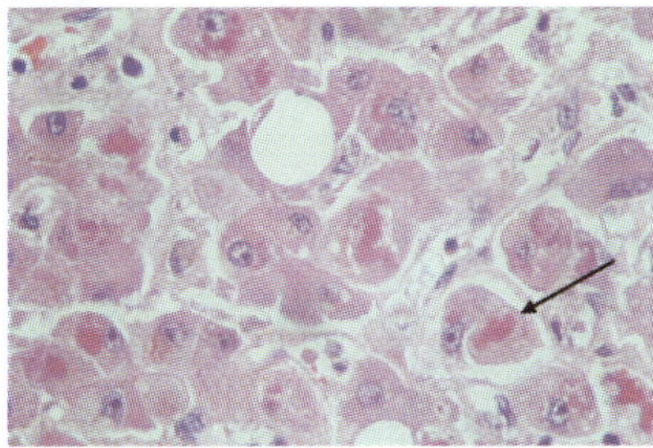

a. Eosinophilic aggregates of prekeratin
b. Intranuclear inclusions
c. Best visualized with Masson trichrome
d. Also seen in Indian childhood cirrhosis

38. **Identify the RBC shown in the figure:**

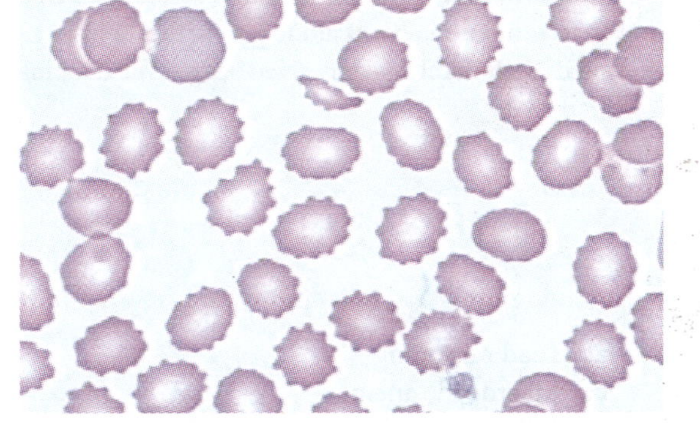

a. Acanthocyte b. Echinocyte
c. Schistocyte d. Spherocyte

39. A 6-year-old boy presents with acute abdomen and non-healing ulcer on medial malleolus. Peripheral smear is shown. The most likely cause of this condition is:

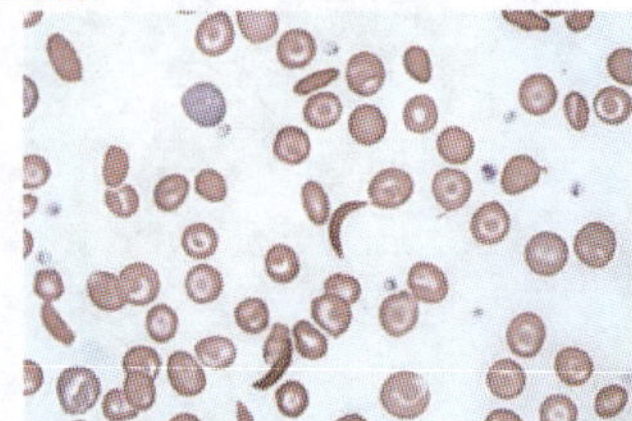

a. Trinucleotide repeat
b. Antibody to RBC membrane
c. Substitution of single amino acid base
d. Genomic imprinting

40. What is your diagnosis on the basis of image given?

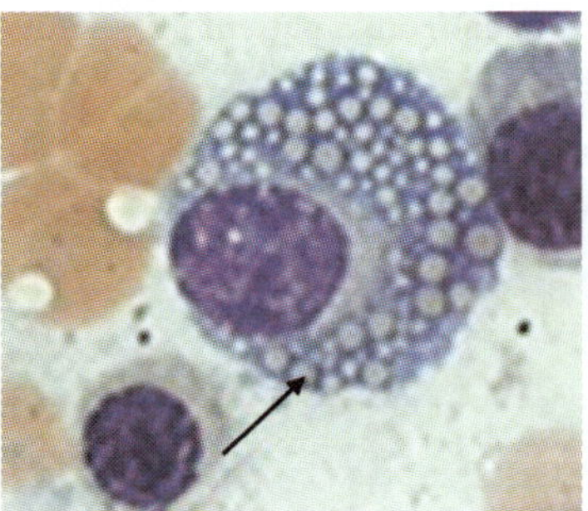

a. Langerhans cell histiocytosis
b. Plasmacytoma
c. Viral encephalitis
d. Leukemia

41. A 45-year-old person presents with complaint of paresthesia in hand and feet with progressive spastic weakness. On examination absent ankle jerk with Babinski sign is noted. Peripheral smear is given below. The diagnosis is:

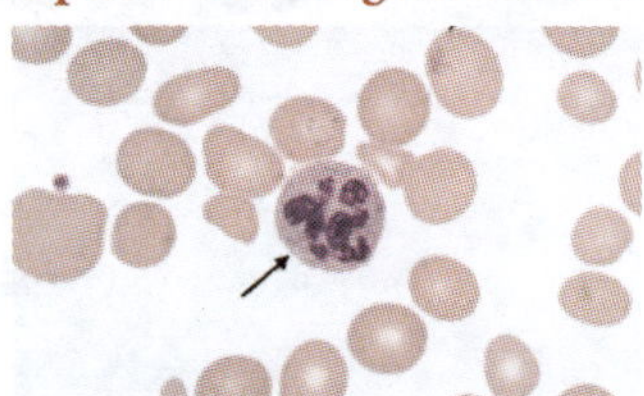

a. Lead poisoning
b. Macrocytic anemia
c. Miller fisher syndrome
d. Devic's disease

42. Spot the diagnosis:

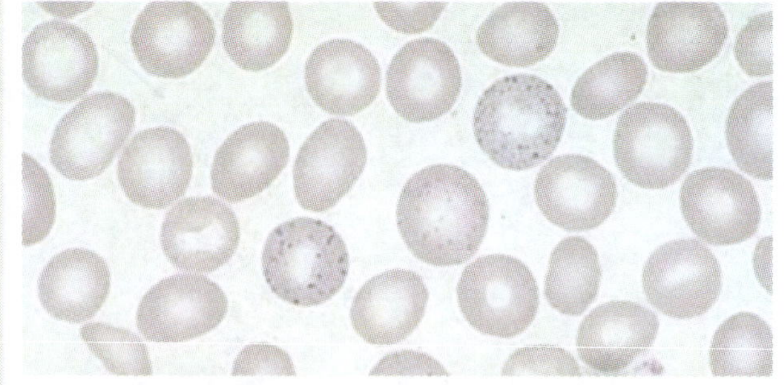

a. Lead poisoning
b. Macrocytic anemia
c. Howell-Jolly bodies
d. Heinz bodies

43. A 6-year-old child presents with lethargy and abdominal pain. Hemoglobin is 8 g% with increased serum iron and increased serum ferritin. Peripheral smear is shown. Which is correct about the image?

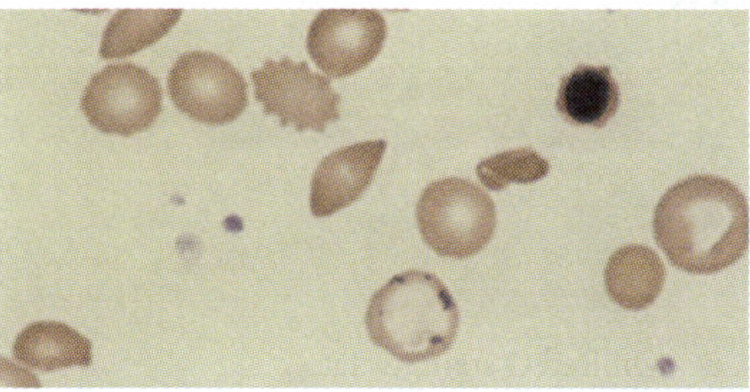

a. Pappenheimer body
b. Heinz body
c. Lead poisoning
d. Howell-Jolly body

44. Which stain is preferred to diagnose these RBC inclusions seen in patients with elevated serum ferritin and serum iron?

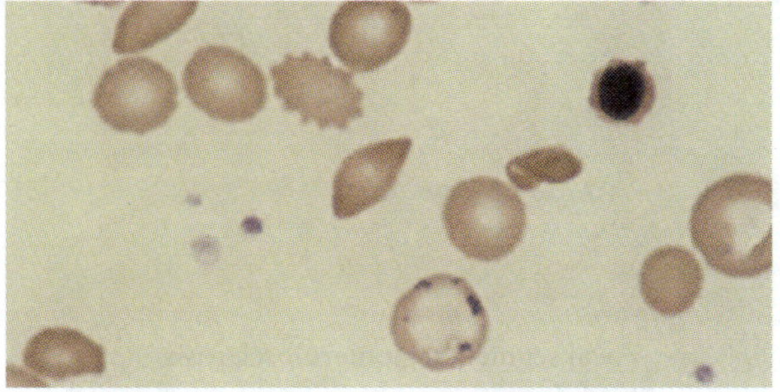

a. Perls stain
b. Rubeanic acid
c. Supravital stain
d. Congo red

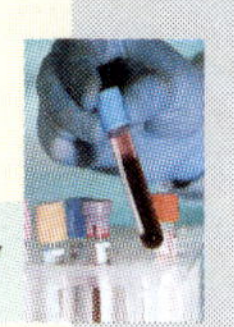

45. The following RBC inclusion is composed of:

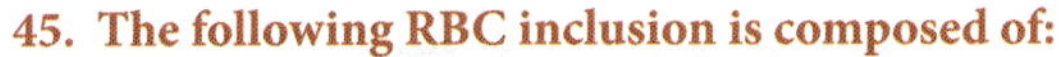

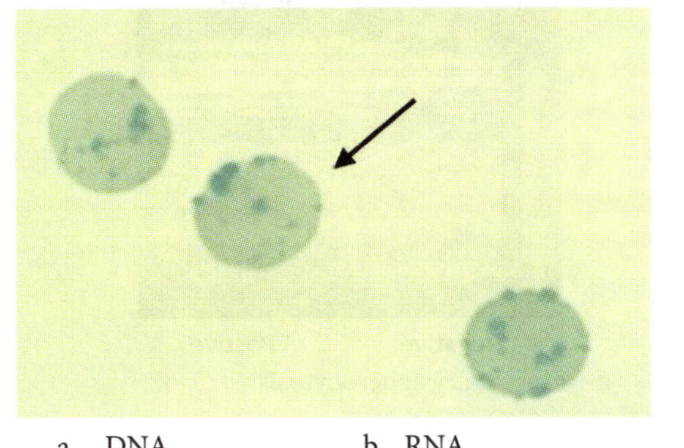

a. DNA
b. RNA
c. Iron
d. Denatured hemoglobin

46. The following RBC inclusions are seen in:

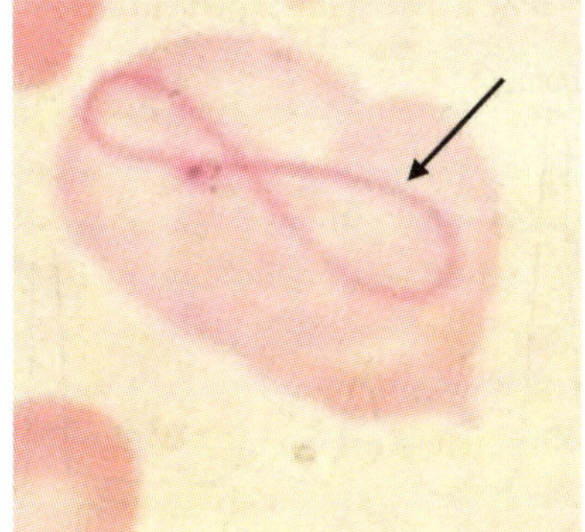

a. HbH disease
b. Hemoglobin Barts
c. Pernicious anemia
d. Malaria

47. The following image shows presence of:

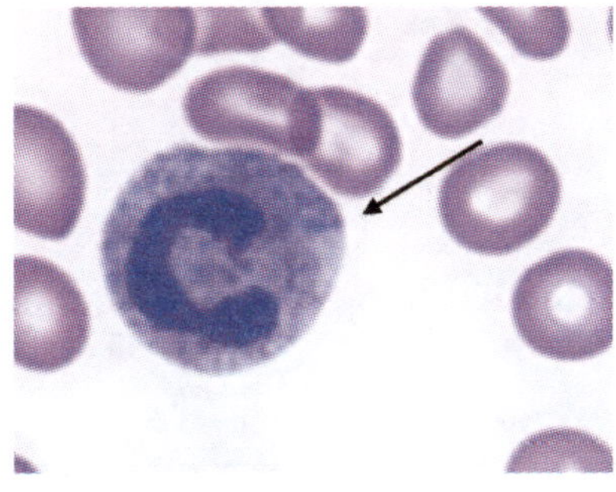

a. Dohle bodies
b. Toxic granules
c. Critical green inclusions
d. Normal inclusions

48. A 70-year-old man presents with painless cervical lymphadenopathy with progressive pallor and petechiae on ankles. Peripheral smear shows presence of:

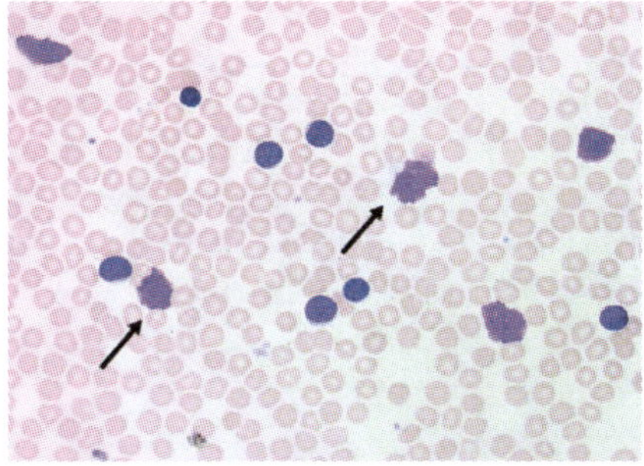

a. Acute ITP
b. Chronic ITP
c. CLL
d. Richter syndrome

49. Which condition is presented in case of following peripheral smear and X-ray spine present with?

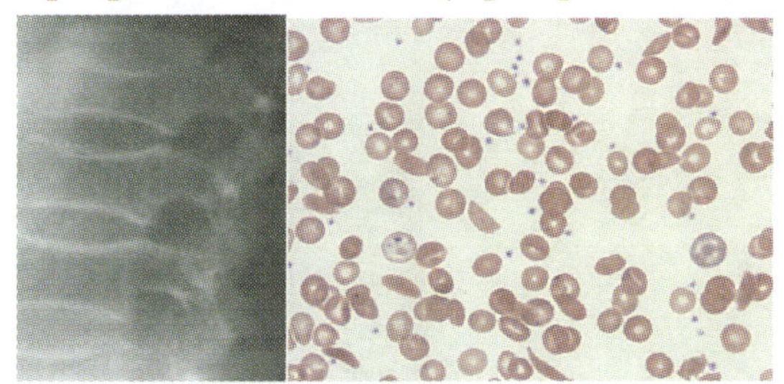

a. Hand Foot syndrome
b. Black urine
c. Elevated haptoglobin
d. Splenomegaly with gall stones

50. Identify the cell:

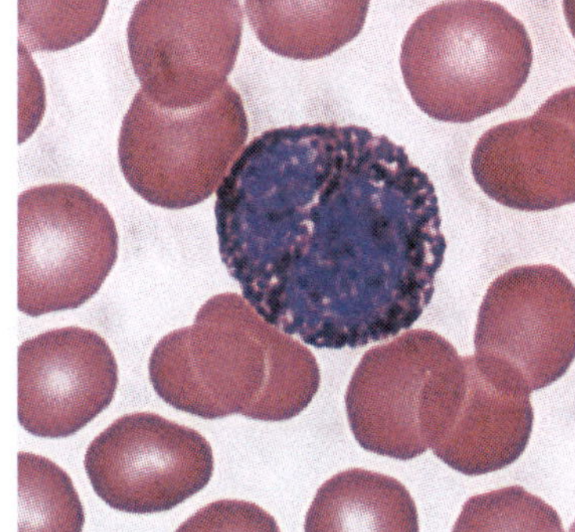

a. Eosinophil
b. Basophil
c. Monocyte
d. Lymphocyte

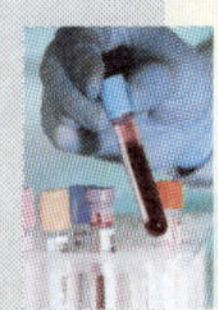
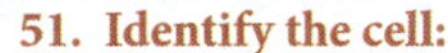

51. Identify the cell:

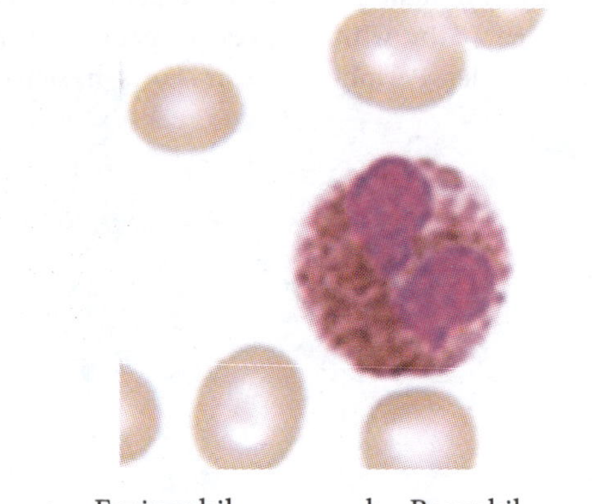

a. Eosinophil
b. Basophil
c. Neutrophil
d. Monocyte

52. Name the test given:

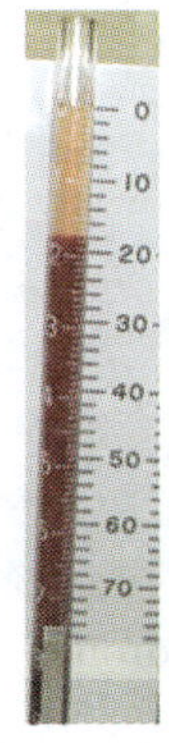

a. Osmotic fragility
b. NESTROFT
c. Sickling test
d. ESR measurement

53. Name the anticoagulant used in the following method:

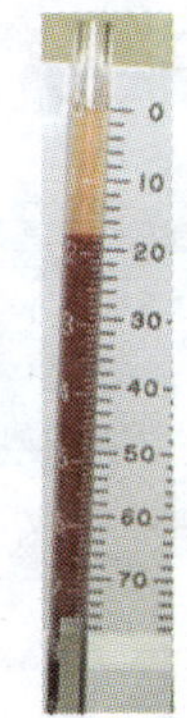

a. EDTA
b. Heparin
c. Trisodium citrate
d. Dalteparin

54. This test is used as a screening tool for:

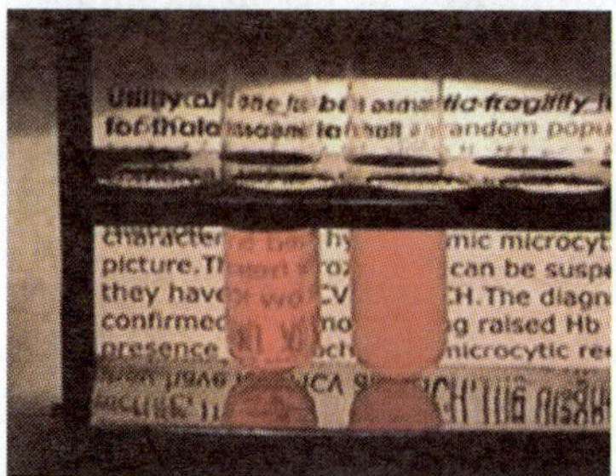

Negative **Postive**

a. Hereditary spherocytosis
b. G6PD
c. Thalassemia
d. Megaloblastic anemia

55. The image shows electrophoresis report of multiple myeloma. The spike is present in:

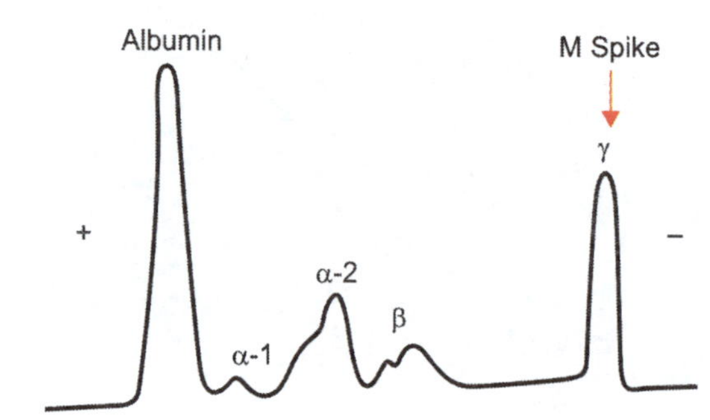

a. Alpha 1 globulin
b. Alpha 2 globulin
c. Beta globulin
d. Gamma globulin

56. The following image shows:

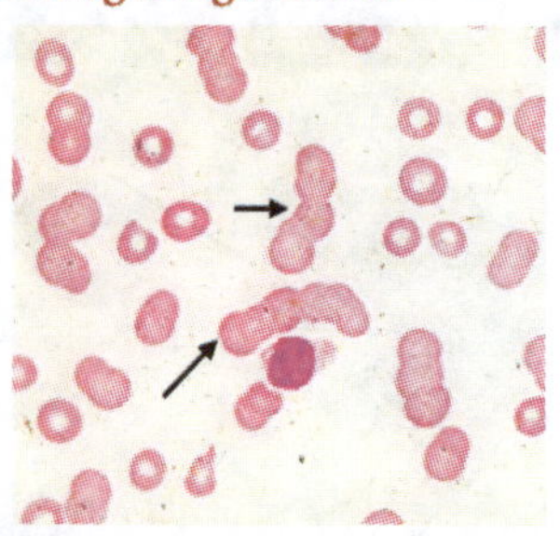

a. Microcytic hypochromic cells
b. Evidence of hemolysis
c. Sickling crisis
d. Rouleaux formation

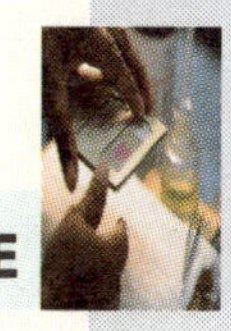

57. Comment on the histopathological specimen:

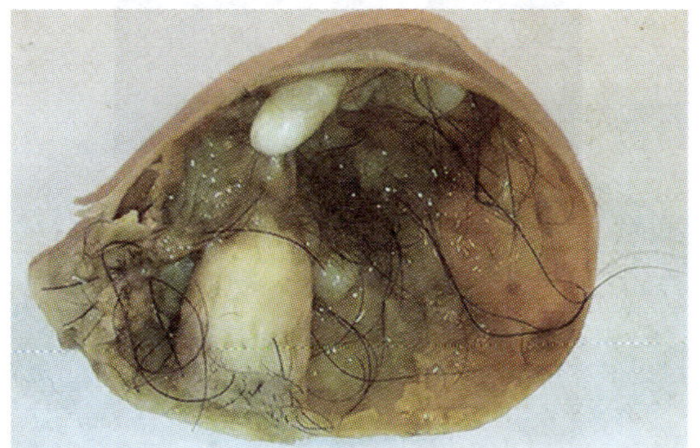

a. Teratoma b. Rhabdomyoma
c. Rhabdomyosarcoma d. Neuroblastoma

58. What is the most likely diagnosis on the basis of the given peripheral smear?

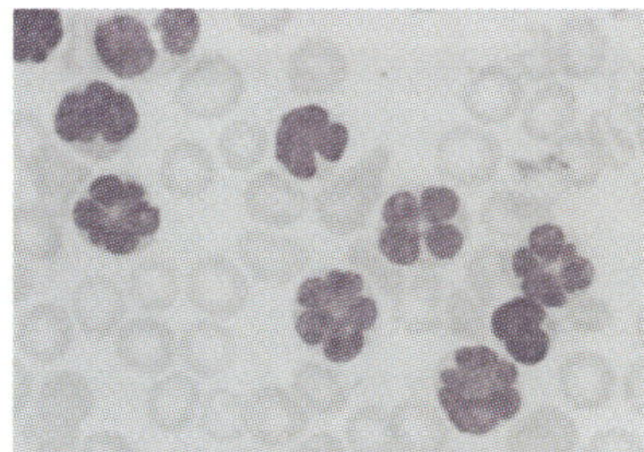

a. Hodgkin lymphoma
b. Diffuse large B cell Lymphoma
c. Adult T cell leukaemia
d. Chronic lymphocytic leukemia

59. The following cells seen in the lymph node are indicative of:

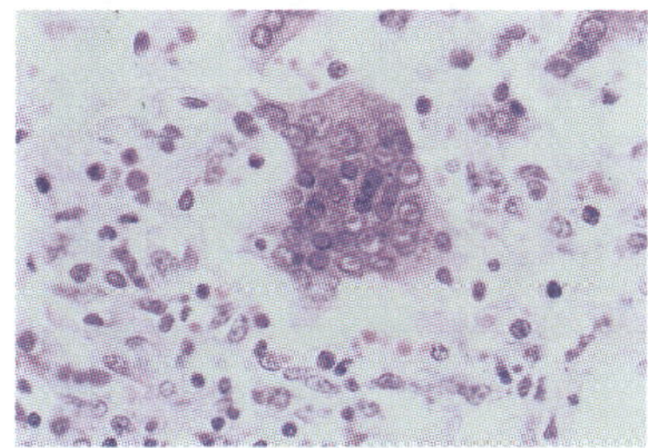

a. Infectious Mononucleosis
b. CMV infection
c. Measles
d. Influenza

60. In which of the following thyroid carcinoma the shown microscopic findings are present?

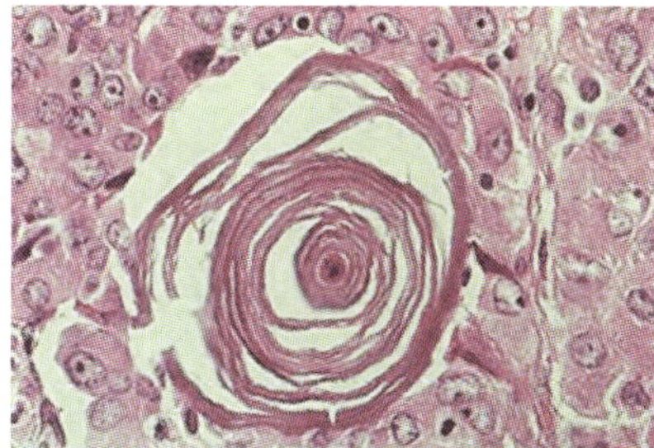

a. Papillary b. Follicular
c. Anaplastic d. Medullary

FORENSIC MEDICINE

61. The following picture shows:

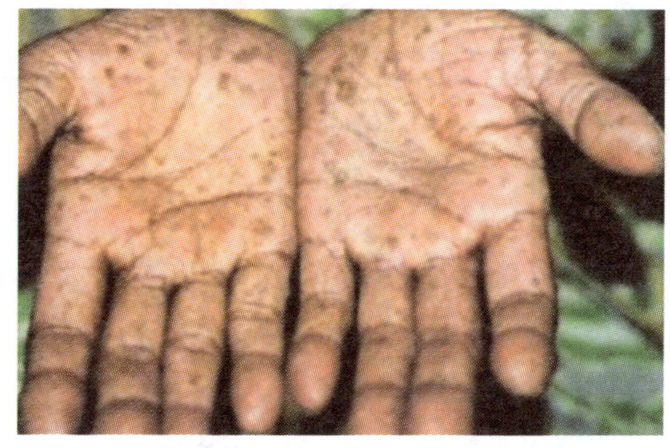

a. Lead poisoning b. Arsenic poisoning
c. Copper poisoning d. Iron poisoning

62. The type of injury shown in the given image is:

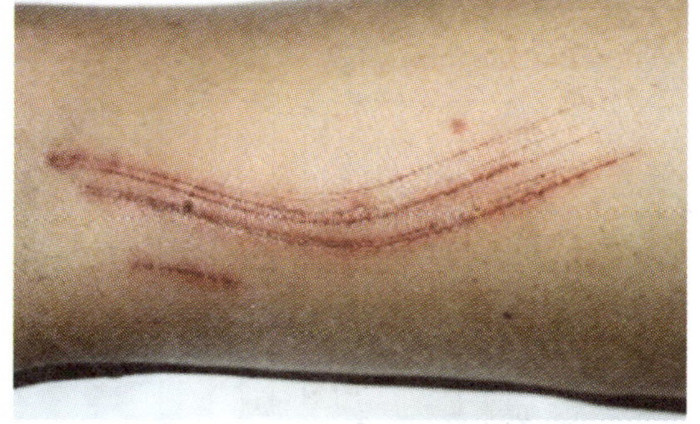

a. Laceration b. Abrasion
c. Chop wound d. Incised wound

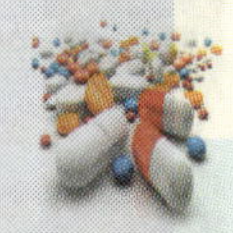

63. There is a history of gunshot injury in a 35-year-old male. Identify the wound shown in the image given below:

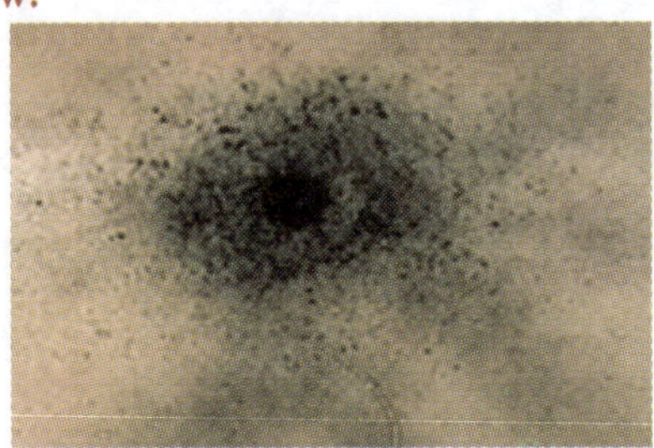

a. Distant shot exit wound
b. Distant shot entry wound
c. Close shot exit wound
d. Close shot entry wound

PREVENTIVE AND SOCIAL MEDICINE (PSM)

64. The following image shows:

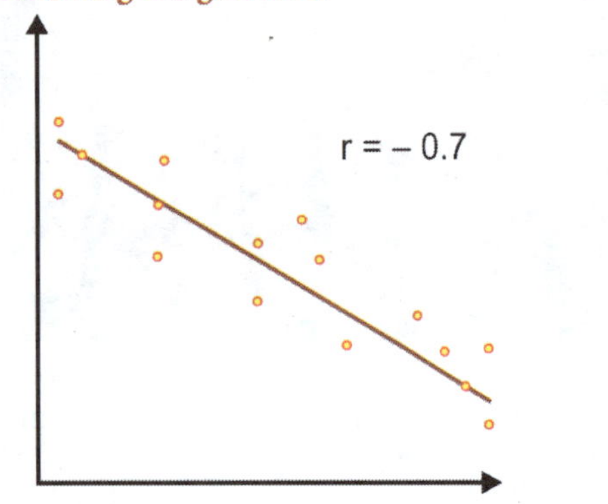

a. Histogram
b. Correlation coefficient
c. Frequency polygon
d. Bar diagram

65. The following image shows:

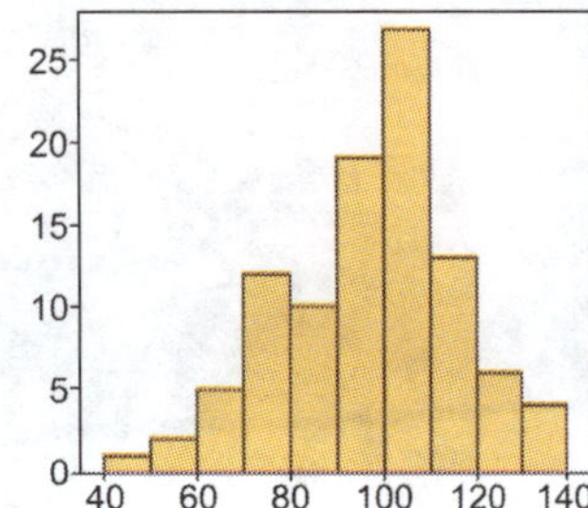

a. Histogram
b. Correlation coefficient
c. Frequency polygon
d. Bar diagram

66. The following image shows presence of:

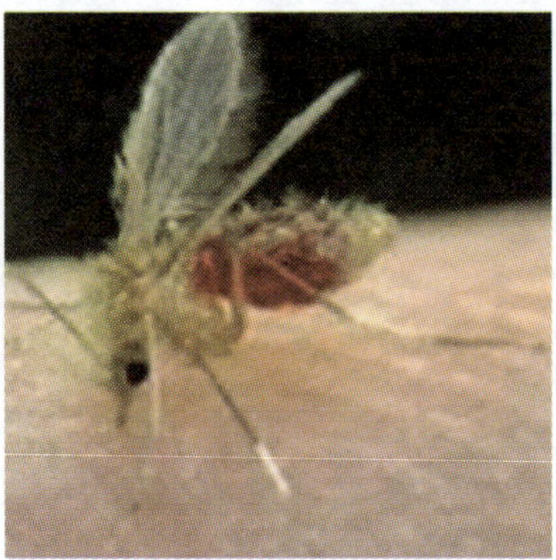

a. Sandfly
b. Aedes
c. Culex
d. Tse Tse Fly

67. The image shows presence of:

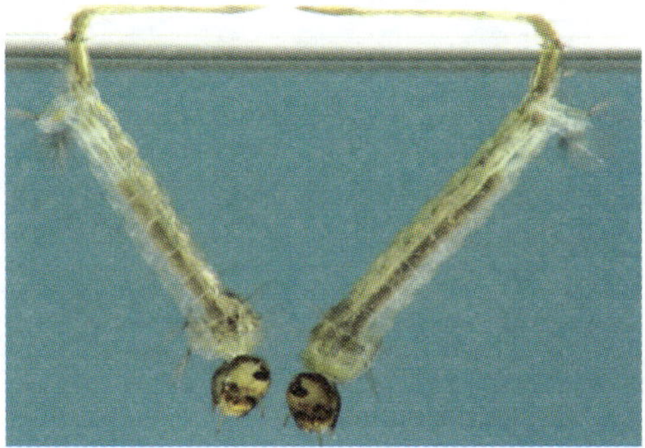

a. Aedes larvae
b. Culex larvae
c. Anopheles larvae
d. Mansonia larva

68. Which of the following organizations is shown below?

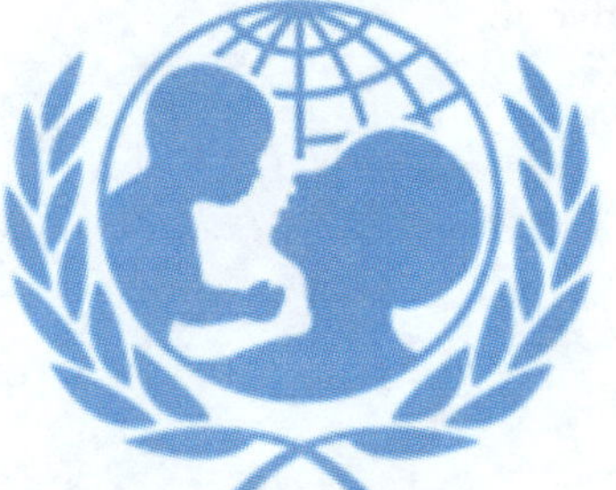

a. World Health Organization
b. UNICEF
c. FAO
d. World Bank

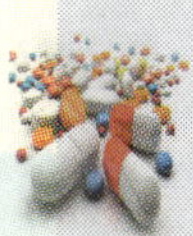

69. The following symbol shows which program of government of India:

a. National Rural Health Mission
b. National Urban Health Mission
c. Reproductive and Child Health Programme
d. A.Y.U.S.H

70. Identify:

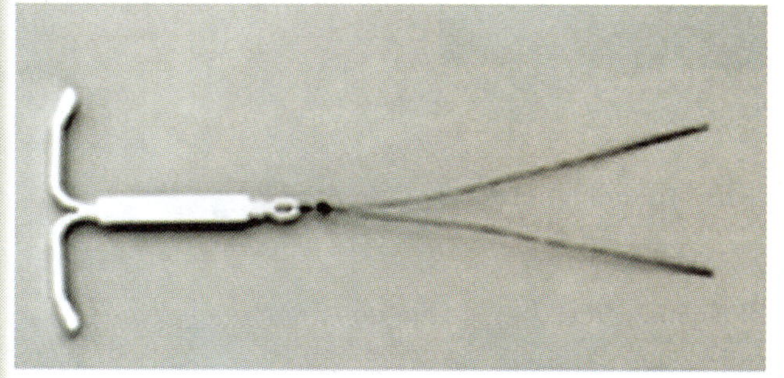

a. Mirena b. Cu T 380 A
c. Para Gard d. Ortho evra

71. Identify the programme from the logo:

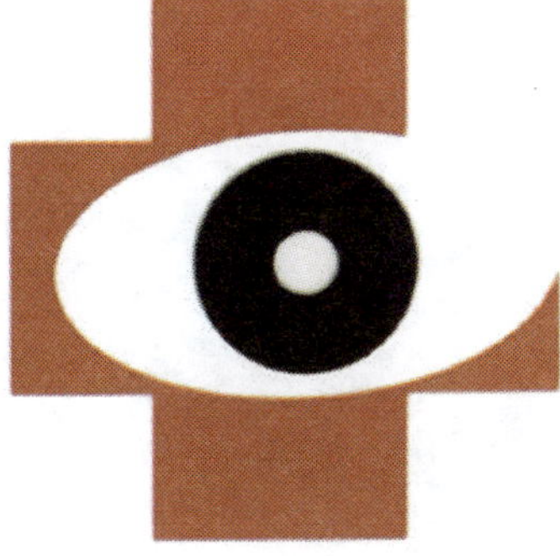

a. NLEP b. ICDS
c. NACO d. NPBCVI

72. Identify the instrument:

a. Bulb thermometer
b. Jacen's thermometer
c. Globe thermometer
d. Kata thermometer

73. The insect shown below is a vector for which of the following diseases:

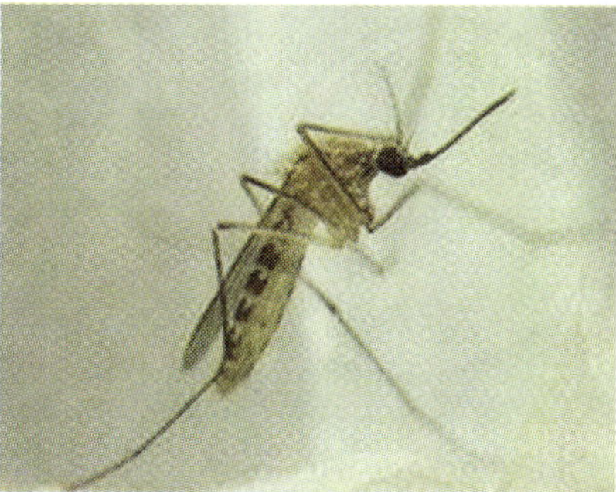

a. Chikungunya b. Malaria
c. Malayan Filariasis d. Japanese Encephalitis

74. The shown organism causes which disease:

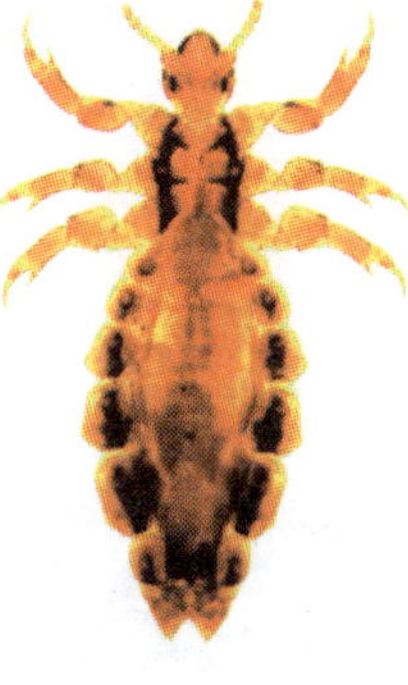

a. Scabies b. Loa Loa
c. Pediculosis Capitis d. Onchocerciasis

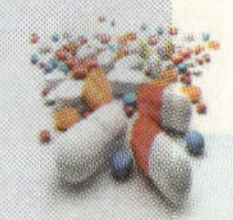

75. Instrument shown in photograph is used to assess:

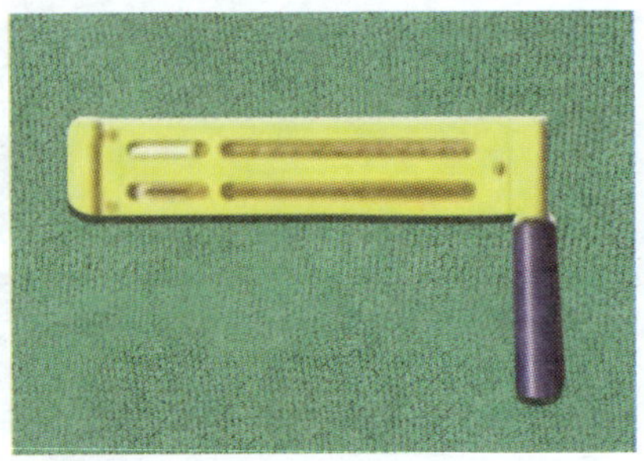

a. Relative humidity of air
b. Environmental heat measurement
c. Cooling power of air
d. Mean radiant temperature of surroundings

76. Identify the instrument:

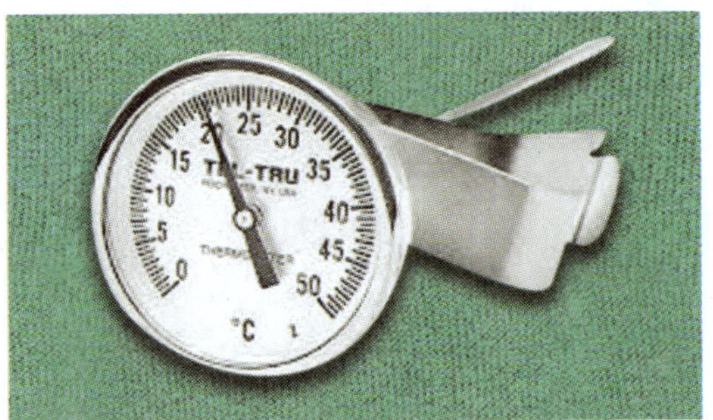

a. Globe thermometer
b. Anemometer
c. Chloroscope
d. Dial thermometer

77. Identify the instrument:

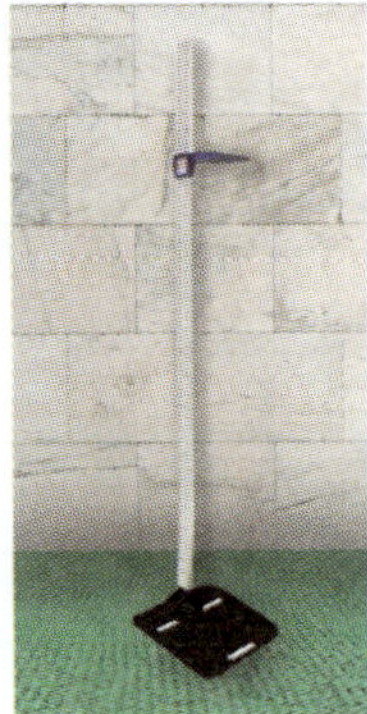

a. Infantometer
b. Anemometer
c. Stadiometer
d. None of these

78. Where is the headquarter of this International Health Agency?

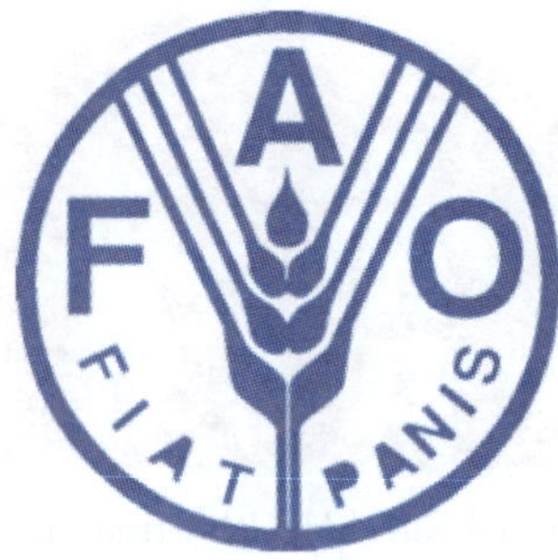

a. Geneva
b. Florida
c. Rome
d. Chennai

79. Where is the headquarter of this organization?

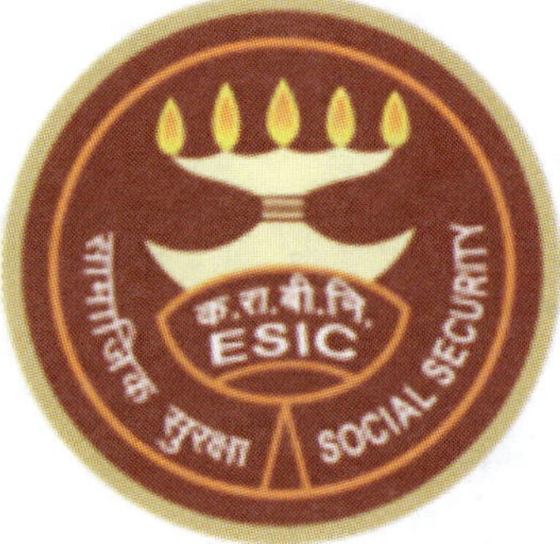

a. Ahmedabad
b. Hyderabad
c. Chennai
d. New Delhi

80. Identify the contraceptive device:

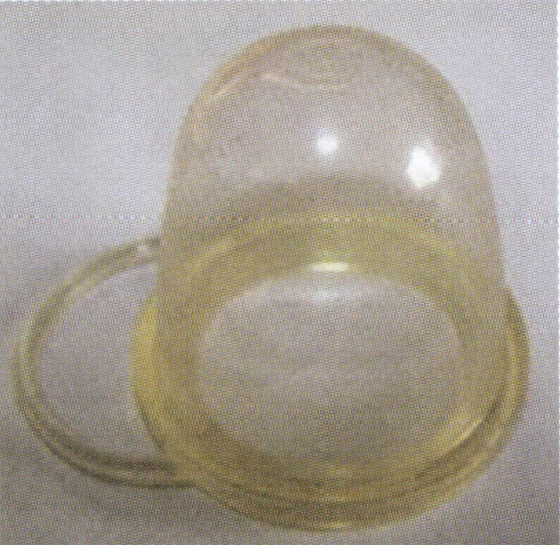

a. Male Condom
b. IUD
c. Cervical cap
d. Vaginal douche

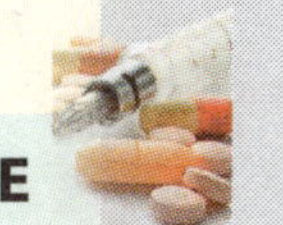

81. Identify the contraceptive shown in the given image:

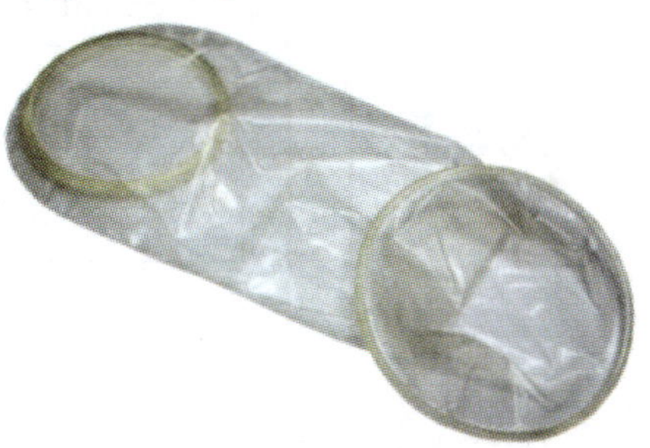

a. Female condom
b. Male condom
c. IUD
d. Copper T

MEDICINE

82. ECG of the patient was done in the ER. Which of the following is the most probable diagnosis:

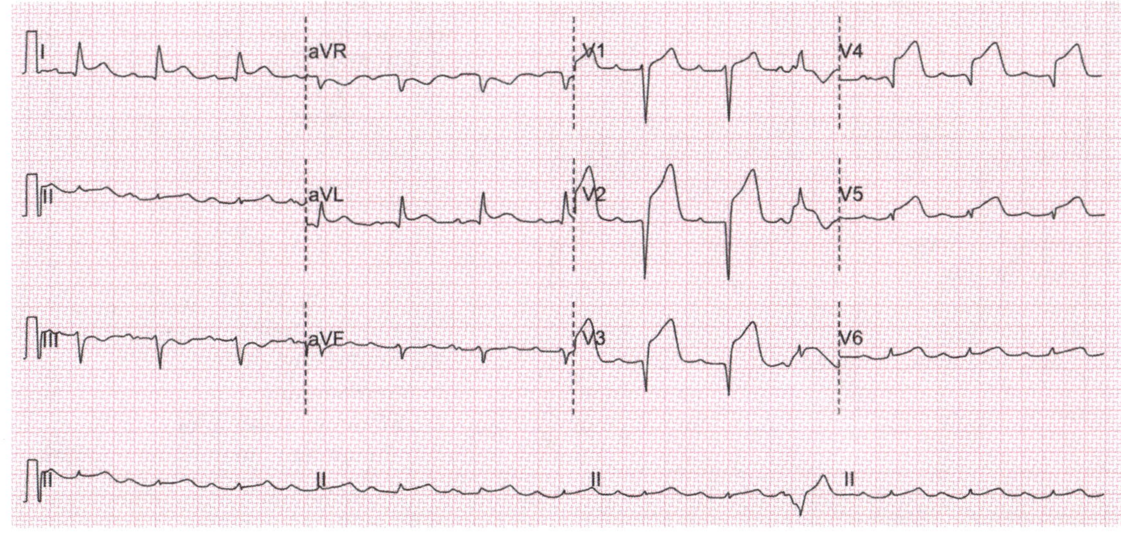

a. Hypoglycemia
b. Hypoglycemic unawareness
c. Anterior wall MI
d. Inferior wall MI

83. A 35-year-old lady has been diagnosed as having anxiety neurosis by her psychiatrist. She came to you for second opinion. Comment on the diagnosis based on ECG:

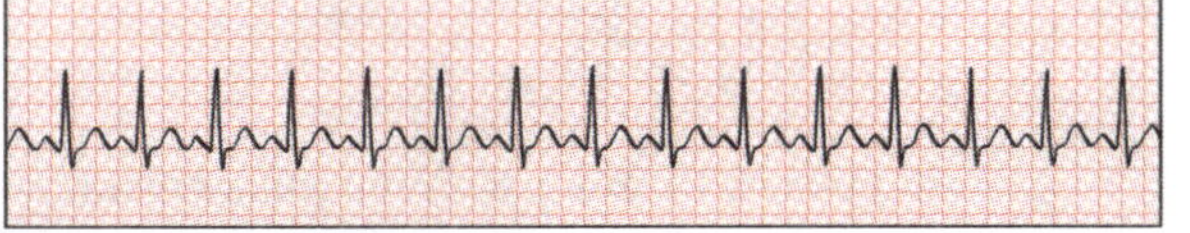

a. Sinus tachycardia
b. WPW syndrome
c. Multifocal atrial tachycardia
d. Atrial fibrillation

84. A 60-year-old patient is having recurrent syncopal attacks post myocardial infarction. The ECG shows:

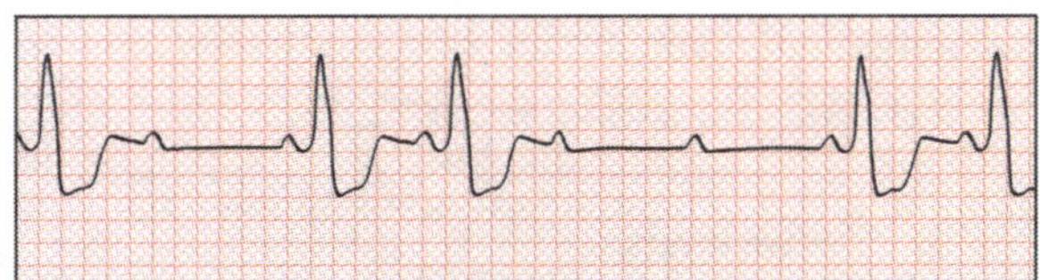

a. Accelerated idioventricular rhythm
b. Ventricular bigeminy
c. Mobitz II heart block
d. Wenckebach phenomenon

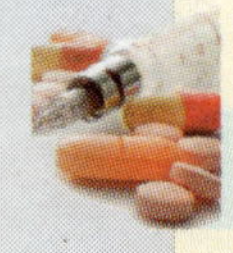

85. Which of the following finding is shown in the chest leads?

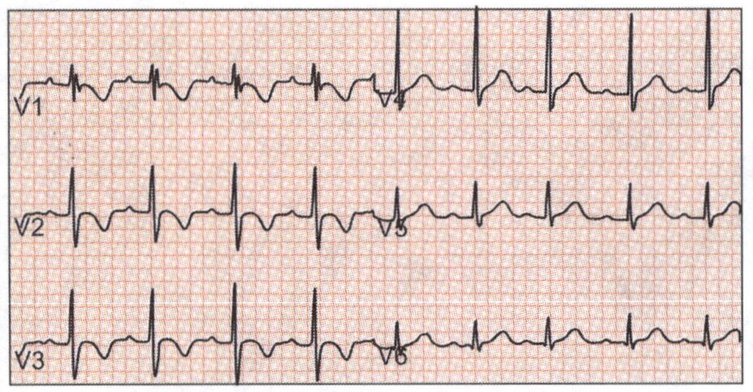

a. Myocardial ischemia b. Myocardial injury
c. Digoxin d. Digoxin toxicity

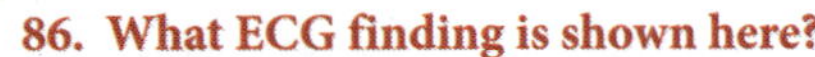

86. What ECG finding is shown here?

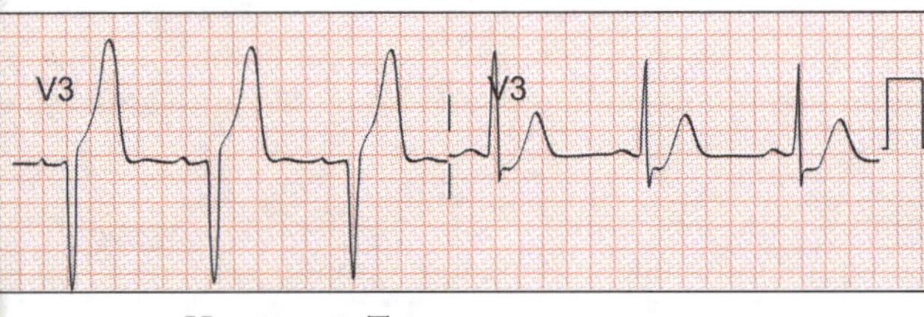

a. Hyperacute T-wave
b. T-wave alterans
c. T-wave inversion
d. Artefact

87. What ECG finding is shown here?

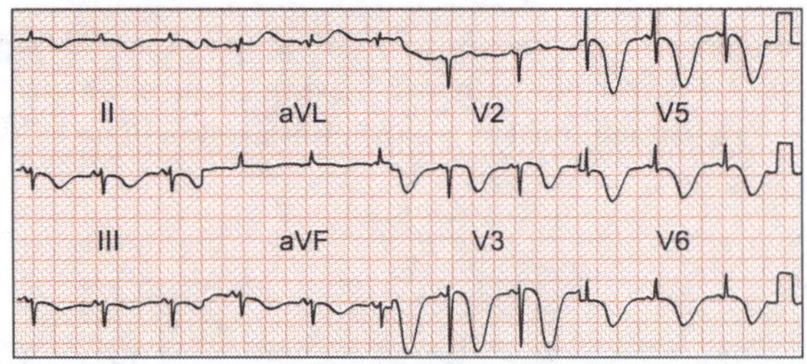

a. T-wave inversion
b. Artifact
c. Premature ventricular complexes
d. Positive U waves

88. A 1-year-old child with CHD is on heart failure treatment. The ECG shows all EXCEPT:

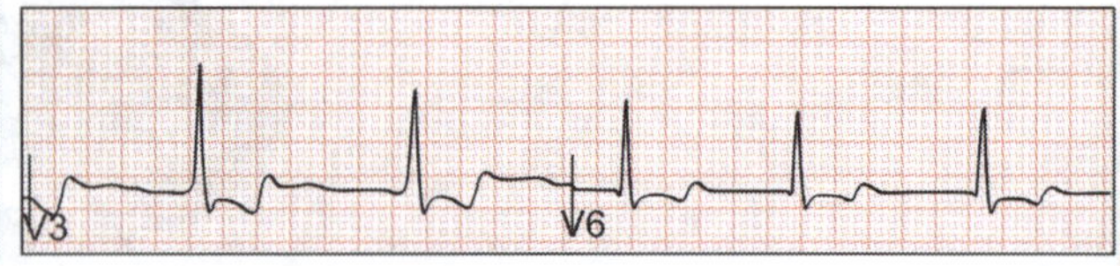

a. Ventricular bigeminy
b. Heart rate of 60 bpm approximately
c. ST depression
d. U wave

89. A 65-year-old man is brought with complaints of breathlessness and chest pain for 18 hours. ECG was done. Which of the following is incorrect:

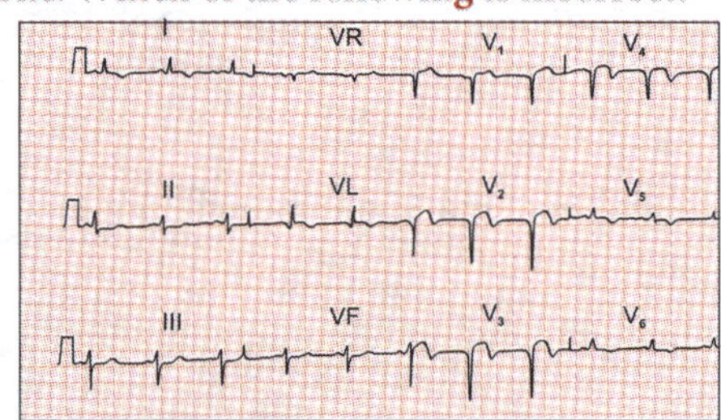

a. Normal sinus rhythm
b. Normal axis
c. ST elevation in V2-V4
d. Premature ventricular contractions

90. A 10-year-old child of valvular heart disease on heart failure treatment, has the following ECG tracing. What is the diagnosis:

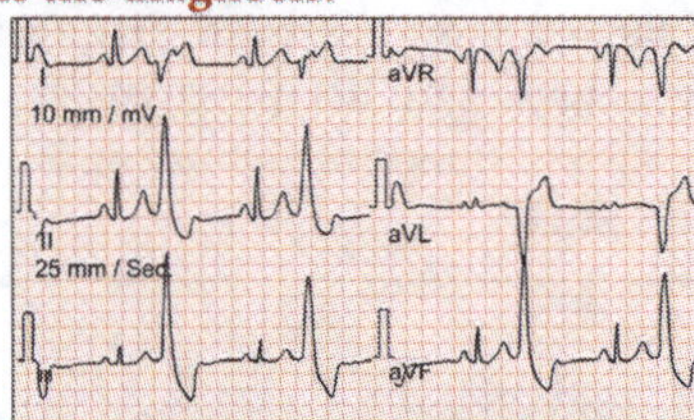

a. Tall tented T wave b. Ventricular bigeminy
c. Non paroxysmal atrial tachycardia with irregular AV block
d. Non paroxysmal atrial tachycardia with regular AV block

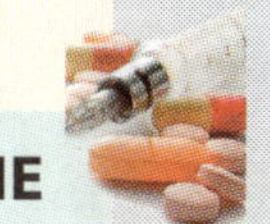

91. A 50-year-old woman with rheumatic heart disease is on medication for heart disease. She feels unwell for most part of the day. Which of the following medicine is responsible for the ECG changes shown below:

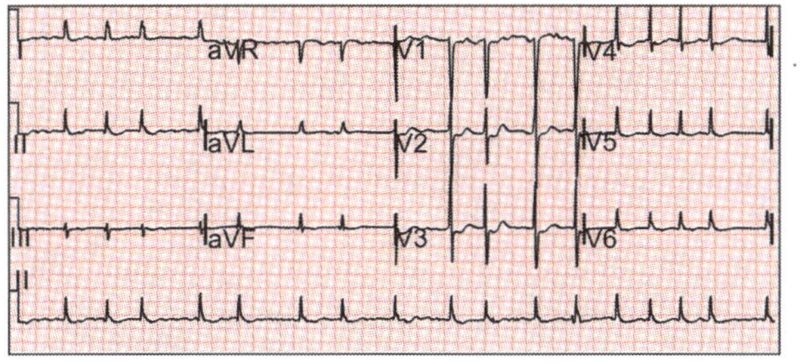

a. ACE inhibitor b. Diuretics
c. Ivabradine d. Digoxin

92. A 25-year-old woman presents with complaints of recurrent episodes of sudden onset palpitations. What does her ECG tracing show:

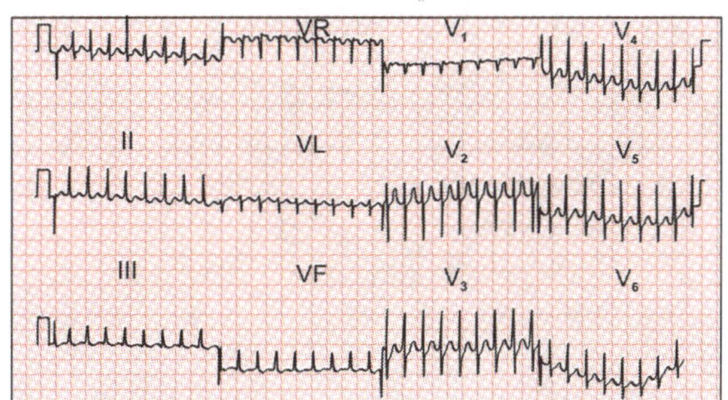

a. Atrial flutter b. Atrial bigeminy
c. PSVT d. Sinus tachycardia

93. A 65-year-old pensioner in ESI dispensary complains of exercise intolerance. On auscultation a systolic murmur grade 3 is heard. What does the ECG show:

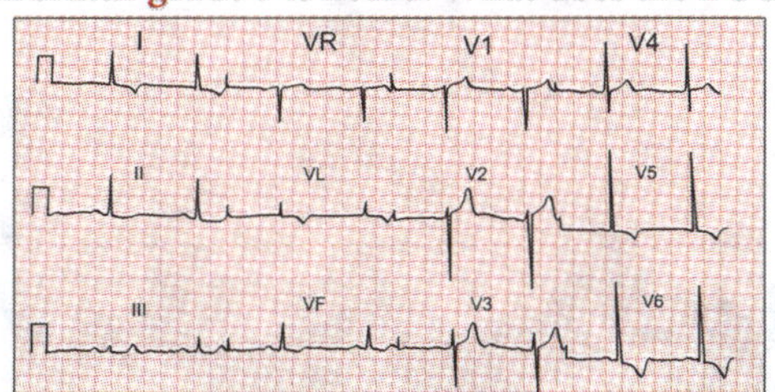

a. Normal tracing
b. Left ventricular hypertrophy
c. Atrial fibrillation
d. Left bundle branch block

94. Identify the ECG given in the figure below:

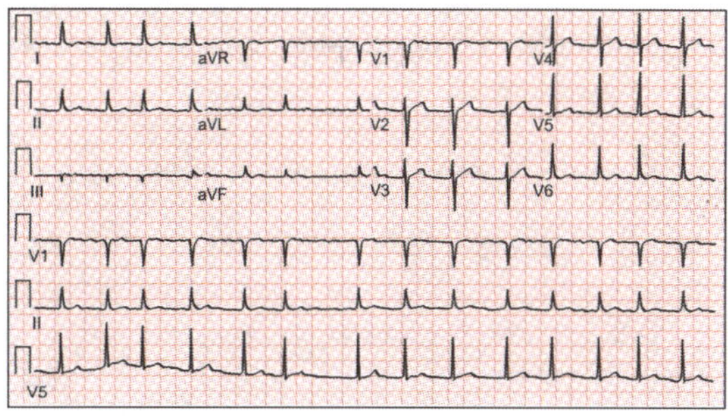

a. Normal sinus rhythm
b. Paroxysmal supraventricular tachycardia
c. Atrial fibrillation
d. Ventricular fibrillation

95. In the ECG shown below which drug will not be given:

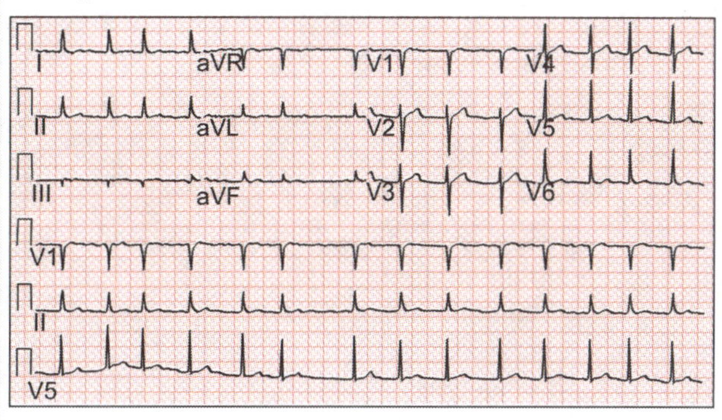

a. Amiodarone b. Adenosine
c. Diltiazem d. Beta blocker

96. A 65-year-old elderly male has history of sweating and chest pain for last 24 hours with the following ECG. Which of the following is not given in managing the patient:

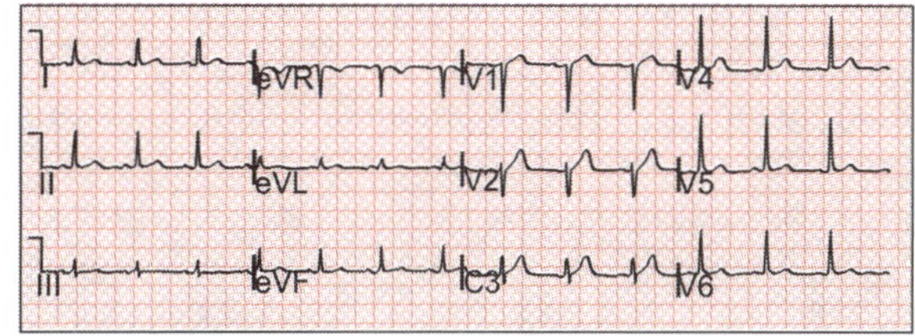

a. Aspirin b. Statin
c. Thrombolytic therapy
d. Morphine

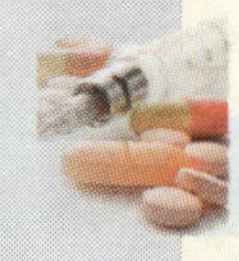

97. A 52-year-old male diabetic patient presents with palpitations to the AIIMS emergency. Urgent ECG was performed. What is the immediate next step in the management:

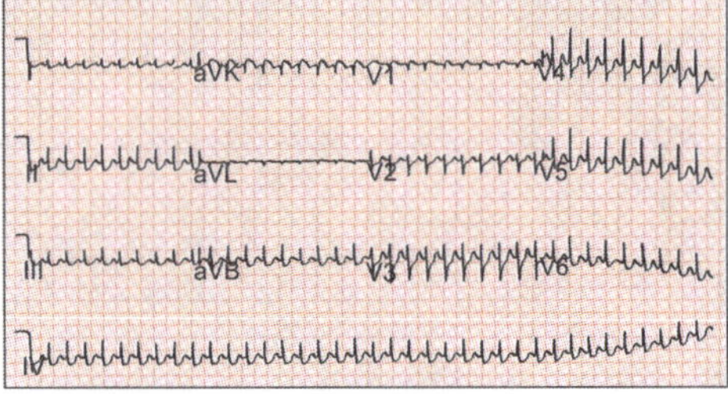

a. Electrical cardioversion
b. Amiodarone
c. Adenosine
d. Primary PCI

98. A 75-year-old male patient presents to the AIIMS emergency with retrosternal chest pain for 6 hours. The following ECG was done. What will be the primary management of the patient:

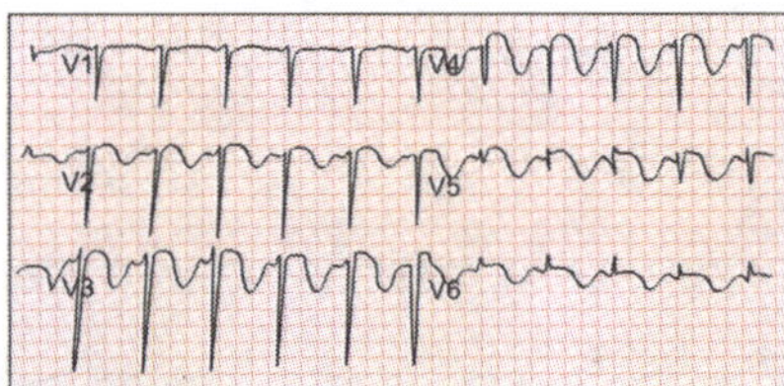

a. Primary PCI
b. Thrombolysis
c. Abciximab
d. Low molecular weight heparin

99. For calculation of rate related (corrected) QT interval, QT interval is divided by √ X:

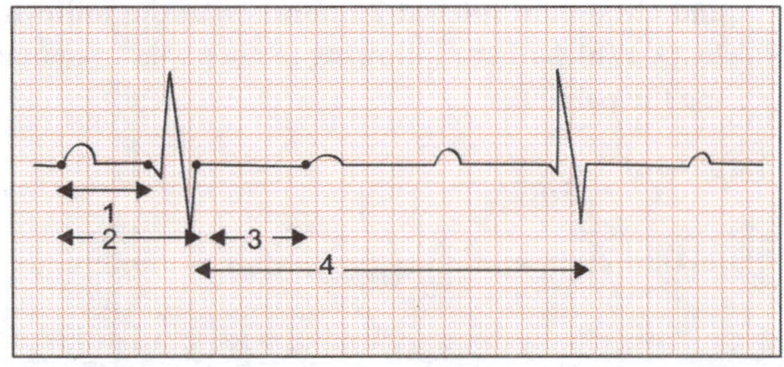

a. 1
b. 2
c. 3
d. 4

100. The marked part of the ECG points to which phase of cardiac action potential:

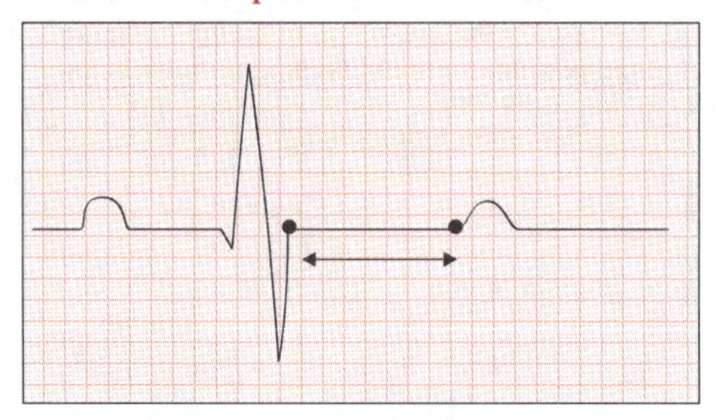

a. Phase 0
b. Phase 1
c. Phase 2
d. Phase 3

101. What does the following ECG show?

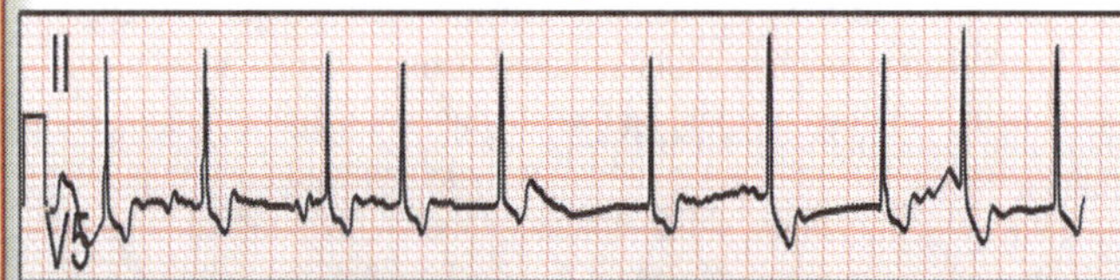

a. Osbourne wave
b. Delta wave
c. Hockey stick sign
d. Epsilon wave

102. In which of the given diseases is this condition observed:

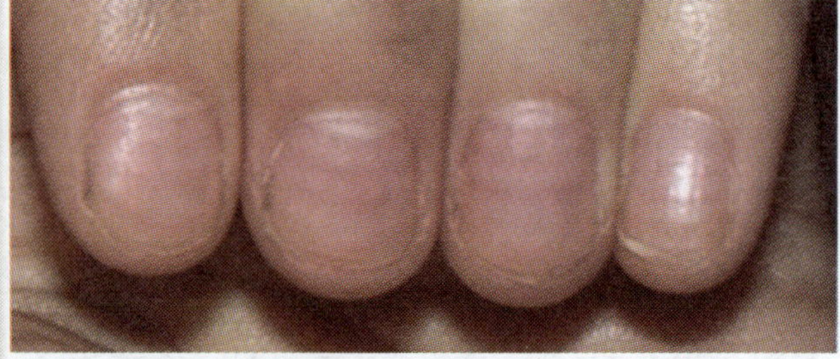

a. Renal failure
b. Thalassemia
c. Liver Cirrhosis
d. Hypoalbuminemia

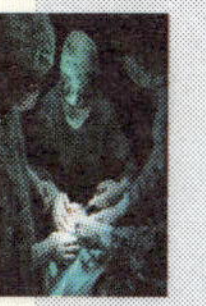

103. The following sign is highly specific for:

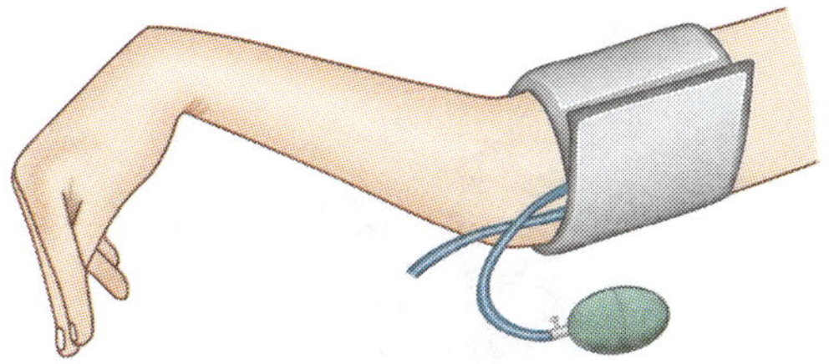

a. Hyperphosphatemia
b. Hypocalcemia
c. Trousseau's syndrome
d. Hypermagnesemia

SURGERY

104. What does the intraoperative photograph depict?

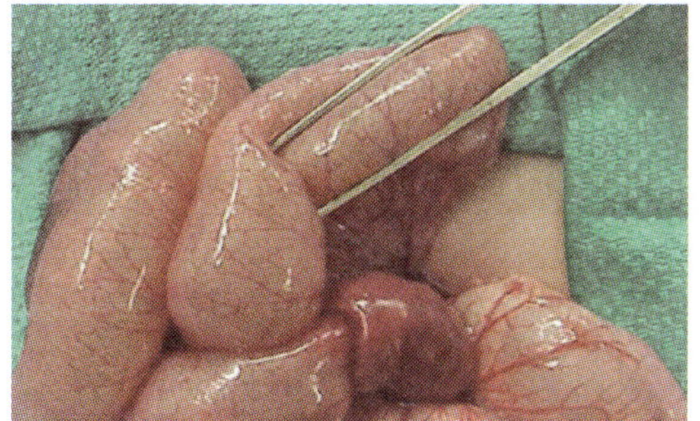

a. Transverse colon
b. Meckel's diverticulum
c. Intussusception
d. Fallopian tube

105. Identify these two surgical instruments:

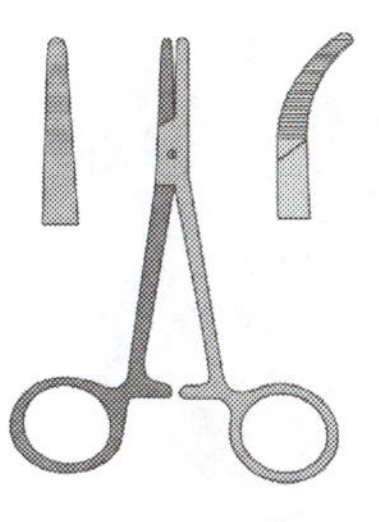
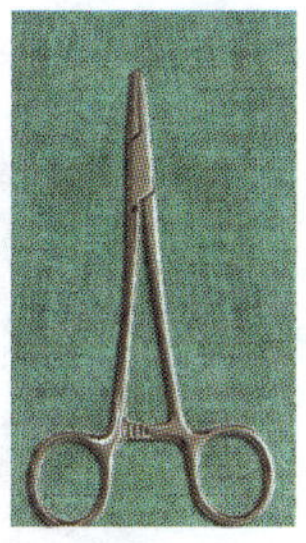

a. Thumb forceps & Sponge Holder
b. Artery Forceps & Needle Holder
c. Sponge Holder & Allis Forceps
d. Needle Holder & Ovum Forceps

106. All are true about the lesion, except:

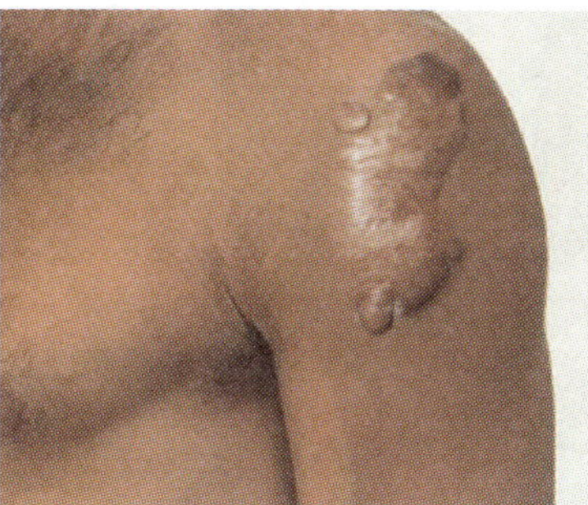

a. Severe itching
b. Claw like process
c. Develops at vaccination sites
d. Collagen bundles are present

107. All are true about the image shown, except:

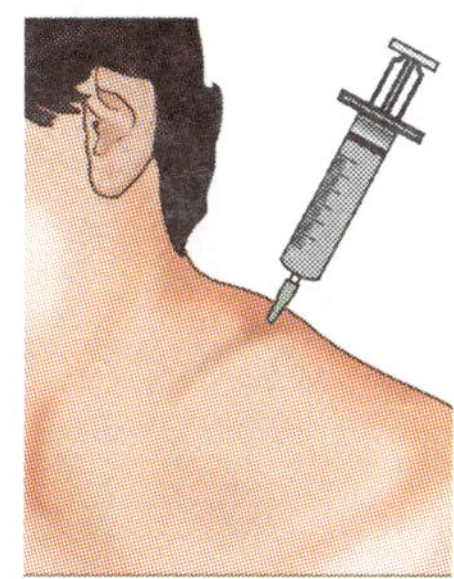

a. Anti-gravity drainage
b. Cold abscess
c. Transillumination test is negative
d. Rubbery consistency of involved lymph nodes

108. All are true about the image shown: except:

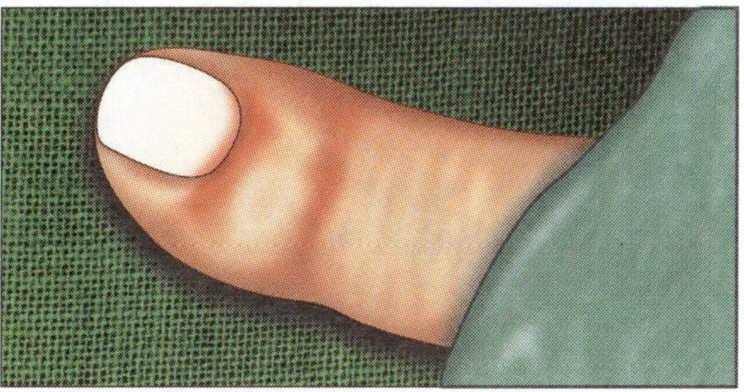

a. Acute paronychia
b. Throbbing pain
c. Ring block with adrenaline used
d. I and D by incising the eponychium

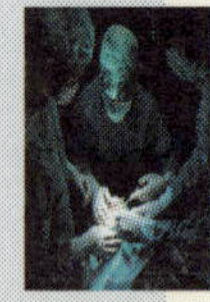

109. Comment on image A and B:

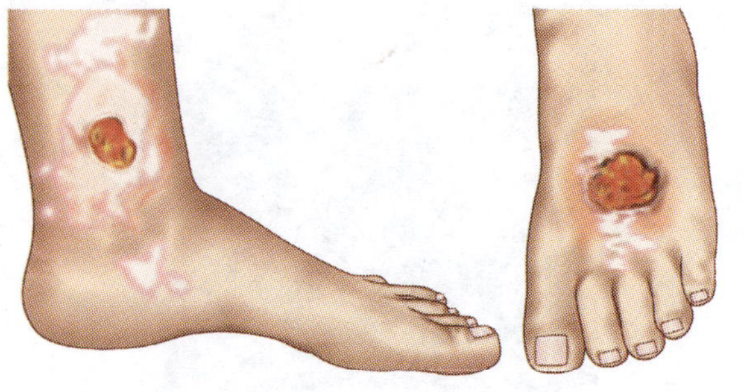

a. A=venous ulcer and B= ischemic ulcer
b. A=arterial ulcer and B= venous ulcer
c. A=neuropathic ulcer and B= arterial ulcer
d. A=Venous ulcer and B= neuropathic ulcer

110. Identify the type of ulcer shown:

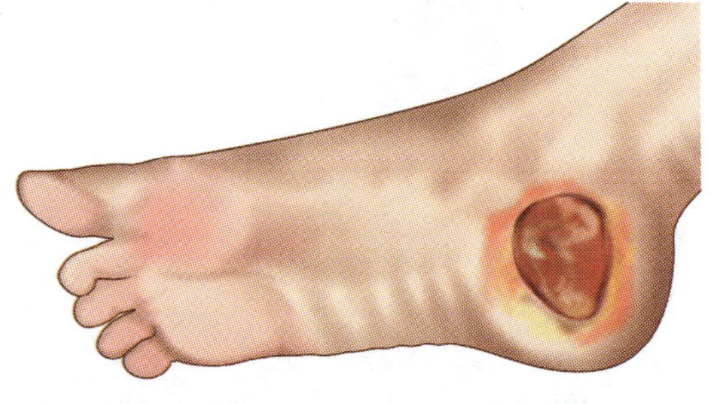

a. Venous ulcer
b. Arterial ulcer
c. Neuropathic ulcer
d. Bazin's ulcer

111. During induction of anesthesia, after giving thiopentone injection a patient develops discoloration of hand. All are true about this condition and its management, except:

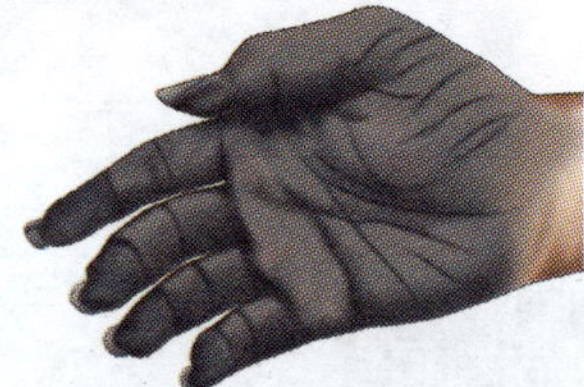

a. Immediately remove the needle in the vessel
b. Inject lignocaine
c. Dilute heparin
d. Intra-arterial thrombolysis

112. A patient presents with ulcer at the site of previous burn site. All are true about the lesion, except:

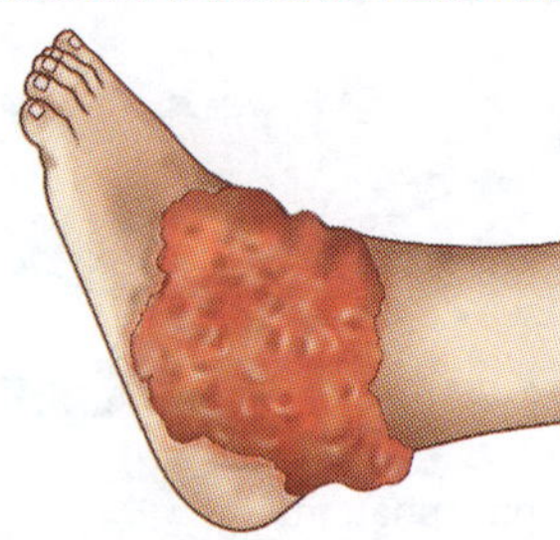

a. Painless scar
b. Cured by surgery
c. Lymphatic metastasis
d. Marjolin' ulcer

113. What is correct about the diagnosis?

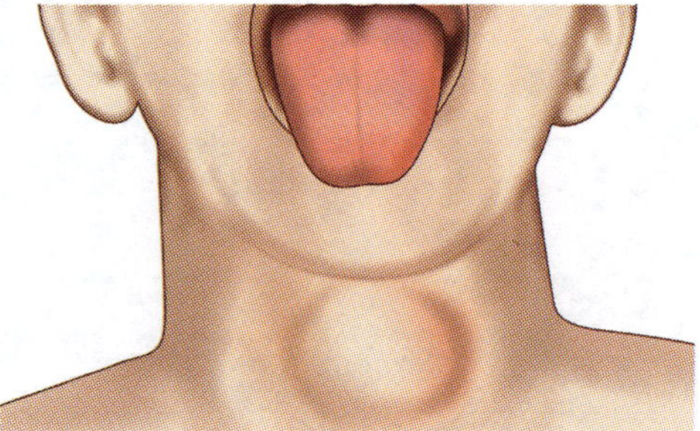

a. Thyroglossal cyst
b. Brachial cyst
c. Cold abscess
d. Carotid body tumor

114. What is true about the image shown?

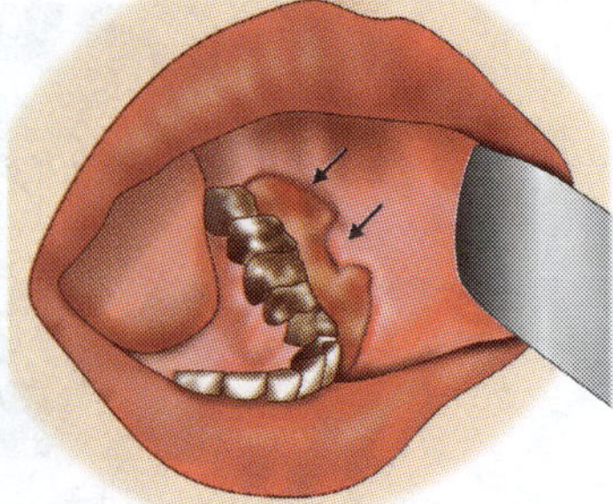

a. Carcinoma alveolar margin
b. Leukoplakia
c. Hyperplastic candidiasis
d. Fibrous epulis

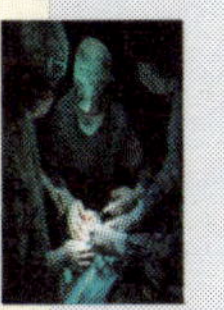

115. Identify the lesion shown in the figure:

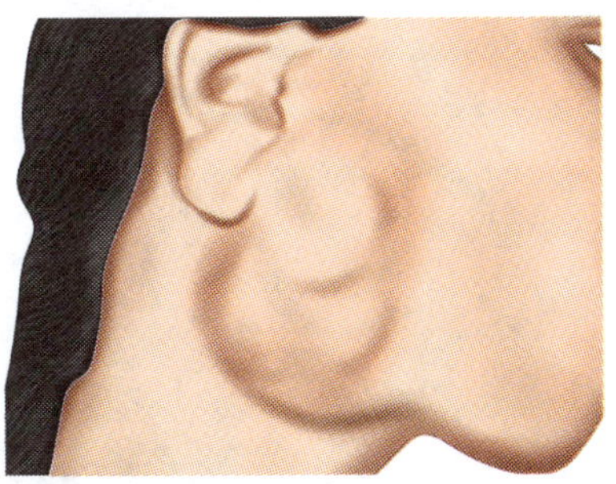

a. Pleomorphic adenoma
b. Mumps
c. Retroauricular lymphadenopathy
d. Sialadenitis

116. All can be seen in this patient, except:

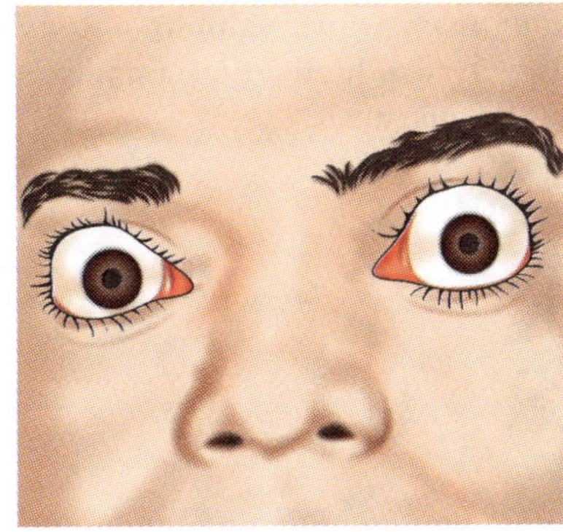

a. Myxedema
b. Dalrymple sign
c. Moist warm hands
d. Constipation

117. All are true about the patient shown in the image EXCEPT?

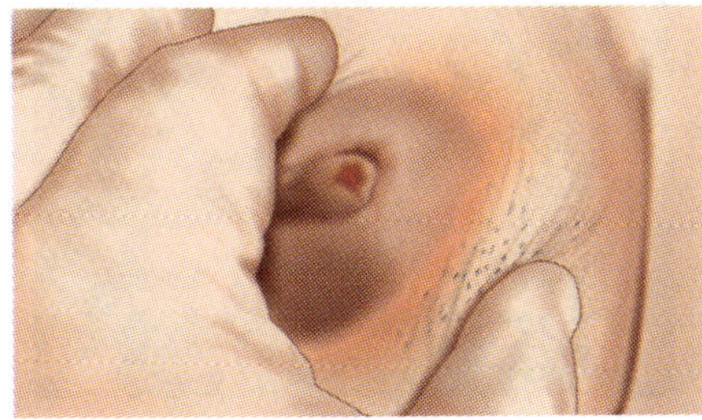

a. Peau d'orange
b. Ulceration of nipple
c. Diagnosis depends on HER2 expression
d. Van Nuys prognostic index

118. A 25-year-old shepherd presents with dragging discomfort in right Hypochondrium and on examination shows presence of enlarged liver 5 cm below costal margins. What is the probable diagnosis:

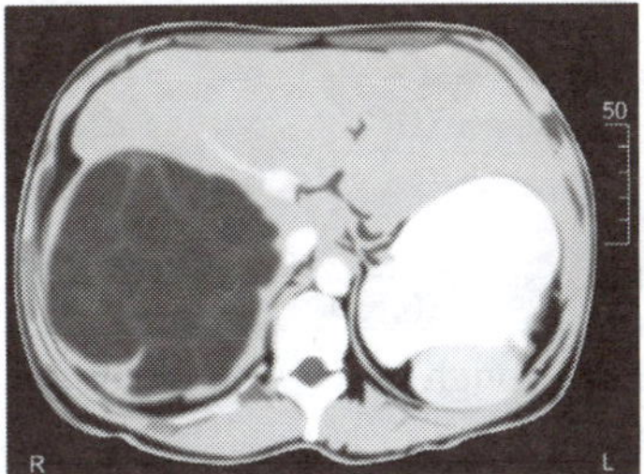

a. Amoebic liver abscess
b. Hydatid cyst
c. Pyogenic liver abscess
d. Hepatic adenoma

119. Which triangle is shown here?

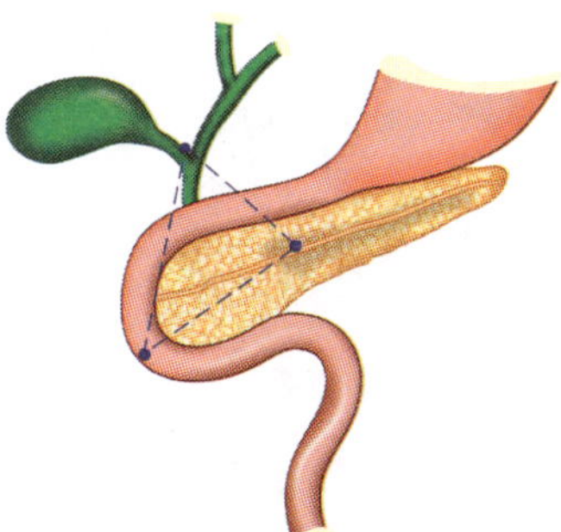

a. Calot's triangle
b. Gastrinoma triangle
c. Hesselbach's is triangle
d. Killian's triangle

120. A 65-year-old grandmother presents with feculent nasogastric aspirate. What is the diagnosis:

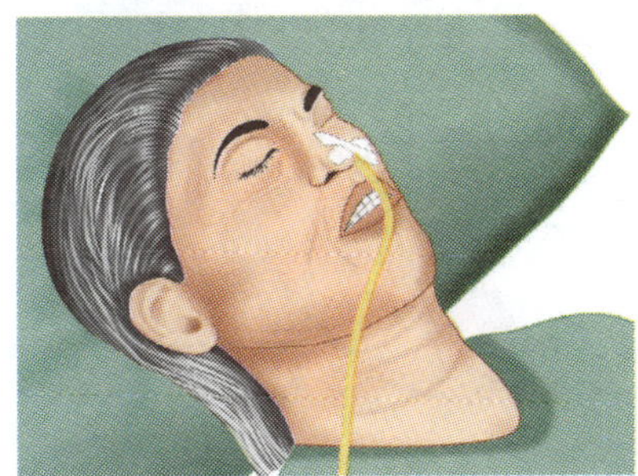

a. Jejunal obstruction
b. Ileal obstruction
c. Diverticulitis
d. Mesenteric ischemia

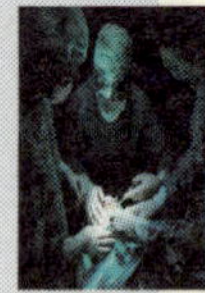

121. The following disease occurs due to all, except:

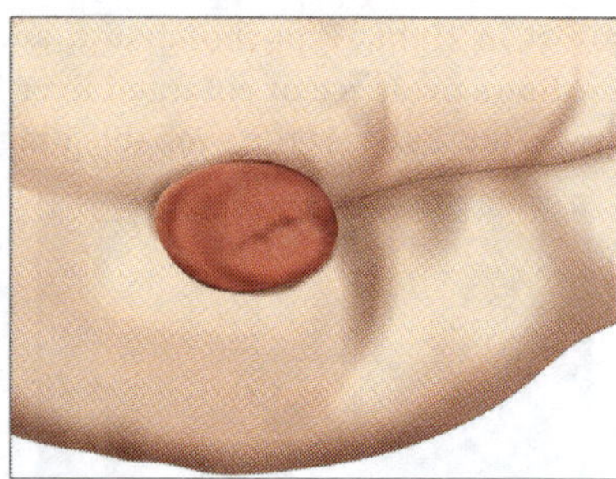

a. Whooping cough
b. Marasmus
c. Obstetric trauma
d. Fistula in ano

122. Which of the following is shown in the image?

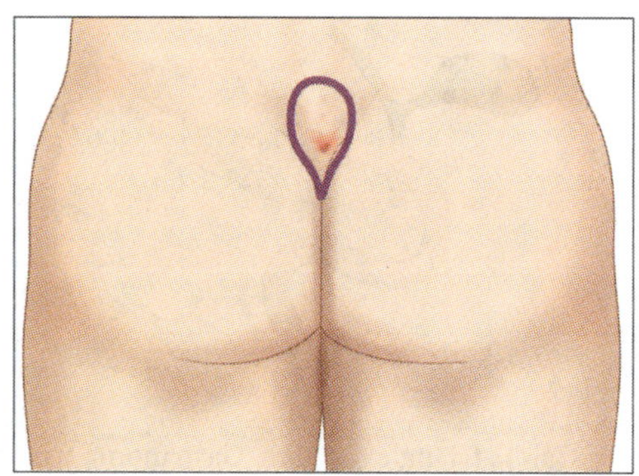

a. Fistula in ano
b. Pilonidal sinus
c. Bowen disease
d. Hidradenitis suppurativa

123. Identify the structure held with artery forceps:

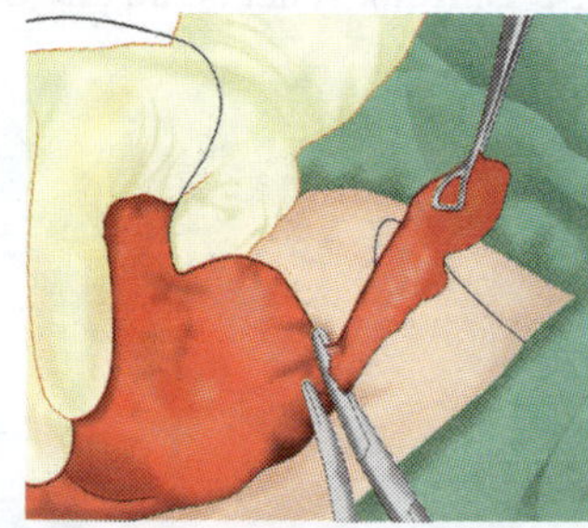

a. Appendix
b. Meckel's diverticulum
c. Zenker's diverticulum
d. Colostomy procedure

124. Which procedure is shown in the image?

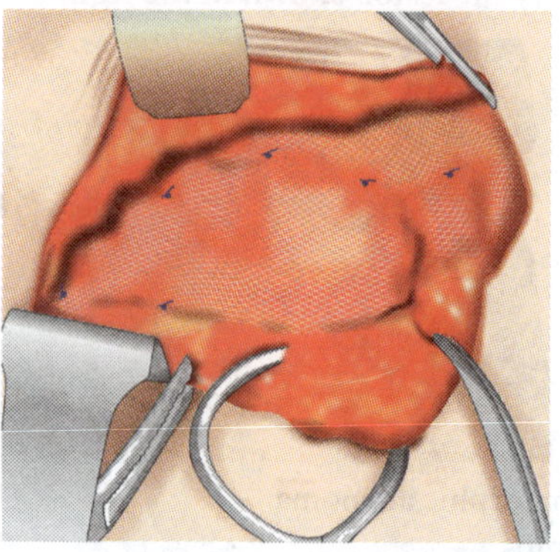

a. Lichtenstein repair
b. Bassini herniorrhaphy
c. Shouldice repair
d. Lord's procedure

125. A 25-year-old presents with dragging pain and testicular mass which exhibits a cough expansile impulse. Trans-illumination impulse is negative. What is the diagnosis:

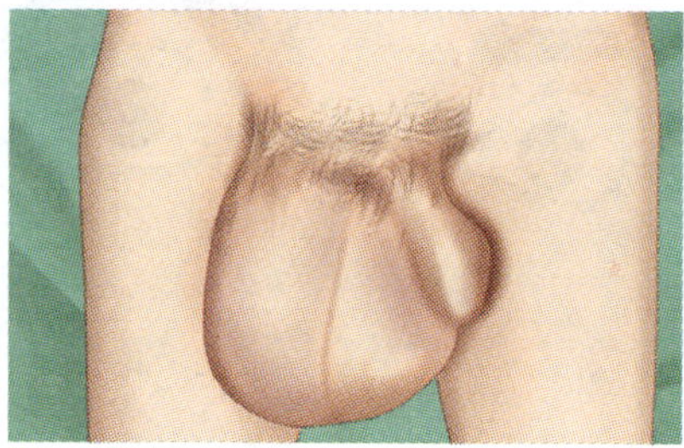

a. Direct inguinal hernia
b. Indirect inguinal hernia
c. Hydrocele
d. Varicocele

126. All are true about the condition shown, except:

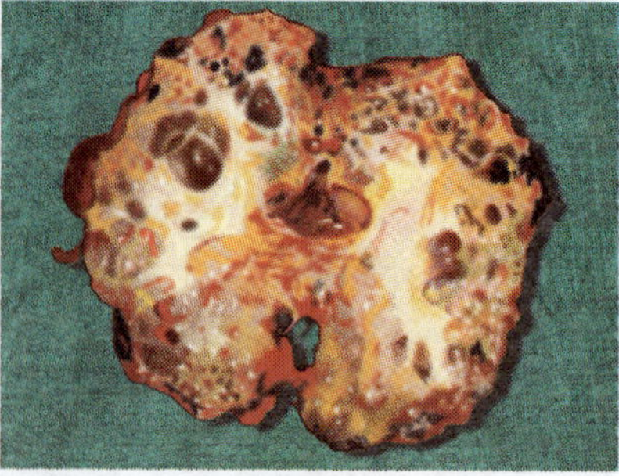

a. Cysts increase in size with age
b. Spider leg deformity
c. Anemia
d. Low Renin due to pressure atrophy of JG apparatus

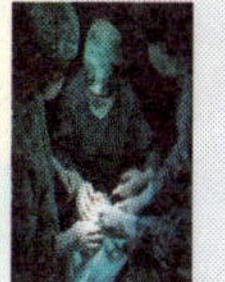

127. All are true due to the conditions shown in the figure, except:

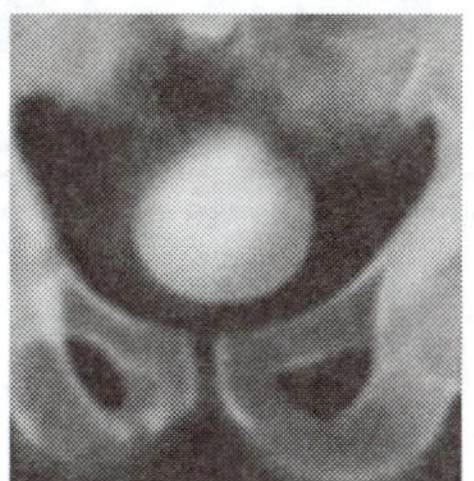

a. Pain at end of micturition referred to the tip of penis
b. Holmium laser
c. Litholapaxy
d. Painless intermittent hematuria

128. The following image shows presence of:

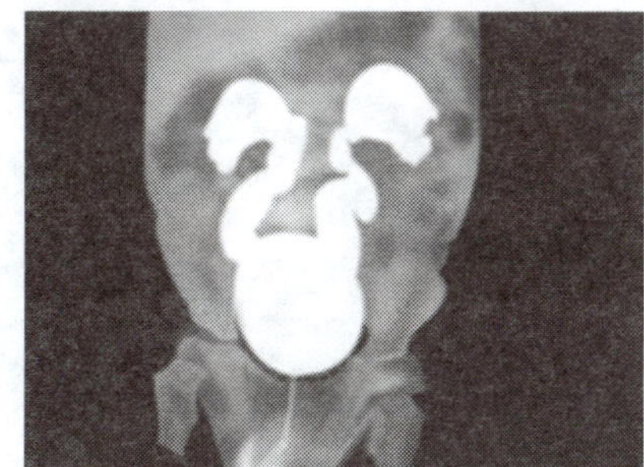

a. Posterior urethral valves
b. Vesico-ureteric reflux
c. Bladder stone
d. Bladder rupture

129. What is incorrect about the image shown?

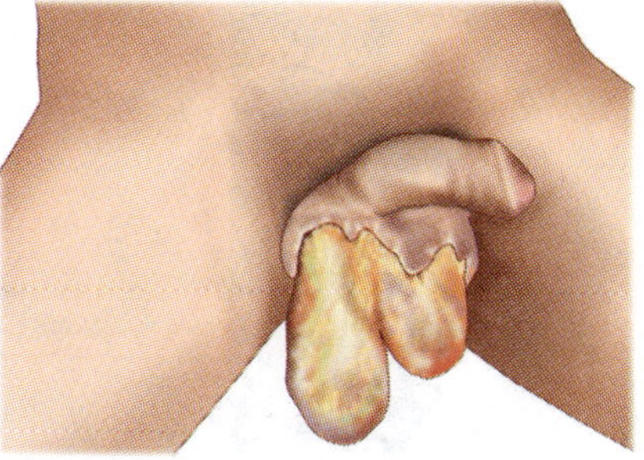

a. Gangrene of scrotum
b. Microaerophilic Hemolytic Streptococci
c. Seen in low socio-economic background
d. Can involve skin of penis

130. The CT chest shows presence of:

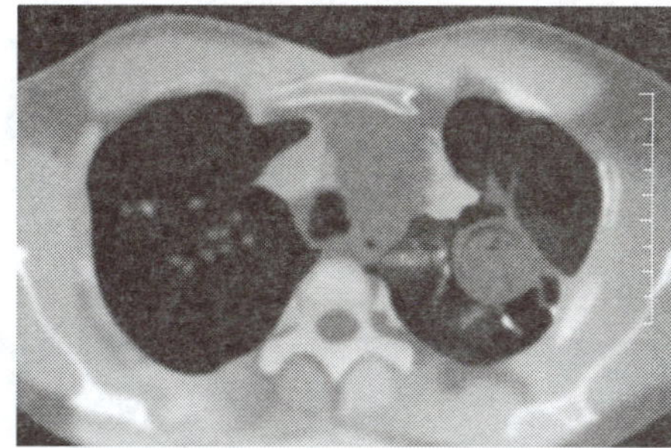

a. Meniscus sign
b. Crescent sign
c. Tree in bud sign
d. Loculated empyema

131. The image shows presence of:

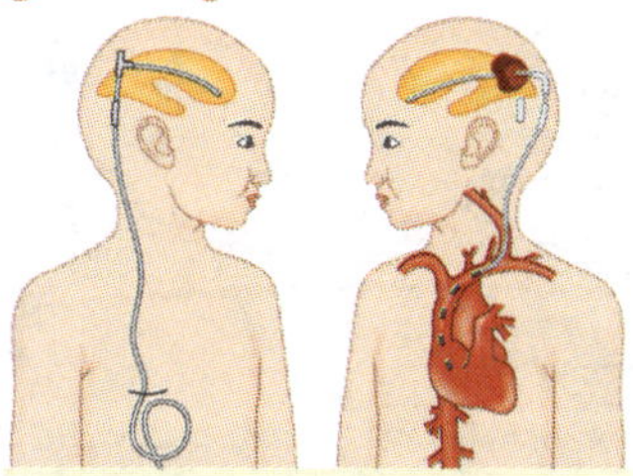

a. A = Ventriculoperitoneal shunt, B = Ventriculo-atrial shunt
b. A = Ventriculo-atrial shunt, B = Ventriculo-peritoneal shunt
c. A = Denver shunt, B = La Veen Shunt
d. A = La Veen Shunt, A = Denver Shunt

132. A 25-year-old patient presents in coma with GCS of 5 and extensor posturing after a bike accident. Which of the following will the best management of the patient:

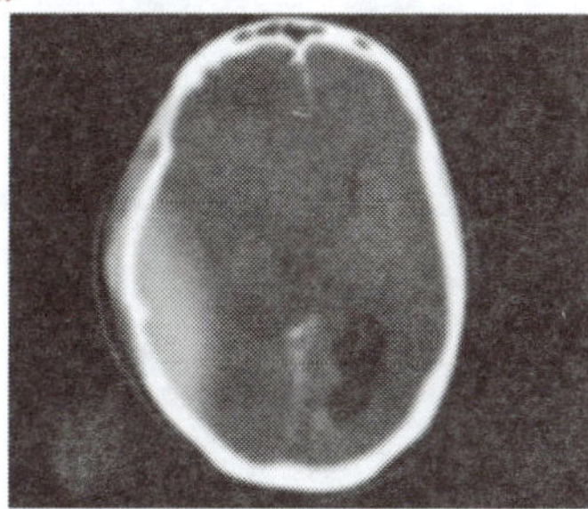

a. Hypertonic saline
b. Thrombolysis
c. Burr hole surgery
d. Hemi-Craniectomy

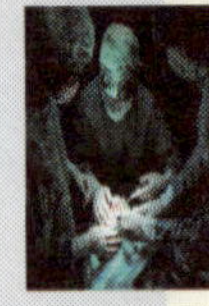

133. Identify the surgical instrument:

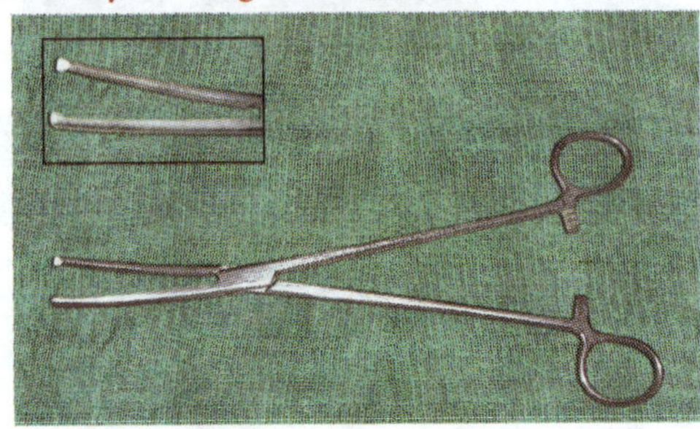

a. Kocher forceps
b. Allis forceps
c. Ovum forceps
d. Artery forceps

136. Identify the image shown:

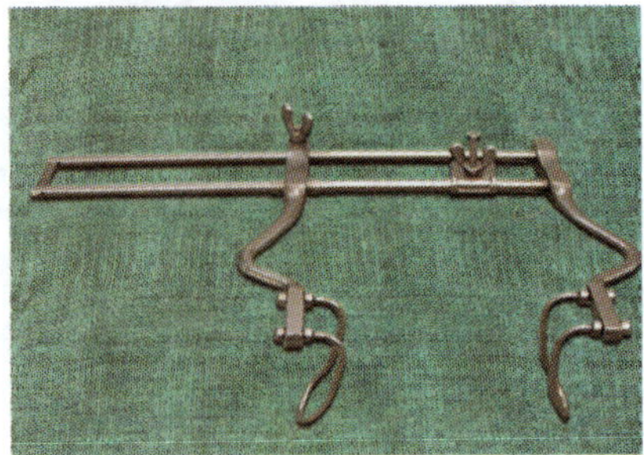

a. Rib Spreader
b. Self-retaining retractor
c. Lister Dilator
d. Male Metallic Catheter

134. Identify the instrument shown:

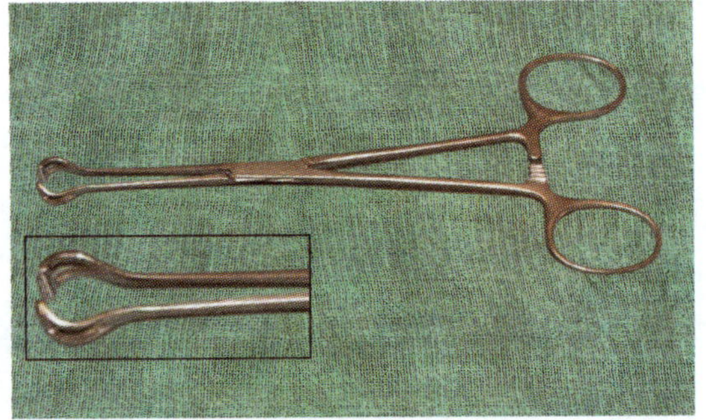

a. Allen forceps
b. Mosquito forceps
c. Babcock forceps
d. Kocher forceps

137. Identify the image shown:

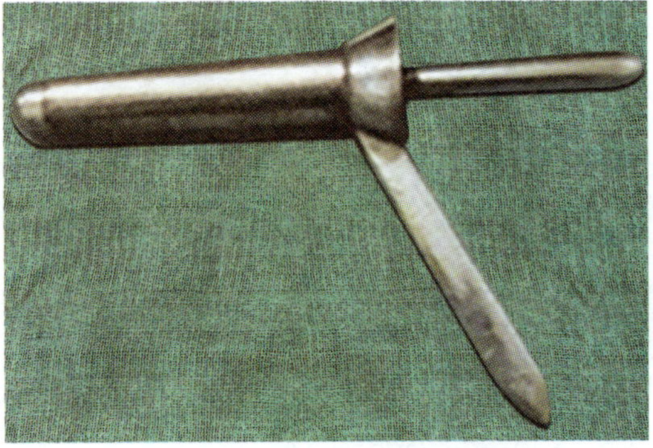

a. Proctoscope
b. Sigmoidoscope
c. Anoscope
d. Colonoscope

135. Identify the instrument shown:

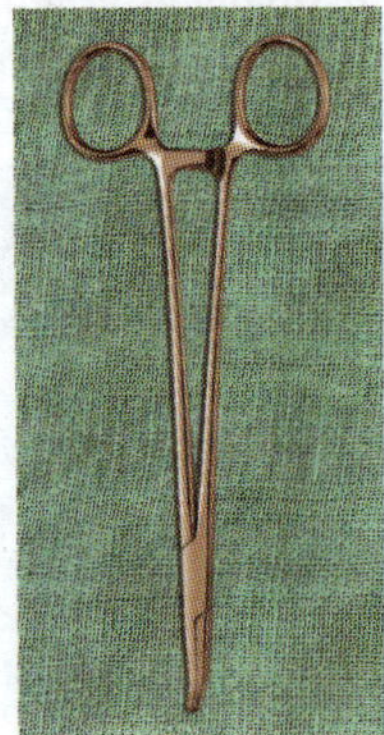

a. Needle holder
b. Cheatles forceps
c. Babcock forceps
d. Kocher forceps

138. Identify the catheter shown in the figure:

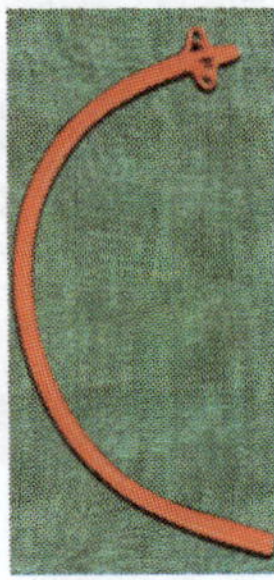

a. Malecot catheter
b. Foley's catheter
c. Red rubber catheter
d. Ryle's tube

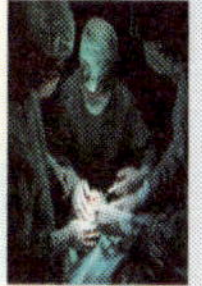

139. Identify the tube shown in the image:

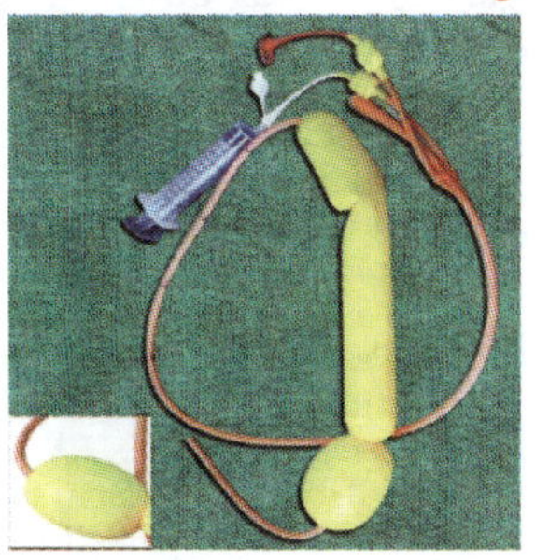

a. Ryle's tube
b. Malecot's Catheter
c. Blakemore Sengstaken Catheter
d. Foley's catheter

140. What is the clinical diagnosis of the patient?

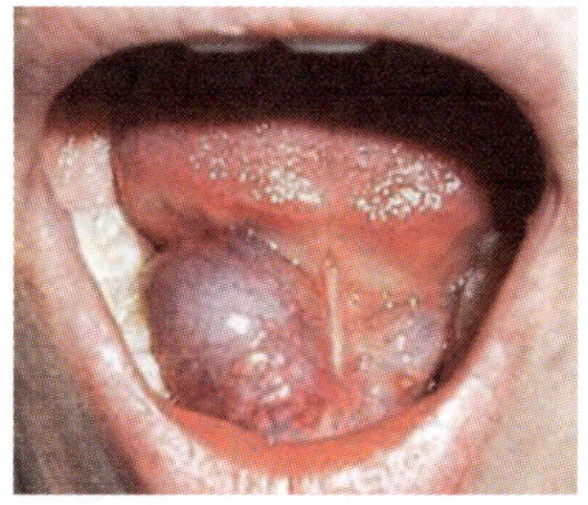

a. Ranula
b. Cystic Hygroma
c. Erythroplakia
d. Epulis

141. The image shows:

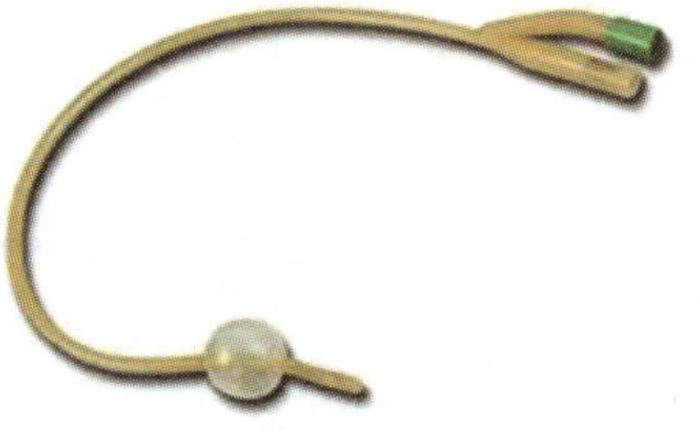

a. Foley's Catheter
b. Swan Ganz catheter
c. Sengstaken Blakemore tube
d. Endotracheal tube

142. Name the retractor:

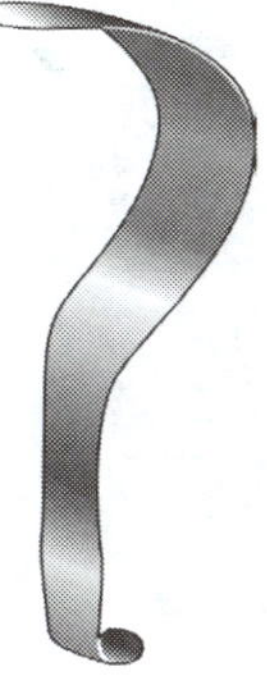

a. Deaver retractor
b. Richardson retractor
c. Malleable retractor
d. Goulet

143. Identify the instrument shown in the image below:

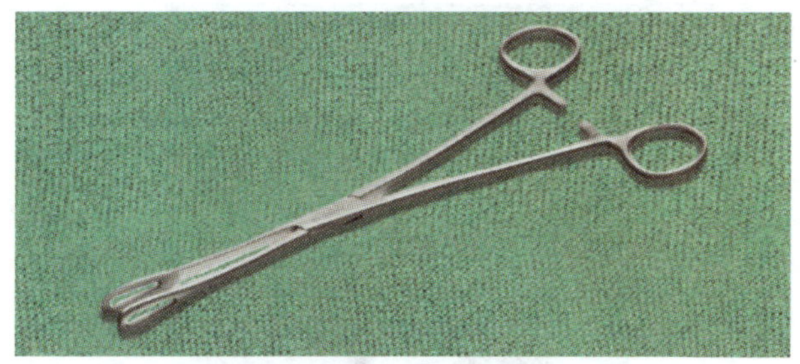

a. Rampley sponge holder
b. Langenbeck's retractor
c. Babcock tissue forceps
d. Needle holder

144. Identify the instrument shown in the image below:

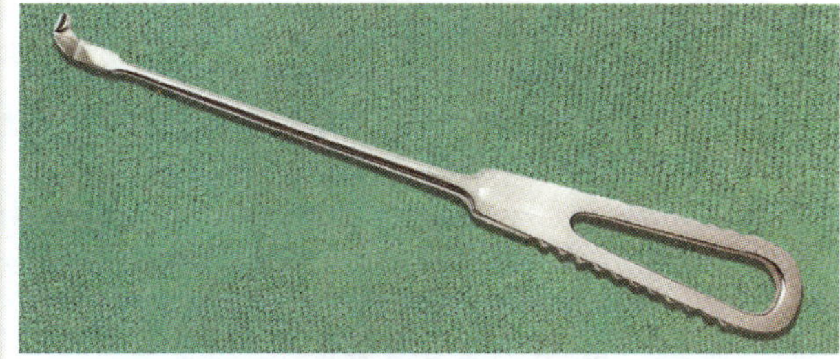

a. Rampley sponge holder
b. Langenbeck's retractor
c. Babcock tissue forceps
d. Needle holder

145. Which type of retractor is shown in the image?

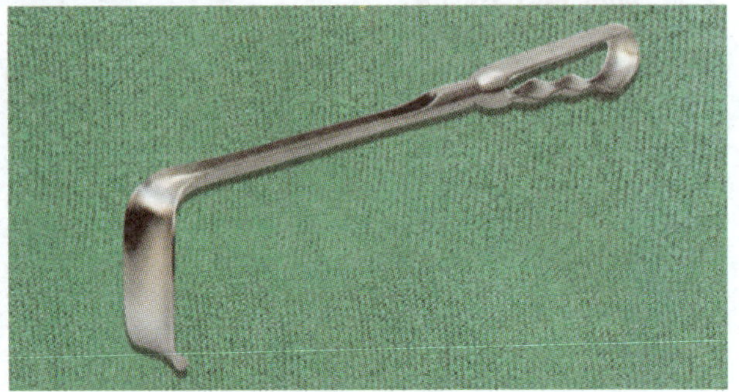

a. Morris retractor
b. Czerny retractor
c. Richardson retractor
d. Lower lid retractor

146. Identify the instrument given below:

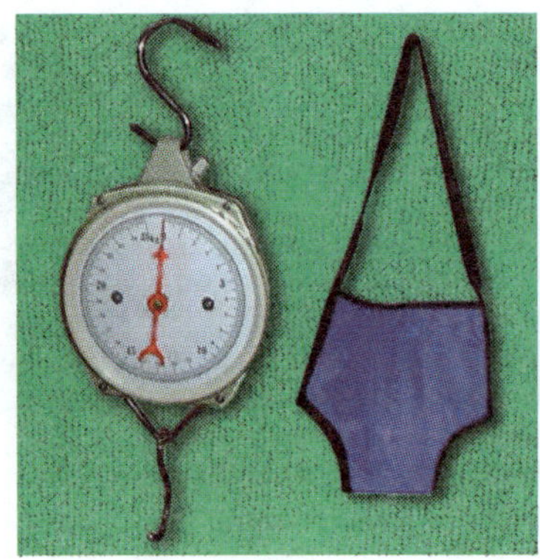

a. Infantometer
b. Sling psychrometer
c. Salter's scale
d. Chloroscope

147. Identify the procedure done for duodenal ulcer:

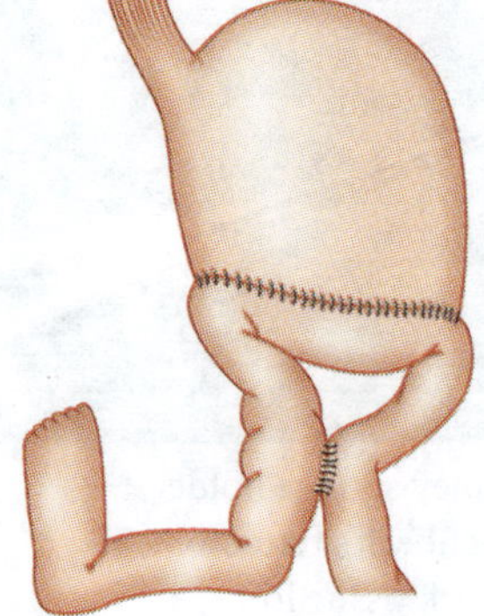

a. Billroth I
b. Billroth II
c. Gastroenterostomy
d. Stamm's Gastrostomy

148. A 30-year-old shepherd presented with painless hepatomegaly. USG was done. What is the clinical diagnosis:

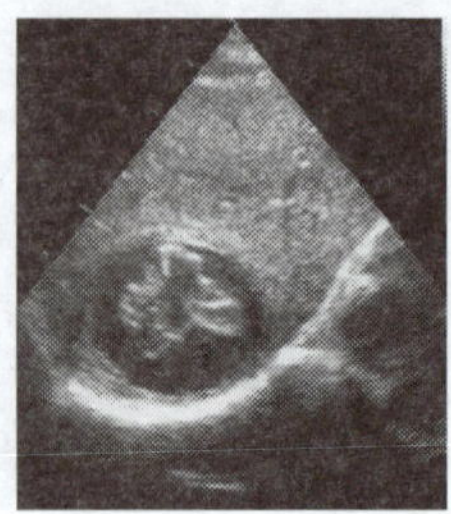

a. Ascariasis
b. Schistosomiasis
c. Entamoeba histolytica
d. Hydatid cyst

149. Diverticulosis appearance on barium enema as shown is called:

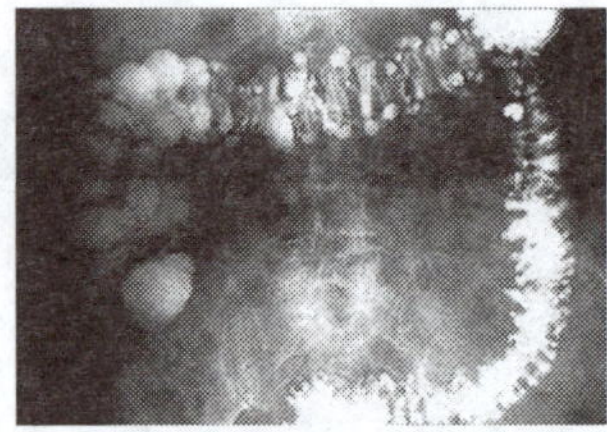

a. Saw tooth appearance
b. Cork screw appearance
c. Bird of prey appearance
d. Claw sign

PEDIATRICS

150. During the clinical examination of a 19-year-old male with a history of chronic respiratory condition, you notice the chest appears as shown in the image below. This is called as:

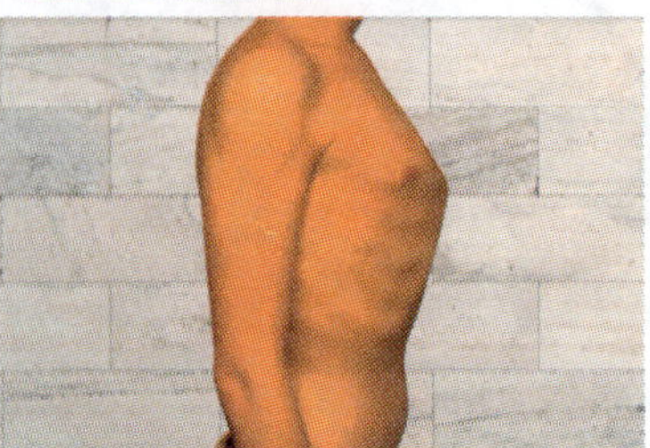

a. Pectus excavatum
b. Pectus carinatum
c. Harrison's sulcus
d. Cobbler's chest

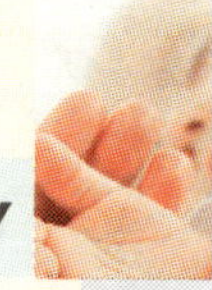

OBSTETRICS AND GYNECOLOGY

151. A 35-year-old lady presents with vaginal discharge. Smears from vaginal discharge show presence of:

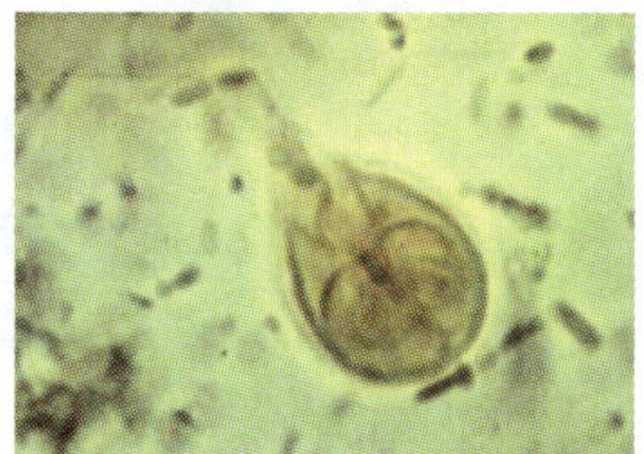

a. Trichomonas
b. Entamoeba histolytica
c. Toxoplasma
d. Giardia

152. Identify the instrument shown below:

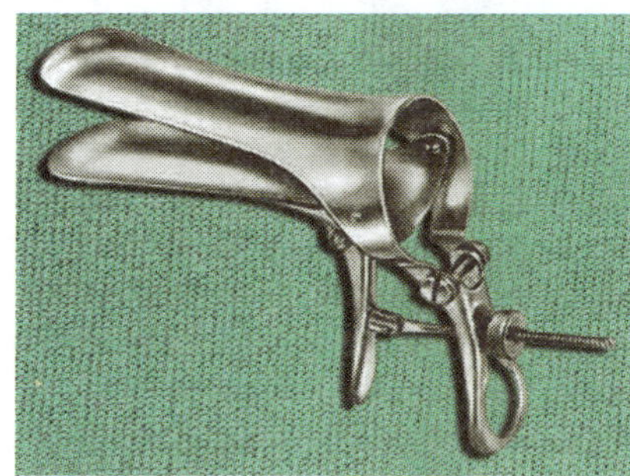

a. Sims speculum
b. Cusco speculum
c. EB curette
d. Deaver's retractor

153. Identify the instruments shown in the figure:

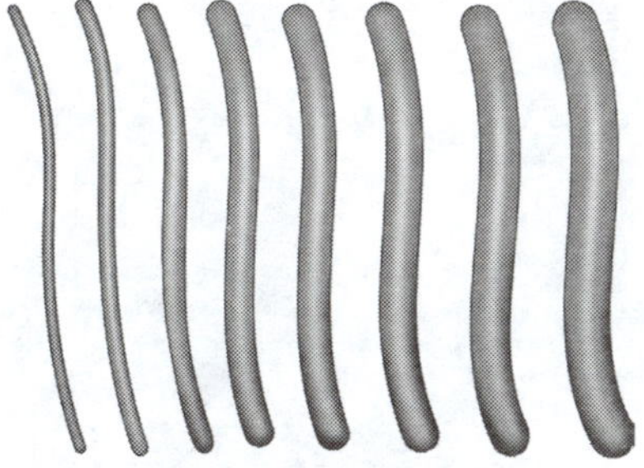

a. Uterine sound
b. Hegar dilator
c. Sims self retaining speculum
d. Interlocking nails

154. The vaginal smear shows presence of:

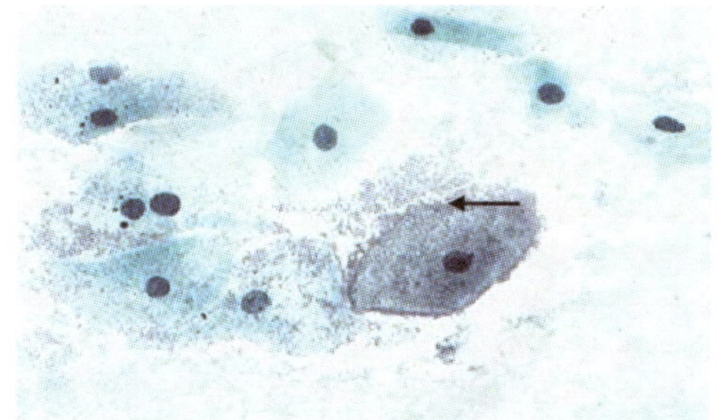

a. Bacterial vaginosis
b. Candidiasis
c. Human papilloma virus
d. Trichomonas vaginalis

155. Least common site of ectopic pregnancy:

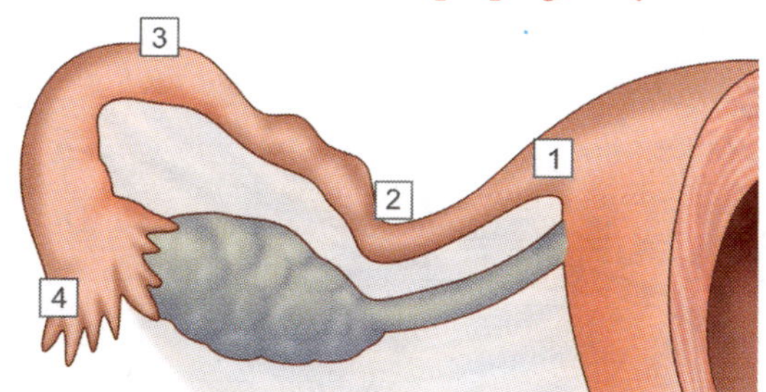

a. Interstitial part
b. Isthmus
c. Ampulla
d. Fimbrial end

156. The HSG report shows:

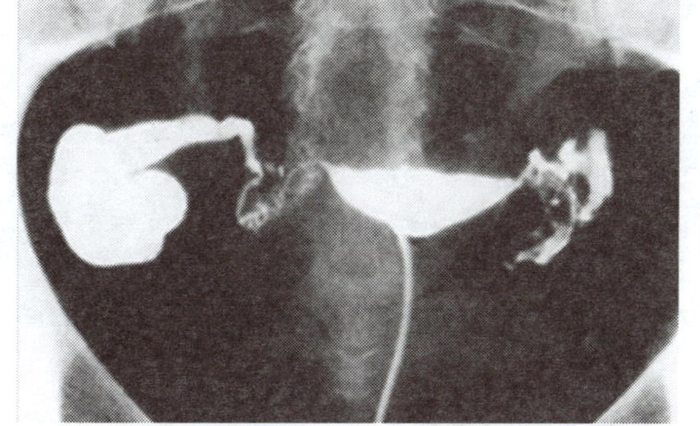

a. Hydrosalpinx
b. Uterus didelphys
c. Adenomyosis
d. Endometriosis

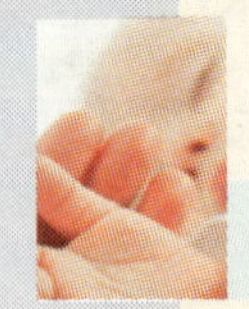

157. The following instrument is called as:

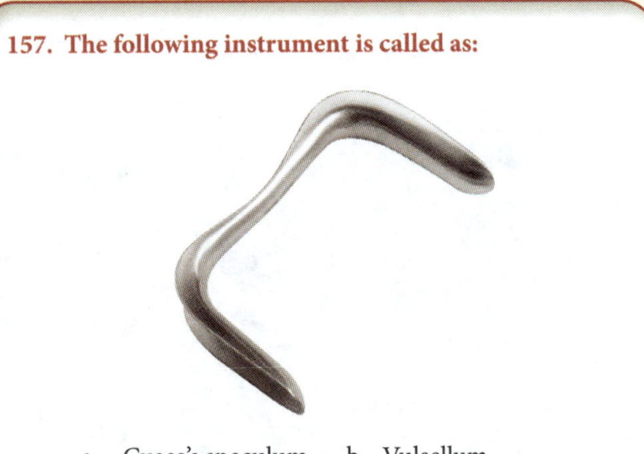

a. Cusco's speculum
b. Vulsellum
c. Sims speculum
d. Vaginal sling

158. Which instrument is shown below?

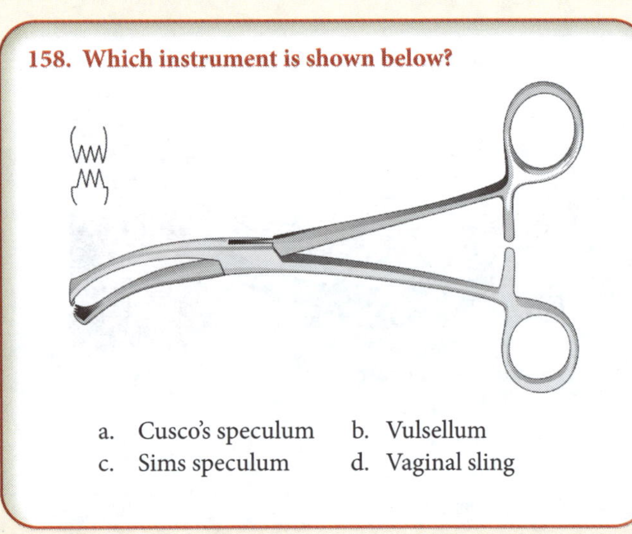

a. Cusco's speculum
b. Vulsellum
c. Sims speculum
d. Vaginal sling

159. The image shows:

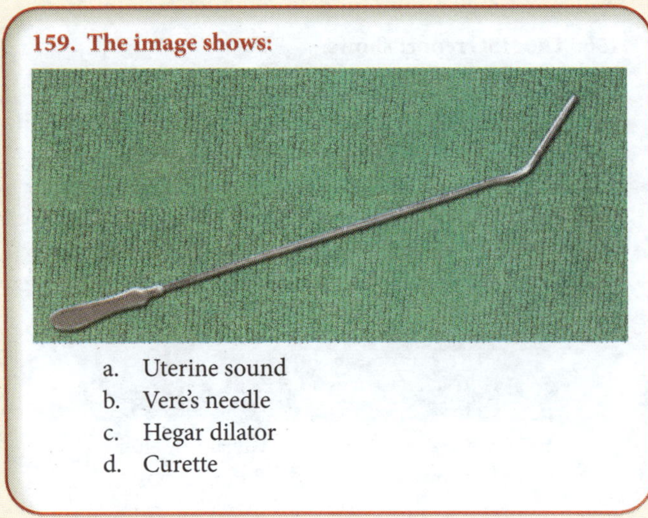

a. Uterine sound
b. Vere's needle
c. Hegar dilator
d. Curette

160. The image shows:

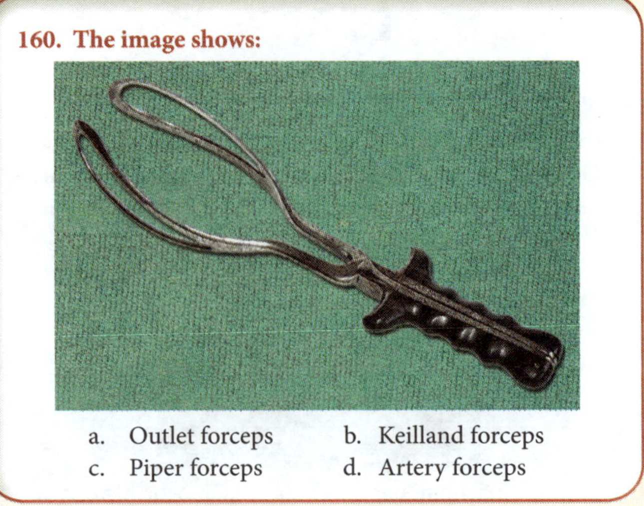

a. Outlet forceps
b. Keilland forceps
c. Piper forceps
d. Artery forceps

161. Identify the image and its use:

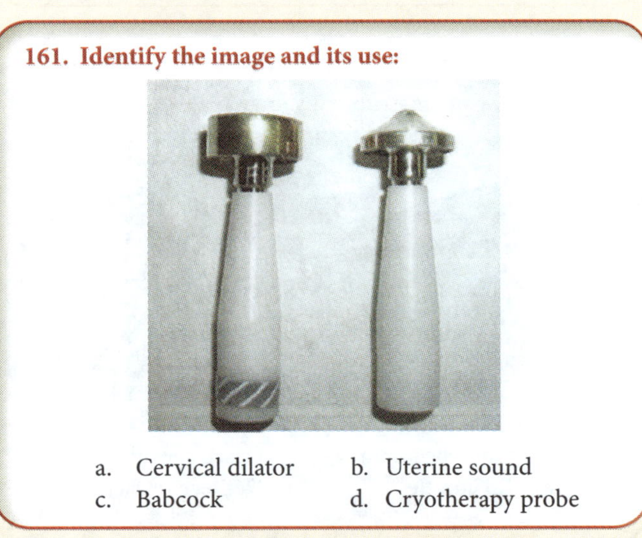

a. Cervical dilator
b. Uterine sound
c. Babcock
d. Cryotherapy probe

162. The following HSG image suggests:

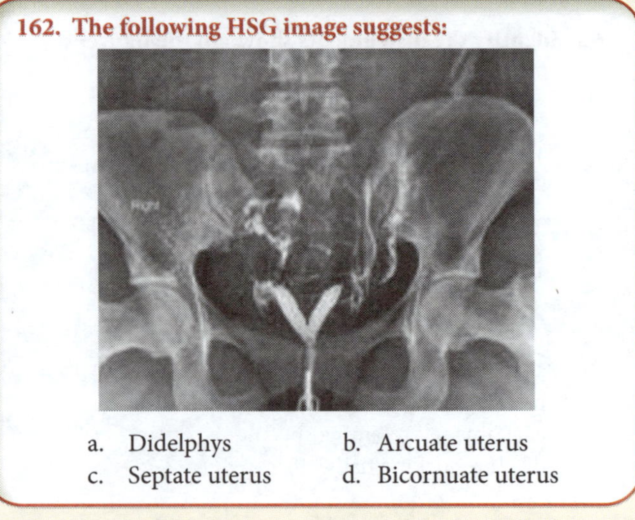

a. Didelphys
b. Arcuate uterus
c. Septate uterus
d. Bicornuate uterus

163. Identify the type of morbidly adherent placenta shown in image:

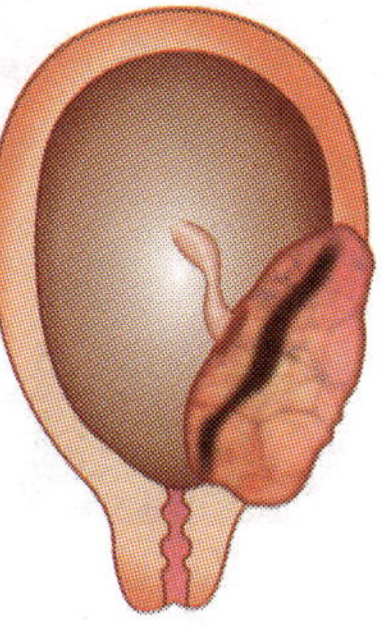

a. Placenta increta
b. Placenta accreta
c. Placenta percreta
d. Total placenta accreta

164. Identify the type of placenta previa as shown in the image below:

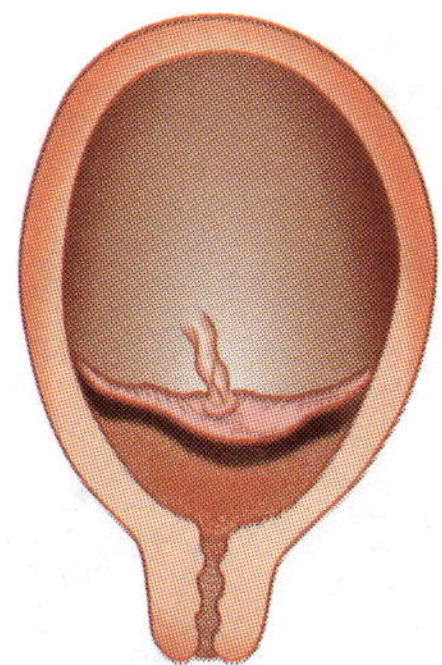

a. I
b. II
c. III
d. IV

165. A 14-year-old presents with cyclical abdomen pain and has not attained menarche yet. Presents with following image. What is the diagnosis?
(Most Recent Question Dec 2019-20)

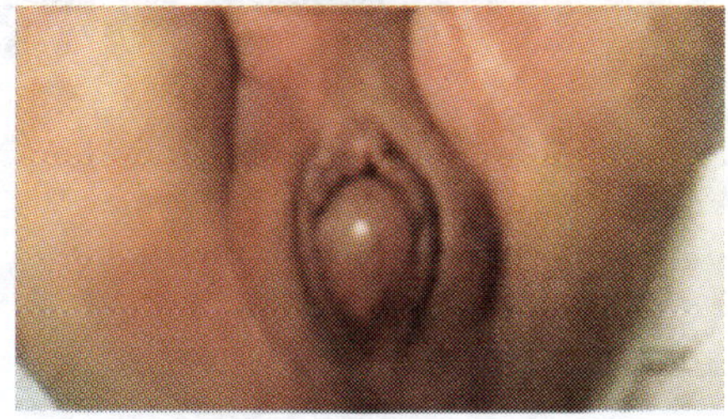

a. Imperforate hymen
b. Prolapse
c. Tumor
d. None of these

166. Procedure being shown in the given image?
(Most Recent Question Dec 2019-20)

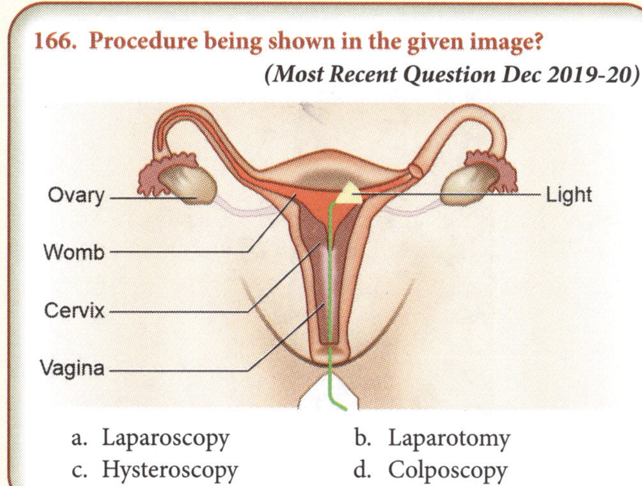

a. Laparoscopy
b. Laparotomy
c. Hysteroscopy
d. Colposcopy

ENT

167. A 21-year-old college student presents with hot potato voice and trismus. Throat examination was done. Clinical diagnosis is:

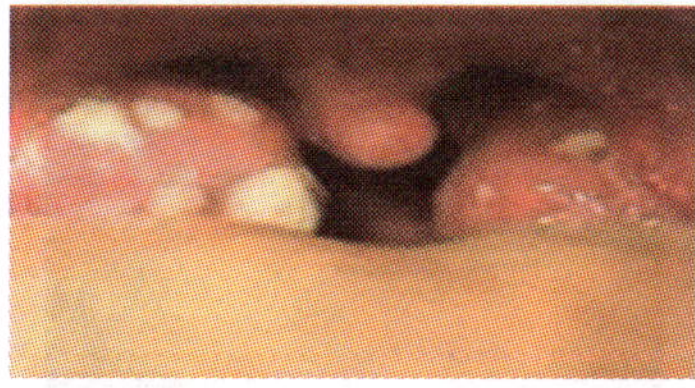

a. Quinsy
b. Epiglottitis
c. Infectious mononucleosis
d. Chronic tonsillitis

168. The shown image is section taken from:

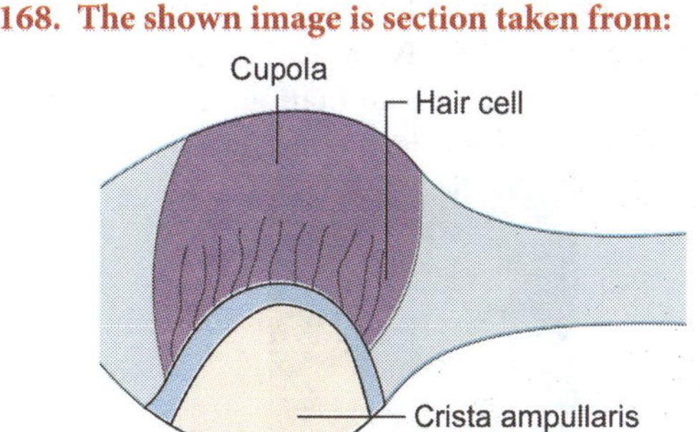

a. Cochlea
b. Vestibule
c. Semicircular canal
d. Bill's bar

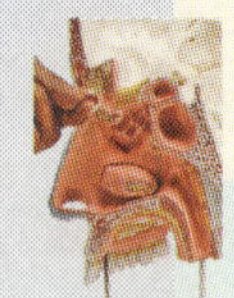

169. **Diagnosis based on your otoscopic finding:**

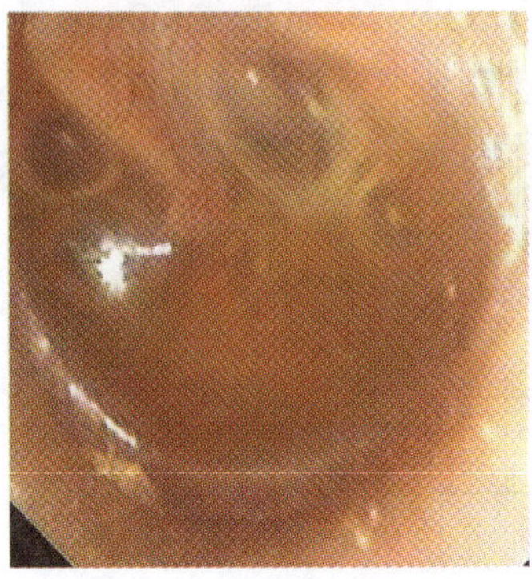

a. Acute otitis media b. Chronic otitis media
c. Serous otitis media d. Serous otitis externa

170. **Diagnosis based on your otoscopic finding:**

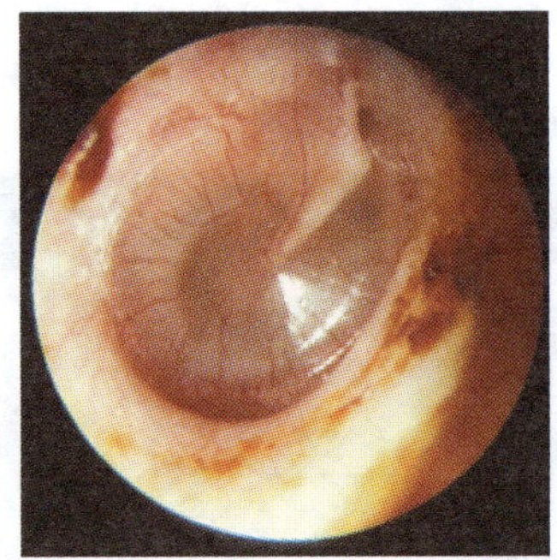

a. Acute otitis media b. Chronic otitis media
c. Serous otitis media d. Serous otitis externa

171. **A 14-year-male from Chhattisgharh presented with swelling of nose which is increasing gradually from last 3-4 months. Upon examination, nose has woody touch. Possible diagnosis:**

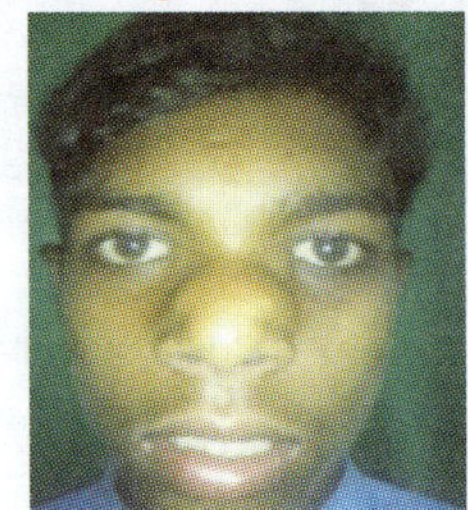

a. Rhinoscleroma b. Rhinophyma
c. Rhinosporidiosis d. Rhinohyperplasia

172. **Diagnosis:**

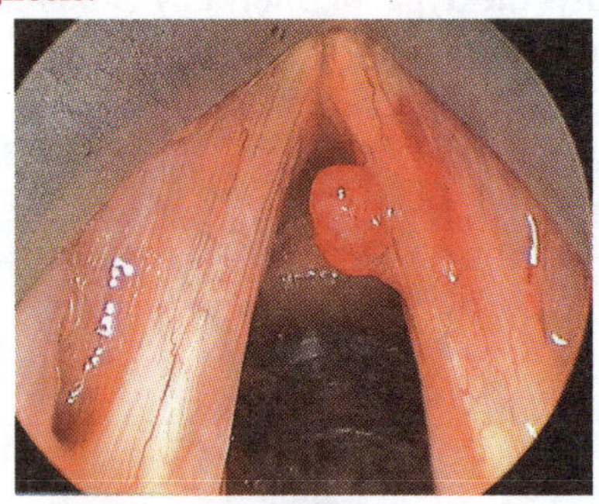

a. Vocal cord nodule
b. Vocal cord polyp
c. Vocal cord granuloma
d. Papilloma

173. **This patient was prepared for surgery. Your senior resident did this marking before proceeding the incision. What is the name of this:**

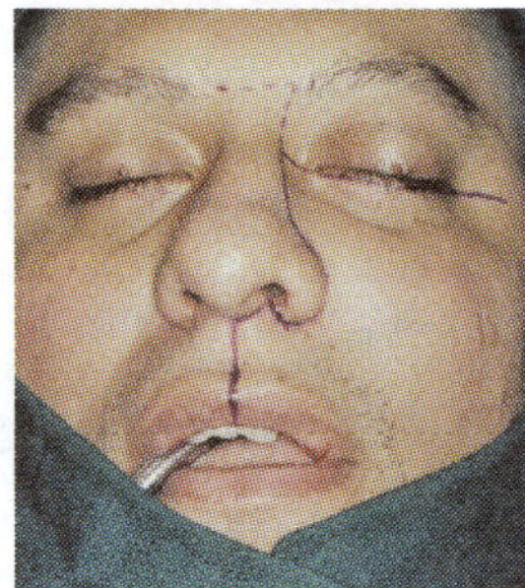

a. Ohngren's line b. Weber fergusson incision
c. Lederman incision d. Frontal sinusotomy

174. **A 13-year-old patient presented with history of recurrent epistaxis. Upon general evaluation you noted the swelling of cheek. Most likely diagnosis:**

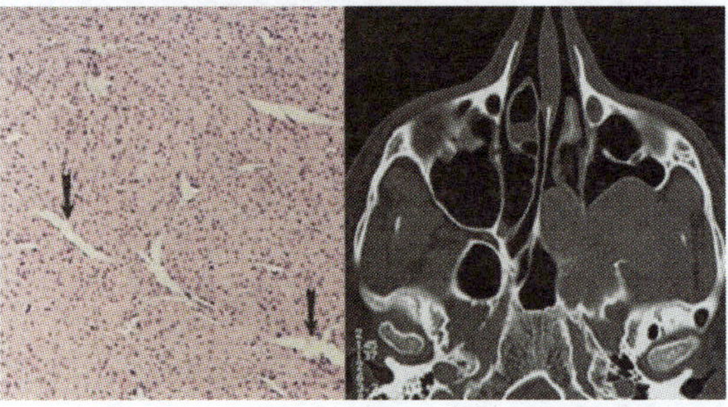

a. Rhinoscleroma b. Angiofibroma
c. Antral polyp d. Ethmoidal polyp

175. The given image is used for:

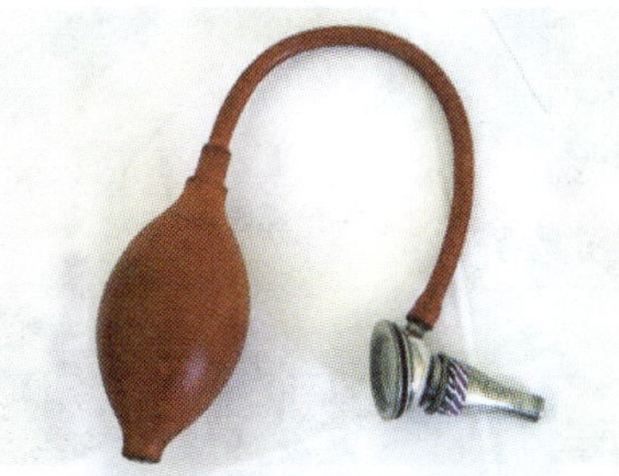

a. Cleaning the external auditory canal
b. Visualizing the whole external ear
c. Packing ear canal or nasal cavity
d. Checking the mobility of tympanic membrane

176. The below given sign is seen in:

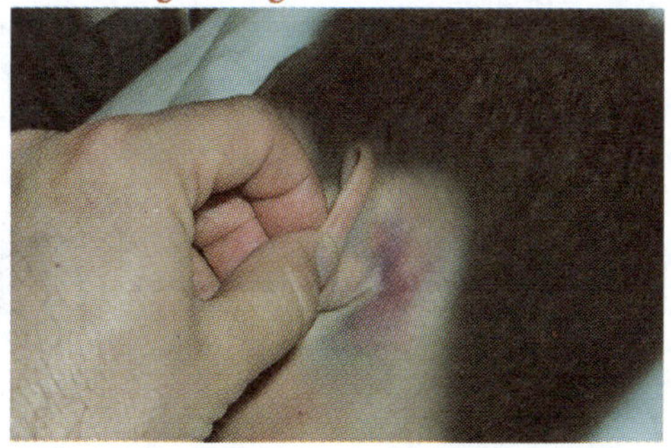

a. Otosclerosis
b. Cholesteatoma
c. Lateral sinus thrombophlebitis
d. Laryngeal pathology

177. Spot diagnosis:

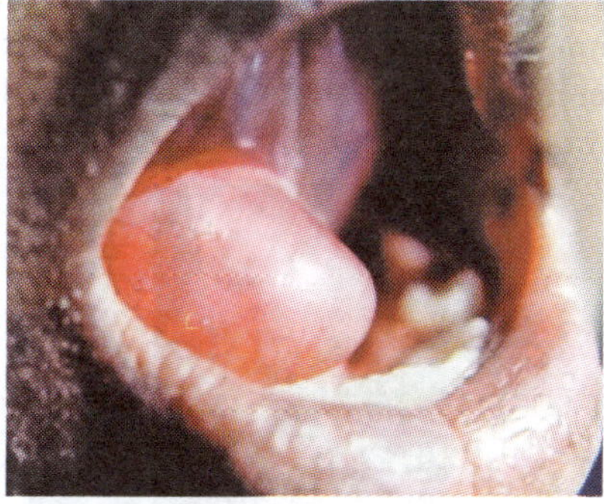

a. Tongue tie
b. Potato tumor
c. Ranula
d. Thyroglossal cyst

178. Identify the shown device:

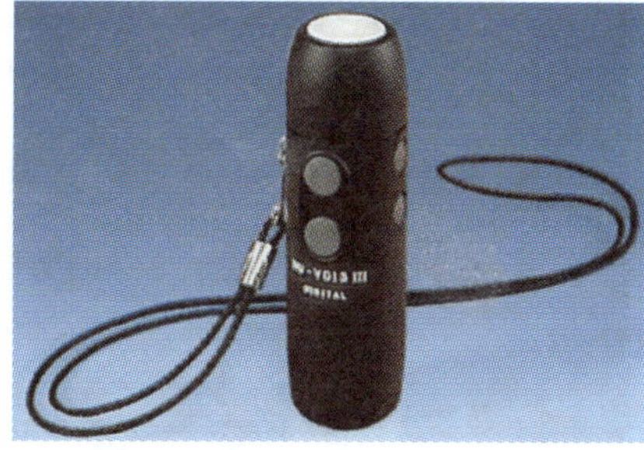

a. Laryngoscopic torch
b. Electrolarynx
c. Transoral pneumatic device
d. Otoscope

ORTHOPEDICS

179. Diagnosis is:

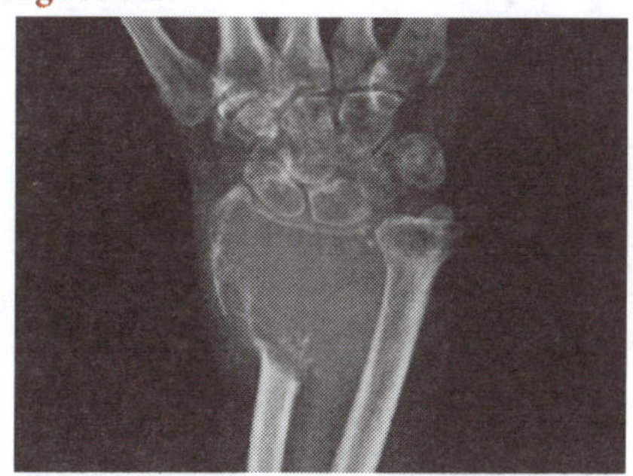

a. Unicameral bone cyst
b. Aneurysmal bone cyst
c. Giant cell tumor
d. Osteosarcoma

180. Diagnosis is:

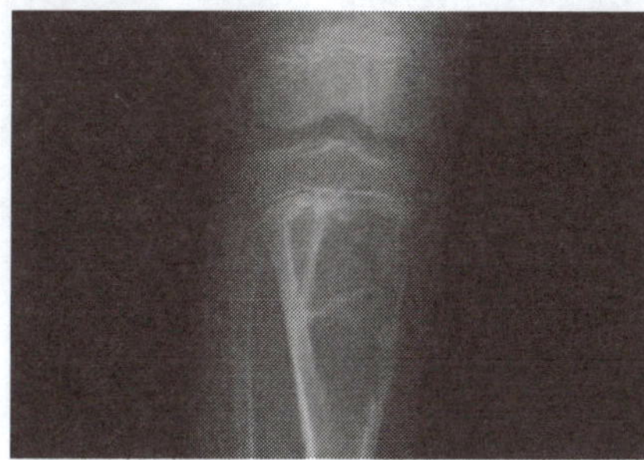

a. Unicameral bone cyst
b. Aneurysmal bone cyst
c. Giant Cell tumor
d. Osteosarcoma

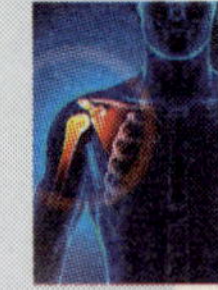

181. Spot diagnosis for foot deformity:

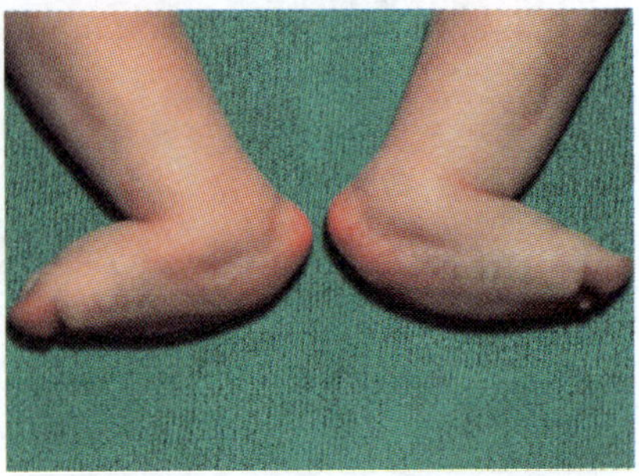

a. CTEV
b. Congenital vertical talus
c. Rocker bottom foot
d. Pes Cavus

182. A 18-year-old male has history of trauma. X-ray is shown below. The diagnosis is:

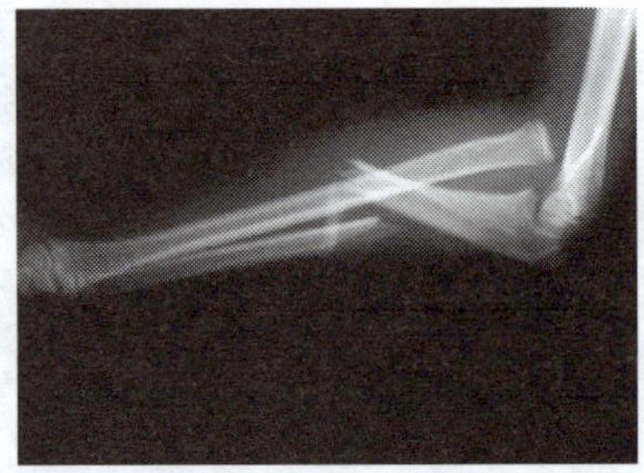

a. Supra-Condylar Fracture
b. Colle's Fracture
c. Galeazzi fracture
d. Monteggia fracture

183. Identify the periosteal reaction:

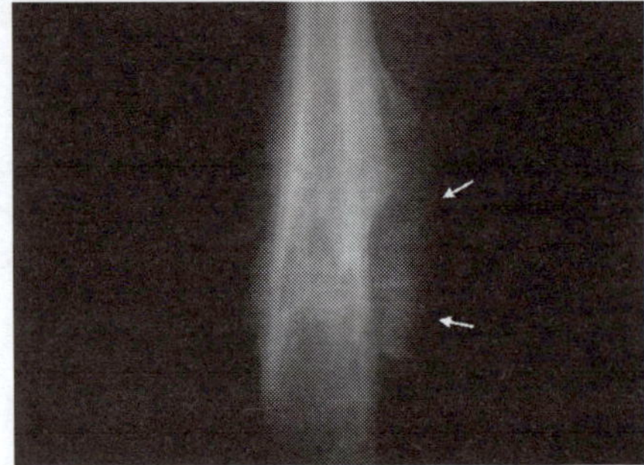

a. Onion peel appearance
b. Codman's Triangle
c. Sun Burst appearance
d. Onion ring appearance

184. The image shows presence of:

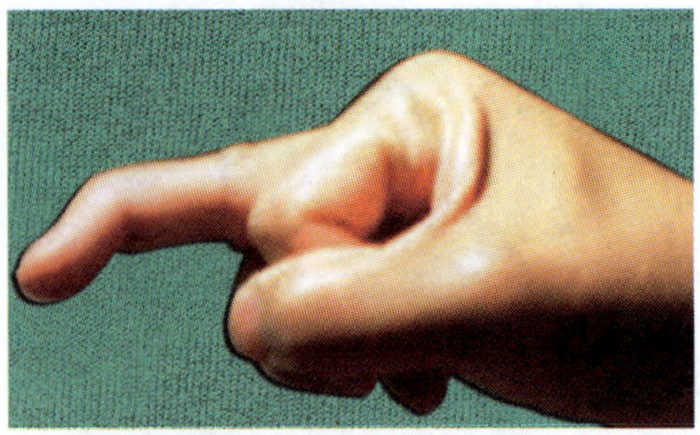

a. Swan neck deformity
b. Boutonniere deformity
c. Mallet finger
d. Dupuytren's contracture

185. The image shows:

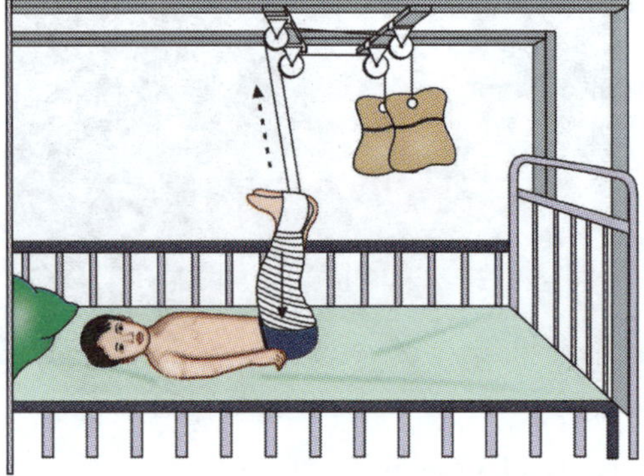

a. Gallow's Traction b. 90–90 traction
c. Russel traction d. Agnes hunt traction

186. A teenage male presented with complaints of pain in the right upper arm and history of trivial fall with no other significant medical history. On X-ray of the upper limb the given finding was observed. The most likely diagnosis is:

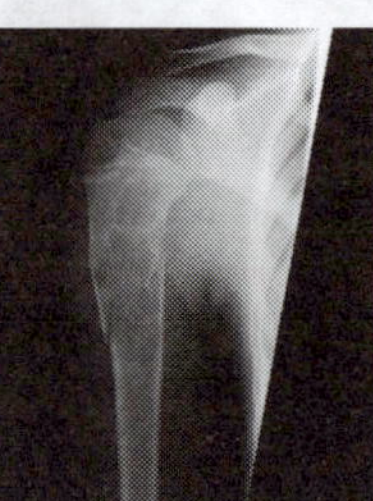

a. Osteosarcoma b. Osteochondroma
c. Simple bone cyst d. Osteoma

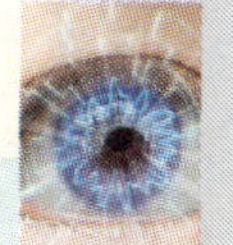

187. The shown splint is used for:

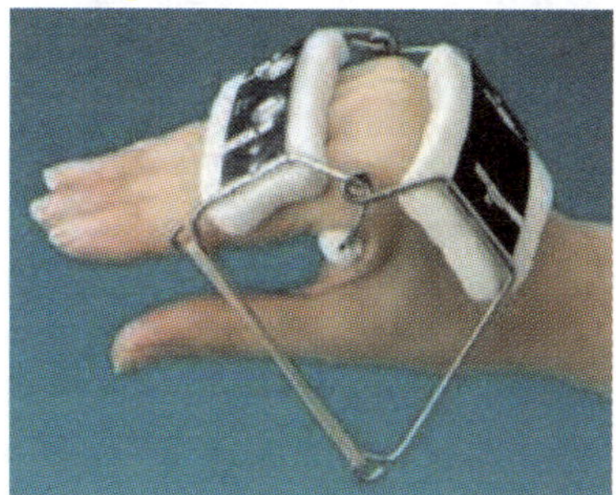

a. Ulnar nerve injury
b. Median nerve injury
c. Both
d. None

188. Spot diagnosis of given X-ray:

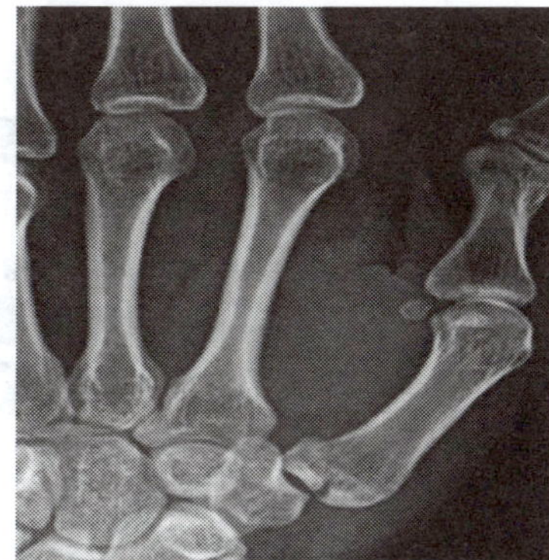

a. Rolando fracture
b. Mallet finger
c. Bennet fracture
d. Boxers fracture

189. A patient presented with complaints of night bone pain. Upon X-ray this is the finding. Most likely diagnosis:

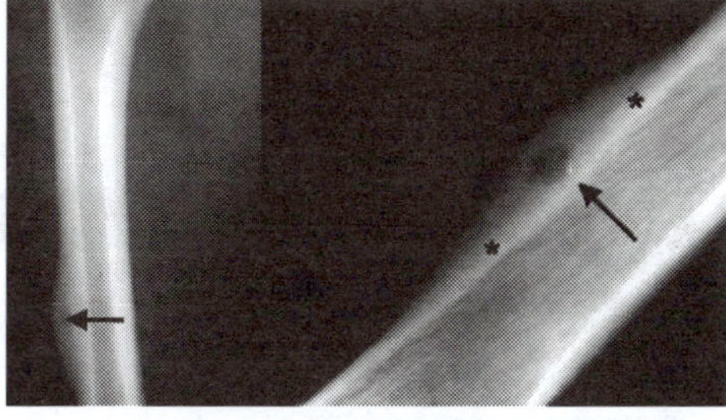

a. Adamantinoma
b. Osteoid osteoma
c. Multiple myeloma
d. Osteochondroma

OPHTHALMOLOGY

190. Which eye abnormality is shown?

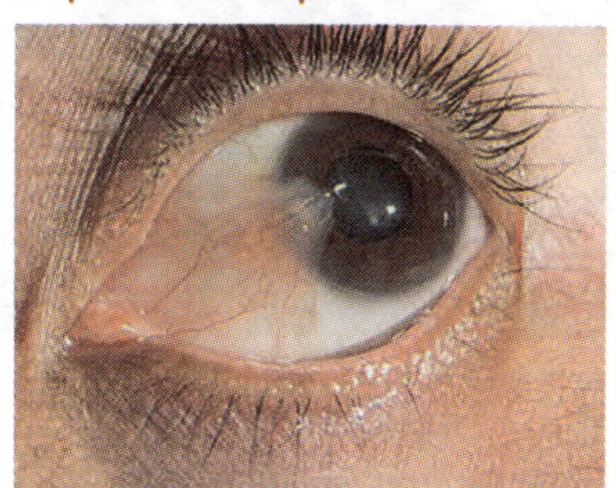

a. Pinguecula
b. Pterygium
c. Keratomalacia
d. Entropion

191. The image shows:

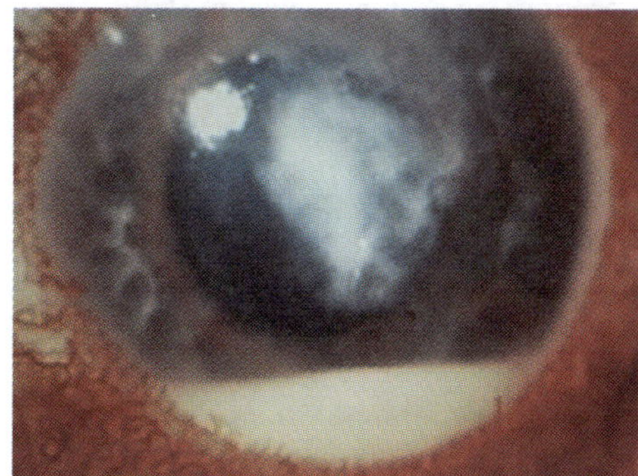

a. Hypopyon
b. Hyphema
c. Stye
d. Chalazion

192. What is the following fundus finding shown below?

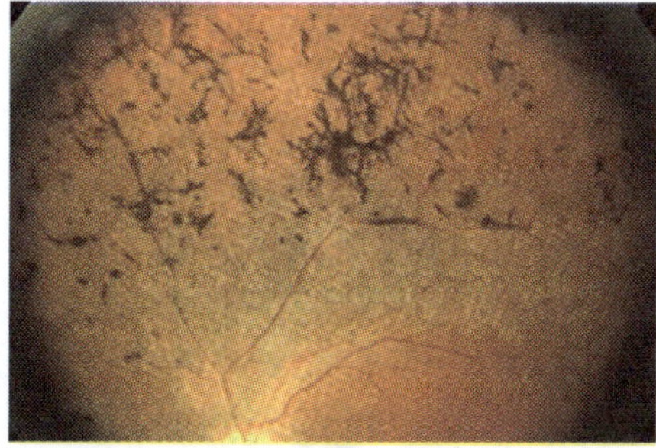

a. Retinitis Pigmentosa
b. Age related macular degeneration
c. Papilledema
d. Papillitis

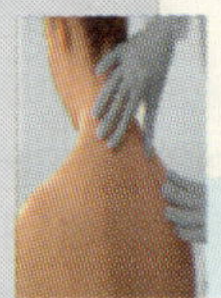

193. The fundus finding shows presence of:

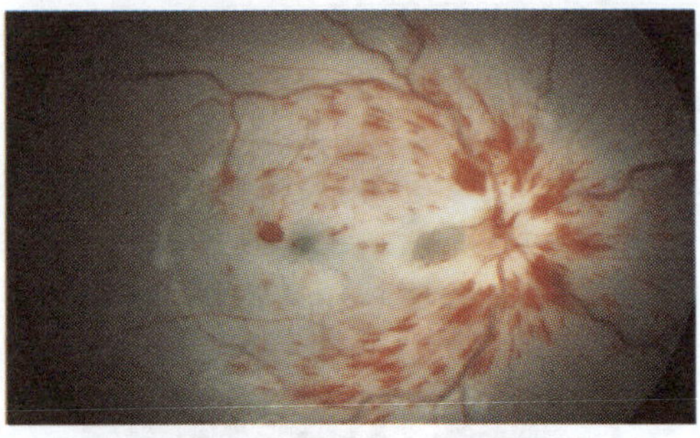

a. Splashed tomato appearance
b. Dot blot hemorrhages
c. Cottage cheese and tomato appearance
d. Cattle trucking appearance

194. A 50-year-old male patient presented to OPD due to progressive decreased vision. Upon investigation, following finding were noted. Possible diagnosis:

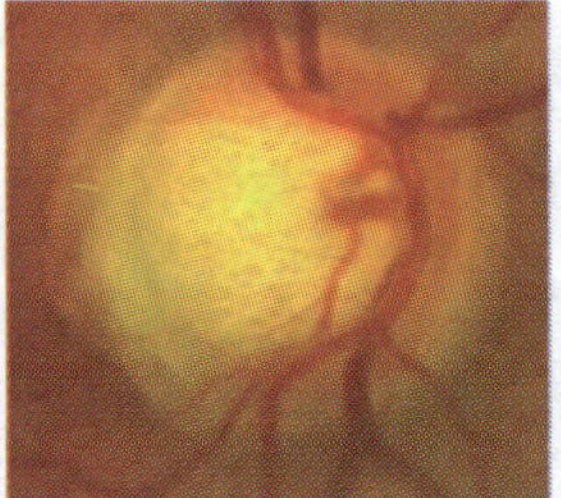

a. Age related macular degeneration
b. Hypertensive retinopathy
c. Retinal detachment
d. Glaucoma

195. This instrument is used for:

a. Checking the correction of astigmatism
b. Differentiating colored halos of cataract and ACG
c. Near vision correction
d. Both A and B

196. The visual field given below represents which of the following:

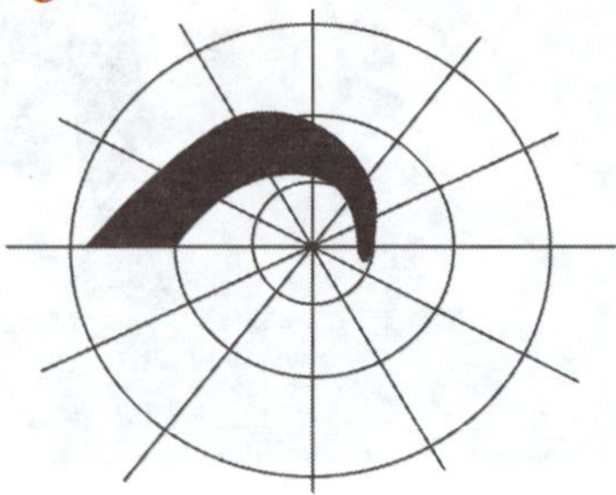

a. Central scotoma
b. Arcuate scotoma
c. Double arcuate scotoma
d. Generalized construction of field

197. The shown instrument is used for diagnosing:

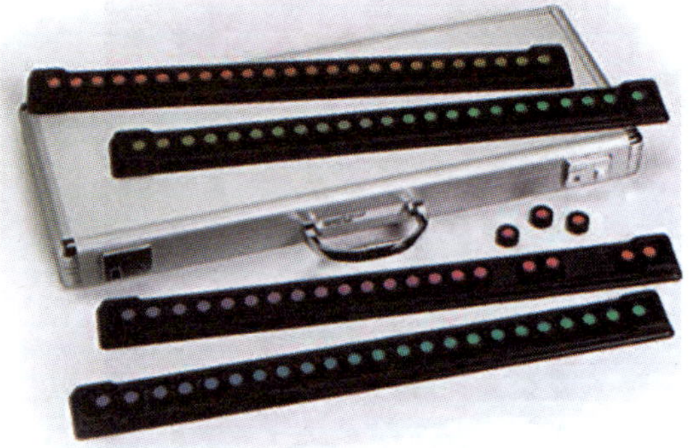

a. Retinal detachment
b. Lenticular opacity
c. Color vision
d. Binocular vision

DERMATOLOGY

198. Identify the instrument:

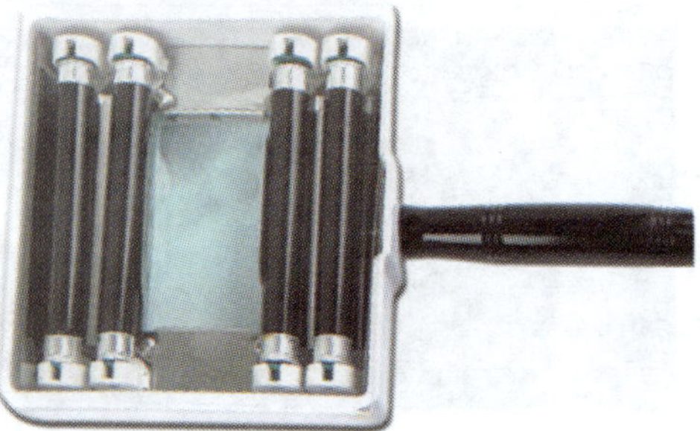

a. Infra-red lamp
b. UV rays lamp
c. Wood lamp
d. Slit lamp

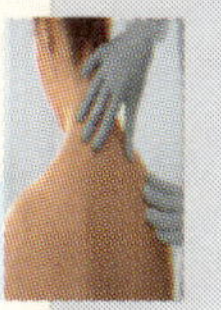

199. This finding is characteristic of:

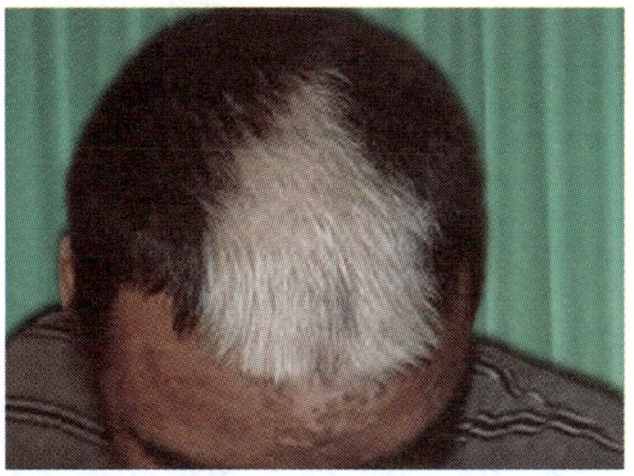

a. Leucoderma b. Piebaldism
c. Nevus anemicus d. Nevus achromicus

200. This test is used for the diagnosis of:

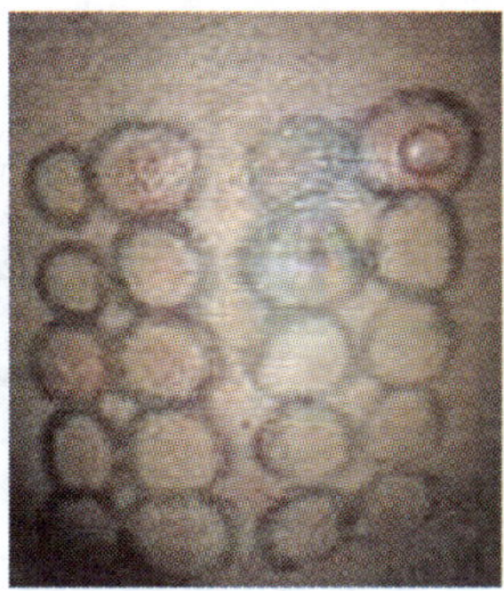

a. Behçet's syndrome b. Contact dermatitis
c. Pyoderma gangrenosum
d. Atopic dermatitis

201. These typical lesions are present in:

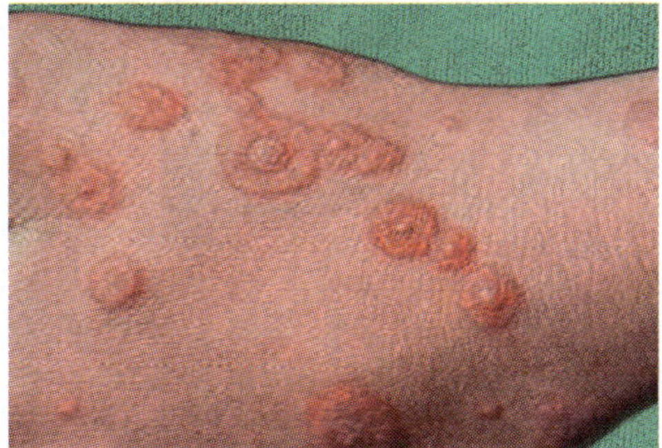

a Pemphigus b. Bullous pemphigoid
c. Erythema multiforme
d. Dermatitis herpetiformis

202. This classical presentation is of:

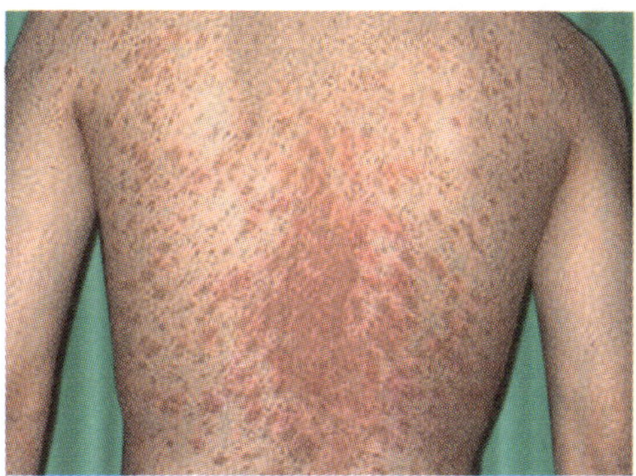

a. Pityriasis rosea b. P. alba
c. P. rubra d. P. versicolor

203. What is the treatment of choice for this condition?

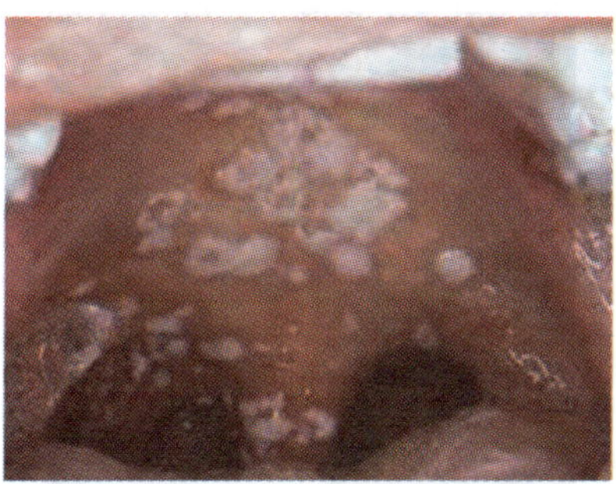

a. Anti-histaminic
b. Steroid
c. Clotrimazole paint
d. Selenium sulphide

204. All are correct about the lesion shown except:

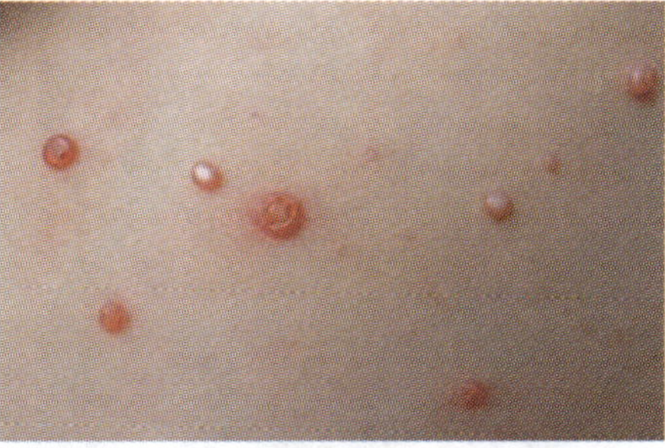

a. Molluscum contagiosum
b. Caused by RNA virus
c. Propagate via auto-inoculation
d. Not seen in soles or palms

205. A patient develops honey colored pustules on the skin. The diagnosis is:

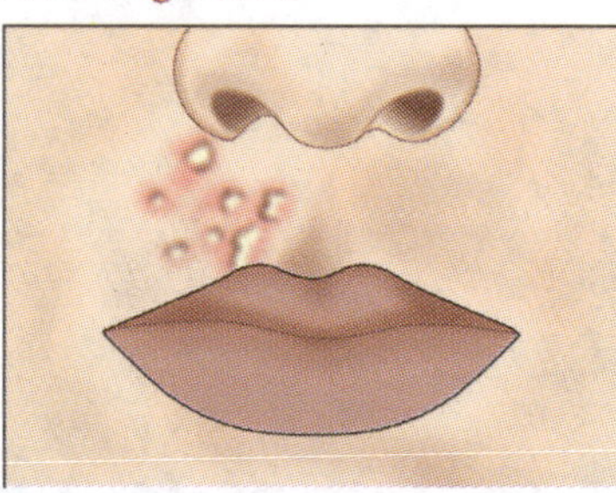

a. Impetigo
b. Staphylococcal scalded skin syndrome
c. Carbuncle
d. Sycosis barbae

206. The image shows:

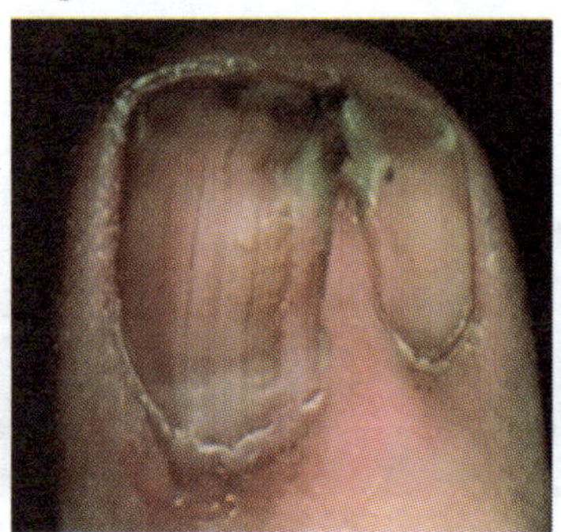

a. Pterygium nail
b. Tinea unguium
c. Botryomycosis
d. Onchomycosis

207. The image shows:

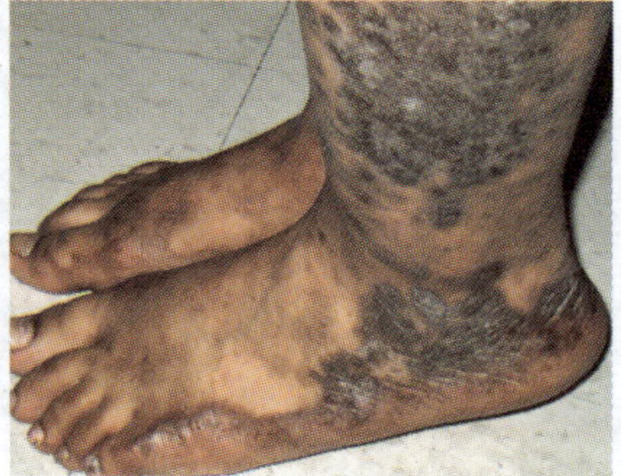

a. Lichen planus
b. Psoriasis
c. Tinea corporis
d. Pityriasis versicolor

208. The image shows which skin lesion:

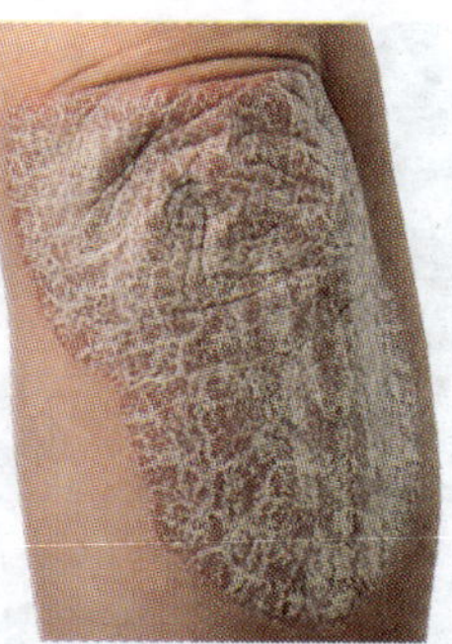

a. Lichen planus
b. Psoriasis
c. Tinea corporis
d. Pityriasis versicolor

209. Multiple painful bleeding ulcers with inguinal bubo is seen with:

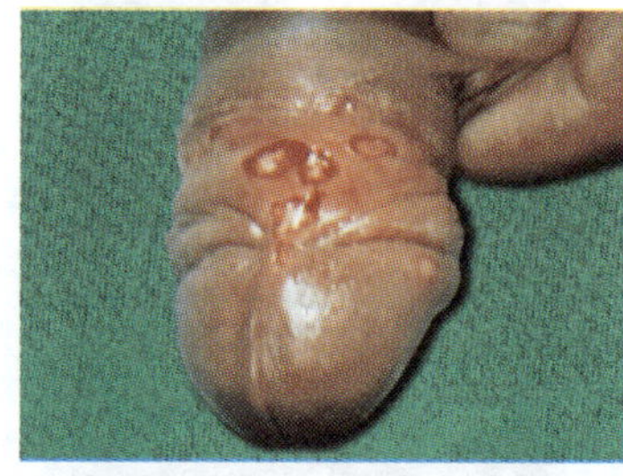

a. Chancre
b. Granuloma inguinale
c. Lymphogranuloma venerum
d. Chancroid

210. All are true about the lesions shown except:

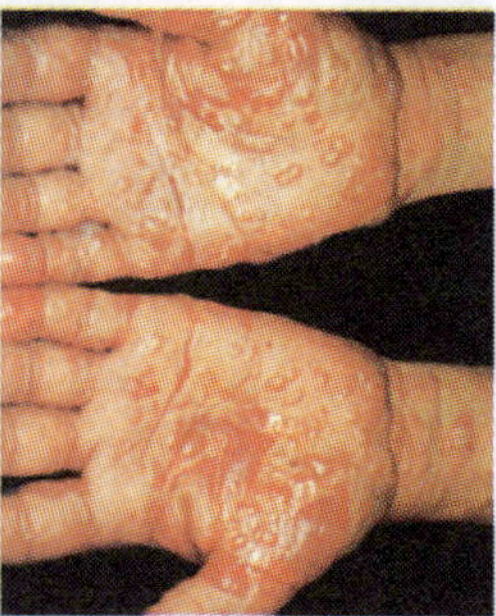

a. Itchy lesions on palms
b. Potent topical steroids resolve most cases
c. Associated with anhidrosis
d. Painful deep seated vesicles

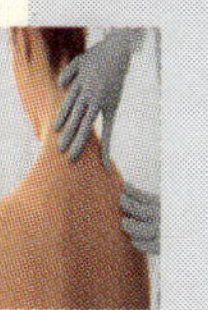

211. The image shows presence of:

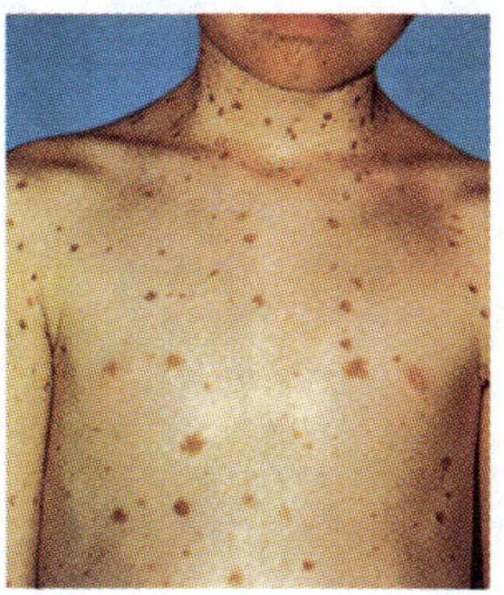

a. Lentiginosis b. Freckles
c. Shagreen patch d. Congenital nevus

212. Identify the type of leprosy based on shown lesion:

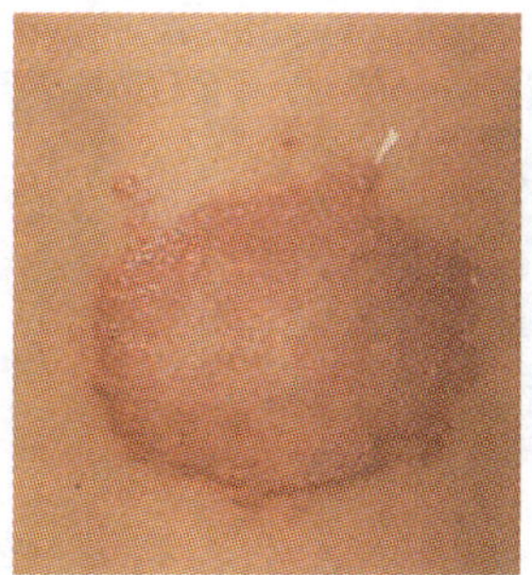

a. Borderline borderline
b. Tuberculoid
c. Borderline tuberculoid
d. Intermediate

213. The given image shows:

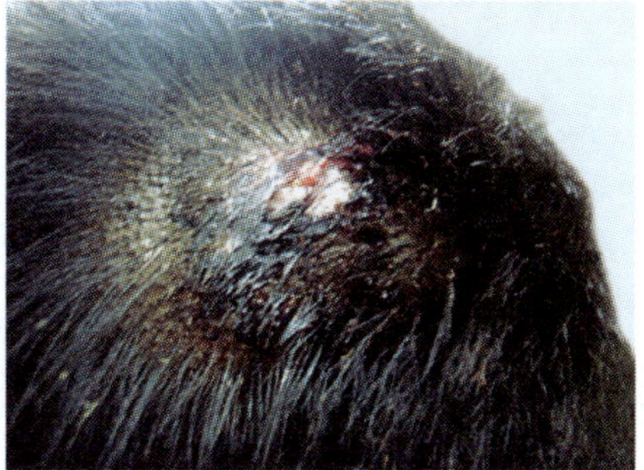

a. Favus b. Kerion
c. Seborrheic d. Scutula

214. Which of the following is not effective against this condition?

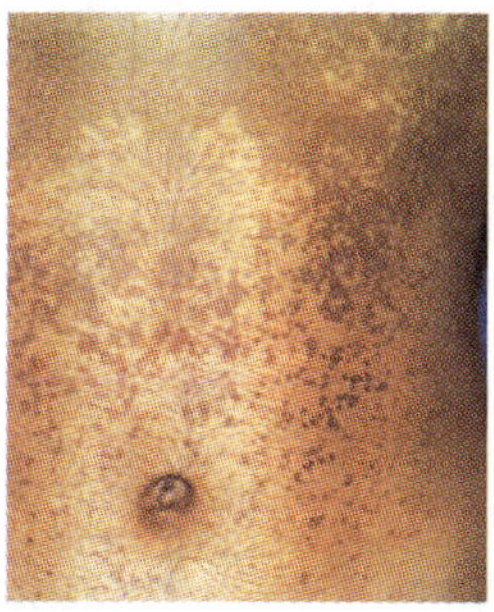

a. Topical ketoconazole b. Griseofulvin
c. Topical selenium sulphide
d. Topical sulfur preparations

215. All are true about the lesion shown *except*:

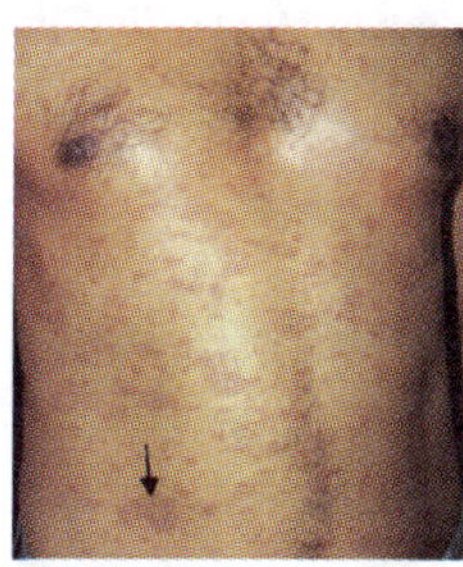

a. HHV-7
b. Herald patch
c. Predominantly occurs on genitals
d. Spontaneous healing

216. A 25-year-old woman presents with skin lesion on left supra-orbital margin. Eye examination is within normal limits. CXR done was normal. Diascopy shows apple jelly nodules. The image shows presence of:

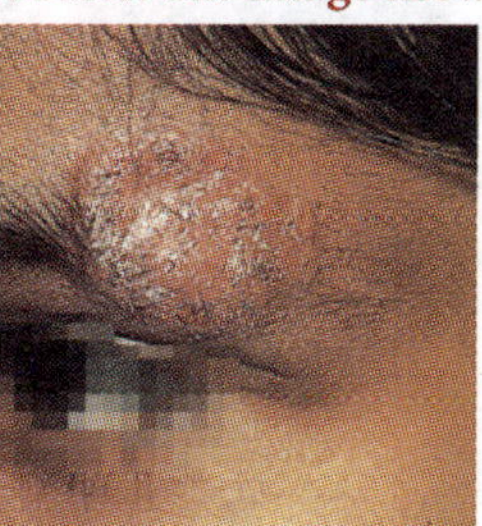

a. Lupus vulgaris b. Lupus Pernio
c. Erythema marginatum
d. Leprosy

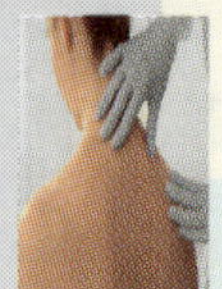

217. The image shows presence of:

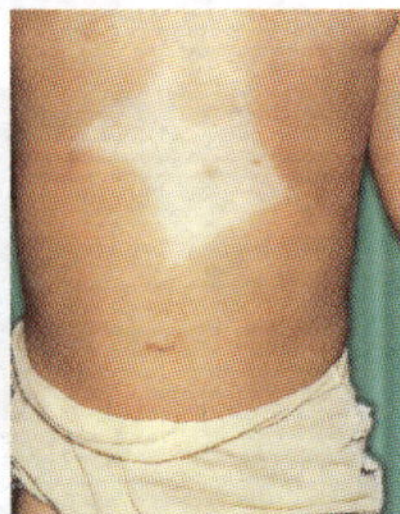

Courtesy: Dermatology by Manish Soni

a. Vitiligo
b. Piebaldism
c. Xeroderma pigmentosum
d. Incontinentia pigmenti

218. A 20-year-old man with history of melena and abdominal pain has pigmentation of lips. Probable diagnosis is:

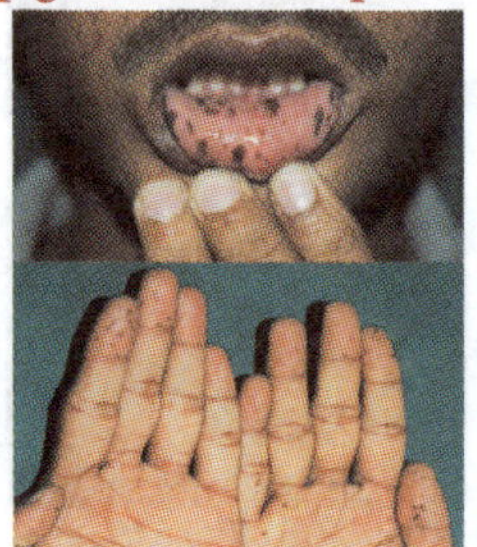

a. Incontinentia pigmenti
b. Cronkhite Canada syndrome
c. Brooke Spiegler syndrome
d. Peutz Jeghers syndrome

219. The image shows presence of:

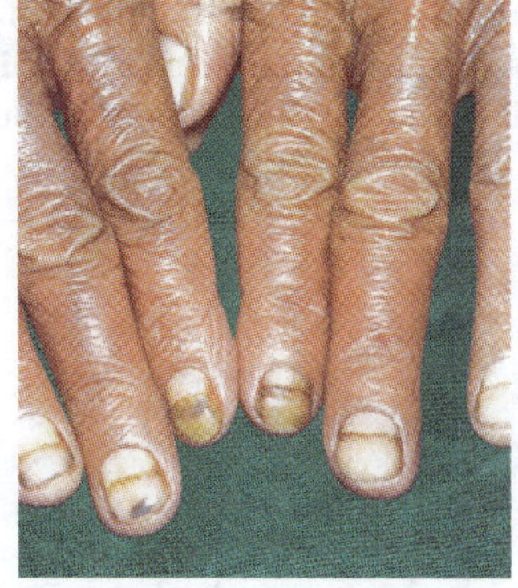

a. Muehrcke's nails b. Lindsay nails
c. Leukonychia d. Beau's lines

220. The image shows presence of:

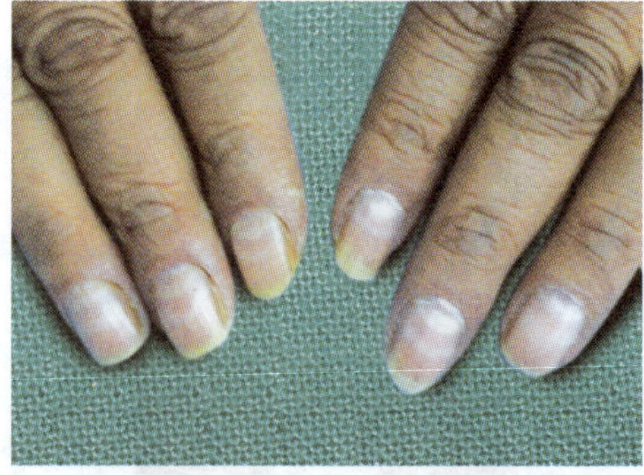

a. Muehrcke's nails b. Lindsay nails
c. Leukonychia d. Beau's lines

221. A 25-year-old young adult female presents with following lesions in axilla, as shown by the arrow:

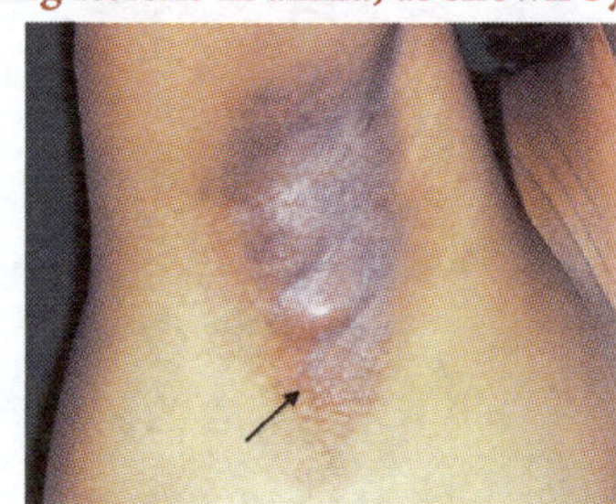

a. Hidradenitis suppurativa
b. Fordyce spot
c. Acne fulminans
d. Acne conglobate

222. The given KOH mount of patient shows:

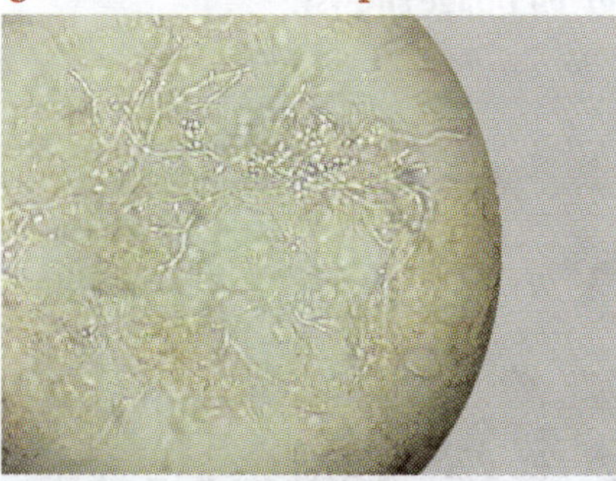

a. Spaghetti and meat ball appearance
b. Budding yeasts and pseudohyphae
c. Clusters of pigmented cells
d. Septate hyphae

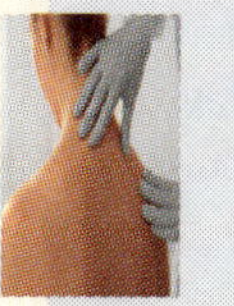

223. These lesions are seen in which of the following:

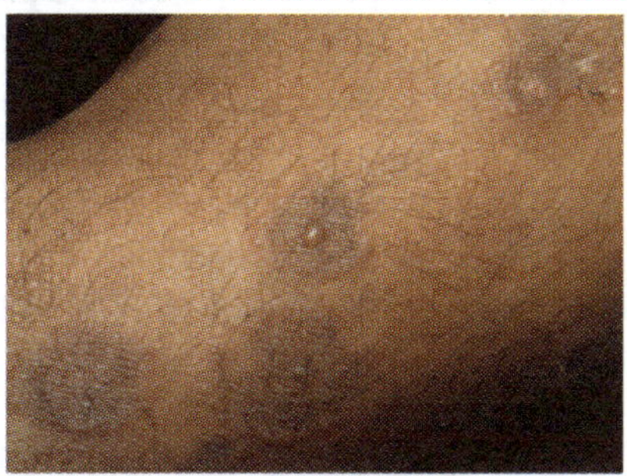

a. Erythema infectiosum
b. Erythema nodosum
c. Erythema induratum
d. Erythema multiforme

224. A 28-year-old lady has asymptomatic dome shaped small lesions on a forehead for last 2 months. She has a 2-year-old daughter with similar lesions. What is the causative agent:

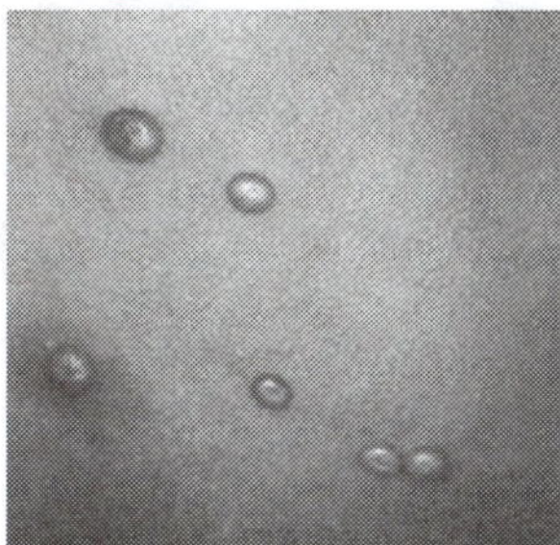

a. Papillomavirus
b. Poxvirus
c. Herpes virus
d. Coxsackie virus

225. A patient after a trip to Bangkok developed fever and perioral vesicles. What is the diagnosis:

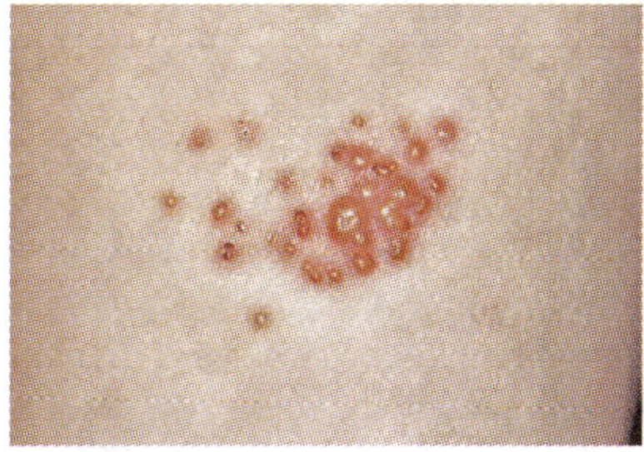

a. Herpes simplex
b. Impetigo
c. Molluscum contagiosum
d. Bullous pemphigoid

226. Identify the lesion:

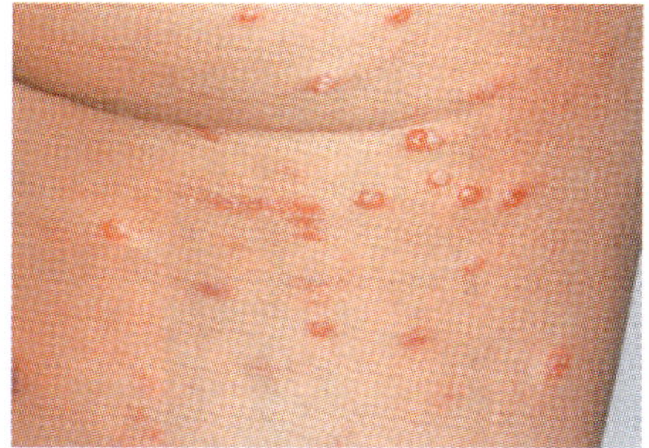

a. Molluscum contagiosum
b. Herpes simplex
c. Pityriasis rosea
d. Gianotti-Crosti syndrome

227. A 13-year-old boy presents with patchy depigmented skin on the right flank and upper thigh in segmental distribution. The depigmentation started 1 year back but has been static for last 4 months. Mother reports use of topical steroids which was ineffective. Diagnosis is:

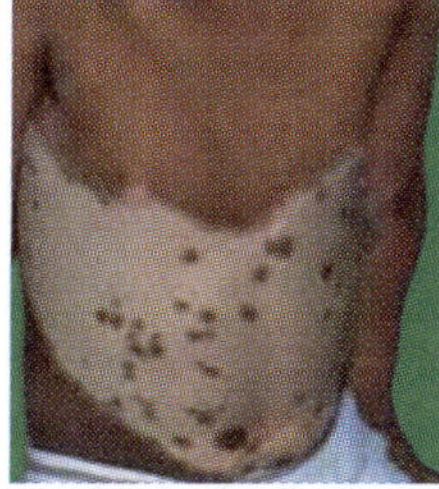

a. Piebaldism
b. Segmental vitiligo
c. Hypomelanosis of Ito
d. Hypopigmented streaks

228. Identify the lesion:

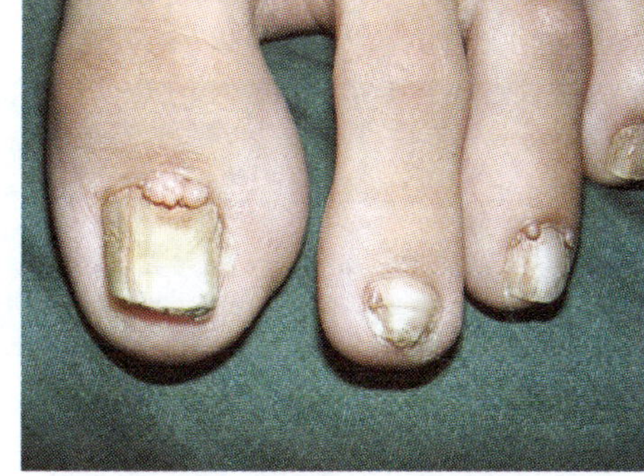

a. Koenen tumor
b. Onychomycosis
c. Onychodystrophy
d. Onychogryphosis

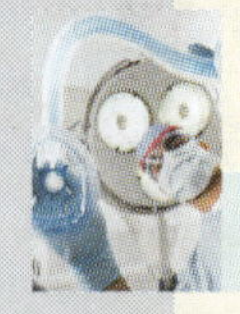

229. All of the following statements regarding this image are true, *except*:

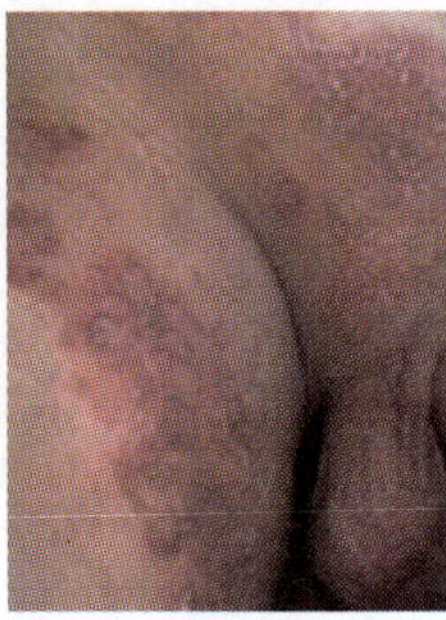

a. Dhobi itch
b. Jock itch
c. More common in tropics
d. Caused by *Candida*

232. The diagrams of a correctly positioned proseal-type Laryngeal Mask Airway is provided below. Above what site is the arrow marked area of the airway positioned:

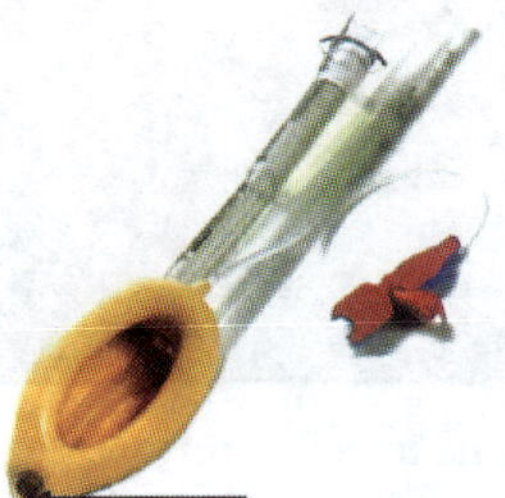

a. Carina
b. Upper end of trachea
c. Vocal cords
d. Above esophagus

ANESTHESIA

230. The image shows which cylinder:

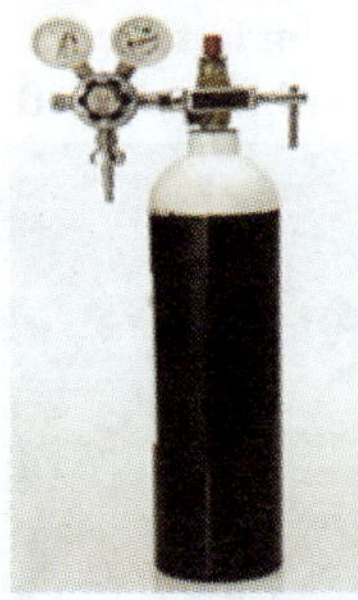

a. Oxygen Cylinder
b. Nitrous oxide cylinder
c. Cyclopropane cylinder
d. Halothane cylinder

231. Name the following instrument used in giving anesthesia:

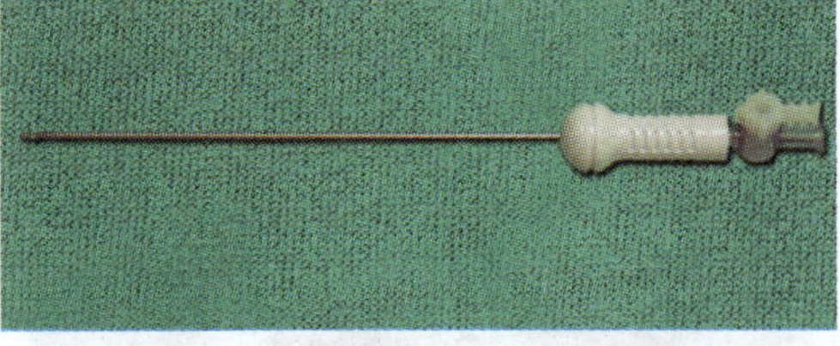

a. Intravenous regional anesthesia access needle
b. Vere's Needle
c. Lumbar puncture needle
d. Hypodermic needle

233. The following procedure is being performed. Identify the markings:

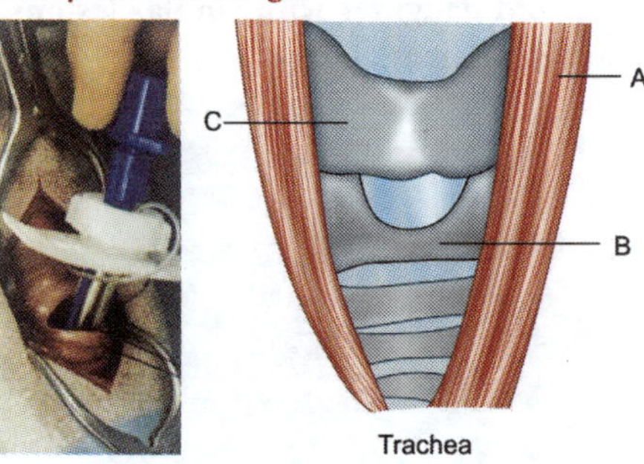

a. A = Sternomastoid muscle, B = Cricoid cartilage, C = T Thyroid cartilage
b. A = Cricoid cartilage, B = Sternomastoid muscle, C = Thyroid cartilage
c. A = Thyroid cartilage, B = Cricoid cartilage, C = Sternomastoid muscle
d. A = Sternomastoid muscle, B = Thyroid cartilage, C = Cricoid cartilage

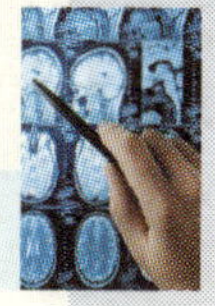

234. All are correct about the image shown except:

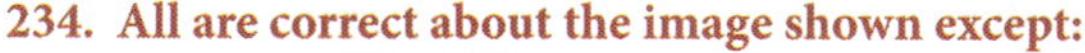

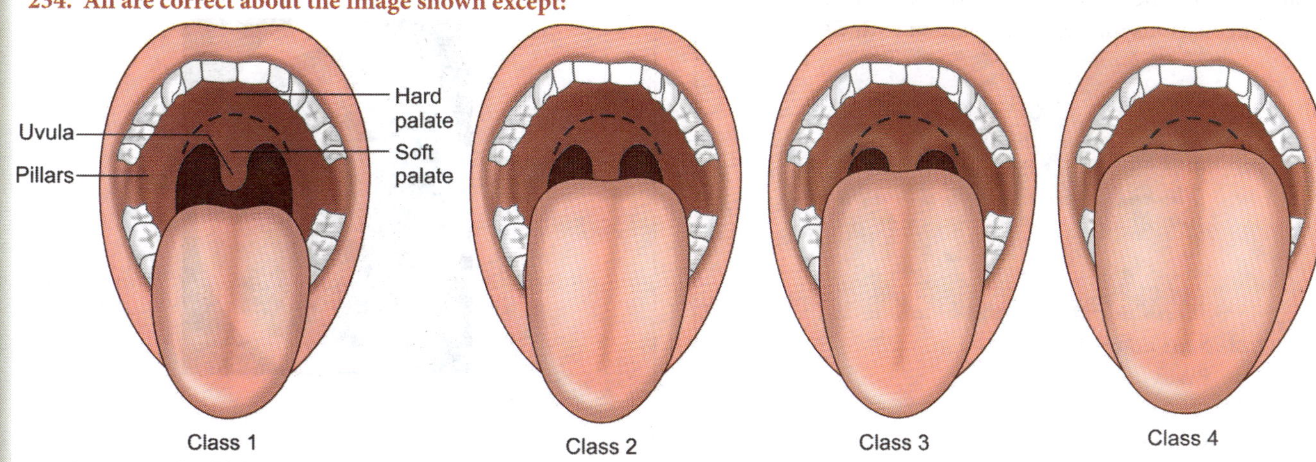

a. Mallampati classification
b. Helps in identifying cases with difficult orotracheal intubation
c. Not influenced by tongue mobility and size
d. Has limited utility in patients reduced neck extension

235. What is the size of this shown pink color canula? ***(2018)***

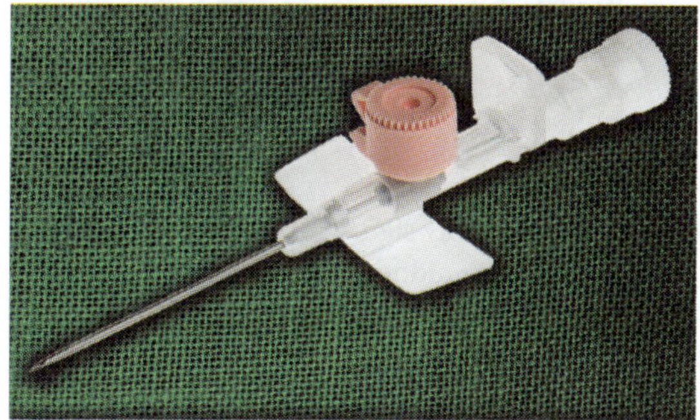

a. 16G b. 18G
c. 20G d. 22G

236. Identify the instrument shown in the image below:

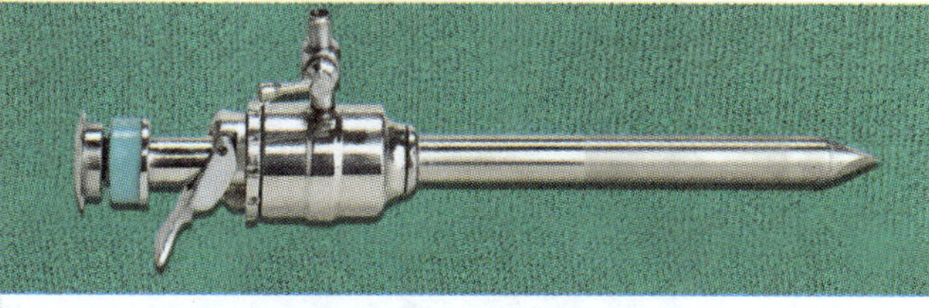

a. SILS port
b. Laparoscopic trocar
c. Deaver retractor
d. Periosteal elevator

RADIOLOGY

237. Comment on the diagnosis: ***(Most Recent Question 2019)***

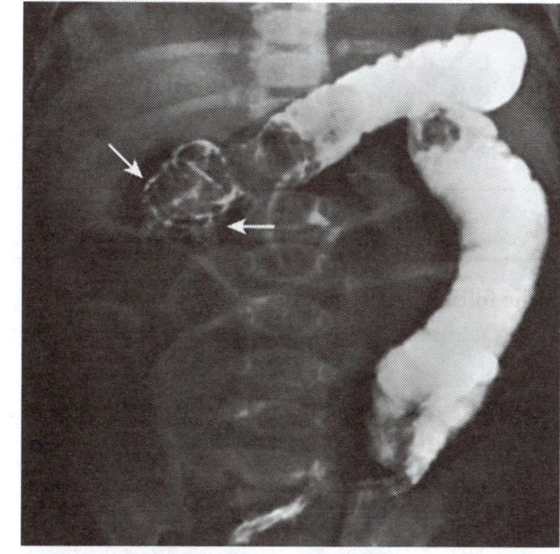

a. Intussusception
b. Malrotation
c. Duodenal atresia
d. Ileal atresia

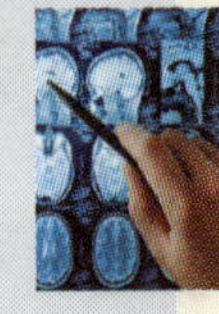

238. Identify the lesion shown in the CT head of an unconscious unresponsive patient with GCS of 5:

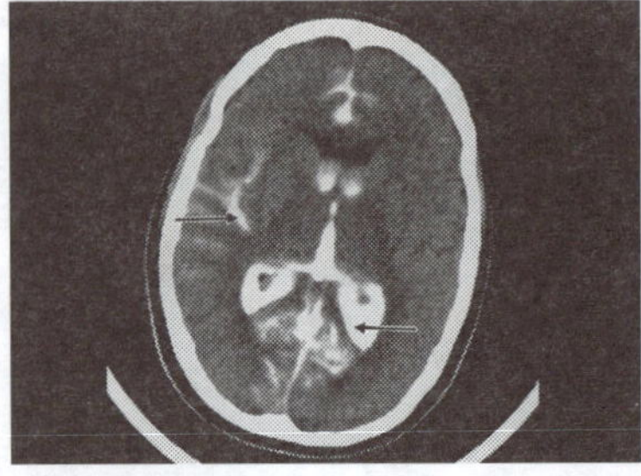

a. SAH and IVH
b. Brain tumor
c. Hydrocephalus
d. Extradural and subdural hemorrhage

239. Identify the lesion shown in the CT head of an unconscious unresponsive patient with GCS of 5:

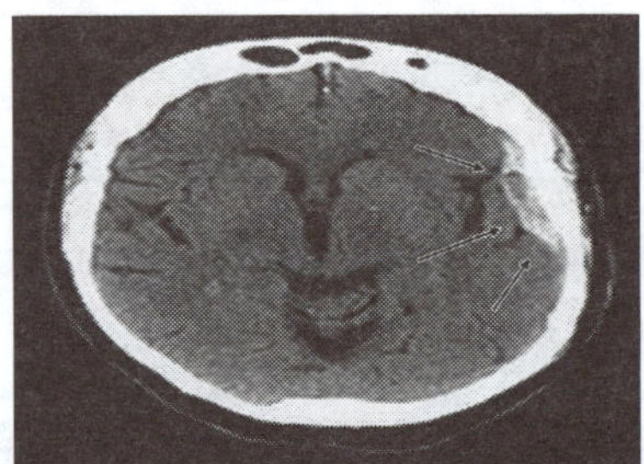

a. Extradural hemorrhage
b. Subdural hemorrhage
c. Subarachnoid hemorrhage
d. Intraventricular hemorrhage

240. The following CT shows:

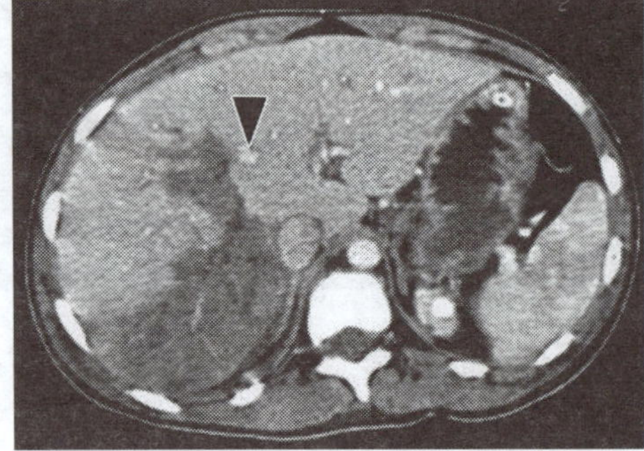

a. Liver laceration
b. Kidney cyst
c. Pancreas contusion
d. Perforation peritonitis

241. CT head shows:

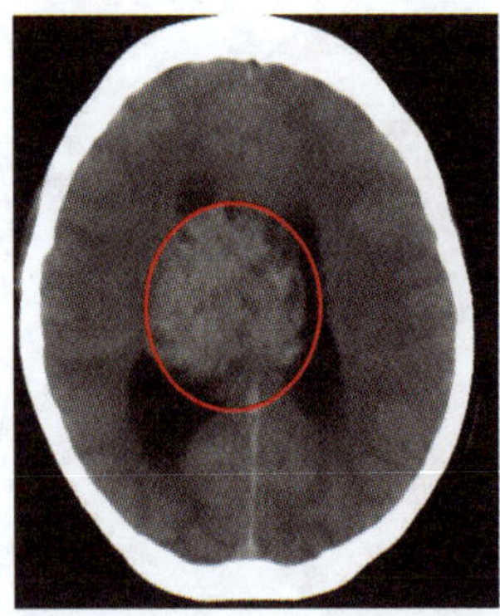

a. Brain tumor
b. Brain infarction
c. S.A.H
d. I.V.H

242. The following IVP shows presence of:

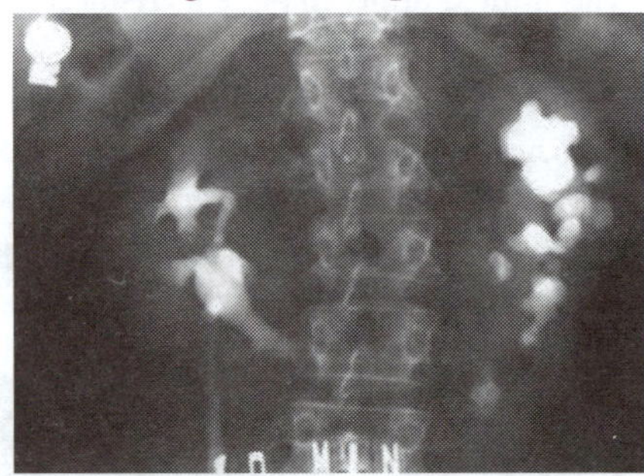

a. Drooping lily sign
b. Horseshoe kidney
c. Duplication of kidney
d. Normal scan

243. The cholangiogram shows:

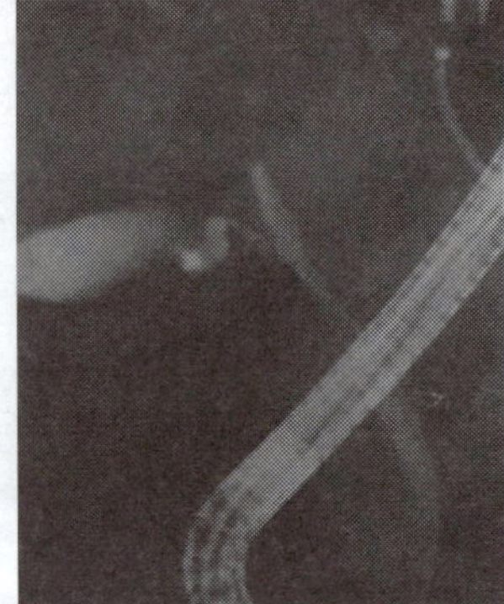

a. Klatskin tumor
b. Gall stones
c. Choledocholithiasis
d. Porcelain gallbladder

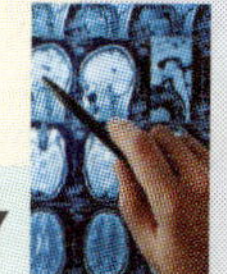

244. A 3-year-old non-vaccinated child presented with fever and fast breathing. His mother told that he has recently developed measles rash. CXR shown below is indicative of which infection:

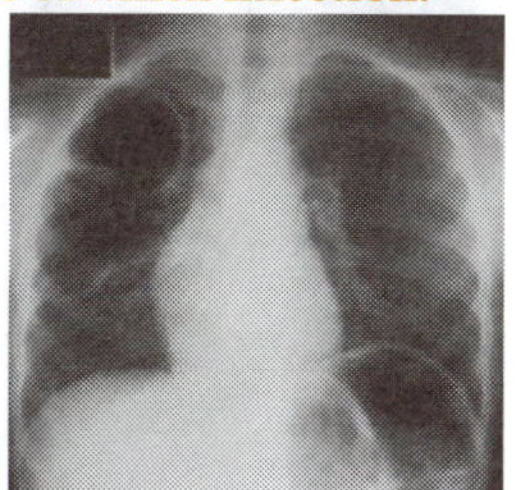

a. Staphylococcus aureus b. Staphylococcal albus
c. Streptococcal pneumoniae
d. Streptococcal viridans

245. A neonate with Down syndrome is having bilious vomiting:

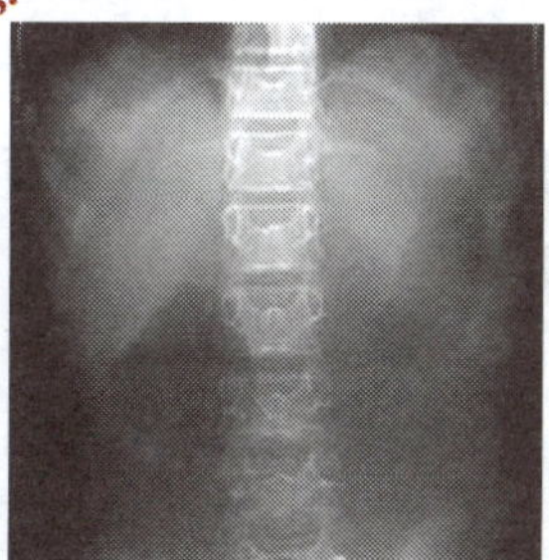

a. Duodenal atresia
b. Congenital hypertrophic pyloric stenosis
c. Ileal atresia
d. Anorectal malformation

246. A 40-year-old intravenous drug abuser presents with Vomiting, Jaundice and Right Hypochondrium pain. USG abdomen shows presence of:

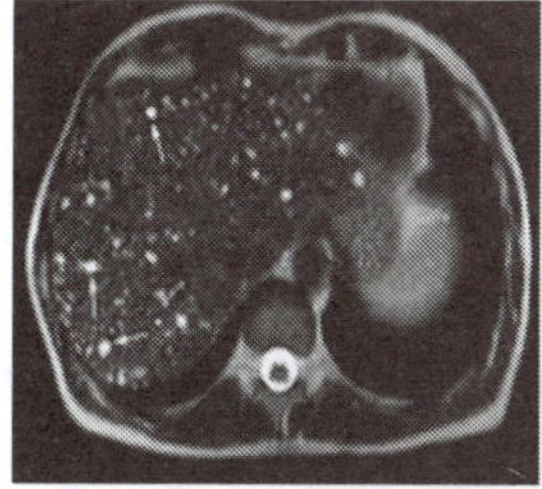
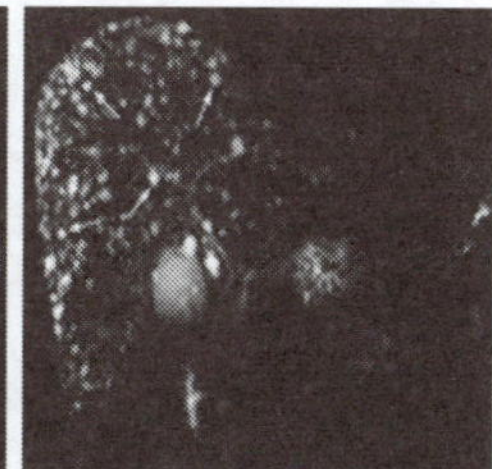

a. Amoebic liver abscess
b. Acute viral hepatitis
c. Acute cholecystitis
d. Hepatocellular carcinoma

247. Neonate with respiratory distress 6 hours after birth. CXR was performed. Diagnosis is:

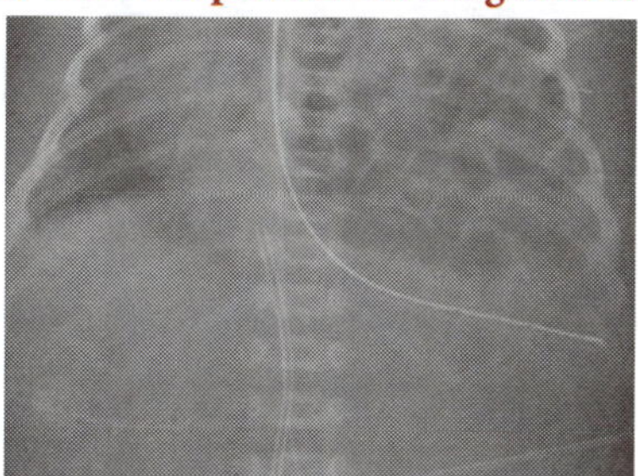

a. Meconium aspiration syndrome
b. Congenital pneumonia
c. Bochdalek hernia
d. Transient tachypnea of newborn

248. A 3 days old neonate with abdominal distention and non-passage of stool. The X-ray done shown below is called:

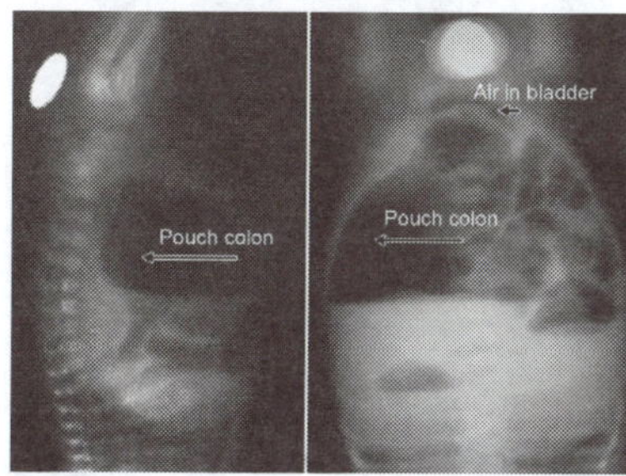

a. Invertogram b. Infantogram
c. Babygram
d. Double contrast barium study

249. Neonate with anoxic spells and single S2. CXR shows all EXCEPT:

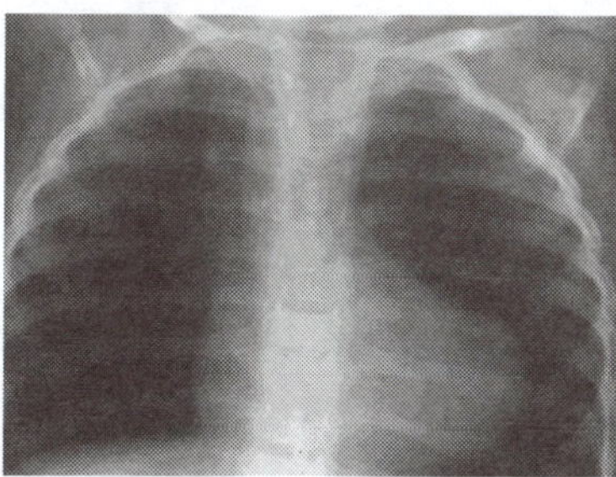

a. Boot shaped heart
b. Pulmonary plethora
c. Right sided aortic arch
d. Right ventricular hypertrophy

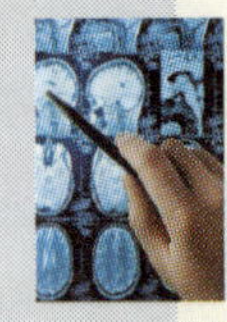

250. In the shown image, what is the marked line with B is which fissure: ***(2018)***

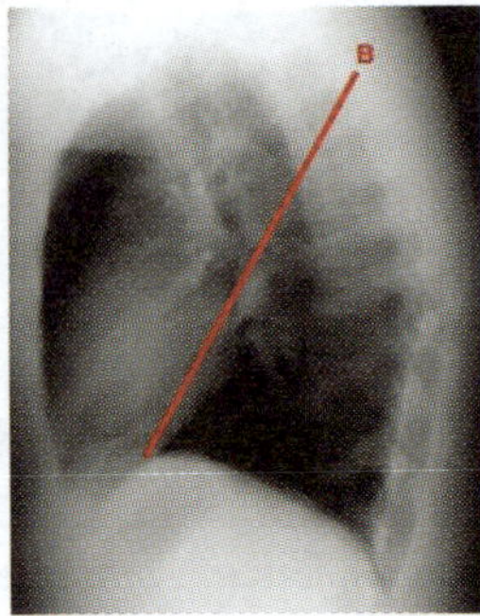

a. Minor fissure
b. Major fissure
c. Transverse fissure
d. Azygous fissure

251. The marked structure in chest X-ray is: ***(2018)***

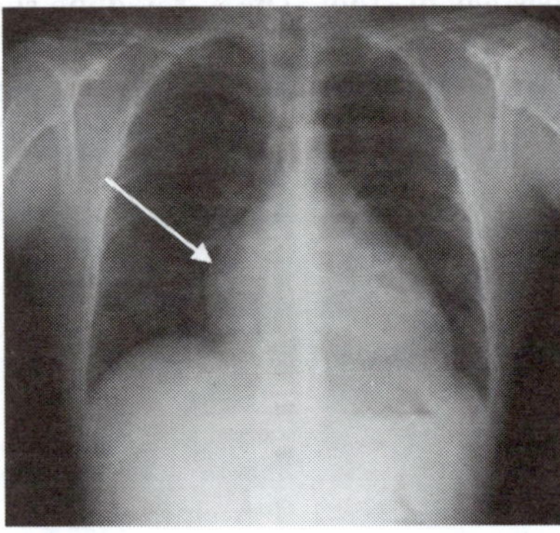

a. Inferior vena cava
b. Right atrium
c. Right ventricle
d. Superior vena cava

252. In the shown X-ray what is the name of structure marked: ***(2018)***

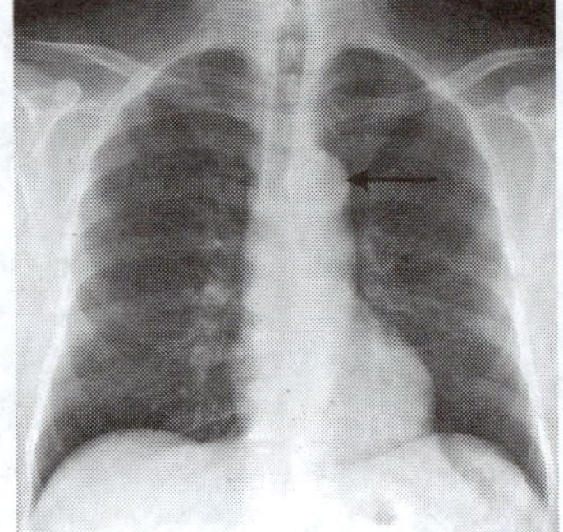

a. Aortic knob
b. Left atrium
c. SVC
d. Pulmonary trunk

253. The following appearance of esophagus in barium swallow is seen in which of the following conditions?

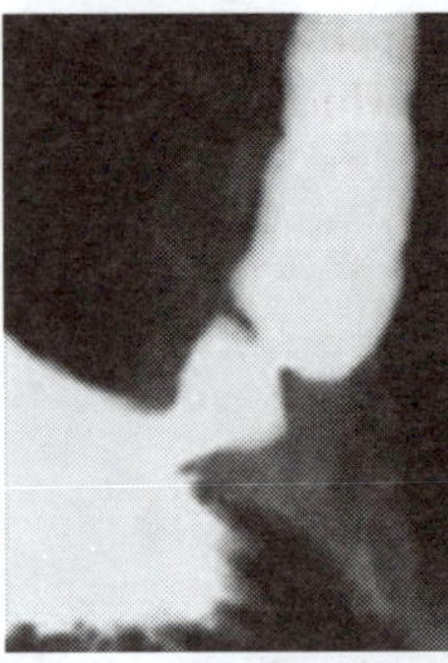

a. Schatzki ring
b. Scleroderma
c. Achalasia cardia
d. Carcinoma esophagus

254. A 2-year-old child was playing on floor and developed sudden breathlessness, wheezing and decreased breath sound in the right lung. CXR shows following finding. Diagnosis:

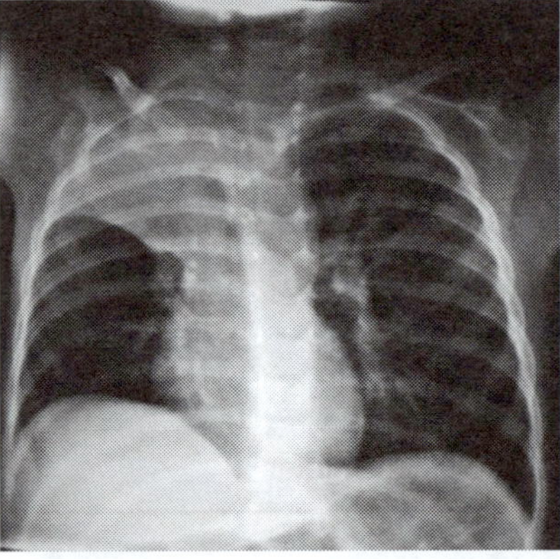

a. Pneumothorax
b. Pneumonia
c. Foreign body aspiration
d. Bronchial asthma

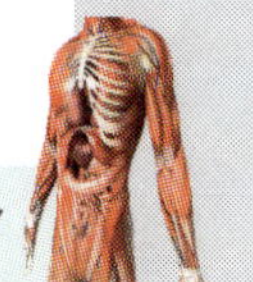

ANSWERS WITH EXPLANATIONS

ANATOMY

1. Ans. (a) Pituitary

2. Ans. (a) Long thoracic nerve

Nerve involved	Muscle
Long thoracic nerve	Serratus anterior
Musculocutaneous nerve	Coracobrachialis muscle
Lateral anterior thoracic nerve	Pectoralis major muscle
Thoracodorsal Nerve	Latissimus dorsi

3. Ans. (a) Coracoacromial ligament

- The image shows a ligament *extending* from the coracoid process to the acromion process.

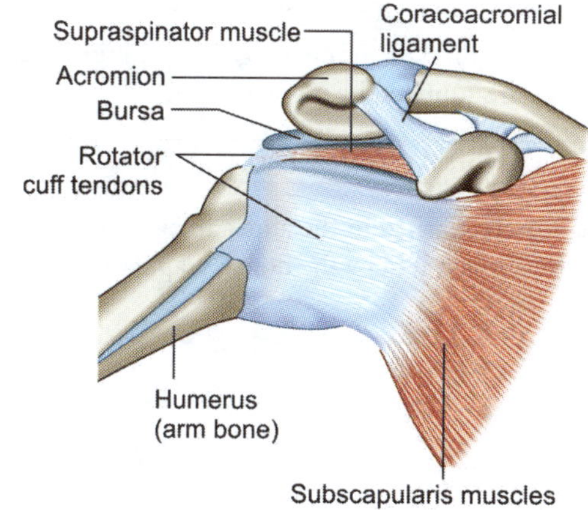

4. Ans. (c) Sural nerve

The image shows sural nerve.

5. Ans. (d) Nerve originates from nerve roots L5-S2

- The image shows pain in the distribution of sciatic nerve, which can occur due to disc prolapse. Such pain is worsened on standing.
- *Arterial claudication pain is worsened on walking.*
- *The sciatic nerve originates from lumbosacral plexus L4-S3*
  - Tibial division
    - Originates from anterior preaxial branches of L4, L5, S1, S2, S3
  - Peroneal division
    - Originates from postaxial branches of L4, L5, S1, S2

6. Ans. (d) All of these

Mnemonic for Branches for External Carotid Artery

Some anatomists like freaking out poor medical students

S : superior thyroid artery
A : ascending pharyngeal artery
L : lingual artery
F : facial artery
O : occipital artery

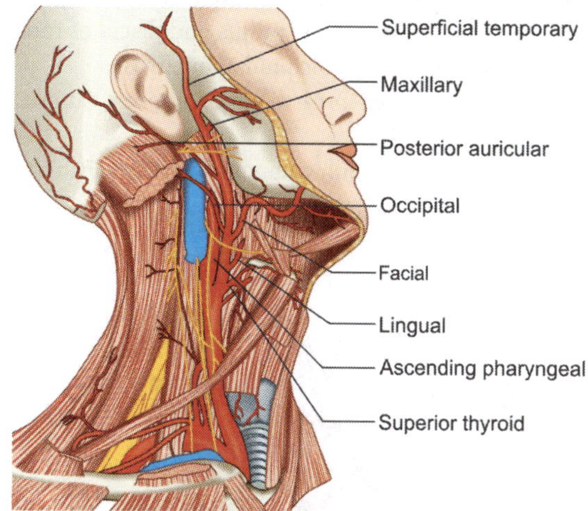

P : posterior auricular artery
M : maxillary artery
S : superficial temporal artery

7. Ans. (b) B

The following diagram and its branches should be remembered.

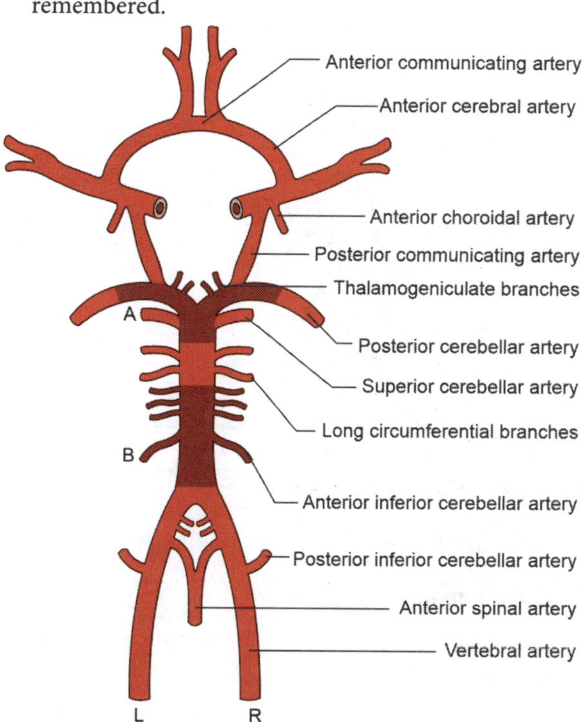

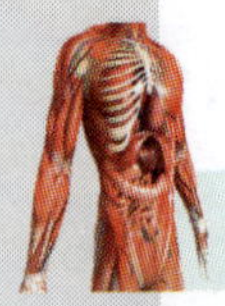

8. Ans. (c) Radial tuberosity

- The shown muscle in the image is biceps brachii muscle, which is inserted at radial tuberosity and at fascia of forearm.

Biceps Brachii

- **Origin**
- **Short head:** Tip or coracoid process of scapula
  Long head: Supraglenoid tubercle of scapula
- **Insertion:** Tuberosity or radius and fascia of radius and fascia of forearm via bicipital aponeurosis
- **Action:** Supinates forearm and, when it is supine, flexes forearm
- **Innervation:** Musculocutaneous nerve (C5 and **C6**)

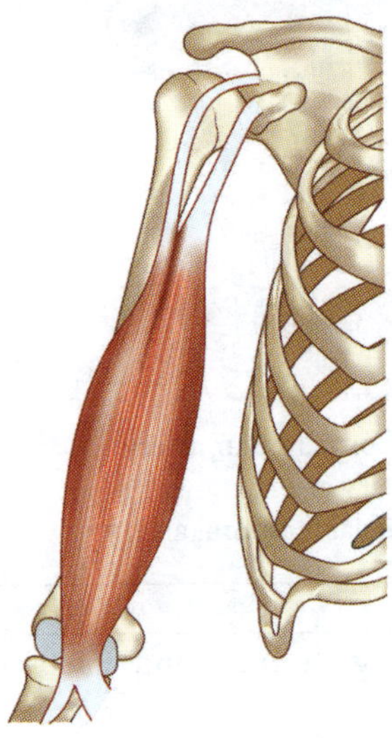

9. Ans. (b) Pterion

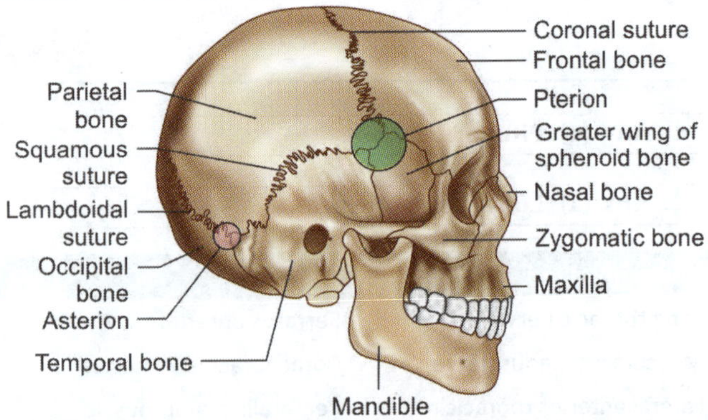

10. Ans. (c) Extensor carpi radialis longus

The arrow shows extensor carpi radialis longus muscle.

11. Ans. (a) Median nerve

- The area marked in the image are the lumbricals.
- They are supplied by median nerve.

12. Ans. (a) Dorsal scapular nerve

The muscle marked in the above image is levator scapulae, which is innervated by the dorsal scapular nerve.

13. Ans. (a) Popeye sign

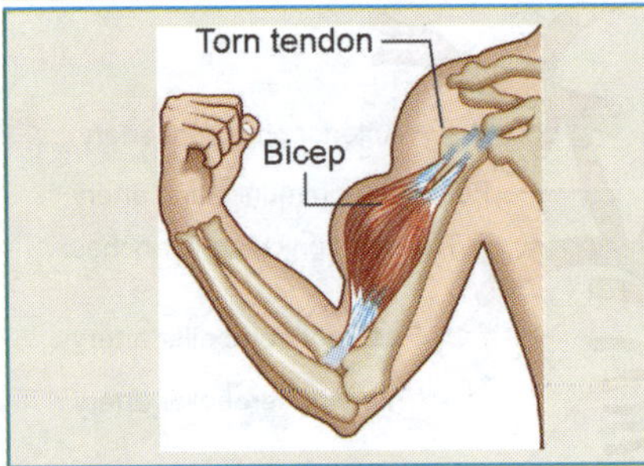

- The sign shown in the image is Popeye sign, which occurs due to the rupture of the tendon of the long head of biceps brachii.
- On flexing the elbow, the characteristic deformity appears due to the bulging of the muscle belly caused by the contraction of the unrestrained muscles.

14. Ans. (a) Corpus callosum

The body of the corpus callosum arches posteriorly and ends as the thickened posterior portion called the splenium.

15. Ans. (c) Pointing index

The image shows presence of point index with lesion of median nerve. The remaining three choices A, C, D are seen in ulnar nerve damage.

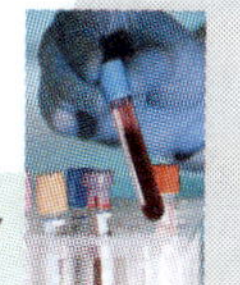

PHYSIOLOGY

16. Ans. (b) B

PR interval (A)	120–200 msec and represents spread of impulse from SAN to AV node
RR interval (C)	Inversely related to heart rate
QT interval (B)	360–440 msec and represents ventricular depolarization and repolarization

17. Ans. (a) Cheyne stokes breathing

Repeated sequence of gradual onset of apnea followed by restoration of respiration; this pattern is defined as Cheyne stokes respiration.

Physiological Causes

- Sleep
- Voluntary hyperventilation
- High altitude

Pathological Causes

- Left ventricular failure
- Uremia
- Brain damage

PHARMACOLOGY

18. Ans. (c) Dexamethasone

- Steroids are associated with cataract formation:
  - Topical steroid causes: Glaucoma
  - Systemic steroid causes: Cataract

19. Ans. (c) Pilocarpine

- The shown delivery system is ocusert.
- It is used for continuous delivery of pilocarpine in glaucoma patients.

20. Ans. (d) Pioglitazone

- The shown image is macular edema. It is caused by PPAR-gamma agonist like Pioglitazone, Rosiglitazone, Troglitazone.

21. Ans. (b) Labetalol

- The shown image is of gum hypertrophy.
- It can be caused by anti-epileptic agent like phenytoin and anti-hypertensive agent like nifedipine and other calcium channel blockers.
- Other agents associated with gum hypertrophy: Tacrolimus, cyclosporine, valproate, barbiturate.

22. Ans. (b) Bleomycin

- The shown image is of flagellate dermatitis. It is associated with anti-cancer agent bleomycin.

PATHOLOGY

23. Ans. (a) Howell-Jolly bodies

- The image shows presence of Howell-Jolly bodies which are dense blue circular inclusions representing nuclear remnants. The presence of Howell-Jolly bodies implies defective splenic function.

24. Ans. (b) Reed Sternberg cell

The image shows presence of Reed Sternberg cell with bilobed nucleus and prominent nucleoli which lead to prominent owl eye appearance.

25. Ans. (b) Myeloblast

- The image shows presence of Myeloblasts and you can see the Auer rods in the cytoplasm of these cells. (Arrow marked)

26. Ans. (a) Gaucher cell

- The image shows presence of an enlarged macrophage showing crumpled tissue paper appearance of cytoplasm. The cell contains undigested glucocerebroside.
- Reed-Sternberg cell is found in Hodgkin's lymphoma
- Anitschkow cell is seen in rheumatic fever
  - Popcorn cell is seen in nodular lymphocyte predominant variety of Hodgkin lymphoma.

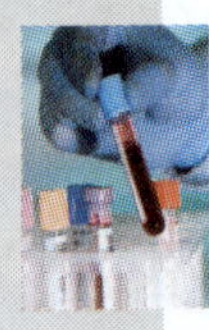

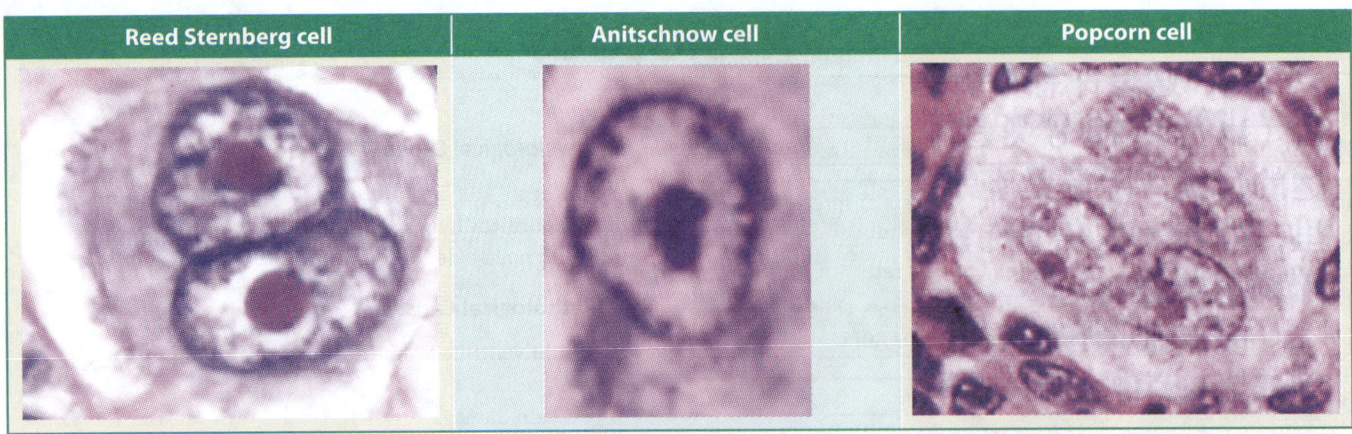

27. Ans. (b) Thalassemia

The image shows a child with prominent cheek bones due to marrow expansion. The peripheral smear shows presence of target cells (Notice the target in the centre of RBC).

28. Ans. (a) Hairy cell leukemia

The image shows presence of immature B cell with hairy projection on the surface.

29. Ans. (b) Schistocyte

Notice the projection on the edge of the RBC.

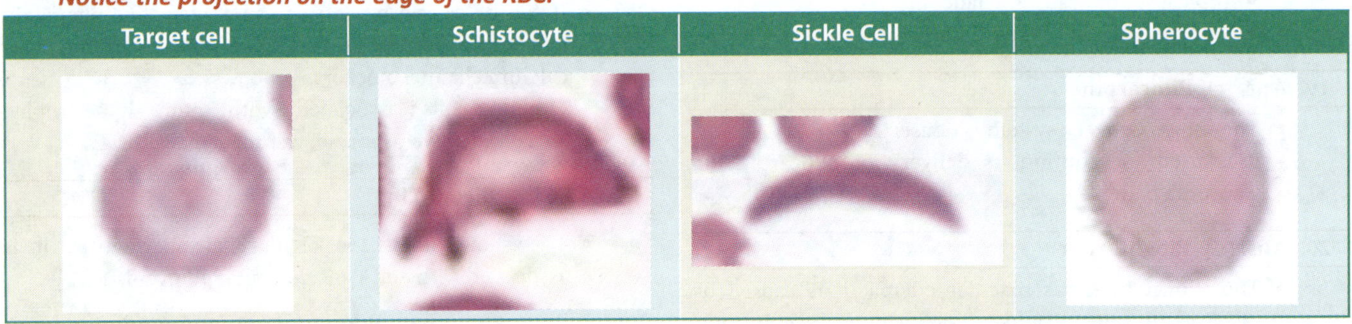

30. Ans. (a) Lipofuscin in cardiac tissue

Ref: Page 25, Harsh Mohan, 7th ed.

- The image shows presence of *wear and tear ligament* which is lipofuscin. It is a yellowish brown pigment accumulating in central part of cells around the nuclei.
- By electron microscopy it is *intralysosomal* electron dense granules in *perinuclear location.*
- It can be seen in:

> - Myocardial fibers and is associated with wasting and hence called as brown atrophy.
> - Intraneuronal in senile dementia
> - Leydig cells of testis
> - Hepatocytes

31. Ans. (b) Hyaline arteriosclerosis

Ref: Harsh Mohan, 7th ed. pg. 372

The image shows an *eosinophilic hyaline material* in tunica media and intima. The lumen of blood vessel is narrowed. This is suggestive of diagnosis of hyaline arteriosclerosis.

32. Ans. (b) Hyperplastic arteriosclerosis

Ref: Harsh Mohan, 7th ed. pg. 372

The image shows *loosely placed concentric layers* in a small artery leading to *onion skin* appearance. The presence of hyperplastic intimal smooth muscle cells with severe intimal sclerosis leads to narrowed blood vessel.

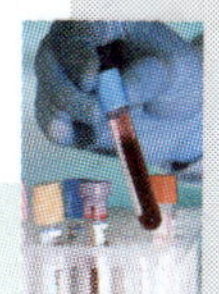

33. Ans. (c) Caseous necrosis

Ref: Pocket Companion to Robbins, 9th ed. pg. 6

The image shows eosinophilic amorphous deposit at 12 o' clock position with surrounding infiltrate showing langhans type giant cell with nuclei arranged in horse shoe pattern. This is seen in caseous necrosis.

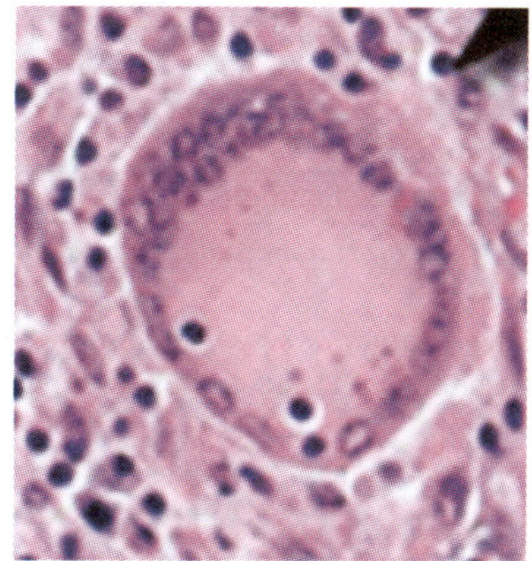

34. Ans. (b) Noncardiogenic pulmonary edema

Ref: Pocket Companion to Robbins, 9th ed. pg. 79

- The image shows lung specimen stained with Oil Red O stain and clinical history is *consistent with fat embolism.*
- Non-cardiogenic pulmonary edema is seen with ARDS and not fat embolism.

35. Ans. (b) Nodular glomerulosclerosis

Ref: Harsh Mohan, 7th ed. pg. 665

- The image shows presence of *intense eosinophilic deposits in nodular fashion all over glomerulus* leading to compression of glomerular capillaries which are hardly visible. This is seen in nodular glomerulosclerosis.
- The lesion shown is also called Kimmelstiel-Wilson change and is specific for type 1 diabetes or islet cell antibody positive diabetes.

36. Ans. (d) Nutmeg liver

Ref: Harsh Mohan, 7th ed. pg. 92

- The specimen shows presence of *mottled appearance of liver* where dark congestion is noted. This is diagnostic of nutmeg liver.
- Dubin-Johnson has a black liver texture and is therefore ruled out.
- Postnecrotic cirrhosis has visible scarring on surface and is therefore ruled out
- Miliary tuberculosis (TB) will show studded appearance.

37. Ans. (b) Intranuclear inclusions

Ref: Harsh Mohan, 7th ed. pg. 607

- The image shows Mallory hyaline body which is marked as X. These are eosinophilic, *intracytoplasmic inclusions* in perinuclear location with swollen and ballooned hepatocytes.
- They are formed from aggregates of cytoskeletal intermediate filaments called prekeratin.
- Aniline Blue and Masson trichrome which are connective tissue stains are best for visualization of Mallory hyaline bodies.
- Conditions that exhibit Mallory hyaline bodies are—I WILL STAY SOBER

- **I**ndian childhood cirrhosis
- **W**ilson disease
- **S**urgery (Intestinal bypass)
- **F**ocal **no**dular hyperplasia
- **B**iliary cirrhosis (primary)
- **H**epatocellular carcinoma

38. Ans. (b) Echinocyte

Ref: Oski's Pediatric Hematology, 7th ed. pg. 773

- The image shows presence of spiculated red cells with uniform projections over the entire circumference of cell. This is an echinocyte.
- In contrast acanthocytes have only few spicules of varying size that project irregularly from cell surface.

Acanthocyte	Echinocyte
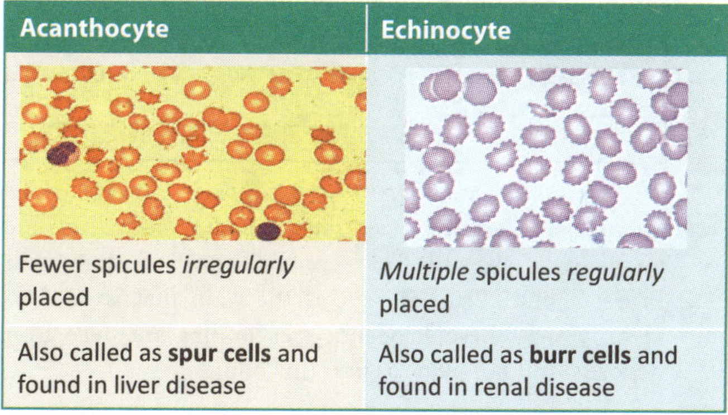	
Fewer spicules *irregularly* placed	*Multiple* spicules *regularly* placed
Also called as **spur cells** and found in liver disease	Also called as **burr cells** and found in renal disease

39. Ans. (c) Substitution of single amino acid base

Ref: Robbins, 8th ed. pg. 645-647

Point mutation in 6th codon of β-globin that leads to replacement of glutamate by valine residue.

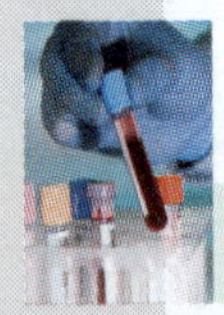

40. Ans. (b) Plasmacytoma

Ref: pg. 364, Harsh Mohan, 7th ed. and Bone Marrow Pathology by Bain 4th ed. pg. 50

The image shows presence of *Mott cells* which are plasma cells characterized by an accumulation of multiple Russell bodies, globular cytoplasmic inclusions composed of immunoglobulin.

41. Ans. (b) Macrocytic anemia

Ref: Chapter 26, Wintrobe's Hematology, 12th ed.

The image shown reveals the following findings:

- *Marked variation* in size and shape of RBC.
- *Macrocytes are seen* and have a wide central pale area. Immature RBC with bluish cytoplasm is noted in middle.

- The combination of clinical findings and reports mentioned in the question point to diagnosis of B_{12} deficiency
- Loss of reflexes due to an associated peripheral neuropathy in a patient who also has Babinski signs is an important diagnostic clue.

42. Ans. (a) Lead poisoning

Ref: Harsh Mohan, Textbook of Pathology, 7th ed. pg. 236

The image shows basophilic stippling of red blood cells. The causes are:

Mnemonic: **LUNATIC**
- **L**ead poisoning
- **U**nstable hemoglobin
- **N**ucleotidase deficiency
- **A**nemia due to B_{12} deficiency
- **T**halassemia
- **I**nfections
- **C**irrhosis

The closest answer Pappenheimer bodies are basophilic erythrocytic inclusions that are usually located at the periphery of the cell. They contain iron and stain with Prussian blue. Prussian blue is the stain that is used to identify that these Pappenheimer bodies are pure iron deposits, and not heme as in Heinz bodies.

43. Ans. (a) Pappenheimer body

Ref: Harsh Mohan, Textbook of Pathology, 7th ed. pg. 277

- The image shows presence of *Pappenheimer bodies* which are basophilic erythrocytic inclusions that are usually located at the periphery of the cell.
- They are composed of *ferritin aggregates* and stain on Romanowsky stain because of clumps of ribosomes which are precipitated with iron containing organelles.

44. Ans. (a) Perl stain

Ref: Harsh Mohan, Textbook of Pathology, 7th ed. pg. 98

- The image shows presence of *blue deposits called Pappenheimer bodies* and they contain iron and stain with perls' Prussian blue.
- Ferric iron deposits in tissue react with the soluble ferrocyanide in the stain, to form insoluble *Prussian blue dye* (a complex hydrated ferric ferrocyanide substance) *in situ.*

45. Ans. (d) Denatured hemoglobin

Ref: Harsh Mohan, Textbook of Pathology, 7th ed. pg. 287

- The image shows a *supra vital stain showing Heinz bodies* seen in G6PD and are composed up of denatured hemoglobin.
- *Heinz bodies,* are clinically detectable by staining with supravital dyes such as crystal violet. Removal of these inclusions by the spleen generates pitted, rigid RBCs that have shortened life spans.
- *Causes of Heinz bodies (not seen on Romanowsky stain)*

- Glucose 6 phosphatase dehydrogenase deficiency
- Glutathione synthetase deficiency
- Drugs
- Toxins
- Unstable hemoglobins

TABLE: Summary of Inclusion in RBC's

Inclusion	Composition
Howell-Jolly body	DNA
Basophilic stippling	RNA remnants
Siderotic granules/ Pappenheimer bodies	Iron
Heinz bodies	Denatured hemoglobin

46. Ans. (c) Pernicious anemia

Ref: Clinical Hematology Turgeon, 4th ed. pg. 104

- The image shows *Cabot ring* which may result in part from abnormalities in metabolism of both iron and arginine-rich histone that are known to occur in pernicious anemia.
- *Cabot rings are usually seen in postsplenectomy and pernicious anemia patients.*

47. Ans. (a) Dohle bodies

Ref: Nathan and Oski Hematology of Children, 7th ed. pg. 1637

The image shows pale blue bodies in cytoplasm of neutrophil which appears in bacterial infections. They are called Dohle bodies.

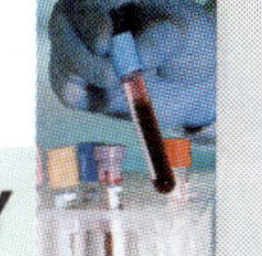

TABLE: Causes of Dohle bodies

- Infections
- Burns
- Cancer
- Massive trauma
- Prolonged use of cyclophosphamide
- May hegglin anomaly

Critical green inclusions in neutrophils are seen in severe liver disease.

48. Ans. (c) CLL

***Ref:** Harsh Mohan, Textbook of Pathology, 7th ed. pg. 355-56*

- The image shows peripheral blood smear showing many *"smudge" or "basket" cells,* nuclear remnants of cells damaged by the physical shear stress of making the blood smear.
- The clinical presentation and peripheral smear favour diagnosis of CLL.

49. Ans. (a) Hand-Foot sydrome

***Ref:** Harsh Mohan, Textbook of Pathology, 7th ed. pg. 294–96*

The X-ray spine shows *fish shaped vertebra* with peripheral smear showing sickle shaped RBC's. The presence of sickling crisis lead to *Hand-Foot syndrome* is characterized by painful infarcts of the digits and dactylitis.

50. Ans. (b) Basophil

***Ref:** Harsh Mohan, Textbook of Pathology, 7th ed. pg. 294–96*

The image shows a white blood cell with blue granules in the cytoplasm indicative of basophil.

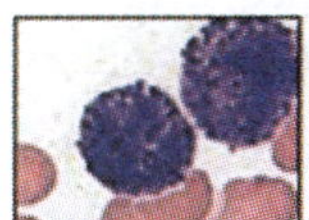
Basophil
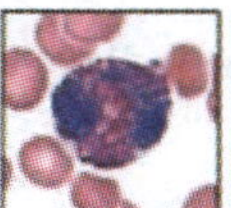
Eosinophil
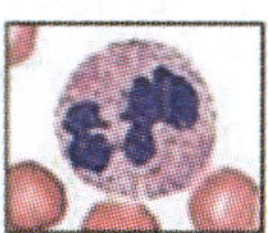
Neutrophil
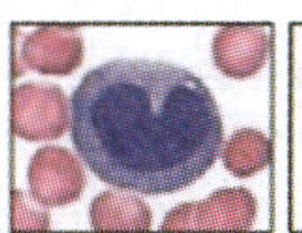
Monocyte
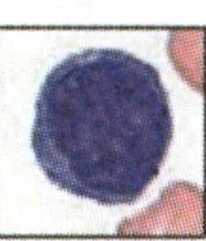
Lymphocyte

51. Ans. (a) Eosinophil

***Ref:** Harsh Mohan, Textbook of Pathology, 7th ed. pg. 129*

The image shows a white blood cell with pink granules in the cytoplasm indicative of eosinophil.

52. Ans. (d) ESR measurement

***Ref:** Wintrobe's Hematology, 12th ed. pg. 16*

This method uses Wintrobe's tube, a narrow glass tube closed at the lower end only. The Wintrobe's tube has a **length of 11 cm** and **internal diameter of 2.5 mm**. It contains 0.7–1 mL of blood. The marking is 0 at the top and 10 at the bottom for ESR. This tube can also be used for PCV. The marking is 10 at the top and 0 at the bottom for PCV.

53. Ans. (a) EDTA

***Ref:** Wintrobe's Hematology,12th ed. pg. 16*

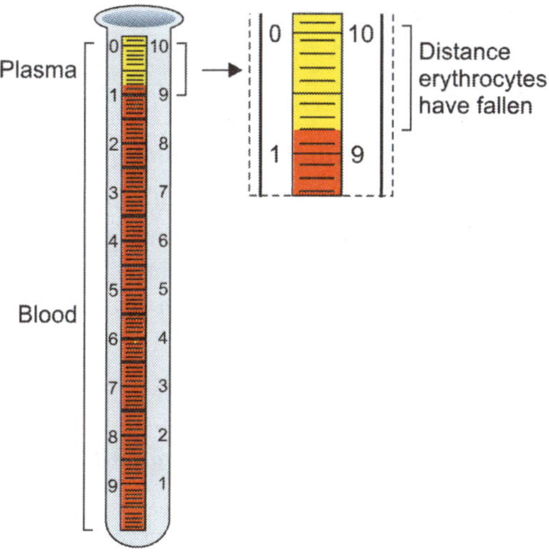

Requirements:

- Anticoagulated blood (EDTA, double oxalate)
- Pasteur pipette
- Timer
- Wintrobe's tube
- Wintrobe's stand

54. Ans. (c) Thalassemia

***Ref:** Harsh Mohan Textbook of Pathology, 7th ed. pg. 292 and Wintrobe's Hematology, 13th ed. pg. 610*

- The image shows performance of *Naked eye single tube, osmotic fragility test.* Notice that in control sample on right side, the fine print of newspaper can be acknowledged.
- However in the left sided sample, *osmotic fragility is reduced* leading to turbidity, leading to opacification of sample and the fine print of the newspaper cannot be read.
- This test is a *screening test for thalassemia* following which high performance liquid chromatography is done.

55. Ans. (d) Gamma globulin

Ref: Chapter 99, Wintrobe's Hematology, 12th ed.

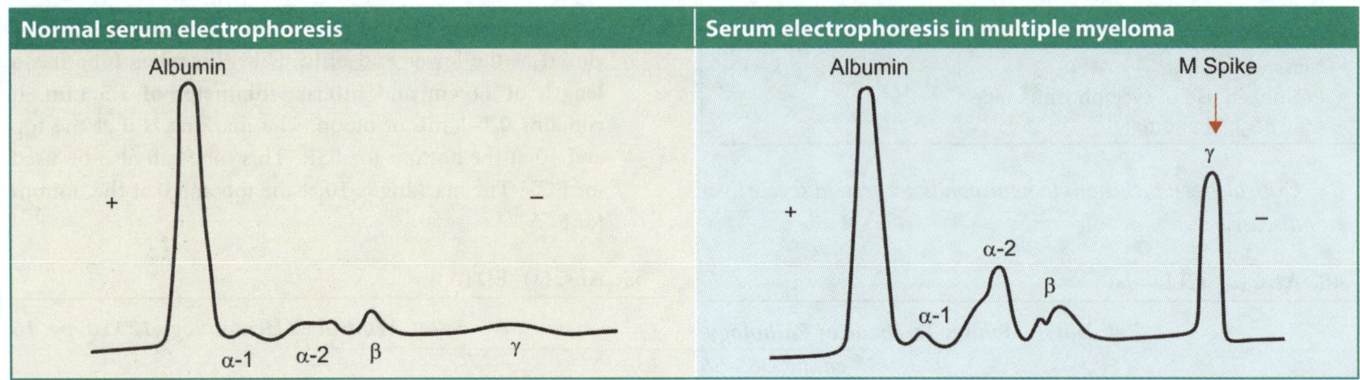

56. Ans. (d) Rouleaux formation

Ref: Wintrobe's Haematology, 13th ed. pg. 593

Rouleaux formation is associated with *increased positively charged proteins* usually fibrinogen or gamma globulins. The positively charged proteins neutralize the negatively charged RBC allowing them to form stacks in the form of stacks of four or more cells.

57. Ans. (a) Teratoma

Ref: Robbins and Cotran Atlas of Pathology, 3rd ed. pg. 356

- Teratomas are made up of a variety of parenchymal cell types representing more than 1 germ layer and often all 3 germ layers.
- Cells differentiate along various germ lines, essentially recapitulating any tissue of the body. Examples include hair, teeth, fat, skin, muscle, and endocrine tissue.
- Arising from totipotential cells, these tumors typically are midline or paraxial.
- The **most common location is sacrococcygeal** (57%).
- Because they arise from totipotential cells, they are encountered commonly in the gonads (29%).
- The **most common gonadal location is the ovary**, although they also occur somewhat less frequently in the testes.

58. Ans. (c) Adult T cell Leukaemia

- Adult T-cell/Leukemia (ATLL). The tumor cell shown on the image has typical multilobated nuclei also known as 'cloverleaf' or 'flower cells'.
- ATLL is CD4+ and is only observed in adults infected by HTLV-1.

59. Ans. (c) Measles

The given slide is pathognomonic for measles. This is a slide of a lymph node biopsy showing a Warthin-Finkeldey giant cell (grapelike clusters of inclusion bodies) with large germinal centers, and randomly distributed multinucleate giant cells (Warthin-Finkeldey cells) which have eosinophilic nuclear and cytoplasmic inclusion bodies.

60. Ans. (a) Papillary

Psammoma bodies are seen in papillary carcinoma of thyroid. Psammoma bodies are concentrically calcified structures often present within the cores of papillae in papillary carcinoma of the thyroid.

FORENSIC MEDICINE

61. Ans. (b) Arsenic Poisoning

62. Ans. (b) Abrasion

- An abrasion is a type of open wound that is caused by the skin rubbing against a rough surface. It may be called a scrape or a graze. When an abrasion is caused by the skin sliding across hard ground, it may be called road rash.

- Elbows
- Knees
- Shins
- Ankles

63. Ans. (d) Close shot entry wound

There is burning, blackening, tattooing around the wound. Shape is circular.

Abrasion collar, grease collar and singeing are seen in closed shot injury.

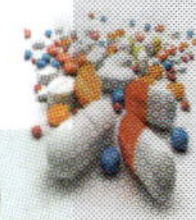

PREVENTIVE AND SOCIAL MEDICINE (PSM)

64. Ans. (b) Correlation coefficient

r – 0.4 | r – 0 | r – 0.4

Positive correlation | No Correlation | Negative

65. Ans. (a) Histogram

66. Ans. (a) Sandfly

67. Ans. (a) Aedes Larvae

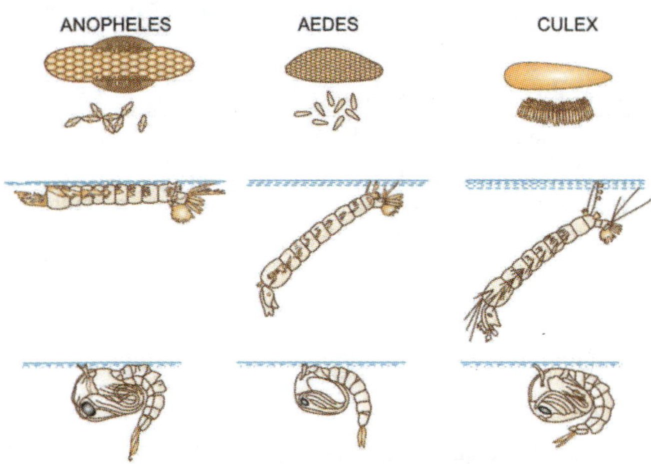

68. Ans. (b) UNICEF

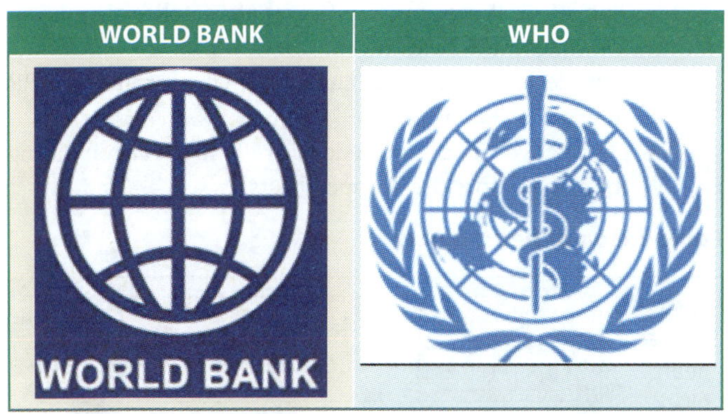

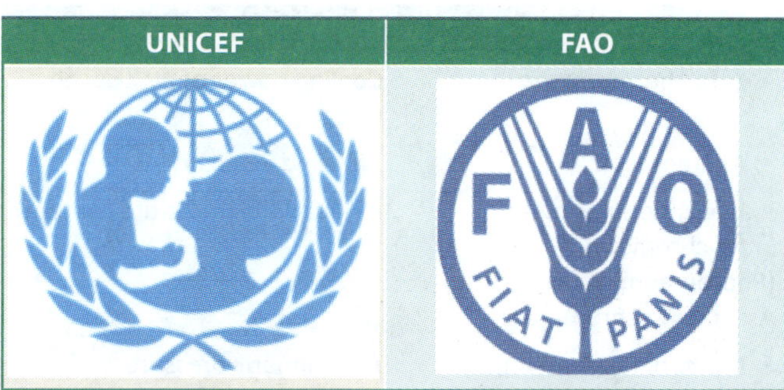

69. Ans. (a) National Rural Health Mission

70. Ans. (a) Mirena

The image shows presence of Mirena. It is a long acting reversible contraceptive, which contains Levonorgestrel and hence has a dual benefit of hormonal action and local action of intrauterine device.

71. Ans. (d) NPBCVI

The logo shown above belongs to National Programme for Control of Blindness and Visual Impairment (NPCBVI). The goal is to reduce the prevalence of blindness to 0.3 % by 2020.

72. Ans. (d) Kata thermometer

The kata thermometer is a heated-alcohol thermometer; the time it takes to cool is measured and used to determine air current. It is useful for measuring low speeds in studies of air circulation.

73. Ans. (d) Japanese Encephalitis

- The vector shown in the image is of Culex species of mosquito.
- It is a vector for Japanese Encephalitis (JE) and Bancoftian Filariasis.

74. Ans. (c) Pediculosis Capitis

- The image is of adult female head louse which causes pediculosis capitis. Louse eggs or nits, are attached near the base of a host hair shaft. It is usually asymptomatic.
- Pruritus due to hypersensitivity to the louse's saliva is common.
- The treatment is permethrin 1%.

75. Ans. (a) Relative humidity of air

INSTRUMENTS USED IN AIR PARAMETERS

Instrument	Use
• Kata Thermometer	Cooling power of air, Low air velocity
• Anemometer	Air/wind velocity
• Hygrometer, Sling Psychrometer (Photograph) Assman Psychrometer	Air humidity (moisture content)
• Mercurial Barometer	Atmospheric pressure
• Aneroid Barometer	Atmospheric pressure
• Wind Vane	Air/wind direction

76. Ans. (d) Dial thermometer

A dial thermometer is used for cold chain temperature monitoring. The purpose of cold-chain monitoring equipment is to keep track of the temperature to which vaccine and diluent are exposed during transportation and storage.

77. Ans. (c) Stadiometer

A stadiometer is a piece of medical equipment used for measuring human height. It is usually constructed out of a ruler and a sliding horizontal headpiece which is adjusted to rest on the top of the head. Stadiometers are used in routine medical examinations and also clinical tests and experiments.

78. Ans. (c) Rome

The Food and Agriculture Organization (FAO) is a specialized agency of the United Nations that leads international efforts to defeat hunger. Its headquarters is in Rome, Italy.

79. Ans. (d) New Delhi

Employees' State Insurance is a self-financing social security and health insurance scheme for Indian workers. The fund is managed by the Employees' State Insurance Corporation according to rules and regulations stipulated in the ESI Act 1948. Its headquarters is located in New Delhi, India.

80. Ans. (c) Cervical cap

The cervical cap is a form of barrier contraception. A cervical cap fits over the cervix and blocks sperm from entering the uterus through the external orifice of the uterus, called the os.

81. Ans. (a) Female condom

The female condom, also known as femidom, covers the cervix, entire vagina and the external genitalia. Hence it is highly protective against AIDS and STD. It has a failure rate of 5-15 per 100-woman years.

MEDICINE

82. Ans. (c) Anterior wall MI

ECG shows presence of ST elevation from V2-V5 diagnostic of anterior wall MI.

83. (a) Sinus tachycardia

Ref: Harrison, 19th ed. pg. 1477

- The ECG shows normal sinus rhythm with heart rate of >100 bpm.
- P waves are normal height and duration. PR interval is 120 msec and QRS duration is 80 msec.
- The findings are diagnostic of sinus tachycardia
- Sinus tachycardia is subdivided into physiological and non-physiological.
- *Inappropriate sinus tachycardia* causes the sinus rate to increase spontaneously at rest or out of proportion to physiological stress or exertion. Affected patients are usually females. Misdiagnosis with anxiety disorder is common.

84. Ans. (c) Mobitz II heart block

Ref: Harrison, 19th ed. pg. 1472

- The ECG shows more P waves than QRS complexes. This suggests a heart block.
- P wave is upright and has a normal morphology. PR interval is 200 msec.
- Dropped beats are present with PR interval remaining the same before the dropped beats.

Comparison of heart blocks

First degree heart block	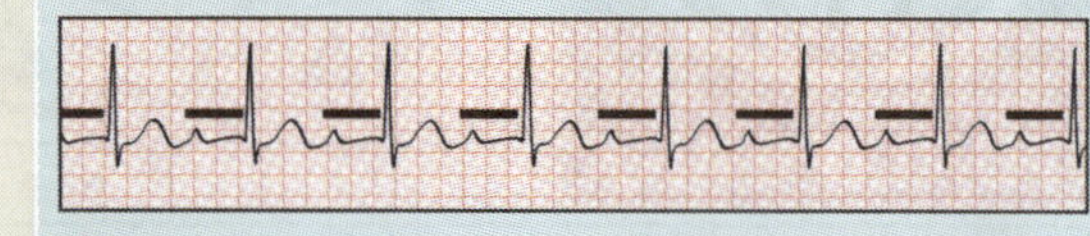 PR interval is prolonged but there are no dropped beats

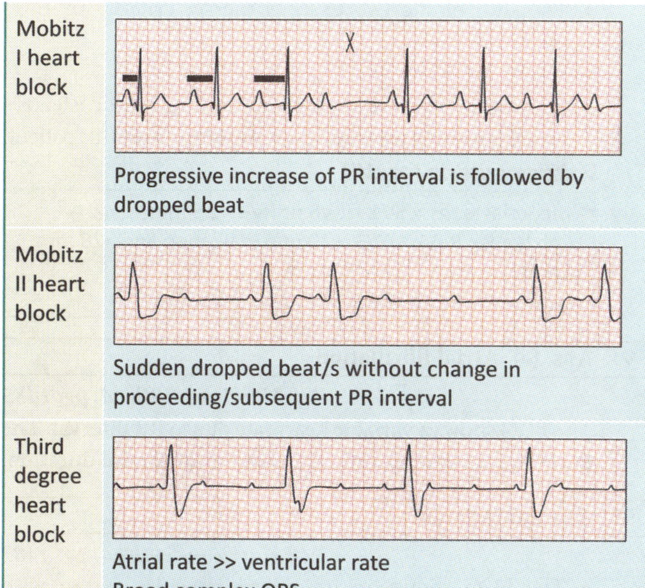

Mobitz I heart block	Progressive increase of PR interval is followed by dropped beat
Mobitz II heart block	Sudden dropped beat/s without change in proceeding/subsequent PR interval
Third degree heart block	Atrial rate >> ventricular rate Broad complex QRS

85. Ans. (a) Myocardial ischemia

Ref: Harrison, 19th ed. pg. 1455-56

- The T-wave is upright in all leads except aVR and V1. In the strip provided, notice the predominant T-wave inversion in V1-V4. This is seen in myocardial ischemia.

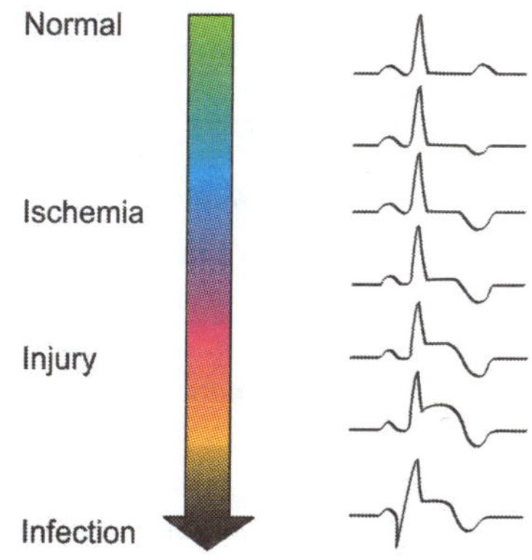

- Diagnosis of myocardial injury needs elevated cardiac biomarkers
- Digoxin leads to ST segment depression
- Digoxin toxicity leads to ventricular bigeminy.

Causes of T-wave inversion:

- Normal in children
- Myocardial ischemia
- Bundle branch block
- Ventricular hypertrophy
- Pulmonary embolism
- Hypertrophic obstructive cardiomyopathy
- Raised intracranial pressure

86. Ans. (a) Hyperacute T-wave

Ref: ACLS Study Guide, 5th ed. pg. 229

The ECG shows presence of large T waves.
They are relatively broad, and are not pointed when compared to Tall tented T waves of hyperkalemia.

Hyperkalemia	Hyperacute ischemia	Normal variant
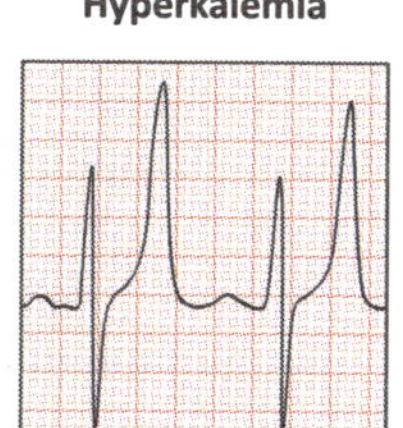	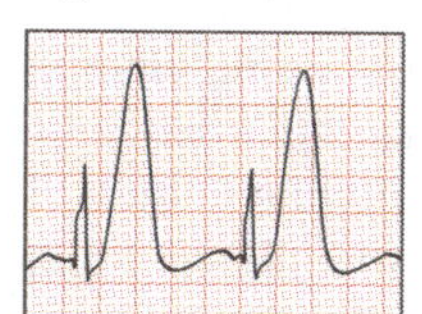	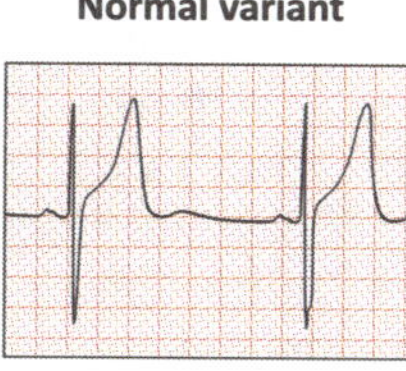
Symmetric, narrow-based, pointed, tenting	Symmetric, broad-based, not tented, not pointed QT interval tends to be long	Asymmetric and not narrow

87. Ans. (a) T wave inversion

Ref: Braunwald, 10th ed. pg. 146 and Harrison, 19th ed. pg. 1457

Heart rate is 60 bpm with left axis deviation. *Deep symmetrical T-wave inversion* is noted in the chest leads.

88. Ans. (a) Ventricular bigeminy

Ref: Harrison, 19th ed. Chapter 269e

Child on CHF treatment implies digoxin being used and possibility of digoxin toxicity
The ECG strip shows heart rate of approximately 60 bpm.
ST segment depression (hockey stick sign) is seen followed by positive deflection of U waves.
Abnormalities of U-wave

Prominent U waves	Inverted U waves
Bradycardia Hypokalemia Hypocalcemia Hypomagnesemia Hypothermia Raised ICP HOCM LVH	Myocardial ischemia HTN Cardiomyopathy

89. Ans. (d) Premature ventricular contractions

Ref: Harrison, 19th ed. pg. 1457

The ECG shows normal sinus rhythm with heart rate of 75 bpm with normal axis.
Raised ST segment in lead V2-V4 and inverted T waves in lead I, aVL, V2-V4 are seen.

90. Ans. (b) Ventricular bigeminy

Ref: Practical Cardiology, 2nd ed. pg. 214

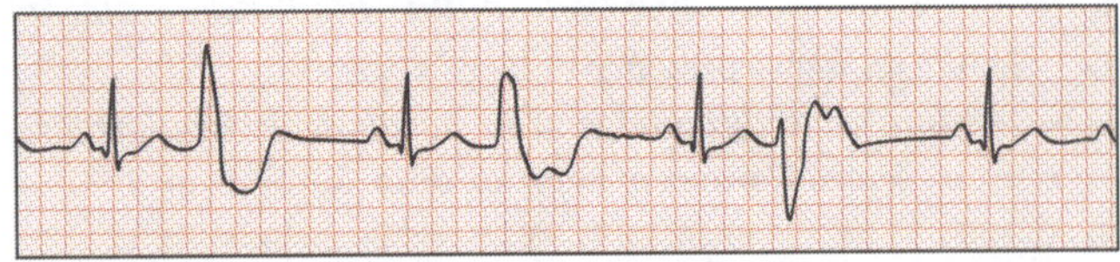

Heart rate of the patient is 50 bpm.

The tracing shows normal sinus rhythm alternating with premature ventricular contraction. This is diagnostic of ventricular bigeminy which is the most common arrhythmia seen with digoxin toxicity.

91. Ans. (d) Digoxin

Ref: Harrison, 19th ed. pg. 1457

- The ECG shows irregular heart rhythm with absent P waves. This is diagnostic of atrial fibrillation.
- Also seen is down-sloping ST segment depression pronounced in V2-V3 and in the rhythm strip.
- This patient of rheumatic heart disease is in atrial fibrillation for which she would have been put on digoxin by her physician.
- The combination of extra-cardiac side effects of digoxin and atrial fibrillation hemodynamic effects would explain the general unwell being of the patient.
- ACE inhibitor can lead to hyperkalemia and diuretics can lead to hypokalemia. However, ECG changes of potassium deficit/excess are not seen.

92. Ans. (c) PSVT

Ref: Harrison, 19th ed. pg. 1480-81

- The findings of the ECG are heart rate of 200 bpm. P waves are not visible.
- The axis is normal with narrow qRS complexes.
- This could either be junctional tachycardia or atrio-ventricular nodal re-entrant tachycardia.
- Taking into consideration the age of the patient the incidence of junctional tachycardia can explain the patient experiencing multiple episodes in the past.

93. Ans. (b) Left ventricular hypertrophy

Ref: Harrison, 19th ed. pg. 1454

- The ECG shows normal sinus rhythm with heart rate of 50 bpm.
- The axis is normal.
- R wave height in lead V5 is 30 mm and S wave depth in lead V1 is 20 mm.
- The sum of the two exceeds the set criteria for LVH mentioned below.
- Inverted T waves are seen in I, aVL, V5-V6.
- Echocardiography is needed to confirm aortic stenosis which is causing left ventricular hypertrophy in this patient.

Voltage criteria for LVH

Precordial leads = SV1 + RV5 or RV6 > 35 mm
Limb leads= RaVL + SV3 > 20 mm in women and >28 mm in men
Not very accurate in obese and athletes

94. Ans. (c) Atrial fibrillation

Ref: Harrison, 19th ed. pg. 1485

The ECG shows a variable heart rate due to RR interval. The P waves are not seen and QRS complex is normal duration.

95. Ans. (b) Adenosine

Ref: Harrison, 19th ed. pg. 1487

- The ECG shows an irregularly irregular rythm with absent P waves, which is seen in Atrial Fibrillation.
- *Serious rhythm degeneration and even death* can occur when *adenosine is inadvertently given to patients of atrial fibrillation/flutter.* This is since the concealed accessory pathway with become unmasked.
- As adenosine will increase the AV nodal delay the accessory pathway will lead to conversion of atrial fibrillation to ventricular fibrillation. This is because the current will now travel preferentially via the accessory pathway.

96. Ans. (c) Thrombolytic therapy

Ref: Harrison, 19th ed. pg. 1595

- The following ECG shows heart rate of 80 bpm with normal axis. P wave is normal with normal duration QRS seen after each P wave. T waves are hyper-acute in leads V2-V5 with simultaneous presence of ST segment elevation in chest leads V2-V5.
- This is diagnostic of STEMI involving anterior wall and the vessel blocked in left anterior descending artery.
- The symptoms of chest pain and diaphoresis are explained by the ECG findings of the pain.
- Now ideal treatment of STEMI is PCI or thrombolysis.
- Since PCI is not in choices we need to consider thrombolysis for the patient but it is *indicated only within 12 hours of onset of MI.*
- In this question the patient presented late and hence *we will treat with aspirin to prevent future MI episode, Statin to stabilize the vulnerable plaques and morphine to calm the patient and reduce pulmonary edema.*
- *E.C.G changes in acute infarction*

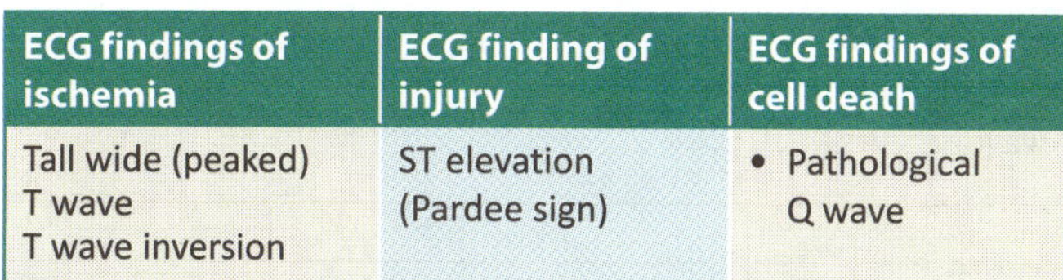

ECG findings of ischemia	ECG finding of injury	ECG findings of cell death
Tall wide (peaked) T wave T wave inversion	ST elevation (Pardee sign)	• Pathological Q wave

ST Elevation MI Management:
- Nitrates
- Morphine
- Oxygen
- Aspirin
- Start adjunctive treatment
- Beta Blockers (IV)
- Nitroglycerine (IV)
- Heparin (IV)
- Reperfusion therapy is the definitive treatment of choice if patient present <12 hours.
  - Thrombolysis (Streptokinase) Door to needle time < 30 minutes
  - Early primary PCI (Cath lab equipped hospital) Door to balloon time < 90 minutes

97. Ans. (c) Adenosine

Ref: Harrison, 19th ed. pg. 1479

- The ECG is showing heart rate of 200/min.
- Axis is normal.
- Rhythm is regular with absence of P waves.
- Narrow complex QRS (<0.08 sec) is present. P waves buried in the preceding T wave.
- This is seen in paroxysmal supraventricular tachycardia.
- The first line management is adenosine 6 mg intravenously.
- In case the patient is having hemodynamic compromise, electrical cardioversion needs to be done.

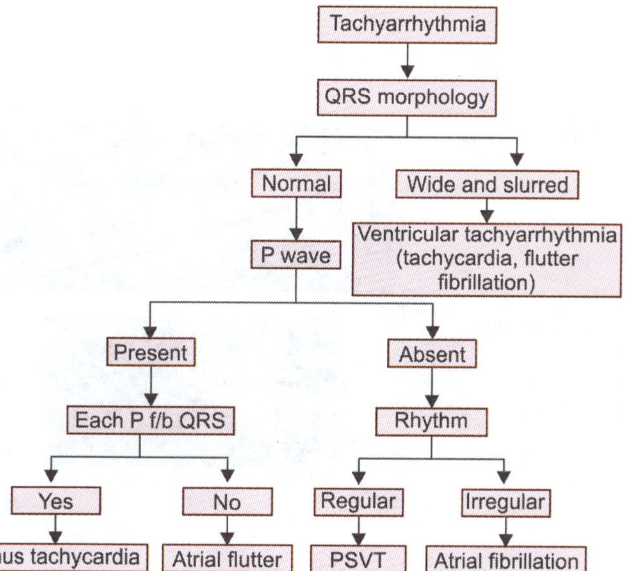

98. Ans. (a) Primary PCI

Ref: Figure 295-4, Harrison, 19th ed. pg. 1604

- The ECG shows heart rate of about 120/min.
- T wave inversion is present from V2-V6
- ST segment elevation >2 mm in noted from V4-V6 exhibiting the traditional Pardee sign
- *STEMI is best managed with primary PCI with first medical contact to device time to be kept <90 minutes*
- If the patient is seen in non PCI capable hospital DIDO time should be less than 30 minutes for thrombolysis.

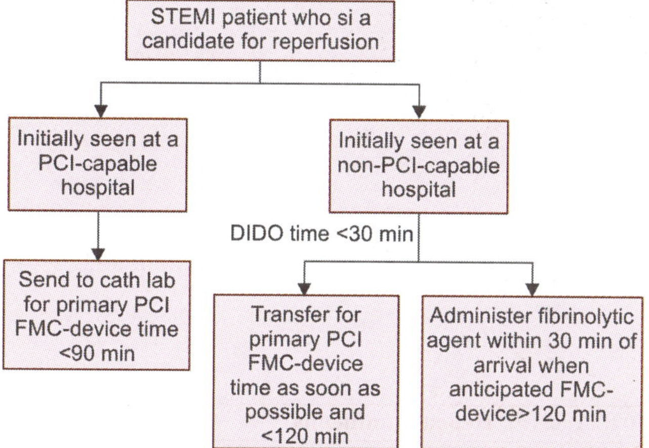

- The patient can be transferred from non PCI capable hospital to PCI capable hospital in case the first medical contact to device time is less than 120 minutes.
- In the question there is no mention of any PCI/ non PCI capable hospital.
- Due to paucity of transport facilities in India, the concept of transfer from non PCI to PCI capable center with performance of PCI within 120 minutes looks impossible.

99. Ans. (d) 4

Ref: Harrison, 19th ed. pg. 1451

- Corrected QT is defined as QT interval divided by √ R-R interval
- R-R interval in ECG is 4.

Markings in the ECG given:

1. is PR interval
2. is PJ interval
3. is ST segment
4. is RR interval

100. Ans. (c) Phase 2

Ref: Harrison, 19th ed. pg. 1451

- The marked part of the ECG is the isoelectric ST segment which corresponds to the plateau, phase 2 of cardiac action potential

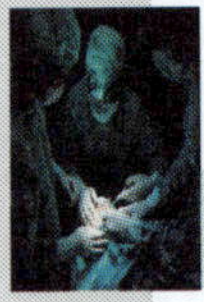

- The rapid upstroke (phase 0) action potential corresponds to onset of QRS.
- Plateau (phase 2) corresponds to isoelectric ST segment.
- Active repolarization (phase 3) corresponds to inscription of T-wave.

101. Ans. (c) Hockey stick sign

Ref: Practical Cardiology, 2nd ed. pg. 125

The image shows rhythm strip exhibiting a variable heart rate with ST segment depression. P-wave is absent with narrow complex. The patient was probably having atrial fibrillation and was started on digoxin which resulted in ST segment depression highlighted below.

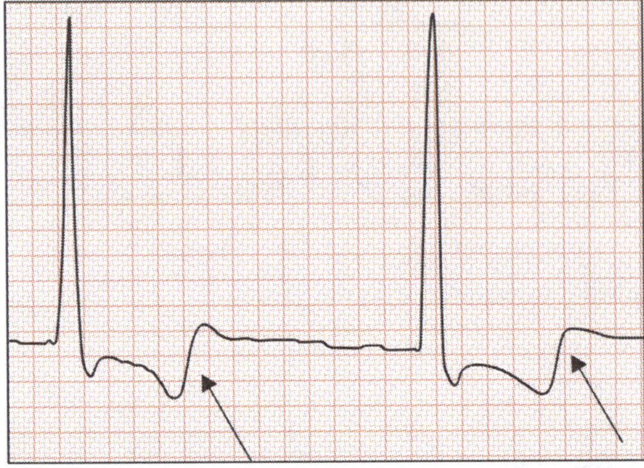

102. Ans. (d) Hypoalbuminemia

Based on the given clinical scenario the most likely diagnosis here is Hypoalbuminemia. The nail finding shown in image is Muehrcke's lines which are white transverse lines.

103. Ans. (b) Hypocalcemia

The image shows Trousseau sign, elicited in hypocalcemia when the ionized calcium level is 1.75–2.25 mmol/L. Trousseau's sign is carpopedal spasm caused by inflating the blood-pressure cuff to a level above systolic pressure for 3 minutes.

SURGERY

104. Ans. (c) Intussusception

Ref: Schwartz 10th ed. pg. pg. 1234

The intraoperative picture shows presence of intussusception.

- Most common lead point causing intussusception in children = Meckel's Diverticulum
- Most common type of intussusception in children = Ileo-colic (Post Rota virus diarrhea)
- Most common lead point causing intussusception in Adults = Polyp (Villous Adenoma)
- Most common type of intussusception in adults= Colo-colic
- Most common small bowel tumor in children causing intussusception = lymphoma

105. Ans. (b) Artery Forceps & Needle Holder

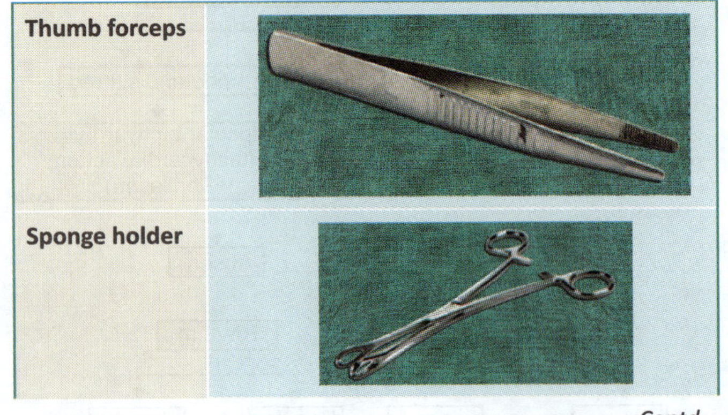

Contd...

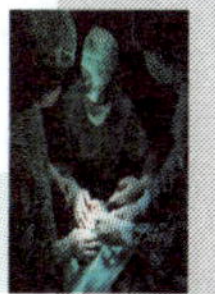

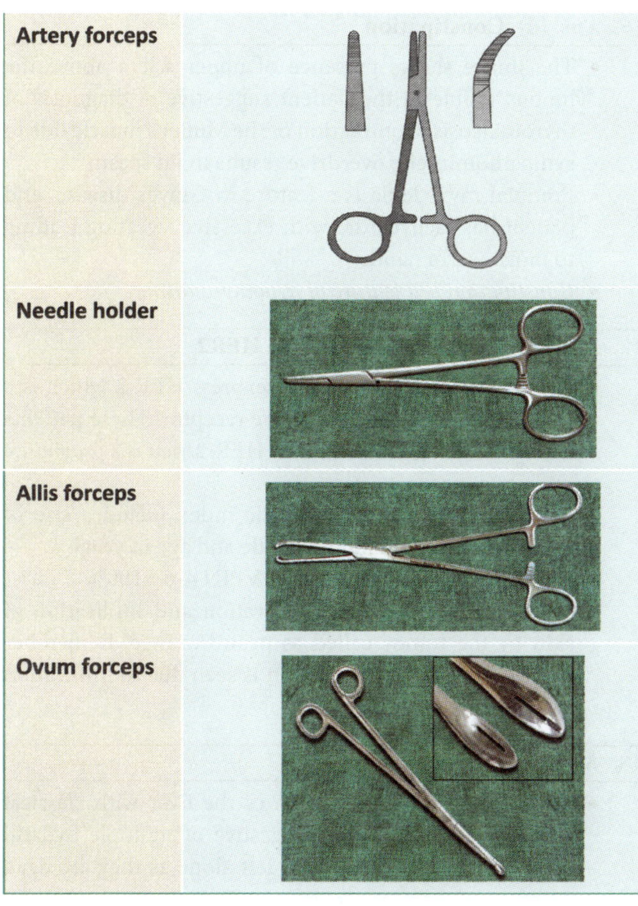

106. Ans. (d) Collagen bundles are present

The picture shows presence of keloid, which is called so as it extends to normal tissues with its claw like processes.

Hypertrophic scar	Keloid
Itching not present or mild	Severe itching and worsens after 1 year
Never crosses boundaries of original incision	Extends to normal tissues and has claw like lesions
Occurs at original site of incision and has minimal vascularity	Occurs at vaccination sites, injection and incision sites and piercing sites.
Occurs due to hypertrophy of mature fibroblasts with minimal blood vessels	*Immature fibroblasts with immature blood vessels and exhibits high tendency to recur and collagen bundles are absent.*

107. Ans. (d) Rubbery consistency of involved lymph nodes

The image shows anti gravity drainage of a cold abscess being done. The upper deep cervical lymph nodes are usually involved. On palpation matting of lymph nodes is characterstic feature while the rubbery consistency of lymph nodes is seen in Hodgkins lymphoma.

Cold Abscess Features are

- No local rise of temperature
- No redness
- Transillumination test is negative
- On sternocleidomastoid contraction test, it becomes less prominent indicating it is deep to deep fascia.

108. Ans. (c) Ring block with adrenaline used

- The image shows presence of commonest hand infection which is acute paronychia. It occurs due to trimming of nail or ingrown toe nail. The infection starts in subcuticular area and spreads all around as eponychium is adherent to nail base.
- *Use of digital block and I and D is done by incising the eponychium. Adrenaline is not used for infiltration in the finger, penis and ear lobule.*

109. Ans. (a) Venous ulcer; (b) Arterial ulcer

- Image A shows presence of ulcer on lateral aspect of leg with granulation tissue present
- Image B shows presence of ulcer on dorsal aspect of foot with wet gangrene visible.
- Neuropathic ulcer in diabetes can occur on the heel or pressure point in the sole of the foot

Characteristics of Arterial and Venous Ulcer

Venous ulcer	Ischemic ulcer
Occur at medial or lateral aspect of leg	Dorsum of foot Typical arterial ulcers occur on tips of toes
Single and oval	Irregular
Superficial and does not penetrate deep fascia	Deep ulcer and penetrates the deep Fascia
Pigmentation present	Pigmentation present

110. Ans. (c) Neuropathic ulcer

Venous ulcer	Occurs above medial or lateral malleolus with granulation tissue and surrounding pigmentation
Arterial ulcer	Occurs on toes with poor peripheral pulses
Neuropathic ulcer	Occurs on heel
Bazin's ulcer	Occurs in obese young females in ankle region with abnormal amount of subcutaneous fat. Lesions begin as erythematous purplish nodules which rupture producing non healing ulcer

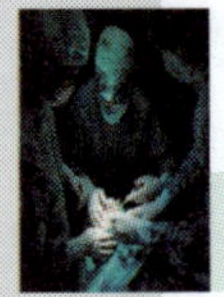

111. Ans. (a) Immediately remove the needle in the vessel

This is a case of inadvertent intra-arterial injection of thiopentone into one of the high division of brachial artery resulting in blanching and severe pain in the hand. Steps to be followed are

- *Do not remove* the needle
- Inject 5 ml of 1% lignocaine or 2 % papaverine
- Intra-arterial dilute heparin
- Intra-arterial streptokinase
- Brachial plexus block to reduce sympathetic activity induced spasm of blood vessels

112. Ans. (c) Lymphatic metastasis

- The image shows presence of marjolin's ulcer which grows very slowly and develops at the site of previous burn site or varicose ulcer, snake bite scar or osteomyelitis scar.
- It is painless scar and does not exhibit metastasis. It is cured by surgery and radiotherapy is not useful.

113. Ans. (a) Thyroglossal Cyst

The image shows presence of midline swelling which is moving with movement of the tongue. The most common site is sub-hyoid cyst. It is a cystic fluctuant trans-illumination negative swelling and moves as it is attached to hyoid bone.

114. Ans. (a) Carcinoma alveolar margin

- The image shows presence of staining of teeth, with an exophytic lesion with everted margins suggestive of diagnosis of a malignancy.
- Leukoplakia is a white patch in the mouth that cannot be scraped off.
- Hyperplastic candida involves the commissures of the mouth with candida invasion and shows no response to drugs, surgery and laser.
- Fibrous epulis is a fibroma arising from periodontal membrane and is slow growing without any ulceration.

115. Ans. (a) Pleomorphic adenoma

- The image shows a nodular growth at location of parotid gland and also notice the ear lobule of the patient is elevated with obliterated retromandibular groove.
- In mumps bilateral parotid enlargement is seen and does not have a bosselated appearance.
- Sialadenitis occurs due to stones and is more common in submandibular gland (80% of stones occur in submandibular gland). Even if parotid is involved bosselated or nodular appearance is suggestive of a tumor.

116. Ans. (d) Constipation

- The image shows presence of upper sclera above the limbus visible in the patient suggestive of diagnosis of thyrotoxicosis. Contraction of the Muller's muscle due to sympathomimetic overdrive results in lid spasm.
- Pretibial myxedema is a feature in Grave's disease, and patient has tachycardia with excessive sweating leading to moist warm hands.
- *Constipation is a feature of hypothyroidism.*

117. Ans. (c) Diagnosis depends on HER2

- 25% of all breast cancers overexpress HER-2 which is a transmembrane tyrosine kinase receptor. These patients should be given Trastuzumab. HER-2/neu is a *prognostic and not a diagnostic marker.*
- Modified Van Nuys prognostic index includes size of tumor, margins, pathology grade and age in years.
- 5 year disease free survival for VPIN 4-6 =100%
- The image shows nipple ulceration and infiltration of skin by the tumor called as peau'd orange. Remember puckering or dimpling of skin is seen due to infiltration of ligaments of cooper.

118. Ans. (b) Hydatid cyst

- The image shows a CT scan of the liver with classical Cart wheel appearance, suggestive of multiple hydatid cysts. The calcified cysts are left alone as they are dead cysts.
- Medical treatment with Albendazole for 21 days is given and surgery is done in case of symptomatic cysts or asymptomatic patient with cyst> 5cm or a non-calcified infected cyst.

119. Ans. (b) Gastrinoma triangle

The image shows gastrinoma triangle where ZES gastrinoma is located. The boundaries are from the *confluence* of cystic duct and Common hepatic duct, *confluence* of second and third part of duodenum and *junction* of neck and body of pancreas.

Hesselbach triangle

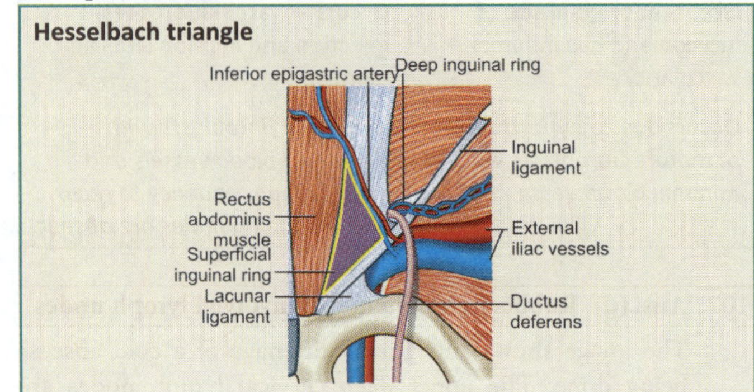

Contd...

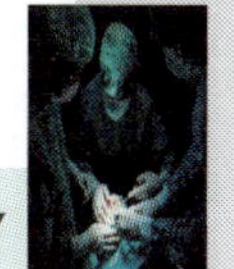

Triangular area on the inferior aspect of the anterior abdominal wall within the groin. Its boundaries are:
- Base is the inguinal ligament
- Lateral border is formed by the inferior epigastric vessels
- Medial border is the lateral edge of the rectus sheath.

Calot's triangle

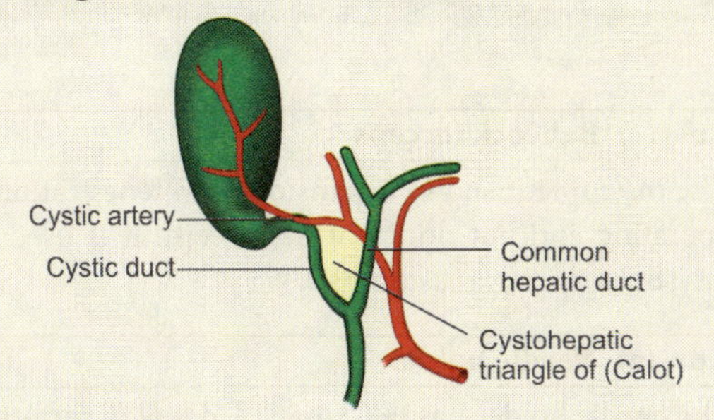

- Triangle formed by cystic duct, common hepatic duct and base of liver and contains the cystic artery.

Killian triangle
- Site for Zenker Diverticulum

120. Ans. (b) Ileal obstruction

- Vomiting of feculent contents indicates terminal ileal obstruction. It does not contain fecal matter but contains terminal ileal contents which undergo bacterial degradation and fermentation resulting in smell of fecal matter.
- Jejunal obstruction results in bilious vomiting while diverticultis produces hematochezia.
- Mesenteric ischemia will lead to abdominal angina.

121. Ans. (d) Fistula in ano

- The image shows presence of rectal prolapse and occurs due to habitual constipation undeveloped sacral curve, whooping cough, marasmus and torn perineum in obstetric trauma

122. Ans. (b) Pilonidal sinus

- The image shows a presence of external sinus opening just above the anal verge in midline over the coccyx. This is diagnostic of pilonidal sinus.
- Methylene blue shall be injected to demonstrate the branches of the sinus followed by excision
- Fistula of ano is located around the anal orifice and is due to infection of the anal glands.
- It is squamous cell carcinoma in situ of the anus, and is the precursor to the invasive squamous cell carcinoma. It is associated with HPV type 16 and 18.
- Hidradenitis suppurativa is recurrent suppuration of apocrine glands in the skin, resulting in multiple abscesses which rupture causing *multiple sinuses.*

123. Ans. (a) Appendix

- *The structure shown is closer to caecumis appendix whereas Meckel's Diverticulum is seen about 60 cm from the ileo-caecal junction.*
- *Intra-operatively, appendix can be identified by tracing Taenia Coli which converges onto the base of the appendix.*

124. Ans. (a) Lichtenstein repair

- The image shows polypropylene mesh which is used in hernia repair called as *Lichtenstein repair.*
- Bassini repair is a herniotomy with approximation of posterior wall of inguinal canal; by suturing the conjoined tendon above to the inguinal ligament below by using interrupted non absorbable suture material such as nylon.
- Shouldice method is method of tensionless repair in three layers where in the above image only a mesh can be seen.
- Lord's procedure is ruled out as it is done for hydrocele.

125. Ans. (b) Indirect inguinal hernia

- Direct inguinal hernia pushes through the posterior wall and hence it is *unusual for it to descend into the scrotum.* It is common in elderly whereas the patient is only 25 years of age.
- Expansile impulse on coughing is diagnostic of hernia and indirect hernia can occur in any age group and is mainly unilateral.
- Trans-illumination test is positive in vaginal hydrocele and impulse on coughing is absent.

126. Ans. (d) Low Renin due to pressure atrophy of JG apparatus

- The picture shows autosomal dominant polycystic kidneys in which there is progressive enlargement of cysts with new ones developing with age. The IVU shows a spider leg deformity of the calyces.
- The damage to the kidney results in decrease in amount of erythropoietin leading to normocytic normochromic anemia.
- The damage to the kidney results in development of reduction in GFR and positive feedback to R.A.A.S system results in increase in renin levels as well as high Blood pressure.

127. Ans. (d) Painless intermittent hematuria

- The image shows presence of large vesical calculus. The stone is more common in males and shows pain aggravated by jumping or jolting and is referred to tip of penis at the end of urination.
- Laser lithotripsy (Holmium Laser) can break most large stones and ultrasound lithotripsy is very safe but only for small stones.

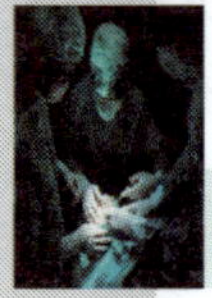

- In litholaplaxy, the stone is grasped firmly and broken while the small fragments are evacuated by using a evacuator

128. Ans. (b) Vesico-ureteric reflux

- The image shows presence of Vesico-ureteric Reflux with dye from the bladder refluxing into the tortuous dilated ureters. This is seen with stage V of V.U.R.
- The investigation of choice is MCU: Micturating Cystourethrography

129. Ans. (a) Gangrene of testis

- The diagnosis is Fournier gangrene characterized by extensive gangrene of scrotal skin. The sloughed skin exposes the testicles. In some cases the gangrene can involve the skin of penis, anterior abdominal wall.
- *The testis is not involved as it has a thick tunica albuginea.*

130. Ans. (b) Crescent sign

- The CT scan shows an air crescent sign with rim of air surrounding the aspergilloma or fungus ball caused by aspergillus species. The fungus settles in the cavity which is pre-existing and grows into a ball.
- Meniscus sign is seen in pleural effusion while tree in bud appearance is seen in pneumocystis carinii infection and tuberculosis.
- Loculated empyema would in the periphery of lung.

131. Ans. (a) A = Ventriculoperitoneal shunt, B = Ventriculo-atrial shunt

La Veen and Denver shunts are used in portal Hypertension and start from peritoneal cavity and hence choice C and D are ruled out.

132. Ans. (c) Burr Hole surgery

The image shows presence of extra-dural haemorrhage due to presence of biconvex lenticular opacity. Due to risk of brain herniation leading to death best management will be burr hole surgery.

133. Ans. (a) Kocher forceps

- The forceps has serrations with a sharp tooth at the tip which differentiates it from artery forceps. It is used to hold tough structures like aponeurosis, fascia.
- Allis forceps has a ratchet and has triangular expansion at the tip where serrations are present.

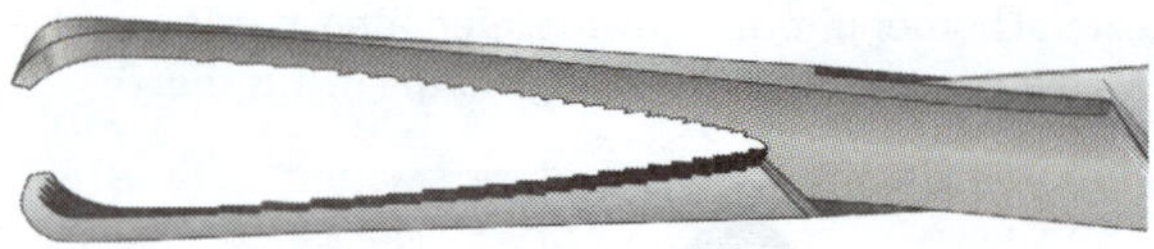

134. Ans. (c) Babcock forceps

The instrument shows expansion with fenestrations at the operating end but does not have teeth. It is used to hold intestines during anastomosis.

135. Ans. (a) Needle holder

The needle holder has two small blades with serrations and is used to hold curved needles which are used to suture the parts.

136. Ans. (b) Self-retaining catheter

The image shows presence of strong heavy instrument used to spread the laparotomy wound and is called as self-retaining retractor.

137. Ans. (a) Proctoscope

The image shows a proctoscope with outer sheath and inner blunt part called as obturator. It is used to diagnose hemorrhoids, carcinoma rectum or rectal ulcers.

138. Ans. (a) Malecot catheter

The image shows a red rubber catheter with a flower shaped ending to ensure that it is a self-retaining catheter. This is used to drain an amoebic liver abscess

139. Ans. (c) Blackmore sengastaken catheter

It is a double balloon and triple lumen tube used for control of bleeding esophageal varices.

140. Ans. (a) Ranula

Ranula is a pseudocyst that is associated with mucus extravasation into the surrounding soft tissues. These lesions occur as the result of trauma or obstruction to the salivary gland excretory duct and spillage of mucin into the surrounding soft tissues.

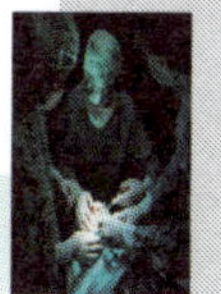

141. Ans. (a) Foley catheter

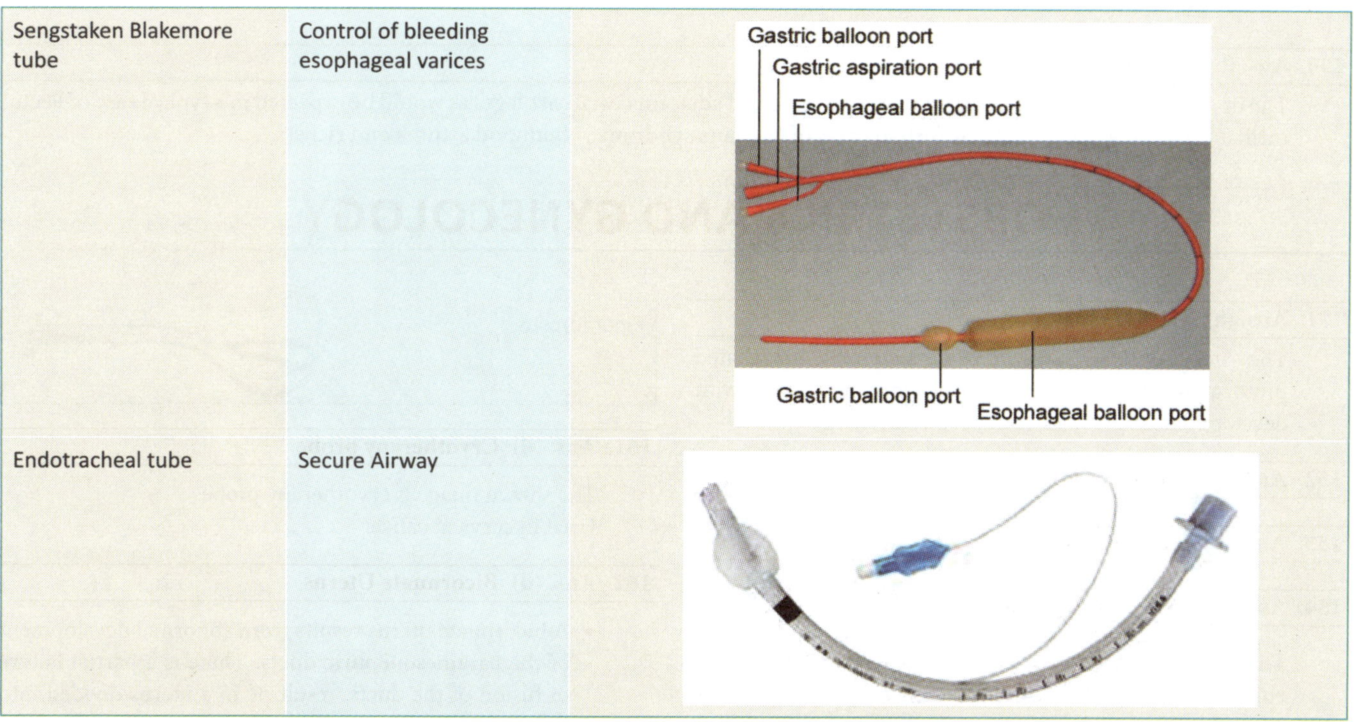

Sengstaken Blakemore tube	Control of bleeding esophageal varices	
Endotracheal tube	Secure Airway	

142. Ans. (a) Deaver retractor

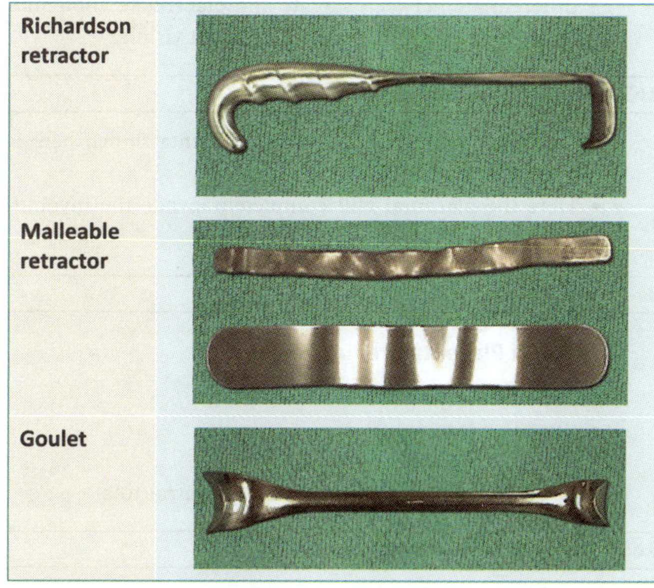

Richardson retractor	
Malleable retractor	
Goulet	

143. Ans. (a) Rampley sponge holder

It is used for holding gauze/sponge for painting the surgical area

144. Ans. (b) Langenback's retractor

It has 90° angle at one end and used for retraction of superficial tissue.

145. Ans. (c) Richardson retractor

Richardson retractor is a 9-1/2" long retractor that can be used during procedures, such as chest or abdominal, to grasp soft tissue using the curved blade.

146. Ans. (c) Salter's scale

Salter's scale is a field instrument used for measurement of body weight. The spring hanging scale (SALTER) is commonly used for taking weight of children under 9 years. This scale can weigh up to 25 kg.

147. Ans. (b) Billroth II

Image shows Billroth II procedure.

- The jejunum is anastomosed to the posterior, dependent, wall of the stomach.
- Two-thirds of the stomach is removed, the duodenal stump is closed and the stomach anastomosed to the jejunum.

148. Ans. (d) Hydatid cyst

- The shown USG image is water lily sign.
- It is seen in hydatid cyst

149. Ans. (a) Saw tooth appearance

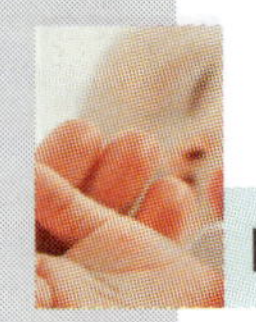

PEDIATRICS

150. Ans. (b) Pectus Carinatum

The image shows forward protrusion of the sternum and adjacent costal cartilages as would be expected in a typical case of Pectus carinatum (Pigeon Chest). This is seen in cases of Marfan's syndrome, childhood asthma and rickets.

OBSTETRICS AND GYNECOLOGY

151. Ans. (a) Trichomonas

The image shows presence of anaerobic flagellated protozoan parasite, which causes vaginitis in women with development of greenish malodorous discharge.

152. Ans. (b) Cusco speculum

153. Ans. (b) Hegar dilator

154. Ans. (a) Bacterial vaginosis

The image shows *presence of clue cells* which are vaginal epithelial cells, coated with bacteria. The patient presents with whitish vaginal discharge with a fishy odor.

155. Ans. (a) Interstitial part

The image shows a fallopian tube with ovary seen close to the fimbrial end of the tube. The chances of ectopic pregnancy is highest in ampulla (choice c), and least in interstitial part (Choice a).

156. Ans. (a) Hydrosalpinx

157. Ans. (c) Sims speculum

158. Ans. (b) Vulsellum

159. Ans. (a) Uterine sound

160. Ans. (a) Outlet forceps

Keilland forceps	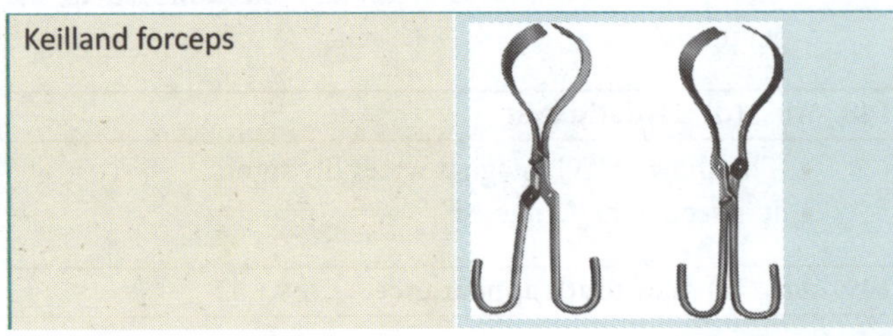

Contd...

Piper forceps	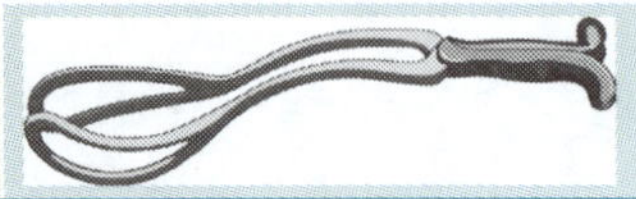

161. Ans. (d) Cryotherapy probe

The shown image is cryotherapy probe.
Used in cervical cancer

162. Ans. (d) Bicornuate Uterus

- A bicornuate uterus results from abnormal development of the paramesonephric ducts. There is a partial failure of fusion of the ducts, resulting in a uterus divided into two horns.
- A divided uterus can be seen, but it is difficult to differentiate between septate and bicornuate anomalies since the uterine fundal contour is not visible.

163. Ans. (c) Placenta percreta

- The type of morbidly adherent placenta shown here is Placenta percreta.
- Here the placental villi completely invade the myometrium.

164. Ans. (d) IV

Types of Placenta Previa

- Type I- low lying
- Type II- marginal
- Type III- partial/incomplete
- Type IV- complete placenta previa/central/total

165. Ans. (a) Imperforate hymen

Ref: Berek and Novak's Gynecology, 16th ed. pg. 427, 455

- An imperforate hymen is a congenital disorder (due to failure of lateral fusion) where a hymen without an opening completely obstructs the vagina.
- It is most often diagnosed in adolescent girls when menstrual blood accumulates in the vagina or in uterus.

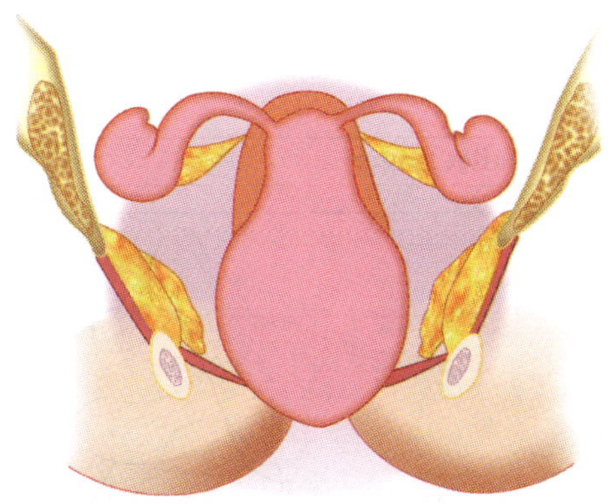

FIGURE: Imperforate hymen causing haematocolpos, haematometra and haematosalpinx

166. Ans. (c) Hysteroscopy

Ref: Berek and Novak's Gynecology, 16th ed. pg. 533, 571

- Hysteroscopy is a procedure that allows a doctor to look inside the uterus in order to diagnose and treat causes of abnormal bleeding.
- It is done using a hysteroscope, a thin lighted tube that is inserted into the vagina to examine the cervix and inside of the uterus.

ENT

167. Ans. (a) Quinsy

- The image shows a deviated uvula indicating a Peri-tonsillar abscess and clinical history of hot potato voice confirms the diagnosis of quinsy

168. Ans. (c) Semicircular canal

169. Ans. (c) Serous otitis media

- During otoscopy, fluid level with air bubble is very suggestive of Glue ear/serous otitis media.

170. Ans. (a) Acute otitis media

- Upon otoscopy, red congested tympanic membrane with fluid level is suggestive of acute suppurative otitis media.
- The shown image shows cart wheel appearance which is due to dilatation of vessels of tympanic membrane due to inflammation.

171. Ans. (a) Rhinoscleroma

- Woody nose is seen in granulomatous stage of rhinoscleroma.

172. Ans. (b) Vocal cord polyp

- The shown image is vocal cord polyp.
- Site: Junction of anterior 1/3rd and posterior 2/3rd
- Most common site is junction of anterior 1/3rd and posterior 2/3rd

173. Ans. (b) Weber fergusson incision

- The shown incision line is weber fergusson incision.
- It is done for maxillectomy in maxillary sinus carcinoma.

174. Ans. (b) Angiofibroma

- The shown case and radiological image is diagnostic of Juvenile nasopharyngeal carcinoma.
- The shown HPE image shows endothelial lining which is also a finding of angiofibroma.

175. Ans. (d) Checking the mobility of tympanic membrane

The shown image is of **siegel speculum** which is used for checking the mobility of tympanic membrane.

176. Ans. (c) Lateral sinus thrombophlebitis

- The shown sign is known as **Griesinger sign**, which is mastoid emissary vein thrombosis seen in case of lateral sinus thrombophlebitis.

177. Ans. (c) Ranula

- The shown image is ranula. It is retention cyst of sublingual gland.

178. Ans. (c) Transoral pneumatic device

- The shown device is transoral pneumatic device, used for voice production.
- It is also known as electrolarynx.
- Vibrating disc held against soft tissue of neck and a low pitch sound is produced in hypopharynx → later modulated into speech by tongue, lip, teeth and palate.

ORTHOPEDICS

179. Ans. (c) Giant cell tumor

The image shows X-ray of wrist joint with presence of Soap Bubble appearance.
Soap bubble appear once is seen in Adamantinoma (MC site of Adamantinoma: Tibia > mandible)

"Soap Bubble appearance as a term" is to be remembered also for:

- Hydronephrosis
- Osteoclastoma (Giant cell tumor)
- Meconium ileus

180. Ans. (b) Aneurysmal bone cyst

- The image shows X-ray of the knee joint with presence of multiple lytic lesions suggestive of aneurysmal bone cyst.
- Unicameral bone Cyst is more common in upper humerus.

181. Ans. (c) Rocker bottom foot

The image shows convexity at the sole of the foot sole. In CTEV the bilateral feet and toes point inwards facing each other.

182. Ans. (d) Monteggia fracture

- The image shows X-ray of the Elbow joint with fracture of upper ulna diagnostic of Monteggia Fracture.
- Galeazzi fracture is an isolated fracture of the junction of the distal third and middle third of the radius with associated subluxation or dislocation of the distal radio-ulnar joint

183. Ans. (c) Sunburst appearance

- The image shows a sun burst appearance lesion which grows rapidly but steadily, and the periosteum will not have enough time to lay down thin shell of bone.
- Therefore in such cases, the tiny fibers that connect the periosteum to the bone (Sharpey's fibers) become stretched out perpendicular to the bone. When these fibers ossify, they produce a pattern sometimes called "sunburst" periosteal reaction.
- It is usually seen in osteosarcoma, but can also be seen in other bone malignancies.

184. Ans. (c) Mallet finger

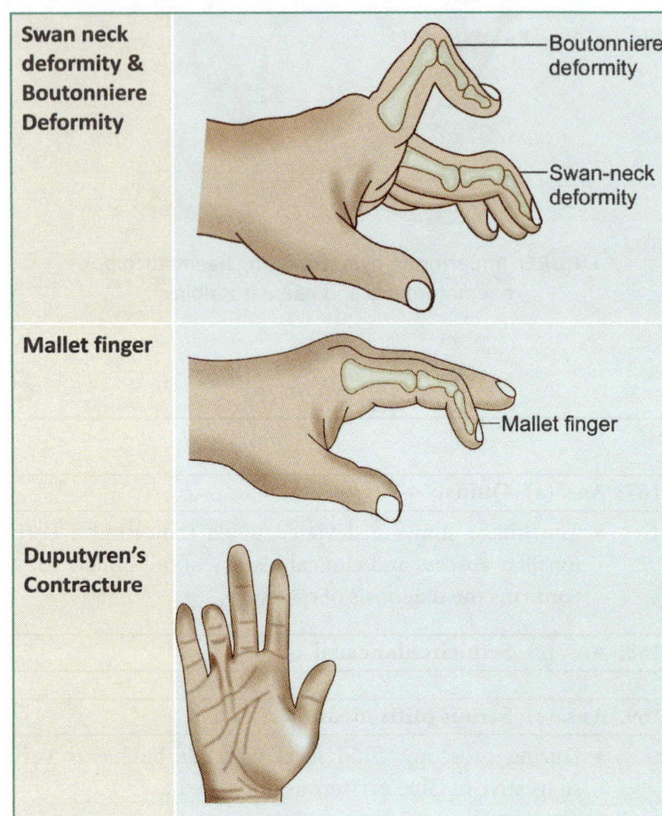

185. Ans. (a) Gallow's Traction

Gallow's traction	Fracture shaft of femur in children <2 years
90–90 traction	Fracture shaft femur in children
Russel traction	Conventional skin traction
Agnes hunt traction	Hip deformity

186. Ans. (c) Simple bone cyst

The image shows fallen leaf sign and the most likely diagnosis here is Simple bone cyst. Simple bone cysts are common benign non-neoplastic lucent bony lesions that are seen mainly in childhood and typically remain asymptomatic.

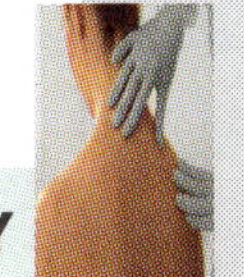

187. Ans. (c) Both

The shown splint is knuckle bender splint used in median nerve injury and can also be used in ulnar nerve injury.

188. Ans. (c) Bennet fracture

- The shown image shows articular fracture of first carpometacarpal joint. It is also known as Bennet fracture.
- **Bennet fracture:** Due to forced abduction; base of thumb fracture
- **Rolando fracture:** Intra-articular comminuted # of base of 1st metacarpal.
- **Boxer's fracture:** 5th metacarpal neck fracture

189. Ans. (b) Osteoid osteoma

- Seed/nidu in cortex is very typical finding of osteoid osteoma

OPHTHALMOLOGY

190. Ans. (b) Pterygium

191. Ans. (a) Hypopyon

192. Ans. (a) Retinitis pigmentosa

The image shows a fundus with bony spicules and a pale disc with thinned out blood vessels suggestive of diagnosis of Retinitis Pigmentosa.

193. Ans. (b) Dot blot haemorrhages

The fundus shows dot in the middle and blotted ink appearance of fundus haemorrhage suggestive of diagnosis of diabetic retinopathy.

194. Ans. (d) Glaucoma

- The given image is of **Laminar dot sign** which is an advanced glaucomatous change in the optic disc.

195. Ans. (d) Both A and B

- The shown image is stenopic slit.
- When placed in front of eye, it allows clearest vision.
- In cataract the colored halo split up and unite while using stenopic slit, however in ACG the colored halo doesn't split
- It has nothing to do with near vision.

196. Ans. (b) Arcuate scotoma

Arcuate scotoma is classical scene in glaucoma. The shape of an Arc is seen in the picture given above. This is the arcuate scotoma.

197. Ans. (c) Color vision

- The shown instrument is FM 100 hue.
- It is most sensitive investigation for diagnosing color vision.

DERMATOLOGY

198. Ans. (c) Wood's Lamp

- Woods lamp emits long-wave UV radiation (UVR), also called black light.
- This is generated by a high pressure mercury arc fitted with a compound filter made of barium silicate with 9% nickel oxide, the "Wood's filter."
- This filter is opaque to all light rays except a band between 320 and 400 nm with a peak at 365 nm.
- The output of Wood's lamp is generally low (<1 mw/ cm^2). The fluorescence of normal skin is very faint or absent.
- It is useful for diagnosis of tinea capitis, Pityriasis Versicolor, Erythrasma, Acne vulgaris, Vitiligo and Porphyria.

199. Ans. (b) Piebaldism

It is an autosomal dominant disorder with melanocyte development defect. The presenting feature which is shown in the image is a white forelock of hair and multiple hypo-pigmented macules.

200. Ans. (b) Contact dermatitis

201. Ans. (c) Erythema multiforme

The image shows presence of target lesions diagnostic of Erythema Multiforme.

202. Ans. (a) Pityriasis rosea

The Picture shows inverted Christmas tree appearance of lesions suggestive of diagnosis of Pityriasis rosea.

The essential clinical features are the following:

- Discrete circular or oval lesions
- Scaling on Most Lesions
- Peripheral Collarette scaling with central clearance on at least two lesions.

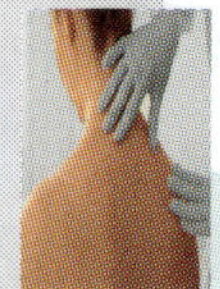

203. Ans. (c) Clotrimazole paint

The image shows presence of oral thrush caused by candida Albicans, and is best managed by topical application of Clotrimazole.

204. Ans. (b) Caused by RNA virus

- The image shows lesion of molluscum contagiosum which are lesions are flesh-colored, dome-shaped, and pearly in appearance. They are often 1–5 mm in diameter, with a dimpled center. *The lesions are caused by pox virus which is a DNA virus.*
- Molluscum contagiosum is most common in children who become infected through direct skin-to-skin contact or indirect skin contact with fomites, such as bath towels, sponges and are commonly seen in intertriginous areas.

205. Ans. (a) Impetigo

The usual organism is streptococcus pyogenes > *Staphylococcus aureus*

206. Ans. (a) Pterygium nail

- The image shows a triangular or wing like appearance in the middle of the nail. Pterygium forms if there is scar tissue in the nail matrix.
- Since the nail matrix at that particular site cannot manufacture nail plate, the proximal nail fold skin grows out with the skin of the nail bed, giving rise to the triangular formation.

207. Ans. (a) Lichen planus

- The image shows presence of purple polygonal plaques on the legs and dorsum of feet of the patient diagnostic of lichen planus.
- "6 Ps" of lichen planus: planar (flat-topped), purple, polygonal, pruritic, papules, and plaques

208. Ans. (b) Psoriasis

209. Ans. (d) Chancroid

210. Ans. (c) Associated with anhidrosis

Ref: Bhutani's Colour Atlas, 6th ed. pg. 105

- The image shows presence of vesicular sago like grains on palms and sides of fingers diagnostic of pompholyx.
- It is associated with hyperhidrosis and more common in summers.

211. Ans. (a) Lentiginosis

Ref: Bhutani's Atlas of Dermatology, 6th ed. pg. 332-33

- The image shows presence of irregular dark macules all over the trunk, neck of the patient. This is seen with lentiginosis.
- Freckles are seen on sun exposed parts of the body with ill-defined edges and darken on sunlight exposure.
- Shagreen patch has *peau d'orange* appearance and is single lesion usually in patients of tuberous sclerosis.
- Congenital nevi have pigmented macules which become nodular and are bilaterally symmetrical.

212. Ans. (c) Borderline tuberculoid

- The shown image is a case of borderline tuberculoid (BT) based on Ridley Jopling classification. They are usually single or few around 3–10 at times.
- It is characterized by well-defined borders but with areas of poor definition (serrated), known as **satellite lesions** near margins.
- In this type of leprosy following characters are seen:
  - Sensation: Significant hypoesthesia
  - Hair: Significant loss
  - Surface: Significant dry or sometimes scaly
  - Size: From large to small

213. Ans. (b) Kerion

Ref: IAP Atlas, 2nd ed. pg. 378

- The image shows a boggy swelling with plaques that drain serous fluid causing crusting in hair.
- This is diagnostic of kerion. In this condition, hair can be easily pulled out.
- Favus causes yellow colored scutula and scarring alopecia.

214. Ans. (b) Griseofulvin

Ref: Bhutani's Colour Atlas, 6th ed. pg. 17

- The image shows presence of discrete hypopigmented scaly macules on anterior abdominal wall and chest suggestive of diagnosis of pityriasis versicolor.

Management of Pityriasis Versicolor

- Lotions or shampoos containing sulfur, salicylic acid, or selenium sulfide will clear the infection if used daily for 1–2 weeks and then weekly thereafter.
- Treatment with some oral antifungal agents is also effective, but they do not provide lasting results and they are not FDA-approved for this indication.
- Ketoconazole, itraconazole and fluconazole are used.
- Griseofulvin is not effective, and terbinafine is not reliably effective for tinea versicolor.

215. Ans. (c) Predominantly occur on genitals

Ref: Bhutani's Colour Atlas, 6th ed. pg. 155

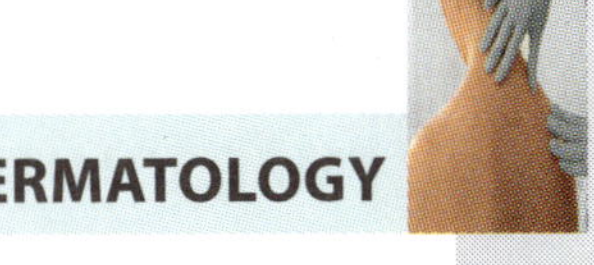

The image shows multiple erythematous plaques on the trunk with herald patch (marked with arrow) in the right iliac fossa. Pityriasis rosea has a viral etiology and is caused by HHV-7.

216. Ans. (a) Lupus vulgaris

Ref: Bhutani's Colour Atlas, 6th ed. pg. 73

- The image shows presence of erythematous brown macule on left supraorbital margin. Since CXR is normal, sarcoidosis is less likely.
- Diascopy should nail the diagnosis in favour of lupus vulgaris with apple jelly appearance.
- Lupus vulgaris is seen in patients with good immunity.

217. Ans. (b) Piebaldism

Ref: Bhutani's Atlas of Dermatology, 6th ed. pg. 307

- The image shows depigmented areas on ventral aspect of trunk with multiple islands exhibiting hyperpigmentation. The image on the right shows a white forelock of hair. Thus the diagnosis is piebaldism.
- The pattern of inheritance is autosomal dominant with defective gene located to chromosome 4.
- It occurs due to defective migration and differentiation of melanoblasts from neural crest.

218. Ans. (d) Peutz Jeghers syndrome

Ref: Bhutani's Atlas of Dermatology, 6th ed. pg. 306

The image shows presence of lentiginosis around lips and fingers. The history of melena points to concomitant GIT lesion. This is seen in Peutz Jehgers syndrome characterized by hamartomatous polyps mostly located in jejunum.

219. Ans. (d) Beau's lines

Ref: Bhutani's Atlas of Dermatology, 6th ed. pg. 277

- The image shows presence of transverse ridges in each of the nails which has occurred due to temporary cessation of nail plate growth.
- The color of proximal and distal part is same, effectively ruling out choice (b) Lindsay nails where the proximal half is white and distal half is pink/brown or red.
- Choice (a) Muehrcke's nails is ruled out as it has white bands parallel to lunula with intervening pink area.
- Choice (c), Leukonychia is ruled out as it has a uniform pallor of nail bed and the nail appears white.

220. Ans. (a) Muehrcke's nails

Ref: Bhutani's Atlas of Dermatology, 6th ed. pg. 277

The image shows Muehrcke's nails characterized by white bands which run parallel to lunula. This is seen in nutritional deficiency states (Hypoalbuminemia) and goes across the entire nail plate. The intervening normal area is pink interspersed with white bands.

221. Ans. (a) Hidradenitis suppurativa

Ref: Bhutani's Atlas of Dermatology, 6th ed. pg. 266

- **Hidradenitis suppurativa:** Keratin obstruction of apocrine duct extending into hair follicles. Lesions similar to acne but in apocrine area hence called inverse acne.
- Most common site is axilla.
- Rx retinoids, broad spectrum antibiotics
- **For fordyce disease:** Keratin obstruction of apocrine duct lesser than hidradenitis
- Only in flammatory papules in apocrine area
- **Acne conglobata:** Nodules and discharging sinus on buttocks, chest back. Rx oral steroids, oral isotretinoin.
- **Fordyce spot:** Ectopic sebaceous buccal gland.
- Site upper lips > Mucosa.

222. Ans. (b) Budding yeasts and pseudohyphae

Ref: Bhutani Atlas of Dermatology, 6th ed. pg. 29

The image shows KOH mount showing pseudohyphae in branching pattern and budding yeasts seen in *candida* infection.

223. Ans. (d) Erythema multiforme

Ref: Bhutani Atlas of Dermatology, 6th ed. pg. 77-78

The image shows presence of target lesions suggestive of erythema multiforme which is acute, self-limited, and is considered to be a type IV hypersensitivity reaction associated with certain infections, medications, and other triggers. The papules evolve into pathognomonic target or iris lesions that appear within a 72-hour period and begin on the extremities.

224. Ans. (b) Poxvirus

Ref: Bhutani Atlas of Dermatology, 6th ed. pg. 45-46

- The image shows multiple, rounded, dome-shaped, pink, waxy papules that are umbilicated and contain a caseous plug. The diagnosis is Molluscum contagiosum and is caused by pox virus.
- Molluscum contagiosum is most common in children who become infected through direct skin-to-skin contact or indirect skin contact with fomites.

225. Ans. (a) Herpes simplex

Ref: Bhutani Atlas of Dermatology, 6th ed. pg. 48-49

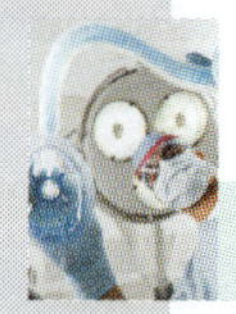

- Notice the grouped vesicles with lesions showing umbilication which is a presentation of primary herpes gingivostomatitis.
- Primary episode is quite distressing for the patient with fever, constitutional symptoms and small eroded painful lesions on lips oral mucosa and perioral area.
- Impetigo presents with honey colored crusts on the skin and is ruled out.
- Molluscum contagiosum is caused by pox virus infection and produces crops of dome shaped papules with umbilicated center which are asymptomatic.
- In the given question the patient has fever and location of vesicles is perioral and a trip to a place known for sex tourism favors diagnosis of herpes simplex.

226. Ans. (a) Molluscum contagiosum

Ref: Bhutani Atlas of Dermatology, 6th ed. pg. 45-46

227. Ans. (b) Segmental vitiligo

Ref: Bhutani Atlas of Dermatology, 6th ed. pg. 209

- Vitiligo is an acquired autoimmune condition targeting melanocytes and presents with localized or widespread white depigmented patches. Thyroid dysfunction is the most common association.
- Piebaldism is an autosomal dominant condition characterized by white forelock and circumscribed depigmented patches affecting the body. It is caused by a defect in proliferation and migration of melanocytes during embryogenesis. Unlike vitiligo, it is congenital and nonprogressive. In the question the depigmentation started at age the of 12 years and the patient presented at 13 years.
- Nevoid hypomelanosis is characterized by hypopigmented patches or streaks which follow the lines of Blaschko. They are present at birth and may develop in the first 2 years of life.

228. Ans. (a) Koenen tumor

Ref: Bhutani Atlas of Dermatology, 6th ed. p-299

Koenen tumor is seen in tuberous sclerosis and is subungual fibroma.
Tuberous sclerosis is inherited as an autosomal dominant trait with variable penetrance and a prevalence of 1/6,000 people. Molecular genetic studies have identified two foci for the TS complex. The *TSC1* gene is located on chromosome 9q34, and the *TSC2* gene is on chromosome 16p13.

229. Ans. (d) Caused by *Candida*

Ref: Bhutani Atlas of Dermatology, 6th ed. pg. 19

The image shows tinea cruris-ringworm of the groin which is also called as "jock's itch"/"Dhobi itch". It is common in the tropics.

ANESTHESIA

230. Ans. (a) Oxygen cylinder

	Body color	Shoulder color
Oxygen	Black	White
Nitrous oxide	Blue	Blue
Carbon dioxide	Grey	Grey
Air	Grey	White/black quarters
Entonox	Blue	Alternate blue and white quarter shoulder
Helium	Brown	Brown

231. Ans. (b) Veres needle

It is used to create pneumoperitoneum before laparoscopic surgery for insufflation of carbon Dioxide.

232. Ans. (d) Above esophagus

233. Ans. (a) Sternomastoid muscle, B = Cricoid cartilage, C = Thyroid cartilage

234. Ans. (c) Not influenced by tongue mobility and size

235. Ans. (c) 20G

- The shown pink canula is 20G in size with flow rate of 55–60 mL/min.
- The canula is ~1mm in diameter and 32 in length.

Theoretical Maximum flow rates		
Colour	Gauge	Flow
Yellow	24G	13 ml/min
Blue	22G	30 ml/min
Pink	20G	55 ml/min
Green	18G	80-100 ml/min
White	17G	135 ml/min
Grey	16G	180 ml/min
Orange or Brown	14G	270 ml/min

236. Ans. (b) laparoscopic trocar

It is used to insert laparoscopic instruments into cavity.

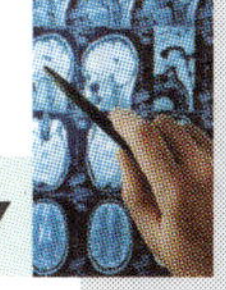

RADIOLOGY

237. Ans. (a) Intussusception

Ref: Nelson 20th ed. pg. 1813

The image shows presence of "coiled spring" sign which is seen when an intussusception has occurred. These ring shadows represent contrast reflux within the lumen between the walls of the intussusceptum and intussuscipiens.

238. Ans. (a) SAH and IVH

The NCCT shows presence of hyperdensity in the area of slyian fissure (right side black arrow) indicating Subarachnoid hemorrhage. The presence of hyperdensity in ventricles indicated concomitant intraventricular hemorrhage (left side white arrow).

239. Ans. (b) Subdural hemorrhage

The concavo convex bleed is marked by three arrows indicating, subdural hemorrhage.

240. Ans. (a) Liver laceration

The image shows a hematoma seen in the posterior part of liver (black area).

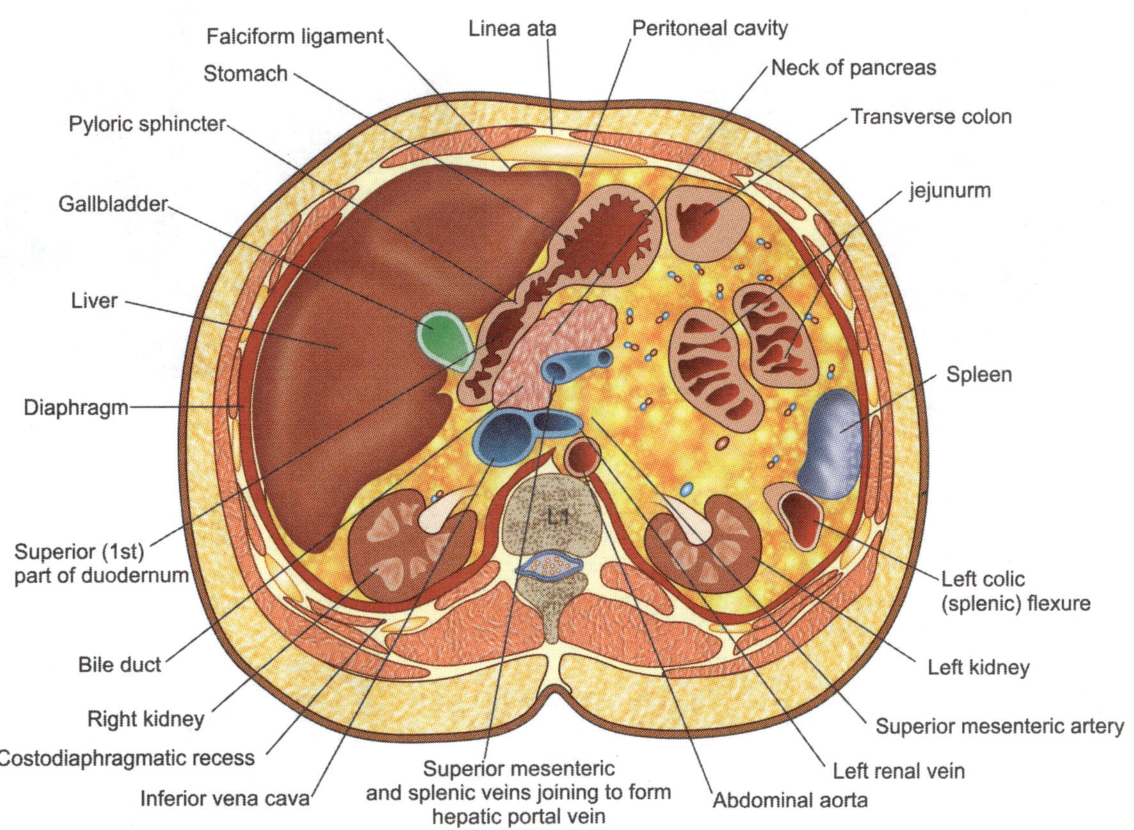

241. Ans. (a) Brain tumor

The image shows a brain tumor obliterating the ventricular system.

242. Ans. (b) Horseshoe kidney

243. Ans. (a) Klastskin tumor

The image shows the endoscope in the middle and the biliary tree. You can notice the contrast in gall bladder (9 o'clock) and cystic duct where it is meeting the common hepatic duct. However the left and right hepatic ducts are not visible indicating a tumor causing obstruction to flow of contrast.

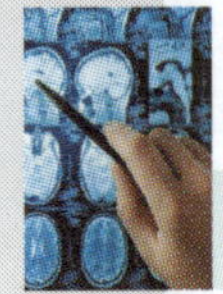

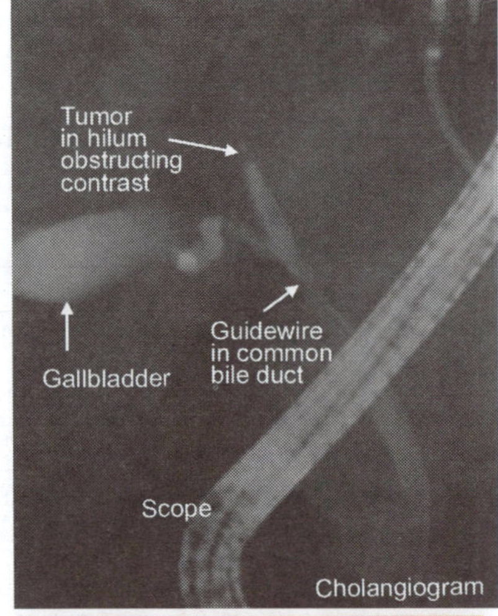

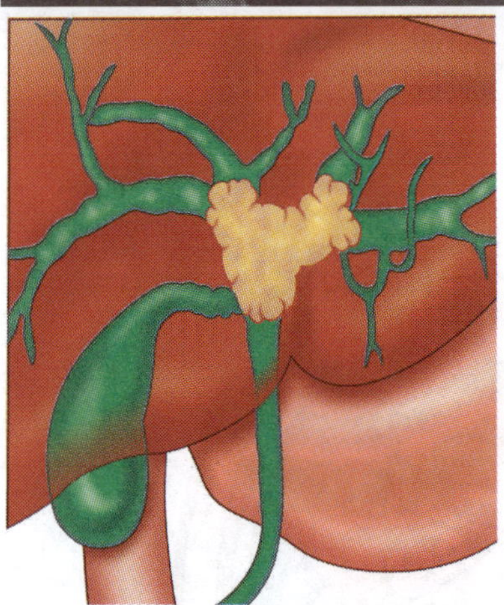

244. Ans. (a) Staphylococcus aureus

The Chest X-ray shows a cystic cavity in right upper zone indicative of infection with a virulent organism. In setting of recovery from measles the organism responsible is *Staphylococcus aureus.*

245. Ans. (a) Duodenal atresia

The image shows presence of double bubble appearance suggestive of diagnosis of duodenal atresia. About 8% of children with Down syndrome are born with duodenal atresia which presents with bilious vomiting.

246. Ans. (b) Acute viral hepatitis

USG Abdomen shows presence of starry sky pattern of the liver, diagnostic of acute viral hepatitis

247. Ans. (c) Bochdalek hernia

The chest X-ray shows loops of bowel on left side of chest indicating congenital diaphragmatic hernia/Bochdalek hernia.

248. Ans. (a) Invertogram

The image shows an invertogram which is an X-ray of neonate taken upside down with a coin placed at the anus of the child as a radiological marker. This is done to evaluate a child with anorectal malformations.

249. Ans. (b) Pulmonary plethora

The CXR shows an enlarged heart with boot shaped configuration and reduced vascularity of lungs. The clinical diagnosis is Tetralogy of Fallot, and due to subpulmonic stenosis it presents with pulmonic oligemia.

250. Ans. (b) Major fissure

- The shown image shows major fissure or oblique fissure.

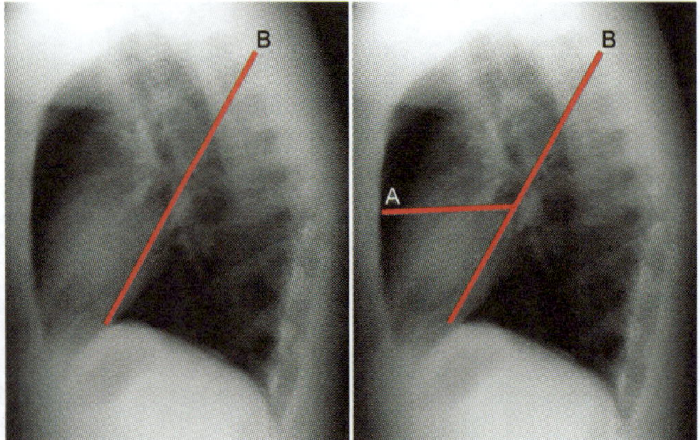

B: Major fissure L Lung | A: Minor Fissure R Ling
B: Major fissure L Lung

251. Ans. (b) Right atrium

- The structure marked in the given chest X-ray is right atrium
- Note down the markings in image

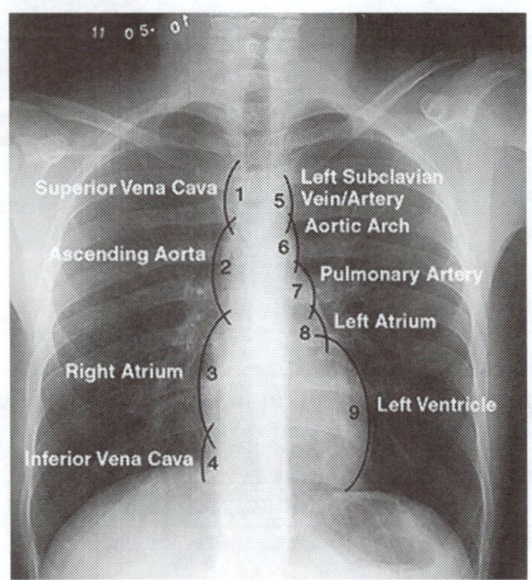

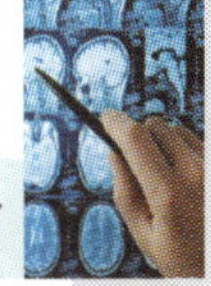

252. Ans. (a) Aortic knob

- The arrow in this X-ray points at aortic knob
- Follow the X-ray markings shown below

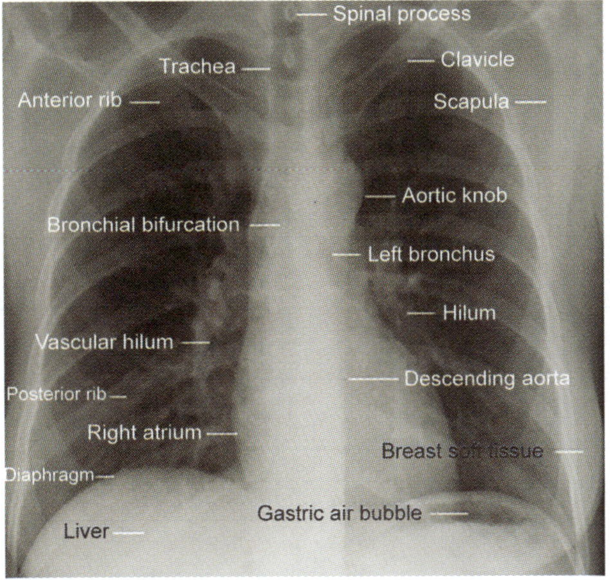

253. Ans. (a) Schatzki ring

The barium swallow shows a narrowing at lower 1/3rd of esophagus which is a feature of Schatzki Ring.

254. Ans. (c) Foreign body aspiration

- Foreign body aspiration can cause collapse of upper lobe of lung.
- The typical X-ray finding here I shifting fissure sign and increased opacity of upper lobe of lung (due to crowding of vasculature).

Notes

A Complete NEXT-Centric Approach

FMGE SOLUTIONS

For **Foreign Medical Graduates** Appearing for *Indian Medical Registration*

AddOn Booklet

Includes Important Key Points of all 19 Subjects for LMR

Deepak Marwah
Director
Medicine Buster Classes

Siraj Ahmad
Faculty (Pharmacology)
AllenNEXT

CBS Publishers and Distributors Pvt Ltd

• New Delhi • Bengaluru • Chennai • Kochi • Kolkata • Lucknow
• Mumbai • Hyderabad • Nagpur • Patna • Pune • Vijayawada

Booklet Contents

KEY POINTS

ANATOMY

IMPORTANT RECENT POINTS (INCLUDES LATEST QS)

- Upper lateral cutaneous nerve is a branch of: **Axillary nerve**
- An injury to anatomical snuff box causes fracture of this bone: **Scaphoid**
- Muscle of arm causing flexion, adduction and medial rotation: **Pectoralis Major**
- Testicular artery is a branch of: **Abdominal aorta**
- Inferior scapular angle lies at which level: **T8**
- Muscle causing adduction at hip joint: **Gluteus medius**
- Deep inguinal ring is formed in: **Transversalis fascia**
- Nerve damage that can cause hypothenar muscle wasting and loss of sensation of medial one and half digits: **Ulnar nerve**
- Failure of closure of rostral neuropore at 25th day leads to: **Anencephaly**
- Parotid gland is supplied by this nerve: **Glossopharyngeal nerve**
- Killian's Dehiscence is formed due to: **Inferior constrictor muscle**
- Muscle biceps brachii inserts into: **Radial tuberosity**
- Nerve supplying area between great toe and 2nd toe: **Deep Peroneal nerve**
- Dermatome supplying area of nipples: **T4**
- Dermatome Supplying area of umbilicus: **T10**
- Retraction of scapula is done by: **Middle fibers of trapezius muscle**
- Nerve supplying cornea: **Trigeminal nerve**
- Longest extraocular muscle: **Superior Oblique (7.7 cm)**
- Shortest extraocular muscle: **Medial rectus (5.5 cm)**

TABLE: Important bone and their nutrient arteries

Bone	Nutrient artery
Femur	Branch of Femoral artery → **Profunda femoris artery**
Tibia	Posterior tibial artery
Fibula	Branch of posterior tibial artery → **Peroneal artery**
Clavicle	Subscapular artery
Radius and Ulna	Anterior interosseous artery
Humerus	Profunda brachii artery

Contd...

TABLE: Branches of subcalvian artery

1st part	**VIT-CD** • Vertebral artery • Internal mammary artery • Thyrocervical trunk
2nd part	Costocervical trunk
3rd part	Dorsal scapular artery

TABLE: Weight of some important organs

Organ	Weight
• Pituitary	0.5–0.6 gram (500–600 mg)
• Brain	Males: 1.4 kg Females: 1.27 kg
• Thyroid gland	20–40 gram
• Kidney	130–160 gram
• Adrenal gland	5–6 gram
• Prostate gland	15–20 gram

TABLE: Length of important anatomical structure

Organ	Length
• Fallopian tube	**10–12 cm**
• Bile duct • Appendix • Gallbladder	**8 cm** **Mn: BAG**
• Spinal cord • Thoracic duct • Transverse colon • Umbilical cord • Femur • Deferens (Vas Deferens)	**45 cm** ***Mn: STTUFeD***

Contd...

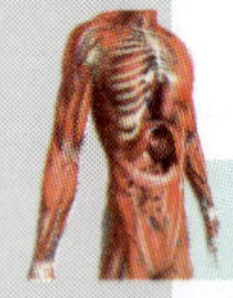

Organ	Length
• Sigmoid colon • Esophagus • Duodenum • Descending colon • Ureter • Urethra (male)	**25 cm** *Mn: SEDDUU*
• Inguinal canal • Optic nerve • Urethra (Female)	**4 cm** *Mn: I lOve U*

TABLE: Glands of face and their duct

Gland	Duct	Nerve	Devel-opment	Acini histology
Parotid gland	Stensen duct (opens opposite to upper 2nd molar)	**CN V** (auriculotemporal branch)	Ectodermal	Serous acini
Submandibular gland	Wharton's duct (open on sides of frenulum at the floor of mouth)	**CN VII** (chorda tympani branch)	Endodermal	Mixed (serous > Mucinous)
Sublingual gland	Bartholin's and Rivinus duct (open at floor of mouth)	**CN VII** (chorda tympani branch)	Endodermal	Mixed (Mucinous > serous)

OFTEN ASKED ONES

• Most frequently fractured bone of body	**Clavicle**
• First bone to ossify	**Clavicle**
• Only long bone which has no medullary cavity	**Clavicle**
• All long bone ossify in cartilage EXCEPT clavicle. *It ossifies in membrane*	**Clavicle**
• Most frequently dislocated carpal bone	**Lunate**
• Most frequently fractured carpal bone	**Scaphoid**
• Nerve supply of deltoid	**Axillary nerve**
• MC fractured carpal bone	**Scaphoid (boat shaped)- 2nd MC site of avascular necrosis**
• Ape thumb deformity	**Median nerve (opponens pollicis muscle paralyzed)**
• Musician's nerve	**Ulnar nerve (root value C8, T1)**
• Labourer's nerve/eye of the hand	**Median nerve**
• Root value of radial nerve	**C5 to T1 (C5, C6, C7, C8, T1)**
• Winging of scapula	**Long thoracic nerve (serratus anterior muscle paralyzed)**
• Police man tip hand/porter's tip hand	**Erb's paralysis**
• Klumpke's paralysis	**Damage to C8 and T1**
• Strongest ligament of body	**Iliofemoral ligament**
• Longest muscle of body	**Sartorius (aka tailor's muscle)**
• Nerve supply of gluteus maximus	**INFERIOR gluteal N. (L5, S1, S2)** *Mn: 512*
• Nerve supply of gluteus medius and minimus	**SUPERIOR gluteal N. (L4, L5, S1)** *Mn: 451*
• Vessel used in coronary artery bypass graft (CABG)	**Internal Mammary Artery**
• Muscle which is known as peripheral heart	**Soleus**
• Locking of the knee by	**Quadriceps femoris muscle (occurs at last stage of extension)**
• Unlocking of the knee by	**Popliteus muscle (occurs at first stage of flexion)**
• Sternal angle and bifurcation of trachea at	**T4 level**
• Arch of aorta begins and terminates at	**T4 level**
• Police man of abdominal cavity	**Greater omentum**
• Muscle of horror	**Platysma**
• Nerve supply of upper eyelid and TIP of nose	**V1 (ophthalmic branch of trigeminal)**
• Most commonly nerve paralyzed	**Facial N (longest intraosseous course)**
• Emergency tracheostomy at	**Tracheal ring 2–3**
• Ova released in form of	**Secondary oocyte**
• Blastocyst formation	**5th day after fertilization**
• Implantation occurs	**6th day after fertilization, completes on 10th day.**
• Liver has 8 segments.	**Caudate lobe-segment 1; Quadrate lobe-segment 4**

Contd...

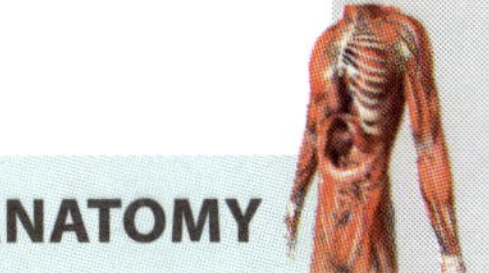

• Narrowest part of esophagus	**Cricopharynx at the root of neck**
• Test which is done to check gluteus medius and minimus	**Trendelenburg test**
• Trigone of bladder develops	**From mesonephric duct (mesodermal in origin)**
• Pouch of Douglas	**Between rectum and uterus**
• Parotid gland duct	**Stensen's duct**
• Submandibular gland duct	**Wharton's duct**
• Muscle which opens Eusta-chian tube while yawning	**Tensor veli palatini and levator veli palatini**
• Ovarian artery/testicular artery is a branch of	**Abdominal aorta**
• Most common fracture of humerus	**Supracondylar fracture**
• Muscle not attached to apex of orbit	**Inferior oblique**
• Which bone does not contribute to Medial wall of orbit	**Zygoma**
• Which layer of scalp is vascular	**Subcutaneous tissue**
• Magendie foramen drains CSF from:	**4th ventricle**
• Closure of neural tube begins at	**Cervical end (if choice given is "multiple sites" then it is the best answer)**
• Junction of anterior and posterior horn of lateral ventricle is called:	**Trigone and lateral ventricle**
• Infection of CNS spreads in inner ear through	**Cochlear Aqueduct**
• Posterior communicating artery is a branch of	**Middle Cerebral Artery**
• The chorda tympani nerve arises from	**Facial nerve**
• Broca's area is located in	**Inferior frontal gyrus**
• Lower angle of scapula lies at	**Level of T 7**
• Nerve injured with fracture of surgical neck of humerus	**Axillary**
• Nerve injured with fracture of shaft of humerus	**Radial**
• Nerve injured with fracture of medial humeral epicondyle	**Ulnar**
• Muscle that initiates abduction of arm	**Supraspinatus**
• Most commonly torn tendon of rotator cuff	**Supraspinatus**
• "Claw" hand is due to paralysis of which muscle group	**Lumbricals**

Contd...

• Innervation to nail bed of ring finger	**Ulnar and median**
• Innervation to nail bed of middle finger	**Median nerve**
• Dermatome of thumb	**C6**
• Spinal levels of axillary nerve	**C5 and C6**

GOLDEN POINTS

- Sprengel's deformity is associated with this bone: **Scapula (failure of normal scapular descent during development)**
- Largest branch of brachial plexus: **Radial nerve**
- Largest branch of lumbar plexus: **Femoral nerve**
- Erb's point anatomical location at junction of: **C5, C6**
- Klumpke's paralysis involves: **C8, T1**
- This nerve injury can cause wasting of intrinsic muscles of hand: **Ulnar nerve**
- Guyon's canal is in relation to this nerve: **Ulnar nerve**
- Paralysis of this muscle can cause "Dropped shoulder": **Trapezius**
- Power grip of hand is mainly due to: **Long Flexors**
- Cephalic veins drain into: **Axillary vein**
- Upper outer quadrant of breast is drained by this lymphatic: **Anterior axillary**
- Main blood supply of the femoral head: **Medial circumflex femoral artery**
- Nutrient artery of the femur: **Profunda femoris artery**
- Nutrient artery of tibia: **Posterior tibial artery**
- Nutrient artery to fibula: **Peroneal artery**
- Ligament which supports talus: **Spring ligament**
- Strongest flexors of the hip: **Psoas major and iliacus muscle (iliopsoas muscle)**
- Chief nerve of medial compartment of thigh: **Obturator nerve**
- Nerve root value of sciatic nerve: **L4, 5, S1, 2, 3**
- Nerve root of posterior cutaneous nerve of thigh: **S1, 2, 3**
- Nerve root value of pudendal nerve: **S2, 3, 4**
- Nerve root value of medial cutaneous nerve of thigh: **L2, L3**
- Hunterian perforators also known as adductor canal perforators are seen in: **Mid-thigh**
- Triceps surae nerve is: **Gastroc-soleus**
- Pressure change in calf compartment during heel touch phase of walking: **Remains same (no change in pressure)**
- Motor nerve supply of diaphragm: **Phrenic nerve**
- **Sensory nerve supply of diaphragm:**
  - Central part: Phrenic nerve
  - Peripheral part: Lower 6 intercostal nerves

Contd...

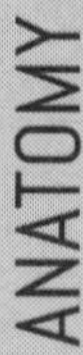

- Most common site of morgagni hernia: **Posterolateral part of diaphragm (*Right anterior being the most common site*)**
- Intercostobrachial nerve is a branch of: **2nd intercostal nerve**
- Azygos lobe is a part of this organ: **Lung**
- **Trautmann's triangle** (transmits infection from temporal bone to cerebellum):
  - Bony labyrinth (anteriorly)
  - Sigmoid sinus (posteriorly)
  - Superior petrosal sinus (above)
- **Triangle of safety** (an important landmark of chest tube insertion)
  - Anterior border of latissimus dorsi
  - Lateral border of pectoralis major
  - Imaginary horizontal level of the nipple
- Triangle of Doom
  - Medially: Vas Deferens
  - Laterally: Gonadal vessels
  - Posteriorly: Peritoneal edge
- **Triangle of Doom contains:** External iliac vessels, Deep circumflex iliac vein, femoral nerve and genital branch of genitofemoral nerve
- **Triangle of pain** (contain femoral branch of genitofemoral nerve, lateral cutaneous nerve of thigh)
  - Medially: Gonadal vessels
  - Laterally: Iliopubic tract
- **Passaro (Gastrinoma) triangle:** Seen at upper abdomen
  - Apex: Junction of cystic duct and CBD
  - Inferior part: Junction of D2 and D3
  - Left lateral point: Pancreatic neck & Body junction
- **Koch's triangle** is formed by:
  - Superiorly: Tendon of todaro
  - Inferiorly: Tricuspid valve septal leaflet
  - Basally: Coronary sinus orifice
- Koch's triangle is a part of: **AV node**
- Blood supply of the Koch's triangle: **Right coronary artery**
- Blood supply of SA node: **Right coronary artery**
- Valve guarding coronary sinus: **Thebesian valve**
- Thoracic duct is also known as: **Van horne canal, Pecquet duct**
- Transtubercular plane lies at which level: **L5**
- Length of inguinal canal: **4 cm**
- Cisterna chyli is situated in: **Abdomen**
- Labia majora is developed from: **Genital swelling**
- Helicine artery is a branch of: **Deep artery of penis**
- Nerve supply of perineum is: **Pudendal nerve**
- Anatomical support of prostrate is: **Pubococcygeus**
- Blood supply of liver: **80% portal vein, 20% hepatic artery**
- Stave cells are seen in: **Spleen**

Contd...

- Most common congenital anomaly of pancreas: **Pancreas divisum**
- Ligament which contains splenic artery: **Splenorenal ligament**
- Angle of mandible is supplied by: **Greater auricular nerve**
- Tip of nose is supplied by: **Ophthalmic nerve (external nasal branch)**
- Metopic suture: **Separates two half of the frontal bone**
- Metopic suture closes at: **6 years**
- Muscle of grinning: **Risorius muscle**
- Common carotid artery bifurcates at: **C4 level (at upper border of thyroid cartilage)**
- Middle meningeal artery is a branch of: **Maxillary artery (1st part of maxillary artery)**
- Anterior choroidal artery is a branch of: **Internal carotid artery**
- Chassaignac tubercle is: **Carotid tubercle on C6 vertebra**
- Ligament of berry function: **Connects thyroid lobe to cricoid lobe**
- Herring bodies are seen in: **Posterior pituitary (ADH and oxytocin both stored here)**
- Otic ganglion supplies this gland: **Parotid gland**
- Gerlach tonsil is also named as: **Tubal tonsil**
- Passavant's ridge is formed by: **Palatopharyngeus and superior constrictor muscle**
- Gillette space corresponds to: **Retropharyngeal space**
- Smallest cranial nerve: **Trochlear nerve**
- Broca's area located at: **Posterior end of inferior frontal gyrus (Area 44, 45)**
- Wernicke's area is located at: **Inferior frontal gyrus (Area 22)**
- Organs devoid of lymphatics: **Brain, choroid, internal ear, glottis**
- Most prominent spinous process in the spine? **Vertebra prominens (C7)**
- Muscles comprise the erector spinae? **Iliocostalis, Longissimus, Spinalis**
- Pairs of spinal nerves exit from the spinal cord? **31 pairs**
- Region where the manubrium and the body of the sternum articulate? **Sternal angle of Louis.**
- Muscles are innervated by the axillary nerve? **Deltoid and teres minor**
- Foot drop is caused by damage to which nerve? **Common peroneal nerve**
- Artery of the anterior compartment of the leg? **Anterior tibial artery**
- Nerve supplying the lateral compartment of the leg? **Superficial peroneal nerve**

Contd...

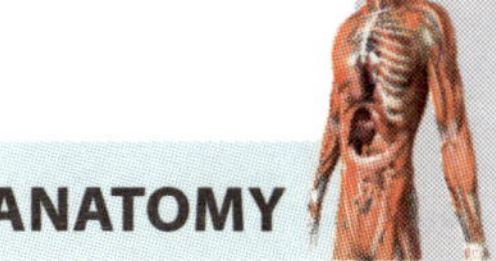

- What is the prominent "bump" on the lateral aspect of the knee? **Head of the fibula**
- What is the part of the lung that extends above the level of the first rib? **The cupula**
- Right lung has how many lobes? **Three**
- Left lung has how many lobes. **Two**
- What is the only valve in the heart that has two cusps? **Mitral (bicuspid) valve**
- Which vein travels with the right coronary artery? **Small cardiac vein**
- What attaches the cusps of the valves to the papillary muscles in the heart? **Chordae tendineae**
- First branch off the abdominal artery? **Inferior phrenic artery**
- At what vertebral level is the hyoid bone found? **C3**
- Ophthalmic artery is a branch of? **Internal carotid artery**
- Where does the inferior mesenteric vein drain? **The splenic vein**
- The folds of the mucosa of the stomach are known as? **Rugae**
- Mucosal folds of small intestine starting 2nd part of duodenum: **Valvulae conniventes also known as Kerckring folds**
- Artery of the embryonic foregut? **Celiac artery**
- **Portal triad** comprised of? **1. Common bile duct 2. Hepatic artery 3. Portal vein**
- Structure which separate the anatomic right and left lobes of the liver? **Ligamentum teres and ligamentum venosum**
- Rectouterine pouch is also known as? **Pouch of Douglas**
- Broad ligament of the uterus is comprised of: **1. Mesosalpinx 2. Mesovarium 3. Mesometrium**
- What two muscles are tested to see if CN XI is intact? **Trapezius and sternocleidomastoid**
- Only organ in the body supplied by preganglionic sympathetic fibers? **Adrenal medulla**
- Location of seminal vesicle? **On the posterior aspect of the urinary bladder**
- Opening of parotid (Stenson's) duct in the oral cavity? **Opposite the second upper molar tooth**
- Function of the arachnoid granulations in brain? **Resorb CSF into the blood**
- Only muscle of the tongue not innervated by the hypoglossal nerve? **Palatoglossus**
- Fundus of stomach is supplied mainly by: **Splenic artery**
- Content of anatomical snuff box: **Radial artery**
- Ovarian artery is a branch of: **Abdominal aorta**

Contd...

- **Ventral Branches of Abdominal Aorta:**
  - Celiac trunk
  - Superior mesenteric artery
  - Inferior mesenteric artery
- Direct branch of Inferior mesenteric artery: **Superior rectal artery**
- Left adrenal gland is **crescentic/semilunar**
- Right adrenal gland is **pyramidal** in shape
- The average weight of adrenal gland: **4–6 g**
- **Structures and level of piercing in diaphragm: *(Mn: I ate, 10 Eggs, At 12)***
  - IVC: T8
  - Esophagus: T10
  - Aorta: T12
- Base of the heart is formed by: **Left atrium**
- Nerve supplying serratus anterior muscle: **Long thoracic nerve**
- Inferior vena cava formed at: **L5 level**
- Muller muscle supplied by which nerve: **Sympathetic nerve**
- Arnold nerve is a branch of: **Vagus Nerve**
- Left gonadal vein drain into: **IVC**
- Muscle of upper limb which cover both elbow and shoulder joint: **Long head of triceps brachii**
- **Supination and pronation** of upper limb is due to: **Radioulnar joint**
- Efferent cremasteric reflex is carried by: **Genitofemoral nerve**
- Collecting duct is derived from: **Ureteric bud**
- Most common fracture of humerus- **Supracondylar fracture**
- **Police man** of abdominal cavity- **Greater omentum**
- Nerve supply of upper eyelid and TIP of nose- **V1 (ophthalmic branch of trigeminal).**
- Disc are NOT found between: **C1 and C2; Sacrum-Coccyx**
- Critical vascular zone of spinal cord: **T4–T9**
- Extension of artery of Adamkiewicz is between: **T9–T11**
- Filum terminale is derived from: **Pia mater**

TABLE: Cranial nerves in a nutshell

• Largest cranial nerve	Trigeminal Nerve (CN V)
• Smallest cranial nerve	Trochlear nerve (CN IV)
• Longest intracranial course	Trochlear nerve (CN IV)
• The only cranial nerve to emerge from the dorsal surface of the Brain stem	Trochlear N
• Cranial N. with longest intraosseous course	Facial nerve (CN VII)
• Most common cranial nerve involved in Raised ICT	Abducens N (CN VI)

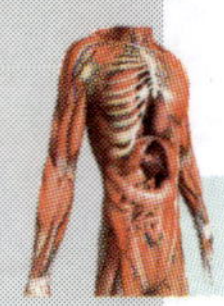

TABLE: Important vertebral levels (also mentioned inside in explanations section)

• Bifurcation of common carotid artery	C3
• Thyroid Cartilage	C5
• Cricoid Cartilage	C6
• Arch of Aorta	T4
• Tracheal bifurcation (standing)	T6
• Xiphoid process	T9
• Transpyloric plane	L1
• Origin of renal artery	L2
• Subcostal plane	L3
• Bifurcation of abdominal aorta	L4
• Transtubercular plane	L5
• Formation of IVC	L5

TABLE: Ribs at a glance

Rib nomenclature	Rib number
• False ribs	8–12
• True ribs also known as vertebrosternal ribs	1–7th ribs
• Floating ribs	11th and 12th
• Typical ribs	3rd to 9th *(individual identification is not possible)*
• Atypical ribs	1st, 2nd, 10th, 11th, 12th *(can be identified individually)*
• Longest rib	7th rib
Strongest rib Shortest rib Widest rib	1st rib
Most oblique rib	9th rib

TABLE: Deep tendon reflexes and their spinal cord level

Reflex/Jerk	Spinal level	Nerve Involved
Biceps Jerk	C5-6	Musculocutaneous
Brachioradialis	C5-6	Radial
Supinator	C5-6	Radial
Triceps	C7-8	Radial
Knee/patella jerk	L3-4	Femoral
Ankle jerk	S1-2	Tibial

TABLE: Normal prostrate anatomy: Has 5 lobes

Lobe	Importance
Anterior	–
Posterior	MC site of prostrate CA
Median	MC site for BPH
Lateral-2	Site for prostatic adenoma in elderly

STRUCTURE WITH NO LYMPHATICS (BASEC)

- Brain & spinal cord
- Articular cartilage
- Splenic pulp, bone marrow
- Epidermis, Hairs, Nails
- Cornea

FASCIA

- Membranous layer of superficials fascia of perineum: **COLLES FASCIA**
- Deep fascia of thighs: **FASCIA LATA**
- Deep fascia of penis: **BUCK'S FASCIA**
- Separates post surface of prostate from rectum: **FASCIA OF DENOVILLIER**
- Condensation of pelvic fascia behind rectum: **FASCIA OF WALDAYER**
- Below umbilicus superf. Fatty layer: **FASCIA OF CAMPER**
- Below umbilicus deep membraneous layer: **FASCIA OF SCARPA**

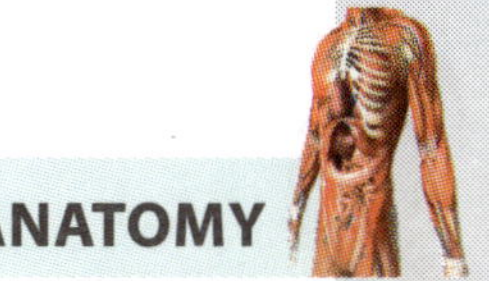

"Since there are multiple questions on aortic and iliac branches, here's the summarized table for the ease of creating an image".

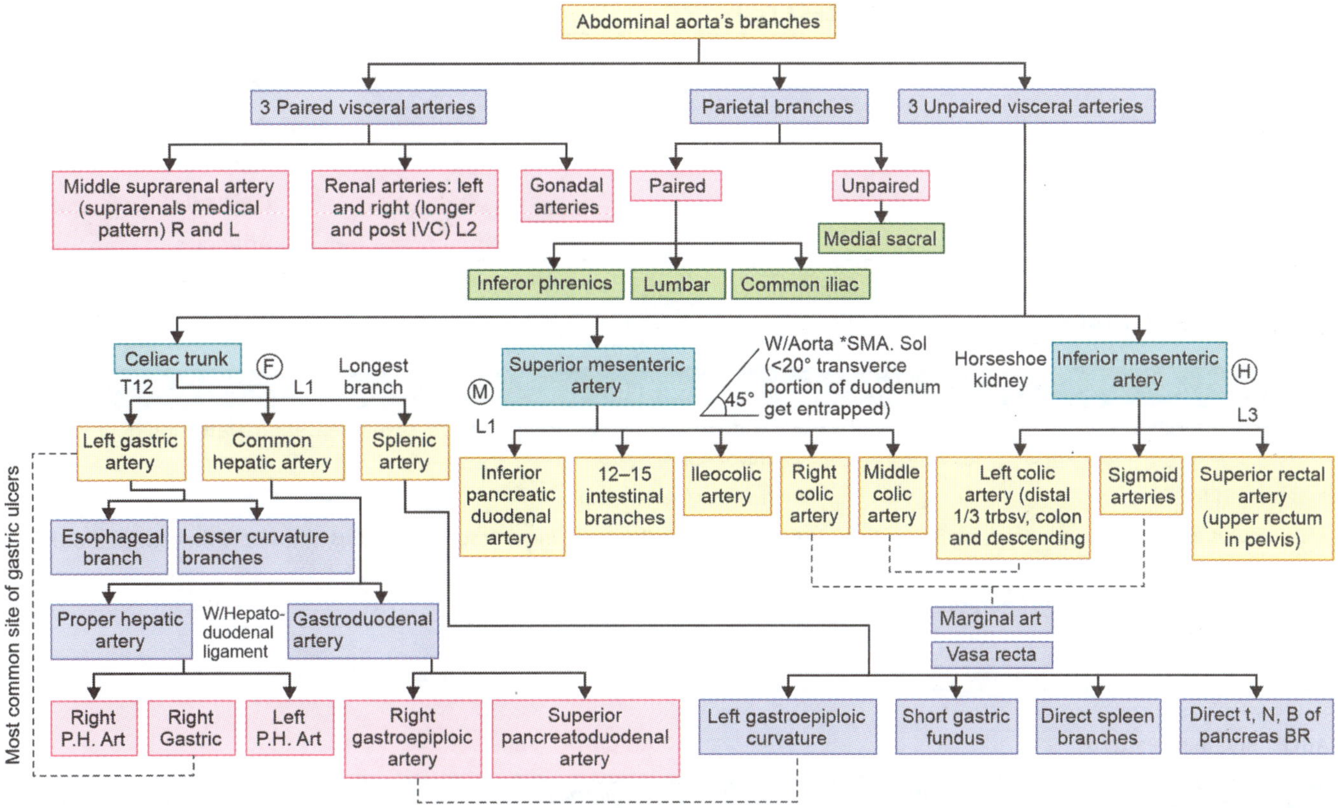

Abdominal aorta's branches
3 Paired visceral arteries
Parietal branches
3 Unpaired visceral arteries
Middle suprarenal artery (suprarenals medical pattern) R and L
Renal arteries: left and right (longer and post IVC) L2
Gonadal arteries
Paired
Unpaired
Medial sacral
Inferor phrenics
Lumbar
Common iliac
Celiac trunk
F
T12
L1
Longest branch
Superior mesenteric artery
M
L1
W/Aorta *SMA. Sol (<20° transverce portion of duodenum get entrapped)
45°
Horseshoe kidney
Inferior mesenteric artery
H
L3
Left gastric artery
Common hepatic artery
Splenic artery
Most common site of gastric ulcers
Esophageal branch
Lesser curvature branches
Proper hepatic artery
W/Hepato-duodenal ligament
Gastroduodenal artery
Right P.H. Art
Right Gastric
Left P.H. Art
Right gastroepiploic artery
Superior pancreatoduodenal artery
Inferior pancreatic duodenal artery
12–15 intestinal branches
Ileocolic artery
Right colic artery
Middle colic artery
Left colic artery (distal 1/3 trbsv, colon and descending
Sigmoid arteries
Superior rectal artery (upper rectum in pelvis)
Marginal art
Vasa recta
Left gastroepiploic curvature
Short gastric fundus
Direct spleen branches
Direct t, N, B of pancreas BR

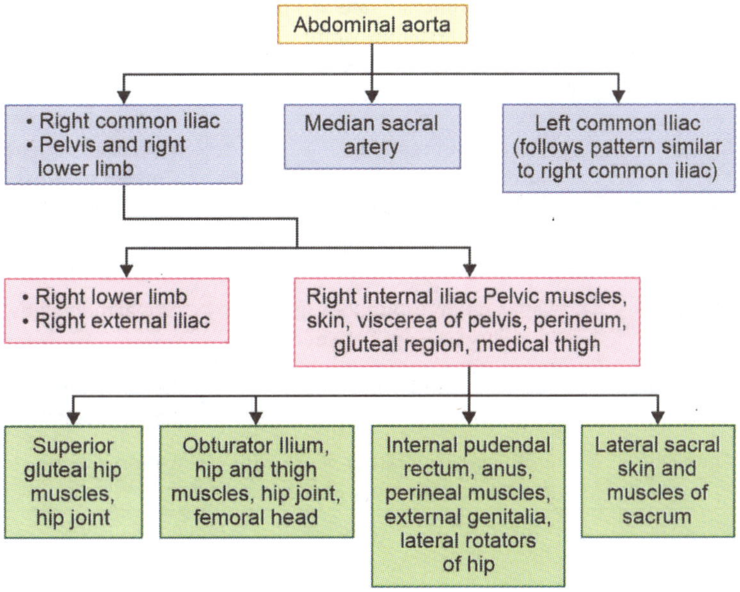

Abdominal aorta
- Right common iliac
- Pelvis and right lower limb

Median sacral artery
Left common Iliac (follows pattern similar to right common iliac)
- Right lower limb
- Right external iliac

Right internal iliac Pelvic muscles, skin, viscerea of pelvis, perineum, gluteal region, medical thigh
Superior gluteal hip muscles, hip joint
Obturator Ilium, hip and thigh muscles, hip joint, femoral head
Internal pudendal rectum, anus, perineal muscles, external genitalia, lateral rotators of hip
Lateral sacral skin and muscles of sacrum

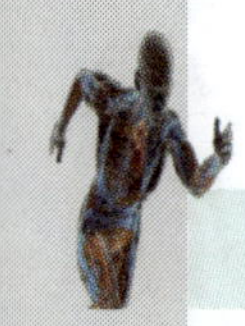

PHYSIOLOGY

IMPORTANT RECENT POINTS (INCLUDES LATEST QS)

Histamine is produced by	Mast cell
Prolactin is inhibited by	Dopamine
Highest percent of blood is present in this vessel	Veins
Maximum surface area for this vessel	Capillaries
Maximum resistance for this vessel	Arterioles

SENSORY SPINAL TRACTS

0.75	Sensation carried
• Ventral/anterior STT	• Crude touch/itching, tickle pressure, sexual sensation, Detection of pressure (Barognosis)
• Lateral STT	• Pin prick/pain, temp
• Fasciculus gracilis (medial) sacral, lumbar region	• Fine touch, vibration, fine pressure, conscious proprioception, stereognosis, 2-point discrimina
• Fasciculus cuneatus (lateral) (thoracic, cervical region)	• Vibration joint/position sense
• CST	• Smoothness and coordination of movt (Skilled movements)

TABLE: Breathing Patterns

	Condition	Description	Causes
	Eupnea Tachypnea Bradypnea	Normal breathing rate and pattern Increased respiratory rate Decreased respiratory rate	Fever, anxiety, exercise, shock Sleep, drugs, metabolic disorder, head injury, stroke
	Apnea Hyperpnea Cheyne-Stokes	Absence of breathing Normal rate, but deep respirations Gradual increases and decreases in respirations with periods of apnea	Deceased patient, head injury, stroke Emotional stress, diabetic ketoacidosis Increasing intracranial pressure, brain stem injury
	Biot's	Rapid, deep respirations (gasps) with short pauses between sets	Spinal meningitis, many CNS causes, head injury
	Kussmaul's	Tachypnea and hyperpnea	Renal failure, metabolic acidosis, diabetic ketoacidosis
	Apneustic	Prolonged inspiratory phase with shortened expiratory phase	Lesion in brain stem

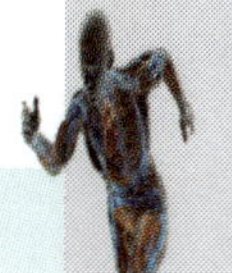

CUTANEOUS MECHANORECEPTORS

Four Types of Mechanoreceptors for Sensing Touch and Pressure

- **Meissner's corpuscles:** Texture and slow vibrations (5-40 Hz)
- **Merkel's cell (slow adapting):** Sustained pressure and touch
- **Ruffini corpuscles (slow adapting):** Sustained pressure
- **Pacinian corpuscles (rapidly adapting):** Deep pressure and fast vibrations (60–300 Hz)

Mechanoreceptors/Exteroceptors

Type of receptor	Location	Sensory modality	Nerve fibres
Non-encapsulated receptors			
Free nerve ending	Epidermis, cornea, gut, dermis, ligaments, joint capsules, bone, dental pulp	Pain, crude touch, pressure, heat/cold	AδC
Merkel disc	Hairless skin	Touch	Aβ
Hair follicle receptors	Hairy skin	Light movement on skin (Touch)	Aβ
Meissner's corpuscles	Dermal papillae in finger tips (skin of palm/sole), Basis of **BRAILLE**, Topognosis, Texture	Fine well localized touch, tactile, Vibration <80Hz	Aβ
Pacinian corpuscles	Dermis ligaments, joint capsules, peritoneum, ext. genitalia	Fast Vibration, Deep pressure	Aβ
Ruffini ending	Dermis of hairy skin	Stretch (sustained pressure)	Aβ
NM spindles	Skeletal muscle	Stretch–muscle length	Aα Aβ
Neurotendinous spindles	Tendons	Compression-muscle tension	Aα

NOCICEPTORS

- **Mechanical nociceptors:** Respond to strong pressure from a sharp object
- **Thermal nociceptors:** Activated by skin temperature above 42°C or severe cold

Contd...

- **Chemical nociceptors:** Responds to various chemical such as bradykinin, Histamine, high acidity
- **Polymodal nociceptors:** Responds to combination of these stimuli

PAIN FIBERS

Impulses from nociceptors transmitted via two fibers:

- **A delta fibers-thin myelinated (2–5 um in diameter):** Release glutamate and is responsible for **First pain/Fast pain/Epicritic pain. Localized, superficial pain.**
- **C fibers- Unmyelinated (0.4–1.2 um in diameter):** Release a combination of glutamate and substance P and is responsible **for second pain/slow pain/Protopathic pain. Dull, poorly localized, Visceral pain.**

SOMATOSENSORY PATHWAYS AND THEIR PRIMARY FUNCTION

- **Dorsal column pathway:** Fine touch, vibration and proprioception, two point discrimination
- **Ventrolateral spinothalamic tract:** Pain and temperature, Crude touch, Detection of pressure (**Barognosis**)
- **Spinocerebellar tract:** Skilled movement
- **Corticospinal tract:** Tone and pressure (anterior CST), fine skill movement, precision (lateral CST)

TABLE: Cell cycle

- **Order of cell cycle:** G1 → S → G2 → M → G1 → G0
- DNA and centromere doubling seen in this phase of cell cycle: **S phase**
- Cell division/doubling of cell seen in this phase of cell cycle: **M phase**
- **Cell hypertrophy is due to:** Arrest of cell cycle before G2 phase (S–G2 phase)
- **Cell hyperplasia is due to:** Arrest of cell cycle before going into quiescent phase (G0) → Increase in number of cells
- Most sensitive phase of cell cycle for radiation injury: **G2-M phase**

TABLE: Cell and cell membrane

Thickness: **7–10 nm**
Main constituent is the **protein.** Protein: **50–60%** Lipid: **30–40%**
Protein: **Lipid ratio is 2:1**
Lipids are regular but asymetrically arranged.
Membrane lipids are **amphiphatic.**
They are arranged as a **bilayer.**
Signal transduction and enzyme activation are the functions of **Phospholipid part.**

Contd...

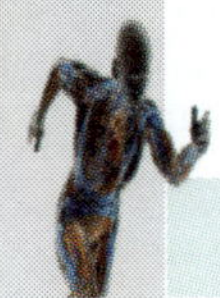

The Fluidity of the cell membrane is increased by **Poly unsaturated fatty acids.**

RBC membrane is especially having **spectrin** (maintains integrity) and **glycophorin.**

Lipid bilayer acts as a **gel.**

Resting membrane potential is due to: K^+

Resting membrane potential is close to **isoelectric potential of:** Cl^- (i.e. –70 mV)

IPSP is due to **Cl^- influx or K^+ efflux or both**

EPSP is due to **Na influx**

For action potential; threshold stimulus is required

Nerve conduction follows All or None phenomenon.

Action Potential

Axon hillock and initial axon segment has the lowest threshold potential in a **nerve fiber.**

Nerve impulse travels in the direction only at synapse.

RMP is due to - **Potassium**

IPSP is due to **Chloride/K^+**

Amplitude is due to **Na^+**

Equilibrium potential of an ion is calculated by: **Nernst equation**

Nernst potential across cell membrane
For K^+ ion: –90 mV
For Na^+ ion: +60 mB
For Cl^- ion: –70 mV

TABLE: Cell organelles

Nissl bodies: Group of ribosomes in neurons which are utilized for protein synthesis

Synthesis of lipids occurs in **Agranular Endoplasmic Reticulum.**

Synthesis of proteins occurs in **Rough ER.**

Intracellular sorting and packing is done in **Golgi complex.**

Cell shape and motility are a function of **Microtubules.**

Catabolism of H_2O_2 is a function of **Peroxisomes.**

Site of ATP synthesis is **Mitochondria.**

GOLDEN POINTS

- Pacinian corpuscles consist of unmyelinated endings with a sensory nerve fiber of 2 um in diameter
- Surfactant is produced by: **Type II cells (Granular pneumocytes)**
- Alveoli are mainly lined by: **Type I cells (95% surface area)**
- Type II alveolar cells make up only 5% of surface area, they represent approximately 60% of epithelial cells in alveoli

Contd...

- Brunner gland secretes: **Alkaline mucus**
- Pyloric gland secretes: **Thin viscid Mucus (protects stomach wall from digestion by gastric enzymes)**
- Part of intestine secreting enteropeptidase: **Duodenum (activates trypsinogen)**
- Most abundant form of vitamin D in plasma: **25-Hydroxyvitamin D [25 (OH)D]**
- Vitamin D form found in skin: **7-Dehydrocholesterol**
- Upon exposure to UV light 7-dehydrocholesterol is converted to Vitamin D3 (Cholecalciferol)
- Most common form of supplemental vitamin A used: **Al-trans retinyl acetate**
- Largest protein in body: **Titin**
- Volume remained in lung after normal expiration: **Functional residual capacity**
- Volatile acids in plasma is buffered by: **Hemoglobin**
- Vibration sense is carried by: **Pacinian corpuscles**
- Bohr's effect: **OHDC is inversely proportional to both acidity and to concentration of CO_2**
- Haldane effect: **Oxygenation of blood in the lungs displaces carbon dioxide from hemoglobin which increases the removal of carbon dioxide**
- Heart rate if Purkinje fibers became the pacemaker of the heart: **15–40 bpm**
- If SA node discharges at 0.00s, when will it normally arrive at the AV bundle (bundle of His): **0.12 second (0.03 from atria + 0.09 from AV node)**
- Structure with the slowest rate of conduction of the cardiac action potential: **AV bundle**
- Frank starling law of the heart: **Increase in venous return causes increased cardiac output**
- Mean systemic filling pressure: **7 mm Hg**
- Nephrons reaches to adult value at: **36 weeks gestation**
- Below this age BP of 120/80 is considered as hypertension: **<12 years**
- In newborn, renal tubular concentrating capacity reaches adult value at: **1 year**
- Normal GFR as adult value is reached at: **2 years**
- Best method of estimating creatinine assay: **Enzyme assay**

Total body water is **60–70%** of total body weight

- **2/3rd** of fluid is Intra Cellular Fluid; **1/3rd** is Extra Cellular Fluid.
- Evans blue dye is used to measure: **Plasma volume**
- Normal pH of blood: **7.35–7.45**
- Normal plasma protein ratio: **1.7:1**
- Life span of normal RBC: **120 days**

Contd...

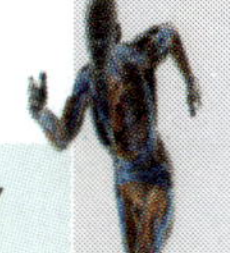

- Platelets are stored at: **Room temperature**
- Mentzer index: **Used to differentiate iron deficiency anemia from beta thalassemia**

TABLE: Measurement of body fluid

Total body water *Mn: DATA*	D_2O (Deuterium oxide/heavy water)- MC used Aminopyrene, Tritium oxide, Antipyrine,
ECF volume *Mn: No SIM*	Sucrose Insulin (most accurate) Mannitol Na^+ Thiosulfate
ICF volume	**Indirect method:** ICF = TBW – ECF *(best done by D_2O – Inulin)*
Interstitial fluid	**Indirect method: ISF = ECF – Plasma volume**
Plasma volume *Mn: AB-P*	Albumin (Radiolabeled I^{125}), Evans Blue
Total blood volume	Plasma volume x 100/100-Hct

TABLE: Na^+ K^+ ATPase pump

- Na^+ K^+ ATPase pump is an active, electrogenic pump moves 3 Na^+ ions outside and in place 2 K^+ ions inside utilizing ATP. It helps in intrusion of K^+.
- It accounts for 20% of energy utilized by cells.
- Thus its coupling ratio is 3:2
- Extracellular binding site is Ouabain binding site
- Its activity is inhibited by ouabain and related cardiac glycosides (digitalis)
- It is a P type ATPase (super family of cation transporters)
- Also called E1/E2 type ATPase responsible for carrying ions across cell membranes.
- **Type:** Heterodimer heterogeneous (α & β subunit)

It is an example of active transport
- Generation of Action Potential by
- Nerve cells not neuroglia
- Muscles
- Contractile tissue
- Glands

TABLE: Important RMP

RBC	**–12 mV**
Rods & cones	**–40 mV**
SA node	**–55 mV**
Smooth muscle	**–50 to –60 mV**
Cardiac muscle (Single Fiber)	**–85 to –95 mV**
Skeletal muscle	**–90 mV**
Nerve fibre	**–90 mV**
Inner hair cells	**–150 mV**

Contd...

TABLE: Neurotransmitters

Purines
- Adenosine
- ATP

Lipids and Gases
- Nitric oxide (NO)
- Carbon monoxide
- Cannabinoids

Biogenic Amines
- Catecholamines: Dopamine, norepinephrine and epinephrine
- Indolamines
- Serotonin and Histamine

Amino Acids
- GABA
- Glycine
- Aspartate
- Glutamate

Neuropeptides
- Substance P
- Endorphins and Enkephalins
- Somatostatin, gastrin, cholecystokinin, oxytocin, vasopressin, luteinizing hormone releasing hormone (LHRH)

TABLE: Blood brain barrier (BBB)

- Membranes are generally **asymmetrical**
- Plasma membranes is composed mainly of **proteins**
- Protein content: **55%**
- Phospholipid: **25% × 42%,** 3% carbohydrate
- Function of phospholipid is **transduction of signals and enzyme activation.**
- Lipids and Proteins in cell membrane interact by **Hydrogen bonds.**
- Fluidity of membranes depends in **lipid content.**
- **Saturated fatty acids** increase transition temperature and decrease fluidity
- **Unsaturated Fatty acids** decrease transition temperature and increase fluidity
- Cerebral blood vessels are unique in that the junctions between vascular endothelial cells are nearly fused. The paucity of pores is responsible for what is termed the **Blood Brain Barrier**
- The lipid barrier allows the passage of lipid soluble substances but restrict movements of those that are ionized or have large molecular weight.
- CO_2, O_2 and lipid soluble substances (such as most anesthetics) freely enter the brain, whereas most ions, proteins and large substances such as mannitol penetrate poorly.

Contd...

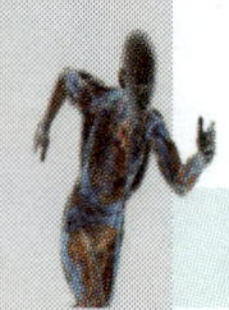

- Water moves freely across the BBB.
- **Mannitol** an osmotically active substance that does not normally cross the BBB, cause a sustained decrease in brain water content and is often used to decrease brain volume.
- BBB may be disrupted by severe Hypertension, tumors, trauma, stroke, infection, marked hypercapnia, hypoxia and sustained seizure activity.

TABLE: Important tests

Decline in serum Ca^{2+} levels show signs of increasing neuromuscular hyperexcitability followed by hypocalcemic tetany.
Lab values: Decreased serum Ca^{2+}
Increased serum phosphate
Decreased urinary Phosphate excretion

Clinical tests for endocrine abnormalities: Radioimmunoassays for T4, T3, TSH, cortisol, Ca^{2+}, etc.

Glucose Tolerance test: Check a fasting blood sugar level, then have patient drink a 75 g glucose solution. Re-draw blood at 30 min, 1 hr., and 2 hrs. If blood glucose level is >200 mg/dL at 2 hours, then highly suggestive of diabetes.

Dexamethasone suppression test: Dexamethasone, a synthetic steroid, is given to the patient at 11 p.m. The following day blood samples are collected at 4 p.m. and 11 p.m. The normal response is a decrease in circulating adrenal steroid hormones. Those with Cushing's will have continued elevated levels.

Radioiodine injection: Hyperthyroidism will show an increase uptake.

TABLE: Cells of stomach and their function

- G cells secretes - **Gastrin**
- I cells secretes - **CCK**
- S cells secretes - **Secretin**
- D cells secretes - **Somatostatin**
- Parietal cells secretes - **Intrinsic factor**
- Chief cells secretes - **Pepsin**

IMPORTANT PHYSIOLOGICAL FACTS

In nephron most of the reabsorption occurs at which portion: **PCT** (~75%)

Length of proximal convoluted tubule: **15 mm**

Length of distal convoluted tubule: **5 mm**

Length of collecting duct: **20 mm**

Location of macula densa: **DCT**

ADH produced by- **Supraoptic nucleus of hypothalamus**

Oxytocin produced by: Paraventricular nucleus of hypothalamus

Teeth grinding is seen in which stage of sleep: **NREM II**

Contd...

Night terror is seen in which stage of NREM: **Stage III & IV**

Sleep walking is seen in which stage of NREM: **Stage III & IV**

Other name of alpha wave: **Berger wave (discovered by Hans Berger)**

Best test for sleep disorder: **Polysomnography**

Bohr's effect: Fall in pH due to increase **pCO_2**, decreases oxygen affinity of Hb
Haldane effect: Binding of O_2 to Hb reduces affinity of Hb to **CO_2**.

Most important stimulus for central chemoreceptor: **↑ $PaCO_2$ (Inc CO_2, Dec O2)**

Most important stimulus for peripheral chemoreceptor: **↓ PO_2, ↑ CO_2**

The partial pressure of O_2 (PaO_2) at sea level: **160 mm Hg.**
The partial pressure of CO_2 (pCO_2) at sea level: **0.23 mm Hg.**
Mean pulmonary arterial pressure: **16 mm Hg**

Mean pulmonary capillary pressure averages about: **7 mm Hg.**
Mean pressure in the aorta: **100 mm Hg.**
GLUT receptor located on sperm: **GLUT 5**

Alpha cells of pancreas secretes: **Glucagon**
Beta cells of pancreas secretes: **Insulin and amylin**
Delta cells of pancreas secretes: **Somatostatin**

Starch is hydrolyzed in mouth by: **Ptylin**

TABLE: Sleep waves

Wave *(Mn: D-TAB)*	Condition	Frequency
• Delta wave	Deep sleep	0.5–3 Hz
• Theta wave	Light sleep	4–7 Hz
• Alpha wave	Relaxed, awake	8–13 Hz
• Beta wave	Excited, active	14–30 Hz

TABLE: Sleep stages

Stage	EEG waves	Eye movement
Awake/alert	Beta (eye open) Alpha (eye closed)	Irregular
I-NREM	Alpha + Theta waves	Burst of rolling
II-NREM	Theta waves Sleep spindles K- complex	Alpha like burst
III-NREM	Theta, Delta synchronization	Fixed
IV-NREM	Delta (slowest wave)	Fixed
REM (paradoxical sleep)	Mixed frequency, Low voltage (theta, alpha > Beta)	Darting movements Active dreaming (+) Nightmares

TABLE: Important reflexes

Reflex	Stimulus	Response
Cushing reflex	Inc ICT (>33 mm Hg)	Inc BP, Bradypnea, Bradycardia
Bainbridge reflex	Atrial distention due to rapid infusion of blood/ Saline	Reflex tachycardia
Bezold-Jarisch coronary chemoreflex	5HT injection, Nicotine in coronary artery	Apnea, ↓BP, ↓HR
Hering-Breuer inflation reflex	Steady lung inflation	↑ Expiration
Hering-Breuer inflation reflex	Marked deflation of lung	↓ Expiration

TABLE: Muscle fiber types

Type I	Type II
Oxidative, slow fibers	Glycolytic, fast fibers
Easily excited	Difficult to excite
Less fatigability	More fatigability
Slow glycogen depletion	Fast glycogen depletion
Used in marathon runner	Used in sprinter (100 meter) runner
Major fuel: **ATP**	Major fuel: **Phosphate**

BIOCHEMISTRY

AMINO ACID CLASSIFICATION

• **Simple**	Glycine, Alanine
• **Branched chain**	Leucine, Isoleucine, Valine
• **Sulphur containing**	Cysteine, Methionine
• **Hydroxyl containing**	Serine, Threonine
• **Amide**	Glutamine, Asparagine
• **Acidic AA**	Aspartic acid, Glutamic acid
• **Basic AA**	Histidine, Arginine, Lysine
• **-OH containing**	Serine, Threonine, Tyrosine
• **Serine analog drugs**	Cycloserine, Azaserine

IMPORTANT RECENT POINTS (INCLUDES LATEST QS)

Wernicke encephalopathy is due to deficiency of	• Thiamine
Strenuous exercise is not done in this glycogen storage disease	• Mc Ardle disease
Vitamin which is most potent anti-oxidant	• Vitamin E

Contd...

Vitamin which helps in iron absorption	• Vitamin C
AA that accelerate ageing	• Homocysteine
AA that decreases ageing	• Cysteine, Taurine
Bend in DNA structure	• Glycine
AA which absorbs UV light	• Tryptophan (Max), Tyrosine, Phenylalanine
MC type of albinism	• OCA 2 (Oculocutaneous Albinism type II)

- Keshan disease is due to deficiency of: **Selenium**
- Kashin-Beck disease: **Due to excess of selenium**
- Menkes disease: **Due to deficiency of copper**
- Acrodermatitis enteropathica: **Due to deficiency of zinc (AR condition)**
- Vitamin having only animal source: **Vitamin B_{12}**
- Vitamin having antioxidant property: **Vitamin E**
- Physiological uncoupler: **Thyroid hormones, unconjugated bilirubin, long chain fatty acid**
- Sickle cell anemia is caused by point mutation in β globin chain
- At 6th position the hydrophilic **glutamic acid gets replaced with valine** (Hydrophobic)
- Hyperammonemia type 1 is due to deficiency of this enzyme: **Carbamoyl Phosphate Synthase I**
- Tomcat urine smell is seen in: **Multiple carboxylase deficiency**
- Boiled cabbage urine smell is seen in: **Hypermethioninemia**
- Smallest and simplest amino acid: **Glycine**
- Storage form of folate: **N-methyl folate**
- Energy for the urea cycle come from: **Fat metabolism**
- Precursor of all sphingolipids: **Ceramide**
- Type of bilirubin is found in neonatal jaundice: **Indirect or unconjugated**
- This amino acid is a phenol: **Tyrosine**
- This vitamin is an important component of rhodopsin: **Vitamin A**
- Part of the 30s ribosome binds to the Shine-Dalgarno sequence: **16s subunit**
- This test is used to determine whether a gene is expressed: **Northern blotting**
- This complex of the ETC contains Cu^{+}: **Complex 4**
- Inhibitors of complex IV of the ETC: **1. Cyanide, 2. CO, 3. Azide**
- Gluconeogenesis is inhibited by: **Insulin**
- **Gluconeogenesis** occurs in both cytoplasm and mitochondria
- Mercaptopurine is – **Nucleotide analogue**

Contd...

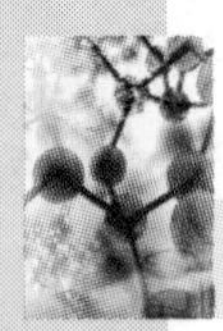

- Source of ATP in RBC cell: **EMP pathway**
- Net ATP produced in anaerobic glycolysis: **2 ATP**
- Net ATP produced in aerobic glycolysis: **7 ATP**
- Cancer cells derive nutrition from **glycolysis.**
- Allosteric inhibition is seen in: **G-6-P, F-6-P**
- Erythrocytes lack **mitochondria** (all the cell organelles)
- Fluoroacetate inhibits aconitase enzyme: **Non-competitive reaction**
- Arsenite inhibits alpha-**Ketoglutarate dehydrogenase** enzyme–**Noncompetitive reaction.**
- Malonate inhibits succinate dehydrogenase enzyme–**Competitive reaction**
- Internal respiration is **exergonic** and **catabolic** and it uses **cytochromes b, c1, c, a, a3**
- Von Gierke's disease is due to **G-6-P Deficiency**
- Pompe's disease lysosomal a1-4, a1-6 glucosidase acid maltase deficiency.
- **Mc Ardle's disease** is muscle phosphorylase deficiency.
- **Acetyl CoA** is not a substrate for gluconeogenesis and cannot be converted back to glucose directly.
- **Gaucher disease** is due to Beta Glucocerebrosidase deficiency.
- Foam cells and sphingomyelinase deficiency is seen in **Niemann-Pick disease**
- Type 1 familial hypolipoprotinemia is due to deficiency of **lipoprotein lipase deficiency.**
- Palmitoleic acid is derivative of which family: **ω7 family**
- Lipoprotein which transport cholesterol from liver to plasma: **VLDL**
- Most important apoprotein in HDL: **Apo A-I**
- Most important apoprotein in chylomicrons: **Apo B-48**
- De novo synthesis of fatty acids occurs in the **cytosol**
- Malic enzyme forms malic acid from pyruvic acid in the presence of **CO_2 & NADPH.**
- Long chain fatty acid penetrate the inner mitochondrial membrane only in combination with **carnitine.**
- Beta-oxidation of odd chain fatty acid produces **acetyl CoA propionyl CoA.**
- Refsum's disease occurs due to deficiency of **phytanic alpha oxidase.**
- Alkaptonuria deficiency is: **Homogentisate oxidase**
- **Liver** is the only organ which produces ketone bodies (but never utilizes it)
- **Gout** is metabolic disorder of purine metabolism.
- Mutation in sickle cell disease: **Base pair substitution**
- **LDL** has maximum cholesterol content

Contd...

- Conversion of norepinephrine to epinephrine: **Demethylation**
- Enzyme required for demethylation: **Phenylethanolamine-N-methyltransferase**
- Enzyme is used to convert phenylalanine to tyrosine: **Phenylalanine hydroxylase**
- Beta oxidation of odd chain fatty acid produces: **Acetyl CoA and Propionyl CoA**
- Complete HGPRT deficiency cause **Lesch-Nyhan syndrome**
- Partial HGPRT deficiency causes **Kelley-Seegmiller syndrome**
- Normal growth require **proto-oncogenes** not oncogenes
- DNA ligase and primase are used in **DNA replication**
- The **sigma sub unit** enables RNA polymerase to recognize promoter regions on DNA.
- **Template** is required for protein and nucleic acid synthesis
- Alzheimer's, cystic fibrosis and prion diseases occur due to **protein misfolding**
- **Microsatellites** are tandem repeats of one to six nucleotide scattered throughout the genome.
- After digestion by restriction endonucleases the DNA ends can be ligated by **DNA-ligase.**
- **DNA microarrays** is used for detection in DNA sequences and Gene expression.
- Proline and glycine have the least tendency to form **Alpha-helix.**
- Structural proteins are usually fibrous proteins, transport and functional protein are usually **globular**
- Simple globular proteins are **albumin and globulin.**
- Adenyl cyclase, guanylate cyclase and glycogen synthase enzymes are activated by **calcium and calmodulin.**
- **Phenylketonuria** is caused by deficiency of phenylalanine hydroxylase & dihydrobiopterin reductase.
- **Alkaptonuria** is due to defective homogentisate 1, 2-dioxygenase.
- Maple syrup urine disease is deficiency of branched chain **alpha keto acid dehydrogenase.**
- **Succinyl CoA** is formed by valine, isoleusine, methionine.
- **Niacin** in biologically active form of NAD+ & NADP+.
- **Vit A** intoxication leads to demineralization of bone, hypercalcemia, hyperostosis.
- **ATP** is used in a set of reactions that converts chemical energy into light energy.
- **Cobalt** containing vit B12 is found only in food of animal origin and is absorbed from distal ileum.
- **Vitamin B12** & **folic acid** supplements treat pernicious anemia by increasing DNA synthesis in bone marrow
- Niacin sparing amino acid: **Tryptophan**

Contd...

- Which bases are purine? **Adenine and Guanine**
- Which bases are pyrimidines? **Cytosine, Uracil, Thymine**
- What enzyme is deficient in Severe Combined Immunodeficiency Disease (SCID)?
- Adenosine Deaminase
- The start codon AUG codes for which amino acid? **Methionine**
- Which RNA is the most abundant?: **rRNA – (Mn: r = rampant)**
- Which RNA is the longest? **mRNA – (Mn: M = massive)**
- Which RNA is the smallest? **tRNA – (Mn: t = tiny)**
- Which organelle is the site for labeling specific proteins for the lysosome? **Golgi apparatus**
- What type of collagen makes the basement membrane? **Type IV**
- Collagen is loaded with tons of which amino acids? **Proline and Lysine**
- What enzyme is deficient in Fructose Intolerance? **Aldolase B**
- What enzyme is deficient in Essential Fructosuria? **Fructokinase**
- **Tyrosinemia types and Enzyme defect**
  - **I: Fumarylacetoacetate hydroxylase** *(hepatorenal)*
  - **II: tyrosine transaminase** *(oculocutaneous)*
  - **III: PHPP hydroxylase** *(neonatal)*

• **Nitisinone** acts by inhibiting this enzyme • Tyrosine → PHPP → Homogentisic acid	**Parahydroxyphenyl Pyruvate Hydroxylase To treat hereditary tyrosinemia type I, Alkaptonuria**
• Folate trap is due to deficiency of	**B_{12}**
• Folate trap increases the risk of this disease	**Acute coronary syndrome**
• **Calcium** acts as cofactor for which enzymes	**Lipase, Lecithinase**
• **Copper** acts as cofactor for this enzyme	**Cyt C oxidase, Lysil oxidase, AA oxidase, SOD, Tyrosinase**
• **Iron** acts as cofactor for this enzyme	**Succinate DeH**
• **Zinc** acts as cofactor for these enzymes	**ALD, ALP, ALA dehydratase, carbonic anhydrase, LDH**

TABLE: Special group attached with amino acids

Amino acid	Special group
Arginine	Guanidinium
Phenylalanine	Benzene
Tyrosine	Phenol
Histidine	Imidazole
Proline	Pyrrolidine
Methionine	Thioether linkage
Tryptophan	Indole
Cysteine	Thioalcohol (-SH)

TABLE: Pathways and their rate limiting enzymes

Pathway	Rate limiting enzyme
• **Glycolysis**	*Phosphofructokinase*
• **Glycogenesis**	*Glycogen synthase*
• **Glycogenolysis**	*Phosphorylase*
• **Cholesterol synthesis**	*HMG - COA Reductase*
• **Ketone body formation**	*HMG - COA synthase*
• **Bile acid synthesis**	*7-a-hydroxylase*
• **Fatty acid synthesis**	*Acetyl COA carboxylase*
• **Uric acid synthesis**	*Xanthine oxidase*
• **Urea cycle**	*CPS I*
• **Pyrimidine synthesis**	*CPS II*

TABLE: Cycles and their location

Mitochondria Mn: KEBOK	Cytoplasm	Both mitochondria and cytoplasm
Krebs cycle	Glycolysis	Gluconeogenesis
ETC	Glycogenesis	Urea synthesis
Bet oxidation of FA	Glycogenolysis	Heme synthesis
Oxidative phosphorylation	HMP Shunt	
Ketogenesis	FA synthesis	
	Cholesterol synthesis	
	Bile acid/Salt synthesis	

TABLE: GLUT receptors, their location and function

Receptor	Location on tissue	Function
GLUT 1	Brain, kidney, colon, placenta, RBC	Glucose uptake
GLUT 2	Liver, pancreatic beta cell, small intestine, Kidney	Rapid uptake or release of glucose
GLUT 3	Brain, kidney and placenta	Glucose uptake
GLUT 4	Heart, skeletal muscles, adipose tissue	Insulin-stimulated glucose uptake
GLUT 5	Small intestine	Absorption of glucose

Contd...

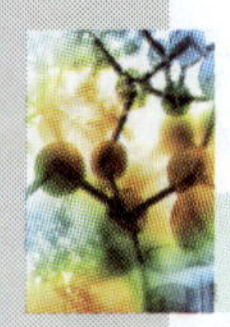

TABLE: Lysosomal storage disease and deficient enzymes

- Hurler's syndrome: **Alpha-L-iduronidase deficiency**
- Hunter's syndrome: **Iduronate-2-sulfatase deficiency**
- Gaucher's: **Glucocerebrosidase deficiency**
- Farber's disease: **Ceramidase deficiency**
- Fabry disease: **Alpha Galactosidase-A**
- Tay-sachs: **Hexosaminidase A deficiency**
- Sandhoff disease: **β-Hexosaminidase A and B**
- Metachromatic leukodystrophy: **Arylsulfatase A enzyme deficiency**
- Krabbe disease: **Galactocerebrosidase**

MAJOR APOLIPOPROTEINS

- **Chylomicron:** A, B48, CII, E *(least protein, max size, max density)*
- **VLDL:** Apo B100, CII, E
- **LDL:** Apo B100
- **HDL:** Apo A1

TABLE: Source of energy during starvation

STAGE	I	II	III
Duration	1st 2–3 days	Up to 2 weeks (longest)	<1 week
Energy source	Carbohydrate	Fats	Proteins
Metabolism	Initially Glycogenolysis then gluconeogenesis	Lipolysis and ketone body formation	Breakdown of protein

TABLE: Amino acid at a glance: Total AA = 20 in number

Essential AA (8): *Can't be synthesized. (Mn: TV TILL 8 PM)*	**Semi-essential AA:** *Can be synthesized under normal condition as per demand.*	**Non-Essential AA:** *synthesized in body readily*
Threonine, Valine, Tryptophan, Isoleucine, Lysine, Leucine, Phenylalanine, Methionine	Histidine Arginine	The remaining 10 AA are Non-essential.

TABLE: Vitamin B, their other names and disease entities due to deficiency

Vitamin	Other name	Deficiency causes
Vit B1	Thiamine	***Beriberi,*** *Wernicke's encephalopathy*
Vit B2	Riboflavin	Angular stomatitis, cheilosis, dermatitis, Glossitis
Vit B_3	Niacin	Pellagra (4D's- Dementia, Diarrhea, Dermatitis, Death)
Vit B_5	Pantothenic acid	Burning foot syndrome, Leiner disease
Vit B_6	Pyridoxine	Peripheral neuropathy, Sideroblastic anemia, Pellagra, Homocystinuria, Hartnup disease
Vit B_7	Biotin	Multiple carboxylase deficiency
Vit B_9	Folic acid	Megaloblastic anemia, Neural tube defect
Vit B_{12}	Cyano-cobalamin	Megaloblastic anemia, subacute combined degeneration (SACD)

Contd...

TABLE: Forms of Vitamin K

Feature	Vitamin K1	Vitamin K2	Vitamin K3
Aka	Phylloquinone	Menaquinone	Menadione
Source	Several green vegetables and prepared synthetically	Synthesized by GI bacteria, supplies 50% human requirement	Synthetic, Analog of 1, 4-naphthoquinone
Solubility	Fat soluble	Fat soluble	Diphosphate salt is Water soluble

TABLE: Urea cycle and their associated enzyme defect

Disease condition	Enzyme defect
• Hyperammonemia I	CPS I defect
• Hyperammonemia II	OTC defect
• Citrullinemia I	Argininosuccinate synthase
• Argininosuccinic aciduria	Argininosuccinate lyase
• Hyperargininemia	Arginase
• HHH Syndrome	Ornithine transporter defect

TABLE: Inborn error of metabolism and urine odor

IEM	Urine odor
• Swimming pool	Hawkinsinuria
• PKU	Mousy/musty
• Glutaric acidemia	Sweaty feet, acrid
• Isovaleric acidemia	Sweaty feet, acrid
• MSUD	Maple syrup
• Hypermethioninemia	Boiled cabbage
• Trimethylaminuria	Rotting fish
• Tyrosinemia	Boiled cabbage, rancid butter

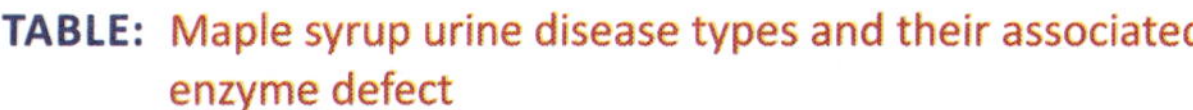

TABLE: Maple syrup urine disease types and their associated enzyme defect

Gene	Component	MSUD types
E1a	Branched chain alpha keto acid decarboxylase	Type Ia MSUD
E1b	Branched chain alpha keto acid decarboxylase	Type Ib MSUD
E2	Dihydrolipoyl transacylase	Type II MSUD
E3	Dihydrolipoamide dehydrogenase	Type III MSUD

TABLE: Inhibitors of electron transport chain

Complex	Inhibitors
• **Complex I**	Rotenone, Piericidin A, Amobarbital
• **Complex II**	Malonate, TTFA
• **Complex III**	BAL, Antimycin A, Naphthoquinone
• **Complex IV**	Na azide, HCN, CO
• **Complex V**	Atractyloside, Oligomycin

TABLE: Important tests and their application

- **Murexide test:** Uric acid
- **Rothera test:** Ketone body

Contd...

- **Biuret test:** Detect maximum 2 peptide bond
- **Hopkins cole test**: Tryptophan
- **Millions test:** Tyrosine
- **Gerhardt test:** Acetoacetic acid
- **Hay test:** Bile salt
- **Fouchet's test:** Bile pigment
- **Ehrlich test:** Urobilinogen
- **Molisch test:** for CHO
- **Guthrie $FeCl_3$ test:** PKU
- **Ames test:** Carcinogenicity due to salmonella typhimurium

TABLE: Must know points about porphyria

- MC type of porphyria: **Porphyria cutanea tarda**
- MC acute porphyria: **Acute intermittent porphyria**
- MC porphyria in child: **Erythropoietic protoporphyria**
- Erythropoietic porphyria: **Usual clinical presentation photosensitivity**
- Hepatic porphyria with cutaneous manifestation: **PCT**

FLOWCHART: Porphyria and their enzyme defect

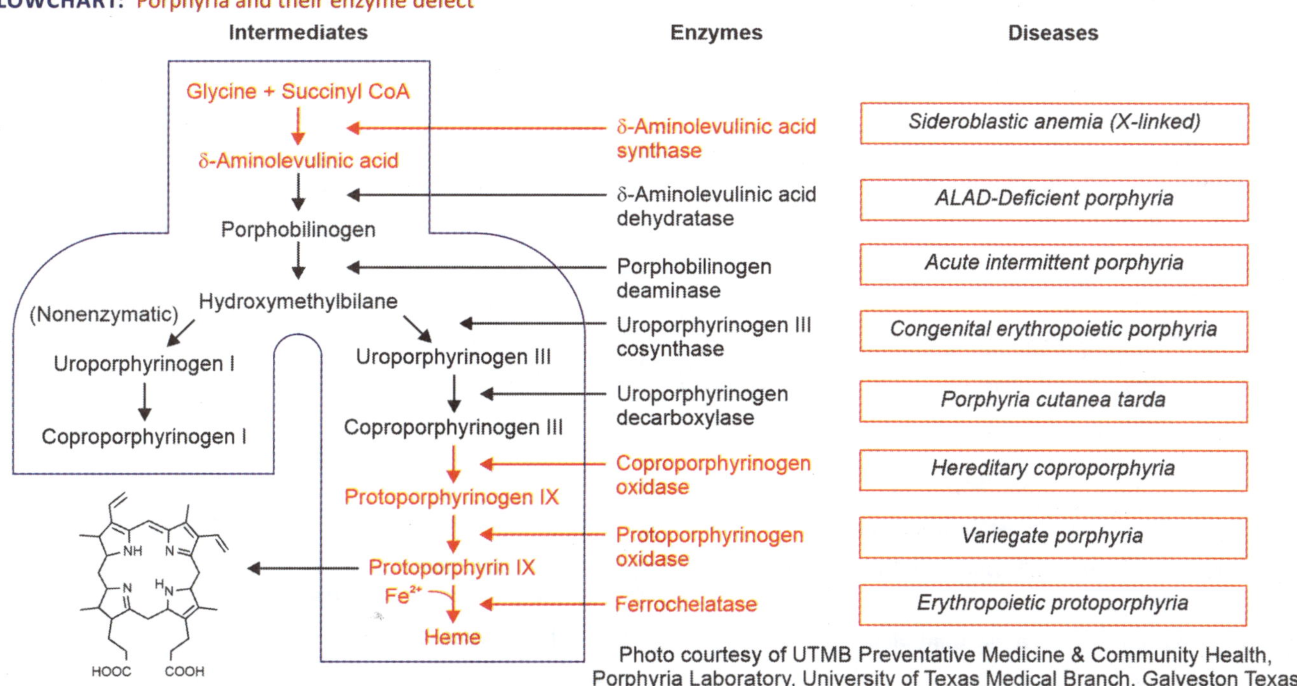

Photo courtesy of UTMB Preventative Medicine & Community Health, Porphyria Laboratory, University of Texas Medical Branch, Galveston Texas

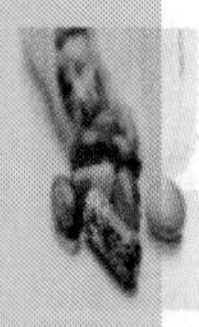

PHARMACOLOGY

IMPORTANT RECENT POINTS (INCLUDES LATEST QS)

- Phase of clinical trial which recruits healthy human volunteers: **Phase 0 and Phase 1**
- Clinical trial to assess safety and non-toxicity: **Phase I**
- Number of patients in Phase II clinical trial: **Up to 200**
- Phase which is dealing with microdosing: **Phase 0**
- Phase V clinical trial is: **Pharmacoepidemiology**
- **Maximum** parasympathetic outflow by which cranial nerve: **CN-X**
- 100% Bioavailability is seen with this route: **I.V. route**
- **Area under curve** denotes: **Extent of absorption**
- **Bioavailability** is the fraction of administered drug that reaches the systemic circulation in the unchanged form.
- **Absorption and first pass mechanism** are two important Determinants of bioavailability.
- Shortest acting steroid: **Hydrocortisone**
- Formoterol and Indacaterol: **Long acting β_2 agonist (Bronchodilator)**
- Antiepileptic with highest teratogenic potential: **Sodium Valproate**
- Drug of choice for cardiogenic shock: **Dobutamine**
- DOC for neurogenic diabetes insipidus: **Desmopressin**
- Shortest acting mydriatic agent: **Tropicamide (t½: 6 hrs)**
- Cycloplegic agent of choice in child: **Atropine 1% ointment**
- Fastest acting insulin: Insulin **Aspart, Lispro, Gluilisine**
- Peakless insulin: **Glargine, Detemir, Degludec**
- Physiological antagonist of Histamine: **Adrenaline**
- Preferred agent for treatment of ventricular arrhythmia: **Lignocaine**
- DOC for diabetic diarrhea: **Clonidine**
- DOC for brucellosis: **Doxycycline**
- DOC for Schistosomiasis: **Praziquantel**
- DOC for nasal carriers of MRSA: **Mupirocin**
- DOC for motion sickness: **Hyoscine/Scopolamine**
- Side effect of aminoglycoside: **Nm blockade, Nephrotoxicity and Ototoxicity**
- DOC for malignant hyperthermia: **Dantrolene**
- **Etomidate**: Cardiostable anesthetic
- Cevimeline is used for: **Xerostomia in Sjögren's syndrome**

Contd...

- Urine should be alkalinized for acidic drug poisoning and acidified for **basic drug poisoning.**
- Drugs having **steep DRC** have narrow therapeutic index
- **Pharmacovigilance** is the science and activities relating to the detection, assessment, understanding and prevention of adverse effect of any other possible drug related problems.
- **Ach** is the principle neurotransmitter at neuromuscular junctions as well as pre-ganglionic fibers.
- Rate limiting step in the **biosynthesis of ach: Uptake of choline**
- Most common sympatholytic drug for causing first dose effect: **selective alpha-1 blocker (e.g., Prazosin)**
- Irreversible alpha-1 adrenoceptor antagonist: **Phenoxybenzamine (DOC for pheochromocytoma)**
- Retrograde ejaculation is a known side effect of: **Alpha 1 blockers (Prazosin, Phentolamine)**
- Vasomotor reversal of dale is seen due to: **Alpha blocker followed by Epinephrine**
- Beta blocker which releases Nitric oxide: **Celiprolol, Nebivolol, Nipradilol** *(CNN)*
- DOC for beta blocker poisoning: **Glucagon**
- DOC for organophosphate poisoning: **Atropine**
- DOC for atropine poisoning: **Physostigmine**
- Pin-point pupil is seen in poisoning with: ***(Mn: POMP)*** Pontine hemorrhage, Organophosphate, Morphine and Phenol poisoning
- **Streptomycin** is contraindicated throughout pregnancy
- Low molecular weight heparin affects which factor: **Factor Xa >> IIa**
- All ACE inhibitors are prodrug EXCEPT **Captopril and Lisinopril**
- **Febuxostat:** Anti-gout and Xanthine Oxidase inhibitor
- **Drugs causing disulfiram like reaction:**
- Griseofulvin, Metronidazole, Chlorpropamide, Cefoperazone, Cefotetan, Moxalactam, Procarbazine
- **Atropine** is the antidote for–Organophosphate and carbamate poisoning.
- **Oximes** are used for Organophosphate poisoning only. Not for carbonate
- Cystoid macular edema in aphakic is caused by **Dipivefrine**.
- New drug approved for over active bladder stimulating β_3 receptors – **Mirabegron, Vibegron**
- DOC for narcolepsy – **Modafinil Topical**
- Antidepressant used for smoking cessation: **Bupropion**
- Treatment of alopecia in males – **Minoxidil/Topical**

Contd...

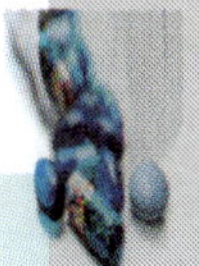

- Vasopressor of choice in pregnancy – **Ephedrine**
- Most cardio selective Beta blocker – **Nebivolol**
- Longest acting Beta blocker – **Nadolol**
- Maximum membrane stabilizing activity Beta blocker – **Propanolol**
- Earliest appearing adverse effect of digitalis – **Nausea and vomiting**
- Only oral inotropic drug- **Digoxin**
- Most widely used Beta blocker for Congestive heart failure – **Carvedilol**
- **Beta Blockers With Partial Agonistic Activity** (*Remembered as COntain Partial Agonistic Activity*)**:** Celiprolol, Oxprenolol, Pindolol, Alprenolol, Acebutolol
- MOA of hyoscine – **M3 blocker**
- **Mannitol** – Indicated in cerebral edema and is contraindicated in cerebral hemorrhage
- Oral mannitol side effect – **Osmotic diarrhea**
- Zileuton – **5-LOX inhibitor**
- Selective COX-2 inhibitor: **Etoricoxib**
- **Sodium Cromoglycate** – Mast cell stabilizer
- Common adverse effect of β_2 agonist (e.g.: Salbutamol) – **Tachycardia, Tremor**
- **Abciximab** – GpIIb/IIIa blocker. Inhibits platelet cross-linking
- DOC for GIST & CML– **Imatinib mesylate**
- DOC Benign Prostatic hypertrophy: **Tamsulosin (SHT1a#)**
- MOA finasteride – **5 alpha reductase inhibitor**
- Long acting somatostatin analogue – **Octreotide**
- Funny current blocker drug: **Ivabradine (If #). Used in angina**
- Phosphodiesterase 3 inhibitor used in heart failure: **Amrinone, Milrinone (inodilator)**
- Recently approved PDE3 inhibitor which is also a myocardial Calcium sensitizer: **Levosimendan**
- Cerebroselective calcium channel blocker: **Nimodipine (DOC for SAH)**
- Ranolazine is recently approved for: **Angina (Late Nat influx inhibitor)**
- Mechanism of action of **Fasudil**: **Rho kinase inhibitor**
- **Edaravone** is recently approved drug for: **Amyotrophic lateral sclerosis**
- **Aducanumab Lecanemab** is an agentt for: **Alzheimer's disease**
- **Livedo reticularis is** side effect of antiparkinsonian drug: **Amantadine**
- Gender specific side effect of valproate: **PCOS**

Contd...

TABLE: Drugs metabolized by acetylation → Causes SLE

These drugs are remembered as CHIPS-ABC drugs:
• Clonazepam
• Hydralazine
• Isoniazid
• Procainamide, PAS
• Sulfonamides
• Acebutolol, Amrinone, ASA
• Benzocaine
• Caffeine

TABLE: Drugs which are enzyme inducers and enzyme inhibitors

Enzyme inducers	Enzyme inhibitors
• Griseofulvin • Phenytoin • Rifampicin • Smoking • Carbamazepine • Phenobarbitone • Barbiturate • DDT	• Phenylbutazone • Erythromycin • Allopurinol, Amiodarone • Ciprofloxacin • Omeprazole • Cimetidine • Ketoconazole • Valproate
Remembered as: *GPRS Cell Phone Battery Dead*	*Mn: PEACOCK Vala*

TABLE: Anti-muscarinic drugs used in ophthalmology

Drug	Duration of effect (days)
Atropine (Preferred in Pediatrics)	7–10
Scopolamine	3–7
Homatropine	1–3
Cyclopentolate	1
Tropicamide (Preferred in adults)	0.25 days (6 hrs)

TABLE: Side effect of antiepileptic drugs

Drug	Side effect
• Na + Valproate	Hepatotoxicity, Reversible Alopecia, Weight Gain, Tremor, PCOS, Most teratogenic (neural tube defect)
• Phenytoin	Gum hypertrophy, Fetal hydantoin syndrome, megaloblastic anemia
• Carbamazepine	Bone marrow suppression, agranulocytosis, SJS
• Topiramate	Renal stone, Weight loss, ACG
• Zonisamide	Renal stone, Weight loss
• Vigabatrin	Visual field defect, Weight gain

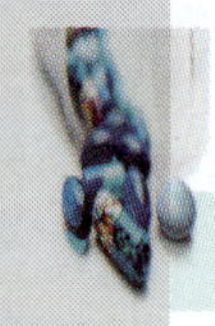

TABLE: Drugs of choice ***for some commonly asked malignancies: (Harrison 19th ed.)***

Malignancy	First line drugs
Chronic Lymphocytic leukaemia	Fludarabine
Chronic Myeloid leukaemia	Imatinib
Hairy cell leukemia	Cladribine
Multiple myeloma	Bortezomib
Choriocarcinoma	Methotrexate
Prostate carcinoma	Bicalutamide/Flutamide

TABLE: Some common side effects of anti-CA drugs

- **Busulfan & Bleomycin** – Pulmonary Fibrosis
- **Doxorubicin & Daunorubicin:** Cardiotoxicity
- **Cisplatin** – Ototoxic, Nephrotoxic, Vomiting
- **Vincristine & Vinblastine** – Peripheral Neuropathy
- **Ifosfamide, Cyclophosphamide:** Hemorrhagic cystitis
- **6 Mercaptopurine:** Hepatotoxicity

SOME IMPORTANT DRUG OF CHOICE

DOC for acute asthma	**Salbutamol**
DOC for nephrogenic diabetes insipidus	**Thiazides (Chlorthalidone)**
DOC for central diabetes insipidus	**Desmopressin**
DOC for morning sickness	**Doxylamine**
DOC for cisplatin induced vomiting	**Ondansetron**
DOC for delayed vomiting due to cisplatin	**Aprepitant (Subtance R #)**
DOC for motion sickness	**Hyoscine**
DOC for levodopa induced vomiting	**Domperidone**
DOC for hypertensive emergencies	**Nicardipine I/V**
DOC for hypertensive emergency in pregnancy	**Labetalol**
DOC for anaphylactic shock	**Adrenaline (1:1000 1/M) 0.5 mL**
DOC for cardiogenic shock with oliguria	**Dopamine**
DOC for carcinoma pancreas	**Gemcitabine**
DOC for hairy cell leukemia	**Cladribine**
DOC for CLL	**Fludarabine**
Drug of choice for cyclophosphamide induced hemorrhagic cystitis	**Mesna**
DOC for glioma	**Nitrosourea**
DOC colorectal cancer	**5 FU**

Contd...

Disulfiram like reaction by anti-cancer drug	**Procarbazine**
Hodgkin's new Regimen (ABVD)	**Adriamycin Bleomycin Vinblastine Dacarbazine**
Non-Hodgkin's Lymphoma Regimen (R-CHOP)	**+/– Rituximab Cyclophosphamide Hydroxydaunorubicin (doxorubicin) Oncovin (Vincristine) Prednisolone**
DOC for liver fluke	**Triclabendazole**
DOC for Dog tape worm/ Echi. Granulosus	**Albendazole**
DOC for Filarial worm	**Diethylcarbamazine (DEC)**
DOC for strongyloides and onchocerca	**Ivermectin**
Oral DOC for scabies	**Ivermectin**
DOC for scabies	**5% Permethrin**
DOC for Platyhelminthes	**Praziquantel or Niclosamide**
Oral DOC for kala-azar	**Miltefosine**
DOC for Chagas disease	**Benznidazole**
DOC for dermatophytosis	**Terbinafine**
DOC for candida	**Fluconazole**
DOC for Aspergillosis	**Voriconazole**
DOC for P. vivax	**Chloroquine**
TOC for P. falciparum	**ACT**
DOC for cerebral malaria	**Artesunate I/V**
DOC for cerebral malaria during pregnancy	**Quinine + Clindamycin**
DOC in Alzheimer's disease	**Donepezil**
Drug used in for Alzheimer's disorder	**Galantamine Rivastigmine Donepezil (DOC) Memantine**
DOC for OCD	**Fluoxetine**
Newly diagnosed Parkinson disease patient should be started first on:	**Rasagiline** *(due to its neuroprotective action- Studies)*
DOC for parkinsonism in young	**Ropinirole and Pramipexole**
DOC for drug induced parkinsonism	**Benzhexol**
DOC for paroxysmal supra ventricular tachycardia	**Adenosine**

Contd...

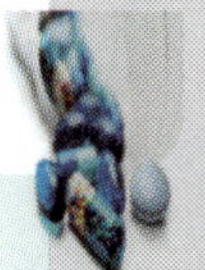

DOC for Supraventricular Tachycardia	**Verapamil**
DOC for Atrial Fibrillation	**Esmolol**
DOC for digitalis induced ventricular arrhythmia	**Lignocaine**
DOC for torsades de pointes	**$MgSO_4$**
DOC for morphine poisoning	**Naloxone**
DOC for alcohol withdrawal syndrome	**Benzodiazepines (Chlordiazepoxide)**
DOC for mania	**Lithium**

TABLE: Drug of choice for different seizures

Absence seizures (petit mal)	Ethosuximide
GTCS (Grand mal)	Lamotrigine > Na^+ Valproate
Focal seizure	Carbamazepine
Myoclonic seizures	Na^+ Valproate > Lamotrigine
Infantile/salaam seizure	ACTH
Infantile spasm with tuberous sclerosis	Vigabatrin
Febrile seizures	Midazolam; Diazepam (per rectal)
Status epilepticus	Lorazepam (IV)
Eclamptic seizure	Magnesium sulfate
Seizure during pregnancy	Levetiracetam
Neonatal seizure	Phenobarbitone

TABLE: Diuretics their MOA and site of action

Diuretic class	Drugs	MOA	Site of action
Osmotic diuretic	Mannitol	Inhibit water and solute reabsorption	All part of tubule, but mainly proximal tubule
Loop diuretics	Furosemide Torsemide	Inhibit Na^+-K^+-2 Cl co-transport	Thick ascending loop of Henle
Thiazide diuretic	Hydrochlorothiazide Benzthiazide Chlorthalidone Indapamide	Inhibit Na^+- Cl^- co-transport	Distal tubule
K^+ sparing diuretic	Spironolactone Triamterene Amiloride	Decrease Na^+ reabsorption Decrease K^+ secretion	Collecting tubule
Carbonic anhydrase inhibitor	Acetazolamide	Inhibit H^+ secretion and HCO_3 reabsorption, which reduces Na^+ reabsorption	Proximal tubule

TABLE: Typical antipsychotics and its action on its D receptor

Typical antipsychotics	
Strong D2 blocker	Haloperidol-*has maximum risk of EPS* Droperidol
Weak D2 blocker	Chlorpromazine Thioridazine – *has minimum risk of EPS*
Intermediate D2 blocker	Fluphenazine Prochlorperazine

TABLE: Antimicrobials with their mechanism of action

Drugs which inhibit cell wall formation	Drugs which inhibit protein synthesis
Cycloserine Vancomycin Fosfomycin Bacitracin Beta lactam	<u>T</u>etracycline <u>C</u>hloramphenicol <u>M</u>acrolides (Erythro, Clarithro, Azithro) <u>C</u>lindamycin <u>S</u>treptogramins (Quinupristin + dalfopristin)
Remembered as: <u>Cell Vall oF Bacteria</u>	<u>T</u>he <u>C</u>hild <u>M</u>ay <u>C</u>limb <u>S</u>tairs

TABLE: Antimicrobials and their side effects

Antimicrobial drugs	Side effects
Chloramphenicol	• Bone marrow suppression • Grey baby syndrome
Tetracycline	• Teeth discoloration and bone growth suppression • Phototoxicity • Fanconi syndrome (in case of expired tetracycline) • Vestibular dysfunction
Vancomycin	• Red man syndrome • Nephrotoxic and ototoxic
Clindamycin	• Pseudomembranous colitis
Erythromycin estolate	• Cholestasis
Aminoglycosides	• Nephrotoxicity and Ototoxicity

TABLE: Choice of drugs for common problems during pregnancy/ safe and unsafe drugs during pregnancy

Drug class (condition)	Unsafe drugs	Safer alternative
Antibacterials	Fluoroquinolones Tetracycline Doxycycline Chloramphenicol Streptomycin Kanamycin Tobramycin	Penicillin G; Ampicillin Amoxicillin-Clavulanate Cloxacillin, Piperacillin Cephalosporins Erythromycin

Contd...

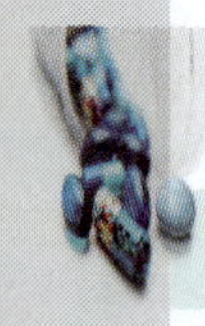

Drug class (condition)	Unsafe drugs	Safer alternative
Antitubercular	Pyrazinamide, Ethambutol Streptomycin	Isoniazid Rifampicin
Anti hypertensives	ACE inhibitors Angiotensin (R) blocker Diuretics Propranolol and Na^+ nitroprusside	Methyldopa Hydralazine Atenolol, Metoprolol, Pindolol Nifedipine
Antithyroid drugs	Carbimazole Radioactive iodine Iodide	Propylthiouracil (PTU)

TABLE: Recommended doses of antitubercular drug

Drug	Daily dose	
	mg/kg	For >50 kg
Isoniazid (H)	5 (4-6)	300 mg
Rifampin €	10 (8-12)	600 mg
Pyrazinamide (Z)	25 (20-30)	1500 mg
Ethambutol (E)	15 (15-20)	1000 mg

TABLE: Important side effects of antitubercular drugs

Peripheral neuropathy (*due to vit B6 deficiency*): **Isoniazid**
Orange color urine- **Rifampicin**
Flu-like symptoms- **Rifampicin**
Hyperuricemia/gout- **Pyrazinamide**
Optic neuritis/Red green color blindness- **Ethambutol**
Nephrotoxic, Ototoxic, Neuromuscular Junction Blocker- **Streptomycin**
Most hepatotoxic ATT: **Pyrazinamide**
Hypothyroidism: **Ethionamide and PAS**
Psychotic symptoms: **Cycloserine**

TABLE: Antiplatelet drugs and their target of inhibition

Antiplatelet drugs	Target of inhibition
Aspirin	Inhibit TXA_2 (Thromboxane A_2) release
Terutroban	TXA_2 receptor blocker

Contd...

Antiplatelet drugs	Target of inhibition
Clopidogrel and Ticlopidine	Inhibit ADP receptor P2Y12 irreversibly
Cangrelor, Ticagrelor	Reversible inhibitor of P_2Y_{12}
Abciximab Tirofiban Eptifibatide	Inhibit GP IIb/IIIa
Atopaxar, Vorapaxar	Thrombin Inhibitor/PAR inhibitor
Heparin	AT3 mediated IIa and Xa inhibition
Low molecular weight heparin (Enoxaparin, Dalteparin, Tinzaparin)	AT3 mediated Xa >> IIa inhibition
Fondaparinux	AT3 mediated Xa inhibition
Hirudin, Lepirudin	Direct thrombin inhibitor

TABLE: Oral hypoglycemic agents

Drugs		Remark
Oral glucose-lowering agents		
Biguanides (Metformin)	• Therapy of type 2 diabetes • Usually initial agent in type 2 diabetes	• Reduce hepatic glucose production • Weight neutral • Do not cause hypoglycemia • Adverse events include diarrhea, nausea, lactic acidosis (black-box warning) • Use cautiously in renal insufficiency, • Avoid use in patents with hepatic dysfunction
α-Glucosidase inhibitors Acarbose, miglitol, voglibose	• Therapy of type 2 diabetes	• Reduce carbohydrate breakdown in GI tract • **Adverse effects:** GI flatulence, elevated liver function tests • Can be combined with other agents • Relatively modest glucose lowering
Dipeptidyl peptidase 4 inhibitors Sitagliptin, Saxagliptin, Linagliptin, Alogliptin, Vildagliptin	• Therapy of type 2 diabetes	• Prolong action of GLP-1; Promotes insulin secretion • Can be combined with other agents • Relatively modest glucose lowering

Contd...

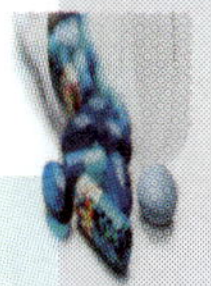

Drugs		Remark
Insulin secretagogues: Sulfonylureas **Second generation:** Glyburide, Glibenclamide, Glipizide, and other	• Therapy of type 2 diabetes	• Stimulate insulin secretion • Major adverse events is hypoglycemia • Adjustments needed in renal/liver disease • 2nd gen are more potent, may have better safety profile than first-generation agents. • Can be combined with other agents • Modest weight gain
Insulin secretagogues-nonsulfonylureas Repaglinide, nateglinide	• Therapy of type 2 diabetes	• Increase insulin secretion, quicker onset and shorter duration than sulfonylureas • Major adverse event: Hypoglycemia
SLGT2 inhibitors Canagliflozin, Dapagliflozin, Empagliflozin	• Therapy of type 2 diabetes	• Prevent glucose reabsorption and promote renal glucose excretion • Mild weight loss and BP reduction • Do not cause hypoglycemia • May increase rate of lower urinary tract and genital mycotic infections, hypotension, and DKA
Thiazolidinediones Rosiglitazone, Pioglitazone	• Therapy of type 2 diabetes	• Increase insulin sensitivity • Adverse effects: Peripheral edema, CHF, weight gain, fractures, macular edema • Use with caution in CHF, liver disease
GLP-1 agonists (SC) Albiglutide, dulaglutide, exenatide, liraglutide Semaglutide (PO)	• Therapy of type 2 diabetes	• Increase Insulin secretion, Decrease gastric emptying, Decrease glucagon • Injected subcutaneously • Often associated with weight loss • Adverse events include nausea • Do not use with agents that decrease GI motility • Risk of hypoglycemia with insulin

Contd...

Drugs		Remark
Amylin analogue Pramlintide (SC)	• Adjunctive therapy with insulin in type 1 and type 2 diabetes	• Slows gastric emptying, decreases glucagon • Injected subcutaneously • Decrease postprandial glycemia • Often associated with weight loss • Risk of hypoglycemia with insulin

TABLE: Hypolipidemic drugs

Drug	Mechanism of action
Statins (simvastatin, rosuvastatin)	HMG-CoA reductase inhibitor
Fibrates (clofibrate, fenofibrate, gemfibrozil)	PPAR-alpha agonist
Cholestyramine, colestipol, colesevelam	Bile acid sequestrant
Ezetimibe	Inhibit cholesterol absorption (NPC_1L_1)
Alirocumab, Evolocumab	PCK-K9 inhibitor
Lomitapide	Microsomal TG transfer protein inhibitor
Torcetrapib, anacetrapib	Cholesteryl Ester Transfer Protein inhibitor
Mipomersen	Apolipoprotein B 100 synthesis inhibitor
Volanesorsen	Apolipoprotein C-III synthesis inhibitor

TABLE: Targeted anti-CA therapy

Class	Drugs	Use
Proteosome inhibitor	BORTEZOMIB, CARFILZOMIB, IXAZOMIB It inhibits NF-KB which does the cell division	**Multiple myeloma**
PARP inhibitor	OLAPARIB, RUCAPARIB, NIRAPARIB	**BRCA # Ovarian CA**
CDK inhibitor	Inhibits CDK 4 and 6 both	**Breast CA**
Tyrosine kinase inhibitor	**Imatinib**	**DOC for CML & GIST**
	Lapatinib	**Breast CA**
	Sorafenib	**Hepatocellular CA**
	Sunitinib	**Renal cell CA**
	Vandetanib	Medullary CA thyroid

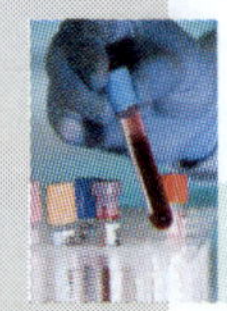

IMPORTANT MAB AND THEIR USE

• Palivizumab	RSV
• Eculizumab	PNH
• Omalizumab, Mepolizumab, Reslizumab	Bronchial asthma
• Daratumumab, isatuximab	MM
• Cetuximab	Recurrent head & neck CA
• Rituximab (anti-CD20)	CLL, RA, ITP, SLE, NHL, AIHA

DRUG USED IN MEDICALECTOMIES

• Labyrinthectomy	Gentamicin
• Adernalectomy	Mitotane, Metyrapone, Aminoglutetheimide, Ketocon
• Prostatectomy (Androgen Ablation)	Bicalutamide (LHRH agonist)
• Castration (orchidectomy/ oophorectomy)	GnRH analogue (Goserelin, Buserelin, Leuprolide)
• Pancreatectomy	Streptozotocin, Alloxan

AGENTS USED IN GOUT AND RHEUMATOID ARTHRITIS

• DOC for acute gouty arthritis	• **NSAIDS (except Aspirin)**
• DOC for chronic gout	• **DOC: Allopurinol (Xanthine oxidase inhibitor)** • **Febuxostat (if allergy w/ Allopurinol)**
• Uricosuric agent used in gouty arthritis	• **Probenecid, Sulfinpyrazone, Lesinurad, Benzbromarone**
• DOC for Rheumatoid arthritis	• **Mtx**
• Calcineurin inhibitor causing gum hypertrophy and Hirsutism	• **Cyclosporine**
• Fastest acting anti rheumatoid agent	• **Leflunomide**
• **TNFα inhibitor**	• Adalimumab, certolizumab, Etanercept, Infliximab, Golimumab
• IL-1 R#	• ANAKINRA
• IL-2#	• DACLIZUMAB • BASILIXIMAB
• IL-6 R#	• TOCILIZUMAB, SARILUMAB
• **Costimulation inhibitor**	• Abatacept • Belatacept (b/w CD 80 & 28)
• **Calcineurin inhibitor:**	• **Cyclosporine, Tacrolimus**
• **Mtor inhibitor**	• **SIROLIMUS, EVEROLIMUS**

PATHOLOGY

IMPORTANT RECENT POINTS (INCLUDES LATEST QS)

• Number of DNA base pairs in human genome	**3.2 billion DNA Base pairs**
• Total Number of genome that is encoding protein in human	**20,000**
• Mobile genetic element/Jumping genes	**Transposons (1/3rd of human genome)**
• Person to person variation (susceptibility to diseases, drug action) in genome	**1.5% (represents 15 million base pairs)**
• MC forms of DNA variation	**SNP and CNV (single nucleotide polymorphism and Copy number variation)**
• Function of PDGF	**Chemotactic for neutrophils, macrophages** **Stimulate proliferation of fibroblast** **Stimulate ECM protein synthesis**
• MC adhesion molecule for Diapedesis	**PECAM/CD 31**
• VEGF that stimulate embryonic vessel development	**VEGF-B**
• VEGF that causes Lymphangiogenesis	**VEGF-C and D**
• Maximum volume of cell contributed by	**Cytosol (54%)**
• Number of mitochondria/cell	**1700**
• Most abundant glycoprotein in basement membrane	**Laminin**

IMPORTANT POINTS ON NECROSIS

• MC type of necrosis/cell death due to sudden occlusion of blood supply	Coagulative necrosis
• Primary mechanism of coagulative necrosis	Denaturation of I/C proteins
• Primary mechanism of liquifactive necrosis	Enzymatic digestion of cell
• Solid organ where ischemic necrosis is liquefactive	Brain
• Variants of coagulative necrosis	Caseous necrosis, gangrene

Contd...

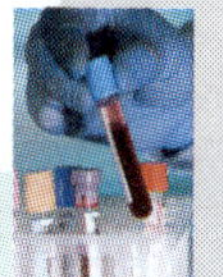

• Caseous necrosis is caused by	TB (most common), syphilis, fungal (Histoplasmosis, Coccidioidomycosis)
• Malignant hypertension causes this type of necrosis	Fibrinoid necrosis

NECROPTOSIS VS PYROPTOSIS

• **Necroptosis** (programmed necrosis)	• Resembles necrosis morphologically and apoptosis mechanistically • Caspase independent programmed cell death → Triggered from signaling by RIP1 and RIP3 complex → reduces mt.ATP gen, production of ROS, inc permeability of lysosomal membrane → cellular swelling and membrane damage **Necroptosis is seen in: (RAPS)** • Reperfusion injury • Acute pancreatitis • Parkinson's disease • Steatohepatitis • Backup defence against CMV (they encode caspase inhibitors)
• **Pyroptosis**	• Occurs in cells infected with microbes • Involves activation of caspase-1 → Activate IL-1 • IL 1 and IL11 → causes cell death of infected death • Characterized by swelling of cells, loss of plasma membrane integrity, and release of inflammatory mediators

GOLDEN POINTS

Most common mediastinal tumor: Thymoma (anterior mediastinum)

Most common middle mediastinal tumor: Lymphoma

Most common middle mediastinal mass: Pericardial cyst

Cancer associated with Epstein-Barr virus:
- Nasopharyngeal Carcinoma
- Burkitt's lymphoma
- Hodgkin's disease

Caseous necrosis is seen in organ in which organ: Lung (Tuberculosis)

Viral infection causing genial CA: HPV

Trilateral retinoblastoma involves: Bilateral eye retinoblastoma plus pinealoblastoma

Most common source of brain metastasis: Lung

Contd...

Thyroid CA associated with pheocromocytoma and hyperparathyroidism: Medullary cancer thyroid (MEN IIa)

India ink is used for diagnosing: Cryptococcus neoformans

Patau syndrome is: Trisomy 13

Edward syndrome: Trisomy 18

Down syndrome: Trisomy 21

Pitting is: Removal of nuclei from old RBC's by the spleen without destroying the cell, and the cell send back plasma circulation.

Culling is defined as: Removal of abnormal RBC form the blood by spleen

Removal of worm out and abnormal RBC's and platelets from the bloodstream by phagocyte cells in the spleen is: Phagocytosis

Highly aggressive lung cancer with rapid doubling capability and metastasis: Small cell lung CA

Type of necrosis seen in Brain pathology: Liquefactive necrosis

MC urinary bladder CA: Transitional cell CA

GITTRE CELLS are modified CNS macrophages

Acrocentric chromosomes are: 13, 14, 15, 21, 22, Y

Pregnancy tumor of gums: Granuloma pyogenicum

Grawitz tumor is also known as Hypernephroma/RCC

HPE finding of type IV lupus nephritis: Wire loop lesions

Noonan syndrome has phenotype similar to: Turner syndrome

Largest gene: Dystrophin gene

Partial trisomy of chromosome 22: Cat eye syndrome

Garland triad aka 1-2-3 sign is suggestive of: Thoracic sarcoidosis

Coast of California sign is seen in: Neurofibromatosis

Accordion sign seen in: Pseudomembranous colitis

Rosenthal fibers in affected brain is characteristic of-Alexander's disease

Bear paw sign is seen in: Xanthogranulomatous pyelonephritis

Subendothelial Deposits are seen in SLE patients

- Necroptosis resembles necrosis morphologically and apoptosis mechanistically as a form of programmed cell death.
- Necroptosis is triggered by ligation of TNFR1, and viral proteins of RNA and DNA viruses.

- Pyroptosis occurs in cells infected by microbes. It involves activation of caspase-1 which cleaves the precursor form of IL-1 to generate biologically active IL-1. Caspase-1 along with closely related caspase-11 also cause death of the infected cell.

- Autophagy is an adaptive response to enhanced nutrient deprivation and involves sequestration of cellular organelles into cytoplasmic autophagic vacuoles (autophagosomes) that fuse with lysosomes and digest the enclosed material.

Contd...

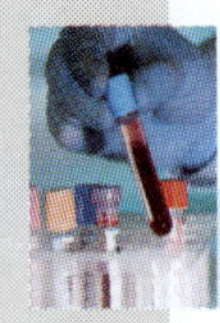

- Location of selectins
  - **L- selectin:** Leucocytes, monocytes, T cell, B cell
  - **E selectin:** Endothelium activated by cytokines
  - **P selectin:** endothelium activated by cytokines (TNF, IL1), Histamine, platelets

Chédiak-Higashi syndrome: Decreased leukocyte functions because of mutations affecting protein involved in lysosomal membrane traffic

Chronic granulomatous disease: Due to decreased oxidative burst

TABLE: Classification of Ehlers-Danlos syndromes

EDS Type	Clinical findings	Inheritance
Classic (VII)	Skin and joint hypermobility, atrophic scars, easy bruising	Autosomal dominant
Hypermobility (III)	Joint hypermobility, pain, dislocations	Autosomal dominant
Vascular (IV)	Thin skin, arterial or uterine rupture, bruising, small joint hyperextensibility	Autosomal dominant
Kyphoscoliosis (VI)	Hypotonia, joint laxity, congenital scoliosis, ocular fragility	Autosomal dominant
Arthrochalasis (VIIa, b)	Severe joint hypermobility, skin changes (mild), scoliosis, bruising	Autosomal dominant
Dermatosparaxis (VIIc)	Severe skin fragility, cutis laxa, bruising	Autosomal dominant

TABLE: Examples of trinucleotide repeat mutations

Disease	Repeated nucleotide	Number of repeats
Fragile X syndrome	CGG	55-200 (pre); >230 (full)
Friedreich ataxia	GAA	34-80 (pre); >100 (full)
Myotonic dystrophy	CTG	34-80 (pre); >100 (full)
Spinobulbar muscular atrophy (Kennedy disease)	CAG	38-62
Huntington disease	CAG	36-121

TABLE: Mechanisms of hypersensitivity reactions

Type	Immune mechanisms	Prototypical disorders
Immediate (type I) hypersensitivity	Production of IgE antibody → immediate release or vasoactive amines and other mediators from mast cells; later recruitment of inflammatory cells	Anaphylaxis; allergies; bronchial asthma (atopic forms)
Antibody-mediated (type II) hypersensitivity	Production of IgG → binds to antigen on target cell or tissue → phagocytosis or lysis or target cell by activated complement or Fc receptors; recruitment or leukocytes	Autoimmune hemolytic anemia; goodpasture syndrome
Immune complex—mediated (type III) hypersensitivity	Deposition of antigen-antibody complexes → complement activation → recruitment of leukocytes by complement products and Fc receptors → release of enzymes and other toxic molecules	Systemic lupus erythematosus; some forms of glomerulonephritis; serum sickness; Arthus reaction
Cell-mediated (type IV) hypersensitivity	Activated T lymphocytes → (1) release of cytokines, inflammation and macrophage activation; (2) T cell-mediated cytotoxicity	Contact dermatitis; multiple sclerosis; type 1 diabetes; tuberculosis

NEPHROPATHY AND HPE FINDINGS

HPE finding	Associated abnormality
Subepithelial Humps	Acute Poststreptococcal Glomerulonephritis
Linear Subendothelial deposits	Goodpasture syndrome (Type II)
Mesangial deposits	IgA Nephropathy
Spike and dome shaped deposits	Membranous nephropathy
Subendothelial humps	Membranoproliferative glomerulonephritis
Holly leaf mesangial deposits	FSGS

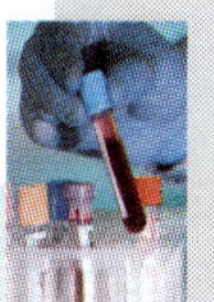

MEN SYNDROMES

Type (Chromosomal location)	Tumors	Remark
MEN 1 (11q13)	• Parathyroid adenoma (90%) • Entropancreatic tumors (30-70%) • Pituitary adenoma (15-50%)	• Overall MC type of MEN1 is Parathyroid adenoma • MC enteropancreatic tumor is: Gastrinoma (>50%) • VIPoma is least common type of enteropancreatic tumor (<1%) • MCC of pituitary adenoma is Prolactinoma
MEN 2A	• Medullary CA thyroid (90%) • Pheochromocytoma (10-50%) • Parathyroid adenoma (>25%)	
MEN 2B Aka MEN 3	• Medullary CA thyroid (>90%) • Pheochromocytoma (>50%) • Associated abnormalities (40-50%) • Mucosal neuroma • Marfanoid habitus • Megacolon • Medullated corneal nerve fibers	
MEN 4	• Parathyroid adenoma • Pituitary adenoma • Reproductive organ tumors *(testicular cancers, neuroendocrine cervical CA).*	

IMPORTANT POINTS

- Most common cause of cell injury is – **Hypoxia**
- Most common cause of hypoxia – **Ischemia**
- Most common and sensitive cells in the body damaged due to hypoxia – **Neurons**
- Cytochrome C plays an important role in: **Apoptosis**
- Not a cellular adaptation: **Necrosis.**
- Barrett's esophagus is an example of: **Metaplasia.**
- Myelin figures are derived from: **Damaged cell membrane.**
- H_2O_2 is produced as well as destroyed in: **Peroxisome.**
- **CNS** – liquefactive necrosis (only solid organ where liquefactive necrosis seen)
- **TB**- caseous necrosis
- Most characteristic **feature of apoptosis** – Absence of inflammation and intact cell membrane

Contd...

- Important indicator of free radical injury – **Lipofuscin** (alveolar wall)
- Myositis ossificans – Connective tissue metaplasia
- Most common site for metastatic calcification – **Lungs**
- **Haber-Weiss reaction is:** Generation of free radical from H_2O_2.
- **Fenton Reaction** – $H_2O_2 + Fe^{2+} \rightarrow Fe^{2+} + OH + OH$
- The most common fixative for light microscope is – **10% neutral buffered formalin**
- The most common fixative for electron microscope is – **Glutaraldehyde**
- Hall mark of acute inflammation – **Increased vascular permeability**
- Formation of endothelial gaps – **Mechanism of increased vascular permeability**
- Rolling of neutrophils done by – **Selectins**
- Leukocytes with giant granules in peripheral blood smear seen in – **Chédiak–Higashi syndrome**
- Eosinophils have major basic protein which is toxic to **parasites**
- Most important chemical mediators of acute inflammation – **Histamine**
- Most potent **microbicidal system** – oxygen dependent MPO system, NADPH oxidase/Respiratory burst
- Most important fibrogenic agent → **TGF – beta**
- **SRS** – A components – LTB4 & LTC4
- Most common complement deficiency associated with **Streptococcal septicemia** and **lupus** like syndrome in children – Deficiency of C2
- Chemotactic for neutrophils – **IL 8**
- Most common type of inflammation - **Catarrhal inflammation**
- **Vitamin K** dependent clotting factors – 2, 7, 9, 10, protein C & S
- **Functions of bradykinin**
  - Contraction of smooth muscles (bronchospasm, vasospasm of muscular arteries)
  - Pain
  - Dilation of the venules
- Monocytes and macrophages are the primary leukocytes in **chronic inflammation**
- Epithelioid cells are macrophages activated by **INF – Gamma**
- Granulation tissue is the hallmark of – **Fibrogenic repair**
- Severe generalized edema is called – **Anasarca**
- Hemosiderin laden macrophages (heart failure cells) found in **Lung**
- **Bernard–Soulier syndrome** – A defect in the glycoprotein factor results in defective platelet adhesion

Contd...

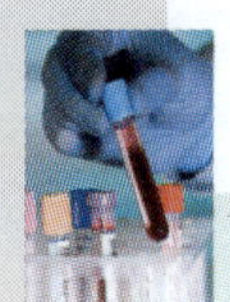

- **Virchow triad** – Endothelial cell injury + alteration of blood flow+ hypercoagulability
- **Thrombin** is procoagulant but thrombin-thrombomodulin complex is anticoagulant
- Most common inherited cause of hypercoagulability – **Leiden mutation** (factor 5 mutation)
- **Lines of Zahn** are produced by the alternating pale layers of platelets mixed with some fibrin and dark layers containing more red cells
- Most common site for **DVT – Deep veins below the knee**
- **Chargaff's rule** – amount of purine is equal to pyrimidine (A + G = C + T)
- Most common death in Marfan syndrome – **Aortic Dissection**
- Autosomal recessive diseases are most common type of mendelian mode of inheritance
- **In AR inheritance**, both parents must have mutant gene
- Essential amino acid in PKU – **Tyrosine**
- **Uniparental Disomy** – Should be suspected in an individual manifesting a recessive disorder, where only one parent is a carrier
- **PGF2a is a vasoconstrictor** where PGD2, PGE2 are vasodilators
- The chief cell responsible for scar contraction is **myofibroblast**
- **Heart failure cells are:** Hemosiderin laden macrophages.
- Heart failure cells seen in: **Lungs**
- Platelet aggregation requires: **Glycoprotein IIb-IIIa**
- Fibrin is degraded by: **Plasmin**
- **Virchow's triad of thrombosis include:** Vascular (endothelial) injury; abnormal blood flow (stasis or turbulence); hypercoagulability.
- Virchow's fifth sign of inflammation is: **Loss of function**
- **Leiden factor is:** Mutated factor V.
- Most common source of embolism: **DVT (deep vein thrombosis)**.
- **Red aka hemorrhagic infarcts are seen in:** Ovary, lung, small intestine.
- **Pale aka white infarcts are seen in:** Heart, spleen, liver, kidney, brain.
- In inflammation Rubor is due to: **Arteriolar dilatation**.
- **Hallmark of acute inflammation:** Increased vascular permeability.
- Which Cells primarily involved in acute inflammation: **Neutrophils**.
- Major microcirculation involved in acute inflammation: **Venules**.
- Cell-matrix adhesion is mediated by: **Integrins**.

Contd...

- Major cells which are involved in chronic inflammation: **Macrophages.**
- **Life span of neutrophils:** 4–8 hours (in blood) and 2–5 days (in tissues).
- Phagocytic cells in brain (CNS): **Microglia.**
- Oxygen dependent killing in phagocytes is through: **NADPH oxidase.**
- **Chédiak–Higashi syndrome** is a defect of: **Phagocytosis.**
- Most abundant glycoprotein in basement membrane: **Laminin.**
- **Warthin finkeldey** giant cells are seen in measles
- **Reed–sternberg cells** seen in **hodgkin's lymphoma**
- Most common site for keloid – **Sternum**
- Triplet repeat of CCG nucleotides seen in-**Fragile X syndrome**
- There is presence of CAG repeats associated with – **Huntington's chorea**
- **Gonadal/Germline mosaicism** seen in – osteogenesis imperfecta and tuberous sclerosis
- Diagnosis of choice for **Fragile X Syndrome** – PCR
- White spots on the iris known as brushfield spots seen in **Down syndrome**
- Mitotic non-disjunction is responsible for development of **mosaicism**
- Patients of Down syndrome having predisposition for **Hirschsprung's disease, duodenal atresia** and **Alzheimer's disease.**
- **Robertsonian translocation** seen in about 4% cases of Down syndrome
- **AML M7** variety is associated with Down syndrome
- Maternal meiotic non-dysjunction is most common cause of **down syndrome**
- **Triple test and Quadruple screen** test is used for screening of Downs syndrome at 15–20 weeks of pregnancy
- Maternal serum of alpha fetoprotein + estriol + hCG are the components of triple test this are low in **Edward syndrome**
- **AFP** is increased in neural tube defects but reduced in Edward and down syndromes
- **Patau syndrome** is trisomy 13, features are polydactyly cleft lip and holoprosencephaly.
- **Edward syndrome** is trisomy 18, features are micrognathia overlapping flexed fingers.
- **Cat eye syndrome** is a partial trisomy of chromosome 22 and is coined due to the particular appearance of the ventricular colobomas in the eyes.
- **Klinefelter syndrome** is male chromosomal disorder of chromosome 47, XXY, there is decrease in testosterone and inhibin but increase in LH and FSH.

Contd...

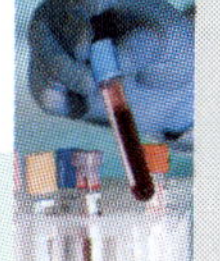

- **Noonan syndrome** is autosomal congenital disorder mostly mutation in genes on chromosome 12.
- Trisomy 7 mostly occur due to mitotic non – Disjunction.
- Trisomy 18 is more commonly seen in **2nd meiotic division**.
- **Lyon's hypothesis** says inactivation of either maternal or paternal x chromosome among all the cells of blastocyst by about 16th day of embryonic life
- **Barr bodies** are absent in normal males and turner syndrome but female has 1 Barr body.
- Benign tumor developing from all three germ layers – **Teratoma**
- Lesion with normal differentiation at abnormal site – **Choristoma**
- Hallmark of malignant transformation – **Anaplasia**
- **Hamartoma** – Abnormal differentiation in normal site
- **Malignant tumors** have upregulation of telomerase activity
- HNPCC is AD but is due to defective **DNA repair**
- Cell cycle sequence **G1-S-G2-M-G0**
- The initiation of DNA replication involve the formation of an active complex between **Cyclin E** and **CDK2**
- The main mediator that propels the cell beyond prophase is – **Cyclin B CDK1 complex**
- Proto-oncogenes were discovered by **Harold Varmus** and **Michael Bishop**
- The point mutation of **Ras family gene** is the single most common abnormality of oncogenes in human tumors
- **MYC** is associated with conflict model in carcinogenesis
- **K-RAS**- Colon, lung & pancreatic tumors
- **N-RAS** – Melanoma, AML
- **H-RAS** – Bladder and kidney tumors
- **C-MYC** – Burkitt's lymphoma
- **L-MYC** – Small cell lung cancer
- **N-MYC** – Neuroblastoma
- **RB gene** was the first tumor suppressor gene to be discovered
- **RB gene** is present on chromosome 13q14
- Retinoblastoma is associated with **Knudsen two hit hypothesis**
- **P53 gene** is the most commonly mutated gene in human cancer
- The nonmutated P53 gene is also called as – **Wild type**
- **Toll – like** receptor causes the activation of NF – Kappa beta and AP-1
- **CD45** is also called a leukocyte common antigen (LCA)
- Antigen presenting cells include – B-cells macrophages and dendritic cells
- HEV are lined by simple cuboidal cells as opposite to regular venules lined by **endothelial cells**.

Contd...

- Pan B cell – **CD 19**
- **Isotype switching** – Change in the class of the antibody produced by the plasma cell
- **IgM** and **IgG** are responsible for activation of classical pathway
- **IgA, IgE** and **IgD** are responsible for activation of alternate pathway
- **NK cells** are unique as they are capable of direct cell lysis
- **MHC is** located on short arm of chromosome 6
- **MHC 1** molecule is present on all the nucleated cells and platelets
- **MHC 2** molecule is present on all the APC'S (Antigen Presenting Cells)

• Crumpled tissue paper app	• Gaucher's disease (massive splenomegaly)
• Hunner ulcer	• Interstitial cystitis
• Cushing ulcer	• Stomach ulcer due to raised ICP
• Curling ulcer	• Ulcer in D1 portion d/t burns
• Cameron ulcer	• Hiatus hernia

IMPORTANT ONE LINERS

- Foam Cells are: **Lipid Laden Macrophages**
- Artery not involved in atherosclerosis: **Pulmonary trunk**.
- Most common cause of aortic aneurysm: **Atherosclerosis**.
- Infection causing atherosclerosis: **Chlamydia pneumoniae, herpes virus (CMV)**.
- Tree bark calcification is seen in: **Syphilitic aneurysm**.
- Pulseless disease is: **Takayasu arteritis**.
- Most common benign vascular tumor: **Hemangioma**.
- Kaposi's sarcoma is associated with: **HHV-8**.
- Characteristic of rheumatic carditis: **Pancarditis**.
- Most commonly involved valve in Rheumatic fever: **Mitral valve**.
- McCallum plaque is seen in: **Rheumatic carditis** (on left atrium).
- Most common cause of constrictive pericarditis: **TB**.
- Gitter cells are: **Microglia**
- Maximum decrease in CSF chloride: **TB meningitis**.
- Characteristic pathological feature of parkinsonism: **Lewy bodies**.
- Most common cause of intracerebral (intraparenchymal) hemorrhage: **Hypertension**.
- Important features of **Dandy-Walker syndrome**: Agenesis of cerebellar vermis and corpus callosum, cystic enlargement of 4th ventricle, hydrocephalus.

Contd...

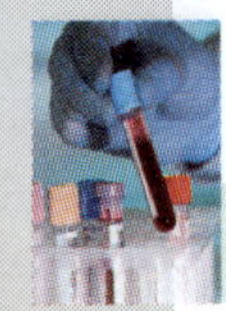

- Most common cerebellar tumor in children: **Astrocytoma**
- Most common cerebellar tumor in children: **Astrocytoma**
- Wermer's syndrome is: **MEN-I**.
- Sipple's syndrome is: **MEN-IIA**.
- Orphan Annie eye nuclei is characteristic of this thyroid CA: **Papillary thyroid carcinoma**.
- Most common thyroid carcinoma: **Papillary carcinoma**.
- Weight range of adrenal in Cushing's disease: **25-40 gm**.
- **Nesidioblastoma** is due to: Hyperplasia of pancreatic beta cells.
- Tadpole cells are seen in: **Rhabdomyosarcoma**.
- Brown tumor of bone is seen in: **Hyperparathyroidism**.
- Most common mutation in Ewing's sarcoma: **Translocation** t 11:22.
- Tophus is pathognomonic for: **Gout**.
- Bilateral breast cancer: **Lobular carcinoma**.
- Most common breast cancer: **Invasive ductal carcinoma.**
- Most common gene involved in breast cancer (overall): **P53.**
- Most common gene involved in familial breast cancer: **BRCA-1.**
- Call-Exner bodies are seen in: **Granulosa-theca cell tumor.**
- Most common testicular tumor and testicular germ cell tumor: **Seminoma.**
- Definitive marker for hepatoblastoma: **AFP**.
- Canals of herring are present in: **Liver.**
- 'Comet tail artefact' with thickening of gallbladder wall: **Adenomyomatosis**.
- 'Onion skin' fibrosis of bile duct is seen in: **Primary sclerosing cholangitis**.
- **Nutmeg liver is seen in:** Right sided heart failure (chronic passive congestion).
- **Rate limiting step in bilirubin metabolism**: Excretion of conjugated bilirubin into canaliculi.
- **Most common site of intestinal amebiasis**: Cecum and ascending colon.
- Pipe-stem appearance is seen in: **Ulcerative colitis**.

Contd...

- Most specific marker of GIST: **C-Kit (CD 117)**.
- Most common site of GIST: **Stomach**.
- Most common site of gastric carcinoma: **Pylorus and antrum**.
- **Most common complication of peptic ulcer:** GI bleeding (e.g. Haematemesis).
- **Most common site of peptic ulcer:** 1st part of duodenum.
- **Most common symptoms of bladder cancer:** Painless hematuria.
- Michaelis-Gutmann bodies are seen in: **Malakoplakia**.
- Kimmelstiel-Wilson lesion is characteristic of: **Diabetic nephropathy**.
- **Hallmark of IgA nephropathy:** Hematuria after 1-2 days of an upper respiratory tract infection.
- Most common cause of nephrotic syndrome in adults: **Membranous GN**.
- Crescent formation is characteristic of: **RPGN**.
- Most common cause of nephritic syndrome: **RPGN**.
- Tamm–Horsfall protein is produced by: **Loop of Henle**.
- Carcinoid tumors arise from: **Enterochromaffin cells**.
- Marker of squamous cell carcinoma of lung: **Cytokeratin**.
- Most common lung carcinoma: **Adenocarcinoma**.
- Potato nodes are seen in: **Sarcoidosis**.
- Bilateral hilar lymphadenopathy with non-caseating granuloma: **Sarcoidosis**.
- Most common form of emphysema seen clinically: **Centriacinar emphysema** (centrilobular emphysema).

HEPATITIS

Mnemonic for failure: causes of acute liver

- A: Acetaminophen, hepatitis A, autoimmune hepatitis
- B: Hepatitis B
- C: Hepatitis C, cryptogenic
- D: Drugs/toxins, hepatitis D
- E: Hepatitis E, esoteric causes (Wilson disease, Budd-Chiari)
- F: Fatty change of the microvesicular type (fatty liver of pregnancy, valproate, tetracycline, Reye syndrome)

TABLE: The hepatitis viruses

Virus	Hepatitis A	Hepatitis B	Hepatitis C	Hepatitis D	Hepatitis E
Type of virus	ssRNA	Partially dsDNA	ssRNA	Circular defective ssRNS	ssRNA
Viral family	Hepatovirus; related to picornavirus	Hepadnavirus	Flaviviridae	Subviral particle in Delta Viridae family	Hepevirus
Route of transmission	Fecal-oral (contaminated food or water)	Parenteral, sexual contact, perinatal	Parenteral; intranasal cocaine use is a risk factor	Parenteral	Fecal-oral

Contd...

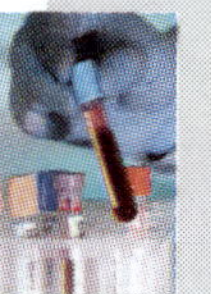

Virus	Hepatitis A	Hepatitis B	Hepatitis C	Hepatitis D	Hepatitis E
Mean Incubation period	2–6 weeks	2–26 weeks (mean 8 weeks)	4–26 weeks (mean 9 weeks)	Same as HBV	4–5 weeks
Frequency of chronic liver disease	Never	5%–10%	>80%	10% (co-infection); 90%–100% for superinfection	In Immunocompro-mised hosts only
Diagnosis	Detection of serum IgM antibody	Detection of HBsAg or antibody to HBcAg; PCR for HBV DNA	3rd-generation ELISA for antibody detection; PCR for HCV RNA	Detection of IgM and IgG antibodies; HDV RNA serum; HDAg In liver	Detection of serum IgM and 10 antibodies; PCR for HEV RNA

TABLE: Hereditary hyperbilirubinemia

Disorder	Inheritance	Defects in bilirubin metabolism	Liver pathology	Clinical course
Unconjugated hyperbilirubinemia				
Crigler-Najjar syndrome type I	Autosomal recessive	Absent UGT1A1 activity	None	Fetal in neonatal period
Crigler-Najjar syndrome type II	Autosomal dominant with variable penetrance	Decreased UGT1A1 activity	None	Generally mild, occasional kernicterus
Gilbert syndrome	Autosomal recessive	Decreased UGT1A1 activity	None	Innocuous
Conjugated hyperbilirubinemia				
Dubin-Johnson syndrome	Autosomal recessive	Impaired biliary excretion of bilirubin glucuronides due to mutation in canalicular multidrug resistance protein 2 (MRP2)	Pigmented cytoplasmic globules	Innocuous
Rotor syndrome	Autosomal recessive	Decreased hepatic uptake and storage? Decreased biliary excretion?	None	Innocuous

UGT1A1, Uridine diphosphate-glucuronyl transferase family, peptide A1

TABLE: Hodgkin's Lymphoma

	Classical				Non-Cl:
	Nodular sclerosis	Mixed cellularity	Lymphocyte rich	Lymphocyte depleted	Lymphocyte predominant
Incidence	MC type	MC type in India		a/w HIV	
RS cell	Variant = lacunar cell	Max no. of RS cell	**Least no. of RS cell**	3 types of RS cell	Popcorn cell
CD marker	15 + and 30+	15 + and 30+	15 + and 30+ CD 20-ve	15 + and 30+	CD 20+ 15 and 30 -ve
Prognosis	Excellent	Very good	Good to Excellent	Poor	Excellent

TABLE: Types of Graft Rejection

	Acute	Hyperacute	Chronic
Duration	5 days to 3 months	Immediately within minutes or hours	Occurs after months or years
Mechanism	Involves humoral (antibodies) and Cellular (T cell) rejection	Due to preformed antibodies (humoral)	Involves T cell (cellular rejection)
Hypersensitivity	IV	II	IV and III

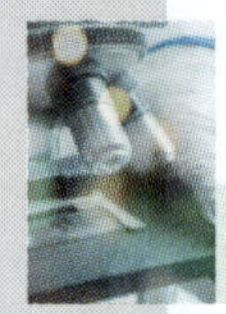

GOLDEN POINTS

• Antoni A and B	Schwannoma, Sarcoidosis, Sporotrichosis (Gardner's disease)
• Asteroid body	Sporotrichosis
• Azzopardi effect	Oat cell lung CA
• Banana bodies	Farber disease (Dec Ceramidase)
• Birbeck granules	Histiocytosis X
• Cigar bodies	Sporotrichosis
• Caterpillar cell/ Anitschnow cell	Aschoff Nodule (RF)
• Caterpillar body	Porphyria
• Civatte bodies	Lichen planus
• Councilman body	Acute viral hepatitis, YF
• Donovan body	Granuloma inguinale
• Dutcher body	Multiple myeloma
• Guarneri body	Small pox
• Gamma gandy body	Portal HTN, sickle cell disease
• Globi bodies	Leprosy
• Globoid cell	Krabbe disease
• Hirano bodies	Alzheimer's
• Hurthle cell	Hashimoto's thyroiditis
• Kamino bodies	Nevus
• Marquee bodies	Kala-azar-Leishmania donovani
• Odland bodies	Normal skin body
• Orphan annie nuclei	Papillary CA thyroid
• Psamomma bodies	Papillary CA thyroid, Serous cystadenoma, Meningioma (PSM)
• Russell bodies	MM
• Schaumann bodies	Sarcoidosis
• Zellballen bodies	Chemodectoma/Paraganglioma

MICROBIOLOGY AND PARASITOLOGY

TABLE: Culture media

VR media	V. cholerae alkaline peptone water
Stuart transport medium	Resp. specimen
Enrichment media	Selenite F broth, Salmonella, Shigella
Enriched media	Blood agar chocolate agar
Selective media	Wilson Blair medium Salmonella
Potassium tellurite blood agar	C. diphtheriae

TABLE: Staining method

Z–N stain	Acid fast stain for mycobacteria, Nocardia
Kinyoun stain	Cold acid fast stain cryptosporidium parvum, Mycobact, Nocardia
Albert stain	Metachromatic stain for C. diphtheriae

TABLE: Colony appearance

• Thumb print app	Bordetella pertussis
• School of red fish	H. ducreyi (Chancroid)
• Fried egg colony	Mycoplasma hominis
• Poached egg colony	C. diphtheriae (Mitis) In tellurite agar
• Frog head colony	C. diphtheriae (intermedius)
• Nagler reaction	Cl. perfringens
• Medusa head	Bacillus anthracis
• Draughtsman colony	Strep. pneumoniae

TABLE: Agglutination tests and their uses

Agglutination test	Used mainly for
Direct agglutination test	Determination of blood group Bacterial agglutination test for serotyping and serogrouping. **E.g.: Vibrio Cholera, Salmonella Sp.**
Slide agglutination test	Used for serotyping of salmonella **VDRL for syphilis**
Tube agglutination test	Aka standard agglutination test. Used for serological diagnosis of typhoid, brucellosis and typhus fever. **E.g.: Widal Test, *Weil–Felix reaction,* and Kahn test**
Passive agglutination test	Rheumatoid factor **ANA for SLE** Antibody to Trichinella spiralis and antibody to group A strep.

RECENT

- Sporulation of bacteria seen in which phase: **Stationary phase**
- Doubling of bacteria seen in this phase: **Exponential phase**
- Bacterial cell wall is made up of: **Peptidoglycan**
- Fungal cell wall is made up of: **Chitin**
- Eukaryotic ribosomes are **80s ribosomes** (60s + 40s subunits)
- Prokaryotic ribosomes are **70s ribosomes** (50s + 30s subunits)
- **Staph. aureus** is the most common organism causing hospital acquired wound infections/surgical wounds
- **Hot air oven utilizes** 180°C for 1 hour, used for lab glass wares/glass syringes
- **Autoclaving**-attain temperature of 122°C under 15lb/sq inch pressure
- **Formaldehyde** gas is used for fumigation of OT/labs/rooms/ woollen blankets
- **Bacillus stearothermophilus** is a thermophile organism whose spores are extremely heat resistant.

Contd...

- **Bacillus subtilis** is the biological indicator for testing dry heat sterilizers, ethylene oxide sterilizers
- **Bacillus subtilis** is used in Guthrie test
- **Clostridium botulinum** spores are the most heat resistant organism and require 120°C 4 min or 100°C 330 min
- Proteus strains are used as antigens for **Weil–Felix reactions**
- **Classical pathway** is activated by IgM, IgG and immune complexes
- **Alternate pathway** is activated by bacterial endotoxin, zymogen, IgA and IgG4, cobra venom
- Most important **opsonizing complement-C3b**
- Most important chemotactic: **C5a**
- Proinflammatory cytokines that are present with dominance of **CMI-IL2, INF gamma, TNF alpha, IL1**
- Anti-inflammatory cytokines that are present with dominance of humoral immunity: **IL4, 5, 6, 10**
- Bruton agammaglobulinemia is X linked disease characterized by defective opsonization due to deficiency of **opsonizing antibodies**
- **Ataxia telangiectasia** is AR disorder characterized by triad of *cerebellar ataxia + oculocutaneous telangiectasia and immunodeficiency.
- **Chédiak–Higashi syndrome:** AR disorder associated with mutation in LYST gene
- **SCID**- due to lack of combined T cell, B cell, NK cells
- Most common primary tumor of anterior mediastinum is **Thymoma**
- **Nagler's reaction** is seen in clostridium perfringens, it is due to alpha toxin
- Most common species of pseudomonas causing intravenous catheter related infection: **Pseudomonas maltophilia**
- Most common organism implicated in osteomyelitis: **Staph. aureus**
- Most common cause of Hand foot mouth disease- **coxsackievirus A16**
- Most common viruses implicated in encephalitis- **Echoviruses**
- **Leptospirosis**-triad of fever, jaundice, renal failure,
- Gas gangrene most commonly caused by clostridium **perfringens (clostridium welchii)**
- Pikes media is transport media for **streptococcus pyogenes**
- Culture media for corynebacterium diphtheriae is - **Loeffler's serum slope**
- Culture media for neisseria gonorrhoeae is - **Thayer Martin medium**
- Fir tree appearance of colonies on culture shown by - **Bacillus anthrax**

Contd...

- Daisy head appearance of colonies on culture shown by **C. diphtheria**
- Fried egg colonies- **Mycoplasma**
- HACEK group of organisms
  - **H**-haemophilus species
  - **A**-actinobacillus actinomycetemcomitans
  - **C**-cardiobacterium hominis
  - **E**-eikenella corrodens
  - **K**-kingella kingae
- Weil Felix reaction is used for diagnosis of rickettsial disease
- **Toxins inhibiting protein synthesis:** Diphtheria, pseudomonas, shiga toxin
- MCC of traveler's diarrhea - **ETEC**
- Sereny test is an invasive test for Shigella
- Causative organism for trench fever - **Bartonella Quintana**
- **Mycoplasma** are also known as PPLO/eaton agent
- All DNA viruses are usually double stranded except **parvovirus (single stranded)**
- All RNA viruses are single stranded except **reovirus**
- Largest virus-pox virus, smallest virus-**parvovirus**
- HP body seen in: **Molluscum contagiosum**
- Negri bodies: **Rabies**
- Small pox- **Guarnieri bodies**
- **Primary infection with VZV** in non immune individuals causes-Chicken pox. Reinfection with VZV in immunocompromised individuals causes-herpes zoster (shingles)
- Swimming pool conjunctivitis - **Adenovirus** type 3, 7, 14
- Enterovirus 70- causes acute **Hemorrhagic conjunctivitis.**
- MCC of diarrhea in infants - **Rotavirus**
- Genital warts - **HPV 6, 11**
- **Antigenic drift in influenza** is due to point mutation under selection pressure of community
- **Antigenic shift in influenza** is due to genetic reassortment of human with avian/animal viruses → antigenic variations
- Yeast like organism-**Candida**
- Septate hyphae is seen in **Aspergillus**
- Most common fungal infection seen in immunocompetent host - **Aspergillus**
- Most common opportunistic fungal infection in HIV/AIDS patient - **Candida**
- Prominent polysaccharide capsule is seen in **Cryptococcus**
- Most common fungus producing meningitis in immunocompromised host is **Cryptococcus**
- Only rickettsia which can be cultured is - **R. Quintana**

Contd...

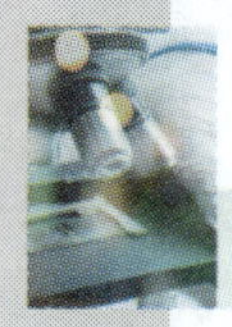

- Enterotoxins are not produced by - **Streptococcus**
- Casoni test is done in case of - **Hydatid cyst**
- Most common Protozoan parasite is **toxoplasma gondii**
- Mega esophagus is seen in **Chagas' disease**
- Smallest tapeworm - **echinococcus granulosus**
- Dwarf tapeworm is **H. nana**
- Longest tapeworm - **T. saginata**
- Cutaneous larva migrans- are caused by Ancylostoma **Braziliense**
- Bile stained eggs in stool is seen in ascaris, trichuris
- **Dumbbell** shaped eggs seen in case of: **Trichuris trichiura**
- Not commonly seen in ascariasis - **Anemia**
- Cystic stage is not seen in - **Trichomonas vaginalis.**
- Cellulitis is caused by: **Streptococcus**
- Pyoderma most commonly caused by staph aureus
- Cetrimide agar isolate which of the following bacteria: **Pseudomonas**
- Thayer martin agar is for: **N. meningitis**
- Traveller's diarrhea is caused by: **ETEC**
- HUS is caused by which strain of E. coli: **EHEC (0157: H7)**
- Incubation period of Diphtheria: **2–5 days**
- IP of chicken pox-**10-21 days**
- Infectious period of chicken pox is 2 days before to 5 days after the onset of rash
- Which protein attached to surface of bacteria and phagocytized: **Antibody**
- Food poisoning 2 hours after intake of food: **Staph. aureus**

TABLE: Some important motilities to note

Tumbling motility	Listeria
Swarming motility	Proteus
Gliding motility	P. aeruginosa, mycoplasma
Darting motility	Campylobacter, Vibrio Cholera
Falling leaf motility	Giardia
Shooting star motility	Vibrio
Cork screw motility	T. pallidum
Lashing motility	Borrelia

TABLE: Various shapes of bacteria

Shape	Associated bacteria
Club shape	Cornyebacteria
Lanceolate	Pneumococci
Half-moon/lens	Meningococci

Contd...

Shape	Associated bacteria
Kidney shape	Gonnococci
Comma	Vibrio and campylobacter
Drumstick appearance	Clostridium tetani
Chinese letter pattern	Corynebacterium diphtheria
D-shaped	Neisseria meningitides
Kidney shaped appearance	N. Gonorrhoeae
Flame shaped appearance	Strep. pneumoniae

TABLE: Types of food poisoning caused by bacillus cereus

Diarrhea type-main symptom	Emetic type-main symptom
Associated with wide range of food intake including meat, puddings etc. **I.P.** 8–16 hours Occurs due to heat labile enterotoxin	*Associated with intake of Chinese fried rice* **I.P.** 1–5 hours Due to pre-formed, heat stable toxin

TABLE: Clostridium microbes that causes food poisoning

Clostridium perfringens type A: Gastroenteritis
Clostridium perfringens type C: Necrotising enteritis
Clostridium botulinum: Botulism
Clostridium difficile: Acute colitis

TABLE: Viral inclusion bodies and their sites

Intracytoplasmic	Intranuclear	Intracytoplasmic + Intranuclear
Negri bodies in Rabies **Guarnieri bodies** in Small pox **Henderson-Peterson bodies** in Molluscum contagiosum	**Cowdry type A in Herpes simplex virus** and Varicella zoster virus and Torres bodies in Yellow fever **Cowdry type B** in Polio and adenovirus	**Warthin finkeldey bodies** in *Measles*

TABLE: Rickettsial diseases, their causative agents and vector

Disease	Cause	Vector
Epidemic typhus	R. prowazekii	Louse
Endemic typhus	R. typhi	Rat flea
Scrub Typhus	R. tsutsugamushi	Trombiculid mite
Indian tick typhus	R. conorii	Tick
RMSF	R. rickettsia	Tick
Trench fever	Bartonella quintana	None
Q fever	Coxiella	None but rarely soft tick

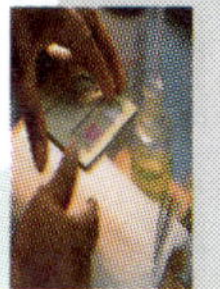

TABLE: Some or important points about immunoglobulin (Ig)

Ig having maximum molecular weight: **IgM**
First antibody produced by newborn: **IgM**
All immunoglobulin are heat stable except: **IgE**
Ig present in **breast milk: IgA**
Ig present **in oral cavity: IgA**
Ig with **maximum half-life: IgG**
Ig with **minimum half-life: IgE**
Ig having **maximum serum concentration: IgG**
Ig having **least serum concentration: IgE**

TEST FOR HIV
- Ser. Elisa – (Screening)
- Western blot – (Confirmatory)
- PCR RNA – IOC
- PCR DNA – IOC for window period
- Viral culture – Efficiency of antiviral

PARASITIC EGGS

Bile stained	Non-bile stained
• Ascaris • Trichuris	• Necator americanus • Enterobius vermicularis • H. nana • Ancylostoma duodenale

FLOATING VS NON FLOATING EGGS IN SATURATED SALT SOLUTION

Floats (FATEH)	Sink/Doesn't Float (STUF)
• Fertilized eggs of Ascaris • Ancylostoma duodenale • Trichuris trichiura • Enterobius vermicularis • H. nana	• Strongyloides stercoralis • Taenia solium/saginata • Unfertilized eggs of ascaris • Fasciola hepatica

TABLE: Important to know

• Sclerotic bodies are seen in	**Chromoblastomycosis**
• Organism present as cluster of round yeast cell with short, stout hyphae which is branched or curved	**Tinea nigra**
• Culture colonies are creamy white, smooth and with yeast odour	**Candida albicans**
• Culture shows round colonies with "cut-glass" appearance in transmitted light/inverted Fir tree app:	**Bacillus anthrax**
• Largest protozoa	**Syringammina Fragilissima (20 cm)**
• Largest liver fluke	**Fascioloides magna**
• Largest nematode	**Ascaris**

FORENSIC MEDICINE

IMPORTANT RECENT POINTS (INCLUDES LATEST QS)

Blood stain specific test: **Hemin test**
Plaintiff is: A person who files case in civil court
Grounds for MTP (Act 1971): • **Therapeutic:** Risk to pregnant women • **Eugenic:** Risk for child to be born • **Humanitarian:** Pregnancy caused by rape • **Socioeconomic:** Pregnancy due to contraceptive failure
Most common type of finger print: **Loops**
Postponement of hanging of pregnant lady is defined by which CrPC: **416**
IPC for marital rape: **IPC 376 A**
Declaration of Geneva is related with: **Hippocratic oath**
Declaration of Helsinki: Ethical principles for medical research involving human subjects
Declaration of Tokyo: International guidelines for physicians concerning torture and other cruel, inhuman or degrading treatment or punishment in relation to detention and imprisonment
Declaration of Lisbon: **Deals with the rights of the patient**
Declaration of Malta: **Hunger strikers**
Blanket consent is taken: **While admission to do any surgery**
Best bone specimen for sex differentiation: **Pelvis**
Davidson bodies is used to determine: **Sex**
Pearson formula is used for: **Stature**
Rugoscopy is study of: **Palate prints**
Locard system is: **Poroscopy**
Galton's system is used for: **Dactylography**
Instantaneous rigors is seen in: **Cadaveric spasm**
Time of floating of dead body in drowning in summer: **24 hours**
For toxicology sampling, best site for blood collection: **Femoral vein**
Hara-kiri is suicide by stabbing in: **Abdomen**
In blast injury which organ injured first: **Tympanic membrane > Lung**
Kennedy phenomenon is seen in: **Gunshot injury**
Pond's fracture is commonly seen in which age group: **Children**
Telefono is: **Beating on ears**
Outer covering of diatom is made of: **Silica**
Raygat's test is used for: **Specific gravity of lung**
Latte's crust of blood stain is used to detect: **Blood group**
Angel dust is: **Phencyclidine**

Contd...

Borax is: **Gastrointestinal irritant**

Widmark's formula helps in measurement of blood level of: **Alcohol**

McEwan's sign is seen in: **Alcoholic intoxication**

White vitriol is: **Zinc sulfate**

Blue vitriol is: **Copper sulfate**

Lee-Jones test is used for: **Cyanide**

Trousseau sign is positive in which poisoning: **Oxalic acid**

Odor of cyanide is: **Bitter almond**

Sexual asphyxia is associated with – **Masochism & Transvestism**

Arborescent or Filigree burns (Lichtenberg's flowers pattern) are seen in – **lightening**

Crocodile/Flash burns/joule burns/arc eye burn are seen in- **Electrocution**

Poisoning which does not affect diffusion at tissue level – **Curare** (It affects conduction at N-M level)

Chicken fat clot is never a characteristic feature of **antemortem wounds**

Defense attitude/boxer's attitude/pugilistic attitude is seen in **burns**

Gettler's test is used in death due to drowning

Podogram – study of footprints

Finger printing bureau of the world was established at writer's building at Calcutta in year 1897

Rounded (horse shoe shaped) nasal openings, orbits, palate: **Mongols**
Triangular (narrow & elongated) nasal openings, orbits, palate: **Europeans**
Quadrangular (square or rectangular) nasal openings, orbits, palate: **Negros**

Bertillon system (anthropometry) is applicable after age of **21 years**

Quetelet's rule of biological variation: No two hands have similar finger prints

Criminals may attempt to **mutilate finger prints** by applying CO_2 now, corrosive agents, burns, eroding against hard surface

Infrared photography: Makes old tattoos readily visible

First temporary teeth to appear is lower central incisor, first permanent (secondary) teeth to appear is 1st molar.

Angle of mandible is obtuse in infancy and old age.

Heart shaped pelvic inlet is seen in males & is widest in its posterior part, in females it is oval, widest most anteriorly than in males.

Whiplash injury results from acute hyperextension of cervical spine in region C4-C6 vertebrae

Ring fracture is any fracture round the foramen magnum

Brush burn/Friction burn/gravel rash are type of graze

Contd...

Gun powder a term usually used for black power consists of pot nitrate: 75%, charcoal: 15 %, sulphur: 10%

MC organ to be damaged in under water blast is **Gastrointestinal tract.**

Zenker's degeneration: Electrical injury produced in muscle

Cause of death in judicial hanging is **fracture of C2-3 or C3-4 vertebrae**

Frequency of hyoid fracture: Throttling > strangulation > Hanging.

Most reliable micro-chemical test for detecting blood in both recent & old stains: **Spectroscopic test**

Res Ipsa Loquitur: Thing or facts speak for itself

Corpus delicti: Body of offense.

Novus actus interveniens: A person is not only responsible for his action but also for logical consequences of actions.
Atavism: The child does not resemble its parents but its grand-parents.

Autopsy of the spinal cord is most commonly done through posterior approach

Subpoena/Summon: A document compelling attendance.

Albuminuria is seen with krait bite; **Hematuria** is seen in viper bite; **Myoglobinuria** is seen in sea snakes

Fatal period in drowning:
Death in fresh water: 4-5 minutes
Death in salt water: 8-10 minutes

Barberio's test is used for identification of: **Semen**

Test to distinguish human vs. animal blood - **Precipitin Test.**

Snake bite:
Cobra & krait: Neurotoxic
Sea snake: Myotoxic
Viper: Vasculotoxic, Hemotoxic

TABLE: Some important IPC's on Hurt (very potential topic)

Sec 319	Hurt
Sec 320	Grievous hurt
Sec 321	Voluntarily causing hurt
Sec 322	Voluntarily causing grievous hurt
Sec 325	Punishment for voluntarily causing grievous hurt
Sec 326	Punishment for voluntarily causing grievous hurt by a dangerous weapon

GOLDEN POINTS

Dowry death investigation is done by: **Magistrate**

IPC for perjury: **IPC 191**

Punishment for perjury: **IPC 193**

Contd...

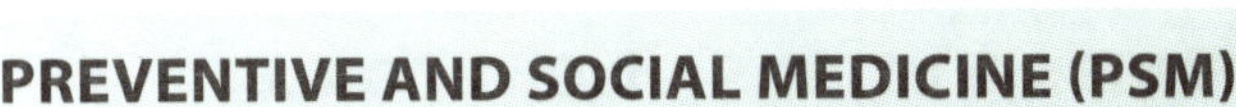

Sexual gratification by contact. Ex: rubbing genitalia on another person: **Frotteurism**
Blood alcohol level while driving: **30 mg%**
Phytobezoar is: **Intake of indigestible plant materials**
A female forges to have a child, whereas she doesn't have. It is **Suppositious child**
A child who is born to an unmarried women: **Illegitimate child**

TABLE: Types of hair on basis of medulla

Ladder or lattice type: **Animals**
Discontinuous type: **Animals**
Interrupted type: **White race, Caucasians**
Fragmented type: **Fetus, newborn**

TABLE: Different metallic poisoning and their effect on hair and skin

Poisoning	Color of hair and skin
Arsenic (As)	• Yellow color of skin, hair & mucous membrane • Milk rose (Brownish pigmentation)/Rain drop pigmentation • Black foot disease
Copper (Cu)	• Jaundiced skin • Green - Blue skin, hair & perspiration • Green – Purple line on gums
Mercury (Hg)	• Blue-black line on gums with jaw necrosis and loosening of tooth • Brown deposits on anterior lens capsule (mercurialentis) • Acrodynia (pink disease)
Lead (Pb)	• Blue stippled burtonian line on gums, especially on upper jaw.

TABLE: Poisoning and organ preserved

Poisoning	Organ preserved
Strychnine poisoning	Spinal cord (entire length)
Pesticides and Insecticides poisoning	Fat
CO, Cyanide, Organophosphates, Opiates, Barbiturates, Alkaloids and Strychnine poisoning *(Mn: COOBAS)*	Brain
Arsenic, Radium and Thallium poisoning *(Mn: ART)*	Bone

TABLE: Poisoning and their Antidote

Poisoning	Antidote/treatment
Oxalic acid (ink remover)	Calcium gluconate
Phosphorus	Copper sulfate
Organophosphorus	Atropine
Datura	Physostigmine
Arsenic	BAL, DMSA
Mercury	BAL, DMSA
Lead (Plumbism)	EDTA, DMSA
Methyl Alcohol	Fomepizole/Ethyl alcohol
Opium (Afeem)	Naloxone
Heroine/Brown sugar/ Junk/ Smack	Amyl nitrite
Bhang/Ganja/Charas	Diazepam
Strychnine	Diazepam
Copper	D-Penicillamine
Cyanide	Hydroxocobalamin

TABLE: Gun powders types and its constituent

Black gun powder	Smokeless powder
Consists of: Potassium nitrate 75% Sulfur 10% Charcoal 15%	**Consists of:** • *Nitrocellulose* (single base; gun cotton) • Nitroglycerine + Nitrocellulose • Nitroglycerine + Nitrocellulose + Nitroguanidine (triple base)

PREVENTIVE AND SOCIAL MEDICINE (PSM)

UPDATES IN PSM

• WHO theme for 2023	Health for all
• Ayushman Bharat Programme (ABP)	Health protection scheme (covers insurance of 5L)
• 2 major initiatives under ABP	Health and Wellness centre, National Health Protection Scheme
• Aim of health and wellness Centre	"bring health care closer to home" (1.5 L in number)
• Nobel prize in physiology to Jeffrey C Hall et al	Discovery of molecular mechanism controlling circadian rhythm
• Definition of blindness	Person unable to count fingers from 3 meter distance
• NPCB now new term	NPCB and Visual impairment

Contd...

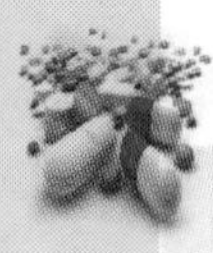

• Goal to reduce blindness by 2020	0.3% (now 1%)
• HDI	0.633
• GFR	2.3
• Sex ratio in India	1020/1000
• Age 0–6 years sex ratio	919/1000
• Highest sex ratio	Kerala (1084)
• Birth and death rate	16.1 and 6.6 respectively
• What is PENCIL portal	Electronic platform for effective enforcement for no child labor under ministry of labour and Employment
• 2 new contraceptives launched by health ministry	Antara (Inj) and Chhaya (pill) MPA: Methylprogesterone Acetate
• JEET program	Joint Effort for Elimination of TB
• SAPNA model	A local school going girl, a role model for leprosy elimination (MEENA- UNICEF)
• World malaria day	25 April 2019
• Mosquirix vaccine (RTS,S)	First approved malaria vaccine (available in Malawi for 5 mo to 2 years child)
• Pre-exposure prophylaxis if rabies	I/D: 2 site on 0 and 7 day IM: 1 site on 0 and 7 day
• Rabies Ig is given in this category of bite	Category III
• Td vaccine advantage	Freeze and heat resistant, open vial policy is applicable. Shelf life-24–36 month
• Characteristics of mentally healthy person	• Feels comfortable, secure and adequate about himself • Feels right towards other • Able to meet demands of life
• NITI Aayog *(replaced planning commission on 1st Jan 2015)*	**National Institution for Transforming India** • Provides a critical directional and strategic input into the development process. "Think tank" • Monitor and evaluate the implementation of programmes • Focus on technology upgradation and capacity building
• 3 years action agenda of NITI Aayog (2018-19 to 2019-20)	• The Aayog was told to prepare: • 15 year vision, 7 year strategy and Three Year Action agenda documents

Contd...

• Proposed ICD 11 to be presented in 2019 contains how many chapters	26
• EYE strategy for	Elimination Yellow Fever Epidemic (by WHO, UNICEF)

IMPORTANT ONE LINERS

Father of Medicine/First true Epidemiologist – **Hippocrates**
'Epidemiological Triad' comprises of – Agent, Host and Environment
Extermination of organism is – **Eradication**
Action taken prior to onset of disease is - **Primary Prevention**
Early diagnosis and treatment – **Secondary Prevention**
Ivory Towers of disease – **Large hospitals**
Prevalence is a ratio not rate
Total no of deaths/total no of cases – **Case fatality**
Observe deaths/expected deaths is – **Standardized mortality ratio (SMR)**
Cohort study is forward looking/prospective study
Relative risk is incidence among exposed/incidence among non-exposed
Framingham heart study is a cohort study
First case to come to notice of investigator is **index case**
Gap between primary case and secondary case is **serial interval**
First vaccine to be discovered is **smallpox vaccine** (Edward Jenner)
Risk of cold chain failure is greatest at- **subcenter/village level**
Bleaching powder – 33% available chlorine
Most effective sterilizing agent is – **Autoclaving**
Sensitivity identifies – true positives, specificity identifies - True Negative.
Usefulness of a screening test is given by – **Sensitivity**
Koplik's spots are diagnostic of – **Measles** (upper 2nd molar)
DOTS is – Directly Observed Treatment, Short Course Chemo-therapy
HBeAg is marker of – Infectivity/Viral replication
SARS is caused be – Corona virus
DANISH 1331 strain for – BCG vaccine
Chandlers Index for hookworms is – Average number of Eggs/g of stool
Only communicable disease of man that is always fatal – **Rabies**
Slim disease is – **AIDS**
MC cause of heart disease in 5-30 years old is – **Rheumatic** fever

Contd...

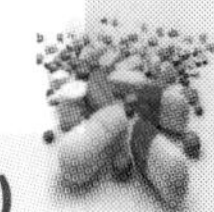

WHO blindness is - **<3/60**
Prevalence of blindness in India – **1%**
MC complaint of IUD insertion is – **bleeding**
MTP Act, 1971 was passed in – **April 1972**
3 most important MCH problems – **Malnutrition, Infection** and **Unregulated fertility**
Tocopherols are – **Vitamin E**
Richest source of vitamin-C – **Amla** (Indian Gooseberry)
Adult Pregnant females are anemic if – **Hb < 11 g%**
IQ calculation by = Mental Age/Chronological Age × 100
Disinfecting action of chlorine is due to – **Hypochlorous acid**
Residual level of chlorine in water – **0.5 mg × Contact period 1 hr**
Paris green is a – **Stomach Poison**
Sickness benefit under ESI Act, 1948 – **91 days**
World Health day – **7th April**
17 D strain – **Yellow fever vaccine**
DOC for lymphogranuloma venereum – **Doxycycline**
Hepatitis A & E transmission – **Faecal-oral route**
DOC cholera in pregnancy – **Azithromycin**
Tourniquet test (dengue) is +ve - >20 petechial spots/sq. inch in cubital fossa
8th Day Disease – **Tetanus neonatorum**
The Factory Act and ESI Act were passed in – **1948**
No plant source for vitamins – **B_{12} and D**
Milk is poor in – **Vit C and iron**
Multi-purpose Workers introduced by - **Kartar Singh Committee**
DOTS Plus refers to – **MDR TB treatment (Cat. IV)**
Midday meal program provides – **1/3 calories and ½ proteins**
MC side effect of Depot contraceptives – **Irregular menstrual bleeding**
Q-fever is caused by **Coxiella burnetii**
Carcinoma protected by OCP's – **Ovarian carcinoma**
Mortality is included in – **NRR** (Net reproduction rate)
Health worker in Malaria control must visit all houses every – **Fortnight**
Hepatitis B vaccine is type of – **killed vaccine**
Vaccine strain for swine flu vaccine in India – **A7/California**/2009
Normal IQ is – 90 to 109
Amplifier host of Japanese encephalitis – **Pigs**
In ORS, Na^+ absorption is due to – **Glucose**
Plasmodium discovered by – **Laveran**
MDR TB is – Resistance to INH and Rifampicin

Contd...

Denominator of GFR – Women in reproductive age group (15-49 years)
Most abundant Ig in breast milk – **IgA**
Most important step after disaster – **Chlorination of water**
Category 9 biomedical waste is – **Incineration ash**
Rural health Scheme was recommended by – **Srivastava Committee**
In DOTS diagnosis is based on – **Sputum smears**
Maximum tolerable sound level to human ears – **85 dB**
Wasted sharps biochemical waste disposed in – **Translucent**
OPV vaccine doses in immunization program including booster dose – **5**
Least priority color in triage – **Black**
Marc Koska discovered – K1 auto-disable syringes
Sufficiency of pasteurization is tested by – **Phosphatase test**
MC organism of food poisoning – **Staphylococcus**
1994 epidemic in India was – **Plague**
Father of Modern Toxicology – **Mathieu Orfila**
Main aim of vision 2020 – **Eliminate avoidable blindness**
Doors + windows area in school area - >25% floor area
Web of causation proposed by – **McMahon and Pugh**
Prophylactic treatment of rheumatic heart disease – **Benzathine penicillin**
Ambulatory patients in triage – **Cat III (Green)**
MDG Goal 4 is to reduce child mortality by – **Two-thirds by 2015**
Blood screening before transfusion – **HIV/HBV/HCV/Malaria/ Syphilis**
Failure rate of condoms – **2-14 per HWY**
India is in Demographic cycle – **Stage 3** (Declining Birth rate and Declining Death rate)
Avian influenza DOC – **Oseltamivir 150 mg BD × 5 days**
Normal distribution curve is – **Bell shaped symmetric**
MPW is located at – **Subcenter level**
International Conference at Alma-Ata (1978) gave concept of – **primary health care**
MC disorder to be screened in neonates – **Neonatal hypothyroidism**
Richest source of vit-A/D is – **Halibut liver oil**
Under RNTCP, Case finding is – **Passive**
Yaws is caused by- **Treponema pertenue**
For every 1 clinical case of Poliomyelitis, there are – **1000 sub-clinical cases**
Small Pox was declared Eradicated on- **8th May, 1980**

Contd...

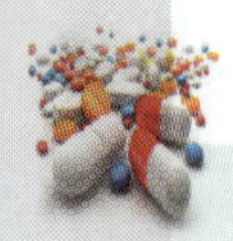

Only Non-steroidal OCP – **Centchroman (Saheli)**
MCC of blindness – **Cataract**
Elimination level for leprosy – **<1/10, 000**
Polio stool samples are transported in – **Reverse cold chain (+2°C to +8°C)**
Reverse smoking causes: **Carcinoma of hard palate**
ORS solution should be used within – **24 hours**
Year of great divide: **1921**
MCC of MMR in India: **Postpartum hemorrhage** MC direct cause of MMR: **PPH** MC indirect cause of MMR: **Anemia**
Gap between primary case and secondary case: **Serial interval**
Total amount of iron given during the pregnancy: **1000 mg**
Best contraceptive for a lactating female: **Progesterone only pill**
Ebola virus is spread by: **Through contact of body fluids**
Vitamin D richest source is: **Fish liver oil**
Chronic malnutrition is assessed by: **Height/age**
Refrigerated breast milk can be kept for: **24 hours**
In cholera epidemic which step should be first taken: **Safe water supply and sanitation**
Toxin in Epidemic dropsy is: **Sanguinarine**
Beds in CHC: **40**
Iodized salt is given in an area endemic of Goiter. Type of prevention: **Specific protection**
Graph showing Sharp rise and sharp fall in number of cases: **Point source epidemics**
Changes in occurrence of a disease over a long period of time: **Secular trend**
Lead time: **Delay between initiation and completion of a process**

TABLE: Levels of prevention

Level of prevention	Timing	Mode of prevention
Primordial	Before emergence of risk factor	–
Primary	Risk factor present but NO disease yet	Health promotion Specific protection
Secondary	When probably Disease has started	Early diagnosis Treatment
Tertiary	Disease in progression	Disability limitation Rehabilitation

TABLE: Vaccines and their associated strain

Vaccine	Strain
Anti HIV	Ankara strain *(under trial)*
Anti-malarial	Lytic cocktail (SPF 66)
BCG	DANISH 1331
Japanese Encephalitis	Nakayama Strain (killed) SA 14-14-2 (live)- Currently used
Killed H1N1	California strain
Measles	Edmonston strain
Mumps	Jeryl Lynn Strain
Rabies	Fixed viral strain
Rubella	RA 27/3 strain
Varicella	Oka strain
Yellow fever	17 D strain

Contd...

TABLE: Some common infectious diseases and their incubation period

Disease	Causative organism	Incubation period
Mumps	RNA Myxovirus	14 to 21 days
Influenza	Orthomyxovirus	18 to 72 hours
Measles (Rubella)	RNA Paramyxovirus	10 to 14 days
Chickenpox	Human Herpes Virus 3	14 to 16 days

TABLE: Common mosquitos and their associated diseases

Anopheles (Sophisticated mosquito)	Culex (nuisance mosquito)	Aedes (tiger mosquito)	Mansonoides
Malaria	• Japanese encephalitis • West Nile fever • *Bancroftian filariasis* • Viral hemorrhagic	• Yellow fever • Rift valley fever • Chikungu-nya fever • Dengue • Dengue haemor-rhagic fever	• Brugian filariasis

TABLE: Some national health programs and their respective years

National Mental Health Programme: **1987**
National Family Planning Programme: **1951**
National Tuberculosis Programme (NTP): **1962**
Revised National TB Control Programme (RNTCP): **1992**
National AIDS Control Programme (NACP): **1987**
National Malaria Control Programme (NMCP): **1953**
National Leprosy Control Program: **1955**
Integrated Child Development Services scheme (ICDS): **1975**
National Programme for Control of Blindness (NPCB): **1976**

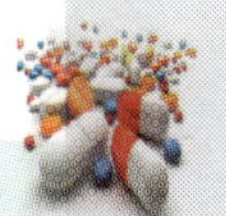

TABLE: IQ scoring of mental retardation

Mental status	IQ range
Normal IQ	70 and below
Mild mental retardation	50–69
Moderate MR	35–49
Severe MR	21–34
Profound MR	20 and below

TABLE: Food adulteration diseases and their toxins

Disease	Toxin	Adulterant
Lathyrism	BOAA	Khesari Dal
Epidemic dropsy	*Sanguinarine*	*Argemone oil*
Endemic ascites	Pyrrolizidine alkaloids	Crotalaria seeds
Ergotism	Ergot/clavine alkaloids	Claviceps fusiformis
Aflatoxicosis	Aflatoxins	Aspergillus flavus

TABLE: Interpretation of Chandler's index

Average number of eggs/g of stool	Interpretation
<200	No significance
200–250	Potential danger
250–300	Minor public health problem
>300	Major public health problem

MODIFIED KUPPUSWAMI SCALE

It includes 3 components:

- Education status of head
- Occupation status of head
- Income per capita.

Total score of 3 components	Socioeconomic class
26–29	Upper
16–25	Upper-middle
11–15	Lower-middle
05–10	Upper-lower
03–04	Lower

TABLE: Triage color code and their significance

Category	Color	Remarks/steps
Category 1	Red	**Highest priority -** Patient immediate resuscitations or lifesaving surgery (0 to 6 hours)
Category 2	Yellow/ blue	High possible resuscitation or life-saving surgery (within 6 to 24 hours)
Category 3	Green	Ambulatory/low minor injuries; non-life threating
Category 4	Black	Dead, Moribund; least priority

TABLE: Biomedical waste management

Color Category	Type of biomedical waste	Treatment options
Yellow	• Human & animal anatomical waste • Soiled waste (with blood, body fluid) • Expired/Discarded/ cytotoxic medicine • Chemical waste • Chemical liquid waste • Discarded linen, mattress, beddings contaminated with blood or body fluids	Incineration/Deep burial Non-chlorinated chemical disinfection
Red	• Recyclable contaminated waste ▪ Disposable items such as tubes, bottles, IV sets, urine bags, syringes without needle, gloves	Autoclaving or microwaving/ hydroclaving followed by shredding
White/ Translucent *(puncture/ leak proof container)*	• Waste sharps including metals: Needles, blades or any contaminated sharp object	Autoclaving or dry heat sterilization followed by shredding and mutilation
Blue	• Glassware: Included medicine vials except those contaminated with cytotoxic waste • Metallic body implants	Disinfection (by soaking waste with detergent and sodium hypochlorite)/ Autoclaving/ Microwaving/ Hydroclaving

INSTRUMENT OF IMPORTANCE PUBLIC HEALTH

Instruments	Use
• Ice Lined Refrigerator	Cold chain temperature maintenance
• Dial Thermometer	Cold chain temperature monitoring
• Horrocks apparatus	Chlorine demand estimation in water
• Chloroscope	Measuring level of residual chlorine in drinking water

Contd...

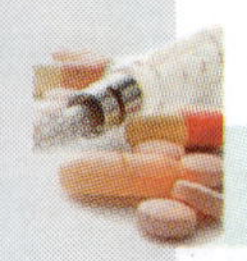

Instruments	Use
• Winchester Quart/ Quart Bottle	Assess physical & chemical quality of drinking water
• Kata Thermometer	Assess cooling power and velocity of air
• Psychrometer	Humidity
• Anemometer	Assess air & wind velocity
• Hygrometer/Sling Psychrometer	Assess air humidity
• Salter's Scale	Field instrument to assess lbw
• Stadiometer	Height of adult
• Shakir's Tape	Mid arm circumference

MEDICINE

SPECIFIC GRAVITY

• Specific gravity of ascitic fluid/Edema	<1.012 (transudate); >1.020 (exudate)
• Effusion fluid	<1.016 (transudate); >1.016 (exudate)
• Urine	1.015–1.025
• Hydatid fluid	1.005–1.009

TABLE: Classification of weight status and disease risk

Classification	Body mass Index (kg/m^2)	Obesity class	Disease risk
Under weight	<18.5	–	–
Healthy weight	18.5–24.9	–	–
Over weight	25.0–29.9	–	Increased
Obesity	30.0–39.9	I	High
Obesity	35.0–39.9	II	Very high
Extreme obesity	≥40	III	Extremely high

TABLE Ethnic-specific cut point values for waist circumference

Ethnic group	Waist circumference
Europeans	
Men	>94 cm (>37 in)
Women	>80 cm (>31.5 in)
South Asians and Chinese	
Men	>90 cm (>35 in)
Women	>80 cm (>31.5 in)
Japanese	
Men	>85 cm (>33.5 in)
Women	>90 cm (>35 in)

TREMORS

• Physiological tremors	Anxiety, Fright (8–12 Hz)
• Resting tremor, Pin rolling	PD (4–6 Hz)
• Intentional tremor	Cerebellar lesion <4 Hz
• Essential/Fine tremor	Hyperthyroidism Rosenbach sign: Fine tremor of closed eyelids
• Flapping tremor/Asterixis	Hepatic and metabolic tremor
• Perioral tremor	Rabbit synd. General paresis of insane

IMPORTANT POINTS

Most common type of headache: **Tension headache**
Most common type of headache in males: **Cluster headache**
Most common type of seizure in neonate: **Subtle seizure**
Most common type of seizure in adults: **GTCS**
Most common cause of meningitis in neonate: **Klebsiella > Staph. Aureus**
Most common primary malignant brain tumor: **Glioma**
Most common benign brain tumor: **Meningioma**
IOC for Addison's disease: **ACTH stimulation test**
IOC Conn's syndrome: **Aldosterone renin ratio**
Congenital adrenal hyperplasia: **21a- Hydroxylase**
Best test for short term control of diabetes: **Serum Fructosamine**
Curschmann's spirals are seen in **Bronchial asthma**
Pink frothy sputum is seen in **Pulmonary edema**
Most common cause of acute bacterial endocarditis: ***Staph aureus***
Most common cause of sub-acute bacterial endocarditis: ***Step viridans***
Most common cause of prosthetic valve endocarditis: **CONS**
Libman sacks endocarditis is seen with: **SLE**
Strongest layer of GIT: **Sub mucosal layer**
Pacemaker of GIT: **Cells of Cajal**
Most common cause of hemoptysis: **Pulmonary TB**
Most common cause of hematemesis: **PUD**
IOC of GERD: **24-hour pH monitoring**
Marker of eradication of H. Pylori: **Urea breath test**
DOC of IBD: **Sulfasalazine**
Hepatitis B antigen first to appear in blood: **HBsAg**
Hepatitis B antigen which never appears in blood: **HBcAg**
Pseudochylous ascites is seen in: **Malignant ascites**
Pseudo-lymphoma is seen in: **Sjögren's syndrome**

Contd...

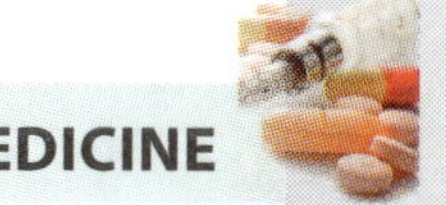

Most common type of nephrotic syndrome in adults: **Focal segmental glomerulosclerosis**

Most common type of nephrotic syndrome in children: **Minimal change disease**

Most sensitive marker of SLE: **ANA (Antinuclear antibody)**

Investigation of choice for SLE: **ds- DNA**

Antibody causing psychosis in SLE: **Anti-Ribosomal-P antibody**

IOC for antiphospholipid antibody syndrome: **Anti-β2 Glyco-protein antibody**

Earliest clinical feature of scleroderma: **Raynaud's phenomenon**

Interstitial pneumonia is most frequently due to influenza virus

Bulging fissure on CXR is seen in: **Klebsiella pneumonia**

Most common site of Bronchiectasis: **Left Lower lobe**

Most common clinical presentation of lung CA: **Cough**

Glucose fever is relates with: **Aldosterone**

Partial pressure of oxygen in alveoli: **103 mm Hg**

CSF glucose compared to blood glucose: 60–70% of concentration of blood

Resistant hypertension: **Resistance to 3 or more anti-hypertensive drugs including thiazides**

Antibody incriminated in causing Henoch-Schonlein purpura: **IgA**

Iron is absorbed from: **Duodenum with fast clearance**

Thalassemia: Autosomal Recessive

Diarrhea can present with hypokalemia and Metabolic acidosis

Seborrheic dermatitis, cellulitis, alopecia and apathy is seen in: **Biotin deficiency**

RBC cast is present in: **Acute Glomerulonephritis**

In Wilson disease, chelation is done by: **Trientine**

In hemochromatosis, all organs are affected except: **CNS**

CNS bleed in boxers: **Subdural hemorrhage**

LE cells are seen in: **SLE**

Emphysema seen due to chronic smoking: **Centriacinar emphysema**

Wegener's granulomatosis is diagnosed by: **c-ANCA**

DOC for enteric fever: **Ceftriaxone**

DOC for listeria meningitis: **Ampicillin**

DOC for Herpes simplex encephalitis: **Acyclovir**

Mottling of lung is seen in: **Silicosis**

Antibody in Goodpasture syndrome: **Anti-GBM**

Most common Callum patch in rheumatic heart disease is seen in: **Left Atrium**

Canon A wave is seen in: **Complete Heart Block**

Most common cause of mitral stenosis: **Rheumatic fever**

Contd...

In case of severe MS how much left atrial pressure required to maintain a normal cardiac output: **~25 mm Hg**

Malar flush with **pinched and blue facies** are clinical findings in case of: **Severe Mitral stenosis**

Carvallo's sign is seen in: Functional tricuspid regurgitation (TR) secondary to severe pulmonary hypertension

Carvallo's sign: Functional TR may be audible along the left sternal border. **This murmur is usually louder during inspiration and diminishes during forced expiration**

TABLE: Congenital heart diseases and their CXR finding

Total anomalous pulmonary venous connection	Figure of 8 or snowman heart
Transposition of great arteries	Egg on side appearance
TOF	Boot shaped heart
Ebstein anomaly	Box shaped heart
Coarctation of aorta	'3' sign

TABLE In HIV positive individuals/AIDS

Most common malignancy	Kaposi sarcoma (70%)
Most common cause of seizures	HIV encephalopathy > Cerebral toxoplasmosis
Most common fungal infection	Cryptococcus neoformans
Most common lymphoma (NHL)	B- cell immunoblastic lymphoma (CMS lymphoma)
Most common cause of blindness	CMV retinitis
Most common eye lesions	Cotton wool spots, HIV keratitis
Most common opportunistic infection	Pneumocystis carinii (Tuberculosis in India)
Most common CXR finding in TB with HIV	Miliary shadows
Most common electrolyte abnormality	Hyponatremia, SIADH

TABLE: ECG basics

ECG finding	Significance
P wave	Atrial depolarization
QRS	Ventricular depolarization
T wave	Ventricular repolarization
U wave	Delayed repolarization of papillary muscles
PR interval	Spread of impulse from SAN to AVN
ST segment	Isoelectric segment

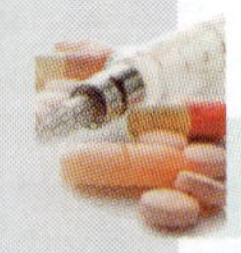

TABLE: S1 heart sounds and its variables

Loud S1	Soft S1	Variable S1	Reversed split S1
Normal in children Anemia Pregnancy Sinus tachycardia Thyrotoxicosis, Beriberi AV fistula Mitral and tricuspid stenosis Short PR interval	Sinus bradycardia Prolonged PR interval Severe MR Chronic severe MR Acute MI Myocarditis Ventricular aneurysm Cardiomyopathy Calcified MS	AV dissociation Atrial fibrillation Complete heart block Multiple ectopics Ventricular tachycardia Atrial flutter with varying block	Mitral stenosis Left atrial myxoma Left bundle branch block

TABLE: Heart sounds and murmurs

Mid-systolic murmur	Pansystolic murmur	Late systolic murmur	Early diastolic murmur	Mid-diastolic murmur	Continuous murmurs
AS PS HOCM TOF ASD	MR VSD TR	MVP OCM	AR PR Graham Steell murmur (pulmonary incompetence due to pulmonary HT and MS)	MS Austin flint (aortic regurgitation) TS Carey-Coombs murmur (Rheumatic fever)	PDA Coronary AV fistula ASD Mammary souffle Anomalous left coronary artery Ruptured aneurysm of sinus of Valsalva Proximal coronary artery stenosis Aortopulmonary window

TABLE Mediastinal masses: Most common lesions are

Anterior mediastinum	Middle mediastinum	Posterior mediastinum
Thymoma Lymphomas Teratomatous neoplasms Thyroid masses	Pericardial cyst *(Most common mediastinal mass)* Lymphoma *(MC mediastinal tumor)* Vascular masses Granulomatous disease Bronchogenic cysts	Neurogenic tumors (Overall MC) Meningoceles Meningomyeloceles Gastroenteric cysts Esophageal diverticula

TABLE: Anemia and their causes

Microcytic Hypochromic anemia	Normocytic Normochromic	Macrocytic anemia
Sideroblastic anemia Iron deficiency Thalassemia Anemia of chronic disease Lead poisoning	CRF A.I.H.A HL/NHL C.L.L Aplastic anemia	CLD Hypothyroidism Aplastic anemia Decrease B_{12} and Folic acid level

TABLE: Extravascular and intravascular hemolysis

Extravascular hemolysis	Intravascular hemolysis
Hereditary Spherocytosis Thalassemia Sickle cell anemia	Cold agglutinin syndrome G6PD (XLR)
Haptoglobin level normal	Haptoglobin level decreases or absent

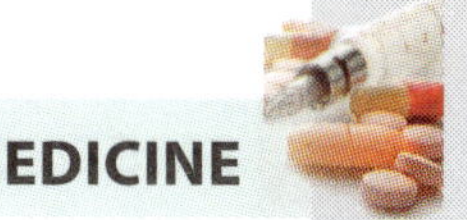

TABLE: Common hematological malignancies

Disease	Finding	IOC	TOC
Polycythemia vera	Hb >19 gm%	Urinary erythropoietin level	Venesection (phlebotomy)
CML	Ph (9:22)	Flow cytometry	Imatinib
Essential thrombocytosis	Platelets conc: ↑↑	Platelets conc:	Hydroxyurea
Myelofibrosis	Tear drop RBC	BM Biopsy	BM Tx

TABLE: Intracranial bleed and their CT findings

Subdural hematoma	Concavo-convex bleed hyper-density
Extradural hemorrhage	Biconvex /flame shaped hyper-density
Subarachnoid hemorrhage	Intraventricular bleed/blood in sylvian fissure
Intraparenchymal bleed	Mostly a lesion or hyperdensity in basal ganglia secondary to hypertension.

TABLE: CSF findings in common infections

CSF	Normal	Acute bacterial meningitis	Tubercular meningitis	Viral meningitis	Guillain–Barré syndrome	Fungal meningitis
Pressure	50–180 mm H_2O	Increased	Increased	Increased	Normal	Elevated
Color	Clear	Turbid	Straw	Clear	Normal	
Cells	0–4 lymphocytes/cu.mm	>1000	>100	>25	Normal	25–500
Sugar	2/3rd of blood sugar	Decreased	Decreased	Normal	Normal	Low
Protein	15–45 mg %	Increased	Increased	Increased	Increased *(albumin-cytological disassociation)*	Normal/ elevated

TABLE: Differences between lower and upper motor neuron lesion

	LMN	UMN	Extra pyramidal damage
TONE	Decreased tone/flaccidity	Increased spasticity	Decreased rigidity
DTR	Areflexia	Brisk reflex	Normal
Special features	Fasciculations + wasting	Babinski's sign + No wasting	Chorea, athetosis, hemiballismus
Superficial reflex	Present	Absent	–
Example	Motor neuron disease	Cerebral malaria	Punch drunk syndrome

TABLE: Modified Jones criteria

Major criteria	Minor criteria	Essential criteria
Carditis	Fever	ASO titer >333 IU for children 5–15 years
Arthritis	Arthralgia	Throat swab positive for group A beta hemolytic streptococcus
Sydenham chorea	Laboratory parameters Increased PR interval CRP positive Leukocytosis Increased ESR	2015 update is discussed in cardiology section in Medicine
Erythema marginatum		
Subcutaneous nodules		

TABLE: Hormonal levels in some common adrenal pathologies

Aldosterone	↑Conn's ↓Addison's
Cortisol	↑Cushing syndrome
Sex sterioids	↑Congenital adrenal hyperplasia ↓Hypogonadism

TABLE: Common infections and their causative organism

Infection	Causative organism
Lobar pneumonia/Community acquired Pneumonia	Pneumococcus
Nosocomial pneumonia	*Staph. aureus*
HIV associated pneumonia	*P. Jiroveci*
Meningitis adults (sporadic)	Pneumococcus
Meningitis adults (epidemic)	*Neisseria meningitidis*

TABLE: Anion gaps

Normal anion gap *(Mn: FUSED CAR)*	Increased anion gap *(Mn: MUDPILES)*	Decreased anion gap *(Mn: BPH-M)*
F- Fistula pancreatic **U-**Ureterosigmoidos-tomy **S-** Small bowel fistula **E-** Extra chloride **D-** Diarrhea **C-** Carbonic anhydrase Inhibitor *(acetazolamide)* **A-** Adrenal insufficiency **R-** Renal tubular acidosis	**M** - Methanol **U** - Uremia **D** - DKA/AKA/SKA *(diabetic/alcoholic/ starvation)* **P** - Paraldehyde / phenformin **I** - Iron / INH **L** - Lactic acidosis **E** - Ethylene glycol **S** - Salicylates	Bromide intoxication Plasma cell dyscrasia Hypoalbumine-mia Monoclonal protein

TABLE: Important casts

Hyaline cast: Present normally in urine
RBC cast: Seen in acute glomerulonephritis
WBC cast: Seen in acute interstitial nephritis, pyelo nephritis
Brood granular casts: Seen in chronic renal failure

TABLE: Tumor markers

Tumor markers	Cancer	Non-neoplastic conditions
Hormones		
Human chorionic gonadotropin	Gestational trophoblastic disease, gonadal gem cell tumor	Pregnancy
Calcitonin	Medullary cancer of the thyroid	
Catecholamines	Pheochromocytoma	
Oncofetal antigens		
α Fetoprotein	Hepatocellular carcinoma, gonadal germ cell tumor	Cirrhosis hepatitis
Carcinoembry-onic antigen	Adenocarcinomas of the colon, pancreas, lung, breast, ovary	Pancreatitis, hepatitis, inflammatory bowel disease, smoking
Enzymes		
Prostatic acid phosphatase	Prostate cancer	Prostatitis, prostatic hypertrophy
Neuron-specific enolase	Small-cell cancer of the lung, neuroblastoma	

Contd...

Tumor markers	Cancer	Non-neoplastic conditions
Lactate dehydrogenase	Lymphoma, Ewing's sarcoma	Hepatitis, hemolytic anemia, many others
Tumor-associated proteins		
Prostate-specific antigen	Prostate cancer	Prostatitis, prostatic hypertrophy
Monoclonal immunoglobulin	Myeloma	Infection, MGUS
CA-125	Ovarian cancer, some lymphomas	Menstruation, peritonitis, pregnancy
CA 19–9	Colon, pancreatic, breast cancer	Pancreatitis, ulcerative colitis
CD30	Hodgkin's disease anaplastic large-cell lymphoma	–
CD 25	Hairy cell leukemia, adult T cell leukemia/ lymphoma	–

TABLE: Suspected carcinogens

Tumor markers	Cancer
Carcinogens	Associated cancer of neoplasm
Alkylating agents	Acute myeloide leukemia, bladder cancer
Androgens	Prostate cancer
Aromatic amines (dyes)	Bladder cancer
Arsenic	Cancer of the lung, skin
Benzene	Acute myelocytic leukemia
Chromium	Lung cancer
Diethylstilbestrol (prenatal)	Vaginal cancer (clear cell)
Epstein-Barr virus	Burkitt's lymphoma, nasal T cell lymphoma
Estrogens	Cancer of the endometrium, liver, breast
Ethyl alcohol	Cancer of the breast, liver esophagus, head and neck
Helicobacter pylori	Gastric cancer, gastric MALT lymphoma
Hepatitis B or C virus	Liver cancer
Human immunodeficiency virus	Non-hodgkin's lymphoma, kaposi's sarcoma, squamous cell carcinomas (especially of the urogenital tract)
Human papilloma virus	Cancers of the cervix, anus, oropharynx

Contd...

Tumor markers	Cancer
Human T cell lymphotropic virus type 1 (HTLY-1)	Adult T cell leukemia/lymphoma
Immunosuppressive agents (azathioprine cyclosporine, glucocorticoids)	Non-hodgkin's lymphoma
Ionizing radiation (therapeutic or diagnostic)	Breast, bladder, thyroid, soft tissue, bone, hematopoietic and many more
Nitrogen mustard gas	Cancer of the lung, head and neck, nasal sinuses
Nickel dust	Cancer of the lung, nasal sinuses
Phenacetin	Cancer of the renal pelvis and bladder
Polycyclic hydrocarbons	Cancer of the lung, skin (especially squamous cell carcinoma of scrotal skin)
Radon gas	Lung cancer
Schistosomiasis	Bladder cancer (squamous cell)
Sunlight (ultraviolet)	Skin cancer (squamous cell and melanoma)
Tobacco (including smokeless)	Cancer of the upper aerodigestive tract, bladder
Vinyl chloride	Liver cancer (angiosarcoma)
Agents that are thought to act as cancer initiators and/or promoters	

TABLE: A comparison of syndromes of obesity—hypogonadism and mental retardation

	Syndrome	
Feature	**Prader-Willi**	**Laurence-Moon-Biedl**
Inheritance	Sporadic; two-thirds have defect	Autosomal recessive
Stature	Short	Normal; infrequently short
Obesity	Generalized Moderate of severe onset 1–3 years	Generalized Early onset, 1–2 years
Craniofacies	Narrow bifrontal diameter almond-shaped eyes strabismus v-shaped mouth high-arched palate	Not distinctive

Contd...

	Syndrome	
Feature	**Prader-Willi**	**Laurence-Moon-Biedl**
Limbs	Small hands and feet hypotonia	Polydactyly
Reproductive status	1° Hypogonadism	1° Hypogonadism
Other features	Enamel hypoplasia Hyperphagia Temper tantrums Nasal speech	
Mental retardation	Mild to moderate	

IMPORTANT TO KNOW

• Light's criteria is used to determine	Exudative vs transudative pleural fluid
• MCC of transudative pleura effusion	CHF
• MCC of exudative pleural Effusion	TB
• Comprehension and Fluency and in Broca's and Wernicke's aphasia	BCWF **Broca:** Comprehension preserved **Wernicke:** Fluency preserved
• Triad of Miller Fisher syndrome	Ophthalmoplegia Areflexia Ataxia
• Oligoclonal IgG • Bands in CSF	Multiple sclerosis (MRI: Dawson fingers)
• Charcot's triad	Intentional tremor, Nystagmus, Dysarthria (IND)
• Charcot triad of Ascending cholangitis	RUQ pain, fever, jaundice
• Ashleaf spot, Shagreen patch seen in	Tuberous sclerosis
• Vogt triad of tuberous sclerosis	Seizure, MR, facial angiofibroma
• Anti Histone A/B is specific for	Drug induced lupus
• McGinn white sign is seen in	Pulm Embolism (S1Q3T3)
• Sputum containing charcot-leyden crystal, curschmann spirals, Creola bodies	Bronchial Asthma
• Current jelly sputum	Klebsiella pneumoniae
• Giant cell/Hecht's pneumonia is seen in	Measles

Contd...

• Austin flint murmur is heard in	Severe AR
• Osborn wave/ J wave is seen in	Hypothermia
• ST segment in ECG	End to S to beginning of T
• ECG finding of digitalis toxicity	T wave inversion, Inverse check mark sign
• Wenckebach phenomenon is seen in	2nd degree heart block (Mobitz 1) Seen in digitalis toxicity, B# toxicity
• Murmur which is increased in valsalva maneuver	HOCM, MVP
• Aschoff bodies are pathognomonic of this condition	RF
• D Xylose test is used for	Malabsorption (pancreatic vs intestinal cause)
• Fulminant hepatitis rate is maximum in	Hep D superinfection
• Diuretic which can cause barter syndrome	Furosemide
• Nephrocalcinosis is a feature of this type of RTA	Type I
• Hyperkalemia is feature of this type of RTA	Type IV
• MM, Fanconi synd, Wilson's disease can cause this RTA	Type II (MC type of RTA)
• RIFLE criteria is used for	Acute kidney injury
• Reid index is used in	Chronic bronchitis (>0.4)
• MC cause of BUDDCHIARI syndrome –	Polycythemia vera
• MC symptom of portal hypertension –	GI bleeding
• Most specific tumor marker of HCC –	Alpha fetoprotein
• MC renal lesion associated with HCV-MPGN -1	MPGN
• MC GN associated with HIV	FSGS
• MC cause of nephrotic syndrome in adult	MGN
• MC type of MI	Ant wall MI
• MC type of HIV in India	HIV 1 subtype C
• MC organ affected in amyloidosis	Kidney
• MC cause of death in amyloidosis	Restrictive cardiomyopathy
• First enzyme rise in MI	Heart fatty acid binding protein > Myoglobin

Contd...

• First enzyme to be elevated in MI	Troponin I
• Most important biomarker for diagnosing MI	Trop I
• MC type of stroke	Embolic
• MC site of hemorrhagic stroke	Putamen
• MC type of fistula in CD	Colocolic
• MC type of incontinence in LMN bladder	Over flow incontinence
• MC type of incontinence in UMN balder	Urge incontinence
• Ankle Jerk in UMNL	Brisk (and absent in LMNL)
• MC cause of cardiac tamponade	Neoplastic disease, idiopathic pericarditis, uremia
• MC nerve affected intracranial aneurysm	III
• MC nerve involved in increased ICP	VI
• MC complication of hemodialysis	Hypotension and increased CV mortality
• Least common RCC	Chromophobe renal carcinoma
• MCC of chr. renal failure	DM nephropathy
• MCC of HTN	Essential HTN
• MCC Of Glomerulonephritis	Ig A nephropathy

CHANNELOPATHIES

Disease	Ion channel involved
• Hypokalemic periodic paralysis type I	Slow Ca+ channel
• Hyperkalemic periodic paralysis	Na^+
• Cystic fibrosis, Myotonia congenita	Cl^-
• Episodic ataxia-1	K^+ channel
• Episodic ataxia-2, Malignant hyperthermia	Ca^+ channel

SURGERY

IMPORTANT RECENT POINTS (INCLUDES LATEST QS)

Most common site for polymazia is **axilla**

Amazia refers to absence of stromal and glandular part of breast but presence of nipple and areola

Tietze disease: Costochondritis, MC involves 2nd costal cartilage

Mondor's disease – Superficial thrombophlebitis of veins over chest wall and upper abdominal wall

Fibrocystic disease of breast is usually B/L and common in younger women

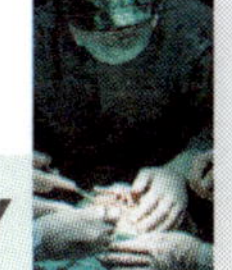

GOLDEN POINTS

Mastitis
MC organism: ***Staph aureus***
Rx – modified Hiltons method
IOC – USG

Breast cyst
Well defined **lump**
IOC – USG GUIDED FNAC
Rx – USG guided aspiration

Fibroadenoma
MC benign **tumor of breast**
Highly mobile – **Breast mouse**
MC breast tumor in females less than **30 yrs of age**
Firm in consistency
Upon mammography: Popcorn calcification
IOC- FNAC
Rx – Excision

Nipple discharge
Bloody – Duct papilloma (MCC)
Greenish / grumous – Duct ectasia (MCC)
Milky – Galactorrhea (MCC pathologically)
Serous – Fibro cystic disease of breast (MCC)

Duct ectasia
IOC - Mammography Rx – Hadfield's operation

Duct papilloma
IOC - Mammography Rx - Microdochectomy

Cystosarcoma phyllodes
Huge lump Irregular and variable consistency IOC –FNAC Rx- benign – Wide local excision Malignant – Simple mastectomy

Breast cancer
Genetic – BRCA 1, BRCA 2, P53 (Li-Fraumeni syndrome) **IOC** – Mammography Ductal carcinoma in situ **MC** non-invasive breast cancer **MC** comedo cell pattern **IOC** - Incisional biopsy **Rx** - Simple mastectomy

TABLES: Types of mastectomy

Simple or total mastectomy	Removal of breast tissue, nipple-areola complex, and skin
Extended simple mastectomy	Simple mastectomy + removal of level I axillary LNs.
Modified radical mastectomy	Removes all breast tissue and skin, nipple areola complex, pectoralis major and minor muscles and the level, I, II and III axillary LNs,
Extended radical mastectomy	Radical mastectomy + Removal or internal mammary, LNs
Super radical mastectomy	Radical mastectomy + Removal of internal mammary, mediastinal and supraclavicular LNs

3 IMPORTANT TYPES OF MRM

Patey's	Pectoralis minor removed to dissect level III LN
Auchincloss's	Preservation of both pectoralis major and minor. Level I and II LN dissection
Scanlon's	Pectoralis minor divided to remove level III LN

Note: *Structure NOT removed in radical mastectomy: Supraclavicular LN*

Bile and gallbladder facts
Maximum capacity gall bladder - **50 mL** Concentration of bile: **5-10 times** Production of bile: **40 mL/hr** Terminal ileum absorbs – **B_{12} & bile salts**

Congenital choledochal cyst
Cyst like dilatation of biliary tree due to weakness of wall
Type 1 is most common
Type 4 is Caroli's disease

Contd...

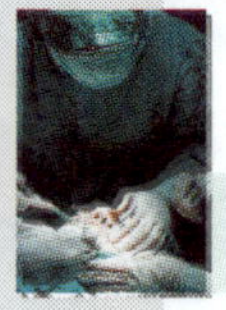

Congenital choledochal cyst
IOC – MRCP
Rx: Excision

Cholelithiasis
Pigmented stones: Hemolytic anemia MC cause
Predisposing factor 5f's – fatty, forty, female, fertile and flatulence
IOC-USG abdomen
Rx-laparoscopic cholecystectomy

Acute cholecystitis
IOC – HIDA scan
Rx - Conservative

Chronic cholecystitis
IOC-USG
Rx-Laparoscopy cholecystectomy

Mucocele of gallbladder
Stone in Hartmann's pouch cannot cause mucocele
C/f–lump in Right Upper Quadrant
IOC–USG
Rx-Laparoscopic cholecystectomy

Empyema/pyocele
Clinical feature-Tender lump + fever
IOC–USG
Rx-Cholecystectomy +/- antibiotics

Pneumobilia
Air from D1 passes in gall bladder through fistula, presence of air in biliary tree
Management: Ileostomy with extraction of stone

Acalculous cholecystitis
Cause-Typhoid infection, trauma, septicemia, DM
IOC–HIDA scan
Rx-Usg guided drainage + Antibiotics

Saint's triad
Gallstones
Hiatus hernia
Diverticulosis

Rigler's triad
Small bowel obstruction
Gas within Gall Bladder and or bile ducts
Ectopic gallstone

TABLE: Gallstones

10% gallstones – Radio opaque
90% gallstones – Radio lucent
Gallstones – Mercedes Benz sign, sea gull sign
Limey bile – Sequestration of calcium salts in bile after gradual obstruction of CBD

TABLE: Important tumor staging and classification

Chang staging	Medulloblastoma
Masaoka staging	Thymoma
Shimada index	Neuroblastoma
Rees	Ellsworth classification, Esson prognostic index Retinoblastoma
Bloom–Richardson classification	CA breast
Noguchi's classification	Adenocarcinoma lung
Sullivan modification of MacFarlane system	Adrenocortical CA
Gleason score	CA prostrate
Nevin staging	CA GB
Duke staging	Colorectal ca
Robson staging	RCC
Jackson score	CA penis

Most common Nodes involved:
CA penis: Inguinal nodes
CA testis: Para-aortic LN
On right: Inter aorto-caval LN
On left: Para-aortic LN
CA bladder: Obturator LN
CA prostrate: Obturator LN

MUST KNOW FACTS

Nigro regimen is used for: **Anal Canal CA**

TOC for Duodenal Atresia, Annular pancreas: **Duodenoduodenostomy**

TOC for superior mesenteric artery syndrome: **Duodenojejunostomy**

Contd...

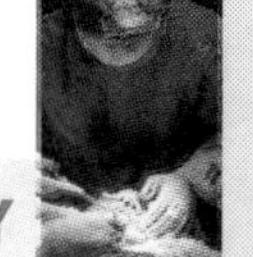

Length of these instruments:
- Proctoscope 10–12 cm
- Rigid Sigmoidoscope: 25 cm
- Flexible sigmoidoscope: 60 cm
- Colonoscope: 160 cm

Intracranial bleed:
EDH: Due to tear of middle meningeal artery, appear biconvex on CT, **lucid interval** is present.
SDH: Due to rupture of bridging veins, appear crescentic or concavo - Convex on CT.
Duret hemorrhage is small area of bleeding in ventral and para median part of upper brain stem. Diagnosis: CT or MRI

Bilateral grade 4 or 5 VUR is better treated surgically with ureteric reimplantation.

Berry aneurysm is the most common intra cranial aneurysm

Young women on OCP's are predisposed to **stroke due to venous thrombosis** of sagittal sinus or small cortical veins

Major causes of delayed neurological deficit after CVA: re-rupture, hydrocephalus, vasospasm, hyponatremia.

Commonly used preparation of mannitol: **20% solution, 0.25 g/kg is given IV bolus**

Primary brain injury occurs at the time of injury, secondary brain occurs at some time after impact

MC tumors of brain: **Metastatic/Secondaries**

MC posterior fossa tumor in children: **Astrocytoma**

MC site of Medulloblastoma: **Vermis**

MC spinal tumor: **Metastatic**

MC primary spinal tumor: **Nerve sheath tumor**

MC intra medullary tumor: **Astrocytoma**

MC site of primary spinal tumor: **Intradural extramedullary**

The term " dumbbell" lesion is used to describe **neurofibroma**

Acoustic neuroma can arise from any nerve except optic and olfactory nerve.

Common uses of **stereotactic radiosurgery: Metastatic** tumors, benign lesions of cranial nerve, A-V malformations, trigeminal neuralgia.

Struma ovarii: Benign ovarian tumor containing thyroid tissue, some patients develop thyrotoxicosis.

Lingual thyroid: rounded swelling developed at the back of the tongue at the foramen cecum.

Refetoff syndrome: End organ resistance to T4

Father of thyroid surgery: Theodor Kocher.

The **external laryngeal** nerve runs close to superior thyroid artery and **recurrent laryngeal nerve runs** close to inferior thyroid artery.

Wolff-chaikoff effect: Iodine induced hypothyroidism

Jod-Basedow effect: Iodine induced hyper thyroidism

Contd...

MC site of thyroglossal cyst: **Sub hyoid.**

Acute suppurative thyroiditis is rare seen in children & caused by streptococcus & anaerobes.

Hashimoto's thyroiditis or Struma Lymphomatosa is MC inflammatory disorder of thyroid and leading cause of hypothyroidism. Auto antibodies are produced against Tg, TPO, TSH-R.

Grave's disease (Diffuse toxic goiter): MC cause of hyperthyroidism caused by stimulatory autoantibodies to TSH–R.

Toxic adenoma (Plummer's disease): Single hyper functioning nodule typically occurs in young patients.

Thyroid storm (Thyrotoxic crisis): It is an emergency due to decompensated hyperthyroidism.

Thyroglossal fistula is never congenital

MC postoperative complication after thyroidectomy: **Hemorrhage.**

MC benign tumor of thyroid gland: **Follicular adenoma.**

Papillary carcinoma: MC carcinoma of thyroid associated with history of radiation exposure. It has best prognosis.

Predisposing factor for long standing goiter: **Follicular carcinoma of thyroid.**

Anaplastic CA of thyroid: MC carcinoma with worst prognosis, neck gets frozen with hard fixed mass.

Medullary carcinoma of thyroid is associated with RET oncogene; tumor marker: Calcitonin.

Sub- Acute thyroiditis/granulomatous thyroiditis/de quervain's thyroiditis is associated with viral infection & can occur as a consequence of viral infection. Only painful condition of thyroid

Pemberton's sign is MC associated with Retrosternal goiter.

MC type of kidney stone (85%) is **calcium oxalate.**

Xanthine & uric acid stone are radio lucent.

Struvite stones composed of Ca^+, NH_3, Mg $(PO)_4$ and best treated by **PCNL + ESWL.**

Randall's plaques are soft tissue calcification found in the deep renal medulla.

Infectious stones are more common in females.

Stone in upper ureter: Pain referred to testis.

Stone in mid ureter: Pain referred along iliohypogastric nerve to iliac fossa, mimicking appendicitis.

Stone in lower ureter: Pain referred along ilioinguinal nerve to thigh, scrotum and perineum.

Acidic urine is seen in **calcium oxalate, cystine, uric acid.**

Alkaline urine is seen in **calcium phosphate, struvite.**

NCCT is most sensitive investigation for renal calculi.

If Stone <2 cm treatment is **ESWL.**

Stone >2 cm treatment is **PCNL.**

MC cause of ureteric obstruction is **Stone.**

Contd...

MC cause of ureteric colic in hematuria is **Clot**.

Pyelonephritis MC caused by E coli
Clinical feature: Fever, flank pain, vomiting and 80 – 90% of patients have diabetes.

Pyonephrosis MC cause is renal stone
Clinical feature: Anemia, fever, swelling in loin.

M. Tuberculosis reaches the genitourinary organs by hematogenous route from lungs.

Intermittent hydronephrosis (dietl's crisis) associated with swelling in the loin.

MC type of RCC mainly sporadic is **clear cell carcinoma**.

RCC/VHL syndrome: MC sites of distant metastasis are lungs> bone> liver > brain.

MC primary renal tumor of childhood is **wilm's tumor.**

Transitional cell carcinoma accounts for 90% of upper urinary tract cancers.

ADPKD associated with cyst in all sites except brain.

Most common gas produced in intestinal obstruction: N_2

Most common gas produced in Clostridial infection: H_2S

MC gas used to create pneumoperitoneum in laparoscopy: CO_2

MC cause of upper G.I bleeding: **Peptic ulcer**

MC cause of lower G.I bleeding: **Non-specific ulcers**

MCC of jejunostomy feeding: **Diarrhea**

MC site of aortic rupture: **Ligamentum arteriosum**

MCC of leg ulcer: **Venous ulcer**

MC site of fasciotomy: **Calf**

Best treatment for subaponeurotic hematoma: **I & D**

Hardy was first surgeon to do proximal ureteric implantation

Grayhack shunt is shunt for priapism made between corpora cavernosa & corpora spongiosa

TABLE: Strawberry Q' forms

- Strawberry gingivitis: **Wegeners granulomatosis**
- Strawberry cervix: **Trichomonas vaginalis**
- Strawberry gallbladder: **Cholesterolosis**
- Strawberry nasal mucosa: **Sarcoidosis**
- Strawberry nasal mass: **Rhinosporidiosis**
- Strawberry tongue: **Kawasaki disease**

Some most common neoplasm

MC childhood tumor - **Leukemia**
MC childhood leukemia - **ALL**
MC solid tumor of childhood - **Brain tumor**
MC tumor of infancy - **Neuroblastoma**
MC abdominal tumor of child - **Neuroblastoma**

THE SURGICAL MOST COMMON LIST

What is/are the most common.

- MC Cause of acute prostatitis is **E. coli.**
- MC Reason to get treatment for BPH is **symptomatic relief**.
- MC Location for prostate CA is in the **peripheral zone of the prostate gland.**
- MC Renal anomaly is **horseshoe kidney**
- MC Renal inflammatory disorder is **pyelonephritis**
- MC Renal tumor is **renal cell carcinoma**
- MC Source of renal neoplasm is **metastasis**.
- MC Surgery performed on males is **circumcision**
- MC Cause of erectile dysfunction is **vasogenic**
- MC Motility disorder of the esophagus is **achalasia cardia**
- MC Site of peptic ulcer disease is **the first part of the duodenum**
- MC Cause of surgical abdomen is **acute appendicitis.**
- MC Causes of appendix obstruction in the young is **mesenteric lymphadenitis or lymphoid hyperplasia**
- MC Causes of appendix obstruction in older patients is **fecolith and foreign body**.
- MC Tumor of the appendix is **carcinoid**.
- MC Benign tumor of the small bowel is **leiomyoma**.
- MC Primary tumor of the small bowel **adenocarcinoma**.
- MC Malignant tumors of the small bowel are **adenocarcinoma, carcinoid, and lymphoma**.
- MC Small bowel malignancy of children is **lymphoma**.
- MC Surgical condition of the small bowel is **obstruction secondary to adhesions**
- MC Anaerobe in the colon is ***Bacteroides* fragilis**
- MC Site for metastases from the colon is **the liver**.
- MC Location of colonic obstruction is the **sigmoid colon**.
- MC Cause of colonic obstruction is **adenocarcinoma**.
- MC Site of volvulus is the **sigmoid colon**.
- MC Site of bile duct carcinoma is the **bifurcation of the common hepatic ducts**.
- MC Causes of acute pancreatitis are alcohol consumption and biliary calculi.
- **MC Causes of death in a patient** with pancreatitis are respiratory distress, cardiovascular collapse, coagulopathy and hemorrhage.
- **MC Local complications of acute pancreatitis are paralytic** ileus, sterile peripancreatic fluid collection, and pancreatic abscess.
- MC Best **diagnostic imaging technique** for prostate CA is TRUS

Contd...

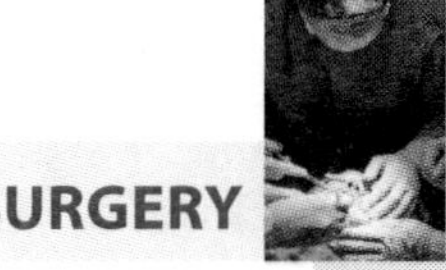

- MC site of carcinoma in oral cavity – **Bucco alveolar complex**
- MC oral cancer – **squamous cell carcinoma**
- Carcinoma tongue MC site – **lateral middle 1/3**
- Carcinoma oral cavity best prognosis – **carcinoma lip**
- MC site of peptic ulcer diseases – **first part of duodenum**
- Second most common site of PUD – **anteropyloric junction**
- Third most site of PUD – **laser curvature of antrum and pylorus**
- MC site of carcinoma stomach – **esophago gastric junction and cardia**
- Maximum conc. of H. pylori – **antrum**
- MC complication of PUD – **Bleeding**
- MC cause of death in PUD – **Perforation**
- Second MC site of gastric carcinoma – **anteropyloric junction**
- MC gastric carcinoma – **adeno carcinoma (histological type)**
- MC benign tumor in small intestine – **adenoma (Ileum)**
- MC malignant tumor in small intestine – **adeno carcinoma (deodeno jejunal junction)**
- MC site of carcinoid tumor in body – **bronchus**
- MC site of carcinoid in intestine – **ileum**
- MC hormone release in carcinoid – **5 HT**
- MC symptom of carcinoid – **flushing and diarrhea**
- MC type of intestinal polyp – **Hyperplastic polyp**
- MC site colorectal carcinoma – **rectum and sigmoid**
- MC effected by metastasis form of colorectal carcinoma – **Liver**
- MC presenting symptom of congenital pyloric stenosis – **vomiting (metabolic alkalosis)**
- MC used surgery in India for duodenal ulcer – **trunkalvegotomoy + drainage**
- MC cause of pernicious anemia – **vitamin B12**
- MC affected part of stomach in pernicious anemia – **fundus and body**
- MC site of leimyomas in GIT – **Stomach**
- MC type of benign tumor of stomach – **leimyomas**
- MC hallmark of Whipplies disease – **SI mucosa macrophages**
- MC test in small intestine malabsorption – **D- xylose absorption test**
- MC CNS manifestation in Whipplies disease - **Dementia**
- MC cause of persistent symptoms of celiac disease – **control intake of gluten**
- MC cause of massive bleeding through PR (55 yrs) - **diverticulosis**
- MC cause painless maroon colored stool - **diverticulosis**
- MC long term affect of radiation on GIT – **telangiectasis**

Contd...

- MC site of polyp in GIT - **small intestine**
- MC site for Hamartomatous polyp – **small intestine**
- MC site for polyp in Peutz-Jeghers syndrome – **small intestine**
- MC site for polyp in juvenile polyposis – **large intestine**
- MC cause of acute of loss vision – **acute pancreatitis (Purtscher's retinopathy)**
- MC cause of complication of pancreatic pseudocyst – **body and tail of pancreas**
- MC presentation of ZES-PUD+ diarrhea
- MC site of PUD in ZES - **Duodeno bulb (second part of duodenal)**
- MC tumor associated with neurofibroma-1—**optic glioma**
- MC tumor associated with NF-2 – **acoustic neuroma**
- PAUD E ORANGE is seen in – **carcinoma of breast**
- PAUD E ORANGE is due to – **lymphatic obstruction**
- MCC of UTI- **E. coli**
- MCC of renal stone – **Ca+ Oxalate**
- MCC Ca+ oxalate stone – **idiopathic hypercalcemia**
- MCC stag horn calculus- **roteus infection**
- ADPKD cysts not seen in – **lung and brain**
- Best treatment for formed abscess: **I/D**
- Best treatment for TB/cold abscess: **ATT**
- MCC of mycotic aneurysm: **Staph aureus**
- Selmonosky triad is seen in: **Thoracic outlet synd (supraclavicular tenderness, hand paleness on elevation, weakness of 4th and 5th finger)**
- Thrombophlebitis of superficial veins of breast: **Mondor's disease**
- Absence of nipple from breast is condition known as: **Athelia**
- MC type of diaphragmatic hernia: **Posterolateral hernia of Bochdalek**
- Hourglass stomach is seen in: **Pyloric stenosis**
- Cullen sign is seen in: **Hemoperitoneum (periumbilical)**
- Gray turner sign: **Dark bluish/greenish discoloration of flank**
- Karydaki/Bascom's procedure is done in: **Pilonodal sinus**
- Scoring/criteria used in acute pancreatitis: **APACHE score (bed side), Balthazar score (CT severity index), Ranson's criteria**
- Kehr sign is seen in: **Splenic rupture**
- Intra-op fluid of choice for irrigation in BPH: **1.5% isotonic Glycine**
- Post op fluid of choice for irrigation: **0.9% NS**
- For cutting umbilical cord of a newborn baby blade used is: **No. 10**
- Use of fogarty catheter: removal of fresh clot embolus in artery

Contd...

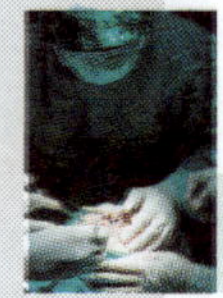

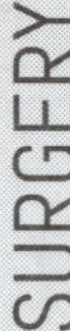

- Needle used for bone marrow biopsy: **Jamshidi Needle**
- Cleft lip corrected at this age and weight: **10 weeks age/10 pounds weight (Millard criteria)**
- Ogilvie syndrome is: **Acute pseudo colonic obstruction**

TABLE: Salivary gland tumors

Pleomorphic adenoma
- Overall most common tumor of salivary gland
- MC benign salivary gland tumor
- MC tumor of major salivary glands
- MC site is parotid tail (superficial lobe)

Warthin's tumor
- 2nd MC benign tumor of parotid gland
- MC malignant tumor of parotid gland: **Mucoepidermoid CA**
- 2nd MC malignant tumor of parotid gland: **Adenoid cystic CA**
- Most common organism associated with sialadenitis: ***Staph. aureus* and *Strep. viridans***
- Most common salivary gland associated with sialolithiasis: **submandibular gland *(80 %) > Parotid gland (20%)***

What is/are the most common...
MC Complication of spinal anesthesia is posture-related headache one day after anesthesia, probably secondary to CSF leakage.
MC Indication for nasogastric tube placement is: **gastric decompression.**
MC Reason for recurrent post-operative ulcer disease is **inadequate vagotomy.**

MISCELLANEOUS

The most common...
MC Suture is over and over.
MC Cause of **hypercalcemia** in a surgical patient is primary and secondary hyperparathyroidism and metastatic bone disease.
MC Cause of **hypermagnesemia** secondary to renal failure.
MC NSAID that decreases platelet function is **aspirin.**
MC Cause of hypovolemic shock is **hemorrhage.**
MC Toe problem is **ingrown toe nails.**
MC Cause of death in children and adults less than 35 years of age is **trauma.**
MC Injury to the thoracic cage is **rib fracture.**
MC Hernia in both sexes and all age groups is **bilateral inguinal hernia.**
MC Causes of true aneurysm are acquired **atherosclerosis, congenital fibromuscular dysplasia (Marfans)**
MC Cause of spontaneous, bloody unilateral nipple discharge is **intraductal papilloma.**
MC Cause of hypercalcemia is **hyperparathyroidism**

Contd...

The most common...
MC Cause of pre-sinusoidal portal hypertension is **schistosomiasis.**
MC Appliance for compression of bleeding esophageal varices is the **Sengstaken-Blakemore tube.**
MC Cause of secondary hypersplenism is **portal hypertension.**
MC Type of primary liver cancer is **hepatoma.**
MC Benign liver tumor is **hemangioma**
MC Indication for splenectomy is **splenic injury.**
MC Cause of spontaneous splenic rupture is **malaria > mononucleosis.**
MC Hemolytic anemia to respond to splenectomy is **congenital hereditary spherocytosis.**
Indication for aortic/bifemoral bypass graft is **bilateral iliac obstruction**
Cause of renovascular hypertension in children is **fibromuscular dysplasia.**
Site of embolic occlusion is **the femoral artery.**
Benign type of melanoma is **superficial lentigo malignant melanoma**
The variant of Hodgkin's Disease with the best prognosis is **lymphocyte predominant**
The variant of Hodgkin's Disease with the worst prognosis is **lymphocyte depleted**

SOME NAMED SURGERIES

• Patey's operation	Parotidectomy, mastectomy
• Commando operation	CA tongue (Post 1/3rd)
• Nissen's fundoplication, Toupet's partial fundoplication, Belsey mark, Hills	GERD
• Ramsted's operation	Congenital Hypertrophic Obstructive Pyloric Stenosis
• Allison's repair	Hiatus hernia
• Hartmann's operation	Hydrocele (small, medium sized)
• Lords operation	Hydrocele (large sized)

IMPORTANT SIGNS

Chvostek's sign	Contraction of facial m/s (masseter spasm) elicited by tapping the facial n. anterior to ear.

Contd...

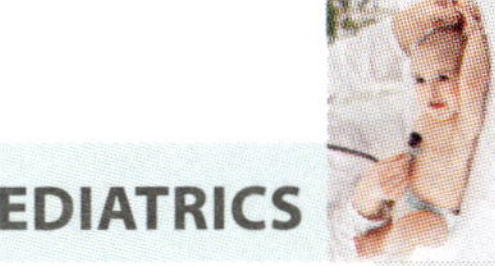

Homan's sign	Calf tenderness may be exaggerated by passive dorsiflexion of ankle
Hamman's sign	Mediastinal crunch seen in esophagus rupture.
Trousseau's Phenomenon/ sign *(Carpopedal spasm elicited by occlusion of brachial artery with a BP cuff for 3 minutes)*	Seen in hypocalcemia (hypoparathyroidism, alkalotic or latent tetany, hypomagnesemia, hypo and hyperkalemia).
Troisier's sign	Enlargement of Virchow's nodes (left supraclavicular LN) in occult gastric carcinoma etc.
Trousseau's sign	Seen in migratory superficial thrombophlebitis (as in pancreatic CA).
Tinel's sign	Tingling sensation on percussion. It indicates partial lesion or beginning of regeneration of nerve

PEDIATRICS

IMPORTANT RECENT POINTS (INCLUDES LATEST QS)

Infant usually doubles his birth length by **4 ½ yrs of age.**
Most full term infants regain their birth weight by the age of **10 days.**
Central incisors is first to develop and second molar is last to develop in primary dentition.
The circumference of head and chest are almost same by the age of **9 months** to 1 year.
IGF-2 **stimulates fetal growth.**
First sign of sexual maturation is enlargement of breast in females and testes in boys.
Malnutrition measurement Acute malnutrition – Weight for height Chronic malnutrition – Height for age
Most vulnerable period of organogenesis is b/w 18-55 days of gestation.
Most common epileptic drug causing Neural tube defects- **Valproate**
Hyperbilirubinemia in girl babies – Oxytocin induced to mother
Closure of ductus arteriosus in preterm baby – indomethacin
Most common complication during vaginal delivery in diabetic mother – **Shoulder dystocia**
Highest risk of transmission of Hepatitis – At the time of delivery.

Contd...

Triad of Congenital Rubella – Deafness + cataract + heart defect (PDA)
Triad of congenital Syphilis – Deafness + interstitial keratitis + Hutchinson's teeth
Triad of Toxoplasmosis – Chorioretinitis + intracranial calcification + hydrocephalus
Most common congenital infection is **CMV**
Most common organism causing fetal malformation – **Rubella**
Recurrent abortions and IUGR are usually–not seen in – **Syphilis**
Sabin field man dye test is used to detect immunoglobulin G in toxoplasmosis
Most of the new born pass urine by **12 hours of age** and almost all of them do so by **48 hrs**
Fetal adrenal cortex is largest organ of fetus.
Most common manifestation of acute hypoxemia in a new born- **bradycardia, cardiac systole.**
Early conjugated NNHB with direct bilirubin more than 0.5 mg/dl is noted as neonatal syphilis.
Vitamin E has role in prevention of **PBD** and **ROP.**
Protein required in a new born – **100 kcal/kg**
Breast milk does not provide immunity against **pertussis.**
Minimum time of breast feeding per episode – **15-20 min.**
Vitamin absent in breast milk – Vitamin C > Vitamin D
Mature Breast milk by **day 7.**
Lacta albumin in breast milk is easily digestible and causes soft/ Golden yellow color stool.
Sucking + swallowing – **34 weeks.**
Earliest fetal breathing movements – **11-16 weeks**
Flag sign – **Kwashiorkor**
Chipmunk facies in case of – **Thalassemia**
Monkey facies in case of– **Marasmus**
Most common cause of congenital hydrocephalus – **Aqueductal stenosis**

TABLE: Development of fetus according to age

Social smile develops by **2 months**
Head control develops by **3 months**
4 months – Hand regard
5 months – Ulnar grasp
Child can sit with support by **5 months**
5 months – Lumbar control, Tripod position
7 months – Palmar grasp
7 months – Stranger anxiety

Contd...

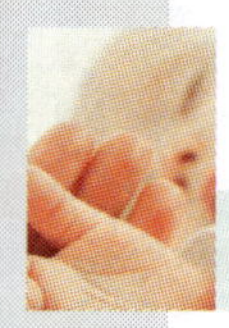

9 months – Wave bye bye

Pincer grasp develops by **9 months** (9-11 months)

Mature pincer grasp at **12 months**

24 months – Can speak in a sentence

2 years - Dry by day

3 years – Dry by night

Can draw- at:
- **Circle:** 3 years
- **Square:** 4 years
- **Triangle:** 5 year

36 months – Climb upstairs with alternate feet

Child knows his full name, gender, eats without spilling, dress without supervision- **5 years**

Tells age and sex, uses pronouns, handedness by **3 years**

Child stands without support by **1 year**

Child can build tower of 3 cubes at **15 months**

Child can go up and downstairs with one step at a time by **2 years**.

Parachute reflex develops during **9th** month of life.

A child can skip by the age of **5 years**

TABLE: Fetal birth weight according to maturity

ELBW: < 1 kg

VLBW: < 1.5 kg

LBW: < 10th percentile (<2-5 kg)

Preterm: < 37 weeks

Post-term: >42 weeks

Early sign of puberty in male is enlargement of testes. In females it is determined by: **Thelarche**

Anemia for an infant at Hemoglobin less than **12 gm%**

In neonatal sepsis, acute phase reactant: **CRP**

Acyanotic congenital heart disease: **ASD, VSD, PDA**

Cyanotic congenital heart disease: **TGA, TOF, TAPVR**

TABLE: Apgar score and its interpretation

	Score 0	Score 1	Score 2
Appearance	Blue or pale all over	Blue at extremities	Pink all over
Pulse rate	Absent	<100	>100
(Grimace) Reflex irritability	No response	Grimace	Cry or pull away when stimulated
Activity	None	Some flexion	Flexed arms and legs that resist extension
Respiratory effort	Absent	Weak, irregular, gasping	Strong, lusty cry
Total score: 10	No distress: 7–10	Mild distress: 4–6	Severe distress: 0–3

Contd...

TABLE: Triple test parameter and its value in different congenital defects

Triple test parameters	Alpha feto protein	Unconjugated estriol	Beta hCG
Down syndrome	Low	Low	High
Edward syndrome	Low	Low	Low
Neural tube defects Omphalocele, multiple gestation	High	Not applicable	Not applicable

GOLDEN POINTS

- MC enzyme deficiency in CAH -21 alpha HYDROXYLASE
- MC teratogenic effect of steroid-Cleft lip & palate
- MC childhood solid tumor other than brain tumor-Neuroblastoma & germ cell tumor
- MC tumor of newborn-Sacrococygeal teratoma
- MC malignancy in newborn----Neuroblastoma
- MC intrarenal tumor in newborn-mesoblastic nephroma
- MC abdominal mass in neonate-Multicystic kidney
- MC cell seen in broncholitis- Clara cell
- MCC of bronchiolitis –RSV
- Upper segment and lower segment ratio becomes equal at this age: 7 Years
- Most common cause of short stature in childhood in India: Constitutional
- Physiological weight loss in a preterm baby is upto: 15%
- Best indication for successful resuscitation in an Indian child: Inc Heart rate
- Earliest clinical feature of neonatal sepsis: Poor feeding
- Mode of heating in a radiant warmer: Radiation

OBSTETRICS AND GYNECOLOGY

EMBRYOLOGY OF UTERUS

- Mullerian duct present in both sexes and appear at 6 weeks.
- Mullerian duct disappear in male fetus at 8–9 weeks.
- Remnant of mullerian duct in male are- utriculus masculinus, appendix of testis.

Contd...

- Male internal genitalia develop from mesonephric duct/ wolfian duct.
- Remnant of wolfian duct in female – epoophoron (cranial part), paraoophoron (caudal end), gartner duct
- All the remanant of wolfian duct are present in borad ligament.
- 15–20 epoophoron join to form gartner duct
- Mullerian duct give rise to- fallopian tube,uterus,cervix,vagina (upper 2/3) (mesodermal origin)
- Lower 1/3 of vagina is derived from rogenital sinus (endodermal origin)

ANATOMICAL FACTS

- Water under bridge- point where uterine artery(bridge) crosses over the ureter
- Water under the bridge is the most common site for ureter injury.
- This point is 2 cm lateral to cervix and 1.5 cm lateral to internal os.
- During mestruation blood is lost from spiral artery, hence menstrual blood is arterial blood not venous
- Shape of uterus: Pyriform
- **Cavity: Triangular shape cavity on coronal section (Slit shape cavity on sagittal section)**
- Volume:
- 10cc- non pregnant
- 5000cc –term pregnancy (volume of uterus=volume of adult blood approximately

Weight of uterus	• Nullipara- 50-70 gram • Multipara- 80 gram • Term pregnancy- 1 kg • Immediately after delivery-1 kg

TABLE: Supports of the genital organs

Level I	Uterosacral ligaments and cardinal ligaments support the uterus and vaginal vault
Level II	Pelvic facias and paracolpos which connects the vagina to the white line on the lateral pelvic wall through arcus tendinous
Level III	Levator ani muscles support the lower one third of vagina

IMPORTANT ONE LINERS

Tubal blockage is most commonly seen with this infection: **Chlamydia**

Fulminant hepatitis in pregnancy most commonly caused by: **HEV**

Constipation in pregnancy is due to this hormone: **Progesterone**

According to American fertility society classification system, unicornuate uterus is classified under this class: **Class II**

Contd...

Type of molar pregnancy in which fetal tissue is formed: **Partial H Mole**

T shaped uterus seen due to this drug exposure: **Diethylstilbestrol (DES)**

Stage of Cervix cancer reaching involving bladder and rectum: **Stage IVa**

Fruit juice which can prevent UTI: **Cranberry juice (due to its anti-adhesion property)**

Tip of iceberg sign on USG: **Dermoid cyst of ovary**

Karman cannula is used for: **Endometrial aspiration**

In this stage of ovarian carcinoma both ovaries are involved and but the capsule is intact: **IB**

Ovarian Capsule is first involved in this stage of ovarian CA: **Ic**

- MC clinical presentation of genital T. B-**Infertility**
- MC change in fibroid-**Hyaline degeneration**
- MC complication of TAH–**Bleeding**
- MC regime is used inchoriocarcinoma–**MAC regime**
- MC site of metastasis of choriocarcinoma–**Lung**
- MCC of infertility–**Tubalfactor**
- MC C Of tubal disease–**PID**
- MC presentation of treated genital T.B–**Ectopic pregnancy**
- MC complication of ECV is–**fetal distress**
- MC fetal complication of forceps application–**asphyxia**
- MC complication of MTP produce is bleeding–**due to**

Incomplete evacuation

- MC type of episiotomy–**mediolateral**
- MC complication of forceps application–**extension of episiotomy**
- MC site for ectopic pregnancy–**Ampulla**
- MC cause of congenital anomaly in baby of diabetic mother–**sacralegenesis**
- MC congenital anamoly in baby of diabetic mother–**neuraltube defect**
- MC problem seen in baby born to diabetic mother–**hypoglycemia**
- MC problem associated in delivery of macrosomia baby–**shoulder dystocia**
- MC cause of PPH–**Uterine atony**
- MC type of PPH–**Primary PPH**
- MC maternal complication of twin vaginal delivery–**atonic PPH**
- MC cause of secondary PPH is–**retained placental bits**
- MC reason for caesarian hysterectomy–**atonic PPH**
- MC indication of forcep is–**prolong second stage of labour**
- MC cancer cervix is squamous cell carcinoma-**95%**

Contd...

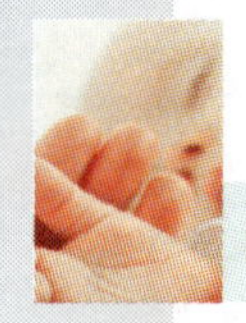

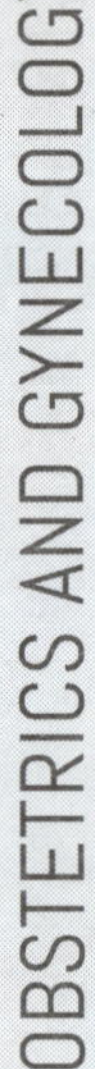

- Most important support of uterus-**cardinal ligament**
- Ovlation occure at 14th day before menstration.
- Endomterium before ovulation is k/a proliferative endometrium.
- Proliferative endometrium is due to effect of estrogen.
- Endomterium after ovulation is k/a secretory endometrium.
- Secretory endometrium is due to effect of progesterone.
- Major source of progesterone in non pregnant female is carpus luteum,hence secretory phase is also k/a luteal phase.

TABLE: Indications of conization

Diagnostic	• Entire squamocolumnar junction not visible, large lesion • Endocervical CIN • Microinvasion suspected • Discrepancy between cytology and colposcopy
Therapeutic	In INC II, III
Methods	• Cone biopsy • LLETZ, LEEP (loop electrosurgical excision procedure), NETZ

TABLE: Bethesda system of cytology reporting

Satisfactory cytology—endocervical cells seen
Unsatisfactory

- **Squamous cell abnormalities**
  Atypical squamous cells (ASC)
  - Ascus—atypical cells of undetermined significance
  - ASC-H—cannot rule out high-grade lesion
  - Low-grade squamous intra epithelial lesion (LSIL)—includes CIN I
  - High-grade squamous intraepithelial lesion (HSIL)—includes CIN II, III
  - Squamous cell carcinoma
- **Glandular abnormalities**
  Atypical glandular cells
  Adenocarcinoma in situ
  Adenocarcinoma
- **Other malignant neoplasma**

GOLDEN POINTS

Main support of uterus is **cardinal ligament (aka transverse cervical ligament).**

Broad ligament, infundibulopelvic ligament, ovarian ligaments–**Does not support uterus.**

Most imp muscle of pelvic floor - **Levator ani.**

Uterus, fallopian tube, cervix and upper 2/3 vagina arise from-**mullerian duct/paramesonephric duct (mesodermal origin)**

Contd...

Lower 1/3 vagina - **Urogenital sinus** (endodermal origin)

Weight of pregnant term uterus - **1 kg**

Wt of uterus immediately after delivery - **1 kg**

Volume of nulliparous uterus = 10 mL, term uterus = 5 liters

Round ligament and ovarian ligaments arise from **gubernaculum.**

Uterus shows both **hypertrophy** and **hyperplasia** during pregnancy.

Endometrium of pregnancy is called **decidua.**

Thickness of endometrium
- After menses = .5 mm
- Mid cycle = 2–3 mm
- Luteal phase = 5-6 mm
- At time of implantation = 10–12 mm

Thickness of endometrium is taken at body near fundus by **USG.**

Water under bridge-ureter crossed by **uterine artery.**

Ratio of cervix to corpus:
- 1:1 - At birth, menopause
- 1:2 - Post-menarche
- 1:3 - Reproductive life
- 2:1 - Pre-menarche

Shape of cervix-round (nullipara), transverse slit like-after deliver/multipara

pH of vagina in adult women - 4–5.5

Vaginal secretions are—cervical secretion, bartholin duct secretion (during coitus)

Epithelial lining-FT (ciliated columnar), uterus (columnar), endocx (high columnar), ectocx (squamous), vagina (st. squamous)

MC CA
- Fallopian tube - Adenocarcinoma
- Uterus - Adenocarcinoma
- Cervix - Squamous cell CA
- Vagina - Squamous cell CA
- Vulva - Squamous cell CA

Sentinel LN used for vulva CA (which is superficial inguinal LN).

Bartholin's cyst - MC cyst of vulva, MC due to obstruction and gonococcus infection, causes fluctuant non tender swelling, at Anterior 2/3rd and posterior 1/3rd of junction between labia minova and Hymen.
Rx-Marsupialization

Length of fallopian tube: **10-12 cm.**

Genital tubercle forms - **Clitoris** (in female), **penis** (in male)

Genital swelling – **Labia majora** (f), **scrotum** (m)

1st polar body - **Released at ovulation.**

2nd polar body-**released after fertilization.**

Ovarian cycle initiated by - **FSH**

Ovulation is due to - *LH* surge, which is due to high level of *estrogen*.

Contd...

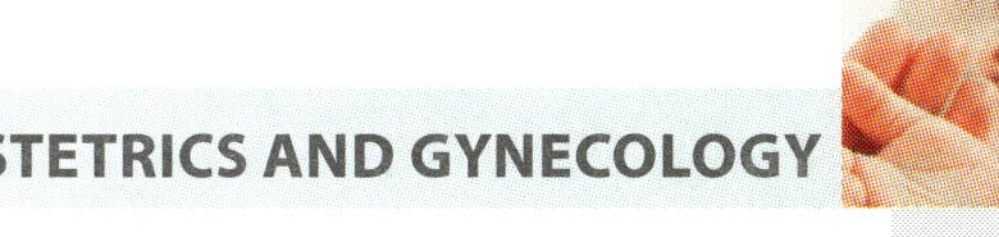

To cause ovulation in ART inj ***hCG*** is given.

In ART after HCG inj-ovulation occus after **36 hrs**.

Ovulation occurs at **14th day** (irrespective of cycle length)

Carpus luteum (CL) secrets-progesterone (**Mainly**), estrogen, relaxin, inhibin A

Life span of CL - **14 day**

Max function/peak activity of CL- *8th day after* ovulation/22nd day of Cycle.

Steroidogenesis of CL maintained by **LH**

Luteolysis of CL prevented by - **hCG**

Telescoping of glands, pseudostratification - **Proliferative/ estrogenic phase**

Ist Histopathological evidence of ovulation-Sub **nucleolar vacuolation**.

Cork screw glands, stromal edema- **late secretory/progesterone phase**.

MC cause of 1° amenorrhea-**gonadal dysgenesis** (Turner syndrome)

MC cause of 2° amenorrhea-**ovulatory dysfunction** (PCOD)

Amenorrhea, absent uterus, normal sec sexual characters - **Mullerian agenesis**

Triad of MRKH s* - Mullerian agenesis, renal anomalies, skeletal anomalies.

Amenorrhoea, absent uterus, absent/dec pubic hair-androgen insensitivity s*/testicular feminization s* (XY (s* = syndrome)

BEST test to differentiate MRKH s* vs AIS - **Karyotyping**.

AIS (androgen insensitivity s*)- risk of gonadoblastoma in undescended testis.

MCC cause of Asherman's*- Vigorous curettage done for PPH.

TOC for **Asherman's*** - Hysteroscopic adhesiolysis + IUCD + high dose estrogen.

Imperforated hymen - C/o Amenorrhea, bluish bulging membrane in vagina.

Imperforated hymen-hematocolpos, hematometra, cyclic ab pain. T/t by cruciate incision.

Premature ovarian failure-FSH>40 IU on 2 separate occasion (1 month apart), at age <40 years.

MC used test of ovarian reserve- **sr** FSH (done at day 3)

Streak gonad, high FSH, hypogonadotropic hypogonadism- **Turner syndrome**

Inability to conceive even after 1 yr of unprotected intercourse - **Infertility**.

MC female factor for infertility - **PCOD**

MC male factor for infertility - **Psychogenic**.

Contd...

Test of ovulation - Sr progesterone level (BEST, done at day 21), TVS (MC USED), endometrial biopsy, cervical mucus, vaginal cytology, basal body temp.

Peri-ovulatory follicle/follicle rupture at - **18-20 mm**

Peri ovulatory uterus show- **Trilaminar sign**.

1st stage of labor - Onset of true labor pain to full cx dilation (i.e. 10 cm)

4th stage of labor - 1 hour observation (post delivery)

True labor pain-progressive dilation, effacement, show, contraction increase in duration frequency and intensity.

1st stage – Nullipara (12 hr), multipara (8 hrs)

Prolonged 1st stage- nulli (20 hrs), multi (14 hrs)

Rate of cervical dilation in active stage
1.2 cm/hr - Nulliparous
1.5 cm/hr - Multiparous

Rate of descent:
1 cm/hr - Nulliparous
2 cm/hr – Multiparous

MCC of unstable lie - **Placenta previa.**

MC type of pelvis in female - **Gynecoid (50%)**.

Least common type of pelvis – **Platypelloid (<5%)**.

Pelvis is classified on the basis of **inlet of pelvis.**

Tri-radiate pelvis (VIT D def), rachitic pelvis (rickets)

Vaginal delivery is never possible in naegle's and robert's pelvis.

Slow progress of labor is called **dystocia**.

Contracted inlet- when AP diameter <10 cm.

Contracted midcavity- when interischial diameter <8 cm.

Contracted outlet- when intertuberous diameter <8 cm.

Best predictor for CPD- trial of labor.

Best method to do pelvic assessment – MRI > pelvimetry (manual)

Pacemaker of uterine contraction-at cornu (right > left)

Adequate uterine contraction- 200-220 Monte Video Unit.

MVU- no of contraction in *10 min* × pressure generated in 1 contraction in mm Hg.

Arrest of labor-no change in cervical dilation even after 2 hours of adequate uterine contractions.t/t is LSCS.

MCC cause of vesico vaginal fistula in developing countries- **Obstructed labor.**

Rx for obstructed labor-**LSCS**.

Obstructed labor with IUD- **LSCS** (no role of destructive procedure at all).

MC position of fetal head when it enters pelvis - **LOA (left occipito anterior)**

Contd...

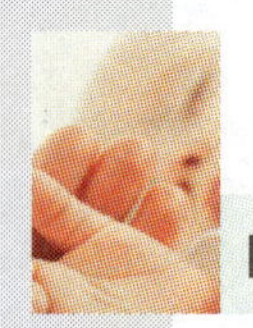

Direct op position seen in **Anthropoid pelvis**.

MCC of face/brow presentation - **Anencephaly**.

Face/ brow presentation/transverse lie- mcc associated with which type of pelvis-**platypelloid**.

Rx of face presentation - VD (if mentum anterior), LSCS (if mentum post).

Longest diameter of fetal head- mentovertical (14 cm) - Brow presentation.

Rx of brow-CS, no role of VD (vaginal delivery).

Grid iron feel - Transverse lie.

Rib cage as presenting part/shoulder presentation-**transverse lie**.

Rx of transverse lie - **LSCS**

MCC of breech- **prematurity/preterm**.

MC type - **Frank breech**.

Worst prognosis/max cord prolapse among breech -**Footling breech.**

Highest risk of cord prolapse among all malpresentation-**trans. Lie**

Stargazer baby-footling breech with hyperextended neck.

Oogonia and spermatogonia are derived from yolk sac.

Folds of Hoboken-umbilical artery.

Day 21-fetal circulation is 1st intact/functional/separated from mother circulation.

MC presentation **cephalic**, MC presenting **part vertex**.

Living ligature-middle layer of myometrium.

MCC of 1* PPH - Uterine atony

MCC of 2* PPH - Retained placental tissue

Syntometrine- oxytocin + methergine

Early cord clamping - HIV/Rh - /baby has heart ds/preterm/ premature

MCC of uterine rupture - Previous CS

MCC of APH- Abruptio placenta (1/200 preg), Placenta previa (1/300)

Most imp risk factor for both (AP, PP) - Previous history of the same.

Placenta Previa: Painless, causeless, bright-red, nontender uterus, normal FHS

Abruptio Placenta-painful, h/o trauma, dark altered blood, tender tense uterus, dec FHS

IOC for placenta previa (PP) & abruptio placenta (AP) - **USG**.

Paget's classification used for: **Abruptio placenta**

Macafee's regimen is used for: **Placenta Previa** - (for conservative management).

Contd...

DOC for lung maturity - Betamethasone 12 mg, IM, 2 doses, 24 hours apart.

Indication for CS in Placenta Previa - Mother unstable, fetal distress, type 3 & 4

Management of Abruptio Placentae - Always termination of pregnancy.

Indication of CS in Abruptio Placentae - Mother unstable, fetal distress.

IOC for adherent placenta - MRI, Rx- **Hysterectomy**.

DOC for chronic hypertension (in preg)- **Methyl dopa**.

DOC for pre-eclampsia - **Labetalol 100 mg bd**

DOC for eclampsia - **$MgSO_4$**

DOC for DM in preg- Insulin. (only FDA approved oral hypoglycemic - Glyburide)

MTP ACT - **Year 1971**.

MTP- opinion of 2 doctors needed if **POG > 12 weeks**.

Minimum age for MTP consent - **18 years**.

Time of cerclage operation - **12-14 weeks**

Decidul cast- pathognomic of ectopic pregnancy.

Recurrent abortion with isolated rise of APTT - **Lupus anticoagulant**.

MCC of thrombocytopenia in preg - **Benign gestational > idiopathic**.

MCC drug used for 2nd Tm abortion - **Prostaglandins**

Rubin criteria is used for-**cervical ectopic**.

Spiegelberg criteria-ovarian ectopic, studdiford - **Abdominal ectopic.**

Follow up of a case of ectopic/molar preg - **Serial hCG level.**

Most consistent finding in ectopic pregnancy - **Pain**
Most consistent sign of ectopic pregnancy - **Tenderness**

MC non tubal site for ectopic - **Ovary**.

Overall, MC ovarian tumor: **Epithelial cell tumor**

Most common germ cell ovarian tumor: **Teratoma**

Most common Malignant germ cell ovarian tumor: **Dysgerminoma**

Menstrual blood stored in vagina: **Hematocolpos**

In a diabetic mother, most common fetal complication will be: Congenital heart disease

In Brow presentation, head of the fetus: **Partial Extension**

Recurrence of hydatidiform mole accessed by: **β-hCG level**

Mechanism of action of combined OCP: **Prevent release of ovum from ovary**

Placental circulation is established by: **21 days**

Primary treatment for hirsutism in PCOD: **Combined OCP**

Oxygenated blood from placenta goes to fetal heart via: **Ductus venosus**

Contd...

Pace maker of uterine contraction is located at: **Tubal ostia**

Treatment of choice of Acute hydramnios with fetal distress in pregnancy: **Amniocentesis**

Cardiac activity in fetus can be assessed via transabdominal scan by: **6 weeks**

Umbilical cord attached to the margin of placenta: **Battledore Placenta**

TABLE: Diameter of fetal skull

Diameters	Measurement (in cm)	Presentation
Suboccipito-bregmatic	9.5 cm	Vertex
Suboccipito-frontal	10 cm	Vertex
Occipito-frontal	11.5 cm	Vertex
Mento-vertical: Extend from mid-point of chin to the highest point on the saggital suture	14 cm	Brow
Submento-vertical	11.5 cm	Face
Submento-bregmatic	9.5 cm	Face

TABLE: Important vessels and their remnants

Ductus venosus	Ligamentum venosum
Ductus arteriosus	Ligamentum arteriosum
Umbilical arteries	Medial umbilical artery
Left umbilical vein	Ligamentum teres of liver

TABLE: Gestational age and fundal height landmark

Gestational age	Fundal height landmark
12 weeks	Pubic symphysis
24 weeks	Umbilicus
36 weeks	Xiphoid Process of sternum
37–40 weeks	Regression of fundal height between 36 and 32 cm

TABLE: Uterine pressure in a nutshell

Period	Contraction pressure
During the first 30 weeks	20 mm Hg
First stage of labor	40–50 mm Hg
2nd stage of labor	100–120 mm Hg
3rd stage of labor	100–120 mm Hg
Contraction felt clinically	> 10 mm Hg
Contraction associated with pain	15 mm Hg
Pressure required for distending lower uterine segment	15 mm Hg

TABLE: Stages of labor and their respective duration

Stages of Labor	Duration	
	Primipara	Multipara
Stage I: From uterine contraction to full cervical dilatation (10 cm)	12 hours	6 hours
Stage II: Full dilatation to delivery of baby	2 hours	30 minutes
Stage III: Delivery of baby to placental delivery	15 minutes	15 minutes
Stage IV: 1 hour post partum to rule out PPH and vulvar hematoma.	1 hour	1 hour

TABLE: Examination signs during pregnancy

Signs	At AOG
Palmer's sign: Regular and rhythmic uterine contraction	4-8 weeks
Vaginal sign: Softened vaginal wall with copious mucoid discharge	6th week
Goodell's sign: Cervix feels soft and congested	6th week
Hegar's sign: Uterus is enlarged and soft; cervix empty.	6-10 weeks
Osiander sign: Increased pulsation at lateral fornices	8th week
Chadwick's sign or Jacquemier's sign: Dusky hue of the vestibule and anterior vaginal wall (due to local vascular congestion)	8th week
Piskacek's sign: Asymmetrical enlargement of the uterus if there is lateral implantation	8th week

TABLE: Types of abortion and its examination and USG findings

Abortion	Size of uterus	Cervix OS	USG finding
Threatened	Equal to AOG	Closed	Fetus alive
Missed	Smaller than AOG	Closed	Dead fetus
Incomplete	Smaller than AOG	Open	Retained products of conception
Complete	Smaller than AOG	Closed	Uterine cavity empty

TABLE: Division of zygote and types of twinning

Division of zygote on/ after	Types of twining
72 hours/3 days	Dichorionic, Diamniotic
Between 4 and 8 days	Diamniotic, Monochorionic (DAMC)
Between 8 and 12 days	Monoamniotic, Monochorionic (MAMC)
>12 days	Siamese, Conjoined Twins

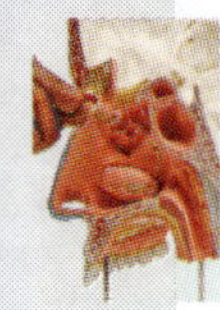

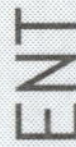

TABLE: Types of prior uterine incisions and risk of uterine rupture

Prior incision	Rupture rate (percentage)
1. Classical	4–9%
2. T-shaped	4–9%
3. Low-vertical	1–7%
4. Low-transverse	0.2–1.5%

TABLE: Ovarian tumor at a glance

Overall, MC ovarian tumor: **Epithelial cell tumor**
Overall, MC benign tumor of the ovary: **Dermoid cyst**
MC benign epithelial tumor of the ovary: **Serous cystadenoma**
MC malignant ovarian tumor: **Serous cystadenocarcinoma**
MC germ cell tumor: Mature Teratoma (Dermoid Cyst)
Most common ovarian tumor associated with pregnancy: **Dermoid Cyst**
Most common ovarian tumor which undergo torsion: **Dermoid cyst**
MC malignant germ cell tumor: **Dysgerminoma**
Ovarian tumor mostly in young age: **Dysgerminoma**
Ovarian tumor metastasized to contralateral ovary: **Granulosa cell tumor**

TABLE: Ovarian tumors and their HPE findings

Ovarian tumor	HPE characteristics
Serous cystadenoma	Psamomma bodies
Clear cell tumor	Hobnail cell
Yolk sac tumor	Schiller duval bodies
Granulosa cell tumor	Call exner bodies
Krukenberg tumor	Signet ring cell

ENT

IMPORTANT RECENT POINTS (INCLUDES LATEST QS)

- Auricle is derived from which Branchial arch: **I & II**
- Stapes is derived from which Branchial arch: **II**
- Hyoid bone is derived from: **Branchial arch II & III**
- Auricle is made of how many cartilages: **1 (yellow elastic cartilage)**
- Area of auricle devoid of cartilage: **Lobule and Incisura terminalis**
- Eustachian tube length – 36 mm **(lateral 1/3 is bony and medial 2/3 is cartilage)**
- External auditory canal length – **24 mm (outer 1/3 is cartilage and inner 2/3rd is bony)**
- Layer of tympanic membrane: **3 layers**

Contd...

- Functional area of tympanic membrane: **45–55 mm²**
- Lever ratio between handle of malleus and long process of incus is – **1.3: 1**
- Ear ossicle which has no muscle attachment: **Incus**
- Origin of tensor tympani muscle on which wall: **Anterior wall (from canal of tensor tympani)**
- Origin of stapedius muscle on which wall: **Posterior wall (Tip of pyramid)**
- While cochlear implant, electrode is placed at: **Scala tympani**
- While cochlear implant, electrode is passed via: **Round window**
- Tuning fork most commonly used for this frequency: **512 Hz**
- Otoacoustic emissions arise from: **Outer cells**
- Best test for screening of hearing in newborn: **Otoacoustic emission**
- Roll over phenomena seen in **Retrocochlear Lesion**
- Bills bar location: **Inner ear**
- Bills bar separates which structure in inner ear: **Facial nerve and Superior vestibular nerve**
- Macewen's triangle or suprameatal triangle is landmark of **mastoid antrum**.
- Organ of Corti contains endolymph, hair cells, and supporting **cells Hansen's and Deiter's cell**
- Otolith membrane of macula is made up of **Ca $(CO)_3$** crystals.
- Hamartoma of auricle may result **in cauliflower ear.**
- Most common organism causing cauliflower ear: ***Stap aureus***
- Perichondritis of the auricle m/c pathogen is **pseudomonas**
- Normal hearing capacity is from 20 Hz to 20, 000 Hz.
- Moderately severe hearing loss: **56–70 dB**
- Noise induced hearing loss seen maximum at: **5–6 khz**
- **Hennebert sign** is seen in: Meniere's disease
- In case of BPPV, which semicircular canal affected: **Posterior semi-circular canal**
- Acute otitis media most commonly caused by: **Streptococcus pneumonia**
- Bullous myringitis is most commonly caused by: **Adenovirus**
- Wax softened by $NaHCO_3$ solution and syringing by sterile water at body temperature.
- Furunculosis of external ear caused by **staphylococcus.**
- Malignant otitis externa caused by **pseudomonas** seen in diabetics and immune compromised.
- **Central perforation of TM:** Safe CSOM
- **Peripheral perforation of TM** – Unsafe CSOM
- In keratosis obturans external ear canal is filled up by: **Cholesteatoma mass.**

Contd...

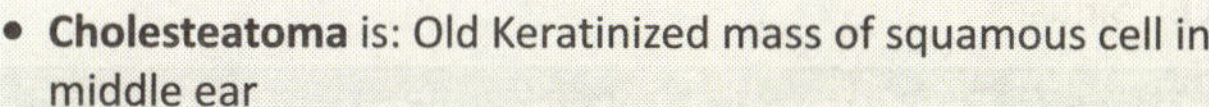

- **Cholesteatoma** is: Old Keratinized mass of squamous cell in middle ear
- **MC site congenital cholesteatoma** - Petrous part of temporal bone
- **MC site of acquired cholesteatoma** – Prussack's space or attic area
- Most **common complication** of CSOM is **brain abscess**
- Most **common intracranial manifestation** of late chronic otitis media: **Brain abscess**
- Most common **extracranial** complication of CSOM: **Mastoiditis**
- Most common organism causing mastoiditis: group A beta hemolytic streptococcus
- Pulsatile tinnitus is seen in **Glomus Tumor**
- Pulsatile otorrhea (aka Lighthouse sign) seen in– ASOM
- **Grommet:** Small tube to drain middle ear
- Most common quadrant preferred for insertion of grommet: **Antero-inferior quadrant**
- Fluctuating hearing loss is seen in – **Ménière's Disease**
- Most common cause of sensorineural hearing loss – **Presbycusis**
- **Paracusis willisii:** Patient hears better in noisy environment. Seen in case of otosclerosis
- Cohort notch at 2000 Hz seen in **Otosclerosis**
- Loudness of sound is measured by its **Intensity**
- Glomus tumor is a tumor of **paraganglionic cells**
- **Phelp's sign**-Glomus tumor (glomus jugulare)
- Cranial nerve involved in Gradenigo's syndrome: **5th & 6th cranial nerve**
- 3 D's of Gradenigo's syndrome: **Diplopia, Deep pain, Discharge**
- Lyre sign is seen in **Carotid Body** tumor
- Most common tumor of CP angle: **Vestibular schwannoma aka Acoustic neuroma**
- Osteomeatal complex is an important landmark during **FESS**
- Chronic dacryocystitis and mucocele of lacrimal sac are treated by **Dacryocystorhinostomy**
- **Osteomeatal complex includes** – middle meatus, uncinate process and ethmoidal bulla
- Most common site of epistaxis – **Little's area**
- Nasal septum perforation can be a side effect of antiangiogenesis drugs like – **Bevacizumab**
- This illicit drug abuse can cause septal perforation: **Cocaine**
- MC type of DNS present with epistaxis: **Spur**
- Mikulicz cell upon HPE in case of– **Rhinoscleroma**
- Most common organism causing rhinoscleroma: **Klebsiella Rhinoscleromatis**

Contd...

- Most common organism causing Rhinosporidiosis: **Rhinosporidiosis seeberi**
- Most common sinusitis in children – **Ethmoidal**
- Most common sinusitis in adults – **Maxillary**
- Polyp in adults most commonly arises from which sinus: **Ethmoid sinus**
- Polyp in child most commonly arises from which sinus: **Maxillary sinus**
- Best treatment for polyp: FESS
- **Vidian Neurectomy** is done for: Vasomotor Rhinitis
- Recurrent facial nerve paralysis seen in **Melkerson Rosenthal Syndrome**
- Frog sign, antral sign– **Juvenile angiofibroma**
- Characteristic feature of Juvenile angiofibroma: **Recurrent severe epistaxis in adolescent male.**
- Caldwell-Luc's operation is done for: **Maxillary sinusitis**
- Young's operation is surgical procedure for: **Atrophic rhinitis**
- Most common bone fractured on face: **Nasal septal fracture**
- MC site of fracture on mandible: **Condylar neck**
- **Reinke's space** – seen in glottis area. Often affected by edema causes polypoid degeneration of vocal cords.
- Narrowest portion of larynx in adult: **Glottis**
- Narrowest portion of larynx in child: **Subglottis**
- Intrinsic muscles of larynx is mainly supplied by: **Recurrent laryngeal nerve**
- Only intrinsic laryngeal muscle NOT supplied by RLN: **Cricothyroid muscle**
- Nerve supplying cricothyroid muscle: **Superior laryngeal nerve (external branch)**
- Abductor of vocal cord: **Posterior cricoarytenoid**
- Most common site of vocal cord nodule: **Anterior 1/3rd and Posterior 2/3rd**
- MCC of vocal cord nodule/Singer's nodule: **Vocal abuse**
- Thumb sign on X-ray neck- **acute epiglottitis**
- Steeple sign in X-ray neck: **Croup**
- Most common organism causing acute epiglottitis: **H. influenza B**
- Most common organism causing croup: **Parainfluenza Type I & II**
- Key hole glottis is seen in: **Phonasthenia**
- Omega shaped glottis: **Laryngomalacia**
- Turban epiglottis is seen in this case: **TB larynx**
- Mouse nibbled appearance of vocal cord: **TB larynx**
- Most common risk factor for CA larynx: **Smoking**
- Laryngeal papillomatosis most commonly caused by: **HPV 6 & 11**

Contd...

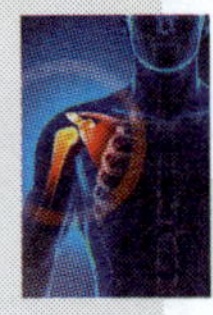

- **Montgomery tube –** silicon tracheal tube used for surgical management of tracheal stenosis
- **Mobius syndrome:** Bilateral facial nerve paralysis associated with abducens nerve palsy (patients unable to smile and unable to move their eyes from side to side)
- **Choanal atresia:** Persistence of bucconasal membrane; UL > BL
- In choanal atresia membrane is most commonly comprised of: **Bone**
- **McGovern's procedure:** In case of Choanal atresia (placing a wide bore nipple in baby's mouth)
- **Ludwig angina:** Airway obstruction due to laryngeal edema

KNOW THE MOST COMMON

MC benign lesion of the ear is **actinic keratosis**

MC location of **epistaxis in children** is anterior, often traumatic.

MC tumor of the paranasal sinuses is **osteoma**

MC infectious disease in humans is **acute viral rhinitis**

MC noninfectious cause of rhinitis is **allergic** (about 20% of population).

MC medical cause of rhinitis is **decongestant abuse**

MC orbital infection is acute **ethmoidal sinusitis**

MC fungal infection of the oral cavity is **moniliasis.**

MC benign neoplasm of the oral cavity and pharynx is **squamous papilloma.**

MC malignant neoplasm of the oral cavity and pharynx is **squamous cell carcinoma.**

MC benign neoplasm of the parotid gland in children is **hemangioma**

MC malignant neoplasm of the parotid gland is **mucoepidermoid carcinoma**

MC malignant neoplasm of salivary glands (except parotid) is **adenoid cystic carcinoma.**

MC cause of stridor in infant is **laryngomalacia**

MC inflammatory condition of the larynx in adults is **acute laryngitis.**

MC benign tumor of the larynx in children is **squamous papilloma**

MC malignant tumor of the larynx is **squamous cell carcinoma**

MC etiologies of neck masses in children are **congenital and inflammatory.**

MC etiology of neck masses in adults is **neoplasm.**

MC **benign neck tumors** are lipoma and neurogenic tumors (schwannoma, neurofibroma).

MC malignant lateral neck masses in children are **lymphoma and rhabdomyosarcoma.**

MC the **cricoarytenoid muscles** are the only ones that **Abduct the vocal cords.**

TABLE: Sinuses

Sinus	Condition at Birth	Adult size	First radiological evidence
Maxillary	+ (6–8 mL)	15 years	4–5 months
Ethmoid	+	12 years	1 year
Frontal	–	20 years	6 years
Sphenoid	–	15 years	4 years

TABLE: Larynx anatomy

	Adult larynx	Pediatric larynx
Location	C3 – C6	High in neck At rest: C3 or C4 While swallowing: C1 or C2
Cartilage	Soft	Softer
Thyroid cartilage	Elevated at thyroid angle	Flat
Shape	Cylindrical	Conical
Length of vocal cord	Female: 15–19 mm Male: 17–23 mm	Female: 6 mm Male: 8 mm

TABLE: Male vs female larynx

Male	Female
Length = 44 mm	36 mm
AP = 43 mm	41 mm
Transverse: 36 mm	26 mm

ORTHOPEDICS

IMPORTANT RECENT POINTS (INCLUDES LATEST QS)

Term orthopedics was coined by **Nicolas Andry.**

Bone within bone appearance is seen in **osteopetrosis**

Short 4th and 5th metacarpal is seen in **pseudo hypoparathyroidism.**

Frankel's line and Wimberger's ring seen in **scurvy.**

Rocker bottom foot is seen in congenital vertical talus and incorrection of CTEV.

Kienbock's disease is avascular necrosis of **lunate.**

Codfish vertebrae is seen in osteoporosis

Triple arthrodesis includes talonavicular, talocalcaneal, calcaneocuboid fusion.

Intra-articular calcification is seen in Charcot's joints.

Quadriceps femoris is main extensor of knee joint.

Contd...

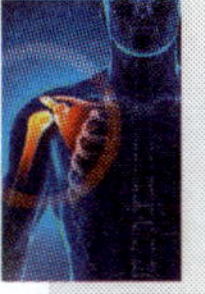

Knuckle-blender splint: Claw hand

Cock up splint is used for radial nerve palsy.

Locking of knee is seen in bucket handle tear of meniscus.

Mallet finger is avulsion of base of distal phalanx.

Maximum weight for skeletal traction is 20 kg

Chauffeur's fracture involves radial styloid.

K-wire is used for cerclage and fore arm bone fixation.

Barton's fracture involve fracture distal end radius with wrist sublaxation.

Scaphoid is treated by glass holding cast.

MCC of bony ankylosis is pyogenic arthritis.

Onion peeling is seen in Ewing's sarcoma.

MC bone to fracture on face is **nasal bone**

MC site of fracture of mandible is **neck of condyle.**

Earliest X-ray finding of Osteomyelitis: **Periosteal reaction**

Drug of choice for acute gouty arthritis: **Indomethacin**

Deformities in RA
Swan-neck deformity: Hyperextension of the PIP joint with flexion of the DIP joint.
Boutonnière deformity: Flexion of the PIP joint with hyperextension of the DIP joint.
Z-line deformity

Deformities in OA:
- Bouchard's node: Node at PIP
- Heberden node: Node at DIP

COMMON FRACTURES AND INJURIES

Fracture	Description
Bankart's fracture	Fracture of anterior glenoid associated with anterior shoulder dislocation
Bennett's fracture	Intra-articular fracture of base of Thumb metacarpal
Boxer's fracture	Fracture of neck of little metacarpal
Bumper fracture	Compression fracture of lateral tibial plateau
Burst fracture	It is a comminuted fracture of the vertebral body where fragments "burst out" in different directions
Chauffeur's #	Intra-articular fracture of radial styloid
Colles' fracture	Distal radius fracture with dorsal angulation, im- impaction and radial drift
Chance fracture aka seat-belt fracture	The fracture line running horizontally through the body of the vertebra and through, the posterior elements
Dashboard fracture	A fracture of posterior lip of the acetabulum, often associated with posterior dislocation of the hip
Duverney fracture	Isolated fracture of the iliac wing
Galeazzi fracture	Radius shaft fracture with dislocation of distal radio-**ulnar joint**
Gosselin fracture	V-shaped distal tibia fracture extending into the tibial plafond
Hangman's #	Fracture of both pedicles of C2
Hill–Sachs fracture	Impacted posterior humeral head fracture occurring during anterior shoulder dislocation
Jefferson fracture	Fracture of first cervical vertebra
Jones fracture	Fracture of base of 5th metatarsal extending into intermetatarsal joint
Lisfranc fracture	Fracture dislocation of midfoot
March fracture	Stress fracture of 2nd and 3rd metatarsal shaft
Monteggia fracture	Proximal ulna fracture with dislocation of radial head
Moore's fracture	Distal radius fracture with ulnar dislocation and entrapment of styloid process under annular ligament
Pipkin fracture-dislocation	Posterior dislocation of hip with avulsion fracture of Fragment of femoral head by the ligamentum teres
Pott's fracture	Bimalleolar fracture of the ankle
Cotton's fracture	Trimalleolar ankle fracture
Rolando fracture	Extra-articular comminuted fracture of base of first metacarpal
Runner's fracture	Stress fracture of distal fibula 3–8 cm above the lateral malleolus
Salter–Harris #	Fractures involving a growth plate
Shepherd's fracture	Fracture of the lateral tubercle of the posterior process of the talus
Smith's fracture	Distal radius fracture with volar displacement
Straddle fracture	Bilateral superior and inferior pubic-rani fracture
Whiplash injury	Cervical spine injury where sudden flexion followed by hyperextension takes place

Contd...

TABLE: Static stabilizer vs dynamic stabilizer of shoulder joint

Static stabilizer	Dynamic stabilizer
Glenoid labrum **Glenohumeral ligament** **Negative pressure in glenoid cavity**	Supraspinatus Infraspinatus Teres minor Subscapularis

TABLE: Shoulders pathology and nerve involved

Ant. Shoulder dislocation	Axillary nerve
Surgical neck humerus #	Axillary nerve
Humerus shaft #	Radial nerve
Supracondylar #	Anterior interosseous nerve > median nerve
Cubitus valgus	Tardy ulnar nerve palsy
Medial condyle humerus #	Ulnar nerve

TABLE: Different splint and their uses

Splint	Used in
Knuckle bender splint	Ulnar nerve
Aeroplane splint	Brachial plexus injury
Dennis brown splint	CTEV
Bohler Braun splint	Fracture femur (anywhere from neck to supracondylar region)
Turn buckle splint	VIC (Volkmann ischemic contracture)

SOME IMPORTANT SIGNS AND TESTS

Adson's test: For thoracic outlet syndrome

Allen's test: For testing patency of radial and ulnar arteries

Alli's test: For CDH

Anvil test: For testing tenderness of the spine

Ape thumb: For median nerve injury

Apley's grinding test: For meniscus injury

Apprehension test: For recurrent dislocation for the shoulder

Barlow's test: For CDH

Galeazzi sign: For CDH
Galeazzi fracture: *Radius* shaft fracture with dislocation of distal radioulnar joint

Blue sclera: Osteogenesis imperfect

Bryant's test: For anterior dislocation of the shoulder

Callaways' test: For anterior dislocation of the shoulder

Chvostek's sign: For tetany

Claw hand: For ulnar nerve injury

Contd...

Coin test: For dorso-lumbar tuberculosis of spine

Cozen's test: For tennis elbow

Drawer test: For ACL and PCL injuries
Anterior: For ACL injury
Posterior: For PCL injury

Finkelstein's test: For de Quervain's tenovaginitis

Foot drop: For common peroneal nerve injury

Froment's sign: For ulnar nerve injury

Gaenslen's test: For SI joint involvement

Gower's sign: For muscular dystrophy

Hamilton–ruler test: For anterior dislocation of the shoulder

Kanavel's sign: For infection in ulnar bursa

Lasegue's test: For disc prolapse

Lachman test: For ACL injury

Ludloff's sign: For avulsion of lesser trochanter

McMurray's test: For meniscus injury

Naffziger's test: Disc prolapse

Ober's test: For tight iliotibial band (e.g. in polio)

O'Donoghue triad: Triad of MCL, ACL & medial meniscus injuries occurring together

Ortolani's test: For CDH

Pivot-shift test: For ACL injury

Policeman tip: For Erb's palsy

Sulcus sign: For inferior dislocation of the shoulder

Thomas's test: For hip flexion deformity

Trendelenburg's test: For unstable hip due to any injury?

IMPORTANT CLASSIFICATION

Neer's: For upper end of humerus fractures

Gustilo: For open fractures

Salter and Harris: For epiphyseal injuries

Lauge Hansen's: For ankle injuries

Pauwel's: For fractures neck of the femur

Garden's: For fractures neck of the femur

Winquist: Femur fracture

Milch: lateral condylar fracture

Campbell: Clavicle fracture

Tile's/Young → Pelvic bone fracture

Thompson and Epstein: Post Hip dislocation

Rockwood: Acromioclavicular Joint injury

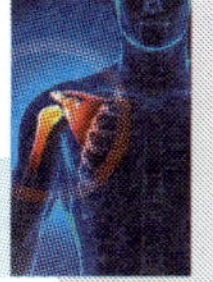

RADIOLOGICAL SIGNS

Special views
Judet views: For acetabular fracture
Oblique view of the wrist: For fracture scaphoid
Mortise view: For ankle injuries
Sunset view: For patella - Femoral dysplasia
Von Rosen view: For CDH
Shenton's line: Hip X-ray

Angle
Carrying angle: Elbow
Pauwel's angle: Fracture neck of the femur
Bohler's angle: Fracture of the calcaneum
Kite's angle: Angle in CTEV
Neck-shaft angle: Of the femoral neck

Classic features
Wormian bones: Osteogenesis imperfecta
Sun-ray appearance: Osteosarcoma
Soap-bubble appearance: Osteoclastoma
Onion-peel appearance: Ewing's Sarcoma
Shepherd-Crook deformity: Fibrous dysplasia
Risser's sign: Epiphysis of iliac bone
Aneurysmal sign: TB spine (anterior type)
Tonguing of vertebra: Morquio-Brails disease
Trethowan's sign: Slipped capital femoral epiphysis
Sagging rope sign: Perthe's disease
Patchy calcification: Chondrosarcoma
Fabella: Sesamoid bone in the lateral head of gastrocnemius
Spondylosis: Degenerative spine disease

GAITS

- **Antalgic gait:** Occurs in painful condition of lower limb
- **Trendelenburg gait**: Occurs in an unstable hip due to CDH, gluteus medius weakness, etc.
- **Stiff hip gait:** Occurs in ankylosis of the hip
- **Duck waddling gait:** Occurs in bilateral CDH
- **Scissoring gait:** Occurs in CP
- **High stepping gait:** Occurs in foot drop
- **Circumduction gait:** Occurs in hemiplegia
- **Charlie-Chaplin gait:** Occurs in tibial torsion
- **Sailor's gait:** Occurs in bilateral CDH

ORTHOPEDICS—THE MOST COMMON LIST

- Location of hip fracture is at the femoral neck and intertrochanter.
- Sprained ligament is the anterior talofibular ligament.
- Foci of acute hematogenous osteomyelitis are the metaphases of long bones secondary to turbulent flow.
- Variety of osteoporosis is the involutional type, often seen in post-menopausal women.
- Musculoskeletal morbidity in the elderly is osteoarthritis.
- The most movable joint is the glenohumeral joint.
- The strongest bone segment is the femoral shaft.

BONE INFECTION—MOST COMMON

- Most common organism causing acute osteomyelitis: ***Staph. aureus***
- MCC of osteomyelitis in **sickle cell anemia patient: Salmonella**
- MCC of osteomyelitis in **IV drug abuser: Pseudomonas**
- MC organism causing osteomyelitis in **open foot injury: Pseudomonas**
- MC organism causing osteomyelitis in **HIV patient: Staph. Aureus**
- MC organism causing osteomyelitis in case of **animal bite: Pasteurella Multocida**
- MC organism causing osteomyelitis in case of **human bite: Eikenella Corrodens**

TABLE: Radiological appearance of some common bone tumors

- **Sun burst appearance:** Osteosarcoma
- **Nidu/Seed in cortex:** Osteoid osteoma
- **Onion skin appearance:** Ewing's sarcoma
- **Exostosis (cartilage cap):** Osteochondroma
- **Soap bubble appearance:** Giant cell tumor/Osteoclastoma

Tumor	Site
Solitary bone cyst	Upper end of humerus
Aneurysmal bone cyst	Lower limb metaphysis
Osteochondroma	Distal femur
Osteoid osteoma	Femur
Osteoblastoma	Vertebrae
Osteoma	Skull, facial bones
Enchondroma	Short bones of hand
Chordoma	Sacrum
Adamantinoma	Tibial

Contd...

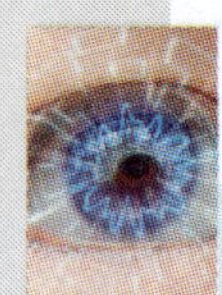

Tumor	Site
Ameloblastoma	Mandible
Osteoclastoma	Lower end femur
Fibrous dysplasia	Polyostotic – craniofacial Monostotic – upper femur
Multiple myeloma	Lumbar vertebrae
Osteosarcoma	Lower end femur
Ewings's sarcoma	Femur
Chondrosarcoma	Pelvis
Secondary tumors	Dorsal vertebrae

Some important facts

- **MC type of ant. shoulder D/L:** Subcoracoid (head lies below coracoid process)
- **Blounts disease:** Dysplasia of proximal posteromedial tibial epiphysis
- **Steinberg and Walker Murdoch sign:** Marfans syndrome
- **MC translocation in Ewing's:** t(11:22)
- **David letterman sign/Terry Thomas sign:** Scapholunate dislocation
- **Game keeper's thumb:** Torn ulnar collateral ligament after injury to thumb MCP joint
- **Booadie's Abscess:** Subacute OM
- **Kanavel Sign:** Tenosynovitis
- **Heberden node and Bouchard Node:** OA
- **Swan neck and Boutonniere deformity:** RA
- **Bag of bone sign:** Charcot's Joint (in DM)
- **IOC for CDH:** MRI
- **Screening for CDH:** USG
- **Trethowan's sign:** SCFE
- **Wimberger corner sign:** Cong. Syphillis
- **Froment sign:** Ulnar nerve palsy
- **Phalen test +ve:** Carpal tunnel syndrome
- **Meralgia paresthetica:** Lat cutaneous nerve of thigh
- **Cheiralgia paresthetica:** Superficial radial nerve

OPHTHALMOLOGY

EYEBALL AT BIRTH

- **AP diameter:** 16.5 mm (adult size 24 mm by 7–8 years)
- **Corneal diameter:** 10 mm (adult size 11.7 mm 2 years)
- Newborn hypermetropic by 2–3 D

Contd...

- Fixation starts at 1 month. Completed by 6 mo
- Macula fully developed by—4–6 mo
- Fusional reflex and accommodation well developed by 4–6 mo
- 3D depth perception/stereopsis—6 years

LENS

- Grow throughout the year
- **Diameter:** 9–10 mm
- **Thickness:** 3.5–5 mm
- **Weight:** 135 mg to 255 mg
- **Total dioptric power:** 18 D (16D – 20D)
- **Refractive index:** 1.39
- **Accommodative power:** 14–16 D at birth; 7–8 D at 25 years and 1–2 D at 50 year

IMPORTANT POINTS

Length of eyeball: **24 mm**

Volume of orbit: **30 ml**

Weight of eyeball: **7 gram**

Volume of eyeball: **6 ml**

Anterior chamber: **Between iris and cornea (posterior wall)**
Posterior chamber: **Between lens and iris**

Deep anterior chamber in: **Young, Male and Myopes**
Shallow anterior chamber in: **Elderly, female and hypermetropes**

DDO (distant direct ophthalmoscope): **Performed at a distance 22 cm (20–28 cm)**

Direct ophthalmoscope: Done closest to patient
Image is Direct, Erect and Virtual; magnified by 15 times

Indirect ophthalmoscope: Performed at a distance of 1 m Image is real (true), inverted; magnified by 5 times

Slit lamp is the best investigation method for diagnosis of vitreous opacities

Functional assessment of optic nerve is done by **Perimetry**.

Acuity for distant vision is tested by - **Snellen chart**

Acuity for near vision is tested by - **Jaeger type cards**

Ishihara chart is used for: **Color blindness**

Retinoscopy
- Done at a distance 1m. If reflex moves in:
- **Same direction** - Emmetropia, hypermetropia, myopia<1D
- **Opposite direction** – Myopia >1D
- **No movement** - Myopia -1D

Field of vision is tested by - Perimetry, Bjerrum's screen, confrontation method

Finchams test: Differentiates colored halos of acute congestive glaucoma from that of acute conjunctivitis

Contd...

Gonioscope: The angle of anterior chamber can be examined with the help of a Gonioscope and slit lamp.

Tonometry: Used for accurate determination of IOT (intraocular tension)

Arden index: It the ratio between light peak to dark trough. Normally it is 1.85

Ring scotoma: Seen in retinitis pigmentosa, glaucoma (double arcuate scotoma)

Roth spots- white centered retinal hemorrhages
Seen in **Leukemia, SABE, DM**

Lens develop from **surface ectoderm**

Lower and lateral walls of orbit are derived from **visceral mesoderm**

Total refractive power of eye is **58-60 D (Avg-58.6)**

Total refractive power of cornea **43.78D +/- 1.86D**

Normal cup-disc ratio-**1:3**

Maximum refractive index is **at center of lens (1.40)**

Newborn eye is short axial length is 17.5 mm generally hypermetropic +2.5D and fovea is immature.

Critical period for the development of fixation of eye reflexes is 2-4 months

Glycolysis is the main route of metabolism of glucose in the lens.

IOT ranges from **10-20 mmHg**

Optic disc - Depressed area of optic disc contains no rods/cones is therefore insensitive to light and called physiological blind spot.

CME (cystoid macular edema)- shows flower petal appearance of fundus.

Ink-blot pattern and smoke-stake patterns is seen in: **CSR** (central serous retinopathy).

CRAO - Cattle truck appearance of retinal veins, cherry red spots.

Aphakia produces high degree of hypermetropia

Frequent changes of presbyopic glasses is an early symptom of- **primary open angle glaucoma.**

First sign of cavernous involvement/raised ICT IS 6th CN palsy.

Structures passing through optic foramen are - **Optic nerve and ophthalmic artery**

Bielschowsky sign is for superior oblique palsy.

Sea saw nystagmus of Maddox - Found in para chiasmal lesion.

Argyll-Robertson pupil Light reflex absent, accommodation reflex present Seen in Neurosyphilis, DM, syringomyelia, disseminated sclerosis.

Horner's syndrome: Triad of MIOSIS, IPSILATERAL PTOSIS, ANHYDROSIS.

Marcus gunn pupil is diagnostic of-acute retrobulbar neuritis (optic neuritis)

Parvocellular pathway - Located on layers 3, 4, 5, 6 of retina

Contd...

Most common cause of viral conjunctivitis-**Adeno virus**

Most common cause of bilateral conjunctivitis in neonates within 3-5 days - ***Neisseria gonorrhoea.***

Most common cause of severe keratoconjunctivitis in contact lens user - **Acanthamoeba**

Most characteristic lesion of HSV recurrent infection is **the-dendritic ulcer (dendritic keratitis)**

Trachoma-leading preventable cause of blindness

SAFE strategy used for trachoma - Surgery, Antibiotics, Facial hygiene, Environmental change

Corneal transparency is maintained by - **Descemet membrane**

Donor cornea from **cadaveric eye** can be used 6 hours of death. It is stored in **Mc Kaufmanns media** for 4 days.

Corneal ulcers - Ulcer Serpens is due to pseudomonas.

LASIK is absolutely contraindicated in keratoconus

Most common fungus infecting lids - **Candida albicans.**

Posterior staphyloma is due to ectasia at posterior pole, seen in myopia

Anterior staphyloma is due to ectasia of cornea at anterior pole, seen in corneal ulcer perforation.

Sympathetic ophthalmia: retrolental flare is the first sign, Dalen Fuchs nodules

Lens capsule is thinnest at posterior pole.

Ascorbic acid in lens is derived from myo inositol phosphate.

Snow flake/snow storm cataract - Seen in diabetes

Oil drop cataract - Seen in galactosemia

Sunflower cataract - Seen in Wilson's disease

Bread crumb appearance - Seen in complicated cataract

Most common complication of morgagnian cataract- **Phacolytic glaucoma.**

Supero temporal dislocation of lens - Seen in Marfans syndrome

Infero nasal dislocation of lens-seen in **homocystinuria.**

Antero inferior dislocation of lens-**Weill marchesani syndrome**.

Hard contact lenses and IOL lens are made up of **PMMA**

Soft contact lenses are made up of **HEMA (Hydroxyethyl Methacrylate), Silicon Hydrogel**

Earliest filed defects in glaucoma - Central/para central scotoma in bjerrums area.

Most effective surgery for congenital or infantile glaucoma is **goniotomy or trabeculotomy**.

Aphakia - Absence of crystalline lens.power of Aphakic eye is 44 D

Most radioresistant structure in retina-**ganglion cell layer**.

Cotton wool spots (cytoid bodies) are due to focal ischemia in the nerve fiber layer, found in HIV retinopathy.

Contd...

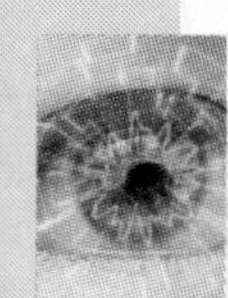

Flame shaped hemorrhages found in - **Hypertensive and arteriosclerosis retinopathy**.

Field defect in toxic amblyopia - **Centroceacal scotoma.**

TOC for paralytic squint-**surgery**

TOC for amblyopia with unilateral strabismus - **Conventional occlusion (of normal eye)**

TOC for accommodative squint-**correction of refractive errors**.

TOC for concomitant squint-**orthoptic exercises**

Most common intraocular foreign bodies - **Chips of iron and steel.**

Most common cause of intermittent proptosis-**orbital varix** (varicose vein in the eye)

In children:
Most common intraocular tumor - Retinoblastoma
Most common intra orbital tumor - Rhabdomyosarcoma

In adults
MC intraocular tumor - **Malignant melanoma of choroid**
MC intra orbital tumor – **Cavernous Hemangioma**
MC tumor which metastasize to eye - **Neuroblastoma**
MC tumor of eyelids **basal cell carcinoma**
MC tumor of lacrimal gland - **Benign mixed tumor**

Mutations in retinoblastoma are seen at 13q14

MC presentation in retinoblastoma - leukocoria > strabismus.

Vitreous is composed of type II collagen+hyluronic acid.

Trichiasis: Is mis directed eye lashes.
Madarosis: Loss of eye lashes/eyebrows
Tylosis: Thickening of lid margin
Blepharitis: **Inflammation of eyelid**

Fastest acting mydriatic and cycloplegic -**Tropicamide**
Shortest acting mydriatic and cycloplegic -**Tropicamide**
Shortest acting mydriatic without cycloplegia-**phenylephrine**.

MC congenital color blindness - **Green (deuteranopia)**

MC cause of blindness in AIDS patients - **CMV retinitis.**

MC cause of blindness worldwide - **Cataract**
MC cause of blindness in India - **Cataract**
MC cause of ocular morbidity - **Refractive errors**
MC cause of ocular morbidity in youngs - **Refractive errors**
MC cause of preventable blindness in children - **Vit A deficiency**

Tear production starts at 6 months

MC ocular manifestation of measles - **Vit A deficiency**

Corneal nerve is visible in-**leprosy, keratoconus.**

Bluish discoloration of sclera - **osteitis deformans.**

MC cause of sudden unilateral loss of vision - **Optic neuritis**

MC treatment modality for acute angle closure glaucoma-**Laser iridotomy**

Contd...

Not seen in herpes zoster opthalmicus-**sclero-keratitis**

Worth 4 dot test is done for: **Binocular vision**

Jack in a box is seen in: **Aphakia**

Tranta's dot, Ropy discharge is seen in: **Vernal conjunctivitis**

Interstitial keratitis is seen in: **Syphilis**

Side effect of oral steroid: **Cataract**

Side effect of topical steroid: **Glaucoma**

D/Dx of color haloes:
- ACG
- Cataract
- Mucopurulent conjunctivitis (Not in angular)
- Vertically fixed mid-dilated pupil seen in: ACG

RECENT ONE'S

MCC of blindness in India: **Cataract**

Retrolental Flare is seen in: **Sympathetic Ophthalmitis**

Ipsilateral CN 3 palsy can lead to: **Weber syndrome**

Most radiosensitive layer of retina: **Rods and cones**

Most radioresistant layer of retina: **Ganglion cell layer**

Ascorbic acid in lens is transported by: **Myoinositol**

Orbital floor is formed by: **Maxillary bone and palatine bone**

MC complication after lens extraction in PHPV: **Vitrous Hemorrhage**

Cornea can be harvested: **Till 6 hours after death**

Alcaftadine trail used this concentration of drug: **0.25%**

Definition of blindness according to WHO: **<3/60**

Vossius ring in eye is due to: **Blunt trauma**

Alkali injury in eye causes: **Symblepharon**

Ankyloblepharon: Upper and lower lid margin fusion

Titmus fly test is for: **Stereopsis**

Jack in the box phenomenon: **Aphakia**

Anterior lenticonus: **Alport syndrome**

Posterior lenticonus: **Lowe syndrome**

Dalen fuch's nodule is seen in: **Sympathetic ophthalmitis**

Buphthalmos is seen in: **Congenital glaucoma (AR condition)**

Krukenberg spindle is seen in: **Pigmentary glaucoma (iris pigment on cornea)**

IOC for indirect ophthalmoscopy: **Indirect ophtha**

Flame shaped hemorrhages are hallmark of: **Hypertensive retinopathy**

Flower petal appearance upon fluorescein angiography: **Cystoid macular edema**

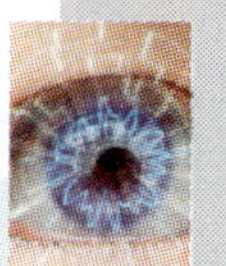

OPHTHALMOLOGY—MOST COMMON LIST

WHAT IS/ARE THE MOST COMMON

- MC Refractive surgery is radial keratotomy
- MC Type of glaucoma is chronic open -Angle glaucoma.
- MC Glaucoma-related surgical procedure is trabeculectomy.
- MC Cause of blindness: **Cataract**
- MC etiology of visual loss in patients with diabetes mellitus is macular edema.
- MC Cause of proptosis in children is: **Orbital Cellulitis**
- MC Cause of proptosis in adults is **Grave's Disease.**
- MC Cause of red eye is **Conjunctivitis.**
- MC Cause of ocular venous occlusion is **glaucoma.**
- MC Indication for corneal treatment: **Pseudophakic bullous keratopathy**

TABLE: CN, their respective nucleus location and their function

Cranial nerve	Nucleus location	Function
Oculomotor III	Upper midbrain	Eyeball movements: Extrinsic ocular muscles
Trochlear IV	Lower midbrain	Eyeball movements: Extrinsic ocular muscles
Abducens VI	Pons	Eyeball movements: Extrinsic ocular muscles
Hypoglossal XII	Medulla	Tongue muscles and movements

TABLE: Few Instruments which are used for ocular examination

Measurement parameter	Instruments used
Corneal thickness	Pachymeter
Corneal curvature	Keratometer
Angle of anterior chamber	Gonioscope
Corneal surface	Placido disc
Corneal endothelium	Specular microscope
Direct ophthalmoscope Remembered as: "DEV"	Routine fundus examination. *"Image formed is Erect and Virtual and magnified, 15 times"*
Indirect ophthalmoscope	For assessment of retinal detachment and other peripheral retinal lesions. *The image is real, inverted and magnified 5 times.*
Perimetry	Optic nerve function

Aqueous humor physiology

- **Protein:** conc less than plasma
- **Glucose:** less than plasma (used by cornea and lens as they are avascular)
- **Acid:** Lactic, Pyruvic, Ascorbic. Conc higher than plasma
- **pH:** 7.2 (lower than plasma)
- **Formed by:** Diffusion (10%), Ultrafiltration: 20% and Active transport: 70%

Must Know Facts

Types of nystagmus	**Staphyloma:** *an ectatic condition of the eyeball w/ herniation of uveal tissue.*	Proptosis
• **Downbeat:** arnold chiari malformation • **Ocular bobbing-** downbeat ff by slow upbeat: Pontine lesion • **See saw:** Optic chiasma lesion	• **Anterior:** corneal ulcer • **Posterior:** Pathological myopia • **Intercalary:** trauma at limbus • **Ciliary:** Scleritis	• **Sequence of ms involved:** IR > MR > SR> LR • **MCC of B/L proptosis:** thyroid ophthalmopathy • **MCC of U/L proptosis:** thyroid Ophth... • **MCC of B/L proptosis in child:** orbital cellulitis • **MCC of U/L proptosis in child:** ALL

TABLE: WHO classification of xerophthalmia

Class	Signs
X1A	Conjunctival xerosis
X1B	Conjunctival xerosis with bitot's spot
X2	Corneal xerosis
X3A	Corneal xerosis with ulceration
X3B	Keratomalacia

TABLE: Swimming pool related infections

Disease	Causative agent
Swimming pool conjunctivitis	*C. trachomatis*
Swimming pool granuloma	*Mycobacterium marinum*
Swimmer's itch	*Schistosoma mansoni* *S. japonicum*
• Swimmer's ear	*Pseudomonas/Staphylococcus aureus* (Mixed)
• Swimming pool folliculitis	*Pseudomonas*

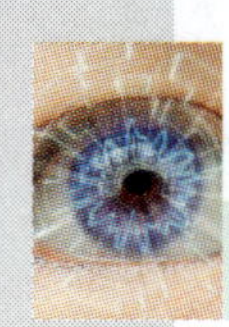

TABLE: Eye discharge and possible etiological agent

Discharge	Etiological agent
Purulent/mucopurulent	Bacterial conjunctivitis
Watery	Viral conjunctivitis
Ropy	Allergic conjunctivitis
Mucopurulent	Chlamydial conjunctivitis

Causes of Painless and Painful Loss of Vision

Sudden painless loss of vision	Sudden painful loss of vision
Vascular occlusion (CRAO, CRVO) *Retinal detachment* *Vitreous hemorrhage* Ischemic optic neuropathy	Acute iridocyclitis Chemical injuries Mechanical injuries Acute congestive glaucoma Optic neuritis
Gradual painless loss of vision	Gradual painful loss of vision
Progressive pterygium involving the pupil Corneal degeneration Corneal dystrophy Developmental cataracts Senile cataracts Optic atrophy Chorioretinal degeneration Age- related macular degeneration *Diabetic retinopathy* Refractive errors Papilloedema & Papillitis	Chronic iridocyclitis Corneal ulceration Chronic simple glaucoma

Cherry red spot of retina is seen in—

- CRAO
- Trauma (Blunt trauma, Berlin's edema)
- Neimann pick disease
- Gaucher's disease
- Tay – Sach's disease
- Sand hoff's disease

Mnemonic: Cherry Tree Never Grow Tall in Sand.

TABLE: Comparison of anterior, intermediate and posterior uveitis

	Anterior	Intermediate	Posterior
Aka	Iridocyclitis	Pars Planitis	Chorioretinitis
Cause	Idiopathic	Idiopathic	Toxoplasmosis
Clinical feature	Sudden painless loss of vision	Floaters	Sudden painless loss of vision
Cells	WBC's Keratic precipitate	Snowballs/ snowbanks	Headlight in fog appearance
Treatment	Topical steroids **DOC:** Cycloplegics	Inj: Triamcinolone	Antimicrobials Systemic steroids

TABLE: Types of cataract and their causes

Type of cataract	Cause
Snow flake/snow storm cataract	Diabetes mellitus/ Down's syndrome
Sunflower/Petals of flower cataract	Wilson's disease Chalcosis (mild reaction to copper) Penetrating trauma (with retention to copper)
Blue dot cortical cataract	Atopic dermatitis Myotonic dystrophy
Vossius ring/Rosette shaped cataract	Blunt trauma
Christmas tree cataract	Myotonic dystrophy
Oil drop cataract **Dust like lenticular opacity**	Galactosemia
Breadcrumb appearance **Polychromatic lusture** **Rainbow cataract**	Complicated cataract/ Secondary cataract
Morgagnian cataract	Hypermature senile cataract

TABLE: Points to know about treatment of glaucoma

First line DOC for ACG: **Mannitol**
TOC for ACG: **Laser iridotomy**
DOC for OAG: PG analogue **(Latanoprost)**
Most powerful anti glaucoma drug: **Latanoprost**
DOC for OAG in India - **Timolol**
Safest anti-glaucoma for children - **Dorzolamide**

TABLE: Lesion in the optic pathway and the type of blindness

Unilateral optic nerve lesion: Unilateral blindness

Binasal hemianopia: Bitemporal optic chiasma lesion. Two different lesions compressing the chiasma from the lateral parts.

Bitemporal hemianopia: Binasal retinal damaged → optic chiasmal lesion. Most common lesion is *pituitary adenoma.*

Homonymous hemianopia: Lesion at optic tract AND optic radiation

Contd...

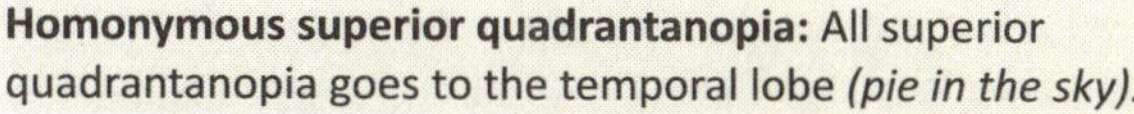

Homonymous superior quadrantanopia: All superior quadrantanopia goes to the temporal lobe *(pie in the sky)*.

Homonymous inferior quadrantanopia: All inferior quadrantanopia goes to the parietal lobe *(Pie on the floor)*.

Homonymous hemianopia w/macular sparing: Lesion in occipital cortex lesion.

Important Nodules

• Dalen fuch nodule	Sympathetic ophthalmitis
• Koeppes nodule	Granulomatous anterior uveitis
• Liesh nodule	NF – 1 and Von Ricklinghausen syndrome
• Foster fuch nodule	Myopia *Foster fuch spot: High myopia*
• Koeppes nodules	Granulomatous uveitis
• Iris nodules	Hansen's disease, NF, fuch heterochromatic iridocyclitis

Must Know

Lesion of the occipital lobe causes: Homonymous hemianopia with macular sparing

- Optic tract lesion causes: Homonymous hemianopia
- Right homonymous hemianopia is due to lesion at: Left optic tract
- Characteristic field defect in pituitary tumor: Bitemporal Hemianopia
- This condition can cause isolated 3rd CN palsy with pupillary sparing: Diabetic Neuropathy, Vascular diseases and Hypertension

DERMATOLOGY

DERMATOLOGY— AT A GLANCE

Average weight of skin: **~ 4 kg**

Normal skin turnover **4–5 weeks**

Skin turnover period in case of psoriasis: **4 days**

Epidermis is compared of **4 layers**-Stratum Basale/germinatum, Stratum spinosum, Stratum granulosum, Stratum corneum.

Dermis is composed of collagen, elastic fibers, sweat/sebaceous glands.

Tzanck smear – Useful in diagnosis of herpes lesion (HSV/VZV multinucleate giant cells)

Tzanck test – Used to differentiate viral lesions of skin from pemphigus.

Body Odor is due to: **Apocrine Gland**

MUST KNOW FACTS

• Cell cycle of keratinocytes	311 hours (28 days)
• Growth rate of scalp hair	0.37 mm/day (90% hair in Anagen phase all time)
• Nail growth rate	**Finger nail:** 1 cm/3 month (0.1 mm/d) **Toe nail:** 1 cm/9 month
• Keratin involved in Epidemolysis bullous simplex	K5 and K14
• Dermis thinnest at	Eyelid and Penis (0.3 mm)
• Type VII collagen defect at basement membrane zone	Epidermolysis bullosa Aquisita
• LIGA disease (Linear IgA bullous disease) due to	BP Ag2
• Bullous pemphigoid is due to this BMZ defect	BP Ag1 and 2
• Herpes gestationis is due this BMZ defect	BP Ag2
• Defect in Hereditary angioedema	C1 esterase inhibitor absent
• Patch test type of HPS reaction	Type IV
• MCC of tinea Unguium	T. Rubrum
• MCC of tinea Mannum	T. Rubrum
• Buddha ears are feature of	Leprosy
• Nevus of ota is seen at this site	Face and Sclera
• Nevus of Ito	Scapular region/Back
• Becker's lesion	Macular lesion + hair
• Sausage digits are seen in	Psoriatic arthritis
• Dermatitis herpetiformis	Celiac sprue *(anti epidermal transglutaminase A/B)*
• Heliotrope rash/Gottron papule/ Mechanic hand is seen in	Dermatomyositis (anti Jo-1 A/b)
• Elephantiasis face is a feature of	Plexiform NF
• Piebaldism+ increased interpupillary distance+ sensory neural deafness	Waardenburg syndrome
• Occlusion due to staph epidermidis in eccrine gland	Miliaria
• Fordyce spot	Ectopic sebaceous gland
• Epidermolysis bullosa simplex	Trauma induced blisters
• Epidermolysis bullosa dystrophica	Absent collagen since birth
• Dilapidated brick wall appearance scene in	Hailey Hailey disease

Contd...

• Row of tombstone appearance and fishnet pattern seen in	Pemphigus vulgaris
• Desmoglein involved in pemphigus foliaceous	DSG 1
• Desmoglein involved pemphigus vulgaris	DSG 3

COLOR ON WOOD LAMP'S LIGHT

- **Pseudomonas, psoriasis** – Pale blue color
- ***Corynebacterium minutissimum*** (erythrasma) – Coral red color
- **Erythrasma**- Coral red
- **Tuberous sclerosis** – Ash leaf spots (blue white)
- **Vitiligo** – Chalky white
- **Porphyria cutanea** tarda – Pinkish red (urine)
- **Tinea versicolor** – Golden fluorescence
- **Pityriasis versicolor**: Yellow
- **Squamous cell carcinoma** – Red fluorescence
- **Burrow of scabies**: Green

Fungi which give fluorescence in wood's light are– ***M. Canis, M. audouinii, T. schoenleinii.***

KOH preparation – Used for diagnosis of Tinea infections

Köbner's isomorphic phenomena seen in:
- Psoriasis
- Lichen planus, lichen nitidus, lichen sclerosus
- Vitiligo
- Kaposi sarcoma
- Pityriasis rubra pilaris
- Necrobiosis lipoidica

Pseudo-isomorphic phenomenon is seen in – **Pityriasis Rubra Pilaris (PRP), molluscum contagiosum, warts**

Nikolsky's sign is seen in–
- Pemphigus
- Staphylococcal scalded skin syndrome (SSSS)
- Toxic shock syndrome
- Porphyria

Pseudo-Nikolsky's sign seen in:
- Toxic epidermal necrolysis
- Steven Johnson syndrome
- Erythema multiforme

Dermatomal involvement is seen in–**Herpes zoster**.

Painful lesions are seen in–**Herpes infection**

Painless lesions are seen in–**Dermatitis herpetiformis (itchy lesions), pemphigoid, pemphigus, erythema multiforme.**

Sub-epidermal lesions are seen in–**Dermatitis herpetiformis, pemphigoid, erythema multiforme.**

Intraepidermal lesions are seen in–**Herpes, pemphigus.**

Contd...

Lesions involving oral mucosa are seen in–**Secondary and congenital syphilis, pemphigus, Peutz Jegher syndrome, lichen planus.**

MC type of warts–**Verruca vulgaris/common warts.**

MC site of common warts–**Dorsum of hand/finger**

Condyloma acuminate (venereal warts) is associated with HPV 16 and 11.

TOC for anogenital warts in pregnancy is **cryotherapy/laser.**

Molluscum contagiosum is due to infection with pox virus.

Extra-genital molluscal lesions are marker of AIDS in adults.

Darier white disease is Autosomal dominant characterized by warty papules and plaques in seborrheic sites.

Dowling Degos disease is autosomal dominant genodermatosis.

MC bacterial skin infection in children is **Impetigo** in which Honey colored crusts are seen.

MC site of Impetigo is **face**.

MC cause of Impetigo is ***Staphylococcus aureus.***

Bullous **pemphigoid** is also known as Senile pemphigoid.

Treatment of bullous pemphigoid is **prednisolone in low doses.**

MC type of pemphigus is **P. vulgaris while the rarest** is **P. vegetans**

P. vulgaris has worst prognosis.

P. vulgaris is diagnosed by **Tzanck** TEST, Fish-net pattern of IgG in epidermis in direct immunofluorescence.

Dermatitis Herpetiformis is recurrent papulovesicular disease with pruritus. Associated with HLA-B8 or DRW3

Max-Joseph spaces, are artificial sub epidermal clefts, often seen in lichen ruber variants of Lichen planus.

Psoriatic arthropathy treated with **Methotrexate (DOC)**

Pityriasis rosea–First feature is Herald patch usually over trunk or upper arm, thigh.

Christmas tree/fir tree pattern seen in **pityriasis rosea.**

Pityriasis versicolor/tinea versicolor caused be **Malassezia** furfur.

"Spaghetti & Meatball" appearance or "Banana & grape" appearance on KOH microscopy: **Pityriasis versicolor**

In **pityriasis rubra** pilaris isolated patches of normal skin are also seen.

Hyperpigmentation is seen in diseases like:
- Addison's disease
- Nelson syndrome
- Hyperthyroidism
- Cushing syndrome
- Ectopic ACTH syndrome
- Freckles

Contd...

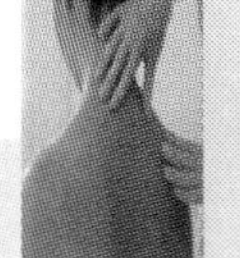

Hypopigmentation is seen in diseases like:
- Vitiligo, piebaldism
- Nevus anemicus
- Nevus depigmentosus
- Pityriasis
- Scleroderma
- Sarcoidosis

Nevus ota, ito, mongolian spots, café au lait spots are causes of local **hypopigmentation.**

Pruritis is hallmark of Atopic dermatitis in which dennie's line and Monk's crawl are seen.

MC presentation of Contact dermatitis is hand **eczema.**

MC cause of air-borne contact dermatitis in India is Allergic Contact Dermatitis due to plant **Parthenium.**

Nummular eczema (discoid dermatitis) is circular/oval coin like pruritic lesions over trunk/extensor surface of limbs in middle age males (M>F).

Asteatotic/xerotic eczema (Winter itch) is inflammatory dermatitis with fine cracks. Seen in summer and involves lower legs in elderly.

Cradle Cap is seen in **Seborrheic Dermatitis.**

Pseudomonas aeruginosa is the MC organism which causes Ecthyma gangrenosum.

Pyoderma Gangrenosum is diagnosed clinically (Morphology of lesions).

MC cause of **Erythema Multiforme** is HSV while MC drug causing it is sulfonamides.

Erythema nodosum is due to infections like streptococcal infection, TB, Leprosy (LL).

Darier sign is seen **Urticaria Pigmentosa.**

Steven Johnson Syndrome is characterized by blisters and epidermal detachment.

In tinea capitis infection of scalp is caused by **trichophyton tonsurans.**

Infection of foot (athlete foot) is caused by **T. rubrum.**

Pistia line is seen in Scarlet fever.

Beau's line is seen in psoriatic arthropathy.

Swimmer's itch – **Bilharziasis/Schistosomiasis.**

Dhobi's/Jock itch – **Tinea cruris.**

Ground itch – **nematode larvae**

Barber's itch **Syncosis barbae**

Itch mite – **Acarus scabiei** (which transmits Scabies)

Scabies is caused by mite **'Sarcoptes scabiei".**

Contd...

Pediculosis is caused by **Pediculosis corporis.**

TB-skin caused by **Mycobacterium tuberculosis bovis** and under some conditions by BCG.

Fox-fordyce disease involves axilla and pubis.

Fordyce spots are ectopic sebaceous glands in neonates.

Retinoic acid is DOC in Acne vulgaris, comedonal acne, nodulocystic acne, pustular acne.

Exclamation marks are seen in **Alopecia Areata.**

Half and half nail sign is seen in **Uremia.**

Koilonychia is seen in Iron Deficiency Anemia.

Pterygium, anonychia, pitting is seen in **lichen planus.**

Onycholysis, ridging, pitting, thimble nails are seen in **psoriasis.**

Café-au-lait spots are seen in:
- Neurofibromatosis
- Albright's syndrome & Fibrous dysplasia.
- Watson's syndrome
- Leopard syndrome
- Fanconi's anemia

Leonine facies are seen in:
- LL-Leprosy
- Paget's disease of bone
- Fibrous dysplasia
- Hyperphosphatemia.

Pinch purpura is seen in Primary systemic amyloidosis, EDS, Scurvy.

MC route of transmission of Syphilis is sexual and sometimes transmitted by **BT, transplacental.**

DOC for syphilitic chancre (hard sore) is **BPG 2.4 million U single i.m. dose**

DOC for chancroid (soft sore) is **Single dose of Azithromycin** (or i/m ceftriaxone).

DOC for Lymphogranuloma venereum/inguinale is **Doxycycline or erythromycin for 2 weeks.**

DOC for Donovanosis is **Azithromycin**

Satellite lesions are seen in BT.

Inverted saucer shaped ulcers are seen in **Borderline leprosy.**

Virchow cell is diagnostic of lepromatous leprosy.

Most commonly involved nerve in leprosy: **Ulnar nerve**

Radial nerve is involved last in leprosy but if it is involved complications are more serious.

- Target/iris lesion is seen in: Erythema Multiforme
- Annular herald patch is seen in: Pityriasis Rosea
- Pityriasis Alba is a type of: Atopic Eczema
- Pityriasis Versicolor is caused by: Malassezia Furfur
- Erythrasma is caused by: Corynebacterium Minutissimum

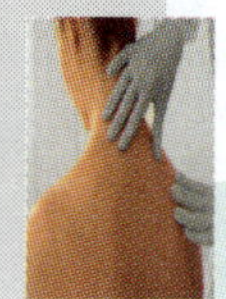

TABLE: Pathologies arising due to obstruction of sweat gland appendage

Obstruction of eccrine sweat gland ducts: Miliaria **Obstruction of apocrine sweat gland ducts:** Fox fordyce spot/ disease also known as Apocrine Miliaria **MC site of fox fordyce spot:** Axilla **MC age group of fox fordyce spot:** 13–35 years ***(Females are MC affected).*** **Fordice spot** are ectopic sebaceous glands.
Classical features of Acrodermatitis Enteropathica include: ***(Mnemonic-"DEAL")*** • **D**iarrhea, Depression • **E**czematous erosive dermatitis • **A**lopecia (non scarring), **A**pathetic look • **L**ethargy, irritability, whining & crying.

TABLE: Difference between pemphigus and pemphigoid bullae

Features	Pemphigus	Pemphigoid
Row of Tomb stone	Present	Absent
Nikolsky Sign	Present	Absent
Bullae location	Intraepidermal – flaccid Bullae	Subepidermal & tense Bullae
Mucosa involvement	Present (common)	Absent or less common
Acantholysis	Present	Absent
Prognosis	Poor	Good

TABLE: The ringworm genera

Trichophyton	Microsporum	Epidermophyton
Infects skin, hair & nail Infecting species include: Trichophyton rubrum mentagrophytes Violaceum Verrucosum schoenleinii	*Infects skin and hair* but does not involve nails Several infecting species include: Microsporum audouinii, M. gypseum and M. canis	*Infect skin & nails* but does not involve hair Only infecting species is Epidermophyton floccosum.
Mnemonic: ***TSH-N (Trichophyton infects Skin, Hair and Nail)*** ***MSH (Microsporum infects Skin and Hair)*** ***ESN (Epidermophyton infects Skin and Nail)***		

TABLE: Causes of genital ulcer

Bacterial	Viral	Parasitic	Non-infectious
Haemophilus ducreyi Treponema pallidum Chlamydia trachomatis Donovanosis balanitis	Herpes simplex Varicella zoster EBV Cytomegalovirus	Sarcoptes scabiei Phthirus pubis Entamoeba histolytica Trichomonas vaginalis	Trauma Pyoderma gangrenosum Reiter's syndrome Wegner's Neoplasms

TABLE: Warts and its associated disease

Warts	Seen in
Plane wart	Verruca plana
Filiform wart	Verruca filiformis
Plantar wart	Verruca plantaris or myrmecia wart
Venereal wart	Condylomata accuminata
Massive wart	Buschke–Löwenstein tumor
Condyloma lata	Treponema Pallidum

TABLE: Differences between syphilis, chancroid and LGV

Disease	Ulcer	Lymph node
Syphilis	Painless	Painless
Chancroid	Painful	Painful
LGV	Painless	Painful (Bubo)

TABLE: Differences between type 1 and type 2 lepra reaction

Type I Leprae Reaction: Reversal reaction	Type II Leprae R: Erythema nodosum leprosum
Type IV delayed HPS reaction	Type III HPS (Jarisch-Herxheimer) reaction
Found in TT (tuberculoid type)	Found in LL (Lepromatous Leprosy)
Thalidomide has no role	Thalidomide is most effective drug.
DOC is corticosteroid	DOC is corticosteroid

IMPORTANT SIGNS

• Carpet Tack Sign	DLE
• Chandelier's sign:	PID in women.
• Antenna sign:	Seen in Keratosis Pilaris
• Buttonholing sign:	NF 1

Contd...

• Dimpling sigri	Dermatofibrosarcoma protuberans
• Asboe Hansen sign	Pemphigus
• Nikolsky sign	Pemphigus, SSSS, TEN
• Auspitz sign/Grattage test	Psoriasis

MUST KNOW TERMS

• Persistence of nuclei in stratum spinosum	Parakeratosis
• Increase in keratinocyte population of spinous layer with thickening of the epidermis	Acanthosis
• Increase in keratinocytes with formation of projections from the surface of the skin	Papillomatosis (Ex: Wart)

ANESTHESIA

IMPORTANT RECENT POINTS (INCLUDES LATEST QS)

- **Guedels stages of ether anesthesia**
  - Stage 1 analgesia
  - Stage 2 delirium
  - Stage 3 surgical anesthesia
  - Stage 4 medullary paralysis.
- Nitric oxide produces second gas effect and fink phenomenon.
- Direct measurement of BP done in **Radial artery.**
- Neuromuscular monitoring performed at **ulnar nerve.**
- Sufentanil is most potent opioid.
- Remifentanil is shortest acting opiod.
- **Alfentanil** is opiod of choice for day care surgery
- Muscle relaxant of choice in shock: **Pancuronium**
- Most cardiostable anesthetic agent: **Etomidate**
- Most cardiostable inhalational agent **Isoflurane**
- Most cerebroprotective inhalational agent **Sevoflurane**
- Whitacre and Sprotte procedure is used for: **Spinal anesthesia**
- **Successful sign of spinal anesthesia:** Flaccid and engorged penis (Reason: Nervi ergentis paralysis)
- **Sequence of block by local anesthesia:** Temperature (cold > Hot) – pain – touch – deep pressure – proprioception
- Nerve fiber Sensitivity to pressure: **A > B > C**
- Nerve fiber sensitivity to hypoxia: **B > A > C**
- Nerve fiber sensitivity to LA: **A gamma, A Delta > Aα & Aβ**
- Anesthetic agents contraindicated in porphyria: **Pentazocine, Etomidate, Thiopentone (PET)**
  - DOC in such condition: **Propofol**
- Protein intake in ICU : **1–1.5 g/kg/day**
- Most common ophthalmic complication during anesthesia: **Corneal abrasion.**

Contd...

- History of postdural puncture headache is not a contraindication of epidural block
- **Flat Capnogram seen in:**
  - Accidental extubation
  - Dissociation of anesthetic tube
  - Mechanical ventilation failing
- O_2 content of anesthetic mixture: **33%**
- Preanesthetic drug which causes longest amnesia: **Lorazepam**
- Anesthetic with least decrease in systemic vascular resistance: **Halothane**
- MC anaesthetic agent causes Malignant hyperthermia: **Sch**
- LA having highest incidence of malignant hyperthermia: **Lignocaine**
- Inhalational test having highest incidence of malignant hyperthermia: **Halothane**
- Malignant hyperthermia is caused by: **Ryanodine receptor**
- Dextrose fluid is never used for resuscitation
- Opioid given as transdermal: **Fentanyl**

PIN INDEX AND COLOR CODING OF COMMONLY USED GASES

Gas	Color code		Pin index position
	Body	Shoulder	
Air	Grey	White/black quartered	1, 5
Oxygen	Black	White	2, 5
Nitrous oxide	Blue	Blue	3, 5
CO_2	Gray	Gray	1, 6
Helium	Brown	Brown	2, 5

GOLDEN POINTS

AMBU Bag stands for Artificial Maneuver Breathing Unit.

Cyclopropane cylinder is **orange**

ENTONOX cylinder color: **Blue body w/blue and white shoulder**

Spinal cord extents **from medulla oblongata to lower border** of L1 in adults and lower border of L3 in infants and neonates.

Structures pierced by spinal needle:
Skin → Subcutaneous tissue → supraspinatus ligament → interspinous ligament → Ligamentum flavum → Dura mater → Arachnoid space

Spinal block/sub arachnoid block is given in L3–L4 interspace in adults and L4–L5 in children.

Postdural puncture headache presents 12–24 hours of spinal block.

Contd...

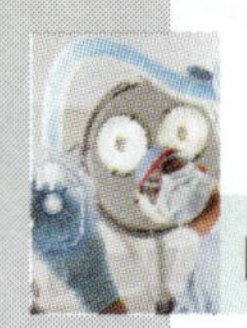

Epidural block is given between dura mater and ligamentum flavum.

Commonly used needle for epidural block is **Tuohys Needle**.

DOC for laryngeal mask insertion is **propofol**

Mallampati grading is used for assessment of size of tongue for laryngoscopy, also for assessment of difficult airway during orotracheal/nasotracheal intubation

Capnography is monitoring of $EtCO_2$ (end tidal CO_2) and it's waveform, normally it is 35–45 mm Hg

Normal CVP is **4–7 cm H_2O** (3–12 mm Hg is the range)

Seldinger technique is used for catheterization of vein (guide wire technique for central access)

Inotrope of choice for intra operative management of right heart failure due to pulmonary hypertension: **Dobutamine and Milrinone**

Potency of inhalational agent is determined by **MAC (minimum alveolar concentration)**

Methoxyflurane is most potent while **N_2O** is minimum in potency

ENTONOX- 50:50 mixture of **N_2O** and **O_2**, cylinder is blue colored with white shoulder

Induction agent of choice in children **Sevoflurane**

Fastest acting induction agent-**Desflurane**

Bupivacaine is most Cardiotoxic LA

Longest acting LA: **Dibucaine**

Most commonly used LA: **Lignocaine**

Local anesthetic which causes methemoglobinemia: **Benzocaine, Prilocaine, Lignocaine (BPL)**

Most common LA which causes Methemoglobinemia: **Prilocaine**

Thiopentone sodium causes reverse coronary steal phenomenon.

Ketamine produces Dissociative anesthesia

Diazepam causes retrograde amnesia

Anesthesia of choice in day care surgery-**Propofol**

Shortest acting depolarizing muscle relaxant: **Succinylcholine**

Shortest acting NDMR *(Non-depolarizing muscle relaxant)*- **Gantacurium (5-10 min) > Mivacurium (10-15 min)**

Fastest acting NDMR - **Rocuronium**

Longest acting NDMR – **Doxacurium (120 min)**

MC used SMR (skeletal muscle relaxant) in routine surgery -**Vecuronium**

MC used method of brachial plexus block is **supraclavicular block.**

Mendelson syndrome: regurgitation of gastric contents causes aspiration pneumonitis

Selliks maneuver: to prevent regurgitation, pressure is applied on cricoid cartilage which compresses esophagus against vertebral column.

Contd...

Drug not useful for induction in infants - **Morphine**

Muscle relaxant of choice in renal failure: **Atracurium**

Muscle relaxant of choice in renal and, or hepatic failure: **Cis-atracurium**

Hoffman elimination is seen in which muscle relaxant: **Atracurium, Cis-atracurium**

Boyle's Machine operates on: **Continuous flow principle**

Venturi mask:
- High flow oxygen delivery device
- Maximum oxygen delivered is 60%

Maximum oxygen delivered by nasal cannula: **44%**

Mapleson circuits type A is Also known as **Magills circuit**
Mapleson circuit type E is known as Ayres T piece best suited for **neonates.**

TABLE: Ester and amides

Ester *(one 'I' in name)*	**Amides** *(2 'I' in name)*
Cocaine Benzocaine Chloroprocaine Tetracaine	Lignocaine Bupivacaine Prilocaine Dibucaine Etidocaine
Remember: Amide group of LA contain "2 i" in their name	

CLASSIFICATION OF MUSCLE RELAXANTS

Neuromuscular blocking agent	
Depolarizing (Non-competitive) MR	Non-depolarizing (Competitive) MR
Suxamethonium/succinyl choline/Scoline Decamethonium	All others, For eg: Gallamine, D-tubocurarine, Atracurium, Mivacurium Ve/ Pan/ro-curonium

ANESTHETIC DOC

Condition	**DOC**
• Day care	Propofol (i/v), Desflurane (inhalation)
• Epilepsy	Thiopentone
• Neurosurgery	Isoflurane, Thipentone
• Renal failure/hepatic failure	Isoflurane Cis-atracurium (M/R)

Contd...

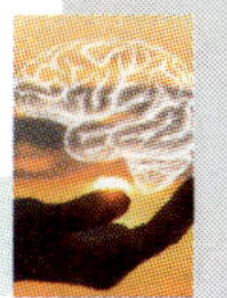

Condition	DOC
• ECT (Electro convulsive therapy)	Methohexital
• Bronchial asthma, COPD	Ketamine (i/v), Halothane (inhalational)
• Aneurysm surgery , IHD	Etomidate
• Cardiac surgery (preserved LV function)	Isoflurane
• Cardiac surgery (poor LV function	Opioid
• CHD: Lt to right shunt	Isoflurane/ sevoflurane
• Cyanotic HD: Rt to left shunt	Ketamine
• CHF, Shock	Ketamine
• Inhalational agent for induction in children	Sevoflurane
• IVRA (I.V Regional Anesthesia)	Prilocaine > Lignocaine
• TIVA (Total I.V. Anesthesia)	Propofol + Remifentanil

PSYCHIATRY

PSYCHIATRY—AT A GLANCE

Van Gogh syndrome: Dramatic self-mutilation occurring in schizophrenia

Squeeze technique is used for: **Premature ejaculation**

Schizophrenia is a thought disorder

Prevalence of schizophrenia: **1%**

Insight is absent in schizophrenia, mood disorder, delusional disorder

Dementia is not seen in schizophrenia

Not seen in schizophrenia: **Intellectual impairment**

Delusion of Fragmentary–delirium, hebephrenic schizophrenia.

Milieu therapy/family therapy/Therapeutic community – **in schizophrenia**

Drug of choice of schizophrenia: **Olanzapine**

Clozapine is particularly effective in **resistance schizophrenia**

Depersonalization & derealization usually occur together & are seen in – depression, anxiety, schizophrenia, epilepsy.

Pseudo-community, split personality seen in schizophrenia

Contd...

Morbid jealousy – Mood disorder, alcoholism, drug abuse, epilepsy, schizophrenia

Ambulatory schizophrenia and pseudoneurotic schizophrenia are now included in border line personality disorder.

TABLE: Neurotransmitter levels

Disease	Related neurotransmitter
Schizophrenia	Increased serotonin and Dopamine Decreased Glutamate
Depression	Decreased serotonin, NA, Dopamine
OCD	Decreased serotonin
Alzheimer's disease	Decreased Ach

TABLE: Prognostic factor of schizophrenia

Good prognostic factor	Bad prognostic factor
Female sex Acute onset (late onset) No family history of schizophrenia History of depressive order Premorbid personality	Male sex Gradual onset (early onset) Family history of schizophrenia Emotional blunting

DEPRESSION

- Depression is the **most common psychiatric disorder** in hospitalized patients.
- MC psychiatric illness: **Anxiety**
- **Nihilistic delusion and delusion of guilt** and poverty – Seen in depression.
- Depression is the MC psychiatric disorder in: **Hypothyroidism, AIDS, patients on ocp's, postpartum psychosis**
- OCD leads to **secondary depression**
- DOC for manic depressive disorder: **Lithium**
- Long term use of lithium can cause: **Hypothyroidism**
- **Pseudo depression & nihilistic delusion** are seen in depression.

IMPORTANT POINTS

Insomnia is seen in this withdrawal: **Alcohol withdrawal**

Hypersomnia is seen in **cocaine withdrawal**

Kubler Ross classified 5 stages of death: Denial → Anger → Bargain → Despair → Acceptance.

Super ego: Based on moral principle. Ego ideal. E.g.: Mother Teresa, Mahatma Gandhi (idealistic thing)

Ego: Based on reality

Instinct: Inborn, based on principle of pleasure, maternal/ paternal instincts

Contd...

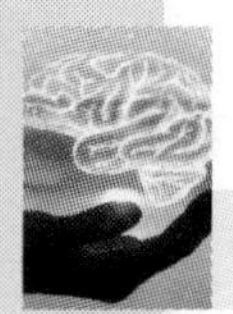

Fibromyalgia is not a somatoform disorder.

CBT does not include: **Interpretation**

Not a defense mechanism – **Transference, derailment**

Generalized anxiety disorder is not an indication for lithium

Angel dust is **Phencyclidine it** produce catatonic syndrome

REM Sleep is characterized by PGO spikes.

NREM stage 2 is characterized by sleep spindles and k-complex.

Muscle hypotonia is most characteristic REM sleep which differentiate it from wakefulness.

Classical tetrad of **Narcolepsy**: Sleep attacks, cataplexy, hypnogogic hallucinations, sleep paralysis.

Illusion: False perception of external object which has real existence.

Impulse: Irresistible desire

Obsessions: Recurrent, irrational, intrusive, ego-dystonic and ego-alien ideas.

Overall most common type of hallucination: **Auditory hallucination**

Visual hallucination are mc seen in organic disease

Tactile hallucination are seen in chronic amphetamine poisoning.

Synaesthesia: Stimulus in one modality & hallucination in other modality
Delusion is not a feature **of conversion disorder.**

Delusion of Grandiosity – **MANIA**

Othello syndrome – Jealousy (infidelity)

Induced delusional disorder – Sharing of delusions b/w usually two or occasionally more persons.

Concrete thinking stage **2-7 years**

MC mental disorder in children – **Neurosis**

MC form of pica is **Geophagia.**

Fear of death most commonly at age of **5 years**

Age of onset in **Autism** < 2 ½ years, there is a marked impairment of language

Rett's syndrome
Occurs exclusively in girls
A neuropsychiatric illness, with normal head circumference at birth
Characterized by: Midline hand winging/hand washing stereotypies

In Asperger's syndrome language is normal AND no delay **in cognitive development** *(remember Shahrukh Khan in movie- My Name is Khan)*

Treatment of choice for Hypochondriasis, somatoform disorder Anxiety neurosis, Hysteria – **Supportive Psychotherapy**

Contd...

Treatment of choice for phobia – **Behavior therapy**

Treatment of choice Gilles de la Tourette's syndrome – **Clonidine/ Haloperidol**

EPS are NOT seen with **clozapine**

Akathisia is most common with haloperidol. It is treated by propranolol

Antidepressant which can be used in t/t of nocturnal enuresis, ADHD, chronic pain: **Imipramine**

Patients of anorexia nervosa are vulnerable to sudden death due to ventricular **arrhythmias**

Delirium is most common organic disorder

Drugs inducing delirium: Alcohol, heroin, morphine, cannabis, cocaine, LSD.

Psychosis may occur in pregnancy, postpartum, epilepsy

Main symptom of Korsakoff psychosis: **Confabulation**

In late phase profound anterograde amnesia & milder retrograde amnesia is found in **delirium & dementia**

In acute delirium sun downing phenomenon is present.

In Korsakoff's psychosis immediate & remote memory is usually retained

Amotivation is lethargy, apathy, loss of interest, anergia, reduced drive, lac of ambition seen in chronic cannabis abuse.

Anxiety is most common psychiatric symptom & generalized anxiety disorder in general population.

Splitting is a defense mechanism against **BPD.**

Sensate focus technique is used for t/t of impotency

Master's and Johnson's technique is most popular t/t method for psycho sexual dysfunction in which both partners are treated together.

Excessive sexual drive is called satyrism in men and nymphomania in female.

Visual hallucination is characteristic of alcohol withdrawal.

Most important dependency producing derivatives are **morphine & heroin.**

ECT most effective in the treatment of major depression with **psychosis, delusion, or suicidal tendency.**

ECT is never indicated in cyclothymia, Dysthymia, Chronic Schizophrenia (with negative symptoms)

MC complication of direct (modified) ECT: **Fracture T4-T8 spine.**

MC complication of modified ECT: Anterograde & Retro Grade amnesia more of retrograde type.

Alcohol is the most common substance abused in India and worldwide.

Most common illicit drug/substance abused: **Cannabis > Amphetamine**
(2nd MC).

Contd...

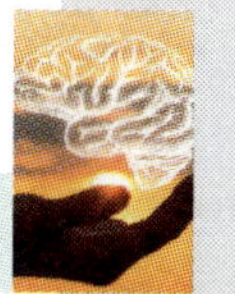

DOC for prophylaxis of bipolar disorder - **Lithium**
DOC for mania: **Lithium**
Therapeutic level of lithium: 0.8 – 1.2 mEq/L
Toxicity seen after >1.5 mEq/L
Most common side effect of lithium: **Tremor**
Most common cause of impotency in male: **Psychogenic**

Antipsychotics

Recently approved sublingual antipsychotic: **Asenapine**
Most common side effect of typical antipsychotic: **Extrapyramidal symptoms (EPS), Hyperprolactinemia**
Most common EPS: **Akathisia**
MC side effect of atypical antipsychotics: **Metabolic/Lipodystrophy syndrome (Weight gain, Inc glucose, altered lipid profile)**
Atypicals with least weight gain: **Aripiprazole, Ziprasidone**
Atypicals with max weight gain: **Clozapine, Olanzopine, Quetiapine**
Atypicals with least risk of EPS: **Clozapine**
Typical with least EPS: **Chlorpromazine and Thioridazine**
Typicals with max risk of EPS: **Haloperidol**
Atypicals associated with cardiac arrhythmia: **Sertindole, Zotepine**
Most potent atypical antipsychotic: **Risperidone**
Atypicals with maximum risk of hyperprolactinemia: **Risperidone**
Atypical antipsychotic causing corneal opacity: **Chlorpromazine and Thioridazine**
Known side effects of clozapine: **Agranulocytosis, Sialorrhea, Sedation, weight gain, Inc. risk of DM**

TABLE: Eating disorder

	Anorexia nervosa	Bulimia nervosa
Feature	Refusal to maintain body weight above a minimal normal	Irresistible craving for food with episodes of over eating in less time (Binge eating)
Method of weight control		Attempts to counter act the effects of over eating by self-induced vomiting: Purgative abuse, Periods of starvations Appetite suppressants
Ritualized exercise	Common	Rare

Contd...

	Anorexia nervosa	Bulimia nervosa
Amenorrhea	100%	50%
Decreased Vital aBP, ¯Pulse	Common	Uncommon
Hypothermia	Common	Rare
Skin changes (hirsutism)	Common	Rare
Medical Complications	Hypokalemia Cardiac arrhythmias	Hypokalemia Cardiac arrhythmias

FEATURE OF CORTICAL & SUBCORTICAL DEMENTIA

Features	Cortical dementia	Subcortical dementia
Site	Cortex (frontal, parietal, temporal, occipital, hippocampus)	Subcortical grey matter
Memory impairment	Severe, early Recall helped very little by cues	Mild to moderate Recall helped partially by cues & recognition tasks
Mathematical skills	Impaired early (Acalculia)	Preserved
Language	Early, Dysphasia (Aphasia)	Normal & Anomia (in severe cases)
Speech	Articulate until late	Dysarthria
Personality	Indifferent	Apathetic, inert

TABLE: Appearance of alcohol withdrawal symptoms

Time	Symptoms
6–12 hours	Minor withdrawal symptoms: Insomnia, tremulousness, anxiety, GIT upset, headache, diaphoresis, palpitations, anorexia
12–24 hours	Alcoholic hallucinosis; visual, auditory, or tactile hallucination
24–48 hours	*Withdrawal seizures:* generalized tonic-clonic seizures
48–72 hours	Delirium tremens; visual hallucinations, disorientation, *tachycardia*, hypertension, low-grade fever, agitation, diaphoresis

TABLE: Substance abuse and its characteristic clinical feature

Substance	Characteristic clinical feature
Cocaine	Magnus symptoms (cocaine bugs or Tactile hallucination)

Contd...

Substance	Characteristic clinical feature
Cannabis	Run Amok Amotivational syndrome Flash backs
Alcohol	Mc-Evan's sign Morbid jealousy
LSD	Bad Trips Flash backs
Amphetamine	Paranoid Hallucinatory syndrome (like paranoid schizophrenia)
Phencyclidine (Angel dust)	Dissociative anesthesia

Therapeutic Modes for Diseases

• Milieu therapy Therapeutic community/ family therapy	In Schizophrenia
• Bio feedback, Jacobson's relaxation technique, Autohypnosis	In type A behavior/personality (Psychosomatic disorder)
• Semens Seqeeze tech (Masters & Johnson's)	In premature ejaculation
• Abreaction therapy (Amytal interview)	In hysteria & d/g of catatonic syndrome. (Interview with mute, stupor)
• Systemic desensitization	TOC in Phobias, OCD
• Aversion therapy	Alcohol dependence, transvestism, homosexuality, hysteria
• Flooding:	Phobias

Types of Personality

	Clinical features	Increased risk of
Type A	Ambitious, achievement oriented people, often high-achieving career oriented "workaholics", impatient	Coronary heart diseases
Type B	Easy going relaxed individuals	–
Type C	No assertive at all and they always suppress their own desires	Depression, cancer
Type D	Distressed	CHD patient has ↑ Mortality & recurrence from MI

RADIOLOGY

IMPORTANT RECENT POINTS (INCLUDES LATEST QS)

- Father of radiology/X-ray: **W.C. Roentgen** (Discovered on 8 November, 1895)
- Father of USG: **John Wild**
- Father of Obstetrical USG: **Ion Donald**
- Father of Doppler: **Doppler John**
- Father of CT Scan: **Godfrey Hounsfield**
- Father of MRI: **Laterbuer and Mansfield**

Components of X-ray machine:
- Cathode-tungsten
- Anode-tungsten
- Anode in mammography: Molybdenum
- Filter- Al, or Al + Cu or Mo
- Collimator- Pb (Lead)

Radiation Units
- Unit of radiation exposure - **Roentgen** (SI = Coulomb/kg)
- Unit of absorbed radiation - **RAD** (SI = GRAY)
- Unit of biologic effectiveness - **Rem** (SI = Sievert)

Normal distance from which a chest **X-ray** is performed: 180 cm (6 ft")

Thickness of lead jacket – **0.5 mm**

Best X-rays are performed in: **60 – 90 kVp**

Minimal amount of pleural fluid required to detect pleural effusion on CXR– **100 – 200 mL**

Best X-ray view to detect minimal effusion is – **Lateral decubitus view of the same side.**

Best investigation to detect minimal fluid – **USG**

FAST Scan is: Focussed Assessment with Sonography for Trauma. Assess four main area to detect fluid in pericardium, RUQ (Morrison pouch), LUQ (Perisplenic), Pelvic area.

Best view to see normal chest- Right lung-LAO; Left lung- RAO

Major part of the radiological hilar shadow – **Pulmonary artery**

In anterior segment of upper lobe is uncommon in **secondary TB.**

Water lily sign or Camalote sign is seen in – **Hydatid lung**

Hounsfield unit of:
- Bone: +1000
- Blood: +40 to +50
- Water: 0
- Fat: - 50 to – 100
- Air: - 1000

IOC for bronchiectasis – **HRCT**

Signet-ring sign is seen in **Bronchiectasis**

MC thoracic manifestation of rheumatoid arthritis – **Pleural effusion**

Egg shell calcification is seen in Silicosis, Sarcoidosis

Contd...

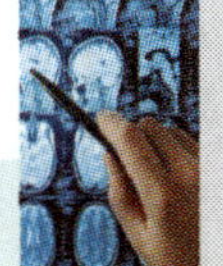

Bat wing appearance on CXR is seen in **Pulmonary edema.**

X-ray signs of Pulmonary embolism- Fleischner's sign, Knuckle sign, Palla's sign.

V/Q mismatch is a sign of pulmonary infarct.

Gold standard investigation of Pulmonary embolism – **Pulmonary angiography**

Golden S sign is seen in **Bronchogenic carcinoma.**

Cannon ball appearance is seen in – **Lung metastasis**

Pop Corn calcification is seen in **Pulmonary Hamartoma**

Bronchial atresia more common in **Left upper lobe.**

Poland syndrome on CXR: **Unilateral hyperlucent lung**

IOC for aortic dissection: **MRI**

Rim sign is seen in: Massive hydronephrosis

Money bag or leather bottle or flask shaped heart is seen in **Pericardial effusion.**

Most sensitive investigation of Pericardial effusion – **Echocardiography-15 ml** can be detected

Pruned tree appearance – Pulmonary arterial hypertension

IOC for Aortic dissection – **MRI**

Champagne glass appearance – **Achondroplasia**

IOC for cardiac tamponade, Pericardial effusion – **2D Echo**

Molten candle wax appearance seen in - **Melorheostosis**

Telephone handle long bones seen in – **Thanatophoric Dwarfism**

Metacarpal sign – Pseudohypoparathyroidism, Turner's syndrome

Pepper-pot skull seen in – **Hyperparathyroidism**

Looser's zones or pseudofractures is the hallmark feature of – **Osteomalacia.**

Rugger jersey spine seen in Renal osteodystrophy, **Osteopetrosis**

Hair on end or crew cut or hair brush appearance seen in – **Thalassemia**

Earliest change in thalassemia – Widening of short bones of hand.

Flask shaped femora seen in- **Thalassemia**

Cotton wool skull seen in – **Paget's disease**

Tram track appearance on skull X-ray: **Sturge weber syndrome**

Most common intracranial calcification: **Pineal Calcification**

Basal ganglia calcification is seen in this condition: Wilson's disease

Erlenmeyer Flask deformity seen in – Metaphyseal dysplasia, Osteopetrosis, Thalassemia

Earliest seen in **Osteomyelitis**- Soft tissue swelling and loss of soft tissue planes.

Hot cross Bun Skull seen in – **Congenital syphilis**

Celery stalk appearance – **Congenital Rubella**

Contd...

Bone most commonly involved in osteoarthritis – **Patella**

Earliest appearance see in rheumatoid arthritis is – **Periarticular soft tissue swelling**

Cup and pencil appearance seen in **Psoriasis**

Bamboo spine, Romanus sign, Dagger sign, Squaring of vertebrae seen in – **Ankylosing spondylitis**

Codmans triangle, Sunray appearance seen in **Osteosarcoma**
Onion peel appearance seen in – **Ewing's sarcoma**

Trap door sign, Fallen fragment sign seen in- **Simple Bone Cyst**

Soap bubble appearance seen in – Giant cell tumor or **Osteoclastoma**

Shepherd Crook deformity femur, Ground glass appearance on X-ray is feature of – **Fibrous Dysplasia.**

Corduroy Cloth appearance on X-ray, Polka dot appearance on CT – **Hemangioma**

Rain drop appearance, punched out lesions on skull is seen in – **Multiple Myeloma**

Inverted napoleon hat sign on AP view, Scotty dog appearance seen in **Spondylolisthesis**

Barium is better for evaluation of motility disorders and for cricopharyngeal dysphagia than endoscopic evaluation.

Pencil tip or bird beak tapering seen in **Achalasia Cardia**

Corkscrew Esophagus seen in – **Diffuse esophageal spasm**

Initial investigation for Hypertrophic Pyloric Stenosis – **USG**

String sign, apple core appearance, Beak sign on barium is seen in – **Hypertrophic Pyloric Stenosis.**

Carman's meniscus sign seen in Malignant ulcer

Double bubble appearance seen in Duodenal atresia, Annular pancreas

Triple bubble sign seen in – **Jejunal atresia**

If coin accidently ingested in esophagus, it will be oriented in coronal plane whereas coins Trachea is oriented saggittally.

Half-life of 18-FDG: **110 minutes**

Best test for avascular necrosis of bone: **MRI**

MC type of ASD in down's syndrome: **Ostium primum**

Overall, MC type of ASD: **Ostium primum**

Widening of C loop of duodenum on barium study: **CA pancreas head**

Double duct sign is seen in: **Periampullary carcinoma**

IOC for acute pancreatitis: **CECT**

In chest X-ray Lordotic view is used for:

- **Lung apex pathology**
- Best view for middle lobe examination
- Interlobar fissural examination

Contd...

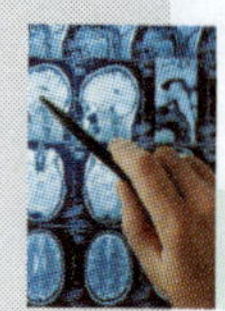

IOC for posterior urethral valve: **VCUG (Voiding Cystourethrogram)**

- **Comet tail app on HRCT:** Round Atelectasis
- Hallmark of ureteric TB: **corkscrew ureter**
- Moth eaten calyces on IVP: **Renal TB**
- Ulcer crater sign and Hampton's line: Benign gastric ulcer
- Double atrial shadow is seen in: **LA enlargement**
- Signs of pneumoperitoneum: saddle bag/Mustache/Cupola/ Falciform lig sign/Rigler sign/urachus sign
- IVP-Spider leg app/swiss cheese appearance: **PCKD**
- IOC for pulm embolism: **CT angiography**
- Chamber enlarged in Ebstein anomaly → All chambers
- MC ASD: **Septum secundum**
- Bulging fissure sign: **Klebsiella Pn**
- CXR finding of Pulm embolism: **Westermark sign, Palla sign, Hampton hump, Fleischner sign**
- Dye used in Bronchography: **Dianosil**
- Scan done for parathyroid adenoma: **Sestamibi scan**
- Radioactive agent used in treatment for ascites: **Gold**
- First sign of radiation exposure: **Erythema**

TABLE: Congenital cardiac conditions and its radiological findings

Lutembacher Syndrome- Congenital ASD with Acquired MS.
Figure of 3 appearance seen in – **Coarctation of Aorta**
Boot shaped heart or Cor-en-sabot seen in – **Tetralogy of Fallot**
Box shaped heart on CXR – **Ebstein anomaly**
Figure of 8 appearance or Snowman appearance seen in – **TAPVC**
Egg on side appearance seen in **TGA**
Most common type of VSD – **Perimembranous**
Most common type of ASD – **Ostium secundum**
Hilar dance on fluoroscopy – **ASD**

TABLE: Some important half-life of radionuclides

Gold-198: 2.7 days
Iodine- 123: 13.3 hours
Iodine-131: 8 days
Phosphorus-32: 14.3 days
Yttrium 90: 64 hours
Cobalt-60: 5.26 years
Caesium-137: 30 years
Radium-226: 1620 years

REMEMBER THESE IMPORTANT RADIOLOGICAL SIGNS IN UROLOGY

Spider leg appearance → **Polycystic kidney**
Cobra head appearance → **Ureterocele**
Flower vase appearance of ureters → **Horseshoe kidney**
Sandy patches → **Schistosomiasis of bladder**
Soap bubble appearance → **Hydronephrosis**
Golf hole ureter → **TB bladder**
String of purse appearance: **Ureteric TB**

TABLE: Conditions where 'Hair on End Appearance' is seen: ***Mnemonic: HI NEST***

- Hereditary spherocytosis
- Iron deficiency anemia
- Neuroblastoma
- Enzyme deficiency (e.g. G-6-P deficiency causing hemolytic anemia)
- Sickle cell disease
- Thalassemia major

TABLE: Radiological findings and their respective pathology

Barium enema findings	Associated pathology
Apple core deformity **Irregular filling defect**	Colon CA
Lead pipe appearance **Loss of haustrations**	Ulcerative colitis
String sign of kantor **Raspberry thorn ulcers**	Crohn's disease
Smooth irregular filling defects	Colonic polyps
Dilated proximal zone with narrow distal zone of coning	Hirschsprung disease
Saw tooth appearance **Champagne glass sign**	Diverticulosis of colon
Thumb print sign	Ischemic colitis
Claw sign **Coiled spring sign**	Intussusception
Bird beak sign, Ace of spades	Volvulus
Bird beak appearance	Achalasia cardia
Rat tail appearance	Esophageal CA
Corkscrew appearance **Nut cracker esophagus** **Curling esophagus**	Diffuse esophageal spasm
String sign	Congenital hypertrophic pyloric stenosis
Inverted 3 sign of Forsberg **Widening of C loop of duodenum/** **Antral pad sign.**	Pancreas head CA
Coffee bean sign	Sigmoid volvulus

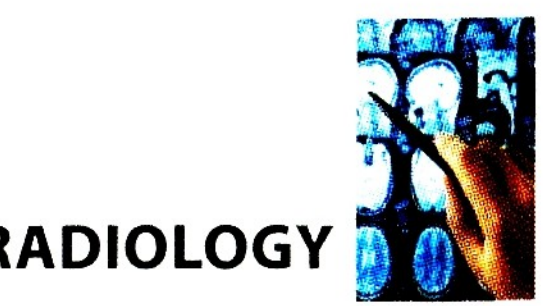

MRI Head Appearances

• Eye of the tiger	Hallervorden spatz disease
• Face of giant panda	Wilson's disease
• Racing car app	Corpus callosum agenesis
• Humming bird sign, Mickey mouse app	PSP (Progressive Supranuclear Palsy)
• Hot cross bun sign	MSA (Multiple System Atrophy)
• Molar tooth app	Joubert syndrome
• Figure of 8 app	Lissencephaly

TABLE: Radiation exposure in different investigations

Procedure	Mean effective dose (mSv)
• Chest X-ray (PA View)	0.02
• Chest X-ray (PA + Lateral view)	0.1
• Mammogram	0.4
• Abdomen X-ray	0.7
• HSG	0.9–1.3
• CT Brain	2.2
• IVP	3
• ERCP	4
• Coronary angiography	7 (2–16)
• Barium enema	8 (2–18)
• CT Colonography	6
• CT Abdomen and Pelvis	10
• Thallium scan	16.9

Notes